SPECIAL FEATURES—cont'd

Client Education Guides

Continued on inside back cover

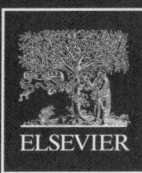

ELSEVIER

evolve

The Latest *Evolution* in Learning.

Evolve provides online access to free learning resources and activities designed specifically for the textbook you are using in your class. The resources will provide you with information that enhances the material covered in the book and much more.

Visit the Web address listed below to start your learning evolution today!

▶▶ *LOGIN: http://evolve.elsevier.com/Black/medsurg/*

Evolve Student Learning Resources for Black and Hawks: *Medical-Surgical Nursing: Clinical Management for Positive Outcomes,* 7th edition, offers the following features:

- **Open-Book Quizzes:** Each chapter includes interactive self-assessment tools such as multiple choice, fill-in-the-blank, and matching with instant scoring and feedback at the click of a button. Crossword puzzles provide a fun and effective way to reinforce chapter key terms.
- **WebLinks:** An exciting resource that lets you link to hundreds of websites carefully chosen to supplement the content of the textbook. The WebLinks are regularly updated, with new ones added as they develop.
- **Concept Map Creator:** An exciting tool that walks you through the thinking process of creating individualized Concept Maps, from initial diagnoses to interventions to outcomes to a completed plan of care.
- **Additional Resources:** Content comes alive with health assessment animations and videos, a glossary of audio pronunciations, a Fluid & Electrolyte self-study module, and more!
- **Enhanced Web Content:** Discussions of Case Management, Diversity in Health Care, and Ethical Issues in Nursing enhance the wealth of content included in the text. Appendixes, Clinical Pathways, Spanish Assessment phrases and Spanish Client Education Guides provide useful tools for clinical practice. Care Plans, Bridges to Home Health Care, Complementary and Alternative Therapies, Case Studies, and Thinking Critically discussions all serve to reinforce the text content.

Think outside the book... *evolve.*

The CD-ROM included with every copy of *Medical-Surgical Nursing: Clinical Management for Positive Outcomes,* 7th edition, features:

- **Open-Book Quizzes** to test your knowledge with interactive exercises and crossword puzzles
- **Additional Resources** to bring the content alive with health assessment animations and videos and a Fluid & Electrolyte self-study module
- **Case Studies** followed by interactive learning activities and a care plan
- **Discussions for Thinking Critically Questions**

Medical-Surgical Nursing

Clinical Management for Positive Outcomes

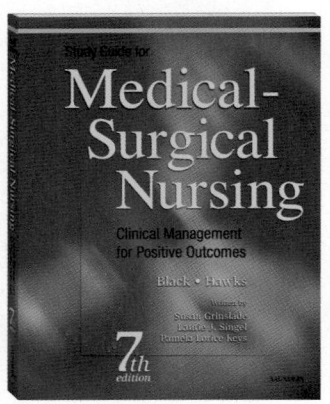
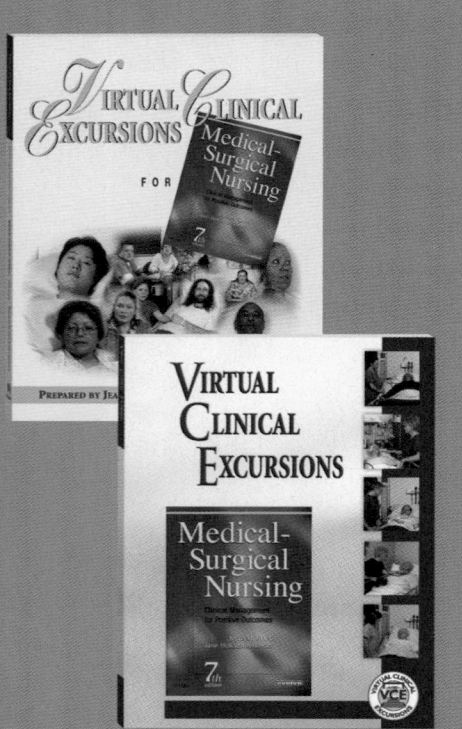
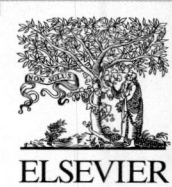

Medical-Surgical Nursing

Clinical Management for Positive Outcomes

7th edition

Joyce M. Black, PhD, RN, CPSN, CWCN
Associate Professor
College of Nursing
University of Nebraska Medical Center
Omaha, Nebraska

Jane Hokanson Hawks, DNSc, RN, BC
Professor of Nursing
Midland Lutheran College
Fremont, Nebraska

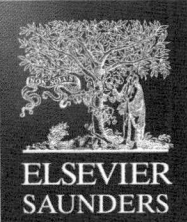

ELSEVIER
SAUNDERS

Volume 2

ELSEVIER
SAUNDERS

11830 Westline Industrial Drive
St. Louis, Missouri 63146

NOTICE

Nursing is an ever-changing field. Standard safety precautions must be followed, but as new research and clinical experience broaden our knowledge, changes in treatment and drug therapy may become necessary or appropriate. Readers are advised to check the most current product information provided by the manufacturer of each drug to be administered to verify the recommended dose, the method and duration of administration, and contraindications. It is the responsibility of the licensed prescriber, relying on experience and knowledge of the patient, to determine dosages and the best treatment for each individual patient. Neither the publisher nor the author assumes any liability for any injury and/or damage to persons or property arising from this publication.

Previous editions copyrighted 2001, 1997, 1993, 1987, 1980, 1974.

International Standard Book Number 0-7216-0220-7 (Single Volume)
0-7216-0221-5 (2-Volume Set)

Executive Publisher: Barbara Cullen
Senior Developmental Editor: Victoria Bruno
Developmental Editor: Adrienne Simon
Publishing Services Manager: Deborah L. Vogel
Senior Project Manager: Jodi M. Willard
Senior Designer: Kathi Gosche

Printed in China

Last digit is the print number: 9 8 7 6 5 4 3 2

*When I walked into the hospital, I used to see a sign that said,
"Enter in to learn, go forth to serve." Therefore this book
is dedicated to those students and patients who taught me the
value of caring and teaching, and I hope they can serve others
through my efforts here. I appreciate the quiet contributions of
my colleagues. And I thank my family—Steve, Jon, Katy,
and Tricia—for their ongoing understanding of the
considerable strain on my time and energy.*
J.M.B.

*To the patients, nurses, students, and faculty I learn from;
to my parents, Esther and the late Charles Hokanson, who
helped me become the person I am; and to my husband,
Edward, and my daughter, Jennifer, whose support
and understanding remain constant.*
J.H.H.

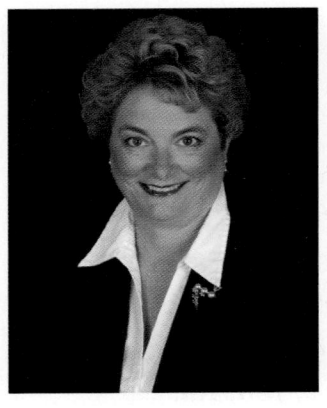

Joyce M. Black, PhD, RN, CPSN, CWCN, is an Associate Professor at the University of Nebraska Medical Center College of Nursing in the Adult Health and Illness Department. She teaches junior-level nursing students in medical-surgical nursing and supervises the research activities of several graduate students. Dr. Black received her Doctorate from the University of Nebraska Medical Center College of Nursing in Omaha, Nebraska, in 1999; her Master of Science in Nursing degree from the University of Nebraska Medical Center College of Nursing in 1981; her Bachelor of Science in Nursing degree from Winona State University in Winona, Minnesota; and her Associate's degree in Nursing from Rochester Community College in Rochester, Minnesota.

Dr. Black has had several years of clinical experience as a medical-surgical nurse at Saint Mary's Hospital in Rochester, Minnesota, which is affiliated with the Mayo Clinic. Her clinical practice has been in orthopedics, critical care, burn care, respiratory diseases, wound care, and plastic surgery. She is certified by the American Society of Plastic Surgical Nurses and by the Wound, Ostomy and Continence Nurses Society. Dr. Black also serves as the editor of *Plastic Surgical Nursing* and as a member of the Board of Directors for the National Pressure Ulcer Advisory Panel. Her area of research is in deep tissue injury, pressure ulcers, and wound healing.

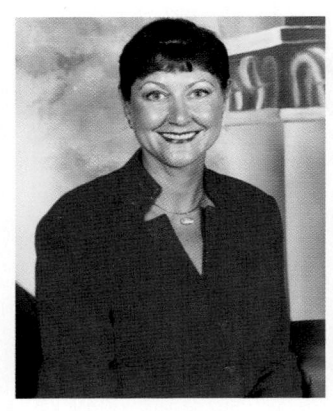

Jane Hokanson Hawks, DNSc, RN, BC, is a Professor of Nursing at Midland Lutheran College, Fremont, Nebraska. She teaches sophomore students in medical-surgical nursing and senior students in advanced medical-surgical nursing and nursing management. Dr. Hawks received her Doctorate of Nursing Science in collegiate nursing education from Widener University in Chester, Pennsylvania; her Master of Science in Nursing degree in medical-surgical nursing and nursing administration from the University of Nebraska Medical Center College of Nursing in Omaha, Nebraska; and her Bachelor of Science in Nursing degree from St. Olaf College in Northfield, Minnesota.

Dr. Hawks has worked in and has taught medical-surgical nursing for more than 26 years. She has practiced in a variety of areas, including critical care, renal transplantation, orthopedics, general surgery, and urology. She serves as the editor of *Urologic Nursing.* Her areas of research include empowerment, mentoring, nursing education, active teaching strategies, and alcoholism. She and her colleagues developed the NANDA nursing diagnosis Altered Family Process: Alcoholism (now known as Dysfunctional Family Processes: Alcoholism). Dr. Hawks co-authored *Mentoring for Mission: Nurturing New Faculty at Church-Related Colleges,* which was published in 2003 and funded through a grant from the Lilly Fellows Foundation.

Section Editors

Robert G. Carroll, PhD
Professor,
Department of Physiology,
Brody School of Medicine,
East Carolina University,
Greenville, North Carolina

Annabelle M. Keene, MSN, RN, BC
School Nurse,
Bellevue Public Schools,
Bellevue, Nebraska;
Formerly, Associate Professor,
College of Saint Mary,
Omaha, Nebraska

Sheila Melander, DSN, RN, ACNP-C, FCCM
Professor,
School of Nursing,
University of Tennessee at Memphis,
Memphis, Tennessee;
Cardiovascular Acute Care Nurse Practitioner,
Owensboro, Kentucky

Contributors

Mary A. Allen, MS, RN
Medical Officer/Nurse Consultant,
National Institute of Allergy and Infectious Diseases,
National Institutes of Health,
Bethesda, Maryland

Donna M. Barker, MS, APN/CNS, ONC
Clinical Nurse Specialist, Orthopedics,
Barrington, Illinois

Francie Bernier, MSN, BSN, RNC
Doctoral Student,
University of Virginia,
School of Nursing,
Charlottesville, Virginia;
Clinical Education Specialist,
Hollister, Inc.,
Libertyville, Illinois

Meg Blair, MSN, RN, CEN
Assistant Professor,
Nebraska Methodist College;
Staff Nurse,
Emergency Department,
Creighton University Medical Center,
Omaha, Nebraska

Lisa Bowman, MSN, RN, CRNP, CNRN
Nurse Practitioner,
Clinical Research Coordinator,
Thomas Jefferson University Hospital,
Philadelphia, Pennsylvania

Patricia C. Buchsel, MSN, BSN, FAAN
Chief Operating Officer,
Creative Cancer Concepts, Inc.,
Rockwall, Texas;
Clinical Faculty,
School of Nursing,
University of Washington,
Seattle, Washington

Andrea R. Cain, BSN, RN
Registered Nurse,
Gupta & Mills Cardiology,
Owensboro, Kentucky

Candace Cantwell, RD, RN, CNSD
Clinical Nurse,
Medical Intensive Care Unit,
University of Pennsylvania Medical Center,
Philadelphia, Pennsylvania

Robert G. Carroll, PhD
Professor,
Department of Physiology,
Brody School of Medicine,
East Carolina University,
Greenville, North Carolina

Verna Benner Carson, PhD, MS, APRN/PMH
National Director of RESTORE Behavioral Health,
Tender Loving Care Home Health Care,
Lake Success, New York;
Formerly, Associate Professor,
School of Nursing,
University of Maryland,
Baltimore, Maryland

Linda K. Clarke, MS, RN, CORLN
Head and Neck Nurse Specialist,
Greater Baltimore Medical Center,
Baltimore, Maryland

Charlene Compher, PhD, RD, FAAN
Assistant Professor in Nutrition Science,
School of Nursing,
University of Pennsylvania,
Philadelphia, Pennsylvania

Linda Carman Copel, PhD, RN, CS, DAPA
Associate Professor,
College of Nursing,
Villanova University,
Villanova, Pennsylvania

Tricia C. Corbett, MSPH
Clinical Instructor,
School of Nursing,
University of Washington,
Seattle, Washington

Pamela Cornwell, MA, RN
Assistant Director of Patient Care Services,
Shriners Hospitals for Children,
Sacramento, California

Melissa Craft, MS, RN, AOCN
Assistant Clinical Professor,
University of Oklahoma,
Oklahoma City, Oklahoma;
Oncology Clinical Nurse Specialist,
Breast Imaging of Oklahoma,
Edmund, Oklahoma

Sherill Nones Cronin, PhD, RN, C
Professor of Nursing,
Director, MSN Program,
Bellarmine University;
Nurse Researcher,
Jewish Hospital,
Louisville, Kentucky

Susan L. Dean-Baar, PhD, RN, CRRN, FAAN
Associate Professor,
Associate Dean for Academic Affairs,
School of Nursing,
University of Wisconsin at Milwaukee,
Milwaukee, Wisconsin

Jean Elizabeth DeMartinis, PhD, APRN (FNP-C)
Associate Clinical Professor,
Creighton University,
Omaha, Nebraska;
Cardiology and Prevention Specialist,
Nurse Practitioner,
MidAmerica Cardiovascular Institute,
Omaha, Nebraska

Peggy Doheny, PhD, RN, ONC
Professor,
College of Nursing,
Kent State University,
Kent, Ohio

Charlotte Eliopoulos, PhD, RNC, MPH, ND
President,
Health Education Network,
Glen Arm, Maryland

James A. Fain, PhD, RN, BC-ADM, FAAN
Associate Professor,
Associate Dean for Academic Programs,
Graduate School of Nursing,
University of Massachusetts at Worcester,
Worcester, Massachusetts

Kathryn Fiandt, DNS, MSN, BSN, FNP, BC
Associate Professor,
University of Nebraska Medical Center;
Clinical Director,
University of Nebraska Medical Center,
Family Health Care Center,
Omaha, Nebraska

Mary L. Fisher, PhD, RN, CNAA, BC
Associate Professor,
School of Nursing,
University of Indiana;
PRN Staff Nurse,
St. Vincent Health Services,
Indianapolis, Indiana

Nancy J. Girard, PhD, MSN, RN, FAAN
Associate Professor,
Chair,
Acute Nursing Care Department,
School of Nursing,
University of Texas Health Sciences Center at San
    Antonio,
San Antonio, Texas

Mikel Gray, PhD, CUNP, CCCN, FAAN
Nurse Practitioner,
Department of Urology;
Professor,
School of Nursing,
University of Virginia,
Charlottesville, Virginia

Catherine Gregory, MSN, BSN, PNP, PALS, ABLS
Pediatric Nurse Practitioner,
Burn Surgery,
Shriners Hospital for Children,
Sacramento, California

Sheila A. Haas, PhD, RN
Dean and Professor,
Marcella Niehoff School of Nursing,
Loyola University at Chicago,
Chicago, Illinois

Diana P. Hackbarth, PhD, RN
Professor,
Marcella Niehoff School of Nursing,
Loyola University at Chicago,
Chicago, Illinois

Margie J. Hansen, PhD, MSN, BSN, RN
Clinical Associate Professor of Nursing,
University of North Dakota,
Grand Forks, North Dakota

Karen A. Hanson, MS, RN, CNP
Nurse Practitioner,
Division of Gastroenterology and Hepatology,
Mayo Clinic,
Rochester, Minnesota

Debra E. Heidrich, MSN, RN, AOCN, CHPN
Guest Lecturer,
Wright State University,
Dayton, Ohio

Esther A. Hellman, PhD, MS, BSN
Assistant Professor,
Creighton University School of Nursing,
Omaha, Nebraska

Beverly E. Holland, MSN, RN, RhD, ARNP
Adult Nurse Practitioner,
Tabler Group, Mental Health Services,
Louisville, Kentucky

Rhonda Holloway, MBA, RN, NP
Private Practice,
Denver, Colorado

Roberta A. Jorgensen, MS, BSN
Gastrointestinal Nurse Coordinator,
Mayo Clinic,
Rochester, Minnesota

Esperanza Villanueva Joyce, EdD, CNS, RN
Nursing Dean and Professor,
Our Lady of the Lake College,
Baton Rouge, Louisiana

Annabelle M. Keene, MSN, RN, BC
School Nurse,
Bellevue Public Schools,
Bellevue, Nebraska;
Formerly, Associate Professor,
College of Saint Mary,
Omaha, Nebraska

Patricia A. Keresztes, PhD, CCRN
Assistant Professor of Nursing,
Purdue University Calumet,
Hammond, Indiana

Helene J. Krouse, PhD, APRN, BC, CORLN, FAAN
Professor,
Assistant Dean for Adult Health,
College of Nursing,
Wayne State University,
Detroit, Michigan

Kim K. Kuebler, MN, RN, ANP-CS
Clinical Coordinator, Oncology,
Emory University Hospital,
Atlanta, Georgia

Judi L. Kuric, PhD, MSN, RN, APRN-BC, CRRN-A, CNRN
Assistant Professor,
University of Southern Indiana;
Acute Care Nurse Practitioner,
Neuro Rehab Solutions,
Evansville, Indiana

Louise Nelson LaFramboise, PhD, RN
Assistant Professor,
College of Nursing,
University of Nebraska Medical Center,
Omaha, Nebraska

Joan M. Lappe, PhD, RN
Professor,
Creighton University School of Nursing,
Omaha, Nebraska

Anne M. Larson, PhD, MS, BA, BC-ANA
Professor of Nursing,
Midland Lutheran College,
Fremont, Nebraska;
Registered Nurse on call, Intensive Care Unit,
Alegent Health,
Immanuel Medical Center,
Omaha, Nebraska

Mira Lessick, PhD, MSN, BSN, RN
Associate Professor,
University of Toledo,
Toledo, Ohio

Patricia A. MacDonald, BSN, RN, NP
Consultant, Rheumatology,
University of Chicago,
Chicago, Illinois

Donna W. Markey, MSN, RN, ACNP-CS
Instructor,
School of Nursing;
Nurse Practitioner,
Digestive Health Center,
Oregon Health and Sciences University,
Portland, Oregon

Karen S. Martin, MSN, RN, FAAN
Health Care Consultant,
Martin Associates,
Omaha, Nebraska

Cynthia McCurren, PhD, MSN, BSN, RN
Associate Professor,
Associate Dean,
School of Nursing,
University of Louisville,
Louisville, Kentucky

Norma D. McNair, MSN, RN, CCRN, CNRN, APRN-BC
Assistant Clinical Professor,
School of Nursing,
University of California at Los Angeles;
Clinical Nurse Specialist,
Neuroscience/Orthopedics,
University of California at Los Angeles Medical Center,
Los Angeles, California

Patricia Meier, MA, BSN, AOCN
Staff Nurse,
Mercy General Health Partners,
Muskegon, Michigan

Sheila Melander, DSN, RN, ACNP-C, FCCM
Professor,
School of Nursing,
University of Tennessee at Memphis,
Memphis, Tennessee;
Cardiovascular Acute Care Nurse Practitioner,
Owensboro, Kentucky

Lindsay Ann Middelton, BSN, RN, CGC
Genetic Counselor,
Clinical Research Nurse,
National Institutes of Health,
National Cancer Institute,
Urology Oncology Branch,
Bethesda, Maryland

*Melanie S. Minton, MBA, BSN, RN, CNRN
Lead Business Faculty,
LeTourneau University,
Houston, Texas;
Director and Educator,
Neuroscience Nursing,
Memorial Hermann Memorial City Hospital,
Houston, Texas

Kim Miracle, MSN, RN, C
Clinical Nurse Specialist,
Outcomes Manager,
Jewish Hospital,
Louisville, Kentucky

Anita E. Molzahn, PhD, MN, BScN, RN
Professor,
School of Nursing,
University of Victoria,
Victoria, British Columbia,
Canada

---

*Deceased.

Mark Moyad, MD, MPH
Phil F. Jenkins Director of Complementary Medicine,
Urologic Oncology,
Clinical Cancer Researcher/Consultant,
University of Michigan,
Ann Arbor, Michigan

Elizabeth A. Murphy-Blake, MSEd, MSN, APRN-C,
FNP-C
Nurse Practitioner,
Veterans Administration Medical Center,
Omaha, Nebraska

Susan Newton, MS, BSN, RN, AOCN
Field Manager,
Oncology Nursing,
Ortho Biotech Oncology,
Bridgewater, New Jersey

Noreen Heer Nicol, MS, BS, RN, FNP
Clinical Senior Instructor,
School of Nursing,
University of Colorado,
Denver, Colorado;
Affiliate Assistant Professor,
School of Nursing,
University of Northern Colorado,
Greeley, Colorado;
Chief Clinical Officer,
National Jewish Medical and Research Center,
Denver, Colorado

Cheryl M. Noetscher, RN, BSN, MS
Manager,
Care Management,
St. Joseph's Hospital Health Center,
Syracuse, New York

Barbara B. Ott, PhD, RN
Associate Professor,
Villanova University,
Villanova, Pennsylvania

Jeannine M. Petit, MSN, BSN, CNRN, GNP-C
Nurse Practitioner,
Neurology Department,
Medical College of Wisconsin,
Milwaukee, Wisconsin

Mary Ellen Pike, MSN, BSN, RN
Assistant Professor,
Bellarmine University,
Louisville, Kentucky

Kathleen A. Popelka, DNSc, CFNP
Nurse Practitioner,
Women Veteran Manager,
Veterans Administration Medical Center,
Omaha, Nebraska

Sharon R. Redding, MN, RN
Associate Professor of Nursing,
College of Saint Mary;
Staff Nurse,
Alegent Bergan Mercy Medical Center,
Omaha, Nebraska

Marlene Reimer, PhD, RN, CNN(C)
Professor,
Faculty of Nursing,
University of Calgary,
Calgary, Alberta,
Canada

Dottie Roberts, MSN, MACI, CMSRN, RN, BC, ONC
Clinical Nurse Specialist,
Rehabilitative/Medical Services,
Palmetto Baptist Medical Center,
Columbia, South Carolina

M. Lynn Rodgers, MSN, RNC, CCRN, CNRN,
ACNP-BC
Acute Care Nurse Practitioner,
Deaconess Hospital,
Evansville, Indiana

Helen Murdock Rogers, DNSc, RN
Associate Professor,
Chairperson,
Nursing Department,
Worcester State College,
Worcester, Massachusetts

Vicki M. Ross, PhD(C), RN
Doctoral Candidate,
University of Kansas,
Kansas City, Kansas

Linda M. Scott, MS, CRNP
Nurse Practitioner,
The National Institutes of Health,
Bethesda, Maryland

Carol A. Sedlak, PhD, RN, ONC
Associate Professor,
College of Nursing,
Kent State University,
Kent, Ohio

Judy Selfridge-Thomas, MSN, RN, CEN, FNP
Nurse Practitioner,
Department of Emergency Medicine,
St. Mary Medical Center,
Long Beach, California;
San Pedro Peninsula Hospital,
San Pedro, California

Nancy Shoemaker, MS, APRN/PMH
Preceptor, Graduate Nursing Students,
School of Nursing,
University of Maryland;
Nurse Psychotherapist,
University of Maryland Fayette Street Clinic,
Baltimore, Maryland

Mary Sieggreen, MSN, APN, NP, CUN
Associate Professor,
Clinical Nursing,
Wayne State University;
Vascular Nurse Practitioner,
Harpen University Hospital,
Detroit Medical Center,
Detroit, Michigan

Karen A. Sikorksi, MS, BSN, APN
Clinical Nurse Specialist, Pain,
OSF Saint Anthony Medical Center,
Rockford, Illinois

Sarah C. Smith, MA, BS, RN, CRNO
Advanced Practice Nurse,
Educational Associate,
Department of Ophthalmology and Visual Sciences,
University of Iowa Health Care,
Oxford, Iowa

Dianne M. Smolen, PhD, RN, C, CNS
Professor and Director, Continuing Nursing Education,
School of Nursing,
Medical College of Ohio,
Toledo, Ohio

**Christine Stewart-Amidei, MSN, RN, CNRN,
　CCRN, CS**
Advanced Practice Nurse,
Neurosurgery,
University of Chicago,
Chicago, Illinois

Nancy Evans Stoner, MSN, RN, CNSN
Clinical Nurse Specialist,
Nutrition Support,
University of Pennsylvania Medical Center,
Philadelphia, Pennsylvania

Janice Tazbir, MS, CCRN
Associate Professor of Nursing,
Purdue University Calumet,
Hammond, Indiana;
Staff RN, Intensive Care Unit,
University of Chicago,
Chicago, Illinois

Amy Verst, MSN, RN, CPNP, ATC
Assistant Professor,
Bellarmine University,
Louisville, Kentucky

Carol Weber, PhD, MSN, BSN, RN
Professor of Nursing,
Regis University,
Denver, Colorado

Ann H. White, PhD, RN
Associate Professor of Nursing,
University of Southern Indiana,
Evansville, Indiana

Bernadette White, MSN, RN, APRNc, HTP
Assistant Professor,
Creighton University School of Nursing,
Omaha, Nebraska

Connie White-Williams, MSN, RN, FNP
Affiliate Faculty,
Cardiothoracic Transplant Coordinator,
University of Alabama at Birmingham,
Birmingham, Alabama

Nancy L. York, MSN, RN
Assistant Professor,
Lansing School of Nursing and Health Sciences,
Bellarmine University,
Louisville, Kentucky

Reviewers

Mike Aldridge, BSN, RN, CCRN
Children's Hospital of Austin,
Austin, Texas

Gwen Anderson, PhD, RN
San Diego State University,
San Diego, California

Carol Pappas Appel, MSN, RN, CNP, AOCN
Barbara Ann Karmanos Cancer Institute,
Detroit, Michigan

Rebecca S. Appleton, PhD, RN
Marshall University,
Huntington, West Virginia

Susan B. Battistoni, PhD, RN
Salisbury University,
Salisbury, Maryland

Susan Birkhead, BSN, MPH
Samaritan Hospital,
Troy, New York

Jonathan S. Black, BS
University of Nebraska Medical Center,
Omaha, Nebraska

Terry Butkus, MSN, RN, FNP
University of Nebraska Medical Center,
Omaha, Nebraska

Elizabeth M. Carson, EdD, MS, RN
Saint Anthony College of Nursing,
Rockford, Illinois

Janet E. Cuddigan, PhD, RN
University of Nebraska Medical Center,
Omaha, Nebraska

R. Eric Doerfler, MSN, NP
Nightingale Health Centers, Inc.,
Harrisburg, Pennsylvania

Diane K. Dressler, MSN, RN, CCRN
Marquette University,
Milwaukee, Wisconsin

Rebecca Ann Fountain, MSN, RN
University of Texas at Tyler,
Tyler, Texas

Joy L. Haagsma, MSN, RN
Cape Cod Community College,
West Barnstable, Massachusetts

Linda E. Hein, MSN, RN, CNS, HNC, CHTP,
  Reiki Master
Veterans Administration Medical Center,
Portland, Oregon;
Private Practice,
Vancouver, Washington

Robbie Helmich Henson, PhD, RN
Oklahoma Baptist University,
Shawnee, Oklahoma

Karen L. Heys, MN, RN
Everett Community College,
Everett, Washington

Sadie Pauline Hutson, MSN, RN, CRNP
University of Pennsylvania,
Philadelphia, Pennsylvania

Molly Ann Hoffman Jalufka, BSN, RNC, TNCC
The Victoria College,
Gonzales, Texas

Jennifer Kane, BSN, RN
Massachusetts General Hospital,
Boston, Massachusetts

Joan A. Masters, PhD, RN, GNP
Northeastern University,
Boston, Massachusetts

Sharon J. Olsen, MS, RN, AOCN
Johns Hopkins University,
Baltimore, Maryland

Debra L. Schutte, PhD, RN
University of Iowa,
Iowa City, Iowa

Lynda Shand, PhD, MA, RN
College of New Rochelle,
New Rochelle, New York

Julie A. Slack, MSN, RN
Mohave Community College,
Kingman, Arizona

Judith Blanche Sweet, MS, RN, FNP
University of California at San Francisco,
San Francisco, California

Scott Carter Thigpen, MSN, RN, CCRN, CEN
South Georgia College,
Douglas, Georgia

Peggy Tidikis-Menck, PhD, RN
University of Nebraska Medical Center,
Omaha, Nebraska

Susan C. Vaughn, MSN(C), BSN, RN
Gentiva Health Services,
Charlotte, North Carolina

Rosalee C. Yeaworth, PhD, RN, FAAN
University of Nebraska Medical Center,
Omaha, Nebraska

Preface

It is our conviction that a book is not a static document. Certainly, a book—bound and printed—portrays health care at a given moment in time. By making the seventh edition of *Medical-Surgical Nursing* a web-enhanced textbook, we are able to provide instructors and students with a guide to delivering safe and appropriate nursing care as well as with enhanced resources from the web that are constantly changing and reflective of day-to-day changes in health care. To that end, we see this book as a "work in progress." Future editions will continue to improve, and we appreciate your comments, questions, and corrections to guide our ongoing work. We can improve only with your input. We also realize that educators and students must share in the task of bringing the book to life.

PHILOSOPHY AND APPROACH

This textbook grows out of the belief that nurses and physicians do not compete with each other but instead collaborate to reach certain outcomes in cooperation with the client and family. Nonetheless, nursing and medicine are separate disciplines. Consequently, nursing and medical content are not intermingled in this text. However, because nursing and medicine are collaborative efforts, it is often difficult for nursing students to understand one without having an understanding of the other. We therefore present thorough coverage of both nursing management and medical management.

With the increased emphasis on outcomes in health care, we have organized client care under the heading of Outcome Management. Several headings appear under this heading, including Medical Management, Nursing Management of the Medical Client, Surgical Management, and Nursing Management of the Surgical Client, as appropriate.

In this text, we use the nursing process to describe nursing management, but we do not apply the nursing process to every disorder. Instead, we have designated the nursing process for major or prototypical disorders. Within the presentation of the nursing process for those disorders, we have developed nursing diagnoses and collaborative problems, as appropriate, with their own outcomes and interventions. Collaborative problems define those client problems that cannot be resolved through independent nursing actions; they are potential complications that may develop because of a disorder, surgical procedure, or nonsurgical treatment. Collaborative problems complete the picture of nursing care and eliminate the need to force-fit every client problem into the framework of a nursing diagnosis. We have written Outcomes and Interventions sections for *each* identified nursing diagnosis and collaborative problem because we have found from our teaching experience that students cannot easily pull apart lists of diagnoses followed by lists of outcomes and interventions and then rebuild them into care plans.

ORGANIZATION

This edition is organized from simple to complex and from common to uncommon disorders. The early portion of the text focuses on the care of clients usually assigned to beginning students. The book then progresses to address the care of clients with more complex disorders, which are more commonly taught in upper division classes.

The format of the text has remained the same but is now divided into 18 units. The first five units are devoted to content that is applicable to all medical-surgical clients. The material in this first portion of the book will guide the student in learning to provide comprehensive care regardless of the specific diagnosis or problem. Concepts that span medical-surgical practice, such as health promotion, care delivery settings, physical assessment, complementary and alternative therapies, fluid and electrolyte balance, genetics, infectious diseases, pain, palliative care, perioperative care, and oncology, are found in this portion of the book. The remainder of the text is divided into common responses to health disorders. These units begin with a review of anatomy and physiology, followed by a chapter on health and diagnostic assessment; one or more "nursing care" chapters then present the nursing care of clients with specific disorders. We have added two new Anatomy and Physiology Reviews to address physiologic genomics and arousal, pain, and conscious awareness. A brief description of each unit is described below.

Unit 1 discusses health promotion and self-care and includes chapters related to health promotion in both middle-aged and older adults. Chapter 4 discusses history taking, physical assessment, and diagnostic testing. Chapter 5 is a new chapter that provides an overview of complementary and alternative therapies.

Unit 2 presents an overview of nursing and health care today. Chapter 6 describes the "stakeholders" in health care delivery, because medical-surgical nurses (not just managers) in all areas of practice must become increasingly aware of how health care is financed. Because the practice of medical-surgical nursing is not confined to certain areas, this edition contains more material on nursing care and philosophy in various care settings. Chapters 7 through 12 address nursing care in ambulatory, acute, intensive care, home health, long-term care, and rehabilitation settings. A new chapter on intensive care and rehabilitation nursing can be used to orient new students to these care settings.

Unit 3 looks at concepts that provide the foundations of care for medical-surgical clients, including separate chapters on fluid and electrolyte disorders. Other chapters address acid-base disorders and the surgical experience.

Unit 4 discusses physiologic concepts basic to medical-surgical nursing care. The unit begins with a new genetics chapter (Chapter 17) and continues with chapters related to cancer, infectious disorders, and wound healing.

Unit 5 covers psychosocial concepts basic to medical-surgical nursing care. The unit begins with a chapter on pain management and continues with chapters on palliative care, sleep and rest disorders, psychosocial and mental health concerns, and substance abuse.

Units 6 through 17 focus on the management of clients with specific disorders. Each unit begins with a structure and function overview of the pertinent body systems, followed by a nursing assessment chapter. The structure and function overview has been shortened and redesigned, and more artwork has been added for each body system.

In general, the discussion of specific disorders includes headings for Etiology, Pathophysiology, Clinical Manifestations, and Outcome Management. Because increasingly more nursing care is being directed toward health promotion, in this edition we have added content that focuses on health promotion, health maintenance, and health restoration to the Etiology topics in the disorders chapters. To emphasize the importance of understanding pathophysiology and its relationship to the treatment of a disorder, we have incorporated headings in the management sections that will help the student see the relationship between the pathophysiologic changes and specific strategies to promote positive outcomes in nursing management. The term *clinical manifestations* has been selected to encompass signs and symptoms along with diagnostic findings. The term *manifestations* replaces "signs and symptoms" in all chapters except one; in Chapter 23 on palliative care, *symptom management* is the preferred term.

Unit 18 presents the care of clients with multisystem disorders. Chapter 82 looks at organ donation issues, the transplantation process, quality-of-life issues, and specific interventions for clients requiring organ transplantation. Shock and multisystem disorders are discussed in Chapter 83. Chapter 84 examines the basic concepts of triage, ethical issues, and maintaining the chain of custody of medicolegal evidence. Chapter 84

also organizes emergency conditions by various nursing diagnoses identified and treated.

Hallmark Features

A completely new design focuses on guiding the reader to the Evolve website, where a wealth of supplemental content resides. Each chapter opens with a listing of web enhancements, which introduces the reader to that chapter's features on the Evolve website. All of the web features—including features that begin in the text and continue on the Evolve website with interactive exercises and bonus material—contain a reference within the text and are designated with an **evolve** icon in the margin. The following is a list of our hallmark features, including a description and the location of the feature:

- **Concept Maps** are flowcharts linking pathophysiological processes, clinical manifestations, and medical and nursing interventions. This feature appears throughout the text.
- **Case Studies** present complex client scenarios with in-depth detail—most with multiple clinical problems. This feature contains an introduction in the text; the Evolve website contains the body of the case study and the discussions, multiple-choice questions, and a nursing care plan.
- **Client Education Guides** act as examples to help students teach clients how to collaborate in their own care; these guides are worded in client-centered language. Some guides appear on the Evolve website, and others remain in the text for this edition. All Client Education Guides are translated into Spanish and appear on the Evolve website.
- **Care Plans** present nursing care using the nursing process format and highlight both nursing diagnoses and collaborative problems, expected outcomes, interventions with rationales, and evaluations. Some care plans appear on the Evolve website, but the majority remain in the text for this edition.
- **Bridge to Home Health Care** boxes describe specific applications and strategies for medical-surgical care in the home. Some bridges appear on the Evolve website, and others remain in the text for this edition.
- **Management and Delegation** boxes present the primary concerns nurses need to address when delegating care activities to unlicensed assistive personnel. This feature appears in the text and includes new topics such as Delegation in Health Care Delivery, Postoperative Care: Vital Signs, and Management of Clients with Vascular Disorders.
- **Bridge to Critical Care** boxes are an integrated feature to highlight major critical care concerns. This feature appears in the text and now includes a new bridge on defibrillation.
- **Critical Monitoring** boxes highlight those clinical manifestations that must be reported to the physi-

cian without delay. This feature appears throughout the text. New Critical Monitoring features for this edition include Ruptured Abdominal Aortic Aneurysm, Acute Pulmonary Edema, Digoxin Toxicity, Angina from Impending Myocardial Infarction, Headache, and Myasthenic and Cholinergic Crises in Clients with Myasthenia Gravis.

- **Physical Assessment Findings in the Healthy Adult** serve both to remind students of the relevant normal findings for each body system and to demonstrate how to chart those findings with clinical precision. This feature appears in the text.
- **Diversity in Health Care** boxes are focused discussions of health and illness related to particular populations. This feature appears on the Evolve website.
- **Ethical Issues in Nursing** boxes feature an ethical dilemma in the form of a question, with the discussion immediately following. This feature remains on the Evolve website for this edition.
- **Case Management** boxes, written by a practicing case manager, present key coordination and anticipatory issues under consistent headings of Assess, Advocate, and Prevent Readmission, thus linking nursing care with client-focused case management. This feature appears on the Evolve website.
- **Clinical Pathways** are excerpted from actual pathways used in specific hospitals. They are accompanied by a guide to show what should occur during specific times in the pathway and how to stay on track when caring for the client. This feature appears on the Evolve website.
- **Thinking Critically Questions** conclude each nursing care chapter. This feature presents short, typical client scenarios and pose questions about what actions to take. Discussions for all the questions are provided on the Evolve website.
- **NOC boxes** appear in chapters that contain nursing diagnoses content. The chapter opens with the appropriate suggested NOC outcome labels for the nursing diagnoses presented in the body of the text, thus emphasizing the importance of outcomes at the outset of the chapter.
- **Anatomy and Physiology Reviews** introduce each body system unit and provide a brief review of the relevant anatomy and physiology of the body system.
- **Appendixes** on Religious Beliefs and Practices Affecting Health Care, A Health History Format That Integrates the Assessment of Functional Health Patterns, and Laboratory Values of Clinical Importance in Medical-Surgical Nursing appear on the Evolve website.

NEW CONTENT AND FEATURES

In addition to the hallmark features listed in the previous section, the seventh edition includes six new boxed features, as well as a new and unique icon. This edition also features four new chapters and two new Anatomy and Physiology Reviews.

Four New Chapters

- **Complementary and Alternative Therapies** (Chapter 5) discusses why people choose alternative therapies and issues related to discussing complementary and alternative therapies with clients. The chapter provides students with the necessary understanding of complementary and alternative therapy.
- **Critical Care** (Chapter 9) provides a basic understanding of the topic of critical care, an area in which medical-surgical nurses are exposed.
- **Rehabilitation** (Chapter 12) provides a basic understanding of the topic of rehabilitation, an area in which medical-surgical nurses are exposed.
- **Genetics** (Chapter 17) discusses basic concepts of genes, chromosomes, and DNA, as well as the nursing role in genetic care. The chapter provides a basic understanding of molecular genetics and principles of human genetics in order to function effectively in today's health care arena.

Two New Anatomy and Physiology Reviews

Physiologic Genomics (Unit 4) is the unit opener for chapters on genetics, perspectives in oncology, cancer, wounds, and infectious disorders. It prepares the student for the chapters in the unit.

Arousal, Pain, and Conscious Awareness (Unit 5) is the unit opener for chapters on pain, palliative care, sleep, psychosocial, and substance abuse. It prepares the student for the chapters in the unit.

New Features

- **Web enhancements boxes** appear on each chapter opener and list the chapter features that appear on the Evolve website.
- **Integrating Pharmacology** boxes explain and explore common classifications of medications that are routinely used to treat a specific condition. These features help students understand how medications can be synergistically used for disease management. This feature appears throughout the text.
- **Genetic Links** boxes "link" a disease with its corresponding genetics. This feature provides the student with the description, genetics, diagnosis/testing, and management of a specific disease and appears throughout the text.
- **Terrorism Alert** boxes provide cutting-edge material on bioterrorism. They aid the student in recognizing the clinical manifestations and diseases associated with bioterrorism. This feature appears throughout the text.
- **Evidence-Based Practice in Action** boxes have been revamped for this edition. Applicable management chapters will feature these boxes in the text and

present a synopsis of the research with 4 to 5 supporting article summaries.

- **Evidence-based** content is noted in the margin by an **EB** icon. This icon introduces the concept of evidence-based (research-based) practice and provides numerous practical examples of how it relates to nursing practice.
- **Complementary and Alternative Therapy** boxes have been completely rewritten for this edition and present nontraditional therapies used by clients and health care providers to treat various conditions. They discuss alternative and complimentary therapies related to specific diseases or body systems. Some boxes are featured in the text, and others appear on the Evolve website.
- **Spanish Assessment Phrases** are listed on the Evolve website.
- **NIC, NOC, NANDA** appendixes located on the Evolve website list all of the labels for NIC and NOC as well as NANDA diagnoses.

ANCILLARY PACKAGE

Student Ancillaries

The **Evolve website** is available at http://evolve.elsevier.com/Black/medsurg/ and features a wealth of assets:

- New **Evolve Learning Resources,** which provide students with open-book quizzes that consist of crossword puzzles, multiple-choice questions, matching questions, and fill-in-the-blank questions for each chapter. Students are prompted at both the beginning and end of each chapter to take advantage of these resources.
- **Special Features,** which include Web-Only Features that appear on the Evolve website (Appendixes, Case Management, Clinical Pathways, Diversity in Health Care, Ethical Issues in Nursing, and Spanish Assessment Phrases); Web-Partial Features, with some features appearing in the text and others appearing on the Evolve website (Bridge to Home Health Care, Care Plans, Client Education Guides, Complementary and Alternative Therapy); and Web-Enhanced Features that start in the text and continue on the Evolve website (Case Studies, Concept Maps, and Thinking Critically).
- **Case Studies** and their accompanying discussions, multiple-choice questions, and a nursing care plan.
- Discussions for the **Thinking Critically** questions.
- Online **Concept Map Creator,** which is a one-of-a-kind program that allows students to create customized concept maps. Students are prompted to enter the following client data: medical diagnosis, pathophysiology, risk factors, clinical manifestations, nursing diagnoses, collaborative problems,

expected outcomes, and nursing interventions. The program then generates a concept map in two formats: (1) a graphic "map" that clearly illustrates the relationships among various client data and components of the nursing process, and (2) a tabular word processing file that students may print and use to record client responses/evaluation data, thereby completing the nursing process.

- **Fluid and Electrolyte Module,** which is a user-friendly tutorial that helps students master the difficult concepts of fluid and electrolyte balance and imbalance. This self-paced program includes animations to help illustrate important concepts, and an accessible and inviting user interface helps make the program easy to navigate. The program is divided into five sections: an introduction, three sections on fluid and electrolyte balance and imbalance, and a quiz section with approximately 75 questions to test students on information learned throughout the program.
- Seventy-five **Animations, Video Clips, and Audio Clips** on anatomy assessment, physical examination including heart sounds to visually supplement medical-surgical nursing.
- More than 45 bonus **Health Assessment Full-Color Images** covering all body systems.
- **Audio Pronunciations** for more than 250 words.
- **Content Updates** from the authors.
- **WebLinks** for each chapter.

The **new Student CD-ROM** packaged with the text contains the following:

- **Open book quizzes** consisting of crossword puzzles, multiple-choice questions, matching questions, and fill-in-the blank questions for each chapter give students the chance to assess their understanding of the chapter.
- The **Fluid and Electrolyte Learning Module** gives the student a self-guided opportunity to learn and master this complex content.
- **Case Studies** with discussions, multiple-choice questions, and a nursing care plan provide real-life examples of clients with complex problems.
- **Anatomy and Physiology animations** that demonstrate complex processes to help students grasp underlying concepts.
- Discussions for the **Thinking Critically** questions give students an opportunity to compare their responses to those of the authors.

The **Virtual Clinical Excursion** workbook/CD-ROM guides students through a multi-floor virtual hospital to care for highly complex and diverse clients. Students will be able to collect client data from various sources (reports, charts, medication administration record, and short video clips and audio clips of nurse-client interactions); work with data entry and retrieval screens; record client data; analyze and interpret data to reach conclusions about complex problems; listen to a report and itemize a client's problems and high-priority concerns; administer medications; and more.

The **Study Guide** is in the traditional print format text but is completely rewritten for this edition. It contains exercises such as compare and contrast similar disorders or clinical manifestations, short answer, reflective (why instead of what), diagram of treatment (e.g., ask where drugs should be placed), best practices, application questions (specific client, not a case study), drug dosages (from IV to oral), decipher what's wrong with sample documentation, sample interventions, keeping skills sharp (safety, drug dosage/math, communication/assessment), and concept map exercises.

Instructor Ancillaries

The **Instructor's Resource** is available both online and on CD-ROM! Instructors also have access to the student resources. The Instructor's Resource includes the following helpful aids:

- **Instructor's Manual (IM)** consists of critical points to emphasize and facilitate student learning for both the classroom and the clinical setting. The classroom activities include Review Activity, Class Assignments, Lecture/Discussion, Guest Speakers, Group Activities, and Concept Map Activity (if applicable). The clinical activities include Skills Laboratory, Clinical Site Activities, and Clinical Conference Activities.
- The **PowerPoint Presentation** consists of approximately 1500 lecture slides, providing instructors with text lecture slides for each unit.
- The computerized **Test Bank** has approximately 2500 questions, including more than 400 questions in the new NCLEX alternate item format. Each test question includes a rationale, Nursing Process step, Cognitive Level, NCLEX category of client needs, and text reference.
- The **Image Collection** consists of more than 800 full-color images from the text and other sources.
- This resource will also contain **WebLinks** to various related websites.

The **Evolve Course Management System** is an interactive learning environment that works in coordination with **Medical-Surgical Nursing, 7th Edition,** to provide Internet-based course management tools you can use to reinforce and expand on the concepts you deliver in class. You can use Evolve to:

- Publish your class syllabus, outline, and lecture notes.
- Set up "virtual office hours" and e-mail communication.
- Share important dates and information through the online class *Calendar*.
- Encourage student participation through *Chat Rooms* and *Discussion Boards*.

ACKNOWLEDGMENTS

We have been asked several times, "Isn't a revision a lot less work than a new book?" You would think so, but it's amazing—a revision is no less work than a new book.

A project of this size certainly could not be accomplished without the collaboration of many people. First and foremost, we recognize the importance of the clinical expertise of our many contributing authors, which enables us to present a new edition that continues to be the "gold standard" for textbooks of medical-surgical nursing. We would also like to thank the special feature contributors.

There are also many people at Elsevier who have made this monumental task a "do-able" task. Thank you, Barbara Nelson Cullen, Executive Publisher, for your ongoing encouragement, help, and support. Thank you, Victoria Bruno, Senior Developmental Editor and Adrienne Simon, Developmental Editor, for your help and day-to-day management, keeping us on track to meet the production schedule. Your organization made this project move well. Thanks also to Victoria for hiring the ancillary writers and developing all the ancillaries, including the Evolve website. Thank you, Catherine Ott, Senior Editorial Assistant, for handling the countless administrative tasks associated with the publication of the book and ancillaries, as well as for coordinating the peer reviews of the book. Thank you, Graphic World, for providing wonderful full-color illustrations. Thank you, Jodi Willard, Senior Project Manager, for keeping the book on schedule and for making this aspect of the book publication go smoothly. Finally, we want to thank *you*—educators and students—for allowing us to join you in the teaching and learning of medical-surgical nursing. We trust that you will find the seventh edition of *Medical-Surgical Nursing: Clinical Management for Positive Outcomes* a valuable asset.

Joyce M. Black and Jane Hokanson Hawks

Contents

6 Mobility Disorders
Anatomy and Physiology Review: The Musculoskeletal System, 588
Robert G. Carroll

27 Assessment of the Musculoskeletal System, 565
Peggy Doheny
Carol A. Sedlak

28 Management of Clients with Musculoskeletal Disorders, 579
Dottie Roberts
Joan M. Lappe

29 Management of Clients with Musculoskeletal Trauma or Overuse, 619
Dottie Roberts

7 Nutritional Disorders
Anatomy and Physiology Review: The Nutritional (Gastrointestinal) System, 658
Robert G. Carroll

30 Assessment of Nutrition and the Digestive System, 668
Vicki M. Ross

35 Management of Clients with Intestinal Disorders, 807

Helen Murdock Rogers

36 Management of Clients with Urinary Disorders, 857

Francie Bernier

37 Management of Clients with Renal Disorders, 913

Anita E. Molzahn

**12 Circulatory Disorders
     Anatomy and Physiology Review:
     The Circulatory System, 1468**
Robert G. Carroll

**13 Cardiac Disorders
     Anatomy and Physiology Review:
     The Heart, 1548**
Robert G. Carroll

18   Multisystem Disorders

82   Management of Clients Requiring Transplantation, 2425
Connie White-Williams

83   Management of Clients with Shock and Multisystem Disorders, 2443
Louise Nelson LaFramboise

84   Management of Clients in the Emergency Department, 2479
Judy Selfridge-Thomas

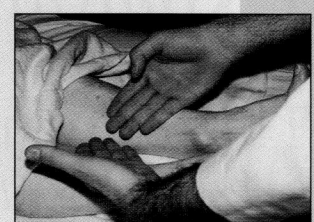

Integumentary Disorders

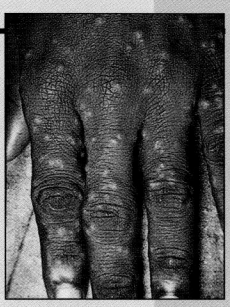

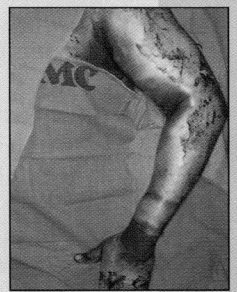

Anatomy and Physiology Review

The Integumentary System
Robert G. Carroll

The integument, or skin, makes up 15% to 20% of the body's weight. Intact skin is the body's primary defense system. It protects us from invasion by organisms, helps to regulate body temperature, manufactures vitamins, and provides our external appearance. Skin has three primary layers (i.e., *epidermis,* or outer layer; the *dermis,* or inner layer; and the *hypodermis,* or subcutaneous layer) as well as epidermal appendages (i.e., eccrine glands, apocrine glands, sebaceous glands, hair follicles, and nails).

The skin is the most prominent organ containing *epithelium,* which is composed of cells that provide a continuous barrier between the body contents and the outside environment. Epithelial cells also cover the gastrointestinal (GI) tract, pulmonary airways and alveoli, renal tubules and the urinary system, and the ducts that empty onto the surface of the skin (lumen) of the GI and respiratory systems. Epithelial cells allow the selective transport of ions, nutrients, and metabolic wastes and have a permeability to water that is partially regulated. Epithelial cells are joined to each other through tight junctions and express different populations of protein transporters on the apical side (generally facing a lumen) and the basolateral (facing the blood, or serosal) side. The functional significance of epithelial transport is covered in the GI and renal chapters (see the Anatomy and Physiology Review for Units 7 and 8).

STRUCTURE OF THE INTEGUMENTARY SYSTEM
EPIDERMIS

The epidermis is the thin, stratified outer skin layer that is in direct contact with the external environment (Figure U11-1). The thickness of the epidermis ranges from 0.04 mm on the eyelids to 1.6 mm on the palms and soles. *Desmosomes* (points of intercellular attachment that are vital for cell-to-cell adhesion) are found in the epidermis. *Keratinocytes,* the principal cells of the epidermis, produce *keratin* in a complex process. The cells begin in the basal cell layer and change constantly, moving upward through the epidermis. On the surface, they are sloughed off or lost by abrasion. Thus the epidermis constantly regenerates itself, providing a tough keratinized barrier.

Skin color reflects both the production of pigment granules *(melanin)* by melanocytes and, in light-skinned people, the presence of blood *(hemoglobin).* Skin color reflects a combination of four basic colors:

- Exogenously formed carotenoids (yellow)
- Melanin (brown)
- Oxygenated hemoglobin in arterioles and capillaries (red)
- Reduced hemoglobin in venules (blue)

Melanin plays the largest role in skin color; it is produced in the epidermis and in corresponding layers of the hair follicle. Although melanin is not produced in the dermis, it can be deposited in the dermis from the epidermis through various processes (such as inflammation).

Melanosomes are granules in melanocytes that synthesize melanin. Skin color differences result from the size and quantity of melanosomes as well as from the rate of melanin production. In natives of equatorial Africa, there is an increase in the size and number of melanosomes (not melanocytes) as well as increased melanin production. The melanosomes are large, discrete, and dispersed. In natives of northern Europe, the melanosomes are small and aggregated, producing less melanin. Sun exposure initially increases the size and functional activity of both melanocytes and melanosomes. With chronic sun exposure, there is an increase in the concentration of melanocytes as well as in size and functional activity. The presence of melanin limits the penetration of sun rays into the skin and protects against sunburn and the development of ultraviolet light-induced skin carcinomas.

Epidermal Appendages

Epidermal appendages are down growths of epidermis into the dermis. They consist of eccrine glands, apocrine units, sebaceous glands, hair, and nails.

Glands

Eccrine glands produce sweat and play an important role in thermoregulation. They are found throughout

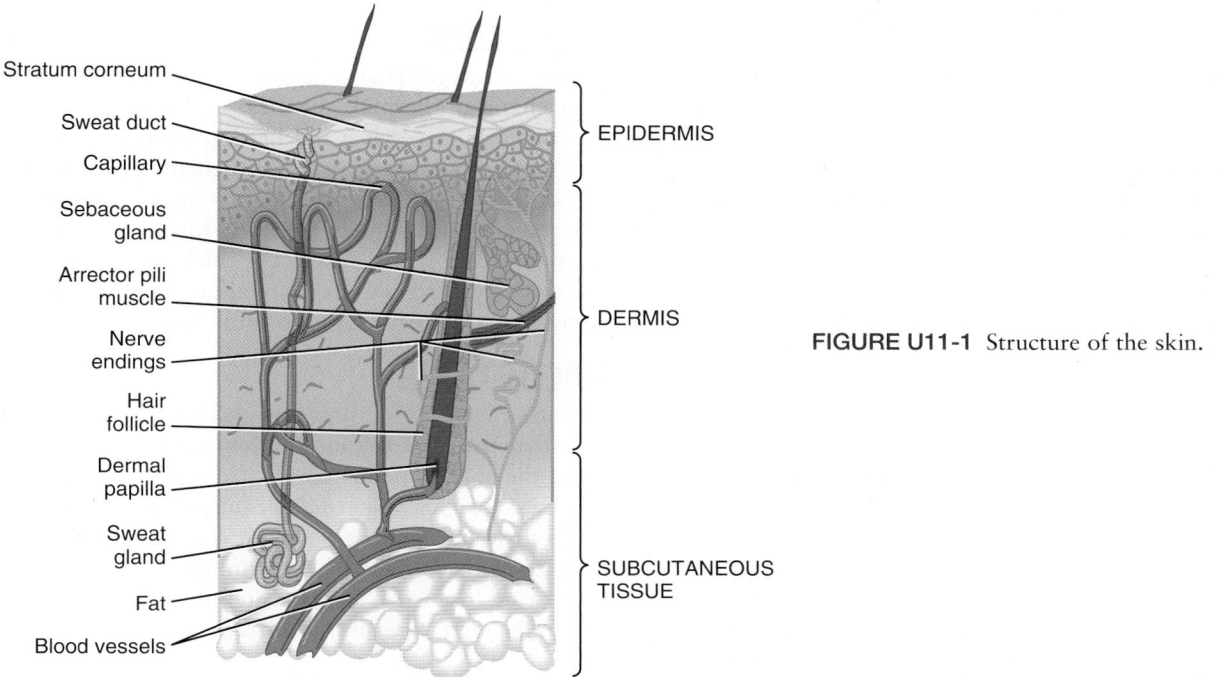

Stratum corneum

Sweat duct

Capillary

Sebaceous gland

Arrector pili muscle

Nerve endings

Hair follicle

Dermal papilla

Sweat gland

Fat

Blood vessels

EPIDERMIS

DERMIS

SUBCUTANEOUS TISSUE

FIGURE U11-1 Structure of the skin.

the skin except on the vermilion border (junction of the pink area of the lip with the surrounding skin), the ears, nail bed, glans penis, and labia minora. They are more numerous on the palms, soles, forehead, and axillae. Sweat is similar to plasma but is more dilute. Eccrine gland secretion is stimulated by heat as well as by exercise and emotional stress. Eccrine glands exit the body independently of the hair shaft (see Figure U11-1).

Apocrine glands occur primarily in the axillae, breast areolae, anogenital area, ear canals, and eyelids. In lower-order animals, apocrine secretions function as sexual attractants *(pheromones)*, and the apocrine secretion musk is used as a perfume base. The role, if any, in humans is not established. Mediated by adrenergic innervation, apocrine glands secrete a milky substance that becomes odoriferous when altered by skin surface bacteria. These glands do not function until puberty, and they require a high output of sex hormone for activity.

Sebaceous glands are found throughout the skin except on the palms and soles and are most abundant on the face, scalp, upper back, and chest. They are associated with hair follicles that open onto the skin surface, where *sebum* (a mixture of sebaceous gland-produced lipids and epidermal cell-derived lipids) is released. Sebum has a lubricating function and bactericidal activity. Androgen is responsible for sebaceous gland development. In utero androgen causes neonatal acne; after puberty sebum production can cause acne in adolescents.

Hair and Nails

Hair is a nonviable protein end product found on all skin surfaces except the palms and soles. Each hair follicle functions as an independent unit and goes through intermittent stages of development. Hair develops from the mitotic activity of the hair bulb. The rate of hair growth varies in different parts of the body. In a typical adult scalp, 85% to 90% of hairs are in an *anagen* (growth) phase. The remainder are in a *telogen* (rest) phase. About 50 to 100 hairs are lost each day. As a rule, the growing phase of hair on the eyebrows, trunk, and extremities does not exceed 6 months. Its resting phase is 3 to 4 months.

Hair form (straight or curly) depends on the shape of the hair in cross-section. Straight hair has a round cross-section; curly hair has an oval or ribbon-like cross-section. Curved follicles also affect the curliness of hair. Melanocytes in the bulb determine hair color. Hair follicles usually occur with sebaceous glands, and together they form a *pilosebaceous unit. Arrector pili* muscles of the dermis attach to hair follicles and elevate the hairs when body temperature falls, producing "goose bumps."

Nails are horny scales of epidermis. The nail matrix is the source of specialized, nonkeratinized cells. They differentiate into keratinized cells, which make up the nail protein. The matrix for nail formation is located in the proximal nail bed. It grows forward from the nail fold to cover the nail bed. Fingernails grow about 0.1 mm each day; complete reproduction takes 100 to 150 days. Toenails grow one third as fast as fingernails do. A damaged nail matrix, which may result from trauma or aggressive manicuring, produces a distorted nail. Nails are also sensitive to physiologic changes; for instance, they grow more slowly in cold weather and during periods of illness.

Nails and hair consist of keratinized and, therefore, "dead" cells. The ingestion of gelatin has not been shown to increase nail growth or strength.

DERMIS

The dermis, a dense layer of tissue beneath the epidermis, gives the skin most of its substance and structure. It varies from 1 to 4 mm in thickness and is thickest over the back. The dermis contains fibroblasts, macrophages, mast cells, and lymphocytes, which promote wound healing. The skin's lymphatic, vascular, and nerve supplies, which maintain equilibrium in the skin, are in the dermis.

The dermis is divided into two parts: papillary and reticular. The papillary dermis, which contains increased amounts of collagen, blood vessels, sweat glands, and elastin, is in contact with the epidermis. The *reticular* dermis also contains collagen but with increased amounts of mature elastic tissue. The dermis houses many specialized cells, blood vessels, and nerves.

The epidermis and dermis meet at the *dermoepidermal junction*. This area contains wave-like projections from the dermis called *papillae* (or rete pegs), which correspond to reciprocal structures in the epidermis. The *subepidermal basement membrane zone* is a semipermeable filter that permits fluid exchange of components such as nutrients, metabolites, and waste products.

HYPODERMIS

The *subcutaneous layer* is a specialized layer of connective tissue. It is sometimes called the *adipose layer* because of its fat content. This layer is absent in some sites, such as the eyelids, scrotum, areola, and tibia. Age, heredity, and many other factors influence the thickness of the subcutaneous layer. Subcutaneous fat is generally thickest on the back and buttocks, giving shape and contour over the bone. This layer functions as insulation from extremes of hot and cold, as a cushion to trauma, and as a source of energy and hormone metabolism.

FUNCTION OF THE INTEGUMENTARY SYSTEM

The skin is a morphologically complex structure that serves several functions essential to life. The skin differs anatomically and physiologically in various areas of the body. Functions of the skin include protection, maintenance of homeostasis, thermoregulation, sensory reception, vitamin synthesis, and processing of antigenic substances.

PROTECTION

The skin protects the body against many forms of trauma (e.g., mechanical, thermal, chemical, radiant). The intact tough epidermal layer is a mechanical barrier. Bacteria, foreign matter, other organisms, and chemicals penetrate it with difficulty. The oily and slightly acid secretions of its sebaceous glands protect the body further by limiting the growth of many organisms. The thickened skin of the palms and soles provides additional covering to absorb the constant use of or trauma to these areas.

HOMEOSTASIS

Skin forms a barrier that prevents excessive loss of water and electrolytes from the internal environment and also prevents the subcutaneous tissues from drying out. The effectiveness of this impermeable membrane is readily recognized when one observes the extreme loss of fluids that occurs with damage to the skin, as with burns and other injuries. Insensible loss of water and electrolytes occurs only through pores in this effective barrier.

THERMOREGULATION

Body temperature represents the balance between heat generation and heat loss processes. The skin, with its ability to alter the rate of heat loss, is the major point of regulation of body temperature. The rate of heat loss depends primarily on the surface temperature of the skin, which is in turn a function of the skin's blood flow. The blood flow of the skin varies in response to changes in the body's core temperature and to changes in temperature of the external environment.

The flow of blood to the skin is derived in two processes. Direct perfusion is from capillary beds entering in lateral directions. Skin is also perfused vertically from vessels that enter from the muscle and fascia supporting it.

In general, the vessels dilate during warm temperatures and constrict during cold. The hypothalamus is partly responsible for regulating skin blood flow, particularly to the extremities, the face, ears, and the tip of the nose. Maintenance of the thermal balance allows the internal temperature of the body to remain at approximately 37° C (98.6° F).

Under severe heat stress, increased cutaneous blood flow is inadequate to dissipate the thermal load. Eccrine glands produce sweat, and cooling is enhanced by fluid evaporation from the skin. Eccrine gland innervation is unique in that these sympathetic cholinergic nerves use acetylcholine (rather than norepinephrine) as the neurotransmitter. Sweating significantly enhances the body's capacity for thermoregulation.

SENSORY RECEPTION

Apart from sight and hearing, the major human sensory apparatus is in the skin. Sensory fibers responsible for pain, touch, and temperature form a complex network in the dermis. This information is transmitted to the spinal cord and is relayed to the somatosensory cortex, where the information is integrated into a somatotopic representation of the body.

The skin contains specialized receptors to detect discriminative touch and pressure. *Touch* (flutter) is sensed by Meissner's corpuscles; *pressure,* by Merkel cells and Ruffini endings; *vibration,* by Pacinian corpuscles; and *hair movement,* by hair follicle endings. Together these receptors communicate information to the somatosensory cortex via the dorsal column pathways.

A second grouping of nerves communicates information about temperature and pain to the somatosensory cortex via the anterolateral pathways. *Temperature* is sensed by specific thermoreceptors in the epidermis, and *pain* is sensed by free nerve endings throughout the epidermal, dermal, and hypodermal layers. The speed of conduction of pain information to the cortex results in a functional division. "Fast" pain is well localized and has a short latency. "Slow" pain is more diffuse, has a longer latency, and is more difficult to endure.

The density of receptors determines the sensitivity of the skin. For example, two-point discrimination is most acute on the skin of the fingers and face, where the highest density of touch receptors occurs. In contrast, the skin on the back has a low density of touch receptors, and the ability to localize touch is therefore reduced.

VITAMIN D PRODUCTION

The epidermis is involved in synthesis of vitamin D. In the presence of sunlight or ultraviolet radiation, a sterol found on the malpighian cells is converted to form cholecalciferol (vitamin D_3). Vitamin D_3 assists in the absorption of calcium and phosphate from ingested foods.

PROCESSING OF ANTIGENIC SUBSTANCES

Langerhans cells are scattered among the keratinocytes located primarily in the epidermis; however, they can also be seen in the dermis. These cells originate in the bone marrow and migrate to the epidermis. Langerhans cells play a role in the cell-mediated immune responses of the skin through antigen presentation.

Cells in both the epidermis and dermis of the skin are important in the immune function. Skin is now recognized not only as a physical barrier but also as a participant in immunologically mediated defense against various antigens. These specialized cells include Langerhans cells and keratinocytes located in the epidermis and lymphocytes located in the dermis. An antigen entering immunologically competent skin is likely to encounter a coordinated response of Langerhans and T cells to neutralize its effect. An antigen entering diseased skin can induce and elicit immune responses. These reactions may be involved in the pathogenesis of many inflammatory skin diseases.

DERMATOLOGIC CARE

As the largest and most visible organ of the body, the skin plays a major role in our physical and mental health and protects us from an array of natural and man-made attacks. Yet the skin is rarely taken as seriously as other organ systems, such as the heart and the lung. In both outpatient and inpatient practice settings, as a nurse you have a unique opportunity to affect a client's dermatologic care. You can teach clients to appreciate the skin's important role and to recognize that some skin conditions are indeed life threatening. For example, forecasts indicated that by the year 2000 as many as 1 in 75 Americans would be afflicted by malignant melanoma, a skin cancer that is often fatal. In the United States today, one person dies every hour from skin cancer. Also, burn injuries continue despite advances in fireproofing homes and clothes. Pressure ulcers, a serious alteration in skin integrity, pose a growing concern as the older population increases and may result in 60,000 deaths per year.

APPEARANCE AND SELF-ESTEEM

Skin is integral to self-image and self-esteem. Each client's unique appearance is established through the skin. The skin was once thought to reflect the normal "aging process" and how that aging process affected the genetic skin types we inherit. We now know that skin type more likely reflects the cumulative amount of sun exposure over a lifetime. It is hoped that with education, untanned skin will once again be viewed as attractive and healthy. Cosmetic surgery should not be considered a procedure for vanity but a procedure to enhance self-esteem.

Today's society has a long-standing prejudice that needs to be dispelled regarding impaired skin. Historically, skin diseases were perceived as divine punishment for being spiritually and physically "unclean." Subtle punishment for skin diseases still exists because of ignorance. For example, a woman with atopic dermatitis may sit isolated and shunned in a waiting room because others view eczematous lesions as contagious. A server at a restaurant may be encouraged to work in the back of the kitchen so that customers will not notice the healed burn scars on his or her hands and body. Vitiligo, loss of pigment in the skin, is sometimes mislabeled "white leprosy," and so on. Clients who have visible chronic skin problems often withdraw from social situations and have altered interpersonal relationships and increased social isolation. When these clients seek professional care for skin problems, psychosocial as well as physical concerns need to be met.

Another function of skin, hair, and nails is to provide an outward appearance or *cosmetic adornment.* The appearance of our skin, hair, and nails is crucial to our psychosocial well-being and can affect our experiences positively or negatively. Skin disorders are often a major cause of morbidity because we live in a beauty-conscious society. Health care providers must be acutely aware of the role of the skin in a person's self-esteem and ability to function in relationships.

EFFECTS OF AGING

The skin undergoes numerous changes that can be seen and felt throughout the life span. Many of these changes are natural, unchangeable, and harmless. Some may be bothersome or painful and are treated until there is an acceptable resolution or acceptance of the condition. Other skin changes may go unnoticed or might not be bothersome because they are slow growing, such as senile keratosis. Table U11-1 lists some age-associated changes.

Adolescence

During puberty, hormone secretion stimulates the maturation of hair follicles, sebaceous glands, and apocrine and eccrine units in certain body areas. Hair follicles on the face (males), pubic region, and axillae activate to produce coarse terminal hairs. Normal changes may bother teenagers, but adolescents must be cautioned about the potential for irritating the skin with excessive use of over-the-counter products.

New nevi can appear after adolescence. At any age, raised, pigmented lesions that bleed or change in color or size should be assessed by a physician to determine whether they require only minor care or removal because of early malignant changes.

Adulthood

Temporary *hormonal changes* account for some adult skin changes. Pregnancy and birth control pills may alter hormonal status and thus change skin structures that are hormonally linked. Pregnancy may cause changes in hair growth patterns and a temporary thinning of hair after pregnancy.

Heredity and exposure to environmental factors, such as sun, tobacco, alcohol, and chemicals, play a major role in many of the skin changes that occur in adults. Some lesions (i.e., seborrheic keratosis and acrochordons) may be removed for cosmetic reasons, if desired, or if physically irritating. Actinic keratoses (because of their premalignant status) and sebaceous cysts (because of their infectious potential) need to be assessed and may be removed.

Older Adulthood

The skin of older people reflects the cumulative influence of environmental insults, decreased circulation, and diminished function of various skin structures. As the stratum corneum becomes thinner, the skin reacts

TABLE U11-1	Common Skin Changes Associated with Aging
Skin Change	**Description**
Adolescence	
Folliculitis	Hair follicle inflammation
Acne	Inflammation of pilosebaceous follicle
Increased perspiration	Response to heat, emotional stress, exercise
Apocrine secretion	Related to sex hormone activity
Skin irritation	Often caused by overuse of over-the-counter skin products
Pigmented nevi	Benign cluster melanocyte-like cells
Adulthood	
Melasma	Blotchy hyperpigmentation
Alopecia	Baldness (hormonal and genetic factors)
Excessive facial or body hair	Androgen-related problem in women
Actinic keratosis	Slightly raised, red papules (premalignant)
Sebaceous cyst	Enclosed cyst in dermis (potentially infectious)
Acrochordon	Small, flesh-colored papule
Older Adulthood	
Xerosis	Dry skin (decreased natural oils and sweat)
Wrinkling	Natural change affected by many factors (e.g., loss of elasticity and subcutaneous fat, sun exposure, gravity, cigarette smoking)
Skin tears	Epidermal thinning; seen most in clients using oral corticosteroids
Senile lentigenes	Black or brown flat lesions ("liver spots")
Seborrheic keratosis	Harmless raised black or brown spots or wart-like growths
Cherry angiomas	Dilated blood vessels that form loops

more readily to minor changes in humidity, temperature, and other irritants. The skin also becomes more transparent. Hair loss is often noticeable on the trunk, pubic area, axillae, and limbs. Loss of pigment causes gray hair. Nails become brittle and may yellow or thicken. Skin may be leathery from overexposure to ultraviolet light. There is no known treatment for past overexposure; protection from ultraviolet light is the only preventive measure.

CONCLUSIONS

The skin is the largest and most visible organ of the body. Anatomically, the skin is divided into (1) the epidermis (outer layer), (2) the dermis (inner layer), and (3) the hypodermis (subcutaneous layer). The skin serves many functions. It is the first line of defense against many forms of trauma. Skin maintains body temperature, prevents water loss, and provides sensations of touch, temperature, and pain. Skin also produces vitamin D and recognizes antigens. Finally, healthy skin is aesthetically pleasing.

BIBLIOGRAPHY

1. Berne, R., et al. (2004). *Physiology* (5th ed.). St. Louis: Mosby.
2. Kierszenbaum, A.L. (2002). *Histology and cell biology: An introduction to pathology.* St. Louis, Mosby.
3. Guyton, A., & Hall, J. (2001). *Textbook of medical physiology* (10th ed.). Philadelphia: W.B. Saunders.
4. Silverthorn, D. (2001). *Human physiology* (2nd ed). Saddle River, NJ: Prentice Hall.

Chapter 50

Assessment of the Integumentary System

Noreen Heer Nicol

Assessment of skin disorders is a complex process because many skin disorders undergo a characteristic evolution. Observation is often required on more than one occasion for diagnosis. Additionally, diagnosis may require the information provided by a complete history, physical examination, laboratory tests, and histopathologic analysis. A complete health history assists in the diagnosis of integumentary disorders, such as occupationally related contact dermatitis, or in revealing psychosocial aspects of skin disorders. The medication history is important because side effects of certain medications can cause skin changes. The physical examination can confirm integumentary disorders as well as reveal disorders that the client may have omitted during the history.

HISTORY

The history includes questions about the chief complaint and current manifestations, medications, allergies, occupation, travel, habits, past health history, family health history, psychosocial history, and a review of systems.

Current Health

Chief Complaint

The most common problems related to the integument are itching *(pruritus),* dryness, rashes, lesions, *ecchymoses* (small hemorrhagic patches), lumps, masses, and cosmetic appearance. The onset, duration, and suspected trigger of each manifestation should be discussed. Ask about changes in the skin, hair, and nails that may be related to the chief complaint. Sample questions that elicit pertinent information related to the presenting dermatologic problem are listed in Table 50-1.

Symptom Analysis

Conduct a symptom analysis, including the factors noted in Table 50-1. Sexual history may be significant if the differential diagnosis includes a sexually transmitted disease (STD) (see Chapters 39 and 43). Persistent itching or pruritus is a manifestation that frequently brings

TABLE 50-1	*Dermatologic Assessment History: Sample Questions*
Information Needed	**Questions**
Chief complaint	"Please tell me what brings you here today."
Definition of problem (onset, location)	"Tell me more about the problem. Where did it start? Have you noticed this problem before?"
Duration	"When did it start? Does it come and go? Has it changed? Has it become better or worse?"
Accompanying manifestations	"Did you have any feelings—such as fatigue, nausea, skin tightness, skin burning—before this problem started? Does it itch?"
Evolution of lesion or eruption	"How does it feel now? Are you experiencing any discomfort? Do you feel tenderness, tightness? Does clothing irritate your skin? Do you have any problems sleeping? Does it limit any of your activities? Has it interfered with your normal daily routine?"
Aggravating and relieving factors	"Have you noticed if the problem worsens after any of these activities: eating particular foods? Using cosmetics? Using soaps? Wearing clothing? Do changes in temperature or climate affect the problem? Does it worsen or improve with changes in season? Are you more comfortable when warm or when cool?"
Medical intervention	"Did you see a health care provider about this? Were you told what the problem was? Was any treatment recommended? Did it help?"
Self-treatment	"What have you tried to do on your own to get relief? What did you use? What over-the-counter medications or home remedies have you tried? What do you do yourself that helps the problem?"
Compliance and treatment factors	"How often were you able to apply or take prescribed medication? Were you able to complete the prescribed treatment? How did you use the medication? (How did you apply it? How did you take it? For how long? Why did you stop?)"

clients to a health care provider. Note whether the itching is associated with skin lesions and whether it is localized or generalized. Persistent itching without associated lesions could suggest significant systemic disease such as biliary obstruction, diabetes mellitus, uremia, lymphoma, or hyperthyroidism. If pruritus is associated with skin lesions, consider scabies, many types of dermatitis, psoriasis, xerosis, and dermatophytosis in the diagnostic process.

Past Health History

Various systemic diseases are characterized by cutaneous manifestations. Does the client have other systemic disorders relevant to the skin (immunologic, endocrine, collagen, vascular, renal, or hepatic conditions)? Ask about childhood diseases, and find out about the vaccination status. Previous trauma and surgical intervention may explain unusual lesions or their location. A history of past allergic reactions to foods or medications is important for avoiding inadvertent reaction through readministration.

Medications

Note prescription and over-the-counter medications that the client is currently taking or has recently finished. Complications from these products can range from nuisance skin rashes to rare or life-threatening events. Medication reactions can be limited to the skin or may be part of a systemic process. The most common type of allergic drug reactions is cutaneous. Fortunately, most of these skin reactions are *morbilliform* (measles-like rash) or maculopapular without blistering or pustulation. These eruptions can be caused by many drugs, including penicillins, sulfonamides, nevirapine, and anti-seizure medications. Sensitivity to antibiotics or other drugs in the form of a drug rash may not occur until the end of a routine course of therapy or with subsequent exposures. Photosensitizing drugs (phenothiazines, tetracycline, diuretics, sulfonamides) may cause a sunburn-like rash in areas of sun exposure.[9a] Topical preparations may include preservatives or active ingredients that are known sensitizers that frequently produce an eczematous rash. The most commonly encountered are neomycin, benzocaine, and diphenhydramine hydrochloride. Oral corticosteroids (prednisone), if used at high doses or routinely, can cause acne breakouts, thinning of skin, stretch marks, and many other systemic side effects.

Complementary and alternative medicine has grown in the United States, particularly as Americans seek self-empowerment to manage their own care. It is important for providers to realize that clients may be anxious to try these products, especially if they suffer from chronic skin disorders such as atopic dermatitis, psoriasis, or wounds. Some components of these medications are beneficial, but for others scientific evidence is lacking. When possible, clients need to be educated about these modalities and their possible adverse physiologic and immunologic side effects. Aloe vera *(A. barbadensis, A. ferox, A. africana, A. spicata)* is promoted for the relief of eczema and psoriasis and to aid in wound healing. Chamomile *(Matricaria recutita, Chamaemelum nobile)*, comfrey *(Symphytum officinale)*, evening primrose *(Oenothera biennis)*, gotu kola *(Centella asiatica)*, and Oregon grape *(Mahonia aquifolium)* have similar uses. Although these products in pure forms or in high quantities may have pharmacologic activities such as antiseptic, diaphoretic, diuretic, or analgesic effects, the effect of diluted topical formulas is not known.[2] Care must also be taken to watch how clients administer products. A pointed example is arnica *(Arnica fulgens, A. montana, A. latifolia, A. cordifolia)*. When used as an antiseptic and antipyretic agent (usually as a soak or poultice), arnica is safe, but it can be fatal when taken orally. The answer to future use of these products is the need for more high-quality evidence-based studies.

Allergies

Ask the client about allergies to medications, foods, inhalants, latex, and other chemicals. Does the ingestion of certain foods cause itching, burning, or eruption of rashes? Does contact with pollens, inhalants, or animals result in hives?

There is a difference between allergy and irritation. *Allergy* is an immunologic response that happens consistently with exposure. *Irritation* can occur unpredictably. Inquire about substances that may cause local skin irritation or lesions on direct contact, such as textiles or metals. Wool is irritating to most people. Jewelry that contains nickel can cause skin discoloration, irritation, rash, or other problems in people who are sensitive to this metal.[16]

Family Health History

A family health history helps to determine genetic predisposition to skin disorders as well as a predisposition to parasitic or other conditions related to the family's lifestyle and living environment. Many dermatologic disorders or systemic disorders with a dermatologic presentation have a genetic or familial component. Genetically transmitted dermatologic conditions include *alopecia* (loss of patches of hair), *ichthyosis* (thickened, scaly skin), atopic dermatitis, and psoriasis. Systemic diseases with dermatologic manifestations include diabetes mellitus, blood dyscrasia, and collagen-vascular diseases (lupus erythematosus). Other diseases, such as scabies, are likely to be passed on to family members because of close and frequent exposure.

Psychosocial History

Psychosocial factors that influence dermatologic disorders often play a large role, particularly in long-term and chronic processes. Skin disease can greatly affect lifestyle and self-image. Cultural and familial influences in caring for a particular disorder may conflict with prescribed therapies. Misconceptions about skin problems (that acne lesions can be scrubbed away) need to be determined and corrected. Visually or physically disabling chronic skin diseases have been associated with chronic unemployment, poor mental health, and even suicide. Assess the client's sexual history, which can help alert to or explain the presence of tissue trauma or lesions caused by STDs (see Chapters 39 and 43).

Do not overlook socioeconomic factors. Compliance with outlined therapies and return for follow-up care are influenced by social expectations and the ability to pay for medications or treatments. When recommending therapies or medications, consider the impact on the client's day-to-day routine as well as the type of prescription insurance plan. Many topical therapies—whether or not they are covered by insurance—are expensive, and expense affects compliance.

Occupation and Travel

Occupational history is important because a large number of skin problems are caused or worsened by exposure to irritants and chemicals in the home and work environment. Learn what substances the client comes in contact with and to what extent. For example, chronic flaring of hand eczema may be caused by the use of certain glues and glazes in a hobby project, total body rash by chemical mists penetrating nonprotective gear at the work site, or hand rash by latex glove allergies.

The travel history can be helpful, especially if it includes hiking or exposure to outdoor agents that result in dermatologic disorders, such as poison ivy, poison sumac, poison oak, or Lyme disease. Ask about recent exposure to ticks, other insects, or infections.

Habits

Inquire about the client's habits. Determine the frequency of hygiene practices, the products used (soaps, lotions, abrasives), and whether cosmetics are used. Record the products used, including brand names. Inquire whether there have been any changes in clothing or bedding, and discuss how these items are cleaned.

Does the client engage in recreational activities that involve prolonged exposure to the sun, unusual cold, or other conditions that could damage the integument? For example, does the client visit tanning salons? More than one million people use tanning salons each day, and federal regulation of salons is limited. Advise clients that exposure leads to premature aging, increased risk of skin cancer, risk of corneal burns if eye guards are not worn, exacerbation of photosensitivity disorders, and increased development of lentigines (age spots) and other types of photodamage.

Review of Systems

Obtain a complete history of the skin. Specifically, ask about past problems with unusual itching, dryness, lesions, rashes, lumps, ecchymoses, and masses. Has the client had problems with moles or other lesions, especially if they have undergone changes in size, shape, or color? A more complete list of questions for the review of systems appears on the website for this textbook.

PHYSICAL EXAMINATION

Examine the skin as thoroughly as any other body organ. This procedure cannot be done properly in the hall or at a quick glance, which the health care provider is often requested to do. Use inspection, palpation, and olfaction to assess hair, nails, and skin. Effective assessment requires knowledge, awareness, and practice in describing the skin of people of all ages, ethnicities, and different lifestyles and in recognizing normal and abnormal skin changes (see the Physical Assessment Findings in the Healthy Adult feature on The Integumentary System below for a description of normal conditions of the integumentary system).

PHYSICAL ASSESSMENT FINDINGS IN THE HEALTHY ADULT

The Integumentary System

Inspection

Skin. Even skin tones, darker on exposed areas of face, neck, arms, and lower legs; lighter on trunk and back. Small tan freckles scattered over face and arms. Scars, striae absent.

Hair and Scalp. Hair evenly distributed over scalp. Clean, without nits or lice. No dandruff, scaling, or scalp lesions. Axillae and legs probably shaved; pubic hair distributed as inverted triangle from symphysis pubis to perineum (female). Pubic hair distributed in diamond pattern from below umbilicus to perineum (male).

Nails. Regular, smooth, oval shape. Pink nail beds. Cuticles manicured, clean. Nail bed angle 160 degrees (no clubbing).

Palpation

Skin. Warm, well hydrated, smooth, elastic, nontender. No lesions, masses, or lumps.

Hair and Scalp. Hair non-oily, even textured, resilient. Scalp smooth, intact, nontender.

Nails. Firm without tenderness or bogginess. Rapid blanch response.

Terminology

The terms routinely used in dermatology have been referred to as a "foreign language" and have been known to inhibit use of the correct terminology for skin disorders by health care providers. Use of standardized terminology often leads to differential diagnosis. This section clarifies some commonly used dermatologic terms and should assist the reader in recognizing and describing skin disorders. Table 50-2 is a glossary of commonly used dermatologic terms.

Types of Lesions

Examination and making the correct diagnosis of skin disorders depend on identifying skin lesions or changes. Two major types of lesions are distinguished: *primary* and *secondary* lesions.

The primary lesion is the first lesion to appear on the skin and has a visually recognizable structure. Figure 50-1 depicts nine primary lesions: macule, papule, plaque, nodule, wheal, vesicle, bulla, cyst, and pustule. Frequently, the health care provider does not see a primary lesion but sees only secondary lesions; the health care provider then must depend on the client's description of "how it looked when it first appeared." An in-depth look should be made to find a primary lesion because these are often key to clarifying the diagnosis.

When a primary lesion undergoes changes, it becomes a secondary lesion. These alterations, brought about by the client or by the client's environment, often occur in the epidermal layer. The changes may result from many factors, including scratching, rubbing, medication, natural disease progression, or processes of involution and healing. Figure 50-2 presents nine secondary lesions: scale, crust, erosion, deep ulcer, scar, lichenification, excoriation, fissure, and atrophy.

Examination Environment

The best setting for conducting a dermatologic assessment is a well-lighted, private room with moderate temperature and neutral, white, or cream-colored walls. Excessive warmth can produce changes in skin color (redness) by causing vasodilatation. Colored walls can affect normal skin hue (color). For a complete examination, ask the client to undress and provide a gown. Explain that all skin surfaces will be examined. Have a second health care provider in the room during a total body examination. Avoid unnecessary exposure during the examination. Have warm hands to avoid stimulation of the skin and to add to the client's overall comfort.

Depth of Examination

The examination is systematic and as complete as appropriate. A total-body skin examination involves assessment of the hair, scalp, nails, mucous membranes, and skin, including the axillae, areas in skinfolds,

TABLE 50-2	*Glossary of Dermatologic Terms*

Actinic	Pertaining to ultraviolet light (UVL)	**Hypopigmentation**	Decreased pigmentation
Amelanotic	Without pigment	**Indurated**	Hard (tissue)
Circinate (pronounced *sir-sin-ate*)	Circular	**Intertrigo**	Irritation of body areas with opposing skinfolds that are subject to friction
Circumscribed	Limited to a certain area by sharply defined border	**Lesion**	Detectable change from normal skin structure
Coalesce	To merge one with another	**Maceration**	Tissue softening or disintegration from excessive moisture
Comedo	Plug in a skin duct containing keratin (open, blackhead; closed, whitehead)	**Milia**	Small, white papules
Cytotoxic	Toxic to cells	**Perioral**	Around the mouth
Dermatome	Area of skin supplied by a single dorsal nerve root	**Periungual**	Under the nail plate
Dermatophyte	Fungus that enters the skin's surface, causing infection	**Pigmentation**	Degree of skin or mucous membrane color
Desquamation	Scaling, peeling of epidermis	**Plantar**	Pertaining to sole of the foot
Discoid	Coin-like	**Polymorphic**	Existing in many forms
Eczematous	General term for disease process characterized by scaling, weeping, crusting, and inflammation	**Pruritus**	Itching
		Punctate	Pinpoint or dot-shaped
		Sclerosis	Hardening or induration of skin
Erythema	Redness	**Sebum**	Lipid excretion produced by sebaceous glands
Exacerbation	Worsening of disease state	**Tautness**	Degree of skin tightness
Exfoliative	Shedding of skin in fairly large quantities	**Texture**	Tactile or visual skin characteristics (coarseness, dryness)
Folliculitis	Hair follicle inflammation	**Ultraviolet light (UVL)**	Electromagnetic radiation from the sun (wavelengths 4-400 nm)
Guttate	Small, water drop–sized lesions, usually widespread	**Urticaria**	Wheals (hives)
Hives	Spontaneously occurring wheals	**Verruca**	Lesion characterized by surface roughness (wart)
Hyperkeratosis	Thickening of stratum corneum, usually from repeated pressure or friction	**Wheal**	Lesion found in hives
Hyperpigmentation	Increased or excessive skin pigmentation (melanin), causing an area of skin to be darker than surrounding areas		

external genitalia, webs between toes and fingers, palms of hands, and soles of feet. Begin at the head, and proceed to the toes. General changes can alter total-body skin color (jaundice, cyanosis, pallor), thickness, turgor, temperature, and vascularity (purpura, petechiae). General findings can suggest systemic disease and may require complete physical examination and appropriate evaluation. The diagnosis of skin disorders is accomplished by careful observation and evaluation of individual lesions. This discussion is limited to assessment of hair, scalp, nails, and skin lesions.

Although you may examine the client's integument over the complete body surface at one time, this is usually not done in the screening examination. Instead, integument assessment is integrated as each body region is examined. For the purpose of discussion, however, assessment of the integument is presented as a separate body system. Significant or abnormal findings are commonly reported as part of each regional assessment rather than being reported separately.

Considerations in Ethnic Populations

As the demographics of the United States continue to change, the background and skills of the health care providers must continue to expand. Providers must learn to distinguish between normal and pathologic dermatologic variations in all ethnic populations, including Asians, African Americans, and Hispanics, as well as Caucasians (e.g., recognizing how inflammation, erythema, or follicular reactivity can appear in different skin pigments). In-

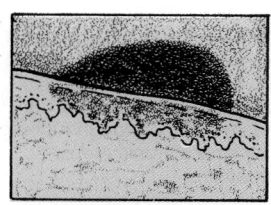

MACULE: Skin color change without elevation, i.e., flat (freckles or petechia). Described as a "patch" if greater than 1 cm (vitiligo).

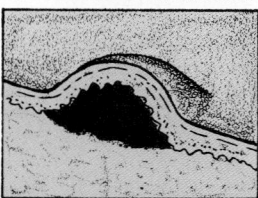

PAPULE: Elevated, solid lesion of less than 1 cm, varying in color (warts or elevated nevus).

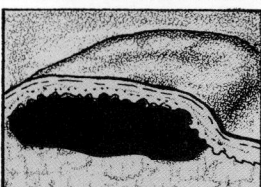

PLAQUE: Raised, flat lesion formed from merging papules or nodules.

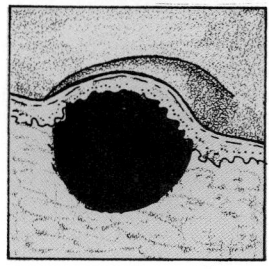

NODULE: Larger than a papule. Raised solid lesion extending deeper into the dermis. A large nodule is referred to as a tumor.

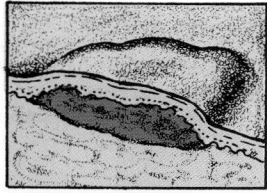

WHEAL (hive): Fleeting skin elevation that is irregularly shaped because of edema (mosquito bite or urticaria).

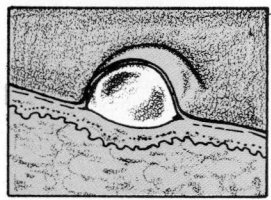

VESICLE (blister): Elevated, sharply defined lesion containing serous fluid. Usually less than 1 cm (blister, chickenpox, or herpes simplex).

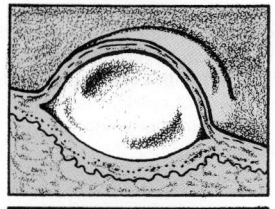

BULLA (plural, *bullae*): Large, elevated, fluid-filled lesion greater than 1 cm (partial-thickness burn).

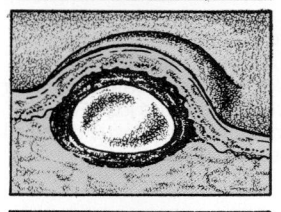

CYST: Elevated, thick-walled lesion containing fluid or semisolid matter.

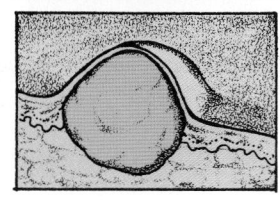

PUSTULE: Elevated lesion less than 1 cm containing purulent material. Lesions larger than 1 cm are described as boils, abscesses, or furuncles (acne or impetigo).

FIGURE 50-1 Primary lesions: visually recognizable structural changes in the skin that have specific characteristics.

flammation is underrecognized in dark-skinned people because erythema is difficult to assess. In diseases such as atopic dermatitis, nummular eczema, pityriasis rosea, or sarcoidosis, follicular accentuation is clearly visible in darker-skinned people. Post-inflammatory hyperpigmentation may persist longer after the disease has cleared in dark-pigmented skin than in fair-skinned people. In addition to appreciating physical differences in the skin of various ethnic populations, one must learn to value the social customs, traditional beliefs, mistrust, and fear that may influence adherence to treatment regimens.

Inspection and Palpation

Hair and Scalp

Examine the hair distribution patterns for symmetry and distribution according to the client's age and sexual development. Fine hair covers much of the body and is the same color as scalp hair. Increased distribution occurs normally in the axillae and pubic area. Having excess body hair is known as *hirsutism*.

Inspect the hair and scalp under good light. Wear gloves while examining open lesions or if you suspect infestation with lice. Inspect and palpate the hair for distribution, thickness, texture, lubrication, and signs of infestation or infection. Because natural hair color varies greatly, ask the client whether hair dye is used because it alters the hair's texture. Hair should be resilient and distributed evenly over the scalp. Individual hair shafts can range from thin and fine to thick and coarse; the shape of hair fibers can be straight, curly, or wavy. Texture and lubrication are affected by the type of hair care products used (harsh shampoo, curling irons, or hair dryers) as well as by a protein-deficient diet or severe health problems, which tend to leave hair dry and brittle. Hair loss or thinning *(alopecia)* can result from genetic predisposition to baldness or a health problem, such as recent chemotherapy or a thyroid disorder.

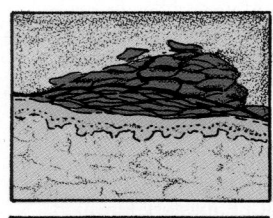

SCALE: Dried fragments of sloughed epidermal cells, irregular in shape and size and white, tan, yellow, or silver in color (dandruff, dry skin, or psoriasis).

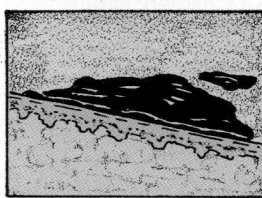
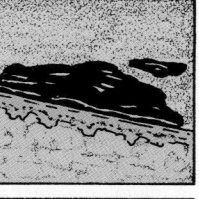

CRUST: Dried serum, sebum, blood, or pus on skin surface producing a temporary barrier to the environment (impetigo).

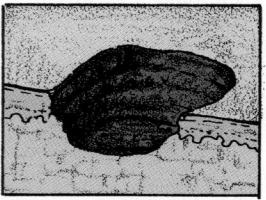

EROSION: A moist, demarcated, depressed area due to loss of partial- or full-thickness epidermis. Basal layer of epidermis remains intact (ruptured chickenpox vesicle).

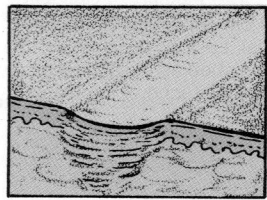

ULCER: Irregularly shaped, exudative, depressed lesion in which entire epidermis and all or part of dermis are lost. Results from trauma and tissue destruction (pressure ulcer).

SCAR: Mark left on skin after healing. Replacement of destroyed tissue by scar tissue.

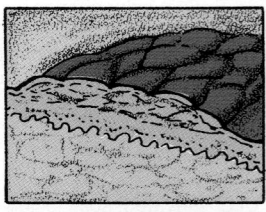

LICHENIFICATION: Epidermal thickening resulting in elevated plaque with accentuated skin markings. Usually results from repeated injury through rubbing or scratching (chronic atopic dermatitis).

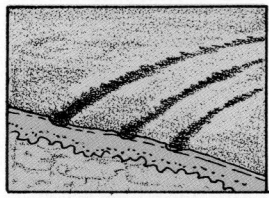

EXCORIATION: Superficial, linear abrasion of epidermis. Visible sign of itching caused by rubbing or scratching (atopic dermatitis).

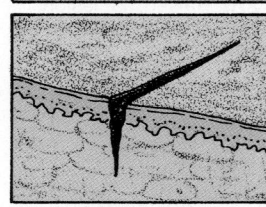

FISSURE: Deep linear split through epidermis into dermis (tinea pedis).

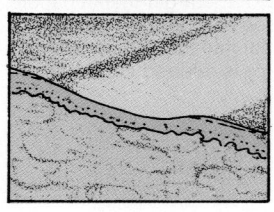

ATROPHY: Wasting of epidermis in which skin appears thin and transparent, or of dermis in which there is a depressed area (arterial insufficiency).

FIGURE 50-2 Secondary lesions: primary lesions that have changed because of the natural progression of the lesion or because of physical change (scratching, irritation, or secondary infection).

Inspect and palpate the scalp for lesions, excoriations (from scratching), lumps, or bruises, which should be absent. Examine hair shafts for the presence of nits, which are the eggs of the human head louse *(Pediculus humanus capitis)* and appear as particles of oval dandruff. Adult lice often bite the scalp behind the ears and along the back of the neck, which results in pustular lesions. It may be difficult to see adult lice on the scalp; they are very small (1 to 2 mm) and have gray-white bodies.

If you see lesions, describe them and ask the client about recent trauma or injury to the head. If the client has not already provided information during the health history interview, conduct a symptom analysis.

Nails

Inspect the client's nails for color, shape, texture, integrity, and thickness (Table 50-3). The nails reflect the client's overall health, indicating nutrition and respiratory status.

Color and Shape. The nail plate is usually transparent and colorless and, when viewed from the side, has a convex shape. The vascular bed underlying the nail plate gives the nail its color. The color is pink in white clients and darker in dark-skinned clients. A hemoglobin deficiency is seen in the nail bed as pallor, and decreased arterial circulation appears as cyanosis.

Perform a *blanch test* by palpating the nail beds to assess capillary refill. Press the nail bed firmly for 5 seconds, and then quickly release while observing the rate of color return to the nail bed. Color should return within 3 to 5 seconds in healthy individuals. Document the results of the blanch test as "rapid" or "sluggish" capillary refill. When palpated, the nail bed feels firm with no softness (bogginess) or tenderness.

TABLE 50-3	*Assessing the Nails*	
Assessment Finding	**Description**	
Normal nail About 160°	Nail shape is convex, and nail plate angle is approximately 160°	
Beau's line Beau's line	Horizontal depression in nail plate; depressions can occur singly or in multiples Cause: Nail growth is disturbed temporarily; related to systemic illness (infection) or direct injury to the nail root	
Splinter hemorrhages	Linear (vertical) red or brown streaks in the nail bed Cause: Minor trauma to the nail bed; subacute bacterial endocarditis; trichinosis	
Paronychia	Inflammation of the skinfold at the nail margin Cause: Trauma; skin infection at the nail base	
Spoon shape	Nail shape is concave as the nail curves upward from the nail bed Cause: Use of strong detergents; iron deficiency anemia; syphilis	
Clubbing	Increased angle between nail plate and nail base Cause: Long-standing hypoxia	

Texture. Texture should be smooth; healthy nails are of uniform thickness with no signs of dryness, softness, brittleness, splitting, peeling, ridges, or pitting. The *angle* formed between the nail plate and the posterior nailfold is about 160 degrees without separation (see Table 50-3). Changes in nail shape and nail bed angle can indicate health problems. Clubbing of the nails refers to an increase of more than 160 degrees in the angle between the nail plate and nail base. The base of a clubbed nail is spongy and soft on palpation. These changes result from **EB** hypoxia (diminished tissue oxygenation). Nail clubbing commonly occurs in clients with congenital heart defects or chronic lung disease.

Integrity. The tissue surrounding the nail should appear intact without signs of inflammation, jagged edges (hangnail), or dryness. Inferior or lateral nailfold inflam-

mation is a sign of paronychia (nailfold infection). If these abnormalities are noted, ask the client about nail care habits such as biting or cutting cuticles.

Thickness. While examining the fingers and toes, you may note common abnormalities such as calluses or corns. A *callus* is a flat, painless thickening of a circumscribed area of skin. Calluses usually occur on the hands and feet. A *corn* is a horny induration and thickening of the skin caused by friction and pressure and is often painful.

Skin

Color. Assess overall skin color during the health history interview. Conduct a more thorough assessment as you proceed through the remainder of the physical examination. Observe the client's face and visible skin surfaces for color tones, which should be congruent with the stated race. Abnormal findings include pallor (paleness), a flushed or ruddy complexion, cyanosis (blue cast), jaundice (yellow cast), and areas of irregular pigmentation. Normal variation occurs from one region of the body to another, particularly in areas protected from the sun and exposure by clothing; these areas are lighter. Overall color should be uniform. Skin tone may range over a variety of colors, including light ivory to deep brown or blue-black, yellow to olive, or light pink to dark, ruddy pink.

Areas that are less pigmented reveal abnormal findings more readily than more heavily pigmented surfaces. For example, *pallor* is best seen in the buccal (mouth) mucosa, especially in clients with dark skin. *Cyanosis* is evident more readily in less pigmented areas, such as the nail beds, lips, and palms. *Jaundice* sharply contrasts with the white of the sclera, especially in dark-skinned clients who have more carotene deposits. Jaundice is best assessed in dark-skinned clients by inspecting color changes in the hard palate.

Examine local areas of color change closely. *Hyperpigmentation* describes areas of increased pigmentation; *hypopigmentation* describes areas of decreased pigmentation. Skin color also results from the circulation; an increased blood supply may lead to the redness of inflammation *(rubor)*, whereas extreme pallor may be a result of anemia or impeded arterial circulation to the area.

Moisture. Moisture refers to the skin's hydration level. Overall skin moisture in healthy individuals can be described as well hydrated. Skin moisture often reflects ambient temperature and humidity levels. Moistness usually occurs in intertriginous areas (where skin touches skin), such as the axillae and groin. Skin that feels overly moist and cool (clammy) or overly dry, scaling, or cracked is abnormal.

Temperature. Assess temperature with the dorsum of the hand. The skin should feel uniformly warm because it reflects circulation. Compare areas of hypothermia or hyperthermia with the same areas on the opposite side (Figure 50-3).

Texture. Palpate *texture* by stroking the skin lightly with the fingertips. The skin should feel smooth, soft, and resilient. There should be no areas of lumps or unusual thickening or thinning *(atrophy)*.

Turgor. Turgor, a reflection of the skin's elasticity and hydration status, is measured by the time needed for the skin and underlying tissue to return to their original contour after being "pinched up." Lightly pinch the skin over the forearm between the thumb and index finger, and then release it. Skin with normal turgor is mobile and elastic and should return to baseline contour within 3 seconds. If the skin remains elevated (tented) for more than 3 seconds, turgor is decreased. Turgor decreases with age as the skin loses elasticity. Assessment of turgor is discussed in Chapter 4.

Edema. Palpate for *edema* (fluid retention), particularly if areas of taut, shiny skin are noted. Edema refers to a collection of fluid in underlying tissues that separate the skin's surface from pigmented and vascular layers, resulting in a blanched appearance. It is an abnormal finding. Palpate edematous areas for consistency, temperature, shape (extent), tenderness, and mobility. Assess and describe edematous areas using the technique described in Chapter 53. Areas examined for edema include those over the sacrum (especially in bedridden clients), the feet, the ankles, and the shins (over the tibia).

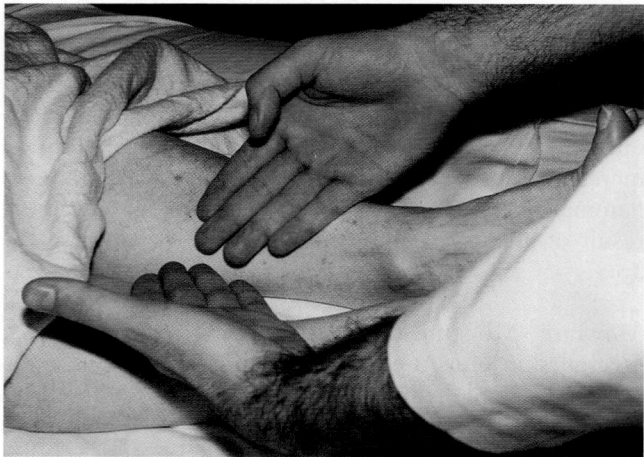

FIGURE 50-3 Assessing skin temperature uses the backs of the hands for the most accurate assessment. (Courtesy of Mary Sieggreen.)

Tenderness. Tenderness is an abnormal finding and is elicited with palpation. No areas of tenderness should be found in a healthy, uninjured client.

Odor. The skin should be free of pungent odors. Odors, when noted, are usually present in the axillae and skinfolds or in open wounds and are related to the presence of bacteria on the skin, inadequate hygiene, or infection. Assess odor in open wounds after cleansing the wound because odor can be related to the drainage itself or to the type of dressing used (hydrocolloid).

Lesions. Inspect the skin for detectable lesions. Assess and describe lesions in an orderly fashion: location, distribution, size, arrangement, color, configuration, secondary changes, and presence of drainage. Palpate skin lesions to determine the characteristics of contour (flat, raised, or depressed), size (using a measuring device), consistency (firm, soft), mobility, and tenderness. Lesions can be mobile or immobile (fixed to underlying tissue). Photographing lesions of concern is an excellent way to document changes over time.

Location, Distribution, and Size. *Location* is described in reference to anatomic landmarks. Measure the lesions for *size* to help classify their type (macule, papule). If multiple lesions are present, the *distribution pattern* can be helpful in determining the diagnosis. Note the extent of the lesions. Lesions can be (1) localized (confined to a specific area), (2) regional, or (3) generalized (present over a large surface). Compare sides bilaterally to determine whether lesions are symmetrical or asymmetrical. Another commonly noted distribution is on sun-exposed areas. Certain diseases feature a classic lesion distribution; for example, lesions of herpes zoster follow along a nerve root dermatome. Table 50-4 presents common configurations and distributions. Figure 50-4 depicts the locations of common skin disorders found during physical examination.

Arrangement. The *arrangement* refers to the pattern of nearby lesions. Two of the typical patterns are *linear* and *satellite,* which can also be helpful in confirming diagnosis. Linear lesions appear in a straight line (scabies). Satellite lesions appear as small peripheral lesions around a central larger lesion (diaper candidiasis).

Color. Skin lesions are found in a wide variety of colors; they may be skin-colored, brown, red, yellow, tan, or blue. Color can be influenced by many factors, including the client's normal skin hue, which may make accurate description difficult. Slight color changes can best be assessed in areas having the least amount of natural pigmentation and those with superficial capillary beds (buccal membrane of the mouth, mucosa, lips, nail beds, ocular conjunctiva, palms, and soles). These areas

TABLE 50-4	*Terminology for Skin Lesion Configuration and Distribution*
Description	

Configuration*

Annular	Ring-shaped
Iris	Concentric rings, "bull's eyes"
Gyrate	Spiral-shaped
Linear	Forming a line
Nummular	Coin-like
Polymorphous	Occurring in several forms
Punctate	Marked by points or dots
Serpiginous	Snake-like

Distribution†

Solitary	Single lesion
Satellite	Single lesion occurring in close proximity to but separate from a large group of lesions
Grouped	Clustered
Confluent	Merged together
Diffuse	Widely distributed
Discrete	Separate from other lesions
Generalized	Diffusely distributed
Localized	Limited, clearly defined
Symmetrical	Bilaterally distributed
Asymmetrical	Unilaterally distributed
Zosteriform	Band-like distribution of lesions along a dermatome

*Position of lesions relative to other lesions.
†Grouping, or pattern, of lesions over entire skin surface.

are especially important in assessing darkly pigmented skin.

Configuration. The term *configuration* refers to the shape or the outline of the lesion. Most lesions are circular. The term *nummular* is used for a circular lesion that is the size of a large coin (nummular eczema). *Annular* describes lesions with an active ring-shaped border and some central clearing (granuloma annulare). Table 50-4 shows other configurations that may be found during assessment.

Skin Self-Examination

Although it is crucial that all health care providers learn to perform an accurate and complete assessment of the skin, it is more important to teach every individual how to do a skin self-examination. Routine self-examination greatly lowers individual risk for severe skin disorders, such as skin cancer. Teach clients to examine their entire bodies to look for any changes in the skin or in their moles or skin lesions. See the Client Education Guide feature on Skin Self-Examination in Chapter 51.

Danger signals to look for are the *ABCDs* of melanoma:

- *A, Asymmetry:* one half is unlike the other half
- *B, Border:* irregular, scalloped, or poorly circumscribed border
- *C, Color:* varied from one area to another, shades of two colors, or changing colors
- *D, Diameter:* larger than 6 mm as a rule (diameter of a Number 2 pencil eraser)

See also the Physical Assessment Findings in the Healthy Adult feature on The Integumentary System on p. 1379. Encourage clients to visit their health care provider for further evaluation of any suspicious-looking lesions.

DIAGNOSTIC TESTS

Before a diagnostic skin procedure (or treatment), perform an assessment and document the findings. Nursing intervention for diagnostic procedures includes explaining the procedure to the client and his or her significant others and allowing them to ask questions and express concerns. Explain appropriate wound care and indications of possible side effects and complications that should be reported, such as prolonged bleeding or infection (indicated by swelling, redness, drainage, increased discomfort, or temperature elevation).

Provide instructions (preferably written) for follow-up care as well as follow-up appointment and telephone number. Documentation of diagnostic procedures (exactly what was done and by whom) and the specific location of the lesion must be completed by appropriate personnel.

Skin Culture and Sensitivity

Bacterial, fungal, and certain viral infections of the skin can be confirmed by culture. Because of the cost and delay in getting results, culture is usually reserved for infections that have been unresponsive to routine care. Clients who have had frequent courses of systemic antibiotics and still experience bacterial skin infections are candidates for a culture and sensitivity test to determine which antibiotic is indicated for treatment.

Potassium Hydroxide Examination and Fungal Culture

Fungal infection of skin, hair, or nails can be confirmed by microscopic identification or culture of scrapings from the area or both. Any area of scaly dermatitis may be scraped for this test. Typical sites are the scalp, intertriginous areas (between the toes, axillae, groin, under or between the breasts, abdominal folds), and the nailfold.

Fine scales from the edge of the site are scraped with a No. 15 scalpel blade or the edge of a glass slide onto a second glass slide. A drop of 10% to 20% potassium hy-

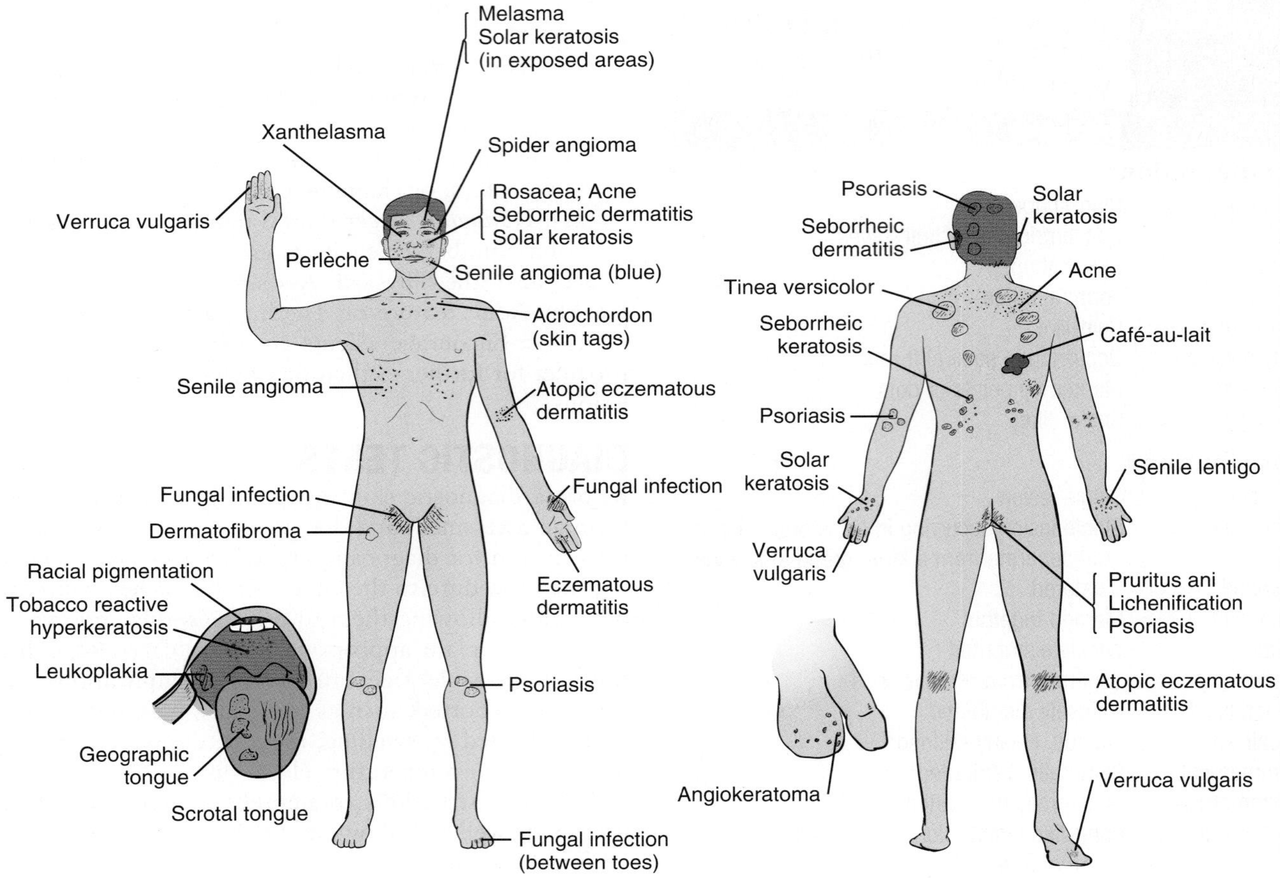

Melasma
Solar keratosis
(in exposed areas)

Xanthelasma

Spider angioma

Rosacea; Acne
Seborrheic dermatitis
Solar keratosis

Verruca vulgaris

Perlèche

Senile angioma (blue)

Acrochordon
(skin tags)

Senile angioma

Atopic eczematous
dermatitis

Fungal infection

Fungal infection

Dermatofibroma

Racial pigmentation

Tobacco reactive
hyperkeratosis

Leukoplakia

Eczematous
dermatitis

Geographic
tongue

Psoriasis

Scrotal tongue

Fungal infection
(between toes)

Psoriasis

Solar
keratosis

Seborrheic
dermatitis

Acne

Tinea versicolor

Seborrheic
keratosis

Café-au-lait

Psoriasis

Solar
keratosis

Senile lentigo

Verruca
vulgaris

Pruritus ani
Lichenification
Psoriasis

Atopic eczematous
dermatitis

Angiokeratoma

Verruca vulgaris

FIGURE 50-4 Common disorders encountered during physical examination of the skin.

droxide is added to the scale, and a coverslip is placed over the specimen. Gentle pressure is applied to the coverslip to flatten the scales. The slide may be gently heated to dissolve the keratin or the cells more quickly. The scrapings are examined under the microscope. For a culture, scrapings from a suspicious lesion are implanted in the appropriate culture medium. For a nail culture, an altered, dystrophic nail is snipped and implanted in the medium. Debris from the nail's subungual area is less suitable for culture.

Tzanck's Smear

Tzanck's smear is used for microscopic assessment of fluids and cells from vesicles or bullae. The presence of multinucleated giant cells establishes a diagnosis of viral infection, such as herpes simplex or herpes zoster infection. An intact, recently evolved vesicle top is removed, and its base is scraped with a scalpel or small curet. The debris is smeared onto a labeled slide and sent for cytologic assessment.

Scabies Scraping

The most difficult part of the test for scabies is selecting an unscratched lesion from which to take the specimen. Often several areas need to be prepared. When visible, a linear

burrow is sampled to look for the mite, its eggs, or feces. The top of the lesion is shaved off with a no. 15 scalpel blade or removed by curette. The specimens are placed on a microscope slide, covered with immersion oil and a coverslip, and examined under low power on the microscope. Local anesthesia is not necessary, and fine bleeding is expected. Some discomfort occurs when the lesion is opened.

Wood's Light Examination

Wood's light ("black light") uses a high-pressure mercury lamp that transmits long-wave ultraviolet light (UVA), or 360 nm; it has limited diagnostic uses. For example, Wood's light can (1) detect few superficial fungal and bacterial skin infections, (2) delineate pigmentary disorders by highlighting the degree of contrast between lesions and normal skin color, and (3) accentuate the contrast between hypopigmented and totally amelanotic areas. It is important to recognize that the most common types of fungi do not fluoresce, and for years this test has been of questionable use in diagnosing fungus.[2a] Wood's light examination is done in a darkened room. The procedure is painless.

Patch Testing

Patch testing is done to attempt to identify substances that produce allergic skin responses.[5,16] It is a painless procedure, and a skilled evaluator must be on hand to read and interpret the results. Patch testing is often done to differentiate between an *irritant* contact dermatitis and an *allergic* contact dermatitis. Small amounts of various substances or allergens are applied to the skin using a commercially prepared tape containing the allergens, or allergens are placed on aluminum disks on a special tape. The client and his or her significant others need to understand that whereas potential allergic substances (allergens) can produce inflammatory skin reactions, compounds of low concentration are used to prevent possible excessive irritation.

Patch testing should not be performed if acute dermatitis is present or if the client is taking substantial amounts of oral steroids; the potential allergen might worsen the dermatitis.

The tape must be worn for 48 hours without disturbing the patches; then it is removed. Interpretations are made at 48, 72, and 96 hours and sometimes at 1 week. A specific eczematous response at the test site with erythema, papules, or small vesicles indicates a positive reaction and confirms an allergic contact sensitivity to the substance on the disk. Counseling regarding allergen avoidance in a positive test or the meaning of the negative result is a critical part of the test.[5]

Biopsy

Skin biopsy refers to the removal of a skin tissue specimen for histologic (cellular microscopic) assessment. There are two types: dermal punch and surgical excision. In both procedures, local anesthesia is used. Small-gauge (26- to 30-gauge) needles are recommended to limit trauma to the skin.

Depending on the size and location of the biopsy specimen and the skill of the practitioner, the procedure is usually quick and almost painless. The most common source of pain is the initial administration of local anesthetic. The specimen is placed in a preservative such as formalin solution, properly identified, and sent for pathologic assessment. Use clean or sterile technique as appropriate to dress or cover the biopsy site.

Punch Biopsy

For a dermal punch biopsy, a circular instrument with a sharp cutting edge is used to remove a specimen of skin that includes epidermal, dermal, and subcutaneous tissue. This method is used to obtain a biopsy specimen of a well-developed, mature lesion. An appropriate-sized punch is chosen (from 3 to 6 mm). The skin site is cleaned, and a local anesthetic is injected. Skin surrounding the lesion is stretched taut, and the punch is pressed firmly downward into the skin site (Figure 50-5, *A*). The instrument is rotated back and forth in a cutting motion that frees the specimen from surrounding tissue. The specimen is then gently grasped with a tissue forceps

or needle, and its base is severed with scissors or a scalpel blade (Figure 50-5, *B*).

Depending on the size of the specimen, hemostasis can be achieved with pressure or application of Monsel's solution or aluminum chloride solution. The oval defect (Figure 50-5, *C*) may be closed with a 4-0 or 5-0 silk or nylon suture to produce a linear scar. Sutures are removed after about 7 to 14 days (with facial biopsies, 3 to 5 days).

Surgical Excision Biopsy

The surgical excision biopsy is used (1) when it is necessary to excise a lesion completely (when full skin thick-

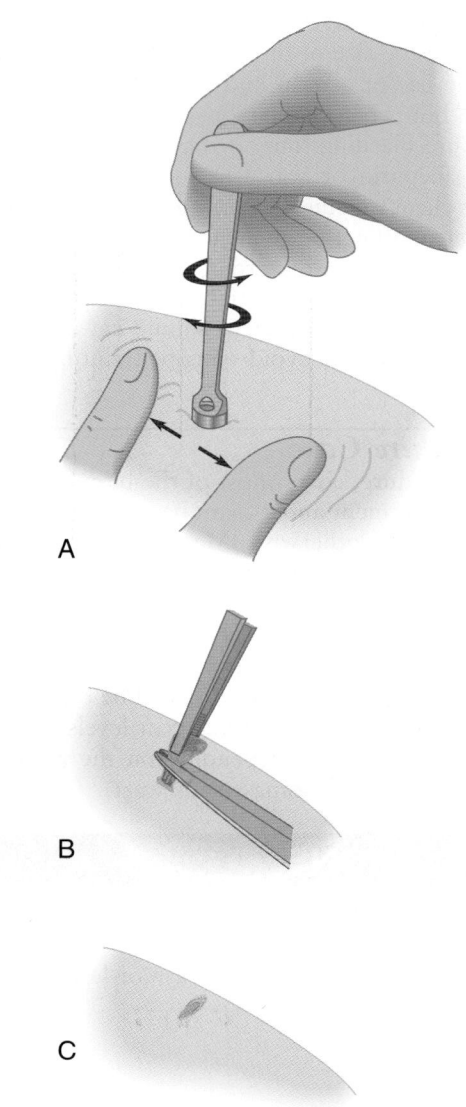

FIGURE 50-5 Skin *punch* biopsy. **A,** A tissue specimen is obtained with the instrument pressed down firmly on the skin. The specimen is freed from surrounding tissue by a rotary back-and-forth cutting motion. **B,** The specimen base is severed with tissue scissors. **C,** Appearance of the biopsy area before closing sutures applied.

ness is needed), (2) when a lesion's borders are indistinct from surrounding skin, or (3) when there is a recurrent or aggressive cancer, such as malignant melanoma. The site is cleansed, the excisional lines are marked with a gentian violet pen, and local anesthetic is administered. The lesion is excised with a scalpel by means of a variety of surgical techniques; a commonly used technique is an elliptical incision.

Hemostasis is achieved with pressure and ligation (suturing closed) of superficial vessels. The incision is closed with sutures. The suture site is rinsed with saline-dampened gauze. A pressure dressing of sterile nonadhering gauze is applied and taped in place.

Preprocedure Care

Depending on the size of the excision, instruct the client to avoid the use of aspirin and products containing aspirin for 48 hours before the biopsy to avoid a prolonged postprocedure bleeding time. If the client is taking anticoagulants (heparin or warfarin), notify the physician. Review the client's medical history for systemic disorders such as liver malfunction, which affects clotting time. If the client has a history of cardiac valve replacement, be sure that prophylactic antibiotics are prescribed. Obtain an informed consent. The client should eat a light meal before the procedure to avoid syncope (fainting).

Postprocedure Care

After the procedure, cover most of the biopsy sites with an antibiotic ointment and a clean bandage or dry dressing unless ordered otherwise. Many nonadhesive types of dressings are available and may be preferable for clients who have fragile or sensitive skin. Remind the client that follow-up assessment is necessary, and plan a follow-up appointment for suture removal. Tell the client how and when biopsy results will be reported. Remember that individuals have different levels of anxiety about the biopsy results, depending on the anticipated possible outcome (melanoma versus wart).

CONCLUSIONS

The skin is the largest organ in the body, and it presents many health care challenges. The key to assessment of the skin or to the assessment of a rash or lesion is use of a comprehensive, systematic approach. Remember, the current view does not tell the whole story; multiple assessments over time or anticipating the changes that came before or those that will occur next will be important.

BIBLIOGRAPHY

1. Berger, T.G., James, W.D., & Odom, R.B. (2000). *Andrews' diseases of the skin: Clinical dermatology* (9th ed.). Philadelphia: W.B. Saunders.
2. Bielory, L., & Kanuga, M. (2002). Complementary and alternative interventions in atopic dermatitis. *Immunology and Allergy Clinics of North America: Atopic Dermatitis, 22*(1), 153-173.
2a. Bradley, B., et al. (1996). Tinea capitis today: What nurses need to know about identifying and managing fungal infections of the scalp in the school setting. *The Journal of School Nursing, 12*(5), S1-S16.
3. Callen, J.P. (2000). *Color atlas of dermatology* (2nd ed.). Philadelphia: W.B. Saunders.
4. Champion, R.H. (1998). *Rook, Wilkinson, & Ebling textbook of dermatology* (6th ed.). Oxford: Blackwell Science.
5. DeLeo, V.A., Elsner, P., & Marks, J.G. (2002). *Contact and occupational dermatology* (3rd ed.). St. Louis: Mosby.
6. Fitzpatrick, T.B., Johnson, R.A., & Wolff, K. (2001). *Color atlas and synopsis of clinical dermatology: Common and serious diseases* (4th ed.). New York: McGraw-Hill.
7. Freedberg, I.M., Eisen, A.Z., & Wolff, K. (2003). *Fitzpatrick's dermatology in general medicine* (6th ed.). New York: McGraw-Hill.
8. Gilchrest, B.A. (2002). *Geriatric dermatology part II.* Philadelphia: W.B. Saunders.
9. Greaves, M.W., & Leung, D.Y.M. (2000). *Allergic skin disease: A multidisciplinary approach.* New York: Marcel Dekker.
9a. Gruchalla, R.S. (2003). Drug allergy. *Journal of Allergy and Clinical Immunology, 111*(2), S548-S549.
10. Hill, M.J. (2003). *Dermatology nursing essentials: A core curriculum—Dermatology Nurses' Association* (2nd ed.). Pitman, NJ: Anthony J. Jannetti.
11. Jarvis, C. (2000). *Physical examination and health assessment* (3rd ed.). Philadelphia: W.B. Saunders.
12. Johnson, B.L., Moy, R.L., & White, G.M. (1998). *Ethnic skin: Medical and surgical.* St. Louis: Mosby.
13. Lane, A.T., Morelli, J.G., & Weston, W.L. (2002). *Color textbook of pediatric dermatology* (3rd ed.). St. Louis: Mosby.
14. Lookingbill, D.P., & Marks, J.G. (2000). *Principles of dermatology* (3rd ed.). Philadelphia: W.B. Saunders.
15. Nicol, N.H. (2001). Alteration in the integument in children. In J. McCance & S. Huether (Eds.), *Pathophysiology: The biologic basics for disease in adults and children* (4th ed.). St. Louis: Mosby.
16. Nicol, N.H., Ruszkowski, A.M., & Moore, J.A. (1995). Contact dermatitis and the role of patch testing in its diagnosis and management. *Dermatology Nursing, 7*(2), S5-S7.

Chapter 51

Management of Clients with Integumentary Disorders

Noreen Heer Nicol
Joyce M. Black

evolve

Web Enhancements

Care Plan
The Client with Atopic Dermatitis
Case Management
The Client with Impaired Skin Integrity
Client Education Guide
Skin Self-Examination (Spanish Translation)
Topical Corticosteroids (Spanish Translation)

http://evolve.elsevier.com/Black/medsurg/

Simple Guidelines to Help Protect You from the Damaging Rays of the Sun (English Version and Spanish Translation)
Postoperative Care After Rhinoplasty (English Version and Spanish Translation)
Appendix C
Laboratory Values of Clinical Importance in Medical-Surgical Nursing

The skin is the largest and most visible organ of the body. Thus disorders of the skin offer the nurse an opportunity to provide care that makes a noticeable and rewarding difference to clients. Anger, frustration, depression, and anxiety are commonly experienced by clients with skin disorders, particularly those with chronic dermatoses. Clients can become embarrassed about their appearance and shun socializing. For other clients, skin lesions can offer secondary gains. Excitability and arousal of the central nervous system from an emotional upset can intensify the vasomotor and sweat responses in the skin, leading to the *itch-scratch-itch* or *flare cycle* (see Pruritus). In some instances, picking and scratching is used as an expression of anger, because typically it gets an immediate response from those nearby. The added dimension of family hostility, rejection, and guilt can damage the family structure and the client's self-esteem.

Learning about the acute or chronic nature of the given disorder, the exacerbating factors, and the management measures that can control it is important for both the client and family members (see the Genetics Links feature on Examples of Genetic Disorders Involving the Skin on p. 1390). Maintaining physical and emotional health is important. Counseling and other psychosocial interventions are often helpful in dealing with the frustrations of visible disease, especially for adolescents and young adults who may consider the dermatoses disfiguring. Evaluation to determine need for medical management of depression or other psychosocial issues is important, especially with significant chronic disorders.

The educational needs of people affected by skin disease are vast. Health care providers need to consistently provide information that includes detailed skin care plans, general disease information, and availability of client-oriented support organizations as well as updates on encouraging research results (see the Client Education Guide feature on Skin Self-Examination on p. 1391). Many new therapies are now available for chronic skin diseases such as psoriasis, atopic dermatitis, and vitiligo. It behooves health care providers to stay current with new therapies to assist clients in obtaining information and treatment advances. Clients tend to for-

evolve *Be sure to check out the bonus material on the Evolve website and the CD-ROM, including free self-assessment exercises.*
http://evolve.elsevier.com/Black/medsurg/

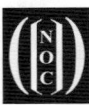

Nursing Outcomes Classification (NOC)
for Nursing Diagnoses—Clients with Integumentary Disorders

Acute Pain and Chronic Pain
Comfort Level
Pain Control
Pain: Disruptive Effects
Pain Level

Anxiety
Aggression Control
Anxiety Control
Coping
Impulse Control
Self-Mutilation Restraint
Social Interaction Skills

Chronic Low Self-Esteem
Self-Esteem

Disturbed Body Image
Body Image
Grief Resolution
Psychosocial Adjustment: Life Change
Self-Esteem

Disturbed Sleep Pattern
Anxiety Control
Rest
Sleep
Well-Being

Fear
Fear Control

Impaired Skin Integrity
Tissue Integrity: Skin and Mucous
  Membranes
Wound Healing: Primary Intention
Wound Healing: Secondary Intention

Ineffective Therapeutic Regimen Management
Compliance Behavior
Knowledge: Treatment Regimen
Participation: Health Care Decisions
Treatment Behavior: Illness and Injury

Ineffective Tissue Perfusion
Sensory Function: Cutaneous
Tissue Perfusion: Peripheral

Risk for Impaired Skin Integrity
Immobility Consequences: Physiologic
Nutritional Status
Nutritional Status: Biochemical
  Measures
Physical Aging Status
Risk Detection
Tissue Integrity: Skin and Mucous
  Membranes
Wound Healing: Primary Intention
Wound Healing: Secondary Intention

Risk for Infection
Immobility Consequences: Physiologic
Immune Status
Immunization Behavior
Knowledge: Infection Control
Risk Control
Risk Detection

GENETICS LINKS

Examples of Genetic Disorders Involving the Skin

Disorder	Skin Features	Inheritance	Metabolic/Gene Defect	Genetic Testing Available
Neurofibromatosis, type 1	Dermal neurofibromas, multiple café-au-lait spots, axillary and inguinal freckling	AD	Mutation in the NF1 gene on chromosome 17	Yes
Tuberous sclerosis	Hypomelanotic macules, facial angiofibromas, shagreen patches, fibrous facial plaques	AD	Mutation in the TSC1 gene on chromosome 9; TSC2 gene on chromosome 16	Yes
Oculocutaneous albinism, type 1	Hypo-pigmentation of skin, hair, and eyes	AR	Mutation in the tyrosinase gene, TYR, on chromosome 11	Yes
Waardenburg syndrome	Hypo-pigmentation of skin and hair; white forelock; premature gray hair	AD	Mutation in the PAX3 gene on chromosome 2	Yes
Fabry disease	Vascular cutaneous lesions (angio-keratomas)	XR	Mutation in the GLA gene on chromosome X; deficient activity of the enzyme α-galactosidase (α- Gal A)	Yes
Bloom syndrome	Sun-sensitive, telangiectatic, hypo- and hyper-pigmented skin; predisposition to cancer	AR	Mutation in the BLM gene on chromosome 15	Yes

AD, Autosomal dominant; *AR,* autosomal recessive; *XR,* X-linked recessive.

get or confuse important skin care treatment programs without written instructions. Clearly outlining the skin care recommendations orally and in writing is essential for increased compliance and good outcomes.

COMMON DERMATOLOGIC INTERVENTIONS

The skin's large surface area allows the absorption, penetration, and permeation of topically applied preparations. The factors that determine how well these processes occur include the client's age, the size of the affected region, the condition of the stratum corneum, the cutaneous blood supply, the molecular weight of the drug, and the medication vehicle (the word *vehicle* is used here to mean the substance containing the medication or the form in which the medication is delivered). Topical therapy can be used to do the following:

- Restore hydration
- Alleviate clinical manifestations
- Reduce inflammation
- Protect the skin
- Reduce scale and callus
- Clean and debride
- Eradicate infection

Topical medications are chosen both for the action of the active ingredients (which are delivered directly to the

---

CLIENT EDUCATION GUIDE

Skin Self-Examination

You will need a bright light, a full-length mirror, a hand mirror, two chairs or stools, a blow dryer, body maps, and a pencil.

A. Examine your face—especially the nose, lips, mouth, and ears—front and back. Use one or both mirrors to get a clear view.

B. Thoroughly inspect your scalp, using a blow dryer and mirror to expose each section to view. Get a friend or family member to help, if you can.

C. Check your hands carefully: palms and backs, between the fingers, and under the fingernails. Continue up the wrists to examine both the front and back of your forearms.

D. Standing in front of the full-length mirror, begin at the elbows and scan all sides of your upper arms. Do not forget the underarms.

E. Next, focus on the neck, chest, and torso. Women should lift breasts to view the underside.

F. With your back to the full-length mirror, use the hand mirror to inspect the back of your neck, shoulders, upper back, and any part of the back of your upper arms you could not view previously.

G. Still using both mirrors, scan your lower back, buttocks, and backs of both legs.

H. Sit down; prop each leg in turn on the other stool or chair. Use the hand mirror to examine the genitals. Check front and sides of both legs, thigh to shin; ankles; and tops of feet, between toes, and under toenails. Examine soles of the feet and the heels.

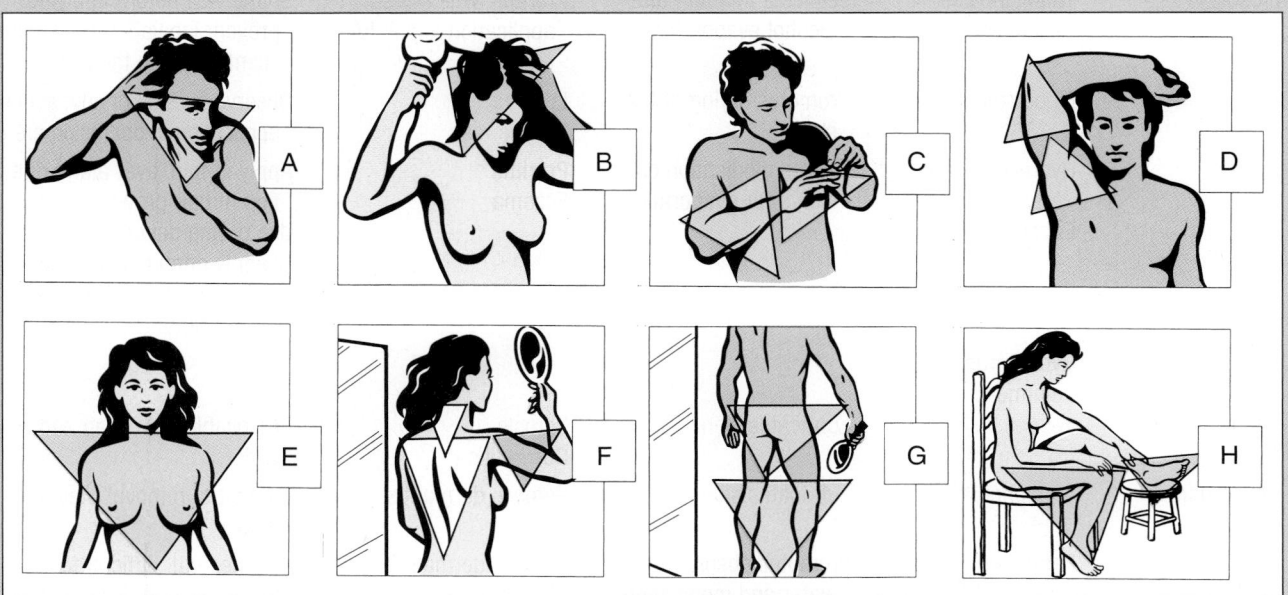

From The Skin Cancer Foundation (1992). *Skin cancer. If you can spot it, you can stop it.* New York: Author.

skin surface) and for the vehicle. Topical medications have many different actions and cover a large spectrum of drug categories, including anti-infective, corticosteroid, antipruritic, and the newer nonsteroidal topical immunomodulators.

TOPICAL VEHICLES

Examples of various topical medication vehicles are ointments, creams, gels, lotions, solutions, and powders (Table 51-1). Ointments are more occlusive, providing better delivery of the medication by preventing water loss from the skin. Use ointments cautiously with excessive heat or humidity because occlusion may result in increased itching or skin infection. When the weather is hot and humid, creams may be better tolerated. Although creams spread more easily than ointments, they are less occlusive, leading to increased skin drying in some people because of the evaporative property of the water. Creams also can be water based with ethyl alcohol and not be as drying as creams have been in the past. Sprays and lotions are available for use on the scalp and other hairy areas. The various ingredients used to formulate the different bases may be irritating to the skin, and care must be taken when recommending any product.

Both the active ingredient and the vehicle must be appropriate for the condition being treated. For acute dermatoses (i.e., weeping, blistering lesions), an aqueous (water-based) compound provides a drying effect. A greasy vehicle has the opposite effect; it promotes lubrication and occlusion and helps treat the dryness and

TABLE 51-1	*Topical Medication Vehicles*			
Category	**Examples**	**Action**	**Use**	**Nursing Implications**
Powders	Talc, cornstarch	Leaves a film of powder May absorb fluid	Intertriginous dermatitis	Dry surface before applying to prevent caking; reapply often
Lotions				
Suspension-based	Calamine lotion	Leaves a thin film of powder as water evaporates	Pruritus	Shake lotions well before applying Observe for overdrying of skin Apply in long, even strokes along direction of hair growth
Solutions	Salicylic acid	Leaves a film of powder as alcohol base evaporates	Warts, acne	Shake well before applying; observe for skin overdrying and drying and tightness of skin due to alcohol Apply as for suspension
Aerosols	Triamcinolone acetonide aerosol	Leaves a thin film after alcohol evaporates	Pruritus, when direct application is painful	Shake well before applying; prevent inhalation by turning client's face to the side
Gels	Fluocinonide gel	Promotes drying of the skin	Eczema Pruritic rash	Observe for skin drying; avoid application to open skin areas
Creams	Hydrocortisone cream Eucerin	Leaves medication on skin after evaporation	Pruritus Eczema	Apply in thin layer along direction of hair growth Use during daytime Reapply often because perspiration or drainage may remove preparation
Ointments	Hydrocortisone ointment			
Water-in-oil	—	Lubricates skin	Xerosis Dermatitis	Removable with soap and water
Absorbent	Aquaphor	Lubricates skin	Xerosis, dermatitis	Difficult to remove; may feel greasy
Water-repellent	Petrolatum	Promotes absorption of water and medication	Xerosis, dermatitis	Retains heat, difficult to remove; observe for maceration; avoid use in hair-bearing areas

scaling caused by chronic dermatosis. Differences in skin permeability also influence the effectiveness of topical medications. For example, absorption is increased in inflamed skin. Depending on the medication and the specific condition, topical medication may be applied to localized lesions or to larger skin surfaces. When increased absorption of the medication is needed, topical medication may be prescribed for application under an occlusive dressing (Table 51-2). Ointments, creams, and gels have greatly increased absorption if they are applied to skin that is wet.

Wound Dressings

Application of wound dressings remains important in the treatment of wounds, ulcers, and recalcitrant dermatitis. Wound dressings create an optimal environment for healing. Ulcers and denuded skin heal more quickly when kept moist by an occlusive or semiocclusive dressing because regenerating epithelium migrates more easily across a moist surface. These wounds are also less painful when kept moist, and absorption of topical medications is enhanced.

The clinician is challenged to understand the properties of the hundreds of wound care dressings on the market. Wound dressing materials include film, hydrocolloid, hydrogel, foam, alginates, and gauze, among others. The recent introduction of silver-impregnated wound dressings is a significant advantage in the topical treatment of infected wounds.

Ideally, with all wound dressings, the area of damaged skin decreases, granulation tissue forms, and manifestations of inflammation are reduced. Treatment may continue for weeks until improvement occurs. Instruct the client and family members to keep the dressing intact and to notify the primary health care provider if there is an increased level of drainage, pain, or foul odors that may indicate the presence of an infection. Routine follow-up examination is very important in wound care.

Soaks and Wet Wraps

Soaks serve several purposes. Moisture softens dry epidermis, which aids in removal of crusts. Removal of cellular skin debris promotes healing and improves absorption of topical medication. The risk of infection is reduced by removal of necrotic tissue and occlusive crusts. Cooling also results from the gradual evaporation of water and has an anti-inflammatory effect, thus relieving itching (pruritus).

Soaks can be accomplished by either soaking the affected area or bathing for 15 to 20 minutes in warm water. The agent added to the soaks is the least important aspect of this therapy. Addition of substances such as colloidal oatmeal (Aveeno) or starch to the bath water may be soothing for some people but does nothing to increase water absorption. Coal tar preparations (Balnetar, T/Derm) have an anti-inflammatory effect and can be helpful in some eczematous and psoriatic conditions. Aluminum acetate (Burow's solution), aluminum sulfate and calcium acetate (Domeboro), and povidone-iodine (Betadine) are also effective antibacterial substances; however, they have drying effects and may cause increased stinging and noncompliance. Bath oils are not recommended because they give the client a false sense of lubrication and make the soaking area very slippery.

After soaking, clients should remove excess water by gently patting the skin with a soft towel. Then they should immediately apply the recommended occlusive substance. Immediate application of this substance to damp skin is the most important detail, because if the occlusive barrier is not provided within 3 to 5 minutes, evaporation begins to occur.

To seal in the water, use occlusives such as white petrolatum (Vaseline) or petrolatum with mineral oil and wool wax alcohol (Aquaphor ointment). Occlusives can be greasy and may be cosmetically unacceptable to some people. Clients may prefer creams or lotions because

---

TABLE 51-2	*Occlusive Dressings for Increased Absorption of Medication*
Purpose/Desired Effect	**Nursing Implications**
Produces airtight barrier, usually with plastic film	Clean skin site of debris and "old" medication before applying prescribed topical medication.
Enhances absorption of topically applied medication (e.g., corticosteroids, keratolytics) by preventing evaporation	Apply topical medication while skin is still damp.
Increases stratum corneum rehydration	Apply plastic film (e.g., Saran wrap) snugly.
Softens hyperkeratotic areas by moisture retention	Use plastic bags for feet, polyethylene gloves for hands, plastic shower cap for scalp.
	Press air out; seal borders with paper tape.
	Leave dressing intact for 2-12 hr (as prescribed), then remove and gently cleanse the site.
	Observe and document complications—maceration, oozing, signs of secondary fungal or bacterial infection, folliculitis.
	Striae, nonhealing ulcerations, telangiectases, erythema, and skin atrophy may develop with prolonged use in conjunction with topical corticosteroids.

they are cosmetically pleasing products. Lotions and even creams may be irritating and drying because of the evaporative property of the water and the substances used as preservatives, solubilizers, and fragrances.

Wet wraps used immediately after soaking and occlusion can optimize hydration and topical therapy; this also promotes cooling of the skin. Wet wraps and occlusion can be applied in various ways. The location and severity of lesions often determine the choices. Total-body wet wraps can be accomplished by putting on wet pajamas or wet long underwear followed by dry pajamas or a dry or plastic sweat suit. The hands and feet can be covered with wet tube socks or wet cotton gloves followed by dry tube socks. Any extremity or the trunk can be covered with wet rolled (e.g., Kerlix) gauze and occluded with elastic bandages or by pieces of tube sock, wet followed by dry. The face can be wrapped with two layers of wet Kerlix gauze, followed by two layers of dry Kerlix gauze held in place with elasticized netting or other tubular dressings; holes are cut out for the eyes, nose, and mouth (Figure 51-1). If the dressing becomes dry, it should be rewetted before removal because debridement by the wet-to-dry method produces tissue damage and pain. Gentle debridement usually still occurs if dressings are removed when damp.

ULTRAVIOLET LIGHT THERAPY

Artificially reproduced forms of ultraviolet light (UVL) are used therapeutically with topical or systemic photosensitizing drugs to cause desquamation (shedding or peeling of the epidermis). Ultraviolet A (UVA) light and ultraviolet B (UVB) light are used to treat diseases re-

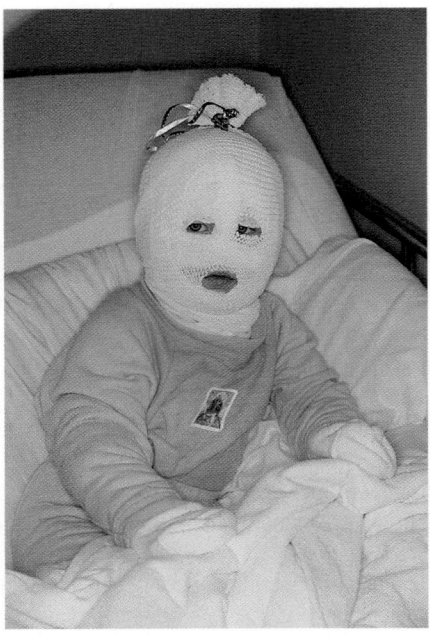

FIGURE 51-1 Wet wraps applied to the entire body.

sponsive to UVL, such as psoriasis, vitiligo, cutaneous T-cell lymphoma, uremic pruritus, and chronic eczematous eruptions. At present, three treatment modalities involve UVL: (1) UVA; (2) broadband and narrowband UVB; and (3) photochemotherapy, or PUVA (psoralen plus UVA). Initially, many of these regimens are given two or three times a week with the frequency decreased to two to four times per month for maintenance.

Obtaining a complete history and physical examination in every client before initiation of any UVL therapy is very important. One must take care to include the complete medication history, because the client may be taking one or more of the many photosensitizing drugs (e.g., thiazide diuretics, tetracycline). Ask clients specifically about previous herpes simplex infections, which can be stimulated by UVL. Pretreatment assessment includes identifying solar energy–induced skin malignancies, premalignant lesions, cataracts, or lupus erythematosus and any additional photodamage. Potential benefit must be weighed against potential risk.

A complete ophthalmologic examination before treatment begins is important and should be performed yearly during long-term treatment. A history of cataract formation is a potential contraindication to PUVA therapy. Clients who exhibit early cataract changes need extra photoprotective measures (e.g., the complete occlusion provided by goggles or PUVA glasses) and more frequent ophthalmologic assessments (every 3 to 6 months). The skin changes of lupus erythematosus (LE) are worsened by sun exposure, and phototherapy is thus contraindicated. If LE is suspected, an antinuclear antibody (ANA) test should be obtained to rule out this condition before therapy is initiated.

Because UVL treatments add to the cumulative effects of natural and artificial UVL, minimize exposure to the head, face, and male genitalia to reduce the risk of skin neoplasms through shielding techniques. Periodic assessments must be done throughout the course of therapy for manifestations of actinic damage (e.g., severe wrinkling, "tissue paper" transparency) or cutaneous malignancy. All phototherapy should be administered by qualified and well-trained dermatologic personnel. Use of home UVL equipment and tanning salons should be considered only when the client has no access to qualified dermatologic personnel. Numerous risks and significantly diminished responses are associated with home and salon therapy.

Ultraviolet B Therapy

UVB therapy requires no oral medications and is usually the first-line UVL therapy used before progression to PUVA. Types of UVB therapy include (1) broadband or narrowband UVB treatment as monotherapy and (2) broadband or narrowband UVB in combination with topicals (tar, anthralin, calcipotriene, corticosteroids, or tazarotene). The topical agents anthralin and tar used with UVB are mainly of historical interest because they have generally been replaced by newer developments that are reimbursable and that are not as time-consuming.

Photochemotherapy

Photochemotherapy (PUVA) combines oral or topical 8-methoxypsoralen with UVA. PUVA is used to treat severe, unresponsive forms of psoriasis, atopic dermatitis, cutaneous T-cell lymphoma, graft-versus-host disease, and alopecia areata or vitiligo. The potent systemic photosensitizing medications (psoralens) used in PUVA increase skin sensitivity to long-wave UVL (UVA). In conjunction with exposure to artificially reproduced forms of UVA light, these medications induce repigmentation (melanin production) in vitiligo and have an antimitotic effect and reduce T-cell population in psoriasis and cutaneous T-cell lymphoma.

Dosage is determined by body weight. The medication is taken orally with food to minimize nausea 60 to 90 minutes before UVA irradiation. Topical medication is used to treat localized sites and clients in whom systemic administration is contraindicated.

The skin and eyes must be protected from ambient UVL irradiation from the time psoralens are ingested until 8 hours after taking the photosensitizing medication. The client should (1) wear protective clothing, such as long sleeves, (2) apply sunscreen to exposed skin, (3) minimize natural skin exposure with topical psoralen, and (4) wear both UVA and UVB protective eyewear for 24 hours after taking the medication when outside or in an automobile.

■ COMMON SKIN DISORDERS
PRURITUS

Pruritus (itching), one of the most common manifestations of skin problems, is a symptom, not a disease. It has been defined as an unpleasant skin sensation, resulting in a strong desire to scratch, and is localized to or generalized over a body area. Pruritus can lead to damage if scratching injures the skin's protective barrier, increasing risk for infection and scarring. Relieving this manifestation, especially for chronically ill clients, is a nursing challenge because of its common occurrence, detrimental effect on skin health, and the major effect it may have on quality of life.

Pruritus can be a secondary clinical manifestation of conditions ranging from dry skin to severe systemic disease. Systemic diseases that can cause generalized and severe pruritus include chickenpox, liver and renal failure, diabetes mellitus, drug hypersensitivity reaction, intestinal parasites, leukemia, and lymphoma.

Stimulation of itching can be initiated through irritation by almost any chemical or physical substance, or allergic reaction, especially if skin is damaged. Once the

itch sensation is established, the client has an almost uncontrollable urge to scratch; and scratching leads to further skin damage and increased inflammation. Pruritus therefore worsens, and the urge to scratch is also intensified. Thus the itch-scratch-itch cycle develops. To minimize skin trauma caused by scratching, clients should keep fingernails short, smooth, and clean.

The client usually volunteers subjective reports of the degree and location of itching. Listen carefully to the client's description of the severity and location of pruritus, and seek information about how pruritus interferes with activities of daily living. Objective manifestations include excoriations and other secondary skin changes such as lichenification. Document all assessment findings.

Appropriate management of itching requires a complete assessment that attempts to discover the underlying cause and knowledge of appropriate therapeutic modalities for treatment. Dry skin may be either the source of pruritus or a contributing factor, and good hydration is often helpful (see Xerotic Eczema), in addition to any other topical therapy. One bath or shower per day for 15 to 20 minutes with warm water and a mild soap is recommended, immediately followed by the application of a sealing emollient, with or without other topical medications, to prevent evaporation of water from the hydrated epidermis (see Soaks and Wet Wraps). Other topical medications often added to emollients to help alleviate itching include menthol (0.25% to 0.5%), camphor (0.25% to 0.5%), urea (10% to 20%), and lactic acid (12%). Camphor and menthol produce a cooling effect. Urea and lactic acid moisturize scaly skin by drawing moisture into the cell structure of the stratum corneum. Topically applied antihistamines and anesthetics are relatively ineffective and are best avoided because they can be potent allergic sensitizers. The sensitizing effect is especially pronounced if these products are used on inflamed skin. Use of topical corticosteroids should be reserved for the treatment of specific steroid-responsive dermatoses. Long-term application of topical steroids, especially on skin not affected with an eczematous condition, may result in thinning of the skin, striae, telangiectases, and easy bruising.

Systemic antihistaminic agents are most helpful in disorders in which histamine is the principal mediator but may be of benefit through a sedative or even placebo effect. A trial of a histamine$_1$ (H$_1$) blocker (hydroxyzine, diphenhydramine, cetirizine) is appropriate either on a regular schedule or as indicated for itching. Tricyclic antidepressants (TCAs) have a high binding capacity for H$_1$ receptors and may be helpful in clients who would benefit from their antidepressant as well as antipruritic effect.

Older clients may have difficulty in following through with frequent bathing or showering because of decreased mobility. In such clients, when hydration cannot precede the application of moisturizers, more frequent application and use of more hydrating products may be needed.

In addition, older clients may have difficulty applying the needed topical agents properly, and assistive personnel may be required to ensure proper therapy. Oral sedating antihistamines should be administered carefully, with use of small doses initially, because many older people have a very low tolerance of these agents and may experience severe drowsiness, especially at the initiation of therapy.

ECZEMATOUS DISORDERS

Eczema is not a specific disease. *Dermatitis* and *eczema* are terms that may be used interchangeably to describe a group of disorders with a characteristic clinical appearance. The following are some examples of eczema or dermatitis:

- *Allergic contact dermatitis* (eruptions from allergy to poison ivy, sumac, or oak or a proven allergen)
- *Irritant dermatitis* (eruption from direct contact with irritating substances, which can be almost anything including cosmetics, chemicals, dyes, or detergents)
- *Nummular eczema* (appearance of coin-shaped, oozing, crusting patches)
- *Seborrheic dermatitis* (yellowish pink scaling of the scalp, face, and trunk)
- *Stasis dermatitis* (eruption resulting from peripheral venous disorders)
- *Atopic dermatitis* (characteristic distribution of eczema in persons with a family history of asthma, hay fever, or eczema)

Eczema/dermatitis has three primary stages; the condition may be limited to any one of the three stages, or the three stages may coexist.

- *Acute dermatitis* is characterized by extensive erosions with serous exudate or by intensely pruritic, erythematous papules and vesicles on a background of erythema.
- *Subacute dermatitis* is characterized by erythematous, excoriated, scaling papules or plaques that are either grouped or scattered over erythematous skin; the scaling may be so fine and diffuse that the skin acquires a silvery sheen.
- *Chronic dermatitis* is characterized by thickened skin and increased skin marking secondary to rubbing and scratching (lichenification); excoriated papules, fibrotic papules, and nodules (prurigo nodularis); and postinflammatory hyperpigmentation and hypopigmentation.

ATOPIC DERMATITIS

Atopic dermatitis is a common, chronic, relapsing, pruritic type of eczema. The word "atopic" refers to a familial tendency for excess inflammation in the skin, linings of the nose, and lungs. It often runs in families. These families may have allergies such as hay fever and asthma, but can also have sensitive skin and a history of eruptions called atopic dermatitis. Even though most people with atopic dermatitis have family members with similar problems, some clients may be the only ones in their families bothered by this condition. Associated allergic disorders include asthma, allergic rhinitis (hay fever), and atopic dermatitis.

Etiology

Atopic dermatitis is the most common chronic skin disorder in young children, affecting 10% to 20% of children in the United States. It is a genetically based disorder for which there is no cure. Most clients with atopic dermatitis have a personal or family history of asthma, hay fever, eczema, or food allergies. The prevalence of this disease is increasing. Allergic rhinitis or asthma eventually develops in approximately half of clients with atopic dermatitis, often as they outgrow their atopic dermatitis.

Pathophysiology

A number of immunoregulatory abnormalities have been described in atopic dermatitis.[10] Atopic dermatitis appears to be caused by dysfunction of skin T cells. A complex chain of events leads to T-cell activation and proliferation, resulting in the release of cytokines and inflammatory mediators, leading to the clinical manifestation of atopic dermatitis. With an increased understanding of these complex immune mechanisms, attempts have been made to shift atopic dermatitis therapy from primarily symptomatic relief to a more specific immunomodulatory approach. Compared with normal skin, the dry skin of atopic dermatitis has reduced water-binding capacity, higher rate of transepidermal water loss, and decreased water content. Water loss leads to further drying and cracking of the skin, which leads to more itching. Rubbing and scratching of itchy skin are responsible for many of the changes seen in the skin.

Clinical Manifestations

Atopic dermatitis begins in many clients during infancy. The dermatitis is usually of acute onset, with a red, oozing, crusting rash. Over time, the skin tends to show the chronic form of dermatitis, with thickened dry texture, brownish-gray color, and scales. The rash tends to become localized to the large folds of the extremities as the client becomes older (Figure 51-2). It is found mainly on elbow bends, the backs of the knees, the neck, the eyelids, and the backs of the hands and feet. Hand and foot dermatitis becomes a significant problem in some adults.

Pruritus is the major clinical manifestation of atopic dermatitis and causes the greatest morbidity. The condition may be mild and self-limiting, or it may be intense, provoking scratching that results in severely excoriated lesions, infection, and scarring.

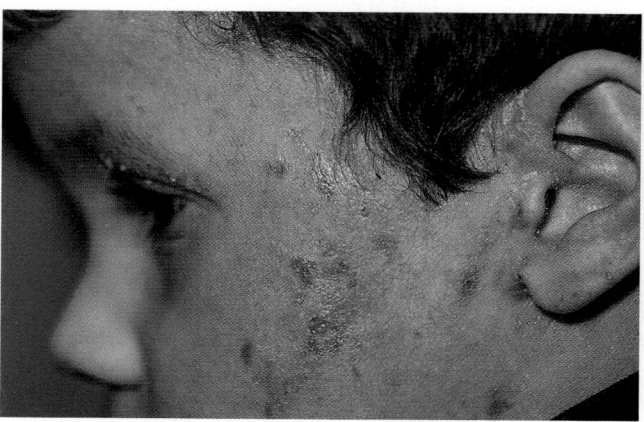

FIGURE 51-2 Atopic dermatitis. Intense pruritus leads to scratching and open lesions.

Complications

Clients with atopic dermatitis tend to experience viral, bacterial, and fungal skin infections. It is not clear whether these cutaneous infections arise secondary to a disruption of normal barrier function or are due to reduced local immunity. Honey-colored crusting, extensive serous weeping, folliculitis, pyoderma, and furunculosis indicate bacterial infection, usually secondary to *Staphylococcus aureus* colonization in clients with atopic dermatitis. Clients with atopic dermatitis are frequently heavily colonized with *S. aureus*. Superficial fungal infections may also appear more frequently. The most common viral infection is herpes simplex, which tends to spread locally or become generalized.

Outcome Management

The goal of therapy is to break the inflammatory cycle that causes excess drying and cracking as well as the itching and scratching.[30] The health care team's understanding of each client's disease pattern and the discovery and reduction of exacerbating factors are crucial to effective management of this chronic disorder.

■ Medical Management

Hydrate the Skin. Hydration is the key to management but is often difficult to achieve. Management begins with daily skin care that hydrates and lubricates the skin. Soaks followed by application of occlusive substances are usually prescribed (see Soaks and Wet Wraps).

Remove Allergens. Allergens, food, aeroallergens, and emotional stresses may be inciting factors in this disorder. Clients should avoid exposure to substances for which there is a positive result on allergy testing that correlates with history of precipitating dermatitis. Stringent restrictions on lifestyle and activities are unjustified. Air-conditioning may help reduce aeroallergen exposure at home and in the workplace. It is important to identify and eliminate triggers that cause the atopic dermatitis to flare. Many of these triggering factors are the same irritants that contribute to generalized pruritus (see Pruritus).

Dietary management of atopic dermatitis has continued to be controversial. Food allergies in the causation of atopic dermatitis seem to be more significant in certain populations of young children and infants. The most common allergens appear to be eggs, cow's milk, soy, wheat, nuts, and fish. Proven allergens are avoided. People with food allergies must be taught to read labels. Care must be taken to avoid malnutrition when any type of restrictive diet is used.

Occlusives, emollients, topical corticosteroids, nonsteroidal topical immunomodulators, and tar preparations all can be employed in various combinations to control atopic dermatitis. The use of topical medications is an important component of therapy for eczema. The nonsteroidal topical immunomodulators (TIMs) are a class of dermatologic drugs introduced in early 2001, and the first new drug class to treat atopic dermatitis since steroids were introduced as a new drug class more than 40 years ago. Tacrolimus ointment 0.1% and 0.03% (Protopic) was the first TIM approved by the Federal Drug Administration (FDA) and is indicated for the treatment of moderate to severe atopic dermatitis. The second TIM, pimecrolimus cream 1% (Elidel), was introduced in 2002 and is indicated for the treatment of mild to moderate atopic dermatitis. Nonsteroidal topical immunomodulators are skin selective and have a higher molecular weight than steroids. They penetrate the skin less as the skin heals during treatment. There is minimal systemic absorption, so these drugs cause no systemic immunosuppression; they have not been shown to be associated with any of the steroid side effects. These newer agents have been shown to be safe, even when used intermittently over the long term; a burning or itching sensation is the primary adverse event reported in trials. These agents are also applied to affected areas once or twice daily. Given their positive safety profile, the TIMs represent an important development in the dermatologic treatment of atopic dermatitis and, possibly, other inflammatory skin diseases. Using these new drugs in combination with other current skin treatments is under evaluation.

These preparations are best absorbed into hydrated skin or by using wet wraps and occlusion. Topical agents containing chemicals or drugs with the potential to cause skin eruptions are avoided.

Systemic medications may include antibiotics and antihistaminics (see Pruritus). The use of a systemic corticosteroid is rarely warranted in atopic dermatitis. Although systemic steroids can be a "quick and easy cure," they should be avoided in this chronic, non–life-threatening disorder. Although there may be dramatic improvement with their use, the recurrence of dermatitis after their discontinuation is equally dramatic. The side effects of long-term systemic steroid use are both unpleasant (moon face and buffalo hump) and dangerous (adrenal suppression, delayed healing). If a short-term course of oral steroid therapy is given, it is important to taper the dosage as the drug is discontinued. Intensified skin care should also be instituted during the taper to suppress flaring of the dermatitis.

Various therapeutic approaches are becoming available. Results have been promising with the use of the nonsteroidal topical immunomodulators, and other experimental modalities are in trial. Clients with severe, recalcitrant disease should be made aware of research advances and encouraged to participate in trials, when possible, to give them a sense of hope.

■ Nursing Management of the Medical Client

Assess the client with atopic dermatitis for bathing habits, use of moisturizers, medication regimen, exposure to known allergens, environmental exposure, and history of skin eruptions. Nursing management is presented in the Care Plan feature on The Client with Atopic Dermatitis on the website.

■ Modifications for Older Clients

Dermatitis is a common skin disorder in the older population. It may be caused by venous insufficiency, allergens, irritants, or underlying malignancy such as leukemia or lymphoma. Because older adults often take many medications, the potential for dermatitis from drug-drug interactions is increased. The fragility of the skin as a result of the flattened epidermal-dermal junction and loss of dermis should be considered in planning any form of treatment.

XEROTIC ECZEMA

Xerotic (dry) skin lacks moisture in the top layer of the skin. Xerotic eczema may present as erythematous, scaling, and finely cracked skin. Xerosis occurs in patches and may involve any skin surface. It is common in the older population. If xerosis is severe, the skin is tight, itchy, and painful. Water loss causes xerotic chapping and fissures. The problem may be accentuated by use of drying skin cleansers, soaps, disinfectants, and solvents and infrequent use of moisturizers. Environmental factors play a large role, especially those that increase water loss in the stratum corneum. Any factors that decrease the relative humidity exacerbate this condition, such as cold or dry winter air, especially in artificially heated rooms.

Management includes hydration and moisturizing the skin plus avoiding irritating factors. Teaching the client correct daily skin care is essential to treating this condition (see Soaks and Wet Wraps). Clients known to have xerosis every winter are advised to increase moisturization before severe weather starts.

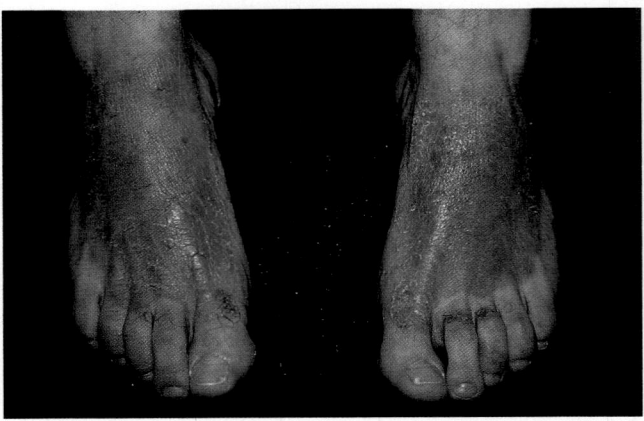

FIGURE 51-3 Contact dermatitis. Note the distinct line of erythema.

CONTACT DERMATITIS

Contact dermatitis is an inflammatory response of the skin. There are two types based on the etiology: irritant or allergic. Irritant contact dermatitis (ICD) is most common and is from exposure to anything that produces a chemical or physical irritant response. Allergic contact dermatitis (ACD) is a delayed hypersensitivity reaction resulting from contact with an allergen. This hypersensitivity reaction is an immune-mediated response by previously sensitized lymphocytes to a specific allergen. Common allergens are poison ivy, nickel, bacitracin, and formaldehyde.

The two conditions are difficult to distinguish. Clinical manifestations begin at the site of exposure with itching, stinging, erythema, and edema, which may extend to involve more distant sites. Manifestations may develop within an hour of contact or as late as 7 to 14 days after contact and may range from mild erythema to vesicles to ulceration (Figure 51-3). With even brief contact of the substance with the skin, an allergic response is possible. For example, contact with poison ivy may have happened quickly and the allergen washed off. However, areas of dermatitis may continue to appear for many days following the initial exposure.

Management begins with identification of the causative agent. First, question the client about recent exposure to plants, chemicals, metals, and the like. Pain and itching may be controlled with topical medication or wet dressings (see Soaks and Wet Wraps). Antihistaminic agents and topical or systemic steroids may be required (see the Client Education Guide feature on Topical Corticosteroids on p. 1399). Patch testing is a test done to attempt to determine the specific agent. Each patch in a standardized test panel (TRUE test [thin-layer, rapid-use epicutaneous test]) contains a substance that is known to be some of the most common causes of allergic contact dermatitis. When these tests elicit a positive reaction, much can be done to teach the client about what to avoid (see Chapter 50).

CLIENT EDUCATION GUIDE
Topical Corticosteroids

Corticosteroids are still among the most commonly used medications for treatment of a variety of dermatologic conditions. Corticosteroids can also be injected directly into the lesion, applied topically, or given systemically. Attempts to diagnose the condition before any corticosteroid use are important because the effects of the medication can mask or change the clinical manifestations. Topical corticosteroids work through broad mechanisms, including anti-inflammatory, antimitotic, immunosuppressant, and vasoconstrictive actions. The effectiveness of these agents largely depends on the potency of the agent used and the degree of absorption through the skin. The greater the potency of a steroid, however, the greater the safety concerns. Skin hydration just before application increases absorption and effectiveness.

Topical steroids range in potency from low to high. Low-potency topical steroids are now available in over-the-counter (OTC) formulations (e.g., hydrocortisone, 0.5% or 1%) and in prescription strength (e.g., desonide, alclometasone). Generally, low-potency steroids are safe to use for longer periods of time and even on thin-skinned areas like the face, groin, or axilla. Prolonged use should still be monitored. Medium-potency (e.g., triamcinolone, fluocinolone) to high-potency (e.g., halcinonide, fluocinonide) corticosteroids should be used with caution and for short periods of time and not on the face, groin, or axilla. High-

potency or super high-potency (e.g., betamethasone dipropionate, clobetasol) steroids should be reserved for use on acute or resistant dermatoses (e.g., contact dermatitis) or areas with thick plaque such as in psoriasis.

Clients should know the strength of the topical steroid they are using and its potential side effects. The lowest potency corticosteroid that is effective should be used. Side effects are more likely with prolonged use of medium-potency to high-potency topical corticosteroids. The most common side effect is skin atrophy, which presents as thin or shiny skin with increased prominence of blood vessels, telangiectases, and easy bruising. Other possible side effects include acne-like conditions, folliculitis, hypopigmentation, delayed wound healing, and striae.

Clients must clearly understand how, when, and where to use topical steroids. Properly applying the medication evenly and sparingly once or twice daily to the affected areas can eliminate many potential problems. More frequent application increases the chance of side effects, makes the therapy more costly, and does not usually increase effectiveness. The condition can recur if treatment is stopped abruptly. When the skin disease disappears or comes under good control, a tar preparation, moisturizer, or other topical preparation may be substituted for the topical steroid.

INTERTRIGO

Intertrigo is a superficial inflammatory dermatitis that occurs between two apposed (touching) skin surfaces. Inadequate ventilation, friction, heat, and moisture buildup result in maceration, erosions, fissures, itching, and burning. Intertrigo is common in hot, humid weather in neck creases, axillae, antecubital fossae, the perineum, finger and toe webs, and abdominal skinfolds and beneath the breasts, particularly in obese clients. One of the most common causes of intertrigo is contamination with body fluids, as occurs in urinary incontinence. Secondary bacterial or *Candida albicans* infection may occur. Whenever candidiasis is present, a careful evaluation is indicated. In an otherwise healthy person, candidiasis is a self-limiting disease that responds well to topical antifungal therapy; however, it can be the presenting manifestation of underlying systemic disease affecting the endocrine system (e.g., diabetes) or the immune system (e.g., immunodeficiency syndromes).

Treatment of intertrigo is to eliminate maceration by promoting drying and to aerate the body skinfolds. For mobile clients, review environmental changes that promote drying of the body folds, such as wearing loose-fitting cotton-blend clothing or periodic removal of clothing to dry off. Instruct clients to avoid tight-fitting clothing

such as jeans and activities that promote sweating. Care recommendations depend on the degree of involvement and the overall condition of the skin. If the skin is still intact, recommendations include washing the area gently with tap water twice daily and then rinsing and drying the area, followed by liberal application of a talc-containing powder or a cellulose-containing powder (e.g., Zeasorb) for extra absorption. Avoid using cornstarch, in pure form, because it encourages *C. albicans* overgrowth.

If inflammation is present, a low-potency topical corticosteroid in a nonocclusive vehicle (e.g., hydrocortisone 1.0% or 2.5% cream or lotion) or a combination steroid-antibiotic-antifungal agent (Vytone 1%) may initially be helpful, but long-term use should be avoided (see the Client Education Guide feature on Topical Corticosteroids, above). Apply cool, wet soaks with tap water or Burrow's solution (an antiseptic) three to four times daily for removal of exudate if secondary infection is present. Applying folded gauze or clean cotton handkerchiefs in skinfolds promotes healing by keeping skin surfaces apart.

STASIS DERMATITIS

Stasis dermatitis is characterized by the development of areas of very dry, dark skin and sometimes shallow ulcers on the lower legs, primarily as a result of venous insufficiency (Figure 51-4). The dermatitis is treated with moisturizing agents and antihistamines; antifungal preparations may also be helpful. When fragile skin ulcerations are present, the wound is called a *venous stasis ulcer.* The treatment of these wounds is discussed in Chapter 55.

PSORIASIS VULGARIS

Psoriasis vulgaris is a chronic, recurrent, erythematous, inflammatory disorder with a worldwide distribution. The prevalence varies according to race and geographic location. Psoriasis occurs equally in both genders, usually commencing in the early 20s to 40s. The Latin *vulgaris* (from *vulgus,* or "the public") means "common." It is a genetic systemic disease with an immunologic basis that manifests in the skin and joints.

Pathophysiology

T cells are a type of white blood cell that normally wards off foreign invaders and fights infection. In psoriasis, however, T cells are mistakenly activated and trigger other immune responses that speed up the growth cycle of skin cells. A normal skin cell matures and falls off the body's surface in 28 to 30 days, but a psoriatic skin cell takes only 3 to 4 days to mature and move to the surface. Instead of falling off (shedding), the cells pile up and form lesions. Understanding that this is a chronic immune-mediated disease has led to the development of therapies targeted at immune and inflammatory pathways that are safer and more effective than previous therapies.[26]

Clinical Manifestations

The epidermis thickens with extra skin cells, and blood vessels dilate with increased blood supply to nourish those cells. At the surface, skin cells pile up. Dead cells create a white, flaky layer of silvery white scales over the patch of inflamed skin.

The eruptions (usually in a symmetrical distribution) commonly occur on the scalp, elbows, knees, genital, and sacral regions (Figure 51-5). Lesions may develop at the site of an injury, which is known as *Koebner's phenomenon.* A generalized eruption may occur with severe psoriasis vulgaris. Another type is palmar plantar psoriasis, which can be pustular or of a plaque type and only affects the palms and soles. In a rare form of psoriasis, known as *pustular psoriasis,* generalized, sterile cutaneous pustules are produced. Severe systemic involvement can be fatal. Up to one third of clients with moderate to severe psoriasis have psoriatic arthritis, which primarily affects the distal joints and may be deforming. Nail dystrophies and pitting occur frequently.

Outcome Management

The course of psoriasis vulgaris is unpredictable. It can be controlled with aggressive therapies but cannot be cured. Exacerbations and remissions are common. As with other chronic diseases, changes in physical and emotional health can precede flares. The goals of medical management of psoriasis are to decrease the T-cell counts in the epidermis, control the rate of epidermal cell turnover, and monitor for complications of therapy.

■ Medical Management

Suppress T-Cell Activation. Mild psoriasis may be treated locally with natural sunlight or topical therapy, including calcipotriene, tazarotene, or topical corticosteroids, or with occasional use of intralesional corticosteroids (see the Client Education Guide feature on Topical Corticosteroids on p. 1399). Injecting small, dilute amounts of corticosteroids (e.g., triamcinolone acetonide) into or just beneath a lesion gives a high drug concentration at the injection site. Systemic steroids are contraindicated in psoriasis. Keratolytic agents (e.g., salicylic acid) may remove scale and allow greater penetra-

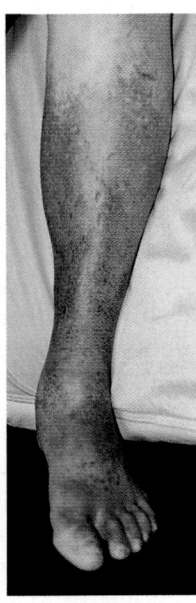

FIGURE 51-4 Stasis dermatitis. Note the dark, stained, shiny skin on the leg as well as the absence of hair.

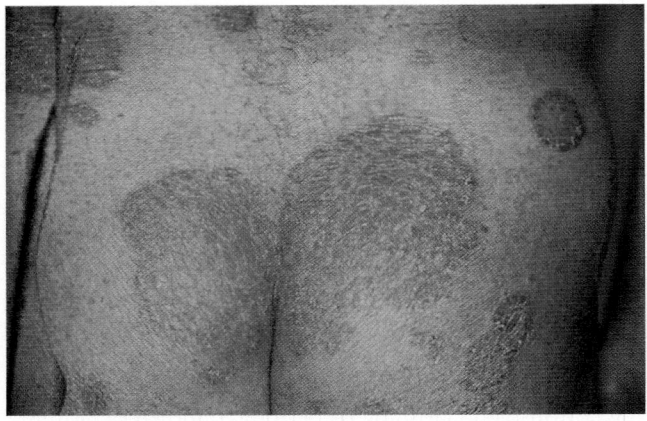

FIGURE 51-5 Plaque psoriasis of the buttocks.

tion of topical agents. Anthralin reduces mitotic action in the cell and is an effective topical agent for treatment of psoriasis with widespread discrete lesions consisting primarily of thick plaques, but it is rarely used in the United States because of its complicated protocol.

The more conventional psoriasis therapies such as UVA and UVB (see Ultraviolet Light Therapy), methotrexate, and cyclosporine, have all been found to be anti–T-cell agents. Recent advances in monoclonal antibody technology and the application of these new immunomodulatory biologics have changed the treatment of psoriasis.

Areas that are difficult to treat, such as the scalp and nails, remain a challenge. Scalp care in psoriasis consists of reducing scales and treating inflammation. Clients are instructed to avoid picking and scratching. Use of steroids and oil vehicles under occlusion is often necessary to enhance percutaneous absorption; on the scalp, a plastic shower cap can be used for this purpose. Other products such as tars, medicated shampoos, and non-steroidal treatments also play an important role in scalp care. There is no consistently effective treatment of psoriatic involvement of the nails. Tazarotene is showing promising results in reducing nail dystrophy. However, the scalp and nails do improve with clearing of psoriasis on the body surface.

Systemic treatment in oral and injectable forms are being increasingly prescribed for psoriasis affecting 10% or more of the body surface area. The most common systemic agents include acitretin (Soriatane), methotrexate, cyclosporine, and the new biologics including etanercept, alefacept, efalizumab, and infliximab, which block the activation of T cells and prevent the migration of T cells into the skin with promising results and minimal complications.[24]

Monitor for Complications. Complications include the potential side effects of the treatments and the progression of the disorder. Potential localized side effects of corticosteroids include atrophy, hypopigmentation, infection, and, rarely, ulceration. The side effects of Soriatane are similar to those of the oral retinoids and requires many special precautions (see Acne Vulgaris).

Methotrexate is potentially toxic to the renal, hepatic, and hematopoietic systems. Thus baseline assessment (e.g., blood chemistry, complete blood count, liver biopsy) is important before this medication is started. During treatment, periodic assessments are needed, including biopsy of the liver. If any serious side effects develop, such as bone marrow depression (decreased white blood cell and platelet count) or gastrointestinal tract bleeding, treatment is discontinued. To limit potential liver damage, advise the client not to consume alcohol throughout therapy. Because methotrexate may cause chromosomal abnormalities, effective birth control methods are important for both women and men before and during treatment and for 3 months after completing methotrexate. Nausea, the most common side effect, can be limited by taking methotrexate with food, using prophylactic antiemetics, and adding supplemental folic acid.

Cyclosporine (Neoral and Gengraf) is approved for up to 1 year in managing chronic plaque psoriasis. It is most often used as a rescue drug with severe flares, especially when clients are erythrodermic. Renal function can be impaired with subsequent hypertension. Therefore renal and metabolic functions as well as blood pressure must be monitored closely. Many drugs are contraindicated with cyclosporine, necessitating constant interaction between the client and the nurse.

Biologic drugs are the newest drugs in managing psoriasis and psoriatic arthritis. This class of drugs is injected or infused into the client. These agents also require specific monitoring. Combination therapy, rotational therapy, and sequential therapy have all been used for psoriasis in attempts to achieve greater efficiency and greater safety

■ Self-Care

Assist the client in coping with an altered self-concept. The appearance of skin lesions may make the client feel "dirty" or untouchable. Because open lesions are at high risk for secondary infection, the client should be taught to keep the creams or ointments on and to keep the area clean and dry. To keep psoriasis in remission, the client needs to control the causative factors. Adequate rest, nutrition, and exercise promote health. Stress should be minimized, and illness and infection should be treated early.

ACNE VULGARIS

Acne is an inflammatory skin disease affecting the tiny pores that cover the face, arms, back, and chest and the oil glands attached to them. The lesions are called *comedones,* or most commonly "zits." Numerous topical and systemic drugs are available for the treatment of acne vulgaris. Acne is common in teenagers; refer to a pediatric nursing textbook for further discussion.

ACNE ROSACEA

Acne rosacea is a chronic inflammatory skin eruption characterized by erythema, papules, pustules, and telangiectases. It occurs on the face, especially the cheeks and over the bridge of the nose. Unlike with acne vulgaris, comedones are generally not seen. The onset is insidious, usually occurring between 30 and 50 years of age, and women are affected more frequently than men. It is more common in fair-skinned people with a history of easy facial flushing. Precipitating factors that appear to make the flushing worse include tea, coffee, alcohol (especially wine), caffeine-containing products, sunlight, extremes of hot and cold, spicy foods, and emotional stress.

Sebaceous hyperplasia of the nose (rhinophyma) often develops after many years of chronic acne rosacea. This condition results from chronic inflammation with an increase in the amount of connective tissue and may be mistaken for an indication of excessive alcohol consumption. Ocular changes such as eyelid inflammation and conjunctivitis may occur.

Avoidance of the stimuli that trigger acne rosacea may be sufficient for management of mild forms of the disorder. Instruct clients to avoid factors that provoke facial vasodilation. Treatment of rosacea is sometimes difficult. The topical agents generally used include antibiotics, metronidazole (MetroGel), and retinoids. Systemic drugs include antibiotics, isotretinoin, and metronidazole, but the pros and cons of using these must be weighed.

SKIN TEARS

Skin tears are wounds resulting from the separation of epidermis from the underlying connective tissue. The most common sites for skin tears, in order of frequency, are the forearm, hand, elbow, and upper arm. Skin tears are most common in older adults as a result of a thinning of the epidermis, a flattening of the dermal-epidermal junction, and reduced adhesion of the dermis to the epidermis. They are very common in clients who have taken long-term oral steroids for conditions like emphysema. Skin tears often result from trauma such as falls and injury from wheelchair handles or brakes or injury that incurred during transfer to a chair. Even though the actual skin damage is minor, families and residents are disturbed by the presence of skin tears, often perceiving the injury as resulting from abuse.

Outcome Management

For tears with small to moderate losses of epidermal tissue, irrigate the wound with normal saline to remove blood or debris. Replace any flaps of epidermis and secure with strips of tape. Cover the open wound with nonocclusive, moisture-retentive dressing, such as petrolatum-impregnated gauze or opaque foam dressing. Do not use adherent clear dressings; when these dressings are removed, the skin can tear again. Prevention is important. Use protective gloves on the client's hands and soft armrests on wheelchairs, and train caregivers in proper transfer techniques (e.g., use of transfer belts). Daily assessment by unlicensed assistive personnel is critical to identify lesions early (see the Management and Delegation feature on Skin Inspection, below).

MANAGEMENT AND DELEGATION

Skin Inspection

Unlicensed assistive personnel frequently are in the position to observe the skin of clients as they assist with various activities of daily living and provide assistance with personal hygiene. Be sure to fully delineate their role in identifying and reporting skin abnormalities. Reportable findings are listed as follows.

Bruising or a change in skin color. Ecchymosis, erythema, jaundice, and pallor may indicate a serious disease process or acute tissue injury. Identification of these changes in skin color by unlicensed assistive personnel should be immediately reported to you for thorough assessment and intervention. Redness overlying bony structures may indicate prolonged or undue pressure. Unlicensed assistive personnel should ensure pressure relief by assisting the client with frequent position changes.

Lumps. Assess any skin lesion or growth in further detail.

Dry, scaling, or cracked skin. Dry skin may indicate dehydration or other integumentary disorders. You may delegate the application of over-the-counter lotions to unlicensed assistive personnel if the skin is not broken. Some clients may need specific lubricants or medications prescribed by a physician; therefore have any findings of dry skin reported to you.

Skin that feels excessively moist and cool or excessively warm. It is appropriate for unlicensed assistive personnel to cover clients with extra bedding if they feel cool or to offer cool compresses for warm skin (see Chapter 29). Localized areas of warmth may indicate underlying processes that need prompt attention. Clearly communicate that any of these findings should be immediately reported to you for prompt assessment and intervention.

Any break in the skin with drainage or bleeding. You may delegate the application of sterile gauze to the surface of the skin to unlicensed assistive personnel for the purpose of containing drainage (see Chapter 16). Skin tears should be treated with nonstick dressings. Assess such skin abnormalities promptly after identification by unlicensed assistive personnel.

Taught or shiny skin. This finding may indicate fluid shifting from the intravascular space. Such skin is susceptible to breakdown and infection. Employ proactive measures to prevent any undue pressure or damage to the skin. Assess the area carefully, and report any unknown disorders or significant change to a physician. Elevate the area to decrease swelling if present.

Client complaints of itching or tenderness. Instruct unlicensed assistive personnel identifying such client complaints to communicate these findings to you promptly. Assess the client for potential allergic reaction, an underlying tissue pathologic process, or the need for additional analgesics.

Rashes. New rashes or other skin eruptions sometimes suggest allergic reactions. Instruct that such findings be reported to you promptly.

You are ultimately responsible for thorough, ongoing assessment and evaluation of integument.

PRESSURE ULCERS

A pressure ulcer is any lesion on the skin caused by un-relieved pressure and resulting in damage to underlying tissue. Pressure ulcers occur commonly in areas subject to high pressure from body weight on bony prominences. Pressure ulcers have also been called "bed sores" and "decubitus ulcers." The word *decubitus* comes from the Latin *decumbere,* which means to lie down. The ulcers were so named because they are common in bedridden clients.

Etiology and Risk Factors

Pressure ulcers develop when soft tissue (skin, subcutaneous tissue, and muscle) are compressed between a bony prominence and a firm surface for a prolonged period of time. Therefore immobility and inactivity are major risk factors. In bedridden clients, infrequent turning and repositioning or lack of padding between surfaces that touch (e.g., knees) may lead to tissue damage. In addition, clients in bed are often positioned in semi-Fowler's position to facilitate breathing or eating. This position increases the risk of ulcers on the sacrum and heels. The ischia are common sites of pressure ulcers in chairbound clients, especially if they sit erect in the chair. The length of time of exposure to pressure before skin breakdown varies among clients; in very debilitated clients, permanent tissue damage can result in less than 2 hours. Cognitive or sensory impairments also increase risk because the client cannot recognize the need to turn or move.

Protein-calorie malnutrition is another major risk factor. Malnourished clients have poor skin integrity, and their skin is damaged easily. In addition, incontinence, friction, and skin shearing can also lead to breakdown. These factors reduce the tolerance the skin has for pressure.

The reported incidence (number of new cases per year) of pressure ulcers in acute care facilities ranges from 2.7% to 29.5%. The prevalence (number of cases at one point in time) in acute care settings ranges from 3.5% to 29.5%. Several populations are at increased risk. Quadriplegic clients, older adults with femoral fractures, and clients in critical care units have the highest risk. Prevention of pressure ulcers begins with identifying the client at risk. Risk factors can be determined by assessing sensory perception, moisture, activity, mobility, nutrition, friction, and shear. Risk for pressure ulcers can be expressed numerically by using an instrument to appraise risk such as the Braden or Norton tool (see later discussion).

Pathophysiology

Continuous pressure on soft tissues between bony prominences and support surfaces (mattress, chair) compresses capillaries and occludes blood flow. If the pressure is relieved, a brief period of rebound capillary dilation (called *reactive hyperemia*) occurs, and there is no tissue damage. If pressure is not relieved, microthrombi form in capillaries and completely occlude blood flow. A blister may form initially. Damage to underlying tissues creates a necrotic area of tissue. The necrotic tissue undergoes the process of inflammation as the body tries to get rid of it and ready the tissue for healing.

Healing occurs through secondary intention. Granulation tissue fills the base of the wound. Contraction of the ulcer edges closes the wound. Eventually, epithelial cells cover the wound. Stage III and IV pressure ulcers often require debridement and surgery to close the wound. Scar tissue predominates in ulcers healed without surgery.

Clinical Manifestations

The clinical manifestations of pressure ulcers have been described in four stages (Figure 51-6). Some pressure ulcers cannot be staged because the wound is covered with eschar and the bottom of the ulcer cannot be seen. Another form of ulcers that cannot be staged is deep tissue injuries, in which the tissue looks bruised over a bony prominence or has broken blisters. Ulcers most commonly occur on the sacrum, heel, greater trochanter (Figure 51-7), and ischial tuberosities. The ulcer may or may not be covered with devitalized tissue, which can be yellow, white, brown, or black.

With pressure ulcers, few additional diagnostic assessments are required. Sometimes osteomyelitis is present in deep wounds. Bone scans are used for confirming this problem. If malnutrition is suspected as a cause, serum protein, albumin, or prealbumin levels may be monitored. It is important to distinguish pressure ulcers from other wounds, such as arterial or venous ulcers. See Chapter 55 for a discussion of these wounds.

Outcome Management
■ Medical Management

Management of the client with a pressure ulcer begins with a complete history and physical examination. There are many causes of delayed wound healing, and delayed healing of pressure ulcers may be the result of other health problems. The goal of medical management is to heal the wound by relieving the pressure over the lesion or decreasing tissue load, cleaning and dressing the wound, and improving nutrition. In addition, the ulcer is monitored for healing, and the client is monitored for complications.

Manage Tissue Load. The term *tissue load* refers to the distribution of pressure, friction, and shear on the tissues. Interventions are designed to decrease tissue load and thereby decrease pressure. Increasing the frequency of turning helps disperse pressure over time. Clients

Stage I

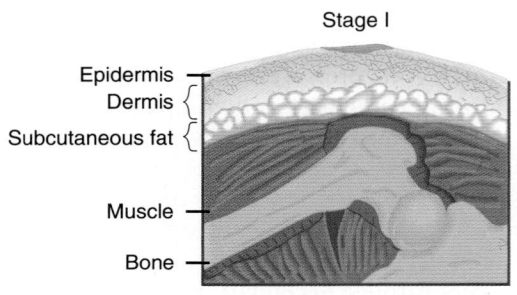

Epidermis
Dermis
Subcutaneous fat
Muscle
Bone

Non-blanching erythema of intact skin;
the heralding lesion of skin ulceration

Stage II

Epidermis
Dermis
Subcutaneous fat
Muscle
Bone

Partial-thickness skin loss involving
epidermis and/or dermis. The ulcer is
superficial and presents clinically as an
abrasion, blister, or shallow crater.

Stage III

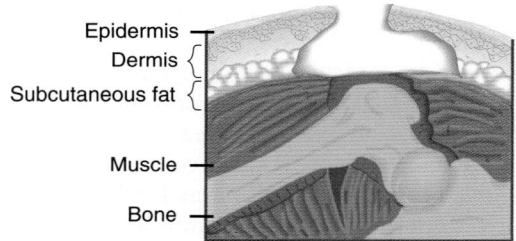

Epidermis
Dermis
Subcutaneous fat
Muscle
Bone

Full-thickness skin loss involving damage
or necrosis of subcutaneous tissue, which
may extend down to, but not through, the
underlying fascia. The ulcer presents
clinically as a deep crater with or without
undermining of adjacent tissue.

Stage IV

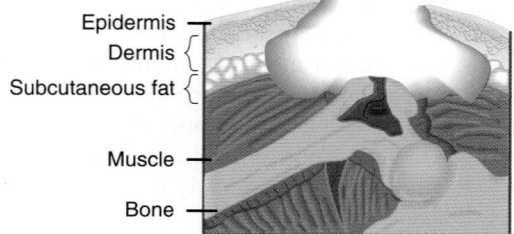

Epidermis
Dermis
Subcutaneous fat
Muscle
Bone

Full-thickness skin loss with extensive
destruction, tissue necrosis, or damage
to muscle, bone, or supporting structures
(e.g., tendon, joint capsule, etc.)

FIGURE 51-6 Stages of pressure ulcers.

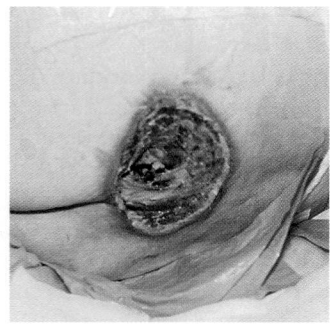

FIGURE 51-7 Common sites for pressure ulcers. Stage IV pressure ulcer on the sacrum. The center of the ulcer contains necrotic tissue that needs to be debrided.

should not lie on a pressure ulcer. If the ulcer is on the sacrum, sitting should be reduced to 1 to 2 hours at a time and only for meals. Restricting blood flow to a wound delays healing. Special low-pressure beds may be required for clients with multiple pressure ulcers (Figure 51-8). If the client can turn or be repositioned so as not to lie on a pressure ulcer, a pressure-reducing overlay may be placed on the mattress. These devices can be compressed by the client's weight, and rendered ineffective. Check for bottoming out when using overlay mattresses (Figure 51-9). Heels should be elevated from the bed by placing pillows under the calf or using pressure reduction boots. Chair cushions should be used if the client is sitting in a chair or getting up to a chair; 4 inches of foam is effective. Specialty cushions also exist for wheelchair-dependent clients.

Provide Ulcer Care. Moist, devitalized tissue supports bacterial growth. Therefore devitalized tissue must be removed from the ulcer. Several forms of debridement can be used depending on the client's goals and the type of wound. *Sharp debridement* is the use of a scalpel to excise devitalized thick, adherent eschar; this form of debridement is completed in the operating room by the physician. *Conservative sharp* debridement is carried out at the bedside using a scalpel and forceps to remove loose necrotic tissue. This form of debridement is done by trained personnel. *Mechanical debridement* is the use of wet-to-dry dressings, hydrotherapy, and high-pressure wound irrigation to soften and remove devitalized tissues. *Enzymatic debridement* is the use of topical debriding agents to dissolve the collagen anchors that hold the necrotic slough tissue to the wound bed. *Biodebridement* is the use of sterile larvae (maggots), which secrete enzymes that digest wound tissue. Finally, *autolytic debridement* involves the use of synthetic dressings to cover an ulcer, allowing enzymes in the wound bed to digest the devitalized tissues. This form of debridement is the slowest and is usually reserved for clients who can-

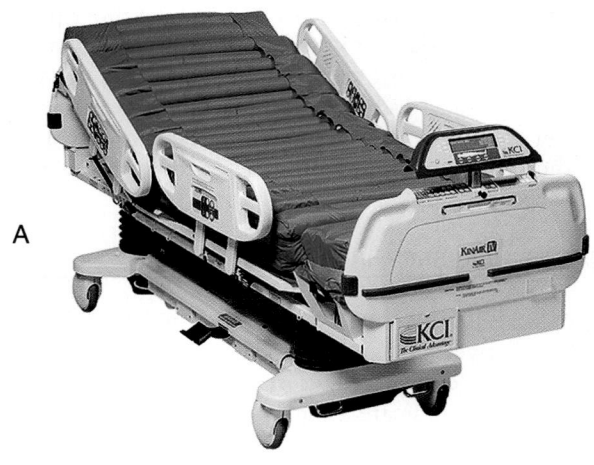

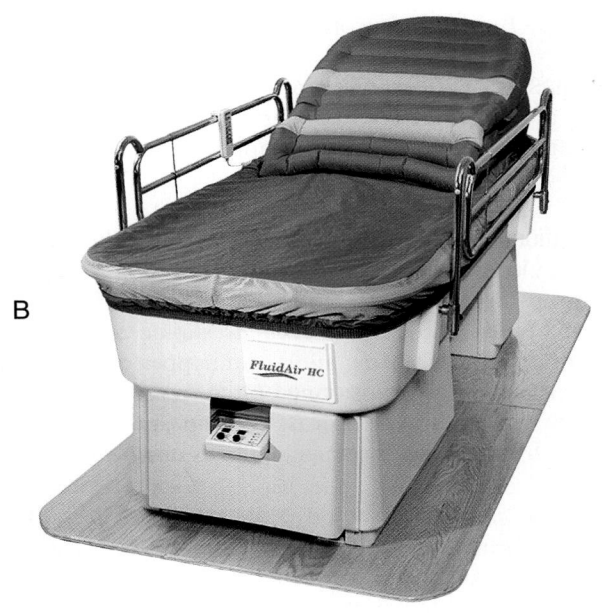

FIGURE 51-8 Pressure reduction surfaces. **A,** KinAir beds provide controlled air suspension to redistribute body weight away from bony prominences. **B,** FluidAir beds use air flow and bead fluidization. Both of these beds are covered with Gore-Tex fabric, which resists tearing. This fabric is also waterproof and acts as a barrier against bacteria. (Courtesy of Kinetic Concepts, Inc., San Antonio, TX.)

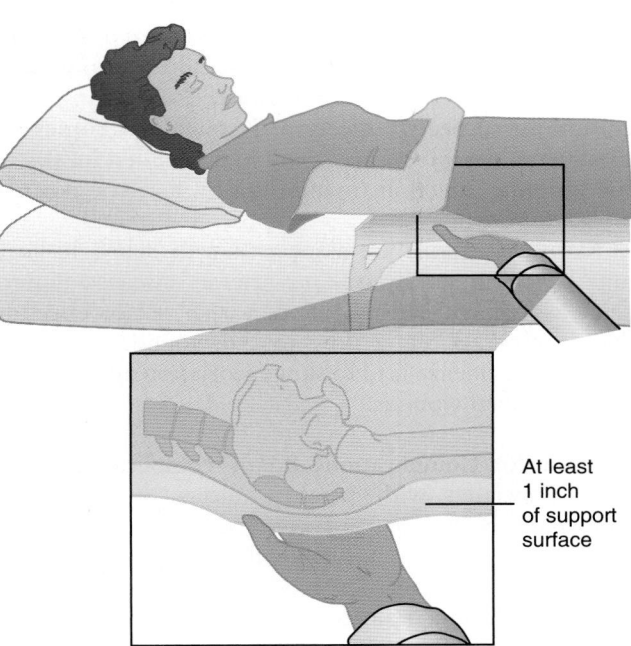

At least 1 inch of support surface

FIGURE 51-9 Assessment of pressure relief ("bottoming out"). Slide your hand (palm up and fingers flat) under the support surface, just under the pressure point. Do not flex your fingers. With adequate support, there will be at least 1 inch of uncompressed support surface between your hand and the client's body. (Modified from Gaymar Industries, Inc., Orchard Park, NY.)

not tolerate the other forms. Some ulcers should not be debrided: ulcers on limbs where perfusion is insufficient to support healing and dry, stable eschar on heels. All forms of debridement (except autolytic) are painful; the client should be given analgesics before beginning.

Improve Nutrition. The association of malnutrition with pressure ulcer formation and delayed healing is clear. In fact, many clinicians believe that pressure ulcers are a specific indicator of malnutrition. If the client's serum albumin or prealbumin concentration is low, if the client is not eating, or if the client's body weight is less than 80% of ideal, consider nutritional supplementation. If the client has no gastrointestinal disorders and can swallow, provide oral supplements. Some clinicians use the phrase "if the gut works, use it" to summarize this recommendation. If the client cannot swallow without aspiration, tube feeding may be required. If the client has gastrointestinal problems, consider total parenteral nutrition. These more aggressive forms of feeding must be compatible with the client's wishes. Monitor nutritional status (as described previously) every 3 months. Body weight should be assessed every 1 to 4 weeks.

Monitor Healing. If the ulcer does not heal within 2 weeks despite adequate nutrition, pressure reduction, daily cleaning, and use of appropriate dressings, the ulcer may be infected. An infected pressure ulcer looks like any other infected wound, with foul-smelling drainage, increasing size, increasing pain in the wound, and fever or elevation in white blood cell count. Older clients do not invariably demonstrate all of the manifestations of infection and are at risk for development of confusion; therefore vigilance in assessing the ulcer for changes is critical. If infection is suspected, a 2-week trial of topical antibiotics is considered. Swab cultures are not appropriate for diagnosis of infection in the ulcer. All pressure ulcers are colonized (covered with surface bacteria), and a swab culture grows only organisms that colonize the surface. Use a quantitative culture for suspected infection. Systemic antibiotics are used when the infection cannot be controlled locally or for systemic infection (manifested by fever or positive blood cultures).

Many conditions are associated with delays in healing. Diabetes, paralysis, and arterial diseases require close assessment because of increased risk of infection due to reduced blood flow to the wound. Urine and bowel incontinence lead to skin excoriation and can contaminate open wounds.

Monitor for Complications. Many complications have been associated with pressure ulcers, including osteomyelitis, bacteremia and sepsis, and cellulitis. Wounds with osteomyelitis do not generally heal; if they do heal, they soon open again. The wound may become increasingly painful and drainage may be foul, often infected with *S. aureus*, *Enterobacter* species, and *Pseudomonas* species. Sepsis can follow osteomyelitis; confusion, reduced levels of consciousness, fever, hypotension, elevated white blood cell count, and other manifestations of septic shock may develop.

The word *cellulitis* literally means "inflammation of the cells." It generally indicates an acute spreading infection of the dermis and subcutaneous tissues, resulting in pain, erythema, edema, and warmth. Associated red streaking visible in skin proximal to the area of cellulitis is characteristic of ascending lymphangitis. Cellulitis characterized by violaceous color and bullae suggests infection with *Streptococcus pneumoniae* (pneumococcus).

■ Nursing Management of the Medical Client
Assessment

All clients should be assessed for risk of pressure ulcers on admission and then daily, depending upon the client's condition. Less frequent assessment may be done if the client's condition is stable. The assessment of the client at high risk for development of pressure ulcers should identify any specific risk factors. The Braden scale (Figure 51-10) is an assessment tool that assists the nurse in predicting which clients are at greatest risk. Assess laboratory data on hemoglobin, hematocrit, albumin, total protein, and lymphocytes.

If the client has a pressure ulcer, it must be recorded on admission to the facility. Note objective data about the pressure ulcer (i.e., stage, size, depth, wound bed appearance, drainage, and condition of periulcer tissue). Reassessment of the ulcer is completed each time dressings are changed or sooner if the ulcer shows manifestations of deterioration. Analyses of the trends in healing are an important step in assessment. Consider whether the ulcer

is increasing in size or depth or is developing more purulent drainage or odor, or whether the periulcer tissue is showing manifestations of deterioration. These changes in the pressure ulcer indicate that it is deteriorating and a change in treatment is needed. The physician or wound nurse should be notified, unless the agency protocol allows independent changes in treatment.

Diagnosis, Outcomes, Intervention

Diagnosis: Risk for Impaired Skin Integrity. Clients who score between 12 and 16 on the Braden risk assessment scale are considered at risk for pressure ulcers. Scores below 12 indicate a high risk. This nursing diagnosis is written as *Risk for Impaired Skin Integrity related to malnutrition and unrelieved pressure as evidenced by Braden risk score*.

Outcomes. The client will experience a reduction in the risk of impairment of skin integrity, as evidenced by no actual tissue breakdown and no persistent reddened areas.

Interventions. Preventive measures to reduce the risk of pressure ulcers cannot be overemphasized (Box 51-1). Interventions are chosen to match the specific risk factors present (Table 51-3). If the client is supine or in semi-Fowler's position, shearing injury can happen quickly and the client should be repositioned often to reduce the risk of injury to the sacral area. It is also important to elevate the heels from the bed by placing pillows under the calves.

Evaluation. Outcomes should be met in 24 to 48 hours. Recall that skin integrity can be impaired in just 2 hours. Therefore several hours are needed to determine whether skin injury occurred before risk reduction measures were implemented. If so, a more aggressive prevention plan is needed.

Diagnosis: Impaired Skin Integrity. If the client has a pressure ulcer, state the nursing diagnosis as *Impaired Skin Integrity related to pressure ulcer secondary to prolonged immobility, malnutrition, and unrelieved pressure as evidenced by (add description of the ulcer)*.

Outcomes. The client will experience healing of the ulcer, as evidenced by development of granulation tissue and decreasing ulcer size. Do not use lower stages of pressure ulcers to describe healing. For example, do not state a stage IV will heal to a stage III. The body does not heal by regeneration of tissue but, rather, by scar tissue. For clients who are terminally ill, outcomes such as healing may not be appropriate. For these clients, outcomes of pain management, comfort, or reducing risk of infection may be more appropriate.

RISK PREDICTORS FOR SKIN BREAKDOWN

Patient's Name _____   Evaluator's Name _____

SENSORY PERCEPTION ability to respond to discomfort	**1. Completely limited:** Unresponsive to painful stimuli, either because of state of unconsciousness or severe sensory impairment, which limits ability to feel pain over most of body surface	**2. Very limited:** Responds only to painful stimuli (but not verbal commands) by opening eyes or flexing extremities. Cannot communicate discomfort verbally, OR has a sensory impairment which limits the ability to feel pain or discomfort over one half of body surface	**3. Slightly limited:** Responds to verbal commands by opening eyes and obeying some commands, but cannot always communicate discomfort or need to be turned, OR has some sensory impairment which limits ability to feel pain or discomfort in one or two extremities.	**4. No impairment:** Responds to verbal commands by obeying. Can communicate needs accurately. Has no sensory deficit which would limit ability to feel pain or discomfort
MOISTURE degree to which skin is exposed to moisture	**1. Very Moist:** Skin is kept moist almost constantly by perspiration and urine. Dampness is detected every time patient is moved or turned. Linen must be changed more than one time each shift	**2. Occasionally Moist:** Skin is frequently, but not always kept moist, linen must be changed two to three times every 24 hours	**3. Rarely Moist:** Skin is rarely moist more than three to four times a week, but linen does require changing at that time	**4. Never Moist:** Perspiration and incontinence are never a problem linen changed at routine intervals only
ACTIVITY degree of physical activity	**1. Bedfast:** Confined to bed	**2. Chairfast:** Ability to walk severely impaired or nonexistent and must be assisted into chair or wheelchair. Is confined to chair or wheelchair when not in bed	**3. Walks occasionally:** Walks occasionally during day, but for very short distances, with or without assistance. Spends majority of each shift in bed or chair	**4. Walks frequently:** Walks a moderate distance at least once every 1 to 2 hours during waking hours
MOBILITY ability to change and control body position	**1. Completely Immobile:** Unable to make even slight changes in position without assistance	**2. Very limited:** Makes occasional slight changes in position without help but unable to make frequent or significant changes in position independently	**3. Slightly limited:** Makes frequent though slight changes in position without assistance but unable to make or maintain major changes in position independently	**4. No limitations:** Makes major and frequent changes in position without assistance
NUTRITION usual food intake pattern	**1. Very Poor:** Never eats a complete meal. Rarely eats more than 1/3 of any food offered. Intake of protein is negligible. Takes even fluids poorly. Does not take a liquid dietary supplement, OR is NPO and/or maintained on clear liquids or IV for more than 5 days	**2. Probably Inadequate:** Rarely eats a complete meal and generally eats only about one half of any food offered. Protein intake is poor. Occasionally will take a liquid dietary supplement, OR receiving less than optimum amount of liquid diet or tube feeding	**3. Adequate:** Eats over half of most meals. Eats moderate amount of protein source one to two times daily. Occasionally will refuse a meal. Will usually take a dietary supplement if offered OR is on a tube feeding or TPN regimen which probably meets most of nutritional needs	**4. Excellent:** Eats most of every meal. Never refuses a meal. Frequently eats between meals. Does not require a dietary supplementation
FRICTION AND SHEAR	**1. Problem:** Requires moderate to maximum assistance in moving. Complete lifting without sliding against sheets is impossible. Frequently slides down in bed or chair, requiring frequent repositioning with maximum assistance. Either spasticity, contractures or agitation leads to almost constant friction	**2. Potential Problem:** Moves feebly Independently or requires minimum assistance. Skin probably slides against bedsheets or chair to some extent when movement occurs. Maintains relatively good position in chair or bed most of time but occasionally slides down	**3. No Apparent Problem:** Moves in bed and in chair independently and has sufficient muscle strength to lift up completely during move. Maintains good position in bed or chair at all times	

Key: 16, minimum risk; 13–14, moderate risk; 12 or less, high risk; NPO, nothing by mouth; IV, intravenously; TPN, total parenteral nutrition.

FIGURE 51-10 The Braden Scale for evaluation of risk of pressure ulcers. (Courtesy of Barbara Braden and Nancy Bergstrom. ©1988.)

BOX 51-1 *Prevention of Pressure Ulcers*

- Perform a systematic skin inspection for all clients at risk at least once a day, giving particular attention to the bony prominences.
- Document results of skin inspection.
- Cleanse the skin at the time of soiling and at routine intervals. The frequency of skin cleaning should be individualized according to need and client preference.
- Avoid hot water; use a mild cleaning agent that minimizes irritation and dryness of the skin. During the cleaning process, take care to minimize the force and friction applied to the skin.
- Minimize environmental factors leading to skin drying, such as low humidity (<40%) and exposure to cold. Treat dry skin with moisturizers.
- Avoid massage over bony prominences, which may be harmful.
- Minimize skin exposure to moisture from incontinence, perspiration, or wound drainage. When these sources of moisture cannot be controlled, apply underpads or briefs that are made of materials that absorb moisture and present a quick-drying surface to the skin. Topical agents that act as barriers to moisture can also be used.
- Minimize skin injury due to friction and shear forces through proper positioning, transferring, and turning techniques. In addition, help reduce friction injuries by the use of lubricants (e.g., cornstarch and creams), protective films (e.g., transparent film dressings and skin sealants), protective dressings (e.g., hydrocolloids), and protective padding.
- When apparently well-nourished clients do not have an adequate dietary intake of protein or calories, caregivers should first attempt to discover the factors compromising intake and offer support with eating. Other nutritional supplements or support may be needed. If dietary intake remains inadequate and if consistent with overall goals of therapy, consider more aggressive nutritional intervention (enteral or parenteral feedings).
- For nutritionally compromised clients, implement a plan of nutritional support or supplementation that meets individual needs and is consistent with the overall goals of therapy.
- If the potential exists for improving the client's mobility and activity status, institute rehabilitation efforts if these measures are consistent with the overall goals of therapy. Maintaining current activity level, mobility, and range of motion is an appropriate goal for most clients.
- Use a written schedule for systematically turning and repositioning the client.
- For clients in bed, use pillows to keep bony prominences (such as knees or ankles) from direct contact with one another.
- For clients in bed who are completely immobile, the care plan should include the use of devices that totally relieve pressure on the heels, most commonly by raising the heels off the bed. Do not use doughnut-type devices; they tend to cause pressure ulcers, not prevent them.
- When the side-lying position is used in bed, avoid positioning the client directly on the trochanter.
- Maintain the head of the bed at the lowest degree of elevation consistent with medical conditions and other restrictions. Limit the amount of time during which the head of the bed is elevated.
- Use a lifting device (trapeze, bed linen) to move, rather than drag, clients in bed who cannot assist during transfers and position changes.
- Place at-risk clients on a pressure-reducing device, such as a foam, static air, alternating air, or water mattress.
- Ensure that any person at risk for a pressure ulcer avoids uninterrupted sitting in chair or wheelchair. The client should be repositioned, with appropriate shifts of the points under pressure, at least every hour. Teach clients who are able to shift their weight every 15 minutes.
- For chair-bound clients, select a pressure-reducing device, such as one made of foam, air, or a combination of these. Do not use a doughnut-type device.
- When positioning chair-bound clients, consider postural alignment, distribution of weight, balance and stability, and pressure relief.
- Provide a written plan for the use of positioning devices and schedules to help chair-bound clients.

Interventions. Consistency in the nursing care provided is an important aspect of interventions directed at achieving wound healing. It is important to develop scientific protocols in ulcer care and to use them consistently. It is also important to give one protocol time to work before changing to another. See Box 51-2 and Chapter 20 for information on wound healing.

Reducing the risk of pressure ulcer development and identifying early manifestations of pressure ulcers are frequently delegated to unlicensed assistive personnel (see the Management and Delegation feature on Care of Clients with Pressure Ulcers on p. 1410). Case managers often assist in managing care between facilities. When preparing for discharge to home, case managers assist with advocating and preventing readmission (see the Case Management feature on The Client with Impaired Skin Integrity on the website).

Evaluation. As the wound heals, assess the degree of outcome attainment every 3 to 4 days. Allow 2 weeks before changing the plan of care, unless the ulcer is deteriorating.

■ Self-Care

The clients at high risk for development of pressure ulcers who are going home should be referred to a home

TABLE 51-3	*Interventions to Reduce Pressure Ulcer Risk Based on Braden Subscale Scores*		
	Score 3	**Score 2**	**Score 1**
Sensory perceptual	Remind client to turn self and remain in off-loaded positions. Examine the position of paralyzed limbs to be certain they are not trapped or pinned and do not rest on each other. Elevate heels from bed.	Inspect skin every shift. Protect client from self-injury on side rails, opposite limb, tubing, devices/monitors.	Assess all bony prominences (occiput, scapulae, elbows, heels). If positioned with head-of-bed elevated for tube feeding, position in 30-degree lateral position rather than supine.
Activity	Place bed setting on prevention mode.	Use padding of at least 4 inches of foam in wheelchair. Reposition wheelchair-bound clients every 2 hours. Float heels from bed.	Depending on other factors (e.g., whether this client can turn at all),consider an upscaled bed. Float heels from bed.
Mobility	Use side rails and trapeze to facilitate self movement.	Turn every 2 hours or more often and inspect bony prominences for manifestations of skin breakdown.	Turn every 2 hours. Consider an upscaled bed if other factors are present.
Moisture	Keep clean and dry between episodes of incontinence. Use skin protectant sprays, wipes, or lotions to protect skin.	Consider urinary tract infection as cause of incontinence. Consider infectious forms of diarrhea. Consider side effects of medications or tube feeding as cause of diarrhea. Obtain order for antifungal powder if rash between skinfolds appears fungal.	Consider placing an indwelling catheter if excoriation is severe. Consider a rectal bag if fecal incontinence is frequent. Monitor for dehydration from fluid loss. Apply skin protectant creams to excoriated areas. Avoid using plastic incontinence pads on specialty beds.
Nutrition	Offer oral supplements to diet. Monitor weight weekly.	Dietary consultation. Assess condition of mouth and ability to swallow. Monitor oral intake, consider calorie count.	Offer tube feeding or hyperalimentation if such is within the goals of the client or family.
Friction/shear	N/A	Apply lotions and creams to abraded areas. Apply cotton sleeves, socks, or heel and elbow protectors. Consider treatment for agitation or spasms.	Apply adhesive dressings to abraded areas. If head of bed is elevated, monitor sacrum and heels closely for shear injury Treat early manifestations of shear with protective dressings.

health agency before discharge from the acute care facility so that devices to reduce pressure can be obtained for home use. The family and the client need to understand the importance of frequent turning. A client who is wheelchair-bound and has arm function should be taught to lift the body, using the arms, off the chair twice every hour for repositioning. A client who is incontinent needs to wear protective pads to absorb the urine or stool and should be assessed often. The U.S. Department of Health and Human Services has developed a "patient guide" for preventing and treating pressure ulcers.[6,7]

If the client is going home with an unhealed ulcer, the client and one or more family members must be taught wound care, wound assessment, and in some cases the administration of intravenous (IV) antibiotics. Teach these interventions before the day of discharge, so that return demonstrations can be used to evaluate learning. In addition, procurement of equipment is often necessary, which takes time. Community nurses need to be involved early in the planning for the discharge of the client with an ulcer. The Bridge to Home Health Care feature on Managing Pressure Ulcers on p. 1411 describes ways to help the client and family manage pressure ulcers.

BOX 51-2 *Interventions for Treatment of Pressure Ulcers*

- Continue to reduce risk of pressure ulcers using appropriate interventions.
- Assess and manage pain associated with the ulcer and its care.
- Position the client to stay off the ulcer. If there is no turning surface without a pressure ulcer, use a pressure reduction bed and continue to turn the client. Do not rely on the bed exclusively to move the client. The client still needs to be repositioned. Establish a written turning schedule, and post it according to agency policy.
- Elevate heels off the bed by using pillows or foam boots. Fleece heel covers do not relieve pressure, but they can reduce friction.
- Maintain the head of the bed at the lowest elevation consistent with the client's medical condition. If the client must have the head elevated to prevent aspiration, reposition into a 30-degree lateral position. Use a seat cushion in the chair, and assess for sacral ulcers daily. For dyspneic clients, position erect and assess for sacral and ischial ulcers daily.
- Use support cushions (4 inches of foam, gels, flotation cushions) for the wheelchair-bound client or for any client who prefers to sit. Teach wheelchair-bound clients to reposition themselves every 15 minutes.
- Use support surfaces for clients with multiple ulcers or when there is no position for the client that does not place the client on an ulcer. Consider upgrading the support surface for those who are not able to keep off the ulcer surface. Begin with a dynamic surface or mattress overlay. Progress to low-air-loss beds or air-fluidized beds if the ulcer does not heal. Check for bottoming out beneath the mattress. Place your hand between the mattress and the bed. If you feel less than an inch between the client's body and the mattress surface, the support is not adequate.
- Ensure adequate dietary intake to prevent malnutrition and delayed healing. Review the dietitian's recommendations for caloric and protein needs. Communicate these recommendations to the physician as needed.
- Provide oral supplementation, tube feeding, or hyperalimentation to achieve positive nitrogen balance. For many clients, the decision not to eat is an important one that can give a sense of control over some aspect of existence. However, pressure ulcers cannot heal in clients with severe malnutrition.
- Supplement the diet with vitamins and minerals. Vitamin C and zinc are commonly prescribed to support wound healing in clients who are not taking in adequate calories.
- Remove devitalized tissue from the wound bed. Begin by cleansing the ulcer bed with normal saline, then use the appropriate technique for debridement. Once the ulcer is free of devitalized tissue, apply dressings that keep the wound bed moist and the surrounding skin dry. Do not use occlusive dressings on ulcers that may be infected.
- Prevent the ulcer from being exposed to urine and feces. Use indwelling catheters and topical creams or dressings to prevent contamination.
- Follow body substance isolation precautions; use clean gloves and clean dressings for wound care.
- Monitor healing. If the ulcer does not show signs of healing in 2 weeks or if manifestations of infection develop, the treatments must change to reduce the risk of sepsis and osteomyelitis.

MANAGEMENT AND DELEGATION

Care of Clients with Pressure Ulcers

When working with unlicensed assistive personnel in the care of clients with pressure ulcers, help them to keep the following points in mind:

- Report any areas of skin redness that do not disappear after pressure relief.
- Report any development of foul odor or drainage from pressure ulcers.
- Reposition the client *at least* every 2 hours. Even a small shift in the client's body weight may be sufficient, but it must be done every 2 hours at a minimum.
- *Do not position the client on the ulcer.* If an ulcer is on the client's trunk, use a dynamic or overlay mattress. However, the use of these support surfaces does not eliminate the need for turning.

- If the client is wheelchair-bound, ensure that the padding provides adequate pressure relief by checking for "bottoming out."
- Keep all pressure off the client's heels. Use small pillows or foam padding to prevent direct contact.
- Keep the head of the bed at the lowest elevation to reduce shear and friction on the skin of the client's lower back.
- Keep the client's skin dry.

Even though you have delegated the skin care of these clients, you are still accountable for their skin condition. Assess the entire skin surface every day. Ask for help in turning the client so that you can see the client's heels and sacrum. Use an assessment guide such as the Braden Scale to determine the risk of further ulceration.

BRIDGE TO HOME HEALTH CARE
Managing Pressure Ulcers

For the client with pressure ulcers, a smooth transition from hospital to home care requires planning, preparation, and communication. For example, it may take a home health nurse several days to obtain special wound care supplies or pressure relief devices not ordinarily stocked by the home health agency. If a pressure relief bed or mattress overlay is required, the agency then contacts a durable medical equipment company and arranges delivery at a predetermined time. To facilitate the transition from hospital care, the home health agency should be notified of the referral before the client's discharge from the hospital and should receive specific instructions per physician orders for wound cleansing, dressing materials, and frequency of dressing changes. In addition, sending a day's supplies home with the client helps to minimize disruption in the wound treatment regimen.

Clients who have stage IV or draining, infected pressure ulcers may initially require daily skilled nursing visits. However, as the infection is treated and drainage subsides, the frequency of skilled nursing visits is usually decreased and the family member or informal caregiver is taught to perform the dressing change. Caregivers should participate in or at least observe dressing change procedures in the hospital, and should receive information about turning and other aspects of care. The earlier the caregiver is introduced to prevention and treatment goals, the faster the client can reach the desired clinical outcome. Hospital nurses can significantly enhance the continuity of care by coordinating educational efforts with the home health agency. The home health nurse should obtain copies of any teaching materials distributed in the hospital. Older adults are often fearful of leaving the security of an inpatient setting; therefore reinforcing familiar teaching materials and wound care procedures helps to ensure a more seamless transition from inpatient to outpatient management.

Maintaining equipment and supplies is more difficult in the home than in inpatient settings. Estimate the needed amount of skin and wound care supplies, and arrange for delivery in a timely manner. Establish an intercommunication sheet in the home that flags a change in wound care orders for other members of the health care team. Leave specific directions for product use, especially when more than one product is being used. *Normal saline* can be made by using the following recipe: mix 8 teaspoons of salt in 1 gallon of bottled or boiled water. Do not use water from an outdoor well.

Adapting the home environment to meet the needs of the client and family members or other caregivers requires creativity and skill. Note the conditions under which the client spends prolonged periods of time. Any firm, unyielding surface can contribute to development of a pressure ulcer in unusual body areas. Sitting on ridged, corded edges of chairs or stools or a firm toilet seat for extended periods can restrict blood flow, leading to pressure ulcer development.

The limitations of older clients and their older caregivers pose additional changes. For example, it may not be possible for a debilitated client to be turned as often as needed during the night to relieve pressure over bony prominences. Frequent turning schedules usually result in increased anxiety and sleep deprivation for older caregivers. Accurately assessing the client's risk category and using an effective pressure-relieving mattress overlay can help to reduce the physical demands for caregivers and increase the possibility that the client can receive needed care and remain at home.

■ Surgical Management

Surgical repair is frequently performed on stage III and stage IV ulcers, on ulcers greater than 2 cm in diameter, and in clients who can tolerate surgery. In stage III ulcers, undamaged tissue near the wound is rotated to cover the ulcer. In stage IV ulcers, musculocutaneous flaps are often used (see later discussion).

PRECANCEROUS CHANGES IN THE SKIN

Precursors to cancer of the skin include damage from recurrent skin trauma and various skin lesions. To understand the role of prevention of skin cancer, these precursor conditions are discussed first. *Photodamage* refers to a spectrum of medical conditions caused by the sun. The spectrum includes sunburn, spider veins (telangiectasias), rough, thick skin, fine and deep wrinkling, actinic keratoses, and carcinomas.

SUNBURN

Sunburn is an acute inflammatory skin response that occurs as a reaction to excessive exposure to sunlight. Dermatopathologic changes include the production of epidermal cells that exhibit cytoplasmic and nuclear changes. These changes are cumulative over the life span and lead to an increased incidence of skin cancer with aging.

A first-degree sunburn produces mild, tender erythema followed by desquamation (peeling), which heals without scarring. Second-degree sunburn causes more extreme erythema and edema, and blistering results from damage to the epidermal cells. Deep sunburn is uncommon unless it is induced by artificial sources such as tanning lamps or booths. Deep sunburn produces burns (see Chapter 52).

Prevention is the best approach to management of sunburn. Client teaching emphasizing sun protection should never be omitted when caring for the sunburned client. For a list of specific precautions, see the Client Education Guide feature on Simple Guidelines to Help Protect You from the Damaging Rays of the Sun on the web site.

Treating sunburn involves decreasing inflammation and rehydrating the damaged skin. For localized, *superficial, partial-thickness* sunburn, use cool tap water soaks for 20 minutes or until the skin is cool. This measure limits skin destruction, prevents edema, and potentially reduces blisters. Tepid tap water baths are indicated for large sunburned areas. After a bath or soak, apply water-based emollients, lotions, foams, gels, or sprays, preferably refrigerated for an additional cooling effect. Emollients should also be applied throughout the day to soothe the skin and relieve dryness. Lotions, foams, or sprays containing camphor and menthol (e.g., Sarna) can also be beneficial. Avoid the use of OTC remedies containing local anesthetics—such as benzocaine, dibucaine (Nupercaine), or lidocaine (Xylocaine)—because they are rarely effective and have the potential to induce contact sensitivity.

For *partial-thickness* sunburn, apply continuous cool, normal saline soaks or soaking baths to reduce oozing and edema. Very large blisters may be aspirated and dressed with sterile dressings. Avoid debridement unless there is evidence of secondary bacterial infection. Silver sulfadiazine may be prescribed.

Prostaglandin inhibitors (nonsteroidal anti-inflammatory drugs [NSAIDs]) may be used to reduce erythema and inflammation in adults. Topical corticosteroids may be prescribed to be used sparingly in nonocclusive vehicles (lotion, spray, gel) for their vasoconstrictive effects. Systemic corticosteroids are prescribed only for clients with extensive, painful burns, but their use has declined because they seem to offer little efficacy when given in a reasonable dose range.

ACTINIC KERATOSIS

Actinic keratosis, the most common epithelial precancerous lesion in Caucasians, is primarily caused by sun exposure. It affects nearly 100% of older white adults. There is a small but definite risk of malignant degeneration and subsequent metastatic potential in neglected lesions.

Actinic keratosis most frequently occurs in areas of chronic, usually high-intensity sun exposure including the face, the tops of the ears, the back of the neck, the forearms, the backs of the hands, and the chest. The clinical appearance of actinic keratoses is varied. The typical lesion is an irregularly shaped, flat, slightly erythematous macule or papule with indistinct borders and an overlying hard keratotic scale or horn that feels rough or sharp to palpation. In some cases, the erythema or the horn may be absent. This scale can be periodically shed or peeled off, but then it regrows. The lesion varies in size from the size of a pinhead to several centimeters across and is often more easily palpated than observed. Single lesions may be seen, but more often they appear in groups on a background of sun-damaged skin.

Outcome Management
■ Medical Management

Topical application of fluorouracil (Carac, Efudex, and Fluoroplex), a topical antineoplastic, is currently one of the best approaches to treatment of widespread actinic damage with multiple lesions. The advantage is that large areas of widespread disease can be treated at the same time. Use not only removes the majority of premalignant and superficial malignant lesions that can be seen but also uncovers and destroys clinically undetectable lesions of this type. However, the major disadvantage is the therapeutic inflammatory response that often accompanies successful treatment. This response sequence is erythema usually followed by vesiculation, erosion, ulcerations, necrosis, and epithelialization.

The medication should be applied twice daily with a gloved hand, carefully avoiding eyes, folds around nose, mouth, and scrotum. Medication should be continued until the inflammatory response reaches the erosion, necrosis, and ulceration stage, at which time the medication should be stopped. The usual duration of therapy is 2 to 4 weeks; by then, the client may experience extreme discomfort requiring pain medication. At the time these products are stopped, topical corticosteroid creams may be applied to reduce inflammation and provide the client with additional pain reduction. Complete healing of the lesions may not be evident for 1 to 2 months after cessation of therapy.

■ Surgical Management

Cryotherapy. Cryotherapy using liquid nitrogen is a common treatment for single lesions or for small numbers of actinic keratoses. Liquid nitrogen is usually applied with a cotton-tipped applicator or spraying device (Figure 51-11, *A*). No local anesthetic is required but the freezing process is associated with a small amount of discomfort, which may linger afterward. Intermittent application of a warm, damp wash cloth to the site may bring relief. Freezing frequently results in inflammation with blister formation, and blister care should be reviewed with the client. Care must be taken to avoid overfreezing the site, which may result in scarring.

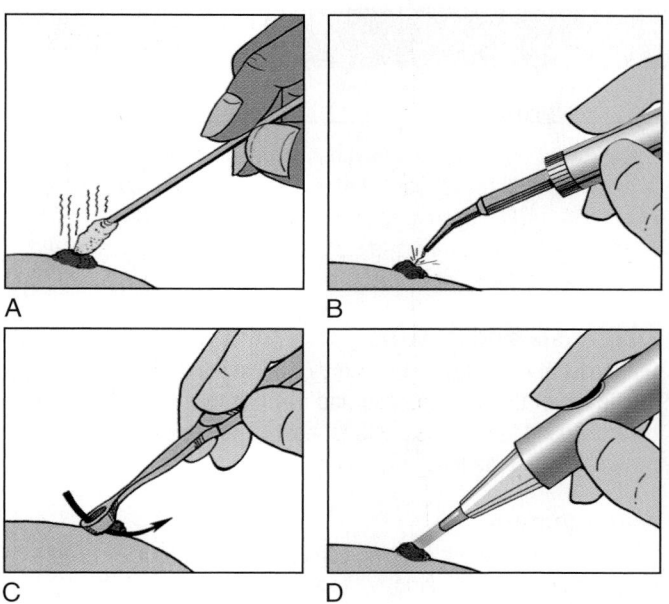

FIGURE 51-11 Methods for destroying skin lesions. **A,** Cryotherapy. Liquid nitrogen is applied with a saturated cotton-tipped applicator directly to the lesion or sprayed on. This causes tissue destruction by freezing. **B,** Electrodesiccation. Tissue is destroyed by heat from an electrical current; note the gloved hand. **C,** Curettage. A curet (cutting instrument) removes tissue by scraping or scooping; note the gloved hand. **D,** The laser removes tissue by vaporizing it.

Electrodesiccation and Curettage. Electrodesiccation produces superficial destruction. The procedure may be done using local anesthesia (see Figure 51-11, *B*). The tissue is destroyed by mechanical disruption of cells and heat. The tissue is removed by scraping or scooping with a loop-shaped instrument called a curet (see Figure 51-11, *C*). This method can provide tissue for histologic diagnosis if needed. The curetted areas usually heal quickly, with adequate wound care resulting in a small white permanent scar. The wound site should be kept moist with a less sensitizing topical antibiotic ointment such as bacitracin.

Laser Excision. Laser uses light energy to vaporize lesions (see Figure 51-11, *D*). Depending upon the wavelength of the light, various portions of the cell are heated. Tissue is not available for histologic examination. Local anesthesia is used.

Punch or Excisional Biopsy. Punch or excisional biopsy is indicated for lesions that are large or have other characteristics of a cutaneous malignancy (induration, erythema, erosion). It is often difficult to distinguish a large actinic keratosis from a squamous cell carcinoma without histologic diagnosis. Biopsy should also be done on lesions that persist after adequate treatment. Local anesthesia is used for the biopsy procedure and allows elec-

trodesiccation to be done painlessly after biopsy. Excisional biopsy requires primary closure of the site and may be a more extensive procedure than the lesion warrants; however, it ensures more complete removal of the growth (see Chapter 50).

SKIN CANCER

Skin cancer is the most common cancer in the United States, and the number of new skin cancers and the number of skin cancer deaths are increasing at alarming rates. Skin cancer is a malignant condition caused by uncontrolled growth and spread of abnormal cells in a specific layer of the skin. The several different kinds of skin cancer are distinguished by the types of cells involved. The three most common types are (1) basal cell carcinoma, (2) squamous cell carcinoma, and (3) malignant melanoma. More than 90% of all skin cancers fall into the first two classifications. Both basal cell carcinoma and squamous cell carcinoma are slow-growing tumors with a cure rate of 95% or greater after early treatment.

Etiology and Risk Factors

The cause of skin cancer is well known. Prolonged or intermittent, repeated exposure to UVL radiation from the sun, especially when it results in sunburn and blistering, plays a key role in the induction of skin cancer, especially malignant melanoma. Most non-melanoma skin cancers occur on parts of the body unprotected by clothing (face, neck, forearms, and backs of hands) and in people who have received considerable exposure to sunlight. All people are at risk of skin cancer regardless of skin tone and hair color, although some are at much greater risk than others. In general, people with red, blond, or light brown hair with light complexions or freckles, many of Celtic or Scandinavian origin, are most susceptible; blacks and Asians are least susceptible. See the Genetic Links feature on Oculocutaneous Albinism Type 1 on p. 1414.

All clients should be taught to look for new moles or lesions and to evaluate them for danger signs of cancer. Danger signals in moles (pigmented nevi) are presented in Box 51-3. Suspicious lesions should be examined by a physician.

The pattern of reaction to acute sun exposure can be correlated with the development of actinic keratosis and skin cancer. People who never tan and always burn after 1 to 2 hours of midday summer sun are most susceptible. People who burn once or twice at the beginning of summer and then tan are somewhat less susceptible. Those who never burn and always tan are the least susceptible. The most severely affected people usually have a history of long-term occupational (farmers, construction workers, surveyors, sailors) or recreational (swimmers, skiers, surfers, sunbathers) sun exposure.

GENETICS LINKS

Oculocutaneous Albinism Type 1 (OCA1)

Description

An autosomal recessive disorder characterized by reduced synthesis of melanin in the skin, hair, and eyes, and associated with characteristic ocular findings. Ocular findings include nystagmus, reduced iris and retinal pigment, foveal hypoplasia with reduced visual acuity, and misrouting of the optic nerves, producing alternating strabismus and reduced stereoscopic vision. There are two categories of OCA1: OCA1A (most common), associated with absent melanin synthesis in all tissue, and OCA1B, associated with varying amounts of melanin synthesis in the skin, hair, and eyes. Clients with OCA1A have white hair, white skin that does not tan, and blue, fully translucent irises. Clients with OCA1B have white or light yellow hair that darkens with age, white skin that gradually develops some generalized pigment, and blue irises that may change color with age to green/hazel or brown/tan.

Genetics

OCA1 is caused by mutations in the tyrosinase gene, TYR, located on chromosome 11. Molecular genetic testing of the TYR gene is clinically available. The carrier rate for OCA1 is approximately 1 in 100 in most populations throughout the world. OCA1 is an autosomal recessive disorder, and offspring of carrier parents have a 25% chance of being affected with OCA1, a 50% chance of being a carrier, and a 25% chance of being unaffected and not a carrier.

Diagnosis and Testing

Diagnosis of OCA1 is established by clinical features of hypopigmentation of the skin and hair and eye findings. Genetic testing is rarely used in diagnosis and is most commonly used for carrier detection in genetic counseling.

Management

A critical aspect of the ongoing care of clients with OCA1 is ophthalmologic care, including, for example, correction of refractive errors (e.g., myopia, hyperopia, astigmatism) to improve visual acuity and annual eye examination. Skin care is dictated by the amount of skin pigment and cutaneous response to sunlight. Clients with OCA1A need to be protected from sun exposure with clothing and sunscreens.

BOX 51-3	*Danger Signals Suggestive of Malignant Transformation of Moles*

- *Change in color,* especially red, white, and blue; sudden darkening; mottled shades of brown or black
- *Change in diameter,* especially sudden increase
- *Change in outline,* especially development of irregular margins
- *Change in surface characteristics,* especially scaliness, erosion, oozing, crusting, bleeding, ulceration, development of a mushrooming mass on the surface of the lesion
- *Change in consistency,* especially softening or friability
- *Change in symptoms,* especially pruritus
- *Change in shape,* especially irregular elevation from a previously flat condition
- *Change in surrounding skin,* especially "leaking" of pigment from the lesion into surrounding skin or pigmented "satellite" lesions

BASAL CELL CARCINOMA

Basal cell carcinoma (BCC), the most common form of skin cancer, is a malignant epithelial tumor of the skin that arises from the basal cells in the epidermis. The tumor is usually painless and slow growing, generally appearing on sun-exposed skin of the face, ears, head, neck, or hands. Occasionally, basal cell carcinoma may appear on the trunk, especially the upper back and chest. The majority of cases are caused by chronic overexposure to UVL radiation, and only a few cases can be linked to arsenic, burns, scars, exposure to radiation, or genetic predisposition. Clinical and histologic findings are used to identify the tumor.

The most common clinical presentation of basal cell carcinoma is the nodular lesion (Figure 51-12). This is a dome-shaped papule with a well-defined border having a classic "pearly" texture. Basal cell carcinoma has this flesh-colored "pearly" or shiny appearance because it does not keratinize. Telangiectatic vessels frequently overlie the lesion. As the lesion enlarges, the center may flatten or ulcerate, but the border is still raised, giving a "rolled-edge" appearance.

Although basal cell carcinomas almost never metastasize, they can be locally destructive and invasive through tissue. This is particularly true on the face, where a lesion can invade deep structures with resultant loss of an eye or ear or the nose. If untreated, the tumor can invade through bone and brain. If the tumor is identified and treated early, local excision or even nonexcisional destruction is usually curative.

Clients who have had one basal cell carcinoma are at risk for development of another. Recurrences of previously treated basal cell carcinomas are also possible but

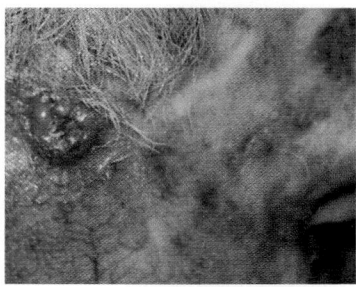

FIGURE 51-12 Basal cell carcinoma characterized by rolled edges and a crater in the center of the lesion. Scars are from previous destruction of skin cancers.

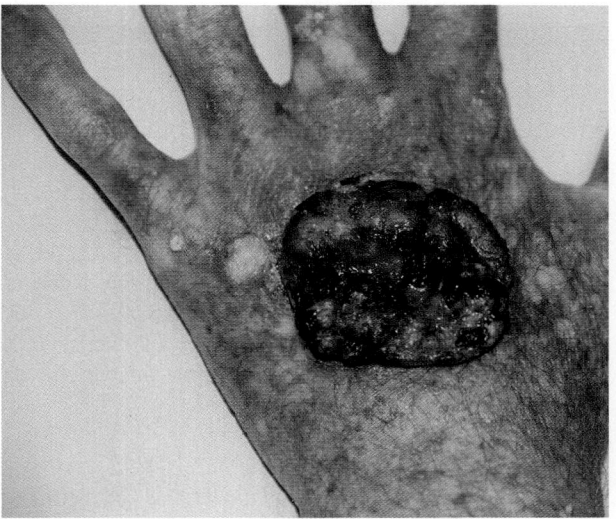

FIGURE 51-13 Squamous cell carcinoma on the hand.

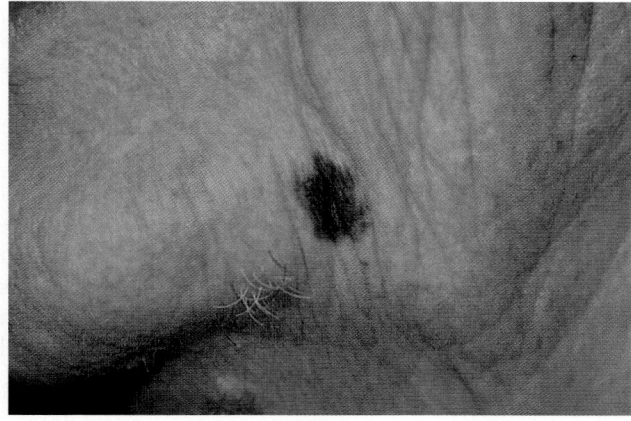

FIGURE 51-14 Superficial spreading melanoma.

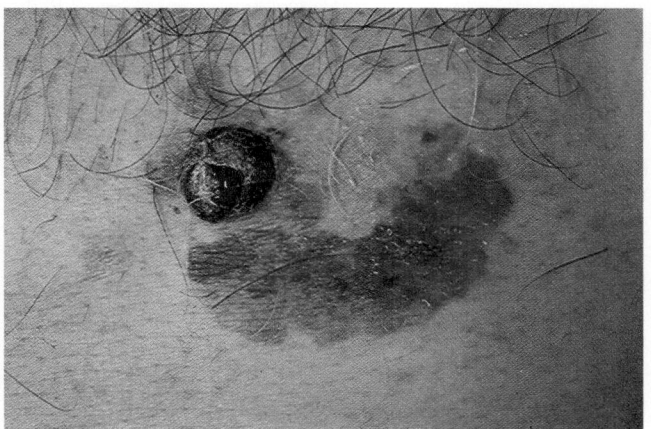

FIGURE 51-15 Nodular melanoma with satellite lesions.

more unusual; recurrence is generally noted within the first 2 years after removal or therapy.

SQUAMOUS CELL CARCINOMA

Squamous cell carcinoma (SCC) (Figure 51-13) is the second most common skin cancer in Caucasians. It is a tumor of the epidermal keratinocytes and rarely occurs in dark-skinned people. It is found on areas often exposed to the sun, typically the rim of the ear, the face, the lips and mouth, and the backs of the hands.

Squamous cell carcinoma is more difficult to characterize than basal cell carcinoma. The tumor is poorly marginated; the edge often blends into surrounding sun-damaged skin. Squamous cell carcinoma may present as an ulcer, a flat red area, a cutaneous horn, an indurated plaque, or a hyperkeratotic papule or nodule. Often it presents as a red- to skin-colored papule surmounted by varying amounts of scale.

The lesions grow more rapidly than does basal cell carcinoma. These tumors are potentially dangerous because they may infiltrate surrounding structures and metastasize to lymph nodes, with a fatal outcome.

MALIGNANT MELANOMA

Malignant melanoma (Figures 51-14 and 51-15) is a cancer of melanocytes; it is the deadliest form of skin cancer. The incidence of melanoma is increasing, such that currently about 1 in 100 persons in the United States can expect to develop this cancer in a lifetime. The incidence of and death rate from melanoma are increasing worldwide. In countries populated with fair-skinned white people, the incidence of melanoma and the mortality rate have risen increased 7% to 15% per year, more than doubling during the 1990s.

Exposure to UVL continues to be one of the most important causes of malignant melanoma. What causes melanocytes to transform to melanoma cells is poorly understood. Primary cutaneous melanoma may develop in precursor melanocytic nevi (common acquired, congenital, and atypical or dysplastic types), although more than 50% of cases are believed to arise without a preexisting pigmented lesion. Melanoma is multifactorial and appears to be related to multiple risk factors including (1) fair complexion, (2) excessive childhood sun exposure and blistering childhood sunburns, (3) increased number of common acquired and dysplastic moles, (4) family history of melanoma, and (5) presence of a changing mole on the skin. The suspicion of melanoma is based on history as well as the clinical appearance.

Clinical Manifestations

The cardinal clinical manifestation of melanoma is a change in a skin lesion observed over a period of months. If a lesion grows so fast that it doubles in size in 10 days, it is usually an inflammation. If a lesion changes so slowly that neither the client nor family is sure of a change, it is usually benign. Changes that may signal melanoma are called the A, B, C, D changes in moles:

- Asymmetry
- Border notching
- Color variegation with black, brown, red, or white hue
- Diameter greater than 6 mm

Other changes include doubling size in 3 to 8 months, bleeding, itching, ulceration, a change in color, or development of a palpable lymph node. Four types of melanoma are presented in Table 51-4. The tumor can metastasize, usually to the brain, lungs, bones, liver, and skin, and is ultimately fatal.

Outcome Management

Management is directed at removing the tumor, if possible. Survival is directly related to the depth of tumor invasion: 10-year survival is greater than 90% if the tumor is less than 1 mm in depth, but if the tumor is larger than 4 mm in depth, 10-year survival decreases to only 40%. Microscopic ulceration is the next most important ad-

verse prognostic pathologic feature. Clinically, metastatic melanoma is universally fatal. It is therefore extremely important for a malignant melanoma to be diagnosed early according to the ABCD rules.

■ Medical Management

Medical management begins with a high level of suspicion for any type of skin cancer but specifically for melanoma. The need for early detection cannot be overemphasized. Any indication, whether it is a confirmed risk factor or a suspicious lesion, is adequate reason for referral. Clients with localized cutaneous disease have been treated with adjuvant chemotherapy, nonspe-

---

COMPLEMENTARY AND ALTERNATIVE THERAPY

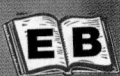

Chemoprevention of Melanoma

A recent review of chemoprevention studies for melanoma found that several interventions could reduce the risk or the recurrence of melanoma. These include higher intakes of polyunsaturated fatty acids (such as fish oil), vitamin E from food, normal levels of selenium, green tea, soy, and nonsteroidal anti-inflammatory drugs, or NSAIDs. More research is needed, but this is interesting initial data.

Reference
Demierre, M-F., & Nathanson, L. (2003). Chemoprevention of melanoma: An unexplored strategy. *Journal of Clinical Oncology, 21,* 158-165.

TABLE 51-4	*Types of Melanoma*	
Tumor Type	**General Information**	**Clinical Manifestations**
Superficial spreading melanoma (SSM)	The most common form of melanoma; slowly changing lesion with more rapid growth just before diagnosis	Deeply pigmented area contained within a brown nevus (freckle); usually flat and asymmetrical; as lesion grows, color changes may occur, ranging from jet black to dark blue to pale gray or white; looks lacy; lesions may have areas of no color; usually 2 cm wide
Nodular melanoma (NM)	Second most common form of melanoma; more aggressive tumor than SSM, with shorter clinical onset time	Common on the trunk, head, and neck; usually 1-2 cm in diameter; often begins in normal skin, rather than in a pre-existing lesion; dark and more uniform in color; may resemble a blood blister or hemangioma; dome-shaped with sharp borders
Lentigo maligna melanoma (LMM)	Fairly uncommon tumor; typically appears on the face of white women; usually has been present for long period of time (5-15 yr)	Generally a large, flat lesion that looks like a stain on the skin; typically tan with various shades of brown; metastasis less common
Acral-lentiginous melanoma (ALM)	Commonly occurs on palms and soles; more common in dark-skinned people; usually occurs in older adults; may evolve over a few months to years	Large lesion, about 3 cm in diameter; resembles LMM (a tan or brown flat lesion on the palm or sole); can be misdiagnosed as a corn; ulceration is common; likely to metastasize

cific passive immunotherapy, radiation therapy, and biologic therapy. No increase in survival has been reported with these adjunctive therapies. Adjuvant interferon (IFN) alfa-2b and various experimental melanoma vaccines show promise in individuals with high-risk primary cutaneous melanoma and those with regional nodal disease. Melanoma vaccines are being investigated for therapeutic use. A variety of vaccines targeting melanoma cell antigens are in the clinical trial phase. See the Complementary and Alternative Therapy feature on Chemoprevention of Melanoma on p. 1416 for interventions that could reduce the risk or recurrence of melanoma.

■ Surgical Management

Treatment of all skin cancers requires removal of the lesion. The margins of the resected specimen must be free of tumor to a specified distance (depending on the type of skin cancer) to guarantee full removal.

A special surgical technique primarily used for the removal of skin malignancies such as basal cell carcinoma and squamous cell carcinoma is *Mohs' surgery,* which is also indicated for primary lesions in areas in which preservation of normal skin is necessary (e.g., eyelids, pinna, nasolabial folds). The technique involves a series of excisions with careful microscopic tissue assessment to "map" the presence or absence of malignant cells within each specimen. The procedure may be lengthy. After all tumor tissue is removed, the wound is closed with sutures or a flap, or is allowed to close by secondary intention.

Basal cell carcinomas and squamous cell carcinomas can also be excised and the surgical wound closed primarily (with skin edges sewn together) or with a skin flap. The advantage of this technique is that it requires much less time, and the scar is controllable as a fine line. The tumor is completely excised with adequate margins of tumor-free tissue. If there is doubt about adequacy of margins, the specimen is sent for pathologic diagnosis (by permanent section technique).

The treatment of malignant melanoma is wide local excision. Surgical excision begins with biopsy to determine the stage of the cancer. Excisional biopsy is the removal of the lesion and a narrow margin of normal-appearing tissue. The tumor is excised with a 1- to 2-cm margin of normal-appearing tissue. The margin width is based on the type of melanoma. The surgical wound is closed either primarily or with grafts or flaps.

Surgeons differ on the timing of the definitive surgery. Some surgeons excise the lesion after frozen section examination while the client is still on the operating table. Other surgeons wait for the results of permanent section pathologic diagnosis and then proceed with definitive treatment. The final excision is usually completed within 1 week of biopsy. Although there is a theoretical risk of tumor spread during biopsy, there is no convincing evidence that waiting 1 to even 6 weeks after biopsy jeop-

ardizes the outcome. In fact, sometimes the delay gives the client time to prepare for surgery, both physically and psychologically.

Most clients with metastatic melanoma live less than 1 year. Currently, there is no cure for metastatic melanoma, but some of the new developments in clinical trials may change currently accepted treatments. A treatment plan is formulated on the basis of several factors: site of the tumor, number of metastases, rate of tumor growth, previous treatments, response to treatment, and the age, general health, and desires of the client. Some treatments include surgery to remove metastatic lesions, radiation therapy, chemotherapy, and local hyperthermia. Alternatively, the client can opt for no further treatment.

CUTANEOUS T-CELL LYMPHOMA (MYCOSIS FUNGOIDES)

Cutaneous T-cell lymphoma (CTCL), or mycosis fungoides, is a malignant disease involving the T helper cells. Malignant T cells in the blood migrate to the skin, where they have an affinity for the epidermis. The malignant cells continue to grow and change, eventually moving into the dermis. The cause is not known, and the course is unpredictable, varying with the type of presentation.

The three distinct clinical presentations are patch, plaque, and tumor. Clinical manifestations include eversion of the eyelids and hyperkeratosis of the palms and soles, often with fissuring. Finally, the plaques form tumors that ultimately ulcerate. Tumors can also develop spontaneously in previously unaffected areas, and eventual visceral or organ involvement ensues. This disease is often described as a slow-growing but highly disfiguring debilitating cancer. Clients often feel desperate by the time diagnosis is confirmed, which adds to the psychological difficulties. The tumor presentation carries the worst prognosis, with a survival period of 3 years or less.

CTCL is extremely difficult to diagnose and is often misdiagnosed. In its early stages, CTCL can clinically mimic eczematous processes. The initial erythematous papules resemble those in other eczematous conditions, including psoriasis and atopic dermatitis. The original eruptions of CTCL may be either transitory or of prolonged duration and sometimes are pruritic.

Outcome Management

Control of pruritus is essential at all stages and is accomplished by rehydration of the skin, various dry skin therapies (see Xerotic Eczema), topical corticosteroids, and PUVA therapy (see Ultraviolet Light Therapy). Prevention of secondary infections is important. Nitrogen mustard and other chemotherapy agents are administered topically. Daily application of chemotherapeutic agents often constitutes the initial treatment. Photophoresis, a treatment involving the removal of small amounts of blood that is irradiated and then returned to the body, is used frequently in more advanced stages. To-tal-body electron beam therapy with or without adjuvant chemotherapy is an aggressive approach often used.

The primary systemic drug was formerly intravenous methotrexate. With advances in treatment, newer drugs have replaced methotrexate: one is denileukin diftitox (Ontak) used primarily in the treatment of persistent or recurrent CTCL. This agent has produced sustained regression of the tumors, in some cases for longer than 2 years. Fatalities remain extremely high in this disease as a result of progression to systemic involvement.

BULLOUS DISORDERS: PEMPHIGUS

Pemphigus is a chronic disorder that results in the development of blisters (bullae). It is fairly uncommon in the general population, but the incidence is increased in Jewish and Mediterranean peoples. There are several types: pemphigus vulgaris, pemphigus foliaceus, and pemphigus erythematosus. This discussion focuses on pemphigus vulgaris, the most common type.

Pemphigus is an autoimmune disease caused by circulating immunoglobulin G (IgG) autoantibodies. These autoantibodies react with the intracellular cement—the substance that holds epidermal cells together. The reaction causes intraepidermal bulla (blister) formation and acantholysis (loss of cohesion between epidermal cells).

Clinical manifestations include flaccid bullae that rupture easily, emitting a foul-smelling drainage and leaving crusted, denuded skin. Nikolsky's sign is the result when the epidermis can be rubbed off by slight friction or injury; this sign is a hallmark of pemphigus. Even slight pressure on an intact blister may cause it to spread to adjacent skin. The lesions are common on the face, back, chest, groin, and umbilicus.

Outcome Management

Management includes large doses of steroids and immunosuppressives. Plasmapheresis has been of some benefit in the treatment of pemphigus. If a large proportion of the skin is denuded, management is similar to that for a burn-injured client. The client is at increased risk for infection, fluid and electrolyte imbalance, and stress response complications (i.e., stress ulcers, body system failure). In addition, nursing management focuses on self-concept and pain management. Potassium permanganate baths may be used to reduce the risk of infection, control the odor of the drainage, and ease the pain.

INFECTIOUS DISORDERS

Several organisms lead to skin infections and infestations. Common skin infections are described in Table 51-5 (see also the Terrorism Alert feature on Smallpox on p. 1420). A few are discussed in detail here.

ERYSIPELAS AND CELLULITIS

Erysipelas is an acute, intensely erythematous infection with clearly demarcated raised margins that is often associated with lymphatic streaking. Fever and leukocytosis (elevated white blood cell count) are present. The initial lesion is small, elevated, and bright red. The involved area spreads peripherally to become a plaque with sharp, indurated borders. Lesions are most common on the face and extremities. Recurrence in the same area is common, possibly because of underlying lymphatic obstruction. Uncomplicated erysipelas remains confined primarily to the lymphatics and subcutaneous tissues. The usual causative agent is beta-hemolytic group A streptococci, which often responds to treatment with penicillin.

Cellulitis is a skin infection extending into the deeper dermis and subcutaneous tissues that results in deep, red erythema without sharp borders that spreads widely through tissue spaces (Figure 51-16). The skin is erythematous, edematous, tender, and sometimes nodular. *Streptococcus pyogenes* is the usual cause of this infection, although other pathogens may be responsible. Lymphangitis may occur; if cellulitis is untreated, gangrene, metastatic abscesses, and sepsis result.

At increased risk for erysipelas and cellulitis are older adults and clients with lowered resistance from diabetes, malnutrition, steroid therapy, or the presence of wounds or ulcers. Other predisposing factors include the presence of edema and other cutaneous inflammation or wounds (e.g., tinea, eczema, burns, trauma). There is a tendency for recurrence, especially at sites of lymphatic obstruction.

Erysipelas and cellulitis are treated by either oral or IV antibiotics that are effective against both streptococci and *S. aureus*. Before antibiotics are administered, a wound specimen for culture and sensitivity testing should be obtained, although culture rarely yields the causative organism. Soaks may reduce edema and inflammation. The enzymes that facilitate a rapid spread of infection also seem to produce other significant manifestations such as high fever, tachycardia, confusion, and hypotension; appropriate interventions should be undertaken if these occur. Monitor the client's temperature and administer prescribed antipyretic medication. Prevent cross-contamination by teaching the client proper hand-washing technique and careful handling of soiled linen, clothing, dressings, and so forth. Standard precautions should be used as appropriate. Close follow-up evaluation is necessary.

HERPES ZOSTER (SHINGLES)

Herpes zoster (Figure 51-17), or shingles, is an infection caused by the reactivation of the varicella zoster virus in clients who have had chickenpox. Although zoster is

TABLE 51-5 *Common Skin Infections and Infestations*

Disease with Causative Organism	Clinical Manifestations	Management
Parasitic		
Scabies: *Sarcoptes scabiei*	Multiple straight or wavy thread-like lines beneath the skin, itching	Application of a scabicide with re-treatment in 1 wk to kill residual eggs. All clothing and linen should be washed and dried in hot cycles or dry cleaned.
Lice: *Pediculus humanus, Phthirus pubis*	Intense itching; scratch marks may be evident	Application of pediculicides. For *head lice,* the shampoo should be worked into dry hair until it is saturated. A fine-toothed comb should be used to remove dead lice and nits. Brushes and combs should be washed in pediculicide also. For *body lice,* a pediculicide lotion is applied to involved body areas. Clothing should be washed and dried in hot cycles or dry cleaned. Other items can be stored in plastic bags for 30-35 days. Family members, close contacts, and sexual partners should also be treated.
Bacterial		
Impetigo: group A streptococci, staphylococci	Pruritic vesicle or pustule that breaks and leaves a thick honey-colored crust	Antibiotics given until culture results available include erythromycin or dicloxacillin. Mupirocin is preferable to oral antibiotics when lesions are limited to small, localized area. Teach control of contagion; infection is contagious as long as skin lesions are present. Use thorough hand-washing, separate laundry for client's linens, and separate washing of client's dishes.
Folliculitis, furuncles, carbuncles: *Staphylococcus aureus*	White pustules on forehead, chest, upper back, neck, thighs, groin, and axillae; furuncles are deeper inflamed nodules; carbuncles are interconnected furuncles and often rupture, expelling purulent, foul-smelling thick drainage	Localized folliculitis is treated with warm compresses, gentle washing, and topical antibiotics. Furuncles are treated as for folliculitis with incision and drainage (I&D) to avoid rupture. Carbuncles are treated with systemic antibiotics and I&D. Instruct client to use disposable razors to avoid reinfection. Reduce spread of infection by careful hand-washing and separate laundry of linens.
Fungal		
Candidiasis: *Candida albicans*	Appearance depends on location; in the *mouth,* infection is called thrush and appears as white plaques with an underlying red base with fissures on corners of the mouth; *skin* lesions are pruritic, red, and moist with eroded scales, commonly found in the axilla and gluteal, perianal, and interdigital folds; *vaginal* thrush causes intense itching and a cheesy drainage	Eliminate or control predisposing factors such as antibiotics (which alter the flora), malnutrition, diabetes, immunosuppression, pregnancy, or birth control pills. Use topical antifungal powders and creams. Keep the skin dry and the environment cool.
Tinea: variety of dermatophytes (tinea corporis, on body; tinea capitis, on scalp; tinea cruris, jock itch; tinea pedis, athlete's foot)	*Tinea corporis:* round red macules and papules with scales—lesions have advancing borders and healing centers; *tinea capitis:* patchy hair loss, inflammation, scales, and folliculitis; *tinea cruris:* red lesions with raised borders; *tinea pedis:* scaling, maceration, pain, and vesicles	Infection is controlled with antifungal solutions and creams. Acute lesions may require wet dressings, keratolytic agents, or both to remove the scales. Client is taught to reduce risk by thoroughly drying after a bath or shower, wearing absorbent underwear and socks, applying talc to intertriginous areas, and wearing open shoes during warm weather.

TABLE 51-5 Common Skin Infections and Infestations—cont'd

Disease with Causative Organism	Clinical Manifestations	Management
Viral		
Herpes simplex: herpes simplex virus	Vesicles preceded by sensation of itching or burning; clear exudate from vesicles, followed by crusting; common to the nose, lips, cheeks, ears, and genitalia	No cure is available. Treatment includes pain relief and topical anesthetics. Acyclovir, and antiviral drug, may decrease viral shedding and hasten healing. Avoiding the sun and using sunscreens reduce recurrent lesions on the lips. Reduce contagiousness by using frequent hand-washing, not picking at lesions, avoiding sexual intercourse and kissing while lesions are active, and not sharing lipsticks. Try to identify (and avoid or control) personal triggers for lesions.
Warts: human papillomavirus	Rough, fresh, or gray-colored skin protrusion	Numerous therapies, some with over-the-counter medication. May require electrodesiccation or cryosurgery. Intralesional injections of cytotoxic drugs may also be used. No treatment is also an acceptable option.

TERRORISM ALERT

Smallpox

Smallpox is a serious, contagious, and sometimes fatal infectious disease caused by the variola virus. Smallpox outbreaks have occurred from time to time for thousands of years, but the disease has been eradicated after a successful worldwide vaccination program. The last case of smallpox in the United States was in 1949 and the last naturally occurring case in the world was in Somalia in 1977. After the disease was eliminated from the world, routine vaccination against smallpox among the general public was stopped because it was no longer necessary for prevention. Except for laboratory stockpiles, the variola virus has been eliminated. However, there is heightened concern that the variola virus might be used as an agent of bioterrorism.

Smallpox normally spreads from contact with infected persons. Generally, direct and fairly prolonged face-to-face contact is required to spread smallpox from one person to another. Smallpox also can be spread through direct contact with infected body fluids or contaminated objects such as bedding or clothing. Indirect spread is less common. Rarely, smallpox has been spread by virus carried in the air in enclosed settings such as buildings, buses, and trains. Smallpox is not known to be transmitted by insects or animals.

There are two clinical forms of smallpox. *Variola major* is the severe and most common form of smallpox, with a more extensive rash and higher fever. *Variola minor* is a less common presentation of smallpox, and a much less severe disease, with death rates historically of 1% or less. There is no specific treatment for smallpox disease, although some medications are in laboratory trials; currently, the only prevention is vaccination.

The first phase of smallpox is an incubation period of 7 to 17 days after exposure to the virus. The person is not contagious nor does he or she feel ill. The first manifestations of smallpox include fever, headache, muscle pain, and malaise (weakness, tiredness) over a 2- to 4-day timeframe. A person with smallpox becomes most contagious with the onset of rash on the tongue and mouth. As the lesions open, the virus enters the mouth and airway, and the person is highly contagious. The rash spreads throughout the body over the next 2 to 3 days. The pox areas become pustular, eventually form a crust, and then a scab. A person is contagious until the last smallpox scab falls off.

It is important to distinguish smallpox from other diseases that have skin eruptions, such as chickenpox. Persons with smallpox report a fever 1 to 4 days before the skin eruptions, all skin eruptions are at the small stage of development, and the skin lesions are deep-seated, round, and pustular that may be draining purulent, thick fluid. The person may recall that the first lesions were in the mouth and that they evolved over 2 to 3 days. Suspicious cases should be isolated and reported to the Centers for Disease Control and Prevention (CDC).

There is a detailed nationwide smallpox preparedness program to protect Americans against smallpox used as a biological weapon. This program includes the creation of preparedness teams that are ready to respond to a smallpox attack on the United States. Members of these teams—health care and public health workers—are being vaccinated so that they might safely protect others in the event of a smallpox outbreak.

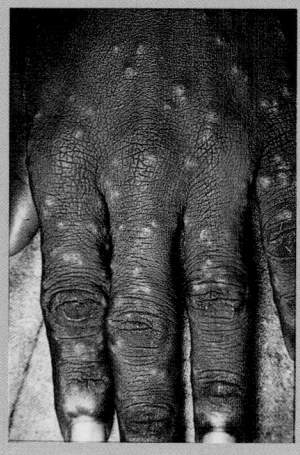

Data from Henderson, D.A. (1999). Smallpox as a biological weapon: Medical and public health management. *Journal of the American Medical Association 281*, 2127-2137.

much less communicable than varicella, people who have not had chickenpox are at risk after exposure to a person with herpes zoster. An increased incidence of herpes zoster is seen in clients with lymphoma, leukemia, or acquired immunodeficiency syndrome, probably because of their decreased immunologic response.

Diagnostic tests may not be necessary because of the specific characteristics of herpes zoster; however, a

Tzanck test demonstrates multinucleated giant cells (see Chapter 50), and a viral culture is also helpful.

The primary lesion of zoster is a vesicle. The classic presentation is grouped vesicles on an erythematous base along a dermatome. The vesicles appear 1 to 2 days after onset of pain and itching at the site. Occasionally, only papules appear and not vesicles. Because they follow nerve pathways, the lesions do not cross the body's midline; however, rarely, the nerves of both sides may be involved. Herpes zoster lesions evolve into ulcers on the superficial mucous membrane.

The eruption generally clears in about 2 weeks, unless the period between the pain and the eruption is longer than 2 days. In such cases, a prolonged convalescence may be expected. Residual pain, called *postherpetic neuralgia*, and itching are the major complications with herpes zoster. The pain may be constant or intermittent and may range from light burning to a deep visceral sensation. The duration of the pain can be weeks or months to years. In older clients, the pain generally lasts months to years. Another potential complication is loss of sight when herpes zoster involves the facial or acoustic nerve. Involvement of the ophthalmic branch of the facial nerve requires close medical attention to avoid ocular damage.

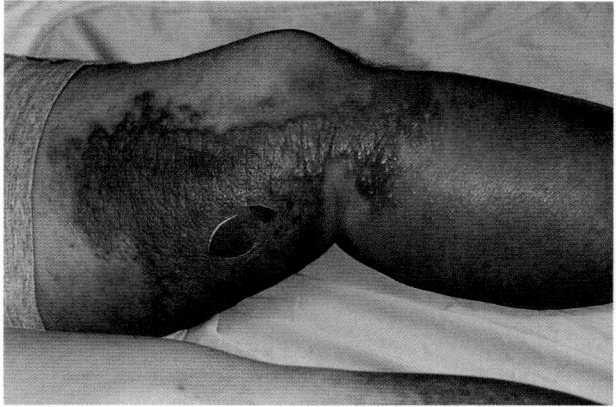

FIGURE 51-16 Cellulitis in a client with long-standing diabetes and stasis dermatitis.

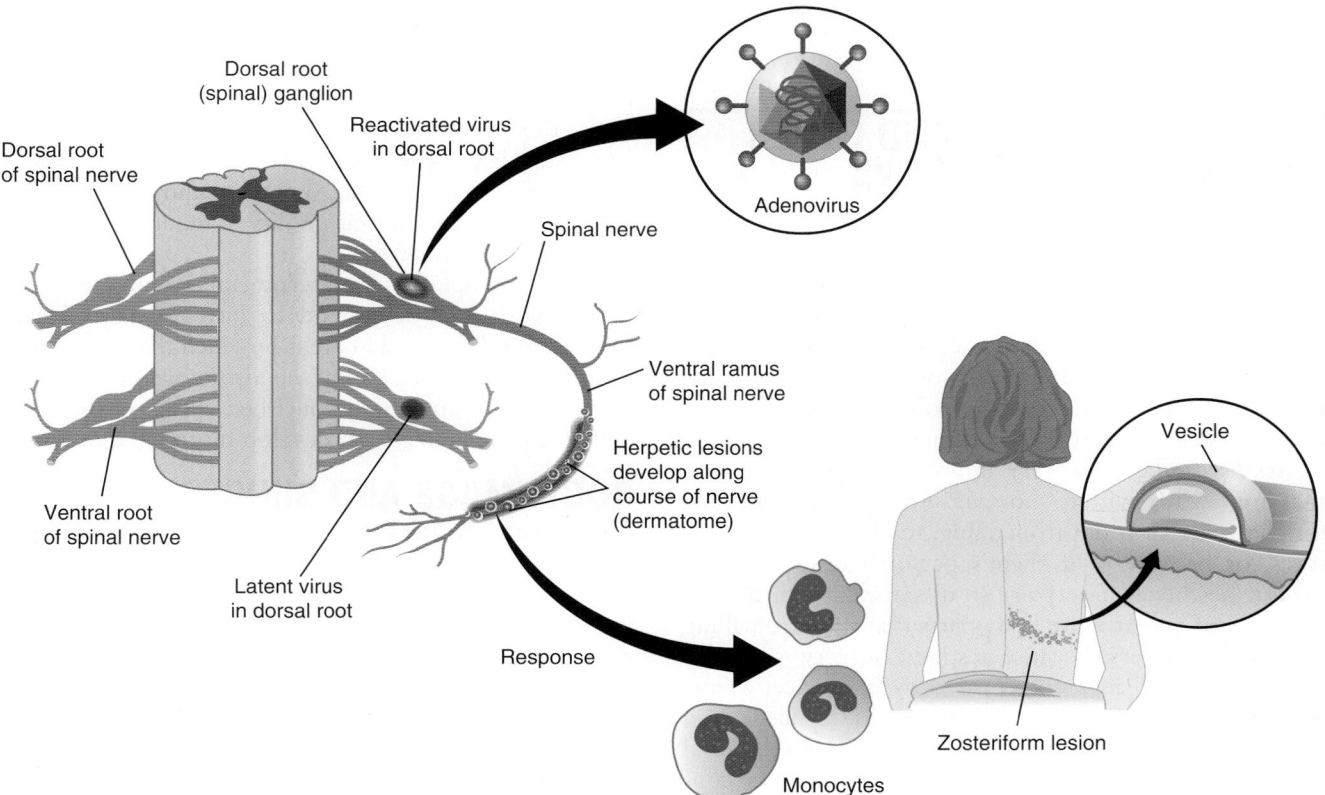

FIGURE 51-17 Pathophysiology of herpes zoster. The dormant herpes virus is reactivated causing vesicular lesions along the dermatome.

Outcome Management

The primary goals of therapy are to limit extent, duration, and severity of pain and rash in primary dermatome, prevent spread of disease, and prevent postherpetic neuralgia. Treatment for herpes zoster is administration of antiviral medications such as acyclovir (Zovirax), famciclovir (Famvir), and valacyclovir (Valtrex). The newer antiviral agents often have more convenient dosing schedules. Antivirals, when started early in the course of the disease, reduce acute pain and accelerate healing of the lesions. Studies suggest that early oral antiviral therapy may assist in reducing postherpetic neuralgia. Analgesics and sedatives are prescribed for pain reduction.

Topical therapy is primarily symptomatic: applications of cool compresses, use of cooling antipruritic preparations (see Table 51-1), cornstarch or baking soda, and measures to prevent secondary infection. If pain is present, the client's normal pain tolerance and current pain level must be assessed. Systemic analgesics are usually required, and occasionally opioids; however, in chronic pain, use of these agents raises the possibility of addiction. Assess the effectiveness and side effects of prescribed analgesics. Because postherpetic neuralgia can last a long time, the client and significant others need continued intervention and support. Chronic pain management may include the use of tricyclic antidepressants, phenothiazines, and other local physical modalities such as electrical stimulating units.

■ PLASTIC SURGERY AND OTHER COSMETIC/RESTORATIVE PROCEDURES

Plastic surgery is the surgical subspecialty that concentrates on the restoration of function and form to body structures damaged by trauma, transformed by the aging process, changed by disease processes (such as skin cancer), or malformed as a result of congenital defects. Plastic surgery can be divided into two major areas: (1) aesthetic (cosmetic) and (2) reconstructive.

Aesthetic plastic surgery improves physical features that are already within "normal" range. It is performed for changes that result from aging, to alter inherited features, or because of a client's personal desire. Clients seeking aesthetic surgery are so dissatisfied with the appearance of one or more body parts that they are willing to undergo surgery. Because aesthetic surgery is considered "cosmetic," it is not covered by insurance; clients pay out of pocket. Most clients are enthusiastic and happy because the surgery is a culmination of a personal desire that they may have held for a long time. In contrast, other clients may or may not have social support for their decision. The client may feel vain, embarrassed, or guilty about taking health care away from "people who really need it." Become sensitive to these feelings in the client, and be comfortable with a person's normal desires to feel good about the way he or she looks.

Reconstructive surgery attempts to restore a more normal appearance or function in a person who has an abnormal body part or in whom a body part is missing. The abnormality may be a result of injury or disease, it may be congenital, or it may be the cause of other medical problems. People undergoing reconstructive surgery are typically motivated to try to gain increased function of body parts and to improve their appearance. Although they may hope that plastic surgery will make them "normal," they usually know this may be unrealistic. Such clients are often struggling with diverse emotions: hope for a future without disease recurrence, eagerness to see final surgical results, anxiety over the surgery itself and impending postoperative pain, and weariness of the illness. The client having reconstructive surgery does have the advantage of social approval. Inasmuch as such a client is seen as a victim, society, as represented by either individuals or institutions, often provides treatment or makes appeals for payment of the operations.

Because of the significant impact of plastic surgery procedures on body image and self-esteem, psychological care is imperative. Plastic surgery is not only an operation on the skin; it reaches into the psyche of the person undergoing the surgery.

Minimal postoperative scarring is the hallmark of successful plastic surgery. It is important to understand that no surgery can be done without creating a scar. Plastic surgery is conducted to minimize scars, so at times it seems that surgery can be done without scars. The quality of scarring is affected by many variables, such as the client's age, general health, skin type, and healing ability. Surgical technique and the quality of wound care also affect the healing process.

Blacks, people of Mediterranean origin, and other people with dark skin tend to have more noticeable scars. Wounds located in areas in which the tissue moves as it heals (e.g., over joints) are also more susceptible to scarring. The skin of malnourished clients heals slowly, and the wounds may also develop more obvious scars.

BODY IMAGE AND SURGERY

The desire to be attractive or beautiful is present in people of all cultures, but the perception of what is attractive varies. The importance of physical appearance varies from person to person; however, it is an integral part of the sense of self. The desire to want to physically resemble one's peers reasonably closely—for instance, to have acceptably "normal" facial features—is a normal desire. A significant portion of any deformity rests in the client's perception of the abnormality. Perceptions develop in part from body image. Body image describes a person's perception of his or her body—how the person *thinks* he or she looks, rather than an objective assessment of the person's characteristics. Body image is a factor in determining self-image, self-concept, and self-esteem. People with a positive body image display more confidence and interact more easily with others. Body image changes continually, depending on individual expectations and feedback from others.

A person with a physical deformity, real or perceived, can have a severely damaged body image. Even the usual processes of aging can be detrimental to body image. A self-perception of "getting old" can impair self-confidence, affect behavior, and interfere with interactions in society. Body image is an important factor in the nursing assessment of the client having plastic surgery.

The client's ability to cope with a temporary or permanent or a perceived or actual disfigurement is also assessed. Assess the client's coping mechanisms. Some coping mechanisms may be effective; others may be ineffective. Men may have more difficulty expressing their feelings about their appearance than that typically noted in women. Listen to the client, be alert for positive and negative self-statements, and note the degree of anxiety and fear. Evaluate the client's willingness or unwilling-

ness to touch or look at involved body areas and the client's comfort with being near other people.

Techniques for working with clients who have alterations in body image are presented in Box 51-4.

FACIAL REJUVENATING PROCEDURES

In childhood, skin is very elastic and is supported at maximum distention by adipose tissue ("baby fat"). During aging, the skin loses elasticity and the subcutaneous fat diminishes and changes character. Skinfolds and wrinkles become increasingly noticeable. Tissue around the eyes and jaw line sags, producing a drooping, tired, weary, or worried expression. The rate of skin change varies among people. Weight loss, habitual sun exposure, genetic tendencies, and alcohol and tobacco use affect the speed and character of the changes.

Facial Resurfacing

Skin Peels

Various products (alpha-hydroxy acid, glycolic acid, trichloroacetic acid) can be used to lift superficial layers

---

BOX 51-4   *Supporting the Client Who Has a Changed Body Image*

Many clients undergoing plastic surgery experience some form of body image alteration. Clients may experience body image changes before surgery due to disease or injury, They may also have problems after surgery from edema, bruising, or less than desired results. Try to anticipate these problems and work with the client as soon as possible to facilitate needed adjustments. You may want to work with the nursing diagnosis of *Risk for Disturbed Body Image* or *Situational Low Self-Esteem related to perceived or actual disfigurement and changes in self-concept.* The expected outcome must be tailored to the client but may include improved self-image with incorporation of the changed body part into the body image, as evidenced by effective coping and appropriate use of defense mechanisms; verbalizing feelings comfortably and appropriately; expressing satisfaction with the changed body image; having the ability to openly verbalize feelings; making positive statements about self; having a normal level of anxiety and normal fears; comfortably looking at self in mirror and/or touching the deformed body area, healed surgical site, or other scars; being able to be with others comfortably; and having no indications of depression.

Some interventions that you may find effective with clients who are experiencing body image disturbances include the following:

• Continue to assess apparent self-concept, coping methods, defense mechanisms, degree of anxiety, and fears frequently.
• Assist the client to explore and express feelings; do not use phrases such as "I know how you feel." These empty phrases build barriers to communication, whereas statements such

as "you are angry" or "you seem depressed," for example, identify the feeling.
• Be sensitive to the client's feelings and needs.
• Acknowledge the client's feelings.
• Present reality; building false hope is detrimental (reality need not be brutal, however).
• Healing is unpredictable; refer questions about healing to the surgeon.
• Do not force the client to view or touch himself or herself; gently assist the client to look at and touch the deformity or healed surgical site (help incorporate it into the client's self-concept and body image).
• Encourage the client to begin meeting in public to begin desensitization to the reactions of others, such as by taking walks in halls; desensitization begins in safe environments and proceeds to new situations, prepare the client for stares and remarks.
• Discuss others' reaction to the client; support grief reactions.
• If the client has a facial deformity, prepare visitors and family members before they see the client.
• Look for vocal expressions or hand gestures in cases of facial disfigurement; facial expression may be limited in clients with extensive facial scars or skin grafts.
• Refer the client and family to local support groups, such as About Face.
• Assist the client with techniques to camouflage scars; licensed aestheticians can assist with make-up choices and techniques.

of skin and remove fine wrinkles from the skin. These products are usually applied in an office setting with the client awake. The best candidates are those clients with fair skin and fine wrinkles. Trained nurses perform the peel procedure. Most skin peel procedures require a regimen of skin care before treatment. Care after the peel includes application of skin moisturizers, use of hydrocortisone to reduce edema and erythema, gentle cleansing, and use of sunscreen. The client often resumes the pre-peel skin regimen after the peel. Hyperpigmentation is the most common complication.

Laser Resurfacing

Laser treatment creates a shallow burn injury to the skin. Laser treatment requires sedation or use of topical anesthetics such as eutectic mixture of local anesthetic (EMLA). Postoperative edema can be reduced somewhat with ice packs and oral corticosteroids for 48 hours. Some clients also experience a burn sensation for 12 to 18 hours after treatment. The skin reepithelializes in about 5 to 10 days, depending on the depth of the injury. Sun-blocking agents are a must, in that hyperpigmentation can develop.

Dermabrasion

Dermabrasion is a process of sanding the surface layers of skin on cheeks and forehead with an electric rotating brush to smooth out pitting and surface blemishes. This operation is the preferred treatment for depressed acne scars and other deep scars. Local anesthesia with sedation is used. The abraded surfaces are covered with antibiotic ointment and gauze. After removal of the gauze, the facial skin weeps serous fluid for 5 to 7 days. Once the weeping stops and new skin has appeared, the client can apply make-up to camouflage the redness. The redness fades over the following 6 weeks.

Dermal Fillers

Soft-tissue augmentation has become a popular means of addressing contour defects that result from aging, photodamage, trauma or scarification, or disease. Several products can be used (e.g., autologous fat, collagen, hyaluronic acid) to fill in small wrinkles or depressed blemishes in the skin. The client's reaction to collagen is tested before treatment, because some people experience induration (hard, raised area) and swelling at the injection site. Clients with autoimmune disorders are not candidates for collagen injection.

Botulinum Injections

Botulinum Toxin Type A (Botox) can be injected to temporarily improve the appearance of moderate to severe frown lines between the eyebrows (glabellar lines). Botox is a protein produced by the bacterium *Clostridium botulinum*. Small doses of the toxin are injected into the affected muscles and block the release of the chemical acetylcholine that would otherwise signal the muscle to contract. The toxin thus paralyzes or weakens the injected muscle for up to 120 days. Following injection, some clients report headache, respiratory infection, flu syndrome, blepharoptosis (droopy eyelids), and nausea. Less frequent adverse reactions include pain in the face, redness at the injection site, and muscle weakness.

Rhytidectomy (Face Lift)

A rhytidectomy *(face lift)* may restore a more youthful appearance to the face (perhaps from 5 to 10 years younger) by removing wrinkled skin from the forehead and around the eyes and mouth (Figure 51-18). Rhytidectomy does not result in removal of all of the wrinkles of the face. Clients may require acid peeling for fine perioral wrinkles (see the following discussion).

Rhytidectomy is usually performed on an outpatient basis with the client under general anesthesia, or using local anesthesia with IV sedation. Incisions are made from the temple along the ear and out into the hair-bearing scalp behind the ear. Through the incisions, excess facial skin is undermined and pulled back toward the ear. *Undermining* is a surgical technique in which the skin is separated from underlying structures.

Postoperatively, the client is placed in the Fowler's position to reduce the risk of edema. Cold compresses can also be used to reduce swelling and bleeding. Suction drains are used to eliminate dead space and remove wound drainage. Drains are removed in 24 to 48 hours, when drainage has subsided. Facial movement (talking and chewing) should be limited. Localized increases in blood pressure should be avoided by keeping the head elevated; any prescribed antihypertensive medications should also be resumed. Coughing also increases blood pressure and should be avoided (by not operating on clients with colds) or treated if it manifests after surgery.

Complications include hematomas, which can cause tissue necrosis and must be surgically removed. Hematoma formation occurs most often in people who smoke or have pre-existing hypertension. Postoperative nausea and vomiting can also increase bleeding and hematoma formation. Hematoma development is first noted as increasing facial asymmetry associated with pain or tightness on one side of the face. Increasing drainage and changes in facial sensation should also be reported.

Blepharoplasty

Blepharoplasty is the surgical removal of excess skin and periorbital fat from the upper or lower eyelid. Blepharoplasty is usually performed on an outpatient basis. Gen-

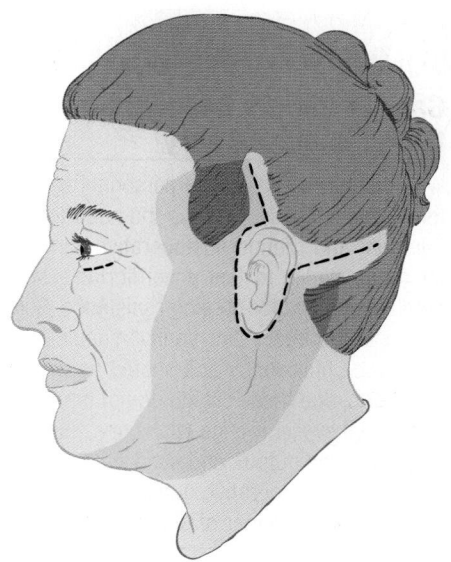

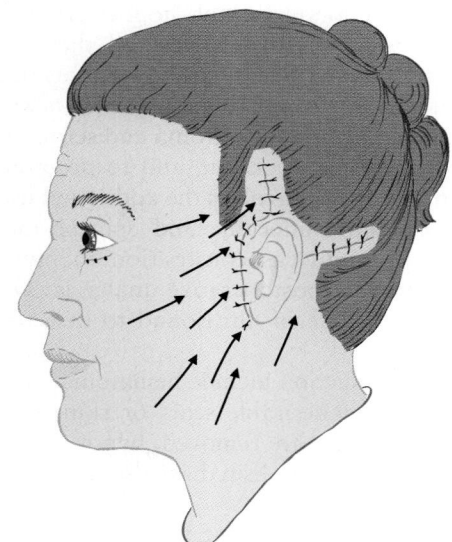

A Before face lift and blepharoplasty

B After face lift and blepharoplasty

FIGURE 51-18 Face lift (rhytidectomy) and blepharoplasty. Face lifts enable removal of large wrinkles and folds of skin from the face and neck. **A,** Area in pink shows amount of tissue that is undermined (lifted from the fascial connection) and moved during a face lift. For the face lift, the incision lines go around the ear and into the hair-bearing scalp; other incisions may also be used. Note also the incision line beneath the eyelid for the blepharoplasty, which enables removal of excess eyelid tissue. **B,** The postoperative near-final result, with tightened facial skin and neck folds.

eral or local anesthesia with sedation can be used. Wide elliptical incisions are made on the upper eyelids. The excised wedge of excess tissue is lifted off, and herniated fat is removed. A lower-lid blepharoplasty incision is placed $\frac{1}{8}$-inch below the edge of the eyelid.

Assess preoperative near and distant vision in each eye by asking the client to read from a book and from something in the distance while one eye is covered. These baseline data are crucial to assess postoperative visual changes. An ophthalmologic examination is indicated before surgery if vision problems are noted.

After blepharoplasty, the head is elevated to reduce edema. Iced normal saline compresses or patches are applied to the eyes as prescribed. Activity is limited for 1 week to reduce blood pressure elevations that often lead to increased edema and ecchymosis (bruising). Normally, severe pain is not experienced after blepharoplasty. An itching sensation, similar to that associated with dry eyes, is usually experienced as a result of slight corneal swelling. This can be prevented with cold wet dressings.

Rhinoplasty

Rhinoplasty is the surgical correction of nasal deformities. This procedure is frequently performed as an outpatient procedure using either local anesthesia and sedation or general anesthesia. Incisions are made inside the nose to reshape the dorsum, ala, or internal cartilage. After surgery, the inside of the nose may be packed and an external splint applied.

Preoperative nursing care focuses on teaching the client to breathe through the mouth after surgery and to not touch the nose. Postoperatively, assess for bleeding. While the client is sleepy from the anesthesia, excessive swallowing may be the only manifestation of bleeding. Examine the back of the throat with a flashlight to look for blood. Some bleeding is normal down the back of the throat and on the nasal packs and dressings. The nurse promptly reports excessive bleeding to the surgeon. The head of the bed is kept elevated to control postoperative edema. Nasal packing can be very uncomfortable. Pain management is important and can usually be achieved with oral analgesics (e.g., codeine, acetaminophen). Aspirin is avoided for 1 week before and 3 weeks after surgery. (See the Client Education Guide feature on Postoperative Care After Rhinoplasty on the website.)   *evolve*

BODY-CONTOURING SURGERY (LIPECTOMY)

Body-contouring surgical procedures (lipectomy) remove excess fatty tissue, skinfolds, or subcutaneous fat from various body parts, including the abdomen, thighs, arms, and buttocks.

Liposuction

Liposuction is a technique used (1) to aspirate fatty tissue from areas of the body resistant to diet and exercise (lipodystrophy), (2) to contour flaps, and (3) to remove lipomas (benign fatty tumors). A blunt, hollow cannula is inserted through very small incisions and then attached to a powerful suction machine that vacuums out adipose tissue. After surgery, compression garments are used to prevent fluid collection (hematoma and seroma), to maintain the desired body contour, and to promote healing. Tumescent technique involves the additional use of large volumes of dilute lidocaine and epinephrine. These medications promote vasoconstriction to minimize bleeding and provide postoperative analgesia. Ultrasonic lipectomy is the use of ultrasound to ease the removal of fat.[1,2]

Complications of liposuction include hematoma, skin necrosis, infection, and undesirable scars or skin dimpling. If large volumes of fat are removed, hypovolemia may develop. Pulmonary embolism has also been reported.

After liposuction, assess the client for hypovolemia and electrolyte imbalance (manifested by syncope, dizziness, and abnormal blood values). If drains are used, monitor the quantity and quality of drainage. Ice and oral analgesics are effective in managing postoperative pain. Dressings usually remain in place for at least 24 hours. Nurses must ensure that dressings remain smooth and uniform; otherwise, contour irregularities can result. Sometimes the client wears a compression garment for several weeks postoperatively.

Clients may gradually resume normal activity except for strenuous exercise. It may be 4 to 6 weeks before the client works up to the preoperative level of exercise. Resuming activity too rapidly may result in soreness and swelling. Bruising is common after liposuction and may take weeks to disappear completely.

Many clients expect the results of liposuction to be immediate. Usually up to 6 months is required for final results to be apparent after edema subsides and subcutaneous tissue heals. Reinforce that results may not be apparent for 6 months following surgery. This period of time is required for complete resolution of edema and reconnection of soft tissues.

Abdominoplasty

Abdominoplasty is the removal of excess abdominal skin and fat and the repair and tightening of separated abdominal muscles. An incision is made across the lower abdomen, and tissue is undermined to the costal margin. The excess skin and fatty tissue are excised and recontoured. The umbilical stalk is detached and reattached once the overlying skin is in its proper position.

After surgery, inspect the incision line for manifestations of pallor or lack of capillary refill. The operative site can swell, with resulting impairment of capillary blood supply. Smoking is prohibited, because nicotine further restricts blood flow to the skin. Tension on the suture line must be minimized; therefore the client must lie in semi-Fowler's position with the knees flexed (a contouring position). The client also needs to walk in a "hunched-over"

MANAGEMENT AND DELEGATION

Care of Clients Recovering from Plastic Surgery

When unlicensed assistive personnel are caring for clients after plastic surgery, reinforce the need for adequate pain management and routine postoperative care. It is not uncommon for these clients to feel uncomfortable about asking for pain medications and for nursing assistance. Some people have the notion that surgery "for vanity" should hurt a little. This is a dangerous philosophy and should not be condoned. Any incision hurts, and these clients do not differ in their need for pain control. Likewise, routine vital signs, pulmonary care, monitoring intake and output, and encouraging ambulation are routine aspects of postoperative nursing care. Withholding care is not an acceptable manner of providing care.

position until the swelling decreases and abdominal skin relaxes. Teach the client postoperative pain management techniques. Abdominoplasty is an abdominal operation and produces significant postoperative discomfort. Adequate analgesia and other pain-relieving measures are essential. Reinforce to unlicensed personnel that these clients require usual postoperative care (see the Management and Delegation feature on Care of Clients Recovering from Plastic Surgery, above).

Panniculectomy

In people who have experienced major weight loss, excess loose skin and subcutaneous tissue may develop over the abdomen, thighs, and arms, hanging in large folds. The folds of tissue are called *pannus*, and panniculectomy is the surgical removal of these tissue folds. As much as 10 pounds of redundant tissue has been surgically removed during one of these operations. Clearly, this operation is not for the cure of the client's obesity, but it can offer some positive gains in self-esteem and reduction in health-related problems.

Postoperative care is usually focused on reducing stress on the long suture lines. For example, place the client in the Fowler's position after abdominal panniculectomy. Monitor the suture lines closely for manifestations of nonhealing. Fatty tissue is poorly perfused, and the client may have pre-existing diet-induced malnutrition. During the healing phase, the client needs to consume adequate amounts of protein and carbohydrate to heal. Other tissue folds must be treated for intertriginous dermatitis (see earlier discussion on Intertrigo).

RECONSTRUCTIVE PLASTIC SURGERY

One of the greatest challenges in plastic surgery is the reconstruction of deformities. Skin grafting is discussed in Chapter 52. This section discusses flap surgery.

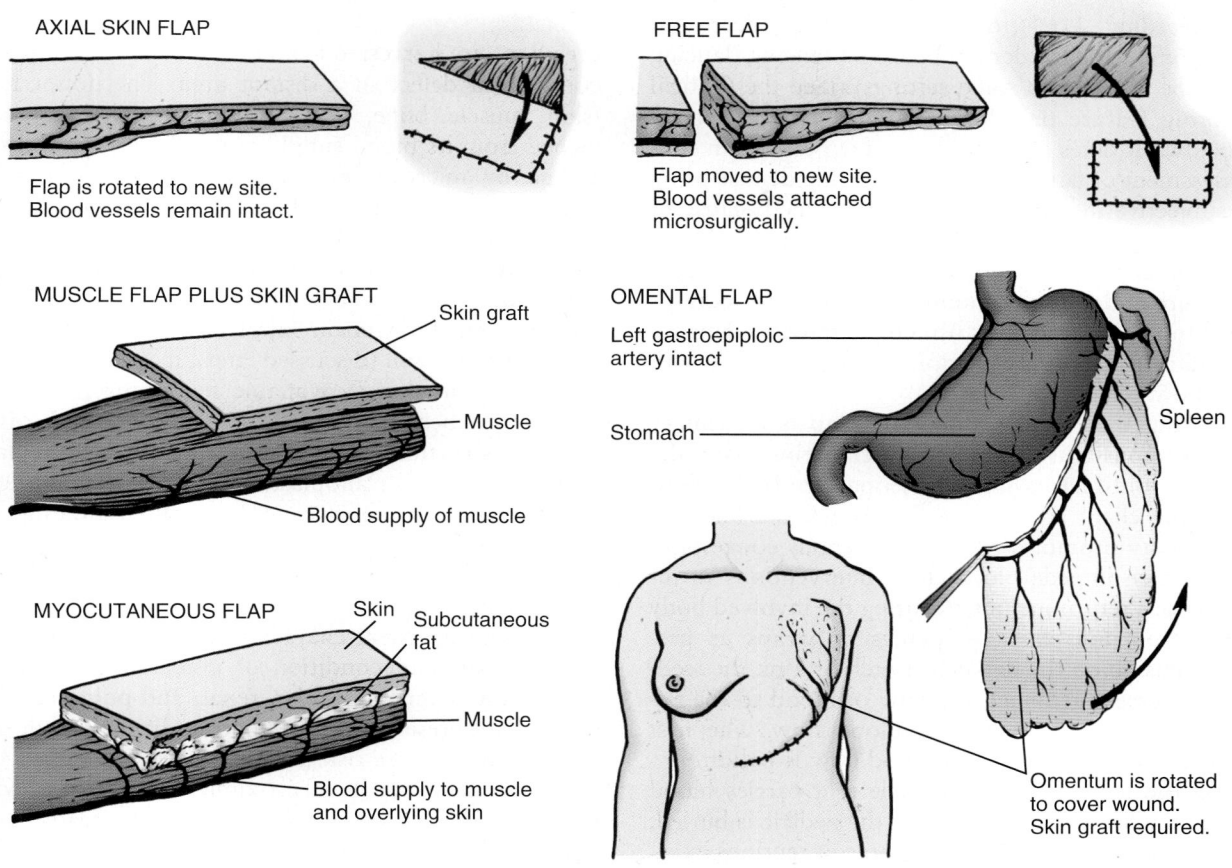

AXIAL SKIN FLAP

Flap is rotated to new site.
Blood vessels remain intact.

FREE FLAP

Flap moved to new site.
Blood vessels attached
microsurgically.

MUSCLE FLAP PLUS SKIN GRAFT

Skin graft
Muscle
Blood supply of muscle

MYOCUTANEOUS FLAP

Skin   Subcutaneous
fat
Muscle
Blood supply to muscle
and overlying skin

OMENTAL FLAP

Left gastroepiploic
artery intact
Stomach
Spleen
Omentum is rotated
to cover wound.
Skin graft required.

FIGURE 51-19 Common flaps.

Flaps are areas of tissue raised from one area of the body without being completely detached, so that the blood supply is intact; the flap is transferred (e.g., by rotation) to adjacent areas. Flaps of tissue can also be transferred to distant areas, where a blood supply is reestablished; these are called *free flaps* and are discussed later. Local flaps are rotated or advanced to reconstruct an adjacent defect (Figure 51-19). Preservation of the nutrient blood vessels is paramount to flap survival. The tissue attachment containing these vessels is sometimes called the *pedicle,* because in the past, flaps were moved from site to site with a visible portion of tissue that "carried" the flap to the recipient site. This style of flap can be seen in the deltopectoral flaps used to repair neck resection tissue loss. Flaps are also used to cover extensive wounds from pressure ulcers and long-standing defects from osteomyelitis.

Skin Flaps

Skin flaps are sections of skin rotated from their origin to cover a defect. Common uses of skin flaps to reconstruct a neck after excision of cancer (deltopectoral flap) or the face (rotation flap). Occasionally skin flaps are used to close pressure ulcers on the pelvis. Blood flow to the flap must be protected. Avoid securing dressings or tracheotomy ties across the flap.

Musculocutaneous Flaps

Flaps comprising both muscle and skin are called *musculocutaneous flaps.* They are commonly used to fill in defects where muscle is missing or where muscle can provide ample blood flow to heal osteomyelitis. These flaps are named by the muscle of origin. For example, large trochanteric pressure ulcers can be repaired with tensor fasciae latae flaps, named for the tensor fasciae latae muscle of the lateral thigh. Intrathoracic muscle flaps used for chest wall reconstruction include serratus anterior, latissimus dorsi, and pectoralis muscles.

Nursing care centers on maintaining perfusion and reducing tissue injury to the flap. You may choose to design your nursing care under the nursing diagnosis of *Risk for Ineffective Tissue Perfusion related to tissue transfer.*

The outcome is that the client will maintain effective peripheral tissue perfusion, as evidenced by usual color of skin, no pallor or cyanosis, warm and dry skin, blanching (capillary refill) in 3 to 5 seconds, no edema or blebs, intact incisions, and controllable pain.

The flap is monitored for color, capillary refill, and dermal bleeding. Look for pallor, coolness, decreased capillary refill, or dark dermal blood on lancing (lancing may not be allowed in some settings). (See the Critical Monitoring feature on Musculocutaneous Reconstruction, below.) It takes a fair amount of experience in clinical assessment of flaps to predict early flap demise using these subjective methods. Findings can vary because of oxygen content of the blood, capillary dilation, blood flow, and skin pigmentation. Therefore in complex flaps, temperature and Doppler monitors are used to monitor circulation. The extremity is usually elevated to improve venous return as long as elevation does not interfere with arterial flow.

Protecting the blood supply to a flap is a primary nursing responsibility. Nursing interventions are designed to avoid factors that can jeopardize blood flow. Position the client so that the flap is relaxed and elevated. Gravity promotes edema and venous congestion, both of which impede blood flow. Interventions to increase venous return include elevating the involved body part and applying elastic stockings or wraps as prescribed. Tension on the flap can stretch or kink the feeding blood vessels, reducing the flow of blood to the tissues. A blood clot can restrict blood flow. The first manifestation of compromised blood flow is pallor.

Know the location of the pedicle that carries blood vessels to the flap. Most of the time the pedicle is buried, and little can be done to harm it. Some exceptions exist, though. When skin flaps are used, such as the deltopectoral flap, the pedicle is visible. Tracheostomy ties should not be tied tightly around the flap; otherwise, circulation to the distal portions will be compromised. When the breast is reconstructed after mastectomy with a latissimus dorsi flap, the pedicle is located in the ipsilateral axilla. The client cannot lie on the ipsilateral side.

Hydrate the client well, if prescribed, to help perfuse the flap. Maintain any postoperative splints to prevent tension on vessels. Limit the use of caffeine by the client and prohibit the use of nicotine by the client and by visitors.

Problems due to impaired arterial supply are apparent early after surgery. Altered perfusion due to venous obstruction may not be evident for a few hours.

Free Flaps

Free flaps are harvested from one area of the body to reconstruct a defect in a distant area. The donor tissue (skin, muscle, bone, or a combination of these) is detached from its blood supply at the donor site and reattached by microvascular anastomosis to arteries and veins at the recipient site. The development of microvascular techniques has made it possible to reconstruct defects that were previously untreatable. Before surgical reconstruction, a flap can be prefabricated to build exactly what is needed for repair. Supplemental techniques, such as tissue expansion (discussed later), may be used to augment the skin that is available for closure. Other advances have been made in the areas of bone and soft tissue reconstruction. Bone has traditionally been replaced with bone grafts or alloplastic materials. More recently, osteoinductive proteins capable of differentiating into bone were discovered. These proteins can be combined with muscle flaps, and the tissue then is transformed into useful bone.

Preoperative client characteristics to consider include health status and condition of potential donor tissue. Diabetes and cardiovascular, renal, and pulmonary disease do not present absolute contraindications, but these diseases do increase risk of flap failure. The vessels used for a flap must not be in proximity to sites of previous trauma or irradiation. After trauma, widespread changes occur in the walls and perivascular tissues of the major vascular bundles. These changes have been labeled as *post-traumatic vessel disease* (PTVD). Vessels with PTVD are more difficult to dissect, are easily damaged, and have little resistance against clots. Donor sites are chosen according to guidelines presented previously. The donor site pedicle is deliberately planned so that the flap can comfortably reach the recipient site.

Free Flap Failure

When all goes well, the advantages of free flaps are obvious. Nevertheless, the phantom called *free flap failure* looms large, limiting use of the procedure. Thrombosis is the most common cause of failure. After surgery, the free flap site is seldom dressed, so that clinical assessments can be performed. Several techniques have been developed in large clinical trials, but no consensus exists as to which is the best technique. The ideal monitoring system would provide a continuous recording of flap perfusion or flap metabolism. It should monitor both visible and buried tissues. Finally, the data should be easily interpreted by nursing personnel and junior medical staff.

Assess for trends in color, texture, and temperature of the flap, as well as Doppler pulses and drainage from wound drains. Other postoperative care includes maintaining adequate hydration, keeping the client warm,

CRITICAL MONITORING

Musculocutaneous Reconstruction

Report the following findings immediately:

- Development of coolness in the flap
- Development of duskiness or pallor in the flap
- Slowing of capillary refill in the flap
- Loss of pulses (palpable or detected by Doppler) in the flap
- Increasing pain in the flap

managing pain, and allowing only appropriate activities. Clients may express some concern with the decision to salvage a body part or may fear that the flap will fail and amputation will be required. The nurse needs to be supportive of the decision for surgery and allow time for expression of fears.

SKIN EXPANSION

Skin expansion is a technique used to increase the amount of local tissue available to reconstruct a defect. An inflatable silicone balloon is placed under the skin or muscle flap adjacent to a defect. The expander is inflated sequentially over several weeks or months to stretch the overlying tissue. When tissue is sufficient to resurface the adjacent defect, the balloon is removed and the flap is contoured (shaped) and advanced to cover the defect.

LASERS

The laser (*l*ight *a*mplification by *s*timulated *e*mission of *r*adiation) is a coagulating, vaporizing, and cutting instrument. A precise beam of laser light is directed onto tissue. The light is converted into heat energy that is absorbed by the cells. The heat vaporizes the cells. The advantages of laser surgery include precision and accuracy of cell destruction, reduced bleeding and swelling, and, sometimes, less postoperative pain. Operating time may be longer, but tissue damage is less, and the postoperative infection rate is lower.

Laser light can be of different colors and wavelengths. Each is absorbed differently depending on cell pigment and water content. The carbon dioxide (CO_2) laser is primarily a cutting and vaporizing tool. Its energy is absorbed by the water in cells, so it penetrates tissue only superficially. The CO_2 laser is used primarily to excise or vaporize lesions such as warts, keloids, and vascular lesions. Argon, copper vapor, and pulsed-dye laser energy are preferentially absorbed by hemoglobin and are used primarily for coagulation. These types of lasers are used to treat birthmarks (e.g., port-wine stain), superficial vascular lesions, and pigmented lesions.

Laser energy generates intense heat, and clients experience a burning sensation or a pin-prick sensation. The tissue reaction can be similar to that of a second-degree burn with blistering. Ointment applied to the affected area for 2 to 4 weeks keeps the tissue moist until healing is complete. It is also essential that the area treated with laser energy be protected from sun exposure for several weeks.

Laser treatment to remove large pigmented lesions may require many operations. A single application may address only a small portion of the lesion, and the results are appreciated slowly as the site heals. Clients must be prepared for the length of time required and the inconvenience of multiple procedures.

REPAIR OF TRAUMATIC INJURIES

Facial Fractures

Fractures can occur in the individual bones of the face: the nasal bones, orbit, malar prominence, mandible, or maxilla (Figure 51-20). The client with facial fractures has often been involved in an automobile accident or an assault or has suffered a sports injury. Pain, improper bite (malocclusion), swelling, bruising, diplopia (double vision), facial asymmetry, enophthalmos (sunken eye), and exophthalmos (bulging eye) are clinical manifestations of facial fractures. Diagnostic assessment includes x-ray studies.

Life-threatening problems (e.g., airway obstruction, hemorrhage, or cervical spine injury) that may accompany facial trauma must be managed immediately. Because of proximity of the injury to the airway, assess airway patency and breath sounds every 2 hours (more

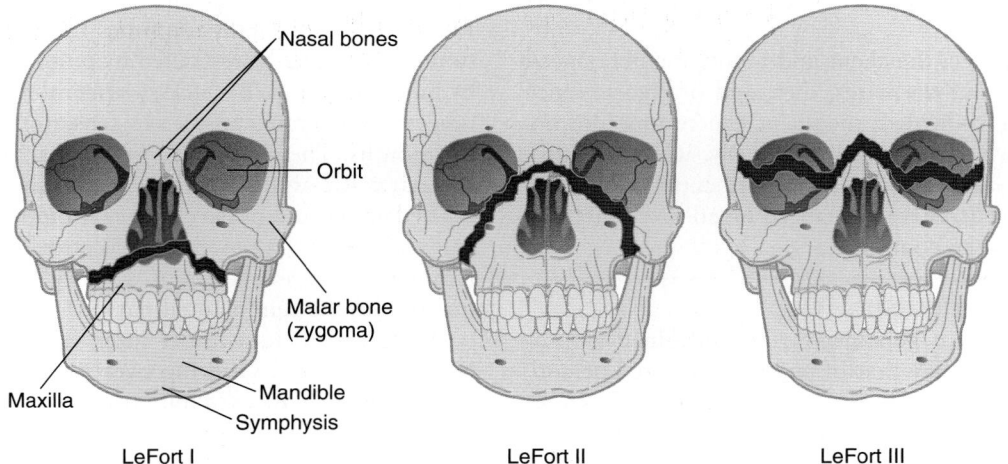

FIGURE 51-20 LeFort fractures. *LeFort I:* transverse fracture of the alveolar process separating the upper dental arch from the maxilla; *LeFort II:* fracture of the mid face, maxilla, and orbits; *LeFort III:* fracture of the orbits that leads to craniofacial dissociation.

often if bleeding is present). Place suction equipment at the bedside. Teach the client to breathe through the nose. Trying to open the mouth may dislocate the fracture.

Repair of facial fractures can be delayed for up to 3 weeks and still achieve good results. Like all fractures, facial fractures must be reduced, stabilized, and immobilized to ensure proper healing. Methods vary according to the location of the fractures.

 When the client has intermaxillary wiring, wire cutters should be in the client's possession at all times. If airway problems develop that cannot be managed with suction, the wires that secure the upper and lower jaws should be cut. The nurse and the client need to be informed about which wires should be cut. These are the only wires that attach the top and bottom teeth. Do not try to cut off the bands attached to the teeth.

A liquefied diet is used until the wires are removed. Without adequate nutrition, clients can lose 10 to 20 pounds during convalescence. Instruct the client how to "blenderize" food and to maintain an adequate balance of carbohydrates, fat, protein, and calories. Milkshakes can be made with a wide variety of foods. High-calorie food supplements can augment the regular diet, and liquid multivitamins may be useful. Alcoholic and carbonated beverages can cause nausea and can fizz and foam in the back of the throat, leading to airway problems; they are to be avoided.

Oral hygiene aids in healing of oral wounds, prevents infection and destruction of teeth and gums, increases comfort, and enhances self-esteem. Rinsing the mouth with water or a mouthwash followed by use of an oral irrigation device on low pressure removes particles from the front of the mouth while the tissues are still tender. Once the initial swelling and tenderness subside, the teeth must be brushed and the mouth rinsed after every meal and at bedtime. Pieces of dental wax can be placed on the open ends of the wires if they irritate buccal surfaces.

Before discharge, the client and family members need to be taught about the wires, diet, and oral care. Once the incisions have healed, the client can resume normal activities. However, as noted previously, while the jaws are wired, the client must carry a wire cutter and know which wires to cut. A well-balanced blenderized diet and oral care should be continued.

Traumatic Amputations

Immediate care of a person who has sustained a traumatic amputation, like that of any other injured person, focuses on life-saving activities (see Chapter 84). Hemorrhage is controlled with direct pressure on the bleeding points. Tourniquets and cautery are not used because they may damage surrounding tissue, so that reimplantation becomes impossible. All amputated parts, including small pieces of tissue, are sent to the health care

facility with the injured person. As soon as possible, these parts are (1) rinsed with sterile normal saline, (2) wrapped in sterile wet gauze, (3) sealed in a watertight bag, and (4) placed on ice. Cooling the amputated part reduces metabolism, increasing the time the part can survive without blood. For example, an amputated finger can survive for 18 hours if effectively cooled. Although the part is rinsed with normal saline, it is never stored in normal saline or on dry ice, or frozen, which causes extensive cellular damage.

Reimplantation surgery is performed using a regional block or with the client under general anesthesia. An operating microscope guides the surgical reattachment of arteries, veins, tendons, and nerves. With severe injuries, such an operation may take 12 to 18 hours. After surgery, incisions are dressed, the extremity is immobilized with casts or splints, and the entire extremity is elevated.

After reimplantation, the client requires careful, frequent nursing assessment (every 15 minutes) including documentation of the reimplanted part's color, temperature, and capillary refill. Arterial or venous blood flow in the reimplanted part may become blocked; if the problem is not immediately corrected surgically, the part will die. Toes and fingertips are usually left uncovered for assessment. Doppler assessments help monitor pulses in the part. Temperature probes are often placed on the extremity. The surgeon usually states the ideal temperature range for reimplantations. A temperature decrease of 2° C or more in an hour or a decline to 32° C (89.6° F) demands immediate attention and is promptly reported to the surgeon. A temperature of 34° to 36° C (93.2° to 96.5° F) is considered excellent for a reimplanted finger. Aspirin is usually prescribed to reduce blood-clotting tendencies. Because anesthesia time is prolonged (18 to 24 hours), nursing care also focuses on monitoring recovery from anesthesia.

An active rehabilitation program usually begins 2 weeks after injury and continues for months. Joint motion initially may be restricted by pins through joints and by bulky dressings. Because peripheral nerves take a long time to regenerate, protective sensation may be absent for months. The client must be careful to avoid injuring the part. Rehabilitation is accomplished through prescribed active and passive range-of-motion exercises several times each day. A final indication of the success of reimplantation is return of sensory and motor nerve function in the reimplanted part.

Psychosocial adjustment after reimplantation varies with each person. Grieving over the loss of appearance and function of the extremity (the reimplanted part never achieves normal complete function and appearance) is a normal reaction that requires support. Many clients have dreams about their injury. Dreams that depict the tragedy again are normal. Dreams that depict harm of a greater magnitude than was actually experienced by the client are abnormal, and the client who has such dreams should be counseled by a psychologist. Praise and encouragement during rehabilitation are helpful.[4]

Teach the client to avoid activities and substances that cause vasoconstriction (which precipitates necrosis) for 2 weeks after surgery (e.g., tobacco, nicotine, cocaine, amphetamines). Exposure to air conditioning is also harmful. Advise the client to avoid cold and chilling (such as by wearing extra clothing and having the car prewarmed before entering to prevent vasoconstriction).

NAIL DISORDERS

Disorders of the nail can indicate any of several dermatologic processes. Potential causes include an infection of the nail (e.g., paronychia), a fungal infection of the nail (e.g., onychomycosis), a dermatologic disease with prominent nail changes (e.g., psoriasis), or pigmentary abnormalities of the nail (as in melanoma).

Unguis incarnatus (ingrown nail) is one of the most common nail conditions and is caused by improper nail trimming and by wearing tight or ill-fitting shoes. It primarily involves the great toe. A painful, warm inflammatory reaction results from excessive lateral growth of the nail into the nailfold. The nail acts as a foreign body, promoting granulation tissue. Decrease inflammation with warm soaks for 20 minutes several times a day. If the problem is minor, lifting the lateral portion of the nail by inserting a cotton wick prevents contact with the nailfold. Sometimes, the involved segment of the nailfold needs to be excised.

Paronychia, or infection around the nail, is characterized by red, shiny skin often associated with painful swelling. These infections frequently result from trauma, picking at the nail, or disorders such as dermatitis. Often these sites become secondarily infected with bacteria or fungi, which later involve the nail. As with ingrown toenail, warm soaks three or more times a day may reduce pressure and pain; however, incision and drainage of inflamed sites is frequently required. Samples for appropriate cultures of the purulent material and the nail should be obtained.

Onychomycosis refers to any fungal infection of the nail, whether due to dermatophytes or candidiasis. Prescribed topical or systemic antibiotic or antifungal therapy, with emphasis for compliance is important. Unfortunately, even with good compliance, recurrence of fungal infections in nails is frequent.

Clients should understand the importance of reducing trauma and irritation to involved nails by (1) trimming nails straight across to reduce further trauma, (2) avoiding overmanicuring or self-induced trauma, (3) limiting harsh chemical irritants such as abrasive cleansers and drying nail products, and (4) keeping the nails dry.

CONCLUSIONS

Skin disorders range from those that are a mere nuisance (such as dry skin) to life-threatening disorders (such as melanoma). Nurses frequently manage skin disorders independently; therefore a thorough knowledge of the use of topical medications and therapies is crucial. Because much of the needed skin care is provided by the client or a family member, the nurse must use excellent teaching skills to convey the necessary self-care information.

THINKING CRITICALLY *evolve*

1. You are caring for an older woman who has had a stroke that left her with residual paralysis on the left side. She also has a pressure ulcer on the left trochanter, in part because she lies on her left side all the time. While caring for her on Monday, you convince her to sit in a chair and to lie on her right side. When you care for her again on Thursday, the ulcer is twice as large and deeper. She refuses to turn to the right and says "I like lying on my left side." What can you do to help this client?

   Factors to Consider. What pressure-reduction methods should be instituted? Is there any harm in lying on a pressure ulcer? Why might she be at increased risk because of malnutrition?

2. The client is a 72-year-old white man who had undergone a wide excisional biopsy on his forearm to rule out squamous cell carcinoma. The next day the client calls the office complaining of pain at the surgery site. What additional questions need to be asked? What potential interventions might be necessary?

   Factors to Consider. What clinical manifestations would indicate an infection is present? Is age a factor in wound healing?

3. The client is an otherwise healthy 41-year-old woman who presented to the clinic with a week-long history of intensely itchy, erythematous red lesions under her breasts. The rash appears to be spreading,

---

evolve **Did you remember to check out the bonus material on the Evolve website and the CD-ROM, including free self-assessment exercises?**

http://evolve.elsevier.com/Black/medsurg/

and the centers of some of the lesions are seen to contain tiny pustules. In addition, the woman complains of a 12-pound weight loss over the past 6 months despite always feeling hungry and thirsty. She denies any medical problems and reports that she does not currently take systemic or topical medications.

Factors to Consider. What is the common cause of intertriginous dermatitis? What diagnostic study can determine the cause of the problem? What endocrine disorder is suggested by the history of skin rash, thirst, and weight loss?

Discussions for these questions can be found on the website and the CD-ROM.

BIBLIOGRAPHY

1. Aly, R., Bayles, C., & Forney, R. (2001). Treatments for common superficial fungal infections. *Dermatology Nursing, 13*(2), 91-101.

2. American Society of Plastic and Reconstructive Surgical Nurses. (1996). *Core curriculum for plastic and reconstructive surgical nurses* (2nd ed.). Pitman, NJ: Author.

3. Ayello, E.A., & Franz, R.A. (2003). Pressure ulcer prevention and treatment: Competency-based nursing curricula. *Dermatology Nursing, 15*(1), 44-55.

4. Berger, T.G., James, W.D., & Odom, R.B. (2000). *Andrews' diseases of the skin: Clinical dermatology* (9th ed.). Philadelphia: W. B. Saunders.

 5. Bergstrom, N., & Braden, B. (1987). The Braden Scale for predicting pressure sore risk. *Nursing Research, 36*(4), 205-210.

 6. Bergstrom, N., et al. (1994). *Treatment of pressure ulcers: Clinical practice guideline No. 15.* Rockville, MD: U.S. Department of Health and Human Services, Public Health Service, Agency for Health Care Policy and Research. AHCPR Pub. No. 95-0652.

 7. Bergstrom, N., et al. (1992). *Pressure ulcers in adults: Prediction and prevention.* Rockville, MD: U.S. Department of Health and Human Services, Public Health Service, Agency for Health Care Policy and Research. AHCPR Pub. No. 95-0050.

8. Bielory, L., & Kanuga, M. (2002). Complementary and alternative interventions in atopic dermatitis. In M. Boguniewicz (Ed.), *Immunology and Allergy Clinics of North America: Atopic Dermatitis, 22*(1), 153-173.

9. Black, J. (2000). Improving outcomes in the elderly after pressure ulcer repair. *Plastic Surgical Nursing 20* (3), 139-143, 170.

10. Boguniewicz, M., et al. (2003). Evolution in the treatment of atopic dermatitis: New approaches to managing a chronic skin disease. *Dermatology Nursing* (suppl.), *15* (4):3-19.

 11. Boguniewicz M., & Leung D.Y.M. (2001). Pathophysiologic mechanisms in atopic dermatitis. *Seminars in Cutaneous Medicine and Surgery, 20*(4), 217-225.

12. Boguniewicz M., & Nicol N.H. (2002). Conventional therapy for atopic dermatitis. In M. Boguniewicz (Ed.), *Immunology and allergy clinics of North America, atopic dermatitis* (pp. 107-124). Philadelphia: W. B. Saunders.

13. Bratcher, C., & Stover, B. (2001). Varicella-zoster virus: Infection, control, and prevention. *American Journal of Infection Control, 26*(3), 369-381.

14. Callen, J.P. (2000). *Color atlas of dermatology* (2nd ed.). Philadelphia: W. B. Saunders.

15. Camisa, C., & Warner, M. (1998). Treatment of pemphigus. *Dermatology Nursing, 10*(2), 115-118, 123-131.

16. DeLeo, V.A., Elsner, P., & Marks, J.G. Jr. (2002). *Contact & occupational dermatology* (3rd ed.). St. Louis: Mosby.

17. Duvic, M., et al. (2003). Analysis of long-term outcomes of combined modality therapy for cutaneous T-cell lymphoma. *Journal of the American Academy of Dermatology, 51*(1), 35-54.

18. Freedberg, I.M., Eisen, A.Z., & Wolff, K. (2003). *Fitzpatrick's dermatology in general medicine* (6th ed.). New York: McGraw-Hill, Health Professions Division.

19. Gilchrest, B.A. (2002). *Geriatric dermatology part II.* Philadelphia: W. B. Saunders.

20. Greaves, M.W., & Leung, D.Y.M. (2000). *Allergic skin disease: A multidisciplinary approach.* New York: Marcel Dekker.

21. Heddens, C. (2001). Belt lipectomy: Procedure and outcomes. *Plastic Surgical Nursing 21*(4), 185-189, 199.

22. Hill, M.J. (2003). *Dermatology nursing essentials: A core curriculum—Dermatology Nurses' Association* (2nd ed.) Pitman, NJ: Anthony J. Jannetti.

23. Kanzler, M.H., & Swetter, S.M. (2003). Malignant melanoma. *Journal of the American Academy of Dermatology, 48*(5), 781-783.

24. Leone, G., Rolston, K., & Spaulding, G. (2003). Alefacept for chronic plaque psoriasis: A selective therapy with long-lasting disease remissions and an encouraging safety profile. *Dermatology Nursing, 15*(3), 216-220.

25. Madison, L.K. (2001). Shingles update: Common questions in caring for a patient with shingles. *Dermatology Nursing, 13*(1), 51-55.

26. Menter, M.A. (Ed.). (2003). Psoriasis for the clinician: A new therapeutics era ("the biologics") beckons. *Journal of the American Academy of Dermatology, 51*(suppl.), 39-142.

26a. Naeyaert, J.M, & Brochez, L. (2003). Dysplastic nevi. *New England Journal of Medicine, 349*(23), 2233-2240.

27. Nicol N.H. (2003). Dermatitis/eczemas. In MJ Hill (Ed.), *Dermatologic nursing essentials: A core curriculum* (2nd ed., pp. 103-116). Pitman, NJ: Anthony J. Jannetti.

28. Nicol N.H. (2000). Managing atopic dermatitis in children and adults. *Nurse Practitioner, 25,* 58-79.

29. Nicol N.H., & Baumeister L. (1997). Topical corticosteroid therapy: Considerations for prescribing and use. *Lippincott's Primary Care Practice, 1*(1), 62-69.

30. Nicol, N.H., Boguniewicz, M. (1999). Understanding and treating atopic dermatitis. *Nurse Practitioner Forum 10*(2), 48-55.

31. Noel, S., & Strohl, R. (2002). The management of high-risk melanoma: Staging, treatment, and nursing issues. *Dermatology Nursing, 14*(6), 363-371.

32. Nunley, J.R. (2000). Cutaneous manifestations of HIV and HCV. *Dermatology Nursing, 12*(3), 163-173.

33. Pinnell, S.R. (2003). Cutaneous photodamage, oxidative stress, and topical antioxidant protection. *Journal of the American Academy of Dermatology, 48*(1), 1-22.

34. Smith, P., Black, J., & Black, S. (1999). Infected pressure ulcers in the long-term care facility. *Infection Control and Hospital Epidemiology, 20*(5), 358-361.

35. Stulberg, D.L., Penrod, M.A., & Blatny, R.A. (2002). Common bacterial skin infections. *American Family Physician, 66*(1), 119-124.

36. Trioa, C. (2002). Promoting positive outcomes in obese patients. *Plastic Surgical Nursing 22*(1), 10-17, 28.

Chapter 52

Management of Clients with Burn Injury

Pamela Cornwell
Catherine Gregory

evolve

Web Enhancements

http://evolve.elsevier.com/Black/medsurg/

Ethical Issues in Nursing
Should the Severely Burned Client Be Allowed to Refuse Treatment?

Appendix C
Laboratory Values of Clinical Importance in Medical-Surgical Nursing

Injuries that result from direct contact with or exposure to any thermal, chemical, or radiation source are termed *burns*. Burn injuries occur when energy from a heat source is transferred to the tissues of the body. The depth of injury is related to the temperature and the duration of exposure or contact.

Burn care has improved in recent decades, resulting in a lower mortality rate for victims of burn injuries.[41] Dedicated burn centers have been established in which multidisciplinary burn team members work together to care for the burn client and family. Advances in prehospital and inpatient care have contributed to survival. However, despite these advances, many people are still injured and die each year from burns. In the United States, estimates range from 1.4 to 2 million burn injuries each year, resulting in 45,000 hospitalizations and 4,500 deaths annually.[5,43]

Etiology

Burn injuries are categorized according to the mechanism of injury.

Thermal Burns

Thermal burns are caused by exposure to or contact with flame, hot liquids, semiliquids (e.g., steam), semi-solids (e.g., tar), or hot objects. Specific examples of thermal burns are those sustained in residential fires, explosive automobile accidents, scald injuries, clothing ignition, and ignition of poorly stored flammable liquids.

Chemical Burns

Chemical burns are caused by tissue contact with strong acids, alkalis, or organic compounds. The concentration, volume, and type of chemical, as well as the duration of contact, determine the severity of a chemical injury. Chemical burns can result from contact with certain household cleaning agents and various chemicals used in industry, agriculture, and the military. Chemical injuries to the eyes and inhalation of chemical fumes are particularly serious.

Electrical Burns

Electrical burn injuries are caused by heat that is generated by the electrical energy as it passes through the body. Electrical injuries can result from contact with exposed or faulty electrical wiring or high-voltage power lines. People struck by lightning also sustain electrical injury.

The extent of injury is influenced by the duration of contact, the intensity of the current (voltage), the type of

evolve Be sure to check out the bonus material on the Evolve website and the CD-ROM, including free self-assessment exercises.
http://evolve.elsevier.com/Black/medsurg/

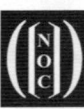

Nursing Outcomes Classification (NOC)
for Nursing Diagnoses—Clients with Burns

Acute Pain and Chronic Pain
Comfort Level
Pain Control
Pain: Disruptive Effects
Pain Level
Risk for Infection
Immobility Consequences: Physiologic
Immune Status
Knowledge: Infection Control
Treatment Behavior: Illness or Injury

Deficient Fluid Volume
Electrolyte and Acid-Base Balance
Fluid Balance
Hydration
Nutritional Status: Food and Fluid
  Intake

Deficient Knowledge
Knowledge: Health Resources
Knowledge: Illness Care
Knowledge: Infection Control
Knowledge: Medication
Knowledge: Personal Safety
Knowledge: Prescribed Activity
Knowledge: Treatment Procedures
Knowledge: Treatment Regimen

Disabled Family Coping
Family Coping
Family Normalization

Disturbed Personal Identity
Self-Esteem
Body Image
Hope
Mood Equilibrium

Hypothermia
Thermoregulation

Imbalanced Nutrition: Less Than Body Requirements
Nutritional Status
Nutritional Status: Food and Fluid
  Intake
Nutritional Status: Nutrient Intake

Impaired Gas Exchange
Electrolyte and Acid-Base Balance
Respiratory Status Gas Exchange
Respiratory Status: Ventilation
Tissue Perfusion: Pulmonary

Impaired Physical Mobility
Ambulation: Walking
Ambulation: Wheelchair
Body Positioning: Self-Initiated
Joint Movement: Active
Mobility Level
Transfer Performance

Impaired Skin Integrity
Tissue Integrity: Skin and Mucous
  Membranes

Wound Healing: Primary Intention
Wound Healing: Secondary Intention

Impaired Tissue Integrity
Tissue Integrity: Skin and Mucous
  Membranes

Ineffective Airway Clearance
Aspiration Control
Respiratory Status: Airway Patency
Respiratory Status: Gas Exchange
Respiratory Status: Ventilation

Ineffective Tissue Perfusion: Peripheral
Sensory Function: Cutaneous
Tissue Integrity: Skin and Mucous
  Membranes
Tissue Perfusion: Peripheral

Ineffective Tissue Perfusion: Renal
Electrolyte and Acid-Base Balance
Fluid Balance
Hydration
Urinary Elimination
Vital Signs Status

Risk for Infection
Immune Status
Tissue Integrity: Skin and Mucous
  Membranes

---

current (direct or alternating), the pathway of the current, and the resistance of the tissues as the electrical current passes through the body. Contact with electrical current of greater than 40 volts is potentially dangerous; however, current of greater than 1000 volts is considered to be high-voltage current and is associated with extensive tissue damage.[16]

Radiation Burns

Radiation burns are the least common type of burn injury and are caused by exposure to a radioactive source. These types of injuries have been associated with nuclear radiation accidents, the use of ionizing radiation in industry, and therapeutic irradiation. Sunburn, from prolonged exposure to ultraviolet rays (solar radiation), is also considered to be a type of radiation burn.

The amount of radioactive energy received after exposure depends on the distance the person is from the source of the radiation, the strength of the radiation source, the duration of exposure, the extent of body surface area exposed, and the amount of shielding between the source and the person. An acute localized radiation injury appears similar to a cutaneous thermal injury and

is characterized by skin erythema, edema, and pain. In contrast, whole-body radiation exposure manifestations may begin with nausea, vomiting, diarrhea, and fatigue, continuing with a headache and fever within hours of exposure. As time proceeds, hemopoietic and gastrointestinal complications are seen. The severity of manifestations is dose-dependent.[43]

Inhalation Injury

Exposure to asphyxiants and smoke commonly occurs with flame injuries, particularly if the victim was trapped in an enclosed, smoke-filled space (e.g., in a residential fire). Victims who die at the scene of a fire usually do so as a result of hypoxia and carbon monoxide poisoning.[12]

The pulmonary pathophysiologic changes that occur with inhalation injury are multifactorial and relate to the severity and type of smoke or gases inhaled. Exposure to asphyxiants, smoke poisoning, and direct thermal (heat) injury to lung tissue constitute the three facets of an inhalation injury. However, not all of these injury components may be present in the client suffering from an inhalation injury.[10,50]

Risk Factors

Data collected from the National Burn Information Exchange reveal that 75% of all burn injuries result from the actions of the victim, with many of these injuries occurring in the home environment. Most at risk to suffer serious burn injuries are young children, older adults, and people with mental or physical limitations.[43] College students are also at risk due to lack of awareness, cooking in dormitory rooms, and rigging things together.

Contact with scalding liquids is the leading cause of burn injury.[12] Toddlers (children 2 to 4 years of age) suffer more scald injuries than persons in any other age group. Scald injuries are frequently the result of mishaps in the performance of everyday tasks such as bathing and cooking. Overturned coffeepots, cooking pans spilling hot liquid and grease, overheated foods, liquids cooked in microwave ovens, and hot tap water have been identified as specific causes.[49] To reduce the incidence of scald injuries, the Consumer Products Safety Commission and Underwriters Laboratory has recommended that the maximum temperature on the thermostats of hot water heaters be lowered and that a warning label identifying the potential for injury be affixed to hot water heaters. Legislation requiring public buildings to lower water temperature to 120° F (48.8° C) has been successful in reducing scald injuries.[41] In addition, a thermostatic control system (antiscald device) has been developed that, when installed at the faucet or shower head, shuts off the flow of water when the temperature rises above a predetermined temperature, typically 119° F (48.3° C).

Direct contact with flame in the young adult (17 to 25 years of age) is the second leading cause of burn injury.[12] Flame injuries that are frequently seen in this category are burns to the hands and face that result from an explosion of flammable liquid, known as flash burns. Actions such as using gasoline to start or accelerate a fire and priming a carburetor on an automobile or boat can result in flash explosions.

Clothing ignition during routine meal preparation has also been cited as a leading cause of burn injury, particularly in the older population.[49] Synthetic fabrics are especially dangerous, because they melt and adhere to the skin, causing prolonged contact with the heat. Another age group at risk for clothing ignition is the pediatric population. During the early 1970s, the fatality rate among young children burned from ignition of sleepwear was significant. In 1975 it was mandated that children's sleepwear, sizes 0 to 6X, pass a standard flame test. This action significantly lowered mortality associated with children's clothing ignition.[45] The mandate for sleepwear to pass a flame test has since been repealed, and testing is no longer be required. Since the repeal, Wilson and Bailie[55] have reported a rash of clothing-related flame burns occurring in 2- to 11-year-old girls. See Box 52-1 for burn injury prevention in the home.

Structural fires account for only 5% of burn-related hospital admissions; however, they are responsible for the greatest number of burn-related deaths.[12] Approximately 30% of all burn-related deaths are a result of structural fires,[10] seemingly from the associated smoke inhalation.[50] Ignition from cigarettes is the nation's largest single cause of all fire deaths.[6] In approximately 10% of cases of residential fire deaths, the fires were caused by children playing with matches or other ignition sources.[41] Additionally, faulty chimneys, flue vents, fixed heating units, fireplaces, central heating systems, wood-burning stoves, ignition of wood-shingled roofs, as well as human error, all have been implicated as causes of residential fires that have resulted in deaths.

Of primary importance in reducing injuries and deaths from residential fires is the presence of a working smoke detector and fire extinguisher. It has been estimated that the risk of dying in a residential fire is reduced 50% when an operating smoke detector is in place.[6]

Pathophysiology

The pathophysiologic changes that occur following a cutaneous burn injury depend on the extent or size of the burn. For smaller burns, the body's response to injury is localized to the burned area. However, with more extensive burns (i.e., involving 25% or more of the total body surface area [TBSA]), the body's response to injury is systemic and proportional to the extent of the injury.[43] The clinical manifestations of burn trauma evolve in dramatic fashion over the postinjury clinical course. Extensive burn injuries affect all major systems of the body. The systemic response to burn injury is typically biphasic, characterized by early hypofunction followed later by hyperfunction of each of the organ systems.

BOX 52-1 *Residential Burn Injury Prevention Recommendations*

In the kitchen:
- Turn pot handles toward the back of the stove.
- Purchase a stove with controls on the front or side to reduce the likelihood of clothing ignition as one reaches across the hot elements.
- Place a screen around any heating appliance to function as a barrier.

In the home:
- Adjust the thermostat setting on the water heater to produce a temperature no higher than 120° F (48.8° C).
- Install water temperature–regulating valves (anti-scald device) that obstruct the flow of water when the water temperature exceeds a preset level.

Direct Injury to the Skin

With direct injury to the skin, heat from an external source is conducted to the skin, where it denatures (devitalizes) the cells. The amount of damage depends on the length of exposure to the heat and the temperature. At sustained temperatures of 40° to 44° C (104° F to 111.2° F), various cellular enzyme systems and cellular systems fail. The sodium-potassium pump fails, which leads to cellular edema. As the temperature rises to 44° C, cell necrosis occurs. In addition, free radicals are produced, increasing cell damage. The processes of cellular damage continue until the heat source is withdrawn and cooling processes return the cell temperature to a tolerable range.

Protein destruction occurs in tissues destroyed by heat. The directly damaged skin is coagulated and fully destroyed. This area of burned tissue is called the *zone of coagulation* (Figure 52-1) and represents the area of direct heat injury. In surrounding skin, which has been exposed to heat, the tissue is edematous and has impaired blood flow. This middle zone is called the *zone of stasis* and consists of skin that initially is viable but may also eventually die of ischemia. The outer ring of tissue injury is called the *zone of hyperemia* and consists of tissue that is inflamed and vasodilated.

Some types of burn create unique patterns of injury. In electrical injuries, heat is generated as the electricity travels through the body, resulting in internal tissue damage.[20] The concept of "the tip of the iceberg" is helpful to understand these injuries. For instance, only a very small percentage of total injury from an electrical burn can be seen from the body's surface. Cutaneous burn injuries may appear negligible, but muscle and soft tissue damage may be extensive, particularly with high-voltage electrical injuries. The voltage, type of current (direct or alternating), contact site, and duration of contact are important considerations because they may affect morbidity. Electricity seeks ground as it exits the body; en route, it creates heat and may pass though vital organs. Alternating current (AC) is more dangerous than direct current (DC). AC produces more heat-related injury and is often associated with cardiopulmonary arrest, ventricular fibrillation, tetanic muscle contractions, and long bone or vertebral compression fracture. The risk of acute renal failure is noteworthy in clients following an electrical injury. Hemoglobin, released from heat-damaged erythrocytes together with myoglobin, the protein that supplies muscles with oxygen, is released in significant quantities into the bloodstream after deep burn injuries involving muscle damage. These substances pass through the glomeruli and are excreted in urine. However, these materials may precipitate and obstruct the renal tubules, causing renal damage unless a brisk urine output is maintained.[43] In addition, victims of electrical injuries may have fallen from the point of electrical contact and sustained associated injuries. Cataract formation is also associated with high-voltage electrical injury, especially when contact points are on the head or neck. In chemical burns, systemic toxic effects may result from cutaneous absorption of the offending agent. Organ failure and even death have resulted from prolonged contact with and absorption of different chemicals.

Fluid Shifts

Immediately following a burn injury, vasoactive substances (catecholamines, histamine, serotonin, leukotrienes, kinins, and prostaglandins) are released from the injured tissues.[23] These substances initiate changes in capillary integrity, allowing plasma to seep into surrounding tissues (Figure 52-2). Direct damage to vessels from heat further increases capillary permeability, which permits sodium ions to enter the cell and potassium ions to exit. The overall effect of these changes is creation of an osmotic gradient, which leads to increases in intercellular and interstitial fluid and further depletes intravascular fluid volumes. The vasoactive substances exert their effects both locally (in the area of injury) and systemically. The burn-injured client's hemodynamic balance, metabolism, and immune status are altered.

The body responds initially by shunting blood toward the brain and heart and away from all other body organs. Prolonged lack of blood flow to these other organs is detrimental. The degree of damage that results depends on the basal needs of the body organ. Some organs can survive for only a few hours without nutrient

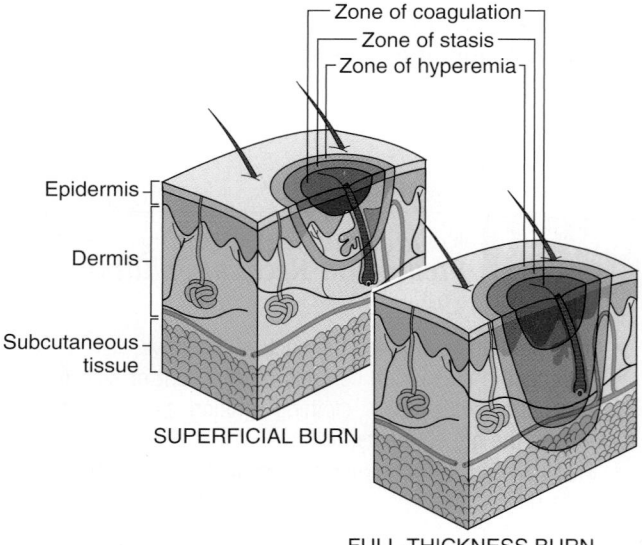

FIGURE 52-1 Zone of tissue injury. The zone of coagulation is the center of the burn wound and represents actual tissue damage. The zone of stasis is the surrounding area and represents areas of potential tissue loss. The outer ring is the zone of hyperemia and is unburned tissue that is inflamed.

blood supply. The lack of renal blood flow decreases glomerular filtration rate, leading to oliguria (low urine output).[43] If fluid resuscitation is delayed or inadequate, hypovolemia progresses, and acute renal failure may occur. However, with adequate fluid resuscitation and an increase in cardiac output, renal blood flow returns to normal. After resuscitation, the body begins to reabsorb the edema fluid and eliminate it through diuresis.

Blood flow to the mesenteric bed is also diminished initially, leading to the development of intestinal ileus and gastrointestinal dysfunction in clients with burns of greater than 25% TBSA.[41] With the reduction in blood flow to the gastric mucosa, ischemic changes to the upper gastrointestinal tract occur, which slows production of the protective mucous lining, resulting in small, superficial erosions to the stomach and duodenum. If the gastrointestinal tract is left untreated and unprotected by antacids or histamine H_2-receptor antagonists, the erosions can progress to ulcerations—called *Curling's ulcers* in burn injured clients—and gastrointestinal bleeding.

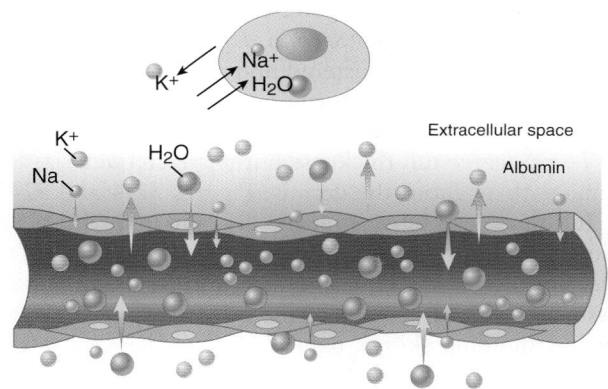

Fluid and electrolyte shift during burn shock

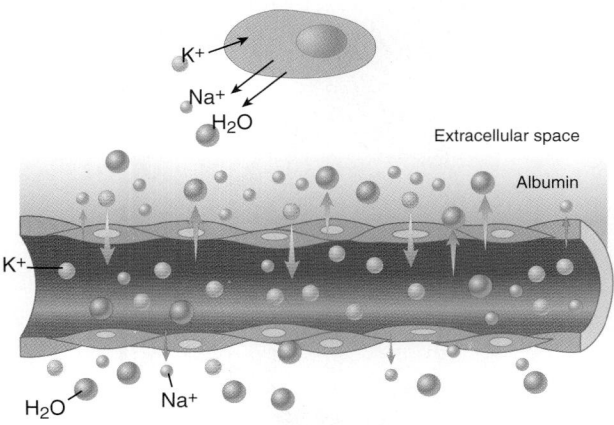

Fluid and electrolyte shift after burn shock

FIGURE 52-2 Changes in capillary permeability allow plasma to seep into interstitial spaces. In addition, the sodium pump fails and sodium remains in the cell. There is a corresponding increase in serum potassium.

Pulmonary System

Minute ventilation is often normal or slightly decreased early after a burn injury. Following fluid resuscitation, an increase in minute ventilation—manifested by hyperventilation—may occur especially if the client is fearful, anxious, or in pain. This hyperventilation is the result of an increase in both respiratory rate and tidal volume and appears to be the result of the hypermetabolism that is seen after burn injury. It typically peaks in the second postinjury week and then gradually returns to normal as the burn wound heals or is closed by grafting.[41]

Pulmonary vascular resistance may increase slightly, and lung compliance may decrease. The changes in lung compliance cause a proportionate increase in the work of breathing; however, these changes are typically small, and in the absence of any pulmonary parenchymal (tissue) damage, they require no specialized treatment.

Inhalation Injury. Exposure to asphyxiants is the most common cause of early mortality from inhalation injury.[12] Carbon monoxide (CO), a common asphyxiant, is produced when organic substances (e.g., wood or coal) burn. It is a colorless, odorless, and tasteless gas that has an affinity for the body's hemoglobin that is 200 times greater than that of oxygen. With inhalation of CO, the oxygen molecules are displaced, and CO binds to hemoglobin to form carboxyhemoglobin (COHb). Tissue hypoxia occurs from an overall decrease in the blood's oxygen-delivering capability.

Direct heat injury to the upper airway results from inhalation of the air heated by fire. The heat immediately produces injury to the airway, which results in edema, erythema, and ulceration. Thermal burns to the lower airways of the pulmonary system are rare because of the protective reflex closure of the glottis and the ability of the respiratory tract to exchange heat effectively. However, thermal burns to the lower airways can occur with the inhalation of steam or explosive gases or with aspiration of scalding liquids.

Smoke poisoning results from the inhalation of the byproducts of combustion: noxious chemicals and particulate matter. The pulmonary response includes a localized inflammatory reaction, a decrease in bronchial ciliary action, and a decrease in alveolar surfactant. Mucosal edema occurs in the smaller airways. After several hours, sloughing of the tracheobronchial epithelium may occur, and hemorrhagic tracheobronchitis may develop. Adult (acute) respiratory distress syndrome may follow.[12]

Myocardial Depression

Some research investigators have suggested that a myocardial depressant factor exists and circulates in the early postinjury period. More recently, a combination of inflammatory mediators and hormones has been suggested as the cause of myocardial depression occurring after the injury.

Altered Skin Integrity

The burn wound itself exhibits pathophysiologic changes caused by disruption of the skin and alterations to the tissue beneath the surface. The skin, nerve endings, sweat glands, and hair follicles injured by burn lose normal functioning. Most important, the skin's barrier function is lost. Intact skin normally keeps bacteria from entering the body and body fluids from seeping out, controls evaporation, and maintains body warmth. With destruction of the skin in burn injury, mechanisms for maintaining normal body temperature can be altered, the risk of infection from invasion of bacteria increases, and evaporative water loss increases. Depending on the depth of the injury, nerve endings either become exposed, resulting in pain and discomfort until wound closure, or are damaged, leaving the innervated area insensate, with potential for permanent impairment of ability to sense touch, pressure, and pain.

Immunosuppression

Immune system function is depressed following burn injury. Depression of lymphocyte activity, a decrease in immunoglobulin production, suppression of complement activity, and an alteration in neutrophil and macrophage functioning are evident following extensive burn injuries. In addition, the burn injury disrupts the body's primary barrier to infection, the skin. Together these changes result in an increased risk of infection and life-threatening sepsis.

Psychological Response

Numerous psychological and emotional responses to burn injuries have been identified, ranging from fear to psychosis.[7] A victim's response is influenced by age, per-sonality, cultural and ethnic background, the extent and location of the injury, and the resulting impact on body image. In addition, separation from family and friends during hospitalization and the change in the client's normal role and responsibilities affect the reaction to burn trauma. Four stages in the psychosocial response to burn trauma have been described: (1) impact, (2) retreat or withdrawal, (3) acknowledgment, and (4) the reconstructive period.[25]

Clinical Manifestations

Degree of Injury

Depending on the skin layers damaged, burn wounds are termed either *partial-thickness* burns or *full-thickness* burns. Burn wounds are also classified as first-, second-, third-, or fourth-degree burns. Partial-thickness burns involve injury to the epidermis and portions of the dermis (Figure 52-3). *First-degree* partial-thickness burns are superficial and painful and appear red. They heal on their own by epidermal cell regeneration within about 3 to 7 days. Sunburn is a good example of a first-degree partial-thickness burn. *Second-degree* partial-thickness burns appear wet or blistered and are extremely painful but can heal on their own (that is, without skin grafting) if they are small and do not become infected.

Third-degree full-thickness burns are characterized by damage throughout the dermis (Figures 52-4 and 52-5). A full-thickness burn appears dry and may be black, brown, white, or ivory. The denatured skin is called *eschar* (pronounced "ES-car"). The burned tissue is painless as a result of damage to the nerve endings; however, the surrounding skin is painful. Unless the area is very small (the size of a half-dollar), the full-thickness burn

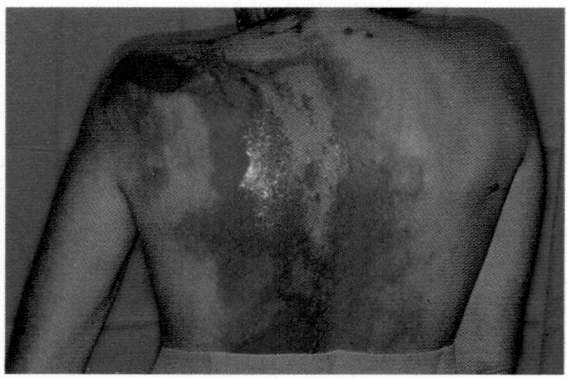

FIGURE 52-3 Partial-thickness burn injury (second-degree burn).

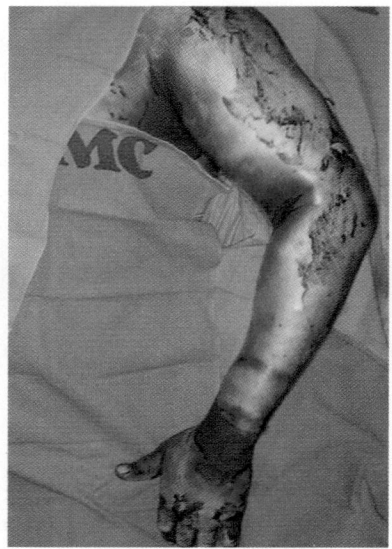

FIGURE 52-4 Full-thickness burn injury (third-degree burn).

must be skin-grafted to heal. The appearance of the burn relative to the depth of injury is described in Figure 52-6.

Fourth-degree full-thickness burns involve skin, fat, muscle, and sometimes bone. The skin appears charred or may be completely burned away. Areas of a fourth-

degree burn require extensive surgical debridement and grafting. Amputations are common in these deep injuries.

In addition to altered physical appearance, the loss of skin leads to other problems. Hypothermia results from loss of body heat through the burn wound and is characterized by a core body temperature below 98.6° F. Hypothermia is extremely harmful because it leads to shivering, which in turn increases oxygen consumption and caloric demands.

The evaporative water loss through the burn contributes to the client's diminished fluid volume and compromised hydration status. Evaporative losses not compensated for by fluid replacement are evidenced by a low blood pressure, decreased urine output, dry mucous membranes, and poor skin turgor.

Fluid and Electrolyte Imbalance

Hyponatremia, hypernatremia, and hyperkalemia are common electrolyte abnormalities that affect the burn-injured client at different points in the recovery process. Extensive burns (greater than 25% TBSA) result in generalized body edema affecting both burned and non-burned tissues and in a decrease in circulating intravascular blood volume (Figure 52-7).[12,45] Hematocrit levels are elevated in the first 24 hours after injury, demonstrating hemoconcentration from the loss of intravascular fluid. In addition, evaporative fluid losses through the burn wound are 4 to 20 times greater than normal and remain elevated until complete wound closure is ob-

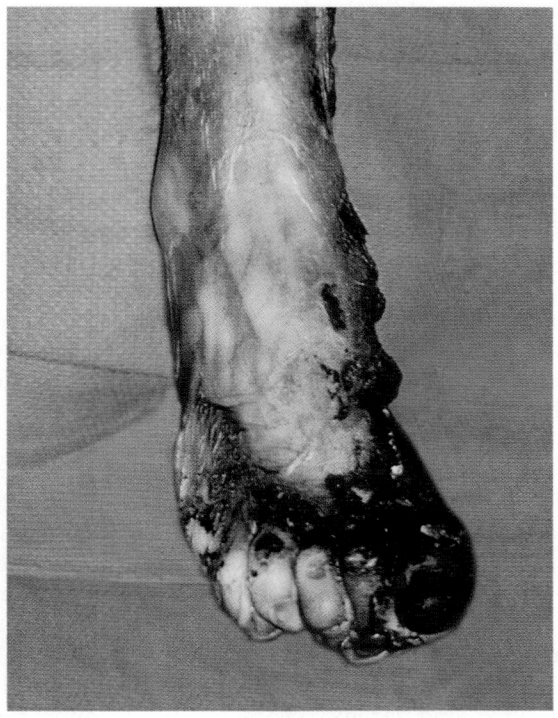

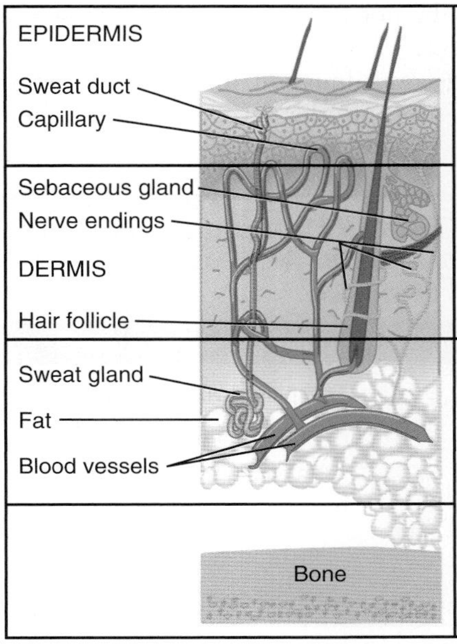

FIGURE 52-5 Full-thickness burn injury (fourth-degree burn).

			WOUND APPEARANCE	WOUND SENSATION	COURSE OF HEALING
EPIDERMIS Sweat duct Capillary	PARTIAL-THICKNESS BURN	1st-degree	Epidermis remains intact and without blisters. Erythema; skin blanches with pressure.	Painful	Discomfort lasts 48-72 hours. Desquamation in 3-7 days
Sebaceous gland Nerve endings DERMIS Hair follicle		2nd-degree	Wet, shiny, weeping surface Blisters Wound blanches with pressure.	Painful Very sensitive to touch, air currents	Superficial partial-thickness burn heals in < 21 days. Deep partial-thickness burn requires > 21 days for healing. Healing rates vary with burn depth and presence/absence of infection.
Sweat gland Fat Blood vessels	FULL-THICKNESS BURN	3rd-degree	Color variable (i.e., deep red, white, black, brown) Surface dry Thrombosed vessels visible No blanching	Insensate (↓ pinprick sensation)	Autografting required for healing
Bone		4th-degree	Color variable Charring visible in deepest areas Extremity movement limited	Insensate	Amputation of extremities likely Autografting required for healing

FIGURE 52-6 Burn injury classification according to depth of injury.

tained. The result is a decrease in organ perfusion. If the intravascular space is not replenished with intravenous (IV) fluids, hypovolemic (burn) shock and, ultimately, death ensue for the victim of an extensive burn.[2,12,23,33,52]

Urine output for the adult client receiving insufficient fluid replacement following a major burn injury diminishes to less than 0.5 ml/kg/hr. Physical findings of the urine sample demonstrate dehydration, characterized by dark amber, concentrated urine and elevated specific gravity. Laboratory tests reveal elevated blood urea nitrogen (BUN) levels until the client is adequately hydrated.

Manifestations of decreased gastrointestinal motility following major burn injuries include the absence of bowel sounds, stool, or flatus; nausea and vomiting; and abdominal distention. After adequate fluid resuscitation,

gastrointestinal motility returns, signaled by a return of hunger and appetite, bowel sounds, flatus, and stool production.

At approximately 18 to 36 hours after burn injury, capillary membrane integrity begins to be restored. The initial increase in hematocrit seen early after injury falls to below normal by the third or fourth day after injury owing to red blood cell loss and damage incurred at the time of injury. Over the ensuing days and weeks, the body begins to reabsorb the edema fluid, and the excess fluid is excreted via diuresis (see Figure 52-7).

Alterations in Respiration

The client may exhibit tachypnea following the burn injury. Arterial blood gas analysis may demonstrate a relatively normal arterial partial pressure of oxygen (PaO_2), with oxygen saturation lower than expected relative to the PO_2. Diagnosis is made by measuring the COHb level in the blood. The clinical manifestations of acute CO poisoning are directly related to the level of COHb saturation and relative degree of tissue hypoxia (Table 52-1). The onset of clinical manifestations typically does not occur until COHb levels reach 15%. Initial manifestations are related to decreased cerebral tissue oxygenation and are neurologic in nature. The neurologic problems caused by CO exposure can lead to progressive and permanent cerebral dysfunction.

Thermal burns to the upper airways (mouth, nasopharynx, and larynx) characteristically appear erythematous and edematous, with mucosal blisters or ulcerations. Increasing mucosal edema can lead to upper airway obstruction, typically between the first 24 and 48 hours after injury. Clinical manifestations, including stridor, dyspnea, increased work of breathing, and eventually cyanosis, may be noted when critical narrowing of the airway is present.[10,26,39]

Physical findings on admission indicative of smoke exposure include soot on the face and nares, facial

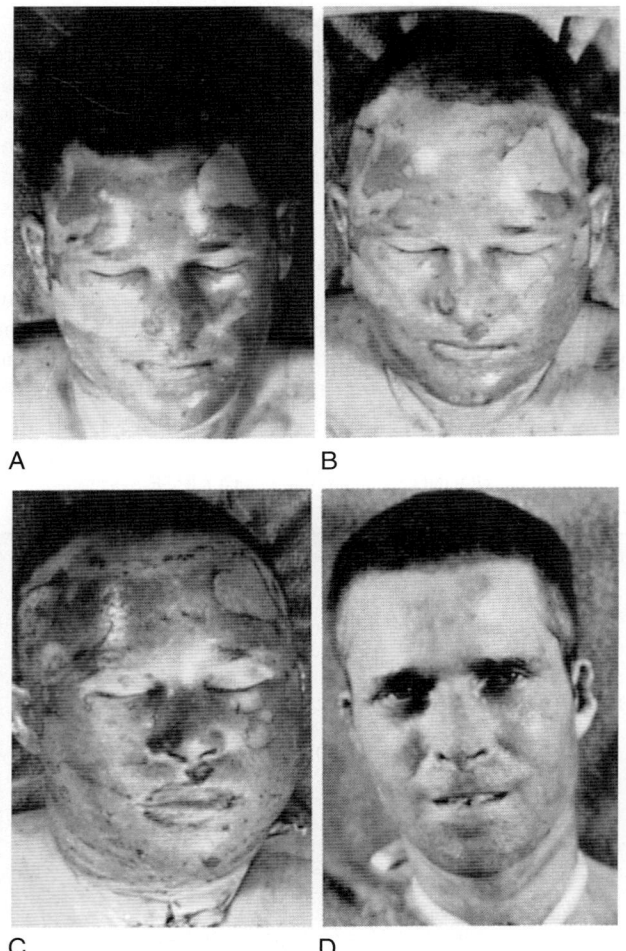

FIGURE 52-7 Edema formation after a burn injury to the face and neck. Edema worsens over the first 24 to 48 hours after burn injury. **A,** At 3 hours after burn. **B,** At 8 hours after the burn. **C,** At 24 hours after burn, when edema has typically maximized. **D,** Complete healing after 40 days. (From Artz, C.P., et al. [1979]. *Burns: A team approach*. Philadelphia: W.B. Saunders.)

TABLE 52-1	*Clinical Manifestations of Carbon Monoxide (CO) Poisoning*
CO Level (%)	**Clinical Manifestations**
5-10	Impaired visual acuity
11-20	Flushing, headache
21-30	Nausea, impaired dexterity
31-40	Vomiting, dizziness, syncope
41-50	Tachypnea, tachycardia
>50	Coma, death

Modified from Cioffi, W.G., & Rue, L.W. (1991). Diagnosis and treatment of inhalation injuries. *Critical Care Clinics of North America, 3*(2), 195.

burns, soot in the sputum, coughing, and wheezing. The manifestations of tracheobronchitis typically do not present until 24 to 48 hours after injury. Early manifestations consist of bronchospasm evidenced as wheezing and bronchorrhea. Lung compliance is decreased, causing an increased work of breathing. Impaired clearance of secretions accentuates the problem. Normally, ventilation and perfusion are matched by equal volumes of air and blood at the alveolar-capillary level. The client with smoke inhalation exhibits pathophysiologic changes that reduce alveolar ventilation, causing a ventilation-perfusion ($\dot{V}/\dot{Q}$) mismatch, which in turn impairs gas exchange.[13,28]

Decreased Cardiac Output

Following a major burn injury, heart rate and peripheral vascular resistance increase in response to the release of catecholamines and to the relative hypovolemia, but initial cardiac output decreases (hypofunction). At approximately 24 hours after burn injury in clients receiving adequate fluid resuscitation, cardiac output returns to normal and then increases (2 to 2.5 times normal) to meet the hypermetabolic needs of the body (hyperfunction). This change in cardiac output occurs even before circulating intravascular volume levels are restored to normal. Arterial blood pressure is normal or slightly elevated unless severe hypovolemia exists. The decreased cardiac output seen initially after burn injury is evidenced by a decreased blood pressure, decreased urine output, weak peripheral pulses, and if monitored via a pulmonary artery catheter, a cardiac output less than 4 L/min, cardiac index of less than 2.5 L/min, and systemic vascular resistance of less than 900 dynes.[6,12]

Pain Responses

The client experiences substantial pain as a result of the burn wound and exposed nerve endings from lack of skin integrity.[28,30] Burn victims typically describe two types of pain resulting from their injury: background pain and procedural pain. Background pain is experienced when the client is at rest or engages in non–procedure-related activities, such as shifting position in bed, or with chest or abdominal wall movements that occur with deep breathing or coughing. Background pain is described as continuous in nature and low in intensity, typically lasting for the duration of the clinical course.[11] Procedural pain is experienced during the performance of therapeutic measures commonly used in burn care. Nearly 52% of clients report moderate to severe pain during burn wound debridement.[13] Procedural pain is described as acute and high in intensity. Clinical responses to pain may include an increase in blood pressure, heart rate, and respiratory rate and dilated pupils, rigid muscle tone, and guarded positioning.

Altered Level of Consciousness

Rarely do burn-injured clients suffer neurologic damage. The client with a major burn injury is most often awake and alert on admission to the hospital. If agitation develops in the immediate postinjury period, the client may be suffering from hypoxemia or hypovolemia and needs further assessment for identifying the origin of these changes. When an alteration in level of consciousness is present, it is most often related to neurologic trauma (e.g., fall, motor vehicle accident), impaired perfusion to the brain, hypoxemia (as from a closed-space fire), inhalation injury (as from exposure to asphyxiates or other toxic materials from the fire), electrical burn injury, or the effects of drugs present in the body at the time of injury.

Clients with associated head trauma may have scalp lacerations, swelling, tenderness, or ecchymosis. Level of consciousness may fluctuate between intervals of lucidity followed by rapid deterioration. Pupils may be of unequal size. Neurologic manifestations may include headache, dizziness, memory loss, confusion or loss of consciousness, disorientation, visual changes, hallucinations, combativeness, and coma.

Psychological Alterations

The period of *impact* begins immediately after injury and is characterized by shock, disbelief, and feelings of being overwhelmed. The client and family members may be aware of what is happening but may be coping with the situation poorly. During this period, families of critically ill clients have a need for assurance, proximity to the injured person, and information. Specifically, families want to know how the client is being treated, specific facts about the client's progress, and why certain procedures are being done.

Retreat is characterized by repression, withdrawal, denial, and suppression. Although seemingly destructive, these coping strategies may be protective in that they allow the client to maintain an intact psyche.

The third phase, *acknowledgment,* begins when the client accepts the injury and the resultant change in body image. Mourning of actual or perceived losses may be apparent. During this phase, clients may benefit from meeting with other burn-injured clients in one-on-one contact or group support meetings.

The final phase, the *reconstructive period,* begins when the client and family accept the limitations imposed by the injury and begin to plan realistically for the future.

Outcome Management

The burn client undergoes a wide range of physiologic and metabolic changes in response to the burn injury. To accomplish the best outcomes, it is essential to have a clear understanding of the pathophysiologic process and the necessary treatment modifications needed over the entire course of burn treatment. Three distinct periods or phases of treatment can be defined in the care of the seriously burned client: the emergent, the acute, and the rehabilitation phases.

EMERGENT PHASE

The emergent phase of burn injury consists of the time between the initial injury and 36 to 48 hours after injury. This phase ends when fluid resuscitation is complete. During this phase, life-threatening airway and breathing problems are of major concern. It is also characterized by the development of hypovolemia, which results as capillaries leak fluid from the intravascular spaces into the interstitial spaces, causing edema. Although the fluid remains in the body, it is unable to contribute to maintaining adequate circulation, because it is no longer in the vascular space. The burn itself, except for initial assessment of severity and depth and, in certain cases, a procedure (escharotomy) performed to restore perfusion to areas exhibiting circulatory compromise, is of less immediate concern. The adequacy of initial treatment of pulmonary and circulatory abnormalities sets the stage for subsequent management. Any early management error leads to a dramatic increase in morbidity and mortality during the subsequent injury phases.

Management of the burn client begins at the scene of the accident. The first step should be to remove the victim from the area of immediate danger, followed by stopping the burning process. Basic life support measures should be implemented during transport of the client to the hospital.

■ Medical Management in the Emergent Phase of Burn Injury

Assess Burn Severity. The American Burn Association has published a severity classification schedule for burn injuries (Table 52-2). These guidelines are intended to assist the clinician in determining injury severity for the burn client. This classification schedule separates injuries into major, moderate, and minor categories. Clients with major burns are usually transferred to a specialized burn care facility after local emergency treatment has been provided. Clients with moderate burns can usually be managed on an inpatient basis at the receiving hospital. Clients with minor burns usually receive initial care in the emergency department and are then discharged for follow-up care on an outpatient basis.

The severity of a burn injury is classified according to the risk of mortality and the risk of cosmetic or functional disability. Several factors influence injury severity.

Burn Depth. The deeper the burn wound, the more serious the injury. Deep partial-thickness and full-thickness burns are more likely to become infected, have more

TABLE 52-2	*American Burn Association Severity Classification for Burn Injuries*

Major Burn Injury
25% TBSA burn in adults <40 yr of age
20% TBSA burn in adults >40 yr of age
20% TBSA burn in children <10 yr of age

or

Burns involving the face, eyes, ears, hands, feet, and perineum likely to result in functional or cosmetic disability

or

High-voltage electrical burn injury

or

All burn injuries with concomitant inhalation injury or major trauma

Moderate Burn Injury
15%-25% TBSA burn in adults <40 yr of age
10%-20% TBSA burn in adults >40 yr of age
10%-20% TBSA burn in children <10 yr of age

with

Less than 10% TBSA full-thickness burn without cosmetic or functional risk to the face, eyes, ears, hands, feet, or perineum

Minor Burn Injury
<15% TBSA burn in adults <40 yr of age
<10% TBSA burn in adults >40 yr of age
<10% TBSA burn in children <10 yr of age

with

<2% TBSA full-thickness burn and no cosmetic or functional risk to the face, eyes, ears, hands, feet, or perineum

Modified from American Burn Association. (1984). Guidelines for service standards and severity classification in the treatment of burn injury. *American College of Surgeons Bulletin, 69*(10), 24-28.
TBSA, Total body surface area.

profound systemic effects, and are more frequently associated with contractures.

Burn Size. The size of a burn (percentage of injured skin, excluding first-degree burns) is determined by one of two techniques: (1) the rule of 9s and (2) an age-specific burn diagram or chart.[31] Burn size is expressed as a percentage of TBSA. The *rule of 9s* was introduced in the late 1940s as a quick assessment tool for estimating burn size. The basis of the rule is that the body is divided into anatomic sections, each of which represents 9%, or a multiple of 9%, of the TBSA (Figure 52-8). This method is easy and requires no diagrams to determine the percentage of TBSA injured. Therefore it is frequently used in emergency departments, where initial triage occurs. A *burn diagram* charts the percentages for body segments

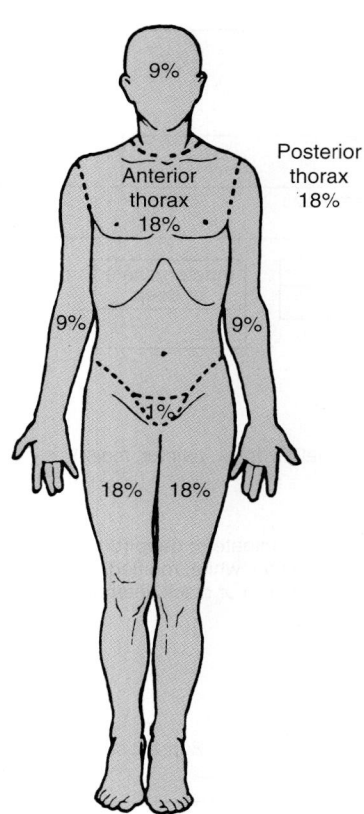

FIGURE 52-8 The rule of 9s provides a quick method for estimating the extent of a burn injury in the adult.

according to age and provides a more accurate estimate of burn size (Figure 52-9). It should be noted that the extent of burn injury is most accurate after initial debridement and should therefore be verified again at that time.

Burn Location. With burns of the head, neck, and chest, associated pulmonary complications are frequent. When burns involve the face, associated injuries often include corneal abrasions. Burns of the ears are susceptible to auricular chondritis, infection, and further loss of tissue. Management of burns of the hands and joints often requires intense physical and occupational therapy, with the potential for major loss of work time and for permanent physical and vocational disability. Burns involving the perineal area are susceptible to infection owing to autocontamination by urine and feces. Circumferential burns of extremities may produce a tourniquet-like effect, leading to distal vascular compromise. Circumferential thorax burns may lead to inadequate chest wall expansion and pulmonary insufficiency.

Age. The client's age affects the severity and outcome of the burn. Mortality rates are higher for children younger than 4 years, particularly in newborns and infants up to 1 year of age, and for clients older than 65 years.[6,12,49] High mortality and morbidity rates in the

older burn-injured client result from the combination of age-related functional impairments (slower reaction time, impaired judgment, and decreased mobility), living alone, environmental hazards, and significant preburn morbidity. Compounding this vulnerability to burn injury is the thinning of the skin and atrophy of skin appendages that occur with aging.

General Health. Debilitating cardiac, pulmonary, endocrine, and renal disease—specifically, cardiopulmonary insufficiency, diabetes, alcoholism-related disease, and renal failure—have been observed to influence the client's response to injury and treatment.[40] The mortality rate for clients with pre-existing cardiac disorders is 3.5 to 4 times higher than that for burn-injured clients without cardiac disorders. Alcoholic clients with burn injury have a threefold increase in mortality rate over that of nonalcoholic clients with burns. In addition, alcoholic clients who survive their burn injury have longer hospital stays and more complications. The increased morbidity among clients with burn injury who are alcoholic may be related to impaired immune function. Obese clients with burn injury are also at increased risk owing to cardiopulmonary complications.

Mechanism of Injury. The mechanism of injury is another factor used to determine the severity of injury. In general, special attention to this aspect of the injury is required for any electrical or chemical burn injury or any burn associated with inhalation injury. The client, people at the scene of the injury, and emergency medical personnel may have important information that could help in determining the severity of the burn. Useful information includes the time of injury, the level of the client's consciousness at the scene, whether the injury occurred in an enclosed or open space, the presence of associated trauma, and the specific mechanism of injury. If the victim has suffered a chemical burn, knowledge of the offending agent, its concentration, the duration of exposure, and whether irrigation was initiated at the scene is useful. For victims of electrical injuries, knowledge of the electrical source, type of current, and the current voltage is useful in determining the extent of the injury. Information concerning the client's past medical history as well as his or her general health should be obtained. Specifically, information regarding cardiac, pulmonary, endocrine, or renal disease should be obtained because it may have implications for treatment. Known allergies should also be identified, as should any current medication regimen.

Treat Minor Burns. Care of the client with minor burn injuries is frequently provided on an ambulatory or outpatient basis. In making the decision about whether to manage a client as an outpatient, the seriousness of the injury must first be assessed. As outlined in Table 52-2, a minor burn injury in the adult is generally considered to be less

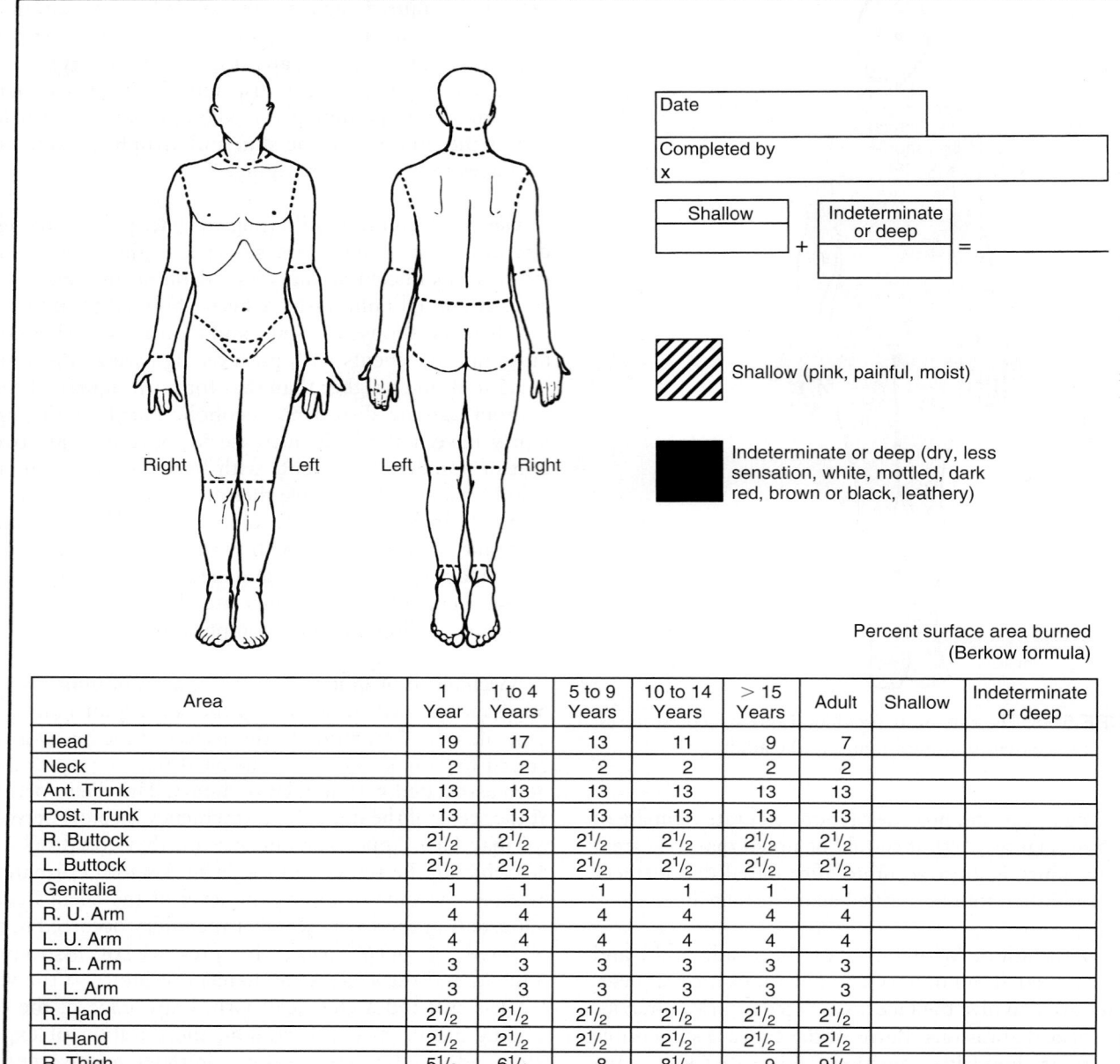

Area	1 Year	1 to 4 Years	5 to 9 Years	10 to 14 Years	> 15 Years	Adult	Shallow	Indeterminate or deep
Head	19	17	13	11	9	7		
Neck	2	2	2	2	2	2		
Ant. Trunk	13	13	13	13	13	13		
Post. Trunk	13	13	13	13	13	13		
R. Buttock	2½	2½	2½	2½	2½	2½		
L. Buttock	2½	2½	2½	2½	2½	2½		
Genitalia	1	1	1	1	1	1		
R. U. Arm	4	4	4	4	4	4		
L. U. Arm	4	4	4	4	4	4		
R. L. Arm	3	3	3	3	3	3		
L. L. Arm	3	3	3	3	3	3		
R. Hand	2½	2½	2½	2½	2½	2½		
L. Hand	2½	2½	2½	2½	2½	2½		
R. Thigh	5½	6½	8	8½	9	9½		
L. Thigh	5½	6½	8	8½	9	9½		
R. Leg	5	5	5½	6	6½	7		
L. Leg	5	5	5½	6	6½	7		
R. Foot	3½	3½	3½	3½	3½	3½		
L. Foot	3½	3½	3½	3½	3½	3½		
Total								

FIGURE 52-9 A sample chart for recording the extent and depth of a burn injury using the Berkow formula. To estimate burn extent using this chart, the nurse outlines the injured areas, excluding first-degree burns. Shallow (second-degree) burns are designated by parallel lines, and deeper (third-degree and fourth-degree) burns are designated by shading in the appropriate areas. The percentage of each injured anatomic area is then estimated using the age-specific table. Total body surface area burn is then calculated.

than 15% TBSA in clients younger than 40 years of age or 10% TBSA in clients older than 40 years, without a risk of cosmetic or functional impairment or disability.[3] In addition, the client or caregiver's ability to perform wound care in the home environment must be considered. Medical care of the minor burn includes wound evaluation and initial care, tetanus immunization, and pain management. While providing initial wound care, the nurse is responsible for teaching home wound care and the clinical manifestations of infection that necessitate further medical care. Other teaching needs include the need to perform active range-of-motion (ROM) exercises to maintain normal joint function and to decrease edema formation. The need for any follow-up evaluations or treatments should be confirmed with the client at this time.

Treat Major Burns. The medical goals for burn care depend on the phase of care. Initial goals are saving life, maintaining and protecting the airway, and restoring hemodynamic stability. Later goals are replacement of missing skin, promoting healing, and assessing and correcting complications.

Monitor Airway and Breathing. The adequacy of the airway and breathing should take prime importance during the emergent phase of burn injury.[10,14,19,25] The oropharynx should be inspected for evidence of ery-thema, blisters, or ulcerations, and the need for endotracheal intubation should be considered. If inhalation injury is suspected, administration of 100% oxygen via a tight-fitting facemask continues until COHb levels fall below 15%.[10] Hyperbaric oxygen is also considered with any exposure to CO. If breathing appears to be compromised by tight circumferential trunk burns, bilateral escharotomies of the trunk may be necessary to relieve ventilatory compromise.

Prevent Burn Shock. In adults with burn injuries affecting more than 15% TBSA, IV fluid resuscitation is generally required.[2] Two peripheral large-bore IV lines placed through nonburned skin, proximal to any extremity burns, is recommended. IV lines may be placed through burned skin if necessary; however, these lines should be secured with a suture. For clients with extensive burns or limited peripheral IV access sites, cannulation of a central vein (subclavian, internal or external jugular, or femoral) by a physician may be necessary.

Fluid resuscitation is used to minimize the deleterious effects of the fluid shifts. The goal of fluid resuscitation is to maintain vital organ perfusion while avoiding the complication of inadequate or excessive fluids. Several formulas used to calculate fluid requirements are listed in Table 52-3. In the calculation of fluid infusion rates, the time of injury, not the time at which fluid resuscita-

TABLE 52-3	*Fluid Resuscitation Formulas Used in Burn Care*					
	First 24 Hours			**Second 24 Hours**		
Formula Name	**Electrolyte-Containing Solution**	**Colloid-Containing Solution**	**Dextrose in Water**	**Electrolyte-Containing Solution**	**Colloid-Containing Solution**	**Dextrose in Water**
Evans	Normal saline 1 ml/kg/% burn	1 ml/kg/% burn	2000 ml	½ of first 24-hr requirement	½ of first 24-hr requirement	2000 ml
Brooke	Lactated Ringer's 1.5 ml/kg/% burn	0.5 ml/kg/% burn	2000 ml	½-¾ of first 24-hr requirement	½-¾ of first 24-hr requirement	2000 ml
Modified Brooke	Lactated Ringer's 2 ml/kg/% burn	None	None	None	0.3-0.5 ml/kg/% burn	Titrate to maintain urine output
Parkland	Lactated Ringer's 4 ml/kg/% burn	None	None	None	0.3-0.5 ml/kg/% burn	Titrate to maintain urine output
Hypertonic saline solution	Fluid containing 250 mEq of sodium/L to maintain hourly urine output of 70 ml in adults	None	None	Same solution to maintain hourly urine output of 30 ml in adults	None	None

Modified from Rue, L.W., & Cioffi, W.G., Jr. (1991). Resuscitation of thermally injured patients. *Critical Care Nursing Clinics of North America 3*(2), 185; and Wachtel, T.L., & Fortune, J.B. (1983). Fluid resuscitation for burn shock. In T.L. Wachtel et al. (Eds.), *Current topics in burn care* (p. 44). Rockville, MD: Aspen Publishers.

tion was initiated, serves as time zero. Thus if a burned client is delayed 2 hours in reaching an emergency department, those 2 hours must be considered in any calculation of needed fluid.

Although each formula is different, fluid management during the first 24 hours after burn injury generally includes the infusion of balanced salt solution, typically lactated Ringer's solution. The exact amount of fluid is based on the client's weight and the extent of injury. Other factors to be considered include the presence of an inhalation injury, a delay in initiation of resuscitation, and deep tissue damage. These factors tend to increase the amount of IV fluid required for adequate resuscitation above the calculated amount.[9] With the exception of the Evans and Brooke formulas, colloid-containing solutions are not given during this period because of the changes in capillary integrity that allow leakage of protein-rich fluid (e.g., albumin) into the interstitial space, resulting in the formation of additional edematous fluid. During the second 24 hours after burn injury, colloid-containing solutions are administered, along with 5% dextrose and water in varying amounts. It is important to remember that all resuscitation formulas are only guides and that fluid resuscitation volumes should be adjusted according to the client's physiologic response. Adequacy of fluid resuscitation is based on urine output when hemodynamic monitoring is not used. An indwelling urethral catheter connected to a closed drainage system should be placed to measure hourly urine production and to guide IV fluid replacement.

Vital signs are used to provide a baseline of information as well as additional data for determining the adequacy of fluid resuscitation. Baseline laboratory studies should include blood glucose, BUN, serum creatinine, serum electrolytes, and hematocrit levels. Arterial blood gas and COHb levels should also be obtained, particularly if an inhalation injury is suspected. A chest x-ray film should be obtained for all clients with extensive burns or inhalation injury. Other laboratory tests in addition to the radiographic study should be performed in all clients with associated trauma, as indicated. Depending on the circumstance of the injury, an alcohol or drug screen may be appropriate. Continuous electrocardiographic (ECG) monitoring should be initiated in all clients with major burn injuries, particularly those who have suffered a high-voltage electrical injury or who have a history of cardiac ischemia.

Prevent Aspiration. Many burn centers advocate the placement of a nasogastric tube for management of unresponsive clients and clients with burns of 20% to 25% TBSA or more, to prevent emesis and reduce the risk of aspiration. Gastrointestinal dysfunction results from the intestinal ileus that develops almost universally in clients during the early post–burn injury period.[25] All oral fluids should be restricted at this time.

Minimize Pain. Pain management for the client with a moderate or major burn is achieved through the administration of IV opioids, typically morphine sulfate. In the adult, small doses are given and repeated in 5- to 10-minute intervals until pain appears to be under control. The intramuscular and subcutaneous routes are *not* used during this phase because absorption from the soft tissues is unreliable during the emergent period, when peripheral perfusion is sporadic. The oral route for pain medication administration is not used owing to the likelihood of gastrointestinal dysfunction.

Clients presenting to emergency departments with minor burn injuries often are initially given small doses of IV opioids (e.g., morphine sulfate). Oral analgesic agents are then prescribed for outpatient use.

Wound Care

Stop the Burning Process. All burn wound care begins at the scene of the injury. Flame and scald burns should be cooled by submerging small burns in cool water until the sensation of burning stops. Major burn victims should have an initial "wet down" at the scene to stop the burning process, but not be submerged in water. Smoldering clothing should be carefully removed, and the client should be covered with a blanket to preserve body heat. Ideally, treatment of chemical burn wounds also begins at the scene of the injury. All clothing should be promptly removed; any chemical powder should be brushed off the skin. Wet chemical burns should be irrigated continuously with copious amounts of water[10] for at least 20 minutes. Neutralizing agents are not recommended because the neutralizing reaction causes heat, which results in further tissue damage.

For chemical eye injuries, irrigate the eyes with a gentle stream of normal saline, flushing both the injured eye and the conjunctiva. It is recommended to irrigate the eyes from the inner canthus outward, to avoid washing any chemicals down the tear duct or toward the other eye.

Electrical burn care also includes stopping the burning process. It is important to remember to shut off any power source before approaching the victim. Early care is directed at assessment of the entire person, owing to the potential path of the electricity through the body (e.g., dysrhythmias, fractures).

Immediate Care. If transfer to a burn center will be accomplished within 12 hours of injury, wound care should consist of covering the wound with sterile towels and placing clean dry sheets and blankets over the client. Unless transport time to the receiving medical facility is prolonged, debridement and application of topical antimicrobial agents are unnecessary. Definitive wound care begins following inpatient admission to the hospital.

Wound care for burns consists of cleansing, debridement, removal of any damaging agents (e.g., chemicals, tar), and application of an appropriate topical agent and a dressing. Burn wounds should be washed with a mild soap and rinsed thoroughly with warm water. Loose, nonviable tissue should be carefully trimmed away, and any hair should be shaved to within a 1-inch margin around the burn wound.

The removal of tar or asphalt is easily accomplished with the use of a citrus-petroleum product such as Medisol (Orange-Sol, Inc., Chandler, AZ) or with mineral oil and a petroleum-based antibiotic ointment such as bacitracin or polymyxin-neomycin-bacitracin (Neosporin).

Clients with minor burns are generally taught wound care and discharged home with instructions to continue wound care twice daily and return to the outpatient clinic or their private physician for follow-up assessment and care.

Prevent Tetanus. Burns, even minor ones, are susceptible to tetanus. The current protocol for tetanus immunization in clients with minor burns is the same as in clients with any other type of trauma.[8] Clients who have been previously immunized against tetanus, but not within the past 5 years, should receive a tetanus toxoid booster. For clients who have not been immunized, tetanus immunoglobulin (a passive immunizing agent) and the first of a series of active immunizations with tetanus toxoid should be administered.

Prevent Tissue Ischemia. Circumferential burns of the extremities may compromise circulation in the affected limb. Elevating injured extremities above the level of the heart and active exercise help to reduce dependent edema formation. However, circulatory compromise may still occur. Therefore frequent assessment of distal extremity perfusion is necessary. Doppler flowmeter assessment of the palmar arch vessels (for the upper extremity) and the posterior tibial artery (for the lower extremity) provides the most precise indication of peripheral perfusion and should be performed regularly during the resuscitation period. The absence of flow or the progressive diminution of the Doppler flowmeter signal intensity is an indication that perfusion is impaired.

An escharotomy is the appropriate treatment for circulatory compromise due to constricting, circumferential burns (Figure 52-10).[16] A midlateral or midmedial incision of the involved extremity is made from the most proximal to the most distal extent of the full-thickness burn. The depth of the incision is limited to the eschar. It is generally performed at the bedside without local or general anesthesia, because full-thickness burns are insensate. However, viable tissue beneath the escharotomy may bleed if cut, and then the client may feel pain. Bleeding can be controlled with pressure, suture ligation, or electrocautery. Pain control is achieved with IV opioid

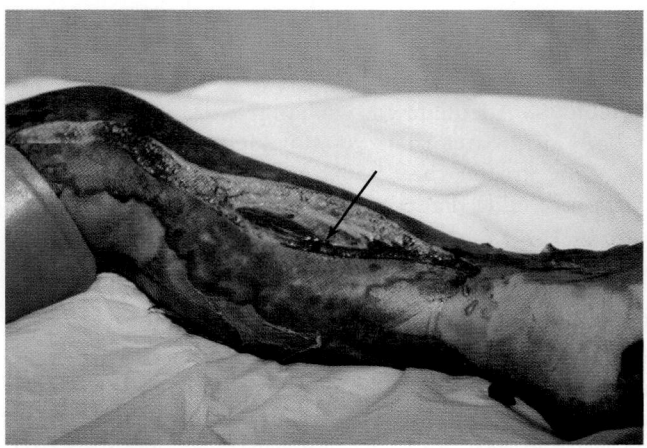

FIGURE 52-10 Escharotomy. Incision is made through the constricting burn eschar to permit expansion of the underlying subcutaneous tissues as edema forms.

administration. After escharotomy, the burn wound can be dressed with topical antimicrobial creams and gauze dressings.

If adequate tissue perfusion does not return following escharotomy, a fasciotomy may be necessary. This procedure, in which the fascia is incised, is performed in the operating room with the client under general anesthesia. A fasciotomy is usually necessary only in injuries caused by high-voltage electricity or those with concomitant crush injury.

Transport to a Burn Facility. Consideration of transfer to a specialized burn care facility is appropriate for all clients with major burn injuries (see Table 52-2). Prompt contact with the receiving burn center is important to facilitate a smooth transfer. All copies of medical records, which should include all fluids and medications given, hourly urine output values, and vital signs, must accompany the client. The client's burn wounds should simply be covered with a sterile sheet and blankets. The burn center performs a complete assessment of the wounds; therefore it is best if topical care has not been initiated.

■ Nursing Management of the Medical Client in the Emergent Phase of Burn Care
Assessment

Because the body's immediate physiologic responses to burn injury can either be life-threatening or lead to significant morbidity, prudent nursing assessment during the emergent phase of burn injury is crucial.

Diagnosis, Outcomes, Interventions

Diagnosis: Impaired Gas Exchange. Effective gas exchange may become impaired when clients have experienced smoke inhalation because of tracheobronchial swelling, the presence of carbonaceous debris in the airway, or CO poisoning.

Outcomes. Adequate gas exchange will be evidenced by a PaO_2 of greater than 90 mm Hg; oxygen saturation (SaO_2) of greater than 95%, arterial partial pressure of carbon dioxide ($PaCO_2$) of 35 to 45 mm Hg; respiratory rate of 16 to 24 breaths/min with a normal pattern and depth; and clear bilateral breath sounds.

Interventions. The client must be frequently assessed for manifestations of respiratory distress such as restlessness, confusion, labored breathing, tachypnea, dyspnea, diminished or adventitious breath sounds, tachycardia, decrease in PaO_2 and SaO_2, and cyanosis. Monitor SaO_2 continuously in clients with major burns during the emergent phase of burn injury. Draw and monitor arterial blood gas and COHb levels per physician order. Report changes in the client's condition immediately.

Instruct the client on the use of the incentive spirometer to encourage deep breathing every 2 hours. Elevate the head of the bed to facilitate lung expansion and to reduce facial edema.

Diagnosis: Ineffective Airway Clearance.
Because of the occurrence of airway epidermal sloughing, increase in secretions, inflammation and swelling of the nasopharyngeal mucous membranes from smoke irritation, and depressed ciliary action from inhalation injury, the client becomes at risk for *Ineffective Airway Clearance*.

Outcomes. Clients will have an effective airway clearance, as evidenced by clear bilateral breath sounds, clear to white pulmonary secretions, effective mobilization of pulmonary secretions, and unlabored respiration with a respiratory rate of 16 to 24 breaths/min.

Interventions. A thorough pulmonary assessment should be performed every 1 to 2 hours during the first 24 hours after injury, and every 2 to 4 hours the second 24 hours after injury, evaluating breath sounds, rate and depth of respirations, and level of consciousness. Be alert to a declining respiratory status as evidenced by crackles, rhonchi, stridor, labored breathing, dyspnea, tachypnea, restlessness, or a decreasing level of consciousness. Report significant findings promptly. Have the client turn, cough, and deep-breathe every 1 to 2 hours for 24 hours and then every 2 to 4 hours. Place an oral suctioning device within the client's reach for independent use. Perform endotracheal or nasotracheal suction as needed. Assess and document the character and amount of secretions.

Diagnosis: Deficient Fluid Volume.
The client with a major burn injury is at risk for hypovolemia, most significantly during the first 36 hours after burn injury. The *Deficient Fluid Volume* is directly related to the increased capillary leakage and fluid shift from the intravascular to the interstitial space after the burn insult.

Outcomes. The client will have improved fluid balance, as evidenced by a urine output of 0.5 to 1 ml/kg/hr, clear sensorium, pulse rate less than 120 beats/min, absence of dysrhythmias, adequate amplitude of peripheral pulses (2+ or better), and blood pressure within the expected range for age and medical history.

Interventions. Assess the client for manifestations of hypovolemia every hour for 36 hours, including tachycardia, decreased blood pressure, decreased amplitude of peripheral pulses, urine output of less than 0.5 ml/kg/hr, thirst, and dry mucous membranes. Report significant findings.

Carefully monitor and document intake and output, administering fluid therapy as prescribed; titrate the infusion every hour to maintain urine output between 0.5 and 1 ml/kg/hr. Large volumes of fluid may be required initially to produce adequate urine volumes.

Monitor serum electrolyte and hematocrit values. Hyponatremia, hyperkalemia, and elevated hematocrit levels are common findings during the emergent phase. As the circulation is restored, levels should return to normal values.

Diagnosis: Ineffective Tissue Perfusion: Renal.
Clients who have suffered deep burn and tissue injury, such as in electrical injury or crush injuries, and those in whom adequate fluid resuscitation has not been achieved are at risk for renal failure. Myoglobin and hemoglobin released from the damaged muscles and red blood cells that precipitate in the renal tubules can create acute tubular necrosis.

Outcomes. The client with evidence of deep tissue injury will maintain a urine output of 75 to 100 ml/hr, or 1 ml/kg/hr, or higher, until the pigment load has decreased.

Interventions. Monitor and document hourly output and urine color. A dark brown or red color is indicative of the presence of hemochromogens. Send urine samples for myoglobin or hemoglobin assay per physician order to provide quantitative information for documentation of the client's condition. Ensure that the catheter is patent, because the tubing may become plugged with hemochromogens. Administer IV fluids per physician orders. Hemochromogens must be flushed from the body; therefore the rate of fluid administration is based on maintaining an hourly urine output of 1 ml/kg/hr or greater.

Diagnosis: Ineffective Tissue Perfusion: Peripheral.
The client may exhibit *Ineffective Peripheral Tissue Perfusion* as a result of constricting circumferential burns.

Outcomes. The client will have adequate peripheral perfusion, as evidenced by the presence of pulses on palpation or Doppler flowmeter assessment, capillary refill time for unburned skin of less than 2 seconds, absence of numbness or tingling, and absence of increased pain with active ROM exercises.

Interventions. Remove all constricting jewelry and clothing, because constricting items may compromise circulation as edema formation ensues. Limit the use of the blood pressure cuff on the affected extremity, because the cuff can reduce arterial inflow and venous return. Elevate the burned extremity above the level of the heart to promote venous return and to prevent excessive dependent edema formation.

Monitor arterial pulses by palpation or with the use of an ultrasonic flow detector (Doppler flowmeter) hourly for up to 72 hours after burn injury. Pulses will diminish with circulation impairments. Assess capillary refill of unburned skin on the affected extremity; capillary refill will be prolonged with impaired circulation. Encourage ROM exercises, and assess the level of pain associated with efforts. Increasing pain with movement is a result of tissue ischemia. When pain is not present, increased movement of the affected area will promote venous return and assist in decreasing edema.

If tissue perfusion is threatened, anticipate and prepare the client for an escharotomy. Once the underlying tissue edema has exceeded the expansion ability of the burned skin, an escharotomy will be needed to restore perfusion. After the procedure is complete, recheck for restoration of circulation by assessing pulses, color, movement, and sensation of the affected extremity. Anticipate some bleeding after escharotomy, because the tissue beneath the eschar bleeds. Bleeding can be controlled by electrocautery or suturing by the physician. Continue to observe and assess the extremity after the procedure.

Diagnosis: Risk for Infection. The burn-injured client faces an increased *Risk for Infection* related to inadequate primary and secondary defenses resulting from traumatized tissue, bacterial proliferation in burn wounds, and an immunocompromised status.

Outcomes. The client will remain free from significant burn wound microbial invasion, as evidenced by quantitative wound cultures containing less than 100,000 colony-forming units (CFUs)/g. In addition, core body temperature will be maintained between 99.6° and 101° F (37.5° C to 38.3° C); there will be no swelling, redness, or purulence present at IV line insertion sites; and results of blood, urine, and sputum cultures will be negative.

Interventions. Tetanus prophylaxis should be administered per physician order, because the anaerobic environment beneath eschar is ideal for tetanus organism growth. Intramuscular or IV antibiotic therapy is not used because the area of potential infection is avascular and would not be reached by antibiotics. Antimicrobial agents are used to deter the growth of bacteria on the surface of the wound.

It is essential to maintain infection control techniques at all times during the client's hospitalization to prevent cross-contamination. Ensure aseptic technique when administering care to burned areas and performing invasive techniques. Enforce strict hand-washing, and instruct family members or significant others on infection control measures.

When wound care is performed, it is important to debride the wound of loose, nonviable tissue, which serves as a medium for bacterial growth. Hair within and around a wound should be shaved (with the exception of eyebrows and eyelashes), because hair is contaminated and prevents adherence of the burn cream. Apply a topical therapeutic agent (an antimicrobial) and loose gauze dressings.

Diagnosis: Impaired Physical Mobility. The client's mobility during the emergent phase of burn injury is impaired by tissue edema, pain, and dressings.

Outcomes. The outcomes related to physical mobility are measured throughout the hospitalization and recovery process. The long-term outcome goal is return of the client to maximum independence in performance of activities of daily living (ADL) with minimum disability and disfigurement. Although this outcome is demonstrated long after the emergent phase, it is important to initiate care on the day of admission and to follow through continually throughout hospitalization.

Interventions. Encourage the client to participate in self-care and ROM exercises at the earliest time possible. The time of the emergency department visit is not too soon to help motivate the client and to overcome fear and dependence related to the injury. Additionally, during early postinjury fluid shifts, increasing movement helps to improve circulation and decrease edema. Consult with occupational and physical therapists for initial assessment and follow-up care throughout the hospitalization.

Diagnosis: Disabled Family Coping. Because of the urgent and critical nature of the injury, the client and family are at risk for ineffective coping skills.

Outcomes. Family members and significant others will have accurate information about the immediate status of the client, as evidenced by their ability to verbalize an understanding of the client's injury and treatment goals. Support services will be provided as needed.

Interventions. It is important to prepare family members or significant others for their first visit with the client after injury. Provide a simple explanation of procedures and equipment, communicate the extent of the burn, and describe changes in the client's appearance. For impending client transfer, provide family members or significant others with support services to assist with travel arrangements. Providing support at this time will help to reduce their anxiety during the client's transfer. Families of clients remaining in the facility should be provided with information that meets their basic needs (e.g., information about lodging, location of cafeteria, parking).

ACUTE PHASE

The acute phase of recovery following a major burn begins when the client is hemodynamically stable, capillary integrity is restored, and diuresis has begun. This is generally 48 to 72 hours after the time of injury. Many of the same principles of care outlined for the emergent phase apply to the acute phase; however, more emphasis is placed on restorative therapies. The acute phase continues until wound closure is achieved.

■ Medical Management in the Acute Phase of Burn Injury

Prevent Infection. Infection control is a major component of burn management. An infection control policy is necessary for managing burn-injured clients to control the transmission of microorganisms that can lead to infection or colonization.[16,53] Standard precautions should be followed in caring for all clients with burn injuries; however, specific infection control practices and isolation techniques exist for all burn centers. These practices include the use of gloves, caps, masks, shoe covers, scrub clothes, and plastic aprons. Strict hand-washing is stressed to reduce the incidence of cross-contamination

between clients and is the single most important means of preventing the spread of infection. Staff and visitors are generally prevented from client contact if they have any skin, gastrointestinal, or respiratory tract infections. See Box 52-2 for basic infection control strategies. All visitors as well as health care providers from other departments should be oriented to established infection control practices before their first contact with the burn-injured client.

Provide Metabolic Support. Maintenance of adequate nutrition during the acute phase of burn care is essential in promoting wound healing and preventing infection.[18] Basal metabolic rates may be 40% to 100% higher than normal levels, depending on the extent of the burn. This response is thought to be the result of a resetting of the homeostatic "thermostat" of the hypothalamic-pituitary-adrenal axis, leading to an increase in heat production. Metabolic rates decrease as wound coverage is achieved.

Aggressive nutritional support is required to meet the increased energy requirements necessary to promote healing and to prevent the untoward effects of catabolism.[15] Several different formulas (Table 52-4) are currently used to estimate energy requirements by factoring different indices: weight, gender, age, extent of burn, and amount of activity. Additional support is generally indicated for the burn-injured client with any of the following: 30% or greater TBSA burn, clinical course requiring multiple operations, need for mechanical ventilatory support, compromised mental status, and poor preinjury nutritional state. Methods for delivering nutritional support include oral intake, enteral tube feedings, peripheral parenteral nutrition, and total parenteral nutrition, which may be used alone or in combination. The preferred feeding route is oral or enteral[29]; however, the decision of how to best meet the client's nutritional needs

---

| **BOX 52-2** | *Basic Principles of Infection Control* |

1. Thorough hand-washing should be done before and after each contact with the burn-injured client.
2. Protective garb (aprons or gowns) should be donned before each contact and promptly discarded after leaving the bedside or room.
3. Gloves should be changed when they become contaminated with secretions or fluids from one anatomic site before contact with another site.
4. Equipment, materials, and surfaces are considered contaminated for the individual client and should be properly decontaminated before use with another client.

From Weber, J.M., & Tompkins, D.M. (1993). Improving survival: Infection control and burns. *AACN Clinical Issues in Critical Care Nursing 4*(2), 418-419.

| **TABLE 52-4** | *Energy Calculation Formulas Used for the Burn-Injured Adult* |

Formula/Author Name	Formula for Daily Caloric Expenditure Estimate
Curreri	(25 kcal/kg body weight) + (40 kcal × % TBSA burn)
Modified Harris-Benedict	RMR × Activity factor × Injury factor
U.S. Army Institute of Surgical Research	[Age- and Gender-specific BMR × (0.89142 + 0.01335 × % TBSA burn) × m² × 24 × Activity factor]

TBSA, Total body surface area; *RMR,* resting metabolic rate; *BMR,* basal metabolic rate.

should be individualized. Typically, parenteral nutrition is reserved for clients with a prolonged ileus or for those in whom enteral feedings fail to meet nutritional needs.

Minimize Pain. Pain continues to be a significant problem throughout the client's hospitalization. During the acute phase of injury, an attempt is made to find the right combination of medications and interventions to minimize the discomfort and pain associated with the injury. As in the emergent phase, the most common approach to pain control is with the use of pharmacologic agents. However, in addition to the opioids used during the emergent phase, other modalities may be used during the acute phase of burn injury to help alleviate the client's pain. Patient-controlled analgesia devices, inhalation analgesics such as nitrous oxide, oral analgesic "pain cocktails," and opioid agonist-antagonist agents may be beneficial during the acute phase of burn injury.[28] Nonsteroidal anti-inflammatory agents (NSAIDs) are also prescribed for the treatment of mild to moderate pain. When NSAIDs are used, extra precautions must be taken to prevent gastric ulceration.

Nonpharmacologic modalities used to treat burn-related pain include hypnosis, guided imagery, art and play therapy, relaxation techniques, distraction, biofeedback, and music therapy. These modalities have been found to be effective in decreasing anxiety, thereby decreasing the perception of pain. They are often used as adjunctive therapies to the pharmacologic treatment of burn pain.[28]

Provide Wound Care. Care of the burn wound is ultimately aimed at promoting wound healing. Daily wound care involves cleansing, debridement of eschar (devitalized tissue), and dressing of the wound.

Wound Cleansing. The practice of hydrotherapy remains a mainstay of burn treatment plans for cleansing the wounds. This is accomplished by immersion, showering, or spraying (Figure 52-11). A hydrotherapy session of 30 minutes or less is optimal for clients with acute burns. Longer time periods may increase sodium loss (water is hypotonic) through the burn wound and may promote heat loss, pain, and stress. During hydrotherapy, the wounds are gently washed using any one of a variety of solutions. Care should be taken to minimize bleeding and to maintain body temperature during this procedure. To prevent cross contamination between clients, single-use plastic hydrotherapy tub liners are available. Clients excluded from hydrotherapy are generally those who are hemodynamically unstable and those with new skin grafts. If hydrotherapy is not used, wounds are washed and rinsed while the client is in bed, before the application of antimicrobial agents.

Debridement. Burn wound debridement involves the removal of the eschar. This promotes wound healing by preventing bacterial proliferation in and under the eschar. Debridement of the burn wound is accomplished through mechanical, enzymatic, or surgical means.

Mechanical debridement can be accomplished with careful use of scissors and forceps to lift and trim away loose eschar. Hydrotherapy softens and loosens eschar so that it is more easily removed. Wet-to-dry dressing changes are another effective means of mechanical debridement. Coarse gauze dressings are saturated with a prescribed solution, wrung out until the dressing is slightly moist, and applied to the wound. The dressing is left in place to dry. Typically 6 to 8 hours later the gauze is carefully removed from the wound, mechanically lifting drainage, exudate, and loose necrotic tissue that has dried on to the gauze. Mechanical debridement of the burn wound can be extremely painful; therefore effective pain management is paramount.

Enzymatic debridement involves the application of commercially prepared proteolytic and fibrinolytic topical enzymes to the burn wound, which facilitates eschar removal. These agents require a moist environment to be effective and are applied directly to the burn wound. Enzymatic debridement is not widely practiced, because several serious side effects are associated with use of these agents.[33] As the enzyme digests necrotic tissue, it also opens up thrombosed blood vessels. This causes some oozing of blood from the blood vessels and creates a site for bacteria to enter the bloodstream. Bacteremia, pain, and bleeding can occur; therefore if enzymatic debridement is used, the client should be assessed for complications continuously throughout the course of treatment. The use of enzymatic debridement agents is contraindicated for wounds communicating with major

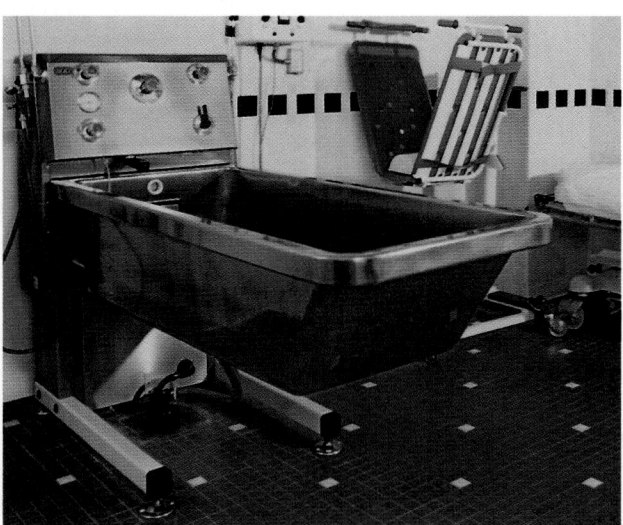

FIGURE 52-11 A low-boy whirlpool tank is used for immersion hydrotherapy treatment of burn wounds. (Courtesy of Shriners Hospitals for Children of Northern California.)

body cavities and for wounds with exposed nerves or nervous tissue.

Surgical debridement of the burn wound involves excision of the eschar and coverage of the wound. Early surgical excision begins during the first week after injury, once the client is hemodynamically stable. Advantages of early excision include early mobilization, reduction of pain (which is otherwise experienced with repeated dressing changes), early wound closure (which reduces

the potential for wound infection), and reduced length of hospitalization.[15,37] A disadvantage of early excision is the risk of excising viable tissue that may heal with time.

Two techniques of surgical debridement are currently used. In *tangential* excision, very thin layers of eschar are sequentially shaved until viable tissue is reached. *Fascial* excision involves removing the burn tissue and underlying fat down to fascia. This technique is frequently used for debridement of very deep burns.

TABLE 52-5   *Topical Antimicrobial Agents Used in Burn Care*

Agent	Antimicrobial Spectrum	Application	Side Effects	Nursing Considerations
Water-Based Creams				
1% silver sulfadiazine	Broad spectrum; effective against some fungi and yeast	2 times daily, 1/16-inch thickness Gauze dressing not required	Transient leukopenia typically appearing after 2 or 3 days of treatment Macular rash	Do not store in warm environment (e.g., warm client room)
Mafenide acetate	Broad spectrum; little antifungal activity	2 times daily, 1/16-inch thickness Gauze dressing not required	Hyperchloremic metabolic acidosis from bicarbonate diuresis due to the inhibition of carbonic anhydrase Pain/burning sensation on application to superficial burns Maculopapular rash	Assess for side effects Assess adequacy of pain management; if pain and discomfort continue, consider other topical treatments Use cautiously in clients with acute renal failure
Solutions				
5% mafenide acetate	Broad spectrum	Gauze dressing required, moistened with solution for application to the wound	Pain on application Pruritus Rash Fungal colonization	Assess for side effects Assess adequacy of pain management
0.5% silver nitrate	Broad spectrum; effective against *Candida* species	Multiple layers of gauze dressing required, moistened with solution for application to the wound	Hyponatremia Hypochloremia Hypokalemia Hypocalcemia	Check serum electrolytes daily Penetrates eschar poorly Remoisten dressings every 2 hours to avoid wound desiccation Protect the environment; stains everything a blackish-brown color
Petroleum-Based Ointments				
Polymyxin B	Gram-negative organisms	Apply as needed in a thin layer; gauze dressing not used unless clothing protection is needed	Hypersensitivity (rash) Overgrowth of non-susceptible organisms including fungi	Assess for side effects
Neomycin sulfate	Predominantly gram-negative organisms			
Bacitracin	Predominantly gram-positive organisms			

Topical Antimicrobial Treatment. Deep partial-thickness or full-thickness burn wounds are treated initially with topical antimicrobial agents. These agents are applied once or twice daily following cleansing, debridement, and inspection of the wound. The nurse assesses for eschar separation, the presence of granulation tissue or reepithelialization, and manifestations of infection. The most commonly used topical antimicrobial agents are listed in Table 52-5. Although no single agent is used universally, many burn centers choose silver sulfadiazine cream as the initial topical agent.

Burn wounds are treated using either an open or a closed dressing technique. For the *open method,* the antimicrobial cream is applied with a gloved hand (Figure 52-12) and the wound is left open to the air without gauze dressings. The cream is reapplied as needed, although formal reapplication is necessary every 12 hours in keeping with the duration of activity of the agent. The advantages of the open method include increased visualization of the wound, greater freedom for mobility and joint motion, and simplicity in wound care. The disadvantages include an increased chance of hypothermia from exposure.

In the *closed method* of wound care, gauze dressing is impregnated with antimicrobial cream and applied to the wound. To prevent circulatory compromise in extremity burns, the gauze should be wrapped from the most distal portion of the extremity in a proximal direction. The advantages of the closed method are decreases in evaporative fluid and heat loss from the wound surface. In addition, gauze dressings may aid in debridement. The disadvantages of gauze dressings are mobility limitations and a potential decrease in effectiveness of

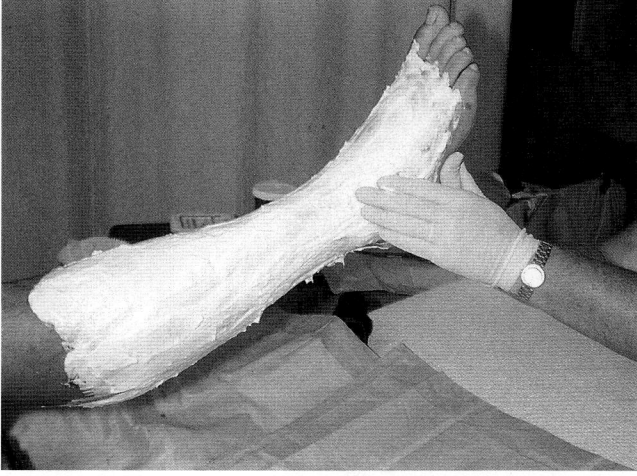

FIGURE 52-12 Silver sulfadiazine, a common antimicrobial cream used in burn care, is applied to the burn wound using a sterile, gloved hand. (Courtesy of the University of Washington Burn Center, Harborview Medical Center, Seattle.)

ROM exercises. Wound assessment is also limited to the times at which dressing changes are performed.

Temporary wound coverings (skin substitutes) are frequently used as a kind of wound "dressing." Table 52-6 outlines the most common biologic, biosynthetic, and synthetic wound coverings available. These products are temporary wound coverings, and each has specific indications.[17,42,48] The character of the wound (depth of injury, amount of exudate, location of the wound on the body, and phase of recovery) and treatment goals are considered in choosing the most appropriate wound covering.

Maximize Function. Maintenance of optimal physical functioning in the client with a burn injury is a challenge for the entire team. Nurses work closely with occupational and physical therapists to identify the rehabilitative needs of the burn-injured client. An individualized program of splinting, positioning, exercise, ambulation, performance of ADL, and pressure therapy should be implemented in the acute phase of recovery to maximize functional recovery and cosmetic outcome. Therapeutic goals at this stage in recovery are to prevent early contracture formation and to maintain soft tissue length.

Wound contracture and hypertrophic scarring are two major problems for the burn-injured client. Wound contractures are typically more severe with extensive burns. Areas seemingly predisposed to contracture are the hands, head and neck, and axilla. Measures used to prevent and treat wound contractures include therapeutic positioning, ROM exercises, splinting, and client and family education.

Table 52-7 lists corrective and therapeutic techniques for positioning clients with specific areas of burn injury during periods of inactivity or immobilization. Allowing the burn-injured client to assume a position of comfort most often contributes to contracture formation. Therefore proper positioning, both in and out of bed, should be maintained for the burn-injured client. These tech- niques place affected body parts in positions that are in opposition to positions of potential contracture or deformity. The natural tendency with healing and immobility is for muscles and joints to contract into a shortened, flexed position. Thus, for example, to reduce the risk of neck contractures, the use of pillows—which place the neck in flexion—is not allowed.

Active ROM exercises are prescribed early in the acute phase of recovery to promote resolution of edema and to maintain strength and joint function. In addition, ADL can be effective in maintaining function and ROM. Ambulation also maintains strength and ROM of the lower extremities and should begin as soon as the client is physiologically stable. Passive ROM and stretching exercises should be included as part of the daily treatment plan if the client is unable to perform active ROM exercises.

TABLE 52-6 *Temporary Wound Coverings Used in Burn Care*

Category/Examples	Description	Indications	Nursing Considerations
Biologic			
Amnion	Amniotic membranes collected from human placentas	To protect partial-thickness burns To protect granulation tissue before autograft application	Cover dressing is changed every 48 hours with amnion.
Allograft homograft	Donated human cadaver skin harvested within 24 hours after death	To debride exudative wounds To cover excised wound and test for receptivity before autograft application To cover and protect meshed autografts	Observe for wound exudate and signs of infection that may be indicative of a wound infection beneath the allograft/xenograft.
Xenograft heterograft	Porcine skin is harvested after slaughter, then cryopreserved or lyophilized for storage	To promote healing of clean, superficial partial-thickness wounds	Xenograft over granulation tissue is changed every 2-5 days. For superficial wounds, ensure that the wound is clean and well rinsed; apply xenograft with slight overlapping of edges to allow for shrinkage; trim away xenograft when skin beneath it has healed.
Biosynthetic			
Biobrane (Bertek Pharmaceuticals, Morgantown, WV)	Nylon fabric bonded to a silicone rubber membrane containing collagenous porcine peptides	Donor site dressing Protective cover over meshed autografts To promote healing of clean superficial partial-thickness wounds	Secure to the surrounding intact skin by staples, skin closure strips, tape, or sutures and then wrap with a gauze dressing; this outer dressing can be removed by 48 hours to check for adherence of the Biobrane; once adherence has occurred, the tape, sutures, and staples can be removed; the Biobrane can then be left exposed to the air. New and healing donor sites of the legs require support during ambulation; the figure-eight elastic (Ace) bandage wrapping technique is recommended to minimize trauma to newly formed capillaries. Assess for infection beneath the fabric and at wound periphery.

Product	Description	Indication	Nursing Considerations
Integra (Integra Life Sciences, Plainsboro, NJ)	Bilaminate substitute composed of collagen (dermal analog) and a Silastic covering (epidermal analog) The dermal analog is allowed to incorporate into the wound, becoming permanent	For application to excised wounds	The Silastic portion is removed after 2-3 days, providing a wound bed for placement of a very thin split-thickness skin graft. Assess for infection. Protect the site from mechanical shearing forces.
Calcium alginates (Curasorb, Tyco Health Care/Kendall Co, Mansfield, MA; Kalginate, DeRoyal Textiles, Camden, SC)	Dressing material derived from brown seaweeds (alginate) and calcium/sodium salts	Donor site dressing. To promote healing of superficial partial-thickness wounds (contraindicated in full-thickness wounds)	To apply, irrigate wound with a physiologic solution, apply calcium alginate dressing to the wound, and cover with an absorptive dressing. The entire dressing should be changed when the outer dressing is saturated with drainage.
Transparent films (Bioclusive, Johnson & Johnson, Arlington, TX; Op-Site, Smith & Nephew, Memphis, TN)	Hypoallergenic film dressing that is occlusive, waterproof, and permeable to moisture vapor	Donor site dressing. To promote healing of clean, small, superficial partial-thickness wounds	Use a margin of intact skin around the entire wound or donor site to adequately secure the dressing. Assess for pooling exudate; if significant exudate forms that threatens the integrity of the closed dressing, drain the exudate aseptically with a small-gauge needle and syringe; seal hole with a film patch.
Non-adhering gauze (Aquaphor gauze, Beiersdorf Inc. Norwalk, CT; Xeroform gauze, Sherwood Medical, St. Louis)	Fine-mesh gauze impregnated with ointment	Donor site dressing. To cover meshed autografts. To cover fragile, newly healed epithelium	Dressing material over donor site should remain intact until healed beneath (10-14 days). New and healing donor sites of the legs require support during ambulation; the figure-eight (Ace) wrapping technique is recommended to minimize trauma to newly formed capillaries.

TABLE 52-7	*Therapeutic Positioning for the Burn-Injured Client*	
Burned Area	**Therapeutic Position**	**Positioning Techniques**
Neck		
Anterior	Extension	No pillow Small towel roll beneath shoulders to promote neck extension
Circumferential	Neutral toward extension	No pillow
Posterior or asymmetrical	Neutral	No pillow
Shoulder/axilla	Arm abduction to 90-110 degrees	Splinting Arms positioned away from the body and supported on arm troughs
Elbow	Arm extension	Elbow splint Elbows positioned in extension with slight bend at the elbow (no more than 10 degrees of elbow flexion) Arms supported on arm troughs with the forearm in slight pronation
Hand		
Wrist	Wrist extension	Hand splint
MCP	MCP flexion at 90 degrees	Hand splint
PIP/DIP	PIP/DIP extension	Hand splint
Thumb	Thumb abduction	Hand splint with thumb abduction
Finger web spaces	Finger abduction	Web spacers of foam, silicone products, or custom-fitted pressure garments to decrease webbing formation
Hip	Hip extension	Supine with the head of bed flat and legs extended Trochanter roll to maintain neutral hip rotation (toes should be pointing toward the ceiling) Prone positioning
Knee	Knee extension	Supine with knees extended (toes should be pointing toward the ceiling) Prone positioning with feet extended over the end of the mattress Sitting in chair with legs extended and elevated Knee splint
Ankle	Neutral	Padded footboard Ankle positioning devices (avoid heel cord tightening)—provide heel protection to prevent pressure sore development

MCP, Metacarpal interphalangeal joint(s); *PIP/DIP,* proximal/distal interphalangeal joint(s).

Splints are used to maintain proper joint position and to prevent or correct contractures. Two types of splints are frequently used. A *static splint* immobilizes the joint. Static splints do not replace exercise and are frequently applied for periods of immobilization or during sleeping hours or are used for clients who cannot maintain proper positioning. In contrast, *dynamic splints* exercise the affected joint. Care must be taken to ensure that all splints fit properly and do not apply excessive pressure, which may lead to further tissue or nerve damage.

Provide Psychological Support. The longest period of adjustment occurs during the acute phase. The burn-injured adult may demonstrate a variety of emotional and psychological responses. Anxiety and fearfulness related to potential disfigurement and perceived changes in role and identity plague the client during this time period. Depression, withdrawal, and regression may result.[7]

The client may begin discussing the burn injury or accident, recounting significant events and searching for the meaning of what has happened.[1] Allowing the expression of these worries and validating that they are "normal" are essential in providing support. Staff members need to actively listen and to allow the client to talk about the accident. Detailed and repetitious recounting of the injury is useful in desensitizing clients to the horror of what has happened and in decreasing nightmares.[7]

Clients who have little information about specific treatment procedures, potential associated discomfort or pain, and available resources or options for pain management typically react with anxiety and a heightened pain response. Providing the client with information about what will occur during a particular procedure or what is expected over the course of recovery is a concept known as *providing preparatory information*. This technique is a psychologically based method that has proved successful in reducing pain and anxiety during certain procedures.[1,7] To enhance the client's sense of personal control, teaching should include education about various coping mechanisms and the use of nonpharmacologic methods for pain control.

Involving clients in their own care helps them to feel some control over the situation at hand. Clients can be encouraged to participate in wound care (e.g., bathing, simple debridement, dressing application) and physical therapy (e.g., active versus passive ROM exercises, application of splints and pressure garments). These interventions have been found to be effective in supporting the client's psychological needs.

■ Nursing Management of the Medical Client in the Acute Phase of Burn Injury
Assessment

Once fluid balance is achieved, the client moves into the acute phase of burn care. During this phase, closure of the wounds becomes one of the major foci of care. Wounds should be assessed every 2 to 3 days by the same personnel so that subtle changes in the wound can be recognized. Of course, the wound is also inspected with each dressing change. Other areas of assessment include respiratory condition; pain control, nutritional status and stress ulceration, mobility and contractures, and psychological adjustments by both the client and the family.

Diagnosis, Outcomes, Interventions

Diagnosis: Impaired Gas Exchange. Note that the consequences of smoke inhalation may not be fully appreciated until the acute phase of burn care. The decreased ciliary action in the airways leads to a high risk for infection (which usually is not manifested until day 3 or 4 after the burn injury), which is demonstrated first by tracheobronchitis and is followed by bronchopneumonia.

Outcomes. The client will have improved gas exchange, as evidenced by unlabored respirations, a respiratory rate of 16 to 24 breaths/min, PaO_2 of greater than 90 mm Hg, $PaCO_2$ of 35 to 45 mm Hg, SaO_2 greater than 95%, and clear bilateral breath sounds.

Interventions. Interventions continue unchanged from the emergent phase of injury. Comprehensive respiratory assessment and preventive pulmonary toilet should be performed every 2 hours.

Diagnosis: Ineffective Airway Clearance. Upper airway and facial edema caused by heat-induced tissue and mucosal damage begins to resolve between 2 and 4 days after injury with superficial burns. Full-thickness injuries, however, resolve more slowly, making *Ineffective Airway Clearance* a problem that may last well into the acute phase of treatment.

Outcomes. The client will have effective airway clearance, as evidenced by clear bilateral breath sounds, clear to white pulmonary secretions, effective mobilization of pulmonary secretions, and unlabored breathing.

Interventions. Continue interventions begun in the emergent phase of treatment. Pulmonary toilet including turning, coughing, and deep-breathing, use of an incentive spirometer every 2 to 4 hours while the client is awake, and endotracheal suctioning as needed facilitates clearance of secretions and sputum. Leave an oral suctioning device within the client's reach for independent use.

Diagnosis: Hypothermia. Clients remain at risk for loss of body heat through burn injuries until wound closure is complete. During dressing changes, clients are especially at risk for becoming hypothermic.

Outcomes. The client will maintain a core body temperature between 99.6° and 101° F (37.5° and 38.3° C).

Interventions. To help prevent the loss of heat from open wounds that occurs as a result of evaporation, limit hydrotherapy treatment sessions to 30 minutes or less with water temperatures of 98° to 102° F (36.6° C to 38.8° C). Cover the client with warm blankets after the hydrother- apy session, exposing only limited areas of body surface during topical agent and dressing application. Provide heat lamps or heat shields and increase the ambient temperature in the treatment room or in the client's room if the client exhibits subnormal temperatures.

Diagnosis: Risk for Infection. During the acute phase of injury, infection remains an ongoing risk owing to inadequate primary and secondary defenses resulting from traumatized tissue, bacterial proliferation in the burn wound, presence of invasive lines or urinary catheters, and an immunocompromised status.[24]

Outcomes. The client will have no significant burn wound microbial invasion, as evidenced by quantitative wound cultures containing less than 100,000 CFUs/g. In addition, the client will maintain core body temperature at 99.6° to

101° F; will demonstrate evidence of no swelling, redness, or purulence at invasive line insertion sites; and will have negative results on blood, urine, and sputum cultures.

Interventions. Continue to follow infection control policy for burn-injured clients in an effort to prevent cross-contamination. Assess for clinical manifestations of infection in the burn wound: discoloration of wounds (e.g., brown, black, or hemorrhagic), drainage, odor, delayed healing, or spongy eschar. As in the emergent phase, provide meticulous wound care in an aseptic fashion, cleaning and rinsing the wound, and debriding loose nonviable tissue to discourage bacterial growth. Apply a topical antimicrobial agent to the wound to decrease the risk for local wound infection. Continue to shave or cut body hair around wound margins until wound closure.

Observe for clinical indicators of sepsis: headache, chills, anorexia, nausea, changes in vital signs, hyperglycemia and glycosuria, paralytic ileus, and confusion, restlessness, or hallucinations. Assess for manifestations of infection at the catheter insertion site. Obtain cultures per physician order, and administer antibiotics and antipyretics as prescribed.

Collaborative Problem: Risk for Stress Ulceration.
Stress ulcers can occur at any time after a burn injury. The assessment and preventive treatment started in the emergent phase of injury should continue until wound coverage is completed.

Outcomes. The nurse will monitor for manifestations of gastrointestinal bleeding and will maintain gastric pH greater than 5.

Interventions. Monitor and document gastric pH values and heme content every 2 hours while the client's nasogastric tube is in place. Administer antacids or H_2 blockers per physician order to reduce the gastric acid content, because high acid levels may lead to bleeding. Monitor stools for occult blood.

Diagnosis: Imbalanced Nutrition: Less Than Body Requirements.
The burn-injured client must maintain adequate protein and caloric intake to meet metabolic demands for wound healing.

Outcomes. The client will have adequate nutrition, as evidenced by maintenance of 85% to 90% of preburn weight and healing of burn wounds, donor sites, and skin grafts.

Interventions. Caloric needs are based on preinjury weight. Obtain a daily weight to assess whether caloric needs are being met and to provide documentation for staff to follow trends. Assess eating habits and patterns, and identify food preferences and food allergies. Order

meals high in calories and proteins. Encourage family members or significant others to bring favorite foods from home. Provide nutritious supplements between meals.

Document daily caloric intake, and consult with the dietitian to perform a nutritional assessment. Consider other methods to meet caloric needs such as tube feeding or total parenteral feeding, because oral feeding may not provide adequate calories for healing.

Performing oral hygiene during each nursing shift and as needed helps to prevent stomatitis and enhance appetite. Provide an aesthetically pleasing environment that is conducive to eating. Schedule treatments to provide for uninterrupted meal times. Allow a period of rest before meal times if the client has endured a painful procedure or treatment, because pain will decrease appetite.

Diagnosis: Acute Pain.
The client can be expected to experience a significant amount of pain during the acute burn phase. The pain experienced during this phase of recovery is directly associated with the burn wound and donor sites, wound care procedures, and ROM exercises.

Outcomes. The client will verbalize a level of acceptable pain control.

Interventions. Continue to frequently assess for pain, and administer appropriate opioids and anxiolytics. Time the administration of medications so that the client receives the benefit of the drug's peak performance during painful procedures, and evaluate the effectiveness of interventions as initiated during the emergent burn phase.

During the acute phase, nonpharmacologic interventions should be initiated to enhance medication effects and to assist in controlling pain. Explore the benefits of relaxation techniques, guided imagery, music therapy, distraction, and biofeedback.

Diagnosis: Impaired Physical Mobility.
Impaired Physical Mobility during the acute phase of burn treatment is related to pain, the presence of dressings and splints, surgical procedures, and wound contractures.

Outcomes. The client will maintain soft tissue length, as evidenced by maintaining ROM without manifestations of early contracture formation.

Interventions. The main interventions during the acute phase of injury are splinting, positioning, and ROM exercises. Collaboration with physical and occupational therapists is essential for guidance in an individualized program for each client.

Optimal positioning of the client involves continuing use of anticontracture positions. Maintaining burned areas in a position of physiologic function by either splinting or positioning will help to prevent or reduce contracture development.

Encourage the client to participate in ADL, to ambulate, and to spend time sitting up in a chair. These activities will not only improve mobility but also assist in moving the client toward independence.

Diagnosis: Disturbed Personal Identity.
During the acute burn phase, the client recognizes the extent of injury and realizes that his or her body is changed forever. Depression, grief, fear, and anxiety confront the client.

Outcomes. The client will acknowledge body changes and demonstrate movement toward incorporating these changes into the self-concept. The client will not exhibit maladaptive responses such as severe depression.

Interventions. The client should be expected to experience emotional lability in progress through recovery. Staff members should provide an accepting atmosphere for the client, although the client should be assisted to exercise control over any destructive behaviors. Family members or significant others should be involved in care as much as possible to demonstrate continued support for the client. Staff members should be available to provide information about the appearance of burns and grafts and to explain changes that can be expected over time (up to 1 year). Providing information helps to reduce misconceptions and can give hope that the painful procedures can produce good results.

Diagnosis: Disabled Family Coping.
Recognize that families often imagine that the survival of the family unit is threatened following a member's injury. Normal coping mechanisms become overwhelmed.

Outcomes. Family members will demonstrate coping strategies, as evidenced by verbalizing realistic expectations for client outcomes, expressing knowledge of the goals of treatment regimen, interacting appropriately with the client, and demonstrating decreased emotional stress.

Interventions. Once beyond the emergent phase, it is important to provide the family members or significant others with information about what to expect for the burn-injured client in the future. It is helpful to provide families with daily updates regarding changes in the client's condition. This assists in maintaining realistic perceptions of the client's progress. Assist the family in finding ways to nurture the client and to participate in some aspects of care. These measures not only assure the client of the family's love and acceptance but also allow family members or significant others to regain some feelings of control. It may also be useful to introduce the family members to the local burn support group. Burn survivors and their families can provide emotional support and validation and can reinforce the concept that it is possible to survive burns and live acceptable happy lives.

■ Surgical Management in the Acute Phase of Burn Injury

Definitive wound care for full-thickness burns is accomplished by *autografting*, the surgical removal of a superficial layer of the client's own unburned skin, which is subsequently grafted to the excised or clean and granulating burn wound. Because the epidermis is split (in layers) rather than taken in full, these grafts are referred to as *split-thickness grafts*. This procedure is performed in the operating room while the client is under general anesthesia. Autografts can be applied either as a sheet *(sheet graft)* or in a meshed form *(meshed graft)*.

A sheet autograft is applied to the excised wound bed without alteration in its integrity. Sheet autografts are frequently used to graft burns in visible areas.

In contrast, a meshed autograft contains many little slits that allow for expansion of the donor skin. Meshing permits coverage of larger areas of irregularly shaped wounds and allows for drainage from a bleeding wound bed. When healed, the meshed pattern of the autograft remains visible. Therefore meshed grafts are used on hidden body areas. When a thicker layer of skin is removed, consisting of the epidermis and the dermis, this is referred to as a *full-thickness graft*. For all autografts, the area of the body from which the skin was removed is referred to as the *donor site* (Figure 52-13).

Graft adherence is dependent on the formation of a fibrin bond between the recipient bed and the graft.[35] There are no vascular connections between the graft and the wound bed immediately after surgery. The graft is held in place only by weak fibrin bonds and is nourished by the diffusion of serum from the wound bed. The graft begins to stabilize after 3 days as a fibrovascular and col-

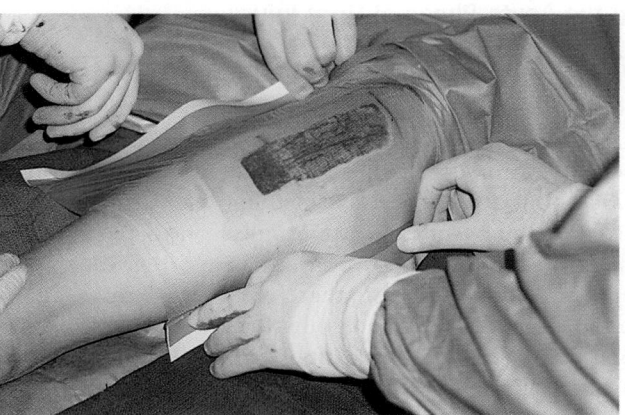

FIGURE 52-13 Harvesting donor skin from the lateral portion of the client's thigh.

lagen network form and provide durability to the graft. A bleeding wound bed, hematoma formation, or shearing of the graft disrupts formation of this bond between graft and bed. Care must be taken during the postoperative period to assess for bleeding, remove accumulated serum beneath sheet grafts (as described next in the discussion on nursing management of the surgical client), and prevent unwanted movement and shearing of autografts.[34]

Various types of dressings are used to cover donor sites, depending on the size, location, and condition of adjacent skin or tissue. However, despite the differences in dressings, the donor site wound requires the same meticulous care as for other partial-thickness wounds, to expedite healing and prevent infection. If the donor site becomes infected, the dressing should be gently removed or soaked off. The wound can then be thoroughly cleansed and an antimicrobial agent applied. Once the donor site has healed, lubricating lotions can be applied to soften the area and reduce itching. Donor sites can be reused after they are healed.

Cultured *epithelial autografting* is a technique for closure of massive burn wounds.[34,36] The process of autologous epithelial cell growth begins with taking a full-thickness skin specimen from an uninjured body site. This specimen is sent to a specialized laboratory for culture and growth. Typically, in 3 to 4 weeks, several sheets of cultured epithelial autografts are ready for application. In the operating room, the cultured epithelial autograft sheets are carefully applied to an excised and nonbleeding wound bed and are secured in place with staples. Dressings are applied and moistened with an antibiotic solution shown to be nontoxic to the cultured epithelial autografts.

Reports demonstrating the success of cultured epithelial autografts in the treatment of massive burn wounds have been limited. Both early and late cultured epithelial autograft loss due to mechanical shearing, nutritional imbalance, infection, or an autoimmune response have been reported.[49]

Nursing Management of the Surgical Client in the Acute Phase of Burn Injury

Preoperative Care
Routine care of clients undergoing surgery is discussed in Chapter 16. Specific preoperative care of the client scheduled for debridement includes providing information about areas to be debrided and plans for pain control. Debridement cases are usually considered contaminated in the operating room and are often done at the end of the surgical list; therefore clients may wait for many hours before undergoing the scheduled procedure. Specific orders for medications to be given or withheld, and the time to begin *nil per os* (NPO) (i.e., nothing by mouth) status should be obtained.

Before skin grafting, clients need information on the type of skin graft to be used, the location of the donor site, the postoperative plans for pain control, and the need for

immobility and elevation of the graft site. Fears over scarring should be addressed; in general, scarring cannot be predicted because scar tissue requires a full year to mature. Both debridement and grafting can be multiple procedures, and clients may become anxious over repeated surgical procedures. Severe anxiety should be communicated to the surgeon and anesthesia personnel.

Postoperative Care
Routine postoperative care is discussed in Chapter 16. Care specific to debrided wounds includes assessment of bleeding and pain control. Many clients report more pain in donor sites (owing to exposed nerve endings) than in recipient sites. Skin-grafted sites must be immobilized to promote adherence of the graft to the wound bed. Various techniques are used, including suture, staples, tape, and dressings. Blebs of serum should be removed from graft sites using a small needle and cotton-tipped applicator or making a slit in the graft with a scalpel or sharp scissors. Skin-grafted sites are elevated to prevent edema, in which the swelling of edematous tissue lifts the graft from the wound bed. Bed rest may be prescribed. If the graft is on the lower legs, the client should typically not walk until postoperative day 7 to be certain the graft has appropriately adhered.

REHABILITATION PHASE
The rehabilitation phase of recovery represents the final phase of burn care and encompasses the time from wound closure to discharge and beyond. In order for the best outcomes to be achieved, caregivers must understand the consequences of burn injury, and treatment for rehabilitation must begin from the day of injury. Rehabilitation should overlap the acute care phase and last well beyond the acute inpatient hospitalization. Ultimately, a burn rehabilitation program is designed for maximal functional and emotional recovery. Measures to promote wound healing, to prevent or minimize deformities and hypertrophic scarring, to increase physical strength and function, to promote emotional support, and to provide education are a part of the ongoing rehabilitation phase.

See the Bridge to Home Health Care feature on Managing After Burns on p. 1461.

■ Medical Management in the Rehabilitation Phase of Burn Injury
Minimize Functional Loss. Early wound excision helps minimize short-term and long-term functional loss by closing the wound, minimizing infection, and eliminating wound pain. A skin graft, although more elastic than eschar, still does not have normal elasticity. The resultant wound stiffness must be counterbalanced with aggressive therapy and splinting.

Exercise, splinting, and positioning continue through all phases of burn injury; however, it is during this phase

BRIDGE TO HOME HEALTH CARE
Managing After Burns

When admitting the burn-injured client to home health services, remember that each case is unique and involves detailed treatment instructions. Include the client's and family members' responses to the client's discharge from the hospital and to the client's being home in the nursing assessment. If clients require assistance with activities of daily living (ADL), they will need a primary caregiver to provide both emotional support and direct care. This person is a critical member of the health care delivery team.

Work with the client and the primary caregiver to set up a place in the home for dressing changes and storage of needed dressing materials that limits the possibility of contamination. This area should be comfortable, relaxing, and off-limits to family pets. If possible, select a room that clients do not use for other activities, especially sleeping, so that they do not associate these activities with pain from dressing changes. The dressing materials and an up-to-date wound care plan can be neatly organized and stored in a sealed plastic box or plastic bag. Supplies should be ordered on a weekly basis in quantities that can be used for one dressing change. In some agencies, prepackaged wound care kits provide an excellent method of infection control and significantly reduce the amount of waste.

Although dressing changes and physical therapy can be painful experiences for the client, both are essential for recovery. Identify ways to decrease the pain or the length of time during which pain will occur. Work with the physical therapist, the client, and the family to determine the best schedule for these activities. Consider scheduling joint visits if this would improve the care given to the client. Instruct a family member to give prescribed pain medications 1 hour before the scheduled dressing change to provide the best relief for the client. While changing dressings, use soft music or relaxation techniques, and involve the client and family as much as possible. These strategies offer a sense of control and can decrease the client's perception of pain.

Unless mechanical debridement of the wound is necessary, the dressings should not stick to the wound bed. Avoid removing dried-on dressings because they cause unnecessary pain. If the dressings are sticking, soak them off with normal saline, or after obtaining the physician's approval, remove them in the shower. Collaborate with the primary physician or a wound care nurse to obtain an appropriate moisture-retentive dressing to reduce or eliminate pain with dressing changes.

Rehabilitation of people who have suffered burn injury involves more than dressing changes and physical therapy. It is also important to consider the psychological stress of the initial injury, scarring, and surgical procedures and other treatments as well as the financial burden from loss of work time and the lengthy recovery period. Evaluate the need of the client and family members for referrals to local agencies that offer social, counseling, financial, and spiritual services as well as support groups. Such services may be essential in order for clients and their families to cope with the traumatic life event that a major burn injury with its sequelae represents.

---

that the importance of these efforts becomes paramount. These measures are crucial to the client's progression to optimal functional independence.

Hypertrophic scarring, which results from an overabundant deposition of collagen in the healed burn wound, can be minimized with the use of massage and pressure therapy.[38] Constant pressure applied to healing burn wounds has been found to reduce the scarring process. Several commercially available products provide the constant, even pressure that is required. Although hypertrophic scarring usually does not peak until several months after the injury, it is important to plan ahead before the onset of loss of function. By the rehabilitation phase of injury, the client should be measured for custom-fit burn scar support garments for any area that did not heal within 3 weeks of injury[38] (Figure 52-14).

Provide Psychosocial Support. In this, the last phase of burn injury, during which the wounds are almost healed and specific plans are made for hospital discharge, the client must face numerous issues and overcome many concerns. Self-image issues, pain, physical limitations, and fear of rejection represent only a few of the issues the client must deal with as discharge nears.[7] During this time, it is important to maintain good communication with the client. It is beneficial to the client for the staff to encourage independence and carry the message that survivors can find ways to achieve whatever goals they set for themselves. Pain control and anxiety prevention continue to require assessment and medical management as needed. Psychosocial assistance for the client and family members or significant others should carry through from admission to discharge.

■ Nursing Management of the Medical Client in the Rehabilitation Phase of Burn Injury
Assessment

Once the client's burns are nearly healed, the focus becomes preparing the client and family for discharge to a home setting and self-care (for some clients, other set-

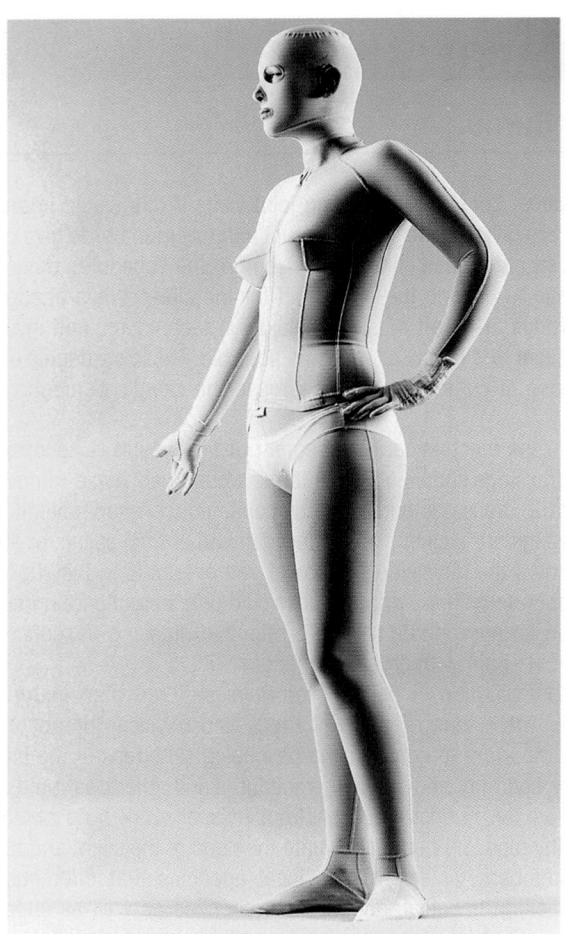

FIGURE 52-14 The model is wearing custom-fitted antiscar support garment. When worn 23 hours a day, this garment is effective in providing pressure over healing burn wounds. Pressure therapy helps to minimize the development of hypertrophic scarring. (Courtesy of Medical Z Corporation, San Antonio, TX.)

tings will be used). Nurses will assess the client's and family's comprehension of teaching and ability to perform needed care. Nurses will also determine the best methods to teach the client and family. The client's psychological status and need for vocational rehabilitation will be addressed during this final phase.

Diagnosis, Outcomes, Interventions

Diagnosis: Impaired Physical Mobility.
During the rehabilitation phase of burn injury, the client's physical mobility and ability to provide self-care are impaired by the presence of dressings, pain, scarring, contracture, and muscle atrophy.

Outcomes. The client will have improved physical mobility, as evidenced by maximum independence in performance of ADL, with minimum disability and disfigurement.

Interventions. The physical and occupational therapy consultations initiated in the early phases of burn injury are especially important for continued treatment in the rehabilitation phase as the client works toward functional independence. Typically, the therapist provides an individualized rehabilitation schedule as well as needed assistive devices for the client.

Motivate the client to participate in self-care activity such as brushing teeth and self-feeding, because this increased activity will not only improve mobility but also lessen dependence. Provide assistive devices furnished by therapy consultants to assist the client with any limitations. Expect tasks to take longer when the client works independently. Allow adequate time for the client to complete the undertaking. Self-confidence will be gained with independent functioning regardless of the time spent.

Encourage active ROM every 2 to 4 hours while the client is awake unless contraindicated because of a recent grafting procedure. Increased activity prevents muscle atrophy, tendon adherence, joint stiffness, and capsular tightness. Help the client to ambulate to promote muscle strength and cardiopulmonary reserve. Provide passive exercise and stretching if the client is unable to actively participate (e.g., if the client is comatose or paralyzed).

Wrap donor sites on both burned and unburned legs with elastic bandage wraps (Ace bandages), using a figure-eight technique, before placing the limbs in a dependent position. The support will decrease capillary venous stasis, which impairs wound healing. Explain the rationale for activities to the client and family members, because understanding improves compliance. Avoid the position of comfort, and maintain burned areas in the position of physiologic function, within the client's limit of endurance. Continue to follow the splinting and positioning regimen recommended in the therapy consultation.

Diagnosis: Acute Pain and Chronic Pain.
Pain experienced during the rehabilitation phase of burn injury is typically associated with wound care and therapeutic activity, particularly ROM exercises.

Outcomes. The client will have an acceptable level of comfort, as evidenced by verbalizing relief or control of pain or discomfort and actively participating in care.

Interventions. Formulate a plan for controlling the client's pain based on an assessment of the client's response to pain and documentation of previous successful treatment regimens. As in the earlier phases of injury, allow adequate time for the onset of the medication for maximum benefits of the medication (5 minutes for the IV route; 20 to 30 minutes for the oral route). Non- pharmacologic methods of pain control, such as relaxation techniques, music therapy, guided imagery, distraction, and hypnosis, may improve the client's comfort, even if such methods were not successful in early phases of injury. As described earlier, effective communication assists in decreasing the client's anxiety. In preparation for impending discharge, the client should at some point during the rehabilitation phase progress to analgesia given only by the oral route.

Diagnosis: Disturbed Personal Identity.
The client is at risk for self-esteem disturbances related to threatened or actual change in body image, physical loss, and loss of role responsibilities.

Outcomes. The client will develop improved self-esteem, as evidenced by making social contact with others outside the immediate family, developing effective coping mechanisms throughout the stages of recovery, and verbalizing feelings about self-concept.

Interventions. Allowing time for two-way communication with the client is especially important during this phase of injury. Provide an atmosphere of acceptance as the client tries various coping strategies to deal with the injury. Provide honest and accurate information about the client's projected appearance to reduce misconceptions that he or she may have.

Assess the need for limit setting for maladaptive behavior. Consult with burn team members to establish such limits and to formulate a treatment plan for such behaviors; explain limit setting to family members or significant others and assist them to maintain the same limits. Promote the client's self-confidence by providing information about the progress made, and support the client's role in care and treatment, providing encouragement and positive reinforcement.

Encourage family members to interact with the client, because this encouragement facilitates societal reintegration. During this phase of recovery, encourage the client to interact with others outside the facility. Use of a family day pass during this time is useful. Help to prepare the client for social interaction after discharge by discussing potential situations and how the client might deal with them. Such preparation provides rehearsal of events and reduces anxiety.

Diagnosis: Impaired Skin Integrity.
The expectation is that by the time the client reaches the rehabilitation phase of burn injury, the majority of wounds will be either healed or grafted. The new skin over areas of donor site, graft, and healed burn is characteristically very thin, with disrupted oil glands. The skin therefore is fragile; it becomes very dry and shears or cracks easily; and it is prone to infection.

Outcomes. The client will have intact skin with no evidence of infection, breakdown, or blistering.

Interventions. Daily wound and skin care should continue throughout hospitalization. Clean burned areas, grafts, and donor sites daily with a mild soap (without fragrance) and water. Rinse thoroughly to remove the soap. After cleaning, the healed skin should be lubricated with a nonirritating, alcohol-free moisturizer. Itching associated with dry skin can be minimized with application of the moisturizer at least three times a day. Avoid any shearing of tissue with dressings, clothing, or splints.

Diagnosis: Deficient Knowledge.
The burn-injured client or a family member or significant other must have knowledge of important treatment modalities that need continuation after discharge from the hospital.

Outcomes. The client or a family member or significant other will verbalize knowledge and demonstrate techniques that facilitate continued wound healing and limb mobility.

Interventions. Demonstrate and discuss the following skin care interventions with the client and appropriate family member or significant other: daily skin and wound care and dressing instructions if any; lubrication of grafts, donor sites, and healed burn wounds using an alcohol-free skin moisturizer at least three times daily; wearing pressure dressings or garments for 23 hours daily; and complete avoidance of direct sunlight for 1 year after injury owing to increased sensitivity to ultraviolet rays.

Review current medications and the dosage, precautions, and potential side effects. Discuss nutritional needs and the benefits of diets with adequate protein and calories.

Provide information on support groups or peers and counseling as needed for adjustment to life outside the hospital setting. Stress the need for follow-up care, and provide appointment dates and times if these have been established.

CONCLUSIONS

Nursing care of the burn-injured client is both complex and challenging. The psychological and physical trauma sustained following a burn injury can be devastating for both the victim and family members or significant others. Having a thorough understanding of the pathophysiologic changes that occur after a burn, knowing what to expect clinically as a result of the injury, and becoming familiar with the standards of care will guide nursing care to promote positive outcomes. As a key member of the burn team, you are responsible for an individualized plan of care that reflects the client's changing needs during progression through the different phases of recovery. Priority issues and care change as the client moves from the critical emergent phase into and, ultimately, through the rehabilitation period.

THINKING CRITICALLY *evolve*

1. You are working on the night shift in your hospital's burn center and receive a call that a client is in transport via ambulance to your unit. He will be a direct admission and bypass the emergency department. The telephone report reveals that the client was found unconscious on the floor of the bedroom. He is covered with soot and has obvious burns on his face, arms, and torso. An intravenous line of lactated Ringer's solution was started and is running wide open. Oxygen is being administered via face mask. On admission, the client is received lying in the supine position on a gurney. He is restless, confused, and combative. He appears anxious and in pain. The eyebrows, eyelashes, and hair are singed. There is soot in the nares and mouth and on the tongue. His voice is raspy, and he is coughing up thick black sputum. Breath sounds are scattered crackles; oxygen saturation is 75%. A face mask is in place but was disconnected from the oxygen tank while the client was being moved onto the burn center gurney.

Heart rate is 142 beats/min, with sinus tachycardia. Respiratory rate is 40 breaths/min and labored. Blood pressure is 144/88 mm Hg; temperature is 35° C. Bowel sounds are absent. There is thick, white leathery eschar on the chest, neck, left and right arm, and hands. The skin of the face and back are pink, moist, and blistered. The body from the waist to the feet is unburned. An IV line is infusing the LR right saphenous vein. Weight is 85 kg. What priorities should be set for the client's care? What interventions should be undertaken?

Factors to Consider. What is the client's respiratory status? Do the physical examination and history provided by the ambulance crew give any clues to his respiratory status? What should you consider when administering pain medication or anxiolytics to this client? What is the client's fluid volume status? How will you monitor fluid resuscitation?

2. It is now 7 days after the injury and the client has just returned to the unit after receiving grafts on his chest, neck, bilateral arms, hands, and axillae. Donor skin was taken circumferentially from both thighs. What assessments should you perform? What interventions should be undertaken?

Factors to Consider. What factors disrupt graft adherence? What can you do to help prevent contracture formation?

3. It is now 2 months since the client was injured and the team begins to discuss discharge plans. The client tells you that he does not want to go home and does not want to talk any more about discharge. What can you do to help the client?

Factors to Consider. What concerns might a burn survivor face upon discharge from the hospital? What professional resources might be helpful in addressing this situation? What lay resources might be helpful?

Discussions for these questions can be found on the website and the CD-ROM.

BIBLIOGRAPHY

1. Adcock, R., Boeve, S., & Patterson, D. (1998). Psychological and emotional recovery. In G.J. Carrougher (Ed.), *Burn care and therapy* (pp. 329-347). St. Louis: Mosby.
2. Ahrns, K.S., & Harkins, D.R. (1999). Initial resuscitation after burn injury: Therapies, strategies, and controversies. *AACN Clinical Issues in Critical Care Nursing, 10*(1), 46-60.
3. American Burn Association. (1984). Guidelines for service standards and severity classification in the treatment of burn injuries. *Bulletin of the American College of Surgeons, 69*(10), 24-28.
4. American Burn Association. (2002). The fire safe cigarette [online]. Available: http://www.ameriburn.org.
5. American Burn Association (2002). Burn incidence and treatment in the US: 2000 fact sheet [online]. Available: http://www.ameriburn.org/pub/Burn%20Incidence%20Fact%Sheet.htm.
6. Barillo, D.J., & Goode, R. (1996). Fire fatality study: Demographics of fire victims. *Burns, 22*(2), 85-88.
7. Blakeney, P., et al. (2002). Psychosocial recovery and reintegration of patients with burn injuries. In D.N. Herndon (Ed.), *Total burn care* (pp. 783-797). London: W. B. Saunders.
8. Carrougher, G.J. (1999). Inhalation injury. *AACN Clinical Issues in Critical Care Nursing, 10*(1), 367-376.
9. Carrougher, G.J. (1998). Burn wound assessment and topical treatment. In G.J. Carrougher (Ed.), *Burn care and therapy* (pp. 133-159). St. Louis: Mosby.
10. Cioffi, W.G. (1998). Inhalation injury. In G.J. Carrougher (Ed.), *Burn care and therapy* (pp. 35-59). St. Louis: Mosby.
11. Davis, S.T., & Sheely-Adolphson, P. (1997). Psychosocial interventions: Pharmacologic and psychologic modalities. *Nursing Clinics of North America, 32*(2), 331-340.
12. Demling, R.H. (1998). *Burn trauma*. New York: Thieme.
13. Everett, J. J. (1994). Pain assessment from patients with burns and their nurses. *Journal of Burn Care and Rehabilitation, 15*(2), 194-198.
14. Gordon, M., & Winfree, J. (1998). Fluid resuscitation after a major burn. In G.J. Carrougher (Ed.), *Burn care and therapy* (pp. 107-126). St. Louis: Mosby.

evolve **Did you remember to check out the bonus material on the Evolve website and the CD-ROM, including free self-assessment exercises?**

http://evolve.elsevier.com/Black/medsurg/

15. Gottschlich, M., & Jenkins, M. (1998). Metabolic consequences and nutritional needs. In G.J. Carrougher (Ed.), *Burn care and therapy* (pp. 213-226). St. Louis: Mosby.

16. Greenfield, E., & McManus, A. (1997). Infectious complications. Prevention strategies for their control. *Nursing Clinics of North America, 32*(2), 297-308.

17. Hansbrough, J., & Franco, E. (1998). Skin replacements. *Clinics in Plastic Surgery, 25*(3), 407-423.

18. Harris, B., & Gelfand, J. (1995). The immune response to trauma. *Seminars in Pediatric Surgery, 4*(2), 77-81.

19. Hildreth, M., & Gottschlich, M. (1996). Nutritional support of the burned patient. In D.N. Herndon (Ed.), *Total burn care* (pp. 237-245). London: W. B. Saunders.

20. Jain, S., & Bandi, V. (1999). Electrical and lightning injuries. *Critical Care Clinics, 15*(2), 319-329.

21. Jordan, B., & Barillo, D. (1998). Prehospital care and transport. In G.J. Carrougher (Ed.), *Burn care and therapy* (pp. 61-88). St. Louis: Mosby.

22. Kirn, D.S., & Luce, E.A. (1997). Early excision and grafting versus conservative management of burns in the elderly. *Plastic and Reconstructive Surgery, 9*, 1013-1017.

23. Kramer, G., Lund, T., & Herndon, D. (2002). Pathophysiology of burn shock and burn edema. In D.N. Herndon (Ed.), *Total burn care* (pp. 78-87). London: W. B. Saunders.

 24. LeBoucher, J., & Cynober, L. (1997). Protein metabolism and therapy in burn injury. *Annals of Nutrition and Metabolism, 41*, 69-82.

25. Lee, J. (1970). Emotional reactions to trauma. *Nursing Clinics of North America, 5*(4), 577-587.

26. Lee-Chiong, T. (1999). Smoke inhalation injury. When to suspect and how to treat. *Postgraduate Medicine, 105*(2), 55-62.

27. Lim, J., Rehmar, S., & Elmore, P. (1998). Rapid response: Care of burn victims. *AAOHN Journal, 46*(4), 169-178.

28. Marvin, J. (1998). Management of pain and anxiety. In G.J. Carrougher (Ed.), *Burn care and therapy* (pp. 167-179). St. Louis: Mosby.

29. Mayes, T. (1997). Enteral nutrition for the burn patient. *Nutrition in Clinical Practice, 12*(1), S43-S45.

30. Meyer, W., et al. (2002). Pain response and pain control. In D.N. Herndon (Ed.), *Total burn care* (pp. 747-765). London: W. B. Saunders.

31. Mlcak, R., Buffalo, M. (2002). Prehospital management, transport and emergency care. In D.N. Herndon (Ed.), *Total burn care* (pp. 67-77). London: W. B. Saunders.

32. Monafo, W. (1996). Initial management of burns. *New England Journal of Medicine, 335*(21), 1581-1586.

33. Monafo, W. (1996). Wound care. In D.N. Herndon (Ed.), *Total burn care* (pp. 88-97). London: W.B. Saunders.

34. Mozingo, D. (1998). Surgical management. In G.J. Carrougher (Ed.), *Burn care and therapy* (pp. 233-246). St. Louis: Mosby.

35. Muller, M., & Herndon, D. (2002). Operative wound management. In D.N. Herndon (Ed.), *Total burn care* (pp. 170-182). London: W. B. Saunders.

 36. Munster, A. (1996). Cultured skin for massive burns. *Annals of Surgery, 224*(3), 372-377.

37. Oman, K., & Reilly, E. (1998). Initial assessment and care in the emergency department. In G.J. Carrougher (Ed.), *Burn care and therapy* (pp. 89-101). St. Louis: Mosby.

38. Pessina, M., & Ellis, S. (1997). Rehabilitation. *Nursing Clinics of North America, 32*(2), 365-373.

39. Pruitt, B., & Cioffi, W. (1995). Diagnosis and treatment of smoke inhalation. *Journal of Intensive Care Medicine, 10*(3), 117-127.

40. Pruitt, B., & Goodwin, C. (1995). Thermal injury. In J.H. Davis & G.F. Sheldon (Eds.), *Clinical surgery*. St. Louis: Mosby.

41. Pruitt, B., Goodwin, C., & Mason, A. (2002). Epidemiological, demographic and outcome characteristics of burn injury. In D.N. Herndon (Ed.), *Total burn care* (pp. 16-30). London: W. B. Saunders.

42. Rose, J.K., et al. (1997). Allograft is superior to topical anti- microbial therapy in the treatment of partial-thickness scald burns in children. *Journal of Burn Care and Rehabilitation, 18*(4), 338-341.

43. Rutan, R. (1998). Physiologic response to cutaneous burn injury. In G.J. Carrougher (Ed.), *Burn care and therapy* (pp. 1-28). St. Louis: Mosby.

44. Saffle, J., & Hildreth, M. (2002). Metabolic support of the burned patient. In D.N. Herndon (Ed.), *Total burn care* (pp. 271-287). London: W. B. Saunders.

45. Sakurai, H., Traber, L., & Traber, D. (1998). Altered systemic organ blood flow after combined injury with burn and smoke inhalation. *Shock, 3*(5), 369-374.

46. Shankowsky, H.A., Callioux, L.S., & Tredget, E.E. (1994). North America survey of hydrotherapy in modern burn care. *Journal of Burn Care and Rehabilitation, 15*(2), 143-146.

47. Sheridan, R., & Tompkins, R. (2002). Alternative wound coverings. In D.N. Herndon (Ed.), *Total burn care* (pp. 212-218). London: W. B. Saunders.

48. Smith, D. (1995). Use of Biobrane in wound management. *Journal of Burn Care and Rehabilitation, 16*(3), 317-320.

49. Thompkins, R.M., & Carrougher, G.J. (1998). Burn prevention. In G.J. Carrougher (Ed.), *Burn care and therapy* (pp. 497-522). St. Louis: Mosby.

50. Traber, D., & Polland, V. (1996). Pathophysiology of inhalation injury. In D.N. Herndon (Ed.), *Total burn care* (pp. 175-183). London: W. B. Saunders.

51. Ward, R.S. (1998). Physical rehabilitation. In G.J. Carrougher (Ed.), *Burn care and therapy* (pp. 293-320). St. Louis: Mosby.

52. Warden, G.D. (2002). Fluid resuscitation and early management. In D.N. Herndon (Ed.), *Total burn care* (pp. 88-97). London: W. B. Saunders.

53. Weber, J. (1998). Epidemiology of infections and strategies for control. In G.J. Carrougher (Ed.), *Burn care and therapy* (pp. 185-206). St. Louis: Mosby.

54. Williams, W. (2002). Pathophysiology of the burn wound. In D.N. Herndon (Ed.), *Total burn care* (pp. 514-522). London: W. B. Saunders.

55. Wilson, D., & Bailie, F. (1999). Night attire burns in young girls: The return of an old adversary. *Burns, 25* (3), 269-271.

Unit 12

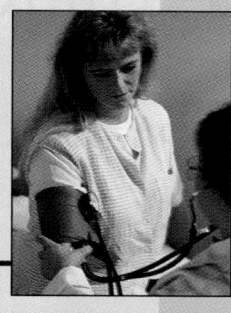

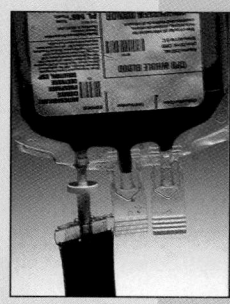

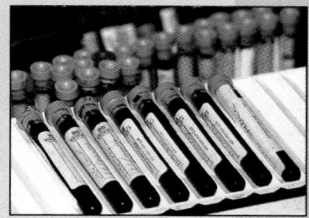

Circulatory Disorders

Anatomy and Physiology Review

The Circulatory System

Robert G. Carroll

The vascular system is a vast network of vessels through which blood circulates in the body. The major functions of the cardiovascular system—delivery of nutrients to tissues and removal of metabolic wastes—are accomplished in the capillaries. Blood leaving the ventricles is distributed through arteries and arterioles, in progressively smaller branches to the capillaries (a *divergent* pattern, like a river to a delta). Blood leaving the capillaries follows progressively larger venules and veins on its way back to the atria (a *convergent* pattern, like tributaries flowing into a river).

The anatomic arrangement of blood vessels allows regulation of blood flow at the individual tissue level so that blood flow delivery can be proportional to the tissue's metabolic needs. Because the volume of blood flowing from the arteries to the capillaries is a major determinant of blood pressure, the blood pressure control systems also include control of arteriolar diameter by the sympathetic nervous system and circulating hormones.

STRUCTURES OF THE VASCULAR SYSTEM

Two series of blood vessels—the systemic and the pulmonary circulations—distribute blood to the capillaries and return blood to the heart. Blood exiting the left ventricle enters the *systemic circulation*, passing progressively through the aorta, arteries, arterioles, capillaries, venules, veins, and finally the vena cava before entering the right atrium (Figure U12-1). For the *pulmonary circulation*, blood flows from the right ventricle into the pulmonary artery, then passes through arterioles, pulmonary capillaries, and venules before returning to the pulmonary vein and the left atrium.

GENERAL BLOOD VESSEL STRUCTURE

The anatomic division of blood vessels into arteries, arterioles, capillaries, venules, and veins is based on the presence of up to three histologic layers (Figure U12-2):

1. The *tunica intima* (innermost layer) consists of endothelial cells that separate the blood from the extravascular spaces. The tightness of the junctions between the endothelial cells varies among tissues. For example, the very tight junctions of cerebral capillaries restrict movement of some drugs to brain cells (the blood-brain barrier). In contrast, the endothelial cell holes and relatively loose junctions in the liver and spleen allow easy transit between the blood and tissue spaces in those organs. The endothelium has surface proteins, or *adhesion molecules,* that facilitate the attachment of white blood cells and their movement from the circulation to the tissues. The endothelium generates substances such as endothelial-derived relaxing factor (EDRF, or nitric oxide), allowing nitroglycerin, friction, and stress to cause vasodilation. Damage to the endothelium may allow blood to enter the middle layer of a blood vessel, creating an aneurysm.

2. The *tunica media* (middle layer) consists of elastic connective tissue and smooth muscle cells. Particularly in the aorta and large arteries, the elastic tissue contributes to the shape of the arterial pressure pulse. Smooth muscle contraction regulates the diameter of the vessel and causes a change in blood flow and blood pressure. Smooth muscle is normally partially contracted because of sympathetic nerve activity. Smooth muscle contraction can also be regulated by circulating hormones and (in the smaller vessels) by tissue metabolic factors.

3. The *tunica adventitia* (outermost layer) consists of a relatively thin layer of connective tissue that provides shape for the blood vessels. This layer also houses the *vasa vasorum*, the small arteries and veins that provide nutrients to the cells of the blood vessel.

VASCULAR SEGMENTS

Arteries and Arterioles

Arteries, particularly the aorta, have an extensive elastic tissue layer that accounts for the difference between arterial pressure (120/80 mm Hg) and left ventricular pressure (120/10 mm Hg). The elastic tissue stretches during ventricular ejection, storing energy. When the aortic

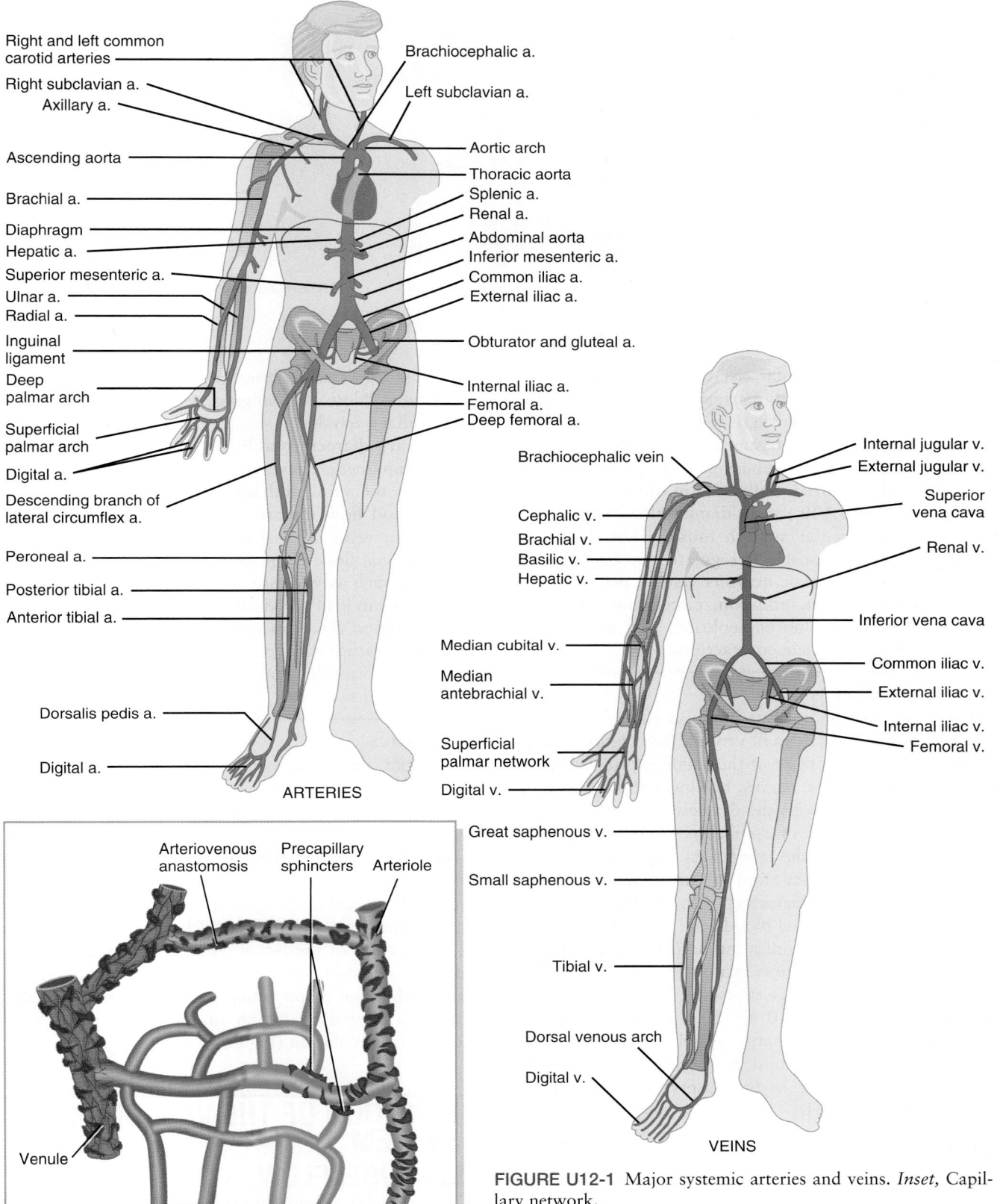

Right and left common carotid arteries

Brachiocephalic a.

Right subclavian a.

Left subclavian a.

Axillary a.

Aortic arch

Ascending aorta

Thoracic aorta

Brachial a.

Splenic a.

Diaphragm

Renal a.

Hepatic a.

Abdominal aorta

Inferior mesenteric a.

Superior mesenteric a.

Common iliac a.

Ulnar a.

External iliac a.

Radial a.

Inguinal ligament

Obturator and gluteal a.

Deep palmar arch

Internal iliac a.

Femoral a.

Superficial palmar arch

Deep femoral a.

Digital a.

Descending branch of lateral circumflex a.

Brachiocephalic vein

Internal jugular v.

External jugular v.

Cephalic v.

Superior vena cava

Brachial v.

Basilic v.

Renal v.

Hepatic v.

Peroneal a.

Inferior vena cava

Posterior tibial a.

Median cubital v.

Anterior tibial a.

Common iliac v.

Median antebrachial v.

External iliac v.

Internal iliac v.

Femoral v.

Superficial palmar network

Dorsalis pedis a.

Digital v.

Digital a.

ARTERIES

Great saphenous v.

Arteriovenous anastomosis

Precapillary sphincters

Arteriole

Small saphenous v.

Tibial v.

Venule

Dorsal venous arch

Digital v.

VEINS

True capillaries

FIGURE U12-1 Major systemic arteries and veins. *Inset,* Capillary network.

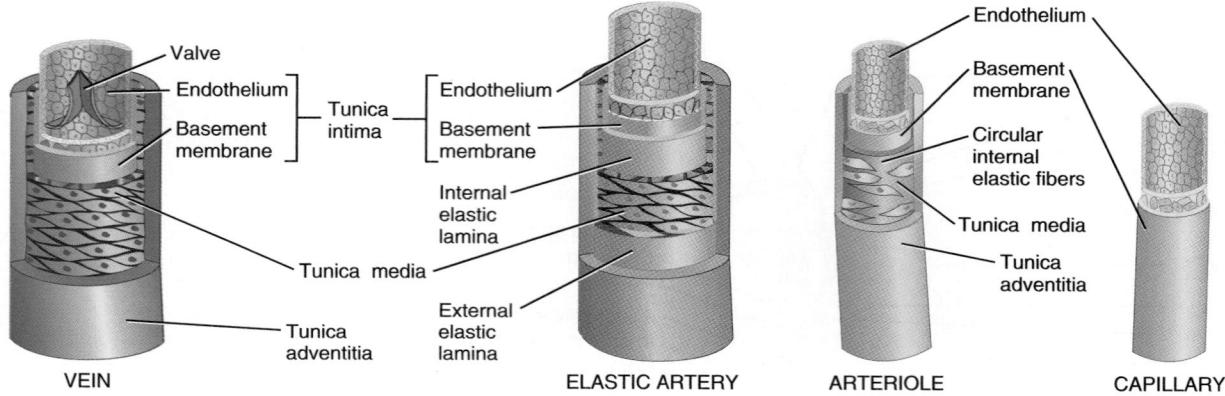

FIGURE U12-2 Structure of blood vessels.

valve closes and ventricular ejection stops, recoil of the elastic tissue slows the fall of arterial pressure during the interval until the next period of ventricular ejection. The efficiency of the elastic tissue decreases with age and with atherosclerosis, contributing to the rise in systolic arterial blood pressure usually seen in older adults.

Arterioles (5 to 100 μm in diameter) contain a high proportion of vascular smooth muscle. The degree of contraction of this muscle is regulated by background activity of the autonomic nervous system, primarily the sympathetic nerves. In addition, circulating hormones such as epinephrine, norepinephrine, and angiotensin can cause smooth muscle contraction.

Microcirculation

The microcirculation consists of the small arterioles, the capillary beds, and the small venules (see Figure U12-1, *inset*). The smooth muscle of the small arterioles is contracted by sympathetic nerves, but local factors become increasingly important as the diameter of the vessel decreases. The *precapillary sphincters* (the last band of smooth muscle before the capillaries) respond only to local factors. Blood passes from the arterioles into capillaries (5 to 10 μm in diameter). The capillary diameter approaches that of the red blood cell (7 μm in diameter). Capillaries have only a tunica intima (see Figure U12-2), and the small wall thickness facilitates exchange by diffusion. In tissues such as the skin, blood also passes through *metarterioles* (10 to 100 μm in diameter). Metarterioles are not exchange vessels but serve a separate role. Decreased blood flow through cutaneous metarterioles helps the body conserve heat; increased flow enhances heat loss.

Venules and Veins

Venules (10 to 100 μm in diameter) collect drainage from the capillaries in a convergent flow pattern. Venule smooth muscle is innervated by sympathetic nerves. Along with the veins, venules serve as capacitance (volume storage) areas, containing up to 75% of the circulating blood volume. Permeability of the postcapillary venules is regulated by hormones such as histamine and bradykinin. Note that angiogenesis is initiated in the postcapillary venules.

Veins are characterized by high volume and low pressure. Sympathetic nerve activity constricts the smooth muscle of the veins and helps move blood toward the heart. Blood flow toward the heart is also assisted by gravity (for veins in the head) and valves that ensure a unidirectional flow. Damage to venous valves can cause swellings, such as varicose veins, and lack of leg muscle movement can lead to venous stasis and clotting. During exercise, blood flow toward the heart is assisted by the drop in intrathoracic pressure during deep respiration and by extravascular compression of veins in the exercising skeletal muscle.

Lymphatics

Lymphatics are a network of endothelial tubes that merge to form two large systems that enter the vena cava. Terminal lymphatics lack tight junctions, allowing large proteins (and metastasizing cancer cells) to enter the circulatory system through the lymphatic system. In the gastrointestinal tract, lymphatics allow digested fats to enter the circulation. Lymph is propelled by (1) massaging from adjacent muscle, (2) tissue pressure, and (3) contraction of the lymph vessels. Valves ensure that the flow of lymph, which over 24 hours is a volume equal to the total blood volume, is toward the vena cava. Lymph is filtered in lymph nodes before progressing back to the circulation (Figure U12-3).

▌FUNCTION OF THE VASCULAR SYSTEM
PRESSURE, FLOW, AND RESISTANCE

The relationship of arterial pressure, cardiac output, and total peripheral resistance is shown by the following equation:

$$Q = \frac{\Delta P}{R}$$

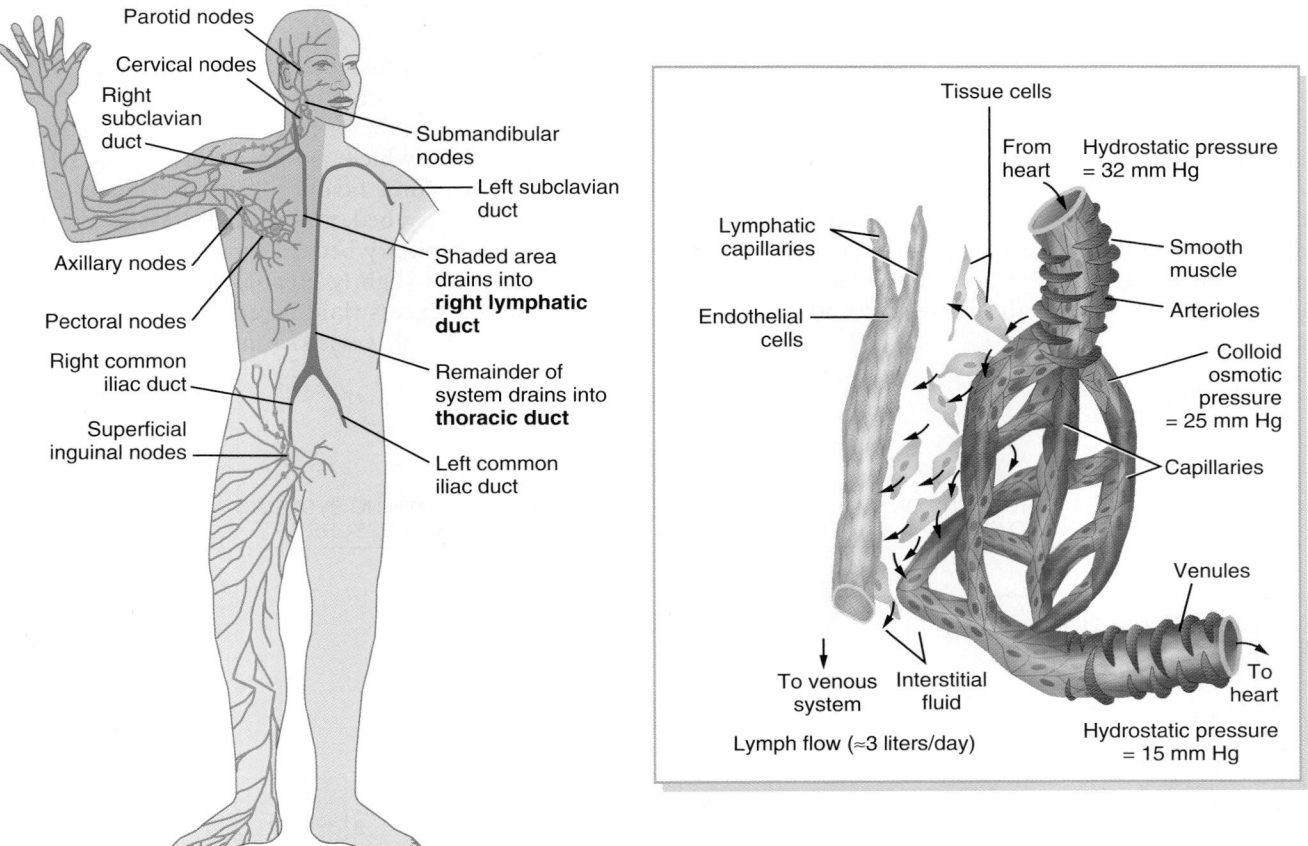

FIGURE U12-3 Major lymphatic vessels and drainage. *Inset,* Fluid exchange at the capillary bed. The primary driving force to move fluids from the capillary is *hydrostatic pressure.* The primary pulling force to bring fluids back into the vessel is *colloid osmotic pressure* from the proteins in the capillary fluids (e.g., albumin). The hydrostatic pressure at the arterial end of the capillary is 32 mm Hg. As the fluid moves through the capillary, the pressure falls. Because proteins do not move across the capillary endothelium, colloid osmotic pressure is constant at 25 mm Hg. Thus at the arterial end the hydrostatic pressure is greater than the colloid osmotic pressure, and fluids then move into interstitial spaces. The opposite is true at the venous end where pressure falls to 15 mm Hg. The hydrostatic pressure is lower than the colloid osmotic pressure, and fluids thus return to the capillary. There is a net loss of fluids out of the capillary (~3 L/day). This fluid is absorbed by the lymphatic system and is returned to circulation at the lymphatic duct.

Or

$$\text{Flow} = \frac{\text{Pressure Gradient}}{\text{Resistance}}$$

In the body, arterial *pressure* is regulated. A decrease in arterial pressure is corrected by a reflex increase in cardiac output and an increase in total peripheral resistance, both mediated by an increase in sympathetic nervous system activity. For a capillary bed, however, *flow* is regulated. If flow is too low, the arteriole dilates and the decrease in resistance allows flow to increase.

Resistance in the vascular system can be affected by (1) the radius of the vessel, (2) fluid viscosity, and (3) the length of the vessel. Of these, vessel radius is the most powerful mechanism for controlling resistance and the

one that is physiologically important. If the radius of the vessel decreases to one half the starting value, resistance to flow increases 16-fold. The body utilizes vascular smooth muscle to alter the diameter of arteries and arterioles and therefore to regulate both pressure and flow. Occasionally, changes in blood viscosity can alter resistance, particularly when the hematocrit is increased *(polycythemia)* or decreased *(anemia).* Resistance increases as viscosity increases and decreases as viscosity decreases.

CAPILLARY EXCHANGE

Exchange of nutrients and wastes between the blood and the tissues is the primary purpose of the cardiovascular system. The movement of nutrients from the blood to the tissue and removal of metabolic wastes are driven by diffusion, filtration, and pinocytosis.

Diffusion

Diffusion is quantitatively the most important process. The rate of diffusion is enhanced by (1) increasing the surface area available for exchange, (2) increasing the concentration gradient, and (3) decreasing the distance that a compound must travel. In tissues such as exercising skeletal muscle, an increase in the number of perfused capillaries enhances the delivery of nutrients to the tissues.

Filtration

Fluid movement across the capillary depends on the balance of the hydrostatic pressure gradient (which favors filtration) and the oncotic pressure gradient from plasma proteins (which favors reabsorption) (Figure U12-4). The net force favors filtration at the arteriolar end of the capillary bed, and reabsorption at the venular end of the capillary bed. In most capillary beds, the volume filtered is slightly greater than the volume absorbed, and the excess fluid is removed from the tissue spaces by the lymph vessels. *Edema* (accumulation of

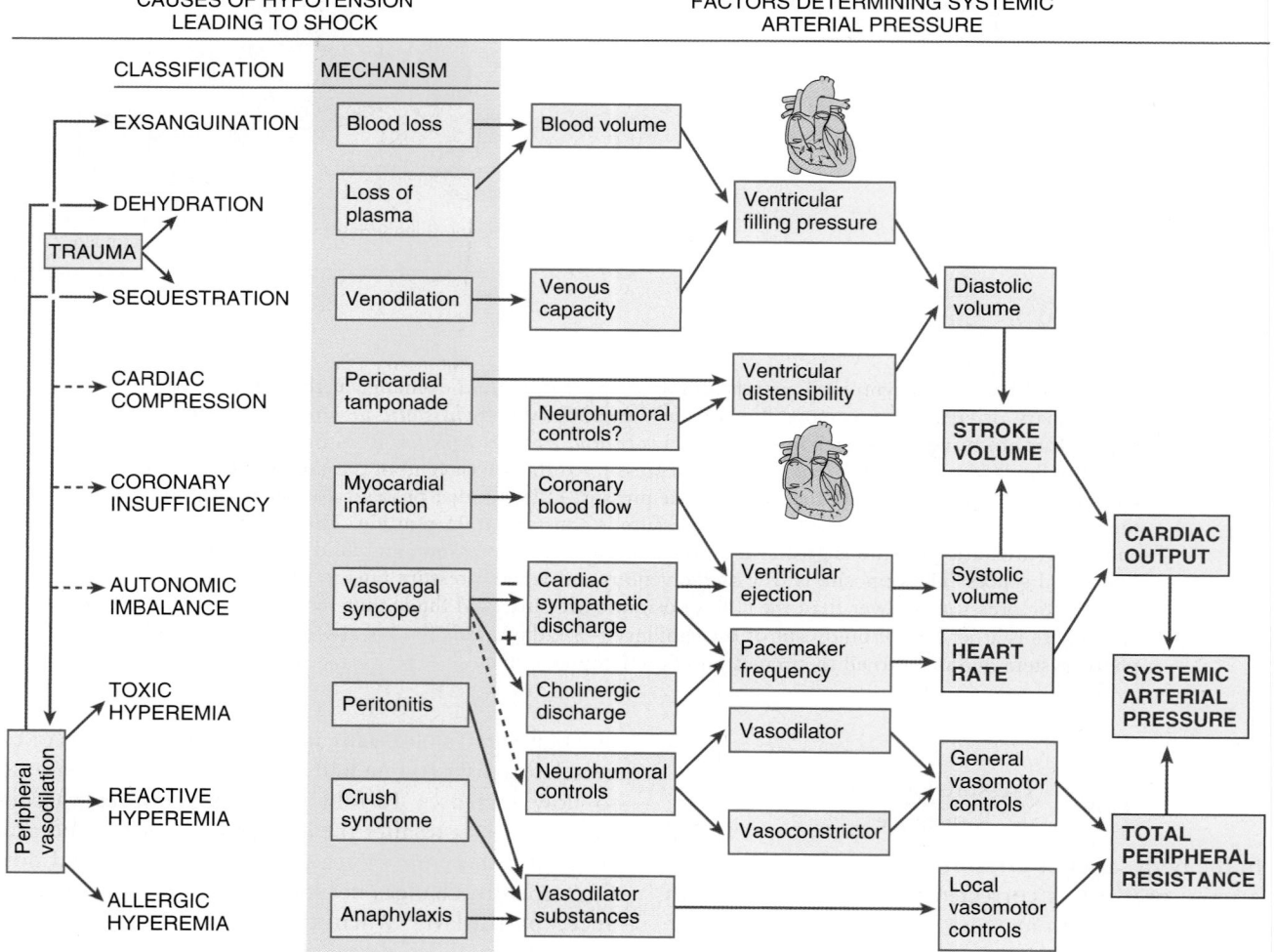

FIGURE U12-4 Control of arterial pressure. Arterial blood pressure is determined by several factors. *Right,* Systemic arterial blood pressure is controlled by two major factors: cardiac output and total peripheral vascular resistance. Cardiac output is also a function of two factors: stroke volume and heart rate. Reading the diagram from the right, you will find the factors that govern each step. Each bifurcation represents possible compensatory mechanisms. *Far left,* Disorders that can lead to shock. (Modified from Rushmer, R.F. [1976]. *Cardiovascular dynamics* [p. 207]. Philadelphia: W.B. Saunders.)

fluid in the tissue spaces) occurs because of (1) increased filtration, (2) decreased reabsorption, or (3) impaired lymph drainage.

Pinocytosis

Pinocytosis is the movement of vesicles, especially from outside the cell to inside the cell. Pinocytosis is thought to be important only as a route for large proteins to cross the capillary wall.

CARDIOVASCULAR CONTROL

Much like the power and water supply systems in a city, the distribution of blood flow in the body depends on a sufficient driving pressure (arterial pressure), allowing the end users (capillary beds) to determine how much of the resource to utilize. Cardiovascular control is best described in terms of (1) regulation of arterial pressure and (2) local regulation of tissue blood flow.

Regulation of Arterial Pressure

The normal arterial pressure is maintained by a negative feedback mechanism called the *baroreceptor reflex* (Figure U12-5). A decrease in blood pressure activates the sympathetic nervous system, increasing cardiac output (heart rate, venoconstriction for venous return, and cardiac contractility) and increasing peripheral resistance to trap blood within the arteries, and restores arterial blood pressure.

Baroreceptor control of blood pressure is augmented by volume-sensitive receptors in the low-pressure atria and veins, which control renal fluid balance, and endocrine vasoconstrictor agents such as angiotensin II, antidiuretic hormone (ADH), and norepinephrine. Chronic regulation of blood pressure depends on the volume of blood in the system and, ultimately, is tied to renal regulation of body fluid balance.

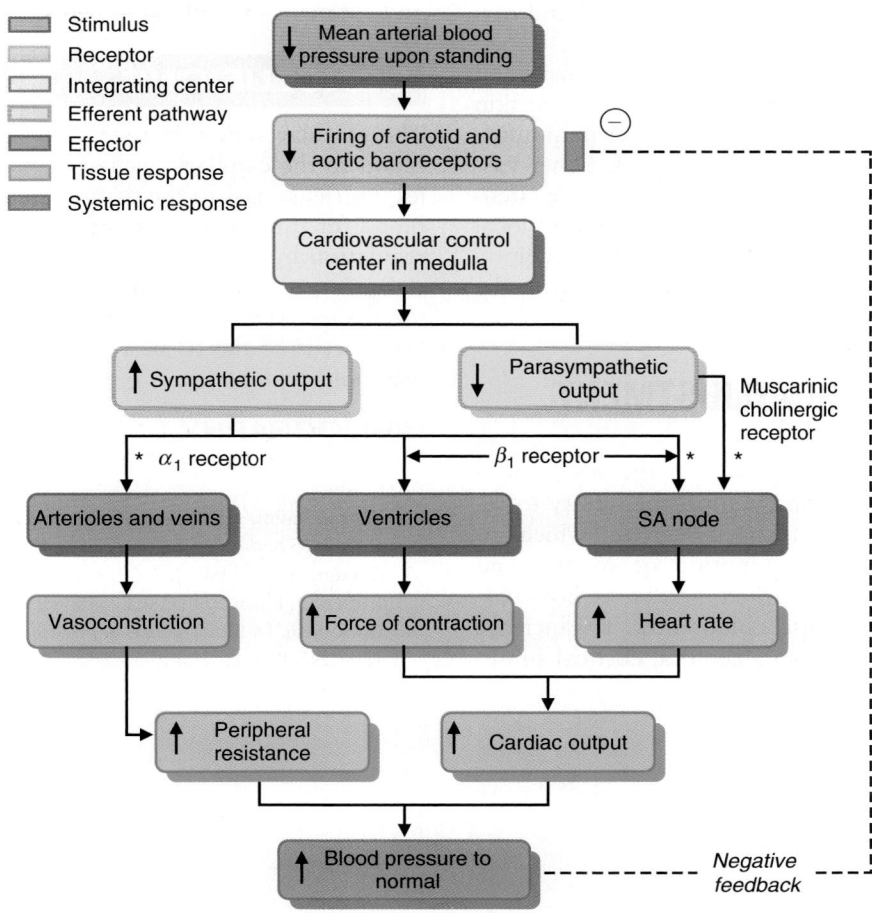

FIGURE U12-5 Baroreceptor control of blood pressure. When baroreceptors sense a drop in blood pressure, they elicit an increase in sympathetic nervous system activity and a decrease in parasympathetic activity. The resultant vasoconstriction, increase in heart rate, and increase in ventricular contractility help to restore blood pressure to the starting point. SA, sinoatrial. (Modified from Silverthorn D. [2001]. *Human physiology* [2nd ed.]. Upper Saddle River, NJ: Prentice Hall.)

Chemoreceptors in the carotid body and aortic body are associated primarily with respiratory control but can elicit cardiovascular responses. A drop in arterial O_2, an increase in arterial CO_2, or a drop in arterial pH can elicit a sympathetic response similar to that caused by a drop in arterial blood pressure

Local Regulation of Blood Flow

If arterial pressure is sufficient, tissues can regulate their blood flow to match their metabolic needs. If blood flow is inadequate, metabolites such as carbon dioxide, adenosine, potassium, and acids accumulate, acting as vasodilators of the arteriolar smooth muscle only of that local area. The resulting increase in blood flow washes out the metabolites and diminishes the vasodilator stimulus. This control system allows tissue blood flow to increase as tissue metabolic activity increases and accounts for the period of increased blood flow that follows a period of occlusion. In the long term, inadequate blood flow to a tissue can cause the growth of new capillaries, again matching blood flow to the tissue's metabolic needs. Blood flow to tissues such as the brain and myocardium is dominated by local control.

At the other extreme of regulation, cutaneous blood flow responds primarily to neural control. Because skin blood flow is tied to thermoregulation rather than nutrition, metabolic control is poorly developed. Other vascular beds, such as the kidney and the splanchnic circulation, respond both to sympathetic control and to local control. During increased sympathetic activity, blood flow to these tissues is decreased and is shunted to the brain and the myocardium.

CARDIOVASCULAR ADJUSTMENT TO EXERCISE

Cardiovascular control must balance the need for a steady arterial blood pressure against the ability to respond to a physiologic challenge. Exercise, which increases skeletal muscle consumption of oxygen and other nutrients, requires a marked increase in both cardiac output and skeletal muscle blood flow. The increase in cardiac output results from a cerebral cortical stimulation of the medullary cardiovascular center and activation of the sympathetic nervous system. The increased cardiac output requires an increased venous return, accomplished both by the arteriolar dilation of the skeletal muscle beds and by a sympathetic-mediated venous constriction. In rhythmic activity such as running, compression of the veins by the contracting skeletal muscle along with the negative intrathoracic pressure from breathing assists the flow of venous blood toward the heart.

The increased cardiac output is preferentially directed to the exercising muscles (including the heart). Local factors in the exercising muscles cause a vasodilation of those vascular beds. The sympathetic activity constricts the arteriolar smooth muscle of the nonexercising vascular beds, such as the gastrointestinal tract, the kidney, and the nonworking muscles. Cerebral blood flow remains unchanged because that vascular bed is regulated primarily by local control. Cutaneous blood flow may be diminished initially but increases as the heat generated by the exercising muscles raises body core temperature, and cutaneous vasodilation helps to cool the body.

CONCLUSIONS

The vascular system is a series of vessels that transport blood to the capillary exchange vessels. In the capillaries, nutrients pass to the tissues and wastes pass into the blood for transport to excretory organs. Blood pressure regulation by the baroreceptor reflex ensures that arterial pressure remains sufficient to propel blood toward the tissues. Tissue blood flow is controlled by the metabolic needs of the tissues, and it increases when tissue metabolism increases.

BIBLIOGRAPHY

1. Berne, R., & Levy, M. (1998). *Physiology* (4th ed.). St. Louis: Mosby.
2. Kierszenbaum, A.L. (2002). *Histology and cell biology: An introduction to pathology.* St. Louis, Mosby.
3. Guyton, A., & Hall, J. (2001). *Textbook of medical physiology* (10th ed.). Philadelphia: W.B. Saunders.
4. Silverthorn, D. (2001). *Human physiology* (2nd ed). Upper Saddle River, NJ: Prentice Hall.

Assessment of the Vascular System

Mary Sieggreen

Peripheral vascular disease is common among older and diabetic clients. It is characterized by disturbances of blood flow through the peripheral vessels. These disturbances eventually damage tissues as a result of ischemia, excessive accumulation of waste and fluid, or both. Damage can be due to any disorder that narrows, obstructs, or injures blood vessels, thus impeding blood flow. Without intervention, damage may progress to the point of tissue or organ death. Assessment of the peripheral vascular system includes data collection through the health history, physical examination, and diagnostic tests when indicated.

HISTORY

When assessing the client, note risk factors for atherosclerosis (see Chapter 54), diabetes (see Chapter 47), and cardiac (see Chapters 56 and 60) as well as arterial, venous (see Chapter 55), and lymphatic disorders. Some clients are reluctant to mention what they believe to be minor manifestations (swelling, intermittent discomfort). Consequently, perform a careful assessment, ask specific questions skillfully, and be alert for information that may indicate early manifestations of insidious conditions.

Studies have found that the effects of peripheral arterial disease (PAD) have significant psychosocial and emotional consequences. Assessment of quality of life as well as functional changes and symptom manifestations is needed to establish effective interventions. Seven themes emerged from one study[10] designed to evaluate the effects of PAD from clients' perspectives. The themes are (1) PAD diagnosis and management, (2) symptom experience, (3) limitations in physical functioning, (4) limitations in social functioning, (5) compromise of self, (6) uncertainty and fear, and (7) adaptation (Table 53-1).

Biographical and Demographic Data

Biographical data include the client's age. Atherosclerosis (hardening of the arteries) is more prevalent in older people. Venous disease, although also more prevalent in older clients, may be identified in younger people. Ask about occupation, and clarify whether the occupation increases the risk for vascular disease. If the client is retired, ask about previous employment history.

Current Health

Ask about frequency and duration of clinical manifestations that may indicate a vascular disorder. The following section describes the typical chief complaints of clients who have arterial and venous disorders.

 evolve Be sure to check out the bonus material on the Evolve website and the CD-ROM, including free self-assessment exercises.
http://evolve.elsevier.com/Black/medsurg/

Chief Complaint

Arterial Disorders. In arterial insufficiency of the lower extremities, the chief complaint is often cramping leg pain in the calf muscles during ambulation that disappears with 1 to 2 minutes of rest. The pain is called *intermittent claudication.* The pain occurs in the muscle group distal to the diseased artery (see Chapter 55).

Intermittent claudication results from inadequate tissue oxygenation *(ischemia)* due to arterial stenosis, usually secondary to atherosclerosis. It is a pathologic process similar to angina. Claudication is predictable and reproducible, which means that (1) the client can walk the same distance each time before pain occurs and (2) the pain occurs each time that this distance is walked.

As an artery becomes more stenosed, the pain may become more severe. When clients report distal forefoot burning, numbness or tingling, pain at rest, or pain that awakens them during the night *(rest pain)*, urgent attention is needed. This pain is related to arterial disease and exacerbated by decreased cardiac output during sleep. The relative leg elevation while in a supine position decreases blood flow through stenosed arteries. Pain is relieved when the client stands because gravity pulls the blood toward the feet. Even during non-sleep hours, elevation of the legs decreases blood flow and increases pain. Clients may report that they sleep upright with the legs dependent (below heart level) to control pain.

Ask about precipitating factors, duration and persistence of the discomfort, the manner of its onset, and associated manifestations. Document the activity required to cause pain. The extent of disease involvement can be gauged by the distance the client is able to walk without pain, or *claudication distance.* For example, one client may be able to walk only one block before experiencing pain, whereas another may be able to walk six blocks.

Disorders of the aorta and iliac vessels can lead to impotence. If a male client has aortoiliac disease, ask about problems with penile erection. Sexuality may be a sensitive issue; ask questions carefully to elicit areas of concern or problems (see Chapters 4 and 39).

Venous Disorders. Chronic venous disease has an insidious onset. Many clients do not recall any precipitating event. There may be a positive family history for venous disease, a job history involving many hours of standing in one place, or multiple pregnancies. Obesity may be a factor. In contrast to the pain in arterial disorders, pain in

TABLE 53-1	*Themes, Definitions, and Characteristics of Peripheral Arterial Disease*	
PAD diagnosis and management	Challenges and frustrations experienced by patients as they receive diagnosis and learn to manage PAD	Patient and clinician delay in diagnosis Lack of control Lack of knowledge Smoking addiction
Symptom experience	Physical discomfort experienced with daily activities by patients with PAD	Cramping Aching Burning Fatigue
Limitation in physical functioning	Inability to meet the required or desired level of physical demands of life as a result of PAD	Walking impairment Limitation of activities
Limitation in social functioning	Inability to meet the desired or required social demands of life as a result of PAD	Social isolation or inadequacy Being a burden to family Role and employment limitations
Compromise of self	Limitation in physical or social functioning that directly affects the "core" or ego of the individual, compromising sense of "wholeness"	Premature aging Feeling abnormal Unfulfilled desire Loss of self
Uncertainty and fear	The fragile (or obscured) anticipation of a future impaired by PAD	Fear of loss of function or independence Fear of amputation Fear of death
Adaptation	The ability to adapt physically, socially, and emotionally to the effects of PAD	Adjustment Flexibility

From Treat-Jacobson, D., et al. (2002). A patient-derived perspective of health-related quality of life with peripheral arterial disease. *Journal of Nursing Scholarship, 34*(1), 55-60. Used with permission of Sigma Theta Tau International.
PAD, Peripheral arterial disease.

chronic venous disease has a slow onset and is not associated with exercise or rest. Clients may also have varicose veins and a history of phlebitis. In these clients, the leg veins have been subjected to increased pressure and return of venous blood has been obstructed. Vein walls are compliant and distend with increased pressure. Valves become incompetent because the distended wall prevents the valve leaflets from meeting each other when they close. An *incompetent vein* allows the column of blood to flow backward, increasing the hydrostatic pressure in the venous end of the capillary. This increase in pressure against the vein wall moves fluid from the intravascular to the interstitial space, causing edema. As the process continues, blood flow slows and tissues become hypoxic (lacking in oxygen). The client may report a feeling of heaviness in the legs or nighttime cramping. Exercise and elevation generally relieve the discomfort and swelling because venous return of blood is improved.

In more severe forms of chronic venous disorders, lower extremity edema may be the initial complaint. Edema worsens toward the end of the day and diminishes after nighttime leg elevation. Pitting edema (see later discussion of edema) may be seen at first, but as the edema becomes more chronic, tissue sclerosis develops and the tissue becomes more difficult to compress.

Initial skin changes noted with chronic venous disorders may include erythema (redness), followed in the late stages by lipodermatosclerosis (brawny, thick, darkly pigmented skin). The skin becomes dry and flaky, which leads to itching and scratching. Continued irritation results in stasis dermatitis, and the skin eventually ulcerates. Ulcers develop in the lower third of the leg, most commonly above the medial malleolus, where venous pressure is highest and there are more perforator veins 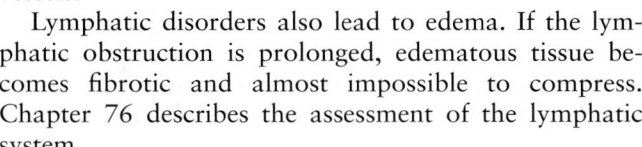 than elsewhere in the leg. Chronic venous edema and sclerotic subcutaneous tissue may compress the lymph vessels.

Lymphatic disorders also lead to edema. If the lymphatic obstruction is prolonged, edematous tissue becomes fibrotic and almost impossible to compress. Chapter 76 describes the assessment of the lymphatic system.

Symptom Analysis

Vascular disease may be arterial, venous, or lymphatic. Table 53-2 compares the clinical manifestations of arterial and venous disorders in the lower extremities.
The client who has venous disease may report chronic aching pain in the legs when they are in a dependent position. Chronic venous insufficiency produces the following manifestations:

- Edema
- Dependent cyanosis
- Brown discoloration of the skin at the ankle
- Ulcers
- Pruritus

Skin temperature remains normal or slightly elevated and pulses are present, although they may be difficult to palpate through the edema.

Chronic arterial insufficiency produces the following manifestations:

- Decrease or absence of arterial pulses
- Thin, shiny, hairless skin

TABLE 53-2	Clinical Manifestations in Lower Extremity Disorders	
Manifestation	**Arterial Disorder**	**Venous Disorder**
Pain	Intermittent claudication; rest pain may be present, or pain may worsen with elevation	Aching, heaviness Exercise and elevation decrease pain Nocturnal cramping Heaviness in the legs at the end of the day
Skin	Absence of hair in chronic condition; thin, shiny skin Thick toenails if fungal infection is present	Brown discoloration Normal toenails
Color	Pale with dependent rubor	Brown discoloration; dependent cyanosis
Temperature	Cool	No change, or may be warmer than unaffected areas
Sensation	Decreased; tingling, numbness may be present	Pruritus may be present
Pulses	Decreased to absent	Present, but may be difficult to palpate if edema is present
Edema	May be present but usually absent	Present, worse at end of day, improved with elevation
Muscle mass	Reduced in chronic disease	Unaffected in pure venous disease
Ulcers	Small, painful ulcers on pressure points, points of trauma, between toes, or distal most point, especially lateral malleolus and toes	Broad, shallow, slightly painful ulcers of the ankle and lower leg; surrounding skin is brown, fibrotic

- Thick, ridged toenails
- Cool skin temperature
- Pain with ambulation (claudication)
- Pain with leg elevation, or at night (rest pain)

The skin is pale when the legs are elevated above heart level and dusky red after they are placed in a dependent position *(dependent rubor)*. Edema is not usually present in pure arterial insufficiency. There may be ulcers from trauma, over pressure points, or on the tips of toes.

Past Health History

Note any history of vascular impairment. Inquire about changes that indicate vasospastic disorders, such as changes in color or temperature of digits. Ask specifically whether the client has a history of hypertension, diabetes, stroke, transient ischemic attacks (TIAs), changes in vision, pain in legs during activity, leg cramps, phlebitis, venous or arterial blood clots, pulmonary emboli, edema, varicose veins, leg ulcers, or extremities that are cold, pale, or blue. Question any previous history of frostbite, which increases risk of vasospasm. Visual changes and TIAs may indicate carotid artery disease. Ask about any past medical tests, operations, or treatments involving the vascular system and about any previous treatment for diabetes mellitus, collagen disorders, or hypertension.

In addition, note medications that the client takes, including over-the-counter drugs and herbal remedies. Some medications increase risk for vascular disorders (birth control pills). Herbal remedies have not been tested under the rigorous science of the Food and Drug Administration and are therefore usually not recommended by licensed health care providers. Herbals may cause unintended effects if the client is taking other medications.

Herbal remedies used to self-treat peripheral vascular disorders include those for hypertension, varicose veins, atherosclerosis, and vascular spasm. Herbs with antihypertensive action include garlic *(Allium sativum)*, hawthorn *(Crataegus oxyacantha)*, kudzu *(Pueraria lobata)*, nettle *(Urtica dioica)*, onion *(Allium cepa)*, purslane *(Portulaca oleracea)*, reishi mushroom *(Ganoderma lucidum)*, and valerian *(Valeriana officinalis)*. Garlic is also thought to be preventive for atherosclerosis. *Ginkgo biloba* is used for varicose veins, obliterative arterial disease of the lower extremities, and intermittent claudication. Horse chestnut *(Aesculus hippocastanum)* and butcher's broom *(Ruscus aculeatus)* are used for varicose veins and phlebitis, and valerian is used as an antispasmodic. Spices with possible antihypertensive effects include basil, black pepper, fennel, and tarragon.

Note allergies, especially to iodine. Iodine is found in contrast agents used in diagnostic testing for vascular disorders.

Family Health History

The family health history helps determine risk factors and provides clues about reported and observed manifestations. Note any family history of diabetes, hypertension, coronary artery disease, collagen diseases, and peripheral vascular disease.

Psychosocial History

Record the occupational history. If the client's occupation is unfamiliar to you, ask questions about the number of hours spent in various positions or activities (standing, prolonged sitting, walking, using vibrating machinery). In addition, some occupations involve contact with chemicals or are associated with cold or wet environments; note these also.

Find out whether the client smokes or has ever used any tobacco products. Ask about the use of prescription and over-the-counter nicotine products. Nicotine in any form is a potent vasoconstrictor.

Determine the client's nutrient and fluid intake (see Chapters 4 and 30). Ask about the usual intake of protein and calories. Also ask about sodium, cholesterol, and fat intake.

Assess the client's activity, rest, and sleep habits. Assess the extent to which clinical manifestations interfere with activities of daily living. Obtaining information about the frequency and duration of manifestations, precipitating activities, and their influence on daily life enables determination of disease severity. Assessment of the client's stress level, emotional state, and coping mechanisms (including the use of tobacco products, alcohol, or recreational drugs) is important.

Remain sensitive to the emotional effect of peripheral vascular disorders. Clients who have visible lesions may be embarrassed. Clients may have concern about the inability to perform self-care and about changes in role and sexual performance. Fear of amputation or functional loss may be significant.[10]

Review of Systems

Review each body system as it relates to peripheral vascular disorders. Inquire about headaches, dizziness, TIAs, stroke, visual disturbances, hypertension, diabetes, pulmonary emboli, phlebitis, blood clots, leg pain or cramps, varicose veins, leg or foot ulcers, and cold hands or feet. Also see Chapter 4 for additional information about the review of systems.

PHYSICAL EXAMINATION

Physical examination of the vascular system involves inspection, palpation, and auscultation. Before starting the physical examination, prepare the environment. Natural lighting is the best because it allows assessment of subtleties in skin color. Warm the room to minimize cutaneous vasoconstriction. A quiet room is helpful for auscultating the low-pitched sounds commonly found in blood vessels. Clients who are free of vascular disorders display characteristics such as those described in the Physical Assessment Findings in the Healthy Adult feature on The Peripheral Vascular System, below.

Inspection

Observe the extremities, noting skin color, hair distribution, nail beds and capillary refill, presence of muscle atrophy or edema, venous pattern, and ulcers. These are reviewed in detail next. Compare one side with the other. Begin with the head and upper extremities, and proceed toward the legs and feet.

Skin Color

A range of normal skin color is noted among people. Localized areas of cyanosis, rubor, or pallor are easily noticed in a person with fair skin (Figure 53-1) but are more difficult to see in a person with darker skin tones (Figure 53-2). For all clients, changes in skin color are best assessed by comparison with the contralateral limb. Ischemic pallor may be detected by comparing the palms of the hands, the soles of the feet, or the nail beds. Clients with arterial disorders may have pale extremities and cyanotic (blue-tinged) or red extremities with venous disorders.

Hair Distribution

Lack of hair growth may indicate chronically inadequate circulation to an area. This sign must be correlated with other manifestations of arterial insufficiency. It is not a valid indicator of acute arterial insufficiency.

Capillary Refill

Capillary refill time is an evaluation of peripheral perfusion and cardiac output. This assessment is usually completed while pulses are assessed. Depress the nail bed or the pad of the toe or finger until it blanches or becomes pale (Figure 53-3). Release pressure on the blanched area, and note the length of time for usual skin color to return. Capillaries usually refill in a fraction of a second, but "normal" times range up to 3 seconds for color return. With diminished blood flow, the return to the baseline color is delayed and a refill time of more than 3 seconds is sometimes called "sluggish." Note whether the room in which you are conducting the test is cold, because external temperatures can delay capillary refill.

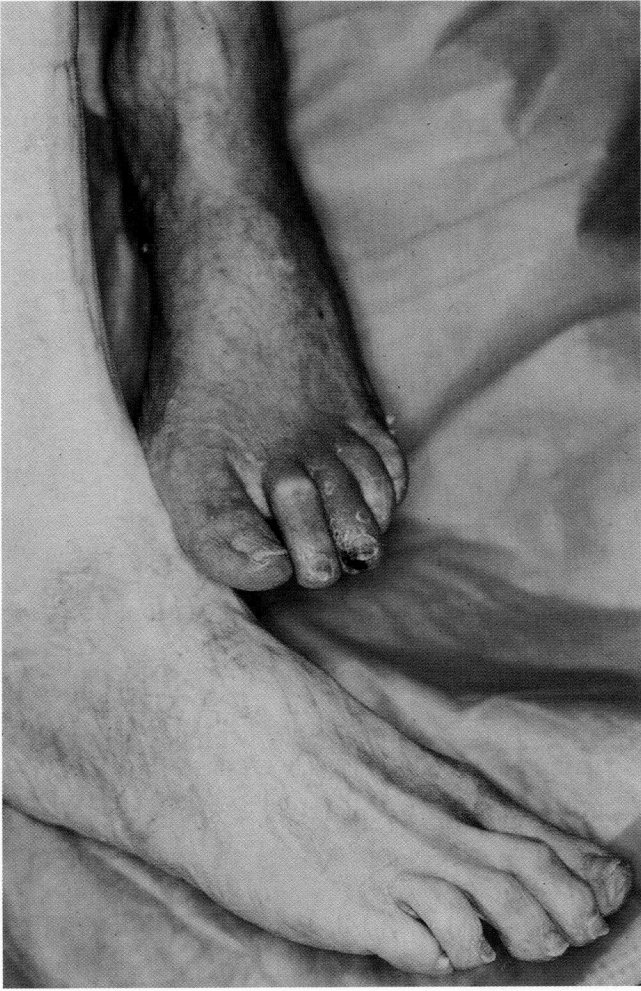

FIGURE 53-1 Dependent rubor is noted as a ruddy color in severe arterial insufficiency in this white client's left leg just minutes before amputation. (Note area of ulceration and necrosis on the third toe.)

PHYSICAL ASSESSMENT FINDINGS IN THE HEALTHY ADULT

The Peripheral Vascular System

Inspection

Extremities of even contour, without edema. Even hair distribution; symmetrical venous pattern. Varicosities, skin lesions, and ulcers absent. Capillaries refill in less than 3 seconds on blanching.

Palpation

Extremities warm and dry without areas of localized heat or tenderness. Pulses (temporal, carotid, brachial, radial, ulnar, femoral, popliteal, posterior tibial, dorsalis pedis) are bilaterally equal and regular. No aneurysmal dilation of aorta.

Auscultation

Blood pressures equal in contralateral extremities. Orthostatic hypotension absent. No bruits.

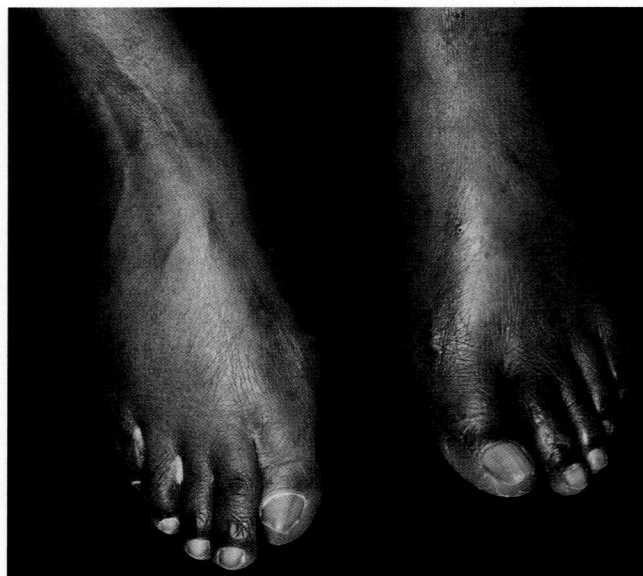

FIGURE 53-2 Dependent rubor in dark skin (which can be difficult to see) in the client's left foot has a reddish hue when compared with the unaffected right foot.

Muscle Atrophy

There can be many reasons for muscle atrophy in an extremity. If atrophy is noted, it may represent long-standing arterial insufficiency. Measure the muscle circumference, and compare it with that of the muscle on the opposite side.

Edema

To assess edema of the leg, push with your thumb on the skin over the client's foot or tibia for 5 seconds. If the skin is edematous, an indentation or pit will remain (thus the term *pitting edema*). Edema is often graded; however, scales used to grade edema are not universal. Because there is no established standard, it is most accurate to describe the edema as *present* or *absent, pitting* or *non-pitting* (Figure 53-4).

Edema resulting from cardiac disease is generally bilateral and occurs in dependent areas (in the legs of a client who is ambulatory and the sacrum of a client who is bedridden). Unilateral edema is usually caused by occlusion of a deep vein. Long-standing edema destroys the structure of the skin and the subcutaneous tissue and is easily recognized from its fibrotic appearance and firm texture.

Venous Pattern

Varicosities may indicate superficial or deep venous insufficiency. Note the presence, location, and distribution of *telangiectasias,* or "spider veins."

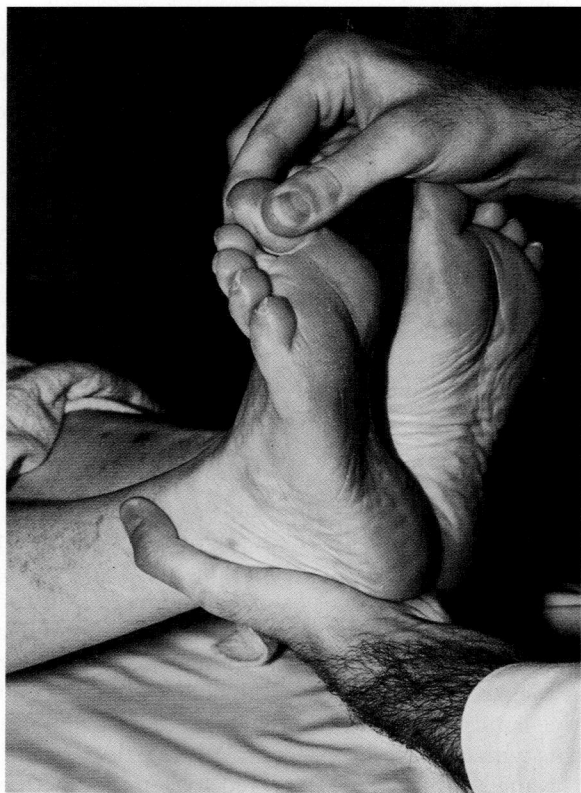

FIGURE 53-3 Determine capillary refill time by compressing the great toe and then releasing pressure. Count the number of seconds required for color to return to the skin.

Ulcers

Note the presence of skin lesions or scar tissue (indicating healed ulcers); fissures of the feet and ulcers of the ankles and heels may be signs of arterial insufficiency. Tissue necrosis (see Figure 53-1) and gangrene may be present with severe arterial disease. Examine between the toes for moist ulcers penetrating into the web spaces (Figure 53-5).

Note the presence of other lesions, such as *angiomas* (benign tumors of blood and lymph vessels) and *petechiae* (small, purplish spots on the skin from several causes, including hemorrhage).

Additional Inspections

If arterial or venous disease is suspected but not confirmed, additional assessments can be performed, such as elevation pallor and Trendelenburg's test.

Elevation Pallor. If arterial insufficiency is suspected, perform the test for elevation pallor. Because leg elevation can cause pain, perform this test only when needed. Note the degree of pallor at rest, and use the test only to

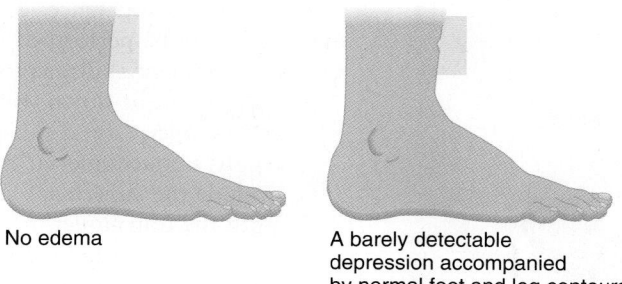

No edema

A barely detectable
depression accompanied
by normal foot and leg contours

A deeper depression
(less than 5 mm) accompanied
by normal foot and leg contours

A deep depression
(5 to 10 mm) accompanied
by foot and leg swelling

An even deeper depression
(more than 1 cm) accompanied by
severe foot and leg swelling

FIGURE 53-4 To assess peripheral edema, press a finger into the skin over the client's tibia. Note the presence, depth, and persistence of any resulting depression. Use descriptive terms to record your findings.

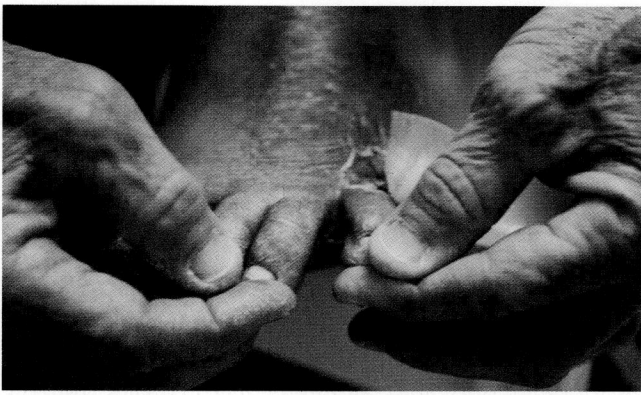

FIGURE 53-5 Carefully examine the web spaces for ulcers or maceration when assessing the foot.

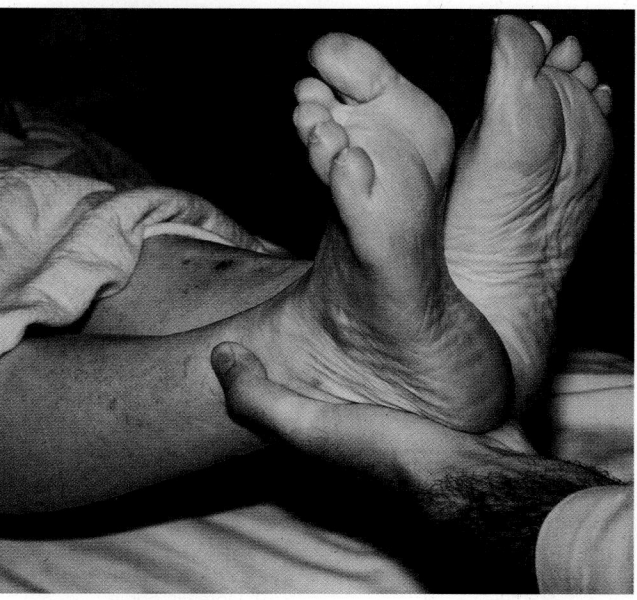

FIGURE 53-6 Assess for elevation pallor if arterial insufficiency is suspected.

determine the severity of ischemia. Perform the test as follows:

1. Elevate the legs 30 cm (12 inches) (Figure 53-6). Pallor occurring within 60 seconds indicates arterial insufficiency.
2. Have the client dangle the legs from the side of the bed or examination table. Normally, the color returns within 10 seconds. Severe arterial insufficiency causes an exaggerated color change of dependent rubor.

Brodie Trendelenburg Tourniquet Test. Intended to help detect abnormal venous filling time, Trendelenburg's test reveals valvular incompetence of the deep veins. Superficial varicose veins are easy to recognize. They appear as dilated, tortuous (twisted) veins. This test helps confirm

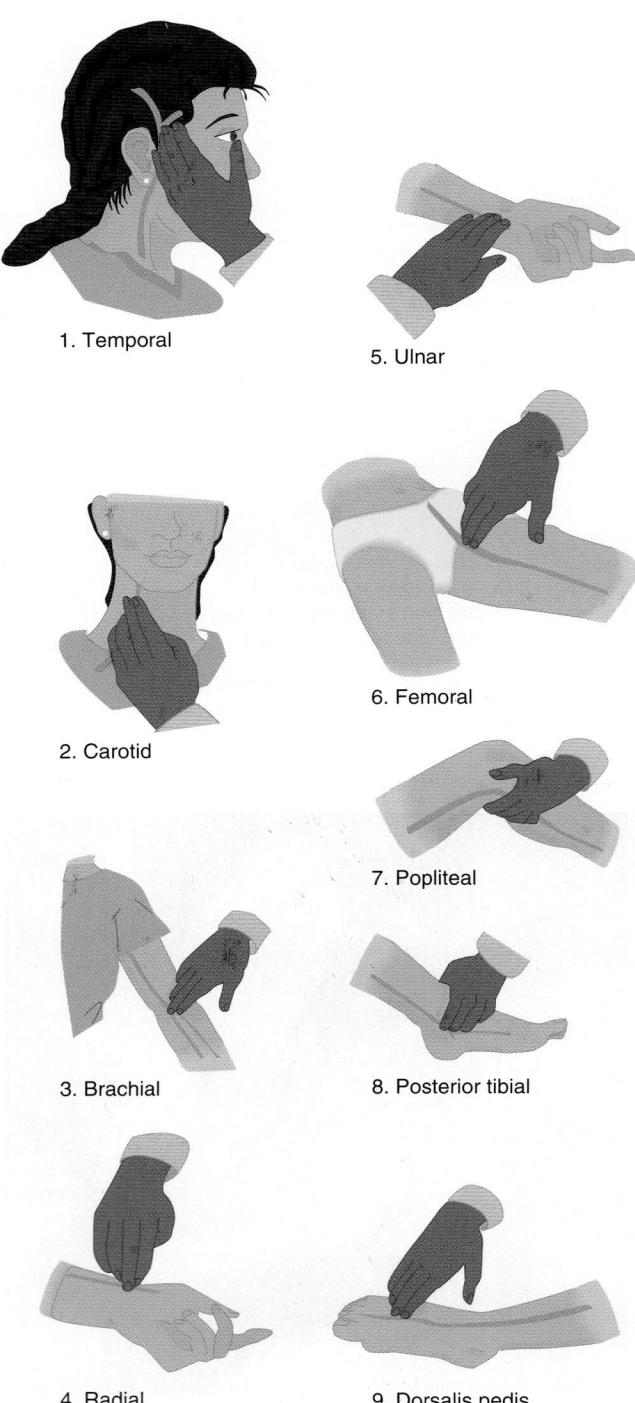

FIGURE 53-7 Assess pulses bilaterally from head to toe, comparing one side to the other for amplitude, rhythm, and symmetry. To prevent possible carotid sinus massage, do not palpate carotid pulses simultaneously. The carotid sinus is nerve tissue, located in the wall of the carotid artery, that helps regulate blood pressure. Massaging over this area may cause sinus bradycardia or syncope.

leg vein valve competence. This noninvasive assessment maneuver may be performed by nurses who possess advanced assessment skills, as follows:

1. Have client lie down with the leg elevated until the veins empty.
2. Apply a tourniquet at midthigh snugly enough to occlude the superficial veins.
3. With the tourniquet in place, help the client stand.
4. Note the time required for the veins to fill from below. Veins usually fill in about 30 seconds.
5. After 60 seconds, release the tourniquet. Normally, when the tourniquet is released, no further blood fills the veins. Additional blood flowing into the vein from above indicates that a valve is incompetent and has allowed back-flow of blood.

Palpation

Temperature

Palpate the arms and legs with the dorsal surface of your hand, and note the temperature (see Chapter 50). Temperature should be similar in contralateral limbs. Vasoconstriction produces cold, pale skin. Bilateral vasoconstriction may be caused by smoking, environmental temperature, anxiety, or generalized arterial disease. Unilateral or localized arterial vasoconstriction indicates arterial disease. Venous disorders may cause an increase in local skin temperature.

Pulses

Palpate pulses by placing the first three fingers of your dominant hand along the length of the selected artery. Apply gentle pressure against the artery, followed by a gradual release. Palpate temporal, carotid, brachial, radial, and ulnar pulses (upper extremities), and femoral, popliteal, posterior tibial, and dorsalis pedis pulses (lower extremities), as shown in Figure 53-7. Palpate pulses bilaterally and simultaneously, except for the carotid pulse (Figure 53-8). Palpate carotid pulses separately to avoid stimulation of the carotid sinus, which may produce bradycardia or sinus arrest. Assess the ulnar pulse during Allen's test, as described later.

Palpate the abdominal aortic pulse by placing the palm of your hand over the upper abdomen just beneath the sternum while the client is supine. Use gentle pressure to push the abdomen downward. When you feel the aortic pulse, cup your fingers and thumb together to determine the width of the aorta (Figure 53-9). You can use both hands if the client is large. When using both hands, place the lateral side of your right hand just left of the midline of the abdomen. Palpate using gentle pressure on the side of the aorta. Then place your left hand to the right of the abdominal midline. Estimate the width of the aorta as it pulsates toward your hands. In very obese clients, you may not be able to feel the aorta.

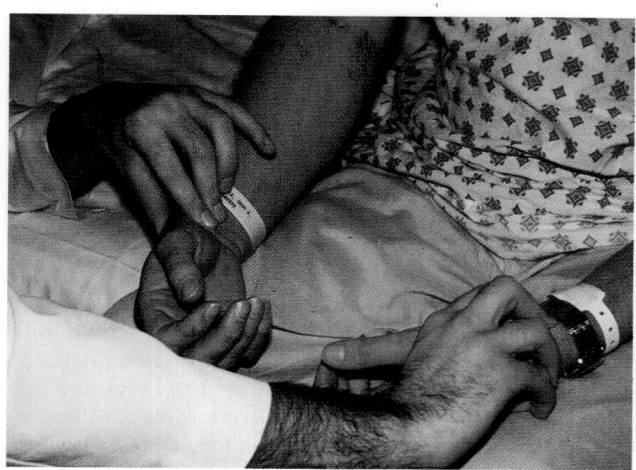

FIGURE 53-8 Palpating radial pulses.

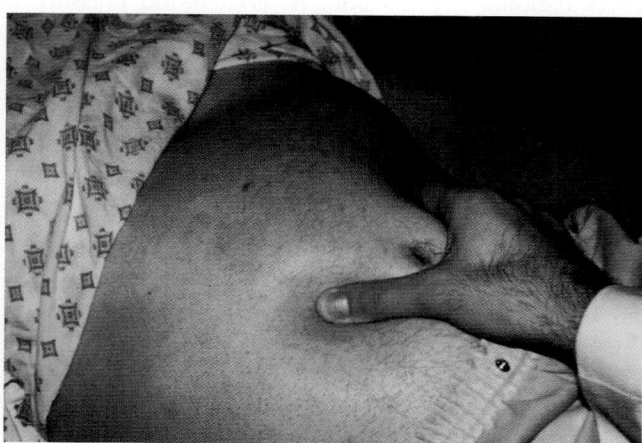

FIGURE 53-9 Palpate the abdomen for aortic aneurysm.

Always note the rhythm, amplitude, and symmetry of pulses. Compare peripheral pulses on the two sides for rate, rhythm, and quality. There are no standard numerical grades or rating scales for pulses. It is most accurate to describe the pulse as *palpable* (or present), *diminished* (weak), *absent*, or *aneurysmal* (easily palpable, bounding).

Note whether a pulse feels unequal on the two sides. The dorsalis pedis pulse is congenitally absent in approximately 10% to 17% of the normal adult population. The posterior tibial pulse is absent congenitally in 9% of the black adult population of the United States. In older clients, dorsalis pedis and posterior tibial pulses may be more difficult to palpate. If they are found, mark the site with a pen to facilitate later examinations. Clients who have arterial grafts may have palpable pulses along the length of the graft.

If there is any question about the presence of a specific pulse, position your hand below the pulse you are seeking, then attempt to palpate the client's pulse again. This position reduces the chance of mistaking your pulse for that of the client by establishing the difference between the two pulses.

Palpate the course of veins to determine fascial defects, which feel like small indentations. These represent incompetent perforator veins.

Allen's Test

Blood flow to the hand is supplied by both the ulnar and the radial arteries, which join at the volar arch in the palm. Allen's test is used to assess the patency of the radial and ulnar arteries distal to the wrist. It is commonly performed before arterial blood samples are drawn for analysis (see Chapter 15) or before an arterial line is inserted (see Chapter 57). Perform Allen's test as follows:

1. Ask the client to make a tight fist while you compress the radial and ulnar arteries.

2. Have the client open the hand, which should be pale and mottled.
3. Release the pressure on the radial artery while continuing to compress the ulnar artery. If the client's hand regains full color within about 6 seconds, the radial artery has normal patency.
4. Repeat steps 1 to 3, this time releasing the pressure on the ulnar artery to assess its patency.

If the client's hand remains pale during either portion of the test, the artery being tested may be occluded. Allen's test is shown in Chapter 61.

Homans' Sign

The test for Homans' sign involves gently compressing the gastrocnemius muscle of the calf and asking the client whether this maneuver causes pain or tenderness. The test can also be performed by quickly dorsiflexing the foot (pointing the toes downward); calf pain that occurs with this maneuver is a positive finding of Homans' sign.

Homans' sign is an unreliable test for deep venous thrombosis and is no longer used. Studies indicate that only about 35% of people with deep venous thrombosis (DVT) have a positive response to Homans' test. Superficial phlebitis, Achilles' tendinitis, and plantar muscle injury can also elicit a positive Homans' sign. Therefore 50% of the people who display a positive response to Homans' test do not have DVT. Doppler studies (see later discussion) are more accurate and should be used to confirm the diagnosis of deep vein thrombosis.

Auscultation

Limb Blood Pressure

The measurement of arterial blood pressure is the most commonly performed noninvasive test of cardiac and vascular function. It may be the best single indicator of arterial perfusion. Arterial stenosis or occlusion produces regional hypotension. Arterial blood pressure is measured with a sphygmomanometer and a properly fitting cuff. For an accurate reading, place the cuff on the client's arm at the level of the heart; it should be wide enough to transmit pressure to the center of the arm and long enough to encircle the arm firmly. Auscultate the blood pressure in both arms. A difference of a few points between readings is normal. A difference of 20 mm Hg between extremity readings may indicate aortic dissection or subclavian artery stenosis. Document asymmetrical readings. All subsequent blood pressure measurements should be performed on the arm with the higher reading. Measure blood pressure while the client is in supine, sitting, and standing positions when possible, and document the position of the client and the site used for each reading. Note *orthostatic* (positional) changes in blood pressure.

Auscultate over the carotid artery, aorta, and renal, femoral, and popliteal arteries to assess for the presence of bruits. A *bruit* is a "whooshing" sound that may be soft or loud; it results from turbulent blood flow from vessel wall irregularities. The presence of a bruit indicates some arterial narrowing. These arterial sounds are best heard with the bell of the stethoscope.

DIAGNOSTIC TESTS

Noninvasive Vascular Laboratory Techniques

Noninvasive diagnostic techniques have assumed an increasingly important role in the management of vascular disorders. Noninvasive diagnostic tests provide reliable, objective data that can be used to evaluate the extent of vascular disease. Variables include blood flow velocity, blood flow abnormality, and some measure of functional limitations.

Doppler Ultrasonography

Hand-held Doppler ultrasonographic instruments permit assessment of arterial disease through (1) evaluation of audible arterial signals or (2) measurement of limb blood pressures (Figure 53-10). Doppler ultrasonography is simple and inexpensive, but the technique may not detect minor disease, and it is less accurate than duplex scanning (see later discussion). There is no special client preparation for this test.

Brightness-mode (*B-mode*) ultrasound refers to the creation of a two-dimensional image from ultrasound waves. It can be used to assess the size and compressibility of a vessel, flow patterns, the presence or absence of thrombus, and valve function.

Ankle-Brachial Index

The ankle-brachial index (ABI) is a commonly used parameter for overall evaluation of extremity status. There is no special preparation for this test.

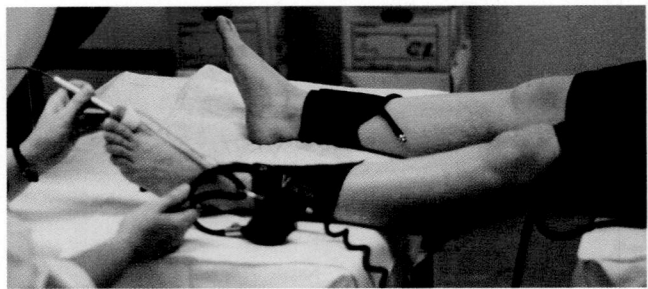

FIGURE 53-10 The ankle-brachial index (ABI) measures the pressures of the dorsalis pedis and posterior tibial arteries. In this photograph, a Doppler probe is used to check toe pressures in a client with diabetes. Ankle pressures may be erroneously high because of calcification in the vessel wall.

The client assumes a supine position, and a regular arm blood pressure cuff is applied to the leg above the malleolus. Doppler probes are used to identify the systolic end-point at both the dorsalis pedis and the posterior tibial sites (see Figure 53-7). The higher of the two pressures is used as the indication of ankle blood pressure status for that foot. This number is then divided by the higher of the two brachial systolic artery pressures by means of the following formula:

$$\text{Ankle-brachial index} = \frac{\text{Systolic ankle pressure}}{\text{Higher systolic brachial pressure}}$$

A systolic ankle pressure of 60 mm Hg with a systolic brachial pressure of 120 mm Hg yields an ABI of 0.5. In normal circulation, ankle pressure is the same as or higher than the brachial pressure. Thus an ABI of 1 or more is considered a normal finding; the client with an ABI of 0.5 to 0.8 typically experiences claudication, and the client with an ABI of 0.4 or less typically experiences rest pain.

In the presence of diabetes, the ABI is artificially elevated because of calcification, which prevents vessel wall compression. A toe-brachial index (TBI) is more reliable in clients who have diabetes (see Figure 53-10) because the toe arteries are less likely to have calcification.

Ultrasonic Duplex Scanning

Ultrasonic duplex scanners are used to (1) localize vascular obstruction, (2) evaluate the degree of stenosis, and (3) determine the presence or absence of vascular reflux (backward flow). This anatomic and physiologic test evaluates the hemodynamic effects of arterial lesions. It is also the most sensitive and specific noninvasive modality for detecting DVT. Both an ultrasound image of the vessel and a Doppler audible signal and waveform are provided. The visual ultrasound data allow more specific localization of stenosis than simple pressure or waveform techniques. No special client preparation is required.

Air Plethysmography

Air plethysmography (APG) uses a pneumatic plethysmograph to measure volume changes in the legs. Venous reflux, venous obstruction, calf muscle pump function, and venous volume can be measured. A large cuff is applied to the client's calf, and a known volume of air is instilled to calibrate the cuff. Venous volume, ejection fraction, and residual volume fractions are then measured.

Impedance Plethysmography

Impedance plethysmography (IPG) and photoplethysmography (PPG) are also used to measure venous blood volume changes in the extremities. During the procedure, electrodes from a plethysmograph are applied to a limb along with a pressure cuff. As pressure is increased, electrical resistance is increased; thus the quality of venous blood flow is demonstrated.

Inform the client about the purpose of the procedure. Explain that a technique similar to blood pressure measurement will be used. The client must be able to assume a supine position with the involved extremity elevated above the level of the heart.

Exercise Testing

Exercise or stress testing provides an objective measurement of the severity of intermittent claudication. It suggests the extent to which intermittent claudication interferes with the client's lifestyle. The most commonly used method for stress testing is the *treadmill exercise test*. This test is similar to that used for clients who have had a myocardial infarction, except that walking speed is usually 1.5 to 2 miles per hour (mph) with a grade elevation of 10% to 20% and a time limit of 5 minutes. A client who can walk 5 minutes is considered mildly symptomatic; a walking time of 1 minute represents severe disease.

Performance on the treadmill test is also gauged by measurement of ankle systolic pressure. In asymptomatic clients, the time required for return to pre-exercise ankle pressure is usually less than 3 minutes with a decline from baseline of 20% or less. In clients with intermittent claudication, recovery time is longer; ankle pressure is usually less than 50 mm Hg and may be unrecordable during recovery.

The client undergoing stress testing should wear loose-fitting clothes and comfortable walking shoes. Explain the procedure so that the client knows what to expect. Inform the client that exercise will be stopped at the maximal level of exertion or when clinical manifestations become disabling.

Computed Tomography

Computed tomography (CT) provides a cross-section of vessel walls and other structures. CT scans can be used in the diagnosis of abdominal aortic aneurysms and postoperative complications, such as graft infection, graft occlusion, hemorrhage, and abscess. Chapter 4 covers client preparation during CT.

Magnetic Resonance Imaging

Magnetic resonance imaging (MRI) is used to detect tissue changes, such as tumors, aneurysms, and DVT, in the pelvic iliac veins and leg veins (see Chapter 4). Blood flow in an extremity is evaluated, with the limb to be examined placed in a cradle-like support in a flow cylinder.

In the future, MRI techniques likely will supply much of the information that currently is available only with invasive angiography. Although MRI does not require ionizing radiation or injection into the arterial system, the expense and time necessary limit its use for routine screening and follow-up.

Magnetic Resonance Angiography

Magnetic resonance angiography (MRA) uses magnetic imaging techniques to access blood vessels. The advantage of this technique is that the images are not obscured by bone, bowel gas, fat, or vascular calcification. The vessel anatomy is displayed as a three-dimensional angiogram. MRA can be used to measure blood flow volume and blood viscosity. It is a noninvasive modality. The disadvantages are its limited availability, its cost, and the need for the client to hold still during the procedure. MRA cannot be used for people who have cardiac pacemakers or intracranial aneurysm clips.

Invasive Techniques

Angiography

Contrast angiography is the most invasive of the diagnostic procedures for arterial disorders and poses the greatest risk for the client. It is frequently performed before a vascular operation and can be used intraoperatively to evaluate the results of an operation.

Procedure

The procedure involves injecting a contrast agent into the arterial system and performing radiographic studies. Angiography is performed in an interventional laboratory or a special procedures room in the radiology department. The procedure is performed under sterile conditions. Local anesthesia is given at the injection site, and a catheter is placed percutaneously. After injection of a contrast agent through the catheter, fluoroscopy may be performed. Serial pictures of the dye movement are taken by cameras positioned over the study field (see Chapter 4).

Preprocedure Care

Explain the procedure, and obtain an informed consent. The client is given nothing by mouth (NPO) for 2 to 6 hours before the procedure. A mild sedative may be used.

Postprocedure Care

Nursing care after angiography usually involves routine postprocedural orders, including the following:

1. Frequent assessment of vital signs and neurologic function and distal pulse checks, with particular attention to the extremity that has been punctured.
2. Assessment of the puncture site for hematoma (bruising) and of the appearance of the extremity distal to the puncture site.
3. Bed rest for 6 to 8 hours, with the punctured extremity kept in straight alignment for a transfemoral approach. Use of a transaxillary approach, while not preferred and used only when the femoral site is inaccessible, does not require postprocedure bed rest.
4. Continuous intravenous (IV) hydration for 6 to 8 hours to assist with contrast excretion. Encourage oral fluid intake.
5. Assessment of blood urea nitrogen (BUN) and creatinine levels the next day.
6. Resumption of preprocedure diet and medications. If the client was receiving heparin, its administration may not be resumed until sealing of the puncture site has been confirmed.

Also assess motor and sensory function in the affected extremity (see Chapter 69). Bleeding can compress nerves and result in permanent neurologic deficits (especially if the brachial plexus is compressed following a transaxillary approach). Report changes in neurologic function of an extremity immediately because these require emergency attention by the physician.

Pain at the injection site is fairly common and can usually be managed with mild analgesics. Severe pain or pain distal to the puncture site requires further assessment of peripheral pulses, neurovascular assessment, and palpation for masses, which may indicate a hematoma. Notify the physician of abnormal assessment data.

Complications of angiography, in addition to allergic reaction to the contrast medium, include thrombi, vessel wall perforation, emboli, renal failure, and pseudo-aneurysm. *Pseudoaneurysm* is a significant complication and may extend the inpatient stay. A pseudoaneurysm is caused by blood leaking outside the vessel wall but within a contained area adjacent to the artery. There is a persistent communication between the artery and the fluid mass. Pseudoaneurysms generally result from arterial trauma (after arterial puncture). They provide a site for potential infection, can be a source of emboli, or may cause intravascular thrombosis. Pseudoaneurysms can become enlarged, compress an adjacent structure, and even rupture, although rupture is rare.

Venography

Venography, performed in a manner similar to that for angiography, is used to examine the venous system. Venograms can be used to detect DVT and other abnormalities, such as incompetent valves. This diagnostic test is performed less frequently than in the past. Newer, noninvasive vascular laboratory studies pose less risk, are more accurate, and provide functional information.

Vascular Endoscopy (Angioscopy)

Vascular endoscopy permits imaging of intra-arterial disease with the use of fiberoptic technology. Images are in color and in three dimensions. Equipment consists of a flexible fiberoptic angioscope, a light source, an irrigation system, a camera, a video recorder, and a monitor. The major advantage of angioscopy is the internal visualization of the vessel lumen. This enables identification of thrombus (blood clot), plaque, hemorrhage, ulceration, or embolus (clot that has broken off from a thrombus and lodged in a more distal artery). Angioscopes can be used to remove debris from vessels and to check the integrity of an anastomosis (suture line that connects a vessel grafted to a native vessel) from within a vessel. They may also be used to remove venous valves in preparation for use of the vein as a bypass graft.

Complications of vascular endoscopy are rare but may include intimal damage, vessel spasm, thrombosis or embolism, perforation, fluid overload, and infection. Postprocedure care is similar to that for clients who have undergone angiography.

Intravascular Ultrasonography

Intravascular ultrasonography provides information about the atherosclerotic intima beneath the luminal surface. It can thus determine the thickness of the arterial wall and can distinguish thrombus and calcium from vascular tissue, allowing more exact removal of lesions. One current limiting factor is the need for specialized interpretation of the scans.

CONCLUSIONS

Vascular assessment requires inspection, palpation, and auscultation skills. Knowledge of anatomy is critical for correct performance of assessments. Diagnostic modalities can range from simple noninvasive tests to complex, sophisticated, invasive technology. A clear understanding of the indications for diagnostic tests and interpretation of the findings assists the clinical decision-making.

BIBLIOGRAPHY

1. Fahey, V. (2004). Clinical assessment of the vascular system. In V.A. Fahey (Ed.). *Vascular nursing* (4th ed.). Philadelphia: W. B. Saunders.

2. Franks, P.J., et al. (1999). Quality of life in a randomized trial in venous leg ulceration. *Phlebology, 14(3),* 95-99.
3. Herbert, L.M. (1997). *Caring for the vascular patient.* New York: Churchill Livingstone.
4. Hirsch, A.T. (Ed.). (2001). Primary care series: Peripheral arterial disease and intermittent claudication: A compilation of the American Journal of Medicine Continuing Education Series. An office based approach to the diagnosis and treatment of peripheral arterial disease. *Excerpta Medica.* Philadelphia: Elsevier.
5. Hirsch, A.T., et al. (2001). Peripheral arterial disease detection, awareness, and treatment in primary care. *Journal of the American Medical Association, 11(286),* 1317-1324.
6. Jaff, M.R., & Hiatt, W.R. (2001). Clinical and vascular laboratory evaluation of peripheral arterial disease. In W.R. Hiatt, A.T. Hirsch, & J.G. Regensteiner (Eds.). *Peripheral arterial disease handbook* (pp. 81-94). Boca Raton, FL: CRC Press.
7. Moore, W.S. (Ed.) (2002). *Vascular surgery: A comprehensive review* (6th ed.). Philadelphia: W. B. Saunders.
8. Rutherford, R.B. (Ed.) (2000). *Vascular surgery* (5th ed.). Philadelphia: W. B. Saunders.
9. Sloan, H., & Wills, E.M. (1999). Ankle-brachial index: Calculating your patient's vascular risks. *Nursing, 99(10),* 58-59.
10. Treat-Jacobson, D., et al. (2002). A patient-derived perspective of health-related quality of life with peripheral arterial disease. *Journal of Nursing Scholarship, 34(1),* 55-60.
11. Treat-Jacobson, D., & Walsh, M.E. (2003). Treating patients with peripheral arterial disease and claudication. *Journal of Vascular Nursing, 21(1),* 5-14.

Chapter 54

Management of Clients with Hypertensive Disorders

Jean Elizabeth DeMartinis

evolve

Web Enhancements

http://evolve.elsevier.com/Black/medsurg/

Client Education Guide
Low-Sodium Diet (English Version and Spanish Translation)
Low-Fat, Low-Cholesterol Diet (English Version and Spanish Translation)
Calorie-Restriction Diet (English Version and Spanish Translation)

Concept Map
Understanding Hypertension and Its Treatment
Appendix C
Laboratory Values of Clinical Importance in Medical-Surgical Nursing

HYPERTENSION

Arterial hypertension, simply put, is high blood pressure. It is defined as a persistent elevation of the systolic blood pressure (SBP) at a level of 140 mm Hg or higher and diastolic blood pressure (DBP) at a level of 90 mm Hg or higher. The National Institute of Health's Seventh Report of the Joint National Committee on Detection, Evaluation, and Treatment of High Blood Pressure (JNC VII) and the Centers for Disease Control and Prevention (CDC) publications *Healthy People 2000* and *Healthy People 2010* have documented the advances made over the last few decades in the prevention, detection, and treatment of hypertension.[21,28] Members of the public have become more knowledgeable about high blood pressure, are more likely to visit a health care provider for hypertension, and are more likely to comply with medical advice. The use of increasingly effective antihypertensive agents has also dramatically reduced the mortality rate associated with hypertension. The percentage of people who receive treatment for hypertension has increased from 31% to 55% and of those with controlled hypertension from 10% to 29%. Ultimately the combined effects of these measures have contributed to a 60% decline in stroke and a 53% decline in the mortality rate from coronary artery disease.[6,10,16] These impressive gains have been seen across all age groups, in both men and women, and in special populations.

The JNC VII and *Healthy People 2010,* however, also document some disturbing current trends. After years of decline, the mortality rates for coronary heart disease and stroke leveled off and have begun to rise again. The prevalence of hypertension is on the rise, and control rates are variable, with the majority of this population undercontrolled.[4] Arterial hypertension affects more than 50 million persons—one in four—in the United States, with the highest rates of occurrence among older adults, African Americans, less educated people, and lower socioeconomic groups. Estimates are that only 25% of all people with hypertension have blood pressure controlled at a target level, that is, below 140/90 mm Hg, relative to specific target levels for special populations. Lack of client compliance and providers' continued ignorance of the need to prescribe and manage complex holistic treatment protocols are cited as the two major factors that have contributed to this abysmal decline in improved client outcomes.[1,6,10,17,21,28]

evolve *Be sure to check out the bonus material on the Evolve website and the CD-ROM, including free self-assessment exercises.*

http://evolve.elsevier.com/Black/medsurg/

Nursing Outcomes Classification (NOC)
for Nursing Diagnoses—Clients with Hypertensive Disorders

Imbalanced Nutrition: More than Body Requirements
  Nutritional Status: Food and Fluid
    Intake
  Nutritional Status: Nutrient Intake
  Weight Control
Ineffective Health Maintenance
  Health Belief: Perceived Resources
  Health-Promoting Behavior
  Health-Seeking Behavior
  Knowledge: Health Behaviors

Knowledge: Health Promotion
Knowledge: Health Resources
Participation: Health Care Decisions
Psychosocial Adjustment: Life Changes
Risk Detection
Self-direction of Care
Social Support
Treatment Behavior: Illness or Injury
Ineffective Therapeutic Regimen Management (Individual)
  Compliance Behavior

Knowledge: Treatment Regimen
Participation: Health Care Decisions
Noncompliance
  Adherence Behavior
  Compliance Behavior
  Symptom Control
  Treatment Behavior: Illness or Injury

Coronary events such as a "heart attack" are still the most common result of hypertension.[13] Increased blood pressure level is related to increased severity of atherosclerosis, stroke, nephropathy, peripheral vascular disease, aortic aneurysms, and heart failure. Nearly all people with heart failure have antecedent hypertension. If hypertension is left untreated, nearly half of hypertensive clients will die of heart disease, a third will die of stroke, and the remaining 10% to 15% will die of renal failure. Hypertension is also a "silent factor" in the etiology of many deaths attributed to stroke or heart attacks.[10,13,16]

These disturbing trends indicate the need for renewed vigor in the battle against hypertension. Hypertension-related morbidity and mortality rates will not decrease until providers appreciate the need for changes in existing treatment protocols that are based on quantifiable client outcomes. The *Healthy People 2000/2010* guidelines are prevention focused, and the JNC VII guidelines are also now primarily prevention focused and strongly recommend the use of nonpharmaceutical as well as pharmaceutical measures to prevent and treat hypertension.[21,28] (See the Evidence-Based Practice in Action feature on New Guidelines for Hypertension Prevention and Management on p. 1491.) Nurses are faced with a profound urgency to enhance public and professional education toward this end and to translate the results of research into improved practice.[1,4,10] An ambitious, but nevertheless feasible, goal is the diagnosis and treatment of hypertension in all affected people in the United States.

Types of Hypertensive Disease, Etiology, and Severity

Hypertension is characterized by type, cause, and severity (Box 54-1).[3,10,13,16,21,23] People with hypertensive disease have either combined SBP and DBP elevations in pressure or isolated systolic pressure elevation alone. The blood pressure remains elevated and continues to rise over time because of a persistent, progressive increase in peripheral arterial resistance. The persistent rise in arterial resistance is due to inappropriate renal retention of salt and water or abnormalities of or within the vessel wall. The severity of the condition directly relates to the number and magnitude of risk factors present, the length of time for which these risk factors have been present, and the presence of accompanying disease states.

Epidemiology and Risk Factors

Primary *(essential)* hypertension constitutes more than 90% of all cases of hypertension. Fewer than 5% to 8% of adult hypertensive clients have secondary hypertension; however, hypertension, regardless of type, results from an array of genetic and environmental factors. The following text discusses the major nonmodifiable and modifiable risk factors that contribute to the development of hypertension. There is necessarily some overlap between categories.[10,13,21]

Secondary hypertension is an elevation in blood pressure from an identifiable disease, such as renal failure. *Malignant* hypertension, now referred to as *resistant or persistent severe* hypertension, is a sustained elevation in blood pressure combined with end-organ damage.

Nonmodifiable Risk Factors[10,21,28]

Family History. Hypertension is thought to be polygenic and multifactorial—that is, in any person with a family history of hypertension, several genes may interact with each other and the environment to cause the blood pressure to elevate over time. The genetic predisposition that makes certain families more susceptible to hypertension may be related to an elevation in intracellular sodium levels and to lowered potassium-to-sodium ratios, which are found more often in blacks than in other groups. Clients with parents who have hypertension are at greater risk for hypertension at a younger age.

📖 EVIDENCE-BASED PRACTICE IN ACTION

New Guidelines for Hypertension Prevention and Management

The "Seventh Report of the Joint National Committee on Prevention, Detection, Evaluation, and Treatment of High Blood Pressure" provides a new guideline for hypertension prevention and management. The following are the report's key messages:

- In persons older than 50 years, systolic blood pressure greater than 140 mm Hg is a much more important cardiovascular disease (CVD) risk factor than diastolic blood pressure.
- The risk of CVD beginning at 115/75 mm Hg doubles with each increment of 20/10 mm Hg; individuals who are normotensive at age 55 have a 90% lifetime risk for developing hypertension.
- Individuals with a systolic blood pressure of 120-139 mm Hg or a diastolic blood pressure of 80-89 mm Hg should be considered as prehypertensive and require health-promoting lifestyle modifications to prevent CVD.
- Thiazide-type diuretics should be used in drug treatment for most patients with uncomplicated hypertension, either alone or combined with drugs from other classes. Certain high-risk conditions are compelling indications for the initial use of other antihypertensive drug classes (angiotensin-converting enzyme inhibitors, angiotensin receptor blockers, beta-blockers, calcium channel blockers).

- Most patients with hypertension will require two or more antihypertensive medications to achieve goal blood pressure (<140/90 mm Hg, or <130/80 mm Hg for patients with diabetes or chronic kidney disease).
- If blood pressure is >20/10 mm Hg above goal blood pressure, consideration should be given to initiating therapy with two agents, one of which usually should be a thiazide-type diuretic.
- The most effective therapy prescribed by the most careful clinician will control hypertension only if patients are motivated. Motivation improves when patients have positive experiences with, and trust in, the clinician. Empathy builds trust and is a potent motivator.
- In presenting these guidelines, the committee recognizes that the responsible physician's judgment remains paramount.

From National High Blood Pressure Education Program, National Institutes of Health, National Heart, Lung, and Blood Institute. (2003). *The Seventh Report of the Joint National Committee on Detection, Evaluation, and Treatment of High Blood Pressure.* Bethesda, MD: U.S. Government Printing Office.

BOX 54-1   *Types of Hypertension*

Primary hypertension—also known as *essential* or idiopathic hypertension. The etiology is a multifactorial, with no identifiable cause, but several interacting homeostatic forces are generally involved concomitantly. Most cases of combined systolic and diastolic elevation fall into this category. Severity of sequelae increases as the blood pressure, both systolic and diastolic, increases.

Secondary hypertension—results from an identifiable cause. Various specific disease states or problems are responsible for the elevation in blood pressure (see Box 54-2), and underlying causes may be correctable. Therefore it is important to isolate the root of the problem so that the most appropriate treatment regimen can be prescribed. Severity depends on underlying causes, personal and environmental factors, and duration of concurrent disease states.

"White coat hypertension"—defined as hypertension in people who are actually normotensive except when their blood pressure is measured by a health care professional. An intermittent vasovagal response accounts for the transient elevation in blood pressure. Differentiation between this diagnosis and essential or secondary hypertension is crucial so that the latter can be treated effectively. Treating this false hypertension produces significant hypotension and severe deleterious sequelae. However, the converse is also true; essential or secondary hypertension disguised as "white coat" hypertension and left undiagnosed and untreated can have ominous consequences over time.

Isolated systolic hypertension (ISH)—occurs when the systolic blood pressure is 140 mm Hg or higher but the diastolic blood pressure remains less than 90 mm Hg. It is thought to emerge because of increased cardiac output or atherosclerosis-induced changes in blood vessel compliance or both in older adults. The likelihood of the development of ISH increases with advancing age, as does the severity of ISH.

Persistent severe hypertension or resistant hypertension (formerly called malignant hypertension)—characterized by a diastolic blood pressure above 110 to 120 mm Hg. It results when hypertension is left untreated or is unresponsive to treatment and becomes a truly severe emergency condition as the pressure continues to rise unchecked.

Age. Primary hypertension typically appears between the ages of 30 and 50 years. The incidence of hypertension increases with age; 50% to 60% of clients older than 60 years have a blood pressure over 140/90 mm Hg. Epidemiologic studies, however, have shown a poorer prognosis in clients whose hypertension began at a young age. Isolated systolic hypertension occurs primarily in people older than 50 years, with almost 24% of all people affected by age 80 years. Among older adults, SBP readings are a better predictor of possible future events such as coronary heart disease, stroke, heart failure, and renal disease than are DBP readings.

Gender. The overall incidence of hypertension is higher in men than in women until about age 55 years. Between the ages of 55 and 74 years, the risk in men and that in women are almost equal; then, after age 74 years, women are at greater risk.

Ethnicity. Mortality statistics indicate that the death rate for adults with hypertension is lowest for white women at 4.7%; white men have the next lowest rate at 6.3%, and black men have the next lowest at 22.5%; the death rate is highest for black women at 29.3%. The reason for the increased prevalence of hypertension among blacks is unclear, but the increase has been attributed to lower renin levels, greater sensitivity to vasopressin, higher salt intake, and greater environmental stress.

Modifiable Risk Factors[1,6,8,10,13]

Stress. Because stress is a matter of perception, people's interpretations of events are what create most stressors and stress responses. Environmental factors or events, personality characteristics, and physiologic phenomena may either cause or set the stage for the mobilization of the stress response. Stressors such as noise, infection, inflammation, pain, decreased oxygen supply, heat, cold, trauma, prolonged exertion, responses to life events, obesity, old age, drugs, disease, surgery, and medical treatment can elicit the stress response. These noxious stimuli are perceived by a person as a threat or as capable of causing harm; subsequently, a psychophysiologic "fight-or-flight" response is initiated in the body.

Stress increases peripheral vascular resistance and cardiac output and stimulates sympathetic nervous system activity. Over time hypertension can develop. Chronic stress, when it is not stopped, will aggravate existing physical and emotional instability, further exacerbating the response. If stress arousal becomes excessive or prolonged, target organ dysfunction or disease will result. A report from the American Institute of Stress estimates that 60% to 90% of all primary care visits involve stress-related complaints.

Obesity. Obesity, especially in the upper body (giving an "apple" shape), with increased amounts of fat about the midriff, waist, and abdomen, is associated with subsequent development of hypertension.[1,6,10,13,21] People who are overweight but carry most of the excess weight in the buttocks, hips, and thighs (giving them a "pear" shape) are at far less risk for development of hypertension secondary to increased weight alone.

Nutrients. Sodium consumption can be an important factor in the development of essential hypertension. A high-salt diet may induce excessive release of natriuretic hormone, which may indirectly increase blood pressure. Sodium loading also stimulates vasopressor mechanisms within the central nervous system (CNS). Studies also show that low dietary intake of calcium, potassium, and magnesium can contribute to the development of hypertension.

Substance Abuse. Cigarette smoking, heavy alcohol consumption, and some illicit drug use all are risk factors for hypertension.[1,6,10,13,14] The nicotine in cigarette smoke and drugs such as cocaine cause an immediate rise in blood pressure that is dose dependent; however, *habitual* use of these substances has been implicated in an increased incidence of hypertension over time. The incidence of hypertension is also higher among people who drink more than 3 ounces of ethanol per day. The impact of caffeine is controversial. Caffeine raises blood pressure acutely but does not produce sustained effects.

Pathophysiology

Primary (Essential) Hypertension

The exact pathologic underpinnings of primary hypertension remain to be established. Any factor that produces an alteration in peripheral vascular resistance, heart rate, or stroke volume affects systemic arterial blood pressure. Four control systems play a major role in maintaining blood pressure[12]: (1) the arterial baroreceptor and chemoreceptors system, (2) regulation of body fluid volume, (3) the renin-angiotensin system, and (4) vascular autoregulation. Hypotheses derived to explain the onset of primary hypertension in people at risk propose that a defect or malfunction must exist in some or all of these systems. Probably no single defect causes essential hypertension in all affected people.

Arterial baroreceptors and chemoreceptors work reflexively to control blood pressure (Figure 54-1). Baroreceptors, major stretch receptors, are found in the carotid sinus, aorta, and wall of the left ventricle. They monitor the level of arterial pressure and counteract increases through vasodilatation and slowing of the heart rate via the vagus nerve. Chemoreceptors, located in the medulla and carotid and aortic bodies, are sensitive to changes in concentrations of oxygen, carbon dioxide, and hydrogen ions (pH) in the blood. A decrease in arterial oxygen concentration or pH causes a reflexive rise in pressure, whereas an increase in carbon dioxide concentration causes a decrease in blood pressure. The major reflex response is to changes in oxygen saturation, and effects of changes in pH and carbon dioxide are minor.

The role of the arterial baroreceptors and chemoreceptors in hypertension is not well understood. The stretch receptors may become desensitized because they must continue to "reset" as prolonged, sustained increases in pressure continue. Chemoreceptor autoregula-

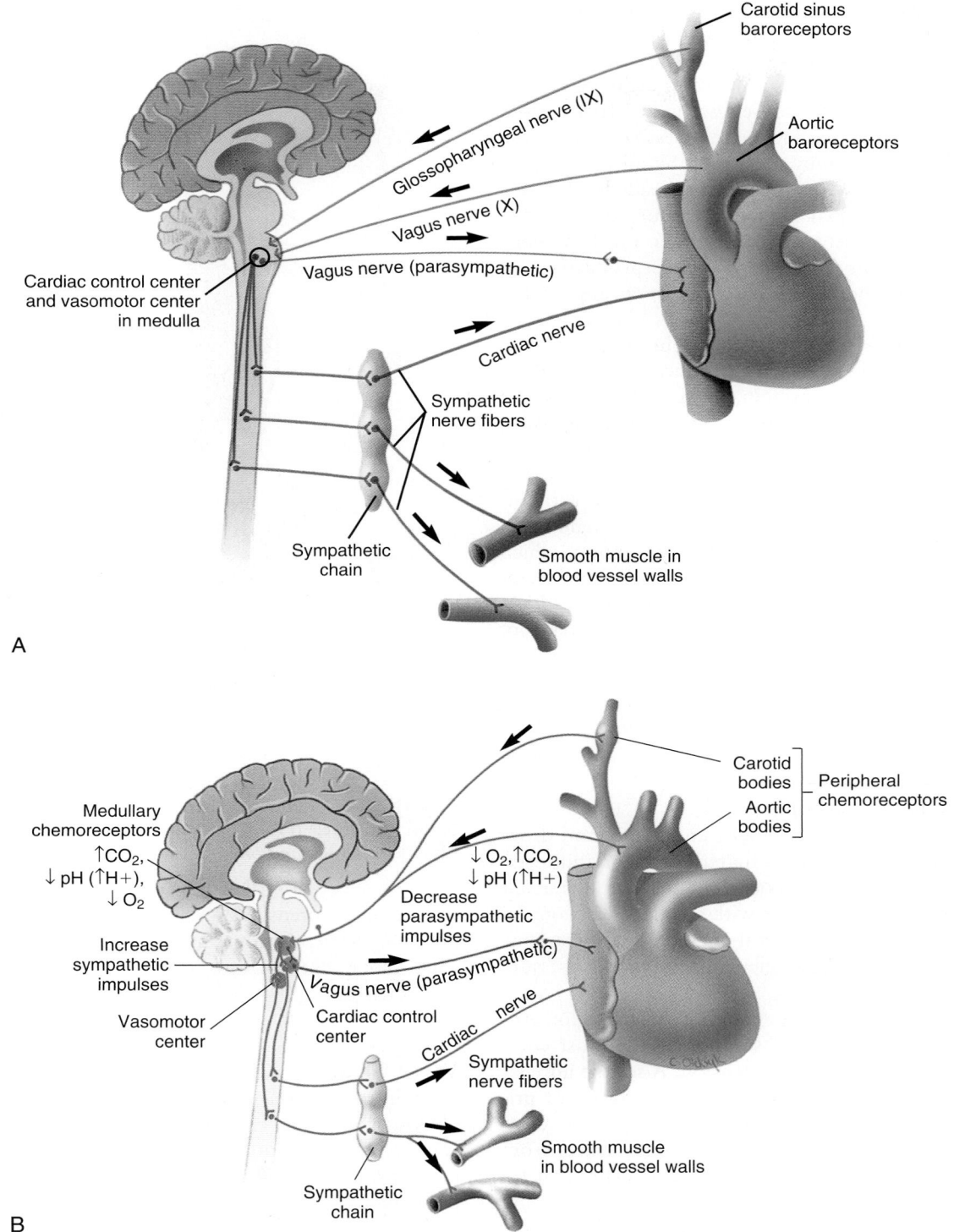

FIGURE 54-1 Baroreceptor and chemoreceptor reflex control of blood pressure. **A,** Baroreceptor reflexes. Baroreceptors located in the carotid sinuses and aortic arch detect changes in blood pressure. The heart rate can be decreased by the parasympathetic system; heart rate and stroke volume can be increased by the sympathetic system. The sympathetic system also can constrict or dilate blood vessels. **B,** Chemoreceptor reflexes. Chemoreceptors located in the medulla oblongata and in the carotid and aortic bodies detect changes in blood oxygen, carbon dioxide, or pH. In response the vasomotor center can cause vasoconstriction or dilation of blood vessels by the sympathetic system, and the cardioregulatory center can cause changes in the pumping activity of the heart through the parasympathetic and sympathetic systems. (From Seeley, R.R., Stephens, T.D., & Tate, P. [1995]. *Anatomy and physiology* [3rd ed.]. St. Louis, MO: Mosby).

tion may be altered as blood volume rises, and sympathetic overstimulation becomes apparent.

Changes in fluid volume affect systemic arterial pressure. Thus an abnormality in the transport of sodium in the renal tubules may cause essential hypertension. When sodium and water levels are excessive, total blood volume increases, thereby increasing blood pressure. In functional kidneys, a rise in pressure leads to diuresis. Pathologic changes that alter the pressure threshold at which kidneys excrete salt and water alter systemic blood pressure. In addition, the overproduction of sodium-retaining hormones has been implicated in hypertension.

Renin and angiotensin play a role in blood pressure regulation. *Renin* is an enzyme produced by the kidney that catalyzes a plasma protein substrate to split off angiotensin I, which is removed by a converting enzyme to the lung to form angiotensin II and then angiotensin III (Figure 54-2). Angiotensin II and III act as vasoconstrictors and also stimulate aldosterone release. With increased sympathetic nervous system activity, angiotensin II and III also seem to inhibit sodium excretion, which results in elevated blood pressure. Increased renin secretion has been investigated as a cause of increased peripheral vascular resistance in primary hypertension. Hypertension may also develop from deficiencies in vasodilator substances, such as prostaglandins, from congenital abnormalities in resistance vessels (arterioles) or from defects in neuroendocrine secretion.

Secondary Hypertension

Many renal, vascular, neurologic, endocrine, and drug- and food-induced problems that directly or indirectly negatively affect the kidneys can result in serious insult to these organs that interferes with sodium excretion, renal perfusion, or the renin-angiotensin-aldosterone mechanism, leading to an elevation in blood pressure over time (Box 54-2).

Chronic renal disease, mainly chronic glomerulonephritis and renal artery stenosis, is the most common cause of secondary hypertension. Also, the adrenal glands cause secondary hypertension as a result of primary excesses of aldosterone, cortisol, and catecholamines. Primary aldosteronism usually arises from solitary benign adenomas of the adrenal cortex that release excess aldosterone. Excess aldosterone causes renal retention of sodium and water, expands blood volume, and elevates blood pressure. *Pheochromocytoma,* a small tumor of the adrenal medulla, can cause dramatic hypertension because of the release of excessive amounts of epinephrine and norepinephrine. Other adrenocortical problems can result in excess production of cortisol (Cushing's syndrome). Clients with Cushing's syndrome have an 80% risk for development of hypertension. Cortisol increases blood pressure by increasing renal sodium

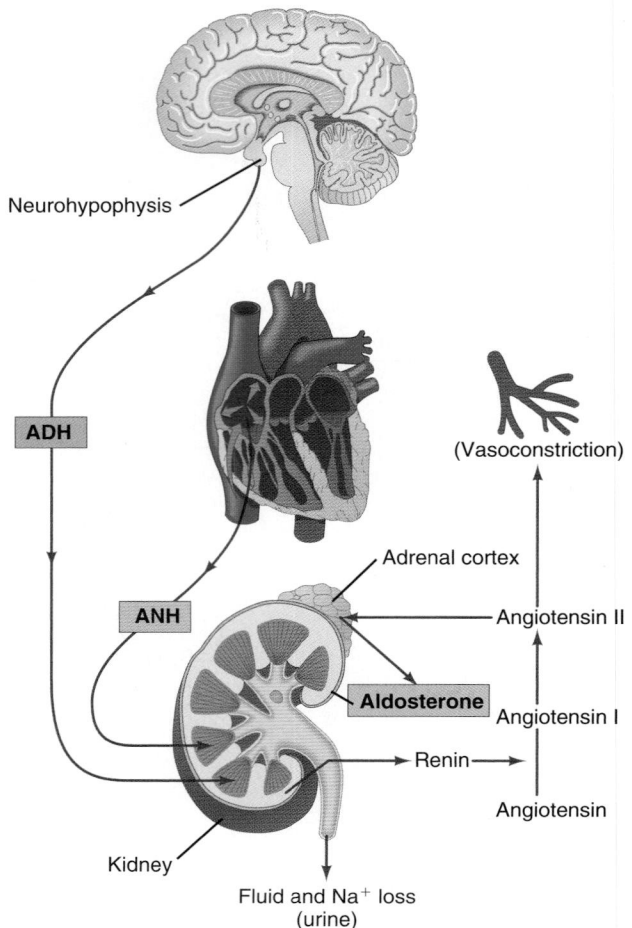

FIGURE 54-2 Renin-angiotensin-aldosterone regulation of blood pressure. (From Thibodeau, G.A., & Patton, K.T. [2003]. *Anatomy and physiology* [5th ed.] St. Louis: Mosby.)

retention, angiotensin II levels, and vascular reactivity to norepinephrine. Chronic stress induces prolonged elevated blood levels of catecholamines, certain hormones, and cortisol.

Vessel Changes

Early in the course of development of hypertension, no obvious pathologic changes in the blood vessels and organs may be seen other than intermittent elevations of blood pressure *(labile hypertension).* Slowly, widespread pathologic changes take place in both the large and small blood vessels and in the heart, kidneys, and brain.[12]

The large vessels, such as the aorta, coronary arteries, basilar artery to the brain, and peripheral vessels in the limbs, become sclerotic, tortuous, and weak. Their lumina narrow, with resultant decreased blood flow to the heart, brain, and lower extremities. As the damage continues, large vessels may become occluded or may hemorrhage, causing infarction of the tissue supplied by the vessel that has suddenly been robbed of its blood supply.

BOX 54-2 *Causes of Secondary Hypertension*

Acute Stress
Alcoholism
Acute alcohol withdrawal
Burns
Chronic intermittent vasovagal response
Hyperventilation
Hypoglycemia
Psychogenic

Vascular Disorders
Arteriosclerosis
Coarctation of the aorta
Increased intravascular volume
Sickle cell crisis

Dissecting Aortic Aneurysm

Endocrine Disorders
Acromegaly
Adrenal disorders
  Cortical
    Cushing's syndrome
    Primary aldosteronism
  Medullary
    Pancreatitis
    Pheochromocytoma
Hypothyroidism
Hyperthyroidism

Neurologic Disorders
Autonomic dysreflexia
Increased intracranial pressure
  Brain tumor
  Encephalitis
  Respiratory acidosis
Sleep apnea

Medications
Abrupt medication withdrawal
Amphetamine use
Anabolic and adrenogenic steroids
Antihistamine/decongestants
Cocaine use
Cyclosporine
Ergot alkaloids
Erythropoietin
Glucocorticoids
Heavy metal poisons (lead, arsenic)
Mineralocorticoids
Monoamine oxidase inhibitors
NSAIDs
Oral contraceptives
Sympathomimetics
  Ephedrine
  Phenylephrine
Tricyclic antidepressants

Problems with Pregnancy
Pregnancy-induced hypertension
Eclampsia

Renal Disorders
Renal artery stenosis
Renal parenchymal disease
  Acute glomerulonephritis
  Chronic pyelonephritis
  Connective tissue diseases
  Diabetic nephropathy
  Hydronephrosis
  Polycystic disease
Renin-producing tumors
Renovascular diseases
  Atherosclerosis
  Vasculitis

Severe Anemia

Tyramine-Containing Foods
Aged cheeses (especially cheddar)
Beer, wine
Chicken liver
Yeast extract

From National High Blood Pressure Education Program, National Institutes of Health, and National Heart, Lung, and Blood Institute (2003). *The Seventh Report of the Joint National Committee on Detection, Evaluation, and Treatment of High Blood Pressure.* Bethesda, MD: U.S. Government Printing Office.

Small vessel damage, equally dangerous, causes structural changes in the heart, kidneys, and brain. Elevated DBP damages the intimal lining of the small vessels. Because of intimal damage, fibrin accumulates in the vessels, local edema develops, and intravascular clotting may occur. The net results of these changes are (1) a decreased blood supply to the tissues of the heart, brain, kidneys, and retina; (2) progressive functional impairment of these organs; and (3) finally, as a consequence of the chronic ischemia, infarction of the tissue supplied by these vessels, originating in much the same way as with occlusion of the large vessels.

Clinical Manifestations

In the early stages of development of hypertension, no clinical manifestations are noted by clients or practitioners. Eventually the blood pressure will rise, and if it is not "caught" during a routine screening, clients will remain unaware that their blood pressure is elevated. If the condition is left undiagnosed, the blood pressure will continue to rise, clinical manifestations will become apparent, and clients will eventually report to a provider's office with complaints of persistent headaches, fatigue, dizziness, palpitations, flushing, blurred or double vision, or epistaxis.[4,10,13]

Assessment of the client with hypertension involves the following three main objectives:
- To assess lifestyle and ascertain the presence of other cardiovascular risk factors or concomitant disorders that can affect prognosis and guide treatment
- To identify the type of hypertension (primary or secondary) and identifiable causes
- To determine the presence or absence of target organ involvement

Clinicians can obtain information relevant to these areas from the history, physical examination, and laboratory studies (Box 54-3).[9,10,21] The diagnosis of hypertension is made when, after the seated client has been allowed to rest for at least 5 minutes, the average of two or more readings separated by at least 2 minutes is 140 mm Hg or higher for the SBP and 90 mm Hg or higher for the DBP. Follow-up examinations are scheduled to diagnose or rule out the presence of hypertension, unless first-visit measurement averages fall into either stage 2 or 3. In such cases, the client is diagnosed with hypertension on the basis of the first-visit measurements, and a temporary management plan is implemented to bring the blood pressure down immediately or in a short time. Careful differentiation of primary from secondary causes

of the high blood pressure must precede any long-term management plan.

Hypertension is classified into a prehypertension category and two stages according to blood pressure readings (Table 54-1).[21] It is important to identify "prehypertensive" values because this range of blood pressures is as-

---

BOX 54-3 *Assessment of the Client with Hypertension*

History

Note the following points when interviewing the hypertensive client:

- Family history of hypertension, diabetes mellitus, cardiovascular disease, hyperlipidemia, or renal disease; smoking; stress; obesity; or sedentary lifestyle
- Previous documentation of high blood pressure, including age at onset, level of elevation, and currently prescribed medical regimen
- History of all prescribed and over-the-counter medications and the client's exact compliance with taking the medications. NOTE: Medications that may either raise blood pressure or interfere with the effectiveness of antihypertensive medications include oral contraceptives, steroids, non-steroidal anti-inflammatory drugs, nasal decongestants, appetite suppressants, cyclosporine, tricyclic antidepressants, monoamine oxidase inhibitors, and erythropoietin
- History of any disease or trauma to target organs
- Results and side effects of previous antihypertensive therapy
- Clinical manifestations of cardiovascular disorders, such as angina, dyspnea, or claudication
- History of or recent weight gain, exercise activities, sodium intake, fat intake, alcohol use, and smoking
- Psychosocial and environmental factors (e.g., emotional stress, cultural food practices, economic status) that may influence blood pressure control

Physical Examination

Physical assessment should include an accurate determination of blood pressure as well as an evaluation of target organs:

- Vital signs and weight
- Blood pressure—because blood pressure is variable and can be affected by multiple factors, it should be measured so that readings are representative of the client's usual level; the following techniques are strongly recommended:

   The client should be seated with the arm bared, supported, and positioned at heart level. The client should not have smoked tobacco or ingested caffeine within the previous 30 minutes.

   Measurement should begin after at least 5 minutes of quiet rest. The client's back should be supported, and both feet should be flat on the floor with the legs uncrossed. The client should not speak while the blood pressure is being monitored.

   Use of the appropriate cuff size will ensure an accurate measurement. The rubber bladder should encircle at least 80% of the limb being measured. The bladder's width should be one-third to one-half the circumference of the limb. Several sizes of cuffs (e.g., child, adult, large adult) should be available.

- Measurements should be taken with a mercury sphygmomanometer, a recently calibrated aneroid manometer, or a validated electronic device.
- Postural blood pressures should be measured and recorded according to position and arm used, including lying, sitting, and standing measurements from both arms.

   Both systolic and diastolic blood pressures should be recorded. The disappearance of sound (phase V) should be used for the diastolic reading.

   Two or more readings should be averaged. If the first two readings differ by more than 5 mm Hg, additional readings should be obtained.

- Funduscopic examination for retinal arteriolar narrowing, hemorrhages, exudates, and papilledema
- Examination of the neck for distended veins, carotid bruits, and enlarged thyroid
- Auscultation of the heart for increased heart rate, dysrhythmias, enlargement, precordial impulses, murmurs, and S3 and S4 heart sounds
- Examination of the abdomen for bruits, aortic dilation, and enlarged kidneys
- Examination of extremities for diminished or absent peripheral pulses, edema, and bilateral inequality of pulses
- Neurologic evaluation for signs of cerebral thrombosis or hemorrhage

Laboratory Studies

Studies used in the routine evaluation of hypertension include a complete blood count, urinalysis, determinations of serum potassium and sodium levels, fasting blood glucose level, serum cholesterol level, blood urea nitrogen and serum creatinine levels, electrocardiogram, and chest radiography. These rests provide useful information in determining the severity of vascular disease, the extent of target organ damage, and the possible causes of hypertension. Clients with the potential for secondary hypertension may need more extensive studies.

sociated with an increased risk of hypertension. Clients who are classified as prehypertensive, particularly those who have additional risk factors, should be informed that they are at twice the risk of developing hypertension than those with values lower than 120/80 mm Hg and that they should institute appropriate lifestyle modifications to address the problem immediately.

Risk Stratification

Risk stratification (Table 54-2)[21] of clients with hypertension is accomplished after assessing each individual for the type and number of major risk factors and the presence or absence of target organ damage (TOD) or clinical cardiovascular disease (CCD). Target organs, sometimes called *end organs*, are the body organs likely to be damaged by untreated disease (e.g., brain, eyes, kidneys).

Outcome Management

The goal of management is to control arterial blood pressure below 140 mm Hg SBP and 90 mm Hg DBP and lower if tolerated to lower than 120 mm Hg SBP and lower than 80 mm Hg DBP while modifying and controlling risk factors. For clients with diabetes or progressive renal disease, goal is 130/80 mm Hg (or to

TABLE 54-1	*Classification and Management of Blood Pressure for Adults**					
				Initial Drug Therapy	
BP Classification	**SBP* mm Hg**	**DBP* mm Hg**	**Lifestyle Modification**	**Without Compelling Indication**	**With Compelling Indications**
Normal	<120	and <80	Encourage		
Prehypertension	120-139	or 80-89	Yes	No antihypertensive drug indicated.	Drug(s) for compelling indications.‡
Stage 1 Hypertension	140-159	or 90-99	Yes	Thiazide-type diuretics for most. May consider ACEI, ARB, BB, CCB, or combination.	Drug(s) for the compelling indications.‡
Stage 2 Hypertension	≥160	or ≥100	Yes	Two-drug combination for most† (usually thiazide-type diuretic and ACEI or ARB or BB or CCB).	Other antihypertensive drugs (diuretics, ACEI, ARB, BB, CCB) as needed.

From National High Blood Pressure Education Program, National Institutes of Health, National Heart, Lung and Blood Institute. (2003). *The Seventh Report of the Joint National Committee on Detection, Evaluation, and Treatment of High Blood Pressure.* Bethesda, MD: U.S. Government Printing Office.

DBP, Diastolic blood pressure; *SBP,* systolic blood pressure; *ACEI,* angiotensin converting enzyme inhibitor; *ARB,* angiotensin receptor blocker; *BB,* beta-blocker; *CCB,* calcium channel blocker.

* Treatment determined by highest BP category.

† Initial combined therapy should be used cautiously in those at risk for orthostatic hypotension.

‡ Treat patients with chronic kidney disease or diabetes to BP goal of <130/80 mm Hg.

TABLE 54-2	*Cardiovascular Risk Stratification*

Major Risk Factors

Hypertension*	Physical inactivity	Family history of cardiovascular disease:
Smoking	Dyslipidemia*	women under age 65 or men under
Age (>55 for men; >65 for women)	Gender (men and postmenopausal	age 55
Diabetes mellitus*	women)	Microalbuminuria or estimated GFR <60
	Obesity (BMI ≥30)*	ml/min

Target Organ Damage/Clinical Cardiovascular Disease (TOD/CCD)

Heart diseases	Stroke or transient ischemic attack
Left ventricular hypertrophy	Nephropathy
Angina/prior myocardial infarction	Peripheral arterial disease
Prior coronary revascularization	Retinopathy
Heart failure	

Modified from National High Blood Pressure Education Program, National Institutes of Health, National Heart, Lung, and Blood Institutes. (2003). *The Seventh Report of the Joint National Committee on Detection, Evaluation, and Treatment of High Blood Pressure.* Bethesda, MD: U.S. Government Printing Office.

*Components of metabolic syndrome

125/75 mm Hg for clients with renal disease and proteinuria >1 g/24 hr).[21]

The most pronounced positive client outcomes have resulted from a systematic, multifactorial, multidisciplinary team approach for primary and secondary prevention and management of hypertension using diverse qualified health care professionals.[1,6,8,10] Multidisciplinary teams can provide the most comprehensive, cost-effective care of clients with a multitude of prevention and management needs, including those related to the prevention, diagnosis, and management of hypertension.

Long-term compliance and adherence has emerged as the most essential element in reducing morbidity and mortality rates associated with hypertension.[1,6,10,17,21,28] Unfortunately, poor compliance with or adherence to antihypertensive therapy persists as one of the most frustrating blocks to effective therapeutic management and is often due to clients' belief systems and values. Poor compliance or adherence is the reason that more than two thirds of clients with hypertension do not have adequate control of their blood pressure. For example, clients may choose not to have the initial prescription filled; successfully initiate therapy only to abandon it after a few weeks or months; or comply with only part of the regimen, thus failing to achieve optimal control.

Normalizing Arterial Pressure

The ultimate factors in evaluating whether the correct choice of treatment regimen has been made are as follows: the desired "control" blood pressure is reached, treatment choices are tolerated and safe, and the client is willing to *commit* to the regimen over the long term.

Lifestyle Modifications.[1,6,8,10,13,23] Strong research evidence has illustrated conclusively that lifestyle modifications are effective in lowering blood pressure and reducing cardiovascular risk factors at little overall cost and with minimal risk. According to the JNC VII (Figure 54-3),[21] lifestyle modifications are suggested as definitive first-line therapy for some clients, at least for the first 6 to 12 months after the initial diagnosis.

Lifestyle modification is also strongly encouraged as adjunctive therapy for all clients with hypertension who are receiving pharmacologic therapy. Continued healthy lifestyle practices, along with pharmacologic therapy, can reduce the number and dosage of antihypertensive medications needed to manage the condition.

Weight Reduction. Excess body weight, exhibited by a body mass index (BMI)—weight in kilograms divided by

FIGURE 54-3 Algorithm for treatment of hypertension. *ACEI,* Angiotensin-converting enzyme inhibitor; *ARB,* angiotensin receptor blocker; *BB,* beta-blocker; *CCB,* calcium channel blocker; *DBP,* diastolic blood pressure; *SBP,* systolic blood pressure. (From National High Blood Pressure Education Program, National Institutes of Health, National Heart, Lung and Blood Institute. [2003]. *The Seventh Report of the Joint National Committee on Detection, Evaluation, and Treatment of High Blood Pressure.* Bethesda, MD: U.S. Government Printing Office.)

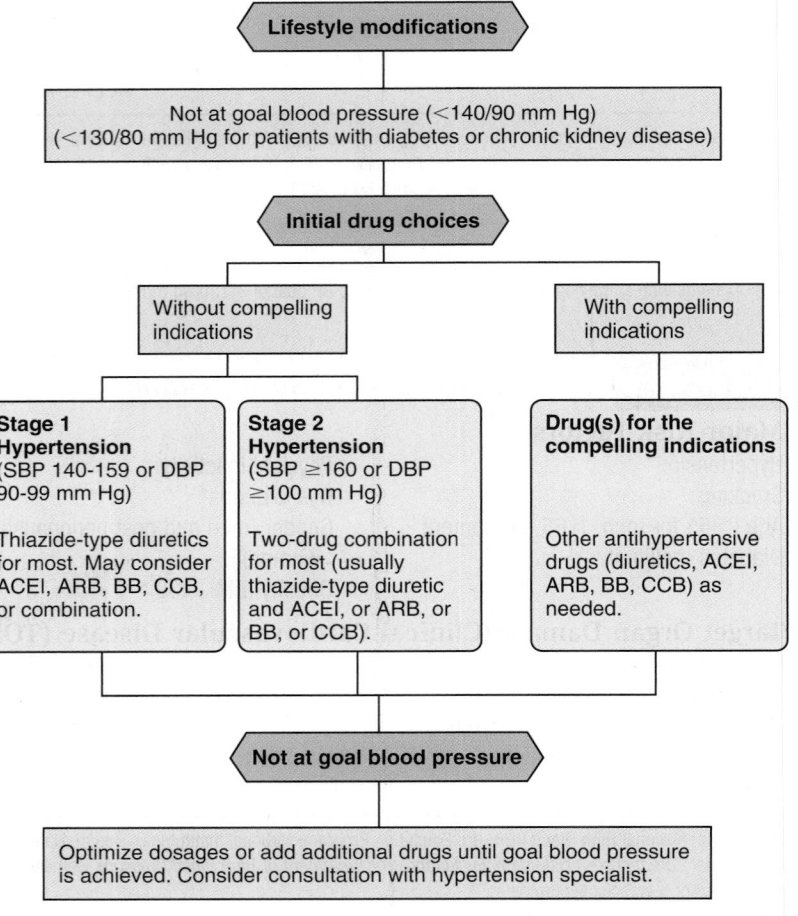

height in meters squared—of 27 or greater, correlates closely with elevated blood pressure. Also, excess body fat accumulated in the torso with a waist circumference of 35 inches or greater for women and 40 inches or greater for men has been associated with an increased risk for hypertension. For many people with hypertension whose body weight is more than 10% greater than ideal, weight reduction of as little as 10 pounds can lower blood pressure. Weight reduction also enhances the effectiveness of antihypertensive medications. Therefore reassess the client's blood pressure during weight loss, and make appropriate changes in pharmacologic interventions as needed.

Sodium Restriction. An estimated 40% of people with hypertension are sodium sensitive. A moderate restriction of sodium intake to 2.3 g of sodium, or 6 g of salt, can be used to lower blood pressure in some cases of stage 1 hypertension. The amount of medication otherwise needed may be decreased if sodium intake is lowered. In addition, this moderate sodium restriction may reduce the degree of potassium depletion that often accompanies diuretic therapy.

Dietary Fat Modification. Modification of dietary intake of fat by decreasing the fraction of saturated fat and increasing that of polyunsaturated fat has little, if any, effect on decreasing blood pressure but can decrease the cholesterol level significantly. Because dyslipidemia is a major risk factor in the development of coronary artery disease, diet therapy aimed at reducing lipids is an important adjunct to any total dietary regimen. In addition to the usual recommendations for sensible eating following the food pyramid (see Chapter 2), the Dietary Approaches to Stop Hypertension (DASH) diet (Table 54-3), which is rich in fruits, vegetables, nuts, and low-fat dairy foods with reduced saturated and total fats, should be recommended for clients who need a more structured, fat-limited dietary intervention.[22,27]

Exercise. A regular program of aerobic exercise adequate to achieve at least a moderate level of physical fitness facilitates cardiovascular conditioning and can aid the obese hypertensive client in weight reduction and reduce the risk for cardiovascular disease and all-cause mortality. Blood pressure can be reduced with moderate-intensity (as low as 40% to 60% of maximum oxygen consumption) physical activity, such as a brisk walk (about 2.5 to 3 mph) for 30 to 45 minutes most days of the week.

Weight training using *light* weights is a positive addition to any exercise regimen; however, lifting *heavy* weights can be harmful because blood pressure rises, sometimes to high levels, with the vasovagal response that occurs during an intense isometric muscle contraction. Advise hypertensive clients to initiate exercise pro-

grams gradually, slowly increasing the intensity and the duration of activity as the body adjusts and becomes more conditioned with ongoing professional surveillance.

Alcohol Restriction. The consumption of more than 1 ounce of alcohol per day is associated with a higher prevalence of hypertension, poor adherence to antihypertensive therapy, and occasionally refractory hypertension. Carefully assess alcohol intake. Advise clients who do drink alcohol to do so in moderation (i.e., no more than 1 ounce of ethanol per day for men and 0.5 ounce for women). There is 1 ounce (30 ml) of ethanol in 2 ounces (60 ml) of 100-proof whiskey, in 10 ounces (300 ml) of wine, or in 24 ounces (720 ml) of beer.

Caffeine Restriction. Although acute ingestion of caffeine may raise blood pressure, chronic moderate caffeine ingestion appears to have no significant effect on blood pressure. Therefore caffeine restriction is not necessary unless cardiac response or other excessive sensitivity to caffeine is present.

Relaxation Techniques. A variety of relaxation therapies, including transcendental meditation, yoga, biofeedback, progressive muscle relaxation, and psychotherapy, can reduce blood pressure in hypertensive clients, at least transiently. Although each modality has its advocates, none has been conclusively shown to be either practical for the majority of hypertensive clients or effective in maintaining a significant long-term effect.[1,6,8,10,16]

Smoking Cessation.[10,14] Although smoking has not been statistically linked to the development of hypertension, nicotine definitely increases the heart rate and produces peripheral vasoconstriction, which does raise arterial blood pressure for a short time during and after smoking. Smoking cessation is strongly recommended, however, to reduce the client's risk for cancer, pulmonary disease, and cardiovascular disease. Smokers appear to have a higher frequency of malignant hypertension and subarachnoid hemorrhage. In addition, risk reduction brought about by antihypertensive therapy may not be as great in smokers as in nonsmokers.

Potassium Supplementation. The high ratio of sodium to potassium in the modern diet has been held responsible for the development of hypertension; however, even though potassium supplements may lower blood pressure, they are too costly and potentially too hazardous for routine use. A reduction in the consumption of high-sodium, low-potassium processed foods with an increase in consumption of low-sodium, high-potassium natural foods may be all that is needed for maximum benefits.

Pharmacologic Intervention. Once a decision has been made to use pharmacologic intervention, any one of sev-

TABLE 54-3   *Dietary Approaches to Stop Hypertension (DASH) Diet*

The DASH eating plan shown below is based on 2000 calories per day. Depending on your caloric needs your number of daily servings in a food group may vary from those listed. This eating plan is from the "Dietary Approaches to Stop Hypertension" (DASH) clinical study supported by the National Institutes of Health. The DASH combination diet lowered blood pressure and so may help prevent and control high blood pressure.

Food Group	Daily Servings (Number)	Serving Size	Examples	Significance of Each Food Group to DASH Diet Pattern
Grains and grain products	7-8	1 slice bread; ½ cup dry cereal; ½ cup cooked rice, pasta, or cereal*	Whole wheat breads, English muffin, pita bread, bagel, cereals and fiber, grits, oatmeal	Major source of energy and fiber
Vegetables	4-5	1 cup raw, leafy vegetable; ½ cup cooked vegetable; 6 oz vegetable juice	Tomatoes, potatoes, carrots, peas, squash, broccoli, turnip greens, collards, kale, spinach, artichokes, beans, sweet potatoes	Rich sources of potassium, magnesium, and fiber
Fruits	4-5	6 oz fruit juice, 1 medium fruit; ¼ cup dried fruit; ½ cup fresh, frozen, or canned fruit	Apricots, bananas, dates, grapes, oranges, orange juice, grapefruit, grapefruit juice, mangoes, melons, peaches, pineapples, prunes, raisins, strawberries, tangerines	Important sources of potassium, magnesium, and fiber
Low fat or nonfat dairy foods	2-3	8 oz milk; 1 cup yogurt; 1.5 oz cheese	Skim or 1% milk, skim or low-fat buttermilk, nonfat or low-fat yogurt, part skim mozzarella cheese, nonfat cheese	Major sources of calcium and protein
Meats, poultry, fish	2 or less	3 oz cooked meats, poultry, or fish	Select only lean; trim away visible fats; broil, roast, or boil, instead of frying; remove skin from poultry	Rich sources of protein and magnesium
Nuts, seeds, and legumes	4-5/wk	1.5 oz or ⅓ cup nuts; ½ oz or 2 tbsp seeds; ½ cup cooked dry beans	Almonds, filberts, mixed nuts, peanuts, walnuts, sunflower seeds, kidney beans, lentils and peas	Rich sources of energy, magnesium, potassium, protein, and fiber
Fats and oils†	2-3	1 tsp soft margarine; 1 tbsp low-fat mayonnaise; 2 tbsp light salad dressing; 1 tsp vegetable oil	Soft margarine, low-fat mayonnaise, light salad dressing; Vegetable oil (such as olive, corn, canola, or safflower)	Besides considering the fats added to foods, choose foods that contain less fat
Sweets	5/wk	1 tbsp sugar; 1 tbsp jelly or jam; ½ oz jelly beans; 8 oz lemonade	Maple syrup, sugar, jelly, jam, fruit-flavored gelatin, jelly beans, hard candy, fruit punch, sorbet ices	Sweets should be low in fat

Modified from Kolasa, K.M. (1999). Dietary Approaches to Stop Hypertension (DASH) in clinical practice: A primary care experience. *Clinical Cardiology, 22*(7 suppl), III-16-22.
*Serving sizes vary between ½ and 1¼ cups. Check the nutrition label.
†Fat content changes per serving size of fats and oil. For example, 1 tbsp regular salad dressing equals 1 serving. 1 tbsp low-fat dressing equals ½ serving. 1 tbsp fat-free dressing equals zero servings.

eral drugs from seven major drug classes can be used.[3,12,21,24] Table 54-1 and Figure 54-3 outline initial and ongoing treatment suggestions that are internationally recognized and supported by results of major worldwide, randomized, long-term clinical trials. Prevention-based healthy lifestyle change with the addition of pharmacologic therapy as indicated is the preferred treatment regimen for those clients in stages 1 and 2.

Antihypertensive medications can be classified into the following categories: diuretics, alpha- and beta-adrenergic antagonists [beta-blocker (BB)], vasodilators, calcium antagonists [calcium channel blocker (CCB)], angiotensin-converting enzyme (ACE) inhibitors, and angiotensin receptor blockers (ARB). Diuretics and BBs will continue to be first-line choices if there are no indications for another type of drug; however, there are compelling and specific indications for various agents in certain conditions.[2, 3, 5,12,19,21,24,30]

If therapy is chosen carefully, more than half of mild hypertension cases can be controlled with one or two drugs. Most clients, however, will require two or more drugs to achieve goal blood pressure.

Provider Responsibilities[2,3,5,10,12,19,21,24,30]

The goal of antihypertensive therapy is to control blood pressure with a minimum of side effects. Clinicians must be currently knowledgeable regarding drug choices and must be able to extrapolate potential side effects or negative effects quickly and effectively to manage clients' blood pressures most successfully, especially if concomitant conditions exist. Refer to a pharmacologic text for detailed descriptions of each drug or drug combination and its actions and side effects. Refer to Box 54-4 and the Concept Map feature on Understanding Hypertension and Its Treatment on p. 1502.[10,16,24]

If more than one drug is necessary, several combination therapies have proved effective. For example, the combination of a diuretic with a beta-adrenergic blocker or other adrenergic inhibitor has been effective in both blacks and whites, in contrast to the responses to the individual drugs, whereas blacks respond less well to beta-adrenergic blockers alone or as first-line treatment. The combination of a diuretic with an ACE inhibitor or a CCB **EB** has additive effects on blood pressure. Finally, combination drugs can be less expensive than the individual drugs, and the need for only one drug may improve compliance in a client who does not like "taking so many pills."

Reducing the number and amounts of antihypertensive medications should be considered once a client's blood pressure has been controlled effectively for at least 1 year. Medication dosages must be decreased slowly and progressively until the lowest effective dosages are reached and maintained. Regular follow-up evaluation is essential if drug therapy has been completely stopped secondary to success of weight loss or other lifestyle

change practices because blood pressure can rise again over time.

■ Nursing Management[8,10,13,16,18]
Assessment

The many sequelae of untreated hypertension can be prevented, or the severity of such problems reduced, if hypertension is well managed. Client education and understanding are crucial to successful management.

Diagnosis, Outcomes, and Interventions

Diagnosis: Ineffective Therapeutic Regimen Management (Individual). Use the nursing diagnosis *Ineffective Therapeutic Regimen Management (Individual)* to identify the learning needs of the newly diagnosed hypertensive client. The nursing diagnosis can be written *Risk for Ineffective Therapeutic Regimen Management (Individual) related to a new diagnosis, no previous learning about the disease process, potential consequences, the rationale for intervention, and proper administration of prescribed medications.*

Outcomes. The client and significant others will demonstrate knowledge required for self-care as evidenced by (1) describing hypertension and its associated risk factors; (2) discussing the importance of lifelong medical follow-up; (3) listing the prescribed medications, including drug name, rationale for use, dose, frequency, potential side effects, and measures to minimize side effects; and (4) demonstrating the proper technique for blood pressure monitoring at home.

CONCEPT MAP *evolve*

Understanding Hypertension and Its Treatment

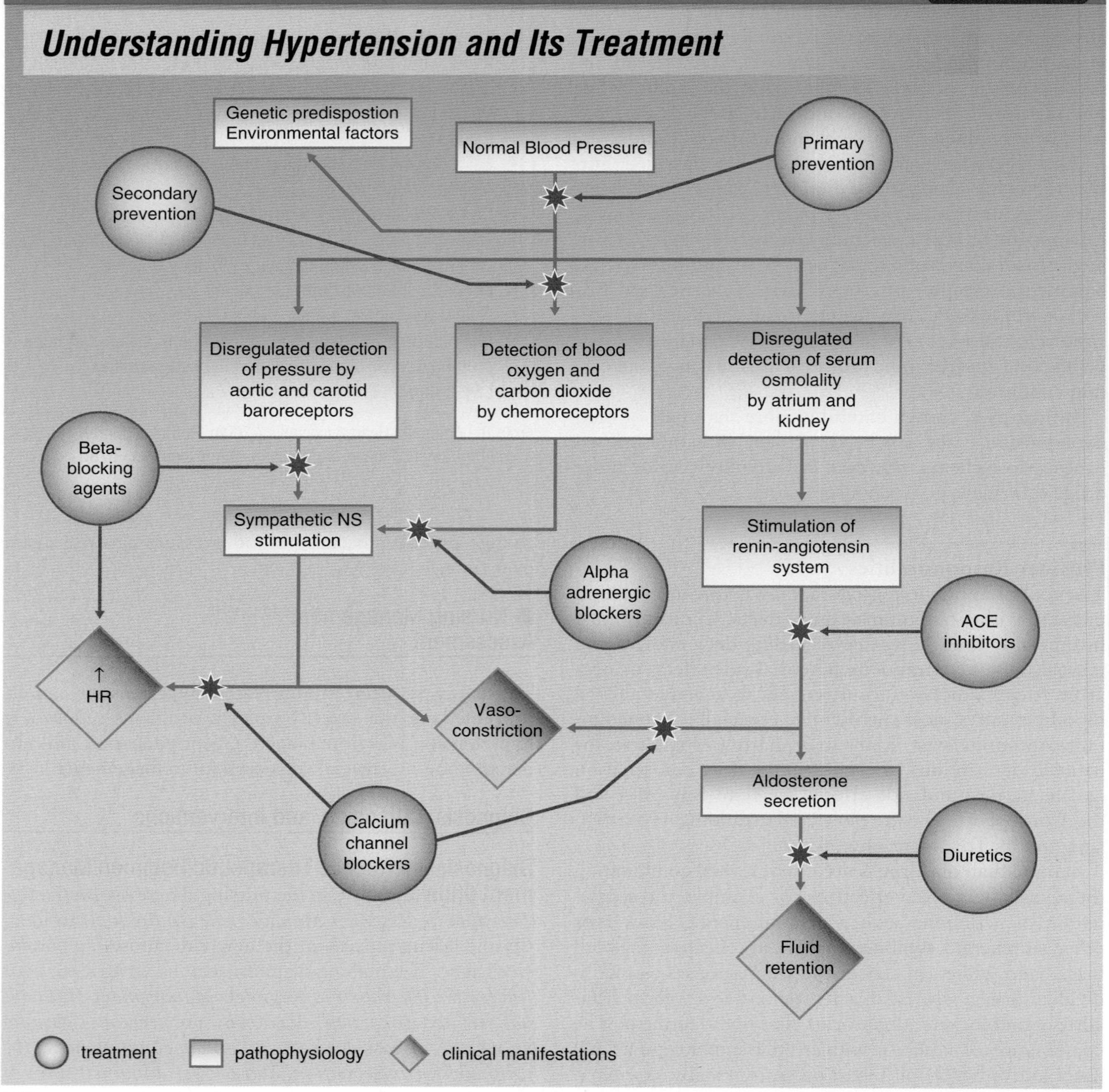

Genetic predispostion
Environmental factors

Normal Blood Pressure

Primary prevention

Secondary prevention

Disregulated detection of pressure by aortic and carotid baroreceptors

Detection of blood oxygen and carbon dioxide by chemoreceptors

Disregulated detection of serum osmolality by atrium and kidney

Beta-blocking agents

Sympathetic NS stimulation

Alpha adrenergic blockers

Stimulation of renin-angiotensin system

ACE inhibitors

↑ HR

Vaso-constriction

Calcium channel blockers

Aldosterone secretion

Diuretics

Fluid retention

○ treatment   ▢ pathophysiology   ◇ clinical manifestations

Different categories of antihypertensive medications are often used to control blood pressure. *ACE,* Angiotensin-converting enzyme; *HR,* heart rate; *NS,* nervous system.

Interventions. Because of the chronicity of hypertension and its dangerous complications, clients with hypertension need clear, practical, and realistic learning guidelines. Guidelines should include information about hypertension and its management. Use written materials with clear illustrations for teaching the client with newly diagnosed hypertension about the condition. Teach the client to measure blood pressure at home at least once a week and to record the findings in a diary.

Inform clients of their blood pressure reading, and advise them of the need for periodic remeasuring. When working with most clients, the examiner should refer to hypertension as *high blood pressure* to help avoid confusion. Many clients unfamiliar with medical terms may believe that hypertension denotes a state of being "hypertense"—that is, being worried or agitated. For these clients, the term *high blood pressure* more accurately conveys the nature of the health problem.

Diagnosis: Imbalanced Nutrition: More Than Body Requirements. Dietary adjustments can reduce the severity of hypertension and in some cases reduce the need for medication. Client teaching about and assessment of needed changes constitute an important aspect of nursing care. Write the nursing diagnosis as *Imbalanced Nutrition: More Than Body Requirements related to high sodium, fat, and total calorie intake.*

Outcomes. The client will demonstrate knowledge of and adherence to the nutritional regimen as evidenced by describing specific dietary modifications, including sodium, fat, and calorie restrictions and their rationales by reduction in levels of urine sodium and blood cholesterol and by losing weight. (See the Client Education Guide features on Low-Sodium Diet, on Low-Fat, Low-Cholesterol Diet, and on Calorie-Restriction Diet on the *evolve* website.)

Interventions. The two most important aspects of dietary intervention for hypertension are weight reduction (for overweight clients) and mild to moderate sodium restriction.[21,27] Therefore advise the client with hypertension to eat a diet low in salt, calories, cholesterol, and saturated fat.[7,15,18,20,25,26] Discuss the prescribed diet with the household members who prepare food. If possible, enlist the aid of a dietitian to provide detailed dietary instructions. Before dietary intervention begins, assess the client's patterns of food intake; lifestyle; food preferences; and ethnic, social, cultural, and financial influences. A highly individualized approach to dietary counseling is crucial to client compliance and adherence.

Restrict Sodium. Sodium is a hidden ingredient in many processed foods, beverages (including water from certain sources), and over-the-counter drugs (particularly antacids, cough remedies, and laxatives). It cannot be seen and often is not tasted. The average adult daily intake of salt is 5 to 15 g, but the therapeutic effects of sodium reduction on blood pressure do not occur until salt intake is reduced to 6 g/day or lower. Low-salt diets can be difficult to adhere to, at least initially. Reassure the client that dietary adherence becomes easier as the palate adjusts to decreased salt over several weeks to months. After the client becomes fully accustomed to the low-salt diet, unsalted foods usually cease to taste bland.

Reduce Fat and Cholesterol. Hypertension and high serum cholesterol (>250 mg/dl) are linked as risk factors in the development of coronary artery disease.[7,15,18,20,25,26] The level of serum cholesterol is determined in part by the consumption of cholesterol, saturated and polyunsaturated fats, and total calories. Cholesterol is contained in animal fats and dairy products. Saturated fats occur predominantly in animal fats and tropical oils

(e.g., coconut and palm oils). Unsaturated fats predominate in most plant-derived fats. Polyunsaturated fats occur predominantly in vegetable and seed oils. A diet low in saturated fats and high in polyunsaturated fats is beneficial in reducing blood pressure. (See the DASH diet in Table 54-3.) Not all clients with hypertension need to lose weight. As discussed previously, only people with a BMI greater than 27 should consider the need to lose weight. Ideally the rate of weight loss should be no more than 0.5 kg (about a pound) a week. Advise the average adult with hypertension to reduce caloric intake by at least 250 calories/day. Caution the client to avoid over-the-counter appetite suppressants because these preparations often contain sympathomimetic agents, which elevate blood pressure.

Diagnosis: Ineffective Health Maintenance. Exercise is like dietary management: A regular exercise program can lower blood pressure in hypertensive clients. This nursing diagnosis can be written as *Ineffective Health Maintenance related to a lack of regular exercise regimen.*

Outcomes. The client will begin and maintain an appropriate exercise program as evidenced by self-report, demonstration of the ability to monitor heart rate during exercise, sensation of reduced physical and emotional stress, and reduced blood pressure.

Interventions. Exercise programs can heighten the client's sense of well-being, provide an outlet for emotional tensions, and raise the levels of high-density lipoproteins (HDLs) relative to total blood cholesterol. Elevated HDL levels are associated with a decreased risk of cardiovascular morbidity and mortality. Instruct the client, however, to avoid heavy weight-lifting, isometric exercises, and other activities inappropriate to the client's physical limitations. A modest but consistent exercise program provides greater benefits than those obtainable with spurts of strenuous activity mixed with periods of inactivity. A gradually increasing program of aerobic activity such as walking, jogging, or swimming can thus be recommended.

Maximal heart rate is calculated by subtracting the client's age from 220. Before advising and initiating an exercise prescription for your client, a qualified specialist must conduct a careful performance evaluation.[1,6,8,10]

Diagnosis: Risk for Noncompliance. Many aspects of hypertension management set the stage for noncompliance.[4,6,13,17,23] Several factors related to specific drug use, including side effects, interference with lifestyle, cost, and inconvenience of physician visits and taking prescribed medications, play an important role in noncompliance. Assess the reasons for noncompliance, and then state the nursing diagnosis as *Risk for Noncompliance related to a lack of understanding about the seriousness of high blood pressure, cost of therapy, side effects of* *medications, complexity of management,* or *multiple changes in lifestyle.*

Outcomes. The client will actively participate in creating a treatment plan, describing the underlying causes of hypertension and self-care strategies, adhering to scheduled follow-up appointments, describing the actions and side effects of current medications, and expressing commitment to and self-responsibility for controlling hypertension.

Interventions. The greatest problem in the management of chronic hypertension involves the client's lack of adherence to nonpharmacologic and pharmacologic interventions. An estimated 40% to 60% of clients with hypertension fail to comply with prescribed therapy. There are several reasons why hypertensive clients do not follow prescribed regimens:

1. The asymptomatic nature of the disease tends to minimize the perceived seriousness of the problem and importance of intervention.
2. Therapeutic regimens often demand difficult lifestyle changes, such as low-sodium diets, weight loss, and smoking cessation.
3. Many hypertensive agents produce annoying side effects, and clients who require antihypertensive medication may consider the intervention worse than the disease.
4. The high cost of medications and the inconvenience of obtaining health care also contribute to noncompliance.

Nursing interventions for promoting compliance with the antihypertensive treatment regimen include individualizing care, ensuring adequate follow-up, communicating often with the client, and teaching the client and his or her family. Compliance usually improves dramatically when the client understands the causative factors underlying hypertension as well as the consequences of inadequate intervention and health maintenance (Box 54-5).

Evaluation

Medications can bring blood pressure down quickly. The remainder of interventions, such as stress management, exercise, and smoking cessation, are more difficult to implement and maintain. Expect the client to struggle with compliance with all the necessary changes. Ask specific questions in a nonjudgmental manner. As needed, recommend involvement in various self-help groups, such as smoking cessation groups.

■ Modifications for Older Clients

Hypertension is one of the most prevalent cardiovascular diseases among older adults, and because of their advanced age, these clients are more likely to suffer from end-organ damage secondary to chronically elevated pressure.[10,21] Blood pressure readings in older adults show

---

BOX 54-5   *Stepped-Care Approach to Management of Hypertension*

Step 1: Implement lifestyle modifications:
Weight reduction
Moderation of alcohol intake
Regular aerobic physical activity
Reduction of sodium intake with maintenance of adequate intake of potassium, calcium, and magnesium
Decreased intake of saturated fats and cholesterol
Smoking cessation

If there is inadequate blood pressure control, move to step 2.

Step 2: Continue lifestyle modifications and make initial pharmacologic selection; diuretics or beta-blockers are recommended because of studies that demonstrate reduced morbidity and mortality. If co-morbid conditions exist, evidence supports the use of other drugs as first-line therapy.

• Start with lowest therapeutic dose of a long-acting drug given once daily, then titrate dose.
• Low-dose combination drugs may be appropriate.

If there is inadequate blood pressure control, move to step 3.

Step 3:   Increase drug dose.
OR
Substitute another drug if no response or side effects become apparent.
OR
Add second drug from a different class or a diuretic if not already used, particularly if there is an inadequate response but initial drug well tolerated and at maximum dose.

If there is inadequate blood pressure control, move to step 4.

Step 4: Add second or third drug if not already prescribed; continue to add medications from other classes; consider referral to a hypertensive specialist.

From the Joint National Committee. (2003). The Seventh Report of the Joint National Committee on the Detection, Evaluation, and Treatment of High Blood Pressure. Bethesda, MD: U.S. Government Printing Office.

---

greater variability from one measurement to the next than seen in younger clients; therefore the diagnosis is made after several readings. Recent research findings indicate a need to treat hypertension in older people, regardless of whether both the SBP *and* DBP are involved or there is evidence of only isolated systolic hypertension. Older adults are more likely to experience adverse reactions to antihypertensive drugs and are monitored closely for evidence of such reactions; they are given detailed advice on the specifics of their medication regimens; and the clinical course of the disease is carefully followed.

The ultimate goal of antihypertensive therapy in older adults is not to try to lower the pressure to "normal" values but rather to lower the pressure gradually to a level sufficient to eliminate target organ damage and to minimize the risk of hypoperfusion. "Start low and go slow" is the principle followed for prescribing medications to the older adult. Too rapid a reduction in blood pressure in older clients, particularly those with chronic hypertension, may produce cerebral hypoperfusion that manifests by decreased mental status, weakness, and dizziness. These changes may appear at measured blood pressures still above the upper limit of normal.

HYPERTENSIVE CRISES: URGENCY VERSUS EMERGENCY[10,21]

Elevated blood pressure alone, in the absence of clinical manifestations or new or progressive target organ damage, rarely requires *emergency* therapy. In most cases the hypertensive crisis really constitutes a hypertensive *urgency* in which a severe elevation in blood pressure has been reached but there is mild or no acute target organ damage. Hypertensive urgencies include cases in which it is desirable to reduce blood pressure within a few hours to 24 hours. Clinicians treat urgent situations primarily with oral medications in an outpatient setting with close follow-up.

Malignant hypertension, a seldom-used term today, constitutes a true medical emergency and is currently referred to as *resistant or persistent severe hypertension.* The seriousness of the crisis correlates not so much with the level of blood pressure elevation as with the extent of target organ damage. Clients who qualify for emergent care are hospitalized, given intravenous medications, and monitored closely for at least 12 to 24 hours.

Without treatment persistent severe hypertension results in a 90% mortality rate within 1 year secondary to renal or heart failure, stroke, myocardial infarction, or aortic dissection. The most common cause of persistent severe hypertension is untreated hypertension. Other causes include eclampsia, dissecting aortic aneurysm, pyelonephritis, sudden catecholamine release (as from a pheochromocytoma), drug or toxic substance ingestion or exposure, and food and drug interactions (e.g., between a monoamine oxidase inhibitor [MAO] and aged cheese).

Clinical manifestations include those of hypertensive encephalopathy evidenced by restlessness, changes in level of consciousness (e.g., confusion, somnolence, lethargy, memory defects, coma, seizures), blurred vision, dizziness, headache, nausea, and vomiting. Assessment may also reveal renal insufficiency, proteinuria, hematuria, urinary sediment casts, hemolytic anemia, left ventricular failure, and pulmonary edema. Severe headache may be occipital or anterior in location, is steady and throbbing, and is often worse in the morning. Visual blurring, reduced visual acuity, and even blindness can occur. Acute renal failure, rapid vascular deterioration, and stroke can also develop.

Outcome Management

The initial goal of therapy in hypertensive crisis is to reduce mean arterial pressure by no more than 25% within the first minutes to 2 hours. Then a reduction in blood pressure toward 160/100 mm Hg is accomplished over the next 2 to 6 hours. Blood pressure is monitored frequently (every 5 to 15 minutes, depending on the drug and the route of administration used), and medications are titrated to manage the course of blood pressure reduction. It is essential to avoid excessive falls in blood pressure, which can precipitate renal, cerebral, or coronary ischemia. Consequently restoration of normal blood pressure must be done slowly and with care. Once the client is out of immediate danger, oral medications are adjusted while vital signs are monitored continuously, and changes in drug therapy regimens are made if necessary. NOTE: Although sublingual administration of nifedipine had been widely used to reduce blood pressure in an urgent situation, it is no longer considered appropriate therapy because of several reports of severe adverse effects from its use.

COMMUNITY SCREENING AND SELF-CARE

Public Health Initiative

Research showing the importance of normalized blood pressure for clients' optimum health led to the introduction by the National Heart, Lung and Blood Institute (NHLBI) of the National High Blood Pressure Education Program (NHBPEP) in 1972.[25] The NHBPEP is the first large-scale public outreach and education campaign to reduce high blood pressure. Its promotion of the detection, treatment, and control of high blood pressure has been credited with influencing the dramatic increase in the public's understanding of hypertension and its role in heart attacks and strokes.

The prevention and treatment of hypertension continue to be a major public health concern in the United States.[7,15,20-22,25,28] Prevention of hypertension and early discovery of new cases depend on a broader national public health effort. With guidance from the *Healthy People 2000/2010* initiatives, this national effort has begun. In addition to the diligent work of the NHBPEP, government support is increasing, and nationwide attention and assistance from business and industry, labor organizations, health care institutions, voluntary associations, and local communities are also on the rise. For example, the JNC VII guideline endorses the American Public Health Association (APHA) resolution challenging food manufacturers and restaurants to reduce sodium in foods by 50% over the next decade.

The following are the revised goals of the national public health plan:

- To prevent the rise of blood pressure with age
- To decrease the existing prevalence of hypertension
- To increase hypertension awareness and detection
- To improve control of hypertension
- To reduce cardiovascular risks
- To increase recognition of the importance of controlled isolated systolic hypertension
- To improve recognition of the importance of the persistence and damage from high-normal blood pressures
- To reduce ethnic, socioeconomic, and regional variations in hypertension
- To improve opportunities for treatment
- To enhance community programs

Managed Care and Community Screening

Because high blood pressure is so common, its management requires a major commitment from clinicians and managed care organizations.[29] Managed care programs offer the opportunity for a coordinated systematic, multifactorial, multidisciplinary approach to care. Nurse-managed clinics offer attractive opportunities to improve adherence and outcomes.

Hypertensive clients usually learn of their condition through incidental screening in health care facilities or through organized community screening in public settings (e.g., shopping malls, schools, the workplace). Nurses are actively involved in both approaches. About 80% of Americans come into contact with some aspect of the health care system at least once a year (e.g., in a health care provider's office, clinic, or hospital). Each encounter with the health care system presents an opportunity for incidental blood pressure screening. Blood pressure measurement should be a routine procedure at every initial encounter with a health care practitioner and annually thereafter.

Organized community screening programs help to assess the remaining 20% of Americans not in contact with any part of the health care system.[29] Such programs identify not only clients with untreated hypertension but also those who have discontinued intervention or whose hypertension is not adequately controlled by current intervention. In addition, screening programs provide an opportunity to educate the public. It is particularly important to screen members of high-risk "target groups," such as black and older populations. Community services need to keep target groups in mind when choosing the setting for blood pressure screenings. Practitioners who take blood pressure readings need to inform clients in writing of their blood pressure and its significance and, if necessary, the importance of follow-up evalua-

tion. Culturally and linguistically appropriate counseling by health care providers is important to those efforts.

Self-Measurement of Blood Pressure

Measurement of blood pressure outside a health care provider's office can provide valuable information for initial evaluation and subsequent follow-up of people with hypertension. Most drug, medical supply, and grocery stores provide standardized blood pressure monitors that their customers can use at no cost. These monitoring stations are generally located near the pharmacy or medical supplies department. Such stores also usually carry a variety of self-measurement blood pressure devices for home use. Choosing a monitoring device may be confusing for some people; however, several models of accurate and appropriate electronic or aneroid-type sphygmomanometers are available. Most insurance packages cover the cost of a home blood pressure unit, and these devices are generally easy to use.

Manual and electronic arm cuffs are the most accurate. Finger and wrist monitors are available but have proved inaccurate in standardized testing. Periodically, the accuracy of the instrument used in the home should be checked by comparing home readings with those obtained in the health care provider's office, at a "health fair," or in a community nursing clinic.

SYNCOPE

Syncope (fainting) is defined as generalized muscle weakness and an inability to stand erect accompanied by loss of consciousness.[11] It is a good measure of cardiovascular status because it may indicate decreased cardiac output, fluid volume deficits, or defects in cerebral tissue perfusion.

Syncope is a common occurrence when a person tries to stand after being bedridden for a while. This form of syncope, called *postural hypotension*, can be seen in clients attempting to ambulate the first few times after surgery, in clients who have been on prolonged bed rest, and in clients who have dysrhythmias. When a person moves quickly to a standing position, blood normally pools in the lower legs. The arterial pressure receptors in the aortic arch detect the fall in cardiac output that occurs with the lack of venous return, and they increase sympathetic tone to compress arterioles to improve venous return. If the sympathetic response is not adequate or is blocked by medication, the person becomes dizzy because of the decreased cerebral perfusion. All medications taken to reduce blood pressure have the potential to cause orthostatic hypotension or postural hypotension—some more than others, such as potent diuretics, alpha$_1$-receptor blockers, and vasodilators.

When a client reports dizziness or is at risk of syncope because of medication use or prolonged bed rest, assess fluid volume status and check the pulse for irregularities.

If syncope develops, it usually can be managed by having the client move slowly to a sitting position and rest a moment before standing. If the client becomes dizzy, instruct him or her to breathe deeply and to keep both eyes open. Syncope should resolve within moments. If it is prolonged, place the client supine, use leg exercises to improve venous return, and wait until the blood pressure returns to a normotensive state. Confused clients who do not wait for syncope to resolve before walking are at risk for falls. Bed alarms may be needed.

CONCLUSIONS

New coalitions between health care providers and individual communities are forming to focus on the prevention and management of hypertension throughout all stages of life. Support from the community and greater use of technology such as the Internet will play an increasingly greater role in promoting long-term adherence to lifestyle and pharmacologic regimens. Achieving long-term control of blood pressure risk factors requires that the same interest and attention given to initial evaluation and treatment decisions also be given to long-term lifestyle management issues. In addition, JNC VII has taken a strong stance toward mandating better pharmacologic control of high blood pressure. In their report, JNC VII stated that clinicians' failure to titrate or combine medications, despite knowing that a client's blood pressure is not at goal, represents clinical inertia and must be overcome.[21]

THINKING CRITICALLY *evolve*

1. A 50-year-old obese black man arrives at your clinic with persistent elevated blood pressure. He has had hypertension for 7 months. Despite attempts at lifestyle management, his blood pressure has continued to rise. He was started on a regimen of antihypertensive medication 1 month ago and has returned to the clinic today for a follow-up visit. His blood pressure is higher than it was initially. What might explain his continued elevated blood pressure?

Factors to Consider. What other history and physical examination data should you obtain to analyze this case more effectively? When and how long should lifestyle modifications alone be encouraged? How long does it take for various medications to be effective? What diseases worsen hypertension? What psychosocial factors affect compliance with or adherence to a treatment regimen? What modifications in the pharmacologic treatment plan, if any, would be most appropriate at this time?

Discussions for these questions can be found on the website and the CD-ROM.

BIBLIOGRAPHY

1. Ades, P.A. (2001). Cardiac rehabilitation and secondary preven- tion of coronary heart disease. *New England Journal of Medicine* 345, 892-902.
2. Agodoa, L.Y., et al. (2001). Effect of ramipril vs amlodipine on re- nal outcomes in hypertensive nephrosclerosis: A randomized control trial (AASK). *Journal of the American Medical Association, 285*, 2719-2728.
3. Basile, J.N. (2001). Hypertension 2001: How will JNC VII be different from JNC VI? *Southern Medical Journal, 94*, 889-890.
4. Berlowitz, D.R., Ash, A.S., & Hickey, E.C. (1998). Inadequate management of blood pressure in a hypertensive population. *New England Journal of Medicine, 339*, 1957-1963.
5. Brenner, B.M., et al. (2001). Effects of losartan on renal and car- diovascular outcomes in patients with type 2 diabetes and nephropathy. *New England Journal of Medicine, 345*, 861-869.
6. Cardiac Rehabilitation Guideline Panel. *Cardiac rehabilitation.* AHCPR Pub. No. 96-0672. Rockville, MD: Agency for Health Care Policy and Research, Public Health Services, U.S. Department of Health and Human Services.
7. Davidson, M.H. (2002). Strategies to improve adult treatment panel III guideline adherence and patient compliance. *The American Journal of Cardiology (Suppl. 89)*, 8C-22C.
8. DeMartinis, J. (2001). Relaxation and stress management. In D. Robinson, & C.P. Kish (Eds.), *Core concepts in advanced practice nursing.* St. Louis, MO: Mosby.
9. DeMartinis, J. (2003). Principles and methods of the basic physical examination. In R. Jones & R. Rospond (Eds.), *Patient assessment in pharmacy practice.* Baltimore, MD: Lippincott Williams & Wilkins.
10. DeMartinis, J.E., Uphold, C.R., & Graham, M.V. (2003). Cardiovascular problems. In C.R. Uphold & M.V. Graham (Eds.), *Clinical guidelines in adult health* (3rd ed.). Gainesville, FL: Barmarrae Books.
11. Epperly, T.D., & Fogarty, J.P. (2001). Syncope. In M.B. Mengel & L.P. Schwiebert (Eds.), *Ambulatory medicine: The primary care of families* (3rd ed.). New York: Lange Medical Books/McGraw-Hill.
12. Furberg, C.D., et al (2001). Clinical implications of recent findings from the antihypertensive and lipid-lowering treatment to prevent heart attack trial (ALLHAT) and other studies of hypertension. *Annals of Internal Medicine, 135*, 1074-1078.
13. Glasser, S.P. (2001). Hypertension syndrome and cardiovascular events: High blood pressure is only one risk factor. *Postgraduate Medicine, 110* (5), 29-36.
14. Hirsch, A.T., et al. (1997). The role of tobacco cessation, antiplatelet and lipid-lowering therapies in the treatment of peripheral arterial disease. *Vascular Medicine, 2*, 252-256.

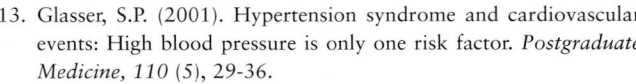 *Did you remember to check out the bonus material on the Evolve website and the CD-ROM, including free self-assessment exercises?*

http://evolve.elsevier.com/Black/medsurg/

15. Isaacsohn, J., et al. (2002). The impact of the national cholesterol education program adult treatment panel III guidelines on drug development. *The American Journal of Cardiology (Suppl) 89,* 45C-49C.

16. Kershaw, G.R. (2001). Comprehensive management of hypertension and its complications. In R. Becker & J. Alpert (Eds.), *Cardiovascular medicine: Practice and management.* New York: Arnold.

 17. Kyngas, H., & Lahdenpera, T. (1999). Compliance of patients with hypertension and associated factors. *Journal of Advanced Nursing, 29* (4), 832-839.

18. McGowan, M.P. (2002). Lipid-lowering therapy in women: new treatment options. *Cardiology Review, December,* 1-12.

 19. Michels, K.B., et al. (1998). Prospective study of calcium-channel blocker use, cardiovascular disease, and total mortality among hypertensive women: the Nurses' Health Study. *Circulation, 97,* 1540-1548.

20. National Cholesterol Education Program (NCEP), National Institutes of Health, National Heart, Lung, and Blood Institute. (2001). *Executive summary of the third report of the National Cholesterol Education Program (NCEP) Expert Panel on detection, evaluation, and treatment of high blood cholesterol in adults (Adult Treatment Panel III).* (NIH Publication no. 01-3305). Bethesda, MD: U.S. Government Printing Office.

21. National High Blood Pressure Education Program, National Institutes of Health, National Heart, Lung and Blood Institute. (2003). *The Seventh Report of the Joint National Committee on Detection, Evaluation, and Treatment of High Blood Pressure.* Bethesda, MD: U.S. Government Printing Office.

22. Nutrition Committee of the AHA. (2000). AHA dietary guidelines: Revision 2000: A statement for healthcare professionals from the nutrition committee of the American Heart Association. *Circulation, 102,* 2284-2299.

23. Ockene, J.K., & Ockene, I.S. (2001). Primary prevention of cardiovascular disease: helping patients change lifestyle behaviors. In R. Becker & J. Alpert (Eds.), *Cardiovascular medicine: Practice and management.* New York: Arnold.

24. Opie, L. (2001*). Drugs for the heart* (3rd ed.). Philadelphia, W.B. Saunders.

25. Pasternak, R. (2002). Adult treatment panel II versus adult treatment panel III: What has changed and why? *American Journal of Cardiology (Suppl) 89,* 3C-7C.

26. Rader, D. (2002). Lipid disorders. In E.J. Topol (Ed.), *Textbook of cardiovascular medicine* (2nd ed.). Philadelphia: Lippincott Williams & Wilkins.

27. Sacks, F.M., Svetkey, L.P., & Vollmer, W.M. (2001). Effects on blood pressure of reduced dietary sodium and the dietary approaches to stop hypertension (DASH) diet. *New England Journal of Medicine, 344,* 3-10.

28. U.S. Department of Health and Human Services. (2000). *Healthy people 2010: National health promotion and disease prevention objectives.* Washington, DC: Public Health Service.

29. Wang, C., & Abbott, L.J. (1998). Development of a community-based diabetes and hypertension preventive program. *Public Health Nursing, 15* (6), 406-414.

30. Whelton, A.W., and SUCCESS VI Study Group (2001). Cyclooxygenase-2-specific inhibitors and cardiorenal function: a randomized, controlled trial of celecoxib and rofecoxib in older hypertensive osteoarthritis patients. *American Journal of Therapeutics, 8* (2), 85-95.

Chapter 55

Management of Clients with Vascular Disorders

Joyce M. Black

evolve

Web Enhancements

http://evolve.elsevier.com/Black/medsurg/

Client Education Guide
  Foot Care (Spanish Translation)
  Stump and Prosthesis Care (Spanish Translation)

Appendix C
  Laboratory Values of Clinical Importance in Medical-Surgical
  Nursing

PERIPHERAL ARTERY DISORDERS

Peripheral vascular disease (PVD) includes disorders of the arterial, venous, and lymphatic systems. In clinical settings, the term *PVD* is usually used to describe peripheral arterial disease. PVD is increasingly common and has the potential to cause loss of limb or, occasionally, life.

Etiology and Risk Factors

Peripheral arterial occlusive diseases are primarily caused by atherosclerosis, a process that slowly occludes the arterial flow of blood. The atherosclerotic process gradually may progress to complete occlusion of medium and large arteries. Primary risk factors for atherosclerosis include diabetes, smoking, and elevated blood lipid levels. Phlebitis, surgery, and autoimmune disease are other risk factors. Clients with PVD often have other health problems seen with atherosclerosis, such as coronary artery disease, myocardial infarction, atrial fibrillation, carotid stenosis, stroke, or renal disease.

The lower limbs are more susceptible to arterial occlusive disorders and atherosclerosis than are the upper limbs, whose natural collateral system is less susceptible to such disorders. The most common locations for stenosis supplying a lower extremity are the aortoiliac bifur-

cation and the femoral bifurcation (Figure 55-1). In general, stenoses occur at bifurcations in arteries.

Arteries can be occluded acutely from embolism, thrombosis, trauma, vasospasm, or edema. Multiple factors increase risk of thromboses including obesity, sepsis, hypotension, low cardiac output, aneurysms, aortic dissection, bypass grafts, and underlying atherosclerotic narrowing of the arterial lumen. Emboli, the most common cause of sudden ischemia, usually are of cardiac origin during periods of atrial fibrillation, but they also can originate from proximal atheroma, tumor, or foreign objects. Emboli tend to lodge at artery bifurcations or in areas where vessels abruptly narrow such as the femoral artery bifurcation.

Clinical manifestations of chronic arterial occlusion may not appear for 20 to 40 years. Claudication, usually insidious in onset, generally occurs in men, although there is an increased incidence in women after menopause. Usually, claudication strikes men in their sixth or seventh decade. Nearly half of clients who experience claudication also have associated severe coronary artery disease.

Pathophysiology

The progressive nature of atherosclerosis slowly starves the tissues of oxygenated blood. Collateral arterioles develop to attempt to compensate for the occluded arterial

evolve **Be sure to check out the bonus material on the Evolve website and the CD-ROM, including free self-assessment exercises.**
http://evolve.elsevier.com/Black/medsurg/

Nursing Outcomes Classification (NOC)
for Nursing Diagnoses—Clients with Vascular Disorders

Acute Pain or Chronic Pain
Comfort Level
Pain Control
Pain: Disruptive Effects
Pain Level
Anxiety
Anxiety Control
Coping
Deficient Knowledge
Knowledge Deficit: Disease Process
Knowledge Deficit: Health Behaviors
Knowledge Deficit: Health Resources
Knowledge: Medication
Knowledge Deficit: Illness
Knowledge: Prescribed Activity
Knowledge Deficit: Treatment
  Procedure(s)
Knowledge: Treatment Regimen
Delayed Surgical Recovery
Endurance
Infection Status
Self-Care: Activities of Daily Living
  (ADL)
Wound Healing: Primary Intention
Wound Healing: Secondary Intention

Health-Seeking Behaviors
Adherence Behaviors
Health Beliefs
Health Promoting Behavior
Health-Seeking Behavior
Knowledge: Health Promotion
Knowledge: Health Resources
Impaired Gas Exchange
Electrolyte and Acid-Base Balance
Respiratory Status: Gas Exchange
Respiratory Status: Ventilation
Tissue Perfusion: Pulmonary
Impaired Physical Mobility
Ambulation: Walking
Body Positioning: Self-Initiated
Immobility Consequences: Physiologic
Mobility Level
Transfer Performance
Ineffective Coping (Individual)
Coping
Role Performance
Ineffective Tissue Perfusion
Pain Level
Tissue Perfusion: Cardiac

Tissue Perfusion: Peripheral
Vital Signs Status
Risk for Activity Intolerance
Health Beliefs: Perceived Control
Mood Equilibrium
Nutritional Status: Energy
Symptom Control
Symptom Severity
Risk for Deficient Fluid Volume
Bowel Elimination
Electrolyte and Acid-Base Balance
Fluid Balance
Hydration
Nutritional Status: Food and Fluid
  Intake
Urinary Elimination
Risk for Impaired Skin Integrity
Immobility Consequences: Physiologic
Nutritional Status
Physical Aging Status
Risk Control
Risk Detection
Tissue Integrity: Skin and Mucous
  Membranes
Tissue Perfusion: Peripheral

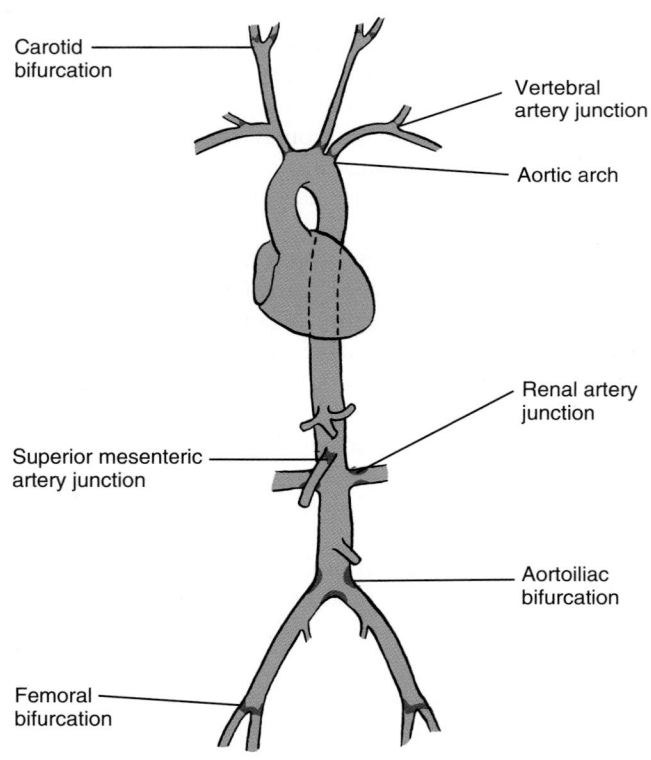

FIGURE 55-1 Major sites of peripheral atherosclerotic occlusive disease.

supply. However, collateral vessels develop slowly. During the interim, vasodilation and anaerobic pathways are used to meet oxygen and nutrient demands. Vasodilation has a limited effect because arteries that become oxygen-deprived quickly become maximally dilated. Cellular anaerobic metabolism tries to meet the basic requirements, but the waste products of lactic and pyruvic acid build up quickly, are extremely toxic, and are excreted slowly.

The physiologic effect of any given stenosis is variable because it is determined not only by the degree of narrowing, but also by the amount of collateral vessels that have developed. However, continued lack of arterial flow eventually results in pain. The pain is called *intermittent claudication* and is analogous to anginal pain. Intermittent claudication occurs when a muscle is forced to work without an adequate blood supply to meet its metabolic demands.

Clinical Manifestations
The most important subjective manifestations of chronic arterial occlusive disease are *intermittent claudication* and *rest pain*. The client typically reports pain described as tightening pressure in the calves or buttocks or a sharp cramp or burning sensation that occurs during

walking and disappears with rest. Claudication also may present as the hip or leg "giving out" after a certain period of exertion. The pain of claudication usually does not occur with sitting or standing.

Intermittent claudication is influenced by the speed or incline of the walk, conditions that increase the demand for oxygen by muscles of the legs. The more rapid the speed or the greater the incline, the faster claudication occurs. The client's exercise tolerance generally decreases over time; episodes of claudication occur with less exertion. Claudication response is constant, reproducible, and not positional. Reproducible means that the client who walks the same distance at the same speed and incline has manifestations at the same distance each time. The client who cannot walk the length of a house because of leg pain one day but can walk indefinitely the next day does not have intermittent claudication.

Paresthesias with exertion indicate ischemia of the peripheral nerves because of the phenomenon of *arterial steal*. This phenomenon occurs as arterioles of the muscles are maximally dilated because of hypoxia. To meet muscular metabolic needs, these arterioles steal from cutaneous and peripheral nerve vessels, which results in coldness and a pins-and-needles sensation.

PVD can occur along any portion of the arterial system. Aortoiliac stenosis and occlusion result in hip, thigh, and buttock claudication with absent or diminished femoral and distal pulses (Figure 55-2). In males, impotence is also part of the syndrome, known as *Leriche syndrome*. Dependent rubor is common when aortoiliac and femoropopliteal disorders are combined. A superficial femoral artery and popliteal occlusion leads to calf claudication, which may improve, stay the same, or potentially progress to rest pain. Popliteal artery disease and stenosis in the anterior or posterior tibial artery results in claudication in the distal leg and foot.

Lower extremity pain may also occur in several other disorders unrelated to arterial disease. Other conditions that cause a similar type of pain include arthritis, lumbar disk protrusion, neuritis, and muscle cramps. However, the pain of other conditions is not consistent, reproducible, or positional.

Objective data associated with arterial insufficiency include weak or absent peripheral pulses, low ankle-brachial index (ABI) scores (see Chapter 53), dependent rubor and pallor with elevation, hypertrophied toenails, coolness of the skin, hairlessness of the extremity, tissue atrophy, ulceration, and gangrene (Figure 55-3). Dependent rubor is a dusky, purplish discoloration of the foot and leg when the foot is placed in a dependent position. This *dependent rubor* changes to white pallor when the leg is elevated. Other manifestations of arterial insufficiency are listed in Table 55-1.

As the disease progresses, clinical manifestations become more severe. The development of pain at rest, usually occurring at night when the client lies supine, indicates limb-threatening disease. Usually described as a dull, deep pain in the toes or forefoot, this sensation awakens the client from sleep and may cause him or her to hang the foot over the side of the bed or get up and walk around for relief. The client may start to sleep in a chair with legs dependent. Placing the leg in a dependent position provides increased gravitational supply of blood. This often results in a moderate degree of lower extremity edema. The affected foot usually demonstrates dependent rubor. Ischemic rest pain often is exacerbated by poor cardiac output. PVD may also be acutely compounded by either emboli or thrombi. Many people live daily with PVD; however, in settings such as acute limb

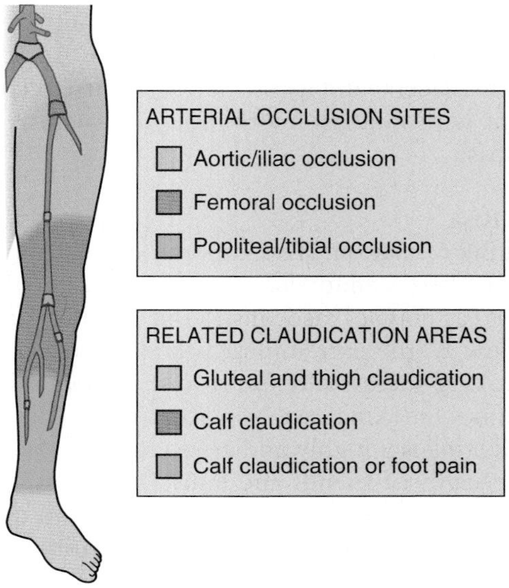

ARTERIAL OCCLUSION SITES
- ☐ Aortic/iliac occlusion
- ☐ Femoral occlusion
- ☐ Popliteal/tibial occlusion

RELATED CLAUDICATION AREAS
- ☐ Gluteal and thigh claudication
- ☐ Calf claudication
- ☐ Calf claudication or foot pain

FIGURE 55-2 Occlusion of the arterial system at various locations leads to a specific pattern of claudication in distal tissues.

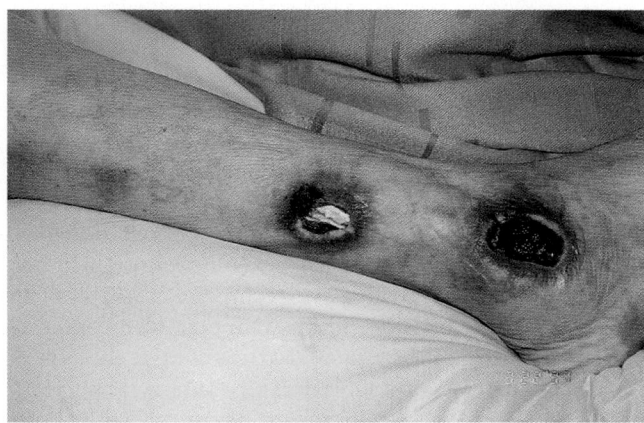

FIGURE 55-3 Arterial ulcers of the foot. Note the pale, hairless appearance of the leg and the smooth, round shape of the ulcers.

TABLE 55-1	*Manifestations of Arterial Insufficiency*
Type of Data	**Manifestations**
Subjective	Exertional pain
	Nocturnal pain
	Ischemic rest pain
	Claudication manifestations
	Foot, calf, thigh, or buttock pain
	Pain worse with exertion
	Pain relieved with several minutes rest
	Pain relieved with dependent position
Objective	Decreased skin temperature
	Shiny skin
	Skin hairless over lower extremity (e.g., shin)
	Dystrophic toenails
	Distal extremity color change with position
	Skin pallor when leg elevated
	Skin rubor when leg dependent
	Bilateral leg diminished pulses throughout
	Slow wound healing in legs
	Impotence

ischemia, the disease can be life-threatening and can require emergency intervention to minimize morbidity and mortality.

Physical manifestations of PVD include pulselessness of the dorsalis pedis artery and pallor of the legs. The skin may have a shiny appearance and the nails are often thick and brittle. Poorly healing injuries or ulcers in the extremities may be present (see later discussion). Mottling, paralysis, and paresthesias tend to occur in limb-threatening conditions and prompt care to restore blood flow is required. The physician should be made aware of these findings.

Laboratory findings may include abnormal hemoglobin levels and elevated urea nitrogen, creatinine, and sodium, which might lead to worsening of peripheral perfusion. Risk factors for the development of vascular disease (lipid profile, coagulation tests) may also be abnormal, reflecting atherosclerosis. An elevated level of total homocysteine (tHcy) in blood is emerging as a prevalent and strong risk factor for atherosclerotic vascular disease in the coronary, cerebral, and peripheral vessels, and for arterial and venous thromboembolism.

Diagnostic evaluation of the lower extremity includes both noninvasive and invasive techniques. ABI can be measured at the bedside. Using Doppler ultrasonography, the pressure at the brachial artery and at the posterior tibialis artery is measured. The ankle systolic pressure is divided by the brachial pressure, with both measured in the supine position. Normally, the ratio is more than 1. In severe disease, it is less than 0.5. Comparison with ABI in the opposite extremity is helpful to

determine the degree of ischemia. ABI is not accurate in diabetes using the ankle pulsation; pulsation in the great toe can be used instead.

Doppler ultrasound studies can determine the quality of blood flow. Upper extremities are evaluated over the axillary, brachial, ulnar, and radial arteries. Lower extremities are evaluated over the femoral, popliteal, dorsalis pedis, and posterior tibial arteries. The shape of the waveform (i.e., monophasic, biphasic, triphasic) provides data on the presence of disease. A monophasic waveform can indicate proximal stenosis or occlusion in the iliac vessels. The biphasic or triphasic waveform is normal and occurs when the main blood vessels in the leg are elastic and dilated by the increased pressure during systole.

Transcutaneous oximetry measures tissue levels of oxygen and carbon dioxide, providing data on impairments of flow in both large and small vessels.

Treadmill examination, a form of lower extremity stress testing, measures the decrease of arterial pressure with ambulation and the rapidity with which it returns to baseline. Color flow imaging visualizes the blood flow in the vessels and records pressures within the vessel.

Arteriography is the definitive examination when surgery is being considered. Arteriography reveals the lumen of the blood vessels. It is not a measurement of actual blood flow like the noninvasive assessment, but instead shows the outline of the contrast media within the lumen. Use of contrast media, however, contributes to risk of many potential complications.

Outcome Management
■ Medical Management

The goals of medical management are to reduce the risk of progressive arterial disease, to promote arterial flow, and to save the limb for clients with intermittent claudication and non–limb-threatening ischemia. Additionally, medical management may be the only course of action in the client with multiple morbidities and who is a poor surgical risk.

Reduce Risk

Smoking Cessation. The importance of stopping cigarette smoking cannot be overemphasized. Cigarette smoke is a potent vasoconstrictor, further impairing blood flow to the extremities. Clients who are able to stop smoking successfully improve their treadmill walking distance. Smoking cessation is extremely difficult, because nicotine is a highly addictive chemical. Social support, especially of friends and family members, seems to be an important factor in assisting smokers to quit their habit. Pharmacologic measures may be instituted by the primary care provider, if necessary. Educate clients about the dangers of cigarette smoke, encourage them to stop, act as role models for nonsmoking, and support policies to prohibit smoking in the workplace. Primary care providers should question clients each time they visit about their desire to quit and the need to quit.

Skin Care. Supportive measures include meticulous care of the feet, which should be kept clean and protected against excessive drying with moisturizing creams. Well-fitting and protective shoes are advised to reduce trauma. Sandals and shoes made of synthetic materials that do not "breathe" should be avoided. Elastic support hose should be avoided, because they reduce blood flow to the skin. In clients with ischemia at rest, "shock blocks" under the head of the bed together with a canopy over the feet may improve perfusion pressure and ameliorate some of the rest pain.

Exercise. A prescribed moderate program of exercise and rest helps increase collateral circulation and improve conditioning. Several studies have shown that clients involved in an exercise program generally feel better and can slowly improve their walking distance. Clients are instructed to walk 30 to 45 minutes every day, as long as no skin ulcerations are present. The exercise program should begin slowly with the client stopping at the onset of pain and progress gradually until the client has substantially lengthened walking distances. For obese and chronically ill clients, it is important that an exercise program (1) be individually tailored to the client's abilities, goals, interests, and resources and (2) be written with specific instructions. Most clients can significantly increase their walking distance, and many can avoid surgery if they exercise regularly and stop smoking.

Dietary Changes. Clients are advised and counseled to reduce body weight by following a low-fat, low-cholesterol diet containing more fruits and vegetables. Interventions for lowering blood lipid levels are recommended for clients with hyperlipidemia. The initial steps for lowering cholesterol is to reduce calorie intake to achieve ideal body weight. If weight loss is seen as improbable, the client should try to maintain current weight.

The next major step is to reduce the total fat intake in the diet to 30% or less of total calories. Saturated fat intake should be reduced. The most common sources of saturated fat in the American diet are red meat, fried foods, and dairy products, especially whole milk and cheese. Increasing the quantity of fish and poultry and changing to skim milk and nonfat cheese may be sufficient to meet saturated fat recommendations.

The third major goal is to reduce intake of cholesterol, which is found in egg yolks, organ meats, shellfish, and animal meats. Increasing dietary fiber, especially soluble fiber, such as that found in oats, lentils, and beans, has a beneficial effect on lipid levels. Fast foods, snack foods, and restaurant dining account for a large amount of the increased fat intake in the United States. Dietary counseling by a registered dietitian is a helpful intervention for clients and families who are attempting to change eating habits.

Promote Arterial Flow. Pentoxifylline (Trental) has been reported to decrease blood viscosity and increase red cell flexibility, thereby increasing peripheral blood flow. Several studies have shown that pentoxifylline increases the duration of exercise in clients with claudication. Cilostazol has also been shown to increase walking distance. It works as a vasodilator and has antiplatelet properties. Platelet inhibitors, aspirin, and Clopidogrel, are used to reduce the risk of embolism in clients with PVD. New medications including L-arginine, which is the precursor of the endothelium-dependent vasodilator, nitric oxide, and vasodilator prostaglandins are being studied.

In severe cases of arterial insufficiency, the physician may order reverse Trendelenburg position be used by elevating the head of the client's bed to be elevated on 6-inch blocks (either constructed or use heavy books such as encyclopedias) so that blood from the heart flows more easily to the extremities whenever the client sleeps or rests. Fleece boots may also be used to keep the feet warm and protected from injury. Float the heels from the bed to prevent pressure ulcers.

■ Nursing Management of the Medical Client Assessment

The history should include questions regarding arterial disease, surgery, medications, and ulcerations. Because of the chronic nature of the problem, perform a psychosocial assessment. Clients may have feelings of powerlessness. Some clients are not aware of chest pain, shortness of breath, or fatigue because their attention is focused on leg discomfort. Question them carefully about these discomforts. Medical or surgical intervention may reduce pain and thus improve walking ability.

The physical examination should include peripheral pulses (begin with dorsalis pedis, then proceed proximally to the posterior tibial, popliteal, and femoral until a pulse is found), ABI, quality of arterial flow assessed with a hand-held Doppler instrument, notations of skin color, skin temperature, and level of hair on the leg, and assessment of skin integrity (including the presence of ulcers, darkened areas of skin, tinea pedis, thickened nails), capillary refill time, and the presence of venous filling when the foot is dependent.

See the Management and Delegation feature on Management of Clients with Vascular Disorders on p. 1514.

Diagnosis, Outcomes, Interventions

Diagnosis: Ineffective Tissue Perfusion. The ideal nursing diagnosis for clients with arterial disorders is *Ineffective Tissue Perfusion.* Write the diagnosis as *Ineffective Tis-*

MANAGEMENT AND DELEGATION

Management of Clients with Vascular Disorders

Clients with peripheral vascular disorders require frequent monitoring and observation of the neurovascular status (NV) of their affected extremities. Following your initial assessment of the NV status in an affected extremity, you may deem it appropriate to delegate the routine monitoring and recording of NV status to an unlicensed assistant.

Your baseline assessment establishes the NV status including skin temperature, color, presence and location of pulses, sensation, and skin integrity. Skin integrity, especially overlying bony prominences like the heels, ankles, and elbows, are at especially high risk for compromise and breakdown and bear close assessment. Pulses are best noted by marking their location with a waterproof marker, noting whether they are palpable or audible by Doppler.

You will implement interventions to minimize pressure and swelling to the affected extremity. Once you have established a baseline and implemented protective measures, you may deem it appropriate to delegate ongoing monitoring and recording on NV status to an unlicensed assistant.

Inform your assistants of the initial findings and instruct them to notify you of any changes in skin color or temperature, quality or detection of pulses, altered sensation (e.g., "pins and needles"), or client report of pain in the extremity. Assistants can help ensure protective measures are maintained by providing heel protectors, sheepskin and other pressure-reducing devices, a bed cradle to keep bed linens off lower extremities, or pillows for elevation of upper or lower extremities.

Perform ongoing assessment of your client as your institution and the client's clinical condition dictates. Changes in assessment may necessitate a change in delegation considerations. Vascular clients may have postoperative dressings on their affected extremities. Delegation considerations in the care of postoperative clients are described in Chapter 16 and apply in this population as well.

sue Perfusion related to interruption of blood flow secondary to arterial occlusion.

Outcomes. The client will maintain adequate peripheral tissue perfusion to affected extremities as evidenced by improvement from baseline of skin color, skin temperature, pulses, and level of pain.

Interventions

Promote Arterial Flow. Position clients with arterial disease so that blood flows toward the legs and feet. In milder cases, clients can benefit from simply sitting for periods of time with their feet flat on the floor. If reverse Trendelenburg position is used, assess for dependent edema. Remind clients with arterial insufficiency to avoid raising their feet above heart level unless the physician has specifically prescribed this as an exercise.

Prevent Vasoconstriction. Explain the dangers of smoking to the client who uses tobacco. Encourage the client to stop smoking completely. The client who realizes that smoking literally threatens life and limbs may develop sufficient motivation to abstain permanently. Help the client locate therapy groups or biofeedback training. Do not advise the use of nicotine patches. Patches provide continuous administration of nicotine and thereby can cause continuous vasospasm.

Encourage the client to avoid stressful situations and to relax, both mentally and physically. Counseling services may be indicated for nervous, "high-strung" clients. Offer information regarding stress reduction classes. Involve significant others.

Prevent the client from becoming chilled. Stockings should be worn to keep the legs warm. Clients should wear protective clothing in layers during cold weather, warm their cars before entering them, and follow winter driving precautions (e.g., not running out of gas).

Diagnosis: Acute Pain. Intermittent claudication is caused by ischemia. The nursing diagnosis can be written *Acute Pain related to inadequate arterial blood supply to the legs.*

Outcomes. The client will experience increased comfort, as evidenced by self-report and demonstrated knowledge of pain reduction measures, both pharmacologic and nonpharmacologic.

Interventions. The pain of ischemia is usually chronic, continuous, and difficult to relieve. Arterial leg ulcers are exquisitely painful. Because of pain, clients with arterial disorders are often depressed and irritable. Pain limits their activities, disturbs their sleep, saps their energy, and has a demoralizing emotional effect. Thus pain must be reduced if the client is to rest and improve.

Help clients assess and plan ways of correcting the position of their beds at home. The head of the bed can be elevated to promote blood flow to the legs. Remind the client with arterial insufficiency of the following points:

- Avoid standing in one position for more than a few minutes.
- Avoid crossing the legs at the knees.
- In general, seek the most comfortable position.
- Watch for and report edema.

Any measure that increases circulation to the extremities helps alleviate ischemic pain. Although pain also can be subdued by analgesics, interventions that augment circulation are best. When strong analgesics, such as morphine, are necessary around the clock, the client may require amputation. Amputation can improve the

CLIENT EDUCATION GUIDE
Foot Care

Client Instructions

Daily Hygiene
- Do not soak your feet; use mild soap and a washcloth to clean them.
- Dry well between your toes.
- Check water temperature with a bath thermometer or your elbow, not your toes, to prevent burns; 32.2° to 35° C (90° to 95° F) is safe.
- Gently rub corns or calluses. Avoid cutting, digging, or using harsh commercial products.

Daily Inspection and Lubrication
- Use good lighting.
- Put on your glasses or contacts, if you wear them.
- Promptly report ulcerations, redness, calluses, blisters, or cracking of the skin on the feet or thickening of the nails to the physician.
- Rub soothing lotions or lanolin on your hands, feet, legs, and arms to prevent dryness.
- Do not use lotion on sores or between your toes.
- Do not use perfumed lotions.
- Dust your feet lightly with cornstarch if they sweat.

Care of Toenails
- Use clippers, not scissors or razor blades.
- Cut straight across the nail.
- Do not perform "bathroom surgery."
- If your eyesight is poor or if you are unable to reach your toes, find qualified assistance.
- Place lamb's wool between overlapping toes.

Proper Footwear
- Never go barefoot, not even at the beach or at home.
- Avoid high heels and shoes with pointed toes.

- Make sure nothing is in your shoes before putting them on your feet.
- Avoid tight socks and shoes.
- Wear cotton socks for absorbency. Change your socks daily.
- Alternate several pairs of comfortable, firm, well-made shoes during the week.
- Avoid shoes that cause your feet to perspire (for example, canvas shoes and rubber boots).
- Make sure that your shoes and slippers fit well and are sturdy enough to prevent foot injury.

Safety
- Avoid sunburn.
- Avoid scratching insect bites on your legs to prevent creating open lesions.
- Do not use heating pads.
- Wear adequate foot protection on cold days.
- Turn on the lights before entering a dark hallway or room.
- Avoid sitting with your legs crossed.
- Use a cane or walker, if indicated.
- When in doubt, ask for help. Have telephone numbers of people who can assist you at hand.

Activity
- Walking is good, but get your physician's permission before beginning a regular program.
- Do not walk if you have open ulcerations.
- Walk until pain begins, stop and rest, then begin again.
- Elevate your feet if they swell.
- Find a nurse and a physician who will get to know you and your foot problems and will take the time to talk with you when you need help.

quality of life by diminishing pain and improving mobility with a prosthesis.

Diagnosis: Risk for Impaired Skin Integrity.
Because of altered peripheral tissue perfusion, the client is at risk of arterial ulceration and skin infection. Write the diagnosis as *Risk for Impaired Skin Integrity related to decreased peripheral circulation.* If the client has an arterial ulcer, this diagnosis can still be used for the remaining intact skin.

Outcomes. The client will reduce risk of skin impairment as evidenced by maintaining soft skin, protecting skin from trauma, and showing no signs of skin injury. If the client has an open wound, see later information in this chapter.

Interventions. Prevent injury to the extremities, particularly the feet. Excellent foot care should be an integral part of the daily routine of clients with peripheral vascular disorders, because prevention is easier to initiate and maintain than is correction. See the Client Education Guide feature on Foot Care, above.

Diagnosis: Risk for Activity Intolerance.
Intermittent claudication may greatly deter activity. This common nursing diagnosis is written as *Risk for Activity Intolerance related to leg pain after walking.*

Outcomes. The client will develop appropriate levels of activity free from pain and excess fatigue, as evidenced by normal vital signs, absence of pain, and verbalized understanding of benefits of gradual increase in activity and exercise.

Interventions. When assisting the client with a walking program, assert that *pain* should be the guide to the amount of activity to be undertaken. Intermittent claudication signals that the muscles and tissues of the legs are not receiving enough oxygen. Before the client begins a walking program, take a careful history and perform a physical assessment. Establish a cardiopulmonary profile and carefully examine the client's feet and legs to locate 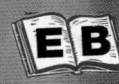 open ulcerations or anatomic deformities. The client should have sturdy shoes to prevent foot trauma.

Although exercise helps most clients with vascular disorders, some clients must not exercise. These clients have leg ulcers, pain at rest, cellulitis, deep vein thrombosis, or gangrene. Exercise and activity increase the metabolic needs of tissues and, consequently, tissue requirements for oxygenated blood. Thus clients with tissue breakdown or necrosis must remain for a period on complete bed rest. Even minimal activity raises the oxygen requirements of the tissues above that which damaged arteries can provide.

Diagnosis: Deficient Knowledge.

The nursing diagnosis *Deficient Knowledge* can be used as a guide to teaching the client about a walking program. State the nursing diagnosis as *Deficient Knowledge related to walking program as evidenced by no previous experience.*

Outcomes. The client will develop and follow a progressive walking program.

Interventions. Remind clients that at first it may be painful to walk any distance and that they may need to stop frequently to rest. They should walk through the pain as much as possible without causing undue distress. Encourage them to walk in enclosed shopping malls in the winter for safety from falls on icy pavement and to avoid vasoconstriction from the environment. In the summer, walking in the malls helps avoid heat exhaustion or stress on other conditions such as heart disease. It is important to stress that small increments of exercise increase are not dramatic, but rather are evidence of improvement. Even improvement to the point of being able to shop in the grocery store is a cause for celebration.

Diagnosis: Health-Seeking Behaviors.

Health conscious clients may request information about self-improvement and interventions to reduce the severity of manifestations. Write the nursing diagnosis as *Health-Seeking Behaviors related to lack of knowledge about the role of exercise, weight reduction, and smoking cessation in management of arterial disease.*

Outcomes. The client will begin and maintain the chosen health promotion program, as evidenced by demon-

COMPLEMENTARY AND ALTERNATIVE THERAPY

Vitamin E Supplements and Peripheral Vascular Disease

Recent data on the ability of vitamin E supplements to reduce the risk of cardiovascular disease have not shown a positive effect. For example, the Heart Outcomes Prevention Evaluation (HOPE) trial was a 4.5-year randomized controlled clinical trial of vitamin E or placebo in 9541 clients aged 55 years or older with a history of coronary artery disease (CAD), stroke, peripheral vascular disease, or diabetes and other cardiovascular disease risk factors. No difference was noted between vitamin E (400 international units/day) and placebo for the outcomes of stroke, death, or other cardiac outcomes for these high-risk clients.

Reference

Yusuf, S., et al. (2000). Vitamin E supplementation and cardiovascular events in high-risk patients. The Heart Outcomes Prevention Evaluation (HOPE) study investigators. *New England Journal of Medicine, 342,* 154-160.

strated knowledge of the specific activities of the program, regular evaluation of goals against performance, and verbalized feelings of increased well-being.

Interventions. Instruct the client in areas of concern or interest. Refer to the nonpharmacologic intervention methods described earlier. See also the Complementary and Alternative Therapy features on Vitamin E Supplements and Peripheral Vascular Disease and on Antioxidant Vitamins to Reduce Cardiovascular Disease above and on p. 1517. Refer the client to groups in the community if available. The client with intermittent claudication caused by arterial disease should be routinely re-examined at least every 3 months for progression of disease.

Evaluation

Arterial disorders are chronic, so do not expect to see reversal of the problems. Write outcomes that allow for time and client adjustments.

■ Modifications for Older Clients

Age-related changes and impairments of physiologic function along with arterial disease affect the nursing diagnoses of *Activity Intolerance* (possibly increased), *Altered Peripheral Tissue Perfusion* (possibly reduced), and *Pain.* Recognition of pain may be complicated by physical or cognitive impairments, ongoing drug therapy, and psychosocial factors (e.g., depression or social isolation). Additionally, sight reduction and flexibility limitations may prevent or decrease self-care. Sight reduction may

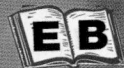
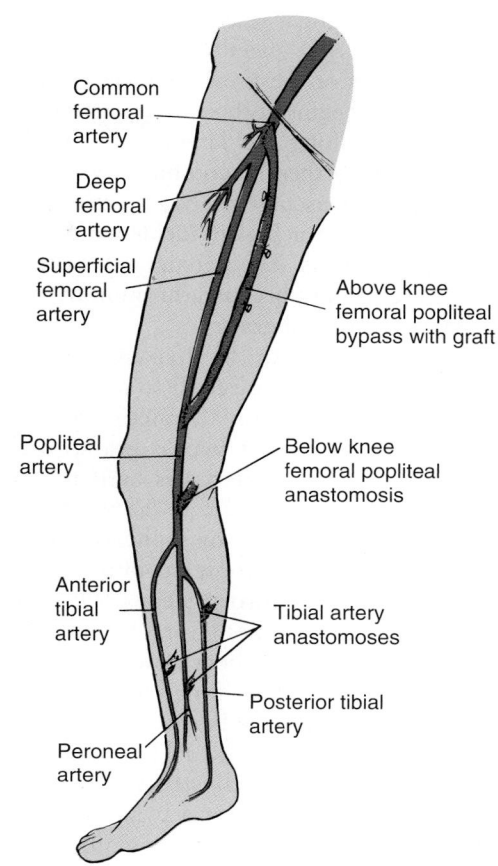

FIGURE 55-4 Femoral artery bypass grafts. The anastomosis can be to any one of three tibial arteries. (From Fahey, V.A. [2004]. *Vascular nursing* (4th ed.). Philadelphia: W.B. Saunders.)

increase risks for falls or other injury, which may be disastrous in the client with impaired circulation.

■ Surgical Management

Surgical management of PVD is called *revascularization* and is reserved for clients with progressive, severe, or disabling manifestations including ischemia at rest. Angiography is commonly used before surgery to mark the level of inflow or areas of obstruction. Revascularization can be done through endovascular techniques or surgical reconstruction with grafting.

Endovascular Interventions. Endovascular procedures include angioplasty, atherectomy, and stent placement. The goal is to operate from within the artery to remove partial or total blockages. Most of the procedures can be done in the radiology department or in cardiac catheterization laboratories. Many of these procedures can be performed through small puncture wounds under local anesthesia with sedation. The client recovers quickly and costs are reduced. Preprocedural and post-procedural care is discussed in Chapter 53.

Arterial Bypass. Arterial bypass operations are used to revascularize limbs. Selecting the client for surgery follows careful history and physical and diagnostic assessments, including arteriography. Arteriography provides a necessary road map to indicate the level of obstruction,

because it is essential to reconstruct the arterial inflow to the legs before correcting the outflow. This process prevents newly placed bypass grafts from thrombosing because of inadequate blood supply to the graft. During the operation, the surgeon assesses inflow, and after it is ascertained that inflow to the femoral system is adequate, a distal site is chosen for outflow.

Improvements in vascular surgery have provided outstanding examples of long-term limb salvage in clients who in the past would have required amputation. Current data indicate that revascularization should be the first option considered in clients with critical limb ischemia. This recommendation is based on the following observations: (1) previous revascularization does not raise the level of amputation, (2) mortality rates for amputation are at least as high as for arterial bypass, and (3) there is no difference in cost between amputation and successful bypass.

Various locations along the arterial system can be reconstructed. Femoral artery bypass grafting or axillobifemoral reconstruction (Figure 55-4) is used if the aortoiliac segment is obstructed. The patency rates of aortobifemoral grafts is 90% at 5 years.

Axillofemoral grafting is reserved for people who have increased operative risk, usually because of their cardiopulmonary status or the presence of intra-abdominal infection. The graft begins at the axillary artery and travels subcutaneously along the lateral chest wall to the femoral artery. It may then be combined with a femorofemoral graft to revascularize both extremities. Axillofemoral grafts have a higher incidence of occlusion than aortofemoral grafts. The patency rates are 60% to 70% at 5 years, in part because thrombi are easily removed from axillofemoral grafts.

The femoral artery can be bypassed with grafts anastomosed (surgically connected) to any one of three lower leg arteries (posterior tibial, anterior tibial, or peroneal artery). The success of bypass grafts of the legs depends largely on what material is used for grafting. The client's own saphenous vein is the most successful grafting material. Up to 80% of saphenous vein grafts are patent after 5 years; in contrast, only 30% of synthetic material (polytetrafluoroethylene [PTFE]) is patent after the same length of time. (Gore-Tex is a common brand name for PTFE.) The client's own saphenous vein is not always large enough or long enough for the surgery, however, or it may have been removed during another operation. In these cases, PTFE is used. In situ grafts can also be used for reconstruction. In situ grafting uses the client's own vein for a bypass of the artery. A section of vein is anastomosed proximally and distally and then the valves are disabled. The vein then acts as an artery.

Clots in the graft are a major complication after surgery. Clots cause immediate impairment in blood flow and the limb becomes cool, pale, painful, and pulseless. Anticoagulant medications (e.g., low-molecular-weight heparin, heparin sodium) or antiplatelet aggregates (e.g., aspirin and Plavix) can be used prophylactically. If graft becomes occluded, fibrinolytics may be used depending on the amount of time that has lapsed since surgery (due to marked risk of bleeding). (See Chapter 58.)

■ Nursing Management of the Surgical Client

Preoperative Care

Preoperatively, obtain baseline vital signs and document the character of peripheral pulses, comparing one side to the other. Know exactly which pulses are palpable and which pulses can be assessed only with the Doppler. To assist with postoperative assessment, mark with ink the sites where peripheral pulses can be palpated. A lack of pulses postoperatively can be considered an occlusion if the nature of the pulses before surgery was not recorded.

As with any preoperative assessment, perform careful cardiac and pulmonary evaluation. Even though the incision for a femoral artery bypass is peripheral and major complications are infrequent, the client probably has other manifestations of atherosclerosis (such as heart and kidney disease) that may complicate the surgery. If the operation is not an emergency, malnutrition can be reversed and open wounds cleaned. The client should have a complete medical evaluation and hypertension should be controlled. Report to the surgeon or anesthesia department any blood pressure reading outside of normal parameters or well above the client's normal. All infections (e.g., tooth abscesses, urinary tract infections, respiratory infections) must be resolved, especially if the a synthetic graft is planned.

Before the client goes to surgery, it is common to begin administration of intravenous fluids, insert a urinary catheter, and weigh the client. In addition, broad-spectrum antibiotics normally are administered.

The client and family are taught the various procedures involved and are offered psychological support. First assess the client's readiness and desire to learn about the surgery. The importance of maintaining medication routine is to be stressed with appropriate guidance from the physician or anesthesia department.

Postoperative Care

The client is placed on bed rest for the evening after surgery, with the leg flat in bed. The leg is wrapped with light dressings or a fleece vascular boot. See the Care Plan feature on Postoperative Care of the Client Who Has Had Arterial Bypass Surgery of the Lower Extremity on pp. 1519 to 1521 for a description of the remainder of nursing care of the client.

Complications. Bleeding may develop along the suture line and can indicate a disruption in the suture line, pseudoaneurysm formation, or a slipped ligature (suture). These problems require additional surgery. Reclotting of the graft is also possible. Peripheral tissue perfusion is monitored and noninvasive follow-up studies are performed to assess patency.

Infection is not a common complication after bypass surgery, but it can occur, especially when synthetic grafting material is used. Because infection in a synthetic graft necessitates its removal, infection often results in the loss of a limb. Poorly nourished clients appear to be at highest risk of infection and delayed healing.

Compartment syndrome may also develop from swelling around the fascial compartments of the leg. In addition to loss of sensation and function, muscle cells can die and release myoglobin, which can cause acute tubular necrosis in the kidney. The manifestations of compartment syndrome include pain out of proportion to the surgery, a tense swollen leg and pain with muscle stretching, and decreased sensation. A change involving any of these manifestations or change in the color of the urine to rusty brown should be reported immediately.

CARE PLAN

Postoperative Care of the Client Who Has Had Arterial Bypass Surgery of the Lower Extremity

Nursing Diagnosis. Risk for Deficient Fluid Volume related to hemorrhage, hematoma, third spacing of fluid, or diuresis from contrast given during angiography.

Outcomes. The client will maintain adequate vascular fluid volume as evidenced by:
- Hemodynamic stability
- Urine output 0.5 ml/kg/hr
- Warm, dry skin
- Being alert, awake
- No excess drainage on dressings
- Intake that equals output
- Stable hemoglobin and hematocrit

Interventions	Rationales
1. Observe the client for an increase in pulse, decrease in blood pressure, anxiety, restlessness, pallor, cyanosis, thirst, oliguria, clammy skin, venous collapse, and decreasing level of consciousness.	1. Hemorrhagic shock can develop from surgical or postoperative blood loss. Blood is shunted from peripheral stores because of the effect of epinephrine.
2. Check the client's dressings for excessive drainage.	2. Incision drainage first appears on dressings.
3. Assess the client's pulmonary artery pressures and cardiac output if parameters are available.	3. Pulmonary artery pressures and cardiac output parameters are reliable indicators of hemodynamic stability.
4. Check the client's daily weights; monitor intake and output closely.	4. Intake should equal output. Weight is a reliable indicator of fluid balance.
5. Check hematocrit and hemoglobin values and notify the physician if they are abnormal.	5. Hematocrit and hemoglobin normally fall slightly because of surgical blood loss. Transfusion may be required.
6. Check the client's creatinine level after angiography.	6. Contrast is excreted by the kidneys.

Evaluation. This outcome should be attainable within 24 hours.

Nursing Diagnosis. Acute Pain related to surgical incision.

Outcomes. The client verbalizes and demonstrates an increased level of comfort as evidenced by reporting less severe pain on a 1-10 scale, using less analgesia, and ambulating increasing distances.

Interventions	Rationales
1. Assess the client's level of pain: type, duration, and location.	1. Baseline data to evaluate the effectiveness of treatment and a guide to choice of analgesia provided.
2. Medicate with prescribed analgesics based on level of pain and prior effectiveness.	2. Analgesia is provided to obtain comfort, using the previous response to analgesia and current level of pain to guide the decision.
3. Evaluate the effectiveness of pain medication after each administration.	3. Determines the adequacy of analgesias.
4. Teach the client how pain will be controlled.	4. Clients can participate in pain management by notifying the nurse prior to intense pain and by using patient-controlled analgesia (PCA) devices.
5. Position the leg to promote blood flow and keep the leg warm.	5. Arterial inflow is aided by supine position and warmth.

Evaluation. Acute pain should subside over 48 to 72 hours.

Continued.

CARE PLAN

Postoperative Care of the Client Who Has Had Arterial Bypass Surgery of the Lower Extremity—cont'd

Nursing Diagnosis. Impaired Physical Mobility related to a surgical procedure, pain, or nerve injury secondary to ischemia.

Outcomes. The client will have increasing physical mobility as evidenced by maintaining intact motor function, avoiding potential complications of immobility, and demonstrating the use of adaptive devices to increase mobility.

Interventions	Rationales
1. Assess the causative factors for immobility and the client's range of motion and ability to ambulate.	1. Mobility can be facilitated once the cause is known.
2. Encourage range of motion while the client is in bed.	2. These activities promote venous return and muscle strength.
3. Ambulate increasing distances daily. Monitor tolerance of ambulation.	3. Ambulation increases muscle strength and endurance. Monitor for balance, stamina, and unsteady gait if muscle atrophy is present.
4. Request a physical therapy consult when appropriate.	4. Assistive devices may be necessary for ambulation.
5. Encourage independence in the client's activities of daily living.	5. Independence improves both physical and psychological recovery.

Evaluation. Outcomes related to mobility may require several days, depending on initial physical status.

Nursing Diagnosis. Risk for Impaired Skin Integrity related to altered circulation, altered nutritional state, infection, and surgical procedures.

Outcomes. The client will maintain adequate skin integrity as evidenced by incisional healing and no open skin areas.

Interventions	Rationales
1. Inspect the client's lower extremities on daily basis, including foot drop.	1. Early detection of ulceration will allow treatment of early lesions.
2. Assess the sensory and motor function of the client's extremities.	2. Compartment syndrome may develop because of bleeding or edema.
3. Monitor the client for low-grade fever, elevated white blood cell count, any drainage from the wound, and graft exposure at each shift.	3. These are clinical manifestations of wound infection.
4. Monitor the client's nutritional status and albumin level. Obtain a dietitian's consultation, if necessary.	4. Malnutrition is the most common cause of delayed healing.
5. Provide proper skin care using lanolin-based creams.	5. Soft skin does not crack open.
6. Protect the client's lower extremities from trauma.	6. Tissue perfusion is decreased and injured sites heal poorly.
7. Use fleece vascular boots when appropriate.	7. Boots protect the skin from breakdown and keep the legs warm.
8. Elevate heels from the bed.	8. Pressure ulcers on the heels may be slow to heal due to poor circulation.
9. Avoid using tape on the skin below the client's knee.	9. Tape burns from tape removal may be slow to heal.
10. Observe strict aseptic technique during dressing changes.	10. Aseptic technique reduces the risk of infection.
11. Instruct the client to inspect feet and incisions daily. (See Client Education Guide on Foot Care.)	11. Circulation to the legs and feet is impaired from arteriosclerosis. Daily assessment and proper care can lead to early intervention.

Evaluation. Expect the wound to heal slowly over 10 days if arteriosclerosis is extensive.

CARE PLAN

Nursing Diagnosis. Risk for Ineffective Tissue Perfusion related to graft thrombosis, compartment syndrome, progressive arterial disease, or inadequate anticoagulation.

Outcomes. The client will maintain adequate tissue perfusion to the lower extremities as evidenced by full pedal pulses, intact sensory and motor function, and minimal swelling.

Interventions	Rationales
1. Assess the client's pedal pulses every hour for 24 hours, then every shift, unless otherwise ordered. Obtain Doppler pressures per doctor's orders. Compare to baseline.	1. Pedal pulses indicate graft patency.
2. Assess the sensory and motor function of the client's extremities.	2. Compartment syndrome may develop because of bleeding.
3. Assess the client's leg for hematoma or severe swelling.	3. Severe swelling may impede the flow through the graft.
4. Monitor creatine phosphokinase levels when appropriate.	4. Enzymes are released from ischemic muscle.
5. Observe for a change in color and the presence of red blood cells in the client's urine.	5. These manifestations may be caused by a release of myoglobin secondary to muscle ischemia.
6. Report any unexpected deviation in perfusion to the physician.	6. Early reporting allows early intervention.
7. Avoid raising the knee section of the gatch bed and placing pillows under the client's knees.	7. Pressure may increase the risk of thrombosis.

Evaluation. Outcomes related to tissue perfusion should be met within 48 hours.

■ Self-Care

Most clients are discharged to home. Because activity was limited by claudication before surgery, the client needs to begin regular permissible exercise, including climbing stairs and going out of doors. The client is taught that swelling of the operative leg is normal. Elastic wraps can be used when the client is ambulating, but they should not be worn continuously.

AMPUTATION

Amputation is the oldest operation known to man, existing before recorded history. Early amputations were done as punishment for crime. Today's amputations are used to treat injuries, cancers, overwhelming limb gangrene, and limb-threatening arterial disease or rest pain. Amputation is common; nearly 2 million people in the United States have undergone amputations. Even though prosthetic devices can restore a reasonable degree of function after amputation, the visible loss engenders an additional emotional component that may not occur with other surgeries.

For many years, amputation was performed with an apology and often a sense of failure. Recently there has been increasing media publicity featuring amputees who have "overcome their handicap" and returned to mainstream society. There are organizations of amputee skiers, golfers, and runners. Publicity has removed much of the old stigma.

Clients with peripheral vascular disease are the most frequent candidates for amputation of the lower extremities. Diabetes mellitus is a major etiology of arterial occlusion and has been associated with more than 55% of major amputations in clients with lower extremity occlusive disease. Traumatic injuries are also a common cause of amputation.

Preoperative Assessment

Usual preoperative assessment is performed (see Chapter 16). In addition, a rehabilitation team designs an individualized care plan focusing on the whole client rather than on a diseased or missing limb. Before amputation, the surgeon and rehabilitative team consider the following:

- *The client's physical condition.* The following physical conditions may predicate the rehabilitation potential: the age of the client, the ability to become ambulatory or remain ambulatory, the comprehension level of the client, the willingness of the client to participate in a rehabilitation program, and the condition of preexisting conditions (e.g., chronic and progressive mental deterioration, advancing neurologic problems, chronic obstructive pulmonary disease, or cardiac disease with heart failure or angina). Ideally, clients should attain independent function with the use of a prosthesis.

- *The type of amputation to be performed.* There are two types of amputation procedures: the open, or guillotine, amputation and the closed, or "flap," amputation. The major indication for guillotine amputation is infection. In open amputation, the surgeon does not close the stump with a skin flap immediately but leaves it open, allowing the wound to drain freely. Antibiotics are used. Once the infection is completely eradicated, the client undergoes another operation for stump closure.

   During a "flap" amputation, the surgeon closes or covers the stump with a flap of skin sutured over the end of the stump. This type of amputation is the most common and performed when there is no evidence of infection and, consequently, no need for open drainage. However, the surgeon may insert small drains to promote wound healing.

- *The level of amputation required.* The level of amputation for any extremity should be as distal as possible (Figure 55-5). Arteriography is used to guide the decision about the level of amputation. Clients with below-knee amputations (even bilateral) more successfully achieve independent function with a prosthesis than do those with above-knee amputations (see Figure 55-5).

- *The client's general attitude toward amputation.* Attitude toward amputation depends to a large

degree on the client's age and maturity. Young clients may resist amputation even though it would greatly improve their function. For some, the thought of amputation dramatically conflicts with their ideal self-image. Conversely, some clients who suffer from the pain of chronic ischemia may welcome amputation. These clients are often more concerned with removing the source of their pain than they are with altering their body image or function.

Diagnostic assessments include the usual preoperative blood studies and radiographs. In addition, the client may have arteriography to determine the level of blood flow in the extremity. Doppler studies are used to measure blood flow velocity, and transcutaneous tissue oxygen levels may also be measured (see Chapter 53). These studies assist with determining the level of amputation that are most likely to heal.

Phantom Limb Sensation. Phantom sensations are feelings that the amputated part is still present. Although these sensations are often referred to as phantom pain, not all of the sensations are painful. The client may describe sensations of warmth, cold, itching, or pain, especially in amputated fingers or toes. *Phantom sensations* are caused by intact peripheral nerves proximal to the amputation site that carried messages between the brain and the now amputated part. These sensations are normal, and the client should be prepared for them. Phantom sensations often are felt immediately after surgery and their frequency gradually decreases over the next 2 years.

Another condition called *phantom pain* is a form of central pain. The client reports actual pain. The pain is usually burning, cramping, squeezing, or shooting in nature. Phantom pain is less well understood and may occur in a large percentage of clients. It is thought to be caused by a combination of physiologic and psychological components. However, no research has identified a link between phantom pain and any clinical psychological disorder. Phantom pain occurs most often in clients who had pain in the limb before the amputation. Interventions that may reduce phantom pain include range-of-motion exercises, visual imaging, and other interventions for chronic pain (see Chapter 22).

Preoperative Care
Assessment

Perform the usual preoperative assessments (see Chapter 16). In addition, support the client and family through their pain, suffering, and decision-making as the client is prepared physically and psychologically for amputation. If the amputation is being done for an infectious process, administer antibiotics and monitor for sepsis (changes in

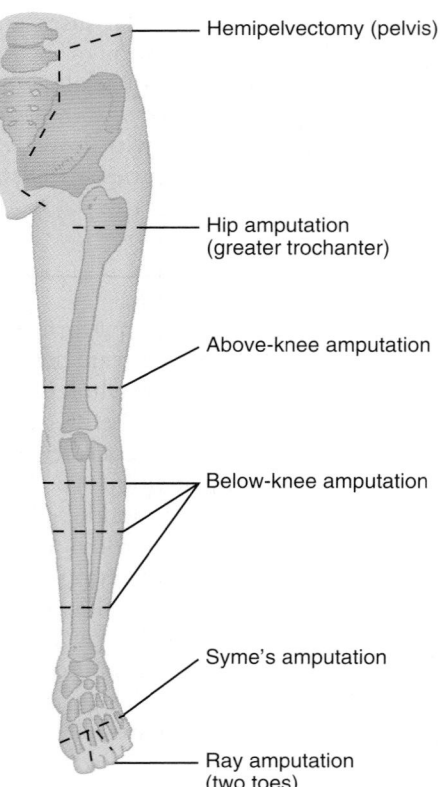

Hemipelvectomy (pelvis)

Hip amputation (greater trochanter)

Above-knee amputation

Below-knee amputation

Syme's amputation

Ray amputation (two toes)

FIGURE 55-5 Common sites of lower extremity amputation.

mental status, fever and chills, increasing pain or odor from the wound, elevated white blood cell count). If the client has an infection in the leg to be amputated, it is important that the remaining leg is not wounded and also infected. Ulcers on the heel are hazardous and the legs should be elevated to remove all pressure from the heel. Diabetic clients need close monitoring of blood glucose levels because infection makes blood glucose regulation erratic. Maintaining or promoting strength in the upper arms facilitates rehabilitation. Teach the client to use the trapeze and side rails for independent movement in bed. Maintain or promote nutrition to aid in healing. Older adults may have several problems that can lead to malnutrition. Ask the dietitian to evaluate the nutrient intake and offer suggestions to meet caloric and protein needs.

Diagnosis, Outcomes, Interventions

Diagnosis: Risk for Delayed Surgical Recovery.
Some clients require amputation on an emergent basis; for those clients the usual preoperative care to stabilize health conditions cannot occur. The need for emergent surgery can create a risk for delayed recovery. State this nursing diagnosis as *Risk for Delayed Surgical Recovery related to preexisting health conditions.*

Outcomes. The risk for delayed surgical recovery will be minimized.

Interventions. Clients with diabetes mellitus are a high-risk surgical group and require frequent assessment of their blood glucose. Blood glucose is normalized using frequent (e.g., four times daily) blood testing and sliding scale insulin. Clients with ulcerated legs or osteomyelitis may be treated with wound packing, antibiotics, and leg elevation with bed rest. Malnourished clients are nourished with foods high in protein or tube feeding. They also may benefit from vitamin and mineral supplements. Severely anemic clients may require iron preparations and blood transfusions. Dehydrated clients should receive preoperative intravenous fluids to restore fluid balance.

Diagnosis: Anxiety.
Clients may fear amputation because it destroys a familiar body image, imposes physical and social limitations, and temporarily upsets personal lifestyle. Such fears and anxiety must be resolved during the preoperative period to ensure successful postoperative recovery. Depending on the reason for the amputation, fear may lead the client to experience anticipatory grief. State this nursing diagnosis as *Anxiety related to impending loss of limb, change in mobility, loss of independence, pain, changes in body image, fear about feelings after amputation.* Other nursing diagnoses may also be appropriate, such as ineffective individual coping, self-esteem disturbance, or body image disturbance.

Outcomes. The client will have reduced anxiety as evidenced by openly discussing feelings and expressing reduced anxiety before surgery.

Interventions. Establish open, honest communication. Allow free expression of fears and negative feelings about the loss of a limb. Ask significant others how they feel about the amputation and how they perceive the client to be responding. The social worker or psychologist may need to be involved if the client is responding poorly.

The client may also be anxious about unknown consequences and sensations after the amputation. Provide and reinforce information. Most clients feel less anxious when they know what to expect on awakening from surgery. Prepare the client for *phantom limb sensation.* Most clients with new amputations experience the peculiar sensation that their missing limb is still present. This phantom limb sensation may or may not be painful. Also, it may either disappear within hours after surgery or persist for years. To avoid misunderstandings, inform clients that phantom limb sensations occur and are normal.

Diagnosis: Acute Pain.
The client may experience severe to moderate pain before surgery. The nursing diagnosis of *Acute Pain related to ischemia of the limb* is used.

Outcomes. The client will have improved comfort as evidenced by statements of reduced pain, use of reduced doses of opioids (e.g., pain is controlled without increasing dosage), ability to move about comfortably, and ability to sleep or rest.

Interventions. Administer prescribed analgesics as necessary to reduce pain. Intervene with supportive measures. For example, use footboards and cradles to avoid pressure on injured or ischemic limbs. Keep ischemic limbs warm with wraps or fleece vascular boots.

Diagnosis: Deficient Knowledge.
A common nursing diagnosis for clients having surgery is *Deficient Knowledge related to expectations after surgery.*

Outcomes. The client will express an understanding of the usual postoperative regimens.

Interventions. Clients want to know what to expect after surgery and what will be expected of them by health care professionals. Emphasize that the client is the most important member of the rehabilitation team. To achieve independence, teach the client about the following:
- Exercising legs and arms several times a day
- Strictly limiting weight-bearing (for leg amputations) until instructed otherwise
- Learning the intricacies of stump and prosthesis care
- Mastering the use of the prosthesis

Postoperative Care

After the operation is completed, the surgeon applies a small amount of fluffed gauze over the end of the stump. A rigid dressing (usually a cast) is applied, distributing pressure evenly over the end of the stump. The cast protects the stump from injury and reduces swelling by gently compressing the tissues. The socket of the distal end of the cast connects to a pylon. A pylon is an adjustable rigid support, the proximal end of which attaches to the below-knee socket or to the knee unit of an above-knee prosthesis. The distal end connects to a foot-ankle assembly. The rigid dressing is usually changed three to four times before application of a permanent prosthesis. Cast changes are necessary because the stump tends to shrink as it heals and, consequently, is no longer adequately compressed by the original cast.

Edema is controlled by elevating the stump for the first 24 hours after surgery. Then, the stump is placed flat on the bed to reduce hip contracture. Edema is also controlled by stump wrapping techniques. In below-knee amputations, the knee is immobilized to eliminate joint flexion. A trapeze and overbed frame are attached to the bed to assist the client to develop upper arm and shoulder strength.

Assessment

Following an amputation, the usual postoperative care is given. Look for bleeding or oozing. Outline the drainage, including the time on the temporary prosthesis or soft dressing. If drains were placed in the wound, carefully monitor the amount and type of drainage.

Postoperative management of acute pain is essential. Acute surgical pain assessment and management is like those techniques used for other postoperative clients. To prevent increased pain, the nurse handles the stump carefully when assessing the site or drainage beneath the stump or dressings.

Due to preexistent conditions such as diabetes, open infected wounds, and decreased perfusion, the client remains at high risk for infection. The nurse monitors the client and the wound for manifestations of wound infection, which usually develops about 72 hours after surgery. Broad-spectrum antibiotics are usually prescribed for several days after surgery, until there is indication that the wound is healing.

Diagnosis, Outcomes, Interventions

Diagnosis: Acute Pain. Following amputation, phantom limb sensation is often present. State this nursing diagnosis as either *Acute Pain related to phantom sensation in amputated limb* or *Anxiety related to phantom sensation in amputated limb*.

Outcomes. The client will express an understanding of the sensations present and will recognize that they are normal and usually diminish in time.

Interventions. Empathetically reinforce the idea that phantom sensation is usual and, more importantly, subsides in time. It is not helpful to correct the client, telling him or her that the limb cannot be hurting because it is absent.

Diagnosis: Ineffective Coping. For clients with some chronic disorders, such as diabetes, the amputation may signal further losses in their battle. These clients may express anger openly or covertly. Many clients express depression after amputation. The client may cry easily, eat little, sleep poorly or sleep more, or avoid interactions with others. Many times depression is a reaction to the fear that the he or she will never walk again, and therefore early ambulation is therapeutic. State the nursing diagnosis as *Ineffective Coping related to reaction/ response to change in body image, fear over loss of independence*.

Outcomes. The client will openly verbalize fears about changes in body image and loss of independence, and will begin to speak optimistically and realistically about the future.

Interventions. The nurse listens to the client and confronts misconceptions about the rehabilitation. If it is possible, the nurse arranges for the client to meet with another amputee.

The client may express concerns that it will be impossible to return to a previous lifestyle, including job, leisure activities, or intimate relationships. With advancements in prosthetic devices, many clients can have both functional and aesthetic prosthetic devices.

Some clients feel the use of the word "stump" to be distasteful and report feeling like they are part of a tree. Use of other terms may be controversial, however, if they encourage or support denial of the problem. Some rehabilitation specialists use the phrase "residual limb" instead.

Diagnosis: Deficient Knowledge. Clients require information and time to learn all the new information about the care of the stump and the prosthesis. Use the nursing diagnosis *Deficient Knowledge related to gait training, care of the stump, care of the prosthesis*.

Intervention

The Prosthesis. The most common prosthesis for clients with a below-the-knee amputation is a patellar tendon-bearing limb prosthesis. The interior of the prosthesis contacts all surfaces of the stump and weight-bearing is on several areas. Clients with above-the-knee amputation are

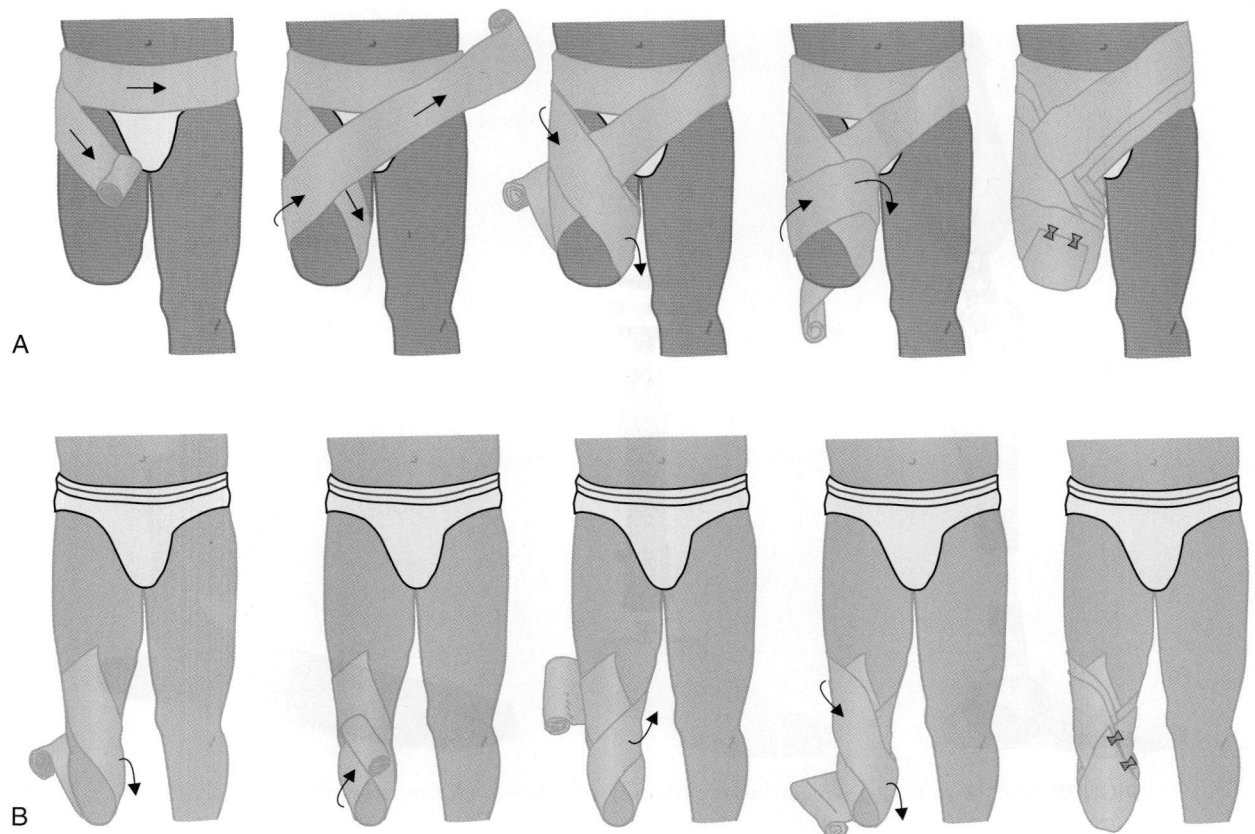

FIGURE 55-6 Common methods of stump wrapping. **A,** For an above-knee stump, two bandages are required. **B,** For a below-knee stump, one bandage is usually sufficient.

fitted with either a quadrilateral socket or an ischial containment prosthesis. Weight is borne on the ischial tuberosity or the soft tissues of the proximal stump, respectively.

Prostheses for the upper extremity consist of a hook or hand device, a harness to supply force to the hand, and a socket for attachment. The client coping with an upper extremity amputation must be highly motivated to master the prosthesis and achieve independence. For successful rehabilitation, the client must integrate the prosthetic arm and hand into the total body image.

Cosmetic prostheses are primarily used to enhance self-esteem and make reentry into society minus a limb more tolerable for clients who are not candidates for a functioning prosthesis. Because the construction of cosmetic prostheses does not allow weight-bearing, caution the client never to attempt transfers or ambulation with a cosmetic prosthesis.

Immediate prosthetic fitting is not always possible. However, anyone with a new amputation who is capable of ambulating should receive a temporary prosthesis as soon as possible after surgery. When a conventional delayed prosthesis fitting is anticipated, the client returns from surgery with the stump dressed and covered with elastic bandages or stump socks (Figure 55-6). When the sutures are removed 2 to 3 weeks after surgery, the surgeon or prosthetist fits the client with a provisional temporary prosthesis made of plaster of Paris or plastic. A permanent prosthesis is fitted once the stump is healed and molded (Figure 55-7).

Gait Training. Physical mobility will be compromised for the client who has just experienced an amputation. Amputating a limb displaces the center of gravity, normally located just below the umbilicus. A client coping with an amputation must relearn balance because the prosthesis, however similar, will not be an exact replica in weight and movement of the lost limb. Adapting to a change in the center of gravity occurs slowly but progressively until the conscious effort of maintaining balance comes under unconscious control. Physically, the client increases strength and endurance with regularly scheduled exercise, controls weight-bearing until the wound completely heals, and practices ambulating with the new prosthesis until a skillful, automatic gait is developed. Physical therapists usually work with the client twice daily for strengthening and gait training.

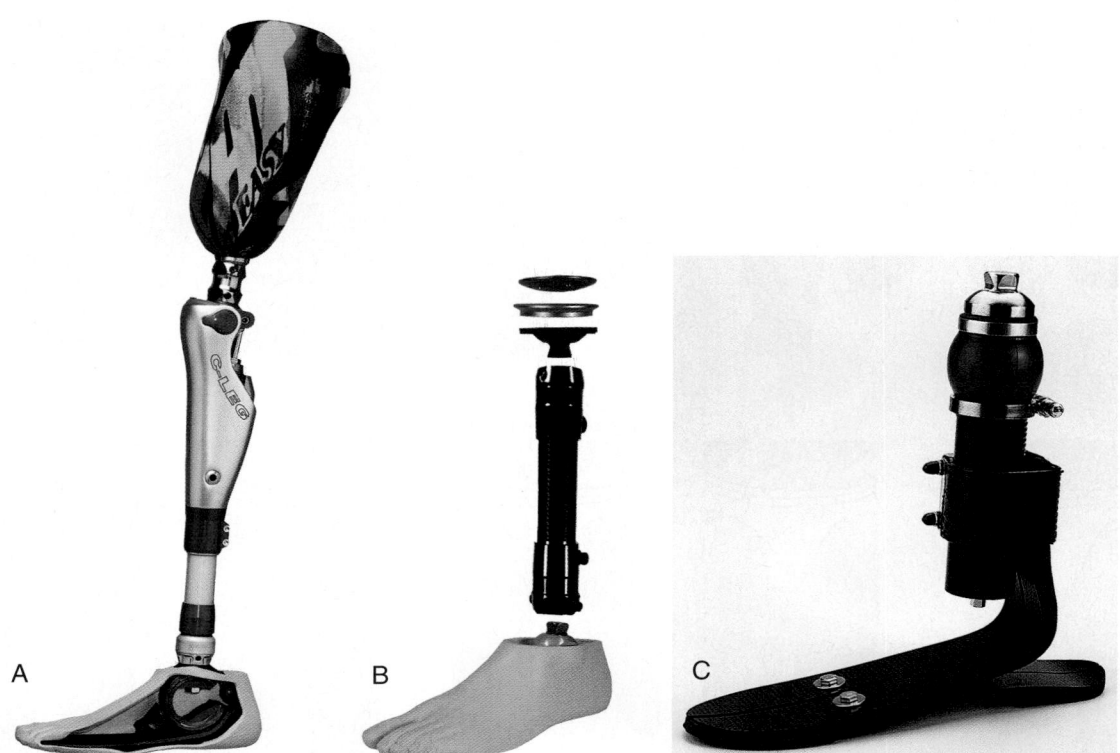

FIGURE 55-7 **A** to **C**, Permanent lower-extremity prostheses. (**A** Courtesy of Otto Bock Health Care, Minneapolis, MN; **B** courtesy of Endolite, Centerville, OH; **C** courtesy of Ossur, Reykjavik, Iceland.)

When the prosthesis is not worn (e.g., during the night), turning also requires a readaptation in body balance. Consequently, the client may need assistance while turning until the new center of gravity is comfortable.

■ Self-Care

When making discharge plans for the client with a new amputation (and probably a prosthesis), consider the client's ambulatory level and the tasks with which the client may need help. Frequently, by the time clients with amputations are aware of their changed circumstances, they are at home, alone, and without the informed and professional advice that can prepare them for their altered lives. Schedule home visits from community health care nurses until such clients have adjusted to their new situation and feel reasonably comfortable and confident in their ability to provide self-care.

See the Client Education Guide feature on Stump and Prosthesis Care on p. 1527 for suggestions of care in the health care facility or at home for clients who have had lower limb amputation.

Traumatic Amputation

Not all amputations are planned. Some clients suffer traumatic loss of limb due to farm machinery accidents, chain saw accidents, or automobile accidents. Some-times the amputated limb can be replanted because usually both the client and the limb were healthy up to the time of injury. It is important to properly store and transport the amputated limb before replantation. The limb should be wrapped in a cloth, placed in a plastic bag, and then placed on ice. The limb or digit itself should not come in contact with ice or water to prevent direct tissue damage. No promises should be made to the client about the ability to successfully replant an amputated limb before evaluation by the replantation surgery team. Individuals whose limbs were amputated because of trauma have had no time before surgery to grieve the loss or adjust to their perceived alterations in body image. They may express sadness or anger, or they may show a strong determination not to let the amputation alter their ability to function. Outcomes after replantation vary with the complexity of repair required and the amount of tissue replanted. Months of rehabilitation are required; the peripheral nerve repairs itself very slowly.

ACUTE ARTERIAL OCCLUSION

Acute occlusion of an artery may be caused by trauma, embolism, or thrombosis and may occur in a healthy or diseased artery. About 90% of acute occlusion occurs in the lower limbs. In arterial embolism, the wall of the ar-

CLIENT EDUCATION GUIDE
Stump and Prosthesis Care

Stump Care
- Inspect the stump daily for redness, blistering, or abrasions.
- Use a mirror to examine all sides and aspects of the stump. Skin breakdown on the stump is extremely serious because it interferes with prosthesis training and may prolong hospitalization and recovery. If you have diabetes mellitus, you are particularly susceptible to skin complications, because changes in sensation may obliterate your awareness of stump pain.
- Perform meticulous daily hygiene. Wash the stump with a mild soap, then carefully rinse and dry it. Apply nothing to the stump after it is bathed. Alcohol dries and cracks the skin, whereas oils and creams soften the skin too much for safe prosthesis use.
- Wear woolen stump socks over the stump for cleanliness and comfort. Wash woolen socks in cool water and mild soap to prevent shrinkage. To prevent stretching, wash socks gently. Dry stump socks flat on a towel. Replace torn socks; mending creates wrinkles that irritate the skin.
- Put on the prosthesis immediately when arising and keep it on all day (once the wound has healed completely) to reduce stump swelling.
- Continue prescribed exercises to prevent weakness.

Prosthesis Care
- Remove sweat and dirt from the prosthesis socket daily by wiping the inside of the socket with a damp soapy cloth. To remove the soap, use a clean damp cloth. Dry the prosthesis socket thoroughly.
- Never attempt to adjust or mechanically alter the prosthesis. If problems develop, consult the prosthetist.
- Schedule a yearly appointment with the prosthetist.

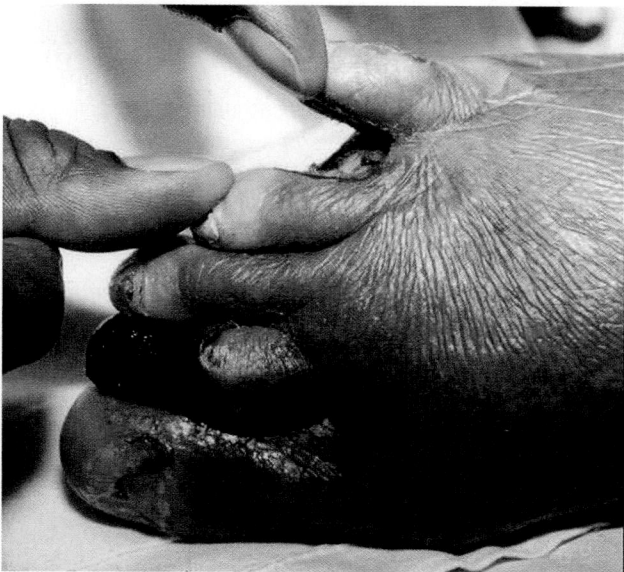

FIGURE 55-8 Distal necrosis of toes from arterial embolization.

topenia, inherited coagulation disorders, disseminated intravascular coagulation, or polycythemia vera may also occur.

The circulatory changes that follow arterial occlusion and that predict the outcome are complex and depend on a variety of factors. Acute occlusion produces a decrease in mean and pulse pressures in the distal arteries and a decrease in tissue perfusion and oxygenation. In a normal artery, blood flow is restored by collateral channels, but with acute emboli, collateral vessels have not had time to develop.

It is important to differentiate between arterial thrombosis and arterial embolism. Acute arterial thrombosis is usually caused by arterial obstruction from a blood clot that forms in an artery that has been damaged by atherosclerosis. Arterial thrombosis may also develop in an arterial aneurysm, especially aneurysms that form in the popliteal artery. Arterial emboli form in the terminal end of an artery and lead to distinct areas of necrotic tissue (Figure 55-8).

The classic manifestations of acute ischemia caused by peripheral thrombus or embolism, which are known as the *six P's* shown in Box 55-1. Muscle necrosis may start as early as 2 to 3 hours after occlusion. Paresthesias indicate advanced damage. Complete paralysis with stiffness of muscles and joints (rigor mortis) indicates irreversible damage. The leg must be amputated to prevent systemic reaction to the products of massive muscle destruction and systemic sepsis.

Outcome Management
Surgery is required to correct arterial embolism. Arterial emboli can be removed by an embolectomy.

tery is often healthy; the obstruction in the artery arises most frequently from a thrombus within the heart. Etiologies include atrial fibrillation, myocardial infarction, prosthetic heart valves, and rheumatic heart disease. Sometimes, portions of a blood clot, such as platelet emboli, which form at points of turbulence and then lodge at a bifurcation, can initiate a thrombus. Atheromatous emboli sometimes block small arteries. In the lower extremity, more than half of the emboli lodge in either the superficial femoral or the popliteal artery. Other noncardiac sources of emboli are laminated clot in an abdominal aortic aneurysm or peripheral aneurysm and up to 20% are from an unidentified source. Most of these emboli lodge in the lower extremities. About 15% travel to the arms. Arterial thrombosis is usually superimposed on atherosclerosis and consequently develops in a damaged vessel; however, coagulopathy from heparin-induced thrombocy-

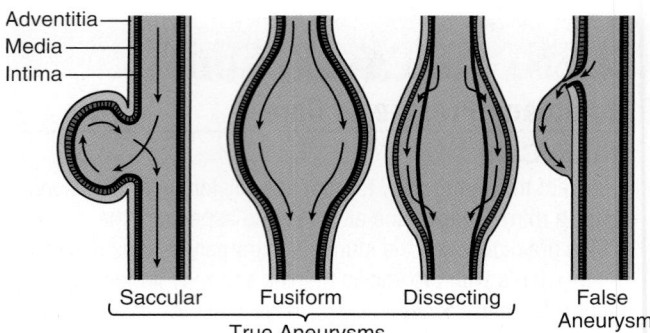

FIGURE 55-9 Classification of aneurysms. In a true aneurysm, layers of the vessel wall dilate in one of the following ways: *saccular,* a unilateral outpouching; *fusiform,* a bilateral outpouching; or *dissecting,* a bilateral outpouching in which layers of the vessel wall separate, creating a cavity. In a false aneurysm, the wall ruptures, and a blood clot is retained in an outpouching of tissue, or there is a connection between a vein and an artery that does not close.

Surgery for thrombosis usually involves an arterial reconstructive procedure for revascularization of the leg. If the decision is made to remove the occluding embolus or thrombus, surgery should be performed as quickly as possible, generally under local anesthesia. If hours have elapsed since the occlusion occurred, the viability of the limb determines whether embolectomy should be attempted.

If surgery is not performed immediately, anticoagulants are used to reduce the risk of further occlusion. Heparin is usually continued for a minimum of 2 to 7 days, after which a change to an oral anticoagulant may be made. The prevailing practice is to treat all clients who have a definite source of embolism and who have satisfactorily recovered from the acute episode of occlusion with long-term anticoagulant therapy. Fibrinolytic agents may also be used to dissolve a thrombus or embolus (see Chapter 60 for discussion of their use).

While decisions about surgery are being made, put the client to bed in a comfortable, warm room. Protect the limb from pressure and other trauma and keep it at room temperature, neither warm nor chilled. The best position for the limb is level or slightly dependent.

ARTERIAL ULCERS

Areas of an ischemic foot or leg subjected to pressure or minor trauma may have skin breakdown. The usual sites of arterial ulcers are the medial and lateral metatarsal heads and the tip of the toes. The ulcers are painful, which distinguishes them from the achy or "heavy" sensation of venous stasis ulcers. Arterial ulcers also have a sharp edge and pale base, and often are surrounded by atrophic tissue (see Figure 55-3). In contrast, venous stasis ulcers are irregular and have a red healthy base (see later discussion).

Once an ulcer develops, it tends to heal poorly, if at all (especially in diabetics). Without adequate blood flow, the damaged tissues fail to receive needed oxygen, nutrients, antibodies, and protective leukocytes, and the

process of tissue damage continues. Eventually, the client may be forced to undergo limb amputation.

Although skin grafting may ultimately be required to cover the site of arterial ischemic leg ulcers (once the ulcerated area is free from infection and granulation tissue is evident), intervention for the skin lesion does not cure the underlying disease. Most ulcers require revascularization to heal. Arterial bypass surgery improves circulation when the client has an aortoiliac or femoropopliteal occlusion. For this surgery to be successful, however, the arteries in the leg must be healthy enough to carry sufficient blood to the foot once the block has been removed or bypassed.

General intervention involves keeping the area of ulceration clean and free from pressure and irritation. Bed rest reduces the oxygen needs of the impaired tissues. Debridement is performed only when the client has reasonable blood flow to heal the wound. Dry intact eschar should be left in place. If surgical debridement is necessary, a qualified health care provider should perform this procedure. After revascularization, if the ulcer bed is clean and granulating, healing is enhanced with moist dressings.

ANEURYSMS

An aneurysm is a permanent localized dilation, stretching, or ballooning of an artery to around 50% increase in the size (Figure 55-9). The exact cause is unknown, but risk factors include atherosclerosis and hypertension. Abdominal aortic aneurysm may be caused by infection, congenital weakening of the connective tissue component of the artery wall (e.g., Marfan's disease or Ehlers-Danlos syndrome), mycotic (fungal) infections, or rarely by trauma. The most common locations for arteriosclerotic aneurysms are the thoracic and abdominal

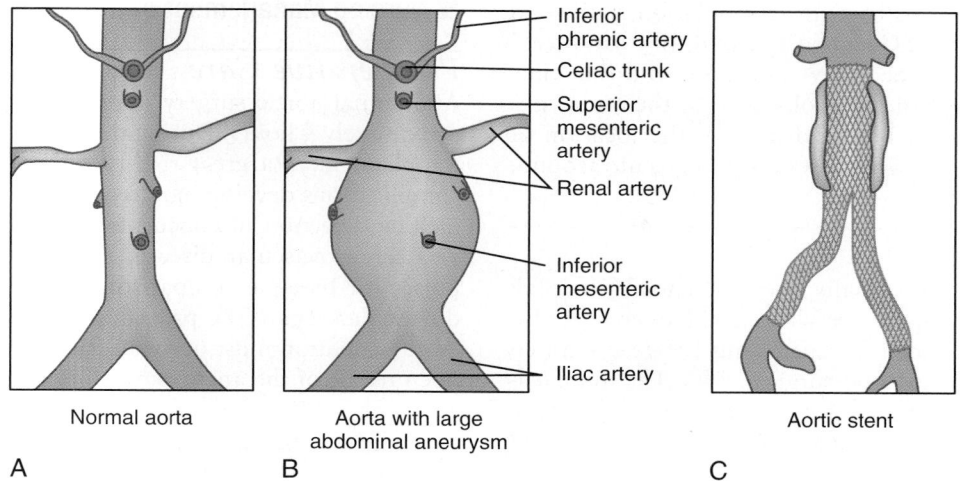

FIGURE 55-10 A, Normal aorta. **B,** An abdominal aortic aneurysm. **C,** A bifurcated synthetic graft in place.

aorta, the iliac arteries, and the femoral and popliteal arteries.

Aneurysms are designated as being either *venous* or *arterial*. They are also described according to the specific vessel that they affect (e.g., abdominal aortic aneurysm).

Aneurysms are also labeled by their shape and size (see Figure 55-9). True aneurysms contain all three layers of the arterial wall (intima, media, and adventitia); saccular aneurysms have a neck or mouth. Fusiform aneurysms involve the entire circumference of the vessel. A dissecting aneurysm is not a true aneurysm, but rather is a hematoma in the arterial wall that separates the layers of the arterial wall. A *pseudoaneurysm,* or false aneurysm, results from the development of a sac around a hematoma that maintains a communication with the lumen of an artery whose wall has been ruptured or penetrated.

ABDOMINAL AORTIC ANEURYSMS

Abdominal aortic aneurysms (Figure 55-10, *B*) are the most common type of aneurysm. They are seen most often in men 40 to 70 years of age. Most abdominal aneurysms are asymptomatic; discovery is usually made on physical or x-ray examination of the abdomen or lower spine for other reasons. When the aneurysm reaches about 5 cm in diameter, it can usually be palpated, except in obese clients. Smaller aneurysms and aneurysms in obese clients may be more difficult to confirm. The most common clinical manifestation is the client's awareness of a pulsating mass in the abdomen, with or without pain, followed by abdominal pain and back pain. Groin pain and flank pain may be experienced because of increasing pressure on other structures. Sometimes mottling of the extremities or distal emboli in the feet alert the clinician to a source in the abdomen. Ultrasonography and computed tomography (CT) scan are the most accurate diagnostic tools.

Outcome Management
■ Medical Management

Surgery is usually not performed on clients with an asymptomatic abdominal aortic aneurysm smaller than 4 to 5 cm. Every 6 months, an ultrasonographic examination is indicated to determine whether any change in the size has occurred. Antihypertensive medications are usually prescribed if indicated.

■ Surgical Management

Surgical resection of the aneurysm and creation of a new artery are the definitive treatments for aneurysm. There are two types of surgery, endovascular surgery and traditional surgery through an abdominal incision.

Endovascular Procedures. Endovascular procedures are a newer method for nonemergency treatment to repair abdominal aortic aneurysm. Two small incisions are made in the groin, and a vascular graft is guided into the aorta (see Figure 55-10, *C*). At the tip of the catheter are a deflated balloon and a tightly wrapped polyester cloth graft. When properly positioned, the graft is secured in place by inflating the balloon and opening the graft to the diameter needed to prevent blood flow into the aneurysm. The balloon is then deflated and removed along with the catheter. At each end of the graft are hooks that help secure it to the inner walls of the aorta. The graft allows blood flow to continue through the aorta to the arteries in the pelvis and legs, without filling the aneurysm.

Postprocedure Care

The usual postoperative care is provided. Assess the surgical sites for swelling and pain (hematoma) and bleeding. Monitor peripheral perfusion closely, comparing findings to baseline. Ambulation is allowed the day after surgery. Clients may ask if they can "feel" the hooks in the aorta. They should be told that they will not be able to feel the hooks because the aorta cannot sense the hooks. Before dismissal, the location of the graft may be confirmed with CT scan, ultrasound, or x-ray study.

Aneurysm Repair

Surgical repair is usually recommended for all aneurysms greater than 6 cm wide. Elective repair is also generally recommended for aneurysms between 4 and 6 cm in clients who are good surgical risks. The more traditional surgical technique for aneurysm repair is done through a midline incision that extends from the xiphoid process to the symphysis pubis. The aneurysm is exposed, the aorta is clamped just above and below the aneurysm to stop the flow of blood, the aneurysm is opened, and a Dacron graft is placed within the aneurysm. The aneurysm sac is then wrapped around the graft to protect it (see Figure 55-10, C).

Complications

Abdominal aortic aneurysm repair is considered a major operation, and many specific postoperative complications can develop. Complications after abdominal aortic aneurysm repair are generally caused by underlying coronary artery disease and chronic obstructive pulmonary disease. These conditions decrease metabolism of anesthetic, increase the risk of postoperative atelectasis, and decrease the client's tolerance of hemodynamic changes from blood loss and fluid shifts.

To reduce the risk of acute myocardial infarction, one of the most serious complications, clients may undergo coronary artery bypass before aneurysm repair.

Prerenal failure can develop for several reasons. The kidney can sustain ischemia from decreased aortic blood flow, decreased cardiac output, emboli, inadequate hydration, or the need for clamps on the aorta above the renal arteries during surgery.

Emboli can also develop and lodge in the arteries of the lower extremities or mesentery. Clinical manifestations include those of acute occlusion in the leg. Bowel necrosis is exhibited as fever, leukocytosis, ileus, diarrhea, and abdominal pain.

The spinal cord can also become ischemic, resulting in paraplegia, rectal and urinary incontinence, or loss of pain and temperature sensation. Spinal cord ischemia tends to occur more commonly when an abdominal aortic aneurysm has ruptured.

Changes in sexual function may also develop fol- lowing repair of an abdominal aortic aneurysm. Retrograde ejaculation occurs in about two thirds of male clients, and loss of potency occurs in one third of males who have undergone repair of abdominal aortic aneurysm.

■ Nursing Management of the Surgical Client

Preoperative Care

Abdominal aortic surgery is major surgery; it lasts approximately 4 hours. During the hours under anesthesia, the client faces a great risk of pulmonary and cardiac complications developing. Preoperative assessment must include detection of concurrent coronary artery disease and cerebrovascular disease. Also assess all peripheral pulses for baseline comparison postoperatively. For endovascular repair, the procedure is much shorter. Standard evaluation must occur because the potential for an open repair of the aneurysm still exists.

Postoperative Care
Assessment

Following surgery, clients usually return to an intensive care unit. A comprehensive postoperative assessment of the client after open surgical repair for abdominal aortic aneurysm repair is essential. Potential complications are many, because of the seriousness of the problem and the complexity of the repair. Even though extracorporeal perfusion (cardiopulmonary bypass) is not needed for the surgery, arterial flow to tissues distal to the aneurysm is reduced during the time required to perform the surgery because the aorta is clamped.

Diagnosis, Outcomes, Interventions

Collaborative Problem: Risk for Hemorrhage. Because of the risk of bleeding at the graft site, the client is at risk for hemorrhage. Use the collaborative problem *Risk for Hemorrhage.* You can also use the nursing diagnosis *Risk for Deficient Fluid Volume,* but recognize that the "fluid" that can be lost is blood.

Outcomes. The nurse will monitor for manifestations of hemorrhage and notify the physician if any manifestations occur.

Interventions. Monitor the client for increase in pulse rate, decrease in blood pressure, clammy skin, anxiety, restlessness, decreasing levels of consciousness, pallor, cyanosis, thirst, oliguria (urine output less than 0.5 ml/kg/hr), increase in abdominal girth, increased chest tube output greater than 100 ml/hr for 3 hours, and back pain (from retroperitoneal bleeding). Monitor central venous pressure, left atrial pressure, pulmonary artery pressure, and pulmonary capillary wedge pressure continuously. Assess for changes indicating hypovolemia. Report any of these manifestations immediately.

Diagnosis: Risk for Impaired Gas Exchange. The large abdominal incision impairs deep inspiration and usually reduced effective coughing. Write the nursing diagnosis as *Risk for Impaired Gas Exchange related to ineffective cough secondary to pain from large incision.*

Outcomes. The client will have improved gas exchange as evidenced by oxygen saturation or PaO_2 greater than 95%, increasing effectiveness in coughing, and clearing of lung sounds.

Interventions. Monitor settings on ventilator to ensure that client is adequately oxygenated. Assess lung sounds every 1 to 2 hours. Report any adventitious sounds. Monitor oxygen saturation continuously. Report any desaturation. After extubation, assist with coughing by using incentive spirometry, provide splinting pillows before coughing, encourage ambulation, and provide adequate analgesia.

Diagnosis: Risk for Ineffecive Tissue Perfusion. During the operation, the aorta is clamped to stop bleeding while the graft is placed. During that time, peripheral tissues are not perfused. The graft site can also become occluded with thrombus. In addition, the client often has preexisting arterial disease. Write the nursing diagnosis as *Risk for Ineffective Tissue Perfusion related to temporary decrease in blood supply.*

Outcomes. The client will maintain adequate tissue perfusion as evidenced by pedal pulses, warm feet, capillary refill of less than 5 seconds, absence of numbness or tingling, and ability to dorsiflex and plantar flex both feet equally.

Interventions. Assess dorsalis pedis and posterior tibial pulses every hour for 24 hours. Report changes in pulse quality or absent pulses (assess with Doppler if needed). Assess dorsiflexion and plantar flexion and sensation (needles-and-pins sensation) every hour for 24 hours. Inspect lower extremities for mottling, cyanosis, coolness, or numbness every 4 hours.

Diagnosis: Acute Pain. Abdominal aortic aneurysm repair necessitates a long incision. Write this common postoperative diagnosis as *Acute Pain related to surgical incision.*

Outcomes. The client will have increased comfort as evidenced by self-report of decreasing levels of pain, use of decreasing amounts of opioid analgesics for pain control, and ambulating or coughing without extreme pain.

Interventions. Opioids are usually provided via a patient-controlled analgesia system or through an epidural catheter. Assess the degree of pain often, and record the baseline level of pain and the degree to which pain is reduced by medications or other interventions. When

changing to an oral route for pain management, plan to pretreat the pain with oral medications 30 minutes or more before discontinuing the infusion.

Collaborative Problem: Risk for Ischemia of the Bowel. If the client undergoes extensive aortic procedures that involve clamping the mesenteric vessels, ischemic colitis can develop. In addition, the inferior mesenteric artery can embolize. The lack of blood supply can lead to ischemia and ileus.

Outcomes. The nurse will monitor the client for abdominal distention, diarrhea, severe abdominal pain, sudden elevations in white blood cell count, and bowel sounds.

Interventions. Maintain accurate intake and output and analyze data hourly for 24 hours. Notify physician if urine output goes below 0.5 ml/kg/hr. Assess urine specific gravity and daily weight. Monitor blood urea nitrogen and creatinine levels. Assess bowel sounds every 4 hours. Keep the client NPO (nothing by mouth) and provide oral care every 2 to 4 hours. Provide routine nasogastric (NG) tube care and assess nares for tissue impairment. Perform guaiac tests of NG drainage every 4 hours or if bleeding is suspected (i.e., drainage has dark, coffee-ground appearance or is bright red).

Collaborative Problem: Risk for Spinal Cord Ischemia. A rare but devastating effect of aortic abdominal aneurysm repair is spinal cord ischemia leading to paralysis, with or without bowel and bladder involvement. It appears to be most common in clients who have suprarenal aortic reconstruction.

Outcomes. The nurse will monitor for manifestations of spinal cord damage and report any abnormal data.

Implementation. Monitor ability to move lower extremities (dorsiflexion and plantar flexion) and sensation in both legs every 1 to 2 hours.

■ Self-Care

Most clients who require abdominal aortic aneurysm repair have significant degrees of arterial disease. Many of the postoperative instructions should address care of clients with arterial disorders, which is discussed earlier. Review all medications to be used by the client to be certain that he or she understands their purpose, schedule, and side effects. Instruct the client about incision care and manifestations of infection.

The client should ambulate as tolerated, including climbing stairs and walking outdoors. If leg swelling develops, the leg should be wrapped in elastic bandages or support stockings should be used. Activities that involve lifting heavy objects, usually more than 15 to 20 lb, are not permitted for 6 to 12 weeks postoperatively. Activities that involve pushing, pulling, or straining may also be restricted. Driving may also be restricted because of postoperative weakness and decreased response time.

The client can resume sexual activity in about 4 to 6 weeks, when he or she is able to walk without shortness of breath (e.g., two flights of stairs). The risk of impotence in male clients should be discussed before discharge. Causes vary from pre-existing aortoiliac disease or diabetes to side effects from aortic cross-clamping. Referral may be appropriate if the client is amenable.

Rupture of an Abdominal Aortic Aneurysm

Rupture of an abdominal aortic aneurysm (AAA) is a catastrophe. Rupture occurs most often in aneurysms 5 cm or more in diameter; an abdominal aneurysm measuring 6 cm or more in diameter has a 20% chance of rupturing in 1 year. Less than 50% of people with a ruptured abdominal aortic aneurysm survive.

See the Critical Monitoring feature on Ruptured Abdominal Aortic Aneurysm below for clinical manifestations.

Surgery is the only intervention for clients with ruptured abdominal aortic aneurysm. New surgical and grafting techniques and faster methods for transport (e.g., helicopters) permit rapid resection of ruptured abdominal aortic aneurysm. However, even with advances in surgery, the operative mortality rate for repair of ruptured abdominal aneurysm may be as high as 50%. Care of the client following emergency repair of a ruptured AAA is the same as elective repair, except that the client has more hemodynamic instability due to preoperative blood loss and ischemic organ disease.

AORTIC DISSECTION

Aortic dissection is the longitudinal splitting of the medial (muscular) layer of the aorta by blood flowing through it. It is the most common catastrophe involving the aorta. Dissection occurs following a tear in the intima, or inner lining, of the aorta, which allows blood to dissect between it and the medial layer. As the dissection progresses, blood flow through the arterial branches of the aorta becomes blocked, and blood flow to the organs that are served by these branches is reduced. Aortic dissections occur more often in men between 50 and 70 years of age, most of whom are hypertensive. Aortic dissections differ from aneurysms in that a false lumen is formed by separation of the intima from the medial layers of the aorta. An aneurysm is a dilation of the entire aortic wall.

Etiology and Classification

The exact cause of dissection is not known. The medial layer of the aorta can become necrotic and thereby lose strength. Clients with Marfan's syndrome (a hereditary condition of connective tissue that predisposes it to aneurysm formation) have a high incidence of dissection. Blunt trauma to the chest wall, such as impact on the steering wheel during a car accident, can also lead to tearing of the aorta.

Dissections are classified by the anatomic location using the Stanford classification system. There are two types of dissections: type A and type B. Type A involves the ascending aorta; type B does not. This system also helps delineate treatment. Usually, type A dissections require surgery, whereas type B dissections may be managed medically under most conditions.

Clinical Manifestations

Abrupt, excruciating pain is the most common presenting manifestation in clients with aortic dissection. Clients describe the pain as ripping or knife-like tearing sensations that radiate to the back, abdomen, extremities, or anterior part of the chest. Hypertension is a common finding, although the client looks "shocky," is sweating profusely, is severely apprehensive, and has diminished peripheral pulses. Other manifestations from decreased perfusion include unequal pulses, different blood pressures in the arms, paraplegia or hemiplegia, decreased urine output or hematuria, mental status changes, and chest pain. A murmur of aortic regurgitation can be heard if the dissection proceeds proximally.

Chest radiograph reveals a widened mediastinum and may show fractured ribs. Transesophageal echocardiogram can be used to determine the size, shape, and location of the tear. Laboratory tests during emergency settings are usually not helpful, except for hemoglobin and hematocrit assays to calculate blood loss and transfusion needs. If the client's condition is stable, helical CT or magnetic resonance imaging can be used to determine the extent of the dissection.

Complications

Cardiac tamponade can develop when the client has dissection of the ascending aortic arch. This life-threatening complication occurs when blood escapes from the area

---

CRITICAL MONITORING

Ruptured Abdominal Aortic Aneurysm

- Pulsating sensation in the abdomen
- Severe, sudden, persistent or constant pain in the abdomen
    Pain is not colicky or spasmodic
    Pain radiates to groin, lower back, buttocks, or legs
- Abdominal rigidity
- Manifestations of shock
    Pallor
    Tachycardia with hypotension
    Dry skin and mouth
    Excessive thirst
    Anxiety

of dissection into the pericardial sac. Clients have pulsus paradoxus, muffled heart sounds, narrowed pulse pressure, and distended neck veins. Pulsus paradoxus occurs when beats are weaker in amplitude during inspiration and stronger with expiration. Blood pressure readings decrease more than 10 mm Hg during inspiration and increase with expiration.

Because the dissection decreases blood supply to many vital organs, ischemic changes in many organs can develop. The spinal cord, kidneys, and abdominal organs are most commonly affected. Ischemia of the spinal cord can lead to manifestations ranging from weakness to paralysis. Renal ischemia can lead to oliguria. Ileus is the most common manifestation of decreased bowel perfusion.

Management

Emergency management is directed at lowering the blood pressure to decrease the force of the blood tearing the aorta. Potent vasodilators, such as nitroprusside, are used to quickly reduce blood pressure. Beta-blockers can also be used to decrease myocardial contractility.

If the client's condition is stable, management is directed at pain reduction, blood transfusion (as needed), and management of heart failure (as needed). Pain levels are used as a guide for needed treatment. Pain subsides when the dissection stabilizes.

Surgery is used for clients whose condition is unstable, in whom severe heart failure develops, who have leaking blood, or who have occlusion of arteries to major organs. During surgery, the torn area is resected and repaired with synthetic graft materials. The operation is similar to that for repair of AAA.

Nursing care is directed at reducing blood pressure. The client is kept at bed rest in a semi-Fowler's position. Unnecessary environmental stresses (e.g., noise) should be minimized. Use opioids to reduce pain; tranquilizers may also be needed. If the client is receiving potent antihypertensive agents, blood pressure should be monitored continuously with an arterial line. Usually the desired parameters for blood pressure are maintained by titrating the vasodilators. Observe the client often for manifestations of further tearing or rupture. Monitor peripheral pulses, level of anxiety, level of pain, and pulse pressure and check for pulsus paradoxus.

If the client is being managed medically, teach the client about the need for antihypertensive agents and beta-blocker drugs. The client and family should understand that, if pain returns, they should immediately return to the emergency department.

RAYNAUD'S SYNDROME

Raynaud's syndrome is a condition in which the small arteries and arterioles constrict in response to various stimuli. It is classified as either vasospastic or obstructive. Manifestations of vasospastic Raynaud's syndrome can be induced by cold, nicotine, caffeine, and stress. Obstructive Raynaud's syndrome is often found in association with autoimmune disorders such as systemic lupus erythematosus, scleroderma, or rheumatoid arthritis.

Raynaud's syndrome may be a benign primary disorder (previously called *Raynaud's disease*) or secondary to another disease or underlying cause (previously called *Raynaud's phenomenon*). Manifestations of both types are the same.

Clinical Manifestations

Raynaud's syndrome causes classic color changes in the hands. Exposure to causative stimuli leads to spasm of the digital arteries, which results in pallor. The resulting tissue hypoxia causes the arteries to dilate slightly. Because they carry mainly deoxygenated hemoglobin, the fingers look cyanotic. Finally, rubor develops when arterial spasms stop completely. Criteria for diagnosing primary Raynaud's disease include (1) manifestations for at least 2 years, (2) intermittent attacks of pallor or cyanosis of the digits by exposure to cold or from emotional stimuli, (3) bilateral or symmetrical involvement, (4) no evidence of occlusive disease in the digital arteries or of any systemic disease that might be the cause of the changes, and (5) gangrene, which (when it occurs) is limited to the skin of the tips of the digits

Noninvasive blood flow studies to determine finger pressures both before and after cold challenge may be necessary. Occasionally, the presence of vasospasm during examination makes the use of cold challenge unnecessary.

Outcome Management

Conservative measures are essential. These measures include keeping hands and feet warm and dry, protecting all parts of the body from cold exposure to prevent reflex sympathetic vasoconstriction of the digits, and cessation of tobacco use. Biofeedback has been of help to some clients.

Medication is used when the vasospastic attacks interfere with the client's ability to work or to perform activities of daily living. Medications are used to induce smooth muscle relaxation, to relieve spasm, and to increase arterial flow. Calcium antagonists, such as nifedipine, are the drugs of first choice because they have been shown to decrease the frequency, duration, and intensity of vasospastic attacks. Medications may be necessary only during the winter months. Individuals who rarely go out in the cold weather may take medications prophylactically 1 to 2 hours before exposure to the cold.

The manifestations of Raynaud's syndrome may be alarming, so reassure the client that the condition is not likely to lead to a serious disability. Advise the client to stay warm by wearing wool gloves and turtleneck sweaters, turning up the thermostat at home if necessary, and staying out of drafts. Teach the client to warm up a cold car before driving. Body core heating is important to prevent chilling and the shunting of blood from the extremities to the trunk. Encourage clients to limit their intake of caffeine or chocolate. They must stop smoking to control the disease. Stress can also bring on vasospasm, so stress management workshops and biofeedback programs may be beneficial. Also, teach the client about any prescribed medications.

BUERGER'S DISEASE (THROMBOANGIITIS OBLITERANS)

Buerger's disease (thromboangiitis obliterans) is an inflammatory disease of the small and medium-sized arteries and veins of the extremities. It is often seen in men and appears to be directly related to smoking. Many clients have a hypersensitivity reaction to intradermal injection of tobacco products, so there may also be an autoimmune element as well. Raynaud's phenomenon, ulcers, and pain are typically seen.

Pain is the outstanding clinical manifestation. Clients have digital ulcerations and pain from ischemia. The pain may be accompanied by manifestations of ischemia, such as color or temperature changes in the fingers. Cold sensitivity, with color changes and pain, may be another early manifestations. Various types of lower extremity paresthesias may occur. Claudication type pain is common with pain in the arch of the foot. Pulsations in the posterior tibial and dorsalis pedis arteries are weak or absent. In advanced cases, the extremities may be abnormally red or cyanotic, particularly when dependent.

Ulceration and gangrene are frequent complications and may occur early in the course of the disease. These lesions can appear spontaneously from migratory superficial thrombophlebitis but can also follow trauma. Gangrene usually occurs in one extremity at a time. Edema of the legs is fairly common in advanced cases. Changes in the nails and skin appear, and segmental thrombophlebitis affects the smaller veins in about 40% of clients. The primary diagnostic study is leg arteriography. Biopsy may also be used; inflammatory lesions are usually noted.

Outcome Management

The goals for management include arresting progress of the disease, producing vasodilation, relieving pain and providing emotional support.

The need for smoking cessation must be clearly and unequivocally conveyed to the client and family. Information about programs to promote abstinence from tobacco should be provided. Because of vasoconstriction, the client should be taught to avoid exposure to cold. Work-related exposure to cold should be considered.

For clients with rest pain and ischemic lesions, adequate pain control is essential. Vasodilation by calcium-channel blockers may be used. Ulcerations need wound care to facilitate healing. Amputation should be deferred until conservative interventions have failed. Thromboangiitis is usually not life-threatening. It does, however, result in disability from pain and amputation.

SUBCLAVIAN STEAL SYNDROME

Subclavian steal syndrome produces arm ischemia arising from subclavian artery blockage. The arm is perfused from the vertebral artery as blood is taken from the brain to supply the arm. The most prevalent physical finding is a significant difference in blood pressure of the right and left arms (usually 20 mm Hg or more). Other manifestations include dizziness and syncope when the arm is exercised. Arm paresthesias and bruit in the supraclavicular fossa are present. Many times the client is not symptomatic and no intervention is necessary. Intervention is surgical, by carotid-subclavian bypass, transluminal dilation of the subclavian artery, or endarterectomy of the subclavian artery.

THORACIC OUTLET SYNDROMES

Thoracic outlet syndromes are a group of disorders that produce manifestations affecting the neck, shoulder, and upper extremities by compression or mechanical irritation of the brachial plexus, subclavian artery, or subclavian vein as these structures pass through the thoracic outlet. Aching or throbbing pain and paresthesias of the neck and upper limb are the most prominent clinical manifestations. In more than half of the clients, the manifestations appear to follow a hyperextension injury to the neck or upper back. Intervention is usually nonsurgical and involves physical therapy. The syndrome in some clients has been treated by surgical removal of the first rib, but this intervention is controversial.

Arterial thoracic outlet syndromes result from chronic compression of the subclavian artery. This leads to the formation of intimal and mural thrombus and, eventually, to peripheral embolization. This type of syndrome is more serious because it frequently results in severe ischemia of the upper extremity. Diagnosis is made by arteriography; treatment is the surgical excision of the anatomic abnormality and removal of the emboli.

Venous thoracic outlet syndrome is caused by external compression of the axillosubclavian vein that results in thrombosis. The primary manifestations are sudden swelling, pain, and cyanosis of the upper extremity. Management is conservative and includes arm elevation and anticoagulation, thrombectomy, or thrombolytic therapy.

VENOUS DISORDERS

Venous disorders can be separated into acute and chronic conditions. Chronic venous disorders can be further separated into varicose vein formation and chronic venous insufficiency. Acute venous disorders include thromboembolism. Acute venous disorders are discussed first.

ACUTE VENOUS DISORDERS

Acute venous disorders are caused by thrombus (clot) formation that obstructs venous flow. Blockage may occur in either the superficial or the deep veins.

THROMBOPHLEBITIS

Superficial thrombophlebitis is usually an easily diagnosed condition; it may iatrogenic, resulting from intravenous catheters or infusion of caustic solutions. Deep vein thrombosis (DVT) is thrombophlebitis of the deep veins. DVT is a common disorder, more so in women than in men, and among hospitalized clients. DVT develops in approximately one third of clients older than 40 years who have had major surgery, orthopedic surgery, or an acute myocardial infarction. In addition, clients with cancer or family history of clotting disorders are at high risk.

Etiology and Risk Factors

There are many risk factors for the development of venous thrombosis (Box 55-2). Thrombus formation is usually attributed to Virchow's triad: (1) venous stasis, (2) hypercoagulability, and (3) injury to the venous wall. At least two of the three conditions must be present for thrombi to form.

Venous stasis is usually caused by immobilization or lack of use of the calf muscle pump. Other conditions that may cause stasis are age older than 40 years, surgery, immobility, prolonged travel, stroke, obesity, pregnancy, paralysis, and heart disease such as heart failure,

myocardial infarction, and cardiomyopathy. Some of the highest risk clients are those having orthopedic surgery.

Hypercoagulability often accompanies malignant neoplasms (especially visceral and ovarian tumors). Dehydration and blood dyscrasias may raise the platelet count, decrease fibrinolysis, increase the clotting factors, or increase the viscosity of the blood. Oral contraceptives and hematologic disorders may also increase the coagulability of the blood.

Conditions that may cause vein wall trauma are intravenous injections, fractures and dislocations, severe blows to an area, chemical injury from sclerosing agents, contrast x-ray studies, certain antibiotics (such as chlortetracycline), and thromboangiitis obliterans (Buerger's disease). The resulting damage to the vein wall attracts platelets, and blood debris accumulates. Platelets do not stick to an intact endothelium. This injury, in combination with low blood flow and a hypercoagulable state, results in thrombus formation.

Pathophysiology

Usually, venous return is aided by the calf muscle pump. When the legs are inactive or the pump is ineffective, blood pools by gravity in the veins (Figure 55-11). Thrombus development is a local process. It begins by platelet adherence to the endothelium. Several factors

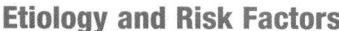

| **BOX 55-2** | *Common Conditions Associated with Venous Thrombosis and Thromboembolism* |

- Age >40 years
- Surgery requiring more than 30 minutes of general, spinal, or epidural anesthesia
- Postoperative edema in the pelvis
- Prolonged position of hip flexion
- Venous stasis (bed rest, prolonged travel, stroke)
- Previous deep vein thrombosis
- Cardiac disease (heart failure, myocardial infarction, cardiomyopathy)
- Pregnancy
- Trauma, especially of the lower extremities
- Estrogen therapy or oral contraceptives
- Malignancy
- Obesity
- Family history of clotting disorders

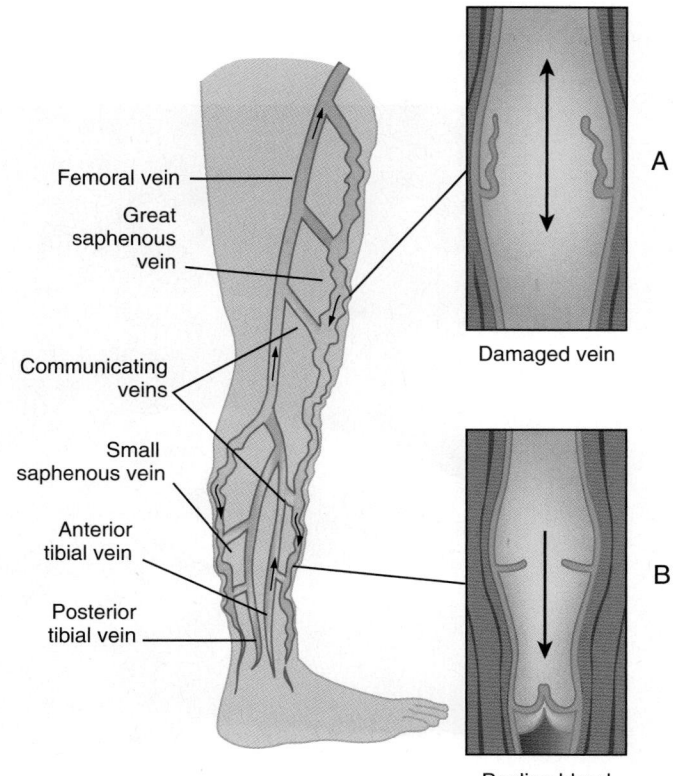

FIGURE 55-11 Venous return from the legs. **A,** Normal flow. **B,** Varicosities and retrograde venous flow.

promote platelet aggregation, including thrombin, fibrin, activated factor X, and catecholamines. In addition, where the platelets adhere to collagen, adenosine diphosphate (ADP) is released. ADP is also released from the damaged tissues and disrupted platelets. ADP produces platelet aggregation that results in a platelet plug. Probably 24 to 48 hours after formation, thrombi undergo lysis or become organized and adhere to the vessel wall, a process that diminishes the risk of embolization.

Deep vein thrombi vary from 1 mm in diameter to long tubular masses filling main veins. Small thrombi are found commonly in the pocket of deep vein valves. As thrombi become larger in diameter and length, they obstruct the veins. If a thrombus occludes a major vein (e.g., femoral, vena cava, axillary), the venous pressure and volume increase distally. Conversely, if a thrombus occludes a deep small vein (e.g., tibial, popliteal), collateral venous channels usually relieve the increased venous pressure and volume. The resulting inflammatory process can destroy the valves of the veins; thus venous insufficiency and postphlebitic syndrome are initiated.

Newly formed thrombi may embolize and travel. Pulmonary emboli, most of which start as thrombi in the large deep veins of the legs, are an acute and potentially lethal complication of DVT. Pulmonary embolism (PE) is discussed in Chapter 63.

Prevention

Due to the frequency of DVT and the risk of PE, prevention is imperative. Prevention is geared toward reversing the three risk factors by promoting venous return, treating hypercoagulability, and reducing risk of injury to the venous wall.

Venous stasis is improved by any activity that causes the leg muscles to contract; passive or active contraction promotes venous return. Leg exercises and ambulation promote venous return. Passive leg muscle contraction occurs by using intermittent sequential compression devices (SCDs) (Figure 55-12). These devices are applied after surgery and care used until the client is ambulatory. Research has shown that SCDs are clinically effective in reducing the incidence of DVT. It is also a good alternative for clients who cannot tolerate anticoagulation. These devices should *not* be used in clients with known DVT. Other methods of promoting venous return include elevating the foot of the bed, applying compression stockings, using motorized foot compressive devices, and providing passive range-of-motion exercises. Encouraging postoperative deep-breathing exercises promotes thoracic pull as a result of the negative thoracic pressure on venous stores in the legs.

Pharmacologic prevention directed at reducing the hypercoagulability includes warfarin, platelet antiaggre-

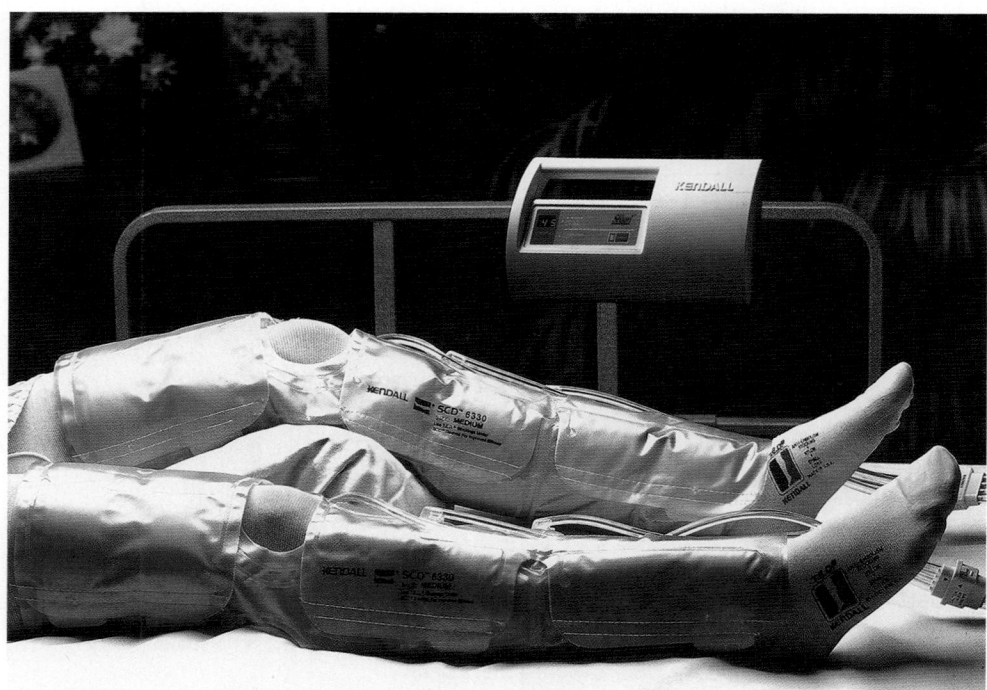

FIGURE 55-12 Pneumatic compression devices, such as the Kendall sequential compression device, are commonly used to prevent deep vein thrombosis in high-risk clients. (Courtesy of Kendall Company, Mansfield, MA.)

gation agents (aspirin being the most common), heparin, and low-molecular-weight heparin. Other methods to reduce coagulation include preventing the venous blood from pooling. Avoid using pillows under the client's knees postoperatively. Teach the client to avoid sitting or standing in one position for prolonged periods.

Measures to prevent injury to the vein wall include avoidance of infiltration during intravenous therapy, pressure on the calf veins during prolonged surgery, trauma to veins in procedures requiring prolonged positioning (delivery, colonoscopy). In addition, access ports should be used in clients requiring multiple intravenous punctures.

Clinical Manifestations and Diagnostic Findings

Clinical manifestations of superficial thrombophlebitis include redness (rubor), induration, warmth (calor), and tenderness (dolor) along a vein. Discomfort may be relieved by applying heat. Activity should be encouraged, and a supportive wrap or stocking should be applied.

The clinical manifestations of DVT are less distinctive; about half of clients are asymptomatic. The most common clinical manifestation is unilateral leg swelling. Other clinical manifestations include pain, redness or warmth of the leg, dilated veins, and low-grade fever. The first clinical manifestation may be PE. Clients may have thrombi in both legs even though the manifestations are unilateral, but this is more common in the client with malignancy.

Homans' sign—discomfort in the upper calf during forced dorsiflexion of the foot—is commonly assessed during physical examination, but findings are insensitive and nonspecific. Homans' sign is present in less than one third of clients with documented DVT. In addition, more than 50% of clients with a positive Homans' sign do not have venous thrombosis. For example, shin splints from running creates a positive Homans' sign without DVT.

Venous duplex scanning has become the primary diagnostic test for DVT because it allows visualization of the vein, which provides a reliable diagnosis of venous thrombus. Venography, the previous gold standard of diagnosis, results in exposure to contrast and is seldom used.

The D-dimer blood test is being used more frequently in evaluation of DVT. The D-dimer is a product of fibrin degradation and is indicative of fibrinolysis, which occurs with thrombosis. Recent studies seem to indicate that the use of the D-dimer, a risk assessment score, and duplex imaging are excellent at predicting and diagnosing DVT in an asymptomatic population.

Plethysmographic examination of the venous system is seldom used, although records of these studies may be found in client records.

Outcome Management
■ Medical Management

The goals of medical management are to detect the thrombus early, prevent extension or embolization of the thrombus, and prevent further thrombus formation.

Superficial thrombophlebitis can be managed with local measures, such as warm packs and elevation of the extremity. Ambulation is encouraged. Sometimes anti-inflammatory medications are required. Clients are encouraged to be seen in follow-up, because an extension of a superficial phlebitis can result in a DVT.

Anticoagulation. Anticoagulant therapy is designed to prevent initiation or extension of thrombi by inhibiting the synthesis of clotting factors or by accelerating their inactivation. Anticoagulant agents do not break up or dissolve clots; they prevent new clots from forming. Various agents that can be used for anticoagulation are discussed in the Integrating Pharmacology feature on Anticoagulant Therapy for the Prevention and Treatment of Deep Vein Thrombosis on p. 1538.

■ Nursing Management of the Medical Client

Goals of nursing management are to prevent existing thrombi from becoming emboli and to prevent new thrombi from forming. Nurses also closely monitor the effect of anticoagulant medications.

Promote Venous Return. Elevation of the legs above the level of the heart facilitates blood flow by the force of gravity. The increase of blood flow prevents venous stasis and the formation of new thrombi. Elevation of the legs also decreases venous pressure, which in turn reduces edema and pain. Elevate the foot of the bed 6 inches (Trendelenburg's position), with a slight knee bend to prevent popliteal pressure. The veins of the legs should be level with the right atrium. The head of the bed may be raised to facilitate eating and bathing. Various forms of elastic support are used to promote venous return. Elastic bandages are advantageous for clients with large or misshapen legs. Apply elastic wraps snugly from toe to groin. Rewrap them every 4 to 8 hours. If compression stockings are prescribed, they must be fitted correctly and removed for a short time every day. Bathe the legs and inspect them closely for manifestations of skin breakdown while the stockings are off.

Reduce Discomfort. Elevation of the extremity, and application of warm packs usually reduce discomfort. Some clients need a mild sedative or analgesic.

Monitor Anticoagulant Therapy. Most physicians use an algorithm to adjust the dose of heparin based on the client's PTT levels. Blood is sampled every 4 to 8 hours for PTT or INR and the dose is adjusted accordingly. Warfarin therapy requires the PT or INR be drawn on a regular basis. Low-molecular-weight heparin requires no testing. When invasive studies are necessary (e.g., arterial blood gas analyses), apply pressure for 30 minutes to the puncture site.

Bleeding can occur in any client receiving anticoagulation. The client should also be observed for frank

INTEGRATING PHARMACOLOGY

Anticoagulant Therapy for the Prevention and Treatment of Deep Vein Thrombosis

Anticoagulation prevents the extension of the original thrombus and the development of new thrombi while the existing thrombus is lysed naturally by fibrinolysis. Oral warfarin (Coumadin) and parenterally administered heparin have been the mainstays of anticoagulant therapy since the 1940s. Even though it is well known that these medications are effective, they have several undesirable characteristics, such as unpredictability in dosage required for therapeutic effect, the need for careful laboratory monitoring, and the potential for life-threatening toxicity.

Acute deep vein thrombosis (DVT) is treated with continuous intravenous heparin or injected low-molecular-weight heparin (LMWH). Heparin is normally administered according to the blood levels of activated partial thromboplastin time (aPPT or PTT), which is maintained at either more than 60 seconds or at a level 1.5 to 2.5 times a baseline established before the beginning of therapy. Heparin is usually infused in the range of 700 to 1400 units/hr. When the client has marked elevated PTT levels, frequent assessment of bleeding or bruising and institution of bleeding precautions are important. Bleeding precautions include avoidance of injections, brushing teeth with a soft sponge device, supervision with ambulation to prevent falls, and increasing intake of fiber and fluids to prevent straining and constipation. Heparin has a short half-life of 4 hours and can be quickly reversed with protamine. Heparin has increased effects when simultaneously administered with other anticoagulants. Therefore a full list of prescribed and over-the-counter medications must be reviewed for potential drug-drug interactions.

LMWH has been available for the past decade. LMWHs are longer acting, homogeneous molecules, with a reliable dose-response curve requiring little or no monitoring, but they are much more expensive than heparin. The action of heparin and the LMWHs are similar. Both bind to antithrombin III, increasing its activity and inhibiting thrombin and other factors. Whereas the anticoagulant function of heparin can be measured through PTT, no such blood test is available for LMWH. This may seem like a drawback for LMWHs, but the reason that standard heparin therapy must be monitored is because heparin has an unpredictable bioavailability and pharmacokinetics, particularly when administered subcutaneously. LMWHs, however, have extremely high bioavailability. The same bleeding precautions and drug-drug interactions apply with LMWH.

Coumadin (warfarin or coumarin) is an oral anticoagulant. It is often used as a long-term anticoagulant after the acute DVT has been treated with injectable forms of heparin. Coumadin has a long half-life (3 to 5 days). Therefore the drug must be stopped for 3 days before any invasive procedure is done. Coumadin is prescribed based on International Normalized Ratio (INR) levels, the recommended therapeutic range is 2 to 2.5. Coumadin can also be prescribed based on prothrombin (ProTime) levels, but there is variation from one laboratory to another, so INR levels are becoming more common, especially with long-term use of warfarin (Coumadin). For hospitalized clients, warfarin (Coumadin) is administered in the afternoon or early evening. This schedule allows for dose adjustments based on daily INR or ProTime results. Warfarin (Coumadin) can be reversed with injections of vitamin K (phytonadione). The therapeutic effect of warfarin (Coumadin) is altered by a host of medications and foods, and in clients with liver disease. Potential drug-drug and drug-food interactions should be reviewed by a pharmacist if the intended response (e.g., changes in INR) is not seen as predicted.

Prevention of Deep Vein Thrombosis

Several medications can be used to prevent DVT. Standard heparin is increased by adjusting the dose to maintain the aPTT ratio in the upper normal range. An average dose is 5000 units given subcutaneously in the abdomen twice daily. LMWH is also given subcutaneously. Subcutaneous injection of anticoagulants can lead to bruising at the injection sites. Clients and families should be taught that this is an expected response and does not indicate active bleeding. The development of painful masses in the abdomen should be reported and may indicate more active bleeding.

The use of antiplatelet drugs, aspirin, and nonsteroidal anti-inflammatory drugs may have a place in the prevention of DVT postoperatively or once conventional anticoagulant therapy for DVT has been concluded, although there is still debate on this topic.

---

bleeding in the urine, tarry or frank blood in the stool, bleeding with brushing the teeth, easy subcutaneous bruising, and flank pain.

Monitor for Pulmonary Embolism. PE is an acute and potentially lethal complication of DVT. Tachypnea is the most common manifestation of PE. Pleuritic chest pain can also occur. It is often sudden and aggravated by breathing. Pleuritic pain is caused by an inflammatory reaction of the lung parenchyma or by pulmonary in-

farction or ischemia caused by obstruction of small pulmonary arterial branches.

Other clinical manifestations may include cough without bringing up blood, diaphoresis, dyspnea, crackles, wheezing, and apprehension. Hemoptysis can occur as a result of pulmonary infarction or atelectasis may produce alveolar hemorrhage. Because of the seriousness of PE, promptly notify the physician of these clinical manifestations. Document the lack of manifestations or PE in clients with DVT to provide evidence of monitoring for the condition. PE is fully discussed in Chapter 63.

■ Surgical Management

Surgical treatment of thrombophlebitis is aimed at reducing PE by inserting a filter into the vena cava to filter the blood before it reaches the lungs (see Chapter 63). Thrombectomy can also be performed, but it is not common.

■ Self-Care

Prevention is the key to managing DVT. Therefore teach the client about risk factors of DVT and how to avoid them. Continue teaching with explanations of medications being taken, actions, doses, timing, adverse effects, and importance of monitoring coagulation status. Begin teaching on the first day of heparinization, discussing reasons for anticoagulants. Clients need to know who to contact and how to reach a health care provider in case problems develop. Inform the client about the monitoring required while on anticoagulation.

After thrombosis of a deep calf vein, clients should wear elastic support for at least 3 to 6 months and probably for life. Elastic support compresses the superficial veins when the client walks, and blood flow in the larger veins is increased while venous pressure is kept to a minimum. Standing and sitting are not allowed for long periods during the acute phase so as not to increase the hydrostatic pressure in the capillaries, which promotes edema. Encourage walking and exercises in bed to decrease venous pressure and promote blood flow.

CHRONIC VENOUS DISORDERS

VARICOSE VEINS

Varicose veins are permanently distended veins that develop from the loss of valvular competence. Faulty valves elevate venous pressure causing distention and tortuosity of the superficial veins. The greater and lesser saphenous veins and perforator veins in the ankle are common sites of varicosities.

Varicose veins may be either primary or secondary. Primary varicose veins often result from a congenital or familial predisposition that leads to loss of elasticity of the vein wall. Secondary varicosities occur when trauma, obstruction, DVT, or inflammation causes damage to valves.

Varicose veins affect a large percentage of the adult population. An estimated 24 million Americans have varicose veins. The prevalence increases with age and peaks between the fifth and sixth decades of life. Varicose veins are more common in women; however, the gender ratio decreases with advancing age and almost disappears in clients older than 70 years. Prolonged standing has been implicated as a cause of varicose veins, but epidemiologic studies have not demonstrated an association between standing at work and an increased incidence of varicose veins.

Clients with varicose veins often complain of aching, a feeling of heaviness in the legs, itching, moderate swelling, and, frequently, the unsightly appearance of their legs. Severity of discomfort is difficult to assess and does not seem related to the size of varicosities. A superficial inflammation may occasionally develop along the path of the varicose vein. To assess for varicose veins, carefully examine both of the client's legs in good lighting. Varicosities appear as dilated, tortuous skin veins (Figure 55-13).

Outcome Management
■ Medical Management

In early stages of varicose veins, the goal is to reduce venous pooling, prevent complications, and improve comfort levels. The simplest form of treatment is the application of below-the-knee compression stockings or elastic wraps. These stockings are designed to apply the greatest amount of pressure over the ankle.

■ Nursing Management of the Medical Client

The client should be taught that varicose veins are a chronic problem. Even though they do not subside,

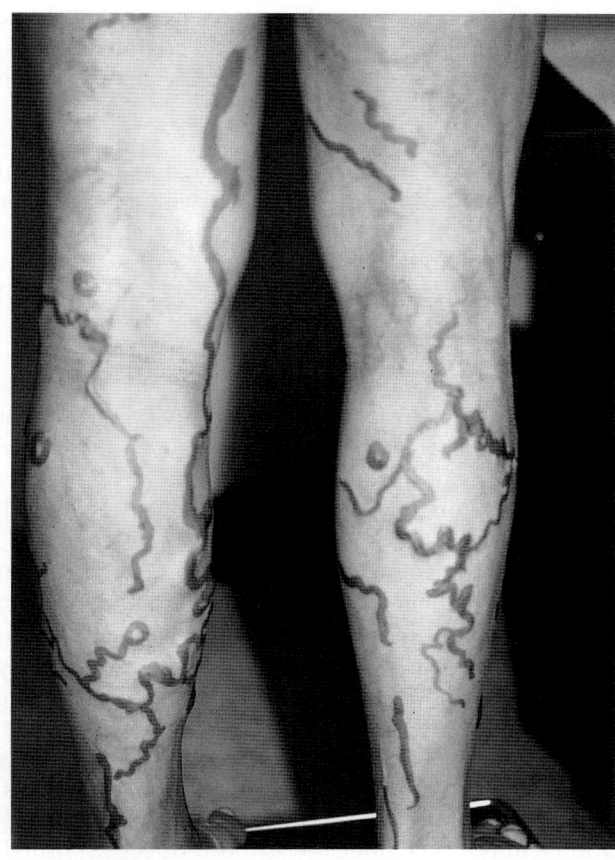

FIGURE 55-13 Varicose veins marked with a pen on the legs. Note the tortuous pattern.

various activities can help prevent ulceration or new varicosities. The client should avoid standing still in one position for extended periods of time. Legs should be elevated when seated and, if swelling is present, legs should be elevated higher than the heart. Elastic stockings or support hose should be worn to help with venous blood return. Fitting elastic stockings is important. Many clients with venous disease have misshapen legs and standard stockings do not fit them well, being too tight in the ankle. Custom stockings may be needed. Elastic wraps need to be wrapped twice daily so that that greatest pressure is at the ankle, with lesser pressure gradually applied to the level of the knee.

■ Surgical Management

Sclerotherapy. Sclerotherapy is the injection of a sclerosing agent into varicose veins. The agent damages the vein and endothelium, causing an aseptic thrombosis that closes the vein. Application of pressure causes the vein walls to grow together. Sclerotherapy is usually performed for cosmetic reasons, but it may relieve the discomfort of both short segments of varicosities and spider veins. It is most effective in closing small, residual varicosities after surgical intervention for varicose veins. (Sclerotherapy is contraindicated before such surgery, because it makes vein stripping more difficult.) Within minutes after injection of the sclerosing agent, elastic compression and active walking should commence. Elastic bandages are worn for 1 to 3 weeks, from morning to night (but not 24 hours a day).

Vein Ligation and Stripping. Surgical management of varicose veins consists of ligation (tying off) of the greater saphenous vein with its tributaries at the saphenofemoral junction, combined with removal of the saphenous vein (stripping) and ligation of incompetent perforator veins. Removal of the vein is performed through multiple, short incisions. An incision is made at the ankle over the saphenous vein and a nylon wire is threaded up the vein to the groin. The wire is brought out through the groin, capped, and then the wire and vein are pulled out through the ankle incision. If the perforator veins alone are ligated, it may be done through multiple small endoscopic incisions.

Elastic compression bandages are applied from foot to groin. The client is rarely hospitalized overnight. Complications are infrequent and include bleeding, infection, and nerve damage. Hemorrhage most commonly occurs at the surgical wound site in the groin. Bleeding comes primarily from the stripped canal. The risk of serious bleeding can be decreased by carefully wrapping the leg from foot to groin and by applying compression, especially to the upper thigh and groin. Some discoloration and bruising along the stripped tract are normal.

Saphenous nerve damage may occur with surgery. In the distal third of the leg, the saphenous nerve runs close to the saphenous vein. Thus risk of nerve injury increases when the distal part of the vein is involved. DVT, embolism, and infection are rare following varicose vein surgery, especially if postoperative precautions (e.g., bandaging, movement, exercise) are taken.

Saphenofemoral Ligation. Some clients require only tying off of the junction of the saphenous and the femoral vein at the groin. This involves one short incision, often local anesthesia, and no hospital stay. Postoperative care is the same.

■ Nursing Management of the Surgical Client

Routine postoperative assessment and care are provided. Specific care includes maintaining firm elastic pressure over the whole limb, reducing the risk of thrombophlebitis by promoting regular movement and exercise of the legs, and improving venous return by elevating the foot of the bed 6 to 9 inches so that the legs are above the heart level when the client is in bed. The client ambulates for short periods, starting immediately after surgery. Clients should walk rather than stand or sit. After ambulation, elevate the client's legs again.

CHRONIC VENOUS INSUFFICIENCY

Chronic venous insufficiency is also known as *postphlebitic syndrome* and follows most severe cases of DVT. Chronic venous insufficiency results from dysfunctional valves that reduce venous return, which thus increases venous pressure and causes venous stasis. Because existing valves are destroyed, venous blood flow is bidirectional, resulting in inefficient venous outflow. The net effect of this change is that the weight of the venous blood column from the right atrium is transmitted along the full length of the veins. Very high venous pressure is exerted at the ankle and the venules become the final pathway for the highest venous pressure. The current theory is that the abnormal capillaries lead to extravasation of red cells, activation of endothelial cells, and white cell trapping. The end result is capillary thrombosis. Skin ulcerations also occur.

Chronic venous insufficiency is marked by the following characteristics:

- Chronically swollen legs
- Thick, coarse, brownish skin around the ankles (referred to as the "gaiter" area)
- Venous stasis ulceration (Figure 55-14)
- Itchy, scaly skin

Management

Goals of management are to increase venous blood return and to decrease venous pressure. Antigravity measures increase blood return to the heart. They include elevating the client's legs above the heart level and avoiding prolonged standing or sitting. Advise the client to avoid the following:

- Crossing the legs

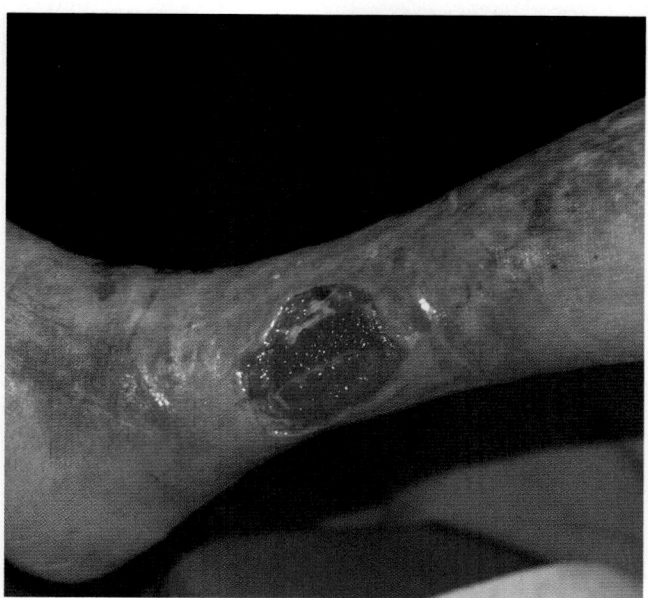

FIGURE 55-14 Venous stasis ulcers usually develop in the lower outer leg, appear irregular, and have a beefy red base. Note the dark stained skin from venous disease.

- Sitting in chairs that are too high to allow the feet to touch the floor or that are too deep (and press on the popliteal area)
- Wearing garters or tightly rolled socks or stockings
- Sources of pressure above the legs (e.g., tight girdles)

Encourage the client to sleep with the foot of the bed elevated 6 inches. At least one third of every 24 hours should be spent with the feet and legs elevated above the heart.

The Bridge to Home Health Care feature on Managing Peripheral Vascular Disease on p. 1542 describes how increased venous pressure on the tissues of the leg can be counteracted by the compression of elastic support hose. Ideally, this support should just balance the increased venous pressure. Thus hose should be fitted individually to the client's legs. Measurements of the ankle and calf circumference and from 1 inch below the knee or 1 inch below the groin to the bottom of the foot are usually taken. Measure after the client has been recumbent and leg edema is minimal. Stockings that extend above the knee often bind the popliteal space and act as a tourniquet, especially when the knee is bent. Knee-length elastic stockings are preferable. Elastic wraps are often preferable for clients who have periods of leg swelling. Apply the elastic wrap using a graded technique, placing more tension on the lower leg. The problem with elastic wraps is that they only maintain their elastic properties for a few washings (with a few exceptions), and clients tend to use them long past their effective compression. Additionally, wraps often are not used properly and do not exert adequate compression.

VENOUS STASIS ULCERATION

Venous stasis ulceration is the end stage of chronic venous insufficiency. Prolonged venous pressure slows nutrient blood flow, which deprives cells of needed oxygen, glucose, and other substances. Skin of the lower legs ulcerates, causing a stasis ulcer, which occurs as a result of stasis of blood. It is characteristically located in the malleolar or gaiter (lower third of the leg) area (see Figure 55-14). It is important to determine the cause of the ulcer before beginning treatment. Determining whether arterial disease is present is imperative; compression devices are contraindicated in arterial disease because they can restrict arterial inflow of blood.

Management of venous stasis ulceration includes leg elevation, wound care, moist dressings, and support stockings. Gravity is the major enemy of venous stasis disease. The client should rest with his or her legs elevated 6 inches. Regular walking is encouraged.

When ulcers are present, cultures are often obtained of painful, odorous, or weeping wounds to rule out infection. Antibiotics may be required to treat infection or cellulitis. Local wound care is essential and should be provided by a health care provider familiar with the disease process. Some ulcers require debridement of eschar (see Chapter 16).

To clean the ulcer, use normal saline. Clean the dry scaly skin around the ulcer and on the leg with saline or mild soaps. Gently clean the area and apply a lanolin-containing lotion every day to keep skin moist and supple. Avoid lotions containing alcohol and perfumes because they dry and irritate the skin. Protect granulation tissue with saline gel dressings or antibiotic ointments. Cover with a nonadherent dressing that does not accumulate heat or humidity at the wound bed. Monitor for sensitivity to topical agents, seen as blistering, itching, and erythema on the treated areas. If the ulcer is large and heavily exuding, more frequent dressing changes, with absorptive dressings, are required.

No topical treatment is adequate without compression. Graduated compression systems, with adequate padding capable of sustaining compression for at least a week, should be the first line of treatment for uncomplicated venous leg ulcers with an ABI ≥0.8. Stockings are the easiest to apply, although soiling may be a problem. In addition, stockings do not fit abnormally shaped legs or those clients with dressings over the ulcer. Elastic wraps can be adjusted for size. Elastic wraps must be wrapped with the most tension at the foot and ankle and rewrapped twice daily.

An Unna boot is a popular form of bandage impregnated with calamine, zinc oxide, and glycerin. When wrapped snugly around the leg, it provides excellent compression during ambulation and applies minimal pressure during limb elevation. An Unna boot is a permeable dressing that can be applied directly over skin ulcers, thereby allowing drainage of exudate. It creates a

---

BRIDGE TO HOME HEALTH CARE
Managing Peripheral Vascular Disease

Many clients who are referred to home health agencies or clinics that serve older people have peripheral vascular disease. Consider what you can do to help clients prevent further complications through assessment and evaluation, blood pressure monitoring, health education, and reporting changes in your clients' status to their physicians.

Assessment

Inspect clients for temperature variations; color changes in the skin; dorsal and ankle foot pulses; extremity size comparisons; shiny, taunt, hairless, or blistered skin; diminished toenail growth and color change; pain with palpation, dependent position, or weight-bearing; and skin breakdown and ulcerations. As part of the assessment, measure the calves, ankles, and feet correctly, as the involved areas of edema indicate. Use a monofilament (thin plastic filament) test for sensation and dorsiflexion and plantiflexion of the great toe (proprioception), especially for diabetic clients. The loss of touch sensation may require special foot protection. The loss of proprioception of the foot (position perception) indicates the need to discourage or stop driving. For many clients, this news is very traumatic. You may want to discuss this safety recommendation with a family member or significant other. Be prepared to problem-solve transportation alternatives.

Use the correct cuff size when monitoring the blood pressure. You may need to travel with a child, adult, and large cuff or have all sizes in the clinics. For consistency, document the cuff size and position. Discuss the benefits of self-monitoring devices with clients. Because clients may have decreased hand strength or arthritis, they may have difficulty pumping the bulb of a par-

tially automatic cuff. Fully automatic, one-button devices are reasonably accurate and may be better options. When your clients have checkups, suggest that they take their blood pressure equipment along and compare their readings with those obtained at the clinic. Instruct them to record and share their list of self-recorded measurements with you and their physician, a strategy that is helpful for blood pressure management.

Education

Health education is an essential component of the care you provide. It is important for clients to avoid smoking, wearing constrictive clothing, and applying excessive heat to their extremities. Clients need information about elevating their legs and performing daily foot hygiene. They may be able to reduce lower extremity edema by wearing properly fitted antiembolic hose or compression socks (Sigvarus or TEDS); home health clients need physicians' orders. Before ready-made compression socks are bought, measure the heel to knee or heel to thigh and the largest calf circumference; the cost ranges from $8 to $15. Before purchasing custom-ordered antiembolic socks, clients need a prescription and are measured by a supply company; these socks cost up to several hundred dollars. Clients need to exercise caution when using compression socks. Most ready-made ones lose significant compression after 6 to 12 months and need to be replaced. When possible, use the "open toe" design to prevent excess pressure on the toes, especially with diabetic clients. The nylon content in these socks causes moisture retention and leads to skin maceration in clients who have poor circulation. The socks should not be worn around-the-clock.

---

moist and warm interface between the ulcerated skin and the bandage. It can be changed on a weekly or biweekly basis; the client wears the boot without interruption and thereby improves compliance. Disadvantages of the Unna boot include allergy, skin irritation, discomfort, difficulty in bathing, and pain while changing the boot. The Unna boot has been shown to achieve healing rates of 70%.

Skin grafting is rarely necessary to achieve healing. Surgery to remove incompetent varicose veins or incompetent perforator veins may also be necessary.

LYMPHATIC DISORDERS
LYMPHEDEMA

Lymphedema is an accumulation of lymphatic fluid in the interstitial tissue that causes swelling, most often in

the arms or legs, and occasionally in other parts of the body. Lymphedema can develop when lymphatic vessels are missing or impaired (primary), or when lymph vessels are damaged or lymph nodes removed (secondary). Lymphedema should not be confused with edema resulting from venous insufficiency, which is not lymphedema.

When the impairment becomes so great that the lymphatic fluid exceeds the lymphatic transport capacity, an abnormal amount of protein-rich fluid collects in the tissues of the affected area. Left untreated, this stagnant, protein-rich fluid not only causes tissue channels to increase in size and number, but also reduces oxygen availability in the transport system, interferes with wound healing, and provides a culture medium for bacteria that can result in lymphangitis (infection).

Primary lymphedema may be classified according to age at onset: congenital (present at birth), praecox

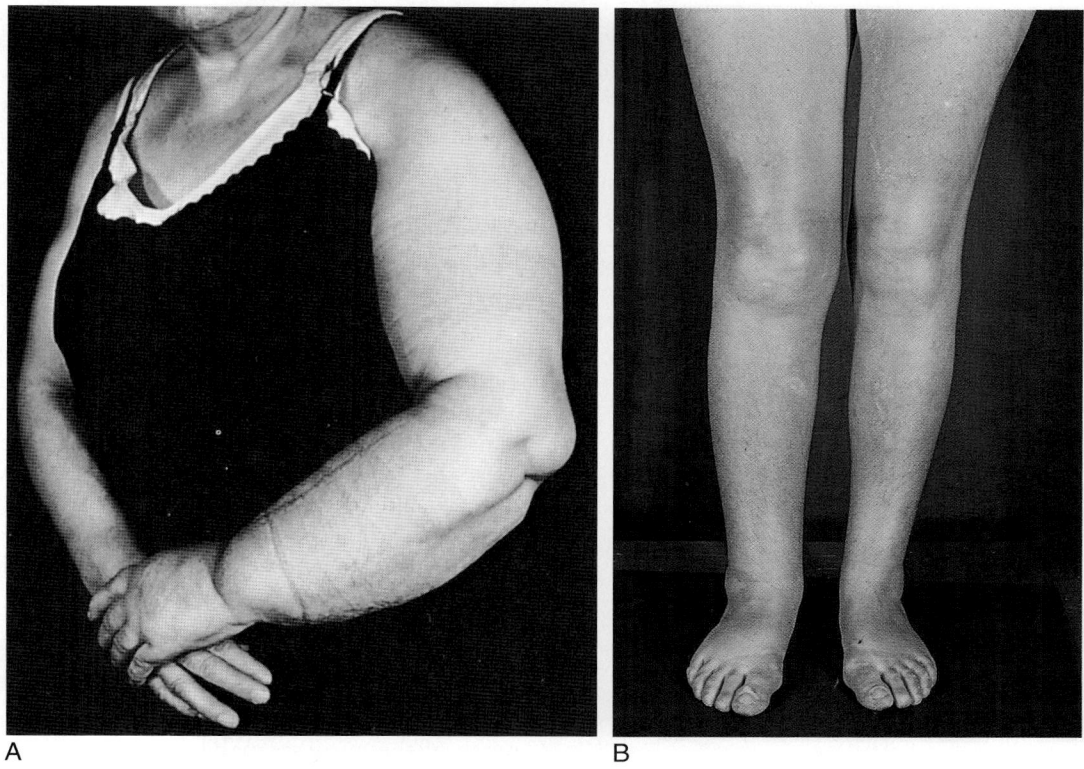

FIGURE 55-15 Types of lymphedema. **A,** Secondary lymphedema of the arm following mastectomy. **B,** Primary lymphedema.

(before age 35 years), or tarda (after age 35 years). Congenital and familial lymphedema is also called *Milroy's disease.* It is inherited as an autosomal dominant trait.

Secondary lymphedema occurs because of some damage or obstruction to the lymph system by another disease process or by a procedure: trauma, neoplasms (primary or metastatic), filariasis, inflammation, surgical excision, or high doses of radiation. Postoperative lymphedema is usually seen after surgical excision of axillary, inguinal, or iliac nodes. These operations are usually performed as a prophylactic or therapeutic treatment for metastatic tumor. For example, lymphedema of the arm is encountered after mastectomy (Figure 55-15, *A*). Radiation in moderate amounts does not appear to damage the lymph vessels. However, heavy radiation for a particularly resistant tumor usually leads to lymphatic obstruction.

Of the primary forms, lymphedema praecox encompasses the largest group of clients; it peaks in the teenage years and is more common in females than in males. The edema usually appears spontaneously and without known cause (see Figure 55-15, *B*).

Filariasis, caused by the filarial nematode *Wuchereria bancrofti* (and others), is one of the most common diseases in undeveloped nations; it is transmitted by mosquitoes from human to human. The living embryos (mi-crofilariae) of the adult worms are found in the bloodstream. The larvae migrate to the lymphatics, where they mature into adult worms. Adult worms in the lymph nodes and lymphatics lead to obstruction, lymphedema, and elephantiasis.

Lymphedema secondary to neoplasms in the lymph nodes is common. The malignant disease may be primary (lymphoma or Hodgkin's disease) or metastatic from another site.

Clinical Manifestations

Primary lymphedema presents as bilateral mild edema of ankles and legs in women at puberty or shortly after puberty, unilateral edema of the entire leg in men and women (Figure 55-16), or bilateral edema present at birth or early age. The skin of clients with congenital lymphedema contains vesicles (blisters) filled with lymph. A dull, heavy sensation is present, but actual pain is absent. Elevation of the limb and rest in bed cause a reduction but not disappearance of the sensation. Smooth skin becomes roughened; the edema is nonpitting. Acute lymphangitis and cellulitis are infrequent. Ulceration of the skin does not occur. However, the limb becomes greatly enlarged, uncomfortable, and unsightly (see Figure 55-16). Lymphedema can be diagnosed with isotopic lymphography, lymphangiography, and phlebography.

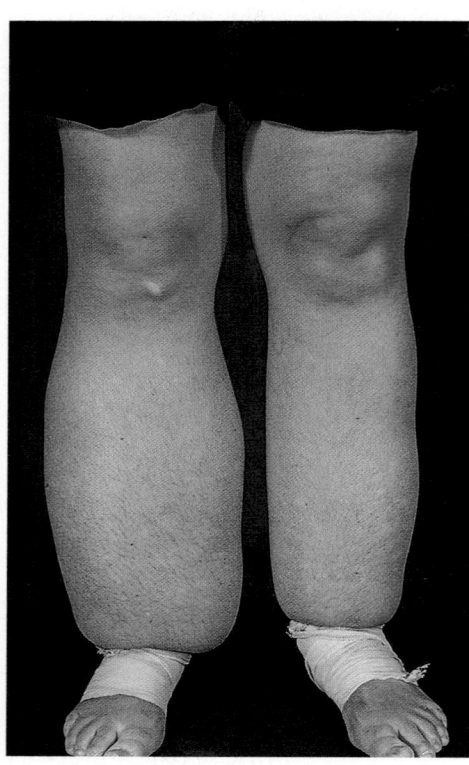

FIGURE 55-16 Severe lymphedema. The client's feet were bandaged so that shoes could be worn.

Management

There is no known cure for lymphedema once the swelling appears. The goal of treatment is to remove as much fluid as possible from the affected extremity and to maintain as normal-appearing an extremity as possible.

Physical therapy for arm or leg lymphedema involves mechanical or manual squeezing of the tissue in order to press the stagnant lymphatic fluid to the proximal part of the limb. This is followed by specific active and passive exercises to transport the lymph farther into the lymphatic system and finally into the bloodstream. Many pneumatic pumping devices for intermittent compression are available. Diuretics may also be prescribed. Elastic stockings or sleeves are used to maintain the effects of the pneumatic pump.

To reduce the swelling, the extremity is elevated above the right atrium. Pneumatic pumps may be used to reduce the extremity size. If pumps are used, teach the client how to apply the device, the frequency of application, and the reasons for its use. When stockings are used, ascertain that the stockings fit and do not gather behind the knee. Activity such as walking, rather than sitting or standing, should be promoted. For bedridden clients, teach bed exercises to promote venous and lymphatic return and to maintain muscle strength.

The client with lymphedema is at high risk for infection. The affected extremity is monitored for clinical manifestations of infection such as redness, warmth, and pain. Meticulous skin care is given to the extremity using mild soaps and lotions. Skin should be gently dried, especially between creases of skin. Nails are kept trimmed. Skin should be lubricated to maintain its suppleness; avoid using products with alcohol, dyes, lanolin, mineral oil, petroleum products, talc, or perfumes. Chemical hair removers and regular razors are not used. If shaving is desired, a well-maintained electric razor should be used. Hot water should be avoided.

Clients with lymphedema may suffer from disturbances in self-concept because of the visibility of their deformity. Encourage the client to discuss these feelings and help the client understand that such feelings are normal. Variations in clothing style may be suggested to disguise the deformity. When caring for clients with lymph disorders, remember that these clients must cope with difficult, chronic diseases. Take time to give emotional support to the client and the family. Emphasize the possible need for lifelong follow-up.

CONCLUSIONS

Clients with vascular diseases can challenge a broad range of the nurse's capability and skill, from monitoring a client with rupture of an abdominal aortic aneurysm in an intensive care unit, to performing and teaching meticulous foot care, to educating and counseling a client to make significant lifestyle changes. Vascular diseases involve a broad spectrum of arterial, venous, and lymphatic problems. Nursing care for clients with arterial disorders centers on promoting circulation and adequate tissue perfusion, protecting against skin breakdown and injury, managing pain, and encouraging positive lifestyle changes. Limb amputation requires particularly sensitive assessment, teaching, and counseling skills. Nursing care for clients with venous disorders focuses on monitoring therapeutic regimens such as thrombolytic therapy, controlling and preventing thrombus formation, and promoting circulation by increasing venous blood return and decreasing venous pressure. Nursing care for lymphedema is palliative.

THINKING CRITICALLY *evolve*

1. The client is admitted to the hospital for the care of leg ulcers. He is homeless and usually wanders the streets, sleeping on external heating grates in the sidewalk. He has large, irregularly shaped ulcers covered with thick, yellow, devitalized tissue. The ulcers are weeping and his stockings have adhered to the ulcers. What type of ulcers are present? What type of wound care will he need? How can he continue to do wound care after discharge?

Factors to Consider. How are arterial and venous ulcers distinguished? Is it important to remove the devitalized tissue? If so, how? How does his lifestyle influence his recovery?

2. A middle-aged man enters the emergency department with complaints of a painful leg. The pain began about 3 hours before he noted a very rapid heartbeat. You note that his leg and foot are cold and white. What may have happened? What other factors need to be addressed in relation to his leg? What are the possible treatments available? What might his post-hospital instructions include?

Factors to Consider. How do you determine the acuteness of the tissue insult? What are the potential outcomes if you delay treatment? What might be the source of emboli, and how can this be assessed?

Discussions for these questions can be found on the website and the CD-ROM.

BIBLIOGRAPHY

1. Aquila, A.M. (2001). Deep venous thrombosis. *Journal of Cardiovascular Nursing 15* (4), 25-44.
2. Bryant, C., et al. (2002). Abdominal aortic aneurysm repair: A look at the first 24 hours. *Journal of Perianesthesia Nursing 17* (3), 164-169.
3. Ennis, W.J., & Meneses, P. (2003). Standard, appropriate and advanced care and medical-legal considerations: Venous ulcerations. *Wounds 15* (4), 107-122.
4. Falanga, V. (1997). Venous ulceration: assessment, classification and management. In D. Krasner & D. Kane (Eds.), *Chronic wound care* (2nd ed., pp. 165-171). Wayne, PA: Health Management Publications, Inc.
5. Frost-Rude, J.A., et al. (2000). Buerger's disease. *Journal of Vascular Nursing 18* (4), 128-130.
6. Hafner, J., et al. (2000). Leg ulcers in peripheral arterial disease: Impaired wound healing above the threshold of chronic critical limb ischemia. *Journal of the American Academy of Dermatology 43* (6), 1001-1008.
7. Hayes, J.M. (2002). Graduated compression stockings: Updating practice, improving compliance. *MedSurg Nursing 11* (4), 163-166.
8. Holloway, G.A. (1997). Arterial ulcers: assessment, classification and management. In D. Krasner & D. Kane (Eds.), *Chronic wound care* (2nd ed., pp. 158-164). Wayne, PA: Health Management Publications, Inc.
9. Lewis, C.D. (2001). Peripheral arterial disease of the lower extremity. *Journal of Cardiovascular Nursing, 15*(4), 45-63.
10. Jones, M.A., et al. (2000). Endovascular grafting for repair of abdominal aortic aneurysm. *Critical Care Nurse 20* (4), 38-48.
11. Nelson E.A., et al. (2003). Compression for preventing recurrence of venous ulcers. *Cochrane Review The Cochrane Library,* (2). Oxford: Update Software.
12. Rudolph, D. (2001). Standards of care for venous leg ulcers: Compression therapy and moist wound healing. *Journal of Vascular Nursing 19* (1), 20-27.
13. Treat-Jacobson, D. (2003). Treating patients with peripheral arterial disease and claudication. *Journal of Vascular Nursing 21* (1), 5-14.

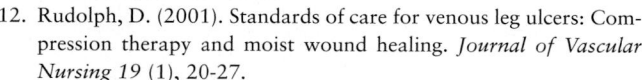

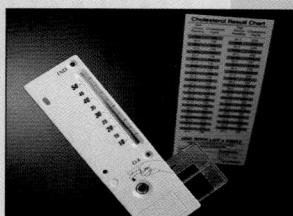

Unit 13

Cardiac Disorders

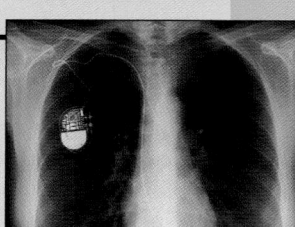

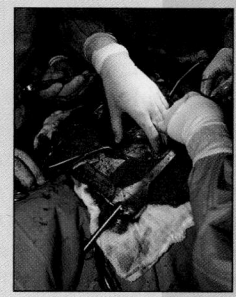

Anatomy and Physiology Review

The Heart

Robert G. Carroll

The human heart, through rhythmic contraction, provides the pressure necessary to propel blood through the body. Blood flow is essential to deliver nutrients to the tissues of the body and to transport metabolic wastes, including heat, to removal sites. The presence of an arterial pulse, caused by the beating of the heart, is appropriately designated as a vital sign.

The heart weighs about 300 g and is located within the mediastinum; it is cone-shaped and tilted forward and to the left. Because of its orientation during fetal development, the apex of the heart (tip of the cone) is at its bottom and lies left of the midline. The base is at the top, where the great vessels enter the heart, and lies posterior to the sternum. The heart consists of four chambers: two smaller atria at the top (the base) of the heart and two larger ventricles at the apex. A band of fibrous tissue separates the atria from the ventricles and seats the four cardiac valves. A muscular septum separates the right from the left atrium and the right from the left ventricle. Table U13-1 describes the basic structures and their functions.

Functionally, the heart is actually two pumps working simultaneously (Figure U13-1). The right atrium and right ventricle generate the pressure to propel the oxygen-poor blood through the pulmonic circulation; the left atrium and left ventricle propel oxygen-rich blood to the remainder of the body through the systemic circulation. At rest, each side of the heart pumps approximately 5000 ml (5 L) of blood per minute *(cardiac output)*. This is accomplished by a contraction frequency *(heart rate)* of 72 beats/min, with each contraction ejecting a volume of 70 ml *(stroke volume)* into the arterial system. Cardiac output can increase five-fold during exercise as a result of increases in both heart rate and stroke volume.

STRUCTURE OF THE HEART
LAYERS OF THE HEART

The heart consists of three distinct layers of tissue: endocardium, myocardium, and epicardium (Figure U13-2, *inset*). The *endocardium* (innermost layer) consists of thin endothelial tissue lining the inner chambers and the heart valves. The *myocardium* (middle layer) consists of striated muscle fibers forming interlaced bundles and is the actual contracting muscle of the heart. The *epicardium* or *visceral pericardium* covers the outer surface of the heart. It closely adheres to the heart and to the first several centimeters of the pulmonary artery and aorta.

The visceral pericardium is encased by the *parietal pericardium,* a tough, loose-fitting, fibrous outer membrane that is attached anteriorly to the lower half of the sternum, posteriorly to the thoracic vertebrae and inferiorly to the diaphragm. Between the visceral pericardium and the parietal pericardium is the *pericardial space,* which holds 5 to 20 ml of pericardial fluid. This fluid lubricates the pericardial surfaces as they slide over each other when the heart beats. Excessive fluid accumulation in the pericardial space can diminish the filling of the ventricles *(cardiac tamponade)*.

CHAMBERS OF THE HEART

The heart consists of four chambers: two upper collecting chambers *(atria)* and two lower pumping chambers *(ventricles)* (see Figure U13-2). A muscular wall *(septum)* separates the chambers of the right side from those of the left side. The *right atrium* receives deoxygenated blood from the body. The blood moves to the *right ventricle*, which pumps it to the lungs against low resistance. The *left atrium* receives oxygenated blood from the lungs. The blood flows into the *left ventricle* (the heart's largest, most muscular chamber), which pumps it against high resistance into the systemic circulation.

CARDIAC VALVES

The cardiac valves are delicate, flexible structures that consist of endothelium covered by fibrous tissue. They permit only unidirectional blood flow through the heart. The valves open and close passively, determined by pressure gradients between the cardiac chambers (Figure U13-3). "Leaky" valves that do not seal when closed are called *regurgitant* or *insufficient*. "Stiff" valves that cannot open completely are called *stenotic*.

TABLE U13-1	*The Heart: Its Structure and Functions*
Structure	**Function**
Pericardium	Two-layered sac that encases and protects the heart
Atrium	Upper, receiving chambers of the heart
Right atrium	Receives deoxygenated systemic blood via superior and inferior vena cava; blood passes to the right ventricle
Left atrium	Receives oxygenated blood from the lungs; blood passes to the left ventricle
Ventricles	Lower, pumping chambers of the heart
Right ventricle	Receives blood from atrium via the tricuspid valve; pumps it to the pulmonary circulation
Left ventricle	Receives blood from atrium via the bicuspid (mitral) valve; pumps it to the systemic circulation
Cardiac valves	Prevent backflow of blood
Tricuspid and bicuspid (mitral) valves	Prevent backflow from right ventricle to right atrium and from left ventricle to left atrium, respectively
Semilunar valves	Prevent backflow from pulmonary artery to right ventricle *(pulmonary semilunar)* and from aorta to left ventricle *(aortic semilunar)*
Coronary arteries (common pattern)	Provide blood supply to the heart
Right coronary artery	Perfuses right atrium, right ventricle, inferior portion of the left ventricle and posterior septal wall, SA node, and AV node
Left coronary artery	
Left anterior descending artery	Supplies blood to anterior wall of left ventricle, anterior ventricular septum, and apex of left ventricle
Circumflex artery	Provides blood to left atrium, lateral and posterior surfaces of left ventricle, occasionally the posterior interventricular septum; sometimes supplies SA and AV nodes
SA node	"Pacemaker" node; initiates heartbeat by generating an electrical impulse
AV node	Normal pathway for impulses originating in the atria to be conducted to ventricles; can be a secondary pacemaker
Bundle of His, bundle branches, Purkinje's fibers	Rapidly transmit cardiac action potentials to enable synchronous contraction of ventricles

AV, Atrioventricular; *SA,* sinoatrial.

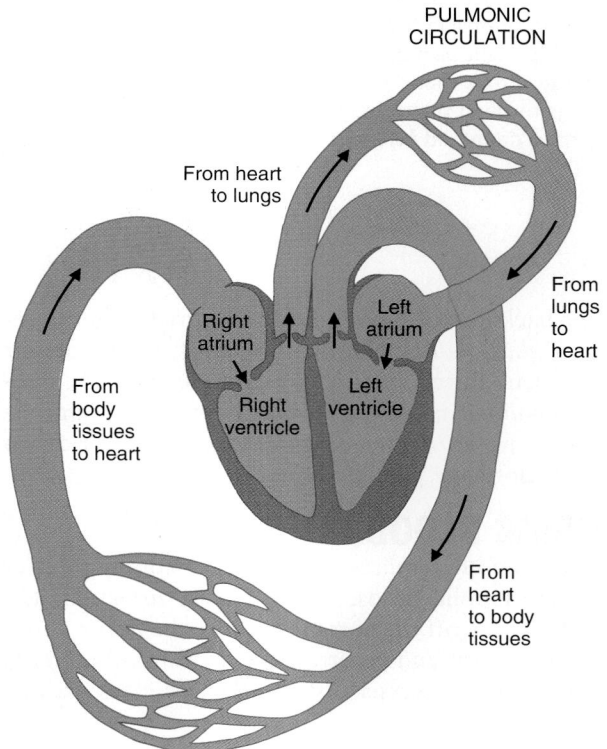

PULMONIC
CIRCULATION

From heart
to lungs

From
lungs
to
heart

Right
atrium

Left
atrium

From
body
tissues
to heart

Right
ventricle

Left
ventricle

From
heart
to body
tissues

SYSTEMIC CIRCULATION

FIGURE U13-1 Functions of the heart. In the peripheral capillaries in systemic circulation, blood oxygen is exchanged for carbon dioxide. The oxygen-poor blood returns to the right atrium and right ventricle to be pumped into the lungs, where carbon dioxide is exchanged for oxygen. Oxygen-rich blood from the lungs enters the left atrium and left ventricle of the heart to be pumped once again into the systemic circulation.

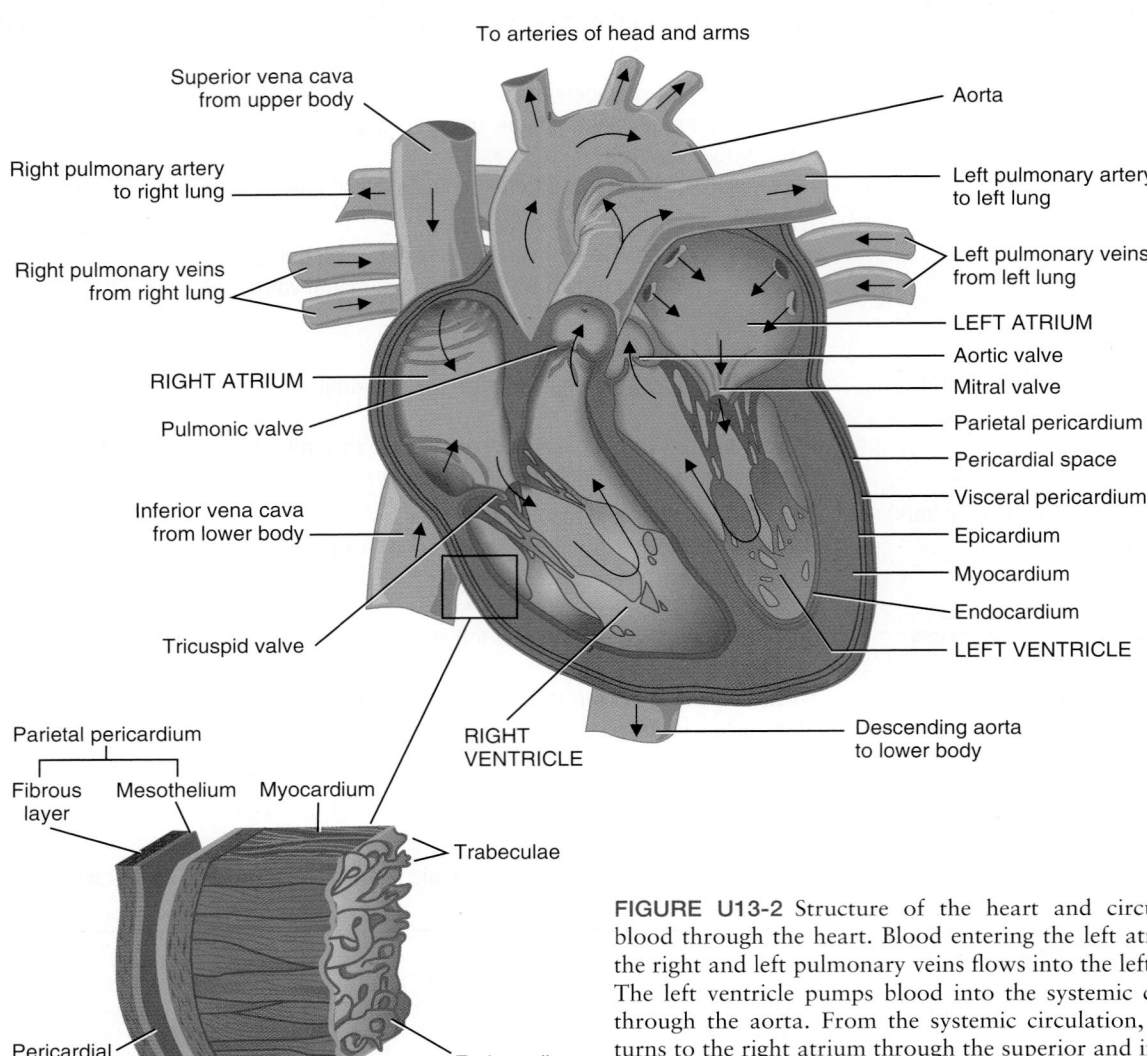

To arteries of head and arms

Superior vena cava
from upper body

Right pulmonary artery
to right lung

Right pulmonary veins
from right lung

RIGHT ATRIUM

Pulmonic valve

Inferior vena cava
from lower body

Tricuspid valve

Aorta

Left pulmonary artery
to left lung

Left pulmonary veins
from left lung

LEFT ATRIUM

Aortic valve

Mitral valve

Parietal pericardium

Pericardial space

Visceral pericardium

Epicardium

Myocardium

Endocardium

LEFT VENTRICLE

Descending aorta
to lower body

RIGHT
VENTRICLE

Parietal pericardium

Fibrous
layer

Mesothelium

Myocardium

Trabeculae

Pericardial
space

Endocardium

Mesothelium

Fibrous
layer

Visceral pericardium
(Epicardium)

FIGURE U13-2 Structure of the heart and circulation of blood through the heart. Blood entering the left atrium from the right and left pulmonary veins flows into the left ventricle. The left ventricle pumps blood into the systemic circulation through the aorta. From the systemic circulation, blood returns to the right atrium through the superior and inferior venae cavae. From there, the right ventricle pumps blood into the lungs through the right and left pulmonary arteries. *Inset*, The pericardium and layers of the heart.

Cardiac valves are of two types: (1) atrioventricular (AV) and (2) semilunar (see Table U13-1). *Atrioventricular valves* lie between the atria and ventricles. The *tricuspid valve,* on the right side, is composed of three leaflets. The *mitral (bicuspid) valve,* on the left, is composed of two. Attached to the edges of the AV valves are strong, fibrous filaments called *chordae tendineae,* which arise from papillary muscles on the ventricular walls. The papillary muscles and chordae tendineae work together to prevent the AV valves from bulging back into the atria during ventricular contraction *(systole).*

The *semilunar valves* consist of three cup-like cusps that open during ventricular contraction and close to prevent backflow of blood into the ventricles during relaxation *(diastole).* Unlike the AV valves, the semilunar valves open during ventricular contraction. The *pulmonic semilunar valve* (right ventricle to pulmonary artery) and the *aortic semilunar valve* (left ventricle to aorta) do not have papillary muscles.

CARDIAC BLOOD SUPPLY

The heart muscle requires a rich oxygen supply to meet its own metabolic needs. The *coronary arteries* (right and left) branch off the aorta just above the aortic valve, encircle the heart, and penetrate the myocardium (Figure U13-4). Coronary vessel distribution can vary greatly,

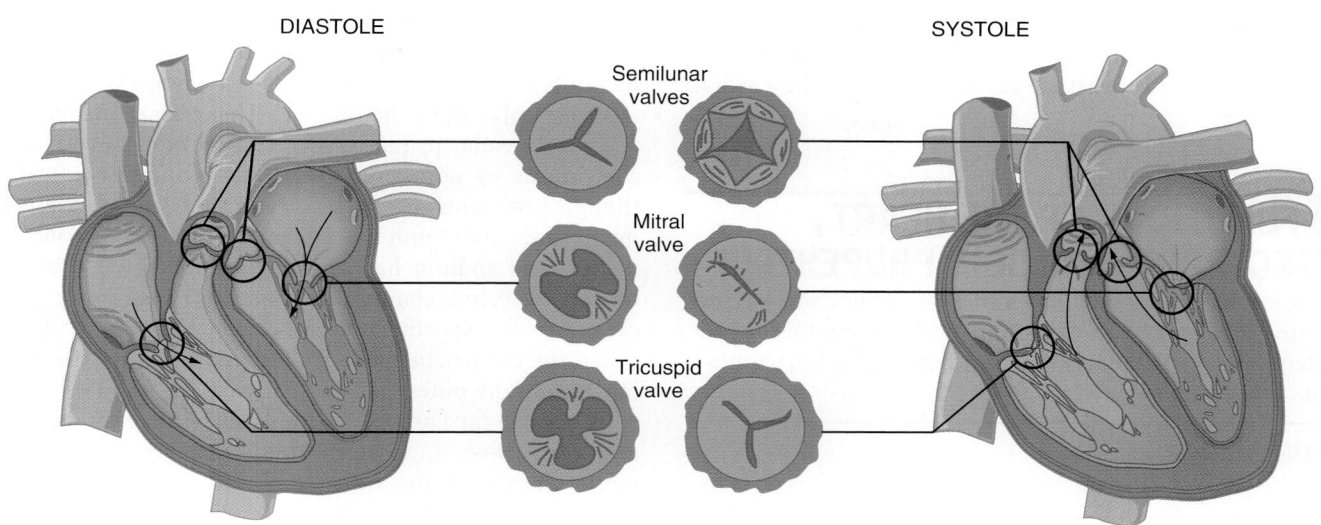

FIGURE U13-3 Valves of the heart. The semilunar, mitral, and tricuspid valves are shown as they appear during diastole, or ventricular filling *(left)*, and during systole, or ventricular emptying *(right)*.

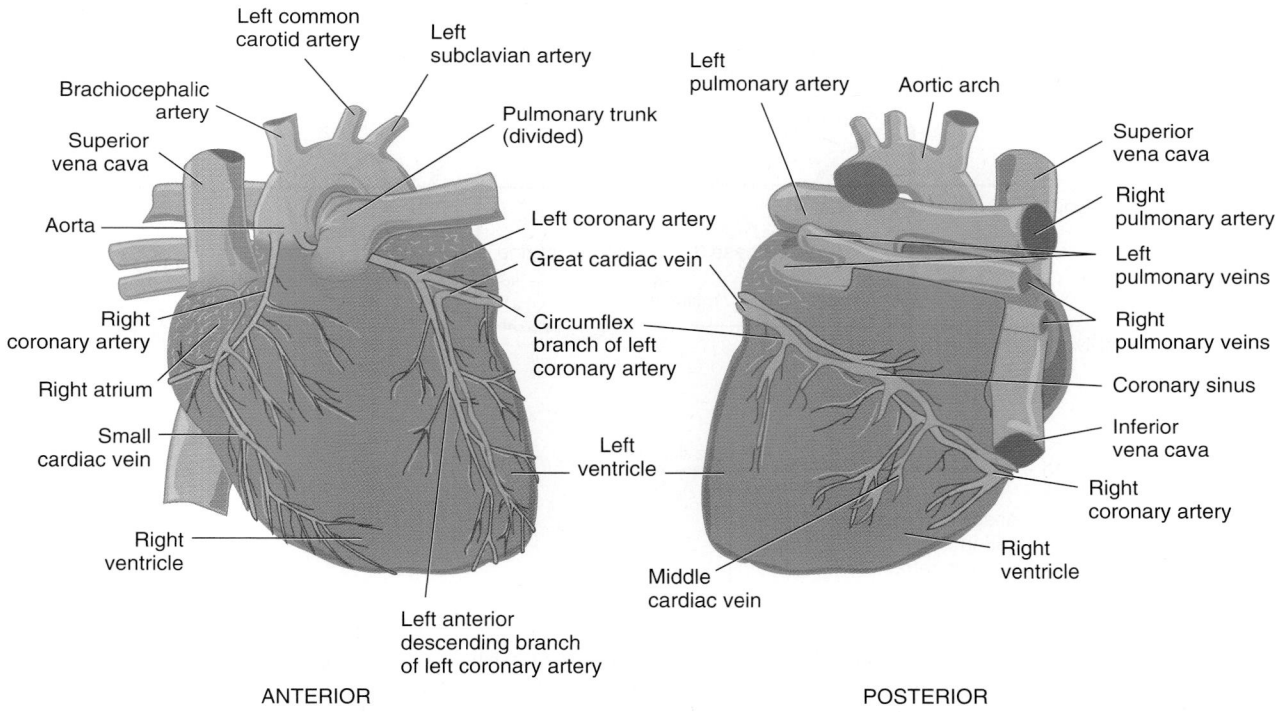

FIGURE U13-4 The coronary arteries. The right and left coronary arteries branch off the aorta just above the aortic valve; they normally supply the myocardium with oxygenated blood.

but the pattern described in Table U13-1 is the most common.

Contraction of the muscle of the left ventricle generates enough extravascular pressure to occlude the coronary blood vessels and prevent blood flow to the muscle of the heart during ventricular systole. Thus 75% of the

coronary artery blood flow occurs during diastole, when the heart is relaxed and resistance is low. For adequate blood flow through the coronary arteries, the diastolic blood pressure must be at least 60 mm Hg. Coronary blood flow increases with increased heart work load (i.e., exercise). The coronary veins return blood from most of the myocardium to the coronary sinus of the right atrium. Some areas, particularly on the right side of the heart, drain directly into the cardiac chambers.

FUNCTIONS OF THE HEART ELECTROPHYSIOLOGIC PROPERTIES

The electrophysiologic properties of cardiac muscle regulate the heart rate and rhythm. These properties include excitability, automaticity, contractility, refractoriness, and conductivity.

Excitability

The ability of cardiac muscle cells to depolarize in response to a stimulus—*excitability*—is influenced by hormones, electrolytes, nutrition, oxygen supply, medications, infection, and autonomic nerve activity.

In myocardial cells, as in other types of muscle and neurons, differences in intracellular and extracellular ion concentrations create electrical and concentration gradients for ionic movement across the semipermeable cell membrane. At rest, the inside of a myocardial cell is more negative than the outside. This *resting membrane potential* results primarily from the differences in concentrations of potassium (K^+) and sodium (Na^+). Although both ions are present on either side of the cell membrane, potassium has a greater intracellular concentration and sodium has a greater extracellular concentration. Selective channels can increase membrane permeability for specific ions, allowing the ion to move down the electrochemical gradient and to alter the resting membrane potential.

When the cardiac cell is stimulated to a certain threshold, a sequence of ion permeability changes cause a dramatic change in the transmembrane potential, this is known as an *action potential* (Figure U13-5, *A*). The action potential consists of depolarization and repolarization phases. The electrocardiogram (ECG) reflects currents generated during the depolarization and repolarization of regions of the heart.

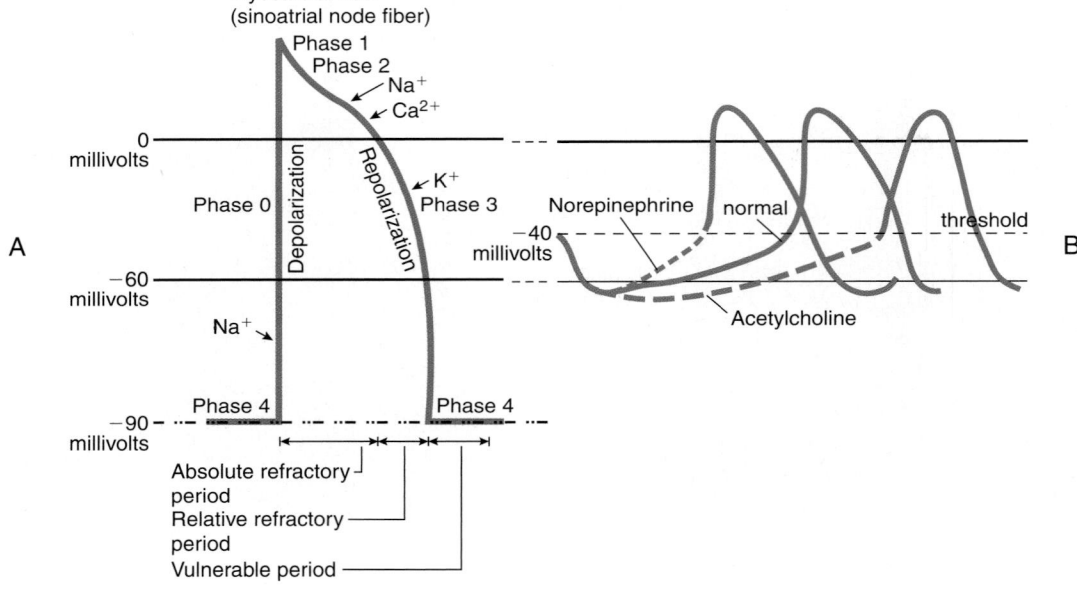

FIGURE U13-5 Action potential. **A,** The action potential of cardiac cells has five phases: *Phase 0:* Sodium permeability increases through fast sodium channels, and cell depolarization (contraction) begins. *Phase 1:* The fast sodium channels close. *Phase 2:* Some sodium and calcium permeability remains through slow Na^+/Ca^{2+} channels. *Phase 3:* Potassium permeability increases in the cell. *Phase 4:* The cell returns to its resting potential, sodium is pumped out of the cell, and potassium is pumped into the cell through the cell's sodium-potassium pump. In all cardiac cells, a period occurs during which the cells cannot be stimulated to fire another action potential. During the end of the action potential, the membrane is relatively refractory and can be reexcited only by a larger than usual stimulus. Immediately after the action potential, the membrane has transitory hyperexcitability and is said to be in a vulnerable state. **B,** The sympathetic neurotransmitter norepinephrine increases slow channel activity, allowing cells to reach threshold more rapidly (increased heart rate). Conversely, the parasympathetic neurotransmitter acetylcholine *(dashed line)* increases potassium permeability, moving the cell membrane potential away from threshold, and causes the cell to reach threshold more slowly (decreased heart rate). Calcium channel blockers slow the heart rate by decreasing slow channel activity.

Depolarization is caused by an increase in cell membrane permeability to sodium. The cell returns to its resting (relaxed) state during *repolarization*. Sodium permeability drops sharply, and potassium permeability increases, returning the membrane to the negative resting potential. In the process of depolarization and repolarization, small amounts of sodium leak into the cell and potassium leaks outward. The cell compensates for this by actively pumping sodium back out and potassium inward (Na-K ATPase).

Other ions, such as calcium and chloride, also play a role in the action potential and the contraction it causes. For the heart, calcium is especially important because it initiates contraction. During depolarization, myocardial cell membrane permeability to calcium increases and calcium moves into the cell. This inward Ca^{2+} triggers the release of more calcium stored in the sarcoplasmic reticulum (see Contractility). As the intracellular concentration of calcium increases, calcium reacts with contractile elements and myocardial muscle fibers contract.

Automaticity (Rhythmicity)

The ability of cardiac pacemaker cells to initiate an impulse spontaneously and repetitively, without external neurohormonal control, is known as *automaticity,* or *rhythmicity.* Given the proper conditions, the heart can continue to beat outside the body. In contrast, skeletal muscle must be stimulated by a nerve to depolarize and contract. The sinoatrial (SA) node pacemaker cells have the highest rate of automaticity of all cardiac cells. The conduction tissue area with the highest automaticity, or rate of spontaneous depolarization, assumes the role of pacemaker (see Chapter 59). SA node cell automaticity is due to changes in ionic permeability of the membrane. Even at rest, a decreasing potassium permeability and increasing slow channel permeability (for Na^+ and Ca^{2+} ions) move the cell membrane potential more positively toward threshold voltage. When threshold is reached, the cell initiates an action potential. Norepinephrine and acetylcholine cause heart rate to increase and decrease, respectively (Figure U13-5, *B*). The rate of spontaneous depolarization can also be affected by other hormones, body temperature, drugs, and disease.

Contractility

The heart muscle is composed of long, narrow cells or fibers. Cardiac muscle fibers, like striated skeletal muscle, contain myofibrils, Z bands, sarcomeres, sarcolemmas, sarcoplasm, and sarcoplasmic reticulum. Contraction results from the same sliding filament mechanism described for skeletal muscle (see the Unit 6 Anatomy and Physiology Review).

The action potential initiates the muscle contraction by releasing calcium through the T tubules of the cell membrane. The calcium reaches the sarcoplasmic reticulum, causing additional calcium release. The intracellu-lar calcium diffuses to myofibrils, where it binds with troponin. When the actin filaments become activated by calcium, the heads of the cross-bridges from the myosin filaments immediately become attracted to the active sites of the actin. Contraction then occurs by power stroke repetition. After contraction, free calcium ions are actively pumped back into the sarcoplasmic reticulum, and muscle relaxation begins.

One important difference between cardiac and skeletal muscle is that cardiac muscle needs extracellular calcium. All the calcium involved in skeletal muscle comes from the sarcoplasmic reticulum. In cardiac muscle, however, extracellular calcium enters through the T tubules and triggers the release of more calcium from the sarcoplasmic reticulum. Because of this, calcium channel blockers can alter contraction of the heart, but not the contraction of skeletal muscle.

Refractoriness

Refractoriness is the heart's inability to respond to a new stimulus while still in a state of depolarization from an earlier stimulus. Refractoriness develops when the sodium channels of the cardiac cell membrane become inactivated and unexcitable during an action potential. Thus the heart muscle does not respond to restimulation, preventing the possibility of tetanic contractions that are seen in skeletal muscle.

Refractoriness occurs in two periods (see Figure U13-5, *A*). The *absolute refractory period* occurs during depolarization and the first part of repolarization. During this period, cardiac cells do not respond to any stimuli, however strong. The *relative refractory period* occurs in the final stages of repolarization; refractoriness diminishes and a stronger-than-normal stimulus can excite the heart muscle to contract. At the end of the refractory period, there is a transient hyperexcitability *(vulnerable period)*. The sodium channels are reset and the cardiac cells can again conduct action potentials.

Normally, the ventricles have an absolute refractory period of 0.25 to 0.3 seconds, which approximates the duration of the action potential. The relative refractory period for the ventricles lasts about 0.05 seconds. The atria have a refractory period of about 0.15 seconds, and they can therefore contract rhythmically much more quickly than the ventricles. The duration of the action potential and the refractory period are not fixed, however; both can shorten as heart rate increases.

Conductivity

Conductivity is the ability of heart muscle fibers to propagate electrical impulses along and across cell membranes. The heart muscle must conduct the action potential from its origin throughout the heart both rapidly and smoothly so that the atria and ventricles contract as a unit. Intercalated disks join adjacent myocardial cells, allowing the action potential to travel over the entire muscle mass (Figure U13-6); however, the fibrous band of tissue that separates the atria and ventricles lacks intercalated disks. Thus the atria are isolated electrically from the ventricles except for the only normal conduction pathway, the atrioventricular node. The conduction system consists of the following major parts:

- Sinoatrial (SA) node
- AV node
- Bundle of His and bundle branches
- Purkinje fibers

The *SA node,* or *pacemaker,* is located at the junction of the superior vena cava and right atrium. Under normal circumstances, the SA node initiates electrical impulses (heartbeats) approximately 60 to 100 times per minute, but it can adjust its rate. Three internodal and one interatrial tract carry the wave of depolarization through the right atrium to the AV node and to the left atrium, respectively. The sympathetic and parasympathetic nervous systems regulate the SA node. Any myocardial tissue that generates impulses at a higher rate than the SA node can become an abnormal pacemaker.

The (AV) node, or *AV junction,* is located in the lower aspect of the atrial septum. The AV node can be a secondary cardiac pacemaker, but it normally receives electrical impulses from the SA node and is the only pathway for conducting impulses from the atria to the ventricles. Within the AV node, the impulse is delayed 0.07 second while the atria contract. This delay enables atrial contraction to be completed before the ventricles contract.

The common *bundle of His* in the interventricular septum is relatively short, branching into right and left segments. The *right bundle branch* (RBB) courses down the right side of the interventricular septum. The *left bundle branch* (LBB) bifurcates into anterior and posterior fascicles, both of which extend into the left ventricle. The right and left bundle branches terminate in Purkinje fibers.

Purkinje fibers are a diffuse network of conducting strands beneath the ventricular endocardium; they rapidly spread the wave of depolarization through the ventricles. Activation of the ventricles begins in the septum and then moves from the apex of the heart upward. Within the ventricular walls, depolarization proceeds from endocardium to epicardium. Repolarization occurs in each cell and does not involve the conduction system. Repolarization occurs in reverse order, so that the last cells to depolarize are the first to repolarize. The action potentials of Purkinje fibers have the longest duration, and their repolarization is occasionally seen as a U wave of the electrocardiogram (ECG).

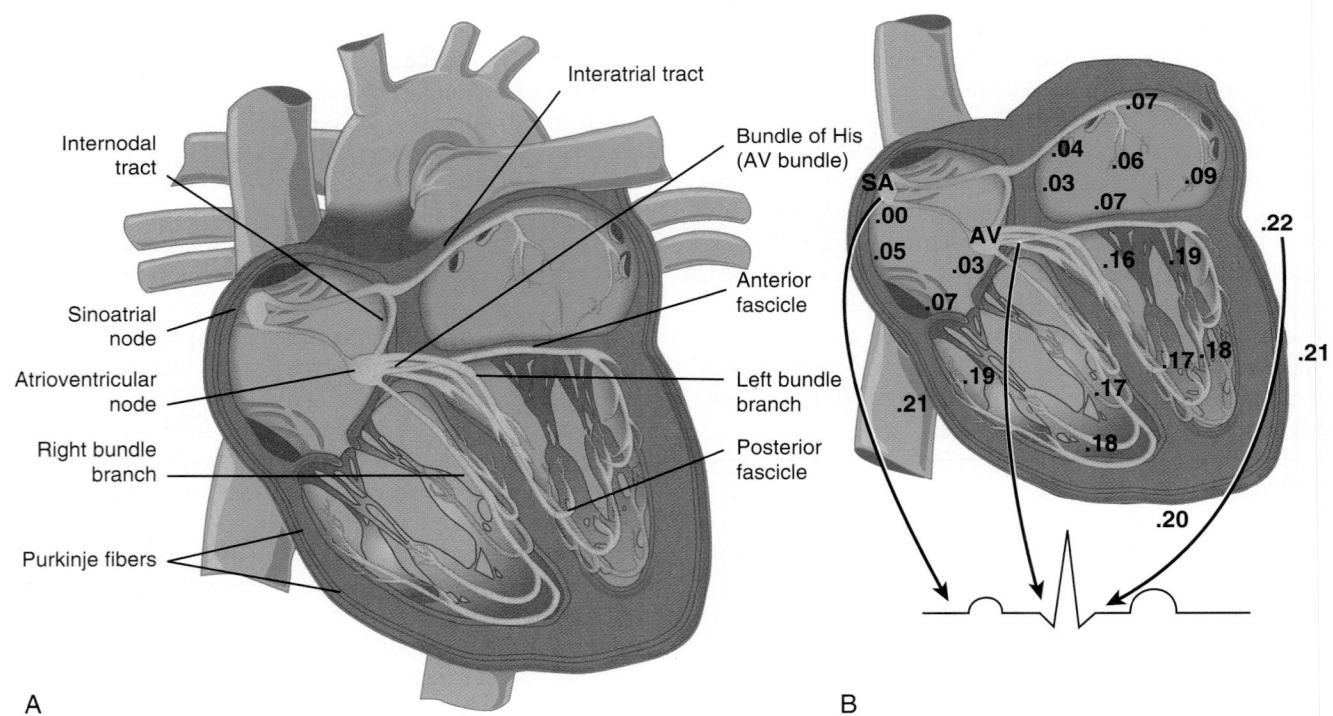

FIGURE U13-6 A, The cardiac conduction system. **B,** Transmission of the cardiac impulse through the heart, showing the time of appearance (in fractions of a second) of the impulse in different parts of the heart. (**B,** Modified from Guyton, A.C., & Hall, J.E. [2001]. *Textbook of medical physiology* [10th ed.]. Philadelphia: W.B. Saunders.)

CARDIAC CYCLE

One cardiac cycle (Figure U13-7) is equivalent to one complete heartbeat. The sequence of events in the cardiac cycle is divided into two parts: ventricular *systole* (contraction) and ventricular *diastole* (relaxation). The cardiac cycle normally begins with the spontaneous depolarization of the pacemaker cells of the SA node and ends following the filling of the relaxed ventricles.

Atrial Systole

Depolarization of the SA node spreads through the atria, both cell to cell and using the internodal and interatrial pathways. Depolarization of the atrial cells (P wave of the ECG) allows calcium entry, followed by contraction and pressure generation (a wave of the venous pressure tracing). Contraction of the atria propels a small amount of blood into the ventricles.

Ventricular Systole

Following a delay at the AV node, the wave of depolarization enters the ventricles, where it is spread rapidly by the bundle branches and Purkinje fibers (QRS complex of the ECG). Following depolarization, calcium enters, initiating contraction of the ventricle. In the *isovolumic contraction phase,* the ventricles begin to contract, closing the AV valves and building up pressure within the

ventricles. As the AV valves close, the first heart sound (S_1) is heard. Because the aortic and pulmonic valves remain closed at this point, no blood leaves the ventricle. The *ejection phase* begins when pressure in the ventricles exceeds the aortic and pulmonic pressures. The semilunar valves open, and the ventricles pump blood into the systemic and pulmonary circulations.

Ventricular Diastole

In early diastole, as the ventricles begin to relax, aortic and pulmonary artery pressures exceed ventricular pressures, and the semilunar valves close. The valve closure causes the second heart sound (S_2). The AV valves remain closed, and no blood moves in or out of the ventricles. This is called *isovolumic relaxation.* As the ventricles continue to relax, pressure in the ventricles falls below that of the atria, the AV valves open, allowing blood that has been pooling in the atria to flow into the ventricles (*ventricular filling*). When the ventricles have filled passively, the cardiac cycle is ready to begin again.

Extra Heart Sounds

The ventricular wall must expand to accommodate rapid ventricular filling. If ventricular wall compliance is decreased (as in heart failure or valvular regurgitation), structures within the ventricular wall vibrate and a third heart sound (S_3) may be heard. An S_3 heart sound may

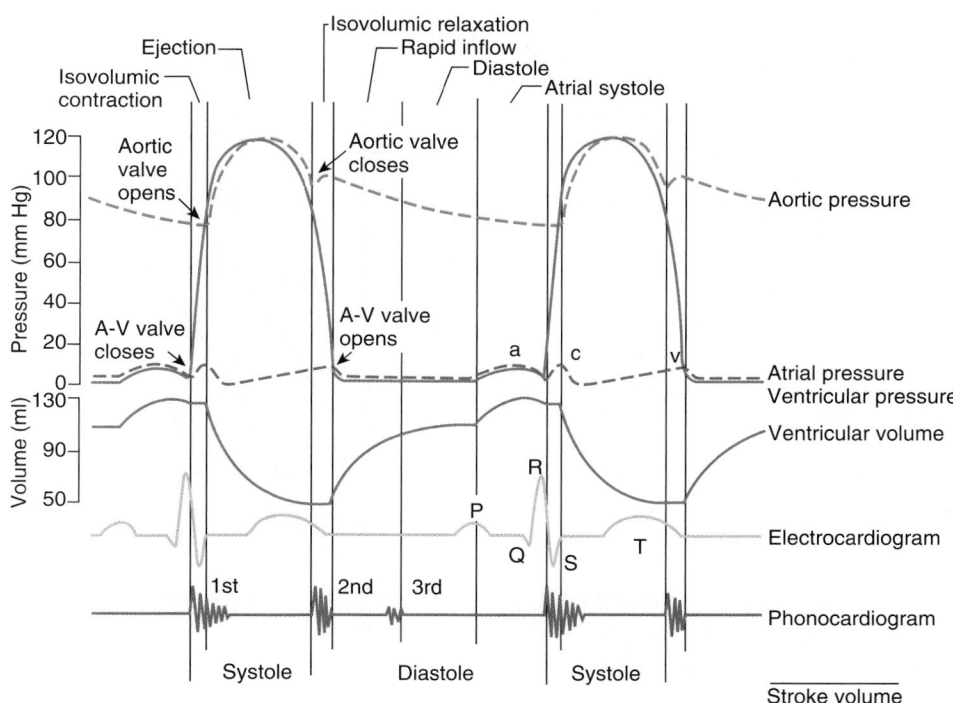

FIGURE U13-7 Changes that occur during the cardiac cycle in left atrial pressure, left ventricular pressure, aortic pressure, ventricular volume, the electrocardiogram, and the phonocardiogram. (From Guyton, A.C., & Hall, J.E. [2001]. *Textbook of medical physiology* [10th ed.]. Philadelphia: W.B. Saunders.)

be a normal finding in people younger than age 30 years. During the last phase of ventricular diastole, atrial contraction (atrial systole or atrial kick) occurs, contributing 5% to 30% more blood volume to the ventricles.

A fourth heart sound (S_4) may be heard on atrial systole if resistance to active ventricular filling is present. This is not a normal finding. It may be a result of hypertrophy, disease, or injury of the ventricular wall.

CARDIAC OUTPUT AND CARDIAC INDEX

Cardiac output (CO) is the volume of blood ejected per minute by rhythmic ventricular contraction. At the end of ventricular diastole (and atrial kick), each ventricle contains approximately 140 ml of blood (end-diastolic volume [EDV]). Normally, during systole, the heart ejects approximately half of its EDV. The volume ejected with each contraction (heartbeat) of the ventricle is the stroke volume. Cardiac output can be calculated as follows:

$$CO = [EDV - ESV] \times HR$$

where ESV is the end-systolic volume, and HR is the heart rate.

Cardiac output averages between 4 and 8 L/min in adults. For a normal 150-pound (70-kg) adult at rest, cardiac output is 5 to 6 L/min. Adjustments in either stroke volume or heart rate can compensate for fluctuations in the other, or both can rise or fall.

Cardiac output is commonly measured by thermodilution with the use of a pulmonary artery (Swan-Ganz) catheter. Several other approaches can also be used, such as obtaining heart rate from an ECG and stroke volume through ventricular imaging techniques.

Clinicians compute the *cardiac index* (CI) from the cardiac output to compensate for individual differences in body size:

$$CI = \frac{Cardiac\ output}{Body\ surface\ area}$$

The normal cardiac index is 2.5 to 4 L/min/m². Stroke volume has a major influence on cardiac output and is determined by (1) preload, (2) afterload, and (3) the contractile state of the heart.

Preload

Preload is the myocardial fiber length of the left ventricle at end diastole. It is determined by the EDV. The Frank-Starling law of the heart states that the greater the resting myocardial fiber length, or stretch, the greater its force of contraction. Preload therefore increases when increased EDV (e.g., from increased venous return) subjects myocardial fibers to greater stretch. The ventricles respond with a greater force of contraction, producing a larger stroke volume and increased cardiac output. This

phenomenon, however, has limits (Figure U13-8), such as the greatly distended ventricles characteristic of heart failure.

Afterload

Afterload is the resistance to left ventricular ejection. More specifically, it is the amount of pressure required by the left ventricle to open the aortic valve during systole and to eject blood. Afterload directly relates to arterial blood pressure and the characteristics of the valves. If arterial blood pressure is high, the heart must work harder to pump blood into the circulation. Stroke volume is inversely related to afterload. For example, if afterload increases because of peripheral vasoconstriction (which increases arterial blood pressure), myocardial fiber shortening is reduced and ejections are less effective. Then the ventricles cannot eject a normal stroke volume.

Contractile State

The contractile *(inotropic)* state refers to the vigor of contraction generated by the myocardium regardless of its blood volume (preload). Unlike skeletal muscle, the myocardium can alter contractile velocity and therefore force. The rate of cross-bridge cycling in the myocardium is calcium dependent, and agents that increase intracellular calcium thus increase contractile force. For example, sympathetic stimulation increases myocardial contractility and ventricular pressure, thereby ejecting

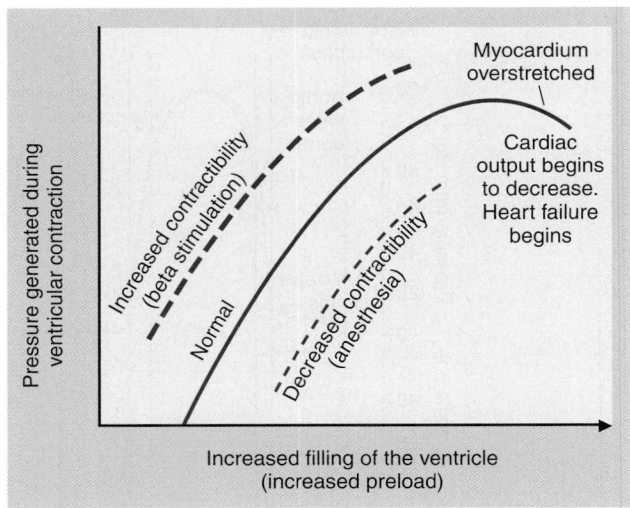

FIGURE U13-8 According to the Frank-Starling law, the more the left ventricle fills with blood (preload), the greater the quantity of blood ejected into the aorta. If the left ventricle fills to such an extent that it overdistends the myocardium *(arrow)*, however, cardiac output begins to decrease and the heart begins to fail. Agents that change contractility can shift this relationship. Norepinephrine increases contractility (+ inotrope) and improves cardiac performance; anesthesia decreases contractility (− inotrope) and impairs cardiac performance.

blood more rapidly and increasing stroke volume. Metabolic abnormalities (e.g., hypoxemia) and metabolic acidosis decrease myocardial contractility, therefore reducing stroke volume (see Figure U13-8).

Cardiac Pressures

With the use of a pulmonary artery pressure (Swan-Ganz) catheter, pressures in the right atrium, right ventricle, and pulmonary artery can be measured. Inflation of a balloon at the catheter tip allows measurement of pulmonary capillary wedge pressure (PCWP), an estimate of left atrial pressure. Assuming normal aortic valve function, arterial systolic pressure reflects left ventricular systolic pressure. These pressures are useful in determining factors that characterize cardiac performance, such as preload, afterload, volume, filling pressures, and resistance. Normal cardiac pressures are shown in Figure U13-9.

HEART RATE

The normal heart rate is 60 to 100 beats/min. *Sinus tachycardia* is a rate of more than 100 beats/min; *sinus bradycardia* is a rate of fewer than 60 beats/min. (The *sinus* in these terms indicates that the impulse arose in the sinoatrial node, the normal pacemaker region of the heart.) The intrinsic heart rate is 90 beats/min. At rest, the heart rate of 70 beats/min reflects the dominant control by the parasympathetic nervous system. Variations in heartbeat can be caused by exercise, the size of the client, age, hormones, temperature, blood pressure, anxiety, stress, and pain.

ARTERIAL PRESSURE

Arterial pressure (see the Unit 12 Anatomy and Physiology Review) is the pressure of blood against arterial walls. *Systolic pressure* is the maximum pressure of the blood exerted against the artery walls when the heart contracts (normally 100 to 140 mm Hg). *Diastolic pressure* is the force of blood exerted against the artery walls during the heart's relaxation (or filling) phase (normally 60 to 90 mm Hg). *Blood pressure* is expressed as systolic pressure/diastolic pressure (e.g., 120/80). Cardiac output is a key determinant of arterial pressure (see Figure U12-4).

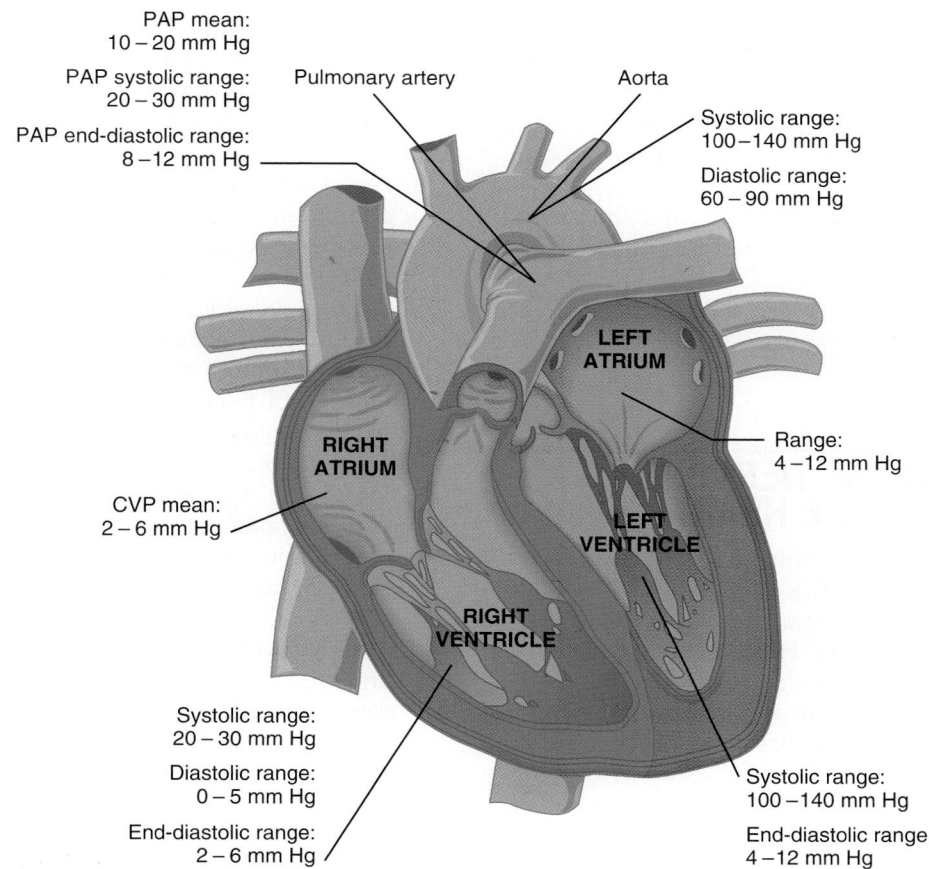

PAP mean:
10 – 20 mm Hg

PAP systolic range:
20 – 30 mm Hg

PAP end-diastolic range:
8 – 12 mm Hg

Pulmonary artery

Aorta

Systolic range:
100 – 140 mm Hg

Diastolic range:
60 – 90 mm Hg

LEFT ATRIUM

RIGHT ATRIUM

Range:
4 – 12 mm Hg

CVP mean:
2 – 6 mm Hg

LEFT VENTRICLE

RIGHT VENTRICLE

Systolic range:
20 – 30 mm Hg

Diastolic range:
0 – 5 mm Hg

End-diastolic range:
2 – 6 mm Hg

Systolic range:
100 – 140 mm Hg

End-diastolic range:
4 – 12 mm Hg

FIGURE U13-9 Normal pressures in the cardiac chambers and associated major blood vessels. *CVP,* Central venous pressure; *PAP,* Pulmonary artery pressure.

Baroreceptors, Stretch Receptors, and Chemoreceptors

Changes in sympathetic and parasympathetic activity occur in response to messages sent from sensory receptors in various parts of the body. Important receptors in cardiovascular reflexes include (1) arterial baroreceptors, (2) stretch-sensitive cardiopulmonary receptors of the atria and veins, and (3) chemoreceptors.

Baroreceptors (pressoreceptors) are stretch-sensitive nerve endings affected by changes in arterial blood pressure. They are located in the walls of the aortic arch and carotid sinuses. Increases in arterial pressure stimulate baroreceptors, which send impulses to the medulla oblongata, resulting in heart rate and arterial pressure decreases (the *vagal response*). When arterial pressure decreases, baroreceptors receive less stretch and thus send fewer impulses to the medulla oblongata (see Figure U12-5). Then sympathetic-mediated increase in heart rate and vasoconstriction occurs.

Cardiopulmonary stretch receptors are located in terminal sections of the vena cava and the atria. These receptors respond to length changes, which reflect circulatory volume status. When blood pressure decreases in the vena cava and the right atrium (e.g., hypovolemia), stretch receptors send fewer impulses than usual to the central nervous system (CNS). This process results in a sympathetic response, particularly to the kidney, to enhance salt and water retention. These changes also stimulate release of antidiuretic hormone (ADH) from the posterior pituitary. Hypervolemia produces the opposite effects.

Chemoreceptors, found in the aortic arch and carotid bodies, are primarily sensitive to increased carbon dioxide and decreased arterial pH (acidemia) and secondarily sensitive to hypoxemia. When these changes occur, chemoreceptors transmit impulses to the CNS to increase heart rate.

THE AUTONOMIC NERVOUS SYSTEM AND THE HEART

The autonomic nervous system (ANS) is the effector limb of the baroreceptor reflex and plays an important role in regulating the following:

- Heart rate (chronotropic effect)
- Myocardial contractility (inotropic effect)
- AV node conduction velocity (dromotropic effect)
- Peripheral vascular resistance (arteriole constriction and dilation)
- Venous return (venule and vein constriction and dilation)

The two subdivisions of the ANS (sympathetic and parasympathetic) generally exert opposing influences and balance their activities to promote cardiovascular adaptation to internal and external demands. ANS responses are involuntary.

Parasympathetic nerves arise from the dorsal motor nucleus of the vagus nerve, located in the medulla oblongata. They innervate the SA node atria, AV node, and to a lesser extent the ventricles and Purkinje system. When stimulated, parasympathetic nerve endings release the neurotransmitter acetylcholine, which produces inhibitory effects by binding to muscarinic receptors. Parasympathetic stimulation decreases the rate of SA node firing, thus lowering heart rate; atrial conductivity lessens as well.

Sympathetic nerve fibers originate between the first and fifth thoracic vertebrae and terminate in all areas of the heart. With stimulation, the nerve endings release the neurotransmitter norepinephrine and produce the following effects: (1) increased heart rate, (2) increased conduction speed through the AV node, (3) increased atrial and ventricular contractility, and (4) peripheral vasoconstriction, by binding to adrenergic receptors, activating G proteins, and opening ionic channels.

The sympathetic nervous system influences adrenal activity. The adrenal medulla responds to stimulation by secreting catecholamines (norepinephrine and epinephrine) into the circulation. Norepinephrine and epinephrine interact with adrenergic receptors found within cell membranes of the heart and blood vessels. The response to stimulation depends on the type and location of adrenergic receptors involved. The five types of receptors follow:

1. *Alpha$_1$-adrenergic receptors* are located in peripheral arteries and veins. When stimulated, alpha receptors produce a dramatic vasoconstrictive response.
2. *Alpha$_2$-adrenergic receptors* are located in several tissues. Their actions include contraction of some vascular smooth muscle, inhibition of lipolysis, inhibition of neurotransmission, and promotion of platelet aggregation.
3. *Beta$_1$-adrenergic receptors* are predominantly located in the heart. When stimulated, beta$_1$-receptors cause an increase in heart rate, AV node conduction, and myocardial contractility. This may result in increased cardiac output and blood pressure.
4. *Beta$_2$-adrenergic receptors* are found in the arterial and bronchial walls. Stimulation of beta$_2$-receptors causes smooth muscles to dilate, producing vasodilation of arterial vessels and bronchodilation.
5. *Beta$_3$-adrenergic receptors* are found in adipose tissue, where they promote lipolysis. Indirectly, this may assist cardiac performance because the myocardium can utilize fatty acids as metabolic fuels. Currently, no direct cardiac role for beta$_3$-adrenoreceptors has been identified.

Hormonal and Other Influences

In addition to epinephrine and norepinephrine from the adrenal medulla, several other hormones regulate cardiac output indirectly by controlling body fluid volume (and thus venous pressure and venous return). The most important hormones include ADH and the renin-angiotensin-aldosterone mechanism.

Other factors also influence cardiac activity and blood pressure. For example, cerebral cortical input from anger, fear, pain, or excitement can augment the effects of the sympathetic nervous system.

EFFECTS OF AGING

At birth, the neonate ventricles are of equal size; however, the vascular changes associated with birth lead to a decrease in pulmonary vascular resistance and pressure and an increase in systemic vascular resistance and pressure. During childhood, the greater work of the left ventricle to eject its cardiac output into the high pressure systemic circulation causes a hypertrophy of the left ventricular muscle, which is characteristic of the adult heart. The heart muscle also undergoes changes with further aging that lead to dilation of the cardiac chambers and lessening of contractility. This has little effect on stroke volume, but it reduces cardiac reserve. Coronary arteries become thickened and rigid. These changes decrease the ability of the heart to respond to additional demands and increase the likelihood of coronary artery disease. Heart valves may thicken and become incompetent, resulting in a systolic ejection murmur.

CONCLUSIONS

Although the heart can be viewed simply as a pump, this remarkable, durable organ is much more than that. The heart is a continuously beating organ that never rests. It moves blood throughout the body to oxygenate cells for energy. It propels blood through its four chambers in one direction, from right to left. Left ventricular contraction moves blood into the arteries under high pressure. This pressure propels blood through the systemic circulation.

Heart disease remains the major cause of death and involves disorders both of structure and of function of the heart. These disorders are studied in the following chapters.

BIBLIOGRAPHY

1. Berne, R., and Levy, M. (1998). *Physiology* (4th ed.). St. Louis: Mosby.
2. Kierszenbaum, A.L. (2002). *Histology and cell biology: an introduction to pathology.* St. Louis, Mosby.
3. Guyton, A., and Hall, J. (2001). *Textbook of medical physiology* (10th ed.). Philadelphia: W.B. Saunders.
4. Silverthorn, D. (2001). *Human physiology* (2nd ed). Saddle River, NJ: Prentice Hall.

Chapter 56

Assessment of the Cardiac System

Kathleen A. Popelka

Since 1900, cardiovascular disease (CVD) has been the number one cause of death in the United States. In 1999, CVD accounted for 40.1% of all deaths, or 1 in every 2.5 deaths, in the United States. CVD is the leading cause of illness and death for both white and black men and women in the United States. Looking at specific age groups, CVD is the leading cause of illness and death for people 65 years of age and older, the second leading cause of death for people 0 to 14 years of age and 25 to 64 years of age, and the fourth leading cause of death for people 15 to 24 years of age. Even though there has been a decline in heart disease mortality rates, the number of women's deaths caused by CVD is declining more slowly than men's mortality rates. Research has shown differences in men and women's risk factors, presentations, and treatment of coronary artery disease.[1-3,7]

According to World Health Organization estimates, 17 million people worldwide die of CVD each year. In 1999, CVD contributed to one third of global deaths. Of all CVD deaths, 78% occurred in low and middle income countries. By 2010, CVD is estimated to be the leading cause of death in developing countries. Heart disease has no geographical, gender, or socioeconomic boundaries.[3] CVD affects individuals in their peak midlife years, disrupting the future of the families dependent on them and undermining the development of nations by depriving them of workers in their most productive years.

The prevalence and complications of CVD have significant implications for nurses using their physical assessment skills. Assessment of the cardiovascular system involves incorporating data from history taking, relating the information to the physical examination and diagnostic tests, and correlating the data with the underlying pathophysiology.

HISTORY

The history of CVD is inseparable from the client's total health history. Important information may be overlooked unless previous illnesses, manifestations, habits, lifestyle, socioeconomic considerations, and family history are examined. Table 56-1 summarizes common risk factors for CVD. Significant cardiovascular data are obtained by assessment of the following areas: risk factor analysis, biographical and demographic data, current health, past health history, family health history, psychosocial history, and review of systems.

evolve Be sure to check out the bonus material on the Evolve website and the CD-ROM, including free self-assessment exercises.

http://evolve.elsevier.com/Black/medsurg/

TABLE 56-1   *Risk Factor Analysis for Cardiovascular Disease*

Risk Factor	High Risk	Highest Risk
Gender and age	Women after menopause	Men older than 60
Family history of high blood pressure	Two blood relatives	Three or more blood relatives
Family history of heart attack	One relative, before age 60	Two relatives, before age 60
Family history of diabetes	One or more relatives with type 1 diabetes	One or more relatives with type 2 diabetes
Blood pressure† (degree of control somewhat modifiable)	Systolic: 160-200 mm Hg Diastolic: 90-110 mm Hg	Systolic: >200 mm Hg Diastolic: >110 mm Hg
Diabetes† (degree of control somewhat modifiable), HbA1c <7%	Type 1 diabetes uncontrolled or type 2 diabetes controlled	Type 2 diabetes uncontrolled
Weight* BMI 18.5-24.9 Kg/m² Waist circumference <40 inches (men) <35 inches (women)	30%-40% overweight	50% or more overweight
Cholesterol level† HDL-C >40 mg/dl	240-280	Over 280
LDL-C <100 mg/dl	100-129 mg/dl	130 mg/dl
Serum triglycerides, fasting† <150	200-499	Over 500
Percentage of fat in diet†	30%-50%	Over 50%
Frequency of recreational exercise*	Minimal	No activity
Frequency of occupational exercise*	Minimal	Sedentary occupation
Cigarette smoking*	20-40 per day	Over 40 per day
Stress at home*	High	Extremely high
Stress at work†	High	Extremely high
Behavior pattern (especially men)†	Type A	Type A
Use of oral contraceptives (women)†	Younger than 40 and use oral contraceptives	Older than 40 and use oral contraceptives
Air pollution†	Moderate	High
Sleep patterns*	More than 8 hr sleep a night	4-6 hr sleep a night

*Modifable risk factors.
†Possibly modifiable risk factors.

Risk Factor Analysis

The American Heart Association recommends that health care providers routinely assess a client's general risk of CVD beginning at age 20. The AHA guidelines also recommend that providers calculate the risk of de-veloping CVD in the next 10 years for people age 40 and older or for anyone who has multiple risk factors. Risk factor screening includes measuring blood pressure, body mass index, waist circumference, and pulse at least every 2 years; obtaining a cholesterol profile and doing glucose testing at least every 5 years beginning at age 20; and obtaining a smoking history.[1-3,7]

To urge Americans to reduce their risk for heart disease, the AHA is introducing a new theme entitled "Taking It Personally" as a part of a national education campaign. When it comes to heart disease, people need to think "It can happen to me." People need to learn their own risk factors, including the ones that cannot be changed such as age and personal history, so that attention can be focused on the risk factors that can be changed, such as cholesterol level.

The 2001 National Cholesterol Education Program Adult Treatment Panel III (ATP III) guidelines high-lighted several modifiable and nonmodifiable major risk factors for coronary heart disease (CHD). Serum lipid levels are among the most important modifiable risk factors, and the cardiovascular benefit of lowering lipid levels is well defined.[11,22]

During the interview, be alert for data indicating the presence of CVD. Particular features to ask about are breathlessness, chest pain, palpitation, and claudication. Note whether the client has ever had an illness or problem related to the heart or blood vessels, such as an enlarged heart, heart murmur, rheumatic heart, heart attack, or heart failure. When reviewing the demographic data, ask whether the client has not been accepted for the armed services or sports, not passed an insurance examination, or had a high rating on an insurance examination.

While conducting the symptom analysis and review of systems, note statements about the following: chest discomfort or pain; shortness of breath on exertion or while sleeping; ankle swelling; dizzy spells; fainting spells; palpitations or rapid heartbeats; unexplained fatigue; coughing at night; coughing up blood; and cramps or pain in the calves, thighs, or hips while walking that is relieved by rest.

Must the client sleep on more than one pillow to breathe comfortably at night? Does the client need to arise several times during the night to urinate? Does the client have tender or swollen calves or varicose veins? These questions screen for the presence of heart disease that is producing physiologic impairment.[4,13,25,27] With the exclusion of chest pain and palpitations, the manifestations are all traceable to the secondary effects of heart disease on other organs, particularly the lungs, brain, kidneys, and blood vessels.

Tailor questions to the client, depending on the manifestations, prior illnesses, physical findings, and other information gathered to help determine possible causes. Of all the CVDs tracked by the AHA, the following are considered to be major[1,7]:

- Ischemic CHD
- Hypertensive disease
- Rheumatic fever or rheumatic heart disease
- Stroke

Classification of the functional severity of illness is also important. Although there is a rough correlation between severity of heart disease, manifestations, and client limitations, the pathophysiologic impairment does not always correlate closely with the manifestations. This lack of correlation is sometimes true even with far advanced heart disease. Diagnostic studies and the client's actual capacities and limitations warrant further investigation.

Ask about current activities and limitations. Do any activities bring on shortness of breath, chest discomfort, fatigue, or dizziness? How far can the client walk, run, and climb steps? Can the client complete housework, mow the lawn, participate in sports, shop, do a full day's work, or have sexual intercourse?[4,13,25,27]

Evaluation of previous treatments, medications, and surgical and nonsurgical interventions provides a foundation for further therapeutic regimens. Ascertain whether the client understood and followed previously prescribed medical regimens. Clients are often said not to respond to therapy when, in reality, they do not take the medications correctly. Diets are commonly not adhered to as prescribed. Confusion about the use, frequency, and amount of different medications or the expense is the cause of noncompliance and of the lack of expected improvement. Question the client's understanding of the illness so that appropriate education can be initiated, corrected, or reinforced.

Biographical and Demographic Data

Biographical and demographic data include name, age, gender, place of birth, race, marital status, occupation, and ethnic background. Alterations in health may have caused changes in the main provider's occupation and status within the family. There are known transcultural considerations regarding heart disease and stroke among culturally diverse individuals. Economic transition, urbanization, industrialization, and globalization bring about lifestyle changes that promote heart disease. Risk factors include tobacco use, physical inactivity, and unhealthy diet.

Mortality from heart disease for Native Americans is twice as high as that for all Americans. Black men are nearly twice as likely to die of stroke as white men. Among American adults age 20 and older, the estimated prevalence of coronary heart disease is 7.2% for the general population, 7.5% for non-Hispanic whites, 6.9% for non-Hispanic blacks, and 5.6% for Mexican Americans.[1,7] The age-adjusted prevalence of CVD in adults for non-Hispanic whites is 30% for men and 23.8% for women; for non-Hispanic blacks it is 40.5% for men and 39.6% for women; and for Mexican Americans it is 28.8% for men and 26.6% for women.[3]

There are greater CVD risk factors among black and Mexican American women than among white women of comparable socioeconomic status (SES). The greater differences in both ethnicity and SES underscore the critical need to improve screening, early detection, and treatment of CVD-related conditions for black and Mexican American women, as well as for women of lower SES in all ethnic groups.[1,7]

Among American Indians and Alaskan natives age 18 and older, 63.7% of men and 61.4% of women have at least one CVD risk factor (hypertension, current cigarette smoking, high serum cholesterol, obesity, or diabetes). If data on physical activity had been included in this analysis, the prevalence of risk factors probably would have been greater.[1,7]

Surveys show that most women are far more afraid of breast cancer than of CVD, even though 1 in 30 women's deaths is attributable to breast cancer whereas 1 in 2.4 is caused by CVD.

Current Health

Documenting the progression of the first manifestations to the current complaints or problems helps organize the history and reveals the sequence of events that led the client to seek help.

Chief Complaint

Inquire about the chief complaint or complaints to establish priorities for intervention and to evaluate how well the client understands the presenting condition.

Common clinical manifestations of CVD are listed in Box 56-1.[4,13,24,25,27] There may be more than one major manifestation. When this occurs, assess them in order of importance.

Symptom Analysis

Conduct a symptom analysis to evaluate and clarify the chief complaint. Following are the more common cardiac manifestations.

Chest Pain. Chest pain is one of the most important manifestations of cardiac disease. It may result from pulmonary, intestinal, gallbladder, or musculoskeletal disorders. *Angina pectoris* is the true manifestation of coronary artery disease. Angina is caused by myocardium ischemia (hypoxia), an imbalance of oxygen supply and demand as the coronary arteries support myocardial tissue. Because chest pain is caused by a number of conditions, it is highly variable. Evaluate chest pain and its cause with a careful symptom analysis. Table 56-2 compares selected cardiac, pulmonary, gastrointestinal, musculoskeletal, neurologic, and anxiety-related conditions in relation to chest pain.[4,13,20,24,25,27] Table 56-3 compares gender differences in manifestations associated with angina.

Timing. Note the time the pain begins and ends to determine the duration of discomfort. Several intermittent small episodes of chest pain are not considered as one long period of pain. Generally, the pain of myocardial infarction lasts longer than 30 minutes or until intervention is begun. Conversely, angina is usually relieved within 5 to 15 minutes by rest, with or without the use of vasodilator drugs such as nitroglycerin. Angina pectoris rarely lasts less than 1 minute or more than 15 minutes in the absence of myocardial infarction or persistent dysrhythmias (abnormal heart rhythms).[13]

Quality. Chest pain may be described as a "strange feeling," indigestion, a dull heavy pressure, burning, crushing, constricting, aching, stabbing, or tightness.

Angina pectoris characteristically has a crescendo (gradually increasing) pattern at onset. Pain described as "shooting" or "stabbing" and reaching maximum intensity virtually instantaneously is often not angina but musculoskeletal or neural in origin.[13]

Quantity. To better quantify chest pain, ask the client to use a scale of 1 (least severe) to 10 (most severe). This recorded scale can then be used to compare future episodes of chest pain. For example, the client may report 10/10 for pain on admission and then report 3/10 for pain after administration of a vasodilating medication.

Location. The site of discomfort provides additional information for determining its cause. Anginal pain is ordinarily retrosternal, felt slightly to the left of the midline or partly under the sternum. The chest pain of myocardial ischemia tends to radiate bilaterally across the chest into the arms, left greater than right, and into the neck and lower jaw. Occasionally, radiation to the back or occiput is noted. Chest pain may be diffuse, localized, or so minor that clients dismiss true ischemic pain or possible infarction. Painless or atypical presentation of myocardial infarction occurs in up to 30% of clients, particularly in diabetic and older clients.[13,16,27]

Precipitating or Aggravating Factors. The pain may be associated with certain factors or conditions. Emotional or sexual excitement, temperature extremes, exertion, deep sleep, position changes, deep breathing, straining during bowel movements, or eating may trigger the onset of chest pain.

Relieving Factors. Anginal pain may be reduced by rest, vasodilator drugs such as nitroglycerin, oxygen, and a change in position. Chest pain that is not reduced by these interventions and lasts 20 minutes or longer highly suggests myocardial infarction.[13,27]

Associated Manifestations. Ask the client whether other manifestations accompany the onset of chest pain, for example, anxiousness, shortness of breath, nausea, vomiting, diaphoresis (perspiration), vertigo, palpitations, or a feeling of impending doom. Pain associated with transmural Q-wave infarction is usually more severe and longer lasting than angina and is often associated with nausea, vomiting, and diaphoresis. Myocardial infarction is frequently accompanied by manifestations of sustained left ventricular dysfunction (*dyspnea* [labored breathing] and *orthopnea* [difficult breathing except in an upright position]) and evidence of autonomic nervous system hyperactivity (tachycardia, diaphoresis, bradycardia).[13,27]

Irregularities of Heart Rhythm—Palpitations. The word *palpitation* is derived from the Latin *palpitare,* which

TABLE 56-2	*Differential Assessment of Chest Pain*		
Condition	**Location**	**Quality**	**Quantity**
Angina pectoris	Substernal or retrosternal region; radiates to neck, jaw, epigastrium, shoulders, arms (especially left)	Pressure, burning, squeezing, tight heaviness, indigestion	Moderate to severe
Coronary insufficiency	Same as angina	Same as angina	Increasingly severe
Myocardial infarction	Precordial, substernal; may radiate like angina	Heaviness, crushing pressure, burning, constriction	Severe, sometimes mild (in 30% of clients)
Pericarditis	Usually begins over sternum and may radiate to neck and down left upper extremity	Sharp, stabbing, knife-like	Moderate to severe
Dissecting aortic aneurysm	Anterior chest; radiates to thoracic area of back; may be abdominal; pain shifts in chest	Tearing	Excruciating, tearing, knife-like
Mitral valve prolapse syndrome	Usually not substernal; sometimes radiates to the left arm, back, jaw	Stabbing, sharp, sticky quality, "kick"	Variable; generally mild but can become severe
Pulmonary embolism (many pulmonary emboli do not produce chest pain)	Substernal, "anginal"	Deep, crushing; if pulmonary infection, may be pleuritic	Can be absent, mild, or severe
Spontaneous pneumothorax	Unilateral	Sharp, well localized, stabbing	Moderate, severe
Pneumonia with pleurisy	Localized over area of consolidation	Sharp, grabbing aching	Variable
Gastrointestinal disorders (esophageal reflux)	Lower substernal area, epigastric, right or left upper quadrant	Burning, colic-like aching, tightness, pressure	Moderate to severe
Musculoskeletal disorders	Variable	Aching	Variable
Neurologic disorders (herpes zoster)	Dermatomal in distribution	Aching, constant burning, pins and needles, sharp	Moderate, severe
Psychogenic states (depression, self-gain, or attention-seeking)	Usually localized to a point	Vague, burning, diffuse	Mild to moderate, disabling

Modified from Andreoli, K., et al. (1987). *Comprehensive cardiac care* (6th ed., pp. 54-55). St. Louis: Mosby; Seller, R.H. (1996). *Differential diagnosis of common complaints* (3rd ed., pp. 57-68). Philadelphia: W.B. Saunders; and Hill, B., & Geraci, S.A. (1998). A diagnostic approach to chest pain based on history and ancillary evaluation. *Nurse Practitioner, 23*(2), 20-45.

CVA, Cerebrovascular accident; P_2, pulmonic second sound; S_2, second heart sound; S_4, fourth heart sound.

Timing	Aggravating and Relieving Factors	Associated Manifestations
<10 min	Aggravated by exertion, cold, stress, or after meals; relieved by rest or nitroglycerin; atypical (Prinzmetal's) angina may be unrelated to activity and caused by coronary artery spasm	Sinus tachycardia, bradycardia, S_4, paradoxical split S_2 during pain episode
>10 min	Same as angina, with gradually decreasing tolerance for exertion	Same as angina
Sudden onset; lasting longer than 15 min	Unrelieved	Dyspnea, sweating, weakness, nausea, vomiting, severe anxiety
Lasts many hours to days	Aggravated by deep breathing, rotating chest or supine position; relieved by sitting up and leaning forward	Fever, infection, pericardial friction rub, syncope, dyspnea, orthopnea
Sudden onset, lasts for hours	Unrelated to anything	Lower blood pressure in one arm, absent pulses, stroke, dyspnea, murmur of aortic insufficiency, pulsus paradoxus, stridor; myocardial infarction can occur
Sudden, recurrent	Not related to exertion, not relieved by nitroglycerin or rest	Variable palpitations, dysrhythmias, dizziness, syncope, dyspnea, late systolic or pansystolic murmur
Sudden onset; lasts minutes to <1 hr	May be aggravated by breathing	Fever, tachypnea, tachycardia, hypotension, elevated jugular venous pressure, right ventricular lift, accentuated pulmonary valve (P_2) sound during S_2, occasional murmur of tricuspid insufficiency and right ventricular S_4; with infarction usually in the presence of heart failure; crackles, pleural rub, hemoptysis, clinical phlebitis present in minority of cases
Sudden onset; lasts many hours	Painful breathing	Dyspnea, shock, tension pneumothorax
Sudden	Painful breathing	Dyspnea, cough, fever, hemoptysis, crackles, occasional pleural rub
Waves, continuous radiation	Precipitated by recumbency, large meals, alcohol ingestion	Nausea, regurgitation, food intolerance, melena, hematemesis, jaundice
Short or long duration Prolonged period of time	History of muscle exertion, viral illness	Tender to pressure or movement
Unassociated with external events	Aggravated by systemic stress	Pain before rash, vesicles
Varies; usually very brief	Situational anger, depression, anxiety	Sighing, chest wall tenderness, fatigue, dyspnea, anorexia

TABLE 56-3	Gender Differences in Manifestations Associated with Angina	
Rank in Frequency	**Among Women**	**Among Men**
1	Fatigue	Rest pain
2	Rest pain	Fatigue
3	Weakness	Shortness of breath
4	Shortness of breath	Weakness
5	Dizziness	Arm pain
5	Arm pain	Dizziness
7	Nausea	Sweating
8	Back pain	Neck pain
9	Loss of appetite	Nausea
10	Neck pain	Heartburn
11	Sweating	Palpitations
12	Heartburn	Throat pain
13	PND	Back pain
14	Palpitations	Loss of appetite
15	Jaw pain	Jaw pain
16	Throat pain	PND
17	Toothache	Toothache

From Penque, S., et al. (1998). Women and coronary artery disease: Relationship between descriptors of signs and symptoms and diagnostic and treatment course. *American Journal of Critical Care, 7*(3), 175-182.
PND, Paroxysmal nocturnal dyspnea.

BOX 56-2   Common Causes of Palpitations

Dysrhythmias
1. Bradydysrhythmias
   a. Heart block
   b. Sinus arrest
2. Extrasystoles
   a. Premature atrial contractions (PACs)
   b. Premature nodal contractions
   c. Premature ventricular contractions (PVCs)
3. Tachydysrhythmias
   a. Atrial fibrillation
   b. Atrial flutter
   c. Multifocal atrial tachycardia
   d. Paroxysmal supraventricular tachycardia
   e. Ventricular tachycardia

Other
1. Anemia
2. Anxiety states
3. Caffeine
4. Drugs
   a. Antidepressants
   b. Bronchodilators
   c. Digitalis
5. Fever
6. Hyperthyroidism
7. Hypoglycemia
8. Perimenopausal
9. Pheochromocytoma
10. Smoking
11. Thyrotoxicosis

means "to throb." *Palpitations* are uncomfortable sensations in the chest associated with a wide range of dysrhythmias (Box 56-2). They are common and do not necessarily indicate serious heart disease. A palpitation is a sensation of rapid heartbeats, skipping, irregularity, thumping, or pounding and may be accompanied by anxiousness.

Tachycardia (rapid heart rate), increased force of myocardial contraction (as can occur with ingestion of caffeine or with emotional or physical stress), or premature ventricular beats may cause palpitations. Any condition in which there is an increased stroke volume, as in aortic regurgitation, may be associated with a sensation of forceful contraction.

The onset and termination of palpitations are often abrupt. Question the client about (1) medications, (2) the frequency of palpitations, precipitating factors, and aggravating or relieving factors, and (3) any manifestations such as dizziness or shortness of breath associated with the onset of the palpitations. See Box 56-2 for common causes of palpitations.[13,27]

Respiratory Manifestations—Dyspnea. *Dyspnea* is defined as shortness of breath or labored breathing. Like chest pain, this common manifestation affects clients with cardiac and pulmonary disorders. *Acute dyspnea* may occur with a fever, exposure to high altitude, acute

pulmonary edema, hyperventilation, anemia, pneumonia, pneumothorax, pulmonary emboli, and airway obstruction. *Chronic dyspnea* also may occur in clients experiencing anxiety, depression, left ventricular heart failure, pulmonary disease, pleural effusion, asthma, obesity, poor physical fitness, and various psychosomatic conditions.

Although dyspnea can develop in any form of heart disease, it usually occurs with cardiac enlargement and other pathologic, cardiovascular, structural, and physiologic changes. Dyspnea develops when the left ventricle fails to function and the lungs become congested with fluid.[13,20,28]

There are several forms of dyspnea: exertional dyspnea, orthopnea, and paroxysmal nocturnal dyspnea.

Exertional Dyspnea. This is the most common form of cardiac-related dyspnea. Also known as *dyspnea on exertion,*[9] it occurs during mild to moderate exercise or activity and disappears with rest. If severe, exertional dyspnea can greatly limit activity tolerance. Ask the client to describe the degree of activity that typically precipitates the onset of dyspnea, for example, walking up one flight of stairs or walking to the mailbox. Noncardiac conditions such as obesity, poor physical conditioning, anemia, asthma, and obstructions of the nasal passages may also lead to dyspnea after mild exercise.

Orthopnea. Orthopnea (difficult breathing except when sitting erect or standing) results from an increase in hydrostatic pressure in the lungs when the person is lying flat and is relieved when the person assumes an upright or semivertical position. It consists of a cough and dyspnea in clients with left ventricular failure or mitral valve disease. Clients with orthopnea need to use two or more pillows when lying down. Clients with severe obstructive lung disease, especially acute asthma, also cannot lie flat comfortably.

Ask clients what actions they take to facilitate breathing. Do they sit up in a chair or dangle their feet at the bedside? What position do they sleep in? How many pillows do they sleep with? Record the degree of head elevation required to breathe. Orthopnea usually indicates a more serious compromise of the cardiovascular system than does exertional dyspnea.[13,20,27]

Paroxysmal Nocturnal Dyspnea. Paroxysmal nocturnal dyspnea is dyspnea during sleep that awakens the sleeper with a "terrifying breathing attack." It commonly occurs 2 to 3 hours after the person goes to bed and is relieved when the person assumes an upright position. The dyspnea usually does not recur after the client goes back to sleep. Episodes can be mild, or they can be severe with wheezing, coughing, gasping, and apprehension. Some episodes associated with severe left ventricular failure progress to pulmonary edema.[13,20,27]

Syncope. Syncope, or fainting, is a transient loss of consciousness related to inadequate cerebral perfusion. Certain cardiac disorders, especially cardiac dysrhythmias (irregular heart rhythms), can precipitate a sudden decrease in cardiac output. Valvular disorders may also lead to an adverse change in circulatory hemodynamics and cause syncope or vertigo. Clients who are susceptible to syncopal episodes (those with Stokes-Adams syndrome) should wear Medic-Alert bracelets to inform emergency health care providers.[13,27]

Fatigue. Easy fatigability on mild exertion is a frequent problem for clients experiencing cardiac disease; it is a common manifestation of decreased cardiac output. Progressive deterioration of activity tolerance results from the heart's inability to pump an effective volume of blood to meet the varying metabolic demands of the body. Fatigue, however, is not specific for cardiac problems. The most common causes of fatigue are anemia, anxiety, chronic diseases, depression, and thyroid dysfunction.[13,20,27]

Weight Gain and Dependent Edema. As the heart fails, or the blood volume expands, fluid accumulates. A client may notice weight gain, shortness of breath, swelling of the lower extremities, or a combination of these. An increase in body weight of 3 pounds or more within 24 hours results from fluid rather than body mass changes. Body weight is a sensitive indicator of water and sodium retention and increases even before edema occurs. The client with heart failure has symmetrical edema of the lower extremities that worsens as the day progresses. Daily weight measurement is important for clients with cardiac problems. Changes in weight should be reported to the health care provider.[13,27]

Other Associated Manifestations. *Cyanosis* is a subtle bluish discoloration. Cyanosis from birth is associated with congenital heart lesions. *Differential cyanosis* is related to a right-to-left shunt through a patent ductus arteriosus (PDA). In right-to-left shunting resulting from pulmonary hypertension, blood in the pulmonary artery (PA) crosses the PDA, which is located below the carotid and left subclavian arteries; deoxygenated blood is pumped to the lower extremity, producing cyanosis in only that location. *Peripheral cyanosis* is due to increased oxygen extraction in states of low cardiac output and is seen in cooler areas of the body such as the nail beds and the outer surfaces of the lips.

Clubbing of the fingernails is seen in association with significant cardiopulmonary disease.[13]

Hemoptysis refers to coughing up of blood. A careful description of hemoptysis is essential because it can include clots of blood as well as blood-tinged sputum. Recurrent episodes of hemoptysis may result from mitral stenosis and pulmonary causes.[13]

Past Health History

Ask the client about the following areas: childhood and infectious diseases, immunizations, major illnesses and hospitalizations, medications, and allergies.

Childhood and Infectious Diseases

In addition to the usual information about common childhood diseases and immunizations, ask about the client's experiences with rheumatic fever, scarlet fever, and severe streptococcal infections. These conditions are associated with structural mitral valve disease. Investigate known or corrected congenital anomalies (atrial or ventricular septal defect, persistent PDA, tetralogy of Fallot, Eisenmenger's syndrome).[4,13,27]

Immunizations

Clients with chronic conditions, such as cardiovascular disorders, should be vaccinated yearly against influenza. Indications for the pneumococcal polysaccharide vaccine are similar to those for the influenza vaccine. Revaccination is recommended every 6 to 10 years.[18]

Major Illnesses and Hospitalizations

Note conditions that influence the client's current cardiovascular performance, that is, diabetes mellitus, chronic obstructive lung disease, kidney disease, anemia, hypertension, stroke, gout, thrombophlebitis (vein inflammation associated with thrombus formation), collagen diseases, and bleeding disorders. Explore previous hospitalizations, surgical procedures, obstetric history, and outpatient interventions. Inquire about previous cardiovascular diagnostic studies, such as an electrocardiogram (ECG), exercise stress test, and echocardiogram. The results of such studies provide baseline data for comparative analysis when later studies are performed.[13,27]

Medications

Evaluate the use of prescription medications, over-the-counter medications, herbals, and recreational drugs. Whenever possible, use brand names or simple descriptors instead of generic names. For example, ask clients whether they are currently taking "water pills," "heart pills," or "blood pressure" medications.

Numerous medications can affect the cardiovascular system. Ask specifically about the use of antihypertensives, diuretics, vasodilators (nitroglycerin), cardiotonic drugs (digoxin), anticoagulants, bronchodilators, contraceptives, hormones, and steroids. Noncardiac medications can have profound secondary effects on cardiovascular performance. For example, tricyclic antidepressants and other psychotropic medications can potentiate dysrhythmias. Oral contraceptives increase the incidence of thrombophlebitis.[14] Steroid use increases fluid retention and may cause hypertension. Various antineoplastic agents may be cardiotoxic, causing dysrhythmias and cardiomyopathy. Elevated levels of thyroid hormones can result in thyrotoxicosis and a resultant hyperdynamic cardiovascular state (bounding pulses, palpitations, tachycardia). Decreased levels of thyroid hormone (hypothyroidism) may explain a client's dyspnea on exertion, fatigue, decreased cardiac output, and heart failure.[19,23,27]

Discuss the use of recreational drugs. Cocaine toxicity is a major threat to the cardiovascular system. The systemic sympathomimetic effects of cocaine result in a "fight-or-flight" reaction that increases heart rate, contractility, blood glucose levels, and peripheral vasoconstriction. Cocaine can potentiate the effects of circulating catecholamines (epinephrine and norepinephrine), resulting in sudden death.

Finally, discuss the use of over-the-counter drugs such as aspirin, cold remedies, and vitamins. Note the dose and times of administration. Ask about use of herbal remedies. Herbs are used for cardiac disorders such as angina, dysrhythmias, and heart disease and for related disorders such as high blood pressure (BP) and peripheral vascular disease.[19,23,27]

Antianginal herbs include angelica *(Angelica archangelica)*, bilberry *(Vaccinium myrtillus)*, evening primrose *(Oenothera biennis)*, flaxseed *(Linum usitatissimum)*, garlic *(Allium sativum)*, ginger *(Zingiber officinale)*, hawthorn *(Crataegus laevigata)*, khella *(Ammi majus)*, kudzu *(Pueraria lobata)*, onion *(Allium cepa)*, purslane *(Portulaca oleracea)*, Sichuan lovage *(Ligusticum chuanxiong)*, and willow *(Salix)*. Some of these herbs are anticoagulants (evening primrose, garlic, Sichuan lovage, willow). Others are vasodilators (bilberry, hawthorn, khella, kudzu). Some have calcium-channel blocking action (angelica). Hawthorne, garlic, bilberry, evening primrose, and flaxseed can lower BP and cholesterol levels. Antioxidants include ginger and purslane.[19,23]

Herbs known to have antidysrhythmic action include angelica, astragalus *(Astragalus)*, barberry *(Berberis vulgaris)*, canola *(Brassica)*, cinchona *(Cinchona)*, gingko *(Gingko biloba)*, hawthorn, horehound *(Marrubium vulgare)*, khella, motherwort *(Leonurus cardiaca)*, purslane, reishi *(Ganoderma lucidum)*, Scotch broom *(Cytisus scoparius)*, and valerian *(Valeriana officinalis)*. Gingko has been used in the treatment of intermittent claudication, vertigo, tinnitus, and organic brain syndrome.[19,23]

Other herbs used for heart disease include chicory *(Cichorium intybus)*, grapeseed *(Vitis vinifera)*, olive *(Olea europaea)*, peanut *(Arachis hypogaea)*, pigweed *(Amaranthus)*, and rosemary *(Rosmarinus officinalis)*. Chicory has digitalis-like properties. Red grape and olive products protect against heart attack. Pigweed is high in omega-3 fatty acids, preventing blood clots that can trigger a heart attack. Peanut and rosemary are antioxidants. Hawthorne is used for mild to moderate heart failure. It inhibits vasoconstriction and dilates blood vessels.[19,23]

In addition to the types and names of the medications the client takes, ask how many pills and how often they are taken. Is the client currently taking these medications? Clients with cardiac disease occasionally stop taking prescribed medications because they (1) are taking too many pills, (2) are experiencing unwanted side effects, (3) believe that the problem has resolved, or (4) worry about the cost. A client may neglect to take prescribed diuretics because "it makes me go to the bathroom all the time." Clients who take antihypertensive medications may stop taking them when their BP reaches a normal range because they perceive that the problem has resolved. Careful questioning can identify areas for client teaching.

Review for substance abuse, including cigarette smoking and use of alcohol or street drugs. Determine the pack-year history (number of cigarette packs smoked per day multiplied by the number of years smoked) of tobacco abuse and the history of alcohol consumption and dependence. If the client is not smoking currently, does he or she use a nicotine inhalation system or a nicotine transdermal product or chew nicotine gum or smokeless tobacco? All nicotine products have a vasoconstrictive effect on the heart and vessels.

Allergies

Note and describe any environmental, food, or drug allergies. Clearly document the manifestations of an allergic reaction, such as rashes, itching, or anaphylaxis (a sudden severe allergic reaction).

Family Health History

Ask about prolonged contact with a communicable disease or the effect of a family member's illness on the client. Specifically, inquire about a family history of heart disease, high BP, stroke, diabetes, or kidney disease. A detailed health history of the client's family can provide insight into possible genetic, environmental, and lifestyle conditions contributing to a cardiac condition. Note nonmodifiable cardiac risk factors such as heredity, age, gender, and race.

Genetic factors contribute to four traits that increase the incidence of atherosclerosis: hypertension, dyslipidemia, diabetes, and obesity. Modifiable risk factors, when corrected, significantly reduce the likelihood of a cardiac event. Modifying risk factors includes reducing stress, losing weight, reducing cholesterol levels, stopping tobacco abuse, and becoming more physically active.[1,8,16,17,21,28]

Psychosocial History

The psychosocial history includes data on lifestyle, household members, marital status, children, relationships with significant others, education, military service, religious beliefs (in relation to perceptions of health and treatment), the living environment, employment, and hobbies. Note data that help identify support systems and coping mechanisms. Psychosocial data provide information about risk factors for the development of CHD (see Chapter 60). Background information can be used to formulate a plan to assist the client in making necessary lifestyle adaptations to promote health and lessen disease.

Occupation

Inquire about all occupations the client has had and the duration of each job worked. The present occupation may be relevant to the significance of the disease; that is, coronary artery disease or dysrhythmias may be incompatible with continuing a career as an airline pilot or

truck driver. The amount of perceived job-related stress may need to be evaluated; stress is a modifiable risk factor for CVD.

Geographic Location

Where one lives is significantly related to death caused by cardiac events. The American Heart Association categorizes age-adjusted death rates for total CVD, CHD, and stroke by state (Box 56-3).

Environment

Ask the client about the following:
* The home, such as safety issues, type of dwelling (number of steps), state of repair, exits for fire, heating and cooling adequacy
* Mode of transportation
* Access to public transportation
* The neighborhood, in regard to noise, pollution, and violence
* Access to family and friends, grocery store, a pharmacy, laundry, church, and health care facilities

BOX 56-3	*Death Rates from Total Cardiovascular Disease, United States (2002)*
Death Rate per 100,000 Population	**State**
289.4 to 325	Alaska, Arizona, Colorado, Hawaii, Idaho, Massachusetts, Minnesota, Montana, New Mexico, Oregon, Puerto Rico, Utah, Washington
325.1 to 347.8	California, Connecticut, Florida, Iowa, Kansas, Maine, Nebraska, North Dakota, South Dakota, Vermont, Wisconsin, Wyoming
348.5 to 388.6	Delaware, District of Columbia, Illinois, Indiana, Maryland, Nevada, New Hampshire, New Jersey, New York, North Carolina, Ohio, Pennsylvania, Rhode Island, Texas, Virginia
388.8 to 465.4	Alabama, Arkansas, Georgia, Kentucky, Louisiana, Michigan, Mississippi, Missouri, Oklahoma, South Carolina, Tennessee, West Virginia

Total cardiovascular diseases are defined here as ICD/9 390-459. (From American Heart Association [2002]. *Heart and stroke statistical update [12/01];* and National Center for Health Statistics [NCHS] compressed mortality file for the years 1996 to 1998. Age adjustments are based on the 2002 standards.)

After a stroke or with deteriorating cardiac function and output, a client may need assistance or environmental adjustments to live safely and fully and meet daily needs.

Exercise

Ask about the type and amount of exercise routinely engaged in during an average week before and after the onset of current manifestations. Research confirms that a sedentary lifestyle potentiates the lethality of myocardial infarction, and it is considered a significant risk factor in the development of coronary artery disease.

Effective, routine aerobic exercise is thought to lower the likelihood of a coronary event. Aerobic exercise includes such activities as swimming, jogging, brisk walking, bicycling, and rowing.

To be beneficial, aerobic exercise should raise the heart rate from 50% to 100% of baseline (depending on age and prior physical conditioning) for at least 30 minutes three to five times a week. Along with general body conditioning, this form of exercise increases the heart's efficiency in using oxygen. Advise clients who are older than 40 years of age or who have a history of CVD to consult their physician before beginning an exercise program.[13,27]

Nutrition

Assess excess or deficit caloric intake and the client's approximate intake of foods high in sodium, cholesterol, saturated fat, and caffeine. Although these are common components of the average American diet, they have been linked to the development of atherosclerosis and hypertensive disease. Elevated serum cholesterol levels are associated with coronary artery disease. This correlation diminishes with age but still remains. Elevated serum triglyceride levels are positively related to the development of coronary artery disease, especially in women.

Examine not only daily food habits but also attitudes toward food and resistance to therapeutic alterations in diet. Cultural beliefs and economic status greatly affect food choices. Consider these factors before recommending dietary changes. Identify and include the primary food purchaser and preparer in dietary instruction.[1,2,8,15,26,28]

Results from the Dietary Approaches to Stop Hypertension (DASH) study have established that a diet abundant in fruits, vegetables, and low-fat dairy products and low in cholesterol and total and saturated fat reduces BP significantly. These changes occurred in the absence of weight loss or fluid restriction. A subgroup analysis of that study suggested that although all groups benefited significantly in terms of systolic BP reduction, two subgroups gained the most from adopting these dietary changes in daily life.[26] The DASH diet resulted in (1) lower systolic BP in African Americans than in whites (lowered by 6.8 versus 3 mm Hg) and (2) an even lower systolic BP in clients with hypertension than in those with high-normal BP (lowered by 11.4 versus 3.4 mm Hg).[26]

Habits

If the client smokes, inquire about the duration of the smoking habit and the number of cigarettes smoked daily. Cigarette smoking increases the risk of coronary artery disease and worsens hypertension. Nicotine, a major ingredient in cigarettes, causes peripheral vasoconstriction, increasing resistance to left ventricular emptying and thus increasing the myocardial workload. Smoking increases the mortality rate of middle-aged clients with coronary artery disease and greatly potentiates the development of peripheral vascular disease. The death rate for coronary heart disease is 70% greater in cigarette smokers than in nonsmokers. Several years after stopping smoking, clients have a death rate from heart attack almost as low as that of people who never smoked.[3,4]

Evidence that caffeine and alcohol ingestion increases the risk of atherosclerosis is inconclusive. Nevertheless, caffeine is a stimulant that, in excessive amounts, can increase heart rate and BP and contribute to palpitations, both of which can raise the myocardial workload and precipitate angina pectoris, heart failure, and some dysrhythmias. Therefore assess caffeine intake and caution those with known heart disease to limit caffeine intake to the equivalent of two 8-oz cups of coffee per day.

Researchers state that only excessive alcohol intake has deleterious effects on the cardiovascular system and its performance. An intake of 100 g of pure (100%) al- cohol may slightly increase BP and heart rate. This amount is approximately equal to three beers or one mixed drink. Alcoholism, in contrast, has been associated with the development of hypertension and damage to the heart muscle, leading to cardiomyopathy. Ask about the client's approximate daily and weekly alcohol consumption (see Chapter 2). Keep in mind that the alcoholic client may lie about the type and amount consumed.

Review of Systems

Ask about past problems involving the cardiovascular system, including chest pain, palpitations, fatigue, edema, shortness of breath, orthopnea, wheezing, fainting (syncope), weight gain, heart murmurs, hypertension, paroxysmal nocturnal dyspnea, and history of rheumatic fever.

Cardiovascular problems also affect the pulmonary, renal, and neurologic systems. Ask about productive cough, decreased urination, dark or concentrated urine, edema of the legs, dizzy spells, and memory loss.[4,5,13,25,27]

PHYSICAL EXAMINATION

The cardiac physical examination includes the following:

- A general inspection
- Assessment of BP, arterial pulses, and jugular venous pulse
- Percussion, palpation, and auscultation of the heart
- Evaluation for edema

The client is supine. Stand at the client's right side. The head of the bed or examination table may be elevated slightly for comfort. Proceed in logical fashion from head to foot. Necessary equipment includes a stethoscope with diaphragm and bell, a penlight, ruler, and an applicator stick. Ensure a woman's privacy by keeping her breasts draped. The female left breast overrides part of the area examined in a cardiac examination. Gently displace the breast upward, or ask the woman to hold it out of the way.[4,13,27] See the Physical Assessment Findings in the Healthy Adult feature on The Cardiovascular System, below.

PHYSICAL ASSESSMENT FINDINGS IN THE HEALTHY ADULT

The Cardiovascular System

Inspection

Skin color even; capillary refill less than 3 seconds. Thorax symmetrical, without visible lifts or point of maximal impulse (PMI). Jugular venous distention absent with client at 45-degree angle. Lower extremity superficial vessels without tortuosity upon standing.

Palpation

Skin warm. PMI palpable in fifth intercostal space at left midclavicular line, approximately 1 cm in diameter. Forceful thrusts, heaves, and pulsations absent. No palpable thrills. Abdominal aorta pulsations slightly palpable over epigastrium without lateral radiation. Carotid and peripheral pulses equal and readily palpable bilaterally. Evidence of unimpeded arterial flow and venous return to upper and lower extremities. No edema evident.

Percussion

Right heart border not discerned.

Auscultation

S_1 and S_2 heard without splitting. Apical rate, 72 beats/min, regular. Murmurs and extra heart sounds absent.

General Appearance

Begin with inspection. Much may be learned through simple observation. Look at the client and consider the following:

- Does the client lie quietly, or is there restlessness or continual moving about?
- Can the client lie flat, or is only an upright, erect position tolerated?
- Does the facial expression reflect pain or obvious manifestations of respiratory distress?
- Are there manifestations of significant cyanosis or pallor?
- Can the client answer questions without dyspnea during the interview?

Level of Consciousness

Note the client's general *level of consciousness* (LOC). The level of consciousness reflects the adequacy of cerebral perfusion and oxygenation. Also assess whether the client manifests appropriate behavior for the surroundings:

- What is the client's affect?
- Are there obvious manifestations of anxiety, fear, depression, or anger?
- How does the client react to those in the immediate vicinity, including significant others?

Assessment of general appearance and level of consciousness provides an initial composite picture of the client and indicates the level of comfort and distress.

Weight Management

Measure the client's weight, height, and waist circumference, and calculate body mass index (BMI). The desirable weight, defined as BMI range of 21 to 25 kg/m² (BMI of 25 kg/m² corresponds to 110% of desirable body weight). A desirable waist circumference for women is no more than 35 inches or 88 cm and for men is less than 40 inches or 102 cm.[1,15] See Chapter 30 for further discussion of nutritional assessment.

Head, Neck, Nails, and Skin

When examining the head, pay particular attention to the eyes, ear lobes, lips, and buccal mucosa. Examine the eyes for *arcus senilis* (a light gray ring around the iris, possibly caused by cholesterol deposits) and *xanthelasma* (yellow raised plaques around the eyelids resulting from lipid deposits). Both findings are common in older clients but may indicate a predisposition to atherosclerosis.

Observe the skin and mucous membranes for abnormalities such as central or peripheral *cyanosis*. The presence of a bluish tinge or duskiness is indicative of central cyanosis, indicating poor arterial circulation. Central cyanosis indicates serious heart or lung disease in which hemoglobin is not fully saturated with oxygen. Peripheral cyanosis, seen in lips, ear lobes, and nail beds, suggests peripheral vasoconstriction.

Assess *capillary refill* (circulation) by putting slight pressure on a nail bed until it blanches (see Chapter 53). Quickly release the pressure. When circulation is adequate, nail color returns to baseline in less than 2 seconds. Always check capillary refill before using pulse oximetry; if capillary refill is abnormal, pulse oximetry findings are inaccurate.

Check fingers for *clubbing,* in which the distal tips of the fingers become bulbous and the angle between the base of the nail and the skin next to the cuticle increases from the normal 160 to 180 degrees or more (see Chapter 50). In addition, the nails feel soft and spongy. Finger clubbing is associated with pulmonary and cardiovascular disease. Splinter hemorrhages of the nail are classically associated with subacute bacterial endocarditis.

Assess *skin turgor* (elasticity) by lifting a fold of skin over the sternum or lower arms and releasing it (see Chapter 50). Normal skin immediately returns to the baseline position, but skin with decreased turgor stays pinched (tenting) for up to 30 seconds. Decreased skin turgor occurs with dehydration, volume depletion, rapid weight loss, and advanced age. The temperature of the skin may reflect cardiac disease. Severe anemia, beriberi, and thyrotoxicosis tend to make the skin warmer; intermittent claudication (leg pain related to peripheral vascular disease) is associated with coolness of the lower extremity compared with the upper extremity.[4,5,13,25,27]

Edema

Edema occurs in right-sided heart failure when the excess intravascular volume begins to increase capillary hydrostatic pressure and forces fluid into the interstitium.

Inspect dependent areas for edema. In the mobile client, edema is best seen in the feet, ankles, and lower legs. In the chair-ridden or bedridden client, edema may be palpated over the sacrum, abdomen, or scapula. Assess the severity of edema by pressing a thumb or finger carefully into the area. A depression that does not rapidly resume its original contour is noted as orthostatic, or pitting, edema. Because there is a wide discrepancy in edema grading scales, record the actual amount of time in seconds for the indentation to resolve (see Chapter 53).[4,13,25,27]

Blood Pressure

Measure BP in both arms initially to rule out dissecting aortic aneurysm, coarctation of the aorta, vascular obstruction, vascular outlet syndromes, and errors in measurement. If the arms are inaccessible, obtain pressures from the thighs and popliteal arteries or the calves and posterior tibial arteries. When pressures are difficult to auscultate, systolic pressures can be determined through palpation or by Doppler ultrasonography.

When recording measurements, note both systolic and diastolic pressures, for example, 120/70 mm Hg. The muffling of Korotkoff's sounds may also be included and recorded as 120/80/70 mm Hg. The American Heart Association recommends recording the point at which the sound disappears (fifth Korotkoff sound) as the diastolic pressure in adults. Also, record the arm in which the measurement was taken and the client's position at the time of the reading.

The American Heart Association recommendations for BP to prevent heart attack and stroke are as follows: BP maintained below 140/90 mm Hg; below 130/85 mm Hg for people with kidney damage or heart failure; or below 130/80 mm Hg for people with diabetes.[1] More recent data recommend lower BP values as treatment goals because the risk of CVD, beginning at 115/75 mm Hg, doubles with each increment of 20/10 mm Hg.[21] The report concluded that a systolic BP of more than 140 mm Hg in persons older than 50 years is a much more important CVD risk factor than elevated diastolic BP and that individuals with a systolic BP of 120 to 139 mm Hg or a diastolic BP of 80 to 89 mm Hg should be con- sidered prehypertensive and require health-promoting lifestyle modifications to prevent CVD.[21]

Postural Blood Pressure

Perform a postural BP reading when an extracellular volume depletion or decreased vascular tone is suspected. Note the client's position at the time of the reading (Figure 56-1).

Paradoxical Blood Pressure (Pulsus Paradoxus)

Pulsus paradoxus is an abnormal decrease in systolic BP of more than 10 mm Hg during inspiration. It is fre-

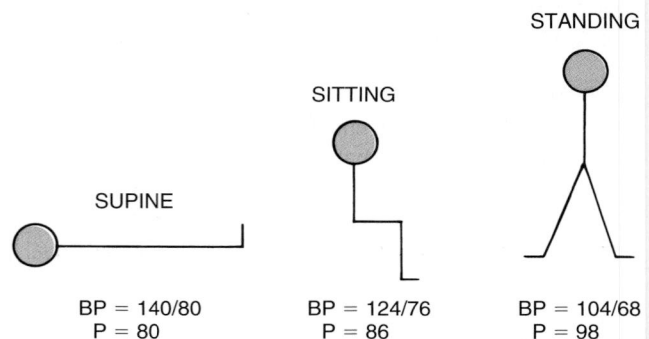

SUPINE
BP = 140/80
P = 80

SITTING
BP = 124/76
P = 86

STANDING
BP = 104/68
P = 98

FIGURE 56-1 Recording postural blood pressure (BP). After measuring the client's BP and pulse in the supine position, leave the BP cuff in place and help the client sit. Then measure the BP within 15 to 30 seconds. Help the client stand, and measure again. Postural hypotension is indicated by a BP decrease of more than 10 to 15 mm Hg systolic pressure and more than 10 mm Hg diastolic pressure. Postural hypotension is typically accompanied by a 10% to 20% increase in heart rate (pulse).

quently found in clients with pericardial tamponade, constrictive pericarditis (inflammation of the pericardial sac), and pulmonary hypertension.

Use a sphygmomanometer and stethoscope to assess for a paradoxical pulse over the brachial artery. Instruct the client to breathe normally. Inflate the cuff 20 mm Hg above the systolic BP. Slowly deflate the cuff (1 to 2 mm Hg/sec), and listen for Korotkoff's sounds to occur only during expiration. (Sounds are first heard during expiration and then during inspiration.) Continue deflating the cuff until Korotkoff's sounds are heard equally well during inspiration and expiration.

The paradoxical pressure is the difference between the BP when the sounds are first heard during expiration and the BP when the sounds are heard on both expiration and inspiration. Normally, this difference is less than 10 mm Hg. If the client is breathing normally and the systolic difference is greater than 10 mm Hg, cardiac compression, such as cardiac tamponade, may be present.

Pulse

Pulse characteristics can vary. If the pulse is irregular, assess for a pulse deficit by taking apical and radial pulses simultaneously, noting differences in rate. Peripheral pulse assessment is discussed in Chapter 53.

Respirations

Note the rate, rhythm, depth, and quality of the breathing pattern. Variations in the respiratory rate and character may indicate heart failure or pulmonary edema. Auscultate the lungs for the presence of crackles, rhonchi (dry rattling), or other abnormal breath sounds (see Chapter 61). Severe left ventricular failure may produce pulmonary congestion and resultant frothy sputum with deep respiratory efforts.

Head and Neck

Neck Veins

Neck vein distention can be used to estimate *central venous pressure* (CVP). The amount of distention reflects pressure and volume changes in the right atrium. The internal jugular veins, although more difficult to detect than the external jugular veins, are more reliable indicators of CVP. The external jugular vein engorges easily with only slight provocation, for example, by holding the breath, twisting the neck, and being constricted by clothing (except in weight lifters, football players, and professional speakers and singers, who have overdeveloped neck muscle tendons). The vessels are prominent and visible but soft and compressible.

A relaxed supine position with the head of the bed inclined between 15 and 30 degrees maximizes jugular vein prominence. Clients who have greatly increased right atrial pressure may require head elevation from 45 to 90 degrees. Support the client's head with a small pil-

low and avoid sharp neck flexion. Turn the client's head slightly away from you. Loosen or remove clothing that compresses the neck or upper thorax. Tangential (oblique) lighting enhances the appearance of the vein. Observe both sides of the neck. The internal jugular vein lies deep to the sternocleidomastoid muscle and runs parallel along its length to the jaw and ear lobe. Identify the pulsations of the internal jugular. Use the external jugular vein if the internal jugular is not visible.

Note the highest point at which the internal jugular pulses can be seen (the *meniscus*). The *sternal angle* (manubrial joint) is a reference point to measure the height of venous pulsation, approximately 4 to 5 cm above the center of the right atrium. Use a centimeter ruler to measure the vertical distance between the sternal angle and the point of highest venous pulsations. See Figure 56-2.

The value is usually less than 3 or 4 cm above the sternal angle when the head of the bed is elevated 30 to 40 degrees. Higher values indicate increased right atrial or right ventricular pressure, as seen in right ventricular failure, tricuspid regurgitation, and pericardial tamponade. Flat jugular veins in a supine client suggest extracellular volume depletion. Unilateral distention may indicate vessel obstruction on that side.

The timing and amplitude of the jugular vein pulsations may also be assessed to evaluate right-sided heart function, tricuspid valve performance, and the presence of certain dysrhythmias.[4,13,20,25,27]

Carotid Arteries

Carotid artery examination indicates the adequacy of stroke volume and the patency of the arteries. Using your fingertips, gently palpate the carotid arteries one side at a time. Check and compare the rate, rhythm, and

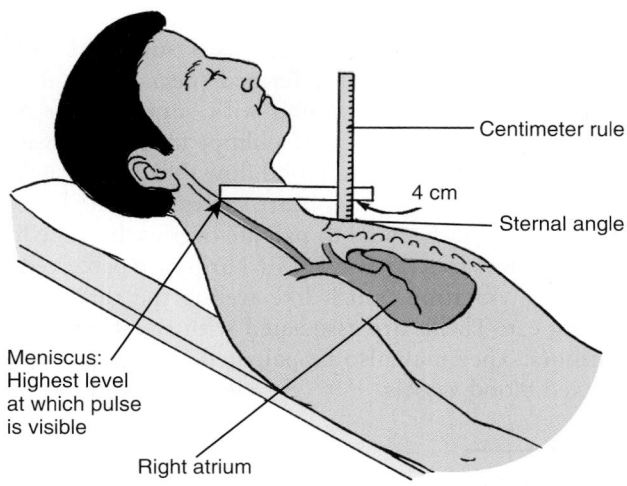

Centimeter rule

4 cm

Sternal angle

Meniscus: Highest level at which pulse is visible

Right atrium

FIGURE 56-2 Estimation of jugular vein measurement to assess central venous pressure.

amplitude of the pulses. Note whether a *bruit* (a blowing sound) is present by listening with the diaphragm of a stethoscope over the arteries while the client holds the breath. Tracheal breath sounds are heard while respiration is ongoing. A bruit generally indicates that the carotid artery has narrowed. Bruits typically result from atherosclerosis or radiation of sounds from an aortic valve murmur.[13,20,25,27]

Chest

Precordium

Perform inspection and palpation of the precordium together to determine the presence of normal and abnormal pulsations. Ideally, the client should be supine with the chest exposed. The left lateral position allows the heart to move closer to the chest wall, accentuating precordial movements and certain heart sounds. Good lighting and a warm, quiet environment are essential. Stand at the client's right side and observe the anterior chest for size, shape, symmetry of movement, and any evident pulsations. Record the location of pulsation in relation to the intercostal space and the midclavicular line. Confirm your observation with palpation. When palpating, use the fingers and palm of the hand.

The *point of maximum intensity* (PMI) or apical impulse is usually seen at the apex. The PMI is associated with left ventricular contraction and should appear at the fifth intercostal space medial to the left midclavicular line. It may be prominent in thin people and obscured in those who are obese or have large breasts. When palpated, the PMI is a single, faint, instantaneous tap beneath the fingers, no more than 2 cm in diameter. The left lateral recumbent position may enhance locating the PMI, but its position is displaced. With left ventricular enlargement and aneurysm, the PMI is more diffuse, sustained, and displaced downward and to the left of the midclavicular line.

Right ventricular enlargement can produce an abnormal pulsation that may be seen as a sustained thrust along the left sternal border. Termed *"heaves" or "lifts,"* these pulsations may be found with various disorders, such as valvular disease and pulmonary hypertension. *Thrills* represent turbulent blood flow through the heart, especially across abnormal heart valves. Use the heel or ulnar surface of the hand to palpate over each of the five cardiac landmarks (Figure 56-3). Thrills are perceived as a rushing vibration, much like feeling the throat of a purring cat. Thrills are associated with significant heart murmurs. They may also be palpated over partially obstructed blood vessels.[4,13,20,25,27]

Heart Sounds

Auscultation of the precordium yields valuable information about normal or abnormal heart rate and rhythm,

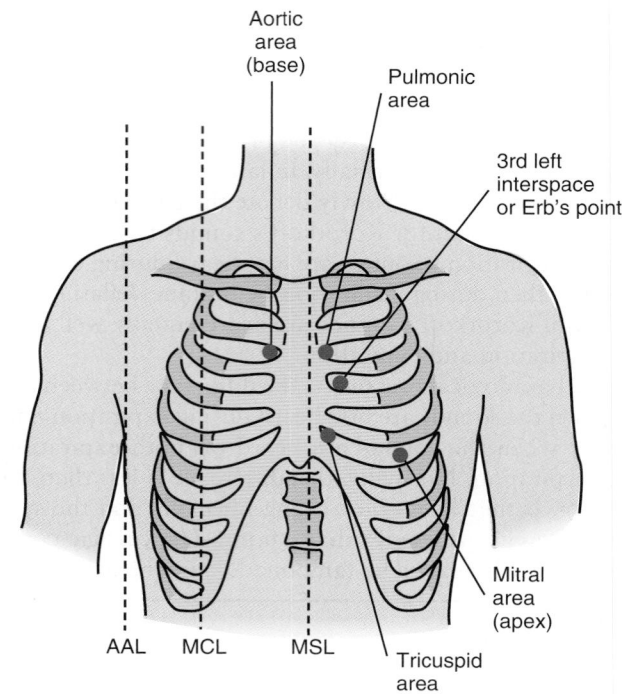

FIGURE 56-3 Cardiac auscultatory sites. S_1 is heard loudest at mitral and tricuspid areas. S_2 is heard loudest at aortic and pulmonic areas. S_3 and S_4 are heard best at the mitral area. *AAL,* Anterior axillary line; *MCL,* midclavicular line; *MSL,* midsternal line.

ventricular filling, and blood flow across heart valves. Assessment of heart sounds is a sophisticated skill, requiring study of heart sound characteristics and extensive clinical practice. To become skilled, you must be thoroughly familiar with normal cardiac sounds. With practice and experience, you will be able to detect abnormal heart sounds.

Discerning abnormal heart sounds is difficult even for skilled practitioners under ideal circumstances. The sensitivity of the human ear decreases sharply when the frequency of sound vibrations is below 1000 Hz. Most cardiac murmurs and sounds are below that frequency. A reliable stethoscope is necessary. Use the bell to hear low-pitched sounds and the diaphragm to hear high-pitched sounds. Always warm the chest piece before placing it on the client's skin.

The environment is key to successful auscultation. The surroundings should be warm and quiet. An exposed chest is ideal, but prevent shivering, which can greatly distort heart sound transmission. Instruct the client to breathe through the nose while supine. The left lateral position may facilitate auscultation. An upright position, leaning forward and holding the breath after exhalation, helps when assessing early diastolic murmurs and pericardial friction rubs.

Always use a systematic approach when evaluating heart sounds. Methods vary. Develop your own routine to ensure a thorough assessment each time you perform cardiac auscultation.

Examination of heart sounds may progress from the base (right second intercostal space) of the heart to the apex or from the apex to the base. Whichever approach you use, pay special attention to each of the precordial locations diagrammed in Figure 56-3. Each area corresponds to a specific valvular outflow tract. Concentrate on one component of the cardiac cycle at a time, that is, the first heart sound (S_1), then the second heart sound (S_2), and so on. It is difficult to assess everything at one time. As many as three or four abnormalities may occur simultaneously. Listen to several complete cardiac cycles at each of the five precordial areas. Listen carefully, noting the quality (crisp or muffled), intensity (loud or soft), rhythm (irregular or regular), and presence of extra sounds (murmurs, gallops, rubs, or clicks). Repeat this process using the bell over each of the precordial areas.[4,13,20,25,27]

Normal Heart Sounds. The *first heart sound* (S_1) is linked to closure of the mitral and tricuspid valves (atrioventricular [AV] valves). It marks the onset of systole (ventricular contraction). It is heard best with the diaphragm at the apex (the mitral valve area) and left lower sternal border (the tricuspid valve area). S_1 results from abrupt closure of the AV valves, which causes some blood turbulence and vibration of structures within the ventricles. This vibration is transmitted across the chest wall as a heart sound. Phonetically, if both heart sounds are appreciated as "lub-dup," S_1 is "lub." Although closure of both mitral and tricuspid valves is heard as a single sound, the mitral valve closes a fraction of a second earlier.

The intensity of S_1 may vary in certain pathologic conditions. Diseased and stiffened AV valves (as seen in rheumatic heart disease) may augment S_1; rhythms of asynchrony between the atria and ventricles (as in atrial fibrillation and AV block) cause varying intensity of S_1. If you are not sure which sound is S_1, check the carotid artery for a pulsation or look for the upstroke of the R wave in the QRS complex (described later) on the ECG monitor.

The *second heart sound* (S_2) is related to closure of the pulmonic and aortic (semilunar) valves and is heard best with the diaphragm at the aortic area. Phonetically, it is the "dup" of the heart sounds. It signifies the end of systole and the onset of diastole (ventricular filling). At the base of the heart, normal S_2 is always louder than S_1, whereas both sounds are usually of nearly equal intensity at the left sternal border over Erb's point. Usually, S_1 is the louder of the two sounds at the apex and occurs just after or along with the carotid pulse.[4,13,20,25,27]

Knowing the usual quality of sounds that occur over the precordium can help distinguish between S_1 and S_2 during rapid heart rates. Simultaneous palpation of the carotid pulse during auscultation also helps discriminate sounds. Carotid pulsation occurs with systole or S_1. Figure 56-4 shows the relationship of heart sounds to events during the cardiac cycle.

Physiologic (normal) *splitting of S_2* occurs during inspiration. Normal splitting results from delayed closure of the pulmonic valve. During S_2, both the aortic and pulmonic components of S_2 (A_2 and P_2) can be heard. Inspiration creates negative pressure within the thoracic cavity, "pulling" blood from the periphery into the right side of the heart. Because of this transient augmentation of venous return, right ventricular volume increases and emptying is delayed, delaying pulmonic valve closure. The "split-second heart sound" is best heard over the pulmonic and mitral areas. The two components of S_2 occur so close together that the pause between them produces a phonetic gap similar to the "pl" sound in the word "split." If a split S_2 is heard when the client is sitting or during expiration, it usually indicates right ventricular failure or other cardiac disease.[13,20,25,27]

Abnormal Heart Sounds. Many abnormal heart sounds may indicate a serious heart disorder or change in cardiac function. You may not be able to label each abnormality, but with a thorough understanding of the normal sounds, you should be able to recognize various abnormal sounds and refer the problem to the physician.

Pathologic Splitting of S_2. A wide splitting of S_2 may be heard during both inspiration and expiration, with an increase during inspiration. This form of splitting occurs in right bundle branch block and is related to delay in depolarization of the right ventricle and late closure of the pulmonic valve. Fixed splitting is the hallmark of atrial septal defect. This form of S_2 split is continuous and does not vary with respirations. Fixed splitting occurs because the emptying of the right ventricle is prolonged. Paradoxical splitting results from a delay in closure of the aortic valve because of aortic stenosis, left bundle branch block, or patent ductus arteriosus. In paradoxical splitting, the S_2 split is heard during expiration rather than inspiration.[4,13]

Gallops. Diastolic filling sounds or *gallops* (S_3 and S_4) occur during the two phases of ventricular filling. Sudden changes of inflow volume cause vibrations of the valves and ventricular supporting structures, producing low-pitched sounds that occur either early (S_3) or late (S_4) in diastole. Such sounds can originate in either side of the heart. These extra heart sounds create a triplet rhythm, acoustically mimicking a horse's gallop. For that reason, the term "gallop" is often used to denote these heart sounds.

A gallop sound that occurs in early diastole, during passive, rapid filling of the ventricles, is known as the

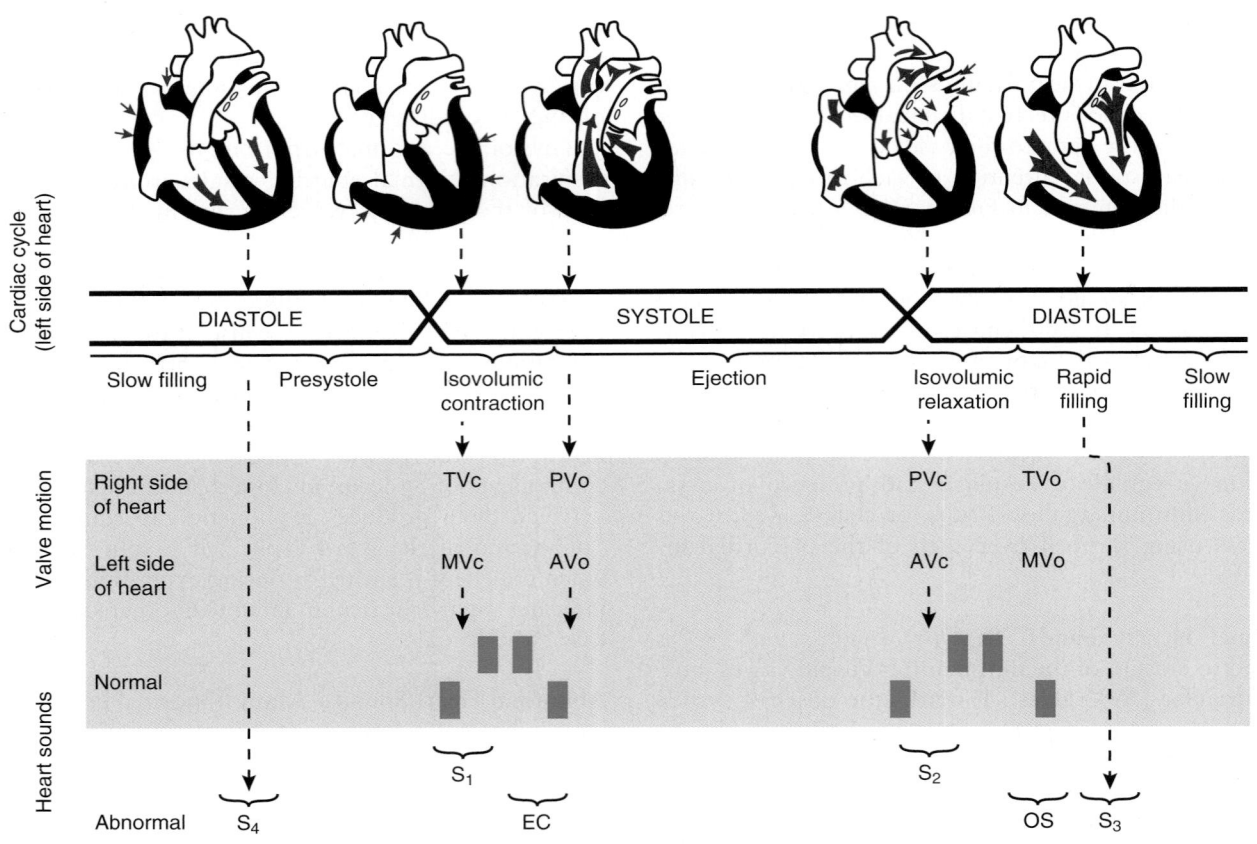

FIGURE 56-4 Relationship of heart sounds to events during the cardiac cycle. Understanding heart sounds is facilitated when they are correlated with cardiac cycle events and valvular movements. *MVc,* Mitral valve closing; *TVc,* tricuspid valve closing; *PVo,* pulmonic valve opening; *AVo,* aortic valve opening; *AVc,* aortic valve closing; *PVc,* pulmonic valve closing; *TVo,* tricuspid valve opening; *MVo,* mitral valve opening; *EC,* ejection click; *OS,* opening snap.

third heart sound (S_3). It is heard best with the bell at the apex and with the client in the left lateral recumbent position. An S_3 immediately follows S_2 and is a dull, low-pitched sound. An S_3 gallop is considered a normal finding in children and young adults. In adults older than 30 years of age, an S_3 is considered characteristic of left ventricular dysfunction.[4,13]

Clinical conditions associated with an S_3 gallop are those that precipitate heart failure, such as myocardial infarction and valvular incompetence. Third heart sounds arising in the left ventricle are best heard at the apex, with the client on the left side. Right ventricular gallops are best detected along the left sternal border, with the client supine.

A *fourth heart sound,* or S_4 *gallop,* occurs in the later stage of diastole, during atrial contraction and active filling of the ventricles. This soft, low-pitched sound is heard immediately before S_1 and is also referred to as an *atrial gallop.* An atrial gallop is found most commonly in disorders involving increased stiffness of the ventricle, such as ventricular hypertrophy, ischemia, and fibrosis. These conditions are often associated with elevated dias-

tolic ventricular pressures and a vigorous atrial contraction. The ventricles become resistant to filling, and the structures within the ventricles vibrate in response to the added blood input during the "atrial kick."

The presence of S_4 may result from myocardial infarction (transient S_4), hypertension, hypertrophy, fibrosis, cardiomyopathy, cor pulmonale, aortic stenosis, or pulmonic stenosis. S_4 is never heard in the absence of atrial contraction (atrial fibrillation). S_4 is heard best with the bell of the stethoscope at the apex, with the client in the supine, left lateral position.[4,13,25,27]

Quadruple Rhythm. At times a quadruple rhythm is noted when both S_3 and S_4 are audible. Clients with this unusual heart sound often have tachycardia, which causes the diastolic filling sounds to fuse, forming a *summation gallop* that may be louder than S_1 or S_2. It can be heard best at the apex and resembles the sound of a galloping horse.

Clicks. Clicks are extracardiac sounds that can be heard any time during the cardiac cycle in clients with

TABLE 56-4	*Characteristics of Murmurs*
Characteristic	**Description**
Location	Area where the murmur is best heard
Loudness	Graded on a six-point scale from I (barely audible) to VI (audible without stethoscope)
Pitch	Classified as either high or low; describe quality as musical, harsh, blowing, or buzzing
Place and duration	When the murmur occurs during the cardiac cycle: early, middle, or late; holosystolic or pansystolic murmurs are heard during the entire systolic phase; an ejection murmur is best heard during midsystole
Quality	A murmur's sound pattern; a *crescendo* starts low and grows louder; a *decrescendo* starts loud and gets softer; a *crescendo-decrescendo* starts softly, becomes loud, and then becomes soft again; a *plateau* is a consistent sound
Radiation	Sound migration to other parts of the body; for example, aortic murmurs often radiate to the carotid arteries, and mitral murmurs radiate to the axilla
Timing	Refers to whether the murmur occurs in systole or diastole; systolic murmurs, unlike diastolic murmurs, are harmless
Variations	Changes that occur with movement or interruption of normal respirations

Modified from Alexander, R.W., et al. (Eds.). (1998). *Hurst's the heart* (9th ed.). New York: McGraw-Hill; and O'Hanlon-Nickols, T. (1997). The adult cardiovascular system. *American Journal of Nursing, 97*(12), 34-40.

aortic stenosis, valve prolapse, or prosthetic valves. There are three basic types of clicks[4,13,20,25,27]:

1. *Click.* A *simple click* occurs during systole and is usually caused by a prolapsed mitral valve.
2. *Ejection sound.* An *ejection click* is a high-pitched sound heard in systole. It can be associated with either opening of the semilunar valves or prolapse (inversion) of the mitral valve. Ejection clicks heard during early systole usually result from sudden tensing of the aortic or pulmonic root at the peak of systolic ejection. They are often the result of high ventricular pressure generated in order to open a rigid, calcified aortic valve. Middle to late systolic clicks are more likely to be due to a benign form of mitral insufficiency (regurgitation). When a billowing mitral valve allows prolapse of the leaflets into the left atrium, a click can be heard as the chordae tendineae act as a tether and prohibit further leaflet excursion into the atria.
3. *Opening snap.* Valves normally open silently, but when they become calcified or rigid from disease, greater pressure is required to force them open. When they do "pop" open, they produce a characteristic sound. Opening snaps occur with the opening of a stenotic mitral and (rarely) tricuspid valve. The resulting sound is brief, high-pitched, and of a snapping quality. It is heard early in diastole at the apex using a diaphragm.

Pericardial Friction Rub. A pericardial friction rub is produced by inflammation of the pericardial sac (pericarditis). The roughened parietal and visceral layers of the pericardium rub against each other during cardiac motion. The sound has three components corresponding to cardiac activity: ventricular systole, ventricular diastole, and atrial systole.

A pericardial friction rub is best detected with the diaphragm at the apex and along the left sternal border. It may be accentuated when a person leans forward or lies prone and exhales. Friction rubs produce a sound that is described as "to and fro," scratchy, grating, rasping, and much like "squeaky leather." Friction rubs may be present during the first week after myocardial infarction or after open heart surgery. Differentiate a pericardial friction rub from a pleural friction rub by noting the timing of the rub in relation to breathing. Pleural friction rubs are heard during inspiration. Pericardial friction rubs are heard throughout the respiratory cycle.

Murmurs. Murmurs are heard as a consequence of turbulent blood flow through the heart and large vessels. Turbulent blood flow produces vibrations in the heart and great vessels that can be detected as a blowing or swooshing sound. Murmurs are caused by (1) increased rate or velocity of blood flow, (2) abnormal forward or backward flow across stenosed or incompetent valves, (3) flow into a dilated chamber, or (4) flow through an abnormal passage between heart chambers. Bruits are due to turbulence in vessels. Murmurs are best heard with the bell of the stethoscope when the client is in the left lateral recumbent position. Table 56-4 describes the characteristics of murmurs. Box 56-4 gives the scale for grading the loudness of murmurs.

Systolic murmurs, also called "benign" murmurs, are often caused by vigorous myocardial contraction or strong blood flow. They are common in children, adults

BOX 56-4	*Grading of Heart Murmurs**
Grade I	Faint; heard after listener has "tuned in"
Grade II	Faint murmur heard immediately
Grade III	Moderately loud, with accompanying thrill
Grade IV	Loud
Grade V	Very loud; heard only with the stethoscope
Grade VI	Very loud; heard without the stethoscope

*Heart murmurs are graded on a scale of 1 to 6 (I to VI).

younger than 50 years of age, and pregnant women. All diastolic murmurs are pathologic and are produced by mitral and tricuspid valve stenosis or aortic or pulmonic insufficiency. Table 56-5 presents a comparison of selected heart murmurs.[4,13,20,25,27]

Lungs

Because the cardiovascular and respiratory systems are intimately related, assessment of the cardiovascular system must include evaluation of the respiratory system. The respiratory assessment is discussed in Chapter 61. Common respiratory findings related to CVD are as follows.

Tachypnea. Tachypnea, or rapid respirations, is often associated with pain and anxiety accompanying myocardial ischemic pain. Tachypnea is also a common compensatory mechanism in heart failure and pulmonary edema.

Crackles. Crackles frequently signal left ventricular failure and usually occur just after the onset of an S_3 gallop. As pulmonary capillary pressure increases because of the backward pressure of left ventricular failure, fluid shifts into the intra-alveolar spaces and crackles can be auscultated. Crackles may also result from atelectasis (incomplete lung expansion) related to limited chest wall excursion during prolonged bed rest, chest splinting from pain, and the effects of sedatives and opioids. Crackles are high-pitched, noncontinuous sounds. Crackles are best heard at the lung bases (because of gravitational effects on the fluid) during late inspiration.[4]

Blood-Tinged Sputum. Pink, frothy sputum may indicate acute pulmonary edema. This manifestation accompanies diffuse pulmonary crackles and denotes serious left ventricular failure. Frank hemoptysis may be associated with pulmonary embolus. A cough frequently occurs with hemoptysis.

Cheyne-Stokes Respirations. Cheyne-Stokes respirations are characterized by abnormal periods of deep breathing alternating with periods of apnea. They are a common finding in heart failure, anemia, and brain damage (from anoxic encephalopathy).

Abdomen

Examination of the abdomen provides information regarding cardiac competence. Abdominal assessment is described in Chapters 30 and 44. Overweight and obesity are associated with insulin resistance. However, the presence of abdominal obesity is more highly correlated with metabolic risk factors than is an elevated BMI. Therefore the simple measure of waist circumference is recommended to identify the body weight component of the metabolic syndrome.[1,8,10]

Inspection and Palpation

Inspection may reveal abdominal distention. Palpation may confirm the presence of *ascites* (fluid accumulation in the peritoneal cavity) and an enlarged liver. Both of these findings indicate liver failure, which can be a sequela (result) of chronic right ventricular failure. In addition, you may elicit a hepatojugular reflex in the client with right ventricular distention.

After assessing for jugular vein distention, apply mild pressure with one hand over the liver for 1 minute. An increase in jugular vein distention during and immediately after liver compression indicates chronically elevated right ventricular pressure.

Auscultation

Auscultation can yield the following clues about cardiovascular function. Decreased bowel sounds may accompany potassium (K^+) depletion. Potassium depletion can complicate long-term diuretic use without sufficient potassium replacement. Increased bowel sounds, indicative of hypermotility, may result from laxative use or may be a side effect of certain antidysrhythmic agents (such as quinidine). Loud bruits, heard with the bell just over or above the umbilicus, may indicate an aortic obstruction or aortic aneurysm (the latter can be detected by a palpable abdominal pulsation). Bruits heard over the upper midline or toward the back typically arise from renal arterial stenosis.

DIAGNOSTIC TESTS

The following are the four most common types of diagnostic procedures used in the diagnosis of CVD:

- Laboratory tests
- Graphic procedures (ECG)
- Radiographic (x-ray) studies
- Hemodynamic studies

Nursing responsibilities in diagnostic testing include the following:

- Explaining the purpose and the procedure and answering any questions

TABLE 56-5 *Heart Murmurs*

Type of Heart Sound	Origin	Preferred Method of Auscultation
Systolic murmurs Ejection type 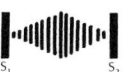	Systolic ejection murmurs are associated with forward blood flow during ventricular contraction across stenotic aortic or pulmonic valves.	Use the stethoscope diaphragm. Ejection murmurs are typically of medium pitch and harsh quality and may be associated with early ejection click. Aortic ejection murmurs are best heard over aortic valve and radiate into the neck, down the left sternal border, and occasionally to the apex. May be accompanied by decreased S_2. Pulmonic ejection murmurs are heard best over pulmonic valve, and they radiate toward left shoulder and left neck vessels. May be accompanied by a wide split S_2.
Pansystolic regurgitant murmurs 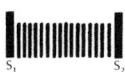	Pansystolic murmurs occur when blood regurgitates through incompetent mitral and tricuspid valves (AV valves) or ventricular septal defect as pressures rise during systole and blood seeks chambers of lower pressure. Damage to valve leaflets, papillary muscles, and chordae tendineae results in mitral valve insufficiency (blood regurgitates from left ventricle to left atrium) and tricuspid valve insufficiency (blood regurgitates from right ventricle to right atrium). Ventricular septal defect results in blood regurgitation from left ventricle to right ventricle.	All regurgitant murmurs are high-pitched, and those of AV valve incompetence have blowing quality. Mitral regurgitant murmurs are heard at apex, radiate into left axilla, and may be accompanied by ejection click and signs of left ventricular failure. Tricuspid regurgitant murmurs are heard loudest over the tricuspid area and radiate into the sternum. Ventricular septal defects are usually loud, harsh, and heard best over left sternal border in fourth, fifth, and sixth intercostal spaces and radiate over the precordium but not the axilla.
Early systolic murmurs 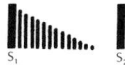	Early systolic (innocent) murmurs are associated with high cardiac outputs, as blood flow velocity is increased across normal semilunar valves. Causes include anemia, tachycardia, thyrotoxicosis, and fever. Murmur disappears with correction of underlying condition. Normal variant in children.	These are best heard with bell over base of heart or along lower left sternal border. Are usually no greater than grade II, are of medium pitch, and have a blowing quality. Intensity may increase during inspiration with client in left recumbent position or with increased heart rates.
Late systolic murmurs 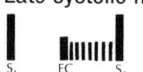	These imply mild mitral regurgitation as mitral valve balloons into left atrium late in ventricular systole.	Best heard with diaphragm of stethoscope over apex and are often preceded by midsystolic or late systolic ejection click.
Diastolic murmurs Early diastolic murmur 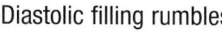	These (decrescendo murmurs) are usually caused by semilunar valve insufficiency, with regurgitation resulting from valvular deformity or dilation of valvular ring. Are heard immediately after S_2 and then diminish in intensity as pressure in aorta or pulmonary artery falls and ventricles fill.	Heard best with diaphragm at base of heart while the client leans forward in deep expiration. Are high-pitched and blowing and radiate down left sternal border, perhaps to apex or down right sternal border. Accompanying signs of heart failure may be present.
Diastolic filling rumbles	Caused by blood flows across stenotic AV valves (more often mitral). May also occur during augmented blood flow across normal AV valves. Murmur has two phases, becoming louder as the blood flow from the atrium to ventricle increases with passive ventricular filling just after AV valve opening and again during atrial contraction (presystole).	With the bell, this murmur is heard over only a small area at and just medial to the apex. Exercise and a left lateral position of the client increase the intensity of the sound. It is a low-pitched, rumbling sound often accompanied by an augmented S_1 and an opening snap.

Modified from Huang, S.L., et al. (1989). *Coronary care nursing* (2nd ed., p. 19). Philadelphia: W.B. Saunders; and Alexander, R.W., et al. (Eds.). (1998). *Hurst's the heart* (9th ed.) New York: McGraw-Hill.
AV, Atrioventricular.

- Witnessing signing of the consent form
- Scheduling the test
- Providing any necessary preliminary care (adjustments in medications and special diets)
- Promoting maximal emotional and physical comfort

After the procedure, review instructions for home care, returning to work, and general aftercare.[9,12,27]

Laboratory Tests

Laboratory test data are used to (1) diagnose a variety of cardiovascular ailments (myocardial infarction), (2) screen people considered at risk for CVD, (3) determine baseline values, (4) identify concurrent disorders (diabetes mellitus, electrolyte imbalance) that may affect treatment, and (5) evaluate the effectiveness of intervention. Tests that are more commonly used to determine cardiovascular function and disease are discussed here.

Prepare the client for the laboratory test by explaining the procedure. Determine whether the client should fast or refrain from intake of a particular substance before blood is drawn; if so, provide clear instructions. Determination of therapeutic levels of specific medications may require documenting the last time the drug was taken by the client to correlate with the laboratory value. Ask whether the client is taking any blood thinners such as warfarin sodium (Coumadin), which delays coagulation and would require a longer time to hold pressure over the venipuncture site.

Handle blood samples carefully. Gently invert laboratory tubes to prevent clotting of specimens for a complete blood count (CBC). Avoid vigorous handling of specimens, which may lead to hemolysis and falsely elevated levels of intracellular ions, such as potassium and magnesium. Apply pressure to the puncture site until bleeding stops. Assess the site for hematoma formation.[9,12,27]

Complete Blood Cell Count

The *red blood cell (RBC) count* or *erythrocyte count* is usually decreased in rheumatic fever and infective endocarditis. The count is usually increased in heart diseases characterized by inadequate tissue oxygenation, for example, right-to-left congenital shunts and heart conditions accompanied by obstructive lung disease.

Measuring the packed cell volume, or *hematocrit,* is the easiest way to ascertain the concentration of red blood cells in the blood. An elevated hematocrit can result from obstructive lung disease and conditions of vascular volume depletion with hemoconcentration (hypovolemic shock and excessive diuresis). Decreases in hematocrit and hemoglobin indicate anemia, which is commonly caused by hemorrhage, hemolysis (from prosthetic valves), and chronic disease states. Clients with anemia have a significant reduction in red blood cell

mass and a decrease in oxygen-carrying capacity. Anemia can be manifest as angina or it can exacerbate heart failure and produce heart murmurs.

The *white blood cell (WBC) count* is elevated in infectious and inflammatory diseases of the heart (infective endocarditis and pericarditis). It is also elevated after myocardial infarction because large numbers of WBCs are necessary to dispose of the necrotic tissue resulting from the infarction.

Cardiac Enzymes

Enzymes are special proteins that catalyze chemical reactions in living cells. Cardiac enzymes are present in high concentrations in myocardial tissue. Tissue damage causes release of enzymes from their intracellular storage areas. For example, myocardial infarction causes cellular anoxia, which alters membrane permeability and causes spillage of enzymes into the surrounding tissue. This leakage of enzymes can be detected by rising plasma levels. Cardiac enzyme levels reflect myocardial integrity or infarction (cellular death).

Myoglobin is a useful marker of myocardial necrosis that is rapidly released from the circulation within 1 to 2 hours of infarction. Its release allows very early detection, but its short half-life makes it less useful in clients who present several hours after onset. Measurement of myoglobin levels is not recommended if there is evidence of muscle damage, trauma, or renal failure because of the greater potential for false-positive test results in these circumstances.[9,12,27]

The enzymes most commonly used to detect myocardial infarction are *creatine kinase* (CK) and *lactic acid dehydrogenase* (LDH). Serum elevations of these two enzymes occur in sequence after myocardial insult. Because these enzymes are also found in other organs and tissues (skeletal muscle and liver), cardiac specificity must be determined by measuring isoenzyme activity. *Isoenzymes* are various forms of CK and LDH, identified by a process known as electrophoresis.

There are three isoenzymes of CK:

- CK-MM (skeletal muscle)
- CK-MB (myocardial muscle)
- CK-BB (brain)

Elevated CK-MB indicates myocardial damage. Plasma MB is significantly elevated within 6 to 8 hours of the onset of manifestations of myocardial infarction, maximal levels are reached between 14 and 36 hours, and levels return to normal after 48 to 72 hours. Samples should be taken immediately on admission and every 6 to 8 hours for the first 24 hours. Diagnosis of injury requires no fewer than two samples separated by at least 4 hours.

Of the five isoenzymes for LDH (numbered 1 to 5), only LDH_1 and LDH_2 are cardiac-specific. If the serum concentration of LDH_1 is higher than the concentration of LDH₂, the pattern is said to have "flipped," signifying myocardial necrosis. Eighty percent of clients have elevations in LDH within 48 hours after myocardial infarction.

The use of *troponin* has led to increased specificity in the detection of myocardial infarction. Troponin has three components: I, C, and T. Troponin I modulates the contractile state, troponin C binds calcium, and troponin T binds I and C. Although troponin is present in all striated muscle, troponin components in cardiac muscle have different amino acid sequences. Therefore antibodies against cardiac troponins I and T are very specific. Elevated levels of troponin I are as sensitive as CK-MB for the detection of myocardial injury. They correlate highly with the development of new areas of regional dysfunction determined by echocardiography and correlate in a linear fashion with the development of complications. Troponins are useful for diagnosis after 4 to 6 hours have elapsed. Once present, troponin I persists for 4 to 7 days.[9,12,13,25,27]

Because of their higher specificity for myocardial injury, troponins can be used to exclude myocardial infarction when CK-MB may be falsely positive, as in athletes, clients with skeletal trauma, and after direct-current (DC) cardioversion, or when CK totals may be high and MB missed, as in the postoperative state.

As well as indicating myocardial damage, elevations in serum cardiac enzymes can reveal the timing of the acute cardiac event (see Chapter 60).

Blood Coagulation Tests

Blood coagulation tests are used to examine the ability of blood to clot. Evaluate coagulation tests such as *prothrombin time* and *partial thromboplastin time* in people with a greater tendency to form thrombi (clients with atrial fibrillation, infective endocarditis, or prosthetic valves). Research has shown an increase in coagulation factors during and after a myocardial infarction. Therefore the client is at greater risk for thrombophlebitis and extension of clots in the coronary artery. Coagulation studies are ordered to guide dosage of antithrombotic drugs. Chapter 76 discusses coagulation tests in detail.

Serum Lipids

Clinical evidence provided by epidemiologic and angiographic studies show that an elevated blood cholesterol is a major risk factor in the development of atherosclerosis. Coronary heart disease is secondary to atherosclerosis and accumulation of lipids within the arterial wall, which is associated with inflammation and vascular remodeling. The cholesterol-containing lipid fraction most closely associated with atherogenesis is low-density lipoprotein cholesterol (LDL-C). Coronary heart disease

risk increases as blood levels of LDL-C increase. A second lipid fraction that plays a major role in determining CHD risk is high-density lipoprotein cholesterol (HDL-C). An inverse relationship exists between HDL-C and CHD incidence. These lipids are composed of fatty substances that are insoluble in water. They are derived from fats in the diet or synthesized in the liver. The lipid profile shows serum cholesterol, triglyceride, and lipoprotein levels and is used to assess the risk for development of coronary artery disease. Serum lipids are discussed in Chapter 53.

C-Reactive Protein

Elevation of C-reactive protein (CRP), an acute-phase protein measure of the presence and degree of inflammation, has been linked to future cardiovascular risks, which include stroke, myocardial infarction, and cardiovascular death. Atherosclerosis is in part a chronic low-grade inflammatory condition. Plasma markers of inflammation, such as CRP, are strong independent predictors of future coronary events in seemingly healthy persons. The CRP may be a marker for events involving atherosclerotic plaque rupture and acute thrombosis than for events primarily involving progression of lesional stenosis.

Serum Electrolytes

Fluid and electrolyte regulation may be affected by cardiovascular disorders. Electrolyte balance is also altered by certain medications. In addition, electrolyte levels can alter cardiac muscle contraction. Chapters 13 and 14 describe fluids and electrolytes.

Potassium. The serum potassium level decreases as a result of diuretic therapy, vomiting, diarrhea, and alkalosis. *Hypokalemia* (abnormally low potassium) increases cardiac electrical instability, the occurrence of ventricular dysrhythmias, and the risk of digitalis toxicity. A characteristic change on the ECG is a U wave. A high serum potassium level is usually associated with kidney and endocrine disorders. *Hyperkalemia* can lead to a tall T wave on the ECG, asystole, and ventricular dysrhythmias.

Sodium. The serum sodium level reflects water balance and may decrease (*hyponatremia*, indicating water excess) with heart failure, stress, excessive intravenous (IV) infusion of hypotonic fluids, and vomiting. Extensive use of diuretics and severely restricted sodium intake also lower serum sodium.

Calcium. Calcium is considered an important mediator of many cardiovascular functions because of its effect on cardiac excitability, contractility, and vascular tone. The serum calcium level decreases as a result of multiple transfusions of citrated blood, renal failure, alkalosis, and laxative and antacid abuse (phosphate excess). *Hypocalcemia* can lead to serious ventricular dysrhythmias, a prolonged QT interval, and cardiac arrest. *Hypercalcemia* occurs with thiazide diuretic use, acidosis, adrenal insufficiency, immobility, and vitamin D excess. Hypercalcemia shortens the QT interval and causes AV block, tachycardia, bradycardia, digitalis hypersensitivity, and cardiac arrest.

Magnesium. Magnesium helps regulate intracellular metabolism, activates essential enzymes, and aids transport of sodium and potassium across the cell membrane. It plays a vital role in neuromuscular excitability.

Hypomagnesemia may result from prolonged use of diuretics, malnutrition, chronic alcoholism, severe diarrhea, and dehydration. Manifestations include mental apathy, facial tics, leg cramps, respiratory depression, and severe cardiac dysrhythmias, including ventricular tachycardia and fibrillation. *Hypermagnesemia* may develop in the client with chronic renal failure. Manifestations include profound muscle weakness, hyporeflexia, hypotension, and bradycardia with a prolonged PR interval and wide QRS complex.

Phosphorus. Most extracellular phosphorus is present in the bone with calcium (85% of the body's total phosphorus). A small amount of phosphorus is found in intracellular fluid. There it helps regulate energy formation (adenosine triphosphate [ATP]) and maintain acid-base balance and neuromuscular excitability. Phosphate levels are inversely related to calcium levels as the kidneys retain or excrete one or the other. Interpret the two levels together.

Hypophosphatemia may result from hyperparathyroidism, diabetic ketoacidosis, prolonged use of IV dextrose infusions, or renal tubular acidosis. Manifestations of hypophosphatemia include bleeding, decreased WBC levels, muscular weakness (including respiratory muscles), and nausea and vomiting.

Hyperphosphatemia usually occurs in clients with chronic renal failure or skeletal disease (including healing fractures) and those undergoing chemotherapy. Manifestations are similar to those of hypocalcemia, with muscle tetany being the most common finding.

Blood Urea Nitrogen and Creatinine

Blood urea nitrogen (BUN) and serum creatinine are indicators of renal function, specifically the ability of the kidney to excrete urea and protein. They are elevated in kidney diseases, during water and saline depletion, and in cardiac disorders that adversely affect renal circulation, for example, heart failure and cardiogenic shock. Elevated levels are also associated with diabetes, hyper-

tension, and the aging process and are used as a laboratory test in cardiovascular risk analysis.

Blood Glucose

Diabetes mellitus is a major risk factor for the development of atherosclerosis. In addition, the stress of an acute cardiac event can greatly elevate blood glucose, causing unstable *hyperglycemia* in clients with latent diabetes mellitus. For these reasons, blood glucose is routinely assessed in all clients with acute cardiovascular disorders.

The American Heart Association recommends normal fasting blood glucose to be less than 110 mg/dl. Diabetic appropriate hypoglycemic therapy aims to achieve near-normal fasting blood glucose, as indicated by HbA1c less than 7% to prevent heart attack and stroke.[1,6]

Electrocardiogram

Procedure

The ECG is an essential tool in evaluating the heart rhythm. Electrocardiography detects and amplifies the very small electrical potential changes between different points on the surface of the body as the myocardial cells depolarize and repolarize, causing the heart to contract. The same electrical impulses spread outward from the heart to the skin, where they can be detected by electrodes attached to the skin. The ECG displays the electrical action of the heart.

There are several types of ECGs: continuous monitoring, 12-lead, signal-averaged, and Holter monitoring. Analysis of ECG waveforms allows identification of disorders of cardiac rate, rhythm, and conduction.

ECG is a common noninvasive test. It is performed for clients older than 40 years of age before surgery to detect any unknown heart disease and is frequently used for clients with known or suspected heart disease.

Preprocedure Care

Prepare the client for a 12-lead ECG or continuous monitoring. Explain that the test helps evaluate the heart's function by recording its electrical activity. The steps required for ECG monitoring are (1) attaching the electrodes to the client's skin, (2) connecting the electrodes to the monitor by a cable, and (3) adjusting the monitor to obtain a readable ECG. During the procedure, advise the client to lie still, breathe normally, and refrain from talking. Record the client's age, height, and weight, and note any cardiac medications being taken.[4,27]

Postprocedure Care

After the procedure, disconnect the equipment. If using conductive gel, wipe the gel from the client's skin. If using conductive stickers, remove them unless serial ECG readings are to be done. If serial ECGs are ordered, leave the stickers in place to ensure consistent lead placement.

Continuous Electrocardiogram Monitoring

For the client who is undergoing continuous ECG monitoring, adjust the monitor by setting the alarms for desired high and low rates. Reassure the client that the equipment does not cause electrical shock or hurt. Clients receiving telemetry are monitored continuously with radiofrequency waves rather than by direct cable attachment. They can get up and move about their rooms or walk in the halls while their heart rhythm is monitored.

Attaching the Electrodes. Electrodes detect electrical impulses from the heart on the skin. Unless the signal is detected accurately, ECG monitoring has little value. The most common electrodes are disk-type or floating electrodes, which are separated from the skin by a spacer filled with conductive gel. The gel improves the signal by reducing local electrical interference on the skin. An adhesive ring surrounds the gel. Peel the paper backing off the pad and apply the electrode to the skin. Three electrodes are required for continuous ECG monitoring. Two of these detect the heart's activity; the third is an electrical ground.

Attach the electrodes to the lead wires before applying them to the chest wall. This process makes it unnecessary to apply pressure to the electrode, which could hurt the client and squeeze the gel outward, reducing contact.

Thorough skin preparation improves impulse conduction. Clean the areas where electrodes are to be applied. Wipe the skin with alcohol, and allow it to air-dry before applying the electrodes. If the client has a lot of chest hair, clip the hair to improve contact.

Position the electrodes on the chest wall by selecting locations that will provide the clearest ECG waveforms. Two common positions are (1) the conventional position and (2) the modified chest lead position (Figure 56-5). The lead II waveform (shown) is the most common rhythm strip lead. MCL$_1$ (shown), V$_1$, and V$_6$ are more helpful for detecting dysrhythmia. When close monitoring of ST segments is essential, such as after cardiac bypass surgery, thrombolytic therapy, or coronary angioplasty, the lead most closely associated with the area of involved heart muscle should be monitored. Change electrodes if the tracing is unclear, the electrodes become dry, or skin contact is lost. Electrodes should be routinely changed every 48 hours to avoid skin irritation and to ensure that electrode gel is sufficient for clear conduction.

Connecting the Monitor. The electrodes are connected to the monitor by lead wires, which are 12 to 18 inches long. One end snaps onto the electrode, and the other end is attached to a cable that is connected to the monitor. The cable has a receptacle for the attachment of each wire. The receptacle and lead wires are color-coded to facilitate connection.

Adjusting the Monitor. The ECG pattern should be clear and distinct. If the pattern is not clear, recheck the first steps. Monitor adjustments depend on the brand of monitor in use. Refer to the operating instructions for assistance.

Setting the Alarms. Set alarm limits appropriately to signal any acute changes. Many monitors have default alarm settings. Verify these for each client. If there are no default settings or institutional standards, alarm limits should be set approximately 20 beats above and below the client's typical heart rate.

At times, false alarms may occur because of poor electrode contact or client movement. Occasionally, the alarm limits are set too far apart (40 to 180 beats/min) or, even worse, the alarms are turned off completely. This practice defeats the purpose of the alarm system and should never be adopted.

Electrocardiogram Tracings

When continuous ECG monitoring is used, assess the heart rhythm hourly. Log rhythm strips into the medical record routinely as well as when dysrhythmias are noted. Dysrhythmias are discussed in Chapter 59.

The impulse waves, recorded by the ECG machine on graph paper, are arbitrarily designated by the letters P, Q, R, S, and T. The QRS letters are generally referred to as the QRS complex. Figure 56-6 depicts the typical ECG pattern formed by these waves.

The components of the ECG are defined as follows:
- The P wave represents depolarization of the atria.
- The PR interval represents the time it takes for the impulse to spread from the atria to the ventricles.
- The QRS complex represents depolarization of the ventricles.
- The T wave represents repolarization of the ventricles.
- The ST segment indicates that ventricular depolarization is complete and repolarization is about to begin.
- The QT interval represents electrical systole and varies with age, gender, heart rate, and medications.
- The U wave is a small wave that sometimes follows the T wave. It may indicate hypokalemia.

An ECG tracing also shows the voltage of the waves and the duration of both the waves and the intervals. ECG graph paper is divided into horizontal lines and vertical lines, large squares and small squares. Voltage is represented on the vertical axis of the ECG paper. Each

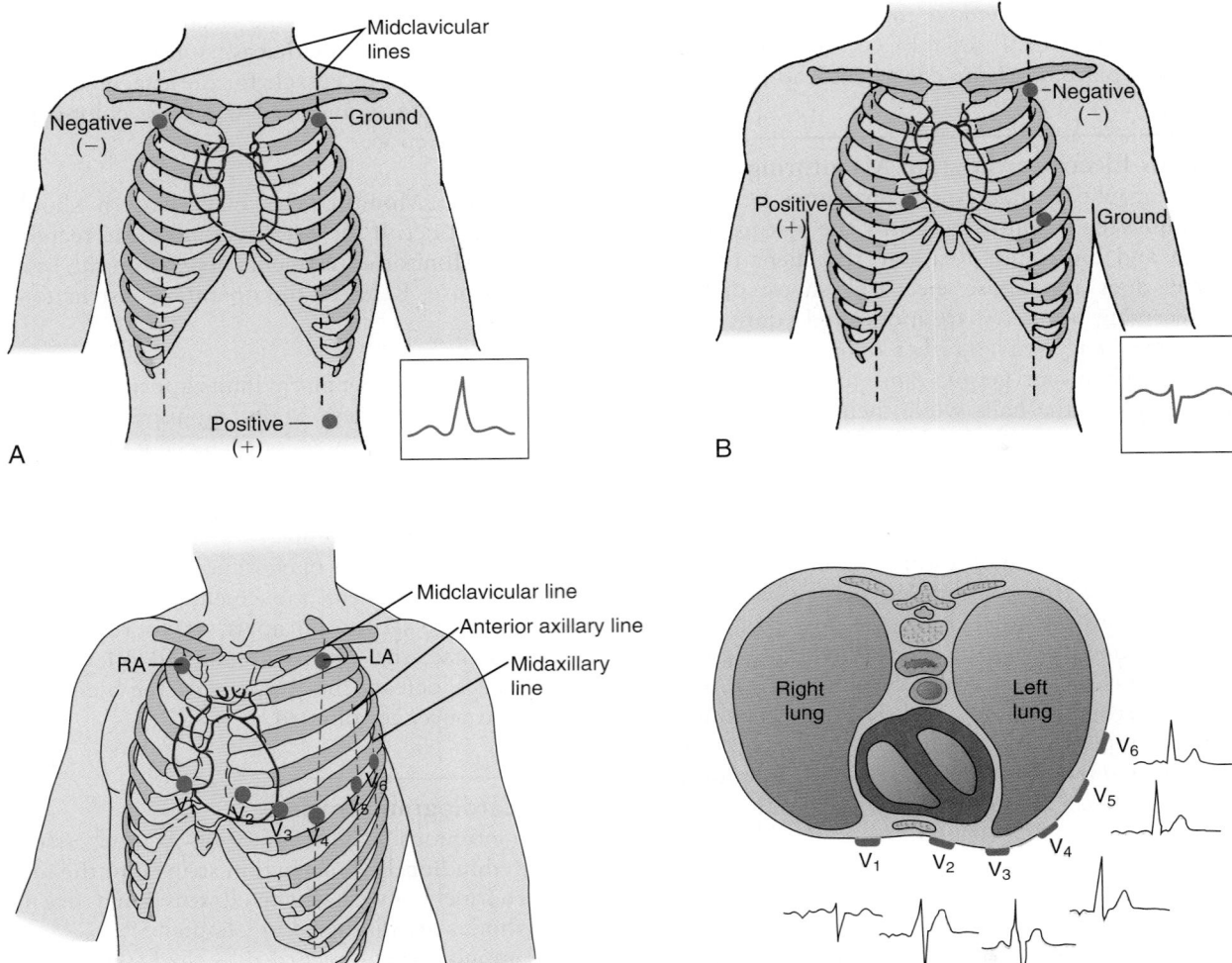

FIGURE 56-5 Common positions for continuous monitoring lead placement. **A,** Lead II. Positive electrode—left leg; negative electrode—right arm. **B,** Lead MCL₁. Positive electrode—fourth ICS at right sternal border; negative electrode—below left clavicle at MCL. **C,** Five lead system. RA electrode—below right clavicle at MCL. LA electrode—below left clavicle at MCL. RL electrode—right abdomen at MCL. LL electrode—left abdomen at MCL. V₁–V₆ are the precordial or chest leads. V₁—fourth ICS at right sternal border. V₂—fourth ICS at left sternal border. V₃—fourth ICS, midway between left sternal border and MCL. V₄—fifth ICS at left MCL. V₅—Horizontal to V₄, fifth ICS, at the AAL. V₆—Horizontal to V₄ and V₅, at the MAL. **D,** Normal electrocardiographic findings with corresponding chest leads to cross-section at the fourth rib level. *AAL,* Anterior axillary line; *ICS,* intercostals space; *MAL,* midaxillary line; *MCL,* midclavicular line; *RA,* right arm; *RL,* right leg; *LA,* left arm; *LL,* left leg.

small square is 1 mm in height. Five small squares are equivalent to 5 mm, which is equivalent to 0.5 mV. Voltage yields information about the presence and degree of atrial or ventricular hypertrophy. Time is measured on the horizontal axis. Each small square signifies the passage of 0.04 second. Each large square indicates the passage of 0.20 second. By studying the duration of the waves and intervals, the examiner can diagnose abnormal impulse formation and conduction.

Normal time durations for waves and intervals are as follows:
- *P wave:* less than 0.11 second
- *PR interval:* 0.12 to 0.20 second (average, 0.16 second)
- *QRS complex:* 0.04 to 0.11 second
- *QT interval:* in women, up to 0.43 second; in men, up to 0.42 second (normal duration is inversely related to heart rate)

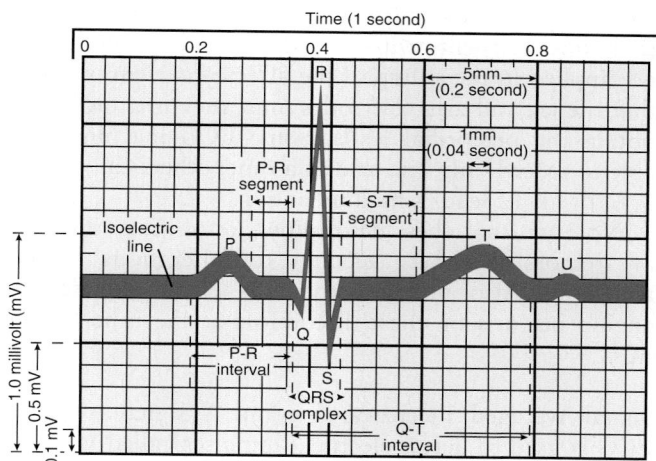

FIGURE 56-6 Normal electrocardiographic (ECG) pattern. The P wave represents depolarization of the atria to the ventricles. The QRS complex represents depolarization of the ventricles, and the T wave represents repolarization of the ventricles. The small U wave is sometimes seen following the T wave. Time and voltage lines of ECG paper: *vertically,* 1 mm = 0.1 mV; 5 mm = 0.5 mV; 10 mm = 1 mV; *horizontally,* one small box = 0.04 second; five small boxes = 0.20 second; 25 small boxes = 1 second.

Because of its normal variation in configuration, more must be said about the QRS complex. The Q wave is always the first downward (negative) deflection of the complex. The R wave is always the first upward (positive) deflection. If there is a negative deflection (below the baseline) after an R wave, it is labeled an S wave. In most instances, a Q wave is not obvious on the ECG of the normal heart. The QRS complex may appear as a mostly positive or mostly negative deflection, depending on the recording electrode used.[9,13,27]

Electrocardiogram Variations

The 12-Lead Electrocardiogram. Indications for a 12-lead ECG are listed in Box 56-5.

The standard ECG has a 12-lead system, offering 12 points of reference for recording the electrical activity of the heart. The 12-lead ECG can be conceptualized as 12 different views of the heart, looking in both horizontal and vertical planes. The standard 12-lead ECG has six *limb* leads (used to view the heart in a frontal or vertical plane) and six *precordial* leads (used to view the heart in a horizontal plane).

The limb leads are composed of three *bipolar* leads (leads I, II, and III) and three *unipolar* leads (leads aVR, aVL, and aVF). The bipolar leads have two electrodes and measure the difference in electrical potential flowing through the heart between two extremities. The unipolar leads compare the electrical potential of a positive elec-

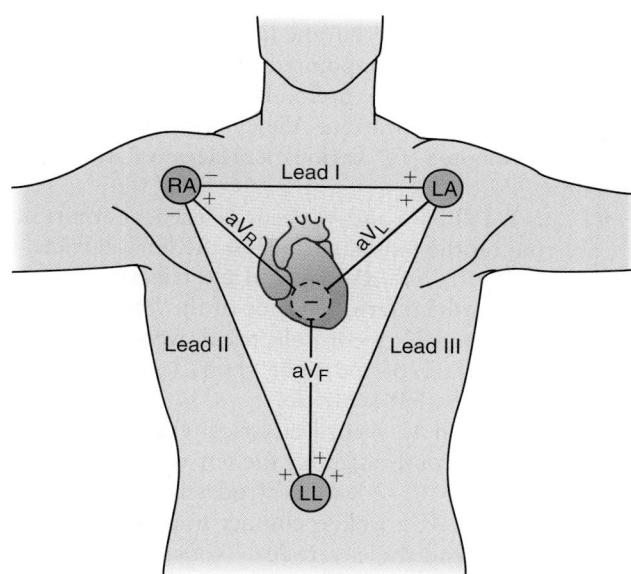

FIGURE 56-7 Standard limb leads. Leads are actually located on the extremities: right arm (RA), left arm (LA), and left leg (LL). The right leg electrode serves as a ground. Leads I, II, and III (Einthoven's triangle) are bipolar, using both a positive and a negative electrode. Leads aV_R, aV_L, and aV_F are augmented unipolar leads that use the calculated center of the heart as their negative electrode.

trode, placed on one limb, and a negative pole within a central terminal that averages the potential of the other two limb leads.

Standard bipolar limb leads are called I, II, and III (Figure 56-7):
- *Lead I* measures the difference in electrical potential between the left arm and right arm.
- *Lead II* measures the difference in potential between the left leg and right arm.
- *Lead III* measures the difference in potential between the left leg and left arm.

Augmented unipolar limb leads are as follows (see Figure 56-7):

- VR measures electrical potential between the center of the heart and the right arm.
- VL measures electrical potential between the center of the heart and the left arm.
- VF measures electrical potential between the center of the heart and the left leg.

The precordial leads (V_1, V_2, V_3, V_4, V_5, and V_6) provide six views of the heart from the anterior and left lateral vantage points. These unipolar leads compare the electrical potential between a positive electrode (in the six different chest locations) and a central, negative terminal that represents an average potential of the three standard limb leads (Figure 56-5, *D*).

Together, the 12 leads permit multidirectional examination of the electrical events in the heart. The location of pathologic change within the heart, which alters electrical activity, can be pinpointed. Table 56-6 correlates the area of infarct with expected ECG changes and coronary artery lesion location. Views from the different leads are oriented to various surfaces of the myocardium:

- Leads I, aVL, V_5, and V_6 record electrical events occurring on the lateral surface of the left ventricle.
- Leads II, III, and aVF record electrical events occurring on the inferior surface of the left ventricle.
- Leads V_1 and V_2 record electrical events occurring on the surface of the right ventricle and anterior surface of the left ventricle.
- Leads V_3 and V_4 record electrical events occurring within the septal region of the left ventricle.

The placement of 12-lead electrodes is shown in Figure 56-5, *A* to *C*. Unbroken contact must be made between the skin and the electrodes. To facilitate contact, the electrodes are placed firmly on the flat surface just above the wrists and ankles. There are many varieties of electrodes: adhesive back, foam, cloth, plastic, and suction cups. In clients with an amputation, the electrodes are applied to the stump of the affected extremity. Note that the leg and arm electrodes must remain attached to obtain the precordial leads. Some ECG machines are able to record only one lead at a time; others can record 3, 6, or all 12 leads simultaneously.

Note unusual chest deformities, respiratory distress, or tremors that may account for alterations in the recording. Also note whether the client experiences angina pectoris or chest discomfort at the time of the ECG.[4,9,13,27]

Signal-Averaged Electrocardiogram. A signal-averaged ECG is used to detect electrical impulses called *late potentials*. These impulses occur during diastole late into the QRS complex and ST segment. This noninvasive test may be done at the bedside and is used to determine whether the client is susceptible to ventricular tachycardia that could result in sudden death. For a signal-averaged ECG, a computer is used to record and process low-level signals that are not detected by a traditional ECG. This technique allows detection of signals that might otherwise be masked by noise that conceals the small electrical events of the heart. Late potentials are multiphasic, low-amplitude, high-frequency spikes that appear after the terminal portion of the QRS complex and extend into the ST segment. They are thought to be generated by delayed activation in an abnormal area of the heart. The presence of late potentials in clients with normal sinus rhythm indicates a risk of ventricular tachycardia and sudden cardiac death.[13]

Holter Monitoring (Ambulatory Electrocardiography). When the client wears a portable Holter monitor, an ECG tracing may be recorded continuously for a day or longer on an outpatient basis, whereas a standard ECG

TABLE 56-6	*Coronary Artery Lesion Location, Area of Infarct, and Electrocardiographic Changes*		
Coronary Artery	**Area of Infarct**	**ECG Leads**	**Dysrhythmias**
LAD	Anterior	V_{2-4}	RBBB, LAH, Mobitz type II, CHB
	Septal	V_{1-2}	
	Anteroseptal	V_{1-4}	
Circumflex	Lateral	I, aVL	Ventricular and possibly SA and AV node conduction disturbances
	Anterolateral	I, aVL, V_{5-6}	
	Inferolateral	aVF, II, III, V_{5-6}	
	Posterior	Reciprocal, V_{1-3}	
RCA	Inferior	II, III, aVF	SA node, AV node, and His bundle conduction disturbances
	Right ventricle	II, III, aVF, V_{4-6R}	

From Alspach, J. G. (Ed.) (1992). *Instructor's resource manual for the AACN core curriculum for critical care nursing.* Philadelphia: W.B. Saunders.
AV, Atrioventricular; *CHB,* complete heart block; *LAD,* left anterior descending; *LAH,* left anterior hemiblock; *RBBB,* right bundle branch block; *RCA,* right coronary artery; *SA,* sinoatrial.

is obtained in a relatively short time. Thus Holter monitoring is used to detect dysrhythmias that may not appear on a routine ECG but occur when the client is ambulating at home or work. Holter monitoring is also useful in evaluating the effectiveness of antidysrhythmic or pacemaker therapy.[13,27] The monitoring system records at preset time intervals and when it senses an unusual event. Clinical indications include, dizziness, pacemaker evaluation, palpitations, and syncope.

To prepare the client, place two to three electrodes on the chest and attach them to the telemetry unit. This unit is not much larger than a beeper and is worn in a sling about the chest or waist. Encourage the client to go about usual daily activities and keep a written account of these activities along with any manifestations that develop. These data are used to document transient dysrhythmias and correlate the client's perceived manifestations with the underlying rhythm.[9,13,27]

Exercise Electrocardiogram (Stress Testing)

Procedure

Exercise tolerance testing defines the body's reaction to measured increases in acute exercise. Changes in heart rate, BP, respirations, and perceived level of exertion provide data for quantitative estimation of cardiovascular conditioning and function. The exercise testing may be used in conjunction with myocardial radionuclide testing. Regardless of the technique used, the optimal exercise testing protocol lasts 6 to 12 minutes and is adjusted to the type of client being tested. The advantages of the exercise test are that it is easily performed, relatively inexpensive, and completely noninvasive. The test helps evaluate the presence, absence, or severity of coronary artery disease, both in clients with known CHD and those initially seen with chest pain of unknown origin. Stress testing is used to evaluate the functional capacity of clients with or without heart disease and can be done serially to evaluate the effectiveness of medical and surgical interventions.

Exercise testing may consist of single or multiple stages. A single-stage test is one in which the exercise workload is constant throughout. Multiple-stage testing involves increasing the exercise workload in increments until a desired point is reached. The incremental increases in workload may occur every 1 to 5 minutes. The duration of testing varies with the type of test being used and the client's tolerance.

There are two major modes of exercise used for stress testing:

1. *Bicycle ergometry* involves a device equipped with a wheel operated by pedals that can be adjusted to increase the resistance to pedaling (multistage testing). It can be used for arm cranking, foot pedaling, or both. Advantages are that this mode of exercise is relatively inexpensive and the equipment is portable. However, frequent recalibration is required and localized muscle group fatigue is often induced.

2. *Treadmill testing* is the most common mode of stress testing, especially when used in conjunction with thallium 201 imaging. The treadmill is a motorized device that has an adjustable conveyer belt able to reach speeds of 1 to 10 miles per hour. The conveyer belt can be adjusted from a horizontal position to a 20% gradient, allowing the client to walk or run on slopes of different angles.[9,13,27]

Preprocedure Care

Before stress testing, inform the client of the purposes and risks of exercise testing and obtain an informed consent. Instruct the client not to eat or smoke for 2 to 3 hours before the test and to dress appropriately for exercise. No strenuous physical efforts should be made for at least 12 hours before testing. Most clients are allowed to take their usual medications unless the physician orders otherwise.

Brief history-taking and physical examination are performed. Obtain a baseline resting ECG immediately before testing. A standing ECG and BP should be recorded to determine vasoregulatory abnormalities, particularly ST-segment depression. Prepare the skin for electrode placement as previously described. Secure electrodes to the chest with tape or a belt. Drape lead wires, cable, and BP cuff to allow maximal freedom of movement. See the Client Education Guide feature on Stress Testing on the website for further client instructions. During the exercise test, the client's BP (taken with an automatically inflating cuff) and ECG are closely monitored by a physician or appropriately trained person.

During the procedure, perform the following:
- Obtain baseline BP, heart rate, and rhythm strip.
- Observe the ECG monitor constantly for changes.
- Record the client's BP, heart rate, rhythm strip, and activity level and time at specified intervals.
- Monitor the client for chest pain, dysrhythmias, ST-segment changes, unexpected changes in BP, or other cardiac manifestations (extreme dyspnea, claudication, vertigo).

A multilead monitoring system is most often used to provide maximal views of the heart wall. The examiner makes frequent observations throughout testing for untoward manifestations related to impaired cardiovascular performance. These include chest pain, ventricular dysrhythmia, extreme dyspnea, claudication (leg pain), vertigo, and a sudden decrease in BP. Reasons for terminating the test are as follows:

1. Chest pain or fatigue
2. Greatly increased heart rate (age-related):
   a. 20 to 29 years: 170 beats/min
   b. 30 to 39 years: 160 beats/min

   c. 40 to 49 years: 150 beats/min

   d. 50 to 59 years: 140 beats/min

   e. 60 to 69 years: 130 beats/min

3. Untoward manifestations of myocardial ischemia or heart failure

4. Failure of systolic BP to increase or a decrease in BP (below resting levels)

5. Sudden development of bradycardia

6. Serious cardiac dysrhythmia

7. Severe hypertension

8. Severe dyspnea

9. ST-segment depression (greater than 2 to 4 mm)

10. Sudden loss of coordination (cerebral ischemia)

Because these manifestations occur with some frequency, an emergency cart containing cardiac drugs and resuscitation equipment is kept close at hand at all times. Clients rarely die because of this procedure, but some may need assistance with resuscitation from dysrhythmias.

A positive exercise test is one that must be terminated before the predicted maximal (or submaximal) limits have been achieved because of manifestations of cardiovascular intolerance. Generally, the earlier these manifestations appear, the more serious the disease. Alterations in the ST segment and T wave on the ECG during exercise and recovery are often considered diagnostic of coronary artery disease because these alterations reflect an imbalance between myocardial oxygen demand and supply. There is, however, controversy about what extent of ST-segment change constitutes an abnormal response to exercise. The most widely held position is that the stress test is positive when the configuration and magnitude of the ST segment fulfill any of the following criteria:

- A 1-mm flat (horizontal) ST-segment depression lasting for 0.08 second
- A 1-mm downsloping ST-segment depression lasting for 0.08 second (this has the highest predictive value)
- A 1.5- to 2-mm upsloping ST-segment depression lasting for 0.08 second (this characteristic alone does not constitute a positive response)

Although the exercise test is helpful as an adjunct diagnostic study for coronary artery disease, it can produce false-positive findings in some cases, especially in women. In some people, ST-segment alterations may occur during exercise even though coronary artery disease is not present. Hyperventilation, certain drugs, and electrolyte imbalances can produce false-positive readings. For this reason, a diagnosis cannot be based on exercise findings alone.

False-negative findings also occur, although with less frequency. Medications such as beta-blocking agents and nitrates can produce false-negative results. Another limitation of the study is that it is absolutely contraindicated for clients with various cardiovascular and noncardiac conditions. See Box 56-6 for contraindications to exercise testing.

Become familiar with the stress testing procedure to provide clear teaching guidelines to clients scheduled for exercise testing. Many clients have misconceptions and unnecessary fears. Although not painful, the procedure can produce great fatigue. Warn the client that this test may trigger chest pain and dyspnea. Along with this warning, explain that the procedure is performed in a controlled environment under close nursing and medical attention. It is essential that the client arrive for the exercise testing appointment relaxed and well rested. Teaching guidelines for stress testing appear in the Client Education Guide feature on the website.[9,13,27]

Postprocedure Care

After the procedure, assist the client to a chair, cart, or bed for recovery. Periodically monitor the client's BP, heart rate, and rhythm strip for at least 15 minutes after test completion or until the ECG returns to baseline.

Electrophysiologic Studies

The electrophysiologic study is an invasive method of recording intracardiac electrical activity. It is used to (1) shed light on the mechanisms of dysrhythmias, (2) differentiate between supraventricular and ventricular dysrhythmias, (3) evaluate sinoatrial (SA) or AV node dys-

---

BOX 56-6 *Contraindications to Exercise Testing*

Acute Cardiovascular Disease

Acute myocardial infarction (usually avoided in clients less than 2 weeks after infarction)

Unstable angina pectoris

Heart failure

Pericarditis

Myocarditis

Endocarditis

Life-threatening dysrhythmias

Thrombophlebitis

Recent systemic embolism

Dissecting or enlarging aneurysm

Others

Severe diseases restricting mobility

Renal failure

Severe pulmonary disruptions

Orthopedic disorders affecting the spine or lower extremities

Neurologic impairment (stroke or paralysis)

Systemic infection

Left ventricular outflow obstruction (aortic stenosis, hypertension, or hypertrophic cardiomyopathy)

function, (4) determine the need for a pacemaker, and (5) evaluate the effect of antidysrhythmic agents used to prevent the occurrence of tachycardias.[9,13,27]

An electrophysiologic catheter has four electrodes at the distal tip that record or stimulate (pace). Under fluoroscopy, the catheter is threaded into the heart via the femoral, basilic, or subclavian vein. The catheter sites selected depend on the purpose of the examination. One catheter is placed at the bundle of His just beneath the AV node as a point of reference. An additional catheter is introduced high in the right atrium. If Wolff-Parkinson-White syndrome is suspected, a catheter may be placed in the coronary sinus. A catheter may also be placed in the right ventricle. During mapping of ventricular tachycardia, a catheter may be introduced into the left ventricle via an artery.

The purpose of the procedure is to reproduce any dysrhythmia so that its origin may be isolated. Ventricular tachycardia is induced by using programmed stimulation to fire an impulse at different times during the cardiac electrical cycle. If dysrhythmia is induced, the client's BP and hemodynamic responses are observed. It is possible to record simultaneously arterial pressure, surface ECGs, and ECGs from intracavitary catheters. The morphology and rate of the induced tachycardia are compared with those of the client's spontaneous ventricular tachycardia. Ventricular tachycardia is often terminated by rapid ventricular decremental pacing. If the tachycardia cannot be stimulated, IV isoproterenol may be infused to simulate stress or exercise, which may produce the tachycardia.

Antidysrhythmic drugs may be administered during the study to evaluate their effect. After the initial antidysrhythmic has been given, induction of ventricular tachycardia is attempted. If ventricular tachycardia is induced, the dosage may be increased or other drugs administered. The electrophysiologic studies are repeated in several days to determine the effectiveness of antidysrhythmic drug therapy.

Frequently, when the irritable focus has been identified (accessory pathway or bundle of His), ablation (destruction) may be performed. Ablation of the irritable focus may be accomplished by the use of radiofrequency waves, direct current, ethyl alcohol, or cryosurgery. Radiofrequency ablation is the most popular method because its effect may be localized, with less damage to surrounding tissue.[9,13,27]

Preprocedure and Postprocedure Care

Preprocedure and postprocedure nursing care of the client undergoing electrophysiologic studies is similar to that of the client undergoing cardiac catheterization. Because these studies attempt, under controlled circumstances, to induce potentially lethal dysrhythmias, it is imperative that emergency drugs, equipment, and a defibrillator be immediately accessible.

Cardiac Diagnostic Imaging

X-ray studies, magnetic resonance imaging (MRI), ultrasonography, and radioisotopes are discussed in Chapter 4. Use of these diagnostic tools to evaluate the heart is discussed next. See Chapter 4 for the preprocedure care and postprocedure care for each of these diagnostic examinations.

Chest X-Ray Studies

Posteroanterior, lateral, and oblique chest x-ray films help determine the size, silhouette, and position of the heart. For the acutely ill client, a portable anteroposterior x-ray study is performed at the bedside. Specific pathologic changes of the heart are difficult to determine with x-ray examination, but anatomic changes in the heart and pulmonary sequelae of various cardiac conditions can be seen. Assessed on x-ray film are valvular and pericardial calcifications; pulmonary congestion (from heart failure); pericardial effusion; and placement of central lines, endotracheal tubes, hemodynamic monitoring devices, and intra-aortic balloon catheters.

Magnetic Resonance Imaging

Although MRI is one of the most expensive noninvasive diagnostic options, a variety of data may be obtained in a single image. MRI provides the best information on chamber size, wall motion, valvular function, and great vessel blood flow without the use of ionizing radiation. MRI is commonly used for examination of the aorta and detection of tumors, aneurysms, masses, cardiomyopathies, and pericardial disease. MRI can show the heart beating and the blood flowing in any direction. All standard quantitative functional indices, except transstenotic gradients, can be obtained from an MRI study.

Information obtained from MRI includes the following:

- Normal morphology and structural changes
- Wall thickness, chamber volumes, valve areas, vessel cross-sections, and extent, location, and size of lesions
- Global and regional biventricular function, including ejection fraction, stroke volume, and cardiac output
- Blood flow quantifications within vessels over the cardiac cycle
- Tissue characterization of paracardiac and intracardiac masses, pericardial effusions, and myocardial infarction

Positron Emission Tomography

The positron emission tomographic (PET) scanner is a diagnostic imaging tool that allows visualization of regional physiologic function and biochemical changes that often separate normal from diseased myocardium. Cellular metabolic information is obtained by mapping regional myocardial glucose metabolism. Combining information from the perfusion and metabolism images provides a thorough assessment of regional cardiac viability. For further discussion of PET, see Chapter 4.

The scanning procedure takes about 2 to 3 hours. An IV radiopharmaceutical, [^{13}N]-ammonia, is administered and a 20-minute blood flow image is begun. An IV injection of glucose follows. Localization of glucose in the myocardium takes about 40 minutes. Final uptake of the tracer is proportional to the glucose metabolic activity of myocardial cells and provides an excellent indication of regional tissue viability.

The following are clinical indications for the use of a PET scan:

- Detection of coronary artery disease
- Assessment of myocardial viability
- Assessment of progression of coronary artery stenosis
- Documentation of collateral coronary circulation
- Differentiation of ischemia from dilated cardiomyopathy

The terms *match* and *mismatch* describe the relationship between the perfusion and metabolism studies. A perfusion study showing poor blood flow and a metabolic study showing decreased glucose uptake of necrotic tissue are described as a *match*. A perfusion study that shows poor blood flow and a metabolic study that shows only stunned viable myocardium that has survived the initial insult are described as a *mismatch*.

Echocardiography

Echocardiography, a noninvasive diagnostic procedure based on the principles of ultrasonography (see Chapter 4), is used to evaluate structural and functional changes in a wide variety of heart ailments. These include mitral valve stenosis and regurgitation, prolapse of mitral valve leaflets, aortic stenosis and insufficiency, hypertropic cardiomyopathy, atrial septal defects, and pericardial effusions.

An echocardiogram is obtained by placing a transducer on several areas of the chest wall. Bursts of ultrasound waves are directed at the part of the heart under investigation. The echocardiogram records the structure and motion of that area in relation to its distance from the anterior chest wall. An ECG is recorded simultaneously on the graph. Two-dimensional echocardiography generates a continuous picture of the beating heart. The images are recorded on videotape for analysis.

Echocardiograms are used to help assess and diagnose pericardial effusion, cardiomyopathy, valvular disorders (including prosthetic valves), cardiac shunts, myocardial ischemia, chamber size, left ventricular function, ventric-

ular aneurysms, and cardiac tumors (atrial myxoma). In addition, they are useful during heart biopsies because the physician can view the heart on a monitor while taking tissue samples.

Transesophageal Echocardiography

Procedure

Transesophageal echocardiography (TEE) yields a higher quality picture of the heart than does regular echocardiography. It is especially useful for clients who have thickened lung tissue or thick chest walls or who are obese. TEE eliminates the interference of the thoracic structures and provides an excellent image of the heart and great vessels from a posterior view. The procedure may also be used intraoperatively, wherein conventional echocardiography is ineffective. Dobutamine stress testing is used in combination with TEE to evaluate clients with suspected coronary artery disease and left ventricular wall motion abnormalities, to estimate ejection fraction and pulmonary wall pressure, and to identify intracardiac myomas.

This combination test involves inserting a flexible endoscope equipped with an ultrasonic transducer tip into the esophagus of a sedated client, administering dobutamine to mimic the effects of exercise (by increasing myocardial oxygen demand through stimulation of beta$_1$ receptors), and recording ultrasonic images of the heart's response. Because the probe is placed behind the heart, it allows the left atrium to be viewed. TEE allows clearer visualization of the heart and its structures and is most useful in diagnosis of cardiac masses, prosthetic valve function, aneurysm, and posterior effusions. The procedure lasts approximately 15 minutes to 1 hour.[9,13,27]

Preprocedure Care

Explain the procedure to the client. Obtain an informed consent. Assure the client that sedation will be used. The client should receive nothing by mouth for 6 to 8 hours before the procedure.

During the procedure, do the following. Administer sedation and topical anesthetic as ordered. If the client has a nasogastric tube in place, remove it before the esophageal scope is inserted. If dobutamine is used, calculate the dose according to the client's weight. To imitate the effects of increasing physical activity, the dose is slowly increased from a baseline infusion of 2.5 to 5 μg/kg/min and thereafter increased in increments of 5 to 10 μg/kg/min up to a maximum of 40 μg/kg/min. Each dose is infused for 5 minutes; images are captured during the final 2 minutes of the infusion. Monitor the client's vital signs, ECG, respiratory status, and pulse oximetry throughout the procedure.

Postprocedure Care

After the procedure, closely monitor vital signs for 30 minutes and record the ECG every 10 minutes. Keep the client fasting until the gag reflex is fully restored. Instruct the client that there may be mild throat discomfort for a day or two and to report significant discomfort or hemoptysis to the physician immediately. Because of the sedation, advise the client not to drive or operate machinery for 24 hours.

Phonocardiography

Phonograms are recordings of audible vibrations from the heart and great vessels. Phonograms are used to assist in determining the timing of cardiac sounds and murmurs. Microphones are placed under elastic straps, usually at the base and apex of the heart. No preparation is required for this assessment.

Myocardial Scintigraphy

Myocardial function, motion, and perfusion may be studied by a method called *scintigraphy,* which involves IV injection of a radioactive isotope. As the isotope is absorbed by the blood cells of the heart muscle, photons are emitted. These photons are detected by an external gamma camera, which produces a radionuclide image. Because these nuclear imaging techniques are relatively noninvasive, they are frequently used as diagnostic tools.

Thallium 201 Scintigraphy. Thallium 201 is the most widely used isotope for myocardial perfusion because of its short half-life (73 hours) and low total body radiation dose. Thallium 201 is a radioactive analog of potassium that is easily extracted by smooth skeletal and cardiac muscle fibers that have the potassium active transport system. Eighty-eight percent of blood-borne ^{201}Tl is taken up on its first pass through the heart. The amount of ^{201}Tl found in the myocardium after an IV injection depends on the regional myocardial perfusion and the efficiency of cellular extraction. Regional perfusion is dependent on coronary artery patency. Areas of the myocardium that receive less blood flow also receive less thallium.

A high concentration of ^{201}Tl is present in well-perfused cells, and a lower concentration remains in the blood, setting up a concentration gradient for diffusion of ^{201}Tl. Infarcted or scarred myocardium does not extract any ^{201}Tl and shows up as "cold spots." If the defective area is ischemic, the cold spots fill in or become "warm" on the delayed images. Infarcts continue to appear cold with little or no perfusion of ^{201}Tl either during a stress test or with delayed images.

The perfusion scanning is performed with a special camera that is capable of showing the source of emitted low-energy photons on a screen. Each photon detected by the camera is recorded on film and a computer screen over a half-hour period. The computer refines and enhances the images and then provides quantitative perfusion information about the myocardial walls.

Thallium 201 imaging can be performed before or after an exercise ECG study or as a resting study only. Ischemic myocardium may be detected by a resting ^{201}Tl study. Two sets of images are obtained 3 hours apart and compared. The ^{201}Tl stress test begins with a graded exercise protocol on a treadmill. The client receives a slow IV infusion of normal saline. The ECG is monitored continuously. About 1 minute before the peak of the stress test, ^{201}Tl is injected intravenously. The client should exercise for the last minute to ensure ^{201}Tl distribution to the heart during 85% maximum stress. The client then cools down and reclines on an examination table for the perfusion scan. Continuous imaging in a 180-degree arc over the chest is performed. The client then waits for 3 hours and returns for repeated films. Before the delayed images are obtained, the client receives additional ^{201}Tl by IV injection. The two sets of images are then carefully compared.

Dipyridamole Thallium 201 Test. This test may be used as an alternative to standard treadmill exercise when the client is not able to achieve a vigorous level of exercise. Dipyridamole serves as a pharmacologic stress agent. It is given IV to dilate the coronary arteries, which would normally dilate during the stress of exercise. Arteries that are narrowed as a result of coronary artery disease do not expand as much as normal arteries. Infusion of dipyridamole for 5 minutes is followed by injection of ^{201}Tl. Thallium 201 travels easily through normal arteries that have dilated and travels less freely through narrowed arteries. At 7 minutes, images are obtained.

Any form of caffeine as well as medications for asthma, such as theophylline or aminophylline, should be omitted before this test. Aminophylline is an antagonist of dipyridamole and may be given slowly IV to reverse any adverse side effects.

Technetium 99m Ventriculography (Multiple-Gated Acquisition Scanning). This test is used to study the motion of the left ventricular wall and measure the ability of the ventricle to eject blood (ejection fraction). If a coronary artery is narrowed, causing ischemia, the segment of the myocardium it serves exhibits diminished wall motion or contractility. In addition, hemodynamic changes may be measured by observing the actual filling and emptying of the cardiac chambers. Changes in cardiac output as well as ejection fraction may be obtained. Multiple gated acquisition (MUGA) scans represent the blood pool within the ventricular and atrial chambers.

Stannous pyrophosphate (PYP) is given IV to allow tagging of the red blood cells with ^{99m}Tc. Approximately

20 minutes after the PYP is injected, the ^{99m}Tc is injected. A heart monitor is then attached, and images are obtained.

MUGA scans use counts from any one of a number of consecutive beats. Multiple serial images are obtained using a gamma camera. The cardiac cycle is broken into intervals, with counts taken during these intervals for a number of beats. These counts are stored and then displayed in a weighted average picture.

If a stress study is to be performed, the client is put on a bicycle ergometer with a gamma camera positioned to project the right and left blood pools. The ECG is monitored continuously. Images are obtained at rest and during each stage of exercise.

First-Pass Cardiac Study

Procedure

During a first-pass study, a single IV injection of ^{99m}Tc is administered and traced as it passes through the heart. Only the initial pass of the ^{99m}Tc through the cardiac chambers is recorded. Ejection fraction and information about ventricular wall motion are obtained. A first-pass study may be performed during exercise or rest.

Preprocedure Care

Before the procedure, ask female clients if they are or may be pregnant because these studies involve radiation exposure (although minimal). Explain the purpose of the procedure, and tell the client what to expect during the procedure. Explain that electrodes will be placed on the chest and an IV line will be inserted for administration of the radioisotope. Generally, total exposure to radiation during these scans is less than or equal to that of one chest x-ray study.

Instruct the client to wear walking shoes if exercise on the treadmill or bicycle is anticipated. Follow the diet protocol of the institution. Some tests may require fasting. A light meal is preferred if the scan is to be performed during exercise because it prevents nausea and stomach cramping during exercise and allows better uptake of the radioisotope. Instruct the client to avoid alcohol and smoking on the day of the procedure.

Check the physician's orders for omission of any medications. Usually, beta-blockers, calcium-channel blockers, and xanthines are prohibited before the procedure. Ensure that the client signs a consent form. During the procedure, ask the client to notify the nurse or technologist of any chest pain (ischemia).

Postprocedure Care

After the procedure, again ask the client to report any chest pain. If the client must return for follow-up scanning, instruct the client to rest between studies.

Cardiac Catheterization

This complex procedure involves insertion of a catheter into the heart and surrounding vessels to obtain detailed information about the structure and performance of the heart, the valves, and the circulatory system. Specifically, cardiac catheterization is performed to do the following:

- Confirm a diagnosis of heart disease and determine the extent to which the disease has affected the structure and function of the heart
- Determine congenital abnormalities
- Obtain a clear picture of cardiac anatomy before heart surgery
- Obtain pressures within the heart chambers and the great vessels (aorta and PA)
- Measure blood oxygen concentration, tension, and saturation within the heart chambers
- Determine cardiac output
- Perform angiography for better coronary artery visualization
- Obtain endocardial biopsy specimens
- Allow infusion of fibrinolytic agents directly into an occluded coronary artery to restore coronary blood flow

Cardiac catheterization is usually performed in the controlled environment of a cardiac catheterization laboratory. Typically, only one side of the heart is catheterized, although it is sometimes necessary to insert the catheter into both sides of the heart. See Chapter 4 for discussions of the preprocedure and postprocedure nursing care and possible complications after cardiac catheterization.[9,13,25,27]

Right-Sided Catheterization. For right-sided cardiac catheterization, the physician inserts a sterile, radiopaque catheter through the antecubital or femoral vein. Under fluoroscopic guidance, the catheter is advanced slowly to the right atrium and right ventricle and is finally wedged in a small branch of the PA. The ECG is continuously monitored during the procedure. Premature ventricular contractions may occur as the catheter is passed through the ventricles. The client may experience fluttering sensations or palpitations as the catheter passes through the heart. If they occur frequently, cardiac output decreases and the physician may need to withdraw the catheter temporarily or order administration of lidocaine (an antidysrhythmic).

Left-Sided Catheterization. This procedure is far more difficult to perform than right-sided catheterization. There are two major methods of catheter introduction. (1) The catheter can be passed retrograde (backward) from the brachial or femoral artery into the aorta and then to the left ventricle. (2) Rarely during right-sided catheterization, the middle or lower third of the atrial septum is punctured and the catheter is passed transseptally into the left atrium.

As the catheter is passed through the venous or arterial system and into various heart chambers, the desired studies are performed. The catheter has several end or side holes that allow blood withdrawal for oxygen analysis from the various cardiac chambers. Pressures can be obtained by attaching the catheter to a transducer with its connecting amplifier and recording device. Radiopaque contrast materials and indicator solutions can be injected via the catheter into the left ventricle to examine the mitral valve, the left ventricular outflow tract, wall motion and thickness, left ventricular end-diastolic volume, and ejection fraction.[9,13,27] The client may experience pain when contrast material is injected and the dye replaces blood flowing through the arteries. The lack of oxygenated blood causes regional cardiac hypoxia.

Angiography

Angiocardiography involves IV injection of contrast material into the heart during cardiac catheterization. Immediately after the injection, a series of x-ray films are obtained that reveal the course of the contrast material as it circulates through the heart, lungs, and great vessels (see Chapter 4).

Cineangiography is a technique in which moving pictures are obtained during cardiac catheterization. The examiner can view the film at both rapid and slow speeds, permitting detailed and unlimited review of the study.

Coronary angiography involves injection of contrast material directly into the coronary arteries (via the coronary ostia) during cardiac catheterization. Table 56-7 outlines the various forms of angiocardiography. See Chapter 4 for preprocedure and postprocedure nursing care.

Hemodynamic Studies

Hemodynamic status is assessed with four parameters: central venous pressure (CVP), pulmonary artery (PA) pressure, cardiac output, and intra-arterial pressure. Each parameter is obtained through an invasive procedure. Critical care nurses perform all of these studies routinely at the bedside. Hemodynamic studies provide a wealth of information reflecting the earliest changes in the circulatory system that are not yet clinically detectable.

Hemodynamic pressure monitoring provides information about blood volume, fluid balance, and how well the heart is pumping. Current technology allows measurement of right atrial pressure (CVP), PA pressures during systole and diastole (reflecting right and left ventricular pressures), and pulmonary capillary wedge pressure (PCWP; an indirect indicator of left ventricular pressure).[9,13,25,27]

TABLE 56-7	*Major Types of Angiocardiography*	
Angiocardiography Procedure	**Method Used**
Right-sided angiocardiography	Contrast medium is injected into the right heart chambers and pulmonary artery by means of a catheter threaded up a vein and into the heart during cardiac catheterization.
Left-sided angiocardiography	Contrast medium is injected into the left side of the heart through a transvenous catheter passed through the atrial septum during cardiac catheterization or via a catheter passed retrograde through an artery into the left side of the heart.
Selective coronary artery angiocardiography	Contrast medium is injected directly into the ostium of each coronary artery via a catheter that is placed retrograde through an artery into the aorta.

The Pulmonary Artery Catheter

Development of the balloon-tipped, flow-directed catheter has enabled continuous direct monitoring of PA pressure (see the Bridge to Critical Care feature on Swan-Ganz Monitoring on pp. 1594 and 1595).

There are many types of PA catheters, with the most commonly used catheter for adults being the quadruple-lumen thermodilution catheter. This PA catheter has four lumina. The proximal lumen terminates in the right atrium, allowing CVP measurement, fluid infusion, and venous access for blood samples. The distal lumen terminates in the PA and measures PA systolic pressure, PA diastolic pressure, PA mean pressure, and PCWP. A small, third lumen is used for inflation and deflation of the balloon. The fourth lumen is the thermistor port and permits measurement of cardiac output. In addition, some catheters have a fifth port for infusion of fluids and capabilities for cardiac pacing and measuring oxygen saturation of the blood.

Inserting the Catheter. Insertion of a PA catheter involves risk for the client. The potential complications are PA infarction, pulmonary embolism, injury to the heart valves, and injury to the myocardium. In addition, while

BRIDGE TO CRITICAL CARE

Swan-Ganz Monitoring (PA Catheter)

Positioning the Swan-Ganz Catheter

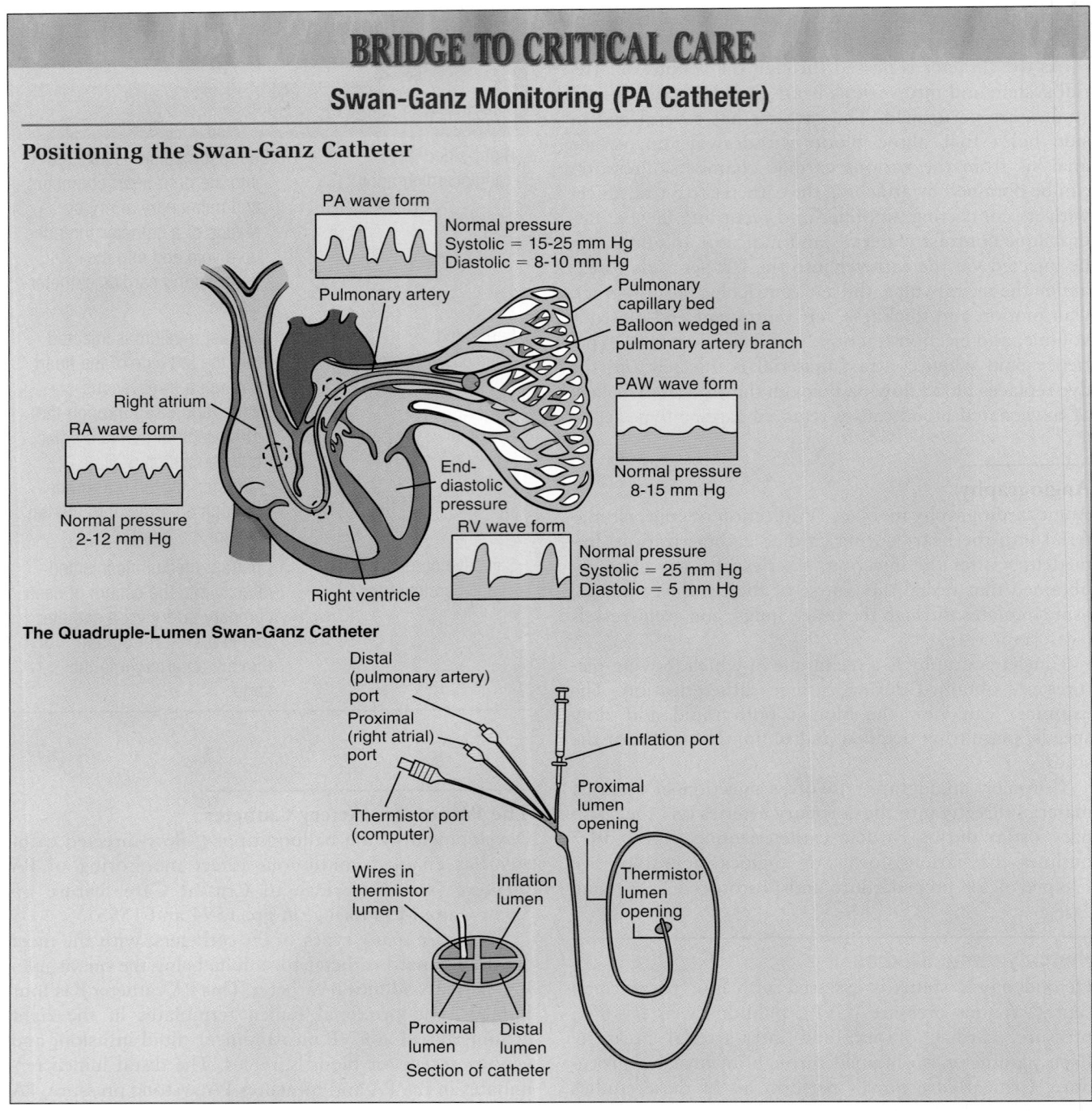

PA wave form
Normal pressure
Systolic = 15-25 mm Hg
Diastolic = 8-10 mm Hg

Pulmonary artery

Pulmonary capillary bed

Balloon wedged in a pulmonary artery branch

PAW wave form
Normal pressure
8-15 mm Hg

Right atrium

RA wave form
Normal pressure
2-12 mm Hg

End-diastolic pressure

RV wave form
Normal pressure
Systolic = 25 mm Hg
Diastolic = 5 mm Hg

Right ventricle

The Quadruple-Lumen Swan-Ganz Catheter

Distal (pulmonary artery) port

Proximal (right atrial) port

Inflation port

Proximal lumen opening

Thermistor port (computer)

Wires in thermistor lumen

Inflation lumen

Thermistor lumen opening

Proximal lumen

Distal lumen

Section of catheter

the catheter is in place, the heart valves are unable to close completely.

PA monitoring must be carried out in a critical care unit under careful scrutiny of an experienced nursing staff. Before insertion of the catheter, explain to the client that (1) the procedure may be uncomfortable but not painful, and (2) a local anesthetic will be given at the catheter insertion site. Support of the critically ill client at this time helps promote cooperation and lessen anxiety.

The physician inserts the PA flow-directed catheter at the bedside via percutaneous puncture of the brachial, subclavian, jugular, or femoral vein using sterile technique. The catheter is connected to a transducer and a fluid-filled pressure monitoring system. Pressure levels and fluctuations are monitored both graphically and by numerical display.

The inflated balloon follows the direction of blood flow through the right ventricle into the PA, where it fi-

BRIDGE TO CRITICAL CARE
Swan-Ganz Monitoring (PA Catheter)—cont'd

Measuring Cardiac Output by Thermodilution

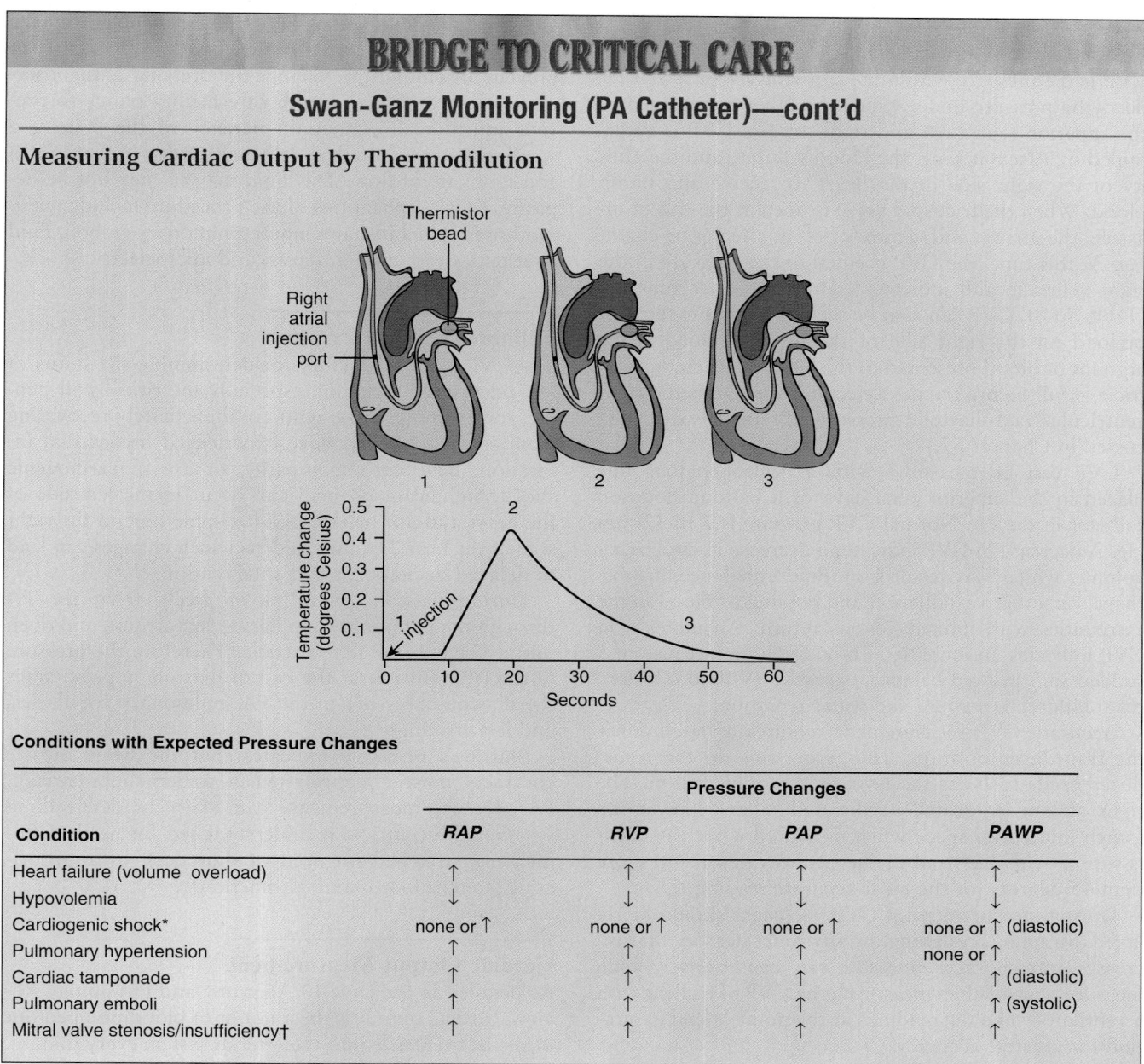

Conditions with Expected Pressure Changes

Condition	Pressure Changes			
	RAP	**RVP**	**PAP**	**PAWP**
Heart failure (volume overload)	↑	↑	↑	↑
Hypovolemia	↓	↓	↓	↓
Cardiogenic shock*	none or ↑	none or ↑	none or ↑	none or ↑ (diastolic)
Pulmonary hypertension	↑	↑	↑	none or ↑
Cardiac tamponade	↑	↑	↑	↑ (diastolic)
Pulmonary emboli	↑	↑	↑	↑ (systolic)
Mitral valve stenosis/insufficiency†	↑	↑	↑	↑

PAP, Pulmonary artery pressure; *PAWP*, pulmonary artery wedge pressure; *RAP*, right atrial pressure; *RVP*, right ventricular pressure.
*Pressure readings depend on the heart's ability to handle circulating volume. Chronic lung disease elevates all readings.
†Mitral valve disease produces unreliable pressure readings.

nally wedges in the right or left branch of the PA. Clinicians can follow the path of the balloon by observing waveforms and pressure readings on the monitor (see the Bridge to Critical Care feature on Swan-Ganz Monitoring on p. 1594 and above).

When wedged, the catheter is "pointing" indirectly at the left end-diastolic pressure. Therefore PCWP is the most accurate, although indirect, indicator of left ventricular end-diastolic pressure or left ventricular *preload* available at the bedside. The normal PCWP is 8 to 13 mm Hg. Ele-

vations of PCWP (greater than 18 to 20 mm Hg) indicate increased left ventricular pressure, as seen in left ventricular failure, and may coincide with the onset of pulmonary congestion. Pressures climbing to more than 30 mm Hg generally herald the onset of pulmonary edema. Conversely, low PCWP suggests insufficient volume and pressure in the left ventricle, as seen in hypovolemic shock. Pressure changes commonly related to various cardiac conditions are shown in the Bridge to Critical Care feature above.

Central Venous Pressure

CVP is the pressure within the superior vena cava. It reflects the pressure under which the blood is returned to the superior vena cava and right atrium. CVP is determined by vascular tone, the blood volume, and the ability of the right side of the heart to receive and pump blood. When the tricuspid valve is open at the end of diastole, the atrium and ventricle are, in effect, one chamber. At this time, the CVP is equal to the pressure in the right ventricle and indicates right ventricular function (Table 56-8). CVP can also be seen as a measurement of preload on the right side of the heart. Preload is the amount of blood presented to the heart or when the ventricle is full before the next ejection. Preload is the right ventricular end-diastolic pressure. (Preload is also discussed in Chapter 57.)

CVP can be measured with a central venous line placed in the superior vena cava or a balloon flotation catheter in the PA. Normal CVP pressure is 2 to 12 mm Hg. A decrease in CVP indicates a decrease in circulating volume, which may result from fluid imbalance, hemorrhage, or severe vasodilation and pooling of blood in the extremities with limited venous return. An increase in CVP indicates an increase in blood volume because of a sudden shift in fluid balance, excessive IV fluid infusion, renal failure, or sodium and water retention.

Accurate CVP measurement requires a baseline for the transducer position. The zero point on the transducer needs to be at the level of the right atrium. The right atrium is located at the midaxillary line at the fourth intercostal space when measured while the client is supine with the head of the bed elevated to no more than 45 degrees for the most accurate reading.

During measurement of CVP, the client should be relaxed. Straining, coughing, or any other activity that increases intrathoracic pressure can cause falsely high measurements. When measuring the CVP of a client with a ventilator, take the readings at the point of end expiration for greatest accuracy.

Check the connections between the catheter and the attachments frequently to ensure that they are secure (to prevent air embolism). Change the dressing at the insertion site according to health care facility policy to prevent infection. To maintain patency of the system, a small amount of fluid is delivered under pressure at a constant rate of flow. This fluid may or may not be heparinized. Complications of the procedure include pneumothorax, phlebitis, air emboli, pulmonary emboli, fluid overload, dysrhythmia, sepsis, and microelectric shock.

Pulmonary Artery Pressure

The CVP is unsatisfactory for determining the status of left-sided heart function, especially in critically ill people, for example, those who are immediately recovering from cardiac surgery, have experienced myocardial infarction, have cardiomyopathy, or are in cardiogenic shock. Significant changes can occur in the left side of the heart and not be reflected for some time in the right side of the heart. Failure to detect such changes can lead to delayed or inappropriate intervention.

During diastole, blood flows freely from the PA through the pulmonary capillaries, left atrium, and open mitral valve to the left ventricle. Therefore the pressure in the left ventricle at the end of diastole approximates the diastolic pressure in the PA, pulmonary capillaries, and left atrium.

Starling's principle indicates that the heart muscle contracts most effectively when under slight stretch. PA pressure measurements can assist in determining whether the ventricle is understretched (in need of fluids), overstretched (in need or diuretics), or appropriately stretched (at maximal function).

Cardiac Output Measurement

As detailed in the Unit 13 Anatomy and Physiology Review, cardiac output is the amount of blood pumped out of the left ventricle into the arterial system every minute.

TABLE 56-8	*Assessing Central Venous Pressure Readings*	
To Assess	**Increased CVP (>11 cm H_2O)**	**Decreased CVP (<3 cm H_2O)**
Right-sided heart hemodynamics	Right heart failure (including chronic heart failure, LVF) Constrictive pericarditis Cardiac tamponade Valvular stenosis Pulmonary hypertension	Early LVF
Blood volume	↑ Circulating volume	↓ Circulating volume
Vascular tone	Vasoconstriction Hypertension	Vasodilation, peripheral pooling Septic shock

Modified from Huang, S.H., et al. (1989). *Coronary care nursing* (2nd ed., p. 101). Philadelphia: W.B. Saunders.
LVF, Left ventricular failure.

That is, cardiac output is equal to the stroke volume (volume of blood pumped out with each beat) multiplied by the heart rate. If the stroke volume of the left ventricle is between 50 and 90 ml (average, 70 ml) and the heart rate is 80 beats/min, the normal cardiac output of the left ventricle is approximately 4 to 8 L/min. Table 56-9 lists the conditions that change cardiac output. The cardiac output of the right ventricle is considered equal to that of the left because the right ventricle, although not as muscular as the left ventricle, pumps against less resistance.

Intra-Arterial Pressure Monitoring

Procedure

Systemic intra-arterial monitoring is a common method for obtaining BP measurements in the acutely ill client. This method provides continuous detection of arterial BP via an indwelling catheter. It is of greatest benefit for clients whose cuff BP measurements are undetectable or unreliable, such as those with low cardiac output, fluctuating hemodynamic status, and excessive peripheral vasoconstriction. Note that intra-arterial pressure readings are at least 10 mm Hg greater than cuff BP readings. The intra-arterial line simplifies obtaining blood samples for arterial blood gas and blood studies, minimizing the need for arterial or venous punctures. Major complications of intra-arterial monitoring include hemorrhage caused by loose connections of the monitoring system, hematoma at the insertion site, infection (local or systemic), and embolization of the artery that supplies the distal portion of the cannulated extremity.

TABLE 56-9	*Conditions That Cause a Change in Cardiac Output*
Decrease Cardiac Output	**Increase Cardiac Output**
Acute heart failure	Hypoxia
Pericarditis with effusion	Hyperthyroidism
Old age	Excitement
Arterial hemorrhage	Exercise
Standing motionless, which	Food intake
decreases venous return	Oral and intravenous fluid
to the heart	intake
Myxedema	Early stage of septic shock
Shock	Pregnancy
Valvular heart disease	
Myocardial ischemia	
Dysrhythmias	
Paroxysmal atrial tachycardia (PAT)	
Atrial fibrillation	
Heart block	
Ventricular tachycardia	
Heat stroke	

The physician introduces a short, nonreactive polytetrafluoroethylene (Teflon) catheter into an artery (radial, brachial, axillary, femoral, or dorsalis pedis) using sterile technique.[9,13,25,27]

Preprocedure Care

Informed consent is required. Before catheter insertion, the adequacy of circulation in the selected extremity must be assessed. If the radial artery is chosen as the site for insertion, blood flow to the hand is evaluated with an Allen test to determine ulnar artery patency. Allen's test is described in Chapter 53. If ulnar artery obstruction is suspected, cannulation of the radial artery should not be attempted.

Besides accurate monitoring and recording of arterial pressure, nursing responsibilities focus on preventing complications of arterial cannulation. Do the following. Check all connections frequently to ensure that they remain tight and secure. Evaluate the cannulated extremity for neurovascular function every 2 hours. Assess color, temperature, capillary filling, and sensation distal to the site of cannulation. Check the insertion site for redness or manifestations of infection daily, and change dressing per institutional policy.

Postprocedure Care

After removal of the arterial cannula, maintain firm constant pressure for 5 to 15 minutes over the site of the artery to prevent hematoma formation. Secure a pressure dressing over the site for 12 hours. Monitor for infection (increased redness, warmth, tenderness, and induration at the catheter insertion site, elevated temperature) and neurovascular compromise (pain, paresthesia [abnormal touch sensation], decreased pulse quality, pallor, coolness). Report these complications immediately to the physician.

CONCLUSIONS

Cardiovascular assessment can range from taking blood pressure measurements to monitoring hemodynamic parameters. Learning how to perform adult cardiac assessment takes time and perseverance. Abnormal heart sounds are harder to interpret than normal heart sounds; be persistent and practice frequently. Even though invasive diagnostic tests are more prevalent, you need to be able to evaluate accurately the client's history, BP, and physical assessment. These data are just as important as the results of invasive studies if the nurse is to continue to assess the client effectively, provide primary preventive care, and monitor treatment. Assessment skills and nursing interventions can make a significant difference in the client's quality of life by preventing complications and improving outcomes.

Initial assessment of cardiovascular risks in all adults should begin at age 20 and should be done every 5 years, or yearly if risks are identified. Diet, weight reduction, smoking cessation, and increased physical activity are essential components of a therapeutic approach for both primary and secondary prevention. Client-focused interventions include simplified medication regimens, explicit instructions, reinforcement of adherence, family support, increased visit frequency, and self-monitoring. Approaches that target health care delivery systems include establishing lipid management and hypertension clinics, case management by nurses, telemedicine, collaborative care by pharmacists, and establishing critical care pathways in hospitals.

BIBLIOGRAPHY

 1. American Heart Association. (2002). *AHA guidelines for primary prevention of cardiovascular disease and stroke: 2002 Update,* #71-0226. *Circulation.* Retrieved July 16, 2002. Available: http://www.americanheart.org/.

 2. American Heart Association. (2001). *Biostatistical fact sheet-risk factors, cholesterol and other lipids.* Available http://www.americanheart.org/statistics/biostats/bioch.htm.

 3. American Heart Association. (2002). *2002 Heart and stroke: Statistical update.* Dallas: Author.

4. Bickley, L.S., & Szilagyi, P.G. (2003). *Bates' guide to physical examination and history taking* (8th ed.). Philadelphia: Lippincott Williams & Wilkins.

5. Braunwald, E. (Ed.). (2001). *Essential atlas of heart disease* (2nd ed.). New York: McGraw-Hill.

 6. Centers for Disease Control and Prevention. (2002). *About chronic disease.* From http://www.cdc.gov/nccd-php/about/about.htm.

 7. Centers for Disease Control and Prevention. (2002). *Facts about cardiovascular disease.* From http://www.cdc.gov/od/oc/media/fact/cardiova.htm.

 8. Cui, J., et al. (2002). Genes and family environment explain correlations between blood pressure and body mass index. *Hypertension, 40*(1), 7-12.

9. Darovic, G.O. (2002). *Hemodynamic monitoring: Invasive and noninvasive clinical application* (3rd ed.). Philadelphia: W. B. Saunders.

 10. Ebrahim, S., & Davy-Smith, G. (2001). Multiple risk factor interventions for primary prevention of coronary heart disease (Cochrane review). Available: http://www.cochrane.org/cochrane/rvabstr/ab00156.htm. Accessed April 19, 2001.

 11. Expert Panel on Detection, Evaluation, and Treatment of High Blood Cholesterol in Adults. (May 2001). *Third report of the National Cholesterol Education Program (NCEP).* (NIH Publication 01-3670.) Washington, DC: National Heart, Lung, and Blood Institute.

12. Fischbach, F. (2000). *A manual of laboratory & diagnostic tests* (6th ed.). Philadelphia: J. B. Lippincott.

13. Fuster, V., et al. (Eds.). (2001). *Hurst's the heart* (10th ed.). New York: McGraw-Hill.

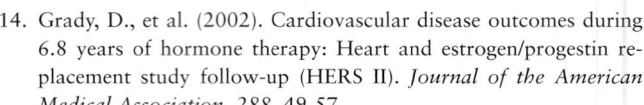 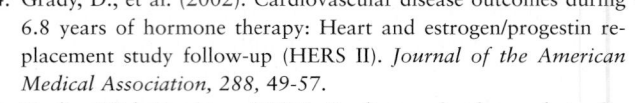 14. Grady, D., et al. (2002). Cardiovascular disease outcomes during 6.8 years of hormone therapy: Heart and estrogen/progestin replacement study follow-up (HERS II). *Journal of the American Medical Association, 288,* 49-57.

15. Healing With Nutrition. (2002). *Cardiovascular disease facts, disease prevention and treatment strategies.* Retrieved September 19, 2002, from http://www.healingwithnutrition.com/cdisease/cardiovascular/cardiovascular.html.

 16. Hochman, J.S., et al. (1999). Sex, clinical presentation, and outcomes in patients with acute coronary syndromes. *The New England Journal of Medicine, 341*(4), 226-232.

 17. Hunt, S.C., et al. (2002). Genome scans for blood pressure and hypertension: The National Heart, Lung, and Blood Institute family heart study. *Hypertension, 40*(1), 1-6.

 18. Immunization Action Coalition. (August 2002). *Summary of recommendations for adult immunization.* St. Paul, MN: Author.

19. Libster, M. (2002). *Delmar's integrative herb guide for nurses.* Clifton Park, NY: Delmar Thomson Learning.

20. McCance, K.L., & Huether, S.E. (Eds.). (2002). *Pathophysiology: The biologic basis for disease in adults and children* (4th ed.). St. Louis: Mosby.

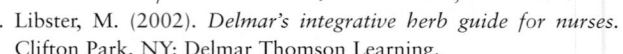 21. National Heart, Lung, and Blood Institute Joint National Committee on Prevention, Detection, Evaluation, and Treatment of High Blood Pressure. (2003). The seventh report of the Joint National Committee on Prevention, Detection, Evaluation and Treatment of High Blood Pressure: The JNC-7 report. *Journal of the American Medical Association, 289*(19), 2560-2572.

 22. National Institutes of Health. (2001). *ATP III guidelines at-at-glance quick desk reference.* (NIH Publication No. 01-3305.) Washington, DC: U.S. Department of Health and Human Services.

23. Nursing Drug Handbook Series. (2001). *Nursing herbal medicine handbook.* Springhouse, PA: Springhouse.

24. Seller, R.H. (2000). *Differential diagnosis of common complaints* (4th ed.). Philadelphia: W. B. Saunders.

25. Stillwell, S.B. (2002). *Critical care nursing reference* (3rd ed.). St. Louis: Mosby.

 26. Svetkey, L.P., et al. (1999). Effects of dietary patterns on blood pressure: Subgroup analysis of the Dietary Approaches to Stop Hypertension (DASH) randomized clinical trial. *Archives of Internal Medicine, 159*(3), 285-293.

27. Urden, L.D., et al. (2002). *Thelan's critical care nursing: Diagnosis and management (*4th ed.). St. Louis: Mosby.

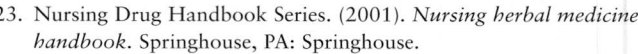 28. Williams, C.L., et al. (2002). Cardiovascular health in children: A statement for health professionals from the Committee on Atherosclerosis, Hypertension, and Obesity in the Young (AHOY) of the Council on Cardiovascular Disease in the Young. American Heart Association. *Circulation, 106*(1), 143-160.

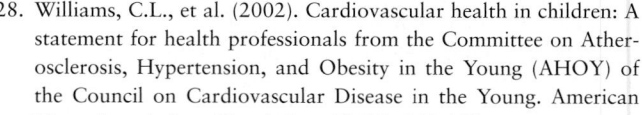 **evolve** *Did you remember to check out the bonus material on the Evolve website and the CD-ROM, including free self-assessment exercises?*
http://evolve.elsevier.com/Black/medsurg/

Chapter 57

Management of Clients with Structural Cardiac Disorders

Barbara B. Ott

Adequate tissue perfusion is essential to good health and even to life. Perfusion to tissues is critical for their function, and inadequate tissue perfusion from cardiac disorders often leads to confusion or anxiety related to the brain's continual need for glucose and blood and muscle pain resulting from the muscles' continual need for blood. This chapter focuses on the cardiac disorders that affect the structure of the heart and impair cardiac pumping. Failure to pump blood can result in inadequate tissue perfusion.

VALVULAR HEART DISEASE

When heart valves that normally move blood progressively through the heart cannot fully open or fully close, perfusion of the heart and distal tissues is impaired. A stenosed valve may impede the flow of blood from one chamber to the next; an insufficient (incompetent) valve may allow blood to regurgitate (flow backward) (Table 57-1). The aortic and mitral valves become dysfunctional more often than do the pulmonary and tricuspid valves. This change occurs because the left side of the heart is a system of higher pressures compared with the lower pressures in the pulmonary circulation.

Valvular heart disease remains fairly common in the United States even though the incidence is steadily decreasing as the incidence of rheumatic fever decreases. Mitral valve prolapse syndrome is one of the most common cardiac abnormalities; as much as 5% of the population is affected, and women are affected more often than men.[5]

MITRAL VALVE DISEASE

Stenosis of the mitral valve leaflets obstructs the flow of blood from the atrium to the ventricle. Regurgitation occurs when the valve is stenotic and allows blood to leak back from ventricle to atrium. In *mitral valve prolapse* (see later discussion), one or both of the valve leaflets bulge into the left atrium during ventricular systole. Usually a benign disorder, prolapse may progress to a stage of pronounced regurgitation and ventricular dilation. Although it is often an isolated abnormality, this syndrome is associated with a number of other conditions, such as endocarditis, myocarditis, atherosclerosis, systemic lupus erythematosus, muscular dystrophy,

---

evolve *Be sure to check out the bonus material on the Evolve website and the CD-ROM, including free self-assessment exercises.*
http://evolve.elsevier.com/Black/medsurg/

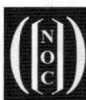 **Nursing Outcomes Classification (NOC)**
for Nursing Diagnoses—Clients with Structural Cardiac Disorders

Activity Intolerance
　Activity Tolerance
　Endurance
　Energy Conservation
Chronic Pain
　Comfort Level
　Pain Control
　Pain: Disruptive Effects
Decreased Cardiac Output
　Cardiac Pump Effectiveness
　Circulation Status
　Tissue Perfusion: Gastrointestinal
　Tissue Perfusion: Peripheral
　Vital Signs Status

Imbalanced Nutrition: Less Than Body Requirements
　Nutritional Status: Food and Fluid
　　Intake
Impaired Gas Exchange
　Respiratory Status: Ventilation
　Tissue Perfusion: Pulmonary
　Vital Signs Status
Impaired Physical Mobility
　Ambulation: Walking
　Joint Movement: Active
　Mobility Level
Risk for Ineffective Airway Clearance
　Aspiration Control

Respiratory Status: Airway Patency
Respiratory Status: Ventilation
Risk for Ineffective Therapeutic Regimen Management: Individuals
　Compliance Behavior
　Participation: Health Care Decisions
Risk for Ineffective Tissue Perfusion: Cerebral
　Neurological Status: Consciousness
　Tissue Perfusion: Cerebral
Risk for Infection
　Immune Status
　Tissue Integrity: Skin and Mucous
　　Membranes

TABLE 57-1　*Mitral and Aortic Valve Stenosis and Regurgitation*

A stenotic valve does not open normally and therefore prevents forward flow of blood.	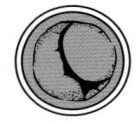 Normal valve (closed)	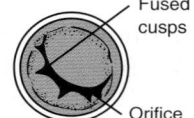 Stenosed valve (open) — Fused cusps, Orifice	A leaky valve allows blood to regurgitate backwards into the chamber it came from.	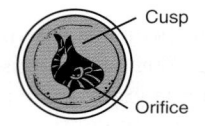 Normal valve (open) — Cusp, Orifice	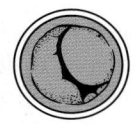 Normal valve (closed)

Mitral Valve Stenosis	**Manifestations**	**Mitral Valve Regurgitation/ Prolapse**	**Manifestations**
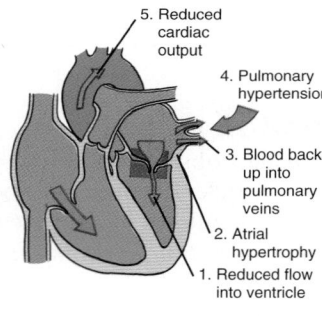 5. Reduced cardiac output 4. Pulmonary hypertension 3. Blood backs up into pulmonary veins 2. Atrial hypertrophy 1. Reduced flow into ventricle	Decreased exercise tolerance Dyspnea, orthopnea Paroxysmal nocturnal dyspnea Mild hemoptysis Low pitched, diastolic murmur Accentuated S1 opening snap Atrial fibrillation	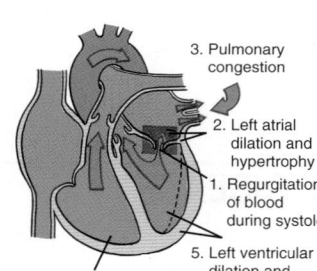 3. Pulmonary congestion 2. Left atrial dilation and hypertrophy 1. Regurgitation of blood during systole 5. Left ventricular dilation and hypertrophy 4. Right ventricular failure	Weakness, fatigue Dyspnea with exertion Palpitations Left ventricular failure Orthopnea Blowing, high pitched pansystolic murmur with radiation to axilla
Aortic Valve Stenosis	**Manifestations**	**Aortic Valve Regurgitation**	**Manifestations**
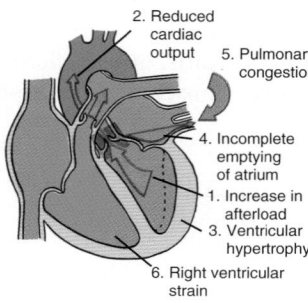 2. Reduced cardiac output 5. Pulmonary congestion 4. Incomplete emptying of atrium 1. Increase in afterload 3. Ventricular hypertrophy 6. Right ventricular strain	Dyspnea on exertion Exercise intolerance Syncope Angina Left ventricular failure Palpitations Systolic murmur with diminished second heart sounds	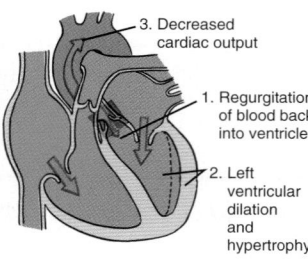 3. Decreased cardiac output 1. Regurgitation of blood back into ventricle 2. Left ventricular dilation and hypertrophy	Fatigue Dyspnea on exertion Palpitations Prominent pulsations in the neck High pitched, blowing diastolic murmur radiating to the sternal border Water hammer pulse (swift collapse of diastolic pulse)

acromegaly, and cardiac sarcoidosis. In addition, a genetic component may be present.

Etiology and Risk Factors

Factors that lead to the development of acquired valvular disease include myocardial ischemia, acute rheumatic fever, infectious endocarditis, and connective tissue abnormalities. Rheumatic heart disease, the most common cause of mitral stenosis, is preventable. Community health nurses working in health care centers or schools can often detect people with beta-hemolytic streptococcal infections (the precursor to rheumatic heart disease). Refer these clients for appropriate diagnosis and intervention.[17]

Pathophysiology

Myocardial ischemia from coronary artery disease affects the mitral valve in many ways. Ischemia leads to loss of contractility, which affects mitral valve performance. Portions of the papillary muscle are fed by the coronary vessels, and when the vessels cannot provide blood flow to the myocardium, the leaflets may also not be supplied.

Acquired valvular dysfunction can also be caused by inflammation of the endocardium resulting from acute rheumatic fever or infectious endocarditis. The inflammation causes the valve leaflets and chordae tendineae to become fibrous. The chordae tendineae shorten, which narrows the outflow tract.

In the client with valvular stenosis, the valve orifice narrows, and the valve leaflets (cusps) may become fused or thickened in such a way that the valve cannot open freely. With valvular insufficiency, scarring and retraction of the valve leaflets result in incomplete closure. Either problem increases the heart's workload. Valvular stenosis subjects the chamber behind the stenotic valve to greater stress (e.g., the left ventricle in aortic stenosis) because the heart must generate more pressure to force blood through the narrowed opening. In the client with valvular insufficiency, the chambers in front and behind the valve are taxed.

The heart may be able to compensate for the additional strain through dilation and eventual hypertrophy for a while. If valvular damage worsens, however, without intervention the heart eventually fails.

Mitral Stenosis

As the mitral valve becomes calcified and immobile, the valvular orifice narrows, which prevents normal passage of blood from the left atrium to the left ventricle. The valve orifice normally measures 4 to 6 cm², but when the orifice is mildly stenosed, it is reduced to 2 cm². This mild stenosis allows blood to flow from the left atrium to the left ventricle only if increased pressure is generated.

In critical stenosis the obstruction of blood flow across the mitral valve during diastolic filling creates a pressure gradient of about 20 mm Hg between the left atrium and the left ventricle.[5] Therefore the pressure in the left atrium is elevated to about 25 mm Hg. The elevated left atrial pressure in turn raises the pulmonary venous and pulmonary capillary pressures. The left atrium hypertrophies to accommodate the increase in pressure and volume, and the right ventricle hypertrophies because of the chronic pulmonary hypertension. Right ventricular failure can result, and inadequate filling of the left ventricle (preload) can result in reduced cardiac output[5] (see Table 57-1).

Mitral Regurgitation

Mitral regurgitation occurs during systole, when much pressure is generated within the left ventricle to eject it forward into the aorta. When the mitral valve does not close, blood flows backward into the left atrium. The backward flow of blood causes left atrial and left ventricular enlargement. The left atrium dilates and hypertrophies in response to the large volume of blood it is receiving during systole. The left ventricle also hypertrophies in response to the large amount of blood lost to the left atrium to pump harder to preserve cardiac output. This hypertrophy of the left ventricle eventually leads to left ventricular failure (see Table 57-1).

Over time the increase in blood to the left atrium causes a rise in left atrial pressure. This pressure is reflected backward into the pulmonary venous and arterial system. With continued high pressures, right-sided heart failure can develop.

Mitral Valve Prolapse

Mitral valve prolapse occurs when the anterior and posterior cusps of the mitral valve billow upward into the atrium during systolic contraction. The chordae tendineae lengthen, allowing the valve cusps to stretch upward. The cusps may be enlarged and thickened. Mitral valve prolapse is often accompanied by mitral regurgitation, causing backward flow of blood into the atrium during systole.

Clinical Manifestations

The clinical manifestations of mitral valvular heart disease may appear gradually or suddenly. Auscultation will reveal a typical pattern of murmur. It is important to note where on the chest wall the murmur is heard best and during what phase of the cardiac cycle it occurs. Asking the client to hold his or her breath may help to distinguish the murmur from respiratory sounds.

Mitral Stenosis

Manifestations of mitral stenosis are usually insidious, occurring over several years after the infection. Clients often report decreased exercise tolerance, dyspnea, orthopnea, and paroxysmal nocturnal dyspnea. On auscultation a loud first heart sound is heard and then an opening "snap" that ushers in a low-pitched, rumbling diastolic murmur. The opening snap is best heard at the apex with the diaphragm of the stethoscope. The diastolic murmur is best heard at the apex using the bell of the stethoscope while the client is in a left lateral recumbent position. Manifestations of right-sided heart failure may also be present.

Atrial fibrillation is a common finding in clients with mitral stenosis. During episodes of atrial fibrillation, the pulse becomes irregular and faint and the blood pressure often drops. Hemoptysis is also seen frequently.[6] Ineffective atrial contractions allow some stagnation of blood in the left atrium and encourage the formation of mural thrombi. These thrombi easily break away and travel as emboli throughout the arterial system, causing tissue infarction. These areas appear as dark areas or areas of necrotic tissue, especially on the toes, where vessels are small.

Mitral Regurgitation

Clients with mitral regurgitation may be asymptomatic until cardiac output falls. Reduced cardiac output first leads to fatigue and dyspnea. Clinical manifestations gradually increase to include orthopnea, paroxysmal nocturnal dyspnea, and peripheral edema. Pulmonary manifestations are less severe than in mitral stenosis because changes in the mean pulmonary capillary pressure are less exaggerated. When the right side of the heart is affected, the manifestations are the same as in mitral stenosis.

Auscultation reveals a blowing, high-pitched systolic murmur with radiation to the left axilla, heard best at the apex. The first heart sound may be diminished, and often a splitting of the second sound is heard. Severe regurgitation is associated with a third heart sound (S_3). Vital signs are usually normal unless mitral regurgitation is severe. Atrial fibrillation is common in clients with this condition; however, emboli and hemoptysis occur far less often than in mitral stenosis.

Mitral Valve Prolapse

It is not uncommon for clients with mitral valve prolapse to be completely asymptomatic. In a healthy client physical examination may reveal a regurgitant murmur or a midsystolic click on auscultation. Manifestations may be vague; if present, they include tachycardia, lightheadedness, syncope, fatigue, weakness, dyspnea, chest discomfort, anxiety, and palpitations related to dysrhythmias.[7] Minimal morbidity and mortality are associated with mitral valve prolapse, and clinically clients have no physical limitations.

Various diagnostic assessments are used to detect valvular lesions or structural heart changes. These studies include echocardiography, chest radiography, stress tests, and cardiac catheterization.[7]

Outcome Management

The goals of treatment for the asymptomatic client are to prevent beta-hemolytic streptococcus infection, which could lead to infective endocarditis (see the Evidence-Based Practice in Action feature on Preventing Bacterial Endocarditis on p. 1615). The prognosis is good for this group of clients. The goals of medical management of the symptomatic clients are to maintain cardiac output and activity tolerance. When cardiac output falls or the client is unable to tolerate simple activities, the valve can be surgically replaced.

Mitral Stenosis

Heart failure is treated with oral diuretics and a sodium-restricted diet. Digitalis is useful in clients with atrial fibrillation for slowing the ventricular heart rate. Beta-blockers may decrease the heart rate and therefore increase exercise tolerance. Anticoagulants are helpful in reducing the risk of embolus. A client with untreated mitral stenosis can progress from having mild disability to severe disability in less than 10 years.[7]

Mitral Regurgitation

The client should restrict physical activities that produce fatigue and dyspnea. Reducing sodium intake and promoting sodium excretion with diuretics can lessen the work of the heart. Nitrates, digitalis, and angiotensin-converting enzyme (ACE) inhibitors have brought about hemodynamic improvement and symptomatic relief in clients with chronic mitral regurgitation.[7]

Mitral Valve Prolapse

Treatment of mitral valve prolapse depends on the manifestations. Beta-blockers are helpful in relieving syncope, palpitations, and chest pain. Aspirin can also help to prevent transient ischemic attacks. For preventing infective endocarditis, the client may receive antibiotics prophylactically before any invasive procedures are performed.[7]

AORTIC VALVE DISEASE

The aortic valve is the last valve through which blood flows before entering systemic circulation. In *aortic stenosis* the orifice of the aortic valve becomes narrowed, which causes a decrease in the blood flow from the left ventricle into the aorta and systemic circulation. This obstruction to flow creates a resistance to ejection and increased pressure in the left ventricle. *Aortic regurgita-*

tion (aortic insufficiency) allows blood to leak back from the aorta into the left ventricle. During systole blood that is ejected into the aorta reenters the left ventricle. To maintain normal pressures, the left ventricle hypertrophies. Both aortic stenosis and regurgitation overwork the left ventricle. Aortic valve disease is far less common than mitral valve disease but often occurs in conjunction with mitral valve disease. A dilation of the ascending aorta, or aortic root disease, is also quite common.[6,7]

Etiology and Risk Factors

Aortic stenosis can be caused by several congenital defects of the aortic valve and by two degenerative processes: (1) calcification of the valve in older adults and (2) retraction and stiffening of the valve from rheumatic fever. As the population in the United States ages, the incidence of aortic stenosis from calcification has been rising.[7]

Aortic regurgitation is most often a result of infectious disorders such as rheumatic fever, syphilis, and infective endocarditis. Connective tissue disorders can also lead to aortic regurgitation.

Pathophysiology

Aortic Stenosis

When aortic stenosis is present, the pressure within the left ventricle rises as the blood is ejected through the narrowed opening. A pressure gradient develops between the left ventricle and the aorta. The elevated pressure in the left ventricle during systole causes the ventricle to hypertrophy. Dilation of the left ventricle occurs over time when the contractility of the hypertrophied muscle deteriorates. Eventually dilation and hypertrophy of the left ventricle are unable to maintain adequate cardiac output, resulting in elevated left ventricular end-diastolic pressure, decreased cardiac output, and increased pulmonary hypertension (see Table 57-1).

Aortic Regurgitation

Aortic regurgitation is a diastolic event in which blood that is propelled forward into the aorta regurgitates back into the left ventricle through an incompetent valve. The backward flow of blood causes abnormal filling and a volume overload of the left ventricle. The magnitude of the overload depends on the severity of the incompetence; however, a small incompetent area can result in significant aortic regurgitation over time.

Because the left ventricle receives blood from both the atrium and the systemic circulation, aortic regurgitation gradually increases left ventricular end-diastolic volume. Left ventricular stroke volume is increased to produce an effective forward-moving volume into the systemic circulation. Compensatory dilation of the left ventricle occurs, but the increase in left ventricular end-diastolic

pressure is minimal.[7] The compensatory mechanisms of dilation and hypertrophy help to maintain an adequate cardiac output. As the condition progresses and the contractile state of the myocardium declines, however, cardiac output declines (see Table 57-1).

Clinical Manifestations

Aortic Stenosis

Clinical manifestations of aortic stenosis tend to occur gradually and late in the course of the disease. Usually a long latent period in which the client is asymptomatic occurs. Manifestations begin to appear as the obstruction and ventricular pressure increase to critical levels. *Angina pectoris* (chest pain) is a frequent finding in about 66% of clients.[7] The character of the angina is similar to that in clients with coronary artery disease, and pain is commonly brought on by exertion and relieved by rest. Myocardial oxygen consumption is higher in clients with aortic stenosis because of the hypertrophy of the left ventricle, and this probably accounts for the angina.

Syncope, another common clinical manifestation, also occurs during exertion because of a fixed cardiac output during a period of increased demand.[6] Syncope at rest may be due to dysrhythmias. Exertional dyspnea, paroxysmal nocturnal dyspnea, and pulmonary edema occur with increasing pulmonary venous hypertension attributable to left ventricular failure. In severe aortic stenosis, additional manifestations may include palpitations, fatigue, and visual disturbances. On auscultation the systolic murmur may be associated with a diminished second heart sound and an early ejection click. A systolic thrill is present over the aortic areas.

Aortic Regurgitation

Clients with chronic severe aortic regurgitation may be asymptomatic for a long time. During this time the left ventricle gradually enlarges. Clients may complain of an uncomfortable awareness of the heartbeat and palpitations because of the large left ventricular stroke volume with rapid diastolic runoff. Clients may also have prominent pulsations in the neck and even head-bobbing with each heartbeat. Sinus tachycardia or premature ventricular contractions may make palpitations more pronounced.

On physical examination, low systolic blood pressure may be due to the large stroke volume and a decreased diastolic blood pressure resulting from the regurgitation and distal runoff. Carotid artery pulsations may be exaggerated. The arterial pulse pressure widens, and palpable pulse amplitude increases, often noted as a sudden sharp pulse, followed by a swift collapse of the diastolic pulse (Corrigan's or water-hammer pulse). Auscultation reveals a soft, high-pitched, blowing decrescendo diastolic murmur heard best at the second right intercostal space and radiating to the left sternal border. Noninvasive assessment of clients with Doppler echocardiography should be performed at intervals.[7]

Outcome Management
■ Medical Management

The goals of medical management are to maintain or improve cardiac function and activity tolerance. When the client reaches the maximum benefit from medications, surgery may be warranted. Aortic valve surgery may be necessary if angina or heart failure develops even though the client has been on medications.

Aortic Stenosis. Prophylactic antibiotics may be given on an individual basis for invasive medical or dental procedures for the prevention of infective endocarditis (see the Evidence-Based Practice in Action feature on Preventing Bacterial Endocarditis on p. 1615. Digitalis and diuretics usually used for ventricular failure must be used with caution.[5] Beta-blockers are not usually ordered because they can depress myocardial function and induce left ventricular failure. Cardiac dysrhythmias should be treated pharmacologically. Advise clients with known or suspected critical obstruction of the aortic valve to avoid vigorous physical activity. Clients with mild obstruction may continue exercise if it is tolerated. The prognosis for clients with symptomatic aortic stenosis is poor without surgical intervention. The incidence of sudden death rises once myocardial failure develops.[5]

Aortic Regurgitation. Medical intervention for aortic regurgitation is the same as for aortic stenosis: relief of manifestations of heart failure and prevention of infection in the already deformed aortic cusps. Prompt surgical treatment is indicated when there is left ventricular failure.[7]

TRICUSPID VALVE DISEASE

Tricuspid stenosis, or *regurgitation*, usually develops from rheumatic fever or in combination with other structural disorders of the heart.[7] Because the tricuspid valve is on the right side of the heart, the major hemodynamic alterations are decreased cardiac output and increased right atrial pressure. The inability of the right atrium to propel blood across the stenosed valve may account for these changes. With *tricuspid regurgitation*, the pressure in the right atrium is also elevated because of regurgitation of the blood volume in the right ventricle back into the right atrium during systole.

Clinical manifestations of tricuspid stenosis are dyspnea and fatigue, pulsations in the neck, and peripheral edema and weight loss. Physical assessment reveals prominent waves in the neck veins as the atrium vigorously contracts against the stenotic valve. A diastolic murmur is heard best along the left lower sternal border.

The murmur increases with inspiration. The ECG reveals tall, tented P waves. Tricuspid insufficiency causes hepatic congestion and peripheral edema. Often atrial fibrillation is present, and jugular waves are evident. The murmur is holosystolic along the left sternal border.

Tricuspid stenosis usually responds well to diuretics and digitalis therapy. If the leaflets are severely stenotic, surgery may be required. Surgery for tricuspid regurgitation, however, may not be necessary unless pulmonary hypertension is present.

PULMONIC VALVE DISEASE

Abnormalities of the *pulmonic valve* are usually congenital defects. Few lesions develop after birth. Pulmonary hypertension, caused by mitral stenosis, pulmonary emboli, or chronic lung disease, can precipitate functional pulmonary regurgitation. Pulmonic stenosis and regurgitation lead to a decrease in cardiac output because blood does not reach the left side of the heart in adequate supply for metabolic demands. Pulmonic regurgitation may lead to dyspnea and fatigue. The murmur is a high-pitched diastolic blow along the left sternal border. No significant changes in the ECG are noted. Pulmonic stenosis causes similar clinical manifestations, but the murmur is often a crescendo-decrescendo type. Right-sided heart failure can also develop. Intervention focuses on ameliorating the underlying cause and treating right-sided heart failure.

Outcome Management
■ Nursing Management of the Medical Client

Nursing assessment should address the type, severity, and progress of the valvular disorder; the presence of fatigue; clinical manifestations of heart failure; heart rhythm (including ECG); vital signs; auscultation and palpation of the heart; the client's support systems; and the degree of knowledge that the client and his or her family have concerning the nature of and intervention in the disorder.

The main focus of nursing intervention in valvular heart disease is to help the client maintain a normal cardiac output, thereby preventing manifestations of heart failure, venous congestion, and inadequate tissue perfusion. To evaluate the effectiveness of therapeutic interventions, perform ongoing hemodynamic assessment. Monitor vital signs closely every 1 to 4 hours. A decrease in cardiac output is manifested in a compensatory rise in the heart rate, a drop in blood pressure, or a decrease in urine output. Carefully auscultate the chest every 4 hours to identify the presence of abnormal breath sounds (crackles, rhonchi) or heart gallops (S_3, S_4).

■ Self-Care

Clients with valvular heart disease require lifelong management. With a sincere desire to understand and accept each client's response to chronic illness, you can help these clients adapt to difficult lifestyle changes and achieve a positive sense of well-being.

Clients may find it difficult to cope physically and psychosocially after hospital discharge. The chronicity of valvular heart disease and its potential complications can create an atmosphere of uncertainty, fear, and frustration. Take time to help the client identify support people, personal strengths, and coping strategies. Assess how the client handles frustration or anger and which activities are particularly relaxing. Address the client's fears and misconceptions. In some cases counseling referrals may help. Stress the importance of follow-up physical examinations and intervention.

Before discharge prepare detailed teaching materials for the client and family concerning the therapeutic regimen, the disease process, factors contributing to manifestations, and the rationale for intervention. Give information about the prescribed medications. Frequently prescribed medications include digoxin, quinidine, diuretics, beta-blockers, potassium supplements, anticoagulants, and sometimes prophylactic antibiotics. Explain their rationale, dosages, side effects, and special considerations in their use.

Review the exercise prescriptions with the client. Clients with aortic stenosis often require activity restrictions. The client should demonstrate ability to pace activity, verbalize improvement in fatigue, and accept activity restrictions.

Address dietary restrictions, and plan interdisciplinary follow-up. Make sure the client knows whom to call when questions arise.

◼ Surgical Management

Symptomatic clients are considered for surgical repair. Indications for valve replacement include the following:
1. Progressive impairment of cardiac function due to scarring and thickening of the valve with either impaired narrowing of the valvular opening (*stenosis*), or incomplete closure (*insufficiency, regurgitation*)
2. Gradual enlargement of the heart with manifestations of decreased activity, shortness of breath, and heart failure.

Procedures. Valves can be reconstructed or replaced. Valve reconstruction can be accomplished if the preoperative assessment indicates that the valve is pliable. If the valve is not pliable, valve replacement is necessary. In clients with mitral regurgitation, valve reconstruction or annuloplasty may be done, which may include the use of a flexible ring that is sewn into the valve for stabilization. Aortic stenosis may be surgically treated with valve replacement or balloon aortic valvuloplasty. In the valvuloplasty procedure, a catheter with a balloon is used to dilate the valve orifice. Surgery for the client with aortic regurgitation is not always the treatment of choice but may be considered.

Artificial cardiac valves are continuing to show improvements in design, safety, function, and durability. Mechanical and tissue prosthetic valves are available. The overall advantages and disadvantages of tissue and mechanical valves are almost equal. Mechanical valves are durable, but blood tends to clot on them, and anticoagulant therapy is therefore necessary. Fortunately, some of the newer artificial valves have reduced rates of thrombus. Tissue valves do not require anticoagulation therapy, but they are less durable. Tissue valves may degenerate or calcify or develop structural abnormalities. The rate of the tissue valve failure is 30% in 10 years, with the rate accelerating over the following 10 years.[5] Some physicians recommend mechanical valves in clients younger than 65 or 70 years of age and tissue valves in clients 70 years or older.[7] Artificial valves are shown in Figure 57-1. The type of valve prosthesis used is based on a number of considerations. The surgeon primarily considers (1) the durability of the valve and (2) the client's tolerance of anticoagulation. Therefore if the client has a preoperative history of bleeding or noncompliance with pharmacologic regimens, a tissue valve may be preferable.

Techniques for valve replacement can include the usual sternotomy approach. Advances in valvular surgery include the use of robotic techniques and minimally invasive surgery. Aortic valve replacement incisions are performed through a mini-sternotomy, in which an incision is made from the sternal notch to the third intercostal space. Mitral valve replacement/repair incisions are performed through a right parasternal incision in which small portions of the third and fourth costal cartilages are excised, a limited thoracotomy, or a partial sternotomy. These techniques reduce the size of the incisions and length of recovery.

Mitral valve repair is becoming more common because it carries relatively few complications, good long-term survival, and low hospital mortality.[22] Surgical intervention is considered for aortic stenosis when the pressure gradient is greater than 50 mm Hg or the valve orifice is less than 0.8 cm². Surgical replacement of the incompetent valve provides the only effective long-term intervention for aortic regurgitation. A high percentage of clients with aortic regurgitation and aortic stenosis show striking clinical improvement with valve replacement.[7] Nursing management of the client after heart surgery is discussed in Chapter 58.

Balloon Valvuloplasty. Sometimes it is possible to open the valves without resorting to open heart surgery. Balloon valvuloplasty is a procedure in which a narrowed heart valve is stretched open (Figure 57-2). The procedure is performed in a cardiac catheterization laboratory and takes up to 4 hours. The client is usually awake but given local anesthesia and sedation. A catheter with a collapsed balloon at the tip, called a

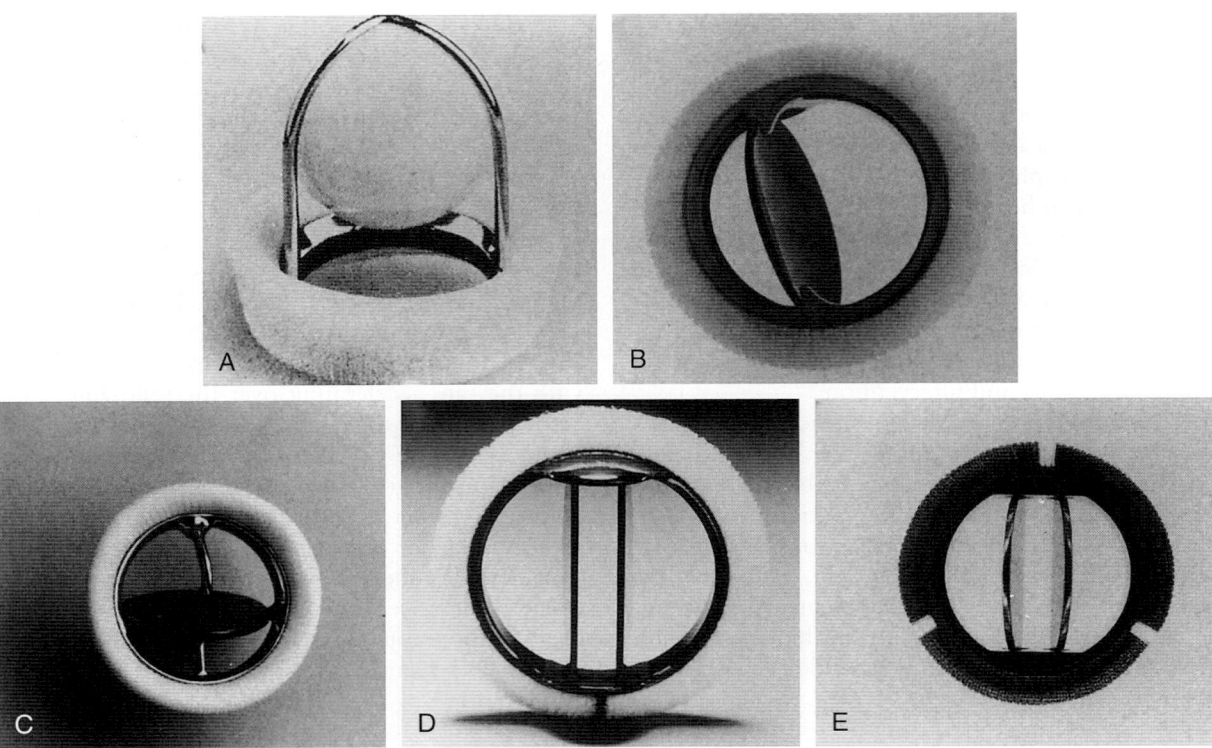

FIGURE 57-1 Prosthetic heart valves. **A,** Starr-Edwards cage and ball valve with a cloth sewing ring and bare struts. **B,** Omniscience valve. **C,** Medtronic-Hall valve. **D,** St. Jude valve. **E,** Carbomedics bileaflet valve. (From Cohn, L.H. [1995]. Aortic valve prostheses. *Cardiology Review 2,* 219.)

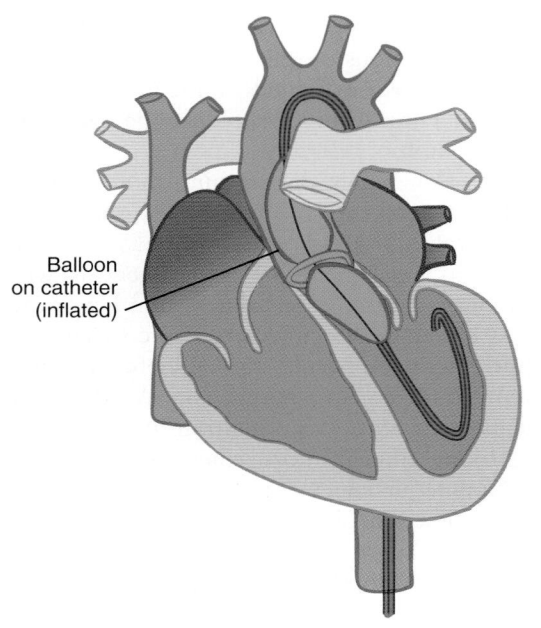

Aortic Valve Balloonoplasty

FIGURE 57-2 Balloon valvuloplasty is a procedure used to stretch stenotic valves.

sheath, is inserted into an artery or vein in the leg. This catheter is then advanced into the heart and across the narrowed valve. The deflated balloon is positioned in the valve opening and then is inflated repeatedly. The inflated balloon widens the valve's opening by splitting the valve leaflets apart. Once the valve is widened, the balloon-tipped catheter is removed. The other catheter remains in place for 6 to 12 hours because in some cases the procedure must be repeated.

The insertion site, which will be covered by a sandbag, is observed for bleeding until the catheter is removed. Intravenous fluids will be given to help eliminate the x-ray dye; intravenous blood thinners or other medications to dilate the coronary arteries may be given. Pain medication is provided. The sheath is removed when clotting time has normalized. For at least 30 minutes after removal of the catheter, direct pressure is applied to the site of insertion; after this a pressure dressing will be applied to reduce the risk of hematoma. The client remains at bed rest for 2 to 4 hours, and bleeding at the site or hematoma development is monitored often. The client is generally discharged by the following day.

The main risk of stretching a mitral valve is for the valve to become severely leaky. A mild increase in the amount of leak *(regurgitation)* is common with the procedure. In about 5% of clients, however, the valve becomes significantly leaky and will require replacement in 6 months. In about 2% of clients this is necessary as an emergency during the valvuloplasty procedure.

CARDIOMYOPATHY

Cardiomyopathy (Figure 57-3) is a heart muscle disorder of unknown cause *(idiopathic).* Of the three major types, *dilated (congestive) cardiomyopathy* is the most common form (i.e., about 60% of all cases). This form is characterized by ventricular dilation, contractile dysfunction, and heart failure. *Hypertrophic cardiomyopathy* has also been called hypertrophic subaortic stenosis, *idiopathic* hypertrophic subaortic stenosis, and asymmetrical septal hypertrophy. It is enlargement and stiffness of the left ventricle from disproportionate thickening of the interventricular septum, compared with the free wall of the ventricle. *Restrictive cardiomyopathy,* rare in Western countries, leads to impaired diastolic filling and endocardial scarring.

The risk of cardiomyopathy increases in clients who chronically ingest excessive amounts of alcohol, are pregnant, have systemic hypertension, and have had some forms of infections. Table 57-2 compares the diagnostic data for the three types of idiopathic cardiomyopathy. These forms of cardiomyopathy are described separately.

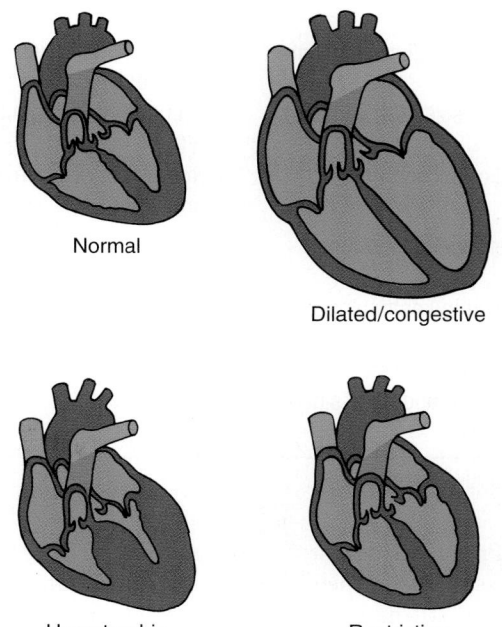

Normal

Dilated/congestive

Hypertrophic

Restrictive

FIGURE 57-3 The three types of cardiomyopathy.

DILATED CARDIOMYOPATHY

In dilated cardiomyopathy usually both the left and right ventricles dilate, the myocardial fibers degenerate, and fibrotic tissue replaces viable tissue. Fibrotic tissue is not pliable, which leads to reduced contractility and decreased stroke volume and low cardiac output, with a compensatory increase in heart rate. These changes eventually lead to heart failure accompanied by lethal ventricular dysrhythmias. The combination of ventricular dilation and ineffective myocardial contractility also increases the risk of blood pooling within the heart and subsequent clot formation. Many clients (75%) with idiopathic dilated cardiomyopathy die within 5 years after the onset of manifestations.[21]

Some forms of dilated cardiomyopathy are idiopathic. Other etiologic mechanisms include viral myocarditis, infections, metabolic problems, toxins, pregnancy, neuromuscular disorders, connective tissue disorders, and genetic predisposition (20% of cases).[21] Dilated cardiomyopathy associated with pregnancy can disappear. Spontaneous rapid improvement occurs in some women and early fatality in others. The clinical manifestations of dilated cardiomyopathy are presented in Table 57-2.

Management

Treatment is similar to that for heart failure. Inotropic agents are used to enhance myocardial contractility and to unload the heart. Nitroglycerin as a vasodilator can be used to decrease preload and afterload. Diuretics and sodium-restricted diets are used to decrease pulmonary congestion and to reduce fluid overload. Anticoagulants may help to prevent clots and emboli. Antidysrhythmic agents may help suppress ventricular irritability. In appropriate candidates implantation of the automatic internal cardiac defibrillator may be used to prevent sudden cardiac death.[21]

Rest improves cardiac function. Most clients experience severe activity intolerance during the later stages of the disease, which automatically limits their activities. During the earlier stages, however, most clients find it difficult to accept rigidly imposed restrictions on activity. Clients should avoid poorly tolerated activities. Advise clients that physical and emotional stress exacerbate the disease. Because alcohol depresses myocardial contractility, the client should abstain from drinking alcoholic beverages.

Only transplantation and specific vasodilator therapy (hydralazine plus nitrates) have resulted in prolonged life. Heart transplantation shows a 5-year survival of greater than 70% in appropriately selected clients.[21]

HYPERTROPHIC CARDIOMYOPATHY

The disproportionate thickening of the interventricular septum in hypertrophic cardiomyopathy leads to wall rigidity and thereby increases resistance to blood flow

TABLE 57-2	*Diagnostic Data for the Three Types of Cardiomyopathy*		
	Dilated	**Restrictive**	**Hypertrophic**
Manifestations	Heart failure, particularly left-sided Fatigue and weakness Systemic or pulmonary emboli	Dyspnea, fatigue Right-sided heart failure manifestations of systemic disease (e.g., amyloidosis, iron storage disease)	Dyspnea, angina pectoris Fatigue, syncope, palpitations Paroxysmal nocturnal dyspnea
Physical examination	Moderate to severe cardiomegaly: S_3 and S_4 Atrioventricular valve regurgitation, especially mitral Hypotension	Mild to moderate cardiomegaly: S_3 or S_4 Atrioventricular valve regurgitation; inspiratory increase in venous pressure (Kussmaul's sign)	Mild cardiomegaly Apical systolic thrill and heave; brisk carotid upstroke S_4 common Systolic murmur that increases with a Valsalva maneuver
Chest x-ray study	Moderate to marked cardiac enlargement, especially left ventricular pulmonary venous hypertension	Mild cardiac enlargement Pulmonary venous hypertension Mild to moderate cardiac enlargement	Left atrial enlargement
Electrocardiogram	Sinus tachycardia Atrial and ventricular dysrhythmias ST-segment and T-wave abnormalities Intraventricular conduction defects	Low voltage Intraventricular conduction defects Atrioventricular conduction defects	Left ventricular hypertrophy ST-segment and T-wave abnormalities Abnormal Q waves Atrial and ventricular dysrhythmias
Echocardiogram	Left ventricular dilation and dysfunction Abnormal diastolic mitral valve motion secondary to abnormal compliance and filling pressures	Increased left ventricular wall thickness and mass Small or normal-sized left ventricular cavity Normal systolic function Pericardial effusion	Asymmetrical septal hypertrophy Narrow left ventricular outflow tract Systolic anterior motion of the mitral valve Small or normal-sized left ventricle
Radionuclide studies	Left ventricular dilation and dysfunction (RVG)	Infiltration of myocardium (thallium 201 scan) Small or normal-sized left ventricle (RVG) Normal systolic function (RVG)	Small or normal-sized left ventricle (RVG) Vigorous systolic function (RVG) Asymmetrical septal hypertrophy (RVG ^{201}Tl scan)
Cardiac catheterization	Left ventricular enlargement and dysfunction Mitral/tricuspid regurgitation Elevated left-sided and often right-sided filling pressures Diminished cardiac output	Diminished left ventricular compliance Square root sign in ventricular pressure recordings Preserved systolic function Elevated left-sided and right-sided filling pressures	Diminished left ventricular compliance Mitral regurgitation Vigorous systolic function Dynamic left ventricular outflow gradient

From Braunwald, E. (2001). *Heart disease: A textbook of cardiovascular medicine* (6th ed.). Philadelphia: W.B. Saunders.
RVG, Radionuclide ventriculogram.

from the left atrium. There is also obstruction of left ventricular outflow. In its severest form, the left ventricular wall reaches tremendous dimensions and encroaches on the left ventricular chamber, which becomes small and elongated. Septal hypertrophy may obstruct the left ventricular outflow tract during sys-

tole. Frequently diastolic dysfunction in the form of stiffness of the left ventricle occurs during diastolic filling. This stiffness raises left ventricular end-diastolic pressure, which eventually results in elevation of left atrial, pulmonary venous, and pulmonary capillary pressures.

Hypertrophic cardiomyopathy appears to be a genetically transmitted disease (~50% of cases).[21] It can also be idiopathic, caused by hypertension or hypoparathyroidism. It appears most often in young adults, both men and women.

The clinical manifestations most commonly manifest in late adolescence or early adulthood but may appear at any age. Many clients with hypertrophic cardiomyopathy are asymptomatic and can lead long lives. They often have relatives with incapacitating manifestations of the disease. Sadly, sudden death is frequently the first clinical manifestation of the disease in asymptomatic clients. Sudden death appears more often in younger clients (i.e., less than 30 years of age, family history of sudden death, genetic abnormalities, and syncope, especially in children) and, if the presence of the disease is known, may be avoided by elimination of strenuous exercise.

The most common manifestation is dyspnea, which occurs in up to 90% of clients.[21] Dyspnea is due to the high pulmonary pressures produced by the elevated left ventricular end-diastolic pressure. Table 57-1 presents the remainder of clinical manifestations.

Management

The goals of intervention for hypertrophic cardiomyopathy are to alleviate manifestations, prevent complications, and reduce the risk of sudden death. These goals can be accomplished by reducing ventricular contractility and relieving left ventricular outflow obstruction. Beta-adrenergic blocking agents and calcium channel blocking medications reduce the heart rate, which lowers the myocardial contractility and oxygen consumption and prevents dysrhythmias. With decreased vigor of ventricular contraction, outflow obstruction diminishes. Beta-adrenergic blockade also reduces the heart rate (which further reduces myocardial workload) and prevents dysrhythmias.

Medications that decrease preload (e.g., nitrates, diuretics, morphine) and that increase contractility (e.g., isoproterenol, dopamine, digitalis) should be avoided. Anticoagulants are used if the client is in atrial fibrillation. The client is at risk for endocarditis and should follow the prophylactic care for that condition. Alcohol should be avoided because its vasodilation properties can exacerbate an outflow problem.

RESTRICTIVE CARDIOMYOPATHY

Any infiltrative process of the heart that results in fibrosis and thickening can cause restrictive cardiomyopathy. The most frequently associated disease is *amyloidosis* (deposition of eosinophilic fibrous protein in the heart). Other disorders include glycogen storage disease, hemochromatosis, and sarcoidosis. Fibrotic infiltrations into the myocardium, endocardium, and subendo-

cardium cause the ventricles to lose their ability to stretch. The excessively rigid ventricular walls impair filling during diastole; however, contractility with systole is usually normal. Filling pressures increase, and cardiac output falls. Eventually cardiac failure and mild ventricular hypertrophy occur. As cardiac output falls and intraventricular pressures rise, manifestations of heart failure appear. Table 57-1 presents the clinical manifestations. In severe or end-stage restrictive cardiomyopathy, the clinical manifestations are almost indistinguishable from chronic constrictive pericarditis. It is important to distinguish between the two problems because surgery can be used to treat cardiomyopathy.

Management

At present no specific interventions have been established for restrictive cardiomyopathy. Intervention aims at diminishing heart failure. A pacemaker, diuretics, vasodilators, and salt restriction may help accomplish this goal.[21] Digitalis may help in some forms of restrictive cardiomyopathy.

Death attributable to dysrhythmia may occur suddenly, or a more progressive course may be followed by eventual, intractable heart failure. The prognosis depends largely on the underlying cause. Unfortunately, intervention rarely results in long-term improvement.[21]

SURGICAL PROCEDURES

Surgical procedures have been developed for hypertrophic cardiomyopathy procedures to reduce the outflow gradient. *Myotomy* is the surgical incision into or resection of a portion of the ventricular septum. The excision of fibrotic endocardium is successful in a limited number of clients with restrictive cardiomyopathy. Surgical ablation can reduce some dysrhythmias.

Heart Transplantation

Cardiac transplantation is now a standard and effective treatment for clients with end-stage cardiac disease. In 2001, 2201 hearts were transplanted in the United States. About 80% of clients with heart transplants are still living 2 years after the operation.

Potential candidates must be evaluated and screened. Their cardiac status is evaluated to determine the need for the heart transplant. The candidates are also evaluated for underlying conditions that predispose to an unfavorable outcome. Box 57-1 shows the selection criteria for heart transplantation.

Finding a donor can be difficult. In heart transplantation the healthy heart must come from a fresh cadaver. This differs from renal transplant, in which a family member can be a donor. Timing is crucial because it is difficult to keep the donor heart alive for long periods before it is given to the recipient.

The current *orthotopic technique* retains a large portion of the right and left atrium in the recipient and implants the donor heart to the atria (Figure 57-4). Cardiopulmonary bypass is used during the operation (see Chapter 58). Temporary pacemaker wires and chest drainage catheters are inserted. Another type of procedure, the *heterotopic technique*, is performed only rarely. The donor heart is placed parallel to the recipient's heart. The right side of the client's heart can continue to function while the dysfunctional left side of the heart is bypassed.

Assisted Circulation and Mechanical Hearts

About 4000 clients in the United States are waiting to receive a heart transplant, but only about 2400 donated hearts are received each year. Clients who are waiting for a heart donor and transplant are at great risk of dying before a heart becomes available. During this waiting period, a ventricular assist device (VAD) may be inserted to keep these clients alive. These high-tech machines help the failing heart to pump blood throughout the body, bridging the time until a donor heart becomes available. In some cases the machine allows the heart to rest and recover so that the VAD can be removed and the client no longer needs a transplant. (See the Bridge to Critical Care feature on Left Ventricular Assist Devices on p. 1611.)

■ Management of the Surgical Client

Management of the postoperative client is discussed in Chapter 58. Specific issues in transplantation include immunosuppression and recognition and treatment of rejection if it occurs. Immunosuppression treatment relies on several drugs: cyclosporine, prednisone, methylprednisolone, azathioprine, and OKT2 monoclonal antibodies. OKT2 monoclonal antibodies suppress the activity or T lymphocytes, the cells mainly responsible for transplant rejection. Drug therapy is adjusted to give the max-

---

BOX 57-1	*Indications and Contraindications for Heart Transplant*

Indications

Heart failure from coronary artery disease
Cardiomyopathy
Heart-valve disease
Severe congenital heart disease
Life-threatening dysrhythmias that do not respond to other therapy

Contraindications

Age over 70 years
Irreversible renal, hepatic or pulmonary disease
Type 1 diabetes with end-organ disease
Active infection
Recent cancer with uncertain prognosis
Psychiatric illness or poor medical compliance
Systemic disease with significantly limited survival

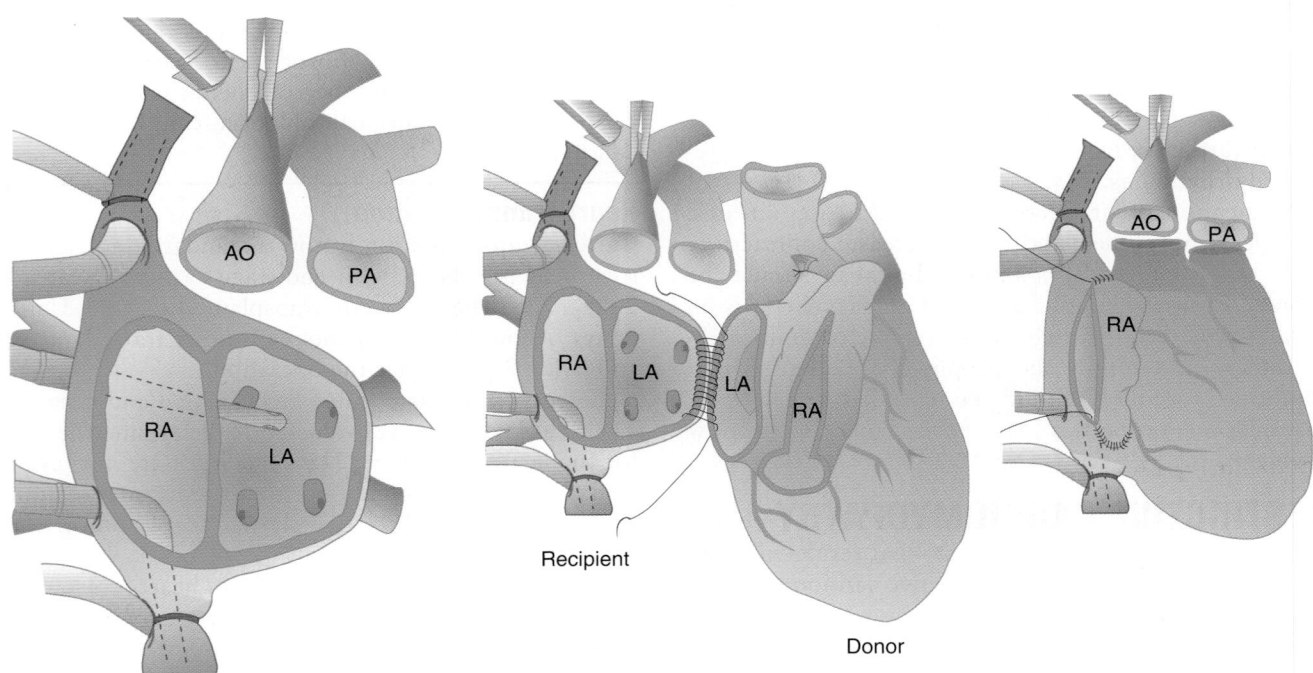

FIGURE 57-4 Orthoptic technique of heart transplantation. *AO*, Aorta, *PA*, pulmonary artery, *RA*, right atrium, *LA*, left atrium.

BRIDGE TO CRITICAL CARE

Left Ventricular Assist Devices

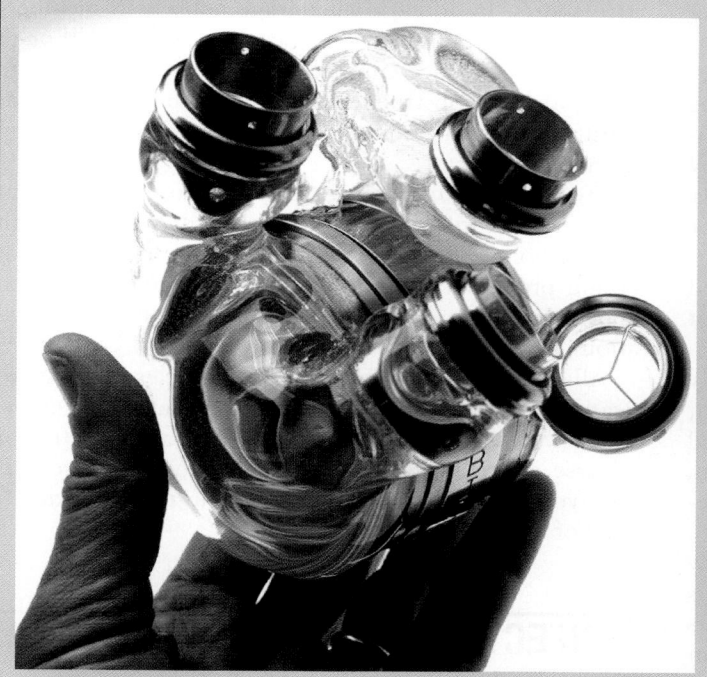

AbioCor pump. (Courtesy of Abiomed, Danvers, MA.)

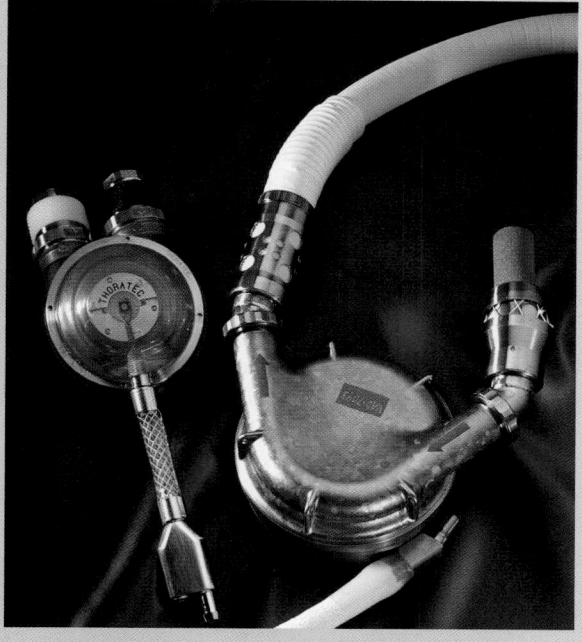

HeartMate Left Ventricular Assist Device. (Courtesy of Thoratec, Pleasanton, CA.)

Indications

Transplant-ready clients who are in danger of dying before a donor heart is available

Heart failure not responsive to standard cardiac treatments

Heart failure following various forms of heart surgery

Devices

Consist of a pump, which is implanted in the abdominal wall and connected to the left ventricle of the heart. Although the ventricle may be too weak to pump blood to the entire body, the pump draws blood from the ventricle and, in turn, propels it out to the rest of the body.

Pneumatic: External pulsatile pump that uses a pressurized sac to propel blood.

Electric: An electrical line attached to the device connects to a portable, external controller, which fits onto the client's belt and operates and monitors the pump. Clients carry reserve battery packs on their belt or shoulder bag so they can change the batteries every 3 to 4 hours, a procedure like changing the batteries in a cell phone.

Placement

The surgeon connects the VAD to the bottom of the heart and the main heart artery (aorta). Blood then flows into the heart and out the aorta by means of a small electrically or pneumatically driven motor that is part of the VAD. A tube is passed through the client's skin. The tube connects to a controller and a battery pack that the client wears or carries. This allows the client to be fully mobile with the device in place.

Complications

Infection, especially pneumonia related to immobility

Bleeding from anticoagulant use

Right-sided heart failure

Thromboembolism

Device malfunction

Nursing Precautions

Monitor cardiac output and hemodynamic status

Perform range-of-motion exercises to maintain muscle strength and joint flexibility

Monitor lung sounds; suction airway or assist client to deep breath and cough

Monitor level of anticoagulation, especially during weaning

Monitor for specific device-related problems

Educate about how to change batteries, reportable problems if client is ambulatory

Data from Mahmood, A.K., et al., (2000). Critical review of current left ventricular assist devices. *Perfusion 15,* 399, 420-432.

imum amount of immunosuppression with the minimum amount of side effects using an individualistic regimen. The risk of acute rejection is highest soon after transplantation and decreases dramatically after 3 months. Even with this intensive regimen, almost all heart-transplant recipients experience some acute rejection during the first postoperative year.

The most reliable technique for assessing organ rejection is the endomyocardial biopsy, which enables identification of the diffuse interstitial infiltrate associated with rejection. If rejection develops pulse therapy with methylprednisolone is used. High doses are given for 3 consecutive days and then gradually reduced over the next 2 weeks. Because of the side effects of increased steroid therapy, the client must be monitored carefully for infections. If the steroid therapy has not been successful in reversing the rejection, equine antithymocyte globulin or OKT3 monoclonal antibody therapy may be used. Some clients have persistent recurrent rejection episodes, which may be treated with total lymphoid irradiation. Over the long term, survival and rehabilitation can be expected in most recipients.

Outcomes of heart transplantation depend on how quickly the transplant can be performed once a donor is found. There is a 10% to 20% mortality rate for clients on the waiting list. As of 2000, 84% of heart transplant clients survived 1 year and 77% survived 3 years.[2] Heart transplant recipients who die after the procedure usually do so within the first 30 days postoperatively. Clients at greatest risk are those who deteriorate rapidly before the transplant procedure. Infection, cardiac failure, or rejection is usually the cause of death.

■ Nursing Management

Management of the client with dilated cardiomyopathy is outlined in the Care Plan feature on The Client with Dilated Cardiomyopathy on the website. In addition, clients who are acutely or chronically ill with cardiomyopathy require strong psychosocial support. The uncertain and serious consequences of the disease create fear and anxiety. The chronic nature of the disorder can deplete coping resources, leaving clients with feelings of helplessness and hopelessness. As physical capabilities diminish, feelings of inadequacy, frustration, and poor self-esteem grow. Clients may become irritable, angry, withdrawn, or dependent.

Even though the prognosis is often poor, you can help clients who suffer from this debilitating disorder to maintain hope and dignity. Encouragement, a caring touch, a listening ear, and attainable goals can promote a high quality of life. Create an environment in which clients can openly express concerns and acknowledge fears. Acceptance, empathy, and kindness can help clients with cardiomyopathies to adopt more successful coping strategies.

■ Self-Care

With hypertrophic cardiomyopathy, syncope or sudden death may follow physical exertion. Therefore warn the client with hypertrophic cardiomyopathy to avoid strenuous physical exercise such as running or active competitive sports. In addition encourage household members to learn cardiopulmonary resuscitation (CPR). Although chest pain often accompanies this disease, nitroglycerin can worsen the obstruction; clinicians can therefore treat chest pain with reduced activity and beta-blocking agents.

Hypertrophic cardiomyopathy predisposes the client to the risk of infective endocarditis. Advise clients with this cardiomyopathy to check with their physician about taking prophylactic antibiotics before and after dental and surgical procedures because American Heart Association guidelines have changed.[2]

All clients with cardiomyopathy need clear, honest education concerning the disease and its cause and intervention. Both you and the client must be watchful for adverse effects of therapy. Clients with restrictive cardiomyopathy are especially vulnerable to the toxic effects of digitalis (see Chapter 58).[3]

■ INFECTIOUS DISORDERS

Bacteria and other microbes are found in abundance in our environment. The heart can become infected by these microbes, a process that prompts an inflammatory response. Involvement of the heart can be lethal during the acute stage or lead to structural damage.

RHEUMATIC FEVER

Rheumatic fever is a diffuse inflammatory disease characterized by a delayed response to an infection by group A beta-hemolytic streptococci (GAS) in the tonsillopharyngeal area. Although this infection remains common, the incidence of rheumatic fever has declined dramatically to about 2 per 100,000 people in the United States. This decline is due to an emphasis on prevention. The incidence in developing countries is about 100 per 100,000 people.[3]

Etiology and Risk Factors

Rheumatic fever develops in only a relatively small percentage of people (3%), even after a virulent bout of streptococcal infection; there is therefore some evidence of host predisposition. There is also a familial predisposition to the disease.[13] Once rheumatic fever is acquired, the client becomes more susceptible than the general population to recurrent infection. Poor hygiene, crowding, and poverty are risk factors for acute rheumatic fever. If appropriate antibiotic therapy for group A beta-hemolytic streptococcal infection is given within the first 9 days, rheumatic fever can usually be prevented.[3]

Prevention is the best treatment. The most effective measures against rheumatic fever are probably socioeconomic. In the affluent neighborhoods of Western cities, where there is spacious housing with no crowding, the incidence of rheumatic fever is low. Identification of high-risk persons is also important. Nurses can help to identify mitral valve prolapse (see earlier discussion) early to prevent valvular disease. Nurses in community settings can identify those with beta-hemolytic streptococcal infections and refer clients for appropriate diagnosis and medical management.

Pathophysiology

Rheumatic fever initiates a diffuse, proliferative, and exudative inflammatory process involving all layers of the heart, joints, subcutaneous tissue, central nervous system (CNS), and skin. Although the cellular disease process is not clear, the mechanism is probably an abnormal humoral and cell-mediated response to streptococcal cell membrane antigens. These antigens bind to receptors on the heart, other tissues, and joints, which begins the autoimmune response. The inflammatory process often produces permanent and severe heart damage. Complications of rheumatic fever include valvular disorders, cardiomegaly, and heart failure. These complications may be fatal.

All layers of the heart swell, a condition called *carditis*. The inflamed myocardium may have areas of necrosis, called *Aschoff's bodies*. These areas are minuscule nodules with localized fibrin deposits surrounded by areas of necrosis in the myocardium. Endocardial inflammation causes swelling of the valve leaflets, which leads to valve dysfunction and murmurs. Small bacterial vegetations form on the valve tissues. Rough eroded areas of the valves attract platelets, which adhere and form platelet-fibrin clumps that eventually scar and shorten the valve. The valves lose their elasticity, and cardiac function is impaired.

First the damaged valve may become scared and stenosed, increasing the cardiac workload because higher pressure must be generated to propel blood through the narrow valve. Second the valve leaflets may become so short that they cannot close securely. As a result blood *regurgitates* (leaks backward) through the damaged valve into the chamber from which it was ejected. Both valvular stenosis and regurgitation eventually cause heart failure from the high workload.

Clinical Manifestations

The clinical manifestations of rheumatic fever are related to the inflammatory response. Many of the common clinical manifestations are also associated with other disorders. The clinical manifestations of rheumatic fever usually last about 3 months.

Major manifestations include the following:

- *Carditis* is the most destructive consequence of this disease. Characteristics include a significant murmur, cardiomegaly, pericarditis that produces a significant friction rub, and heart failure. Chest pain resulting from pericardial inflammation may be present. Sometimes myocardial involvement that produces atrioventricular (AV) conduction defects or atrial fibrillation occurs.
- *Arthritis*, a prominent finding, is painful and migratory. It most often affects the larger joints, such as the ankles, knees, elbows, shoulders, and wrists. The arthritis may or may not be symmetrical. If the client takes aspirin early in the course of the disease, arthritis manifestations may not be as apparent. Joint manifestations may last hours or days.
- *Chorea*, a disorder of the CNS, is manifested by sudden, irregular, aimless, involuntary movements. Chorea disappears without treatment and produces no permanent sequelae.
- *Erythema marginatum* is an unusual rash that is seen primarily on the trunk. The lesions are crescent-shaped and have clear centers. The rash is transitory and its appearance may change in minutes or hours.
- *Subcutaneous nodules* are small, painless, firm nodules that adhere loosely to the tendon sheaths, especially in knees, knuckles, and elbows. They are usually evident only during the first week or so and generally only in children.

Minor manifestations include the following:

- *Fever*, with a temperature of 38° C (100.4° F) or higher, alternates with normal temperature. Weakness, malaise, weight loss, and anorexia probably develop as a result of fever, pain, and the general debilitation associated with serious illness.
- *Arthralgia*, pain in one or more joints without the presence of arthritis is common.

A positive throat culture for group A beta-hemolytic streptococci can help to confirm the diagnosis. An elevated white blood cell (WBC) count, erythrocyte sedimentation rate (ESR), and C-reactive protein may indicate inflammation. An ECG or echocardiogram can help to confirm rhythm problems and structural changes.[3]

The diagnosis is made by the presence of major manifestations; the Jones criteria (Box 57-2) and abnormal laboratory findings are used to make the diagnosis.

Outcome Management
■ Medical Management

The goals of medical management include (1) eradicating infection, (2) maximizing cardiac output, and (3) promoting comfort.

Eradicate Infection. The first priority is to eradicate the streptococcal infection. Usually this can be accomplished with oral administration of penicillin. For penicillin-allergic clients, erythromycin is usually prescribed. The client typically takes prophylactic agents for rheumatic

---

BOX 57-2 *Jones Criteria for the Diagnosis of Rheumatic Fever**

Major Manifestations
1. Carditis
2. Polyarthritis
3. Chorea
4. Erythema marginatum
5. Subcutaneous nodules

Minor Manifestations
1. Clinical findings
   a. Previous rheumatic fever or rheumatic heart disease
   b. Arthralgia
   c. Fever
2. Laboratory findings
   a. Elevated acute phase reactants
      (1) Erythrocyte sedimentation rate
      (2) C-reactive protein
      (3) Leukocytosis
   b. Prolonged P-R interval

Evidence of Group A Streptococcal Infection
1. Positive throat culture for Strep A
2. Elevated or rising anti-streptococcal antibody titer
3. Recent scarlet fever

Modified from Special Writing Group of the American Heart Association. (1992). Guidelines for the diagnosis of rheumatic fever: Jones criteria. 1992 update. *Journal of the American Heart Association, 268*(15), 2069-2072.

*In some instances, rheumatic fever can be diagnosed without fulfillment of Jones criteria.

EB fever for 5 years after the initial attack. After 5 years recurrences are rare and prophylaxis continues only in high-risk clients.[13] Clients who have had rheumatic fever remain vulnerable to bacterial endocarditis. Therefore in addition to the antibiotics they take to prevent rheumatic fever recurrence, they must be referred for evaluation for possible prophylactic medications before and after any surgical procedure or dental work. Specific evaluation for prophylaxis medication must be individualized according to recommendations by the American **EB** Heart Association.[10] (See the Evidence-Based Practice in Action feature on Preventing Bacterial Endocarditis on p. 1615.) Careful monitoring for side effects of multiple cardiac drugs that may be prescribed for clients with valvular disease is essential.

Maximize Cardiac Output. Corticosteroids are used to treat carditis, especially if heart failure is evident. If heart failure develops, treatment, including cardiac glycosides and diuretics, is effective.

Promote Comfort. Clients with arthritic manifestations obtain clinical relief with salicylates; however, be-

cause these drugs can result in a misdiagnosis, a firm diagnosis should be in place before salicylates are given. Bed rest is usually prescribed to reduce cardiac effort until evidence of inflammation has subsided. For clients with rheumatic valvular heart disease, bacterial endocarditis prophylaxis may be necessary (see Infective Endocarditis).

■ Nursing Management of the Medical Client Assessment

Nursing assessment involves gathering baseline and ongoing subjective and objective data. Assess vital signs to reveal the presence of fever, tachycardia, and stability of blood pressure. Vital signs are also used as a measure of activity tolerance. Auscultate heart sounds for the presence of a friction rub, and palpate peripheral pulses. A baseline ECG is used to determine whether heart block is present. Assess baseline nutritional and hydration data.

Assess psychosocial data about the client's feelings regarding restrictions of activity, support systems, coping strategies, level of discomfort, and knowledge (both the client's and his or her family's) concerning the nature of, and intervention for, rheumatic fever.

Diagnosis, Outcomes, Interventions

Diagnosis: Activity Intolerance. A reduced cardiac reserve and enforced bed rest can quickly lead to activity intolerance. The nursing diagnosis statement would be *Activity Intolerance related to reduced cardiac reserve and enforced bed rest.*

Outcomes. The client will have improved tolerance of activity and progress toward an optimal level of physical activity tolerance based on underlying cardiovascular status and psychosocial readiness as evidenced by the ability to (1) pace activity, (2) verbalize improvement in fatigue, (3) express acceptance of any imposed activity restrictions, and (4) steadily increase activity level to include climbing one flight of stairs without chest pain or without ECG changes, while the heart rate remains under 90 beats/min.

Interventions. Bed rest is important in the acute phase because it reduces myocardial oxygen demand and usually continues until the following criteria are met:
- Temperature remains normal without use of salicylates
- Resting pulse remains under 100 beats/min
- ECG tracings show no manifestations of myocardial damage
- ESR returns to normal
- Pericardial friction rub is not present

Once ambulatory the client must still be careful not to overdo. Assess the client's stamina and response to

EB EVIDENCE-BASED PRACTICE IN ACTION

Preventing Bacterial Endocarditis

Although bacterial endocarditis is relatively uncommon, it remains a life-threatening infection responsible for substantial morbidity and mortality.[5] Patients with cardiac conditions were placed into categories of high, moderate, or negligible risk based on the potential outcome if they were to develop endocarditis.[5] The American Heart Association (AHA) has established guidelines for antibiotic prophylaxis to prevent bacterial endocarditis in patients who are at high risk.[1] Prophylactic antibiotics are administered according to the risk associated with various procedures. Risk for bacteremia is highest with dental extractions and oral surgical procedures, moderate for procedures affecting the genitourinary tract, and lowest for gastrointestinal diagnostic procedures.[2]

Successful prophylaxis depends on patient adherence. If patients do not understand the reason for prophylaxis and implications for their health, they may not adhere to the regimen. Nurses can play a key role in preventing bacterial endocarditis in patients at high risk by teaching patients and their families the significance of prophylactic antibiotic treatment.[3] An informal chart review in a cardiology clinic in Canada by Lynch[4] revealed a poor understanding of bacterial endocarditis prevention among high-risk pediatric patients and their families despite efforts by physicians to discuss the importance of this issue. Lynch points out that these findings are not surprising considering the information patients and families are given when a heart lesion is diagnosed. It is understandable that their recall of bacterial endocarditis prophylaxis might be poor.

Nurses are often in the ideal position to convey appropriate information to patients about their disease process and available prevention measures. Lynch[4] and Estlow[3] offer examples of teaching modules for promoting awareness of effective bacterial endocarditis prophylaxis in children. The teaching package must be understandable, concise, and logical. Nurses possess the education necessary to provide teaching in the most effective manner with content based on the most current medical recommendations. This intervention can result in favorable outcomes such as decreased incidence of bacterial endocarditis, decreased cost for treatment through disease prevention, and decreased morbidity and mortality associated with the disease.

Further research is needed to compare patient outcomes and prophylaxis compliance in patients who have received intense nursing instruction compared to those patients who have not had the benefit of such intervention. With the present cost constraints on health care services, research is also needed to quantify the cost-benefit for improved outcomes in preventing bacterial endocarditis when extensive teaching is provided to patients and their families.

Implications for nursing practice include the need for nurses to possess strong patient teaching skills, allocation of adequate nursing hours to provide patient teaching, and evaluation methods to measure patient outcomes and validate the need for patient education provided by qualified nurses.

References

1. Dajani, A.S., et al. (1997). Prevention of bacterial endocarditis: Recommendations by the American Heart Association. *Journal of the American Medical Association, 277*(22), 1794-1801.
2. Durack, D.T. (1995). Prevention of infective endocarditis. *New England Journal of Medicine, 332*(1), 38-44.
3. Estlow, M.M. (1998). Prevention of infective endocarditis in the pediatric congenital heart population. *Pediatric Nursing, 24*(3), 205-212.
4. Lynch, L.I. (1999). A teaching module: Promoting awareness of effective bacterial endocarditis prophylaxis in children. *Pediatric Nursing, 25*(6), 621-626.
5. Taubert, K.A., & Dajani, A.S. (1998). Preventing bacterial endocarditis: American Heart Association guidelines. *American Family Physician, 57*(3), 457-469.

exercise to gauge the degree of gradual activity progression. Assess vital signs before and after exercise. After 3 to 5 minutes of rest, reassess vital signs. The client should reduce or discontinue activity if chest pain, vertigo, dyspnea, confusion, a drop in blood pressure, or an irregular pulse develops. The length of activity restriction depends on whether carditis develops and on the extent of permanent heart damage. Restrictions may extend for months. In severe cases of rheumatic carditis, clients may be forced to undergo restrictions on a permanent basis. Encourage a gradual increase in activity within the limits of the client's condition.

The client experiencing chorea requires sedatives, bed rest, and protection from self-injury. A carefully planned and supervised activity schedule should be maintained and evaluated.

Diagnosis: Chronic Pain. The inflammatory response in the joints can lead to pain. The nursing diagnosis statement would be *Chronic Pain related to the inflammatory response in the joints.*

Outcomes. The client will experience increased comfort as evidenced by (1) reports of restful sleep and reduced discomfort, (2) expression of joint pain reduction, (3) reduced use of pain medications, and (4) a relaxed body posture and a calm facial expression.

Interventions. Obtain a clear description of the pain or discomfort. Identify the source of greatest discomfort as a focus for intervention. Administer analgesics as needed. Balance rest and activity according to the degree of pain and activity tolerance. Other pain interventions are discussed in Chapter 22.

Diagnosis: Imbalanced Nutrition: Less Than Body Requirements. Hypermetabolism seen with fever and inflammation and other factors in rheumatic fever can lead to protein calorie malnutrition. This nursing diagnosis is stated as *Imbalanced Nutrition: Less than Body Requirements, related to fever, inflammation, anorexia, and fatigue.*

Outcomes. The client will maintain or restore adequate nutritional balance as evidenced by (1) the resumption of body weight before the illness or no further weight loss, (2) consumption of 75% or more of each meal served, (3) normal serum albumin or prealbumin, and (4) a positive nitrogen balance.

Interventions. A high-protein, high-carbohydrate diet helps maintain adequate nutrition in the presence of fever and infection. Hypermetabolic states (fever and infection) can induce a catabolic state, thus delaying healing. Vitamin and mineral supplements may also benefit the client. Oral hygiene every 4 hours; small, attractive meal servings; and foods that are not overly rich, sweet, or greasy stimulate the appetite. Adequate fluid intake prevents dehydration resulting from fever. If the client shows manifestations of severe carditis or heart failure, sodium and fluids must be restricted. Daily weights can serve as an indication of nutritional and fluid status.

Diagnosis: Risk for Ineffective Therapeutic Regimen Management (Individuals). Following rheumatic fever, the client must follow a lifelong regimen to reduce the risk of rheumatic heart disease. This nursing diagnosis is stated as *Risk for Ineffective Therapeutic Regimen Management (Individuals) related to a need for lifelong therapy.*

Outcomes. The client and his or her family will demonstrate adequate knowledge of rheumatic fever and its cause, course, and therapy as evidenced by the ability to describe accurately the causes and process of rheumatic fever, its clinical manifestations, its prevention, and the rationale for prescribed interventions.

Interventions. Today streptococcal infections do not have to develop into rheumatic fever if the client seeks immediate assessment and begins antibiotics. Clients who have recovered from an episode of rheumatic fever can avoid subsequent attacks by taking prophylactic doses of antibiotics and observing good health practices. Because repeated attacks may lead to serious heart disease and permanent cardiac disability, it is important to emphasize means of avoiding subsequent attacks.

Instruct the client about how to reduce exposure to streptococcal infection as follows:

1. Take good care of the teeth and gums, and obtain prompt dental care for cavities and gingivitis. Pro-

phylactic medication may be needed before invasive dental procedures, and individualized evaluation for prophylaxis medication is needed.[10]

2. Avoid people who have an upper respiratory infection or who have had a recent streptococcal infection.

3. Notify the physician if any manifestations of streptococcal sore throat *(pharyngitis)* develop. It is extremely important to begin antibiotic therapy promptly for any infection. The clinical manifestations include fever (102° to 104° F), chills, sore throat, and enlarged, painful lymph nodes. Advise clients who have had rheumatic fever that they must guard against infections for the rest of their lives to avoid development of heart disease.

Evaluation

Rheumatic fever is treated over 10 days. Expect activity tolerance to improve once fever and pain are controlled. Altered nutrition may require more than 2 weeks to show improvement, depending on the severity of anorexia and fever.

INFECTIVE ENDOCARDITIS

Endocarditis is an inflammatory process of the endocardium, especially the valves. This disorder carries high morbidity and mortality rates, but outcomes can be improved greatly with rapid diagnosis and effective treatment.

Many different terms and classifications are used to describe infective endocarditis. Some are defined in the following list:

- *Subacute bacterial endocarditis* (SBE): develops gradually over several weeks or months; usually caused by organisms of low virulence, such as *Streptococcus viridans,* which has a limited ability to infect other tissues
- *Acute bacterial endocarditis:* develops over days or weeks with an erratic course and earlier development of complications; commonly caused by *Staphylococcus aureus,* which is capable of infecting other body tissues
- *Native valve endocarditis:* an infection of a previously normal or damaged valve
- *Prosthetic valve endocarditis:* an infection of a prosthetic valve
- *Nonbacterial thrombotic endocarditis:* caused by sterile thrombotic lesions (often aggregates of platelets), which may develop in people with cancer or other chronic diseases

Changes in the population at risk are altering the classic picture of endocarditis. The incidence is continuing to rise. Each year, about 15,000 to 20,000 new cases are appearing. Infective endocarditis (IE) is now the fourth leading cause of life-threatening infectious disease syndromes.[3] IE occurs more often in men, and the median age of clients has risen from 30 to 40 years in the early antibiotic era to 47 to 64 years in recent decades.[12] The average age of clients with IE among drug abusers is 27 to 37 years. Fewer clients are being seen with the classic physical manifestations of advanced endocarditis, such as Osler's nodes, finger clubbing, or Roth's spots (see Clinical Manifestations). The proportion of cases caused by gram-negative bacilli, fungi, and other unusual microbes is increasing.

The changes are traced to several notable alterations in the population. The increased incidence of endocarditis caused by yeasts and fungi is attributable to the increased number of persons with valve prostheses, to the increased number of persons using intravenous (IV) drugs, and rising use of long-term antimicrobial therapy or immunosuppression. Nosocomial infections are now the cause of up to 29% of all cases.[12]

The decreased incidence of rheumatic fever results in a lower incidence of endocarditis, whereas the number of children surviving congenital heart disease results in an increased incidence. The growing population of older adults also leads to an increase in the number of endocarditis episodes.

Etiology and Risk Factors

Common infecting organisms include staphylococci (*S. aureus, S. faecalis, S. epidermidis*), streptococci, *Escherichia coli*, gram-negative organisms (*Klebsiella, Pseudomonas, Serratia marcescens*), fungi (*Candida, Aspergillus*) and HACEK organisms (*Haemophilus parainfluenzae, Haemophilus aphrophilus, Actinobacillus actinomycetemcomitans, Cardiobacterium hominis, Eikenella* species, and *Kingella* species). These organisms enter the body through the oral cavity after dental procedures, mouth or tooth abscesses, oral irrigations, or oral irritations from dental floss or bridgework. The upper respiratory tract is another port of entry following surgery, intubations, or infections. Direct exposure of the bloodstream to organisms can occur with prolonged IV catheters, hemodialysis catheters, and IV drug use. Procedures involving the gastrointestinal and genitourinary tracts (e.g., barium enemas, sigmoidoscopy, colonoscopy, percutaneous liver biopsy, catheterization, urethrotomy, prostatectomy, cystoscopy) have been associated with infective endocarditis.

Reproductive conditions have also been linked (e.g., delivery of a newborn, abortion, intrauterine devices, pelvic inflammatory diseases). Defective heart valves causing changes in blood flow and pressures encourage the proliferation of vegetations. Open heart surgery to replace damaged valves increases the risk of endocarditis. Fortunately, coronary artery bypass grafting (CABG), one of the most frequently performed surgical procedures in the United States, carries a low risk of infective endocarditis because the endocardium is not invaded during the operation.

Circulating microorganisms in the bloodstream attach to the endocardial surface and multiply. Usually multiplication of these organisms requires a rough or abnormal endocardium. IV drug abusers may be injecting particulate matter into the bloodstream, causing damage to the previously normal endocardium that allows the organism to adhere, thereby initiating acute bacterial endocarditis.

Pathophysiology

Microorganisms enter the bloodstream in many ways. Once the colonization process begins on the endothelium, replication occurs and bacterial colonies form within layers of platelets and fibrin. As the colonies become entangled within the tight layers of fibrin and platelets, the colony becomes less and less vulnerable to the body's defense mechanisms. The bacteria stimulate the humoral immune system to produce nonspecific antibodies, but the bacteria are protected by the fibrin-platelet aggregation. It is not uncommon for these vegetations to form clots that travel to other organs, forming abscesses. The vegetations can severely damage heart valves by perforating and deforming the valve leaflets (Figure 57-5). Extensions of the bacteria may invade the aorta or pericardium. The amount of damage depends on the type and virulence of the organisms causing the infection.

Many complications are possible. Heart failure may develop as a result of structural valvular damage. Arterial emboli can occur from the vegetation. Systemic

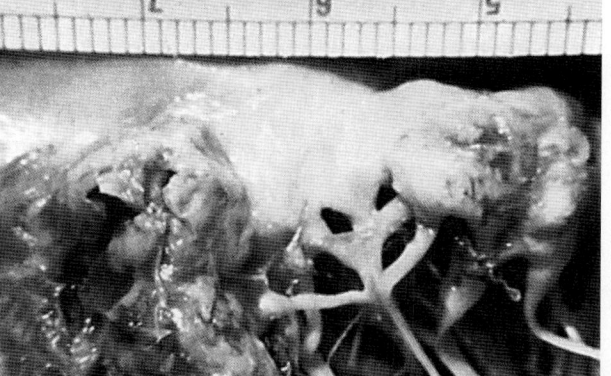

FIGURE 57-5 Vegetations of the heart valves resulting from infective endocarditis. Large vegetations were present on the leaflets of the mitral valve. (From Braunwald, E. [2001]. *Heart disease: A textbook of cardiovascular medicine* [6th ed.] Philadelphia: W.B. Saunders.)

embolization occurs in 30% to 40% of clients with left-sided infective endocarditis.[12] Common infarction sites are the kidney, spleen, and brain. Pulmonary embolus is associated with right-sided infective endocarditis. Emboli can also travel to the brain and produce myriad manifestations. Occasionally immune complex glomerulonephritis will develop. Renal function usually returns to normal after the infection has been controlled.

Clinical Manifestations

Clinical manifestations of infective endocarditis include those related to the infectious process, embolization, and the immune response.

Clinical manifestations related to the infection include fever, chills alternating with sweats, malaise, weakness, anorexia, weight loss, pallor, backache, and splenomegaly.[12] Clients may report feeling as though they have the flu, with headaches and musculoskeletal aching. In acute infection, clients appear very ill. Fever, chills, and prostration are so severe that hospital admission is usually necessary within a few days.

Cardiac murmurs eventually develop, but they may be absent in the early stages of infection. In clients with pre-existing valvular disease, new murmurs may be heard. Heart failure may develop suddenly in either acute or subacute endocarditis. Mechanical complications include perforation of a valve leaflet, rupture of one of the chordae tendineae, or development of a functional stenosis from the obstruction of blood flow by large vegetations.

Clinical manifestations related to embolization can occur in any part of the body. They are presented in the following list in order from head to toe:

- Stroke, transient ischemic attacks, aphasia, or ataxia
- Loss of vision from embolization to the brain or retinal artery
- Petechiae on the neck, conjunctiva, chest, abdomen, and mouth
- Roth's spots—a white or yellow center surrounded by a bright-red, irregular halo seen by ophthalmoscope
- Myocardial infarction, which may develop as a result of coronary artery embolism
- Pulmonary embolus
- Splinter hemorrhages, which look like tiny splinters under the nail
- Osler's nodes—painful, erythematous, pea-sized nodules on tips of the fingers and toes resulting from inflammation around a small, infected embolus
- Finger clubbing, although less common today, may occur in clients with long-standing infective endocarditis; pathogenesis remains unclear
- Janeway's lesions—flat, small, nontender red spots on the palms of the hands and the soles of the feet

- Evidence of an immunologic reaction to infection, including arthralgia, proteinuria, hematuria, casts, and acidosis

Because the clinical manifestations of endocarditis are numerous and often nonspecific, several modalities are used for the differential medical diagnosis. Blood cultures for bacteria, fungus, and yeast are the most important diagnostic tests. Blood cultures should be obtained for all clients with both fever and heart murmur. ECGs and echocardiograms should be done on admission to the hospital and repeated during the hospital stay.[14] A chest x-ray study is useful in identifying early heart failure. A complete blood count (CBC) and other routine diagnostic procedures are also helpful.

Diagnosis is confirmed by clinical manifestations, blood cultures, and echocardiography. The Duke criteria can assist with diagnosis and classification (Table 57-3).

Outcome Management
■ Medical Management

The chief aims of management are to eradicate the infecting organism and to treat the complications. The advent of antimicrobial therapy has changed this infection from one that was almost always fatal to one that is rarely fatal. The choice of antibiotic depends on the organism involved. Penicillin and gentamicin are commonly used. Because of resistive strains of bacteria, other antibiotics might be needed. Therapy is usually administered by the IV route and continued for 4 to 6 weeks. Drug administration is usually begun in the hospital but is occasionally continued at home with extensive discharge planning and education. The American Heart Association offers recommendations for prophylaxis for infective endocarditis. Compliance with the regimen over a lifetime is important.

Occasionally, after the infection is under control (negative blood cultures, absence of fever, and normal WBC count), it may be necessary for the client to undergo heart-valve replacement for reversal of newly developed heart failure. Complications that could have developed as a result of the infecting organism warrant careful evaluation.

■ Nursing Management of the Medical Client

Nursing assessment focuses on gathering data about the client's hemodynamic stability (particularly the presence of a new heart murmur and embolic complications), level of comfort, coping ability, support from significant others, and potential for self-care.

Administer IV antibiotics as prescribed. Antibiotics relieve much discomfort within a few days. Treat fever, when present, with rest, cooling measures, forced fluids, and sometimes salicylates. As with most infectious processes, encourage the client to eat a nutritious diet, drink sufficient fluids, and rest mentally and physically.

The client may need to be hospitalized or transferred to a setting that can provide IV medications for 2 to 6

TABLE 57-3	*Diagnosis of Infective Endocarditis*

Definitive Infective Endocarditis

Pathologic criteria

Microorganisms: demonstrated by culture or histology in a vegetation, *or* in a vegetation that has embolized, *or* in an intracardiac abscess, *or*

Pathological lesions: vegetation or intracardiac abscess present, confirmed by histology showing active endocarditis

Clinical criteria, using specific definitions listed below

Two major criteria, *or*

One major and three minor criteria, *or*

Five minor criteria

Possible Infective Endocarditis

Findings consistent with infective endocarditis that fall short of definite endocarditis but are not rejected

Rejected

Firm alternative diagnosis for manifestations of endocarditis, *or*

Sustained resolution of manifestations of endocarditis, with antibiotic therapy for 4 days or less, *or*

No pathologic evidence of infective endocarditis at surgery or autopsy, after antibiotic therapy for 4 days or less

Criteria for Diagnosis of Infective Endocarditis

Major Criteria

Positive blood culture

Typical microorganism for infective endocarditis from two separate blood cultures

Viridans streptococci, *Streptococcus bovis,* HACEK group *or*

Community-acquired *Staphylococcus aureus* or enterococci in the absence of a primary focus, *or*

Persistently positive blood culture, defined as recovery of a microorganism consistent with infective endocarditis from:

Blood cultures drawn more than 12 hr apart, *or*

All of three or a majority of four or more separate blood cultures, with first and last drawn at least 1 hr apart

Evidence of endocardial involvement

Positive echocardiogram

Oscillating intracardiac mass, on valve or supporting structures, *or* in the path of regurgitant jets, *or* on implanted material, in the absence of an alternative anatomical explanation, *or*

Abscess, *or*

New partial dehiscence of prosthetic valve, *or*

New valvular regurgitation (increase or change in preexisting murmur not sufficient)

Minor Criteria

Predisposition: predisposing heart condition *or* intravenous drug use

Fever ≥38.0° C (100.4° F)

Vascular phenomena: major arterial emboli, septic pulmonary infarcts, mycotic aneurysm, intracranial hemorrhage, conjunctival hemorrhages, Janeway's lesions

Immunologic phenomena: glomerulonephritis, Osler's nodes, Roth's spots, rheumatoid factor

Microbiologic evidence: positive blood culture but not meeting major criteria as noted previously* *or* serologic evidence of active infection with organism consistent with infective endocarditis

Echocardiogram: consistent with infective endocarditis but not meeting major criteria

Modified from Durack, D.T., Lukes, A.S., Bright, D.K. (1994). New criteria for diagnosis of infective endocarditis: Utilization of specific echocardiographic findings. *American Journal of Medicine, 96,* 200.

*Excluding single positive cultures for coagulase-negative staphylococci and organisms that do not cause endocarditis.

weeks if home care is not an option. Do not enforce complete bed rest unless fever or manifestations of heart damage develop. Auscultate the heart every 8 hours for murmurs. Assess for rapid pulse, easy fatigability, dyspnea, restlessness, manifestations of heart failure, and embolic manifestations. Document these manifestations if they occur, and report them to the physician.

When the client's condition improves, plan and implement a progressive activity schedule and a teaching plan (see the Client Education Guide feature on Infective *evolve* Endocarditis on the website). As activity increases, monitor the client's physical response to exercise. For example, assess blood pressure, heart rate, diaphoresis, vertigo, and weakness.

■ Self-Care

The trend toward early hospital discharge has changed the course of treatment for clients with infective endocarditis.

IV therapy may now be routinely given in the home. Clients who are alert, cooperative, and reasonably stable and who want to return home may be allowed to do so. Typically the nurse, pharmacist, and physician teach the techniques of self-administered IV antibiotics. Before discharge, the client must demonstrate the knowledge and technique required. The physician's office or home health care nurses often monitor the client's progress.

Home IV antibiotic therapy offers many benefits. It is less costly than hospital care, motivates clients to become active participants in their own care, reestablishes a more normal lifestyle, and promotes a sense of control that aids in psychosocial and physiologic recovery. To be effective, this program calls for exceptional communication and cooperation between members of the health care team and the client.

Invasive procedures, especially dental work, increase the risk of endocarditis. Oral antibiotics are advised before most dental procedures are performed (Box 57-3). Other invasive diagnostic and surgical procedures also require antibiotics.

MYOCARDITIS

Myocarditis is an inflammation of the myocardial wall. It can be caused by almost any bacterial, viral, or parasitic organism as well as by radiation, toxic agents such as lead, and drugs such as lithium and cocaine. Myocarditis affects people of all ages and may be acute or chronic. An immunodeficient person is at greater risk for myocarditis. Frequently, the inflammation is not limited to the myocardium but extends to the pericardium, with production of an associated pericarditis. The incidence is not possible to ascertain[17] and varies with the client's age and with various etiologic agents.

In the United States, most cases of myocarditis are due to viral infections. Viruses associated with this disorder include coxsackievirus A and B, mumps, influenza virus serotypes A and B, rubella virus, measles virus, adenoviruses, echoviruses, cytomegalovirus, and Epstein-Barr virus. Other causes include bacterial, fungal, rickettsial, spirochetal, helminthic, and protozoal infections.[21] Myocarditis can also be caused by hypersensitivity immune reactions seen with acute rheumatic fever and postcardiotomy syndrome, toxins and chemicals such as alcohol, large doses of radiation therapy to the chest for the treatment of malignancy, and parasitic infections, including Chagas' disease and toxoplasmosis.

Myocardial damage from acute myocarditis is usually the result of the direct invasion or the toxic effects of the microorganism in cardiac myocytes. This can cause an alteration in cellular energy systems and cellular damage. Endomyocardial biopsies are used in diagnosis of the viral infection.[21]

Usually myocarditis involves both ventricles. If myocardial contractility is impaired, ventricular diastolic pressures and volumes may be elevated to maintain stroke volume. Disruptions leading to cardiac dysrhythmias can decrease cardiac output.

Clinical Manifestations

Clinical manifestations vary widely, and there may be no clinical manifestations at all. The health history may reveal a recent upper respiratory infection, viral pharyngitis, or tonsillitis. The most frequent manifestations, however, are fatigue, dyspnea, palpitations, and chest pain. The client often experiences chest pain as a mild continuous pressure or soreness in the chest. Thus the chest pain of myocarditis can be distinguished from the effort-induced pain of angina pectoris. Tachycardia, if present, may be disproportionate to the degree of fever, exertion, or illness.[21] Dysrhythmias can also occur, sometimes producing a fatal circulatory collapse. A pericardial friction rub may occur if the client has pericarditis.

If myocardial involvement becomes extensive or prolonged, myofibril degeneration can produce heart failure, with pulmonary congestion, dyspnea, neck-vein distention, peripheral edema, and cardiomegaly. Recurrent myocarditis can produce cardiomyopathy. Possible complications include heart failure, dilated cardiomyopathy, and sudden death from lethal dysrhythmias or rupture of a myocardial aneurysm.[21]

The chest x-ray may show an enlarged cardiac silhouette resulting from ventricular enlargement or pericardial effusion. Blood tests may show a moderate leukocytosis and elevated cardiac enzymes. Echocardiography is helpful in determining heart chamber size and ventricular functioning. Gallium scan shows regional wall abnormalities, dilated ventricles, and hypokinesis of the left ventricle. ECG abnormalities and elevated serum levels of cardiac enzymes are helpful in the diagnosis. The ECG may show a bundle branch block or complete AV heart block, ST-segment elevation, or T-wave flattening.

Outcome Management

Clients with acute myocarditis are usually admitted to the hospital for observation. Clients with pericardial effusion, dysrhythmias, heart failure, or hypotension are usually admitted to the intensive care unit (ICU). Medical management begins with specific therapy for the underlying infection. Bed rest is suggested to decrease cardiac work. Supplemental oxygen may be prescribed for clients with low cardiac output or dysrhythmias. Immunosuppressive therapy is being investigated.[29] Antipyretic agents are helpful for the fever and its hemodynamic effects, which result in increased myocardial workload. Clients who remain at home may use Holter monitoring, which provides continuous surveillance of the client's heart rhythm. In most cases myocarditis is self-limiting and uncomplicated.[21] Although most clients recover rapidly, some have recurrent or chronic myocarditis and some become very ill and die.

Nursing management for the client experiencing myocarditis is essentially the same as that provided to clients with infective endocarditis and rheumatic fever. Review those sections in this chapter.

Teaching begins when acute manifestations have subsided and the client has demonstrated physical and emotional readiness. Teach clients how to monitor their pulse rate and rhythm. Instruct them to report any sudden changes in heart rate, rhythm, or palpitations immediately. Encourage family members to take CPR training, which can be obtained from such groups as the local fire department, the American Red Cross, or the American Heart Association. Educating family members about CPR can enhance their sense of preparedness for an emergency.

Because the myocardial infectious process resolves slowly and late complications can occur, advise clients to continue self-monitoring and to schedule clinical follow-up appointments, even after apparent recovery.

The potential of lethal dysrhythmias may frighten **EB** the client and his or her significant others. The client who is experiencing extreme anxiety, fear, and ineffective coping may manifest insomnia, tearfulness, somatic complaints, an inability to problem-solve, and agitation. Determine with the client (and family) the specific focus of anxiety. Clarify any misconceptions. Speak slowly and calmly, and focus on the present situation, giving feedback about current reality. Encourage the use of relaxation techniques to help allay stress. Schedule activities around periods of undisturbed sleep.

BOX 57-4	*Causes of Pericarditis*

Infections
  Viral: coxsackie, influenza
  Bacterial: tuberculosis, staphylococcus, streptococcus, meningococcus, pneumococcus
  Parasitic
  Fungal
Myocardial injury
  Myocardial infarction (Dressler's syndrome)
  Cardiac trauma: blunt or penetrating
  Post cardiac surgery
  Hypersensitivity
Collagen diseases
  Rheumatic fever
  Scleroderma
  Systemic lupus erythematosus
  Rheumatoid arthritis
Drug reaction
  Procainamide
  Methysergide
  Hydralazine
Radiation therapy
Cobalt therapy
Metabolic disorders
  Uremia
  Myxedema
Chronic anemia
Neoplasm: lymphoma
Aortic dissection

PERICARDITIS

Pericarditis may be either acute or chronic *(recurrent)*. It is not known why pericarditis may be an acute illness in some clients and recurrent in others.

ACUTE PERICARDITIS

Acute pericarditis is a syndrome resulting from inflammation of the parietal and visceral pericardium. Because of the proximity of the pericardium to the pleura, lungs, sternum, diaphragm, and myocardium, pericarditis may be a consequence of a number of inflammatory or infectious processes (Box 57-4). Acute pericarditis is usually viral (idiopathic) in origin.

Agents or processes causing pericardial inflammation create an exudate of fibrin, WBCs, and endothelial cells. The exudate covers the pericardium and causes further inflammation of the surrounding pleura and tissues. The fibrinous exudate may localize to one region of the heart, or it may be generalized. Acute pericarditis may be either *dry* (fibrinous) or *exudative*. Under normal conditions the pericardial sac contains about 50 ml of clear, serous-like fluid. Volumes from 100 to 3000 ml of serofibrinous exudate can accumulate with pericarditis. The exudate accumulates in the pericardial sac, causing cardiac tamponade that restricts cardiac filling and emptying (see later discussion on tamponade). Without prompt treatment, shock and death can result from decreased cardiac output.

Dry pericarditis can occur after a common viral infection, myocardial infarction, tuberculosis, bacteremia, or renal failure. Delicate adhesions form within the pericardial space along with serous fibrin deposition, hemorrhage, and calcification. Adhesions may eventually obliterate the pericardial sac. Inflammation of the pericardium frequently penetrates the myocardium to some degree, which produces myopericarditis.

Although chest pain is common, the nature of this pain varies. Sometimes the pain is similar to that of myocardial infarction; at other times it mimics the pain of pleurisy. The pain is exacerbated with respiration and rotating the trunk but usually does not radiate to the arms. Sitting up often relieves the pain.

Pericardial *friction rub* is a classic objective manifestation of acute pericarditis. The rub is produced by inflamed, roughened pericardial layers that create friction as their surfaces rub together during heart movement. Auscultation over the precordium reveals a scratchy, leathery, or creaky sound that is heard anywhere over the precordium but most frequently at the third inter-costal space left of the sternal border. The rub is best heard with the diaphragm of the stethoscope and with the client holding his or her breath (to eliminate the breath sounds). In some clients the sound is best heard with the client sitting up. Pericardial friction rubs vary in intensity from hour to hour and from day to day.

Fever is another common finding in clients with pericarditis. The temperature may rise to 39.4° C (103° F). Chills, malaise, joint pain, anorexia, nausea, and weight loss accompany the fever. Dyspnea and chest pain can potentiate anxiety. An increase in heart rate usually corresponds to the degree of fever and anxiety.

The ECG may indicate tachycardia, but with underlying heart disease or uremia, bradycardia can occur. Laboratory studies show an elevated ESR and may show an elevated WBC count. Cardiac enzymes are usually normal but may be elevated.

Outcome Management

When the cause of acute pericarditis is known, treatment of the cause can be planned accordingly. If no causal agent is known, symptomatic intervention for acute dry pericarditis is provided. Clients may be hospitalized for diagnosis and for the treatment of complications.[20] Pain and fever, usually self-limited, may be eased by aspirin given in the maximally tolerated doses. Nonsteroidal anti-inflammatory drugs (NSAID) may also be prescribed. Stronger analgesia, such as morphine sulfate, may be necessary if chest pain becomes severe.

If acute pericarditis is present after a myocardial infarction, reassure the client that the pain experienced with pericarditis does not mean that another infarction is occurring. If the client becomes anxious, worrying about the cause of the pain, oxygen demand increases and myocardial ischemia may develop.

The focus of nursing care related to pericarditis is the same as that described for the other inflammatory cardiac diseases discussed in this chapter. Nursing assessment of the client with pericarditis also includes scrutiny for the presence of pericardial tamponade (pulsus paradoxus, distended neck veins). Vigilant assessment is necessary. Provide reassurance about the temporary nature of the disease.

ACUTE PERICARDITIS WITH EFFUSION

Acute pericarditis with effusion results when fluid accumulates within the pericardial sac. Rapid or excessive fluid accumulations may compress the heart and reduce ventricular filling and cardiac output. When fluid accumulates slowly, the fibrous pericardium is better able to stretch and accommodate its presence. Clients can tolerate 1 to 2 L of fluid without an increase in intrapericardial pressure if accumulation is slow; however, the normal unstretched pericardial sac can accommodate the rapid addition of only 80 to 200 ml of fluid without a decrease in cardiac output.[20]

Pericardial effusion may be asymptomatic. If dry pericarditis precedes the condition, the friction rub may disappear. Fever may develop. Heart sounds may be muffled because the pericardial fluid accumulates between the stethoscope and the heart valves and chambers quieting the heart sounds.

Pulsus paradoxus can be present. If the client has normal breathing and a systolic difference greater than 10 mm Hg, evaluation for cardiac compression and possibly cardiac tamponade should be performed.[4]

Echocardiography is the most accurate technique for evaluating pericardial effusion.[4] This test is sensitive enough to detect as little as 20 ml of pericardial fluid. Pericardiocentesis is not indicated unless there is evidence of cardiac compression caused by cardiac tamponade (see Cardiac Tamponade). If pericardial effusion is present, an enlarged cardiac silhouette is seen on the chest radiograph.

Care of the client with pericardial effusion is similar to the plan of intervention for dry pericarditis. Bed rest, analgesia, and proper positioning can help to alleviate manifestations. Psychological support is important.

CHRONIC CONSTRICTIVE PERICARDITIS

Chronic constrictive pericarditis is a chronic inflammatory condition in which the pericardium changes into a thick, fibrous band of tissue. This tissue encircles, encases, and compresses the heart, preventing proper ventricular filling and emptying. Cardiac failure eventually results from this slow compression.

This condition usually begins with an episode of acute pericarditis characterized by fibrin deposition, often with pericardial effusion. In most cases the visceral and parietal layers become completely fused. The heavily fibrosed pericardium restricts diastolic filling in all chambers and decreases systolic ejection.

Clinical manifestations include right ventricular failure first, followed by decreased cardiac output manifesting as fatigue on exertion, dyspnea, leg edema, ascites, low pulse pressure, distended neck veins, and delayed capillary refill time.[12] Constrictive pericarditis is a progressive disease without spontaneous reversal of manifestations.

Medical treatment includes digitalis, diuretics, and sodium restriction to relieve manifestations of right ventricular failure. Surgical intervention involves the excision of the damaged pericardium *(pericardiectomy)* and should be performed early in the course of the disease.[19]

CARDIAC TAMPONADE

Cardiac tamponade is a life-threatening complication caused by accumulation of fluid in the pericardium. This fluid, which can be blood, pus, or air in the pericardial sac, accumulates fast enough and in sufficient quantity to compress the heart and restrict blood flow in and out of the ventricles. This is a cardiac emergency.

Large or rapidly accumulating effusions raise the intrapericardial pressure to a point at which venous blood cannot flow into the heart, which decreases ventricular filling. As a result, venous pressure rises and cardiac output and arterial blood pressure fall. A narrowing pulse pressure signals cardiac tamponade. The heart attempts to compensate by beating rapidly (tachycardia), but tachycardia cannot sustain cardiac output for long. Prompt intervention is necessary to prevent shock and death.

Hypotension, tachycardia, jugular venous distention, cyanosis of lips and nails, dyspnea, muffled heart sounds, diaphoresis, and paradoxical pulse (a decrease in systolic arterial pulsation exceeding 10 mm Hg, during inspiration) are present. The client may be comfortable and quiet one minute and then restless with a feeling of impending doom. Clients may panic when fluid accumulates rapidly as a result of seriously reduced cardiac output. Slowly developing tamponade is characterized by manifestations that resemble those of heart failure: nonspecific ECG changes, decreased voltage, and visualization of fluid in the pericardial sac on echocardiogram (see the Critical Monitoring feature on Cardiac Tamponade, below.)

Immediate intervention is required. The emergency intervention of choice is *pericardiocentesis,* a procedure in which fluid or air is aspirated from the pericardial sac (Figure 57-6). This procedure relieves pressure on the heart, thereby improving cardiac function and perhaps saving the client's life. Pericardiocentesis is performed with a soft catheter to reduce the risk of cardiac lacerations.

CRITICAL MONITORING

Cardiac Tamponade

Report the following manifestations of cardiac tamponade immediately!

- Elevated venous pressure (increased central venous pressure)
- Distended neck veins
- Kussmaul's sign (distended neck veins on inspiration)
- Hypotension
- Narrowed pulse pressure
- Tachycardia
- Dyspnea
- Restlessness, anxiety
- Cyanosis of lips and nails
- Diaphoresis
- Muffled heart sounds
- Pulsus paradoxus
- Decreased friction rub
- Decreased QRS voltage and electrical alternans

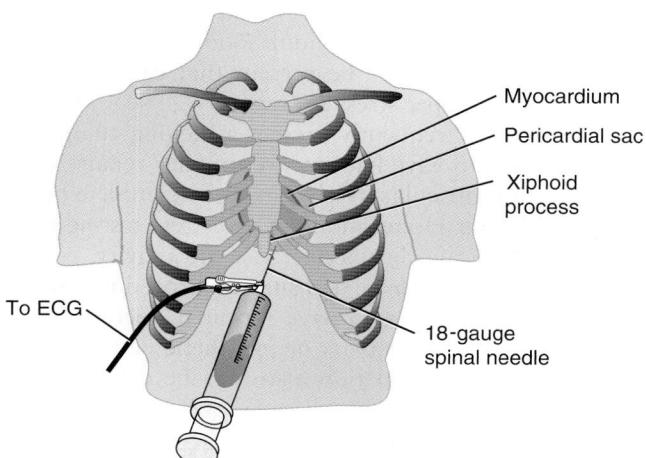

FIGURE 57-6 Pericardiocentesis to remove blood from pericardial sac during tamponade. *ECG,* Electrocardiogram.

CONGENITAL DISORDERS

Congenital heart disorders result from faulty development of cardiac structures in utero. Congenital disorders include septal defects, vessel stenosis, abnormally positioned vessels, and patency of the ductus arteriosus. Advances in the medical and surgical treatment of people with congenital heart disease have assisted an ever-growing number of clients to survive to adulthood. As this number grows, medical and nursing support has grown also.

With today's available treatments, about 85% of children with congenital heart disease will survive to adulthood.[10] Therefore we can expect to see more adults with congenital defects in the future.[10] Each congenital defect brings its own morbidity and mortality statistics; in general, however, people with less complex defects will have a longer survival than those with more complex defects (the course for such defects is still uncertain).

Operations may be palliative or corrective. Most adult clients today underwent their surgical procedures many years ago during the developmental phase of these interventions. Their course would probably be quite different from that followed today. Because many refinements in surgical techniques continue to be developed, clinical outcomes vary significantly.

Many people with a congenital heart defect have remained asymptomatic; others have had varying levels of functional ability. Clients may have both residual problems (those not corrected or improved at surgical repair) and sequelae (results of the surgery). Common lifelong problems include the risk of infective endocarditis in clients with artificial valves or with suture repair of an atrial septal defect. It is not uncommon for a client with a repaired coarctation of the aorta to find that the aorta has gradually become narrowed again. In such cases hypertension may develop. Clients who as children underwent repair for cyanotic defects tend to experience sequelae and complications in adulthood. Some degree of exercise intolerance may be present that can be better managed after proper stress testing.

Dysrhythmias frequently present a lifelong complication. Clients who have had intraventricular repairs may present with ventricular dysrhythmias or complete heart block. A 24-hour Holter monitor and stress testing may help to evaluate the client's tolerance for activity.

Many people who have had surgical procedures as infants and children had to have repeated operations as they "outgrew" their repairs or prosthetic devices. Our growing geriatric population also may be experiencing unknown late consequences of congenital heart disease or surgical repair. It is important to encourage these people to participate in long-term follow-up.

Your role as a nurse who is caring for the adult with congenital heart disease varies with the setting; however, you play an integral role in helping these clients to achieve optimal health and functioning. Nursing assessment, intervention, education, and follow-up are directed toward improving functional levels, managing medications, psychosocial adjustment, and preventing complications.

CONCLUSIONS

The client with a cardiac disorder frequently has activity intolerance, decreased cardiac output, and ineffective coping because of the seriousness of the disorder. Nurses must be skilled in the physical and psychosocial aspects of disease when providing care.

THINKING CRITICALLY *evolve*

1. A 45-year-old man arrives in the emergency department after an automobile accident. Initially he does not complain about himself, but then he is more concerned about his daughter, who was injured in the accident. Neither the child nor the client were wearing seat belts when their car was struck from behind. While sitting at his daughter's bedside in the emergency department, the client becomes increasingly anxious; his respiratory rate increases, and he becomes restless. The vital signs reveal a blood pressure of 88/72 mm Hg, pulse of 118 beats/min, and respirations of 28 breaths/min. What other assessments are needed to rule out cardiac tamponade? What intervention will relieve pressure on the heart and improve cardiac function?

Factors to Consider. What are the clinical manifestations of cardiac tamponade? How is cardiac output affected by cardiac tamponade?

2. The client is a 60-year-old man with dilated cardiomyopathy. His prognosis is very poor. He is able to tolerate only minimal amounts of activity—using the bedside commode, feeding himself, and shaving himself in bed. Today he continues to be short of breath but seems particularly withdrawn. Repeated physical assessment to identify cardiovascular status shows no change in assessment findings. He continues to take his medications at the proper dosages. His physician

evolve **Did you remember to check out the bonus material on the Evolve website and the CD-ROM, including free self-assessment exercises?**
http://evolve.elsevier.com/Black/medsurg/

thinks these medications are at their maximal levels. Repeated psychosocial assessment would show that the client is withdrawn because he is anxious that his physical condition will worsen and that he will be hospitalized and placed on a ventilator again, which he does not wish to happen. He was terrified the last time this was done, and he sees no purpose in just prolonging his dying. What nursing actions might help your client?

Factors to Consider. What are the clinical manifestations of cardiomyopathy? What are the psychological considerations for the client's care?

3. A 52-year-old man with a lengthy history of mitral valve prolapse is recovering from kidney transplantation surgery. This is his fourth postoperative day, and he and his spouse are asking questions about care at home. What priorities for client education should be established?

Factors to Consider. What complication is associated with mitral valve prolapse? How does the medication regimen following transplantation surgery further place the client at risk?

Discussions for these questions can be found on the website and the CD-ROM.

BIBLIOGRAPHY

 1. American Heart Association. (2002). Dietary/weight loss supplements: AHA recommendations. Dallas, TX: American Heart Association.

2. American Health Association. (2002). 2002 Heart and stroke statistical update. Dallas, TX: American Heart Association.

3. Bayer, A.S., et al. (1998). AHA Scientific statement: Diagnosis and management of infective endocarditis and its complications. *Circulation, 98,* 2936-2948.

4. Bickley, L.S., & Szilagyi, P.G. (2003). *Bates' guide to physical examination and history taking* (8th ed.). Philadelphia: Lippincott Williams & Wilkins.

5. Braunwald, E. (1997). Valvular heart disease. In E. Braunwald (Ed.), *Heart disease* (pp. 1007-1076). Philadelphia: W.B. Saunders.

6. Braunwald, E. (1997). Valvular heart disease. In E. Braunwald (Ed.), *Heart disease* (pp. 1007-1076). Philadelphia: W.B. Saunders.

7. Braunwald, E. (1997). Valvular heart disease. In E. Braunwald (Ed.), *Heart disease* (pp. 1007-1076). Philadelphia: W.B. Saunders.

8. Dajani, A.S. (1997). Rheumatic fever. In E. Braunwald (Ed.), *Heart disease* (pp. 1769-1775). Philadelphia: W.B. Saunders.

9. Dajani, A.S. (1997). Prevention of bacterial endocarditis: Recommendations by the American Heart Association. *Journal of the American Medical Association, 277*(22), 1794-1801.

10. Findlow, D., & Doyle, E. (1997). Congenital heart disease in adults. *British Journal of Anesthesia, 78,* 416-430.

11. Futterman, L.G., & Lemberg, L. (1995). New indications for dual chamber pacing: Hypertrophic and dilated cardiomyopathy. *American Journal of Critical Care, 4*(1), 82-87.

12. Karchmer, A.W. (1997). Infective endocarditis. In E. Braunwald (Ed.), *Heart disease* (pp. 1077-1104). Philadelphia: W.B. Saunders.

13. Kawai, C. (1999). From myocarditis to cardiomyopathy: Mechanisms of inflammation and cell death. *Circulation, 99*(8), 1091-1100.

14. Lashley, F.R. (1999). Genetic testing, screening, and counseling issues in cardiovascular disease. *Journal of Cardiovascular Nursing, 13*(4), 110-126.

15. Lawrie, G.M. (1998). Mitral valve repair vs. replacement. *Cardiology Clinics, 16*(3), 437-448.

16. Lorell, B.H. (1997). Pericardial diseases. In E. Braunwald (Ed.), *Heart disease* (pp. 1478-1534). Philadelphia: W.B. Saunders.

17. McLachlan, J., Reddy, P., & Ratts, T.E. (1998). Mitral valve prolapse: A common diagnosis in women. *Journal of the Louisiana State Medical Society, 150,* 92-96.

18. Micevski, V. (1999). The use of molecular technologies for the detection of enteroviral ribonucleic acid in myocarditis. *Journal of Cardiovascular Nursing, 13*(4), 78-90.

19. Myers, R.B., & Spodick, D.H. (1999). Constrictive pericarditis: Clinical and pathophysiologic characteristics. *American Heart Journal, 138,* 219-232.

20. Sparacino, P.A. (1999). Cardiac infections: Medical and surgical therapies. *Journal of Cardiovascular Nursing, 13*(2), 49-65.

21. Wynne, J., & Braunwald, E. (2001). The cardiomyopathies and myocarditises. In E. Braunwald (Ed.), *Harrison's principles of internal medicine* (15th ed., pp. 1359-1365). New York: McGraw Hill.

Chapter 58

Management of Clients with Functional Cardiac Disorders

Janice Tazbir
Patricia A. Keresztes

---

evolve

Web Enhancements

http://evolve.elsevier.com/Black/medsurg/

Case Management
Heart Failure
Clinical Pathway
Coronary Bypass Grafting
Complementary and Alternative Therapy
Indo-Mediterranean Diet and Heart Disease Reduction
Eggs and Heart Disease
Do All Fish Products Prevent Heart Disease?
Nuts and the Risk of Sudden Cardiac Death

Elevated Homocysteine Levels and Heart Disease
Aspirin to Reduce the Risk of Coronary Artery Disease
Moderate Lifestyle Change and Coronary Artery Disease
Prayer for Health Benefits
Appendix C
Laboratory Values of Clinical Importance in Medical-Surgical
Nursing

Normal functioning of the heart is based on a balance between oxygen supply and oxygen demand. To function as an effective pump, the heart muscle must be adequately supplied with blood from the coronary arteries. In *coronary heart disease* (CHD) atherosclerosis develops in the coronary arteries, causing them to become narrowed or blocked. When a coronary artery is narrowed or blocked, blood flow to the area of the heart supplied by that artery is reduced. If the remaining blood flow is inadequate to meet the oxygen demand of the heart, the area may become ischemic and injured and myocardial infarction (MI) may result. In addition the heart may fail to pump sufficient blood supply to the other organs and tissues in the body. Over time, changes resulting from CHD may lead to the development of chronic heart failure.

The term *coronary heart disease,* also called *coronary artery disease* or *ischemic heart disease,* refers to diseases of the heart that result from a decrease in blood supply to the heart muscle. This chapter reviews the risk factors, etiology, pathophysiology, clinical manifestations, and medical and nursing interventions for two major disorders of cardiac function: CHD and heart failure. The related conditions of angina pectoris and myocardial infarction (MI) are discussed in Chapter 60.

CORONARY HEART DISEASE

Currently CHD is the single largest killer of both men and women in the United States, affecting more than 12 million people.[4] Although these numbers seem high, the death rate from CHD decreased by 24% from 1989 to 1999. Contributing to this decline in the death rate are factors such as improved technology for diagnosis and treatment, the use of thrombolytic drugs in acute MI, improved interventional therapies and surgical techniques, and modification of risk factors in populations at risk.

---

 evolve Be sure to check out the bonus material on the Evolve website and the CD-ROM, including free self-assessment exercises.
http://evolve.elsevier.com/Black/medsurg/

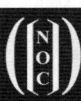

Nursing Outcomes Classification (NOC)
for Nursing Diagnoses—Clients with Functional Cardiac Disorders

Acute Pain
Comfort Level
Pain Control
Pain Level
Decreased Cardiac Output
Cardiac Pump Effectiveness
Circulation Status
Tissue Perfusion: Abdominal Organs
Vital Signs Status
Excess Fluid Volume
Electrolyte and Acid-Base Balance
Fluid Balance
Hydration

Impaired Gas Exchange
Electrolyte and Acid/Base Balance
Respiratory Status: Ventilation
Ineffective Airway Clearance
Respiratory Status: Airway Patency
Respiratory Status: Gas Exchange
Respiratory Status: Ventilation
Ineffective Tissue Perfusion
Sensory Function: Cutaneous
Tissue Perfusion: Peripheral
Tissue Perfusion: Pulmonary
Risk for Activity Intolerance
Activity Tolerance
Endurance

Energy Conservation
Self-Care: Activities of Daily Living
Self-Care: Instrumental Activities of
Daily Living
Risk for Anxiety
Anxiety Control
Coping
Risk for Impaired Skin Integrity
Tissue Integrity: Skin and Mucous
Membranes
Risk for Infection
Tissue Integrity: Skin
Wound Healing: Primary Intention

American Indians, and native Hawaiians.[5] Reduction of risk is a based on control of the modifiable risk factors.

BOX 58-1	*Risk Factors for Coronary Heart Disease*

Nonmodifiable Major Risk Factors
Heredity, including race
Age
Gender

Modifiable Major Risk Factors
Cigarette smoking
Hypertension
Elevated serum cholesterol
Diabetes mellitus
Physical inactivity
Obesity

Contributing Risk Factors
Stress
Homocysteine level

Etiology and Risk Factors

Although CHD claims more lives each year than any other disease, its causes are poorly understood. Clinical evidence suggests that many factors contribute to the onset of atherosclerosis. Risk factors that precipitate CHD can be presented in two categories: modifiable and nonmodifiable risk factors (Box 58-1). The more risk factors a person has, the greater the risk of CHD. Although risk factors influence the development of CHD in all people, the importance of selected risk factors may vary by gender and race. Compared with the rate in whites, the risk of heart disease is higher among Mexican Americans,

Nonmodifiable Risk Factors

Heredity (Including Race). Children whose parents had heart disease are at higher risk for CHD. This increased risk is related to genetic predisposition to hypertension, elevated lipid levels, diabetes, and obesity; all of these conditions increase the risk of CHD.

For people 35 to 74 years of age, the age-adjusted death rate from CHD for African-American women is 72% higher than that for white women and native Americans. The prevalence of CHD is lowest among Mexican Americans.[6]

Increasing Age. Age influences both the risk and the severity of CHD. Symptomatic CHD appears predominantly in people older than 40 years of age, and four of five people who die of CHD are age 65 years or older. Angina and MI, however, can occur in a person's 30s and even in one's 20s. At older ages women who have heart attacks are twice as likely as men to die of heart attack.[5]

Gender. Coronary heart disease is the number-one killer of both men and women. In 1999 mortality from CHD was almost equal for men and women. Although men are at higher risk for heart attacks at younger ages, the risk for women increases significantly at menopause, so that CHD rates in women after menopause are two to three times that of women the same age before menopause. Women who take oral contraceptives and who smoke or have high blood pressure are at greater risk for CHD. Women with an early menopause are also at higher risk than are women with a normal or late menopause.[3,5]

Two lifestyle changes during the past two decades may be responsible for the increased incidence of CHD among women. More women (many with full responsibility for the household and children) have entered the work force, and more women have begun to smoke tobacco at an earlier age.

Modifiable Risk Factors

Smoking, hypertension, elevated serum cholesterol levels, physical inactivity, obesity, and diabetes mellitus constitute the modifiable risk factors for CHD. These factors can be modified or reduced by treatment.

Smoking. Both active and passive smoking have been strongly implicated as a risk factor in the development of CHD. Smoking triples the risk of heart attack in women and doubles the risk of heart attack in men. It also doubles the risk of dying from a heart attack and may quadruple the risk of sudden death. Nonsmokers who are exposed to second-hand tobacco smoke at home or work may also have a higher mortality rate from CHD. This risk is reduced to that of nonsmokers within 5 to 10 years after smoking cessation.[3]

Tar, nicotine, and carbon monoxide contribute to the damage. Tar contains hydrocarbons and other carcinogenic substances. Nicotine increases the release of epinephrine and norepinephrine, which results in peripheral vasoconstriction, elevated blood pressure and heart rate, greater oxygen consumption, and increased likelihood of dysrhythmias. In addition, nicotine activates platelets and stimulates smooth-muscle-cell proliferation in the arterial walls. Carbon monoxide reduces the amount of blood available to the intima of the vessel wall and increases the permeability of the endothelium.

Hypertension. High blood pressure afflicts nearly 50 million American adults and children. It increases the workload of the heart by increasing afterload, enlarging and weakening the left ventricle over time. As blood pressure increases, the risk of a serious cardiovascular event also escalates. When clients have hypertension, obesity, tobacco use, high cholesterol levels, and diabetes, the risk of heart attack increases significantly.

Compared with whites, African Americans have hypertension at an earlier age and it is more severe at any age. Consequently the rate of heart disease in African Americans is 1.5 times greater than that of whites Americans. Although hypertension cannot always be prevented, it should be treated to lower the risk of CHD and premature death.[3,5]

Elevated Serum Cholesterol Levels. The risk of CHD increases as blood cholesterol levels increase. This risk increases further when other risk factors are present. In

adults total cholesterol levels of 240 mg/dl are classified as "high" and levels ranging from 200 to 239 mg/dl are classified as "borderline high." At young and middle ages, men have higher cholesterol levels. In women cholesterol levels continue to increase up to about age 70.[3]

Cholesterol, a sterol found in animal tissue, circulates in the blood in combination with triglycerides and protein-bound phospholipids. This complex is called a *lipoprotein.* There are four basic groups of lipoproteins, all produced in the intestinal wall. Elevation of lipoproteins is called *hyperlipoproteinemia.* Elevation of lipids, a component of lipoproteins, is called *hyperlipidemia.* Lipoproteins and their functions are as follows:

- Chylomicrons primarily transport dietary triglycerides and cholesterol.
- Very-low-density lipoproteins (VLDLs) mainly transport triglycerides synthesized by the liver.
- Low-density lipoproteins (LDLs) have the highest concentration of cholesterol and transport endogenous cholesterol to body cells.
- High-density lipoproteins (HDLs) have the lowest concentration of cholesterol and transport endogenous cholesterol to body cells.

People with high levels of HDL in proportion to LDL are at lower risk for CHD than people with a low HDL-LDL ratio. High concentrations of HDL seem to protect against the development of CHD. Experts believe that the cholesterol in HDL, in contrast to that in LDL, does not become incorporated into the fatty plaques that develop in the lining of the artery wall. The ratio of total cholesterol to HDL or of LDL to HDL is the best test for predicting the risk of CHD. Exercise and low-fat, low-cholesterol diets increase the amount of HDL in the blood. The following are the current recommendations for cholesterol and lipoproteins:

- Total blood cholesterol <200 mg/dl
- LDL <160 if fewer than two other risk factors (<130 mg/dl if two or more risk factors)
- HDL >40 mg/dl

Triglycerides are not an independent risk factor in men, but their significance in women is unknown; however, the combination of a high triglyceride level and a low HDL level seems to be a more important predictor of CHD in women than in men. The Consensus Panel Statement from the American Heart Association (AHA) recommends that triglyceride levels be below 150 mg/dl.[3]

In the average American diet, about 45% of the total calories come from fat. This level exceeds that recommended in the AHA Step 1 Diet. Dietary fat comes in many forms and "disguises." A high intake of cholesterol and saturated fats is associated with the development of CHD, whereas a proportional intake of polyunsaturated and monounsaturated fats is linked with lower risk (see the Complementary and Alternative Therapy features on Mediterranean Diets and Cardiovascular Disease and on Low-Carbohydrate Diets and Weight

COMPLEMENTARY AND ALTERNATIVE THERAPY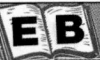

Mediterranean Diets and Cardiovascular Disease

A traditional Mediterranean diet may reduce the risk of dying from cardiovascular disease and cancer. Researchers evaluated more than 22,000 apparently healthy individuals aged 22 to 86 in Greece. Participants were rated on how closely they followed a Mediterranean diet. This type of diet is traditionally high in fruits and vegetables, legumes, nuts, cereal grains, olive oil (monounsaturated fat), and contains moderate amounts of fish, dairy (mostly cheese and yogurt), and alcohol and is low in saturated fat. Adherence to the diet was measured on a scale of 0 (did not follow the diet closely) to 9 (strictly followed the diet). After about 4 years of follow-up, the researchers found that the more closely individuals adhered to the diet, the lower their risk of death, including death from cardiovascular disease and cancer (about a 25% decrease for every 2-point increase on the scale). Thus a greater adherence to the traditional Mediterranean diet was associated with a significant reduction in total mortality.[2]

The first clinical-trial evidence in support of the health benefits of the Mediterranean diet came from the Lyon Diet Heart Study, in which 605 clients with a previous MI were randomly assigned to a Mediterranean diet or a control diet similar to the AHA Step I Diet. Clients in the Mediterranean diet arm were encouraged to eat more fruits, vegetables, and fish; to eat less red meat; and to replace butter and cream with margarine high in alpha-linolenic acid (canola-oil-based margarine). After a mean follow-up of 27 months, the trial was stopped because of a 73% reduction in coronary events and a 70% reduction in all-cause or total mortality in the Mediterranean diet arm of the study.[1]

References

de Lorgeril, M., et al. (1994). Mediterranean alpha-linolenic acid-rich diet in secondary prevention of coronary heart disease. *Lancet, 343,* 1454-1459.

Trichopoulou, A., et al. (2003). Adherence to a Mediterranean diet and survival in a Greek population. *New England Journal of Medicine, 348,* 2599-2608.

COMPLEMENTARY AND ALTERNATIVE THERAPY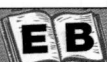

Low-Carbohydrate Diets and Weight Loss and Cardiovascular Disease Markers

Low-carbohydrate diets seem to be gaining a lot of attention; however, few randomized clinical trials have been conducted to determine their effectiveness. Two recent small and short trials were conducted. The first trial randomly assigned 132 severely obese individuals with a mean BMI of 43 and a high prevalence of diabetes (39%) or the metabolic syndrome (43%) to a low-carbohydrate diet (30 g or less per day) or a low-fat, low-calorie diet. A total of 79 individuals completed the 6-month study.[2] The second study was a 1-year trial involving 63 obese men and women assigned to an Atkins diet (low carbohydrate) or low fat low calorie diet.[1]

Both studies found a significantly greater weight loss with the low-carbohydrate versus the low-fat diet during the first 6 months (mean reduction, 6-7 kg versus 2-3 kg). The difference (4 kg in both studies) in weight loss overall was not great, however, and a large number of participants could not follow either diet over time (about 40% of the individuals in both studies dropped out). In fact, there was no longer a significant difference in weight loss in the second study after 12 months was completed. In both studies the reduction in serum triglycerides in the low carbohydrate group was significant but was probably a reflection of greater initial weight loss, but reducing carbohydrates can also reduce triglycerides. No significant change in bad cholesterol (LDL) was found between the two groups or two studies, and the greater increase in good cholesterol (HDL) in the low-carbohydrate groups is probably a reflection of greater intakes of saturated fat, which is not necessarily healthy.

The potential complication(s) of following a diet that is low in carbohydrate (high in protein) is unknown. Some researchers believe this type of diet increases the risk of kidney stones and can be dangerous for individuals with renal or liver disease (high protein) and may increase the risk of heart disease over the long term because of higher saturated fat intake and lower intakes of natural vitamins and minerals. Nonetheless, these two studies were beneficial in showing that at least for the short term, the low-carbohydrate diet may help in reducing weight and in reducing cardiovascular disease markers. The dropout rate and difficulty in achieving long lasting results demonstrate that this type of diet, along with other diets, comes with a big "catch."

References

Foster, G., et al. (2003). A randomized trial of a low-carbohydrate diet for obesity. *New England Journal of Medicine, 348,* 2082-2090.

Samaha, F., et al. (2003). A low-carbohydrate as compared with a low-fat diet in severe obesity. *New England Journal of Medicine, 348,* 2074-2081.

Loss and Cardiovascular Disease Markers on p. 1630). The AHA Step 1 Diet contains no more than 30% of calories from fat, 55% from carbohydrate (at least half of which should be complex), and 15% from protein. When fat intake does not exceed 30% of total calories, the expected rise in triglyceride levels from a high carbohydrate diet is minimal. Saturated fats should account for no more than 10% of caloric intake.

See the Complementary and Alternative Therapy features on Indo-Mediterranean Diet and Heart Disease Reduction, on Eggs and Heart Disease, on Do All Fish Products Prevent Heart Disease?, and on Nuts and the Risk of Sudden Cardiac Death on the website.

Physical Inactivity. In the United States about 25% of adults report no leisure-time physical activity, even though regular aerobic exercise is important in preventing heart and blood vessel disease. The Framingham Study demonstrated an inverse relationship between exercise and the risk of CHD. Those who exercise reduce their risk of CHD because they have (1) higher HDL levels; (2) lower LDL cholesterol, triglyceride, and blood glucose levels; (3) greater insulin sensitivity; (4) lower blood pressure; and (5) lower body mass index.[7] The AHA recommends 30 to 60 minutes of physical activity on most days of the week.

Obesity. Obesity places an extra burden on the heart, requiring the muscle to work harder to pump enough blood to support added tissue mass. In addition obesity increases the risk for CHD because it is often associated with elevated serum cholesterol and triglyceride levels, high blood pressure, and diabetes.[39]

Distribution of body fat is also important. A waist measurement is a way to estimate fat. For men a high-risk waistline measurement is more than 40 inches, and for women a high-risk waist measurement is more than 35 inches. Body mass index (BMI) is another measure to estimate body fat. A BMI from 18.5 to 24.9 is considered healthy. People can lower their heart disease risk by losing as little as 10 to 20 pounds.[5] An alternating pattern of weight gain and weight loss, however, is associated with an increased risk for CHD.

Diabetes. The prevalence of diabetes is increasing rapidly, with 20% of those in middle adult years and 35% of the entire older population having some degree of abnormal glucose tolerance. Contributing to this is the increased frequency of obesity and sedentary lifestyles. A fasting blood glucose level of more than 126 mg/dl or a routine blood glucose level of 180 mg/dl and glucosuria signals the presence of diabetes and represents an increased risk for CHD. Clients with diabetes have a 2- to 8-fold higher prevalence, incidence, and mortality from all forms of CHD.[4]

Contributing Risk Factors

Response to Stress. A person's response to stress may contribute to the development of CHD. Some researchers have reported a relationship between CHD risk and stress levels, health behaviors, and socioeconomic status. Stress appears to increase CHD risk through its effect on major risk factors. For example, some people respond to stress by overeating or by starting or increasing smoking. Stress is also associated with elevated blood pressure. Although stress is unavoidable in modern life, an excessive response to stress can be a health hazard. Significant stressors include major changes in residence, occupation, or socioeconomic status.

Homocysteine Levels. Researchers have reported that elevated levels of plasma homocysteine (an amino acid produced by the body) are associated with an increased risk of CHD (see the Complementary and Alternative Therapy feature on Elevated Homocysteine Levels and Heart Disease on the website). Scientists do not know whether homocysteine directly or indirectly increases CHD risk, however, because homocysteine levels are related to renal function, smoking, fibrinogen, and C-reactive protein (CRP). Elevated homocysteine levels can be reduced by treatment with folic acid, vitamin B_6, and vitamin B_{12}. Experts currently recommend that homocysteine levels be measured in people with a history of premature CHD, stroke, or both in the absence of other risk factors.[7,11]

Inflammatory Responses. A newly identified risk factor currently being researched is the presence of any chronic inflammatory state that leads to an increase in the body's production of CRP. Too much CRP tends to destabilize plaque inside artery walls. When plaque lesions crack or break, a clot is formed and this may lead to heart attack. Researchers have discovered that a high CRP is a marker for coronary disease. This means that clients with chronic inflammatory diseases, such as arthritis, lupus, and autoimmune deficiency, may be at higher risk for heart attack.

Menopause. The incidence of CHD markedly increases among women after menopause. Before menopause estrogen is thought to protect against CHD risk by raising HDL and lowering LDL levels. Epidemiologic studies have shown that the loss of natural estrogen as women age may be associated with increases in total and LDL cholesterol and a gradually increasing CHD risk. If menopause is caused by surgical removal of the uterus and ovaries, the risks of CHD and MI increase.

For primary prevention of CHD, data are insufficient to support hormone replacement therapy (HRT). Randomized clinical trials are currently under way to guide clinical recommendations for HRT.[25,26]

Evidence regarding the role of estrogen-replacement therapy (ERT) for women with diagnosed CHD is conflicting. Observational studies indicate that ERT is beneficial for women with diagnosed CHD; however, recent results from a large multicenter clinical trial show an increase in cardiovascular events after 1 year of treatment with estrogen and progesterone therapy but a decrease in cardiovascular events in years 4 and 5.[19] Additional research is being conducted in this area.[26,27]

TABLE 58-1   *Progression of Atherosclerosis, Clinical Manifestations, and Associated Lesions*

Type and Characteristics	Earliest Onset	Clinical Manifestation	Illustration
Phase I			

Type I (initial lesion)
   Isolated macrophage foam cells
   Intimal thickening located near
     bifurcations of artery
	Infancy and childhood	Clinically silent	Intima / Media / Adventitia / Adaptive thickening (smooth muscle)

Type II (fatty streak)
   No decrease in lumen
   Flat, fatty streaks
   Lipid accumulation with clusters
     of macrophage foam cells
	Infancy and childhood	Clinically silent	Macrophage foam cells

Type III (preatheroma)
   Raised fatty streaks
   Lipid-filled foam cells and
     smooth muscle cells
	From third decade on	Clinically silent	Extracellular lipids

Phase II			

Type IV (atheroma)
   Disturbed intimal structure with
     extracellular lipid and fibrous
     tissue in core
   Small to moderate decreases in
     lumen
	From third decade on	Clinically silent	Core of extracelluar lipid

Type Va (fibroatheroma)
   Lipid core with fibrotic layer
   Multiple lipid cores and fibrotic
     layers
	From fourth decade on	Va is usually clinically silent, whereas Vb may be associated with chronic stable angina	Fibrous thickening

Phase III			

Type VI (complicated lesion)
   Plaque rupture
   Mural thrombus with partial oc-
     clusion of lumen
	From fourth decade on	Angina pectoris due to partial occlusion of vessel	Thrombus / Fissure and hematoma

Phase IV			

Type VI lesion
   Same as above except greater
     degree of occlusion
	From fourth decade on	Acute syndromes, unstable angina, myo-cardial infarction, sudden death	

TABLE 58-1	*Progression of Atherosclerosis, Clinical Manifestations, and Associated Lesions—cont'd*		
Type and Characteristics	**Earliest Onset**	**Clinical Manifestation**	**Illustration**
Phase V *Type Vb-c* Complicated plaques from phase III become calcified (Vb) or fibrotic (Vc)	From fourth decade on	Stable angina	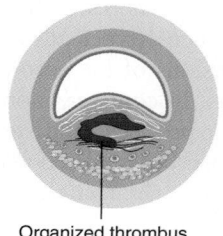 Organized thrombus covered over by fibrous or calcified tissue

Pathophysiology

Atherosclerosis primarily affects the intima of the arterial wall and normally takes years to develop. When clinical manifestations develop, atherosclerosis is usually well advanced. Atherosclerosis develops in five phases that include six progressive types of lesions (Table 58-1).[40]

Phase 1 is present in most people 30 years of age and younger and is characterized by clinically silent lesions of types I through III that do not appreciably thicken the arterial wall or narrow the arterial lumen. *Type I* lesions are microscopic adaptations of smooth muscle and occur most often near branches in the arteries. Type I lesions progress and mature into *type II* lesions.[15,16] *Type III* lesions, known as *intermediate* lesions, develop during one's 20s. These lesions surround the smooth-muscle cells. Type III lesions are also referred to as *pre-atheromas* because they form the bridge between early and advanced lesions. In phase 1, the progression of lesions is predictable, characteristic, and uniform.[17,40]

Phase 2, characterized by type IV and V lesions, represents the development of vulnerable plaques. The *type IV* lesion, also called an *atheroma,* is characterized by further changes in the intimal structure caused by the accumulation of large amounts of extracellular lipids and fibrous tissue localized into a lipid core. The lipid core thickens the artery wall but often does not narrow the lumen of the artery. The periphery of type IV lesions is vulnerable to rupture, which may lead to rapid progression to more severe lesions.

When new fibrous connective tissue forms a thin protective cap over the atheroma, the lesion is classified as *type V.* These lesions are further subdivided into types Va, Vb, and Vc. *Type Va* lesions contain irregularly stacked multiple layers of lipid cores separated by thick layers of fibrous connective tissue. These lesions may rapidly progress to a *type VI* lesion or continue to develop into stenotic plaques that eventually occlude the entire lumen of the artery.[14] A type V lesion that contains

calcium in the lipid core and other parts of the lesion is referred to as *type Vb.* The absence of a lipid core, with minimal lipid deposition in other parts of the lesion, is characteristic of a *type Vc* lesion. *Type Vc* lesions are often seen in arteries in the legs.[17,40]

Phase 3 is marked by the acute disruption of type IV and V lesions that causes thrombus formation and the development of a type VI lesion *(complicated).* If thrombus formation during phase 3 does not limit the flow of blood through the artery, these events are often asymptomatic. The net result of phase 3 is a rapid increase in plaque size that may result in stable angina. If the thrombus reduces or significantly blocks flow through the artery *(phase IV),* an acute coronary syndrome such as unstable angina, MI, or sudden cardiac death often results (see Chapter 60). Type VI lesions are characterized by a core that contains extracellular lipids, tissue factor, collagen, platelets, thrombin, and fibrin. These lesions may also be associated with disruption of the plaque surface, hematoma or hemorrhage into the plaque, and thrombosis.[17,40]

Phase 5 follows a phase 3 or 4 event and occurs when the thrombus over the disrupted plaque begins to calcify (type Vb lesion) or fibrose (type Vc lesion), forming a chronic stenotic lesion. The phase 5 lesion often contains organizing thrombi from several earlier episodes of plaque disruption, ulceration, hemorrhage, and organization. As the phase 5 lesion progresses, it occludes a greater portion of the arterial lumen and eventually may lead to total occlusion. Phase 5 lesions are associated with chronic stable angina and are often accompanied by the development of collateral circulation.[17,40]

Collateral circulation is the presence of more than one artery supplying a muscle. Normally some collateral circulation is present in the coronary arteries, especially in older people. Collateral vessels develop when the blood flow through an artery progressively decreases and causes ischemia to the muscle. Extra blood vessels develop to meet the metabolic demands of the muscle. The development of collateral circulation takes time. Therefore an occlusion of a coronary artery in a younger person is more likely to be lethal because there are no collateral arteries present to supply the myocardium with blood.

For many years researchers thought that the more obstructive lesions (types Vb and Vc) were responsible for most occlusions of the coronary arteries and acute coronary events. In contrast, more recent studies suggest that lesions that produce mild stenosis (types IV and Va) are more frequently associated with rapid progression to coronary occlusion. In fact nearly 60% to 70% of all acute coronary syndromes occur in arteries with mild (<50% stenosis) or moderate (50% to 70% stenosis) occlusion. It is thought that this occurs because less occlusive lesions are more vulnerable to plaque rupture and thrombosis.[40,45] Plaque disruption is thought to result from external stresses on the vessel and internal changes that increase plaque fragility. Physical forces that exert external pressure on the atherosclerotic plaques, such as blood and pulse pressures, heart contraction, vasospasm, and shear stress may trigger plaque rupture.[45] Internal factors, such as inflammation, may increase plaque vulnerability.

Systemic infections of *Chlamydia pneumoniae* and *Helicobacter pylori* have been linked to the development of atherosclerosis and are thought to contribute to plaque instability because they activate the inflammatory response. Treatment of these infections with antibiotics has been found to improve the prognosis after an acute coronary event.[18] Researchers are investigating methods to detect vulnerable plaques and are evaluating the effectiveness of interventions designed to stabilize atherosclerotic plaques.

Clinical Manifestations

Atherosclerosis by itself does not necessarily produce subjective clinical manifestations. For manifestations to develop, there must be a critical deficit in the blood supply to the heart in proportion to the demands for oxygen and nutrients; in other words, a supply-and-demand imbalance must exist. When atherosclerosis progresses slowly, the collateral circulation that develops generally can meet the heart's demands. Thus whether manifestations of CHD develop depends on the total blood supply to the myocardium (by way of the coronary arteries and collateral circulation) and not solely on the condition of the coronary arteries.

Rapid progression of atherosclerotic lesions (type VI) may cause ischemia and may result in the development of acute coronary syndromes of unstable angina, MI, and sudden cardiac death. Slow progression of atherosclerotic lesions (types Vb and Vc) is associated with stable coronary artery disease and the clinical manifestation of chronic stable angina. These lesions usually cause ischemia during periods when myocardial oxygen demand increases.[17] Angina, MI, and sudden cardiac death are discussed in Chapter 60.

Techniques to determine the extent of CHD and identify the affected vessels include the electrocardiogram (ECG); B-mode ultrasonography; Doppler flow studies; intravascular ultrasound; electron-beam computed tomography; and thallium, sestamibi, or echocardiographic stress tests (see Chapter 60).

Outcome Management
■ Medical Management

The primary goals that guide the medical management of a client with CHD are reducing and controlling risk factors and restoring blood supply to the myocardium.

Reduce Risk Factors. Prevention, rather than treatment, is the goal with regard to CHD. Modification of risk factors can significantly improve prognosis even after an acute coronary event.[18] Recent findings indicate reducing risk factors may limit and even prevent the progression of CHD by increasing the stability of atherosclerotic plaques, decreasing thrombogenicity, and limiting external stress on the vessel.[5] For people without diagnosed CHD, the goal of medical treatment is to prevent the development of risk factors and clinical disease. Cessation of cigarette smoking; participating in regular exercise; and controlling blood pressure, diabetes, cholesterol levels, and weight can reduce the risk of CHD.[5]

Primary and secondary prevention goals are in place for all the major risk factors. Ideally primary prevention should begin with promoting healthy lifestyles in children. Primary care should include family-oriented education about the risk factors, review of the family history, and modification of risk factors. For clients with diagnosed CHD, the goals of prevention are to (1) reduce the incidence of subsequent coronary events, (2) decrease the need for treatments such as angioplasty and coronary artery bypass graft (CABG) surgery, (3) extend overall survival, and (4) improve the quality of life.

People should stop smoking and avoid contact with secondary smoke. Health professionals should provide counseling, nicotine replacement, and referrals to smoking-cessation programs for clients who smoke. Blood pressure should be measured at least every 2 years in adults, and clients should be encouraged to control blood pressure by maintaining ideal weight, exercising regularly, moderating alcohol intake, and following a moderately low sodium diet (see the Complementary and Alternative Therapy feature on Alcohol or Which Type of Alcohol to Reduce the Risk of Heart Disease on p. 1635). Blood pressure should be below 140/90 mm Hg (<130/85 mm Hg for those with heart failure, diabetes, or renal insufficiency). Antihypertensive therapy should begin if blood pressure exceeds 140/90 mm Hg after 6 months of lifestyle modification or if the initial blood pressure exceeds 160/100 mm Hg (130/85 mm Hg for those with heart failure, diabetes, or renal insufficiency).[5,7]

Total, LDL, and HDL cholesterol should be measured annually for adults older than 20 years of age. The fol-

COMPLEMENTARY AND ALTERNATIVE THERAPY

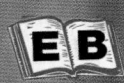

Alcohol or Which Type of Alcohol to Reduce the Risk of Heart Disease

Researchers studied the association of alcohol ingestion with the risk of MI among more than 38,000 male health professionals who were free of cardiovascular disease and cancer at baseline. Alcohol consumption and type of alcohol were documented every 4 years using a food-frequency questionnaire. After 12 years of follow-up, the total number of MIs was 1418. Compared with men who consumed alcohol less than once a week, men who consumed alcohol 3 or 4 or 5 to 7 days per week had a 32% and 37% reduction of MI. The risk was similar in men who consumed less than 10 g of alcohol per drinking day and those who consumed 30 g or more (a single alcoholic drink contains 11 to 14 g of alcohol). No single type of alcoholic beverage provided an additional benefit. In other words, red wine, white wine, beer, and liquor were similar in their effect. Therefore moderate drinking was associated with a reduced risk of MI. The problem with this large study is that although alcohol in moderation seems to reduce the risk of dying from a MI, researchers are not sure whether or not it reduces the risk of all-cause mortality (this needs to be studied). Regardless, for now moderate consumption reduces the risk of death from cardiovascular disease.

Reference
Mukamal, K., et al. (2003). Roles of drinking pattern and type of alcohol consumed in coronary heart disease in men. *New England Journal of Medicine, 348,* 109-118.

COMPLEMENTARY AND ALTERNATIVE THERAPY

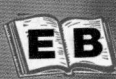

Guggulipid Supplements for the Treatment of High Cholesterol

Herbal extracts of *Commiphora mukul* (guggul) have been used in Asia as cholesterol-lowering agents, and their popularity seems to be increasing in the United States. A recent study determined the short-term safety and efficacy of two doses of a standardized guggul extract (guggulipid, containing 2.5% guggulsterones) in healthy adults with high cholesterol eating a typical Western diet. A total of 103 adults were studied for 8 weeks. The intervention was an oral three times daily dose of standard guggulipid (1000 mg), high-dose guggulipid (2000 mg), or matching placebo. Placebo clients ($n = 36$) had a decrease in LDL-C of 5%, whereas the standard-dose of guggulipid ($n = 33$) and high-dose guggulipid ($n = 34$) increased LDL-C by 4% and 5%. No significant changes were noted in levels of total cholesterol, HDL-C, triglycerides, or VLDL-C with guggulipid. Guggulipid was generally well tolerated, but six clients who received this supplement developed a hypersensitivity rash compared with none in the placebo group. Therefore in this short-term study, this supplement does not appear to reduce cholesterol and may cause a hypersensitivity reaction in some clients.

Reference
Szapary, P., et al. (2003). Guggulipid for the treatment of hypercholesterolemia: A randomized controlled trial. *Journal of the American Medical Association, 290,* 765-772.

COMPLEMENTARY AND ALTERNATIVE THERAPY

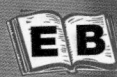

Red Yeast Rice Supplements to Reduce Cholesterol

Chinese red yeast rice supplements have been available on the U.S. market for several years, and currently they have been involved in litigation because some companies argue that this natural supplement has a similar structure to cholesterol-lowering drugs (statins). This supplement was tested against a placebo in 83 individuals (46 men, 37 women). A total of 2.4 g of red yeast rice or placebo was given daily for 3 months. Total cholesterol, LDL, and triglycerides decreased compared with placebo. Total cholesterol had the largest reduction, with an average decrease of 45 mg/dl. No effect was seen of this supplement on HDL (good cholesterol) levels. No apparent adverse effects were seen with this supplement, but this study was of short duration.

Reference
Ashley, J., et al. (1999). Cholesterol-lowering effects of a proprietary Chinese red-yeast-rice dietary supplement. *American Journal of Clinical Nutrition, 69,* 231-236.

---

lowing are the primary prevention goals for cholesterol management:

- LDL <160 mg/dl if no risk factors or only one risk factor
- LDL <130 mg/dl if two or more risk factors
- HDL >40 mg/dl
- Triglycerides <150 mg/dl

The following are the secondary prevention goals for cholesterol management:

- LDL <100 mg/dl
- HDL >40 mg/dl
- Triglycerides <150 mg/dl

The AHA Step 1 Diet should be recommended for clients who are unable to meet the primary prevention goals, and the Step 2 Diet should be recommended for those with CHD who do not meet the recommended goals (see the Complementary and Alternative Therapy features on Guggulipid Supplements for the Treatment of High Cholesterol and on Red Yeast Rice Supplements to Reduce Cholesterol, above and at right). In addition, drug therapy is recommended for clients who do not meet the recommended goals for cholesterol management.[9,39] See

COMPLEMENTARY AND ALTERNATIVE THERAPY

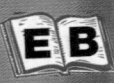

Statin Drugs and Dietary Supplements

The largest randomized trial of statin drugs in combination with supplements included 160 individuals studied over 3 years. The supplement combination included 800 international units of vitamin E plus 100 µg of selenium plus 1000 mg of vitamin C and 25 mg of beta-carotene with or without a statin drug plus niacin. Simvastatin plus niacin provided a marked clinical angiographically measurable benefit in clients with coronary disease and low HDL levels. The group taking the supplement combination plus the statin drug experienced a significant reduction in HDL (or "good cholesterol") compared with the group that took the statin drug alone. Further study is needed to determine whether the desired effects of statin drugs are diminished when taken in combination with antioxidant vitamin supplements.

Reference

Brown, B.G., et al. (2001). Simvastatin and niacin, antioxidant vitamins, or the combination for the prevention of coronary disease. *New England Journal of Medicine, 345,*1583-1592.

COMPLEMENTARY AND ALTERNATIVE THERAPY

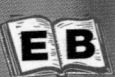

Diet versus Statin Therapy for High Cholesterol

A preliminary recent study randomly assigned 55 healthy hyperlipidemic men and women to receive one of three treatments: a very low-saturated-fat diet based on low-fat dairy foods and whole-grain cereals (control arm); the same diet plus 20 mg daily of lovastatin (statin group); or a diet with a high intake of plant sterols, soy protein, soluble fibers, and almonds (dietary portfolio group). The data were based on 46 clients who completed the 4-week study. The researchers reported that the statin and dietary portfolio treatment arms had about a 30% decrease in LDL ("bad cholesterol") versus an 8% reduction the control group. Although a longer and larger trial is needed, this unique study suggests that over a short period, individuals willing to go a more directed dietary change could potentially reduce their cholesterol as much as some cholesterol-lowering drugs; however, cholesterol lowering drugs are still the treatment of choice for clients who cannot significantly reduce their cholesterol levels with diet and physical activity over a period of 3 to 6 months.

Reference

Jenkins, D., et al. (2003). Effects of a dietary portfolio of cholesterol-lowering foods vs lovastatin on serum lipids and c-reactive protein. *Journal of the American Medical Association, 290,* 502-510.

COMPLEMENTARY AND ALTERNATIVE THERAPY

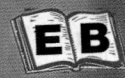

Lifting Weights and Coronary Heart Disease in Men

A cohort of 44,452 men enrolled in the Health Professionals' Follow-up Study were followed up at 2-year intervals from 1986 to 1998. Men who trained with weights for 30 minutes or more per week had a 23% risk reduction in coronary heart disease compared with men who did not train with weights ($P = 0.03$ for trend). In summary, researchers found that total physical activity, running, weight training, and walking were each associated with a reduced risk of coronary heart disease.

Reference

Tanasescu, M., et al. (2002). Exercise type and intensity in relation to coronary heart disease in men. *Journal of the American Medical Association, 288,* 1994-2000.

the Complementary and Alternative Therapy features on Statin Drugs and Dietary Supplements and on Diet versus Statin Therapy for High Cholesterol at left.

During routine physical examinations, health professionals should determine the client's activity level and participation in exercise. Clients should be encouraged to exercise three to four times weekly for 30 to 60 minutes and to increase their physical activity in daily life (see the Complementary and Alternative Therapy feature on Lifting Weights and Coronary Heart Disease in Men, above). An exercise test may be needed to guide an exercise prescription for clients with confirmed CHD.[5,7]

Clients should be encouraged to maintain ideal body weight as indicated by a BMI between 21 and 25 kg/m² and a waist circumference less than 40 inches in men and 36 inches in women. Height, weight, BMI, and waist-to-hip ratio should be measured at each visit. People with BMI and waist circumferences higher than those recommended should be counseled regarding weight management and physical activity.[5,7]

Fasting blood glucose should be maintained near normal levels in clients with diabetes mellitus. Hypoglycemic therapy should be used to achieve normal fasting blood glucose as indicated by hemoglobin A_{1c} (HbA_{1c}). Other risk factors should be treated aggressively.[6,9]

Hormone-replacement therapy should be considered for all postmenopausal women without diagnosed CHD, particularly if they have multiple risk factors. The decision about HRT, however, should be made by considering the risks for breast cancer, gallbladder disease, thromboembolic disease, and endometrial cancer.[5] Estrogen-progesterone therapy reportedly increases cardiovascular events in women with diagnosed CHD during the first year of treatment but decreases events in the fourth and fifth years. Consequently, initiating estrogen-progesterone therapy for women with confirmed CHD is

INTEGRATING PHARMACOLOGY

Preventive Pharmacology for Coronary Heart Disease

Several medications can be prescribed to prevent the development or progression of coronary heart disease. They include the statins to reduce elevated LDL levels and antiplatelet aggregates to reduce the risk of clotting in narrowed vessels

Statins

A reduction in elevated LDL levels can significantly reduce coronary events in individuals without CHD. Lipid-lowering drug therapy for primary CHD prevention is most clearly indicated when two or more CHD risk factors are present and the LDL remains higher than 160 mg/dl after an adequate dietary trial. In addition clients with LDL levels higher than 160 mg/dl and with one other strong risk factor (diabetes, smoking, or a family history of early CHD) may also be candidates for drug therapy. For clients with elevated risk due to sudden cardiac death in family members and elevated LDL levels, drug treatment may be beneficial.

Educating the client about the need to take this medication for a lifetime is important. Noticeable effects will not be seen and may lead clients to discontinue the medication without informing their care provider. If cost is an issue, consider prescribing half-pill doses or recommending ingestion of grapefruit juice when the drug is taken to increase drug absorption. Follow-up assessment of serum lipids is important to monitor progress. Clients should be taught that the medication must be taken every day indefinitely to maximize benefit, noting that the LDL level returns to the pretreatment level soon after the medication is discontinued. Dietary adjustments must also be continued.

Antiplatelet Aggregating Agents

Aspirin in low doses is the best known agent for the prevention of coronary heart disease. Aspirin's benefits include reducing the coagulability of blood so that it can flow more freely through tight, narrow vessels. Aspirin is also an antiinflammatory agent and can reduce the inflammatory process, which destabilizes plaque inside artery walls. A risk factor with the consumption of aspirin is that clients may take the medication because it is readily available without prescription believing it could not harm them. Aspirin should not be used by clients with allergy to aspirin or other salicylates, asthma, uncontrolled high blood pressure, severe liver or kidney disease, excess alcohol consumption, or bleeding disorders. Persons taking other medications that affect bleeding or clotting also should not take aspirin.

---

not recommended. For women with CHD who have already been receiving ERT for more than 1 year, continuing therapy is recommended until the results of additional research are known.[26,27]

Additional management strategies are recommended for clients with diagnosed CHD. These include the use of antiplatelet therapies such as acetylsalicylic acid (aspirin), heparin, and low-molecular-weight heparin if it is not contraindicated.[5,17] Aspirin reduces the risk of fatal or nonfatal MI by 71% during the acute phase, by 60% at 3 months, and by 52% at 2 years[17] (see the Complementary and Alternative Therapy feature on Aspirin to Reduce the Risk of Coronary Artery Disease on the website). Adjunctive therapies, such as angiotensin-converting enzyme (ACE) inhibitors, beta-blockers, and nitrates, are also recommended.[5,7,17]

Glycoprotein IIb/IIIa receptor antagonists are the most recent pharmacologic treatment for secondary prevention of CHD. These drugs prevent platelet aggregation in acute coronary syndromes, and when combined with aspirin they decrease the incidence of recurrent cardiac events.[17] The therapeutic effects, adverse responses, and nursing implications of pharmacologic agents used in the primary prevention of CHD are outlined in the Integrating Pharmacology feature on Preventive Pharmacology for Coronary Heart Disease, above.

Restore Blood Supply. For some clients even aggressive management of risk factors fails to prevent coronary oc-clusion. Various techniques have been developed to open the vessels and restore blood flow through the coronary arteries. Percutaneous coronary interventions (PCI) includes percutaneous luminal coronary angioplasty, rotational atherectomy, directional antrectomy, laser angioplasty, and implantation of intracoronary stents. The American College of Cardiology, along with the AHA, issues guidelines for the use of PCI and reports on all procedures collectively. More than 500,000 PCI procedures are performed yearly. The use of PTCA alone has decreased dramatically, whereas the use of percutaneous transluminal coronary angioplasty (PCTA) with placement of intracoronary stents has dramatically increased. Stents have been shown to reduce late restenosis in coronary arteries. The use of GPIIb/IIIa platelet receptor antagonists has also improved outcomes of PCI. PCI is recommended for clients with mild angina, single or multivessel coronary artery disease, unstable angina, and acute MI and following thrombolytic therapy.[38] These procedures are performed in a "catheterization laboratory," which is outfitted with high-resolution fluoroscopy and x-ray.

Percutaneous Transluminal Coronary Angioplasty. Percutaneous transluminal coronary angioplasty is a technique in which a balloon-tipped catheter is usually inserted into the femoral artery (although the brachial or radial artery can be used) and threaded under x-ray guidance into a blocked coronary artery. The balloon is inflated several times to reshape the lumen by stretching it and flattening the atherosclerotic plaque against the arterial wall (analogous to making footprints in the snow), thus opening the artery (Figure 58-1). PTCA is less invasive and less expensive than open heart surgery and therefore is an attractive alternative.[38]

Directional Coronary Atherectomy. Directional coronary atherectomy (DCA) reduces coronary stenosis by excising and removing atheromatous plaque. The DCA cutter consists of a catheter that contains a rigid cylindrical housing with a central rotating blade (Figure 58-1, E). The blade shaves off the atherosclerotic material and deposits it in the nose cone of the housing for later histopathologic study. DCA is appropriate for lesions in medium to large coronary arteries located in the proximal or middle portions of the vessel. It is not recommended for use with tortuous vessels, distal lesions, or heavily calcified lesions.

Intracoronary Stents. Intracoronary stents were originally designed to reduce restenosis and abrupt closure of coronary vessels resulting from complications of coronary angioplasty. They are now used instead of PTCA to eliminate the risk of acute closure and to improve long-term patency. Several different stent designs are available, but most are balloon-expandable or self-expandable tubes that, when placed in a coronary artery, act as a mechanical scaffold to reopen the blocked artery (Figure 58-1, C). Coronary stents are made of numerous materials, ranging from stainless steel to bioabsorbable compounds. The procedure for placing a stent is similar to that for PTCA. Once the coronary lesion is identified by angiography, the balloon catheter bearing the stent is inserted into the coronary artery and the stent is positioned at the site of the occlusion. A major concern related to stent placement is the prevention of acute thrombosis, especially during the first several weeks after the procedure. The use of GPIIb/IIIA platelet receptor antagonists has decreased the risk of thrombus formation following stent placement. New technology, including the use of intracoronary gamma and beta radiation with stent placement, has reduced restenosis rates by 3% to 50%. A new type of stent that slowly releases an immunosuppressant or antibiotic agent to reduce restenosis is being investigated.[38,42]

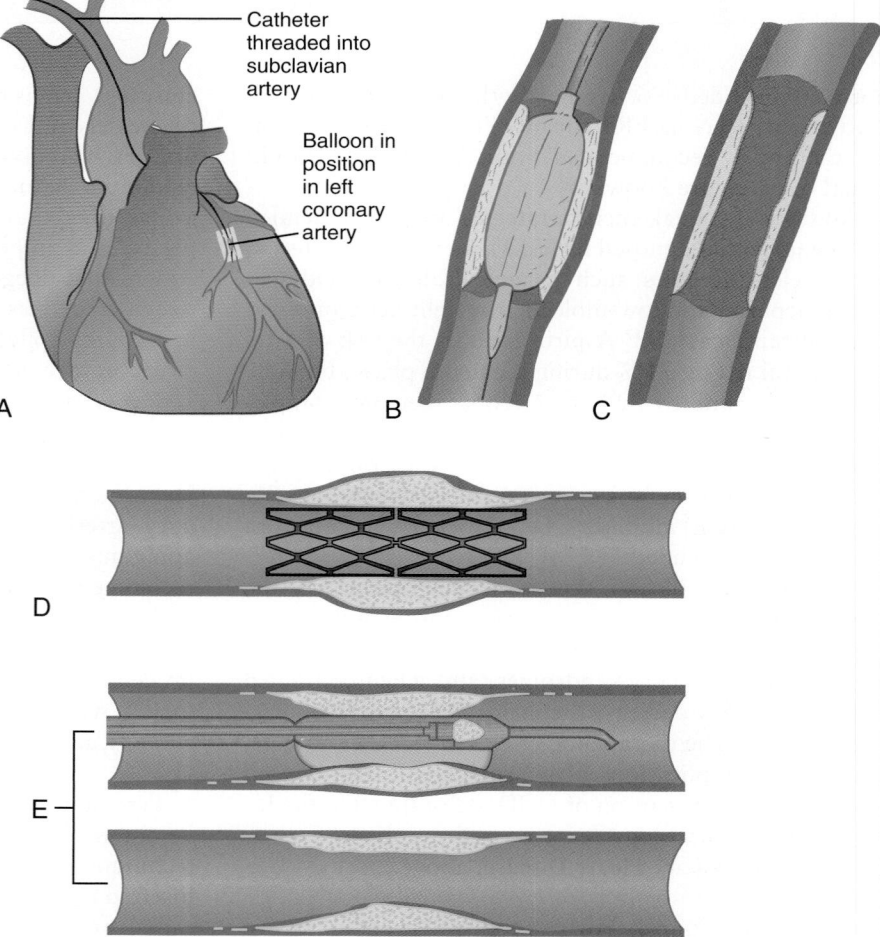

FIGURE 58-1 Interventional cardiology can be performed to open occluded coronary arteries. **A,** Percutaneous transluminal coronary angioplasty (PTCA). **B,** The balloon-tipped catheter is centered in the lesion and expanded to compress the blockage. **C,** The artery is restored to its original diameter. **D,** Placement of a coronary artery stent at the site of the lesion. **E,** Atherectomy. If the plaque has hardened and become calcified, atherectomy can be used to pulverize the material. Some catheters are fitted with a laser that dissolves the lesions.

Catheter threaded into subclavian artery

Balloon in position in left coronary artery

The three components of cardiopulmonary bypass are hemodilution, hypothermia, and anticoagulation. Hemodilution occurs as the client's blood becomes diluted with the isotonic crystalloid solution used to prime the bypass machine. Hypothermia (28° C to 36° C) is used to reduce tissue oxygen requirements by approximately 50% to protect the organs from ischemic injury. Anticoagulation is necessary to prevent coagulation in the bypass machine once the client's blood comes into contact with the surfaces in the machine. These three components contribute to the clinical sequelae and the complications associated with cardiopulmonary bypass, including coagulopathies. Excessive bleeding after cardiac surgery is related to the hemodilution and excessive activation of the hemostatic system because blood cells are injured as they contact the bypass machine. The risk of complications is high when the duration of cardiopulmonary bypass exceeds 2 hours and dramatically increases whenever bypass persists beyond 3 to 4 hours. This proportional increase in complications is attributed to the increase in blood trauma, altered capillary membrane permeability, and subsequent tissue anoxia.

Coronary Artery Bypass Graft. Coronary artery bypass graft surgery involves the bypass of a blockage in one or more of the coronary arteries using the saphenous veins, mammary artery, or radial artery as conduits or replacement vessels. Before surgery, coronary angiography precisely locates lesions and points of narrowing within the coronary arteries.

During traditional CABG surgery, a median sternotomy incision is made through the sternum so that the heart and aorta can be seen. The client is placed on cardiopulmonary bypass (CPB) or the "heart-lung machine" while the bypasses are performed. After being connected to the bypass, the heart is stopped *(cardioplegia)* using a solution of iced saline containing potassium. After the bypasses have been performed, the client is taken off of the machine, and the heart takes over again. All bypasses were originally performed using saphenous veins from the leg as the new conduit. The distal end of the vein is sutured to the aorta, and the proximal end is sewn to the coronary vessel distal to the blockage (Figure 58-2). The veins are reversed so that their valves do not interfere with blood flow.

Today the saphenous vein is used less often. More commonly, the internal mammary artery (IMA) is grafted to a coronary artery. It is more routinely used to revascularize the portion of the myocardium supplied by the left anterior descending (LAD) artery. The disadvantage of the IMA is that more time is required to remove it and the mammary artery is shorter. An advantage is that IMA grafts have a greater chance of remaining patent. Radial arteries have been used as an alternative to saphenous vein grafts.[15] The radial artery is frequently used in clients having repeat CABG and when radiation therapy to the chest makes it impossible to use the IMA. The radial artery has had excellent patency rates.[15,33]

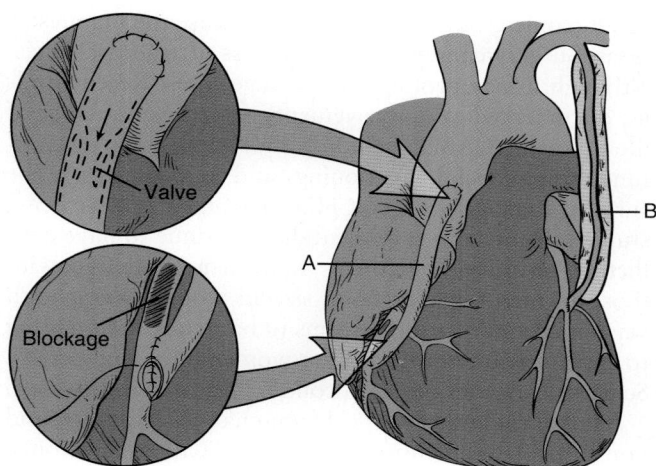

FIGURE 58-2 Coronary artery bypass grafting (CABG). **A,** A section of saphenous vein is harvested from the leg and anastomosed (upside down, because of its directional valves) to a coronary artery to bypass an area of occlusion on the right coronary artery. **B,** Bypass of the left coronary artery with internal mammary artery.

Three different types of "less invasive" CABG surgery are also performed: (1) off-bypass CABG performed through a median sternotomy with a smaller incision; (2) minimally invasive direct CABG (MID-CABG) performed through a left anterior thoracotomy without cardiopulmonary bypass; and port-access CABG with femoral-to-femoral bypass and cardioplegia with a limited incision. Many institutions are performing MID-CABG surgery.

In off-bypass CABG, the surgery is performed on a beating heart after a reduction in cardiac motion with several different medications and devices. The benefit of this type of CABG surgery is the avoidance of the use of CPB because of the many potential complications of CPB.[15]

For clients who need revascularization of the anterior coronary arteries, MIDCABG is a less invasive approach. The IMAs are used as conduits, and the client does not to be placed on CPB. MIDCABG surgery is less costly than traditional CABG surgery and is associated with fewer postoperative complications. A small study comparing outcomes in CABG to minimally invasive bypass procedures found were fewer reported cardiac and pulmonary complications in the minimally invasive group.[46]

In studies comparing CABG with and without CPB, the advantages of surgery on a beating heart have been documented. These advantages include a decrease in mortality, in postoperative need for mechanical ventilation, in pulmonary complications, and in the incidence of stroke and atrial fibrillation.[23] Clients who benefit from this type of CABG include those who refuse transfusions of blood and blood products and those with advanced respiratory disease, impaired renal function, and heavily calcified aortas.[10]

Outcomes. Surgical methods only ease the manifestations. Surgery cannot halt the process of atherosclerosis, although it may prolong life in some cases. Recent studies documented an improvement in perceived quality of life following CABG, including improvements in physical functioning, social functioning, and mood states.[38] The surgical management of CHD in women is also being studied. Data from several studies continue to have conflicting results of outcomes in women compared with those in men. Smaller body size in women along with smaller coronary arteries seems to be a consistent finding to explain poorer outcomes for women following CABG. Scientists are continuing to conduct research in this area.

The development of calcium-channel blockers and nonsurgical interventions such as PTCA, atherectomy, and stents have reduced the number of CABG surgical procedures being performed. Survival rates using CABG have not been significantly better than those of medically treated clients. CABG nevertheless remains a common procedure; and, because it can reduce angina in 80% to 90% of clients who do not respond to medical management, it will continue to be an important intervention in the management of CHD. Benefits from CABG surgery also include prolongation of life, increased exercise tolerance, reduced need for medication, and ability to resume former activities.

Complications. Possible complications of CABG surgery include the following:
- Postoperative bleeding
- Wound infection and dehiscence
- Intraoperative stroke
- MI
- Blood clots
- Multiple organ system failure
- Death

Complications resulting from persistent hypotension are cerebral ischemia, renal shutdown, myocardial infarction, and shock. To correct these complications, the surgeon may use a mechanical device to support the failing heart if medications are unsuccessful.

The intra-aortic balloon pump (IABP) is a counterpulsation device that supports the failing heart by increasing coronary artery perfusion during diastole and reducing afterload. It consists of a sausage-shaped balloon catheter that is passed through the femoral artery and positioned in the descending thoracic aorta just distal to the subclavian artery. The catheter is attached to a power console that inflates and deflates the balloon in time with the heart.

The balloon is inflated during diastole; blood is pushed back into the aorta, and coronary artery perfusion is improved.

The balloon is deflated during systole; resistance is decreased, and the workload of the heart is thus reduced (see the Bridge to Critical Care feature on Intra-Aortic Balloon Pumping on p. 1643). The timing of the balloon inflations and deflations is critical. A nurse educated in the use of the balloon pump is assigned to care for the client. Monitoring the effects of the pumping on the client's vital signs requires special skills.

■ Nursing Management Before Cardiac Surgery

Clients may have experienced cardiopulmonary clinical manifestations for varying amounts of time. Some clients will have had cardiac disease for months or years. Others may have had their first manifestations of heart disease today and already be on their way to surgery.

Note the client's psychological readiness for surgery and his or her reaction to the need for heart surgery. The client may initially experience shock and grief over the impending surgery. Chief concerns may be helplessness and fear of disability or death.

The psychological preparation of the cardiac surgery client is very important. Many hospitals throughout the United States have extensive preoperative education programs that greatly reduce client and family anxiety. Such a program should include a thorough explanation of the preoperative, intraoperative, and postoperative procedures. Also helpful is the introduction of the client to involved health care team members and the health care facility environment. Box 58-2 provides a list of topics for education. Your institution probably has written material for you to use.

Allow clients to tell you in their own words about their heart problem and the surgery. Correct any misconceptions, using pictures and a model of the heart. Clients tend to ask the greatest number of questions about what will happen to them in the recovery room and intensive care unit (ICU).

Explain that they will awaken from the anesthetic with a chest tube in place. Discuss the ventilator that will assist the client's breathing for the first 8 to 24 hours. Remind clients that during this time they will be unable to talk. Explain that an IV line for fluid or blood will be inserted in an arm and that various equipment that continuously monitors vital signs will be attached to their skin.

Answer questions concerning the necessity of using blood products. Use these facts to respond to concerns about transfusion. Postoperative blood transfusions are used only as needed; blood is screened carefully, and there is little risk of contracting blood-borne illnesses. Emphasize that although the client will experience pain, the pain will be swiftly reduced by medication and comfort measures.

Finally, explain that the client will be awakened frequently in the ICU for vital nursing assessments and interventions. Give examples of scheduled activities: vital signs every 15 minutes; temperature every 2 hours; frequent turning, coughing, and deep breathing; blood drawn for tests every morning.

Clients also need information concerning discharge from the ICU and health care facility. Explain the average length of stay in the ICU, the room to which the

Intra-Aortic Balloon Pumping—Counterpulsation Device

When the left ventricle fails to support adequate circulation and perfusion, an intra-aortic balloon pumping (IABP) device can be used to augment coronary artery filling and decrease left ventricular workload. A polyethylene balloon is inserted via the femoral artery into the descending thoracic aorta distal to the left subclavian artery and connected to an external pneumatic pumping system. The pump inflates the balloon with helium or carbon dioxide during diastole and deflates it during systole. The inflation-deflation cycle is triggered by the client's ECG, specifically by the R wave, which signals the beginning of systole. Balloon inflation during diastole augments coronary artery filling. Systolic balloon deflation decreases afterload.

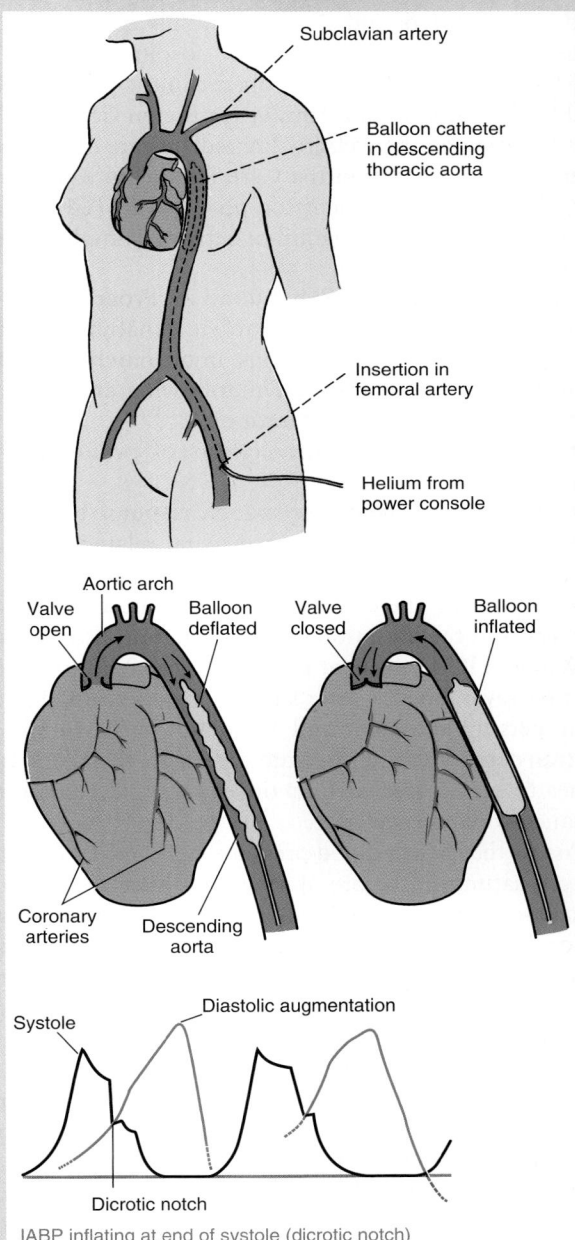

IABP inflating at end of systole (dicrotic notch)
Blood pressure waves

The IABP device is used in clients with cardiogenic shock, septic shock, acute anterior myocardial infarction (MI), complications following MI, angioplasty with MI, ventricular dysrhythmias with ischemia, left ventricular failure, unstable angina refractory to medications, and low cardiac output after surgery.

Guidelines for Management

1. Select an ECG lead that optimizes the R wave.
2. Time the IABP device using an arterial waveform.
3. Monitor perfusion in the extremity with IABP.
4. Monitor perfusion in arms (catheter can occlude subclavian artery)
5. Monitor arterial pressures (which should improve).
6. Monitor urine output (the catheter can occlude the renal artery).
7. Keep the affected limb straight to prevent dislodgment of the catheter.
8. Monitor for balloon rupture and misplacement (loss of augmentation, wrinkled appearance in safety chamber, blood in tubing).
9. Monitor for bleeding resulting from anticoagulant use.
10. Monitor for aortic dissection (acute back, retroperitoneal, testicular or chest pain, decreased pulses, variations in blood pressure between arms, decreased cardiac output, tachycardia, decreased filling pressures, decreased hemoglobin, decreased hematocrit).
11. Monitor skin integrity on the sacrum, the coccyx, and the heels.
12. Do not elevate the head of the bed above 15 degrees.
13. Clarify or reinforce the client's and family's understanding of the IABP device.

Complications

- Dissection of the femoral or iliac artery or aorta
- Bleeding
- Plaque dislodgment, which can cause embolization
- Balloon rupture
- Arterial occlusion with limb ischemia or neuropathy
- Mechanical destruction of red blood cells
- Inability to wean from the IABP device
- Hematoma at the insertion site
- Mesenteric/renal ischemia (catheter too low)
- Arm ischemia (catheter too high)

Weaning

- The ratio of IABP-assisted beats to unassisted beats is decreased from 1:1 to 1:2 based on the following parameters:
- Heart rate <110 beats/min
- No dysrhythmias
- Mean arterial pressure >70 mm Hg without vasopressors
- Pulmonary arterial wedge pressure <18 mm Hg
- Cardiac index >2.5
- Capillary refill >3 sec
- Urine output >0.5 ml/kg/min
- SVO_2 between 70% and 80%

BOX 58-2 *Guidelines to Preparing the Client Undergoing Cardiac Surgery*

Plan teaching well in advance of the surgical date, if possible. By the time of surgery, the client should be prepared by the following:

1. Describe the surgical procedure:
   a. All steps, including heart-lung machine
   b. Review of anatomy and physiology of heart and valves
   c. Brief definition of unfamiliar technical terms
   d. Length of time in surgery and approximate time of first visit by family
   e. Giving the client pictures of the heart and involved valve for future reference
2. Describe the intensive care unit (ICU) environment and monitoring equipment:
   a. Cardiac monitor and alarm
   b. Endotracheal (ET) tube and projected length of time with ET tube in place
   c. Mechanical ventilator and alarm
   d. Suctioning procedure
   e. Arterial line and automatic blood pressure cuff
   f. Any limitation on visits from family
   g. Chest tubes or mediastinal tubes
   h. Nasogastric tube and length of NPO (nothing by mouth) status
   i. Urinary catheter
   j. High noise level in ICU
   k. Multiple intravenous lines and fluids
3. Describe preoperative preparation:
   a. Showering with antimicrobial soap
   b. Shaving of chest, abdomen, neck, and groin
   c. Special cardiac studies: echocardiogram, electrocardiogram, cardiac catheterization
4. Describe comfort measures:
   a. Pain reduction
   b. Turning, range-of-motion exercises
   c. Out of bed next morning
   d. Medication for sleep, if needed

---

client will return from the ICU, the average length of stay in the health care facility, and the diet and activities permitted once the client returns home. Be general in the discussion. Remember, many unforeseen events can arise and greatly alter the postoperative course.

Give verbal and written information concerning health care facility services, rules, and regulations; visiting hours; the chaplain's name and visiting hours (if appropriate); and the names of the clinical nurse-specialists and other health care professionals who can be contacted for information. Most clients benefit from a tour of the recovery room and ICU. If they are not physically able to participate in a tour, audiovisual material is helpful.

Familiarize the client with the equipment that will be used in the ICU (e.g., chest drainage tubes, oxygen apparatus, ventilators, cardiac monitors, IV setups). Reassure the client that lights and alarm noises are part of the critical care environment and are not indicators that something is wrong.

■ Nursing Management of the Surgical Client

Many hospitals have initiated rapid recovery programs for cardiac surgery clients that reduce the hospital stay to 4 days. Clients are initially cared for in intensive care unit (ICU). With rapid recovery programs, most of the client's recovery takes place in the home, with the client and family assuming primary responsibility for many aspects of care. Discharge planning begins at the time of admission, activity progression in the postoperative period is accelerated, and client and family education continues on a daily basis throughout hospitalization.

Many hospitals have developed clinical pathways for CABG. See the Clinical Pathway feature on Coronary Bypass Grafting on the website. Immediate care of the client *evolve* after CABG is shown in the Care Plan feature on Coronary Bypass Surgical Clients on pp. 1645 to 1648. In addition, a three-phase program of activity is implemented.

Phase 1 (In-Hospital) Rehabilitation Programs. Most CABG clients participate in cardiac rehabilitation following surgery. Phase 1 begins immediately after the client returns from surgery. The following are the goals of phase 1 inpatient rehabilitation:
- To prevent the negative effects of prolonged bed rest
- To assess the client's physiologic response to exercise
- To manage the psychosocial issues related to recovery from CABG surgery
- To educate the client and family concerning recovery and the adoption of risk reduction behaviors

While in ICU the client is turned every 2 hours during the first several hours after surgery. Once extubated, the client gets up in a chair and ambulates in the room. After transfer to the intermediate care unit, the client continues to walk three or four times a day, increasing the distance walked each time.

Assess the client's blood pressure, heart rate, ECG, and oxygen saturation before, during, and after activity. Systolic blood pressure should not increase more than 20 mm Hg or decrease more than 10 to 15 mm Hg after exercise. Heart rate should not increase more than 20 beats/min above resting, and no significant dysrhythmias should occur. Activity levels will be reduced if clients have adverse physiologic responses (e.g., tachycardia, dysrhythmias, pain) to exercise. Clients are seated for all meals. Research has demonstrated that early mobilization improves cardiac function and benefits the client psychologically.

Education for a healthier lifestyle is an important part of each phase of cardiac rehabilitation. The emphasis in

CARE PLAN

Coronary Bypass Surgical Clients

Nursing Diagnosis. Decreased Cardiac Output related to alterations in preload/afterload/contractility/heart rate.

Outcomes. The client will have improved cardiac output as evidenced by stable blood pressure with decreasing need for vasoactive medications, normal sinus rhythm without pacing, clear lung sounds, warm/dry skin, preoperative mental status, urine output greater or equal to 0.5 ml/kg/hr without medical diuresis, and palpable peripheral pulses.

Interventions	Rationales
1. Assess hemodynamic parameters (heart rate, CVP, RAP, BP, SVR, PAP, PCWP, CO) continuously or according to protocol for CO/CI.	1. Monitoring allows for early intervention.
2. Monitor potassium and magnesium levels.	2. Hypokalemia and hypomagnesemia can lead to ventricular dysrhythmias.
3. Monitor weight daily and calculate change.	3. Body weight is a reliable indicator of fluid volume. Compare findings to previous weights.
4. Monitor for peripheral edema.	4. Peripheral edema may develop with dilutional hypoproteinemia or heart failure.
5. Monitor I & O hourly.	5. Hourly assessment allows for rapid adjustments in fluids to prevent hypotension and maintain renal perfusion.
6. Monitor heart sounds every 4 hours.	6. A ventricular gallop (S_3) is an early sign of heart failure. S_4 may indicate decreased ventricular compliance.
7. Administer prescribed fluids, packed red blood cells, or colloids.	7. Hypovolemia is a common cause of low cardiac output. These fluids/proteins increase circulating fluid volume.
8. Administer prescribed vasodilators (specify).	8. Reducing afterload reduces stress on the left ventricle.
9. Warm the client to reduce shivering.	9. Shivering from intraoperative hypothermia leads to vasoconstriction and increases afterload. Hypothermia can lead to depressed contractility.
10. Administer inotropic medications as prescribed (specify).	10. Inotropic medications enhance myocardial contractility, leading to improved cardiac output by more complete emptying of the ventricles.
11. Monitor the ECG and arterial blood pressure to verify timing and effect of balloon counterpulsations (IABP). (See also the Bridge to Critical Care feature on IABP on p. 1643.)	11. IABP must receive a signal to identify the beginning of a new cardiac cycle. Dysrhythmias may affect the timing of balloon deflation and inflation. MAP should remain approximately on 80 mm Hg on IABP.
12. Protect external pacemaker wires from water and accidental exposure to electricity by placing them in a rubber glove.	12. Static electricity and water can cause the pacer wires to conduct electricity.

Nursing Diagnosis. Impaired Gas Exchange related to ventilation/perfusion mismatch or intrapulmonary shunting.

Outcomes. The client will have adequate gas exchange as evidenced by PaO_2 >90, $PaCO_2$ <35, pH between 7.35 and 7.45, and oxygen saturation >90%.

Interventions	Rationales
1. Monitor oxygen saturation continuously.	1. Continuous monitoring allows for early intervention.
2. Monitor results of ABGs; report abnormal or unexpected findings to the surgeon.	2. Hypoxemia or acidosis may require modification in ventilation parameters.

BP, Blood pressure, *CI,* cardiac index; *CO,* cardiac output; *CVP,* central venous pressure; *IABP,* intraaortic balloon pump; *MAP,* mean arterial pressure; *PADP,* pulmonary artery diastolic pressure; *PAP,* pulmonary artery pressure; *PAWP,* pulmonary artery wedge pressure; *PCWP,* pulmonary capillary wedge pressure; *RAP,* right atrial pressure; *SVR,* systemic vascular resistance.

Continued

Coronary Bypass Surgical Clients—cont'd

Interventions	Rationales
3. Monitor settings on ventilator, position of ET tube, lung sounds, and response to mechanical ventilation.	3. Supplemental oxygen is not adequate to facilitate transport of oxygen across the alveolar membrane when intrapulmonary shunting exists. Mechanical ventilation is used with positive pressure to facilitate alveolar ventilation. The ET tube must remain at the carina; its position within the airway is monitored by confirming placement.
4. Securely tape or hold the ET tube in place.	4. Securing the ET tube allows the client to be moved in bed without dislodgement.
5. Use an oral bite block. (See also Bridge to Home Health Care feature on Living with a Ventilator on the website.)	5. Bite blocks prevent obstruction of the tube from biting.

Evaluation. The goals of this care plan may be short-term. Early extubation (within 3 to 8 hours after surgery) is becoming more common in clients undergoing elective CABG. Clients who are hemodynamically stable, have minimal pericardial bleeding, and are normothermic are the best candidates.

Nursing Diagnosis. Ineffective Airway Clearance related to retained secretions and excess secretions.

Interventions	Rationales
1. Monitor lung sounds.	1. Fluids in the alveoli accumulate as a result of atelectasis and dilutional hypoproteinemia.
2. Monitor coughing effort.	2. After extubation, coughing is used to clear the airways. Because of incisional pain, many clients cough poorly.
3. Administer supplemental oxygen to maintain oxygen saturation levels above 93%.	3. Oxygen saturation levels over 93% equate to 90% arterial blood saturation, which is adequate in most clients.
4. Maintain comfort using prescribed opioids.	4. Pain control can facilitate adequate coughing.
5. Splint the incision with "heart pillows" or pillows.	5. Splinting the incision before coughing promotes more intense coughing efforts.
6. Ambulate when tolerated.	6. Respiratory effort is increased with ambulation; therefore deep breathing occurs.
7. Teach proper use of the incentive spirometer (ICS) once extubated. Demonstrate as needed.	7. Correct use of ICS encourages sustained inspiration to open alveoli.

Evaluation. Expect this outcome to be met after 4 to 5 days; clearing the chest of secretions requires time and client effort.

Collaborative Problem. Risk of Hemorrhage related to inadequate hemostasis, disruption of suture lines, or coagulopathy.

Outcomes. The nurse will monitor for the bleeding in excess of expectations (should be less than 70 ml/hr).

Interventions	Rationales
1. Monitor mediastinal chest tubes for output hourly.	1. Hourly assessment of output and total output is analyzed. Clients with IMA grafts are at increased risk of bleeding because of the surgical resection needed.
2. Report excess volumes and/or institute prescribed treatments for blood loss.	2. Agents such as protamine (to reverse heparin), aminocaproic acid (inhibits lysis of clots by blocking the conversion of plasminogen to plasmin), fresh-frozen plasma, platelets, and fluids may be used to restore volume.

BP, Blood pressure, *CI,* cardiac index; *CO,* cardiac output; *CVP,* central venous pressure; *IABP,* intraaortic balloon pump; *MAP,* mean arterial pressure; *PADP,* pulmonary artery diastolic pressure; *PAP,* pulmonary artery pressure; *PAWP,* pulmonary artery wedge pressure; *PCWP,* pulmonary capillary wedge pressure; *RAP,* right atrial pressure; *SVR,* systemic vascular resistance.

CARE PLAN

Interventions	Rationales
3. Retransfuse blood from mediastinum as ordered.	3. Autotransfusion is one mechanism of using the client's own blood, which is collecting in the autotransfusion reservoir, for transfusion.
4. Keep chest tubes positioned without kinks and/or gently strip them (per agency or physician protocol).	4. Maintain patency of the tube. Aggressive chest tube stripping can lead to bleeding by dislodging small clots.

5. Monitor for manifestations of cardiac tamponade:
  Elevated CVP, PADP, PAOP
  Decreased CO, BP
  Pulsus paradoxus
  Muffled heart sounds
  Sudden cessation of chest tube drainage
	5. Cardiac tamponade, which is the collection of blood/fluid in the pericardial sac, can severely restrict ventricular filling.

Evaluation. The risk of bleeding is highest in the first 24 hours after surgery.

Nursing Diagnosis. Acute Pain related to tissue trauma secondary to sternotomy and leg incision.

Outcomes. The client will report comfort based on tolerable pain levels.

Interventions	Rationales
1. Monitor reported level or pain	1. Reported pain levels are the most accurate method of describing the intensity of pain.
2. Assess the nature of the pain.	2. Angina must be differentiated from incisional pain. Clients with IMA grafts will often have chest wall pain. Saphenous vein graft harvest incisions are often reported as quite painful.
3. Administer ordered opioids for surgical pain by prescribed route management to meet client goal.	3. Treatment of acute pain reduces sympathetic stimulation, which increases cardiac workload. Pain control also enhances recovery.
4. Premedicate before activities such as ambulation and coughing.	4. Premedication assists the client to fully participate.

Evaluation. Expect pain levels to be highest for the first 48 hours after surgery.

Collaborative Problem. Risk of Postcardiotomy Delirium or Stroke.

Outcome. The nurse will monitor for the return of baseline levels of consciousness and mental acuity.

Interventions	Rationales
1. Monitor for return of consciousness when removed from sedating medications.	1. Neurologic examination is accurate only if the client is awake and able to participate.
2. Assess neurologic status every shift. Compare current level of mental acuity to baseline levels. Report any deviations to surgeon.	2. Baseline levels of mental acuity provide a comparison. Early intervention for stroke may limit permanent damage.
3. Reorient frequently to setting, timing, and procedures being performed.	3. Delirium is short-term, and reorientation is helpful to assist the client in restructuring thoughts.
4. Explain all procedures, using a calm and clear voice.	4. The environment of an ICU may threaten the confused client. Explanations also build trust and gain cooperation.
5. Secure all invasive lines and tubes.	5. Disoriented clients may accidentally pull or remove lines. Accidental dislodgement may injure the client and/or require replacement of the device.
6. Administer sedative medications cautiously.	6. Mild sedation may help prevent injury. However, the use of sedation in older adults may increase agitation.

Continued

CARE PLAN

Coronary Bypass Surgical Clients—cont'd

Interventions	Rationales
7. Avoid restraints in lieu of other methods to prevent self-injury.	7. Physical restraints may increase agitation.
8. Explain that changes in mental acuity, agitation, confusion, and/or hallucinations are temporary (as applies).	8. Transient changes in acuity are usually due to decreased cerebral perfusion and microemboli during the cardiac bypass pump run. Discussion of permanent changes is left to the neurologist.
9. Organize nursing care to provide time for sleep. Limit environmental noise as much as possible.	9. Sleep deprivation may increase confusion.
10. Liberalize visitation time with family.	10. Familiar voices and faces will help with reorientation.

Evaluation. Once the sedative effects of the medications and anesthetics wear off, mental acuity of baseline levels should return.

Nursing Diagnosis. Risk for Infection related to sternotomy incision, diabetes, and obesity.

Outcomes. The client will have decreased risk of infection as evidenced by primary healing of the sternotomy incision.

Interventions	Rationales
1. Monitor temperature hourly initially, and every 4 hours once stable.	1. Fever over 38.3° C (101° F) may indicate atelectasis early in recovery. Later fever may indicate sternal wound infection or infective endocarditis.
2. Monitor incision for signs of delayed primary healing.	2. Erythema, pain, drainage, or opening of the sternal margin are signs of delayed healing.
3. Administer insulin drip as ordered to control blood glucose levels to desired values as ordered.	3. Blood glucose levels over 200 mg/dl create ineffective phagocytosis and increase the risk of infection.
4. Apply a front-closing brassiere or other supportive dressings for obese woman clients.	4. Pendulous breasts can create tension on the suture lines and impair sternotomy healing.
5. Collaborate with the dietician to ensure that a diet of adequate calories and protein is delivered.	5. Protein and calorie needs increase after major stress and are needed for wound healing.
6. Administer antibiotics as prescribed (specify).	6. Antibiotics reduce the risk of surgical site infection.

Evaluation. Incisions should heal by primary intention in 7 to 10 days.

BP, Blood pressure, *CI,* cardiac index; *CO,* cardiac output; *CVP,* central venous pressure; *IABP,* intraaortic balloon pump; *MAP,* mean arterial pressure; *PADP,* pulmonary artery diastolic pressure; *PAP,* pulmonary artery pressure; *PAWP,* pulmonary artery wedge pressure; *PCWP,* pulmonary capillary wedge pressure; *RAP,* right atrial pressure; *SVR,* systemic vascular resistance.

phase 1 is on the identification and modification of reversible risk factors to prevent further deleterious cardiac events.[9]

Self-Care. Before hospital discharge, instruct the client and family (or significant other) about medication actions and side effects, dietary restrictions, physical activity restrictions and progression, and incisional care. Because it is not always possible to anticipate all the problems clients may encounter the first few days at home, instruct the client whom to call when there is an emergency or when there are questions or concerns. If possible, introduce the client to the home health nurse who will be supervising home care. Following discharge, the home health care nurse provides additional education and counseling and assesses the client for complications.[38,47,53] In addition, instruct the client on how to assess response to exercise and activity.[9]

Before discharge, a low-level symptom-limited exercise test may be performed to evaluate the client's ability to perform activities of daily living (ADL) and exercise. The test results are used to prescribe a safe and effective exercise program for the first few weeks at home and serve as a basis for the initial exercise prescription in phase 2.

Phase 2 (Outpatient Exercise Training) Rehabilitation Programs. Outpatient (phase 2) exercise training usually takes place in a facility that provides continuous ECG monitoring, emergency equipment, and medically supervised exercise. Outpatient treatment usually begins 10 to 14 days after discharge and requires physician referral. The following are the goals of phase 2:

- To restore clients to a desirable exercise capacity appropriate to their health status, lifestyle, and occupation
- To provide additional education and support to the client and family for adoption of risk-reduction behaviors
- To meet the psychosocial needs of clients and families, restore confidence, and minimize anxiety and depression
- To promote early identification of medical problems through close observation and monitoring of clients during exercise
- To assist clients in returning to occupational and leisure activities

Exercise therapy is conducted three times weekly for 2 to 3 months. The duration of the aerobic exercise session ranges from 20 to 40 minutes at an intensity of 70% to 85% of the baseline exercise heart rate. During each exercise session, blood pressure, heart rate, respiratory rate, and ECG are monitored before, during, and after exercise. Activity levels are increased gradually, based on the client's response. A nutritionist may counsel clients about proper diet, and a psychologist or social worker may counsel clients about stress management and adoption of other risk prevention behaviors.

At the end of the program, clients are given a symptom-limited exercise test and are reevaluated. Decisions regarding progression to a phase 3 or home program are based on the client's results of the stress test, ability to self-monitor his or her response to exercise, the client's stability, and psychological or emotional status. Periodic evaluations are scheduled so that activity progression and cardiopulmonary function can be assessed.[9]

Phase 3 (Community) Rehabilitation Programs. Phase 3 programs are conducted in community settings, such as a "Y" or a health club. The following are the goals of phase 3:

- To maintain and, if possible, increase exercise capacity
- To institute long-term follow-up of risk-reduction behavior change
- To encourage clients to take responsibility for continuing lifestyle changes

Exercise consists of walking, jogging, weight training, and recreational games. Clients are usually not monitored while exercising, although some facilities obtain exercise ECGs on a monthly basis. Clients are responsible for monitoring their own heart rate response to exercise, although blood pressure can be taken by program personnel if indicated.[9]

Home Exercise Rehabilitation Programs. For CABG clients a home exercise program is usually prescribed in conjunction with or in place of the outpatient program. Clients are given detailed exercise instructions and are told to keep a log of heart rates, perceived exertion rates, exercise parameters, and any problems that occur during the home program. Cardiac rehabilitation staff members or the client's physician should analyze the data and adjust the home exercise program if necessary. Once clients reach their optimal level of functional capacity, they are instructed to continue to exercise at least three times weekly so that cardiopulmonary exercise capacity can be maintained.

■ Modifications for Older Clients

More than half of all CABG procedures are performed on people older than 65 years of age, and 71% of them are performed on men.[3] Older clients have a postoperative recovery similar to that for younger clients, but the pace is slower and they typically remain hospitalized an average of 2 to 4 days longer. They also have a higher mortality rate.

Postoperative complications that are more prevalent in older clients include dysrhythmias related to aged sinoatrial node cells, drug toxicity associated with impaired hepatic and renal perfusion, multiple drug interactions, and decreased physical stamina. These complications contribute to a 15-day mean length of hospital stay for clients older than 80 years of age.

During the first and second weeks after discharge, depression, fatigue, incisional chest discomfort, dyspnea, and anorexia are common. By the fourth to fifth weeks, older clients report improved mood, comfort, and appetite. At 1 year, almost all (93%) clients are pleased with the outcome and improved quality of life.

HEART FAILURE

Despite aggressive medical and surgical treatment, CHD may eventually lead to the development of heart failure. Heart failure is a significant cardiac functional disorder that can result in reduced oxygen delivery to the body's organs and tissues. Heart failure affects about 5 million people in the United States, with 500,000 new cases diagnosed each year. In contrast to decreases in mortality rates associated with other cardiovascular diseases, the incidence of heart failure and the mortality associated with it have increased steadily since 1975.[20] Annually about 300,000 clients die from direct or indirect consequences of heart failure, and the number of deaths attributed to heart failure has increased 6-fold over the past 40 years.

Heart failure can affect both women and men, although the mortality is higher among women.[4,21] There are also racial differences; at all ages death rates are higher in African Americans than in non-Hispanic whites. Heart failure is primarily a disease of older adults, affecting 6% to 10% of those over 65 years of age. It is also the leading cause of hospitalization in older people.[3,20]

Heart failure is a physiologic state in which the heart cannot pump enough blood to meet the metabolic needs of the body (determined as oxygen consumption). Heart failure results from changes in systolic or diastolic function of the left ventricle. The heart fails when, because of intrinsic disease or structural defects, it cannot handle a normal blood volume or, in the absence of disease, cannot tolerate a sudden expansion in blood volume (e.g., during exercise). Heart failure is not a disease itself; instead, the term refers to a clinical syndrome characterized by manifestations of volume overload, inadequate tissue perfusion, and poor exercise tolerance. Whatever the cause, pump failure results in hypoperfusion of tissue, followed by pulmonary and systemic venous congestion. Because heart failure causes vascular congestion, it is often called *congestive heart failure,* although most cardiac specialists no longer use this term. Other terms used to denote heart failure include *cardiac decompensation, cardiac insufficiency,* and *ventricular failure.*

Etiology and Risk Factors

The performance of the heart depends on four essential components:

- Contractility (inotropic state) of the muscle
- Preload (amount of blood in the ventricle at the end of diastole)
- Afterload (the pressure against which the left ventricle ejects)
- Heart rate

Table 58-2 defines the terms commonly used to describe cardiac function. Adverse changes in these determinants of myocardial performance ultimately cause the heart to fail. CHD is the primary cause of heart failure in two thirds of clients with decreased ventricular dysfunction; however, heart failure can also be caused by other disorders. The causes of heart failure can be divided into three subgroups (Table 58-3):[20]

- Abnormal loading conditions
- Abnormal muscle function
- Conditions or diseases that limit ventricular filling

Abnormal Loading Conditions

Abnormal loading is associated with any condition that increases either the pressure or the volume load of the ventricle. The effect of increasing volume on the ventricle can be explained by the analogy that the heart muscle is like a stretched rubber band. When the rubber band is stretched, it contracts with more force. The heart muscle does the same. Venous return stretches the heart and improves contractility. When the rubber band is over-stretched, however, it becomes limp and cannot

TABLE 58-2	Terms Used to Describe Cardiac Function
Term	**Function**
Afterload	Force that the ventricle must develop during systole to eject the stroke volume
Cardiac output	Stroke volume × heart rate
Inotropic state	A measure of contractility
Preload	Stretch of myocardial fibers at end-diastole
Stroke volume	The amount of blood ejected from the ventricle with each contraction

contract. Likewise, when the heart is overloaded with blood, excessive stretch and decreased contraction occur. Overload develops because blood does not leave the ventricles during contraction. Therefore cardiac workload increases in an effort to move blood.

Preload refers to the stretch of the ventricular myocardial fibers just before ventricular contraction. The load or stretch placed on the ventricular fibers corresponds to the end-diastolic ventricular volume and pressure. Preload is determined by the condition of the heart valves (especially the mitral valve), blood volume, ventricular wall compliance, and venous tone. Table 58-3 lists conditions that increase preload. Increased preload usually increases contractility (more stretch on the rubber band) and stretch because of filling pressures from venous return and previous volume. Stretch and filling pressures may rise beyond the capabilities of the normally compliant heart. This increased preload lessens the force and efficiency of ventricular contraction. Cardiac output decreases. Under the strain of this load, the heart will fail.

Increased pressure load in the ventricle is related to *afterload,* the amount of tension the heart must generate to overcome systemic pressure and to allow adequate ventricular emptying. Thus afterload indicates how hard the heart must pump to force blood into circulation. The tone of systemic arterioles, the elasticity of the aorta and large arteries, the size and thickness of the ventricle, the presence of aortic stenosis, and the viscosity of the blood all determine afterload. High peripheral vascular resistance and high blood pressure force the ventricle to work harder to eject blood (see Table 58-3). Subjected to prolonged high pressures, the ventricle eventually fails.[20]

Abnormal Muscle Function

Disorders that impair the contractile function of the myocardial fibrils and reduce ventricular filling and stroke volume affect the cardiac muscle's ability to pump effectively (see Table 58-3).

Myocardial fibrils are injured during an MI, and during the healing phase some of the heart muscle is re-

TABLE 58-3	*Etiology of Heart Failure*		
Abnormal Loading Conditions		**Abnormal Muscle Function**	**Limited Ventricular Filling**

Conditions That Increase Preload

Regurgitation of mitral or tricuspid valve
Hypervolemia
Congenital defects (left-to-right shunts)
Ventricular septal defect
Atrial septal defect
Patent ductus arteriosus

Abnormal Muscle Function

Myocardial infarction
Myocarditis
Cardiomyopathy
Ventricular aneurysm
Long-term alcohol consumption
Coronary heart disease
Metabolic heart disease
Endocrine heart disease

Limited Ventricular Filling

Mitral or tricuspid stenosis
Cardiac tamponade
Constrictive pericarditis
Hypertrophic obstructive cardiomyopathy

Conditions That Increase Afterload

Hypertension, pulmonary or systemic
Aortic or pulmonic stenosis
High peripheral vascular resistance

---

placed by noncontracting scar tissue. Scar tissue does not move during contraction, and the ventricles pump less efficiently. Some degree of heart failure, either chronic or transient, appears in more than half of clients after MI.

Certain conditions externally compress the heart, thereby limiting ventricular filling and myocardial contractility. Disorders that greatly restrict cardiac chamber filling and myocardial fiber stretch include *constrictive pericarditis,* an inflammatory and fibrotic process of the pericardial sac; and *cardiac tamponade,* which involves the accumulation of fluid or blood within the pericardial sac. Because the pericardium encloses all four heart chambers, compression of the heart both decreases diastolic relaxation, thereby elevating diastolic pressure, and hampers forward blood flow through the heart.

Conditions That Precipitate Heart Failure

Some clients have pre-existing mild to moderate heart disease with no evidence of heart failure. In these clients adequate cardiac output depends on functional compensatory mechanisms. When the heart undergoes undue stress, these compensatory mechanisms may prove inadequate and the heart fails.

Heart failure can be precipitated by conditions that increase cardiac and systemic oxygen demand, reduce the ability of the heart to contract, or increase the workload of the heart (Box 58-3).

Pathophysiology

The healthy heart can meet the demands for oxygen delivery through the use of cardiac reserve. *Cardiac reserve* is the heart's ability to increase output in response to stress. The normal heart can increase its output up to five times the resting level. The failing heart, even at rest, however, is pumping near its capacity and thus has lost much of its reserve. The compromised heart has a lim-

BOX 58-3	*Conditions That Precipitate Heart Failure*

- Dysrhythmias, especially tachycardia
- Systemic infections (sepsis)
- Anemia
- Thyroid disorders
- Pulmonary embolism
- Thiamine deficiency
- Chronic pulmonary diseases
- Medication dose changes
- Physical or emotional stress
- Endocarditis, myocarditis, or pericarditis
- Fluid retention from medication or salt intake
- A new cardiac condition

ited ability to respond to the body's needs for increased output in situations of stress.

When cardiac output is not sufficient to meet the metabolic needs of the body, compensatory mechanisms, including neurohormonal responses, become activated. These mechanisms initially help to improve contraction and maintain integrity of the circulation but, if continued, lead to abnormal cardiac muscle growth and reconfiguration (remodeling) of the heart. The compensatory responses to a decrease in cardiac output are ventricular dilation, increased sympathetic nervous system stimulation, and activation of the renin-angiotensin system.

Ventricular Dilation

Ventricular dilation refers to lengthening of the muscle fibers that increases the volume in the heart chambers. Dilation causes an increase in preload, and thus cardiac output, because a stretched muscle contracts more forcefully (Starling's law); however, dilation has limits as a compensatory mechanism. Muscle fibers, if stretched beyond a certain point, become ineffective. Second, a dilated heart requires more oxygen. Thus the dilated heart with a normal coronary blood flow can suffer from a lack of oxygen. Hypoxia of the heart further decreases the muscle's ability to contract.[20,24]

Increased Sympathetic Nervous System Stimulation

Sympathetic activity produces venous and arteriolar constriction, tachycardia, and increased myocardial contractility, all of which work to increase cardiac output and improve delivery of oxygen and nutrients to tissues. This compensatory effect occurs at the cost of increasing peripheral vascular resistance (afterload) and myocardial workload, however. In addition, sympathetic stimulation reduces renal blood flow and stimulates the renin-angiotensin system.[12,16,24]

Stimulation of the Renin-Angiotensin System

When blood flow through the renal artery is decreased, the baroreceptor reflex is stimulated and renin is released into the bloodstream. Renin interacts with angiotensinogen to produce angiotensin I. When angiotensin I comes into contact with ACE, it is converted to angiotensin II, a potent vasoconstrictor. Angiotensin II increases arterial vasoconstriction, promotes the release of norepinephrine from sympathetic nerve endings, and stimulates the adrenal medulla to secrete aldosterone, which enhances sodium and water absorption. Stimulation of the renin-angiotensin system causes plasma volume to expand and preload to increase.

Cardiac compensation exists when the initial compensatory mechanisms of ventricular dilation, sympathetic nervous system stimulation, and renin-angiotensin system stimulation succeed in maintaining an adequate cardiac output and oxygen delivery to the tissues in the presence of pathologic changes. Once cardiac output is restored, the body produces counterregulatory substances that restore cardiovascular homeostasis. If underlying pathologic changes are not corrected, prolonged activation of the compensatory mechanisms eventually leads to changes in the function of the myocardial cell and excess production of the neurohormones. These processes are responsible for the transition from compensated to decompensated heart failure. At this point manifestations of heart failure develop because the heart cannot maintain adequate circulation.[12,16,24]

When compensatory mechanisms fail, the amount of blood remaining in the left ventricle at the end of diastole increases. This increase in residual blood in turn decreases the ventricle's capacity to receive blood from the left atrium. The left atrium, having to work harder to eject blood, dilates and hypertrophies. It is unable to re-

ceive the full amount of incoming blood from the pulmonary veins, and left atrial pressure increases; this leads to pulmonary edema (Figure 58-3). Left ventricular failure (LVF) results.

The right ventricle, because of the increased pressure in the pulmonary vascular system, must now dilate and hypertrophy to meet its increased workload. It too eventually fails. Engorgement of the venous system then extends backward to produce congestion in the gastrointestinal tract, liver, viscera, kidneys, legs, and sacrum; edema is the main manifestation. Right ventricular failure (RVF) results. RVF usually follows LVF, although occasionally it may develop independently.

Decompensated Heart Failure

Remodeling. Several structural changes, known as *remodeling,* occur in the ventricle during decompensated heart failure. Remodeling is thought to result from hypertrophy of the myocardial cells and sustained activation of the neurohormonal compensatory systems. Recall that one of the initial compensatory responses to a decrease in cardiac output is dilation of the ventricle. This dilation increases cardiac output but also increases wall stress in the ventricle. To reduce wall stress, the myocardial cells hypertrophy, resulting in a thickening of

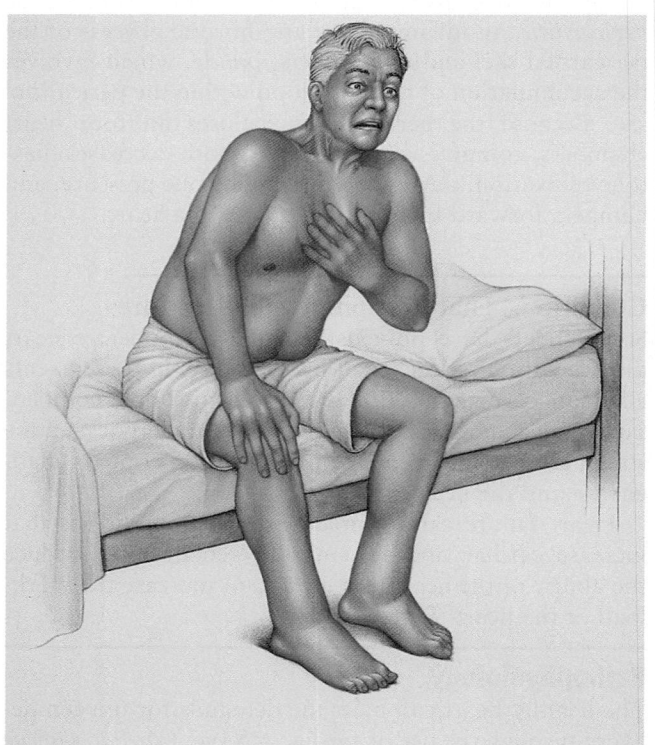

FIGURE 58-3 Appearance of a client with both right-sided and left-sided heart failure. (From *Mayo Clinic Health letter* [1997], *15*:1-3. Mayo Foundation for Medical Education and Research, Rochester, MN. By permission of Mayo Foundation.)

the ventricular wall. According to Laplace's law, an increase in wall thickness reduces wall stress.

When used over time, these compensatory responses produce changes in the structure, function, and gene expression of the myocardial cell. Changes in the myocardial cells eventually increase failure by reducing myocardial contractility, increasing ventricular wall stress, and increasing oxygen demand. In addition to increasing myocardial dysfunction, the genetically abnormal myocytes die prematurely and at an accelerated rate through the process of *apoptosis* (programmed cell death). Apoptosis affects cells scattered throughout the myocardium and causes a further reduction in cardiac function.[12,16,20,24]

Sustained Neurohormonal Activation. Remodeling changes continue to increase wall stress and further stimulate neurohormonal activity. Long-term sympathetic activation exerts a direct toxic effect on the heart that promotes myocyte hypertrophy and apoptosis. Prolonged activation of the renin-angiotensin system also stimulates myocyte hypertrophy and myocardial fibrosis. This creates a self-perpetuating cycle of cell death and further hypertrophy.[16,24]

In addition, if renal artery pressure falls, a lowered glomerular filtration rate (GFR) increases retention of sodium and water. In response to a continued reduction in renal blood flow, the renin-angiotensin-aldosterone mechanism is activated. Aldosterone, released from the adrenal cortex, promotes further retention of sodium and water by the renal tubule. This results in an expansion in blood volume of up to 30% and edema. As the sodium concentration in the extracellular fluid increases, so does the osmotic pressure of the plasma. The hypothalamus responds to the higher osmotic pressure by releasing antidiuretic hormone (ADH) from the posterior pituitary. This in turn promotes renal tubular reabsorption of water. Aldosterone, however, is more important than ADH in the production of edema because it promotes sodium retention.[16,20,24]

Clinical Manifestations

The manifestations of heart failure depend on the specific ventricle involved, the precipitating causes of failure, the degree of impairment, the rate of progression, the duration of the failure, and the client's underlying condition. Manifestations of pulmonary congestion and edema dominate the clinical picture of LVF; RVF is associated with manifestations of abdominal organ distention and peripheral edema.[16,24] Heart failure has been classified into several stages based on a client's functional ability and clinical manifestations (Box 58-4).

Types of Heart Failure

Heart failure may be categorized as (1) LVF versus RVF, (2) backward versus forward, and (3) high output versus low output.[1]

BOX 58-4	*New York Heart Association Classification of Cardiovascular Disability*

Class I

No limitation on physical activity. Ordinary physical activity does not cause undue fatigue, palpitation, dyspnea, or anginal pain.

Class II

Slight limitation of physical activity. Comfortable at rest, but ordinary physical activity results in fatigue, palpitation, dyspnea, or anginal pain.

Class III

Marked limitation of physical activity. Comfortable at rest, but less than ordinary physical activity causes fatigue, palpitation, dyspnea, or anginal pain.

Class IV

Unable to carry any physical activity without discomfort. Symptoms of cardiac insufficiency or of the anginal syndrome may be present even at rest. If any physical activity is undertaken, discomfort is increased.

From Konstam, M., et al. (1994). *Heart failure: Evaluation and care of patients with left-ventricular systolic dysfunction. Clinical practice guideline No. 11* (AHCPR Pub. No. 94-0612). Rockville, MD: Agency for Health Care Policy and Research, Public Health Service, U.S. Department of Health and Human Services.

Left Ventricular Versus Right Ventricular Failure. The theory of LVF versus RVF is based on the fact that fluid accumulates behind the chamber that fails first. Because the circulatory system is a closed circuit, however, impairments of one ventricle commonly progress to failure of the other. This is referred to as *ventricular interdependence.* Figure 58-4 depicts clinical manifestations that differentiate LVF from RVF.

Left Ventricular Failure. Left ventricular failure causes either pulmonary congestion or a disturbance in the respiratory control mechanisms. These problems in turn precipitate respiratory distress. The degree of distress varies with the client's position, activity, and level of stress.

Dyspnea (difficult breathing) is a subjective problem, and it does not always correlate with the extent of heart failure. Because breathing is usually effortless at rest, the feeling of breathlessness can mean anything from an awareness of breathing to extreme distress. An apprehensive client with only moderate ventricular failure may be more aware of dyspnea than a client with advanced disease. To some degree, exertional dyspnea occurs in all clients. Therefore elicit from the client a description of the degree of exertion that results in the sensation of breathlessness. The mechanism of dyspnea may be related to the decrease in the lung's air volume

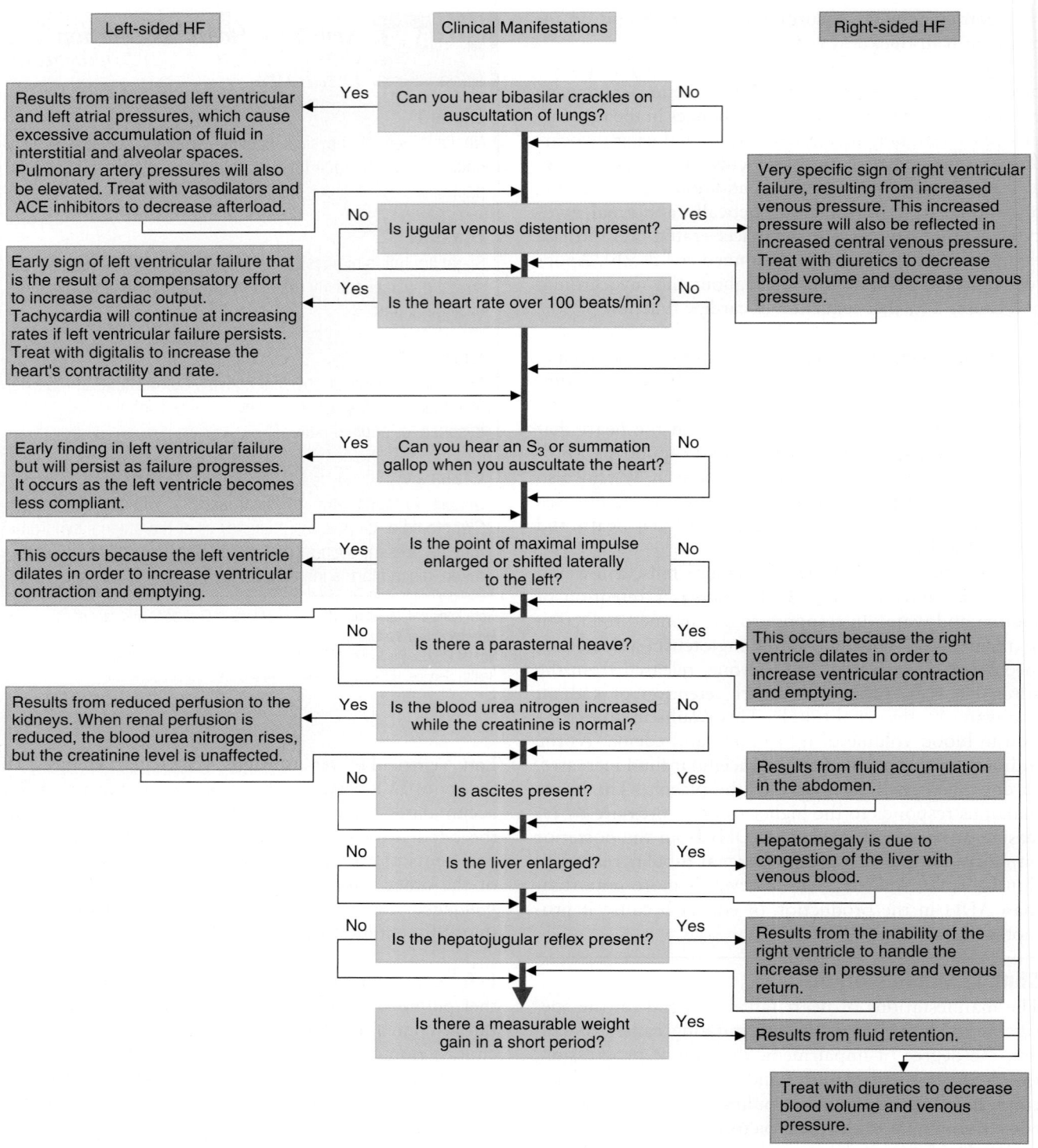

FIGURE 58-4 Clinical manifestations of left-sided and right-sided heart failure. *HF,* Heart failure.

(vital capacity) as air is displaced by blood or interstitial fluid. Pulmonary congestion can eventually reduce the vital capacity of the lungs to 1500 ml or less.

Orthopnea is a more advanced stage of dyspnea. The client often assumes a "three-point position," sitting up with both hands on the knees and leaning forward. Orthopnea develops because the supine position increases the amount of blood returning from the lower extremities to the heart and lungs (preload). The client learns to avoid respiratory distress at night by supporting the head and thorax on pillows. In severe heart failure, the client may resort to sleeping upright in a chair.

Paroxysmal nocturnal dyspnea (PND) resembles the frightening sensation of suffocation. The client suddenly awakens with the feeling of severe suffocation and seeks relief by sitting upright or opening a window for a "breath of fresh air." Respirations may be labored and wheezing *(cardiac asthma)*. PND represents an acute exacerbation of pulmonary congestion. It stems from a combination of increased venous return to the lungs during recumbency and suppression of the respiratory center to sensory input from the lungs during sleep. Once the client is upright, relief from the attack of PND may not occur for 30 minutes or longer.

Cheyne-Stokes respirations sometimes occur in clients with severe forms of heart failure. Cheyne-Stokes respirations probably result from the prolonged circulation time between the pulmonary circulation and the central nervous system (CNS).

Cough is a common manifestation of LVF. The cough, often hacking, may produce large amounts of frothy, blood-tinged sputum. The client coughs because a large amount of fluid is trapped in the pulmonary tree, irritating the lung mucosa. On auscultation bilateral crackles may be heard.

Cardiovascular manifestations also denote LVF. Inspecting and palpating the precordium may reveal an enlarged or left laterally displaced apical impulse. This occurs because the left ventricle dilates in an effort to supplement ventricular contraction and emptying. Heart gallop (S_3 or S_4) sounds may be an early finding in heart failure as the left ventricle becomes less compliant and its walls vibrate in response to filling during diastole. The appearance of pulsus alternans (alternating strong and weak heartbeats) may also herald the onset of LVF.

Cerebral hypoxia may occur as a result of a decrease in cardiac output, causing inadequate brain perfusion. Depressed cerebral function can cause anxiety, irritability, restlessness, confusion, impaired memory, bad dreams, and insomnia. Impaired ventilation with resultant hypercapnia may also be a precipitant.

Fatigue and muscular weakness are often associated with LVF. Inadequate cardiac output leads to hypoxic tissue and slowed removal of metabolic wastes, which in turn cause the client to tire easily. Disturbances in sleep and rest patterns may worsen fatigue.

Renal changes can occur in both RVF and LVF but are more striking in LVF. Nocturia occurs early in heart failure. During the day the client is upright, blood flow is away from the kidneys, and the formation of urine is reduced. At night urine formation increases as blood flow to the kidneys improves. Nocturia may interfere with effective sleep patterns, which may contribute to fatigue. As cardiac output declines, decreased renal blood flow may result in oliguria, a late manifestation of heart failure.

Complications of Left Ventricular Failure. Acute pulmonary edema, a medical emergency, usually results from LVF. In clients with severe cardiac decompensation, the capillary pressure within the lungs becomes so elevated that fluid is pushed from the circulating blood into the interstitium and then into the alveoli, bronchioles, and bronchi. The resulting pulmonary edema, if untreated, may cause death from suffocation. Clients with pulmonary edema literally drown in their own fluids. The dramatic manifestations of acute pulmonary edema terrify the client and his or her significant others. See the Critical Monitoring feature on Acute Pulmonary Edema below for typical manifestations.

Right Ventricular Failure. When right ventricle functioning decreases, peripheral edema and venous congestion of the organs develop. Liver enlargement *(hepatomegaly)* and abdominal pain occur as the liver becomes congested with venous blood. If this occurs rapidly, stretching of the capsule surrounding the liver causes severe discomfort. The client may notice either a constant aching or a sharp pain in the right upper quad-

CRITICAL MONITORING

Acute Pulmonary Edema

- Severe dyspnea
- Orthopnea
- Pallor
- Tachycardia
- Expectoration of large amounts of frothy, blood-tinged sputum
- Fear
- Wheezing
- Sweating
- Bubbling respirations
- Cyanosis
- Nasal flaring
- Use of accessory breathing muscles
- Tachypnea
- Vasoconstriction
- Hypoxia in ABG findings

rant. In chronic heart failure, abdominal tenderness generally disappears.

In severe RVF, the lobules of the liver may become so congested with venous blood that they become anoxic. Anoxia leads to necrosis of the lobules. In long-standing heart failure, these necrotic areas may become fibrotic and then sclerotic. As a result a condition called *cardiac cirrhosis* develops, manifested by ascites and jaundice.

In chronic heart failure, the increased workload of the heart and the extreme work of breathing increase the metabolic demands of the body. Anorexia, nausea, and bloating develop secondary to venous congestion of the gastrointestinal tract. The combination of increased metabolic needs and decreased caloric intake results in a marked wasting of tissue mass, called *cardiac cachexia.* Anorexia and nausea may also result from digitalis toxicity.

Dependent edema is one of the early manifestations of RVF. Venous congestion in the peripheral vascular beds causes increased hydrostatic capillary pressure. Capillary hydrostatic pressure overwhelms the opposing pressure of plasma proteins, and fluid shifts out of the capillary beds and into the interstitial spaces, with resultant pitting edema. Edema is usually symmetrical and occurs in the dependent parts of the body, where venous pressure is highest. In ambulatory clients edema begins in the feet and ankles and moves up the lower legs. It is most noticeable at the end of the day and often subsides after a night's rest. In the recumbent client, pitting edema may develop in the presacral area and, as it worsens, progress to the genital region and medial thighs. Concurrent jugular vein distention differentiates the edema of heart failure from that of lymphatic obstruction, cirrhosis, and hypoproteinemia.

Anasarca, a late manifestation in heart failure, is substantial and generalized edema. It can involve the upper extremities, genital area, and thoracic and abdominal walls. Cyanosis of the nail beds appears as venous congestion reduces peripheral blood flow.

Clients with heart failure often feel anxious, frightened, and depressed. Almost all clients realize that the heart is a vital organ and that when the heart begins to fail, health also fails. As the course of the disease progresses and manifestations worsen, the client may have an overwhelming fear of permanent disability and death. Clients express their fears in varying ways: nightmares, insomnia, acute anxiety, depression, or withdrawal from reality.

Backward Versus Forward Failure. The clinical presentation of heart failure arises from inadequate cardiac output, the pooling of blood behind the failing chamber, or both. *Backward* failure focuses on the ventricle's inability to eject completely, which increases ventricular filling pressures, causing venous and pulmonary congestion. *Forward* failure is a problem of inadequate perfusion. It results when reduced contractility produces a de-

crease in stroke volume and cardiac output. As cardiac output falls, blood flow to vital organs and peripheral tissues diminishes. This causes mental confusion, muscular weakness, and renal retention of sodium and water. Each of these types of failure is usually present to some degree in the client with heart failure.[1,41]

High-Output Versus Low-Output Failure. *High-output* failure occurs when the heart, despite normal-output to high-output levels, is simply not able to meet the accelerated needs of the body. Causes include sepsis, Paget's disease, beriberi, anemia, thyrotoxicosis, arteriovenous fistula, and pregnancy.

Low-output failure occurs in most forms of heart disease, resulting in hypoperfusion of tissue cells. The underlying disorder is related not to increased metabolic needs of the tissues but to poor ventricular pumping action and a low cardiac output.

Acute Versus Chronic Heart Failure. The onset of heart failure may be *acute,* as when a client experiences an MI, or *gradual,* as in chronic heart failure. In chronic heart faiure, there is a progression of compensatory events: a decrease in contractility, neurohormonal activation, increased preload and afterload, and finally cardiac remodeling.[3]

Diagnostic Findings

The diagnosis of heart failure rests primarily on presenting manifestations and pertinent data from the client's health history. Diagnostic studies assist in determining the underlying cause and the degree of heart failure. A new laboratory measurement of B-type natriuretic peptide (BNP) is now included in the diagnosis of heart failure. Additional studies include an echocardiogram, chest x-ray, and ECG.

B-type natriuretic peptide is a protein secreted from the ventricles in response to overload, such as occurs in heart failure. As the degree of heart failure worsens, the level of BNP secreted into the blood increases. Higher levels of BNP are correlated with a diagnosis of heart failure.[13]

Two-dimensional (2-D) echocardiogram, coupled with Doppler flow studies, provides information about cardiac chamber size and ventricular function. These tests aids in assessing myocardial, valvular, congenital, endocardial, and pericardial heart disease,[3] allowing the clinician to determine whether the dysfunction is systolic or diastolic.

In LVF, chest x-ray often depicts an enlarged cardiac silhouette, pulmonary and venous congestion, and interstitial edema. On x-ray interstitial edema produces images called Kerley's B lines. Pleural effusions may develop and generally reflect biventricular failure.

Arterial blood gas analysis is performed. Early heart failure with pulmonary edema may lead to respiratory alkalosis that is due to hyperventilation. As the disorder progresses and oxygenation becomes more impaired, acidosis develops. Pulse oximetry values show decreased oxygen levels.

Liver enzymes may reflect the degree of liver failure. Elevated blood urea nitrogen (BUN) and creatinine levels reflect decreased renal perfusion.

An ECG may give clues to the cause of LVF. Abnormalities in the ECG arise from the underlying cardiac disorder and from therapeutic agents. It may demonstrate evidence of a prior MI, dysrhythmias, or left ventricular dysfunction.

Outcome Management
■ Medical Management

When clients experience acute heart failure, the body compensates in many ways. The short-term effects from these compensatory mechanisms are beneficial and directed toward restoration of normal cardiac output. If cardiac output continues to decline, however, these same compensatory mechanisms become counterproductive and lead to progressive deterioration in cardiac function.

The use of various drugs is typically the mode of therapy for the treatment of heart failure; however, mechanical devices may provide respite for the heart in acute failure. The most common devices are ventricular assist devices (see later discussion) and counterpulsation (see Chapter 59). The goals of the management are to improve ventricular pump performance, reduce myocardial workload, and prevent further heart failure by affecting the process of cardiac remodeling.

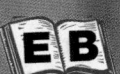 See the Complementary and Alternative Therapy features on Hawthorn Extract for Treating Heart Failure and on CoQ10 Supplements and Congestive Heart Failure, below.

Improve Ventricular Pump Performance

Supplemental Oxygen. High concentrations of oxygen by mask or cannula are provided to relieve hypoxia and dyspnea and to improve oxygen-carbon dioxide exchange. For hypoxemia, partial rebreather masks with a flow rate of 8 to 10 L/min can be used to deliver oxygen concentrations of 40% to 70%. A non-rebreathing mask can achieve even higher oxygen concentrations. If these methods do not raise the arterial oxygen tension (Pao_2) above 60 mm Hg, the client may need intubation and ventilatory management. Intubation also provides a route for removing secretions from the bronchi. If severe bronchospasm or bronchoconstriction occurs, bronchodilators are given. The heart rhythm is monitored because some bronchodilators may lead to dysrhythmias.

Digoxin. Digoxin exerts a direct and beneficial effect on myocardial contraction in the failing heart. Improved cardiac output enhances kidney perfusion, which may create a mild diuresis of sodium and water. Digoxin does not appear to have an effect on long-term mortality in clients with heart failure.[1] It is used in clients who remain symptomatic despite ACE inhibitor and beta-blocker therapy. It is very effective in heart failure associated with low cardiac output caused by ischemic, rheumatic, hypertensive, or congenital heart disease. Digoxin therapy may also be initiated to control the ventricular response in atrial fibrillation, the most common dysrhythmia in heart failure. Digoxin is not given for heart failure associated with high cardiac output states, such as anemia and thyrotoxicosis. Digoxin is contraindicated in constrictive pericarditis or cardiac tamponade and should be used with caution in clients who

---

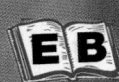

COMPLEMENTARY AND ALTERNATIVE THERAPY

Hawthorn Extract for Treating Heart Failure

A meta-analysis was conducted on 13 trials that met the inclusion criteria for this study. In most studies, hawthorn was used as an adjunct to conventional treatment of heart failure. A variety of parameters improved with hawthorn treatment, and clinical manifestations such as dyspnea and fatigue improved significantly with hawthorn versus placebo. Reported side effects were minimal but included: nausea, dizziness, and cardiac and gastrointestinal complaints. The conclusion of the meta-analysis suggests a significant benefit of hawthorn extract as a potential adjunctive treatment for chronic heart failure.

Reference

Pittler, M., Schmidt, K., & Ernst, E. (2003). Hawthorn extract for treating chronic heart failure: Meta-analysis of randomized trials. *American Journal of Medicine, 114,* 665-674.

COMPLEMENTARY AND ALTERNATIVE THERAPY

CoQ10 Supplements and Congestive Heart Failure

The research on CoQ10 supplements for heart failure has been mixed, and more placebo-controlled trials are needed; however, researchers conducted such a trial on 46 clients (39 men, 7 women) with congestive heart failure. Individuals took either a 200 mg/day CoQ10 supplement or placebo for 6 months. Although the blood levels of CoQ10 increased dramatically in those who took the supplement, no beneficial effect over placebo was observed. CoQ10 did not affect the ejection fraction, peak oxygen consumption, or exercise duration in clients with heart failure who were also receiving standard medical therapy.

Reference

Khatta, M., et al. (2000). The effect of coenzyme Q10 in patients with congestive heart failure. *Annals of Internal Medicine, 132,* 636-640.

have had acute MI because it increases myocardial oxygen demand.

Digoxin has a narrow therapeutic index, and toxicity occurs in about one in five clients. Clients at risk for the toxic effects of digoxin are older adults; those with advanced heart disease, severe dysrhythmias, or acute MI; and those concurrently using quinidine, verapamil, and amiodarone. Digoxin dosage may need to be reduced if the client is taking any of these medications. Digoxin toxicity is more prevalent when the serum concentration is equal to or greater than 2 μg/L, serum potassium is less than 3 mEq/L, or serum magnesium is low. Digoxin toxicity may be a life-threatening condition (see the Critical Monitoring feature on Digoxin Toxicity below).

Inotropes. Inotropic agents such as dopamine, dobutamine, and amrinone may be ordered for clients with severe low-output heart failure. These medications facilitate myocardial contractility and enhance stroke volume.

Dopamine is a naturally occurring catecholamine with alpha-adrenergic, beta-adrenergic, and dopaminergic activity. Dopamine, given in small doses (<4 μg/kg/min), stimulates the dopaminergic receptors in the renal, mesenteric, cerebral, and coronary vascular beds. Vasodilation in the kidney is especially advantageous, leading to improved GFR, urine output, and excretion of sodium.

The alpha-adrenergic and beta-adrenergic receptors in the vasculature and myocardium are affected by mod-

---

CRITICAL MONITORING

Digoxin Toxicity

Digoxin remains a common medication for clients in heart failure because it increases ventricular contractility and emptying by slowing the heart rate, which promotes ventricular filling. Digoxin preparations, however, have a narrow window of therapeutic efficacy, and toxicity from digitalis is not uncommon. Nurses play a significant role in early detection of the subtle manifestations of digitalis toxicity. The diagnosis of digoxin toxicity remains a clinical challenge, in part because therapeutic and toxic digoxin concentrations overlap from one individual to another.

Several causes are known:
- Deteriorating renal function, especially in clients with hyperthyroid conditions
- Dehydration
- Electrolyte imbalances, especially potassium and magnesium imbalances
- Myocardial ischemia
- Acidosis
- Medication interactions:
    Amiloride
    Amiodarone
    Amphotericin B
    Calcium-channel blockers
    Hydrochlorothiazide and other loop diuretics
    Indomethacin
    Propafenone
    Quinidine
    Quinine
    Spironolactone
    Triamterene

Clinical Manifestations

Nausea, vomiting, diarrhea
Anorexia
Palpitations
Irregular heart block, bradycardia and junctional tachycardia
Confusion

Lethargy, ataxia
Visual changes (unusual)
- Halos or rings of light around objects
- Seeing lights or bright spots
- Changes in color perception, especially yellow green
- Blind spots in vision
- Diagnosis

Serum levels of digitalis are used to determine whether toxicity is present. A key factor in determining digoxin toxicity is whether or not blood is drawn at least 6 hours after the last digoxin dose, which ensures that adequate distribution of the drug has been achieved before blood sampling. Blood levels would not be elevated in acute forms of toxicity, such as overdose. Toxic plasma levels are over 2.4 ng/ml.

Treatment

Because of its long half life of 38 to 48 hours, treatment is directed at removing the drug. Acute toxicity can be treated with gastric lavage, activated charcoal to limit absorption, or digoxin-Fab fragments (Digibind), which is an antidote. Digibind is composed of digoxin-specific antibody fragments prepared from the immunoglobulin G (IgG) of sheep immunized with digoxin. The smaller Fab fragment avidly binds digoxin but is minimally immunogenic in humans and is excreted renally. Clients are admitted to an ICU for cardiac monitoring. Factors that led to the toxicity are addressed.

Prevention

Assess potential drug-drug interactions
Assess for manifestations of toxicity
Assess electrolyte levels (potassium, magnesium)
Hold the medication if the heart rate below 60 beats/min or a new dysrhythmia has developed
Push IV digoxin slowly over 5 minutes
Schedule serum digoxin levels to be drawn at least 4 hours after an intravenous (IV) dose and 6 hours after an oral dose

erate doses of dopamine (4 to 8 μg/kg/min). The results are increases in heart rate, stroke volume, and cardiac output. Alpha-adrenergic effects, such as intense vasoconstriction, dominate when dopamine is given in doses larger than 10 μg/kg/min. Although dopamine may improve cardiac output, it may do so at the expense of the myocardium by leading to tachycardia, which increases myocardial oxygen demands and decreases myocardial oxygen supply. This change may prove costly to the already ischemic myocardium. Moderate doses of dopamine also restrict blood flow to the kidney.

Another inotropic agent, dobutamine, is a synthetic derivative of dopamine that produces strong beta-stimulatory effects within the myocardium; it increases heart rate, atrioventricular (AV) conduction, and myocardial contractility. Dobutamine is capable of increasing cardiac output without increasing myocardial oxygen demands or reducing coronary blood flow.

Amrinone is also used to increase cardiac output in severe heart failure. In addition to the positive inotropic effects, amrinone increases renal blood flow and GFR.

Reduce Workload

Reduce Afterload. Vasodilating agents have become an increasingly important intervention in clients with heart failure. Vasodilators vary in their mechanisms of action, which include the following:

- Direct dilation of veins
- Dilation of arterioles
- Combined action on veins and arterioles
- Inhibition of ACE

Direct Dilation of Veins. Venous dilators relax venous smooth muscle and increase the capacity of the systemic venous bed; blood is "trapped" in the veins, and venous return to the heart is decreased. This increased venous capacity reduces preload. Examples include nitroglycerin and isosorbide dinitrate.

Dilation of Arterioles. Arteriolar dilators reduce systemic arteriolar tone, which decreases peripheral vascular resistance and afterload. Reduction in afterload reduces the left ventricular workload and increases cardiac output. Improved renal perfusion may initiate diuresis. ACE inhibitors are commonly used.

Combined Action on Veins and Arterioles. Combined venous and arteriolar dilators decrease both preload and afterload. Sodium nitroprusside helps to manage severe heart failure. A potent vasodilator, sodium nitroprusside relaxes the smooth muscles of both veins and arterioles. It does not directly affect the heart muscle or heart rate.

Inhibition of Angiotensin-Converting Enzyme Inhibitors. Angiotensin-converting-enzyme inhibitors are now considered first-choice treatment and are the cornerstone of heart-failure drug therapy. ACE inhibitors have proved to slow the progression of heart failure by reducing remodeling changes in the heart. ACE inhibitors reduce afterload by blocking the production of angiotensin, a potent vasoconstrictor. They also increase re-

nal blood flow and decrease renal vascular resistance, which enhances diuresis. Side effects include orthostatic hypotension, persistent cough and kidney problems, skin rashes, an altered sense of taste, and hyperkalemia. Potassium levels should be monitored, especially if diuretics or potassium supplements are being used.[20,28]

Beta-adrenergic antagonists (beta-blockers) are used to inhibit the effects of the sympathetic nervous system. They increase clinical improvement and decrease mortality. These findings are apparent when clients are concurrently receiving ACE inhibitory therapy, suggesting that the combination of two agents that have inhibitory effects on two neurohormonal systems may have an additive effect.[1]

Nesiritide (recombinant human BNP) is a newer medication for the treatment of heart failure. Nesiritide mimics BNP secreted by the ventricles during heart failure, producing vasodilation and diuresis. The medication is given intravenously, and blood pressure response is closely monitored.

Reduce Preload. Diuretics enhance renal excretion of sodium and water, which reduces circulating blood volume, diminishes preload, and lessens systemic and pulmonary congestion. Table 58-4 describes the characteristics of a commonly used diuretic. Although they are effective, diuretics should be administered cautiously because of their side effect profile. Diuretics can produce mild to severe electrolyte imbalance. Hypokalemia, a particularly dangerous problem, potentiates digitalis toxicity and can cause myocardial weakness and cardiac dysrhythmias. Moreover, vigorous diuresis may produce hypovolemia and hypotension, jeopardizing cardiac output. Many people find it best to take diuretics in the morning so that trips to the bathroom to urinate happen during the day. Taking diuretics in the evening or at night often results in interrupted sleep because the urge to empty the bladder continues for hours.

Position the Client. The client is placed in a high Fowler position or chair to reduce pulmonary venous congestion and to relieve the dyspnea. The legs are maintained in a dependent position as much as possible. Even though the legs are edematous, they should not be elevated. Elevating the legs increases venous return rapidly.

Reduce Fluid Retention. Controlling sodium and water retention improves cardiac performance. Sodium restrictions are placed on the diet to prevent, control, or eliminate edema. Diets with 2 to 4 g of sodium are usually prescribed (Table 58-5).

From the use of some loop diuretics, potassium is lost via the kidneys, which can lead to dysrhythmias and electrolyte imbalances. Hypokalemia sensitizes the myocardium to digitalis and therefore predisposes the client to digitalis toxicity. Potassium supplements and adequate dietary potassium are important.

TABLE 58-4 *Nursing Implications for Medications Used in Heart Failure*

Class (Example)	Assessing Therapeutic Responses	Assessing Adverse Responses	Nursing Implications
Decreases Myocardial Workload			
Diuretic (furosemide)	Urine output should increase. The reduction in circulating volume decreases central venous pressures, pulmonary congestion, and peripheral edema. It may also decrease systemic blood pressure.	Clients may experience orthostatic hypotension, hypokalemia, electrolyte imbalance, blurred vision, headache, loss of appetite, hearing loss, and stomach cramps and pain.	Monitor electrolytes, intake and output, weight, blood pressure, and renal function. Intravenous (IV) administration should not exceed 0.5 mg/kg/min, and hearing loss is possible with high doses. Teach clients to rise slowly to avoid orthostatic hypotension.
Venous vasodilator (nitroglycerin)	Reducing peripheral resistance decreases blood pressure, and the reduction in preload may decrease the heart rate and pulmonary congestion. Vasodilation of coronary vessels should keep clients free of anginal pain.	Clients may experience flushing, weakness, headache, postural hypotension, dizziness, and reflex tachycardia.	Monitor clients for hypotension. Ointment and patches should be rotated daily, and clients may need a nitrate-free interval to avoid tolerance. Avoid getting ointment on the fingers. IV nitroglycerin should be in glass bottles with tubing specific for nitroglycerin. If a client is receiving continuous IV nitroglycerin, the blood pressure and heart rate should be continually monitored.
Vein and arteriole dilator (sodium nitroprusside)	The peripheral vasodilation decreases the blood pressure. The decrease in afterload increases cardiac output by enhancing contractility.	Clients may experience hypotension, sweating, palpitations, restlessness, headache, nausea, and vomiting. Cyanide toxicity is possible in clients with decreased liver function, and thiocyanate toxicity is possible in clients with decreased kidney function or anyone who has prolonged use of nitroprusside. Signs of thiocyanate toxicity include psychoses, blurred vision, tinnitus, and seizures. Signs of cyanide toxicity include metabolic acidosis, tachycardia, decreased pulse and reflexes, and coma.	Solution must be mixed with 5% dextrose in water (D_5W) and wrapped with opaque material to protect it from light. Blue color indicates almost complete degradation to cyanide. Constant blood pressure and heart rate monitoring is necessary. Monitor acid/base status, because acidosis can be the earliest indicator of cyanide toxicity. Monitor thiocyanate levels if infusion is for more than 3 days or if the dose is more than 4 mg/kg/min.
Angiotensin-converting enzyme (ACE) inhibitor (captopril)	The decrease in afterload increases cardiac output by enhancing contractility. The neurohormonal effects include inhibition of ACE and vasodilation and a decrease in systemic blood pressure.	Clients may experience oliguria, chest pain, palpitations, insomnia, dizziness, fatigue, nausea, vomiting, maculopapular rash, and cough.	Monitor blood pressure. Administer 1 hr before meals. Two weeks of therapy may be necessary before the full therapeutic effect is achieved. May increase blood urea nitrogen, creatinine, liver enzymes, and potassium levels. If given concurrently with digoxin, it may cause an increase in digoxin levels.

Drug	Action	Side Effects	Nursing Implications
Beta-adrenergic antagonist (atenolol)	The effects of blockade of beta-adrenergic receptors are seen clinically by decreased heart rate, blood pressure, and cardiac output. The neurohormonal response inhibits the sympathetic nervous system that causes vasodilation and decreasing automaticity in the heart. Clinically, this decreases blood pressure and the heart rate and the incidence of dysrhythmias.	Clients may experience bronchoconstriction, severe bradycardia, or hypotension. They may also experience atrioventricular conduction abnormalities, dizziness, confusion, constipation or diarrhea, and vomiting. Male clients may experience impotence.	Clients must be instructed not to stop taking medication abruptly because they may experience angina. The drug should not be given in clients with a history of bronchospastic pulmonary disease. If the client is diabetic, it may potentiate hypoglycemia. The nurse must monitor the heart rate, rhythm, and blood pressure frequently and assess pulmonary status for bronchoconstriction.
Cardiac glycoside (digoxin)	The increased contractility increases cardiac output. Suppression of the atrioventricular node decreases the heart rate.	The client may experience nausea, vomiting, abdominal pain, diarrhea, anorexia, bradycardia, dysrhythmias, drowsiness, fatigue, and visual disturbances. Digoxin toxicity is a potentially fatal condition and must be assessed for whenever a client is on digoxin therapy.	Always take apical pulse for 1 minute and hold if the rate is under 60 beat/min or if the pulse is newly irregular. The most recent digoxin and electrolyte levels must be assessed before administration. IV doses should be given over 5 minutes. Serum levels should be drawn no sooner than 4 hr after an IV dose and 6 hr after an oral dose.
Inotrope (dobutamine)	The enhanced myocardial contractility increases cardiac output and may increase the heart rate and blood pressure.	Clients may experience anginal pain, increased heart rate, palpitations, premature ventricular beats, paresthesia, headache, nausea, and vomiting. Extravasation should be avoided; if present, treat with phentolamine.	Monitor the electrocardiogram and blood pressure continuously. Observe for hypertension and tachycardia. Use a central line for administration if possible. Observe the IV site frequently.
Inotrope (dopamine)	The enhanced myocardial contractility increases the systolic blood pressure, heart rate, and cardiac output. Improved circulation to renal vascular beds results in increased urine output in low to moderate doses.	The client may experience palpitations, cardiac dysrhythmias, tachycardia, vasoconstriction, or hypotension. Extravasation should be avoided; if present, treat with phentolamine.	Continuous monitoring of blood pressure and heart rate is necessary. In higher doses, observe for decreases in urine output, cool extremities, and decreased pulses. The IV site must be monitored frequently to avoid extravasation. Central lines are preferred, especially in clients with occlusive vascular disease or diabetic endarteritis. The hemodynamic effects are dose dependent.

Data from Armstrong L.L. (Ed.) (1998). *The University of Chicago Hospitals Formulary of Accepted Drugs.* Hudson, OH: Lexi-Comp.

TABLE 58-5	*Sodium Content of Selected Foods*

Foods Low in Sodium

Dairy products	Skim milk, eggs, cottage cheese, cream cheese, ice cream
Meats*	Turkey, chicken, veal, lamb, liver, fresh fish, tuna packed in water (meats should be unprocessed)
Fruits and vegetables*	Any fresh or frozen food in this group
Beverages	Any juice (except tomato or V8 brand vegetable), coffee, tea, bottled water
Breads	Some breads and cereals
Seasonings	Garlic, onion, bay leaf, pepper, dill, nutmeg, rosemary, allspice, thyme, sage, caraway, cinnamon, almond and vanilla extract, fresh dried herbs
Fats	Margarine, oils, shortening, unsalted salad dressings
Desserts	Sherbet, fruit ice, gelatin, fruit drinks
Miscellaneous	Unbuttered, unsalted popcorn; unsalted nuts; vinegar

Foods High in Sodium

Milk and dairy products	Aged, hard cheese; pasteurized, processed cheese; buttermilk
Meats	Sausage, frankfurters, ham, bacon, corned beef; all smoked, pickled, or cured meats; canned meats, salami, most luncheon meats, beef jerky; frozen "TV" dinners
Fruits and vegetables	Pickled or canned fruits and vegetables, olives, sauerkraut, pickles
Breads and cereals	Salted crackers, macaroni and cheese, pretzels, rye rolls, pizza, commercial pancake mixes
Beverages	Tomato juice, V8 vegetable juice, beef broth, bouillon
Fats	Commercial salad dressings, dips and party spreads, peanut butter
Seasonings	Garlic, celery, or onion salt; Accent, monosodium glutamate (MSG), meat tenderizer, soy sauce, ketchup, steak sauce, mustard, canned soup
Desserts	Fruit pies, doughnuts, cakes, commercial puddings
Miscellaneous	Baking soda, baking powder, salted popcorn, salted nuts, potato chips

*Food sources high in potassium.

It is usually not necessary to restrict fluid intake in clients with mild or moderate heart failure. In more advanced cases, however, it is beneficial to limit water to 1000 ml/day (1 L/day). The reason is that excessive water intake tends to dilute the amount of sodium in body fluids and may produce a low-salt syndrome (*hyponatremia*). Hyponatremia is characterized by lethargy and weakness; it results more often from the combination of a restricted sodium diet, increased sodium loss during diuresis, and excessive water intake.

Use Ventricular Assist Devices. Advances continue to be made in perfecting methods of mechanical ventricular support. The goal of mechanical circulatory support is to decompress the hypokinetic ventricle, decrease myocardial workload, reduce oxygen demands, and maintain adequate systemic perfusion to sustain end-organ function. In the client with heart failure, the two most common options are ventricular assist devices (VADs) as a bridge to transplantation and as permanent support.[32] VADs have the capability to support circulation, either partially or totally, until the heart recovers or is replaced. Devices may be right ventricular, left ventricular, or biventricular VADs. Complications of any VAD include bleeding, hemolysis, thromboembolism, infection, and multiorgan failure.[6,16,41] (See the Bridge to Critical Care feature on Left Ventricular Assist Devices on p. 1611.)

Traditionally non-pulsatile pumps have been used as VADs. Difficulties with these devices include end-organ dysfunction, thromboembolic complications, and the need for full anticoagulation. Their use in clients with heart failure is diminishing because better technology has become available. These pumps can be used for a relatively short period of about 10 days.

Total artificial hearts provide complete control of the cardiovascular system and allow total mobility. Their use is limited in smaller people because the device may not fit the client's small body. Complications include infection, thromboembolism, and the possibility of mechanical failure. Initially total artificial hearts were limited to people awaiting transplantation. Currently these devices are being used when there are contraindications to transplantation, such as advanced age.[41]

Extracorporeal membrane oxygenation (ECMO) systems are widely used for short-term hemodynamic stabilization. These devices remove blood from the inferior vena cava to a centrifugal pump that pumps the blood to an oxygenator. The oxygenated blood is returned to the client via the femoral artery. Long-term use (<48 hours) does not promote recovery. In addition, bleeding is a concern because anticoagulation therapy is needed.

Reduce Stress and Risk of Injury. In addition to improving ventricular pump performance and reducing myocardial workload, the client also needs to reduce physical and emotional stress. Sometimes clinicians overlook rest as an intervention to diminish the workload of the heart. The proper use of rest as the initial step in management offers many benefits. Rest can promote diuresis, slow the heart rate, and relieve dyspnea, all of which allow more conservative use of pharmacologic agents (e.g., ACE inhibitors, diuretics, beta-blockers).

Whether the physician prescribes complete, modified bed rest depends on the seriousness of the client's condition. The physician may prescribe a mild sedative or small doses of barbiturates and tranquilizers to promote rest and overcome problems of restlessness, insomnia, and anxiety.

The client may also be at risk for injury because of immobility. The client should be confined to bed only long enough to regain cardiac reserve but not so long as to promote complications of immobility. Give the client confined to bed rest specific guidelines to prevent the harmful effects of immobility. Clients should perform passive leg exercises several times daily to prevent venous stasis, which may lead to the formation of venous thrombi and pulmonary emboli. Anticoagulant therapy prevents these potentially deadly complications.

■ Nursing Management of the Medical Client

The following are the goals of nursing management for the client with heart failure:

- To monitor for reduced cardiac output
- To maintain adequate fluid balance
- To reduce myocardial workload
- To assess response to medical therapies
- To educate the client about self-care after discharge (see the Bridge to Home Health Care feature on Managing Heart Failure, below)

Consider the psychosocial effect of heart failure on the client and family. Nursing diagnoses that may apply to the client with heart failure are discussed in the Care Plan feature on The Client with Heart Failure on pp. 1664 to 1668.

Text continued on p. 1668

BRIDGE TO HOME HEALTH CARE

Managing Heart Failure

One third of all clients hospitalized for heart failure are readmitted within 90 days of discharge. Problems with self-monitoring techniques, medication, and diet are the primary reasons. Home health and outpatient care nurses can make a positive difference in readmission rates through nursing interventions.

Review clients' cardiovascular history, disease etiology, and medical management plan to guide your assessment. Auscultate the heart and lungs during each visit, and look for manifestations of fluid accumulation. Measure blood pressure with both the client sitting and standing. If blood pressure decreases significantly and the client experiences lightheadedness or dizziness, it may be necessary to adjust diuretic or vasoactive medications. Worsening cardiac status or drug toxicities can cause changes in pulse rate or rhythm.

Clients may experience unique manifestations such as fullness in their ears, increased urination at night, and chest heaviness. The client, family members, and informal caregivers need to be educated about the correlation between manifestations and clinical status. Evaluate changes in the prevalence and severity of manifestations. The assessment can include measuring intake and output, abdominal girth and lower extremities, and weight. Instruct clients to call you or their physicians if they lose or gain 2 to 3 pounds in 1 day or 5 to 7 pounds in 1 week. When manifestations are noted and cardiac decompensation is detected early, heart failure can be managed successfully in non-institutional outpatient settings.

Use various techniques to help clients manage their medications. Write the medication schedule clearly, and suggest reminder systems such as pill boxes. Examine all pill bottles for the drug name, strength, expiration date, and available refills. Re-view brand versus generic labeling to minimize confusion and prevent drug administration errors. Simplify dosing frequencies; by limiting doses to twice a day (bid), three times a day (tid), or four times a day (qid), medication administration can be associated with daily routines such as meals and bedtime. Flexible dose times can promote drug tolerance and increase accurate administration. Discourage the use of over-the-counter medications because of the potential for drug interactions.

Limiting sodium intake to 2000 mg a day can help prevent fluid retention. Rarely do clients need to restrict fluid intake to less than 2000 ml/day. Evaluate the client's appetite, meal frequency, portion sizes, and food preferences, and provide appropriate health education. If possible, open cupboards and the refrigerator to gain insight into the client's eating patterns. Suggest a food diary to assess intake accurately. Teach clients, family members, and informal caregivers how to distinguish the sodium content of foods by reading food labels.

Because a client's functional status is often severely impaired, explain energy-conservation techniques before initiating limited mobility and aerobic routines. Even the most severely affected client may benefit from chair exercises done in a sitting position. Instruct clients to keep an activity log to demonstrate their progress toward activity goals. Clients should perceive their activities as only somewhat hard to do and should not participate in activities that worsen their manifestations or produce fatigue.

Clients who have chronic illnesses, including heart failure, often have feelings of depression. Consider whether clients need psychosocial and financial assistance. Antidepressant medications benefit some clients and improve their sense of well-being.

CARE PLAN

The Client with Heart Failure

Nursing Diagnosis. Decreased Cardiac Output related to heart failure or dysrhythmias or both.

Outcomes. The client will have an increase in cardiac output as evidenced by regular cardiac rhythm, heart rate, blood pressure, respirations, and urine output within normal limits.

Interventions	Rationales
1. Assess blood pressure for hypotension or hypertension and respiratory rate for tachypnea q 1 hr (more or less frequently, depending on the client's stability).	1. Hypotension may indicate decreased cardiac output and may lead to a decrease in coronary artery perfusion. Hypertension may be caused by chronic vasoconstriction or may indicate fear or anxiety, and increased respiratory rate may indicate fatigue or increased pulmonary congestion.
2. Assess heart rate and rhythm q 1 hr for tachycardia, or continue monitoring for the presence of dysrhythmias.	2. Tachycardia can increase myocardial and oxygen demands and may be a compensatory mechanism related to the decreased cardiac output (increased heart rate to compensate for decrease in stroke volume). Ventricular enlargement decreases conduction of cardiac impulses and may lead to dysrhythmias. Dysrhythmias further compromise cardiac output by reducing ventricular filling time and myocardial contractility and by increasing myocardial oxygen demands. Common dysrhythmias include premature atrial contractions (PACs), premature ventricular contractions (PVCs), and paroxysmal atrial tachycardia (PAT). Ventricular dysrhythmias must be watched for because they can increase the chance of sudden death.
3. Document rhythm strips q 8 hr and if dysrhythmias occur. Measure and note rate, QRS, PR, and QT intervals and ST segment with each strip and note any deviations from baseline.	3. Documentation of rhythm confirms rhythm and gives a baseline for changes. Changes in the ST segment may indicate myocardial ischemia, which may be present because of decreased coronary artery perfusion.
4. Report dysrhythmias to the physician, or follow protocol for emergency treatment.	4. Dysrhythmias can decrease cardiac output and may lead to life-threatening dysrhythmias.
5. Auscultate heart rate q 2 hr for changes in heart sounds such as murmurs, S_3, or S_4.	5. Delayed filling time, incomplete ejection, and structural changes within the heart and fluid overload may cause abnormal heart sounds detected by auscultation. S_3 may indicate a noncompliant or stiff ventricle, and S_4 may indicate a weak, overdistended ventricle.
6. Monitor lung sounds q 2 hr for adventitious sounds such as crackles and for the presence of coughing.	6. Increased ventricular pressures are transmitted back to the pulmonary circulation, increasing pulmonary capillary hydrostatic pressure and exceeding oncotic pressure fluid moving within the alveolar septum and are evidenced by the auscultation of crackles, increased shortness of breath, and sputum production. This indicates a further decrease in cardiac output and the possibility of the development of pulmonary edema. Coughing can be caused by the increased fluid in the lungs or by angiotensin-converting enzyme (ACE) inhibitors.
7. Monitor intake and output (I & O) and analyze findings q 8 hr and as required (PRN). Note color and amount of urine q 2 hr and PRN.	7. If intake exceeds output, the client is at risk for fluid overload and may not be able to clear fluids because of a decompensating heart. Dark, concentrated urine and oliguria may reflect a decrease in renal perfusion. Diuresis is expected in clients receiving diuretic therapy.

CARE PLAN

Interventions	Rationales
8. Assess for changes in mental status.	8. Change in mental status may indicate decreased cerebral perfusion or hypoxia.
9. Assess peripheral pulses for strength and quality and for pulsus alternans.	9. Decreased strength of peripheral pulses is often found in clients with decreased cardiac output, and a further decrease in pulses from baseline may indicate further cardiac failure. Pulsus alternans may be detected and indicates severe heart failure.
10. Administer prescribed medications and evaluate responses.	10. Prescribed medications are utilized to increase contractility and decrease preload or afterload, and their responses must be evaluated. Therapeutic levels must be monitored. Clients need to be monitored for potential side effects.
11. Encourage physical and psychological rest.	11. Increased physical or mental strain can increase myocardial and oxygen demands.
12. Encourage clients to eat small meals and rest afterward.	12. Larger meals increase myocardial workload and may cause vagal stimulation, which may lead to bradycardia.

Evaluation. Following the administration of ACE inhibitors and diuretics, dyspnea should improve. Heart failure is a chronic disorder and complete resolution is not possible; expect small gains in cardiac output in the days that follow.

Nursing Diagnosis. Excess Fluid Volume related to reduced glomerular filtration, decreased cardiac output, increased antidiuretic hormone (ADH) and aldosterone production, and sodium and water retention.

Outcomes. The client will demonstrate adequate fluid balance as evidenced by output equal to or exceeding intake, clearing breath sounds, and decreasing edema.

Interventions	Rationales
1. Monitor I & O q 4 hr (more or less frequently depending on client's status).	1. I & O balance reflects fluid status.
2. Weigh clients daily.	2. Body weight is a sensitive indicator of fluid balance and an increase indicates fluid volume excess.
3. Assess for presence of peripheral edema.	3. Heart failure causes venous congestion, resulting in increased capillary pressure. When hydrostatic pressure exceeds interstitial pressure, fluids leak out of the capillaries and present as edema in the legs, sacrum, and scrotum.
4. Assess for jugular vein distention, hepatomegaly, and abdominal pain.	4. Elevated volumes in the venae cavae occur as right atrium preload increase from inadequate emptying from right atrium and are transmitted to the jugular vein and manifest as distention; they can also be the cause of hepatomegaly, splenomegaly, and abdominal pain.
5. Follow low-sodium diet or fluid restriction.	5. Decreased systemic blood pressure can trigger renin, leading to a cascade of events that ends with stimulation of aldosterone, which causes increased renal tubular absorption of sodium. Low-sodium diet helps prevent increased sodium retention, which decreases water retention. Fluid restriction may be used to decrease fluid intake, hence decreasing fluid volume excess.
6. Auscultate breath sounds q 2 hr and prn for the presence of crackles and monitor for sputum production.	6. When increased pulmonary capillary hydrostatic pressure exceeds oncotic pressure, fluid moves within the alveolar septum and is evidenced by the auscultation of crackles. Frothy, pink-tinged sputum is an indicator that the client is developing the life-threatening complication of pulmonary edema.

Continued

CARE PLAN

The Client with Heart Failure—cont'd

Interventions	Rationales
7. Administer diuretic therapy as ordered and evaluate effectiveness of the therapy.	7. Diuretics are commonly prescribed to promote the diuresis of accumulated fluid. The nurse should expect an increase in urine output, improved breathing, and weight loss after the client receives diuretic therapy

Evaluation. After administration of diuretics, expect profound urine output if the client has reasonable cardiac output. Weight loss and output should stabilize in 2 to 3 days. Expect fairly rapid improvement in peripheral edema.

Nursing Diagnosis. Impaired Gas Exchange related to fluid in alveoli.

Outcomes. The client will have improved gas exchange as evidenced by decreased dyspnea, no cyanosis, normal arterial blood gases, and a decrease in pulmonary congestion on auscultation.

Interventions	Rationales
1. Auscultate breath sounds q 2 hr.	1. Auscultation of crackles may indicate pulmonary congestion.
2. Encourage the client to turn, cough, and deep breathe and use the incentive spirometer q 2 hr.	2. This will help facilitate oxygen delivery and clear the airways.
3. Administer oxygen as ordered. Monitor for the development of dry nasal mucous membranes and skin changes from the oxygen tubing.	3. Oxygen therapy will improve oxygenation by increasing the amount of oxygen available for delivery. Administration of non-humidified oxygen and dry and injure nasal membranes. Tubing pulled tightly can lead to pressure ulcers on the face and ears.
4. Assess respiratory rate and rhythm q 2 hr and PRN.	4. Increased respiratory rate indicates difficulty with oxygenation, and a decreased respiratory rate may indicate impending respiratory failure.
5. Assess for cyanosis q 4 hr and prn.	5. Circumoral cyanosis or cyanosis to the finger tips or end of nose indicates hypoxia from lack of oxygen in peripheral tissues.
6. Position the client to facilitate breathing and observe for paroxysmal nocturnal dyspnea.	6. Fowler position and orthopneic positioning facilitate diaphragmatic excursion. Paroxysmal nocturnal dyspnea may occur because as the client assumes a supine position, venous return to the heart is increased. This increase in return increases preload and will increase pulmonary capillary hydrostatic pressure and lead to pulmonary alveolar edema.
7. Monitor pulse oximetry. Move the probe to ensure good contact with the skin or ear.	7. A low SaO_2 reflects hypoxia.
8. Obtain arterial blood gases if ordered.	8. Arterial blood gases indicate whether the client has hypoxia, acidosis, or both.
9. Administer diuretic therapy as ordered, and monitor for effectiveness.	9. Diuretics promote fluid loss in the alveoli as well as systemically.

Evaluation. Expect dyspnea to improve rapidly once the diuresis has occurred unless the client has significant lung disease from other problems. Because the lung is a low-pressure area, the redevelopment of edema in the lung can occur quickly and continued monitoring is important.

Nursing Diagnosis. Ineffective Tissue Perfusion related to decreased cardiac output.

Outcomes. The client will have adequate tissue perfusion as evidenced by warm, dry skin, peripheral pulses, and adequate urine output.

CARE PLAN

Interventions	Rationales
1. Note color and temperature of the skin q 4 hr.	1. Cool, pale skin is indicative of decreased peripheral tissue perfusion.
2. Monitor peripheral pulses q 4 hr.	2. Decreased pulses are indicative of decreased tissue perfusion from vasoconstriction of the vessels.
3. Provide a warm environment.	3. A warm environment promotes vasodilatation, which decreases preload and promotes tissue perfusion.
4. Encourage active range of motion.	4. Range of motion helps decrease venous pooling and promotes tissue perfusion.
5. Monitor urine output q 4 hr.	5. Decreased perfusion to the kidneys may result in oliguria.
6. Protect the skin from trauma by applying cotton socks or fleece boots.	6. Poorly perfused skin heals slowly, if at all once injured.

Evaluation. Once cardiac output is improved, expect peripheral blood flow to improve slightly. Pre-existing atherosclerosis will prevent the skin from making dramatic improvement, but the client should return to baseline condition.

Nursing Diagnosis. Risk for Activity Intolerance related to decreased cardiac output.

Outcomes. The client will have improved levels of activity without dyspnea.

Interventions	Rationales
1. Space nursing activities.	1. Clustering activities increases myocardial demand and may cause extreme fatigue.
2. Schedule rest periods.	2. Rest periods help alleviate fatigue and decrease myocardial workload.
3. Monitor the client's response to activities.	3. Dyspnea, tachycardia, angina, diaphoresis, dysrhythmias, and hypotension are all indicative that the activity required more myocardial demand than the body was able to compensate for. Assess vital signs before and after an activity. The time it requires for the vital signs to return to baseline indicates the degree of cardiac deconditioning.
4. Increase activity as ordered or according to the rehabilitation nurse's directions.	4. Gradually and appropriately increasing physical activity may help the client gain cardiac conditioning and improve activity tolerance.
5. Instruct the client to avoid activities that increase cardiac workload.	5. Activities such as stair climbing, working with arms above the head, or sustained arm movement may cause extreme fatigue and demand more cardiac output than the body can supply.

Evaluation. The client will perform spaced activities without dyspnea and will gradually increase activity tolerance. This goal will require time; deconditioning due to marked dyspnea often prevents rapid improvement.

Nursing Diagnosis. Risk for Impaired Skin Integrity related to decreased tissue perfusion and activities.

Outcomes. The client will have reduced risk of skin impairment.

Interventions	Rationales
1. Reposition the client q 2 hr.	1. Changing position frequently deters the formation of pressure ulcers by decreasing the amount of time of pressure on any given area.
2. Provide a therapeutic mattress or bed while the client is in bed.	2. Pressure-reduction mattresses and beds are available to decrease the pressure on the sacrum when the client is in bed.

Continued

CARE PLAN

The Client with Heart Failure—cont'd

Interventions	Rationales
3. Assess the skin, especially bony prominences, for redness each shift and as needed. Use protective devices if redness is noted.	3. Redness is indicative of increased pressure to an area and is the first sign of breakdown. Risk areas include the sacrum, coccyx, heels, elbows, and back of the head.
4. Float the heels from the bed if the client has little spontaneous leg movement.	4. The posterior prominence of the heels makes them high risk for breakdown in clients positioned in Fowler's position.
5. Assist the client with morning care and lubricate the skin.	5. Clients may have difficulty providing themselves with adequate skin care, and the nurse must ensure the skin is clean and has proper moisture to prevent cracking.

Evaluation. Intact skin should remain intact.

Nursing Diagnosis. Risk for Anxiety related to decreased cardiac output, hypoxia, diagnosis of heart failure, and fear of death or debilitation.

Outcomes. The client will not exhibit manifestations of anxiety and will be able to express concerns.

Interventions	Rationales
1. Provide a calm environment.	1. A calm environment decreases additional anxiety.
2. Explain in advance all procedures and routine regimens.	2. By providing information in advance, the client will not feel anxious about the routine care being provided.
3. Encourage the client to ask questions.	3. By encouraging the client to ask questions, the nurse is providing an open forum for discussion with the client.
4. Provide emotional support to clients and their significant others.	4. Allowing clients and their support systems to vent fears and anxiety, the nurse assists them in decreasing anxiety.
5. Encourage the client to use additional support systems.	5. Additional support people such as religious leaders, social workers, counselors, and clinical nurse specialists may increase the client's support system and decrease anxiety.

Evaluation. Anxiety should improve once dyspnea improves. Concerns over deteriorations in health will require additional time for discussion and may require changes in living arrangements.

■ Surgical Management for Heart Failure

Heart Transplantation. When the heart is irreversibly damaged and no longer functions adequately and when the client is at risk of dying, cardiac transplantation and the use of an artificial heart to assist or replace the failing heart are measures of last resort. With the development of cyclosporine, and more recently FK-506 and mycophenolate mofetil, and with improvements in the procurement and preservation of donor hearts, cardiac transplantation has become an accepted therapeutic procedure. One-year survival rates after transplantation are greater than 85%. Although transplantation may not be appropriate for all clients, it may be the only option available to some. Heart transplantation is discussed in Chapter 57.

Cardiomyoplasty. For clients with low cardiac output who are not candidates for cardiac transplantation, a procedure called *cardiomyoplasty* may support the failing heart. This procedure involves wrapping the latissimus dorsi muscle around the heart and electrostimulating it in synchrony with ventricular systole.

Immediate postoperative care is similar to that of any cardiac surgery client. Continuous cardiac and hemodynamic monitoring is initiated. Inotropic and vasopressor agents are administered to maintain cardiac output until the pulse generator is activated (within 2 to 3 weeks). Because the muscle flap obliterates the left upper lobe and can reduce vital capacity by as much as 20%, aggressive pulmonary hygiene and judicious pain management are essential to prevent atelectasis or pneumonia.

In addition an upper-extremity exercise regimen is prescribed.

■ Modifications for Older Clients

Heart failure is becoming increasingly a disorder of the very old. Cardiac decompensation can be triggered by seemingly minor illnesses and dietary indiscretions. Medications commonly used by older people may have an impact on heart performance even though they pose little risk of interaction with cardiovascular medications. Nonsteroidal anti-inflammatory drugs (NSAIDs) tend to worsen heart disease because they promote sodium retention; tricyclic antidepressants (TCAs) and neuroleptic agents lead to orthostatic hypotension. Conversely cardiac performance can affect the medication's action. The development of RVF can markedly increase the prothrombin time and thereby increase the action of anticoagulants.[45] See the Case Management feature on Heart Failure on the website. Continuous monitoring of homebound clients with heart failure can be facilitated by computer-assisted programs. Nurse researchers are studying the effect of daily interaction via the computer with heart failure clients.[22]

CONCLUSIONS

Disorders of cardiac function are the leading causes of death in the industrialized world. It is imperative that you fully understand the care of clients with heart disease to improve the outcomes and quality of life and to reduce morbidity and mortality. CHD is the precursor to several problems. Your role is to educate the client about risk reduction. Heart failure is a frequent end-point of cardiac disease. It is important to maximize cardiac output and reduce system demands on the heart.

THINKING CRITICALLY *evolve*

1. Your client is a 67-year-old man with newly diagnosed insulin-dependent diabetes in end-stage heart failure. The client was recently released from the hospital. You are to begin intravenous dobutamine therapy during this initial home visit. What assessment should be made before initiating dobutamine therapy? What other assessment interventions might be done?

Factors to Consider. How does heart failure respond to the administration of dobutamine? What teaching or learning needs might be assessed in the client?

2. A 70-year-old man is scheduled for a coronary artery bypass graft. What postoperative complications are most prevalent in older adults?

Factors to Consider. How is CABG surgery accomplished? Why is the CABG surgery a popular option?

Discussions for these questions can be found on the website and the CD-ROM.

BIBLIOGRAPHY

1. Ades, P. (2001). Cardiac rehabilitation and secondary prevention of coronary heart disease. *New England Journal of Medicine, 345* (12), 892-900
1a. Albert, N. (1999). Heart failure: The physiologic basis for current therapeutic concepts. *Critical Care Nurse, 19*(suppl 6), 2-13.
2. Allen, B., et al. (1999). Comparison of transmyocardial revascularization with medical therapy in patients with refractory angina. *New England Journal of Medicine, 341,* 1029-1036.
3. American Heart Association. (2003). *Heart and stroke facts.* Dallas: Author.
4. American Heart Association. (2002). *2002 Heart and stroke facts statistical update.* Dallas: Author.
5. American Heart Association. (1999). *Scientific statement on prevention of cardiovascular diseases.* Dallas: Author.
6. Aregenziano, M., et al. (1997). The influence of infection on survival and successful transplantation in patients with left ventricular assist devices. *Journal of Heart and Lung Transplantation, 16,* 822-831.
7. Assmann, G., et al. (1999). Coronary heart disease: Reducing the risk. *Arteriosclerosis, Thrombosis, and Vascular Biology, 19,* 1819-1824.
8. Baig, M.K., et al. (1998). The pathophysiology of advanced heart failure. *Heart and Lung, 28,* 87-97.
9. Balady, G., et al. (2000). Core components of cardiac rehabilitation/secondary prevention programs. *Circulation, 102,* 1069-1073,
10. Chen-Scarabelli, C. (2002). Beating heart coronary artery bypass graft surgery: Indications, advantages, and limitations. *Critical Care Nurse, 22* (5), 44-58
11. Coffey, M., Crowder, G., & Cheek, D. (2003). Reducing coronary artery disease by decreasing homocysteine levels. *Critical Care Nursing, 23* (1), 25-30.
12. Collins, A. (2001). More than a pump: The endocrine functions of the heart. *American Journal of Critical Care, 10* (2) 94-96.
13. Dao, Q., et al. (1999). Utility of B-type natriuretic peptide in the diagnosis of chronic heart failure in an urgent care setting. *Journal of the American College of Cardiology, 37,* 379-385.
14. Doering, L.V. (1999). Pathophysiology of acute coronary syndromes leading to acute myocardial infarction. *Journal of Cardiovascular Nursing, 13*(3), 1-20.
15. Eagle, K., et al. (1999). ACC/AHA guidelines for coronary artery bypass graft surgery: Executive summary and recommendations. *Circulation, 100,* 1464-1480.
16. Epstein, F. (1999). Hormones and hemodynamics in heart failure. *New England Journal of Medicine, 341*(8), 577-585

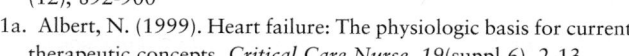

evolve **Did you remember to check out the bonus material on the Evolve website and the CD-ROM, including free self-assessment exercises?**
http://evolve.elsevier.com/Black/medsurg/

17. Fischer, A., et al. (1999). Thrombosis and coagulation abnormalities in the acute coronary syndromes. *Cardiology Clinics, 17,* 283-294.

18. Gustein, D.E., & Fuster, V. (1998). Pathophysiologic bases for adjunctive therapies in the treatment and secondary prevention of acute myocardial infarction. *Clinical Cardiology, 21,* 161-168.

 19. Hulley, S., et al. & the Heart and Estrogen/Progestin Replacement Study (HERS) Research Group. (1998). Randomized trial of estrogen plus progestin for secondary prevention of coronary heart disease in postmenopausal women. *Journal of the American Medical Association, 280,* 605-613.

20. Hunt, S., et al. (2001). ACC/AHA guidelines for the evaluation and management of chronic heart failure in the adult: Executive summary. *Circulation, 104,* 2996-3007.

 21. Konstam, M., et al. (1994). *Heart failure: Evaluation and care of patients with left ventricular systolic dysfunction.* Clinical practice guideline no. 11 (AHCPR Pub. No. 94-0612). Rockville, MD: Agency for Health Care Policy and Research, Public Health Service, U.S. Department of Health and Human Services.

 22. LaFramboise, L., et al. (2003). Comparison of health buddy with traditional approaches to heart failure management. *Family and Community Health, 26*(4), 275-288.

23. Lorenz, B., & Coyle, K. (2002). Coronary artery bypass graft surgery without cardiopulmonary bypass: A review and nursing implications. *Critical Care Nurse, 22*(1), 51-60.

24. MacKlin, M. (2001). Managing heart failure: A case study approach. *Critical Care Nurse, 21*(2), 36-51.

 25. Maglish, B.L., et al. (1999). Outcomes improvement following minimally invasive direct coronary artery bypass surgery. *Critical Care Nursing Clinics of North America, 11*(2), 177-208.

26. Mosca, L., et al. (2001). Hormone replacement therapy and cardiovascular diseases. *Circulation, 104,* 499-503

27. Mosca, L., et al. (1999). Guide to preventive cardiology for women. *Circulation, 99,* 2480-2484.

 28. Packer, M., & Cohn, J.N. (1999) Consensus recommendation for the management of chronic heart failure. *American Journal of Cardiology, 83,* 1A-38A.

29. Parson, C. (1999). Evidence based clinical outcome management in interventional cardiology. *Critical Care Nursing Clinics of North America, 11*(2), 143-157.

 30. Pasternak, R., et al. (2002). ACC/HA/NHLBI clinical advisory on the use and safety of statins. *Circulation, 106,* 1024-1028

31. Piano, M., Bondmass, M., & Schwertz, D. (1998). The molecular and cellular pathophysiology of heart failure. *Heart and Lung, 27,* 3-19.

32. Poirier, V. (1997). The Heartmate left ventricular assist system: Worldwide clinical results. *European Journal of Cardio-Thoracic Surgery, 11,* 539-544.

33. Reger, T., & Vargas, G. (1999). The return of the radial artery in CABG. *American Journal of Nursing 99* (9), 26-32.

 34. Ross, A., & Ostrow, L. (2001). Subjectively perceived quality of life after coronary artery bypass surgery. *American Journal of Critical Care, 10* (1) 11-16.

35. Scherr, K., Jensen, L., & Koshal, A. (1999). Mechanical circulation as a bridge to cardiac transplantation: Toward the 21st century. *American Journal of Critical Care, 8,* 324-335.

36. Shah, P.K. (1996). Pathophysiology of plaque rupture and the concept of plaque stabilization. *Cardiology Clinics, 14*(1), 17-28.

37. Smith, A., & Brown, C. (2003). New advances and novel treatments in heart failure. *Critical Care Nurse Supplement* 11-20.

 38. Smith, S., et al. (2001) ACC-AHA guidelines for percutaneous coronary intervention (revision of the 1993 PTCA guidelines)— Executive summary. *Circulation 103,* 3019-3041.

 39. St. Joer, S., et al. (2001). Dietary protein and weight reduction: A statement for healthcare professionals from the nutrition committee on nutrition, physical activity, and metabolism of the American Heart Association. *Circulation, 104,* 1869-1874.

 40. Stary, H.C., et al. (1995). A definition of advanced types of atherosclerotic lesions and a histological classification of atherosclerosis. *Circulation, 92,* 1355-1374.

 41. Stevenson, L., & Kormos, R. (2001). A definition of advanced types of arthrosclerotic lesions and a histological classification of atherosclerosis. *Circulation 92,* 1355-1374.

42. Taccetta-Chapnick, M. (2002). Using carvedilol to treat heart failure. *Critical Care Nurse, 22*(2), 36-58.

 43. Teirsteine, P., et al. (2000). Three-year clinical and angiographic follow-up after intracoronary radiation. *Circulation, 101,* 360-370.

 44. Wenger, N.K. (1999). Women, myocardial infarction, and coronary revascularization. *Cardiology in Review, 7,* 117-120.

 45. Zhou, J., et al. (1999). Plaque pathology and coronary thrombosis in the pathogenesis of acute coronary syndromes. *Scandinavian Journal of Clinical and Laboratory Investigation, 59* (suppl 230), 3-11.

46. Zimmerman, L., et al. (2002). Comparison of recovery patterns for patients undergoing coronary artery bypass grafting and minimally invasive direct coronary artery bypass in the early discharge period. *Progress in Cardiovascular Nursing, 17*(3), 132-141.

Chapter 59

Management of Clients with Dysrhythmias

Andrea R. Cain
Sheila Melander

evolve

Web Enhancements

Client Education Guide
  The Client with a Permanent Pacemaker (Spanish Translation)
Ethical Issues in Nursing
  What Is Your Role in a "Do Not Resuscitate" Decision?

http://evolve.elsevier.com/Black/medsurg/

Appendix C
  Laboratory Values of Clinical Importance in Medical-Surgical Nursing

The heart is endowed with a specialized system for generating rhythmic electrical impulses and for conducting these impulses rapidly throughout the heart to cause contraction of the heart muscle. When this system functions normally, the atria contract about one sixth of a second ahead of the ventricles. This orderly electrical activity must precede contraction to provide adequate cardiac output for perfusion of all body organs and tissues.

The rhythmic and conduction systems of the heart are susceptible to damage by heart disease, especially by ischemia of the heart tissues resulting from decreased coronary artery blood flow. The consequence is often a bizarre heart rhythm or abnormal sequence of contraction through the heart chambers. The abnormal rhythms, called *dysrhythmias* (or *arrhythmias*), can severely decrease the heart's ability to pump effectively, even to the extent of causing death.

Before reading about dysrhythmias, you may want to review the electrical conduction system of the heart in the Unit 13 Anatomy and Physiology Review and the electrocardiogram (ECG) in Chapter 56.

A *normal sinus rhythm* is a heart rhythm that begins in the sinoatrial (SA) node, is between 60 and 100 beats/min, and has normal intervals and no aberrant or ectopic beats (Figure 59-1). Characteristics of normal sinus rhythm are shown in Table 59-1.

DYSRHYTHMIAS

Dysrhythmias (abnormal heart rhythms) are common in people with cardiac disorders but also occur in people with normal hearts. Dysrhythmias are often detected because of associated manifestations of dizziness, palpitations, and syncope. Abnormalities in conduction are dangerous because of reduced cardiac output, which can lead to impaired cerebral perfusion. The most serious complication of a dysrhythmia is sudden death.[5,9] Because seconds can literally make the difference between life and death for the person who is experiencing a serious dysrhythmia, evaluating responsiveness, quickly activating the emergency medical service (EMS), and initiating cardiopulmonary resuscitation (CPR) can determine the outcome.

Etiology and Risk Factors

Dysrhythmias result from disturbances in three major mechanisms: (1) automaticity, (2) conduction, and (3) problems with reentry of impulses.[17,22]

evolve *Be sure to check out the bonus material on the Evolve website and the CD-ROM, including free self-assessment exercises.*
http://evolve.elsevier.com/Black/medsurg/

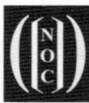

Nursing Outcomes Classification (NOC)
for Nursing Diagnoses—Clients with Dysrhythmias

Acute Pain and Chronic Pain	Anxiety	Decreased Cardiac Output
Pain Management	Anxiety Control	Circulation Status
Pain Control	Coping	Vital Signs Status

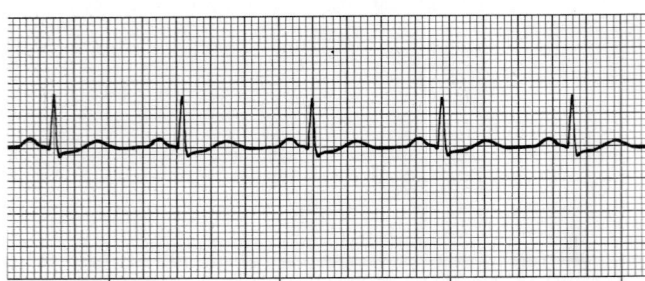

FIGURE 59-1 Normal sinus rhythm as seen on an electrocardiogram (ECG) strip. Note the regular R-R interval, a rate of 80 beats/min, and a P-R interval of 0.16 second.

TABLE 59-1	Characteristics of Normal Sinus Rhythms
Rhythm	Regular, P-P intervals and R-R intervals may vary as much as 3 mm and still be considered regular
Rate	60-100 beats/min
P waves	One P wave preceding each QRS complex
P-R interval	0.12-0.20 sec, consistent with each complex
QRS complex	0.04-0.10 sec, consistent with each complex
Q-T interval	<0.40 sec

Disturbances in Automaticity

The term *automaticity* is used to describe alterations in the normal heart rates produced by various pacemaker cells in the myocardium. Recall that the SA node is the pacemaker of the heart because it possesses the highest level of automaticity. It normally produces a rhythm of 60 to 100 beats/min. The SA node is regulated by the nervous system through the vagus nerve. Sympathetic stimulation increases the rate of firing; lack of sympathetic stimulation or vagal stimulation (which is parasympathetic) decreases the rate.

Under a variety of circumstances, cardiac cells in any part of the heart, whether they are latent pacemaker cells or non-pacemaker myocardial cells, may take on the role of a pacemaker and start generating extraneous electrical impulses. When impulses begin from other sites, the sites are called *ectopic* pacemakers. For instance, if the SA node fails to fire, other sites in the atria can fire. If the atria do not initiate a beat, it can begin in the AV node; if the AV node does not initiate a beat, one can start in the ventricles. When an ectopic pacemaker initiates a beat, the appearance of the ECG differs from the way it looks with a normal sinus rhythm beat.

This fail-safe mechanism is crucial during heart disease. Latent pacemaker cells in the atrioventricular (AV) junction usually assume the role of pacemaker of the heart but at a slower rate (40 to 60 beats/min). Such a pacemaker is called an *escape* pacemaker. If the AV junc-

tion cannot take over as the pacemaker because of disease, an escape pacemaker in the electrical conduction system below the AV junction (i.e., in the bundle branches or Purkinje fibers) may take over at a still lower rate (<40 beats/min). In general, the farther the escape pacemaker is from the SA node, the slower it generates electrical impulses.

These impulses can also occur prematurely—before the SA node would normally fire again. Premature impulses occur when the heart is ischemic, as with coronary artery disease. Ischemia can develop with myocardial infarction (MI), or heart failure, and is characterized by areas of calcification along different points in the heart. Irritation of the AV node, Purkinje system, or myocardium from drugs, nicotine, or caffeine can also produce rhythm changes.

Each of these areas of myocardium (atria, AV node, ventricles) has its own intrinsic rate:

- Sinus node, 60 to 100 beats/min
- Atria, 60 to 100 beats/min
- AV node, 40 to 60 beats/min
- Ventricles, 20 to 40 beats/min

Latent pacemaker cells can also fire at increased rates beyond their inherent rate. When rates exceed these values, the rhythm is called *accelerated* and is classified as a problem of "altered automaticity." For example, an accelerated junctional tachycardia can develop with a rate higher than 60 beats/min (the inherent AV node rate). Abnormal automaticity is commonly caused by ischemia, hyperkalemia, hypocalcemia, hypoxia, increased catecholamine levels, digitalis toxicity, and administration of atropine. A rhythm faster than the intrinsic rate

The authors would like to thank Maribeth Guzzo for her contribution to this chapter in the sixth edition of *Medical-Surgical Nursing*.

is called *tachycardia.* A rhythm slower than the intrinsic rate is called *bradycardia.* Therefore sinus bradycardia is identified as a heart rate below 60 beats/min and sinus tachycardia is defined as a heart rate above 100 beats/min.

Disturbances in Conduction

Conduction is the speed the impulse travels through the sinus node, AV node, and Purkinje fibers. Conduction may be either too rapid or too slow. Blocks that slow or stop an impulse can occur anywhere along the pathway. Blocks can result from ischemia of the tissues, scarring and compression of conduction pathways, inflammation of the AV node, extreme vagal stimulation of the heart, electrolyte imbalances, increased atrial preload, digitalis toxicity, beta-blocking agents, impaired cellular metabolism, MI (especially inferior), and valvular surgery.

Blocks result in ECG changes in appearance. Because the blocked impulse needs more time to travel to its destination, the wave is wider than normal. Disturbances in conduction can also lead to decreased cardiac output and life-threatening dysrhythmias.

Reentry of Impulses

Reentry is the activation of muscle for a second time by the same impulse. The waves of electrical impulse are not extinguished but persist because of a combination of slow conduction and blocks. Therefore the conduction system is delayed or blocked (or both) in one or more segments while being transmitted normally through the rest of this system.

A problem occurs when some cells have been repolarized sufficiently so that they can prematurely depolarize again, producing ectopic beats and rhythms. Hyperkalemia and myocardial ischemia are the two most common causes of delay or block in the conduction system responsible for the reentry mechanism. The reentry mechanism can result in atrial fibrillation (AFib) and ventricular fibrillation (VFib).

Risk Factors

Understanding which client populations are at risk for development of abnormal heart rhythms can be useful in preventing and correcting these abnormalities. Myocardial ischemia, hypoxia, autonomic nervous system imbalances, lactic acidosis, electrolyte imbalances, drug toxicity, and hemodynamic abnormalities are risk factors for dysrhythmias.

Pathophysiology

The significance of all dysrhythmias is their effect on cardiac output and cerebral or vascular perfusion. During normal sinus rhythm, the atria fill and stretch the ventri-

cles with about 30% more blood. This process is called the *atrial kick.* The extra stretch improves the contractility of the ventricles and thereby increases cardiac output. When the impulse starts in the AV node or in the ventricles, atrial and ventricular contraction are no longer coordinated. Atrial kick is lost and cardiac output falls. For example, during contractions initiated in the ventricle, the impulse begins in the ventricle and travels backward up the heart. As a result the atria fill the ventricles while they are contracting or even afterward. Obviously the efficiency of the heart as a pump is restricted during dysrhythmias, and the clinical manifestations are due to changes in cardiac output.

Clinical Manifestations

The reduced cardiac output leads to clinical manifestations of palpitations, dizziness or syncope, pallor, diaphoresis, altered mentation (restlessness and agitation to lethargy and coma), hypotension, sluggish capillary refill, swelling of the extremities, and diminished urine output. Palpitations, dizziness, and syncope are the clinical manifestations that are most effectively evaluated by ambulatory ECG monitoring. The client wears a portable ECG monitor and manually records (writes down) worrisome manifestations, and the correlation of manifestations to the heart rhythm can then be assessed. Shortness of breath, chest pain, and fatigue may also be caused by dysrhythmias; however, these manifestations are more commonly seen in myocardial ischemia and heart failure.

Depending on the type of dysrhythmia, physical assessment findings may reveal (1) a heart rate below 50 or above 140 beats/min; (2) an extremely irregular heart rhythm or pulse; (3) a first heart sound that varies in intensity; (4) sudden appearance of heart failure, shock, and angina pectoris; and (5) a slow, regular heart rate that does not change with activity or medications such as atropine or epinephrine.

Diagnostic findings include ECG abnormalities. The key to dysrhythmia interpretation is the analysis of the form and interrelations of the P wave, the P-R interval, and the QRS complex. The ECG should be analyzed with respect to its rate, rhythm, and site of the dominant pacemaker as well as the configuration of the P and QRS waves. Remember, any ECG findings should be correlated with clinical observations of the client; that is, treat the client, not the monitor.

You will find it necessary to develop a method of analyzing ECG strips that allows you consistently to identify the rhythm demonstrated. The analysis of rhythms is one of two types: sight reading or paper analysis. Sight readers analyze ECGs by looking at the whole rhythm. Much experience and continual, regular viewing of rhythm strips are required for this technique, which is of little use to the beginner. Health care providers with less experience need to develop a method of ECG analysis (Box 59-1).

BOX 59-1 *Electrocardiographic Interpretation of Dysrhythmias*

There are seven basic steps to assist you in the identification of dysrhythmias. The electrocardiogram (ECG) should be studied in an *orderly* fashion as follows:

Step 1. Calculate the heart rate. The simplest method for obtaining the rate is to count the number of R waves in a 6-inch strip of the ECG tracing (which equals 6 seconds). Multiply this sum by 10 to get the rate per minute (beats/min). Because the ECG paper is marked into 3-inch intervals (at the top margin), the approximate heart rate can be rapidly calculated.

Another method is to count the number of large squares between R waves. Find an R wave crossing a large square. Count the number of large squares until the next R wave. The approximate heart rate is as follows:

- 1 large square = 300 beats/min
- 2 large squares = 150 beats/min
- 3 large squares = 100 beats/min
- 4 large squares = 75 beats/min
- 5 large squares = 60 beats/min
- 6 large squares = 50 beats/min
- 7 large squares = 43 beats/min
- 8 large squares = 37 beats/min
- 9 large squares = 33 beats/min
- 10 large squares = 30 beats/min

Step 2. Measure the regularity (rhythm) of the R waves (ventricular rhythm). This can be done by gross observation or actual measurement of the intervals (R-R).

If the R waves occur at regular intervals (variance <0.12 second between beats), the ventricular rhythm is normal. When there are differences in R-R intervals (>0.12 second), the ventricular rhythm is said to be irregular. The division of ventricular rhythm into regular and irregular categories assists in identifying the mechanism of many dysrhythmias.

Note atrial regularity and measure the atrial rate. Measure the regularity (rhythm) of the P waves (P-P). Use the previously described method, but calculate the distance between the same point on two consecutive P waves.

Step 3. Examine the P waves. If P waves are present and precede each QRS complex, the heartbeat originates in the sinus node and a sinus rhythm exists. The absence of P waves or an abnormality in their position with respect to the QRS complex indicates that the impulse started outside the sinoatrial node and that an ectopic pacemaker is in command.

Step 4. Measure the P-R interval. Normally this interval should be between 0.12 and 0.20 second. Prolongation or reduction of this interval beyond these limits indicates a defect in the conduction system between the atria and the ventricles.

Step 5. Measure the duration of the QRS complex. If the width between the onset of the Q wave and the completion of the S wave is greater than 0.12 second (three fine lines on the paper), an intraventricular conduction defect exists.

Step 6. Examine the ST segment. Normally this segment is isoelectric, meaning it is neither elevated nor depressed because the positive and negative forces are equally balanced during this period. Elevation or depression of the ST segment indicates an abnormality in the onset of recovery of the ventricular muscle, usually because of injury (e.g., acute myocardial infarction).

Step 7. Examine the T wave. Normally the T wave is upright and one third the height of the QRS complex. Any condition that interferes with normal repolarization (e.g., myocardial ischemia) may cause the T waves to invert. An abnormally high serum potassium level causes the T wave to become very tall, sometimes the height of the QRS complex.

Outcome Management

The goal of management is to control or ablate the dysrhythmia and reduce potential complications from it. The specific management of dysrhythmias depends on the type and on the client's response to it. All dysrhythmias can reduce cardiac output, which can cause a client to have no manifestations or to have many. Rhythm disturbances resulting in syncope, near-syncope, or sudden death warrant further evaluation. Ventricular dysrhythmias can be life-threatening, demanding immediate treatment. This chapter reviews dysrhythmias and their management, progressing from problems arising (1) in the atria, (2) in the AV junction, and (3) in the ventricles.

ATRIAL DYSRHYTHMIAS DISTURBANCES IN AUTOMATICITY

Sinus Tachycardia

Sinus tachycardia is characterized by a rapid, regular rhythm at a rate of 100 to 180 beats/min with a normal P wave and QRS complex (Figure 59-2, *A*). It often occurs in response to an increase in sympathetic stimulation or decreased vagal (parasympathetic) stimulation. Causes include the following:

- Fever
- Emotional and physical stress
- Heart failure
- Fluid volume loss
- Hyperthyroidism
- Hypercalcemia
- Medications, including, atropine, nitrates, epinephrine, and isoproterenol
- Caffeine
- Nicotine
- Exercise

Most clients do not experience clinical manifestations except for occasional palpitations; however, the clinical manifestations depend on the heart rate and its effect on cardiac output. Between these quick beats, there is little time for ventricular filling and atrial contraction. Clients with underlying heart disease may not tolerate the in-

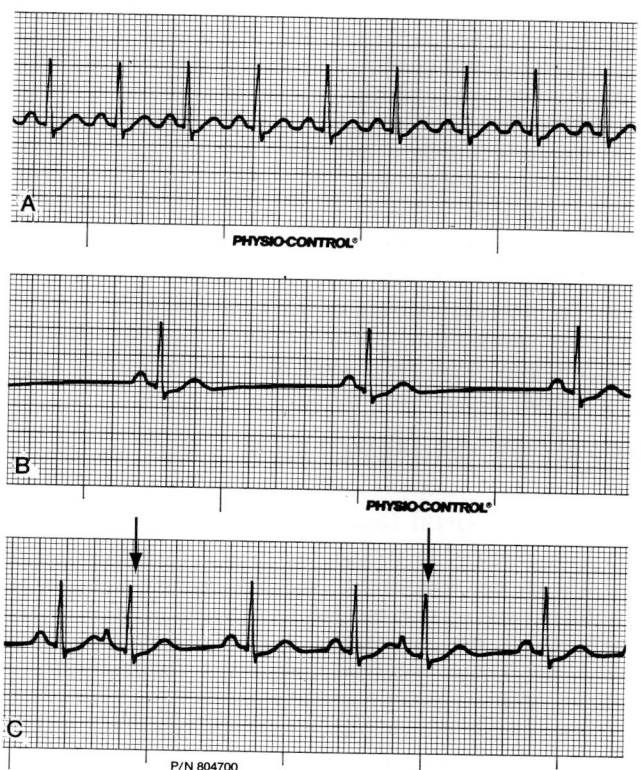

FIGURE 59-2 Atrial dysrhythmias. **A,** Sinus tachycardia—regular R-R interval, rate 125 beats/min; P-R interval, 0.16 second. **B,** Sinus bradycardia—regular R-R interval, rate 40 beats/min; P-R interval, 0.16. **C,** Premature atrial contractions. The second and fifth beats are premature atrial contractions (PACs). Note the difference in the appearance of the P wave and the shortened R-R interval.

creased myocardial workload and reduced coronary artery filling time that accompanies the increased heart rate. These clients may experience hypotension and *angina pectoris* (chest pain).

Management focuses on alleviating the underlying cause and reducing further demands on the heart. Medications such as digitalis, beta-adrenergic blocking agents (e.g., propranolol), and calcium-channel blockers, **EB** may be prescribed.[1,5] Bed rest is ordered to reduce metabolic demand. Oxygen may be prescribed to supply the myocardium adequately.

Sinus Bradycardia

Sinus bradycardia occurs when the SA node fires at a rate of less than 60 times per minute. The P wave and QRS complex are normal (Figure 59-2, *B*). Sinus bradycardia may result from the following:

- Increased vagal (parasympathetic) tone, as occurs with Valsalva's maneuver (e.g., straining while moving the bowels)
- Drugs (especially digitalis, propranolol, or verapamil)

- MI (most often inferior MI)
- Hyperkalemia
- Various diseases, such as hypothyroidism, myxedema, and obstructive jaundice

In some people, sinus bradycardia is a normal condition. Athletes often have sinus bradycardia because their heart is an effective pump with a greater than normal stroke volume. Because cardiac output is the product of stroke volume and heart rate, the heart rate decreases, and yet cardiac output is adequate.

Clients may be asymptomatic; when manifestations do develop, it is because cardiac output is decreased. Fatigue, hypotension, lightheadedness, syncope, shortness of breath, decreased level of consciousness, pulmonary congestion, or heart failure may develop. The slowed rate of SA discharge may allow junctional or ventricular pacemakers to take over, thereby producing ectopic beats.

The aim of management is to correct the underlying cause of sinus bradycardia, and the goal of intervention is to increase the heart rate just enough to relieve manifestations but not enough to cause tachycardia. The intervention sequence for treating symptomatic bradycardia is atropine, transcutaneous pacing if available, dopamine, epinephrine, and isoproterenol or insertion of a temporary transvenous pacemaker.[5,23,32]

Sinus Dysrhythmia

Sinus dysrhythmia is characterized by phasic changes in the automaticity of the SA node, which cause it to fire at varying speeds. The heart rate generally ranges between 60 and 100 beats/min. The ECG shows a normal P wave, P-R interval, and QRS complex; the only abnormality is an irregular P-P interval.

Sinus dysrhythmia may develop from alterations in vagal tone and in response to delayed atrial filling with inhalation. During inspiration, venous return to the right atrium is delayed because of increased intrathoracic pressure. In quiet respiration, the heart rate can decrease about 5%; with deep inspiration, the rate can decrease up to 30%.

Clients with sinus dysrhythmia do not usually require intervention other than alleviation of the underlying cause. Cardiac output is not affected.

Premature Atrial Contractions

Premature atrial contractions (PACs) are early beats arising from ectopic atrial foci, interrupting the normal rhythm. They commonly result from enhanced automaticity of the atrial muscle and can occur in both normal and diseased hearts. PACs are associated with valvular disease and atrial chamber enlargement; they may also be seen with stress, fatigue, alcohol, smoking, coronary artery disease (CAD), cardiac ischemia, heart failure, cardioactive medications (digitalis, quinidine, procainamide), pulmonary congestion, and pulmonary hypertension. Frequent PACs may mark the onset of AFib or heart failure or may reflect electrolyte imbalances.

In clients with PACs, P waves are premature and differ from the normal sinus P wave in appearance, size, or shape (Figure 59-2, C). Premature beats from any ectopic focus can be palpated as skipped or irregular beats. The client who experiences numerous PACs may note palpitations, or "missed beats." PACs are usually benign; however, if the client has increasing numbers of "skipped beats" or feels palpitations often, the problem should be evaluated. Intervention usually focuses on correcting the underlying cause and may include administration of quinidine or procainamide.

DISTURBANCES IN CONDUCTION

Sinoatrial Node Conduction Defects

Under certain circumstances, the impulse from the SA node is either (1) not generated in the SA node *(SA arrest)* or (2) not conducted from the SA node *(sinus exit block)*. Causes of SA node conduction abnormalities include the following:

- Conditions that increase vagal tone
- Coronary artery disease
- MI
- Digitalis and calcium-channel blocker toxicity
- Hypertensive disease
- Tissue hypoxia
- Scarring of intra-atrial pathways
- Electrolyte imbalances

During *SA arrest,* neither the atria nor the ventricles are stimulated, resulting in a pause in the rhythm. An entire PQRST complex will be missing for one or more cycles. After the pause of sinus arrest, a new pacemaker focus assumes the pacing responsibility. The new pacer paces the heart at its inherent rate, which is usually slower than the original SA node rate. The new pacer site is often another atrial focus, but the junction or ventricle can also assume pacing responsibility.

During *sinus exit block,* a conduction delay occurs between the sinus node and the atrial muscle. Unlike the rhythm in SA arrest, the rhythm of SA node discharge in sinus exist block remains constant and uninterrupted. The ECG characteristically displays a normal sinus rhythm interrupted intermittently by pauses. This creates a pattern of pauses that, when measured, comprises multiples of the underlying P-P interval. Sinus arrest differs from SA exit block in that the SA node at times does not fire at all. The result is the occurrence of pauses that are longer and not a multiple of the underlying P-P interval. These pauses are also frequently terminated by escape ectopic beats. Sinus arrest often is associated with a more serious prognosis.

The client usually remains asymptomatic, depending on the duration and frequency of the pauses; however, lengthy pauses can cause lightheadedness or syncope. Intervention is unnecessary unless the client becomes symptomatic and exhibits manifestations of decreased cardiac output. An irregular pulse can be palpated or auscultated. Clinicians can only infer impulse formation within the SA node from the appearance of P waves, which reflect atrial depolarization.

Intervention may include administration of a vagolytic (atropine) or a sympathomimetic (isoproterenol) agent to increase the rate of SA node firing. If pharmacologic measures fail, a pacemaker may be required. Finally, the physician must determine and treat the underlying cause of the dysrhythmia.[1,5,18]

REENTRY OF IMPULSES

Paroxysmal Atrial Tachycardia

Paroxysmal atrial tachycardia (PAT) is the sudden onset and sudden termination of a rapid firing from an ectopic atrial pacemaker (Figure 59-3, A). PAT is due to the reentry phenomenon. This process allows (1) the atrial impulses to travel down less refractory conduction pathways to the bundle of His and (2) retrograde conduction through previously refractory parallel fibers. A circular circuit for rapid repetitive depolarizations results from these events.

Occasionally PAT appears in clients with a normal heart but most commonly develops in clients with cardiac disease. Common cardiac problems precipitating PAT include the following:

- MI
- Cardiomyopathy
- Extreme emotions
- Caffeine ingestion
- Fatigue
- Smoking
- Excessive alcohol intake

Less common causes include rheumatic heart disease, valvular disease, pulmonary emboli, cor pulmonale, thyrotoxicosis, digitalis toxicity (PAT with block), and cardiac surgery.

Clinicians identify PAT by three or more consecutive atrial ectopic beats occurring at a rate greater than 150 beats/min alternating with normal sinus rhythm. The P waves are usually upright, narrow, and peaked in lead II. At faster atrial rates, the P waves may become lost in the preceding T wave. The P-R intervals may be normal; however, rapid atrial rates may overcome the conduction limits of the AV node, causing varying degrees of AV block. Atrial tachycardia with 2:1 block (i.e., two P waves for every QRS complex) most often results from digitalis toxicity. The QRS complexes are usually normal, although aberrant ventricular conduction may occur at very rapid atrial rates or when a conduction defect exists within the ventricle.

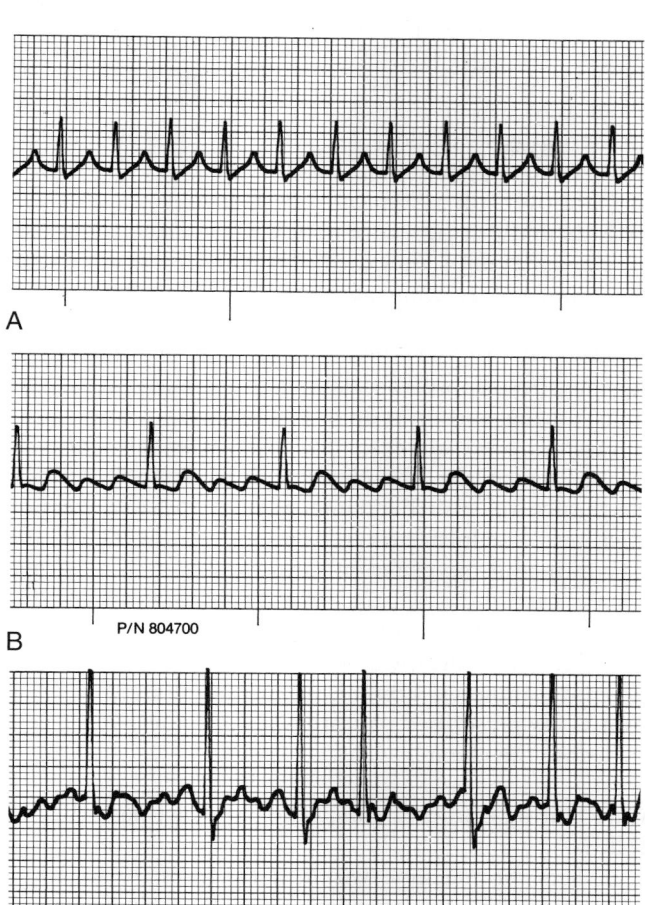

A

B   P/N 804700

C

FIGURE 59-3 **A,** Paroxysmal atrial tachycardia (PAT). The rate is rapid, about 175 beats/min. The P wave is not distinguishable, but the QRS complex is narrow, indicating that the impulse began above the atrioventricular node. **B,** Atrial flutter. Note the saw-toothed appearance of the P waves. There are three P waves for every QRS complex, indicating a 3:1 block. Atrial rate is 75 beats/min. **C,** Atrial fibrillation is identifiable by a chaotic P wave, not one clear P wave, and an irregular R-R interval.

Paroxysmal atrial tachycardia decreases ventricular filling time and mean arterial pressure and also increases myocardial oxygen demand. Clients may report palpitations and lightheadedness.

Management varies with the severity of manifestations. Clients with extremely rapid heart rates or significant underlying cardiovascular disease may experience syncope and heart failure. In such instances, heart rate must be immediately reduced. Any maneuver that stimulates the vagus nerve can successfully terminate PAT or increase AV block. The vagus nerve can be stimulated by carotid sinus massage and Valsalva's maneuver (bearing down). Useful pharmacologic agents include adenosine, verapamil, and beta-blockers. Sedatives may also be used to reduce sympathetic stimulation. The physician may also use cardioversion (see later discussion) as an effective means of terminating PAT if medications and vagal stimulation are not effective.

Ablation procedures that destroy a part of the reentrant path are being more widely used (see later discussion). Such procedures can result in a long-term cure in selected clients.[1,15,16,20]

Atrial Flutter

Atrial flutter is a dysrhythmia arising in an ectopic pacemaker or the site of a rapid reentry circuit in the atria, characterized by rapid "saw-toothed" atrial wave formations and usually by a slower, regular ventricular response. Atrial flutter differs from PAT in that it produces a much more rapid atrial rate. The P waves are actually inverted or bidirectional, producing a "picket fence" or saw-toothed pattern of "flutter waves" (Figure 59-3, *B*). The atrial rate generally ranges from 220 to 350 beats/min. The AV node cannot conduct all the atrial impulses that bombard it; that is, the AV node blocks a 1:1 conduction. Therefore the ventricular rate is always slower than the atrial rate. Thus the pulse, which reflects the ventricular rate, may be normal even though the atrial rate may be quite rapid. The ratio of atrial to ventricular beats may be constant (2:1, 3:1, 4:1, and 7:1, and so forth), or it may vary. A variable degree of block produces an irregular ventricular rhythm.

Atrial flutter most commonly occurs in association with organic diseases such as CAD, mitral valve disease, pulmonary embolus (PE), and hyperthyroidism. In addition it may occur after cardiac surgery. The client may sense occasional palpitations and chest pain, especially when rapid ventricular rates exist.

Intervention aims at controlling rapid ventricular rates. Cardioversion is used (see later discussion). Medications used include digitalis, quinidine, verapamil, propranolol, and procainamide, especially if cardioversion is not successful. Carotid sinus massage helps to slow the ventricular response temporarily so that flutter waves can be identified.[1,5,18]

Atrial Fibrillation

Atrial fibrillation is characterized by rapid, chaotic atrial depolarization from a reentry disorder. Ectopic atrial foci produce impulses between 400 and 700 beats/min. At extremely rapid rates, however, the entire atrium may not be able to recover from one depolarization wave before the next begins, resulting in mechanical and electrical disorganization of the atria. As with atrial flutter, the AV node is bombarded with more impulses than it can conduct. Most of these impulses are blocked; however, as a result of the erratic atrial impulses, the ventricular rhythm is very irregular. The ventricular rate ranges from 160 to 180 beats/min.

Examination of the ECG reveals erratic or no identifiable P waves and underlying ventricular rhythm that appears to be irregular and undulating (Figure 59-3, C). Because of atrial disorganization, no "atrial kick" occurs. This loss of additional blood volume can decrease cardiac output by as much as 20% to 30%. With increasing ventricular rates, cardiac output declines even further and may result in angina pectoris, heart failure, and shock.

Atrial fibrillation may be associated with sick sinus syndrome, hypoxia, increased atrial pressure, pericarditis, and many other conditions. Clients may be asymptomatic, or they may note an irregular pulse and palpitations. The client may have a pulse deficit between apical and radial pulses.

Mural thrombi formation can severely complicate the condition. Blood pools in the "quivering" atria because of lack of adequate contraction of atrial muscle. This blood can clot, which increases the potential for cerebral and pulmonary vascular emboli. Most clients with sudden onset of AFib are given anticoagulants to reduce risk of stroke and PE until the impulses are controlled.

Outcome Management

The initial treatment goal is to control the rate of impulses with the administration of drugs such as diltiazem, verapamil, beta-blockers, or digoxin. Chemical cardioversion, usually after a period of anticoagulation therapy, can then be attempted with procainamide or quinidine. Electrical cardioversion is the third therapeutic option.

Electrical Cardioversion

Cardioversion, most often an elective procedure, involves the use of a synchronized direct current (DC) electrical countershock that depolarizes all the myocardial cells simultaneously, allowing the SA node to resume the pacemaker role. The electrical discharge is synchronized with or triggered by the client's QRS complex for avoidance of accidental discharge during the repolarization phase when the ventricle is vulnerable to the development of VFib. A QRS complex must be present for successful conversion of the dysrhythmia.

Low voltages (50 to 100 J) are tried initially. If the attempt is unsuccessful, cardioversion using larger voltages can be repeated. Only specially trained physicians can perform this procedure.[1,15]

Cardioversion is used to treat AFib, atrial flutter, and supraventricular tachycardia (see later discussion) that is resistant to medication, and it is used in ventricular tachycardia in an unstable client. The unstable client may be hypotensive or dyspneic; may be experiencing chest pain; or may have evidence of heart failure, MI, or ischemia. Analgesia or sedation may be provided before the electrical shock.

Care Before Cardioversion. The physician evaluates the ECG to identify the type of dysrhythmia present. The client must sign an informed consent, after which the intervention is scheduled. The client and family must receive a full explanation of cardioversion.

Cardioversion is typically performed at the client's bedside in the critical care unit. If a life-threatening dysrhythmia develops after cardioversion, emergency equipment and trained clinicians must be in the room.

If the client has been taking a digitalis preparation, a therapeutic drug level must be present. Digitalis toxicity may predispose the client to ventricular dysrhythmias during cardioversion. In addition, a low serum potassium level increases the risk of lethal dysrhythmias. Premedicate the client with prescribed antidysrhythmics to ensure maintenance of post-conversion rhythms. Administer oxygen before cardioversion, and discontinue if oxygenation saturation is within normal limits. Keep the client on NPO (fasting) status for several hours before cardioversion. Start an intravenous (IV) line for medication delivery. To reduce fear and to promote amnesia, administer an antianxiety medication IV as prescribed. Anesthesia personnel are present to sedate the client.

Care During Cardioversion. The physician performs the following steps:

1. Sets the machine within a range of 50 to 200 J (more or less, depending on the underlying impedances)
2. Turns the synchronizer switch to "on" to deliver the shock during the QRS complex, not on the down slope of the T wave
3. Lubricates the paddles and places them exactly as described for defibrillation
4. Calls for all health care personnel to stand back from the bed
5. While standing back from the bed, depresses and holds the buttons on the paddles until the shock is delivered

Newer equipment for cardioversion includes adhesive skin paddles attached to the client's chest and back.

Care After Cardioversion. Clinicians immediately assess the ECG and pulse after the procedure. In some cases VFib or ventricular tachycardia occurs, demanding emergency action. Monitor the client's ECG rhythm and vital signs continuously for at least 2 hours, and carefully assess for rhythm changes and complications. A successful response to cardioversion resolves the dysrhythmia and restores normal sinus rhythm. The client's airway is protected until sedation lightens. With a good response and no complications, the client may be discharged later that day when fully awake and able to eat.

ATRIOVENTRICULAR JUNCTIONAL DYSRHYTHMIAS

If the SA node fails to fire and an impulse is not initiated in other ectopic sites in the atria, the AV junction is the next pacemaker for the heart. An impulse begins in the junction and simultaneously spreads up to the atria and down into the ventricles. During junctional rhythms, cardiac output decreases as a result of a lack of atrial kick to the ventricles. Junctional rhythms are not dependable for a long-term cardiac pacemaker because the intrinsic rate is slow and more irritable ectopic foci may fire, such as from the ventricles. Consider junctional rhythms to be a warning or forerunner of more serious dysrhythmias.

Two major types of dysrhythmias arise in the AV junction:

- Disturbances in automaticity, with the AV junctional tissue assuming the role of the pacemaker
- Disturbances in conduction, with the AV junction blocking impulses journeying from the atria to the ventricles

Both types of dysrhythmias can result from ischemia or trauma in the area of the AV junction (i.e., after MI or cardiac surgery). Digitalis toxicity, quinidine toxicity, and hyperkalemia may also cause junctional dysrhythmias.

Junctional rhythms produce abnormal upward direction of impulse (e.g., in lead II the P waves are inverted) because the impulse is traveling through the atria in a direction opposite that found in normal sinus rhythm. Also, the P-R interval shortens to less than 0.12 second. The impulse may spread through the atria at the same time that the ventricles are being activated by the AV junction. In this instance, the P wave would be buried in the QRS complex and not observed on the ECG. Also, the atria may contract after the ventricles. In this case the P wave would follow the QRS complex. The QRS complex is normal if ventricular conduction is normal.

DISTURBANCES IN AUTOMATICITY

The major junctional dysrhythmias caused by changes in automaticity are (1) premature junctional contractions (PJCs), (2) junctional escape rhythm, and (3) junctional tachycardias. As with PACs, an ectopic focus in the AV junctional tissue may develop increased automaticity and discharge prematurely, initiating depolarization of the heart.

Premature Junctional Contractions

A PJC is the single, early firing of a junctional ectopic focus (Figure 59-4). PJCs are slower as a result of lower intrinsic rates. Usually clients can tolerate junctional rhythms without loss of cardiac output, although clients with severe forms of cardiac disease may not because of decreased cardiac output.

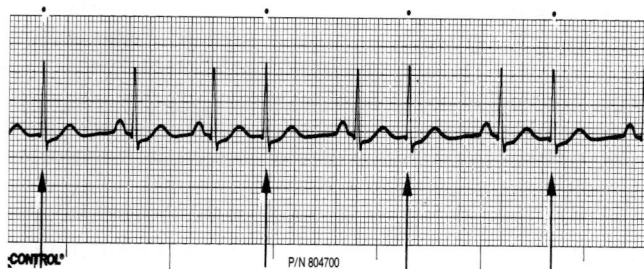

FIGURE 59-4 A premature junctional contraction. The beats marked with *arrows* are premature junctional contractions. Note the absence of a P wave but otherwise normal deflection, indicating that the impulse was initiated above the ventricles.

Paroxysmal Junctional Tachycardia

A junctional rhythm with a rate that exceeds 60 beats/min is termed a *junctional tachycardia.* It usually stops and starts abruptly, thereby acquiring the name *paroxysmal junctional tachycardia,* or PJT. The usual rate is 140 to 220 beats/min.

Causes of PJT include metabolic imbalances and increased sympathetic stimulation. Rapid ventricular rates can lead to left ventricular failure resulting from increased myocardial oxygen demand and decreased blood supply. PJT that cannot be distinguished from PAT on the ECG is called *supraventricular tachycardia* (SVT).

Management of rapid junctional rhythms begins with vagal stimulation, such as carotid sinus massage. If clinical manifestations develop, treatment consists of pharmacologic agents and cardioversion. Common medica- tions include propranolol, quinidine, and digitalis. Evaluation of digitalis intoxication and potassium levels may also be indicated.[1,18]

DISTURBANCES IN CONDUCTION

The second group of disturbances arising in the area of the AV junction includes AV block. Impulses passing through the AV junction are blocked to varying degrees. Therefore the conduction of impulses from the atria to the ventricles slows or stops entirely, depending on the degree of the AV block. Normally the impulse coming from the SA node is delayed at the AV junction for less than 0.20 second before traveling on to the bundle of His. If the AV junction has been damaged by ischemia, rheumatic fever, or drug toxicity, impulses are delayed or completely blocked at the AV junction for abnormally long periods.

First-Degree Atrioventricular Block

First-degree AV block is a delay in passage of the impulse from atria to ventricles. This delay usually occurs at the level of the AV node. The rhythm is regular, and each P wave is followed by a QRS complex; however, the P-R interval is prolonged beyond the normal 0.20 second. The P-R interval usually remains constant (Figure 59-5, A). This characteristic is an important differentiation between first-degree AV block and other AV blocks. This block is often associated with CAD, increased vagal tone, and congenital anomalies and may also result from digitalis administration.

First-degree AV block, existing alone as the only abnormal feature of a client's ECG, produces no clinical manifestations and requires no intervention. If the block is a result of digitalis, the medication may be discontinued. Because first-degree AV block can progress to a higher-degree AV block, the client requires observation and ECG monitoring.[1,18]

Second-Degree Atrioventricular Block

In a client with second-degree AV block, a more serious form of conduction delay in the heart, some impulses are conducted and others are blocked. Second-degree block results in intermittently dropped QRS complexes. Atrial depolarization continues without disturbance, and normal-appearing P waves occur at regular intervals. Second-degree AV block does not usually affect conduction through the ventricles, and QRS complexes appear normal in configuration. Second-degree AV block develops from CAD, digitalis toxicity, rheumatic fever, viral infections, and inferior-wall MI.

Second-degree AV block is subdivided into two additional types: Mobitz type I (Wenckebach phenomenon) and Mobitz type II.

Mobitz Type I Block (Wenckebach Phenomenon)

The Mobitz type I form of second-degree block is caused by an abnormally long refractory period. The level of block occurs at the AV node. On the ECG the P-R interval gradually lengthens until a P wave is not conducted (Figure 59-5, B). This is the mildest form of second-degree heart block. This dysrhythmia is due to increased vagal tone, digoxin administration, or congenital anomalies.

Mobitz type I does not usually result in clinical manifestations because the ventricular rate is adequate; however, the client may have an irregular pulse. Vertigo, weakness, or other manifestations of low cardiac output may be experienced if the ventricular rate drops precipitously.

Intervention is not required as long as the ventricular rate remains adequate for perfusion. The client is assessed for progression to a higher (more serious) degree of block. Clinicians focus primarily on managing the underlying cause. Intervention, if needed, is similar to that described for Mobitz type II block.[1,18]

Mobitz Type II Block

Mobitz type II block occurs in the presence of a long absolute refractory period with little or no relative refractory period. The level of block is below the AV node, usually a consequence of a block within the His bundle system. The P waves are normal and are followed by normal QRS complexes at regular intervals until suddenly a QRS complex is dropped (Figure 59-5, C). Mobitz type II blocks result from ischemia, digitalis, or quinidine toxicity or from anterior-wall MI.

Mobitz type II, a more serious condition than Mobitz type I, may progress to third-degree AV block, especially in clients with an anterior wall MI. Clients with second-degree AV block require close ECG monitoring for possible progression to complete heart block.

Interventions include (1) administration of atropine and isoproterenol (which speed the rate of impulse conduction), (2) insertion of a temporary or permanent pacemaker, and (3) withholding cardiac depressant drugs (e.g., digitalis). Second-degree block, which occurs after MI, particularly an inferior MI, may be reversible as the injury of ischemia heals.[1,18]

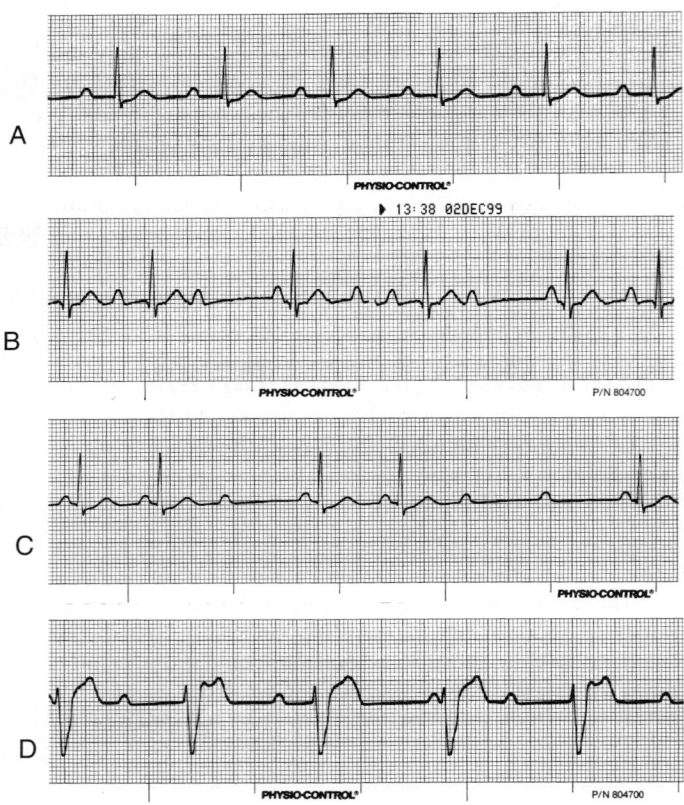

FIGURE 59-5 Junctional dysrhythmias. **A,** First-degree atrioventricular (AV) block. **B,** Second-degree AV block (Mobitz type I, Wenckebach phenomenon; note the regularly occurring P waves and the increasing P-R intervals). **C,** Second-degree AV block (Mobitz type II). **D,** Third-degree AV block (note variable P-R interval and lack of association of the P wave with the QRS complex).

Third-Degree Atrioventricular Block

Third-degree AV block is the complete absence of conduction of the electrical impulses due to a block in the AV node, bundle of His, or bundle branches. Third-degree heart block is sometimes called *AV dissociation* or complete heart block because the two halves of the heart are working independently of each other. The atria are paced by the SA node, but because the message is blocked, the ventricles are being paced by a ventricular ectopic pacemaker (Figure 59-5, *D*). The atrial rate is always equal to or faster than the ventricular in complete heart block. The ventricular rate is typically 40 to 60 beats/min.

Other features of the ECG in third-degree heart block include (1) regular P-P intervals, (2) regular R-R intervals, (3) an absence of meaningful or consistent P-R intervals, and (4) normal-appearing P waves. The greatest danger inherent in third-degree AV block is ventricular standstill or asystole, characterized by the Stokes-Adams attack. If a focus in the ventricles does not initiate a heartbeat, asystole will lead to immediate loss of consciousness and in some cases even death.

Third-degree AV block results from a variety of causes, including the following:

- Fibrotic or degenerative changes in the conduction system
- MI (especially anterior wall MI)
- Congenital anomalies
- Cardiac surgery
- Myocarditis
- Viral infections of the conduction system
- Drug toxicity (digitalis, beta-blockers, calcium-channel blockers)
- Trauma
- Cardiomyopathy
- Lyme disease

The slow ventricular rate leads to decreased cardiac output and circulatory impairment. Clients may experience hypotension, angina pectoris, and heart failure.

The major interventions in complete heart block are atropine, transcutaneous pacing, catecholamine infusions (dopamine or epinephrine), and transvenous pacemaker. If asystole develops, CPR is used until a pacemaker can be inserted. Isoproterenol is rarely indicated.[1,5,18]

Bundle-Branch Block

Bundle-branch block indicates that conduction is impaired in one of the bundle branches (distal to the bundle of His), and thus the ventricles do not depolarize simultaneously. The abnormal conduction pathway through the ventricles is causing a wide or notched QRS complex. The defect may result from the following:

- Myocardial fibrosis
- Chronic CAD
- MI

- Cardiomyopathies
- Inflammation
- Pulmonary embolism
- Severe left ventricular hypertrophy
- Congenital anomalies

These disturbances of conduction through the ventricles result in either a right bundle-branch block (RBBB) or a left bundle branch block (LBBB). Because of its association with left ventricular disease, LBBB carries a worse prognosis. The left bundle branch is composed of anterior and posterior fascicles (small bundles), and one or both fascicles may be involved.

No specific intervention for this conduction defect has been established; however, if RBBB exists along with block in one of the fascicles of the left bundle, the one remaining fascicle represents the only conduction pathway to the ventricles. Therefore in this situation, a pacemaker is required.[1,18]

VENTRICULAR DYSRHYTHMIAS

Ventricular dysrhythmias arise below the level of the AV junction. Like dysrhythmias in the atria or junction, dysrhythmias in the ventricles are caused by abnormalities of automaticity or conduction. Ventricular dysrhythmias are generally more serious and life-threatening than atrial or junctional dysrhythmias because ventricular dysrhythmias more commonly develop in association with intrinsic heart disease. Also, ventricular dysrhythmias usually cause greater hemodynamic compromise (e.g., hypotension, heart failure, shock). The independent contraction of the ventricles results in a reduced stroke volume and therefore a reduced cardiac output. Rapid ventricular rates prevent optimal filling of the ventricular chambers and reduce stroke volume even further. At rates of less than 40 contractions per minute, cardiac output is simply not sufficient to support the body's vital functions.

The ECG tracing of a client with ventricular dysrhythmias reveals wide and bizarre QRS complexes. Normally impulses traverse the ventricles via the shortest, most efficient route. This normal pathway results in a narrow QRS complex. When an impulse originates in the ventricles, however, the impulse follows an abnormal pathway through the ventricular muscle tissue. This abnormality appears as a wide (>0.12 second) complex on the ECG.

DISTURBANCES IN AUTOMATICITY

Dysrhythmias resulting from problems in automaticity are characterized by ectopic impulses, which result from either myocardial irritability or the phenomenon of reentry. The following are the three ventricular dysrhythmias:

- Premature ventricular contractions (PVCs)
- Ventricular tachycardia (VT)
- Torsades de pointes

Premature Ventricular Contractions

Premature ventricular contractions, also called *ventricular premature beats*, are the most common of all dysrhythmias other than those of the sinus node. They are usually caused by the firing of an irritable pacemaker in the ventricle. PVCs result from enhanced ventricular automaticity or reentry. Factors promoting PVCs are listed in Box 59-2.

Premature ventricular contractions produce easily recognized ECG changes. They occur earlier than the expected beat of the underlying rhythm and are usually followed by a compensatory pause. On the ECG an unusually wide and bizarre QRS appears, interrupting the underlying rhythm (Figure 59-6, *A*).

Isolated PVCs are usually not treated. If the client becomes symptomatic because of decreased cardiac output, lidocaine or any of the other class I antidysrhythmics can be given to treat PVCs. In clients with acute MI, the development of PVCs indicates that the myocardium is ischemic; in such instances, ectopic foci become irritated and fire more often.

In the following situations PVCs are considered dangerous:

- Frequent (>6/min)
- Coupled with normal beats (bigeminy)
- Multiform (Figure 59-6, *B*)
- In pairs after every third beat (trigeminy) (Figure 59-6, *C*)
- A result of acute MI
- On the T wave (Figure 59-6, *D*)

Clinicians refer to "falling on the T wave" as the R-on-T phenomenon. The downward slope of the T wave is the most vulnerable period of the cardiac cycle. If the heart is stimulated at this time, it often cannot respond to the stimulus in an organized fashion because the muscle fibers are in various stages of repolarization. Therefore

PVCs that occur during this vulnerable period can precipitate the more life-threatening dysrhythmias of ventricular tachycardia (VTach) (Figure 59-6, *E*) and Vfib.

Outcome Management of Nonthreatening Dysrhythmias

■ Medical Management

Suppress Irritable Foci. Management of dangerous PVCs involves the administration of antidysrhythmic agents that have myocardial depressant actions. In acute situations the clinician may administer class I and class

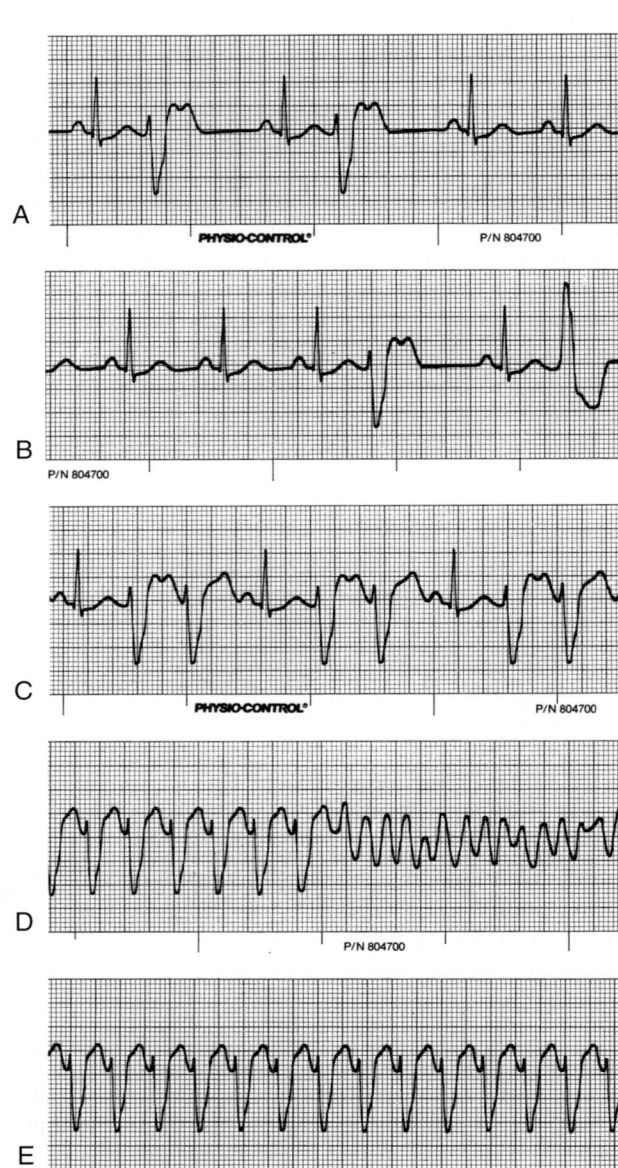

FIGURE 59-6 Ventricular dysrhythmias. **A,** Beats 2 and 4 are unifocal premature ventricular contractions (PVCs). **B,** Multifocal PVCs. **C,** Paired PVCs. **D,** R-on-T phenomenon, leading to ventricular fibrillation. **E,** Ventricular tachycardia.

BOX 59-2	*Causes of Premature Ventricular Contractions*

- Myocardial hypoxia
- Hypokalemia
- Hypocalcemia
- Acidosis
- Alcohol
- Caffeine
- Nicotine
- Coronary artery disease
- Heart failure
- Toxic agents (e.g., digitalis, tricyclic antidepressants)
- Exercise
- Hypermetabolic states
- Intracardiac catheters

II antidysrhythmic agents intravenously (IV), followed by a continuous IV drip. The Integrating Pharmacology feature on Toxicity and Antidysrhythmic Agents on p. 1684 describes a variety of antidysrhythmic agents.[1,18,19]

Improve Myocardial Oxygen. Oxygen is an essential component of dysrhythmia management, especially for dysrhythmias that result from irritable foci in an ischemic myocardium. These include PVCs and other ventricular dysrhythmias. Oxygen should be given to all clients at risk of ventricular dysrhythmias, such as those with chest pain or hypoxemia or during cardiac arrest.

■ Nursing Management of the Medical Client

Assessment

Assess the client for clinical manifestations of decreased cardiac output. Monitor the ECG continuously for patterns of PVCs that indicate further deterioration (e.g., PVCs moving closer to the preceding T wave).

Diagnosis, Planning, Interventions

Diagnosis: Decreased Cardiac Output.

Dysrhythmias often lead to decreased ventricular filling as a result of the rapid rate or from not being coordinated to allow for atrial kick. Express this common nursing diagnosis as *Decreased Cardiac Output related to decreased ventricular filling time secondary to (name the rhythm).*

Outcomes. The client will have an adequate cardiac output as evidenced by (1) return of normal heart rate, rhythm, palpable pulse, and blood pressure to baseline levels; (2) return of level of consciousness to baseline value; (3) warm, dry skin; (4) clear lung sounds; (4) the absence of S_3 or S_4; (5) the absence of dysrhythmias; and (6) adequate urine output.

Interventions. Monitor heart rate and rhythm and vital signs continuously, aided by the computer as needed. Assess skin temperature, lung sounds, heart sounds, and peripheral pulses every 2 to 4 hours. Monitor laboratory studies, especially if an MI is suspected. Give antidysrhythmic medications according to orders. Use blood levels as a guide to dosage. Many medications, especially antidysrhythmics, can rise to toxic levels, especially if the client has a pre-existing liver, renal, or electrolyte disorder. Do not attempt to memorize the Pharmacology Box; rather, commit a few drugs to memory (amiodarone, lidocaine, verapamil, and sotalol). These medications can be administered orally or by continuous IV infusion. You must be diligent in monitoring for the intended effect and side effects of the medication.

Maintain a quiet atmosphere, and administer analgesics to control pain. Stimulation can lead to increased levels of catecholamine release and may trigger tachycardias and increased oxygen demand.

Apply oxygen with nasal prongs to supplement serum levels. Hypoxia can lead to further myocardial ischemia and dysrhythmias.

If life-threatening dysrhythmias develop, many nurses are trained to use defibrillation for the client. Other emergency interventions include CPR, various medications, and preparation of the client for a transcutaneous or permanent pacemaker (See the Bridge to Critical Care feature on Defibrillation on p. 1685).

Diagnosis: Anxiety.

The risk of death from sudden onset of life-threatening dysrhythmias weighs heavily on most clients. Express this nursing diagnosis as *Anxiety related to fear about unknown outcome.*

Outcomes. The client will experience a reduced level of anxiety as evidenced by (1) a report of feeling less anxious and not voicing feelings of helplessness or hopelessness, (2) an increased ability to sleep and rest, (3) a return of the heart rate to baseline level, and (4) a reduction of dyspnea.

Interventions. Identify the client's anxiety and assist the client in discussing sources of fear. Clarify misconceptions. Commonly the client or a member of the family has had a heart condition, and the client's ability to cope may be directly influenced by that experience.

Explain the equipment present in the room. Most rooms are stocked with several types of equipment, and its presence does not always indicate the severity of the client's condition.

Remain with the client, and tell the client and family what is happening now and what will be happening (e.g., blood will be drawn soon).

Finally, explore the usual coping methods with the client. Positive coping methods are usually supported; discuss maladaptive coping mechanisms, and suggest substitutions. For example, smoking may be a common coping mechanism, but it is not permitted with cardiac disorders or in most hospitals. Therefore if smoking is the client's coping mechanism when stressed, a substitute would need to be found, such as nicotine patches or chewing gum. Be aware that these patches can actually increase nicotine levels because they provide constant levels of the drug. Light smokers require less nicotine. Adjust the dose of the patch, beginning with the lowest levels. Patches can also cause nasal constriction.

Evaluation

The degree of expected outcome attainment is assessed hourly (or more often) if the client has life-threatening dysrhythmias. Dysrhythmias are treated promptly and

INTEGRATING PHARMACOLOGY

Toxicity and Antidysrhythmic Agents

Numerous antidysrhythmic agents are used to treat and prevent disturbances in cardiac rhythms. Antidysrhythmic drugs have and will continue to have a significant role in decreasing the incidence of sudden cardiac death. Unfortunately antidysrhythmic drugs also can also lead to dysrhythmias at both therapeutic and toxic drug concentrations. See Chapter 58 for a discussion of digoxin toxicity.

Class I: Sodium-Channel Blockers

All class I agents block fast sodium channels and reduce the rate of rise of the action potential (phase 0) in certain cells. They inhibit depolarization of neuronal cells, thereby producing local anesthesia. They inhibit depolarization in atrial, ventricular, and Purkinje myocytes, thereby decreasing conduction velocity and automaticity. Class I agents are further categorized as A, B, or C subclasses based on the degree of sodium channel blockade and effects on repolarization. Class IA agents prolong action potential duration and produce moderate slowing of cardiac conduction; prolongation of action potential duration occurs from blockade of outward rectifying potassium channels. Class IB agents shorten the duration of action potentials and selectively depress cardiac conduction in ischemic cells. Class IC agents have little effect on the potential duration of action potentials but markedly depress cardiac conduction (potent sodium-channel blockers).

Procainamide is a commonly used class IA medication used to treat sustained ventricular dysrhythmias. At toxic levels it leads to prolongation of QT interval and QRS complex. Other toxic manifestations include gastrointestinal disturbances, headache, mild hypotension, rash, insomnia, dizziness, ataxia, hallucinations, and weakness.

Lidocaine is a class 1B agent, used for suppression of VTach or dysrhythmias associated with cardiac surgery. Evidence supporting the efficacy of lidocaine is lacking at this time. ACLS protocol recommends other antidysrhythmics, such as amiodarone, as a better choice. Lidocaine blocks sodium channels and shortens action potential. Side effects are blurred vision, tinnitus, drowsiness, nausea or vomiting, lightheadedness, confusion, hypotension, and atrioventricular block.

Class II: Beta-Adrenergic Blockers

Class II: Beta-adrenergic blockers indirectly block calcium-channel opening and block the ability of catecholamines to cause dysrhythmias. Beta-blockers are used to treat hypertension and myocardial infarction. They are also used to treat migraine headaches, essential tremors, thyrotoxicosis, glaucoma, anxiety, and various other disorders. As a result of their expanded use, the incidence of overdose with these agents has also increased. Manifestations of beta-blocker overdose are related to blocking sympathetic beta-adrenergic receptors. Seizures have been reported.

Class III: Potassium Channel Blockers

Class III: Potassium channel blockers prolong refractoriness and delay repolarization by blocking potassium channels; they have little direct effect on sodium channels. Amiodarone is commonly used to suppress dysrhythmias. Toxic effects include photosensitivity, neurotoxicity, hyperthyroidism, heart failure, complete heart block, pulmonary fibrosis, skin pigmentation (blue nail coloration), and corneal deposits. It may induce QT prolongation.

Class IV: Calcium-Channel Blockers

Class IV: Calcium-channel blockers slow sinoatrial node pacemaker cell and atrioventricular conduction by direct blockade of L-type voltage-gated calcium channels. Calcium-channel blocker overdose is rapidly emerging as the most lethal prescription drug ingestion. Overdose by short-acting agents is characterized by rapid progression to cardiac arrest. Overdose by extended-relief formulations result in delayed onset of dysrhythmias, shock, sudden cardiac collapse, and bowel ischemia.

As in the case of any client with suspected or known acute poisoning, attempt to obtain the original medication containers, pill counts, the quantity that may have been ingested, approximate time of ingestion, and a report of any potential co-ingestants. To clarify the role of the antidysrhythmic agent, ask the client the following:

• What were the indications for starting the drug?
• How long has the client used this medication?
• How do the manifestations correlate with the initiation of drug therapy?
• Is the client compliant with the drug regimen? Does the client take any extra doses?
• What other medications has the client begun recently? Include nonprescription and herbal medications as well.

From Cummings, R. (2001). *ACLS provider manual.* Dallas, TX: American Heart Association; Asselin, M.E., & Cullen, H.A. (2002). A new beat for BLS and ACLS guidelines. *Nursing Management, 33*(2),31-38; Ophie, L.H., & Marcus, F.I. (2001). Antiarrhythmic drugs. In L.H. Ophie (Ed.), *Drugs for the heart* (5th ed.). Philadelphia: W.B. Saunders; and Miller, J.M., & Zipes, D.P. (2001). Management of the patient with cardiac arrhythmias. In E. Braunwald (Ed.), *Heart disease* (6th ed.). Philadelphia: W.B. Saunders.

usually stop quickly once treatment is begun. Clients with recalcitrant dysrhythmias may require several medications. Anxiety sometimes abates quickly but usually requires several days. Some clients remain anxious for their entire hospital stay.

Ventricular Tachycardia

Ventricular tachycardia (VTach or VT) is a life-threatening dysrhythmia that occurs when an irritable ectopic focus in the ventricles takes over as the pacemaker. It occurs in the presence of significant cardiac disease, such as in clients with CAD, cardiomyopathy, mitral valve prolapse, heart failure, acute MI with hypoxia and acidosis, and digitalis toxicity.

Ventricular tachycardia is characterized by rapidly occurring series of PVCs (three or more) with no normal beats in between (Figure 59-6, *E*). P waves are absent, and the P-R interval is absent. The QRS complex is wide (>0.12 second) and bizarre. The ventricular rate ranges between 100 and 220 beats/min, usually 130 to 170 beats/min. The ventricular rhythm is slightly irregular. VT produces a very low cardiac output that can quickly lead to cerebral and myocardial ischemia. At any time, VT can develop into VFib.

Clients with VT commonly express feelings of impending death.

Sustained but hemodynamically stable VT is initially treated with antidysrhythmics (i.e., lidocaine, procainamide, or bretylium). Cardioversion may be required for conversion to sinus rhythm (see earlier discussion). When the client is unconscious and in VT, it is not time for medications; it is time to defibrillate. The physician may also order IV antidysrhythmic agents, usually lidocaine. Another drug gaining favor is magnesium sulfate, particularly if the client has low magnesium levels.[1,2,5,13,18]

Torsades de Pointes

Torsades de pointes is a form of VT in which the QRS complexes appear to be constantly changing. Delayed repolarization of the ventricle is revealed as a prolonged Q-T interval and a broad flat T wave in the preceding sinus rhythm. The rhythm is regular or irregular with a ventricular rate of 150 to 300 beats/min (Figure 59-7, *B*). The QRS complex is wide and bizarre.

Torsades de pointes is usually a result of drug toxicity (procainamide, quinidine, disopyramide) or electrolyte imbalances (hypokalemia or hypomagnesemia) (see the

---

BRIDGE TO CRITICAL CARE

Defibrillation

When a client is in ventricular fibrillation or pulseless ventricular tachycardia, the nurse must be able to safely and effectively use an automatic external defibrillator (AED) or conventional (manual) defibrillator (monophasic or biphasic).

Guidelines for Use of an Automatic External Defibrillator (AED)

1. Turn the power on the AED device.
2. Attach cables to the adhesive defibrillator pads.
3. Peel paper from pads and attach pads to the client's chest at the upper right sternal border and the cardiac apex.
4. Place the AED in analyze mode.
5. Announce loudly, "Analyzing rhythm, stand clear!"
6. If VF/VT is present, the AED will charge to the appropriate joules and signal that a shock is indicated.
7. Announce, "Shock is indicated, stand clear!"
8. Confirm that no one is touching the client.
9. Press the shock button when indicated.
10. Repeat the analyze and shock steps until VF/VT is no longer present. The device will signal "No shock indicated."
11. For each set of three shocks, provide 1 minute of CPR.

Guidelines for the Use of Conventional Defibrillators (Monophasic and Biphasic)

1. Turn on the defibrillator.
2. Select energy level at 200 J for monophasic defibrillation.
3. Set the lead switch to paddles.
4. Apply gel on the paddles or use conductor pads, and place on the client's chest (at 2nd right intercostal space and at the anterior axillary line in the 5th left intercostal space).
5. Look at the monitor display, and assess the cardiac rhythm. If VF/VT is present, proceed to the next step.
6. Press the charge button on the apex paddle (the right hand).
7. When the defibrillator is fully charged, state loudly, "Shocking on three, all clear!"
8. Chant "Shocking on three. One, I'm clear. Two, you're clear. Three, all clear!"
9. Apply 25 pounds of pressure with both paddles, and press the discharge button on both paddles simultaneously.
10. Look at the monitor display. If VF/VT is still present, immediately recharge the defibrillator.
11. Shock at 200 J to 300 J, then at 360 J. Always remember to make sure the client's surroundings are clear, repeating the chant and assessing for safety each time before shocking.

From Cummings, R. (2001). *ACLS provider manual.* Dallas, TX: American Heart Association.

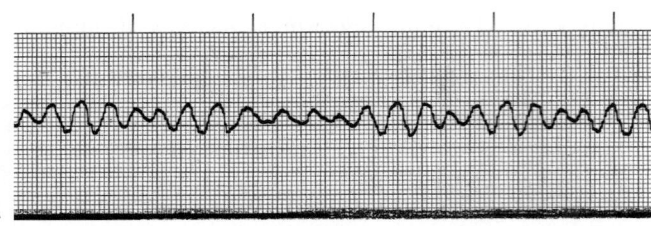

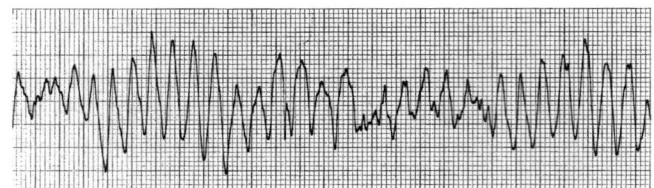

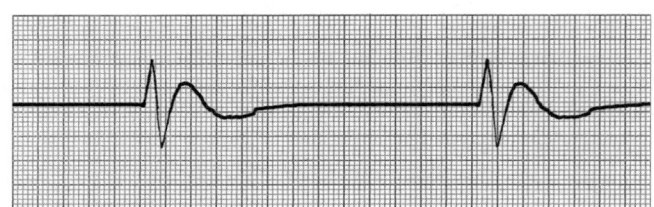

FIGURE 59-7 A, Coarse ventricular fibrillation. **B,** Torsades de pointes. **C,** Ventricular asystole in a dying heart. (B from Phillips, R.E., & Feeney, M.K. [1990]. *The cardiac rhythms: A systematic approach to interpretation* [3rd ed., p. 393]. Philadelphia: W.B. Saunders.)

Genetic Links feature on Long Q-T Syndrome at right). Clinical manifestations begin with palpitations and syncope. This rhythm often precedes VFib and sudden death.

Torsades de pointes is treated only if the Q-T interval is prolonged with temporary overdrive ventricular or atrial pacing. Discontinuation of offending agents is also crucial. IV magnesium sulfate is considered the treatment of choice.[1,2,13,18]

Pre-Excitation Syndromes

Pre-excitation syndromes occur when part or all of the ventricle is reentered by a depolarization wave traveling down a congenital or acquired accessory conducting pathway between the atrium and ventricle.

An accessory pathway is abnormal conductive tissue connecting the atria and ventricle. Normally the AV node is the only connection between the atria and ventricles and controls (blocks) rapid atrial rates that prevent rapid ventricular rates (e.g., AFib). When accessory pathways are present, there is nothing to block rapid atrial rates, and ventricular rates soar.

Of the several types of disorders in this category, *Wolff-Parkinson-White syndrome* (WPW) appears most frequently. In clients with WPW, attacks of very rapid supraventricular dysrhythmias suddenly develop. Most

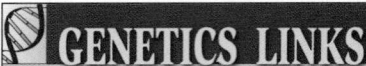

GENETICS LINKS

Long Q-T Syndrome*

Description

Long Q-T syndrome (LQT) produces episodic tachydysrhythmias including *torsades de pointes* (TdP), which may eventually lead to ventricular fibrillation. The most common manifestation of LQT is syncope typically occurring without warning. Undetected or untreated ventricular fibrillation may result in premature sudden death.

Genetics

LQT is inherited in an autosomal-dominant pattern of inheritance with most individuals (90%) inheriting the gene from an affected parent. Offspring of an affected parent have a 50% chance of inheriting the disease-causing mutation. LQT is caused by mutations in one of five known genes associated with this disorder: *KCNQ1, KCNH2, SCN5A, KCNE1,* and *KCNE2.* A family history of syncope, sudden death, or successful reversal of cardiac arrest may be suspicious of LQT syndrome.

Diagnosis/Genetic Testing

LQT syndrome produces a prolongation of the QT interval and T-wave abnormalities, which can be determined clinically by electrocardiography. Clinical molecular genetic testing of the five genes associated with LQT may also make the diagnosis of LQT. About 30% of clinically affected families do not have a detectable mutation in one of these five genes. It is thought that one of more genes, not yet identified, may be responsible.

Management

Most affected individuals live normal lifestyles. Management is focused on client education, avoidance of triggering events, beta-blockers, pacemakers, and ready availability of external defibrillators.

*Also known as Romano Ward syndrome (RWS).

adults with WPW have normal hearts, but if the tachydysrhythmias occur persistently, myocardial fatigue and ventricular failure may result.

Clients with WPW do not require intervention unless they experience recurring tachydysrhythmias. In this instance, the physician may elect to use vagotonic maneuvers, cardioversion, adenosine, amiodarone (Cordarone), esmolol administration, or chemical, mechanical, or radiofrequency ablation. Ablation is an interventional procedure that destroys the accessory pathway.

Interventional Medical Management

Ablating Conduction Pathways. A variety of procedures can be used to treat dysrhythmias when medications are not successful in bringing about conversion of the abnormal rhythm to a normal rhythm. Interventions include (1) chemical and mechanical ablation and (2) radiofrequency of the abnormal pathway. These procedures involve risk to normal conduction tissue, and a pacemaker may be needed either temporarily or permanently.[15,16]

Chemical Ablation. Alcohol or phenol is inserted into involved areas of the myocardium through an angioplasty catheter. Test injections with saline or lidocaine are given to determine whether the dysrhythmia ceases before the final injection. Postprocedural care is the same as for angioplasty.

Mechanical Ablation. The abnormal pathway is surgically removed or treated with a cryoprobe to interrupt its effect on heart rhythms. SVT, AFib, atrial flutter, and WPW syndrome may be treated with this method when the client does not respond to medication. Before the procedure the myocardium is mapped to determine whether other forms of surgery (e.g., coronary bypass grafting, valve replacement) might correct the dysrhythmia. Mapping also isolates the area to be treated. The procedure may be performed through open-heart or closed-heart methods.

Postprocedure care and recovery are similar to those following cardiac catheterization.

Radiofrequency Ablation. Radiofrequency catheter ablation (RFA) is used primarily for SVT associated with WPW or AV nodal reentry, although it has also been used successfully to treat refractory VT. A steerable pacing catheter directs low-power, high-frequency current to a localized accessory pathway and necroses a small portion of the heart. When this current is applied, the temperature of the contact tissue rises, water is driven out, and coagulation necrosis results. The amount of tissue injury depends on the amount of energy delivered (5 to 50 W), the length of time it is delivered (10 to 90 seconds), and the resistance at the end of the catheter. RFA produces lesions that are smaller and more controllable than DC catheter ablation lesions.

The major advantage of RFA is the high rate of success (99% at some centers) and low morbidity. RFA is more successful than conventional medical therapies or DC ablation but equal in success to surgical treatment.

Although RFA is a relatively safe procedure, some complications can occur:

- Cardiac tamponade (1%)
- Deep vein thrombosis (1%)
- Trauma to vessel (1%)
- Transient ischemic attack or stroke (0.5%)
- Perforation of AV leaflet (extremely rare)
- Hematoma at introducer site (common)
- Unintentional AV block requiring pacemaker implantation (up to 10%)

Postprocedure nursing care and recovery are similar to those following cardiac catheterization. Specific nursing responsibilities include (1) preprocedure education of client and family, (2) interventions to reduce anxiety before and during the RFA procedure, (3) monitoring of vital signs and lower-extremity perfusion during and after the procedure, and (4) discharge instructions. Clients are usually discharged within 24 hours after RFA and are instructed to resume normal activities gradually but to avoid strenuous activities for 7 to 10 days. ECGs are obtained routinely at 1, 3, 6, and 9 months after RFA. Aspirin, 325 mg, is prescribed for 14 days after RFA to prevent clot formation and platelet aggregation at the ablation site.[9,10]

REENTRY OF IMPULSES

Ventricular Fibrillation

Ventricular fibrillation is a life-threatening dysrhythmia characterized by extremely rapid, erratic impulse formation and conduction. This lethal dysrhythmia causes abrupt cessation of effective cardiac output. It usually results from severe myocardial damage, hypothermia, R-on-T phenomenon, hypoxia, contact with high-voltage electricity, electrolyte imbalance, or toxicity from quinidine, procainamide, or digitalis.

The ECG tracing displays bizarre fibrillatory wave patterns, and it is impossible to identify P waves, QRS complexes, or T waves (Figure 59-7, A). VFib may be either coarse or fine. Untreated, the deflections become smaller, and eventually all ventricular activity ceases. Death results within minutes without immediate intervention (i.e., defibrillation, CPR, and medications).

When VFib appears, the clinician must immediately initiate CPR until the defibrillator is engaged. Defibrillate up to three times if needed. Defibrillation can be performed by nurses who have advanced training (see Defibrillation). A standard pattern of energy and current is used. Defibrillation begins with 200 joules (J); if not successful, it is advanced to 300 J, and then to 360 J. With persistent VFib, epinephrine is given and the clinician defibrillates at 360 J. Other medications are alternated with defibrillation (lidocaine, magnesium sulfate, sodium bicarbonate), depending on the client's cardiac rhythm and electrolyte and acid-base balance.[1,2,18]

DISTURBANCES IN CONDUCTION

Ventricular Asystole

Ventricular asystole (cardiac standstill) represents the total absence of ventricular electrical activity (Figure 59-7, C). The client has no palpable pulse (no cardiac output), and a rhythm is absent if the client is monitored. The occurrence of sudden ventricular asystole in a conscious person results in faintness, followed within seconds by loss of consciousness, seizures, and apnea. If the dysrhythmia remains untreated, death ensues. Ventricular asystole must be treated immediately.

Cardiac standstill can occur as a primary event, or it may follow VFib or pulseless electrical activity. Asystole can occur also in clients with complete heart block (CHB) in whom there is no escape pacemaker. Possible causes include the following:

- Hypoxia
- Hyperkalemia and hypokalemia
- Pre-existing acidosis
- Drug overdose
- Hypothermia

The treatment of choice consists of CPR, epinephrine, atropine, transcutaneous pacing, and correction of the cause.[1,2,17,18]

Pulseless Electrical Activity

Pulseless electrical activity represents the presence of some electrical activity in the heart, as seen on the monitor, other than VFib or VT; however, a pulse cannot be detected by palpation of any artery. Common causes include cardiac tamponade, massive pulmonary embolus, tension pneumothorax, and severe hypovolemia.

Rapid searching for the cause is imperative. Until the cause is located, CPR is initiated and fluid volume restored.

OUTCOME MANAGEMENT OF LIFE-THREATENING DYSRHYTHMIAS
■ Medical Management

The goal of management is to stop the dysrhythmia immediately and to restore normal sinus rhythm. Remember, because there is inadequate or no perfusion of blood during these dysrhythmias, CPR is performed. Finally the cause of the dysrhythmia is identified and treated.

Life-threatening dysrhythmias can often be effectively controlled by defibrillation. The most crucial element for survival after cardiac arrest is the time interval from collapse to care, especially defibrillation. With each passing minute, the chances of survival decline as much as 10%. Electrical intervention can (1) abruptly stop the heart's erratic electrical discharge or (2) resume the flow of electrical current where there is none. Methods of electrical therapy include defibrillation and cardioversion (see earlier discussion).

Defibrillation. The use of defibrillation delivers an electrical current (shock) of preset voltage to the heart through paddles placed on the chest wall (closed chest procedure). This current causes the entire myocardium to depolarize completely at the moment of shock, thus producing transient asystole and allowing the heart's intrinsic pacemakers to regain control. The amount of energy required to produce this effect is determined largely by the client's *transthoracic impedance,* or resistance to current flow. Because of this factor, the amount of energy

that reaches the heart is less than the amount that the defibrillator is charged to deliver.[1,10,12]

The procedure is associated with potential hazards, particularly myocardial damage. The higher the amount of energy or frequency of the shocks, the greater the risk of injury. Advances in the equipment now allow measurement of transthoracic impedance. Once impedance is determined, the defibrillator automatically selects the amount of current needed that can restore rhythm and cardiac output. It is expected this mode of defibrillation will reduce the risk of complications.[1,16]

The degree of transthoracic resistance depends on several variables:

1. *Energy level.* The higher the energy level that is selected, the more current will follow.
2. *Number and frequency of shocks.* The more shocks administered and the shorter the time between them, the lower the transthoracic resistance.
3. *Ventilation phase.* Resistance is lower when shocks are delivered during exhalation, when there is less air (and therefore smaller diameter) in the lungs.
4. *Paddle size.* The larger the paddle, the lower the resistance.
5. *Chest size.* The smaller the distance between the defibrillator electrodes once they are in place, the lower the resistance.
6. *Paddle-skin interface material.* Conductive material between the skin and paddles reduces transthoracic impedance.
7. *Paddle pressure.* Applying firm pressure increases contact between the skin and the paddles, helping to overcome transthoracic resistance. Exert about 25 pounds of pressure on each paddle.
8. *Paddle placement.* Place one paddle on the upper chest, to the right of the sternum; place the other paddle on the lower left chest, to the left of the nipple, with the center of the paddle in the midaxillary line.

If the client has a permanent pacemaker or an internal cardiac defibrillator, place the paddles at least 5 inches away from the generator to avoid damaging it. If a temporary pacing system is in use, disconnect the pacing lead from the pulse generator immediately before defibrillation and reconnect it after the shock.[1,4,12]

Most defibrillators can be used to perform either *synchronized* cardioversion or *unsynchronized* cardioversion (commonly called *defibrillation*). Defibrillation is always indicated in VFib and is also used in VT when the client is unconscious and pulseless. Specially trained nurses, emergency medical technicians, and physicians perform this procedure in acute settings.

Care Before Defibrillation. Immediately before defibrillation, assess the client's responsiveness and do the following:

1. If the client is not responsive, activate the EMS system.

2. Call for the defibrillator.
3. Assess the client's airway, breathing, and circulation (ABCs). Open the airway. Look, listen, and feel.
4. If the client is not breathing, give two slow breaths.
5. Assess the client's circulation; if no pulse is present, start CPR.
6. Perform CPR until the defibrillator is in place.
7. Check the ECG to verify the presence of VFib or pulseless VT.
8. Check leads for any loose connections.
9. Remove any nitroglycerin patch.

On confirmation of the emergency, the code alarm is given over the health care facility intercom system or to pagers to summon the emergency team (e.g., "Code 99, Dr. Blue"). In the meantime, CPR measures are started by the first person to arrive on the scene. The clinician turns on the defibrillator and sets it at 200 J. In the presence of VFib, the synchronous mode must not be used. Start an IV line as needed for administration of resuscitation medications. Intubation is completed with oxygen supplementation.

Care During Defibrillation. When VFib develops, clinicians must attempt defibrillation at the earliest opportunity. The paddles are lubricated with electrode paste or conducting pads to enhance conduction and prevent burning of the skin. The paste should not extend beyond the paddles, and the paddles must lie flat against the body to avoid burns. The clinician places the paddles firmly against the chest. A transverse (anterolateral) position for paddle placement is used. One paddle is placed at the second intercostal space, at the right of the sternum, and the other paddle is positioned at the fifth intercostal space on the anterior axillary line (Figure 59-8).

To ensure safe defibrillation, people who perform defibrillation must always announce when they are about to shock. The phrase "One. I'm clear. Two. You're clear. Three. All clear" is recommended. Because electricity is carried along metal devices and the client, all personnel, including the clinician administering the shock, must stand back from the bed. Open chest defibrillation occurs when electrical current is applied directly to the heart.

Care After Defibrillation. The clinician immediately assesses the ECG and pulse after defibrillation. If the first countershock is unsuccessful, immediate defibrillation must be performed again at a higher energy level (300 and 360 J). Defibrillation may be applied up to three times (200, 300, 360 J) if needed for persistent VFib or pulseless VT. Defibrillators are frequently equipped with paddles that can monitor the ECG, even immediately after defibrillation. Therefore if the paddles are left in place after the shock has been delivered, the cardiac response can be quickly evaluated.

If the three defibrillations have not been successful, CPR should be continued. A member of the health care

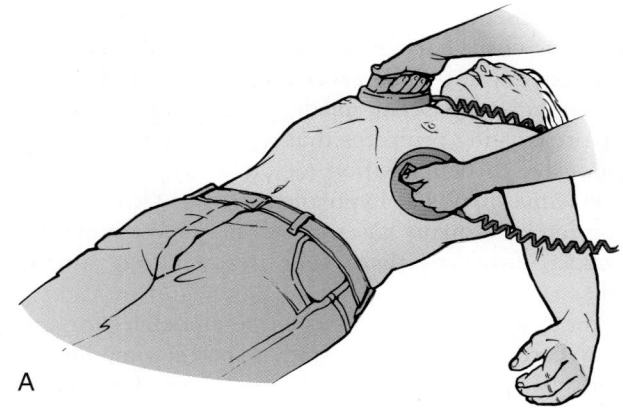

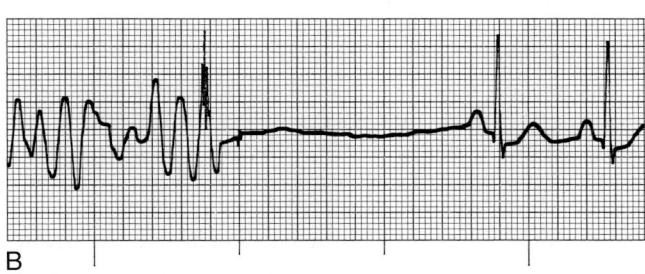

FIGURE 59-8 A, Anterolateral paddle placement for external countershock. External paddles are placed at the second right intercostal space and at the anterior axillary line in the fifth left intercostal space. **B,** Ventricular fibrillation converted to normal sinus rhythm.

team administers appropriate medications again before the next defibrillation attempt. A successful response is indicated by cessation of fibrillation, restoration of sinus rhythm, and palpation of a regular pulse. After successful defibrillation, continuous ECG monitoring is required. The client's vital signs and neurologic status must also be continuously assessed.

For clients with a pacemaker or an automatic implantable cardioverter-defibrillator (AICD), a programmer-analyzer should be available to examine the system for damage and erroneous reprogramming after defibrillation. Continue to monitor for pacemaker malfunction for at least the next 24 hours.

In documenting the outcome of defibrillation, record the following points:

• Preprocedure rhythm
• Times and voltage of shocks delivered
• Post-defibrillation rhythm pattern
• Names, times of administration, and doses of administered medications
• Other hemodynamic data available before, during, and after defibrillation

Termination of Resuscitation. In general, if an organized rhythm and pulse have not returned, the Advanced Cardiac Life Support team leader can cease efforts to resuscitate clients from confirmed and persistent asystole when the client has received successful endotracheal intubation, successful IV access, suitable basic CPR, and all rhythm-appropriate medications. Always consider any pre-existing problems that may make the client less responsive to defibrillation (acidosis, hypokalemia, hyperkalemia, hypoxia, hypovolemia), and treat them appropriately. In many cases clients may have other, noncardiac, disorders that make resuscitation attempts futile.

The American Heart Association guidelines for emergency cardiac care do not state a specific time limit beyond which rescuers cannot have a successful resuscitation. Cardiac arrests in special situations such as hypothermia, electrocution, and drug overdose present exceptions to any rules. Special situations call for common sense and clinical judgment.[1,5]

 Television portrayal of defibrillation and CPR contributes to many misconceptions about these treatments. One article discusses whether the information on television provides accurate information.[6] Three television shows were viewed (*ER, Chicago Hope,* and *Rescue 911).* The cause of the cardiac arrest, the demographics of the client, the underlying illness, and the outcomes were recorded. A total of 97 episodes of the three shows were reviewed. Of the 60 clients who received CPR, 46 (77%) survived the immediate cardiac arrest. Survival rates for CPR on these television programs are much higher than the highest rates reported in the literature. Most people resuscitated were children, teenagers, and young adults. In the hospital, cardiac arrest is most common in older adults. On television, most cardiac arrests have been caused by trauma; in reality, most cardiac arrests are due to heart disease. During the same episodes, 37 people died. In only eight of the situations in which people died was there any discussion about the use of CPR or reference to "do-not-resuscitate" orders.

Clients participate in discussions about their health care today more than ever before. Many people have few resources from which to hear about acute care. Consequently images in the media strongly shape the public's belief about medical care, illness, and death. The portrayal of CPR and death on three popular programs has been misleading. Misrepresentation of CPR on television may lead people to misinterpret the outcomes seen there as real life. Nurses need to be able to clarify misconceptions.

Automated External Defibrillator. An automated external defibrillator (AED) delivers electrical shocks to a client after it identifies VT or VFib. The device is attached to the client with adhesive sternal-apex pads on flexible cables, which allows "hands-free" defibrillation, a feature available with conventional defibrillation as well. AEDs also have an internal microprocessor-based detection system that analyzes the rhythm for the characteristics of VFib or VT. When VFib or VT is present, the AED "advises" the operator to deliver a shock.

Automated external devices are "automated" in the sense that the device—not the operator—analyzes the rhythm and determines the presence of VFib or VT.[1,5] The most common cause of unconsciousness in an adult is VFib. Defibrillation is the only effective treatment. AEDs are thus common in emergency response units and have been placed in many public setting because of the ease in using them.

■ Surgical Management

Clients with persistent heart rhythm problems may benefit from implanted devices to control their rhythm.

Controlling Abnormal Impulses

Automatic Implantable Cardioverter-Defibrillator. The automatic implantable cardioverter-defibrillator (AICD) consists of a pulse generator and a sensor that continuously monitors heart rhythm. When the device detects a dysrhythmia, it automatically delivers a countershock. For VFib the AICD gives an electrical countershock within 15 to 20 seconds. It can also detect and treat VT with cardioversion. Compared with external defibrillation, this implanted system does not require as much energy because less energy is lost when the impulse is applied directly to the heart. In addition, a back-up pacemaker helps to control the rhythm.

The AICD is usually implanted surgically into a pouch below the left clavicle or into the abdominal cavity for two types of conditions[1,8]:
1. Survival of one or more episodes of sudden cardiac death resulting from VT or VFib
2. Recurrent, refractory, life-threatening ventricular dysrhythmias that can develop into VT or VFib, or both, despite antidysrhythmic therapy

Clients who require AICDs have a great deal of anxiety. Anxiety can develop from past episodes of near death as well as from feelings of not ever being able to die. Other clients may fear that the AICD will not be able to reverse the dysrhythmia. Be sensitive to these thoughts, and facilitate their discussion.[1,4,12]

Restoring Impulse Generation

Pacemakers. Pacemakers provide an artificial SA node or Purkinje system. Pacemakers can be *permanent* or *temporary.*

An artificial pacemaker is indicated if the conduction system fails to transmit impulses from the sinus node to the ventricles, to generate an impulse spontaneously, or to maintain primary control of the pacing function of the heart. Many conditions can affect the ability of the heart's conduction system to function normally, creating circumstances that warrant pacing (Box 59-3). Pacemakers can be used temporarily or prophylactically un-

BOX 59-3 *Conditions That May Necessitate a Pacemaker*

- Ablation
- Acute myocardial infarction
- Autonomic nervous system failure
- Cardiac surgery
- Drug toxicity (antidysrhythmics)
- Electrolyte imbalance
- Myocardial ischemia

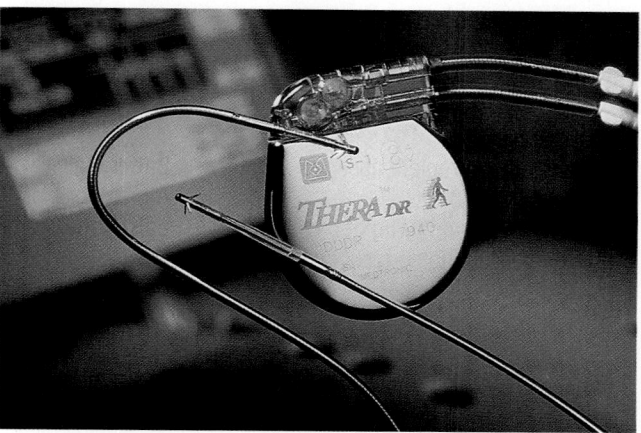

FIGURE 59-9 A permanent pacemaker (pulse generator). (Courtesy of Medtronic, Inc., Minneapolis, MN.)

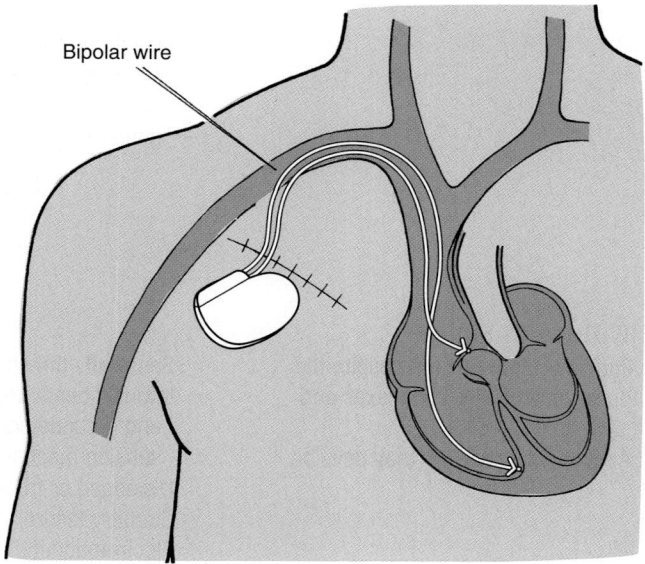

Bipolar wire

FIGURE 59-10 Transvenous temporary endocardial pacing is routine for most cardiac surgical procedures. This can be established by insertion of electrode wires through a vein (subclavian or internal jugular) and into the right atrium or right ventricle. Temporary pacing wires can also be advanced through pulmonary artery catheters. (From Urden, L.D., Stacy, K.M., & Lough, M.E. [Eds.], *Thelan's critical care nursing: Diagnosis and management* [4th ed.]. St. Louis: Mosby.)

til the condition underlying the disturbance resolves. Pacemakers also can be used on a permanent basis if the client's condition persists despite adequate therapy.

An artificial pacemaker is intended to provide a physiologic back-up for the heart during failure of the conduction system to depolarize the myocardium and maintain adequate cardiac output. When cardiac output is diminished because of lack of depolarization of the ventricles, artificial pacing can provide the necessary stimulus directly to the atria or ventricles, or both, to bring about contraction. If cardiac output is compromised because an ectopic pacemaker is causing the ventricles to depolarize and contract at a rate that does not promote adequate ventricular filling, artificial pacing competes with the ectopic pacemaker to assume the primary pacing function of the heart.

Pacemaker Design. An artificial pacemaker provides an external source of energy for impulse formation and delivery and stimulation of myocardial tissue. Whereas numerous pacemaker models are available, each with unique capabilities, every pacemaker consists of a pulse generator with circuitry, the lead, and the electrode system.

The pulse generator is essentially the pacemaker's power source. It houses the electronic circuitry responsible for sending out appropriately timed signals and for sensing cardiac activity. The output circuit controls the current pulse delivery rate, pulse duration, and refractory period. The sensing circuit is responsible for identifying and analyzing any spontaneous intrinsic electrical activity and responding appropriately.

The pulse generator can be external or internal. The external unit is designed for temporary pacing, primarily for support of transient dysrhythmias that impair cardiac output.

The unit is the size of a small transistor radio and operates by dry-cell batteries (Figure 59-9). It has dials for the adjustment of power, rate of discharge, and mode. The pulse generator can also be permanently implanted. The surgeon places the permanent pulse generator into a small tunnel burrowed within the subcutaneous tissue below the right (Figure 59-10) or left clavicle or in the abdominal cavity. The pulse generator is a small—about the size of a stethoscope head—hermetically sealed (to prevent exposure to body fluids) lithium battery. Pace-

maker generators can be reprogrammed after insertion as needed.

The lead delivers the electrical impulse from the pulse generator to the myocardium. The leads consist of flexible conductive wires enclosed by insulating material. The electrode is the end of the lead that delivers the impulse directly to the myocardial wall. It is usually made of platinum-iridium, a highly conductive material that also deters the adherence of platelets. This system not only delivers electrical impulses but also relays informa-

TABLE 59-2	Pacemaker Malfunctions and Nursing Interventions	
Problem	**Possible Cause**	**Nursing Interventions***
Failure to Pace Properly Intermittent or complete absence of pacing artifact Rapid, inappropriate firing of pacemaker (pacemaker-mediated tachycardia)	Battery failure A break or loose connection anywhere along the system Pulse generator failure Circuitry failure "Oversensing" or "undersensing" by the pacemaker	Replace pulse generator. Replace battery unit. Check and tighten all connections between pulse generator and leads. Reduce or increase sensitivity threshold of pacemaker unit. Assess client's tolerance of pacemaker failure; have emergency drugs on hand; perform CPR as indicated.
Failure to Capture Pacing artifact present but not followed by a QRS complex or P wave	Increased pacing threshold; can be related to electrolyte imbalance, ischemia, drug toxicity, perforation, or excessive fibrosis of tissue at electrode site Lead displacement due to migration, or idle manipulation of pulse generator ("twiddler's syndrome")	Increase voltage by 1-2 mA (temporary pacemaker). Increase amplitude of pacemaker output/pulse width. Reposition client to either side in attempt to improve contact of electrode with endocardium; in temporary pacemaker, try moving arm if lead wire is inserted in antecubital area. Obtain chest film to determine pacemaker position. Have emergency drugs on hand; initiate CPR if necessary.
Failure to Sense Pacing artifact present despite the presence of QRS complexes and P waves A competitive rhythm may develop	Sensitivity threshold set too low Intrinsic beats are of too-low voltage and go undetected by pacemaker's sensing mechanism Dislodged or fractured lead Circuitry failure Electromagnetic interference	Increase sensitivity threshold on pulse generator. Reposition client. If client's intrinsic rhythm or rate is adequate, turn off pacemaker. Increase pacing rate to overdrive client's intrinsic heart rate. Give antidysrhythmics to decrease ectopy. Notify physician. Obtain chest x-ray to determine electrode placement.
Oversensing Results from the inappropriate sensing of extraneous electrical signals or myopotentials (which should be ignored)	Sensitivity threshold set too high T wave sensing myopotentials Electromagnetic interference Two leads touching	Decrease sensitivity threshold. Correct conditions that produce large T waves.

Modified from Huang, S.H., et al. (1989). *Coronary care nursing* (2nd ed.). Philadelphia: W. B. Saunders; and Urden, L.D., Stacy, K.M., & Lough, M.E. (Eds.), *Thelan's critical care nursing: Diagnosis and management* (4th ed.). St. Louis: Mosby.
CPR, Cardiopulmonary resuscitation.
*For all problems document malfunction by an electrocardiogram. If the pacemaker is programmable, have the reprogramming machine available. Monitor the client's tolerance to pacemaker malfunction (vital signs, chest pain).

tion about spontaneous intracardiac signals back to the sensing circuit within the pulse generator.

Electrodes can be *unipolar* or *bipolar*. Unipolar designs incorporate the cardiac electrode as the negative terminal of the electrical circuit; the metallic shell or second wire of the impulse generator is the positive electrode. Bipolar systems use two wires, each ending in an electrode a short distance apart.

Single-chamber pacemakers pace either the ventricles or atria; *dual-chamber* pacemakers pace both the ventricles and atria.

Pacemaker Methods. Impulses can be delivered to myocardial tissue by three major modes of artificial pacing: external, epicardial, and endocardial.

External (Transcutaneous) Pacing. The heart is stimulated through large, gelled electrode pads placed anteriorly and posteriorly and connected to an external transcutaneous pacemaker. Transcutaneous pacing is the treatment of choice in emergency cardiac care because it can be started quickly while a temporary transvenous pacemaker is being inserted or as prophylaxis against dysrhythmias. It is also the least invasive pacing technique. Because no vascular puncture is needed for electrode placement, transcutaneous pacing is preferred in clients who are receiving anticoagulation therapy or who might require thrombolytic therapy.

Because the anterior electrode is placed to the left of the sternum and centered close to the point of maximal impulse (PMI), excessive chest hair must be clipped or shaved to ensure good contact, or alternative pacing electrode positions must be used. The pacing device is usually activated at a rate of 80 beats/min. Electrical capture is characterized by widening of the QRS complex and broadening of the T wave. Many clients feel extreme discomfort with each paced beat; this is a significant limitation to transcutaneous pacing.

Opioid analgesia and sedation may be given to clients who are conscious or who regain consciousness to reduce discomfort and anxiety. Additional complications of external transcutaneous pacing can include skin burns, muscle twitching, psychological reactions, failure to "capture" (inability of the impulse to initiate a contraction), and failure to "sense" (inability of the pacemaker to sense intrinsic electrical activity) (Table 59-2).

Epicardial (Transthoracic) Pacing. With this method of artificial pacing, the electrical energy travels through lead wires from an external pulse generator through the thoracic musculature directly to the epicardial surface of the heart. Epicardial pacing is most commonly used during and immediately after open-heart surgery because there is direct access to the epicardium at this time. Some occasional complications include lead dislodgment, microshock, cardiac tamponade, infection, psychological reactions, failure to capture, and failure to sense.

Endocardial (Transvenous) Pacing. Endocardial pacing is the most common mode of pacing the heart in emergency situations. The surgeon inserts the pacing

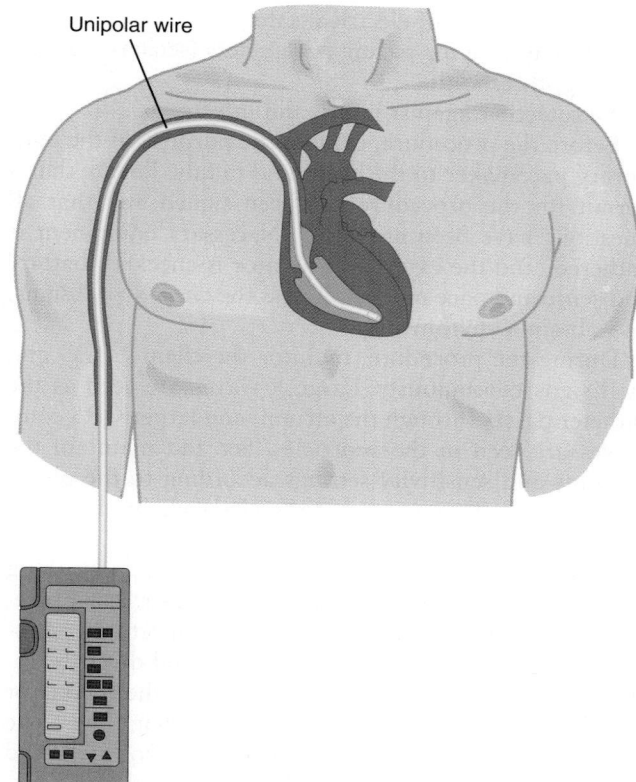

Unipolar wire

FIGURE 59-11 A temporary endocardial pacemaker.

electrode via the transvenous route (the antecubital, femoral, jugular, or subclavian vein) and then threads the electrode into the right atrium or right ventricle so that it comes into direct contact with the endocardium. This procedure can be done at the bedside under fluoroscopic control or in a cardiovascular laboratory.

Major drawbacks include thrombophlebitis, infection at the insertion site, sepsis from nonsterile technique, increased chance of lead displacement as the client changes position, and the discomfort of having the extremity nearest the insertion site immobilized (Figure 59-11). Other additional complications occasionally seen are pacer-induced dysrhythmias, hiccups, abdominal twitching, myocardial irritability, perforation of chamber or septum, failure to capture, and failure to sense.

Temporary Pacing. Temporary pacing can be used in emergent or elective situations that require limited, short-term pacing (<2 weeks). The pulse generator is external. Temporary pacemakers can be applied transcutaneously and can be inserted transthoracically or, more commonly, transvenously.

Although the principles of cardiac pacing are the same for temporary and permanent pacemakers, each type presents distinct issues for nurses to assess and to teach to the client and family. Clients with a temporary pacemaker need the following:

- An explanation about the pacemaker
- Monitoring for response to the pacemaker

- Maintenance of electrical safety
- Monitoring for pacing parameters (sensing, capturing, threshold)
- Protection against injury and infection

Before the procedure, explain the purpose of the temporary pacemaker to the client and family. Ensure that a permit for the procedure has been signed and that all questions have been answered. Necessary equipment is gathered, and the external generator is checked (battery and sense and pace modes). Assess the client's vital signs, and obtain a rhythm strip.

During the procedure, monitor the client's ECG and vital signs continuously. Large P waves are seen as the catheter passes through the atrium, and larger QRS complexes are seen in the ventricles. Set and maintain the stimulus and sensitivity settings according to the physician's orders. Tape or suture the electrode at the insertion site.

After the procedure assess vital signs routinely along with heart rhythm and emotional reactions to the procedure and pacing. Secure and check all connections. Monitor battery and control settings. Clean and dress the incision site according to protocols. Keep the generator dry and protect the controls from mishandling. The client must be protected from electrical microshocks and electromagnetic interference. Wear rubber gloves when exposed wires are handled. Check electrical equipment for adequate grounding. Limit the motion of the extremity at the insertion site. Stabilize the arm, catheter, and pacemaker to an arm board and avoid movement of the arm above shoulder level. Do not lift the client from under the arm. If the leg is the insertion site, limit its motion, especially hip flexion and outward rotation.

In addition to protecting the client from injury, monitor pacemaker function. Document the location and type of pacing lead. Note the pacing mode, stimulus threshold, sensitivity setting, pacing rate and intervals,

and intrinsic rhythm. Pacing intervals are shown in Figure 59-12.

Permanent Pacing. Permanent pacing is indicated for chronic or recurrent dysrhythmias that are severe, unresponsive to antidysrhythmic medication, and caused by AV block or sinus node malfunction. The need for permanent pacemakers is confirmed through ECGs, electrophysiology studies, and Holter monitoring. Indications for permanent pacemakers have been grouped into three classes. Class I criteria are identified in Box 59-4.[7]

Clinical manifestations that are directly attributable to the slow heart rate include transient dizziness, lightheadedness, near syncope or frank syncope as manifestations of transient cerebral ischemia, and more generalized manifestations such as marked exercise intolerance or frank heart failure.[5,18]

Pacemaker Modes. There are two basic types of pacemakers:

1. *Fixed-rate* (non-demand or asynchronous). Fixed-rate pacemakers are designed to fire constantly as a

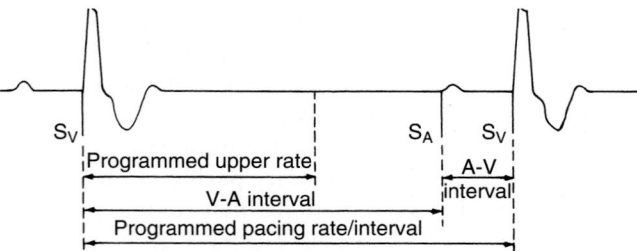

S_A = Atrial stimulus
S_V = Ventricular stimulus

FIGURE 59-12 Pacing intervals. The atrioventricular (A-V, delay) interval can be thought of as an artificial P-R interval. The programmed pacing rate, or *interval*, is also called the ventriculoventricular (V-V) interval. Ventricular pacing occurs if intrinsic ventricular activity does not occur within the V-V interval. (From *Symbiotics series: Selecting the DDD patient* [1984]. Minneapolis: Medtronic.)

BOX 59-4 *Clinical Conditions That Warrant Permanent Pacemakers (Class I Criteria)*

A. Third-degree and advanced second-degree atrioventricular (AV) block associated with the following complications:
  1. Symptomatic bradycardia (including heart failure)
  2. Arrhythmias and other medical conditions that require drugs that result in symptomatic bradycardia.
  3. Documented periods of asystole greater than or equal to 3 seconds or any escape rate less than 40 beats/min in an awake, symptom-free client
  4. After catheter ablation of the AV junction
  5. Postoperative AV block that is not expected to resolve after cardiac surgery
B. Alternating bundle-branch block
C. Sinus node dysfunction with symptomatic bradycardia, including frequent pauses

From Gregoratos, G., et al. ACC/AHA/NASPE 2002 guideline update for implantation of cardiac pacemakers and antiarrhythmic devices: Summary article: A report to the American College of Cardiology/American Heart Association Task Force on Practice Guidelines (ACC/AHA/NASPE Committee to update the 1998 Pacemaker guidelines). *Circulation, 106,* 2145-2161.

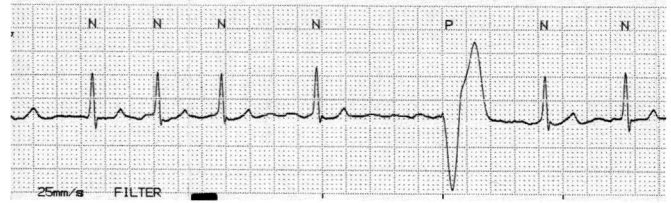

FIGURE 59-13 Demand pacing. The pacemaker initiates an electrical impulse when the sinus node fails to pace the heart.

preset rate without regard to the electrical activity of the client's heart. This mode of pacing is appropriate in the absence of any electrical activity *(asystole)* but is dangerous in the presence of an intrinsic rhythm because of the potential of the pacemaker to fire during the vulnerable period of repolarization and initiate lethal ventricular dysrhythmias.

2. *Demand* pacemakers contain a device that senses the heart's electrical activity and fires at a present rate only when the heart's electrical activity drops below a predetermined rate level (Figure 59-13).

In addition to a variety of capabilities, permanent pacemakers now have special programmable and anti-tachydysrhythmic functions that are quite complex. To communicate all the functions of the individual pacemakers, international codes were developed. Pacemakers are identified with a five-digit letter code. Although the last two letters contain pertinent information, commonly a pacemaker is referred to only by its first three letters (Box 59-5).

Pacemaker Function. Because there are many types of pacemakers with more than 250 programs, the general functions are discussed first. A simple demand pac-

---

BOX 59-5 *Classification System for Pacemakers*

First Letter: Chamber Paced
Indicates which chamber(s) of the heart will be stimulated:
V = Ventricle
A = Atrium
D = Dual-chamber (both atria and ventricles stimulated)

Second Letter: Chamber Sensed
Indicates the chamber(s) of the heart in which the lead is capable of recognizing intrinsic electrical activity:
V = Ventricle
A = Atrium
D = Dual-chamber (sensing capabilities in atria and ventricles)
O = No sensing capability

Third Letter: Mode of Response
Indicates how the pacemaker will act based on the information it senses:
T = Triggered (may have energy output triggered)
I = Inhibited (pacing output inhibited by intrinsic activity)
D = Dual-chamber (may be either inhibiting or triggering of both chambers)

Fourth Letter: Programmable Functions
Indicates ability to change function once the pacemaker has been implanted:
P = Programmable for one or two functions
M = Multiprogrammable ability to change functions other than the rate or output

Fifth Letter: Tachydysrhythmic Functions
Indicates specific methods of interrupting tachydysrhythmias:
B = Bursts of pacing
N = Normal rate competition
S = Scanning

Examples
Pacing Modes Within Single-Chamber Pacemakers
Atrial demand pacemaker (AAI). A pacemaker that senses spontaneously occurring P waves and paces the atria when they do not appear.

Atrial fixed-rate pacemaker (AOO). A pacemaker that paces the atria and does not sense.
Ventricular demand pacemaker (VVI). A pacemaker that senses spontaneously occurring QRS complexes and paces the ventricles when they do not appear.
Ventricular fixed-rate pacemaker (VOO). A pacemaker that paces the ventricles and does not sense.

Pacing Modes Within Dual-Chamber Pacemakers
Atrial synchronous ventricular pacemaker (VDD). A pacemaker that senses spontaneously occurring P waves and QRS complexes and paces the ventricles when QRS complexes fail to appear after spontaneously occurring P waves, as in complete atrioventricular (AV) block. In this type of pacemaker, the pacing of ventricles is synchronized with the P waves so that the ventricular contractions follow the atrial contractions in a normal sequence. A major benefit is that it permits the heart rate to vary, and AV synchrony occurs, depending on the physiologic demands of the body. A built-in safety mechanism causes ventricular depolarizations to occur at a fixed rate should atrial rates become too fast.
AV synchronous pacemaker (VAT). A pacemaker that has ventricular pacing, atrial sensing, and triggered response to sensing. The ventricular pacing stimulus will fire at a set time after sensing a spontaneous atrial depolarization.
AV sequential pacemaker (DVI). A pacemaker that senses spontaneously occurring QRS complexes and paces both the atria and ventricles (the atria first, followed by the ventricles after a short delay) when QRS complexes do not appear.
AV sequential fixed-rate pacemaker (DOO). A pacemaker that paces both the atria and ventricles but does not sense.
Optimal sequential pacemaker (DDD). A pacemaker that senses spontaneously occurring P waves and QRS complexes and (1) paces the atria when P waves fail to appear, as in sick sinus syndrome; and (2) paces the ventricles when QRS complexes fail to appear after spontaneously occurring or paced P waves. In this type of pacemaker, like the VDD pacemaker, the pacing of ventricles is synchronized with the P waves so that the ventricular contractions follow the atrial contractions in a normal sequence.

ing system works in the following manner. The cardiac cycle normally begins with the client's own beat. The pacemaker's sensor senses whether the intrinsic beat has occurred; if not, the pacer sends out an impulse to begin myocardial depolarization through a pulse generator. The impulse generator is said to "capture" the myocardium and thereby maintain heart rhythm.

For a predetermined amount of time after the pacemaker impulse, the pacemaker cannot sense incoming signals. This feature prevents the pacer from sensing its own generated electrical current and from acting again. The *refractory period* is followed by the *noise-sampling period*. If any electromagnetic interference is sensed during this phase, the pacemaker goes into a fixed-rate mode of operation and remains in this mode until the source of interference is removed. At the end of the noise-sampling period, the *alert period* begins and the cycle starts again. If a PVC or PAC occurs during the alert period, the pacemaker can sense it and start its cycle again without emitting any impulse.

Electrocardiography of Paced Beats. The ECG appearance of a paced rhythm differs from that of a normal sinus rhythm. A pacing artifact is seen. With atrial pacing, a P wave follows the artifact but is hidden in some leads. Examination of leads II and V_1 is best for deciding whether a P wave follows a pacer spike. The QRS complex appears normal with atrial pacing; the impulse travels through usual conduction systems.

The ECG with ventricular pacing shows an abnormal QRS complex because the impulse begins in the ventricle. With right ventricular endocardial pacing, a pseudo-LBBB wave is created on ECG. If the left ventricle is paced, a pseudo-RBBB is created.

Assess the ECG strip for pacer spikes followed by the expected appearance of a P wave or QRS complex. Spikes not followed by depolarization waves or paced beats that appear too early or too late may signal pacemaker failure.

Pacemaker Failure. Malfunctions can occur in the pacemaker's sensor or pulse generator. Complications associated with the components of the pacemaker system itself (see Table 59-2) may include the following:

1. *Failure to sense*—an inability of the sensor to detect the client's intrinsic beats; as a result, the pacemaker sends out impulses too early (Figure 59-14, *A*). The failure may be due to improper position of the catheter, tip or lead dislodgment, battery failure, the sensitivity being set too low, or a fractured wire in the catheter.
2. *Failure to pace*—a malfunction of the pulse generator. The ECG shows an absence of any impulse (Figure 59-14, *B*). Component failure to discharge (pace) can be due to battery failure, lead dislodgment, fracture of the lead wire inside the catheter, disconnections between catheter and generator, or a sensing malfunction.

3. *Failure to capture*—a disorder in the pacemaker electrodes; the impulse does not generate depolarization (Figure 59-14, *C*). This complication can result from low voltage, battery failure, faulty connections between the pulse generator and catheter, improper position of the catheter, catheter wire fracture, fibrosis at the catheter tip, or a catheter fracture.

Clinical manifestations associated with pacemaker malfunctioning include syncope, bradycardia or tachycardia, and palpitations. When these manifestations occur, the malfunctioning leads or pacemaker must be replaced.

Teach the client and family how to care for the pacemaker and the precautions to follow (see the Client Education Guide feature on the Client with a Permanent Pacemaker on p. 1697).[3,9]

■ Nursing Management of Clients with Pacemakers
Assessment

Assess the client for *subjective* clinical manifestations of dysrhythmias and alterations in cardiac output: palpitations, syncope, fatigue, shortness of breath, chest pain, or skipped beats felt in the chest. The client may also feel

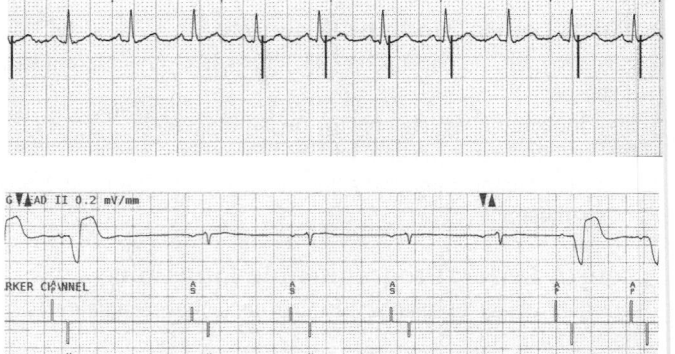

A

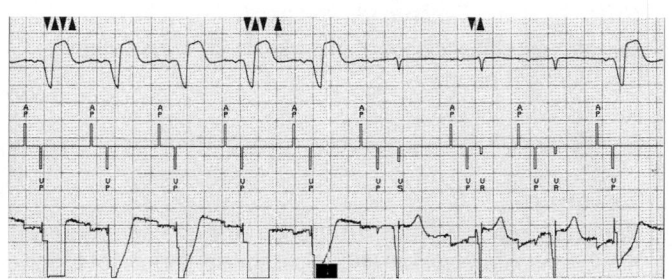

B

C

FIGURE 59-14 Pacemaker failures. **A,** Failure to sense. **B,** Failure to pace. **C,** Failure to capture.

anxiety about the heart disorder and may manifest nervousness, fear, sleeplessness, uncertainty, or hopelessness. *Objective* clinical manifestations may include diaphoresis, pallor or cyanosis, variations in radial and apical pulses such as bradycardia or tachycardia, rhythm changes, hypotension, crackles, and decreased mental acuity. The client may be fearful of being left alone. Monitoring is begun, and the heart rhythm is observed continuously by a nurse, a computer, and an ECG technician. Rhythm strips are examined at least every shift.

Explain the purpose of the pacemaker and the experience of having a pacemaker inserted to the client and family. Most permanent pacemakers are inserted transvenously. Try to keep the ECG leads off the possible insertion site. The insertion site is prepared according to hospital policy. A preoperative ECG is obtained, and a patent IV line is maintained. Prophylactic antibiotics may be given.

After insertion, monitor vital signs and pacemaker function. Pain can usually be managed with oral analgesics if the transvenous approach has been used. Initially instruct the client to avoid excessive extension or abduction of the arm on the operative side. Perform passive range-of-motion exercises on the arm.

Obtain paced and nonpaced ECGs. A magnet can be placed over the pulse generator, converting it to a fixed-rate pacing mode, so that the client's intrinsic rhythm can be determined. The location of the pacemaker electrodes is determined by x-ray. The model and serial numbers of the pulse generator and leads, along with the date of implantation and programmed functions of the initial implant, are recorded.

CLIENT EDUCATION GUIDE
The Client with a Permanent Pacemaker

Wound Care

1. Assess your wound daily, and keep the incision clean and dry until it heals.
2. Report any fever, redness, drainage, warmth, discoloration, or swelling to the physician.
3. Avoid constrictive clothing (e.g., tight brassiere straps), which puts excessive pressure on the wound and the pulse generator.
4. Avoid extensive "toying" with the pulse generator because this may cause pacemaker malfunction and local skin inflammation.

Pacemaker Management

1. Take your pulse as instructed by your physician in your wrist or on your neck. You will be taught how to do this before leaving the hospital.
2. Notify the physician if your pulse is slower than the set rate; also report sensations of feeling your heart "racing," beating irregularly, fatigue, or of dizziness.
3. Avoid being near areas with high voltage, magnetic force fields, or radiation; this can cause pacemaker problems.
4. Avoid being near large running motors (gas or electric) and standing near high-tension wires, power plants, radio transmitters, large industrial magnets, and arc welding machines. Riding in a car is safe, but do not bring the pacemaker to within 6 to 12 inches of the distributor coil of a running engine.
5. You can continue to operate safely most appliances and tools that are properly grounded and in good repair, including microwave ovens, televisions, video recorders, AM and FM radios, electric blankets, lawn mowers, leaf blowers, and cars.
6. You can safely operate the following office and light industrial equipment that is properly grounded and in good repair,

such as electric typewriters, copying machines, and personal computers.
7. An airport's metal detector can be triggered by the pacemaker's metal casing and the programming magnet. Mention your pacemaker to security guards. The metal detector itself does not harm the pacemaker.
8. At all times carry a pacemaker identity card (including programming information, pacemaker manufacturer, emergency phone numbers). Wear a medical alert bracelet.
9. Avoid activity that might damage the pulse generator, such as playing football and firing a rifle with the butt end against the affected shoulder.
10. Some stores sell antitheft devices that may affect pacemaker function. If you suddenly become dizzy, move away from the area and notify the store clerk about the pacemaker.
11. If radiation therapy has been prescribed to the area in which the pulse generator was implanted, the pulse generator must be relocated.
12. Do not lift more than 5 to 10 pounds (equivalent to a full grocery sack or a gallon of milk) for the first 6 weeks after surgery. Do not move your arms and shoulders vigorously for the first 6 weeks. Normal activities (including sexual activity) can be resumed in 6 weeks.
13. Discuss with the nurse the purpose, dose, schedule, and possible side effects of prescribed medications. Consult your written information sheets to reinforce learning.
14. Plan to see your physician to test your pacemaker. Your cardiologist periodically will reevaluate pacemaker function and can reprogram it if needed. You may also be able to check your pacemaker by telephone. If this is possible, you will receive instructions.

Transtelephonic Pacemaker Monitoring Special telephone monitoring of the client's ECG may be done from time to time on an outpatient basis. Telephone ECG systems are designed for follow-up monitoring of clients with pacemakers. Via finger tip, wrist, or ankle electrodes, the transmitter detects, amplifies, and converts a client's electrical activity and pacemaker artifacts to frequency-modulated audio tones for transmission, via the telephone, to an ECG receiver. From the transmitted signals, the ECG receiver provides an ECG strip recording and printout of the rate and pulse width of a client's implanted pacemaker.

■ Self-Care

It may be necessary to teach about the nature of the disorder several times because the client's attention span may be shorter than normal as a result of severe anxiety. Before discharge, make certain that clients appreciate the importance of taking antidysrhythmic agents as prescribed. Include details about medication administration, dosage, and side effects in the discharge plan. If discharged too early and in an unstable condition, many clients risk further exacerbations or additional complications. Make sure that nursing discharge criteria are met and documented.

Clients who have experienced cardiac dysrhythmias while at a health care facility may be apprehensive about leaving the facility. Those who have experienced innocuous dysrhythmias may need only calm reassurance and an explanation of the cause of the disorder. Clients with recurring life-threatening dysrhythmias, such as VT, require comprehensive and specialized attention. These clients may have experienced frightening events in the course of their hospitalization.

When a client is at risk for development of a life-threatening dysrhythmia, ascertain whether the client's housemates and significant others know how to perform CPR. Refer them to community agencies that provide CPR training (e.g., the American Heart Association, the American Red Cross, local fire department, local hospital).

Sometimes clients with serious, chronic, or potential dysrhythmias use portable telemetry units for self-monitoring at home after discharge. This allows resumption of daily activities while providing continuous 24-hour surveillance of cardiac rhythm. Nurses are often responsible for instructing clients in the use of these units. Ask the client to keep a diary of daily activities so that clinicians can correlate factors in the client's life that are contributing to the development of dysrhythmias.

Finally, instruct clients about the importance of regular medical follow-up. Advise them to keep regular appointments with their physician after discharge. Explain to the client and his or her significant others about how to obtain emergency medical attention if it becomes necessary.

Living under the constant threat of sudden death provokes anxiety, depression, and occasionally dependent behavior. In some cases psychological counseling can bolster coping resources. Recommend community and private counseling services for the client and his or her significant others.

CONCLUSIONS

Common dysrhythmias usually do not interfere with everyday activities. In fact most people with dysrhythmias lead a productive and relatively normal life. Clients need to follow a prescribed medical regimen, to take medications as directed, to report any manifestations and side effects, and to be aware of the importance of continued medical care.

THINKING CRITICALLY *evolve*

1. You are walking with a client in the hospital. He is recovering from an MI. A dysrhythmia develops. What assessments should you perform? What care does the client need?

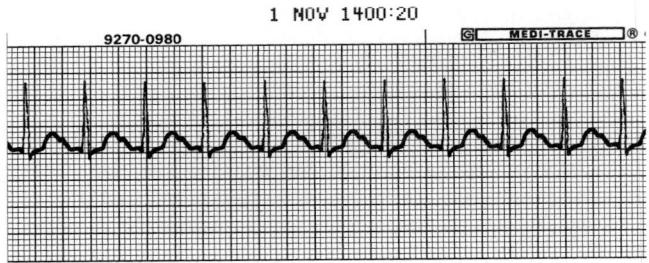

Factors to Consider. What is the usual heart rhythm response to activity? How can you assess if your client is tolerating this rhythm? How should the client be returned to his room?

2. An 82-year-old woman is brought to the emergency department by her son after losing consciousness and hitting her head after falling. She is now awake and states that she has been having periods of dizziness and blackouts for the past few weeks. During your physical examination, you notice what appears to be

a pacemaker device implanted under her left clavicle. What additional assessments should you make? What information should you obtain about the pacemaker? **Factors to Consider.** What might have happened to the pacemaker during the fall? Could a faulty pacemaker be responsible for the loss of consciousness?

Discussions for these questions can be found on the website and the CD-ROM.

BIBLIOGRAPHY

1. American Heart Association. (2000). *Handbook of emergency cardiac care for health care providers 1996.* Dallas: Author.

2. Asselin, M.E., & Cullen, H.A. (2002). A new beat for BLS and ACLS guidelines. *Nursing Management, 33*(2),31-38.

3. Busch, M., & Haskin, J. (2000). Pacemakers and implantable defibrillators. In S. Woods, et al. (Eds.), *Cardiac nursing* (4th ed.). Philadelphia: J.B. Lippincott.

4. Conover, M.B. (2003). *Understanding electrocardiography* (8th ed.). St. Louis: Mosby.

5. Cummings, R. (2001). *ACLS provider manual.* Dallas, TX: American Heart Association.

6. Diem, S., Lantos, J., & Tukley, J. (1996). Cardiopulmonary resuscitation on television: Miracles or misinformation. *New England Journal of Medicine, 334*(12), 1578-1582.

7. Gregoratos, G., et al. (2002). ACC/AHA/NASPE 2002 Guideline update for implantation of cardiac pacemakers and antiarrhythmia devices: Summary article: A report of the American College of Cardiology/American Heart Association task force on practice guidelines (ACC/AHA/NASPE Committee to update the 1998 pacemaker guidelines). *Circulation, 106,* 2145-2161.

8. Hayes, D.L., & Zipes, D.P. (2001). Cardiac pacemakers and cardioverter-defibrillators. In E. Braunwald (Ed.), *Heart Disease* (6th ed.). Philadelphia: W.B. Saunders.

9. Hudak, C., Gallo, B., & Morton. P. (1997). Patient management: Cardiovascular system. In C. Hudak, et al. (Eds.), *Critical care nursing: A holistic approach* (8th ed.). Philadelphia: Lippincott.

10. Main, C. (2000). Cardiac electrophysiology procedures. In S. Woods, et al. (Eds.), *Cardiac nursing* (4th ed.). Philadelphia: Lippincott.

11. Mair, M. (2003). Monophasic and biphasic defibrillators: The evolving technology of cardiac defibrillation. *American Journal of Nursing, 103*(8), 58-60.

12. Massie, B.M., & Amidon, T.A. (2004). Disturbances in rate and rhythm. In L.M. Tierney, et al. (Eds.), *Current medical diagnosis and treatment* (43rd ed.). Stamford, CT: Appleton and Lange.

13. Massie, B.M., & Amidon, T.A. (2004). Conduction disturbances. In L.M. Tierney et al. (Eds.), *Current medical diagnosis and treatment* (43rd ed.). Stamford, CT: Appleton and Lange.

14. Mattoni, T. (2003). Performance of an automatic external cardioverter-defibrillator algorithm in the discrimination of supraventricular from ventricular tachycardia. *American Journal of Cardiology, 91,* 1323-1326.

15. Miller, J.M., & Zipes, D.P. (2001). Management of the patient with cardiac arrhythmias. In E. Braunwald (Ed.), *Heart disease* (6th ed.). Philadelphia: W.B. Saunders.

16. Morady, F. (1999). Radio-frequency ablation as treatment for cardiac arrhythmias. *New England Journal of Medicine, 34*(7), 534-544.

17. Myerburg, R.J., & Castellanos, A. (2001). Cardiac arrest and sudden cardiac death. In E. Braunwald (Ed.), *Heart disease* (6th ed.). Philadelphia: W.B. Saunders.

18. Olgin, J.E., & Zipes, D.P. (2001). Specific arrhythmias: Diagnosis and treatment. In E. Braunwald (Ed.), *Heart disease,* (6th ed.). Philadelphia: W.B. Saunders.

19. Ophie, L.H., & Marcus, F.I. (2001). Antiarrhythmic drugs. In L.H. Ophie (Ed.), *Drugs for the heart* (5th ed.). Philadelphia: W.B. Saunders.

20. Ozcan, C., et. al. (2001). Long-term survival after ablation of the atrioventricular node and implantation of a permanent pacemaker in patients with atrial fibrillation. *New England Journal of Medicine, 344*(14), 1043-1051.

21. Rakel, R.E. (1992). *Conn's current therapy.* Philadelphia: W.B. Saunders.

22. Tchou, P.J. (2002). Ventricular tachycardia. In E. Topol (Ed.), *Textbook of cardiovascular medicine* (2nd ed.). Philadelphia: Lippincott.

23. Thelan, L.A., et al. (1998). Temporary pacemakers. In L.A. Thelan, et al. (Eds.), *Critical care nursing: Diagnosis and management* (3rd ed.). St. Louis: Mosby.

24. Thelan, L.A., et al. (1998). Implantable cardioverter defibrillator. In L.A. Thelan, et al. (Eds.), *Critical care nursing: Diagnosis and management* (3rd ed.). St. Louis: Mosby.

Management of Clients with Myocardial Infarction

Janice Tazbir
Patricia A. Keresztes

---

evolve

Web Enhancements

http://evolve.elsevier.com/Black/medsurg/

Case Management
  Acute Myocardial Infarction
Case Study
  Cardiogenic Shock, Tachycardia, and Heart Failure
Concept Map
  Understanding Myocardial Infarction and Its Treatment

Tables
  Differential Diagnosis of Chest Pain
Appendix C
  Laboratory Values of Clinical Importance in Medical-Surgical Nursing

---

The heart requires a balance between oxygen supply and oxygen demand in order to function properly. The integrity of the coronary arteries is an important determinant of oxygen supply to the heart muscle. Any disorder that reduces the lumen of one of the coronary arteries may cause a decrease in blood flow and oxygen delivery to the area of the myocardium supplied by that vessel and lead to acute coronary syndromes of angina, acute myocardial infarction (AMI), and sudden cardiac death. Coronary heart disease (CHD) is the primary underlying cause of these syndromes and is the single largest killer of American men and women.[1]

The clinical syndromes associated with CHD are familiar to most Americans. Almost every day, the news media covers a story on a celebrity who has suffered from or was treated for chest pain, heart attack, or cardiac arrest. Turn on any television hospital drama and you will see someone seeking treatment for an episode of chest pain. Many of us also have had personal experience with CHD through the illness of a relative or close friend.

It is estimated that 1 million Americans will have a new or recurrent acute coronary syndrome this year. Acute coronary syndromes are responsible for more than 250,000 deaths annually and result from a progressive atherosclerotic process that culminates in rupture of atherosclerotic plaques and thrombus formation.[1] This chapter reviews the risk factors, pathophysiology, clinical manifestations, and medical and nursing interventions for the acute coronary syndromes of angina pectoris (a type of chest pain) and AMI.

ANGINA PECTORIS

Angina pectoris is chest pain resulting from myocardial ischemia (inadequate blood supply to the myocardium).[1] It is a common manifestation of CHD and affects about 6,400,000 Americans—2,400,000 men and 4,000,000 women. According to the Framingham Heart Study, approximately 400,000 new cases of angina occur each year.[13,24] Angina can also occur in clients with normal coronary arteries, but it is less common. Clients with

---

evolve Be sure to check out the bonus material on the Evolve website and the CD-ROM, including free self-assessment exercises.
http://evolve.elsevier.com/Black/medsurg/

Nursing Outcomes Classification (NOC)
for Nursing Diagnoses—Clients with Myocardial Infarction

Acute Pain
  Comfort Level
  Pain Control
  Pain: Disruptive Effects
  Pain Level
Anxiety and Fear
  Anxiety Control
  Coping
  Fear Control
Decreased Cardiac Output
  Cardiac Pump Effectiveness
  Circulation Status
  Vital Signs Status
Excess Fluid Volume
  Electrolyte and Acid-Base Balance
  Fluid Balance
  Hydration
Impaired Gas Exchange
  Electrolyte and Acid-Base Balance

  Respiratory Status: Ventilation
Ineffective Health Maintenance
  Health Promoting Behavior
  Health Seeking Behavior
  Knowledge: Health Behaviors
  Participation: Health Care Decisions
  Psychosocial Adjustment: Life Change
  Self-Direction of Care
Ineffective Tissue Perfusion (Cardiopulmonary)
  Pain Level
  Tissue Perfusion: Cardiac
Powerlessness
  Depression Control
  Depression Level
  Health Beliefs: Perceived Ability to Perform
  Health Beliefs: Perceived Control
  Health Beliefs: Perceived Resources

Risk for Activity Intolerance
  Cardiac Pump Effectiveness
  Circulation Status
  Energy Conservation
  Knowledge: Prescribed Activity
Risk for Constipation
  Bowel Elimination
  Mobility Level
  Nutritional Status: Food and Fluid Intake
Risk for Impaired Skin Integrity
  Immobility Consequences: Physiologic
  Tissue Integrity: Skin and Mucous Membranes
  Tissue Perfusion: Peripheral
Risk for Injury
  Risk Control

CRITICAL MONITORING

Angina from Impending Myocardial Infarction

- Continuous, enduring, severe chest pain lasts more than 20 minutes.
- Pain is usually felt in the retrosternal area, possibly radiating to the arms (the pain is most common in the left shoulder and arm), back, neck, or lower jaw.
- Pain is described as squeezing, pressing, or a sensation of heaviness.
- Deep breathing or changing posture does not change the severity of the pain.
- Pain may occur in the upper abdomen, accompanied by nausea and vomiting.
- Pain is relieved by nitroglycerin; pain is not relieved by antacids or food.
- ECG often shows ischemic changes.
- Chest radiograph is normal for client.

aortic stenosis, hypertension, and hypertrophic cardiomyopathy can have angina pectoris.

Etiology and Risk Factors

Angina pectoris is associated with atherosclerotic lesions and is a manifestation of CHD (see Chapter 58). Angina can be caused either by chronic or acute blockage of a coronary artery or by coronary artery spasm. Chronic blockages are associated with fixed calcified (type Vb) or fibrotic (type Vc) atherosclerotic lesions that occlude more than 75% of the vessel lumen.[9]

When fixed blockages are present in the coronary arteries, conditions that increase myocardial oxygen demand (e.g., physical exertion, emotion, exposure to cold) may precipitate episodes of angina. Because the severely stenosed arteries cannot deliver enough oxygen to meet the increased demand, ischemia results.[2] In contrast, acute blockage of a coronary artery results from rupture or disruption of vulnerable atherosclerotic plaques that cause platelet aggregation and thrombus formation (see Etiology under Myocardial Infarction).[1] Acute blockages are associated with unstable angina and AMI.

Primary prevention is through the lifelong commitment to reducing the risk factors of CHD (see Chapter 58). Secondary prevention is through recognition and early treatment of anginal attacks (see the Critical Monitoring feature on Angina from Impending Myocardial Infarction at left). Tertiary prevention is resolution of angina before myocardial damage occurs.

Pathophysiology

Three coronary arteries normally supply the myocardium with blood to meet its metabolic needs during varying workloads. The right coronary artery supplies arterial blood to the right side of the heart, the left coronary artery divides into the left circumflex, which feeds the posterior heart muscle, and the anterior descending artery, which supplies the anterior myocardium, especially the left ventricle. The coronary vessels are usually efficient and perfuse the myocardium during diastole.

When the heart needs more blood, the vessels dilate. As the vessels become lined and eventually occluded with atherosclerotic plaques and thrombi, the vessels can no longer dilate properly.[9]

If the coronary vessels slowly become occluded, other vessels develop to provide the myocardium with needed arterial blood. These vessels are called collateral vessels.

Myocardial ischemia develops if the blood supply through the coronary vessels or oxygen content of the blood is not adequate to meet metabolic demands. Disorders of the coronary vessels, the circulation, or the blood may lead to deficits in supply.

Disorders of the coronary vessels include atherosclerosis, arterial spasm, and coronary arteritis. Atherosclerosis increases resistance to flow. Arterial spasm also increases resistance. Coronary *arteritis* is inflammation of the coronary arteries caused by infection or autoimmune disease.

Disorders of circulation include hypotension and aortic stenosis and insufficiency. Hypotension may be a result of spinal anesthesia, potent antihypertensive drugs, blood loss, or other factors that result in decreased blood return to the heart. Aortic valve stenosis or insufficiency results in decreased filling pressure of the coronary arteries.

Blood disorders include anemia, hypoxemia, and polycythemia. Anemia and hypoxemia result in decreased oxygen flow to the myocardium. Polycythemia increases blood viscosity, which slows blood flow through the coronary arteries.

The opposite of supply is demand, and increased demands can be placed on the heart. Conditions that increase demands on the myocardium are those that increase cardiac output or increase myocardial need for oxygen (Box 60-1).

Myocardial ischemia occurs when either supply or demand is altered. In some people, the coronary arteries can supply adequate blood when the person is at rest; when the person attempts activity or is taxed in some other manner, however, angina develops. Myocardial cells become ischemic within 10 seconds of coronary artery occlusion. After several minutes of ischemia, the pumping function of the heart is reduced. The reduction in pumping deprives the ischemic cells of needed oxygen and glucose. The cells convert to anaerobic metabolism, which leaves lactic acid as a waste product. As lactic acid accumulates, pain develops. Angina pectoris is transient, lasting for only 3 to 5 minutes.[2,13] If blood flow is restored, no permanent myocardial damage occurs.

Clinical Manifestations

Characteristics of Angina

Angina is a clinical syndrome characterized by discomfort in the chest, jaw, shoulder, back, or arm. Angina pectoris produces transient paroxysmal attacks of sub-

---

BOX 60-1   *Factors Influencing Myocardial Supply and Demand*

Factors That Decrease Supply

Coronary Vessel Disorders
Atherosclerosis
Arterial spasm
Coronary arteritis

Circulation Disorders
Hypotension
Aortic stenosis
Aortic insufficiency

Blood Disorders
Anemia
Hypoxemia
Polycythemia

Factors That Increase Demand

Increased Cardiac Output
Exercise
Emotion
Digestion of a large meal
Anemia
Hyperthyroidism

Increased Myocardial Need for Oxygen
Damaged myocardium
Myocardial hypertrophy
Aortic stenosis
Aortic insufficiency
Diastolic hypertension
Thyrotoxicosis
Strong emotions
Heavy exertion

---

sternal or precordial pain with the following characteristics[13]:

- *Onset.* Angina can develop quickly or slowly. Some clients ignore the chest pain, thinking that it will go away or that it is indigestion. Ask what the client was doing when the pain began.
- *Location.* Nearly 90% of clients experience the pain as retrosternal or slightly to the left of the sternum.
- *Radiation.* The pain usually radiates to the left shoulder and upper arm and may then travel down the inner aspect of the left arm to the elbow, wrist, and fourth and fifth fingers. The pain may also radiate to the right shoulder, neck, jaw, or epigastric region. On occasion, the pain may be felt only in the area of radiation and not in the chest. Rarely is the pain localized to any one single small area over the precordium.

- *Duration*. Angina usually lasts less than 5 minutes. However, attacks precipitated by a heavy meal or extreme anger may last 15 to 20 minutes.
- *Sensation*. Clients describe the pain of angina as squeezing, burning, pressing, choking, aching, or bursting pressure. The client often says the pain feels like gas, heartburn, or indigestion. Clients do not describe anginal pain as sharp or knife-like.[13]
- *Severity*. The pain of angina is usually mild or moderate in severity. It is often called "discomfort," not "pain." Rarely is the pain described as "severe."
- *Associated characteristics*. Other manifestations that may accompany the pain include dyspnea, pallor, sweating, faintness, palpitations, dizziness, and digestive disturbances.
- *Atypical presentation*. Women, older adults, and clients with diabetes may have atypical presentations of CHD that are equivalent to angina. In women, CHD may be manifested as epigastric pain, dyspnea, or back pain, whereas the older adults frequently experience dyspnea, fatigue, or syncope.[2]
- *Relieving and aggravating factors*. Angina is aggravated by continued activity, and most anginal attacks quickly subside with the administration of nitroglycerin and rest. The typical "exertion-pain, rest-relief" pattern is the major clue to the diagnosis of angina pectoris.
- *Treatment*. Has the client treated the pain with nitroglycerin? Did it work? Angina should subside after nitroglycerin use.

An important aspect of assessing angina is to determine quickly and accurately that the pain is indeed angina. Other conditions also lead to chest pain, such as pulmonary embolism, pleurisy, and pneumonia (see the table on Differential Diagnosis of Chest Pain on the website).

As vessels become lined with atherosclerotic plaques, plaques may be disrupted and thrombi may form, leading to clinical manifestations of inadequate blood supply in the tissues supplied by these vessels. Problems such as stroke, claudication, and angina develop. Stroke is described in Chapter 72 and claudication is discussed in Chapter 55.

Patterns of Angina

Classic angina pectoris can be subdivided into the following basic patterns:

- *Stable angina*. Stable angina is paroxysmal chest pain or discomfort triggered by a predictable degree of exertion (e.g., walking 20 feet) or emotion. Characteristically, a stable pattern of onset, duration, severity, and relieving factors is present.[11,14] Normally, stable angina is relieved with rest or nitroglycerin, or both.
- *Unstable angina*. Unstable angina (preinfarction angina, crescendo angina, or intermittent coronary syndrome) is paroxysmal chest pain triggered by an unpredictable degree of exertion or emotion, which may occur at night. Unstable angina attacks characteristically increase in number, duration, and severity over time. If unstable angina occurs, it must be treated as a medical emergency with the client receiving immediate medical attention.[5,13]
- *Variant angina*. Variant angina (*Prinzmetal's angina*) is chest discomfort similar to classic angina but of longer duration; it may occur while the client is at rest. These attacks tend to happen between midnight and 8 AM. Variant angina results from coronary artery spasm and may be associated with elevation of the ST segment on the electrocardiogram (ECG).
- *Nocturnal angina*. Nocturnal angina is possibly associated with rapid eye movement (REM) sleep during dreaming.
- *Angina decubitus*. Angina decubitus is paroxysmal chest pain that occurs when the client reclines and lessens when the client sits or stands up.
- *Intractable angina*. Intractable angina is chronic incapacitating angina that is unresponsive to intervention.
- *Postinfarction angina*. Pain occurs after MI, when residual ischemia may cause episodes of angina.

Diagnostic Tests

Initial laboratory testing and noninvasive testing of clients suspected of having angina include resting ECG, chest radiography, hemoglobin, fasting glucose, and fasting lipid profile.[13] Further testing is based on initial results of these and individual risk factors for CHD. The following modalities are described in Chapter 56.

Electrocardiography. The ECG tracings remain normal in more than 50% of clients with angina pectoris at rest. An ECG recorded in the presence of pain may document transient ischemic attacks with ST-segment elevation or depression. An ECG recorded during an episode of pain also suggests coronary artery involvement and the extent of cardiac muscle affected by the ischemic event.[28]

Exercise Electrocardiography. During a *stress test*, the client exercises on a treadmill or stationary bicycle until reaching 85% of maximal heart rate. ECG or vital sign changes may indicate ischemia.[28] Exercise electrocardiography is less sensitive in women and older adults.

Radioisotope Imaging. Various nuclear imaging techniques are used to evaluate myocardial muscle. Regions of poor perfusion or ischemia appear as areas of diminished or absent activity (cold spots).

Electron-Beam (Ultrafast) Computed Tomography (EBCT). This noninvasive method enables detection of the amount of calcium in coronary arteries. Because calcification occurs with atherosclerotic plaque formation, measurement of coronary calcium may reflect the extent of coronary atherosclerosis. High coronary calcium values have been associated with obstructive coronary disease.

Coronary Angiography. Angiography remains the most accurate in diagnosing the percentage of blockage in coronary arteries due to atherosclerosis.

Chest X-Ray. Chest x-rays are an inexpensive technique that allows detection of cardiomegaly and noncardiac causes of chest pain (e.g., pleuritis or pneumonia).

Outcome Management

The aims of therapy in the treatment of chronic stable angina are to reduce manifestations and ultimately to reduce the risk of mortality and morbid events. These goals are accomplished through (1) antianginal pharmacologic intervention, (2) education and risk factor modification to control or eliminate known cardiovascular risk factors, and (3) in some instances, revascularization through interventional cardiology or coronary artery bypass graft (CABG) surgery.[13] Smoking cessation after 1 year decreases the risk of CHD by 50%, a 10% reduction in cholesterol lowers the risk of CHD by 20%, and a 6-mm reduction in diastolic blood pressure lowers the risk of CHD by 10%.[1,2] The American Heart Association (AHA) recommends that people with angina control their modifiable risk factors and seek prompt treatment for episodes of chest pain. The mnemonic "A, B, C, D, E" is promoted for health care professionals and clients alike in aiding to reduce manifestations and control risk factors[1,2]:

- *A* for aspirin and antianginal therapy
- *B* for beta-blocker therapy and blood pressure control
- *C* for cigarettes and cholesterol
- *D* for diet and diabetes
- *E* for education and exercise

Clients with chronic stable angina (CSA) are usually managed effectively with risk factor reduction and pharmacologic therapy. Revascularization through interventional cardiology procedures or CABG surgery is reserved for these clients with triple-vessel or left main coronary artery disease, with left ventricular dysfunction, or whose manifestations are not adequately controlled by pharmacologic therapy.[1,2,13] Revascularization is used most often for clients with unstable angina or AMI.[1,12,26] Interventional cardiology procedures and CABG are discussed in Chapter 58.

■ Medical Management

Medical management of clients with angina pectoris focuses on three goals: (1) relieve the acute pain, (2) restore coronary blood flow, and (3) prevent further attacks to reduce the risk of AMI.[13]

The diagnosis of angina pectoris is confirmed by history and various tests. Obtain a complete history of the pain and its pattern. Clients are encouraged to describe the pain in their own words. Record a complete analysis of manifestations. This description provides a baseline that can be used in ongoing care.

Most physical findings are transient. The client exhibits pallor or has cold, clammy skin. Tachycardia and hypertension may be recorded. Pulsus alternans (the force of each beat varies) may be present at the onset of ischemic attacks. On auscultation, an S_3 or S_4 gallop or a paradoxical split of S_2 may be noted. If mitral regurgitation is present because of ischemia of the papillary muscle, a murmur can be heard.

Relieve Acute Pain and Restore Coronary Blood Flow. The primary goal of pharmacologic treatment of angina is to balance myocardial oxygen supply and demand by altering the various components of the process, thereby increasing oxygen supply to the myocardium or reducing myocardial oxygen demand. The components of myocardial oxygen consumption that can be pharmacologically treated are (1) blood pressure, (2) heart rate, (3) contractility, and (4) left ventricular volume. Drugs used in the treatment of angina and associated nursing implications are listed in the Integrating Pharmacology feature on Treatment of Angina on p. 1706.

The major types of medications used to treat the acute attack in angina pectoris are as follows:

1. *Opiate analgesics* are used to relieve or reduce acute pain.
2. *Vasodilators* help reduce acute pain and prevent further attacks by widening the diameter of coronary arteries and increasing the supply of oxygen to the myocardium. *Nitroglycerin,* a *short-acting* nitrate, has been the treatment of choice against anginal attacks since 1867. Administered sublingually, per tablet, or via translingual spray, nitroglycerin helps relieve or reduce anginal pain within 1 to 2 minutes. *Long-acting* nitrates, given orally or transdermally, help maintain coronary artery vasodilation, thereby promoting greater flow of blood and oxygen to the heart muscle.
3. *Beta-adrenergic blockers* help reduce the workload of the heart, decrease myocardial oxygen demand, and may decrease the number of anginal attacks.
4. *Calcium-channel blockers* are used to dilate coronary arteries, thereby increasing oxygen supply to the myocardium.
5. *Antiplatelet* agents inhibit platelet aggregation and reduce coagulability, thus preventing clot formation.

Prevent Further Attacks. Education and counseling regarding modification of risk factors are necessary to re-

INTEGRATING PHARMACOLOGY

Treatment of Angina

Angina is ischemic pain in the myocardium. The medications used to treat acute angina episodes are vasodilators designed to restore arterial flow (supply) or reduce oxygen consumption (demand).

Nitroglycerin is the most common medication used and should be given to clients with known ischemic heart disease who report manifestations of angina. Because of its potent vasodilatory effect, assess the blood pressure before beginning treatment and 5 minutes after each dose. The most common practice is to give three doses of sublingual nitroglycerin 5 minutes apart as long as the client does not become severely hypotensive. If the pain is not relieved, notify the physician immediately; morphine may be required. If the client does not have a history of ischemic heart disease, collect a thorough assessment of the pain and notify the physician immediately if there are any indications of serious forms of chest pain. Some physicians order simultaneous liquid antacids and nitroglycerin to reduce both cardiac and gastrointestinal pain. If the medications are given 5 minutes apart, it may help with clinical decision making about the cause of the pain. Concurrent use of sildenafil (Viagra) may cause severe hypotension and death.

Clients with long-standing angina may also use topical nitroglycerin of extended-release forms. These forms of nitroglycerin provide continuous vasodilation. Tolerance to the medication can develop, especially in doses with longer half-lives, hence topical nitroglycerin is removed during the night to restore efficacy. Assessment of nocturnal angina, especially during REM sleep, is needed.

A second method of controlling pain is to reduce the myocardial need for oxygen. Beta-blocking agents reduce myocardial oxygen consumption by controlling the high-oxygen demands from the effects of the sympathetic nervous system. Original forms of beta-blocking agents contained both $beta_1$ and $beta_2$ antagonists and therefore could prompt bronchoconstriction. Newer forms are selective $beta_1$ antagonists only.

Aspirin is commonly used in acute events and to promote blood flow through narrowed and tortuous coronary arteries, where slowed blood is likely to clot and prevent forward flow of blood. Aspirin prevents platelets from aggregating (collecting) by blocking prostaglandin synthesis. Aspirin is irritating to the gastrointestinal tract and should be given with food. It also leads to increased bleeding risk from all invasive procedures. Concurrent use of other medications that also slow clotting must be carefully monitored.

Other medications for the treatment of angina are the same as the medications used for the treatment of coronary artery disease. See Chapter 58.

---

duce the progression of CHD and to prevent further attacks. Recommendations should follow the guidelines established by the AHA for primary and secondary prevention of CHD.[1] Specific recommendations for risk factor modification are described in Chapter 58.

■ Nursing Management of the Medical Client

Relieve/Reduce Acute Pain and Restore Coronary Blood Flow. In addition to documenting the clinical manifestations of angina, ascertain how long the client has had angina, whether risk factors for CHD are present, and the client's emotional reaction to chest pain. Start cardiac monitoring, obtain a 12-lead ECG, and control ongoing angina.[8,10,18,19] Until the angina is controlled and coronary blood flow is reestablished, the client is at risk for myocardial damage from myocardial ischemia. If the client reports angina, assess the pain and ask the client whether the pain is the same as that experienced in the past. Note new characteristics or increased pain. The phrase "all patients with chest pain get MONA" is used to guide treatment of clients with chest pain[8]:

- *M*, morphine sulfate
- *O*, oxygen therapy
- *N*, nitrates
- *A*, aspirin

Give sublingual nitroglycerin tablets or spray as prescribed. Nitroglycerin dilates coronary arteries, reducing pain and restoring coronary blood flow. Because nitroglycerin causes vasodilation and hypotension, monitor blood pressure. If the pain is not relieved after three nitroglycerin tablets, each taken 5 minutes apart, or after morphine, notify the physician. In addition, an environment that provides rest and security as well as allays fear and anxiety helps reduce pain. Oxygen therapy is used to ensure adequate oxygenation. Aspirin is given for its antiplatelet activities.

Prevent Further Attacks Through Self-Care. The client must be knowledgeable about the care of episodes of angina and how to reduce the risk factors that exacerbate the process. Use the following information to help clients control risk factors for angina pectoris.

1. Educate the client to avoid activities or habits that precipitate angina (eating large meals, drinking coffee, smoking, exercising too strenuously, going out in cold weather, being exposed to excessive stress). If an attack begins, the client should stop the activity and sit down. An antianginal medication (e.g., nitroglycerin) should be taken. Three pills can be taken sublingually 5 minutes apart. If the pain does

not subside, worsens, or radiates, the client should take an aspirin.[11] The client should call "911" and explain that he or she is experiencing chest pain; the client would then be taken promptly to the emergency department. Stress this point, because if the client is experiencing an AMI, the sooner treatment is initiated, the lower the mortality rate.[1,6,8,10,29,34] Family members should not drive the client to the hospital because of the risk for sudden death precipitated by ventricular fibrillation. If the client is taken by ambulance, defibrillators are available in case of ventricular fibrillation.

2. Explain the importance of daily management of hypertension. Advise the client to take daily medication even if no clinical manifestations are evident (see Chapter 54).

3. Encourage and help plan a regular program of daily exercise to promote improved coronary circulation and weight management.

4. Instruct clients who smoke to quit smoking at once. Smoking cigarettes raises carboxyhemoglobin levels in the blood, which reduces the amount of oxygen available to the myocardium.[4,32] Clients with angina pectoris exposed for 2 hours to cigarette smoke demonstrate elevations in carboxyhemoglobin concentration, decreased exercise time, increased heart rate, and elevated blood pressure. Advise clients to avoid "passive smoking" (i.e., being with a smoker or in a smoke-filled room).[33]

5. Urge overweight clients to lose excess weight. Explain that weight reduction may also reduce blood pressure, cholesterol, and the incidence of adult onset diabetes. Encourage them to eat small meals, avoid high-calorie and high-cholesterol diets, abstain from gas-forming foods, and rest for short periods after meals. In addition, recommend a high-fiber diet, which not only may prevent constipation and other intestinal tract ailments but also may decrease the number and severity of anginal attacks. Diets high in fiber may also help lower serum cholesterol and triglyceride levels. CHD is less common among clients with a high intake of dietary fiber than in those with a low intake. High-fiber diets can also decrease hypertension.[4,32]

6. Help the client who leads an active, hectic life to adjust activities to a level below that which precipitates anginal attacks. Encourage brief rest periods throughout the working day, an early bedtime, and longer or more frequent vacations. Advise clients who are anxious and nervous to consider counseling. Relaxation techniques may also be used.

ACUTE MYOCARDIAL INFARCTION

Acute coronary syndrome refers to the clinical manifestations that are compatible with AMI. An AMI is also known as a heart attack, coronary occlusion, or simply a "coronary," which is a life-threatening condition characterized by the formation of localized necrotic areas within the myocardium. AMI usually follows the sudden occlusion of a coronary artery and the abrupt cessation of blood and oxygen flow to the heart muscle. Because the heart muscle must function continuously, blockage of blood to the muscle and the development of necrotic areas can be lethal.[26,29]

Every 29 seconds an American suffers a coronary event and approximately every 1 minute someone dies of a coronary event.[1] Every year about 1.1 million Americans have AMIs.[1] Indeed, AMI is the leading cause of death in America and is responsible for an estimated 529,000 deaths each year.[1,2,6] About 250,000 people a year die before they reach the hospital.[1] Studies indicate that half of all AMI victims wait more than 2 hours before getting help.[2,34] On the basis of data from the Framingham study, about 45% of all AMIs occur in people younger than age 65 years and 5% occur in those younger than age 40.[24] Eighty-five percent of people who die of AMI are 65 years of age or older.[2] Women have higher in-hospital mortality rates than men.[31] The difference may result from differences in treatment for men and women. In one study of women with AMI, aspirin, beta-blocking drugs, coronary thrombolysis, acute cardiac catheterization, percutaneous transluminal coronary angioplasty (PTCA), and CABG surgery were used less often than in men with AMI.[31] Death rates for CHD are higher for African Americans, Hispanics, and American Indians than for Caucasians.[1]

Etiology and Risk Factors

The most common cause of AMI is complete or nearly complete occlusion of a coronary artery, usually precipitated by rupture of a vulnerable atherosclerotic plaque and subsequent thrombus formation.[9] Plaque rupture can be precipitated by both internal and external factors.

Internal factors include plaque characteristics, such as the size and consistency of the lipid core and the thickness of the fibrous cap as well as conditions to which it is exposed, such as coagulation status and degree of arterial vasoconstriction. Vulnerable plaques most frequently occur in areas with less than 70% stenosis and are characterized by an eccentric shape with an irregular border, a large, thin lipid core, and a thin, fibrous cap.[9]

External factors result from actions of the client or from external conditions that affect the client. Strenuous physical activity and severe emotional stress, such as anger, increase sympathetic activity, which in turn increases hemodynamic stress that may lead to plaque rupture. At the same time, sympathetic activity increases myocardial oxygen demand. Scientists have reported that external factors, such as exposure to cold and time of day, also affect plaque rupture. Acute coronary events occur more frequently with exposure to cold and during the morning hours. Researchers hypothesize that the sudden increases in sympathetic activity associated with these factors may contribute to plaque rupture.[5,28] The role of inflammation in triggering plaque rupture is currently being studied.[20]

Regardless of the cause, rupture of the atherosclerotic plaque results in (1) exposure of the plaque's lipid-rich core to flowing blood, (2) seepage of blood into the plaque, causing it to expand, (3) triggering of thrombus formation, and (4) partial or complete occlusion of the coronary artery. *Unstable angina* is associated with short-term partial occlusion of a coronary artery, whereas AMI results from significant or complete occlusion of a coronary artery that lasts more than 1 hour.[9] When blood flow ceases abruptly, the myocardial tissue supplied by that artery dies. Coronary artery spasm can also cause acute occlusion. The risk factors that predispose a client to a heart attack are the same as for all forms of CHD (see Chapter 58).

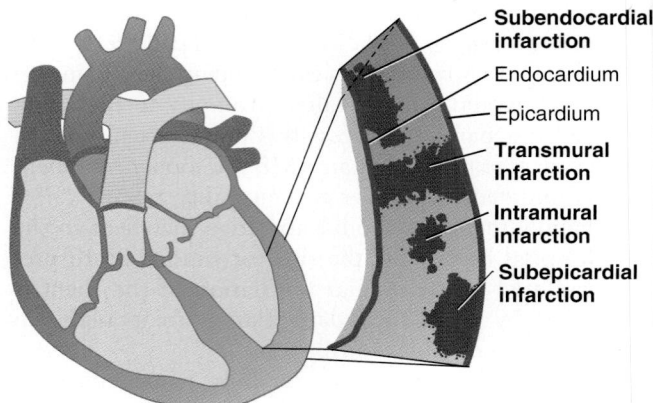

FIGURE 60-1 Depth of infarction in the wall of the ventricle. Subendocardial, intramural, and subepicardial injuries are only in one layer. Transmural infarction extends through all three layers.

Pathophysiology

AMI can be considered the end-point of CHD. Unlike the temporary ischemia that occurs with angina, prolonged unrelieved ischemia causes irreversible damage to the myocardium. Cardiac cells can withstand ischemia for about 15 minutes before they die. Because the myocardium is metabolically active, manifestations of ischemia can be seen within 8 to 10 seconds of decreased blood flow. When the heart does not receive blood and oxygen, it converts to *anaerobic metabolism,* creating less adenosine triphosphate (ATP) and more lactic acid as a by-product.[28] Myocardial cells are very sensitive to changes in pH and become less functional. Acidosis causes the myocardium to become more vulnerable to the effects of the lysosomal enzymes within the cell. Acidosis leads to conduction system disorders, and dysrhythmias develop. Contractility is also reduced, decreasing the heart's ability to pump. As the myocardial cells necrose, intracellular enzymes are introduced into the bloodstream, where they can be detected by laboratory tests.

Figure 60-1 illustrates the depth of various types of infarctions in the wall of the ventricle. Cellular necrosis occurs in one layer of myocardial tissue in subendocardial, intramural, and subepicardial infarctions. In a transmural infarction, cellular necrosis is present in all three layers of myocardial tissue. The infarct site is called the *zone of infarction and necrosis.* Around it is a zone of hypoxic injury also called a penumbra. This zone can return to normal but may also become necrotic if blood flow is not restored. The outermost zone is called the *zone of ischemia;* damage to this area is reversible.

Transmural infarctions cause changes in the architecture of the left ventricle, called *remodeling,* which can result in acute or chronic heart failure. Within the first few hours of AMI, the necrotic area stretches in a process called *infarct expansion.* This expansion is furthered by

the neurohormonal activation that occurs with AMI.[8] Increased heart rate, ventricular dilation, and activation of the renin-angiotensin system increasing preload all occur during AMI and can further "remodeling."[8,21,25,27] This expansion may continue for up to 6 weeks after an AMI and is accompanied by progressive thinning and lengthening of infarcted and noninfarcted areas. The gene expression of remodeled cardiac cells changes, causing permanent structural changes to the heart. This remodeling results in left ventricular dysfunction and produces increases in ventricular volumes and pressures. Remodeling may continue for years after an AMI and may result in chronic heart failure (see Chapter 58).[9,25,27]

The most common site of an AMI is the *anterior wall* of the left ventricle near the apex, resulting from thrombosis of the descending branch of the left coronary artery (Figure 60-2). Other common sites are (1) the *posterior wall* of the left ventricle near the base and behind the posterior cusp of the mitral valve and (2) the *inferior (diaphragmatic) surface* of the heart. Infarction of the posterior left ventricle results from occlusion of the right coronary artery or circumflex branch of the left coronary artery. An inferior infarction occurs when the right coronary artery is occluded. In nearly 25% of inferior wall AMIs, the right ventricle is the site of infarction. Atrial infarctions develop less than 5% of the time. See the Concept Map on Understanding Myocardial Infarction and Its Treatment on p. 1710.

Clinical Manifestations

The clinical manifestations associated with AMI result from ischemia of the heart muscle and the decrease in function and acidosis associated with it. The major clinical manifestation of AMI is chest pain (Figure 60-3), which is similar to angina pectoris but more severe and unrelieved by nitroglycerin. The pain may radiate to the neck, jaw, shoulder, back, or left arm. The pain also may

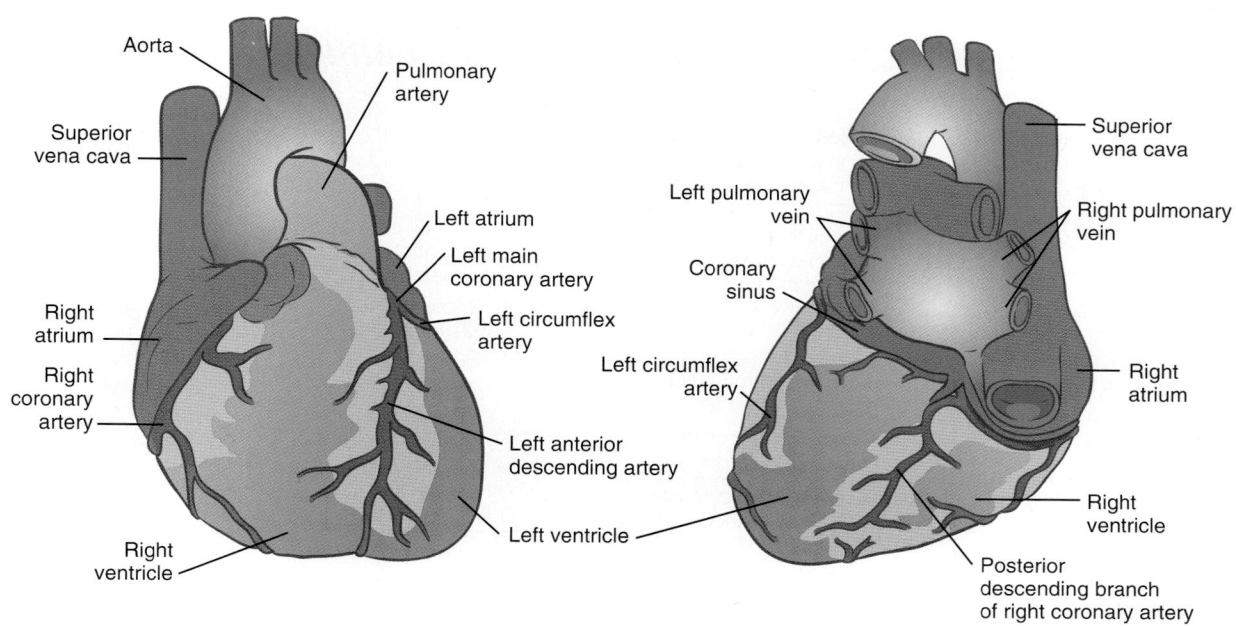

FIGURE 60-2 There are three coronary arteries. The right coronary artery supplies arterial blood to the right side of the heart; the left coronary artery divides into the left circumflex, which feeds the posterior heart muscle and anterior descending artery, which supplies the anterior myocardium

present near the epigastrium, simulating indigestion. AMI may also be associated with less common clinical manifestations, including the following[2]:

- Atypical chest, stomach, back, or abdominal pain
- Nausea or dizziness
- Shortness of breath and difficulty breathing
- Unexplained anxiety, weakness, or fatigue
- Palpitations, cold sweat, or paleness

Women experiencing AMI frequently present with one or more of the less common clinical manifestations.[1]

Diagnostic Evaluation

It is recommended that all clients with a suspected AMI (ischemic-type chest discomfort) ingest aspirin and obtain baseline cardiac serum markers and a 12-lead ECG within 10 minutes of arrival in the emergency department. Recommended methods of identifying acute cardiac ischemia in emergency departments are troponin T serum levels and echocardiography based upon appropriate triage, 30-day survival rates, and cost-effectiveness. The Acute Cardiac Ischemia Time-Insensitive Predictive Instrument (ACI-TIPI), an algorithm based on questions and 12-lead ECG findings, is also accurate and of low cost.[18,26]

Electrocardiography

When blood flow to the heart is decreased, ischemia and necrosis of the heart muscle occur. These conditions are reflected in altered Q wave, ST segment, and T wave on the 12-lead ECG (Figure 60-4). Twelve-lead ECG examines the heart from 12 views, with the view provided from the V_5 lead being the most sensitive in detecting abnormalities. (Figure 60-5). The Q-wave change is significant; normally the Q wave is small or absent. Ischemic tissue produces an elevation in the ST segment and a peaked T wave or inversion of the T wave. ST segment elevation is considered significant if greater than 1 mm. Through the course of an MI, changes occur first in the ST segment, then the T wave, and finally the Q wave. As the myocardium heals, the ST segment and T waves return to normal, but the Q-wave changes persist.[28] However, an ECG can be completely normal in a client with AMI, especially in the early hours following infarct.

The 12-lead ECG can be used to determine the location of the infarct. Leads V_1 and V_2 face the septum of the heart, leads V_3 and V_4 face the anterior wall of the left ventricle, and V_5 and V_6 face the lateral wall of the left ventricle.

Laboratory Tests

Laboratory findings include elevated levels of serum creatine kinase (CK)-MB isoenzyme, myoglobin, cardiac troponin T, and cardiac troponin I. Historically, elevations in lactate dehydrogenase (LDH) M1 isoenzyme, serum aspartate transaminase (AST), leukocytes (leukocytosis), and erythrocyte sedimentation rate (ESR) have aided in the diagnosis of AMI.[15,18,19] The pattern of isoenzyme changes in AMI follows a typical pattern (see Figure 60-6). Knowing the typical pattern allows an estimation of the time of the actual injury.

Understanding Myocardial Infarction and Its Treatment

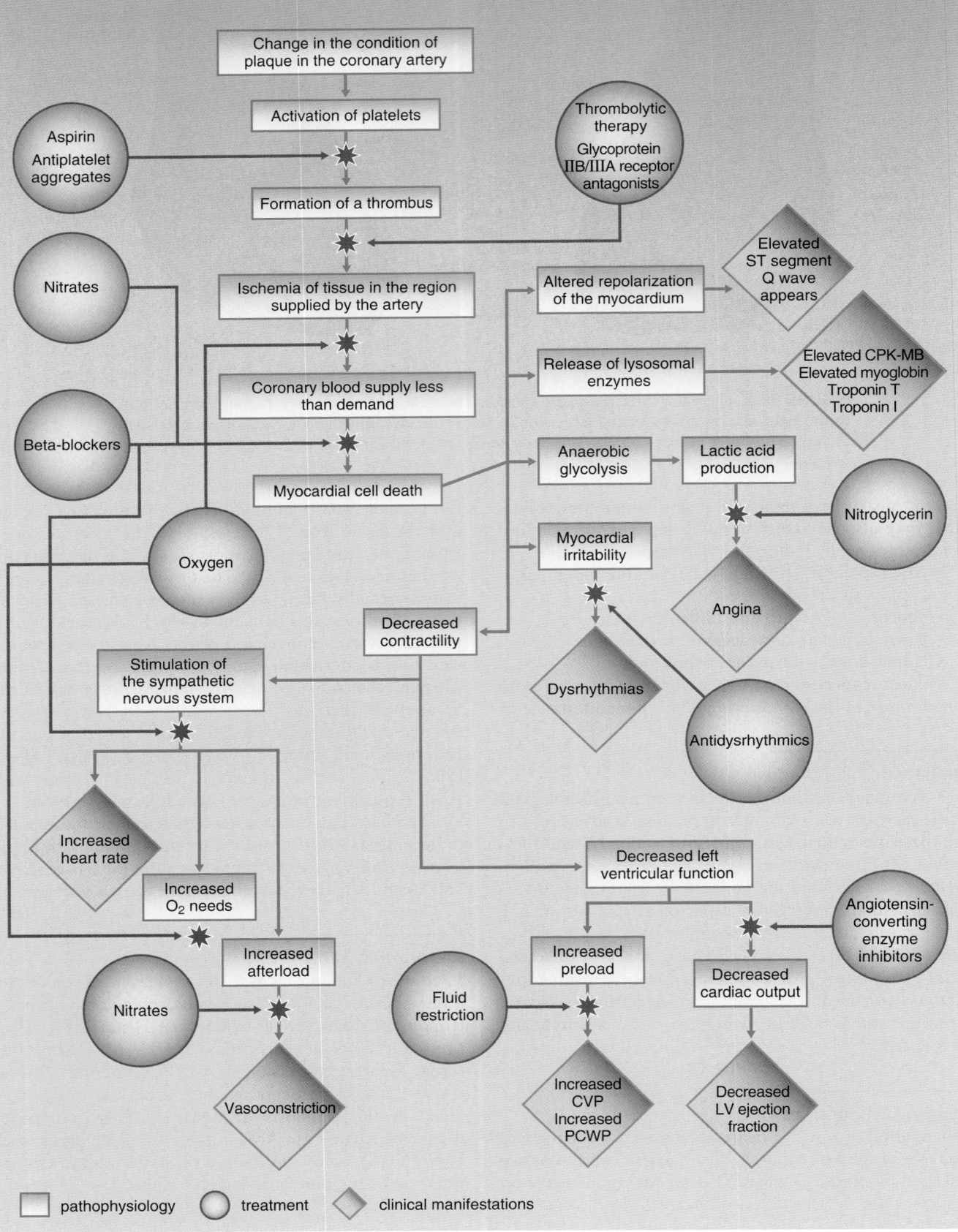

Change in the condition of plaque in the coronary artery

Activation of platelets

Aspirin
Antiplatelet aggregates

Thrombolytic therapy
Glycoprotein IIB/IIIA receptor antagonists

Formation of a thrombus

Nitrates

Ischemia of tissue in the region supplied by the artery

Altered repolarization of the myocardium

Elevated ST segment Q wave appears

Coronary blood supply less than demand

Release of lysosomal enzymes

Elevated CPK-MB Elevated myoglobin Troponin T Troponin I

Beta-blockers

Myocardial cell death

Anaerobic glycolysis

Lactic acid production

Nitroglycerin

Oxygen

Myocardial irritability

Angina

Decreased contractility

Dysrhythmias

Stimulation of the sympathetic nervous system

Antidysrhythmics

Increased heart rate

Increased O₂ needs

Decreased left ventricular function

Angiotensin-converting enzyme inhibitors

Nitrates

Increased afterload

Increased preload

Decreased cardiac output

Fluid restriction

Vasoconstriction

Increased CVP Increased PCWP

Decreased LV ejection fraction

☐ pathophysiology   ◯ treatment   ◇ clinical manifestations

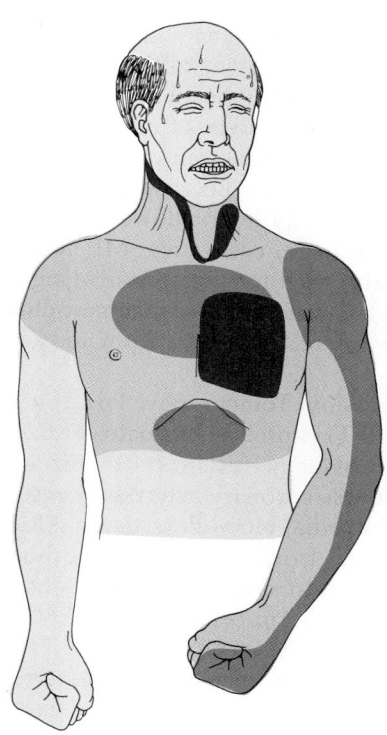

FIGURE 60-3 Possible pain patterns with myocardial infarction. The red area is the most common location of pain. Orange areas are areas of referred pain and the location of pain in women. However, pain can develop in any area of the chest (yellow).

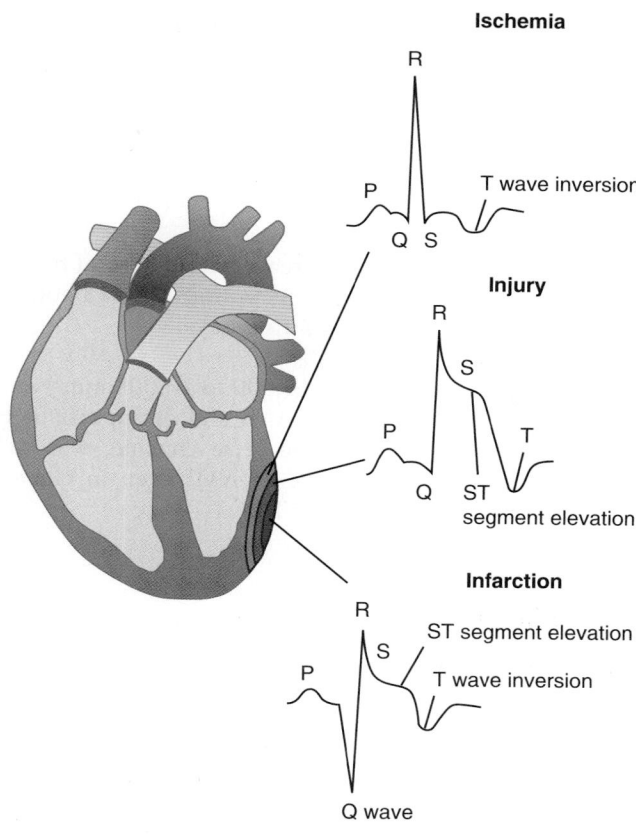

FIGURE 60-4 Zones of hypoxic injury, zone of infarction, zone of necrosis, and the electrocardiographic patterns accompanying these changes during myocardial infarction.

CK-MB. Serum levels of CK-MB (an isoenzyme of CK found primarily in cardiac muscle) increase 3 to 6 hours after the onset of chest pain, peak in 12 to 18 hours, and return to normal levels in 3 to 4 days.

Myoglobin. Myoglobin is a heme protein found in striated muscle fibers. Myoglobin is rapidly released when myocardial muscle tissue is damaged. Because of the rapid release, it can be detected within 2 hours after AMI. Although many other factors can raise the serum myoglobin level (e.g., strenuous exercise, heavy ethanol use), myoglobin is a highly sensitive indicator of AMI if serum levels double when a second sample is drawn within 2 hours of the first. Conversely, it is reliable to exclude the diagnosis of AMI if the levels do not increase every 2 hours. The diagnostic window ends 24 hours after an AMI.[22]

Troponin. The cardiac troponin complex is a basic component of the myocardium that is involved in the contraction of the myocardial muscle. Cardiac troponin T and I are more sensitive to cardiac muscle damage than cardiac troponin C.

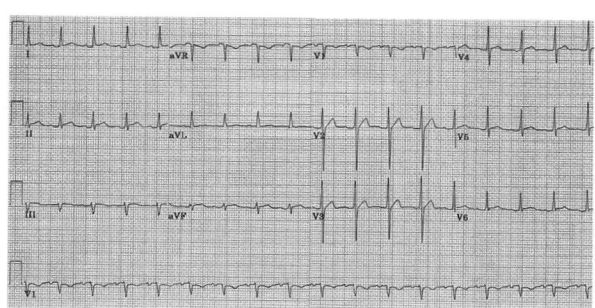

FIGURE 60-5 A 12-lead ECG showing sinus tachycardia and ST elevation consistent with acute myocardial infarction.

Cardiac *troponin T* is similar to CK-MB with regard to sensitivity, and levels increase within 3 to 6 hours after pain has started. Levels remain elevated for 14 to 21 days.[15,22] This is useful (and more accurate than LDH) in confirmation of distant AMI.[15,22]

Cardiac *troponin I* levels increase 7 to 14 hours after AMI. This is a very specific and sensitive indicator of AMI and is not affected by any other disease or injury to any other muscle except cardiac muscle.[15,22] Elevation persists for 5 to 7 days.

LDH. The LDH_1 subunit is plentiful in heart muscle and is released into the serum when myocardial damage occurs. Serum levels of LDH elevate 14 to 24 hours after onset of myocardial damage, peak within 48 to 72 hours, and slowly return to normal over the next 7 to 14 days. Figure 60-6 illustrates the pattern of enzyme changes after AMI.

AST. Serum levels of AST increase within several hours after the onset of chest pain, peak within 12 to 18 hours, and return to normal within 3 to 4 days.

Leukocytosis. Leukocytosis (10,000 to 20,000 mm^3) appears on the second day after AMI and disappears in 1 week. Myeloperoxidase, a leukocyte enzyme, was recently shown to be predictive of AMI even in clients without elevations in troponin T.[7]

Imaging Studies

Radionuclide imaging studies provide information on the presence of coronary artery disease as well as the location of ischemic and infarcted tissue. Cardiac imaging studies have been used to provide information for triage decisions and the management of clients who present to the emergency department with acute chest pain.[6,18,26]

When a client experiences acute chest pain, perfusion imaging with agents such as thallium, sestamibi, and teboroxime can be used to identify ischemic and infarcted tissue. Perfusion imaging is sometimes called "cold spot" imaging because the radioisotope in the bloodstream is not taken up by ischemic or infarcted tissue.

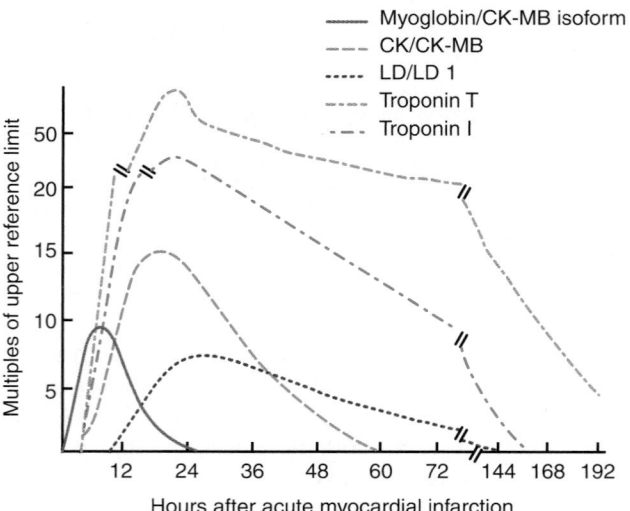

FIGURE 60-6 Isoenzyme alterations in acute myocardial infarction. (From Wong, S.S. [1996.] Strategic utilization of cardiac markers for the diagnosis of acute myocardial infarction. *Annals of Clinical Laboratory Science, 26,* 301-312. Copyright 1996 by the Institute for Clinical Science, Inc.)

Infarct, or "hot spot" imaging, is useful in confirming AMI in clients who present to the hospital several days after an AMI. Technetium 99m–tagged pyrophosphate binds with calcium in areas of myocardial necrosis. Areas of uptake (hot spots) seen on nuclear imaging indicate areas of infarction. Because this test does not give positive results for 24 hours, however, it cannot be used to identify an acute, early-stage MI. Radiolabeled antimyosin is also used for hot spot imaging, but its diagnostic value is limited because it cannot differentiate between a new infarct and a scar from an earlier infarct.

Positron Emission Tomography. Positron emission tomography (PET) is used to evaluate cardiac metabolism and to assess tissue perfusion. It can also be used to detect CHD, assess coronary artery flow reserve, measure absolute myocardial blood flow, detect AMI, and differentiate ischemic from nonischemic cardiomyopathy. It may also be used to assess myocardial viability to determine which clients can benefit from CABG.

Magnetic Resonance Imaging. Magnetic resonance imaging (MRI) helps identify the site and extent of an MI, assess the effects of reperfusion therapy, and differentiate reversible and irreversible tissue injury. Its use as a diagnostic tool for coronary artery disease is increasing, although MRI cannot be used in clients with implanted metallic devices, such as pacemakers or defibrillators. MRI is discussed in Chapter 4.

Echocardiography. Echocardiography is useful in assessing the ability of the heart walls to contract and relax. The transducer is placed on the chest, and images are relayed to a monitor screen. Wall motion is abnormal in ischemic or infarcted areas.[18,28]

Transesophageal Echocardiography. Transesophageal echocardiography (TEE) is an imaging technique in which the transducer is placed against the wall of the esophagus. The image of the myocardium is clearer when the esophageal site is used because no air is between the transducer and the heart. This technique is particularly useful for viewing the posterior wall of the heart.

Outcome Management

Since the advent of coronary care units and devices that aid in promptly recognizing and treating life-threatening dysrhythmias, 70% to 80% of people experiencing an AMI survive the initial attack. Chances for survival greatly diminish with the presence of the following[1,3]:

- Older age (clients 80 years or older have a 60% mortality rate)
- Manifestations of heart failure
- ST-segment depression
- Elevation of cardiac markers

- Hypotension (systolic blood pressure less than 55 mm Hg on admission betokens a 60% mortality rate)
- More than three coronary risk factors
- More than two anginal events within 24 hours

Deaths generally result from severe dysrhythmias, cardiogenic shock, heart failure, rupture of the heart, and recurrent AMI.

Clients who avoid complications after AMI still require 6 to 12 weeks for complete recovery. However, 25% of men and 38% of women die within 1 year after having AMI and 22% of men and 46% of women are disabled with heart failure within 6 years of an AMI.[1]

■ Medical Management

Major goals of care for clients with AMI include the following[26]:

- Initiating prompt care
- Reducing pain
- Delivering successful treatment for the acute pain and reperfusion of the myocardium
- Preventing complications
- Preventing remodeling and heart failure
- Rehabilitating and educating the client and significant others

Treat the Acute Attack Immediately. Clients with manifestations of AMI must receive immediate treatment.[26] Delays may increase damage to the heart and reduce the chance of survival. The goal for treatment of AMI is "door to needle" in less than 30 minutes, or specifically from onset of pain till thrombolytic therapy within 30 minutes or percutaneous angioplasty within 1 hour. Most communities have an emergency medical system (EMS) that responds quickly (call "911"). Until EMS personnel arrive, keep the client quiet and calm. It is recommended that, if conscious, a client chew an aspirin with the onset of manifestations, because mortality is reduced 23% with this action alone.[11]

Many people who experience manifestations of AMI delay calling for help because they misinterpret what they are sensing. Their expectations of what AMI should feel like and their experience are not the same. Many studies have documented an average client delay time that exceeded 7 hours.[34] In women, this delay may even be longer.[31] Community education to "call first, call fast" is important.

While waiting for EMS to arrive, elevate the client's head and loosen any tight clothing around the neck. Once EMS workers arrive, the client is assessed and transported quickly to an emergency department. EMS workers are trained to respond to possible AMI clients with protocols to ensure quick and proper treatment. Sudden death from AMI due to ventricular tachycardia degenerating first to ventricular fibrillation and later to asystole is the most common cause of sudden cardiac

death.[16] The client is given oxygen; an intravenous (IV) line is inserted, and the client is connected to a heart monitor. Portable automatic external defibrillators (AED) are becoming standard on ambulances and can even been seen in public places. These devices can guide amateurs on how to resuscitate a person with chest pain who is having a dysrhythmia. Clients who become unconscious before reaching the emergency department may require defibrillation or cardiopulmonary resuscitation (CPR).

The client experiencing AMI needs immediate admission to a hospital with a coronary care unit if possible. The first 24 hours after AMI is the time of highest risk for sudden death. There is a significant benefit if treatment is administered within the first hour of onset of manifestations.[17] The first hours after the onset of pain is the crucial time frame for salvage of the myocardium. Therefore efforts have been made to decrease the time for initial treatment. All emergency departments treat AMI clients within 30 minutes of presenting to the hospital. The mnemonic 4D's (*d*oor, *d*ata, *d*ecision, and *d*rug), along with treatment algorithms, has been adopted by many emergency departments to treat those with AMI and remains current. Equally important is for everyone to have 911 access for EMS personnel who are trained in triage of chest pain and defibrillation. [26]

Reduce Pain. Upon admission, the client who complains of chest pain is admitted to the emergency department, given oxygen therapy, and placed on ECG monitoring. An IV line is placed, serum cardiac markers are drawn, and a 12-lead ECG is undertaken within 10 minutes.[26] Pain control is a priority, and pain is usually treated with IV morphine. Continued pain is a manifestation of myocardial ischemia. Pain also stimulates the autonomic nervous system and increases preload, which in turn increases myocardial oxygen demand. Oxygen is used to treat tissue hypoxia.

Monitor Heart Rhythm. Because dysrhythmias are common, ECG monitoring is essential and antidysrhythmic medications should be at hand. A two-dimensional echocardiogram and test may be performed in the emergency department to aid in ruling in or ruling out AMI.

Improve Perfusion. The general principles of pharmacologic treatment of AMI consist of anti-ischemic and antithrombotic therapies.[12,30] (See the Integrating Pharmacology feature on Medications for Myocardial Infarction on p. 1714.) Anti-ischemic therapy usually consists of beta-blockade and IV nitroglycerin. Antithrombotic therapy and the combination of different antithrombotic agents are being studied widely. Antithrombotic therapy is usually initiated with the administration of an aspirin if the client has not taken one before reaching the emergency department. Heparin therapy is the next step.

INTEGRATING PHARMACOLOGY

Medications for Myocardial Infarction

The portion of the coronary artery occluded by a thrombus can be opened by using various medications that dissolve the clot or prevent new clots from forming or extending. Non–clot-specific thrombolytic agents (streptokinase, urokinase) can be infused over 60 minutes after the client is premedicated with a steroid and diphenhydramine to prevent allergic responses. For large or anterior infarcts, clot-specific agents are more common forms of plasminogen activator. This medication is given in a bolus followed by an infusion. Several relative and absolute contraindications exist for thrombolytic therapy (see Box 60-2).

Heparin is also used in combination with the thrombolytic to prevent new clot formation. The dose of heparin is based on lean body weight and adjusted to the partial thromboplastin time. Heparin is contraindicated in clients with known bleeding conditions or recent stroke. Low-molecular-weight heparin is more commonly used due to ease of administration.

Preventing platelet aggregation is an important component of therapy. Aspirin continues to be used routinely in coronary angioplasty and to treat clients with myocardial infarction or unstable angina. The advantages of early aspirin administration are clear; it is strongly advised that aspirin be consumed early in care. Glycoprotein (GP) IIb/IIIa serves as the receptor on platelets that permits platelet aggregation. Agents that block this final common pathway by blocking the binding of adhesive proteins to GP IIb/IIIa, termed *GP IIb/IIIa antagonists,* are currently considered the most powerful specific inhibitors of platelet participation in acute thrombosis.

Pain is managed with morphine or intravenous nitroglycerin. Nitroglycerin is a coronary vasodilator used to reduce preload and afterload. Other medications, beta-blockers, ACE inhibitors, and statins are discussed in Chapter 58.

BOX 60-2 *Absolute and Relative Contraindications for Thrombolytic Therapy*

Absolute Contraindications

Previous hemorrhagic stroke at any time
Stroke or other cerebrovascular events with the past year
Known intracranial tumor
Active internal bleeding (except menstruation)
Suspected aortic aneurysm

Relative Contraindications

Severe uncontrolled hypertension at the time of admission blood pressure >180/100 mm Hg)
Other intracranial pathology
Current use of anticoagulants (International Normalized Ratio >23)
Known bleeding problems
Recent trauma (past 2-4 weeks), including head trauma
Prolonged (>10 minutes) or potentially traumatic cardiopulmonary resuscitation
Major surgery (<3 weeks prior)
Nonsuppressible vascular punctures
Recent (past 2-4 weeks) internal bleeding
Prior allergic reaction to streptokinase (if streptokinase planned)
Pregnancy
Active peptic ulcers
History of chronic severe hypertension

Antithrombotic therapy continues with medications that lyse (dissolve) the clot that forms part of the blockage of the coronary artery. Thrombolytic therapy includes streptokinase, urokinase, tissue-type plasminogen activator (t-PA), anisoylated plasminogen-streptokinase activator complex (anistreplase, APSAC), alteplase, urokinase plasminogen activator, and reteplase. For best efficacy, thrombolytic agents should be given within an hour after the onset of chest pain.[26] The choice of thrombolytic agent is not as important as the speed with which it is given.[17] After the thrombolytic agent is administered, IV heparin or a glycoprotein IIb/IIIa is usually continued. All of these thrombolytic agents can be given intravenously.

Not all clients with AMI are suitable candidates for thrombolytic therapy (Box 60-2). History of recent cerebral vascular accident, surgery, pregnancy, or use of anticoagulants are contraindications for thrombolytic ther-

apy. Complications of thrombolytics include bleeding, allergic reactions, and stroke. Successful reperfusion of the coronary arteries is evidenced by (1) return of ECG changes to normal, (2) relief of chest pain, (3) presence of reperfusion dysrhythmias, usually sudden onset of frequent premature ventricular contractions (PVCs) or short runs of PVCs, and (4) a rapid, early peak of the CK-MB isoenzyme ("washout"). If reperfusion is not attained or if the client is not a candidate for thrombolytic therapy, then primary angioplasty, stenting, or CABG may be performed. Interventional cardiology procedures and bypass surgery are discussed in Chapter 58. If ST elevation is present, reperfusion strategies are to be promptly initiated.[26] Guidelines suggest that thrombolytic therapy should be initiated within 30 minutes or PTCA should be initiated within 60 minutes.[26] PTCA may be considered before thrombolytic therapy in institutions that have cardiac surgery capabilities, that have skilled physicians in PCTA, and that perform more than 200 PTCA procedures per year.[26]

Antidysrhythmic agents are initiated. Clinicians begin beta-blockade and angiotensin-converting enzyme (ACE) inhibitors within 72 hours of onset to reduce ventricular remodeling and reduce mortality.[21] Stool

TABLE 60-1   *Clinical Manifestations Based on Location of the Acute Myocardial Infarction*

The classic pattern of ECG changes with AMI begins with an abnormal T wave that is prolonged and peaked. This is followed within minutes by ST-segment elevation in the leads facing the area of injury with reciprocal changes of ST-segment depression in the opposite leads. Q-wave formation follows, and the Q-wave changes only disappear over months. The classic evolution of ST elevation and Q-wave formation is often diagnostic of AMI. Knowledge of the area of the heart with infarct can prevent complications and allow diagnosis of AMI when ECG changes are not present.

Area	ST-Segment Elevation and Q Waves on 12-Lead ECG	Common Dysrhythmias	Other Manifestations	Complications
Left anterior descending (LAD)	V_1-V_6 depending on the branch	Ventricular tachycardia Bundle branch blocks (BBBs) Premature ventricular contractions (PVCs) Atrial fibrillation or flutter	Severe heart failure Low CO, BP Elevated pulmonary artery diastolic pressure (PAD), pulmonary capillary wedge pressure	Cardiogenic shock Myocardial rupture High mortality with this location
Circum-flex/V_5	I, aVL, V_5, V_6 ST depression of V_1 to V_4 (reciprocal)	AV nodal blocks (especially Mobitz 1)	Heart failure and left ventricular dysfunction Bradycardia	Papillary muscle dysfunction Aneurysms
Right circumflex artery (RCA)	II, III and aVF	Premature atrial contractions (PACs) and atrial fibrillation Atrioventricular (AV) block (all types)	Hypotension due to decreased right ventricle ejection, especially when client is given nitroglycerin or morphine sulfate. Requires large volumes of fluids to maintain BP	Ventricular tachycardia/ ventricular fibrillation
Inferior wall	II, III, aVF	Atrial dysrhythmias	Hiccups, nausea, vomiting	Papillary muscle rupture Septal rupture
Anterior wall	V_3, V_4	Second degree AV block Sinus tachycardia		Cardiogenic shock Extension of the infarct to lateral wall
Septal wall	V_1, V_2	Infranodal BBB and second and third degree heart block		Septal rupture
Lateral wall	I, aVL, V_5, V_6	AV nodal blocks		Cardiogenic shock and heart failure
Posterior wall	ST-segment depression V_1-V_4	Bradycardia	Nausea	Papillary muscle dysfunction Aneurysms

BP, Blood pressure; *CO,* cardiac output.

softeners are used to relieve constipation and to lower the risk of bradycardia from straining that stimulates the vagus nerve.

Determine the Location of the Myocardial Infarction. Determining the exact coronary vessel that has infarcted is done through analysis of the 12-lead ECG and is validated with coronary angiography to determine the degree of occlusion (expressed in percentages). Determin-

ing the exact artery that is involved is important so potential complications can be assessed and minimized (Table 60-1). Knowledge of the area of the heart with infarct can prevent complications and allow diagnosis of AMI when ECG changes are not present.

Monitor for Complications. The possibility of death from complications always accompanies an AMI. Thus prime collaborative goals include the prevention of life-threatening complications or at least recognition of them.

Dysrhythmias. Dysrhythmias are the cause of 40% to 50% of deaths after AMI. Ectopic rhythms arise in or near the borders of intensely ischemic and damaged myocardial tissues. Damaged myocardium may also interfere with the conduction system, causing dissociation of the atria and ventricles *(heart block)*. Supraventricular tachycardia (SVT) sometimes occurs as a result of heart failure. Spontaneous or pharmacologic reperfusion of a previously ischemic area may also precipitate ventricular dysrhythmias.

Provide continuous cardiac monitoring and frequent counts of PVCs (many monitoring systems count continuously). Notify the physician if more than six PVCs occur per minute and the client is symptomatic (e.g., hypotension, chest pain). For *dysrhythmias,* provide prompt intervention per protocol or orders. For new-onset, symptomatic *ventricular ectopy* (runs, couplets), administer amiodarone or lidocaine per order or protocol. For *ventricular tachycardia,* administer amiodarone or lidocaine, if pulseless ventricular tachycardia occurs, provide synchronized cardioversion. For *ventricular fibrillation,* provide immediate defibrillation coupled with CPR and administration of epinephrine or vasopressin. For *supraventricular tachycardia (SVT),* administer a vagal maneuver, adenosine, diltiazem, or amiodarone, and prepare for possible elective cardioversion. For *heart block or symptomatic bradycardia,* administer atropine and prepare for use a temporary pacemaker.[8,26] Dysrhythmias are discussed in Chapter 59.

Cardiogenic Shock. Cardiogenic shock accounts for only 9% of deaths from AMI, but more than 70% of clients in whom shock develops die of it.[1] Causes include (1) decreased myocardial contraction with diminished cardiac output, (2) undetected dysrhythmias, and (3) sepsis.

Clinical manifestations include systolic blood pressure significantly below the client's normal range, diaphoresis, rapid pulse, restlessness, cold and clammy skin, and grayish skin color.

Shock can be prevented with rapid relief of pain and sufficient IV fluids to prevent circulatory collapse. It is also vital to identify dysrhythmias rapidly.

Administer vasopressors (dopamine, dobutamine) as prescribed to raise blood pressure by increasing peripheral resistance. In other cases, vasodilators (nitroprusside, nitroglycerin) promote better blood flow in the microcirculation and reduce afterload. Positive inotropic agents (dobutamine, epinephrine, milrinone) increase cardiac contractility and cardiac output and improve tissue perfusion. Administer oxygen therapy and antidysrhythmic agents as prescribed, and continuously monitor arterial and pulmonary artery pressures.[26] Analgesics

such as morphine sulfate should be given to ensure client comfort. Chapter 83 explains shock in detail.

Heart Failure and Pulmonary Edema. The most common cause of in-hospital death in clients with cardiac disorders is heart failure. Heart failure disables 22% of male clients and 46% female clients who experience an AMI and is responsible for one third of deaths after an AMI.[1]

Heart failure may develop at the onset of the infarction or may occur weeks later. Clinical manifestations include dyspnea, orthopnea, weight gain, edema, enlarged tender liver, distended neck veins, and crackles. It is managed by correcting the underlying cause, relieving clinical manifestations, and enhancing cardiac pump performance.[23,25,27] Heart failure is discussed in Chapter 58. See the Case Study feature on Cardiogenic Shock, Tachycardia, and Heart Failure, below.

Pulmonary Embolism. Pulmonary embolism (PE) may develop secondary to phlebitis of the leg or pelvic veins (venous thrombosis) or from atrial flutter or fibrillation. PE occurs in 10% to 20% of clients at some point, during either the acute attack or convalescence. PE is discussed in Chapter 65.

Recurrent Myocardial Infarction. Within 6 years after an initial AMI, 18% of men and 35% of women may experience recurrent MI.[1] Possible causes include overexertion, embolization, and further thrombotic occlusion of a coronary artery by an atheroma. The clinical manifestation is the return of angina. Management is the same as for AMI.

Complications Caused by Myocardial Necrosis. Complications that are due to necrosis of the myo-

---

CASE STUDY *evolve*

Cardiogenic Shock, Tachycardia, and Heart Failure

Mr. Borg is a 70-year-old retired African-American man who was admitted to the emergency department (ED) after arriving by rescue squad. According to his wife, he had been vomiting and experiencing progressive weakness earlier in the day. When the rescue squad arrived at his home, he was in supraventricular tachycardia with a heart rate over 180 beats/min. The squad administered adenosine (Adenocard) 6 mg IV, followed by an additional 12 mg 3 minutes later. En route he denied chest pain or shortness of breath, but he was becoming cyanotic and his heart rhythm was again becoming tachycardic. . . . *Case Study continued on the website and the CD-ROM with discussions, multiple-choice questions, and a nursing care plan.* *evolve*

cardium include ventricular aneurysm, rupture of the heart (*myocardial rupture*), ventricular septal defect (VSD), and ruptured papillary muscle. These complications are infrequent but serious, usually occurring about 5 to 7 days after MI.[28] Weak, friable necrotic myocardial tissue increases vulnerability to these complications (Figure 60-7).

Manifestations of heart failure develop with ventricular aneurysm, rupture of the ventricular septum, and rupture of the papillary muscle. Manifestations of severe mitral insufficiency often develop when the papillary muscle of the left ventricle ruptures. Ventricular dysrhythmias (e.g., frequent PVCs and ventricular tachycardia) occur often in the presence of a ventricular aneurysm (the necrotic tissue is very irritable). Manifestations of cardiac tamponade develop with rupture of the heart.

The goal of treatment is to decrease the workload of the heart and increase the oxygen supply to keep the area of infarction and necrotic tissue as small as possible.

Surgery is performed to (1) excise the ventricular aneurysm, (2) replace the mitral valve if the papillary muscle is ruptured, or (3) repair the VSD. Pericardiocentesis and immediate surgery help relieve cardiac tamponade that occurs after rupture of the heart.

Pericarditis. In up to 28% of clients with an acute transmural MI, early pericarditis develops (within 2 to 4 days). The inflamed area of the infarction rubs against the pericardial surface and causes it to lose its lubricating fluid.[28] A pericardial friction rub can be auscultated across the precordium. The client complains that chest pain is worse with movement, deep inspiration, and cough. The pain of pericarditis is relieved by sitting up and leaning forward.

Frequent assessment may lead to early identification and intervention. Relieve pain with analgesics, such as acetaminophen, nonsteroidal anti-inflammatory drugs (NSAIDs), or other anti-inflammatory agents. Reduce the client's anxiety by differentiating the pain of pericarditis from the pain of AMI.

Dressler's Syndrome (Late Pericarditis). Dressler's syndrome, a form of pericarditis, can occur as late as 6 weeks to months after AMI. Although the etiologic agent is unknown, an autoimmune cause is suggested.[28] The client usually presents with a fever lasting 1 week or longer, pericardial chest pain, pericardial friction rub, and occasionally pleuritis with pleural effusions. This is a self-limiting phenomenon, and no prevention is known. Treatment includes aspirin, prednisone, and opioid analgesics for pain. Anticoagulation therapy may precipitate cardiac tamponade and should be avoided in these clients.

Rehabilitation and Education. Cardiac rehabilitation following AMI is an essential component of professional and personal management. The following are recommendations for managing rehabilitation of clients who have suffered an AMI:

- All clients with cardiovascular disease should adopt a cardioprotective dietary pattern.
- Intensive dietary advice, compliance checks, and long-term follow-up should be given, preferable by a dietitian.
- There is insufficient evidence to recommend nutritional supplements of antioxidant vitamins, minerals, or trace elements for the prevention of cardiovascular disease.
- Fish and fish oil supplements may reduce the risk of sudden cardiac death.
- For overweight and obese clients with CHD, the combination of reduced-energy diet and increased physical activity is recommended.
- Initial goal of weight loss therapy should be to reduce the client's weight by 10%.
- All clients with cardiovascular disease should be advised to quit smoking and should be supported to stop smoking as a priority measure.
- All clients with CHD should consider having standard pharmacotherapy with aspirin, beta-blocker, ACE inhibitor, and a statin unless contraindicated.
- Comprehensive cardiac rehabilitation should embrace a case management approach.[4]

Strengthen the Myocardium. A successful rehabilitation program begins the moment the client enters the coronary care unit for emergency care and continues for

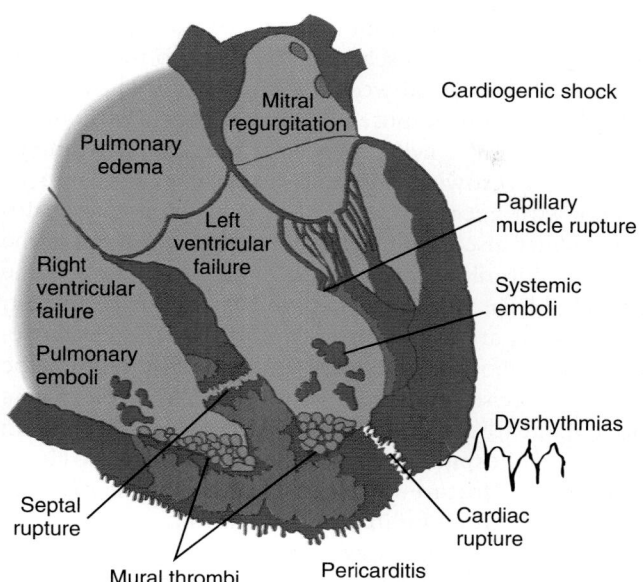

FIGURE 60-7 Major complications of acute myocardial infarction.

months and even years after discharge from the health care facility.[4,32] The overall goal of rehabilitation is to help the client live as full, vital, and productive a life as possible while remaining within the limits of the heart's ability to respond to increases in activity and stress. Six important subgoals of the rehabilitation process are as follows:

- Developing a program of progressive physical activity
- Educating the client and significant others about the cause, prevention, and treatment of CHD
- Helping the client accept the limitations imposed by illness
- Aiding the client in adjusting to changes in occupational goals
- Lessening the exposure to risk factors
- Changing the psychosocial factors adversely affecting recovery from CHD

Cardiac rehabilitation is a comprehensive, long-term program that involves periodic medical evaluation, prescribed exercises, and education and counseling about cardiac risk factor modification.[4,32] Cardiac rehabilitation is a multifactorial program that begins when the client is still hospitalized and continues throughout recovery. Cardiac rehabilitation consists of four phases: phase I (inpatient), phase II (immediate outpatient), phase III (intermediate outpatient), and phase IV (maintenance outpatient).[32]

Phase I (Inpatient). Phase I begins with admission to the coronary care unit. After AMI, clients usually remain on bed rest for less than 24 hours unless complications such as heart failure or dysrhythmias develop. Although the myocardium must rest, bed rest puts the client at risk for hypovolemia, hypoxemia, muscle atrophy, and pulmonary embolus. Thus the client must avoid both invalidism and reckless overexertion. See the Care Plan feature on The Client with Acute Myocardial Infarction on pp. 1719 to 1727. Case managers may also be assigned to coordinate care. See the Case Management feature on Acute Myocardial Infarction on the website.

Provide complete bed rest for the first day or so with use of a bedside commode for bowel movements. Most clients receive a 2-g sodium diet. If the client is nauseated, provide a clear liquid diet until nausea subsides. A coronary care nurse or physiotherapist should start passive exercises. As the client regains strength, have the client sit for brief periods on the side of the bed and dangle the feet. Allow the client to ambulate to a bedside chair for 15 to 20 minutes after the first day if dangling has been tolerated without development of chest pain, dysrhythmias, or hypotension. When the client is transferred from the coronary care unit to an intermediate or regular unit, bathroom privileges and self-care activities are encouraged. Wireless heart monitoring (telemetry) may continue. Allow brief walks in the hall with super-

vision. The length and duration of these walks are increased progressively, working up to 5 to 10 minutes according to the client's endurance. The client loses 10% to 15% of skeletal muscle and contractile strength within the first week of bed rest and 20% to 25% after 3 weeks of bed rest. The client must increase activities gradually to avoid overtaxing the heart as it pumps oxygenated blood to the muscles. The metabolic equivalent test (MET) provides one way of measuring the amount of oxygen needed to perform an activity:

$$1 \text{ MET} = 3.5 \text{ ml O}_2/\text{kg/min}$$

One MET is about equivalent to the oxygen uptake a client requires when resting. Early mobilization activities after AMI should not exceed 1 to 2 METs, as from shaving, washing, and self-feeding. (Later activities can increase to 10 or 11 METs, such as cycling or running.)

With each activity level increase, monitor the heart rate, blood pressure, and fatigue level, adjusting the client's activity level accordingly. During early activities, the heart rate should not increase more than 25% above resting level. Blood pressure must not increase more than 25 mm Hg above normal.

Help the client avoid fatigue. Dyspnea, chest pain, tachycardia, and a sense of exhaustion warn that the client is attempting to do too much. Instruct the client regarding these warning signs of overexertion. Include family members in these discussions; family members may fear that allowing the client to become active again will precipitate another AMI and while attempting to help, they may discourage autonomy.

During phase I, client education should include cardiac anatomy and physiology risk factors and management of CHD, behavioral counseling, and home activities.

Phase II (Immediate Outpatient). If no complications arise, the physician discharges the client to the home by the end of the second week. Nearly 50% of clients after AMI have an uncomplicated hospital course without evidence of angina, heart failure, or major dysrhythmias. There is a growing trend toward early discharge of clients with uncomplicated AMI. A team at one health care facility discharges post-AMI clients at the end of the 4th day but allows clients to go home early only if the household has adequate help and is conducive to rest. Such clients are followed up carefully by trained nurse-clinicians who visit the home and supervise physiologic status, exercise, and diet every other day. Researchers hope that earlier discharge after AMI reduces depression as well as hospital expenses. See the Bridge to Home Health Care feature on Heart-Healthy Living After an Acute Myocardial Infarction on p. 1728.

Resuming sexual activity may be one of the most difficult aspects of returning to normal life after AMI. Sexual intercourse usually may resume 4 to 8 weeks after an AMI. The client should be able to climb two flights of

Text continued on p. 1727

CARE PLAN

The Client with Acute Myocardial Infarction

Nursing Diagnosis. Acute Pain related to myocardial ischemia resulting from coronary artery occlusion with loss or restriction of blood flow to an area of the myocardium and necrosis of the myocardium.

Outcomes. The client will experience improved comfort in the chest, as evidenced by a decrease in the rating of the chest pain, the ability to rest and sleep comfortably, less need for analgesia or nitroglycerin, and reduced anxiety.

Interventions	Rationales
1. Assess the characteristics of chest pain, including location, duration, quality, intensity, presence of radiation, precipitating and alleviating factors, and associated manifestations. Have the client rate pain on a scale of 0 to 10, and document findings in nurses' notes.	1. Pain is an indication of myocardial ischemia. Assisting the client in quantifying pain may differentiate pre-existing and current pain patterns as well as identify complications. Usually a scale of 0 to 10 is used, with 10 being the worst pain and 0 being none.
2. Assess respirations, blood pressure, and heart rate with each episode of chest pain.	2. Respirations may be increased as a result of pain and associated anxiety. Release of stress-induced catecholamines increases heart rate and blood pressure.
3. Obtain a 12-lead electrocardiogram (ECG) on admission, then each time chest pain recurs for evidence of further infarction.	3. Serial ECGs and stat ECGs record changes that can give evidence of further cardiac damage and location of myocardial ischemia.
4. Monitor the response to drug therapy. Notify the physician if pain does not abate within 15 to 20 minutes.	4. Pain control is a priority because it indicates ischemia.
5. Provide care in a calm, efficient manner that reassures the client and minimizes anxiety. Stay with the client until discomfort is relieved.	5. External stimuli may worsen anxiety and cardiac strain and limit coping abilities.
6. Limit visitors as the client requests.	6. Limiting visitors prevents overstimulation and promotes rest.
7. Administer morphine as ordered.	7. Morphine is an opiate analgesic and alters the client's perception of pain and reduces preload time vasoconstriction.
8. Administer nitrates as ordered.	8. Nitrates relax the smooth muscles of coronary blood vessels, decreasing ischemia and hence decreasing pain.

Evaluation. The client should be pain-free within 15 to 20 minutes after administration of drug therapy. The client will verbalize relief of pain and will not exhibit associated manifestations of pain.

Nursing Diagnosis. Ineffective Tissue Perfusion (Cardiopulmonary) related to thrombus in coronary artery, resulting in altered blood flow to myocardial tissue.

Outcomes. The client will demonstrate improved cardiac tissue perfusion, as evidenced by a decrease in the rating of pain and resolving ST segments.

Interventions	Rationales
1. Keep the client on bed rest with a quiet environment.	1. Stress activates the sympathetic nervous system and increases myocardial oxygen needs.
2. Administer oxygen as ordered.	2. Oxygen increases myocardial supply of oxygen.
3. Administer thrombolytics or send the client for angioplasty as ordered.	3. Thrombolytic therapy or angioplasty can break apart the thrombus and increase myocardial tissue perfusion.
4. Monitor ST segments.	4. ST-segment elevation indicates myocardial tissue injury; ST-segment depression indicates decreased myocardial perfusion.

Evaluation. The return of ST segments to baseline is dependent on the degree of ischemia and rapidness of treatment.

Continued

CAREPLAN

The Client with Acute Myocardial Infarction—cont'd

Collaborative Problem. Dysrhythmias related to electrical instability or irritability secondary to ischemia or infarcted tissue, as evidenced by an increase or decrease in heart rate, change in rhythm, and atrial or ventricular dysrhythmias.

Outcomes. The client will have no dysrhythmias, as evidenced by normal sinus rhythm or return to the client's own baseline rhythm.

Interventions	Rationales
1. Teach the client and family about the need for continuous monitoring. Keep alarms on and limits set at all times.	1. Continued monitoring keeps staff aware of rhythm changes. Family anxiety is decreased when explanations are provided.
2. Assess the apical heart rate. Auscultate for change in heart sounds (murmurs, rub, S_3, and S_4).	2. The apical heart rate suggests early cardiac decompensation and potential loss of cardiac output.
3. Document the rhythm strip every shift and prn (as needed) if dysrhythmias occur. Measure the pulse rate, QRS, PR, and QT segments with each strip. Note and report any deviations from the client's baseline values.	3. Dysrhythmias are the most common complication after AMI.
4. Report six or more multifocal premature ventricular contractions (PVCs) per minute to the physician.	4. Multifocal PVCs indicate ventricular irritability, which decreases cardiac output and may lead to life-threatening dysrhythmias.
5. Give antidysrhythmic agents as ordered.	5. Antidysrhythmic drugs reduce myocardial irritability.
6. Monitor the effects of antidysrhythmic agents.	6. The desired results are increased diastolic threshold potential and decreased action potential duration.
7. Monitor serum potassium levels.	7. Altered potassium levels can affect cardiac rhythms.
8. Maintain a patent intravenous (IV) line or heparin lock at all times.	8. This measure is for emergency administration of IV cardiac medications.
9. Monitor ST segments, and document changes.	9. ST depression indicates myocardial ischemia, and ST elevation indicates injury; either may precipitate dysrhythmias.

Evaluation. Within 24 hours of admission, the client's cardiac rhythm will remain stable and the client will exhibit no manifestations of rhythm disturbance.

Nursing Diagnosis. Decreased Cardiac Output related to negative inotropic changes in the heart secondary to myocardial ischemia, injury, or infarction, as evidenced by change in the level of consciousness, weakness, dizziness, loss of peripheral pulses, abnormal heart sounds, hemodynamic compromise, and cardiopulmonary arrest.

Outcomes. The client will have improved cardiac output, as evidenced by normal cardiac rate, rhythm, and hemodynamic parameters, dysrhythmias controlled or absent; and absence of angina.

Interventions	Rationales
Assess for and document the following as evidence of myocardial dysfunction with decreasing cardiac output:	
1. Mental status—be alert to restlessness and decreased responsiveness.	1. Cerebral perfusion is directly related to cardiac output and aortic perfusion pressure and is influenced by hypoxia and electrolyte and acid-base variations.
2. Lung sounds—monitor for crackles and rhonchi.	2. Crackles may develop, reflecting pulmonary congestion related to alterations in myocardial function.
3. Blood pressure—monitor for hypertension or hypotension.	3. Hypotension related to hypoperfusion, vagal stimulation, dysrhythmias, or ventricular dysfunction may occur; it may be related to pain, anxiety, catecholamine release, or pre-existing vascular problems.

CARE PLAN

Interventions	Rationales
4. Heart sounds—note the presence of gallop, murmur, and increased or decreased heart rate.	4. Bradycardia may be present because of vagal stimulation or conduction disturbances related to the area of myocardial injury. Tachycardia may be a compensatory mechanism related to decreased cardiac output. A gallop may be related to fluid volume overload or heart failure, and a murmur may be present if a ruptured chordae tendineae occurred.
5. Urine output—be alert to output less than 0.5 ml/kg/hr.	5. Urine output less than 0.5 ml/kg/hr may reflect reduced renal perfusion and glomerular filtration as a result of reduced cardiac output.
6. Peripheral perfusion—monitor for pallor, mottling, cyanosis, coolness, diaphoresis, and peripheral pulses.	6. Decreased peripheral pulses may indicate a decrease in cardiac output.
7. Monitor arterial blood gas (ABG) levels.	7. Acidosis may cause dysrhythmias and depressed cardiac function and some cardiac medications increase oxygen demand and may cause hypoxia.
8. If a pulmonary artery catheter is used, record hemodynamic parameters every 2 to 4 hours and as required (prn). Be alert to pulmonary capillary wedge pressure (PCWP) greater than 18 mm Hg, cardiac output less than 4 L/min, and cardiac index less than 2.5 L/min.	8. A PCWP greater than 18 mm Hg may indicate fluid volume overload or heart failure. A cardiac output less than 4 L/min and a cardiac index less than 2.5 L/min indicate heart failure or decrease in cardiac output. Use hemodynamic monitoring to assess drug therapy and for prevention or early detection of complications of AMI (i.e., extension, heart failure, cardiogenic shock).
9. Maintain hemodynamic stability by monitoring the effects of beta-blockers and inotropic agents.	9. Assess the effect of drug therapy on myocardial contractility and function.
10. Monitor and assess angina for type severity and duration.	10. Angina indicates myocardial ischemia, which may decrease cardiac output.

Evaluation. Within 2 to 3 days of admission, the client will have normal hemodynamic pressures, normal vital signs, clear breath sounds, no shortness of breath, normal ABG values, and normal sinus rhythm with rate between 60 and 100 beats/min.

Nursing Diagnosis. Impaired Gas Exchange related to decreased cardiac output, as evidenced by cyanosis, impaired capillary refill, reduced arterial oxygen tension (PaO$_2$), and dyspnea.

Outcomes. The client will demonstrate improved gas exchange, as evidenced by absence of cyanosis, brisk capillary refill, absence of dyspnea, and ABG levels within normal limits.

Interventions	Rationales
1. Administer oxygen as ordered; maintain continuous oximetry.	1. Increases amount of oxygen available for myocardial uptake; oximetry measures peripheral oxygen saturation.
2. Monitor ABGs as ordered.	2. The presence of hypoxia indicates a need for supplemental oxygen. Monitoring provides data on the adequacy of tissue perfusion and oxygenation.
3. Continue to assess the client's skin, capillary refill, and level of consciousness every 2 to 4 hours and prn.	3. Cyanosis (circumoral or at extremities) indicates hypoxia. Capillary refill greater than 3 seconds indicates poor perfusion and possibly hypoxia.
4. Assess respiratory status for dyspnea and crackles.	4. Dyspnea may indicate inadequate oxygenation, and the presence of crackles may impair gas exchange because of decreased exchange of oxygen and carbon dioxide through fluid in alveoli.
5. Prepare for intubation and mechanical ventilation if hypoxia increases.	5. With increasing hypoxia, mechanical ventilation may be necessary to oxygenate the client adequately.

Continued

CARE PLAN

The Client with Acute Myocardial Infarction—cont'd

Evaluation. Within 2 to 3 days of admission, client's breath sounds will be clear, and ABG values will be within normal limits.

Collaborative Problem. Risk for Bleeding related to coagulopathies associated with thrombolytic therapy or arterial puncture after angioplasty.

Outcomes. The nurse will monitor for bleeding and reduce bleeding risk. If bleeding does occur, it will be recognized and treated at once.

Interventions	Rationales
1. Obtain coagulation studies as ordered.	1. Coagulation studies can help determine the tendency to bleed.
2. Monitor invasive line sites for active bleeding.	2. Thrombolytic therapy disrupts the normal coagulation process, and bleeding may occur at any invasive site.
3. Inspect all body fluids for presence of blood.	3. Internal bleeding may be manifested in urine, sputum, and gastrointestinal drainage.
4. Hold pressure on any discontinued lines 15 minutes; if arterial, hold for 30 minutes.	4. Pressure is used to achieve hemostasis at catheter sites.
5. If the client has had an angioplasty, monitor puncture sight frequently for hemorrhage.	5. Active bleeding may occur after angioplasty.
6. Observe neurologic status.	6. A change in neurologic status may indicate intracranial bleeding.
7. Avoid intramuscular (IM) injections.	7. IM injections may cause bleeding.
8. Assess for back or flank pain.	8. Flank or back pain may suggest retroperitoneal bleeding.
9. Keep an IV line patent.	9. In case of active bleeding, a patent line must be maintained to transfuse blood products.
10. Maintain an active type and crossmatch on the client.	10. If the client requires blood or blood products, an active type and crossmatch help eliminate any delay in treatment.

Evaluation. The nurse will monitor for and prevent bleeding.

Nursing Diagnosis. Powerlessness related to the hospital environment and anticipated lifestyle changes, as evidenced by verbalized "feelings of doom," crying, and anger.

Outcomes. The client will regain a sense of "control," as evidenced by feeling able to express feelings of powerlessness over the present situation and future outcomes.

Interventions	Rationales
1. Provide opportunities for the client to express feelings about oneself and the illness.	1. These opportunities create a supportive climate and send the message that caregivers are willing to help.
2. Explore reality perceptions, and clarify if necessary.	2. Listening to the client's feelings and words can help the client acquire a more hopeful outlook.
3. Eliminate the unpredictability of events by allowing adequate preparation for tests and procedures.	3. Information helps the client and family feel more hopeful and be more willing to participate in care.
4. Reinforce the client's right to ask questions.	4. Maintain a supportive climate to let the client feel free to ask questions or have information repeated.
5. Allow choices when possible.	5. Self-care allows the client to feel independent.
6. Provide positive reinforcement for increased involvement in self-care.	6. When clients participate in planning for care, they are more likely to feel a sense of control and to follow through with actions.

CARE PLAN

Interventions	Rationales
7. Help the client identify strengths and areas of control.	7. Self-confidence and security come with a sense of control; foster full client participation.

Evaluation. Within 24 hours of admission, client will verbalize a feeling of control over the situation and will actively participate in decisions regarding care.

Nursing Diagnosis. Anxiety and Fear related to hospital admission and fear of death, as evidenced by client and family appearing restless, hostile, or withdrawn; client and family verbalize fatalism or act extremely emotional as if in the grieving process.

Outcomes. The client will have reduced feelings of anxiety and fear, as evidenced by demonstrating appropriate range of feelings and initial manifestations of effective coping (participating in the treatment regimen), being able to rest, and asking fewer questions.

Interventions	Rationales
1. Limit nursing personnel; provide continuity of care.	1. Continuity of care promotes security and development of rapport with and trust of health care providers.
2. Allow and encourage the client and family to ask questions; do not avoid questions. Bring up common concerns.	2. Accurate information about the situation reduces fear, strengthens the client-nurse relationship, and assists the client and family to face the situation realistically.
3. Allow the client and family to verbalize fears.	3. Sharing information elicits support and comfort and can relieve tension and unexpressed worries.
4. Stress that frequent assessments are routine and do not necessarily imply a deteriorating condition.	4. The client may feel reassured after learning that frequent assessments may prevent development of more serious complications.
5. Repeat information as necessary because of the reduced attention span of the client and family.	5. The client's attention span is short, and time perception may be altered. Anxiety decreases learning and attention.
6. Provide a comfortable, quiet environment for the client and family.	6. A comfortable environment enhances coping mechanisms and reduces myocardial workload and oxygen consumption.

Evaluation. Coping is very individualized. Base the timing of outcomes on the client's demonstrated behaviors and statements.

Nursing Diagnosis. Risk for Constipation related to bed rest, pain medications, and NPO (nothing by mouth) or soft diet, as evidenced by subjective feeling of fullness, abdominal cramping, painful defecation, and palpable impaction.

Outcomes. The client will have improved bowel elimination, as evidenced by eliminating a stool without straining or having a vasovagal response (bradycardia).

Interventions	Rationales
1. Ensure that the client has adequate bulk in diet and adequate fluid intake (without violating fluid restrictions).	1. Bulk and fluid within the colon prevent straining.
2. Monitor the effectiveness of softeners or laxatives. Instruct the client on prevention of straining and avoiding the Valsalva (vasovagal) maneuver.	2. Stool softeners decrease the myocardial workload of straining. The Valsalva maneuver causes bradycardia, decreasing cardiac output.
3. Encourage the client to use a bedside commode rather than a bedpan.	3. Use of bedpans necessitates more straining and increases the vasovagal response.

Evaluation. Within 2 to 3 days of admission, client should have normal bowel function.

Continued

CARE PLAN

The Client with Acute Myocardial Infarction—cont'd

Nursing Diagnosis. Ineffective Health Maintenance related to AMI and implications for lifestyle changes.

Outcomes. The client and family will learn about the medical regimen and lifestyle changes, as evidenced by verbalizing an understanding of a heart attack and the necessary lifestyle changes regarding diet, medications, stress reduction, quitting smoking, and cholesterol, weight, and blood pressure reduction.

Interventions	Rationales
1. Explain the following, providing both oral and written instructions: anatomy and functions of heart muscle, coronary arteries, and atherosclerotic process; definition of a "heart attack"; healing process of the heart; and role of collateral circulation.	1. Use of multiple learning methods enhances retention of material; information helps the client understand the underlying problems of overall heart functions.
2. Assist the client with identifying personal risk factors.	2. Risk factor identification is the first step before changes can be implemented.
3. Assist the client in devising a plan for risk factor modification (e.g., diet; smoking cessation; cholesterol, stress, and blood pressure reduction).	3. This information is helpful in providing opportunity for the client to identify risk factors, assume control, and participate in a treatment regimen.
4. Provide guidelines for a diet low in cholesterol and saturated fat. Arrange for dietary consultation before hospital discharge.	4. Consultation with other health professionals enhances client learning from others. Guidelines developed with the client and family before discharge help once they are home.
5. Teach the client and family about medications that will be taken after hospital discharge (name, purpose, dosage, schedule, precautions, potential side effects).	5. The more clients understand the medical regimen and potential side effects, the more adept they will be in monitoring for them.
6. Discuss post-AMI activity progression; arrange for a cardiac rehabilitation consultation.	6. Continued follow-up will let clients know how they are doing; outpatient cardiac rehabilitation supports and assists clients in the lifestyle changes necessary for a healthy recovery and life.
7. Use other professionals to collaborate in the care of the client.	7. Dietitians can assist in diet education; social services can identify assistance in the area; cardiac rehabilitation personnel can assist in exercise regimens; clergy can assist in coping strategies; and support groups can assist in social support.

Evaluation. Adaptation to new self-care strategies is very individualized. Plan the projected time frame once the client's learning style is known.

Nursing Diagnosis. Risk for Activity Intolerance related to an imbalance between oxygen supply and demand, as evidenced by weakness, fatigue, change in vital signs, dysrhythmias, dyspnea, pallor, and diaphoresis.

Outcomes. The client will have improved activity tolerance, as evidenced by participating in desired activities, meeting activities of daily living (ADL), reduced fatigue and weakness, vital signs within normal limits during activity, and absence of cyanosis, diaphoresis, and pain.

Interventions	Rationales
1. Monitor vital signs before and immediately after activity and 3 minutes later. If blood pressure decreases and heart rate increases, cardiac decompensation is suggested and activity should be decreased.	1. Vital signs should return to baseline levels in 3 minutes. The development of cardiac decompensation chest pain or dyspnea may indicate a need for an alteration in exercise regimen or medication.
2. Monitor for tachycardia, dysrhythmias, dyspnea, diaphoresis, weakness, fatigue, or pallor after activity.	2. These indicators of myocardial oxygen deprivation may call for decreased activity, changes in medications, or use of supplemental oxygen.

CARE PLAN

Interventions	Rationales
3. Encourage verbalization of feelings or concerns regarding fatigue or limitations.	3. Knowing limitations prevents exertion and increasing myocardial workload.
4. Provide assistance with self-care activities, and provide frequent rest periods, especially after meals.	4. Large meals may increase myocardial workload and cause vagal stimulation, with resultant bradycardia or ectopic beats; caffeine, a cardiac stimulant, increases heart rate.
5. Increase activity per cardiac rehabilitation nurse and physician orders.	5. Gradual increase in activity increases strength and prevents overexertion, enhances collateral circulation, and restores a normal lifestyle as far as possible.

Evaluation. With stable acute myocardial infarction, the client should progress normally through steps of phase I cardiac rehabilitation without manifestations of exercise intolerance in 3 to 4 days.

Collaborative Problem. Risk for Heart Failure related to disease process, as evidenced by tachycardia, hypotension or hypertension, S_3 or S_4 heart sounds, dysrhythmias, ECG changes, decreased urine output, decreased peripheral pulses, peripheral edema, cool ashen skin, diaphoresis, crackles, jugular vein distention, edema, and chest pain.

Outcomes. The nurse will monitor for clinical manifestations of heart failure by assessing cardiac rate, rhythm, hemodynamic parameters, skin perfusion, renal perfusion, and CNS perfusion.

Interventions	Rationales
1. Auscultate the apical pulse.	1. Atrial (S_3) or ventricular (S_4) gallop rhythms are common and reflect tissue noncompliance or distention of chambers.
2. Assess heart rate and rhythm.	2. Sinus tachycardia, paroxysmal atrial contractions, paroxysmal atrial tachycardia, multifocal atrial tachycardia, and PVCs are commonly seen with heart failure.
3. Document dysrhythmias, if present, as necessary.	3. Dysrhythmias reduce ventricular filling time, decrease myocardial contractility, and increase myocardial oxygen demands, which further compromises cardiac output.
4. Note lung sounds every 2 to 4 hours and as needed.	4. Crackles may develop; ineffective cardiac output causes an increase in venous congestion that transcends to the pulmonary vasculature and leaks into the alveolar tissue, resulting in congestion.
5. Palpate peripheral pulses every 2 to 4 hours and as necessary.	5. Pulses may be weak, thready, or difficult to obtain when cardiac output is decreased.
6. Monitor blood pressure every 2 to 4 hours and as needed.	6. Hypotension related to hypoperfusion, vagal stimulation, or ventricular dysfunction may occur. Hypertension may be related to pain, anxiety, catecholamine release, or pre-existing vascular problems.
7. Inspect skin for pallor, cyanosis, and diaphoresis every 2 to 4 hours and as needed.	7. Pallor is associated with vasoconstriction, reduced cardiac output, and anemia. Cyanosis may develop during severe episodes of pulmonary edema. Dependent areas are often blue or mottled with increased venous congestion.
8. Monitor urine output, noting changes or decreasing output and dark or concentrated urine, every 2 to 4 hours and as needed.	8. Urine output less than 0.5 ml/kg/hr may reflect reduced renal perfusion and glomerular filtration as a result of reduced cardiac output.
9. Assess for chest pain.	9. Chest pain may indicate inadequate cardiac perfusion related to the hypertrophied myocardium.
10. Assess for peripheral edema.	10. In heart failure, especially right-sided, the inability to pump venous blood back to the heart results in venous pooling and increased pressure in the vascular space that leaks in the interstitium, presenting as peripheral edema.

Continued

CARE PLAN

The Client with Acute Myocardial Infarction—cont'd

Interventions	Rationales
11. Assess changes in sensorium.	11. Cerebral perfusion is directly related to cardiac output, and mentation may be a sensitive indicator of deterioration.
12. Provide frequent rest periods.	12. Physical rest decreases the production of catecholamines, which increases heart rate, myocardial oxygen demand, and blood pressure.
13. Instruct the client on avoidance of activities that increase cardiac workload.	13. Avoidance of activities provides an opportunity for myocardial recovery and decreases workload and myocardial oxygen consumption.
14. Provide a bedside commode. Avoid the Valsalva maneuver.	14. The Valsalva maneuver causes bradycardia and temporarily decreases cardiac output.
15. Elevate the client's legs and avoid pressure under the knees. Permit increase in activity as tolerated.	15. This position enhances venous return, reduces dependent swelling, decreases venous stasis, and may reduce the incidence of thrombus and embolus formation.
16. Administer medications as ordered.	16. ACE inhibitors and beta-blockade help reduce the incidence of heart failure after AMI in clinical trials.[21]

Evaluation. The nurse will monitor for heart failure and report manifestations promptly.

Nursing Diagnosis. Excess Fluid Volume related to reduced glomerular filtration rate (GFR), decreased cardiac output, increased antidiuretic hormone (ADH) production, and sodium and water retention, as evidenced by orthopnea, S_3 heart sound, oliguria, edema, jugular neck vein distention, increased weight, increased blood pressure, respiratory distress, and abnormal breath sounds.

Outcomes. The client's fluid volume balance will be adequate, as evidenced by balanced intake and output (I&O), clear or clearing breath sounds, vital signs within normal limits, stable weight, and minimal edema.

Interventions	Rationales
1. Monitor I&O (especially note color, specific gravity, and amount) every 2 to 4 hours, and as needed, and 24-hour totals.	1. Intake greater than output may indicate fluid volume excess. If client receives diuretic therapy, an increase in output is expected.
2. Maintain chair or bed rest in the semi-Fowler position.	2. This position promotes diuresis by recumbency-induced increased GFR and reduced ADH production.
3. Involve the client and family in fluid schedules, especially if there are restrictions, and provide frequent oral care.	3. Involving the client in the therapy regimen may enhance a sense of control and fosters cooperation with restrictions. Fluid restrictions dry the oral mucous membranes.
4. Weigh the client daily.	4. Daily weights can show the increase or decrease in congestion and edema in response to therapy. A gain of 5 pounds represents about 2 L of fluid.
5. Assess for jugular neck vein distention, edema, peripheral pulses, and presence of anasarca.	5. Excessive fluid retention may be demonstrated by venous engorgement and edema formation. Peripheral edema often begins in the feet and ascends upward as heart failure worsens.
6. Auscultate breath sounds. Note adventitious sounds, and monitor for dyspnea or tachypnea.	6. These manifestations of pulmonary congestion reflect increased vascular volume and pulmonary hypertension or worsening of heart failure.
7. Monitor for sudden extreme shortness of breath and feelings of panic.	7. These are manifestations of extreme pulmonary capillary hypertension (pulmonary edema).
8. Palpate for hepatomegaly. Note complaints of right upper quadrant pain or tenderness.	8. Advancing heart failure leads to venous congestion, which results in liver engorgement and altered liver function (i.e., impaired drug metabolism, prolonged drug half-life).

CARE PLAN

Interventions	Rationales
9. Evaluate the effectiveness of diuretics and potassium supplements.	9. Fluid shifts and use of diuretics can alter electrolytes, especially potassium and chloride, which affects cardiac rhythm and contractility.
10. Note increased lethargy, hypotension, and muscle cramping.	10. These are manifestations of hypokalemia and hyponatremia that may occur because of fluid shifts and diuretic therapy.
11. Assess the need for dietary consultation as needed.	11. Restrictions of foods high in sodium may be necessary. The client may need to eat foods enriched with potassium when taking loop diuretics.

Evaluation. Depending on the degree of heart failure, fluid volume excess may be slow to resolve. Initially, there may be a resolution of manifestations after diuresis. Fluid balance adjustments may then be made daily.

Nursing Diagnosis. Risk for Impaired Skin Integrity related to bed rest, edema, and decreased tissue perfusion, as evidenced by reddened areas and the presence of areas of breakdown.

Outcomes. The client will have intact skin integrity, as evidenced by an absence of reddened areas and no areas of breakdown.

Interventions	Rationales
1. Inspect the client's skin; note bony prominences, edema, altered circulation, pigmentation, obesity, and emaciation.	1. Altered skin color in isolated areas suggests damage caused by pressure or decreased circulation.
2. Assist with active or passive range-of-motion (ROM) exercises.	2. ROM exercises enhance venous return. Isometric exercises may adversely affect cardiac output by increasing myocardial work and oxygen consumption.
3. Reposition the client every 2 hours in a bed or chair.	3. Repositioning increases circulation and reduces the time that weight deprives any one area of blood flow.
4. Provide pressure-reducing devices, sheepskin, elbow protectors, and heel elevation if needed.	4. These devices reduce pressure to bone prominences and maintain skin integrity.
5. Assess and provide special air or flotation beds for clients at high risk for pressure ulcers.	5. These beds reduce pressure to skin and may improve circulation.
6. Pad the chair with a pressure reduction pad or 4 inches of foam.	6. Weak clients do not move spontaneously. Pressure reduction surfaces can prevent pressures in excess of capillary filling pressures.

Evaluation. Skin impairment may be evident within 48 hours of admission or a significant change in condition.

stairs before resuming sexual activity. Caution clients not to eat or drink alcoholic beverages immediately before intercourse. Taking nitroglycerin before intercourse may help prevent exertional angina. However, clients cannot take sildenafil (Viagra) while taking nitroglycerin; both medications are vasodilators.

Advise the client to stop smoking. Encourage frequent walks, but warn against strenuous activities, such as shoveling snow. The walking program aims for a goal of 2 miles in less than 60 minutes.

A monitored group program may help the client achieve the best possible physical conditioning. These programs typically last from 10 to 12 weeks and are im-

plemented in a supervised setting. They offer various training devices, such as treadmills, stationary bicycles, and rowing machines. During phase II, the client performs large-muscle exercises for at least 20 to 30 minutes three or four times a week. In addition, clients are trained in warm-up and stretching exercises.[32] During the sessions, cardiac rehabilitation staff monitor cardiac rhythm, heart rate, and blood pressure before exercise, at peak exercise, and during recovery. Clients also report their level of perceived exertion several times during the exercise session.

Some clients may be able to return to work at the end of 8 or 9 weeks if they remain asymptomatic. Clients

BRIDGE TO HOME HEALTH CARE

Heart-Healthy Living After an Acute Myocardial Infarction

The role of the home health nurse is to help clients who had an AMI adjust to their lifestyle by teaching healthy heart living. Focus your teaching on areas that will help clients become responsible for self-care. Assume that you need to repeat health education that was provided in the hospital during the AMI episode. When stress is high, clients usually recall little of what was taught.

Instruct the client and significant other or family member to monitor for clinical manifestations that may indicate extensions and recurrences of the AMI. Clients need to report indigestion, shortness of breath, increased edema, and palpitations. Learning when to call the physician or nurse for these physical problems is important.

Determine what your clients know about their medications. Knowing what the medication is called, its function, the schedule for taking it, and its side effects is required for client safety. Generally, multiple medications are prescribed, and you need to give the client written instructions and information about each medication. Many pharmacists provide a computer printout of medications and interactions for the client to keep. Medication planners that have compartments for various times of day allow the client to prefill medications for a week at a time and may prevent errors.

The convalescence period for the client and family creates anxiety about daily activities. Instruct the client to avoid prolonged baths or showers to prevent vasodilation. Use tepid water and a stool or bath chair in the shower. Encourage the use of energy-conservation techniques, such as keeping the arms at waist level and getting enough rest to prevent fatigue. Routine household activities and mild recreational activities, such as playing golf, are usually permitted.

Climbing more than two flights of stairs and lifting more than 20 pounds are restricted. If clients do not ask about resuming sexual relations, consider introducing the topic. They may be too timid to consult their physicians about this subject.

An appropriate unsupervised exercise is a prescribed indoor walking program. Exercising after a heavy meal or during mild illness is contraindicated. Instruct the client to begin each exercise session with a warm-up period that may last as long as 15 minutes and to end the session with a cool-down period. Walking should be constant and should last long enough to increase blood flow to the muscles.

The client or caregiver should have an emergency plan that includes having someone available to drive if a ride is needed and someone in the home who knows basic cardiopulmonary resuscitation (CPR). A personal emergency response system may be appropriate for clients who live alone. Some emergency response systems are worn around the neck, and the push of a button summons medical assistance. Caregiver stress, communication problems, and fear of the unknown are valid concerns. Community resources and additional information can be obtained by calling the American Heart Association's toll-free number, 800-242-8721.

---

with less physically strenuous jobs can sometimes resume a full-time schedule, but manual laborers may have to work part time or find less taxing work. Occupational evaluations can be done to assess cardiac impairment in relation to job requirements and client skills.[32]

Between the eighth and tenth weeks, the client requires a complete physical examination, including ECG, exercise stress tests, lipid analysis, and chest x-ray study. Clinicians must correct pre-existing health problems that might have contributed to the development of CHD (e.g., hypertension, anemia, hyperthyroidism).

Recovery after AMI may be lengthy and difficult. The client may have undergone surgery or may have been managed medically. In either case, a serious threat to integrity has occurred. Initially after AMI, clients may attempt to prove that they are not seriously ill. Coping strategies include denial and minimization. Some clients conceal the recurrence of chest pain. As recovery continues, clients begin to comprehend that a heart attack has really occurred, to understand why it happened, and to consider its impact on the future. Clients begin the process of life adjustment to find a lifestyle that can be tolerated and maintained while preserving a sense of self-worth. Several strategies are used to regain self-control, such as gauging progress, seeking reassurance, learning about health, and being cautious. Eventually, most clients come to terms with the fact that they will not be living life to the fullest. Clients learn to accept limitations and to refocus on other aspects of life. Some clients are unable to adjust. Sometimes clients find that they have had too many setbacks and are powerless to make changes or gain control. The education and counseling that accompany a structured cardiac rehabilitation program can help improve psychological well-being, social adjustment, and functioning.[32]

Phase III (Intermediate Outpatient). The extended outpatient phase of cardiac rehabilitation lasts from 4 to 6 months. Exercise sessions continue to be supervised, and clients are taught how to monitor their exercise intensity by taking their pulse or, if in a walking program, by counting the number of steps they take in a 15-second interval. Clients with dysrhythmias are monitored more closely, and intermittent rhythm strips may be taken. For clients who prefer to exercise at home, clinicians trained in cardiac rehabilitation can provide detailed, written instructions for a long-term exercise program. Various methods are used to determine the appropriate exercise routines. Periodic evaluation is necessary to assess the client's endurance and tolerance to the prescribed exercise program.

Phase IV (Maintenance Outpatient). Phase IV, the final phase of cardiac rehabilitation, usually takes place in the home or community and is unsupervised. The client maintains a program of regular exercise and other lifestyle modifications to modify cardiac risk. Clients should undergo an exercise testing and risk factor assessment annually.

■ Nursing Management of the Medical Client

The goals of nursing management after AMI are as follows:

- Recognize and treat cardiac ischemia
- Administer thrombolytic therapy as ordered, or ready client for PTCA and observe for complications
- Recognize and treat potentially life-threatening dysrhythmias
- Monitor for complications of reduced cardiac output
- Maintain a therapeutic critical care environment
- Identify the psychosocial impact of AMI on the client and family
- Educate the client in lifestyle changes and rehabilitation

CONCLUSIONS

CHD is a progressive occlusive disorder that commonly results in reduced coronary blood flow. This reduction is manifested clinically by angina and AMI. AMI, permanent damage to the myocardium, may be the first indicator of how serious the heart disease is. Your responsibilities in the care of these clients are to educate them about the warning signs of AMI, to monitor their response to therapy, to prevent complications, and to promote rehabilitation.

THINKING CRITICALLY *evolve*

1. Mrs. Polk, a 62-year-old housewife who cares for her two grandchildren, is admitted to the emergency department with complaints of chest pain. She is diaphoretic and pale and complains of pain "under my left breast that pushes to my back." She rates the pain as an 8 on a scale of 1 to 10. Her ECG shows an elevated ST segment. She is placed on oxygen therapy, and an IV line is inserted. Cardiac serum markers are drawn and sent to the laboratory. Her vital signs are temperature 36.9° C, apical pulse 110 beats/min, and blood pressure 108/68 mm Hg.

Factors to Consider. What additional testing is necessary to rule in or rule out an acute MI? What other information from Mrs. Polk's history might aid in the diagnosis?

2. The physician immediately orders reteplase, a thrombolytic agent, for Mrs. Polk.

Factors to Consider. What information must be obtained from Mrs. Polk to safely initiate thrombolytic therapy?

3. You administer the thrombolytic therapy as ordered. Mrs. Polk states her pain is now a 1 on a scale of 1 to 10. ST segments are resolving, and she is no longer diaphoretic.

Factors to Consider. What effects from the thrombolytic therapy appear to be occurring? Which side effects of the therapy should you anticipate?

4. A client with long-standing coronary artery disease experiences severe chest pain unrelieved by nitroglycerin. He is admitted with an acute MI to the coronary care unit. What are the priorities on admission? What medical treatment may be instituted in the first hours following the infarction?

Factors to Consider. What time frame is considered most crucial to the salvage of myocardial muscle? What care is given to the newly admitted client?

Discussions for these questions can be found on the website and the CD-ROM.

BIBLIOGRAPHY

1. American Heart Association. (2001). *2002 Heart and Stroke Statistical Update.* Dallas, TX: American Heart Association. Available: http://www.americanheart.org/.

2. American Heart Association. (2002). *Heart attack, stroke & cardiac arrest warning signs.* Available: http://www.americanheart.org/.

3. Antman E., et al.(2000). The TIMI risk score for unstable angina/non-ST elevation MI: A method for prognostication and therapeutic decision making. *Journal of the American Medical Association, 284*(7), 876-878.

4. *Best Practice Evidence-based Guideline-Cardiac Rehabilitation.* (2002). *The New Zealand Guideline Group.* Available: http://www.nzgg.org.nz/library/gl-complete/Cardiac-Rehab/index.cfm.

---

evolve Did you remember to check out the bonus material on the Evolve website and the CD-ROM, including free self-assessment exercises?

http://evolve.elsevier.com/Black/medsurg/

5. Beattie, S. (1999). Management of chronic stable angina. *Nurse Practitioner, 24*(5), 44, 49, 53, 56, 59-61.

 6. Braunwald E., et al. (2002). *ACC/AHA 2002 guideline update for the management of patients with unstable angina and non-ST-segment elevation myocardial infarction: A report of the American College of Cardiology/American Heart Association Task force on Practice Guidelines.* Available: http://www.acc.org/clinical/guidelines/unstable/unstable.pdf.

 7. Brennen, M.L., et al. (2003). Prognostic value of myeloperoxidase in patients with chest pain. *New England Journal of Medicine 349*(17), 1595-1604.

8. Cummings, R. (2001). *ACLS provider manual.* Dallas, TX: American Heart Association.

9. Doering, L.V. (1999). Pathophysiology of acute coronary syndromes leading to acute myocardial infarction. *Journal of Cardiovascular Nursing, 13*(3), 1-20.

10. Dracup, K., & Cannon, C. (1999, April). Combination treatment strategies for management of acute myocardial infarction. *Critical Care Nurse Supplement,* 1-17.

 11. Feldman, M., & Cryer, B. (1999). Aspirin absorption rates and platelet inhibition times with 325-mg buffered aspirin tablets (chewed or swallowed intact) and with buffered aspirin solution. *American Journal of Cardiology, 84,* 404-409.

12. Gensini, G., Comeglio, M., & Falai, M. (1999). Advances in antithrombotic therapy of acute myocardial infarction. *American Heart Journal, 138*(2), S171-S176.

 13. Gibbons, R.J., et al. (1999). ACC/AHA/ACP-ASIM guidelines for the management of patients with stable chronic angina: A report of the American College of Cardiology/American Heart Association Task Force on Practice Guidelines (Committee on the Management of Patients with Stable Chronic Angina*). J Am Coll Cardiol, 33*:2092-2197.

14. Goodwin, M., et al. (1999). Early extubation and early activity after open heart surgery. *Critical Care Nurse, 19*(5), 18-26.

15. Hudson, M., et al. (1999). Cardiac markers: Point of care testing. *Clinica Chimica Acta, 28*(4), 223-237.

16. Huikuri, H., et al. (2001). Sudden death due to cardiac arrhythmias. *New England Journal of Medicine, 345*(20), 1473-1482.

17. Kosnik, L. (1999, October). Treatment protocols and pathways: Improving the process of care. *Critical Care Nurse Supplement,* 3-7.

18. Lau, J., et al. (2001). Evaluation of technologies for identifying acute cardiac ischemia in emergency departments. *AHRQ Publication Evidence Report/Technology Assessment Number 26.* Available: http://www.ahrq.gov/.

19. Lee, T.H., & Goldman, L. (2000). Evaluation of the patient with acute chest pain. *New England Journal of Medicine, 342*(16), 1187-1193.

20. Libby, P., Ridker, P., & Maseri, A. (2002). Inflammation and atherosclerosis. *Circulation, 105,* 1135-1143.

21. Moser, D., et al. (1999, October). The role of the critical care nurse in preventing heart failure after acute myocardial infarction. *Critical Care Nurse Supplement,* 11-15.

22. Murphy, M., & Berding, C. (1999). Use of myoglobins and cardiac troponins in the diagnosis of acute myocardial infarction. *Critical Care Nurse, 19*(1), 58-65.

23. O'Connor, C.M., Gattis, W.A., & Swedberg, K. (1999). Current and novel pharmacologic approaches in advanced heart failure. *Heart and Lung, 28,* 227-239.

24. Peeters A, et al. (2002). A cardiovascular life history-a life course analysis of the original Framingham Heart Study cohort. *Eur Heart J, 23*(6), 795-799.

25. Rich, M.W. (1999). Heart failure disease management: A critical review. *Journal of Cardiac Failure, 5*(1), 64-75.

26. Ryan TJ, et al. (1999). *ACC/AHA guidelines for the management* *of patients with acute myocardial infarction: 1999 update. A report of the American College of Cardiology/American Heart Association Task Force on Practice Guidelines (Committee on Management of Acute Myocardial Infarction).* Available: http://www.acc.org.

27. Soran, O., Schneider, V.M., & Feldman, A.M. (1999). Basic therapy for congestive heart failure: Current practice, new prospects. *Journal of Critical Illness, 14*(2), 78-89.

28. Thelan L., et al. (1998). *Critical care nursing: Diagnosis and management* (3rd ed.). St. Louis: Mosby.

29. Thygesen K., et al. (2000). Myocardial infarction redefined. A consensus document of the Joint European Society of Cardiology/American College of Cardiology Committee for the Redefinition of Myocardial Infarction. *J Am Coll Cardiol, 36*(3), 959-969.

30. Verheugt, F. (1999). What an interventional cardiologist should know about the pharmacological treatment of acute myocardial infarction. *Seminars in Interventional Cardiology, 4,* 17-20.

31. Wenger, N.K. (1999). Women, myocardial infarction, and coronary revascularization. *Cardiology in Review, 7,* 117-120.

32. Wenger , N.K., et al. (1995). *Cardiac rehabilitation as secondary* *prevention. Clinical practice guideline: Quick reference guide for clinicians.* No. 17. Rockville, MD: Agency for Health Care Policy and Research and the National Heart, Lung and Blood Institute, Public Health Service, U.S. Department of Health and Human Services.

33. World Health Organization. (1999). Combating the tobacco epidemic. *WHO's World Health Report, 1999.* Geneva Switzerland: World Health Organization.

34. Zerwic, J. (1999). Patient delay in seeking treatment for acute myocardial infarction symptoms. *Journal of Cardiovascular Nursing, 13,* 21-32.

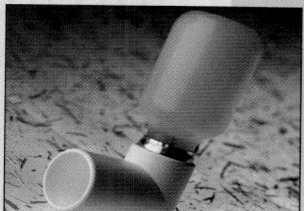

Oxygenation Disorders

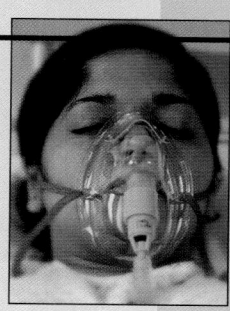

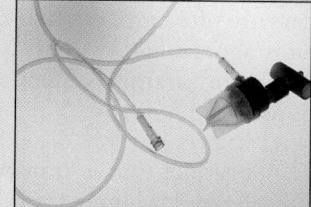

Anatomy and Physiology Review

The Respiratory System

Robert G. Carroll

Our body needs a constant supply of oxygen to support metabolism. The respiratory system brings oxygen through the airways of the lung into the alveoli, where it diffuses into the blood for transport to the tissues. This process is so vital that difficulty in breathing is experienced as a threat to life itself. Whether death is a real possibility or not, people with respiratory disorders are often anxious and fearful that they may die, perhaps agonizingly.

The respiratory system also has other essential functions:

1. Expels carbon dioxide (CO_2), a metabolic waste product that is transported from the tissues to the lungs for elimination.
2. Filters and humidifies air that enters the lungs.
3. Traps particulate matter in the mucus of the airways and propels it toward the mouth for elimination by coughing or swallowing.

An active immune system helps prevent the entry of inhaled pathogens.

Respiratory control is tied most closely to arterial blood and brain CO_2 levels as well as to arterial blood oxygen levels. Respiration is also controlled by higher cortical centers. For example, an increase in ventilation accompanies exercise and keeps arterial blood gases within the normal range.

Respiratory problems are widespread. Acute disorders range from minor inconveniences (colds or flu) to more life-threatening problems (asthma, some types of pneumonia, and chest trauma). Chronic disabling conditions include *chronic airflow limitation* (also called chronic obstructive pulmonary disease), and certain restrictive lung diseases. Chronic respiratory problems affect many people, often causing them to make radical lifestyle changes, such as retiring from work earlier than they wish.

Respiratory problems are associated with many causes: allergies, occupational factors, genetic factors, smoking and tobacco use, infection, neuromuscular disorders, chest abnormalities, trauma, pleural conditions, and pulmonary vascular abnormalities. The most significant factor in chronic respiratory illness and lung cancer is cigarette smoking.

STRUCTURE OF THE RESPIRATORY SYSTEM

UPPER AIRWAYS

The airways are the regions through which air passes on its way to the exchange areas of the lungs. The upper airways consist of the nasal cavities, pharynx, and larynx.

Nasal Cavity

The nose is formed from both bone and cartilage. The nasal bone forms the bridge, and the remainder of the nose is composed of cartilage and connective tissue (Figure U14-1). Each opening of the nose on the face (*nostrils* or *nares*) leads to a cavity *(vestibule)*. The vestibule is lined anteriorly with skin and hair that filter foreign objects and prevent them from being inhaled. The posterior vestibule is lined with a mucous membrane, composed of columnar epithelial cells, and goblet cells that secrete mucus. The mucous membrane extends throughout the airways, and cilia (hair-like projections) propel mucus to the pharynx for elimination by swallowing or coughing. The portion of mucous membrane that is located at the top of the nasal cavity, just beneath the cribriform plate of the ethmoid bone, is specialized *(olfactory)* epithelium, which provides the sense of smell. Because the olfactory epithelium does not lie along the usual path of air movement, smell is enhanced by sniffing.

Along the sides of the vestibule are *turbinates,* mucous membrane–covered projections that contain a rich blood supply from the internal and external carotid arteries. They warm and humidify inspired air.

Paranasal sinuses, open areas within the skull, are named for the bones in which they lie: frontal, ethmoid, sphenoid, and maxillary. Passageways from the paranasal sinuses drain into the nasal cavities. The nasolacrimal ducts, which drain tears from the surface of the eyes, also drain into the nasal cavity.

The mouth is considered part of the upper airway but only because it can be used to deliver air to the lungs when the nose is obstructed or when high volumes of air are needed, such as during exercise. The mouth does not

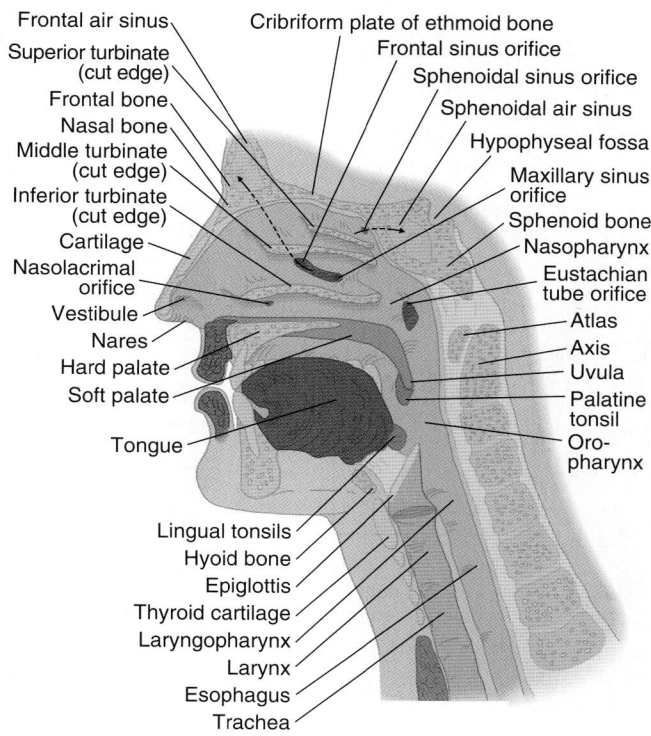

FIGURE U14-1 Structures of the upper airway. Air enters the body through the nares or mouth and is filtered and humidified while passing toward the alveoli. The epiglottis directs air into the trachea during respiration and directs food into the esophagus during swallowing. Dashed arrows indicate passage of air into sinuses.

perform the nasal functions efficiently, especially those of warming, humidifying, and filtering air.

Pharynx

The pharynx is a funnel-shaped tube that extends from the nose to the larynx. It can be divided into three sections.

The *nasopharynx* is located above the margin of the soft palate and receives air from the nasal cavity. From the ear, the eustachian tubes open into the nasopharynx. The pharyngeal tonsils (called *adenoids* when enlarged) are located on the posterior wall of the nasopharynx.

The *oropharynx* serves both respiration and digestion. It receives air from the nasopharynx and food from the oral cavity. Palatine (faucial) tonsils are located along the sides of the posterior mouth, and the lingual tonsils are located at the base of the tongue.

The *laryngopharynx (hypopharynx),* located below the base of the tongue, is the most inferior portion of the pharynx. It connects to the larynx and serves both respiration and digestion.

Larynx

The larynx is commonly called the *voice box.* It connects the upper (pharynx) and lower (trachea) airways. The

larynx lies just anterior to the upper esophagus. Nine cartilages form the larynx: three large unpaired cartilages (epiglottis, thyroid, cricoid) and three smaller paired cartilages (arytenoid, corniculate, cuneiform). The cartilages are attached to the hyoid bone above and below the trachea by muscles and ligaments, all of which prevent the larynx from collapse during inspiration and swallowing.

The larynx consists of the endolarynx and a surrounding triangle-shaped bone and cartilage. The endolarynx is formed by two paired folds of tissue, forming the false and the true vocal cords. The slit between the vocal cords forms the *glottis.* The *epiglottis,* a leaf-shaped structure immediately posterior to the base of the tongue, lies above the larynx. When food or liquids are swallowed, the epiglottis closes over the larynx, protecting the lower airways from aspiration.

The thyroid cartilage protrudes in front of the larynx, forming the "Adam's apple." The cricoid cartilage lies just below the thyroid cartilage and is the anatomic site for an artificial opening into the trachea (tracheostomy, or cricothyroidotomy). The internal portion of the larynx is composed of muscles that assist with swallowing, speaking, and respiration and that contribute to the pitch of the voice. The blood supply to the larynx is through the branches of the thyroid arteries. The nerve supply is through the recurrent laryngeal and superior laryngeal nerves.

LOWER AIRWAYS

The lower airway, or tracheobronchial tree, is composed of the trachea, right and left mainstem bronchi, segmental bronchi, subsegmental bronchi, and terminal bronchioles (Figure U14-2). Smooth muscle, wound in overlapping clockwise and counterclockwise helical bands, is found in all of these structures. This arrangement allows contraction of the smooth muscle to decrease the diameter of the airways, increasing the resistance to air flow. This muscle is subject to spasm in many airway disorders. The lower airways continue to warm, humidify, and filter inspired air as it flows toward the lungs.

Trachea

The trachea (windpipe) extends from the larynx to the level of the seventh thoracic vertebrae, where it divides into two main *(primary)* bronchi. The point at which the trachea divides is called the *carina.* The trachea is a flexible, muscular, 12-cm long air passage with C-shaped cartilaginous rings. Along with all other regions of the lower airways it is lined with pseudostratified columnar epithelium that contains goblet (mucus-secreting) cells and cilia (Figure U14-3). Because the cilia beat upward, they tend to carry foreign particles and excessive mucus away from the lungs to the pharynx. No cilia are present in the alveoli.

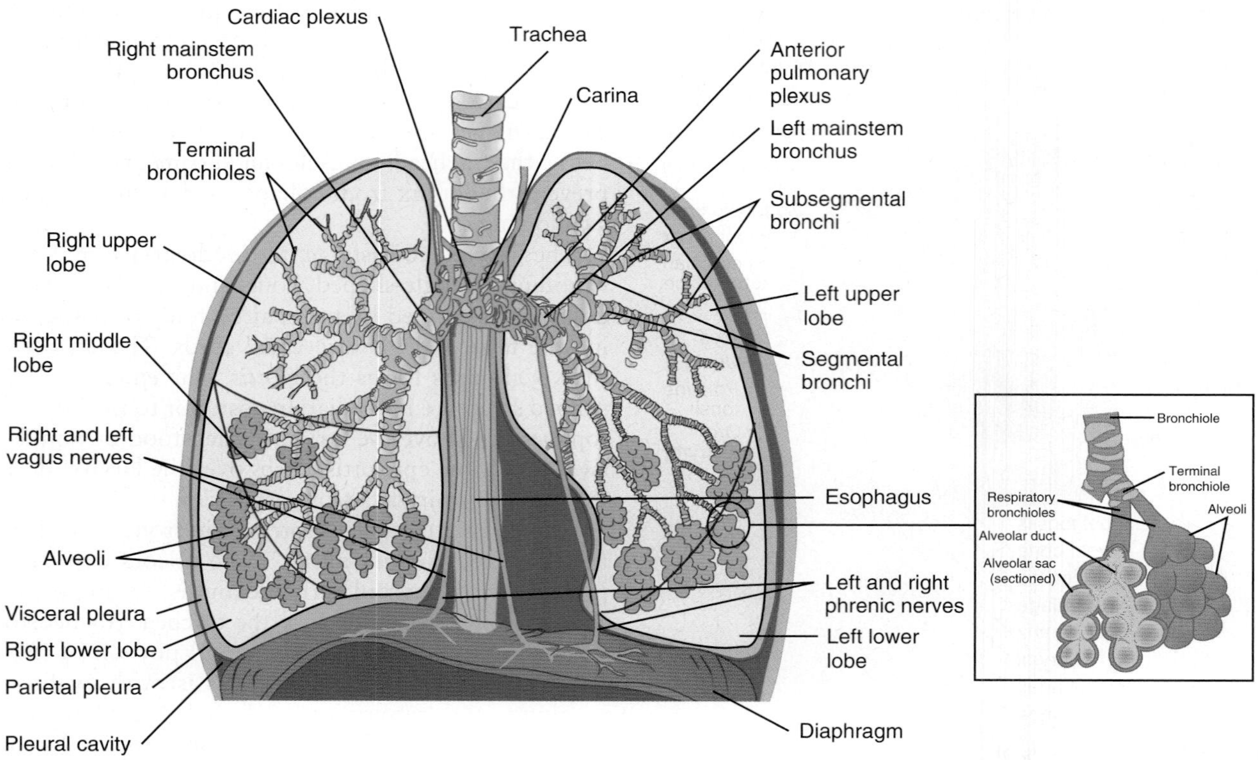

Cardiac plexus

Right mainstem bronchus

Trachea

Carina

Anterior pulmonary plexus

Left mainstem bronchus

Terminal bronchioles

Subsegmental bronchi

Right upper lobe

Left upper lobe

Right middle lobe

Segmental bronchi

Right and left vagus nerves

Esophagus

Alveoli

Left and right phrenic nerves

Visceral pleura

Left lower lobe

Right lower lobe

Parietal pleura

Pleural cavity

Diaphragm

Bronchiole

Terminal bronchiole

Respiratory bronchioles

Alveoli

Alveolar duct

Alveolar sac (sectioned)

FIGURE U14-2 Structures of the lower airways. Air passes from the trachea through bronchi and bronchioles before reaching the alveoli. Cartilage in the bronchi and trachea prevents airway collapse during forced expiration. *Inset:* Gas exchange occurs in the respiratory zone, which consists of the respiratory bronchioles, alveolar ducts, and alveolar sacs.

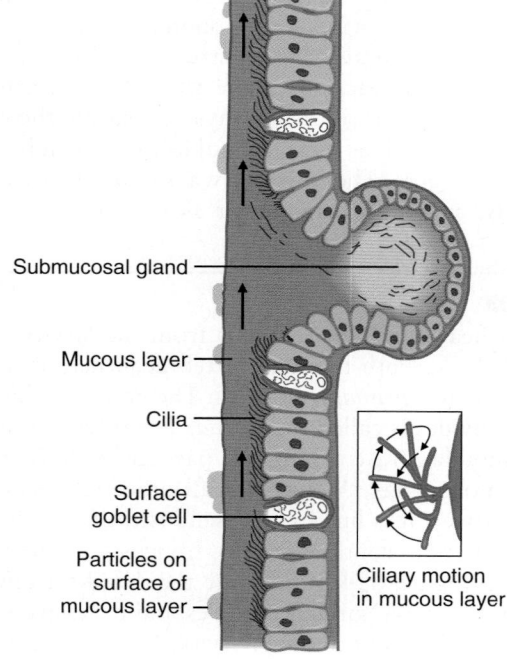

Submucosal gland

Mucous layer

Cilia

Surface goblet cell

Particles on surface of mucous layer

Ciliary motion in mucous layer

FIGURE U14-3 The mucociliary blanket is an important respiratory defense mechanism. Mucus is secreted by surface goblet cells. About 100 ml of mucus is normally secreted each day by the submucosal glands. Mucus covers the epithelial lining of the tracheobronchial tree in two layers: the watery solution layer close to the mucosal surface and the thicker gel layer. The cilia (hair-like projections) beat in an upward direction toward the upper airway. Particulate matter is trapped on the mucous layer and moved upward by the cilia. Debris-laden mucus is then either swallowed or expectorated as sputum.

Bronchi and Bronchioles

The right mainstem bronchus is shorter and wider, extending more vertically downward, than the left mainstem bronchus. Thus foreign bodies are more likely to lodge there than in the left mainstem bronchus. The *segmental* and *subsegmental bronchi* are subdivisions of the main bronchi and spread in an inverted, tree-like formation through each lung. Cartilage surrounds the airway in the bronchi, but the bronchioles (the final pathway to the alveoli) contain no cartilage and thus can collapse and trap air during active exhalation.

The *terminal bronchioles* are the last airways of the conducting system. The area from the nose to the terminal bronchioles does not exchange gas and functions as *anatomic dead space*. The lack of gas exchange means that the first air out of the mouth during exhalation resembles room air, but the last air out (end-tidal air) resembles alveolar air.

LUNGS AND ALVEOLI

Lungs

The lungs lie within the thoracic cavity on either side of the heart (see Figure U14-2). They are cone-shaped, with the apex above the first rib and the base resting on the diaphragm. Each lung is divided into superior and inferior lobes by an oblique fissure. The right lung is further divided by a horizontal fissure, which bounds a middle lobe. The right lung, therefore, has three lobes; the left lobe has only two. In addition to these five lobes, which are visible externally, each lung can be subdivided into about 10 smaller units *(bronchopulmonary segments)*. Each segment represents the portion of the lung that is supplied by a specific tertiary bronchus. These segments are important surgically, because a diseased segment can be resected without the need to remove the entire lobe or lung. The two lungs are separated by a space (the *mediastinum*), where the heart, aorta, vena cava, pulmonary vessels, esophagus, part of the trachea and bronchi, and the thymus gland are located.

The lungs contain gas, blood, thin alveolar walls, and support structures. The alveolar walls contain elastic and collagen fibers; these form a three-dimensional, basket-like structure that allows the lung to inflate in all directions. These fibers are capable of stretching when a pulling force is exerted on them from outside of the body or when they are inflated from within. The elastic recoil helps return the lungs to their resting volume.

Branches of the pulmonary artery provide most of the blood supply to the lungs. The blood is oxygen-poor, but oxygen is supplied by inspired air. The trachea and bronchioles, which are not part of the oxygen exchange surface, receive oxygen-rich blood from branches of the aorta.

Lung Volumes

The lungs of an average 19-year-old man have a total capacity of about 5900 ml. However, a person cannot exhale all the air from the lungs, and about 1200 ml of air always remains, no matter how forceful the expiration. This remaining volume *(residual volume)* prevents the collapse of the lung structures during expiration. The volume of air that moves in and out with each breath is called the *tidal volume*. During quiet breathing, tidal volume is about 500 ml. When a person takes a deep breath, the lung is more fully expanded. The amount of extra air inhaled, beyond the tidal volume, is called the *inspiratory reserve volume;* the extra air that can be exhaled after a normal breath is called the *expiratory reserve volume.*

Lung volumes are often combined into capacities:
- *Total lung capacity* (all four volumes)
- *Vital capacity* (all volumes except residual volume), which is the amount a person can ventilate
- *Functional reserve capacity* (expiratory reserve plus residual volumes)
- *Inspiratory capacity* (tidal volume plus inspiratory reserve volume)

These volumes and capacities are frequently altered by disease. Lung volumes as measured by spirometry are shown in Figure U14-4. (Pulmonary function tests are described in Chapter 61.)

Alveoli

The lung parenchyma, which consists of millions of alveolar units, is the working area of the lung tissue. At birth, a person has approximately 24 million alveoli; by age 8 years, a person has 300 million. The total working alveolar surface area is approximately 750 to 860 square

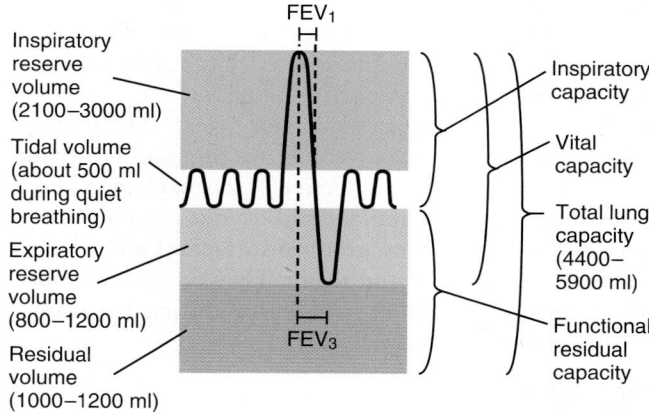

FIGURE U14-4 Lung volumes and capacities as measured by spirometry. The four volumes of the lungs (identified on the left) are combined to form four capacities (identified on the right).

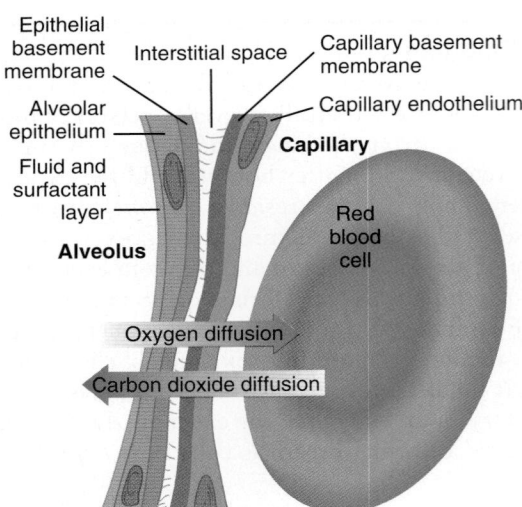

FIGURE U14-5 The ultrastructure of the respiratory membrane where oxygen is exchanged. Accumulation of fluid in the interstitial space (pulmonary edema) diminishes the diffusion of oxygen into the pulmonary capillary.

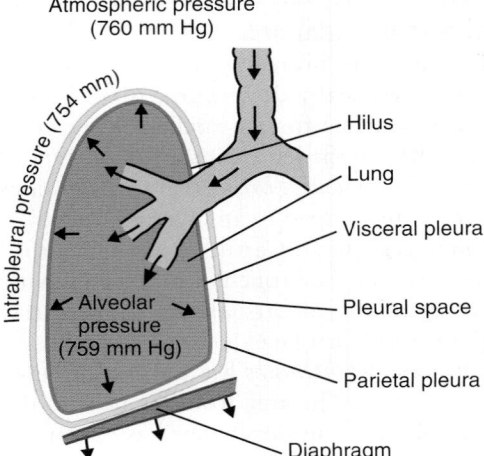

NORMAL INSPIRATION

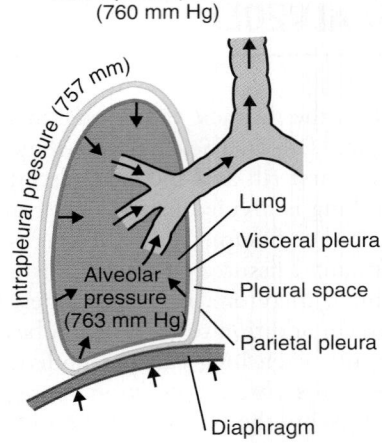

NORMAL EXPIRATION

FIGURE U14-6 Normal inspiration and expiration. Contraction of the diaphragm increases the size of the thoracic cavity, and reduces alveolar pressure to below atmospheric pressure. Relaxation of the diaphragm allows the elastic recoil of the lungs to diminish the size of the thoracic cavity, increasing alveolar pressure to greater than atmospheric.

feet. The blood supply flowing toward the alveoli comes from the right ventricle of the heart.

The entire alveolar unit (respiratory zone) is made up of respiratory bronchioles, alveolar ducts, and alveolar sacs (see Figure U14-2). The alveolar walls are extremely thin, with an almost solid network of interconnecting capillaries. Because of the extensiveness of the capillary system, the flow of blood in the alveolar wall has been described as a "sheet" of flowing blood.

Oxygen and CO_2 are exchanged through a respiratory membrane, about 0.2 mm thick (Figure U14-5). The average diameter of the pulmonary capillary is only about 5 μm, but red blood cells (7 μm in diameter) must squeeze through, actually touching the capillary wall. Thus the distance across which oxygen and CO_2 must diffuse is greatly reduced. Thickening of the respiratory membrane (e.g., with pulmonary edema or fibrosis) may interfere with normal exchange of gases.

The alveolus comprises two cell types: *Type I pneumocytes,* which line the alveolus, are thin and incapable of reproduction but are effective in gas exchange. *Type II pneumocytes* are cuboidal and do not exchange oxygen and CO_2 well. They produce surfactant and are important in lung injury and repair. They differentiate into type I cells; oxygenation is impaired during the transition from type II to type I cells.

THORAX

The bony thorax provides protection for the lungs, heart, and great vessels. The outer shell of the thorax is made up of 12 pairs of ribs. The ribs connect posteriorly to the transverse processes of the thoracic vertebrae of the spine. Anteriorly, the first seven pairs of ribs are at-

tached to the sternum by cartilage. The 8th, 9th, and 10th ribs *(false ribs)* are attached to each other by costal cartilage. The 11th and 12th ribs *(floating ribs)* allow full chest expansion because they are not attached in any way to the sternum.

DIAPHRAGM

Breathing is accomplished by skeletal muscle alteration of the thoracic space. The diaphragm is the primary muscle of breathing and serves as the lower boundary of the thorax (Figure U14-6). The diaphragm is dome-shaped in the relaxed position, with central muscular attachments to the xiphoid process of the sternum and the lower ribs. Contraction of the diaphragm pulls the muscle downward, increasing the thoracic space and inflating the lungs. The nerve supply of the diaphragm (phrenic nerve) comes through the spinal cord at the level of the third cervical vertebra. Thus spinal injuries at C3 or above can impair ventilation.

PLEURAE

The pleurae are serous membranes that enclose the lung in a double-walled sac. The *visceral* pleura covers the lung and the fissures between the lobes of the lung. The *parietal* pleura covers the inside of each hemithorax, the mediastinum, and the top of the diaphragm; it joins the visceral pleura at the *hilus* (a notch in the medial surface of the lung, where the mainstem bronchi, pulmonary blood vessels, and nerves enter the lung).

Normally, no space exists between the pleurae; the *pleural space* is a potential space between the two layers of pleura. A thin film (only a few milliliters) of serous fluid acts as a lubricant in the potential space. The fluid also causes the moist pleural membranes to adhere, creating a pulling force that helps to hold the lungs in an expanded position. The action of the pleurae is analogous to coupling two sheets of glass with a thin film of water. It is extremely difficult to separate the sheets of glass at right angles, yet they readily slide along each other. Because of the nature of this coupling, the movement of the lungs closely follows the movement of the thorax. If air or increased amounts of serous fluid, blood, or pus accumulates in the thoracic space, the lungs are compressed and respiratory difficulties follow. These conditions constitute *pneumothorax* (air in the pleural space) or *hemothorax* (blood in the pleural space).

FUNCTION OF THE RESPIRATORY SYSTEM

The respiratory system enhances gas exchange. Inspiration brings oxygen-rich air into the alveoli. The upper and lower airways filter and humidify inspired air. Gas exchange between the air and the blood occurs in the alveolus. Oxygen diffuses into the blood, and CO_2 diffuses from the blood into the alveolar air. The CO_2-enriched air is removed from the body during expiration. The large number and large surface area of alveoli are necessary to meet both resting and exercise gas exchange requirements.

The thorax and diaphragm alter pressures in the thorax to drive air movement. The movement of air depends on pressure gradients between the atmosphere and the air in the lungs, with air flowing from regions of higher pressure to regions of lower pressure. On inspiration, the dome of the diaphragm flattens and the rib cage lifts. As thoracic and lung volumes increase, alveolar pressure decreases and air moves into the lungs.

Airway resistance also affects air movement and is affected primarily by the diameter of the airways. Decreasing the diameter by half results in a 16-fold increase in airway resistance. Thus a decreased diameter of the airways due to bronchial muscle contraction or to secretions in the airways increases resistance and decreases the rate of air flow. This is a common finding in obstructive airway diseases such as asthma.

During quiet breathing, expiration is usually passive, that is, does not require the use of muscles. The chest wall, in contrast to the lungs, tends to recoil outward. The opposing forces of lung and chest wall create a subatmospheric (negative) force of about −5 cm of water in the intrapleural space at the end of quiet exhalation. Exhalation is also a result of elastic recoil of the lungs.

VENTILATION

Ventilation, the movement of air in and out of the lungs, involves three forces: (1) compliance properties of the lung and the thorax (chest wall), (2) surface tension, and (3) the muscular efforts of inspiratory muscles.

Compliance

Compliance refers to the ease with which the lung expands and indicates the relationship between the volume and the pressure of the lungs. The lungs are elastic structures that tend to recoil to a volume slightly less than *residual volume* (the volume of gas remaining in the lungs after a full exhalation). The force required to distend the lungs is the difference between the alveolar pressure and the intrapleural pressure. Diseases that cause fibrosis of the lungs result in "stiff" lungs with low compliance; stiff lungs require high inspiratory pressures to achieve a set volume of gas. In contrast, diseases such as emphysema that damage the elastic structure of the alveolar walls result in "floppy" lungs with greater compliance. Relatively low pressures can achieve the same volume of air during inspiration, but passive exhalation is impaired.

Surface Tension

Changes in the surface tension of the liquid film lining the alveoli also affect compliance by changing resistance. *Surface tension,* the result of the air-liquid interface at each alveolus, restricts alveolar expansion on inspiration and aids alveolar collapse on expiration. Surfactant produced by type II cells in the alveolar lining lowers surface tension and thus increases compliance and aids ventilation. A deficiency of surfactant results in stiff lungs. Premature babies lacking surfactant may suffer infant respiratory distress syndrome, or hyaline membrane disease.

Muscular Effort

Ventilation also requires muscular effort. For inspiration to occur, the pressure within the alveoli must be less than atmospheric pressure. Contraction of the diaphragm and the external intercostal muscles enlarges the size of the thorax. The external intercostal muscles pull the ribs upward and forward, thus increasing the transverse and anteroposterior diameter. Two accessory muscles of inspiration—the scalene and sternocleidomastoid muscles—elevate the first and second ribs during inspiration to enlarge the upper thorax and stabilize the chest wall. The sternocleidomastoid muscle elevates the sternum. The expanding thorax creates a more negative intrapleural pressure, which expands the lungs. When the alveolar pressure becomes lower than the atmospheric pressure, air flows into the lungs.

During exhalation, the inspiratory muscles relax. The elastic recoil of the lung tissue increases alveolar pressure above atmospheric pressure and causes air to move out of the lungs. Air flow stops when the recoil pressure of the lungs balances the muscular and elastic forces of the chest (see Figure U14-6).

Although expiration is usually passive, forced expiration and coughing employ accessory muscles to decrease the size of the thoracic space and cause expiration. Contraction of the abdominal muscles forces the diaphragm upward to its dome-shaped position. Contraction of the internal intercostal muscles pulls the ribs inward, thus decreasing the anteroposterior diameter of the chest wall.

Work of Breathing

Respiratory muscle contraction represents a significant metabolic load. Tidal volume and respiratory rate are adjusted to minimize the workload on the body. For example, clients with obstructive lung disease use slower but deeper breaths to maintain appropriate alveolar ventilation. Clients with restrictive lung disease use frequent, shallow breaths to maintain alveolar ventilation.

RESPIRATORY CONTROL

Human metabolism is not one of steady state. The oxygen needs of the tissues change with changing metabolic demands. Respiratory control mechanisms match the elimination of CO_2 and supply of oxygen to the metabolic needs. The lungs have no intrinsic control of themselves; instead, they are controlled by the central nervous system.

Central Nervous System Control

The medulla has several levels of respiratory centers. The dorsal respiratory group primarily provides for inspiration. The ventral respiratory group is normally quiet unless increased ventilation is needed or if active exhalation is performed. The pons has an apneustic center, which contains both expiratory and inspiratory neurons. The upper pons contains the pneumotaxic center, which fine-tunes breathing. For example, the pneumotaxic center allows for talking and breathing.

Output from the respiratory neurons, located in the medulla, descends via the ventral and lateral columns of the spinal cord to phrenic motor neurons of the diaphragm and intercostal motor neurons of the intercostal muscles. The result is rhythmic respiratory movements.

The cortex also allows voluntary control of breathing (holding our breath or altering the rate or depth of breathing).

Reflex Control

The cough reflex is a neural reflex stimulated by mechanical stimuli (Table U14-1). Inhaled irritants and mucus (mechanical stimuli) excite rapidly adapting pulmonary stretch receptors concentrated in the region of the carina and the large bronchi. The stimulation of the receptors results in high-velocity expiratory gas flow (cough).

Peripheral Control

Peripheral control of respiration is due to the sensing of partial pressure of oxygen (PO_2) and of partial pressure of CO_2 (PCO_2) in the blood. In the blood, CO_2 is an acid. An increase in PCO_2 causes acidosis, or a decrease in pH. Receptors that are responsive to changes in oxygen,

TABLE U14-1	*Physiologic Elements of a Cough*
Deep inspiration	Inhaled volume of air must be sufficient to increase lung volume, to increase diameter of bronchi and bronchioles, and to move mucus up and out of airways
Inspiratory pause	Pause (inspiratory pause) allows a buildup and distribution of air and pressure distal to mucus
Closed glottis	Intact muscles and nerves supplying larynx required; allows development of high intrapleural pressures, resulting in a high air flow velocity to propel mucus out of airway
Abdominal muscles	Increase intra-abdominal pressure, which forces diaphragm upward to increase intrapleural pressure against closed glottis
Open glottis	After intrapleural pressures increase, glottis opens suddenly to allow a high velocity of air to leave lungs; flow rates may be as high as 300 L/min
Mucus is expelled	Expulsion due to high velocity of air leaving airway

CO_2, and pH are located in the brain and in structures adjacent to blood vessels. Arterial blood oxygen and CO_2 pressures are sensed by receptors in the carotid body and the aortic body. The carotid body receptors are located close to the carotid sinus, and the aortic bodies are located near the aortic arch. Chemoreceptors are also located on the brain side of the blood-brain barrier. These receptors respond only to P_{CO_2} (or pH). An elevated P_{CO_2} in arterial blood is the normal stimulus to increase ventilation. Low levels of partial pressure of oxygen in arterial blood (Pa_{CO_2}) can stimulate ventilation, but only when P_{O_2} drops below 70 mm Hg. There is a powerful synergism between these respiratory stimuli, with the greatest ventilatory drive caused by a simultaneous increase in P_{CO_2} and decrease in P_{O_2}.

GAS EXCHANGE AND TRANSPORT

The exchange of gases occurs between air and blood in the respiratory membrane. Respiration is the exchange of oxygen and CO_2 at the alveolar-capillary level *(external respiration)* and at the tissue-cellular level *(internal respiration)*. During respiration, body tissues are supplied with oxygen for metabolism and CO_2 is released.

In the earth's atmosphere, air contains 20.84% oxygen, 78.62% nitrogen, 0.04% CO_2, and 0.50% water vapor. Each gas exerts a pressure *(partial pressure)* as if it were the only gas present. The sum of the partial pressures is the *barometric pressure*. When a liquid is exposed to a gas, gas enters the liquid in proportion to the individual pressures. P_{O_2} in the alveoli is about 104 mm Hg, and P_{CO_2} is about 40 mm Hg. Venous blood has a P_{O_2} of 40 mm Hg and a P_{CO_2} of about 45 mm Hg. These differences in concentration result in the movement of oxygen into the pulmonary capillary bloodstream and of CO_2 out of the pulmonary capillary bed into the alveoli (Figure U14-7).

The high P_{O_2} gradient between the alveolar air and blood is necessary because oxygen is less soluble than CO_2. Diseases that decrease gas diffusion generally alter oxygen exchange before altering carbon dioxide exchange.

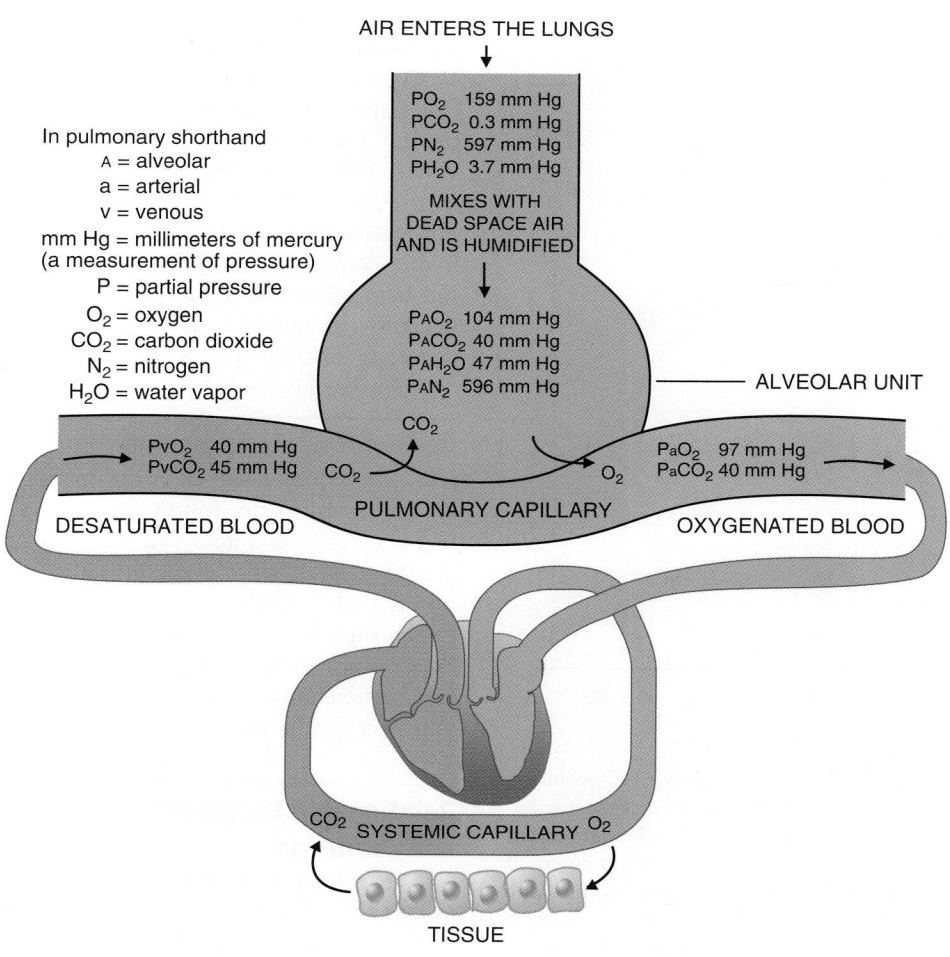

FIGURE U14-7 Partial pressures of gases during normal respiration.

Oxygen Transport

After diffusing into the pulmonary capillaries, oxygen is transported throughout the body by the circulatory system. The oxygen is dissolved in the plasma (3%) or bound in the ferrous iron-containing protein hemoglobin (97%). The combination of hemoglobin and oxygen forms *oxyhemoglobin,* which greatly increases the oxygen content of the blood above that dissolved in plasma. Tissues take up oxygen at varying rates; the rate of oxygen consumption creates an oxygen pressure gradient between the blood and the mitochondria. Carbon monoxide (CO) and other chemicals impair the ability of hemoglobin to transport oxygen in the blood.

The *oxyhemoglobin dissociation curve* represents the relationship between PaO_2 and the saturation of hemoglobin. This saturation reflects the amount of oxygen available to the tissues. For a normal curve, it is assumed that the client's temperature is 37° C, pH is 7.40, and PcO_2 is 40 mm Hg. The oxyhemoglobin dissociation curve is affected by a number of factors, including (1) temperature, (2) pH, (3) PcO_2, (4) enzymes in the red blood cell (2,3-diphosphoglycerate [2,3-DPG]), (5) presence of CO, and (6) abnormal hemoglobin. Changes in affinity of oxygen for hemoglobin cause the oxyhemoglobin to move from its normal contour, or to *shift* (Figure U14-8).

A *shift to the left* of the oxyhemoglobin dissociation curve increases the affinity of the hemoglobin molecule for oxygen. It is easier for oxygen to bind to hemoglobin, but oxygen is not easily released at the tissues. Thus at any PO_2 level, oxygen saturation is greater than normal but tissue hypoxia is present. Clinical situations that diminish the tissue delivery of oxygen include alkalosis, hypocapnia, hypothermia, decreased 2,3-DPG levels, and CO poisoning.

A *shift to the right* indicates an easier release of oxygen at the tissue level but more difficulty in binding in the lungs. This shift protects the body by allowing oxygen attached to hemoglobin to be released in the tissues to maintain adequate tissue oxygenation. Exercise improves the delivery of oxygen to the tissues, as do a number of clinical situations, including acidosis, hypercapnia, hyperthermia, hyperthyroidism (which increases 2,3-DPG), anemia, and chronic hypoxia.

Alternatively, shifts in the oxyhemoglobin dissociation curve can be expressed by a single numerical value, the P_{50}. The P_{50} represents that oxygen partial pressure at which 50% of the hemoglobin is bound to oxygen, that is, the 50% saturation point. If the affinity of hemoglobin for oxygen is decreased (shifted to the right), then a higher oxygen partial pressure is needed to bind 50% of the hemoglobin and the P_{50} is increased. Conversely, a decrease in the P_{50} represents a leftward shift in the curve, or an increase in the affinity of hemoglobin for oxygen (see Figure U14-8).

Carbon Dioxide Transport

CO_2, the waste product of tissue metabolism, is carried by the blood in the following ways: (1) combined with water as carbonic acid (70%), (2) coupled with hemoglobin (23%), or (3) dissolved in plasma (7%). Red blood cells contain the enzyme carbonic anhydrase, which rapidly breaks down CO_2 into hydrogen ions and bicarbonate ions. When venous blood enters the lungs for gas exchange, this reaction reverses, forming CO_2, which is then exhaled.

Relationship Between Ventilation and Perfusion

The relationship between *ventilation* (air flow) and *perfusion* (blood flow) determines the efficiency of gas exchange. Figure U14-9 illustrates ventilation with perfusion (unit of dead space), lack of ventilation of an

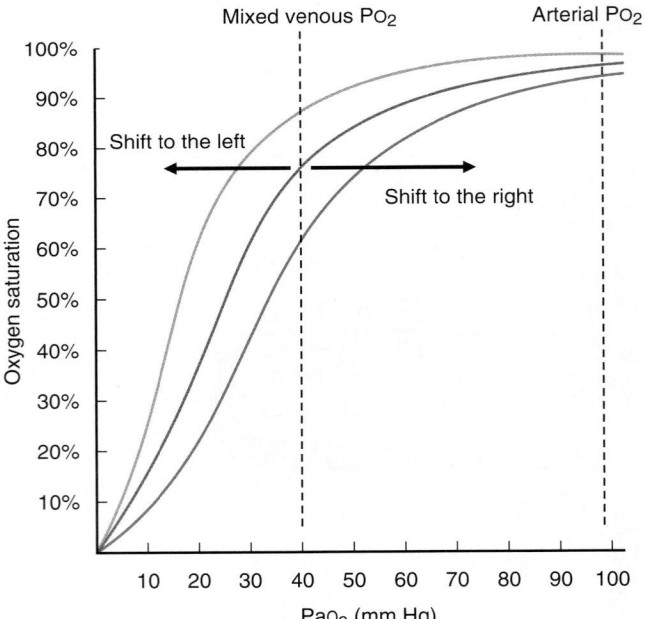

FIGURE U14-8 The normal oxyhemoglobin dissociation curve, showing how changes in the affinity of oxygen for hemoglobin shift the curve to the right or the left. Changes in the PaO_2 at the flattened top portion of the curve result in small changes in oxygen saturation. The opposite is true as the slope of the curve steepens. At the steepest portion of the curve, with the PaO_2 below 60 mm Hg, small changes in the PaO_2 result in large decreases in oxygen saturation.

alveolar unit with continued perfusion (a shunt), and total blockage with collapse of alveoli (atelectasis). Low ventilation/perfusion ($\dot{V}/\dot{Q}$) ratios and high $\dot{V}/\dot{Q}$ ratios both result in lower oxygen delivery to the body.

The ventilation-perfusion balance differs from the top to the base of the lung. Blood flow and (to a lesser extent) ventilation are greater in the more dependent lung segments at the base of the lung. Consequently, the base of the lung has the lowest $\dot{V}/\dot{Q}$ ratio, and the apex of the lung has the highest $\dot{V}/\dot{Q}$ ratio.

The $\dot{V}/\dot{Q}$ balance is controlled at both the airway and vascular levels. Hypoxia, resulting from underventilation of an alveolar region, causes vasoconstriction, which redirects blood to well-ventilated alveoli. CO_2 in the airways dilates the airway smooth muscle. Poorly perfused alveoli have low CO_2 levels, and the resultant airway constriction directs ventilation to better perfused alveoli.

REGULATION OF ACID-BASE BALANCE

The lungs, through gas exchange, have a key role in regulating the acid-base balance of the body. Pulmonary

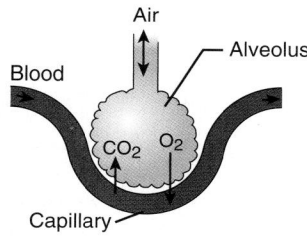

NORMAL
A normally functioning alveolus and normal pulmonary capillary flow. Ventilation and perfusion match.

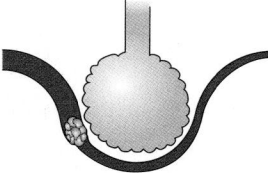

DEAD SPACE UNIT
When there is ventilation without perfusion, a dead space unit exists. Example: Pulmonary embolus preventing blood flow through the pulmonary capillary

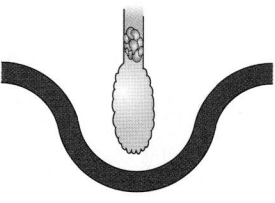

SHUNT UNIT
When there is no ventilation to an alveolar unit but perfusion continues, a shunt unit exists, and unoxygenated blood continues to circulate. Examples: atelectasis, pneumonia. The alveoli collapse.

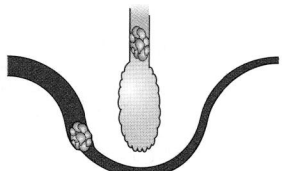

SILENT UNIT
When there is neither ventilation nor perfusion, a silent unit develops. Example: Pulmonary embolus combined with ARDS (adult respiratory distress syndrome). The alveoli collapse.

FIGURE U14-9 Relationships between ventilation (air flow) and perfusion (blood flow).

disorders that change the CO_2 level in the blood cause either respiratory acidemia or respiratory alkalemia. Insufficient ventilation causes *hypercapnia*, a respiratory acidemia caused by retention of excessive amounts of CO_2. Hyperventilation, conversely, causes *hypocapnia*, a respiratory alkalemia due to the low amounts of CO_2 in the blood.

The effectiveness of ventilation is best measured by the P_{CO_2} in the arterial blood (Pa_{CO_2}). Because the respiratory system normally maintains a Pa_{CO_2} between 35 and 45 mm Hg at sea level, a Pa_{CO_2} above this range represents *hypoventilation*. Anesthetic agents, sedatives, and opioids all tend to increase the resting Pa_{CO_2}. (Acid-base balance is detailed in Chapter 15.)

REACTION TO INJURY

The elaborate defense mechanisms of the lungs involve clearance mechanisms, defense by the respiratory epithelium, and immunologic responses in the lungs. Any injury to the lung affects the barrier between the atmosphere and the bloodstream. This barrier, which lies within the alveolar septum, is made up of epithelial (types I and II pneumocytes) and vascular endothelial cells. Injury resulting from airborne or blood-borne agents may increase vascular permeability and cause pulmonary edema. Inflammatory cells (e.g., neutrophils) arrive soon after acute injury. Then the proportion of lymphocytes, monocytes, and macrophages increases.

The basic lung repair processes include lymphatic drainage of excess fluid and phagocytic removal of protein and debris. This action generally restores lung function and structure. More severe injury requires endothelial and epithelial cell regeneration and proliferation of interstitial cells (fibroblasts). Type II cells that are generated for defense eventually differentiate into thin type I cells, which permit gas exchange. The lung's ability to recreate alveolar septa determines the degree to which normal lung function and structure are restored.

Defense by Clearance Mechanisms

The *upper airways* filter particles. Because the nose has a larger surface-volume ratio and a much more tortuous pathway for airflow than the mouth, particle deposition and conditioning of the air are more efficient when a person breathes through the nose. Larger particles (>10 mm) are generally trapped; smaller particles (<1 mm) may readily enter the lower airways.

There are four clearance mechanisms of the lower airways and alveoli:
- Cough (first five to eight bronchial generations)
- Mucociliary system (to terminal bronchioles)
- Macrophages (alveoli and respiratory bronchioles)
- Lymphatics (alveoli and interstitium)

The cough, an automatic protective reflex used to clear the trachea, occurs most rapidly in the clearing process (see Table U14-1). If the swallowing reflex is delayed or absent, a cough may be stimulated to avoid aspiration of particles into the lower airways.

Defense by the Respiratory Epithelium

Unlike the upper and lower airways, the alveoli lack a mucous layer to trap foreign particles and cilia to propel them to the pharynx for elimination. The alveolar lining is made up of flat, membranous pneumocytes (type I cells) and rounded granular (type II) cells. The type II cells are resistant to injury and cover most of the alveolar surface after exposure to infectious agents. Alveolar macrophages, derived from blood monocytes that migrate into the lungs, are also found over the surface of the alveoli. Alveolar macrophages are active phagocytes that remove dead cells and protein and that synthesize and secrete substances that regulate the immune system. They leave the lung by the mucociliary system or the lymphatic system.

Defense by Immunologic Mechanisms

The systemic immune system responds to the lung during inflammatory processes by mobilizing blood neutrophils and monocytes. Recruited thymus-dependent (T) and thymus-independent (B) lymphocytes contribute to local cell-mediated immune reactions and the production of specific antibodies within the alveoli. Cell-mediated immunity is a key determinant in resistance to organisms such as *Mycobacterium tuberculosis* and *Pneumocystis carinii*. Immune mechanisms are generally a host defense function. However, hypersensitivity immune reactions lead to tissue injury and are responsible for clinical conditions such as asthma, granuloma formation, and lung transplant rejection. (Chapter 78 describes types I, II, III, and IV hypersensitivity reactions.)

EFFECTS OF AGING

Most of the changes that occur with aging affect the lower airway. Movement of cilia in the upper airway slows and becomes less effective. This change predisposes older clients to a greater number of respiratory infections.

Lung structure also changes with age. The lungs become rounder as a result of increased anteroposterior diameter, circumference, area, and height of the lung. The proportion of the lung formed by alveolar duct air increases, and alveolar air decreases. Loss of alveolar wall tissue and its elastic tissue fibers is seen. The result is a deterioration of lung function.

The air spaces enlarge, although this is not referred to as emphysema because it is not a result of disease. These changes may be due to environmental pollutants rather than to aging alone. An increased incidence of true emphysema and a greater prevalence of chronic cough and sputum production are seen in older adults. These findings suggest that environmental or occupational pollutants, in addition to the normal aging process, may be a component in the decline of lung function.

CONCLUSIONS

The primary function of the lungs is gas exchange. The physical structure of the airways allows air to be warmed, filtered, and humidified as it enters the body. In the alveolar sacs, oxygen is exchanged for CO_2. The mechanics of breathing are coordinated by the ribs, diaphragm, pleural space, elastic recoil of the lungs, and the nervous system. The respiratory system also helps regulate acid-base balance. Alterations in structure and function can result in various disorders.

BIBLIOGRAPHY

1. Berne, R., & Levy, M. (1998). *Physiology* (4th ed.). St. Louis: Mosby.
2. Kierszenbaum, A.L. (2002). *Histology and cell biology: An introduction to pathology.* St. Louis, Mosby.
3. Guyton, A., & Hall, J. (2001). *Textbook of medical physiology* (10th ed.) Philadelphia: W. B. Saunders.
4. Levitzky, M. (1999). *Pulmonary physiology* (5th ed.). New York: McGraw-Hill.
5. Silverthorn, D. (2001). *Human physiology* (2nd ed.). Saddle River, NJ: Prentice Hall.
6. West, J. (1995). *Respiratory physiology: The essentials* (5th ed.). Baltimore: Williams & Wilkins.
7. West, J. (1997). *Pulmonary pathophysiology: The essentials* (5th ed.). Baltimore: Williams & Wilkins.

Chapter 61

Assessment of the Respiratory System

Amy Verst

GENERAL RESPIRATORY ASSESSMENT

Nurses who care for clients experiencing respiratory disorders perform and interpret a variety of assessment procedures. This chapter discusses the physical assessment and diagnostic procedures for clients who have respiratory disorders. The assessment data are used to plan client care.

HISTORY

A respiratory history contains information about a client's present condition and previous respiratory problems. Interview the client and his or her family, and focus on the clinical manifestations of the chief complaint, events leading up to the current condition, past health history, family history, and psychosocial history.

The detail and time taken for a respiratory history depend on the client's condition (acute, chronic, or emergent). State questions simply using short, easy-to-understand sentences. When necessary, reword questions to clarify statements the client seems not to understand. Ask questions in the context of the client's daily activities. For example, ask the client, Are you able to carry the groceries in from the car? Are you able to make your bed, vacuum the house, bathe yourself, or dress yourself without stopping to rest and catch your breath?

Biographical and Demographic Data

Begin the history by obtaining biographical data. Include the client's name, age, gender, and living situation.

Demographic data are usually recorded on an agency assessment form. Note the client's biologic age and compare it with the client's appearance. Does the client look his or her stated age? Disorders such as lung cancer and chronic lung disorders often make the client appear older. The living situation, whether it be alone, with children, or with significant others, is important in planning the client's discharge.

Current Health

Chief Complaint

The chief complaint helps to establish priorities for intervention and to assess the client's level of understanding of the current condition. Common respiratory complaints include *dyspnea* (difficulty breathing), cough, sputum production, *hemoptysis* (blood-stained sputum), wheezing, *stridor* (a high-pitched respiratory sound), and chest pain. Focus on the manifestations,

FIGURE 61-1 The Visual Analogue Scale of dyspnea. Although the scale can be in the form of either a vertical or a horizontal line, the most commonly used scale consists of a 100-mm horizontal line, like the one shown here.

How short of breath are you right now?

None   Extremely
                                                          Severe

and prioritize questions to elicit a symptom analysis (see Chapter 4).

In emergency or acute situations, simple questions are often all that can be asked until the client is stable and comfortable. Whenever possible, ask the client's significant others for further details.

Take as extensive a respiratory history as the client's condition allows. Detailed questioning provides valuable clues to (1) the client's manifestations, (2) the client's degree of existing respiratory dysfunction, (3) the client's and his or her family's understanding of the condition and its management, and (4) the family's support system and ability to cope with the manifestations and management of the condition on an ongoing basis.

Dyspnea. *Dyspnea* (difficulty breathing) is one of the most common manifestations experienced by clients with pulmonary and cardiac disorders. It is a subjective symptom and a reflection of the client's assessment of the degree of work of breathing he or she exerts for a given task or effort. Clients may define dyspnea as shortness of breath, suffocation, tightness, being winded, or being breathless.

The assessment of dyspnea involves several aspects. The subjective nature of dyspnea makes it difficult to quantify objectively. Several methods are used to assess accurately the level of dyspnea experienced by a client. The Visual Analogue Scale (Figure 61-1) is used to quantify breathlessness in response to particular questions. It is easy to understand, and the amount of dyspnea during various activities can be assessed. The Modified Borg Category Ratio Scale (Table 61-1) is used to rate the intensity of dyspnea. It is simple, and results have been reproduced in several populations.

In addition to a subjective assessment, conduct a symptom analysis to document the characteristics of the dyspnea. Assess all the characteristics because many respiratory and nonrespiratory causes can result in dyspnea.

Cough. Detail the many aspects of the client's *cough* by conducting a symptom analysis. Note when and how the cough began (suddenly or gradually) and how long it has been present. Determine the frequency of the cough and the time of day when the cough is better or worse (early morning, late afternoon, nighttime). Use the client's own words to describe the cough. A cough may be described as hacking, dry, hoarse, congested, barking, wheezy, or bubbling.

TABLE 61-1	The Modified Borg Category-Ratio Scale for Assessment of Dyspnea
Score	**Intensity**
0	Nothing at all
0.5	Very, very slight
1	Very slight
2	Slight
3	Moderate
4	Somewhat severe
5	Severe
6	
7	Very severe
8	
9	Very, very severe
10	Maximal

Modified from Burden, J., et al. (1982). The perception of breathlessness. *American Review of Respiratory Diseases, 126,* 825-828.

Determine which medications or treatments the client has used for the cough (antitussives, codeine, inhalers, nebulizers, rest, sitting up). Find out what precautions are used to prevent the spread of infection (if it is present). Use this opportunity to remind the client about good handwashing technique, proper disposal of soiled tissues, and completion of a full course of antibiotics (if prescribed).

Coughing may lead to stress incontinence; you may want to ask female clients about this embarrassing problem. The incontinence should clear when the coughing subsides; protective padding may be helpful.

Sputum Production. *Sputum* is the substance expelled by coughing or clearing the throat. The tracheobronchial tree normally produces about 3 ounces of mucus a day as part of the normal cleaning mechanism; however, sputum production with coughing is not normal. Question the client about sputum color (clear, yellow, green, rusty, bloody), odor, quality (watery, stringy, frothy, thick), and quantity (teaspoon, tablespoon, cup). Document in the client's medical record any changes in color, odor, quality, or quantity. Ascertain whether sputum is produced only after the client is lying in a certain position. The amount of sputum produced is increased in several disorders; for instance, clients with bronchitis may expectorate several cups of sputum daily.

Sputum may be a secretion from the oral or nasopharyngeal area or sinuses rather than from the tracheobronchial tree. For example, draining sinuses may provoke a productive cough.

Hemoptysis. *Hemoptysis* refers to blood expectorated from the mouth in the form of gross (visible to the naked eye) blood, frankly bloody sputum, or blood-tinged sputum. Attempt to identify the source of the blood—the lungs, a nosebleed, or the stomach. Blood from the lungs is usually bright red because blood in the lungs stimulates an immediate cough reflex. If the blood remains in the lungs for a while, it may turn dark red or brown. Ask the client whether the hemoptysis occurred as a result of forceful coughing. Also obtain an estimate of the amount of blood expectorated (teaspoon, tablespoon, cup).

Pulmonary causes of hemoptysis include chronic bronchitis, bronchiectasis, pulmonary tuberculosis, cystic fibrosis, upper airway necrotizing granulomas, pulmonary embolism, pneumonia, lung cancer, and lung abscesses. Cardiovascular abnormalities, anticoagulants, and immunosuppressive drugs that cause parenchymal (lung tissue) bleeding can also cause hemoptysis.

Wheezing. Wheezing sounds are produced when air passes through partially obstructed or narrowed airways on inspiration or expiration. *Wheezing* may be audible, or it may be heard only with a stethoscope. The client may not complain of wheezing but complain of chest tightness or chest discomfort instead. Ask the client to identify when the wheezing occurs and whether it resolves spontaneously or medication (such as inhaled bronchodilators) is required for relief. Not all wheezing is caused by asthma. Wheezing can be caused by mucosal edema, airway secretions, collapsed airways resulting from loss of elastic tissue, and foreign objects or tumors partially obstructing air flow.

Stridor. *Stridor* is the name given to high-pitched sounds produced when air passes through a partially obstructed or narrowed upper airway on inspiration. Stridor is associated with respiratory distress and can be life-threatening because the airway is compromised. Several conditions can lead to stridor: epiglottitis, sleep *apnea* (cessation of breathing), heart failure, and aspiration. Inquire about changes in voice character, hoarseness, difficulty swallowing, sleep-related disorders such as insomnia, degree of snoring, *hypersomnolence* (excessive sleepiness) in the morning, early morning headaches, weight gain, fluid retention, apnea, and restlessness.

Chest Pain. Chest pain may be associated with pulmonary and cardiac problems, and distinguishing between the two is important. Conduct a complete symptom analysis for any chest pain. *Angina pectoris* (from Latin, pain of the chest) may be associated with de-

creased blood flow to the heart and is a potentially life-threatening problem.

Determine the location, duration, and intensity of the chest pain to provide early clues to the cause. Coughing and pleuritic infections can cause chest pain. Pleuritic chest pain is commonly a sharp, stabbing pain that occurs at one site on the chest wall and increases with chest wall movement or deep breathing. *Retrosternal* (behind the sternum) pain is usually burning, constant, and aching. Pain can also originate in the bony and cartilaginous parts of the thorax.

The characteristics of angina pectoris and other chest pains differ from each other. Cardiac chest pain is usually described as an aching, heavy, squeezing sensation with pressure or tightness in the substernal area. Angina pectoris can also radiate into the neck or arms (see Chapter 56 for comparison of types of chest pain). Ask the client what brings on the pain (activity, coughing, movement) and what relieves the pain (nitroglycerin, splinting the chest wall, heat).

Symptom Analysis

To obtain a complete history of the respiratory system, assess the characteristics of any clinical manifestation. Assessment of these characteristics leads to a comprehensive symptom analysis. When the client describes a specific respiratory manifestation, assess the following factors: onset, location, duration, characteristics/client's perception, aggravating factors, associated manifestations, relieving factors, timing, setting, and severity. Some students can memorize these factors with the mnemonic OLDCARTS.

Onset. When did the manifestations begin? Analyze their duration to determine whether the current symptoms are indicative of an acute problem or exacerbation of a chronic condition.

Location. Note the *location* of the manifestation. Ask the client to identify its exact location. Location is especially important when the complaint is chest pain because it is essential to determine whether the pain is cardiac or respiratory in origin.

Duration. How long has the manifestation been affecting the client? This is the *duration* of the problem. It should be correlated with the onset and timing of the symptoms to determine an acute or chronic condition.

Characteristics/Client's Perception. Describe the *characteristics* of the manifestation in common language. Ask the client to report the amount, size, number, and extent of the chief complaint. Especially with sputum production, ask the client to estimate how much sputum is produced a day—a cup, a tablespoon, or teaspoon.

Avoid using terms such as "a little" or "a lot," which have different meanings among clients and health care providers.

In an assessment of a cough, the cough may be described as tight, loose, dry, hacking, or congested. Have clients describe the characteristics of their cough in their own words. Dyspnea may be described as breathlessness, shortness of air, a band constricting the chest, and so forth. Use the client's own words to note the *client's perception*. Note any unique properties of the complaint. Use a direct quotation to document the client's complaint. For example, the client might report a "catch" in the left posterior chest when taking deep breaths.

Aggravating and Relieving Factors. The *aggravating* and *relieving factors* precipitate, worsen, or alleviate a manifestation. Environmental allergens, such as dog or cat dander, dust mites, mold, and pollen, are often described as aggravating factors. Sitting up or lying down may relieve or exacerbate the manifestation. Medication may also worsen or relieve the manifestation.

Associated Manifestations. *Associated manifestations* occur in conjunction with the chief complaint. Examples include chills, fever, night sweats, anorexia, weight loss, excessive fatigue, anxiety, and hoarseness. You may be able to recognize that chills and fever commonly accompany infectious lung disorders, whereas anorexia and weight loss can occur in clients with disorders that result in dyspnea.

Timing. *Timing* encompasses both the *onset* (the gradual or sudden appearance of the manifestation) and the *period* (days, weeks, months) during which the problem has occurred. Ask the client whether the problem occurs at a specific time of day most frequently, for example, the morning cough or shortness of air associated with lying flat at night.

Setting. In what setting does the manifestation occur most often? The *setting* refers to the time and place or particular situation—physical setting and psychological environment—in which the client experiences the complaint. For example, the client may cough in the morning after smoking a cigarette or complain of respiratory distress at work.

Severity. The client should note the *severity* of the problem. Often a scale of 1 to 10, with 1 being the least and 10 the most, is used to describe pain or distress.

Past Health History

Examine the past health history of the client and family members for data related to the upper and lower respiratory systems (the upper respiratory history and physical examination are discussed later). These systems are common sources of both acute and chronic health problems. Assess clients with chronic conditions for changes in their ongoing respiratory manifestations (cough, dyspnea, sputum production, or wheezes) because these changes provide clues to the cause of the new problem. Include questions about the following areas.

Childhood and Infectious Diseases

In addition to obtaining data regarding common childhood diseases and vaccinations, ask the client about the occurrence of tuberculosis, bronchitis, influenza, asthma, and pneumonia and the frequency of lower respiratory infections after upper respiratory infection. Determine the existence of congenital problems, such as cystic fibrosis and premature birth history. These problems are associated with respiratory complications such as obstructive and restrictive pulmonary disease.

Immunizations

Inquire about vaccination against pneumonia (polyvalent pneumococcal vaccine [Pneumovax]) and influenza. Ask the client to list the dates of these vaccinations. Pneumovax provides lifelong immunity against pneumococcal pneumonia, whereas "flu shots" must be received annually in the fall of the year.

Major Illnesses and Hospitalizations

Ask the client about previous hospitalizations or treatment for respiratory problems. Determine the dates of illnesses or hospitalization, the specific respiratory problem, medical treatment (including surgery, use of a ventilator, and inhalation treatments or oxygen therapy), and the present status of the problem.

Has a chest x-ray film been taken? When? Have other pulmonary diagnostic tests been performed? These test results can provide baseline data for the evaluation of the current problem. Inquire about previous injuries to the mouth, nose, throat, or chest (blunt trauma, fractured ribs, or pneumothorax).

Medications

Obtain detailed information regarding both prescribed and over-the-counter medications, including herbal remedies, because many products affect the respiratory system. The client may have taken antibiotics for respiratory infections, bronchodilators, or steroids. Specify the route of administration (pill, liquid, or inhalation). Many respiratory medications are inhaled through a metered-dose inhaler (MDI) or mini-nebulizer. If an MDI is used, the client may use a spacer to disperse the medication properly. Ask the client to demonstrate use of the MDI and spacer.

Herbal medicines for respiratory problems include remedies for nasal discharge and congestion, cough, sore throat, fever and headache, and immunostimulant effects. *Ephedra (E. sinica, E. vulgaris)* is a stimulant and is illegal in the United States. Expectorants include anise *(Pimpinella anisum)*, coltsfoot *(Tussilago farfara)*, and horehound *(Marrubium vulgare)*. Coltsfoot and horehound are also believed to have antitussive action.

Sore throat remedies include mint *(Mentha piperita* [peppermint], *Mentha spicata* [spearmint]) and slippery elm *(Ulmus rubra)*. Remedies for the fever and headache that may accompany colds and influenza include boneset *(Eupatorium perfoliatum)*, feverfew *(Tanacetum parthenium)*, and white willow *(Salix purpurea, Salix fragilis)*. Stimulants of the immune system, believed to help ward off colds and flu, include *Echinacea (E. angustifolia, E. pallida, E. purpurea)* and goldenseal *(Hydrastis canadensis)*.

Allergies

Question the client about a history of allergies and timing of manifestations to help identify a possible allergic basis for the condition. Ask about precipitating and aggravating factors, such as foods, medications, pollens, smoke, fumes, dust, and animal dander. Sources of molds that may cause allergic manifestations include the water reservoir of a furnace humidifier, air conditioners, and plant soil.

Ask the client to describe the allergic manifestations experienced (chest tightness, wheezing, cough, rhinitis, watery eyes, scratchy throat) and their severity. Determine the age at which allergies first occurred and whether they have become progressively more severe.

Has the client been tested for allergies? When? Are medications (including allergy shots) taken prophylactically or on an as-needed basis to provide symptomatic relief?

Family Health History

Question the client about the family history of respiratory diseases. Identify blood relatives (in regard to *genetically transmitted* diseases) and family members (in regard to *infectious* conditions) who have had asthma, cystic fibrosis, emphysema, chronic obstructive pulmonary disease (COPD), lung cancer, respiratory infections, tuberculosis, or allergies. List the age and cause of death of each deceased family member.

Do any household members smoke cigarettes, pipes, or cigars? Secondary inhalation of smoke often precipitates or worsens respiratory manifestations.

Psychosocial History

Respiratory status is affected by numerous factors that may lead to acute problems or that may affect the client's coping with chronic problems such as COPD. Areas to be assessed are described next.

Occupation

Identify any environmental agents that might be contributing to the client's condition. Ask specifically about the work environment and hobbies. Focus on exposure to dust, asbestos, beryllium, silica, and other toxins or pollutants. Farmers are exposed to airborne particles that may be inhaled, such as grain dust, fertilizers, and animal dander. Hobbies may involve chemicals, heat, dust, and airborne particles from grinding, soldering, or welding.

Geographic Location

Ask about recent travel to areas where respiratory diseases are prevalent, such as Asia (tuberculosis), the Ohio River valley (histoplasmosis), or the San Joaquin valley (valley fever). Polluted city air has also been related to increasing incidence and severity of asthma.

Environment

Ask about the client's living conditions. How many people are in the household? Crowded living conditions increase risk of exposure to infectious respiratory diseases such as tuberculosis and cold viruses. Recent exposure to continuous air conditioning in a hotel or motel setting may be related to Legionnaire's disease.

Assess for environmental hazards such as stairs or poor air circulation. A client with a chronic respiratory condition may have difficulty climbing stairs or breathing unfiltered air.

Habits

Inquire about any history of smoking tobacco products. Calculate the pack-years, which helps quantify the smoking history, as follows:

Years of smoking × Packs smoked per day = Pack-years

Smoking has been associated with decreased ciliary function of the lungs, increased mucus production, and the development of lung cancer. Ask the client about the use of smokeless tobacco (snuff, chewing tobacco) and smoking non-tobacco substances (marijuana and clove cigarettes).

Ask about alcohol use. Ciliary action is slowed by alcohol, which reduces mucus clearance from the lungs. Heavy alcohol ingestion depresses the cough reflex and increases risk of aspiration. Clients who use and abuse recreational drugs are at risk for drug overdose and respiratory failure. Sharing needles increases the risk of human immunodeficiency virus (HIV) infection and the development of acquired immunodeficiency syndrome (AIDS) and opportunistic infections such as *Pneumocystis carinii*.

Exercise

Clients who are active may describe the onset of coughing and wheezing during exercise. These clients need to be further evaluated for exercise-induced asthma before continuing workouts. Clients with chronic respiratory conditions often do not have the lung capacity to sustain even mild forms of exercise and subsequently become dyspneic. Has tolerance for activity decreased or remained stable? Ask the client to describe typical activities, such as walking, light housekeeping chores, or grocery shopping, that are tolerated or, conversely, that result in shortness of breath.

Nutrition

Maintaining a nutritious diet is important for clients with chronic respiratory disease, which can result in decreased lung capacity and greater workload for the lungs and cardiovascular system. The added workload increases caloric expenditure, and weight loss may occur. Clients may become anorectic because of the effects of medications and fatigue. The client may not have enough energy to consume the needed calories to maintain body weight. Ask the client to recall intake for the last 24 hours. Assess the amount of protein, kilocalories, and sodium intake (see Chapter 30).

Review of Systems

Ask the client to describe other manifestations associated with the respiratory system. In addition to cough, dyspnea, sputum production, hemoptysis, wheezing, stridor, and chest pain, include breathlessness, fever, hoarseness, night sweats, anorexia, weight loss, and dependent edema. Upper respiratory manifestations include colds, nasal discharge, postnasal drip, sinus pain and swelling, *epistaxis* (nosebleed), and sinus headaches.

Hypoxia may precipitate subtle neurologic alterations, such as restlessness, fatigue, disorientation, and personality changes. Tachycardia usually accompanies respiratory problems as the body attempts to compensate for decreased oxygen delivery. Stomach upset, nausea, and vomiting can result from accumulation of excess mucus swallowed from draining sinuses. Anorexia and weight loss are seen in many chronic respiratory conditions. Chapter 4 and the website for this textbook contain questions for a review of systems.

PHYSICAL EXAMINATION

Physical examination follows the health history. Use the techniques of inspection, palpation, percussion, and auscultation. Successful examination requires that you be familiar with the anatomic landmarks of the posterior, lateral, and anterior thorax (Figure 61-2). Use these landmarks to locate and visualize the underlying structures, particularly the lobes of the lungs, the heart, and major vessels. Compare the findings on one side of the thorax with those on the other side. Palpation, percussion, and auscultation proceed in a back-and-forth or side-to-side manner so that you continually evaluate findings by using the opposite side as the standard for comparison.

Note the condition and color (pale, red, blue) of the client's skin throughout the examination of the thorax, and record abnormalities. Assess the respiratory rate, depth, and rhythm, if these were not assessed previously with the vital signs during inspection of the thorax (see Chapter 4). Assess the client's level of consciousness and orientation throughout the examination to determine whether gas exchange is adequate. See the Physical Assessment Findings in the Healthy Adult feature on The Respiratory System on p. 1750 for expected respiratory findings.

Inspection

The physical examination begins during the history-taking stage as you observe the client and the client's response to questions. Note any manifestations of respiratory distress at this time: position of comfort, tachypnea (rapid, shallow breathing), gasping, grunting, central cyanosis, open mouth, flared nostrils, dyspnea, the color of facial skin and lips, and the use of accessory muscles. Note the *inspiratory-to-expiratory (I:E) ratio*. Because the normal length of inspiration is half that of expiration, the normal ratio is 1:2. See Figure 61-3.

Observe the client's speech pattern. How many words or sentences can be said before another breath is taken? Clients who are short of breath may be able to say only three or four words before taking another breath. During the physical examination, the client should be bare to the waist while maintaining privacy and warmth. Inspection and palpation, often performed together, are discussed separately.

Head and Neck

Begin inspection with observation of the head and neck for any gross abnormalities that would interfere with respiration. Note the odor of the breath and whether sputum is present. Note nasal flaring, breathing with pursed lips, or cyanosis of the mucous membranes. Record the use of accessory muscles, such as flexion of the sternocleidomastoid muscle.

Chest

Chest Wall Configuration. Continue inspection by observing the chest wall configuration. Observe chest size and contour, and note the *anteroposterior* (AP) diameter. Calculate the ratio of the AP diameter to the transverse (lateral) diameter. The transverse diameter is generally twice the AP diameter (Figure 61-4, *A*).

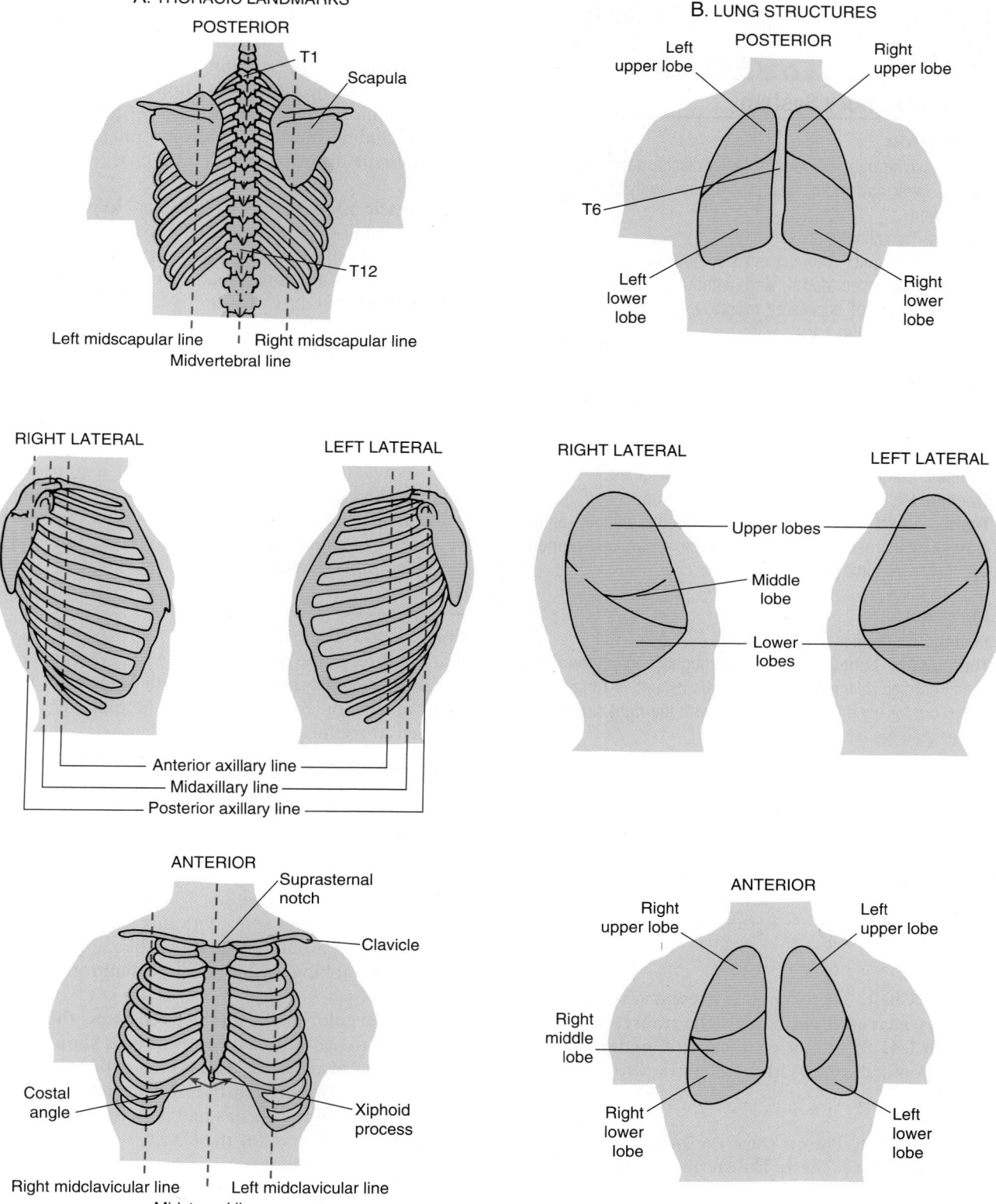

FIGURE 61-2 Thoracic landmarks and underlying lung structures. During chest examination, it is important to document in a universally understood manner the location of unusual or abnormal findings. Use the terminology of thoracic landmarks and lung structure to do so.

PHYSICAL ASSESSMENT FINDINGS IN THE HEALTHY ADULT

The Respiratory System

Inspection

Nose. Nose straight, without flaring or discharge; nares patent; mucosa pink and moist; septum midline, without masses or perforation

Sinuses. Transilluminate

Thorax. Even color; regular, even contour; respirations quiet, unlabored, of even depth, and without retractions, bulges, masses, or use of accessory muscles; anteroposterior-transverse diameter ratio 1:2

Digits. Clubbing absent; nail beds pink; immediate capillary refill on blanching

Palpation

Nose. Nontender, without masses or lesions

Sinuses. Nontender, without swelling or bogginess

Trachea. Midline and mobile without crepitus

Thorax. Chest wall symmetrical, smooth, without lumps, masses, tenderness, or crepitus; thoracic excursion symmetrical; tactile fremitus present

Percussion

Sinuses. Nontender

Thorax and Lungs. Resonant throughout peripheral lung fields; cardiac dullness; diaphragmatic excursion ranges from 3 to 6 cm for each hemidiaphragm, with the right side slightly higher than the left

Auscultation

Thorax and Lungs. Vesicular sounds throughout peripheral lung fields; bronchovesicular sounds over the area of tracheal bifurcation, both anteriorly and posteriorly; bronchial sounds over the trachea anteriorly; adventitious sounds absent; vocal resonance absent

---

Barrel Chest. Barrel chest is present when the AP diameter is increased and equals the transverse diameter (Figure 61-4, *B*). It is a characteristic finding in clients with chronic disorders that interfere with ventilation 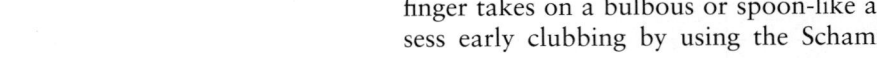 (*emphysema*).

Pigeon Chest. Pigeon chest (*pectus carinatum*) is the opposite of funnel chest. The sternum juts forward and increases the AP diameter (Figure 61-4, *C*). Congenital atrial or ventricular septal defects are the most common cause of pigeon chest, but rickets, Marfan's syndrome, and severe primary kyphoscoliosis may contribute to pigeon chest.

Funnel Chest. Funnel chest (*pectus excavatum*) is a deformity in which the sternum is depressed and the organs that lie below it are compressed (Figure 61-4, *D*). In severe cases, the sternum may actually touch the spinal column. In most cases, however, pectus excavatum is clinically insignificant. Some causes of funnel chest, including Marfan's syndrome and congenital connective tissue disorders, may be serious.

Thoracic Kyphoscoliosis. Thoracic kyphoscoliosis is an accentuation of the normal thoracic curve (Figure 61-4, *E*). The client takes on a hunched-over or hunchback appearance. Causes include congenital defect, osteoporosis secondary to aging, spinal tuberculosis, rheumatoid arthritis, and poor posture over a long period. The underlying lungs are distorted, which can make interpretation of lung findings difficult.

Chest Movement. Observe chest movement during respiration. Normal respiratory rate is 12 to 22 breaths/min. Note the amplitude, or depth of expansion, and rhythm. Abdominal breathing is more apparent in men, whereas women use their thoracic muscles. Note the use of accessory muscles, retractions, symmetry, and any paradoxical movements.

Fingers and Toes

Examination of the fingers and toes may reveal *clubbing*, which may be present in clients with pulmonary fibrosis, lung cancer, or bronchiectasis. Clubbing occurs as a compensatory measure in chronic hypoxia. The physiologic cause of clubbing has not yet been identified, although some hypotheses have been proposed. The body develops collateral circulation around an area of impaired circulation to provide more oxygen to that area. With clubbing, the nail bed loses its normal angle of 160 degrees between the nail plate and the finger, and the angle increases to 180 degrees. The base of the nail bed may feel spongy and soft. With advanced clubbing, the finger takes on a bulbous or spoon-like appearance. Assess early clubbing by using the Schamroth technique (Figure 61-5).

Note the color of the nail beds to assess the status of peripheral tissue oxygenation. Nail beds should be pink and without cyanosis or dusky blue color. Quickly and gently compress (between thumb and index finger) and release several of the client's nail beds on each extremity. Continuously observe for the *blanch response* and *capillary refill*. With compression, the nail bed becomes pale as capillary blood is squeezed from the tissue. On release of the pressure, oxygenated arterial blood fills the capillary bed. Normal capillary refill occurs within 3 seconds; a refill time longer than 3 seconds indicates delayed capillary refill.

RESPIRATORY PATTERN	DESCRIPTION
A. Eupnea (Normal) 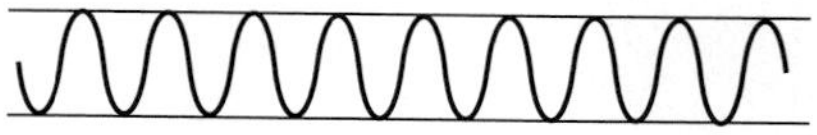	Rate = 12 to 20 breaths/min Depth = Average tidal volume 350-500 ml (adults) Rhythm = Regular, occasional sigh breath deeper than baseline tidal volume I:E Ratio* = 1:2
B. Hyperventilation 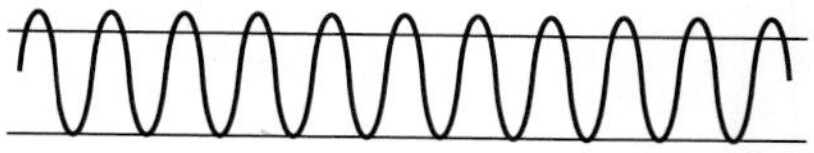	Rate = May increase Depth = Deep—large tidal volumes Rhythm = Usually regular I:E Ratio = Approaches 1:1 Comment = May be associated with CO_2 loss (respiratory alkalosis)
C. Tachypnea 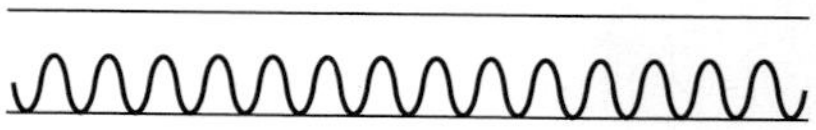	Rate = Rapid Depth = Shallow—small tidal volume with each breath Rhythm = Regular I:E Ratio = Approaches 1:1 Comment = May be associated with CO_2 retention (respiratory acidosis)
D. Bradypnea 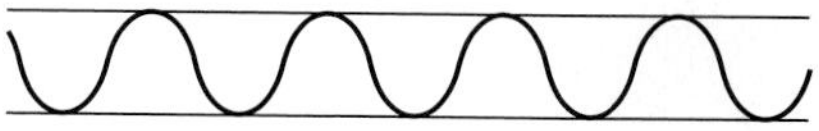	Rate = Slow Depth = Tidal volumes vary depending on the cause Rhythm = Regular I:E Ratio = 1:2
E. Apnea 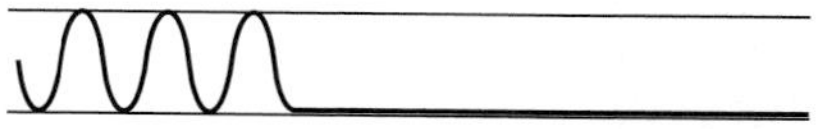	Complete absence of breathing Comment = May be temporary
F. Cheyne-Stokes 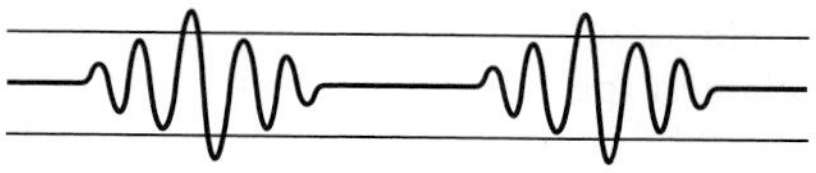	Rate = Variable Depth = Depth of each breath varies in a cyclical pattern: Shallow before and after apnea, deep with hyperventilation Rhythm = Apneic periods alternate with hyperventilation Comment = Regular-irregular—crescendo-decrescendo pattern
G. Biot's 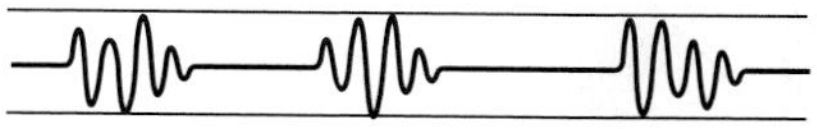	Rate = Variable Depth = Depth variable—predominantly shallow Rhythm = Unpredictable irregularity Comment = Long periods of apnea alternate with breathing periods
H. Kussmaul's 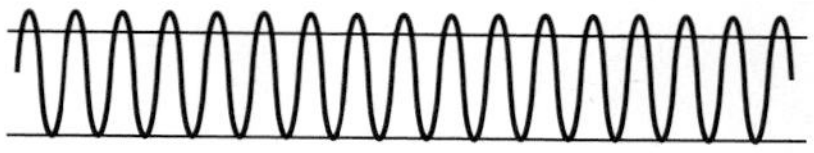	Rate = Rapid Depth = Deep without pauses Rhythm = Regular Comment = Associated with diabetic ketoacidosis
I. Apneustic 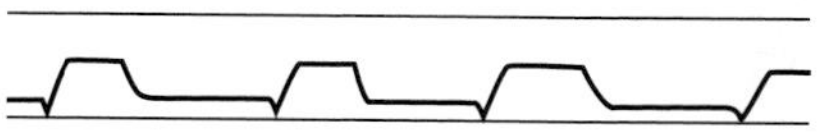	Rate = Rapid Depth = Shallow Comment = Prolonged inspiration followed by short, ineffective expiration

* Inspiration to Expiration (I:E) ratio

FIGURE 61-3 Assessing respiratory patterns.

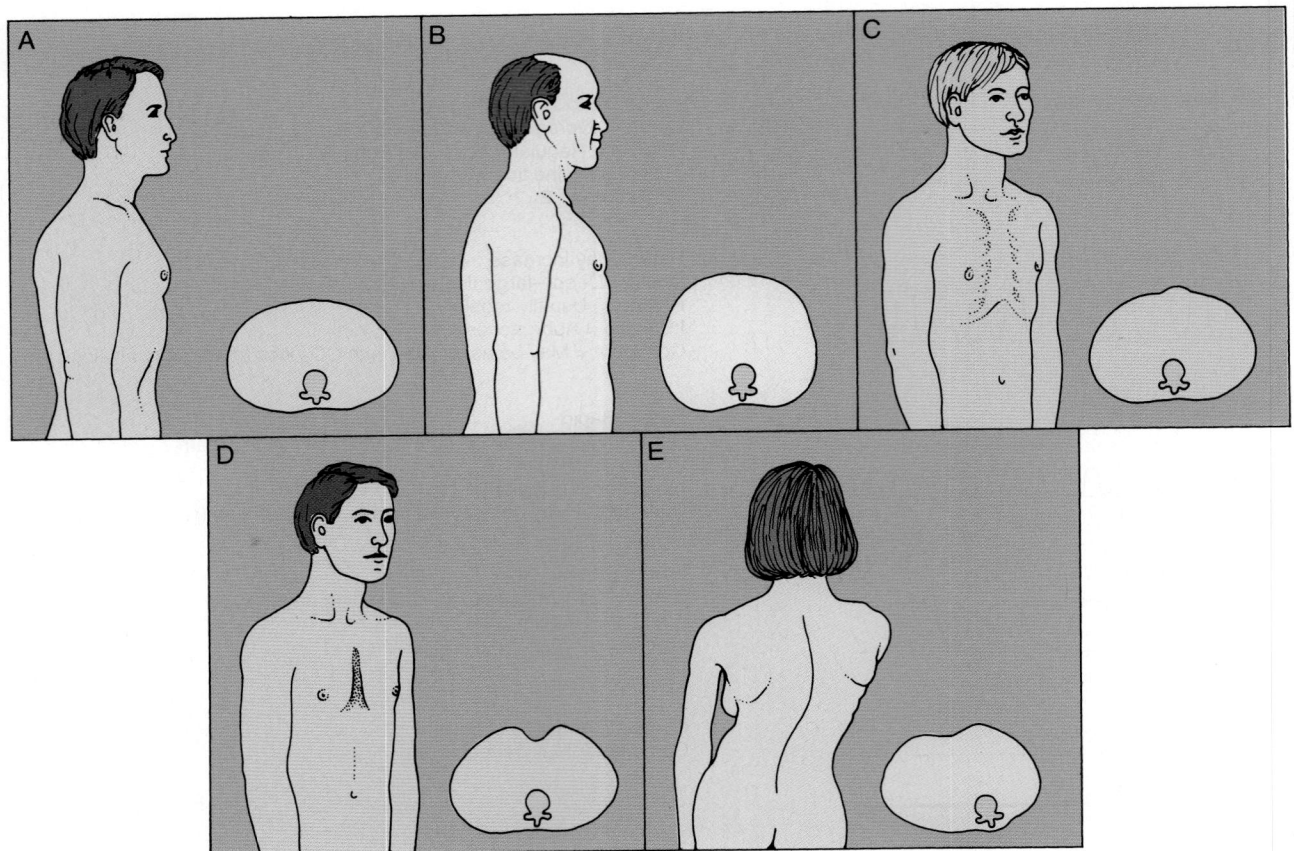

FIGURE 61-4 Chest deformities. **A,** Normal adult, for comparison. The ratio of anteroposterior diameter to transverse diameter can be seen here as 1:2. **B,** Barrel chest. The anteroposterior-transverse diameter ratio is 1:1. **C,** Pigeon chest (pectus carinatum). **D,** Funnel chest (pectus excavatum). **E,** Thoracic kyphoscoliosis.

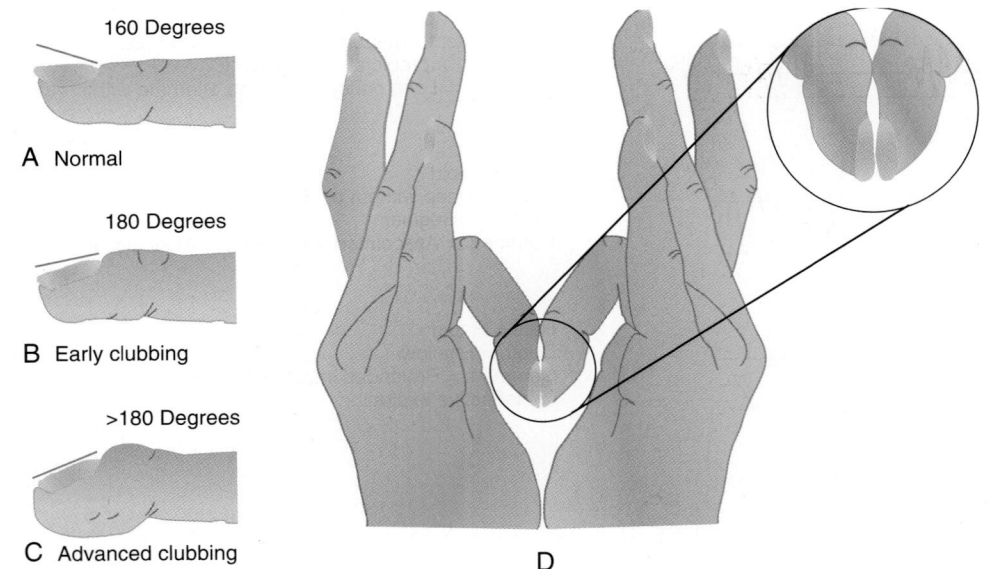

FIGURE 61-5 Clubbing. **A,** A normal digit, with an angle of 160 degrees. **B,** A flattened angle between the nail and the skin, exceeding 180 degrees. **C,** Advanced clubbing with a rounded nail. **D,** Assess clubbing with the use of the Schamroth technique. Instruct the client to place the nails of the fourth (ring) fingers together while extending the other fingers and to hold the hands up. A diamond-shaped space between the nails is a normal finding and indicates the absence of clubbing.

Palpation

Palpation is the use of the hands to feel various structures on and below the surface of the body. The technique of palpation is described in Chapter 4.

Trachea

Gently place the thumb of the palpating hand on one side of the trachea and the remaining fingers on the other side. Move the trachea gently from side to side along its length while palpating for masses, *crepitus* (air in the subcutaneous tissues), or deviation from the midline. The trachea is usually slightly movable and quickly returns to the midline position after displacement. A chest mass, goiter, or an acute chest injury may displace the trachea.

Chest Wall

Palpate the chest wall, holding the heel or ulnar aspect of your hand against the client's chest. During palpation continue the investigation of abnormalities found on inspection. Palpation combined with inspection is particularly effective in assessing whether the movements or thoracic excursion of the chest during inspiration and expiration are symmetrical and equal in amplitude. During palpation assess for crepitus, defects or tenderness of the chest wall, muscle tone, edema, and tactile *fremitus* (the vibration of air movement through the chest wall while the client is speaking).

Thoracic Excursion

During evaluation of thoracic excursion, the client sits upright. Place your hands on the client's posterior chest wall (Figure 61-6). The thumbs oppose each other on either side of the spine, and the fingers face upward and out like butterfly wings. As the client inhales, your hands should move up and out symmetrically. Any asymmetry suggests a disease process in that region.

Tactile Fremitus

Palpate the posterior chest wall while the client says words that produce relatively intense vibrations ("ninety-nine"). The vibrations are transmitted from the larynx via the airways and can be palpated on the chest wall (Figure 61-7). Compare the intensity of vibrations on both sides for symmetry. Stronger vibrations are felt over areas where there is consolidation of the underlying lung (as with pneumonia). Decreased tactile fremitus is usually associated with abnormalities that move the lung farther from the chest wall, such as pleural effusion and pneumothorax.

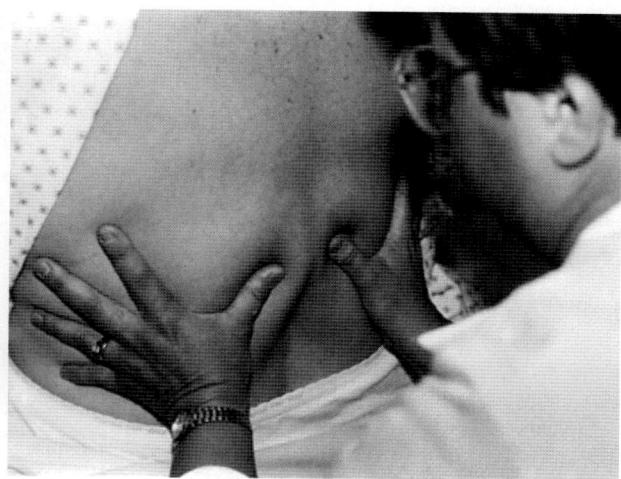

FIGURE 61-6 Assessment of thoracic excursion to determine the degree and symmetry of chest movement.

Percussion

Percussion is an assessment technique of producing sounds by tapping on the chest wall with the hand (see Chapter 4). Tapping on the chest wall between the ribs produces various sounds that are described in relation to their acoustic properties:

- *Resonant* sounds are low-pitched, hollow sounds heard over normal lung tissue.
- *Hyperresonant* sounds indicate an increased amount of air in the lungs or pleural space. These sounds are louder and lower pitched than resonant sounds. Hyperresonant sounds are produced by emphysema and pneumothorax; they are normally heard in children and in very thin adults.
- *Dull* sounds occur over dense lung tissue, such as a tumor or a consolidation. These sounds are thud-like and medium pitched and normally heard over the liver and heart.
- *Flat* notes are soft and high pitched; they result from percussion over airless tissue. This sound can be replicated with percussion of the thigh or bony structures.
- *Tympanic* notes are high, hollow, drum-like sounds heard with percussion over the stomach, a large tension pneumothorax, or a large air-filled chamber (such as the empty stomach).

Figure 61-8 illustrates the location of percussion sounds of the chest.

Begin percussion at the apices and proceed to the bases, moving from the posterior to the lateral and then to the anterior areas (see Figure 61-7). The posterior chest is best percussed with the client in an upright position and with arms crossed to separate the scapulae.

Percussion is also used to assess diaphragmatic excursion. Ask the client to take a deep breath and to hold it as you percuss down the posterior lung field and listen

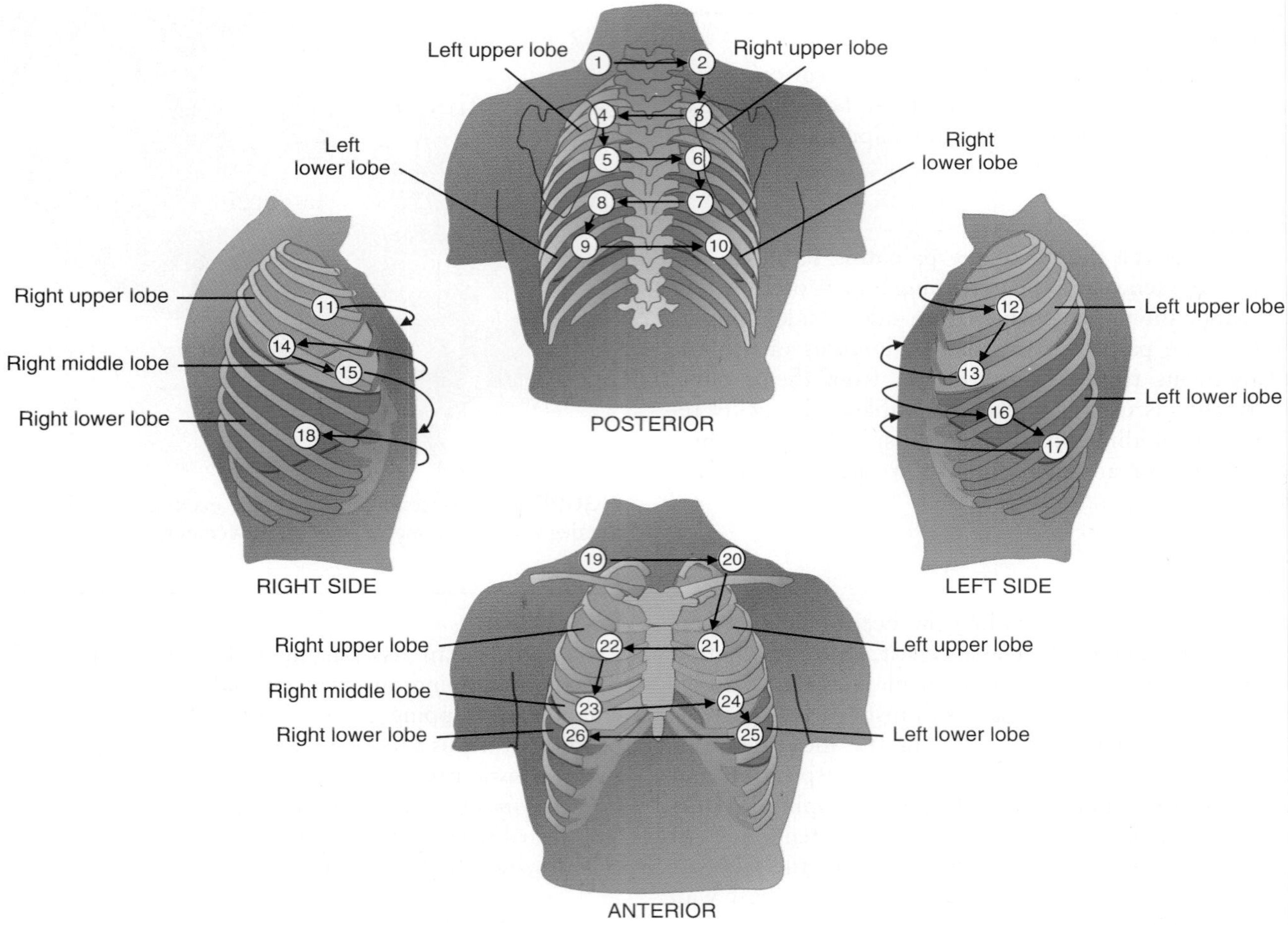

Left upper lobe → ① ② ← Right upper lobe

④ ③

Left lower lobe → ⑤ ⑥ ← Right lower lobe

⑧ ⑦

⑨ ⑩

POSTERIOR

Right upper lobe → ⑪

Right middle lobe → ⑭ ⑮

Right lower lobe → ⑱

RIGHT SIDE

⑫ ← Left upper lobe

⑬

Left lower lobe

⑯

⑰

LEFT SIDE

⑲ ⑳

Right upper lobe → ㉒ ㉑ ← Left upper lobe

Right middle lobe → ㉓ ㉔

Right lower lobe → ㉖ ㉕ ← Left lower lobe

ANTERIOR

FIGURE 61-7 Sequence of palpation, percussion, and auscultation of the thorax (posterior, lateral, and anterior).

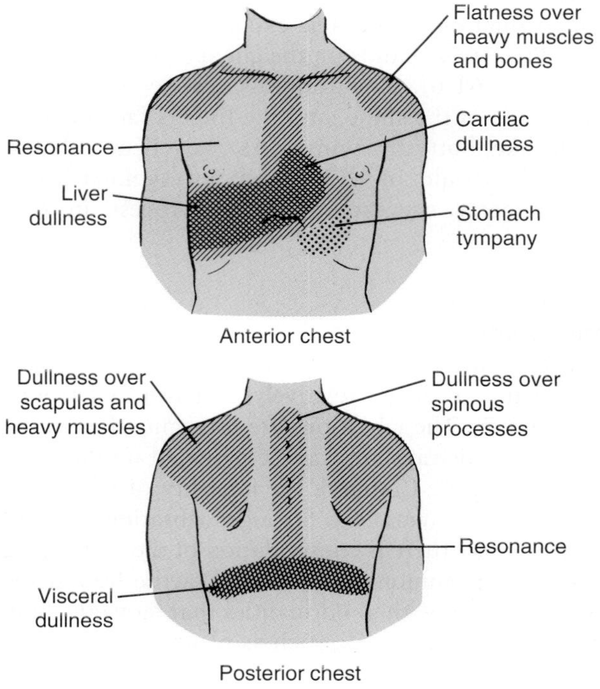

FIGURE 61-8 Location of thoracic percussion sounds and their associated structures.

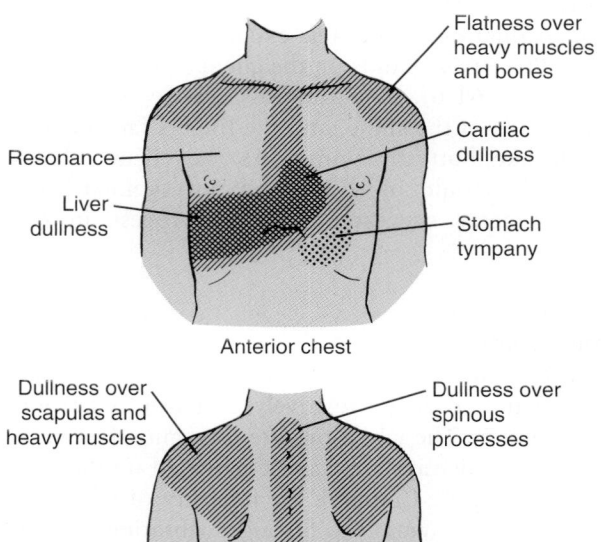

Flatness over heavy muscles and bones

Resonance

Cardiac dullness

Liver dullness

Stomach tympany

Anterior chest

Dullness over scapulas and heavy muscles

Dullness over spinous processes

Resonance

Visceral dullness

Posterior chest

for the percussion note to change from resonant to dull. Mark this area with a pen. The process is repeated after the client exhales, and again the area is marked.

Assess both the right and left sides. The distance between the two marks should be 3 to 6 cm; smaller spans are found in females and larger spans in males. The marks on the right are slightly higher because of the presence of the liver. A client with an elevated diaphragm related to a pathologic process has decreased diaphragmatic excursion.

If the client has lung disease in the lower lobes (consolidation or pleural fluid), the same dull percussion note is heard. When abnormalities are found, other diagnostic tests should be used to assess the problem fully.

Auscultation

Auscultation involves listening to chest sounds with a stethoscope. By listening to the lungs while the client breathes through an open mouth, you can assess the following:

- The character of the breath sounds
- The presence of adventitious sounds (described later)
- The character of the spoken and whispered voice

Figure 61-7 identifies a sequence for auscultation with comparison of sounds from right to left.

Listen to all areas of the lungs over a bare chest; do not listen to lungs over sheets, gowns, or shirts because sounds heard might be from the movement of fabric beneath the stethoscope. At each position, listen at the diaphragm for a full respiratory cycle of inspiration and expiration as the client breathes through the mouth.

Normal Breath Sounds

Breath sounds are noises resulting from the transmission of vibrations produced by the movement of air in the respiratory passages. Be familiar with the sounds created by normal air exchange and their location (Table 61-2). Normal breath sounds (vesicular, bronchial, and bronchovesicular) are heard in the locations identified in Figure 61-9. The sounds are described as follows:

- *Vesicular* breath sounds are heard throughout the chest and heard best in the bases of the lungs. They are low-pitched, soft, "swishing" sounds best heard during inspiration with an I:E ratio of 5:2.
- *Bronchial* breath sounds are heard over the manubrium in the large tracheal airways. Bronchial sounds, heard only anteriorly, are best heard during expiration with an expiratory-to-inspiratory (E:I) ratio of 2:1. These sounds are loud and high-pitched and have a hollow or harsh quality.
- *Bronchovesicular* sounds are heard anteriorly and posteriorly over the central, large airways. They are heard equally during inspiration and expiration and have a tubular or breezy-sounding quality.
- *Absent* or *diminished* breath sounds are confirmed during deep respirations after the client has been instructed to take deep breaths and sounds cannot be heard. "Shallow" breaths may produce diminished sounds in the peripheral lung regions, but "deep" breaths should produce normal vesicular sounds. If absent breath sounds are a new finding, immediate medical attention is required because this finding

TABLE 61-2	*Characteristics of Normal Breath Sounds*				
	Pitch	**Amplitude**	**Duration**	**Quality**	**Normal Location**
Bronchial (tracheal)	High	Loud	Inspiration < expiration	Harsh, hollow, tubular	Trachea and larynx
Bronchovesicular	Moderate	Moderate	Inspiration = expiration	Mixed	Over major bronchi where fewer alveoli are located: posterior, between scapulae, especially on the right; anterior, around the upper sternum in the first and second intercostal spaces
Vesicular	Low	Soft	Inspiration > expiration	Rustling, like the sound of the wind in the trees	Over peripheral lung fields where air flows through smaller bronchioles and alveoli

From Jarvis, C. (2000). *Physical examination and health assessment* (3rd ed.) Philadelphia: W.B. Saunders.

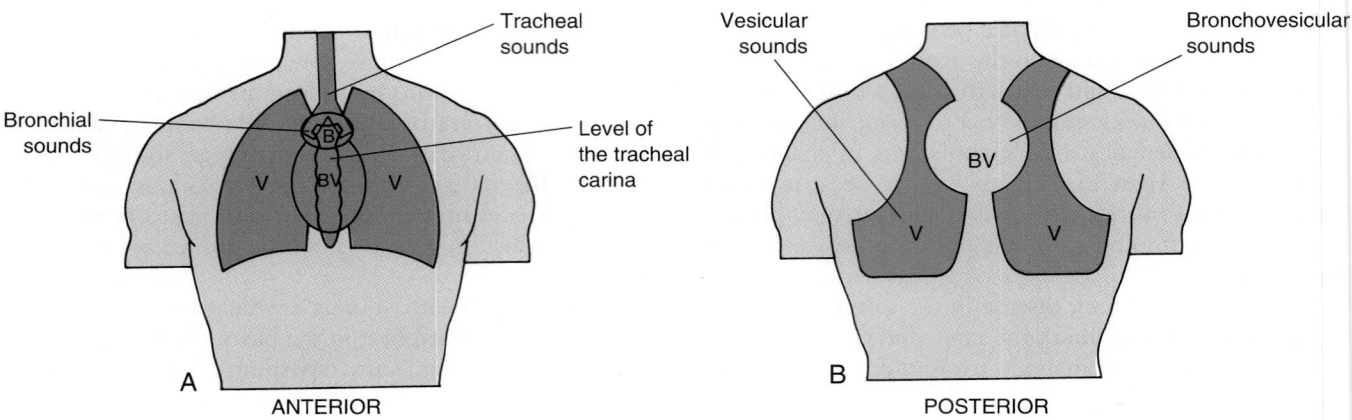

FIGURE 61-9 **A** and **B**, Location of normal breath sounds.

usually indicates pneumothorax or other respiratory emergency.

Adventitious Breath Sounds

Adventitious sounds (Table 61-3) are abnormal sounds superimposed on normal breath sounds. The current American Thoracic Society nomenclature for adventitious sounds is used throughout this chapter. Adventitious sounds include (1) crackles, (2) rhonchi, (3) wheezes, and (4) pleural friction rubs.

Crackles. *Crackles* (formerly called rales) are audible when there is a sudden opening of small airways that contain fluid. The sound of a crackle can be reproduced by rubbing a lock of hair between the thumb and finger close to the ear. Crackles are usually heard during inspiration and do not clear with a cough. Crackles can be found in clients with pulmonary edema, pulmonary fibrosis, or pneumonia.

Rhonchi. *Rhonchi* (also called *gurgles*) occur as the result of air passing through fluid-filled, narrow passages. Diseases in which there is excess mucus production, such as pneumonia, bronchitis, or bronchiectasis, are associated with rhonchi. Rhonchi are usually heard on expiration and may clear with a cough.

Wheezes. A *wheeze* is a continuous musical or hissing noise that results from the passage of air through a narrowed airway. Wheezes are heard during inspiration or expiration or both. Severe wheezes are audible without a stethoscope. Wheezing is commonly associated with asthma and its bronchoconstriction and edema, but foreign bodies can also cause airway narrowing and wheezing.

Pleural Friction Rubs. *Pleural friction rubs* are the result of pleural inflammation often associated with pleurisy, pneumonia, or pleural infarct. A rub is described as a creaking, grating noise similar to that made by two pieces of leather rubbing together. A rub is audible on inspiration and expiration over the area of the inflammation. Chest wall splinting can be associated with a pleural friction rub.

Voice Sounds

Assess voice sounds (vocal resonance) by auscultation if tactile fremitus is abnormal. Auscultation while the client speaks normally reveals muffled and indistinct sounds. The sound is louder medially over the larger airways and softens toward the periphery. Consolidation results in *bronchophony* or increased resonance so that when the client says "ninety-nine," it can be heard clearly.

If bronchophony is present, assess for egophony next. *Egophony* involves a change in the sound of the letter *e* to that of the letter *a*, indicating consolidation. The sound also has a nasal or bleating quality.

A third voice test for consolidation is *whispered pectoriloquy*. Ask the client to whisper "one-two-three." If the words are distinct, the abnormal finding of whispered pectoriloquy is present. Consolidation enhances the transmission of sound vibrations and results from lung tumors, pneumonia, or pulmonary fibrosis.

■ ASSESSMENT OF THE NOSE, PHARYNX, AND SINUSES
HISTORY

Upper respiratory problems can occur alone or progress to lower respiratory complications, such as viral infections.

Current Health

Chief Complaint

The client may present with a current complaint of nosebleeds (epistaxis); sinus infection; hay fever; postnasal

TABLE 61-3 *Adventitious Breath Sounds*

Sound*	Description	Mechanism	Clinical Example
Discontinuous Sounds			
Crackles—fine (rales, crepitations)	Discontinuous, high-pitched, short crackling, popping sounds heard during inspiration that are not cleared by coughing; this sound can be simulated by rolling a strand of hair between the fingers near the ear or by moistening the thumb and index finger and separating them near the ear	Inhaled air collides with previously deflated airways; airways suddenly pop open, creating a crackling sound as gas pressures between the two compartments equalize	*Late inspiratory crackles* occur with restrictive disease: pneumonia, heart failure, and interstitial fibrosis. *Early inspiratory crackles* occur with obstructive disease: chronic bronchitis, asthma, and emphysema
Crackles—coarse (coarse rales)	Loud, low-pitched, bubbling and gurgling sounds that start in early inspiration and may be present in expiration; may decrease somewhat by suctioning or coughing but will reappear shortly; sound like opening a self-fastening tape (Velcro) fastener	Inhaled air collides with secretions in the trachea and large bronchi	Pulmonary edema, pneumonia, pulmonary fibrosis, and in the terminally ill who have a depressed cough reflex
Atelectatic crackles (atelectatic rales)	Sound like fine crackles but do not last and are not pathologic; disappear after the first few breaths; heard in axillae and bases (usually dependent) of lungs	When sections of alveoli are not fully aerated, they deflate and accumulate secretions; crackles are heard when these sections reexpand with a few deep breaths	In aging adults, bedridden people, or in people just aroused from sleep
Pleural friction rub	A very superficial sound that is coarse and low-pitched; it has a grating quality as if two pieces of leather are being rubbed together; sounds just like crackles, but *close* to the ear; sounds louder if the stethoscope is pushed harder onto the chest wall; sound is inspiratory and expiratory	Caused when pleurae become inflamed and lose their normal lubricating fluid; their opposing roughened pleural surfaces rub together during respiration; heard best in the anterolateral wall where there is greatest lung mobility	Pleuritis, accompanied by pain with breathing (rub disappears after a few days if pleural fluid accumulates and separates pleurae)
Continuous Sounds			
Wheeze—high-pitched (sibilant rhonchi)	High-pitched, musical squeaking sounds that predominate in expiration but may occur in both expiration and inspiration	Air squeezed or compressed through passageways narrowed almost to closure by collapsing, swelling, secretions, or tumors; the passageway walls oscillate in apposition between the closed and barely open positions; the resulting sound is similar to a vibrating reed	Obstructive lung disease such as asthma or emphysema
Wheeze—low-pitched (sonorous rhonchi)	Low-pitched, musical snoring, moaning sounds; they are heard throughout the cycle, although they are more prominent on expiration; may clear somewhat by coughing	Air flow obstruction as described by the vibrating reed mechanism above; the pitch of the wheeze cannot be correlated with the size of the passageway that generates it	Bronchitis

Modified from Jarvis, C. (2000). *Physical examination and health assessment* (3rd ed.). Philadelphia: W.B. Saunders.

*Although nothing in clinical practice seems to differ more than the nomenclature of adventitious sounds, most authorities concur on two categories: (1) discontinuous, discrete crackling sounds and (2) continuous, coarse, or musical sounds.

drip; rhinitis; sneezing; or nasal, facial, or referred ear pain. Obstruction by engorged mucous membranes or nasal polyps may occlude the upper airway. Loss of or a decreased sense of smell may accompany manifestations of the common cold and allergies or may signal a more serious neurologic problem.

Inquire whether the client has experienced these manifestations previously and, if so, when and how often. Ask the client to describe self-treatment measures, such as nasal sprays, decongestants, antihistamines, and other over-the-counter and herbal cold and allergy medications. For example, a herbal remedy for hay fever is nettle *(Urtica dioica)*. See the earlier discussion of herbal remedies.

Symptom Analysis

Perform a complete symptom analysis to determine the nature of the problem, including its onset, duration, and severity.

Aggravating and Relieving Factors. Ask the client about factors that alleviate or worsen the manifestations, such as increased humidity, sitting upright, lying supine, weather and seasonal changes, or allergies. Nasal and sinus problems may be allergy related and provoked by pollen, fumes, smoke, animal dander, or dust particles. Nosebleeds may increase during the winter months if mucous membranes are dry because of insufficient humidity.

Associated Manifestations. A foul taste in the mouth, unpleasant breath odor *(halitosis)*, nasal obstruction, and facial pain (particularly over the frontal and maxillary sinuses) may accompany sinusitis. Chronic sinusitis may be accompanied by headache or facial pain present on awakening and diminishing during the day (because the sinuses drain when the client sits or stands).

Past Health History

Ask about past problems with frequent colds, sinus infections, nasal stuffiness, or trauma (fracture). Explore episodes of epistaxis for cause (hypertension), frequency, and treatment (cauterization or nasal packing).

PHYSICAL EXAMINATION

Inspect and palpate the client's nose and sinuses. The structures assessed include the external nose, vestibule, nasal mucosa, septum, turbinates, nasal canals, and sinuses. Function of the first cranial nerve (olfactory) is usually not tested unless a deficit in the sense of smell is reported or suspected.

Nose

External Nose

Inspect and palpate the external nose for deviations from normal alignment, symmetry, color, discharge, nasal flar-

ing, lesions, and tenderness. Normal findings are listed. The skin color over the nose is the same as that of the facial skin. Alignment is straight and symmetrical without deviation from the midline. Discharge from the nares (nostrils) should be absent, and the nares should not flare (spread) with respirations. The client is able to breathe quietly through the nose rather than breathe through the mouth. Masses, lesions, and tenderness are absent.

Check the nasal canals for patency by asking the client to occlude one naris with a finger and to breathe through the open naris while closing the mouth. Repeat this for the opposite naris. The client should be able to breathe without difficulty through both nares. Ask the client to tip the head back, and inspect the outer nares for crusting, bleeding, or dryness, which should be absent.

Internal Nose

Next inspect the vestibules with a penlight while the client's head is tipped back. Normal findings include coarse hairs, a clear passage without discharge, and a midline septum. Further examination of the internal nose requires the use of a nasal speculum and is not conducted unless indicated. If a detailed examination of the internal nose is performed, either attach a nasal speculum tip to the otoscope head or use a metal nasal speculum (Figure 61-10) and penlight for illumination. While the client tips the head back, gently insert the speculum into one naris, taking care not to scrape the mucosa. Inspect one naris at a time.

Hold the speculum correctly, and insert the blades gently about a half-inch into the nostril. Gain additional control of the speculum by resting the index finger of the dominant hand on the side of the client's nose. Steady the client's head with the nondominant hand. Open the blades gently and vertically while avoiding pressure on

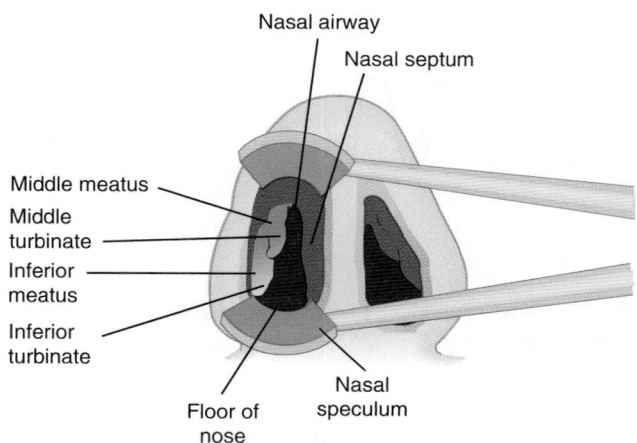

FIGURE 61-10 Internal inspection of the nose with a nasal speculum.

the septum and turbinates. Slowly move the head to inspect all areas of the nasal chamber. Observe the condition of the mucous membrane (pallor, redness, swelling). Normally the mucosa is moist and dark pink without sign of inflammation, pallor, or a blue color. The presence of discharge is abnormal. The septum divides the nasal cavity into halves without deviation, masses, perforation, or exudate. The turbinates are the same color as the mucosa and should be free of exudate, swelling, or inflammation (only the inferior and part of the middle turbinate are visible; the superior part is not). Look for polyps and other masses. Observe mucous plugs for color, consistency, amount, and odor.

Inspection may be hampered by nasal congestion. For adequate inspection, shrinking the nasal mucosa with a topical vasoconstrictor (phenylephrine hydrochloride) may be necessary. When the agent is instilled into the nose, ask the client to say "*e*" and hold the sound. Use of this technique raises the posterior tongue, occludes the upper airway, and prevents the fluid from running into the pharynx.

Nasopharynx

The nasopharynx is best examined with a mirror while the tongue is depressed with a tongue blade or pulled forward and grasped with a gauze sponge. Prevent fogging of the mirror by warming it before putting it into the mouth. Hold the mirror to one side of the uvula, and focus light on it. A small part of the nasopharynx can be observed with a nasal speculum. Specialists may use a nasopharyngoscope to examine the nasopharynx.

Paranasal Sinuses

Assess the paranasal sinuses by (1) inspecting and palpating the soft overlying tissues, (2) observing any nasal secretions (it is possible to determine which sinus is infected according to where discharge appears), and (3) transilluminating the maxillary and frontal sinuses. Palpate and percuss the frontal and maxillary sinuses to assess for swelling and tenderness, which are normally absent.

Palpate the frontal sinuses simultaneously by placing the thumbs above the eyes, just under the bony ridge of the orbits, and apply gentle pressure. Palpate the maxillary sinuses by using either the index and third fingers or thumbs to press gently on each side of the nose just under the zygomatic bones. Use direct percussion over the eyebrows for the frontal sinuses and on either side of the nose below the eyes in line with the pupils for the maxillary sinuses.

Transillumination is a technique used to assess the sinuses further if tenderness is present. Either a penlight or the otoscope handle fitted with a transilluminator head (see Chapter 4) is used. Darken the room. Place the light against the orbital bones immediately below the eyebrows and direct upward. Shield the light source with one hand. Normally a reddish glow appears above the frontal sinus area. Lack of illumination may indicate si-

nus congestion and accumulation of purulent fluid. Assess the maxillary sinuses by placing the light beneath the center of the eyes and the zygomatic bones and directing it down and in toward the roof of the mouth. Ask the client to open the mouth. A glow should appear on the hard palate on the side being illuminated. For a more complete assessment of sinus conditions, radiologic studies may be done. Air, normally present in the sinuses, appears as a dark area on a developed film.

Smell

The senses of taste and smell are closely related. Many conditions affect taste and smell, such as viral infections, normal aging, head injuries, and local obstruction. Some medications can affect smell and taste, such as metronidazole, local anesthetics, clofibrate, some antibiotics, some antineoplastics, allopurinol, phenylbutazone, levodopa, codeine, morphine, carbamazepine, lithium, and trifluoperazine. Smell impairment may be (1) *hyposmia* (a decrease in smell sensitivity) or (2) *anosmia* (bilateral and complete absence of smell sensitivity).

Assess smell by having the client identify various odors. Various substances are placed in individual test tubes (covered to eliminate visual cues). Test each nostril separately; have the client sniff the tubes (first with the eyes closed and then with the eyes open). Document whether the client can (1) perceive each odor and (2) identify each odor accurately.

Smell is perceived mainly via the olfactory nerves, although some smell is perceived through the trigeminal nerves. Trigeminal irritants are perceived even by clients with anosmia. (Therefore a client who claims not to smell trigeminal irritants may be experiencing a conversion hysterical loss of smell rather than hyposmia or anosmia.) A client with a tracheostomy may not be able to smell because of limited upper-airway movement. Olfactory stimulants and trigeminal stimulants commonly used to assess smell are listed in Box 61-1. See Chapter 69 for further discussion of smell assessment.

DIAGNOSTIC TESTS

Diagnostic procedures augment the assessment of clients with respiratory disorders. To clarify which diagnostic test is used when and for what purpose, the tests are discussed here in the framework of what is being evaluated:

BOX 61-1	*Substances Used in Assessing Smell*
Olfactory Stimulants	**Trigeminal Stimulants**
Coffee (instant powder)	Ammonia
Phenylethyl alcohol	Acetone
Almond oil	Menthol
Peppermint	Distilled water
Musk	

functional status, anatomy, or specimens. The diagnostic test may be used for any or all of these reasons. This listing is limited to the most commonly used diagnostic tests.

TESTS TO EVALUATE RESPIRATORY FUNCTION

The diagnostic tests used to evaluate the functional status of the pulmonary system include the following:

- Pulmonary function tests
- Pulse oximetry
- Capnography
- Arterial blood gas (ABG) analysis
- Ventilation-perfusion studies

Pulmonary Function Tests

Pulmonary function tests (PFTs) provide information about respiratory function by measuring lung volumes, lung mechanics, and diffusion capabilities of the lungs (see the Unit 14 Anatomy and Physiology Review). PFTs performed in a pulmonary function laboratory can measure respiratory volumes and capacities. PFTs done outside a laboratory are modified to include ventilation tests of forced expiratory volume, vital capacity, and maximal voluntary ventilation measures. A measure of expiratory flow obtained with a hand-held device is called a *peak flow*. Many clients with asthma use a peak flowmeter (Figure 61-11) at home to monitor changes in their condition and responses to treatment.

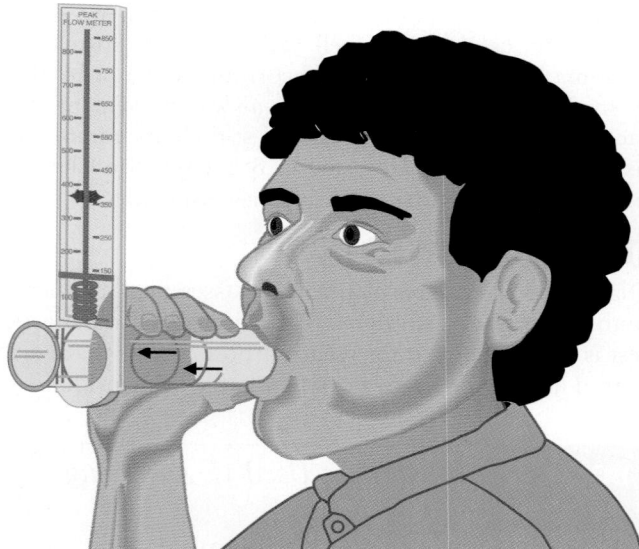

FIGURE 61-11 Use of a peak flowmeter to measure peak expiratory flow volume. The client stands and exhales into the mouthpiece. Normal peak flow values for adults are based on age, gender, height, and underlying lung disorder. Normal values range from 300 to 700 L/min but are best assessed compared against a client's baseline values.

Education about the purpose, procedure, and implications of the test is performed by the nurse and reinforced by the examiner. Explicit instructions for each maneuver are given during the testing. Instruct clients that it is normal to feel short of breath after the test. Clients should not smoke or use a bronchodilator for 6 hours before undergoing a PFT.

Forced Spirometry

The flow and volume capacities of the lungs are measured with forced spirometry. The volume of air inhaled and exhaled is plotted against time during a series of ventilatory maneuvers. Flow volume loops are created as visual patterns. Normal loop spirograms and spirogram patterns with obstructive and restrictive disorders are shown in Figure 61-12. Table 61-4 defines maneuvers used to test lung mechanics.

Lung Volume Determination

Lung volume is measured by a gas dilution technique or body plethysmography. The two most commonly used gas dilution methods are (1) the *open-circuit* nitrogen method and (2) the *closed-circuit* helium method. These tests are most often used to measure functional residual capacity (FRC).

In the open-circuit method, all exhaled gas is collected while the client breathes pure oxygen. Measurement of the total amount of nitrogen washed out from the lungs permits calculation of the volume of gas present in the lungs at the beginning of the maneuver. The open-circuit method also allows assessment of the uniformity of ventilation in the lungs.

When helium is used to test the lungs in the closed-circuit method, the client inhales a mixture of air with a known concentration of helium. Helium does not significantly diffuse into the pulmonary bed. The helium diffuses throughout the air in the breathing box and lungs. The client exhales and is disconnected from the box. Changes in helium concentration in the box are computed to determine the total lung volume.

The body plethysmograph, or *body box*, is a device used to measure lung volumes. The lung volume changes that occur with obstructive and restrictive lung disorders are shown in Table 61-5. While sitting in the airtight box, the client is instructed to perform a panting maneuver. Changes in the box pressure reflect changes in thoracic volume. Clients who cannot pant, who cannot tolerate closed spaces, or who have equipment that would interfere with the procedure cannot be tested by this method.

Diffusion Capacity

Studies of the lung diffusing capacity (DL) or carbon monoxide lung diffusion capacity [DL_{CO}]) measure gas transfer of carbon monoxide (CO) across the alveolar capillary membrane. The DL indicates the ease with which CO diffuses across the alveolar capillary membrane and binds with hemoglobin. (Hemoglobin has 250 times greater affinity for CO than for oxygen.) With normal hemoglobin and normal ventilatory function, the only limiting factor to diffusion of CO is the alveolar capillary membrane. The test involves inhaling room air mixed with 0.3% CO and 10% helium.

In many diseases, such as sarcoidosis, systemic lupus erythematosus, and emphysema, the alveolar membrane is thickened and oxygen transfer and diffusion are impaired, resulting in a decrease in DL. An increased DL is found with exercise, polycythemia, and hypervolemia.

Instruct the client to exhale forcefully, then inhale quickly, and hold the breath for 10 seconds and exhale. A sample of the exhaled air is collected for analysis.

Pulse Oximetry

Procedure

Pulse oximetry is a safe and simple method of assessing oxygenation. It has the advantage that the data are obtained noninvasively and continuously. Previously oxygenation was most commonly assessed by use of ABG determinations. Pulse oximetry was originally used in surgery but has been extended to most acute care settings. In fact, it is so common that it has been called the "fifth vital sign."

The pulse oximeter (Figure 61-13) passes a beam of light through the tissue, and a sensor attached to the finger tip, toe, or ear lobe measures the amount of light absorbed by the oxygen-saturated hemoglobin. The oximeter then gives a reading of the percentage of hemoglobin that is saturated with oxygen (SaO_2). SaO_2 is closely correlated with the saturations obtained from the pulse oximeter if it is above 70%. Table 61-6 provides a quick guide for comparison of SaO_2 and partial pressure of arterial oxygen (PaO_2).

Limitations of pulse oximetry are still present despite the advancement of the technology. Motion at the sensor site changes light absorption. The motion mimics the pulsatile motion of blood, and because the detector cannot distinguish between movement of blood and movement of the finger, results can be inaccurate. Hypotension, hypothermia, and vasoconstriction reduce arterial blood flow to the sensor; keeping the finger warm may help with this problem. Sensors for the nose can also be

FIGURE 61-12 A normal flow volume loop pattern and patterns for obstructive and restrictive lung disease. (From Kersten, L.D., et al. [1989]. *Respiratory nursing* [p. 382]. Philadelphia: W.B. Saunders.)

LOOP SPIROGRAM PATTERNS AND EXPLANATION

NORMAL PATTERN

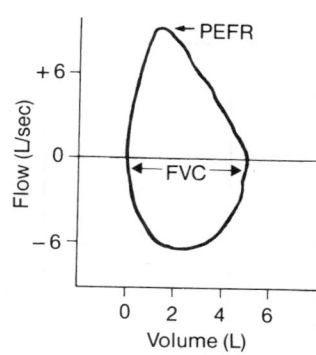

The expiratory curve shows a straight line decrease in flow after peak flow (PEFR). The inspiratory curve has a normal rounded pattern.

OBSTRUCTIVE PATTERN

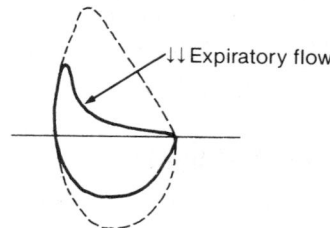

The expiratory curve shows scooping at low lung volumes (minimal to mild obstruction). As obstruction increases, the scooping becomes more marked and is accompanied by a decreased $FEF_{50\%}$ (mild to moderate obstruction).

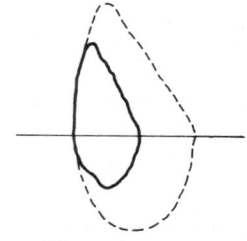

The expiratory curve shows a sudden decrease in PEFR in an "index finger" pattern, followed by a nearly horizontal line.

The inspiratory curve is normal, except for absolute decreases in flow rates.

RESTRICTIVE PATTERN

The entire loop resembles a miniature normal flow-volume loop. The FVC is markedly reduced. The expiratory curve shows a straight line decrease in flow with decreasing lung volumes. Peak flow rates may be normal, increased, or decreased, depending on the degree of respiratory impairment.

*The dotted lines represent the boundaries of the normal flow-volume loop.

TABLE 61-4   *Pulmonary Function Test (PFT) Components*

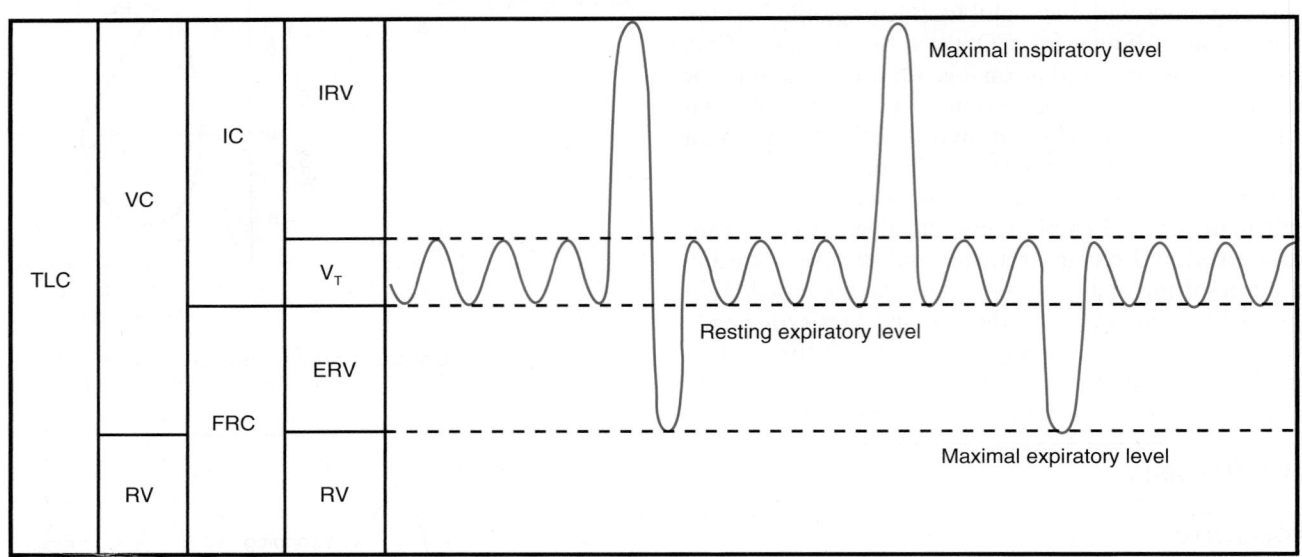

Lung Volumes and Capacities

VC	Vital capacity	Volume of air that is measured during a slow, maximal expiration after a maximal inspiration; normal range varies with age, gender, and body size
IC	Inspiratory capacity	Largest volume of air that can be inhaled from resting expiratory volume
ERV	Expiratory reserve volume	Largest volume of air exhaled from resting end-expiratory level
FRC	Functional residual capacity	Volume of air remaining in lungs at resting end-expiratory level
IRV	Inspiratory reserve volume	Volume of air that can be inhaled from a tidal volume level
RV	Residual volume	Volume of air remaining in the lungs at the end of maximal expiration
TLC	Total lung capacity	Volume of air contained in the lungs after maximal inspiration
V_T	Tidal volume	Volume of air inhaled or exhaled during each respiratory cycle; normal range is 400-700 ml

Lung Mechanics

FVC	Forced vital capacity	Maximal volume of air that can be forcefully expired after a maximal inspiration to total lung capacity
FEV_1	Forced expiratory volume	Volume of air expired during a given time interval (t in seconds) from the beginning of an FVC maneuver
$FEF_{25\%-75\%}$	Forced expiratory flow$_{25\%-75\%}$	Average of flow during the middle half of an FVC maneuver
PEFR	Peak expiratory flow rate	Maximal flow rate attained during an FVC maneuver
MVV	Maximal voluntary ventilation	Largest volume that can be breathed during a 10- to 15-second interval with voluntary effort
MIP	Maximal inspiratory pressure	Greatest negative or subatmospheric pressure that can be generated during inspiration against an occluded airway
MEP	Maximal expiratory pressure	Highest positive pressure than can be generated during a forceful expiratory effort against an occluded airway

monly used. If the client has a tendency to bleed or is receiving anticoagulant medication, pressure is needed for a longer period.

When interpreting the results, note whether the client is receiving oxygen; record the amount and source of oxygen on the laboratory request form. The results are evaluated in light of the oxygen needed. For example, if the PaO_2 is 85 mm Hg with 50% oxygen, the client has a more significant problem with oxygen transport than does a client whose PaO_2 is 85 mm Hg with room air (21% oxygen).

Complications of arterial sampling include bleeding or hematoma formation at the site and injury to the artery and surrounding structures. Report any of these complications to the physician.

Ventilation-Perfusion Lung Scan

Ventilation-perfusion ($\dot{V}/\dot{Q}$) scanning is used to assess lung ventilation and lung perfusion. ($\dot{V}/\dot{Q}$) cans are valuable in identifying pulmonary embolism, pulmonary infarction, emphysema, fibrosis, and bronchiectasis. Quantitative perfusion scans may be helpful in preoperative assessment of clients undergoing surgical resection of thoracic malignancy.

Procedure

The scan consists of two parts, which may be done together or separately: (1) assessment of the distribution of ventilation *(ventilation scan)* and (2) assessment of the pulmonary vasculature *(perfusion scan)*.

Preprocedure Care

Explain the procedure to the client. The test is painless except for local discomfort when radiologic material is injected for the perfusion scan. The client will hear clicking noises during the scan, but the noise is not loud. If the client has dyspnea while lying down, reassure the client that sitting up is possible during the procedure. Radiation exposure is minimal. The client can remain dressed with all metal items removed. The procedure takes 30 to 60 minutes to complete.

Ventilation Scan

Radioactive gas is inhaled and produces an image of the areas where ventilation is occurring. Assessment of the pattern of deposition of radioactive gas in the alveoli is also possible.

Ventilation images are compared with the pictures taken during the perfusion scan. The same amount of radioactivity should be discernible on both ventilation and perfusion pictures. If there are areas in which there is ventilation but little or no perfusion, a pulmonary embolus is suspected. Further assessment may be needed. If there is doubt about the cause of impaired perfusion, pulmonary angiography may be needed.

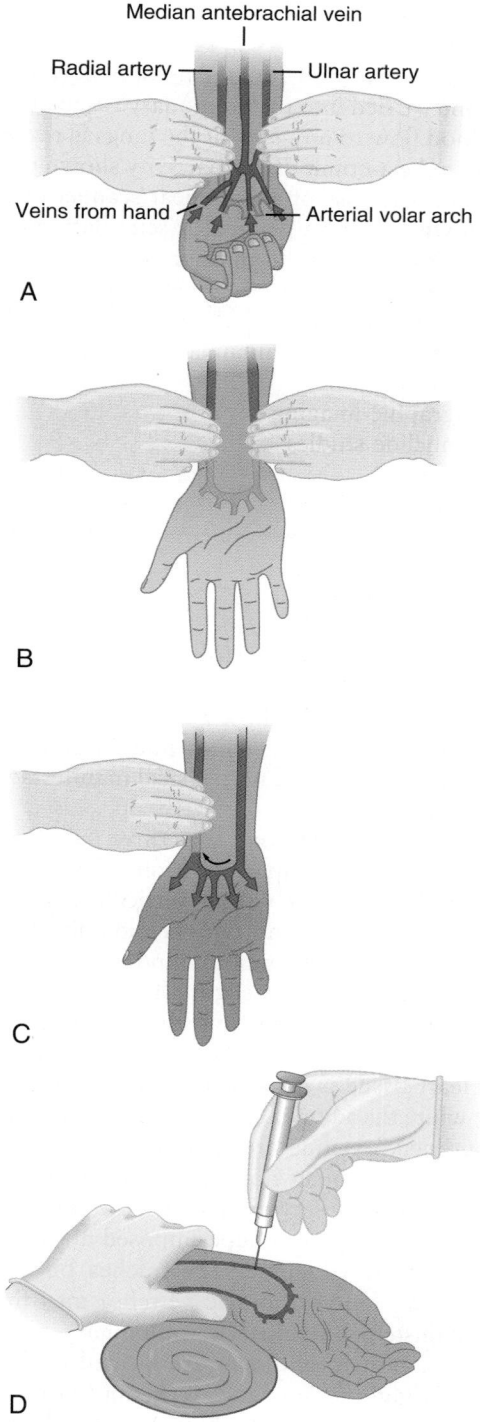

FIGURE 61-14 Obtaining a sample of arterial blood by arterial puncture. First, perform Allen's test, a quick assessment of collateral circulation in the hand. This test is essential before radial artery puncture. **A,** Occlude both the radial and the ulnar arteries with your fingers. Ask the client to close the hand into a fist. **B,** When the client opens the hand with the arteries still occluded, the hand is pale. **C,** When you release either the radial or the ulnar artery, the client's hand should become pink because of collateral circulation. Assess the patency of each of the two arteries in this way, one at a time. **D,** If collateral circulation is adequate, you can draw arterial blood from the radial artery with a heparinized needle and syringe as shown.

Perfusion Scan

Radiologic material (non–iodine-based) is injected intravenously and carried into the pulmonary vasculature. Decreased blood flow to any part of the lungs is revealed as a decrease in the amount of radioactivity shown on either the x-ray film with use of a rectilinear scanner or on Polaroid film with use of a gamma or scintillation camera. Scanning is done in both the anterior and posterior views.

TESTS TO EVALUATE ANATOMIC STRUCTURES

Diagnostic tests used to evaluate anatomic structures include the following:

- Radiographic imaging
- Radionuclide studies
- Endoscopy
- Alveolar lavage

Radiography

Chest X-Ray Studies

Chest x-ray studies provide information about the chest that may not be available through other assessment means and may be able to illustrate graphically the cause of respiratory dysfunction. Chest films may reveal abnormalities when there are no physical manifestations of pulmonary disease.

Chest films show the bony structures (ribs, sternum, clavicles, scapulae, and upper portion of the humerus). The vertebral column is visible vertically through the middle of the thorax. The two hemidiaphragms normally appear rounded, smooth, and sharply defined; the right hemidiaphragm is slightly higher than the left. The junction of the rib cage and the diaphragm, called the *costophrenic angle,* is normally clearly visible and angled. Heart tissue is dense and appears white but less intensely white than bone. Normally the heart shadow is clearly outlined, extends primarily onto the left side of the thorax, and occupies no more than one third of the chest width. Close observation shows the trachea in the upper middle chest almost superimposed above the cervical and thoracic vertebrae. The trachea bifurcates at the level of the fourth thoracic vertebra into the right and left mainstem bronchi. The pulmonary blood vessels, bronchi, and lymph nodes are located in the hilum on both the right and left sides of the mid-thorax. Lung tissue appears black on x-ray film. Vascular lung structures are visible as white, thin, wispy strings fanning out from the hilum (Figure 61-15).

Chest x-ray studies may be performed for the following reasons:

- As part of a routine screening procedure
- When pulmonary disease is suspected
- To monitor the status of respiratory disorders and abnormalities (pleural effusion, atelectasis, tubercular lesions)

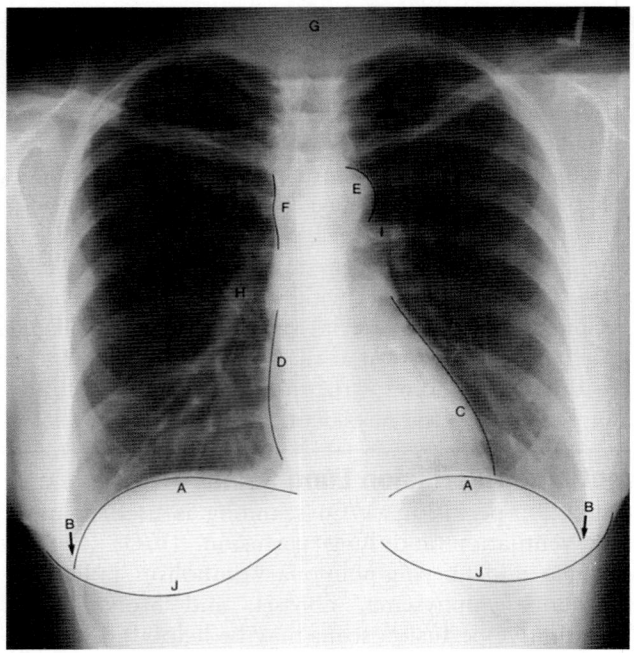

FIGURE 61-15 A normal chest x-ray film taken from the posteroanterior view. The backward L in the upper right corner is placed on the film to indicate the left side of the client's chest. **A,** diaphragm: **B,** costophrenic angle; **C,** left ventricle; **D,** right atrium; **E,** aortic arch; **F,** superior vena cava; **G,** trachea; **H,** right bronchus; **I,** left bronchus; **J,** breast shadows.

- To confirm endotracheal or tracheostomy tube placement
- After traumatic chest injury
- In any other situation in which radiographic information helps in the management of a respiratory problem

Procedure

Routine adult chest x-ray studies are performed with the client standing or sitting facing the x-ray film, with the chest and shoulders in direct contact with the film cassette.

Preprocedure Care

Instruct the client about the need for radiologic testing. The test is painless, and exposure to radiation is minimal. The client must remove all jewelry and underclothes and put on a gown. Assess the client's pregnancy status; pregnant women should not be exposed to radiation. All gonads should be shielded during the study. The test takes 5 to 10 minutes to complete.

Several positions are possible and are described as follows.

Posteroanterior View. The client's shoulders are rotated forward to pull the scapulae away from the lung field.

The x-ray beam penetrates from the back for the posteroanterior (PA) position. The radiograph is usually taken on full inspiration, which causes the diaphragm to move downward. Radiographs taken on expiration are sometimes requested to demonstrate the degree of diaphragm movement or to assist in the assessment and diagnosis of pneumothorax.

Anteroposterior View. For clients who cannot be transported to the radiology department, portable chest radiography may be performed. These radiographs are usually taken with the film placed behind the client and the x-ray beam entering from the front of the chest (the AP position). Because the x-ray beam enters from the front, the heart appears larger than it really is and larger than on a PA view.

Lateral View. The lateral view usually accompanies a standard PA view. It is taken from the right or left side of the chest. The arms are raised above the head, and the side of the chest is placed against the film. The lateral view allows better visualization of the heart and the dome of the diaphragm. In conjunction with a PA film, a lateral radiograph gives a three-dimensional view, allowing more specific identification of the location of an abnormality.

Lateral Decubitus View. The lateral decubitus (from the Latin "lying down") position may be used when it is necessary to determine whether opaque areas on the pleura are due to solid or liquid media. The client lies on the right or left side, depending on which side of the chest is being assessed. In a left lateral decubitus position, the client lies on the left side.

Oblique View. The oblique position is used to visualize behind and around underlying structures. The shoulders are rotated to either the right or left of the film. By turning the client, the examiner can shift the angle at which the x-ray beam passes through the chest. In a right oblique position, the right side is closest to the film. The view may be taken from an anterior or posterior position.

Lordotic View. The lordotic position, which consists of a forward curve of the lumbar spine, is useful if clearer visualization of the upper lung fields is needed. The angle of the cathode x-ray tube is lowered and the beam directed at an upward angle. This angle results in removal of the clavicles and first and second ribs from the field of vision.

Fluoroscopy

Fluoroscopy makes it possible for the chest and intrathoracic structures to be observed while they function dynamically (see Chapter 4). Fluoroscopy is not used routinely; rather, it is used when continuous observation of the thorax is an advantage (observing transbronchial passage of biopsy forceps during bronchoscopy). Other uses for fluoroscopy include the following:

- Observing the diaphragm during inspiration and expiration
- Detecting mediastinal movement during deep breathing
- Assessing the heart, blood vessels, and related structures
- Identifying esophageal abnormalities
- Detecting mediastinal masses

Instruct the client about the need for this painless test. Sometimes a radiopaque (non–iodine-based) contrast agent is administered intravenously to help distinguish the structures being assessed. The client must remove all jewelry and underclothes and put on a gown. The test takes 30 to 45 minutes to complete. Exposure to radiation is minimal, but pregnant women should not be exposed to fluoroscopy.

Images obtained by fluoroscopy are not as clear and definitive as those obtained on a standard chest film. If abnormalities are discovered, still photographs and cinefluorography may be used to obtain a permanent record. Cinefluorographs are motion pictures that allow more leisurely study and restudy of the area photographed without exposing radiology personnel or clients to unnecessary radiation.

Computed Tomography

Computed tomography (CT) provides more sophisticated tomography than is possible with conventional x-ray equipment (see Chapter 4). CT scans are particularly helpful in identifying peripheral (pleural) or mediastinal disorders. Special techniques can be used to view pulmonary nodules. Thin cuts of CT scans are used in diagnosing interstitial lung disorders such as pulmonary fibrosis and bronchiectasis.

Spiral or helical CT scan of the chest is an alternative to the lung scan for identifying pulmonary emboli. Spiral CT is easily and rapidly performed while images are obtained continuously as the client moves through the scanner. The chest can be imaged in less than 30 seconds, allowing the study to be performed with just one breath-hold. Images are clearer because artifact from client motion or breathing is reduced or eliminated (Figure 61-16).

Magnetic Resonance Imaging

Magnetic resonance imaging (MRI) employs magnetic fields rather than radiation to create images of body structures. MRI is used in much the same way as CT, although MRI is more definitive than CT because it creates more detailed images of anatomic structures. See Chapter 4 for a detailed discussion of MRI and client preparation.

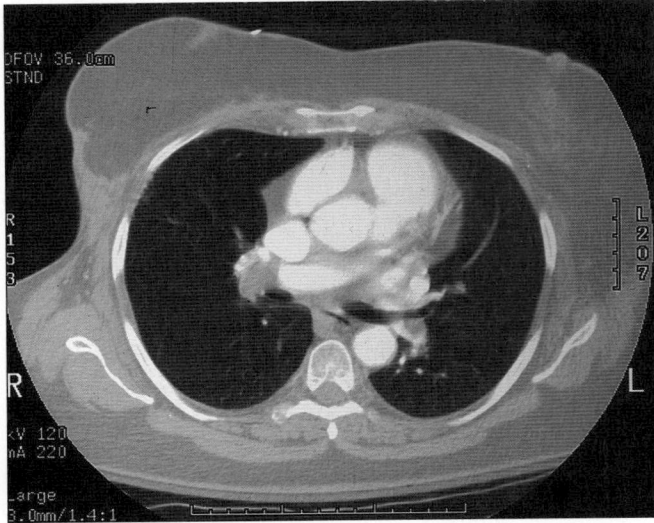

FIGURE 61-16 A spiral CT scan can be used to diagnose pulmonary embolus. This scan shows a pulmonary embolus in the pulmonary artery.

Ultrasonography

Ultrasonic waves (sound waves too high in frequency for a human ear to detect) are used diagnostically to assess various body structures. Ultrasonography may be used in conjunction with other pulmonary diagnostic procedures, such as thoracentesis and pleural biopsy, to assess fluid or fibrotic abnormalities. Ultrasonography is especially helpful and accurate in detecting the amount and location of 50 ml or less of pleural fluid. In comparison, positive detection by chest radiography requires at least 500 ml of liquid. If the technique is used in combination with thoracentesis, the ultrasonographer can determine the best location for needle placement as well as the depth of the fluid. This approach facilitates obtaining an adequate amount of fluid for laboratory analysis without unnecessary puncturing and probing.

The client can either remain dressed or put on a gown (see Chapter 4 for client preparation needed for ultrasonography). The test takes 15 to 30 minutes to complete.

Gallium Scans

Gallium scanning is usually done 24 to 48 hours after intravenous injection of radioactive gallium citrate. Many organs take up radioactive gallium, as do some tumors and areas of inflammation. A gallium scan might be used to distinguish embolism from pneumonitis as the cause of an infiltrate on a chest radiograph. Gallium has an affinity for areas of inflammation, such as those associated with pneumonia; however, little inflammation occurs with a nonseptic pulmonary embolism. Therefore gallium accumulates around pneumonitis but not around a pulmonary embolism. The usefulness of gallium scanning in clinical pulmonary assessment is limited.

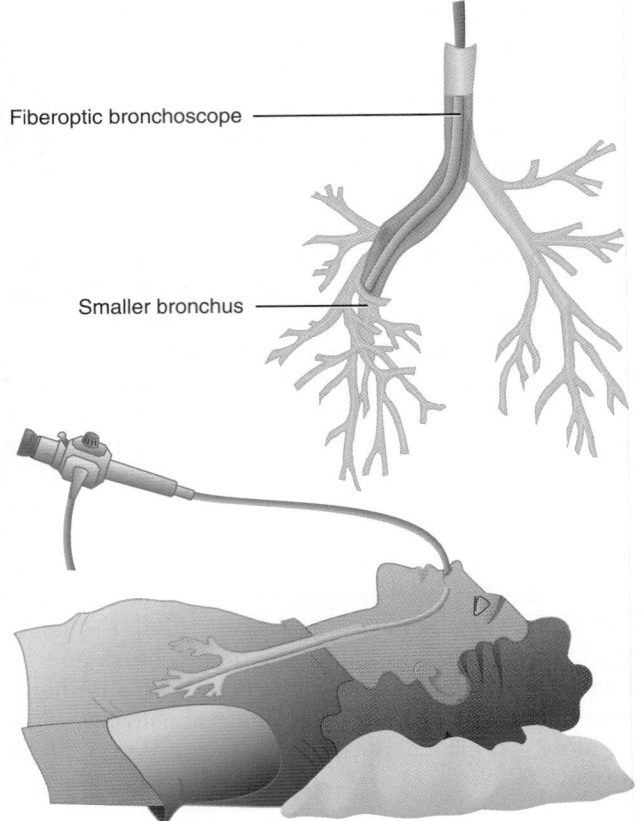

FIGURE 61-17 Bronchoscopy.

Educate the client about the test. The test is painless except for local pain at the injection site. Gallium is not iodine based and produces no side effects. The client returns for serial scans at 24, 48, or 72 hours. Scanning is performed with the client supine. The client may remain dressed but must remove all metal objects. The scan takes 45 to 60 minutes to complete.

Bronchoscopy

Procedure

Bronchoscopy involves passage of a lighted bronchoscope into the bronchial tree (Figure 61-17). It may be performed with rigid steel or flexible fiberoptic instruments. Bronchoscopy may be performed for diagnostic or therapeutic purposes. Diagnostic purposes include the following:

- Examination of tissue
- Further evaluation of a tumor for potential surgical resection
- Collection of tissue specimens for diagnosis
- Evaluation of bleeding sites

Therapeutic bronchoscopy is used to accomplish the following:

- Remove foreign bodies

- Remove thick, viscous secretions
- Treat postoperative atelectasis
- Destroy and remove lesions

Preprocedure Care

Explain the procedure to the client and family, and obtain informed consent. Instruct the client not to eat or drink anything for 6 hours before the test. Explain that the throat may be sore after bronchoscopy and that he or she will experience some initial difficulty in swallowing. Before sedation the client should remove dentures, contact lenses, and other prostheses. The client undresses and puts on a gown. Local anesthesia and intravenous sedation are used to suppress cough and to relieve anxiety. A topical anesthetic agent is also sprayed into the back of the throat. The test takes 30 to 45 minutes to complete.

During the procedure, the client lies supine with the head hyperextended. Monitor vital signs and oxygen saturation, talk to and reassure the client, and assist the physician as necessary.

Postprocedure Care

After the procedure, monitor vital signs according to agency protocol. Observe the client for respiratory distress, including dyspnea, changes in respiratory rate, use of accessory muscles, and changes in or absent lung sounds. Expectorated secretions are inspected for evidence of hemoptysis. Nothing is given by mouth until the cough and swallow reflexes have returned, usually in 1 to 2 hours. When the client can swallow, feeding may begin with ice chips and small sips of water. If sore throat develops, it can be treated with warm saline gargles and throat lozenges once the client's gag reflex has returned.

Lung sounds are monitored for 24 hours. Development of asymmetrical or adventitious sounds should be reported to the physician. Pneumothorax has been noted after bronchoscopy.

Laryngoscopy

Laryngoscopy is visual examination of the larynx and is used to diagnose laryngeal papillomas, nodules, polyps, or cancer. Laryngoscopy can be performed during bronchoscopy or as a separate procedure. Two approaches are used: indirect and direct. Care of the client having a laryngoscopy is similar to that for bronchoscopy.

Indirect Laryngoscopy

Indirect visualization allows inspection of the nasopharynx and posterior soft palate using a small mirror or an instrument resembling a telescope. While the mirror is inserted, slight pressure is applied to the tongue, and the client is instructed to say "a" then "e," which elevates the soft palate (Figure 61-18, A). The instrument should not touch the tongue, or the client will gag. The na-

sopharynx is then inspected for drainage, bleeding, ulceration, or masses.

Direct Laryngoscopy

Direct visualization of the larynx may be accomplished with the use of several different instruments; most devices are lighted endoscopes. The client is instructed to protrude the tongue, and the examiner *gently* holds the tongue with a gauze sponge and pulls it forward. A laryngeal mirror or telescopic endoscope is inserted into the oropharynx; again, contact with the tongue is avoided. The client is instructed to breathe in and out rapidly through the mouth or to "pant like a puppy." Panting decreases the gagging sensation caused by the examination. During quiet respiration, the base of the tongue, epiglottis, and vocal cords are examined for signs of infection or tumor (Figure 61-18, *B*). The client is instructed to vocalize a high-pitched *"eee"* to approximate (close) the vocal cords. The examiner observes the movement of the cords, the color of the mucous membranes, and the presence of any lesions. If the client is unable to cooperate as described, the examination may be performed with a fiberoptic endoscope inserted through the nose (see Figure 61-17).

Alveolar Lavage

Sterile saline can be injected during bronchoscopy to wash tissues. The saline is aspirated and examined for atypical cells. Alveolar lavage may be used in the diagnosis of interstitial lung disease, sarcoidosis, hypersensitivity pneumonitis, and *Pneumocystis carinii* pneumonia. No additional client preparation is needed because this procedure is done during bronchoscopy.

Endoscopic Thoracotomy

Endoscopic thoracotomy is a diagnostic procedure that is an alternative to open-lung biopsy and thoracotomy for pleural surface disorders.

Procedure

Typically three small incisions are made into the middle chest wall. A scope attached to a camera and video projector is inserted through the first incision to inspect tissue; tissues are manipulated, and biopsy specimens are obtained through the other incisions. A chest tube is inserted to promote lung reexpansion. Advantages of the procedure include reduced anesthesia time, less pain, and shortened hospital stay. In addition, biopsy specimens may be obtained from the lower lobes, which is not routinely done during open-lung biopsy procedures.

Preprocedure Care

Instruct the client about the need for this test, and obtain a signed informed consent form. Endoscopic thora-

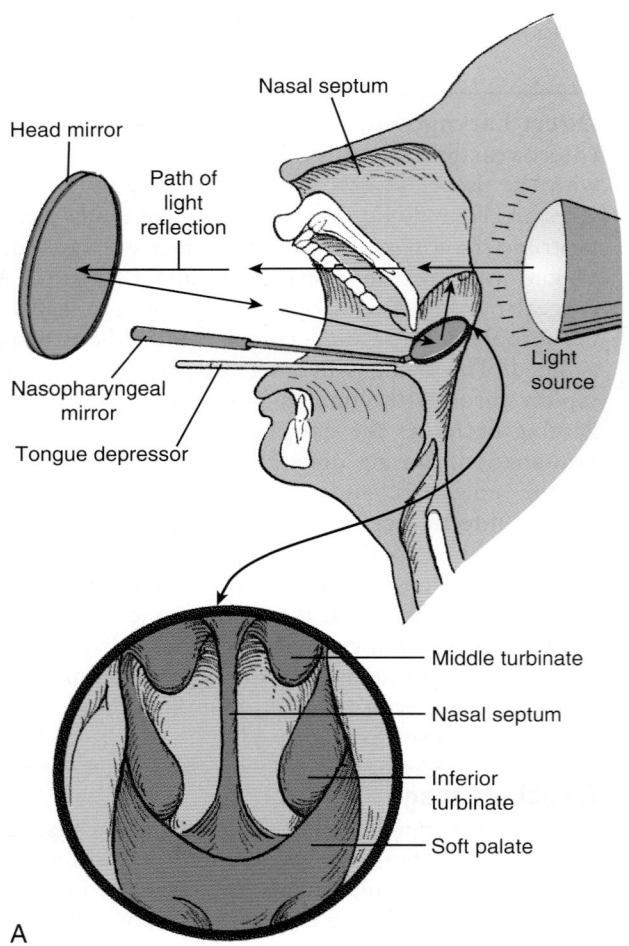

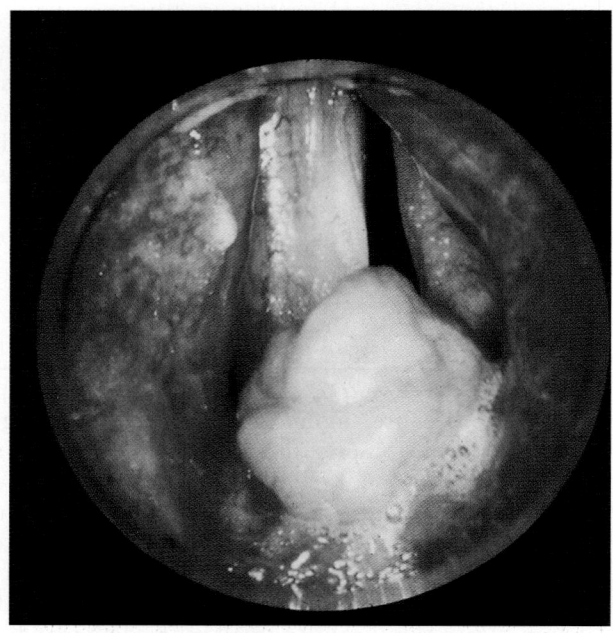

A

B

FIGURE 61-18 Laryngoscopy. **A,** Indirect laryngoscopy enables assessment of the pharynx and buccal cavity and some visualization of the larynx. (Laryngeal structure and function are best assessed by direct visualization, such as with flexible or rigid laryngoscopy or flexible fiberoptic bronchoscopy.) A head mirror, tongue depressor, light source, and small examining mirror are used in the indirect method. The mirror is positioned behind the soft palate after the tongue is depressed. To visualize the larynx, gently grasp the tongue with a gauze sponge and pull it forward. Place the mirror against the soft palate in front of the uvula, and move it gently until the cords are visualized. Have the client vocalize the high-pitched sound *"eee,"* which causes the larynx to move. The larynx is assessed for symmetrical cord motion. **B,** Large granular-cell tumor of the true vocal cord, as seen during laryngoscopy. (From Fu, Y.S., et al. [2001]. *Head and neck pathology—with clinical correlations.* New York: Churchill Livingstone.)

cotomy is a surgical procedure, and general anesthesia is administered (see Chapter 16 for a discussion of the needs of the surgical client). Explain that a chest tube will be in place and that it will be necessary to perform coughing and deep-breathing exercises.

Pulmonary Angiography
Sometimes the vascular structure of the thorax must be assessed. Angiography and other procedures designed to examine specific vascular structures (aortography for the aorta) all use similar techniques.

Pulmonary angiography may be done to detect the following:

- Congenital abnormalities of the pulmonary vascular tree
- Abnormalities of the pulmonary venous circulation
- Acquired diseases of the pulmonary arterial and venous circulation (primary pulmonary arterial hypertension)
- Destructive effects of emphysema
- Potential benefits of resection for bronchogenic carcinoma

- Peripheral pulmonary lesions
- Extent of thromboembolism in the lungs

Procedure

Contrast medium is injected into the vascular system through an indwelling catheter. During pulmonary angiography, the catheter can be inserted either peripherally or directly into the main pulmonary artery or one of its branches. The contrast agent is injected while cinefluorographs or still photographs are taken. (Pulmonary angiography is discussed in Chapter 63.)

Instruct the client about the need for this test, and obtain informed consent. The test is painless and does not involve exposure to radiation. Further preprocedure and postprocedure care of the client is as for angiography (see Chapter 4).

SPECIMEN RECOVERY AND ANALYSIS

The following procedures are used for recovery and analysis of pulmonary specimens:

- Sputum collection
- Thoracentesis
- Biopsy

Sputum Collection

Normally the goblet cells produce 100 ml of mucus a day, but an infectious process can lead to excessive production of mucus (commonly called *sputum*). Assessment of sputum for bacteria, fungus, or cellular elements guides the treatment of an underlying infection.

Procedure

Inspect the sputum for color; quantity; quality; and the presence of blood, food particles, or other unusual contents. If possible sputum should be collected before antimicrobial treatment is begun.

Acid-fast smear and culture specimens are collected in the morning, at which time sputum is more plentiful and concentrated because of pooling through the night. Sputum can be collected by (1) the direct method, (2) the indirect method, or (3) gastric lavage.

Preprocedure Care

Explain the need for and the purpose of this test to the client. When a specimen is obtained by the direct method, the client brushes the teeth to reduce contamination and then coughs into a sputum specimen container. Encourage the client to cough, not spit, to obtain sputum. Inhaling nebulized saline or water can be used to thin the sputum to facilitate expectoration.

Indirect techniques for obtaining sputum consist of a sterile suction catheter with an attached sputum trap. Sputum can also be obtained by transtracheal aspiration.

A puncture is made with a needle through the cricothyroid membrane into the trachea, and sputum is aspirated.

Although gastric lavage is not a common technique for obtaining sputum, it can be used for uncooperative or extremely ill clients. Lavage is based on the assumption that sputum is swallowed during sleep and sometimes after coughing. A nasogastric tube is inserted by appropriate technique. Gastric juice is aspirated with a syringe and sent to the laboratory. The tube is then removed.

The collected sputum is analyzed for Gram's stain, culture, and sensitivity study. Gram's stain is used to classify bacteria as gram-positive or gram-negative and, along with the sputum culture, provides guidelines for appropriate antimicrobial therapy. After Gram's stain, the sputum is incubated for 24 hours or longer on the appropriate culture medium and studied by a microbiologist. Obtaining a specimen for the culture allows further identification of the infecting organism. When the organism is identified, its sensitivity to antibiotic treatment is tested and an appropriate antibiotic is prescribed.

Identification of organisms that cause tuberculosis and similar diseases (acid-fast bacilli) requires tests other than Gram's stain, culture, and sensitivity study.

Regardless of the technique used to obtain the specimen, note the color, consistency, odor, and amount of sputum obtained.

Nose and Throat Cultures

Bacteria in the nose and throat can be identified by culture during assessment of the upper airway. Some bacteria are normally present (streptococci, staphylococci, pneumococci, *Haemophilus influenzae*, and *Klebsiella pneumoniae*). Other organisms are abnormal (those causing diphtheria or tuberculosis).

Swab the nose and throat using a sterile cotton swab. Place the swab in a sterile culture tube. Some laboratories require the swab to be suspended in a tube containing 2 ml of fluid to keep air in the tube moist and prevent evaporation and drying of the specimen. Because the fluid is not a culture medium, the swab should not touch the fluid. If Loeffler's medium is used in the tube (if diphtheria is suspected), the medium should touch the swab. When culture tubes without fluid are used, take the specimen to the laboratory immediately, where the swab is streaked across a culture plate.

Thoracentesis

Procedure

Thoracentesis is performed to drain fluid or air found in the pleural space. Therapeutic thoracentesis removes an accumulation of pleural fluid or air that has caused lung compression and respiratory distress. When the main

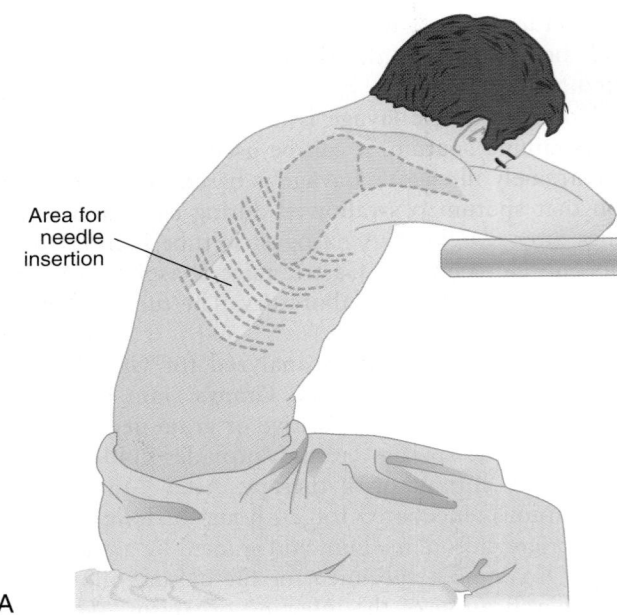

Area for
needle
insertion

A

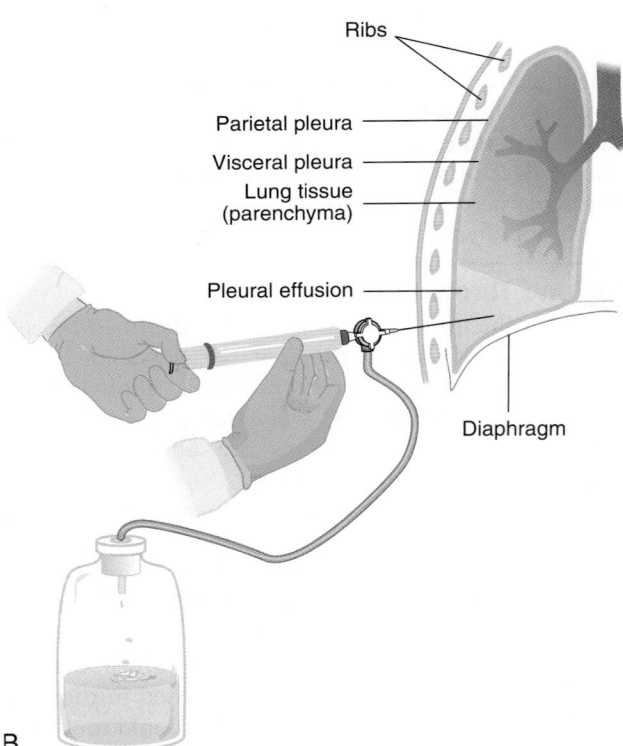

Ribs

Parietal pleura

Visceral pleura

Lung tissue
(parenchyma)

Pleural effusion

Diaphragm

B

FIGURE 61-19 Thoracentesis. **A,** Correct position of the client for the procedure. The arms are raised and crossed. The head rests on the folded arms. This position allows the chest wall to be pulled outward in an expanded position. If an institutional over-bed table is not available, you may leave the client's arms down, but position them toward the client's hips or cross them in front of the chest. **B,** Usual site for insertion of a thoracentesis needle for a right-sided effusion. The actual site varies, depending on the location and volume of the effusion. The needle is kept as far away from the diaphragm as possible but is inserted close to the base of the effusion so that gravity can help with drainage.

goal is to determine the cause of an infection or empyema, diagnostic thoracentesis is performed. The fluid collected is sent to the laboratory for assessment of specific gravity, glucose, protein, and pH; culture; sensitivity study; and cytologic evaluation. The color and consistency of the pleural fluid are also documented.

Preprocedure Care

Obtain informed consent, and instruct the client about the procedure and the need for it. The client must sit upright while leaning over the tray table (Figure 61-19, *A*). In the upright position, pleural fluid accumulates in the base of the thorax. Alternatively place the client in a recumbent position with the arm resting under the head. Insertion of the needle is painful. Explain the importance of holding still during the procedure. Sudden movement may force the needle through the pleural space and injure the visceral pleura or lung parenchyma. State that you will help to hold the client, and provide reassurance. The test takes 5 to 15 minutes to complete.

During the procedure, assist the physician; monitor vital signs; and observe for dyspnea, complaints of difficulty breathing, nausea, or pain.

Postprocedure Care

After the procedure, the client is usually turned onto the unaffected side for 1 hour to facilitate lung expansion. Assess vital signs according to the facility's policy. Carefully assess the respiratory rate and character and the breath sounds. Tachypnea, dyspnea, cyanosis, retractions, or diminished breath sounds, which may indicate pneumothorax, should be reported to the physician.

Record the amount of fluid withdrawn as fluid output. Chest films may be obtained to evaluate the degree of lung reexpansion or pneumothorax. Subcutaneous emphysema may follow this procedure because air in the pleural cavity leaks into subcutaneous tissues. The tissues feel like lumpy paper and crackle when palpated *(crepitus)*. Usually subcutaneous emphysema causes no problem unless it is increasing and constricting vital organs (the trachea). Clients often need reassurance about this disorder.

If the client has pleural effusion related to a malignancy, cytotoxic medications may be inserted into the pleural space after thoracentesis. Some of these agents burn; with others, the client must roll about to have the medication coat the entire pleural space. Review the interventions used with the various medications.

Biopsy

Biopsy specimens may be taken from various respiratory tissues for examination. As mentioned previously, specimens from tracheobronchial structures may be obtained during bronchoscopy. Biopsy specimens of scalene and mediastinal nodes may be obtained (with local anesthesia) for pathologic study, culture, or cytologic assessment.

Pleural Biopsy

Procedure

Pleural biopsies can be performed surgically through a small thoracotomy incision or during thoracentesis with the use of a Cope needle. Needle biopsy is a relatively safe, simple diagnostic procedure that can help to determine the cause of pleural effusions. The needle removes a small fragment of parietal pleura, which is used for microscopic cellular examination and culture. If bacteriologic studies are needed, the biopsy specimen should be obtained before chemotherapy is begun.

Preprocedure Care

Obtain informed consent, and instruct the client about the need for and purpose of the test. Preparation and positioning of a client for pleural biopsy are similar to those for thoracentesis. The test is painful, and the client must hold still. Assist and reassure the client. The test takes 15 to 30 minutes to complete.

Postprocedure Care

Rare complications include temporary pain associated with intercostal nerve injury, pneumothorax, and hemothorax. After the biopsy procedure, observe for indications of complications (dyspnea, pallor, diaphoresis, excessive pain). A pneumothorax associated with needle biopsy may develop. Chest tubes and chest drainage equipment must be available. Follow-up chest x-ray studies are usually done after the procedure. Development of hemothorax is indicated by a substantial increase in fluid in the pleural space and requires immediate thoracentesis.

Lung Biopsy

As with pleural biopsy, lung biopsy may be done by surgical exposure of the lung (open-lung biopsy) with or without endoscopy using a needle designed to remove a core of lung tissue. The tissue is examined for abnormal cellular structure and bacteria. Lung biopsies are most often performed to identify pulmonary tumors or parenchymal changes *(sarcoidosis)*.

Procedure

Needle puncture (aspiration) biopsy of chest lesions is done with fluoroscopy. After a lesion is identified on a chest film and localized by fluoroscopy, topical anesthesia is administered and the needle is inserted through the chest wall into the lung tissue and lesion. A small sample of cells is aspirated for microscopic study, and the needle is withdrawn. Aspiration biopsy may enable definitive diagnosis of malignant neoplasms, granulomas, or other nonmalignant growths. Possible complications of needle aspiration lung biopsy are hemoptysis, hemothorax, and pneumothorax.

Postprocedure Care

After the procedure, examine any sputum closely for evidence of blood. Observe for respiratory distress (may indicate pneumothorax). Monitor the client's vital signs, breath sounds, skin color, and temperature.

CONCLUSIONS

Respiratory assessment begins with obtaining a thorough client history. One of the most essential aspects of history taking is determining the degree of dyspnea and the impact it has on activities of daily living. Note the client's smoking history and occupational risks because they are common risk factors for respiratory disorders. The chest is inspected for obvious deformity and shape. Percussion, palpation, and auscultation assist in locating areas of possible fluid accumulation or consolidation that interfere with breathing.

Chest x-ray studies, bronchoscopy, pulmonary function tests, and ABG analysis are common diagnostic assessments. Educate the client about the diagnostic modalities, and monitor for potential complications after the study.

BIBLIOGRAPHY

1. Bickley, L.S., & Szilagyi, P.G. (2003). *Bates' guide to physical examination and history taking* (8th ed.). Philadelphia: Lippincott Williams & Wilkins.
2. Bourke, S. (2003). *Respiratory medicine* (6th ed.). Malden, MA: Blackwell Publishing.
3. Des Jardins, T.R., & Burton, G.G. (2002). *Clinical manifestations and assessment of respiratory disease* (4th ed.). St. Louis: Mosby.
4. Evans, S., & Scanlon, P. (2003). Current practice in pulmonary function testing. *Mayo Clinic Proceedings, 78,* 758-763.
5. Gold, W.M., Murray, J.F., & Nadel, J.A. (2002). *Atlas of procedures in respiratory medicine.* Philadelphia: W.B. Saunders.

6. Guyton, A.C., & Hall, J.E. (2000). *Textbook of medical physiology* (10th ed.). Philadelphia: W.B. Saunders.

7. Hlastala, M.P., & Berger, A.J. (2001). *Physiology of respiration.* New York: Oxford University Press.

8. Hyatt, R. (2003). *Interpretation of pulmonary function tests: A practical guide* (2nd ed.). Philadelphia: Lippincott Williams & Wilkins.

9. Jarvis, C. (2000). *Physical examination and health assessment* (3rd ed.). Philadelphia: W.B. Saunders.

10. Murray, J.F., & Nadel, J.A. (2000). *The textbook of respiratory medicine* (3rd ed.). Philadelphia: W.B. Saunders.

11. Parshall, M.B., et al. (2001). Reliability and validity of dyspnea sensory quality descriptors in heart failure patients treated in an emergency department. *Heart and Lung: The Journal of Acute and Critical Care, 30*(1), 57-65.

12. Spector, N., & Klein, D. (2001). Chronic critically ill dyspneic patients: Mechanisms and clinical measurement. *AACN Clinical Issues: Advanced practice in acute and critical care, 12*(2), 220-223.

13. West, J. B. (2003). *Pulmonary pathophysiology: The essentials* (6th ed.). Philadelphia: Lippincott Williams & Wilkins.

14. Wyka, K., Matthews, P., & Clark, W. (2002). *Foundations of respiratory care.* Albany, NY: Delmar.

Management of Clients with Upper Airway Disorders

Linda K. Clarke

---

evolve

Web Enhancements

http://evolve.elsevier.com/Black/medsurg/

Bridge to Home Health Care
Living with a Tracheostomy
Client Education Guide
Swallowing Technique After a Partial
Laryngectomy (Spanish Translation)
Care of a Tracheoesophageal Puncture Wound (English
Version and Spanish Translation)

Exercises After Radical Neck Surgery (English Version and
Spanish Translation)
Ethical Issues in Nursing
What Type of Client Education Is Needed for Informed Con-
sent to Radical Procedures?
Appendix C
Laboratory Values of Clinical Importance in Medical-Surgical
Nursing

The initial complaint for clients with disorders of the upper airway is a problem with breathing. Obstructions to nasal breathing are observed in clients with nasal polyps, deviated nasal septum, or nasal fractures. After surgical interventions, nasal breathing continues to be compromised because of postoperative edema. Laryngeal disorders may also result in breathing problems. Tumors of the larynx create obstruction to air entering the trachea, as well as to air being exhaled. Vocal cord paralysis and laryngospasm may also affect the passage of air through the larynx and vocal cords. Clients with epistaxis and sinusitis exhibit nasal bleeding and drainage, respectively, and may have fever and pain. Inflammation associated with these problems results in obstruction to breathing. Surgical intervention and nasal packing further exacerbate breathing problems.

METHODS OF CONTROLLING THE AIRWAY

Airway obstruction can be prevented or treated with many modalities. Antihistamine treatment is discussed in Chapter 78. Intubation to support ventilation and oxy-genation is discussed in Chapter 65. This chapter begins with a discussion of tracheostomy because it is a common method of airway management in hospitalized clients.

Tracheostomy

A *tracheotomy* is a surgical incision into the trachea through overlying skin and muscles for airway management. A *tracheostomy* is the surgical creation of a stoma, or opening, into the trachea through the overlying skin (Figure 62-1). These terms are often used interchangeably. For simplicity, the term *tracheostomy* is used here.

Tracheostomy can be performed as an emergency procedure or as an elective procedure, depending on the indication. A percutaneous tracheostomy can be done at the bedside in critical care units. This method is cost-effective, saves time, and avoids transporting critically ill clients to the operating room.[24] A tracheostomy provides the best route for long-term airway maintenance. There are many indications for this procedure, including the following:

- Relief of acute or chronic upper airway obstruction
- Access for continuous mechanical ventilation

---

evolve *Be sure to check out the bonus material on the Evolve website and the CD-ROM, including free self-assessment exercises.*

http://evolve.elsevier.com/Black/medsurg/

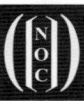

Nursing Outcomes Classification (NOC)
for Nursing Diagnoses—Clients with Upper Airway Disorders

Anxiety and Fear
Anxiety Control
Coping
Fear Control
Social Interaction Skills
Impaired Nutrition: Less Than Body Requirements
Nutritional Status: Food and Fluid Intake
Impaired Verbal Communication
Communication Ability
Communication Ability: Expressive Ability
Ineffective Airway Clearance
Aspiration Control
Respiratory Status: Airway Patency

Risk for Aspiration
Respiratory Status: Gas Exchange
Risk Control
Risk Detection
Risk for Constipation
Hydration
Mobility Level
Nutritional Status: Food and Fluid Intake
Risk Control
Risk Detection
Risk for Impaired Gas Exchange
Respiratory Status: Gas Exchange
Vital Signs Status
Risk for Ineffective Family Therapeutic Regimen Management
Family Functioning

Family Participation in Professional Care
Risk for Ineffective Therapeutic Regimen Management (Individuals)
Compliance Behavior
Knowledge: Treatment Regimen
Risk for Infection
Immobility Consequences: Physiologic
Knowledge: Infection Control
Nutritional Status
Risk Control
Risk Detection
Tissue Integrity: Skin and Mucous Membranes
Wound Healing

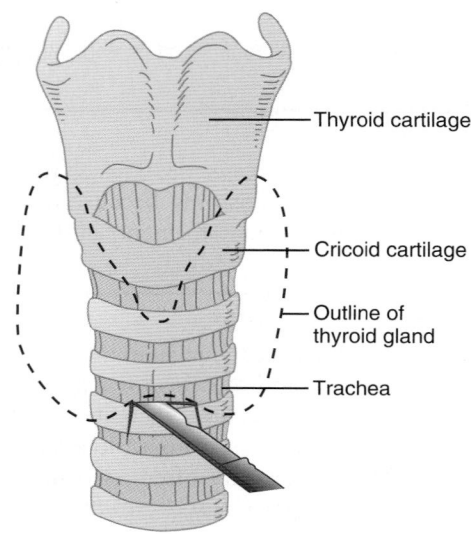

FIGURE 62-1 Incision for a tracheostomy is made through the fibrous tissue above the third tracheal cartilage. Two small vertical incisions create a flap that can be closed later.

- Prevention of aspiration pneumonia
- Promotion of pulmonary hygiene
- Bilateral vocal cord paralysis
- Prolonged endotracheal tube insertion resulting in erosion or pain

A tracheostomy is by far the most satisfactory artificial airway. It bypasses the upper airway and glottis, making stabilization, suction, and the attachment of respiratory equipment much easier than with other types of artificial airways. The client can eat and, with some adjustments, talk.[19,24]

Tracheostomy Tubes

The tracheostomy opening is fitted with a tube to maintain airway patency. Tracheostomy tubes vary in their composition, number of separate parts, shape, and size. Tracheostomy tubes are chosen specifically for each client. Incorrectly fitted tubes can precipitate permanent or life-threatening damage.

The diameter of a tracheostomy tube should be smaller than the trachea so that it lies comfortably within the tracheal lumen. Air should be able to pass between the outer wall of the tracheostomy tube and the tracheal mucosa. Although there is no standard tracheostomy tube sizing system, all packages indicate the inner and outer diameters in millimeters.

The length and curve of a tracheostomy tube are important. Tracheostomy tubes may be long (e.g., Hollinger tube, Shiley single-cannula tube) or short. They may be angled, with the angle ranging from 50 to 90 degrees. Short to moderately short tubes with an angle of about 60 degrees are most often used. A tube must be long enough to avoid dislodgment into paratracheal tissue when the client coughs or turns his or her head. The lower end of a tracheostomy tube should be located above the carina. The curve of the tube must allow the tip to be in a straight line with the trachea, rather than pressing on the anterior or posterior tracheal wall.

Tracheostomy tubes may be cuffed or uncuffed. An inflated cuff permits mechanical ventilation and protects the lower airway by creating a seal between the upper and lower airways (Box 62-1). Tracheostomy cuffs do not hold the tube in place.

Tracheostomy tubes are made of various substances, such as nonreactive plastic, stainless steel, sterling silver,

| BOX 62-1 | *Inflation and Deflation of Tracheostomy Tube Cuff* |

Inflation (Minimal Leak Technique)
Objective
Inflate the cuff with the minimum volume of air required to adequately seal the trachea during positive-pressure ventilation and to prevent aspiration of foreign material while exerting the lowest possible cuff-to-tracheal wall pressure.

Intervention
1. Withdraw all residual air from the cuff.
2. Place 6 ml of air in a syringe.
3. Place the diaphragm of a stethoscope over the client's neck in the area of the tracheostomy tube cuff.
4. On inhalation, slowly inject air through the one-way valve into the pilot line in 1-ml increments.
5. Auscultate the neck area over the cuff.
6. Apply positive pressure to the tracheostomy tube with a manual self-inflating bag. An audible air leak can be heard via the stethoscope unless the cuff is inflated.
7. Continue slowly injecting air until the air leak is no longer present during inhalation.
8. When a leak is no longer auscultated, withdraw a small amount of air from the cuff until a very small leak is heard. This is called a *minimal leak*.
9. Note the amount of air necessary to achieve the minimal leak. This is the *minimal occluding volume* (MOV).
10. Once minimal leak is attained, measure the cuff pressure with a manometer.
11. Routinely measure and document cuff pressures.

Deflation
Objective
Allow air to flow around the tracheostomy tube to permit phonation and to provide an opportunity to blow secretions above the cuff into the oropharynx, where they can be removed by suctioning.

Intervention
Routinely deflating the cuff is not necessary provided that safe cuff inflation and cuff pressure measurements are performed.
1. Remove the ventilator assembly (if present) and attach a self-inflating bag to the 15-mm adapter on the inner cannula.
2. Hyperoxygenate, hyperinflate, and suction the trachea to remove secretions below the cuff. Remove secretions above the cuff by gently applying suction deep into the oropharynx.
3. Insert an empty syringe into the one-way valve, and pull back on the plunger to remove the air in the cuff. At the same time, apply positive pressure with the manual self-inflating bag. This maneuver blows secretions lying directly above the cuff into the mouth, which prevents secretions accumulated above the cuff from draining into the trachea and lower airway.
4. Suction the oropharynx again.
5. If the person is ventilator-dependent, remember that with the cuff "down" or deflated, a portion of ventilation volume will not reach the lungs. Air will escape through the upper airway, which may compromise the person's respiratory status. This volume loss creates an audible leak. Phonation is possible during the exhalation phase of ventilation.

*The same procedure is used for inflation and deflation of endotracheal tube cuffs.

or silicone. Plastic tubes are disposable and used for only one person. Metal tubes may be reused after being sterilized.[24,25]

Universal Tracheostomy Tube. The most common tube is a universal, or standard, tracheostomy tube (Figure 62-2) having three parts: (1) outer cannula with cuff, flange, and pilot tube, (2) inner cannula, and (3) obturator. The parts fit together as one unit and may not be interchanged with other units. Therefore all three parts of each individual set are kept together.

The outer cannula fits in the tracheostomy stoma to keep it open. The outer cannula has a flange or neckplate that fits flush with the neck and has holes on each side to attach the securing tapes or ties. A tracheostomy tube must be secured in place to prevent accidental extubation, excessive motion, or misalignment. Cloth tape or commercially available self-fastening (Velcro) ties may be used.

The obturator is placed into the outer tube before insertion. Its rounded tip smooths the end of the cannula and facilitates nontraumatic insertion of the tube into the stoma. The obturator is removed immediately after insertion to open the tube. Place the obturator in a plastic wrapper and tape it to the head of the client's bed in a conspicuous place. If the tracheostomy tube is accidentally displaced, the obturator can be immediately placed into the outer cannula for quick reinsertion.

Once the obturator is removed, the inner cannula is placed into the outer cannula. Lock it into place to prevent accidental removal (e.g., when the client coughs). Frequent removal and cleaning of the inner cannula is necessary to maintain airway patency. At the distal end, most inner cannulas have a standard 15-mm adapter that fits respiratory therapy and anesthesiology equipment.[24]

Single-Cannula Tracheostomy Tube. A single-cannula tracheostomy tube is slightly longer than a standard, double-cannula tube. Because it does not have an inner cannula that can be cleaned to eliminate secretions, a single-cannula tube should not be used in clients with excessive secretions or difficulty clearing secretions. Clients in whom a single-cannula tube is used must have continuous supplemental humidification to prevent obstruction by accumulated secretions. The longer single-

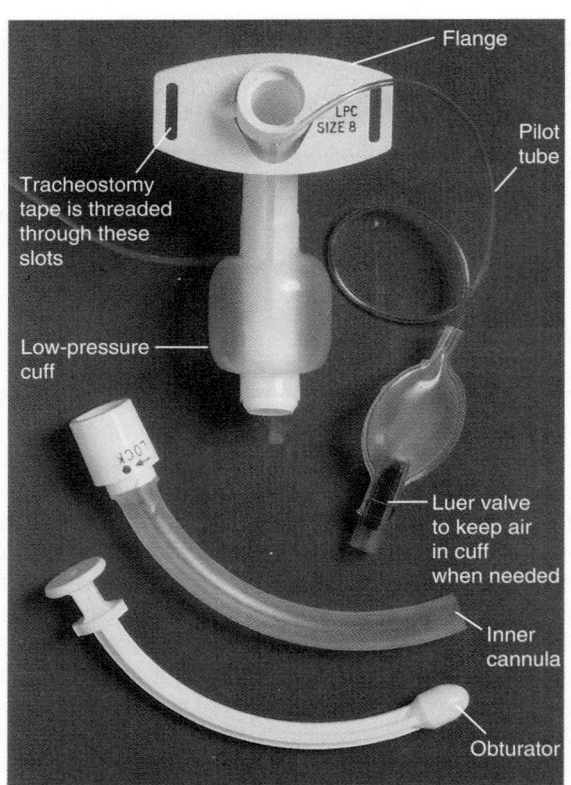

FIGURE 62-2 Parts of a tracheostomy tube. (Courtesy of Shiley, Inc., Irvine, CA.)

cannula tube is used in the client with a thick neck or with an altered airway in whom a standard tracheostomy tube would be too short.[25]

Fenestrated Tracheostomy Tube. A fenestrated tracheostomy tube has one large opening (Latin, *fenestra*), or several small ones, on the curvature of the posterior wall of the outer cannula. Fenestrated tubes have an inner cannula and may be cuffed or cuffless. When the inner cannula is removed, the fenestration permits air to flow through both the upper airway and the tracheostomy opening. This permits speech and more effective coughing. This tube may be used while a client is being weaned from a tracheostomy and for a client in whom use of the tracheostomy is expected to be prolonged. When the inner cannula is in place, the fenestration is closed, and the tube functions as a universal tracheostomy tube. When weaning a mechanically ventilated client, remove the inner cannula and deflate the cuff to allow the client to breathe through the fenestrae and around the tube.[24]

Tracheostomy Speaking Valves. For a "talking tracheostomy," a one-way valve in a plastic **T** piece is attached to the 15-mm end of the inner cannula of a universal tracheostomy tube. This modification permits talking without the need to plug the tracheostomy tube.

The one-way valve allows air (and the aerosol of supplemental humidification and oxygen) to flow into the arm of the **T** piece during inspiration. On exhalation, the one-way valve closes, directing air from the lungs up through the vocal cords and upper airway. Phonation and effective coughing are facilitated by this normal passage of air.

A talking tracheostomy is *never* used unless there is enough room around the tracheostomy tube to permit sufficient air flow for breathing. *Always deflate* a cuffed tracheostomy tube before the client uses the talking tracheostomy adapter. Cuff inflation prevents exhalation, potentially causing suffocation.[24]

Communitrach Tube. The Communitrach tube allows speech by coordination of phonation efforts. Ventilation and phonation are separated because of different air sources. With this device, an air flow tube (that looks like a second pilot tube) runs outside the pilot (main) tube and opens just above the cuff. There is a port at the distal end of the air flow tube. When the port is occluded by a finger and compressed air or oxygen is directed through the air flow tube, a current of air is generated up through the vocal cords. With practice, the client learns to use this air flow for speech, although the "voice" produced in this way does not sound normal. Mucosal irritation may develop from the forced flow of air or oxygen into the upper airway.[24,25]

Tracheostomy Button. Use of a tracheostomy button is sometimes indicated during weaning as an intermediate measure between using a standard tracheostomy tube and extubation. A button is a short, straight, plastic cylinder secured by a flange to the anterior tracheal wall but is not deep enough to enter the tracheal lumen. It has a removable cap with a one-way flap inside that permits inhalation but not exhalation. Exhalation occurs through the normal upper airway. When the cap is on, the client can talk.

A button cannot be used with a ventilator. It replaces a standard tracheostomy tube for people with retained secretions who do not require ventilatory assistance. A button creates less airway resistance than that produced by a plugged standard tracheostomy tube; hence, breathing is easier. Artificial humidification of inspired air is necessary with a button (as with any tracheostomy tube), because the natural airway is bypassed.

Permanent Tracheostomy. Most clients with a permanent tracheostomy use a universal cuffless tracheostomy tube or an Olympic tracheostomy button. For appearance's sake, many people prefer a low-profile inner cannula. This design does not incorporate a 15-mm adapter. Instead, the inner cannula fits into the outer cannula and lies flush with the neck. If the client has had a total laryngectomy, the cut end of the trachea is sutured to the skin, creating a permanent stoma. Once the stoma is healed, most laryngectomy clients do not need a tube.

Metal Tracheostomy Tube. Metal tracheostomy tubes are made of sterling silver or stainless steel. The most popular type is the Jackson tracheostomy tube. Metal tubes are cuffless and most often used in clients who have a permanent tracheostomy or laryngectomy. The inner cannula locks together with the outer cannula. Because metal tubes do not have a standard 15-mm adapter, rapid adaptation to respiratory or anesthesia equipment is impossible unless a specific adapter is available. The Hollinger tube is also made of metal and is similar to the Jackson tube.

Potential Problems Associated with Tracheostomy Tubes and Cuffs

Most tracheostomy tube cuffs are designed to exert a low pressure against the tracheal wall. These cuffs are easily distensible, so that they accept a high volume of air without generating excessive force (i.e., high-volume, low-pressure cuffs). Low cuff pressure is necessary to prevent damage to the tracheal mucosa. The volume of air in the cuff determines the pressure exerted on the tracheal mucosa. Cuff pressures should not exceed 20 cm H_2O. With pressures greater than 42 cm H_2O, circulation to the tracheal mucosa is impaired, resulting in ischemia and necrosis. This is because the normal pressure within tracheal arteries is 42 cm H_2O. In the veins and lymphatic vessels, the normal pressures are 24 cm H_2O and 7 cm H_2O, respectively.

Tracheal damage from cuff pressure is a frequent complication of intubation. Cuffed tubes can cause tracheal damage in as few as 3 to 5 days.

Tracheal Wall Necrosis. Necrosis of the tracheal wall can lead to the formation of an abnormal opening between the posterior trachea and the esophagus. This problem is called *tracheoesophageal fistula*. The fistula allows air to escape into the stomach, causing distention. It also promotes aspiration of gastric contents. Fistulae most often develop when a cuffed tube is used in conjunction with a standard nasogastric (NG) tube. Use of small-lumen NG tubes can decrease the risk of fistula. Necrosis of the anterior trachea can lead to the rare but life-threatening complication of hemorrhage due to erosion into the innominate artery. This complication is manifested as the bleeding in and around or from the tracheostomy or by pulsation of the tracheostomy tube. Immediate intervention is mandatory because exsanguination can occur.[24]

When long-term tracheostomy is required, uncuffed tracheostomy tubes are usually used unless the client is at high risk of aspiration. Some clients who require long-term mechanical ventilation can tolerate uncuffed tracheostomy tubes. Tidal volumes and respiratory rates may be adjusted on the ventilator to produce satisfactory ventilation and arterial blood gas (ABG) concentrations while eliminating the risks associated with the use of tracheostomy tube cuffs.

Tracheal Dilation. Prolonged intubation can lead to dilation of the trachea from the cuff. This complication should be suspected when increasing amounts of air are needed to seal the cuff or when bulging of the tracheal wall is seen on x-ray films.

Tracheal Stenosis. Tracheal stenosis is narrowing of the trachea and may be noted 1 week to 2 years after intubation. It results from chronic inflammation, fibrosis, and necrosis, which cause scar formation in the inflamed trachea. It can also result from excessive movement of the tracheostomy tube from ventilator tubing. The severity of stenosis can be prevented by choosing the right size of tube, maintaining adequate cuff pressure, keeping intubation time short, preventing infection, and reducing movement of the tube. Tracheal stenosis is a potential complication of long-term tracheostomy and may require tracheal resection.[25]

Tracheomalacia. Tracheomalacia is a softening of the trachea resulting from secretions pooling above the cuff and thinning the cartilage. This weakened area of the trachea collapses on deep inspiration, impeding airflow and making it difficult to achieve an adequate seal. This problem can be managed by placing a foam-cuff tracheostomy tube. This tube has a sponge-like consistency. The cuff is foam-filled and self expands with air after insertion, conforming to the size and shape of the client's trachea, and reducing pressure on the tracheal wall.[25]

Airway Obstruction. The flow of air through a tracheostomy tube may become occluded for several reasons. The tracheostomy tube may be misaligned so that its opening lies against the tracheal wall, preventing air flow. Cuff overinflation causes the cuff to herniate over the tip of the tube, obstructing air flow. Without adequate airway care, the inner cannula can become occluded with dried secretions or excessive bronchial secretions.

Infection. Tracheostomies increase the risk of bronchopulmonary infection because they (1) bypass upper airway protective mechanisms (i.e., filtering, warming, and humidifying) and (2) decrease mucociliary transport and coughing, thus increasing retained secretions. Stoma site infection may occur as well. Nosocomial infection is also a potential problem. The lower airway (below the larynx) is normally sterile. Therefore all solutions and equipment entering the trachea must be sterile. Organisms (e.g., *Pseudomonas aeruginosa* and other gram-negative bacteria) grow readily in respiratory equipment, which can then contaminate the lower airway. In addition, some bacteria may colonize a tracheostomy without causing infection.

Changing Tracheostomy Tubes. Recommendations for changing tracheostomy tubes vary. Most physicians and health care facilities have established protocols. Some facilities direct that tracheostomy tubes be changed as often as every week, whereas others allow longer periods between tube changes. Ideally, the tube should be changed at least every 3 to 4 weeks to minimize the risk of infection. Each client has a unique set of circumstances that dictate the frequency of tracheostomy tube changes.

Accidental Decannulation. A tracheostomy tube that is not properly secured may be accidentally dislodged from the stoma. Because most new tracheostomy tubes are sutured in place, decannulation is rare, but it is serious nonetheless. Decannulation may occur while the ties are being changed. Manipulation of a tracheostomy tube or suctioning often produces vigorous coughing, which can expel the tube from the stoma unless the tube is held firmly. With accidental extubation, if the stoma is less than 4 days old, it may close, because a tract is not yet formed. If extubation occurs, call for help immediately and follow the steps in Box 62-2.

Maintain ventilation and oxygenation by bag and mask. If ventilation is impossible, you must reinsert the tube. To do so, deflate the cuff, remove the inner cannula of the tube, insert the obturator in the outer cannula, elevate the person's shoulders with a pillow, and gently hyperextend the neck. You may need to use tracheal dilators (spreaders) to hold the stoma open. Insert the outer cannula with obturator into the client's neck, and immediately remove the obturator. Auscultate for breath sounds. If breath sounds are present, insert the inner cannula and reconnect it to oxygen and ventilation equipment. If the tracheostomy tube cannot be reinserted in 1 minute, call a code for respiratory arrest. Unless the client is breathing adequately, an emergency cricothyroidotomy is necessary (see Chapter 84).

If accidental decannulation occurs once a tract has formed following a tracheostomy, the same procedure is used, but reinsertion of the tube is generally easier. If bleeding occurs or the airway is obstructed, use emergency measures, as indicated earlier.

Subcutaneous Emphysema. Subcutaneous emphysema develops when air escapes from the tracheostomy incision into the tissues, dissects fascial planes under the skin, and accumulates around the face, neck, and upper chest. These areas appear puffy, and slight finger pressure produces a crackling sound and sensation. Generally this is not a serious condition; the air is eventually absorbed.

BOX 62-2 *Accidental Decannulation of Tracheostomy Tube*

Prepare for Potential Decannulation
Keep the following equipment at the client's bedside:
- Extra tracheostomy tubes of the same size and one size smaller
- Obturator belonging to the existing tube
- Tracheal dilator (spreader)
- Oxygen source
- Suction catheters and suction source
- Resuscitation bag

If Extubation Occurs
Call for help.
Hyperextend the client's neck to facilitate tube reinsertion.
Assess the presence of tracheal retention sutures and use them to maintain an airway
- Pull top suture upward and outward.
- Pull lower suture downward and outward.

If retention sutures are not present, insert the tracheal dilator into the tracheostoma to open the airway.
Place the obturator into the outer cannula and reinsert the tracheostomy tube into the tracheostoma. If the replacement tube is cuffed, deflate the cuff before insertion.
Secure the tube with ties or Velcro strap.
Assess tube placement by auscultating for breath sounds. Insert the inner cannula and reconnect oxygen/ventilation equipment.
If the tracheostomy tube cannot be reinserted in 1 minute, call a code.

Weaning, Removal, and Rescue Breathing

Weaning from a Tracheostomy Tube

When continuous mechanical ventilation becomes unnecessary, weaning from a tracheostomy tube begins by deflating the cuff to determine the client's ability to manage secretions without aspirating them. A smaller, uncuffed tube may be inserted to ensure adequate ventilation around the tube. The tube is then plugged briefly to assess the client's ability to breathe through the upper airway. The time is gradually lengthened according to the client's respiratory status, general medical condition, and confidence. Eventually, the tracheostomy tube can be removed. The weaning process takes a variable length of time (typically 2 to 5 days) depending on the client's ability to breathe through the upper airway. If the tracheal opening is still needed for some intervention, an uncuffed tube, a fenestrated tube, or a tracheal button may be used.

Plugging a tracheostomy tube is usually done by inserting a tracheostomy plug (decannulation stopper) into the opening of the outer cannula. This closes off the tracheostomy, allowing air flow and respiration to occur normally through the nose and mouth. *When a cuffed tracheostomy tube is plugged, the cuff must be deflated.* If the cuff remains inflated, ventilation cannot occur, and respiratory arrest could result.[24]

Explain the process to the client and family. Most clients are anxious about weaning because they fear they may not be able to breathe. Constant, supportive observation during weaning is necessary. Encourage the client to begin to think about breathing through the nose again. This breathing is a strange sensation for people who have used a tracheostomy tube for a long time. Explain ways to facilitate optimal respiration and to maintain control of breathing (e.g., inhale slowly and completely through the nose; avoid holding the breath).

ABG analysis and measurement of spontaneous respiratory mechanics (respiratory rate, tidal volume, vital capacity, inspiratory effort, expiratory effort) are important assessments during weaning. Oximetry and other noninvasive assessment modes may also be used once baseline ABG values are established.

During weaning from tracheostomy, assess for indications of respiratory distress or ventilation impairment. Clinical manifestations of problems may include the following:

- Abnormal respiratory rate and pattern
- Use of accessory muscles to assist breathing
- Abnormal pulse and blood pressure
- Abnormal skin and mucous membrane color
- Abnormal ABG levels or oxygen saturation

Remove the tracheostomy plug immediately if any manifestation of respiratory distress or ventilation impairment appears. Also assess the client's quality of phonation and ability to deep-breathe and cough effectively. If oxygen has been administered via the tracheostomy, administer it at the prescribed rate of flow using nasal prongs.

Removing a Tracheostomy Tube

A tracheostomy tube is removed after resumption of normal respirations as indicated by the client's ability to breathe comfortably with the tracheostomy plugged, as well as to cough and raise secretions, and normal ABG values or oxygen saturation. Gradually increase the length of plugging sessions until the client is comfortable and confident with the tube plugged continuously for at least 24 hours.

After a tracheostomy tube is removed, place a dry, sterile dressing over the stoma. Initially, every 8 hours, clean the skin around the stoma, remove mucus with hydrogen peroxide, rinse the area with normal saline, and apply a fresh, dry dressing over the healing stoma. Document the condition of the stoma and the surrounding skin. If either appears irritated or infected, notify the physician. Topical antibiotic ointment may be pre-

scribed. A tracheostomy stoma closes gradually (over a period of several days). As long as the stoma is open, an air leak is present. Instruct the client to place clean fingers firmly over the dressing to facilitate normal speech and coughing.

After extubation, ongoing assessment of respiratory function is necessary. Some complications of tracheostomy, such as tracheal stenosis, can appear months after tracheostomy tube removal.

Performing Rescue Breathing

Emergency rescue breathing in the mouth-to-neck mode (i.e., mouth to tracheostomy or mouth to stoma) may be necessary if a client who has a tracheostomy or laryngectomy experiences respiratory depression or respiratory arrest. If a tracheostomy tube is in place, provide ventilation by attaching a manual self-inflating bag to the standard 15-mm adapter on the inner cannula. Some volume is lost from an uncuffed tube. Adequate ventilation can often be compensated for by altering the usual method of manual inflation (e.g., compress the bag more forcefully and quickly). If the tracheostomy tube is cuffed, inflate the cuff and maintain ventilation at the correct rate—that is, 12 to 16 breaths/min for an adult. If inflation of the cuff impedes ventilation, immediately deflate the cuff, and attempt to compensate for volume loss by compressing the bag more forcefully or quickly. If ventilation continues to be impaired or prevented and you determine the cause is a malfunction in the tube, remove the tube immediately and provide mouth-to-stoma ventilation. Keep the client's nose and mouth closed during mouth-to-stoma rescue breathing to prevent air from escaping through the upper airway.[22]

■ Nursing Management of the Client with a Tracheostomy

Preoperative Care

For clients who are to undergo elective tracheostomy, reinforce education provided by the physician. You may delegate some respiratory assistance tasks to other staff members, as discussed in the Management and Delegation feature on Assisting with Respiratory Care on p. 1782. The client's understanding of the tracheostomy tube may be enhanced by looking at anatomic diagrams and by handling a tracheostomy tube. The postoperative changes in ability to speak and eat should be explained. If the tracheostomy is expected to be permanent, information about living a productive life with modifications in clothing can be provided. A visit by a client with a permanent tracheostomy may be desirable.

When an emergency tracheostomy is needed, precious seconds may be all the time available for teaching. The client may be anxious or even unconscious. Education is often provided to the family in lieu of the client.

MANAGEMENT AND DELEGATION

Assisting with Respiratory Care

Assisting with respiratory care is one of the more controversial areas involving the use of assistive personnel. Opinions differ widely on the role of assistive personnel in caring for clients who need respiratory care. The performance of suctioning in particular is central to this debate. Your clinical facility should provide you with clear guidelines about the role of assistive personnel in this aspect of care.

The following aspects of respiratory care are commonly delegated to unlicensed assistive personnel:

- Setting up of oxygen delivery equipment and suction equipment
- Stocking routine respiratory care supplies at the bedside
- Assisting clients with the use of an incentive spirometer (after client instruction from a nurse or respiratory care clinician)
- Assisting clients with coughing and deep-breathing (after client instruction from a nurse or a respiratory care clinician)
- Performing tracheostomy care
- Measuring and recording peripheral oxygen saturation (SPO_2)

Controversial aspects of respiratory care less commonly delegated to unlicensed assistive personnel are as follows:

- Suctioning via an artificial airway
- Performance of chest physiotherapy to promote the loosening of secretions

Before the delegation of any aspect of respiratory care, consider the following:

- What is the client's respiratory status? Complete a thorough respiratory assessment.
- What is the indication for respiratory care? Is the client's condition stable? A client with acute respiratory compromise should receive your full attention and care; the care of such a client should not be delegated.
- Is your client on oxygen therapy? Oxygen is a type of medication for your client. All guidelines that pertain to medications also apply to oxygen. You may delegate the setup of oxygen delivery equipment to assistive personnel. However, you are responsible to verify that the ordered amount (dose) of oxygen is actually being delivered to the client.
- Has the client been instructed in the use of the incentive spirometer or coughing and deep-breathing exercises? Does the client need reinforcement or reinstruction? Reinforcement can be provided by assistive personnel; education and instruction should always be provided by a registered nurse or a respiratory care clinician.
- Does the client have a *new* artificial airway, such as an oral airway, nasotracheal or endotracheal tube, or tracheostomy? Have you assessed the client during suctioning? How has the client tolerated suctioning previously? Well-tolerated suctioning via an existing artificial airway may be delegated to a skilled assistant, if this is consistent with training and institutional policy.
- Does this client have a new or long-term tracheostomy? A new tracheostomy should always be managed by a registered nurse. The tracheostomy tube that has been placed through a new surgical incision should be evaluated as for any other fresh postoperative site.
- Have the client and family members managed this tracheostomy at home? This is an opportunity to evaluate their sterile technique, to provide reinforcement, and to review instructions with the client and family. After doing so, you may choose to delegate suctioning for this client to assistive personnel.
- Are the assistive personnel aware that suctioning and care of artificial airways are sterile procedures? The sterile technique of assistive personnel should be evaluated intermittently.

Findings that are immediately reportable to you, the registered nurse, should be described for the assistive personnel. These include any change or difficulty that the caregiver or the client experiences during the provision of care, changes in the respiratory rate or pattern, and changes in the consistency, color, and quantity of respiratory secretions.

Postoperative Care
Assessment

After tracheostomy, frequent assessment is required, including monitoring vital signs; assessing amount, color, and consistency of secretions; and observing for indications of shock, hemorrhage, respiratory insufficiency, or complications related to the client's general condition or the surgical intervention.

Diagnosis, Outcomes, Interventions

Diagnosis: Ineffective Airway Clearance. Numerous factors can lead to ineffective airway clearance in clients with tracheostomy—for example, dehydration, fever, anesthesia, anticholinergic drugs, sedatives, and immobility.

Outcomes. The client will have an effective airway clearance, as evidenced by no retained secretions, clear (or clearing) lung sounds, and no fever.

Interventions. Promote airway clearance and pulmonary aeration by changing the client's position frequently, providing humidification and hydration, using sedatives cautiously, and performing frequent hyperinflation and suctioning to promote lung expansion and reduce the risks of atelectasis, pulmonary infection, and ineffective gas exchange. Hyperinflation creates an "artificial sigh," improving lung aeration and facilitating removal of tracheobronchial secretions by enhancing the cough effort. When the client's condition is stabilized sufficiently, coughing may be enhanced by having the client place a finger over the tracheostomy tube opening while attempting to cough. It is important that the client wash his or her hands before doing this. Have the person cough into clean gauze squares and dispose of them carefully. Paper tissues are not recommended for use with a tracheostomy.

Perform Suctioning. When a cuffed tracheostomy tube is used, secretions collect above the cuff. It is difficult to remove such secretions by oropharyngeal suctioning. However, the secretions can be "blown" into the mouth by simultaneously deflating the cuff and giving a deep manual inflation. The client may also be instructed to cough during cuff deflation to expel accumulated secretions through the tracheostomy tube. If the client is unable to produce an effective cough, suction the tracheostomy tube during deflation to prevent aspiration of secretions into the lower airway.

Suction the airway as needed. Use proper technique to reduce mucosal trauma, which can lead to tracheal infection. Mucosal trauma is indicated by tracheal irritation, tracheitis, and bloody tracheal secretions. If tracheal secretions are thick and not easily removed, instill 3 to 5 ml of sterile normal saline into the trachea; the saline reduces viscosity of secretions for easier removal and acts to mechanically stimulate the cough reflex. Instill the saline directly into the tracheostomy tube during inhalation. If the client is unable to cough, suction the airway through the tracheostomy tube. Refer to the Management and Delegation feature, Assisting with Respiratory Care, before delegating activities to unlicensed assistive personnel.

Provide Tracheostomy Care. Tracheostomy care is detailed elsewhere in fundamentals textbooks. Reinsertion of the clean inner cannula is shown in Figure 62-3.

Provide Adequate Hydration. The normal hydrating mechanisms of the upper airway are bypassed by a tracheostomy. Hydration can be provided by an oral, parenteral, or inhalation route. Inhalation techniques include increasing the humidity of room air with a room humidifier and administering aerosols with dry gases such as oxygen.

If humidification is insufficient, the body tries to make up the deficit by taking fluid from body water. The result is inspissated (very thick) mucus, which can compromise airway patency and increases the risk of secretion pooling and subsequent infection. Dried mucus also occludes air passages and leads to atelectasis, pneumonia, and potentially severe gas exchange abnormalities.

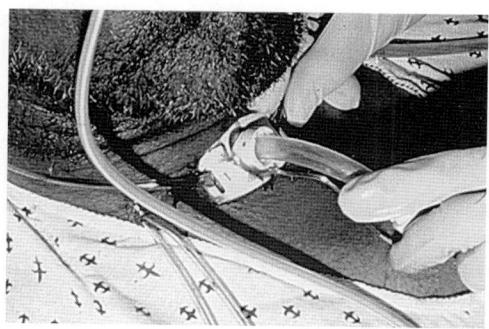

FIGURE 62-3 Reinserting a cleaned inner cannula.

Prevent Tube Movement. Secure a tracheostomy tube in midline tracheal alignment. Support ventilator and aerosol tubing to prevent pulling on the tracheostomy tube. Be careful not to disconnect tubing when turning the client. If cloth tape is used to secure the tube, tie a square knot, allowing room for two fingers to slide comfortably under the tape. Avoid placing the knot over the client's carotid artery or spine. Inspect the skin under the securing tape for skin irritation. When a tracheostomy is required for prolonged periods, the use of fastening devices such as padded straps with self-adhesive fasteners promotes comfort.

Diagnosis: Risk for Impaired Gas Exchange. After tracheostomy, impaired gas exchange may occur because of various factors. Factors affecting oxygen delivery include the following:

- Aspiration of blood, oral secretions, or gastric contents
- Restricted lung expansion from immobility
- Excessive tracheobronchial secretions
- Inability to cough and deep-breathe
- Pre-existing medical conditions (e.g., obesity, fever, inadequate hydration, pneumonia, tracheal injury such as from burns)

Factors affecting the removal of carbon dioxide include (1) the use of sedatives or anesthetic agents, (2) deteriorating level of consciousness, and (3) any other condition potentially affecting ventilatory efficiency and leading to hypoventilation and retention of carbon dioxide.

Outcomes. The client will have adequate gas exchange, as evidenced by maintaining oxygen saturation at greater than 90% (or ABG values within normal limits) and having no manifestations of respiratory distress.

Interventions. Assessment of gas exchange by ABG analysis is important immediately after tracheostomy and whenever there is a change in the client's condition or a change in treatment. Noninvasive monitoring such as pulse oximetry is appropriate once baseline values are established by ABG analysis. If shock or hypotension exists, or if peripheral vasoconstrictive drugs are used, data obtained by transcutaneous monitoring will be incorrect because of vasoconstriction.

Do not allow smoking in the room of a person who has a tracheostomy. Do not use aerosol spray cans (e.g., room deodorizers) near the person. Do not shake bedding or create dust clouds. Be careful when shaving or tending the person's hair that whiskers or hair does not fall into the trachea. Cover the tracheostomy with a thin cloth towel during shaving.

Diagnosis: Risk for Infection. The tracheostomy bypasses normal upper airway protective mechanisms. The client also has an incision. Both areas can become infected.

Outcomes. The client will exhibit no indications of infection, as evidenced by the absence of fever and by having a clean and dry tracheostomy site, healing incisions, and clear sputum.

Interventions. Use aseptic technique when working with the tracheostomy. Careful hand-washing, appropriate use of gloves, use of sterile supplies and solutions, and changing and decontaminating respiratory equipment every 24 hours are essential. Create a "loop" in the aerosol or ventilator tubing assembly; that is, let the tube loop down to catch condensate. Drain water and condensate in the tubing away from the tracheostomy into a receptacle.

Clean and inspect the skin around the stoma and the stoma itself. Observe for indications of irritation, inflammation, skin breakdown, and purulent drainage. If skin or stomal infection does occur, a topical antibacterial ointment may be prescribed.

Tracheostomy dressings (Figure 62-4) are often used, especially in the early postoperative stage. Damp blood and mucus-soaked dressings constitute a perfect medium for the growth of microorganisms. These conditions promote tissue irritation and breakdown. Change dressings whenever they are soiled or damp. Using hydrogen peroxide and cotton-tipped applicators, carefully clean the skin each time the dressing is changed. Rinse with normal saline and dry the area. Do not use plastic-backed or waterproof dressings. Moisture, secretions, and blood may seep behind the dressings, which hold warmth and moisture in. Skin then becomes irritated and macerated.

Diagnosis: Risk for Aspiration. The presence of a tracheostomy increases the risk of aspiration because the tubes tether the larynx, preventing normal upward movement of the larynx and closure by the epiglottis on swallowing.

Outcomes. The client will exhibit no evidence of aspiration—that is, will have clear lung sounds, no fever, and no choking on swallowing.

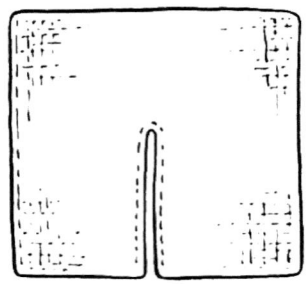
Purchased dressing with pre-cut slit

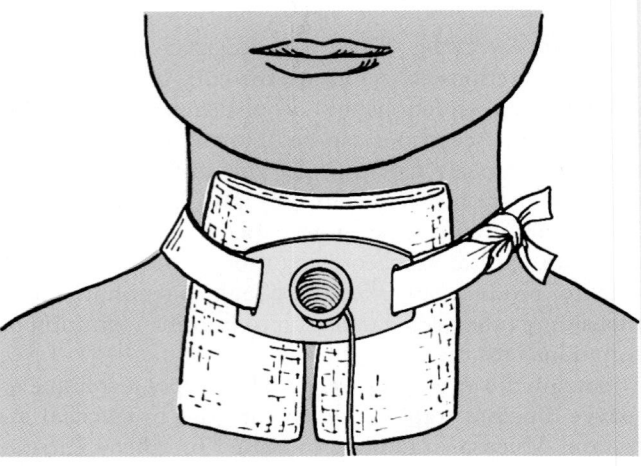

FIGURE 62-4 Tracheostomy dressings. If there is significant bleeding or tracheal secretions, cleaning the skin and changing the dressing frequently may prevent infection and skin breakdown. Manufactured dressing with a precut slit has no fine threads that could unravel and enter the stoma. Place the dressing around the tracheostomy tube with the slit downward, as shown, or upward.

Interventions. Intravenous fluids are usually given during the first 24 hours after tracheostomy. Then, if the client is alert and swallowing and if gag mechanisms are intact, oral intake of fluid and food may be attempted.

If a cuffed endotracheal tube was used before the tracheostomy, assess for the presence of tracheoesophageal fistula before permitting oral feedings. To assess for fistula, give the client a "test swallow" of water (at room temperature) before giving fluid or food. Severe coughing may indicate aspiration or a fistula. Withhold oral food and fluid, and continue feeding by NG tube or other methods. A swallowing evaluation by a speech-language therapist should be considered.

A client in whom normal swallowing is not expected to return for some time, or in whom the swallowing mechanism is permanently impaired (e.g., after a stroke), requires gastrostomy feedings or a permanent feeding tube (see Chapter 32). Tube-feedings may cause reflux, and the nutritive substance may be aspirated into the trachea. Before administering tube-feedings, inflate the cuff of the tracheostomy tube. Leave it inflated for at least 1 hour after feeding. Suction above the cuff before deflating it to remove any tube-feeding material.

When feeding a client with a tracheostomy, have the client sit upright. Often, food and fluids with semisolid consistency (e.g., pudding) are easier to swallow than water. Tipping the chin toward the chest narrows the airway and helps food enter the esophagus. Overinflation of the cuff causes swallowing difficulty. If oral fluid intake is limited, continue intravenous fluids.

Diagnosis: Impaired Verbal Communication.
Because the vocal cords are bypassed by the tracheostomy tube, the client cannot talk. The nursing diagnosis of *Impaired Verbal Communication* may need to be combined with the nursing diagnosis of *Fear* or *Anxiety* if the client feels afraid of not being able to summon help.

Outcomes. The client will have a satisfactory method of communicating with the nursing staff, as evidenced by being able to summon help and have needs met.

Interventions. Make sure the client can always reach an emergency call system to summon help. Be sure all staff members who may be answering the call system are aware that the client is unable to talk. Make a written list of common needs, words, and phrases that the client can point to (e.g., "I want to pass urine," "I am thirsty," or "I have pain") to communicate needs. Provide paper and pencil or a picture communication board to facilitate communication. When possible, assess the client's reading ability preoperatively and select appropriate communication tools to be used postoperatively.

Diagnosis: Risk for Constipation.
When the glottis and vocal cords are bypassed (as with tracheostomy), the client cannot perform a Valsalva maneuver. This deficit impairs the person's ability to defecate.

Outcomes. The client will have regular bowel movements (according to a usual schedule).

Interventions. Assess for most recent bowel movement. Elimination is a frequently overlooked area of client care. Use prescribed stool softeners, laxatives, and even enemas or suppositories as necessary.

Diagnosis: Anxiety and Fear.
Anxiety and fear are due to various factors affecting the client with a tracheostomy—for example, inability to talk, fear of suffocating, anxiety about diagnosis, or fear that the tracheostomy tube will come out.

Outcomes. The client will have decreasing manifestations of anxiety and fear, as evidenced by a pulse rate within normal limits, a calm facial expression, the ability to communicate, and no expressed fears.

Interventions. Frequent observation is essential. Your presence and skilled nursing care are reassuring. Be certain to allow the client adequate time to communicate needs and concerns. Assist the family in reassuring the client that nurses are present and that the client is not alone.

Diagnosis: Risk for Ineffective Therapeutic Regimen Management (Individuals) and Risk for Ineffective Family Therapeutic Regimen Management.
The client and family members need a lot of new information about permanent or long-term tracheostomy care.

Outcomes. Before discharge from the health care facility, the client and significant others will be confident in performing tracheostomy care, suctioning, and preoxygenation and in the use of safety measures, emergency airway management, aerosol therapy, and other aspects of the client's airway maintenance regimen.

Interventions. Learning self-care is important for the client with a permanent tracheostomy. It provides a sense of self-control and reduces dependency on others. The client and significant others should begin performing self-care procedures as soon as possible postoperatively in order to allow sufficient time for learning. Multimedia resources, videotape, and booklets should be used to supplement the demonstrations and teaching. Follow-up telephone calls, contact through the physician's office, and home health nursing care (see the Bridge to Home Health Care feature on Living with a Tracheostomy on the website) are necessary to identify the effectiveness of the teaching.

Significant others must also be able to provide tracheostomy care and other components of airway management. Teach family members how to provide rescue breathing using the information presented previously.

The client and significant others are often anxious about home management. Send home a duplicate tracheostomy tube for use in changing the tube or in the event of accidental decannulation. Close follow-up is essential. Arrange for home equipment and follow-up visits by a home health agency or community health nurse with expertise in caring for people with complex airway needs. Involve a tracheostomy nurse specialist in client teaching when available. Order home health care equipment from medical suppliers who employ respiratory therapists or nurses. Ideally, have the equipment initially delivered to the hospital, so that the client and significant others can learn its use under the supervision of professionals.

Evaluation

Nursing diagnoses related to airway management should be resolvable within a few days. Problems with

BOX 62-3 *Clinical Manifestations of Laryngeal Cancer*

Glottic Tumor

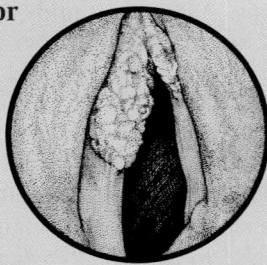

True glottic tumors interfere with normal closure and vibration of the vocal cords

Manifestations

Early: Voice change, hoarseness, hemoptysis

Late: Dyspnea, respiratory obstruction, dysphagia, weight loss, pain

Metastasize: Through regional lymph nodes (rare except in superior or inferior tumors)

Supraglottic Tumor

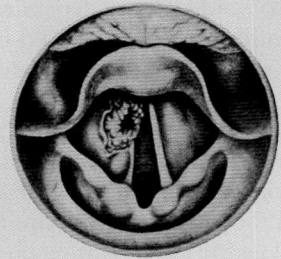

Carcinoma of the false cord partially hiding the true cord

Manifestations

Early: Aspiration on swallowing (especially liquids), persistent unilateral sore throat, foreign-body sensation, dysphagia, weight loss, neck mass, hemoptysis (expectoration of blood)

Late: Dyspnea, pain in the throat or referred to the ear

Subglottic Tumor

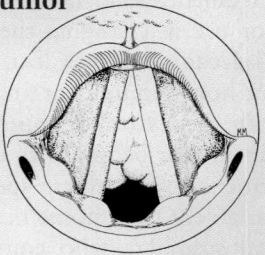

Subglottic polyp; this type of polyp can be single and smooth or lobulated as shown

Manifestations

Early: None

Late: Dyspnea, airway obstruction, dysphagia, weight loss, hemoptysis

Top and bottom figures from DeWeese, D.F., & Saunders, W.H. (1982). *Textbook of otolaryngology* (6th ed). St. Louis: Mosby; middle figure from Del Regato, J.A., et al. (1985). *Ackerman and Del Regato's cancer* (6th ed.). St. Louis: Mosby.

communication, infection, constipation, and eating remain areas of concern and require long-term planning.

NEOPLASTIC DISORDERS
BENIGN TUMORS OF THE LARYNX

Papillomas are one type of benign tumor of the larynx. They are small, wart-like growths believed to be viral in origin. Papillomas may be removed by surgical excision or laser. Surgery must be exact, because the nondiseased portion of the vocal cords needs to be retained for function. Other benign tumors of the larynx are *nodules* and *polyps*. Nodules and polyps frequently occur in people who abuse or overuse their voice.

CANCER OF THE LARYNX

Cancer of the larynx accounts for 2% to 3% of all malignancies. Care of the client with cancer of the larynx presents a unique challenge to the nurse because of the cosmetic and functional deformities commonly resulting from the disorder and its treatment. Benign and early malignant tumors may be treated with limited surgery, and the client recovers with little functional loss. Advanced tumors require extensive treatment, including surgery, radiation treatments, and chemotherapy. When a total laryngectomy is required, postoperatively the client is unable to speak, breathe through the nose or mouth, or eat normally. In addition, the creation of a permanent tracheostoma resulting from surgery has a tremendous impact on the client's functional ability and quality of life.

Laryngeal cancer is classified and treated by its anatomic site. Cancer of the larynx (voice box) may occur on the glottis (true vocal cords), the supraglottic structures (above the vocal cords), or the subglottic structures (below the vocal cords) (Box 62-3).

The American Cancer Society estimates 8900 new cases of laryngeal cancer each year, most occurring in men. However, the incidence of cancer of the larynx in women is increasing.[1] If untreated, cancer of the larynx is inevitably fatal; 90% of untreated people die within 3 years. It is potentially curable if diagnosed and treated early.

Etiology and Risk Factors

The primary etiologic agent in laryngeal cancer is cigarette smoking. Three of four clients in whom laryngeal cancer develops have smoked or currently smoke. Alcohol appears to act synergistically with tobacco to increase the risk of development of a malignant tumor in the upper airway. Additional risk factors include occupational exposure to asbestos, wood dust, mustard gas, and petroleum products and the inhalation of other noxious fumes. Chronic laryngitis and voice abuse may also contribute to the disorder. Research points to a link between tobacco exposure and mutation of the *p53* gene in squamous cell carcinoma of the head and neck.[2,13,21]

Pathophysiology

Squamous cell carcinoma is the most common malignant tumor of the larynx, arising from the membrane lining the respiratory tract. Metastasis from cancer of the glottis is unusual because of the sparse lymphatic drainage from the vocal cords. Cancer elsewhere in the larynx spreads more quickly because there are abundant lymphatic vessels. Metastatic disease often may be palpated as neck masses. Distant metastasis may occur in the lungs. Patterns of spread of head and neck cancer are shown in Figure 62-5.

Clinical Manifestations

The earliest clinical warning signs of laryngeal cancer are dependent on the location of the tumor. In general, hoarseness that lasts longer than 2 weeks should be evaluated. Hoarseness occurs when the tumor invades muscle and cartilage surrounding the larynx, causing fixation of the vocal cords. Most clients wait before seeking a diagnosis for chronic hoarseness.

Tumors on the glottis prevent glottic closure during speech, which causes hoarseness or a voice change. Supraglottic tumors may cause pain in the throat (especially with swallowing), aspiration during swallowing, a sensation of a foreign body in the throat, neck masses, or pain radiating to the ear by way of the glossopharyngeal and vagus nerves. Subglottic tumors have no early manifestations; clinical evidence does not appear until the lesion grows to obstruct the airway.

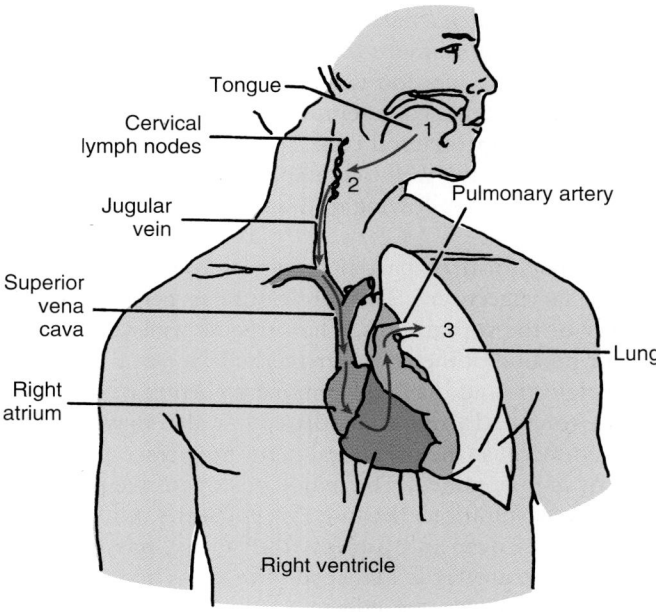

FIGURE 62-5 Pattern of spread of head and neck cancer. (From Black, J. [1991]. Reconstructive surgery in the elderly. *Plastic Surgical Nursing, 11,* 157.)

Diagnostic Findings

The diagnosis of laryngeal cancer is made by visual examination of the larynx using direct or indirect laryngoscopy. The nasopharynx and posterior soft palate are inspected indirectly with a small mirror or an instrument resembling a telescope. While the mirror is inserted, slight pressure is applied to the tongue, and the client is instructed to say "a" and then "e," which elevates the soft palate (see Figure 61-18, *A*). The instrument should not touch the tongue, or the client will gag. The nasopharynx is then inspected for drainage, bleeding, ulceration, or masses. Direct visualization of the larynx may be accomplished with use of several different instruments; most devices used are lighted endoscopes. The client is instructed to protrude the tongue, and the examiner *gently* holds the tongue with a gauze sponge and pulls it forward. A laryngeal mirror or telescopic endoscope is inserted into the oropharynx; again, contact with the tongue is avoided. The client is instructed to breathe in and out rapidly through the mouth, or to "pant like a puppy." Panting decreases the gagging sensation caused by the examination. During quiet respiration, the base of the tongue, epiglottis, and vocal cords are examined for manifestations of infection or tumor (see Figure 61-18, *B*). The client is instructed to vocalize a high-pitched *eee* to approximate (close) the vocal cords. The examiner observes the movement of the cords, the color of the mucous membranes, and the presence of any lesions. If the client is unable to cooperate as described, the examination may be performed with a fiberoptic endoscope inserted through the nose.

Before any definitive treatment for tumor is initiated, a panendoscopy and biopsy should be performed to determine the exact location, size, and extent of the primary tumor. Computed tomography (CT) or magnetic resonance imaging (MRI) is used to assist with this process. Laboratory analysis includes a complete blood count, determination of serum electrolytes including calcium, and kidney and liver function tests. These data help determine the physiologic readiness of the client for surgery. Because the airway will be altered after surgery, the client requires a thorough pulmonary assessment with ABG analysis for identification of any pre-existing pulmonary disorders that would interfere with breathing. Clients who are to undergo partial laryngectomy must have an adequate pulmonary reserve in order to produce an effective cough postoperatively. The operation is associated with an increased risk of aspiration, and the client must be able to cough to rid the airway of aspirated secretions. Finally, for ascertaining possible tumor spread or other primary tumors, a chest radiography and barium swallow study or esophagography are performed.

Once the tumor has been identified and a biopsy performed, the tumor can be staged. Staging has important implications for treatment choice and outcome. It is essential to determine the extent of the primary tumor in order to select the most appropriate intervention. Staging is accomplished by (1) measuring the size of the primary tumor, (2) determining the presence of enlarged lymphatic nodes, and (3) determining the presence of distant metastasis. This system of staging is called the TNM (tumor-node-metastasis) classification system (see Chapter 19).

Outcome Management
■ Medical Management

Tumor Ablation. The goal of client care is ablation of the tumor, with sparing of undiseased tissue when possible. The choice of treatment for glottic cancer depends on the degree of tumor involvement. If the tumor is limited to the true vocal cord, without causing limitation of the cord's movement, radiation therapy is usually the best treatment, with cure rates of 85% to 95%. The radiation dose depends on the size and location of the tumor; it is usually a minimum dose of 5500 to 6000 cGy (*gray* is a more accurate unit than *rad*) over 5 to 7 weeks. Hyperfractionation (delivery of radiation twice a day) may be done to improve tumor control. During radiation therapy, the client needs to be assessed for manifestations of destruction of normal tissue, ability to eat, airway distress, and other side effects. The complications of radiation therapy to the larynx include skin irritation, xerostomia, mucositis, laryngeal edema, and delayed healing. Radiation therapy is discussed in Chapter 19.

Supraglottic tumors may be treated with radiation therapy or a partial laryngectomy, with or without lymph node dissection. Subglottic tumors are usually more advanced carcinomas in which the tumor has spread to surrounding tissues. Metastasis is common. Treatment requires a total laryngectomy with or without radical neck dissection on the same or both sides of the tumor (see later discussion). The operative site may require reconstruction with pectoralis myocutaneous flaps (see Chapter 51).

Chemotherapy alone is not considered to be curative in treating head and neck cancers but it is now integrated into standard therapy for head and neck cancer. It may be administered preoperatively to reduce tumor size, concurrently with radiation therapy, postoperatively to reduce the risk of metastasis, or as palliative treatment. Larynx preservation may be possible with induction chemotherapy followed by radiation. Chemotherapy is generally not effective in advanced laryngeal cancer, but it may control the development of new primary tumors through a process called *chemoprevention*.[21]

Clients with laryngeal tumors often present in a compromised nutritional state due to dysphagia and weight loss. In addition, surgery, radiation therapy, and chemotherapy can directly affect oropharyngeal structures and impair swallowing. Nutritional intervention should begin before treatment to prevent malnutrition, thereby improving the overall prognosis.

■ Nursing Management of the Medical Client

The client undergoing radiation therapy for laryngeal cancer should be taught about the procedure and how to assess for and manage any expected problems at home. Written material is usually best, so that the client and family can refer to it as needed. Skin care for the irradiated site should include the use of prescribed creams and sunscreens, which are "patted" onto the skin; avoiding extremes of temperature; avoiding rough or tight garments; and avoiding rubbing or scratching the area.

■ Surgical Management

The goals of surgical intervention for laryngeal cancer are to (1) remove the cancer, (2) maintain adequate physiologic function of the airway, and (3) achieve a personally acceptable physical appearance. Many clients require tracheostomy for airway management (see earlier discussion). Most clients with advanced laryngeal cancer also have malnutrition from obstruction to swallowing by the tumor, as well as from the effects of the cancer. Before surgery, supplemental nutrition may be provided by NG tube-feedings or gastrostomy feedings. If long-term difficulty in swallowing is anticipated, a gastrostomy tube may be inserted at the time of surgery.

Laser Surgery. Small tumors can often be eradicated with the use of laser. Laser surgery for vocal cord tumors can preserve much of the normal glottis, leaving the client with a usable voice. Sometimes laser surgery is combined with radiation therapy.[21]

Partial Laryngectomy. For cancer involving one true vocal cord, or one cord plus a portion of the other, a partial laryngectomy is feasible. This procedure is also called a vertical partial laryngectomy and involves the removal of half or more of the larynx (Figure 62-6). A horizontal neck incision is made, and the diseased portion of the vocal cord is removed. Sometimes up to one third of the contralateral cord is also removed. This operation is generally well tolerated, and the client has only mild difficulty swallowing and an altered but adequate voice.

Another form of partial laryngectomy is the supraglottic laryngectomy. This procedure is performed for cancer of the supraglottis. The surgeon removes the superior portion of the larynx from the false vocal cords to the epiglottis and may also remove a portion of the base of the tongue. Lymph node dissection also may be performed. Because the true vocal cords are preserved, voice quality is maintained. The major postoperative problem is risk of aspiration, because the epiglottis, which normally closes over and protects the larynx, has been removed. The airway is managed with a tracheostomy after surgery; when the edema subsides in surrounding tissues, the tracheostomy tube can usually be removed and the stoma allowed to heal. The client then needs to be taught how to swallow to avoid aspiration.[8]

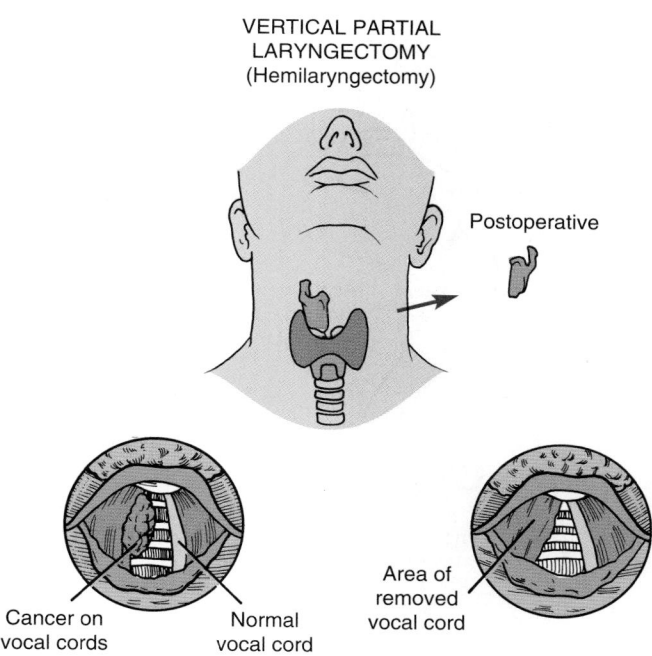

VERTICAL PARTIAL
LARYNGECTOMY
(Hemilaryngectomy)

Postoperative

Cancer on
vocal cords

Normal
vocal cord

Area of
removed
vocal cord

FIGURE 62-6 Technique of partial laryngectomy.

For selected confined transglottic carcinomas, a supra-cricoid partial laryngectomy may be indicated. This conservative procedure preserves functional speech and swallowing without a permanent tracheostomy.

Total Laryngectomy. For large glottic tumors with fixation of the vocal cords, a total laryngectomy is required. The larynx is the connection of the pharynx (upper airway) and the trachea (lower airway) (Figure 62-7, *A*). When the larynx is removed, a permanent opening is made by suturing the trachea to the neck. The esophagus remains attached to the pharynx (Figure 62-7, *B*). Because no air can enter the nose, the client loses the sense of smell. The biggest problem for the client after laryngectomy is loss of voice. The client should be made aware that without surgery, the voice quality worsens as the tumor enlarges, but in any case the loss of voice constitutes a serious psychological issue. Because the trachea and esophagus are permanently separated by surgery, there is no risk of aspiration unless a fistula forms from the trachea to the esophagus. Besides this, the potential complications of the total laryngectomy are the same as for the partial laryngectomy (see earlier discussion).

Cervical Lymph Node Dissection. Metastasis to the cervical lymph nodes is common with tumors of the upper aerodigestive tract. Surgical management of laryngeal tumors often includes neck dissection. Radical neck dissection (also called en bloc) involves the removal of lymphatic drainage channels and nodes, the sternocleidomastoid muscle, the spinal accessory nerve, the jugular vein, and tissue in the submandibular area. A modified radical neck dissection spares the spinal accessory nerve, and a selective neck dissection removes only the lymph nodes within the area of anticipated spread.

Complications. Possible complications after laryngeal surgery are airway obstruction, hemorrhage, carotid artery rupture, and fistula formation. Airway obstruction is due to edema in the surgical site, bleeding into the airway, or loss of airway from a plugged tracheostomy tube. Airway obstruction constitutes an emergency and requires immediate intervention for restoration of the airway.

Hemorrhage is usually the result of inadequate hemostasis during surgery. Some blood-tinged sputum is expected in the tracheal secretions for the first 48 hours, but frank bleeding from the tracheotomy site or tube is a manifestations of hemorrhage and must be reported to the physician immediately. Also assess the client for other manifestations of bleeding such as evident hematoma or unilateral swelling, tachycardia, hypotension, and changes in respiratory patterns.

Carotid artery rupture is usually a late complication and is related to poor condition of the neck tissue. It may be the result of previous radiation therapy to the area, pharyngocutaneous fistula, recurrent tumor, or infection. This condition is also a life-threatening emergency and carries an extremely high mortality rate. Mild bleeding from the oral cavity, neck, or trachea may precede impending rupture by 24 to 48 hours. A pulsating tracheostomy tube may indicate that the tip of the tube is resting on the innominate artery, which may cause injury to the artery and result in hemorrhage.

Fistulae between the hypopharynx and the skin may also develop. Many fistulae heal on their own, but treatment may require surgery, depending on the location and size.

■ Nursing Management of the Surgical Client

Partial Laryngectomy

Preoperative Care
In addition to the usual preoperative assessments, assess the client's nutritional status. Compare current body weight with ideal body weight, usual caloric intake, total lymphocyte count, albumin levels, and hemoglobin value and hematocrit. In addition, assess dentition and the oral cavity. Because many of these clients have abused tobacco and alcohol, the dentition and oral cavity are frequently in poor condition. In addition, if the client is an active alcoholic, plans should consider support through the period of alcohol withdrawal. The ideal plan of care would allow some nutritional support and oral care before surgery. Currently, few clients can be admitted before surgery; therefore such supportive care must be accomplished before hospital admission.

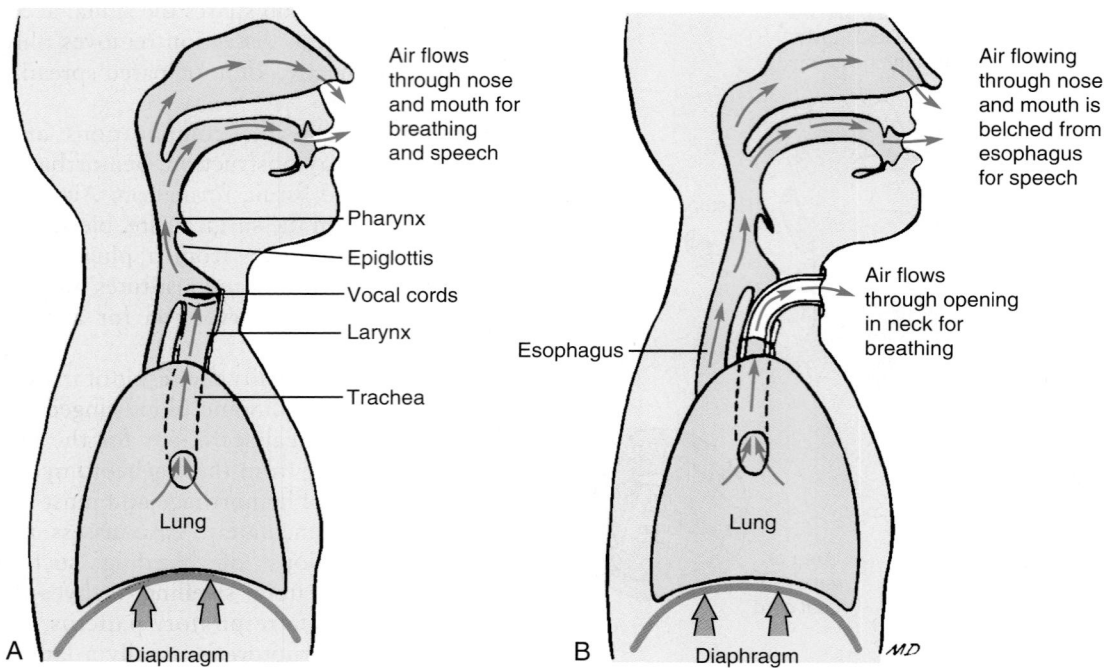

FIGURE 62-7 A, Before laryngectomy, air flow is through the nose and mouth. **B,** After surgical removal of the larynx, a new opening must be made for air passage. The trachea and esophagus are separated.

The client's work history and financial concerns should also be investigated during this initial assessment. Inability to purchase medical insurance or to pay for health care services may account for the client's lack of personal and medical care.

The client's usual coping strategies and family support should also be evaluated. Some degree of cosmetic (aesthetic) change will result after surgery, and the client will be unable to speak for some time. Preoperative plans should consider alternative methods of communication and family support networks. Preoperative education by rehabilitated laryngectomees is important for these **EB** clients.[2]

Because of the multiple problems common in these clients, a team approach to their care is used. Members of the team usually include the primary physician or surgeon, nurses, a social worker, a dietitian, a speech or swallowing therapist, a physical therapist, and home health care nurses. If extensive surgery is required, a plastic surgeon and a maxillofacial prosthodontist may also care for the client during reconstruction.

Postoperative Care
Assessment

In addition to the routine postoperative assessments, after a partial laryngectomy the client needs to undergo careful assessment of the airway, lung sounds, and posi-

tion of the tracheostomy tube, as well as checking for potential complications related to the surgical procedure and the tracheostomy tube (see earlier discussion).

Diagnosis, Outcomes, Interventions

Diagnosis: Risk for Aspiration. Because of the removal of the epiglottis (which normally acts as a trap door to close the airway and prevent aspiration) and because secretions are excessive after surgery, the client is at very high risk for aspiration. This is a priority diagnosis.

Outcomes. The client will have reduced risk of aspiration, as evidenced by clear breath sounds throughout the chest, normal (for age) respiratory rate and rhythm, chest secretions that are clear or only slightly blood-tinged, and ability to cough.

Interventions. In the immediate postoperative period, priority is given to management of the upper airway. The client should be positioned in the semi-Fowler to high Fowler position to decrease edema of the airway, facilitate breathing, and improve comfort.

A cuffed tracheostomy tube is generally inserted during surgery and is maintained for the first several days after surgery to minimize aspiration of secretions and for assisted or controlled ventilation. Secretions collect above the cuff. For removal of secretions, the cuff should be deflated during exhalation. The client should be instructed to cough during deflation of the cuff. If the client cannot cough, suctioning should be used to prevent secretions from being aspirated. The cuff should be reinflated during inspiration.

When the edema has subsided, the tracheostomy tube may be removed. The decannulation process is slow and begins with observation of the client for aspiration, as follows. The cuff of the tube is deflated, and the client is observed for the ability to swallow saliva and other secretions without coughing or requiring additional suctioning. If increased secretions are present through and around the tracheostomy tube, aspiration is occurring and the cuff should be reinflated. If no aspiration is occurring, the tracheostomy tube can be replaced with a smaller, uncuffed tube. If the uncuffed tube is tolerated without aspiration, the tube is capped (plugged) to determine the client's ability to breathe through the upper airway. If the client can breathe through the upper airway for 24 hours, the tracheostomy tube is removed, and the stoma is taped closed and covered with an occlusive dressing.

Diagnosis: Ineffective Airway Clearance.

The physical alteration in the airway and the presence of a tracheostomy tube interfere with normal movement of mucus up and out of the bronchial tree. In addition, as a result of prior smoking, the cilia have become ineffective. *Ineffective Airway Clearance* is also a priority nursing diagnosis for several days.

Outcomes. The client will have improved airway clearance, as evidenced by effortless, quiet respirations at baseline rate and clear breath sounds.

Interventions. The client may have copious secretions because of the presence of the tracheostomy tube, a history of chronic obstructive lung disease, and aspiration. There may also be oral secretions that cannot be swallowed. Oral secretions accumulate because of the disruption of normal airflow, and swallowing may be impaired as a result of surgery. In the alert and conscious client, coughing and deep-breathing mobilize and eliminate many of these secretions. However, in the client who has undergone head and neck surgery and is just emerging from anesthesia, these measures may not be possible. Suctioning of the trachea is needed for the first 24 to 48 hours after surgery. The frequency of suctioning depends on the client's needs, but suctioning every hour or more often is common for the first 24 hours. Sterile technique must be used to avoid introducing microorganisms into the tracheobronchial tree in a client with impaired immune defenses due to malignancy and surgery. (Suctioning techniques can be found in fundamentals of nursing textbooks.)

The inner cannula of the tracheostomy tube should be cleaned as often as necessary to provide a clear airway.

In the immediate postoperative phase, the inner cannula is cleaned after suctioning. Once the client is ambulatory and can handle secretions safely, the cannula can be cleaned three times a day and as necessary.

Chest physiotherapy, ultrasonic nebulization, and aerosol administration of bronchodilators and mucolytics into deeper parts of the respiratory tract for sputum induction are recommended to prevent pulmonary complications. These treatments are performed every 4 hours for the first few days after surgery and then usually decreased to four times a day once the client can ambulate.[24]

Diagnosis: Risk for Impaired Gas Exchange.

Like other postoperative clients, clients with neck surgery have a high risk for atelectasis related to low tidal volume breathing secondary to pain, sedation, and increased mucus production.

Outcomes. The client will have adequate oxygenation, as evidenced by pulse oximetry values above 90%, ABG values within normal limits (that take into consideration any pre-existing lung disorders, such as emphysema), no air hunger, and clear lung sounds.

Interventions. Oxygenation is assessed through ABG analysis or pulse oximetry and the fraction of inspired oxygen (FIO_2) may be adjusted. If the client has pre-existent chronic air flow limitations, oxygen may have to be delivered at lower percentages or not at all. Compressed air with high humidity may be substituted in such cases.

Diagnosis: Impaired Nutrition: Less Than Body Requirements.

A combination of the pre-existing malignancy and swallowing difficulties sets the stage for malnutrition. In addition, concomitant lung disorders and alcoholism, which are common in this population, increase the tendency for malnutrition.

Outcomes. The client will have an improved nutritional status, as evidenced by maintaining baseline body weight or losing less than 5 pounds; consuming adequate fluid, protein, fat, and carbohydrate each 24 hours; swallowing without aspirating or choking; and maintaining hemoglobin, hematocrit, albumin, and total lymphocyte values within normal limits.

Interventions. Immediately after surgery, typically an NG tube is inserted for removal of gastric secretions until postoperative ileus subsides. If long-term difficulty in swallowing is anticipated, a gastrostomy tube may be inserted at the time of surgery. Assess for bowel sounds, passage of flatus, and hunger as manifestations of returning gastrointestinal function. In some clients, tube-feeding with commercial supplements is indicated.

Continually ascertain the correct position of the tube before each feeding. (Techniques for checking feeding tube placement can be found in fundamentals of nursing textbooks.) The tube-feeding can be administered by pump, slow drip, or bolus feeding, depending on the client's tolerance. Aspiration remains a high risk with partial laryngectomy, and precautions to guard the client from this event with its untoward results are critical.

When the epiglottis has been removed, the timing for resumption of oral feeding after a partial laryngectomy is controversial. One approach is to begin oral feedings with the tracheostomy tube in place when edema has subsided and the client is able to swallow secretions. The advantage of this technique is that aspirated liquid can be suctioned. A second technique is to delay oral feeding until the client has been decannulated and the stoma has healed. The advantage of this technique is that with a closed stoma, the client is able to increase intrathoracic pressure and remove any aspirated material through an effective cough.

Whenever the client eats, eating should begin with a nonpourable pureed diet; liquids are reserved until swallowing has been relearned. See the Client Education Guide feature on Swallowing Technique After a Partial Laryngectomy, below. Once swallowing can be accomplished without aspiration, carbonated beverages may be added. Thin liquids should be withheld until the risk of aspiration is minimal.

Diagnosis: Risk for Infection. The loss of primary defenses of the skin and delayed healing due to pre-existing malignancy and malnutrition make *Risk for Infection* a common nursing diagnosis.

CLIENT EDUCATION GUIDE

Swallowing Technique After a Partial Laryngectomy

- Begin with soft or semisolid foods.
- Stay with a nurse or swallowing therapist during meals until you master the technique of swallowing without choking.
- Be patient; learning to swallow again is frustrating.
- Follow these steps in sequence:
1. Take a deep breath.
2. Bear down to close the vocal cords.
3. Place food into your mouth.
4. Swallow.
5. Cough to rid the closed cord of accumulated food particles.
6. Swallow.
7. Cough.
8. Breathe.

Outcomes. The client will have no clinical manifestations of wound infection, as evidenced by continued approximation of incisional edges; decrease in the amount of wound drainage; absence of purulent drainage; absence of redness, swelling, tenderness, or warmth beyond the suture lines; absence of fever; and a white blood cell count within normal limits.

Interventions. During surgery, a wound drain is placed into the surrounding tissues of the neck and attached to constant suction. A closed wound drainage system is attached to the client's gown to prevent accidental dislodgment. Using standard precautions, assess the amount and color of the drainage every 4 hours for the first 24 hours. Assess the wound for manifestations of hematoma or seroma formation by noting whether the amount of drainage is increasing or whether there is a change in the color or consistency of the drainage. Also assess the color of the surgical incisions. If the amount of drainage is decreasing, the drain may be removed by the physician. Dressings are placed over the drain puncture sites on the skin. Small to moderate amounts of serosanguineous drainage should be expected for another 48 to 72 hours.

The suture lines should be cleaned at least twice daily with hydrogen peroxide followed by a water or saline rinse. A thin film of antibiotic ointment may be applied to the suture line to prevent crusting of secretions and promote healing.

Evaluation

Expect the problems with airway management to resolve within a few days. Infection, apart from atelectasis, does not arise for about 72 hours. Nutritional problems and problems with healing may require several weeks to resolve.

■ Self-Care

The client who has undergone partial laryngectomy may be discharged from the hospital before completion of wound healing. If upper airway edema has not subsided, the client is discharged with a temporary tracheostomy. The client and significant others should understand and demonstrate proper care of the tube, including inner cannula care, technique for insertion of the entire tube in case of accidental decannulation, suctioning, humidification techniques, and emergency resuscitation measures.

Once decannulation has been performed, the stoma must be cleansed and an occlusive dressing applied at least once a day. Additional wound care includes cleaning the incision area with hydrogen peroxide and water and applying an antibiotic ointment. All instructions given to the client should be in writing, with additional teaching materials used as available. Ongoing assessment for healing, recurrent tumor, or a new tumor is required.

Total Laryngectomy

The nursing management of the client after a total laryngectomy is the same as the care given to a client with a partial laryngectomy, except for feeding and teaching about permanent stoma care. Clients who have a total laryngectomy have a permanent tracheostomy and need to learn how to speak using alternative methods.

Nutrition. Immediately after surgery, the client's nutrition is supplemented with tube feedings. The client remains on tube feedings until edema has subsided and suture line healing has occurred. When the client can swallow secretions, oral feedings can begin. The diet usually begins with liquid or semi-soft foods and progresses as healing occurs.

Communication. For the first few days after surgery, the client should communicate by writing. If the client is very fatigued, requests such as "I need something for pain" may be expressed by using a communication board so that the client can just point to the statement. Even though the client cannot speak, conversation should still include the client's input through nodding and pointing and not be directed only to others such as the family. Avoiding conversation with the client because of difficulty in communication is demeaning to the client and leads to frustration.

Artificial Larynx. An artificial larynx may be used as early as 3 to 4 days after surgery. These battery-operated speech devices are held alongside the neck or can be adapted with a plastic tube that is inserted in the mouth. The air inside the mouth is vibrated, and the client articulates as usual (Figure 62-8). The speech quality is monotone and mechanical-sounding but intelligible.[8,25]

Esophageal Speech. Esophageal speech is a technique that requires the client to swallow and hold air in the upper esophagus. By controlling the flow of air, the client can pronounce as many as 6 to 10 words before stopping to swallow more air. The voice is deep but is loud and effective once the technique is mastered.[8]

Tracheoesophageal Puncture. Tracheoesophageal puncture (TEP) is a surgical technique that also restores speech (Figure 62-9). A small puncture is made into the upper tracheostoma to the cervical esophagus for creation of a fistula. After the fistula tract has healed, a small one-way valve, or voice prosthesis, is inserted. By occlusion of the prosthesis, air can be shunted into the esophagus and used to produce speech. The TEP may be done concurrently with a total laryngectomy or as a

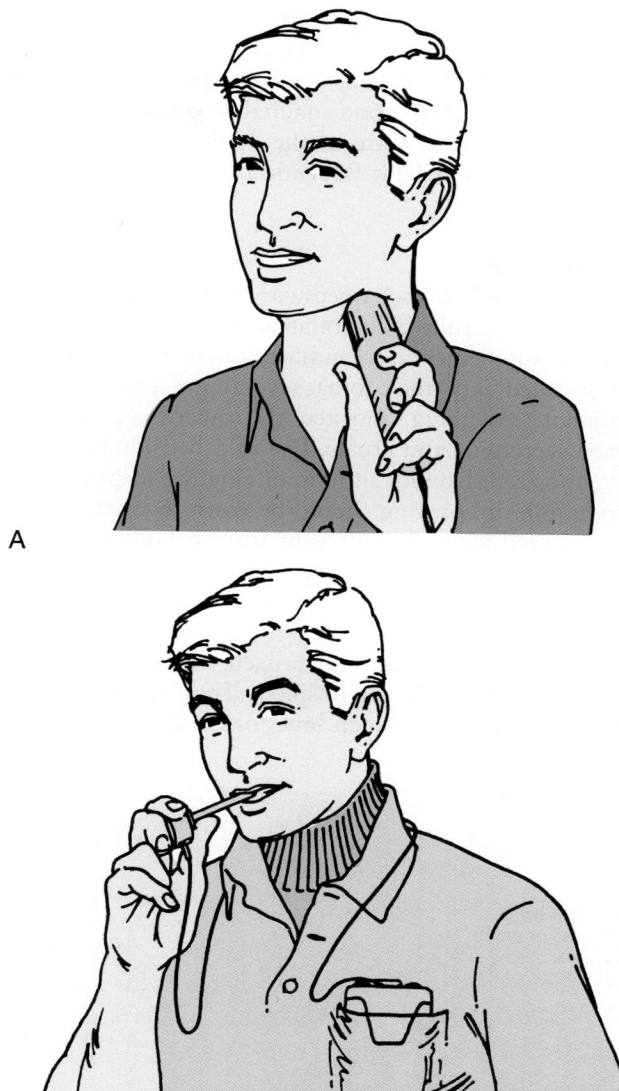

A

B

FIGURE 62-8 Artificial larynx. This hand-held, battery-powered speech aid is placed against the neck. **A,** When the artificial larynx is activated, it creates a vibration that is transmitted to the neck and into the mouth. Words silently formed by the mouth become sounds from the vibrations emitted by the device. Any type of artificial larynx requires muscle and tongue control and hand strength; usually, such a device is not used until immediate postoperative neck tenderness has subsided. **B,** Electronic speech aid allows the client to adjust tone, pitch, and volume. An oral connector permits speech without the necessity of placing the device against the neck. This is an advantage immediately after surgery, when the neck is too sensitive for a neck-vibrating device.

secondary procedure after healing and radiation therapy. These devices require maintenance; therefore only clients who are highly motivated, who are able to perform self-care, and who have good manual dexterity are eligible for this procedure. Care of the TEP surgical wound is presented in the Client Education Guide feature on the website.[8]

■ Self-Care

Clients should be discharged with an extra tracheostomy tube to allow tube changes at home (Figure 62-10). To provide supplemental humidification, normal saline may be instilled into the stoma several times each day to stimulate coughing, moisten the mucosa, and loosen dried secretions and crusts. Use of a bedside humidifier or vaporizer also aids in humidifying the inspired air. A stoma bib or covering should be worn to warm and filter inspired air and to prevent foreign bodies from entering the stoma. These coverings can be purchased, or the client may improvise by using a scarf, necktie, or turtleneck shirt.

The client must be encouraged to continue speech therapy as begun in the hospital. The techniques to restore speech require much time for mastery; the client is

seen by a speech therapist after dismissal from the hospital. Community support groups for clients after laryngectomy such as the Lost Cord Club and the International Association of Laryngectomees offer needed reassurance. Much patience is required by the client and family while the client is relearning to speak. The process is time-consuming and frustrating, and progress may sometimes be slow. Encourage the family to give the client enough time to formulate the words and not speak for the client.

Once the incision has completely healed, the tracheostomy tube is no longer required (Figure 62-11). This process varies but usually takes about 6 to 8 weeks. Occasionally, the tube may be required at night, if the stoma is small or the client does not get adequate air exchange during sleep. Once the tracheostomy tube has

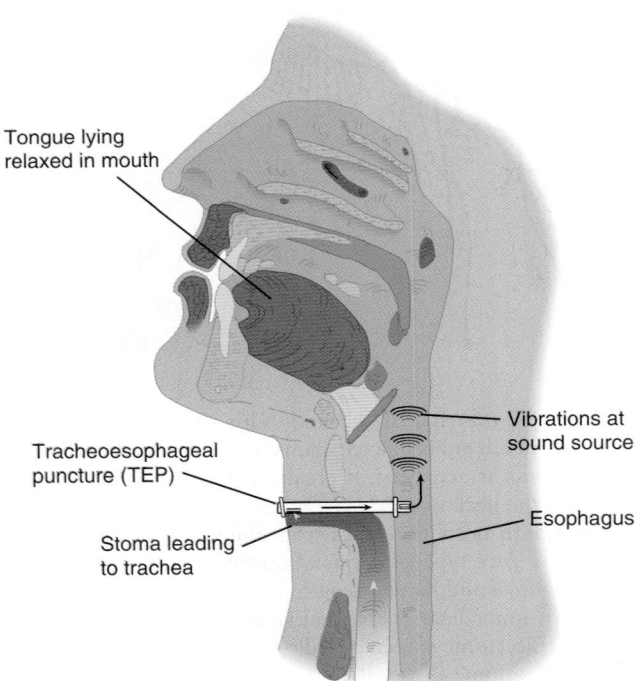

FIGURE 62-9 Tracheoesophageal puncture for voice rehabilitation after laryngectomy. A prosthesis is inserted into a fistula created in the neck. The prosthesis has a one-way valve that permits air to pass into the esophagus but prevents accidental aspiration. To speak, the client occludes the prosthesis with a finger or attachment. Exhaled air is then shunted through the prosthesis, where it vibrates, and exits the mouth as a spoken word.

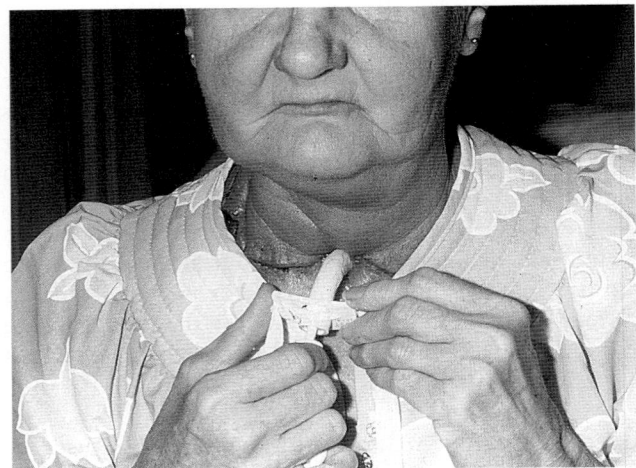

FIGURE 62-10 Insertion of a laryngectomy tube into a permanent tracheostoma. The obturator or guide is inserted into the outer cannula. After the tube is lubricated with water-soluble ointment, the client takes a deep breath and the lubricated tube is inserted. The obturator is removed, and the tube is tied in place.

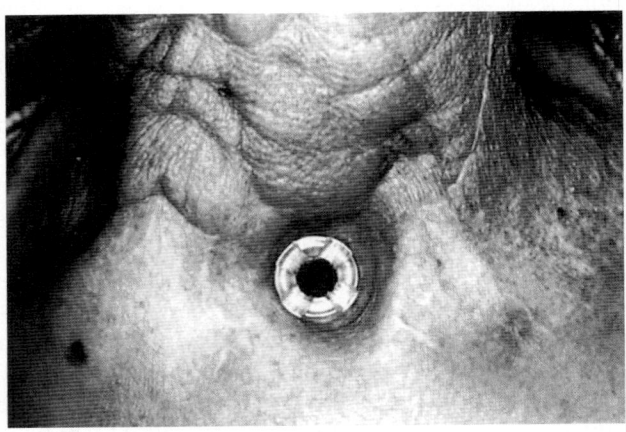

FIGURE 62-11 Healed tracheostomy incision.

been removed, the client can disguise the stoma with clothing and begin to regain a sense of normalcy.

Tub baths or showers are permitted, but the client must use caution to prevent introduction of water into the stoma, aiming the water spray at midchest. Commercial stoma shower covers are available. Water sports are prohibited. If the client fishes, a life preserver must be worn at all times on the boat.

The client should wear a medical alert bracelet and carry an emergency wallet card to identify the fact that resuscitation cannot be performed through the mouth. Information about obtaining these forms of identification is available from the American Cancer Society. The use of mouth-to-stoma rescue breathing is imperative when resuscitation is needed in these clients. Family members should be directed to a community program that teaches mouth-to-stoma resuscitation. For additional security, a wireless "beeper" or automatic response monitoring device can be useful.

The client may require a nutritional plan for the first few weeks at home. The dietitian should work with the client and family to determine the consistency of food easiest to swallow as well as the kinds of foods required to obtain needed protein and calories.

It is essential that the client not smoke so that lung function is preserved and the formation of other aerodigestive tract tumors is prevented. For some clients after laryngectomy, the process of smoking cessation seems pointless. Some clients continue to smoke by inhaling the cigarette smoke through the stoma. The attitude is one of "Why quit now? What else could happen to me?" Use extra support and encouragement with the client, remembering to be an advocate of the client's choice as well as providing assurance that the quality of life after smoking cessation improves.

Follow-up care is important to assess the healing process, to evaluate coping mechanisms, and to examine the client for possible metastasis or new tumors. The client should be taught to report any of the following manifestations to the physician:

- A lump anywhere in the neck or body
- Persistent cough, sore throat, or earache
- Hemoptysis
- Sores around the stoma or within the trachea that do not heal
- Difficulty swallowing or breathing

Neck Dissection

Preoperative Care

Before surgery, the client's understanding of the plans for surgery should be assessed. Determine what the surgeon has told the client and how much information has been retained or lost because of anxiety. In addition, address the fears the client has about the diagnosis of cancer and fears of deformity after surgery. Assist the client to understand the anatomic and physiologic alterations that will occur as a result of radical surgery. Explain to the client and family what to expect after surgery (e.g., placement in the intensive care unit, tracheostomy, drainage tubes) and review postoperative care (e.g., communication techniques to be used if a tracheostomy is to be placed).

The client's support systems and degree of coping should be assessed. If the client is an alcoholic, the use of alcohol may be the usual coping tool. Because alcohol will not be available, assess the other coping mechanisms available to the client, and encourage the client to use them. Sources may include friends and family. Identify new support systems, if needed, such as interaction with people who have had the same surgery or diagnosis.

Postoperative Care

After surgery, the usual postoperative assessments are performed, with special attention given to the airway. Airway patency can be lost as a result of edema of the neck or bleeding within the area. Assess the client for manifestations of airway edema or bleeding. Auscultate lung sounds every 2 hours for the first 24 hours. Report manifestations of airway obstruction immediately.

Place the client in a semi-Fowler position to minimize postoperative edema. Monitor neck drainage for volume and color. Sanguineous or serosanguineous drainage is expected for the first 72 hours after surgery. Once drainage has stopped, the wound drains are removed.

Pressure dressings may be used in the immediate postoperative period, depending on physician preference. If a dressing is used, it should be reinforced as needed and observed for any drainage. If musculocutaneous flaps were needed for coverage, pressure dressings are not used, and special flap care is required. (See Chapter 51 for specific care of flaps.)

If the surgical defect was repaired with musculocutaneous flaps, the flap should be assessed for arterial inflow and venous outflow. Flap temperature, color, and blanching should be noted every hour for the first 24 hours and every 4 hours after that time. Other means of monitoring flap perfusion (Doppler signals) may be used.

Because of the disruption of the sensory nerve fibers from the incisions used, most clients report only minimal pain at the surgical site. If an en bloc radical neck dissection has been performed, postoperative shoulder dysfunction is the rule, with forward rotation and dropping of the shoulder. Sectioning of the spinal accessory nerve during neck dissection also interrupts innervation to the upper trapezius muscle.

Exercises to increase range of motion and muscle strength, shown in the Client Education Guide feature on Exercises After Radial Neck Surgery on the website, are encouraged to prevent a "frozen shoulder" and to restore full movement. If a selective or modified neck dissection has been performed, minimal alterations in range of motion and muscle strength are anticipated. Encourage use of exercise to prevent permanent disability.[3,25]

■ Self-Care

After neck dissection, caution clients about the potential for injury to neck tissue due to lack of sensation. The use of a heating pad or exposure to temperature extremes may result in tissue injury (burns, frostbite) in a client who cannot feel these temperatures. Clients who have a tracheostomy need specific instructions for its management. Explain ongoing evaluations and follow-up.

HEMORRHAGIC, INFECTIOUS, AND INFLAMMATORY DISORDERS

EPISTAXIS

Epistaxis (nosebleed) may result from irritation, trauma, infection, foreign bodies, or tumors. Epistaxis may also be the result of systemic disease (e.g., atherosclerosis, hypertension, blood dyscrasias) or systemic treatment (e.g., chemotherapy or anticoagulants), or it may be idiopathic.[20]

Outcome Management
■ Medical Management

Ninety percent of nosebleeds are anterior, most occurring in children and young adults. Anterior epistaxis is initially treated by assisting the client to a sitting position. Apply pressure by pinching the anterior portion of the nose for a minimum of 5 to 10 minutes. This maneuver is often successful because the most common source of epistaxis is the anterior part of the septum in an area known as Kisselbach's plexus, a venous plexus vulnerable to trauma. In addition, the application of ice compresses to produce vasoconstriction may also reduce bleeding. If more definitive treatment is necessary, anterior epistaxis can usually be controlled by cauterization of the bleeding vessel with applications of silver nitrate. If these measures do not stop the bleeding, nasal packing may be inserted unilaterally or bilaterally. Antibacterial ointment is applied to half-inch gauze, which is then gently but firmly inserted into the anterior nasal cavities to apply pressure to the bleeding vessels. The use of petrolatum gauze packing should be avoided, because it has no antimicrobial properties, and a malodorous discharge may develop within 1 to 2 days of insertion. Nasal packing should remain in place for a minimum of 48 to 72 hours.[20]

Ten percent of nosebleeds are posterior, usually occurring in persons older than 50 years. Posterior bleeding tends to cause increased swallowing of blood, which can be noted in the pharynx. For clients with posterior epistaxis, a *posterior plug* may be necessary in addition to the anterior nasal packing (Figure 62-12). Insertion of a posterior plug is very uncomfortable, and a mild analgesic may be required to reduce anxiety and discomfort. A small, red rubber catheter is passed through the nose into the oropharynx and mouth. A gauze pack is tied to the catheter, and the catheter is withdrawn; this moves the pack into proper placement in the nasopharynx and posterior nose to apply pressure. The nasal cavity is packed with half-inch gauze, and the strings from the posterior pack are tied around a rolled gauze or bolus to maintain its position outside the nasal vestibule. The ties from the oral cavity are taped to the client's face to prevent loosening or dislodgment of the plug. A nasal balloon may be substituted for the traditional nasal pack. When the balloon is inflated with normal saline, pressure is applied to the lateral nasal wall.[20]

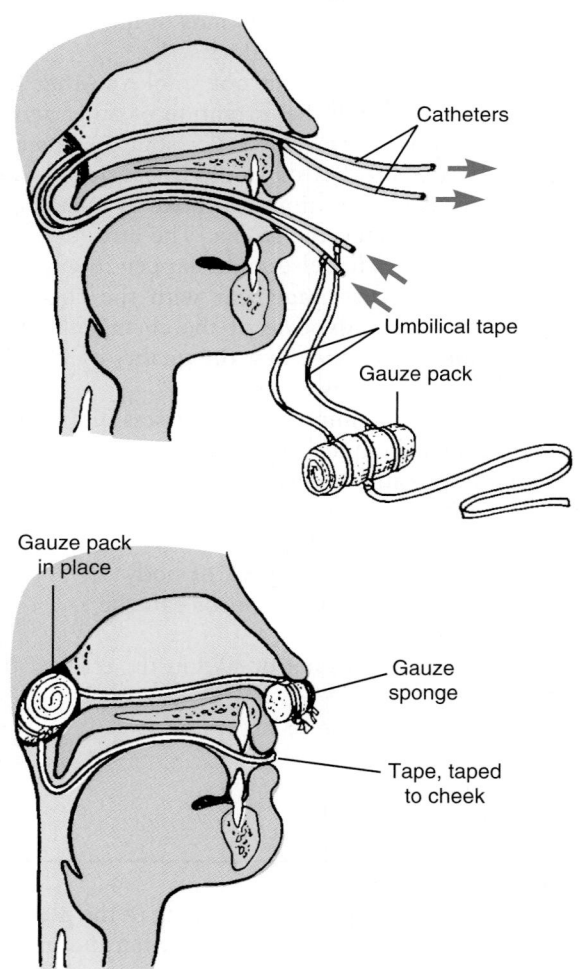

FIGURE 62-12 Instillation of a posterior nasal pack (plug), typically used in an emergency.

■ Nursing Management of the Medical Client

Clients with a posterior plug and anterior nasal packing may be admitted to the hospital and monitored closely for hypoxia. The presence of posterior packing may alter consciousness and respiratory status, especially in older adults. Because hypertension is frequently cited as a risk factor for epistaxis, monitor the client's blood pressure. General comfort measures, such as humidification, the use of a drip pad to collect bloody drainage and mucus, and application of water-soluble ointment around the nares to provide lubrication, help alleviate the discomfort. Monitor the client closely for any manifestations of airway obstruction and bleeding from the anterior or posterior nares. Inspect the oral cavity for the presence of blood, soft palate necrosis, and proper placement of the posterior plug. If the posterior plug is visible, notify the physician for readjustment of the packing. Posterior nasal packs remain in place for 5 days.[9,20] Prophylactic antibiotics are used to prevent toxic shock syndrome and sinusitis.

■ Surgical Management

If anterior and posterior packs fail to control epistaxis, internal maxillary or ethmoidal surgical *artery ligation* may be required. An incision is made in the gum line above the incisor on the affected side, and the maxillary sinus is entered. The artery that supplies the area of bleeding is identified, and a metal clip or suture is used to ligate the artery.

■ Nursing Management of the Surgical Client

The nasal packing inserted to control epistaxis remains in place for a minimum of 24 hours, during which time the client must be observed for additional bleeding, evidence of hypertension or hypotension, and infection. Upon discharge, the client is instructed to minimize activity for approximately 10 days, such as avoiding strenuous exercise; not blowing the nose; sneezing with the mouth open; and not lifting, stooping, or straining. The use of water-soluble ointment around the nares may provide comfort, and mouth rinses of half-strength hydrogen peroxide mixed with water or saline should be provided for oral hygiene. The use of a humidifier or vaporizer adds supplemental moisture to prevent dryness and crusting of secretions.

SINUSITIS

Sinusitis is a common infection that may occur in any of the paranasal sinuses. *Pansinusitis* is infection of more than one sinus. The term *rhinosinusitis* is thought to more accurately describe respiratory manifestations referable to an inflammatory disease of the nose or sinuses. However, the terms *rhinitis* and *sinusitis* may still be used.

Sinusitis is a common medical condition that affects an estimated 35 million people a year.[14] The sinuses are protected against infection by mucociliary action. The normal mucus produced by the sinuses is removed through small openings in the nose called *ostia*. When the ciliary action is impaired or the ostia are obstructed, mucus can accumulate in the sinus, which may then become infected. Blockage of the ostia may be due to a deviated nasal septum, bony abnormalities, congenital malformations, infections, or allergy.

A medical diagnosis of sinusitis is suggested by the client's clinical manifestations and confirmed by x-ray findings. Fever and chills along with headaches and facial pain exacerbated with bending, pain or numbness in the upper teeth, and a purulent or discolored nasal discharge may be present. Sinus radiographs or CT scans may show opacification of the sinus, thickened mucous membranes, and an air-fluid level (due to accumulation of secretions in the sinus), all indicative of sinusitis.

Outcome Management
■ Medical Management

Medical management of sinusitis includes (1) use of the appropriate antibiotic to manage the bacterial infection, (2) decongestants to reduce nasal edema, (3) corticosteroid nasal sprays to reduce mucosal inflammation, and (4) humidification by use of normal saline solution irrigations or a vaporizer or humidifier to prevent nasal crusting and to moisten secretions.

Antral irrigation or sinus lavage may be performed in clients who are not responding to treatment or who have increased purulent exudate in the maxillary sinus. Antral irrigation is performed with the use of a local anesthetic. A trocar (a sharp metal instrument) is inserted through the ostium in the lateral wall of the nose into the sinus. Prepare the client for the procedure with thorough explanations of the anesthetic procedure, the sensation of passage of the trocar through the ostium, and feelings of pressure. Normal saline solution is then injected through the cannula to rinse the sinus of purulent exudate. The client is placed in a sitting position, leaning slightly forward with the mouth open to allow drainage of the irrigating solution through the nose and mouth. A specimen of the exudate may be obtained for culture to determine the causative organism for prescription of an appropriate antibiotic.[15]

■ Surgical Management

Functional Endoscopic Sinus Surgery. If nonoperative measures fail, functional endoscopic sinus surgery (FESS) may be necessary. The major objective of FESS is the reestablishment of sinus ventilation and mucociliary clearance.[15] FEES is usually performed as an outpatient surgical procedure using local anesthesia (with or without conscious sedation) or with the client under general anesthesia. Small fiberoptic endoscopes are passed through the nasal cavity and into the sinuses to allow direct visualization of the sinuses in order to remove diseased tissue and to enlarge sinus ostia (Figure 62-13). A more popular method of performing FESS is with the use of small, powered instruments offering precision and safety in the surgical approach.[15]

Possible complications of FESS include nasal bleeding, pain, scar formation, and rarely, cerebrospinal fluid leak and blindness resulting from intraorbital hematoma formation or direct injury to the optic nerve. After FESS, nasal packing may be inserted to minimize nasal bleeding. Packing is removed within a few hours of the surgical procedure.

Caldwell-Luc Procedure. The Caldwell-Luc procedure is another surgical procedure performed for the management of chronic maxillary sinusitis. An incision is made into the gingival buccal sulcus above the lateral incisor teeth with the client under general anesthesia, or local anesthesia may be used. Through this opening, the diseased mucous membrane is removed. In addition, an opening between the maxillary sinus and lateral nasal wall (nasal antral window) may be created to increase aeration of the sinus and to permit drainage into the nasal cavity.

After the procedure, the maxillary sinus and anterior nasal cavity are packed with half-inch gauze. Because of the packing, nasal breathing is obstructed. The oral cavity must be frequently evaluated for the presence of blood or packing that may have become dislodged, obstructing the pharynx. If packing is present in the pharynx, the visible portion may be held with a hemostat and cut with scissors. Be certain that the hemostat is holding the trimmed gauze; otherwise, it may be aspirated.[9]

External Sphenoethmoidectomy. External sphenoethmoidectomy is a surgical procedure performed to remove diseased mucosa from the sphenoidal or ethmoidal sinus. A small incision is made over the ethmoidal sinus on the lateral nasal bridge, and the diseased mucosa is removed. Nasal and ethmoidal packing is then inserted. An eye pressure patch is usually applied to decrease periorbital edema.[9]

■ Nursing Management of the Surgical Client

After sinus surgery, observe the client for profuse nasal bleeding, respiratory distress, ecchymosis, and orbital and facial edema for the first 24 hours postoperatively. Apply ice compresses to the nose and cheek to minimize edema and control bleeding. Place the client in a semi-Fowler to high Fowler position for 24 to 48 hours after surgery to minimize postoperative edema. The nasal packing is generally removed the morning after surgery; however, antral packing may remain in place for 36 to 72 hours. Give mild analgesics to the client to minimize discomfort postoperatively and before removal of the packing.

Instruct clients to increase fluid intake, which maximizes the water content of secretions. Although there may be some pain, a mild analgesic is usually all that is required. Minor nasal bleeding is expected for 24 to 48 hours after surgery. Use of a drip pad under the nose may eliminate the need for constant wiping (Figure 62-14). Instruct clients to avoid blowing the nose for 7 to 10 days after surgery; tell them to sniff backward or spit, not blow. Teach the client to sneeze only with the

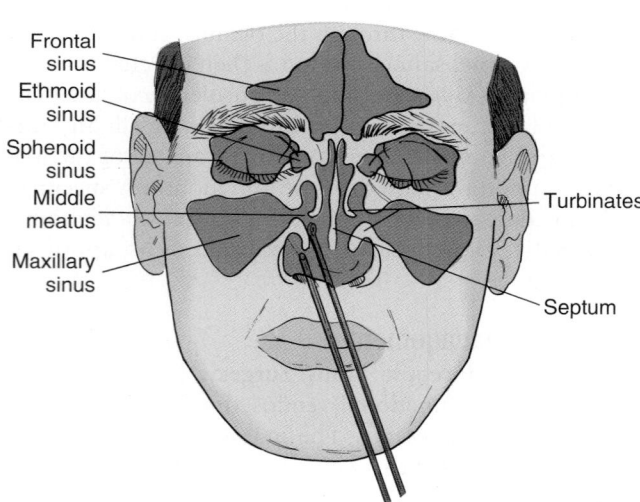

FIGURE 62-13 Functional endoscopic sinus surgery. The middle meatus is the site to which most of the sinuses drain; if it is plugged, drainage is obstructed. With an endoscope, the sinuses can be seen and obstructions removed.

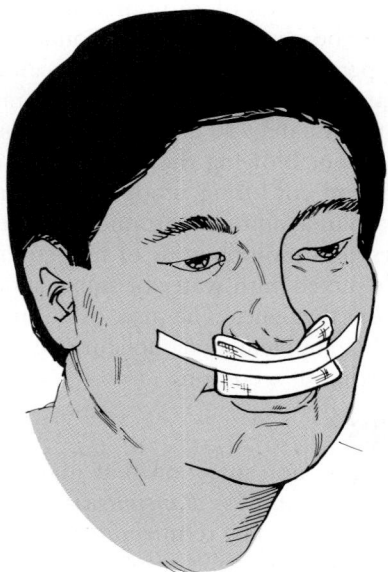

FIGURE 62-14 A nasal drip pad is taped beneath the nares to absorb drainage after nasal or sinus surgery. The usual technique consists of folding 4 × 4 dressings into thirds and taping them in place. These dressings can be changed at the nurse's discretion.

mouth open. Nasal saline sprays may be started 3 to 5 days after surgery to moisten the nasal mucosa. Explain that the client is to engage in minimal physical exercise and to avoid strenuous activity, lifting, and straining for approximately 2 weeks. After FESS, the client needs to return to the physician's office for removal of crusts and debris and examination of the nose.

After a Caldwell-Luc procedure, the client may have temporary numbness of the upper teeth caused by interruption of sensory nerves from the mucosal incision. This abnormality may persist for several weeks.[9]

PHARYNGITIS

Pharyngitis is inflammation of the pharynx (tonsils, palate, uvula) and may be viral, bacterial, or fungal in origin. Beta-hemolytic streptococci are the most common infecting organisms. A culture of the pharyngeal mucosa is sometimes indicated before treatment is started. Clients may complain of a sore throat, difficulty in swallowing, fever, malaise, and cough and have an elevated white blood cell count. Treatment of pharyngitis depends on the causative agent. Both viral pharyngitis and bacterial pharyngitis are contagious by droplet spread. Good hand-washing technique is essential, and the use of a mask may prevent spread. Antibiotics are used to treat the bacterial pharyngitis, antifungal agents are used to treat fungal infections, and use of comfort measures is required for viral types. Bed rest, fluids, warm saline irrigations or gargles, analgesics, and antipyretics are recommended until the clinical manifestations are alleviated.

Chronic pharyngitis (chronic pharyngeal inflammation) is most common in people who habitually use tobacco and alcohol, have a chronic cough, are employed or live in dusty environments, or use their voices excessively. Clinical manifestations vary according to the degree of irritation and inflammation.

ACUTE TONSILLITIS

Tonsillitis is an infection of the tonsils. *Streptococcus* is the most common infecting organism, although tonsillitis can be caused by *Haemophilus influenzae* and other organisms.

The client with tonsillitis reports throat pain, difficulty in swallowing, otalgia (referred pain to the ear), and generalized malaise. Examination discloses an acutely inflamed mucous membrane around the tonsillar area with or without the presence of purulent exudate. In some clients, lymphadenopathy of the cervical lymph nodes may also be present.

Complications from streptococcal tonsillitis include pneumonia, nephritis, osteomyelitis, and rheumatic fever. Acute tonsillitis may become chronic. Acute otitis media, acute rhinitis, acute sinusitis, and peritonsillar abscess or other deep neck abscesses may also develop.

■ Medical Management

Antibiotics are used to treat acute tonsillitis. In addition, the client is instructed to minimize activity, to maximize bed rest, and to increase fluid intake. Saline throat irrigations or gargles may relieve the discomfort. Mild analgesics such as acetaminophen, with or without codeine, may be prescribed.

■ Surgical Management

Surgical removal of the tonsils (tonsillectomy) and the adenoids (adenoidectomy) is collectively called *tonsilloadenectomy,* or T&A. The tonsils and adenoids may be removed separately but are most often removed in the same procedure. Removal of chronically diseased tonsil or adenoid tissue is indicated in the following circumstances:

- Recurrent, incapacitating episodes of acute or chronic tonsillitis
- Tonsillar or adenoid hypertrophy causing obstruction of the airway and impaired swallowing
- Resolution of a peritonsillar abscess
- Repeated ear problems related to eustachian tube obstruction
- Sinus complications

T&A is most often done in children. Tonsillectomy may also be indicated for a carrier of diphtheria, because tonsils may "seed" the body with infectious organisms. Adults with recurrent sore throat, ear pain, or hearing dysfunction, or who snore because of hypertrophied adenoid or tonsillar tissue, may also benefit from this procedure. Although T&A is not as routine as in the past, it is indicated in clients who have repeated episodes of infection. T&A is performed as an outpatient procedure or as a same-day surgery procedure. Tonsillectomy may be performed with the use of either general or local anesthesia, although general anesthesia is more commonly used. Surgical intervention is contraindicated during an acute infection, that is, upper respiratory infection. Other contraindications to T&A include hematologic disorders such as hemophilia, aplastic anemia, purpura, and leukemia.

■ Nursing Management of the Surgical Client

After tonsillectomy, place the client in a lateral decubitus position until the client is awake and alert. This position provides for drainage of blood and other secretions through the nose and mouth. Gently inspect the oropharynx and mouth for fresh blood frequently during the first several hours postoperatively. Monitor vital signs closely. Hemorrhage is the most serious complication after tonsillectomy and is most often seen during the first 12 to 24 hours. If postoperative hemorrhage occurs, resuturing or cauterization of the bleeding vessel is mandatory.

The client should begin taking oral feedings once recovery from anesthesia is complete. Encourage cool fluids and introduce appropriate foods to provide a soft, bland diet, as tolerated. Highly seasoned foods, as well as any food the client finds difficult to swallow, should be avoided.

Pain in the first 7 to 10 postoperative days is common after tonsillectomy. Most clients report generalized throat pain as well as otalgia. Mild analgesics such as acetaminophen with or without codeine may be required to alleviate pain. Increased swallowing of fluids also helps minimize discomfort. Aspirin is contraindicated because of the risk of bleeding associated with its use.

Encourage clients to seek immediate medical attention if bleeding occurs after hospital discharge. Delayed bleeding may occur once the healing membrane separates from the underlying tissue (7 to 10 days postoperatively). The surgical site is usually well healed in 14 to 21 days, and the client should have little difficulty after this time.[17]

CHRONIC TONSILLITIS

The most frequent manifestation of chronic tonsillitis is recurrent sore throat. Between episodes of acute tonsillitis, the throat remains uncomfortable. The tonsils are often enlarged, and if they are infected, a sharp line may be seen between the color of the buccal mucosa and that of the tonsillar pillar. The most reliable indication of chronic tonsillitis is the expression of purulent material from the tonsillar crypts with a wooden tongue blade. Once chronic tonsillitis is diagnosed, surgical removal is recommended. Surgery is contraindicated during acute tonsillar infection, although tonsillectomy may be performed in a client with acute peritonsillar abscess.

PERITONSILLAR ABSCESS (QUINSY)

Peritonsillar abscess (quinsy) may arise from acute streptococcal or staphylococcal tonsillitis. The tissue between the tonsils and the fascia covering the superior constrictor muscles becomes infected, causing extensive swelling of the soft palate and the pharyngeal wall. The uvula may be pushed to one side, and up to half of the pharyngeal opening may be occluded. Pus formation in the fascial space pushes the tonsil forward toward the midline of the throat.

Peritonsillar abscess is typically manifested several days after the onset of acute tonsillitis. As the tonsillitis-related problems begin to resolve, increasing pain develops on one side of the throat and ear. Inflammation and edema create a partial obstruction to swallowing. Often, the client keeps the mouth partially open to allow drooling, rather than attempting painful swallowing. The voice takes on a characteristic "hot potato" or muffled sound. Thick secretions are raised with difficulty.

A peritonsillar abscess may rupture spontaneously. If spontaneous rupture does not occur, surgical intervention may be necessary. With the client in a sitting position (to allow expectoration of pus and blood), an incision is made and the abscess drained.

Topical anesthetic throat sprays, analgesic agents, hot saline throat irrigations (at temperatures of 40.5° to 43.3° C [105° to 110° F]), saline or alkaline mouthwashes or gargles, and ice collars may be used to make the throat more comfortable. Cool and room-temperature fluids are tolerated best. Ingestion of cool to warm soft foods may also be possible. High-dose antibiotics are often prescribed early to avoid the need for incision and drainage. It takes at least 1 month for the infection of a peritonsillar abscess to subside. Usually, a tonsillectomy is performed following resolution of the abscess and infection, to prevent recurrence. However, a "quinsy tonsillectomy" may be performed during the acute infection.[23]

RHINITIS

Rhinitis, or rhinosinusitis, is inflammation of the nasal mucosa. The classic manifestations of rhinitis are increased nasal drainage, nasal congestion, and paroxysmal sneezing. Normally, nasal drainage is composed of clear mucus. If the infection spreads to the sinuses, however, drainage may become yellow or green. Rhinitis may be classified as acute, allergic, vasomotor, or drug-related (rhinitis medicamentosa).

Acute rhinitis is also known as the common cold, or coryza. Acute rhinitis may be bacterial or viral in origin; it is treated symptomatically. Acute rhinitis usually lasts 5 to 7 days, with or without treatment. Common interventions for acute rhinitis are symptomatic and include supplemental humidification, decongestants to reduce the edema of the nasal mucosa, increased fluids to prevent dehydration, and analgesics to relieve the generalized myalgia. Sometimes antibiotics are given to prevent a secondary infection by bacteria.

Allergic rhinitis affects between 15% and 20% of the American population and occurs most often as a seasonal disorder. In addition to obstruction to nasal breathing, the client may also experience irritation of other mucous membranes (e.g., the conjunctiva, causing tearing and edema of the eyelids). There is a broad association between allergic rhinitis and disease affecting other body systems. Treatment is symptomatic. A complete allergy evaluation may be required to determine the offending allergen. Most clients are placed on a desensitization program and instructed to avoid the antigen (substance that causes the allergic reaction); treatment is with antihistamines, steroids, or mast cell–stabilizing sprays.[16]

Vasomotor rhinitis causes the same manifestations as those of acute and allergic rhinitis but has no known cause. Clients with vasomotor rhinitis in whom results of culture and allergy evaluation are negative are given symptomatic treatment. If medications have been prescribed for the treatment of rhinitis (especially nasal sprays), the client must be taught the use of medications, including side effects and possible interactions with other medications.

Rhinitis medicamentosa is caused by abuse or overuse of topical nasal decongestant sprays or intranasal cocaine. These substances initially cause vasoconstriction. When used frequently, however, the initial decongestion is followed by severe mucosal edema. The edema is self-treated with more medication, and the rhinitis becomes cyclic. Management of rhinitis medicamentosa consists of avoidance of the causative agent and evaluation and treatment of the original problem.

LARYNGITIS

Laryngitis may be caused by an inflammatory process or vocal abuse. The laryngeal membrane is continuous with the lining of the upper respiratory tract, and infections in other areas of the nose and throat may include the larynx. Edema of the vocal cords caused by the chronic irritation of an upper respiratory tract infection inhibits the normal mobility of the vocal cords, which causes an abnormal sound.

Laryngitis may also be the result of gastroesophageal reflux disorder (GERD). In this syndrome, the cardiac sphincter between the stomach and the esophagus relaxes, and gastric acid is allowed to enter the esophagus. Reflux of gastric secretions, especially during sleep, may result in the aspiration of gastric secretions into the larynx, causing a chemical irritation or burning of the mucous membrane lining the larynx. Clients with gastroesophageal reflux may complain of hoarseness from the chemical irritation of the gastric acid on the vocal cords, increased mucus production from the body's natural tendency to protect the irritated membrane, foreign body sensation, or sore throat. Chronic cough and asthma may also be associated manifestations of GERD.

Hoarseness is a common manifestation of disorders of the larynx and may be caused by inflammation of the vocal cords, abnormal movements of the vocal cords, or a benign or malignant tumor of the vocal cords. All of these problems interfere with normal mobility of the vocal cords, which produces a change in sound. Abnormal voice may also be the result of vocal abuse. Screaming, shouting, and loud speaking over a period of time may produce edema of the vocal cords and the formation of nodules or polyps—outpouchings of inflamed mucous membranes.

The treatment of laryngitis is aimed at the causative factors. If inflammatory laryngitis is suspected, the inflammation should be treated. Antibiotics may be used if a bacterial infection is suspected. In severe cases, systemic steroids (e.g., methylprednisolone [Medrol]) may be prescribed to reduce inflammation and edema. Supplemental humidification may add increased moisture to liquefy secretions, and mucolytic agents may be prescribed to thin and mobilize mucus. The client with

laryngitis may also be placed on voice rest to allow the edema of the vocal cords to subside without added strain. Caution the client to avoid whispering, which also causes excessive vocal cord strain.

Gastroesophageal reflux is initially treated symptomatically. The client is instructed to elevate the head of the bed 6 to 10 inches to minimize reflux; to avoid lying on the right side; to avoid eating or drinking for 2 to 3 hours before going to sleep; to avoid caffeine, alcohol, and tobacco, which are known to increase gastric secretions; and to use antacids and histamine$_2$ receptor blockers (famotidine [Pepcid], ranitidine [Zantac], omeprazole [Prilosec]) to neutralize and decrease acid production.[3]

Chronic laryngitis may stem from repeated infections, allergy, chronic irritant exposure, long-term voice abuse, or reflux esophagitis of acidic gastric contents. Chronic laryngitis is manifested as a tickling sensation in the throat, voice huskiness, and painful or difficult phonation. Management involves correction or removal of the irritation, in addition to measures to increase comfort. Long-term voice retraining may be necessary if improper use or overuse of the voice is the main cause of chronic laryngitis. This retraining includes (1) learning to use the voice without straining and (2) forming and projecting words to use the diaphragm without shouting.

DIPHTHERIA

Diphtheria is an acute, communicable disease caused by *Corynebacterium diphtheriae*. The incidence of diphtheria has declined in the United States as a result of required vaccination. Diphtheria is a highly contagious disease that is spread easily in populations with poor hygiene, crowding, and limited access to medical care.

Humans are the only natural reservoir for *C. diphtheriae*. This organism colonizes the mucosal surface of the nasopharynx and multiplies. The bacteria release a toxin that causes the tissues to necrose, forming a tough pseudomembrane covering the tonsils and pharyngeal walls. This membrane is difficult to dislodge and causes bleeding if removed. Systemic toxins can damage distal sites such as the heart, nerves, and kidneys.

Diphtheria is spread by aerosolization of the pathogen (droplet infection), and when objects used by diphtheria-infected people, such as eating utensils, towels, or handkerchiefs, are used by others. Healthy people, as well as clients recovering from the disease, may harbor the organism in the throat for 2 to 4 weeks.

The clinical manifestations can range from a single, localized lesion without systemic manifestations to those of a rapidly progressive fatal illness.

The two types of diphtheria are tonsillar and pharyngeal. *Tonsillar* diphtheria is seldom life-threatening, although it can progress rapidly to more fatal forms. A low-grade fever, fatigue, headache, and sore throat are common manifestations.

Pharyngeal diphtheria is the more serious form of diphtheria, especially when a membrane covers the larynx or bronchus. The client is gravely ill, with a weak pulse, restlessness, and confusion. Fever may or may not be present. Because of the location of the membrane, the airway is often obstructed, and the client exhibits stridor and cyanosis. The neck may also be swollen and warm.

Diphtheria is diagnosed by culture of the material with the enzyme-linked immunosorbent assay (ELISA) or the Elek test (toxigenicity test). Gram staining or fluorescent antibody staining may also be performed; these tests yield results more quickly. Although cultures are used to identify the organism, treatment begins immediately, before definitive results have been obtained. Treatment consists of antitoxin administration.

To prevent transmission of the disease, the client is placed in strict isolation. Contacts need to be identified, screened, immunized, and treated. Specimens from all contacts should be obtained for culture. People vaccinated 5 or more years previously should receive a booster dose. People who were never immunized should be given vaccine and antibiotics. During antitoxin administration, observe the client for anaphylaxis; epinephrine is kept at the bedside.

Nursing management focuses on management of the airway obstruction. Suction equipment and a tracheotomy tray should be kept at the bedside. Oxygen is administered. Clients experience pain, especially with swallowing. In addition to analgesia, pain can be reduced by limiting the diet to liquids and soft foods. Throat irrigation and fluids may also help control pain.

OBSTRUCTIONS OF THE UPPER AIRWAY

ACUTE LARYNGEAL EDEMA

Acute laryngeal edema may be associated with inflammation, injury, or anaphylaxis. This condition is manifested by hoarseness and dramatic shortness of breath of acute onset. Dyspnea progresses rapidly, and unless a patent airway is established, respiratory arrest occurs. Endotracheal intubation may be very difficult because the larynx is edematous and is likely to bleed. Emergency tracheostomy may be required. If anaphylaxis is the precipitating cause, subcutaneous epinephrine 1:1000 is given. Intravenous corticosteroids are also used.

CHRONIC LARYNGEAL EDEMA

Chronic laryngeal edema may occur when lymph drainage is obstructed, as with infection or tumor or after radiation therapy. If the edema is significant, an artificial airway may be required (either a tracheostomy or an endotracheal tube). The choice of route depends on the severity of the edema.

LARYNGOSPASM

Laryngospasm (spasm of the laryngeal muscles) may occur (1) after administration of some general anesthetic agents, (2) after repeated and traumatic attempts at endotracheal intubation, (3) as a response to some inhaled agents and foreign material, such as industrial fumes, dusts, and chemicals, and (4) from hypocalcemia.

Management is directed at reestablishing the airway as quickly and efficiently as possible. Administer 100% oxygen until the airway is fully reestablished and the larynx relaxes and spasms stop. Titrate FIO_2 according to ABG or pulse oximetry values. If the laryngospasm persists, paralysis with neuromuscular blocking agents, such as succinylcholine, may be required to allow intubation until the spasm subsides. Manual or mechanical ventilation is then necessary until the effects of the paralyzing agent have worn off. Occasionally, emergency cricothyroidotomy or tracheotomy may be necessary and should not be delayed.

LARYNGEAL PARALYSIS

Laryngeal paralysis may be the result of neck surgery, peripheral disorders, central nervous system (CNS) disorders, tumor, or viral infections or it may be of unknown cause. One of the most common causes of laryngeal paralysis is trauma to the recurrent laryngeal nerve during thyroidectomy. Other causes of laryngeal paralysis are aortic aneurysm; mitral stenosis; thoracic surgery; thyroid gland carcinoma; neck injuries; tuberculosis; tumors of the bronchi, lungs, and mediastinum; metallic poisons (e.g., lead); and infection (e.g., diphtheria). CNS disorders that may lead to laryngeal paralysis include stroke and myasthenia gravis. Bilateral laryngeal paralysis is rare, and when it occurs, the client usually exhibits difficulty in breathing or stridor.

With unilateral vocal cord paralysis (in which only one vocal cord is affected), the airway is usually not impaired and the primary manifestation is hoarseness. The client may have a breathy quality of the voice. Aspiration of food or saliva may occur until the normal, moving cord compensates by approximating the paralyzed cord (bringing the cords together). The client must be observed for manifestations of aspiration such as coughing upon swallowing, ineffective cough, decreased breath sounds, and crackles, rhonchi, or wheezes. The client with bilateral vocal cord paralysis can have a near-normal voice if the vocal cords are paralyzed in the adducted position. However, the major concern is airway compromise, especially on exertion. Dyspnea, intercostal muscle retraction, and stridor may occur with activity or upper airway infections.

If the paralyzed cords are bilaterally adducted, an emergency tracheotomy may be required. Surgery, such as arytenoidectomy, in which one or both arytenoid cartilages are removed and the vocal cords are held in an open position, may be used to open the glottis.

Injection of absorbable sponge (Gelfoam), as a temporary measure, or of polytetrafluoroethylene (Teflon), for permanent correction, may be used if the client with unilateral vocal cord paralysis exhibits manifestations of aspiration or requires strength or projection of the voice. The injected material is placed into the paralyzed cord to add bulk and to allow better approximation with the functioning cord.

Type I thyroplasty is recommended for permanent unilateral vocal cord paralysis. For this procedure, a window is made in the thyroid cartilage through an external incision, and a stent is inserted to move the paralyzed vocal cord into a midline position. The client may show manifestations of airway edema from both the injection and the thyroplasty and should be observed for respiratory distress.

LARYNGEAL INJURY

Laryngeal injury most often results from trauma during a motor vehicle accident, when the driver's neck strikes the steering wheel. Other causes include inhalation of hot gases and aspiration of caustic liquids. If complete airway obstruction does not occur, carefully assess for post-traumatic edema, which may lead to complete obstruction. Few outward manifestations may be present. It is often easy to overlook potential problems in the neck structures while focusing on other, possibly more dramatic injuries. Observe for increased dyspnea, intercostal muscle retraction, neck swelling, laryngeal tenderness, dysphagia, stridor, inability to speak, and change in respiration patterns.

The thyroid cartilage may be fractured. This problem leads to soft tissue and laryngeal edema as well as hematoma formation. If airway obstruction occurs, tracheostomy may be necessary. Indications of a fractured thyroid cartilage include (1) a tender, swollen ecchymotic neck, (2) stridor, (3) cyanosis in some cases, and (4) subcutaneous emphysema in some cases.

Damage to the larynx above the cricoid cartilage may lead to tracheal stenosis. The cricoid cartilage forms the only complete circle of cartilage in the upper airway, and it maintains the open lumen of the upper end of the airway.

CHRONIC AIRWAY OBSTRUCTION
NASAL POLYPS

Nasal polyps are outpouchings of mucous membrane lining the nose or paranasal sinuses and may occur as solitary or multiple lesions. Polyps may be exacerbated by allergic manifestations, although they are not caused by allergies. Most people who have symptomatic polyps seek medical attention for obstruction to nasal breathing.[9]

The medical management of clients with nasal polyps is symptomatic. Attempts are made to reduce the size of the polyps by eliminating or treating the causative factor (i.e., allergy). In many clients, surgery is needed to remove nasal polyps in order to restore nasal breathing before allergy treatment. Nasal polypectomy (removal of nasal polyps) can be done in the physician's office or in the operating room. Nasal polypectomy is usually performed with use of a local anesthetic. The anesthetic (commonly lidocaine with epinephrine) eliminates discomfort while also producing vasoconstriction to minimize bleeding during the procedure. A snare-like instrument is used to remove the polyps. The bleeding sites are cauterized, and intranasal packing is inserted. Intranasal splints can be used to prevent formation of adhesions. The nasal packing is maintained for several hours to minimize the possibility of postoperative bleeding and is generally removed before discharge of the client from the health care facility.

Because of the presence of nasal packing and edema, clients need to breathe through their mouth for the first 24 to 48 hours. The use of humidification, frequent mouth care, and increasing oral fluids help to minimize the dryness and oropharyngeal discomfort. Inspect the oral cavity frequently to evaluate the effectiveness of these measures. Clients with polyps frequently also have asthma (when combined with aspirin allergy, this is called *triad disease*). Asthmatic manifestations may be exacerbated after surgery.[9]

The client is placed in a semi-Fowler to high Fowler position after surgery to minimize edema. In addition, continuous use of ice compresses is recommended for the first 48 hours to reduce edema and to control bleeding. With the proper application of nasal packing at the time of surgery and the use of ice compresses in the immediate postoperative period, nasal bleeding should be minimal. However, the client should be assessed for changes in vital signs and the oropharynx inspected for the presence of blood. Because the nasal packing absorbs anterior bleeding, it is essential to observe the client for posterior nasal bleeding. Manifestations of active posterior bleeding include frequent swallowing and the presence of blood in the throat.

Most clients experience only minimal discomfort after a nasal polypectomy. Mild analgesics may be given for any postoperative discomfort. The use of aspirin and aspirin-containing products should be avoided because of their anticoagulant effects. Instruct the client not to blow his or her nose and to refrain from sneezing if possible. When the stimulus to sneeze cannot be overcome, the client should sneeze through an open mouth.

DEVIATED NASAL SEPTUM
AND NASAL FRACTURE

The nasal septum (the dividing structure of the nose) is usually straight and separates the nose into two equal chambers. After trauma, the septum may become deviated, creating asymmetrical breathing passages. For some clients, the deviation may cause an obstruction to nasal breathing, dryness of the nasal mucosa leading to bleeding, and occasionally a cosmetic deformity. A deviated nasal septum changes the velocity of air, altering normal nasal activity and resulting in dryness, crusting, nasal bleeding, and changes in the membranes lining the nose.

If a nasal fracture occurs, immediate medical management is advised. Within several hours of nasal injury, severe edema may occur, which causes difficulty in reducing the fracture. Immediately after the injury, ice should be applied. A simple nasal fracture may be reduced in an emergency facility with use of local anesthesia. If immediate reduction of the nasal fracture is not possible, it is advisable to wait several days until edema subsides but before healing begins.

For correction of a deviated nasal septum, reconstruction of a cosmetic deformity of the nose, and reduction of a nasal fracture, the principles of surgical management are similar. All three procedures are usually performed with use of local anesthesia combined with mild sedation. Because of the vasoconstrictor properties of local anesthetics, these agents reduce bleeding during and immediately after surgery. Surgery to correct a deviated nasal septum is known as a nasal septoplasty and consists of making an incision on either side of the septum, elevating the mucous membrane, and straightening or removing the offending portion of the cartilage. If a cosmetic deformity is also of concern or if the deformity interferes with septal reconstruction, a rhinoplasty (reconstruction of the external nose) may be done in conjunction with the nasal septoplasty or as a separate procedure. (See also Chapter 51.)

After these three procedures, intranasal packing and internal splints may be used to maintain the position of the septum, to control bleeding, and to prevent hematoma formation. If the client has undergone rhinoplasty or reduction of a nasal fracture, an external splint and a small dressing may also be applied. Postoperative care is directed at airway management, control of edema and hemorrhage, pain reduction, client education, and emotional support. Because of the presence of bilateral nasal packing, clients require the same care as discussed for the client who has undergone nasal polypectomy.[9]

CONCLUSIONS

Disorders of the upper airway range from a simple cold to cancer of the larynx. This chapter presents care of clients most commonly hospitalized with upper airway disorders. Nursing management ranges from assessment of life-threatening airway obstruction to teaching techniques that reduce the spread of infection.

THINKING CRITICALLY *evolve*

1. The client has a temporary tracheostomy after undergoing a supraglottic laryngectomy. On the second postoperative day, the client indicates to you that he is having trouble breathing. How should you evaluate the client and eliminate the problem?
Factors to Consider. What principles are used as the basis of tracheostomy care? How does evaluation of pulse oximetry contribute to decision making for care?

2. You walk into the room of a client who underwent total laryngectomy 12 hours ago. The client is complaining of severe nausea but has not vomited. What are the client's risks following this type of surgery? How should you respond to the present problem?
Factors to Consider. What risks are inherent in the occurrence of tracheal interruption? How well can the client communicate with you at this time?

3. You enter the room of a client in whom a nosebleed has developed. Bright red blood is seeping continuously from the nares, and the client states that it feels like some blood is going down the back of his throat. What is the priority intervention? What are the implications if the bleeding continues?
Factors to Consider. What are the causes of epistaxis? What are the psychological effects of a nosebleed?

Discussions for these questions can be found on the website and the CD-ROM.

BIBLIOGRAPHY

1. American Cancer Society. (2002). *Cancer facts and figures 2002.* Atlanta, GA: Author.
2. Cady, J. (2002). Laryngectomy: Beyond loss of voice: Caring for the patient as a whole. *Clinical Journal of Oncology Nursing,* 6(6), 347-351.
3. Ch'ien, A.P.Y., et al. (2002). Managing gastroesophageal reflux disease. *The Nurse Practitioner: The American Journal of Primary Health Care,* 27(5), 36-53.

4. Devine, P., & Doyle, T. (2001). Brachytherapy for head and neck cancer: A case study. *Clinical Journal of Oncology Nursing, 5*(2), 55-57.

 5. Dropkin, M.J. (1999). Body image and quality of life after head and neck cancer surgery. *Cancer Practice, 7*(6), 309-313.

6. Gaziano, J.E. (2002). Evaluation and management of oropharyngeal dysphagia in head and neck cancer. *Cancer Control, 9*(5), 400-409.

7. Gosselin, T.K., & Pavilonis, H. (2002). Head and neck cancer: Managing xerostomia and other treatment induced side effects. *ORL-Head and Neck Nursing, 20*(4), 15-22.

8. Hahn, M.J., & Jones, A. (2000). *Head and neck nursing.* London: Churchill Livingstone-Harcourt Publishers.

9. Higgins, T.S., et al. (1998). Nasal cavity, paranasal sinuses, nasopharynx conditions and care. In L.L. Harris & M.B. Huntoon (Eds.), *Core curriculum for otorhinolaryngology and head-neck nursing* (pp. 169-206). New Smyrna Beach, FL: Society of Otorhinolaryngology and Head-Neck Nurses.

 10. Ishikawa, Y., & Bach, J.R. (2000). Evolution of mechanical ventilation: Its successes and shortcomings. In D.C. Tippett (Ed.), *Tracheostomy and ventilator dependency: Management of breathing, speaking, and swallowing* (pp. 47-64). New York: Thieme.

11. Jemal, A., et al. (2002). Cancer statistics, 2002. *CA: A Cancer Journal for Clinicians, 52*(1), 23-45.

12. Kearney, K. (2001). Epiglottitis. *American Journal of Nursing, 101*(8), 37-38.

 13. Koch, W.M., et al. (1999). Head and neck cancer in nonsmokers: A distinct clinical and molecular entity. *Laryngoscope, 109,* 1544-1551.

14. Krouse, J.H. (1999). Introduction to sinus disease: I. Anatomy and physiology. *ORL-Head and Neck Nursing, 17*(2), 7-12.

15. Krouse, J.H., & Krouse, H.J. (1999). Introduction to sinus disease: II. Diagnosis and treatment. *ORL-Head and Neck Nursing, 17*(3), 6-16.

16. Krouse, J.H., & Krouse, H.J. (2002). Allergic disease and associated concurrent medical illnesses. *ORL-Head and Neck Nursing, 20*(4), 10-14.

17. McKenna, M. (1999). Postoperative tonsillectomy/adenoidectomy hemorrhage: A retrospective chart review. *ORL-Head and Neck Nursing, 17*(3), 18-21.

18. Schreiber, D. (2001). Trach care at home: A how-to guide. *RN, 64*(7), 43-46.

19. Seay, S.J., & Gay, S.L. (2002). Tracheostomy emergencies. *American Journal of Nursing, 102*(3), 59-63.

20. Sparacino, L.L. (2000). Epistaxis management: What's new and what's noteworthy. *Lippincott's Primary Care Practice, 4*(5), 498-507.

21. Spaulding, M.B. (2002). Recent advances in the treatment of head and neck cancer: A patient care perspective. *ORL-Head and Neck Nursing, 20*(1), 9-18.

22. Stapleton, E.R., et al. (Eds.). (2001). *BLS for healthcare providers.* Dallas: American Heart Association.

23. Steyer, T.E. (2002). Peritonsillar abscess: Diagnosis and treatment. *American Family Physician, 65*(1), 93-96.

24. Tamburri, L.M. (2000). Care of the patient with a tracheostomy. *Orthopedic Nursing, 19*(20), 49-60.

25. Tippett, D.C., & Vogelman, L. (2000). Communication, tracheostomy, and ventilator dependency. In D.C. Tippett (Ed.), *Tracheostomy and ventilator dependency: Management of breathing, speaking, and swallowing* (pp. 93-142). New York: Thieme.

26. Wilkinson, J.M. (2000). *Nursing diagnosis handbook with NIC interventions and NOC outcomes.* Upper Saddle River, NJ: Prentice Hall.

Management of Clients with Lower Airway and Pulmonary Vessel Disorders

Sherill Nones Cronin
Kim Miracle

---

evolve

Web Enhancements

http://evolve.elsevier.com/Black/medsurg/

Case Management
  Chronic Obstructive Pulmonary Disease
  The Older Adult
Case Study
  COPD with Nutritional Concerns
Client Education Guide
  Asthma (Spanish Translation)

Clinical Pathway
  Chronic Obstructive Pulmonary Disease
Concept Map
  Understanding Asthma and Its Treatment
Appendix C
  Laboratory Values of Clinical Importance in Medical-Surgical
  Nursing

A distinguishing feature of lower airway and pulmonary vessel disorders is the presence of dyspnea. *Dyspnea* (shortness of breath) is a subjective experience that results when air flow, oxygen exchange, or both are impaired. The sensation of uncomfortable breathing can be as distressing as pain and can lead to severe functional disability. The intensity and frequency of dyspnea as well as its association with specific activities must be assessed to develop realistic expectations of treatment outcomes (see Evidence-Based Practice in Action feature on The Assessment of Dyspnea on p. 1809). Because the experience of dyspnea is associated with much anxiety, nursing interventions to relieve this manifestation are essential to the care of clients with conditions of the lower airways and pulmonary vessels.

▌DISORDERS OF THE LOWER AIRWAYS

ASTHMA

Asthma is a disorder of the bronchial airways characterized by periods of reversible bronchospasm (spasms of prolonged contraction of the airway). Asthma is often called *reactive airway disease*. This complex disorder involves biochemical, immunologic, endocrine, infectious, autonomic, and psychological factors. Approximately 26 million Americans have been diagnosed with asthma in their lifetime. Of these 26 million, 10.6 million have had an asthma episode in the past 12 months, resulting in nearly 5000 deaths. The financial impact of this disease is also considerable, with an estimated $12.7 billion spent annually in direct care and lost productivity.[2]

---

evolve Be sure to check out the bonus material on the Evolve website and the CD-ROM, including free self-assessment exercises.

http://evolve.elsevier.com/Black/medsurg/

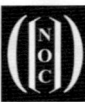

Nursing Outcomes Classification
for Nursing Diagnoses—Clients with Lower Airway and Pulmonary Vessel Disorders

Activity Intolerance
Activity Tolerance
Endurance
Energy Conservation
Self-Care: Activities of Daily Living (ADL)
Self-Care: Instrumental Activities of Daily Living (IADL)

Anxiety
Aggression Control
Anxiety Reduction
Coping
Impulse Control
Social Interaction Skills

Decisional Conflict
Decision Making
Participation: Health Care Decisions

Deficient Knowledge
Knowledge: Disease Process
Knowledge: Energy Conservation
Knowledge: Health Behaviors
Knowledge: Health Resources
Knowledge: Illness Care
Knowledge: Infection Control

Knowledge: Medication
Knowledge: Treatment Regimen

Disturbed Sleep Pattern
Rest
Sleep
Well-Being

Imbalanced Nutrition: Less Than Body Requirements
Nutritional Status
Nutritional Status: Food and Fluid Intake
Nutritional Status: Nutrient Intake
Weight Control

Impaired Gas Exchange
Electrolyte and Acid/Base Balance
Respiratory Status: Gas Exchange
Respiratory Status: Ventilation
Tissue Perfusion: Pulmonary
Vital Signs Status

Ineffective Airway Clearance
Aspiration Control
Respiratory Status: Airway Patency
Respiratory Status: Gas Exchange
Respiratory Status: Ventilation

Ineffective Breathing Pattern
Respiratory Status: Airway Patency
Respiratory Status: Ventilation
Vital Signs Status

Ineffective Coping
Aggression Control
Coping
Decision Making
Impulse Control
Information Processing
Role Performance
Social Support

Interrupted Family Processes
Caregiver Emotional Health
Caregiver Well-Being
Family Coping
Family Normalization

Risk for Infection
Immobility Consequences: Physiologic
Knowledge: Infection Control
Tissue Integrity: Skin and Mucous Membranes

Sexual Dysfunction
Sexual Functioning
Endurance

Etiology and Risk Factors

Asthma occurs in families, which suggests that it is an inherited disorder. Apparently, environmental factors (e.g., viral infection, allergens, pollutants) interact with inherited factors to produce disease. Other inciting factors can include excitatory states (stress, laughing, crying), exercise, changes in temperature, and strong odors. Asthma also is a component of *triad* disease: asthma, nasal polyps, and allergy to aspirin.

Pathophysiology

Asthma involves a chronic inflammatory process that produces mucosal edema, mucus secretion, and airway inflammation (Figure 63-1). When people with asthma are exposed to extrinsic allergens and irritants (e.g., dust, pollen, smoke, mold, medications, foods, respiratory infections), their airways become inflamed, producing shortness of breath, chest tightness, and wheezing. Initial clinical manifestations, termed *early-phase reaction,* develop immediately and last about an hour.

When a client comes in contact with an allergen, immunoglobulin E (IgE) is produced by B lymphocytes. IgE antibodies attach to mast cells and basophils in the bronchial walls. As shown in the Concept Map feature on Understanding Asthma and Its Treatment on p. 1810, the mast cell empties, releasing chemical mediators of in-

flammation, such as histamine, bradykinin, prostaglandins, and slow-reacting substance of anaphylaxis (SRS-A). The substances induce capillary dilation, leading to edema of the airway in an attempt to dilute the allergen and wash it away. They also induce airway constriction in an attempt to close the airway to prevent inhalation of more allergen.

About half of all asthma clients also experience a *delayed (late-phase) reaction.* Although clinical manifestations are the same as in early phase, they do not begin until 4 to 8 hours after exposure and may last for hours or days.

In both phases, the release of chemical mediators produces the airway response. In the late-phase response, however, the mediators attract other inflammatory cells and create a self-sustaining cycle of obstruction and inflammation. This chronic inflammation produces hyperresponsiveness of the airways. This hyperresponsiveness causes subsequent episodes in response not only to specific antigens but also to stimuli, such as physical exertion and breathing cold air. Clinical manifestations may occur with increasing frequency and severity.

Both alpha-adrenergic and beta-adrenergic receptors of the sympathetic nervous system are found in the bronchi. Stimulation of alpha-adrenergic receptors causes bronchoconstriction; conversely, stimulation of

EB EVIDENCE-BASED PRACTICE IN ACTION

The Assessment of Dyspnea

Dyspnea, or "shortness of breath," is one of the most common and significant complaints of clients with disorders of the lower airways. The experience of dyspnea is generally associated with much anxiety and should be consistently evaluated and treated by nurses. Much like pain, however, dyspnea is a subjective experience, which makes it more difficult to assess accurately. Currently, research is helping us to better understand the phenomenon of dyspnea and to identify more effective assessment strategies.

In the clinical setting, it is important to follow the intensity and frequency of dyspnea and the severity of this manifestation with specific activities to evaluate treatment outcomes. Self-rating scales have been easy for clients to use and effective for routine monitoring of dyspnea intensity. One such scale, which is similar to those used to measure pain, the numeric rating scale (NRS) asks clients: "On a scale of 0 to 10, indicate how much shortness of breath you are having right now, with 0 = no shortness of breath and 10 = shortness of breath as bad as can be." Gift and Narsavage[2] found the NRS to be a valid clinical measure of present dyspnea in a study of COPD clients.

Another scale, the modified Borg scale (MBS), is a vertical scale from 0 to 10 in which numbers are anchored with corresponding verbal expressions of progressively increasing dyspnea intensity. Clients rate their dyspnea by selecting the number with the corresponding words that most appropriately describe their sensation of breathlessness. The MBS was found to be an accurate tool for measuring dyspnea in emergency department clients with acute bronchospasm and was easily incorporated into triage and posttreatment assessment practice.[4]

In addition to intensity, assessment of the sensory qualities of dyspnea provides additional data to assist with treatment decisions and evaluation of interventions. Clients' use of descriptors of breathing, such as "heavy," "tight," "suffocating," and "hunger for more air," may help clinicians detect early indications of increasing dyspnea severity and client distress.[5]

Assessment of clients experiencing dyspnea should also include an assessment of fatigue and of their ability to engage in physical activity. Fatigue commonly accompanies the experience of dyspnea, although the underlying mechanism that explains how they are related remains elusive.[3] Dyspnea and physical activity are also highly correlated, although the relationship between fatigue and physical activity is not consistent. It has been hypothesized that as dyspnea increases, physical activity may be limited or avoided. Continued inactivity may result in decreased muscle strength, leading to fatigue due to disuse and degeneration of locomotive muscles. Because of fatigue, clients often further curtail their activity levels. Thus the relationships among dyspnea, fatigue, and physical activity are circular, which should be explained to clients to break the downward spiral.[6]

Finally, a thorough assessment of dyspnea should also include consideration of the client's psychological state. Manifestations that frequently accompany dyspnea, such as anxiety, panic, and helplessness, can be excessive and incapacitating, altering the client's ability to function. Detection and control of these manifestations may be one of the most critical needs of these clients, especially during acute episodes.[1]

References

1. Baker, C.F., & Scholz, J.A. (2002). Coping with symptoms of dyspnea in chronic obstructive pulmonary disease. *Rehabilitation Nursing, 27*(2), 67-74.
2. Gift, A.G., & Narsavage, G. (1998). Validity of the numeric rating scale as a measure of dyspnea. *American Journal of Critical Care, 7*(3), 200-204.
3. Graydon, J.E., et al. (1995). Predictors of functioning of patients with chronic obstructive pulmonary disease. *Heart & Lung, 24*(6), 369-375.
4. Kendrick, K.R., et al. (2000). Usefulness of the modified 0-10 Borg scale in assessing the degree of dyspnea in patients with COPD and asthma. *Journal of Emergency Nursing, 26*(3), 216-222.
5. Parshall, M.B., et al. (2001). Reliability and validity of dyspnea sensory quality descriptors in heart failure patients treated in an emergency department. *Heart & Lung, 30*(1), 57-65.
6. Woo, K. (2000). A pilot study to examine the relationships of dyspnea, physical activity, and fatigue in patients with chronic obstructive pulmonary disease. *Journal of Clinical Nursing, 9*(4), 526-533.

beta-adrenergic receptors causes bronchodilation. Cyclic adenosine monophosphate (cAMP) balances the two receptors. Some theories suggest that asthma may be a result of lack of beta-adrenergic stimulation.

Clinical Manifestations

During asthma attacks, clients are dyspneic and have marked respiratory effort. Manifestations of marked respiratory effort include nasal flaring, pursed-lip breathing, and use of accessory muscles. Cyanosis is a late development.

Auscultation of breath sounds usually reveals wheezing, especially during expiration. The inability to auscultate wheezing in an asthmatic client with acute respiratory distress may be an ominous sign. It may indicate that the small airways are too constricted to allow any air flow. The client may require immediate, aggressive medical intervention. In addition, bronchospasm may lead to almost continuous coughing in an attempt to clear the airway and exhale.

The diagnosis of asthma is based on clinical manifestations, spirometry results, and response to treatment. Spirometry reveals decreased peak expiratory flow rate

Mucous glands
Smooth muscle
Cartilage
NORMAL
Thick mucus in airway
Mucosal edema
Increased mucous glands
Hypertrophied muscle
Narrowed lumen
Cartilage
ASTHMA

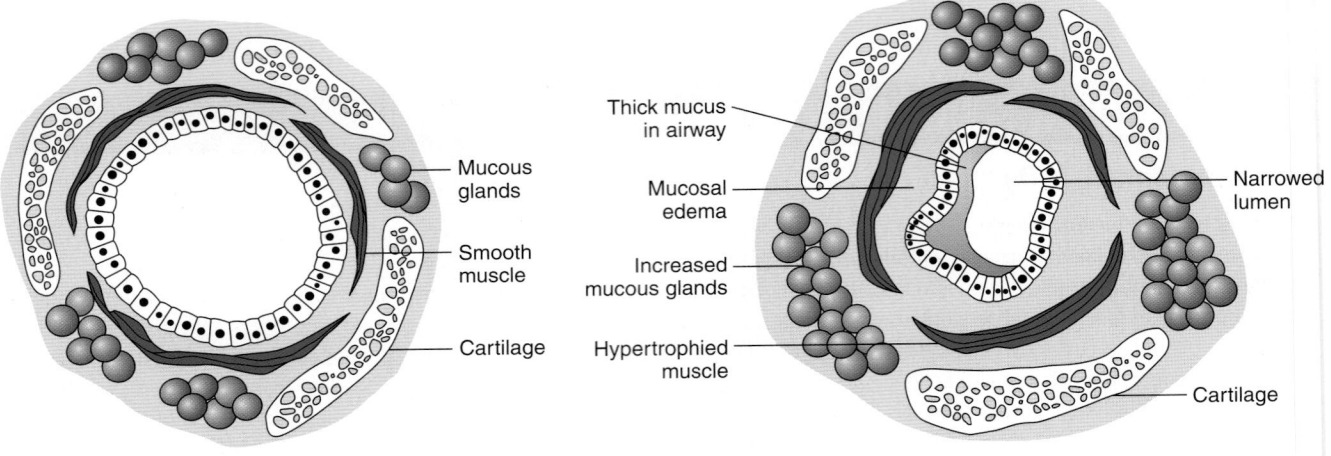

FIGURE 63-1 Common bronchial wall changes in asthma are hypertrophied smooth muscle, edema, mucous gland hypertrophy, and mucus in the lumen. (From Copstead, L.C., & Banasik, J.L. [2000]. *Pathophysiology: Biological and behavioral perspectives*. Philadelphia: W.B. Saunders.)

CONCEPT MAP

Understanding Asthma and Its Treatment

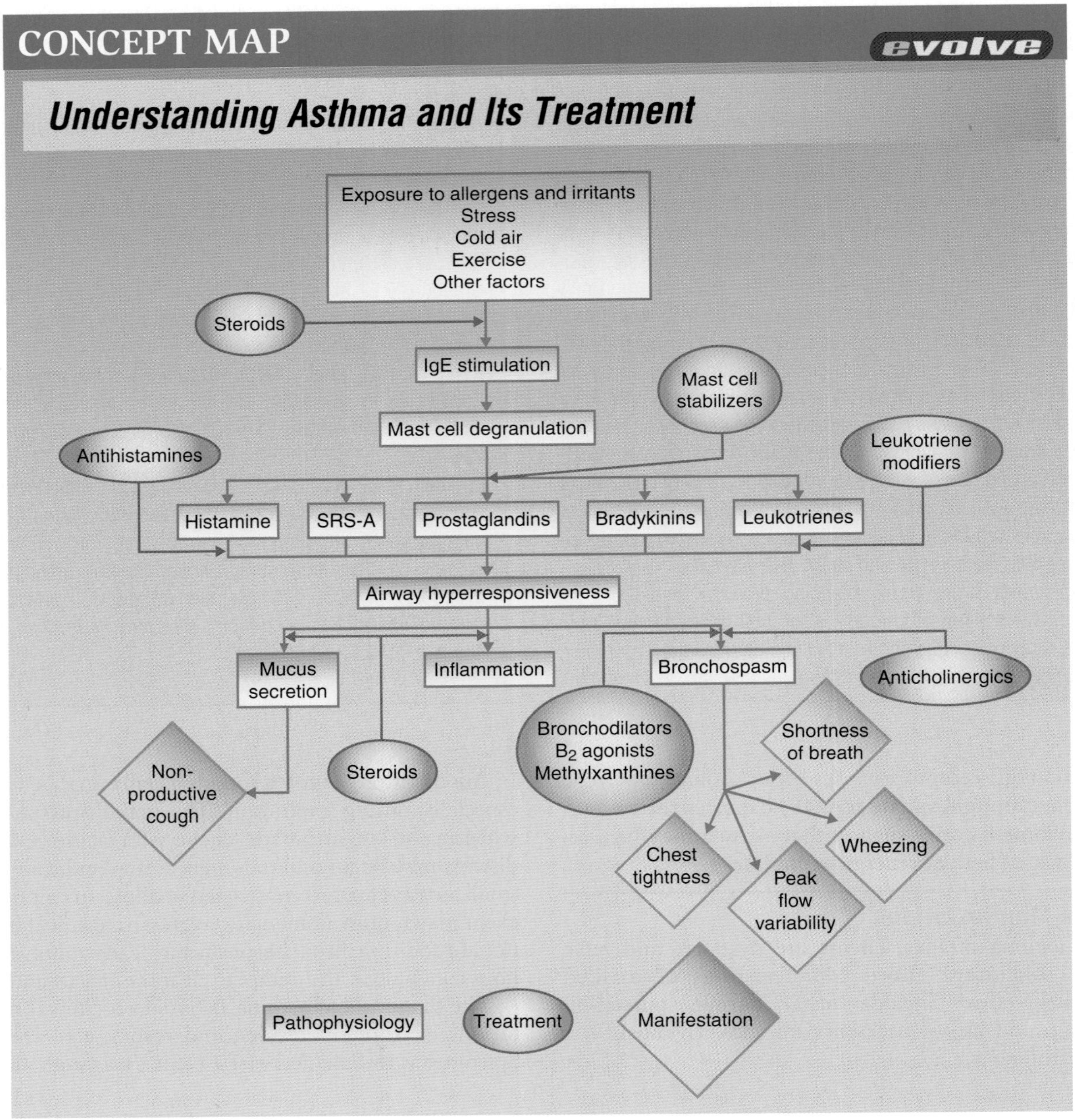

evolve
Exposure to allergens and irritants
Stress
Cold air
Exercise
Other factors
Steroids
IgE stimulation
Mast cell stabilizers
Mast cell degranulation
Antihistamines
Leukotriene modifiers
Histamine
SRS-A
Prostaglandins
Bradykinins
Leukotrienes
Airway hyperresponsiveness
Mucus secretion
Inflammation
Bronchospasm
Anticholinergics
Non-productive cough
Steroids
Bronchodilators
B_2 agonists
Methylxanthines
Shortness of breath
Chest tightness
Peak flow variability
Wheezing
Pathophysiology
Treatment
Manifestation

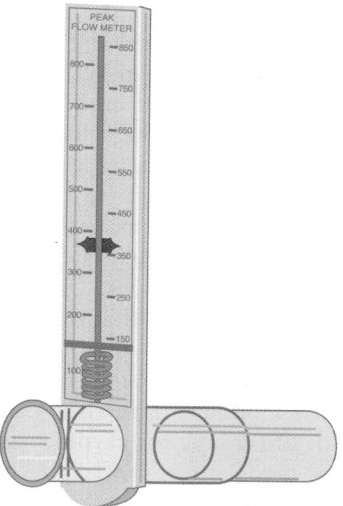

FIGURE 63-2 Peak flowmeters. Several types of portable meters are available for self-monitoring of air flow.

(PEFR), timed forced expiratory volume (FEV), and forced vital capacity (FVC). Functional residual capacity (FRC), total lung capacity (TLC), and residual volume (RV) are increased because air is trapped within the lungs. A 12% improvement in forced expiratory volume in 1 second (FEV_1) after inhaled administration of a beta-agonist bronchodilator implies a reversible air flow

obstruction, that is, by definition, asthma. Figure 63-2 shows a peak flowmeter for monitoring air flow.

Baseline assessment of pulmonary status also may include pulse oximetry and arterial blood gas (ABG) analysis. Pulse oximetry usually reveals low oxygen saturation. ABGs often show some degree of hypoxemia, with elevated partial pressures of arterial carbon dioxide ($PaCO_2$) in severe cases.

Status asthmaticus is a severe, life-threatening complication of asthma. It is an acute episode of bronchospasm that tends to intensify. With severe bronchospasm, the workload of breathing increases 5 to 10 times, which can lead to acute cor pulmonale. When air is trapped, a severe paradoxical pulse (i.e., drop in blood pressure >10 mm Hg during inspiration) develops as venous return is obstructed. Pneumothorax commonly develops. If status asthmaticus continues, hypoxemia worsens and acidosis begins. If the condition is untreated or not reversed, respiratory or cardiac arrest ensues.

Outcome Management
■ Medical Management

Many disorders can cause wheezing, such as sinusitis, gastroesophageal reflux disease (GERD), heart failure, bronchitis, and lung tumors. These conditions are ruled out before an asthma diagnosis is given.

Management of asthma is based on the severity of the disease (Table 63-1) and is directed at reversing airway

TABLE 63-1	*Classifying Asthma Severity*			
	Symptoms		**Nighttime Symptoms**	**Lung Function**
Step 4 Severe persistent	Continual symptoms Limited physical activity Frequent exacerbations		Frequent	FEV_1 or PEF ≤60% predicted PEF variability >30%
Step 3 Moderate persistent	Daily symptoms Daily use of inhaled short-acting beta$_2$ agonist Exacerbations affect activity Exacerbations ≥2 times a week; may last days		>1 time a week	FEV_1 or PEF >60% to <80% predicted PEF variability > 30%
Step 2 Mild persistent	Symptoms >2 times a week but <1 time a day Exacerbations may affect activity		>2 times a month	FEV_1 or PEF ≥80% predicted PEF variability 20%-30%
Step 1 Mild intermittent	Symptoms ≤2 times a week Asymptomatic and normal PEF between exacerbations Exacerbations brief (from a few hours to a few days); intensity may vary		≤2 times a month	FEV_1 or PEF ≥80% predicted PEF variability <20%

Data from National Institutes of Health. (1997). *Guidelines for the diagnosis and management of asthma.* NIH Pub. No. 97-4051. Washington, DC: Author; and National Institutes of Health (2002). *The NAEPP Expert Panel report: Guidelines for the diagnosis and management of asthma—Update on selected topics 2002.* NIH Pub. No. 02-5075. Washington, DC: Author.
FEV$_1$, Forced expiratory volume in 1 second; *PEF,* peak expiratory flow.

EB spasm. The general goals of asthma therapy include the following:

- Prevention of chronic asthma and asthma exacerbations
- Maintenance of normal activity levels
- Maintenance of normal or near-normal lung function
- Minimal or no side effects while receiving optimal medications
- Client satisfaction with asthma care[22]

Emphasis has moved away from episodic treatment of manifestations after they occur to long-term control through inhaled corticosteroids to prevent asthma whenever possible.

Reverse Airway Spasm. A severe asthma episode may constitute a medical emergency. Medical intervention for such episodes is aimed primarily at the following:

- Maintaining a patent airway by relieving bronchospasm and clearing excess or retained secretions
- Maintaining effective gas exchange
- Preventing complications, such as acute respiratory failure and status asthmaticus

Emergency management of the client begins with inhaled beta$_2$ agonists. Beta$_2$ agonists stimulate the beta-adrenergic receptors and dilate the airways. If the spasm does not abate (i.e., if FEV_1 remains <50% of predicted), nebulized atropine sulfate or intravenous (IV) steroids may be given. Atropine is an anticholinergic that blocks the effect of the parasympathetic system. When the vagus nerve is stimulated, bronchial smooth muscle tone increases. If these treatments do not reverse the clinical manifestations, the client usually is admitted to the hospital for further treatment. If the client has an acute asthma attack and no medications are nearby, the attack sometimes can be lessened by *pursed-lip breathing*, which increases pressure in the airways so that they remain open and trapped air can be exhaled more easily.

Supplemental oxygen is indicated if PaO_2 levels decrease to less than 60 mm Hg. Monitor the client closely for clinical manifestations of increasing anxiety, increased work of breathing, and indications of tiring. Endotracheal intubation and mechanical ventilation may be necessary. Sedation, and in rare cases administration of paralytic agents, may be necessary to blunt the client's respiratory effort and to prevent further air trapping and pressure increases. Status asthmaticus is treated with aggressive use of IV corticosteroids and frequent administration of inhaled beta-adrenergic medications to avoid intubation and mechanical ventilation.

Control Inflammation. Mucosal inflammation is controlled through the use of inhaled corticosteroids. Steroids prevent the mast cell from emptying, reducing the edema and spasm.

Mast cell stabilizers and leukotriene modifiers are included in special circumstances.[11] Mast cell stabilizers, such as cromolyn (Nasalcrom, Intal) and nedocromil (Tilade), suppress the release of bronchoconstrictive substances during antigen-antibody reactions. Leukotriene modifiers are used in the treatment of both acute and chronic asthma. The release of leukotrienes into the airways of asthmatic clients causes smooth muscle constriction, increased vascular permeability, edema of the airway mucosa, mucus release, and inhibited mucus clearance. Leukotrienes also attract eosinophils to the airway mucosa, which subsequently promote inflammation. Drugs that block leukotriene receptors mediate the actions of leukotrienes and serve as a useful addition to other therapies during an exacerbation. Leukotriene modifiers have also become an important component of therapy for chronic asthma, offering another class of medications for long-term asthma control. A growing body of evidence indicates that leukotriene modifiers are effective, well tolerated, and have a low risk of adverse effects. Continued research and follow-up are needed.[13]

■ Nursing Management
Assessment

Initially, assess the client for clinical manifestations of airway distress. If present, they constitute an emergency that must be managed before a detailed history of the disease or other health problems is obtained (see the Critical Monitoring feature on Asthma below for a list of manifestations of acute airway distress).

Asking clients to rate dyspnea on a scale of 0 to 10 is an easy and effective measure of present dyspnea and

---

CRITICAL MONITORING

Asthma

Notify the physician if the client still has the following manifestations after treatment for asthma:

- Increased anxiety
- Increased respiratory rate and effort
- Feelings of not being able to "catch one's breath"
- Continued low oxygen saturation
- Wheezing, both inspiratory and expiratory
- Almost continuous nonproductive cough
- Nasal flaring as respiratory distress increases
- Lips pursed while exhaling
- Use of accessory muscles of breathing
- Increasing tachycardia (tachycardia is a normal response to beta-adrenergic drugs)
- Paradoxical pulse as bronchospasm worsens
- Cyanosis and central nervous system depression as late findings

may help to monitor and evaluate dyspnea in clinic and home care settings: "On a scale of 0 to 10, indicate how much shortness of breath you are having right now, with 0 meaning no shortness of breath and 10 meaning shortness of breath as bad as can be."[9]

Determine any known medication allergies so that allergenic medications can be avoided during treatment. Ascertain whether the client has a history of cardiac disease because nonselective beta$_2$ agonists can produce tachycardia and stress a diseased heart.

Once the acute episode is controlled, explore the history of the client's asthma. Assist the client to determine whether there is a pattern to the manifestations. These data may help to identify a trigger that precipitates the asthmatic manifestations. If an extrinsic trigger can be identified, it may be possible to reduce or eliminate it. For example, if the client is allergic to mold, common sources of mold can be avoided. Ask about current medications. Some clients are inadvertently given medications that may induce bronchospasms. For example, a noncardioselective beta-blocker, such as propranolol (Inderal), prescribed for hypertension may cause bronchospasm.

Within the psychosocial domain, ask about the client's ability to manage the asthma and his or her general adaptation to the illness. Denial of the illness can interfere with early treatment. Determine whether the client feels control over the illness and feels capable of managing it. Clients who have this feeling of control show better compliance with treatments. Determine whether the client is experiencing an increased number of stressors. A stressful lifestyle may exacerbate asthma.

Assess the attitude of the family. The family can be a great source of support and can assist the client in recognizing early manifestations. In contrast, an unsupportive family may contribute to denial or may be an additional source of stress to the client. Involve the case manager (see the Case Management feature on Chronic Obstructive Pulmonary Disease on the website).

The client with a new diagnosis of asthma may be asked to assess the home and work environment for likely triggers of the clinical manifestations. In addition, skin testing for allergy may be performed. The presence of pets that shed hair or dander, cigarette smoke, or occupational exposure to other allergens may require some lifestyle changes. In many cases, the pets can remain in the house but cannot sleep with the asthmatic client. Encourage clients to stop smoking, and teach clients and others about the dangers of second-hand smoke. Elimination of irritants is generally performed in a reasonable fashion, such as removing exposure to one allergen at a time. Potential improvements in a client's manifestations that might result from a major lifestyle change, such as job change or loss of a pet, may be offset quickly by the stress felt from such a change.

Diagnosis, Outcomes, Interventions

Diagnosis: Ineffective Breathing Pattern. Because of airway spasm and edema, the client cannot move air in and out of the lungs as needed to maintain adequate tissue oxygenation. The correct nursing diagnosis would be *Ineffective Breathing Pattern related to impaired exhalation and anxiety.* Anxiety with dyspnea is another cause of breathing pattern problems.

Outcomes. The client will have improved breathing patterns, as evidenced by (1) a decreasing respiratory rate to within normal limits; (2) decreased dyspnea, less nasal flaring, and reduced use of accessory muscles; (3) decreased manifestations of anxiety; (4) a return of ABG levels to normal limits; (5) oxygen saturation greater than 95%; and (6) vital capacity measurements within normal limits or greater than 40% of those predicted.

Interventions. Assess the client frequently, observing respiratory rate and depth. Assess the breathing pattern for shortness of breath, pursed-lip breathing, nasal flaring, sternal and intercostal retractions, or a prolonged expiratory phase. During an acute asthma attack, these assessments can be conducted continuously.

Place the client in the Fowler position, and give oxygen as ordered. Monitor ABGs and oxygen saturation levels to determine the effectiveness of treatments. Compare pulmonary function test results with normal levels. The degree of dysfunction assists in planning client activity.

Diagnosis: Ineffective Airway Clearance. The excessive production of mucus and spasm in the airway makes it difficult to keep the airway patent. The nursing diagnosis *Ineffective Airway clearance related to increased production of secretions and bronchospasm* is appropriate.

Outcomes. The client will have effective airway clearance, as evidenced by (1) decreased inspiratory and expiratory wheezing; (2) decreased rhonchi; and (3) decreasing dry, nonproductive cough.

Interventions. If the airway is compromised, the client may require suctioning. Some clients experience asthma episodes as a result of pulmonary infection. Monitor the color and consistency of the sputum, and assist the client to cough effectively. Encourage oral fluids to thin the secretions and to replace fluids lost through rapid respiration. The humidity in the room may be increased slightly. If chest secretions are thick and difficult to expectorate, the client may benefit from postural drainage, lung percussion and vibration, expectorants, and frequent position changes. Give frequent oral care, every 2 to 4 hours, to remove the taste of the secretions and remoisten the oral mucous membranes that have dried from mouth breathing.

Diagnosis: Impaired Gas Exchange. When air is trapped within alveoli, the alveoli are eventually drained of oxygen and the client can become hypoxic. The nursing diagnosis is *Impaired Gas Exchange related to air trapping.*

Outcomes. The client will have adequate gas exchange, as evidenced by (1) decreased inspiratory and expiratory wheezing; (2) decreased rhonchi; (3) oxygen saturation >90%; (4) PaO_2 greater than 60 mm Hg; (5) $PaCO_2$ equal to or less than 45 mm Hg, (6) pH of 7.35 to 7.45; (7) usual skin color (no cyanosis); and (8) decreasing dry, nonproductive cough.

Interventions. Assess lung sounds every hour during acute episodes to determine the adequacy of gas exchange. Assess skin and mucous membrane color for cyanosis. Cyanosis is a late manifestation of hypoxia and an indication of serious gas-exchange problems. Monitor pulse oximetry for oxygen saturation levels. Administer oxygen as ordered to maintain optimal oxygen saturation.

Refer to the Care Plan feature on The Client with Chronic Obstructive Pulmonary Disease on pp. 1824 to 1828 when working with clients with diagnoses of *Activity Intolerance, Anxiety, Imbalanced Nutrition,* or *Disturbed Sleep Pattern.*

Evaluation

Generally, asthma episodes can be reversed quickly if there is no underlying problem, such as infection. Expect the client to be hospitalized only briefly; plan a coordinated approach to assessment and follow-up.

■ Self-Care

The approach to pharmacologic therapy often is referred to as *step care,* meaning that the medications ordered and the frequency of administration are adjusted according to the severity of the client's asthma. Asthma medications are categorized into two major classes: (1) *long-term*–control medications, used to achieve and maintain control of persistent asthma, and (2) *quick-relief* medications, used to treat acute air flow obstruction and its accompanying manifestations. The most effective long-term–control medications are those that reduce inflammation, with inhaled steroids being the most potent. Quick-relief medications include short-acting inhaled beta$_2$ agonists and oral steroids.

For clients who respond poorly to inhaled agents, theophylline and aminophylline are still used at times. These medications are regarded as weak bronchodilators. Wide variations exist in their rates of metabolism, and these medications have a high potential for toxicity; for these reasons, their use is declining. Theophylline lev-

els must be monitored to evaluate effectiveness and possible toxicity.

Figure 63-3 depicts a stepwise approach for managing asthma in adults. All clients with asthma require a short-acting inhaled beta$_2$ agonist as needed for acute manifestations. Clients with mild, moderate, or severe persistent asthma require daily long-term–control medications. The preferred treatment strategy is to start with more intensive therapy to achieve rapid control and then "step down" to the minimum therapy needed for maintenance.

Changes in the treatment plan may be needed as asthma severity and control vary over time. Follow-up visits every 1 to 6 months are recommended to monitor the disease and to maintain control. The presence of one or more indicators of poor control (i.e., awakening at night with dyspnea or coughing, increased use of short-acting inhaled beta$_2$ agonists, urgent care visits) may suggest a need to "step up" therapy. Before increasing medications, however, consider other possible reasons for poor control (Table 63-2).

Nebulized medications can be difficult to learn to use.[30] The client must coordinate inhalation with compression of the metered-dose inhaler canister (Figure 63-4). The Client Education Guide feature on Asthma on p. 1816 provides directions for using an inhaler. Observe the client's use of the nebulizer to ascertain whether the medication is entering the airway.

Through appropriate use of the peak flowmeter and medications, clients with asthma should be able to anticipate most exacerbations and enhance their quality of life. Peak flow values fall about 24 hours before manifestations develop. Clients should be taught to increase their routine medications in anticipation of asthma exacerbations. Many clients can manage their asthma effectively with a thorough action plan to guide their decisions. An action plan for asthma is presented in Figure 63-5. It is recommended that a written plan be used as part of the overall effort to educate the client in self-management.[23]

CHRONIC OBSTRUCTIVE PULMONARY DISEASE

Also known as *chronic obstructive lung disease,* chronic obstructive pulmonary disease (COPD) refers to several disorders that affect the movement of air in and out of the lungs. Although the most important of these—obstructive bronchitis, emphysema, and asthma—may occur in a pure form, they most commonly coexist, with overlapping clinical manifestations. The term *COPD* is commonly used, but some pulmonologists think it is not completely accurate, and the term *chronic air flow limitation* may be used in its place.

COPD can occur as a result of increased airway resistance secondary to bronchial mucosal edema or smooth muscle contraction. It may also be a result of decreased elastic recoil, as seen in emphysema. Elastic re-

Stepwise Approach for Managing Asthma in Adults and Children Older Than 5 Years of Age: Treatment

Classify Severity: Clinical Features Before Treatment or Adequate Control			Medications Required To Maintain Long-Term Control
	Symptoms/Day Symptoms/Night	PEF or FEV$_1$ PEF Variability	Daily Medications
Step 4 **Severe Persistent**	Continual Frequent	≤60% >30%	■ Preferred treatment: – High-dose inhaled corticosteroids AND – Long-acting inhaled beta$_2$-agonists AND, if needed, – Corticosteroid tablets or syrup long term (2 mg/kg/day, generally do not exceed 60 mg/day). (Make repeat attempts to reduce systemic corticosteroids and maintain control with high-dose inhaled corticosteroids.)
Step 3 **Moderate Persistent**	Daily >1 night/week	>60% – <80% >30%	■ Preferred treatment: – Low-to-medium dose inhaled corticosteroids and long-acting inhaled beta$_2$-agonists. ■ Alternative treatment (listed alphabetically): – Increase inhaled corticosteroids within medium-dose range OR – Low-to-medium dose inhaled corticosteroids and either leukotriene modifier or theophylline. If needed (particularly in patients with recurring severe exacerbations): ■ Preferred treatment: – Increase inhaled corticosteroids within medium-dose range and add long-acting inhaled beta$_2$-agonists. ■ Alternative treatment: – Increase inhaled corticosteroids within medium-dose range and add either leukotriene modifier or theophylline.
Step 2 **Mild Persistent**	>2/week but <1 time/day >2 nights/month	≥80% 20%-30%	■ Preferred treatment: – Low-dose inhaled corticosteroids. ■ Alternative treatment (listed alphabetically): cromolyn, leukotriene modifier, nedocromil, OR sustained release theophylline to serum concentration of 5-15 μg/ml.
Step 1 **Mild Intermittent**	≤2 days/week ≤2 nights/month	≥80% <20%	■ No daily medication needed. ■ Severe exacerbations may occur, separated by long periods of normal lung function and no symptoms. A course of systemic corticosteroids is recommended.

Quick Relief **All Patients**	■ Short-acting bronchodilator: 2-4 puffs short-acting inhaled beta$_2$-agonists as needed for symptoms. ■ Intensity of treatment will depend on severity of exacerbation; up to 3 treatments at 20-minute intervals or a single nebulizer treatment as needed. Course of systemic corticosteroids may be needed. ■ Use of short-acting beta$_2$-agonists >2 times a week in intermittent asthma (daily, or increasing use in persistent asthma) may indicate the need to initiate (increase) long-term control therapy.

 Step down
Review treatment every 1 to 6 months; a gradual stepwise reduction in treatment may be possible.

 Step up
If control is not maintained, consider step up. First, review patient medication technique, adherence, and environmental control.

Note
■ The stepwise approach is meant to assist, not replace, the clinical decision making required to meet individual patient needs.
■ Classify severity: assign patient to most severe step in which any feature occurs (PEF is % of personal best; FEV$_1$ is % predicted).
■ Gain control as quickly as possible (consider a short course of systemic corticosteroids); then step down to the least medication necessary to maintain control.
■ Provide education on self-management and controlling environmental factors that make asthma worse (e.g., allergens and irritants).
■ Refer to an asthma specialist if there are difficulties controlling asthma or if step 4 care is required. Referral may be considered if step 3 care is required.

Goals of Therapy: Asthma Control

■ Minimal or no chronic symptoms day or night
■ Minimal or no exacerbations
■ No limitations on activities; no school/work missed
■ Maintain (near) normal pulmonary function
■ Minimal use of short-acting inhaled beta$_2$-agonist (<1 time/day, <1 canister/month)
■ Minimal or no adverse effects from medications

FIGURE 63-3 Stepwise approach for managing asthma in adults and children older than 5 years of age. (From National Institutes of Health [2002]. *The National Asthma Education and Prevention Program Expert Panel report: Guidelines for the diagnosis and management of asthma—Update on selected topics*. NIH Pub. No. 02-5075. Washington, DC: Author.)

TABLE 63-2	*Possible Reasons for Poor Asthma Control—"ICE"*
Inhaler technique	Check client's technique
Compliance	Ask when and how much medication the client is taking
Environment	Ask client whether something in the environment has changed
Also consider	
Alternative diagnosis	Assess client for the presence of concomitant upper respiratory disease or alternative diagnosis

From National Institutes of Health. (1997). *Practical guide for the diagnosis and management of asthma.* NIH Pub. No. 97-4051. Washington, DC: Author.

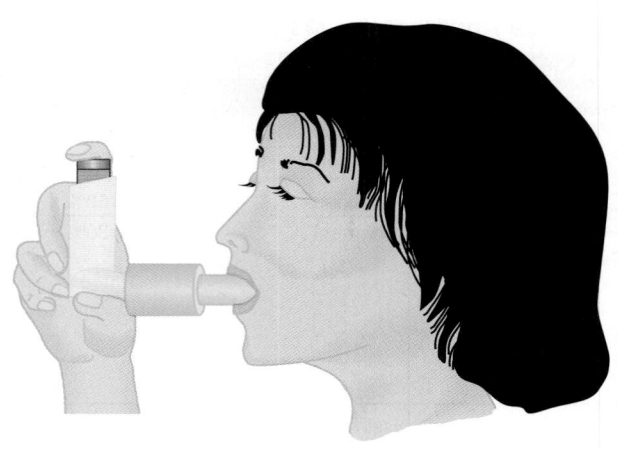

FIGURE 63-4 A client using a metered-dose inhaler with a spacer.

CLIENT EDUCATION GUIDE

Asthma

Client Instructions

Asthma may be triggered by pollen, dust, animal dander, molds, smoke, or other allergens. Learn what triggers your asthma and minimize your exposure to it.

Monitor the pollution index and pollen counts. Limit outdoor activities when these indicators are high.

Take all medications as prescribed by your physician. If you are taking both a bronchodilator and a steroid via inhaler, take the bronchodilator first to open the airways.

Use your peak flowmeter daily.

Follow these directions on how to use a peak flowmeter:
- Attach the mouthpiece and set the pointer to zero (0).
- Stand up and take a deep breath.
- Put the mouthpiece in your mouth, and close your lips tightly around it.
- Blow into the mouthpiece as hard and as fast as you can.
- Record the value and reset the meter.
- Repeat the procedure for a total of three readings.
- Record the highest value on your record sheet.
- Monitor peak flow daily, know your "green zone," when air flow is normal; the "yellow zone," when values have fallen and you need to increase your routine medications; and the "red zone," when you need to increase your rescue medications and notify your doctor

Use these directions for using an inhaler:
- Remove the cap and shake the inhaler well.
- Hold the canister upright with your index finger on the top and your thumb on the bottom.

- Breathe out through your mouth.
- Place the mouthpiece 1 to 2 inches away from your opened mouth (unless using a spacer).
- Begin with a slow, deep breath. As you breathe in, press the canister down with your finger to give yourself one puff of medication.
- Hold your breath in for at least 5 to 10 seconds.
- Slowly breathe out, holding your lips tight (pursed).

If your physician has prescribed more than one puff, wait 1 minute between puffs to let the medication open up the upper airway. That way, the next puff can reach lower into your lungs.

Pursed-lip breathing, progressive muscle relaxation, and tripod positioning (i.e., leaning on your arms positioned in front of you) may improve your breathing during asthma episodes.

Unless your physician has told you to limit fluids, drink 8 to 10 glasses of water every day. Water helps to thin your sputum so that you can cough it up more easily.

Some forms of asthma may be triggered by exercise. Discuss an exercise plan with your physician before starting.

Call your physician if you experience any of the following manifestations:
- Wheezing and shortness of breath, even though you are taking your medications as prescribed
- Fever, muscle aches, chest pain, or thickening of sputum
- Sputum color changes to yellow, green, gray, or red (bloody)
- Problems that may be related to your medications (e.g., rash, itching, swelling, or trouble breathing)

ASTHMA ACTION PLAN FOR _____

Doctor's Name _____ Date _____

Doctor's Phone Number _____

Hospital/Emergency Room Phone Number _____

Take These Long-Term-Control Medicines Each Day (include an anti-inflammatory)

Medicine	How much to take	When to take it

GREEN ZONE: Doing Well

- No cough, wheeze, chest tightness, or shortness of breath during the day or night
- Can do usual activities

And, if a peak flow meter is used,
Peak flow: more than _____
(80% or more of my best peak flow)

My best peak flow is: _____

Before exercise ☐ _____ ☐ 2 or ☐ 4 puffs 5 to 60 minutes before exercise

FIRST ➡ **Add: Quick-Relief Medicine – and keep taking your GREEN ZONE medicine**

YELLOW ZONE: Asthma Is Getting Worse

- Cough, wheeze, chest tightness, or shortness of breath, or
- Waking at night due to asthma, or
- Can do some, but not all, usual activities

-Or-

Peak flow: _____ to _____
(50% - 80% of my best peak flow)

SECOND ➡ ☐ _____ ☐ 2 or ☐ 4 puffs, every 20 minutes for up to 1 hour
(short-acting beta$_2$-agonist) ☐ Nebulizer, once

If your symptoms (and peak flow, if used) return to GREEN ZONE after 1 hour of above treatment:
☐ Take the quick-relief medicine every 4 hours for 1 to 2 days.
-Or-
☐ Double the dose of your inhaled steroid for _____ (7-10) days.

If your symptoms (and peak flow, if used) do not return to GREEN ZONE after 1 hour of above treatment:
☐ Take: _____ ☐ 2 or ☐ 4 puffs or ☐ Nebulizer
(short-acting beta$_2$-agonist)
☐ Add: _____ _____ mg. per day For _____ (3-10) days
(oral steroid)
☐ Call the doctor ☐ before/ ☐ within _____ hours after taking the oral steroid.

RED ZONE: Medical Alert!

- Very short of breath, or
- Quick-relief medicines have not helped, or
- Cannot do usual activities, or
- Symptoms are same or get worse after 24 hours in Yellow Zone

-Or-

Peak flow: less than _____
(50% of my best peak flow)

Take this medicine:

☐ _____ ☐ 4 or ☐ 6 puffs or ☐ Nebulizer
(short-acting beta$_2$-agonist)

☐ _____ _____ mg.
(oral steroid)

Then call your doctor NOW. Go to the hospital or call for an ambulance if:
- You are still in the red zone after 15 minutes AND
- You have not reached your doctor.

DANGER SIGNS

- Trouble walking and talking due to shortness of breath
- Lips or fingernails are blue

➡ ■ Take ☐ 4 or ☐ 6 puffs of your quick-relief medicine AND
■ Go to the hospital or call for an ambulance (_____) NOW!

FIGURE 63-5 Asthma action plan. (From National Institutes of Health. [1997]. *Practical guide for the diagnosis and management of asthma.* NIH Publication no. 97-4053. Washington, DC: Author.)

coil, similar to the recoil of a stretched rubber band, is the force used to passively deflate the lung and exhale. Decreased elastic recoil results in a decreased driving force to empty the lung.

A widespread disorder, COPD affects more than 16 million Americans. It now accounts for 4% of all deaths in the United States, making it the fourth leading cause of death. Caring for clients with COPD has been estimated at $14.5 billion annually in direct care costs alone[12]; however, the burden of COPD is even greater from a global perspective, where it is currently the sixth leading cause of death and the 12th leading cause of morbidity worldwide.[27]

Etiology and Risk Factors

The specific causes of COPD are not clearly understood. The effects of numerous irritants found in cigarette smoke (i.e., stimulation of excess mucus production and coughing, destruction of ciliary function, and inflammation and damage of bronchiolar and alveolar walls), however, make smoking the leading risk factor for COPD development.[16] Chronic respiratory infections, including sinusitis, contribute to development of COPD, as does the aging process. Heredity and genetic predisposition also appear to have a role.

Pathophysiology

COPD is a combination of chronic obstructive bronchitis, emphysema, and asthma. The pathophysiology of bronchitis and emphysema is presented here (see earlier discussion of pathophysiology of asthma).

Chronic Obstructive Bronchitis

Inflammation of the bronchi (chronic obstructive bronchitis) causes increased mucus production and chronic cough. In contrast to those of acute bronchitis, the clinical manifestations of chronic bronchitis continue for at least 3 months of the year for 2 consecutive years. Additionally, if the client has a decreased FEV_1/FVC ratio of less than 75% and chronic bronchitis, the client is said to have chronic *obstructive* bronchitis, indicating that the client has obstructive lung disease combined with chronic cough. Chronic bronchitis is characterized by the following:

- An increase in the size and number of submucous glands in the large bronchi, which increases mucus production
- An increased number of goblet cells, which also secrete mucus
- Impaired ciliary function, which reduces mucus clearance

The lung's mucociliary defenses are impaired, and there is increased susceptibility to infection. When infection occurs, mucus production is greater, and the bronchial walls become inflamed and thickened. Chronic bronchitis initially affects only the larger bronchi, but eventually all the airways are involved. The thick mucus and inflamed bronchi obstruct the airways, especially during expiration. The airways collapse, and air is trapped in the distal portion of the lung. This obstruction leads to reduced alveolar ventilation. An abnormal ventilation/perfusion $\dot{V}/\dot{Q}$ ratio develops, with a corresponding fall in PaO_2. Impaired ventilation may also result in increased levels of $PaCO_2$. As compensation for the hypoxemia, polycythemia (overproduction of erythrocytes) occurs.

Emphysema

Emphysema is a disorder in which the alveolar walls are destroyed. This destruction leads to permanent overdistention of the air spaces. Air passages are obstructed as a result of these changes rather than from mucus production, as in chronic bronchitis. Although the precise cause of emphysema is unknown, research has shown that the enzymes protease and elastase can attack and destroy the connective tissue of the lungs. Emphysema may result from a breakdown in the lung's normal defense mechanisms (alpha₁-antitrypsin [AAT]) against these enzymes. Difficult expiration in emphysema is the result of destruction of the walls (septa) between the alveoli, partial airway collapse, and loss of elastic recoil. As the alveoli and septa collapse, pockets of air form between the alveolar spaces (blebs) and within the lung parenchyma (bullae). This process leads to increased ventilatory dead space from areas that do not participate in gas or blood exchange. The work of breathing is increased because there is less functional lung tissue to exchange oxygen and carbon dioxide. Emphysema causes destruction of the pulmonary capillaries, further decreasing oxygen perfusion and ventilation.

The three types of emphysema are centrilobar, panlobar, and paraseptal (Figure 63-6).

Centrilobular (or *centriacinar*) *emphysema,* the most common type, produces destruction in the bronchioles, usually in the upper lung regions. Inflammation develops in the bronchioles, but usually the alveolar sac remains intact. *Panlobular emphysema* affects both the bronchioles and the alveoli and most commonly involves the lower lung. These forms of emphysema occur most often in smokers.

Paraseptal (or *panacinar*) *emphysema* destroys the alveoli in the lower lobes of the lungs, resulting in isolated blebs along the lung periphery. It is believed to be the likely cause of spontaneous pneumothorax. Paraseptal emphysema occurs in older clients and in clients with an inherited deficiency of AAT. Normally, AAT inhibits the action of enzymes that break down proteins. Clients without AAT are at increased risk for COPD because the walls of the lung are at higher risk for destruction. Cigarette smoking is thought to alter the balance of these enzymes and thus to increase destruction of lung tissue. The treatment of early emphysema with AAT replacement therapy looks promising.

NORMAL LUNGS

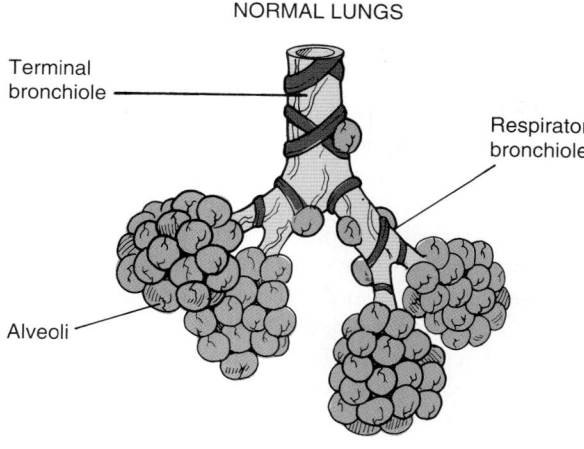

CENTRIACINAR EMPHYSEMA

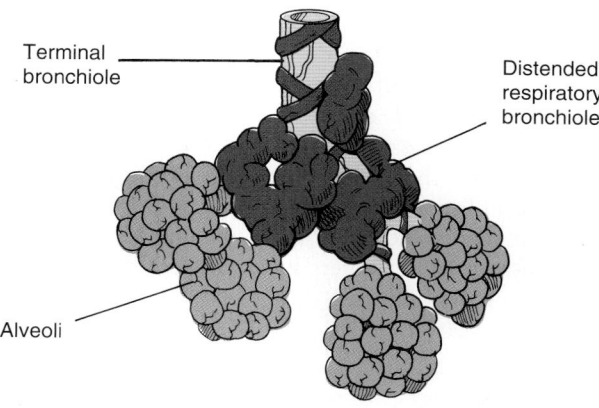

PANACINAR EMPHYSEMA

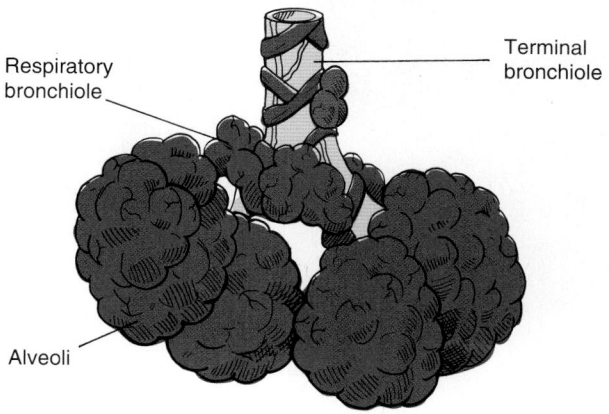

FIGURE 63-6 Types of emphysema.

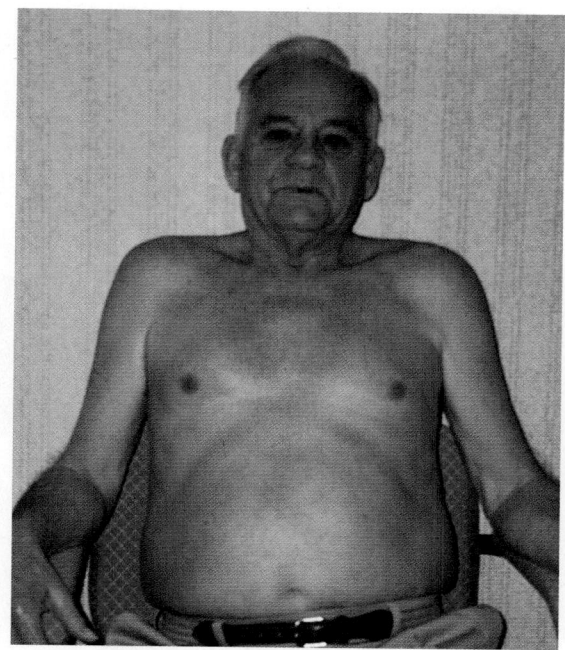

FIGURE 63-7 A client with chronic obstructive bronchitis. Note the stocky build and the presence of pursed-lip breathing and barrel chest. The slight gynecomastia is a side effect of corticosteroid therapy. The client's shoulders are raised because of shortness of breath and increased work of breathing.

prolonged expiration. As the chronic bronchitis progresses, copious amounts of sputum are produced and pulmonary infection is common. The client suffers from chronic hypoxemia and hypercapnia (Figure 63-7). The characteristic sitting position is leaning over a table with shoulder girdle raised. Gait and walking pace correspond to the clients breathing with frequent rest periods to breathe.

Clients who have primary emphysema have progressive dyspnea on exertion that eventually becomes dyspnea at rest (Figure 63-8). The anteroposterior diameter of the chest is enlarged, and the chest has hyperresonant sounds to percussion. Chest films show overinflation and flattened diaphragms (Figure 63-9, *A*). ABGs are usually normal until later stages, when compensated respiratory acidosis is often evident. The client may have an enlarged heart and right ventricular lift. The electrocardiogram (ECG) shows right heart strain pattern and right axis deviation. Other manifestations may be cyanosis around the lips, clubbing of the fingers, and pitting peripheral edema. Noticeable nicotine stains may be apparent on the client's hands. Table 63-3 contrasts common findings in chronic bronchitis and emphysema.

Complications

Respiratory infections commonly develop in clients with COPD. This situation is a result of alterations in the normal respiratory defense mechanisms and decreased immune resistance. Because respiratory status already is

Clinical Manifestations

All three disorders—asthma, chronic bronchitis, and emphysema—are present to some degree in clients with COPD. Clients with chronic obstructive bronchitis as the major disease have a productive cough, decreased exercise tolerance, wheezing, shortness of breath, and

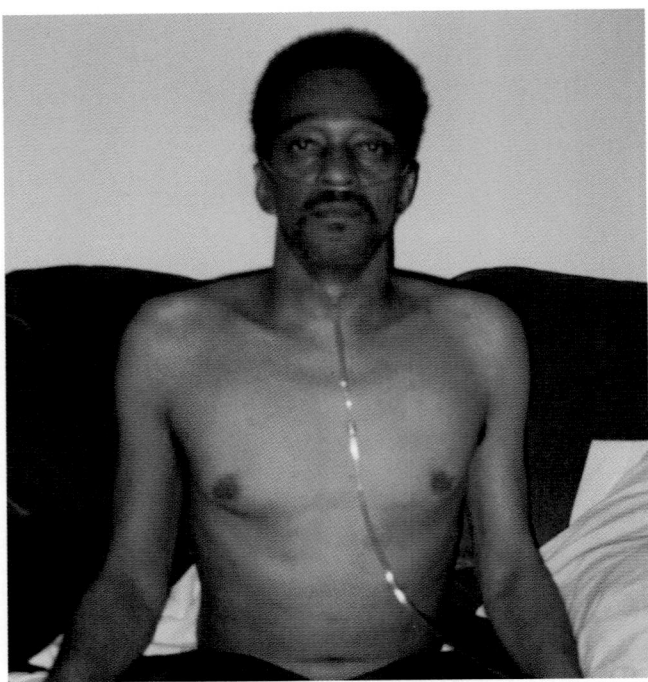

FIGURE 63-8 A client with emphysema. Note the thin appearance and the presence of continuous oxygen therapy. The use of accessory muscles of respiration (neck and shoulder muscles) reflects the client's shortness of breath and increased work of breathing necessary to increase minute ventilation and to maintain adequate arterial blood gas values.

compromised, infection frequently leads to acute respiratory failure and is a common reason for hospitalization (see Chapter 65).

Spontaneous pneumothorax may develop from rupture of an emphysematous bleb. This rupture results in a closed pneumothorax and requires insertion of a chest tube for reexpansion of the lung (see Chapter 64).

Similar to asthma, chronic obstructive bronchitis and emphysema may worsen at night. Clients often report sleep-onset dyspnea and frequent or early-morning awakenings. During sleep, there is a decrease in the muscle tone and activity of the respiratory muscles. This decreased tone leads to hypoventilation, an increase in resistance of the airways, and $\dot{V}/\dot{Q}$ mismatch. Eventually, the client becomes hypoxemic.

Outcome Management
■ Medical Management

The treatment goals for the client with COPD are to improve ventilation, to facilitate the removal of bronchial secretions, to prevent complications, to slow the progression of clinical manifestations, and to promote health maintenance and client management of the disease. At times, the client may receive continuous mechanical ventilation for adequate oxygenation. Ventilator-dependent clients with COPD may be managed in critical care, although some centers have non–critical care areas for clients on ventilators.

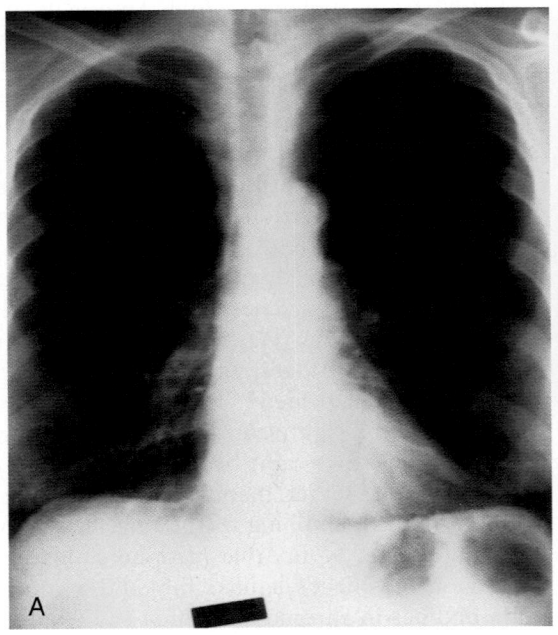
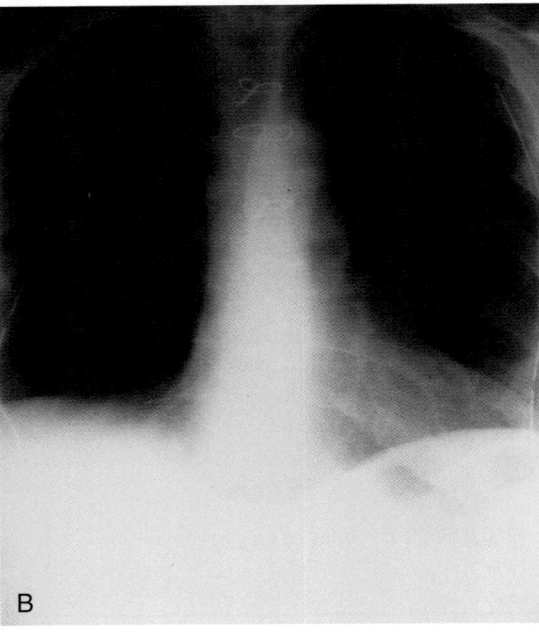

FIGURE 63-9 A, Preoperative chest x-ray of a client with emphysema. Note the flattened diaphragm and the laterally hyperexpanded chest walls. **B,** Postoperative chest x-ray after lung volume reduction surgery. The right side of the diaphragm is rounded and no longer flattened by emphysematous lung tissue. (From Allen, G. [1996]. Surgical treatment of emphysema using bovine pericardium strips. *AORN Journal, 63*(2), 373-388.)

Improve Ventilation. Bronchodilators remain the mainstay in the treatment of COPD.[15] These drugs reduce airway obstruction and may relieve manifestations in COPD. They are usually administered via the inhalation route but in rare occasions may be given orally or administered intravenously.

Of the several types of bronchodilators, beta$_2$ agonists are the most frequently prescribed. They are sympathomimetic drugs that act on the beta$_2$-adrenoceptors in the smooth muscles of the airways and cause bronchodilatation. These drugs may also enhance mucus clearance and improve the endurance of respiratory muscles. Beta$_2$ agonists (e.g., albuterol, metaproterenol) have minimal adverse effects, with rapid onset of action, a peak effect in 60 to 90 minutes, and duration of 3 to 4 hours. Parenteral, oral, and inhalation forms of these drugs are available. The inhalational route is preferred in acute exacerbations because it results in greater bronchodilata-

tion with overall fewer side effects. Side effects that may develop with the use of these drugs are tachycardia, tremor, nervousness, and nausea.

Anticholinergic agents are another type of bronchodilator that is commonly used as part of the treatment regimen. They offer greater bronchodilator effect and fewer side effects than short-acting inhaled beta$_2$ agonists. These drugs work by blocking the cholinergic receptors located in the larger airways, resulting in bronchodilatation. Ipratropium bromide (Atrovent) is the most commonly used drug in this category. When given by metered-dose inhaler, two puffs achieve maximal bronchodilatation in 1.5 to 2 hours and last 4 to 5 hours. Adverse reactions from these drugs include dry mouth, nervousness, dizziness, fatigue, and headache.

Methylxanthines (e.g., theophylline, aminophylline), in both parenteral and oral forms, are also used to treat

TABLE 63-3	*Primary Clinical Manifestations in Chronic Bronchitis and Emphysema*	
Clinical Manifestations	**Chronic Bronchitis**	**Emphysema**

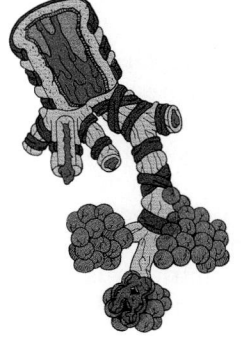

Onset of symptoms	Age 40-50 yr	Age 50-75 yr
Physical appearance	Stocky build with no history of weight loss; use of accessory muscles to breathe in late stages; cyanotic; barrel chest	Cachectic appearance with history of major weight loss; tachypnea and use of accessory muscles to breathe, even in early stages; pink skin color
Chief complaint	Persistent cough and copious sputum production	Persistent shortness of breath with progressive exertional dyspnea
Clinical course	Variable, with exacerbations usually related to respiratory infection	Progressive deterioration
ABGs	Decreased Pao$_2$, increased Paco$_2$	Pao$_2$ normal or slightly decreased; Paco$_2$ low or normal until end stage
Pulmonary function	Small airways affected early (reduced FEF$_{25\%-75\%}$); FEV$_1$ reduced later as airway damage progresses; normal to variable diffusion capacity	Reduced FEF$_{25\%-75\%}$ and FEV$_1$; reduced diffusion capacity because of destruction of alveoli
Associated findings	Frequent episodes of cor pulmonale with dependent edema (especially in late stage); elevated hematocrit	No history of cor pulmonale until very late stage; no edema; on auscultation, diminished breath sounds even with deep breathing

ABGs, Arterial blood gases; *FEF$_{25\%-75\%}$,* forced expiratory flow, midexpiratory phase; *FEV$_1$,* forced expiratory volume in 1 second; *Paco$_2$,* partial pressure of arterial carbon dioxide; *Pao$_2$,* partial pressure of arterial oxygen.

acute exacerbations. In addition to their bronchodilatory properties, methylxanthines enhance mucociliary clearance, stimulate the central respiratory drive, reduce pulmonary vascular resistance, and improve lung function during sleep. The level of benefit achieved with these agents is dose related, but there is no uniform relationship between the drug's effectiveness and serum blood levels. Age, smoking status, circulatory status, and hepatic function are factors that affect metabolism. Toxicity with methylxanthines may occur even at therapeutic levels, so blood levels of these agents need to be monitored closely. Several drugs also interfere with these agents even when administered in therapeutic levels. Side effects may include gastric upset, tachycardia, nausea and vomiting (possible toxicity), tremors, and nervousness.

Corticosteroids are used in the acute management of clients with COPD exacerbations. The exact mechanisms of action of these drugs in obstructive airway disease are poorly understood. They appear to work by reducing airway inflammation and edema while also inhibiting the breakdown of epinephrine by catechol-O-methyltransferase, thereby potentiating the bronchodilatory effect of the catecholamines. If used, corticosteroids should be administered either orally or parenterally, depending on the severity of the exacerbation. They should be used early in the course of treatment because their effect is not apparent for several hours. Clients who show a rapid response to parental steroids can be switched to oral forms on the third or fourth day of treatment, followed by a tapering course. The most common adverse effects are hypertension, peptic ulcer, dysphoria, hyperglycemia, cough, oral thrush, and fragile skin. A short course of corticosteroids may result in few adverse effects, but chronic use is often associated with much higher adverse reaction rates. Clients who require long-term steroids often develop paper-thin skin that tears easily, a round face, thin and sparse hair, delayed wound healing, and a hump between their scapula.

Oxygen is used when the client has severe exertional or resting hypoxemia (PaO_2 <40 mm Hg).[18] Oxygen (1 to 3 L) by nasal cannula may be required to raise the PaO_2 to no less than 60 mm Hg. *Oxygen is used cautiously in clients with emphysema, however. Because of long-standing hypercapnia, the respiratory drive in emphysematous clients is triggered by low oxygen levels rather than increased carbon dioxide levels. The drive to breathe is the opposite of normal in clients with emphysema. If high levels of oxygen are administered to these clients, their respiratory drive can be obliterated and carbon dioxide retention can occur.*

Remove Bronchial Secretions. Pulmonary hygiene is needed to rid the lungs of secretions and to reduce the risk of infection. In the hospital, the client may be treated with nebulized bronchodilators and positive-pressure air flow or positive end-expiratory pressure devices to increase the caliber of the airways. Postural drainage and chest physiotherapy may be prescribed to move the secretions from the small to the large airways, from which they can be expelled.

Promote Exercise. Aerobic exercise is used to enhance cardiovascular fitness and to train respiratory muscles to function more effectively. Exercise does not improve lung function, but respiratory muscles can be strengthened even when the lungs are diseased. Progressively increased walking is the most common form of exercise. Before a walking program is begun, ABGs should be assessed and compared with resting levels. Supplemental oxygen should be used during exercise if the client becomes severely hypoxemic.

Breathing exercises may also be prescribed. Encourage diaphragmatic breathing and pursed-lip breathing, and discourage rapid, shallow *panic* breathing.

Control Complications. Edema and cor pulmonale are treated with diuretics and digitalis. Phlebotomy may be used to reduce blood volume in clients with marked elevations in hematocrit (>60%). Phlebotomy also reduces cardiac workload.

Improve General Health. The most effective way to slow disease progression is for the client to stop smoking. Exposure to known allergens should be minimized. All clients with COPD should avoid high altitudes, and supplemental oxygen may be required for air travel. No specific climate has been shown to alter the course of the disorder.

Adequate nutrition is essential to maintain respiratory muscle strength. Malnutrition is common and contributes to decreased respiratory muscle strength and reduced diaphragmatic mass. Consult a clinical dietitian to assist clients in modifying their diet to meet their caloric needs. Clients with COPD often have difficulty eating because of dyspnea. Offer the client frequent small meals rather than large meals. When the client must be tube-fed, understand that substrate metabolism also may affect lung function. Macronutrients are metabolized to produce carbon dioxide and water. The ratio of carbon dioxide produced to oxygen consumed is the respiratory quotient (RQ). The RQ of carbohydrate oxidation is 1, and the RQ of fat oxidation is 0.7. Excess carbohydrate leads to increased production of carbon dioxide and can lead to respiratory distress. Enteral formulas are designed for pulmonary disease and provide more calories from fat. It is equally important not to overfeed the client with carbohydrates (see the Case Study feature on COPD with Nutritional Concerns on p. 1823).

Adjust oxygen delivery devices so that the mouth is not obstructed but oxygen is delivered through the nose during eating. Calculate the liter flow of the nasal cannula when converting from a mask style (see the formulas in Table 63-4). For example, if a client is using a Venturi oxygen mask at 28%, he or she would receive the same amount of oxygen on 2 L by nasal cannula.

■ Nursing Management of the Medical Client Assessment

The nursing history can ascertain whether the client's clinical manifestations are primarily those of chronic bronchitis, emphysema, or asthma. Determine the client's ability to recognize manifestations that require further care. For example, if a client says, "I knew I was developing an infection and went to the doctor," this statement indicates an understanding of the disorder. In contrast, if a client does not fully understand the reasons for hospitalization, educate the client about COPD. A review of past medical history helps to determine whether the client has other disorders, such as heart disease, that might affect treatment.

Complete a physical examination with an emphasis on the respiratory and cardiac system. Note the degree of dyspnea, the presence of orthopnea, decreased breath sounds, and clinical manifestations of heart failure. Evaluate mental status because confusion and restlessness may be early indicators of increasing hypoxia and hypercapnia. Record the client's baseline oximetry and the level of inspired oxygen. Ask if the client smokes and, if so, if he or she has interest in smoking cessation. Infection is a common cause of exacerbation of COPD. Note the presence of a productive cough, pain with coughing, fever, and the color and consistency of sputum.

Consider the impact of stressors that may have led to exacerbations of COPD. Possible factors include the progressive illness itself, marital or other family problems, and financial concerns. Review the client's usual coping strategies. Determine whether these strategies are working now; if not, why not? Support systems, such as friends and family, also are important components of

psychosocial stability. Determine the reliability of the client's support system.

The psychosocial impact of COPD is significant. Clients commonly have feelings of loss of control over their bodies and their social environment. These responses leave the client socially isolated and depressed and can severely affect quality of life. Psychosocial intervention is important.

A thorough history may need to be delayed until the client is able to breathe comfortably, or it may be taken over short periods of time or obtained through the family. Likewise, the physical examination should not tire the client. Protein-calorie malnutrition may be evident. Consult the dietitian for methods to improve client's intake.

Diagnosis, Outcomes, Intervention

Common nursing diagnoses and interventions for the client with COPD are listed in the Care Plan for the client with COPD. Because COPD is common, many institutions use clinical paths or care maps to guide care. (See the Care Plan feature on The Client with Chronic Obstructive Pulmonary Disease on pp. 1824 to 1828 and the Clinical Pathway feature on Chronic Obstructive Pulmonary Disease on the website).

Evaluation

Dyspnea will be slow to improve. Expect several days for the client to return to baseline levels.

TABLE 63-4	*Converting Low-Flow to High-Flow Oxygen Systems**	
100% Oxygen Flow Rate (L)		**Fio₂ (%)**
Nasal Cannula or Catheter		
1		24
2		28
3		32
4		36
5		40
6		44
Oxygen Mask		
5-6		40
6-7		50
7-8		60
Mask with a Reservoir Bag		
6		60
7		70
8		80
9		90
10		100

Fio_2, Fraction of inspired oxygen.
*A normal ventilatory pattern is assumed.

CASE STUDY   *evolve*

COPD with Nutritional Concerns

Bill Smith is a 55-year-old disabled car salesman who is cared for at home by his wife of 36 years. Bill is being seen in the office today for a routine visit. He reports that he has been coughing up more sputum than normal and that sometimes he feels as if he is choking. Bill's wife also reports that she is afraid he is not getting enough to eat, because she has noticed he has put three more holes in his leather belt to hold up his pants . . . . *Case Study continued on the website and the CD-ROM with discussions, multiple-choice questions, and a nursing care plan.* *evolve*

CARE PLAN

The Client with Chronic Obstructive Pulmonary Disease

Nursing Diagnosis. Impaired Gas Exchange related to decreased ventilation and mucus plugs.

Outcomes. The client will maintain adequate gas exchange as evidenced by arterial blood gas (ABG) values (i.e., PaO_2 of at least 60 mm Hg, pH within normal limits, and $PaCO_2$ at baseline) or oxygen saturation over 90%, mental status at baseline, minimal anxiety.

Interventions	Rationales
1. Regularly monitor the client's respiratory rate and pattern, pulse oximetry, ABG results, and manifestations of hypoxia or hypercapnia. Report significant changes or a lack of response promptly.	1. Prompt recognition of deteriorating respiratory function can reduce potentially lethal outcomes.
2. Administer low-flow oxygen therapy (1 to 3 L/min on 24% to 31% FiO_2) as needed via nasal prongs or a high-flow Venturi mask.	2. Oxygen corrects existing hypoxemia. Excessive increases in oxygen (55% to 70% FiO_2) may diminish respiratory drive and increase carbon dioxide retention further.
3. Assist the client into the high-Fowler position.	3. The upright position allows full lung excursion and enhances air exchange.
4. Administer bronchodilators if ordered. Monitor for side effects.	4. Bronchodilators relax bronchial smooth muscle, facilitating air flow. Common side effects include tremor, tachycardia, and other cardiac dysrhythmias.
5. Use caution when administering opioids, sedatives, and tranquilizers.	5. These medications are respiratory depressants and can further impair ventilation.

Evaluation. Bronchospasm is fairly quickly reversible with inhaled bronchodilators and steroids, but until the underlying trigger is controlled, it may quickly recur.

Nursing Diagnosis. Ineffective Airway Clearance related to excessive secretions and ineffective coughing.

Outcomes. The client will have improved airway clearance as evidenced by effective coughing techniques and a patent airway.

Interventions	Rationales
1. Monitor lung sounds every 4-8 hours and before and after coughing episodes.	1. Rhonchi present in the large airways may impair airway patency.
2. Teach the client to maintain adequate hydration by drinking at least 8 to 10 glasses of fluid per day (if not contraindicated) and increasing the humidity of the ambient air.	2. Hydration helps to thin secretions.
3. Teach and supervise effective coughing techniques.	3. Proper coughing techniques conserve energy, reduce airway collapse, and lessen client frustration.
4. Teach and supervise incentive spirometer techniques 10 times per hour while awake.	4. Incentive spirometer is an objective measure of the depth of inhalation to promote lung expansion.
5. Perform chest physical therapy, if needed, and instruct the client and significant others in these techniques.	5. Chest physical therapy techniques use forces of gravity and motion to facilitate secretion removal.
6. Assess the condition of the oral mucous membranes and perform or offer oral care every 2 hours.	6. Thick secretions line the mouth when the client coughs; oral care removes them.

Evaluation. The client will often require 48 or more hours to clear severely congested lungs.

CARE PLAN

Nursing Diagnosis. Anxiety related to acute breathing difficulties and fear of suffocation.

Outcomes. The client will express an increase in psychological comfort and demonstrate the use of effective coping mechanisms.

Interventions	Rationales
1. Remain with the client during acute episodes of breathing difficulty, and provide care in a calm, reassuring manner.	1. Reassures the client that competent help is available if needed. Anxiety can be contagious; remain calm.
2. Provide a quiet, calm environment.	2. Reduction of external stimuli helps promote relaxation.
3. During acute episodes, open doors and curtains and limit the number of people and unnecessary equipment in the room. Provide a fan if the client perceives a benefit from the moving air.	3. Environmental changes may lessen the client's perceptions of suffocation.
4. Encourage the use of breathing retraining and relaxation techniques.	4. A feeling of self-control and success in facilitating breathing helps reduce anxiety.
5. Give sedatives and tranquilizers with extreme caution. Nonpharmaceutical methods of anxiety reduction are more useful.	5. Oversedation may cause respiratory depression.

Evaluation. Anxiety can usually be controlled quickly but may recur with each episode of dyspnea and requires both short-term and long-term interventions.

Nursing Diagnosis. Activity Intolerance related to inadequate oxygenation and dyspnea.

Outcomes. The client will have improved activity tolerance as evidenced by maintaining a realistic activity level (specify based on underlying condition and baseline activity) and demonstrating energy conservation techniques.

Interventions	Rationales
1. Monitor the severity of dyspnea and oxygen saturation with and following activity.	1. Activity increases the demand for oxygen, and the inability to meet the demand may result in dyspnea and desaturation.
2. Stop or slow any activity that leads to a significant change in respiratory rate, failure of pulse to return to near resting rate within 3 minutes of activity, changes in mental status.	2. Significant changes in respiratory, cardiac, or circulatory status signal activity intolerance.
3. Maintain supplemental oxygen therapy as needed during activity.	3. Supplemental oxygen helps alleviate exercise-induced hypoxemia, thus improving activity tolerance.
4. Schedule active exercise after respiratory therapy or medication (e.g., bronchodilator in metered-dose inhaler).	4. Lung function is maximized during peak periods of treatment and drug effect.
5. Assist the client in scheduling a gradual increase in daily activities and exercise.	5. Gradual increases in physical activity improve respiratory and cardiac conditioning, thus improving activity tolerance.
6. Advise the client to avoid conditions that increase oxygen demand, such as smoking, temperature extremes, excess weight, and stress.	6. These factors increase peripheral vascular resistance, which increases cardiac workload and oxygen requirements.
7. Instruct the client in energy conservation techniques, such as pacing activities throughout the day, interspersed with adequate rest periods, and alternating high-energy and low-energy tasks.	7. Conservation techniques allow the client to accomplish more tasks with a limited energy supply.
8. Teach the client to use pursed-lip and diaphragmatic breathing techniques during activities.	8. Breathing retraining ensures maximal use of available respiratory function. Pursed-lip breathing leaves positive end-expiratory pressure in the lungs and helps keep airways open.

Evaluation. Depending on the degree of underlying lung disease, activity intolerance may be slow to be correctable, and this goal should be long term for complete resolution.

Continued

CARE PLAN

The Client with Chronic Obstructive Pulmonary Disease—cont'd

Nursing Diagnosis. Imbalanced Nutrition: Less Than Body Requirements related to reduced appetite, decreased energy level, and dyspnea.

Outcomes. The client will eat 75% of served foods during the acute phase and maintain body weight within normal limits for gender and body build, and hemoglobin, prealbumin and albumin levels will be within normal ranges.

Interventions	Rationales
1. Assist the client with mouth care before meals and as needed.	1. Coughing and sputum production may impair appetite. Mouth-breathing dries mucous membranes.
2. Advise the client to eat small, frequent meals (e.g., six meals a day) that are high in protein and calories.	2. Large meals may create an excessive feeling of fullness that may make breathing uncomfortable and difficult. High protein and calorie levels are needed to maintain nutritional status in light of the increased work of breathing.
3. Advise the client to avoid gas-producing foods, such as beans and cabbage.	3. Gas-forming foods may cause abdominal bloating and distention and thus impair ventilation.
4. Instruct the client in the use of high-calorie liquid supplements if indicated.	4. Liquid supplements provide high-calorie concentrations in a relatively small volume.
5. Advise hypoxemic clients to use oxygen via nasal cannula during meals.	5. Adequate oxygenation increases the energy available for eating.
6. Suggest methods to make meal preparation more convenient (e.g., Meals on Wheels program).	6. Reducing the energy expenditure of preparation maximizes the energy available for eating.
7. Consult with the dietitian to assist with food choices that reduce the production of carbon dioxide.	7. Clients with carbon dioxide benefit from foods that do not produce excess CO_2.
8. Monitor the client's food intake, weight, and serum hemoglobin, prealbumin and albumin levels.	8. Changes in body weight reflect the degree of nutrition or malnutrition. Hemoglobin, prealbumin, and albumin levels reflect protein intake.

Evaluation. Improving nutrition, lab values, and body weight are long-term goals. During an acute exacerbation of dyspnea, short-term goals such as the amount of dietary intake may be accomplishable.

Nursing Diagnosis. Disturbed Sleep Pattern related to dyspnea and external stimuli.

Outcomes. The client will report feeling adequately rested.

Interventions	Rationales
1. Promote relaxation by providing a darkened, quiet environment; ensuring adequate room ventilation; and following bedtime routines.	1. The hospital environment can interfere with relaxation and sleep. Using established bedtime rituals increases relaxation.
2. Schedule care activities to allow periods of uninterrupted sleep.	2. For most people, completing four to five complete sleep cycles (60 to 90 minutes) per night promotes a feeling of being rested.
3. Avoid the use of "sleeping pills."	3. Many forms of hypnotics, sedatives, and barbiturates impair sleep cycles.
4. Instruct the client in measures to promote sleep:	
a. Plan physical exercise during the day and passive, nonstimulating activities in the evening.	a. Activity increases the need for sleep and contributes to a feeling of tiredness.
b. Avoid stimulants, such as caffeine.	b. Stimulants increase metabolism and inhibit relaxation.
c. Maintain a consistent bedtime and a regular bedtime routine.	c. Consistency promotes relaxation and prevents disruptions of the biologic clock.
d. Eat a high-protein snack before bedtime.	d. Protein digestion produces tryptophan, an amino acid that has a sedative effect.
e. Use relaxation techniques (e.g., meditation, massage, warm bath, warm beverage).	e. Sleep is difficult unless the client is relaxed.

CARE PLAN

f. If the client awakens during the night, suggest a quiet, diverting activity, such as reading, in another room.

g. If dyspnea is severe, a recliner chair or hospital bed may be more comfortable than a regular bed.

f. Frustration over being awake deters sleep efforts further. The bedroom should be associated mentally with sleep to enhance future sleep promotion.

g. The upright position facilitates ventilation.

Evaluation. During acute respiratory problems, sleep may be difficult because of interruptions and dyspnea. Short-term outcomes such as napping may be accomplishable. Long-term plans for sleep may have to be deferred until dyspnea is controlled.

Nursing Diagnosis. Interrupted Family Processes related to chronic illness of a family member.

Outcomes. The family will verbalize their feelings, participate in the care of the ill family member, and seek external resources as needed.

Interventions	Rationales
1. Plan interventions considering the client and significant other as the unit of care. Encourage participation in the planning process.	1. COPD affects not only the client experiencing the condition but also the client's significant others.
2. Assess family communication patterns, and intervene if they are ineffective. Family counseling may be needed.	2. Effective communication helps each member to understand his or her own and others' feelings. Counseling may facilitate healthy interaction.
3. Encourage as wide a social support network as feasible.	3. The use of a wide support group prevents a few family members from being overloaded with responsibility.
4. Encourage the client and family to seek support from other sources (e.g., self-help groups and support groups, such as the Better Breathers clubs sponsored by the American Lung Association).	4. Clients may benefit from opportunities to share common experiences and to learn from others in similar situations.
5. Provide the family with anticipatory guidance as the client's COPD progresses.	5. Knowing what to expect facilitates family adjustment.

Evaluation. Coping with a family member's illness may require weeks or months to accomplish as the family learns to recognize and treat various exacerbations and live through various family events and activities with the disease (e.g., travel).

Nursing Diagnosis. Sexual Dysfunction related to dyspnea, reduced energy, and changes in relationships.

Outcomes. The client will report increased satisfaction with sexual function.

Interventions	Rationales
1. Provide an opportunity for the client to discuss concerns.	1. Many people are embarrassed or reluctant to talk about their sexual concerns.
2. Suggest measures that may facilitate sexual activity (e.g., alternative positions, use of bronchodilator therapy before beginning sexual activity, choosing a time of day when dyspnea is minimal).	2. Such measures can reduce physical exertion and maximize available oxygen levels.
3. Encourage the client and partner to consider alternative forms of sexual expression (e.g., hugging, cuddling, stroking, kissing).	3. Alternative methods require less energy expenditure compared with intercourse.
4. Recommend a professional sex therapist if appropriate.	4. Talking with a skilled professional may assist the client with constructive problem-solving.

Evaluation. During a acute flare-up of dyspnea, the discussion of sexual activity should be introduced when appropriate. Resolution of the problems and issues is a long-term goal.

Continued

CARE PLAN

The Client with Chronic Obstructive Pulmonary Disease—cont'd

Nursing Diagnosis. Risk for Infection related to ineffective pulmonary clearance.

Outcomes. Client will have a decreased risk of infection as evidenced by health promotion behaviors and awareness of manifestations of pulmonary infection.

Interventions	Rationales
1. Teach the client to wash his or her hands after contact with potentially infectious material.	1. Hand-washing is the primary defense against the spread of infection.
2. Encourage the client to obtain a flu vaccination yearly and a pneumococcal vaccination.	2. Vaccination provides immunity for infections.
3. Teach the client and family how to care for and clean respiratory equipment used at home.	3. Water in respiratory equipment is a common source of bacterial growth.
4. Teach the client and family the manifestations of pulmonary infections (change in color or volume of sputum, fever, chills, malaise, productive cough, confusion, increased dyspnea), self-care, and when to call the physician.	4. Early recognition of manifestations can lead to a rapid diagnosis. Self-care with preplanned interventions (e.g., antibiotics) should be understood. Notification of the physician can provide for early treatment.

Evaluation. Risk reduction cannot be measured in a short period of time. Verbal statements of comprehension and plans to follow the instructions should be noted. Sometimes a reduction in the number of acute pulmonary infections or hospitalizations can be measured.

Nursing Diagnosis. Decisional Conflict related to smoking cessation.

Outcomes. The client and family will seriously consider the value of smoking cessation and develop a plan to stop smoking.

Interventions	Rationales
1. Ask the client if he or she was smoking before . hospitalization	1. Validates the frequency of smoking.
2. Advise the client and family on the benefit of smoking cessation.	2. Many clients believe there is no benefit to stopping smoking now. Even though it is difficult to stop, most clients experience less dyspnea within a few weeks.
3. Assess if the client is ready to stop smoking now (or at dismissal).	3. It is important for the client to determine if he or she is willing to try. Family may be helpful by discarding all remaining cigarettes.
4. Assist with plans for counseling and pharmacotherapy.	4. Both cognitive and behavioral strategies are needed and can be provided by therapists.
5. Arrange follow-up care.	5. Many clients benefit from nicotine patches or antidepressant medications to assist with smoking cessation.

Evaluation. Smoking cessation is a difficult problem. A short-term goal would be for the client to value the need to stop. The long-term goal would be the cessation of tobacco use.

Clients with COPD often continue to deteriorate despite medical care. It is difficult to cope with failing health that limits activity and employment. As much as possible, encourage the client to live an active life with daily exercise. The support of significant others is essential.

■ Surgical Management

Surgery is relatively uncommon in the treatment of COPD. At times, bullectomy (removal of large bullae, which compress the lung and add to dead space) may benefit clients with recurrent spontaneous pneumothorax. Lung transplantation may be used to provide relief of disabling manifestations for clients with end-stage COPD, although it does not increase life expectancy.[12]

Lung volume–reduction surgery (LVRS) may provide palliative relief for selected COPD clients. In this procedure, portions of diffusely emphysematous lungs are removed to help restore more normal chest-wall configuration and to improve respiratory mechanics and functional capacity (see Figure 63-9). LVRS may improve quality of life in selected clients.[8] Whether it reduces mortality is uncertain, however, and in some clients it has been shown that this procedure actually increases mortality rate.[21] More data are needed regarding the procedure and its long-term effects, and multicenter studies are under way to evaluate its safety and effectiveness.

■ Nursing Management of the Surgical Client

After surgery, monitor closely the client's ABG values. Chest assessment and radiographs help to determine whether the lungs are expanding. Assess the chest tubes for air leaks and drainage. Intensive pulmonary toilet is essential.[28] Repeated coughing and deep breathing help to prevent pulmonary complications. Many clients have chest physiotherapy every 4 hours and nebulized aerosol treatments. Manage pain aggressively to promote activity and pulmonary hygiene.

After discharge, the client is assessed for adequate ventilation and tissue oxygenation (with pulse oximetry) and progressive wound healing. Pulmonary treatments may continue until lung sounds are clear. The client is weaned from oxygen and placed into a formal pulmonary rehabilitation program.

■ Modifications for Older Clients

The prevalence of COPD rises significantly in people in the middle to late adult years and is a leading cause of hospitalizations in older persons. The older client frequently has other problems that influence the treatment of COPD. For example, the client may have decreased exercise tolerance, impaired nutrition, or a long-standing habit of smoking that retards rehabilitation. Also consider the possibility of drug-drug interactions in older clients. Remember, too, that the older adult has special requirements when chronic conditions are exacerbated (see the Case Management feature on the Older Adult on the website).

■ Self-Care

Pulmonary rehabilitation is designed to reduce the toll of pulmonary disease for the client and the health care system. The goals of pulmonary rehabilitation are to relieve clinical manifestations, to maximize functional level, and to educate clients on how to manage their disease process successfully and maintain an active and independent lifestyle, and to improve quality of life.[19] Clients are taught how to administer medications, what side effects to look for and how to manage them, and the safe and correct use of oxygen. Lower-body exercise (walk-ing, cycling) is commonly prescribed. Upper-body exercise is also used in some cases.

To facilitate self-care and adherence, the client and significant others need thorough information about the disease process. Review the manifestations of impending respiratory problems (e.g., increased confusion or drowsiness), respiratory infection, and right-sided heart failure (e.g., peripheral edema, distended neck veins) so that prompt intervention can be obtained if these complications develop. The need for routine respiratory follow-up should also be discussed. In your teaching, include a discussion of the hazards of infection and ways to decrease personal risk (i.e., avoid crowds during the flu and colds season, clean respiratory equipment well, obtain pneumococcal vaccine every 6 years and flu vaccines yearly). Review the need for lifestyle modifications, especially smoking cessation.[33]

Clients with end-stage lung disease experience significant, intensely distressing manifestations. Whether care is provided in the home or in an extended-care facility, the focus is on minimizing these manifestations and making the client as comfortable as possible (see the Bridge to Home Health Care feature on Conserving Oxygen with Chronic Obstructive Pulmonary Disease on p. 1830).

TRACHEOBRONCHITIS

Acute tracheobronchitis is an inflammation of the mucous membranes of the trachea and the bronchial tree. This disorder commonly follows viral infections of the upper respiratory tract. It may also result from inhalation of noxious or irritating gases and particulate matter (including cigarette smoke), bacterial pneumonia, overvigorous tracheobronchial suctioning, and harsh paroxysms of coughing.

Manifestations include a raw, burning pain over the upper anterior chest wall over the midsternum. Pain is increased with exposure to cold environments, cigarette smoke, cough, and tracheobronchial suctioning. In addition, the client may have a cough that progresses from dry to productive as the irritation increases. Fever, headache, and malaise may be present. Observe for cough-related syncope. Lightheadedness or fainting may occur with forceful coughing spells. Fainting is caused by prolonged elevation of intrapulmonary pressure during the compressive phase of a cough. The increased pressure impairs venous return to the thorax, causing a decrease in cardiac output.

Outcome Management

Treatment is focused on the cause of the cough. Cough suppressants are rarely effective. Antibiotics, bronchodilators, corticosteroids (inhaled and systemic), and anticholinergics are the primary treatments. Sinusitis is a common accompanying finding as well as a cause of tracheobronchitis.

BRIDGE TO HOME HEALTH CARE

Conserving Oxygen with Chronic Obstructive Pulmonary Disease

Clients with chronic obstructive pulmonary disease (COPD) are challenged to make the most of their lives, given their available oxygen.

Usually, home health nurses are primarily responsible for monitoring manifestations; reviewing and reinforcing previously taught oxygen-conservation techniques; giving further instructions; and determining whether referrals to registered dietitians and occupational, physical, or respiratory therapists are needed. Evaluate what your clients already know, and proceed from there. Be certain that your clients understand the importance of using pursed-lip breathing, abdominal breathing, and metered-dose inhalers consistently and correctly. Have them demonstrate their technique.

Help your clients develop an oxygen-conservation plan that allows them to participate in activities that are most important to them. Ask them to keep a simple diary and to record their usual behavior during a 1- or 2-day period that includes all waking hours. When you analyze the diary, identify your clients' priorities. Help them relate specific activity to feelings of dyspnea during the day. In this way, you can teach specific oxygen-conservation techniques and pacing of activities to meet their priorities. To increase comfort, have your clients schedule the use of inhalers before activities and keep them within easy reach.

Encourage clients who are concerned about adequate oxygen for sexual activity to assume passive positions and to allow their partners to be more active. If winded, clients should use massage and other relaxation techniques as part of foreplay.

Adequate nutrition is essential to clients who have COPD; they may be malnourished because of respiratory muscle wasting. The diet may be high in protein and calories and low in carbohydrates. Answer your clients' questions, and determine whether they are willing or able to purchase, prepare, and eat the foods that were suggested. Encourage easy food preparation to prevent fatigue. Use foods that are prepackaged or can be heated in the microwave. Consider home-delivered meals. Use liquid food supplements to increase protein and calories; many brands are available, including some that are specially formulated for people who have pulmonary problems.

Encourage clients to rest just before eating and to follow these suggestions. Eat in a relaxed and quiet area. Small, frequent meals are best. Schedule meals early in the day if fatigue increases as the day continues. Snack frequently. Schedule inhalers after meals because inhaler medications can taint the taste of food and make it more difficult to achieve adequate nutrition.

Clients who have COPD often feel isolated because of their decreased ability to leave their homes. Suggest that they and their families join local support groups where they can share their experiences and feelings about the disease and learn new techniques to improve their quality of life. Many hospitals sponsor groups. Another valuable resource is the American Lung Association, which has local offices throughout the United States; call for information about prevention and the latest developments in treatment.

Priority nursing goals include relief of pain and elimination of the tracheal irritation. Strongly advise the client to stop smoking. Whenever possible, eliminate other irritating gases or substances from the environment. Promote airway clearance by encouraging effective coughing, increased fluid intake, changing positions, and increasing inspired humidity. Inspired humidity may be increased through the use of aerosols. Advise clients to avoid cold air and to cover the mouth and nose before going outdoors.

BRONCHIECTASIS

Bronchiectasis, an extreme form of bronchitis, causes permanent, abnormal dilation and distortion of bronchi and bronchioles. It develops when bronchial walls are weakened by chronic inflammatory changes in the bronchial mucosa and occurs most often after recurrent inflammatory conditions. Any condition producing a narrowing of the lumen of the bronchioles, however, may result in bronchiectasis, including tuberculosis, adenoviral infections, and pneumonia.

Some forms of bronchiectasis are congenital and are associated with cystic fibrosis, sinusitis, dextrocardia (heart located on right side), and alterations in ciliary activity (Kartagener's syndrome). Bronchiectasis is usually localized to a lung lobe or segment rather than generalized throughout the lungs. At times, however, persistent, nonresolving infection may cause the disorder to spread to other parts of the same lung. Diagnosis may be confirmed by chest radiograph, bronchogram, or computed tomography (CT) scan.

Manifestations vary according to the etiologic agent. The main manifestations are cough and purulent sputum production in large quantities. Fever, hemoptysis, nasal stuffiness, and drainage from sinusitis also are common. The client may complain of fatigue and weakness. Clubbing of the fingers may be present.

Outcome Management

Management of bronchiectasis is the same as for COPD. Most clients are managed medically to prevent progression of the disorder and to control clinical manifestations.

Antibiotics, chest physical therapy, hydration, bronchodilators, and oxygen commonly are prescribed. Severe cases may be treated by surgical resection if the pathologic process is well localized in one lobe or two adjacent lobes and when no contraindications to surgery exist.

DISORDERS OF THE PULMONARY VASCULATURE
PULMONARY EMBOLISM

Pulmonary embolism (PE) is an occlusion of a portion of the pulmonary blood vessels by an embolus. An embolus is a clot or other plug (thrombus) that is carried by the bloodstream from its point of origin to a smaller blood vessel, where it obstructs circulation. Depending on its size, an embolus can be lethal. It is estimated that in the United States more than 355,000 people are diagnosed annually for PE, resulting in as many as 240,000 deaths per year.[29]

Etiology and Risk Factors

Virtually all PEs develop from thrombi (clots), most of which originate in the deep calf, femoral, popliteal, or iliac veins. Other sources of emboli include tumors, air, fat, bone marrow, amniotic fluid, septic thrombi, and vegetations on heart valves that develop with endocarditis.

Major operations, especially hip, knee, abdominal, and extensive pelvic procedures, predispose the client to thrombus formation because of the reduced flow of blood through the pelvis. Traveling in cramped quarters or for a long time or sitting for long periods is also associated with stasis and clotting of blood. Preventive measures, such as early ambulation, frequent leg exercises, sequential compression stockings, and anticoagulant prophylaxis, are essential.

Pathophysiology

When emboli travel to the lungs, they lodge in the pulmonary vasculature. The size and number of emboli determine the location. Blood flow is obstructed, leading to decreased perfusion of the section of lung supplied by the vessel. The client continues to ventilate the lung portion, but because the tissue is not perfused, a $\dot{V}/\dot{Q}$ mismatch occurs, resulting in hypoxemia.

If an embolus lodges in a large pulmonary vessel, it increases proximal pulmonary vascular resistance, causes atelectasis, and eventually reduces cardiac output. If the embolus is in a smaller vessel, less dramatic clinical manifestations follow but perfusion is still altered.

The arterioles constrict because of platelet degranulation, accompanied by a release of histamine, serotonin, catecholamines, and prostaglandins. The chemical agents result in bronchial and pulmonary artery constriction. This vasoconstriction probably plays a major role in the hemodynamic instability that follows PE.

Pulmonary embolism can lead to right-sided heart failure. Once the clot lodges, affected blood vessels in the lung collapse. This collapse increases the pressure in the pulmonary vasculature. The increased pressure increases the workload of the right side of the heart, leading to failure. Massive PE of the pulmonary artery can also result in cardiopulmonary collapse from lack of perfusion and resulting hypoxia and acidosis.

Clinical Manifestations

The clinical manifestations of PE are nonspecific and, in some clients, may not appear until late in the event. The most common manifestations of PE are tachypnea, dyspnea, anxiety or fretfulness, and chest pain. Hypoxemia may be present depending on the size of the embolism. Because these clinical manifestations are similar to those seen with myocardial infarction and other cardiovascular illnesses, overdiagnosis is as likely as underdiagnosis. Extensive differential diagnosis often is required. The pain usually experienced with PE is pleuritic in nature, caused by an inflammatory reaction of the lung parenchyma or by pulmonary infarction or ischemia, caused by obstruction of small pulmonary arterial branches. Typical pleuritic chest pain is sudden in onset and exacerbated by breathing. The client is usually dyspneic, especially if the embolus has occluded major arteries or major portions of lung tissue. Apprehension, cough, diaphoresis, syncope, and hemoptysis may occur. The presence of hemoptysis indicates that the infarction or areas of atelectasis have produced alveolar damage.

Respirations typically increase. Crackles, an accentuated second heart sound, tachycardia, and fever may also develop. Less common findings include heart gallops, edema, heart murmur, and cyanosis.

Diagnostic Findings

When PE is suspected, the optimal strategy for diagnosis is an integrated approach that includes a thorough history and physical examination, supplemented by selective diagnostic tests. Pulse oximetry will be low and may be unresponsive to inhaled oxygen. ABG analysis indicates arterial hypoxemia (low PaO_2) and hypocapnia (low $PaCO_2$) in massive PE. Severe respiratory alkalosis may occur. Lactate dehydrogenase (LDH) isoenzymes show an increase in LDH_3 if there is lung tissue injury. A chest radiograph may help to rule out other pulmonary diagnoses.

A noninvasive diagnostic test for PE is the $\dot{V}/\dot{Q}$ lung scan. A radioisotope lung scan is performed by IV injection of particles of human serum albumin that have been labeled with iodine 131 or technetium 99m. These particles are trapped in the pulmonary microvasculature and are distributed according to pulmonary flow. Both lungs are scanned with a scintillation counter, and the amount of radioactivity counted gives an indication of obstruction to flow. A lung scan can be seen in Chapter 61.

An alternative to lung scanning that is being used more frequently is spiral CT scan of the chest. This approach is particularly effective for identifying PE in the proximal pulmonary vascular tree and for clients who are unstable or have limited cardiopulmonary reserve.

Pulmonary angiography remains the definitive means of diagnosis of PE (Figure 63-10). A radiopaque contrast agent is injected into the right atrium and pulmonary artery via a catheter threaded through a peripheral vein. Visualization of any filling defects of the heart and right pulmonary artery is achieved by taking sequential radiographs. Because of the invasive nature of the test, pulmonary angiography typically is reserved for cases in which the index of clinical suspicion is high despite non-diagnostic findings on other tests.

Outcome Management
■ Medical Management

Successful management of PE depends on having a high index of suspicion for manifestations such as dyspnea and anxiety in high-risk clients. Prompt recognition of the condition and immediate treatment are essential. Goals are to stabilize the cardiopulmonary system and reduce the threat of a further PE with anticoagulation therapy or trapping with an umbrella in the vena cava. For some clients, the clot can be lysed.

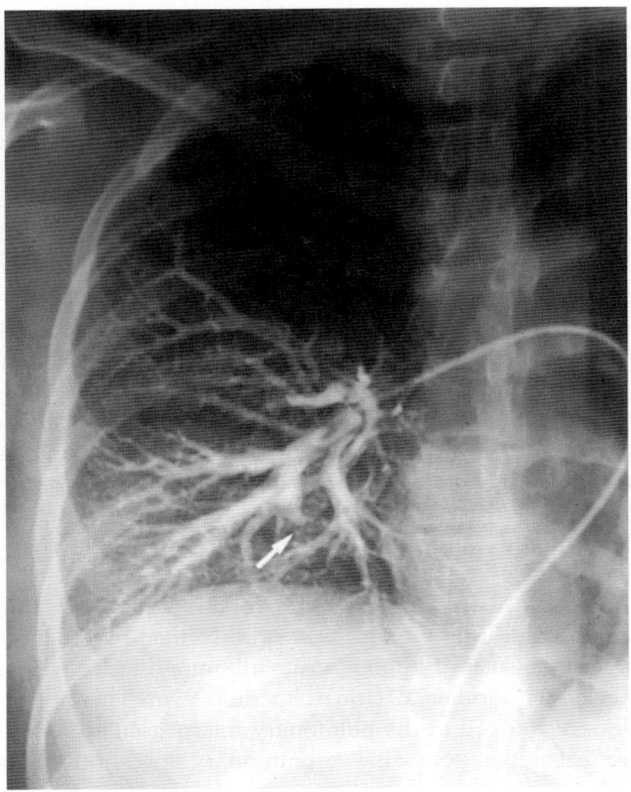

FIGURE 63-10 Angiogram showing a pulmonary embolus (*arrow*).

Stabilizing the Cardiopulmonary System. Maintenance of cardiopulmonary stability is the first priority. Cardiopulmonary support varies with the client's manifestations. Sometimes hypoxemia can be reversed with low-flow oxygen by nasal cannula. Other clients may require endotracheal intubation to maintain PaO_2 greater than 60 mm Hg. Hypotension is treated with fluids. If fluids do not raise the preload (right ventricular end-diastolic pressure) enough to raise blood pressure, inotropic agents may be required. Acidosis, which has a powerful vasoconstricting effect, is corrected with bicarbonate.

Anticoagulant Therapy. Typically, anticoagulation begins with IV standard (unfractionated) heparin sodium to reduce the risk of further clots and to prevent extension of existing clots. *Anticoagulants do not break up existing clots,* but they do prevent extensions of existing clots. Clinical trials have shown that subcutaneously administered low-molecular-weight heparin is as safe and effective as standard heparin in the treatment of hemodynamically stable clients with PE. Anticoagulants are administered until a therapeutic partial thromboplastin time (PTT) is achieved. In general, the initial target International Normalized Ratio should be 2.5 to 3.0. Administration of sodium warfarin is begun about 3 to 5 days before heparin is stopped to provide a transition to oral anticoagulation. Because the half-life of warfarin is long, about 2 to 3 days is required to achieve adequate anticoagulation. Clients are maintained on warfarin for 3 to 6 months.

Fibrinolytic Therapy. The effectiveness of fibrinolytic therapy in the management of a massive PE is not clear, but it may be useful in clients who are hemodynamically unstable. Thrombolytic agents lyse the clots and restore right-sided heart function; however, some clinicians have found that although the clot dissolves, the mortality rate is not improved.

■ Nursing Management of the Medical Client

Monitor the client closely for hypoxemia and respiratory compromise, and assess vital signs and lung sounds frequently. Monitor ABG or oximetry values, and monitor the client for manifestations of right-sided heart failure. Auscultate heart sounds frequently, assessing for murmurs or extra heart sounds. Check for peripheral edema, distended neck veins, and liver engorgement.

To facilitate breathing, elevate the head of the bed and apply oxygen per physician's orders. Because the usual cause of a PE is thrombus from the lower legs, elevate the legs with caution to avoid severe flexure of the hips. Such flexure would slow blood flow and increase the risk of new thrombi.

The client typically experiences fear with the sudden onset of severe chest pain and inability to breathe. Anxiety, restlessness, and apprehension are common. Emotional support can reduce anxiety and lessen dyspnea. Stay with the client and give calm, yet efficient, nursing care.

Analgesics are given as needed to reduce pain and anxiety. Morphine is the most common agent. Anxiety and pain increase oxygen demand and dyspnea. Administer oral care with soft brushes or rinses while oxygen is in use, especially if the client breathes through the mouth.

Once anticoagulation is achieved, watch for manifestations of excess anticoagulation, such as blood in the urine, in the stool, or along the gums or teeth; subcutaneous bruising; or flank pain. When invasive studies, such as ABGs, are necessary, apply pressure to the puncture site for at least 10 minutes. The client is discharged with oral anticoagulation therapy. Instruct the client about side effects, the importance of follow-up to monitor prothrombin times, and precautions to prevent bleeding. Review methods to reduce thrombophlebitis if that was the likely cause of the embolus (see Chapter 55).

■ Surgical Management

Surgical interventions that may be used in treatment of PE include (1) vena cava interruption with the insertion of a filter (Figure 63-11) and (2) pulmonary embolectomy. The Greenfield filter, a basket-like cone of wires bent to look like an umbrella, is the most commonly used filter. The filter is inserted by threading it up the veins in the leg or neck until it reaches the vena cava at the level of the renal arteries. The filter allows blood flow while trapping emboli; however, vena cava filters

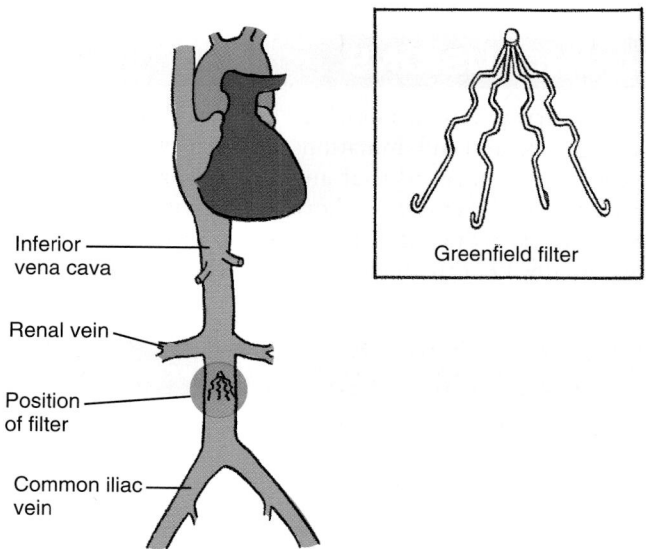

Inferior vena cava

Renal vein

Position of filter

Common iliac vein

Greenfield filter

FIGURE 63-11 Inferior vena cava filters are inserted into the vena cava through the iliac vein, such as the Greenfield filter, prevent emboli from traveling to the lung.

are less effective than anticoagulation and may lead to deep vein thrombosis, and so these generally are used only when anticoagulants are contraindicated or ineffective.[20]

Embolectomy is used in clients with significant hemodynamic instability caused by the embolus, especially those with unstable circulation and contraindications to thrombolytic therapy. An embolectomy involves surgical removal of emboli from the pulmonary arteries by either a thoracotomy or an embolectomy catheter. Newly developed catheters use high-velocity jets of saline to draw the thrombus toward the catheter tip and pulverize it.

VENOUS AIR EMBOLISM

Venous air embolism (VAE) is the entry of air into the venous system. VAE may occur in any condition in which an open vein above the right atrium level is exposed to the atmosphere (e.g., trauma to a vein, insertion or removal of central venous catheters or pulmonary artery catheters, surgical procedures on the head and neck [e.g., craniotomy]), pelvic operations in Trendelenburg position, and during gas insufflation in laparoscopy.

Entry of air into the venous system produces manifestations in the right ventricle, pulmonary circulation, or systemic circulation (if right-to-left shunts are present). Small amounts of air do not produce manifestations because air is removed from the circulation. Large boluses of air (3 to 8 ml/kg) can cause right ventricular outflow obstruction and result in cardiogenic shock and circulatory arrest.

Manifestations develop immediately following embolization and are similar to pulmonary thromboembolism. The severity of manifestations is related to the degree of air entry. Manifestations include dyspnea, chest pain, mill wheel murmur upon auscultation of the heart, tachycardia, hypotension, decreased consciousness, circulatory shock, or sudden death (with severe VAE).

If VAE is suspected, any central line procedure in progress is immediately terminated and the line is clamped. Promptly place the client in Trendelenburg position and rotate toward the left lateral decubitus position. This maneuver helps trap air in the apex of the ventricle, prevents its ejection into the pulmonary arterial system, and maintains right ventricular output. The client is given 100% oxygen, and mechanical ventilation may be needed for significant respiratory distress or refractory hypoxemia. If a central venous catheter is present, aspirate from the distal port and attempt to remove air.

PULMONARY HYPERTENSION

Pulmonary hypertension is defined as a prolonged elevation of the mean pulmonary artery pressure (PAP) above 25 mm Hg at rest (normal, 10 to 20 mm Hg) or above 30 mm Hg during exercise (normal, 20 to 30 mm Hg).

Severe forms of pulmonary hypertension are classified as either *secondary* or *idiopathic (primary)*. Secondary pulmonary hypertension is usually associated with underlying heart or lung disease (e.g., PE, veno-occlusive disease, COPD). The cause of the idiopathic form is, by definition, unclear. It occurs most often in young adults between the ages of 30 and 40 years. Women are affected more often than men.[1] The condition is progressive, leading to right-sided heart failure and severe dyspnea.

Etiology

The pulmonary circulation is generally a low-pressure, low-resistance system. Increased cardiac output in a healthy person, as with exercise, causes minimal elevations in PAP because of the large pulmonary vascular reserve. When pulmonary vasoconstriction is present, however, pressure elevation occurs because the pulmonary vasculature cannot accommodate increased blood flow.

Mild forms of pulmonary hypertension are normally caused by pulmonary vasoconstriction resulting from chronic hypoxia, acidosis, or both. Administration of oxygen, correction of acid-base imbalance, and use of vasodilating medications in selected cases generally return PAP to normal, either completely or partially.

Clinical Manifestations

Clients with mild pulmonary hypertension may be relatively asymptomatic. In moderate to severe forms, the main (and occasionally only) manifestation is dyspnea. Fatigue, syncope, angina-like chest pain, palpitations, and muscular weakness also may occur.

A chest x-ray study shows right ventricular hypertrophy, enlarged pulmonary arteries, prominent hilar vessels, and normal or reduced intrapulmonary vascular markings. Cardiac catheterization provides the most valuable diagnostic measurements.[26] Typical findings include elevated PAP and increased arteriovenous oxygen differences accompanied by normal systemic blood pressure and normal to low cardiac output. Pulmonary wedge pressures (PWPs) remain normal because left ventricular function is typically unchanged.

Outcome Management

The overall prognosis in severe pulmonary hypertension is poor, although treatment options are improving. This disorder has no known cure, but treatment of the underlying cause of secondary pulmonary hypertension may slow its progression. Supportive intervention with supplemental oxygen helps to reduce hypoxemia,

whereas anticoagulants may be used to prevent thromboembolic events.

Vasodilator therapy is the cornerstone of pharmacologic management. First-line vasodilators used for treatment are the calcium channel antagonists nifedipine and diltiazem. For clients who do not respond to these drugs, prostacyclin (epoprostenol) therapy has been used and has been found to improve hemodynamic status and physical manifestations. Prostacyclin is a potent pulmonary vasodilator that also reduces right ventricular dilatation, prevents tricuspid regurgitation from worsening, and has antithrombotic properties related to its effects on platelets. Long-term studies (longer than 12 weeks) show promise for clients on prostacyclin therapy in terms of prolonged survival and improved quality of life.[1] Treatment with prostacyclin is expensive and difficult to manage because it requires long-term, continuous central infusion; however, an oral form of the drug, bosentan, has recently been introduced. Additionally, nitrous oxide is being tested in pulmonary hypertension clients because of its ability to decrease PAP and PVR by increasing pulmonary blood flow. It, too, has shown some promise in improving manifestations.[25] These exciting new avenues of treatment require further research.

Some clients with severe pulmonary hypertension may undergo heart-lung, single, or bilateral-lung transplantation, although data regarding long-term effectiveness are not yet available. In addition, atrial septostomy is an investigational surgical procedure being tested in patents in the early stages of pulmonary hypertension. This procedure involves the creation of intra-atrial right to left shunt to decompress the right atrium and right ventricle and augment left ventricle filling and cardiac output. This helps to increase tissue oxygenation delivery.

CONCLUSIONS

Lower-airway disorders include asthma, chronic air flow limitations, and inflammations of the airways. Nursing care centers on reversal of any airway spasms and education of the client about how to live with the disorder and how to reduce the risk of future problems. PE is a potentially life-threatening disorder that usually can be managed effectively with prompt recognition.

THINKING CRITICALLY *evolve*

1. A 52-year-old woman is being treated at the neighborhood health clinic for chronic bronchitis. Her husband of 30 years smoked two to three packs of ciga-

evolve *Did you remember to check out the bonus material on the Evolve website and the CD-ROM, including free self-assessment exercises?*

http://evolve.elsevier.com/Black/medsurg/

rettes a day. The client never smoked. During this exacerbation, she presents with shortness of breath; wheezing; a deep, throaty, productive cough when she tries to talk; and fatigue. Her blood pressure is 180/90 mm Hg, pulse is 90 beats/min, respirations are 28 breaths/min and labored, and temperature is 99.4° F. She tells you that she tried to shovel the driveway on this cold winter day and did not wear a scarf over her mouth as she usually does. She further states that her inhalers did not seem to help her. She is taking a diuretic for hypertension, with blood pressure controlled at about 160/86 mm Hg. What is your priority nursing action? What teaching is appropriate at this time?

Factors to Consider. What are the clinical manifestations of chronic obstructive emphysema? What nursing assessments are in order?

2. An older client is recovering from pelvic surgery. Because of a previous stroke, she is hemiplegic. She has been on bed rest since the surgery. While the nursing assistant is giving her a bath, she notices the client grimacing as if in pain. The client responds to her question by pointing to her chest and nodding when asked if the pain is severe. The nursing assistant notifies you that the client is in distress. What is the priority assessment?

Factors to Consider. What complications of surgery and resulting bed rest might pose a risk for this client? How would you compare and contrast the clinical manifestations for pneumonia and pulmonary embolus?

3. You enter the room of the client from Question 2 and discover that she is apprehensive. She is trying to hold her breath because it hurts to breathe. She is sweating, and there is frothy sputum on her lips. What nursing interventions are appropriate? What treatment might be ordered?

Factors to Consider. What are the clinical manifestations of pulmonary embolus? What diagnostic studies may be ordered?

Discussions for these questions can be found on the website and the CD-ROM.

BIBLIOGRAPHY

1. Adiutori, D.M. (2000). Primary pulmonary hypertension: A review for advanced practice nurses. *MedSurg Nursing, 9*(5), 255-264.
2. American Lung Association (2002). *Trends in asthma morbidity and mortality.* Available: http://www.lungusa.org/data/asthma/ASTHMAdt.pdf.
3. Baker, C.F., & Scholz, J.A. (2002). Coping with symptoms of dyspnea in chronic obstructive pulmonary disease. *Rehabilitation Nursing, 27*(2), 67-74.
4. Burns, S.M., & Lawson, C. (1999). Pharmacological and ventilatory management of acute asthma exacerbations. *Critical Care Nurse, 19*(4), 39-53.
5. Cheever, K.H., Kitzes, B., & Genthner, D. (1999). Epoprostenol therapy for primary pulmonary hypertension. *Critical Care Nurse, 19*(4), 20-27.
6. Clark, N.M., & Partridge, M.R. (2002). Strengthening asthma education to enhance disease control. *Chest, 121*(5), 1661-1669.
7. Faul, J.L., et al. (1999). Quality of life and lung volume reduction surgery. *American Journal of Critical Care, 8*(6), 359-396.
8. Geddes, D., et al. (2000). Effect of lung-volume reduction surgery in patients with severe emphysema. *New England Journal of Medicine, 343*(4), 239-245.
9. Gift, A.G., & Narsavage, G. (1998). Validity of the numeric rating scale as a measure of dyspnea. *American Journal of Critical Care, 7*(3), 200-204.
10. Graydon, J.E., et al. (1995). Predictors of functioning of patients with chronic obstructive pulmonary disease. *Heart & Lung, 24*(6), 369-375.
11. Hallstrand, T.S., & Fahy, J.V. (2002). Practical management of acute asthma in adults. *Respiratory Care, 47*(2), 171-182.
12. Heffner, J.E. (2002). Chronic obstructive pulmonary disease: On an exponential curve of progress. *Respiratory Care, 47*(5), 586-607.
13. Janson, S., & Lazarus, S.C. (2002). Where do leukotriene modifiers fit in asthma management? *The Nurse Practitioner, 27*(4), 19-29.
14. Kendrick, K.R., et al. (2000). Usefulness of the modified 0-10 Borg scale in assessing the degree of dyspnea in patients with COPD and asthma. *Journal of Emergency Nursing, 26*(3), 216-222.
15. MacIntyre, N.R. (2001). Chronic obstructive pulmonary disease management: The evidence base. *Respiratory Care, 46*(11), 1294-1303.
16. Mannino, D.M. (2001). Chronic obstructive pulmonary disease: Epidemiology and evaluation. *Hospital Physician, 37,* 22-31.
17. Mannino, D.M., et al. (2002). Surveillance for Asthma—United States, 1980-1999. *Morbidity & Mortality Weekly Report, 51*(SS-1), 1-26.
18. McCrory, D.C., et al. (2001). Management of acute exacerbations of COPD: A summary and appraisal of published evidence. *Chest, 119*(4), 1190-1209.
19. McDermott, A. (2002). Pulmonary rehabilitation for patients with COPD. *Professional Nurse, 17*(9), 553-556.
20. Mills, T.D., Chan, O., & Matson, M. (2001). The use of vena caval filters. *Hospital Medicine, 62*(6), 327-331.
21. National Emphysema Treatment Trial Research Group. (2001). Patients at high risk of death after lung-volume-reduction surgery. *New England Journal of Medicine, 345*(15), 1075-1083.
22. National Institutes of Health. (1997). *Guidelines for the diagnosis and management of asthma.* NIH Publication no. 97-4051. Washington, DC: Author.
23. National Institutes of Health (2002). *The National Asthma Education and Prevention Program Expert Panel report: Guidelines for the diagnosis and management of asthma—Update on selected topics.* NIH Publication no. 02-5075. Washington, DC: Author.
24. Parshall, M.B., et al. (2001). Reliability and validity of dyspnea sensory quality descriptors in heart failure patients treated in an emergency department. *Heart & Lung, 30*(1), 57-65.
25. Pesola, G.R., & Pesola, H.R. (2000). Spiral CT diagnosis of pulmonary embolus. *American Journal of Emergency Medicine, 18*(4), 441-443.
26. Phillip, M.C. (2000). Primary pulmonary hypertension. *MedSurg Nursing, 9*(1), 17-20.

27. Rennard, S.I., & Farmer, S.G. (2002). COPD in 2001: A major challenge for medicine, the pharmaceutical industry, and society. *Chest, 121*(5), 113S-115S.

28. Schedel, E.M., & Connolly, M.A. (1999). Lung volume reduction surgery: New hope for emphysema patients. *Dimensions of Critical Care Nursing, 18*(1), 28-34.

29. Streif, M.B. (2000). Vena caval filters: A comprehensive review. *Blood, 15*(12), 3669-3677.

30. Togger, D.A., & Brenner, P.S. (2001). Metered dose inhalers. *American Journal of Nursing, 101*(10), 26-32.

31. Woo, K. (2000). A pilot study to examine the relationships of dyspnea, physical activity, and fatigue in patients with chronic obstructive pulmonary disease. *Journal of Clinical Nursing, 9*(4), 526-533.

32. Wray, B.B. (2001). Asthma: Best treatment options. *Annals of Allergy, Asthma, & Immunology, 87*(1), 9-12.

33. Zampella, M.A. (2003). COPD: Managing flare-ups. *RN, 66,* 14-22.

Management of Clients with Parenchymal and Pleural Disorders

Nancy L. York

𝐞𝐯𝐨𝐥𝐯𝐞

Web Enhancements

Case Management
Pneumonia
Client Education Guide
Tuberculosis (English Version and Spanish Translation)
Clinical Pathway
Pneumonia
Ethical Issues in Nursing
How Should the Decision to End Continuous Mechanical
Ventilation Be Made?

http://evolve.elsevier.com/Black/medsurg/

How Should the Federal Government Regulate Testing for
Tuberculosis?
What Is the Nurse's Obligation When Neuromuscular Blocking
Agents Are Used?
Appendix C
Laboratory Values of Clinical Importance in Medical-Surgical
Nursing

The parenchyma of any organ, in this case the lung, is the tissue essential for the function of the organ. This chapter reviews disorders of the lung parenchyma, such as pneumonia, tuberculosis, cystic fibrosis, and cancer.

ATELECTASIS

Atelectasis is the collapse of lung tissue at any structural level (e.g., segmental, basilar, lobar, or microscopic). It develops when there is interference with the natural forces that promote lung expansion. Such interference may result from a reduction in lung distention forces, inhalation of irritating anesthetics, localized airway obstruction, insufficient pulmonary surfactant, or increased elastic recoil. Examples of each of these causes are given in Box 64-1. Atelectasis is particularly common after surgery, especially upper abdominal or thoracic procedures. Clients who are elderly, obese, or bedridden or who have a history of smoking are also susceptible to atelectasis.

Atelectasis may be diagnosed through physical examination, although generally, it is initially detected on chest radiograph. Some clients are asymptomatic. If significant hypoxemia (low level of oxygen in the blood) is present, however, dyspnea (difficult or labored breathing), tachypnea (rapid breathing), tachycardia (rapid heartbeat), and cyanosis (bluish discoloration of skin and mucous membranes) may occur. Chest auscultation may reveal bronchial or diminished breath sounds and crackles over the involved area. Temperature of less than 101° F (38.3° C) is common. However, older adults with atelectasis typically do not exhibit a fever.

If atelectasis is severe, physical assessment findings include the following:
- A tracheal shift toward the side of the atelectasis
- A decrease in tactile fremitus over the affected lung area
- A dull percussion note over the atelectatic region
- Decreased chest movement on the involved side

None of these manifestations is specific for atelectasis, and the entire clinical picture must always be considered.

𝐞𝐯𝐨𝐥𝐯𝐞 *Be sure to check out the bonus material on the Evolve website and the CD-ROM, including free self-assessment exercises.*

http://evolve.elsevier.com/Black/medsurg/

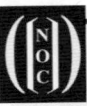

Nursing Outcomes Classification (NOC)
for Nursing Diagnoses—Clients with Parenchymal and Pleural Disorders

Activity Intolerance
Activity Tolerance
Endurance
Acute Pain and Chronic Pain
Comfort Level
Pain: Disruptive Effects
Anxiety
Anxiety Control
Coping
Deficient Knowledge
Knowledge: Disease Process
Knowledge: Health Behaviors
Knowledge: Medication
Knowledge: Treatment Regimen

Disturbed Sleep Pattern
Anxiety Control
Rest
Sleep
Imbalanced Nutrition: Less Than Body Requirements
Nutritional Status
Nutritional Status: Food and Fluid Intake
Impaired Gas Exchange
Respiratory Status: Gas Exchange
Respiratory Status: Ventilation
Impaired Oral Mucous Membrane
Tissue Integrity: Skin and Mucous Membrane

Impaired Physical Mobility
Joint Motion: Active
Ineffective Airway Clearance
Aspiration Control
Respiratory Status: Airway Patency
Ineffective Breathing Pattern
Respiratory Status: Airway Patency
Respiratory Status: Ventilation
Ineffective Coping
Coping
Information Processing
Role Performance
Social Support

BOX 64-1 *Causes of Atelectasis*

Reduction in Lung Distention Forces
Pleural space encroachment (e.g., pneumothorax, pleural effusion, pleural tumor)
Chest wall disorders (e.g., scoliosis, flail chest)
Impaired diaphragmatic movement (e.g., ascites, obesity)
Central nervous system dysfunction (e.g., coma, neuromuscular disorders, oversedation)

Localized Airway Obstruction
Mucus plugging
Foreign body aspiration
Bronchiectasis

Insufficient Pulmonary Surfactant
Respiratory distress syndrome
Inhalation anesthesia
High concentrations of oxygen (oxygen toxicity)
Lung contusion
Aspiration of gastric contents
Smoke inhalation

Increased Elastic Recoil
Interstitial fibrosis (e.g., silicosis, radiation pneumonitis)

One of the primary goals of nursing intervention is to prevent atelectasis in the high-risk client. Frequent position changes and early ambulation help promote drainage of all lung segments. Deep-breathing and effective coughing enhance lung expansion and prevent airway obstruction. Incentive spirometry is an excellent means of encouraging a client to deep-breathe.

If atelectasis develops, treatment is directed toward the underlying cause. If the client becomes hypoxic, oxygen should be administered as prescribed (e.g., per cannula, 1 to 4 L/min). More aggressive measures to maintain airway patency, such as postural drainage, chest physiotherapy, and tracheal suctioning, may also be ordered. If an airway obstruction is causing atelectasis, bronchoscopy may be used to remove the material.

INFECTIOUS DISORDERS
INFLUENZA

The term *flu* is often used inappropriately to describe many clinical manifestations and disorders. *Influenza* refers to an acute viral infection of the respiratory tract. Influenza usually occurs seasonally in epidemic form. People most at risk are very young children, older adults, people living in institutional settings, people with chronic diseases, and health care personnel. The first flu virus was identified in the 1930s. Since then, influenza viruses have been identified as types A, B, and C. Type A is the most prevalent and is associated with the most serious epidemics. Type B outbreaks also can reach epidemic levels, but the disease produced is generally milder than that caused by type A. Type C viruses have never been connected with a large epidemic.

Clinical manifestations of influenza include fever, myalgias (muscular pain), and cough. Influenza predisposes to complications such as viral bronchitis or pneumonia, bacterial pneumonia, and superinfections (infections that occur during the course of antimicrobial therapy). Influenza differs from a common cold primarily in its sudden onset and widespread occurrence within the population. Chest findings are usually negative unless pneumonia results. Conversely, colds have a slow onset of manifestations, usually do not cause fever, have malaise as a major manifestation, and commonly cause nasal manifestations.

Outcome Management

Intervention for influenza is based on manifestations as they arise (i.e., supportive measures to relieve fever, myalgia, and cough). In 1999, two new anti-influenza drugs (zanamivir and oseltamivir) were developed and appear to be extremely effective in preventing massive multiplication of the virus. They must be administered within 24 hours of onset. Rimantadine can be used to treat influenza type A in adults, but it has no effect on type B infections. When taken within 48 hours after the onset of illness, rimantadine reduces the duration of fever and other manifestations and allows clients to return to their daily routines more quickly. These drugs do not, however, replace the need for immunization. Encourage clients at risk for influenza to obtain an annual immunization before the start of the "flu season" each winter. Vaccination controls influenza for many high-risk clients. However, clients who are allergic to eggs or have a history of Guillain-Barré syndrome should not receive an influenza immunization.

Influenza is a communicable disease spread by droplet infection. Prevent the spread of this infection by encouraging clients with influenza to remain at home, practice frequent hand-washing, and cover the nose and mouth when sneezing or coughing.

See the Complementary and Alternative Therapy feature on Vitamin E Supplements and Acute Respiratory Tract Infections in Older Adults at right.

PNEUMONIA

Pneumonia (pneumonitis) is an inflammatory process in lung parenchyma usually associated with a marked increase in interstitial and alveolar fluid. Advances in antibiotic therapy have led to the widespread perception that pneumonia is no longer a major health problem in the United States. However, pneumonia and influenza are currently the sixth most common cause of death for all ages and one of the most common causes in older adults. Among all nosocomial infections, pneumonia is the second most common but has the highest mortality.[6,8]

Etiology and Risk Factors

There are many causes of pneumonia, including bacteria, viruses, mycoplasmas, fungal agents, and protozoa (Table 64-1). Pneumonia may also result from aspiration of food, fluids, or vomitus or from inhalation of toxic or caustic chemicals, smoke, dusts, or gases. Pneumonia may complicate immobility and chronic illnesses. It often follows influenza.

Major risk factors for pneumonia include (1) advanced age, (2) a history of smoking, (3) upper respira-

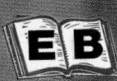

COMPLEMENTARY AND ALTERNATIVE THERAPY

Vitamin E Supplements and Acute Respiratory Tract Infections in Older Adults

Older adults have a potentially increased risk of infectious diseases and related conditions because of reduced immune function. Therefore a randomized controlled trial was conducted to examine the effect of two capsules daily of one of the following: a multivitamin and mineral complex, vitamin E (200 mg/day), a multivitamin-mineral complex plus vitamin E, or a placebo for a maximum of 15 months. The primary outcomes measured were incidence and severity of acute respiratory tract infections. After a median study duration of 441 days, 1024 episodes of acute respiratory tract infections were reported by 68% of the participants. When the treatment groups were compared with the placebo group, results were similar for all aspects of incidence and severity of acute respiratory tract infection, except more clients in the multivitamin-mineral treatment arm experienced a significant reduction in activity restriction (34.8% versus 48.5%; $p = .04$, number needed to treat = 8). Individuals taking either multivitamin-mineral or vitamin E supplementation did not have a reduced incidence rate of acute respiratory tract infections. Interestingly, multivitamin-mineral supplementation had no effect on the severity of infection, whereas vitamin E supplementation was associated with illnesses of significantly greater severity.

Reference

Gratt, J., Schouten, E., & Kok F. (2002). Effect of daily vitamin E and multivitamin-mineral supplementation on acute respiratory tract infections in elderly persons: A randomized controlled trial. *Journal of the American Medical Association, 288,* 715-721.

tory infection, (4) tracheal intubation, (5) prolonged immobility, (6) immunosuppressive therapy, (7) a nonfunctional immune system, (8) malnutrition, (9) dehydration, and (10) chronic disease states, such as diabetes, heart disease, chronic lung disease, renal disease, and cancer. Additional risk factors are exposure to air pollution; altered consciousness (from alcoholism, drug overdose, general anesthesia, or a seizure disorder); inhalation of noxious substances; aspiration of food, liquid, or foreign or gastric material; and residence in institutional settings, where transmission of the disease is more likely. (See the Terrorism Alert feature on Pneumonic Plague on p. 1841.)

Pathophysiology

The feature common to all types of pneumonia is an inflammatory pulmonary response to the offending organism or agent. The defense mechanisms of the lungs lose

TABLE 64-1	*Assessment and Treatment of Pneumonia*
Common Name	**Clinical Manifestations**
Pneumococcal pneumonia (caused by *Streptococcus pneumoniae*)	Sudden onset with a single shaking chill, high fever, stabbing-pleuritic chest pain, malaise, weakness, occasional vomiting, tachypnea, dyspnea, and elevated WBC count Single or multiple lobar consolidation on the chest x-ray film Cough productive of rusty brown or blood-streaked purulent sputum that turns yellow and mucoid
Staphylococcal pneumonia (caused by *Staphylococcus aureus*)	Sudden onset with fever, multiple chills, pleuritic pain, dyspnea, rales, decreased breath sounds, elevated WBC count, and exaggerated cough productive of purulent golden-yellow or blood-streaked sputum Chest x-ray film may show patchy infiltrates, empyema, abscesses, and pneumothorax Disease may start with headache, cough, and myalgia
Influenzal pneumonia (caused by *Haemophilus influenzae*)	Similar to those of pneumococcal pneumonia Cough productive of apple- or lime-green purulent sputum, which may be blood-tinged
Gram-negative bacterial pneumonia (most commonly caused by *Klebsiella pneumoniae*)	Sudden onset with high fever, multiple chills, pleuritic pain, dyspnea, cyanosis, and elevated WBC count Lobar consolidation and cavitation on chest x-ray film Cough productive of red sputum resembling currant jelly (mucoid, sticky, and difficult to expectorate)
Anaerobic bacterial pneumonia, hypostatic pneumonia (caused by normal oral flora)	Insidious onset with low-grade fever, dyspnea, crackles, cyanosis, hypertension, tachycardia, and elevated WBC count Patchy infiltrates in dependent lung segments on chest x-ray film Cough productive of purulent, greenish-yellow, foul-smelling sputum
Legionnaires' disease (caused by *Legionella pneumophila*)	Prodrome of 24-48 hours with fever, headache, and malaise followed by high fever with pulse-temperature dissociation, dyspnea, hypoxia, pleuritic pain, nausea, vomiting, diarrhea, confusion, and elevated WBC count Single or multilobar consolidation and small pleural effusions on chest x-ray film Dry cough productive of scant mucoid or blood-tinged sputum
Mycoplasma pneumonia (caused by *Mycoplasma* microorganisms)	Insidious onset with slowly rising fever, headache, myalgia, malaise, and normal WBC count Pulmonary infiltrate—sometimes extensive—on chest x-ray film Cough productive of scant mucoid sputum Client may show only minimal signs and symptoms
Viral pneumonia (caused by influenza A virus)	Prodrome with headache and myalgia followed by high fever, dyspnea, normal breath sounds with occasional wheezing and crackles, and normal or slightly elevated WBC count Diffuse, patchy infiltrates on chest x-ray film Dry cough with initial mucoid sputum that later turns purulent Cough may be unproductive
Fungal pneumonia (caused by histoplasmosis, blastomycosis, coccidioidomycosis, aspergillosis, candidiasis)	Usually asymptomatic When manifestations occur, they range from brief periods of malaise to severe, life-threatening illness Typical illness resembles influenza
Parasitic pneumonia (caused by protozoa, nematodes, platyhelminths); common organism is *Pneumocystis carinii*	Clients who have *P. carinii* pneumonia are invariably immunocompromised (HIV) Cough, dyspnea, pleuritic chest pain, fever and night sweats, crackles
Aspiration pneumonia (caused by aspiration of gastric contents or food)	Often asymptomatic with minor aspiration Major aspiration may lead to tachypnea, apnea, cyanosis, hypotension, fever, adventitious lung sounds (crackles, rhonchi, wheezing), hypoxemia, respiratory failure, leukocytosis

HIV, Human immunodeficiency virus; *WBC,* white blood cell.

TERRORISM ALERT

Pneumonic Plague

Plague is a disease caused by *Yersinia pestis,* a bacterium found in rodents and their fleas in many areas around the world. This naturally occurring form of plague—also called bubonic plague—leads to skin masses and necrosis and has been responsible for the deaths of thousands of people over time. A variant of plague is the pulmonary form, which is quickly fatal.

Clinical manifestations occur anytime from 1 to 6 days after becoming infected. Once a person has the disease, he or she can spread the bacteria to others in close contact through droplets in the air during coughing or sneezing. The bacteria can be spread before the person even shows manifestations of the disease. Because of the delay between being exposed to the bacteria and becoming ill, people could travel over a large area—possibly infecting others—before showing manifestations of the disease.

Bubonic plague should be suspected when a person develops swollen glands, fever, chills, headache, and extreme exhaustion and has a history of possible exposure to infected rodents, rabbits, or fleas. A person usually becomes ill with bubonic plague 1 to 6 days after being infected.

When bubonic plague is left untreated, plague bacteria invade the bloodstream and can lead to pneumonic plague. Clinical manifestations of pneumonic plague include fever, weakness, and rapidly developing pneumonia with shortness of breath, chest pain, cough, and sometimes bloody or watery sputum. Nausea, vomiting, and abdominal pain may also occur. Without early treatment, pneumonic plague usually leads to respiratory failure, shock, and rapid death. The development of these severe respiration infection manifestations in a group of persons should lead to the consideration of pneumonic plague. The bacterium used in an aerosol terrorism attack could cause the pneumonic form of plague.

Pneumonic plague is treated with antibiotics, which are given within 24 hours of the first manifestations. People in direct and close contact with someone with pneumonic plague should wear tight-fitting disposable surgical masks. Clients with the disease should be isolated and medically supervised for at least the first 48 hours of antibiotic treatment. People who have been exposed to a contagious person can be protected from developing plague by receiving prompt antibiotic treatment.

Data from Inglesby, T.V. (2000). Plague as a biological weapon. *Journal of the American Medical Association, 283,* 2281-2290.

effectiveness and allow organisms to penetrate the sterile lower respiratory tract, where inflammation develops. Disruption of the mechanical defenses of cough and ciliary motility leads to colonization of the lungs and subsequent infection. Inflamed and fluid-filled alveolar sacs cannot exchange oxygen and carbon dioxide effectively. Alveolar exudate tends to consolidate, so it is increasingly difficult to expectorate. Bacterial pneumonia may be associated with significant ventilation-perfusion mismatch as the infection grows.

Clinical Manifestations

The onset of all pneumonias is generally marked by any or all of the following manifestations: fever, chills, sweats, pleuritic chest pain, cough, sputum production, hemoptysis, dyspnea, headache, and fatigue. Older clients may present not with fever or respiratory manifestations but with altered mental status and dehydration.

Chest auscultation reveals bronchial breath sounds over areas of *consolidation* (dense white areas on the chest film). Consolidated lung tissue transmits bronchial sound waves to outer lung fields. Crackling sounds (from fluid in interstitial and alveolar areas) and whispered *pectoriloquy* (transmission of the sound of whispered words through the chest wall) may be heard over affected areas. Tactile fremitus is usually increased over areas of pneumonia, whereas percussion sounds are dulled. Unequal chest wall expansion may occur during inspiration if a large area of lung tissue is involved; this is due to decreased distensibility in the affected area. Table 64-1 lists the clinical manifestations of specific types of pneumonia.

Definitive diagnosis is usually determined through sputum culture analysis and sensitivity or serologic testing. At times, fiberoptic bronchoscopy or transcutaneous needle aspiration or biopsy may be necessary for confirmation. Additional diagnostic testing may consist of (1) skin tests, if tuberculosis or coccidioidomycosis is suspected, (2) blood and urine cultures to assess systemic spread, and (3) transcutaneous oxygen level analysis or arterial blood gas (ABG) measurements to assess the need for supplemental oxygen.

Chest x-ray examination provides information about the location and extent of pneumonia. As previously mentioned, on a chest film, areas of pneumonia appear as consolidation.

Pneumonia may involve one or more lobe segments of the lungs *(segmental pneumonia),* one or more entire lobes *(lobar pneumonia)* (Figure 64-1, *A*), or lobes in both lungs *(bilateral pneumonia).* On the basis of location and radiologic appearance, pneumonias may be classified as bronchopneumonia, interstitial pneumonia, alveolar pneumonia, or necrotizing pneumonia. *Bronchopneumonia* (bronchial pneumonia) (see Figure 64-1, *B*) involves the terminal bronchioles and alveoli. *Interstitial (reticular) pneumonia* involves inflammatory re-

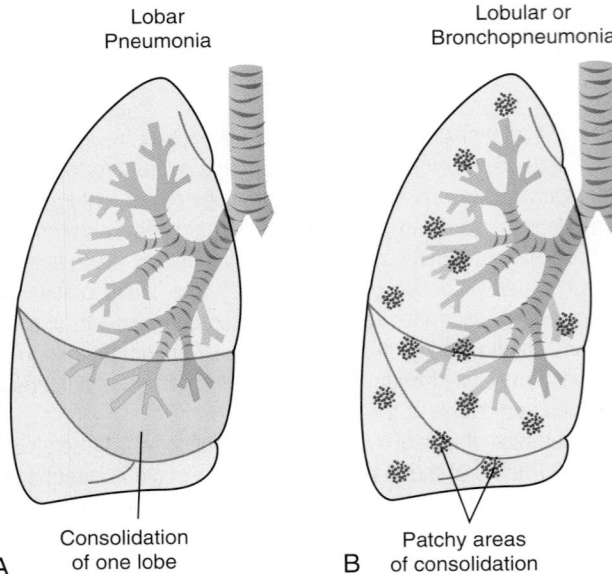

Lobar
Pneumonia

Lobular or
Bronchopneumonia

A Consolidation
of one lobe

B Patchy areas
of consolidation

FIGURE 64-1 Two types of pneumonia. **A,** Lobar pneumonia with consolidation in one lobe of one lung. **B,** Lobular or bronchopneumonia with patchy consolidation throughout lobes of one or both lungs.

sponses within lung tissue surrounding the air spaces or vascular structures rather than the air passages themselves. In *alveolar* (or *acinar*) *pneumonia,* there is fluid accumulation in a lung's distal air spaces. *Necrotizing pneumonia* causes the death of a portion of lung tissue surrounded by viable tissue; x-ray examination may reveal cavity formation at the site of necrosis. Necrotic lung tissue, which does not heal, constitutes a permanent loss of functioning parenchyma.

Outcome Management
■ Medical Management

Treatment of pneumonia should include specific antibiotic therapy, respiratory support as needed, nutritional support, and fluid and electrolyte management. Initial drug therapy should consist of broad-spectrum antibiotics until the specific organism has been identified. Oxygen should be administered as ordered, and bronchodilator medications, postural drainage, chest physiotherapy, and tracheal suctioning may be used to maintain airway patency. See the Clinical Pathway feature on Pneumonia on the website for a Care Map and clinical *evolve* guide to treating pneumonia.

■ Nursing Management of the Medical Client
Assessment

The nursing history should explore the following areas with the client in whom pneumonia is suspected or confirmed:

- Contact with other clients experiencing similar manifestations (suggests viral or mycoplasmal pneumonia)
- Factors suggesting the presence of noninfectious diseases that produce manifestations similar to those of pneumonia (e.g., pulmonary embolism, allergic reaction to drugs or other substances, neoplasm)
- Lowered levels of consciousness, which increase the risk of aspiration
- Presence of tuberculosis or contact with others who have active tuberculosis
- Presence and character of any chest pain
- Presence and character of cough and sputum production

Perform respiratory assessment every 4 hours, including determination of the rate and character of respirations, auscultation of breath sounds, and assessment of skin and nail beds to determine the severity of hypoxia. In addition to the physical examination, transcutaneous oxygen level analysis or ABG measurements may be used to evaluate the need for oxygen support.

Diagnosis, Planning, Interventions

Nursing diagnoses common to pneumonia are described here. Other applicable nursing diagnoses are *Deficient Fluid Volume related to fever, diaphoresis, and mouth breathing; Imbalanced Nutrition: Less Than Body Requirements related to dyspnea; Pain related to frequent coughing;* and *Impaired Oral Mucous Membrane related to mouth breathing and frequent cough.* Collaborative problems include risk of hypoxemia, respiratory failure, and sepsis.

Diagnosis: Ineffective Airway Clearance. The inflammation and increased secretions seen with pneumonia make it difficult to maintain a patent airway. An appropriate nursing diagnosis is *Ineffective Airway Clearance related to excessive secretions and weak cough.*

Outcomes. The client will maintain effective airway clearance, as evidenced by keeping a patent airway and effectively clearing secretions.

Interventions. Take measures to promote airway patency, such as increasing fluid intake, teaching and encouraging effective coughing and deep-breathing techniques, and frequent turning. Clients with an altered level of consciousness should be turned at least every 2 hours and should be placed in side-lying positions, unless contraindicated, to prevent aspiration. Only thickened liquids should be given to clients with dysphagia. Administer bronchodilating medications, if prescribed. If indicated, more aggressive measures to maintain airway patency may be required (e.g., chest physiotherapy, suctioning, artificial airway).

Diagnosis: Ineffective Breathing Pattern. Many clients experience compensatory tachypnea because of an inability to meet metabolic demands. This occurs because affected alveoli cannot effectively exchange oxygen and carbon dioxide. Higher respiratory rates can also develop as a result of chest pain and increased body temperature. An appropriate nursing diagnosis is *Ineffective Breathing Pattern related to tachypnea.*

Outcomes. The client will have improved breathing patterns, as evidenced by (1) a respiratory rate within normal limits, (2) adequate chest expansion, (3) clear breath sounds, and (4) decreased dyspnea.

Interventions. Position the client for comfort and to facilitate breathing (e.g., raise the head of the bed 45 degrees). Teach the client how to splint the chest wall with a pillow for comfort during coughing and about the use of incentive spirometry. Administer prescribed cough suppressants and analgesics; be cautious, however, because opioids may depress respirations more than desired. Routinely monitor respiratory rate and transcutaneous oxygen levels, auscultate the chest, and document findings. Monitor ABG values, and observe for manifestations of hypoxemia, hypercapnia, and acid-base imbalance.

Diagnosis: Activity Intolerance. Depleted energy reserves, due to not eating during periods of dyspnea, and impairment of oxygen and carbon dioxide transport leave little oxygen to meet metabolic demands. An appropriate nursing diagnosis is *Activity Intolerance related to decreased oxygen levels for metabolic demands.*

Outcomes. The client will have improved activity tolerance, as evidenced by an ability to perform activities of daily living and a progressive increase in physical activity without excessive dyspnea and fatigue.

Interventions. Assess the client's baseline activity level and response to activity. Note how well the client tolerates activity by assessing for changes in respiratory and pulse rate, marked dyspnea, fatigue, pallor or cyanosis, and dysrhythmias. Schedule activity after treatments or medications. Use oxygen as needed. Gradually increase activity on the basis of tolerance. Balance activity with adequate rest periods.

Teach the client to avoid conditions that increase oxygen demand, such as smoking, temperature extremes, weight gain, and stress. Pursed-lip and diaphragmatic breathing, which improve air flow, as well as techniques to lower energy use, should be reinforced. Activities that are tiring should be interspersed with rest.

Provide psychological support and a quiet environment to reduce anxiety and promote rest. Regulate nursing care and visitors as warranted by the client's condition.

Pneumonia is a common reason for hospital admission. Many institutions provide care using Care Maps. (See the Case Management feature on Pneumonia on the *evolve* website.)

Evaluation

The level the client will probably attain is monitored every 2 to 3 days. Pneumonia should resolve quickly once the client is receiving antibiotics, as long as there are no immune disorders or malnutrition. Older clients may require additional time to fully recover.

■ Prevention

Prevention is the best defense against the spread of pneumonia. When caring for hospitalized clients, (1) wash hands frequently, (2) use gloves appropriately, (3) encourage fluid intake, (4) turn clients every 2 hours, and (5) control clients' pain so they may breathe deeply and cough adequately. Encourage clients to use their incentive spirometer frequently. Reduce the risk of aspiration in clients with dysphagia by raising the head of the bed to 45 degrees. Furthermore, hold tube feedings when residual volume is high, and stop feeding 1 hour before treatments that require lowering the head of the bed (e.g., x-ray examination, chest physical therapy [CPT]).

■ Self-Care

Clients with pneumonia who are ambulatory but have an ongoing health problem may require hospitalization. For clients with intact defense mechanisms and good general health, recuperation can often take place at home with rest and supportive treatment; the term *walking pneumonia* is sometimes used to describe this situation.

Chest physiotherapy may be performed for a prescribed period. The client is monitored in a clinic setting until the chest radiograph is clear and clinical manifestations abate. Encourage the client to plan for influenza immunization each winter. People who live with the client are also monitored for the onset of pneumonia.

LUNG ABSCESS

Lung abscess is a collection of pus within lung tissue. In its early stages, the abscess resembles a localized pneumonia. If a lung abscess remains unidentified and untreated, tissue necrosis may occur. Lung abscesses are becoming more rare as a result of improved treatment of pneumonia and effective preventive care of clients at high risk for aspiration. Today, abscesses are most often a result of anaerobic bacteria.

Single lung abscesses usually occur distal to a bronchial obstruction. They nearly always create putrid (foul) material. The bronchial obstruction may be due to the following:

- Aspirated foreign material (e.g., vomitus, mucus, teeth, blood, food, or tissue from upper airway surgery)
- Benign or malignant tumors

Multiple lung abscesses can follow pneumonia caused by necrotizing bacteria (such as *Staphylococcus aureus,* which creates necrotic lung tissue). Bacteria may also arise from septic emboli from infected foci, such as septic phlebitis. Immunosuppressed clients and clients who may aspirate foreign material are at high risk for lung abscesses.

Early assessment findings in a client with a lung abscess are the same as those in a client with bronchopneumonia (i.e., chills, fever, pleuritic pain, cough with abundant sputum). The body attempts to wall off the abscess with fibrous tissue. If the attempt is unsuccessful, the abscess ruptures into a bronchus, causing a cough that produces copious amounts of sputum. The sputum is purulent, foul-smelling, and foul-tasting. After bronchial rupture, hemoptysis often occurs. Chest auscultation reveals decreased breath sounds and dullness to percussion over the affected area. Crackles may be present when the abscess drains.

The diagnosis is commonly confirmed by chest radiography or computed tomography (CT) scan. Sputum cultures assist with identification of the organism.

Outcome Management

Antibiotics are prescribed on the basis of culture results. Although bronchoscopy was once believed to be essential in managing lung abscesses, it is now reserved for clients whose disease fails to improve or who may have malignancy. Surgery is seldom needed because of the success of antibiotic therapy.

Caring for a client with a lung abscess is similar to caring for a client experiencing pneumonia (e.g., promoting hydration, teaching effective cough techniques, and administering postural drainage). Lung abscesses produce copious volumes of sputum. Nursing intervention focuses on removing sputum from the lungs through postural drainage and expectoration. Note the color, quantity, quality, and smell of the expectorated material, including the presence of blood. Use gloves when handling articles contaminated with sputum.

The sputum may have a foul taste. Provide frequent opportunities for the client to use mouthwash, brush the teeth, and floss. Because long-term antibiotic administration is usually necessary, observe oral mucous membranes for indications of *Candida albicans* overgrowth (i.e., white patches). Encourage long-term dental care. Oral nystatin (which the client swishes around the mouth and swallows or spits) may be ordered.

Antibiotic therapy for a lung abscess may be needed for 8 weeks or longer. Clients with lung abscesses must understand the importance of compliance with the medication schedule. The entire course of antibiotics must be taken. Teaching about medications should cover (1) the reasons for taking them, (2) specific directions, such as time of day, frequency, and when to take in relation to food, (3) potential side effects, and (4) what to do if side effects occur. Reassessment after the antibiotics course is completed (e.g., with culture of sputum or chest films) is essential to evaluate the effectiveness of treatment.

PULMONARY TUBERCULOSIS

Tuberculosis (TB) is one of the two most prominent mycobacterial diseases known to humankind. The World Health Organization (WHO) currently estimates that 8 million new cases of TB occur yearly with approximately 3 million people dying of the disease.[1] Before the development of anti-TB drugs in the late 1940s, TB was the leading cause of all deaths in the United States. Drug therapy, along with improvements in public health and general living standards, resulted in a marked decline in incidence over the next three decades. However, between 1985 and 1992, the number of reported TB cases increased by 20%. This increase was attributed to the emergence of the human immunodeficiency virus (HIV) epidemic, drug misuse, recent influxes of immigrants from developing countries, and the deterioration of the nation's health care infrastructure.

There are two prevalent public health concerns in the United States related to TB. First is the increase in the number of cases of TB due to infection by multidrug-resistant organisms (MDR-TB), which are extremely difficult to treat. It is believed that resistance develops because people either stop taking their medication once they begin to feel well or are noncompliant with treatment as a result of other health problems, such as substance abuse.

The second public health concern is that clients with HIV infection are particularly susceptible to TB because *Mycobacterium tuberculosis,* the organism causing TB, is an extremely *opportunistic* pathogen. In some HIV-seropositive populations, the TB infection rate is 1000-fold higher than the annual rate in the United States. Clients infected with HIV are at greater risk for acquiring a new infection with rapid progression to active disease or for experiencing reinfection from dormant lesions.

Etiology and Risk Factors

TB is a communicable disease caused by *M. tuberculosis,* an aerobic, acid-fast bacillus (AFB). TB is an airborne infection. In nearly all instances, TB infection is acquired by inhalation of a particle small enough (1 to 5 mm in diameter) to reach the alveolus. Droplets are emitted during coughing, talking, laughing, sneezing, or singing. Infected droplet nuclei may then be inhaled by a susceptible person (host). Before pulmonary infection can occur, the inhaled organisms must resist the lung's defense mechanisms and penetrate lung tissue.

Brief exposure to TB does not usually cause infection. People most commonly infected are those who have repeated close contact with an infected person whose disease is not yet diagnosed. Such people include anyone who has repeated contacts with medically underserved clients, low-income populations, foreign-born people, or residents of long-term care facilities or institutional settings. Other high-risk populations are intravenous drug users, homeless people, and people who are occupationally exposed to active TB (health care workers).

In countries that do not have public health programs and those in which TB commonly occurs in cattle, humans may experience bovine TB after drinking raw milk from infected cattle. This form of TB can be prevented by pasteurizing milk and maintaining tuberculin skin-testing programs for cattle.

Pathophysiology

Primary (First) Infection

The first time a client is infected with TB, the disease is said to be a *primary infection.* Primary TB infections are usually located in the apices of the lungs or near the pleurae of the lower lobes. Although a primary infection may be only microscopic (and hence may not appear on x-ray film), the following sequence of events is typically observed.

A small area of bronchopneumonia develops in the lung tissue. Many of the infecting tubercle bacilli are phagocytosed (ingested) by wandering macrophages. However, before the development of hypersensitivity and immunity, many of the bacilli may survive within these blood cells and may be carried into regional bronchopulmonary (hilar) lymph nodes via the lymphatic system. The bacilli may even spread throughout the body. Thus the infection, although small, spreads rapidly.

The primary infection site may or may not undergo a process of necrotic degeneration *(caseation),* which produces cavities filled with a cheese-like mass of tubercle bacilli, dead white blood cells (WBCs), and necrotic lung tissue. In time, this material liquefies, may drain into the tracheobronchial tree, and may be coughed up. The air-filled cavities remain and may be detected on x-ray study.

Most primary tubercles heal over a period of months by forming scars and then calcified lesions, also known as *Ghon tubercles.* These lesions may contain living bacilli that can be reactivated, even after many years, and cause secondary infection.

Primary TB infections cause the body to develop an allergic reaction to tubercle bacilli or their proteins. This cell-mediated immune response appears in the form of sensitized T cells and is detectable as a positive reaction to a tuberculin skin test. The development of this tuberculin sensitivity occurs in all body cells 2 to 6 weeks after the primary infection. It is maintained as long as living bacilli remain in the body. This acquired immunity usually inhibits further growth of the bacilli and the development of active infection.

The reason active TB disease develops in some clients (instead of being controlled by the acquired immune response and thereby remaining dormant) is poorly under-

stood. However, factors that seem to play a role in the progression from a dormant TB infection to active disease are (1) advanced age, (2) HIV infection, (3) immunosuppression, (4) prolonged corticosteroid therapy, (5) malabsorption syndromes, (6) low body weight (10% or more below ideal weight), (7) substance abuse, (8) presence of other diseases (e.g., diabetes mellitus, end-stage renal disease, or malignancy), and (9) genetic predisposition.

Secondary Infection

In addition to progressive primary disease, reinfection may also lead to a clinical form of active TB, or secondary infection. Primary sites of infection containing TB bacilli may remain latent for years and then may be reactivated if the client's resistance is lowered. Because reinfection is possible and because dormant lesions may be reactivated, it is extremely important for clients who have had a TB infection to be reassessed periodically for new evidence of active disease.

Clinical Manifestations

The detection and diagnosis of TB are achieved through subjective assessment findings and objective test results. The diagnosis can be difficult because TB mimics many other diseases and may occur concurrently with other pulmonary diseases. Nurses and other health care providers should maintain a high index of suspicion for TB in high-risk clients.

The history includes assessing the probability of recent or past exposure to TB as well as the client's occupation, other usual activities, and travel to or residence in countries with a high incidence of TB. A history of exposure to TB is certainly important, but most clients are unaware of exposure. It is advisable to determine whether the client has been previously tested for TB and to obtain the results of that testing.

Figure 64-2 shows the logical progression of the diagnosis and management of TB. Typical findings in pulmonary TB are (1) nonproductive or productive cough, (2) fatigue, (3) anorexia (loss of appetite) and weight loss, (4) low-grade fever, (5) chills and sweats (often at night), (6) dyspnea, (7) hemoptysis, (8) chest pain that may be pleuritic or dull, and (9) chest tightness. Crackles may be present on auscultation.

Primary TB infections may remain unrecognized because they are relatively asymptomatic. Calcified lesions on chest radiograph and a positive skin test reaction are frequently the only indications that a primary TB infection has occurred. Most clients harbor tubercle bacilli for life and never experience active disease because their body defenses are adequate to arrest primary infection. The tubercles heal through fibrosis and calcification. However, infected people face a 10% risk that the primary infection will progress to active disease sometime in their lives. In

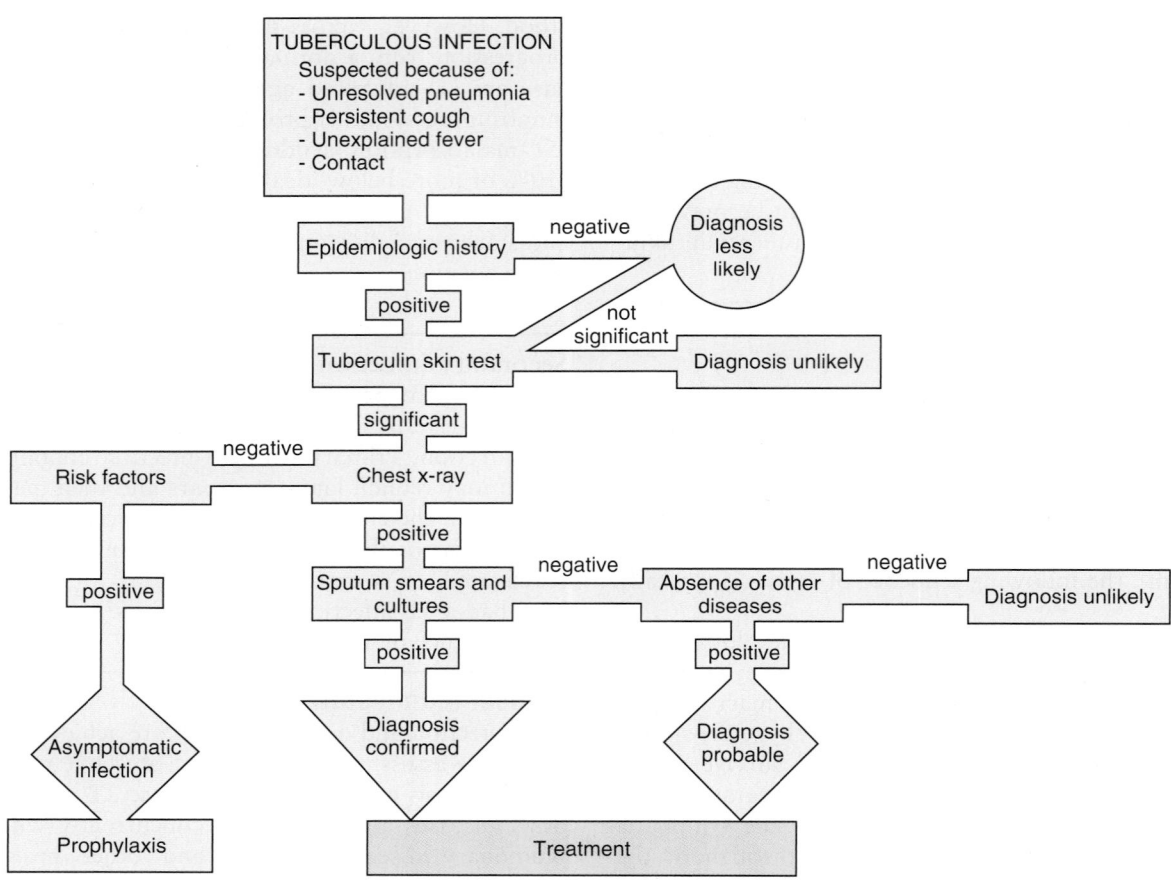

FIGURE 64-2 Algorithm for diagnosis and management of tuberculosis: a logical progression. (Courtesy of the American Lung Association, New York, NY.)

this situation, the primary complex sites progress and worsen, possibly causing cavitation and the spread of active infection, and the client becomes clinically ill.

Diagnostic Findings

Tuberculin Skin Testing

Tuberculin skin testing, typically the Mantoux test, is performed on a routine basis in high-risk groups when active TB is suspected. Mantoux testing uses purified protein derivative (PPD) tuberculin to identify TB infection. A small amount of the derivative is administered intradermally to form a wheal on the lower left forearm. The wheal must be examined ("read") in 48 to 72 hours by a trained professional. The presence of induration, not erythema, indicates a positive test result[25]:

- More than 5 mm of induration is considered a positive result for clients with known or suspected HIV infection, intravenous drug users, people in close contact with a known case of TB, and the client with a chest radiograph suggestive of previous TB.
- More than 10 mm of induration is considered positive for clients in all other high-risk groups.
- Induration of 15 mm or more is considered positive for clients in low-risk groups.

False-positive reactions to tuberculin skin testing can occur in clients who have other mycobacterial infections or who have received the bacille Calmette-Guérin (BCG) vaccination. False-negative reactions are also possible, especially in people who are immunosuppressed or anergic (impaired ability to react to antigens). For these clients, and for anyone who has a positive skin test reaction, the AFB sputum smear examination and chest radiograph are used to identify active disease. It is critical to initiate respiratory isolation of such clients until AFB sputum results are known.

The term *tuberculin converter* refers to a client who does not show radiologic or bacteriologic evidence of pulmonary TB but whose tuberculin skin test "converts" from a known negative reaction to a known positive reaction. The absence of a positive (reactive) tuberculin test result does not always mean that TB is absent.

Acid-Fast Bacillus Smear and Culture

A more definitive diagnosis of TB is made from the AFB smear and culture. Three different sputum specimens should be collected on three consecutive mornings. Sputum AFB smears are not extremely sensitive, but the positive result of a sputum AFB smear confirms active dis-

INTEGRATING PHARMACOLOGY

Tuberculosis Medications

There are five medications that are considered *first-line medications* for the treatment of tuberculosis: isoniazid, rifampin, pyrazinamide, ethambutol, and streptomycin. Isoniazid (INH) and rifampin (RIF) are the two most significant medications; they are highly effective and require a short duration of treatment. These two drugs are typically given together orally over a 6-month to 24-month period to achieve a cure. Pyrazinamide, ethambutol, and streptomycin provide adjunct effects that reduce the risk of acquired drug resistance while accelerating the client's response to treatment.

INH is the single most important drug used in treating TB. It is most frequently administered orally; however, other routes include intramuscular and intravenous administration. INH is low cost and can be given daily or twice or three times weekly. It is metabolized by the liver and should be temporarily discontinued for liver enzymes elevated to three times the normal range if manifestations of hepatic toxicity such as nausea, vomiting, anorexia, fatigue, or jaundice occur. Typically INH is well tolerated by clients; however, the risk of developing hepatitis increases with age, alcohol consumption, and underlying liver disease.

RIF is also a potent antituberculosis medication that can be given either orally or intravenously and is metabolized by the liver. Both INH and RIF are bactericidal and the combination of the two drugs allows action against active, slow, and intermittently growing organisms. A common side effect of RIF is that it colors the body fluids such as urine, sweat, saliva, sputum, and tears orange. Gastrointestinal upset is also a common side effect that can be decreased with dividing the dose in half and taking twice a day with meals instead of once a day. Hepatotoxicity is rare but can occur.

Pyrazinamide is a third medication given to clients because of its effects of eliminating bacteria resistant to INH and RIF. Either ethambutol or streptomycin should also be given to clients until susceptibility to INH and RIF is demonstrated.

Because of the duration of treatment and side effects, noncompliance remains a serious problem. Local and national health initiatives, including providing medications at no cost, have been used to address these issues.

---

ease. A more reliable indicator is a positive culture for *M. tuberculosis*, which does confirm active TB; however, final culture results may not be available for 2 to 12 weeks. Although newer detection tests can generate faster results and show clinical promise, the prevalence of MDR-TB still mandates the use of traditional culture methods for diagnosis.

Outcome Management
■ Medical Management

Most people with newly diagnosed active TB are not hospitalized. If pulmonary TB is diagnosed in the hospitalized client, the client may be kept in the hospital until therapeutic drug levels are established. Some clients with active TB may be hospitalized for the following reasons:

- They are acutely ill.
- Their living situation is considered a high risk.
- They are thought to be noncompliant with therapy.
- They have a history of previous TB and noncompliance, and the disease has been reactivated.
- Concomitant diseases are present and acute.
- Improvement does not occur after treatment.
- The organisms are highly resistant to the usual treatment, requiring second-line or third-line drugs. In this situation, brief hospitalization is necessary to monitor the effects and side effects of the drugs.

Treatment of TB is a long-term process that should be initiated immediately upon suspicion of infection. Clients with a diagnosis of active TB are usually started on a minimum of four medications to ensure elimination of resistant organisms. The dose of some drugs may initially be large because the bacilli are difficult to kill. Treatment continues long enough to eliminate or substantially reduce the number of dormant or semidormant bacilli.

Medications used for TB may include *first-line* and *second-line* agents. First-line agents are almost always initially prescribed until results of culture and sensitivity tests are available. In clients with a previous history of incomplete TB treatment, resistant organisms may have developed and secondary agents are used.

The U.S. Centers for Disease Control and Prevention (CDC) currently recommends a two-phase approach for treatment, consisting of (1) an *induction* phase using four drugs aimed at destroying large numbers of rapidly multiplying organisms and (2) a *continuation* phase, usually using two drugs, directed at eliminating most remaining bacilli.

The recommended basic treatment regimen for previously untreated clients is 2 months of daily doses of isoniazid, rifampin, pyrazinamide, and ethambutol. This treatment is followed with 4 months of isoniazid and rifampin. The length of time a client remains infectious varies. Sputum cultures and clinical responses (absence of fever and dyspnea, reduction in cough) are used to evaluate the effectiveness of the therapy. (See the Integrating Pharmacology feature on Tuberculosis Medications, above.)

If compliance with daily dosing is a problem, some TB protocols call for administration of medications

EB two or three times a week rather than daily. The CDC recommends clients are assigned to receive *directly observed therapy* (DOT) if intermittent dosing is being used. See the Evidence-Based Practice in Action feature on Directly Observed Therapy for Tuberculosis, **EB** below.

Fixed-dose combinations of drugs are also being studied as a means to reduce clients' noncompliance to medical therapy. Two medications being reviewed are Rifamate (a combination of INH and RIF) and Rifater (a combination of INH, RIF, and pyrazinamide). By combining multiple drugs into a single pill it is hoped that clients will be more compliant because of the ease of taking fewer pills less often each day.

If the medication regimen does not seem effective (e.g., worsening manifestations, continued presence of AFB in sputum, increasing infiltrates or cavity formation on radiograph), then the treatment program needs reevaluation and the client's compliance should be assessed. At least two medications (never just one) are added to a failing TB treatment program.

Because medications used to treat TB have potentially serious side effects, baseline studies (depending on the specific drugs prescribed) are performed first. Drug toxicity can limit the treatment of TB. Drug tolerance, drug effect, and drug toxicity depend on factors such as the medication dosage, the time since last dosage, the medication's chemical formula, and the

---

EB EVIDENCE-BASED PRACTICE IN ACTION

Directly Observed Therapy for Tuberculosis

Directly observed therapy (DOT) for tuberculosis (TB) is the practice of health care personnel observing or assisting clients as they take their prescribed medications for 6 months, or until a cure is achieved. In addition, DOT allows health care personnel to provide immediate information and support to clients who require it. This process may be conducted in a variety of settings including a clinic, hospital, client's home, school, workplace, or other convenient location.[1]

Directly observed therapy is the result of increasing nonadherence to the long-term treatment plan for TB. Nonadherence is a major problem facing health care providers and clients, and was a major contributing factor in the resurgence of TB in the 1990s. Clients who do not complete their drug regimen face an increased chance of spreading the disease to others, treatment failure, relapse of disease, emergence of drug-resistant forms of the disease, increased costs of therapy, disability, and even death.

Reasons for nonadherence are many. Factors relating to nonadherence include duration of treatment, medication side effects, and cost. Additionally, as manifestations subside, clients often lose the motivation to continue taking their medications.[5]

Studies have documented the positive outcomes of DOT. Clients who participate in a DOT program demonstrate higher completion rates of therapy, lower relapse rates, less acquired drug resistance, and faster sputum conversion rates (from positive to negative). These outcomes ultimately lead to lower costs of treating TB for the client and society.

A newer approach to DOT includes Deferred DOT (D-DOT), which uses DOT only during the continuation phase (last 4 months) of therapy when intermittent dosing is being used. The assumption of D-DOT is that clients are motivated to take their medications while acutely ill, then become nonadherent once manifestations disappear and dosing is less frequent. Therefore D-DOT is required once clients feel healthy to prevent nonadher-

ence from occurring. D-DOT has demonstrated positive outcomes of high completion rates of therapy, decreased costs associated with therapy, and increased convenience to clients.[2-4]

Implications

DOT is recommended by the Centers for Disease Control and Prevention and is currently the basis for treating tuberculosis in the United States. If properly implemented, DOT can lead to successful cure rates, decrease spreading of the disease, decrease drug-resistant forms of the disease, and decrease costs to society. Nurses need to be aware of the positive outcomes of DOT and be able to educate clients on its purpose and results. Nurses need to conduct careful assessments to identify clients who are at risk or who do not adhere to their prescribed therapy. These clients need to be introduced immediately to DOT therapy until a cure is obtained.

References

1. Bayer, R., et al. (1998). Directly observed therapy and treatment completion for tuberculosis in the United States: Is universal supervised therapy necessary? *American Journal of Public Health, 88*(7), 1052-1058.
2. Burman, W.J., et al. (1997). A cost-effectiveness analysis of directly observed therapy vs. self-administered therapy for treatment of tuberculosis. *Chest, 112*(1), 63-70.
3. Desvarieux, M., et al. (2001). A novel approach to directly observed therapy for tuberculosis in an HIV-endemic area. *American Journal of Public Health, 91*(1), 138-141.
4. Mac, J.T., Doordan, A., & Carr, C.A. (1999). Evaluation of the effectiveness of a directly observed therapy program with Vietnamese tuberculosis patients. *Public Health Nurse, 16*(6), 426-431.
5. McDonnell, M., Turner, J., & Weaver, M.T. (2001). Antecedents of adherence to antituberculosis therapy. *Public Health Nurse, (18)*6, 392-400.

client's age, renal and intestinal function, and compliance with treatment.

■ Nursing Management of the Medical Client

Nursing management of the client with TB includes many interventions already discussed for the client with pneumonia, depending on the specific nursing diagnoses identified. Possible nursing diagnoses for the client with TB are as follows: *Anxiety; Ineffective Airway Clearance; Impaired Gas Exchange; Pain; Imbalanced Nutrition: Less than Body Requirements; Ineffective Coping; Compromised Family Coping; Ineffective Health Maintenance; Deficient Knowledge related to treatment or noncompliance;* and *Disturbed Sleep Pattern.*

Prevention of Transmission. During hospitalization, appropriate infection control and hospital employee health practices are essential. First, early identification of clients with TB is key. High-risk clients and clients with clinical manifestations of pneumonia should be immediately isolated until results of AFB smears and cultures are obtained.

Private respiratory isolation rooms should be available. These rooms should be maintained at negative pressure relative to the hallway; negative pressure keeps room air from flowing out into the hallway when the door is opened, thereby avoiding the spread of infectious particles outside the room. Negative-pressure ventilation sends room air directly to the outside, with at least six air exchanges per hour. Additional equipment, such as ultraviolet lamps (proven to kill mycobacteria) and high-efficiency particulate air (HEPA) filters, may also be used.

Personal protective equipment, called *particulate respirators,* is required for all health care workers entering a TB isolation room. When fitted properly, these respirators filter droplet nuclei; the fit of a particulate respirator should be reassessed if there is a change in the wearer's facial shape.

Monitoring health care workers' TB status is essential. Skin testing should be performed yearly in all health care workers who may be exposed to TB. Semi-annual testing should be completed in high-risk areas or where high rates of TB skin test conversion are occurring.

When a client is found to have TB, public health officials (often nurses) talk with the client and develop a contact list. Everyone with whom the client has had contact is then assessed with a tuberculin skin test and chest radiograph to check for TB infection.

Preventive Therapy. Between 10 and 15 million people in the United States have dormant or asymptomatic TB. Chemoprophylaxis may help many of them avoid active TB and may prevent initial infection in people recently exposed. Isoniazid preventive therapy (IPT) consists of 300 mg of the drug daily for 6 to 12 months. IPT stops the growth of the bacilli, thus preventing active pulmonary or extrapulmonary TB. IPT is recommended for clients who:

- Are newly infected (have converted tuberculin skin test results but no other indication of active disease)
- Live or closely associate with others who have active TB
- Have significant tuberculin skin test reactions and abnormal chest x-ray findings compatible with those of inactive TB
- Have positive tuberculin skin tests and conditions (e.g., steroid therapy, diabetes mellitus, acquired immunodeficiency syndrome [AIDS]) that place them at increased risk for TB
- Are younger than 35 years of age and have significant tuberculin skin test reactions, even though they may have a normal chest radiograph and no other risk factors

■ Self-Care

TB treatment is a long process. Nurses in clinics and public health facilities are often responsible for follow-up assessment and monitoring, including (1) determining medication compliance, (2) understanding the pharmacologic actions of medications, (3) monitoring unwanted side effects, (4) collecting follow-up sputum specimens, (5) obtaining serial chest x-ray studies, and (6) observing for reversal or worsening of initial assessment findings, all of which are part of the ongoing follow-up. It is essential that clients with TB, and their significant others, receive the information summarized in the Client Education Guide feature on Tuberculosis on the website. Providing complete information and ongoing support helps clients understand the long-term recovery process. The more information clients have and the more personal control they feel they have, the more likely they are to comply with treatment.

EXTRAPULMONARY TUBERCULOSIS

Extrapulmonary tuberculosis (XPTB) is TB that occurs anywhere outside the lungs. Pulmonary TB is the most common form of the disease, but after initial invasion, tubercle bacilli can spread throughout the body via the blood and lymph. *M. tuberculosis* thrives in oxygen-rich areas. Highly aerobic sites, such as the renal cortex, bone growth plates, and meninges, are where XPTB most commonly grows. It may also occur in the genitourinary tract, lymph nodes, pleurae, pericardium, abdomen, and endocrine glands.

Widespread dissemination throughout the body *(miliary tuberculosis)* involves the lungs and many other organs. It is more common in clients who are HIV-seropositive or are 50 years or older. Miliary TB may develop from delayed or late dissemination after immune system compromise in older people who were infected with TB many years earlier.

Despite the severity of the disease, XPTB is often difficult to detect. Assessment findings are frequently nondistinct. Weight loss, fatigue, malaise, fever, and night sweats may or may not be present. The only physical finding that is specific for disseminated TB is a granuloma in the choroid of the retina. Clinical manifestations may precede changes in the chest radiograph.

The diagnosis and treatment of XPTB proceed similarly to those of pulmonary TB. However, the treatment period may be longer, and more medications may be used. Treatment depends on the extent, severity, course, and complications of the disease.

NONTUBERCULOUS MYCOBACTERIAL INFECTION

Overview

Nontuberculous mycobacteria (NTM), also known as MOTT (mycobacteria other than tubercle [bacilli]), are responsible for growing numbers of mycobacterial infections. Although NTM infection is still relatively uncommon, the following changes in disease patterns have appeared: (1) more cases, (2) wider geographical distribution, and (3) new groups of vulnerable hosts, most notably, clients with HIV infection.

NTM are widely distributed in nature (i.e., in food, standing fresh water, salt water, animal bedding, soil, animals, and birds), and most clients acquire their infections from environmental sources rather than from other diseased clients. Infection is common in the southeastern part of the United States and more prevalent in rural areas. The most commonly occurring NTM diseases are caused by *Mycobacterium avium* complex, *Mycobacterium kansasii*, and *Mycobacterium fortuitum*. The primary site of NTM disease is the lungs, although extrapulmonary sites (e.g., liver, spleen, lymph nodes, skin, joints) may occur. Disseminated disease with multiple organ involvement is also possible, most commonly in immunosuppressed clients.

Pulmonary NTM disease is similar to TB, although the clinical manifestations may be less severe. Clinical manifestations of the disease include (1) fever, (2) anorexia, (3) night sweats, (4) diarrhea, (5) abdominal pain, and (6) weight loss. Clients with pre-existing bronchopulmonary disease (e.g., bronchiectasis, chronic obstructive pulmonary disease [COPD], or healed pulmonary TB) are at highest risk of pulmonary involvement.

Diagnosis of NTM disease is often difficult because of the widespread distribution of the organisms in the environment. Definitive diagnosis of disease is possible only if NTM are isolated from specimens collected from normally sterile sites (e.g., blood, cerebrospinal fluid, bone marrow, lymph nodes) or through biopsy. However, NTM disease is strongly suspected when (1)

a client presents with a clinical syndrome that is compatible with NTM, (2) no other pathogens can be identified, and (3) repeated sputum cultures reveal large numbers of NTM.

Outcome Management

The same medications used to treat TB are prescribed for NTM disease. However, NTM are considerably more resistant to drugs than *M. tuberculosis*. Consequently, combined drug regimens and longer treatment periods are necessary. Treatment typically consists of three to six different medications and lasts for a minimum of 18 to 24 months beyond conversion of negative sputum cultures.[14] Unsuccessful treatment may result in further lung damage and general debilitation. Regular, daily medication is essential. The more clients understand about the condition and its management, the more likely they will be to complete the full course of medication.

Other aspects of the nursing management of NTM disease are the same as for pulmonary TB (see earlier discussion). Because these diseases are not believed to be transmitted from person to person, however, isolation and measures to control infection, other than good hygiene, are not necessary.

VIRAL PULMONARY INFECTIONS

In spring 2003, a worldwide severe acute respiratory syndrome (SARS) was identified in a unique risk group—previously healthy persons. The majority of clients identified as having SARS were adults in the 25- to 70-year-old age group who were previously healthy. Few suspected cases of SARS were reported among children 15 years of age or younger. The organism, a coronavirus, was also previously unknown. By midsummer, the SARS outbreak was deemed to be under control; however, another outbreak was not seen as being impossible because cases were still being reported.

The incubation period for SARS is typically 2 to 7 days. The illness begins generally with a prodrome of fever (temperature >100.4° F [>38° C]) that is sometimes associated with chills, rigors, headache, diarrhea, malaise, and myalgia. Occasional mild respiratory manifestations are noted.

After 3 to 7 days, a lower respiratory phase begins with the onset of a dry, nonproductive cough or dyspnea, which can progress to hypoxemia requiring mechanical ventilation. The case-fatality rate among persons with illness meeting the current WHO case definition of SARS is approximately 3%.

As the condition progresses, chest radiographs show focal interstitial infiltrates progressing to more generalized, patchy, interstitial infiltrates. In the late stages, chest radiograph has shown areas of consolidation. Laboratory tests reveal leukopenia and thrombocytopenia or low-normal platelet counts. Early in the respiratory phase, elevated creatine phosphokinase levels (as high as 3000 international units/L) and hepatic transaminases (two to six times the upper limits of normal) have been noted. In most clients, renal function has remained normal.

The severity of SARS ranges from mild illness to death. Although a few close contacts of clients with SARS have developed a similar illness, most have remained well. Some close contacts have reported a mild febrile illness without respiratory manifestations, which suggests the illness might not always progress to the respiratory phase.

Treatment regimens have included several antibiotics to presumptively treat known bacterial agents of atypical pneumonia. In several locations, therapy also has included antiviral agents such as oseltamivir or ribavirin. Steroids have also been administered orally or intravenously to clients in combination with ribavirin and other antimicrobials. At present, the most efficacious treatment regimen, if any, is unknown.

FUNGAL PULMONARY INFECTIONS

Most fungi that are pathogenic to humans limit their activities to the skin. However, the spores of some fungi become airborne and can be inhaled into the respiratory tract, causing pulmonary diseases that, in their chronic forms, produce granulomatous conditions similar to TB. The most common of these are coccidioidomycosis and histoplasmosis. Each has a specific geographical distribution and occurs in people living or traveling in the regions where these fungi are found. Person-to-person transmission is virtually unknown. Opportunistic fungal infections occur in clients with impaired immunity including those who require long-term high dose immunosuppressant therapy, have hematologic malignancies, or have undiagnosed HIV. In fact, histoplasmosis is often a sentinel infection, the first hint that a client is HIV infected.[21]

Coccidioidomycosis is found in the Western Hemisphere, primarily in the San Joaquin Valley of California, Utah, Nevada, New Mexico, Arizona, western Texas, and northern Mexico and South America. The disease is most likely to develop in people engaging in desert recreational activities or working in construction or other occupations that involve digging (e.g., archaeology). The disease is mild and self-limiting in 60% of those affected. Such clients either are asymptomatic or have only mild upper respiratory assessment findings. The remaining 40% experience a syndrome similar to influenza, with cough, fever, pleuritic chest pain, myalgias, and arthralgias. *Erythema multiforme,* a flat, red rash that erupts with dark red papules, occurs in some people.

Etiology

The causative organism of *histoplasmosis,* the fungus *Histoplasma capsulatum,* is endemic to the central and eastern portions of North America, most notably the Ohio River, Missouri River, and Mississippi River val-

leys. It is also found in South and Central America, India, and Cyprus. This fungus lives in moist soil of appropriate chemical composition, in mushroom cellars, on the floors of chicken houses and bat caves, and in bird droppings, especially those from starlings, pigeons, and blackbirds.

Clinical Manifestations

As with coccidioidomycosis, *H. capsulatum* infections are usually asymptomatic or mild. Clinical manifestations include fever, fatigue, cough, dyspnea, and weight loss of 1 to 2 months' duration. A few clients may demonstrate disseminated or chronic forms of pulmonary fungal disease and have central nervous system, liver, spleen, gastrointestinal tract, or musculoskeletal involvement. Chronic disease may result in progressive changes similar to those seen with TB, including emphysema-like pulmonary structural changes.

The diagnosis of fungal pulmonary diseases is usually based on history and clinical assessment findings. Skin testing is also used for coccidioidomycosis and can indicate exposure but not active infection. Chest radiographs may show hilar adenopathy (lymph gland enlargement), small areas of infiltrates, or manifestations of pneumonia. Sometimes, cavities and calcified nodules may form, usually remaining in the lungs as permanent indicators of previous infection. In addition to the pathogenic fungi, common fungal spores may cause serious, potentially fatal pulmonary disease in immunocompromised people. These fungi include *Aspergillus, Blastomyces dermatitidis, Candida,* and *Cryptococcus neoformans.*

Outcome Management

Mild, primary forms of fungal pulmonary disease usually do not require treatment. Progressive, disseminated, or chronic forms are usually treated with intravenous amphotericin B until the client is asymptomatic for 7 to 10 days. This fungicidal antibiotic is toxic, and acute reactions (e.g., chills, fever, vomiting, headache, decreased renal function) may occur during its infusion. Antiemetics, antihistamines, antipyretics, or hydrocortisone may be prescribed as premedications. To reduce the common problem of thrombophlebitis at the intravenous site, a small amount of heparin may be added to the infusion. Ketoconazole and fluconazole, less toxic oral medications, may also be used. If the disorder is not responsive to drug therapy, surgical removal of affected areas (e.g., lung cavities) may be necessary.

Nursing management in relation to fungal pulmonary infection consists of (1) providing preventive education to minimize exposure of clients to infectious fungi (i.e., learning to avoid high-risk situations and to recognize early indications of infection) and (2) appropriate support and education for infected clients and their significant others, along with symptomatic management of the disease. Education involves teaching about not only the disease and intervention measures but also reportable indications of complications.

NEOPLASTIC LUNG DISORDERS
MALIGNANT LUNG TUMORS

Lung cancer is malignancy in the epithelium of the respiratory tract. At least a dozen different cell types of tumors are included in the classification of lung cancer. The following are the four major types of lung cancer:

- Small cell carcinoma (oat cell carcinoma)
- Squamous cell carcinoma (epidermoid)
- Adenocarcinoma
- Large cell carcinoma

There is no current effective screening test for lung cancer, and the range of treatment options is limited, resulting in frequent poor prognoses. Lung cancer is the leading cause of cancer deaths in the United States, killing approximately 159,000 Americans yearly.[16] The term *lung cancer* excludes other lung disorders, such as sarcoma, lymphoma, blastoma, and mesothelioma.

Etiology and Risk Factors

Cigarette smoking is by far the most important risk factor for lung cancer. Ninety percent of clients who develop lung cancer are, or have been, smokers. Cigarette smoke contains tar, nicotine, carbon monoxide, formaldehyde, hydrogen cyanide, and benzene. The relative risk of developing lung cancer is increased about 13-fold by active smoking and about 1.5-fold by long-term passive exposure to cigarette smoke. The lung cancer death rate is related to the total amount (often expressed in "cigarette pack-years") of cigarettes smoked, such that the risk is increased 60- to 70-fold for a person smoking two packs a day for 20 years as compared with a non-smoker. Persons who develop lung cancer may have a genetic predisposition. First-degree relatives of persons with lung cancer have a two- to three-fold excess risk of lung cancer or other cancers, many of which are not smoking related. Genetic epidemiologic studies have proposed an association between the P450 enzyme or chromosome fragility genotypes and the development of lung cancer. Age also has a role because lung cancer rarely occurs in people younger than 40 years. Finally, TB and low-level radiation are also risks for lung cancer.

Pathophysiology

Lung cancers are divided into two major categories: (1) small cell lung cancers (SCLCs) and (2) non–small cell lung cancers (NSCLCs), which include squamous cell carcinoma, adenocarcinoma, and large cell carcinoma. The characteristics of each of these types are described in Table 64-2. The cancerous lung tissue cannot exchange oxygen and carbon dioxide and therefore performs no biological function. Furthermore, tumor cells grow and invade surrounding lung tissue. Airways are invaded, obstructing the flow of air. Cancerous cells invade local lymph nodes and the thoracic duct. Significant growth of the tumor and invasion may occur before diagnosis.

In general, survival rates are best for NSCLC, especially with treatment in the early stages. Despite growing knowledge and improving technology, however, overall survival of lung cancer remains low, especially for clients with small cell carcinomas.

Clinical Manifestations

The warning signals of lung cancer are presented in Box 64-2. In many instances, lung cancer may mimic other pulmonary conditions. Extrapulmonary manifestations may occur before pulmonary manifestations. Specific clinical assessment findings vary according to tumor type, location, and extent as well as pre-existing pulmonary health.

Centrally located pulmonary tumors usually obstruct air flow, producing clinical manifestations such as coughing, wheezing, stridor, and dyspnea. As obstruction increases, bronchopulmonary infection often occurs distal to the obstruction. Chest, shoulder, arm, and back pain may develop as the tumor invades the perivascular nerves. Squamous and small cell tumors often cause hemoptysis. Small cell tumors may also extend into the pericardium, causing pericardial effusion and, possibly, tamponade. Cardiac dysrhythmias are also likely.

Peripheral pulmonary tumors often do not produce early assessment findings. In time, pleural pain develops that increases on inspiration, is sharp and severe, and is usually localized. Pleural effusion (see later) also occurs and, along with the pain, limits lung expansion. Only 30% of peripheral lung tumors are successfully categorized by bronchoscopic and cytologic examination.

Pancoast's tumor occurs in the apices of the lungs in both squamous cell and adenocarcinomatous cancers. The tumor is asymptomatic until it extends into surrounding structures. Clinical manifestations are caused by compression of the brachial plexus in the distribution from the eighth cervical nerve to the first two thoracic nerves. This results in arm and shoulder pain on the affected side along with atrophy of the arm and hand muscles. With continuing tumor growth, the ribs over the tumor (usually the first and second ribs) may be invaded, resulting in bone pain. Later, involvement of the cervical sympathetic nerve ganglia may lead to *Horner's syndrome*. This syndrome consists of miosis (contraction of the pupil), partial ptosis (drooping upper eyelid), and anhidrosis (absence of sweating) on the affected side of the face.

Diagnostic Findings

Numerous diagnostic tests may be used to determine the presence and extent of lung cancer. Sputum cytologic

TABLE 64-2	*Overview of Malignant Pulmonary Neoplasms*		
Cell Type	**Approximate Incidence**	**Specific Characteristics**	**Growth Rate**
Epidermoid (squamous cell)	30%-35%	Arises from bronchial epithelium As growth occurs, cavitation may develop in lung distal to tumor; Pancoast's tumor arises in apex and upper lung zones Secondary infections distal to obstructive tumor in bronchioles commonly occur	Slow growth, with metastasis not common If metastasis occurs, usually to lymph, adrenals, and liver
Adenocarcinoma	35%-40%	Majority arises from bronchial mucous gland Often subpleural; rarely cavitates; often arises in previously scarred lung tissue Incidence strongly linked to cigarette smoking Increasing incidence in women Bronchioloalveolar cell carcinoma is a subtype	Slow growth Can metastasize throughout lung or to other organs of the body
Large cell	15%-20%	More often peripheral mass, either single or multiple masses Cavitation common May be located centrally, midlung, or peripherally Rare hilar involvement Often grows to large tumor mass before diagnosis	Slow Metastasis may occur to kidney, liver, and adrenals
Small cell (oat cell)	20%-25%	65%-75% manifest as hilar or central mass May compress bronchi Involvement of diaphragm through paralysis of phrenic nerve and hoarseness through paralysis of recurrent laryngeal nerve Pleural and pericardial effusions and tamponade often seen Does not form cavities	Rapid growth Metastasis to mediastinum and to thoracic and extrathoracic structures occurs early

study and chest radiograph are most commonly used. Bronchoscopy may be used to biopsy a tumor located in the bronchial tree. CT scans provide detailed anatomic assessment of the chest and adjacent lymph nodes. Magnetic resonance imaging (MRI) can provide high-quality images of the lung and mediastinum to assess for tumor invasion. New imaging techniques use monoclonal antibodies that have an affinity for cancer cells. The antibodies are tagged with technetium and injected into the client. They concentrate in the area of tumor and can be detected by single-photon emission computed tomography (SPECT) images.

Percutaneous transthoracic needle biopsy, mediastinoscopy, or direct surgical biopsy may be required to confirm the diagnosis of certain lung cancers. Radionuclide scans may be used to detect metastasis to the bone, liver, or brain (see Chapter 4). Central pulmonary tumors are easiest to locate and identify with fiberoptic

BOX 64-2	*Warning Signals of Lung Cancer*

- Any change in respiratory patterns
- Persistent cough
- Sputum streaked with blood
- Frank hemoptysis
- Rust-colored or purulent sputum
- Unexplained weight loss
- Fatigue
- Chest, shoulder, back, or arm pain
- Recurring episodes of pleural effusion, pneumonia, or bronchitis
- Unexplained dyspnea

bronchoscopy and sputum cytologic study. During bronchoscopy, bronchial washings or brushings are performed to obtain tumor cells for cytologic and pathologic study. Positive tissue diagnosis is possible 90% of the time.

The tumor-node-metastasis (TNM) classification scheme is used for lung cancer staging (Figure 64-3). Staging is performed to provide a guideline for the selection of appropriate therapies and to estimate prognosis. Staging information is valuable in helping clients and their families make treatment decisions and set appropriate short-term and long-term goals.

Metastasis

If tumors spread, by either direct extension or metastasis, further clinical manifestations may result. Direct extension to the recurrent laryngeal nerve produces hoarseness. Compression of the esophagus may cause dysphagia. Invasion or compression of the superior vena cava produces superior vena cava syndrome, a potentially life-threatening emergency. Obstruction of venous blood flow leads to clinical manifestations, including (1) shortness of breath, (2) facial, arm, and trunk swelling, (3) distended neck veins, (4) chest pain, and (5) venous stasis. Immediate palliative surgical treatment may be necessary.

Regional lymph node involvement may produce manifestations caused by impaired lymph drainage. Involvement of the mediastinal lymph nodes may result in vocal cord paralysis, dysphagia, diaphragmatic paralysis on the affected side (due to phrenic nerve compression), vena cava compression, and malignant pleural effusion (see later discussion). Usually, when mediastinal lymph nodes are involved, surgical excision of the pulmonary tumor is no longer possible.

Outcome Management
■ Medical Management

Early Identification. Early detection is the key to improving survival rates for clients with lung cancer. When premalignant changes begin, dysplastic cells are identifiable with fiberoptic bronchoscopy and sputum cytologic studies. At this stage, lesions are potentially curable. However, a tumor must be at least 1 cm in diameter before it is detectable on a chest radiograph; invasion and metastasis have usually already occurred once the tumor reaches this size.

Management of the client with lung cancer depends on tumor type and stage as well as the client's underlying health status. Following diagnosis, primary treatment modalities are surgery, radiation therapy, and chemotherapy.

Radiation Therapy. Radiation therapy (radiotherapy) may be used as a potentially curative treatment in clients with locally advanced disease (1) for whom surgery poses

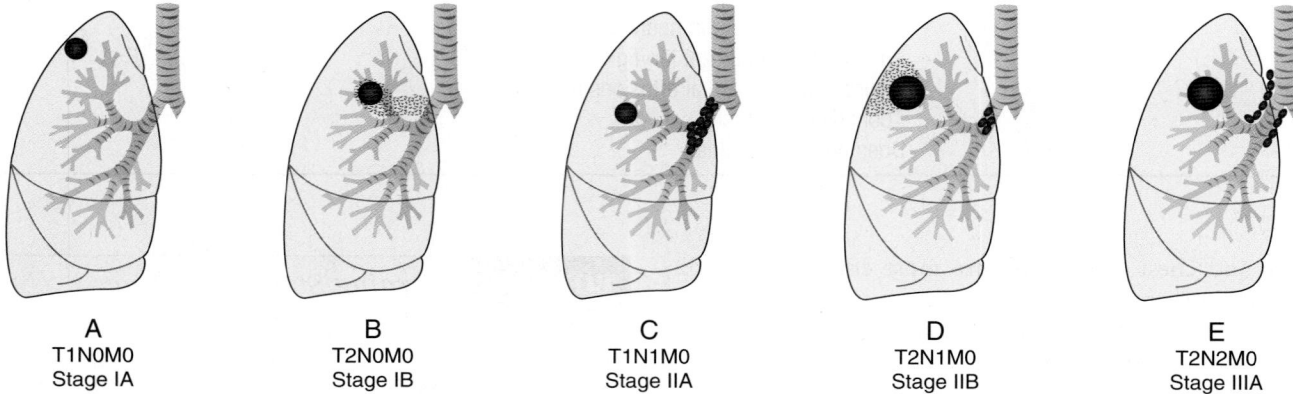

A	B	C	D	E
T1N0M0	T2N0M0	T1N1M0	T2N1M0	T2N2M0
Stage IA	Stage IB	Stage IIA	Stage IIB	Stage IIIA

FIGURE 64-3 Examples of stages of lung cancer by the tumor-node-metastasis (TNM) classification system. **A,** Stage IA—T1N0M0: tumor is 3 cm or less in diameter with no metastases to regional lymph nodes and no distant metastasis. **B,** Stage IB—T2N0M0: tumor is greater than 3 cm in diameter or is any size that either invades the visceral pleura or has associated atelectasis or obstructive pneumonitis extending to the hilar region; however, there are no metastases to lymph nodes or distant metastasis. **C,** Stage IIA—T1N1M0: tumor is 3 cm or less in diameter with metastasis to lymph nodes in the peribronchial or ipsilateral hilar region, or both, without distant metastasis. **D,** Stage IIB—T2N1M0: tumor is greater than 3 cm in diameter or is any size that either invades the visceral pleura or has associated atelectasis or obstructive pneumonitis extending to the hilar region, with metastasis to lymph nodes in the peribronchial or ipsilateral hilar region, or both, without distant metastasis. **E,** Stage IIIA—T2N2M0: tumor is greater than 3 cm in diameter or is any size that either invades the visceral pleura or has associated atelectasis or obstructive pneumonitis extending to the hilar region, with metastasis to ipsilateral mediastinal or subcarinal nodes, without distant metastasis.

an unacceptably high risk, (2) who have technically inoperable tumors, or (3) who refuse thoracotomy. Radiation therapy may also be used in combination with surgery or chemotherapy to improve treatment outcomes.

Radiotherapy is administered over a period of 5 to 6 weeks, either consecutively or in split courses. Doses are limited by the presence of other structures in the treatment area and by normal tissue tolerance. Irreversible fibrotic changes and other pulmonary side effects may occur. To delineate precisely the area to be irradiated, CT scanning is often performed before treatment begins. This method also minimizes tissue damage to surrounding areas.

Radiotherapy may also be used for palliation of manifestations such as pain, shortness of breath, hemoptysis, and obstruction or compression of bronchi, blood vessels, or esophagus. Irradiation of metastases to the brain and bone may reduce the distressing manifestations associated with these sequelae as well.

Chemotherapy. The response of lung cancer to chemotherapy depends on the tumor's cell type. SCLC responds well to chemotherapeutic agents because of its rapid growth rate. Results of clinical trials have demonstrated that long-term survival in clients with SCLC can be improved with intensive combination chemotherapy. As a result, chemotherapy is the cornerstone of management of SCLC.

The effectiveness of chemotherapy in the treatment of NSCLC remains controversial. This modality is commonly used in clients treated with surgery or radiation who experience recurrent disease or distant metastasis. However, large-scale studies have failed to demonstrate significantly improved long-term survival rates for such clients. As a result, the decision to use chemotherapy is usually made on an individual basis, depending on the client's previous history, current condition, and acceptance of the risks and side effects involved.

■ Nursing Management of the Medical Client

Diagnostic Phase. The client who is undergoing diagnostic tests for lung cancer faces an uncertain future. If the diagnosis is confirmed, the client can anticipate a variety of physical difficulties, potentially extensive medical treatment, and many emotional changes. The nursing assessment plays a critical role in developing a plan of care that will provide needed support.

The nursing history should include an exploration of the client's chief complaints, particularly cough (productive or nonproductive), dyspnea, pain, and recurrent infection. Ask the client about the presence of risk factors, such as a smoking history, exposure to occupational respiratory carcinogens, or a family history of the disease. Assess the client's socioeconomic situation and available social support because these factors affect subsequent management options.

Nursing management during the diagnostic phase focuses on emotional support and client education along with required physical care. Help clients maintain a sense of control by keeping them informed about all scheduled tests. Once a diagnosis of lung cancer is confirmed, nursing care must incorporate measures designed to help the client cope with anxiety and fear, family responses, financial considerations, absence from work and social activities, and possible changes in life goals.

Treatment Phase. Nursing care of the client receiving radiation and chemotherapy is detailed in Chapters 18 and 19.

■ Surgical Management

Surgical intervention is the treatment of choice in early-stage NSCLC. Cure is possible if the disease is still localized to the thoracic cavity and no distant metastases are present. However, only 20% to 25% of clients with NSCLC meet these criteria at the time of diagnosis. For clients who successfully undergo surgical resection, the 5-year survival rate is approximately 35% to 40%.[35]

The role of surgical resection in the treatment of SCLC is limited. Surgery may be effective for clients with the early stages of SCLC, as a component of combined modality therapy. For clients with more advanced disease, surgery causes unnecessary risk and stress, with no valid benefits.

The primary aim of surgical resection is to remove the tumor completely while preserving as much of the normal surrounding lung tissue as possible. The extent of the operation depends on the location and size of the pulmonary tumor and the severity of the underlying pathologic process. Clients with pre-existing pulmonary disease may not be able to tolerate extensive removal of lung tissue.

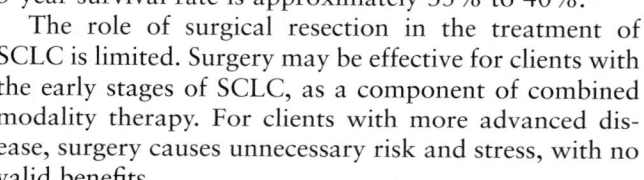

Preoperative Management

Extensive pulmonary function testing may be performed before surgery to determine the client's ability to tolerate the proposed surgical intervention. Clients with impaired pulmonary function may be treated with antibiotics, bronchodilating medications, intermittent positive-pressure breathing procedures, and supervised breathing exercises to improve respiratory efficiency. Clients are encouraged to refrain from smoking during the preoperative period because smoking increases pulmonary secretions and diminishes blood oxygen saturation.

Surgical Procedures

Laser Surgery. One surgical treatment modality is laser therapy. Currently, laser therapy is used as a palliative measure for relief of endobronchial obstructions that are not resectable. Laser procedures do not produce systemic or cumulative toxic effects and are well tolerated. Laser therapy may be given in an outpatient setting. However, for the laser to be used, the tumor mass must be accessible by bronchoscopy. Therefore tumors pressing on bronchial tissue from outside the bronchial lumen are not amenable to laser therapy.

Pulmonary Resection. Complete resection of tumor remains the best chance of cure. Common pulmonary resection procedures are shown in Figure 64-4 and are discussed here.

Wedge Resection. Removal of a small, localized area of diseased tissue near the surface of the lung. Because the resected area is small, pulmonary structure and function are relatively unchanged after healing.

Segmental Resection. Removal of one or more lung segments (a bronchiole and its alveoli). The remaining lung tissue overexpands to fill the previously occupied space.

Lobectomy. Removal of an entire lobe of the lung. Postoperatively, the remaining lung overexpands to fill the open portion of the thoracic space.

Pneumonectomy. Removal of an entire lung. Once the lung is removed, the involved side of the thoracic cavity is an empty space. To reduce the size of the cavity, the surgeon severs the phrenic nerve on the affected side to paralyze the diaphragm in an elevated position. A thoracoplasty, which is the removal of several ribs or portions of ribs to further reduce the thoracic space, may also be performed.

Closed-chest drainage is not used after pneumonectomy. The serous fluid that accumulates postoperatively in the empty thoracic cavity eventually consolidates, which prevents shifts of the mediastinum, heart, and remaining lung.

Chest Tubes. Chest surgery causes a pneumothorax on the operated side. During thoracotomy, the parietal pleura is incised, and the pleural space is entered. Atmospheric air rushes into the pleural space. This changes the normally negative pressure in that pleural space to a positive pressure. As a result, the lung recoils to its unexpanded size and remains collapsed. Chest trauma, such as rib fractures, leads to pneumothorax in the same manner. Chest tubes are usually inserted in an operating room during chest surgery. However, in some emergencies, a chest tube may be inserted in a treatment room or at the bedside.

Two catheters are usually placed in the chest following resectional surgery (except pneumonectomy). One catheter (the upper, or anterior, tube) is placed anteriorly through the second intercostal space to permit the escape of air rising in the pleural space. The other catheter (the lower, or posterior, tube) is placed posteriorly through the eighth or ninth intercostal space in the midaxillary line to drain serosanguineous fluid accumulating in the lower portion of the pleural space. The lower tube may have a larger diameter than the upper tube, to enhance fluid drainage. Chest tubes are brought out of the chest wall through stab wounds or through the incision. The catheters are secured to the client's skin with sutures.

The two chest tubes may be joined to each other with a plastic Y-junction (and then attached to one closed-chest drainage system). However, it is preferable to leave them separate and to attach them to separate drainage systems. This arrangement makes it possible to monitor air and fluid drainage from each tube and, later, to remove a nondraining tube without disrupting the rest of the system. Flexible drainage tubing connects the chest tube to the drainage collection apparatus. Usually, chest tubes are connected to a closed-chest drainage apparatus before the client leaves the operating room.

■ Nursing Management of the Surgical Client

Preoperative Assessment
Preoperative preparation of the client with lung cancer who is to undergo surgery is the same as for any surgical client but with greater emphasis on assessment and

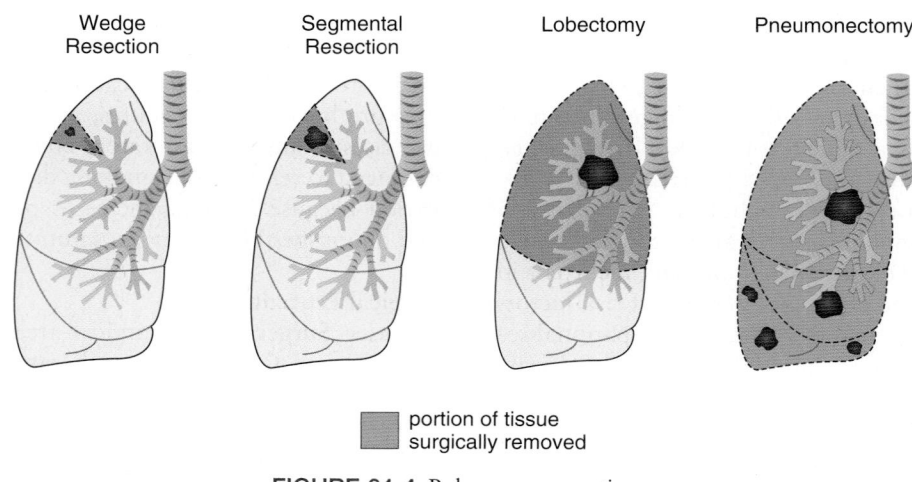

Wedge   Segmental   Lobectomy   Pneumonectomy
Resection   Resection

portion of tissue
surgically removed

FIGURE 64-4 Pulmonary resections.

preparation of the respiratory system (see Chapter 16 for discussion of preoperative nursing care).

Preoperative Care

Nursing interventions during the preoperative period are aimed primarily at reducing the client's anxiety level. Anxiety results from fear of cancer and its prognosis as well as from fear of the surgical procedure and insufficient knowledge of surgical routines and postoperative self-care activities. The client and family are taught about the following issues:

The anticipated surgical procedure: Assess the client's (and family's) understanding, and give further information as needed.

The early postoperative period: Talk specifically about what will be happening to the client and how he or she can participate in recovery activities. Specific explanations should be given about the presence of chest tubes (except with pneumonectomy) and drainage tubes, intubation and mechanical ventilation, oxygen therapy, and available pain reduction measures.

Postoperative exercises: These include (1) respiratory exercises, such as the use of incentive spirometry to maintain effective pulmonary function, (2) splinting techniques to promote effective coughing and deep breathing (Figure 64-5), and (3) leg exercises to prevent thrombophlebitis. All of these exercises should be demonstrated preoperatively, and opportunity should be given for practice and return demonstration.

Postoperative Assessment

During the immediate postoperative period, thorough assessment is essential. Make observations as often as

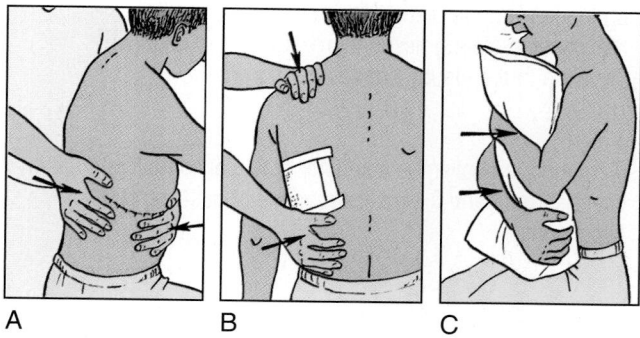

A   B   C

FIGURE 64-5 Splinting techniques to promote effective coughing and deep breathing. Apply firm, even pressure after the client has taken a deep breath and during forced expiratory cough. Do not squeeze the chest or interfere with chest inspiratory expansion. **A,** Place one hand around the client's back and the other around the incisional area. **B,** Support the area below the incision with one hand while exerting downward pressure on the shoulder on the affected side with the other. **C,** Have the person hug a pillow during forced expiratory cough.

the client's condition warrants. Frequency of observations is determined by the following factors:

- Amount of anesthesia received and the client's reaction to it
- Amount of intraoperative blood loss
- The client's preoperative condition (e.g., presence of pre-existing medical conditions, such as COPD, diabetes and heart disorders)
- The client's response to pain
- Facility protocols

Postoperative Care

Nursing interventions are based on careful assessment and appropriate nursing diagnoses. General postoperative nursing measures are applicable (see Chapter 16). See the Care Plan feature on The Client Undergoing Thoracic Surgery on pp. 1858 to 1862 for a discussion of nursing management.

Maintain Closed-Chest Drainage. Clients have closed-chest drainage after all forms of chest surgery (except pneumonectomy) and some forms of chest trauma. In closed-chest drainage, the chest drainage system is airtight, or closed, to prevent the inflow of atmospheric pressure. Historically, closed-chest drainage was performed with the use of a glass bottle water-seal apparatus (one-, two-, or three-bottle setup) with or without controlled mechanical suction. Glass bottle water-seal drainage systems have been replaced with disposable single units, such as the Pleur-Evac, Atrium, or Aqua-Seal (Figure 64-6). However, knowledge of the basic principles of closed-chest drainage aid in understanding any specific system.

Closed-chest drainage after thoracotomy or chest trauma is used to do the following:

- Promote evacuation of air and serosanguineous fluid from the pleural space and prevent the reflux of atmospheric air into the pleural space
- Help reexpand the remaining lung tissue by reestablishing normal negative pressure in the pleural space
- Prevent mediastinal shift and pneumothorax by equalizing pressures on the two sides of the thoracic cavity

Closed drainage systems have three main compartments:

1. The *collection chamber* collects drainage and allows monitoring of the volume, rate, and nature of drainage.
2. The *water-seal chamber* is used as a one-way valve so that air or fluids can drain from the client's chest but not return.
3. The *suction-control chamber* uses suction to promote drainage from the pleural space (at a greater rate than achieved by gravity alone) and assist in reexpanding the lung.

Text continued on p. 1862

CARE PLAN

The Client Undergoing Thoracic Surgery

Collaborative Problem. Potential complications of thoracic surgery: pulmonary edema; respiratory insufficiency; tension pneumothorax and mediastinal shift; subcutaneous emphysema; pulmonary embolus; cardiac dysrhythmias; hemorrhage, hemothorax, and hypovolemic shock; and thrombophlebitis.

Outcomes. The nurse will monitor for respiratory, cardiac, and vascular complications.

Interventions	Rationales

1. Monitor for manifestations of respiratory failure:
  a. Tachypnea and tachycardia
  b. Dyspnea
  c. Use of accessory muscles or retractions
  d. Cyanosis
  e. Decreased pulse oximetry
  f. Decreased Pao_2 levels and increased $Paco_2$ levels
  g. Restlessness
  h. Increase in adventitious breath sounds
	1. Postoperatively, respiratory insufficiency may result from an altered level of consciousness due to anesthesia and pain medications, incomplete lung reinflation, decreased respiratory effort due to chest pain, and inadequate airway clearance.

2. Monitor for manifestations of tension pneumothorax:
  a. Severe dyspnea
  b. Tachypnea and tachycardia
  c. Extreme restlessness and agitation
  d. Progressive cyanosis
  e. Laryngeal and tracheal deviation to unaffected side
  f. Lateral or medial PMI shift
	2. Postoperative tension pneumothorax can result from air leaking through pleural incision lines if closed-chest drainage fails to function properly.

3. Observe for subcutaneous emphysema around incision and in the chest and neck:
  a. Assess progression by periodically marking the chest with a skin-marking pencil at the outer periphery of emphysematous tissue. If neck involvement occurs, measure neck circumference at least every 2 to 4 hours.
  b. Keep emergency tracheostomy tray at bedside
	3. Subcutaneous emphysema may result from air leakage at pulmonary incision site.
	  a. Rapid progression (i.e., an increase of more than a hand's width in 1 hour) may indicate leakage through the bronchial stump.
	
	  b. Severe subcutaneous emphysema in the neck may compress the trachea and may require tracheostomy.

4. Monitor chest tube drainage system:
  a. Amount and color of drainage
  b. Water-seal chamber for tidaling and bubbling
  c. Suction control chamber filled to appropriate level and bubbling
  d. Intact and occlusive dressing at insertion site
	4. Chest tube drainage systems promote evacuation of air and drainage from the pleural space and assist in the reexpansion of lung tissue by reestablishing negative pressure in the pleural space after surgery.

5. Monitor for manifestations of pulmonary embolus:
  a. Chest pain
  b. Dyspnea and tachypnea
  c. Fever
  d. Hemoptysis
  e. Indications of right-sided heart failure
	5. Pulmonary embolism is a serious potential complication after chest surgery and a significant cause of postoperative hypoxemia.

6. Monitor for manifestations of acute pulmonary edema:
  a. Dyspnea
  b. Crackles
  c. Persistent cough
  d. Frothy sputum
  e. Cyanosis
  f. Decreased pulse oximetry reading
	6. Circulatory overload may result from the reduced size of the pulmonary vascular bed due to surgical removal of pulmonary tissue and delayed reexpansion of the affected lung. Additionally, hypoxia increases capillary permeability, causing fluid to enter pulmonary tissue.

$Paco_2$, Partial pressure of arterial carbon dioxide; Pao_2, partial pressure of arterial oxygen; *PMI*, point of maximal impulse; *ROM*, range of motion.

CARE PLAN

Interventions	Rationales
7. Monitor intravenous flow rates. Consult physician if fluid amounts (maintenance plus intermittent medications [e.g., antibiotics]) exceed 125 ml/hr.	7. After chest surgery, intravenous fluids should not exceed 125 ml/hr because of possible circulatory overload.
8. Assess cardiac monitor for the development of cardiac dysrhythmias, particularly atrial fibrillation, atrial flutter, and paroxysmal atrial tachycardia.	8. Cardiac dysrhythmias are fairly common after chest surgery. Rhythm disturbances result from a combination of factors, including increased vagal tone, hypoxia, mediastinal shift, and abnormal blood pH.
9. Assess dressing and incisional area every 4 hours for evidence of bleeding (increase to every 1 to 2 hours if bleeding develops). Assess drainage in closed-chest drainage system for manifestations of bleeding.	9. Blood loss may be great with major thoracic surgery because blood vessels in the thorax are of large diameter and the incision is often large and produces considerable capillary oozing.
10. Monitor for manifestations of hypovolemic shock: 　a. Increased pulse 　b. Decreased blood pressure 　c. Restlessness and decreased level of consciousness 　d. Decreased urine output (<0.5 ml/kg/hr) 　e. Cool, pale, clammy skin 　f. Increased respirations	10. The body compensates for lost blood volume by increasing blood flow (through increased heart rate) to vital organs and decreasing peripheral circulation.
11. Monitor for thrombophlebitis: 　a. Unilateral leg edema 　b. Calf tenderness, redness, unusual warmth	11. Anesthesia and immobility reduce vasomotor tone, leading to decreased venous return and peripheral pooling of blood.
12. Encourage client to perform leg exercises. Discourage placing pillows under knees, crossing the legs, or prolonged sitting. Apply elastic hose or pneumatic compression stockings, if ordered.	12. These measures prevent venous stasis, thus reducing the risk of thrombophlebitis.

Evaluation. The nurse monitors for the development of these complications. Most occur early after surgery, except for pulmonary embolus.

Nursing Diagnosis. Ineffective Airway Clearance related to increased secretions and to decreased coughing effectiveness due to pain.

Outcomes. The client will demonstrate effective airway clearance, as evidenced by clear breath sounds, effective coughing, and adequate air exchange in the lungs.

Interventions	Rationales
1. Once vital signs are stable, place the client in semi-Fowler's position.	1. The upright position enhances lung expansion and facilitates ventilation with minimal effort.
2. Help the client cough and deep breathe at least every 1 or 2 hours during the first 24 to 48 postoperative hours.	2. Increasing the volume of air in lungs promotes expulsion of secretions.
3. Instruct the client to take a deep breath slowly and to hold it for 3 to 5 seconds, then exhale; to take a second breath and then, while exhaling, to cough forcefully twice.	3. Coughing helps move tracheobronchial secretions out of the lung. Deep breathing dilates the airways, stimulates surfactant production, and expands lung tissue.
4. When possible, schedule coughing and deep-breathing sessions at times when pain medication is maximally effective.	4. The less postoperative pain a client experiences, the more effective are coughing and deep breathing.
5. Assess breath sounds before and after coughing. Provide support and reassurance: 　a. Explain that breathing exercises will not damage the lungs or the suture line. 　b. Manually splint the incision area during coughing and deep breathing.	5. This helps in evaluation of coughing effectiveness. 　a. Client's fear of "splitting open" the incision may hamper coughing efforts. 　b. Physical support of the incision is both comforting and reassuring.

Continued

CARE PLAN

The Client Undergoing Thoracic Surgery—cont'd

Interventions	Rationales
c. Offer sips of warm water.	c. Warm water can aid relaxation and produce more effective coughing.
d. Maintain adequate level of hydration and adequate humidity of inspired air.	d. Fluids and moisture help thin secretions, making them easier to expectorate.
e. Monitor results of chest radiographs.	e. Frequent chest films help detect atelectasis and infection.
f. Evaluate the need for suctioning.	f. If coughing is ineffective, suctioning may be required to remove pulmonary secretions. Suctioning should be performed cautiously so that disruption of pulmonary suture lines is avoided.

Evaluation. Outcomes on effective airway clearance require days to achieve.

Nursing Diagnosis. Acute Pain related to surgical procedure.

Outcomes. The client will be more comfortable, as evidenced by verbalizing that discomfort is reduced, using less opioid medication, and moving in bed with less pain.

Interventions	Rationales
1. Assess pain intensity using a self-report measurement tool.	1. Use of a consistent, valid tool promotes communication and evaluation of pain intervention effectiveness.
2. Administer pain medication as ordered.	2. Use of opioids is a common method of postoperative pain control. Opioids bind to opiate receptors, decreasing sensations of pain.
3. Observe for side effects of medication used.	3. Side effects are monitored.
4. Offer and instruct clients to ask for pain medication before pain becomes severe.	4. A preventive approach to pain control provides a more consistent level of relief and reduces client anxiety.
5. Assess medication effectiveness and avoid overmedication.	5. Adequate pain reduction must be obtained. However, overmedication can depress respirations and the cough reflex.
6. Use nonpharmacologic pain reduction measures concurrently.	6. Proper positioning, relaxation techniques, and like measures can augment effects of medications.

Evaluation. Pain will be most acute for 48 to 72 hours postoperatively, requiring opioids for pain control. Expect pain to subside after that time, and offer less potent opioids or analgesics.

Nursing Diagnosis. Impaired Physical Mobility related to pain, muscle dissection, restricted positioning, and chest tubes.

Outcomes. The client will maintain physical mobility in the arm and shoulder, as evidenced by regaining of preoperative arm and shoulder function.

Interventions	Rationales
1. Position client as indicated by phase of recovery and surgical procedure:	1. Repositioning maximizes long expansion and drainage of secretions, promotes ventilation and oxygenation, and enhances comfort.
a. Nonoperative side-lying position may be used until consciousness is regained.	a. This position prevents aspiration.
b. Semi-Fowler's position (head of bed elevated 30 to 45 degrees) is recommended once vital signs are stable.	b. The upright position enhances lung expansion and facilitates chest tube drainage.

Pa_{CO_2}, Partial pressure of arterial carbon dioxide; Pa_{O_2}, partial pressure of arterial oxygen; *PMI*, point of maximal impulse; *ROM*, range of motion.

CARE PLAN

Interventions	Rationales
c. Avoid positioning client on operative side if a wedge resection or segmentectomy has been performed.	c. Lying on the operative side hinders expansion of remaining lung tissue and may accentuate perfusion of poorly ventilated tissue, thus further impeding normal gas exchange.
d. Avoid complete lateral positioning after pneumonectomy.	d. Because the mediastinum is no longer held in place on both sides by lung tissue, extreme turning may cause mediastinal shift and compression of the remaining lung.
2. Gently turn the client every 1 to 2 hours, unless contraindicated.	2. Frequent turning promotes mobilization and drainage of air and fluid from the pleural space. Turning also improves circulation, promotes lung aeration, and enhances comfort.
3. Avoid traction on chest tubes while changing client position. Check for kinking or compression of tubing.	3. Traction may dislodge the chest tubes. Kinking or compression inhibits drainage and reestablishment of negative intrapleural pressure.
4. Encourage regular ambulation, once the client's condition is stable. Maintain supplemental oxygen, if ordered.	4. Early ambulation improves ventilation, circulation, and morale. Oxygen therapy is used to avoid hypoxia.
5. Begin passive ROM exercises of the arm and shoulder on the affected side 4 hours after recovery from anesthesia. Exercises should be performed two times every 4 to 6 hours through the first 24 postoperative hours, with progression to 10 to 20 times every 2 hours.	5. ROM exercises help prevent adhesion formation in the operative area, which can lead to dysfunction syndrome (i.e., "frozen shoulder").
6. Active ROM exercises are begun once the client's condition permits.	6. Active ROM exercises prevent adhesions of the incised muscle layers.
7. Encourage the client to use the arm on the affected side in daily activities (e.g., eating, reaching, grooming). Keep bedside stand on the operative side to encourage reaching. Teach the importance of continued use of the arm after discharge.	7. Regular use of the affected arm and shoulder reduces the possibility of contractures.
8. Carefully assess client's response to activity and exercise. Observe for manifestations of dyspnea and fatigue.	8. It may take time for the client's activity tolerance to increase, because the body must adjust to reduced respiratory capacity after resectional surgery.
9. Allow adequate rest periods between activities.	9. Adequate rest enables the client to cooperate more fully with activities.

Evaluation. Expect the client to be able to turn independently after 24 hours. Improvement in ROM requires a few days, until pain subsides and the chest tube is removed.

Nursing Diagnosis. Risk for Ineffective Coping related to temporary dependence and loss of full respiratory function.

Outcomes. The client will use adaptive coping mechanisms, as evidenced by verbalizing feelings related to emotional state and taking appropriate actions to regain self-care capabilities.

Interventions	Rationales
1. Provide opportunity for client to express feelings.	1. Loss of normal body function and self-care capabilities can lead to feelings of powerlessness, anger, and grief. Open expression of these feelings can help client begin coping.
2. Encourage use of positive coping strategies that have been successful in the past.	2. The use of effective coping actions can decrease feelings of hopelessness and helplessness.
3. Allow client to have as much control over daily activities and decision making as is possible.	3. Active involvement in the plan of care gives the client a sense of control and promotes return to independence.

Continued

CARE PLAN

The Client Undergoing Thoracic Surgery—cont'd

Interventions	Rationales
4. Support and praise all independent activities that promote recovery.	4. Emotional support and encouragement help motivate client to continue progress toward independence.

Evaluation. The use of effective coping mechanisms depends on prior coping strategies. This outcome may be met quickly if the client is able to cope with a diagnosis of cancer and has hope for recovery and a support system. On the contrary, coping in the face of a dreaded diagnosis, fear of pain, little hope for recovery, and limited support systems taxes the client's coping mechanisms.

Nursing Diagnosis. Deficient Knowledge related to self-care after discharge.

Outcomes. Client will be able to state or demonstrate discharge plans.

Interventions	Rationales
1. Provide thorough instruction and preparation for hospital discharge:	1. Thorough understanding promotes compliance and enhances self-care capabilities.
a. Surgical wound and chest tube insertion site care	a. Wound care varies according to condition of incision and client.
b. Continuation of exercise program	b. Continued exercise increases activity tolerance and prevents complications.
c. Precautions regarding activity and environmental irritants	c. Heavy lifting should be avoided. Return to work depends on the client's condition and type of job. However, it is usually possible to return to work within 4 to 6 weeks. Environmental irritants can cause severe coughing episodes.
d. Clinical manifestations to be reported to health care professional	d. Evidence of infection, deteriorating respiratory status, or other complications should be reported promptly.
e. Importance of regular follow-up care	e. The client should be monitored closely for manifestations of surgical complications, recurrence of malignancy, and metastasis.
f. Community agencies that can provide resources, as needed	f. Community resources can facilitate home management.

Evaluation. Client and family must demonstrate understanding of discharge teaching.

Paco₂, Partial pressure of arterial carbon dioxide; *Pao₂*, partial pressure of arterial oxygen; *PMI*, point of maximal impulse; *ROM*, range of motion.

Assess Chest Drainage. Measure *and* document the amount of drainage coming from the pleural space in the collection chamber. This record helps determine the amount of blood loss and the flow rate of drainage from the pleural space. Disposable plastic systems are manufactured with a marked write-on surface on which to record the amount of drainage. Drainage rates and amounts are used in planning blood replacement therapy and assessing the client's status. As much as 500 to 1000 ml of drainage may occur in the first 24 hours after chest surgery. Between 100 and 300 ml of drainage may accumulate during the first 2 hours; after this time, the drainage should lessen. Excessive drainage or a sudden large increase may require further surgery to determine its cause.

Normally, chest drainage is grossly bloody immediately following surgery, but it should not continue to be so for more than several hours. Assess blood loss by monitoring the rising fluid level in the collection chamber. Suspect hemorrhage if the pulse rate becomes rapid and the blood pressure drops. Check fluid in the drainage collection chamber. If the fluid level has not risen, check the tubes for patency. Notify the surgeon if (1) the drainage remains frankly bloody for longer than the first few postoperative hours, (2) bleeding recurs after it has slowed, or (3) there are any other manifestations of hemorrhage.

Assess Water-Seal Function. A water seal provides a one-way valve between atmospheric pressure and sub-

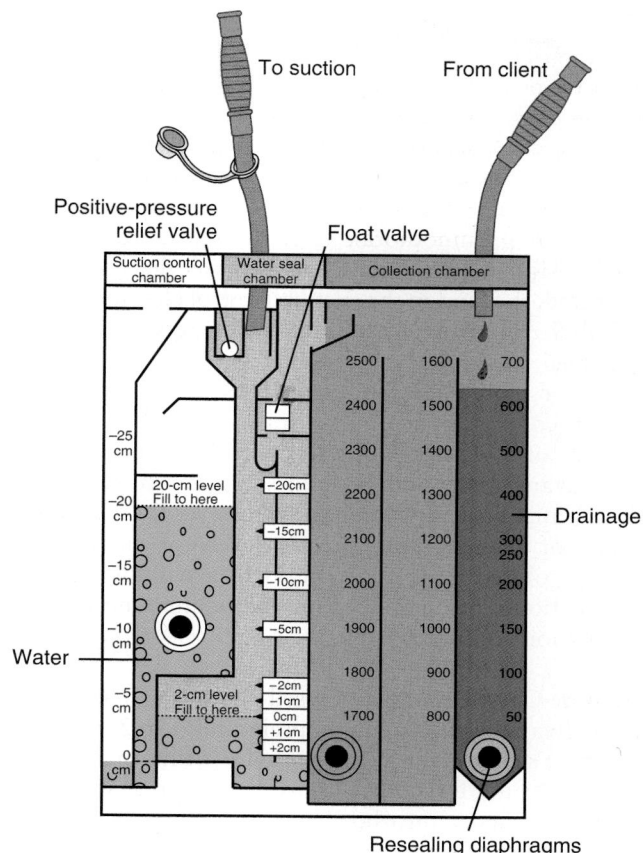

FIGURE 64-6 A commonly used disposable chest drainage system combines the three bottles into a single device. (Courtesy of Deknatel, Fall River, MA.)

atmospheric (negative) intrapleural pressure. It allows air and fluid to leave the intrapleural space but prevents the back-flow of atmospheric air into the chest.

On expiration, air and fluid in the pleural space travel through the drainage tubing. The air bubbles up through the water seal and enters atmospheric air. On inspiration, the water seal prevents atmospheric air from being sucked back into the pleural space (which would collapse the lung). The fluid in the water-seal compartment is not drawn into the chest cavity because the negative pressures generated during inspiration in the intrapleural space are not high enough to pull the fluid through the drainage tubing. However, fluctuation of the fluid occurs during respiration; this fluctuation is called *tidaling* (tidal movement) or *vacillation*.

A closed-chest drainage system must be airtight between the pleural space and the water-seal compartment. Any air leak allows the entry of atmospheric air into the pleural space during inspiration, creating a positive pressure that collapses the lung. All connections within the drainage system must be tight and secure. However, the water-seal chamber itself *must* have an air vent to pro-

vide an escape route for air passing through the water seal from the pleural space.

Observe the Water Seal. Fluid in the water-seal compartment should rise with inspiration and fall with expiration (tidaling). When tidaling is occurring, the drainage tubes are patent and the apparatus is functioning properly. Tidaling stops when the lung has reexpanded or if the chest drainage tubes are kinked or obstructed. If tidaling does not occur:

1. Check to make sure the tubing is not kinked or compressed.
2. Change the client's position.
3. Have the client deep breathe and cough.
4. *If indicated,* milk the tube (see later discussion). If these measures do not restore tidaling, notify the surgeon. (*Note:* Tidaling may not occur or may be minimal in systems not using suction.)

Observe for Bubbling in the Water-Seal Compartment. Bubbling in the water-seal compartment is caused by air passing out of the pleural space into the fluid in the chamber. *Intermittent* bubbling is normal and indicates that the system is accomplishing one of its purposes, that is, removing air from the pleural space.

Continuous bubbling during both inspiration and expiration, however, indicates that air is leaking into the drainage system or pleural cavity. Because air entering the system also enters the pleural space, this situation must be corrected in the following manner:

1. Locate the source of the air leak, and repair it if you can. Begin by inspecting the chest wall where the catheters are inserted.
2. If a chest catheter is loose or has been partially removed, gently squeeze the skin up around the catheter or apply sterile petrolatum gauze around the insertion site. Determine whether this measure stops the continuous bubbling in the chamber.
3. If the air leak continues, check the tubing, inch by inch, and all the connections. A break in the tubing or a loose connection may be found that can be sealed with tape.
4. If the leak still cannot be located, it may be necessary to replace the drainage system.

Rapid bubbling in the absence of an air leak indicates considerable loss of air, as from an incision or tear in the pulmonary pleura. When this occurs, notify the physician *immediately* so that appropriate measures can be taken to prevent collapse of the lung or mediastinal shift, such as (1) application of suction, (2) increase in the amount of suction, or (3) thoracotomy.

When caring for a client with water-seal drainage, find out whether this particular client's water-seal chamber should be bubbling. Having this knowledge facilitates accurate assessment of the drainage pattern (e.g., if intermittent bubbling changes to constant bubbling or if an apparatus that has not been bubbling begins to bubble).

Suction. Suction at 10 to 20 cm H_2O may be applied to a chest drainage system if gravity drainage is not adequate or if a client's cough and respirations are too weak to force air and fluid out of the pleural space through the chest catheters. Additionally, suction may be applied to closed-chest drainage (1) if air is leaking into the pleural space faster than it can be removed by a water-seal apparatus or (2) to speed up the removal of air from the pleural space. Suction is regulated by the height of the water column in the suction chamber. The more fluid in the chamber, the more suction (subatmospheric pressure) is created. Most clients who require a chest tube postoperatively also need suction for 24 to 72 hours.

If there was no water in the chamber, atmospheric air would go straight from the air vent into the suction source as fast as the suction was applied. Passage of the air through water slows it, and the suction force is controlled. Increasing the source of suction only causes more air to travel through the air vent. The suction applied to the client remains stable. An occluded atmospheric air vent is dangerous because it causes the suction to be applied directly to the pleural cavity. A suction force greater than 50 cm H_2O may cause lung damage.

Assess Suction Apparatus Function. Because most suction regulators can create potentially damaging amounts of suction, the amount of suction in the system must be controlled. Proper functioning of a wet suction control compartment is indicated by continuous bubbling in the suction control chamber. Vigorous bubbling does not increase the amount of suction; rather, it causes the water in the bottle to evaporate more rapidly.

Absence of bubbling in a suction control chamber means that the system is not functioning properly and that the correct level of suction is not being maintained. Possible reasons for malfunction of a mechanical suction apparatus include (1) large amounts of air leaking into the pleural space or into the drainage apparatus and (2) mechanical problems in the regulator (suction power source). The most serious problem is air leaking into the pleural space. Check for air leaks by briefly clamping the chest drainage tube close to the client's body and observing the chamber.

If bubbling begins in the suction control chamber, there is nothing wrong with either the drainage apparatus or the regulator. The problem is therefore an air leak into the pleural space around the chest tubes. If the air leak cannot be sealed off (e.g., with petrolatum gauze), notify the surgeon immediately.

If bubbling does not begin in the suction control chamber when the chest catheter is clamped, the problem is in the drainage connections or the regulator. Check the system carefully, looking for loose connections and for air

leaks around compartment tops and in the tubing (e.g., split tubing). Make sure that the tubing is not kinked, is correctly positioned, and has no dependent loops. If the suction power source appears to be causing the problem, obtain another suction canister and regulator.

Because the chest catheter remains clamped during this inspection, observe the client closely for indications of tension pneumothorax (e.g., dyspnea, tachycardia, hypotension, tracheal shift). As soon as the problem is corrected, the fluid in the suction control chamber begins to bubble. Immediately remove the clamps on the chest catheter.

Newer closed-chest drainage systems feature a dry suction column, which uses a spring or dial mechanism in place of a water column to control the suction level. The advantages include ease in setup, no noise of bubbling water, no evaporation of water over time, and provision of higher, more precise levels of suction. An orange-colored indicator appears in a window to indicate suction is being applied instead of bubbling water in the suction control column.

Promote Chest Drainage. Closed-chest drainage systems must always be placed lower (preferably 1 to 2 feet) than the client's chest. Drainage by gravity is thus maintained, and fluid is not forced back into the pleural space. Chest drainage systems must be placed upright on the floor or hung from the foot of the bed.

If the drainage apparatus is on the floor, be careful not to lower a high-low bed or side rails onto it. If a client with closed-chest drainage is to be moved, always keep the chest drainage system below the level of the client's chest.

If the apparatus is placed above the level of the client's chest, even for a moment, fluid from the drainage chamber is siphoned back into the pleural cavity. If absolutely necessary, chest tubes may be double-clamped briefly during momentary movement of the apparatus above the level of the person's chest (e.g., when moving drainage apparatus from one side of the bed to the other if the tubing is not long enough to allow movement around an end of the bed).

Follow positioning orders carefully. If a client can be positioned on the side that has chest tubes, be sure the client is not lying on (compressing or kinking) the catheters or tubing. This may impair drainage, cause retrograde pressure (forcing drainage back into the pleural cavity), and increase the client's discomfort. Coil the drainage tubing (connecting the chest tube to the drainage apparatus) on the client's mattress so that it falls straight to the drainage apparatus, with no dependent loops. Dependent loops of tubing that contain fluid obstruct fluid flow and create back-pressure, thus impairing air or fluid drainage.

Drainage tubing should be neither too short nor too long. Excessive tubing length causes tangling and kinking. However, make sure the tubing is long enough to allow the person to turn and sit up without pulling on the chest tubes. Each time the client is turned or moved, check the chest tubes to make sure they are not being pulled or displaced. Check the drainage tubing to be certain it is properly positioned.

Tube patency is unlikely to be a problem when chest tubes are evacuating only air or when fluid or blood is draining well by gravity. However, if fragments of a blood clot or lung tissue are visible in the tube, use of chest tube clearance techniques *may* be indicated. Traditionally, nurses have manipulated chest tubes by *milking* or *stripping* (Figure 64-7):

- To strip a chest tube, gently compress it, and slide one hand down the tubing, away from the client's chest and toward the drainage system. Stabilize the tubing with the other hand so that the tube will not be pulled on or displaced during stripping.
- To milk a chest tube, compress the tube intermittently using a twisting or squeezing motion.

Theoretically, these techniques dislodge clot material from the tube lumen and propel it toward the drainage collection chamber. However, studies have demonstrated no difference in tube patency with or without such manipulation. Additionally, stripping a chest tube can cause complications because it creates excessive negative in-

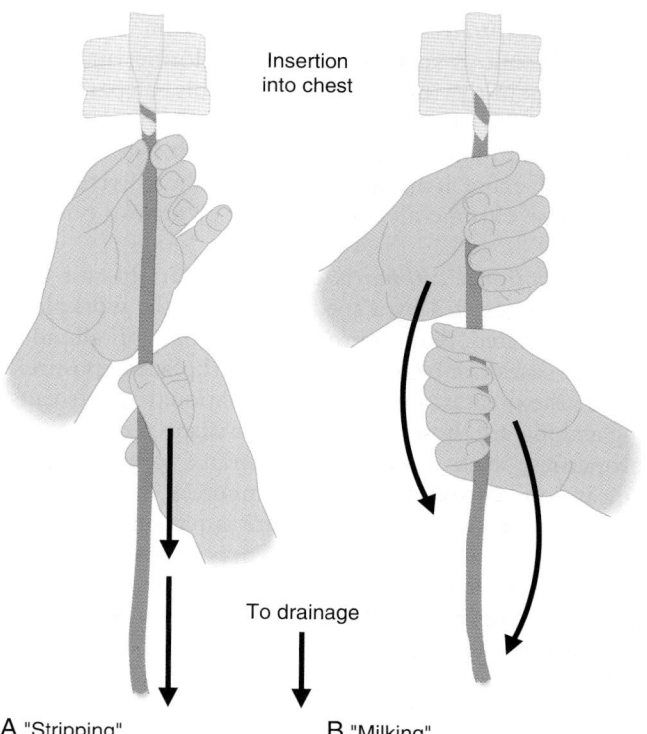

A "Stripping"   B "Milking"

FIGURE 64-7 Stripping (**A**) and milking (**B**) of chest tubes are performed carefully to remove blood clots, but these procedures are not performed routinely.

trapleural pressure (>100 cm H_2O). Therefore these techniques should be used with extreme caution, if at all.

Encourage Activity. Encourage a client with closed-chest drainage to cough and deep breathe frequently. In addition to clearing the bronchi of secretions, these activities promote lung expansion and the expulsion of air and fluid from the pleural space by increasing intrapulmonary and intrapleural pressures.

A client with a chest drainage system can sit up in bed, get in and out of bed, and ambulate without clamping of the chest tubes as long as the apparatus stays upright. Do not exert traction (pull) on the tubing. Various arrangements are used to hold a chest drainage system below waist level during ambulation. The device may be placed in a wheelchair in front of the client. Many disposable units have handles to allow for carrying. If the client's condition warrants, removal of suction during ambulation may be ordered, allowing gravity drainage.

Mobile Chest Tube Drainage Systems. Mobile chest drains (Heimlich valve, Tru-Close thoracic vent, Pneumostat chest drain valve) are smaller chest tubes that use a mechanical one-way valve instead of a water-seal chamber and do not have a suction control chamber. Air is allowed to leave the chest on exhalation through the one-way valve, which then prevents air from reentering on inhalation. Mobile chest drains are used for clients who require a chest tube but do not require suction to reinflate the lung or to drain large amounts of fluid from the pleural cavity. They are used for clients who require long-term treatment for pleural effusions or persistent air leaks. Because of their small size and lack of large drainage collection system, clients are allowed to be more mobile earlier in their recovery.

Clamp Chest Drainage Tubing. In most situations, clamping of chest tubes is contraindicated. When the client has a residual air leak or pneumothorax, clamping the chest tube may precipitate a tension pneumothorax because the air has no escape route. If the tube becomes disconnected, it is best to immediately reattach it to the drainage system or to submerge the end in a bottle of sterile water or saline to reestablish a water seal; therefore one of these sterile solutions should be at the bedside at all times. If fluid is not readily available, it is preferable to leave the tube open because the risk of tension pneumothorax outweighs the consequences of an open tube.

There are occasions, however, when clamping is appropriate, such as the following:

- Assessing a persistent air leak
- Evaluating the client's readiness for removal of the drainage system
- Changing the drainage system

Except when clamping is clearly indicated, *never* clamp chest drainage tubes without an order to do so. If clamps must be used, the best time to apply them is after an expiration. Remove the clamps as soon as possible.

Remove Chest Tubes. The physician determines when to remove chest tubes and closed-chest drainage. One indication is that the lung has reexpanded, as signified by the cessation of fluctuation in the water-seal chamber (if suction is not applied). Chest auscultation, chest percussion, and chest x-ray studies confirm lung reexpansion.

Usually, a lung is fully reexpanded after 2 or 3 postoperative days of chest drainage. Chest tubes are generally left in place and connected to drainage systems for an additional 24 hours after all air and significant fluid drainage have stopped. The tubes may be temporarily clamped to determine how the client will tolerate their removal. Chest tubes may not be removed if the chest is draining more than 50 to 70 ml of fluid daily. The sooner the chest tubes can be removed, the better. Their presence often contributes to postoperative pain and inactivity. The longer the tubes are in place, the greater the risk of infection. Chest tubes used for treatment of empyema (see later discussion) may be in place longer than tubes placed after chest surgery.

Removal of chest tubes can be moderately painful. The prescribed premedication for pain reduction should be administered approximately 30 minutes before the procedure. Assemble equipment as necessary, such as sterile scissors or a suture set to cut sutures securing the tubes, sterile petrolatum gauze, 4-inch × 4-inch gauze to cover the wound, and tape.

If chest tubes are accidentally removed, cover the insertion site with sterile petrolatum gauze and notify the surgeon. Observe the client for respiratory distress by assessing lung sounds every 2 hours because tension pneumothorax may develop. If it does, remove the petrolatum gauze to allow air to escape.

BENIGN LUNG TUMORS

Benign pulmonary neoplasms account for fewer than 10% of all primary pulmonary tumors. The term *benign* may be misleading because these tumors can mechanically interfere with lung function (e.g., obstruction of a major bronchus may occur), depending on the tumor's location. The most common benign lung tumor is the hamartoma, which usually arises in peripheral lung parenchyma. This tumor is more common in older men. Other benign tumor types are fibroma, hemangioma, lipoma, and papilloma.

Benign lung tumors are often difficult to diagnose because clients may be asymptomatic. Unless there is preexisting lung disease or major airway obstruction, pulmonary function study results and ABG values are usually within normal limits. The tumor may be first detected on chest x-ray study. Confirmatory diagnosis usually requires bronchoscopy or, more commonly, thoracotomy. Until the diagnosis is confirmed, most clients are anxious and fearful of the possibility of cancer. Emotional support is an important adjunct to the physical preparation required for diagnostic procedures.

Surgical intervention is the treatment of choice for all benign neoplasms. Tumor removal promptly alleviates any respiratory manifestations that may have resulted from pressure on lung structures. Postoperative management is the same as that after surgical treatment of malignant lung disease.

OCCUPATIONAL LUNG DISEASES

Lung diseases are among the most common occupational health problems. They are caused by the inhalation of various chemicals, dusts, and other particulate matter that are present in certain settings. Not all clients exposed to occupational inhalants experience lung disease. Harmful effects depend on (1) the nature of the exposure, (2) the duration and intensity of the exposure, and (3) the particle size and water solubility of the inhalant. The larger the particle, the lower its probability of reaching the lower respiratory tract. Highly water-soluble inhalants tend to dissolve and react in the upper respiratory tract; poorly soluble substances may travel as far as the alveoli. Clients who are smokers or who have underlying lung disease are at greater risk. The most commonly encountered occupational lung diseases are described in Table 64-3.

Acute respiratory irritation results from the inhalation of chemicals such as ammonia, chlorine, and nitrogen oxides in the form of gases, aerosols, or particulate matter. If such irritants reach the lower airways, alveolar damage and pulmonary edema can result. Although the effects of acute irritants are usually short-lived, some may cause chronic alveolar damage or airway obstruction.

Occupational asthma is defined as variable air flow obstruction caused by a specific agent in the workplace. It is estimated that approximately 10% of all adult asthma cases can be attributed to workplace exposure.[46] By far the greatest number of occupational agents causing asthma are those with known or suspected allergenic properties, such as plant and animal proteins (e.g., wheat flour, cotton, flax, and grain mites). In most cases, the asthma resolves after exposure is terminated. However, hyperactivity of the airways may persist for years.

Hypersensitivity pneumonitis, or allergic alveolitis, is most commonly due to the inhalation of organic antigens of fungal, bacterial, or animal origin. The nature of the exposure and the client's immunologic reactivity determine the pulmonary response. Nonatopic people (i.e., those with no history of allergies) demonstrate a pulmonary response to organic dusts more often than atopic people, although atopic people, too, may exhibit pulmonary reactions.

TABLE 64-3	*Characteristics of Occupational Lung Disease*			
Disease	**Onset of Symptoms**	**Diagnosis**	**Treatment**	**Clinical Course**
Acute respiratory irritation	Immediate—within minutes of exposure Pulmonary edema may be delayed for hours	Consistent history Physical findings of respiratory tract irritation	Avoidance of exposure Respiratory support as needed	Resolves in hours to days Pulmonary edema may last days to weeks
Occupational asthma	Immediate—within minutes of exposure Can be delayed up to 6 hours	PFTs demonstrate reduced rates of FEV_1 to FVC Chest x-ray usually normal	Avoidance of exposure Asthma medication Steroids Bronchodilators	Resolves within hours Permanent loss of physiologic lung function may occur
Hypersensitivity pneumonitis	Within a few hours of exposure	Chest x-ray findings range from normal to fine or diffuse infiltrates PFTs demonstrate a reduction in vital capacity	Avoidance of exposure Steroids	Symptoms typically lessen in 48 hours Chest x-ray and PFT findings may last for weeks to months or may be permanent
Pneumoconiosis	Requires long-term exposure First manifestation often cough progressing to dyspnea	Restrictive pattern on PFTs Chest x-ray with asbestosis shows interstitial markings in lower lobes and with silicosis shows opacities in upper lobes	Avoidance of exposure Cessation of smoking	Gradual worsening with fatigue, loss of appetite, chest pain, respiratory failure, and death

FEV_1, Forced expiratory volume in 1 second; *FVC,* forced vital capacity; *PFTs,* pulmonary function tests.

Pneumoconioses, or the "dust diseases," result from inhalation of minerals, notably silica, coal dust, or asbestos. These diseases are most commonly seen in miners, construction workers, sandblasters, potters, and foundry and quarry workers. Pneumoconioses usually develop gradually over a period of years, eventually leading to diffuse pulmonary fibrosis that diminishes lung capacity and produces restrictive lung disease. Early clinical manifestations are cough and dyspnea on exertion. Chest pain, productive cough, and dyspnea at rest develop as the condition progresses.

Outcome Management

Early detection is one way to prevent progression of occupational lung disease. The respiratory history should consist of (1) a complete occupational history and questions about the actual job performed rather than title or job description, (2) past as well as current occupations, and (3) exposure to organic and inorganic substances in each job. The physical examination should include assessment of respiratory pattern and effort, presence of cough, lung sounds, and other manifestations indicating potential lung disease. Some employers support ongoing assessment programs (e.g., routine pulmonary function studies or chest radiographs) for workers at risk for occupational lung disorders.

Exposure precautions are essential for avoiding permanent pulmonary disability. Safety measures include adequate ventilation, the wearing of masks, and care in the handling of garments worn in dusty environments. If occupational lung disease is significant, the client may qualify for a disability allowance. Refer clients to community resources, such as federal or state departments of labor, if they have questions about their eligibility for such allowances.

Nursing interventions for clients experiencing occupational lung diseases are similar to those for clients with other restrictive lung disorders (see the following discussion). Supportive measures can help clients adjust their lifestyles to their conditions.

RESTRICTIVE LUNG DISORDERS

Restrictive lung disorders constitute a major category of pulmonary problems. The category includes any disorder that limits lung expansion and produces a pattern of abnormal function on pulmonary function tests characterized by a decrease in total lung capacity (TLC). Restrictive lung diseases may result from conditions affecting lung tissues or from extrapulmonary causes. Extrapulmonary causes include neurologic and neuromuscular disorders and disorders affecting the thoracic cage, pleura, and movement of the diaphragm. Obesity may also lead to restrictive lung disorders. Box 64-3 lists restrictive lung disorders.

Manifestations vary according to the cause of the restrictive disorder. For example, kyphosis, scoliosis, and kyphoscoliosis result in changes in the thoracic cage (Figure 64-8). Generally, clients with restrictive lung disease exhibit a rapid, shallow respiratory pattern. Chronic hyperventilation occurs in an effort to overcome the effects of reduced lung volume and compliance. Shortness of breath is experienced, at first only with exertion, but later at rest. ABG measurements reveal alveolar hyperventilation (i.e., reduced partial pressure of arterial carbon dioxide [$PaCO_2$]) during the initial and intermediate phases of the disease process. As the disease progresses, respiratory muscle fatigue may occur, leading to inadequate alveolar ventilation and carbon dioxide retention. Hypoxemia is a common finding, especially in the later stages of restrictive lung disease.

Pulmonary function tests demonstrate impairment of the lungs' bellows action. Commonly, the ratio of forced expiratory volume in 1 second (FEV_1) to forced vital capacity (FVC), or FEV_1/FVC ratio, is normal or increased (i.e., 75% or more of expected values). The FEV_1/FVC ratio by itself is not an absolute indicator of restrictive lung disorders. Reduced TLC is the primary indicator of the disease. TLC is less than 80% of expected value in clients with restrictive lung disease.

Often a specific diagnosis of restrictive lung disease is made only after extensive testing, including chest radiography, biopsy, immunologic testing, and testing to differentiate neurologic dysfunction, such as electromyography and cerebrospinal fluid analysis.

Outcome Management

Management is based on the severity of impairment and the ability to reverse the condition. Clients with spinal deformities may be helped by corrective spinal surgery. Likewise, obese clients breathe better after weight loss. Selected clients may benefit from the use of transtracheal oxygen administration or nighttime mechanical ventilation with a mask or cuirass respirator (a device that covers the chest and moves the chest wall out and back through changes in pressure), especially clients who have postpoliomyelitis syndrome.

The primary goals of nursing management of the client with restrictive lung disease are (1) promotion of adequate oxygenation, (2) maintenance of a patent airway, and (3) achievement of the highest possible functional level. Interventions to attain these goals are similar to those used in the treatment of COPD (see Chapter 63). ABG analysis is important for monitoring oxygen

---

BOX 64-3 *Restrictive Lung Diseases*

Restrictive lung diseases are disorders affecting lung volumes and compliance of either chest wall or lung tissue. Their causes are classified as intrapulmonary or extrapulmonary.

Intrapulmonary
Pulmonary fibrosis
Sarcoidosis and other interstitial lung diseases
Pneumonia
Atelectasis
Pneumoconiosis
Surgical lung resection
Neoplastic disease

Extrapulmonary
Head or spinal cord injury
Amyotrophic lateral sclerosis
Myasthenia gravis
Muscular dystrophy
Congenital chest wall deformity
Acquired chest wall changes (e.g., kyphosis or scoliosis)
Abdominal distention restricting diaphragmatic movement
Sleep disorders
Poliomyelitis
Pleural effusion
Pleurisy
Excessive obesity

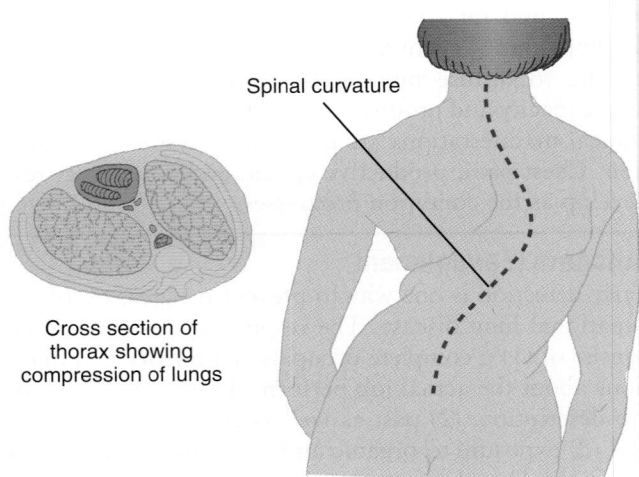

Spinal curvature

Cross section of thorax showing compression of lungs

FIGURE 64-8 Thoracic scoliosis. Note the **S** shape of the spine. These thoracic deformities alter the chest cage space. Lung tissue may be compressed, producing altered lung function (restrictive lung disease).

needs, acid-base balance, and the effects of physical activity. $PaCO_2$ values should be monitored because rising carbon dioxide level is an indicator of impending respiratory failure.

Most restrictive lung disorders are not reversible. End-stage disease is characterized by the development of pulmonary hypertension, cor pulmonale, severe hypoxemia, and eventual respiratory failure. Efforts should be made to maintain the client's functional status and quality of life at as high a level as possible.

CYSTIC FIBROSIS

Cystic fibrosis (CF) is a congenital restrictive lung disorder in which the secretions of the exocrine (mucus-producing) glands are abnormal. This disorder affects the sweat glands, respiratory system, digestive tract (particularly the pancreas), and reproductive tract. CF is the most common inherited genetic disease in the Caucasian population, affecting approximately 30,000 children and adults in the United States.[32,45] CF is an autosomal recessive trait, resulting from mutations at a single gene locus on the long arm of chromosome 7. CF used to be considered a "pediatric problem" because it was fatal in childhood. However, advances in early diagnosis and treatment, including antibiotics, chest physiotherapy, and nutrition programs, have extended the median life expectancy into the early 30s, with maximum survival documented as high as the seventh decade of life.[33,37]

Pathophysiology

The hallmark of CF is the raised transepithelial electric potential difference (PD) detected in airway epithelia. The transepithelial PD reflects components of both the rate of active ion transport and the resistance to ion flow of the superficial epithelium. CF airway epithelia exhibit both raised transport rates (Na^+) and decreased Cl^- permeabilities. These abnormalities in the sodium and chloride transport alter water movement across the membrane, leading to thick secretions of mucoproteins that plug the airway. Furthermore, the mucociliary transport is slowed, which decreases the ability to clear the airways of mucus and leads to stasis of mucus and a medium for infection. Lung infections often develop from *Staphylococcus aureus* and *Pseudomonas aeruginosa* organisms; these organisms seldom infect the lungs of people without CF.

The thick mucus also plugs the glands and ducts of the pancreatic acini, intestinal glands, intrahepatic bile ducts, and the gallbladder, causing dilation and fibrosis. These changes result in decreased production of pancreatic enzymes needed for digestion of carbohydrates, fats, and proteins. Sweat glands, salivary glands, and lacrimal glands are also affected, leading to high concentrations of sodium and chloride in these secretions.

Clinical Manifestations

Usual clinical manifestations are persistent cough that is worse at night and especially upon arising. As CF progresses, the cough becomes productive and then paroxysmal, with gagging and emesis. Recurrent lung infections lead to tenacious purulent, often green sputum. Asthmatic wheezing is common. Because of the pancreatic involvement, clients may have steatorrhea.

Chest radiography shows hyperinflation, and pulmonary function tests reveal increased airway resistance. The airways are hyperreactive and clients often complain of dyspnea with cold air, smoke, and exercise. CF is diagnosed by elevated chloride levels in the sweat. Distal intestinal obstruction can occur, which presents as right lower quadrant pain, loss of appetite, occasional emesis, and often a palpable mass. The syndrome can be confused with appendicitis, which occurs frequently in clients with CF.

Late onset of puberty is common in both males and a female with CF. The delayed maturational pattern is likely secondary to the effects of chronic lung disease and inadequate nutrition on reproductive endocrine function. More than 95% of male clients with CF are azoospermic, reflecting obliteration of the vas deferens that probably reflects defective liquid secretion. Twenty percent of women with CF are infertile as a result of effects of chronic lung disease on the menstrual cycle. Thick, tenacious cervical mucus blocks sperm migration, and there are possible fallopian tube and uterine wall abnormalities in liquid transport. However, more than 90% of completed pregnancies produce viable infants, and women with CF are generally able to breast-feed infants normally.

Outcome Management

The goals of therapy for CF are to ensure a reasonable quality of life for as long as possible and to prevent or slow the decline in pulmonary functioning. They are achieved by removing secretions, improving aeration, and administering antibiotic agents.

Clearing tracheobronchial secretions is promoted by (1) adequate hydration, (2) bronchodilators and mucolytic aerosols, and (3) effective coughing techniques including positive expiratory pressure devices, postural drainage, and chest vibration, percussion, and exercise. Oxygen is used if hypoxemia is present. Sitting erect also facilitates breathing.

Anti-inflammatory agents decrease inflammatory response in the respiratory tract epithelium and improve pulmonary function. Short-term systemic corticosteroids are used during acute exacerbations and nonsteroidal anti-inflammatory drugs are often given long term.

Antibiotic therapy has played an important role in extending the life expectancy of clients with CF. Intravenous antibiotics are essential during acute infections.

Inhaled antibiotics are also being used with more regularity. The choice of antibiotic should be determined by results of sputum culture and sensitivity testing. Sputum should be assessed for color, quality, and quantity. All respiratory equipment should be thoroughly cleaned on a routine basis to prevent reinfection from contaminated equipment.

Persistent pulmonary infection with *Pseudomonas* organisms is common in the end stages of CF. Continuous treatment with large doses of intravenous antibiotics is usually indicated. Moderate to severe hemoptysis can occur if the infection causes erosion of pulmonary blood vessels. Blood replacement and temporary cessation of postural drainage may be required.

Maintenance of adequate nutrition is critical. Most (>90%) clients with CF benefit from pancreatic enzyme replacement. Capsules generally contain between 4000 and 29,000 units of lipase. The dose of enzymes (typically no more than 20,000 units/kg per meal) should be adjusted on the basis of weight gain, abdominal manifestations, and character of stools. Replacement of fat-soluble vitamins, particularly vitamins E and K, is usually required.

New treatments for CF have shown moderate success and are still being studied for long-term effects, including the following:

- Use of synthetically produced DNase, an enzyme that breaks down the deoxyribonucleic acid (DNA) released from neutrophils and causes the "stickiness" of mucus
- Augmentation of the immune defense with supplemental gamma-globulin
- Use of drugs that alter ion movement and thin secretions

Gene therapy is also being evaluated. Gene transfer is possible, but a safe and effective approach for determining long-term success has yet to be demonstrated.[32,37]

Treatment of end-stage disease is primarily concerned with the management of severe complications. Obstruction of the airways leads to a state of hyperinflation. In time, restrictive lung disease is superimposed on the obstructive disease. Pneumothorax (air in the chest cavity) develops in 20% of all adult clients, requiring lung reexpansion with chest tubes.

Over time, pulmonary obstruction leads to chronic hypoxemia, hypercapnia, and acidosis. Pulmonary hypertension and, eventually, cor pulmonale may result. Treatment consists of digitalis, diuretics, and oxygen therapy. Clients with severely reduced lung function (FEV_1 <30% of predicted) whose disease no longer responds to maximal therapy and who are experiencing a decline in quality of life may be candidates for bilateral lung transplantation.

Attention to psychosocial concerns is a nursing priority throughout the course of the disease. In the adult client with CF, psychosocial concerns center on three major areas:

- Disease management (e.g., treatment compliance, sleep disturbance, hemoptysis, nutrition, and hospitalizations)
- Growth and development (e.g., daily activities, work, and sex and reproduction)
- Family relations (e.g., substance abuse, depression, anxiety, and marital problems)

Nursing intervention involves helping clients cope with these problem areas as well as providing emotional support to both clients and their families.

LUNG TRANSPLANTATION

Lung transplantation is appropriate for clients who have end-stage lung disease that is unresponsive to medical therapy and who are experiencing progressive deterioration in health status. This procedure involves replacement of one or both of the diseased lungs with lungs from a cadaver donor. Live donor lobar transplantation has also been performed. The success of lung transplantation has improved significantly since the early 1980s and has become a widely accepted treatment for certain pulmonary diseases, such as emphysema, cystic fibrosis, alpha$_1$-antitrypsin deficiency, drug-induced pulmonary fibrosis, sarcoidosis, and primary pulmonary hypertension. The current 5-year survival rate after transplantation is 44%.[28]

Preoperative Care

Preoperative assessment consists of both medical and psychosocial evaluation. Once the severity of lung disease is established, the client's physical health is assessed to determine candidacy for transplantation. A battery of tests is performed to rule out active infection and to evaluate cardiac, hepatic, hematopoietic, and renal functions. Psychosocial evaluation focuses on assessing the client's history of compliance with medical therapy and medical recommendations as well as his or her ability to cope with stress.[38]

Postoperative Care

Postoperatively, the client is observed for excessive bleeding. Monitor vital signs, hemodynamic pressures, electrocardiogram (ECG), ABG values, urine output, transcutaneous oxygen level analysis, and chest tube drainage. Pulmonary edema may develop in the denervated transplanted lung. Therefore the client may be started on mechanical ventilation with positive end-expiratory pressure (PEEP) for 24 to 48 hours.

Serum electrolytes, complete blood counts, and chest radiographs are obtained at least daily. Fluids are restricted, lung sounds are auscultated, and the severity of peripheral edema is monitored. Pain control is important to allow deep breathing and coughing in addition to chest physiotherapy. Many clients benefit from epidural analgesia. Following extubation, maintain good pain control and help the client cough, deep breathe, and use incentive spirometry to expand the lung.

The client who has received a lung is at high risk for infection and transplant rejection. Isolation is used to decrease inadvertent exposure to pathogens. Laboratory values are monitored, especially the WBC and absolute **EB** neutrophil counts. Monitor the client for clinical manifestations of infection, such as (1) changes in vital signs (especially fever), (2) local infections at intravenous access sites and incision lines, and (3) changes in respiratory status (excessive secretions, tachypnea, dyspnea, fatigue). Rejection of the transplanted lung may manifest as dyspnea, development of infiltrates on chest radiograph, need for ventilatory support, and fatigue.

Following the initial procedure, the client may experience alterations in self-concept related to changes in (1) appearance, from the side effects of medications such as steroids and immunosuppressants, (2) lifestyle, or **EB** (3) work ability and role performance. Be sensitive to these issues, and encourage the client and family to discuss their feelings and explore options.

■ Self-Care

Before discharge from the facility, teach the client about the medication regimen, and stress the need for daily medication despite a lack of manifestations. The client should report fever, dyspnea, cough, new or increased productive sputum, chest pain, reduced exercise tolerance, excessive weight gain, and fatigue to the physician. In addition, the client should begin a pulmonary rehabilitation program.

During follow-up visits, the client is monitored for manifestations of rejection, compliance with immunosuppressive therapy, and progress in functional status.

Lung transplantation offers some hope for extended life to clients with previously fatal conditions. However, it is a frightening and stressful surgery. Clients receiving lung transplants are always critically ill before surgery. In addition, they must undergo a radical, major surgical procedure and endure prolonged intensive care and isolation procedures. People with transplants also must adapt to an altered self-concept. The client and significant others need constant emotional support for achievement of a successful outcome.

Outcomes appear promising. ABG levels improve markedly in unilateral and bilateral lung transplant recipients by 3 months after transplantation. Unilateral lung recipients may continue to have mild hypoxemia **EB** but rarely require supplemental oxygen. Pulmonary function studies have shown that some unilateral graft

recipients can reach 60% to 65% of their predicted FVC and FEV_1 values. The values for bilateral lung recipients often approach normal predicted values, but these clients can have mild restrictive physiology.

Exercise capacity has been the most interesting functional outcome observed in lung transplant recipients. Bilateral and bilateral graft recipients demonstrate marked and similar improvement in distances covered after transplantation. Typically, transplant recipients can walk 100 to 120 m/min within 6 months of transplantation and are generally able to sustain this rate over time. Limitations appear to be related to muscle deconditioning and abnormalities in skeletal muscle oxidative capacity.

■ SARCOIDOSIS

Sarcoidosis is an inflammatory condition that affects many body systems. The disease is characterized by the formation of widespread granulomatous lesions. In addition to lung involvement, which occurs in more than 90% of cases, clients may present with clinical manifestations involving the peripheral lymphatic system, skin, liver, eyes, spleen, bones, salivary glands, joints, nervous system, and heart.[44]

The cause of sarcoidosis remains unknown; it is suggested that a triggering agent (which may be genetic, infectious, immunologic, or toxic) stimulates enhanced cell-mediated immune processes at the site of involvement. A series of interactions between T lymphocytes and monocyte-macrophages leads to the formation of *non-caseating* (i.e., having no cheesy necrotic degeneration) granulomas, which are characteristic of the disease. Granuloma formation may regress with therapy or as a result of the disorder's natural course, but it may also progress to fibrosis and restrictive lung disease. In chronic cases, approximately 10% of clients die of the disease.

As many as half of clients are asymptomatic, and the diagnosis is confirmed by chest radiography.[44] Clients with pulmonary manifestations usually present with a dry cough and shortness of breath. Chest pain, hemoptysis, or pneumothorax may also be present. Systemic manifestations include fatigue, weakness, malaise, weight loss, and fever. A definitive diagnosis of sarcoidosis is made from tissue biopsy. When lung involvement is suspected, bronchoscopy, bronchoalveolar lavage, mediastinoscopy, or open lung biopsy may be performed.

Outcome Management

Medical management is primarily determined by the extent to which the client's life is disturbed by the manifestations experienced. If the client with sarcoidosis is asymptomatic, management involves ongoing assessment for further disease progression, such as chest x-ray studies every 6 months. When manifestations are present, medical treatment usually consists of systemic corticosteroids to suppress the immune process and often leads to dramatic improvement.

Nursing intervention in clients with sarcoidosis is the same as that in clients with other restrictive lung diseases and hypoxemia. Assess for drug side effects, especially adverse responses to corticosteroids (such as weight gain, change in mood, and development of diabetes mellitus). Also assess for manifestations of improvement, such as increased exercise tolerance, disappearance of initial assessment findings, improved pulmonary function studies, and better oxygenation. If assessment findings worsen, document them and notify the physician.

INTERSTITIAL LUNG DISEASE

Interstitial lung diseases (ILDs) comprise a group of diffuse inflammatory lower respiratory tract disorders. The term *interstitial* is used to indicate that the interstitium of the alveolar walls is thickened and usually fibrotic. The alveolar walls thicken as a result of the accumulation of inflammatory cells. The thickened alveolus becomes nonfunctional.

The cause of ILD is not clearly defined. It most commonly develops from idiopathic pulmonary fibrosis, sarcoidosis, and collagen-vascular disorders. ILD can also result from the inhalation of inorganic dust, such as crystalline silica, asbestos, and coal dust, or of organic dust from organisms encountered in farming, use of air conditioning, and animal husbandry. Other possible causes are radiation damage and infectious agents.

Manifestations of ILD are insidious and nonspecific, such as fatigue, progressive dyspnea, dyspnea at rest, and nonproductive cough. Because the clinical manifestations are nonspecific, ILD may remain undiagnosed for years. The client's history plays a major part in diagnosis because it is important to determine the agents to which the client has been exposed. Physical examination may reveal reduced chest expansion, which is reflected as a decrease in TLC. Inspiratory and expiratory crackles are frequently heard. The crackles have a characteristic sound, like the sound of hook-and-loop tape (Velcro) being pulled apart. Clubbing of the finger tips may be present.

Diagnostic assessment includes gallium ventilation-perfusion scans. These scans usually reveal impaired perfusion in the lower lobes and multiple areas of impaired ventilation. The ventilation-perfusion mismatch results in hypoxemia and carbon dioxide retention. Bronchoscopy and biopsy may also be used to confirm ILD.

Outcome Management

Management of a client with ILD is based on the level of respiratory impairment. Inflammation is controlled with corticosteroids. Explain to the client that corticosteroids reduce further impairment but previously injured alveolar-capillary units are permanently damaged. Clients often show subjective improvement while taking steroids, the dosage of which can eventually be tapered and stopped. If the offending agent is known, the initial treatment is to remove the client from exposure to the agent. As the disorder progresses, inhaled corticosteroids and bronchodilators help mobilize secretions and provide oxygen during periods of exercise. Nursing management is the same as that for clients with restrictive lung disorders.

DISORDERS OF THE PLEURA AND PLEURAL SPACE
PLEURAL PAIN

Pleural pain is a common pulmonary manifestation arising from the parietal pleura, which is richly supplied with sensory nerve endings. Pleuritic pain indicates the presence of pleural inflammation (*pleurisy*) caused by pneumonia, pulmonary infarction, pleural effusion (see the following discussion), or pneumothorax, among others. It is often accompanied by a pleural friction rub that is discovered during chest auscultation.

Pleuritic chest pain often develops abruptly and is usually severe enough that the client seeks medical attention. It commonly occurs on only one side of the chest, usually in the lower lateral portions of the chest wall, and is aggravated by deep breathing or coughing. Often the client can point directly to the exact location of the pain. However, pleural pain may also be referred to the neck, shoulder, or abdomen. Because other types of chest pain (e.g., cardiac pain, chest wall pain) may be misinterpreted as pleuritic pain, careful assessment is necessary.

Pleuritic pain may restrict normal respiratory efforts, leading to problems with gas exchange and airway clearance. If pain-relieving measures, including administration of prescribed analgesics, do not relieve the pain, the physician may perform an intercostal nerve block (see Chapter 22).

PLEURAL EFFUSION

Pleural effusion is an accumulation of fluid in the pleural space. Pleural fluid normally seeps continually into the pleural space from the capillaries lining the parietal pleura and is reabsorbed by the visceral pleural capillaries and lymphatic system. Any condition that interferes with either secretion or drainage of this fluid leads to pleural effusion.

Causes of pleural effusion can be grouped into four major categories. They are conditions that do the following:

- Increase systemic hydrostatic pressure (e.g., heart failure)

- Reduce capillary oncotic pressure (e.g., liver or renal failure)
- Increase capillary permeability (e.g., infections or trauma)
- Impair lymphatic function (e.g., lymphatic obstruction due to tumor)

Clinical manifestations depend on the amount of fluid present and the severity of lung compression. If the effusion is small (i.e., 250 ml), its presence may be discovered only on chest x-ray study. With large effusions, lung expansion may be restricted, and the client may experience dyspnea, primarily on exertion, and a dry, nonproductive cough caused by bronchial irritation or mediastinal shift. Tactile fremitus may be decreased or absent, and percussion notes may be dull or flat.

Thoracentesis (see Chapter 61) is used to remove excess pleural fluid. The removed fluid is analyzed to determine whether it is transudate or exudate. *Transudates* are substances that have passed through a membrane or tissue surface. They occur primarily in conditions in which there is protein loss and low protein content (e.g., hypoalbuminemia, cirrhosis, nephrosis) or increased hydrostatic pressure (e.g., heart failure). *Exudates* are substances that have escaped from blood vessels. They contain an accumulation of cells, have a high specific gravity and a high lactate dehydrogenase (LDH) level, and occur in response to malignancies, infections, or inflammatory processes. Exudates occur when there is an increase in capillary permeability. Differentiating between transudates and exudates helps establish a specific diagnosis. Diagnosis may also require analysis of the fluid for white and red blood cells, malignant cells, bacteria, glucose content, pH, and LDH.

Pleural fluid may be (1) hemorrhagic (or bloody), such as when a tumor is present or after trauma or pulmonary embolus with infarction, (2) chylous (or thick and white), such as after lymphatic obstruction or trauma to the thoracic duct, or (3) rich in cholesterol, such as in chronic, recurrent effusions due to tuberculosis or rheumatoid arthritis. If there is a high WBC count and the pleural fluid is purulent, the effusion is called an *empyema*. An empyema of any volume requires drainage and treatment of the infection.

If the pus is not drained, it may become thick and almost solidified or loculated (containing cavities), a condition called *fibrothorax*. Fibrothorax may significantly restrict lung expansion and may require surgical intervention. The procedure, known as *decortication*, involves removal of the restrictive mass of fibrin and inflammatory cells. Decortication is usually not performed until the fibrothorax is relatively solid, so it can be easily removed.

After the procedure, closed-chest drainage with suction is used to reexpand the lung rapidly and fill the pleural space. If the fibrous material has restricted the lung for some time, the lung may not reexpand effectively and further intervention (usually thoracoplasty) may be needed.

RECURRENT PLEURAL EFFUSION

In some cases, pleural effusions may recur despite repeated thoracenteses (e.g., malignancy-induced effusions), with resultant compromise of lung function or persistent pleural pain. Treatment of recurrent effusions is accomplished through obliteration of the pleural space. Methods of obliterating the pleural space are as follows:

Pleurectomy (pleural stripping): Surgical stripping of the parietal pleura away from the visceral pleura, which produces an intense inflammatory reaction that promotes adhesion formation between the two layers during healing.

Pleurodesis: Instillation of a sclerosing substance (e.g., unbuffered tetracycline, nitrogen mustard, talc) into the pleural space via a chest tube to create an inflammatory response that causes the pleura to adhere and sclerose to each other.

Because pleural space obliteration creates permanent changes, the client's existing and predicted postprocedure respiratory status must be carefully evaluated. If a large area is involved, significant alterations in ventilatory mechanics (e.g., deep breathing, coughing) may occur, leading to compromised respiratory function.

After the procedure, closely monitor lung function, including respiratory rate and ventilation pattern. Document alleviation or persistence of pleural pain and watch for indications of a return of the pleural effusion. Pulmonary function studies (see Chapter 61) and ABG measurements should also be performed.

BRONCHOPLEURAL FISTULA

A bronchopleural fistula is a communication between the pleural space and a bronchus. It may occur when an undrained empyema erodes into a bronchus or when the pleural space does not heal spontaneously after removal of a chest tube. A bronchopleural fistula raises the risk of pleural infection and may compromise ventilation and oxygenation.

The management of a client with a bronchopleural fistula is often complex. Bronchopleural fistulae may be slow to heal. The client may be discharged home with a chest tube still in place and connected to a collection system. Teach the client and family how to care for the chest tube and collection system and to recognize both manifestations of irritation at the chest puncture site and changes in chest drainage (e.g., blood) that require the physician to be notified.

METASTATIC PLEURAL TUMORS

Primary tumors in the lungs and other organs often metastasize to the pleura. The primary tumor is usually in a lung but may occur in the breast, ovaries, liver, kidneys, uterus, testicles, or larynx or may result from leukemia or lymphoma. Metastatic pleural disease frequently causes pleural effusions. Assessment findings in malignant pleural effusion are the same as those in pleural effusion from other causes. Diagnosis of pleural effusion is by chest x-ray examination. The source of the effusion is determined from cytologic examination of pleural fluid obtained by thoracentesis. Intervention is the same as for any pleural effusion, along with treatment of the primary malignancy.

DISORDERS OF THE DIAPHRAGM
SUBDIAPHRAGMATIC ABSCESS

A subdiaphragmatic abscess may develop as a result of (1) gastrointestinal perforation, (2) surgery of the upper gastrointestinal system, liver, or biliary tract, (3) abdominal trauma, or (4) other intra-abdominal surgery. A subdiaphragmatic abscess can compromise respiratory status or erode and perforate the diaphragm.

Clinical manifestations include pleuritic pain or pain referred to the shoulder on the affected side. Dyspnea and poor or no diaphragmatic movement are common. Flank pain or tenderness and a palpable abdominal mass in the region of the abscess is noted. The client has fever, anorexia, weight loss, and vomiting. Chest radiograph shows the diaphragm is generally elevated on the affected side. Fluoroscopic studies of diaphragmatic movement reveal limitation or absence of diaphragmatic movement on the affected side. Pleural effusion also commonly occurs. Thoracentesis and analysis of the pleural fluid reveal an exudate.

Subdiaphragmatic abscess are drained and treated with antibiotics. Supportive measures are used to maintain ventilation and respiratory status. An untreated subdiaphragmatic abscess is nearly always fatal. With treatment, the mortality rate is still high but drops to approximately 25%.

DIAPHRAGMATIC PARALYSIS

Bilateral diaphragmatic paralysis almost always causes severe morbidity in adults. The most common causes include high spinal cord injury, thoracic trauma (including cardiac surgery), multiple sclerosis, anterior horn disease, and muscular dystrophy. Unilateral paralysis of the diaphragm is much more common than is bilateral paralysis. The most common cause is nerve invasion from malignancy, usually a bronchogenic carcinoma.

Although the diaphragm is the primary muscle of respiration, its role can be assumed in part by the accessory and abdominal muscles. As a result, diaphragmatic paralysis is often difficult to detect. The diagnosis is suggested by finding an elevated hemidiaphragm on the chest x-ray study and is confirmed by fluoroscopy. During the fluoroscopic procedure, the client

is asked to "sniff." If paralysis is present, the nonparalyzed side of the diaphragm descends during inspiration (the sniff), and the paralyzed side paradoxically rises. Clients with unilateral diaphragmatic paralysis usually experience dyspnea when lying on the affected side. Dyspnea on exertion is not usual unless there is underlying lung disease. Both TLC and vital capacity (VC) are reduced by about 20%. There is also less ventilation to the affected side, and mild hypoxemia occurs because of shifts of ventilation and blood flow. Preexisting lung disease combined with unilateral diaphragmatic paralysis may be disabling, depending on the extent of the lung disease.

The effects of bilateral diaphragmatic paralysis are potentially much more severe than those of unilateral paralysis. However, the problem is often subtle and overlooked, especially if the client has a neuromuscular disorder. Fatigue, disturbed sleep, and morning headache are frequently the only manifestations. A classic manifestation of bilateral paralysis of the diaphragm is increased dyspnea when the client is lying flat on the back (supine). Paradoxical inward abdominal movement during inspiration in the supine position and active use of the accessory muscles of inspiration also occur. The pulmonary effects of bilateral paralysis are pronounced when the client is supine. Functional residual capacity (FRC) is also decreased, as is lung compliance. In the side-lying position, ventilation is preferentially distributed to the uppermost lung tissue and away from blood flow, leading to a significant mismatch of ventilation and perfusion. Severe hypoxemia results. Reduced tidal volume leads to retention of carbon dioxide and respiratory acidosis. Respiratory muscle function decreases during rest and sleep, further compromising respiratory status.

Little can be done to treat diaphragmatic paralysis. Management is aimed at supporting ventilatory function as needed. If the phrenic nerve is intact, a phrenic nerve pacer may be surgically inserted. However, this measure is possible only if the phrenic nerve can be stimulated (its status is tested first during a fluoroscopic procedure). Use of a phrenic nerve pacer is useful primarily for clients with spinal cord injuries.

Nursing management focuses on maintenance of a patent airway and detection of deteriorating gas exchange. Because inspiration is impaired, the client may need assistance to cough and deep breathe effectively. Position the client on the unaffected side in the semisitting or sitting position. Suction as necessary. Increase hydration to liquefy secretions. Administer oxygen as prescribed. If respiratory function declines significantly, the physician and client (or possibly significant others) must decide whether a permanent tracheostomy should be placed and whether mechanical ventilation or other assistance devices (e.g., rocking bed, cuirass respirator) should be used.

CONCLUSIONS

Clients with lung disorders are a challenge to the nurse providing care. In addition to common nursing diagnoses centering on *Impaired Gas Exchange* and *Ineffective Airway Clearance,* the client is often anxious because of the feelings of dyspnea and air hunger. Management of lung disorders consists of methods to open the airway (bronchodilators), clear infection (antibiotics), and improve oxygenation (position, coughing and deep breathing, oxygen).

THINKING CRITICALLY *evolve*

1. Your client, who has undergone thoracotomy, has a pleural chest tube connected to water-seal drainage. While your client is being positioned for a bedside chest radiograph, the drainage tubing is inadvertently disconnected from the chest drainage apparatus. What actions should you take?

Factors to Consider. What happens to the normally negative pressure in the pleural space when it is exposed to room air? Is this a dangerous problem?

2. A client with exertional dyspnea is admitted to the unit with a diagnosis of pleural effusion. He has difficulty breathing during the transfer from the cart to bed. You are asked to prepare the client for a thoracentesis. How would you prioritize care? What preparations are necessary for a thoracentesis?

Factors to Consider. What is the purpose of a thoracentesis? How are complications avoided? What clients are at risk for pleural effusion?

Discussion for these questions can be found on the website and the CD-ROM.

BIBLIOGRAPHY

1. American Thoracic Society. (2000). Diagnostic standards and classification of tuberculosis in adults and children. *American Journal of Respiratory and Critical Care Medicine, 161,* 1376-1395.
2. Blank-Reid, C.A., & Reid, P.C. (1999). Taking the tension out of traumatic pneumothoraxes. *Nursing, 29*(4), 41-46.
3. Boutotte, J.M. (1999). Keeping TB in check. *Nursing, 29*(3), 34-40.
4. Breeding, D.C. (1998). Controlling silica exposures. *Occupational Health and Safety, 67*(10), 178-181.
5. Brogdon, C.F. (1998). Women and cancer. *Journal of Intravenous Nursing, 21*(6), 344-355.

6. Brooks, J. (2001). Postoperative nosocomial pneumonia: Nurse-sensitive interventions. *AACN Clinical Issues, 12*(2), 305-323.
7. Carpenito, L.J. (2000). *Nursing diagnosis: Application to clinical practice* (8th ed.). Philadelphia: J.B. Lippincott.
8. Carroll, P. (1998). Preventing nosocomial pneumonia. *RN, 61*(6), 44-48.
9. Carroll, P. (2002). A guide to mobile chest drains. *RN, 65*(5), 56-60.
10. Centers for Disease Control and Prevention. (2002, August). Treatment of tuberculosis. Retrieved January 19, 2004, from http://www.cdc.gov/mmwr/preview/mmwrhtml/rr5211a1.htm.
11. Chernecky, C., & Shelton, B. (2001). Pulmonary complications in patients with cancer. *American Journal of Nursing, 101*(5), 24A-24H.
12. Clarkson, E.F. (1999). Tuberculosis: An overview. *Journal of Intravenous Nursing, 22*(4), 216-220.
13. Colice, G.L., & Rubins, J.B. (1999). Practical management of pleural effusions. *Postgraduate Medicine, 105*(7), 67-77.
14. Cook, J.L. (1999). Pulmonary nontuberculous mycobacterial infections in immunocompetent patients. *Clinical Laboratory Science, 12*(5), 302-308.
15. D'Epiro, N.W. (1999). Identifying and treating atypical pneumonia. *Patient Care, 33*(14), 175-184.
16. Dest, V.M. (2000). Oncology today: Lung cancer. *RN, 63*(5), 32-38.
17. Doull, I.J. (2001). Recent advances in cystic fibrosis. *Archives of Disabilities in Children, 85,* 62-66.
18. Duquette, S.L., LaLonde, L.C., & Traiger, G.L. (2000). Living-donor lobar lung transplantation: A case study. *Critical Care Nurse, 20*(1), 69-80.
19. Elpern, E.H., & Cheatham, J. (2001). Inpatient care of the adult with an exacerbation of cystic fibrosis. *AACN Clinical Issues, 12*(2), 293-304.
20. Godden, J., & Hiley, G.J. (1998). Managing the patient with a chest drain: A review. *Nursing Standard, 12*(32), 35-39.
21. Graybill, J.R., Kaufmann, C.A., & Patel, R. (1999). Treatment of systemic fungal infections. *Patient Care, 33*(19), 50-72.
22. Harris, J.R., & Miller, T.H. (2000). Preventing nosocomial pneumonia: Evidence-based practice. *Critical Care Nurse, 20*(1), 51-66.
23. Iseman, M.D. (2000). Tuberculosis chemotherapy, including directly observed therapy. In *A clinician's guide to tuberculosis.* Philadelphia: Lippincott Williams & Wilkins.
24. Kemp, C. (1999). Metastatic spread and common symptoms. Part four: Lung cancer, malignant melanoma, multiple myeloma. *American Journal of Hospital Palliative Care, 16*(3), 545-553.
25. King, A.B. (1999). Accurately interpreting PPD skin test results. *Nurse Practitioner, 24*(5), 144-147.
26. King, L. (2001). Minimizing the risk of hospital transmission of pulmonary TB. *Nursing Stand, 16*(4), 45-52.
27. King, M.A., & Tomasic, D.M. (1999). Treating TB today. *RN, 62*(6), 26-31.

evolve Did you remember to check out the bonus material on the Evolve website and the CD-ROM, including free self-assessment exercises?

http://evolve.elsevier.com/Black/medsurg/

28. Lanuza, D.M., & McCabe, M.A. (2001). Care before and after lung transplant and quality of life research. *AACN Clinical Issues, 12*(2), 186-201.

29. Marshall, B.C., & Samuelson, W.M. (1998). Basic therapies in cystic fibrosis: Does standard therapy work? *Clinical Chest Medicine, 19*(3), 457-500.

 30. Maurer, J.R., et al. (1998). International guidelines for the selection of lung transplant candidates. *Heart & Lung, 27*(4), 223-229.

31. McHugh Shuster, P. (1998). Chest tubes: To clamp or not to clamp. *Nurse Educator, 23*(3), 9-13.

32. Moss, R.B. (2001). New approaches to cystic fibrosis. *Hospital Practice, 36*(1), 25-37.

33. Orenstein, D.M., Winnie, G.B., & Altman, H. (2002). Cystic fibrosis: A 2002 update. *Journal of Pediatrics, 140*(2), 156-164.

34. Pass, H.I., et al (Eds.). (2000). *Lung cancer: Principles and Practice*. Philadelphia: Lippincott Williams & Wilkins.

35. Quinn, S. (1999). Lung cancer: The role of the nurse in treatment and prevention. *Nursing Standard, 13*(41), 49-55.

36. Redlich, C.A., & Anwar, M.S. (1998). Occupational asthma: Keys to diagnosis and management. *Journal of Respiratory Disease, 19*(6), 508-519.

37. Rosenstein, B.J., & Zeitlin, P.L. (1998). Cystic fibrosis. *Lancet, 351*(9098), 277-282.

38. Smith, C.M. (1997). Patient selection, evaluation, and preoperative management for lung transplant candidates. *Clinical Chest Medicine, 18*(2), 183-197.

39. Smith, E.L. (1998). Pulmonary metastasis. *Seminars in Oncologic Nursing, 14*(3), 178-186.

40. Stenton, C. (1998). Managing allergic alveolitis. *Practitioner, 242*(1584), 200-204.

41. Taubert, J. (2001). Management of malignant pleural effusion. *Nursing Clinics in North America, 36*(4), 665-683.

42. Vaz, A., et al. (1998). Coccidioidomycosis: An update. *Hospital Practice, 33*(9), 105-120.

43. Veynovich, B., & Barron, D.A. (1999). Manifestations and exacerbation of pulmonary diseases other than obstructive lung disease. *Topics in Emergency Medicine, 21*(4), 44-58.

44. Wiese, T.A., & Iannuzzi, M.C. (2002). Sarcoidosis: A primer on presentation and diagnosis. *Journal of Respiratory Disease, 23*(4), 237-249.

45. Wilmoth, D., et al. (2001). Caring for adults with cystic fibrosis. *Critical Care Nurse, 21*(3), 34-44.

46. Youakim, S. (2001). Work-related asthma. *American Family Physician, 64*(11), 1839-1848.

Chapter 65

Management of Clients with Acute Pulmonary Disorders

Ann H. White

evolve

Web Enhancements

Bridge to Home Health Care
Living with a Ventilator
Concept Map
Understanding ARDS and Its Treatment

http://evolve.elsevier.com/Black/medsurg/

Appendix C
Laboratory Values of Clinical Importance in Medical-Surgical Nursing

RESPIRATORY FAILURE

The most important function of the respiratory system is to provide the body tissues with oxygen and to remove carbon dioxide. The body relies primarily on the central nervous system (CNS), the pulmonary system, the heart, and the vascular system to accomplish effective respiration. Respiratory failure develops when one or more of these systems or organs fail to maintain optimal functioning. If the respiratory failure occurs so rapidly that the compensatory mechanisms cannot accommodate or if the compensatory mechanisms are overwhelmed, acute respiratory failure develops.

Respiratory failure is a broad, nonspecific clinical diagnosis indicating that the respiratory system is unable to supply the oxygen necessary to maintain metabolism or cannot eliminate sufficient carbon dioxide (CO_2). *Acute respiratory failure* is defined as a partial pressure of arterial oxygen (PaO_2) of 5 mm Hg or less on room air or partial pressure of arterial CO_2 ($PaCO_2$) of 50 mm Hg or more. Some experts will also identify a pH of less than or equal to 7.35 as another indication of acute respiratory failure.[13] In clients with chronic hypercapnia, $PaCO_2$ elevations of 5 mm Hg or more from their previously stable levels indicate that acute respiratory failure has been superimposed on chronic respiratory failure.

Acute respiratory failure may be classified as hypoxemic or ventilatory failure. Clients with acute *hypoxemic* respiratory failure have severe arterial hypoxemia and are minimally responsive to supplemental oxygen despite adequate ventilation. Hypoxemic respiratory failure may be caused by diffuse problems such as pulmonary edema; near-drowning; adult (acute) respiratory distress syndrome; or localized problems such as pneumonia, bleeding into the chest, or lung tumors.

Ventilatory or hypercapnic respiratory failure is when the client is unable to support adequate gas exchange that can result from CNS depression, inadequate neuromuscular ability to sustain breathing, or respiratory system overload. Conditions such as acute deterioration of chronic obstructive pulmonary disease (COPD, sometimes called (chronic airflow limitation), and status asthmaticus are other causes of ventilatory failure.

Most clients in acute respiratory failure eventually have an elevated $PaCO_2$ directly related to alveolar hypoventilation from either (1) decreased minute ventilation with normal dead space ventilation or (2) normal or increased minute ventilation with increased dead space ventilation.

---

evolve Be sure to check out the bonus material on the Evolve website and the CD-ROM, including free self-assessment exercises.
http://evolve.elsevier.com/Black/medsurg/

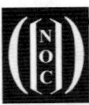

Nursing Outcomes Classification (NOC)
for Nursing Diagnoses—Clients with Acute Pulmonary Disorders

Anxiety
Anxiety Control
Coping
Symptom Control
Excess Fluid Volume
Electrolyte and Acid-Base Balance
Respiratory Status: Ventilation
Fluid Balance
Hydration
Imbalanced Nutrition: Less Than Body Requirements
Nutritional Status
Nutritional Status: Food and Fluid Intake
Nutritional Status: Nutrient Intake
Nutritional Status: Biochemical Measures
Nutritional Status: Energy
Impaired Gas Exchange
Respiratory Status: Gas Exchange

Respiratory Status: Ventilation
Electrolyte & Acid/Base Balance
Tissue Perfusion: Pulmonary
Vital Signs Status
Impaired Oral Mucous Membrane
Oral Health
Tissue Integrity: Skin and Mucous Membranes
Impaired Spontaneous Ventilation
Endurance
Muscle Function
Neurological Status: Central Motor Control
Vital Signs Status
Respiratory Status: Gas Exchange
Respiratory Status: Ventilation
Impaired Verbal Communication
Communication Ability
Communication: Expressive Ability

Communication: Receptive Ability
Ineffective Airway Clearance
Aspiration Control
Respiratory Status: Airway Patency
Respiratory Status: Gas Exchange
Respiratory Status: Ventilation
Ineffective Breathing Pattern
Respiratory Status: Patent Airway
Respiratory Status: Ventilation
Vital Signs Status
Risk for Infection
Immune Status
Risk Control
Tissue Integrity: Skin and Mucous Membranes
Immobility Consequences: Physiological

BOX 65-1 *Causes of Noncardiogenic Pulmonary Edema*

Aspiration of gastric contents, especially if a large amount of HCl is present
Barotrauma (e.g., with PEEP with mechanical ventilation)
Drugs (e.g., after administration of narcotics)
Fluid overload from IV fluids or renal failure
Hypoalbuminemia (e.g., nephrotic syndrome, hepatic disease, malnutrition)
Sepsis
Inhalation of toxic chemicals (e.g., sulfur dioxide, paraquat, phosgene, chlorine, nitrogen oxides)
High altitudes (>8000 ft)
Neurogenic stimulus (e.g., increased intracranial pressure, epileptic seizures, head trauma)
Near-drowning syndrome
Mechanical ventilation, oxygen toxicity, ARDS
Malignancies blocking outflow of lymph within the lungs
Pancreatitis
Pneumonia
Smoke inhalation (e.g., trapped in a burning building)
Unilaterally, after reexpansion of collapsed lung (pneumothorax)

ARDS, Adult (acute) respiratory distress syndrome; *HCl,* hydrochloric acid; *IV,* intravenous; *PEEP,* positive end-expiratory pressure.

In the first category, the clients have normal lungs, but the respiratory status is impaired by drugs or diseases that affect respiration (e.g., neuromuscular disorders). In the second category, the clients have intrinsic lung diseases such as COPD or severe pneumonia with significant lung dam-age that increases the amount of nonfunctional lung tissue, thus increasing dead space (or wasted) ventilation. Even with normal or increased minute ventilation, they cannot "blow off" (exhale) a sufficient amount of CO_2. Further discussion of both types of respiratory failure, the conditions that commonly lead to the problem, and the usual management options follows.

HYPOXEMIC RESPIRATORY FAILURE

PULMONARY EDEMA
Pulmonary edema is the abnormal accumulation of fluid in the interstitial spaces surrounding the alveoli with advancement of fluid accumulation in the alveolar sacs. Pulmonary edema is classified by its underlying causes: *Cardiogenic* causes include left ventricular failure, mitral valve stenosis, cardiogenic shock, hypertension, and cardiomyopathy. *Noncardiogenic* causes are shown in Box 65-1. Pulmonary edema can also develop after catastrophic injury to the CNS, such as head injury; this form of pulmonary edema is called *neurogenic* pulmonary edema.

Etiology
Refer to Chapter 13 for a detailed review of the processes guiding fluid movement. Normally, fluid moves into the interstitial space at the arterial end of the capillary as a result of hydrostatic pressure in the vessel and returns to the venous end of the capillary due to oncotic pressure and increases in interstitial hydrostatic pressure. Fluid in the interstitial spaces of the lungs is not uncommon. It normally escapes from the microcirculation and enters

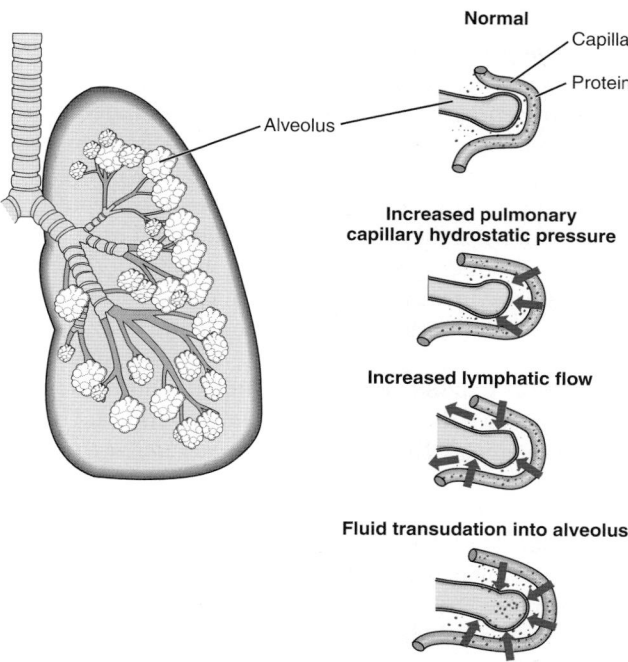

Normal

Capillary

Proteins

Alveolus

Increased pulmonary capillary hydrostatic pressure

Increased lymphatic flow

Fluid transudation into alveolus

FIGURE 65-1 Progression of pulmonary edema. Pulmonary edema occurs when capillary hydrostatic pressure is increased, promoting movement of fluid into the interstitial space of the alveolar-capillary membrane. Initially, increased lymphatic flow removes the excess fluids, but continued leakage eventually overwhelms this mechanism. Gas exchange becomes impaired by the thick membrane. Increasing interstitial fluid pressure ultimately causes leaks into the alveolar sacs, impairing ventilation and gas exchange. (From Hansen, M. [1998]. *Pathophysiology*. Philadelphia: W.B. Saunders.)

the interstitium, providing nutrients for the cells. The residual fluid is returned via the lymphatic system. Increased volume of fluid in the pulmonary arteries from obstruction of forward flow is the most common cause of pulmonary edema. Heart failure is the most common example of the obstruction of forward flow. Lung tumors can obstruct lymphatic flow and can also lead to pulmonary edema.

Pathophysiology

Increased hydrostatic pressure in the pulmonary vessels creates an imbalance in the Starling forces, resulting in an increase of fluid filtration into the interstitial spaces of the lung that exceeds the lymphatic capacity to drain the fluid away. Increasing volumes of fluid leak into the alveolar spaces (Figure 65-1). The lymphatic system attempts to compensate by draining excess interstitial fluid volume through the hilar lymph nodes and back into the vascular system. If this pathway becomes overwhelmed, fluid moves from the pleural interstitium into the alveolar walls. If the alveolar epithelium is damaged, the fluid begins to accumulate in the alveoli. Alveolar edema is a serious late manifestation in the progression of fluid imbalance.

Hypoxemia develops when the alveolar membrane is thickened by fluid that impairs the exchange of oxygen and CO_2. As fluid fills the interstitium and alveolar spaces, lung compliance decreases and oxygen diffusion is impaired. If pulmonary edema has developed because of left ventricular failure, right ventricular failure may occur because the pulmonary artery pressure is elevated. This elevation increases afterload for the right ventricle, resulting in manifestations of right ventricular failure.

Clinical Manifestations

The manifestations of pulmonary edema are due to failure of the regulatory factors guiding fluid movement. Most manifestations are seen in the respiratory system and include marked dyspnea, tachypnea, weak and thready tachycardia, hypertension (if cardiogenic), orthopnea at less than 90 degrees, and the use of accessory muscles. The client's frequent coughing is an attempt to rid the chest of fluid. The sputum is thin and frothy because it is combined with water. If the hydrostatic pressure is very high, small capillaries break and sputum becomes pink tinged. The client may be anxious from dyspnea and restless from hypoxemia. Chest auscultation reveals crackles, wheezes, and the presence of an S_3 heart sound. A heart murmur may be noted if the cause is mitral valve disease. Pulse oximetry readings are commonly less than 85% and arterial blood gas (ABG) determinations may reveal an arterial PaO_2 of less than 50 mm Hg. Respiratory alkalosis is common because of the tachypnea. Pressure in the pulmonary artery and pulmonary artery wedge pressure (PAWP) are elevated. The chest x-ray shows areas of "whiteout" where fluid has replaced air-filled lung tissue, which normally appears black. Right ventricular failure may also be noted, with manifestations of hepatomegaly, jugular venous distention, and peripheral edema.

Outcome Management
■ Medical Management

Medical management concentrates on four areas: (1) correction of hypoxemia, (2) reduction in preload, (3) reduction of afterload, and (4) support of perfusion.

Correct Hypoxemia. It is imperative to maintain adequate oxygenation. Clients with severe pulmonary edema commonly require oxygen therapy at high FiO_2 levels and may require noninvasive positive pressure ventilation (NPPV) such as continuous positive airway pressure (CPAP) or mechanical ventilation if they cannot meet the work of breathing. NPPV is any type of respiratory support that does not require endotracheal tube (ET) intubation.

Reduce Preload. The client is placed in an upright position. Usually, the client does not lie down because of orthopnea and a feeling of choking when supine. Diuretics are prescribed to promote fluid excretion. Nitrates, such as nitroglycerin, are used for their vasodilating properties. Other management strategies consist of treating the underlying condition.

Reduce Afterload. Afterload is reduced to diminish workload on the left ventricle. Antihypertensive agents, including potent agents such as nitroprusside, are prescribed. Morphine is prescribed to reduce the sympathetic nervous system response and to reduce anxiety from the dyspnea.

Support Perfusion. The left ventricle is supported by using inotropic medications such as dobutamine. Urine output is monitored closely to determine whether renal perfusion is adequate. An intra-aortic balloon pump (IABP) may be required with severe heart failure and pulmonary edema (see Chapter 57).

■ Nursing Management
Assessment

The client with pulmonary edema is assessed quickly on admission, concentrating on only the information and assessment findings essential to begin treatment. The client is typically anxious and having significant shortness of breath. Managing the client's anxiety and reducing the dyspnea is imperative. A complete assessment is carried out over the following hours, when the client can breathe more comfortably and answer questions. A baseline weight and lung assessment is essential, because these parameters will assist in determining treatment effectiveness.

Diagnosis, Outcomes, Interventions

Diagnosis: Impaired Gas Exchange. The fluid-filled alveoli retard the exchange of gases. Use the nursing diagnosis *Impaired Gas Exchange related to capillary membrane obstruction from fluid* to plan care.

Outcomes. The client will demonstrate improved gas exchange, as evidenced by rising PaO_2 to 55 or 60 mm Hg, oxygen saturation above 90%, normalizing pH, decreasing anxiety and dyspnea, and fewer crackles and wheezing within 12 hours.

Interventions. Monitor vital signs every 15 minutes initially, until the client is stable. Administer oxygen as ordered using a high-flow rebreather bag to maintain oxygenation. Titrate the actual liter flow of oxygen to maintain saturation above 90%. Continuous assessment is needed because the client may not be able to tolerate the work of breathing and may require NPPV or endotracheal (ET) intubation and mechanical ventilation. NPPV, mechanical ventilation, and intubation equipment should

readily available. To reduce preload, position the client with the legs in a dependent position. Raising edematous legs increases venous return and will stress the overtaxed left ventricle. Preload is reduced with morphine and nitroglycerin. Because perfusion to the skin is often compromised, repositioning is important.

Air hunger can lead to panic and feelings of suffocation. Administering opioids (morphine) and anxiolytics to control both dyspnea and anxiety will relax the client and improve breathing. Stay with the client and use breathing techniques to support the client.

Diagnosis: Excess Fluid Volume. Accumulation of fluid from several causes leads to fluid overload. Use the nursing diagnosis *Excess Fluid Volume related to excess preload*.

Outcomes. The client will demonstrate improved fluid balance, as evidenced by diuresis (input less than output), decreased number of crackles and wheezes, eupnea, weight loss, resolving peripheral edema, and decreased anxiety.

Interventions. Administer a diuretic (furosemide) as prescribed to promote diuresis. Place an indwelling catheter to monitor response to diuretics. Monitor urine output, weight, and potassium levels (potassium loss is a side effect of furosemide). Monitor blood pressure to determine whether the client can maintain perfusion without inotropic support. Because oral fluids are restricted, oral care is completed every 2 hours.

Evaluation

If the previously described interventions are implemented immediately, a fairly rapid response to diuresis and oxygen therapy should be seen.

■ Self-Care
Consider the reasons for development of pulmonary edema when developing a plan for self-care. Clients may need further education on daily weights, dietary choices, and scheduling of medications. Instruct the client and family members on the early manifestations of fluid overload so that early intervention is possible.

ACUTE VENTILATORY FAILURE
Ventilatory failure is the inability of the body to sustain respiratory drive or the inability of the chest wall and muscles to mechanically move air in and out of the lungs. The hallmark of ventilatory failure is an elevated CO_2 level.

Etiology and Risk Factors
In acute ventilatory failure, the respiratory load placed on the lung to exchange oxygen and CO_2 is impaired by

(1) problems of resistance to moving air in and out of the lung, (2) the ability of the lung to expand and contract (elastic recoil), and (3) conditions that increase the production of CO_2 or decrease the surface available for exchange of gases. The competence of the nerves and muscles coordinating the movement of the chest can also be impaired by loss of drive to breathe, impaired transmission of signals to the chest and diaphragm, and muscle fatigue. Conditions that can lead to acute ventilatory failure are listed in Table 65-1.

Pathophysiology

Alveolar ventilation is maintained by the CNS acting through nerves and the muscles of respiration to drive breathing. Failure of alveolar ventilation leads to a ventilation/perfusion ($\dot{V}/\dot{Q}$) mismatch resulting in hypercapnia (rising CO_2 levels) and eventually acidosis develops. Left untreated, acute ventilatory failure leads to death.

Functional residual capacity (FRC) is the volume of air remaining in the lung after normal expiration. In obstructive forms of ventilatory failure, the residual pressure in the chest impairs inhalation and increases the workload of breathing. When end-expiratory alveolar volumes remain above their critical closing point, the alveoli remain open and functioning, allowing oxygen to diffuse into the bloodstream. If alveolar volumes fall below the closing point, the alveoli tend to collapse. When alveoli collapse, no oxygenation or blood flow to the alveoli occurs (Figure 65-2). In acute ventilatory failure, the residual volume and FRC are decreased, resulting in

TABLE 65-1	*Risk Factors for Acute Ventilatory Failure*		
Systems, Structures, and Conditions	**Causes of Respiratory Failure**	**Systems, Structures, and Conditions**	**Causes of Respiratory Failure**
Central nervous system	Drug overdose Pickwickian syndrome Stroke Ondine's curse Cerebral trauma (↑ intracranial pressure) Central sleep apnea Tumors Myxedema	Conducting airways	Epiglottitis Laryngotracheitis Trauma Tracheal stenosis Foreign body aspiration Tumors Asthma Bronchospasm
Peripheral nervous system	Multiple sclerosis Poliomyelitis Amyotrophic lateral sclerosis Guillain-Barré syndrome Botulism Tetanus Drugs Spinal cord injury Myasthenia gravis Electrolyte imbalance	Lungs	Chronic obstructive pulmonary disease Cystic fibrosis Pneumonia Pulmonary emboli Aspiration Inhaled toxins Pulmonary edema Adult (acute) respiratory distress syndrome Interstitial lung disease Near-drowning Inhaled toxins Trauma Radiation pneumonitis Oxygen toxicity
Musculoskeletal and pleural functions	Muscular dystrophy Kyphoscoliosis Flail chest Ankylosing spondylitis Morbid obesity Restrictive pleural diseases Pleural effusion Pneumothorax Hemothorax	Nonpulmonary conditions	Sepsis Myocardial infarction Eclampsia Anaphylaxis Shock Disseminated intravascular coagulation Fat embolism Systemic inflammatory response syndrome

From Bucher, L., & Melander, S. (1999). *Critical care nursing*. Philadelphia: W.B. Saunders.

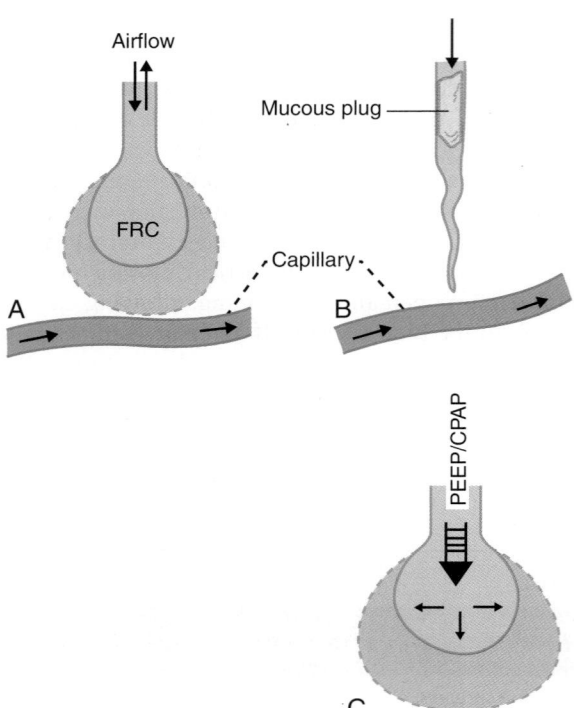

FIGURE 65-2 Effects of positive airway pressure on alveolus. **A,** Normal alveolus. *Dotted line* represents expansion during inspiration. **B,** Collapsed alveolus. Perfusion (continued). **C,** The alveolus is opened by positive pressure. *Dotted line* indicates alveolus during inspiration, and *solid line* indicates end-expiratory alveolar volume. *CPAP,* Continuous positive airway pressure; *FRC,* functional reserve capacity; *PEEP,* peak end-expiratory pressure.

a true intrapulmonary shunt (perfusion without oxygenation) and decreased lung compliance.

Once alveolar collapse occurs, reinflation necessitates very high opening pressures, the generation of which significantly increases the work of breathing. The hypoxemia resulting from alveolar collapse and the increased oxygen consumption caused by the increased work of breathing may severely compromise the client.

Clinical Manifestations

To avoid frank apnea, recognizing impending ventilatory failure is critical. Continuous monitoring of high-risk clients concentrating on changes in respiratory rate, mental status, and patterns of breathing is essential. The hallmark manifestations of hypercapnia are headache and dyspnea. The client may also verbalize that dyspnea is increasing despite treatment. Altered respiratory patterns can herald impending ventilatory failure. The client's respiratory rate can rise to 50 to 60 breaths/min, but the breaths are shallow and impaired by spasm of the airway. The rate can also fall to four to six per minute. Clients become confused, less conversant, and are difficult to arouse. If the cause of ventilatory failure

is obstruction of the airway, the systolic pressure falls during inspiration as a result of intrathoracic resistance. This change, called *pulsus paradoxus,* is present when systolic blood pressure falls more than 10 mm Hg during inspiration. Pulse oximetry indicates steadily decreasing oxygen saturation values, and ABG analysis shows falling PaO_2 and rising $PaCO_2$.

Outcome Management
■ Medical Management

Medical management is directed at reversing bronchospasm, maintaining oxygenation, treating the underlying problem, and providing ventilatory assistance. Mechanical ventilation is not used until other methods of maintaining ventilation have been tried.

Reverse Bronchospasm. Several forms of bronchodilators are used to treat obstructions to airflow in clients with COPD and asthma. These agents include inhaled $beta_2$-selective agonists (albuterol), ipratropium, theophylline, and corticosteroids. If infection is the underlying cause, broad-spectrum antibiotics are given.

Maintain Oxygenation. Oxygen by mask may be adequate to support oxygenation. Using forms of NPPV such as CPAP reduces the workload of breathing by decreasing the force needed to overcome the pressure in the chest. Outcomes after mechanical ventilation with lower tidal volumes may be better than the traditional formula (10 to 15 ml of body weight per kilogram), which sometimes lead to stretch-induced lung injury.[29]

Manage the Underlying Problem. Table 65-1 demonstrates the many causes of ventilatory failure. Some of these causes can be quickly managed, such as reversing drug overdose with naloxone, but others require more aggressive treatment. Supportive therapies are used to reverse or control the underlying problem.

Maintain Ventilation. Initially, NPPV should be used if the client is alert and can maintain the mask over the nose or mouth without becoming claustrophobic. NPPV keeps small airways open and improves gas exchange with the goal being to keep oxygen saturation above 90%. Frequent ABG readings may need to be taken to ensure that adequate oxygenation is being achieved. In some cases, NPPV with a heliox adjunct will support the client and prevent the need for intubation and mechanical ventilation. Heliox is a helium/oxygen mixture (60% to 70% helium/30% to 40% oxygen) that flows easily in constricted areas. Studies have shown that this mixture decreased hypercapnia and airway resistance in COPD clients.[2] If NPPV is not successful, mechanical ventilation is required and helps to minimize the work of breathing while effectively promoting gas exchange (oxygenation and ventilation). The client requires an ar-

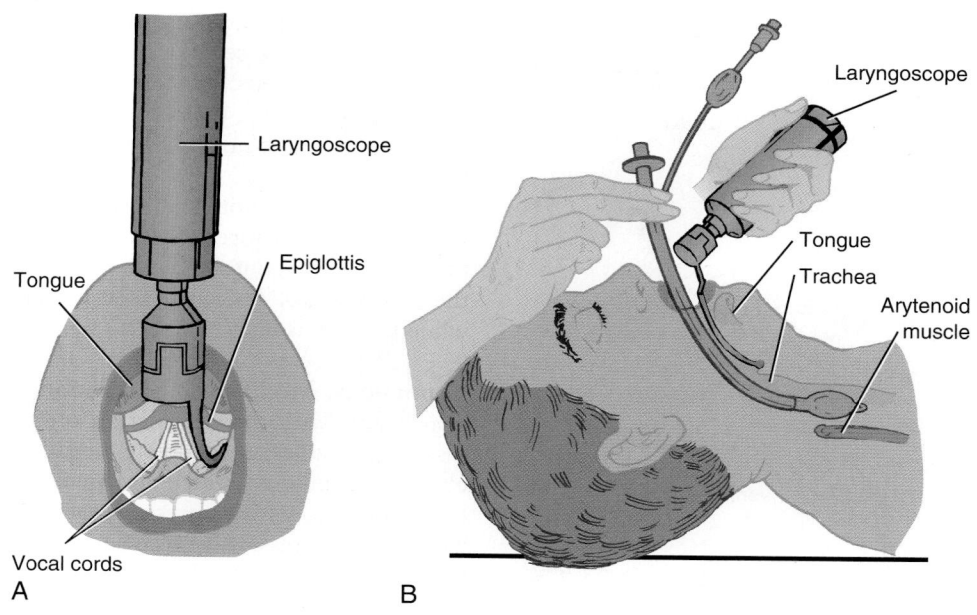

FIGURE 65-3 A, A laryngoscope is used to visualize the vocal cords. **B,** The endotracheal tube is inserted with the client's head extended to align the airway.

tificial airway, usually by ET intubation and the use of positive-pressure ventilation (PPV). If prolonged intubation is required, the ET tube is replaced with a tracheostomy.

Endotracheal Intubation

Intubation. The ET tube is a long, slender, hollow tube usually made of polyvinyl chloride and is inserted into the trachea via the mouth or nose. It passes through the vocal cords, and the distal tip is positioned just above the bifurcation of the main stem of the bronchus (carina). Oral intubation is usually used for short-term airway management. Nasal intubation, a more secure method, is believed to be more comfortable because the tube does not move as much in the airway. However, nasal intubation is not being used in many hospitals because of the risk of sinusitis. Before intubation, the client is supine, and all dental bridgework and plates and loose teeth are removed because these items can be jarred loose and aspirated during the procedure. The client's head is hyperextended, the lower aspect of the neck is flexed, and the mouth is opened (Figure 65-3). This position brings the mouth, pharynx, and larynx into a straight line. A laryngoscope is used to hold the airway open, expose the vocal cords, and serve as a guide for the tube into the trachea. ET tubes are inserted only by fully trained health care team members.

Intubation should not cause or exacerbate hypoxia. If the client's neck and mandible are mobile, the procedure usually takes about 30 seconds. Certain pre-existing conditions such as obesity with a stocky neck, a possible spinal cord injury, or rheumatoid arthritis of the neck

can make intubation difficult. For clients with expected difficulty of intubation, an oxygen mask can be used to provide oxygen through the mouth. An oxygen saturation monitor may also be used to warn of hypoxemia.

A good practice to remember during difficult intubation is to hold your breath while intubation is attempted. If you must stop to breathe before the client is intubated, the intubation is taking too long. Stop the intubation, reoxygenate the client by mask, and reattempt intubation.

Immediately after ET tube insertion, tube placement is verified by auscultation and chest x-ray to ensure aeration of both sides of the chest. Record in the nurses' notes and on the respiratory flow sheet the point at which the tube meets the lips or nostrils by using the numbers listed on the side of the ET tube. If the tube slips, its correct position can be reestablished quickly. Secure the ET tube immediately after intubation with adhesive tape, twill tape, or specially designed ET tube holders (Figure 65-4). Retaping is required only if the tape becomes loose or soiled.

Cuff Inflation. The cuff of an ET tube seals the tube against the tracheal wall to facilitate PPV and protects the respiratory tract from aspiration of foreign material. The amount of air required to seal an ET tube cuff is reflected by the cuff pressure, which is usually maintained at less than 20 mm Hg. Most ET tubes are designed with soft plastic cuffs for use with high volumes of air at low pressures. Cuffs are inflated with a volume of air high enough to seal the trachea while exerting the lowest possible pressure on the tracheal wall. Low cuff pressure is necessary to prevent damage to the tracheal mucosa. Ar-

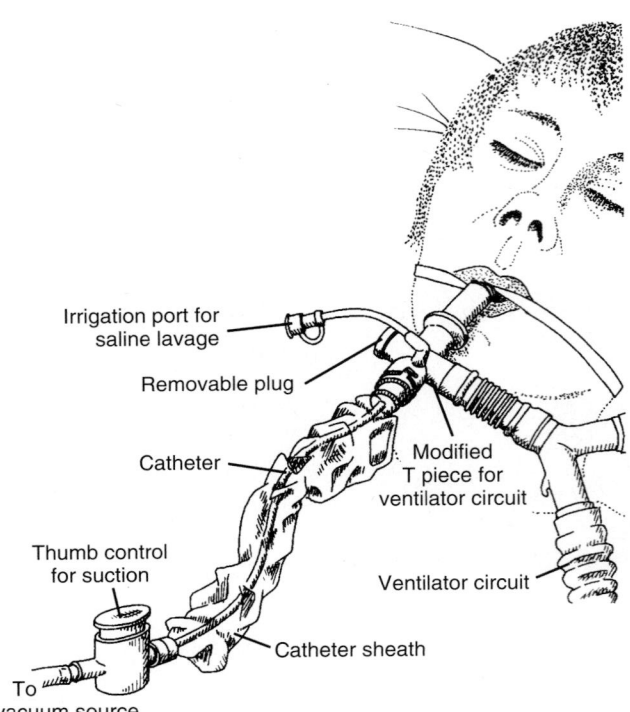

Irrigation port for
saline lavage

Removable plug

Catheter

Modified
T piece for
ventilator circuit

Thumb control
for suction

Ventilator circuit

Catheter sheath

To
vacuum source

FIGURE 65-4 Secured cuffed endotracheal tube with closed tracheal suction system. (From Sill, J.R. [1991]. *Respiratory care certification guide.* St. Louis: Mosby.)

terial pressures in the tracheal wall are approximately 20 to 25 mm Hg; venous pressures are 18 to 20 mm Hg. Therefore cuff pressures greater than 18 to 20 mm Hg impair circulation to the tracheal mucosa and necrosis may develop. Assess cuff pressures every 8 hours or as institutional policy dictates.

The most common method of cuff inflation *(minimal occlusion volume technique)* aims to provide an adequate seal in the trachea at the lowest possible cuff pressure. Slowly inject air into the cuff while auscultating with a stethoscope placed over the larynx (over the cuff) during a positive-pressure breath. At the point when sounds (from air movement) cease, inflation is stopped, indicating that the cuff is sealed against the tracheal wall.

Cuff Deflation. Generally, ET cuffs should remain inflated at all times. If cuff deflation is required for any reason, suction the trachea (with the client being hyperventilated and hyperoxygenated before and during this procedure) and clean the area above the cuff of secretions by gently suctioning deep into the oropharynx. Advance the suction catheter to the end of the ET tube and deflate the cuff while applying suction to the suction catheter so that any secretions lying above the cuff can be removed. If necessary, repeat pharyngeal suctioning.

Cuff Leaks. Cuff leaks can be a major problem. They may be caused by a rupture or tear in the cuff or

pilot system or by a change in ET tube position in the trachea. There are several signs of a leak in or around the ET tube cuff, including the pilot balloon not filling when air is injected, the client can talk when the cuff is inflated, or air is heard leaking during positive pressure breathing.

If the system is not functional, the ET tube may need to be replaced. Before replacement, increasing tidal volume may help maintain ventilation by compensating for the escaping gas. The client is at high risk for aspiration while the cuff is leaking.

Continuous Mechanical Ventilation. Normal respiration begins with the contraction of the diaphragm and respiratory muscles to create negative pressure in the chest: A vacuum is created and air flows in. When a ventilator is used, positive pressure forces air into the lungs. The positive pressure is necessary for gas exchange and to keep alveoli open. Unfortunately, positive pressure forces can also damage the alveoli and may retard venous return and cardiac output.

The goals of continuous mechanical ventilation (CMV) are the following:

- To maintain adequate ventilation
- To deliver precise concentrations of FiO_2
- To deliver adequate tidal volumes to obtain an adequate minute ventilation and oxygenation
- To lessen the work of breathing in those clients who cannot sustain adequate ventilation on their own

Types of Ventilators. Several types of mechanical ventilators are available. A control panel of one ventilator system is shown in Figure 65-5.

Pressure-cycled ventilators deliver a volume of gas to the airway using positive pressure during inspiration. This positive pressure is delivered until the preselected pressure has been reached. When the preset pressure is reached, the machine cycles into exhalation. Pressure-cycled ventilators are used in only a small portion of clients who require CMV.

Volume-cycled (volume-controlled or *volume-limited) ventilators* deliver a preset tidal volume of inspired gas. The tidal volume that has been preselected is delivered to the client regardless of the pressure required to deliver this volume. A pressure limit can be set to prevent the occurrence of dangerously high airway pressures.

Time-cycled ventilators terminate when a preset inspiratory time has elapsed. In most of these devices, a pressure limit is also incorporated.

Flow-cycled ventilators are triggered to stop when a preset flow rate has been achieved.

Modes of Ventilation. The ventilation mode refers to the way the client receives breaths from the ventilator. Table 65-2 describes several conventional modes of CMV.

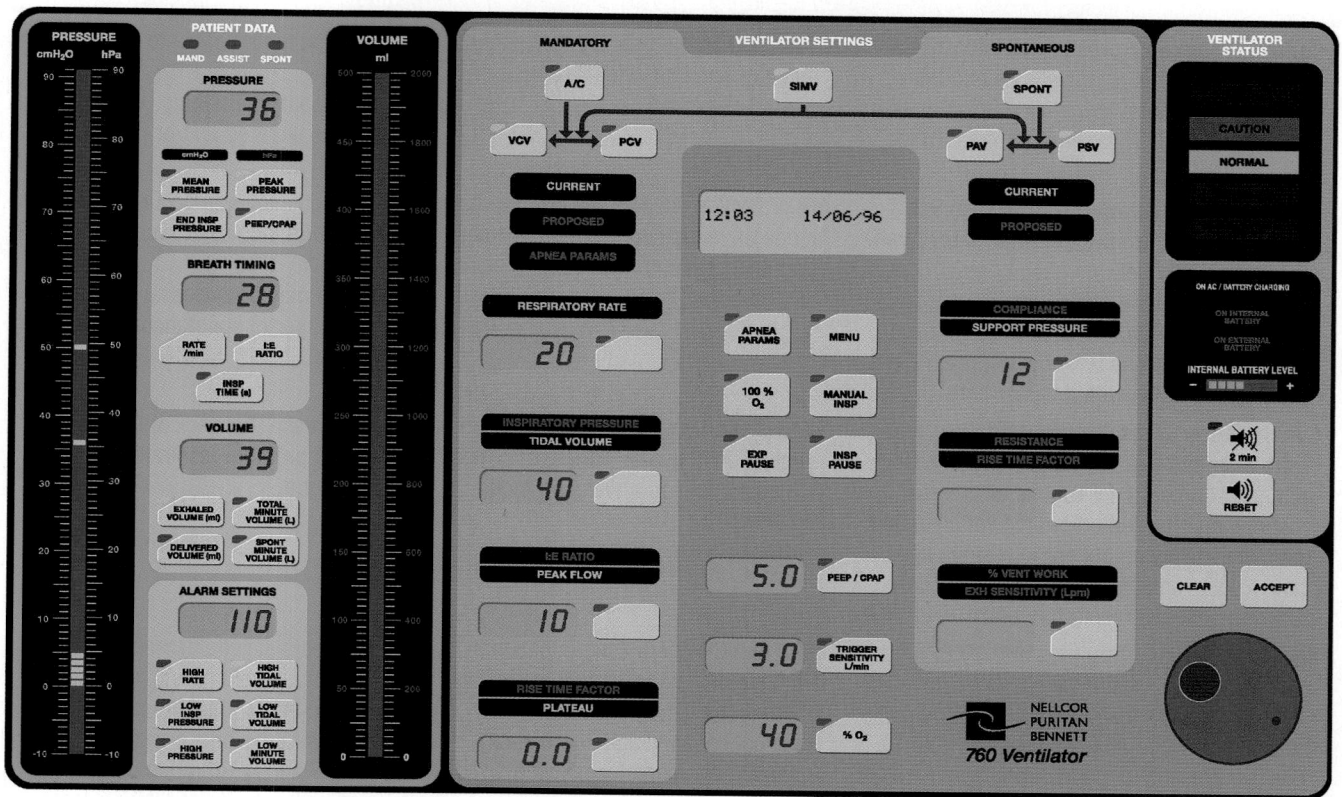

FIGURE 65-5 Nellcor Puritan Bennett 760 Ventilator. (Courtesy of Mallinckrodt, Inc., Nellcor Puritan Bennett Ventilator Division.)

Triggering Mechanisms. All breaths given to the client must be initiated or triggered. Triggering mechanisms can be based on (1) time, (2) negative pressure, (3) flow, or (4) volume.

Time-triggered inhalation is used to manage clients who cannot breathe on their own. The ventilator will trigger a breath after a preset time, serving as a back-up in case a client's own breathing rate falls below a preset value.

Negative pressure inhalation is triggered by the initial negative pressure that begins inspiration. As soon as the client initiates a breath, the ventilator is triggered to produce inhalation. The sensitivity of the system is set to reduce the workload of breathing. Pressure fluctuations (e.g., hiccoughs, leaks) can cause premature triggering.

Flow-triggered inhalation occurs when the client can initiate a breath. The ventilator completes the breath by sensing the flow of air into the chest. This system works well in combination with positive end-expiratory pressure (PEEP).

Volume-triggered ventilation occurs when the ventilator completes the breath to maximize inhaled gas volumes.

Alarms. Ventilators have several alarms to assist with their safe use. See the Bridge to Critical Care feature on Troubleshooting Alarms on p. 1887 for a discussion of the alarm systems most commonly seen with ventilators.

Positive End-Expiratory Pressure/Continuous Positive Airway Pressure. The techniques PEEP and CPAP are applied during expiration to prevent intrathoracic pressures from returning to ambient atmospheric pressure. CPAP is applied to a client with spontaneous respiration; PEEP is applied during mechanical ventilation. CPAP and PEEP are used to apply positive airway pressure that keeps the alveoli open and reduces the amount of shunting with the goal that the FiO_2 may be reduced to the lowest possible level to maintain gas exchange and to prevent oxygen toxicity (Figure 65-2, *C*). This increased pressure also increases FRC and enhances oxygenation as a result of the enlarged surface area that is available for diffusion. Positive pressures of 5 to 20 cm H_2O are typically used in adults. Pressures may be adjusted until the level is found that produces the best PaO_2 without producing adverse effects. This level is called "best PEEP."

Risks of PEEP include overdistention of the alveoli, $\dot{V}/\dot{Q}$ mismatch, subcutaneous emphysema, and decreased cardiac output from increased intrathoracic pressure.

Physiologic Changes After Mechanical Ventilation. Many physiologic changes occur when a client is placed

TABLE 65-2   *Modes of Mechanical Ventilation*

Mode of Ventilation	Clinical Application	Nursing Implications
Control (volume or pressure) ventilation (CV): Delivers gas at preset rate and tidal volume or pressure (depending on selected cycling variable), regardless of patient's inspiratory efforts	CV is used as the primary ventilatory mode in patients who are apneic	Used in patients unable to initiate a breath Spontaneously breathing patients must be sedated and/or paralyzed
Assist-control (volume or pressure) ventilation (A/C) or continuous mandatory ventilation (CMV): Delivers gas at preset tidal volume or pressure (depending on selected cycling variable) in response to patient's inspiratory efforts and will initiate breath if patient fails to do so within preset time	A/C or CMV is used as the primary mode of ventilation in spontaneously breathing patients with weak respiratory muscles	Hyperventilation can occur in patients with increased respiratory rates Sedation may be necessary to limit the number of spontaneous breaths
Synchronous intermittent mandatory (volume or pressure) ventilation (SIMV): Delivers gas at preset tidal volume or pressure (depending on selected cycling variable) and rate while allowing patient to breathe spontaneously); ventilator breaths are synchronized to patient's respiratory effort	SIMV is used both as a primary mode of ventilation in a wide variety of clinical situations and as a weaning mode	May increase the work of breathing and promote respiratory muscle fatigue
Positive end-expiratory pressure (PEEP): Positive pressure applied at the end of expiration of ventilator breaths (used with CV, A/C, and SIMV) **Constant positive airway pressure (CPAP):** Positive pressure applied during spontaneous breaths	PEEP and CPAP are used in patients with hypoxemia refractory to oxygen therapy; they increase functional residual capacity and improve oxygenation by opening collapsed alveoli at end expiration	Side effects include decreased cardiac output, volutrauma, and increased intracranial pressure No ventilator breaths are delivered in PEEP and CPAP mode unless used with CV, A/C, or SIMV
Pressure support ventilation (PSV): Preset positive pressure used to augment patient's inspiratory efforts; patient controls rate, inspiratory flow, and tidal volume	PSV is used as the primary mode of ventilation in patients with stable respiratory drive, is used with SIMV to support spontaneous breaths, and is used as a weaning mode in patients who are difficult to wean	Advantages include increased patient comfort, decreased work of breathing and decreased respiratory muscle fatigue, and promotion of respiratory muscle conditioning
Volume-assured pressure support ventilation (VAPSV): Tidal volume is set to ensure patient receives minimum tidal volume with each pressure support breath		
Independent lung ventilation (ILV): Each lung is ventilated separately	ILV is used in patients with unilateral lung disease, bronchopleural fistulas, and bilateral asymmetric lung disease	Requires a double-lumen endotracheal tube, two ventilators, sedation, and/or pharmacologic paralysis

High-frequency ventilation (HFV): Delivers a small volume of gas at a rapid rate
  High-frequency positive-pressure ventilation (HFPPV): delivers 60-100 breaths/min
  High-frequency jet ventilation (HFJV): delivers 100-600 cycles/min
  High-frequency oscillation (HFO): delivers 900-3000 cycles/min
	HFV is used in situations in which conventional mechanical ventilation compromises hemodynamic stability, with bronchopleural fistulas, during short-term procedures, and with diseases that create a risk of volutrauma	Patients require sedation and/or pharmacologic paralysis
		Inadequate humidification can compromise airway patency
		Assessment of breath sounds is difficult

Inverse ratio ventilation (IRV): Proportion of inspiratory to expiratory time is greater than 1:1; can be initiated using pressure-controlled breaths (PC-IRV) or volume controlled breaths (VC-IRV)	IRV is used in patients with hypoxemia refractory to PEEP; the longer inspiratory time increases functional residual capacity and improves oxygenation by opening collapsed alveoli, and the shorter expiratory time induces auto-PEEP that prevents alveoli from recollapsing	Requires sedation and/or pharmacologic paralysis because of discomfort Increased intrathoracic pressure can result in excessive air trapping and decreased cardiac output

From Urden, L.D., Stacy, K.M., & Lough, M.E. (2002). *Thelan's critical care nursing: diagnosis and management.* (4th ed.) St. Louis: Mosby.

BRIDGE TO CRITICAL CARE

Troubleshooting Alarms

Display Message	Possible Cause	Remedy
HIGH CONTINUOUS PRESSURE	Airway pressure higher than set PEEP plus 15 cm H_2O for more than 15 sec	Check client Check circuit Check ventilator settings and alarm limits
CHECK TUBINGS	Disconnected pressure transducer (expiratory) Blocked pressure transducer (expiratory) Water in expiratory limb of ventilator Wet bacterial filter Clogged bacterial filter	Check ventilator internals on expiratory side Refer to service Replace filter Remove water from tubing and check humidifier settings (i.e., relative humidity) Check heater wires in humidifier (if present)
AIRWAY PRESSURE TOO HIGH *Note:* If airway pressure rises 6 cm H_2O above set upper pressure limit, the safety valve opens. Safety valve also opens if system pressure exceeds 120 cm H_2O.	Kinked or blocked client tubing Mucus or secretion plug in endotrachial tube or in airways Client coughing or fighting ventilator Inspiratory flow rate too high Improper alarm setting	Check client Check ventilator settings and alarm limits
LIMITED PRESSURE *Note:* Alarm is active only in PRVC and VS modes	Kinked or blocked client tubing Mucus or secretion plug in endotrachial tube or in airways Client coughing or fighting ventilator Improper alarm setting Client's lung/thorax compliance decreasing Client's airway resistance increasing	Check client Check ventilator settings and alarm limits
EXPIRED MINUTE VOLUME TOO HIGH	Increased client activity Ventilator self-triggering (autocycling) Improper alarm limit setting Wet flow transducer	Check client Check trigger sensitivity setting Check alarm limit settings Dry the flow transducer
EXPIRED MINUTE VOLUME TOO LOW	Low spontaneous client breathing activity Leakage in cuff Leakage in client circuit Improper alarm limit setting	Check client Check cuff pressure Check client circuit (perform leakage test if necessary) Check pause time and graphics to verify Consider more ventilatory support for client
EXPIRED MINUTE VOLUME DISPLAY READS 0	Flow transducer faulty Circuit disconnected from client	Replace flow transducer Connect Y-piece to client

APNEA ALARM
Note: If in VS, ventilator will revert to PRVC. Back-up rate and time must be set.
	Time between two consecutive inspiratory efforts exceeds:
	  Adult: 20 sec.
	  Pediatric: 15 sec.
	  Neonate: 10 sec.
		Check client
		Check ventilator settings

PEEP/CPAP AND/OR PLATEAU PRESSURE FAILS TO BE MAINTAINED	Leakage in cuff Leakage in client circuit Improper alarm limit setting	Check cuff pressure Check client circuit (perform leakage test if necessary) Check pause time and graphics to verify Consider more ventilatory support for client

Modified from *Servo Ventilator 300 operating manual 8.0* (1996). Solna, Sweden: Siemens-Elema AB.
CPAP, Continuous positive airway pressure; *PEEP,* positive end-expiratory pressure; *PRVC,* pressure-regulated volume control; *VS,* volume support.

on mechanical ventilation. Decreased cardiac output is the most common of these. Normal unassisted respiration begins with subatmospheric pressure. Negative pressure increases during inhalation and decreases during exhalation. Positive pressure applied to the airway has the opposite effect. As positive pressure inflates the lungs the pressure in the thorax builds, decreasing the flow of blood to the vena cava and reducing blood flow to the right atrium of the heart. Exhalation is passive and pressures return to the normal resting subatmospheric level. Blood flow to and from the right ventricle is also decreased if PPV is continued for more than a few minutes. This, in turn, decreases the filling of the left ventricle, leading to a lowered cardiac output. The lowered cardiac output is reflected in the hypotension that clients commonly exhibit immediately after initiating mechanical ventilation. It is imperative that blood pressures be monitored closely.

Positive pressure may also briefly affect the left side of the heart by increased filling and output. This increase is due to the displacement of blood from the pulmonary system into the left ventricle. However, this effect is noted only immediately after institution of PPV.

PPV may lead to stretch injury in the alveoli and the release of inflammatory mediators. To minimize stretch injury, the lowest possible tidal volume and PEEP should be used.

Other body systems are also affected by PPV. During the inspiratory phase, the diaphragm descends into the abdomen, resulting in decreased blood flow to the splanchnic area, leading to ischemia of the gastric mucosa. Ischemia of the gastric mucosa may be one of the reasons that clients receiving PPV for an extended period have a high incidence of gastrointestinal bleeding and stress ulcerations. Decreasing blood flow to the splanchnic region also results in decreased blood flow to the kidneys. Decreased blood flow signals the posterior pituitary gland to increase secretion of vasopressin (antidiuretic hormone [ADH]). Elevated vasopressin levels lead to reabsorption of free water in the renal tubular cells, thereby increasing water retention. Lymphatic flow also decreases.

In addition, PPV can cause neurophysiologic changes. When the oxygenation levels improve in a client with respiratory failure, cerebral oxygenation also improves. A client with compensated *respiratory acidosis* (chronic CO_2 retention) may be adversely affected by positive-pressure breathing because too much CO_2 is exhaled, or "blown off." If acute respiratory alkalosis occurs, the client may exhibit dizziness, lightheadedness, and anxiety. If severe alkalosis persists, convulsions, cardiac dysrhythmias, and cerebral edema may occur. Cerebral edema may also contribute to intensive care unit (ICU) psychosis.

Oxygen toxicity can develop in clients who receive oxygen at concentrations greater than 70% for as little

as 16 to 24 hours. Oxygen free radicals are produced in excess of their normal consumption by antioxidants; oxygen free radicals damage cell membranes, which increases the risk of pulmonary fibrosis. Manifestations of oxygen toxicity include fatigue, lethargy, weakness, restlessness, and nausea and vomiting. Later manifestations include severe dyspnea, coughing, tachycardia, tachypnea, crackles, and cyanosis. Because these manifestations are vague, oxygen concentration is limited to the minimal percentage and amount of time needed to maintain oxygenation.

■ Nursing Management

The nurse coordinates efforts of the health care team, teaches and supports the client and family, monitors the client's response to ventilation, intervenes to maintain oxygenation and ventilation, and ensures that the client's complex needs are met (see the Care Plan feature on The Mechanically Ventilated Client on pp. 1889 to 1893).

Neuromuscular Blocking Agents. Sedation is often necessary to maintain ventilation by creating a synchronous respiratory pattern and reduce oxygen demand. In some clients, paralysis with neuromuscular blocking agents is also needed. The most common agents given are vecuronium (Norcuron) and pancuronium (Pavulon). Because neuromuscular blocking agents do not inhibit pain or awareness, they are combined with a sedative or an anxiolytic agent. Pain medication may also be required if the client has pain. If the client is awake, be aware of the anxiety or fear related to inability to breathe independently.

Several nursing precautions are needed while these neuromuscular blocking agents are administered. Reorient the client often, and explain all procedures because the client can still hear but cannot move or see. Safety is a major concern because the client can not verbalize or identify problems. Specific attention should be given to the eyes to prevent corneal abrasions and other eye injuries. Eye care with lubricating ointment is important.[16]

Suctioning. Because the client loses the ability to cough while on mechanical ventilation and secretions tend to pool and obstruct the airways, suctioning is often required. The client should be suctioned through the ET tube only when needed to prevent hypoxemia and to prevent injury to bronchial and lung tissue. Priorities when suctioning a client include hyperoxygenation before suctioning and maintaining sterile technique including the use of the closed tracheal suction system (see Figure 65-4). Refer to the nursing care plan for additional guidelines for suctioning a client.

Weaning from a Ventilator. The physician decides when to begin gradually removing, or "weaning," the client from CMV. The modes of the ventilator that depend on

Text continued on p. 1893

CARE PLAN

The Mechanically Ventilated Client

Nursing Diagnosis. Impaired Spontaneous Ventilation related to imbalance between ventilatory capacity and ventilatory demand.

Outcomes. The client will have a normal respiratory rate and pattern, return of arterial blood gases (ABGs) and pulse oximetry to normal, decreased dyspnea, absence of air trapping, and no complications after continuous mechanical ventilation (CMV).

Interventions	Rationales
1. Check ventilator settings, FiO_2, alarms, and connections and endotracheal (ET) tube placement (use cm markings) at beginning of each shift, hourly thereafter, and after any changes.	1. Determine baseline values, and validate that settings are accurate. Ensure that alarms are functional.
2. Assess lung sounds every 1-2 hours as indicated.	2. Lung sounds should be present bilaterally (unless a previous change in lung sounds is known).
3. Check placement of the ET tube, and secure the tube.	3. The visible portion of the ET tube should not change. Check previous records for a mark that is visible (in cm). Securing prevents dislodgment.
4. Use a bite block.	4. A bite block prevents the client from chewing on the tube and ET tube compression.
5. Assess for manifestations of skin or mucous membrane irritation every shift.	5. ET tubes can place pressure on the lips and oral mucosa at the ET tube site.
6. Assess for agitation, distress, and "fighting" the ventilator.	6. An incorrect ventilator setup may be providing less air than the client requires.
7. Assess for an obstructed airway. If it is obstructed, manually inflate lungs with a resuscitation bag and 100% oxygen and suction the airway.	7. Airway obstruction with mucus may prevent oxygenation. Providing air to the client is imperative. A common cause of obstruction is retained secretions.
8. Sedate and paralyze the client if ventilator settings and oxygenation are adequate.	8. Sedation and paralysis may be required to prevent mismatch.
9. Medicate the client if pain is indicated.	9. Pain can lead to agitation.
10. Perform passive range-of-motion (ROM) or assisted ROM exercises; transfer the client to a chair when feasible.	10. Immobility leads to decreased respiratory muscle strength.

Evaluation. The timing of goal attainment will vary greatly because of underlying co-morbid conditions. Expect postoperative clients to require CMV for 24 hours or less. Clients with end-stage pulmonary disease may require prolonged ventilatory support.

Nursing Diagnosis. Impaired Gas Exchange and Ineffective Breathing Pattern related to underlying disease process and artificial airway and ventilator system.

Outcomes. The client will have improved gas exchange and breathing pattern, ventilation of both lungs, no manifestations of hypoxemia (O_2 saturation >90%, respiratory rate <24 breaths/min, no restlessness); arterial blood gases (ABGs) and acid-base balance will return to preintubation level or normal values.

Interventions	Rationales
1. Auscultate lung sounds and respiratory rate and pattern every 1 to 2 hours as needed.	1. Auscultation reveals the amount of fluid and secretion in the lungs; validates that the ET tube is placed correctly so that both lungs can be ventilated; determines ventilatory effectiveness.
2. Provide adequate humidity via the ventilator or nebulizer.	2. Replaces the function of the upper airway to warm and humidify the inspired air; thins secretions to facilitate their removal.

Continued

CARE PLAN

The Mechanically Ventilated Client—cont'd

Interventions	Rationales
3. Turn and reposition the client every 2 hours.	3. Both lungs can be fully ventilated; secretions can be mobilized.
4. Monitor ABG values and pulse oximetry.	4. Degree of oxygenation can be indicated; lack of improvement in ABGs may require a change in interventions.

Evaluation. If the client's underlying problem has been corrected by mechanical ventilation, these outcomes will be met quickly. If the client has a pre-existing pulmonary disease or is acutely ill, it may take several days for attainment of outcomes.

Nursing Diagnosis. Ineffective Airway Clearance related to inability to cough and stimulation of increased secretion formation in the lower tracheobronchial tree from the ET tube.

Outcomes. The client will have improved airway clearance, as evidenced by fewer crackles, fewer wheezes, and an absence of fever.

Interventions	Rationales
1. Assess the need for suctioning: noisy, wet respirations; restlessness; increased pulse and respirations; visible mucus bubbling into the ET tube; and an increase in peak airway pressure.	1. Detecting the need for suctioning early can prevent desaturation.
2. Thoroughly explain the procedure before starting, and provide reassurance to the client throughout.	2. Suctioning can be an uncomfortable and frightening experience.
3. Airway suctioning is performed on an "as-needed" basis, not at regularly scheduled intervals.	3. Suctioning can traumatize the airway and mucosa.
4. Select a catheter of appropriate size. The most common sizes for adults are 12 and 14 French.	4. The suction catheter should never exceed half the diameter of an artificial airway or the natural airway it is to enter.
5. Avoid excessive vacuum pressures that may traumatize the airway.	5. The safe range of pressure for adults is 80 to 120 mm Hg.
6. Maintain sterility throughout the procedure. Use closed system for suctioning. Clean gloves can be used for closed suctioning; sterile gloves are needed for open suctioning.	6. Usual cilia clearance and cough are suppressed. Closed systems avoid opening the ET tube and exposing the airway to the environment.
7. Hyperoxygenate before and after each suctioning attempt and after the procedure. Increase the Fio_2 on the ventilator (remember to return to previous setting upon completion) or manually ventilate the client.	7. Providing extra oxygen prevents desaturation from suctioning.
8. Instill saline infrequently and only when secretions are tenacious.	8. Excess saline instillation before suctioning has been associated with pulmonary edema.

Evaluation. The ability to maintain a clear airway will require several days until the underlying problem (e.g., pneumonia) is stabilized and the client's strength returns.

Nursing Diagnosis. Anxiety related to dependence on CMV for breathing

Outcomes. The client will exhibit decreased anxiety as evidenced by reduction in the level of stress or anxiety and decreased feelings of powerlessness.

Interventions	Rationales
1. Develop a means of communication.	1. Communication allows the client to have needs met.
2. Place a nurse-call device within the client's reach.	2. Anxiety is increased when fear of being alone is present.

CARE PLAN

Interventions	Rationales
3. Be available and visible.	3. The client's anxiety is alleviated when not alone.
4. Provide distractions (e.g., television, radio).	4. Anxiety is reduced because the client does not focus on the ventilator and noises.
5. Explain all procedures.	5. The client feels respected and fears are alleviated.
6. Medicate as necessary for anxiety.	6. Antianxiety medications and opioids may be needed, but use them with caution during weaning because these drugs suppress respiratory drive.
7. Provide privacy.	7. Providing privacy demonstrates respect for the client.
8. Respect the client's rights and opinions.	8. The client feels respected and maintains dignity when included in discussion.
9. Provide a calm environment.	9. A frenzied environment engenders anxiety; if the client becomes anxious, ventilation is more difficult and oxygen needs increase.
10. Explain to the client and family that the client's vocal cords have been bypassed, which prevents talking; encourage them to use other modes of communication.	10. Clients can hear and respond even though they cannot talk.

Evaluation. Expect the client to remain moderately anxious while receiving CMV.

Collaborative Problem. High Risk for Complications of CMV and Positive-Pressure Ventilation (PPV).

Outcomes. The nurse will monitor the client for pulmonary barotrauma, cardiovascular depression, inadvertent extubation, and improper positioning of the ET tube.

Interventions	Rationales
1. Assess for acute, increasing, or severe dyspnea; agitation; panic; decreased or absent breath sounds; localized hyperresonance; increased breathing effort; tracheal deviation away from the side with abnormal findings; subcutaneous emphysema; and decreasing Pao_2 levels.	1. Barotrauma can lead to pneumothorax or tension pneumothorax.
2. Assess for an acute or gradual fall in blood pressure, tachycardia (early manifestation), bradycardia (late manifestation), dysrhythmias, weak peripheral pulses, acute or gradual increase in pulmonary capillary wedge pressure (PCWP), and respiratory "swing" (depression) in arterial or pulmonary artery wave forms during inspiration.	2. Cardiovascular depression can occur after an increase in tidal volume, positive end-expiratory pressure (PEEP), continuous positive airway pressure (CPAP), or with hyperinflation; positive pressure decreases venous return and cardiac output because of an increase in intrathoracic pressure.
3. Monitor for manifestations of inadvertent extubation: vocalization, low-pressure alarm, bilateral decrease in upper lobe airway sounds, gastric distention, clinical manifestations of inadequate ventilation; change in length of portion of ET tube that extends beyond the lip. If inadvertent extubation occurs, notify the physician, because reintubation may be necessary; manage ventilation and oxygenation with a self-inflating resuscitation bag.	3. Inadvertent extubation can be obvious, as when the tube is found in the client's hand; it can also be obscure, as when the tube slips into the hypopharynx or esophagus.
4. Keep an intubation tray readily available.	4. Intubation supplies may be needed quickly.

Evaluation. Most complications of PPV occur within 48 hours after intubation. Inadvertent extubation can occur at any time.

Continued

CARE PLAN

The Mechanically Ventilated Client—cont'd

Nursing Diagnosis. Risk for Infection related to impaired primary defenses in respiratory tract.

Outcomes. The client will remain free of infection, as evidenced by clear sputum, no fever, clear lung sounds, no increased difficulty with ventilation (e.g., increased peak inspiratory pressure), white blood cell (WBC) count within normal limits, and respiratory rate less than 24 breaths/min.

Interventions	Rationales
1. Wash your hands thoroughly.	1. Hand-washing reduces spread of infection.
2. Use sterile technique for open suctioning.	2. The respiratory tract is considered sterile.
3. Monitor the client for increased breathing effort, localized changes on auscultation, and changes in Pao_2.	3. Infected lung segments transmit sound differently (more solid) and do not permit gas exchange.
4. Provide oral care every 2 hours.	4. The client's mouth becomes dry, and stomatitis may develop from lack of oral secretions.
5. Drain water from ventilator tubing; do not drain water back into the humidifier.	5. Water may become a source of contamination, especially with *Pseudomonas*.
6. Monitor laboratory values, WBC count, and differential.	6. WBC count increases may indicate pulmonary infection.
7. Monitor sputum for changes in color, consistency, amount, and odor.	7. Infection may cause sputum to increase, darken, thicken, and become malodorous.

Evaluation. Infection usually develops after 72 hours of intubation unless the client is immunosuppressed; then infection develops more rapidly.

Nursing Diagnosis. Imbalanced Nutrition: Less Than Body Requirements related to lack of ability to eat while on a ventilator and to increased metabolic needs.

Outcomes. The client will exhibit adequate nutritional intake, as evidenced by (1) stable weight or weight appropriate to height, (2) intake of adequate calorie levels, (3) no manifestations of catabolism, (4) wound healing, (5) absence of infection, (6) laboratory value within normal limits (prealbumin, total protein, transferrin), and adequate muscle strength to breathe spontaneously.

Interventions	Rationales
1. Provide adequate nutrition (high calorie intake, protein, vitamins, and minerals); provide a nutrition consult as needed.	1. Inadequate nutrition decreases diaphragmatic muscle mass, decreases pulmonary function, and increases mechanical ventilation requirements. Calorie and protein needs are calculated by a dietitian.
2. Begin tube feeding as soon as it is evident that the client will remain on CMV for a length of time (usually 2-3 days).	2. The client should not be allowed to go into a catabolic state.
3. Avoid excessive carbohydrate loads.	3. Carbohydrate loads may increase carbon dioxide production to the point of producing hypercapnia.
4. Weigh the client daily.	4. Changes in body weight are a reliable indicator of nutritional balance.
5. Monitor intake and output.	5. Fluids are still required, and output should match intake.
6. Assess for complications of tube feeding: aspiration, diarrhea, constipation. Feed the client while he or she is sitting upright, with the cuff inflated. Check for residual tube feeding every 4 hours (continuous feeding) or before beginning another feeding (intermittent feeding).	6. Diarrhea is often caused by osmotic changes from an excessive concentration of tube feeding or the use of sorbitol-based elixirs; consider reducing the concentration or changing to crushed pills. Constipation is caused by a lack of free water within the feeding; add 100 ml of water every 4 to 6 hours if allowable.
7. If the client cannot tolerate enteral feeding, consider total parenteral feeding (TPN).	7. Clients with decreased gastrointestinal function may require parenteral nutrition to meet metabolic needs.

CARE PLAN

Interventions	Rationales
8. Monitor bowel sounds.	8. Bowel obstruction and ileus present as changes in bowel sounds.
9. Before tube feeding or between bolus feedings, obtain pH and Hemoccult test every 8 hours.	9. A change in pH may indicate an increased risk of gastric stress ulcer. A positive Hemoccult test indicates bleeding.

Evaluation. Malnutrition is preventable. Expect the client's weight to stabilize (unless there is fluid imbalance).

Nursing Diagnosis. Impaired Verbal Communication related to mute state when the ET tube is in place.

Outcomes. The client will be able to communicate with health care providers in order to have basic needs met.

Interventions	Rationales
1. Help the client develop a means of communication. Keep a pencil and paper pad or a picture board readily available.	1. With an ET tube passing through the vocal cords, the client cannot cough effectively or speak.
2. Be patient and willing to spend time communicating.	2. Prevents feelings of frustration, and reduces anxiety.

Evaluation. Depending on pre-existing problems (language), disease-related problems (confusion), or treatment-related problems (restraints) affecting communication, the timing to develop effective communication may be long or short.

Nursing Diagnosis. Impaired Oral Mucous Membrane related to nothing by mouth (NPO) status.

Outcomes. The client's gums and mouth will remain moist and ulcer-free.

Interventions	Rationales
1. Provide oral hygiene every 2 hours.	1. Oral mucous membranes dry in 2 hours.
2. Moisten the mouth with solutions that do not contain alcohol or lemon.	2. Alcohol and lemon solutions dry mucous membranes.
3. Moisten lips with lubricant.	3. Lubricants prevent drying, cracking, and excoriation.
4. Brush the client's teeth twice daily.	4. Dental caries are prevented by saliva.
5. Suction oral secretions from mouth.	5. Secretions pool in the oropharynx because of the inflated tracheal cuff.
6. Assess for pressure areas at the corner of the mouth from the ET tube.	6. ET tube repositioning may be required.

Evaluation. Oral mucous membranes can be restored to pink and moist within 24 hours. Oral care, however, is an ongoing need.

---

the client's initiating a breath can be used as modes for weaning. The decision is usually based on ABG readings and assessments made by nurses and respiratory therapists. The length of time required for successful weaning generally relates to the underlying disease process and to the client's state of health before the ventilator was used. For example, a young client who is recovering from an overdose of drugs can usually be weaned rapidly, but a client with COPD who develops acute respiratory failure and has little or no pulmonary reserve often takes longer and requires much professional patience and skill. Criteria for weaning are shown in Box 65-2.

Techniques for Weaning. After tapering the client off paralytics and sedatives, weaning from mechanical ventilation can be accomplished in two ways.

"Rapid" Weaning. The rapid (T piece) weaning technique is often used when mechanical ventilation has been instituted only briefly. One example is to start in the morning after the client has had a good night's rest. Place the client in the semi-Fowler position. Reduce the ventilator's respiratory rate to no more than half the original rate. Obtain ABG values in 30 minutes. If these values are at or near baseline level, place the client on a T piece at the same FiO_2. Obtain ABG values in 30 min-

---

BOX 65-2 *Criteria for a Weaning Trial*

Respiratory Criteria
Minute ventilation ≤15/L min
Respiratory rate ≤38 breaths/min
Tidal volume ≥325 ml
Maximum inspiratory pressure ≤ −15 cm H_2O
Fio_2 ≤50%

Other Criteria
Improvement, correction, or stabilization of the active disease process
Nutritional and fluid status sufficient to maintain the increased metabolic needs and demands of spontaneous respiration
Adequate physical strength and mental alertness
Afebrile status (any infections controlled)
Stable cardiovascular, renal, and cerebral status
Optimal levels of arterial blood gases, electrolytes, hemoglobin, and other laboratory tests

---

utes. If the ABGs are again at or near baseline level and the respiratory rate is below 25 to 30 breaths/min, the client may be extubated. Apply a face tent to deliver oxygen and humidity. Some nurse researchers are questioning the practice of beginning a weaning program in the morning. You may see changes in practice in the next few years based on the correlation of circadian rhythms with ideal time frames for weaning.

"Gradual" (Slow) Weaning. This technique is used after prolonged mechanical ventilation or if a neuromuscular disorder is present. The first step is to ascertain whether spontaneous breathing is present. Once spontaneous breathing has been established, slowly reduce the amount of ventilatory support. Continue to reduce ventilatory support until the client can accept full responsibility for his or her own ventilatory requirements. This process may be accomplished through increasingly longer periods on a T piece (followed by periods of CMV support) or by decreasing the rate of intermittent mandatory ventilation (IMV) or synchronized IMV (SIMV) breaths. This technique may take weeks or even months. Patience is crucial.

Difficulties in Weaning. A first weaning attempt may not be successful for several reasons, including decreased muscular strength caused by protein-carbohydrate malnutrition, certain disease processes, or caused by the inability of respiratory muscles to sustain respiratory efforts as a result of disuse after prolonged CMV. Increased work of breathing caused by increased airway resistance, abdominal distention, a small-diameter artificial airway, upper airway obstruction, or unresolved acute lung diseases may also affect the success of first weaning attempt. Other reasons include increased venti-

lation requirements, difficulty managing secretions, and psychological factors, such as fear.

If the first attempt at weaning is not successful, determine the reasons and try to eliminate them in subsequent attempts. Clients who require prolonged ventilatory support and extended periods of weaning often do best in a setting that promotes rehabilitation concepts. These clients can usually be transferred to subacute or long-term acute care facilities.

Extubation. Once the client has been weaned successfully, has demonstrated adequate ventilatory effort, and maintained an acceptable level of consciousness to sustain spontaneous respiration, the ET tube may be removed. ET tubes are removed on physician's orders and only by health care team members qualified to reintubate if necessary. The occurrence of laryngospasm and tracheal edema after extubation may occlude the airway, requiring immediate reintubation.

The ET tube is suctioned, the cuff deflated, and the tube removed. Immediately after extubation, the client is usually given oxygen. Assess the client for manifestations of respiratory distress and hypoxemia, as evidenced by restlessness, irritability, tachycardia, tachypnea. ABGs are obtained and monitored for decreased PaO_2 or increased $PaCO_2$ levels, which indicate an inability to sustain ventilation. If these manifestations are noted, notify the physician and prepare for reintubation.

Some clients are restless and extubate themselves. Because the cuff is not deflated, the tracheal wall can be damaged and bleeding can ensue. In most cases, the client requires reintubation, which must be done swiftly to prevent hypoxemia and to avoid needing to insert the ET tube through swollen tissues. Sometimes, however, the client can be monitored and not reintubated, especially if the time for extubation was approaching.

Dysfunctional Ventilatory Weaning Response. Some clients cannot adjust to lowered levels of mechanical ventilation, and the process of weaning them from the ventilator is delayed. The nursing diagnosis *Dysfunctional Ventilatory Weaning Response related to respiratory muscle fatigue or anxiety* may be used. Manifestations of respiratory muscle fatigue include a respiratory rate more than 30 breaths/min, increased $PaCO_2$, abnormal patterns of breathing, hemodynamic changes such as dysrhythmias, diaphoresis, anxiety, and dyspnea.

An unsuccessful attempt to wean the client may have taken place, resulting in reventilation. When the client cannot sustain ventilation independently, the ventilator is set at full ventilation; the client has no spontaneous breaths and therefore can rest. Once the client has rested, attempts at weaning should begin again. Some clients can never be weaned from mechanical ventilation. Those clients can be managed in less acute care units or at home for many years.

Ventilator-Dependent Clients. Some clients become stable and can be discharged from acute care and return home (see the Bridge to Home Health Care feature on Living with a Ventilator on the website for ways to assist the ventilator-dependent client).

ADULT (ACUTE) RESPIRATORY DISTRESS SYNDROME

Adult (acute) respiratory distress syndrome (ARDS) is a sudden, progressive form of respiratory failure characterized by severe dyspnea, hypoxemia, and diffuse bilateral infiltrates. It follows acute and massive lung injury that results from a variety of clinical states, often occurring in previously healthy persons. The syndrome was first described in 1967 and has been referred to by several terms, including shock lung, wet lung, post-traumatic lung, congestive atelectasis, capillary leak syndrome, and adult hyaline membrane disease. Tremendous advances in the treatment of this condition have occurred over the last two decades.

Etiology and Risk Factors

ARDS develops as a result of ischemia during shock, oxygen toxicity, inhalation of noxious fumes or fluids (e.g., gastric acid), or inflammation from pneumonia or sepsis that traumatizes the alveolar capillary membrane. There may be a direct insult to lung tissue or indirect injuries occurring in other body areas, with inflammatory mediators sent to the lung through the vascular system. Conditions leading to ARDS are listed in Box 65-3. Early recognition and treatment of these conditions may reduce the risk of ARDS.

Pathophysiology

The hallmark of ARDS is a massive inflammatory response by the lungs that increases permeability of the alveolar membrane, with resultant fluid movement into the interstitial and alveolar spaces. This leads to the development of noncardiogenic pulmonary edema, which decreases lung compliance and impairs oxygen transport. Three phases of ARDS have been described[24]:

1. *Phase I (Exudative)* is seen approximately 24 hours after the initial insult and consists of damage to the capillary endothelium and leakage of fluid into the pulmonary interstitium. Microemboli also develop and cause a further increase in pulmonary artery pressures. Inflammatory responses accompany the pulmonary parenchymal damage, leading to the release of toxic mediators, the activation of complement, the mobilization of macrophages, and the release of vasoactive substances from mast cells. There is further damage to the basement membrane, interstitial space, and alveolar epithelium. Fibrin, blood, fluid, and protein exude into the interstitial spaces around the

---

BOX 65-3 *Risk Factors for Adult (Acute) Respiratory Distress Syndrome*

Direct Pulmonary Trauma
Viral, bacterial, or fungal pneumonias
Lung contusion
Fat embolus
Aspiration (e.g., foreign material, drowning, vomitus)
Massive smoke inhalation
Inhaled toxins
Prolonged exposure to high concentrations of oxygen

Indirect Pulmonary Trauma
Sepsis
Shock
Multisystem trauma
Disseminated intravascular coagulation
Pancreatitis
Uremia
Drug overdose
Anaphylaxis
Idiopathic
Prolonged heart bypass surgery
Massive blood transfusions
Pregnancy-induced hypertension
Increased intracranial pressure
Radiation therapy

---

alveoli and increase the distance across the capillary membrane.

2. *Phase 2 (Proliferative)* begins about 7 to 10 days later. Type I and type II alveolar cells are ultimately damaged, resulting in decreased surfactant production, alveolar collapse, and atelectasis leading to further impairment in gas exchange. Significant hypoxemia is present due to decreased surfactant production, intrapulmonary shunting, and $\dot{V}/\dot{Q}$ mismatch.

3. *Phase 3 (Fibrotic)* occurs in about 2 to 3 weeks. There is irreversible deposition of fibrin into the lung, resulting in pulmonary fibrosis, further decreasing lung compliance and worsening hypoxemia. The end result is a significant $\dot{V}/\dot{Q}$ imbalance and profound arterial hypoxemia (see the Concept Map feature on Understanding ARDS and Its Treatment on p. 1896).

Clinical Manifestations

The initial insult of ARDS is followed by a period of apparently normal lung function that may last from 1 to 24 hours. Then hypoxemia rapidly develops and progresses along with decreasing lung compliance and development of diffuse lung infiltrates.

The earliest clinical manifestation of ARDS is usually an increased respiratory rate and profound dyspnea 12 to

CONCEPT MAP

evolve

Understanding ARDS and Its Treatment*

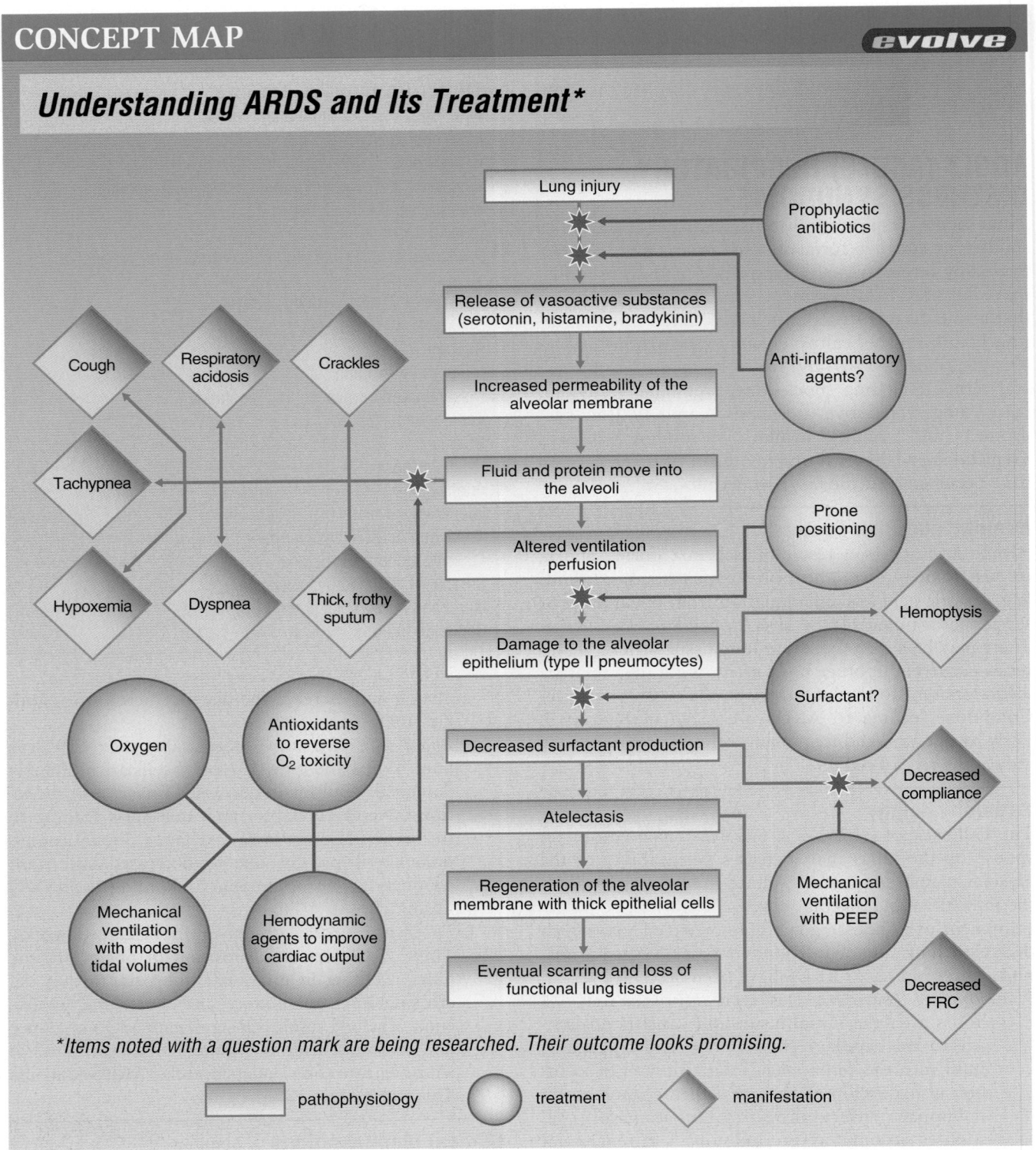

Items noted with a question mark are being researched. Their outcome looks promising.

pathophysiology — treatment — manifestation

24 hours after the initial injury. Breathing becomes increasingly labored; the client may exhibit air hunger and retractions. Chest auscultation may or may not reveal the presence of adventitious sounds. If present, abnormal sounds may range from fine inspiratory crackles to widespread coarse crackles. ABG analysis reveals increasing hypoxemia (PaO_2 <60 mm Hg) that does not respond to increased fraction of inspired oxygen levels (FiO_2 <40%) and compensatory hypocapnia. In the early stages, respiratory alkalosis is present because of hyperventilation. Later, metabolic acidosis develops from increased work of breathing and hypoxemia. The chest x-ray usually demonstrates diffuse, bilateral, and rapidly progressing interstitial or alveolar infiltrates (Figure 65-6).

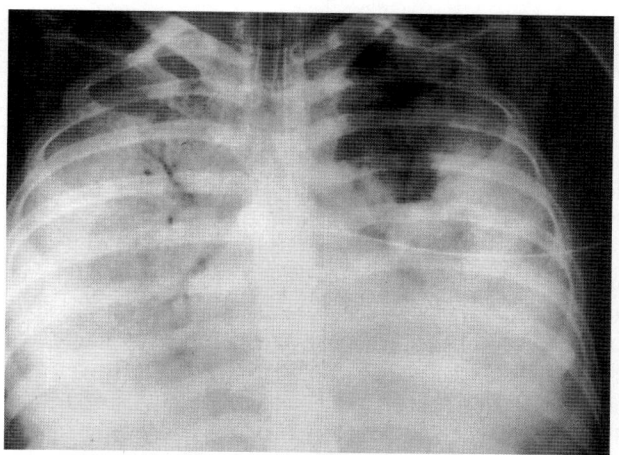

FIGURE 65-6 Adult (acute) respiratory distress syndrome (ARDS). This chest x-ray study shows massive consolidation from pulmonary edema following multisystem trauma. (From Fraser, R.G., et al. [1990]. *Diagnosis of diseases of the chest* [3rd ed., p. 493]. Philadelphia: W.B. Saunders.)

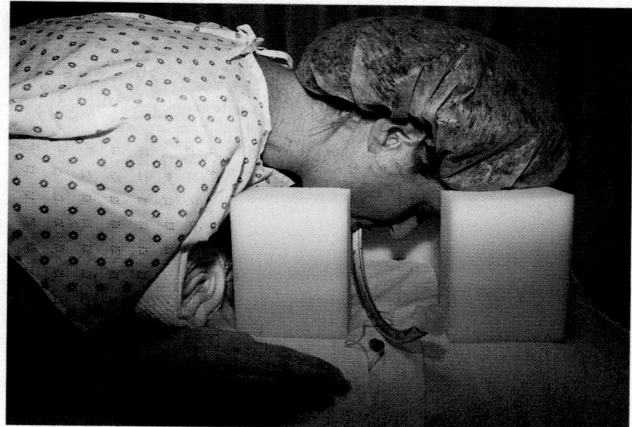

FIGURE 65-7 Use of the prone position to improve ventilation-perfusion. (Courtesy of H.E.A.D. Prone, Inc., Cambridge, MA.)

Recommended diagnostic criteria include acute onset, bilateral infiltrates seen on chest x-rays, ratio of PaO_2 (partial pressure of oxygen) and FiO_2 (fraction of inspired oxygen) less than or equal to 200 mm Hg (regardless of PEEP levels), and PAWP less than or equal to 18 mg Hg.[24] Additional diagnostic tests may be needed based on the underlying cause and include bronchial washing and biopsy to determine whether infection is present.

Outcome Management

The keys to successful management of ARDS are early detection and initiation of treatment. The goals of medical management are (1) respiratory support, (2) maintenance of hemodynamic stability, (3) treatment of the underlying cause, when possible, and (4) prevention of complications.

■ Medical Management

Support Respiration and Ventilation. Mechanical ventilation, ET intubation, and PEEP are usually required to maintain adequate blood oxygen levels. The goal of ventilatory support is to use the least amount of FiO_2 and PEEP possible to maintain oxygen saturation at or above 90% while decreasing the potential of oxygen toxicity. PEEP will also be used to decrease intrapulmonary shunting and to increase lung compliance. Studies have shown that using smaller tidal volumes (permissive hypercapnia) and the least amount of PEEP possible can reduce the risk of lung injury (low levels of CO_2 [hypocapnia] have been shown to decrease lung compliance).[15,19] Additional studies have encouraged the use of inverse ratio ventilation (IRV) as one method of increasing mean airway pressure without creating further peak pressures in the alveolus from PEEP.[6] IRV increases the inspiratory portion of each breath to more than half the respiratory cycle. Because IRV maintains a constant mean arterial pressure through the ventilatory cycle, alveoli stay open and gas exchange

is improved. Other alternative modes of ventilation (e.g., extracorporeal membrane oxygenation [ECMO] and partial liquid ventilation) may be used in some situations but are still considered investigational therapies. Surfactant therapy has been successful for neonates but to date has not had the same results in adults with ARDS.

Nitric oxide (NO) is now being used more often in the treatment of ARDS. NO causes selective vasodilatation in the pulmonary vascular system and is a powerful bronchodilator. Inhaled NO dilates the capillary bed of the lungs, which in turn reduces the pressure in the pulmonary arteries without lowering systemic blood pressure.[25]

Antioxidants, scavengers of oxygen free radicals, are also being used. *N*-acetylcysteine and procysteine have been effective in reducing the degradative effect of the proteases.[6] Pharmacologic efforts to inhibit the substances released by the endotoxins, neutrophils, and macrophages are also being explored. Prostaglandins are also being investigated as a possible treatment therapy for ARDS clients, especially those with sepsis and multiple organ failure.[6]

The prone position has been used to improve oxygenation by changing the distribution of perfusion. The belief is that ARDS does the greatest damage in the dependent parts of the lungs. By placing the client in a prone position, there is a change in the dependent portions of the lung, resulting in increased perfusion to the less damaged portions of the lungs and decreased pulmonary shunting. Prone positioning is also thought to reduce compression of the lung by the heart, improve chest wall compliance, and result in better draining of bronchial secretions.[17] Placing a client in a prone position is a challenge that requires coordination by many health care professionals to turn the client while maintaining equipment patency and decreasing client anxiety. Side effects include hypotension, desaturation, and dysrhythmias, although these appear to be short term. The prone position is shown in Figure 65-7 and is further discussed

📖 EVIDENCE-BASED PRACTICE IN ACTION

Prone Positioning and Adult (Acute) Respiratory Distress Syndrome

Adequate perfusion and ventilation of lung tissue are important to provide adequate oxygenation to tissues and maintain life. Adult (acute) respiratory distress syndrome (ARDS) is typically characterized by decreased lung compliance and severe hypoxia. Using mechanical ventilation has long been accepted as a means to overcome the decreased compliance and to correct the life threatening hypoxia. Additional studies are beginning to investigate the use of prone positioning with mechanical ventilation as another means to improve oxygenation while decreasing some of the complications associated with mechanical ventilation.

A meta-analysis completed by Curley identified 17 primary research studies that investigated the use of prone positioning.[3] Ryan and Pelosi presented findings from 11 studies investigating the use of prone positioning.[4] Although the studies all had different methodologies, each study met the criteria for scientific rigor and investigated the use of prone positioning to improve oxygenation. When combining the results of all 17 studies in the Curley meta-analysis, 69% of the clients (169 of 213 clients) responded positively to being placed in a prone position as demonstrated by an increase in the oxygenation saturation and Fio_2 ratio of 20% or more.[3] The studies reviewed by Ryan and Pelosi identified that 70% of the clients demonstrated improvement in oxygenation.[4] Various reasons were given for the improvements noted, including re-expansion of dependent portions of the lungs leading to atelectasis, changes in the $\dot{V}/\dot{Q}$ ratio, increase in functional residual capacity, and decreasing the amount of venous stasis.[4] As a result, the percentage of oxygen for mechanical ventilation could be decreased, thereby also decreasing the possibility of oxygen toxicity.

Several contraindications to the use of prone positioning included shock, hemorrhage, multiple trauma, spinal injury or instability, pregnancy, increased intracranial pressure, and recent abdominal surgery.[2,4] Both studies also identified complications associated with placing a client in a prone position, including the potential for impaired skin integrity, development of dependent edema in the face and anterior chest wall, damage to the eyes (corneal abrasions and ulcerations), nerve damage, and most importantly potential to dislodge extraneous tubes such as the endotracheal tube, venous and arterial lines, and Foley catheter. Care must be taken to prevent any of these complications. Strategies identified to prevent skin breakdown, eye injury, facial edema, and nerve damage included the use of padded cushions for bony prominences,

reposition the head every 2 hours, place extremities in a functional position, inspect the eyes and skin every 2 hours, and the use of pressure reduction devices.

To prevent loss of a line or the endotracheal tube when turning the client to and from a prone position, the nursing, respiratory therapy, and other health care professionals involved in the care of the client must work together in a coordinated effort for client safety and sense of security. Finally, a protocol must be in place for rapid response in the event the client goes into cardiopulmonary arrest while in the prone position. Another concern identified by the researchers was the use of tube feedings while the client is in the prone position. The increased potential for regurgitation and possible aspiration of feedings or stomach contents into the lungs was mentioned.[1] The need for caloric intake was recognized as important for the critically ill client. If the gastrointestinal function is confirmed, enteral feedings can be used with a client in the prone position with careful monitoring for potential aspiration. None of the studies reported aspiration as a noted complication.

Implications

Additional studies need to be conducted on the effects of prone positioning for clients with adult (acute) respiratory distress syndrome. All the studies reviewed in the meta-analyses had small sample sizes (fewer than 30 clients in any one study). Consistent results of all the studies demonstrated the improved oxygenation of a majority of the clients. Prone positioning has been found to be an effective means to improve oxygenation in clients with adult (acute) respiratory distress syndrome, especially in the early stages of the adult (acute) respiratory distress syndrome when edema in the lungs and atelectasis is apparent.

References

1. Balas, M. (2000). Prone positioning of patients with acute respiratory distress syndrome: Applying research to practice. *Critical Care Nurse, 20*(1), 24-36.
2. Breiburg, A., et al. (2000). Efficacy and safety of prone positioning for patients with acute respiratory distress syndrome. *Journal of Advanced Nursing 32*(4), 922-929.
3. Curley, M. (1999). Prone positioning of patients with acute respiratory distress syndrome: A systematic review. *American Journal of Critical Care, 8*(6), 397-405.
4. Ryan, D., & Pelosi, P. (1996). Prone positioning in acute respiratory distress syndrome. *British Medical Journal, 312,* 860-861.

in the Evidence-Based Practice in Action feature on Prone Positioning and Adult (Acute) Respiratory Distress Syndrome on p. 1898.

Kinetic therapy via continuously rotating beds can also be used to improve ventilation. The constant postural drainage assists in removing airway plugs. To be effective, the movement must be at least 45 degrees from side to side, which is best accomplished by a rotation bed. Shearing of the sacrum may develop, and therefore the client should be completely assessed daily. Beds set to rotate at less than 40 degrees do not provide adequate pressure relief; if used at that degree, turning must also be completed.

Maintain Hemodynamic Stability. Hemodynamic monitoring is used to observe the effect of fluids and degree of pulmonary edema. The use of pharmacologic agents in the treatment of ARDS varies according to the client's underlying disease process. Inotropic agents (e.g., dobutamine) may be indicated to improve cardiac output and to increase systemic blood pressure. Fluids are carefully monitored to prevent further systemic fluid overload.

Treat the Underlying Condition. Antibiotics are administered if suspected or confirmed infection is present. Although controversial, the use of large doses of corticosteroids is also common. The rationale for steroid administration is to reduce inflammatory response and to promote pulmonary membrane stability; however, controlled clinical trials have not demonstrated their effectiveness in ARDS. Indiscriminate use should be avoided.[6]

Monitor for Complications. In addition to lung fibrosis, other complications may arise during supportive management of the client with ARDS, such as cardiac dysrhythmias caused by hypoxemia, oxygen toxicity, renal failure, thrombocytopenia, gastrointestinal bleeding secondary to stress ulcers, sepsis from invasive lines, and disseminated intravascular coagulation (DIC) (see Chapter 77).

Prognosis

The outcome for any one client is difficult to predict. For most of the 1970s and 1980s, mortality rates seemed to be constant at 60% to 70%. In the 1990s, however, rates improved, and current rates are about 40%; however, a 90% mortality rate remains for clients with sepsis or multiple organ failure who develop ARDS.[8]

■ Nursing Management

The principles of nursing management of clients with pulmonary edema and care of the client requiring mechanical ventilation are appropriate in the care of the client with ARDS. Placing a client in prone position clearly is within the realm of nursing. Evaluation of the client's response to treatment as well as careful monitoring for potential complications is essential. Emotional support for the client's family and significant others is also important. The disease can progress very rapidly, leaving family members unprepared for the severity of the client's condition. Clear communications and frequent condition updates are essential to keeping the family adequately informed.

■ CHEST TRAUMA
PATHOPHYSIOLOGY

The chest is a large, exposed portion of the body that is vulnerable to impact injuries. Because the chest houses the heart, lungs, and great vessels, chest trauma frequently produces life-threatening disruptions. Injury to the thoracic cage and its contents can restrict the heart's ability to pump blood or the lungs' ability to exchange air and oxygenate blood. Major dangers associated with chest injuries are internal bleeding and punctured organs.

Chest injuries can range from relatively minor bumps and scrapes to severe crushing or penetrating trauma. Chest injuries may be *penetrating* or *blunt*.[27] Penetrating chest injuries may cause an open chest wound, permitting atmospheric air into the pleural space and disrupting the normal vacuum ventilation mechanism. Penetrating chest injuries may seriously damage the lungs, heart, and other thoracic structures. Blunt injuries are most commonly deceleration injuries associated with motor-vehicle crashes. Blunt chest trauma may also result from falls or blows to the chest.

Initial assessment is directed toward identifying and treating immediate life-threatening conditions. Any client with chest trauma should be considered to have a serious injury until proven otherwise. Airway patency, adequacy of breathing, and circulatory sufficiency (i.e., presence of shock), or ABCs, are always of primary concern. Immobilization of a potential spinal cord injury should also be initiated.

Once initial emergencies have been addressed, assess the client more thoroughly (Box 65-4). A medical history helps to identify any pre-existing conditions that could further complicate the injury. A thorough physical examination should be performed, with care being taken not to focus only on obvious injuries. Information about the accident (obtained from the injured client or witnesses) assists in the diagnosis of regional as well as anatomic injuries. A chest x-ray and electrocardiogram (ECG) are obtained for detection of possible pulmonary or cardiac impairment.

OUTCOME MANAGEMENT

Initial management should focus on airway patency, ventilation, hemorrhage control, stabilization of any thoracic fractures, and immobilization of the spinal column. Clients are typically divided into two categories: stable

---

BOX 65-4 *Chest Trauma: Assessment and Interventions*

1. Assess "ABCs":
   a. Maintain *a*irway, *b*reathing, and *c*irculation.
   b. Ensure adequate air movement.
2. Obtain a quick history:
   a. What happened?
   b. What was the mechanism of injury?
   c. How long ago did it happen?
   d. Where is the pain? Does it radiate?
   e. Is there anything that makes the pain better or worse?
   f. What does the pain feel like?
   g. How severe is the pain on a scale of 1 to 10?
   h. Is there a significant medical history?
3. Perform a quick (1-minute) assessment for:
   a. Shortness of breath and cyanosis
   b. Vital signs
   c. Skin color and temperature
   d. Wound size and location
   e. Paradoxical chest movement
   f. Distended neck veins
   g. Tracheal deviation
   h. Respiratory stridor
   i. Bilateral breath sounds
   j. Use of accessory muscles
   k. Estimated tidal volume
   l. Subcutaneous emphysema
   m. Sucking chest wounds
   n. Heart sounds
   o. Dysrhythmias
4. Quickly intervene:
   a. Administer oxygen.
   b. Cover any open chest wound.
   c. Control flail segment.
   d. Prepare to insert a chest tube.
   e. Initiate a large-bore intravenous line.

---

and unstable. The stable client needs careful and continuous monitoring, and the unstable client requires immediate management of ventilation-perfusion imbalances, shock, and pain.[11]

Ventilation-perfusion imbalances may result from atelectasis, hemopneumothorax, flail chest, aspiration, or pulmonary contusion. Oxygen or mechanical ventilation may be required. General respiratory status (e.g., rate and depth of respirations, chest movement, spontaneous vital volumes) and ABG values should be monitored closely. Deterioration of any of these parameters may indicate previously undetected injury or late-developing complications.

Therapeutic measures such as thoracentesis, chest tube insertion, bronchoscopic aspiration, video-assisted thoracic surgery (VATS), and thoracotomy (see Chapter 64) may be indicated. Management should focus on maintaining effective functioning of any equipment used (e.g., chest drainage system) and supporting the client and significant others to understand the procedures and the rationale for their use.

Monitor continually for clinical manifestations of shock. Shock often results from hypovolemia, but in the chest-injured client it may also be caused by cardiac tamponade, cardiac contusion, flail chest, or tension pneumothorax. Central vascular pressure readings (central venous pressure or pulmonary artery pressure) require careful interpretation. Once the cause of shock is determined, rapid treatment is crucial (see Chapter 83).

Excessive blood loss may further compromise oxygenation. Assess external bleeding carefully, and estimate blood loss. Internal bleeding may result from injuries to the thoracic or abdominal viscera, torn muscles, or fractures. Considerable bleeding (2 L or more) into the pleural space may occur. This is usually detected quickly as hypovolemic shock. Bleeding into areas such as the chest wall (e.g., from torn intercostal muscles) is more difficult to assess. A liter of blood can accumulate between the chest wall muscles without producing much swelling.

Fluid replacement is with blood and blood products, if indicated, or with crystalloid intravenous solutions (e.g., lactated Ringer's solution, normal saline). A chest-injured person may require large quantities of blood replacement. Until the results of typing and crossmatching are available, the client is given O-negative blood. The volume of blood replacement is determined through assessment of clinical findings, hemodynamic measurements, and laboratory results (e.g., hemoglobin and hematocrit). When possible, surgery is delayed until blood volume is restored.

Pain associated with chest injuries may cause the client to breathe rapidly and shallowly, which leads to atelectasis and pooling of tracheobronchial secretions. Analgesics minimize pain, permit periods of rest and relaxation, and allow the client to cough and to take deeper breaths. Opioids are most effective if given via the intravenous route. Intercostal nerve blocks or epidural analgesia may be used in clients with underlying health problems. Splinting the chest may also be helpful.

SPECIFIC CHEST INJURIES

FRACTURED RIBS

Etiology

Rib fractures are common chest injuries, particularly in older adults. Such fractures are usually associated with a blunt injury, such as a fall, a blow to the chest, coughing or sneezing, or the impact of the chest against a steering wheel during rapid deceleration. The fifth through the ninth ribs are most commonly affected.

Clinical Manifestations

Clinical manifestations include (1) localized pain and tenderness over the fracture area on inspiration and palpation, (2) shallow respirations, (3) the client's tendency to hold the chest protectively or to breathe shallowly to minimize chest movements, (4) bruising or surface markings (sometimes present) at the site of injury, (5) protruding bone splinters if the fracture is compound, and (6) a clicking sensation during inspiration when costochondral separation or dislocation is present.

Fractured ribs compromise ventilation by three mechanisms. Pain from the injury causes splinting, shallow breathing, and ineffective cough, which predisposes to atelectasis and pneumonia. Secretions accumulate and obstruct the bronchi, becoming a site of infection; shallow breathing reduces lung compliance. Rib fractures can result in a flail chest, which interferes with the normal physiology of breathing, and bone splinters from fractured ribs may penetrate the lung or pleura, resulting in a pneumothorax or hemothorax. Chest films are carefully reviewed for 24 to 48 hours after injury for indications of these complications. Bright-red sputum may be coughed up if the lung has been penetrated. Continuously assess the client for manifestations of pneumothorax or hemothorax, and report such findings promptly.[10]

Outcome Management

Fractured ribs are generally treated conservatively with good pulmonary physiotherapy, rapid mobilization, and proper pain management. Strapping the ribs with tape is no longer recommended because it restricts deep breathing and can increase the incidence of atelectasis and pneumonia.

Adequate pain control and splinting of the chest during coughing and deep breathing help the client with rib fractures to carry out painful but vital mobilization activities more comfortably. If pain is severe enough to impair ventilation significantly, a local anesthetic solution may be injected at the fracture site itself. Intercostal nerve blocks may also be used.[11] A client with an underlying chest or heart disease (e.g., COPD, heart failure) may benefit particularly from this type of pain management. A chest film should be taken after this procedure to ensure that pneumothorax has not occurred. Hospitalization may be required, especially in older adults, whose vital capacity may be significantly compromised. The pain from fractured ribs usually lasts 5 to 7 days. Complete healing occurs in approximately 6 to 8 weeks.

FRACTURED STERNUM

Sternal fractures usually result from blunt deceleration injuries, such as impact from a steering wheel. About 40% to 60% of the clients with fractured sternums have other major injuries, such as flail chest; pulmonary and myocardial contusions; ruptured aorta, trachea, bronchus, or esophagus; and hemothorax or pneumothorax.[11]

Clinical manifestations include sharp, stabbing pain; swelling and discoloration over the fracture site; and crepitus. The main priority is to control associated injuries. A client with a nondisplaced fracture may need analgesics or intercostal nerve blocks for pain reduction. Surgical fixation may be required for severe sternal fractures.

FLAIL CHEST

Etiology

Severe chest injuries that compress the rib cage often produce a "crushed" chest in which the ribs are pushed in on lung tissue. By definition, a flail chest consists of fractures of two or more adjacent ribs on the same side and, possibly, the sternum, with each bone fractured into two or more segments (Figure 65-8). The flail segment most commonly involves the lateral side of the chest. It is common for the end of a fractured rib to tear the pleura and lung surface (thereby producing *hemopneumothorax*) and for a crushed chest to have a flail segment. Pulmonary edema, pneumonitis, and atelectasis often develop rapidly with a crushed chest when fluids increase and collect at the injured site.

The "flail" segment no longer has bony or cartilaginous connections with the rest of the rib cage. Lacking attachment to the thoracic skeleton, the flail section "floats," moving independently of the chest wall during ventilation. This abnormality disrupts the normal bellows action of the thorax by causing *paradoxical motion*, during which the flail portion of the chest and its underlying lung tissue are (1) "sucked in" with inspiration (instead of expanding outward as normal) and (2) "blown out" with expiration, instead of collapsing normally inward.[11] This alteration in normal chest wall mechanics diminishes the client's ability to achieve an adequate tidal volume and to produce an adequate cough. Hypoventilation and hypoxia may result, leading to respiratory failure. Furthermore, mediastinal structures tend to swing back and forth (mediastinal flutter) with significant paradoxical motion. These swings may seriously affect circulatory dynamics, producing elevated venous pressure, impaired filling of the right side of the heart, and decreased arterial pressure.

In addition, pulmonary contusion occurs, resulting in an accumulation of fluid in the affected alveoli, which leads to intrapulmonary shunting and further hypoxia. The full effects of pulmonary contusion may not be manifested until the height of the body's inflammatory response in 24 to 48 hours.

The client with a flail chest commonly experiences emotional and physical distress while trying to breathe despite excruciating pain. Respirations are usually rapid, shallow, and labored. Paradoxical movement of the chest

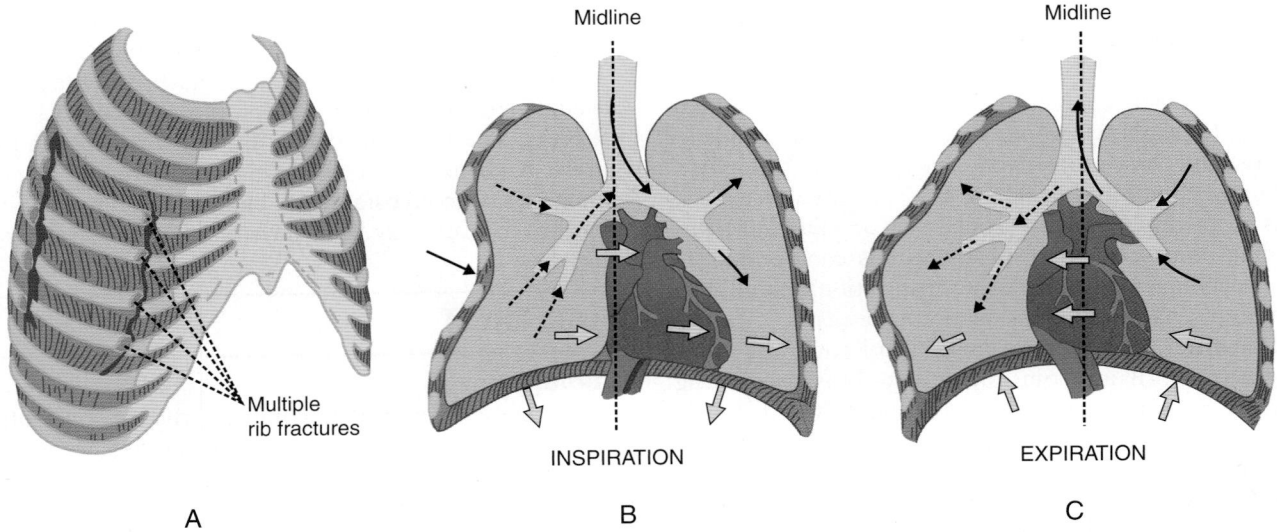

FIGURE 65-8 Flail chest. *Solid and dashed arrows* indicate air movement; *open arrows* indicate structural movement. **A,** A flail chest consists of fractured rib segments that are unattached (free-floating) to the rest of the chest wall. **B,** On inspiration, the flail segment of ribs is sucked inward. The affected lung and mediastinal structures shift to the unaffected side. This compromises the amount of inspired air in the unaffected lung. **C,** On expiration, the flail segment of ribs bellows outward. The affected lung and mediastinal structures shift to the affected side. Some air within the lungs is shunted back and forth between the lungs instead of passing through the upper airway.

wall is usually obvious. Breath sounds are absent or decreased on the affected side and crepitus may be heard or felt at the fracture site. Hypercapnia and hypoxia worsen as the effort necessary to breathe further depletes the already diminished oxygen supply. Frequent assessment of ABGs is needed to monitor respiratory effectiveness and to detect acidosis. Various factors produce metabolic and respiratory acidosis in chest-injured clients.

Outcome Management

Treatment is usually with intubation and mechanical ventilation, which can accomplish the following:

- Restore adequate ventilation, thus reducing hypoxia and hypercapnia
- Decrease paradoxical motion by using positive pressure to stabilize the chest wall internally
- Reduce pain by decreasing movement of the fractured ribs
- Provide an avenue for removal of secretions

Internal stabilization with continuous ventilation may require 21 days or more. Muscle relaxants or musculoskeletal paralyzing agents may be administered to reduce the risk of separation of the healing costochondral junctions.

SPECIFIC PULMONARY INJURIES

PNEUMOTHORAX

Pathophysiology

Pneumothorax is the presence of air in the pleural space that prohibits complete lung expansion. Lung expansion occurs when the pleural lining close to the chest wall and the visceral lining close to the lung maintain negative pressure in the pleural space. When the continuity of this system is lost, the lung collapses, resulting in a pneumothorax.[21] A pneumothorax may be closed or open. In a closed pneumothorax, air may escape into the pleural space from a puncture or tear in an internal respiratory structure such as the bronchus, bronchioles, or alveoli (Figure 65-9, *A*). Fractured ribs may also lead to closed pneumothorax. In an open pneumothorax, air may enter the pleural space directly through a hole in the chest wall or diaphragm (Figure 65-9, *B*).

A pneumothorax may be classified as spontaneous or traumatic, and either classification may result in a tension pneumothorax. A spontaneous pneumothorax may be idiopathic in that no cause can be found (primary) or as a result of another illness in lung such as COPD, tuberculosis, or cancer (secondary). Whereas the chest wall remains intact, a bleb or bullae ruptures, leading to a collapsed lung. A traumatic pneumothorax results in a collapsed lung resulting from either blunt force trauma to the chest wall or the creation of an open sucking chest wound caused by a motor-vehicle accident, gun or knife wound, or a diagnostic procedure such as a thoracentesis. Additional risk factors for developing a pneumothorax are listed in Table 65-3.

A tension pneumothorax develops when air is trapped in the pleural space during inspiration and cannot escape during expiration. The intrapleural pressure becomes greater than the lung tissue pressure, resulting in compression of the lung and surrounding structures.

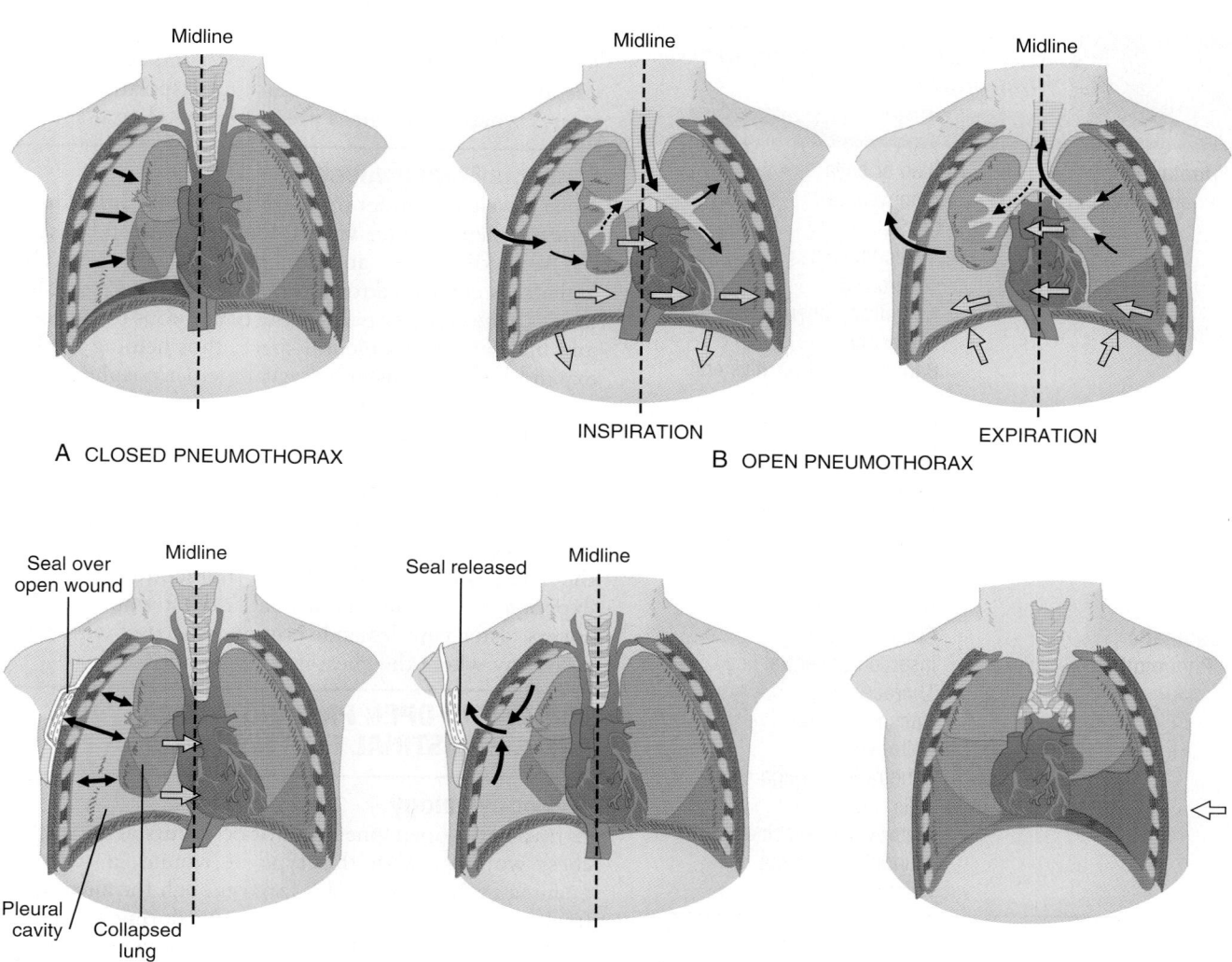

FIGURE 65-9 Pneumothorax. **A,** Closed pneumothorax. The lung collapses as air gathers in the pleural space. **B,** Open pneumothorax (sucking chest wound). *Solid and dashed arrows* indicate air movement; *open arrows* indicate structural movement. A chest wall wound connects the pleural space with atmospheric air. During inspiration, atmospheric air is sucked into the pleural space through the chest wall wound. Positive pressure in the pleural space collapses the lung on the affected side and pushes the mediastinal contents toward the unaffected side. This reduces the volume of air in the unaffected side considerably. During expiration, air escapes through the chest wall wound, lessening positive pressure in the affected side and allowing the mediastinal contents to swing back toward the affected side. Movement of mediastinal structures from side to side is called mediastinal flutter. **C,** Tension pneumothorax. *Left,* If an open pneumothorax is covered (e.g., with a dressing), it forms a seal, resulting in tension pneumothorax with a mediastinal shift. A tear in lung structure continues to allow air into the pleural space. As positive pressure builds in the pleural space, the affected lung collapses, and the mediastinal contents shift to the unaffected side. *Right,* Tension pneumothorax is corrected by removing the seal (e.g., dressing), allowing air trapped in the pleural space to escape. **D,** Massive hemothorax *(arrow)* below the left lung, causing collapse of lung tissue.

TABLE 65-3	*Risk Factors for Developing Pneumothorax*
Type of Pneumothorax	**Risk Factors**
Spontaneous Pneumothorax	Bleb or bulla Emphysema AIDS Cystic fibrosis Tuberculosis Necrotizing pneumonia Malignancy Barotrauma or positive end-expiratory pressure Chest tube malfunction High altitudes Decompression diving injuries Ankylosing spondylitis Lymphangial myxomatosis Cocaine use Menstruation
Traumatic Pneumothorax	Chest surgery Insertion of central line Thoracentesis Gunshot wound Knife wound Penetrating foreign object Falls Motor vehicle accidents Blunt chest trauma Fractured rib

From Bucher, L., & Melander, S. (1999). *Critical care nursing.* Philadelphia: W.B. Saunders.

Clinical Manifestations

Clinical manifestations of *moderate* pneumothorax include tachypnea; dyspnea; sudden sharp pain on the affected side with chest movement, breathing, or coughing; asymmetrical chest expansion; diminished or absent breath sounds on the affected side; hyperresonance (tympany) to percussion on the affected side; restlessness; anxiety; and tachycardia.

Clinical manifestations of *severe* pneumothorax include all the preceding and distended neck veins; point of maximal impulse shift; subcutaneous emphysema; decreased tactile and vocal fremitus; tracheal deviation toward the unaffected side; and progressive cyanosis.

Chest x-ray may reveal a slight tracheal shift away from the affected side and retraction of the lung back from the parietal pleura. On chest x-ray, pneumothorax is expressed as a percentage. For example, a client may have a complete 100% to a partial 10% pneumothorax. The use of percentages allows for evaluation of progress on subsequent x-rays. If pneumothorax is suspected but respiratory distress is too severe to permit x-ray confir-

mation, the physician may insert an 18-gauge needle (emergency thoracentesis) into the second or third intercostal space in the midclavicular line. Aspiration demonstrates whether free air is present in the pleural space.

Outcome Management

Most physicians prefer to insert a chest tube immediately into the pleural space via the fourth intercostal space at the midaxillary or anterior axillary line. The chest catheter is connected to closed chest drainage (see Chapter 64). The catheter permits the continuous escape of air and blood from the pleural space, thus helping the lung expand by reestablishing negative subatmospheric pressure in the pleural space. Sometimes a thoracotomy is done to explore the chest surgically and to repair the site of origin of the pneumothorax or hemothorax. Surgical treatment may also be accomplished through VATS.[21] A thoracoscopy is completed with direct visualization of the defect in the chest that needs to be repaired. Because the VATS is less invasive than a thoracotomy, the client experiences less pain, has a smaller chest wound, and recovers faster with less side effects associated with a thoracotomy where the chest is actually opened.

TRAUMATIC OPEN PNEUMOTHORAX AND MEDIASTINAL FLUTTER

Pathophysiology

A traumatic open pneumothorax occurs with sucking chest wounds. With this type of wound, a traumatic opening in the chest wall is large enough for air to move freely in and out of the chest cavity during ventilation (Figure 65-9, *B*). This abnormal movement of air through the chest wound produces a sucking noise that is audible in a quiet environment. Open sucking chest wounds may result from accidental injuries or surgical trauma. For example, if a chest drainage catheter is accidentally pulled out of a chest, the remaining puncture incision in the chest wall may become a sucking wound.

Outcome Management

When an open sucking chest wound is detected, emergency intervention includes immediately covering the wound securely with anything available. An airtight covering usually prevents tension pneumothorax and pre- serves ventilation of the opposite lung. Do not waste time looking for a sterile gauze petrolatum dressing (the ideal covering for such a wound) if it is not immediately available. Cover the wound with whatever is at hand (e.g., a towel) right away until someone can bring a sterile petrolatum dressing. When possible, fix the temporary dressing firmly in place with several strips of wide tape.

If the client is conscious and cooperative, ask him or her to take a deep breath and to try to blow it out while keeping the mouth and nose closed. This pushing effort against a closed glottis helps push air out through the chest wound and re-expand the lung. When the client does this, apply the dressing before the client inhales again.

Stay with the chest-injured client after a dressing has been applied to a sucking wound. Carefully assess for indications of tension pneumothorax and *mediastinal shift* (contents of mediastinum are pushed to the unaffected side of the chest). These complications may develop if the air leak is in the lung or a bronchus; such a situation allows air to escape into the pleural space. In such instances, closing the chest wall wound with an airtight dressing prevents the outflow of escaping air. Thus an open pneumothorax has been accidentally converted into a tension pneumothorax. If tension pneumothorax appears to be developing after the wound is sealed, immediately unplug the seal to allow the air to escape. Closed chest drainage is necessary to (1) remove the air from the pleural space and (2) allow the lung to re-expand if it is collapsed.

In addition to experiencing dyspnea and collapse of the lung on the affected side, the client with a traumatic open pneumothorax may experience *mediastinal flutter*. This complication results from air rushing in and out of the thoracic cavity on the affected side. With inspiration, the mediastinal structures (heart, trachea, esophagus) and collapsed lung are pushed toward the unaffected side. With expiration, these structures then move back toward the affected side. Fluttering back-and-forth movements of these vital mediastinal structures produce severe cardiopulmonary compromise, which is fatal if not treated promptly.

Chest tubes are inserted on the affected side away from the open wound. Surgical closure of the wound may follow. Supplemental high-flow oxygen should be administered.

TENSION PNEUMOTHORAX AND MEDIASTINAL SHIFT

Although it is dangerous to have air moving in and out of the pleural space with each respiration, the client is at even greater risk when air moves only into the pleural space and cannot move back out (tension pneumothorax). Tension pneumothorax (Figure 65-9, C) is a true emergency. Air enters the pleural space with each inspiration, becomes trapped there, and is not expelled during expiration (i.e., one-way valve effect). Pressure builds in the chest as the accumulation of air in the pleural space increases. Tension pneumothorax most commonly occurs with blunt traumatic injuries and is frequently associated with flail chest injuries.

If untreated, tension pneumothorax collapses the lung on the affected side as intrapleural pressure or tension increases, causing a mediastinal shift (mediastinal contents—heart, trachea, esophagus, great vessels—pushed or "shifted" toward the chest's unaffected side). Medi-

astinal shift may cause (1) compression of the lung in the direction of the shift (i.e., the lung opposite the pneumothorax) and (2) compression, traction, torsion, or kinking of the great vessels; thus blood return to the heart is dangerously impaired. The latter situation causes a subsequent decrease in cardiac output and blood pressure. Tension pneumothorax produces serious circulatory and pulmonary impairment that can be rapidly fatal. This is a high-priority emergency requiring prompt assessment and intervention.

Clinical Manifestations

Clinical manifestations of tension pneumothorax may include (1) marked, severe dyspnea; (2) tachypnea; (3) subcutaneous emphysema in the neck and upper chest; (4) progressive cyanosis; (5) acute chest pain on the affected side; (6) hyperresonance (tympany) upon percussion of the affected side; (7) tachycardia; (8) asymmetrical chest wall movement; (9) diminished or absent breath sounds on the affected side; and (10) extreme restlessness and agitation. Other manifestations include (1) neck vein distention; (2) laryngeal and tracheal deviation or shift to the unaffected side; (3) a feeling of tightness or pressure within the chest; (4) a point of maximal impact (PMI) shift laterally or medially; (5) severe hypotension leading to shock; and (6) muffled heart sounds.

A suspected mediastinal shift may be confirmed by x-ray study. Laryngeal and tracheal deviation toward the unaffected side can be detected by gentle palpation and with x-ray study. ABG analysis demonstrates hypoxia and respiratory alkalosis. When mediastinal shift is severe and not immediately corrected, respiratory acidosis may ensue.

Outcome Management

The immediate intervention is to convert a *tension* pneumothorax into an *open* pneumothorax, a less serious disorder. Large-bore chest tubes (36 to 40 French) are inserted on the affected side at the fifth intercostal space anterior to the midaxillary line. Once tubes are inserted, suction drainage should be established. If a delay in the chest tube insertion is anticipated, a 14- to 18-gauge needle may be inserted into the pleural space of the affected side at the level of the second intercostal space at the midclavicular line. Prompt thoracentesis to remove air may be life saving. As trapped air rushes from a tension pneumothorax, the tension is relieved, the lung should re-expand, and if mediastinal shift is present, it corrects itself. Supplemental oxygen is administered.

HEMOTHORAX

Hemothorax may be present in clients with chest injuries. A small amount of blood (<300 ml) in the pleural space may cause no clinical manifestations and may require no intervention with the blood being reabsorbed spontaneously. Severe hemothorax (1400 to 2500 ml) may be life threatening because of resultant hypovolemia and tension (Figure 65-9, *D*). Massive hemothorax is associated with 50% to 75% mortality.

Clinical manifestations include respiratory distress, shock, and mediastinal shift. There is dullness upon percussion of the affected side. A chest film confirms a diagnosis of hemothorax. If the client is in severe distress, the physician may aspirate blood from the pleural space by inserting a 16-gauge needle into the fifth or sixth intercostal space at the midaxillary line. To drain intrathoracic accumulations of blood, the physician inserts a large-caliber (36 French or larger) chest catheter, which is then connected to a drainage system. An initial drainage of 500 to 1000 ml is considered moderate, and additional treatment may not be required. An initial drainage of more than 1500 ml or continued large amounts of drainage (200 ml/hr) warrants immediate exploratory thoracotomy or the use of VATS to repair the site of active bleeding. Fluid replacement with O-negative blood or autotransfusion of blood should be used.

OTHER TRAUMATIC LUNG EVENTS
NEAR-DROWNING

Clients who initially survive suffocation after submersion in a water or fluid medium are said to have experienced a near-drowning or *immersion syndrome.* Immersion syndrome is the immersion into cold water that leads to cardiac dysrhythmias. Freshwater drowning (i.e., in a swimming pool) is more common than saltwater drowning. Risk factors that increase the potential for near drowning are alcohol or drug ingestion, overestimation of swimming skills, hypothermia, hyperventilation, extreme fatigue, sudden acute illness (seizure or acute myocardial infarction), head or spinal cord injury from a diving mishap, and hypoglycemia.[1,12]

Regardless of the fluid aspirated, the ultimate result is pulmonary edema. Both freshwater and saltwater wash out alveolar surfactant. Freshwater also changes the surface tension of surfactant. The loss of surfactant leads to alveolar collapse, intrapulmonary shunting, decreased lung compliance, and hypoxemia. Poor perfusion and hypoxemia result in acidosis and eventual pulmonary edema. Near drowning also compromises the respiratory system and leads to hypoxia, hypercapnia, cardiac arrest, and severe alterations in fluid-electrolyte balance.

Clinical Manifestations

The client may be unconscious or awake but restless and complaining of chest pain or a headache. Vomiting often occurs. Hypothermia may also be present. Cardiac manifestations include tachycardia, hypotension, and dysrhythmias. Pink frothy sputum indicates that pulmonary edema is already present.

Outcome Management

Begin assessment and interventions with the ABCs. If there is a possibility of spinal cord injury, the spinal column should be immobilized. Basic cardiopulmonary resuscitation (CPR) should be initiated if necessary and continued, especially with hypothermic clients. Resuscitation efforts for client with hypothermia have been successful long after typical CPR time guidelines would indicate to discontinue resuscitation efforts. Attempting to drain the fluid from the lungs is not advised.

Obtain a history of the submersion from the client or someone who has the information needed. Include the length of submersion, temperature of the water, any associated injuries, and type of water. Assess the level of consciousness. Note any respiratory efforts and adventitious sounds. Open the airway while maintaining spinal immobility. Look for manifestations of hypoxia, such as confusion, irritability, lethargy, or unconsciousness. Obtain a complete set of vital signs and assess for any additional injuries that may be present, including associated trauma, spinal cord injury from diving, air embolism from scuba diving, and seizures.

For respiratory insufficiency, intubate and ventilate with 100% oxygen and 5 to 10 cm of PEEP to prevent the alveoli from collapsing. If PEEP is used, slow and cautious removal of PEEP is required. Surfactant levels may remain low for up to 48 to 72 hours especially after freshwater aspiration. If the client is breathing, provide respiratory support with a non-rebreather mask. Oxygen saturation should be maintained above 90%.[9]

Remove the client's wet clothing, and wrap the client in a warm blanket. Core rewarming may be indicated if   the client is hypothermic. Rewarm the client slowly to avoid a rapid influx of metabolites (lactic acid) that may be trapped in the cold extremities.

Once the vital functions are stabilized, correct any acid-base or electrolyte abnormalities. Diagnostic studies include ABG analysis, complete blood count, electrolytes, appropriate toxicology studies if alcohol or drug ingestion is suspected, and a chest film. Clients are at high risk for pulmonary edema even several hours after a near-drowning incident. Monitor neurologic status carefully. A deteriorating level of consciousness may indicate cerebral edema, severe acidosis, or increased hypoxia. Table 65-4 identifies factors associated with near drowning outcomes.

CARBON MONOXIDE POISONING

Etiology and Risk Factors

Carbon monoxide (CO) is a colorless, odorless, tasteless gas that is formed by the incomplete combustion of any carbon fuel. Intoxication by CO is the leading cause of

TABLE 65-4	*Factors Associated with Prediction of Outcome in Near-Drowning*

Factors Suggestive of Favorable Outcome

Submersion time <5 minutes
Immediate resuscitation
CPR given <10 minutes
Spontaneous cardiac rhythm in ED
GCS >6 on arrival at ED
Spontaneous purposeful movement and intact brain stem function at 24 hours

Factors Suggestive of Poor Outcome

Submersion time >10 minutes
No resuscitation within the first 10 minutes
CPR given >25 minutes
Use of cardiotonic medications in the field or ED
GCS score <5
No spontaneous purposeful movements 24 hours after submersion

From Shoemaker, W. C., et al. (2000). *Textbook of critical care* (4th ed.) Philadelphia: W.B. Saunders.
CPR, Cardiopulmonary resuscitation; *ED,* emergency department; *GCS,* Glascow Coma Scale score.

death by poisoning. CO preferentially binds to hemoglobin, with an affinity for hemoglobin 200 to 230 times greater than that of oxygen. CO displaces oxygen, leading to reduced supplies of oxygen in the arterial blood and development of tissue hypoxia. CO also shifts the oxygen-hemoglobin dissociation curve to the left, which further reduces the oxygen levels by decreasing the release of oxygen into the tissues.

Generally, the client gives a history of exposure to CO after being found in an enclosed space in the presence of gases or fire. Faulty furnaces are also associated with CO poisoning. If CO poisoning is due to smoke inhalation, manifestations such as hoarseness, stridor, burns, or soot on the mouth or nose may be present. Sputum may be black because of inhalation of soot.

Clinical Manifestations

Clinical manifestations are vague until levels of CO bound to hemoglobin (carboxyhemoglobin, or COHb) are around 40%. With levels below 20%, manifestations include headache, vertigo, dizziness, nausea, and dyspnea on exertion. Above 20%, the client may have impaired concentration, clumsiness, and throbbing headache. Only when levels exceed 30% are manifestations more evident, including irritability, visual changes, impaired thought, and vomiting. At 40% vital signs

change, and eventually seizures and coma ensue when levels are greater than 50%. The diagnosis is confirmed by measurement of carboxyhemoglobin levels in the blood. Pulse oximetry should not be used because the readings are unreliable because of the detection CO-hemoglobin as oxyhemoglobin.

Outcome Management

Removal of the CO from the body is imperative. When the client is breathing room air, the CO will be removed from the body in about 320 minutes. Administering 100% oxygen will shorten the half-life of CO to 80 minutes. Hyperbaric oxygen may be required to reduce the half-life of CO 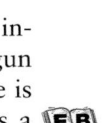 to minutes by forcing it off of the hemoglobin molecule for clients with severe CO poisoning. Hyperbaric oxygen will decrease the half-life of CO to 23 minutes.[18]

Reasons for CO poisoning must be explored and interventions directed at correcting those problems begun before hospital discharge. If the client's home furnace is faulty, it must be repaired. If the CO poisoning was a suicide attempt, crisis counselors should be used. Long-term neurologic and psychiatric consequences may develop, and the clients should be observed and followed up by their usual health care provider.

CONCLUSIONS

Two forms of respiratory failure exist: hypoxemic and ventilatory. Hypoxemic failure includes problems that lead to failure to transport oxygen and CO_2 across the capillary. Ventilatory failure includes disorders that impair neurologic triggers to breath and neuromuscular movement with respiration. Mechanical ventilation is a common method of treatment for both problems. Chest trauma involves life-threatening problems that demand prompt recognition and treatment.

THINKING CRITICALLY *evolve*

1. You are caring for a client who is receiving mechanical ventilation. You have just suctioned the client's airway and begin to leave the room when the high-pressure alarm sounds. What should you do?
Factors to Consider. What changes in the client can trigger the high-pressure alarm? What changes in the ventilator can cause high pressure?

2. You are going to position the client prone to improve ventilation and perfusion. What considerations should be made before, during, and after the prone position is used?

evolve **Did you remember to check out the bonus material on the Evolve website and the CD-ROM, including free self-assessment exercises?**

http://evolve.elsevier.com/Black/medsurg/

Factors to Consider. How can the tubes be moved safely with the client? What complications might occur in a prone position? What procedures cannot be done while the client is prone?

Discussions for these questions can be found on the website and the CD-ROM.

BIBLIOGRAPHY

1. Anas, N., & Lewis, K. (2000). Drowning and near-drowning. In A. Grenvik, et al. (Eds.), *The textbook of critical care* (4th ed., pp. 200-211). Philadelphia: W.B. Saunders.

2. Austan, F., & Polise, M. (2002). Management of respiratory failure with noninvasive positive pressure ventilation and heliox adjunct. *Heart and Lung, 31*(3), 214-218.

3. Balas, M. (2000). Prone positioning of patients with acute respiratory distress syndrome: Applying research to practice. *Critical Care Nurse, 20*(1), 24-36.

4. Brashers, V. (2002). Alterations of pulmonary function. In K. McCance & S Huether (Eds.), *Pathophysiology: The biologic basis for disease in adults and children.* (4th ed., pp. 1118-1120) St. Louis: Mosby.

5. Brochard, L. (2000). Noninvasive ventilation. In A. Grenvik, et al. (Eds.), *The textbook of critical care* (4th ed., pp. 1302-1306). Philadelphia: W.B. Saunders.

6. Brower, R., et al. (2001). Treatment for ARDS [Electronic version]. *Chest, 120*(4), 1347-1367.

7. Burns, S. (1999). Making weaning easier: Pathways and protocols that work. *Nursing Clinics of North America, 11*(4), 465-479.

8. Chesnutt, M., & Prendergast, T. (2003). Lung. In L. Tierney, S. McPhee, & M. Papadakis (Eds.), *Current medical diagnosis and treatment* (pp. 306-311). New York: Lange Medical Books.

9. Cohen, R., & Moelleken, B. (2003). Disorders due to physical agents. In L. Tierney, S. McPhee, & M. Papadakis (Eds.), *Current medical diagnosis and treatment* (pp. 1549-1551). New York: Lange Medical Books.

10. Easter, A. (2001). Management of patients with multiple rib fractures. [Electronic Version] *American Journal of Critical Care, 10*(5), 320-329.

11. Golden, P. (2000). Thoracic trauma [Electronic Version]. *Orthopedic Nursing, 19*(5), 37-47.

12. Goll, C. (2001). Near drowning. In P. Swearingen & J. Hicks Keen (Eds.), *Manual of critical care nursing* (4th ed., pp. 136-140). St. Louis: Mosby.

13. Goll, C. (2001). Acute respiratory failure. In P. Swearingen & J. Hicks Keen (Eds.), *Manual of Critical Care Nursing* (4th ed., pp. 243-246). St. Louis: Mosby.

14. Klein, D. (1999). Prone positioning in patients with acute respiratory distress syndrome: The Vollman Prone Positioner. *Critical Care Nurse, 19*(4), 66-71.

15. Lafferty, J., & Kavanagh, B. (2002). Hypocapnia. *New England Journal of Medicine, 347*(1), 43-53.

16. Lenart, S., & Garrity, J. (2000). Eye care for patients receiving neuromuscular blocking agents or propofol during mechanical ventilation. *American Journal of Critical Care, 9*(3), 188-191.

17. Meade, M., & Herridge, M. (2001). An evidence-based approach to acute respiratory distress syndrome [Electronic version]. *Respiratory Care, 46*(12), 1368-1376.

18. Moon, R., Dear, G., & Stolp, B (2000). Hyperbaric oxygen in critical care. In A. Grenvik et al. (Eds.). *The textbook of critical care* (4th ed., pp. 1534-1535). Philadelphia: W.B. Saunders.

19. Mortelli, M., & Manning, H. (2002). Acute respiratory distress syndrome [Electronic version]. *American Family Physician, 65*(9), 1823-1830.

20. Pierson, D. (2001). The future of respiratory care. *Respiratory Care, 46*(7), 705-718.

21. Rodger, M. (1999). Common respiratory problems: Pulmonary embolism, pneumothorax, and thoracic pulmonary surgery. In L. Bucher & S. Melander (Eds.), *Critical care nursing* (pp. 486-496): Philadelphia: W.B. Saunders.

22. Sakallaris, B. (1999). Acute respiratory failure. In L. Bucher & S. Melander (Eds.) *Critical care nursing* (pp. 411-445): Philadelphia: W.B. Saunders.

23. Sassoon, C., & McGovern, J. (2000). Oxygenation Strategy. In A. Grenvik, et al. (Eds.), *The textbook of critical care* (4th ed., pp. 1308-1323). Philadelphia: W.B. Saunders.

24. Stacy, K. (2002). Pulmonary disorders. In L. Urden, K. Stacy, & M. Lough (Eds.), *Thelan's critical care nursing: diagnosis and management* (4th ed., pp. 551-560, 570-573). St. Louis: Mosby.

25. Stacy, K. (2002). Pulmonary therapeutic management. In L. Urden, K. Stacy, & M. Lough (Eds.), *Thelan's critical care nursing: diagnosis and management* (4th ed., pp. 587-613). St. Louis: Mosby.

26. Staudinger, T., et al. (2001). Comparison of prone positioning and continuous rotation of patients with adult respiratory distress syndrome: Results of a pilot study. *Critical Care Medicine, 29*(1), 51-56.

27. Tarizan, A.J. (2000). Caring for dying patients who have air hunger. *Journal of Nursing Scholarship, 32*(2), 137-143.

28. Taylor, R. & Trottier, S. (2000). Pathophysiology of acute lung injury. In A. Grenvik, et al. (Eds.), *The textbook of critical care* (4th ed., pp. 1382-1390). Philadelphia: W.B. Saunders.

29. The Acute Respiratory Distress Syndrome Network. (2000). Ventilation with lower tidal volumes as compared to traditional tidal volumes for acute lung injury and the acute respiratory distress syndrome. *New England Journal of Medicine, 342*(18), 1301-1308.

30. Voggenreiter, G., et al. (1999). Intermittent prone positioning in the treatment of severe and moderate posttraumatic lung injury. *Critical Care Medicine, 27*(11), 2375-2382.

Sensory Disorders

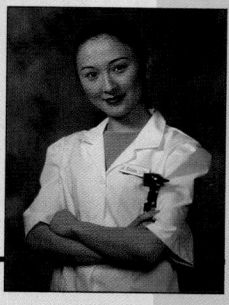

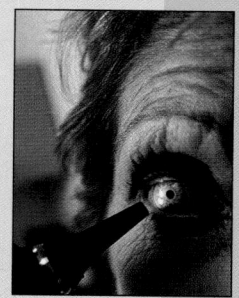

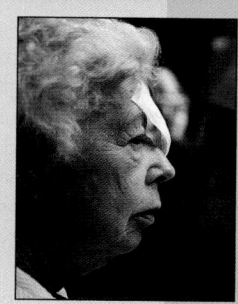

Anatomy and Physiology Review

The Eyes and Ears
Robert G. Carroll

OVERVIEW

The visual, auditory, and olfactory systems are "distance" senses, bringing information about our environment to our perception. Each system detects the intensity and quality of stimuli, encodes and processes this information, and transmits it to the cerebral cortex. Together these senses provide much of the available information about our environment. This review covers vision and hearing; smell is described in Unit 7.

The *visual apparatus* is specialized to detect light. Light passes through the cornea, aqueous humor, lens, and vitreous humor before striking the retina. The visual receptors—rods and cones—encode data about the intensity and wavelength of light. This information is processed and transmitted through nerve cells of the retina, the optic nerve, and the thalamus before arriving at the visual cortex. The information is constructed in the primary and associated visual cortex into a conscious perception.

The *auditory apparatus* is specialized to detect sound. Sound waves pass through the pinna to the ear drum (tympanic membrane), through the bones of the middle ear, and then to the receptors in the cochlea. The auditory hair cells are arranged on the organ of Corti (the end organ for hearing) and are coded to detect the intensity and frequency of sound. This information passes through the auditory nerve through the lateral lemniscus and, finally, to the auditory cortex. Within the primary and secondary auditory cortex, auditory discrimination occurs.

VISUAL SYSTEM
STRUCTURE OF THE VISUAL SYSTEM

External Structures

The visual system is a complex group of structures that includes the eyeballs, muscles, nerves, fat, and bones. The *ocular adnexa* (Figure U15-1, *A*) are the accessory structures of the eye (muscles, fat, and bone) that support and protect it. The bony orbit (eye socket) surrounds and protects most of the eye so that only a small portion is visible. The orbit is formed from portions of the frontal, lacrimal, ethmoid, maxillary, zygomatous, sphenoid, and palatine bones. These bones are thin and fragile and break easily when pressure is applied to the eye (as in a fist fight). In addition to bone, the orbit also contains fat, various connective tissues, blood vessels, and nerves.

The *eyeball* is moved by six ocular muscles, which are attached to the surface of the globe (Figure U15-2) and which move the eye through six cardinal gazes. The four rectus muscles (the medial, lateral, superior, and inferior) move the eyes horizontally and vertically. The two oblique muscles (superior and inferior) rotate the eye in circular movements to allow vision at all angles.

The upper and lower *eyelids* are elastic folds of skin that close to protect the anterior eyeball. When the eyelids close, they distribute tear film, which prevents evaporation and drying of the surface epithelium. The elliptic space between the two open lids is the *palpebral fissure*. The corners of the fissure are called the *canthi*. The medial, or inner, canthus is next to the nose; the lateral, or outer, canthus is the outside corner. Oil-secreting *meibomian glands* are embedded in both upper and lower lids (see Figure U15-1, *B*).

The *lacrimal gland,* in the upper lid over the outer canthus, produces tears that reach the eyeball through secretory ducts. Tiny openings *(puncti)* in both the upper and lower lids at the inner canthus direct tears to the lacrimal sac. The *nasolacrimal duct* directs the flow of tears into the nose. The tear film is composed of lipids secreted by the meibomian glands and dissolved salts, glucose, urea, protein, and lysozyme secreted by the lacrimal glands. The tear film lubricates, cleans, and protects the ocular surface. Mucus, secreted by goblet cells located in the lids, assists these processes.

Internal Structures

The *conjunctiva* is a thin transparent layer of mucous membrane that lines the eyelids and covers the eyeball (see Figure U15-1, *C*). The *cornea* is a transparent avas-

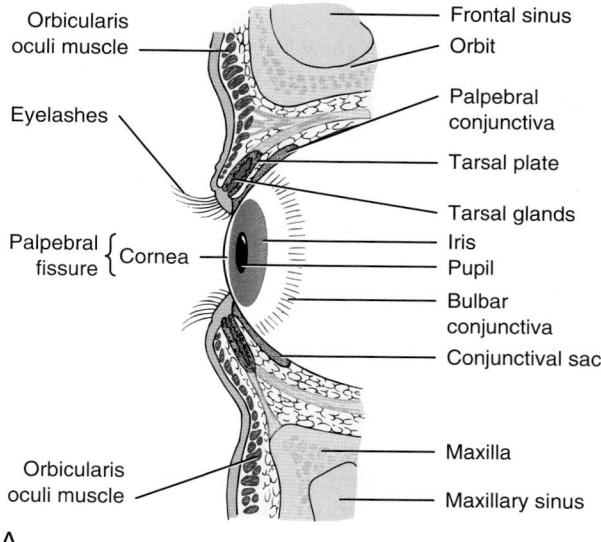

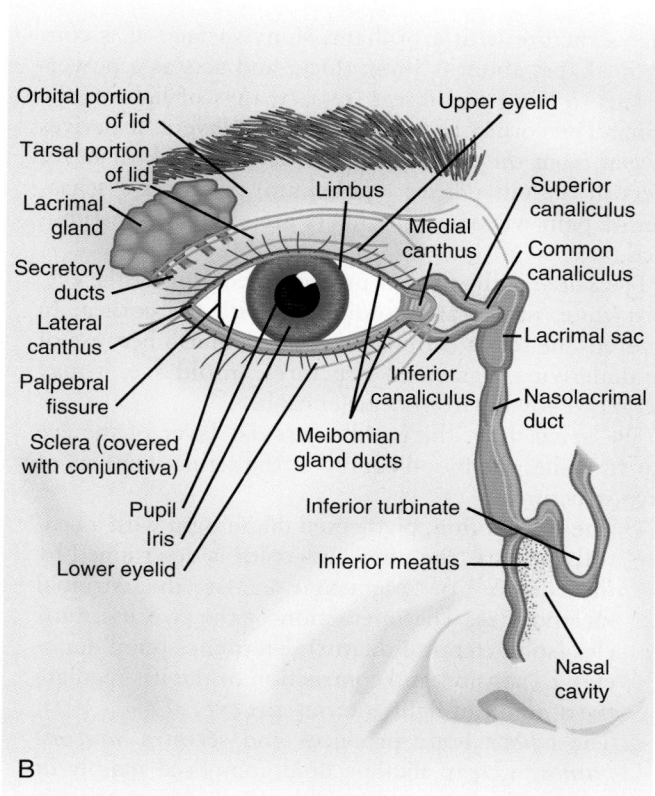

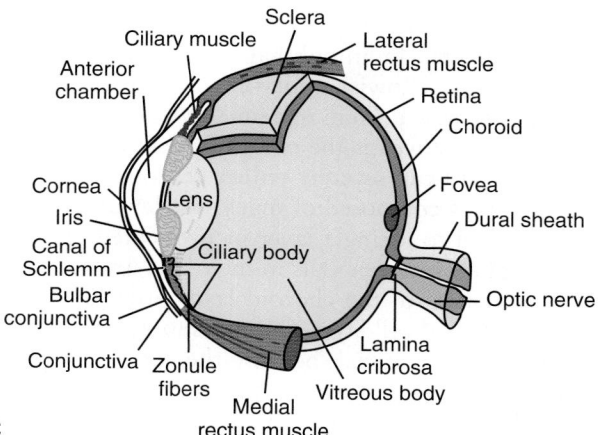

FIGURE U15-1 Surface anatomy of the eye. **A,** Ocular adnexa. **B,** Frontal view of the lacrimal drainage system. **C,** Horizontal section of the eye.

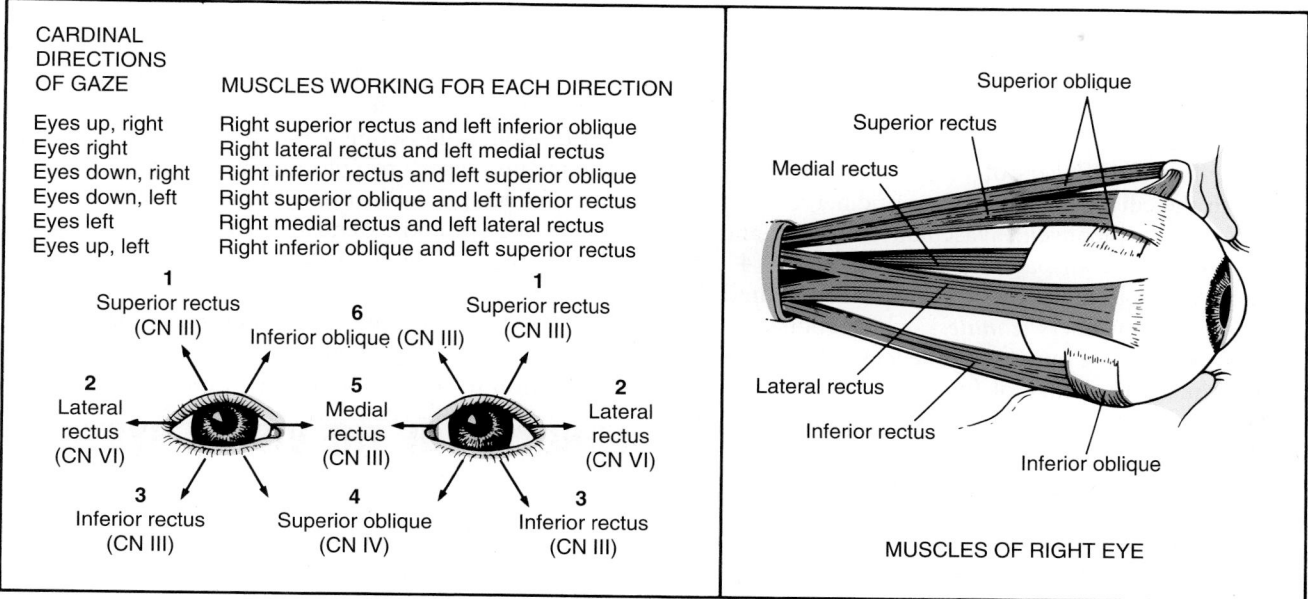

FIGURE U15-2 The six cardinal directions of gaze and the muscles responsible for each.

cular structure with a brilliant, shiny surface. It is convex in shape, about 0.5 mm thick, and acts as a powerful lens to bend and direct (refract) rays of light to the retina. The cornea is composed of five layers. It derives oxygen from the atmosphere. A rich network of nerve fibers in the outer layer (epithelium) produces a sensation of pain whenever the fibers are exposed or stimulated.

The *sclera* is the fibrous protective coating of the eye. It is white, dense, and continuous with the cornea. In children, the sclera is thin and appears bluish because of the underlying pigmented structures. In old age, it may become yellowish from degeneration.

The *uveal tract,* the middle vascular layer of the eye that furnishes the blood supply to the retina, consists of three structures:

1. The *iris* is a thin, pigmented diaphragm with a central aperture, the pupil. Iris color is determined by the degree of pigmentation in the stromal melanocytes. The interaction of the two iris muscles (sphincter and dilator) determines pupil diameter. Expansion and contraction of the iris regulate the amount of light entering the eye.

2. The *ciliary body* produces and secretes *aqueous humor,* a clear alkaline fluid composed mainly of water, which occupies the space between the iris and the cornea (the anterior chamber of the eye). The ciliary body is in direct continuity with the iris and is circular, surrounding the lens. Aqueous humor circulates from the posterior chamber through the pupil into the anterior chamber. The flow continues into the anterior chamber angle and is filtered out through the trabecular meshwork into Schlemm's canal. From there, the aqueous humor is channeled into a capillary network and into episcleral veins. Normal intraocular pressure is maintained as long as there is a balance between the aqueous production and the aqueous humor outflow.

3. The *choroid* is the posterior segment of the uveal tract between the retina and the sclera. It is composed of three layers of vessels and is attached to both the ciliary body and the optic nerve.

The *lens* is a biconvex, avascular, colorless, and almost completely transparent structure, about 4 mm thick and 9 mm in diameter. It is suspended behind the iris by ligamentous fibers (*zonules*), which connect to the ciliary body. The sole purpose of the lens is to focus light on the retina. The change of focus from distant to near is called *accommodation*. There are no pain fibers or blood vessels in the lens. The lens is surrounded by a transparent envelope (the capsule). The lens of the eye consists of about 65% water and 35% protein.

The *vitreous body* is a clear, avascular, jelly-like structure. Vitreous fluid is thick and viscous, and occupies a space called the *vitreous chamber.* It fills the largest cavity of the eye, accounting for two thirds of its volume. It helps maintain the shape and transparency of the eye.

Retina

The retina is a thin, semitransparent layer of nerve tissue that forms the innermost lining of the eye. It consists of 10 distinct layers of highly organized, delicate tissue. The retina contains all the sensory receptors for the transmission of light and is actually part of the brain.

There are two types of retinal receptors: rods and cones. About 125 million *rods* are distributed in the periphery of the retina; they function best in dim light. Damage to these structures results in night blindness. The *cones,* numbering about 6 million and concentrated in the center of the retina, provide resolution of small visual angles, resulting in perception of fine details. They are also responsible for color vision.

The center of the retina (*macula*) is an area about 5 mm in diameter. In an ophthalmoscopic examination, it appears as a yellowish spot with a depressed center, the *fovea.* An area 1.5 mm in diameter where only cones are present, the fovea is the point of finest vision. Damage to the fovea can severely reduce central vision.

The retina is composed of many fine layers of neural tissue attached to a single layer of pigmented epithelial cells. The photoreceptor cells in the retina are nourished by the capillaries of the choroid layer just beneath the pigment epithelial cell layer. Oxygen supply to these delicate structures is crucial, because the conversion of visual stimuli into impulses that the brain records as images requires very active metabolic processes.

Optic Nerve and Neural Pathways

The optic nerve is located at the posterior portion of the eye and transmits visual impulses from the retina to the brain. The head of the optic nerve (*optic disc*) can be seen by ophthalmoscopic examination. The optic nerve contains no sensory receptors (rods or cones) and represents a blind spot in the eye. The nerve emerges from the back of the eye and extends for 25 to 30 mm, traveling through the muscle cone to enter the bony optic foramen, eventually joining the other optic nerve to form the optic chiasm. The optic nerve neurons synapse in the thalamus, and thalamic nerves then transmit the visual information to the occipital lobe of the cortex.

FUNCTION OF THE VISUAL SYSTEM

Vision requires accurate transmission of light to the photoreceptors of the retina, encoding of the wavelength and intensity by the retinal receptors, and interpretation of the coded signals by the visual cortex.

Transmission of Light

Light passes through the cornea, aqueous humor, lens, and vitreous humor before striking the retina. Blood vessels are opaque, and the cornea, lens, and fovea are sparsely vascularized, which enhances light transmission. The cornea and lens refract light, allowing it to converge to a focal point on the fovea of the retina. Refraction at the lens is regulated by contraction of the ciliary muscles.

Near vision is accomplished by contraction of the ciliary muscles, which increases curvature of the lens and brings near objects into focus on the retina. *Far vision* is accomplished by relaxing the ciliary muscles and flattening the lens. With age, lens elasticity decreases, reducing the ability to accommodate for near vision. Visual abnormalities are corrected by placing an appropriate refractor (eye glasses or contact lens) in the light pathway.

Visual Receptors of the Retina: Cones and Rods

Three types of cones are sensitive to specific wavelengths of light, with peak sensitivities in the red, green, and blue wavelengths. Density of the cone receptors is highest in the fovea (the area of highest visual acuity). Bright light causes contraction of the iris, limiting the light entering the eye and focusing the light on the fovea. Exposure to light bleaches retinal photopigments, reducing the receptor responsiveness to subsequent exposure (light adaptation). However, prolonged exposure to dark allows the receptors to recover; cones recover completely in about 5 minutes.

Rods are sensitive to light in the green and yellow wavelengths and impart night *(scotopic)* vision. Rods are distributed throughout the retina, but few rods are in the fovea. In the dark, the iris dilates, admitting light to large portions of the retina. Consequently, night vision is enhanced by looking just to the side of the object of interest. After light exposure, rods recover slowly, taking about 20 minutes to return to peak sensitivity (dark adaptation). Because the rod photopigments are not sensitive to red light, exposure to red light does not interfere with dark adaptation.

Image Processing and the Visual Cortex

Interneurons in the retina process the receptor output and transmit information via the optic nerve to the thalamus. The thalamus processes information about the wavelength and intensity of the light and relays the information to the visual cortex. Visual space in the cortex is completely crossed; objects appearing on the left side of the body are represented on the right visual cortex and vice versa (Figure U15-3). The two eyes work together as one, focusing on the same point in space and fusing their images so that a single mental impression is obtained. The ability of the eyes to fuse two images into a single image is called *binocular vision,* accounting for one aspect of depth perception.

EFFECTS OF AGING ON VISION

Structural Changes

Several age-related changes occur in the structures of the eye and surrounding tissue. Eyebrows and eyelashes turn gray, and skin around the eyelids becomes wrinkled and loose because of loss of muscle tone and elasticity. Loss of orbital fat causes the eyes to sink deeper into the orbit and sometimes limits the upward gaze. Tear secretions may also diminish, resulting in the condition of dry eyes.

The most frequent and significant age-related change in the eye is the formation of a *cataract.* With age, the thickness and density of the lens increase and the lens becomes progressively yellowed and opaque. Throughout the life span, the lens continues to grow by forming new fiber cells. Although the rate of growth gradually diminishes, the accumulation of cells over time contributes to lens density. Loss of transparency also results from molecular deterioration from absorption of ultraviolet radiation. The yellow material is associated with the devel-

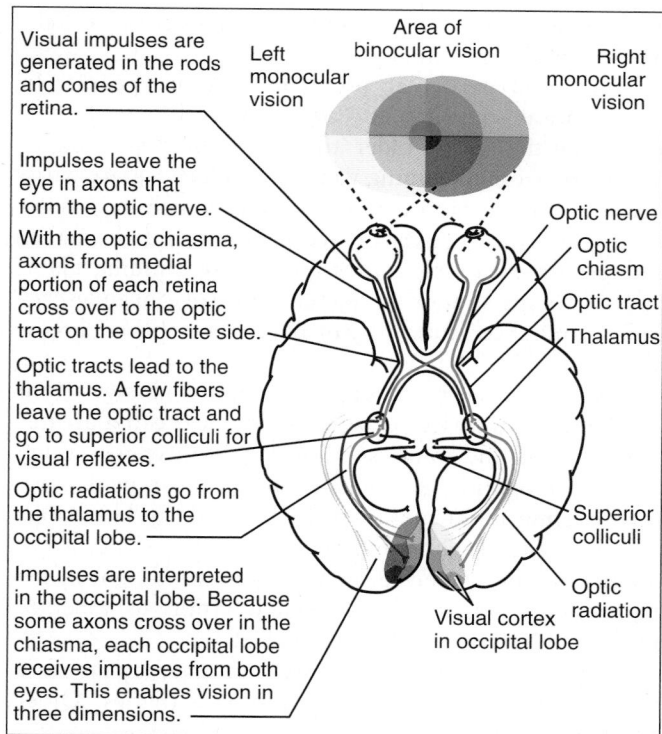

FIGURE U15-3 Visual pathways from the retina to the occipital lobe. The pathway is partially crossed, so that objects in the visual space of one side are interpreted in the contralateral visual cortex.

opment of abnormal fluorescent substances in the aging lens. The lens accommodation diminishes because of ciliary muscle atrophy.

The cells of the inner layer of the cornea (endothelium) decrease in number with age. Because this layer does not reproduce lost cells, the ability of this layer to heal after injury or surgery may be compromised. The corneal reflex also may be diminished or absent. Another phenomenon characteristic of aging is the *arcus senilis,* a grayish yellow ring found on the periphery of the cornea surrounding the iris. This ring is thought to be the result of the accumulation of lipids.

The ciliary body produces less aqueous humor during the aging process, but there is less outflow and intraocular pressure remains relatively stable or increases only slightly. The ciliary muscle tends to atrophy with age, and sometimes connective tissue replaces lost muscle tissue. The loss in muscle action along with lens thickening decreases the focusing ability of the lens. Decreasing ability to focus at near accommodation *(presbyopia)* is common.

Visual Changes

The major visual changes with aging include decreases in (1) visual acuity, (2) tolerance of glare, (3) ability to adapt to dark and light, and (4) peripheral vision. Each of these decreases is related to changes in the eye structure and each affects the quality and intensity of the light able to reach the retina.

Glare is a particular problem for older people. In combination with difficulty adjusting to dark and light, it is often the reason older adults stop driving at night. The lights from oncoming vehicles produce a glare when passing through both cornea and lens, which may make it very difficult to discern objects. Bright sunlight, either indoors or outdoors, causes an equally blinding glare. Indoor rooms should be lighted with soft incandescent lights, and sheer curtains can be used to diffuse bright sunlight.

Because the eye takes longer to adapt to changes from dark to light and vice versa, older people are at a greater risk for falls and injuries. Any place subject to sudden changes in lighting (e.g., inside a theater) can be dangerous. Getting up at night can be particularly hazardous for older adults. However, because red wavelengths are longer and are perceived by the cones, a red light in the bathroom at night allows enough vision to function without interfering with dark vision.

Peripheral vision decreases with age and may interfere with social interactions and physical activities. Older adults suffering from loss of peripheral vision may not notice someone sitting next to them. They may also have difficulty finding objects out of their range of vision.

The iris loses pigment with age, and older people may thus appear to have grayish or light blue eyes. The pupil becomes gradually smaller with age. A decrease in pupil

size results in a smaller amount of light reaching the retina, meaning that the light must pass through the densest, most opaque area of the lens.

AUDITORY SYSTEM
STRUCTURE OF THE AUDITORY SYSTEM

The ear is housed in the *temporal bone* of the skull. The temporal bones are two of the eight cranial bones that form part of the base and lateral wall of the skull. The petrous portion of the temporal bone houses the otic capsule, the densest bone in the body. The temporal bone articulates with the sphenoid, parietal, and occipital bones.

External Ear

The ears are located on each side of the head at approximately eye level. The external ear is divided into the auricle *(pinna)* and the external auditory canal *(ear canal)*. The tympanic membrane *(eardrum)* separates the external ear from the middle ear.

Auricle (Pinna)

The *auricle* (pinna), the conspicuous part of the ear, is attached to the side of the head by skin at approximately a 20- to 30-degree angle. Except for the fat and subcutaneous tissue in the lobule, it is composed mostly of cartilage. The cartilage is held to the skull by small muscles (the posterior, anterior, and superior auricular muscles), which are innervated by a branch of the facial nerve.

The parts of the pinna are illustrated in Figure U15-4. The *helix,* the outer rim of the pinna, leads inferiorly to the lobule. The *concha* is the deepest part, leading to the ear canal. The tragus and antitragus are triangular folds of cartilage that project over the entrance to the ear canal. Hair covers most of the ear, but it is usually rudimentary, except in the region of the tragus and antitragus. Sebaceous glands are also found on the skin surface.

In front of the external opening of the ear is the temporomandibular joint (TMJ). Often, TMJ problems produce referred pain to the ear (otalgia) because of their shared sensory nerve supply.

External Auditory Canal (Ear Canal)

The ear canal extends from the concha of the pinna to the tympanic membrane (see Figure U15-4). This slightly S-shaped canal is approximately 2.5 cm (1 inch) in length and follows an inward, forward, and downward path. The skeleton of cartilage in the outer third is continuous with the cartilage of the pinna. The inner two thirds is a bony canal entering the skull. The lumen of

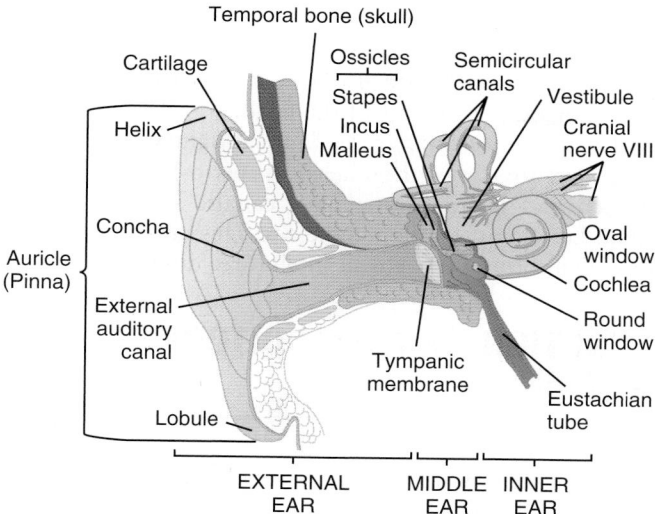

FIGURE U15-4 Anatomy of the ear.

the ear canal is irregularly shaped and is narrowest where the transition from cartilage to bone occurs. The skin covering the cartilage portion is thick, containing sebaceous and ceruminous glands and hair follicles. The sebaceous and ceruminous glands secrete a golden to black substance called *cerumen* (wax). The skin covering the bony portion is very thin.

Tympanic Membrane

The tympanic membrane (eardrum) is an oval disk (approximately 1 cm in diameter); it covers the end of the auditory canal and separates the canal from the middle ear (see Figure U15-4). The eardrum is a thin, translucent, pearly gray membrane obliquely directed downward and inward, so that the posterior part is more accessible than the anterior part.

Middle Ear

The middle ear consists of the middle ear cleft and contents: ossicles, oval and round windows, eustachian tube, and facial nerve (see Figure U15-4). The middle ear lies between the ear canal and the *labyrinth* (inner ear). The middle ear cavity has a mucosal lining.

Ossicles

The middle ear contains the three smallest bones *(ossicles)* of the body, named according to their appearance. The outermost and largest ossicle is the *malleus* (hammer), which is firmly attached to the tympanic membrane. The innermost and smallest ossicle is the *stapes* (stirrup); its footplate occupies the oval window, in direct contact with the perilymph of the inner ear. The *incus* (anvil) lies between the other two and is shaped like a tooth with two roots (see Figure U15-4).

Windows

The middle ear contains two windows, whose names reflect their shape. The *round window* is an opening in the inner ear from which sound vibrations exit. The *oval window* is an opening in the inner ear into which sound vibrations enter. The oval window is not a true window because the footplate of the stapes bone covers it.

Eustachian Tube

The eustachian tube is a narrow channel approximately 35 mm (1½ inches) long and only 1 mm wide at its narrowest end. This tube connects the middle ear to the nasopharynx (see Figure U15-4). The structure consists mostly of fibrous tissue, cartilage, and bone; it extends downward, forward, and inward from each middle ear. The eustachian tube is lined with a mucous membrane that is continuous with the lining of the middle ear at one end and with the nasopharynx at the other end. A small section of this tube, originating in the middle ear, remains permanently open. Otherwise, the walls of the tube lightly oppose or touch each other, closing the tube to both the throat and ear and preventing the sound of normal nasal respiration and of one's own voice from passing up the eustachian tube.

Mastoid Bone

The mastoid section of the temporal bone includes the cone-shaped *mastoid process;* the *mastoid antrum,* a large cavity posteriorly continuous with the middle ear; and the *mastoid air cells,* which extend from the antrum and fill the temporal bone with air pockets.

The mastoid bone is a bony protuberance behind the lower portion of the pinna. The mastoid cavity is close to several important cranial structures: the dura of the temporal lobe, the cerebellar dura, the sigmoid sinus, and the jugular bulb. The middle ear is also bounded by the internal carotid artery. Therefore infection of the middle ear and mastoid cavities can also involve these structures.

Inner Ear (Labyrinth)

The inner ear or labyrinth is located deep within the petrous section of the temporal bone; it contains the sense organs for hearing and balance, which form the eighth cranial nerve (Figure U15-5). The inner ear is a complicated system of intercommunicating chambers and connecting tubes composed of two structures:

1. The *bony labyrinth* is the rigid capsule (otic capsule) that surrounds and protects the delicate membranous labyrinth. The *vestibule* connects the cochlea (for hearing) to the three semicircular canals (for balance). The *cochlea,* which looks like a snail shell with 2½ turns, is approximately 7 mm in diameter at the widest part and is structurally di-

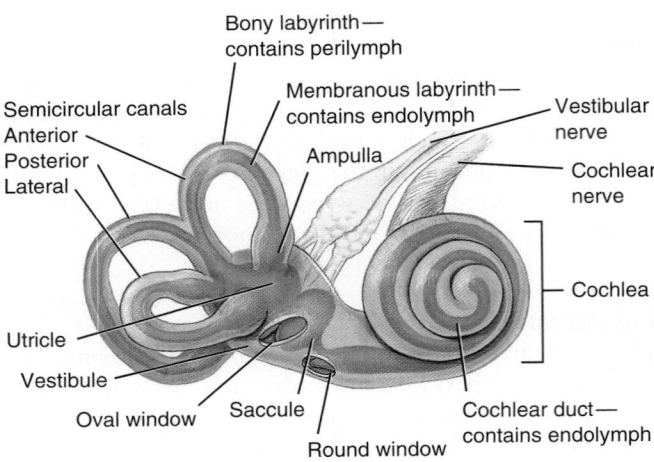

FIGURE U15-5 The labyrinths of the inner ear. (From Applegate, E.J. [2000]. *The anatomy and physiology learning system* [2nd ed.]. Philadelphia: W.B. Saunders.)

vided into three compartments (Figure U15-6). The upper compartment *(scala vestibuli)* leads from the oval window to the apex of the cochlear spiral. The lower compartment *(scala tympani)* leads from the apex of the cochlear spiral to the round window. The *scala media,* which contains the organ of Corti, lies between the scala vestibuli and scala tympani.

2. The *membranous labyrinth,* lying within but not completely filling the bony labyrinth, is bathed in a fluid called *perilymph,* which communicates with the cerebrospinal fluid (CSF) via the cochlear duct. The membranous labyrinth consists of the utricle, the saccule, the semicircular canals, the cochlear duct, and the *organ of Corti* (the end organ for

hearing). The membranous labyrinth contains a different fluid *(endolymph).* This fluid also protects the end organ because it acts as a cushion against abrupt movements of the head.

The three *semicircular canals* are at right angles to each other and are named the anterior (superior), posterior (inferior), and lateral (horizontal) canals. The horizontal canal lies closest to the middle ear. This arrangement allows detection of movement in all three dimensions.

FUNCTION OF THE AUDITORY SYSTEM

External Ear

The ears are a pair of complex sensory organs for both hearing and balance. Their location on either side of the head produces binaural hearing, allows the detection of sound direction, and aids in maintaining equilibrium. The temporal bone provides protection for the organs of hearing and balance. It houses (1) the external and internal auditory canals; (2) the mastoid air cells, which provide an air reservoir for the middle ear; (3) the blood vessels; (4) the facial, vestibular, and auditory nerves; (5) the labyrinth; and (6) the cochlea.

Sound Wave Conduction

The head, pinna, and ear canal act as an integrated system to transmit sound vibrations to the eardrum. Sound is transmitted from the external ear through the middle ear (which amplifies the sound) to the inner ear (see Figure U15-6). The funnel shape of the pinna collects and directs sound to the eardrum.

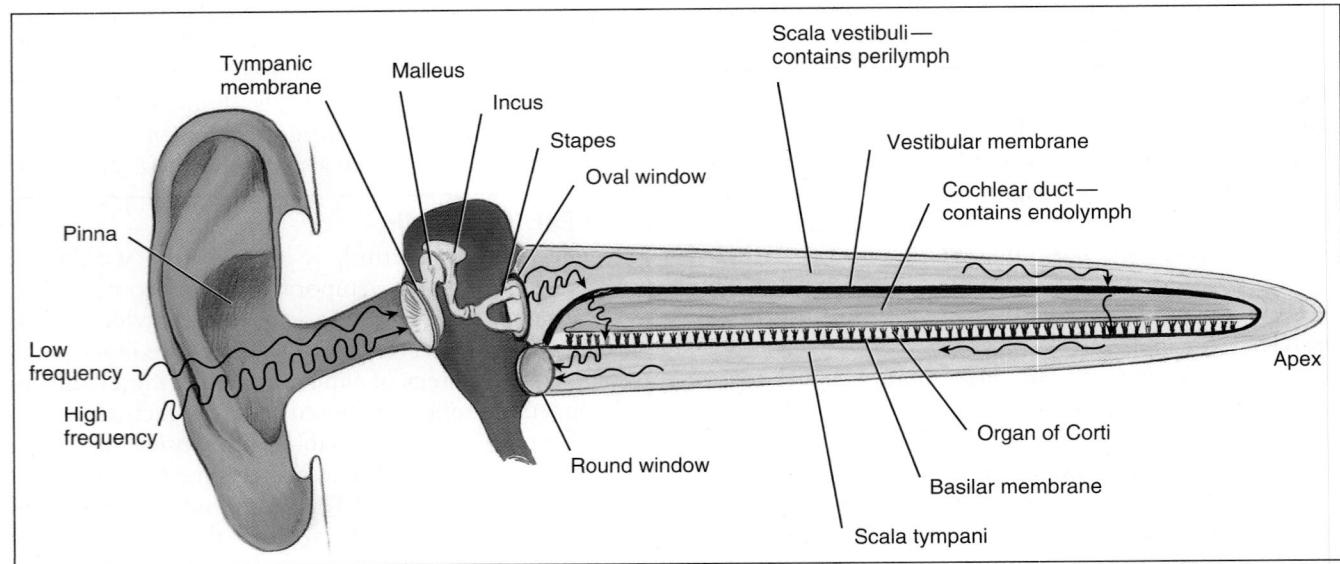

FIGURE U15-6 The uncoiled cochlea, showing the pathway of pressure waves. (From Applegate, E.J. [2000]. *The anatomy and physiology learning system* [2nd ed.]. Philadelphia: W.B. Saunders.)

The tympanic membrane, a common membrane between the external ear canal and the middle ear space, protects the middle ear and conducts sound vibrations from the external ear to the ossicles. The sound pressure applied to the stapes (the smallest ossicle) in the oval window is 22 times greater than the sound pressure exerted on the eardrum. The pressure of the sound vibrations is increased as a result of transmission from a larger area to a smaller area, and the lever effect of the ossicular chain. The sound energy, after transformation, is carried by neural elements to the brain for decoding and, thus, hearing.

Wax Production

Cerumen (wax) protects the ear. Wax is to the ear what tears are to the eyes. The sticky consistency of the wax and the fine hairs of the ear canal help clean the ear canal of foreign matter and protect it from water damage. Impacted cerumen can cause hearing losses in clients of all ages. At times, wax must be mechanically removed.

Middle Ear

Sound Wave Conduction

The ossicles transmit sound vibrations mechanically (see Figure U15-6). The ossicles are held in place by joints, muscles, and ligaments, which also offer some protection from loud sounds. The light weight and the configuration of the ossicles provide an efficient means of transmitting sound vibrations from the air molecules of the external ear to the fluid molecules of the inner ear. Fluids offer more resistance than air and need more force to transmit movement. The ossicular chain produces and magnifies this force in order to move the inner ear fluids.

Ventilation and Pressure Regulation

The eustachian tube provides an air passage from the nasopharynx to the middle ear to equalize pressure on both sides of the eardrum. This tube regulates ventilation and pressure, both of which are necessary for normal hearing. During yawning, swallowing, and sneezing, the eustachian tube is opened by the *tensor veli palatini* muscle. The natural opening and closing of the eustachian tube also allows drainage of exudate from the middle ear mucosa. The tube can be forcibly opened by increasing nasopharyngeal pressure. This act is accomplished by attempting to blow air through the nose while holding the nose closed.

Inner Ear

Hearing

Sound waves are transmitted by the ossicles to the delicate membrane of the oval window (see Figure U15-6).

These vibrations move the perilymph in the scala vestibuli. The perilymph of the scala vestibuli is continuous with that of the scala tympani at the extreme tip of the "snail shell," called the *helicotrema*. The sound energy vibrations enter through the oval window and exit through the round window.

Vibrations in the perilymph of the scala vestibuli are transmitted through the vestibular membrane *(Reissner's membrane)* to the endolymph that fills the cochlear duct. The cochlear duct is located between the scala vestibuli and the scala tympani. The *organ of Corti*, which is bathed in the endolymph, lies on the basilar membrane in a spiral strip from the basal turn near the round window to the apex at the helicotrema. This organ transforms mechanical sound vibrations into neural activity and separates sound into different frequencies. The electrochemical impulse travels via the acoustic nerve to the brain stem. Auditory nerve input from both ears joins at the lateral lemniscus, reducing the possibility of unilateral deafness from central nervous system damage. The auditory nerves ascend through the thalamus to the cortex by a variety of pathways, reaching both the primary and secondary auditory regions of the temporal cortex of the brain. Efferent innervation via the acoustic nerve (eighth cranial nerve) reaches the cochlea and vestibule via the internal auditory canal, which also carries the facial nerve (seventh cranial nerve).

Sound is filtered by the ear components. Human auditory sensitivity ranges from 15 to 20,000 Hz. The auditory canal diminishes the passage of sounds with frequencies greater than 3500 Hz, the higher end of the human voice frequency. The middle ear diminishes passage of sounds with frequencies less than 1000 Hz, the lower end of human voice frequency. The muscles of the middle ear decrease sound transmission by uncoupling the ossicles. For example, contraction of the tensor tympani allows reflex adaptation to a noisy environment. Contraction of the stapedius decreases sound transmission while speaking.

Balance

The *utricle* and *saccule* are vestibular receptors that position the head as it relates to the pull of gravity. The utricle and saccule contain hair cells arranged in sheets (maculae). These hair cells detect changes in linear acceleration, including the force of gravity. The *semicircular canals* are arranged to sense rotational movements, such as movements or changes in position. Each of the semicircular canals connects with the utricle. Where the canals connect with the utricle is an enlarged portion *(ampulla)*. The ampulla contains a cluster of hair cells *(crista)* concerned with dynamic balance. For example, when head position is changed, movement of the endolymph stimulates the hair cells, initiating increased impulses that travel over the vestibular division of the acoustic nerve to the brain. Balance functions in the vestibular system, along with visual cues and musculoskeletal cues, combine to maintain balance. Hearing and balance are partially maintained with the loss of function of one ear.

EFFECTS OF AGING ON HEARING

Many physiologic changes lead to changes in hearing in older people. The hairs become coarser during the aging process; thus retention of wax is more of a problem. *Presbycusis,* a gradual sensorineural loss caused by nerve degeneration in the inner ear or auditory nerve, is a type of hearing loss that occurs with aging, even in people living in a quiet environment. Loss of auditory neurons in the organ of Corti and cochlear hair cell degeneration create an inability to hear high-frequency sounds. There may also be degeneration of the cochlear conductive membrane and decreased blood supply to the cochlea, leading to inability to hear at all (but especially higher) frequencies. Finally, a loss of cortical auditory neurons leads to diminished hearing and speech comprehension.

CONCLUSIONS

Vision and hearing are two senses that allow distance perception of the environment. Because we rely on these senses for communication with those around us, alterations in either sense can have a profound social and emotional impact. Some reductions in the ability to see or to hear are a normal part of age-related changes.

BIBLIOGRAPHY

1. Applegate, E.J. (2000). *The anatomy and physiology learning system* (2nd ed.). Philadelphia: W. B. Saunders.
2. Guyton, A.C., & Hall, J. (2001). *Textbook of medical physiology* (10th ed.). Philadelphia: W. B. Saunders.
3. Kandel, E.R., Schwartz, J.H., & Jessell, T.M. (1999). *Principles of neural science* (4th ed.). Norwalk, CT: Appleton & Lange.
4. McPhee, S.J., et al. (1999). *Pathophysiology of disease.* New York, McGraw-Hill.
5. Nolte, J. (1999). *The human brain* (4th ed.). St. Louis: Mosby.
6. Silverthorn, D. (2001). *Human physiology* (2nd ed.). Upper Saddle River, NJ: Prentice Hall.

Assessment of the Eyes and Ears

Sarah C. Smith
Helene J. Krouse

---

evolve

Web Enhancements

Assessment Terms
English and Spanish
Appendix A
Religious Beliefs and Practices Affecting Health Care

http://evolve.elsevier.com/Black/medsurg/

Appendix B
A Health History Format That Integrates the Assessment of Functional Health Patterns
Appendix C
Laboratory Values of Clinical Importance in Medical-Surgical Nursing

---

ASSESSMENT OF THE EYE

One of the most important considerations in an ocular assessment is that many ophthalmic disorders are asymptomatic. The four most common preventable causes of permanent vision loss in developed nations are (1) *amblyopia* (reduced visual acuity that is not correctable with glasses in the absence of anatomic defects in the eye or visual pathways), (2) diabetic retinopathy, (3) age-related maculopathy, and (4) glaucoma. Routine eye examinations are therefore imperative.

The eye is a unique organ because its external anatomy can be assessed easily. Even the internal eye is visible through the cornea, where blood vessels and central nervous system (CNS) tissue (the retina and optic nerve) can be visualized without the use of x-rays or invasive procedures. The effects of many systemic problems, such as infections, cancer, and vascular and autoimmune disorders, can be detected in an internal eye examination. Clients may voice misconceptions about vision and the eyes (Box 66-1). If you encounter such misconceptions while conducting a physical examination, be prepared to address them.

HISTORY

An ophthalmic history includes (1) demographic data, (2) exploration of current manifestations, (3) past health history, (4) family health history, (5) psychosocial history and lifestyle, and (6) review of systems.

Biographical and Demographic Data

Demographic data relevant to ocular assessment include age and gender. The incidence of cataracts, dry eye, retinal detachment, glaucoma, esotropia (eyes turning inward), and exotropia (eyes turning outward) increases with age. Hereditary color vision deficits are more common in men than in women.

Current Health

Ocular manifestations can be divided into three basic categories: (1) vision, (2) appearance, and (3) sensations of pain and discomfort.

Chief Complaint

The most common chief complaint is a change or loss of vision, but the complaint may also be less specific, such

---

evolve Be sure to check out the bonus material on the Evolve website and the CD-ROM, including free self-assessment exercises.
http://evolve.elsevier.com/Black/medsurg/

BOX 66-1 *Common Misconceptions About Vision and the Eyes*

The following statements are often passed along as "advice." All of the following are false:

1. Reading in the dark is harmful to the eyes.
2. Children will outgrow crossed eyes.
3. A cataract is a film growing over the surface of the eye.
4. Cataracts must "ripen" before they are removed.
5. The surgeon takes out the eye to operate on it.
6. A person with failing eyesight should avoid reading to save the eyes.
7. Children must be cautioned not to sit too close to the television.
8. Wearing someone else's glasses may damage your eyes.
9. Misuse of the eyes in childhood results in the need for glasses later in life.
10. Cataracts can be removed by a laser.
11. Emotional stress increases intraocular pressure.

BOX 66-2 *Red Eye*

Nurses often encounter a client whose chief complaint is a "red eye." The condition causing the eye to be red (engorgement of the conjunctival vessels) may be a subconjunctival hemorrhage that requires no treatment, or it may be a manifestation of a serious eye disorder, which requires immediate attention. Disorders involving red eye include the following:

Conjunctivitis—Bacterial, viral, allergic, and irritative
Herpes simplex keratitis—inflammation of the cornea
Scleritis—inflammation of the sclera
Angle-closure glaucoma—sudden occlusion of the anterior chamber angle by iris tissue
Adnexal disease—stye, dacryocystitis, blepharitis, lid lesions (carcinoma), thyroid disease, and vascular lesions
Subconjunctival hemorrhage—accumulation of blood in the potential space between the conjunctiva and the sclera
Pterygium—abnormal growth of tissue that progresses over the cornea
Keratoconjunctivitis sicca—inflammation associated with lacrimal deficiency
Abrasions and foreign bodies—hyperemic response
Abnormal lid function—Bell's palsy, thyroid ophthalmopathy, or lesions that cause ocular exposure

To evaluate a red eye:
1. Check the client's visual acuity with a Snellen chart.
2. Inspect for a pattern of redness.
3. Observe for the presence of discharge.
4. Using a penlight or slit lamp, observe for corneal opacities.
5. Using fluorescein stain, observe for corneal defects.
6. Examine the anterior chamber for depth, blood cells, or pus.
7. Examine the pupils for irregularity.
8. Check intraocular pressure.
9. Observe for the pressure of proptosis or a lid disorder.

---

as headache or eyestrain. Commonly, the client is unable to verbalize a specific complaint. The chief complaint may be as vague as "something is wrong with my eyes."

Symptom Analysis

Whenever possible, characterize clinical manifestations according to rapidity of onset, location, duration, and characteristics (such as frequency and severity). The circumstances surrounding onset as well as the client's response to treatment are important. Record current eye and systemic medications being used and all other current and past ocular disorders.

Abnormal Vision. Visual changes or loss of vision can be caused by abnormalities in the eye or anywhere along the visual pathway. Considerations include (1) a refractive (focusing) error; (2) interference from lid *ptosis* (drooping eyelid); (3) clouding or interference in the cornea, lens, aqueous or vitreous space; and (4) malfunction of the retina, optic nerve, or intracranial visual pathway.

Glare or halos can result from uncorrected refractive error, scratches on glasses, dilated pupils, corneal edema, or cataract. Flashing or flickering lights may indicate retinal traction or migraine. Floating spots may represent normal vitreous body strands or the pathologic presence of blood, pigment, or inflammatory cells in the vitreous body. *Diplopia* (double vision) may occur in one eye or both and can be caused by refractive correction, muscle imbalance, or neurologic disorders.

Abnormal Appearance. The most common abnormal appearance is a *red eye*. Causes include minor irritation, vascular congestion, subconjunctival hemorrhage, inflammatory disorders, infection, allergy, and trauma (Box 66-2). Other external changes in appearance include growths or lesions, edema, and abnormal position.

Abnormal Sensation. Eye pain is often poorly localized. Nonspecific complaints include eyestrain, pulling, pressure, fullness, or generalized headache. The pain may be periocular, ocular, or retrobulbar (behind the globe). Foreign-body sensation produces a sharp superficial pain that can be relieved by topical anesthesia. Deeper internal aching may indicate glaucoma, inflammation, muscle spasm, or infection. Reflex spasm of the ciliary muscle and iris sphincter that occurs with inflammation may produce brow ache and *photophobia* (sensitivity to light) or a constricted pupil *(miosis)*. Itching is usually a sign of an allergic response. Dryness, burning, grittiness, and mild foreign-body sensation can occur with dry eyes or mild corneal irritation.

Tearing may be due to irritation or an abnormality of the lacrimal system. Increased ocular secretions usually indicate viral or bacterial infections and may also be present in allergic and noninfectious irritations.

Past Health History

The past health history focuses on systemic disorders commonly associated with ocular manifestations, such as diabetes mellitus, arthritis, hypertension, and thyroid disease.

Childhood and Infectious Diseases

Diseases that occur in childhood with possible ocular sequelae include diabetes mellitus, retinoblastoma, thyroid disorders, rheumatoid arthritis, exposure to sexually transmitted diseases (STDs) such as syphilis and acquired immunodeficiency syndrome (AIDS), and muscular dystrophy. Inquire about vaccinations, particularly for measles (rubella).

Major Illnesses and Hospitalizations

In addition to childhood and systemic diseases, ask about hypertension, multiple sclerosis, myasthenia gravis, and adult onset of thyroid disorders, rheumatoid arthritis, and diabetes mellitus. Ocular diseases and structural problems include refractive errors (and corrective lenses used), strabismus, amblyopia, cataracts, glaucoma, and retinal detachment. If the client wears eyeglasses or contact lenses, ask when the last eye examination took place and when the prescription was last changed. Has the client been hospitalized or undergone surgery related to the eyes or brain? Does the client have a history of head trauma or eye trauma related to motor vehicle accidents, sports injury, or other unintentional events?

Medications

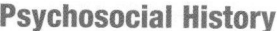

Many medications affect the eyes. Prescription drugs that can affect the eyes include insulin, corticosteroids, oral hypoglycemics, and thyroid replacement hormones. Ask whether the client uses eyedrops, and note the name, dose, and frequency taken. Specifically ask about use of over-the-counter eye drops such as natural tears. Over-the-counter preparations that can dry the ocular surface include antihistamines and decongestants.

Inquire about the use of herbal remedies, dietary supplements such as vitamins, and the consumption of specific foods. Some clients may consume large doses of vitamins A and C and certain foods, believing that these substances will prevent the development of vision problems such as cataracts and macular degeneration. Other

nutrients believed to promote eye health include vitamin E, zinc, lutein, selenium, manganese, copper, and the B vitamins glutathione, niacinamide, and riboflavin.

Allergies

Note any allergies to medications and other substances. Has the client ever had an allergic reaction to eyedrops or other medications that have affected the eyes? Allergic manifestations include eye redness, tearing, and itching. Determine past allergic reactions not only to medications but also to inhalants (dust, chemicals, or pollens) and contactants (cosmetics or pollens).

Family Health History

Because many ocular disorders tend to be familial, ask specifically about strabismus, glaucoma, *myopia* (nearsightedness), and *hyperopia* (farsightedness). Other common familial disorders include migraine, retinoblastoma, macular degeneration, retinitis pigmentosa, sickle cell anemia, keratoconus, and diabetes mellitus. Lack of a family health history does not necessarily rule out the possibility of a genetic disorder. Some clients do not know the ocular history of family members, and some may be embarrassed or hesitant to share the information.

Psychosocial History

Psychosocial history and lifestyle data significant to the ocular health history include occupational hazards, leisure activities and hobbies, and health management behaviors. A driving history can reveal a vision problem. Ask about the nature of the client's work and hobbies. Is the client exposed to irritating fumes, smoke, or airborne particles? Are safety goggles worn in situations in which eye injury could occur from fragments of metal or sand? Is lighting insufficient, harsh, or glaring, leading to eyestrain? Leisure and sports activities associated with increased incidence of eye injury include baseball, racquetball, and contact sports; football is associated with a potential for head trauma. Participation in active outdoor activities, such as gardening, hiking, and cross-country skiing, increases the risk of foreign-body injury, abrasion, or penetrating injury. Does the client wear sunglasses or other protective eye gear when outdoors?

Explore health management behaviors related to the eyes. If the client has a systemic disease that affects the eyes, ask whether the client practices self-care measures. For example, does the diabetic client aggressively manage the disease by attempting to regulate blood glucose levels with diet and medication? If the client wears contact lenses, are the lenses cleaned and stored as recommended? Is the client capable of taking care of the lenses safely?

Visual ability is one of several capabilities necessary for a person to operate a motor vehicle. Use tact when assessing a client who may have impaired vision. Clients may not answer truthfully if they feel that driving privileges will be lost.

Briefly review the client's driving history for information that can indicate a vision deficit. Ask whether driving at night is difficult because of the need to adjust to the glare from oncoming headlights. Does the client have trouble seeing the dashboard instrument panel at night because of dim lighting? Are traffic or street signs difficult to read while driving? Is the client able to drive in conditions of reduced visibility, such as in rain or fog? Do other vehicles, pedestrians, bicyclists, or objects appear unexpectedly in the peripheral vision while the client is looking straight ahead? Has the client had a motor vehicle accident or "close call" within the past year?

The social stigma of blindness underlies the anxiety that clients experience with actual or potential vision loss. Total loss of vision isolates a person within a different reality. Although most clients are successfully rehabilitated, some losses are permanent. Some people, for a variety of reasons, remain socially isolated. The image of a blind person who is pitied and must accept the charity of others is disturbing.

Not all work environments can be adapted for someone who is visually impaired. Clients with actual or potential vision loss may be faced with barriers in their vocations that force an unwanted change. Age may be a major factor in the client's ability to meet this challenge. Self-esteem is closely related to one's roles in a particular lifestyle. Loss of control in personal, family, and work situations can be devastating. The issue of dependence versus independence may also be a factor in the client's ability to cope with the stressors of vision loss.

Review of Systems

The review of systems (ROS) relevant to the eyes includes asking about manifestations such as headaches and problems with sinusitis. Determine whether manifestations occur in association with pain or discomfort, visual changes, swelling, redness, or drainage from the eye. Ask about the time of day and the season of year during which manifestations occur as well as about sensitivity to light. Detailed questions are presented in Chapter 4 and on the website for this textbook.

PHYSICAL EXAMINATION

Your role and scope of practice in ophthalmic assessment and examination vary according to state nurse practice acts, institutions, and employer guidelines. Regardless of the level of responsibility in any practice situation, you must be knowledgeable about ophthalmic clinical manifestations and diagnoses as they relate to the holistic approach to client care.

Examination of the eyes includes assessment of external structures, using inspection and palpation, extraocular movements (EOMs), visual acuity, and visual fields (peripheral vision). If you have advanced clinical assessment skills, you may perform tonometry and examine the internal eye structures with an ophthalmoscope. For an example of an assessment recording, see the Physical Assessment Findings in the Healthy Adult feature on The Eye, below.

Observe the client's body structure and features for obvious deformities and apparent age. For example, the hand deformities or abnormal gait of a client with arthritis may be a clue to the diagnosis of an associated eye disorder of keratoconjunctivitis sicca *(dry-eye syndrome)* in a client who reports itching and burning eyes.

External Eye

External eye structures include the eyebrows, eyelashes, eyelids, the lacrimal apparatus, anterior portion of the eyeballs, conjunctivae, sclerae, corneas, anterior chambers, pupils, and irises. Inspect and palpate these structures while the client sits at eye level.

Eye Position

Assess eye position for symmetry and alignment. Sunken or protruding eyes, such as protrusion of one eye or both eyes *(exophthalmos)*, are an abnormal finding.

PHYSICAL ASSESSMENT FINDINGS IN THE HEALTHY ADULT

The Eye

Inspection

Visual acuity 20/20. Eyebrows full, mobile. Eyelashes curve out and away from eyelids. Ptosis absent. Eyelids without lesions or inflammation. Eyes moist. Palpebral conjunctivae pink; bulbar conjunctivae clear. Scleral color even, without redness. Corneal light reflection symmetrical. PERRLA, directly and consensually. Cornea smooth; lens and anterior chamber clear. Irises evenly colored. EOMs full, without nystagmus. Conjugate movement. No strabismus. Visual fields full to confrontation.

Palpation

Eyeballs firm. Orbits without edema. No regurgitation from puncta. Tenderness absent over lacrimal apparatus.

Funduscopic Examination

Red reflexes visualized. AV ratio approximately 2:3. Vessels without tortuosity, narrowing, pulsation, or nicking. Disc margins clear, no cupping, cup-to-disc ratio 1:3. No evidence of retinal hemorrhage, patches, spots.

AV, Artery-to-vein; *EOM,* extraocular movement; *PERRLA,* pupils equal, round, reactive to light and accommodation.

Eyebrows

Inspect the eyebrows for symmetry, hair distribution, skin conditions, and movement. The eyebrows normally move up and down smoothly under control of the facial nerves. Hair loss of the lateral aspects occurs with aging. The skin may be dry and flaking (dandruff), which is abnormal.

Eyelids and Eyelashes

Examine the eyelids and eyelashes for placement and symmetry. When open, the upper lids rest at the top of the irises and the lower lids at the bottom so that the sclerae are not visible above or below the irises. Sagging of the upper lids that covers part of the pupil *(ptosis)* is abnormal. Ptosis may occur with aging but also results from edema, third cranial nerve disorders, and neuromuscular disorders. Check for effective closure by asking the client to close the eyes. Eyelids that turn inward *(entropion)* or outward *(ectropion)* can result in corneal irritation. Lid eversion and inversion are often related to aging tissues but may result from facial nerve paresis, scarring, or allergies. Elevate the eyebrows to inspect the upper lids for lesions. Inspect the lower lids by asking the client to open the eyes. Examine the skin of the eyelids and orbit by palpating for texture, firmness, mobility, and integrity of the underlying tissues.

Blink Response

Blinking is an involuntary reflex that occurs bilaterally up to 20 times a minute. Rapid, infrequent, or asymmetrical blinking is abnormal.

Eyeballs

Palpate the eyeballs for symmetry and firmness. Instruct the client to close the eyes and look down. Place the tip of the index fingers on the upper eyelids, over the sclerae, and palpate gently. Normally, the eyeballs feel firm and symmetrical, not asymmetrical, hard, or soft. If you have advanced clinical skills, you may perform tonometry to measure intraocular pressure (see Internal Eye under Physical Examination).

Lacrimal Apparatus

Examine the lacrimal apparatus by retracting the upper lid and having the client look down so that part of the lacrimal gland can be visualized. Observe this area for swelling or tenderness. The eye surface should be moist and without excess tearing. Inspect the area between the lower lid and the nose, which should be free of edema. Gently palpate the area over the lower orbit rim near the inner canthus (over the lacrimal sac). No regurgitation of fluid from the sac or puncta should be present.

Conjunctivae and Sclerae

Inspect the conjunctivae and sclerae for color changes, texture, vascularity, lesions, thickness, secretions, and foreign bodies. The bulbar conjunctivae are colorless and transparent, allowing the sclerae to be seen. Small blood vessels may be visible. In white people, the sclerae are white; in people with dark skin, they may appear light yellow. Wear gloves to inspect the palpebral conjunctivae, and wash your hands both before and after this portion of the examination.

Retract the lower eyelids to expose the conjunctivae without applying pressure to the eyeballs. You (or the client) should gently push the lower lids down against the bony orbit while the client looks up. Healthy conjunctivae are pink to light red; paleness or a bright red color is abnormal. If the lower palpebral conjunctivae are normal, the upper palpebral conjunctivae usually are not inspected. If examination is necessary, evert the upper eyelids by gently grasping the eyelashes of the upper lid and pulling down while the client looks down. Place a cotton-tipped applicator just above the lid margin, and turn the upper lid inside out over the applicator. After inspection, return the eyelid to its normal position by gently pulling the eyelashes forward while the client looks up.

Corneal Reflex

The corneal reflex test is performed to assess the function of the fifth (trigeminal) cranial nerve. Instruct the client to keep the eyes open and look straight ahead. Bring a sterile cotton wisp from behind the client and touch it lightly to the cornea. Blinking and tearing indicate that the nerves are intact. Use a separate wisp for each eye. An alternative method is to use a syringe or the bulb from an otoscope to puff air gently across the cornea, eliciting the blink-and-tear response. A client wearing contact lenses may not respond to the same degree as someone who does not wear them because of insensitivity to the stimulus.

Cornea

Inspect the cornea from an oblique angle while shining a penlight on the corneal surface. The irises are easily visible. In older adults, a thin, grayish white ring around the edge of the cornea *(arcus senilis)* may be seen. Abnormalities include surface irregularity and cloudiness *(opacity)*.

Anterior Chamber

Using the same oblique angle and penlight, inspect the anterior chamber while observing the cornea. The chambers should appear clear and transparent with no cloudiness or shadows cast on the irises. The depth of the chamber between the cornea and iris is normally about 3 mm. Shallower or deeper chambers are abnormal; refer the client to an ophthalmologist.

Iris and Pupil

Inspect the iris and the pupil. The iris should light up with oblique lighting from the penlight and should have a consistent color. Bulging or uneven coloring is abnormal. When light shines into the eyes, the iris constricts as the optic nerves are stimulated, causing the pupil to become smaller. Dim lighting causes the pupil to dilate. Inspect the pupils for size, equality, shape, and ability to react to light and accommodation. Pupils are normally black, round, with smooth borders and are the same size. The actual size depends on the level of lighting, the effect of medications that alter iris contractility, changes in intracranial pressure, or lesions impinging on the optic nerve.

Dim the light to test pupil reactions to light and accommodation. Instruct the client to look straight ahead. To test direct response to light, bring the penlight in from the side to shine directly over the center of the pupil. The illuminated pupil should constrict briskly and evenly. Repeat this maneuver on the other eye. Both eyes should react to the same degree. Test consensual response by observing one pupil while the penlight is shone on the opposite pupil. Both pupils should constrict to the same degree, although the consensual response is slightly slower.

Test accommodation by holding the penlight 4 to 6 inches (10 to 15 cm) away from the client's nose. Instruct the client to look first at the penlight, then at the distant wall straight ahead, and then back at the penlight. While the client gazes from near to far and back again, observe the pupils' response to changes in distance. The pupils should dilate when the client looks at the far point and should constrict when the client looks at the near object. Then move the penlight toward the bridge of the client's nose, observing the pupils for convergence and constriction.

Results of the pupil assessment that are normal are recorded as PERRLA (*p*upils *e*qual, *r*ound, and *r*eactive to *l*ight, and *a*ccommodation). Abnormal results include light intolerance (*photophobia*), irregular or unequal pupils or pupils that do not react to light or accommodation. Pupil abnormalities may be caused by neurologic disease, intraocular inflammation, iris adhesions, systemic or ocular medication side effects, or surgical alteration, or they may be benign variations of normal findings.

Ocular Motility

Evaluation of ocular motility provides information about the extraocular muscles; the orbit; the oculomotor, trochlear, and abducens nerves; their brain stem connections; and the cerebral cortex. Ask the client to track a target with both eyes as it is moved in each of the six cardinal directions of gaze (see Figure U15-2). Note the speed, smoothness, range, and symmetry of movements and observe for unsteadiness of fixation (*nystagmus,* where the eyes seem to jiggle).

The eyes normally move parallel to each other, smoothly and in unison. Test the function of the oculomotor, trochlear, and abducens nerves by asking the client to look straight ahead while you stand directly in front. Hold a penlight about 12 inches (30 cm) from the client's eyes. Instruct the client to keep the head still and to follow the penlight's movements with the eyes only. Move the penlight slowly and smoothly through the six cardinal positions of gaze, being careful not to go beyond the client's field of vision. Move the penlight in an orderly manner from the center outward along each of the six directions; pause briefly to observe for nystagmus, and then return to the center. Nystagmus is an involuntary rapid, oscillating movement of the eyeball and is considered an abnormal finding except for slight nystagmus in the extreme lateral gazes (end-point nystagmus). If the eyes do not move in parallel or if the upper eyelid covers more than a tiny portion of the iris, note the conditions as abnormal findings.

Corneal Light Reflex Test. The corneal light reflex test (Hirschberg's test) determines eye alignment. Shine a penlight at the bridge of the client's nose from a distance of 12 to 15 inches (30 to 38 cm) while the client stares straight ahead. Observe where the light reflects from both corneas; the reflection should be symmetrical. Asymmetrical reflection is abnormal and may indicate strabismus, a disorder in which the eye axes cannot be directed to the same object. A constant deviation of ocular alignment is termed *tropia.* Deviation toward the nose is called *esotropia,* a deviation away from the nose is called *exotropia,* and a vertical (up or down) deviation is called *hypertropia and hypotropia,* respectively. Latent deviations are seen only when one eye is covered and are called *phorias (esophoria* and *exophoria).*

Cover-Uncover Test. This test assesses eye muscle function and alignment for tropia and phoria. Ask the client to stare straight ahead at a fixed point about 20 inches (51 cm) away. Cover one of the client's eyes with an opaque card while you observe the uncovered eye for lateral or medial movement as it focuses on the fixed point. There should be no movement. Remove the eye cover, and observe that eye for movement as it focuses on the fixed point; again, there should be no movement. Repeat the maneuvers for the opposite eye. The test may need to be repeated several times to confirm abnormal findings of strabismus.

Vision

Visual Acuity. Testing visual acuity is the standard, routine method used to determine the clarity of the ocular media (cornea, lens, and vitreous) and the function of the visual pathway from the retina to the brain. Although abnormal acuity implies an uncorrected refractive error or pathologic process, normal acuity does not exclude disease of the visual system. Visual acuity is assessed in one eye at a time and then in both eyes together, with the client comfortably seated. Begin with the right eye while covering the left eye with an occluder or opaque card. Test visual acuity with and without corrective lenses. Traditionally visual acuity is measured using the Snellen chart (Figure 66-1, *A*) at a distance of 20 feet; at this distance, rays of light from an object are practically parallel and little effort of accommodation is required. In rooms that measure shorter than 20 feet, mirrors or projection may be used to achieve the required distance. Charts may also be reduced proportionately to compensate for distance. Adaptations may be needed for the client who is illiterate or who does not speak English; variations of the Snellen chart are available for these clients. Numbers and symbols can be used in lieu of letters. There must be adequate lighting for the client to see.

Begin by asking the client to read the smallest line of symbols or letters that is seen. Credit the client for the smallest line of print that is read with more than 50% accuracy. Record the results according to the standardized numbers printed next to the lines on the chart. The sizes of the symbols are identified according to the distances at which they are normally visible. For example, the largest symbols can be read 200 feet away by people with unimpaired vision. The results of visual acuity testing are expressed as a fraction. The numerator denotes the distance the client is from the chart letters, and the denominator denotes the distance from the chart at which a client with normal vision can see the chart letters. Examples of results follow:

- Vision that is 20/20 is normal; that is, the client is able to read at 20 feet what a person with normal vision can read at 20 feet.
- A client with a visual acuity of 20/60 can read at a distance of 20 feet only what a client with normal vision can read at 60 feet.
- The client with *myopia* (nearsightedness) has results of 20/30 or greater, signifying that the client can read at 20 feet only what a person with normal vision can read at 30 feet (or greater).

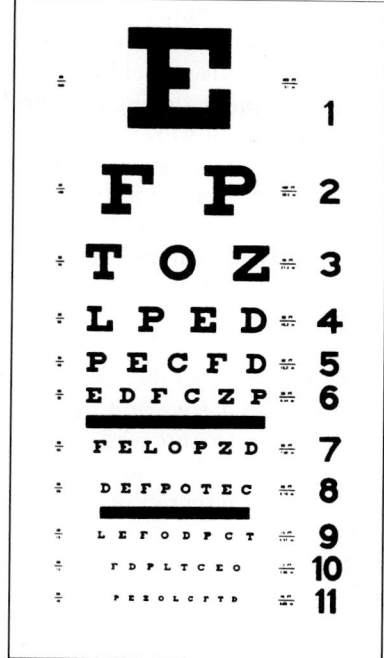

A

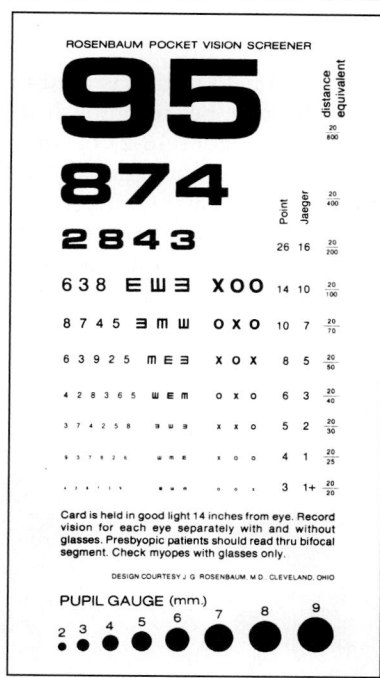

B

FIGURE 66-1 A, Snellen's chart, for assessment of visual acuity. **B,** A Rosenbaum pocket vision screener. The charts are not pictured to scale with respect to one another. (**B** courtesy of SMP Division, Cooper Laboratories [P.R.], Inc., San German, Puerto Rico.)

- *Hyperopia* (farsightedness) results are 20/15 or less; that is, the client can read at 20 feet what a person with normal vision can read at 15 feet (or less).

A result of 20/15 indicates better-than-average visual acuity.

- *Legal blindness* is defined as 20/200 or less with corrected vision (glasses or contact lenses) or less than 20 degrees of visual field in the better eye.

When the client cannot distinguish the largest letter on the chart, ask the client to read the number of fingers held up in front of him or her at a distance of 3 feet (CF = count fingers). If the client cannot distinguish fingers, ask whether the client perceives hand movements (HM = hand motion). Finally, determine whether the client can perceive light (LP = light perception). NLP indicates no light perception.

Test near vision with a card or newsprint held 12 to 14 inches (30 to 36 cm) from the client's eyes (Figure 66-1, *B*). Corrective lenses are worn if they are needed. The client with normal vision can read the material at that distance. Complaints of blurring or attempts by the client to move the card either closer or farther away signal abnormal near vision.

If the client becomes familiar with the letters through repeated examination, have the client read the letters backward. If the client can read most of the letters in a particular line but misses one or two, document the visual acuity as 20/40–2.

Visual Fields. Visual field testing is used to evaluate peripheral vision. It may be accomplished by the *confrontational method* (Figure 66-2) or with a computerized instrument. The confrontational method assumes that the examiner has normal peripheral vision.

The client sits facing you about 2 feet (60 cm) away. The client's eyes and yours should be at the same level. Both you and the client cover the eyes directly opposite to one another with an opaque cover (your right eye and the client's left eye) and stare at each other's uncovered eye. Hold a small object, such as a penlight, in your free hand, holding it equidistant between yourself and the client, just out of view at the periphery of the visual field. Starting with the superior field, slowly bring the penlight down between the client and yourself until the client states that he or she can see it. (You should be able to see the penlight at the same time.)

Repeat this maneuver at 45-degree angles, progressing through the superior, temporal, inferior, and nasal fields until all are tested. You may need to position the penlight slightly behind the client to test the temporal fields adequately. Repeat the test for the other eye. Normal visual fields extend about 50 degrees superiorly, 90 degrees laterally, 70 degrees inferiorly, and 60 degrees medially. Gross visual field defects can be detected; if any are found, refer the client for further examination.

A variety of manual and computerized visual field testing equipment may be used to permit more accurate, reproducible detection and quantification of *scotoma* (an area of decreased visual function). CNS disorders, such as a brain lesion or syphilis, and ocular disorders, such as glaucoma or retinal detachment, can alter visual fields.

Special Testing of Vision

Color Vision. Color vision problems are genetic and can be acquired by both men and women. Men are more often affected with inherited losses in color vision (7%), and women are affected to a lesser degree (0.5%). Nutritional problems, optic nerve disorders, and problems with the fovea centralis can also alter color perception.

Color vision testing is not always part of a routine eye examination. It is used most often in screening people seeking a license to operate a motor vehicle or for employment in which color discrimination is important. A common test involves the use of color plates on which numbers are outlined in primary colors and surrounded by "confusion" colors. The person with color vision problems is unable to recognize the figure. One such test consists of 84 chips of color that are matched in terms of increasing hues.

Central Area Blindness Assessment

The Amsler grid is a 20-cm square that is divided into 5-mm squares with a dot in the center. The grid is used to detect and follow the development of central area blindness *(scotoma),* such as occurs in macular degeneration. The client wears glasses, closes one eye, and holds the grid 12 inches from the face (the usual reading distance). The client fixes vision on the central dot and describes any areas of distortion or absences in the grid.

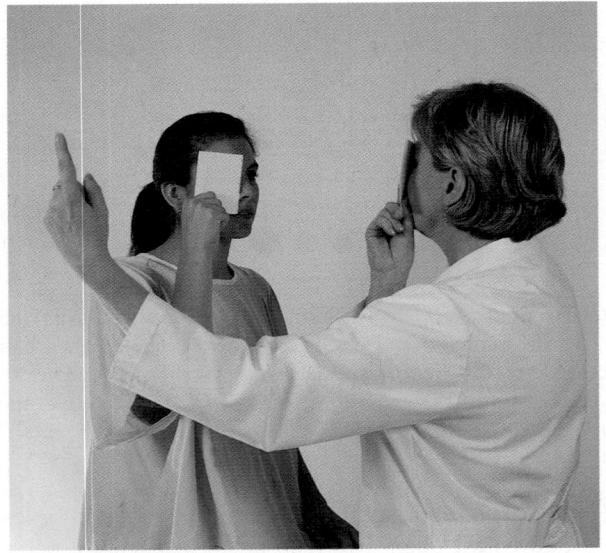

FIGURE 66-2 Confrontational method of assessment of visual fields. (From Jarvis, C. [2000]. *Physical examination and health assessment* [3rd ed.]. Philadelphia: W.B. Saunders.)

Internal Eye

Internal eye structures are visible only with illumination such as that provided by an ophthalmoscope. This instrument is used to inspect the structures posterior to the iris, including the lens and fundus (which includes the retina, retinal vessels, choroid, optic disc, macula, and fovea). Using the ophthalmoscope requires considerable skill and practice.

Direct Ophthalmoscopy

The hand-held direct ophthalmoscope provides a magnified ($\times$15) image of the fundus (posterior portion of the eye) and a detailed view of the disc and retinal vascular bed. Ophthalmoscopy is a part of a general physical examination as well as an ophthalmologic examination. Dilating the eye enhances the view, although a darkened room can cause adequate dilation. The ophthalmoscope is held 1 to 2 inches away from the client's eye and, through a light source and reflective mirrors, the macula, optic disc, and retinal vessels can be examined (Box 66-3 and Figure 66-3). The view may be impaired by a cloudy cornea or the presence of a cataract.

Normally the red reflex is a bright red-orange glow seen through the pupil. The optic disc appears round with well-defined margins (except in the nasal margin) and a creamy pink color. The *physiologic cup* (depressed center of the disc) should be no larger than half the diameter of the optic disc. Retinal veins are darker than arteries and radiate from the disc. Veins are slightly thicker than arteries and should be free of pulsation. Tortuous vessels or straightened arteries are abnormal, as is nicking (the disappearance of a vessel where an artery and vein cross each other so that one vessel looks discontinuous). The retinal background is pink in white people and dark and heavily pigmented in people with a dark complexion. Choroidal vessels may appear as linear orange streaks. A normal retina is shown in Figure 66-3.

The fundus is the only site in the body where the vascular bed may be observed directly. Thus funduscopic examination yields information about many systemic diseases. Abnormal findings include an altered arteriovenous ratio, narrowed arteries, widened veins, pinched-off vessels, abnormal arterial light reflex, excessive tortuosity, numerous arteriovenous nicks, exudates, white patches, and focal hemorrhage.

Indirect Ophthalmoscopy

Indirect ophthalmoscopy provides a stereoscopic picture over a large area of the retina. The light source comes from a head-mounted light. The examiner holds a convex lens in front of the client's eye and, through a viewing device attached to the headband, sees an inverted reversed image. The indirect ophthalmoscope provides for binocular visual inspection with depth perception and permits a wider field of view compared with the direct method.

BOX 66-3	*Guidelines for Using an Ophthalmoscope*

1. Assemble the ophthalmoscope by attaching the head to the handle.
2. Darken the room.
3. Turn on the ophthalmoscope light by depressing the rheostat button and turning the rheostat to the brightest light.
4. Turn the aperture selector to a large round circle of light.
5. Turn the lens selector dial to zero.
6. Instruct the client to stare straight ahead and to focus on a distant object.
7. Leave both of your eyes open during the examination. Learn to suppress visual stimulation from the eye that is not looking through the viewing aperture.
8. Hold the ophthalmoscope while steadying the client's head with your free hand.
9. Approach the client from the side at approximately a 45-degree angle and a distance of 15 inches. Direct the light into the client's pupil.
10. Move slowly closer to the client's eye, keeping the light directed on the pupil. If the client blinks, hold your position steady until the client's eye opens again. At approximately 15 inches, visualize the red reflex, then the anterior chamber. Moving closer, look at the lens. Finally, when very close (1 to 2 inches), vessels of the fundus may be seen.
11. Adjust the lens selector with your index finger to focus on a blood vessel, and follow the vessel into the optic disc.
12. Focus on the disc, adjusting the lens selector as needed to correct for any visual deficits of both you and the client. Once the focus is adjusted, examine the optic disc (for color, margins, shape, and presence of physiologic cup; see Figure 66-5).
13. Follow the major blood vessels from the disc and look for evidence of tortuosity, pulsation, diameter, ratio of arteries to veins (normally 2:3), and areas where arteries and veins cross for signs of nicking.
14. Note the retinal background color. Look for the presence of exudate or hemorrhage.
15. Last, ask the client to look into the light so you can examine the fovea centralis. The fovea may be seen as a tiny bright light in the center of the macula. Only a very brief glimpse is possible because the light is too bright for the client to look at for long.
16. Repeat the examination for the opposite eye.

Tonometry

Tonometry is a method of measuring intraocular fluid pressure with the use of calibrated instruments that in-

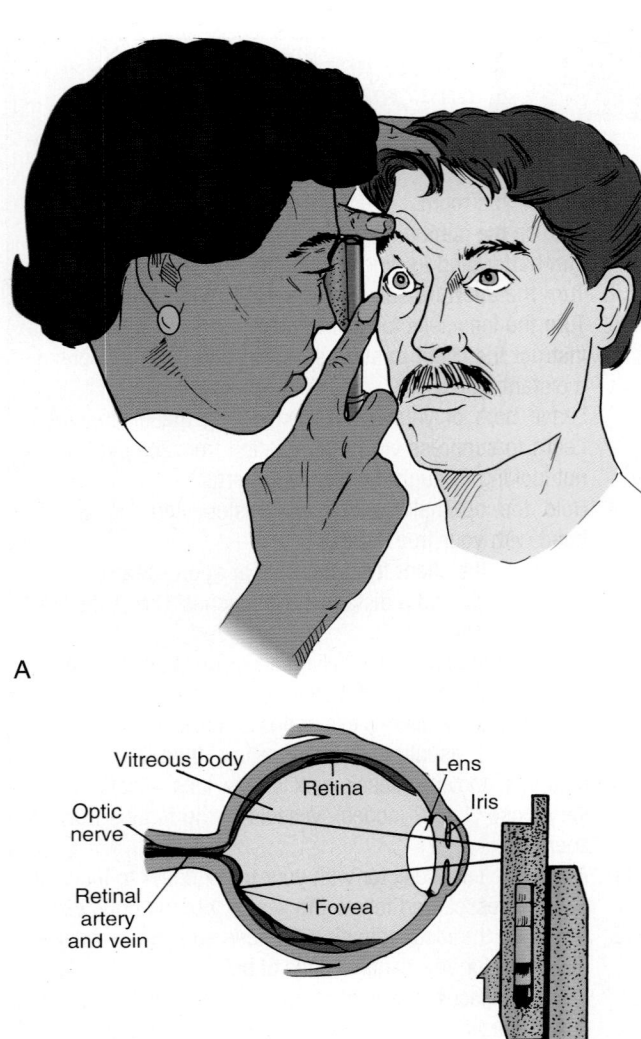

dent or flatten the corneal apex. The eye can be thought of as an enclosed compartment through which there is a constant circulation of aqueous humor, which maintains the shape of the eye with a relatively uniform pressure within the globe. As the pressure increases, the eye becomes firmer and a greater force is required to cause the same amount of indentation. Pressures between 8 and 21 mm Hg are considered within normal range.

The two most common types of tonometers are the hand-held tonometer and applanation tonometer (Figure 66-4). The portable hand-held instrument may be used in an office, clinic, emergency department, or operating room or at the bedside. It measures the amount of tension on the cornea. First the cornea is anesthetized with a topical anesthetic eyedrop. While the client sits and looks straight forward, the Tonopen is held perpendicular to the cornea and tapped several times directly on the cornea. A computer chip in the instrument averages the readings and notes the standard deviation.

An applanation tonometer, which may either be hand-held or attached to a slit-lamp microscope, measures the amount of force required to flatten the corneal apex by a standard amount. Anesthetic eyedrops are also used beforehand.

Intraocular pressure is noted in the client record with a large T. The top number indicates the pressure in the right eye; the bottom number indicates the pressure in the left eye.

FIGURE 66-3 A, The examiner uses the right hand to hold the ophthalmoscope to the right eye to examine the client's right eye. The examiner uses the left hand and left eye when examining the client's left eye. Note the positioning of the examiner's free hand, which is placed to steady the client's head and to slightly retract the eyebrow. **B,** The examiner sees what appears in the angle of light through the viewing aperture. **C,** The actual area of retina visualized depends on the dilation of the pupil. Note the structures that may be examined.

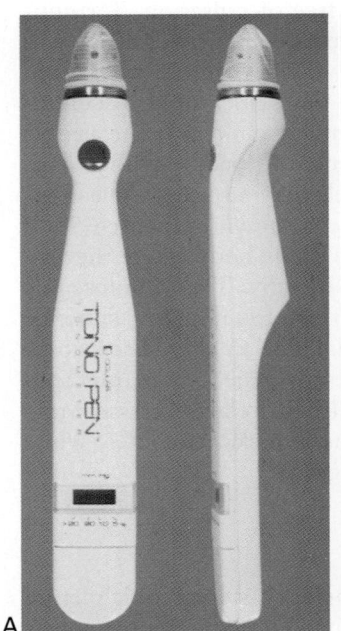 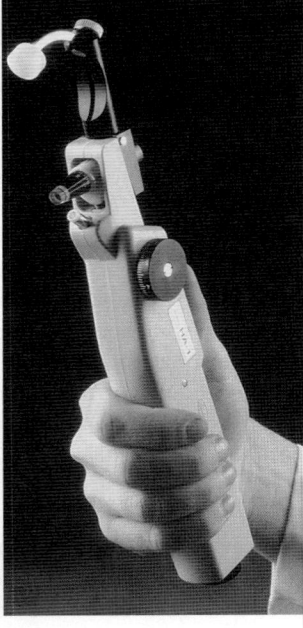

FIGURE 66-4 A, Tonometer seen from two viewpoints. **B,** Hand-held applanation tonometer. (**A** Courtesy of Ophthalmic Photography at the University of Michigan W.K. Kellogg Eye Center, Ann Arbor; **B** Courtesy of Kowa Optimed, Torrance, CA.)

Slit-Lamp Examination

The slit-lamp microscope is used to illuminate and examine the anterior segment of the eye under magnification. A linear slit beam of incandescent light is projected onto the globe, illuminating an optical cross-section of the anterior chamber. The angle of illumination, length, width, and intensity of the light can be adjusted. The client sits, and the head is stabilized by an adjustable chin rest and forehead strap. Details of the lid margins, lashes, conjunctiva, tear film, cornea, iris, lens, and aqueous humor can be studied. At the highest magnification setting, the abnormal presence of red or white blood cells in the aqueous humor can be visualized. The presence of protein *(flare),* an anterior chamber reaction that accompanies intraocular inflammation, may also be detected. Normal aqueous humor is optically clear, without cells or flare. The presence of cells and flare is documented as 1 to 4+.

Fluorescein dye is often used in a slit-lamp examination to highlight corneal irregularities. Sterile paper strips containing fluorescein dye are wetted and touched against the inner surface of the lower lid, instilling the yellow dye into the tear film and onto the corneal surface. A blue filter is attached to the light beam, causing the dye to fluoresce. The dye highlights defects in the cornea.

In addition to the applanation tonometer, several other devices may be attached to the slit lamp to expand the scope of the examination. A gonioscope provides visualization of the anterior chamber angle. The Hruby lens permits examination of the vitreous body and fundus. A pachymeter is used to measure the thickness of the cornea and the anterior chamber.

DIAGNOSTIC TESTS

Fundus Photography

Special retinal cameras are used to document fine details of the fundus for study and future comparison. One of the most common applications is the evaluation of insidious optic nerve changes in clients with glaucoma. Photographs are compared over time to identify subtle changes in disc shape and color (Figure 66-5).

Exophthalmometry

The exophthalmometer is designed to measure the forward protrusion of the eye. This instrument provides a method of evaluating and recording the progression and regression of the prominence of the eye in disorders such as thyroid disease and tumors of the orbit.

Ophthalmic Radiography

X-ray study, tomography, and computed tomography (CT) are useful in the evaluation of orbital and intracranial conditions. Common abnormalities evaluated by these methods include neoplasms, inflammatory masses,

fractures, and extraocular muscle enlargement associated with Graves' disease. Radiography is also useful in the detection of foreign bodies. See also Chapter 4.

Magnetic Resonance Imaging

Magnetic resonance imaging (MRI) allows obtaining multidimensional views without repositioning the client (Figure 66-6). MRI is used to image edema, areas of demyelination, and vascular lesions. The availability of MRI equipment is often limited, however, and the examination is lengthy.

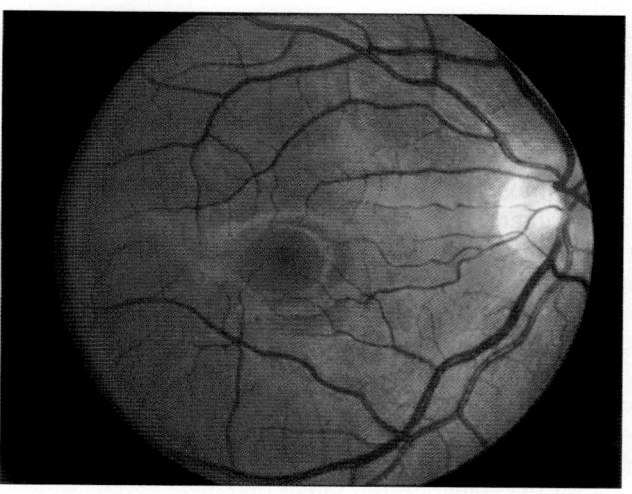

FIGURE 66-5 A normal fundus. (Courtesy of Ophthalmic Photography at the University of Michigan W.K. Kellogg Eye Center, Ann Arbor.)

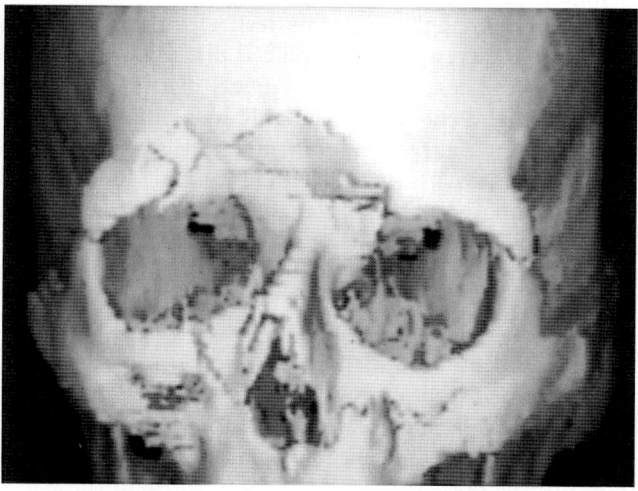

FIGURE 66-6 A magnetic resonance imaging (MRI) scan showing massive facial fractures. Note the three-dimensional appearance obtained with MRI.

Ultrasonography

Ultrasonography uses high-frequency sound waves transmitted through a probe placed directly on the eyeball. As the sound waves bounce back off the various tissue components, they are collected by a receiver and amplified on an oscilloscope screen. Sound waves derived from the most distal structures arrive last, having traveled the farthest. *A-scan* ultrasonography is used to measure axial length, the distance from the cornea to the retina, to determine the refractive power of an intraocular lens in cataract surgery. *B-scan* ultrasonography is used to evaluate the characteristics of a lesion as well as its size and growth over time or the presence of a foreign body.

Ophthalmodynamometry

Ophthalmodynamometry is a test that consists of exerting pressure on the sclera with a spring plunger while the central retinal vessels emerging from the disc through an ophthalmoscope are observed. This instrument gives an approximate measurement of the relative pressures in the central retinal arteries and indirectly assesses carotid arterial flow on either side. Ophthalmodynamometry is indicated in the neurologic evaluation of clients who complain of "blacking out" of vision in one eye *(amaurosis)*, spells of weakness on one side of the body, or other manifestations of cerebral ischemia. A difference of more than 20% in the diastolic pressures between the two eyes suggests insufficiency of the carotid arterial system on the side with the lower pressure.

Electroretinography

An electrical potential exists between the cornea and retina of the eye. Because the retina is neurologic tissue, the retina exhibits certain electrical responses when stimulated by light. Electroretinography (ERG) measures the change in the electrical potential of the eye caused by a diffuse flash of light. For this test, electrodes incorporated into a contact lens are placed directly on the anesthetized eye. Because eye movements disrupt the values of the test, the client must be able to fixate on a target while keeping the eyes still. Normal ERG findings signify functional integrity of the retina. Retinal diseases that can be evaluated with ERG include retinitis pigmentosa (progressive degeneration of photoreceptor cells), massive ischemia, disseminated infection, or toxic effects from drugs or chemicals.

Visual Evoked Response

Visual evoked response (VER) is similar to ERG in that it also measures the electrical potential resulting from a visual stimulus. The entire visual pathway from the retina to the cortex can be evaluated through the placement of electrodes on the scalp. Reduced speed of neuronal conduction, as with demyelination in optic neuri-

tis, results in an abnormal response. Retinal or optic nerve disease can be diagnosed by stimulation of each eye separately.

Fluorescein Angiography

Fundus photography is enhanced by the use of fluorescein dye, whose molecules emit green light when stimulated by blue light. The client sits in front of a retina camera after the pupils are dilated. A small amount of fluorescein dye is injected into an antecubital vein. The dye circulates throughout the body before eventual excretion by the kidneys. As the dye passes through the retinal and choroidal circulation, it can be visualized and photographed because of its ability to fluoresce (Figure 66-7). A rapid sequence of pictures captures the initial rapid perfusion of the retinal and choroidal vessels. Later photos may demonstrate the gradual leakage of dye from abnormal vessels. Changes in blood flow, ischemia, and hemorrhage may be detected. Because it can so precisely delineate areas of abnormality, it is an essential guide for planning laser treatment of retinal vascular disease.

You may administer the intravenous (IV) fluorescein dye injection under an ophthalmologist's direction. First assess the client's general health status and identify any allergies. Allergic reactions to other dye injections, such as for an IV pyelogram (IVP) or cholangiogram, should be considered before the fluorescein injection. Diphenhydramine may be prescribed prophylactically. Although anaphylactic shock is a rare occurrence, emergency

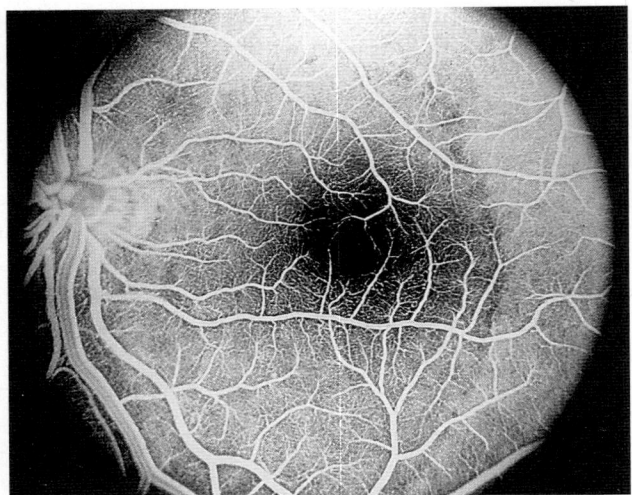

FIGURE 66-7 A normal fluorescein angiogram. The normal pattern of fluorescein angiography can be divided into three phases: (1) The *filling phase* (pictured) takes 8 to 20 seconds. (2) The *recirculation phase* starts 0.5 second after the filling phase and lasts 3 to 5 minutes. (3) The *late phase* lasts 30 to 60 minutes. Photographs are taken before injection, at half-second intervals for 20 seconds, and then at intervals of 5 minutes.

equipment should be located nearby. Occasionally, a client's vasovagal response to the dye may include vertigo, nausea, and momentary loss of consciousness. Obtain consent for the procedure. Explain that during the injection the client may experience a warm sensation. The client will also hear the mechanics of the camera taking rapid-sequence photographs and experience bright flashes of light.

After the examination, encourage the client to increase intake of fluids because the dye is excreted through the kidneys. During the next 24 hours, the urine will be yellowish, and light-complexioned clients may experience a temporary yellow tint to the skin that will fade within a few hours as the dye is excreted. Because the pupils are dilated before the examination, it may be necessary to wear dark glasses for several hours until the pupils can constrict again in the presence of light.

ASSESSMENT OF THE EAR

The otologic history can be an important assessment tool and should be obtained before audiometric testing. Certain behavioral cues can indicate hearing impairment (Box 66-4). Collect significant data by conducting a thorough interview. Include the specific items in the otologic history (Box 66-5).

HISTORY

An otologic history includes demographic data, current clinical manifestations, past health history, family health history, psychosocial history, and review of systems. Ear problems often result from childhood illnesses or abnor-

malities associated with adjacent structures. The history interview is essential for determining current problems related to the ear.

Biographical and Demographic Data

Demographic data relevant to otologic assessment include the client's age. Hearing impairment may occur as a consequence of the aging process (Table 66-1).

Current Health

Chief Complaint

The most common chief complaints include the following:

- Hearing loss
- Pain
- Tinnitus
- Ear drainage
- Loss of balance
- Vertigo
- Dizziness

The client may also complain of associated nausea or vomiting. Complete a symptom analysis to determine the onset, duration, frequency, and precipitating and relieving factors. Explore the client's past health history to determine the chronicity of the problem and the probable cause (see Box 66-5).

Symptom Analysis

Hearing loss may occur suddenly or gradually and can accompany the normal aging processes. The loss may be conductive, sensorineural, or related to a CNS disorder. The client may report an inability to hear certain words or sounds or that sounds are muffled.

Pain may be perceived as a feeling of fullness in the ear. It may be intensified by movement and relieved by holding the head still or by applying heat. Ear pain may occur as a result of related problems of the nose, sinuses, oral cavity, pharynx, or temporomandibular joint (TMJ).

Ear drainage can be bloody (sanguineous), clear (serous), mixed (serosanguineous), or may contain pus (purulent). Drainage may also be accompanied by an odor.

Tinnitus (ringing in the ears) may be reported as high-pitched or low-pitched, roaring, humming, hissing, or loud and persistent. Tinnitus may occur more commonly at certain times of the day and may involve one or both ears.

Loss of balance may be accompanied by vertigo or dizziness. *Vertigo* is a sensation of motion while the person is not moving. A client may feel that either he or she or the room is moving. *Dizziness* is a sensation of unsteadiness and a feeling of movement within the head or lightheadedness.

BOX 66-4	*Clues Suggesting Hearing Impairment*

Any adult who exhibits one or more of the following traits may be experiencing hearing impairment:

- Is irritable, hostile, hypersensitive in intercliental relations
- Has difficulty hearing upper frequency consonants (SI, Sh)
- Complains about people mumbling
- Turns up volume on television
- Asks for frequent repetition and answers questions inappropriately
- Loses sense of humor, becomes grim
- Leans forward to hear better or turns head to preferred side
- Shuns large-group and small-group audience situations
- Shuns areas with increased background noise
- Might appear aloof and "stuck up"
- Complains of ringing in the ears
- Has an unusually soft or loud voice

BOX 66-5 *Otologic History Assessment Guide*

Current Problem

What changes are you having in your hearing?

Do you have any of the following manifestations?

Distortion of hearing	Yes	No
Differences in the pitch of sound	Yes	No
Noise in your ear	Yes	No
Fullness or pressure in your ear	Yes	No
Pain in your ear	Yes	No
Drainage from your ear	Yes	No

Have you ever had a hearing examination?
  If yes, why?
  What were the results?

Use of Hearing Aids

Are you wearing hearing aids now?	Yes	No
Are your hearing aids effective?	Yes	No
How old are your hearing aids?	L __ yr R __ yr	

Associated Problems

Do you have any of the following manifestations?

Head noise or ringing	Yes	No
Feeling dizzy or unsteady	Yes	No
Blurred vision	Yes	No
Double vision	Yes	No
Numbness in the hands or feet	Yes	No
Weakness in the arms or legs	Yes	No
Tingling around the mouth or face	Yes	No
Loss of consciousness or blackouts	Yes	No
Fainting	Yes	No
Convulsions or seizures	Yes	No

Risk Factors

Have you ever worked around loud noises?	Yes	No
How long? _____ yr		
Do you still work around loud noise?	Yes	No
Do you wear ear protection?	Yes	No

Past Health History

Did you have hearing problems as a child?	Yes	No
Did you have frequent ear infections as a child?	Yes	No
Did you ever have a perforation in your eardrum?	Yes	No
Did you ever get hit in the ear?	Yes	No
Have you had ear surgery?	Yes	No

  If yes,

	Date	Operation	Surgeon
Right ear	_____	_____	_____
Left ear	_____	_____	_____

Do you have any food or medication allergies?
  Please list and describe your reaction.

Family History

Do you have family members who were hard of hearing before 50 years of age?
  If yes, explain.

Have any members of your family ever had ear surgery?
  If yes, explain.

TABLE 66-1 *Changes in Auditory Acuity Caused by Aging*

Anatomic Changes	Physiologic Changes
Degeneration of basilar conductive membrane of cochlea	Decreased ability to hear at all frequencies but greater at higher frequencies
Degeneration of cochlear hair cells	Decreased ability to hear high-frequency sounds
Decreased vascularity of cochlea	Loss of hearing equal at all frequencies
Loss of auditory neurons in spiral ganglia of organ of Corti	Loss of ability to hear high-frequency sounds
Loss of cortical auditory neurons	Diminished hearing and speech comprehension

Past Health History

Childhood and Infectious Diseases

Common childhood diseases involving the ears include the following:

- Acute middle ear infections (otitis media)
- Eardrum perforations resulting from otitis media
- Complications of ear infections such as chronic otitis media, frequent upper respiratory tract infection, and acute and chronic sinus infections

Infectious diseases with ear sequelae include mumps, measles, and meningitis. Specifically inquire whether the client has been immunized for mumps, measles, and *Haemophilus influenzae* type b (Hib). A pneumococcal conjugate vaccine shows good promise in preventing initial ear infections and reducing subsequent episodes of acute otitis media in infants and children.[2] In utero exposure to maternal influenza or rubella may result in congenital hearing loss in the child. Premature birth is also associated with hearing problems.

Major Illnesses and Hospitalizations

Inquire about a history of upper respiratory tract infections. Has the client had a tonsillectomy or adenoidectomy? Does the history include ear surgery? Has the client had trauma to the head or ear, such as a severe blow or sustained loud noise exposure or concussion from sudden changes in air pressure (such as may occur in an explosion)? Does the history include chronic eardrum perforation?

Medications

Certain medications can damage the vestibulocochlear nerve (eighth cranial nerve), with resultant hearing loss, tinnitus, or disturbances in equilibrium. Aspirin is a common cause of tinnitus. Other drugs include aminoglycosides, analgesics, salicylates, quinine, chemotherapeutic agents, and antiprotozoal agents (Box 66-6). Obtain a complete medication history for prescription and over-the-counter drugs and herbal remedies.

Review the use of herbal remedies. Ginger *(Zingiber officinale)* is known for its anti-nausea effect and can be used for the relief of motion sickness. Ginkgo biloba *(Ginkgo biloba)* has been used for tinnitus and vertigo.

One popular alternative health treatment used to remove cerumen or ear wax from the ear canals is ear candles. One end of a hollow candle is inserted into the canal and the opposite end is lit with the intent of creating negative pressure in the ear and drawing out the cerumen. Ear candles have not demonstrated any efficacy in removing cerumen from ear canals. Use of ear candles have resulted in a number of complications and injuries, including burns to the auricle and ear canal, occlusion of the ear canal from candle wax, and tympanic membrane perforation. Ask clients about use of ear candles to remove cerumen, and instruct them regarding potential dangers of this alternative treatment.

Allergies

In addition to asking about allergies to medications and other substances, inquire about allergies resulting in nasal stuffiness and congestion. Close proximity of the eustachian tubes to the nasal mucosa may result in edema, which obstructs the flow of air between the middle ear and nose so that air pressure cannot be equalized.

Family Health History

Ask about a history of hearing loss or ear surgery among family members. Determine the age at onset for hearing loss or changes in hearing acuity.

BOX 66-6 *Selected Ototoxic* Drugs*

Aminoglycoside Antibiotics
Streptomycin
Neomycin
Gentamicin
Tobramycin
Amikacin
Kanamycin
Netilmicin

Other Antibiotics
Vancomycin
Viomycin
Polymyxin B
Polymyxin E
Erythromycin
Capreomycin
Chloramphenicol
Minocycline

Other Drugs
Chemotherapeutic agents (bleomycin, cisplatin, nitrogen mustard)
Salicylates
Quinine drugs
Quinidine
Chloroquine

Diuretics
Furosemide
Ethacrynic acid
Acetazolamide
Bumetanide
Mannitol

Chemicals
Metals (lead, mercury, gold, arsenic)
Alcohol
Aniline dyes
Caffeine
Carbon monoxide
Nicotine
Potassium bromate
Povidone-iodine

*Substances toxic to the ear.

Psychosocial History

Psychosocial and lifestyle factors that influence the incidence of hearing impairment include occupational hazards, environmental exposure, and leisure activities and hobbies. Ask about exposure to loud noises (Table 66-2), including the type, frequency, and duration. Is

TABLE 66-2	*Decibel (dB) Ratings and Hazardous Time Exposure of Common Noises*	
Typical Level* (dB)	**Example**	**Dangerous Time Exposure**
0	Lowest sound audible to human ear	
30	Quiet library, soft whisper	
40	Quiet office, living room, bedroom away from traffic	
50	Light traffic at a distance, refrigerator, gentle breeze	
60	Air conditioner at 20 ft, conversation, sewing machine	
70	Busy traffic, noisy restaurant (constant exposure)	Critical level begins
80	Subway, heavy city traffic, alarm clock at 2 ft, factory noise	More than 8 hr
90	Truck traffic, noisy home appliances, shop tools, lawnmower	Less than 8 hr
100	Chain saw, boiler shop, pneumatic drill	2 hr
120	Rock concert in front of speakers, sandblasting, thunderclap	Immediate danger
140	Gunshot blast, jet plane	Any length of exposure time is dangerous
180	Rocket launching pad	Hearing loss is inevitable

Courtesy of American Academy of Otolaryngology—Head and Neck Surgery, Washington, DC.
*Sound levels refer to intensity experienced at typical working distances. Intensity drops 6 dB with every doubling of distance from noise source.

protective ear gear worn? Sound intensity is measured in units known as *decibels (dB)*. Ordinary speech level measures about 50 dB; heavy traffic is about 70 dB; at above 80 dB noise becomes uncomfortable to the human ear. Exposure to levels greater than 85 to 90 dB for months or years causes cochlear damage.

Does the client swim, especially in water that might be contaminated? Has the client had problems with "swimmer's ear"? Does the client use earplugs to prevent water from entering the ear canal? Contaminated water can provoke an external ear infection and, if the tympanic membrane is perforated, may lead to infection in the middle ear.

Explore the client's ear hygiene habits. Does the client put objects into the ear, such as pencils, hairpins, or cotton-tipped applicators? Inserting such objects can traumatize the ear canal and damage or perforate the tympanic membrane.

Review of Systems

The review of systems related to the ear includes asking about problems with the nose, sinuses, mouth, pharynx, and throat. Has the client experienced head trauma, loss of balance, dizziness, or vertigo. Detailed questions for the review of systems are found in Chapter 4 and on the website for this textbook.

PHYSICAL EXAMINATION

Physical examination of the ear includes assessment of hearing acuity, balance, and equilibrium. Because the external ear is completely visible, it is easy to identify anatomic landmarks and to assess abnormalities. The eardrum reveals important information regarding the middle ear. Because much of the middle ear and inner ear is inaccessible to direct examination, however, you must make inferences indirectly by testing auditory and vestibular function. See the Physical Assessment Findings in the Healthy Adult feature on The Ear at left.

Inspection and Palpation

External Ear

Gross examination of both ears should precede individual examination of either ear. Use inspection and palpation to assess the external ear. Note the size, configuration, and angle of attachment to the head. Observe the configuration of the pinna for gross deformity. Note whether the ears protrude and if so the degree of protrusion, the color of the skin of the ears, and whether

---

PHYSICAL ASSESSMENT FINDINGS IN THE HEALTHY ADULT

The Ear

Inspection
Auricles symmetrical, superior portion level with outer canthus of eye. Outer canals clear. Preauricular and postauricular areas without swelling, masses, or lesions. AC > BC, bilaterally. No lateralization. Whisper heard at 3 feet.

Palpation
Tenderness over tragus and mastoid absent. No masses.

Otoscopic Examination
Soft cerumen present in canals. No discharge. TMs intact, gray. Cone of light at 4:00 in right ear and at 7:00 in left ear. Landmarks visualized. No retraction or bulging. TM freely movable with pneumatic pressure.

AC, Air conduction; *BC,* bone conduction; *TM,* tympanic membrane.

additional skin tags are present. The skin of the ear should be smooth and without breaks or inflammation, especially in the crevice behind the ear. Note any lumps, skin lesions, or cysts, and record approximate size and location.

Perform palpation and manipulation of the pinna to detect tenderness, nodules, or *tophi* (small, hard nodules in the helix that are deposits of uric acid crystals characteristic of gout). During palpation, move the pinna, feel the mastoid area, and press on the tragus, noting any pain or discomfort, which may indicate inflammation or infection (see the Physical Assessment Findings in the Healthy Adult feature on The Ear on p. 1934).

Ear Canal

Direct Observation. Inspection of the ear canal is carried out by direct observation, otoscopy, or microscopic examination. For direct observation, ask the adult to tip his or her head slightly to the opposite side while you pull the pinna up, back, and out. Use a penlight to inspect the ear canal for any abnormalities such as extreme narrowing, excessive wax, redness, scaliness, swelling, drainage, cysts, or foreign objects. None of these manifestations should be present. Visualization of the eardrum with this method would be unlikely.

Otoscopy. The eardrum is located at the end of the only skin-lined canal in the body. Proper visualization requires illumination and magnification for accurate assessment. An otoscope is portable, and otoscopic examination is the most commonly used method. An otoscope is a device (Figure 66-8) that consists of a handle, a light source, a magnifying lens, and an attachment for visualizing the ear canal and eardrum. A pneumatic device at-

tached to the otoscope is used for injecting air into the ear canal to test the mobility and integrity of the eardrum.

Specula for the otoscope come in various sizes. Because the diameter of the meatus and the length of the ear canal vary, select the speculum with the largest diameter that fits comfortably into the ear canal. Check the light source for brightness. If the light appears yellowish or dim (like a flashlight with weak batteries), recharge or replace the batteries.

Hold the otoscope with the dominant hand, positioning it so that your hand rests against the client's head (Figure 66-9). If the client moves suddenly, the otoscope will also move, thereby reducing the likelihood of damaging the external canal during examination. With your nondominant hand, pull the pinna up, back, and out (in the adult), thus straightening the ear canal (Figure 66-9, A). While this is done, gently tilt the client's head away from you and insert the speculum slowly and carefully

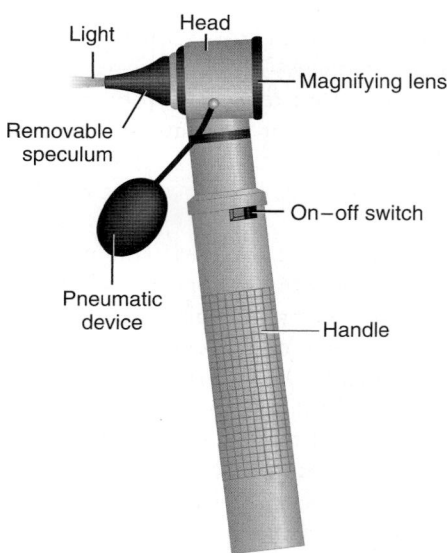

FIGURE 66-8 An otoscope.

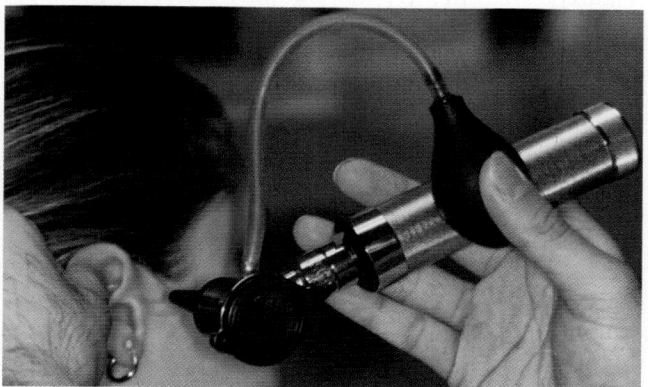

A

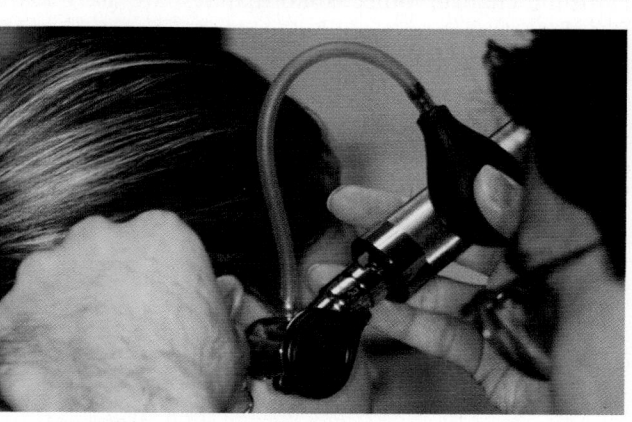

B

FIGURE 66-9 Use of the otoscope. **A,** Hold the otoscope handle between the thumb and fingers. Pull the pinna backward and upward in the adult to straighten the auditory canal. **B,** Carefully insert the speculum into the ear canal while allowing the back of the fingers that hold the otoscope handle to rest against the client's head. If a pneumatic bulb attachment will be used, position the bulb between thumb and otoscope handle to facilitate compression of the pneumatic bulb.

into the ear canal. Bring your eye close to the magnifying lens to visualize the ear canal and eardrum. When a pneumatic bulb is present, advance the otoscope far enough to make a secure seal (Figure 66-9, *B*).

Observe the ear canal while the speculum is entering and leaving. Move the otoscope in a circular fashion to visualize the entire ear canal. Note abnormalities such as extreme narrowing of the ear canal, nodules, redness, scaliness, swelling, drainage, cysts, foreign objects, and excessive wax. Most of these abnormalities will impair visualization of the eardrum. Sometimes the ear canal must be cleaned of wax, dead skin, and other debris. Wax and debris can be removed with a cerumen spoon (wax curet), suction aspirator, or irrigation.

Cerumen should not interfere with the examination when the amount is small. Cerumen is normally present in the external ear and varies in color from light yellow to black. Cerumen that is impacted in the ear canal is a common cause of hearing loss, especially in older people; therefore assess the amount of cerumen present.

Distinguishing landmarks of the normal eardrum (Figure 66-10) are (1) the *annulus,* the fibrous border that attaches the eardrum to the temporal bone; (2) the short process of the malleus, which protrudes into the eardrum superiorly; (3) the long process of the malleus *(manubrium);* (4) the umbo of the malleus, at the point of maximal concavity, which attaches to the center of the eardrum; (5) the *pars flaccida,* a small triangular area above the short process of the malleus; and (6) the *pars tensa,* the remaining and largest portion of the eardrum.

The normal eardrum is slightly conical, translucent, shiny and smooth, and pearly gray. The position of the drumhead is oblique with respect to the ear canal. In the presence of disease, not only does the color of the eardrum change; other abnormalities are also manifested, such as retraction, bulging, or perforation of the eardrum and a white plaque *(tympanosclerosis)* on the eardrum.

Carefully inspect the entire eardrum, including the border *(annulus),* rotating the otoscope as needed. A cone of light reflex should be present on the eardrum in the lower anterior quadrant. The umbo and the long and short processes of the malleus should be easily visible through the eardrum.

Test the mobility of the eardrum by using the pneumatic device of the otoscope to inject a small puff of air into the ear canal. Observe the eardrum for normal movement (see the Physical Assessment Findings in the Healthy Adult feature on The Ear on p. 1934). An adequate seal is important to perform this maneuver accurately.

Tests for Auditory Acuity

Assessment of the middle and inner ear for hearing is accomplished by sophisticated methods of indirect testing (audiometry and vestibular testing). A gross assessment of hearing can be made simply through conversation, by evaluating the logical sequence of replies, and the appropriateness of the responses. Gross assessments can be made at the bedside or in the office.

Test each ear separately to estimate hearing ability. Begin by occluding one of the client's ears with a finger. Then, standing a foot away, whisper two-syllable numbers softly toward the unoccluded ear and ask the client to repeat the numbers. Increase the intensity of your voice from a soft, medium, or loud whisper to a soft, medium, or loud voice. If you suspect that the client is lip-reading, turn the client's face to one side. Ask the client whether hearing is better in one ear than in the other ear. If auditory acuity between the two ears is different, test the ear that hears better first. Next produce noise in the better-hearing ear by rapidly but gently moving the finger in the client's ear canal while the other ear is tested.

Although the ticking of a watch can also be used to test hearing, it produces a higher-pitched sound, which is less relevant to functional hearing compared with the voice test.

The tuning fork also provides a general estimate of hearing loss. A frequency of 512 Hz is recommended. The two major tuning fork tests date from the 19th century and are named after their originators: Weber and Rinne.

Weber Test

The Weber test is used to assess conduction of sound through bone. Set the tuning fork into vibration by striking the tines on your hand. Place the rounded tip of the handle on the center of the client's forehead or nasal bone (Figure 66-11, *A*). Placement on the teeth (even false teeth) is a reliable option. Does the client hear the tone in the center of the head, the right ear, or the left ear? Normally the sound is heard equally in both ears by bone conduction. If there is a sensorineural (nerve) hearing loss in one ear, the sound is heard in the unaffected ear. With a conductive (air conduction) hearing loss, the sound is heard better in the affected ear.

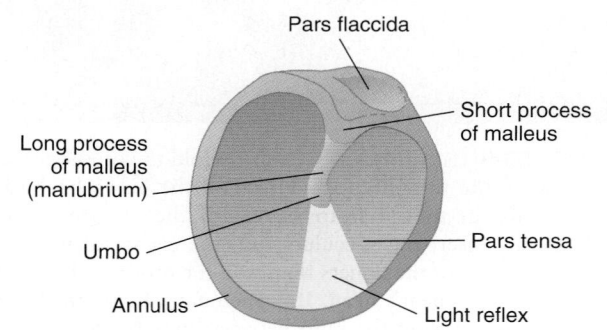

FIGURE 66-10 Normal right eardrum (tympanic membrane).

Pars flaccida

Short process of malleus

Long process of malleus (manubrium)

Umbo

Annulus

Pars tensa

Light reflex

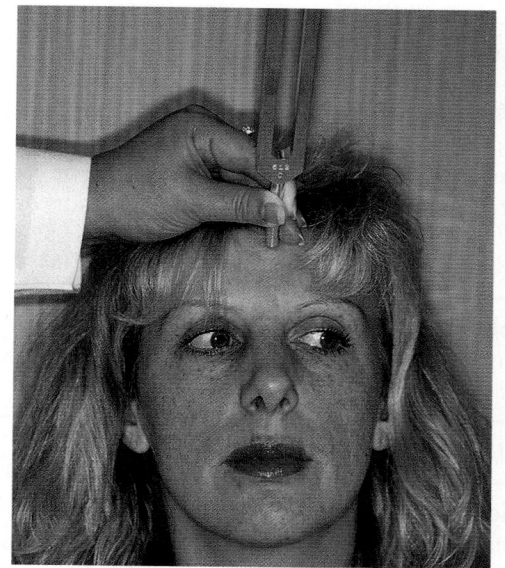

A

FIGURE 66-11 Weber and Rinne tests for hearing impairment. The Weber test detects lateralization of hearing; the Rinne test distinguishes conductive hearing loss from sensorineural hearing loss. Perform the two tests consecutively. **A,** For the Weber test, place a vibrating tuning fork on the client's head to produce a centrally located stimulus. The client should hear the sound equally in both ears. The tone is louder in an ear with unilateral conductive loss and quieter in an ear with unilateral sensorineural loss. **B,** Perform the Rinne test to characterize the unilateral hearing loss as either conductive or sensorineural. Hold a vibrating tuning fork on the mastoid bone. **C,** When the client no longer hears the sound, place the tuning fork about 2 inches from the external ear. When the tone is louder through air than through bone, the positive Rinne test finding indicates either normal hearing or a sensorineural hearing loss. A negative Rinne test finding, or louder bone conduction than air conduction, indicates a conductive loss.

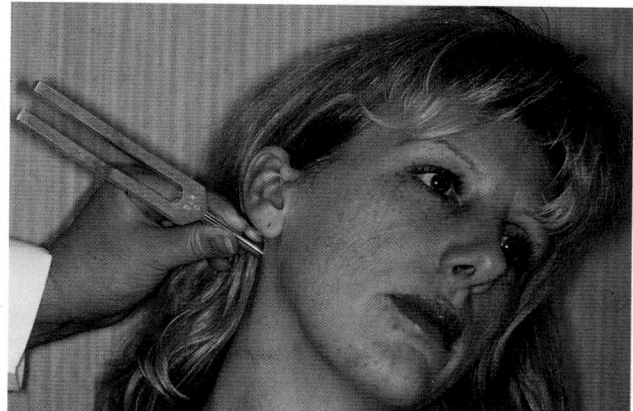

B

from the opening of the ear canal for air conduction (Figure 66-11, *C*). Move the tuning fork when the client no longer hears the sound by bone conduction, and ask the client to indicate whether the tone is louder in front of or behind the ear. Ask the client to state when the tone is no longer heard by air conduction.

Normally sound is heard twice as long or as loud by air conduction than it is by bone conduction. Results are as follows:

- In *normal* hearing, air conduction is greater than bone conduction (a positive Rinne test finding).
- With a *conductive* hearing loss, bone conduction sounds louder or longer than air conduction sounds (a negative Rinne test finding).
- With a *sensorineural* hearing loss, the client hears better by air conduction (a positive Rinne test finding).

Conductive hearing loss results when the pathways of normal sound conduction are blocked. Because vibrations against the mastoid bone can bypass the obstruction, bone conduction lasts longer or sounds louder than air conduction. In *sensorineural* hearing loss, the acoustic nerve is less able to perceive vibrations from either bone or air; therefore normal patterns are reported by the client.

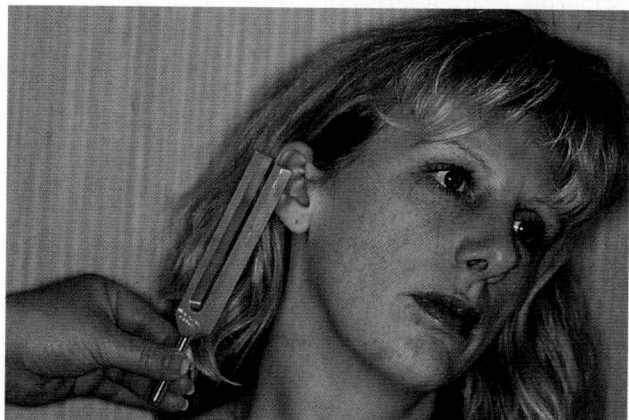

C

Tests for Vestibular Acuity

Romberg Test

Assess the inner ear for balance by performing a Romberg test. The client stands with the feet together, arms by the sides, and eyes closed. Note the ability to maintain an upright posture with only a minimal amount of sway. Stand close to the client to offer balance support if it is needed. If the client loses his or her balance, this is a positive Romberg sign, suggesting a vestibular ear problem or cerebellar ataxia.

Rinne Test

The Rinne test compares air conduction to bone conduction and helps to differentiate conductive from sensorineural hearing loss. Shift the vibrating tuning fork between two positions: first against the mastoid bone for bone conduction (Figure 66-11, *B*) and then 2 inches

A *tandem* Romberg test should also be performed. Instruct the client to walk forward and backward, heel to toe. A peripheral vestibular lesion can cause marked swaying or falling. A client without pathologic vestibular change can usually maintain balance, depending on his or her age.

A *past-pointing test* can also indicate a labyrinthine disorder. While the client is seated, facing you with eyes open, hold out your index finger at the client's shoulder level. Instruct the client to touch your finger with the right index finger. Ask the client to lower the arm, close the eyes, and touch your finger again. Repeat the procedure, testing the client's left index finger. Observe and record the presence or absence as well as the degree and direction, of past-pointing. A labyrinthine disorder can lead to past-pointing when the eyes are closed. Cerebral lesions are indicated when past-pointing occurs whether the eyes are open or closed.

Test for Nystagmus

Nystagmus is involuntary, rhythmic oscillation of the eyes associated with vestibular dysfunction. Nystagmus occurs normally when a client watches a rapidly moving object or looks beyond 30 degrees laterally *(end-point nystagmus)*. To assess for *gaze nystagmus,* place your finger directly in front of the client at eye level. Ask the client to follow (track) the finger without moving the head. Starting at the midline, slowly move your finger toward the client's right ear and then the left ear, but not more than 30 degrees laterally, superiorly, or inferiorly. Observe the client's eyes for any jerking movements. For example, if the eyes jerk quickly to the left, and drift slowly back to the right, the client has left spontaneous *(horizontal)* nystagmus. Nystagmus is named for the direction of the fast phase. Nystagmus can be horizontal, vertical, or rotary.

DIAGNOSTIC TESTS

Tests for Aural Structure

The temporal bone and its structures can be examined easily by radiography (x-ray study). The oldest, but not necessarily most useful, study is x-ray examination of the mastoid bone. More recent radiographic techniques have largely been replaced by imaging studies (see Chapter 4 for more detailed discussion of the following imaging techniques and client preparation).

Computed Tomography

Computed tomography without contrast medium is the most commonly ordered CT scan for imaging of the temporal bone. Contrast is not generally needed because most bony structures are seen well. Contrast may be used to delineate vascular or soft tissue structures.

Magnetic Resonance Imaging

Magnetic resonance imaging reveals membranous organs as well as nerves and blood vessels of the temporal bone. MRI is the test of choice for tumors of the temporal bone. Contrast can be used for enhancement. For certain diagnostic assessments, both MRI and CT scans are obtained.

Arteriography

Arteriography is used to assess vascular abnormalities in the temporal bone.

Tests for Auditory Function

Audiometric Tests

Audiology may be broadly called the science of hearing. Audiometric tests are performed to measure hearing and comprehension. A hearing test is performed in a sound-proof booth by an *audiologist.* An *audiometer* is an electronic instrument used to test hearing by producing sounds of varying pure-tone frequencies between 250 and 8000 Hz and loudness. The unit of measure of hearing, the decibel (dB), is a logarithmic function of sound intensity. The average normal adult has a hearing threshold of 0 to 20 dB hearing loss. The greater the threshold level, the poorer the hearing sensitivity. The client is asked to signal the audiologist by raising a hand or pressing a button when a tone is heard; the responses are plotted on a graph called an *audiogram* (Figure 66-12). Earphones are used for the audiogram.

Normal hearing is a range established nationally by testing the hearing levels of people of all ages. A client with normal hearing ability has 80% or more hearing, depending on his or her age.

Some audiometric tests are performed by computer-assisted instruments. The objective of these special tests is to reveal whether a disorder is in the cochlea, acoustic nerve, or brain stem.

Audiography. The components of hearing are tested through assessment of air conduction, bone conduction, and speech. Air conduction is assessed by presenting tones through the earphones. When the examiner varies the loudness and frequency of tones, a hearing level is established. Bone conduction is assessed by presenting tones through a bone conduction oscillator placed behind the ear on the mastoid bone. The bone conduction level is the level at which the cochlea can hear, bypassing the middle ear structures, and is referred to as the *nerve hearing level.* A difference between air and bone conduction signifies a conductive hearing loss. When air and bone conduction are the same, either normal hearing or a *sensorineural* (nerve) hearing loss exists. Speech evaluation includes (1) *speech reception threshold* (the level of

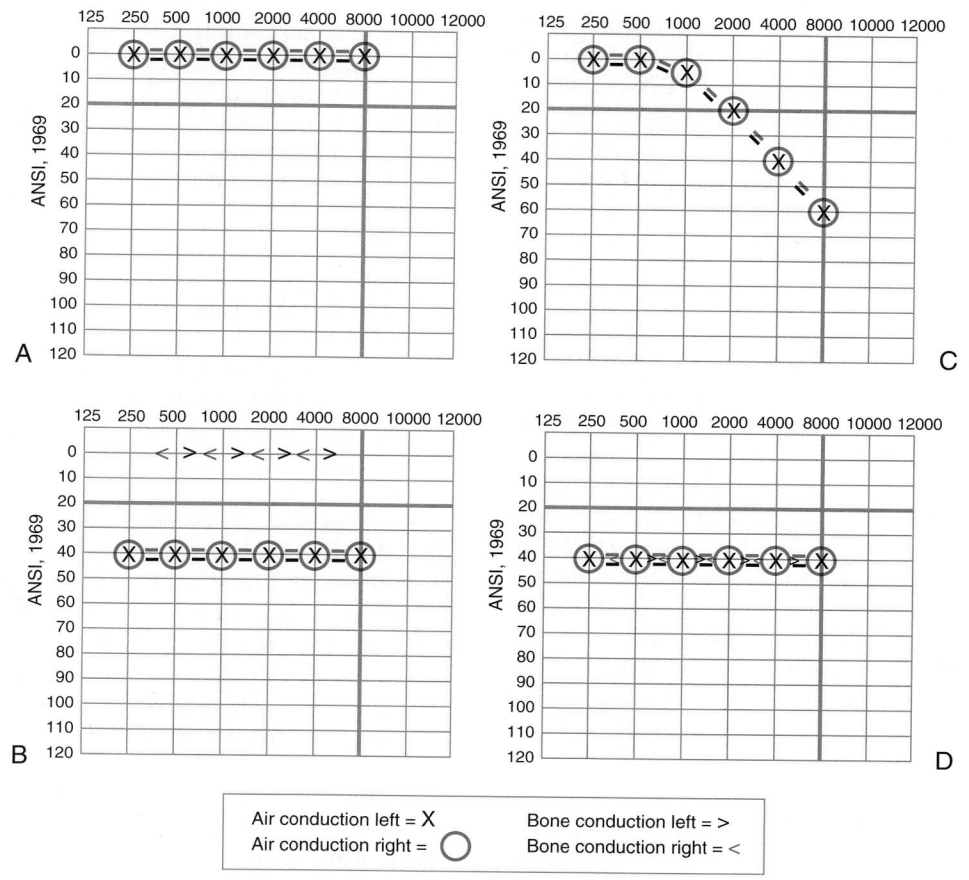

FIGURE 66-12 Audiograms showing types of hearing. **A,** Normal hearing. **B,** Conductive hearing loss. **C,** High-frequency hearing loss. **D,** Sensorineural hearing loss. (Courtesy of Arnold G. Schuring, M.D.)

speech hearing), which serves as a check on the reliability of the air conduction test, and *speech discrimination* (the ability to understand the spoken word).

Tympanometry. A popular test used for differentiating problems in the middle ear is tympanometry, or impedance audiometry. This test measures *compliance* (mobility) and *impedance* (opposition to movement) of the tympanic membrane and ossicles of the middle ear. The examiner applies positive, normal, and negative air pressure into the external meatus and measures the resultant sound energy flow, which is traced on a graph called a *tympanogram.* Abnormalities on the tympanogram reveal dysfunction of the middle ear, eustachian tube, and ossicles. Tympanometry can also be used to measure the stapedial muscle reflex and its decay. This test also indicates the function of the acoustic nerve.

Tests for Brain Stem Response. The auditory brain stem response test is currently one of the most popular approaches to the assessment of the auditory nervous system. By presenting a sound to the ear and measuring the

response (computer averaging) in the brain stem, the examiner can obtain specific diagnostic information. Imaging tests of the head are usually ordered to confirm the abnormality. Brain stem auditory evoked responses (BAERs) can be recorded from scalp electrodes. The early potentials reflect activity in the cochlea, eighth cranial nerve, and brain stem. Later evoked potentials reflect cortical activity. Early evoked responses are used to estimate the magnitude of the hearing loss and differentiate cochlea, eighth cranial nerve, and brain stem lesions.

Electrocochleography. *Electrocochleography* is designed to measure the response of the cochlea and the eighth cranial nerve to acoustic stimulation. Electrodes are placed through the tympanic membrane onto the promontory near the round window or in the ear canal, and an acoustic stimulation is applied. This test is used to evaluate the presence of Ménière's disease or perilymphatic fistula.

Otoacoustic Emissions. *Otoacoustic emissions* (OAEs) are low-level sounds produced by the cochlea that are involved in modulation of the hearing mechanism. OAEs can be recorded spontaneously or can be evoked through stimulation with short bursts of sound. Evoked OAEs can be observed in nearly all normal-hearing people and can therefore serve as a useful screen for hearing acuity, especially in infants. Because they can be measured quickly, they are generally easier to obtain than BAERs, especially in uncooperative and crying infants.

Vestibular Tests

Electronystagmography. The vestibular system can be tested by electrophysiologic means. Although the physical assessment of balance is important, the most common objective measurement of balance is accomplished by electronystagmography (ENG). The ENG instrument was developed to measure nystagmus (involuntary, rapid eye movement) in response to stimulation of the vestibular system. This stimulation includes testing the client at rest in different positions for both the eyes and the head and with different temperatures of air or water in the ear canals, thus stimulating the semicircular canals. The different test results give a recording (electronystagmogram) that reflects the status of each labyrinth and can indicate CNS disorders.

Platform Posturography. *Platform posturography* is another balance test that helps to identify, quantify, and localize the source of balance disorders. The client stands in a tall box-like device while the floor moves. No visual cues are provided, and the response to correcting balance is recorded. Most people correct posture changes with adjustments in muscles (of the feet and ankles). The client is strapped in for safety in case he or she loses balance. This test can help to isolate the etiologic basis of balance disorders as vestibular, visual, or proprioceptive.

Rotary Chair Assessment. Rotary chair or harmonic acceleration can also be used. Rotation of the client in a chair in darkness provides information about vestibular dysfunction and the level of central compensation.

Laboratory Tests

Blood Tests

Blood tests that are diagnostic for systemic abnormalities are only secondarily significant for ear disease. For example, an elevated white blood cell (WBC) count suggests an infection but is not diagnostic of ear disease. In the presence of clinical manifestations of ear infection, and in the absence of other manifestations of infection, however, an elevated WBC count does suggest acute ear infection. Other blood tests are useful for diagnosis of autoimmune diseases and other systemic illnesses that can affect hearing and balance.

Cultures

Drainage samples from the ear canal are sometimes obtained for culture to identify an infecting organism. This is rarely necessary in choosing an antibiotic for acute infections. When long-term drainage is present, such as in chronic otitis media, cultures are more helpful because multiple pathogenic organisms can be present.

Tests for the Presence of Cerebrospinal Fluid

Clear drainage found in the ear presents a dilemma. Is this cerebrospinal fluid (CSF) or serous drainage? A fistula from the inner ear to the middle ear can drain CSF. This pathway can also lead to meningitis by retrograde contamination. Therefore an analysis of clear fluid drainage from the ear or nose is often helpful in the diagnosis.

Tissue Specimens

Biopsy specimens of abnormal tissue from the ear canal or from other tissue harvested during surgery are necessary to rule out a malignancy and to identify unusual problems. In an infected ear, abnormal tissue is readily identified by visual assessment. If the surgeon is in doubt about the findings, a tissue sample is taken for pathologic examination.

CONCLUSIONS

Understanding the complexity of ocular structures and the physiology of vision is essential to providing comprehensive nursing care for clients with ocular disorders. Ophthalmic registered nurses perform the roles of educator, technician, counselor, and coordinator in the diagnostic setting.

Hearing and balance are vital to a person's safety and independence. Understanding the physiology of hearing and balance is essential to providing comprehensive nursing care for clients with ear disorders.

evolve   *Did you remember to check out the bonus material on the Evolve website and the CD-ROM, including free self-assessment exercises?*

http://evolve.elsevier.com/Black/medsurg/

BIBLIOGRAPHY

1. Eagle, R. (1999). *Eye pathology: An atlas and basic text.* Philadelphia: W.B. Saunders.

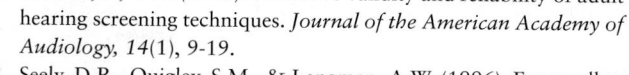 2. Eskola, J., et al. (2001). Efficacy of a pneumococcal conjugate vaccine against acute otitis media. *New England Journal of Medicine, 344*(6), 403-409.

3. Goldblum, K. (Ed.). (2002). *Ophthalmic nursing core curriculum.* Dubuque, IA: Kendall.

4. Harris, L.L., & Huntoon, M.B. (Eds.). (1998). *Core curriculum for otorhinolaryngology and head-neck nursing.* New Smyrna Beach, FL: Society of Otorhinolaryngology and Head-Neck Nurses.

5. Jarvis, C. (2000). *Physical examination and health assessment* (3rd ed.). Philadelphia: W.B. Saunders.

6. Kanski, J. (2003). *Clinical ophthalmology* (5th ed.). Oxford: Butterworth Heinemann.

7. Scudder, S., et al. (2003). Predictive validity and reliability of adult hearing screening techniques. *Journal of the American Academy of Audiology, 14*(1), 9-19.

8. Seely, D.R., Quigley, S.M., & Langman, A.W. (1996). Ear candles: Efficacy and safety. *Laryngoscope, 106,* 1226-1229.

9. Wilson, S., Giddens, J., & Thompson, J. (2001). *Health assessment for nursing practice* (2nd ed.). St. Louis: Mosby.

10. Vaughan, D., Asbury, T., & Riordan-Eva, P. (1999). *General ophthalmology* (15th ed.). Norwalk, CT: Appleton & Lange.

11. Woodson, G. (2001). *Ear, nose and throat disorders in primary care.* Philadelphia: W.B. Saunders.

Chapter 67

Management of Clients with Visual Disorders

Sarah C. Smith

evolve

Web Enhancements

Client Education Guide
Care After Cataract Removal (Spanish Translation)

http://evolve.elsevier.com/Black/medsurg/

Appendix C
Laboratory Values of Clinical Importance in Medical-Surgical Nursing

The role that vision plays in our lives is difficult to define because it is so deeply personal and intimate. It is the connection between the mind and the body and the rest of the world. The visual pathway is a multidimensional system with many structures and processes subject to trauma or disorders. When there is a failure of any part along the visual pathway, the result is loss of vision.

Loss of vision is closely associated with loss of independence. Even simple tasks become difficult to perform without assistance. Seeing what food is being served at the table; selecting clothes for color and design; avoiding objects while walking; and reading books, magazines, or personal mail are no longer possible. The visually impaired person must adapt to this loss to maintain control in the daily affairs of life.

The nursing diagnosis *Disturbed Sensory Perception* is commonly identified for clients with visual problems or impairment. Nursing interventions focus on providing a safe environment and education for self-care. The most important assessment you can make, however, is to address your client's grieving process. Visual impairment is more than a physiologic deficit. It is a loss that has physical, emotional, and spiritual effects on the person afflicted. Even minor changes in vision can provoke feelings of anger and frustration in people who must rely on clear and sharp vision in their work (e.g., airline pilots, artists, photographers, architects). Permanent and profound loss of vision can result in morbid grieving in which an individual is unable to cope with or adapt to life changes.

Surveys have shown that most people are more afraid of going blind than dying of cancer. Although we have made some improvements in the way our society views and provides for people who are physically challenged, blind people are frequently regarded with pity. Loss of vision is a threat to a person's independence, self-esteem, and self-control.

GLAUCOMA

Glaucoma comprises a group of ocular disorders characterized by increased intraocular pressure, optic nerve atrophy, and visual field loss. It is estimated that more than 80,000 people in the United States are blind as a result of glaucoma. The incidence of glaucoma is about 1.5%, and in blacks between ages 45 and 65 years, the prevalence is at least five times that of whites in the same age group. In most cases blindness can be prevented if treatment is begun early.

evolve *Be sure to check out the bonus material on the Evolve website and the CD-ROM, including free self-assessment exercises.*
http://evolve.elsevier.com/Black/medsurg/

Nursing Outcomes Classification (NOC)
for Nursing Diagnoses—Clients with Visual Disorders

Anticipatory Grieving
Coping
Grief Resolution
Psychosocial Adjustment: Life Change
Deficient Knowledge
Knowledge Deficit: Treatment
Procedure

Knowledge Deficit: Regimen
Disturbed Sensory Perception
Anxiety Control
Body Image
Vision Compensation Behavior

Ineffective Therapeutic Regimen Management
Compliance Behavior
Knowledge: Treatment Regimen
Participation: Health Care Regimen
Treatment Behavior: Illness or Injury

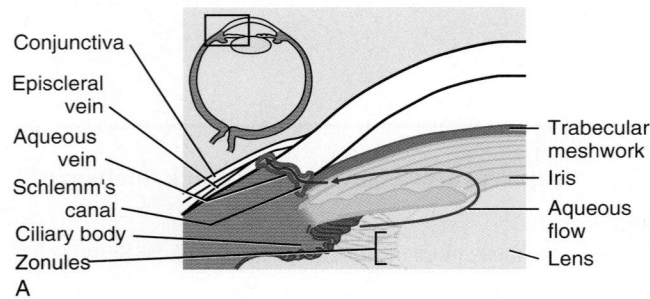

A

Conjunctiva
Episcleral vein
Aqueous vein
Schlemm's canal
Ciliary body
Zonules

Trabecular meshwork
Iris
Aqueous flow
Lens

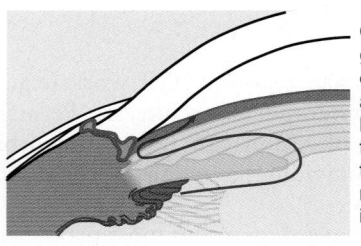

B

Open-angle glaucoma occurs when aqueous humor outflow through the trabecular meshwork is impaired

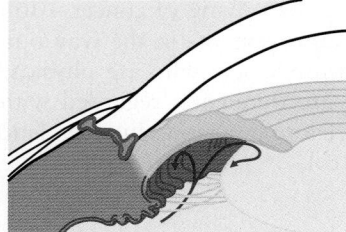

C

Angle-closure glaucoma occurs when the root of the iris occludes the trabecular meshwork

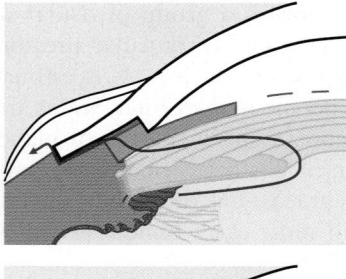

D

Filtering surgery, which provides bypass for aqueous

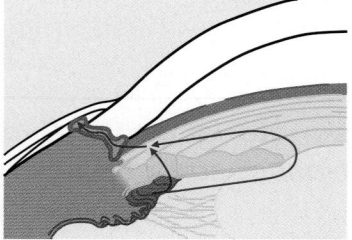

E

Iridectomy restores access of aqueous to the trabecular meshwork

Classification

Many terms are used to describe the various types of glaucoma:

- *Primary* and *secondary glaucoma* refer to whether the cause is the disease alone or another condition.
- *Acute* and *chronic* refer to the onset and duration of the disorder.
- *Open* (wide) and *closed* (narrow) describe the width of the angle between the cornea and the iris (Figure 67-1, *A*). Anatomically narrow anterior-chamber angles predispose people to an acute onset of *angle-closure glaucoma.*

Primary Open-Angle Glaucoma

Primary open-angle glaucoma, the most common form, is a multifactorial disorder that is often genetically determined, bilateral, insidious in onset, and slow to progress. This type of glaucoma is often referred to as the "thief in the night" because no early clinical manifestations are present to alert the client that vision is being lost. Aqueous humor flow is slowed or stopped because of obstruction by the trabecular meshwork (see Figure 67-1, *B*).

Angle-Closure Glaucoma

An acute attack of angle-closure glaucoma can develop only in an eye in which the anterior chamber angle is anatomically narrow. The attack occurs because of a sudden blockage of the anterior angle by the base of the iris (see Figure 67-1, *C*).

Other Forms of Glaucoma

Normal-tension glaucoma resembles primary open-angle glaucoma. In this type of glaucoma, the optic nerve is dam-

FIGURE 67-1 A, Normal flow of aqueous humor. **B,** Open-angle glaucoma occurs when aqueous humor outflow is impaired by the trabecular meshwork. **C,** Angle-closure glaucoma occurs when the root of the iris occludes the trabecular meshwork. Filtering surgery (**D**) and iridectomy (**E**) restore the flow of aqueous humor through the trabecular meshwork.

aged even though intraocular pressure (IOP) is not high. *Secondary glaucoma* may occur as a result of trauma that can disrupt the flow pattern of aqueous humor.

Etiology and Risk Factors

About 90% of primary glaucoma occurs in people with open angles. Because there are no early warning clinical manifestations, it is imperative that regular ophthalmic examinations include tonometry and assessment of the optic nerve head (disc). The most common cause of chronic open-angle glaucoma is degenerative change in the trabecular meshwork, resulting in decreased outflow of aqueous humor. Hypertension, cardiovascular disease, diabetes, and obesity are associated with the development of glaucoma. Increased IOP also results from *uveitis* (inflammation of filtering structures). Encroachment by a rapidly growing tumor and chronic use of topical corticosteroids may also produce manifestations of open-angle glaucoma. Neither the causes of *low-tension glaucoma* nor the reason optic nerves are damaged even though the IOP is "normal" (i.e., between 12 and 22 mm Hg) are not known. People at higher risk for this form of low-tension glaucoma are people with a family history of normal-tension glaucoma, people of Japanese ancestry, and people with a history of systemic heart disease, such as irregular heart rhythm.

Secondary glaucoma develops from edema, eye injury *(hyphema)*, inflammation, tumor, or in advanced cases of cataract or diabetes. Edematous tissue may inhibit the outflow of aqueous humor through the trabecular meshwork. Delayed healing of corneal wound edges may result in epithelial cell growth into the anterior chamber.

Pathophysiology

Intraocular pressure is determined by the rate of aqueous humor production in the ciliary body and the resistance to outflow of aqueous humor from the eye. IOP varies with diurnal cycles (the highest pressure is usually on awakening) and body position (increased when lying down). Normal variations do not usually exceed 2 to 3 mm Hg. IOP and blood pressure are independent of each other, but variations in systemic blood pressure may be associated with corresponding variations in IOP. Increased IOP may result from hyperproduction of aqueous humor or obstruction of outflow. As aqueous fluid builds up in the eye, the increased pressure inhibits blood supply to the optic nerve and the retina. These delicate tissues become ischemic and gradually lose function.

Clinical Manifestations

Acute angle-closure glaucoma causes severe pain and blurred vision or vision loss. Some clients see rainbow halos around lights, and some experience nausea and vomiting. Secondary glaucoma has the same clinical manifestations as acute angle-closure glaucoma. Visual field defects are the result of the loss of blood supply to areas in the retina. The individual response to IOP varies; some clients sustain damage from relatively low pressures, whereas others sustain no damage from high pressure.

An ophthalmoscopic examination shows *atrophy* (pale color) and *cupping* (indentation) of the optic nerve head. The visual field examination is used to determine the extent of peripheral vision loss (see visual fields in Chapter 66). In chronic open-angle glaucoma, a small crescent-shaped *scotoma* (blind spot) appears early in the disease. In acute angle-closure glaucoma, the fields demonstrate larger areas of significant loss of vision.

In clients with angle-closure glaucoma, a slit-lamp examination may demonstrate an erythematous conjunctiva and corneal cloudiness. The aqueous humor in the anterior chamber may also appear *turbid* (hazy), and the pupil may be nonreactive. Increased IOP (>23 mm Hg) indicates the need for further evaluation. Gonioscopy is performed to determine the depth of the anterior chamber angle and to examine the entire circumference of the angle for any abnormal changes in the filtering meshwork.

Outcome Management

The goal of management is to facilitate the outflow of aqueous humor through remaining channels and to maintain IOP within a range that prevents further damage to the optic nerve. If the IOP is very high, it must be reduced to retain vision. If vision is lost, the goals are to restore independence for the client.

■ Medical Management

Reduce Intraocular Pressure (Promote Aqueous Flow). Intraocular pressure can be reduced by increasing the outflow of aqueous fluids. In narrow-angle glaucoma the pupil is constricted using topical miotics or epinephrine, which opens the canal of Schlemm and promotes drainage of aqueous humor. Further, the production of aqueous humor can be reduced by using topical beta-blocker or alpha-adrenergic agents or oral carbonic anhydrase inhibitors. Figure 67-2 shows the sites of action for various drugs.

It is important to avoid mydriatic agents because they dilate the pupil by inhibiting the parasympathetic nervous system and blocking acetylcholine. Cycloplegic agents paralyze the ciliary muscle and the dilator muscle of the iris, causing both pupillary dilation and paralysis of accommodation. These dilating agents are contraindicated in narrow-angle glaucoma because further dilation of the pupil restricts outflow of aqueous humor.

In emergent situations, an oral osmotic diuretic (glycerin [Osmoglyn]) may be administered. Diabetic clients often receive a synthetic glycerin such as isosorbide (Ismotic) to reduce the effect on blood glucose levels. Intravenous (IV) mannitol, a potent osmotic diuretic, may be used to arrest extremely high IOP. It should be used

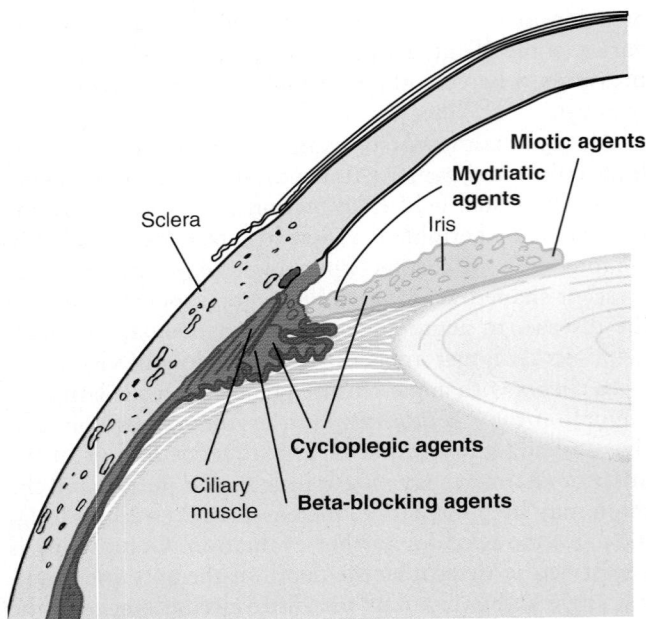

FIGURE 67-2 Sites of action of mydriatic, beta-blocking, cycloplegic, and miotic agents.

only for management of a glaucoma crisis under close nursing and medical supervision.

■ Nursing Management of the Medical Client
Assessment

Nursing assessment includes establishing demographic data of age and race because open-angle glaucoma occurs most often in clients over 40 years of age and in blacks. Determine whether there is a family history of glaucoma or other eye problems and whether the client has had ocular surgery, infections, or trauma. An accurate list of current medications is imperative because over-the-counter medications (such as antihistamines) may dilate the pupil, increasing the risk for angle-closure glaucoma. Always note a history of allergic reactions, particularly to medications or dyes.

Ask the client to describe any changes in vision. Although the manifestations of primary open-angle glaucoma are insidious, the client may describe blind spots in the periphery or an overall decreased visual acuity with loss of contrast sensitivity. Decreased, uncorrectable visual acuity usually occurs when there has been irreversible damage to the optic nerve.

If it has been previously established that the client has visual loss from glaucoma, assess how the client is coping with this loss. Although people adapt to the loss of vision in different ways, they usually manifest grief and loss at any stage of the disease process. Clients may be understandably anxious during examinations because they may fear discovery that further vision loss has occurred. Assess the client's perception of glaucoma and

the effect it has on quality of life. Help the client identify effective coping skills that may have been used in the past.

Diagnosis, Outcomes, Interventions

Diagnosis: Disturbed Sensory Perception. The increased IOP alters the function of the optic nerve, decreasing vision. The nursing diagnosis *Disturbed Sensory Perception (Visual) related to recent loss of vision* may be appropriate if the loss of vision is a new problem for the client.

Outcomes. The client will maintain as much functional vision as possible, report no further loss of vision, adapt to any visual loss, be able to perform activities of daily living (ADL), and recognize clinical manifestations of complications.

Interventions. Reassure the client that although some vision has been lost and cannot be restored, further loss may be prevented by adhering to the treatment plan.

Diagnosis: Anticipatory Grieving. Vision lost to glaucoma is irreparable. Even with the most aggressive medical and surgical management, vision loss may progress. A typical nursing diagnosis would therefore be *Anticipatory Grieving related to loss of vision*. Significant loss of vision represents the need for compromise and adaptation for both the client and his or her family.

Outcomes. The client will express grief, describe the meaning of the loss, and share the grief with significant others.

Interventions. Assess the causative and contributing factors that may delay the work of grieving and promote family cohesiveness. The social stigma of blindness underlies the anxiety that clients experience with actual or potential loss of vision. Total loss of vision isolates a person within a different reality. Although most clients are successfully rehabilitated, some losses are permanent. Also, some people, for a variety of reasons, remain socially isolated. The image of a blind person who is pitied and must accept the charity of others is disturbing.

Use therapeutic communication to express empathy as the client relates expected and actual losses that are due to loss of vision. People with actual or potential loss of vision may be faced with barriers in their vocations that force an unwanted change. Not all jobs and work environments are adaptable for a person who is visually impaired. Age may be a major factor in the person's ability to meet this challenge.

Self-esteem is closely related to the roles of people in their particular lifestyle. Loss of control in personal, family, and work situations can be devastating. The issue of dependence versus independence may also be a factor in the person's ability to cope with the stressors of vision loss.

Collaborative Problem: Risk for Blindness. The risk for blindness from extremely high IOP can be addressed as a collaborative problem.

Outcomes. The nurse will monitor for sudden loss of sight, nausea, or eye pain, quickly administer prescribed medications, try to calm the client, and notify the physician.

Interventions. Glycerin is supplied in a variety of strengths. Check the percentage of the solution closely against what is supplied. If the glycerin is not already flavored, the extreme sweetness and viscosity may be made more palatable by mixing it with equal parts of a tart juice, such as lemon. Serving the solution over cracked ice also makes it more palatable. After 3 hours encourage the intake of water and other liquids to prevent mild to moderate dehydration and make sure the client can get to the bathroom during the diuretic phase.

When infusing mannitol, carefully evaluate the client's cardiovascular and renal status before treatment is begun. Document baseline vital signs before treatment and frequently during the infusion. Because mannitol tends to crystallize, the bottle may need to be warmed before it is administered. Do not use the vial while crystals are present. An in-line micropore filter should also be used to prevent infusion of any crystallized particles.

Although the preservation of vision cannot be guaranteed, it is important to keep the client and family calm. Increased anxiety raises blood pressure, which further raises IOP. Monitor vision, comparing findings to baseline, and report any deterioration or eye pain immediately.

Diagnosis: Risk for Ineffective Therapeutic Regimen Management (Individuals). The regimen for eyedrops and oral medications to control glaucoma ranges from simple to complex. This nursing diagnosis should be stated as *Risk for Ineffective Therapeutic Regimen Management (Individuals) related to complex medication schedule.*

Outcomes. The client will describe the disease process and the regimen for disease control and will relate how the medication routine will be incorporated into ADL.

Interventions. The client may need to instill as many as three or four different eyedrops from one to six times a day. Constricting eyedrops are usually prescribed four times a day, and beta-blockers are usually prescribed every 12 hours; however, the eyedrops may be needed every 4 to 6 hours. The schedule is designed to provide the best possible control of IOP around the clock.

Medications are an integral part of the treatment and care of a client with glaucoma, and nursing inter-

TABLE 67-1	*Teaching the Client About Eyedrops for Glaucoma*
Medication	**Teaching Aspects**
Pilocarpine HCl	Usually given three to four times a day
	A miotic, causing pupillary constriction to open Schlemm's canal
	Space out administration, beginning on awakening and ending at bedtime
	May cause blurred vision after instillation
	Brow ache has been reported
	Consider use of thin gel strips (a timed-release form) to improve compliance
Timolol maleate and other beta-blockers (e.g., levobunolol)	Usually given every 12 hours
	Decreases production of aqueous humor
	Space out administration
	Contraindicated in clients with asthma and chronic obstructive pulmonary disease
	Assess for bradycardia before administration
Carbonic anhydrase inhibitors (e.g., acetazolamide)	Inhibits production of aqueous humor
	Available as tablets and in sustained-release capsules
	Side effects include anorexia and tingling in the hands and feet

ventions must thus be directed at the client's ability to understand and comply with prescribed therapy. First, determine the client's current level of knowledge. Provide necessary information about glaucoma and its treatment in understandable terms. Diagrams may be helpful to the client and his or her significant others. Because treatment for glaucoma is often complex, involving both oral and topical ophthalmic medications, review a written plan of care in large print with the client and family. To maximize compliance, ensure that the plan of care fits into the client's lifestyle.

The administration of eyedrops is a critical component of self-care for the client with glaucoma. After instructing the client and family on the technique of instillation, validate the client's or the family's ability to instill eyedrops properly by asking for a demonstration. Be sure to include discussion of medications and their side effects. Table 67-1 lists additional guidelines for teaching the client about eyedrops.

Evaluation

Independent self-care is the area for evaluation in the medically managed client. Evaluate the client's ability for self-care (a short-term outcome) and compliance with the medical regimen (a long-term outcome).

■ Modifications for Older Clients

Older clients with arthritic or shaking hands have difficulty instilling their own eyedrops. Instruct the client to lie down on a bed or sofa. Tilting the head back can lead to loss of balance. The eyedrop regimen for glaucoma requires accurate timing. Older clients may need visual reminders, such as a check-off list and may also need to use a timer or an alarm clock to help them remember.

■ Surgical Management

When maximal medical therapy fails to halt the progression of visual field loss and optic nerve damage, surgical intervention is recommended. Many procedures are used to improve aqueous humor outflow; however, no operation has been uniformly successful.

Laser Trabeculoplasty. The use of the laser to create an opening in the trabecular meshwork is often indicated before filtering surgery is considered. The laser produces scars in the trabecular meshwork, causing tightening of meshwork fibers. The tightened fibers allow increased outflow of aqueous humor. IOP is reduced through improved outflow in about 80% of cases. The effect of the laser treatment decreases with time, and the procedure may need to be repeated. Medical treatment with topical eyedrops is usually continued.

Trabeculectomy. Trabeculectomy is the creation of an opening through which the aqueous fluid escapes. A half-thickness scleral flap is loosely sutured over the created opening through which the fluid escapes, again resulting in subconjunctival absorption of aqueous humor (see Figure 67-1, *C*).

Filtering Procedures. Operations such as trephination, thermal sclerostomy, and sclerectomy create an outflow channel from the anterior chamber into the subconjunctival space (see Figure 67-1, *D*). Aqueous humor is absorbed through the conjunctival vessels. In about 25% of cases, the opening closes because of scar tissue formation and reoperation is necessary. Such filtering procedures are less successful in young and black clients, who tend to have an increased ability to produce thicker scar tissue. Topical corticosteroids are used postoperatively because their anti-inflammatory action inhibits proliferation of fibroblasts at the surgical site.

Iridectomy. *Iridectomy* is the creation of a new route for the flow of aqueous humor to the trabecular meshwork.

The laser is used to create the new opening in the iris (see Figure 67-1, *E*).

Other Techniques. 5-Fluorouracil (5-FU), mitomycin, and other antimetabolites are sometimes injected subconjunctivally because they also inhibit fibroblast proliferation and thereby reduce postoperative scarring. Ocular implantation devices (e.g., Molteno implant, Baerveldt seton) are sometimes used to control the flow of aqueous humor in clients with complicated types of glaucoma. A device is sutured to the outer surface of the eyeball on the sclera between the ocular muscles. A tiny probe is inserted under the scleral flap directly into the anterior chamber that directs the flow of aqueous humor more posteriorly than in the more common filtering procedures.

Cyclodestructive Procedures. When other surgical procedures have failed, *cyclocryotherapy* (application of a freezing tip) or cyclophotocoagulation may be used to damage the ciliary body and decrease production of aqueous humor.

■ Nursing Management of the Surgical Client

Preoperative Care

Preoperative nursing care includes preparing the client for a surgical procedure that may be performed in either an outpatient or inpatient setting (see Chapter 16).

Laser therapy is most commonly performed in a clinic or office, including the use of a topical anesthetic. Explain both the expected outcome of the procedure and the "popping" sounds and flashing lights that the client will experience. Explain that there will be a waiting period (usually 1 to 2 hours) after the procedure to evaluate a possible rise in IOP. Because of the instability of the IOP, the client should arrange for a friend or family member to accompany him or her and to provide transportation.

Postoperative Care

Following surgery, the eye is covered with a patch and a metal or plastic shield for protection to protect from light and trauma. Instruct the client not to lie on the operative side to avoid pressure on the surgical site. When the effects of perioperative sedation have diminished, the client may walk about and eat as desired.

Frequent monitoring of IOP is necessary because the surgical site is microscopic. Assess the client for continued or increasing pain, nausea, and decreased vision. Follow-up care is needed to monitor for delayed healing. The anterior chamber may fail to heal, or the wound may seal too tightly. Both situations warrant further surgery.

■ Self-Care

The postoperative plan must include client education and evaluation of the home environment and available care. Because the level of independence varies with each client, use information supplied by the client and family or friends to assess how much support may be needed. Although many clients with glaucoma undergo repeated surgical procedures, carefully review the information each time. Client and family education includes the following steps:

1. Manifestations of infection (redness, swelling, drainage, blurred vision, pain)
2. Manifestations of increased IOP (increasing pain, nausea, decrease in vision)
3. The rationale for eye protection (shield or eyeglasses at all times) to protect from light and trauma
4. Medications and eyedrop instillation technique
5. Scheduled return visit date and time
6. Treatment of the surgical site:
   a. Carefully clean the area around the eye with warm tap water and a clean washcloth.
   b. Do not rub or apply pressure over the closed eye, which may damage healing tissue.

CATARACTS

A *cataract* is opacity of the lens. Some degree of cataract formation is to be expected in most people over 70 years of age. Worldwide, cataract is the primary cause of reduced vision and blindness. More than a million cataract operations are now being performed annually in the United States. A person with a normal life span is more likely to undergo a cataract operation than any other major surgical procedure.

The most common cataract is the age-related or senile type. Senile cataracts usually begin around the age of 50 years and consist of cortical, nuclear, or posterior subcapsular opacities, which may coexist in various combinations. In cortical cataracts, spoke-like opacifications are found in the periphery of the lens. They progress slowly, infrequently involve the visual axis, and often do not cause severe loss of vision. Nuclear sclerotic cataracts are a result of a progressive yellowing and hardening of the central lens (nucleus). Most people over age 70 years have some degree of nuclear sclerosis. Posterior subcapsular opacities occur centrally on the posterior lens capsule and cause visual loss early in their development because they lie directly on the visual axis.

Etiology and Risk Factors

The cumulative exposure to ultraviolet light over a person's life span is the single most important risk factor in cataract development. People who live at high altitudes or who work in bright sunlight, such as commercial fishermen, appear to experience cataract formation earlier in life. Glassblowers and welders who do not wear eye protection are also at higher risk.

Cataracts may develop as a result of many other systemic, ocular, and congenital disorders. *Systemic* disorders include diabetes, tetany, myotonic dystrophy, neurodermatitis, galactosemia, Lowe's syndrome, Werner's syndrome, and Down syndrome. *Intraocular* disorders include iridocyclitis, retinitis, retinal detachment, and onchocerciasis. Infections (German measles, mumps, hepatitis, poliomyelitis, chickenpox, infectious mononucleosis) during the first trimester of pregnancy may cause *congenital* cataracts. Blunt trauma, lacerations, foreign bodies, radiation, exposure to infrared light, and chronic use of corticosteroids may also result in cataracts.

Pathophysiology

Cataract formation is characterized chemically by a reduction in oxygen uptake and an initial increase in water content followed by dehydration of the lens. Sodium and calcium contents are increased; potassium, ascorbic acid, and protein contents are decreased. The protein in the lens undergoes numerous age-related changes, including yellowing from formation of fluorescent compounds and molecular changes. These changes, along with the photoabsorption of ultraviolet radiation throughout life, suggest that cataracts may be caused by a photochemical process.

Cataracts progress in a predictable pattern. They begin as immature cataracts that are not completely opaque, and some light is transmitted through them, allowing useful vision. Mature cataracts are completely opaque (the former term for this stage was *ripe*). Vision is significantly reduced. Hypermature cataracts are those in which the lens proteins break down into short-chain polypeptides that leak out through the lens capsule. The pieces of protein are engulfed by macrophages, which may obstruct the trabecular meshwork, causing phacolytic glaucoma.

Clinical Manifestations

Blurred vision, sometimes monocular diplopia (double vision), photophobia (light sensitivity), and glare occur because the opacity of the lens obstructs the reception of light and images by the retina. Clients usually see better in low light, when the pupil is dilated, which allows for vision around a central opacity. There is no complaint of pain. A cloudy lens can be observed (Figure 67-3).

A cataract should be suspected when the red reflex seen with the direct ophthalmoscope is distorted or absent. Although cataracts can usually be easily identified with the direct ophthalmoscope, an accurate determination of the type and extent of the lens change requires a slit-lamp examination.

Outcome Management
■ Surgical Management

There is no known treatment other than surgery that prevents or reduces cataract formation. Of all the fields

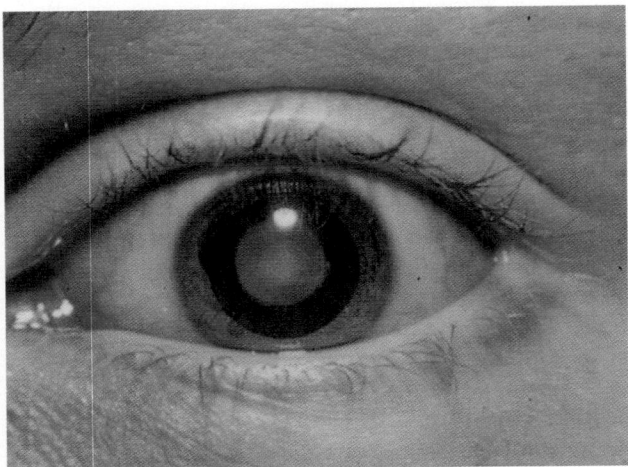

FIGURE 67-3 The cloudy appearance of a lens affected by cataract. (Courtesy of Ophthalmic Photography at the University of Michigan W. K. Kellogg Eye Center, Ann Arbor.)

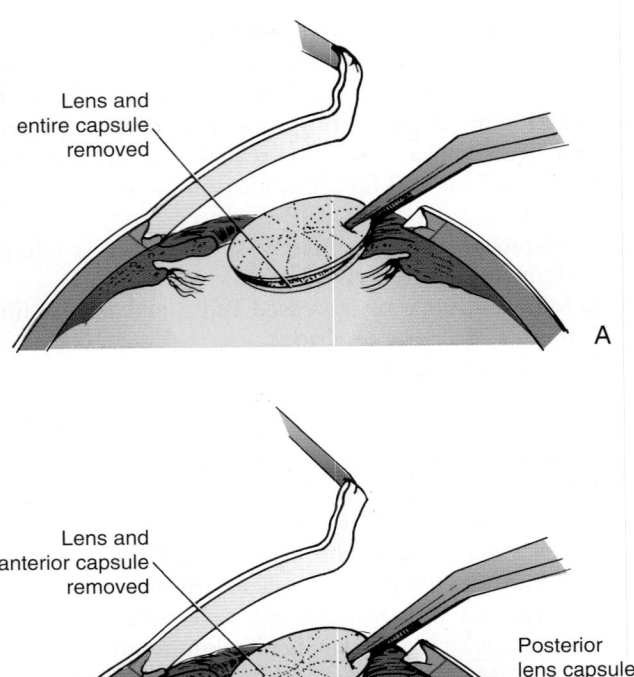

FIGURE 67-4 A, A small incision is made into the cornea for the insertion of the phacoemulsification tip. Using ultrasound, the cataract is dissolved. **B,** An artificial lens is inserted into the eye, which unfolds into place.

of medicine, cataract surgery has been one of the greatest beneficiaries from advances in techniques and technology. When your grandparents had cataract surgery, the cataract had to ripen, during which time vision was dramatically impaired, and then was plucked from the eye. Because no lens replacement was available, large, thick glasses were needed. Today cataract surgery is the most common surgery performed.

Unless other ocular complications or health factors occur, cataract surgery is performed on an outpatient basis. Preoperative eyedrops may include a dilating agent such as tropicamide (Mydriacyl) to facilitate the surgery. A cycloplegic cyclopentolate (Cyclogyl) may also be administered to paralyze the ciliary muscles. Cataract surgery is performed under topical anesthesia using eyedrops or regional anesthesia (retrobulbar injection of local anesthetic solution). The client is often given an intravenous sedative in addition.

The cataract is removed by making a small incision in the cornea. The cataract is broken into microscopic particles using an ultrasonic probe. The use of high-energy sound waves is called *phacoemulsification.* Then a folded intraocular lens (IOL) is inserted through the microincision, then unfolded, and locked into permanent position (Figure 67-4). The small incision is "self-sealing" and usually requires no stitches. It remains tightly closed by the natural outward pressure within the eye. This type of incision heals fast and provides a much more comfortable recuperation.

Complications. *Secondary glaucoma* is one of the major complications that may occur after cataract extraction. As a result of postoperative edema in the ocular tissues, a certain rise in IOP is anticipated and expected. This elevation most often resolves within 24 to 72 hours. If prolonged IOP persists, medical therapy may be necessary.

Postoperative infection, bleeding, macular edema, and wound leaks are also possible. The incidence of retinal detachment is higher in the first 12 months after cataract surgery.

■ Nursing Management of the Surgical Client
Assessment

During the history and physical examination, ask the client about any predisposing factors (trauma, systemic diseases, medications such as corticosteroids, and other ocular problems). Visual acuity (both distant and near) in each eye is documented. Ask the client to describe visual disturbances. The client's visual acuity may be relatively close to normal ranges, and yet the client may experience difficulty in performing ADL. The client's individual perception of the quality of vision is an important factor in determining the need for surgery.

Diagnosis, Outcomes, Interventions

Diagnosis: Disturbed Sensory Perception. An IOL does not provide the same visual acuity as the natural lens of the eye. Although vision may be greatly improved, varying degrees of change in depth perception may remain. In addition, the eye is patched for protection, making vision monocular. Write the nursing diagnosis as *Disturbed Sensory Perception related to lens extraction and replacement and use of eye patch*.

Outcomes. The client will have improved visual perception as evidenced by improved vision or adaptation to changes in visual acuity.

Interventions. Adaptation is the key issue in caring for the client having cataract surgery. Nursing interventions are based on assisting the client to gain or maintain as much independence as possible. Evaluate the client's lifestyle, abilities, and home environment. A 55-year-old client who is an architect and otherwise healthy may have an early cataract removed because it interferes with his work in areas where bright light is used. A 75-year-old diabetic client who is retired and mainly watches television has entirely different needs.

Evaluation

Adaptation to restored normal vision is usually rapid. Adaptation to limited vision requires more time based on individual variations.

■ Self-Care

After cataract surgery, clients are expected to return for a follow-up visit the next morning and again at 1 week and at 1 month. Postoperative care includes observation of the ocular dressing, if present, and assessment of the client's ability to perform ADL at the preoperative level. Nausea and vomiting are no longer expected outcomes of the surgical procedure but, if present, should be reported immediately. Prolonged vomiting may result in increased IOP and wound dehiscence. The eye patch is usually removed the next morning but may be removed after a few hours if the client has limited vision in the other eye. Instruct the client to wear a metal or plastic shield to protect the eye from accidental injury and not to rub the eye. Glasses may be worn during the day. The Client Education Guide feature on Care After Cataract Removal, above, provides instructions to be followed.

Restrictions on postoperative activity vary according to the practice of the ophthalmologist. Generally, the client should avoid heavy lifting (>5 pounds) or straining in the early postoperative period.

Eye care for the client after cataract surgery is the same as that for glaucoma clients (see Glaucoma). Postoperative eye medications may include antibiotics, corticosteroids, or both. Assess the client's or the family's ability to instill eyedrops appropriately. Review the rationale and schedule for the medications with the client and family. Postoperative discomfort should be minimal to moderate and is usually relieved by acetaminophen.

CLIENT EDUCATION GUIDE
Care After Cataract Removal

- Leave the eye patch in place.
- For 24 hours, limit your activity to sitting in a chair, resting in bed, and walking to the bathroom.
- Do not rub your eye.
- You can wear your glasses.
- Do not lift more than 5 pounds (the weight of a gallon of milk).
- Do not strain (or bear down).
- Do not sleep on the side of your body that was operated on.
- Take your eyedrops.
- Take acetaminophen (e.g., Tylenol) as needed for pain or itching.
- DO NOT take aspirin or drugs containing aspirin.
- Report any pain that is unrelieved, redness around the eye, nausea, or vomiting.
- Wear eye shield to protect your eye.

Clients commonly experience an itching sensation after cataract surgery. Instruct the client to report any pain that is unrelieved. Review the clinical manifestations of infection and increased IOP with the client and family.

Depending on the client's age, ability, and availability of assistance, make a referral for home health care if indicated. Adjustment to changes in vision also varies with the individual client.

▍RETINAL DISORDERS
RETINAL DETACHMENT

Retinal detachment is the separation of the retina from the choroid, a membrane dense with blood vessels that is located between the retina and the sclera ("white" of the eye). The retina is a thin layer of light-sensitive tissue that lines the back portion of the eye. When the retina detaches, it is deprived of its blood supply and source of nourishment and loses its ability to function. This can impair vision to the point of blindness.

Rhegmatogenous retinal detachment is the most common type and is due to a retinal hole, liquid in the vitreous body with access to the hole, and subsequent fluid accumulation between the retina and the retinal pigment epithelium. The liquid seeps through the hole and separates the retina from its blood supply. Without intervention, the detachment continues to spread and the detached retina loses the ability to function. It may become increasingly detached over a period of hours to years.

Predisposing factors to retinal detachment include aging, cataract extraction, degeneration of the retina, trauma, severe myopia, previous retinal detachment in the other eye, and a family history of retinal detachment. Retinal holes and tears usually occur from spontaneous vitreous traction, but abnormal adhesions may be present between the retina and vitreous body secondary to diabetic retinopathy, injury, or other ocular disorders. Atrophy of the vitreous body may also result in a retinal tear.

Characteristic clinical manifestations of retinal detachment are described by clients as a shadow or curtain falling across the field of vision. Shadows or black areas in the field of vision are the result of separation of visual receptors from the neural pathway. No pain is associated with a detached retina. The onset is usually sudden and may be accompanied by a burst of black spots or floaters indicating that bleeding has occurred as a result of the detachment. The person may also see flashes of light caused by separation of the retina.

Visual field loss occurs in the opposite quadrant of the actual detachment. For example, a tear in the temporal region, which is affected more frequently, creates a visual defect in the nasal area. The extent of loss of vision is related to the portion of the retina involved. Giant retinal tears involving the entire retina may result in temporary blindness, whereas peripheral tears may not interfere with central vision at all.

The pupil must be widely dilated for a retinal examination. Tell clients that they will experience an extremely bright light and will be asked to change their gaze frequently to facilitate the ophthalmoscopic examination. A scleral depressor also may be used externally on the lid or conjunctiva to assist in rotating the eyeball and to indent the retina for increased viewing ability. Areas of detachment appear bluish gray as opposed to the normal red-pink color. Retinal tears are most often horseshoe shaped but may be round (Figure 67-5).

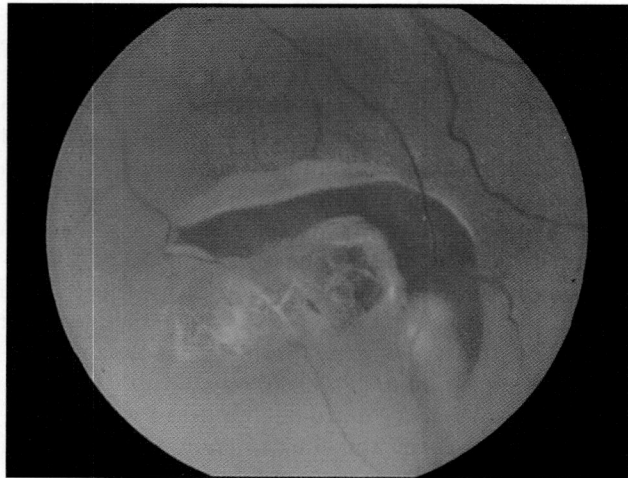

FIGURE 67-5 Bluish gray appearance of areas of retinal detachment. (Courtesy of Ophthalmic Photography at the University of Michigan W. K. Kellogg Eye Center, Ann Arbor.)

Outcome Management
■ Surgical Management

There is no known medical treatment for a detached retina. The goal of surgical repair of retinal detachment is to place the retina back in contact with the choroid and to seal the accompanying holes and breaks. Because retinal detachment repair may take several hours, general anesthesia is commonly used. The pupil must be widely dilated before the operation, and the client may be given a sedative.

Laser Photocoagulation. If the retina is torn or the detachment is slight, a laser can be used to burn the edges of the tear and halt progression. If the detachment is small, the laser can seal the retina against the choroid. Laser surgery is usually performed as an outpatient procedure with the client under local anesthesia.

Cryopexy. Cryopexy uses nitrous oxide to freeze the tissue behind the retinal tear, stimulating scar tissue formation that will seal the edges of the tear. It is usually done as an outpatient procedure with the client under local anesthesia.

Pneumatic Retinopexy. Pneumatic retinopexy is most effective for detachments that occur in the upper portion of the eye. The eye is numbed with local anesthesia, and a small gas bubble is injected into the vitreous body. The bubble rises and presses against the retina, pushing it against the choroid. The gas bubble is slowly absorbed over the next 1 or 2 weeks. Cryopexy or laser is used to seal the retina into place.

Scleral Buckling. The surgical procedure to place the retina back in contact with the choroid is called *scleral buckling* (Figure 67-6). The sclera is actually depressed from the outside by rubber-like silicone (Silastic) sponges or bands that are sutured in place permanently. In addition to the buckling procedure, an intraocular injection of air or sulfur hexafluoride (SF6) gas bubble, or both, may be used to apply pressure on the retina from the inside of the eye. This holds the retina in place by gravitational force during the healing phase. Postoperative positioning of the client maximizes the tamponade effect of the air or gas bubble. The bubble is slowly absorbed.

Postoperative swelling of tissues and cells in the anterior chamber caused by the inflammatory process or compromise of the venous drainage system may result in increased IOP. Because of the fragility of the tissues involved in the repair, re-detachment of the retina may occur at any time. At times, the retina has been separated from its blood supply long enough that, even when reattached, it no longer has useful function and the client's vision does not improve significantly. Postoperative infection is also a risk.

The client should not expect immediate return of vision. Postoperative inflammation and the dilating drops interfere with vision. As healing takes place over weeks and months, vision may improve gradually.

■ Nursing Management

Nursing care focuses on helping the client cope with the fears and reality of loss of vision and to adapt to changes in vision. The client must be aware of the clinical manifestations of further loss of vision.

Following surgery, observe the eye patch for any drainage. Blood loss in retinal detachment surgery is minimal, and only serous drainage is expected on the postoperative dressing. Assess the level of pain and the presence of nausea.

Activity restrictions may be necessary if an air or gas bubble has been injected. The client needs to be positioned so that the bubble can apply maximal pressure on the retina by the force of gravity. This position, usually

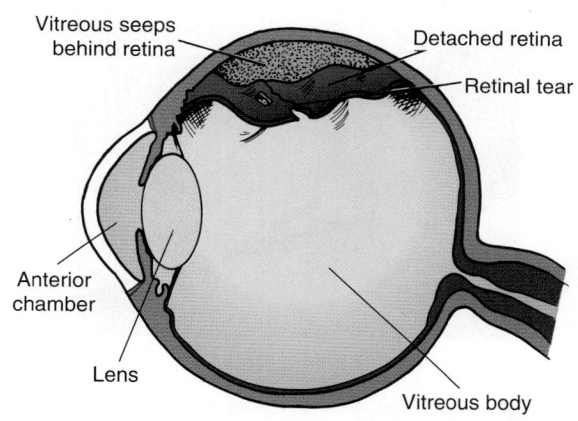

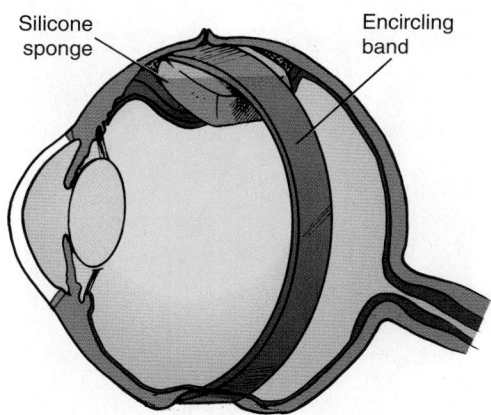

FIGURE 67-6 Scleral buckling to repair a detached retina. A silicone sponge implant is placed over the tear and held in place with an encircling band. When the buckle is tightened, the implant indents the sclera, holding the choroid and retina together.

head down and to one side, is maintained for several days. Provide suggestions for comfort and support with the positioning (pillows under stomach, elbows, or ankles).

Posterior segment surgery, such as scleral buckling procedures, causes considerably more discomfort than anterior segment procedures do. Ocular muscles are separated, and the globe is manipulated to reach the posterior portions of the eyeball. Opioids may be needed during the first 24 hours after surgery. Nausea and vomiting may also require management.

Intravenous (IV) acetazolamide (Diamox) may be used to reduce increased IOP, which is monitored closely during the first 24 hours. Encourage the client to resume a regular diet and fluids as tolerated. The eye patch and shield are removed the next morning. Redness and swelling of the lids and conjunctiva should be expected from the surgical manipulation. After several days, the swelling and ecchymosis of the lids subside, but the conjunctiva may remain red or pink for a few weeks.

Postoperative eye medications generally include an antibiotic-steroid combination eyedrop to prevent infection and reduce inflammation. Cycloplegic agents are prescribed to dilate the pupil and relax the ciliary muscles, which decreases discomfort and helps prevent the formation of iris adhesions to the corneal endothelium (synechiae). Either warm or cold compresses may be applied for comfort several times a day.

■ Self-Care

Because retinal detachment surgery is often performed on an urgent basis, the client rarely has an opportunity to plan for the surgery. Evaluate the home environment, and assist the client and family in preparing for any necessary support. You may need to find help at home for independent living until sight returns or the client adapts to changes in vision. Although the eye patch is usually removed early in the postoperative period, clients commonly have decreased functional vision in the eye. See the Bridge to Home Health Care feature on Coping with Failing Vision on p. 1957 for suggestions on how to assist clients.

Instruct the client to clean the eye with warm tap water using a clean washcloth. Warm compresses may be continued at home. Either an eye shield or glasses should be worn during the day, and the shield should be worn during naps and at night. Advise the client to avoid vigorous activities and heavy lifting during the immediate postoperative period. If an air or gas bubble has been injected, it may take several weeks to be totally absorbed. Clients are advised to avoid air travel during this time because the gas and air expand at high altitudes.

DIABETIC RETINOPATHY

Diabetic retinopathy is a progressive disorder of the retina characterized by microscopic damage to the retinal vessels, resulting in occlusion of the vessels. As a result of inadequate blood supply, sections of the retina deteriorate and vision is permanently lost. Diabetic retinopathy is one of the leading causes of blindness worldwide. All diabetic people are at risk for retinopathy, although there appears to be a strong correlation between incidence and severity of retinopathy and duration of the disease and blood glucose control. About 30% to 40% of the diabetic population has some degree of retinopathy. Clients who have had diabetes for 15 to 20 years have an 80% to 90% risk for development of retinopathy. Recently a genetic predisposition to retinopathy was found in the Asian Indian population with diabetes. Persons with allele 210 bp have increased risk.

The two types of diabetic retinopathy are (1) background (*nonproliferative*) and (2) *proliferative*. In background retinopathy, the retinal vessels are hyperpermeable and weak. The capillaries develop microaneurysms, and the retinal veins become dilated and tortuous. Multiple hemorrhages occur from these defective vessels. Retinal edema is caused by leaking capillaries, and after the serous fluid is absorbed, a yellowish precipitate ("hard exudate") remains. Hemorrhages, exudates, and ischemia contribute to impaired vision, particularly if these occur on or around the macula. Progressive retinal ischemia stimulates the growth of new but ineffective blood vessels. These new and fragile blood vessels proliferate and grow into the vitreous body. These vessels leak, hemorrhage, and undergo fibrous changes that may form bands that pull on the retina, causing detachment. This process is called *proliferative retinopathy* (Figure 67-7). With increasing ischemia, microinfarcts of the nerve fiber layer, called "cotton-wool spots," appear.

Clinical manifestations are quite varied. Clients may report "spiders," "cobwebs," or tiny specks floating in their vision; dark streaks or a red film that blocks vision; vision loss, usually in both eyes, but more so in one eye; blurred vision that may fluctuate; a dark or empty spot in the center of the vision; poor night vision; or difficulty adjusting from bright light to dim light (Figure 67-8).

Outcome Management

The two main treatments for diabetic retinopathy are photocoagulation and vitrectomy. In most cases, these treatments are effective and slow or stop the progression of the disease for some time.

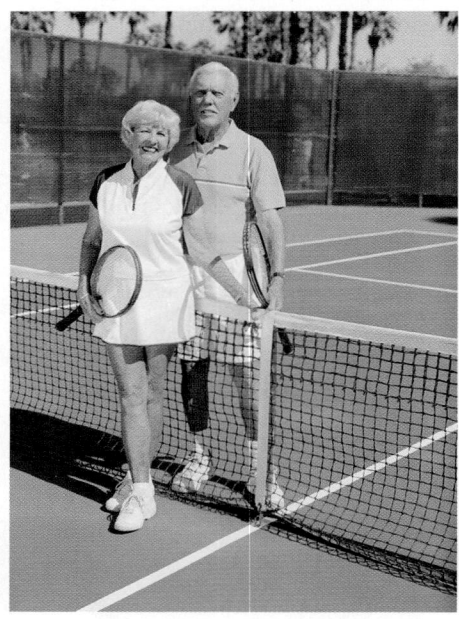

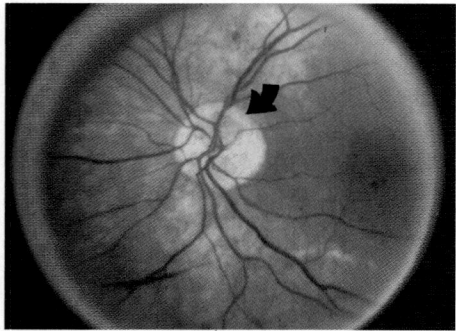

FIGURE 67-7 Proliferative diabetic retinopathy. Neovascularization covers one fourth to one third of the optic disc *(arrow)*. (Standard photograph no. 10A of the Modified Airlee House Classification of Diabetic Retinopathy. Courtesy of the Early Treatment Diabetic Retinopathy Study Research Group.)

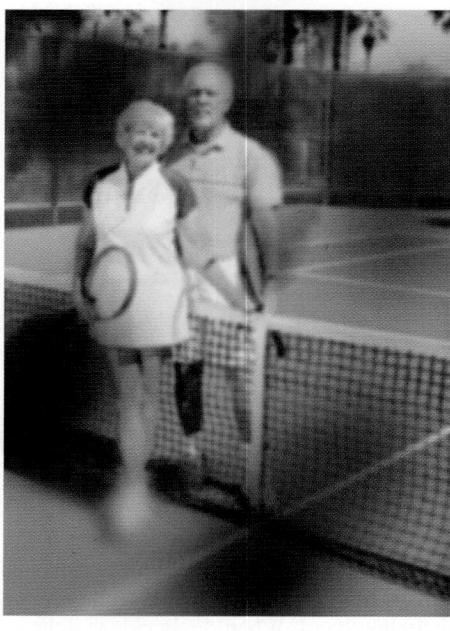

FIGURE 67-8 A, Normal vision. **B,** Vision with diabetic retinopathy.

Photocoagulation

The goal of photocoagulation is to stop the leakage of blood and fluid in the retina and thus slow the progression of diabetic retinopathy. In photocoagulation a high-energy laser beam creates small burns in areas of the retina with abnormal blood vessels to seal any leaks. The procedure can be done as an outpatient under local anesthesia. A medical contact lens is placed on the cornea to help focus laser light on the sections of the retina to be treated. Fluorescein angiographic photographs may serve as maps to show where the laser burns should be placed. For proliferative diabetic retinopathy, panretinal or scatter photocoagulation can be used to treat the entire retina except the macula. The treatment causes the abnormal new blood vessels to shrink and disappear. Thus it reduces the chances of vitreous hemorrhage. Panretinal photocoagulation is usually done in two or more sessions. The treatment significantly reduces the risk of severe vision loss.

Vitrectomy

Vitrectomy is removal of the blood-filled vitreous. A vitreous cutter cuts the tissue and removes it, piece by piece, from the eye. The volume of removed tissue is replaced with saline to maintain the normal shape and pressure of the eye. During a vitrectomy the surgeon may also use a laser probe to perform a procedure called *panretinal photocoagulation* to prevent renewed growth of abnormal blood vessels and bleeding.

Nursing Interventions

Shortly after laser treatment, the client can usually return home driven by someone else. Vision will be blurry for about a day. Mild pain, headache, and sensitivity to light are expected and can be controlled with an eye patch and over-the-counter pain relievers. Immediately following laser surgery to treat macular edema, small spots caused by the laser burns may appear in the visual field. The spots generally fade and disappear with time. Follow-up care should be arranged before the client leaves; new areas of leakage may appear later and may require additional laser treatments.

RETINITIS PIGMENTOSA

Retinitis pigmentosa is a genetic disorder that initially destroys the rods of the eye (see the Genetic Links feature on Retinitis Pigmentosa at right). Because the rods perceive black and white vision, the earliest manifestation is noticed during childhood as night blindness. Over the next several years, manifestations progress until a total loss of peripheral vision occurs. In time, central vision is also lost. No treatment is available to slow or stop this disorder. Genetic counseling is advised.

AGE-RELATED MACULAR DEGENERATION

Age-related macular degeneration (AMD) is a degenerative process that affects the macula and surrounding tissues, resulting in central visual deficits. AMD is found to some degree in most adults over 65 years of age. It is one of the most common causes of visual loss in older people. The exact cause is unknown, but the incidence increases with each decade in people over 50 years of age. It may be hereditary. It has been demonstrated that the blue rays of the spectrum (sunlight or its reflection in the ocean or desert) seem to accelerate macular degeneration more than other rays of the spectrum. There are two types of age-related macular degeneration: (1) nonex-

GENETICS LINKS

Retinitis Pigmentosa

Description

Retinitis pigmentosa (RP) describes a group of inherited disorders in which abnormalities of the photoreceptors (rods and cones) or the retinal pigment epithelium (RPE) of the retina lead to progressive visual loss. Clients initially experience "night blindness" (decreased night vision), followed by constriction of the peripheral visual field and eventually loss of central vision in the advanced stage of the disease. Most clients are legally blind by age 60. The prevalence of RP is approximately 1 in 3,500 to 1 in 4,000 individuals in the United States and Europe; it is considered the most common inherited cause of blindness.

Genetics

RP can be inherited in an autosomal-dominant, autosomal-recessive, or X-linked recessive fashion. The mode of inheritance is determined by family history. To date, at least 34 different genes are known to cause RP; mutations in at least 12 genes cause autosomal-dominant RP, 16 genes cause autosomal recessive RP, and 6 genes cause X-linked RP.

Diagnosis/Testing

The diagnosis of RP is based on documentation of progressive loss in photoreceptor function by electroretinography (ERG) and visual field testing. DNA testing is available for all the cloned genes causing RP on a research basis only. Routine genetic testing for RP is not available in clinical laboratories.

Management

RP is neither preventable nor curable, but therapy with high-dose vitamin A has been suggested to have a possible effect on slowing changes in retinal function. Various optical aids have been promoted for RP clients, and referral to agencies for the visually impaired can assist in providing vocational training, mobility training, and skills for independent living.

udative *(dry)* and (2) exudative *(wet).* Both types are usually bilateral and progressive.

Dry Macular Degeneration

Nonexudative AMD is characterized by atrophy and degeneration of the outer retina and underlying structures. Seventy percent of clients have the dry form, which involves thinning of the macular tissues and disturbances in its pigmentation. Yellowish round spots *(drusen)* may be seen on the retina and macula with an ophthalmoscope. Drusen are deposits of amorphous material from the pigment epithelial cells of the retina. Over time, these spots increase, enlarge, and may calcify.

Wet Macular Degeneration

At the exudative stage of AMD, Bruch's membrane, which lies just beneath the pigment epithelial cell layer of the retina, becomes compromised. Thirty percent have the wet form, which can involve bleeding within and beneath the retina, opaque deposits, and eventually scar tissue. The wet form accounts for 90% of all cases of legal blindness in clients with macular degeneration. It results in serous fluid leaks from the choroid, with accompanying proliferation of choroidal blood vessels. A dome-shaped retinal pigment epithelium may be seen when examining the fundus. These leaks produce a visual effect called *metamorphopsia,* which appears as distorted lines; the center of vision appears more distorted than the rest of the scene. A dark, blurry area or "whiteout" appears in the center of vision. Color perception changes or diminishes. Fundus photography and angiography may be performed on a regular basis to document and evaluate changes.

Outcome Management

Recently research findings have shown that the use of high-dose antioxidant vitamins C and E, beta carotene, and zinc supplements may delay progression of AMD and vision loss. See the Complementary and Alternative Therapy features on Macular Degeneration and Dietary Supplements and on Egg Yolks and Better Vision, below.

Further damage from exudative macular degeneration sometimes may be arrested by the use of argon photocoagulation, even though laser damage to the retina in this area results in a blind spot. Wet AMD can also be treated by injecting verteporfin (Visudyne), which becomes activated with low levels of laser. Retinal transplantation is a new experimental approach to macular degeneration but will require at least 3 to 5 years of clinical research. When the fovea is involved, central vision is lost and the only helpful measures are low-vision aids. Special sunglasses that block out the blue end of the spectrum may decrease the progress of the disease.

The client with AMD is threatened with the loss of central vision (see the Bridge to Home Health Care feature on Coping with Failing Vision on p. 1957). To evaluate changes in vision, teach the client to use the Amsler chart at home. You may assist the client to maximize remaining vision with low-vision aids and community referral to a low-vision specialist and low-vision support groups.

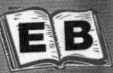

COMPLEMENTARY AND ALTERNATIVE THERAPY

Macular Degeneration and Dietary Supplements

The largest randomized trial (*n* = 3,640) of a combination daily dietary supplement (500 mg vitamin C plus 400 international units vitamin E plus 15 mg beta-carotene plus 80 mg zinc plus 2 mg copper) compared with placebo for macular degeneration found a significant reduction in the risk of disease progression over the 6-year study. The only individuals who benefited, however, were those with intermediate to advanced stages of already diagnosed macular degeneration. Individuals at risk or with early stage macular degeneration did not benefit from taking this supplement over the study period. In addition, the supplement did not have any effect on cataract development or risk.

Reference

Age-Related Eye Disease Study Research Group. (2001). A randomized, placebo-controlled, clinical trial of high-dose supplementation with vitamins C and E, beta carotene, and zinc for age-related macular degeneration and vision loss: AREDS Report no. 8. *Archives of Ophthalmology, 119,* 1417-1435.

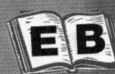

COMPLEMENTARY AND ALTERNATIVE THERAPY

Egg Yolks and Better Vision

Two carotenoids may be deposited in the eye and prevent macular degeneration or cataracts (leading causes of blindness in older adults in the United States). These carotenoids are called lutein and zeaxanthin, and they are found in large amounts in egg yolks. Researchers gave a little more than one egg yolk per day to 11 individuals and found that after a little more than 1 month their levels of these two carotenoids increased significantly in the blood; however, their low-density lipoprotein (LDL, or bad cholesterol) also increased significantly. These carotenoids can also come from dark, green leafy vegetables and corn; however, the body does not seem to absorb it as well as it does with egg yolks. In moderation (several times a week), egg yolks may prevent some eye problems, but clients must pay attention to cholesterol intake.

Reference

Handelman, G., et al. (1999). Lutein and zeaxanthin concentrations in plasma after dietary supplementation with egg yolk. *American Journal of Clinical Nutrition, 70,* 247-251.

RETINAL ARTERY OCCLUSION

Occlusion of the retinal artery or vein can cause loss of vision. The most common causes of occlusion are emboli from atherosclerosis, valvular heart disease, increases in blood viscosity, and spasm in the carotid artery. Retinal artery occlusion causes a sudden, unilateral, painless loss of vision. The severity of the visual loss ranges from total loss, when the central artery is occluded, to a loss of a visual field, when a branch of the artery is blocked. Retinal vein occlusion is due to systemic vascular disorders, venous stasis, hypertension, or increased blood viscosity.

Retinal artery occlusion is an emergency. Management includes intermittent massage of the eyeball by a physician to move an embolus from the central artery into a branch and increased oxygenation (95% oxygen for 10 minutes). Surgery can include anterior chamber paracentesis to reduce IOP and to move the embolus. Anticoagulants are used in the early phases of occlusion.

CORNEAL DISORDERS
CORNEAL DYSTROPHIES

Corneal dystrophies comprise a group of hereditary and acquired disorders of unknown cause, characterized by deposits in the layers of the cornea and alteration of the corneal structure. Corneal dystrophies are associated with all five layers of the cornea. Although the disease usually originates in the inner layers (Descemet's membrane, the stroma, and Bowman's membrane), the degeneration, erosion, and deposits affect all layers. Corneal endothelium constantly removes fluids from the cornea to maintain its clarity. As the endothelial cells are gradually lost, the dystrophy progresses. Once lost, the endothelial cells do not grow back but instead spread out to the fill empty spaces. The pump system becomes less efficient, causing corneal clouding, swelling, and eventually reduced vision.

The most common form, Fuchs' dystrophy, is inherited, usually begins in a person's 20s or 30s, affects more women than men, and is slowly progressive. Fuchs' dystrophy is characterized by deposits that look like warts in Descemet's membrane. Manifestations of early stages of Fuchs' dystrophy are glare and light sensitivity. As the dystrophy progresses, the vision may seem blurred in the morning and sharper later in the day. This happens because the internal layers of the cornea tend to retain more moisture during sleep; this moisture evaporates when the eyes are open. As the dystrophy worsens, the vision becomes continuously blurred.

The cornea is evaluated by slit-lamp examination. Fluorescein staining is used to enhance visualization of surface corneal defects. Corneal scrapings may be taken with a sterile spatula for further staining and micro-

---

BRIDGE TO HOME HEALTH CARE

Coping with Failing Vision

Providing a safe home environment for the client with failing vision is essential. Promoting an autonomous lifestyle is desirable. Assessing the client's ability to remain safely at home is an important responsibility of home health care nurses.

Basic emergency procedures can be implemented by the use of nationwide services such as Lifeline. This service provides a portable electronic device usually worn around the client's neck or wrist. By simply pushing the button, immediate contact is made with emergency personnel. The toll-free phone number is 1-800-852-5433.

Local telephone companies can provide special adaptive equipment for 9-1-1 access. Telephones that can be programmed and have lighted or large numbers are available in most retail stores.

Home safety precautions can be simple. Burns can be prevented by color-coding water faucets. Use red for hot water and blue for cold water. Marking the "Off" dials on stoves and microwave ovens with colored tape or paint reduces the chance of injury.

Adequate lighting is essential. During the day, natural light is preferable. Open drapes or shades to provide ample light. Replace light bulbs with the highest wattage recommended.

Removal of hazards, such as throw rugs, clutter, and unnecessary furniture, can promote unrestricted ambulation. Handrails can be installed in hallways, in bathrooms, and on steps to prevent falls. Equipment such as canes, walkers, raised toilet seats, and bathtub rails promote safety. These items are available at medical supply stores.

Many commercial products are now marketed that can be of great assistance in the home. Pill organizers are clearly marked boxes with the day of the week and the times pills are to be taken. These can be filled by family members for a week at a time. Electronic lamp timers and voice-activated switches will allow the client to function more independently.

Access to a television and a radio is important. Large-print newspapers and reading materials help keep the client in touch with current events. The local library and the American Association for the Blind can provide assistance in obtaining needed items.

Creativity and planning can allow the client to remain at home in a safe environment for as long as possible.

scopic evaluation. Specular microscopy may be used to evaluate the corneal endothelium.

Outcome Management

The goal of treatment is to restore visual clarity for both safety and improved quality of life.

■ Medical Management

Fuchs' dystrophy cannot be cured; however, with certain medications, blurred vision resulting from the corneal swelling can be controlled. Saline eyedrops or ointments are often prescribed to draw fluid from the cornea and reduce swelling. Another simple technique that reduces moisture in the cornea is to hold a hair dryer at arm's length, blowing air into the face with the 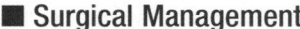 eyes closed. This technique draws moisture from the cornea, temporarily decreases swelling, and improves the vision.

■ Surgical Management

Corneal Transplantation. Corneal transplantation *(keratoplasty)* is the use of donor corneas to improve the clarity of vision. Two depths of keratoplasty are performed. Penetrating keratoplasty indicates full-thickness corneal replacement; lamellar keratoplasty denotes a partial-thickness procedure. Because there is a direct relationship between age and health of the endothelial layer of the cornea, young donor tissue is preferred. Donor eyes are obtained from cadavers, must be enucleated soon after death because of rapid endothelial cell death, and must be stored in a preserving solution. Storage, handling, and coordination of donor tissue with surgeons are provided by a network of state eye-bank associations around the country.

Corneal transplantation surgery is usually performed with the client under local anesthesia. Figure 67-9, *A,* shows the eye after keratoplasty. Unlike cataract surgery, however, visual return after a corneal transplant is relatively slow and typically takes 6 to 12 months. The reason for the slow return of vision is that the sutures holding the new cornea in place tend to distort the vision, and they must be left in place for a considerable time before it is safe to remove them.

Rejection of donor tissue can occur following corneal transplantation from unsuitable storage of donor tissue, dystrophy of the donor's endothelium, surgical trauma, or immunologic rejection. Wound leakage, bleeding into the anterior chamber, glaucoma, cataract, and infection are other complications that may occur. At the first sign of graft rejection, when the cornea becomes cloudy and edematous and when there is an anterior chamber reaction (the presence of white blood cells or protein) (see Figure 67-9, *B*), topical steroids are prescribed in frequent doses to control the inflammatory response and to reverse the rejection reaction. In severe cases, a second transplantation may be necessary.

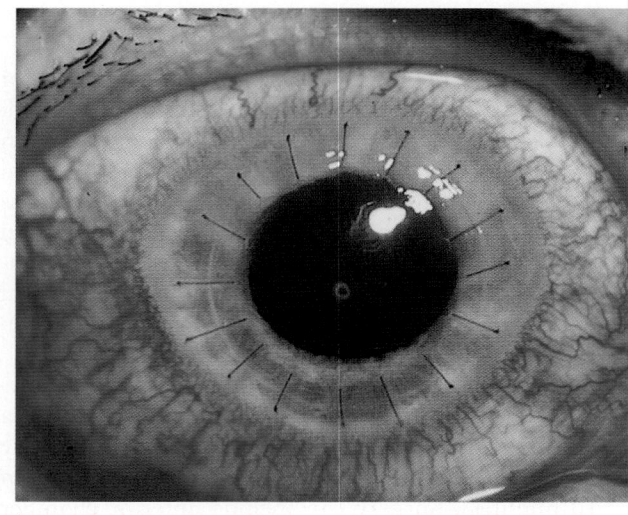

A

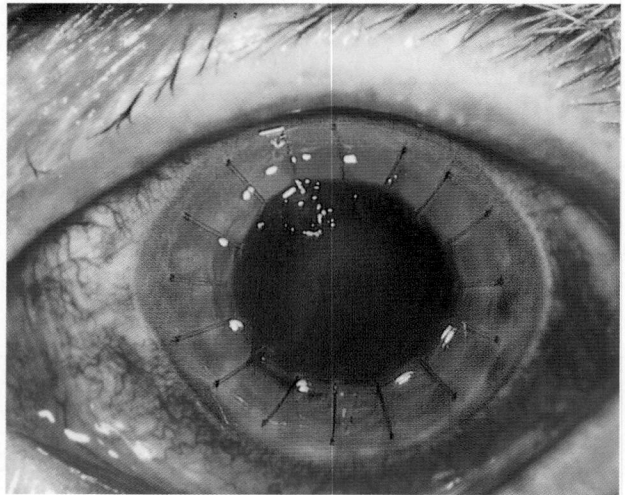

B

FIGURE 67-9 A, Clinical appearance of the eye after keratoplasty. **B,** Acute graft rejection. (Courtesy of Ophthalmic Photography at the University of Michigan W.K. Kellogg Eye Center, Ann Arbor.)

■ Nursing Management of the Postoperative Client

Corneal transplantation is usually performed as outpatient surgery. Postoperatively the client returns from the operating room with an eye patch and protective shield in place. Observe the patch for signs of drainage. No bleeding is expected with this procedure. The client should experience only mild to moderate discomfort, which should be relieved by acetaminophen. Unreduced pain may indicate a rise in IOP and should be reported to the surgeon. Because the eye patch is to be in place until the following morning, assess the client's ability for self-care and reinforce information on the hazards of monocular vision (see Self-Care under Retinal Detachment).

The eye is examined the next morning with the slit lamp. Depending on the extent of preoperative visual limitations, most clients experience improved vision immediately. Instruct clients, however, not to raise their expectations for full vision too high. Vision continues to improve gradually because the healing process may take up to a year or more. Glasses or contact lenses are usually needed to obtain the best result. Many months may be required for restoration of vision, and revisions in the care plan may be needed.

■ Self-Care

Postoperative eyedrops usually include an antibiotic and a corticosteroid. Topical corticosteroid therapy may be needed indefinitely. Discharge instructions include the rationale for the medications and proper instillation technique. It is important for the client to wear eye protection in the form of regular glasses, sunglasses, or a protective shield to prevent injury to the eye. Advise the client never to rub the eye. The area around the eye may be cleaned with warm tap water using a clean washcloth.

Teach the client and family to recognize the clinical manifestations of graft rejection. A mnemonic tool may be useful in teaching the client to remember the signs of graft rejection (RSVP):

- **R** Redness
- **S** Swelling
- **V** Decreased vision
- **P** Pain

Teach the client and family to recognize the signs of increased IOP and infection.

Advise the client to evaluate vision in the eye each day. A picture on the wall or some object in a well-lighted room should be selected as a point of reference. If a change in vision from the day before is noted, the client should reevaluate his or her vision in a few hours. If no improvement is noted or if vision is worse, the client should notify the physician. Because graft rejection may occur at any time (even years) after the surgery, advise the client to make the vision check a routine part of ADL for the rest of his or her life.

CORNEAL INFECTION: KERATITIS

The corneal epithelium is normally an effective barrier against microorganisms. Once it is compromised from disease or trauma, the underlying stromal layer becomes an excellent culture medium for a variety of organisms. Dry eyes or ineffective eyelid closure predisposes the eye to keratitis. Clients who have a systemic collagen disorder, such as rheumatoid arthritis, are particularly susceptible to corneal infections and ulceration. Clients who are comatose are at high risk of injury to the cornea from medical devices or incomplete closure of the eye (Box 67-1).

Clinical manifestations include excess tearing, pain worsened by eyelid movement, sensitivity to light, and indurated sclera. Blurred vision results from the inability of the cornea to provide the proper refractive surface.

BOX 67-1   *Eye Care for Unconscious Clients*

Unconscious, sedated, or paralyzed clients are at high risk of corneal injury because they cannot maintain normal lid closure. Normal lid closure during sleep is provided by tonic contraction of the orbicularis oculi muscle. The use of muscle relaxants reduces the tonic contraction of the muscle and leads only to passive closure of the eye lids. Further, the client may have lost the blink reflex when sedatives are used. Tears quickly evaporate from the eye and increase the risk of injury. Corneal abrasion has been reported in as little as 48 hours.

Eye protection and lubrication are important to preserve sight. The use of eyedrops or ointments are effective in maintaining eye moisture. Films that preserve humidity in the eye can also be used; however, the family may be alarmed by the client's appearance with these products.

Data from Joyce, N. (2002). *Eye care for intensive care patients. A systematic review.* Adelaide, South Africa: The Joanna Briggs Institute for Evidence Based Nursing and Midwifery.

Fluorescein staining of the cornea outlines the affected area, which can be viewed through the slit lamp or with a hand-held flashlight.

Corneal infections may develop into ulcerations that severely compromise the integrity of the eye. Sources of infection include bacteria (e.g., *Staphylococcus aureus*, *Pseudomonas aeruginosa*, *Streptococcus pneumoniae*), fungi *(Candida, Aspergillus)*, viruses (adenovirus, herpes simplex, herpes zoster), and protozoa *(Acanthamoeba)*. *Hypopyon* (a layer of white cells in the anterior chamber) may accompany corneal ulceration.

Outcome Management

The goal of treatment is to eradicate the infection, prevent further injury to the cornea, and promote comfort and healing.

■ Medical Management

Topical antibiotic, antifungal, and antiviral therapy is prescribed, with the frequency of instillation based on the severity of the infection to prevent perforation and to promote healing. Maximal therapy includes the alternating instillation of two broad-spectrum eyedrops every 15 minutes around the clock. As the infection begins to respond to the medication, the frequency of administration is gradually decreased. Systemic IV medication may be prescribed as well.

To aid the healing process, surgical intervention may be necessary. *Tarsorrhaphy* (suturing the eyelid closed) promotes healing by decreasing eyelid blinking and by decreasing evaporation of the corneal tear film. For corneal perforation, a conjunctival flap may be performed to cover the defect. Tissue adhesive, a kind of "super glue," may also be used to seal the perforation. A soft contact lens may be used as a bandage to maintain the seal. Large perforations may require either lamellar (partial-thickness) or penetrating (full-thickness) keratoplasty.

When medical and surgical interventions fail, *enucleation* (removal of the entire eyeball) may be necessary (see Surgical Management under Ocular Melanoma). In some cases, *evisceration* (removal of orbital contents only) may be indicated. The scleral shell is left intact along with the ocular muscles, which allows for improved ocular prosthetic fit and function.

■ Nursing Management

Although the early stages of corneal infection are often managed at home, the client may need to be hospitalized for the management of a severe corneal ulcer. If the client and family have been instilling frequent eyedrops at home, the client may be fatigued from lack of sleep as well as anxious about possible loss of vision. Assess the client's level of discomfort and methods of coping with the stress of pain and lack of sleep. Often at this stage the client is not coping well at all. When eyedrops are given every 15 minutes around the clock, the schedule is a challenge not only for the client but for you as well. Hand-washing is particularly important in this situation and is carried out even if gloves are worn to instill the drops. The threat of losing eyesight compels many clients to watch the clock for fear that you will forget to administer the eyedrops. You can build the client's trust and reduce anxiety by scrupulous adherence to the time schedule.

The client's eye may need to be cleaned frequently because the medications and excessive tears will become dried and the lids will stick together. Warm tap water, applied with soft gauze pads, is used. The combination of tearing, medications, and cleaning may cause the skin of older clients to become excoriated. Antibiotic ophthalmic ointment may be applied to the lower lid margin and cheek to reduce irritation.

Effective sleep and rest are nearly impossible, with interruptions every 15 minutes. The client rarely reaches the deeper stages of sleep, and most experience restless, light sleep in stages 1 and 2. In addition to the eye pain the client may already be experiencing, some eyedrops, such as fortified bacitracin, may cause stinging that lasts several minutes.

You can institute several measures to comfort the client. Outline a daily routine of care, based as much as possible on the client's normal routine at home. Because there are many interruptions to the client's personal time and space, identify at least two periods during the day when the client may rest or nap, with the only interruption being the nurse who comes in to administer the eyedrops. Post a sign on the door to the client's room for privacy during these rest times. You and the client may also agree that you will not open topics of conversation during this time but will quietly

instill the eyedrops. Adopt this same routine during the client's normal nighttime. Some clients are actually able to sleep during instillation of eyedrops at night; however, establish this routine with the client in advance. Older clients, who are accustomed to more stage 2 sleep than younger clients, are able to rest more effec- tively. Because younger clients tend to become confused and irritable more often, speak to the client before touching him or her. Oral analgesics are given at regular intervals, and mild sleeping medications may be helpful at bedtime.

Clients usually become adapted to this regimen of interruptions after the first 48 hours. As the cornea begins to show improvement, the eyedrops may be reduced in frequency to every 30 minutes and then to every hour. Most clients do not notice a great deal of difference in the every-30-minutes routine, but when the routine is reduced to every hour, they begin to sleep more heavily as the body attempts to compensate for lost sleep. At the end of an hour, the client may complain to you that it has seemed like only a few minutes since the last interruption. Intense dreaming may also be experienced during this time.

■ Self-Care

At discharge from the facility, the client should be able to demonstrate how to instill eyedrops properly. The client will also understand the importance of complying with the medication regimen. Instruct the client and family about the clinical manifestations of increasing infections. The eye may continue to be cleaned with warm tap water at home. Assess the home environment if the client's vision is greatly reduced. Referrals for rehabilitation also may be necessary.

■ UVEAL TRACT DISORDERS: UVEITIS

Uveitis is an inflammation of the uveal tract that can affect one or more parts (iris, ciliary body, choroid). Uveitis commonly occurs in its acute form from a hypersensitivity reaction or in its chronic form following microbial infection. Clients complain of pain, blurred vision, and photophobia. There is marked redness of the eye, and the pupil is usually constricted. Cells (white blood cells) and flare (protein), called an *anterior chamber reaction,* are seen in the anterior chamber fluid with the slit lamp.

The primary cause of discomfort in clients with uveitis is ciliary body muscle spasm. A cycloplegic medication such as atropine effectively relieves the spasm, and the dilation of the pupil prevents the inflamed iris from adhering to the lens and the corneal endothelium from forming synechiae. Topical steroid drops are prescribed to reduce the inflammation.

MALIGNANT OCULAR TUMORS OCULAR MELANOMA

Although fewer than 1% of the people in the United States are affected by malignant ocular tumors, treatment of these tumors can be a challenge for both client and nurse. Choroidal melanomas are often detected during a routine ocular examination because there is no pain associated with the development of the tumor. By the time the tumor has grown large enough to obstruct vision, there may be involvement of the macula and metastasis.

Outcome Management

The goal of treatment is to care for the malignancy while preserving the eye.

■ Medical Management

When ocular melanoma is discovered early, radiation therapy alone may be the treatment of choice. Radiation therapy to the eye is accomplished through insertion of a tiny plate or plaque about the size of a dime that holds tiny seeds of radioactive iodine 125. The plaque is sutured to the sclera directly over the site of the tumor. It is left in place for several days, depending on the required dose, and then removed. Both insertion and removal are performed in the operating room. During treatment a lead shield is placed over the eye. Radiation exposure to the nurse who cares for the client is minimal—a small fraction of a chest x-ray study. Despite this extremely low exposure, the routine restrictions for hospital personnel and visitors are implemented for the sake of consistency. Hospitalization for treatment with radioactive iodine is required, depending on regulations.

During the client's hospitalization for this treatment, provide support and encouragement for the client. The plaque is only mildly to moderately uncomfortable, and discomfort should be relieved with acetaminophen. The difficult challenge for clients is confinement to their room with limitations on visitors at a time when support is essential. Eye medications include a cycloplegic agent and an antibiotic-steroid eyedrop.

■ Surgical Management

Enucleation. The goal of surgical removal is to preserve life by removing the tumor. Removal of the entire eyeball (*enucleation*) has been the traditional method of treatment and may be combined with radiation treatments. *Exenteration* (removal of the eyeball and surrounding tissues and bone) may also be necessary. The goal for clients following enucleation is adaptation to monocular vision and return to their former level of independence.

Enucleation is usually performed with the client under general anesthesia, but IV conscious sedation may also be used. The ocular muscles are dissected from the eyeball, which is removed by severing the optic nerve and vessels at the back. An acrylic sphere covered by donor scleral tissue is usually placed within the capsule of tissue that formerly held the eyeball. Scleral tissue encourages fibrovascular ingrowth, which prevents migration and extrusion of the implant. A soft plastic scleral shell is placed in the visible outer portion of the socket as a support until a permanent prosthesis can be made. A newer type of implant, hydroxyapatite, which is made of the same inorganic material present in human bone, is now being used.

Several weeks later a central hole is drilled into the sphere and covering tissues. A peg (which later fits into a depression on the posterior surface of the artificial eye) is then inserted into the hole. The movement of the implant by the muscle cone is transferred directly to the prosthesis. With the artificial eye being primarily supported by the peg instead of the lids and socket tissues, fewer cosmetic and structural complications occur.

■ Nursing Management

The client undergoing enucleation for a malignant tumor is stressed not only by the threat of cancer but also by disfigurement of the face. Assess the client's response, home, and family for support mechanisms. Nursing interventions are focused on assisting the client to grieve for the lost body part and lost vision and to identify coping mechanisms that will facilitate rehabilitation.

Preoperative Care

Assist the client in preparing for the surgical procedure. Most often the client is made aware of the tumor at a routine office visit. Surgery is usually scheduled within a few days. Recognizing that the client is most appropriately in a state of shock and denial, carefully explain the perioperative events. Although it is possible to have an enucleation as an outpatient procedure, the client may stay overnight in the hospital.

Postoperative Care

Provide routine postoperative care. The client returns from the operating room with a pressure dressing over the eye. Assess the dressing for bleeding using standard postoperative routines. Clients are understandably anxious about the removal of the dressing the next morning. Prepare the client by explaining how the eye and conformer will appear. The socket and lids will be swollen, and the white plastic conformer is visible. Determine the client's or the family's ability to care for the wound postoperatively.

Some clients fear that their appearance will frighten others, especially children. In this case, an eye patch may be worn during the 4 to 6 weeks before the prosthesis is fitted but should not be worn continuously. Eventually the eye prosthesis can be worn and looks pleasingly nor-

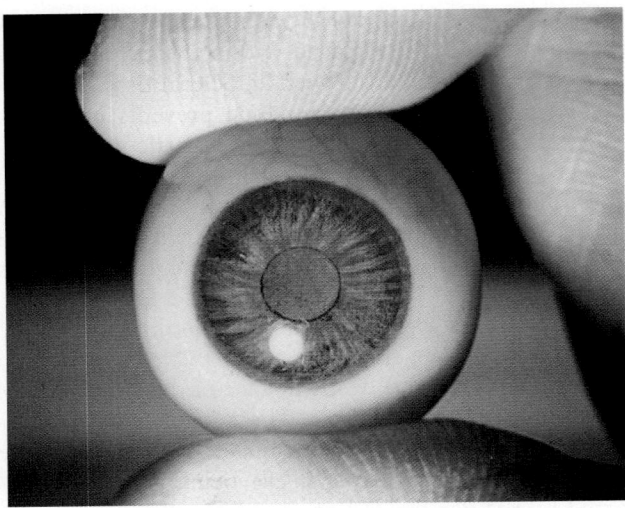

FIGURE 67-10 An ocular prosthesis. (Courtesy of Ophthalmic Photography at the University of Michigan W.K. Kellogg Eye Center, Ann Arbor.)

mal (Figure 67-10). Refer to a fundamentals of nursing textbook for insertion and removal of the prosthesis.

The area around the lids may be cleaned with warm tap water with a clean washcloth. Soap and water should be kept away from the socket. If the plastic conformer accidentally comes out, it should be washed and replaced. Antibiotic ophthalmic ointment is usually ordered to be instilled in the socket once or twice a day.

■ Self-Care

Adjustment to monocular vision is a challenge the client begins to face immediately. Depth perception is altered, and the client needs to exercise caution in walking, crossing streets, and driving. Advise the client to practice ADLs until visual and body adjustments are made.

Emphasize the need for extra precaution with the remaining eye. Eye protection should be worn when engaging in any activity that might even remotely result in an injury. Many clients are advised to wear glasses even if no correction is needed.

■ EYELID TUMORS

Basal cell and squamous cell carcinomas of the lids are the most common malignant tumors of the eyelids. These tumors appear more frequently in people with a fair complexion who have had chronic exposure to the sun. Malignant lid tumors are most often (90% to 95%) of the basal cell type and frequently appear on the lower lid as nodules that gradually enlarge, becoming scaly and ulcerated. Benign tumors of the lids are common and often increase in frequency as people age. *Melanocytic nevi* (moles) and *verrucae* (warts) commonly appear on the lids and lid margins. Xanthelasma appears as yellow,

wrinkled patches, which are actually lipid deposits under the skin of the eyelids. These benign lesions may be removed for cosmetic reasons. Malignant tumors may be removed and treated by various methods, such as electrodesiccation, cryotherapy, and surgery. When the tumor is large, reconstruction may be required.

■ EYELID, LACRIMAL, AND CONJUNCTIVAL DISORDERS
DRY EYE SYNDROME

Dry eye syndrome is a condition in which tear production is inadequate. It most commonly occurs in women between 50 and 60 years of age. Three primary causes are lacrimal gland malfunction, mucin deficiency, and mechanical abnormalities that prevent the spread of tears across the surface of the eye. The lacrimal gland can be genetically malformed or malformed because of injury or infection. Tear production is also decreased in Sjögren's syndrome, an autoimmune disorder that commonly accompanies rheumatoid arthritis. Facial nerve (seventh cranial nerve) palsy disrupts tear production. Mechanical abnormalities include problems with eyelid structure, eyeball extrusion, and misuse of contact lenses. Conjunctivitis and mumps can obstruct the gland. Some medications, such as antihistamines, atropine, and beta-adrenergic blocking agents, decrease tear production.

Manifestations include burning, itching eyes and a sensation of "something" in the eye. The term *keratoconjunctivitis sicca* is used to describe the problem.

Management includes determining the degree of injury to the cornea. Artificial tears (eyedrops and lubricants) can be used. In addition, some clients benefit from using airtight goggles at night to prevent tear evaporation. Postmenopausal women have found some relief from estrogen replacement. Surgery can be used to open the lacrimal duct or to repair lid problems.

Other eyelid, lacrimal, and conjunctival disorders are discussed in Table 67-2.

■ REFRACTIVE DISORDERS

Light is bent (refracted) as it passes through the cornea and lens of the eye. Refractive errors exist when light rays are not focused appropriately on the retina of the eye. Three basic abnormalities of refraction occur in the eye: (1) myopia, (2) hyperopia, and (3) astigmatism. Optical correction is important to distinguish between visual loss caused by disease and visual loss caused by refractive error. *Refractometry* is the measurement of refractive error and should not be confused with *refraction*, the method used to determine which lens or lenses (if any) will most benefit the client.

TABLE 67-2 *Eyelid, Lacrimal, and Conjunctival Disorders*

Disorder	Definition	Appearance	Management
Dacryocystitis	Inflammation of lacrimal gland		Antibiotics, daily massage of the lacrimal system
Hordeolum (stye)	Infection of glands of eyelids	Redness and swelling of a localized area of the eyelid	Warm compresses and antibiotics; may need to be incised and drained
Chalazion	Chronic granuloma of meibomian gland	Painless, localized swelling of the lid margin	If cosmetically distracting, may be surgically removed
Blepharitis	Chronic, bilateral inflammation of eyelids	Itching and burning of the eyes, eyes appear red, scales noted on the lashes	Wash eyelids with baby shampoo, water, and cotton-tipped applicators; antibiotic ointments may be prescribed
Conjunctivitis	Inflammation of conjunctiva from various microorganisms	Redness, tearing, and exudation of eyelid; may progress to eyelid drooping, abnormal tissue growth	Antibiotic eye drops
Entropion	Turning in eyelid margin	Inversion of lower eyelid; dry and irritated eyes	Surgical resection
Ptosis	Drooping of eyelid from several causes	Irritation of eye caused by drying, loss of tears	Artificial tears; surgical correction needed; sometimes glasses used to lift redundant skin
Lagophthalmos	Inadequate closure of eyelids	Irritation of eye caused by drying	Artificial tears, eye shields at night; surgical correction
Absence of blinking	Lack of blinking seen with Parkinson's disease and hyperthyroidism	Blinking fewer than 20 times a minute	Artificial tears; eye shields at night

MYOPIA

Myopia, or *nearsightedness*, is a condition in which the light rays come into focus in front of the retina (Figure 67-11, *A*). In this case the refractive power of the eye is too strong and a concave, or minus, lens is used to focus light rays on the eye. In most cases myopia is caused by an eyeball that is longer than normal, which may be a familial trait. Transient myopia may occur with the administration of a variety of medications (sulfonamides, acetazolamide, salicylates, and steroids) and has been associated with other disorders, such as influenza, typhoid fever, severe dehydration, and large intakes of antacids (for stomach ulcers). Correction is accomplished with eyeglasses or contact lenses.

HYPEROPIA

The hyperopic, or *farsighted*, eye focuses light rays behind the eye, and consequently the image that falls on the retina is blurred (see Figure 67-11, *B*). Vision may be brought into focus by placing a convex, or plus, lens in front of the eye. The lens supplies the magnifying power that the eye is lacking. Hyperopia may be caused by an eyeball that is shorter than normal or a cornea that has less curvature than normal. Because children have a greater ability to accommodate, they are less often affected than adults. Demands for close work and reading usually bring on manifestations of headache or eyestrain. Correction is based on a person's age and individual needs and complaints.

ASTIGMATISM

Astigmatism is a refractive condition in which rays of light are not bent equally by the cornea in all directions so that a point of focus is not attained (see Figure 67-11, *C*). In most instances, astigmatism is caused because the curvature of the cornea is not perfectly spherical. This is the cause of poor vision for both distant and near objects. Astigmatism is corrected with cylindrical lenses.

■ Surgical Management

The following are the three main types of refractive surgery and a new procedure.

Laser in situ keratomileusis (LASIK) is currently the most commonly used corrective surgery for nearsightedness in the United States. An extremely thin layer of the cornea is peeled back for the laser reshaping on the middle layer of the cornea and then put back in place. There

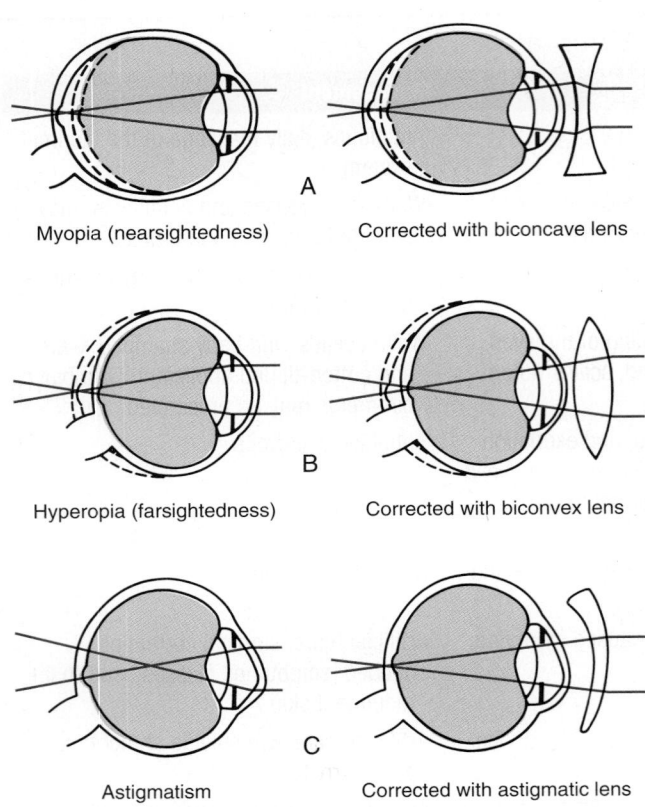

Myopia (nearsightedness) — Corrected with biconcave lens

A

Hyperopia (farsightedness) — Corrected with biconvex lens

B

Astigmatism — Corrected with astigmatic lens

C

FIGURE 67-11 A-C, Common refractive disorders and their correction. *Dashed lines* in **A** and **B** indicate normal eye contour.

is little postoperative discomfort, rapid recovery of clear vision, and quick stabilization of refractive change. LASIK is performed in a surgeon's office or same-day surgery center and does not require a hospital stay. It takes about 10 to 15 minutes per eye. It has a high success rate and low complication rate for low to moderate nearsightedness and may also be used to correct more severe nearsightedness.

Excimer laser photorefractive keratectomy (PRK) uses short-wavelength, high-energy ultraviolet radiation lasers to reshape the corneal surface. In PRK for myopia, the central cornea is flattened with the excimer laser. The same laser may be used to reshape the cornea by making the central curvature steeper to correct hyperopia. It may be used to correct nearsightedness and astigmatism at the same time. PRK is performed on an outpatient basis in a surgeon's office or same-day surgery center. The PRK procedure takes about 30 minutes, most of which is spent teaching the client to hold the eye still. The actual treatment takes less than a minute. Recovery from PRK is longer and more painful than recovery from either radial keratotomy (RK) or LASIK. Vision will be reduced for several days after surgery.

Radial keratotomy (RK) involves making tiny cuts in the cornea, which flatten it and reduce nearsightedness.

In people who have both astigmatism and nearsightedness, the surgeon may make additional cuts to flatten the misshapen part of the cornea that is causing the astigmatism. RK is an outpatient procedure. It is done under local or topical anesthesia in a surgeon's office or same-day surgery center. The operation on one eye takes about 10 to 15 minutes, and the entire process usually takes less than 2 hours, including preparation time, postoperative care, and paperwork. RK is successful and safe for people who have mild to moderate nearsightedness (less than 3 diopters). Although it is still used in some cases, it has been mostly replaced by LASIK and PRK.

Corneal ring implants are clear pieces of acrylic that can be surgically implanted into the cornea. The implants flatten the cornea and thereby reduce nearsightedness. The implants are shaped like crescents or half-circles. Two implants are used for each eye, and the implants are inserted along the sides of the cornea (*corneal periphery*). They do not cover the central portion of the cornea. Corneal ring implants appear to be very effective for correcting mild nearsightedness.

■ Nursing Management of the Surgical Client

Clients are assessed preoperatively for degree of myopia or astigmatism. Clients with a severe case usually cannot achieve full correction. Surgery is performed on an outpatient basis with local anesthesia. Eye protection is used, such as goggles to prevent dry eyes. Vigorous activities, activities that could get water in the eye, and eye makeup are to be avoided.

The eye is treated with steroid eyedrops, and most clients report watering of the eyes and minimal pain. Refraction slowly stabilizes after surgery. There is a period of adjustment during which visual acuity waxes and wanes. Reduced contrast sensitivity in night vision and daytime glare is common. Some clients require re-treatment for scarring that is unresponsive to topical steroids.

OCULAR MANIFESTATIONS OF SYSTEMIC DISORDERS ENDOCRINE DISORDERS: GRAVES' DISEASE

Graves' disease may exist with or without any clinical evidence of thyroid dysfunction. Ocular manifestations include retraction of both upper and lower lids, resulting in a staring or frightened expression (Stellwag's sign), and lid lag (Graefe's sign), the retarded lowering of the upper lid when looking down (Figure 67-12). When the gaze is changed from down to up, the globe then lags behind the upper lid. Other signs are infrequent blinking, marked fine tremor with lid closure, and jerky movements on lid opening.

The globes enlarge because of the increased size of extraocular muscles, edema of tissues, and excess orbital

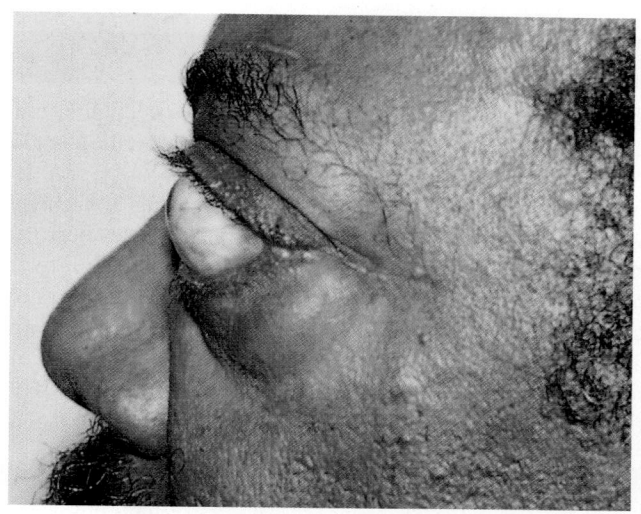

FIGURE 67-12 Graves' exophthalmos. (Courtesy of Ophthalmic Photography at the University of Michigan W.K. Kellogg Eye Center, Ann Arbor.)

fat. The eye develops *proptosis* (forward protrusion of the eyeballs), which is called *exophthalmos*. Subsequent degeneration of muscle tissue leads to fibrosis, which restricts muscle movement, resulting in double vision.

Outcome Management

As a primary measure, adequate control of thyroid abnormalities is essential. Diuretics as well as steroid therapy and radiotherapy may be indicated. Surgical interventions include corrective lid surgery and tarsorrhaphy for lid retraction to protect the cornea. Decompression of the orbit, which usually involves removal of the inferior and medial walls of the orbit, may be necessary to accommodate proliferative orbital fat and enlarged ocular muscles. Ocular muscle surgery may also be indicated. If the surgery is extensive, suction drains may be placed at the operative sites. Drainage is usually serosanguineous. It is important that the client sleep with the head elevated to reduce postoperative swelling.

Advise the client to expect redness, swelling, and ecchymoses around the eyes and lids. In the immediate postoperative period, check the client's visual acuity with a near vision card every hour to monitor the possibility of pressure on the optic nerve (see Thinking Critically). Caution the client to modify normal activities for the first 2 weeks after surgery.

RHEUMATOID AND CONNECTIVE TISSUE DISORDERS

Sjögren's syndrome includes keratoconjunctivitis sicca, a common condition in which tear secretion is reduced in association with a systemic disorder such as rheumatoid arthritis, psoriatic arthritis, connective tissue disorders,

sarcoidosis, or Crohn's disease. Manifestations include ocular irritation and foreign-body sensation. Frequent instillation of lubricating eyedrops or ointment is effective in most cases.

Several ocular problems may be associated with systemic lupus erythematosus (SLE), a connective tissue disorder. The eyelids may be involved, with the discoid lesions characteristic of the disease. Punctate epithelial keratopathy and secondary Sjögren's syndrome may also occur. Retinopathy of SLE produces cotton-wool spots and increased retinal vessel fragility, as in diabetes. Optic neuropathy can also occur.

NEUROLOGIC DISORDERS

About 90% of clients with myasthenia gravis have ocular involvement. In most cases it is the presenting manifestation. *Ptosis* (drooping of the eyelid) is bilateral but may be asymmetrical. Diplopia is frequently in the vertical plane. Nystagmus is also present. Ocular myopathy and cranial nerve palsy may develop later, as may ophthalmoplegia (paralysis of all extraocular muscles). Medical treatment is supportive and includes systemic steroids.

There is also a close association between optic neuritis and multiple sclerosis. About three fourths of women and one third of men with optic neuritis have multiple sclerosis at 15-year follow-up. Typically an attack of optic neuritis starts with acute onset of loss of vision in one eye, with periocular discomfort made worse by movement of the eye. Visual impairment is progressive over 2 weeks and usually resolves after 4 to 6 weeks. Recovery may take longer and may be incomplete. Medical treatment consists of oral, IV, and retrobulbar steroids.

CIRCULATORY DISORDERS

The primary response of retinal arterioles to hypertension is a narrowing. In clients with chronic hypertension, the blood-retina barrier is disrupted in small areas, resulting in increased vascular permeability. Funduscopic examination reveals vasoconstriction, leakage, and arteriosclerosis. Hypertensive retinopathy is graded for severity on a scale of 1 to 4, with 4 the most severe. Systemic hypertension is also associated with an increased risk of retinal vein occlusion. There is no known treatment for retinal vein occlusion.

IMMUNOLOGIC DISORDERS

Ocular complications occur frequently in clients with acquired immunodeficiency syndrome (AIDS). In many cases, it is the presenting ocular manifestations that lead to diagnosis of human immunodeficiency virus (HIV) infection. Cytomegalovirus (CMV) retinitis is the most common opportunistic ocular infection. This sight-threatening condition is often asymptomatic until it is well established, when the client begins to notice visual field loss, "floaters," or other vague vision problems. A unilateral lesion with the appearance of a cotton-wool spot often develops with white irregular borders associated with hemorrhages. Small lesions may be seen beyond the edges. The retina in the center of the lesion becomes thin and tears easily. Loss of vision is involved and central vision is greatly diminished.

Clients with CMV retinitis require long-term IV therapy. Because progression is rapid, early treatment is essential and may prevent involvement of the other eye. Careful monitoring of side effects and response to the medication is imperative.

Other infectious ocular conditions that may occur in people with HIV disease are bacterial corneal ulcers (syphilis, staphylococcosis), fungal corneal ulcers (candidiasis, cryptococcosis, histoplasmosis, sporotrichosis), and protozoan (toxoplasmosis, pneumocystosis) and viral infections (herpes simplex).

Noninfectious ocular manifestations in people with HIV infection include HIV retinopathy and neoplastic processes such as Kaposi's sarcoma and non-Hodgkin's lymphoma, which appear around the ocular adnexa. Direct ophthalmoscopy reveals the presence of cotton-wool spots, retinal hemorrhages, and other microvascular anomalies. The lesions of AIDS retinopathy are indistinguishable from the retinopathy of diabetes or hypertension. They usually occur in the superficial retina and resolve over a period of a few weeks, whereas CMV retinitis lesions will expand. Kaposi's sarcoma and non-Hodgkin's lymphoma present around the eyelids and orbit with diplopia, ptosis, conjunctival edema, or hemorrhage. Diagnosis is confirmed with imaging, needle biopsy, and systemic work-up. Treatment of Kaposi's sarcoma is usually conservative and may include radiotherapy.

LYME DISEASE

Lyme disease *(Borrelia burgdorferi)*, transmitted by the bite of a tick, consists of three stages. The initial stage involves a lesion and erythema around the bite, accompanied by regional lymphadenopathy, malaise, fever, headache, myalgia, arthralgia, and frequently conjunctivitis. Several weeks to months later, the second phase is associated with neurologic and cardiac problems. Along with these problems, there may be cranial nerve palsies, uveitis, optic neuropathy, keratitis, choroiditis, and exudative retinal detachments. Rheumatologic complications may develop in the third stage, which may occur over several years. Tetracycline and penicillin are effective in treating the initial infection and in preventing late complications.

CONCLUSIONS

To provide comprehensive nursing care for clients, it is essential to understand the complexity of ocular structures and the physiology of vision. The specialty practice of ophthalmic nursing is devoted to caring for clients with eye disorders. Ophthalmic registered nurses perform the roles of caregiver, advocate, educator, counselor, technician, coordinator, and researcher. Ophthalmic nursing care not only is directed at those biologic systems that are affected by an actual or potential deficit but also is an integration of how actual or potential visual deficits affect the individual as an entire being.

THINKING CRITICALLY *evolve*

1. Your client is a 72-year-old retired carpenter who has undergone outpatient cataract surgery. He and his wife live an hour away from the surgery center, where they received instructions to call the emergency number if any unusual pain or nausea occurs. They have an appointment to return for a follow-up evaluation the next morning. After supper the client's wife calls to report that her husband has a headache. She says that her husband also has an upset stomach, but she thinks he feels queasy because he ate some spicy food. The client does not want his wife to drive him back at night and thinks she should not have bothered to call because they have an appointment in the morning. How would you proceed? What further assessment data are needed? What are the likely complications following cataract surgery, and what are their clinical manifestations?

Factors to Consider. Might the headache and upset stomach be related to the cataract surgery, or are they likely to be unrelated?

2. Your client, a 55-year-old woman with Graves' ophthalmopathy, has undergone surgery in the late afternoon today for a right orbital decompression. An incisional drain is in place at the right temple with a bulb attached for suction. The surgeon has ordered postoperative vision checks with a near-vision card every hour throughout the night. The surgery lasted more than 3 hours; general anesthesia was used, and the client is still sedated. Her right eye is extremely swollen; she is unable to open it to read the vision card. She winces and cries when her operative eye is touched, and she is so sleepy that she cannot respond

by reading the vision card. What should you do to carry out the surgeon's postoperative orders?

Factors to Consider. Are such severe eye pain and swelling normal postoperative findings? How would you assess the eye? How would you rouse the client to perform these crucial eye assessments?

Discussions for these questions can be found on the website and the CD-ROM.

BIBLIOGRAPHY

1. Age Related Eye Disease Study. (2001). Age-related eye disease study: a randomized, placebo-controlled clinical trial for high dose supplementation with vitamins C, E, and beta carotene for AMD and vision loss. *Archives of Ophthalmology, 119*(10), 1417-1436.

2. Allen, P., & Shepherd, J. (1998). The ophthalmic registered nurse's responsibility to the adult patient with low vision. *Insight, 23*(2), 53.

3. Bresnick, G.H., et al. (2000). A screening approach to the surveillance of patients with diabetes for the presence of vision threatening retinopathy. *Ophthalmology, 107*(1), 19-24.

4. Cooper, J. (1999). Teaching patients in postoperative eye care: the demands of day surgery. *Nursing Standard, 13* (32), 42-46.

5. D'Ambrosio, F. (1999). Assessing disability in the patient with cataracts. *Current Opinion in Ophthalmology, 10*(1), 42.

5a. Diabetic retinopathy. *Diabetes Care, 25*(1), 590-593.

6. Elfervig, L.S., & Elfervig, J.L. (2001). Proliferative diabetic retinopathy. *Insight, 26*(3), 88-93.

7. Elfervig, L.S., & Elfervig, J.L. (1999). Endophthalmitis. *Insight, 24*(3), 99-103.

8. El-Shazly, M., Zeid, M., & Osman, A. (2000). Risk factors for eye complications in patients with diabetes mellitus: development and progression. *Eastern Mediterranean Health Journal, 6*(2/3) 313-325.

9. Emery, J. (1999). Capsular opacification after cataract surgery. *Current Opinion in Ophthalmology, 10*(1), 42.

10. Fishbaugh, J. (1995). Look who's driving now? Visual standards for driver's licensing in the United States. *Insight, 20*(4), 11-20.

11. Garvican, L., Cloves, J., & Gillow, T. (2000). Preservation of sight in diabetes: Developing a national risk reduction program. *Diabetic Medicine, 17*(9), 627-634

12. Goldblum, K. (Ed.). (2002). *Ophthalmic nursing core curriculum.* Dubuque, IA: Kendall Publishing.

13. Halle, C. (2002). Achieve new vision screening objectives. *Nurse Practitioner, 27*(3), 21-22, 25-26.

14. Kanski, J. (1999). *Clinical ophthalmology* (4th ed.). Oxford: Butterworth Heinemann.

15. O'Day, B. (1999). Employment barriers for people with visual impairments. *Journal of Visual Impairment and Blindness, 93*(10), 627-642.

16. Oetting, T.A. (2001). A paradigm shift in cataract surgery: less for the surgeon to do—more for the nurse and technicians to do. *Insight 26*(1), 23-30.

17. Rich, D., Lane, A.M., & Miller, J.W. (2001). Photodynamic therapy—the nurses' role. *Insight 26*(2), 44-48.

18. Rowen, S. (1999). Preoperative and postoperative medications used for cataract surgery. *Current Opinion in Ophthalmology, 10*(1), 29.

19. Smith, S. (2001). The dry eye: an introduction. *Plastic Surgical Nursing, 21*(3), 135-140.

20. Smith, S. (1999). Non-proliferative diabetic retinopathy and macular edema. *Insight, 24*(2), 59-64.

21. Stewart, W. (1999). Perspectives in the medical treatment of glaucoma. *Current Opinion in Ophthalmology, 10*(2), 99.

22. Ticho, B.H., & Dreger, V. (2000). Enuculeation: indications, methods and prosthetic devices. *Insight, 25*(1), 23-28.

23. Vader, L. (1996). The significance of cultural values in vision loss. *American Black Nurses Foundation Journal, 1*(3), 69-71.

24. Vader, L. (2000). Ophthalmic nursing. In N. Burden (Ed.), *Ambulatory surgery nursing.* Philadelphia: W.B. Saunders.

25. Vaughan, D., Asbury, T., & Riordan-Eva, P. (1999). *General ophthalmology* (15th ed.). Norwalk, CT: Appleton & Lange.

26. Whitaker, R., & Whitaker, V. (1999). Glaucoma: What the ophthalmic nurse should know. *Insight, 24*(3), 86.

Management of Clients with Hearing and Balance Disorders

Helene J. Krouse

evolve

Web Enhancements

Care Plan
    The Client with Vertigo
Client Education Guide
    Infection of the Tympanic Membrane, Middle Ear, or Mastoid
    Cavity (English Version and Spanish Translation)

http://evolve.elsevier.com/Black/medsurg/

Precautions After Ear Surgery (Spanish Translation)
Appendix C
Laboratory Values of Clinical Importance in Medical-Surgical
Nursing

HEARING IMPAIRMENT

Hearing impairment ranges from minor difficulty in understanding words or hearing certain sounds to total deafness. Hearing impairment is the nation's primary disability: 1 in 15 Americans is affected. By the year 2050, about one in five clients in the United States will be 55 years or older; of these estimated 58 million people, 26 million are expected to have hearing impairment. Of the 10 million people in the United States with a hearing loss who are now 65 years or older, more than 90% have a sensorineural hearing loss. Because of fear, misinformation, lack of information, and vanity, many clients do not admit that they have a hearing problem. Up to 80% of all hearing impairments are caused by hearing nerve disorders, for which no cure is currently available. Hearing impairments diminish the quality of life for a third of adults between 65 and 75 years of age.

Etiology and Risk Factors

Many factors influence the type and amount of hearing loss. Hearing loss is not an actual disorder but is a clinical manifestation of many possible problems. Both common and uncommon causes of hearing impairment are examined in this chapter. Hearing loss can be classified into three main areas:

- Conductive hearing loss (i.e., otosclerosis, trauma)
- Sensorineural hearing loss (i.e., presbycusis, noise-induced, and sudden hearing loss)
- Mixed hearing loss

Conductive hearing loss results from interference of sound transmission through the external ear and middle ear. It may be caused by (1) anything that blocks the external ear, such as wax, infection, or a foreign body; (2) thickening, retraction, scarring, or perforation of the tympanic membrane; or (3) any pathophysiologic changes in the middle ear that affect or freeze one or more of the ossicles (Figure 68-1).

Sensorineural hearing loss is caused by impairment of the function of the inner ear, the eighth cranial nerve, or the brain. Causes are congenital and hereditary factors, noise injury, aging and degenerative processes, Ménière's disease, and ototoxicity. Systemic disorders, such as autoimmune disease, syphilis, certain collagen disorders, and diabetes, may cause sensorineural hearing losses. Most recently, cigarette smoking and exposure to environmental tobacco smoke have been associated with age-related hearing loss.

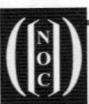

Nursing Outcomes Classification (NOC)
for Nursing Diagnoses—Clients with Hearing and Balance Disorders

Acute Pain
  Comfort Level
  Pain Control
  Pain: Disruptive Effects
  Pain Level
Deficient Knowledge
  Knowledge of Treatment Regimen
Disturbed Sensory Perception: Auditory
  Hearing Compensation Behavior
  Risk Control: Hearing Impairment
Impaired Adjustment
  Acceptance: Health Status
  Participation: Health Care Decisions
  Psychosocial Adjustment: Life Change
  Self-Esteem
  Social Support

Impaired Social Interaction
  Communication Ability
  Social Involvement
Impaired Verbal Communication
  Communication Ability
  Communication Ability: Expressive Ability
Ineffective Coping
  Caregiver Stressors
  Coping
  Quality of Life
  Role Performance
  Social Interaction Skills
  Social Support
Nausea
  Comfort Level
  Hydration

Nutritional Status: Food and Fluid Intake
  Symptom Severity
Risk for Infection
  Immune Status
  Immunization Behavior
  Knowledge: Infection Control
  Risk Control
  Risk Detection
Risk for Injury
  Risk Control: Hearing Impairment
  Safety Behavior: Fall Prevention
Risk for Loneliness
  Family Coping
  Loneliness
  Social Involvement

In a *mixed hearing loss,* conductive and sensorineural hearing components are present simultaneously. A client with a perforated eardrum and presbycusis has both conductive and sensorineural hearing losses.

Conductive Hearing Loss

Ear Obstructions. Obstruction of the ear is most commonly caused by impacted cerumen. Although the ear canal is self-cleaning, cerumen may become impacted from a disorder or from improper cleaning. Older people are more susceptible to cerumen impaction because hair in the ear becomes coarser with age and traps the wax. Some people produce more cerumen in the ear canal and require a regular routine for eliminating excessive buildup of wax in the ear canal. Insertion of cotton-tipped swabs into the ear canal can create further impaction of ear wax or can even traumatize the ear canal or perforate the eardrum.

Ear obstruction can also be caused by a wide array of foreign bodies that fit into the ear canal and impede conduction of sound waves. The most common foreign bodies found in the adult ear are pieces of cotton and insects. Foreign bodies commonly seen in children consist of small toys, beads, insects, and food, such as kernels of corn. Teach clients to avoid inserting hard instruments into the ear and to avoid obstructing the ear canal with objects.

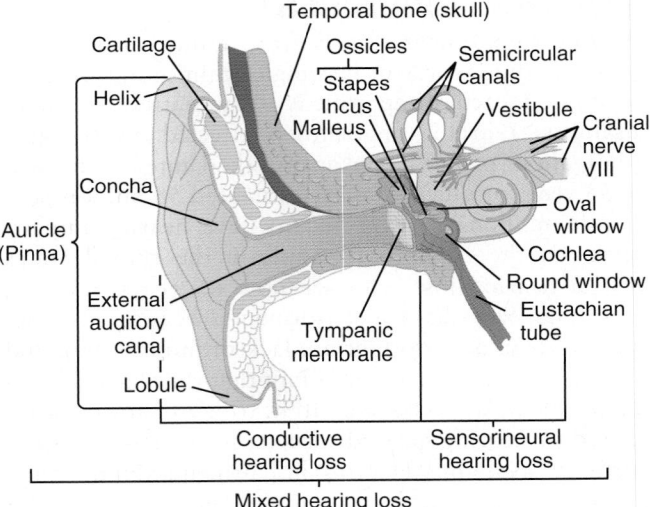

FIGURE 68-1 Hearing loss can result from three causes. Conductive hearing loss occurs in areas of the outer ear when sound is conducted. Sensorineural hearing loss occurs in the inner ear where sound is transmitted by the nerves. In addition, both types can be present, called mixed hearing loss.

Infection. Many infections can lead to hearing loss. An infection of the inner ear, called *labyrinthitis,* can be either viral or bacterial in origin. Viral labyrinthitis can be associated with recent respiratory tract infections, measles, mumps, or rubella. Bacterial labyrinthitis, which is rare, is associated with otitis media or meningitis. Otitis media is a common disorder of the middle ear. Repeated infections or allergic inflammation can lead to fluid accumulation behind the eardrum, causing dampening of the sound being conducted to the inner ear. In addition, drainage, perforation, or scarring of the tympanic membrane can result in a conductive hearing loss. Otitis media and other infectious ear processes are discussed later in the chapter under Otalgia.

Otosclerosis. *Otosclerosis,* or hardening of the inner ear, is a genetic disorder in which repeated resorption and redeposition of abnormal bone gradually leads to fixation of the footplate of the stapes in the oval window (Figure 68-2, *A*). The immobility of the footplate prevents transmission of sound vibration into the inner ear, leading to conductive hearing loss. This disorder occurs twice as often in women and is 10 times more prevalent in whites. The disorder is autosomally dominant with variable penetrance and therefore can be transmitted to offspring if only one parent has the disorder.

Tympanosclerosis. Tympanosclerosis is the result of repeated infection and trauma to the tympanic membrane. It consists of a deposit of collagen and calcium within the middle ear that can harden around the ossicles, causing a conductive hearing loss. Tympanosclerotic deposits can also be found mounded in the middle ear or as plaque on the tympanic membrane.

Trauma to the Tympanic Membrane. The tympanic membrane can be damaged by trauma. Increased pressure from a hand slap, falling in water, sports injuries, cleaning the ear with a sharp instrument, and industrial accidents involving welding sparks can rupture the thin membrane. Trauma to the tympanic membrane from a blast or blunt injury can involve the middle ear, causing a fracture or dislocation of the ossicles and tearing of the tympanic membrane. Also, the facial nerve is vulnerable to trauma. A basilar skull fracture involves the temporal bone and, depending on the fracture site, causes ossicular damage as well as facial nerve paralysis and sensorineural hearing loss. Care of clients with facial fracture is discussed in Chapter 51. When the tympanic membrane is perforated, infection is a concern.

Sensorineural Hearing Loss

Presbycusis. Presbycusis is a progressive hearing loss found predominantly in older people. This degenerative process involves changes in the labyrinthine structures over time. The client initially experiences a decrease in high-frequency sound. At times, *tinnitus,* or the perception of noise in the ear, accompanies this decline in hearing.

Sudden Hearing Loss. Sudden (idiopathic) hearing loss (SHL) is a fairly common condition in which the client

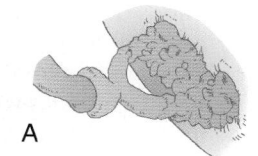

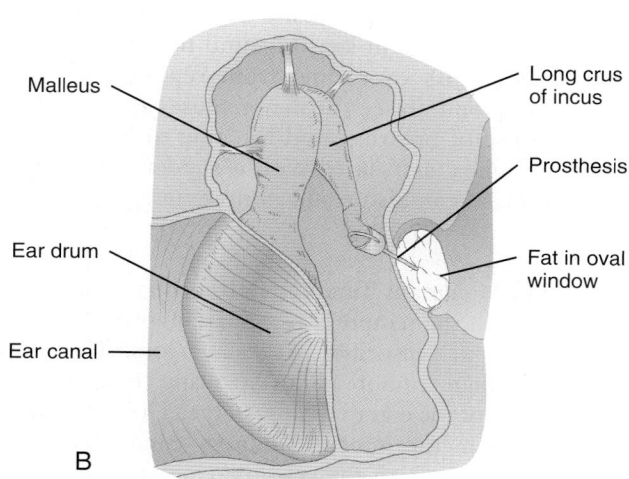

FIGURE 68-2 A, Stapedial otosclerosis. A chain of three ossicles connects the tympanic membrane to the oval window and cochlea. Otosclerosis knits the bone of the middle ear to the stapes, preventing sound transmission from the eardrum to the middle ear. **B,** Stapedectomy removes the ankylosed bone and replaces it.

loses hearing in an ear within minutes or hours. This condition is almost exclusively unilateral. Although the exact cause of sudden sensorineural hearing loss has not been determined, postmortem examinations of temporal bones suggest that the disease involves a viral infection of the inner ear. Prompt early intervention with oral corticosteroids has been shown to at least partially restore the lost hearing in many clients with sudden hearing loss. In the United States alone, about 4000 new cases of sudden hearing loss are reported annually.

Sensorineural hearing loss of abrupt onset can sometimes occur from discrete causes. Some of these specific causes are (1) rapid infectious processes, such as meningitis or mumps; (2) ototoxic agents; (3) trauma; (4) metabolic disturbances; and (5) immunologic disorders. In most cases of SHL, however, no specific cause is found.

Congenital Hearing Loss. Congenital episodes of sensorineural hearing loss are not uncommon. These losses can be severe and present at birth or can develop during childhood or early adulthood and gradually worsen with time. Congenital hearing loss often results in total deafness. It can occur either in a genetic pattern within families or spontaneously. Both autosomal-recessive and autosomal-dominant methods of transmission have been documented. In milder cases of congenital hearing loss, the individual may not be aware of a loss until hearing is screened for work or school. In families with a history of congenital hearing loss, infant screening is essential to allow early detection of the problem and rehabilitation of congenitally deaf infants.

Noise-Induced Hearing Loss. Noise-induced hearing loss is a specific type of sensorineural hearing loss that most often occurs over time from repeated acoustic trauma from loud noise. The major causes are industrial noise, the use of firearms, and listening to loud music. Traumatic injury associated with a sudden loud noise, such as a blast, can also result in noise-induced hearing loss.

Benign and Malignant Tumors. Both benign and malignant tumors of the temporal bone can involve the inner ear and lead to sensorineural hearing loss. The most common benign tumor is an acoustic neuroma or schwannoma of the eighth cranial nerve. The tumor usually develops in the internal auditory canal, the bony channel through which the vestibular nerve passes as it leaves the inner ear. The tumor presses on the nerve, which then sends false signals to the brain. If the vestibular portion of the nerve is compressed, the client is unable to interpret stimuli about position and movement. If the cochlear branch is compressed, the client experiences tinnitus. The first clinical manifestation is often partial or complete sensorineural hearing loss followed by tinnitus. The client may also report dizziness.

Other tumors in the cerebellopontine angle likewise involve the seventh and eighth cranial nerves as they enter the internal acoustic meatus. Malignant tumors invade the entire inner ear, usually spreading from the middle ear and mastoid system.

Ménière's Disease. *Ménière's disease* is a disorder that affects both vestibular and auditory function. It is caused by excess endolymph (clear intracellular fluid in the membranous labyrinth of the inner ear) in the vestibular and semicircular canals. Hearing loss is fluctuant and usually subtle and reversible in the early stages. Later the hearing loss becomes permanent. Although Ménière's disease is associated with sensorineural hearing loss, the most prominent clinical manifestation is *vertigo* (feeling that the surroundings or one's own body is revolving). Therefore it is fully discussed in the section Balance Disorders.

Central Auditory Dysfunction. *Central auditory dysfunction* is a phenomenon whereby the central nervous system (CNS) cannot interpret normal auditory signals. Central auditory dysfunction, also known as *central deafness,* is a rare form of sensorineural hearing loss.

Diseases that alter the CNS, such as strokes and tumors, can cause central deafness.

Mixed Hearing Loss
Some causes of hearing impairment can result in both sensorineural and conductive hearing losses. These types of losses are referred to as *mixed hearing loss.* Clients with mixed hearing loss present with clinical manifestations associated with both sensorineural and conductive hearing losses.

Prevention and Screening
A major nursing responsibility is the identification of hearing impairment in clients in both hospital and community settings. The different types of hearing loss are listed in Box 68-1. Identification of clients at risk for hearing loss and adequate protection of the ears are important to maintain normal function. The American Speech-Language-Hearing Association (ASHA) has recommended specific guidelines for annual hearing screenings for children 3 to 10 years of age who are at risk for hearing impairment.

BOX 68-1 *Types of Hearing Loss*

Air-conduction hearing loss: Loss of hearing through the external and middle ear

Bone-conduction hearing loss: Loss of hearing through the inner ear

Central hearing loss: Loss of hearing from damage to the brain's auditory pathways or auditory center

Conductive hearing loss: Loss of hearing in which air conduction is worse than bone conduction and involves the external and middle ear

Fluctuating hearing loss: A sensorineural hearing loss that varies with time

Functional hearing loss: Loss of hearing for which no organic lesion can be found

Mixed hearing loss: Both sensorineural and conductive hearing loss

Neural hearing loss: A sensorineural hearing loss originating in the eighth cranial nerve or brain stem

Sensorineural hearing loss: Loss of hearing involving the cochlea and hearing nerve; bone and air conduction are equal but diminished

Sensory hearing loss: A sensorineural hearing loss in the cochlea involving the hair cells and nerve endings

Sudden hearing loss: A sensorineural hearing loss with a sudden onset

Conductive hearing loss results from interference with conduction in the external and middle ear; sensorineural hearing loss in the inner ear and mixed hearing loss in all three areas.

Primary prevention is aimed at minimizing the risks from trauma, noise exposure, use of ototoxic drugs, and infectious diseases such as meningitis, mumps, and measles. To reduce the risk of head trauma, young clients should be instructed to wear protective headgear or helmets when participating in sports. People should avoid insertion of hard instruments or objects into the ear canal to prevent obstruction, trauma, or perforation. Individuals in occupations with high noise exposure should be instructed to wear earplugs and to avoid prolonged exposure. Exposure to noise levels in excess of 80 decibels (dB) throughout an 8-hour day is considered excessive and should be avoided. In addition, teenagers need to be aware that listening to extremely loud music in enclosed spaces, such as cars, can contribute to hearing loss.

Secondary prevention involves early detection of hearing impairment through screening and referral of any ear problems. Hearing screenings are important to detect hearing impairment in children that can be related to congenital, infectious, or allergic processes. Hearing tests and ear examinations should be performed in clients 65 years and older and in people experiencing hearing difficulties. When administering drugs with ototoxic side effects, monitor clients for vertigo, lessened hearing acuity, and tinnitus. If any of these manifestations occurs, the client or nurse must stop the ototoxic medication and promptly notify the physician.

Tertiary prevention focuses on maintenance of optimal function through hearing rehabilitation programs, proper use and care of hearing aids, and implementation of coping and communication strategies.

Pathophysiology

Conductive hearing loss is the result of interference of sound transmission into and through the external ear and middle ear. The inner ear is not affected in a pure conductive loss; therefore sound transmission from the inner ear to the brain is normal. Normal movement of sound vibrations through the ear canal, tympanic membrane, or ossicles is impeded because of the nature of the disease process involved in the conductive loss. Sound is perceived as faint or distant, but it remains relatively clear. Most conductive hearing losses are correctable by medical or surgical treatment.

Sensorineural hearing loss, however, results from disease or trauma to the organ of Corti or auditory nerve pathways of the inner ear leading to the brain stem. Normal reception and transmission of sound waves are disrupted. Sound is distorted and faint. Sensorineural hearing losses are usually permanent and are generally not correctable by medical or surgical treatment.

Clinical Manifestations

Most hearing loss is gradual and goes unnoticed by the client until several incidents of communication problems have occurred. Significant others and co-workers are usually aware of the client's hearing problem long before the client realizes or admits to the problem. A small loss of hearing goes unnoticed and does not cause manifestations. Health care providers should be alert for the following manifestations of hearing loss in a client:

- Failure to respond to oral communication
- Inappropriate response to oral communication
- Excessively loud speech
- Abnormal awareness of sounds
- Strained facial expressions
- Tilting of head when listening
- Constant need for clarification of conversation
- Faulty speech articulation
- Listening to radio and television at increased volume

The hearing impaired or "hard-of-hearing" client may repeat the information, even incorrectly, or may ask for clarification. Clients with a hearing loss can also experience distorted or abnormal sounds. Sometimes a sound is heard at different pitches for each ear; this is called *diplacusis*. A sound may cause a rapid increase in loudness; this is called *recruitment*. These abnormal sounds can cause discomfort.

The onset of a conductive hearing loss can be sudden or progressive. In cases of fluid in the middle ear, hearing loss is often bilateral but is usually restored with medical or surgical treatment. In other conductive processes, such as otosclerosis, clinical manifestations consist of slow progressive hearing loss with changes noted even in adolescence. Hearing loss is usually bilateral but may be asymmetrical. Other manifestations are mild tinnitus, recurrent vertigo, and postural imbalance. It is common for the client to speak in a soft voice.

If damage to the tympanic membrane is suspected, such as perforation, examination of the client may reveal a conductive hearing loss and serous drainage in the ear canal. The hearing loss found with a total perforation of the eardrum is approximately 35 dB (one third of the hearing range). With small perforations, no loss may be present. If a perforation is present, damage to the ossicles should be suspected. Diagnostic findings of conductive hearing loss include greater bone conduction than air conduction on the Rinne test. If hearing loss is greater in one ear, Weber's test shows lateralization to the more affected ear. Pure-tone audiometry confirms hearing loss. *Speech discrimination* (understanding of words) is usually maintained.

Noise-induced hearing loss is characterized by a greater loss in the higher frequencies. Sudden or fluctuating hearing losses are recognized as separate disorders from routine sensorineural hearing loss. Although fluctuating losses usually suggest syphilis or Ménière's disease, sudden sensorineural hearing losses are believed to be viral in origin. Recognition of these patterns is important because medical treatment of such disorders can result in significant improvements in hearing.

A characteristic of a severe hearing loss is loss of discrimination. To some clients, a hearing loss feels like a blockage or fullness in the ear or an inability to distinguish the direction of sounds.

Tinnitus accompanies most sensorineural hearing losses and is annoying. *Tinnitus* literally means "ringing" but can actually sound like roaring, the chirping of crickets, or occasionally music. Tinnitus is not a disease but a distressing manifestation, and it is sometimes a warning sign of hearing loss or other, more serious problems. Ear noise that cannot be heard by an observer is classified as *subjective tinnitus,* which is the most common kind. Any ear noise that can be heard by someone other than the client is called *objective tinnitus.* In some clients the tinnitus becomes the problem, and the underlying cause may be forgotten.

The major nursing responsibility in a client with tinnitus is to perform a thorough history and assessment of the onset, frequency, constancy, and level of intensity of the tinnitus. Unilateral tinnitus merits a complete neuro-otologic evaluation with the goal of ruling out the possibility of a tumor, most likely an acoustic neuroma. The nurse must keep in mind that tinnitus is a manifestation of an underlying pathologic process that warrants further referral.

Table 68-1 presents the clinical manifestations of conductive and sensorineural hearing losses. Diagnostic measures include (1) testing for hearing of pure tones on audiometry, (2) speech reception and discrimination, (3) tympanometry, and, (4) sometimes, brain stem auditory evoked responses. Tones are presented using earphones (air conduction) and vibrators (bone conduction). The minimal level at which the client can hear is determined. The *speech reception threshold* is the lowest intensity at which the client can correctly repeat 50% of the words presented. The speech discrimination test is a measure of the client's ability to understand speech when it is presented at a volume that is easily heard.

Outcome Management
■ Medical Management

The goals for medical management of the client with hearing impairment are (1) to restore hearing, (2) to assist hearing, (3) to manage tinnitus, and (4) to implement aural rehabilitation.

Restore Hearing. Hearing loss that results from blockage or fullness in the ear associated with an infectious process may be restored to normal with administration of antibiotics for bacterial infections. In the case of sudden hearing loss, prompt administration of oral corticosteroids is used in an attempt to lessen the progressive hearing loss or to reverse a sudden loss. Antiviral medications have been advocated for sudden sensorineural hearing loss, although they have not been shown in clinical trials to be of additional benefit. If ototoxicity is suspected, the administration of all ototoxic medications is discontinued. Most sensorineural hearing loss cannot be reversed with medical or surgical intervention. Conductive hearing loss, in contrast, is often amenable to surgical correction.

Assist Hearing. Unfortunately, most hearing losses are permanent, and hearing cannot be restored. The use of hearing aids and assistive listening devices can greatly improve the client's ability to communicate and interact with others.

Hearing aids amplify sound in a controlled manner. They are used by both *hearing-impaired* clients (those with slight or moderate hearing loss) and *deaf* clients (those with severe or profound hearing loss). Hearing aids make sound louder but do not improve the quality of sound. Therefore clients with decreased discrimination benefit less from a hearing aid. The hearing aid amplifies all background noises, such as hospital machinery, background conversation in restaurants, footsteps, and department store noises, as well as speech. These noises may mask conversation or confuse the hearing-impaired client, especially one who is an older adult.

A client should undergo a trial period before purchasing a hearing aid to see whether he or she can adapt to its use. In fact, in most states, such a trial period is mandatory. Bilateral (binaural) aids may be desirable.

Several types of hearing aids are available, and they vary according to size and location. Hearing aids can be worn in the following locations:

- In the ear
- In the ear canal
- Behind the ear (postauricular)

TABLE 68-1	*Clinical Manifestations of Conductive and Sensorineural Hearing Losses*	
	Conductive Hearing Loss	**Sensorineural Hearing Loss**
Voice quality	Soft voice	Loud voice
Effect of environmental noise on hearing	Hearing improved	Hearing made worse
Speech discrimination	Good	Poor
Ability to hear on telephone	Good	Poor
Lateralization on Weber's test	To diseased ear	To normal ear
Result of Rinne test	Negative, AC < BC	Positive, AC > BC

AC, Air conduction; *BC,* bone conduction.

• In eyeglasses
• In the middle of the chest (body-worn aid)

Regardless of type, the hearing aid consists of four parts:

1. Microphone to receive sound waves from the air and change sounds into electrical signals
2. Amplifier to increase the strength of electrical signals
3. Receiver (loudspeaker) to change the electrical signals into sound waves
4. Battery to provide the electrical energy needed to operate the hearing aid

On all types of hearing aids except the body-worn type, all four components are housed in one small case. The louder sounds are then directed into the ear through a custom-molded earpiece (Figure 68-3).

The evolution in hearing aid design has led to smaller and more effective aids. Small hearing aids are available that fit into the ear canal. The latest advancement in hearing aids is digital processing. Another advancement is directional microphones, which enhance the voice of a speaker in front of the client and suppress background noise. Programmable hearing aids allow the selection of various amplification patterns by the user and may have some added benefit for clients. Hearing aid technology will continue to advance.

Assistive listening devices help the hearing-impaired client hear the television or radio as well as use the telephone. Stationary devices called *teletypewriters* and a portable instrument called a *telecommunication device for the deaf* (TDD) are used for telephone communication by the profoundly deaf. A flashing light signals the presence of a dial tone, a busy signal, or a ring. When another teletypewriter or TDD is reached, messages are typed and displayed on a screen or printed. Other devices, such as flashing lights that alert a deaf person to a ringing doorbell, alarm clock, or smoke alarm are available. Hearing dogs are trained to be sensitive to certain noises, such as the telephone, doorbells, and crying children. On hearing the sound, a hearing dog moves back and forth between the client and the sound to alert the client.

Manage Tinnitus. Tinnitus can be a distressing disorder associated with the sensorineural hearing loss. Many approaches have been tried to alleviate this problem, including biofeedback, electrostimulation, hypnosis, medication, hearing aids, and tinnitus maskers. They have all met with minimal success. Tinnitus maskers appear similar to hearing aids except that they generate noise. The tinnitus masker is of benefit only while it is being used. Every approach for relief from tinnitus is only moderately successful, at best. Clients should be counseled to avoid unproved treatments for tinnitus. The nurse and the client's family must be alert to manifestations of depression if the tinnitus is chronic. The quality of the spouse's support of the client with tinnitus has been shown to be strongly correlated with role function. In addition, the nurse should be alert to spousal interaction and should facilitate problem-solving as needed.

Implement Aural Rehabilitation. Aural rehabilitation may improve communication if (1) hearing loss is irreversible or is not amenable to surgical intervention or (2) the client elects not to have surgery. The purpose of aural rehabilitation is to maximize the hearing-impaired client's communication skills.

Hearing is one of our primary modes of communication. Rehabilitation is directed toward teaching the client to use the other sense more effectively, those of vision, touch, and vibration, and to maximize the use of any remaining hearing ability. The outcome of rehabilitation is affected by all demographic variables and the severity of impairment. As with other forms of rehabilitation, success depends partly on the client's level of motivation.

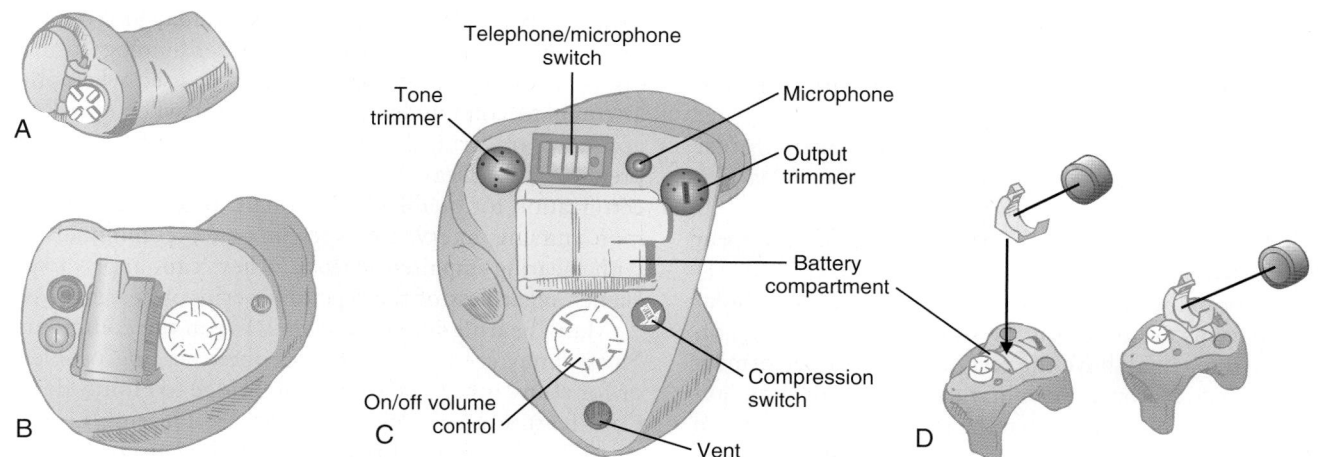

FIGURE 68-3 Types of hearing aids and components. **A,** In-the-canal aid. **B,** In-the-ear aid. **C,** Hearing aid components. **D,** Battery compartment. (Courtesy of Arnold G. Schuring, M.D.)

Speech reading, the current term used for lip reading, is an important means of communication. Speech reading is the process of understanding vocal communication by the integration of lip movements with facial expressions, gestures, environmental clues, and conversation contexts. Speech reading is difficult without auditory cues for several reasons. Many movements for speech are rapid, many sounds are similar (*b, m, p*), and the production of certain sounds in any language is not visible. The hearing-impaired client must guess at a high percentage of words. Knowledge of this fact alone helps the nurse be more understanding of the client who is using this communication approach.

Because of reduced auditory feedback (the inability of hearing-impaired clients to monitor their own speech), the clearness, pitch quality, or rate of the client's speech may deteriorate. These changes may alter the efficiency of communication and reduce the intelligibility of speech. The goal of speech training is to conserve, develop, or prevent deterioration of speech skills.

Last, but still important, is sign language. Sign language allows communication by hand signals that represent different letters of the alphabet, words, and phrases.

■ Nursing Management of the Medical Client

Assessment

The client's ability to communicate may be informally assessed during the history. The nurse should assess the client's ability to follow conversation. During the interview, the nurse should look for answers to the following questions:

1. Does the client admit to having a hearing loss and difficulty communicating, or does he or she blame other people for not speaking clearly?
2. In what settings does the client have more problems with hearing or communicating?
3. Are family members, co-workers, and friends aware of the hearing problem? Are they supportive of the client, making communication easier and including him or her in conversation? Do others feel frustrated or angry when the client cannot hear correctly or does not respond? Does the client feel left out? Embarrassed?
4. Does the client try to understand spoken words? Or does he or she withdraw or refuse to participate, letting others do the talking?
5. Does the client wear a hearing aid? Does it appear to work?

Occasionally, laboratory, radiologic, and vestibular examinations are used for assessment. In an otology office, the nurse may have the responsibility of performing the history, otologic examination, and screening audiometry. The history is often the most important part of the clinical assessment, as previously described (see Box 66-5). The extent of assessment of the sensorineural hearing loss depends on the setting and the nurse's educational preparation and experience. Nurses should be able to inspect the outer ear and grossly assess auditory acuity.

Visualization of the ear canal and tympanic membrane is accomplished with the otoscope. Cerumen in the canal or on the eardrum can interfere with the examination and may need to be removed. The blind removal of ear wax with an ear syringe should be performed only if the ear is free of other abnormalities, such as an infection or perforation of the eardrum.

Impacted accumulations of ear wax may be softened and loosened for removal by alternating instillations of glycerin and hydrogen peroxide eardrops. The eardrops are warmed to body temperature and used daily as directed for 1 to 2 weeks. The ear is then irrigated gently with warm water for removal of the softened wax or cleaned under magnification with a cerumen spoon. Wax on the tympanic membrane should be removed by a otolaryngologist or an advanced-practice nurse in otorhinolaryngology. However, the removal of cerumen can lead to irritation from mildly caustic commercial products.

Diagnosis, Outcomes, Interventions

Diagnosis: Impaired Verbal Communication. Clients who have lost their ability to hear are best managed with the nursing diagnosis *Impaired Verbal Communication related to effects of hearing loss.*

Outcomes. The client will develop effective methods to communicate needs and will be included in conversation.

Interventions. When normal conversation is impossible, writing may be used successfully by clients who have good comprehension of English (or their primary language). Writing may cause frustration when the client's primary language is American Sign Language because it is grammatically different from standard English. Visual aids, such as pictures, diagrams, and models, may also improve the nurse's ability to explain medical terminology or procedures. An expert interpreter should be used when other attempts to communicate have failed or when speed and accuracy are critical. The National Registry of Interpreters for the Deaf (NRID) has local chapters and offers certification for qualified individuals. Box 68-2 lists common nursing interventions to improve communication with hearing-impaired clients. They can apply to all clients, regardless of the type or severity of hearing loss.

Many hearing-impaired clients live in the community. Nurses may see these clients for their hearing problems or for many other problems. The Bridge to Home Health Care feature on Living with a Severe Hearing Loss on p. 1977 addresses approaches to home care of hearing-impaired clients.

BOX 68-2   *Common Nursing Interventions for Hearing-Impaired Clients*

- Get the client's attention by raising your arm or hand.
- Stand with a light on your face; this helps the client to speech-read.
- Talk directly to the client while facing him or her.
- Speak clearly, but do not overaccentuate words.
- Speak in a normal tone; do not shout. Shouting overuses normal speaking movements and so may cause distortion and may be too loud for the client with sensorineural damage. If the client has conductive loss only, it is sometimes helpful to make the voice louder without shouting.
- If the client does not seem to understand what is said, express it differently. Some words are difficult to "see" in speech reading, such as "white" and "red."
- Move closer to the client and toward the better-hearing ear.
- Write out proper names or any statement that you are not sure was understood.
- Do not smile, chew gum, or cover the mouth when talking.
- Remember that a client's inattention may indicate tiredness or lack of understanding.

- Use phrases rather than one-word answers to convey meaning. State the major topic of the discussion first, and then give details.
- Do not show annoyance by careless facial expressions. Clients who are hard of hearing depend more on visual clues for understanding.
- Encourage the use of a hearing aid if it is available; allow the client to adjust it before speaking.
- In a group, repeat important statements, and avoid making asides to others in the group.
- Avoid the use of the intercommunication system because this may distort sound and cause poor communication.
- Do not avoid conversation with a client who has hearing loss. It has been said that to live in a silent world is much more devastating than to live in darkness, and clients with hearing loss appear to have more emotional difficulties than do those who are blind.

BRIDGE TO HOME HEALTH CARE

Living with a Severe Hearing Loss

People are often reluctant to admit that they have a hearing impairment. This reluctance results in difficulty with verbal communication, inability to follow instructions, and social isolation. To maximize communication, reduce background noise (turn off the television or radio), face the person, and speak clearly without shouting. Sometimes the only way to communicate is by writing. Develop written materials for repeated use. Include introduction materials (e.g., your name, your agency's name, the purpose of your visit), reportable problems, and treatment regimens.

In many cases, hearing loss is due to accumulation of cerumen. Use an otoscope to visualize the ear canal. If cerumen is present, a physician may need to remove it. If you are responsible for removing the cerumen, contact the physician to discuss a prescription for an ear irrigation solution, instill the solution, and evaluate the amount and color of drainage.

When people experience a hearing loss, they need a medical evaluation and a hearing aid evaluation. Many older adults are reluctant to wear a hearing aid for various reasons. It is a visual manifestation of an impairment, it is expensive, and it necessitates leaving home for evaluation, fitting, and follow-up appointments. If a client's reluctance is due to cosmetic reasons, show pictures of hearing aids and discuss individuals who wear hearing aids, such as former President George Bush. Newer hearing aids are available that are smaller, less noticeable, and more discreet.

If cost is a problem, consider a referral to a social worker to identify local resources. Currently Medicare pays for the cost of a hearing evaluation and little for the hearing aid; Medicaid usually pays for the hearing aid. Consider other financial resources, such as the American Association of Retired Persons and local hearing aid vendors. When leaving home is a problem, check whether a vendor will make a home visit. If this is not possible, suggest that the client use a head-set amplifier that can be purchased from a local electronics store.

Teaching is an important nursing intervention related to hearing impairment. It involves cleaning the devices and changing the batteries. Also, evaluate the client's ability to use the telephone and answer the door. Local telephone companies can equip the telephone with an adjustable volume control, hearing aid adapters, loud ringing signals, and a telecommunication device for the deaf (TDD). A TDD allows the hearing-impaired individual to communicate by typing information into a specially designed device. To receive information, the receiver must have a specific TDD telephone number. Teach the client with a TDD about TDD telephone numbers for an emergency response, and provide information about the home health agency and community resources.

It is important to involve informal caregivers, significant others, and family members in the management of a hearing impairment. Teach these people to maximize communication with a variety of techniques and adaptive equipment.

Diagnosis: Ineffective Coping. The individual with a loss of hearing goes through the same stages of grieving as others experiencing a loss. Rehabilitation cannot begin until some acceptance of the hearing loss has taken place, leading to the nursing diagnosis *Ineffective Coping related to recent loss of hearing.*

Outcomes. The client will discuss or will demonstrate problem-solving–based coping strategies, as evidenced by the following:

1. Taking the initiative to inform others of the hearing impairment and requesting that they assist with communication by using techniques that promote comprehension
2. Not experiencing feelings of embarrassment, frustration, or withdrawal
3. Not blaming others for failure to communicate effectively
4. Avoiding situations and environments, such as noisy areas, that impair hearing

Interventions. Work with the client and family on methods to enhance communication and thereby enhance coping. Encourage the client to role-play how he or she might tell people about the hearing impairment and indicate what techniques should be used to help hearing. Self-help groups, such as Self-help for Hard of Hearing People (SHHH), located in Bethesda, Maryland, can assist with resources, information, and support for clients and their families.

Diagnosis: Impaired Social Interaction. Clients with hearing losses can experience fears of inadequacy, feelings of inferiority, depression, and varying degrees of stress and isolation. The nursing diagnosis *Impaired Social Interaction related to perceived inability to interact with others secondary to hearing loss* can be used to guide interventions.

Outcomes. The client will exhibit a willingness to be involved in social situations as evidenced by (1) attempting to become a part of social events, (2) conversing with others, (3) indicating lessened feelings of inadequacy, and (4) responding appropriately to questions asked (not fabricating answers to cover hearing loss).

Interventions. The ASHA urges that all clients with hearing impairments *not* be grouped into one category. Each client is unique and has an individual hearing problem. The nurse functions as a role model in accepting the client as an individual and demonstrating effective communication techniques.

Work with the client to enhance coping, encourage continued social involvement, and advocate the use of various organizations to their fullest extent. Many agencies and associations exist for the hearing-impaired client. Services are offered by audiology clinics and sponsored by universities, hospitals, community programs, state or local departments of health, the Department of Veterans Affairs (VA), and national organizations.

Diagnosis: Deficient Knowledge of Managing Hearing Loss. Clients with new hearing aids need information about their care and proper use. Therefore *Deficient Knowledge of managing hearing loss related to lack of previous exposure to a hearing aid* is an important nursing diagnosis.

Outcomes. The client will have greater knowledge about the hearing aid as evidenced by proper use and care of the aid.

Interventions. The hearing aid user should know how to care for the aid (Box 68-3) and what to do if the device does not work. Gain a basic knowledge of the hearing aid to help with insertion for clients who are ill. Encourage the client to use the hearing aid and to store it safely when not using it. Turn the device off before removal to prevent squealing feedback. The maintenance of a hearing aid is becoming less of a problem today. Usually the aid is returned to the dealer for factory repair while the client uses a "loaner" hearing aid. Unlicensed assistive

---

BOX 68-3 *Care of a Hearing Aid*

- Turn the hearing aid off when it is not in use.
- Open the battery compartment at night to avoid accidental drainage of battery power.
- Keep an extra battery available at all times.
- Wash the ear mold frequently (daily if necessary) with mild soap and warm water, and use a pipe cleaner to cleanse the cannula.
- Dry the ear mold completely before reconnecting it to the hearing aid.
- Do not wear the hearing aid when you have an ear infection.

What to Do If the Hearing Aid Fails to Work
- Check the on-off switch.
- Inspect the ear mold for cleanliness.
- Examine the battery for correct insertion.
- Examine the cord plug for correct insertion.
- Examine the cord for breaks.
- Replace the battery, cord, or both, if necessary. The life of batteries varies according to the amount of use and power requirements of the aid. Batteries last 2 to 14 days.
- Check the position of the ear mold in the ear. If the hearing aid "whistles," the volume control is too high, the ear mold is probably not inserted properly into the ear canal, or you need to have a new ear mold made.

personnel often care for clients with hearing aids. Delegation of care of the hearing aid and the hearing-impaired client is shown in the Management and Delegation feature on Hearing Aids, below.

Cost has been cited as a major factor in the non-use of hearing aids. Clients needing financial assistance should be referred to the state department of vocational rehabilitation, the local Lions Club, and, in some states, Medicaid.

Evaluation

A client with a new hearing loss or disorder needs frequent evaluation to determine the severity of hearing loss, coping strategies, and ability to communicate adequately. Because many forms of hearing loss are permanent or progressive, long-term evaluation should also be performed to be certain the client is adapting positively. Also determine whether the client has questions about the equipment used for hearing rehabilitation and the need for further education.

■ Surgical Management

Surgery is usually not warranted for sensorineural hearing loss; however, because mixed, conductive, and sensorineural hearing loss exists, surgery may be performed (1) to restore the conductive hearing loss, (2) to remove tumor, and (3) to assist hearing in profoundly deaf people.

Restore Conductive Hearing. The most common cause of conductive hearing loss is serous otitis media (see later discussion). Although most commonly seen in children, this disorder can occur at any age. In cases of serous otitis media and persistent conductive hearing loss that do not resolve after 2 to 3 months of medical management, an incision into the tympanic membrane and evacuation of fluid can be performed with the client under local or general anesthesia. This procedure, known as *myringotomy,* will restore hearing. It is discussed later in this chapter.

Another type of conductive hearing loss that can be treated medically or corrected surgically results from otosclerosis. Because speech discrimination is usually unimpaired, simple amplification of sound is quite effective. People who are at high risk of otosclerosis or who are not candidates for surgery can be given medications in an attempt to reduce the severity of the bony fusion. Sodium fluoride has been given to replace the hydroxyl ion in bone and decrease resorption. In addition, calcium gluconate and vitamin D have been used to retard bone resorption. If hearing is stable, these minerals and vitamins are given for only 2 years. The clinical efficacy of these medications remains unsubstantiated.

MANAGEMENT AND DELEGATION

Hearing Aids

Caring for hearing aids and helping clients with maintenance of these devices may be delegated to unlicensed assistive personnel. Clients with new hearing aids need individualized teaching provided by you, the registered nurse. You are to evaluate the client's understanding of the instruction. Before delegating hearing aid care, consider the following issues:

The client's learning needs. Are these new hearing aids? Does the client have a new hearing loss disorder? If so, you should instruct the client to care for these devices and provide consistent teaching.

The competency level of the unlicensed assistive personnel who will potentially perform hearing aid care. Unlicensed assistive personnel may not provide the initial instruction but may reinforce the instructions you have provided.

Instruct unlicensed assistive personnel caring for the client with hearing aids to achieve the following:

- Encourage the use of hearing aids and independent care by clients without cognitive impairment.
- Provide safe storage of the hearing aids when not in use (in the client's personal case or another small storage device). If the client is hospitalized, ensure that the case is labeled with the client's name and location.

- Turn the device off when it is not in use. If the aid is to be off for a prolonged duration (such as during the night or sleeping hours), open the battery compartment to avoid additional drainage of battery power.
- Cleanse the ear mold with mild soap and water each day or as needed.
- Completely dry the ear mold before reconnecting it to the hearing aid.
- Help the client insert the ear mold into the ear. If the hearing aid makes a whistling noise, the device is not inserted properly into the ear. At this point, it may be necessary for you to assess more completely placement in the ear canal.
- Allow the client to adjust the volume before speaking.
- Speak clearly in a normal tone to the client. Do not shout.
- Turn off the device before removing it to prevent squealing "feedback."

Findings that are immediately reportable to you are (1) difficulty with placement in the ear, (2) redness or drainage in the ear, (3) mechanical failure of the device, and (4) other issues of concern to the client.

Stapedectomy. Surgical intervention for otosclerosis has been very successful. *Stapedectomy* is a surgical procedure whereby the damaged stapes is removed and replaced with a stainless steel, polytetrafluoroethylene (Teflon) or plastic prosthesis (Figure 68-2, *B*). The oval window is grafted with absorbable gelatin sponge (Gelfoam) or tissue grafts. Stapedectomy was once a common middle ear procedure; however, the pool of clients with otosclerosis is dwindling, and today stapedectomy is performed less and less often.

The client must be free of otitis externa and otitis media before surgery. To reduce the risk of bleeding, the client should use no aspirin or products with aspirin for 1 week before surgery. Preoperative and postoperative audiograms and tympanograms are performed to test hearing acuity levels.

 After surgery the client is often instructed to lie on the nonoperative ear with the head of the bed elevated. This position helps reduce edema and prevent dislodgment of the prosthesis. Antibiotics are prescribed. The packing in the ear canal should not be disturbed. On discharge from the hospital, the client is told to report the acute onset of vertigo. To reduce the risk of development of a perilymph fistula (rupture of the oval window, which permits leakage of perilymph fluid), the client should avoid excessive exercise, straining, and activities that might lead to head trauma. If the client needs to blow the nose, it should be done gently, one nostril at a time. The client should sneeze with the mouth open. No airplane travel is allowed for a month.

Hearing aids may still be required after stapedectomy, and the client's hearing will need to be reevaluated. Complications of the operation include granuloma formation and perilymph fistula. Either complication may result in profound deafness and persistent vertigo. Hearing loss may also develop after surgery from middle ear adhesions or shifting of the prosthesis.

Tumor Excision. Surgery is usually recommended for treatment of acoustic neuroma. Current microsurgical techniques often allow preservation of hearing and usually enable resection of the tumor without injury to the facial nerve. In older clients, especially those with total deafness in the affected ear, a more conservative, nonsurgical approach is sometimes taken because acoustic neuroma is benign and very slow growing.

Assist Hearing in Profound Deafness. Use of implantable hearing devices (IHDs) may be appropriate in certain clients. There are three types of IHDs: cochlear implants, temporal bone stimulators, and middle ear implants.

Cochlear Implants. Cochlear implants provide auditory sensation to clients with severe to profound sensorineural hearing loss who cannot benefit from a hearing aid (Figure 68-4). Preoperative vestibular testing is highly recommended for all clients in whom a cochlear implant is being considered.

The cochlear implant contains a small computer that changes the spoken word to electrical impulses. The impulses are transmitted across the skin to an implanted coil that carries the impulse to the hearing nerve endings in the cochlea by means of an electrode introduced through the round window. The most effective cochlear implants use multiple-frequency channels. In multichannel cochlear implants, up to 22 electrodes are inserted along the cochlear partition. The surgery for insertion of a cochlear implant is similar to mastoid surgery. The success of a cochlear implant varies widely, ranging from minimal improvement in auditory awareness to the ability to understand speech on the telephone.

Temporal Bone Stimulators (Bone Hearing Devices). In some cases of hearing loss, sound can be transmitted by applying a stimulation directly to the temporal bone, thereby transmitting sound through the skull to the inner ear. For clients with a conductive hearing loss, a device is available in which the receiver is implanted under the skin into the skull. The external device transmits the sound through the skin. This device is worn above the ear rather than in the ear canal. Because some conductive hearing losses cannot be surgically repaired, the temporal bone stimulator may provide an alternative rehabilitative method to conventional hearing aids. It is not widely used at present.

Middle Ear Implants (Semi-Implantable Hearing Device). A variety of IHDs devices are being evaluated for sound amplification and quality for individuals with moderate to moderately severe sensorineural hearing loss. However, many challenges have to be met before a workable device is available. This method of hearing aid technology is still in the research stage.

OTALGIA

Otalgia is defined as pain in the ear, or earache. Otalgia can be primary in origin (i.e., coming from a disorder in the ear), infectious, or referred (i.e., coming from a disorder outside the ear). Otalgia from ear pain can be the result of infection in the external or middle ear or of trauma to the ear and head. Referred otalgia can be caused by disorders in the temporomandibular joint (TMJ), cranial nerves, face, scalp, pharynx, tonsils, thyroid, trachea, teeth, or cervical muscles.

Etiology and Risk Factors

Otalgia can be related to infectious processes in the external ear and middle ear. Bacterial contaminants can enter the ear through insertion of unclean articles, such as fingers or toys. Insertion of any sharp objects into the ear canal can traumatize the skin and provide an open

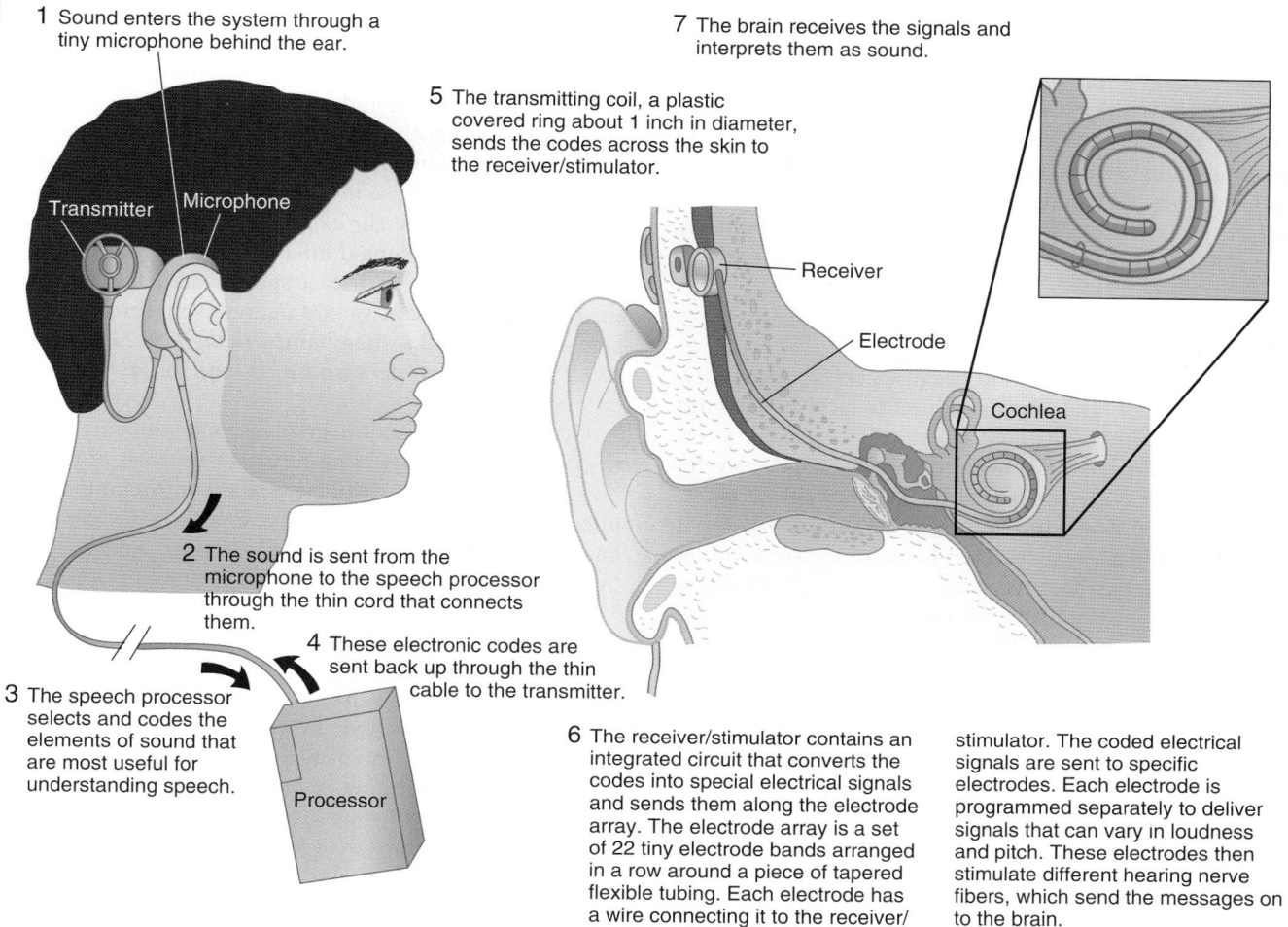

1 Sound enters the system through a tiny microphone behind the ear.

5 The transmitting coil, a plastic covered ring about 1 inch in diameter, sends the codes across the skin to the receiver/stimulator.

7 The brain receives the signals and interprets them as sound.

Transmitter   Microphone

Receiver

Electrode

Cochlea

2 The sound is sent from the microphone to the speech processor through the thin cord that connects them.

4 These electronic codes are sent back up through the thin cable to the transmitter.

3 The speech processor selects and codes the elements of sound that are most useful for understanding speech.

Processor

6 The receiver/stimulator contains an integrated circuit that converts the codes into special electrical signals and sends them along the electrode array. The electrode array is a set of 22 tiny electrode bands arranged in a row around a piece of tapered flexible tubing. Each electrode has a wire connecting it to the receiver/ stimulator. The coded electrical signals are sent to specific electrodes. Each electrode is programmed separately to deliver signals that can vary in loudness and pitch. These electrodes then stimulate different hearing nerve fibers, which send the messages on to the brain.

FIGURE 68-4 Cochlear implant to restore hearing.

medium for infection. Instillation of contaminated solutions into the ear or swimming in polluted water raises the risk for development of ear infection and inflammation. Clients with recent upper respiratory infections, eustachian tube dysfunction, and allergies are also at increased risk for ear infections.

Infectious and neoplastic processes of the pharynx can also cause referred otalgia. It is not uncommon for clients with acute tonsillitis to complain of significant ear pain, even though the ears may be normal on examination. Otalgia following tonsillectomy is universal and is not a manifestation of infection. In clients with unilateral otalgia and a history of smoking, consideration must be given to a neoplastic process of the lateral pharynx, especially if concurrent manifestations, such as hoarseness or dysphagia, are present. Examination of the lower pharynx by means of a fiberoptic endoscope is necessary in the smoker with persistent hoarseness, and referral to an otolaryngologist is indicated.

Trauma to the head, temporal bone, and ear can also result in ear pain. Engaging in contact sports without protective headgear can result in severe trauma to the head, injuring the hearing apparatus. A blow to the ear by an object such as a ball or hand can cause local or diffuse pain in the area. Noise trauma from a blast or loud noise may create a ringing sensation that is perceived as painful and uncomfortable. Nerve damage may be accompanied by an intolerance to even soft sounds, resulting in severe pain. Exposure to extremely hot or cold temperatures can lead to burns or severe frostbite, respectively, of the external ear.

Blockage of the eustachian tube and otalgia can be the result of enlarged adenoid tissue and tonsils in children, middle ear infections often associated with upper respiratory infections, and *barotrauma* (pressure injury to the middle ear). Acute blockage from altitude changes caused by flying or underwater diving will cause middle ear problems. Hyperbaric oxygen treatments can also cause barotrauma. Hyperbaric oxygen treatment is common for carbon monoxide poisoning as well as other disorders. The incidence of barotrauma is increased when an upper respiratory infection is present. *Aerotitis media* is a form of serous otitis media in which fluid or air is trapped in the middle ear during descent in an airplane.

Any long-term blockage of the eustachian tube leads to serous otitis media and a hearing loss.

Mouth and gum pain, TMJ pain, cervical muscle tenderness, and pain from dental work can cause referred pain to the ear. TMJ arthralgia may result from teeth grinding, gum chewing, excessive talking, or biting down on hard objects. The resultant inflammation to this joint can be perceived by the client as an earache. Similarly, stress on the neck muscles can be referred to the ear.

External Ear Trauma

Auricular trauma is common because ears are prominent and unprotected. The pinna is subject to lacerations, blunt injury, abrasions, burns, and frostbite. A special concern with ear trauma is that a hematoma can quickly develop between the skin and cartilage (called *perichondrial hematoma*). The hematoma exerts pressure on the cartilage, impairing its healing. Such hematomas are common after blunt injuries such as occur in wrestling, fighting, or boxing and are responsible for so-called cauliflower ear.

People can often avoid ear trauma by wearing headgear for contact sports, wide-brimmed hats in the summer, and earmuffs or hats in the winter; heavy pierced earrings should not be worn because they can lacerate the lobule.

Foreign Bodies

Surprisingly a wide array of foreign bodies fit into the ear canal. The most common foreign body found in the adult ear is either a piece of cotton or, most annoying, an insect.

Ear pain from obstruction usually results from the buildup of matter in the ear canal, which leads to pressure and pain. Clients may also report decreased hearing, a sense of fullness, a throbbing sensation, and itching. The onset, duration, frequency, and intensity of manifestations should be noted.

Eustachian Tube Disorders

Because the eustachian tube connects the middle ear to the nasopharynx, pharyngeal disorders also cause eustachian tube dysfunction and thus secondary middle ear problems. For example, in children a common disorder is blockage of the eustachian tube by enlarged adenoid tissue. In adults swelling of the mucosa in the eustachian tube during an upper respiratory infection can lead to serous otitis media (see later discussion). For persistent unilateral blocked eustachian tube, a malignant tumor must be ruled out as the cause.

Ear Infections

Otitis Externa. The most common problems found in the external ear are infections, primarily bacterial or fungal. The most frequent infection, called *external otitis*, involves the external ear canal. Infection begins when the protective waxy coating has been damaged by dryness, moisture, or treatment. Infection can lead to edema, which can occlude the canal. External otitis occurs more frequently in the summer than in the winter. The most common form of external otitis is also called *swimmer's ear*, because it is prevalent in clients in whom water remains in the ear canal after swimming. In addition, opportunistic fungal infections are common. When a debilitating systemic disease such as diabetes is present, the external otitis can spread aggressively through cartilage and bone and is then named *malignant external otitis; Pseudomonas aeruginosa* is the usual offending pathogen.

Occasionally infection involves only the cartilage of the pinna (chondritis), with resultant necrosis of the cartilage and loss of the distinctive shape of the pinna if the infection is not treated quickly. Frostbite of the pinna has findings similar to those of infection. Another form of infection is seen as an ear canal furuncle or abscess.

Tympanic Membrane Infection. Infections of the external ear canal can involve the surface of the tympanic membrane. Infection can cause hard deposits in the tympanic membrane, known as *tympanosclerosis* (see discussion of hearing impairment). A specific infection of the tympanic membrane is *bullous myringitis*. This inflammatory disease forms blisters or bullae between the layers of the eardrum, which are extremely painful. It is usually caused by the bacterium *Mycoplasma pneumoniae*. Holes or perforations of the tympanic membrane can be caused by infection and also can be accompanied by drainage.

Tympanic membrane disorders can lead to perforation of the membrane. A perforation may be either acute, as seen in trauma and acute infection, or chronic, as seen in repeated infection. An acute perforation has a better chance of healing spontaneously than does a chronic perforation.

Otitis Media. Otitis media is the most prevalent disorder of the middle ear. It is most common in children but does occur in adults. When an infection is sudden in onset and short in duration, the diagnosis is acute suppurative otitis media. When the infection is repeated, usually causing drainage and perforation, the problem is chronic otitis media. Chronic otitis media is often caused by organisms such as *Pseudomonas, Staphylococcus*, and *Klebsiella*. Anaerobes such as *Bacteroides* have also been identified in culture analysis of specimens from the ear. Infection can cause swelling of the mucosa throughout the middle ear and eustachian tube. At times *serous otitis media* is found in conjunction with upper respiratory infections or allergies.

Chronic otitis media can lead to tympanic membrane retraction, adhesive otitis media, or necrosis of the tympanic membrane (perforations) or of the ossicles. Both problems create a conductive hearing loss. Necrosis of the bone covering of the facial nerve may cause facial paralysis. Because of the anatomy of the temporal bone, middle ear infection can also lead to brain abscesses that are life-threatening if not treated properly. Cholesteatoma, another complication, is discussed below.

Subsequent to infectious otitis media or allergic disease, fluid may form in the middle ear, known as *serous otitis media*. This fluid is formed when a vacuum develops in the middle ear, caused by a blocked eustachian tube. When the swelling subsides, the fluid may be too thick to drain. Tympanometry is a useful diagnostic assessment to distinguish a normal ear from one with a middle ear effusion.

Mastoiditis. The mastoid system is a series of air cells contained within the temporal bone that communicate with the middle ear. Before the discovery of antibiotics, a mastoid infection was a life-threatening event. Now acute mastoiditis is rare, although chronic mastoiditis does sometimes occur. With repeated middle ear infections, the mastoid cavity becomes a significant part of the problem, increasing the amount of drainage. A chronic infection also leads to the development of cholesteatoma (see below).

Drainage from the mastoid cavity via the ear canal is the most likely manifestation to appear. The drainage courses through the middle ear and out the tympanic membrane through a perforation. Tenderness over the mastoid cavity behind the ear points to an infection but usually is caused by an acute exacerbation of chronic mastoiditis rather than an acute mastoiditis. The protrusion of the pinna as a result of swelling over the mastoid may be part of this process.

Cholesteatoma. *Cholesteatoma* is a cyst in the middle ear or mastoid system that is lined with squamous epithelium and filled with keratin debris. Often infection is present in the mass of the cholesteatoma. Although cholesterol granules can be present in the specimen, yielding the term *cholesteatoma*, they are not the primary pathologic process.

Cholesteatoma most often results from chronic otitis media or marginal perforation of the tympanic membrane. Clients have conductive hearing loss and foul-smelling discharge from the ears. Although it is a benign growth, the cholesteatoma causes erosion of the surrounding structures, leading to other problems, such as brain abscesses, vertigo, and facial paralysis. Fortunately, these complications are uncommon.

Other Masses

Benign masses of the external ear canal are usually cysts that arise from a sebaceous gland or, more rarely, from the cerumen glands. Cysts can also be congenital in nature. Bony protrusions seen in the bony portion of the ear canal are called *exostoses*. The skin covering an exostosis is normal. If the skin is red, the mass is usually an abscess. Infectious polyps found in the ear canal arise from either the tympanic membrane or, more commonly, the middle ear, through a hole in the tympanic membrane.

Malignant tumors are also found in the external ear. The cutaneous carcinomas are most often basal cell carcinoma on the pinna and squamous cell carcinoma in the ear canal. If not treated, the carcinomas can invade underlying structures; squamous cell carcinoma may spread throughout the temporal bone. Rare tumors of the cerumen glands are of the adenoma cell type. Masses of the external ear are diagnosed through physical examination and biopsy to rule out malignancy. Surgical excision may be required.

Both benign and malignant tumors can involve the tympanic membrane, but they seldom arise from it; however, an infectious glandular polyp can be isolated to the tympanic membrane. Tumors in the middle ear can be seen through or protrude through the tympanic membrane.

The most common benign growth in the middle ear is an infectious polyp. A facial nerve neuroma is found along the course of the facial nerve. Malignant tumors involving the middle ear can be primary or secondary.

The same tumors that arise in the middle ear can be found in the mastoid cavity. Because the mastoid cavity is connected to other air cells throughout the temporal bone and is close to the brain, malignant tumors at this location carry a poor prognosis.

Pathophysiology

Otalgia related to a problem in the ear is usually the result of an inflammatory process that can be caused by trauma or infection. Inflammation causes chemical mediators to be released into the tissue and the chemotaxis of leukocytes to the damaged area, resulting in tissue edema, pain, heat, and redness. This inflammatory process results in swelling of tissue that impinges on nerve endings and surrounding areas, causing the otalgia. Masses such as tumors grow and press on nearby tissue and nerves, causing pain. Sometimes the infection or mass erodes into tissue and bone as in cholesteatoma and causes further inflammation and pain.

Otalgia can also be caused by referred pain to the ear. In conditions such as TMJ or cervical adenopathy, the pain does not originate in the ear; however, the neuronal pain pathways for these processes cross over and are perceived in the ear. Although the perception of pain in the ear is real, the cause of the pain is not related to a pathologic process in that area.

Clinical Manifestations

In the case of head trauma and damage to the tympanic membrane, clients often report an episode of brief but intense otalgia. Blunt injury to the auricle can result in a blue or reddish purple, tense swelling over the pinna. Perichondrial hematomas can develop and, left untreated, form a hypertrophic scar known as a *cauliflower ear,* which is an occupational hazard for boxers. If the tympanic membrane is ruptured from barotrauma or otitis media, the client often notes a sudden *reduction of pressure and pain.* Pain is not usually elicited on palpation of the external ear; this phenomenon usually provides a differential diagnosis between problems of the external ear and middle ear. Disorders involving the tympanic membrane are painful, perhaps the most painful of all middle ear disorders. Hearing loss may be noted but is often reversible.

Ear pain from obstruction usually results from the buildup of matter in the ear canal, which leads to pressure and pain. Clients may also report decreased hearing, a sense of fullness, a throbbing sensation, and itching. The onset, duration, frequency, and intensity of manifestations should be noted.

Pain in the external ear is the most common clinical manifestation of infection. Pain ranges from mild to severe and is generally unilateral. Pain is more intense when the ear canal is swollen. Painful sites are tender because of the close proximity of bone (a hard surface) when the ear is palpated. A clue to early external otitis is tenderness when the pinna is gently pulled on, in contrast to otitis media, in which touching the ear does not cause pain. A forerunner of pain in external otitis is itching in the ear canal. Inflammation (redness) is easily identified with an otoscope. At different stages of infection, drainage will be found from the ear canal. In early infectious disorders, the drainage may be clear rather than discolored by pus.

Manifestations of otitis media include ear pain and an immobile tympanic membrane. Because the tympanic membrane is a semitransparent membrane, what lies beneath it is visible. It can also become discolored or displaced. Therefore both fluid and infection can be seen in the middle ear. The tympanic membrane may be dull or red instead of the normal pearly gray. The eardrum may be normal, perforated, infected, retracted, or bulging depending on the disease process involved.

In addition, the client may report bubbling, crackling, or popping sensations in the ear, especially during swallowing. There is a sense of fullness in the ear and conductive hearing loss that fluctuates.

Suppurative otitis media is invasion of the middle ear by virulent organisms and formation of pus, often accompanied by purulent *otorrhea* (drainage). Clinical manifestations include intense ear pain, fever, mild to moderate conductive hearing loss, thickened and bulging tympanic membrane, and occasional dizziness.

Outcome Management
■ Medical Management
The goals of medical management are to (1) promote healing, (2) alleviate pain, and (3) restore normal function of the ears.

Promote Healing
Ear Irrigation. The ear is commonly irrigated to cleanse the external auditory canal or to remove impacted wax, debris, or foreign bodies to promote healing. Irrigation is not used in clients with a history or clinical suspicion of perforated eardrum. Ear irrigation is performed as follows.

Warm the irrigating solution (usually water) to body temperature, and place it in the irrigating syringe. Protect the client's clothes with a plastic drape, and place a kidney-shaped basin below the ear to catch the irrigating solution. Have the client sit with the ear to be irrigated toward you and the head tilted toward the other ear. In the adult, pull the external ear upward and backward (or in children pull external ear directly back), and direct the tip of the syringe along the upper wall of the ear canal (Figure 68-5). The canal should not be completely obstructed by the syringe to allow the back-flow of solution.

Sometimes the client is instructed to use a medicinal ear irrigation solution. The most common solution for ear irrigation is boric acid and alcohol, which is obtained by prescription. This solution cleanses the ear of debris and infection and provides a drying agent. A 2- or 3-ounce ear syringe is needed for irrigation. A family member performs the irrigation for the client. Usually the ear irrigation is followed by the use of eardrops.

When charting the ear irrigation, include the type of irrigation solution used and the nature of returned solution regarding amount, texture, color of cerumen, and type of debris. In addition, instruct the client to report pain, vertigo, or nausea during the procedure.

Antibiotics. Local and systemic antibiotics are the cornerstone of preventing and managing infectious

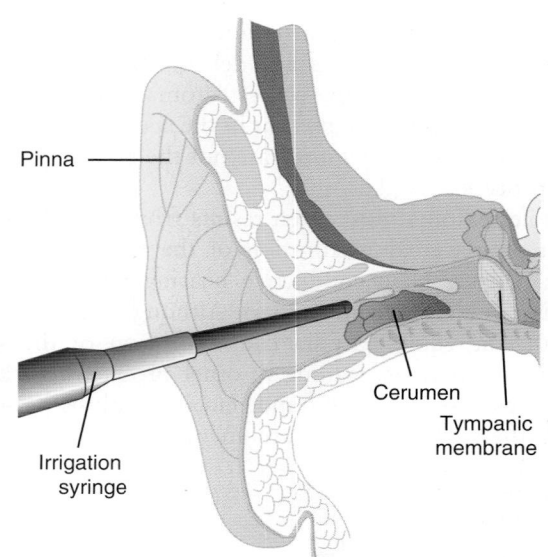

FIGURE 68-5 Ear irrigation. The tip of the syringe is directed along the upper wall of the ear canal.

processes; however, the first rule of treating infection is meticulous cleaning of the site so that the local antibiotic can reach the infected area. Suction, irrigation, or manual removal of matter with a cotton-tipped swab can be used. Regular application of antibiotic-steroid eardrops for a week is required.

If the ear canal is swollen shut, a wick must be inserted to allow the drops to penetrate the canal. Eardrops are placed directly on the wick. Commercially prepared wicks or single pieces of one-fourth-inch gauze can be used. The wick serves not only as a bandage but also as an excellent vehicle to medicate the ear canal. The wick is gently inserted into the ear canal by means of forceps while the external ear is gently pulled upward and backward. The wick is usually slightly less than 1 inch in long (Figure 68-6). The client should lie on the unaffected side for 3 to 5 minutes to allow gravity to promote movement of the medication into the ear canal. If the infection is generalized or severe, systemic antibiotics are used. An infection that involves cartilage has to be treated aggressively and quickly with systemic antibiotics to avoid complications.

With any form of otitis media, appropriate antibiotic therapy may be necessary. If drainage is present, a specimen may be collected for culture analysis and sensitivity testing. Most episodes of acute otitis media, however, do not produce drainage, and the specific bacterial cause need not be identified. Otitis media is generally easily managed, but if it is not treated properly, it can lead to sinusitis, meningitis, and brain abscess because of the proximity of the ear to other tissues.

Suppurative otitis media is managed with systemic antibiotics, topical antibiotic drops, and analgesics. If otitis media becomes chronic, myringotomy may be required to ventilate the middle ear and equalize pressure between the middle ear and external ear. Because infection starts in the middle ear, the problems in the mastoid cavity are avoided by early use of antibiotics with otitis media.

Alleviate Pain. Because external otitis is one of the most painful disorders of the ear, appropriate analgesics are required. Pain persists for 24 to 48 hours after treatment is initiated. Once the swelling and drainage are reduced by treatment, in about 48 hours the pain subsides.

Restore Normal Function and Remove Foreign Bodies. Removal of foreign bodies from the ear canal can be quite difficult. The external auditory canal is an exquisitely sensitive, elliptical, cylinder-like structure. In adults, it is about 24 mm long and has two anatomic points of narrowing. Objects caught behind these narrow points create the greatest problems for removal. If perforation of the tympanic membrane is deemed unlikely and the object is not tightly wedged, you can irrigate the external canal with warm water. Direct the stream of water superiorly and anteriorly into the ear canal and around the object (see Figure 68-5). Water pressure builds up and forces the object outward. It often takes about 200 to 300 ml of water to remove an object. Do not irrigate vegetable foreign proteins, such as beans, because they would swell and become even more difficult to remove.

For removal of a live insect, the ear canal is filled with mineral oil, lidocaine, or an ether-soaked cotton ball, *not water,* to kill or stupefy the insect. Water would cause the insect to swell and become more difficult to remove.

The least traumatic method of removing a foreign body is with the aid of an operating microscope. The nurse should not spend a long time attempting to remove an object from the ear without asking for help. After removing the object, inspect the tympanic membrane and ear canal for manifestations of trauma. If trauma is noted, the client should be treated for external otitis and seen again in 4 to 5 days.

■ Nursing Management of the Medical Client Assessment

When obtaining the history of the pain, ask the client about what events have triggered the ear pain, paying special attention to a recent history of the following:
- Upper respiratory tract infection
- Travel by airplane
- Exposure to loud noises
- Trauma to the head
- Stressors that lead to teeth grinding or dental work

The nurse first observes the external ear for redness, swelling, lumps, scaling, crusting, or drainage, either serous or purulent. During assessment of the external ear, manipulation of the ear is important. If the client

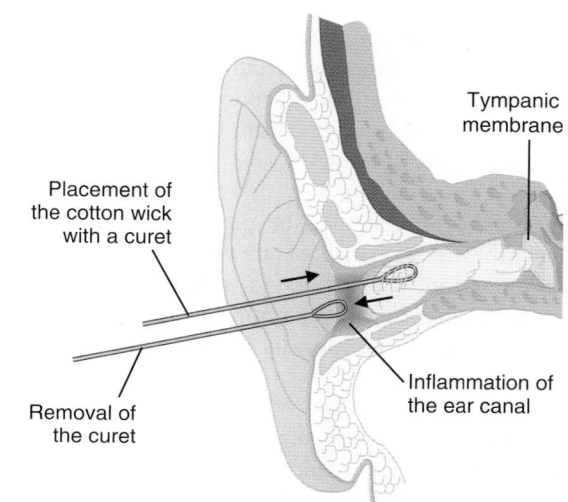

FIGURE 68-6 Administration of antibiotics for otitis externa. A curet with a cotton wick around it is placed in the ear canal. The wick is gently placed in the canal, and an antibiotic or treatment solution is added to the wick.

Tympanic membrane

Placement of the cotton wick with a curet

Removal of the curet

Inflammation of the ear canal

complains of pain when any part of the ear is palpated, an abscess, a lesion, or some kind of inflammatory process of the ear canal is suspected. If an otoscopic examination is performed, care must be taken not to cause the client unnecessary pain. An abscess may be close to the opening of the canal, where the pressure of the speculum may cause greater pain.

During the physical examination, determine the presence of pain with swallowing, neck rotation, palpation of the face and head (over the sinuses), palpation of the mastoid process, and manipulation of the pinna. Assess the TMJ by inserting your index fingers into the external auditory canals and applying pressure anteriorly while the client opens and closes the mouth. TMJ syndrome may cause pain, clicking, or crepitation of the joint during movement.

Diagnosis, Outcomes, Interventions

Diagnosis: Risk for Infection.
Because of tissue damage from trauma, foreign body, or pathogen, the nursing diagnosis *Risk for Infection related to tissue destruction* may be appropriate in the client with otalgia.

Outcomes. The client will have reduced risk of infection or will experience resolution of infection without complications.

Interventions. Monitor for clinical manifestations of infection, and administer antibiotics as prescribed. Other medications, such as antihistamines, decongestants, and steroid nasal sprays, may be ordered to reduce inflammation that can damage tissue. Teach the client to complete the entire prescription of the antibiotic even though manifestations may have cleared (see the Client Education Guide on Infection of the Tympanic Membrane, *evolve* Middle Ear, or Mastoid Cavity on the website).

During an infectious process, instruct the client to avoid getting water in the ear while bathing or showering by using earplugs or placing cotton balls coated with petroleum jelly in the ear canal.

Eardrops may also be prescribed for bacterial or fungal infections, which are often seen in otitis externa. Various irrigations of the mastoid system and middle ear are used for chronic infections along with antibiotic eardrops or powders. In chronic otitis media with discharge, both broad-spectrum oral antibiotics and topical antibiotic drops are used.

Diagnosis: Acute Pain.
Otalgia may be caused by a process in the ear or may be referred from a source outside the ear, resulting in the nursing diagnosis *Acute Pain related to inflammation in the external or middle ear or from referred pain in the head and neck area.*

Outcomes. The client will be able to reduce pain and achieve an acceptable comfort level.

Interventions. Otalgia is managed by treating the primary problem. Comfort can be promoted by using anesthetic ear solutions or systemic analgesics. After the physician has prescribed the analgesic therapy, instruct the client as to the amount, frequency, and duration. Other measures are the application of heat by warm compress, a soft diet, a quiet environment, and positioning of the client with the affected ear down.

The client with TMJ syndrome should avoid chewing and hyperextension of the jaw (e.g., for dental examination and care). He or she should also try to stop grinding the teeth. A specially fitted mouth guard to be worn while sleeping can be helpful in preventing teeth grinding at night.

In the case of eustachian tube dysfunction or barotrauma, teach the client how to facilitate opening of the eustachian tube. Chewing gum, sucking hard candy and swallowing often, yawning, and blowing air out against closed nostrils (Valsalva maneuver) help open the tube.

Evaluation

The positive outcome for the client with otalgia depends on (1) the thoroughness of the instructions provided by the nurse and (2) the client's compliance with the prescribed treatment regimen. Ongoing assessment of the client to achieve resolution of infectious and inflammatory processes contributing to the otalgia are key to effective management.

■ Surgical Management

The surgical treatment of infections involves incision and drainage in the acute phase for abscesses and, at times, for perichondritis. Perichondrial hematomas are incised and drained and then dressed in large, bulky dressings. The most common surgical treatment is excision of cysts and cutaneous carcinomas. For conditions that occlude the ear canal, more extensive surgery that involves removal of bone and skin grafting, known as a *canaloplasty*, is performed.

Myringoplasty. Surgery can be performed on the tympanic membrane with use of an operating microscope for magnification. Closure of a simple perforation is called a *myringoplasty*. If the tympanic membrane needs to be reconstructed, temporalis fascia or other connective tissue can be used.

Tympanoplasty. *Tympanoplasty* is the surgical correction of a perforated tympanic membrane. The four types of corrections are based on medial position of the placement of the graft as follows:

- *Type I:* Graft rests on malleus
- *Type II:* Graft rests on incus
- *Type III:* Graft attaches to head of stapes
- *Type IV:* Graft attaches to footplate of stapes

When the eustachian tube is stable, postoperative hearing results worsen as one proceeds from type I to type IV tympanoplasty. Under favorable conditions, type I tympanoplasty should result in normal or near-normal restoration of conductive hearing loss, whereas type IV should result in approximately a 30-db air-bone gap. In tympanoplasty, a graft is placed to restore the damaged tympanic membrane. The location of the graft depends on the original defect. Sometimes tympanostomy (ventilation) tubes are inserted.

Ossiculoplasty. The surgical procedure of ossicular reconstruction is called *ossiculoplasty*. Various methods of repositioning these tiny ear bones are now in use. In addition, various synthetic prostheses have been used to reconnect the ossicles to carry sound. In an attempt to prevent extrusion of the prostheses, tissue is combined with the prostheses to rebuild the ossicles. This semibiologic method is used in different forms by most otologic surgeons (Figure 68-7).

Laser surgery can be performed in chronic ear disease for a cholesteatoma associated with the stapes.

Myringotomy. An incision into the tympanic membrane through which fluid is removed by suction is called *myringotomy*. To keep the incision open and to prevent a recurrence of fluid, various types of transtympanic tubes can be inserted into the incision. These tubes extrude by themselves in 3 to 12 months and rarely have to be removed. More permanent tubes (T tubes) with larger flanges may be used for clients who require repeated myringotomies.

Mastoidectomy. Radical mastoidectomy removes the contents of the mastoid bone for control of infection and cholesteatoma. Because the radical mastoidectomy sacrifices hearing, a modified radical mastoidectomy was de-

veloped to save the remaining middle ear structures. With the advent of antibiotics, simple mastoidectomy became possible, which maintained a normal-appearing ear canal. Because radical and modified mastoidectomies exteriorize the mastoid cavity to the external ear canal, they are known as *open* or *canal wall–down mastoidectomies*. *Closed* or *canal wall-up mastoidectomies* are simple mastoidectomies with modifications that are performed in conjunction with tympanoplasty and ossiculoplasty to retain or regain hearing. Today even the open mastoidectomy is performed with various tympanoplasties.

■ Nursing Management of the Surgical Client

Preoperative Care
The scope of nursing activities for the client undergoing surgery for otalgia can be as broad as a preoperative assessment performed in an office or clinic or as limited as an assessment performed in the holding area of the surgical suite. Before surgery, an audiogram and tympanogram are obtained to assess preoperative hearing acuity. The client's level of knowledge about the procedure, expectations, and psychosocial readiness for surgery are evaluated along with the physiologic status.

The client undergoing ear surgery should be told what to expect during the procedure because local anesthesia with sedation is often used. Instructions should be given about the duration of the procedure, the estimated length of hospital stay, and immediate postoperative instructions. Often fear of the unknown can be decreased by an understanding of the events that will occur.

Postoperative Care
Pain is not usually a major problem, but mild analgesia may be required. Vertigo or lightheadedness may occur when the client ambulates for the first time. Clients should be supervised when ambulating on the day of surgery to protect them from falling. Some clients who are quite vertiginous exhibit nystagmus (see Chapter 66) from stimulation of the inner ear. The vertigo usually passes very quickly and seldom requires medication.

The ear rarely bleeds after surgery. A small amount of serosanguineous drainage on a cotton ball is expected. After most ear procedures, only a cotton ball is needed in the ear, although a dressing over the ear may be necessary after tympanomastoidectomy. See the Client Education Guide feature on Precautions After Ear Surgery on p. 1988.

Immediate postoperative instructions may include the following:

1. Positioning should be specified, such as the client lying with operated ear up for several hours after surgery.
2. If necessary, the client should blow the nose gently one side at a time.

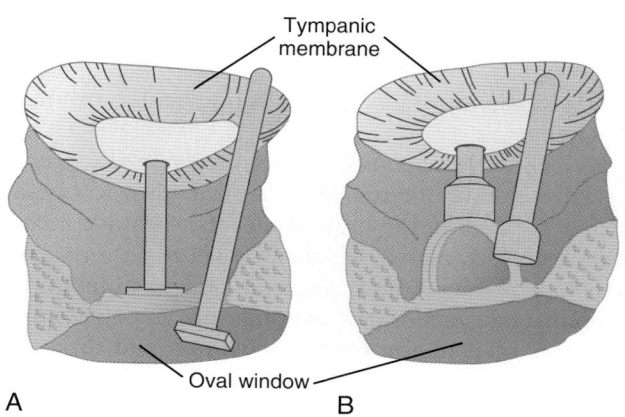

FIGURE 68-7 Middle ear prostheses used for reconstruction. **A,** Ossicle columella prosthesis (total ossicular replacement). **B,** Ossicle cup prosthesis (partial ossicular replacement). (Courtesy of Arnold G. Shuring, M.D.)

Tympanic membrane

Oval window

A   B

CLIENT EDUCATION GUIDE
Precautions After Ear Surgery

To prevent injury and promote healing:
- Continue to blow your nose gently one side at a time and to sneeze or cough with your mouth open for 1 week after surgery.
- Avoid physical activity for 1 week and exercises or sports for 3 weeks after surgery.
- Return to work as recommended, usually 3 to 7 days after surgery (3 weeks if work is strenuous).
- Avoid heavy lifting, especially after stapedectomy.
- Change the cotton ball in your ear daily as prescribed.
- Keep your ear dry for 4 to 6 weeks after surgery.
- Do not shampoo for 1 week after surgery.
- Protect your ear when necessary with two pieces of cotton (outer piece saturated with petroleum jelly).
- Avoid airplane flights for the first week after surgery. For sensation of ear pressure, hold your nose, close your mouth, and swallow to equalize pressure.
- Wear noise defenders in loud environments.
- Report any drainage other than a slight amount of bleeding to the physician.

BOX 68-4   *Disorders Associated with Vertigo and Dizziness*

Peripheral Labyrinthine (Inner Ear) Disorders
Benign paroxysmal positional vertigo (BPPV)
Labyrinthitis
Ménière's disease
Cholesteatoma

Central Nervous System Disorders
Cerebellar lesions
Temporal lobe lesions
Tumors of cranial nerve VIII (e.g., acoustic neuroma)
Stroke
Multiple sclerosis

Systemic Disorders
Diabetes
Postural hypotension
Arthritis
Hypoglycemia
Allergies

---

3. The client should sneeze or cough with the mouth open.
4. Participation in water sports or activities is prohibited.

Normal occurrences in the initial period after ear surgery may include the following:
- Decreased hearing in operated ear from surgical packing (people may sound like they are talking in a barrel)
- Noises in the ear, such as cracking or popping
- Minor earache and discomfort in cheek and jaw
- Ear swelling

BALANCE DISORDERS

As already described, *vertigo* is the perception that either oneself or one's surroundings are moving. The person with vertigo usually remains seated or supine to prevent falling. Vertigo is often described as "dizziness." Dizziness, which can involve feelings of disorientation in space or lightheadedness, is different, however. Vertigo results from imbalance of neural signals from the vestibular system in the ears. The imbalance of signals is interpreted by the brain as constant motion in space.

Disorders of balance and coordination result from problems of the vestibular system and "righting" reflexes. Balance can also be affected by problems outside the vestibular system. Few problems are more private than those involving one's sense of balance. Balance problems may be debilitating and may also cause embarrassing gait problems, which can jeopardize safety. More than 90 million Americans aged 17 years or older have experienced vertigo or a balance problem. Vertigo is second only to chronic pain as the most common manifestation reported in America today.

Etiology and Risk Factors

Although vertigo and dizziness are not synonymous, they both relate to a sense of balance and equilibrium. Dizziness, vertigo, and syncope (fainting) are all manifestations of one of the following types of problems:
- Peripheral vestibular disorders (i.e., labyrinthine or inner ear)
- Central disorders (i.e., medullary, cerebellar, or cortical)
- Systemic disorders (i.e., cardiovascular or metabolic)

Peripheral vestibular disorders involve a disorder in the labyrinth or internal ear. Central disorders result from a problem in the brain or nerves, such as a tumor of the eighth cranial nerve (acoustic neuroma) or stroke. Systemic disorders begin in a nerve or organ outside the cranium (e.g., orthostatic hypotension, hypoglycemia). Examples of common causes of vertigo and dizziness, grouped by etiology, are presented in Box 68-4.

Little can be done to reduce the risk of balance disorders. Clients should be treated early for manifestations of ear problems. Clients at high risk for falling as a result of vertigo should stand up slowly to prevent injury and should keep a light on at all times to enable visual cues to lessen the disequilibrium. Finally, situations that lead to vertigo should be avoided. Motion sickness occurs normally if the provocative stimulus is present. Humans are not evolutionarily adapted to special environmental situations, such as deep-sea diving, high-speed flying, and space travel. Vertigo or dizziness may occur in these environments.

Peripheral Vestibular Disorders

Benign Paroxysmal Positional Vertigo. Benign paroxysmal positional vertigo (BPPV) is a common cause of vertigo. It tends to follow head injury and viral infections of the inner ear. BPPV is due to *cupulolithiasis,* the presence of calcium crystals in the semicircular canals. These crystals are normally deposited on small hair-like structures in the ear called *otoliths,* and they slow responses to head movement. When they are dislodged, head movement creates a hypersensitive response. BPPV is provoked when the head is placed in certain positions, usually hyperextended and to one side. Clinical manifestations usually consist of brief attacks of rotational vertigo, a rapid head tilt to the affected ear, and a lag time of 3 to 6 seconds between change of position and vertigo with nystagmus. It is usually self-limited and resolves spontaneously over weeks to months.

Labyrinthitis (Vestibular Neuronitis). Labyrinthitis is infection or inflammation of the cochlear or vestibular portion of the inner ear or both. Causes are not fully understood, but the syndrome tends to occur in spring and early summer and to be preceded by an upper respiratory infection. A virus has therefore been implicated but has never been isolated. Three classic manifestations are reported: vertigo, nausea, and vomiting. There are no hearing changes. Vertigo is usually sudden in onset; it peaks in 24 to 48 hours and then gradually subsides over 1 to 2 weeks. Supportive treatment is usually given during the wait for the underlying problems to clear.

Ménière's Disease. As mentioned previously, Ménière's disease is caused by excess endolymph in the vestibular and semicircular canals. Normal vestibular activity depends on the stability of fluid pressure. Ménière's disease causes hearing changes and vertigo. It is discussed under Balance Disorders because vertigo is often the most troublesome manifestation in the early stages.

Ménière's disease is an episodic illness that waxes and wanes, often remaining quiescent for many years and then reappearing. A cluster of manifestations develops consisting of (1) paroxysmal whirling vertigo, (2) fluctuating hearing loss, (3) tinnitus, and (4) aural fullness. Only one or two manifestations may be present initially. Vertigo is characterized by remission and relapses without apparent cause, although the manifestations become less severe in time. The initial attacks consist of approximately 30 minutes of intense vertigo, which commonly provokes nausea and vomiting. Remaining stationary reduces vertigo.

A sensorineural hearing loss (see Hearing Impairment) that may be reversible in the early stages is a serious consequence of Ménière's disease. Control of episodes of the disease is usually possible, although a cure is not yet available. Clients are treated with low-sodium diets, diuretics, and balance exercises. Surgery, which is another option, is discussed later.

Central Disorders of Balance

Dizziness may be a manifestation of a transient ischemic attack (TIA) ("small stroke"). A temporary loss of blood flow to the brain leads to several manifestations, depending on the brain area that is not being perfused. Clients can experience momentary losses of consciousness, transient numbness, tingling, weakness, and changes in speech. TIAs should be reported and treated aggressively to prevent true ischemic changes.

Systemic Disorders Leading to Vertigo

Physiologic Vertigo. Physiologic vertigo is involved in common disorders such as motion sickness. In these conditions, vertigo is minimal or absent, but autonomic manifestations are present. Motion sickness leads to perspiration, nausea, vomiting, increased salivation, yawning, and malaise. Physiologic vertigo can usually be suppressed by supplying sensory cues that come from other stimuli. For example, motion sickness from reading in a car can be reduced by looking out the window at the moving environment.

Presbyastasis. A disorder that is recognized more and more is *presbyastasis,* or disequilibrium of aging. Because of the generalized degenerative changes that occur in aging, balance and stability are affected. In addition to the labyrinth, balance also depends on the visual system and the proprioceptive changes in the muscles. Because all three systems are involved in aging, older adults have difficulty with stability, which results in falls and subsequent trauma.

Orthostatic Hypotension. Orthostatic hypotension is a sudden drop in blood pressure and dizziness on sitting or standing. The manifestations noted are lightheadedness and faintness, not vertigo, which is due to inadequate cerebral blood flow. Older adults are at high risk of orthostatic hypotension because of atherosclerosis and the use of medications that lead to diuresis or hypotension (e.g., furosemide, calcium-channel blockers). Orthostasis is diagnosed through assessment of positional blood pressure changes. Clients should be taught to change position slowly, and medications may require adjustment if blood pressure is too low.

Pathophysiology

The body maintains balance and equilibrium by responding to an intricate network of information. The ability to maintain balance depends on the intactness of four systems:

- Vestibular system (the labyrinth or inner ear)
- Visual system (the eyes)
- Proprioceptive system (the somatosensory nerves of joints and muscles)
- Cerebellar system (the coordinator)

The sensations transmitted from the ears, the eyes, and the somatosensory nerves are integrated in the brain stem and cerebellum and perceived in the cerebral cortex. Gradual interference of vestibular input causes compensatory changes that allow the brain to adjust slowly. Quick changes demand more adjustments than can be made. Infections can destroy the nerve and alter transmission of messages. Overproduction of endolymph can slow transmission of messages and lead to the perception that the body is in constant motion. Head trauma can shake free calcium carbonate crystals on the utricular macule and alter endolymph movement.

Clinical Manifestations

Vertigo is the most common clinical manifestation in a client with a balance problem. The clinical manifestations of balance disorders vary widely depending on (1) the cause, (2) the location (one or both ears), (3) the client's age at onset, (4) the extent of the loss of vestibular function, and (5) the rapidity with which damage occurs. Disease in the external ear, middle ear, and inner ear usually leads to vertigo that is sudden, transient, and accompanied by vagal manifestations (e.g., nausea, vomiting, sweating, pallor). The vertigo associated with cerebrovascular lesions does not follow a pattern; however, tinnitus and hearing loss are usually not present.

An important differentiation is whether the vertigo is associated with hearing loss. The close anatomic relationship between the balance and hearing systems sometimes causes the sensation of vertigo in conjunction with a hearing loss. In most instances, vertigo is present without a hearing loss. It is also important to distinguish between vertigo from vestibular problems and other forms of vertigo. Table 68-2 differentiates the two forms of vertigo.

Dizziness is described by clients in such varied terms that it is almost impossible to define. Not all the terms listed here suggest true vertigo. The nurse should record the terms or description the client uses to help find the actual cause. Clinical manifestations are listed in Box 68-5.

Even after the vertigo has abated, anxiety tends to persist. Clients are very worried about having another "attack."

For the client with vertigo, the differential diagnosis may be accomplished by means of a thorough medical assessment, including audiometry, vestibular tests, imag-

---

BOX 68-5	*Clinical Manifestations of Vertigo*

- Staggering
- Giddiness
- Lightheadedness
- Disorientation
- Visual blurring
- Veering in one direction while walking
- Unsteadiness
- Reeling
- Faintness
- Wooziness
- Shakiness

- Instability
- Wobbliness
- Bewilderment
- Confusion
- Being dazed
- Clumsiness
- Sense of floating
- Sense of falling
- Weakness
- Vague feeling of uncertainty

TABLE 68-2	*Vestibular and Nonvestibular Vertigo*	
	Vestibular	**Nonvestibular**
Common descriptions	Spinning (environment moves), on a merry-go-round	Lightheadedness, feeling of being dissociated from body, swimming, giddiness, spinning inside (environment stationary)
Clinical manifestations	Drunkenness, tilting, motion sickness, off balance	
Course of illness	Episodic	Constant
Precipitating factors	Head movement, position change	Stress, hyperventilation, cardiac dysrhythmia, orthostatic hypotension
Associated manifestations	Nausea, vomiting, tinnitus, hearing loss, impaired vision, unsteadiness	Perspiration, pallor, paresthesias, palpitations, syncope, difficulty concentrating, tension headache; anxiety

ing evaluation, and, sometimes laboratory studies. Clients who have had vertigo may become quite anxious when they think about experiencing it again. Because vertigo is only a clinical manifestation, the diagnosis and treatment of the underlying disease are important. Unlike with vision or hearing problems, no single organ is responsible for balance problems. Therefore the diagnosis, treatment, and rehabilitation of the client with a balance problem can be difficult as well as frustrating.

Outcome Management
■ Medical Management

Two main treatment goals guide the medical management of the client with vertigo. They are (1) suppression of the CNS and the vestibular system and (2) vestibular rehabilitation.

Suppress the Central Nervous System and Vestibular System. Treatment of acute vertigo involves several medicines, called *antivertigo agents*. These medicines tend to suppress the balance system or the CNS, allowing recovery over time. They should be used judiciously in clients with BPPV because they slow recovery of function. Other medicines used for specific disorders are antibiotics, steroids, diuretics, tranquilizers, and vitamins.

A recent treatment for manifestations associated with Ménière's disease is the application of low-pressure pulses through the ear canal to the middle ear. This airwave transmission passes through the external and middle ear structures to the fluids in the inner ear. The initial use of this device shows promise in relieving vertigo and improving hearing function during the early stages of Ménière's disease.

Promote Vestibular Rehabilitation. Vestibular rehabilitation is a recognized form of control for vertigo. Because the balance system can compensate, head and total body exercises are performed by the client to hasten compensation. Vestibular rehabilitation consists of exercises that promote vestibular adaptation, habituation, and activities of daily living. Usually physical therapists are involved in structuring this treatment. Vestibular rehabilitation uses all three organ systems that provide balance.

The exercises included in vestibular rehabilitation are performed as follows:

1. While lying in bed, slowly then quickly turn the eyes up, down, and from side to side, and the head forward, backward, and from side to side.
2. Perform the same exercises while sitting; in addition, bend forward and pick up objects from the ground.
3. While standing, perform the previously mentioned exercises; in addition, change from sitting to standing position with the eyes open and then closed, and turn around in between (i.e., change direction as well as position with eyes open and closed).

4. While moving about, walk up and down steps with the eyes open and then closed, or play games involving stooping and stretching, such as basketball.

It is believed that when vertigo is induced by these exercises, a tolerance for it is acquired. Clients should perform these exercises from the time of the acute attack and continue until they are free of manifestations for two consecutive days. Driving a car safely needs to be addressed with clients who have vertigo. Vestibular rehabilitation therapy has been found efficacious in treating vertigo associated with certain types of vestibular deficits. Several studies have found marked improvements in postural stability, walking, and symptom control in clients who have undergone vestibular rehabilitation therapy compared with those who have not participated in this treatment. Appropriateness of this therapy in treating vertigo in older clients has been evaluated in a few studies. Initial findings indicate that vestibular rehabilitation is well tolerated and can be effective treatment for vertigo in the older person. See the Evidence-Based Practice in Action feature on Vestibular Rehabilitation in Older Adults on p. 1992.

A specific intervention strategy that is currently being used involves a series of manipulative interventions known as the *Epley maneuvers*. These maneuvers, which are used specifically for BPPV, are designed to facilitate return of dislodged otoliths to their more normal position within the labyrinth. The Epley maneuvers are essentially a more direct, rapid method to restore normal function and are of variable efficacy.

■ Nursing Management of the Medical Client
Assessment

Nursing assessment of the client with a balance problem should consist of the following areas:

1. A client interview to obtain a health history and specific information about the onset and characteristics of the balance problem and associated hearing problems. Attempt to distinguish the type of vertigo reported, and note aggravating conditions (e.g., head movement)
2. An interview with a family member to determine the effects of the client's balance problem on others
3. Assessment of the effect of the vertigo on the client's performance of the activities of daily living

The importance of the history and interview cannot be overemphasized. An adequate description of vertigo should include information about the onset, exacerbating and alleviating factors, associated clinical manifestations, and predisposing factors in the medical history, as previously described. All clients bring some degree of anxiety regarding this illness to the examination. Balance problems can have devastating effects on a client's behavior. The disruption of the client's routine, the

EB EVIDENCE-BASED PRACTICE IN ACTION

Vestibular Rehabilitation in Older Adults

Vestibular rehabilitation therapy (VRT) provides a comprehensive approach to management of the vertiginous client, which includes exercises that promote stability and alleviate manifestations while improving ones daily functioning. VRT is implemented in phases. Initially the person performs vestibular adaptation exercises to promote compensatory processes in the central nervous system. These adaptation exercises focus on improving stability in different postural positions (supine, sitting, and standing) and facilitating performance of activities of daily living. Habituation exercises are instituted later in the process during the maintenance phase of treatment.[1,2]

A brief vestibular rehabilitation (VR) intervention, used in a primary care setting, reduced manifestations and improved balance and postural control in clients with dizziness and vertigo.[3] Clients with chronic vestibular disorders accompanied by unsteadiness, imbalance, or motion intolerance experienced significant symptom improvement and reduction in falls after receiving VR in weekly sessions designed for daily home use.[4] These two prospective studies, although based on small numbers of clients, provide good initial evidence of the effectiveness of VR in treating clients with vestibular disorders.

The effectiveness of the treatment is related to adherence to the regimen of activities over the rehabilitation period. This involves ongoing support, instruction, and evaluation to obtain benefits from VR in managing vertigo. While performing these exercises, individuals often experience manifestations of vertigo and dizziness and may become unsteady. Older persons commonly experience dizziness and unsteadiness as a result of age-related deterioration of the vestibular system. Along with the physical consequences of gait alteration and disequilibrium, the older person may feel anxious and less confident in functioning independently.[5] Inclusion of general precautions and protective adaptations to prevent falls, such as the use of walkers and handrails, is included in the rehabilitation program, especially with older clients.

A chart review of younger and older adults on VRT revealed overall improvements and beneficial results in both groups unrelated to age differences.[6] Another study examined a combined approach of VR and cognitive behavioral therapy in older clients. There was a significant improvement in walking time and relief of dizziness manifestations but no effect on anxiety or depression.[7] These two studies provide initial support regarding the efficacy of VR in managing vertigo and dizziness in older clients. Improvement in psychological distress was not achieved, but because of the small number of older clients studied, more research is warranted to substantiate or refute the beneficial effects on anxiety and depression.

Implications

Vestibular rehabilitation can be an effective treatment in managing vertigo in certain vestibular disorders. It is beneficial in alleviating manifestations and improving function and activities in older adults. Inclusion of protective measures to reduce the risk of falls and continued support of the client during rehabilitation can improve outcomes. VRT is well tolerated by the older client and seems to be an effective therapy for management of vertigo.

References

1. Herdman, S.J ., Blatt, P.J ., & Schubert, M.C. (2000). Vestibular rehabilitation of patients with vestibular hypofunction or with benign paroxysmal positional vertigo. *Current Opinion in Neurotology, 13,* 39-43.
2. Konnur, M.K. (2000). Vertigo and vestibular rehabilitation. *Journal of Postgraduate Medicine, 46,* 222-223.
3. Yardley, L., et al. (1998). A randomized controlled trial of exercise therapy for dizziness and vertigo in primary care. *The British Journal of General Practice, 48*(429), 1136-1140.
4. Black, F.O., et al. (2000). Outcomes analysis of individualized vestibular rehabilitation protocols. *The American Journal of Otology, 21*(4), 543-551.
5. Matheson, A.J., Darlington, C.L., & Smith, P.F. (1999). Dizziness in the elderly and age-related degeneration of the vestibular system. *New Zealand Journal of Psychology, 28* (1), 10-16.
6. Whitney, S.L., et al. (2002). The effect of age on vestibular rehabilitation outcomes. *Laryngoscope, 112* (10), 1785-1790.
7. Johansson, M., et al. (2001). Randomized controlled trial of vestibular rehabilitation combined with cognitive-behavioral therapy for dizziness in older people. *Otolaryngology-Head and Neck Surgery, 125* (3), 151-156.

severity of the "attacks," and the fear of the unknown can make the client agitated, anxious, or depressed. The nurse must be aware of these feelings and must demonstrate self-confidence, patience, courtesy, and gentleness.

A structured questionnaire such as the one shown in Box 68-6 should be completed by the client. These questions can also be used to facilitate the interview; however, the interview should be guided by client cues. A gross assessment of the client's balance can be made by watching the client's gait. Evidence of instability may be noted if the client touches the wall or walks with a wide-based, waddling gait.

The same inspection, palpation, and otoscopic examination should be performed for the client with a balance problem as was performed for the client with hearing loss (see earlier discussion). The client must be questioned for the loss of hearing and tinnitus, which can accompany a balance problem.

BOX 68-6 *Assessment Guide for Clients with Balance Disorders*

A. When you are dizzy, do you experience any of the following sensations? Please read the entire list first. Then circle the numbers of those sensations that describe what you experience most accurately.
  1. Lightheadedness
  2. Tendency to lose balance or to fall
  3. Objects spinning or turning around you
  4. Sensation that you are turning
  5. Headache
  6. Nausea or vomiting
  7. Pressure in the head

B. Please fill in the blank spaces.
  1. When did the dizziness first occur? _____
  2. Is your vertigo constant? _____
  3. Does it come in attacks? _____
  4. How often do attacks occur? _____
  5. How long are the attacks? _____
  6. Does vertigo occur only in certain positions? _____

       When upright? _____
       When lying flat? _____

Turning to the right? _____
Turning to the left? _____
  7. Have you ever stumbled or fallen because of vertigo? _____
  8. Do you know of anything that will stop the vertigo or make it better? _____
     Make your vertigo worse? _____
     Bring on an attack? _____
  9. Did you ever injure your head? _____
  10. Do you take any medications regularly (e.g., tranquilizers; oral contraceptives; barbiturates; a course of antibiotics, such as streptomycin, neomycin)?

      _____
  11. Do you use tobacco in any form? _____
      Alcohol? _____
  12. Have you worked for long in a noisy environment? _____
  13. Do you suffer easily from motion sickness? _____

Diagnosis, Outcomes, Interventions

Nursing care is detailed in the Care Plan feature on The Client with Vertigo on the website.

■ Surgical Management

About 5% or less of all clients with vertigo undergo surgical intervention.

Endolymphatic Sac Surgery. The endolymphatic sac procedures include decompression and various forms of shunts to the CNS or mastoid cavity. The intent of these procedures is to lessen the fluid pressure within the labyrinth and control the vertigo of Ménière's disease. Forty-four studies have been conducted over the past decade to determine the efficacy of endolymphatic sac procedures. A collective review of the results of 1800 cases of various surgical approaches to the endolymphatic sac found that 22% of clients had improved hearing, 53% had no change in hearing acuity, and 25% had worsened hearing as determined by the established guidelines. Refinement of surgical approaches and outcomes research on these techniques continues to be important.

Labyrinthectomy. *Labyrinthectomy* is a form of surgery designed to destroy the labyrinth and eliminate its abnormal input. It is performed through the oval or round window (membranous limits of cochlear and inner ear). This is a destructive procedure that removes the membranous labyrinth, either subtotally through the oval window or totally through the mastoid bone. Any remaining hearing is sacrificed.

In a nonsurgical approach to labyrinthectomy, an ototoxic drug can be injected through the tympanic membrane into the middle ear to destroy the hair cells of the vestibular system. This procedure is carried out over a series of visits and is designed to decrease the abnormal vestibular signal in the affected ear. A secondary and sometimes unavoidable effect is concurrent cochlear toxicity. Clients are treated until their vestibular manifestations improve significantly, with the goal of preserving as much hearing as possible.

Vestibular Nerve Resection. Vestibular nerve resection is a highly effective procedure performed to alleviate vertigo. Vestibular nerve resection can be performed through the labyrinth (sacrificing hearing) or around the labyrinth (saving hearing). The retrolabyrinthine surgical approach is the most common form of surgical control for vertigo today. This method preserves the inner ear structures and approaches the vestibular nerve from behind the semicircular canal. Alleviation of the client's vertigo is usually immediate. Because of the compensation by all the other structures related to maintaining balance, a client can function with only one labyrinth.

CONCLUSIONS

Nurses caring for clients with hearing and balance problems need to focus on safety and on promoting independence. Many hearing-impaired clients live a normal life with hearing augmentation and aural rehabilitation. Clients who have diminished hearing or balance disorders are at increased risk for injury because of lack of awareness of the risks or from losing balance. Infections of the ears remain common, but excellent antibiotics have reduced the incidence of chronic problems caused by infections. Tumors of the ear are rare, but when they occur, they are quite destructive.

THINKING CRITICALLY *evolve*

1. A middle-aged man comes to the health clinic with ear pain and difficulty hearing. He had some serous drainage 1 day ago but does not recall any recent infection (throat or ear). The problem has persisted intermittently over the past 6 months and is getting progressively more painful and occurring more frequently. If surgery were deemed necessary for this client, how would you prepare him? What discharge teaching might need to be completed for this client after ear surgery?

Factors to Consider. What preoperative assessments are needed? How should equal pressures be maintained on the tympanic membrane? What normal occurrences might the client expect in the initial period following surgery?

2. An older woman reveals a 10-year history of ear infection. She is experiencing sensorineural hearing loss associated with presbycusis, which affects older people. During her clinic appointment, she tells the nurse that her right ear is painful and is keeping her awake at night. She explains that she can hear most sounds, although sounds on the right side seem to be coming through a filter. She has been using her eardrops as directed but has stopped taking her oral antibiotic because she felt better 2 days ago. She requests information about daily medication or a surgical procedure that might alleviate the problem. How should you respond to the client's request? How do age-related changes contribute to her problem?

Factors to Consider. What is the assessment focus for this client? What is the prognosis for the client with presbycusis? What type of teaching does the client require?

Discussions for these questions can be found on the website and the CD-ROM.

BIBLIOGRAPHY

1. Black, F.O., et al. (2000). Outcomes analysis of individualized vestibular rehabilitation protocols. *The American Journal of Otology, 21(4)*, 543-551.
2. Brackmann, D.E., Shelton, C., & Arriaga, M.A. (Eds.). (2001). *Otologic surgery.* Philadelphia: W.B. Saunders.
3. Cruickshanks, K.J., et al. (1998). Cigarette smoking and hearing loss: The epidemiology of hearing loss study. *Journal of the American Medical Association, 279*, 1715-1719.
4. Cummings, C.W., et al. (1998). *Otolaryngology-head and neck surgery* (3rd ed.). St. Louis: Mosby.
5. Densert, B., & Sass, K. (2001). Control of symptoms in patients with Meniere's disease using middle ear pressure applications: Two year follow-up. *Acta Otolaryngology, 121*, 616-621.
6. Fairbanks, D.N.F. (2001). *Antimicrobial therapy in otolaryngology-head and neck surgery* (10th ed.). Alexandria, VA: American Academy of Otolaryngology-Head and Neck Surgery.
7. Francis, H.W., et al. (2002). Impact of cochlear implants on the functional health status of older adults. *Laryngoscope, 112*(8 Pt 1), 1482-1488.
8. Habkerkamp, T.J., & Tanyeri, H.M. (1999). Management of idiopathic sudden sensorineural hearing loss. *The American Journal of Otology, 20*, 587-592.
9. Hanley, K., O'Dowd, T., & Considine, N. (2001). A systematic review of vertigo in primary care. *The British Journal of General Practice, 51*, 666-671.
10. Harris, L.L., & Huntoon, M.B. (Eds.). (1998). *Core curriculum for otorhinolaryngology and head-neck nursing.* New Smyrna Beach, FL: Society of Otorhinolaryngology-Head and Neck Nurses, Inc.
11. Herdman, S.J., Blatt, P.J., & Schubert, M.C. (2000). Vestibular rehabilitation of patients with vestibular hypofunction or with benign paroxysmal positional vertigo. *Current Opinion in Neurotology, 13*, 39-43.
12. Holten, K.B., & Gick, J. (2001). Management of the patient with otitis externa. *Journal of Family Practice, 50(4)*, 353-360.
13. Hough, J.V., et al. (2001). Semi-implantable electromagnetic middle ear hearing device for moderate to severe sensorineural hearing loss. *Otolaryngology Clinics of North America, 34(2)*, 401-416.
14. Johansson, M., et al. (2001). Randomized controlled trial of vestibular rehabilitation combined with cognitive-behavioral therapy for dizziness in older people. *Otolaryngology-Head and Neck Surgery, 125(3)*, 151-156.
15. Karver, S.B. (1998). Otitis media. *Primary Care, 25(3)*, 619-632.
16. Konnur, M.K. (2000). Vertigo and vestibular rehabilitation. *Journal of Postgraduate Medicine, 46*, 222-223.
17. Linstrom, C.J. (1998). Cochlear implantation: Practical information for the generalist. *Primary Care, 25(3)*, 583-612.
18. Matheson, A.J., Darlington, C.L., & Smith, P.F. (1999). Dizziness in the elderly and age-related degeneration of the vestibular system. *New Zealand Journal of Psychology, 28(1)*, 10-16.

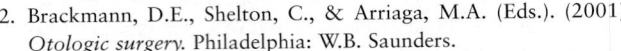

evolve Did you remember to check out the bonus material on the Evolve website and the CD-ROM, including free self-assessment exercises?

19. Palaniappan, R. (2002). Balance disorders in adults: An overview. *Hospital Medicine, 63*(5), 278-281.

20. Roland, P.S. (2001). Chronic external otitis. *Ear, Nose & Throat Journal, 80,* 759-760.

21. Roy, D., & Chopra, R. (2002). Tinnitus: An update. *Journal of the Royal Society of Health, 122*(1), 21-23.

22. Russell, K.E., Coffin, C., & Kenna, M. (1999). Cochlear implants and the deaf child: A nursing perspective. *Pediatric Nursing, 25,* 396-400, 444.

23. Sandhaus, S. (2002). Stop the spinning: Diagnosing and managing vertigo. *Nurse Practitioner, 27*(8), 545-581.

24. Silverman, C.A. (1998). Audiologic assessment and amplification. *Primary Care, 25*(3), 545-581.

 25. Snik, A.F., & Cremers, C.W. (2001). Vibrant semi-implantable hearing device with digital sound processing: Effective gain and speech perception. *Archives in Otolaryngology-Head and Neck Surgery, 127,* 1433-1437.

26. Stark, J., Toppila, E., & Pyykko, I. (1999). Smoking as a risk factor in sensory neural hearing loss among workers exposed to occupational noise. *Acta Otolaryngology, 119,* 302-305.

27. Thai-Van, H., Bounaix, M.J., & Fraysse, B. (2001). Meniere's disease: Pathophysiology and treatment. *Drugs, 61,* 1089-1102.

28. Tucci, D.L., et al. (2002). Treatment of sudden sensorineural hearing loss with systemic steroids and valacyclovir. *Otology and Neurology, 23*(3), 301-308.

29. Waltzman, S.B., et al. (2002). Long-term effects of cochlear implants in children. *Otolaryngology-Head and Neck Surgery, 126,* 505-511.

30. Whitney, S.L., et al. (2002). The effect of age on vestibular rehabilitation outcomes. *Laryngoscope, 112* (10), 1785-1790.

31. Whitney, S.L., & Rossi, M.M. (2000). Efficacy of vestibular rehabilitation. *Otolaryngologic Clinics of North America, 33*(3), 659-672.

32. Whitney, S.L., et al. (2002). The effect of age on vestibular rehabilitation outcomes. *Laryngoscope, 112,* 1785-1790.

33. Yardley, L., et al. (1998). A randomized controlled trial of exercise therapy for dizziness and vertigo in primary care. *The British Journal of General Practice, 48* (429), 1136-1140.

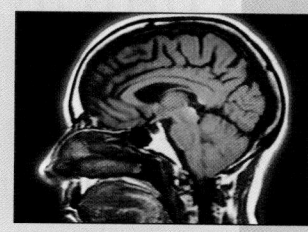

Cognitive and Perceptual Disorders

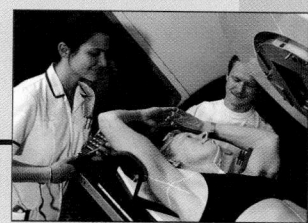

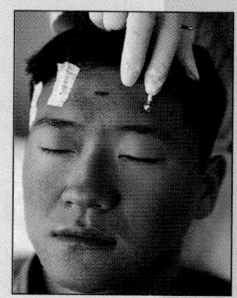

Anatomy and Physiology Review

The Neurologic System

Robert G. Carroll

The nervous system is the body's most organized and complex structural and functional system. It profoundly affects both psychological and physiologic functions. This unit discusses the importance of the nervous system to human functioning and the major consequences of neurologic disorders.

CENTRAL NERVOUS SYSTEM

The brain and spinal cord are known collectively as the *central nervous system* (CNS). The CNS is divided into three major functional divisions:

1. Higher-level brain, or cerebral cortex
2. Lower brain level (basal ganglia, thalamus, hypothalamus, midbrain, pons, medulla, cerebellum)
3. Spinal cord

These structures are protected by a rigid bony encasement, three layers of membranes, a fluid cushion, and a blood-brain or blood–spinal cord barrier.

BRAIN

The brain is the largest and most complex part of the nervous system. It is composed of more than 100 billion neurons and associated fibers. The brain tissues have a gelatin-like consistency. This semi-solid organ weighs about 1400 g (~3 pounds) in the adult human.

Cerebrum

The cerebrum is divided by a deep groove *(longitudinal fissure)* into two sections called *cerebral hemispheres*. A transverse fissure separates the cerebrum from the cerebellum. The outermost layer of the cerebrum, the *cerebral cortex,* is only 2 to 5 mm thick. Directly beneath the cerebral cortex are varying thicknesses of association tracts above the commisural tracts, known as the *corpus callosum* (Figure U16-1).

The cerebral cortex is composed of gray matter (predominantly nerve cell bodies and dendrites) formed into raised convolutions, or *gyri*. About 75% of the neuronal cell bodies in the brain are found in the cortex. The shallow grooves between the gyri *(sulci)* divide the cerebral cortex into five lobes: frontal, parietal, occipital, temporal, and central (insula) (Figure U16-2).

The term *neocortex* is often used to refer to the cerebral cortex. The neocortex includes all the cerebral cortex except the olfactory portions and the hippocampal regions.

Both the left cortex and the right cortex interpret sensory data, store memories, learn, and form concepts; however, each hemisphere dominates the other in many functions. In most people, for example, the *left* cortex has dominance for systematic analysis, language and speech, mathematics, abstraction, and reasoning. The *right* cortex has dominance for assimilation of sensory experiences, such as visual-spatial information, and activities such as dancing, gymnastics, music, and art appreciation.

In the frontal lobes, the precentral gyrus *(motor cortex)* controls voluntary motor activity. Most of these fibers cross to the opposite side of the brain at the medulla and descend via the spinal cord as the *lateral corticospinal tracts*. The area anterior to the precentral gyrus *(premotor area)* is also associated with voluntary motor activities. *Broca's area,* which lies anterior to the primary motor cortex and superior to the lateral sulcus, coordinates the complex muscular activity of the mouth, tongue, and larynx and makes expressive *(motor)* speech possible. Damage to this area leaves the client unable to speak clearly, a disorder called *Broca's aphasia.*

The *prefrontal areas* control (1) attention over time (concentration); (2) motivation; (3) the ability to formulate or select goals; (4) the ability to plan; (5) the ability to initiate, maintain, or terminate actions; (6) the ability to self-monitor, and (7) the ability to use feedback (called *executive functions*). These same areas are thought to contribute to reasoning, problem-solving activities, and emotional stability by inhibiting the limbic areas of the cerebrum (see later discussion).

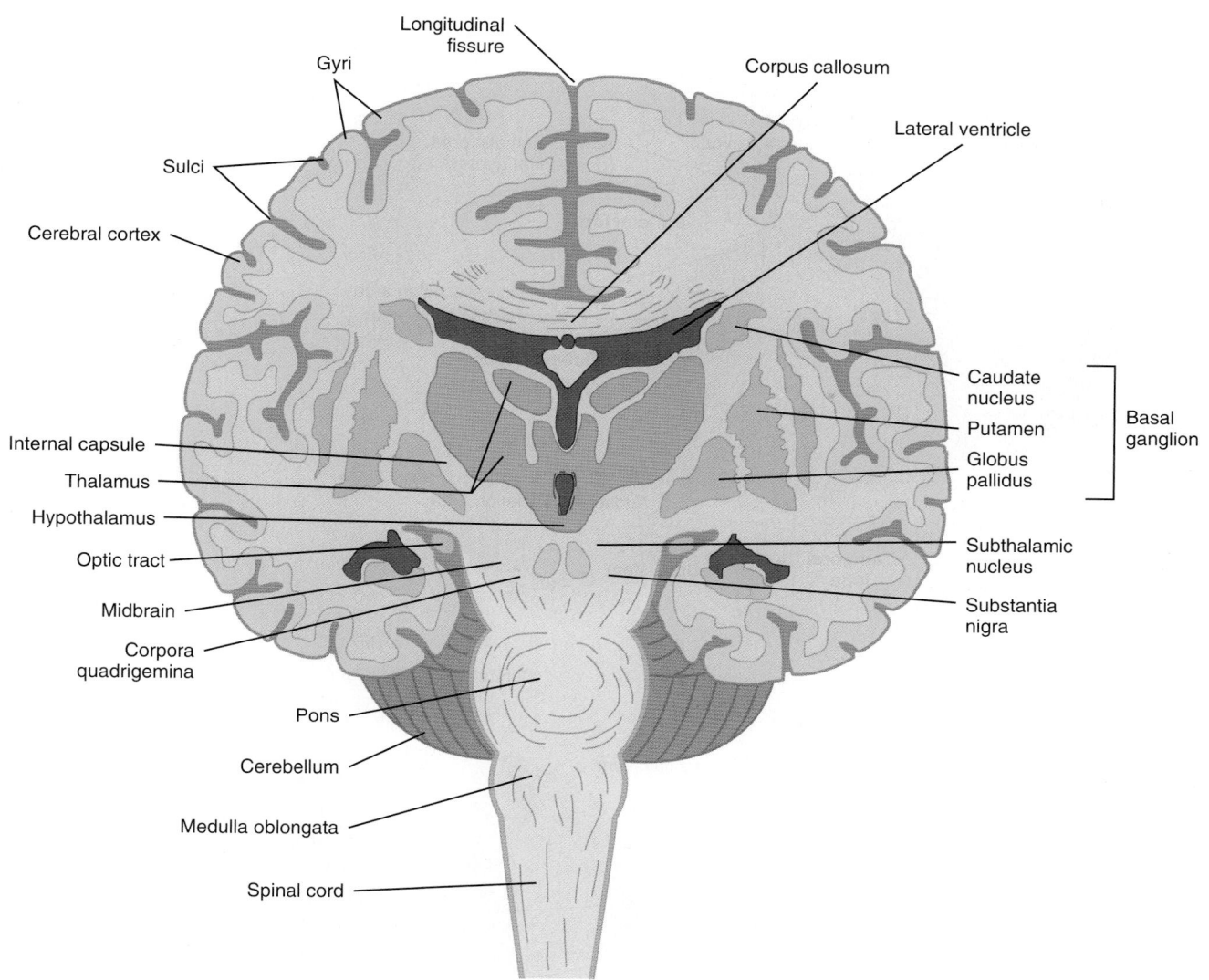

FIGURE U16-1 Structures of the brain (coronal section).

Each *parietal lobe* is located posterior to the central sulcus of Rolando and contains a primary somatic (tactile) receptive area and the somatic (tactile) association areas. The post-central gyrus and the anterior portion of the parietal lobe are the primary receptive (interpretation) areas for tactile sensations (e.g., temperature, touch, pressure). The association areas occupy the remainder of the parietal lobe. Concept formation and abstraction are carried out by the parietal association areas. The right parietal areas are also dominant for spatial orientation and awareness of size and shapes *(stereognosis)* and body position *(proprioception)*. The left parietal areas assist with right-left orientation and mathematics.

Each *occipital lobe* contains a primary visual receptive (interpretation) area and visual association areas. The primary visual cortex is on either side of the calcarine sulcus. The other areas of the occipital cortices are visual association areas. Visual memories are stored in these areas, which contribute to our ability to recognize visually and understand our environment.

Each *temporal lobe* is located under (inferior to) the lateral sulcus. The temporal lobe contains a primary auditory receptive area and secondary auditory association areas. Spoken language memories are stored in the left temporal auditory association areas. All other sound memories that are not language (e.g., music, various animal sounds, other noises) are stored in the right temporal lobe auditory areas. Damage to these areas would leave one unable to understand spoken or written language or to recognize music or other environmental sounds. Cells that facilitate understanding language reside in *Wernicke's area.*

The *central (insula) lobe* is located deep within the lateral sulcus and is surrounded by the frontal, parietal, and temporal lobes. Nerve fibers for taste pass through the parietal lobe to the insular lobe. Many association

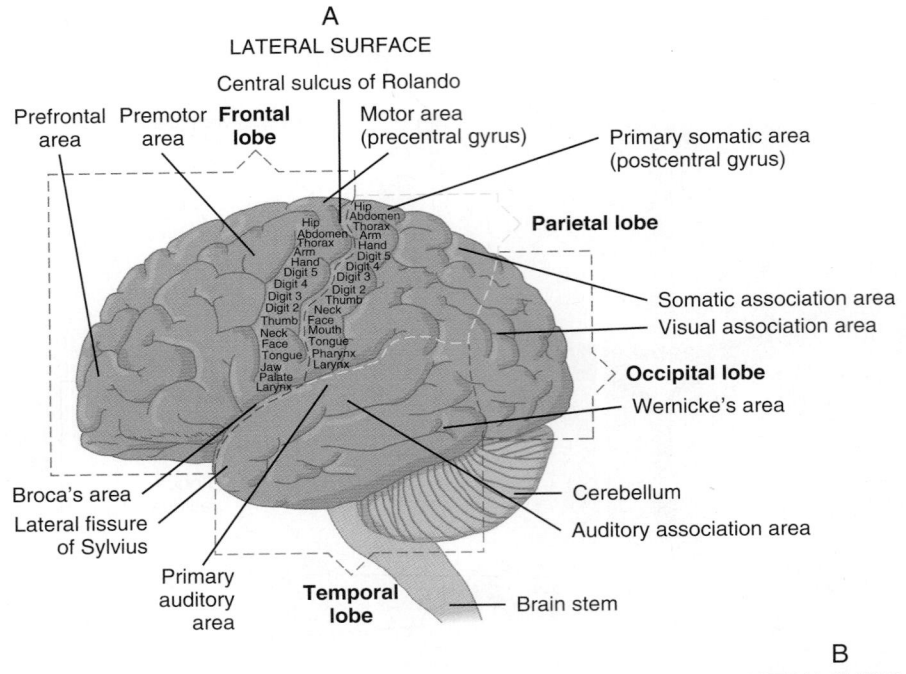

A
LATERAL SURFACE

Central sulcus of Rolando

Prefrontal area Premotor area **Frontal lobe** Motor area (precentral gyrus)

Primary somatic area (postcentral gyrus)

Parietal lobe

Somatic association area
Visual association area

Occipital lobe

Wernicke's area

Broca's area
Lateral fissure of Sylvius

Primary auditory area
Temporal lobe

Cerebellum
Auditory association area

Brain stem

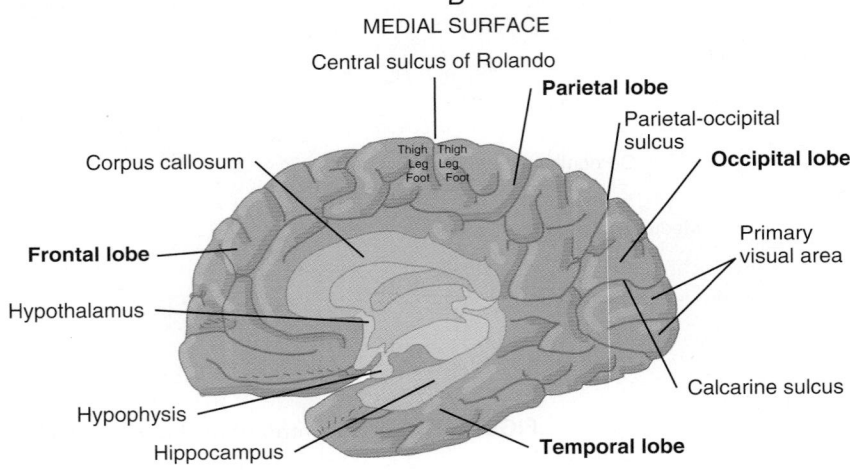

B
MEDIAL SURFACE

Central sulcus of Rolando

Parietal lobe

Parietal-occipital sulcus

Occipital lobe

Corpus callosum

Frontal lobe

Hypothalamus

Hypophysis

Hippocampus

Primary visual area

Calcarine sulcus

Temporal lobe

FIGURE U16-2 The lateral (**A**) and medial (**B**) surfaces of the cerebral cortex. The central lobe is the fifth lobe.

fibers leading to other parts of the cerebral cortex pass through this lobe.

Hippocampus

The hippocampus, a part of the medial section of the temporal lobe, plays an essential role in the process of *memory*, a complex phenomenon. Three levels of memory have been identified:

1. *Short-term (recent) memory* is lost after seconds or minutes.
2. *Intermediate memory* lasts days to weeks and eventually is lost.
3. *Long-term (remote) memory* is stored and lasts a lifetime.

Theories about the physiologic basis of memory suggest that reverberating neuronal messages cause short-term memory and that actual neuronal structural changes lead to long-term memory. The hippocampus assists in the conversion of short-term memory into intermediate and long-term memory in the thalamus. The association fibers of the frontal, parietal, temporal, and occipital lobes as well as the diencephalon are important in long-term memory.[2]

Basal Ganglia

The basal ganglia consist of several structures of subcortical gray matter buried deep in the cerebral hemispheres. These structures include the caudate nucleus, putamen, globus pallidus, substantia nigra, and subthalamic nucleus. The basal ganglia serve as processing stations that link the cerebral cortex to thalamic nuclei. Almost all the motor and sensory fibers connecting the cerebral cortex and the spinal cord travel through the white matter pathways near the caudate nucleus and putamen ganglia. These pathways are known as the *internal capsule*. The basal ganglia, along with the corticospinal tract, are important in controlling complex motor activity.

Diencephalon

The *diencephalon* is composed of the thalamus and the hypothalamus. The paired *thalami* lie between the cerebral hemispheres and superior to the brain stem. Its gray matter surrounds the lateral edges of the third ventricle. The *hypothalamus* forms the floor and portions of the wall of the third ventricle. Other important structures found in and near the diencephalon include (1) the optic tracts and optic chiasm, (2) the pituitary gland on the floor of the diencephalon, and (3) the pineal gland on the roof of the diencephalon.

The thalamus channels all ascending (sensory) information, except smell, to the appropriate cortical cells. The hypothalamus regulates autonomic nervous system (ANS) functions, such as heart rate, blood pressure, water and electrolyte balance, stomach and intestinal motility, glandular activity, body temperature, hunger, body weight, and sleep-wakefulness. It also serves as the regulator of the pituitary gland by releasing factors that stimulate or inhibit pituitary gland output.

Limbic System

The limbic system comprises many nuclei, including parts of the medial portion of the frontal and temporal lobes (hippocampus), thalamus, hypothalamus, and the basal ganglia. It is considered the center for feelings and control of emotional expression (fear, anger, pleasure, sorrow). The limbic system (the temporal lobe component) also receives nerve fibers from the olfactory bulbs and thus plays an essential role in the interpretation of smells.

Brain Stem

The brain stem is composed of the midbrain, pons, and medulla oblongata (Table U16-1). They are composed of ascending pathways, the reticular formation, cranial nerves and their nuclei, and descending autonomic and motor pathways.

Reticular Formation

The reticular formation is composed of a complex network of gray matter (nuclei), ascending reticular pathways, and descending reticular pathways. Its nuclei extend from the superior part of the spinal cord to the

TABLE U16-1	*Brain Stem Structures and Their Functions*	
Structures	**Functions**	
Midbrain		
Corpora quadrigemina		
Superior colliculi	Visual reflexes	
Inferior colliculi	Auditory reflexes	
Cerebral aqueduct		
Origin of CN III and IV		
Ascending sensory pathways		
Reticular formation		
Red nuclei	Motor pathways to spinal cord, cerebellum	
Substantia nigra	Part of basal ganglia	
Descending motor pathways		
Pons		
Fourth ventricle		
Nuclei of inferior colliculus	Auditory processing	
Nuclei of CN V, VI, VII		
Locus ceruleus	Secretes norepinephrine	
Raphe nuclei	Secretes serotonin	
Ascending sensory pathways		
Medical lemniscus, auditory pathway	Discriminitive touch	
Descending motor pathways		
Medial longitudinal fasciculi	Efferent pathway to spinal cord	
Reticular formation		
Respiratory centers		
Pontine nuclei; pontocerebellar fibers		
Medulla Oblongata		
Fourth ventricle		
Central canal		
Raphe nuclei	Secretes serotonin	
Ascending sensory pathways		
Medial lemniscal pathways	Discriminitive tactile pathways	
Spinothalamic and trigeminothalamic tracts	Pain pathways	
	Tactile, temperature	
Lateral lemnisci	Auditory pathways	
Nuclei of CN VIII, IX, X, XI, XII		
Olive and vestibular-cerebellar systems		
Pyramids (corticospinal, corticobulbar, corticopontine)	Voluntary motor	
Reflex centers: respiratory, vasomotor, cardiac, coughing, swallowing, sneezing, vomiting		
Reticular formation		
Descending motor pathways (pyramids)	Voluntary motor	

CN, Cranial nerve.

diencephalon and communicate with the basal ganglia, cerebrum, and cerebellum.

The reticular formation assists in regulation of skeletal motor movement and spinal reflexes. It also filters incoming sensory information to the cerebral cortex. About 99% of sensory information is disregarded as unessential. One component of the reticular formation, the *reticular activating system*, controls the sleep-wake cycle (see Chapter 24) and consciousness.

Cerebellum

The cerebellum is composed of gray and white matter. The *cortex* of the cerebellum is a thin layer of gray matter arranged in parallel long and deep gyri, called *folia*, and separated by cerebellar sulci (Figure U16-3). Deep fissures divide the cerebellum into three lobes, but the functional division of the cerebellum consists of a right and left hemisphere separated by a narrow band of white matter called the *vermis*. An extension of dura mater, the *falx cerebelli*, partially separates the hemispheres.

The cerebellum integrates sensory information related to the position of body parts, coordinates skeletal muscle movement, and regulates muscle tension, which is necessary for balance and posture. Three pairs of nerve tracts *(cerebellar peduncles)* provide the communication pathways. The inferior peduncles are sensory *(afferent)* pathways from the spinal cord and medulla, which carry information related to the position of body parts to the cerebellum. The middle peduncles carry information about voluntary *(purposeful)* motor activities from the cerebral cortex to the cerebellum. The cerebellum also receives sensory input from the receptors in the muscles, tendons, joints, eyes, and inner ear. After this information is integrated and analyzed, the cerebellum sends impulses via the superior peduncles *(efferent pathways)* to the brain stem, thalamus, and cortex.

Most of the tracts in the cerebellum travel through various nuclei without crossing. Therefore the right cerebellar hemisphere predominantly affects the right (ipsilateral) side of the body and vice versa.

SPINAL CORD

The *spinal cord,* that portion of the CNS surrounded and protected by the vertebral column, is continuous with the medulla and lies within the upper two thirds of the *vertebral canal* (the cavity within the vertebral column). The lower spinal cord terminates caudally in a cone-shaped structure known as the *conus medullaris* at the level of the first (L1) and second (L2) lumbar vertebrae. The spinal cord is subdivided into four areas: (1) cervical cord, (2) thoracic cord, (3) lumbar cord, and (4) sacral cord (conus medullaris) (Figure U16-4).

Within the spinal cord, butterfly-shaped gray matter (mostly unmyelinated) is surrounded by mostly myelinated white matter. The white matter consists of *ascending tracts* and *descending tracts* that conduct nerve impulses between the brain and the cells outside the CNS. The cell bodies in the gray matter are grouped into clusters of nuclei and *laminae* (a defined group or column of cells). The tracts in the white matter are arranged into three paired columns: posterior, lateral, and anterior (Figure U16-4, *inset*).

Ascending and Descending Pathways

The *ascending (sensory) pathways* carry sensory information through the spinal cord to the brain. For example the spinothalamic tract carries sensory information from the spinal cord to the thalamus. After synapsing in

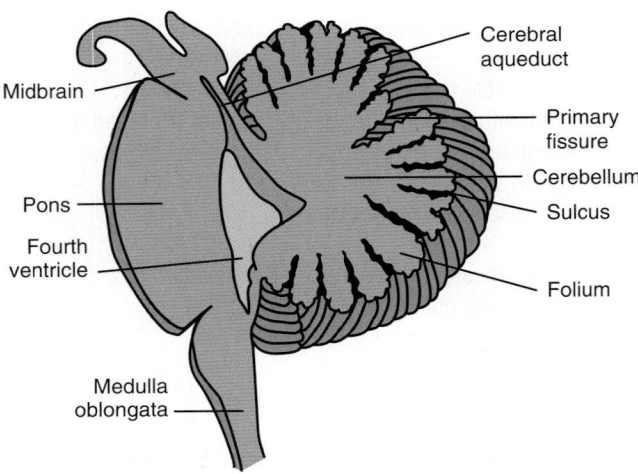

FIGURE U16-3 Sagittal view of the brain stem, fourth ventricle, and cerebellum.

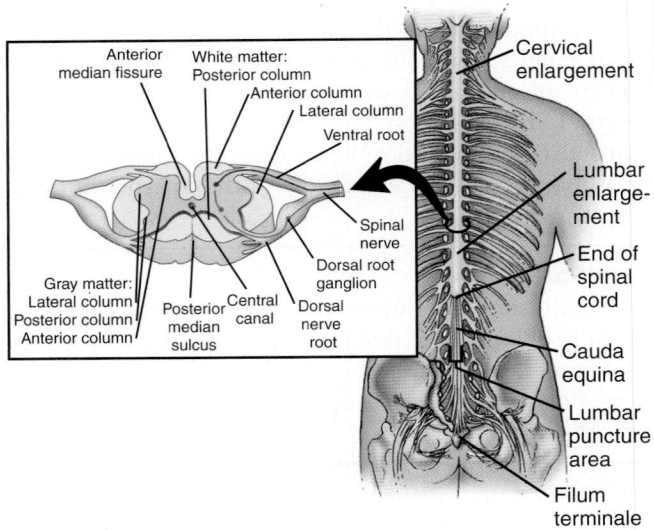

FIGURE U16-4 The spinal cord ends at L-2. *Inset,* Transverse section *(left)* of the spinal cord. (Modified from Thibodeau, G., & Patton, K. [2003]. *Anatomy and physiology* [5th ed., p. 381]. St. Louis: Mosby.)

the thalamus, information is relayed to regions of the brain such as the parietal lobe. *Descending (motor) pathways* carry mostly efferent signals to the spinal cord. The corticospinal tract *(upper motor neuron)* is a descending tract passing from the frontal lobe of the cerebral cortex to the motor neurons of the spinal cord. *Lower motor neurons* are cells that begin in the anterior horn of the spinal cord and pass through the spinal nerves to the muscle cells. *Propriospinal tracts* remain within the cord.

Table U16-2 summarizes the specific functions of the major brain and spinal cord tracts.

Many of the tracts communicating with the cerebral cortex cross (decussate), but not all cross at the same place. The term *contralateral* refers to the opposite side of the body and is used to describe tracts that cross (often at the medulla) and ascend or descend; *ipsilateral* (same-sided) tracts do not cross. For example, sensory tracts (including the anterior spinothalamic, posterior, and anterior spinocerebellar tracts) cross in the medulla as they ascend to the cerebral cortex. Therefore the sensory neurons in the cerebral cortex interpret sensory stimuli from the contralateral side of the body.

The lateral corticospinal spinal tract *(pyramidal tract)* crosses at the medulla as it descends from the frontal lobe of the cerebral cortex to the spinal cord. The poste-

rior spinocerebellar tracts are ipsilateral tracts and thus coordinate muscular function on the same side of the body. The crossing of the lateral spinothalamic tract is unique.

PROTECTIVE AND NUTRITIONAL STRUCTURES

Cranium and Vertebral Column

Eight bones that fuse early in childhood compose the cranium. The fused junctions are called *sutures*. The cranium encloses the brain structures and serves as a source of protection.

The floor, or *basilar plate*, of the cranial vault has three depressions, called *fossae*. The frontal lobes lie in the anterior fossa. The temporal lobes and the base of the diencephalon lie in the middle fossa. The cerebellum rests in the posterior fossa.

The vertebral column, a flexible series of vertebrae, surrounds and protects the spinal cord. It consists of 7 cervical vertebrae, 12 thoracic vertebrae, 5 lumbar vertebrae, 5 sacral vertebrae fused into a sacrum, and 4 coccygeal vertebrae fused into a coccyx. Ligaments hold the vertebrae together, and disks between the vertebrae prevent the bones from rubbing together.

Meninges

The *meninges*, three membranes that envelope the brain and spinal cord, are predominantly for protection (Figure U16-5). Each layer—the pia mater, arachnoid, and dura mater—is a separate membrane.

The *pia mater* is a vascular layer of connective tissue that is so closely connected to the brain and spinal cord that it follows every sulcus and fissure. This layer serves as a supporting structure for blood vessels passing

TABLE U16-2	*Major Nerve Tracts of the Spinal Cord*	
Tract	**Location**	**Function**
Ascending Tracts		
Fasciculus gracilis	Posterior column	Touch, pressure, body movement, position
Fasciculus cuneatus	Posterior column	
Spinothalamic	Lateral and anterior columns	Pain, temperature Light (crude) touch
Spinocerebellar		
Posterior	Lateral column	Coordination of muscle movements
Anterior	Lateral column	
Descending Tracts		
Corticospinal		
Lateral	Lateral column	Voluntary motor
Ventral	Anterior column	Voluntary motor
Reticulospinal		
Anterior	Anterior column	Muscle tone, sweat glands
Medial	Anterior column	
Rubrospinal	Lateral column	Coordination of muscle movements
Lateral	Lateral column	Autonomic nervous system fibers

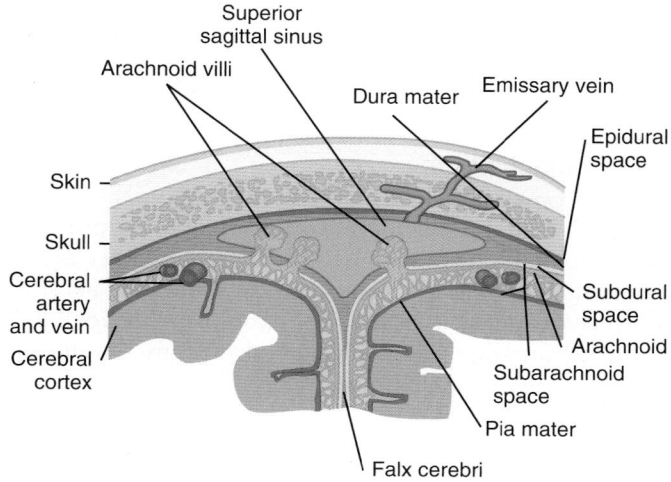

FIGURE U16-5 The meninges (coronal section through the superior sagittal sinus).

through to the tissues of the brain and spinal cord. The pia mater and astrocytes together form the membrane part of the blood-brain barrier (see Blood-Brain Barrier).

The *arachnoid,* a thin layer of connective tissue, extends from the top of each gyrus to the top of the adjacent gyrus; it does not extend into the sulci and fissures. The space between this layer and the pia mater is known as the *subarachnoid space.* Cerebrospinal fluid (CSF) flows through this space.

The cranial *dura mater* is a tough, nonstretchable vascular membrane with two layers. The *outer* dura mater is actually the membrane *(periosteum)* of the cranial bones. The *inner* dura mater forms the plates that separate the two cerebral hemispheres *(falx cerebri),* the cerebrum and the brain stem and cerebellum *(tentorium cerebelli),* and the cerebellar hemispheres *(falx cerebelli).* The tentorium cerebelli is a landmark term that is often used by clinicians to separate parts of the brain; it is often referred to as *tentorium. Supratentorial* refers to the cerebrum and all the structures superior to the tentorium cerebelli; *infratentorial* refers to structures inferior to the tentorium cerebelli: the brain stem and the cerebellum.

Brain spaces that often fill with blood after head trauma include the potential space *(subdural space)* between the inner dura mater and the arachnoid and the *epidural space* between the dura mater and the periosteum.

The meninges anchor the spinal cord. The pia mater, which closely surrounds the spinal cord, continues from the tip of the conus as a thread-like structure *(filum terminale)* to the end of the vertebral column, where it is anchored into the ligament on the posterior side of the coccyx. The *denticulate ligaments* extend laterally from the pia mater to the dura mater to suspend the spinal cord from the dura mater.

Two common spaces that are commonly accessed by physicians are the subarachnoid space (for diagnostic studies) and the epidural space (for delivery of medications). The *subarachnoid space* extends below the level of the spinal cord to the second sacral (S2) vertebral level, and the *epidural space* lies between the dural sheath and the vertebral bones.

Reflex Mechanisms

Our unconscious automatic responses to internal and external stimuli, known as *reflex responses,* provide many homeostatic functions. Although the spinal cord is often thought of as the reflex center, it is not the only site for reflex regulation. Many of the complex reflexes controlling heart rate, breathing, blood pressure, swallowing, sneezing, coughing, and vomiting are found in the brain stem.

Some intrinsic reflex circuits in the spinal cord create patterns of movement (flexion and extension) that are the basis for posture and forward progression. Other reflex circuits are the bases for spinal cord reflexes, which include the myotatic (deep tendon, stretch) reflex, the flexor withdrawal reflex, the crossed extension reflex, and the extensor thrust reflex. Visceral-somatic reflexes can also excite or inhibit the motor neurons, producing changes in muscle tone and even in movement.

Neuromuscular spindles monitor muscle stretch. As a muscle stretches, increased firing of spindles leads to contraction of the same muscle, commonly seen as the *knee-jerk reflex.* The Golgi tendon organs are sensory nerve endings that protect against excessive contraction.

Simple reflexes require only two or three neurons; for example, the *knee-jerk reflex* requires only a sensory and a motor neuron. The *withdrawal reflex* helps prevent or decrease tissue injury when a body part touches a potentially harmful object. The harmful stimuli are sent via the sensory neuron to the interneuron in the spinal cord for interpretation, and the response message is sent via the motor neuron, resulting in the withdrawal response (Figure U16-6).

Cerebrospinal Fluid and the Ventricular System

The CSF is a clear, colorless fluid. About 100 to 160 ml of CSF circulates through the ventricles and within the subarachnoid space. When a person is lying in a horizontal position, the average CSF pressure is 100 to 180 mm Hg.

About two thirds of the CSF is made in the choroid plexus of the four ventricles, primarily in the lateral ventricles. Small amounts are produced by ependymal, arachnoid, and other brain cells. The *choroid plexus* is a network of blood vessels within the pia mater that is in direct contact with the lining of the ventricles. The choroid plexuses together produce about 500 ml of CSF per day. If CSF were allowed to accumulate, it would exert enough pressure to damage the brain. Normally, however, it is absorbed into the blood at the same rate at which it is formed.

The *ventricular system* is a series of cavities within the brain. CSF flows from each of the lateral ventricles via the foramen of Monro into the third ventricle (Figure U16-7). The third ventricle is midline just beneath the fornix. CSF drains from the third ventricle through the aqueduct of Sylvius into the fourth ventricle. The fourth ventricle is located in the brain stem just anterior to the cerebellum. From the fourth ventricle, CSF passes via one of three foramina (two foramina of Luschka and one foramen of Magendie) into a large subarachnoid space that lies behind the medulla and below the cerebellum, called the *cisterna magna.* The cisterna magna is continuous with the subarachnoid space, which surrounds the brain and spinal cord.

Eventually, the CSF circulates upward into the region of the superior sagittal sinus, where it is absorbed across the arachnoid villi. The arachnoid granulations are ex-

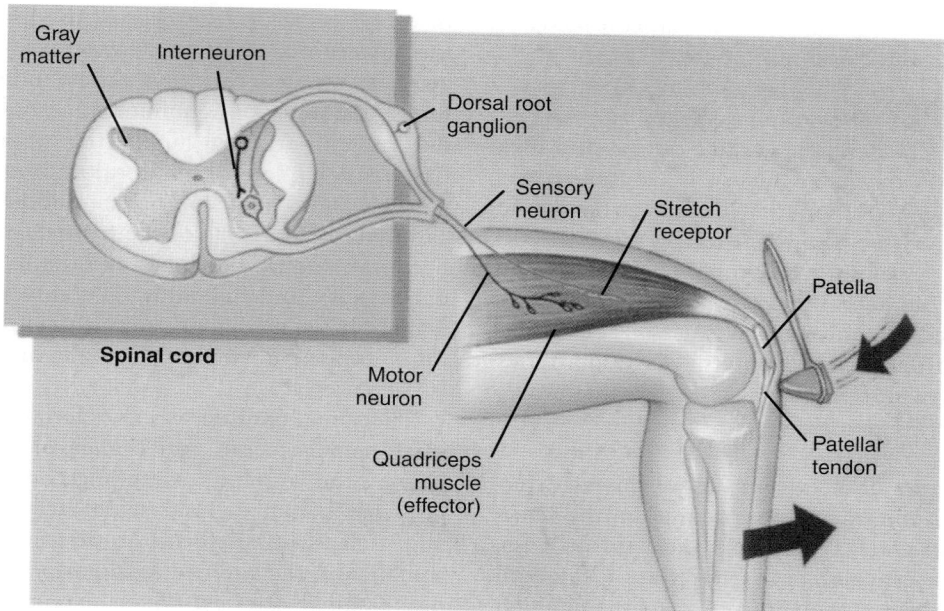

FIGURE U16-6 Patellar reflex and neural pathway involved in the reflex response. (From Thibodeau, G., & Patton, K. [2003]. *Anatomy and physiology* [5th ed., p. 430]. St. Louis: Mosby.)

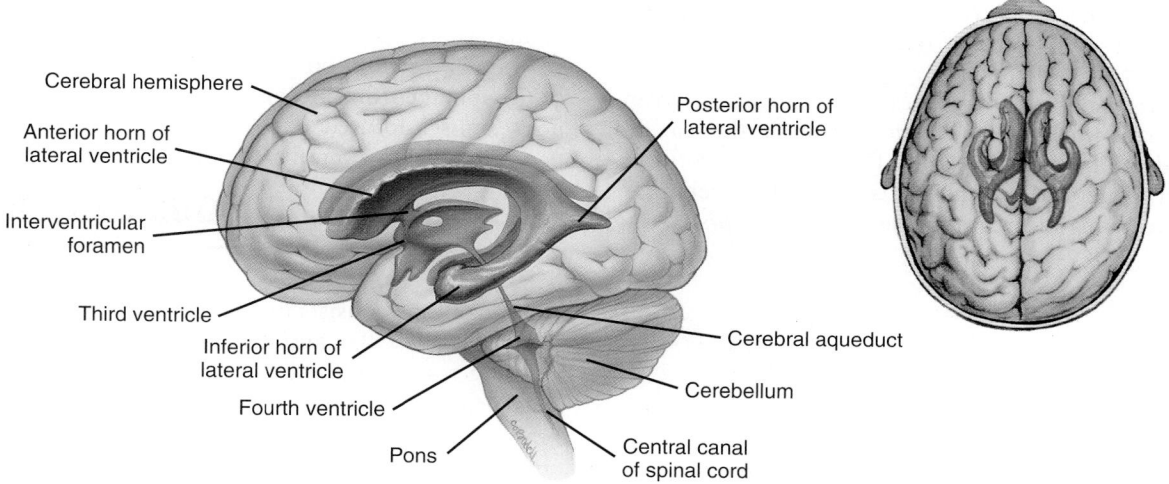

FIGURE U16-7 The ventricles of the brain produce and circulate cerebrospinal fluid. (From Thibodeau, G., & Patton, K. [2003]. *Anatomy and physiology* [5th ed., p. 378]. St. Louis: Mosby.)

tensive tufts of pia-arachnoid that along with the inner dura extend into the superior sagittal sinus and permit one-way flow of CSF into the sinus.

Blood-Brain Barrier

Three brain barriers (blood-brain, blood-CSF, and brain-CSF) primarily regulate and maintain an optimal and stable chemical environment for neurons. Brain barriers are either physical barriers or physiologic processes (transport systems) that slow movement of certain substances from one CNS compartment to another by regulating ion movement between the compartments. Physical barriers include tight junctions of the endothelial cells lining the capillaries, pores of the capillaries of the choroid plexuses, the basement membrane (ependymal cells) next to the choroid plexuses, and the pial-glial membrane.

An intact blood-brain barrier may prevent some drugs from crossing into the brain, a fact that must be considered when medications are prescribed for nervous system disorders. Certain events, including dilutional hyponatremia, acute hypertension, high doses of some anesthetics, vasodilation, and hypercarbia, can increase the permeability of the blood-brain barrier.

BLOOD SUPPLY

The brain requires 20% of the cardiac output and uses 20% of the body's oxygen. Glucose is catabolized or burned for its energy. Gray matter has higher metabolic needs than white matter. The brain receives 750 to 900 ml of blood flow per minute. Blood flow is regulated by levels of carbon dioxide. When carbon dioxide levels rise, a negative feedback mechanism causes vasodilation.

The vertebral arteries and the internal carotid arteries (Figure U16-8) provide the arterial supply to the brain.

Arterial Supply

The *vertebral arteries* branch from the subclavian arteries, travel through the transverse foramina in the cervical vertebrae, and enter the cranial vault through the foramen magnum. The vertebral arteries are located on the anterolateral surface of the medulla. At the junction of the medulla and pons, the vertebral arteries join to form the basilar artery. The basilar artery bifurcates at the midbrain level to form two posterior cerebral arteries. The vertebral artery system supplies the brain stem, the cerebellum, the lower portion of the diencephalon, and the medial and inferior regions of the temporal and occipital lobes.

The *internal carotid arteries* branch from the common carotid arteries and enter through the carotid canals at the base of the skull. The internal carotid arteries bifurcate into the anterior and middle cerebral arteries. Near this bifurcation, the *circle of Willis* (a ring of blood vessels at the base of the brain) is formed by the posterior cerebral arteries, posterior communicating arteries, internal carotid arteries, anterior cerebral arteries, and anterior communicating branches. The internal carotid arteries supply the upper diencephalon, basal ganglia, lateral temporal and occipital lobes, and parietal and frontal lobes. The middle cerebral arteries supply large portions of the frontal, parietal, temporal, occipital, and insular lobes and the basal ganglia, internal capsule, and thalamus. The anterior cerebral arteries supply the medial portions of the frontal and parietal lobes and the upper basal ganglia and internal capsule (see Figure U16-8).

The spinal cord derives its arterial blood supply from small spinal arteries that branch off larger arteries, including the vertebral, ascending cervical, deep cervical, intercostal, lumbar, and sacral arteries. These arteries and their branches form the three main arteries of the spinal cord, the anterior spinal artery, and a pair of posterior spinal arteries, which extend the length of the cord.

Venous Supply

Most of the venous blood from the head returns to the heart through the internal jugular veins, the external jugular veins, and the vertebral veins.

Venous distribution is similar to arterial distribution of the spinal cord. The venous system drains into the venous sinuses located between the dura mater and the periosteum of the vertebral column.

CELLS OF THE NERVOUS SYSTEM

Structure

Nervous tissue consists mainly of *neuroglia* and *neurons* (as well as vascular and some connective tissues). Neurons are responsible for communication, and neuroglial cells provide support for the activity of neurons. The brain and spinal cord constitute the CNS.

Neuroglia

Glial cells, collectively called *neuroglia,* provide structure and support for neurons. They are plentiful, with a ratio of glial cells to neurons high as 50:1. They also control ion concentrations within the extracellular space and contribute to the transport of nutrients, gases, and waste products between neurons and the vascular system and the CSF. Clinically, these cells are responsible for the development of many intracranial tumors. Four types of neuroglial cells exist (Figure U16-9).

In addition to these functions, each type of glial cell has specific functions.

Astrocytes supply nutrients to the neurons. They have specialized contacts with blood vessels in the pial-glial membrane and form part of the blood-brain barrier. As-

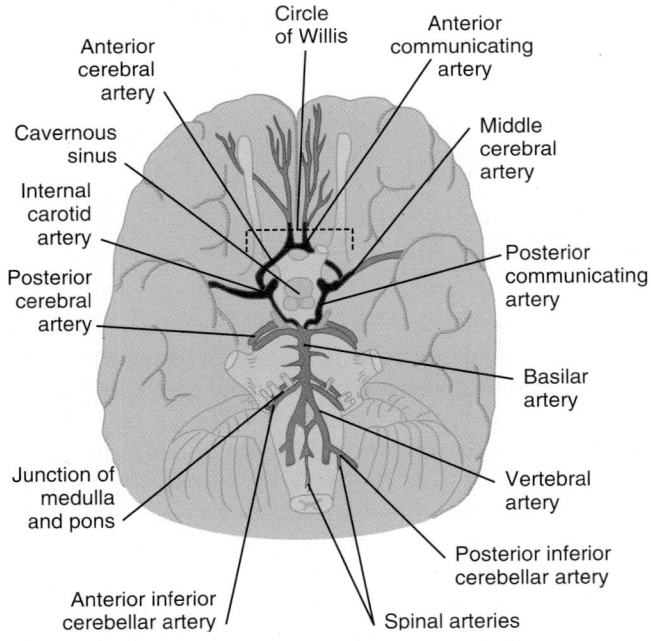

Circle of Willis

Anterior cerebral artery

Cavernous sinus

Internal carotid artery

Posterior cerebral artery

Junction of medulla and pons

Anterior inferior cerebellar artery

Anterior communicating artery

Middle cerebral artery

Posterior communicating artery

Basilar artery

Vertebral artery

Posterior inferior cerebellar artery

Spinal arteries

FIGURE U16-8 Inferior view of the cerebral circulation.

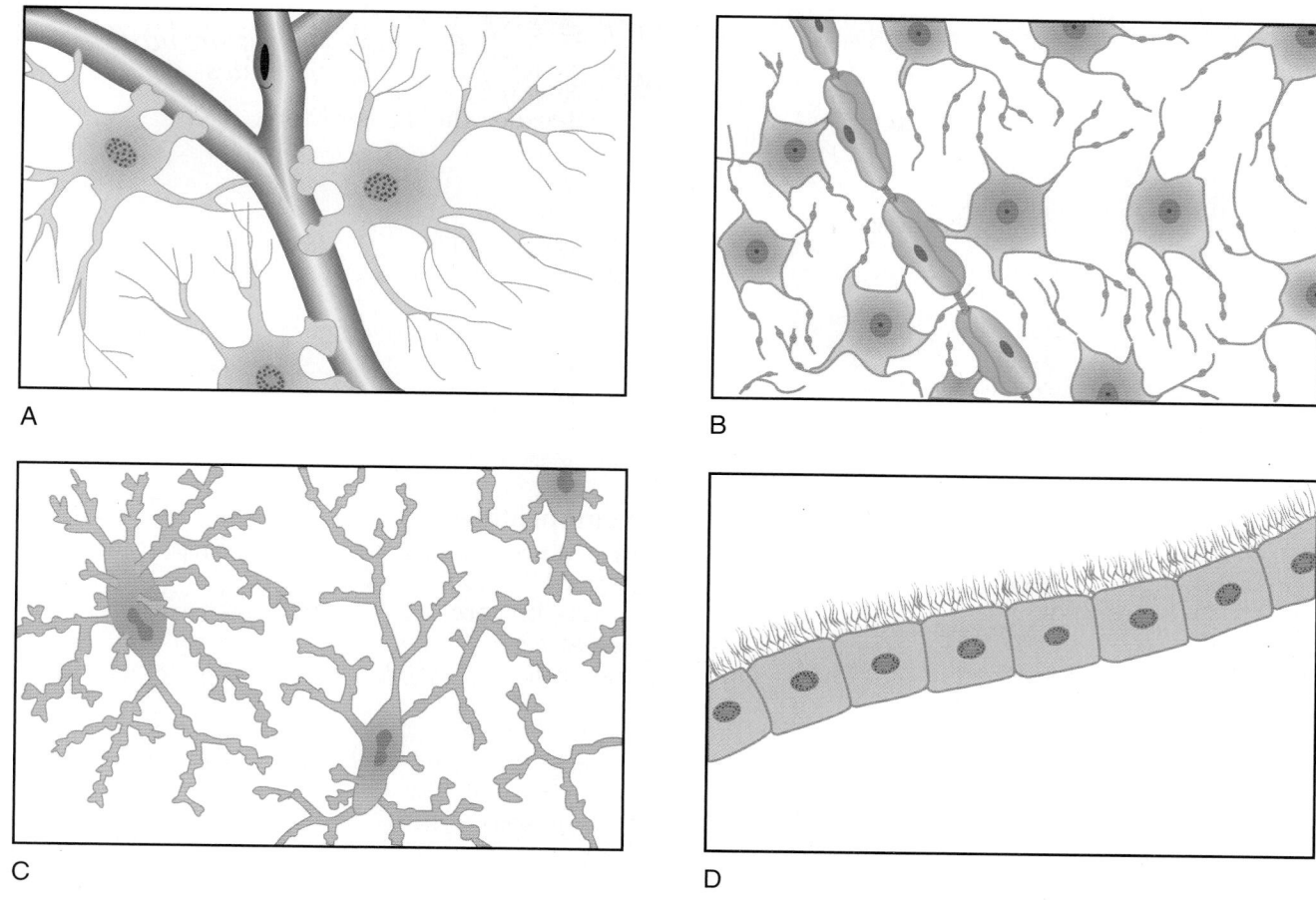

A

B

C

D

FIGURE U16-9 Neuroglial cells. **A,** Astrocytes along the capillary. **B,** Oligodendrocytes along the nerves. **C,** Microglia (phagocytes). **D,** Ependymal cells form a sheet that lines fluid cavities in the brain.

trocytes appear to be the CNS cells that respond to brain trauma by forming scar tissue.

Oligodendrocytes are comparable to the Schwann cells in the PNS. These cells wrap themselves around axons, and the spiraled part of their membrane is referred to as *myelin*. The outermost part of the Schwann cells also make up the *neurilemma*, a sheath that surrounds the myelin sheath. Neurilemma is essential to nerve regeneration (see later discussion).

Microglia are phagocytic scavenger cells and are related to macrophages. They phagocytose products from injured neurons.

Ependymal cells line the ventricles, choroid plexuses, and the central canal that extends through the spinal cord. They create a one-cell-layered membrane that allows regulated diffusion of substances between the interstitial fluid and the CSF.

Neurons

A neuronal cell body *(soma)* is like other cells in that it contains most of the organelles seen in other cells. Unique structures in the neuron include *neurofibrils,*

which are networks of thread-like structures supporting other structures. *Nissl bodies* are dark-staining sections of rough endoplasmic reticulum and are unique to the neuron.

Tree-like *dendrites* carry messages to the neuronal cell body; *axons* carry messages away from the cell body (Figure U16-10).

Three types of neurons exist:

1. *Unipolar* neurons have only one nerve fiber leaving the cell body, but they branch to form a dendrite and axon. Unipolar neurons often send general sensory signals.
2. *Multipolar* neurons have numerous afferent synapses and axons that make multiple synapses.
3. *Bipolar* neurons are often utilized in the pathways of special sensory systems (eyes, nose, and ears).

Synapses, which are crucial to nerve function, are small spaces between neurons and their targets (other neurons, muscles, or glands). As a message travels down the neuron, it reaches a synapse that it must cross to "jump" to the next neuron. There are two types of synapses; *chemical* synapses dominate. In an *electrical synapse,* the electrical nerve impulses of two cells cross

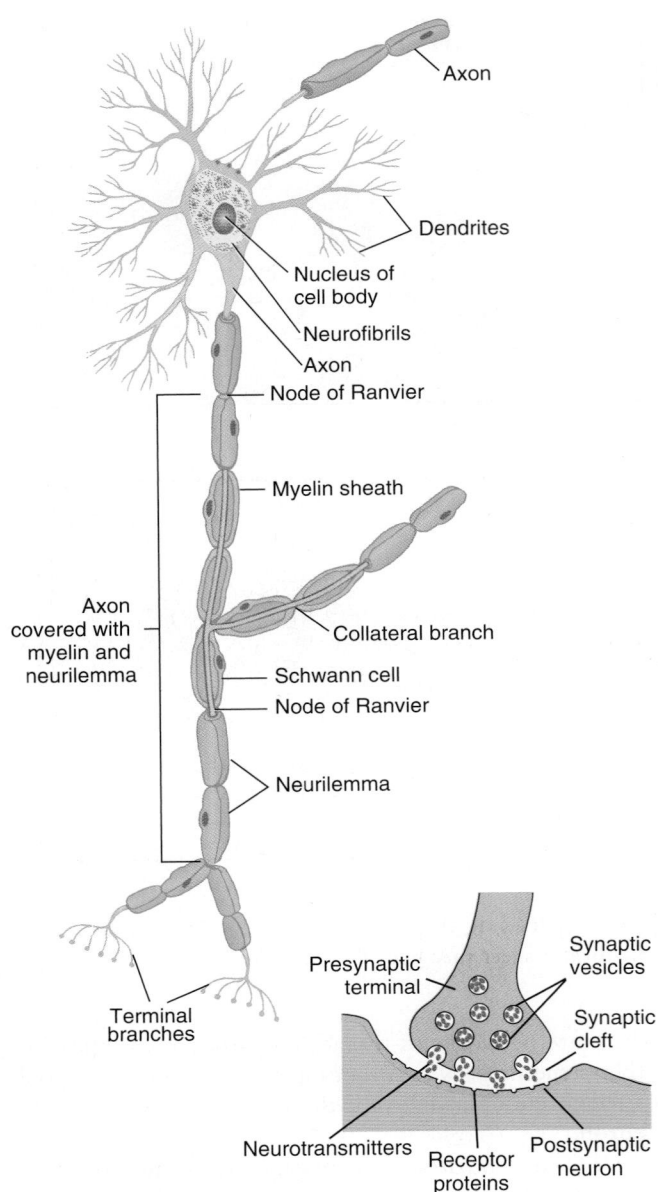

FIGURE U16-10 A neuron (the basic element of the nervous system) and a chemical synapse.

BOX U16-1 *Common Neurotransmitters and Neuropeptides*

Small-Molecule Transmitters
Acetylcholine
Dopamine
Norepinephrine
Epinephrine
Histamine
Serotonin
Gamma-aminobutyric acid (GABA)
Glycine
Glutamate
Aspartate
Nitric oxide

Neuropeptides
Hypothalamic-releasing hormones (thyrotropin, luteinizing, growth)
Pituitary hormones
Beta-endorphin
Enkephalin
Substance P
Gastrin
Insulin
Glucagon
Cholecystokinin
Angiotensin II
Bradykinin
Calcitonin

Modified from Guyton, A.C., & Hall, J.E. (2001). *Textbook of medical physiology* (10th ed.) Philadelphia: W.B. Saunders.

directly through a very small separation (called *gap junctions* or a *nexus*) from the presynaptic to the postsynaptic cell; this type of synapse is found in smooth and cardiac muscle cells.

Chemical substances called *neurotransmitters* are discharged into the space *(cleft)* between two neurons and propel the message onto the next neuron. Transmitters are manufactured in the cell body and transported anterograde to the terminals *(boutons)*, stored, and secreted from the vesicles in the first neuron *(presynaptic neuron)* into the synaptic cleft (see Figure U16-10). The neurotransmitter excites, inhibits, or modifies signals to the second neuron *(postsynaptic neuron)* by interacting with the receptors on its membrane. More than 100 neurotransmitters have been identified. Box U16-1 lists the more common transmitters.

IMPULSE CONDUCTION

Resting Potential
A neuron not conducting a nerve impulse is said to be "resting." Although it is resting, it remains charged and potentially ready to fire. The potential to fire is produced by a difference in electrical charge between the interstitial fluid outside the neuron and the intracellular fluid within (Figure U16-11). The inside of the nerve cell is electrically negative, and the interstitial fluid electrically positive. A resulting membrane potential, measured in millivolts (mV) results from this difference in electrical potential between the two compartments. The *resting membrane potential* (RMP) of neurons is between -45 and -75 mV, somewhat less polarized than the -90 mV RMP of cardiac and skeletal muscle cells.

The cell is *depolarized* when an influx of sodium makes the membrane potential more positive (i.e., rising

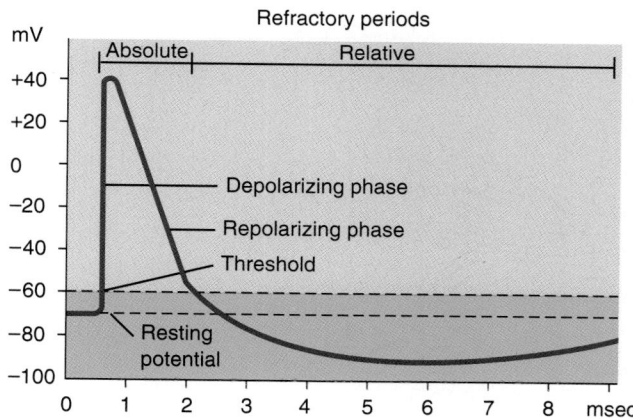

FIGURE U16-11 Generation of nerve impulses. The resting membrane potential is shown at –70 mV.

to zero). In most cells, this is due to an electrical stimulus transmitted by an adjacent cell.

As the membrane potential rises during depolarization, it reaches a specified level *(threshold)*. When threshold is reached, the excited cell is committed to full action potential because the cell follows an all-or-none phenomenon.

Repolarization is the restoration of the membrane polarity, and sodium and potassium are returned to their usual places via the sodium-potassium pump.

After an action potential is generated, no segment of the nerve fiber can conduct another action potential for a brief period of time (<1 ms). This interval is called the *absolute refractory period*. Sodium and potassium are returning to their original locations during this period, and sodium cannot enter the nerve cell. During the next period, called the *relative refractory period*, only a stimulus stronger than the ordinary one can produce an action potential. On average a return to a resting potential takes approximately 10 to 30 ms.

Nerve Impulses

Because neurons are arranged in chain-like pathways, impulses must travel quickly from one cell to another. In nerve cells the impulse begins at the axon. When the action potential reaches the presynaptic knob at the dendrite, the membrane's permeability to calcium increases, allowing increased calcium influx. Calcium promotes fusing of the vesicles with the membrane and release of the neurotransmitters inside. Some neurotransmitters are transported back into the vesicles *(reuptake)*. Others are decomposed by an enzyme process. For example, acetylcholinesterase decomposes acetylcholine at the postsynaptic membrane.

Myelin

Myelin surrounds most large nerve fibers and is separated by nodes of Ranvier. Action potentials are gener-

ated only at the nodes, and thus they skip between them rather than depolarize the entire membrane. This jumping characteristic is known as *saltatory conduction*. Conduction using this process is rapid. Neurons with their axons covered by myelin are called *myelinated nerve fibers*; neurons with little or no myelin are called *unmyelinated nerve fibers*. Myelinated fibers in the CNS constitute the *white matter* in the brain and spinal cord. *Gray matter* consists of cell bodies that are unmyelinated. The speed of the nerve impulse conduction is also related to the diameter of the fiber; the greater the diameter, the faster the impulse.

Receptors

Receptors are biologic transducers that use the stimulus of one form of energy—mechanical, electrical, chemical, thermal or light—to initiate the "electrical" energy of the nerve impulse. Although sensory receptors may be stimulated by more than one form of energy, each receptor is especially sensitive to a particular form of energy.

Receptors exhibit a phenomenon known as *adaptation*, a decreased receptor sensitivity in response to steady continuous stimuli. Slow-adapting receptors can maintain the lower rate of discharge for minutes to even hours. Fast-adapting receptor bursts of impulses terminate less than 1 second after initiation of the stimulus. The mechanism of adaptation is not known.

Receptors respond more effectively to change than to continuous stimulation. This characteristic of nerve "fatigue" is protective.

PERIPHERAL NERVOUS SYSTEM

The PNS includes all neurons other than those in the brain and spinal cord. It consists of pathways of nerve fibers between the CNS and all outlying structures in the body. Included in the PNS are 12 pairs of cranial nerves and 31 pairs of spinal nerves.

Nerves that conduct impulses to the brain and spinal cord are called *sensory (afferent) neurons*. Nerves that conduct impulses away from the brain and spinal cord are called *motor (efferent) neurons*. Most nerves are mixed, having both sensory and motor components.

SPINAL NERVES

The spinal nerves develop from a series of nerve rootlets that collect laterally as spinal roots. Each spinal nerve consists of a *dorsal (sensory) root* and a *ventral (motor) root*, which unite to form a spinal nerve. The dorsal root emerges from the posterolateral cord. The ventral root emerges from the anterolateral spinal cord. There are 31 pairs of spinal nerves: 8 pairs of cervical nerves, 12 pairs of thoracic nerves, 5 pairs of lumbar nerves, 5 pairs of sacral nerves, and usually 1 pair of coccygeal nerves (see Figure U16-4). The specific area of sensory reception for

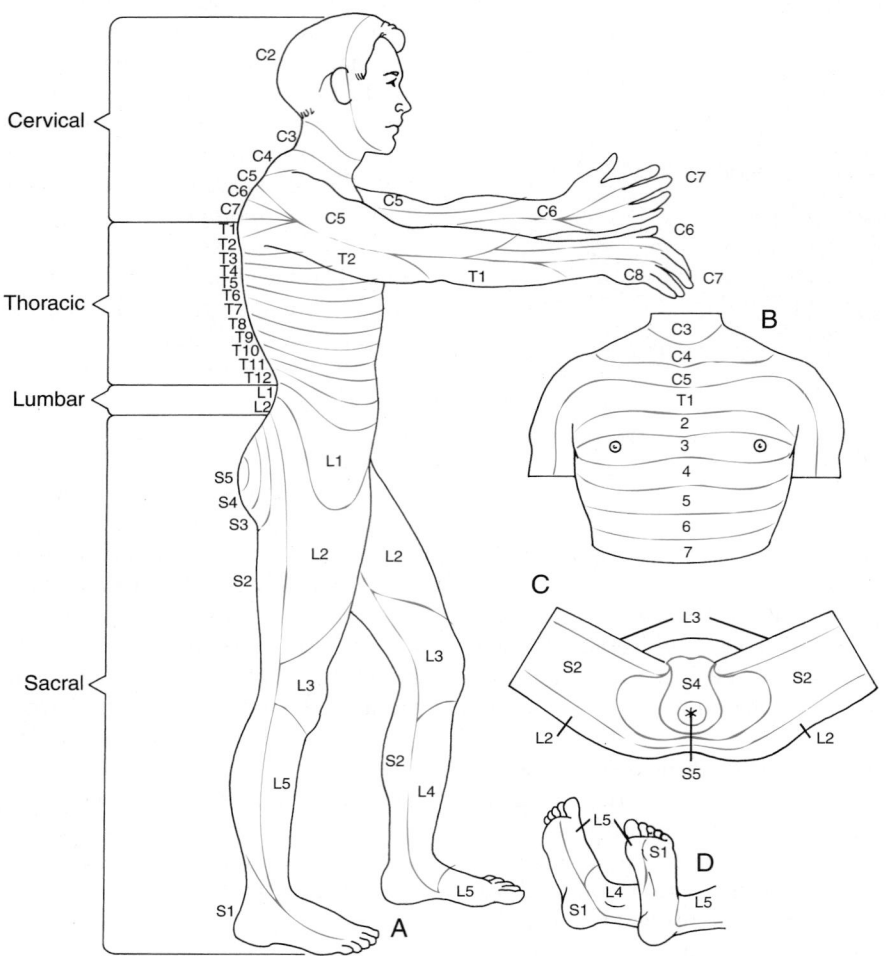

FIGURE U16-12 Dermatomes (segments of the spinal cord) indicate distribution of spinal nerves. *Solid lines* divide the regions of the spinal cord (i.e., cervical, thoracic, lumbar, sacral). *Dotted lines* indicate dermatomes. **A,** Torso and limbs. **B,** Anterior chest. **C,** Perineum. **D,** Feet. Dermatomes are used during assessment to identify specific areas of sensory impairment (e.g., touch, pain, temperature).

each dorsal root is called a *sensory dermatome* (Figure U16-12).

The peripheral nerves that are formed into plexuses have specific names. There are three major plexuses:

1. The *cervical plexus* supplies the muscles and skin of the neck and branches to form the phrenic nerve, which innervates the diaphragm.
2. The *brachial plexus* supplies the muscles and skin of the shoulder, axilla, arm, forearm, and hand. It branches to form the ulnar, median, and radial nerves.
3. The *lumbosacral plexus* supplies sensory and motor impulses to the muscles and skin of the perineum, gluteal region, thighs, legs, and feet. Its many branches include the pudendal, gluteal, femoral, sciatic, tibial, and common fibular nerves.

CRANIAL NERVES

Twelve pairs of cranial nerves arise from the brain. Most of the cranial nerves are composed of both motor and sensory neurons, although a few cranial nerves carry only sensory impulses (Figure U16-13). Except for the olfactory and optic nerves, whose nuclei lie just below the cerebrum, all other cranial nerve nuclei lie within the brain stem. Table U16-3 presents the 12 pairs of cranial nerves.

AUTONOMIC NERVOUS SYSTEM

The autonomic nervous system (ANS) is the part of the PNS that coordinates involuntary activities, such as visceral functions, smooth and cardiac muscle changes, and

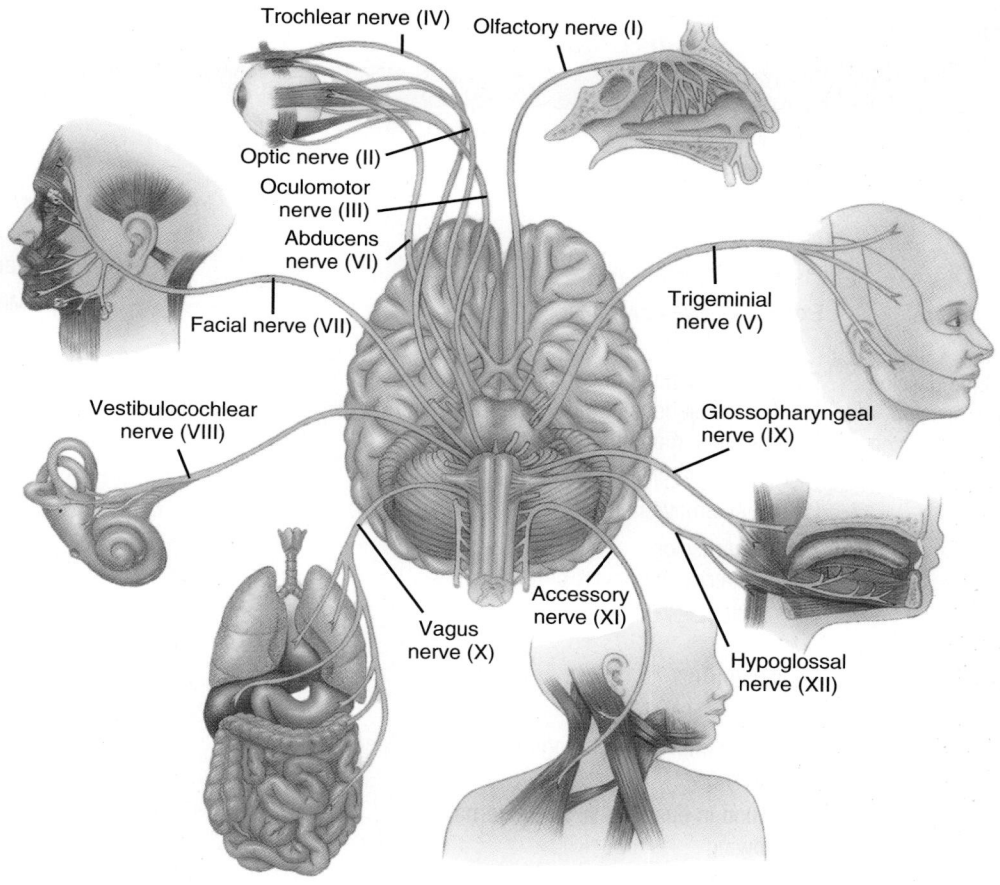

FIGURE U16-13 Ventral surface of the brain showing the attachment of the cranial nerves. (From Thibodeau, G., & Patton, K. [2003]. *Anatomy and physiology* [5th ed., p. 421]. St. Louis: Mosby.)

glandular responses. Although it can function independently, its primary control is from the brain and spinal cord. The ANS has two divisions: the *sympathetic* and *parasympathetic nervous systems.* The efferent ANS fibers travel within some cranial and spinal nerves. These two systems are highly integrated and interact with each other to maintain a stable internal environment.

Unlike the *somatic* neurons, which usually are single neurons linking the CNS to a muscle or gland, the ANS has a *two-neuron chain* leading to the effector organ. The terminal of the first neuron is located in the CNS and synapses with nerve fibers whose cell bodies are within an autonomic ganglion. The axon of the second neuron *(postganglionic fiber)* carries impulses to the target viscera. An exception is the adrenal medulla, which is innervated directly by preganglionic fibers. The medulla is actually composed of postganglionic neurons that secrete epinephrine into the bloodstream during an "adrenaline rush."

The *sympathetic nervous system* coordinates activities used to handle stress and is geared for action as a whole for short periods. The preganglionic neurons of the sym-

pathetic nervous system emerge from the spinal cord via the motor (ventral) roots of the thoracic and upper two lumbar spinal nerves (T1-L2) (Figure U16-14). Preganglionic axons are short; postganglionic axons are long.

The *parasympathetic nervous system* is associated with conservation and restoration of energy stores and is geared to act locally and discretely for a longer duration. The preganglionic fibers emerge from the brain stem via the cranial nerves and from the spinal cord via the sacral spinal nerves at S2-4. These preganglionic fibers have long axons that synapse with the postganglionic neurons in ganglia close to or located within the organs to be innervated. Each postganglionic neuron has a relatively short axon. Most, but not all, organ systems have both parasympathetic and sympathetic innervation. About 75% of the parasympathetic fibers are in the vagus nerve.

Table U16-4 lists the effects of both the sympathetic and parasympathetic nervous systems on different organs. These functions and responses are related to the type of neurotransmitter released. The preganglionic fibers of the sympathetic and parasympathetic nerves

	Name	Function	Type
TABLE U16-3		*Functions and Types of Cranial Nerves*	
I	Olfactory	Olfaction (smell)	Sensory
II	Optic	Vision	Sensory
III	Oculomotor	Extraocular eye movement	Motor
		Elevation of eyelid	
		Pupil constriction	Parasympathetic
IV	Trochlear	Extraocular eye movement	Motor
V	Trigeminal		
	Ophthalmic division	Somatic sensations of cornea, nasal mucous membranes, face	Sensory
	Maxillary division	Somatic sensations of face, oral cavity, anterior two thirds of tongue, teeth	Sensory
	Mandibular division	Somatic sensation of lower face	Sensory
		Mastication (chewing)	Motor
VI	Abducens	Lateral eye movement	Motor
VII	Facial	Facial expression	Motor
		Taste, anterior two thirds of tongue	Sensory
		Salivation	Parasympathetic
VIII	Vestibulocochlear		
	Vestibular	Equilibrium	Sensory
	Cochlear	Hearing	Sensory
IX	Glossopharyngeal	Taste, posterior third of tongue; pharyngeal sensation	Sensory
		Swallowing	Motor
X	Vagus	Sensation in pharynx, larynx, external ear	Sensory
		Swallowing	Motor
		Thoracic and abdominal visceral parasympathetic nervous system activities	Parasympathetic
XI	Spinal accessory	Neck and shoulder movement	Motor
XII	Hypoglossal	Tongue movement	Motor

and the postganglionic fibers of the parasympathetic nerves release acetylcholine. The postganglionic fibers of the sympathetic nerves release norepinephrine. Fibers that secrete acetylcholine are called *cholinergic fibers;* fibers that secrete norepinephrine are called *adrenergic fibers.*

The complexity of the sympathetic and parasympathetic response also depends on the type of receptor that combines with the neurotransmitter. The sympathetic nervous system has four types of receptors: alpha$_1$, alpha$_2$, beta$_1$, and beta$_2$. The parasympathetic nervous system has muscarinic and nicotinic receptors.

EFFECTS OF INJURY ON THE NERVOUS SYSTEM REGENERATION

For many years it was thought that nerve cell bodies were not able to regenerate; however, it appears that CNS cortical neurons do attempt to regenerate. PNS re-generation can occur if only the axon in the PNS is injured. Initially there is breakdown of the myelin sheath and axon. The axon swells and fragments while the myelin sheath disintegrates distal to the injury. The cell body takes up water. Macrophages phagocytose the breakdown products. Neurilemma cells migrate into the emerging space (Figure U16-15).

The injured axon tip forms a new plasma membrane. A few days after injury, sprouts emerge from the tip. Peripheral nerve sprouts enter the distal stump and often come in contact with a *neurilemma cord,* which serves as a guide. The regenerating axon grows along the cord at a rate of 4 mm daily. Later the neurilemma cells encapsulate the regenerating nerve fibers. With time the axon and myelin sheath both thicken. Axons within the CNS sprout and form growing tips but appear unable to sustain the metabolic responses necessary for extensive regeneration. It is believed that the axon tip is not able to penetrate the glial scar formed at the injury site, such as after spinal cord injury.

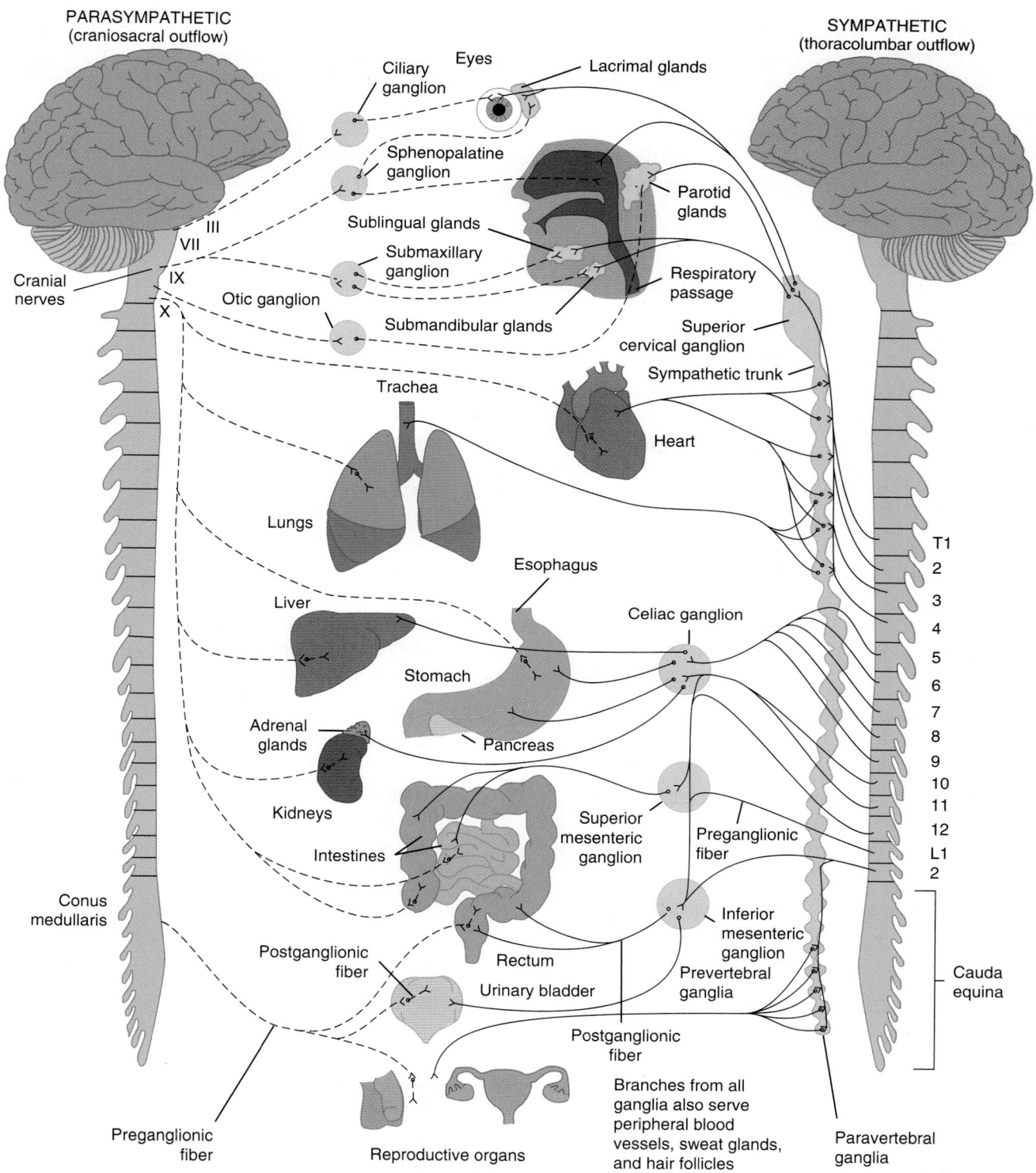

FIGURE U16-14 Autonomic nervous system.

An uninjured axon may sprout a collateral branch at a node of Ranvier that may enter into an adjacent denervated neurilemma cord. Collateral nerve regeneration occurs in both the PNS and the CNS, for example, after peripheral nerve trauma or inflammation of a peripheral nerve, as in Bell's palsy.

EFFECTS OF AGING ON THE NERVOUS SYSTEM

Neurons undergo senescence. Intracellular, cellular, and biochemical changes occur. Lipofuscin accumulates in the cell. Neurofibrillary tangles and senile plaques

TABLE U16-4 *Effects of the Sympathetic and Parasympathetic Nervous Systems on Organs*

Organ	Effect of Sympathetic Stimulation	Effect of Parasympathetic Stimulation
Eye		
Pupil	Dilation (alpha)*	Constriction
Ciliary muscle	Slight relaxation (far vision)	Constriction (near vision)
Glands	Vasoconstriction and slight secretion	Stimulation of copious secretion (containing many enzymes for enzyme-secreting glands)
Nasal		
Lacrimal		
Parotid		
Submandibular		
Gastric		
Pancreatic		
Sweat glands	Copious sweating (cholinergic)	Sweating on palms of hands
Apocrine glands	Thick, odoriferous secretion	None
Heart		
Muscle	Increased rate (beta$_1$)	Slowed rate
	Increased force of contraction (beta$_1$)	Decreased force of contraction (especially of atria)
Coronaries	Dilated (beta$_2$); constricted (alpha)	Dilation
Lungs		
Bronchi	Dilation (beta$_2$)	Constriction
Blood vessels	Mild constriction	? Dilation
Gut		
Lumen	Decreased peristalsis and tone (beta$_2$)	Increased peristalsis and tone
Sphincter	Increased tone (alpha)	Relaxation (most times)
Liver	Gluconeogenesis, glycogenolysis (beta$_2$)	Slight glycogen synthesis
Gallbladder and bile ducts	Relaxation	Contraction
Kidney	Decreased output and renin secretion	None
Bladder		
Detrusor	Relaxation (slight) (beta$_2$)	Contraction
Trigone	Contraction (alpha)	Relaxation
Penis	Ejaculation	Erection
Systemic arterioles		
Abdominal viscera	Constriction (alpha)	None
Muscle	Constriction (alpha)	None
	Dilation (beta$_2$)	
	Dilation (cholinergic)	
Skin	Constriction	None
Blood		
Coagulation	Increase	None
Glucose	Increase	None
Lipids	Increase	None
Basal metabolism	Increase up to 100%	None
Adrenal medullary secretion	Increase	None
Mental activity	Increase	None
Piloerector muscles	Contraction (alpha)	None
Skeletal muscle	Increased glycogenolysis (beta$_2$)	None
	Increased strength	
Fat cells	Lipolysis (beta$_1$)	None

Modified from Guyton, A.C., & Hall, J.E. (2001). *Textbook of medical physiology* (10th ed.). Philadelphia: W.B. Saunders.
*Sympathetic nervous system composed of alpha, beta$_1$, and beta$_2$ receptors.

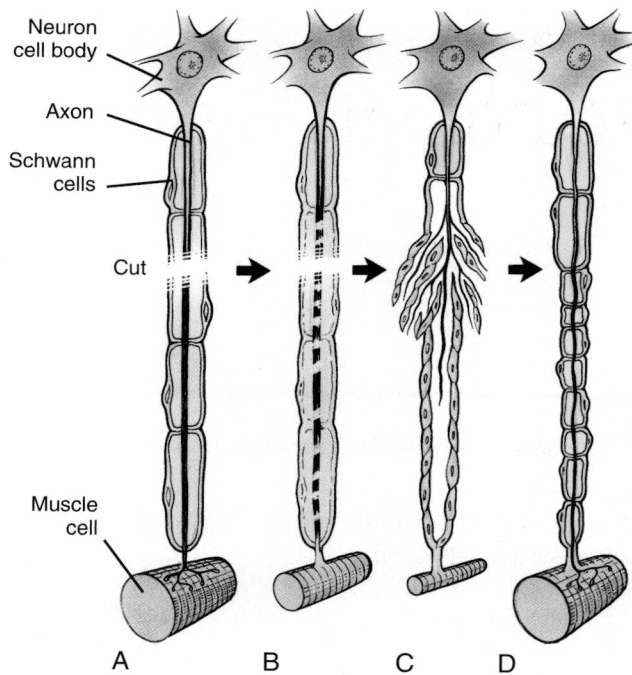

FIGURE U16-15 Regeneration of peripheral nerve tissue. **A,** An injury results in a cut nerve. **B,** Immediately after the injury, the distal portion of the axon degenerates, as does its myelin sheath. **C,** The remaining neurilemma cells tunnel from the point of injury to the effector. New Schwann cells grow within this tunnel, maintaining a path for regrowth of the axon. Meanwhile, several growing fibers reach the tunnel. **D,** The neuron's attachment is reestablished. (From Thibodeau, G., & Patton, K. [2003]. *Anatomy and physiology* [5th ed., p. 353]. St. Louis: Mosby.)

develop. After we reach 30 years of age, neurons decrease in number and neuroglial cells increase in size and number. The number of dendrites decreases, but the intrinsic dendritic changes are quite variable in hippocampal areas of the brain on postmortem examination in the normal aging population. Variations in dendrite length, stability, and growth have been attributed to compensatory response to death of dendrites.

Aging has little effect on sensory and primary memory but causes a decrease in working memory, including longer retrieval times for short-term memory, categorization, and episodic memory. Dendritic changes are quite pronounced in pathologic conditions such as Alzheimer's disease (see Chapter 74). The axons also change in normal aging; their diameters thin, and the number of receptors decreases.

CONCLUSIONS

The nervous system has three major divisions:
1. The CNS regulates higher-level process, such as thought and vital functions.
2. The PNS provides pathways to the CNS.
3. The ANS coordinates involuntary activities such as digestion.

The *neuron* is the structural and functional unit of the nervous system. The typical neuron is composed of a cell body, one axon, and several dendrites. The impulses along the nerve are carried through the action of several electrolytes. Neurotransmitters carry the impulse from neuron to neuron.

BIBLIOGRAPHY

1. Berne, R., et al. (2004). *Physiology* (5th ed.). St. Louis: Mosby-Year Book.
2. Guyton, A.C., & Hall, J.E. (2001). *Textbook of medical physiology* (10th ed.). Philadelphia: W.B. Saunders.
3. Hanson, M. (1998). *Pathophysiology.* Philadelphia: W.B. Saunders.
4. Kandel, E.R., Schwartz, J.H., & Jessel, T.M. (2000). *Principles of neural science* (4th ed.). New York: McGraw-Hill.
5. Thibodeau, G., & Patton, K. (2003). *Anatomy and physiology* (5th ed.). St. Louis: Mosby

Chapter 69

Assessment of the Neurologic System

Jeannine M. Petit

Assessment of a client experiencing a neurologic disorder is a challenge. Neurologic disorders range from simple to complex and can have profound consequences for activities of daily living (ADL) and survival. Neurologic assessment establishes baseline data that are used to compare ongoing assessments, diagnose actual and potential health problems, manage client care, and evaluate the outcome. Because of the complexity of the nervous system, neurologic assessment is both multifaceted and lengthy. The following are the three main components of a neurologic assessment:

- A comprehensive history
- A neurologic physical examination
- General and specific neurodiagnostic studies

Assessment is both anatomic and functional. Continuous observations of the client are made and compared with baseline data. Astute observations are essential because many neurologic changes occur subtly. Nurses collect data on the client's ability to function physically (self-care deficit) and mentally (confusion and altered problem solving). Finally, because many neurologic disorders are serious, the nurse provides skillful, crisis-oriented support for the client and significant others.

This chapter presents basic neurologic assessment procedures. Additional assessment techniques for specific neurologic disorders are discussed throughout Unit 16. Novice practitioners may follow the assessment sequence described in this chapter to avoid missing parts of a complex examination. Advanced clinicians may develop a preferred sequence based on experience. The sequence suggested in Table 69-1 integrates cranial nerve and reflex testing into motor and sensory examinations.

HISTORY

The history consists of biographical data, the chief complaint and symptom analysis, past health history, family health history, psychosocial history, and review of systems.

Biographical and Demographic Data

Biographical data comprise demographic, administrative, and insurance information. Often included are (1) a personal profile or brief description of the client, (2) the source of the history (client or a significant other), and (3) the client's mental status (indicating the reliability of the data). Neurologic problems often affect mental status, sometimes making it difficult to obtain an accurate history directly from the client.

Current Health

Chief Complaint

Obtain a detailed description of the events that have led the client to seek care. Avoid suggesting manifestations to the client, and use open-ended questions.

TABLE 69-1	*Neurologic Assessment Guidelines*			
Functional Category	**Specific Category**	**Area of Nervous System Involved**	**Assessment Technique**	**Examples of Disorders**
1. Consciousness (awareness of self and environment)	Arousal response to verbal, tactile, and visual stimuli	Reticular activating system (mesencephalon, diencephalon) Both hemispheres	Is client alert? What is attention span? Is there normal response to visual and auditory stimuli? Reaction to loud noises, shaking, deep pressure over eye orbits or sternum? Are vital signs, pupils, and reflexes normal?	Elevation: insomnia, agitation, mania, delirium Depression: somnolence, lethargy, semi-coma, coma
2. Mentation	Thinking	Cerebral hemispheres plus specific regional functions	Is client oriented (time, place, person)?	Disorientation
	Insight, judgment, planning	Frontal lobe, with association fibers to other area of cerebrum	Does client recognize implication of illness? Are goals congruent with abilities? How would client respond to given situation (house on fire)?	Lack of judgment, inattention to grooming, appearance, and personal habits
	Fund of information	Basic biologic intellect (frontal lobe) integrated into other areas	Calculation ability, knowledge of current events consistent with educational level. Who is U.S. president?	Impairment—functioning not congruent with level of education
	Memory	Temporal lobe and association to most other areas of cortex		
	Recent	Hippocampus	What did client eat for breakfast? What happened yesterday?	Dementia
	Past	Frontal lobe	Recall past events during taking of history	Lapses of memory for past events may coincide with past CNS problems (trauma, infection, psychic trauma)
	Feeling (affect) (congruence of response to stimulus)	Limbic system (usually involves both hemispheres)	Compare observed with expected reactions. Are emotions labile? Appropriate?	Blunted affect: hysteria, schizophrenia, bilateral frontal lobe lesions
	Perceptual distortions (illusions, hallucinations)	General and specific cortical areas in hallucinations	Observations for behavior indicating perceptual problems.	Irritative lesions of cortex may → hallucinations (occipital cortex → visual, postcentral gyrus → somatic sensation, uncus → smell)

C, Cervical; *CN,* cranial nerve; *CNS,* central nervous system; *L,* lumbar; *S,* sacral; *T,* thoracic.
↑, increase; ↑↑, significantly increased; ↓, decreased; ↓↓, significantly decreased; →, may affect or lead to.

Continued

TABLE 69-1			*Neurologic Assessment Guidelines—cont'd*	

Functional Category	Specific Category	Area of Nervous System Involved	Assessment Technique	Examples of Disorders
3. Language and speech	Dysarthria (defects in articulation, enunciation, and rhythm in speech)	Impairment of muscles of tongue, palate, pharynx, or lips (may be due to ↓ impulses or incoordination) Brain stem, cerebellum, or extraneural causes; CN V, VII, IX, X, XII	Have client repeat a difficult phrase ("Susie sells seashells by the seashore")	Slurring, slowness, indistinctness, nasality, break in normal speech rhythm (speech of intoxication); amyotrophic lateral sclerosis; pseudobulbar palsy; myasthenia gravis; stroke
	Dysphonia (abnormal production of sounds from larynx)	Many extraneural causes Recurrent laryngeal nerve problems (part of vagus); CN X Medulla (area of nucleus of CN X)	Is client's voice hoarse, strained, soft? Whispered voice is intact Use indirect laryngoscopy findings	Parkinsonism, dystonia Compression of recurrent laryngeal nerve by bronchogenic carcinoma of left mainstem bronchus Left atrial hypertrophy Brain stem tumors, occlusion of posterior inferior cerebellar or vertebral artery
	Aphasia (inability to use and understand written and spoken words)	Fluent (receptive) left temporal and parietal lobes (Wernicke's area) Nonfluent (expressive) Broca's area (lateral) inferior portion of frontal lobe of dominant side Global (combined)	Observe vocal expression, written expression, comprehension of spoken and written language, and gesture communication	Stroke of middle cerebral artery Trauma, tumor, abscess, etc., in left temporal and parietal lobe areas Damage to Broca's area or association fibers (stroke, tumor)
	Agnosia (inability to recognize objects or symbols by means of senses)	Primarily in parietal temporal and occipital areas	Sense organs intact? Can the client recognize objects by sight, touch, hearing, etc.?	Stroke
4. Motor function	Expression (facial)	CN VII	Symmetry of smile, frown, raising of eyebrows	Central facial weakness (upper motor neuron dysfunction); weakness of lower half of face Causes: stroke, corticobulbar tract Peripheral facial weakness (lower motor dysfunction); weakness of entire half of face Causes: Bell's palsy, brain stem tumor, fracture of temporal bone

C, Cervical; *CN*, cranial nerve; *CNS*, central nervous system; *L*, lumbar; *S*, sacral; *T*, thoracic.
↑, increase; ↑↑, significantly increased; ↓, decreased; ↓↓, significantly decreased; →, may affect or lead to.

TABLE 69-1	Neurologic Assessment Guidelines—cont'd			
Functional Category	**Specific Category**	**Area of Nervous System Involved**	**Assessment Technique**	**Examples of Disorders**
4. Motor function—cont'd	Eating (chewing, swallowing)	CN V, VII, IX, X, XII	Strength of masticator muscles, gag reflexes, ability to swallow	Tetanus, peripheral spasm of muscle; amyotrophic lateral sclerosis, medullary tumor; pseudobulbar palsy may be associated with dysarthria
	Eye movements	CN III, IV, VI	Extraocular movement, pupil size, reactivity, pupils react equally to accommodation, diplopia, nystagmus	Cerebral peduncle pressure → CN III dysfunction, cavernous sinus thrombus → CN III, IV, VI problem. Muscular problems (myasthenia gravis, hyperthyroid). Horner's syndrome (ptosis, constricted pupil), anisocoria
	Moving	Motor precentral gyrus (pyramidal) and cerebellar systems, basal ganglia, CN XI, spinal cord, upper motor neuron, (brain → spinal cord via corticospinal tract)	Gait, heel-to-toe walking, presence or absence of involuntary movements, coordination, muscle tone, mass, strength, Romberg's test, ability to shrug shoulders and to rise from chair	*Upper motor neuron:* Brain and cord-sparing anterior horn cell. Tone ↑↑ (spastic). Bulk ↓ due to atrophy of disuse. Reflexes ↑↑ due to loss of central inhibition. No fasciculations. Frequent clonus
		Lower motor neuron (motor cells of cranial and spinal nerves and anterior horn cells → peripheral muscles)		*Lower motor neuron:* Segment anterior horn cell peripheral nerve. Tone ↓↓ (flaccid). Bulk ↓ due to tone loss. Reflexes ↓ or absent due to loss of anterior horn cell. Fasciculations. No clonus
		Involves cerebellum		*Cerebellar problem* → loss of coordination and balance

TABLE 69-1	*Neurologic Assessment Guidelines—cont'd*			
Functional Category	**Specific Category**	**Area of Nervous System Involved**	**Assessment Technique**	**Examples of Disorders**
5. Sensory function	Seeing	CN II: optic, occipital lobe	Acuity, visual fields, funduscopy	Field test: loss in retina or optic nerve → loss in eye involved, optic chiasm → bitemporal hemianopsia Optic tract → homonymous hemianopsia, parietal lobe → quadrant problems (inferior), temporal lobe → superior quadrant problems ↑ Intracranial pressure → papilledema (raised disc → hemorrhage)
	Smelling	CN I: temporal lobe (uncus)	Ability to detect familiar odors	Usually ↓ smell due to extraneural causes (upper respiratory infection, allergy, smoking), olfactory groove; meningioma, olfactory hallucinations
	Hearing	CN VIII: cochlear division, temporal lobe	Acuity of hearing, presence or absence of unusual sounds, Weber's and Rinne tests	May have conductive (nerve OK) or neural hearing loss; Ménière's syndrome (tinnitus, hearing loss, vertigo, and nystagmus), basilar skull fracture → otorrhea Brain stem vascular dysfunction or tumors → ↓ hearing
	Taste	CN VII, IX: insular lobe	Ability to differentiate sweet, salt, sour, and bitter	Brain stem or insula lesions → ↓ taste; extraneural causes, smoking, poor oral hygiene

C, Cervical; *CN,* cranial nerve; *CNS,* central nervous system; *L,* lumbar; *S,* sacral; *T,* thoracic.
↑, increase; ↑↑, significantly increased; ↓, decreased; ↓↓, significantly decreased; →, may affect or lead to.

TABLE 69-1	*Neurologic Assessment Guidelines—cont'd*			
Functional Category	**Specific Category**	**Area of Nervous System Involved**	**Assessment Technique**	**Examples of Disorders**
5. Sensory function—cont'd	Feeling (sensory)	Peripheral nerves → Dermatomes → Spinal cord → Tracts (leading to) Pain-temperature-tactile, anterolateral system, proprioception, stereognosis, dorsal roots → thalamus leading to somasthetic area (postcentral gyrus, parietal lobe)	Pain: pinprick Touch: cotton touched to skin Proprioception: check where digit is in space Vibration: place vibrating tuning fork on bony prominence Temperature: test tubes of cold and warm water laid against skin; person identifies whether hot or cold	Polyneuropathy (diabetes, anemia) Spinal cord lesions → dermatome alterations Upper pons → thalamus, contralateral loss Thalamus → contralateral loss + paresthesias Thalamus → cortex → cortical sensory loss
6. Bowel and bladder function	Bowel function	Afferent Spinal nerve S3-5 External sphincter (voluntary control) Internal sphincter Autonomic nervous system Cerebral cortex	Check for fecal impaction or incontinence Check muscle tone	Fecal incontinence with lesions S3-5 Anal anesthesia—conus medullaris and tabes dorsalis May be extraneural causes Loss of inhibitory control (stroke)
	Bladder function	Autonomic nervous system Afferent Spinal nerve T9-L2, S2-4 Pudendal nerve Efferent Spinal nerve T11-L2 External sphincter (voluntary) Spinal nerve S2-4 Cerebral cortex	Feels when bladder is full, complete emptying. Does client have urgency, frequency?	Urinary incontinence Flaccid bladder Spastic bladder Loss of inhibitory control (stroke) May be extraneural causes

Symptom Analysis

Determine the onset and sequence of manifestations and their progress. Describe neurologic disease processes accurately to facilitate the diagnostic process. Ask the client to describe manifestations using his or her own words. Use a symptom analysis to elicit the characteristics and progression of manifestations (see Chapter 4).

The health history guides the physical examination. For example, a complaint of dizziness cues a focus on examination of the eyes, ears (vestibular nerve), and cerebellar function instead of motor and sensory functions. Detailed neurologic examination is indicated when the client reports behavioral changes, altered level of consciousness (LOC), growth and development problems, pain, changes in motor or sensory function, infection, or trauma. Assess for neurologic problems that may be related to other problems, such as alcohol and recreational drug use, metabolic imbalances, and metastatic lesions.

Past Health History

Childhood and Infectious Diseases and Immunizations

Collect data regarding common childhood diseases and immunizations. Diseases associated with neurologic sequelae include rubella, rubeola, cytomegalovirus infection, herpes simplex, influenza, and meningitis. Ask whether the client has completed the recommended immunization schedule. Public health resources provide schedules for childhood immunizations as well as recommendations for travelers to foreign countries.

Major Illnesses and Hospitalizations

A number of major illnesses are associated with neurologic changes, such as diabetes mellitus, pernicious anemia, cancer, infections, and hypertension. Advanced liver disease and renal disease result in metabolic disturbances, fluid and electrolyte imbalances, and acid-base changes that affect mental function. Inquire about hospitalization, injury, or surgery for neurologic system problems, such as head trauma, seizures, stroke, and crushing tissue injury. Has the client undergone a neurologic diagnostic study, such as electroencephalography (EEG), electromyography (EMG), or computed tomography (CT)? Results of such diagnostic studies provide valuable data for future comparison.

Medications

The medication history includes all medicines that the client is taking or has taken, both prescription and over-the-counter, including herbal preparations. Specifically, ask about aspirin and other anticoagulants, anticonvulsants, antidepressants, antihypertensives, central nervous system (CNS) stimulants such as diet pills, and CNS depressants such as opioids, tranquilizers, and sedatives. Diet pills have been linked to stroke.[13] Many preparations for allergies and colds contain ingredients that cause drowsiness. A number of medications may alter the sense of smell, such as antibiotics, antihistamines, decongestants, antihypertensives, bronchodilators, muscle relaxants, and psychiatric agents. Inquire about the current or past use of recreational drugs, the type of drug, and the duration of use.

Common herbal preparations used for neurologic problems are as follows:

- CNS stimulants: betel nut *(Areca catechu)*; ephedra *(Ephedra sinica, E. vulgaris, E. nevadensis),* also known as Ma Huang, and illegal in some areas; nutmeg *(Myristica fragrans).*
- Sedatives/hypnotics: chamomile *(Matricaria recutita, Chamaemelum nobile)*; gotu kola *(Centella asiatica)*; hops *(Humulus lupulus)*; kava kava *(Piper methysticum)*; St. John's wort *(Hypericum perforatum)*; valerian *(Valeriana officinalis).*
- Antidepressives: *Ginkgo biloba*; sage *(Salvia officinalis)*; St. John's wort. Sage can be used as an aid for dizziness, as can *G. biloba. G. biloba* has also been indicated for treating tinnitus, short-term memory loss, and headache.
- Analgesics: cayenne *(Capsicum),* taken internally for headache and toothache or applied externally for neuralgia; feverfew *(Tanacetum parthenium),* used for prevention of migraine and cluster headaches; white willow *(Salix purpurea, S. fragilis, S. daphnoides),* used as an analgesic and antipyretic.
- Antihypertensive or anti-stroke effects: garlic *(Allium sativum)*; *G. biloba*; onion *(Allium cepa)*; reishi mushroom *(Ganoderma lucidum).*

Growth and Development

The growth and development history may help determine whether neurologic dysfunction was present at an early age. The perinatal history may contain data about in utero exposure to viruses (rubella); maternal consumption of alcohol, tobacco, or other drugs; and radiation. Ask whether the client was born at full term. Premature birth increases the risk of neurologic damage from inadequate oxygenation and intracranial bleeding if ventilator support was used. A difficult or prolonged labor and delivery can result in hypoxia or use of forceps for delivery, with consequent central and peripheral neurologic damage.

At what age did the client accomplish major developmental tasks, such as walking and talking? Was the client able to participate in games, sports, and other childhood activities with peers? Did the client have any problems with coordination, balance, or agility?

Family Health History

Ask about a family history of neurologic disorders to determine the presence of genetic risk factors. Inquire about epilepsy, Huntington's disease, amyotrophic lateral sclerosis, muscular dystrophy, hypertension, stroke, mental retardation, and psychiatric disorders.

Psychosocial History

An understanding of personal psychosocial factors (educational background, level of performance, and personality changes) enhances assessment. Inquire about changes that have occurred in daily routines. Ask about changes in sleep patterns, exercise routines, hobbies and recreation, occupation, perceived stressors, and sexual interest and performance. Is there risk of exposure to neurotoxic fumes or chemicals, such as pesticides, paints, or bonding agents (glue), or does the client spend time in an inadequately ventilated living area or workspace?

Review of Systems

Neurologic disorders often subtly affect the ability to function in an integrated fashion. Ask the client to describe any neurologic manifestations, such as behavior changes, mood swings, loss of consciousness, seizures, headaches, dizziness, vertigo, memory deficits, speech or motor function problems (unstable balance or posture, gait changes, tics, tremors), and sensory function problems (vision changes, pain, paresthesia or tingling, paralysis). Significant neurologic assessment data are listed in Box 69-1. Detailed questions for the review of systems can be found on the website.

The client who has a neurologic problem may be unaware of its presence. Attempt to supplement and cor-

roborate the history and review of systems by speaking with a family member or significant other who knows the client well. Ask specifically about mental or physical changes that have been noticed.

PHYSICAL EXAMINATION

The physical examination is intended to detect abnormalities in neurologic functioning. Variations in client age, physical condition, and LOC determine how detailed an examination can be. A comprehensive neurologic examination is described here. Adapt the examination to the client's severity of illness and ability to cooperate. Box 69-2 is a guide for adapting the assessment in various situations. A suggested sequence for the physical examination is as follows:

1. Vital signs
2. Mental status (including language and communication)
3. Head, neck, and back
4. Cranial nerves (including pupils)
5. Motor system (including coordination and gait)
6. Sensory function

BOX 69-1   *Manifestations Related to Neurologic Assessment*

Eye
Vision and visual field loss
Diplopia
Ptosis
Proptosis

Ear, Nose, and Throat
Infections
Hearing loss
Tinnitus
Dizziness
Vertigo
Voice change
Dysphagia
Changes in taste or smell
Experiences of unusual smells

Cardiovascular
Syncope
Palpitations
Hypotension
Hypertension
Vertigo
Transient ischemic attacks
Stroke

Neurologic
Weakness
Numbness

Paresthesias
Headache
Pain
Altered thinking
Speech difficulty
Vomiting
Vertigo
Ataxia
Fainting
Seizures
Any loss of consciousness
Distortions of reality
Use of consciousness-altering drugs
Disorientation to time, place, or person
Altered sleep patterns
Changes in ability to speak, read, or understand language
Changes in memory of recent or remote events
Changes in ability to concentrate

Skin
Hair and nail changes

Musculoskeletal
Tremor
Weakness
Altered coordination
Staggering
Difficulty climbing stairs

BOX 69-2   *The Initial Neurologic Examination in the Clinical Setting*

The sequence in which the neurologic examination is performed and the amount of time devoted to each step are dictated by the client's situation. For example, assessment of the head-injured client in the emergency department requires evaluation of vital signs, pupil reactivity, level of consciousness, and motor response. These clients may not be stable or cooperative enough to allow completion of the cranial nerve and sensory response assessment. Spinal cord–injured clients, however, are usually coherent and able to participate in the sensory examination. The sensory assessment information is essential for documenting changes in the status of spinal cord–injured clients.

As clients become more stable and cooperative, the examination can be performed in more depth and with less frequency. Remember that neurologically impaired clients frequently experience fluctuations in status. Alter the assessment schedule and technique to detect and report these fluctuations.

Following are suggested modifications in the screening neurologic examination that may be made on the basis of the client's initial presentation:

Initial examination for diagnosis and triage:
- Client history based on chief complaint
- Physical examination, including vital signs
- Level of consciousness
- Pupillary response
- Brain stem function (corneal reflex)
- Motor and sensory functions in all four extremities

If the client is conscious and stable:
- Complete baseline neurologic examination
- Focused examinations at prescribed intervals

If the client is conscious and unstable:
- Quick baseline physical assessment
- Frequent focused examinations until client is stable
- Vital signs
- Level of consciousness
- Pupillary response
- Brain stem function
- Motor and sensory functions in extremities
- Spinal cord function

If the patient is unconscious but stable:
- Vital signs
- Level of consciousness and ability to arouse
- Cranial nerve function
- Motor and sensory functions
- Pathologic reflexes

If the patient is unconscious and unstable:
- Vital signs
- Level of consciousness
- Cranial nerve function
- Motor and sensory functions relative to the ability to test for them
- Pathologic reflexes
- Frequent focused examinations on ongoing basis (hourly or more often)

If spinal cord involvement is suspected:
- Motor functions in detail with testing of specific muscle groups
- Sensory function
- Reflexes
- Bowel and bladder functions
- Vital signs

7. Reflexes
8. Autonomic nervous system

Neurologic findings are summarized in the Physical Assessment Findings in the Healthy Adult feature on The Neurologic System on p. 2025.

Vital Signs

Although cortical changes occur first (LOC), initially assess vital signs because neurologic disorders can cause life-threatening changes. Clients who have cervical spinal cord injuries exhibit a classic triad of hypotension, bradycardia, and hypothermia related to the loss of sympathetic nervous system function. Inadequate perfusion of vital organs may result from hypotension if the blood pressure is not sustained.

Changes in vital signs can also accompany the late stages of increased intracranial pressure (ICP). The body attempts to provide an adequate supply of oxygen and glucose to the brain by increasing the blood flow to the brain to compensate for the elevated ICP. *Cushing's response* consists of elevated systolic blood pressure, widened pulse pressure, and bradycardia. Respiratory rate and rhythm can be altered by increased ICP on the brain stem.

Mental Status

Document general data about the client's mental status (LOC, orientation, memory, mood and affect, intellectual performance, judgment and insight, and language and communication). The mental status examination is discussed in Chapter 4.

Level of Consciousness

The LOC is the most sensitive indicator of changes in neurologic status. Consciousness is maintained by the cerebral hemispheres and reticular activating system. Test LOC by using stimuli to determine arousal. Stimuli

PHYSICAL ASSESSMENT FINDINGS IN THE HEALTHY ADULT

The Neurologic System

Inspection

Mental Status. Oriented to person, place, time, and situation. No difficulty recalling recent and past events. Serial 7s deferred. Mood and affect congruent, cooperative, and pleasant. Thought process clear and logical. Demonstrates effective problem-solving. Speech articulate, clear, and fluent.

Head, Neck, and Back. Normocephalic without obvious lesions. Maintains head position. Spine in straight alignment with normal cervical, thoracic, and lumbar curves. Neck and back have full range of motion.

Cranial Nerves.

CN I. Discerns smell of coffee, cinnamon, alcohol.

CN II. Visual acuity per Snellen's chart is OU = 20/20. Visual fields full to confrontation. Optic disc margins sharp, no cupping; cup-to-disc ratio is 1:3. Retina: Arteriovenous ratio is 2:3, without nicking. Fovea visualized.

CN III, CN IV, CN VI. PERRLA, direct and consensual. Accommodation present. EOMs intact without nystagmus or strabismus. Cover-uncover test negative. Corneal light reflections symmetrical.

CN V. Opens and closes mouth; chews, clenches teeth, and moves jaw side to side voluntarily. Sensation intact to forehead, cheeks, and chin. Corneal reflexes present.

CN VII. Face movements symmetrical with smiling, frowning, eyebrow raising, lip pursing, and cheek puffing. Discerns sweet, salty, sour, and bitter tastes (also CN IX).

CN VIII. Gross hearing intact. Whisper heard at 3 ft. Air conduction greater than bone conduction bilaterally.

CN IX and CN X. Tongue and uvula midline. Uvula and soft palate rise in midline with phonation. Gag reflex present bilaterally. Swallows, coughs, and speaks without difficulty.

CN XI. Performs shoulder shrugs. Turns head against resistance. Maintains head position against resistance.

CN XII. Tongue protrudes midline without deviation; pushes side to side with equal strength.

Motor Function. Muscle groups symmetrical. Gross and fine motor coordination intact. Moves all extremities through range of motion. Romberg's test negative. Pronator drift absent. Gait smooth, steady. Maintains balance walking on toes and heels. Rapid alternating movements and point-to-point maneuvers performed without difficulty.

Sensory Function. Sensation to light touch, pain, and vibration intact distally and over trunk, neck, and face. Position sense of fingers and toes intact. Stereognosis and graphesthesia present bilaterally. Two-point discrimination: 2 mm on index fingers. Discerns 2-point simultaneous stimulation.

Palpation

Head, Neck, and Back. Skull without lesions or tenderness; smooth and firm. Neck and paravertebral muscles firm, relaxed, and nontender. No pain or tenderness over spinous processes.

Motor Function. Muscle bulk full and tone firm; strength rated as 5/5 bilaterally.

Percussion

Reflexes. Deep tendon reflexes rated 2+ (on a scale of 0-4+) in triceps, biceps, wrists, knees, and ankles. Plantar reflexes present bilaterally. Abdominal reflexes present in all four quadrants.

Auscultation

Vascular Flow. Absence of bruit over carotid arteries bilaterally.

---

include verbal, visual, tactile, and noxious agents, such as painful pressure.

When assessing LOC, begin by observing spontaneous behavior before using stimuli; then provide stimuli, and make observations regarding the response. Start with a visual cue, such as walking in front of the client or waving hello. If a response is not elicited, provide verbal stimulation. Use touch and painful (noxious) stimuli only if the client does not respond to the milder forms of stimulation.

If a painful stimulus is needed to elicit a response, it should be a central stimulus, such as sternal pressure, supraorbital ridge pressure, or sternocleidomastoid muscle pinch. Although nail bed pressure may be used, it is a peripheral stimulation and may elicit a spinal reflex re-sponse rather than a central, or brain, response. Noxious stimuli are also discussed in Chapter 70.

Document the location and type of stimuli applied along with the client's response so that the results can be accurately compared with those of future examinations. Terms such as "alert," "lethargic," "stuporous," "semicomatose," and "comatose" are vague. Avoid these terms unless your agency has explicit definitions for them to maintain consistency.

The *Glasgow Coma Scale* is an assessment tool designed to note trends in a client's response to stimuli (see Chapter 75). The original Glasgow Coma Scale was developed for use with head-injured clients. Many variations of this scale now exist for use with other client populations.

Orientation

Establish *orientation* to time, place, person, and event (or situation); for instance, ask, What is your name? What year is this? What kind of place is this? Where are you? What brought you to the hospital today?

Memory

Identify gross deficits in long-term and short-term memory with simple tests. Test *long-term memory* when the client relates the past health history. (Of course, another source must be able to validate the data.) Test *short-term memory* by (1) stating three words for the client to remember (red, Broadway, three), (2) asking the client to say the words immediately, and (3) then asking the client to repeat them after a few minutes.

Mood and Affect

Assess mood by asking the client to describe how he or she feels by observing facial expression and from reports of significant others. Facial expression may reveal emotions such as anxiety, distrust, and depression. Is the client's affect appropriate to the situation?

Intellectual Performance

Intellectual performance consists of the fund of knowledge and calculation ability. Ask the client to identify commonly known people, places, current events, and the like. Assess calculation ability by asking the client to count by 7s (*serial 7s*) or 3s. If the client is unable to perform reversed serial 7s, have the client perform simple addition or subtraction ($3 + 4 = ?$, $13 - 5 = ?$).

Judgment and Insight

Judgment and insight include reasoning, abstract thinking, problem solving, and the client's perception of the situation. Assess reasoning, abstract thinking, and problem-solving for indications of major problems with thought content (see Chapter 4).

Listen to how the client answers questions. Are the answers logical? Do they relate to the question? Can the client concentrate and remain focused, or is the client easily distracted? Assess abstract thinking by asking the client to explain a proverb such as "A rolling stone gathers no moss." Evaluate reasoning and problem-solving by describing a situation and asking the client to give a solution. For example, "What would you do if you lost your house keys?" Assess insight and perception by asking the client to give an opinion about what might be the cause of the chief complaint.

Language and Communication

Language and communication assessment tests the ability to express and comprehend one's environment. Grossly evaluate *expression* and *comprehension* during the initial interview. Does the client initiate speech? Is speech fluent and appropriate?

Assess speech quality. Is speech clear and intelligible, or is it garbled because of facial droop or poor dentition? Note the content of speech (orientation, intellect, logic). Assess speech for articulation problems (usually motor disorders) or comprehension or expression problems (aphasic disorders).

Does the client follow verbal commands? Evaluate the client's ability to communicate and understand verbally, in writing, mathematically, and nonverbally.

Comprehension and Expression. Assess comprehension and expression in more depth. Test the *ability to comprehend spoken language* by asking the client to follow basic commands ("Show me your right thumb," "Stick out your tongue"). To determine *comprehension of written language,* ask the client to read several words or sentences and explain them. Write a simple command ("Stick out your tongue"), and have the client read and then perform the command.

Evaluate *expression* as the client responds to questions that require more than a nod or a "yes" or "no" answer. Evaluate speech for flow, choice of words, and completion of phrases or sentences. If the client is expressively aphasic, test comprehension by asking *yes* or *no* questions or by having the client follow simple verbal commands. Assess written expression by having the client write answers to simple questions on paper ("Write your name and address").

Integrated Sensory Functions. *Integrated sensory functions* involving language are often tested with this portion of the neurologic examination. Have the client perform simple addition or subtraction without writing. Ask the client to identify orally common objects, such as a pen, a key, and a watch. These skills require integration of cortical functioning (calculation) and visual recognition with expressive speech.

Head, Neck, and Back

Examine the head, neck, and spine using inspection, palpation, percussion, and auscultation. Tumors, vascular disorders, traumatic disorders, and problems involving the vertebrae and surrounding muscles may be detected.

Inspection

Inspect the head for size, shape, contour, and symmetry. Note any ecchymosis (bruising) around the eyes or behind the ears. Anterior basilar skull fractures often result in "raccoon eyes," with periorbital ecchymosis and, occasionally, drainage of cerebrospinal fluid (CSF) from the nares. Middle fossa basilar skull fractures often result in ecchymosis over the mastoid process behind the ears (Battle's sign) and drainage of blood, CSF, or both from the ears.

Palpation

Palpate the skull lightly for nodules or masses and to supplement inspection findings. Wear gloves if there are open or draining areas. The skull normally feels smooth and firm. Areas of bogginess or depressions are abnormal. Palpation of neck muscles may identify masses or tender areas. Ask the client to flex the neck with the chin touching the chest; look for nuchal (back of the neck) rigidity, which is a manifestation of meningeal irritation.

Inspect and palpate spine alignment. Note any deviation from the normal curvatures. Palpate the paravertebral muscles for masses, tenderness, and spasm (also see Chapter 27).

Percussion

Gentle percussion over the spinous processes may produce pain or tenderness, which are abnormal findings.

Auscultation

Auscultation of major neck and other vessels may reveal bruits or other sounds suggesting an abnormality. Use the bell of the stethoscope to auscultate the carotid arteries. Bruits result from turbulent flow, usually a sign of atherosclerotic disease.

Cranial Nerves

The cranial nerves are referred to by specific name or Roman numeral. Cranial nerve (CN) examination is important for two reasons. First, CN III through CN XII arise in the brain stem. Testing their function provides information about the brain stem and related pathways. Second, three reflexes involving cranial nerves are called *protective reflexes* (corneal, gag, and cough reflexes). The presence or absence of protective reflexes indicates the ability to protect the eye surfaces and airway. This is especially important in unconscious patients.

Normal cranial nerve reflexes require an appropriately received stimulus *(input)* that produces an appropriate response *(output)*. During testing of cranial nerves, the absence of a normal response may indicate (1) failure to receive stimuli (input failure), (2) failure to respond appropriately (output failure), or (3) a combination of input and output failure. Determining which problems exist is often a challenge. For example, vision

is a function of CN II, and pupillary light response is a function of both CN II and CN III (see Figure U16-13; see Table 69-1). The structure and function of the cranial nerves are discussed in the Unit 16 Anatomy and Physiology Review.

Olfactory Nerve (CN I)

The function of CN I is purely sensory. Ask the client to smell and then identify an aromatic, nonirritating odor (coffee, isopropyl alcohol, toothpaste) with each nostril separately and with the eyes closed. Test with several different odors. If the client can perceive any one smell, consider the nerve functional.

Although inability to smell *(anosmia)* may develop in older people, problems such as basal skull fracture or olfactory groove tumor also may be responsible. Other possible causes of anosmia are cribriform plate fracture, an olfactory bulb or a tract tumor, and previous sinus disorders or surgery.

Optic Nerve (CN II)

CN II has a purely sensory function. Assessment of the optic nerve involves the following steps:

1. Inspect the globe for foreign bodies, cataracts, inflammation, or other obvious abnormalities. Details of eye assessment are given in Chapter 66.
2. Test *visual acuity.* Have the client read a newspaper, a sign (from a distance), or a Snellen's chart. Eyeglasses should be worn during the test if the client usually wears them. Refraction errors are not significant in neurologic assessment.
3. Test *visual fields* to determine whether vision is absent in one or more directions or in a portion of the visual field, such as half of the visual field, the middle portion, or both sides. Such losses may indicate various problems and may correlate with the area of the brain involved.
4. Examine the eye fundus with an ophthalmoscope. Gross inspection of the eyes and examination of the fundus can provide information about neurologic disease. Possible causes of abnormal findings include trauma to orbit or eyeball; fracture of optic foramen; diabetic retinopathy; laceration or blood clot in the brain's temporal, parietal, or occipital lobes; and increased ICP *(papilledema).*

Oculomotor (CN III), Trochlear (CN IV), and Abducens (CN VI) Nerves

CN III, CN IV, and CN VI have only motor components. CN III controls pupil constriction and elevation of the upper lid. Pupils should be equal in size and round. In about 20% of the population, *anisocoria* (unequal pupils) is a normal finding. Older clients who have undergone cataract surgery with lens implants may have irregular, nonreactive pupils. This finding does not indicate neurologic damage. Note pupil size before shining a light into the client's eyes. Document each pupil's size and shape.

Approach the pupil from the temporal side while the client looks straight ahead. Test each pupil for both direct and consensual responses (pupillary constriction) to a light. A *direct response* occurs in the eye being tested. A *consensual response* occurs in the other eye. A direct response indicates an intact connection in the midbrain between CN II and the ipsilateral CN III. An intact consensual response indicates a connection between CN II and the contralateral CN III via a connection in the midbrain.

Test *accommodation* (eyes able to focus on both near and far objects) by having the client look across the room (away from the light source) and then at your fingers held about 6 inches from the client's nose. Normally, the lens shape changes and the pupils constrict. The notation *PERRLA* (*p*upils *e*qual, *r*ound, *r*eactive to *l*ight and *a*ccommodation) indicates that these functions are normal. When testing *pupillary light reflex* only (not accommodation), the abbreviation *PERL* (*p*upils *e*qual, *r*eactive to *l*ight) is used.

CN III lies over the edge of the uncal portion of the temporal lobe. Increased ICP or edema causes that area of the brain to shift, and CN III is stretched. This disruption of the CN III pathway causes either a sluggish response or an absence of response to light. This response can be unilateral or bilateral, depending on the site and severity of edema. *Hippus,* the rhythmic constriction and dilation of a pupil, is caused by early compromise of CN III with increased ICP; it is not seen in all clients. Destruction of part of CN III can cause *ptosis* (drooping of the eyelid). Disorders or pressure on a specific side of CN III can cause the ipsilateral pupil to dilate, the eyelid to droop, and the eye to deviate outward.

CN III, CN IV, and CN VI coordinate to control eye movements in all six cardinal directions of gaze (see Chapter 66). Test the function of these nerves by having the client hold the head still and follow your finger or another object as it is moved in all directions of gaze. *Conjugate gaze* allows for the eyes to move in a coordinated effort for binocular vision (two images "merged" into one). *Disconjugate gaze* often occurs as a result of weakness of one or more extraocular muscles. *Diplopia* (double vision) occurs with disconjugate gaze because the two images are not "merged." If a client has diplopia but no muscle weakness can be demonstrated, shine a light so it reflects on both eyes. The area of reflection is normally symmetrical, meaning that the client has a conjugate gaze. In disconjugate gaze, the light's reflection is asymmetrical (not the same in both eyes).

If *extraocular movements* (EOMs) are intact, document as "EOMs intact." Also observe for *nystagmus* (involuntary eye movements), seen as fine, rhythmic eye movements that can be vertical, horizontal, or rotational. Possible causes of abnormal findings include (1) pressure on CN III, CN IV, or CN VI at the brain stem due to fracture of the orbit; (2) increased ICP; and (3) tumor at or trauma to the base of the brain. An inability to look down or to walk down steps because of a visual disturbance might be related to CN IV dysfunction. Inability of an eye to move laterally outward is associated with compression of or damage to CN VI.

Trigeminal Nerve (CN V)

CN V has a motor division and a sensory division. The motor division innervates the muscles of mastication. Test CN V function by asking the client to clamp the jaws shut, open the mouth against resistance, open the mouth widely, move the jaw from side to side, and make chewing movements. A normal CN V allows all these activities. Document any asymmetry in the temporal muscles.

The sensory division mediates all sensations for the entire face, scalp, cornea, and nasal and oral cavities. With the client's eyes closed, test sensations such as pain (sharp point), touch (wisp of cotton), and temperature (hot and cold metal objects) on both sides of the face from the top of the head (vertex) to the chin.

Test the *corneal reflexes* by gently touching the cornea with a sterile wisp of cotton or gently stroking the eyelash. (Omit this test during the screening examination.) The normal response is brisk eyelid blinking. The corneal reflex involves CN V and CN VII. CN V is the afferent (sensory) arc, and CN VII controls closure of the eye (motor). Possible causes of abnormal findings include a tumor at or trauma to the base of the brain, a fracture of the orbit, and trigeminal neuralgia.

Facial Nerve (CN VII)

CN VII has both a motor division and a sensory division. The motor division innervates muscles controlling facial expression. Observe the face for symmetry and the ability to use facial muscles. Ask the client to smile, frown, raise the forehead and eyebrows, tightly close the eyes and resist attempts to open them, whistle, show the teeth, and puff out the cheeks. Test the anterior part of the tongue for taste by asking the client to close the eyes and protrude (stick out) the tongue. Then place a taste substance on one side of the anterior tongue. Have the client keep the tongue protruded while identifying the taste. Ask the client to rinse the mouth or drink a small amount of water before testing the other side. Test taste on each side with sweet, salty, acidic or sour (vinegar or lemon), and bitter (coffee) substances.

Common abnormalities noted with CN VII dysfunction include (1) loss of the nasolabial fold, (2) inability to close the eye and blink reflexively, (3) facial asymmetry, (4) drooling, (5) difficulty swallowing secretions, (6) loss of tearing, and (7) loss of taste on the anterior two thirds of the tongue. Possible causes of abnormal findings are Bell's palsy, temporal bone fracture, and peripheral laceration or contusion of the parotid region.

The lower half of the facial muscles, especially around the mouth, also receive innervation from the voluntary motor area of the frontal lobes. Deficits of lower facial muscles can be related to a lesion in the contralateral frontal lobe (client who has had a stroke and has a flattened nasolabial fold and facial droop on the opposite side retains the ability to close the eyelid on the same side of the face). Deficits on the lower half of the face only are called *central deficits* because the lesion is in the CNS. A deficit involving both the upper face and lower face is called a *peripheral deficit* because the lesion involves CN VII, which is a peripheral nerve.

Vestibulocochlear or Acoustic Nerve (CN VIII)

CN VIII is a sensory nerve with two divisions: cochlear and vestibular. The cochlear nerve permits hearing. Test *auditory acuity* by having the client listen to and report on a whispered voice, rustling fingers, or a tuning fork at various distances from the ear. Test *bone and air conduction* with a tuning fork. Audiometry may be used for a precise assessment.

The vestibular nerve helps maintain equilibrium by coordinating the muscles of the eye, neck, trunk, and extremities. *Equilibrium tests* include Romberg's and caloric tests (oculovestibular reflex) and electronystagmography. (Hearing and equilibrium assessment is described in Chapter 66.) Possible causes of abnormal findings include Ménière's syndrome and acoustic neuroma.

Glossopharyngeal (CN IX) and Vagus (CN X) Nerves

CN IX and CN X have both motor and sensory components. Because of overlapping innervation of the pharynx, assess these nerves together. Ask the client to open the mouth widely and say "Ah." Place a tongue depressor on the first third of the tongue to flatten it and enhance visualization. Observe the position and movement of the uvula and palate. The palate should rise symmetrically with the uvula at the midline. Test the *gag reflex* by gently touching each side of the pharynx with a tongue depressor, which normally elicits a brisk response. Use a small amount of water to assess the ability to swallow. Test the posterior third of the tongue for taste, as with CN VII (perform when testing CN VII). Dysfunction of CN IX includes loss of taste and sensation of the glossopharyngeal nerve.

To test the function of CN X, ask the client to cough and to speak. Damage to CN X causes an ineffective cough and a weak, hoarse voice. To differentiate areas of weakness, ask the client to vocalize different sounds: "kuh-kuh" (soft palate), "mi-mi" (lips), "la-la" (tongue). Possible causes of abnormal findings include brain stem trauma or tumors, neck trauma, and stroke.

Spinal Accessory Nerve (CN XI)

CN XI has only a motor component. It innervates the sternocleidomastoid muscle and the upper portion of the trapezius muscle. Ask the client to (1) elevate the shoulders (with and without resistance), (2) turn (not tilt) the head to one side and then the other, (3) resist attempts to pull the chin back toward the midline, and (4) push the head forward against resistance. Disorders may produce drooping of a shoulder, muscle atrophy, weak shoulder shrug, or weak turn of the head. Possible causes of abnormal findings include neck trauma, radical neck surgery, and torticollis.

Hypoglossal Nerve (CN XII)

CN XII has only a motor component. This nerve innervates the tongue. Ask the client to open the mouth widely, stick out the tongue, and rapidly move the tongue from side to side and in and out. Document any deviation from midline. Assess strength by having the client push the tongue against the inside of the cheek while applying external pressure. Possible causes of abnormal findings include neck trauma associated with major blood vessel damage.

Motor System

Assessing the motor system thoroughly involves numerous procedures. The following discussion focuses on the screening examinations and common abnormalities.

Muscle Size

Inspect all major muscle groups bilaterally for symmetry, hypertrophy, and atrophy.

Muscle Strength

Assess the power in major muscle groups against resistance (see Chapter 27). Assess and rate muscle strength on a 5-point scale in all four extremities, comparing one side with the other, as follows:

5/5 = Normal full strength. Muscle moves actively through the full range of motion against the effects of gravity and applied resistance.

4/5 = Muscle moves actively through the full range of motion against the effect of gravity with weakness to applied resistance.

3/5 = Muscle moves actively against the effect of gravity alone.

2/5 = Muscle moves across a surface but cannot overcome gravity.

1/5 = Muscle contraction is palpable and visible; trace or flicker movement occurs.

0/5 = Muscle contraction or movement is undetectable.

Next test for subtle weakness in upper and lower extremities. For upper extremities, have the client hold the arms straight out in front with the palms up ("like holding a tray"). Ask the client to close the eyes and to maintain the position. A *pronator drift* is said to be present if one arm pronates and falls lower than the other. For the lower extremities, have the client walk on the heels and then on the toes to test dorsiflexion, plantiflexion, and balance.

Assessment of specific muscle groups evaluates deficits in certain areas, such as spinal cord disorders. Disorders of muscle strength may be exhibited as weakness on one side of the body, in both lower extremities, or in both upper and lower extremities.

If asymmetry is detected, ask the client or family whether it is long-standing or recent. Consider the client's age, handedness, and physical condition when interpreting the results of muscle-strength testing. One would not expect the same strength from a physically fit young client as from an older or debilitated client. If abnormalities are found in muscle power, more detailed assessment may be conducted with procedures such as EMG (see later discussion).

Muscle Tone

Assess muscle tone while moving each extremity through its range of passive motion. When tone is decreased *(hypotonicity)*, the muscles are soft, flabby, or flaccid; when tone is increased *(hypertonicity)*, the muscles are resistant to movement, rigid, or spastic. Note the presence of abnormal flexion or extension posture.

Muscle Coordination

Assessment of muscle coordination consists of testing rapid alternating movements, point-to-point maneuvers, and maintenance of truncal balance and head position. Test *rapid alternating movements* by asking the client to touch (approximate) each finger to the thumb quickly in succession. Alternatively, ask the client to pat the thighs first with the palms, then with the back of the hands, and to repeat the patting quickly.

For *point-to-point testing*, hold up an index finger approximately 18 inches from the client. Ask the client first to touch his or her nose with a finger, then touch your index finger, and then touch the nose again. Repeat this several times while you move your index finger to different locations. Perform the test for the client's right and left hands. Test lower-extremity coordination by asking the client to place the heel of the foot below the other knee and then to slide the heel down the shin toward the great toe. Repeat for the other leg.

Assess *truncal balance* with the client sitting. Can the client remain upright without support? Gently push the client to a leaning position. Can the client return to an upright position? Note *head position* by observing the ability to move the head while following your movements.

Disorders related to coordination indicate cerebellar or posterior column lesions. The defining characteristics of cerebellar dysfunction are (1) ataxia, (2) intention tremor (tremor upon nearing the object), (3) nystagmus, (4) ocular dysmetria (inability to gaze on an object), and (5) dysdiadochokinesia (arresting one motor impulse and substituting an opposite one).

Gait and Station

Assess gait and station by having the client stand still, walk, and walk in tandem (one foot in front of the other in a straight line). Walking involves the functions of motor power, sensation, and coordination. The ability to stand quietly with the feet together requires coordination and intact *proprioception* (sense of body position). If the client has difficulty standing, assess further to determine whether the client is weak or unsteady. If the client is weak, protect the client from falling. Box 69-3 includes terms used to describe gait disorders.

BOX 69-3   *Terms Associated with Gait Disorders*

Ataxic Staggering and unsteady.

Double step Alternate steps differing in length or rate.

Dystonic Irregular and nondirective.

Dystrophic or broad-based Legs far apart; weight shifting from side to side (waddling).

Equine High steps.

Festinating Walking on toes at an accelerating pace.

Helicopod Feet (or foot) making a half-circle with each step.

Hemiplegic Paralyzed on one side; paralyzed limb swings outward; foot drags; arm on affected side does not swing freely.

Parkinsonian Short, accelerating steps; shuffling; forward-leaning posture; head, hips, and knees flexed; difficulty starting and stopping.

Scissors Legs crossed while walking with short, slow steps.

Spastic Stiff, short steps; toes catch and drag; legs held together; hips and knees flexed.

Steppage Foot and toes lifted high; heel comes down heavily.

Tabetic High steps; foot slaps down.

Movement

Examine the muscles for fine and gross abnormal movements. Examples of fine movements are *fasciculations* (involuntary ripples or twitches that occur while the client is relaxed), which may indicate lower motor neuron disease. Examples of more grossly abnormal movements, often representing extrapyramidal disease, are described in Box 69-4.

Move all joints through a full range of passive motion. Abnormal findings include pain, joint contractures, and muscle resistance.

Test for *apraxia* (the inability to carry out a learned movement on command in the absence of weakness or paralysis). Ask the client to perform a common activity, such as tying shoes or combing hair. Apraxia is present if a client can follow other commands (indicating intact comprehension), has the motor strength to move the extremity involved, but cannot carry out the command.

Motor Testing of the Unconscious Patient

In this chapter, the term *patient* is used to describe the client who is unconscious and who cannot be an active participant in care. The family is considered the client in these situations.

BOX 69-4   *Abnormal Movements Associated with Extrapyramidal Disease*

Akinesia Reduced body movement in the absence of weakness or paralysis; habitual movements (swinging arms) limited or absent.

Athetosis Gross, writhing, worm-like movements of body, face, or extremities.

Ballismus A form of chorea; involuntary dramatic movements of arms and legs (**hemiballismus** involves only one side).

Bradykinesia Slow movement.

Chorea Discrete, jerky, purposeless movements in distal extremities and face.

Dystonia Prolonged twisting movements or postures.

Myoclonus Sudden muscle contractions of varying intensity that may involve a small part of one extremity or the entire body; may violently fling a client to the floor.

Spasms Involuntary contraction of large muscle groups (arms, legs, neck).

Tic Involuntary movement of groups of muscles in stereotypic patterns; may be physical or psychogenic in origin; pathologic causes of tics include Tourette's syndrome.

Tremors Involuntary trembling or quivering; may vary in direction, amplitude, rhythmicity, parts involved, speed, and timing in relation to rest or activity; types include parkinsonian, essential, and cerebellar.

An unresponsive patient can be tested only for response to painful stimuli (reflex withdrawal of limbs, wincing, grimacing). Although a pain stimulus is used, the response is usually recorded as a motor system response. These responses are often incorporated into the motor scale of the Glasgow Coma Scale. (See Chapter 75 for further information.)

Use deep pain to elicit a sensory response when an unconscious patient is unresponsive to superficial stimuli. Use minimal stimulation to assess cerebral response to pain with techniques such as rubbing the sternum, applying pressure to the orbital rim, or squeezing the sternocleidomastoid muscle. Nail bed pressure may be used; however, the stimulus is a peripheral source of pain and may produce a spinal segment reflex response even in the absence of cerebral function. Document the site and type of stimulus used so that the examination can be adequately reproduced at a later time. Note the patient's response to the noxious stimuli. Box 69-5 describes the most common responses to painful stimuli.

Sensory Function

Sensory assessment involves testing for touch, pain, vibration, position (proprioception), and discrimination. Assessment of hearing, vision, smell, and taste is also sensory assessment. Sensory assessment may identify dermatomes as having normal, absent, reduced, exaggerated, or delayed sensation. Dermatomes are discussed in the Unit 16 Anatomy and Physiology Review.

A complete sensory examination is possible only on a conscious and cooperative client. Always test sensation with the client's eyes closed. Help the client relax and keep warm.

Conduct sensory assessment systematically. Test a particular area of the body, and then test the corresponding area on the other side. Begin testing a selection of dermatomes that represent cervical, thoracic, lumbar, and sacral segments of the spinal cord. If you note a

---

BOX 69-5   *Responses to Painful Stimuli*

Localization: reaches for the source of the stimulus and attempts to push the examiner away

Flexion withdrawal: moves without purpose and may exhibit minimal movement, grimacing, or wincing

Abnormal flexion (decorticate posturing): flexes, adducts, and internally rotates the wrists and arms to the chest and rigidly extends the legs (indicates damage in the corticospinal tracts near the cerebral hemispheres that has left the rubrospinal tract intact)

Abnormal extension (decerebrate posturing): extends and pronates the arms while rigidly extending the legs (indicates damage in the upper brain stem)

No response: no visible reaction to painful stimuli

sensory loss, you can perform a more detailed testing of surrounding dermatomes. Document asymmetrical findings (those varying from one side to the other). If the client has a sensory loss, document the area of loss and where normal sensation begins. Sensation assessment may be documented on a body chart of dermatomes.

Superficial Sensation

Test superficial sensations by stimulating the skin in symmetrical areas on each side of the body according to dermatome distribution. Test *superficial pain* by alternating the sharp and dull ends of a broken cotton applicator. The wooden broken end is pointed enough for testing sharp sensation, yet dull enough not to break the skin. The cotton swab end serves as the dull stimulus. Use a new swab for each client to eliminate concern about cross-contamination from one client to another.

Touch and Pain. Ask the client to close the eyes. Explain that the client will feel a sharp or a dull stimulus. Demonstrate how sharp and dull feel. Touch the client with the dull end of the swab. Then apply a painful stimulus with the pointed end. Move from the fingers to the shoulders. Alternate the two stimuli inconsistently (so that the client cannot predict which is being used), and ask the client to distinguish sharp from dull. Then test from the toes to the thighs. Finally, test the anterior and posterior trunk and the buttocks.

Keep the dermatome pattern in mind while testing. Where there is a loss of the sense of pain, test for awareness of temperature. Otherwise, it is not necessary to test for temperature because pain and temperature sensations travel on related pathways.

Other Modalities. Other modalities for testing superficial sensation in the conscious client include using a cotton wisp to assess *light touch*. Follow the same guidelines as for testing superficial pain sensation, stimulating symmetrical areas of the dermatomes.

Temperature. *Temperature* is not assessed routinely. Perform the test only when pain and light touch responses are abnormal. Use two test tubes, one filled with warm water and one with cold water. Check first to ensure that the warm water is not too hot. Assess each major dermatome symmetrically. Alternatively, use the side of the tuning fork, which is usually cold, to test for awareness of temperature.

Mechanical Sensation

Mechanical sensations are assessed with vibration and proprioception.

Vibration. Use a tuning fork to test for vibration. Place the end of a vibrating tuning fork on a distal bony prominence, such as a finger or great toe joint. Ask the client to indicate when the vibration is felt and when it is no longer felt. Once the client indicates that the sensation has stopped, test your own joint to see whether you can feel vibration. You serve as the control. If the client reports that the sensation has stopped but you can still sense a clear vibration, the client has reduced vibratory sense. If the client does not feel vibration at all, move the tuning fork proximally to test the wrist, elbow, or ankle.

Proprioception. Test proprioception by holding the side of the client's fingertips, then the great toes, between thumb and index finger. As each of the client's fingers and toes are gently flexed and extended, ask the client to state when movement is felt and in what direction. If impairment is detected, test more proximal joints.

Discrimination

Cortical discrimination depends on the ability to integrate and interpret sensory stimuli in the parietal lobe. Included are tests for stereognosis, graphesthesia, extinction phenomenon, and simultaneous two-point stimulation. Box 69-6 lists definitions for abnormalities of sensation.

To test *stereognosis* (discernment of the form and configuration of objects felt, or three-dimensional discrimination), place three small, familiar objects, such as a coin, a key, and a paper clip one at a time in the client's hands. Ask the client to identify each with the eyes closed.

To test *graphesthesia* (recognition of the form and configuration of written symbols), trace different separate letters and numbers on the client's palm with the blunt end of a pen. Ask the client to identify each with the eyes closed. Orient the figures so that they are right-side-up for the client.

BOX 69-6	*Abnormalities of Sensation*

Dysesthesias: well-localized, irritating sensations, such as warmth, cold, itching, tickling, crawling, prickling, and tingling
Paresthesias: distortions of sensory stimuli (light touch may be experienced as burning or painful sensation)
Anesthesia: absence of the sense of touch
Hypoesthesia: reduced sense of touch
Hyperesthesia: pathologic (abnormal) overperception of touch
Analgesia: absence of the sense of pain
Hypalgesia: reduced sense of pain
Hyperalgesia: increased sense of pain
Agraphesthesia: inability to identify symbols traced on the palm when the eyes are closed
Astereognosis: loss of sense of three-dimensional discrimination

To test for the *extinction phenomenon* (simultaneous stimulation), prick the client's skin at the same point on the two sides of the body at the same time. Ask the client to state whether one or two pricks are felt.

To perform *two-point stimulation* (two-point discrimination), simultaneously prick the skin with two pins at varying distances apart to identify the smallest distance at which the client can perceive two pricks. Normal dis-

tances at which two-point discrimination is lost are the upper arms, 75 mm; thighs, 75 mm; back, 40 to 70 mm; chest, 40 mm; forearms, 40 mm; palms, 8 to 12 mm; toes, 3 to 8 mm; fingertips, 2.8 mm; and tongue, 1 mm.

Abnormalities of sensation are defined in Box 69-6, and Figure 69-1 summarizes patterns of sensory loss. Sensory changes are part of the normal aging process. Careful assessment of such changes is the basis of

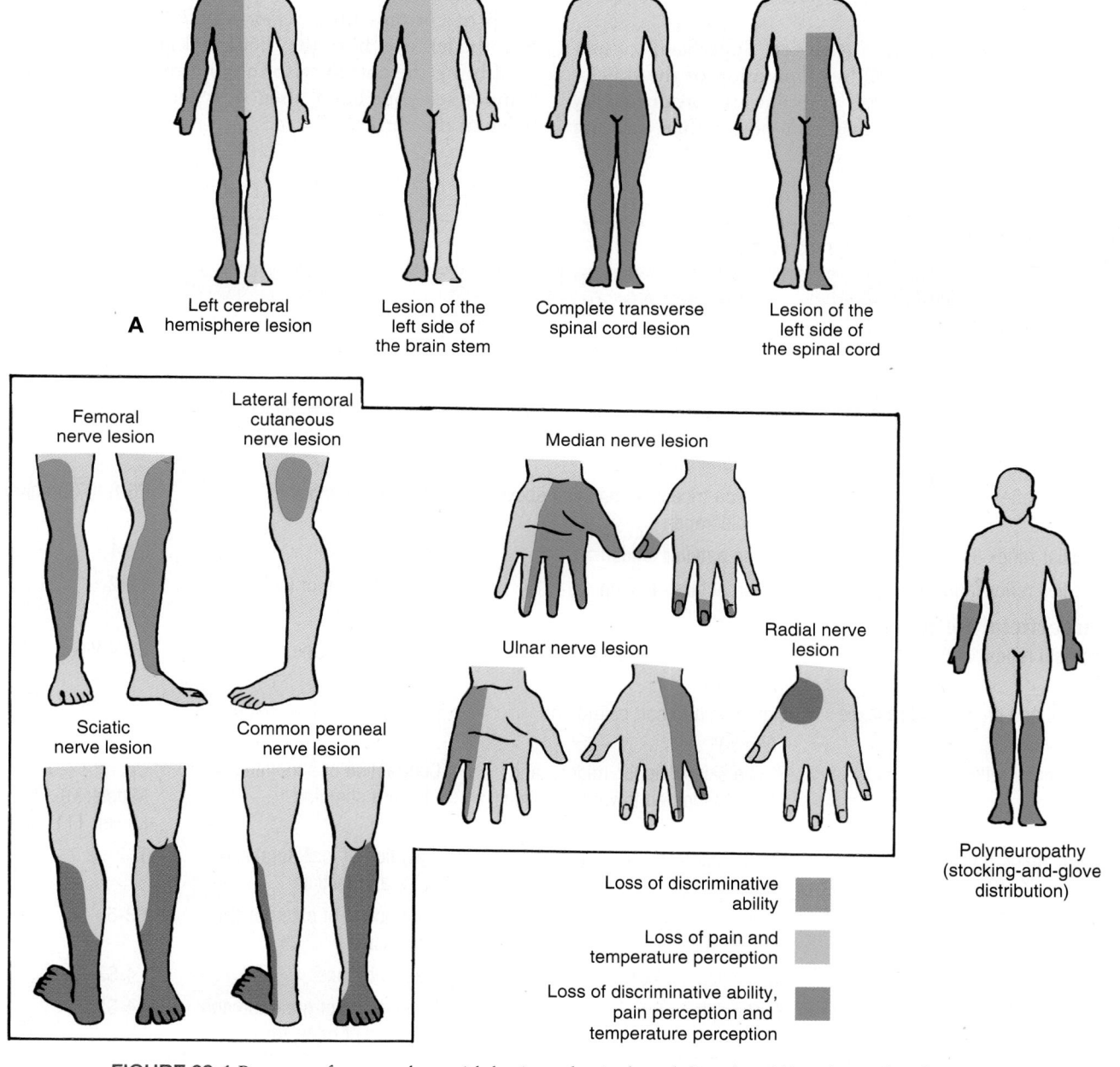

FIGURE 69-1 Patterns of sensory loss with brain and spinal cord disorders (**A**) and peripheral nerve lesions (**B**).

nursing intervention for older clients. Table 69-1 contains guidelines for assessment.

Reflex Activity

Reflex testing evaluates the integrity of specific sensory and motor pathways. Reflex activity assessment, always a part of neurologic assessment, provides information about the nature, location, and progression of neurologic disorders.

Normal Reflexes

Two types of reflexes are normally present: (1) superficial, or cutaneous, reflexes; and (2) deep tendon, or muscle-stretch, reflexes (Table 69-2).

Superficial (Cutaneous) Reflexes. Superficial (cutaneous) reflexes are elicited by stimulation of the skin or mucous membranes. The stimulus is produced by stroking a sensory zone with an object that will not cause damage. Superficial reflexes (abdominal, plantar, corneal, pharyngeal [gag], cremasteric, and anal) are absent in pyramidal tract disorders. For example, they are absent on the affected side after a stroke.

Abdominal Reflex. Lightly stroking the skin on an abdominal quadrant normally contracts the abdominal muscle, moving the umbilicus toward the stimulated side.

Plantar Reflex. Scratching the foot's outer aspect of the plantar surface (outer sole) from the heel toward the toes normally contracts or flexes the toes in clients older than 2 years of age.

Corneal Reflex. Gently touching the cornea with a wisp of cotton causes reflex blinking. For example, to test the left eye, have the client look up and to the right, and bring the cotton wisp in from the side so the client cannot see your hand; then very gently touch the outer edge of the cornea.

TABLE 69-2	*Important Reflexes*		
Reflex	**Assessment Technique**	**Expected Response**	**Pathway Involved**
Tendon Reflexes			
Biceps reflex	A blow on the examiner's thumb placed over the biceps tendon	Flexion of elbow	C5-6
Brachioradialis reflex (supinator)	Styloid process of radius is tapped while forearm is in semiflexion and semipronation	Flexion of elbow, fingers, and hand with supination of forearm	C5-6
Triceps reflex	Strike on triceps tendon just above the olecranon	Extension of elbow	C6-8 (C7 primarily)
Patellar reflex (knee jerk)	Tap on patellar tendon	Leg extends	L2-4
Achilles reflex (ankle jerk)	Tap on Achilles tendon	Plantar flexion of foot	S1-2
Superficial Reflexes			
Corneal reflex	Light touch at the corneoscleral junction	Closure of eyelids	CN V, VII
Palatal and pharyngeal reflexes	Light touch to soft palate and pharynx	Elevation of palate; gagging	CN IX, X
Abdominal reflexes	Stroke skin of upper, middle, and lower abdomen toward umbilicus	Contraction of abdominal wall toward stimulus	Upper: T7-9 Middle: T9-11 Lower: T11-12
Cremasteric reflex	Stroke medial surface of upper thigh	Elevation of ipsilateral scrotum and testicle	T12-L2
Anal reflex	Stroke perianal region	Contraction of external anal sphincter	S3-5
Plantar reflex (normal)	Stroke sole of foot	Flexion of toes	L4-S2
Plantar reflex (pathologic; Babinski's sign)	Stroke sole of foot	Dorsiflexion of great toe and fanning of other toes	L4-S2

Modified from Mitchell, P. A., et al. (1988). *AANN's neuroscience nursing: Phenomena and practice.* Norwalk, CT: Appleton & Lange.
C, Cervical; *CN,* cranial nerve; *L,* lumbar; *S,* sacral; *T,* thoracic.

In an unconscious patient, you can test the corneal reflex by holding the eyelids open and placing a drop of sterile saline on the cornea. This technique prevents inadvertent corneal abrasions.

Pharyngeal (Gag) Reflex. Gentle stimulation with a tongue blade at the back of the throat and pharynx normally produces gagging. The corneal and pharyngeal reflexes are usually assessed with the cranial nerves, discussed earlier.

Cremasteric Reflex. Stroking the inner thigh of a man normally elevates the ipsilateral testicle.

Anal Reflex. Stimulate the perianal skin or gently insert a gloved finger into the rectum. Normal response is contraction of the rectal sphincter.

Deep Tendon (Muscle-Stretch) Reflexes. Deep tendon reflexes are also called muscle-stretch, or myotactic, reflexes because reflex muscle contraction normally results from rapid stretching of the muscle. This is produced by

sharply striking a muscle tendon's point of insertion with a sudden, brief blow of a reflex hammer (Figure 69-2 and Box 69-7).

Reflexes commonly assessed include the biceps, triceps, brachioradialis, patella, and Achilles tendon:
- A *biceps jerk* (forearm flexion) is produced by tapping the biceps brachii tendon.
- A *triceps jerk* (forearm extension) is produced by tapping the triceps brachii tendon at the elbow.
- A *brachioradial jerk* or *supinator reflex* (elbow flexion, supination of forearm, and flexion of fingers and hand) is produced by taping the styloid process of the radius about 1 to 2 inches above the wrist.
- A *knee jerk, quadriceps jerk,* or *patellar reflex* (leg extension) is produced by tapping the quadriceps femoris tendon just below the patella.
- An *ankle jerk* (plantiflexion of the foot) is produced by tapping the Achilles tendon.

Other Normal Reflexes. Some normal reflexes involve structures other than skeletal muscles. For example, reflex mechanisms help maintain respiration and keep

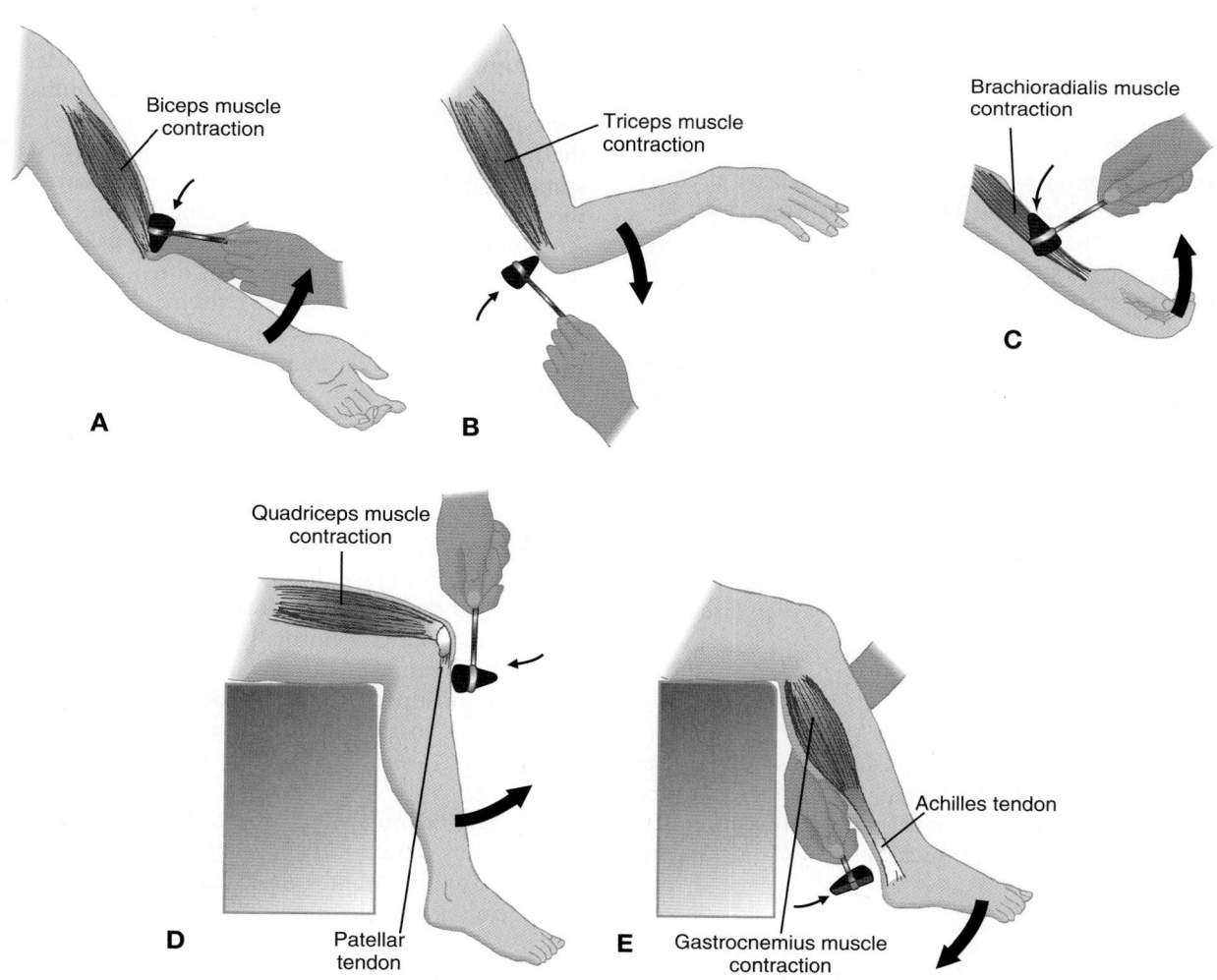

FIGURE 69-2 Deep tendon (muscle-stretch) reflexes. **A,** Biceps jerk (C5-6). **B,** Triceps jerk (C7-8). **C,** Brachioradial jerk (C5-6). **D,** Patellar reflexes (L2-4). **E,** Ankle jerk (S1-2).

BOX 69-7 *Assessing Deep Tendon Reflexes*

Use the following guidelines when assessing deep tendon reflexes:

1. Test deep tendon reflexes with the client either sitting or supine.
2. Support the joint where the tendon is being tested so that the attached muscle is relaxed.
3. Use the pointed end of a triangular reflex hammer to strike over small areas while you place your thumb over the biceps tendon. Use the flat end of the hammer to strike over larger areas, such as the Achilles tendon.
4. Hold the reflex hammer loosely between thumb and fingers so it can swing in an arc.
5. Swing the reflex hammer using only wrist motion, not the arm or elbow.
6. Tap the tendon briskly.
7. Note the speed, force, and amplitude of reflex responses.
8. Compare reflex responses on the two sides of the body.
9. Grade reflexes on a 0 to 4+ scale. Consider the strength of the reflex in relation to the bulk of the muscle mass.

Repeat testing of reflexes graded 0 or 1+ by using the technique of reinforcement (see next phase). Note in the record that *reinforcement* was used. Reinforcement is a maneuver used to enhance deep tendon reflex responses when they are graded 0 or 1+. Reinforcement maneuvers for various deep tendon reflexes are as follows:

1. Ask the client to perform isometric contraction of other muscles, which may increase the generalized reflex response.
2. For the upper extremities, have the client either clench the teeth together or contract the quadriceps muscles (push the thighs against the table).
3. For the lower extremities, have the client lock the fingers together and try to pull them apart at the same time you test the tendon.

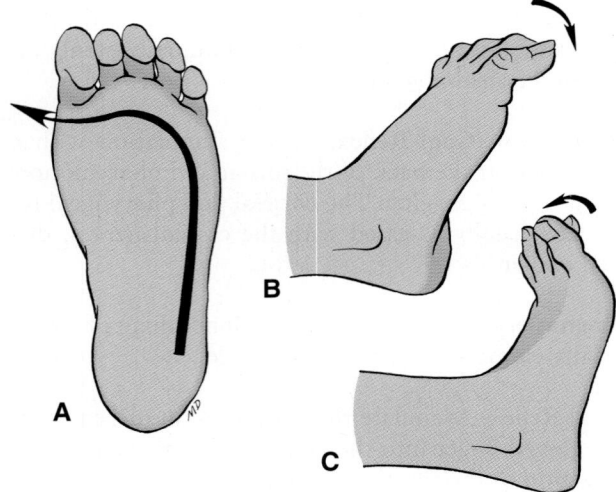

FIGURE 69-3 Babinski's reflex. **A,** Test maneuver: Using a blunt point, scratch the sole of foot as shown. **B,** Normal response (absence of Babinski's response) is plantiflexion of the toes. **C,** Abnormal response (presence of Babinski's response) is dorsiflexion of the big toe and often a fanning of the other toes.

move upward and laterally along the outer border of the sole to the ball of the foot. Continue the stimulus across the ball of the foot (without touching the toes) toward the medial side and off the foot. Alternatively, start the stimulus at the midlateral sole and carry it down toward the heel. A normal response is plantiflexion of the toes. An abnormal response (presence of Babinski's reflex) is dorsiflexion of the great toe and, often, fanning of the other toes (Figure 69-3). In extreme circumstances, a Babinski reflex may be accompanied by dorsiflexion of the foot at the ankle and flexion at the knee and hip (called *triple flexion*).

When exaggerated deep reflexes are present, superficial reflexes are usually diminished or absent and pathologic reflexes (Babinski's reflex) are observed.

Jaw Reflex. The jaw reflex is also called *mandibular reflex* or *jaw jerk*. Have the client relax the mouth, leaving it open slightly. Then tap gently on the lower jaw below the mouth. The jaw normally contracts and closes the mouth as a result of downward tapping. This reflex is absent in most people but may be present in clients who have lesions in the corticobulbar tract above the midpons.

Palm-Chin (Palmomental) Reflex. The palm-chin reflex is produced by vigorous, rapid irritation on the mound of the palm at the thumb's base with a blunt instrument, which causes the chin muscles to pull up on the same side.

Clonus. Clonus consists of rapidly alternating joint flexions and extensions resulting from continuous rhythmic

blood pressure within normal limits. Reflex salivation may follow the taste (or smell) of food. Flashing a light in an eye causes the pupils of both eyes to constrict (*light reflex* or *pupillary reflex;* see also the earlier discussion of cranial nerve assessment).

Abnormal Reflexes

Pathologic reflexes indicate neurologic disorders, often related to the spinal cord or higher centers. These responses include Babinski's, jaw, palm-chin (palmomental), clonus, snout, rooting, sucking, glabella, grasp, and chewing reflexes.

Babinski's Reflex. Test Babinski's reflex by gently scraping the sole of the foot with a blunt object. To elicit the reflex, start the stimulus at the midpoint of the heel, and

contractions of a stretched muscle. This is not like a normal stretch reflex, which typically produces one reflex action. With clonus, the action continues. Support the leg at the knee, and help the client relax the leg. Rapidly flex the foot, and hold it in a flexed position. The flexion stretches the calf muscles and causes repeated "beats" of clonus if this reflex is present.

Snout Reflex. A brisk midline tap above or below the mouth results in pursing of the lips. This reflex is normal in infants but is abnormal in adults.

Rooting Reflex. Stroking the side of the face causes the mouth to open and the head to turn to the stimulated side. This reflex is normal in infants but is abnormal in adults.

Sucking Reflex. Touching the lips with a blunt object results in movement of the tongue, lips, and jaws. This reflex is normal in infants but is abnormal in adults.

Glabella Reflex. Tapping the forehead between the eyebrows results in sustained closure of the eyelids.

Grasp Reflex. Placing an object in the palm of the hand causes the fingers to curl around it.

Chewing Reflex. A tongue blade placed between the teeth results in the tight closing of the jaws.

Grading Reflex Activity

Figure 69-4 shows the grading and documentation of superficial reflexes. Although 1+ or 3+ responses are not considered normal, they may not be significant findings. Asymmetrical responses are more significant. Abnormal reflexes may be present in both neurologic and metabolic disorders. Table 69-2 summarizes important reflexes.

Autonomic Nervous System

The autonomic nervous system cannot be examined directly. The autonomic nervous system innervates many body organs through sympathetic and parasympathetic pathways; thus its function is evaluated by a full body systems assessment. Clinical manifestations of autonomic nervous system disorders occur in many body systems. Unit 16 focuses on neurologic disorders (heatstroke, autonomic dysreflexia). Disorders of other portions of the autonomic system are discussed in the cardiac, urinary, digestive, reproductive, and endocrine units of this book.

The following are examples of activity under autonomic nervous system influence:

- Increased or decreased heart rate
- Peripheral vasoconstriction or vasodilation
- Bronchoconstriction or bronchodilation
- Increased or decreased peristalsis
- Constriction or dilation of the pupil

Review medications the client is taking. Many medications have side effects involving the parasympathetic or sympathetic nervous system.

Functional Assessment

A client who has a neurologic disorder may experience problems that disrupt basic function either permanently or temporarily. Ability to cope effectively with ADL (ability to meet basic needs) is often altered. For example, a client may have problems seeing, hearing, breathing, walking, talking, or eating. Remember, a client with a neurologic disorder may be frustrated just trying to do the things most people take for granted.

Functional assessment can be incorporated into the neurologic examination as well as into the daily care of the client. During the examination, note any deficits the client experiences and how the client manages them. Ask what changes have been made in daily routines to accommodate deficits. Document not only the deficit but also the functional response. Examples include the following:

- *Motor strength of right arm 4/5:* The client reports independence in ADL but notices difficulty in carrying books or groceries with the right arm.
- *Diplopia:* The client uses an eye patch, alternating the side covered every few hours to reduce the headache and nausea caused by diplopia.
- *Right gaze preference:* The client overcomes gaze preference and moves the eyes past the midline to the left when asked. The client turns the head to the left to see visitors enter a room.

Clinical Applications

Initial assessment for diagnosis and triage of the client with a possible neurologic deficit consists of a history, a *brief* physical examination, and a neurologic examination. The *initial* neurologic examination usually includes assessments of the following (see Box 69-2):

- LOC using the Glasgow Coma Scale
- Pupillary response
- Focal motor and sensory abnormalities in all four extremities
- Brain stem function via assessment of protective reflexes (gag, cough, and corneal reflexes)

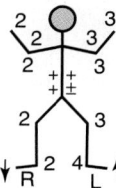

FIGURE 69-4 Documentation of muscle-stretch and superficial reflexes in left hemiparesis. Muscle-stretch reflex grades: 0, absent; 1, diminished; 2, normal; 3, brisker than normal; 4, hyperactive (clonus). Superficial reflex grades: 0, absent; ±, equivocal or barely present; +, normally active.

The initial assessment provides the baseline for comparison when serial assessments are completed. If assessment findings are recorded on a time-oriented flow sheet, changes in status can be quickly identified. The frequency of serial assessments is determined by the diagnosis and may be as often as every 15 minutes. You are responsible for monitoring the client's progress and reporting any unexpected deviations. All clients initially undergo complete neurologic assessment. Serial examinations may focus on deficits or functions that may indicate potential danger (pupillary responses and LOC for suspected increased ICP).

Thorough assessment and reporting of changes in a client serve a major role in determining the plan of care. Often the client's current condition (a decreased level of responsiveness and a change in pupillary reaction) is compared with initial data.

Because nurses are with clients consistently, it is the nurse's responsibility to develop sound assessment skills and to recognize trends in the client's condition that warrant further care. In no other area of practice are subtle changes as important to detect and act on than in the care of the client with a neurologic disorder.

DIAGNOSTIC TESTS

Nursing care for the client who is to undergo diagnostic studies centers on physical and psychological preparation. You must plan the specific assessments that must be made after the study is completed, such as continued neurologic assessment. Determine which components of the neurologic examination you will use in serial assessments before and after the test. These findings will be compared with results of the baseline neurologic examination. Before a diagnostic study, educate the client and family about the purpose of the study, the preparation needed, and the client's role during the test.

After the diagnostic procedures have been performed, assess the client for possible side effects and neurologic changes, and help the client understand the results of the studies, as needed. More information on diagnostic testing can be found in Chapter 4.

Noninvasive Tests of Structure

Skull and Spinal X-Ray Studies

Skull x-ray studies reveal the size and shape of the skull bones, suture separation in infants, fractures or bony defects, erosion, calcification, sella turcica erosion, and pineal gland shift (>12 years of age). Spinal x-ray studies show fractures, dislocation, compressions, curvature, erosion, narrowed spinal cord canal, congenital malformations, neoplasms, and degenerative processes.

The nurse may accompany clients who are confused, combative, or ventilator dependent to the radiology department to assist with client positioning and cooperation during the examination. If a spinal fracture is sus-

pected, the neck is immobilized before the client is moved for the x-ray films. A lateral view of the cervical spine is taken first because the x-ray study can usually be conducted with minimal movement to determine whether fractures have occurred. Multiple views of the cervical spine are needed to rule out fracture. Until the results are known, maintain preprocedure precautions, such as spinal immobilization.

Computed Tomography

Procedure

The primary purpose of CT scanning is to detect intracranial bleeding, space-occupying lesions, cerebral edema, and shifts of brain structures. Infarctions, hydrocephalus, and cerebral atrophy can also be identified. It is especially useful in acute trauma not only to identify the extent of injuries quickly but also because of its ready availability at lower cost than other types of scans. Advances in technology have expanded the uses of CT. Spiral CT utilizes injection of contrast material followed by rapid image sequencing to study movement of the contrast material through the cerebral blood vessels. Xenon CT uses inhaled xenon gas, which is absorbed into the bloodstream, to enhance views that depict regional cerebral blood flow.

Aneurysms and arteriovenous malformations (AVMs) are best detected by angiography. The basilar cisterns and posterior fossa are not as well visualized on CT scans because these areas reveal high-density contrast between bone and air-filled sinuses (Figure 69-5).

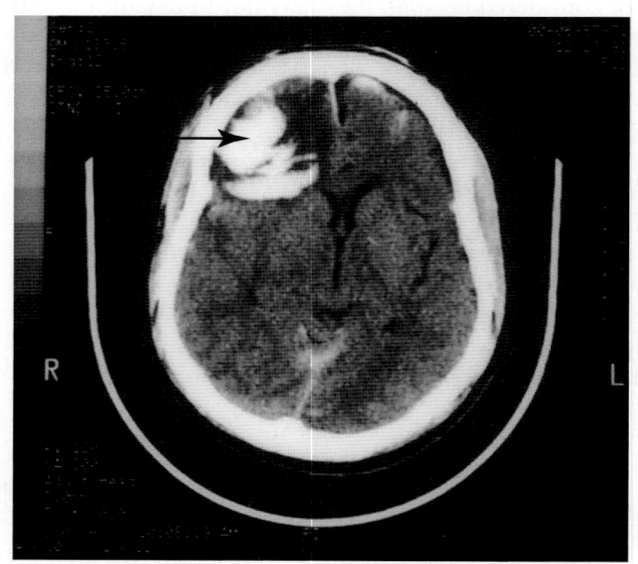

FIGURE 69-5 A computed tomography scan of the head. The brain tissue is gray, and the skull is white. The mass in the left frontal lobe (arrow) is blood from a head injury.

CT scans can be used for stereotactic procedures. Before the scan, a frame is applied to the client's head with pins inserted into the skull. The scan is performed with the frame in place. The computer marks reference measurements on the scan to guide the location of treatment.

Preprocedure Care

Answer any questions the client and family have about the CT scan. Explain that fasting usually is not required for CT of the head. If you think that the client might become nauseated, adjust the intake of food and fluids accordingly. For example, some clients prefer a light meal to reduce nausea, whereas others may prefer an empty stomach before the test.

Explain that a contrast agent may be used. Because some agents are iodine-based, ask whether the client has allergies to iodine or contrast material (see Chapter 4). If the client does not have an intravenous (IV) infusion, IV access will be established before the study begins. Check that informed consent has been obtained before a test in which contrast material will be used.

Postprocedure Care

After the test, assess the client for reactions to contrast media and observe for complications, such as a hematoma at the injection site and signs of IV infiltration of contrast material or fluids. Report infiltration of contrast medium to the radiologist. The client can resume normal activities unless other diagnostic tests are planned.

If a stereotactic frame was used during CT, it is left in place until the stereotactic procedure is completed. The frame may be a source of anxiety, and light sedation may be ordered to help keep the client relaxed.

Serial neurologic examinations are necessary after any testing to evaluate the potential effects on the client's neurologic function from contrast media, transportation to a new environment, or sedation. Assess the client before and after the CT scan.

Magnetic Resonance Imaging

Procedure

Magnetic resonance imaging (MRI) provides more anatomically detailed pictures than are available with CT (Figure 69-6) and has several advantages over CT. MRI can detect disorders in white matter pathways caused by loss of myelin, as in multiple sclerosis, better than CT. MRI can evaluate cerebral infarction within hours of the event; CT would not demonstrate the ischemic stroke for several days. MRI is the scan of choice for congenital brain malformations and spinal cord lesions. MRI with contrast material delineates blood flow through cerebral blood vessels in more detail than is possible with CT.

Preprocedure Care

Teach the client and family about the purpose of the test, what the client will hear and feel during the examination, and the client's role during the test. Before the test, the client should remove all metal-containing objects. IV fluid pumps must be removed immediately before the test. Special MRI-compatible monitoring devices, such as pulse oximeters and electrocardiographic (ECG) leads, can be left in place.

Usually, the client may eat and may take prescribed medications before the examination. If contrast material is to be used, ask whether the client tends to become nauseated easily and adjust the intake of food and fluids accordingly. Chapter 4 details the MRI procedure and client care.

Postprocedure Care

After the test, the client can resume previous activities.

Noninvasive Tests of Function

Magnetic Resonance Spectroscopy

Magnetic resonance spectroscopy (MRS) is a noninvasive MRI method of studying the distribution of chemicals or molecules in the body. MRS can detect abnormal amounts or those that are not normally present. The amount or presence of certain molecules or markers is associated with specific neurodegenerative diseases such

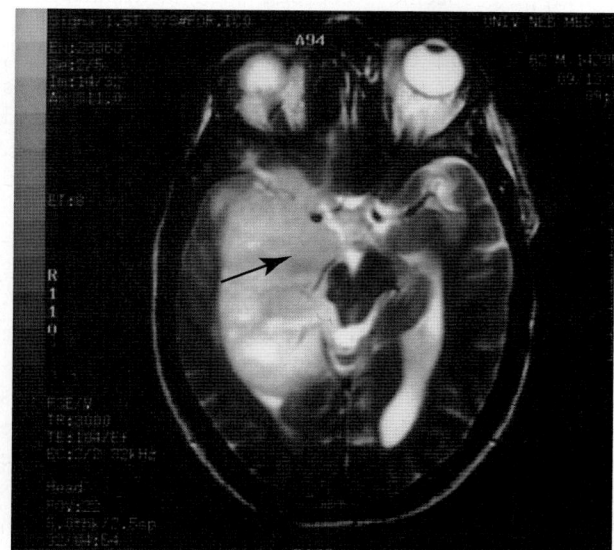

FIGURE 69-6 Magnetic resonance imaging of the head. The eyes are evident at the top of the image. The client has a brain tumor (arrow).

as multiple sclerosis, Huntington's disease, dementia, and disorders of the mitochondria. Nursing care is the same as for MRI.

Functional Magnetic Resonance Imaging

Similar to MRI, functional magnetic resonance imaging (fMRI) uses a strong magnet and radiofrequency waves to produce an image. Instead of lying still and quiet, the client performs cognitive, motor, or sensory tasks during the scan. The client may be asked to recite all the words they can remember that start with a certain letter or press a button at the sound of a noise. Certain areas of the brain are activated with each type of task. The fMRI detects changes in venous blood oxygenation and blood flow in activated areas. Blood flow increases in areas where neuronal activity increases. The fMRI is currently used more for experimental than diagnostic purposes. It increases understanding of the effects stroke, hypoglycemia, and neurodegenerative diseases on specific areas of the brain.

Positron Emission Tomography

Procedure

Positron emission tomography (PET) enables visualization of physiologic function in body areas. Often the function of diseased tissue is different from that of normal tissues. PET has three primary uses:

- Determining the amount of blood flow to specific body tissues
- Revealing how adequately tissues use blood or nutrients, such as oxygen
- Mapping specific receptors, such as medications and neurotransmitters

Cerebral blood flow, cerebral glucose metabolism, and oxygen extraction can be measured by PET. It is used in the diagnosis of stroke, brain tumors, and epilepsy and to chart the progress of Alzheimer's disease, Parkinson's disease, head injury, schizophrenia, and bipolar disorder.

A major disadvantage of PET is its high cost. The procedure requires its own positron to manufacture highenergy radioactive tracers; a PET system can cost $5 million initially. A PET scan is shown in Chapter 4. As a result, a modification of the procedure, called singlephoton emission computed tomography (SPECT), has been developed. SPECT uses less precise but more stable and more commercially available isotopes to measure cerebral blood flow rather than metabolic activity as measured with PET.

The isotope is administered per IV the day before the scan, and the client returns the following day. SPECT uses a rotating camera to track the single proton emitted from radioactive decay. Pictures are taken from multiple views and take about an hour. Only the head is placed in the scanner. The isotope is eliminated from the body in about 2 days. Potassium iodide or potassium perchlorate may be given by mouth prior to the scan to decrease the amount of radioactive iodine taken up by the thyroid gland from the isotope. SPECT is used to analyze blood flow in clients with ischemic stroke, subarachnoid hemorrhage, migraine, Alzheimer's disease, epilepsy, and other neurodegenerative diseases, such as Parkinson's disease.

Preprocedure Care

Educate the client and family about the purpose of the test, what the client will hear and feel, and the client's role during the test. In contrast to CT and MRI equipment, the PET and SPECT scanners are absolutely quiet. Clients may have to fast for 4 hours before the scan. If the client is diabetic, it is preferred that the blood glucose level be below 150 g/dl. Clients who are agitated may require sedation before the scan.

Postprocedure Care

After the test, the client can resume usual activities.

Tests for Vascular Abnormalities

The noninvasive tests described here are useful in assessing cerebrovascular disorders.

Ophthalmodynamometry. Ophthalmodynamometry is used to compare the retinal artery pressures in the eyes. It may help in the diagnosis of extracranial vascular disease. While the retina is observed through an ophthalmoscope, pressure (or suction) is applied to the eyeball with a dynamometer and readings are obtained. A reduction in retinal artery pressure suggests insufficient carotid flow on the ipsilateral side.

Doppler Ultrasonography. Doppler ultrasonography may be used to measure blood flow (including direction and velocity) in the supraorbital region. In clients with occlusion or stenosis of the internal carotid artery, the direction of blood flow is altered (reversed) in the supraorbital artery, a change that may be detected by ultrasonography. Transcranial Doppler studies evaluate arterial flow in the circle of Willis and its major branches.

Doppler Scanning. Doppler scanning combines Doppler ultrasonography with pulsed-wave echocardiography. Visual representation of moving blood is obtained. Assessment of flow through carotid arteries is a common use of Doppler scanning.

Quantitative Spectral Phonoangiography. A noninvasive method of assessing the extent of carotid stenosis, quantitative spectral phonoangiography is spectral analysis of bruits arising from the carotid bifurcation.

Electroencephalogram

An electroencephalogram (EEG) is a measurement of the electrical activity of the superficial layers of the cerebral cortex. The electrical potentials from neuron activity within the brain are recorded in the form of wave patterns. Box 69-8 describes the common types of brain wave patterns.

Procedure

Electrodes are attached to the client's scalp. The waveforms are amplified and recorded on a moving paper strip, much as for an electrocardiogram. The recordings are interpreted according to the characteristics, frequency, and amplitude of brain waves.

If the patient is comatose or unable to be moved, a bedside study can be performed. For routine diagnostic examination, the client is taken to an EEG laboratory, a more controlled environment. The scalp is cleaned, and electrodes are applied to the scalp and ear lobe (for reference) with special conductive gel.

The first portion of the test is performed with the client as relaxed as possible to obtain a baseline recording. Further readings are taken while the client is hyperventilating, sleeping, or viewing flickering lights. Hyperventilation alters acid-base balance (respiratory alkalosis) and decreases cerebral blood flow. Flickering lights may trigger seizures. Sleep may evoke abnormal EEG patterns not present while the client is awake. The client may be kept awake the night preceding the test (sleep-deprived EEG) or may be sedated to induce sleep.

The EEG is used to assess seizure disorders. The results are diffusely abnormal in various metabolic disturbances, toxic conditions (drug overdose), coma, dementias, infections (meningitis and encephalitis), narcolepsy, and insomnia. The EEG may be used in the operating room to monitor cerebral activity during surgery on the blood vessels in the head or neck. Some clients are assessed for seizure activity with the use of a 24-hour ambulatory cassette recording. In situations where the diagnosis is uncertain, the client is hospitalized to videotape the seizure activity while simultaneously connected to the EEG.

Absence of waves on the recording ("flat lines") may be one of the criteria for defining brain death. EEG studies of comatose patients show a high correlation of flat EEGs with death of the client in a coma.

Preprocedure Care

Explain the purpose of the test and the procedure to the client and family. Reassure them that electricity does not enter the brain (shock is not given) and that the machine cannot read minds.

Before EEG is performed, the client's hair must be shampooed. Stimulants (coffee, alcohol, tea, cola, and cigarettes), antidepressants, tranquilizers, and anticonvulsants should be avoided for 24 to 48 hours before the test. Sometimes sleep is withheld. If the client will be asked to sleep for a portion of the test, sleep should be minimized the night before the test. The client will be asked to relax during the test because anxiety can block alpha rhythms and produce artifacts from increased muscle tone in the head and neck. For hospitalized patients, send adequate supplies (IV fluids or oxygen) to the laboratory if they will be needed during the test.

If EEG is being performed to evaluate the possibility of brain death, artifacts must be kept to a minimum. Electrode manipulation, electrical interference, respirator cycling, and someone walking in the room can cause artifacts. Follow agency guidelines when EEG is performed at the bedside.

BOX 69-8	Types of Electrical Brain Waves
Wave Form (Duration)	**Description**
Alpha (8-13 cycles/sec)	Normal; seen during wakeful, relaxed state with eyes closed; disappear during sleep, sudden alerting, attention to environmental stimuli and mental activity; found over occipital and parietal areas
Beta (12-40 cycles/sec)	Fast waves indicating mental or physical activity; prominent over frontal and parietal areas
Theta (4-7 cycles/sec)	Less common in adults than in children; often seen during periods of emotional stress or drowsiness and often characteristic of coma and brain injury; prominent over temporal and parietal areas
Delta (1-4 cycles/sec)	Normal; seen in stage 3 and 4 of sleep (deep sleep)
Sleep spindles (12-14 cycles/sec)	Seen in stage 2 sleep (not rapid eye movement [REM])
Spike and slow waves (variable)	Seen in irritable brain tissue (seizure)

Postprocedure Care

After EEG, the client can resume previous activity, medications, and diet. If seizure activity is possible, follow precautions to avoid seizures. The hair can be washed, and acetone may be used to remove the electrode paste or gel from the scalp and hair.

Evoked Potential Studies

Evoked potential (EP) studies measure evoked potentials or the brain's electrical response to various stimuli. EP studies assess the transit time of afferent pathways of the cerebral hemispheres and the brain stem. Various stimuli are used, such as auditory, somatosensory, and visual. Typical stimuli are flashing lights, buzzing tones, and peripheral nerve stimulation. EP studies can be used to assess blindness, deafness, and brain stem injury. Specific brain signals can be accentuated and others filtered out, allowing assessment of brain waves from other areas.

Evoked potential studies are carried out in the same fashion as EEG studies. EP studies can detect abnormalities in infants, children, and clients who are sedated or paralyzed with neuromuscular blocking agents. Some clinicians believe that EP studies are more reliable than clinical assessments in predicting neurologic recovery from coma or head injury. EP studies are useful as an ancillary test for multiple sclerosis and other neurologic diseases that are difficult to diagnose. Nursing interventions are the same as for the client undergoing an EEG study except in the explanation of the variations between the tests.

Neuropsychological Testing

Neuropsychological testing involves a series of tests to evaluate cortical function by localizing the area and the extent of impairment and determining the rate of progression or recovery. The tests gauge many types of abilities, such as motor, perceptual, language, visuospatial, and cognitive. Test results can provide information regarding the extent of cognitive impairment and the effect it may have on functional ability and can aid in determining decision-making ability for legal and insurance matters. Clinical manifestations, as well as results of neuropsychological evaluations, neurologic examinations, and neurodiagnostic studies, are correlated and used to plan rehabilitation. Serial testing is valuable for monitoring rehabilitative progress and recovery in clients with problems such as head injury, epilepsy, and mild cognitive impairment.

A client may be referred for neuropsychological assessment while in the acute phase or even months after an injury. For example, after a head injury in which the physical neurologic assessment is normal and the EEG reveals only mild generalized abnormalities, the client may complain of being unable to work because of persistent headaches. Test results may be used to make recommendations about treatment, including educational and vocational rehabilitation.

Neuropsychological tests measure deficits in coping skills by assessing these skills directly. They may be helpful when deficits in adaptive abilities are suspected. An individual test may be performed in the case of a disorder with only one specific manifestation, or a complete series of tests with extensive evaluation may require several hours or days of testing. The client's level of performance is compared with scores representing normal performance levels. General measures of intelligence (Wechsler Adult Intelligence Scale) as well as tests of emotional and personal adjustment (the Minnesota Multiphasic Personality Inventory) are used.

Testing may be nonspecific in implicating the presence of brain damage or very narrow in scope with sensitivity for certain areas of the brain. Results may indicate that something is wrong but may be unable to identify the specific problem.

Memory loss is common after head injury and in neurologic disorders. Skills such as reading, which have been stored in the brain over the years, may be retained, in contrast to new learning or short-term memory, which may be impaired. An impaired memory may interfere with the effectiveness of client teaching and the client's ability to learn. A brain-injured client with damage to the limbic system, especially the hippocampus, amygdala, or areas of the temporal and prefrontal lobes, is a candidate for neuropsychological testing to determine memory loss.

Testing can identify problems in cognitive, psychomotor, and affective domains. Left hemisphere lesions impair factual information functions, like problem-solving, decision-making, and judgment. Client and family teaching must be modified to address these deficits.

Both the right and left hemispheres are involved with psychomotor learning. The right hemisphere controls visuospatial abilities, and the left controls verbal instructions and sequencing of activities. Repetition and time are needed for the individual to perform activities automatically. Memory loss that is identified from damage to the right or left hemisphere and is causing affective learning deficits can be improved with role modeling and one-to-one and group therapy. Documentation of client behavior and functional abilities assists the neuropsychologist in following the client's progress and recovery.

Invasive Tests of Structure

Lumbar Puncture

Procedure

In a lumbar puncture (LP), also known as a *spinal tap,* a needle is inserted into the subarachnoid space in the lumbar region of the spine below the level of the spinal cord. CSF can be withdrawn or substances can be injected into this space.

Lumbar puncture is performed for assessment and therapeutic purposes. LP enables assessment of CSF pressure and collection of CSF for evaluation. When meningitis or subarachnoid hemorrhage is suspected, the CSF is examined for white blood cells and blood. Therapeutically, LP is used to administer spinal medications such as analgesics, antispasmotics, chemotherapy, and anesthetics. These medications can also be delivered via continuous infusion pump. In adults, removal of more CSF than is required for analysis helps in the diagnosis of hydrocephalus.

Even though LP is generally a safe procedure, it is associated with potential hazards. The procedure can be uncomfortable. The client feels pressure in the lower back and may experience pain if a nerve root is touched with the needle during insertion. The potential complications of LP are CSF leakage, infection, intervertebral disk damage, and brain herniation.

A space-occupying lesion within the cranium, such as a tumor or bleeding, increases ICP. Therefore LP is not performed in clients with papilledema (a sign of increased ICP), suspected intracranial lesions, increased ICP, or infection of the skin at the puncture site. CT scans are used in these clients to rule out masses before an LP is performed. If an LP were performed in a client with increased ICP, there would be a rapid decrease in CSF pressure around the spinal cord. This change in pressure might allow the structures within the brain to drop (herniate) into the spinal canal. The process of herniation creates pressure on the vital centers in the medulla (cardiac and respiratory centers) and may cause sudden death.

Preprocedure Care

Educate the client and the family about the purpose of LP, what the client will feel, and the client's role during the examination. Obtain an informed consent. If possible, the client should empty the bladder and bowels before the procedure. The client must lie still during the test. Sedation may be ordered before the procedure.

Assemble the necessary equipment in the client's room. Lumbar puncture trays containing all the needed equipment are available. In addition, have laboratory request forms available and a marking pencil to label the samples of spinal fluid.

Intraprocedure Care

Lumbar puncture to remove a sample of CSF is described here; however, the same general principles apply to any LP procedure:

1. Position the client on the side (lateral recumbency) with the back close to the edge of the bed. Place a pillow under the flank so that the spinous processes are horizontal. Use additional pillows between the knees and under the head to keep the spine horizontal.

2. Ask the client to draw the knees up to the abdomen and the chin onto the chest (Figure 69-7). Help the client maintain this curved position to separate and increase space between the vertebrae so that the needle can be inserted more easily. Sudden movement may result in needle displacement.

3. Stand in front of the client, and place one hand behind the client's knees and the other around the neck. Keep the client's upper shoulder from falling forward, thus preventing rotation of the spine. (An alternative position is to have the client sitting up with the head and chest bent toward the knees.)

4. After a local anesthetic is given, the clinician places a small needle into the space between the vertebrae in the lower back. In adults, the needle is inserted about the level of the top of the iliac crests (hip bones) or at the next lower vertebral level (usually between the third and fourth or fourth and fifth lumbar vertebrae). In adults, the spinal cord normally ends at the lower border of the first lumbar vertebra. Thus, the puncture site is low enough to avoid spinal cord injury. If the client has abnormal anatomy or spinal deformities, the LP may need to be performed in the x-ray department with fluoroscopic guidance.

5. The needle bevel is usually held parallel to the longitudinal fibers of the dura. This position limits the size of the dural tear and reduces the risk of CSF leak.

6. Local pain may occur as the needle passes the dura mater. Ask the client to mention additional discomfort, which may indicate misplacement of the needle.

7. When the needle has entered the subarachnoid space, the clinician removes the stylus and attaches a stopcock and manometer to measure CSF pressure. The first stabilized CSF pressure is the *opening pressure.* Normal opening CSF pressure with the client in a horizontal position is 6 to 13 mm Hg (80 to 180 mm H_2O). Pressures exceeding 15 mm Hg (200 mm H_2O) are abnormal. Normally, CSF pressure oscillates (fluctuates) in the manometer, readily responding to coughing, straining, and changes in respiration. If there is a blockage in the spinal canal, the CSF pressure may not oscillate.

8. CSF specimens are collected in a series of small sterile test tubes numbered in sequence of collection (no. 1, no. 2). Two to 3 ml of CSF is collected in each tube; 8 to 10 ml may be removed.

9. The needle is withdrawn, and the clinician places a dry sterile dressing over the puncture site.

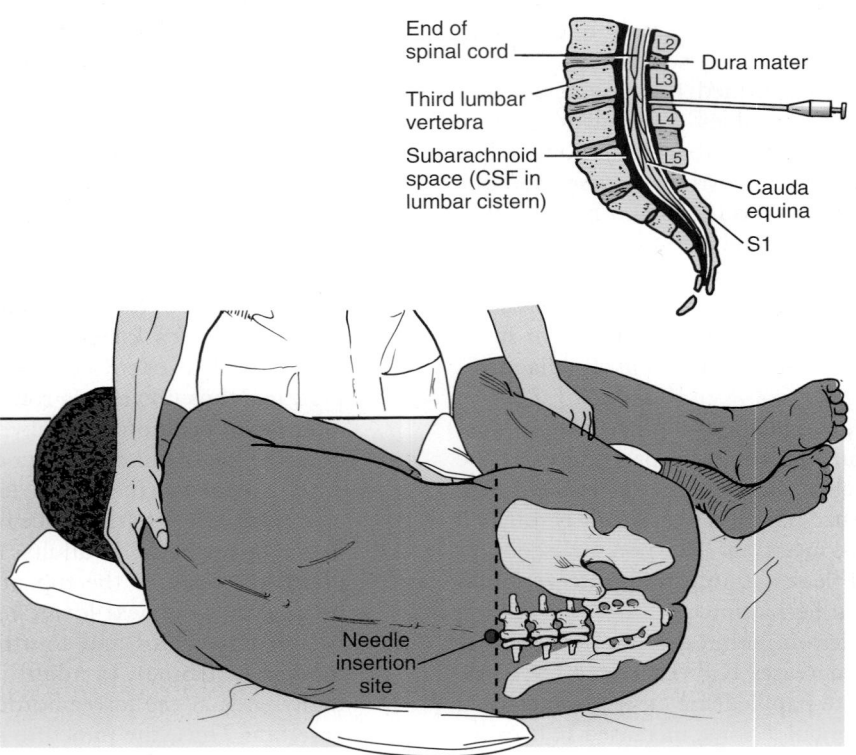

FIGURE 69-7 Lumbar puncture. Position the client laterally, with the knees drawn up to the abdomen and the chin brought down to the chest. This position increases the spaces between the vertebrae. The sterile lumbar puncture needle is inserted as shown, between the third and fourth (or fourth and fifth) vertebrae and enters the subarachnoid space.

In adults, CSF is assessed for cells, chloride, glucose, protein, and lactate dehydrogenase (LDH) as well as pressure. To preserve the specimen for cell count, it should be taken to the laboratory immediately. Other tests that can be performed include serology for syphilis, glutamine, C-reactive protein, and a variety of cell stains. Table 69-3 lists common abnormalities of CSF. The first vial of CSF obtained is not assessed for blood because it may contain blood from the puncture.

Postprocedure Care

Record vital signs after the LP. Lying flat for several hours is sometimes prescribed. The client can eat and drink as before the test. Drinking extra fluids will help restore CSF volume. If the CSF pressure measurement indicated a high ICP, assess the client for decreasing LOC, which would indicate rising ICP.

Post-LP headache (spinal puncture headache, spinal headache) is typically throbbing, bifrontal, and suboccipital and may develop within a few hours to several days after an LP. Post-LP headache occurs in 10% to 25% of clients. The incidence has decreased in recent years as a result of the use of smaller gauge spinal needles. The headache probably occurs because CSF continues to leak through the opening in the dura made by the needle. As a result of the leak, the CSF circulating around the cranium is depleted. The fluid loss allows abnormal movement of the brain inside the skull. When the brain moves, tension is placed on the meninges and venous sinuses, causing pain. The headache is usually relieved when the client lies down and is made worse with sitting up or with a sudden jolt of the head. Such headaches usually disappear within 24 hours but may last for several days.

To reduce the risk of post-LP headache, have the client remain in bed after the examination. Although physician's orders may differ, an average time in bed is 3 hours. Encourage fluids to replace the CSF withdrawn during the test. Once a headache begins, treatment may be bed rest in a dark, quiet room and the administration of analgesics and fluids.

If the headache continues, an epidural blood patch may be required. Blood is withdrawn from the client's vein and injected into the epidural space, usually at the LP site. The blood acts as a fibrin patch to seal the hole in the dura and prevents further CSF leakage. Blood patches cannot be performed in a client who

TABLE 69-3	*Normal Cerebrospinal Fluid (CSF) Values and Significance of Abnormal Values*	
Substance	**Normal Value (Conventional Units)**	**Significance of Abnormal Values**
Blood	None; CSF clear, and colorless	Gross blood is seen in CNS hemorrhage. If the CSF is grossly bloody, other tests may not be able to be performed. Rarely, there are some blood cells in the first tube of CSF collected because of trauma during the tap. The collection of specimens should be marked in sequence so it is possible to determine whether there is more blood in the first tube than in the last tube.
Cells	0-5 mononuclear; can be stained for better visualization	Increased neutrophils may be seen in bacterial or tubercular infections such as bacterial meningitis or cerebral abscess. Lymphocytes may be increased in viral, tubercular, fungal, or syphilitic meningitis. Aerobic fungal pathogens can be cultured.
Glucose	50-75 mg/dl; should be 20 mg less than serum glucose level	Glucose level is lowered in neoplasm, inflammation, and bacterial infections. Be certain to compare CSF glucose with serum glucose. Ideally, a serum specimen should be drawn 30-60 minutes before lumbar puncture, because it takes glucose about 30-60 minutes to diffuse into the CSF.
Protein Albumin	15-45 mg/dl 10-30 mg/dl	Infectious or inflammatory processes that interrupt the blood-brain barrier increase proteins because there is greater diffusion. Elevated levels of tau protein or decreased levels of beta-amyloid seen in Alzheimer's disease. Decreased proteins can be seen when water reabsorption occurs, as with elevated intracranial pressure.
IgG Oligoclonal bands	1-4 mg/dl Absent	IgG and oligoclonal bands (an abnormal type of protein band seen on immunoelectrophoresis) are often present in multiple sclerosis and neurosyphilis.
Pressure	70-180 mm H_2O	Elevated in bacterial meningitis, hydrocephalus, cerebral bleeding, and tumors. Decreased in shock and lesions obstructing spinal canal.

CNS, Central nervous system; *CSF*, cerebrospinal fluid; *IgG*, immunoglobulin G.

has bleeding tendencies or infection at the puncture site.

Myelography

A *myelogram* is an x-ray study in which contrast material is injected into the subarachnoid space to examine the spinal canal. A LP is performed and some CSF is removed. Myelography is used to visualize intradural nerve roots in selected clients in whom MRI cannot be performed.

Cerebral Angiography

A *cerebral angiogram* consists of injection of contrast material into an artery to visualize intracranial circulation (Figure 69-8). Angiography is the procedure used most often to visualize aneurysms, AVMs, major vessel displacement, vascular occlusion, and thrombi. Cerebral angiography is not only invasive, but it is also a procedure in which small errors can result in permanent disability or death. Meticulous attention must be given to the client before, during, and after angiography. Risks associated with the procedure are lessened when the test

is performed by an experienced interventional radiologist using newer, very small catheters.

Procedure

A catheter is inserted into the femoral artery and guided under fluoroscopy into the carotid or vertebral arteries. Once the vessels are reached, the contrast agent is injected and a series of x-ray films is taken from lateral, anteroposterior, and oblique approaches. Sequential views show the movement of the contrast material in the vessels.

After the catheter is removed, a sterile dressing is placed over the puncture site and firm pressure is applied to the site for 10 minutes to prevent hematoma formation. Sandbags and a pressure dressing may be used to provide firm pressure after the first 10 minutes. The injection site may be tender.

Interventional Angiography. A polymer, glue, or small balloons are used to occlude feeding vessels in tumors or AVMs. Blocking the feeding vessels reduces the size and vascularity of the tumor or AVM, thus diminishing the need for, and the complications of, its surgical removal.

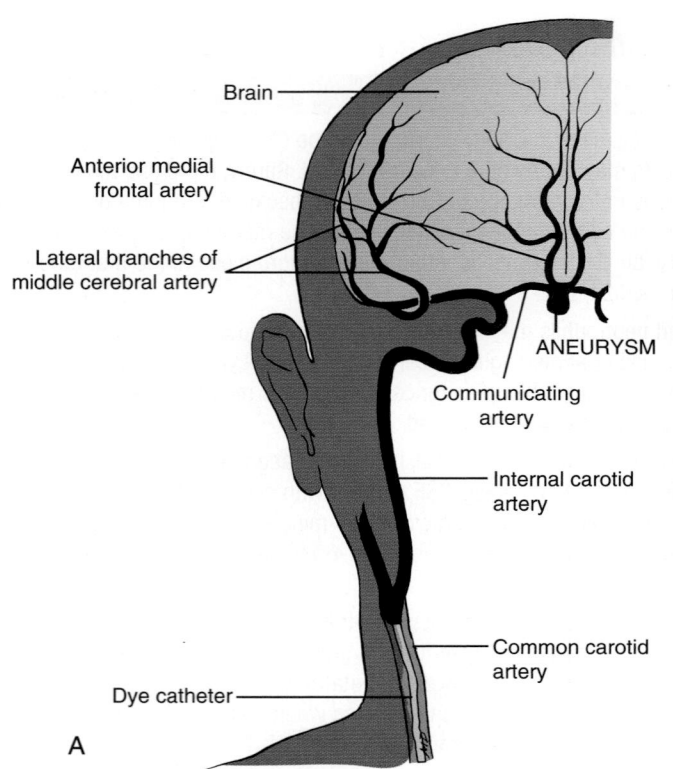

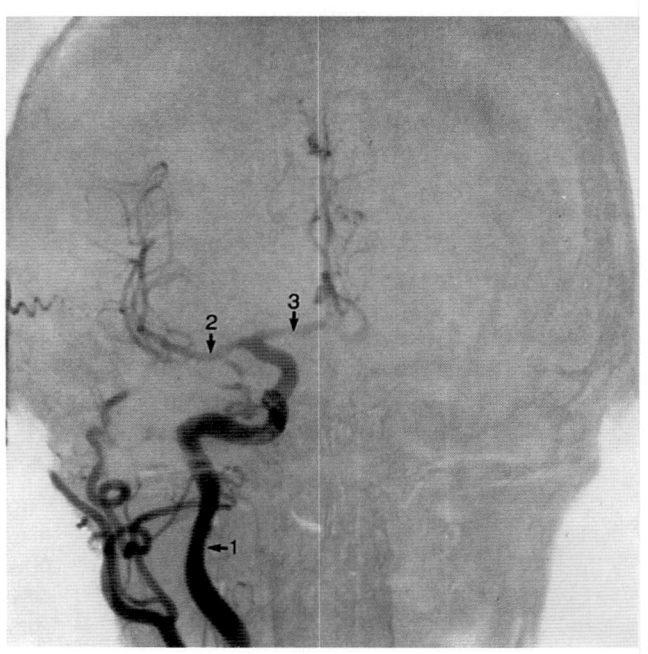

FIGURE 69-8 Cerebral angiography allows x-ray visualization of the brain's vascular system when a contrast dye is injected arterially. **A,** Insertion of dye through a catheter in the common carotid artery, subsequently outlining vessels of the brain. **B,** An angiogram using the subtraction technique. *1,* Internal carotid artery. *2,* Middle cerebral artery. *3,* Middle meningeal artery.

Interventional angiography also enables balloon angioplasty to be performed to expand atherosclerotically narrowed cerebral vessels.

Digital Venous Angiography. Computerized digital video subtraction systems allow visualization of vascular structures. Much less contrast medium is required compared with that needed for cerebral angiography. A central venous line is necessary to inject the contrast medium. Raw data are stored in digital form and can be retrieved at any time. Images with the best vascular visualization are selected and subjected to electronic manipulation to improve image detail.

Indications for digital venous angiography include the following:
- Assessment for transient ischemic attacks
- Serial follow-up evaluations for known carotid stenoses
- Assessment of intracranial tumors
- Postoperative assessment of aneurysms
- Follow-up evaluations after extracranial or intracranial bypass procedures
- Assessment of dural venous sinuses

Three to four venous injections of contrast material are usually required for a complete diagnostic craniocerebral study. The only potential complication is a reaction to the contrast material.

Preprocedure Care

Educate the client and family about the purpose of the test, what the client will experience, and the client's role during the procedure. Before the test, the client may not take anything by mouth for 4 to 6 hours but should be kept well hydrated. IV fluids may be prescribed. Document the neurologic status of the client to serve as a baseline measure after the examination. The client should remove any metal items from the head, such as barrettes and earrings. Report allergies to iodine.

During the test, the client is given an injection of local anesthetic before placement of the catheter. The client may have a warm, flushed feeling when the contrast material is injected. The client is continually assessed for neurologic deterioration while the angiogram is performed.

Postprocedure Care

After the test, assess for complications, which are rare. They include (1) local and systemic allergic reactions to the contrast medium, (2) spasm or occlusion of the vessel by a clot, (3) hemorrhage, and (4) obstructive clot formation above a femoral injection site. Assess for reactions to the contrast material. Spasm or occlusion of the target vessels causes manifestations similar to those of a stroke (see Chapter 72). Clot formation at the injection site also causes ischemic reactions in the affected area. These adverse reactions are usually reversible and rarely cause permanent damage.

Complications vary according to their cause. For example, indications of centrally located reactions include changes in LOC, aphasia, hemiplegia (paralysis of one side of the body), hemiparesis (muscular weakness or partial paralysis of one side of the body), convulsive seizures, and increased focal manifestations. Nausea, vomiting, extremity numbness or weakness, speech disturbances, profuse sweating, and alterations in LOC may indicate a delayed reaction to the contrast material.

After angiography, position the client safely and comfortably and maintain the prescribed bed rest. Clients **EB** undergoing diagnostic angiograms may need to stay in bed only 4 hours. If interventional treatment was performed, the client may have to remain in bed longer.

Check the injection site frequently for bleeding and hematoma formation. Keep the affected extremity straight to prevent vessel kinking and clot formation. As- **EB** sess vital signs (every 15 minutes for 1 hour, then every 30 minutes for 1 hour, then every hour for 4 hours), pulses distal to the puncture site, color and temperature of the extremity, and the ability to move the distal extremity. The client can usually resume a regular diet.

Cerebral Perfusion Studies

When brain death is suspected, cerebral perfusion can be assessed. The patient is injected with technetium 99m (^{99m}Tc), a radioisotope. The ability of ^{99m}Tc to perfuse from blood vessels into brain tissue is assessed with a scanner. In patients who are clinically brain-dead, there is no uptake of the substance by the cerebrum or cerebellum. The radioisotope is injected, and the scanner can be brought to the bedside to evaluate perfusion. Although brain-death can be determined by clinical examination, the perfusion study is used when the clinical findings are clouded by the previous use of long-acting sedative medications.

Invasive Tests of Function

Caloric Testing

The oculovestibular reflex, or *caloric test,* provides information about the function of the vestibular portion of CN VIII and pathways in the pons and midbrain. It aids in the differential diagnosis of brain stem lesions (see also Chapter 70).

The test is performed only in an unconscious patient to determine the presence of brain stem function. Check that the ear canal is patent and that the tympanic membrane is intact. Ice-cold water is introduced into the auditory canal. If brain stem function is intact, the eyes move in a conjugate fashion slowly toward the irrigated side and then quickly move back to midline. With brain stem death, this nystagmus pattern does not occur. Oculovestibular tests are contraindicated for patients with perforated eardrums or with acute labyrinthine disease. As with pupil signs, abnormalities in eye movements help to localize the area of a disorder. They also help to differentiate between structural and metabolic causes of coma.

Peripheral Nerve Studies

Electromyography. Electromyography is used to measure and document electrical currents produced by skeletal muscles, called *muscle action potentials.* Small-needle electrodes are inserted into muscles. The electrical potentials of each muscle are amplified, transmitted to an oscilloscope, and displayed on a screen. The recording can be made audible and documented on paper (Figure 69-9).

In the hands of an experienced electrophysiologist, EMG provides objective diagnostic information for various neuromuscular disorders. EMG can differentiate

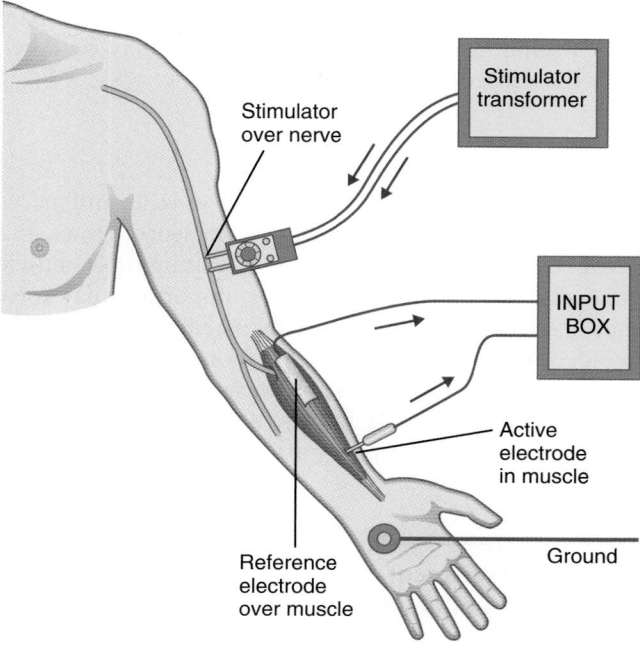

FIGURE 69-9 Electromyography measures and documents electrical currents produced by skeletal muscles. A stimulator is placed over the peripheral nerve being tested. A small pin is inserted into the muscle being assessed for nerve innervation, and a ground wire is placed on the client's skin.

between primary muscle disease and disease secondary to denervation. It helps to identify specific primary muscle diseases. The results may indicate a transmission defect at the neuromuscular junction, such as myasthenia gravis. The procedure can be used to help to differentiate diseases of the anterior horn cells from those primarily of peripheral nerves. Peripheral nerve degeneration and regeneration can be monitored with EMG before clinical manifestations appear.

Nerve Conduction Velocity Study. A nerve conduction velocity study, often performed in conjunction with EMG, is used to evaluate the excitability and conduction velocities of motor and sensory nerves. It is helpful in identifying peripheral nerve disorders. A stimulating electrode and a recording electrode are placed to test specific nerves (usually on a limb). The time required for the passage of a nerve impulse from the point of stimulation to the point of recording is measured precisely. Conduction velocity is calculated. Both motor and sensory modalities can be altered in peripheral nervous system disorders (carpal tunnel syndrome), whereas only motor fibers are affected in chronic disease of the anterior horn cell or motor nerve roots.

Explain the procedure. The client should avoid all stimulants, depressants, and sedatives for 24 hours before the test. There may be discomfort when the electrodes are inserted. There may be a mild electrical shock during the procedure. The client lies flat and may be asked to contract various muscles at specific times during the test. Clients with neuritis may have residual pain after testing. Mild analgesic medications may be taken after the procedure if needed.

Muscle Biopsy

When other tests are inconclusive, muscle and nerve biopsies are used in the diagnosis of neuropathies and myopathies. An EMG is helpful in locating those muscle areas that are most abnormal. It is important that areas that have been traumatized by needle electrodes be avoided when tissue is taken for biopsy. Different techniques are used to obtain the specimens, for example, open incision or needle biopsy. Both muscle and nerve specimens require special preparation. Care of the biopsy site is needed.

Cellular Assessment

With analysis of the human genome, genetic testing has increased in importance in recent years. Chromosome analysis assists diagnosis of some abnormal neurologic conditions and provides the basis for genetic counseling in families with evidence of congenital neurologic malformations and inherited neurologic diseases. Chromosomes can be prepared for microscopic examination from tissue culture of cells obtained from peripheral blood, bone marrow, skin, chorionic villus, and autopsy specimens.

Mental retardation and convulsive seizures may result from neurologic dysfunction associated with inborn errors of metabolism. Diagnosis of carbohydrate and lipid metabolism disorders may require measurements of specific enzyme concentrations in blood cells or in biopsy specimens from brain, muscle, liver, or peripheral nerve cells. Usually, protein metabolism disorders are indicated by increased amounts of particular amino acids in the urine or blood. Postprocedure care is usually directed at anxiety control while the client awaits and receives test results. In some neurodegenerative disorders such as Huntington's disease, neuropsychological testing and counseling are recommended before testing to prepare the client for test results. Several days are required for results to become available.

CONCLUSIONS

Neurologic assessment begins with the history of the disorder and proceeds to the physical examination. The physical examination can be lengthy because of the complexity of the CNS. The neurologic examination consists of assessments of cognition, sensation, motor function, and reflexes. The complexity and length of time required for the assessment may tempt you to omit portions to speed up the process. Before omitting portions, remember that the assessments provide baseline data for further evaluation and legal proof of a client's status. Diagnostic tests include LP, CT, MRI, and angiography. Understanding how a test is performed enables the nurse to provide adequate client preparation and to perform appropriate follow-up assessments.

BIBLIOGRAPHY

1. The American Association for Neuroscience Nurses. (1996). *Core curriculum for neuroscience nursing.* Chicago: Author.
2. Blumenfeld, H. (2002). *Neuroanatomy through clinical cases.* Sunderland, MA: Sinauer Associates.
3. Burns, G. (1999). Functional neuroimaging. *Life Sciences, 65*(24), 2531-2540.
4. Cutrer, F.M., & O'Donnell, A. (1999). Recent advances in functional neuroimaging. *Current Opinions in Neurology 12,* 255-259.
5. Estes, M. (2002). *Health assessment & physical examination* (2nd ed.). Australia: Delmar Thomson Learning.
6. Evans, R.W. (1999). *Diagnostic testing in neurology.* Philadelphia: W.B. Saunders.
7. Evans, R.W. (2003). *Saunders manual of neurologic practice.* Philadelphia: W.B. Saunders.
8. Gilman, S. (1998). Imaging the brain: Part I. *New England Journal of Medicine, 338*(12), 812-820.
9. Gilman, S. (1998). Imaging the brain: Part II. *New England Journal of Medicine, 338*(13), 889-896.
10. Goetz, C. (2003). *Textbook of clinical neurology* (2nd ed.). Philadelphia: W.B. Saunders.

11. Hickey, J.V. (2003). *Clinical practice of neurological and neuro-science nursing* (5th ed.). Philadelphia: Lippincott Williams & Wilkins.

12. Jarvis, C. (2004). *Physical examination and health assessment* (4th ed.). Philadelphia: W.B. Saunders.

13. Kernan, W., et al. (2000). Phenylpropanolamine and the risk of hemorrhagic stroke. *New England Journal of Medicine, 343*(25), 1826-1832.

14. Lynn-McHale, D., & Carlson, K. (Eds.). (2001). *AACN procedure manual for critical care* (4th ed.). Philadelphia: W.B. Saunders.

15. Moore, K., & Agur, A. (2002). *Essential clinical anatomy* (2nd ed.). Philadelphia: Lippincott Williams & Wilkins.

16. Nettina, S.M. (Ed.). (2001). *The Lippincott manual of nursing practice* (7th ed.). Philadelphia: Lippincott Williams & Wilkins.

17. Pagana, K., & Pagana, T. (2002). *Manual of diagnostic and laboratory tests* (2nd ed.). St. Louis: Mosby.

18. Petit, J. (2001). *Primary neurologic care.* St. Louis: Mosby.

19. Swartz, M.H. (2002). *Textbook of physical diagnosis: History and examination* (4th ed.). Philadelphia: W.B. Saunders.

20. Urden, L.D., Stacy, K.M., & Laugh, M.E. (2002). *Thelan's critical care nursing: Diagnosis and management* (4th ed.). St. Louis: Mosby.

Chapter 70

Management of Comatose or Confused Clients

Christine Stewart-Amidei

Perhaps more than any other clients we encounter, clients who are comatose or confused need to be cared for in a holistic manner. All aspects of physiologic and psychological function need to be addressed. Even if clients cannot interact with the environment, the nurse must care for them in a respectful and dignified manner. It is important for family members to see that their loved ones are spoken to and cared for in a professional and caring way.

The brain serves many functions in the body. In contrast to other body systems that monitor and regulate a group of functions, such as the gastrointestinal (GI) tract regulating digestion, the nervous system monitors and regulates all other body systems. Some of these functions are self-protective, including the ability to think, be awake, respond appropriately to the environment, and move about. Other functions are automatic, such as the regulation of body temperature and protective reflex responses. When these protective functions are lost, the clinical manifestations reflect the complexity of the nervous system.

The term *patient* is used in this chapter to describe the client who is comatose. It is assumed that such a client cannot be an active participant in care and that the *family* serves as the *client* in these circumstances.

DISORDERS OF CONSCIOUSNESS

Consciousness is a state of being that has two important aspects: (1) wakefulness and (2) awareness of self, environment, and time. *Awareness of self* means that the patient can identify himself or herself. *Awareness of environment* indicates that the patient can identify his or her present location and reason for being there. *Awareness of time* indicates that a patient knows the date, month, and year and can identify common current facts, such as the name of the President of the United States.

Unconsciousness can be brief, lasting for a few seconds to an hour or so, or sustained, lasting for a few hours or longer. To produce unconsciousness, a disorder must (1) disrupt the ascending reticular activating system, which extends the length of the brain stem and up into the thalamus, (2) significantly disrupt the function of both cerebral hemispheres, or (3) metabolically depress overall brain function, as in a drug overdose.

Coma is a state of sustained unconsciousness in which the patient (1) does not respond to verbal stimuli,

Nursing Outcomes Classification (NOC)
for Nursing Diagnoses—Comatose or Confused Clients

Bowel Incontinence
 Bowel Elimination
 Bowel Continence
Disturbed Sleep Pattern
 Rest
 Sleep
Disturbed Thought Processes
 Cognitive Orientation
 Distorted Thought Control
 Communication Ability
Imbalanced Nutrition: Less than Body Requirements
 Nutritional Status: Nutrient Intake
 Nutritional Status: Biochemical
  Measures
 Nutritional Status: Body Mass
Impaired Oral Mucous Membrane
 Oral Health
 Tissue Integrity: Skin and Mucous
  Membranes
Interrupted Family Processes
 Family Coping
 Family Normalization

Family Participation in Professional
 Care
 Grief Resolution
 Social Support
Risk for Aspiration
 Neurologic Status
 Respiratory Status: Gas Exchange
 Respiratory Status: Ventilation
Risk for Caregiver Role Strain
 Caregiver Emotional Health
 Caregiver Lifestyle Disruption
 Caregiver Performance: Direct Care
 Caregiver Physical Health
 Caregiver Stressors
 Caregiver Home Care Readiness
 Caregiver-Patient Relationship
 Knowledge: Health Resources
 Social Support
Risk for Deficient Fluid Volume
 Electrolyte and Acid-Base Balance
 Hydration
 Nutritional Status: Food and Fluid
  Intake

 Thermoregulation
 Urinary Elimination
**Risk for Disuse Syndrome
(Contractures)**
 Immobility Consequences: Physiologic
 Joint Movement: Passive
 Mobility Level
 Muscle Function
Risk for Impaired Skin Integrity
 Immobility Consequences: Physiologic
 Tissue Integrity: Skin and Mucous
  Membranes
 Tissue Perfusion: Peripheral
Risk for Injury
 Neurologic Status
 Risk Control
 Safety Status: Falls
 Safety Status: Physical Injury
Risk for Suffocation
 Aspiration Control
 Neurologic Status: Consciousness
 Respiratory Status: Gas Exchange

---

(2) may have varying responses to painful stimuli, (3) does not move voluntarily, (4) may have altered respiratory patterns, (5) may have altered pupillary responses to light, and (6) does not blink. In general the longer the coma lasts, the more likely it is irreversible and due to a permanent disorder in the brain structure. Duration of coma is also associated with mortality and outcome; the longer the coma, the higher the mortality rates, and the poorer the neurologic outcome.[9]

Etiology and Risk Factors

Two types of disorders produce coma (Table 70-1):

1. Structural lesions in the brain that place pressure on the brain stem or the structures within the posterior cranial fossa, including the cerebellum, midbrain, pons, and medulla. These types of lesions affect the reticular activating system (RAS).
2. Metabolic disorders and diffuse lesions, which impair wakefulness and awareness by reducing the supply of oxygen and glucose, which are necessary energy substrates, by allowing waste products to accumulate in the brain or by altering other cerebral metabolic processes.

Structural causes of coma include brain tumors, head trauma, and ischemic or hemorrhagic stroke. The brain can be a site for tumors to metastasize from many organs, such as breast and lung, or tumors may arise from the brain itself. Automobile and motorcycle accidents, physical assaults, gunshot wounds, and falls are common causes of head injury. The impact of the initial injury causes damage, but further damage can occur as a result of ischemic consequences of injury. Patients with head injury (see Chapter 75) may also have sustained injury to the chest or airway, which increases the risk of hypoxia. Ischemic stroke occurs with interruption of blood supply to the brain. Hemorrhagic stroke can occur as a consequence of hypertension or from rupture of a vascular anomaly. Ischemia causes swelling of the brain, which if severe, can cause coma. Hemorrhage causes coma by placing pressure on brain tissue.

There are many metabolic causes of coma. The term *metabolic* is used to describe any problem that alters brain metabolism. Most metabolic comas originate in organ systems outside the brain. *Hypoxia* is a common cause of metabolic coma. Blood loss, high altitudes, or carbon monoxide poisoning may deprive the brain of oxygen. *Ischemia,* inadequate tissue levels of oxygen, may occur with cardiac disorders in which cardiac output is decreased, such as cardiac arrest or even fainting. Disorders of the heart, liver, lungs, and kidney may produce coma through the accumulation of metabolic waste products. Many other factors affect brain metabolism, including toxins, hypoglycemia, fever, infections such as encephalitis, and fluid, electrolyte, or acid-base imbal-

TABLE 70-1 *Causes of Altered Consciousness*	
Type of Lesion	**Causes**
Structural brain lesions	
Supratentorial lesions (causes upper brain stem dysfunction)	Cerebral edema
	Brain tumor
	Brain abscess
	Cerebral hemorrhage
	Cerebral infarction (large)
	Epidural hematoma
	Subdural hematoma
Infratentorial lesions (compresses or destroys the reticular formation)	Cerebellar abscess
	Brain stem or cerebellar hemorrhage
	Brain stem or cerebellar infarction
	Brain stem or cerebellar tumor
Metabolic disorders and diffuse lesions	Diseases of other organs, e.g., heart, liver, lungs, endocrine glands, kidney
	Poisons, alcohol and drugs
	Fluid, electrolyte, acid-base imbalances
	Seizures
	Infections (e.g., encephalitis, meningitis)
	Severe nutritional deficiencies
	Hypoglycemia
	Ischemia or anoxia
	Syncope
	Temperature regulation disorders

ances. An overdose or sudden withdrawal of prescribed medication or illicit drugs can also induce coma.

Of note is that coma may be purposely induced as a means to treat neurologic illness. In this situation medication is given to produce coma to rest the brain and hopefully prevent further injury to the brain. Induced or therapeutic coma may be considered for persons with extreme brain swelling secondary to brain injury, stroke, or metabolic disease. Medications used to induce coma include pentobarbital and propofol. Therapeutic coma may be continued for days to a few weeks. Care for patients in induced coma is largely the same as for those who are comatose from some disease process. Full life support in an intensive care setting is required.

Pathophysiology

Consciousness is a complex function controlled by the RAS and its integrated components. The RAS begins in the medulla as the reticular formation (RF) (Figure 70-1). The reticular formation connects to the RAS, which is located in the midbrain, which then connects to the hypothalamus and thalamus. Integrated pathways connect to the cortex via the thalamus and to the limbic system via the hypothalamus. Feedback systems also connect at the brain stem level. The reticular formation produces wakefulness, whereas the RAS and higher con-

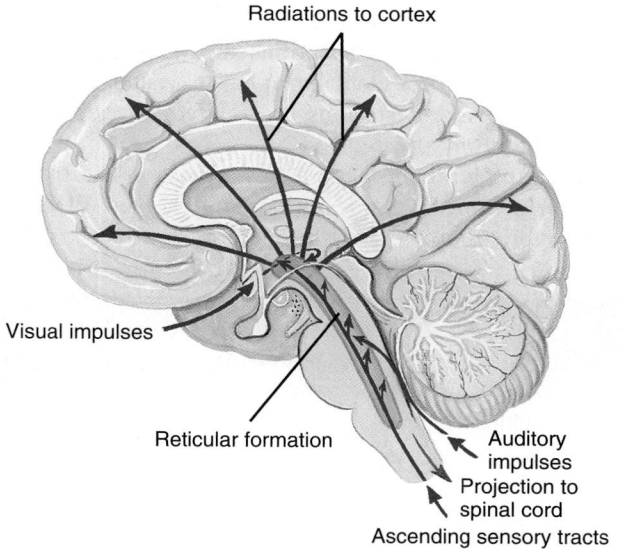

FIGURE 70-1 The reticular activating system (RAS) consists of centers in the brain stem reticular formation along with fibers conducting to the centers from below and fibers conducting from the centers to widespread areas of the cerebral cortex. A functioning RAS is essential for consciousness. (From Thibodeau, G., & Patton, K. [2003]. *Anatomy and physiology* [5th ed., p. 395]. St. Louis: Mosby.)

nections are responsible for awareness of self and the environment. Diffuse cortical connections allow maximum integration of all conscious-related activities.

Disorders that affect any part of the RAS can produce coma. To produce coma a disorder must affect both cerebral hemispheres or the brain stem itself. Disorders affect these areas in one of three ways:

1. Direct compression or destruction of structures responsible for consciousness. A tumor or hemorrhage in the brain stem or swelling in the cerebral hemispheres can cause coma in this manner.
2. Decrease in availability of oxygen or glucose, both of which are needed for cerebral metabolism. Hypoxia and ischemia are the most common causes; without oxygen and glucose, the brain cannot form the chemicals necessary to carry out its functions.
3. Toxic effects of substances on structures of the RAS. Toxic wastes from liver or kidney disease, bacterial invasion from meningitis, and metabolites from drug overdose are examples of such substances.

The causes may overlap. The anatomic location and the severity of the problem determine the depth of coma.

Clinical Manifestations

Supratentorial lesions (located above the dura roofing the cerebellum) cause a fairly predictable set of clinical manifestations (Table 70-2). Such lesions can involve the entire cortical or subcortical level of the brain tissue, as with ischemia. The disorder may also be located in only one hemisphere, as with tumor or hemorrhage. These lesions first produce manifestations such as headache, localized sensorimotor deficits, aphasia, visual loss, and seizures. The manifestations are related to the specific area of the brain affected.

For example, if the patient has a mass in the frontal lobe, early clinical manifestations may consist of headaches, subtle motor deficits (unilateral arm drift), mem-

ory deficits, or partial seizures. *Partial seizures* are seizures that occur in one area of the body, such as the hand. As the lesion expands, manifestations worsen because the lesion places pressure on nearby areas. This pressure may cause a more pronounced unilateral motor deficit (e.g., patient cannot raise the right leg or arm), aphasia, or a deficit in the visual field (blind in one half of the visual field). The patient usually has intact pupillary reflexes (see the Critical Monitoring feature on Manifestations of Changes in Neurologic Status on p. 2059). If the lesion is not detected or cannot be treated and progresses, coma eventually develops. Coma indicates that the lesion has expanded and now compresses structures deep in the brain stem.

Disorders of the infratentorial area (located beneath the dura roofing the cerebellum) cause the patient to lose consciousness suddenly either (1) by directly affecting the RAS or its pathways or (2) by invading the brain stem or reducing its blood supply. Infratentorial lesions may produce unusual respiratory patterns (Table 70-3). The brain stem houses the center for rhythmic breathing. This center's function is lost as consciousness decreases, and the lower brain stem begins to regulate breathing by responding to changes primarily in the carbon dioxide levels as well as in acid-base balance and oxygen levels. The result is a very irregular breathing depth and pattern. The lesion in the brain stem commonly compresses the cranial nerves, and various cranial nerve palsies can be seen, in particular, abnormal eye movements and loss of pupillary reactivity to light. Specific patterns of pupil size and reactivity to light occur when pressure is exerted at various levels (see Table 70-3).

Coma caused by a metabolic disorder more often is manifested as the presence of bilateral or symmetrical findings because the disorder affects the entire brain. The patient usually demonstrates confusion and stupor before any physical manifestations are noticed. Physical manifestations of coma due to a metabolic disorder in-

TABLE 70-2	*Differential Manifestations of Structurally Induced and Metabolic Coma*
Mechanism	**Manifestations**
Supratentorial coma	History of progressive onset; initiating manifestation is usually focal cerebral dysfunction; neurologic manifestations at any given time point to one anatomic area (e.g., frontal lobes, thalamus) Signs of dysfunction progress cephalocaudad Motor manifestations are often symmetrical
Infratentorial coma	History of sudden onset of coma Localizing brain stem manifestations precede or accompany coma onset Cranial nerve palsies "Bizarre" respiratory patterns that appear at coma onset
Metabolic coma	Confusion and stupor commonly precede motor manifestations Motor manifestations are usually symmetrical Pupillary reactions are usually preserved Asterixis, myoclonus, tremor, and seizures are common Acid-base imbalances with hyperventilation or hypoventilation are common

clude tremor, asterixis (flapping tremors of the hands), *myoclonus* (a single, sudden jerking movement), and seizures. Pupillary response is usually normal unless the condition is related to drug overdose. Depending on the underlying cause, acid-base imbalances may be noted. For example, metabolic acidosis would be present in a patient with diabetic coma.

Level of consciousness is the single most important indicator of neurologic function. In the comatose patient, this indicator is lost and other indicators of neurologic function must be evaluated. Information about the time frame of onset, motor response, pupil size and reactivity to light, presence or absence of oculocephalic and oculovestibular responses and other cranial nerve functions, and breathing pattern can localize the level of involvement and determine the depth of coma. For further discussion on these indicators, see Chapter 75.

Diagnostic Findings

The neurologic examination is supplemented by diagnostic testing. Tests identify structural or physiologic abnormalities that affect brain function.

Computed Tomography and Magnetic Resonance Imaging

A computed tomography (CT) or magnetic resonance imaging (MRI) scan usually provides data that indicate whether the cause of the coma is structural. In coma a CT scan is usually performed first because it is quicker. Tumors and areas of bleeding are evident on the scan. In metabolic coma the structures may appear unremarkable, or edema or diffuse nonspecific changes may be seen.

Lumbar Puncture

A lumbar puncture can be performed when it is known, from data provided by the CT or MRI scans, that the patient does not have an expanding intracranial mass. Ob-

taining this information before lumbar puncture is done avoids the risk of herniation caused by sudden changes in cerebrospinal fluid (CSF) pressures (low in the spinal column and high in the ventricles). A lumbar puncture can assist in the diagnosis of infection or bleeding as a cause of coma. The CSF may be cloudy or bloody when the patient has an infection or bleeding into the ventricles or the subarachnoid space.

Electroencephalography

Electroencephalography (EEG) can be used to determine whether the patient is comatose because of continuous seizures. EEG results are abnormal in many patients with coma and do not serve as a clear diagnostic tool. A portion of the general population may have abnormal EEG results as well.

Laboratory Tests

Liver, endocrine, and kidney function may be evaluated through blood tests. A urine or blood toxicology screen may be useful in distinguishing drug-induced coma. Blood oxygenation tests may be used to evaluate for hypoxia. Other laboratory tests specific to the patient's situation may be ordered. Chapter 69 covers specific neurologic diagnostic tests.

Tests for Abnormal Ocular Reflexes

Oculocephalic Response. The oculocephalic response (OCR), also known as *doll's eye reflex,* is movement of the eyes in the direction opposite that in which the head is moved. For example, the doll's eye reflex is considered present if the eyes move to the right when the head is rotated to the left, and vice versa. This test can be performed only in unconscious patients because conscious patients have voluntary control over eye movements. The presence of the doll's eye reflex indicates that brain

TABLE 70-3	*Eye Manifestations and Respiratory Patterns by Level of Involvement in Coma*	
Level of Involvement	**Eye Manifestations**	**Respiratory Pattern**
Supratentorial	Small reactive pupils	Cheyne-Stokes: regular respirations with regular periods of apnea
Upper midbrain	Fixed, dilated pupils (unilateral or bilateral) or midposition fixed pupils	Central neurogenic hyperventilation: regular deep respirations
Upper pons	Midposition fixed or pinpoint pupils	Apneustic breathing: regular but deep inspiration and expiration with regular periods of apnea
Lower pons	Pinpoint pupils	Cluster breathing: clusters of irregular inspiration and expiration between periods of apnea
Medulla	Pinpoint or midposition fixed pupils	Ataxic breathing: completely irregular respirations with apneic periods

stem function is preserved. The reflex is absent or impaired in patients with brain stem problems. The doll's eye test should never be performed in comatose patients with suspected or known cervical spine injury because the head movement required may produce permanent spinal cord damage.

The brain stem in a comatose patient may be functioning even in the absence of the doll's eye reflex. Patients in metabolic coma, except that caused by barbiturate or phenytoin (Dilantin) poisoning, retain ocular reflexes. Other agents and disorders can block the eye's response. Neuromuscular drugs, such as succinylcholine, and Ménière's disease, which destroys the labyrinth in the ear, obliterate the oculocephalic response. In the patient without Ménière's disease or evidence of neuromuscular drugs, however, absence of the oculocephalic response supports the diagnosis of brain death.[4]

Oculovestibular Response. If oculovestibular responses (OCRs) are absent, an OVR (caloric) test can be performed to test cranial nerves III, IV, VI, and VIII (see Chapter 69). A normal response to instillation of iced water into one ear canal is seen as slow, smooth movement of both eyes toward the irrigated ear, followed by fast movement to the opposite side with nystagmus. Instillation of warm water results in slow eye movement away from the irrigated ear, followed by a fast movement to the same side with nystagmus. *Nystagmus* is the involuntary oscillation of the eyeballs; it may be horizontal, vertical, oblique, rotary, or mixed, with various rates of movement.

Failure to produce eye movement and nystagmus with the instillation of warm or cold water into the ear canal indicates an altered brain stem, with a few exceptions. The use of ototoxic drugs, barbiturates, sedatives, phenytoin, or tricyclic antidepressants or the presence of Ménière's disease may produce a false-negative caloric test result. In a patient without these conditions, the absence of an OVR supports the diagnosis of brain death.

Testing the OVR is contraindicated in a patient with a ruptured tympanic membrane (eardrum) or otorrhea (ear discharge). This test is usually performed only in comatose patients because awake patients may vomit in response to the stimulation of cranial nerve VIII.

Outcome Management
■ Medical Management

The goals of medical management are to preserve brain function and to prevent additional brain injury. The primary focus is on maintaining the supply of oxygen and glucose to the brain.

The patient's airway, breathing, and circulation ("ABCs") must be maintained. A nasal or oral airway may be inserted for a short time. If the patient is breathing spontaneously, closely monitor the airway and respirations because the airway may become obstructed and

aspiration may occur as consciousness decreases. If the patient is completely unresponsive or respiratory patterns become ineffective, an endotracheal tube is inserted, with care taken to avoid injury to the cervical spine (see also Chapter 65). Ventilation and supplemental oxygen are given.

Normal cerebral perfusion is promoted through monitoring blood pressure and maintenance of the systolic pressure between 100 and 160 mm Hg. Blood pressures lower or higher than these levels may alter cerebral perfusion pressure. Use of vasoactive agents may be required to keep the systolic pressure at 100 mm Hg or the *mean* systolic blood pressure above 80 mm Hg, or medications may be needed to lower the blood pressure. Blood pressure must be cautiously lowered, however, because high blood pressure may represent a compensatory mechanism to perfuse the brain.

Determine Level of Involvement. Once airway, breathing, and circulation are established, initial assessment of the comatose patient includes evaluation of the following factors:[1,4]

1. Level of consciousness, through observation of response to stimuli.
2. Presence or absence of localizing neurologic manifestations, such as unilateral lack of movement or posturing, indicating focal intracranial disease.
3. Pupil size and reactivity to light.
4. Deep tendon and superficial reflexes (see Chapter 69). Superficial reflex assessment is particularly valuable in comatose patients because it provides objective information about brain stem function in the absence of consciousness. Assess the corneal reflex carefully to avoid corneal abrasion.
5. Response to noxious stimuli. First, loud verbal stimuli and then shaking are performed to produce a response. If none is noted, the examiner applies a painful stimulus, such as pressure to the sternum, nail beds, or supraorbital notch. Care must be taken not to damage skin underlying the areas where pressure is applied. Other aspects of sensory assessment are not possible or are unreliable in comatose patients.
6. Evidence of trauma. Trauma may be the result of coma rather than the cause of it (e.g., a tongue bite may result from a seizure). Examine the ears for ruptured eardrums and otorrhea.
7. Determination of serum oxygenation, blood alcohol, blood urea nitrogen, ammonia, and glucose levels if manifestations suggest a metabolic disorder.
8. History from significant others (or observers of what has happened), if possible.

Reverse Common Causes of Coma. Immediate interventions for the patient in a coma include treatment of common causes of coma while assessment of neurologic status and diagnostic testing continue. For example, after a blood specimen is drawn for testing, intravenous (IV) glucose is given to reverse potential insulin reactions. For comatose patients who appear malnourished, Wernicke's encephalopathy may occur secondary to alcohol abuse. These patients are commonly given thiamine for prevention, especially if they are given glucose.

If the patient is having repetitive seizures, coma and brain damage can follow. The patient is given IV diazepam or lorazepam to stop the seizures. If the patient is not intubated, closely monitor the airway because of the respiratory depressant effects of these medications.

Many metabolic causes of coma lead to acid-base, fluid, and electrolyte imbalances. The patient's acid-base balance should be restored quickly. Fluid imbalances should be restored slowly to prevent rebound fluid shifts into the brain (see Chapter 13). Isotonic saline is usually given if the patient is dehydrated, and fluids are withheld if the patient is fluid overloaded. If cerebral edema is present, osmotic diuretics may be used to promote shifting of extracellular brain fluid back into the plasma. Other medications, such as steroids, barbiturate therapy, and neuromuscular blocking agents, decrease intracranial pressure (ICP) through more indirect means. (Electrolyte imbalances are covered in Chapter 14.)

If infection is suspected, specimens for culture are obtained from the blood, urine, throat, and wounds (if present). Once such specimens have been collected, antibiotics are given. Body temperature should be normalized as much as possible by means of antipyretics, air circulation, and cooling mattresses. Care must be taken to ensure that the patient does not shiver because shivering increases ICP.

Coma from drug overdose may be reversed by specific antidotes if the ingested drug can be identified. Often, however, the specific drug ingested is not known. A urine or blood specimen should be collected for a toxicity screen. Opioid overdose may be reversed with naloxone. Because the duration of action of naloxone is 2 to 3 hours shorter than that of most opioids, naloxone may need to be administered again. Seizures resulting from cocaine overdose can be treated with diazepam. Patients with cocaine overdose often have cardiac dysrhythmias and irregular respirations. Gastric lavage may be used to remove ingested agents, followed by instillation of activated charcoal. In rare circumstances, hemodialysis may be used to remove toxins from the blood.

Structural causes of coma may require surgery to decompress the cranial vault. Burr holes may be created to drain a subdural hematoma. A craniotomy may be performed to remove a tumor, abscess, or intracerebral hematoma. A ventricular catheter or shunt may be placed to relieve hydrocephalus.

To stimulate your thought process, see Thinking Critically at the end of this chapter for the description of a scenario involving a patient with coma from a hypertensive hemorrhage.

Prevent Complications. If the coma is prolonged, initiate enteral feeding to promote nutrition and prevent muscle wasting. Parenteral nutrition may be used if paralytic ileus is present. Take care to avoid hyperglycemia, which can exacerbate brain injury in the presence of ischemia. Brain cells have a high glucose need compared with other cells, however; supplying the cell need without causing brain damage requires a delicate balance.

Prevent the complications of immobility, such as pneumonia and pressure ulcers, with frequent turning or the use of an oscillating bed. Continue to reposition the patient to relieve skin pressure unless the bed provides more than 40 degrees of rotation. The eyes may need to be taped closed to avoid corneal abrasion. Suctioning may be needed to keep the airway clear and prevent pneumonia. Passive range-of-motion exercises keep joints mobile and minimize muscle wasting. Position the extremities in correct alignment to prevent contractures. Use sequential compression stockings to prevent deep venous thrombosis (DVT); low-dose heparin may also be ordered. All these complications are continually assessed for and are treated promptly if they occur.

Outcomes. In the past, little information was available on which to base a prediction about the outcome for a patient in coma. Most of the time, a "wait-and-see" approach was taken. Today the family and the health care team should have some idea of the probable eventual outcome for the patient. It is discouraging and inappropriate to treat a patient vigorously who has no chance of recovery, but it is even more inappropriate to deny treatment to a patient with a reasonable chance of recovery.

Coma after head injury has a statistically better outcome than coma associated with medical illness.[9] About 50% of patients in coma from head injury die, many instantly. Immediate treatment may improve the outcome somewhat for those who reach the hospital. Recovery in traumatic cases is closely linked to age; the younger the patient, the better the recovery. Severely abnormal neuro-ophthalmologic manifestations reflecting brain stem dysfunction imply a poor prognosis; about 90% of patients with such manifestations either die or remain in near-vegetative states.[4]

The absence of pupillary, corneal, or oculovestibular responses during the early stages of coma is highly predictive of mortality or significant morbidity (e.g., persistent vegetative state). The recovery of these responses and a return to purposeful movement correlate with a better prognosis. Patients who lapse into coma as a result of metabolic disorders have an extremely poor prognosis if the coma lasts longer than 1 week.

Some patients in coma awaken slowly and begin to respond normally. They often require physical, occupational, and speech therapy to return to maximal levels of function. Persistent unresponsiveness is caused by damage to any area of the brain that destroys the patient's ability to respond to the environment. The brain stem and cerebellum remain intact, however, so that vital functions, such as heart, lung, and GI functions, continue. Patients can remain unresponsive for years. Significant ethical and legal debates have arisen regarding the maintenance of nutritional intake for such a patient, particularly when a patient's family questions the rationale for artificial feeding.

Coma stimulation, application of planned meaningful, multimodality sensory stimulation, has been suggested as a measure to enhance outcome from coma. Clinical validity of coma stimulation has not been clearly established. The type of stimulation, timing of application, and outcomes measures used vary among studies, making it difficult to determine whether coma stimulation is of benefit.[2] Nonetheless the nurse is encouraged to interact with comatose patients through all their sensory systems.

■ Nursing Management of the Medical Client

Assessment

Frequent, systematic, and objective nursing assessment of the comatose patient, including neurologic status, is essential. Serial observations are important for comparison and to facilitate prompt reporting of even subtle changes in status. Even if assessment findings seem insignificant for long periods, documentation provides an objective pattern and an important baseline for future observations. Assessment of consciousness is most effective when the assessments are performed by a consistent nurse. The neurologic assessment is performed as often as every 15 minutes during the first few hours of coma. Depending on the client's condition, assessments may need to be continued hourly for several days.

The Critical Monitoring feature on Manifestations of Changes in Neurologic Status on p. 2059 lists the neurologic manifestations of a person who is unconscious. Presenting manifestations are ordered according to the degree of seriousness. Remembering these subtle changes in assessment helps in early identification of a patient's improvement or worsening. A decrease in the patient's Glasgow Coma Scale (GCS) score also indicates worsening. The GCS is the most common neurologic assessment tool used in clinical practice (see Chapter 75).

Although neurologic assessment is the priority evaluation, the entire body of a comatose patient must be periodically observed because the patient is unable to offer any specific complaints. Complications of the initial condition causing coma, injuries sustained from other causes, and/or immobility can arise at any time during the course of care. If surgery has been performed, postoperative assessments must be performed as well.

Diagnosis, Outcomes, Interventions

This section describes interventions appropriate for all comatose patients regardless of the cause of the coma.

Interventions specific to particular etiologic factors are described elsewhere (e.g., hepatic coma in Chapter 49, and uremic coma in Chapter 38).

Comatose patients are completely dependent on others because their protective reflexes are impaired. Nursing intervention provides the safety normally afforded by protective reflexes. Coma is often life-threatening and requires aggressive medical intervention. Physicians are concerned with establishing a medical diagnosis and prescribing appropriate treatment; nurses are responsible for meeting basic human needs and preventing the complications associated with coma. Nurses are also responsible for assessing and intervening to reduce ICP.

Altered cerebral tissue perfusion is one of the highest risks for a patient with an altered level of consciousness. This outcome is often seen as a direct consequence of increasing ICP. Nursing management of this problem is described in Chapter 75.

Diagnosis: Risk for Suffocation. Patients who are unconscious cannot swallow because of loss or suppression of the gag or coughing reflex and thus are at risk for suffocation. Airway obstruction is the most common source of harm to patients with decreased consciousness. Write the nursing diagnosis as *Risk for Suffocation related to loss of gag reflex.*

Outcomes. The patient will exhibit no manifestations of accidental suffocation or airway obstruction as evidenced by (1) clear lung sounds; (2) equal lung expansion; and (3) the absence of stridor, cyanosis, and pallor.

Interventions. For initial airway management, an oral airway can be inserted in an unconscious patient. Endotracheal intubation, with the use of a ventilator, may be required to maintain airway patency or improve ventilation.

For extended airway management, a tracheostomy may be required to (1) allow long-term continuous mechanical ventilation, (2) facilitate removal of tracheobronchial secretions, and (3) separate the upper and lower airways (see Chapter 65).

Diagnosis: Risk for Aspiration. The lack of effective airway clearance and gag reflex puts the comatose patient at *very* high risk for aspiration. Write the nursing diagnosis as *Risk for Aspiration related to lack of effective airway clearance and loss of gag reflex.*

Outcomes. The patient will exhibit no manifestations of aspiration as evidenced by (1) clear lung sounds, (2) no stridor, (3) absence of fever, (4) minimal amounts of clear mucus on suctioning, and (5) clear lungs as demonstrated by chest x-ray.

Interventions. Monitor the results of arterial blood gas (ABG) analysis and pulse oximetry to determine the level

CRITICAL MONITORING

Manifestations of Changes in Neurologic Status

"Change" is the key word. Notify the physician whenever there is a change in the client's neurologic status. The following manifestations are listed in the order that indicates a *worsening* in the client's condition. Remember, a client may display a "transient" deterioration in neurologic responses that does not warrant calling a physician. For example, after you have just performed suctioning of the client's airway or have turned the client, you would anticipate a possible change in neurologic status. If you hyperoxygenate the client and ensure proper positioning for venous return from the jugular veins and airway maintenance, however, any manifestations of increased deficit should last only a few seconds or no more than 4 or 5 minutes. Worsening deficit that lasts longer than this increases the risk for irreversible brain injury and requires immediate attention.

Normal

Alert, oriented to person, place, time
Responds appropriately to verbal commands
Eyes open spontaneously with any stimulus, unless in a deep
  sleep

Abnormal; Changes Due to Altered Perfusion of the Cerebral Cortex

Altered level of consciousness
Altered perception of time, then place, and lastly person
Motor deficits (e.g., hemiparesis, hemiplegia)
Speech deficits (e.g., expressive or receptive speech or both)
Memory deficits (e.g., recent, intermediate, remote)
Hyperreflexia
Babinski's sign
Seizures
Decorticate rigidity
Emotional lability
Altered sensory interpretation
Cheyne-Stokes respiration
Headache, nausea, vomiting, papilledema

Abnormal; Changes Due to Altered Perfusion Just Inferior to the Cortex

Pupillary changes: asymmetry of size, shape, or time-
  responsiveness
Loss of reaction to direct light
Visual field changes (e.g., homonymous hemianopsia; see Chapter 72)

Abnormal; Changes Due to Altered Perfusion of the Diencephalon

Altered temperature; first high fevers, then hypothermia
Cheyne-Stokes respiration

Abnormal; Changes Due to Altered Perfusion of the Posterior Pituitary Gland

Diabetes insipidus (decreased antidiuretic hormone)

Abnormal; Changes Due to Altered Perfusion of the Midbrain

Dysfunction of CN III (loss of reaction to indirect or consensual
  light, dysconjugate eye movement)
Dysfunction of CN IV (dysconjugate eye movement)
Central neurogenic hyperventilation

Abnormal; Changes Due to Altered Perfusion of the Upper Pons

Dysfunction of CN V (altered sensory function to cornea, nasal
  membranes, face, oral cavity, tongue, teeth, or altered mastication)
Dysfunction of CN VI (altered lateral eye movement)
Dysfunction of CN VII (altered facial expression, taste, and salivation)
Central neurogenic hyperventilation
Abnormal extension posture
Pinpoint pupils

Abnormal; Changes Due to Altered Perfusion of the Lower Pons

Apneustic breathing
Flaccidity

Abnormal; Changes Due to Altered Perfusion of the Medulla

Dysfunction of CN VIII (altered equilibrium and hearing)
Dysfunction of CN IX (altered taste, pharyngeal sensations, and
  cough and swallowing)
Dysfunction of CN X (altered sensations in pharynx, larynx, external ear, and altered cough and swallowing; altered parasympathetic nervous system functions in thoracic and abdominal viscera)
Dysfunction of CN XI (altered neck and shoulder movement)
Dysfunction of CN XII (altered tongue movement)
Projectile vomiting
Cushing's triad (increased systolic blood pressure, wide pulse
  pressure, bradycardia)
Ataxic (Biot's respiration)

CN, Cranial nerve.

of oxygenation provided by ventilators or oxygen. Assess breath sounds every 1 to 2 hours in acutely ill patients. Keep suctioning equipment available.

Perform tracheobronchial suctioning only as needed to prevent or decrease the accumulation of secretions from immobility, the lack of a cough and sigh reflex, or pneumonia. Not suctioning a person who cannot expectorate his or her own secretions can cause hypoxia and result in neurologic damage. Suctioning should be gentle, and the catheter should not remain in the airway for longer than 10 seconds. While suctioning, observe the cardiac monitor for dysrhythmias (e.g., premature ventricular contractions) secondary to hypoxia. Hyperoxygenating the patient before, during, and after suctioning decreases the risk of dysrhythmias. Hyperoxygenation and limiting the suctioning time to 10 seconds also minimize increased ICP associated with suctioning. Never suction the nasal passages in the patient with a basilar skull fracture because the suction catheter can enter the cranial cavity.

A comatose patient may lack pharyngeal reflexes and be unable to swallow. Pneumonia secondary to aspiration is a common cause of death in unconscious patients. To reduce the risk of aspiration, never give a comatose patient fluids to swallow. Secretions also accumulate in the posterior pharynx and may be aspirated. If the patient is intubated or has a tracheostomy, make sure the cuff is inflated. Suction the upper trachea and posterior pharynx as often as necessary to remove secretions. After tracheal suctioning, the same suction catheter can be used for oral or pharyngeal suctioning, but not vice versa. Also, turn the patient from side to side every 2 hours to facilitate drainage of secretions and prevent pneumonia.

While performing mouth care, place a comatose patient in a lateral position to prevent aspiration. If facial paralysis is present, keep the affected side uppermost. Keep the patient's mouth open by placing an oral airway or bite block between the teeth. Pay close attention to the roof of the mouth in patients who breathe through the mouth for long periods. Crusts of dried mucus may form, break off, and be aspirated. Use of artificial moisturizers may help prevent crust formation; however, frequent oral care is the best prevention.

As consciousness returns and the patient begins to respond to verbal stimuli and has a gag reflex, test the patient's ability to suck and to swallow liquids. Before the test, position the patient in high Fowler's position, and have suction equipment nearby in case it is needed. Use a thick juice, nectar, or ice chips rather than water; liquid of a thick consistency is easier to swallow. Place about 1 teaspoon of liquid into the back of the mouth. Observe for swallowing, and suction as needed to prevent aspiration. If a patient cannot suck through a straw or drink from a glass because of facial paralysis, place fluids in the unaffected side of the mouth with an irriga-

tion syringe. Watch for difficulty in swallowing. Suction as needed.

If there is any question about a patient's ability to swallow, a formal swallowing evaluation should be performed by a speech therapist. Patients who cannot swallow for long periods may require placement of a gastrostomy tube. Many rehabilitation and extended-care facilities require the use of gastrostomy tubes rather than nasogastric (NG) tubes because there is less risk of aspiration with gastrostomy tube feedings.

Patients with impaired swallowing require special instruction. Swallowing can be stimulated by having the patient lean the head forward and, after taking fluid, quickly tip the head backward. Stroking the anterior neck may also promote swallowing.

Once a patient can safely swallow, begin oral nutrition with small liquid feedings, progressing to a soft diet. Discontinue tube feedings only when the patient can take adequate nutrition orally. Many patients are fed orally during the daytime and tube fed at night to maintain adequate nutrition.

When changing from tube feeding to oral feeding, turn off the tube feeding several hours before the meal. This will stimulate the appetite. When a patient begins to eat independently, be reassuring and encouraging. Remind the patient to eat slowly and to swallow after each bite. Position the patient sitting up as tolerated.

Diagnosis: Impaired Oral Mucous Membrane. Several factors can impair oral mucous membranes. The comatose patient usually has an NPO (nothing by mouth) order, is unable to swallow, and breathes through the mouth. A possible nursing diagnosis might be *Impaired Oral Mucous Membrane related to mouth breathing.*

Outcomes. The patient will maintain intact oral mucous membranes as evidenced by oral and nasal mucous membranes that are pink, moist, and without lesions, crusts, or bloody drainage.

Interventions. Using a flashlight and tongue depressor, inspect the patient's mouth every 8 hours. Keep the patient's lips coated with a water-soluble lubricant to prevent encrustation, drying, and cracking. Carefully inspect a paralyzed cheek for crusts or other conditions that require intervention. Provide oral hygiene to prevent excessive drying of oral mucous membranes and complications such as parotitis, aspiration, and respiratory tract infections.

At least twice a day, brush the patient's teeth with a small toothbrush, and rinse the mouth. Clean the oral mucous membranes (especially the roof of the mouth), tongue, and gums with sponge toothbrushes. Avoid using agents that contain lemon or alcohol because they dry the membranes. While performing mouth care in an unconscious patient, suction excess secretions to prevent aspiration. Toothbrushes with suction attachments are now available in many health care agencies.

Nasal passages may become occluded because an unconscious patient is unable to sniff, blow, sneeze, or otherwise clear the nose. To clear the nasal passages of mucus and crust formations, gently swab the nose with an applicator moistened with water or normal saline. Then apply a thin coat of water-soluble lubricant with a cotton-tipped applicator.

Do *not* clean the nasal passages or ears of a patient with a basilar skull fracture. If bleeding occurs from the ears or nose or if CSF (a watery discharge) appears to be draining from these areas, notify the physician.

Diagnosis: Risk for Impaired Skin Integrity.

Normal reflexes reduce the risk of skin ischemia by signaling conscious (even sleeping) persons to shift their body weight. Comatose patients have lost these protective reflexes and are completely immobile. Sometimes patients are agitated and can shear the skin with frequent nonpurposeful movements; this diagnosis also applies to these patients. Write the nursing diagnosis as *Risk for Impaired Skin Integrity related to immobility.*

Outcomes.

The patient will have reduced risk of skin impairment as evidenced by no reddened areas over bony prominences and no areas or manifestations of skin irritation or dryness.

Interventions.

Provide nursing intervention for all self-care needs, including bathing and care of the hair, skin, and nails. Patients often scratch themselves as the depth of unconsciousness lessens; therefore keep the nails trimmed. Patients who are comatose for long periods may be lifted occasionally into a bathtub half-filled with warm water. It may be helpful to apply solutions high in fatty acids (e.g., castile soap, baby oil, or cold cream) daily and to bathe the patient weekly to prevent loss of cutaneous oils as well as skin irritation and dryness.

Perineal care should be performed at least every 8 hours and after every episode of incontinence. If perineal care is not effective for a woman with vaginal discharge or odor, consult the physician about the use of cleansing douches.

When the patient cannot respond to local tissue hypoxia from being in one position for an extended time, the risk of pressure ulcers increases. Patients should be repositioned at least every 2 hours. If repositioning is impossible because of the patient's medical condition, place him or her on a special mattress or bed (Figure 70-2). The use of a special bed, however, does not eliminate the need to pad bony prominences and assess the skin every 4 hours. In addition, meet the nutritional needs of the patient to reduce the risk of pressure ulcers.

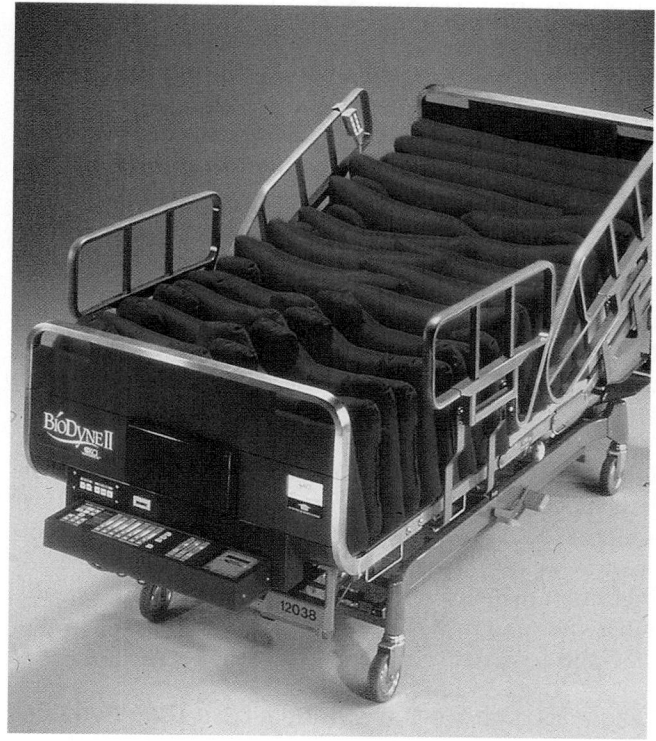

A

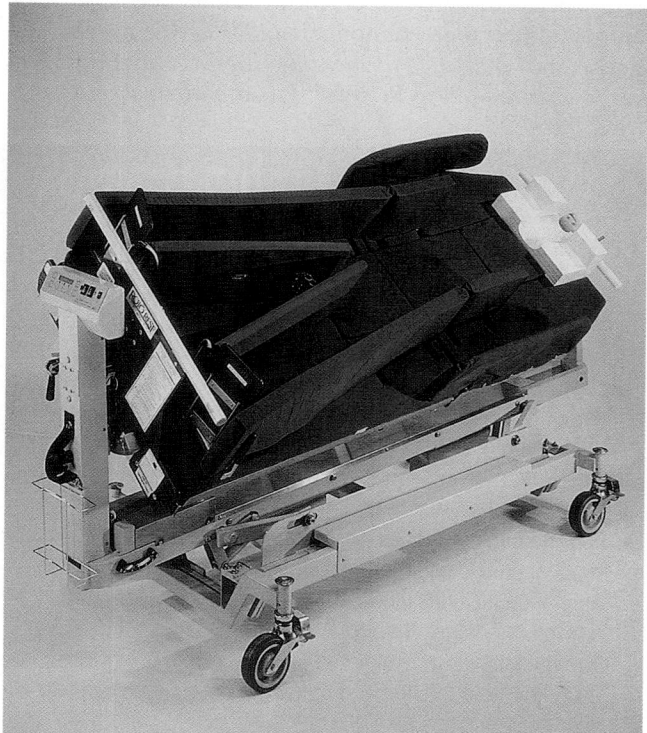

B

FIGURE 70-2 **A,** BioDyne, an oscillating-air support surface. **B,** Roto Rest, an oscillating bed. Both devices are used to prevent tissue hypoxemia and reduce the incidence of nosocomial pneumonia in patients that are unable to move or care for themselves. (Courtesy of Kinetic Concepts, Inc., San Antonio, TX.)

Diagnosis: Risk for Disuse Syndrome (Contractures).
Normal movement and stretch are needed to prevent tightening of one group of muscles. When muscle groups are not used during periods of immobility, joint contractures can develop. Footdrop is of special concern. Write the nursing diagnosis as *Risk for Disuse Syndrome (Contractures) related to no voluntary movement.*

Outcomes. The patient will maintain full range of motion in any joint as evidenced by an absence of contractures. Another outcome could be that the patient will have a reduced risk of contractures as evidenced by (1) a normal range of motion, (2) an absence of flexed arms and legs, and (3) no manifestations of footdrop.

Interventions. Prevent contractures by maintaining the patient's extremities in functional positions with proper support. Hand and forearm splints prevent flexion contracture of the fingers and wrists. Orthotic devices or high-top athletic shoes are used to support the feet. Remove the support devices every 4 hours to perform skin care and passive exercises. Assess the heel closely.

Diagnosis: Imbalanced Nutrition: Less Than Body Requirements.
Comatose patients cannot eat and yet have normal or even increased metabolic needs; so they can quickly become malnourished. Write the nursing diagnosis as *Imbalanced Nutrition: Less Than Body Requirements related to inability to eat and swallow.*

Outcomes. The patient will demonstrate the following manifestations of adequate nutrition: (1) stable weight; (2) adequate calories for age, height, and weight; (3) intake equaling output; (4) healing of incisions and wounds within 12 to 14 days; and (5) hemoglobin, blood urea nitrogen, total lymphocyte count, total protein, and serum albumin values within normal limits for age and gender.

Interventions. Intravenous fluids are begun on admission for comatose patients. Initially the IV site provides access to the circulatory system for the administration of medications. Because fluid intake is restricted and only limited amounts of glucose and few electrolytes are given by the IV route, an IV infusion cannot be considered nutritional support. Consider that 1 liter of solution of 5% dextrose provides only 200 kilocalories!

Just because a patient is comatose, never assume that hunger is not present and that caloric needs are reduced. In fact, the opposite is true; such a patient's caloric needs are usually increased. Nutritional and fluid needs of comatose patients are usually met through enteral feedings because of the risk of aspiration with the oral route. If the patient does not have paralytic ileus or delayed gastric emptying and if bowel sounds are audible, start enteral feedings (see the Management and Delegation feature on Preparing Enteral Nutrition, below).

MANAGEMENT AND DELEGATION

Preparing Enteral Nutrition

Enteral nutrition may be delivered via oral, nasal, gastrostomy, or jejunostomy tubes. Gastrostomy or jejunostomy tubes are most commonly used because they pose a lower risk of aspiration. The delivery of enteral nutrition, including the verification of tube placement, is your responsibility. You may choose to delegate the reconstitution or preparation of enteral feedings to assistive personnel. Before delegating the preparation of tube feeding or refilling the nutrition reservoir bag, consider the following:

- Your abdominal assessment does not reveal abdominal distention, pain, discomfort, or complaints of nausea. Your examination includes verification of tube placement and residual volume of less than 50% of the previous hour's intake. The presence of any of these findings would prompt you to delay the tube feeding and notify the physician of your examination findings.
- You have checked the physician's order for the type and rate of tube feeding to be delivered.
- Instruct assistive personnel in the proper dilution and handling of enteral feeding. (*Hint:* When mixing powdered enteral feedings, always place the powder in the mixing container before the water; this will ensure that the powder dissolves fully.)
- Instruct assistive personnel to place a 4-hour supply of feeding in the reservoir bag and to store the remaining mixture in a refrigerator for future use. Label the storage container with the patient's name, date on which mixture was prepared, and description of mixture.
- Although assistive personnel may prime the pump, you must set the pump and ensure that the flow rate matches the ordered flow rate.
- You are responsible for performing any irrigation of the tube.
- You may delegate care of gastrostomy and jejunostomy tube site to assistive personnel.
- You are responsible for monitoring fluid and nutritional balance via input and output and changes in weight.
- Describe findings that are immediately reportable to you for assistive personnel. They include any difficulty in preparing the enteral feeding and patient complaints of fullness, nausea, or vomiting.
- Verify the competence of assistive personnel in performing these tasks during orientation and annually thereafter.

The nutritional requirements of a patient in coma are complex; a complete nutritional assessment with comparison of height and weight charts, laboratory tests, and clinical examination is essential. There is a marked increase in metabolic needs. Malnutrition increases the morbidity and mortality of neurologically ill patients. Diarrhea and delayed gastric emptying may result from malabsorption. Healing cannot take place in the presence of a negative nitrogen state. Immunodeficiency, with increased risk of infection, sepsis, stress ulcers, weight loss, skeletal-muscle protein wasting, and lung-tissue catabolism, leading to diaphragmatic weakness with respiratory reduction, results from prolonged calorie and protein deprivation. Starvation can lead to death.

Nursing responsibilities in tube feeding of comatose patients are critical because these patients cannot communicate and may have lost protective cough and gag reflexes. The possible complications from enteral feeding, and their prevention, are described in the following list:

1. Vomiting and aspiration if the stomach is overfilled or the head of the patient is below the level of the stomach, such as during chest physiotherapy. When tube feeding a patient, elevate the head of the bed at least 30 degrees to minimize possible aspiration.

2. Delayed gastric emptying. Check residual volumes every 4 hours. If the residual volume is more than 100 ml, delay the feeding for 1 hour and then reassess. Assess bowel sounds, and check for gastric distention; if this complication persists after several hours, notify the physician. If there is a high suspicion that the patient has a bowel obstruction, do not return the gastric residue to the stomach.

3. Tube dislocation into the trachea or lungs, causing aspiration. Some facilities use blue food coloring to tint the formula; then, if suctioned secretions are blue, aspiration is suspected. Comatose patients are often restless. Tape the tube securely to prevent dislodgment. Aspiration may occur if a feeding tube is pulled out during a feeding session or whenever it is unclamped. During feeding sessions, cloth "wristlets" or wrist restraints may be needed.

    Verify NG tube placement by aspirating for gastric contents. Some agency policies and some manufacturers of small-bore tubes require checking tube placement by listening with a stethoscope for "whooshing" while instilling air through the tube. Never tube feed a patient in the supine position unless all other positions are impossible to use. Leave the head of the bed elevated 30 degrees for at least 30 minutes after bolus feedings.

4. Ulcerated or crusted nares due to local pressure from the feeding tube.

5. Tracheoesophageal fistula, that is, breakdown of the anterior esophageal wall from prolonged contact between the NG tube and a tracheostomy tube. This complication is manifested by gastric contents in tracheal secretions. Stop the feeding and notify the physician immediately.

6. Trauma to the gastric mucosa if the tube's distal end hardens, as may happen over time.

7. Fluid volume deficit if hypertonic tube feedings are given. To prevent this problem, ensure that the patient receives approximately 1 ml of fluid for every kilocalorie of feeding. Depending on the agency's policy, this intervention may require consultation with the dietitian or the physician.

8. Constipation or diarrhea, which may develop from the osmolarity of the feeding, the use of liquid medications with a sorbitol base, or a too rapid infusion.

9. Sacral pressure ulcers from continued positioning in the semi-Fowler position. Turn the patient 30 degrees lateral (to the side) with the head of the bed elevated to reduce pressure on the sacrum.

Diagnosis: Risk for Deficient Fluid Volume. The comatose patient cannot drink fluids or respond to normal thirst mechanisms. Such a patient is therefore at *Risk for Deficient Fluid Volume*. Recall that hypertonic tube feedings also increase this risk.

Outcomes. The patient will have reduced risk of deficient fluid volume as evidenced by (1) intake and output being equal for 24, 48, and 72 hours; (2) stable body weight; (3) absence of excessive perspiration, diarrhea, or vomiting; (4) serum glucose, hematocrit, BUN, creatinine, sodium, potassium, and chloride values within normal limits; and (5) moist oral mucous membranes with an absence of tongue furrows.

Interventions. Important aspects in maintaining fluid and electrolyte balance in unconscious patients are (1) accurate documentation of intake and output, (2) daily weights with comparison of trends, and (3) assessment and documentation of conditions that might increase fluid volume deficit (e.g., diaphoresis, polyuria, diarrhea, vomiting, hypertonic tube feedings).

Before fluid and electrolyte intervention is planned for a comatose patient, carefully assess the fluid-electrolyte status. The coma itself may have a fluid or electrolyte cause. Blood tests such as blood glucose, hematocrit, BUN, or creatinine, serum sodium, potassium, chloride, and carbon dioxide measurements help determine fluid and electrolyte status (see Chapters 13 and 14). Dehydration and water intoxication (true hyponatremia) are common causes of electrolyte imbalance associated with coma.

Always avoid overhydration in a patient receiving IV fluids because of the risk of cerebral edema. Diuretics may be prescribed to correct fluid overload and reduce edema. Monitor the response to these medications.

When evaluating the response to any diuretic, empty the indwelling catheter before administering the diuretic. Evaluation of the response should consider the diuretic given, the dose, and the patient's renal status.

Diagnosis: Risk for Injury.

It may not be apparent that the comatose patient is at *Risk for Injury* because he or she does not move. If the coma starts to lighten, however, the patient can move and without protection could fall or be injured. Seizures may also occur, leading to injury. Although loss of the corneal blink reflex, which increases the risk of corneal abrasions, is also a type of injury, it is addressed as a collaborative problem. Nursing interventions for a loss of the corneal blink reflex are discussed in Chapter 67.

Outcomes. The patient will not sustain injury as evidenced by an absence of abrasions or bruises and experiencing no falls from bed.

Interventions. Keep the side rails up on the bed and the bed in the lowest position whenever the patient is not receiving direct care or is unattended. Observe seizure precautions for anyone who has a history of seizure or is at risk of seizure. Protect the patient from injury during seizures or periods of agitation (e.g., use padded side rails, keep the patient's nails short and filed). It is of utmost importance to protect the patient's head. Give the prescribed seizure medication on time to maintain a high seizure threshold. If a dose of the medication is missed for any reason (e.g., vomiting), notify the physician. Antiepileptic medication should not be withheld without a physician order.

Use caution when moving the patient, who cannot voice pain. Give adequate support to the limbs and head when moving or turning the unconscious patient. Limbs without tone may dislocate if they are allowed to fall unsupported. Always turn an unconscious patient toward you or someone else to prevent falls. Protect an unconscious patient from external sources of heat (e.g., heating pads).

Do not restrain the patient unless absolutely necessary because restraint is likely to worsen confused and combative behavior. If restraints are used, they must be released at least every 2 hours for range-of-motion exercises and skin checks. Do not leave unstable patients unattended. Attempt to manage the patient's behaviors without restraints first. "Sitters," hospital volunteers, or family members or friends may be able to provide attendant services. Avoid oversedation because it may alter respirations, which increases ICP and masks changes in a patient's level of consciousness.

Diagnosis: Bowel Incontinence.

Once a paralytic ileus is corrected, the patient will produce feces. Most patients are incontinent because voluntary control is required for the function of the external anal sphincter. Write the nursing diagnosis as *Bowel Incontinence related to inability to respond to normal cues about evacuation*; also consider *High Risk for Impaired Skin Integrity related to fecal incontinence*.

Outcomes. The patient will have reduced fecal incontinence, as evidenced by (1) a bowel movement every 2 to 3 days and (2) no manifestations of fecal impaction.

Interventions. Plan interventions to (1) control bowel movements, (2) maintain the patient's normal elimination schedule, and (3) prevent fecal impaction or constipation. As soon as the patient is able, begin a program of bowel retraining. Maintain a regular schedule, administering stool softeners and suppositories, and performing digital removal of stool at about the same times each day. Examine the abdomen frequently for distention. Constipation and fecal impaction may occur. Small, frequent liquid stools may indicate impaction. If diarrhea or constipation persists, assess for possible causes, such as medications, enteral feedings, and intestinal bacterial infections.

Caution: Consult with the physician before performing digital removal of stool in a patient with an altered level of consciousness. This intervention has been known to induce seizures and may increase ICP. Rectal application of an anesthetic jelly prior to the stimulus decreases this risk.

Diagnosis: Interrupted Family Processes.

Having a family member in a coma is a significant stressor. A possible nursing diagnosis is *Interrupted Family Processes related to uncertain future or impending death of a family member*. Individualize the etiology portion of the diagnosis to fit the specific patient and family.

Outcomes. Family members will exhibit positive coping behaviors as evidenced by (1) showing an ability to solve problems, (2) meeting the needs of other family members, and (3) asking questions about the patient that indicate understanding of previous teaching.

Interventions. The significant others of a comatose patient are often very stressed. It is difficult for family members when they cannot communicate with the patient. The uncertainty of not knowing whether the patient will recover is a major stressor. Include family members in the patient's care to the extent that they can and want to be involved. Family members need information and realistic hope.

It is important for the family to see the patient receiving high-quality, professional, and compassionate nursing care. For example, talk to the patient as though he or she can understand. Initially this behavior will seem awkward, but in time it will feel appropriate. Tell the patient that he or she will be turned to the side, bathed, and so on before performing the task. Depending on the depth of the coma, the patient's sense of hearing may still be intact. Therefore speak to the patient as if he or she can hear, and tell the family to do the same. Comatose patients have awakened and reported that they remember hearing specific voices.

The family is often in a state of shock, needing someone to recognize their needs and help them through this difficult situation. They may experience various conflicting feelings, such as guilt and anger. The Client Education Guide feature on When a Loved One Is in an Altered State of Consciousness on the website suggests ways for the patient's family members to cope with these feelings.

Allow significant others to stay with the patient when and where possible. At times family members may become zealous about attending and may stay at the patient's bedside continuously. Encourage family members to care for themselves also by eating regular meals and obtaining adequate sleep. Have them consider using external support systems (e.g., neighbors and church groups). Tell them they will be telephoned if any significant changes occur in their loved one's status, and ask them to leave a phone number where they can be reached. Encourage family members to phone if they have questions or concerns.

Social workers may be contacted to provide additional support. Some hospitals, especially tertiary care centers, have "family homes," where family members who must travel a long distance to the hospital may stay to be close to the hospital and the patient.

Evaluation

The patient may remain comatose for a few hours or even months. Some comatose patients (e.g., patients with diabetic coma) awaken and make a complete recovery while in the hospital. Therefore some expected outcomes have brief time frames (e.g., airway obstruction), whereas others are prolonged, requiring frequent reevaluation (e.g., family coping). Your evaluation may identify a need for revision of the care plan.

■ Modifications for Older Adults

The older patient in a coma requires the same quality of care as patients in other age groups; however, the older patient is at higher risk for all complications of immobility, especially pressure ulcers and pneumonia. Urinary retention is common in older men because of prostatic enlargement. Finally, fully assess the patient for the common disorders of aging (e.g., diabetes) that might be the cause of the coma.

■ Self-Care

The site to which a patient with coma is discharged from an acute care setting depends on (1) the condition of the patient, (2) the cause of the coma, and (3) the level of available family support. If the patient is recovering from coma, plan for placement in a rehabilitation center. Patients remaining in coma but showing slow recovery may be placed in an extended-care facility until they can participate in rehabilitation.[2,4] Coma stimulation programs, although not readily available, provide an alternative for the patient who is slow to recover.[2]

If the patient is in a coma and is not expected to awaken but may live for a time with nutritional support, placement in a skilled nursing center is common.[4] In these centers, supportive care is given. Family members usually specify how aggressively they wish the patient to be treated in the event of a deterioration in status. Your role in discharge of the comatose patient centers on communication with the receiving nurses and the family. If the patient is ventilator dependent or combative, special consideration is required for transport to the new facility. Provide a complete plan of care.

CONFUSIONAL STATES

Confusion is a mental state marked by alterations in thought and attention deficit, followed by problems in comprehension. It is accompanied by a loss of short-term memory and, often, irritability alternating with drowsiness. Confusion is a common clinical manifestation in many neurologic and metabolic disorders.

Confusion has been shown to increase both morbidity and length of hospital stay. This relationship has major implications in terms of cost containment, especially because people older than 85 years are the fastest-growing age group in the United States.

Etiology and Risk Factors

Confusion has many causes. Common causes of acute confusion are alcohol withdrawal and drug ingestion. Confusion can also follow fever, head injury, and use of anesthetics. Other causes of confusion are decreased cerebral perfusion, hypoxia, hypoglycemia, severe fluid and electrolyte disorders, sepsis, liver or renal failure, poisons, and drug overdose.

Delirium and dementia are classifications of types of confusion. Three features are common to all types of *delirium*[6]:

- A disturbance of consciousness with a reduced ability to focus, sustain, or shift attention
- A change in cognition (memory, language, disorientation) or development of a perceptual disturbance that is not better accounted for by a pre-existing, established, or evolving dementia
- A change that develops over a short time (hours to days) and may fluctuate during the course of the day

Several classifications of delirium have each of the three common features but specific causes. They are (1) delirium related to a general medical condition, (2) delirium resulting from substance intoxication (prescribed drugs, over-the-counter medications, or street drugs), (3) delirium due to substance withdrawal, (4) delirium with multiple causes, and (5) delirium "not otherwise specified."[6]

Sundowning is defined as agitation, confusion, and restlessness that occurs after the sun sets; however, diurnal variations may be responsible for these changes as well.[3]

Dementia is the chronic form of confusion. As with delirium, there are common features in the many types of dementia. They are as follows:

- The development of multiple memory impairments
- One or more of the following cognitive disturbances: *aphasia* (problems with expressing speech or understanding sounds), *apraxia* (inability to convert a thought to action), *agnosia* (inability to recognize objects), and impaired executive functioning
- Significant impairment and decline in social or occupational functioning
- A gradual onset and continuing cognitive decline

The classifications of dementia include the four common features with variable causes and characteristics. There are many subtypes of dementia of the Alzheimer's type. Essentially all other causes, such as central nervous system (CNS) disorders, systemic conditions, substance-induced conditions, depression, and schizophrenia, must be ruled out. The other types of dementia are (1) vascular dementia (multi-infarct), (2) dementia secondary to other general medical conditions, (3) substance-induced persisting dementia, (4) dementia with multiple causes, and (5) dementia "not otherwise specified."[7]

An in-depth discussion of the care related to specific types of delirium and dementia, as well as the memory changes that occur in patients with amnesic disorders and other cognitive disorders not meeting the criteria for any of the preceding classifications, is beyond the scope of this book. The reader should refer to a psychiatric textbook for this information. This discussion focuses on the general care of a patient with confusion, however, because dementia of the Alzheimer's type is a growing problem. Chapter 74 details the pathologic processes and care related to this type of degenerative disease.

Risk factors that lead to confusion vary with the specific etiologic factors. In general, the proper management of various diseases, such as diabetes mellitus, would reduce the incidence of confusion. Disorders such as Alzheimer's disease have no known prevention at this time, although new drugs may slow disease progression. Avoid the use of any medications that contribute to confusion in people who are at risk for confusion.

Pathophysiology

Three mechanisms account for the development of *acute confusion*: (1) damage to the brain with swelling or loss of oxygen, blood, or both (functional disorder); (2) im-

pairment of the action of the nervous system by chemicals or other substances (metabolic disorder); and (3) the rebound overactivity of a previously depressed center in the brain. Chemicals that cross the blood-brain barrier, such as alcohol, impair the metabolism of neuronal cells. When the drug action wears off or the drug is withdrawn from the patient, the lower centers in the brain are overactive. This overactivity accounts for the development of acute confusion, combativeness, and other abnormal behaviors.

Chronic confusional states are due to disorders that cause brain tissue destruction, biochemical imbalances, or compression of the brain. For example, people with Alzheimer's disease lack acetylcholine, a neurotransmitter that is necessary for short-term memory. Other disorders that cause chronic confusion may be inherited; may be secondary to a transmissible agent, as with Creutzfeldt-Jakob disease; or may follow diseases such as encephalitis.

Clinical Manifestations

The earliest manifestation of a brain disorder is a *disorder of attention*. The patient may report the loss of concentration or may appear preoccupied. At the same time, restlessness, emotional lability, insomnia or drowsiness, and vivid nightmares may begin. Patients may appear anxious and may fear that they are "going crazy." As the disorder progresses, stupor and coma develop. Behaviors seen in the patient are reflective not of personality but of the cause of the disorder. For example, barbiturate or alcohol abuse and withdrawal and liver disorders cause agitated delirium. In contrast, anoxia and kidney and lung disorders are associated with a quieter response. Disorders that develop rapidly are more likely to cause an agitated response than those that develop slowly.

Fluctuations in cognition (the ability to think and reason) are common in patients with metabolic brain disorders. Patients may be totally irrational one moment and lucid the next. Some of the fluctuations are caused by the environment. Delirious patients become more disoriented at night, in unfamiliar surroundings, when they hear unfamiliar noises or see unfamiliar people, or when restraints are used. The lack of a window in the room has caused many patients to become disoriented.

Loss of memory for recent events is a hallmark of metabolic brain disorders. The patient commonly has difficulty with both immediate recall and abstract thought. Patients who are delirious quickly lose orientation to time. Normal people can readily recall six or seven digits forward and five or six backward and identify the commonalities between an orange and an apple or a tree and a bush; delirious patients cannot do these things. The patient's general intelligence level can affect the behaviors observed, however. If possible, the patient's level of education should be known before the assessment.

Perceptual errors (e.g., mistaking the nurse for a daughter) as well as hallucinations, illusions, and delusions are common accompaniments of delirium.

Hallucinations are sensations occurring in the absence of external stimuli. A patient may hear, see, feel, smell, or taste something that is not present. The patient may or may not realize that the experience is "not real." Unfortunately, the most common hallucinations involve rodents and unfriendly animals (e.g., snakes, spiders). These visions are terribly frightening.

Illusions differ from hallucinations in that illusions are the misinterpretation of something actually in the environment. For example, if a patient sees a shadow on the drape and mistakes it for a real person, the patient is experiencing an illusion.

Delusions are thoughts or beliefs that have no basis in fact. For example, a patient may think that he or she has been robbed or poisoned when there is no basis for this belief.

No specific diagnostic tests for confusion exist. The patient may undergo CT or MRI scanning to determine whether there is a structural cause for the confusion, such as a tumor or stroke. In addition, a series of laboratory studies may be performed to look for a metabolic cause. Common studies include a complete blood count, electrolyte measurements, determination of vitamin B_{12} and folate levels, thyroid and liver function studies, drug toxicity screening tests, and an EEG. A lumbar puncture may be performed for the analysis of CSF.

Outcome Management
■ Medical Management

In all care settings, the medical management of the confused patient begins by determining the cause of the confusion and correcting it, if possible.[3] When no specific cause is found, the medical management focuses on controlling manifestations. Sometimes medications can be given to calm agitation. Nutritional needs also must be monitored.

■ Nursing Management of the Medical Client
Assessment

A thorough history is required for assessment of the confused patient. The history should include the onset of the confusion, past medical illnesses, work and occupational history, and past injuries. Disorders such as diabetes or liver failure may be out of control and responsible for the confusion. The patient may have been exposed to heavy metals or toxic wastes at work. Record past injuries, especially head injury. Depending on the level of confusion, the patient may not be able to answer each question, and you may need to rely on the family or others who have been with the patient. Review medications, including over-the-counter drugs and nutritional supplements.

Specific questions about the patient's ability to handle routine financial transactions or home safety with tasks such as cooking, dressing, and driving will help determine whether the patient can be safely returned home or is in need of an alternative arrangement. At times the family will report a change in personality, such as apathy, social isolation, disinterest in current events, and irritability. Record these observations because they may be clinical manifestations of Alzheimer's disease or frontal lobe lesions.

The confused patient requires ongoing assessment with the Mini-Mental State Examination (see Chapter 69). This examination is much more sensitive than other tools for serial evaluations of confused patients.[7] Analyze the data collected to determine whether the confusion is improving, worsening, or unchanged.

The confused patient is often combative and argumentative. Observe for factors in the patient's environment that might affect confusion. Assess whether the patient is able to refrain from self-injury or injury to others. If not bedridden, the patient may wander about and become lost or injured if harmful items are not secured (e.g., knives).

Confusion can occur in patients of any age or culture and from variable causes. The nurse's role as a patient advocate supersedes personal bias related to any of these variables.

Diagnosis, Outcomes, Interventions

This section describes interventions appropriate to the confused patient, regardless of the cause, with an emphasis on the issue of safety.

Diagnosis: Disturbed Thought Processes. Use the nursing diagnosis *Disturbed Thought Processes related to failure in memory and lack of self-protective behavior to address needs for safety.*

Outcomes. The patient will have improved thought processes as evidenced by (1) higher scores on the Mini-Mental State Examination; and (2) decreased frequency of hallucinations, illusions, and delusions.

Interventions. The confused patient will benefit from consistency in the environment and care routine. Keep objects, such as the tray table and bedside chair, in the same place. If possible, the same staff member should care for the patient. Give the patient short explanations as events occur, such as "You need an x-ray" and "Please sit in the wheelchair." Saying to a confused patient, "In 2 hours, an x-ray tech will be coming to take you for a CT scan," is useless because such a patient will neither understand nor remember it. Response time may be slowed in confusion; allow the patient time to respond.

Reorient the patient as often as necessary, but use caution about the specific communication used. Patients with chronic untreatable confusion do not benefit from reorientation and may become more agitated when you attempt to reorient them. For example, in one study in which a 92-year-old patient was told repeatedly that her mother or father could not possibly be alive, the patient reacted each time as if it was the first time she had been told and grieved deeply.[7] For these selected patients, avoid reorienting, redirect their thoughts and agitation, or "go along" with the confusion. Of course, when the patient is at risk of injury, safety precautions are foremost. Clocks and calendars in the room also help with reorientation. The use of familiar objects is helpful when a patient's remote memory is intact. For example, the use of a quilt from home on the bed may help the confused patient recognize the bed as his or her own.

Promote reduction of unfamiliar noise because it adds to confusion. The patient's room should be quiet and softly lighted without producing shadows.

Consistency in the care of a patient with confusion requires communication among caregivers. This communication occurs not only through the oral reporting method but also in the care plan and documentation records.

Diagnosis: Risk for Injury.

Confusion greatly increases risk of harm. The patient cannot interpret, or may not be able to respond to, environmental stimuli that precede danger. Write the nursing diagnosis as *Risk for Injury related to the unpredictable behavior and inability to interpret environmental stimuli.*

Outcomes. The patient will have reduced risk of injury and will not injure others.

Interventions. The patient must be protected from self-injury. The patient should be in a room near the nursing station so that assessments can be performed every 30 to 60 minutes. In addition, the bed should be in the low position. Structure the patient's environment to minimize injury; remove any extraneous equipment.

The routine use of physical restraints (e.g., side rails, cloth restraints) or chemical restraints (e.g., medication) is discouraged.[8] The use of side rails and restraints does not guarantee that patients will not fall and often either makes them more agitated or leads to more severe injury when they do fall. Alternatives to restraints include the use of sitters for ongoing observation and placement of the client in an area permitting constant observation, such as the nursing station. Motion detection devices can be applied to the patient or the bed to signal the nursing staff when movement occurs. If all other alternatives have been unsuccessful and restraints are used, make frequent assessments and record the data. Cloth restraints must be removed every 2 hours to assess the skin beneath them and perform range-of-motion exercises. Chemical

restraint (e.g., tranquilizers) can result in greater confusion and tremors (extrapyramidal symptoms).

The patient with brain alteration is not in control of his or her behavior. Behaviors may be unpredictable, irrational, or impulsive, or the patient may be frightened and suspicious. Never "punish" a confused patient for inappropriate behavior or remarks. Instead, remember that these personality changes are a result of brain lesions, and adjust the care plan accordingly. If a patient is agitated, provide reassurance and a calm environment. Redirect or distract the patient. Monitoring systems may be used for patients who wander.

Confused older patients are at increased risk for falls. A formal assessment of the risk of falls should be completed. Some institutions have programs for patients who are at risk for falling or who have fallen. These programs include frequent assessments, routine toilet trips, bed and wandering monitors, and environmental changes (mattress on the floor, use of a lap buddy). Trying to ambulate to the bathroom is a common time for falls, and toilet trips should be offered routinely (every 2 hours).

Diagnosis: Disturbed Sleep Pattern.

A common problem seen in confused patients consists of daytime napping and nighttime hallucinations. This problem is stated as *Disturbed Sleep Pattern related to alterations in usual sleep habits.*

Outcomes. The patient will have improved sleep patterns as evidenced by (1) sleeping 4 to 6 hours continuously at night and (2) not sleeping as often during the day.

Interventions. Plan nighttime interventions to allow 4 to 6 hours of uninterrupted sleep. Recall that a sleep cycle requires 1.5 to 2 hours, and the loss of rapid eye movement (REM) sleep can increase confusion. When you enter the room at night, assess the patient for REM. If REM is present, the patient should be allowed to complete the REM portion of the sleep cycle. You should return later to care for the patient.

Keep the patient active during the day so that there is some fatigue by nighttime. Daytime sleeping is a difficult pattern to break, and the patient may have to be kept awake for this pattern to be reversed. Bedtime routines should be developed. Avoid the use of caffeinated beverages and alcohol, which may prevent sleep. For the older patient, the normal changes in sleep with aging need to be considered, such as the greater use of short naps and less sleep during the night. Sleeping medications are seldom given to the confused patient because they often alter sleep cycles and rob the patient of REM sleep. See Chapter 24 for further information about sleep disorders.

Diagnosis: Risk for Caregiver Role Strain.

The unfamiliar behavior of the confused patient or the stress of providing continual care for the patient at home may increase stress in the family and alter their ability to cope.

This nursing diagnosis is stated as *Risk for Caregiver Role Strain related to long-term, stressful, and complex care required by family member.*

Outcomes. The patient's family members will maintain their own physical and psychological health as evidenced by (1) improved use of support systems, (2) obtaining of adequate equipment to provide care, (3) limited use of addictive substances for coping, (4) interaction with friends and extended family (as desired), and (5) appropriate analysis of the patient's condition.

Interventions. Teach the family to monitor for the effects of confusion. When confusion is a new problem for the patient, the family will be distressed by the behavior. Explain to the family that the patient is not able to control behavior or speech at this time. Assess whether the patient becomes calm or agitated when the family is present, and advise visitations accordingly. If possible, the need for and use of restraints should be explained to the family before they see a patient in restraints. The family may become very upset when they see their loved one "tied" to a bed. Advance explanations can avert some of this reaction. In some instances a patient suffered an injury because the family did not understand the purpose for the restraints and untied them. See the Management and Delegation feature on Physical Restraints, below.

MANAGEMENT AND DELEGATION

Physical Restraints

The use of physical restraints to protect a patient from self-harm or injury or to manage a patient at risk for disruption of medical therapies is a decision made collaboratively between you and the physician and may include consultation with other members of the interdisciplinary team. The serious decision to use physical restraints is made after your comprehensive assessment and evaluation of previous interventions and alternatives.

A clear goal is the use of the least restrictive device for the shortest interval possible. Regulatory agencies consider the use of restraints to be a high-risk intervention. Death and injury have been associated with restraint use in hospital environments. Your clinical site should provide you with clear guidelines regarding the use of restraints and the role of unlicensed assistive personnel in caring for restrained patients.

Before delegating care of the patient in physical restraints, consider the following:

- Have the patient and family been informed and educated regarding the need for restraints to protect the patient? Your education of the patient and family should include standards of care and discussion of what factors lead to discontinuation of restraints.
- Have you assessed the patient to determine the most appropriate type of restraint? The restraint must be the right size. Follow the manufacturer's recommendations for sizing. Never use anything other than a manufactured device that has been approved by the Food and Drug Administration.
- Have you obtained a physician's order for the use of restraints? In addition to the initiation order for restraints, there should be ongoing discussion of the need to continue restraint use with the interdisciplinary team and physician order updates every 24 hours.

Your assessment of the patient's safety and comfort needs must occur at regular intervals as defined by your institution. You are accountable for assessing and documenting the patient's condition, the patient's response to restraints, and the safety and comfort interventions provided.

Consider the following points when delegating components of care to assistive personnel:

- Be clear about the type of restraint being used. In addition to applying restraints according to the manufacturer's instructions, restraints are to be secured only to the bed frame or chair with slip knots.
- Explain that restraints are never used as a punishment.
- Patients with altered mental status experiencing unmet elimination needs may become agitated. Instruct assistive personnel to offer assistance with elimination at regular intervals.
- Provide specific expectations and a time schedule for observation of the patient.
- Instruct on how to remove restraints one at a time in agitated patients.
- How to respond to patients who ask for the restraints to "be cut off" by re-explaining the need for them.

You may delegate these components of care to assistive personnel:

- Assistance with activities of daily living, such as bathing, grooming, and feeding.
- Active or passive range of motion.
- Turning and repositioning the patient. The patient should be instructed to resecure restraints after position changes.

Describe for the assistive personnel the findings that are immediately reportable to you. Such findings may include skin redness or irritation noted at points of contact with the restraint device, changes in color or movement of areas distal to the restraint, the patient's unplanned removal of a restraint, disruption of a medical therapy, and the patient's complaints of discomfort or distress. Verify the competency of assistive personnel in caring for restrained patients during orientation and in an ongoing manner thereafter.

Choosing the placement site for a confused patient being discharged from the hospital varies with the cause of confusion. If the confusion is acute and full recovery is expected, the patient may be able to go home under the care of family members. If the confusion is chronic, the patient needs either care or supervision at home or placement in an extended-care facility. Some communities offer adult day care and respite services that give family members relief from the constant care of the confused person. See Chapter 74 for care of the patient with Alzheimer's disease at home.

Advise the family to have legal counsel determine the patient's competence and the need for guardianship or durable power of attorney. The family may also need to grieve the loss of the patient's previous functional role, personality, companionship, and so on. Assess for evidence of violence in the caregiver and the patient. Caregiver violence is possible, especially if the patient was violent toward the caregiver in the past.

Help the caregiver find respite care and personal time to meet his or her own needs and to learn stress management techniques. Female caregivers are especially vulnerable to social isolation.

Evaluation

Most of the time, confusion will require many months to abate. The diagnosis of a chronic, progressive condition such as Alzheimer's disease or dementia of the Alzheimer's type may require an entire change in care plan prioritization. These conditions are discussed in Chapter 74.

■ Modifications for Older Clients

It is common but incorrect to believe that older people naturally undergo a marked deterioration in mental function. In general, older people have difficulty recalling new information, but their remote memory is intact. In addition, depression occurs in 20% to 30% of older people. Depression may follow the loss of friends, spouse, health, and independence and may lead to manifestations such as memory loss and confusion.

Older adults are particularly at risk for confusion during hospitalization.[3,6] They are dealing not only with the stress of being ill but also with the stress of an unfamiliar environment. Older patients may rely heavily on familiar landmarks and routines to help them maintain an independent lifestyle. These cues are often lost in the hospital or extended-care setting. A large percentage of the population in hospital and extended-care settings are older adults, who typically have other conditions that contribute to confusion. Confusion is best managed by using a team approach and teaching unlicensed assistive personnel to (1) introduce themselves at the beginning of a work shift; (2) use the same time for the patient's sleep, naps, and meals; (3) routinely place the patient on the toilet or commode; (4) talk to the patient about the past; (5) gently redirect lost or wandering patients; and (6) encourage self-care (eating, dressing, and so on).

CONCLUSIONS

Patients who are confused or comatose are vulnerable to many complications, including injury, aspiration, malnutrition, and skin breakdown. Nurses provide a lifeline for these patients, giving protection and promoting normal body functions. The families of these patients require therapeutic management because they face many difficult decisions.

THINKING CRITICALLY *evolve*

1. A 48-year-old man is brought to the emergency department by ambulance. His wife states that he had been shaving in the bathroom when she heard a thud. She found him unresponsive on the floor. How do you intervene?
Factors to Consider. What was the patient's neurologic baseline when he was received in the emergency department? What other clinical manifestations did the client display? Were there any physical manifestations of injury to his head or other parts of his body? Does he have any other significant medical history or allergies?

2. You are caring for a 72-year-old woman who recently underwent repair of a hip fracture. Her husband indicates that she had recently been confused, which led to her falling and fracturing her hip. How do you intervene?
Factors to Consider. What do you include in your assessment? What types of interventions do you need to consider? How do you involve her family?

Discussions for these questions can be found on the website and the CD-ROM.

BIBLIOGRAPHY

1. Bateman, D.E. (2001). Neurologic assessment of coma. *Journal of Neurology, Neurosurgery, Psychiatry, 71*(Suppl 1), i13-17.
2. Davis, A.E., & White, J.J. (1995). Innovative sensory input for the comatose brain-injured patient. *Critical Care Nursing Clinics of North America, 7*(2):351-361.

3. Foreman, M.D., et al. (1999). Standard of practice protocol: Acute confusion/delirium. *Geriatric Nursing 20*(3), 147-152.

4. Hickey, J.V. (2002). Management of the unconscious patient. In *The clinical practice of neurological and neurosurgical nursing* (5th ed., pp. 288-299). Philadelphia: J.B. Lippincott.

5. Hilgers, J. (2003). Comforting a confused patient: learn how simple interventions and diversions can help. *Nursing, 33,* 48-50.

 6. Mentes, J., et al. (1999). Acute confusion indicators: Risk factors and prevalence using MDS data. *Research in Nursing and Health, 22*(2), 95-105.

7. Rapp, C.G. (2001). Acute confusion/delirium protocol. *Journal of Gerontological Nursing, 28*(4), 21-33.

8. Rogers, P.D., & Bocchino, N.L. (1999). Restraint-free care: Is it possible? *American Journal of Nursing, 99*(10), 26-34.

9. Wijdicks, E.F. (2000). Coma in the critically ill: using neurologic findings and clinical context as clues to diagnosis. *Journal of Critical Illness, 15*(11), 609-610, 615-618.

Chapter 71

Management of Clients with Cerebral Disorders

*Melanie S. Minton**

evolve

Web Enhancements

http://evolve.elsevier.com/Black/medsurg/

Client Education Guide
Epilepsy (Spanish Translation)
Migraine Headache (Spanish Translation)

Appendix C
Laboratory Values of Clinical Importance in Medical-Surgical Nursing

---

SEIZURE DISORDERS

In this chapter, an important distinction is made between seizures and epilepsy. A *seizure* is a sudden, abnormal electrical discharge from the brain that results in changes in sensation, behavior, movements, perception, or consciousness. A seizure may occur in isolation or with some acute problem within the central nervous system (CNS), such as a low blood glucose level, drug or alcohol withdrawal, or traumatic brain injury. *Epilepsy* is a chronic disorder of recurrent seizures. An isolated, single seizure does not constitute epilepsy.[21,26,49,51]

EPILEPSY

Epilepsy is derived from the Greek *epilepsia,* meaning "seizure." In early times, epilepsy was viewed as being of divine origin and was called the "sacred disease" because someone with epilepsy was thought to be "seized" or struck down by the gods. An epileptic syndrome is composed of paroxysmal neurologic dysfunction causing recurrent episodes of one or more of the following manifestations: loss of consciousness, convulsive movements or other motor activity, sensory phenomena, and behavioral abnormalities. About 2.3 million Americans are known to have seizures or epilepsy. About 181,000 new

cases of seizures and epilepsy are documented annually.[21,26,50,52]

Etiology and Risk Factors

Epilepsy can be caused by any process that disrupts the stability of the neuronal cell membrane. A variety of conditions are associated with an extremely high likelihood of onset of a chronic seizure disorder. One of the best examples of such conditions is severe, penetrating head trauma, which is associated with up to a 50% risk of the development of epilepsy. This association suggests that the injury results in a long-lasting pathologic change in the CNS that transforms a presumably normal neural network into one that is abnormally hyperexcitable.

The identified mechanism responsible for such malfunction is unknown. Possible theories include neuronal structural impairment, abnormalities involving the sodium-potassium pump, and changes in various neurochemicals.[21,53] Hypersensitive neurons can be found throughout the brain and spinal cord. The neuronal cell membrane appears to be more permeable and more sensitive to various offending factors. An epileptogenic focus may develop at the location of increased cell membrane permeability. The epileptogenic focus may be limited to a specific area or encompass the entire cortical surface.

*Deceased.

---

evolve Be sure to check out the bonus material on the Evolve website and the CD-ROM, including free self-assessment exercises.

http://evolve.elsevier.com/Black/medsurg/

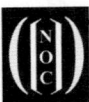

Nursing Outcomes Classification (NOC)
for Nursing Diagnoses—Clients with Cerebral Disorders

Anticipatory Grieving
Aggression Control
Coping
Family Coping
Grief Resolution
Psychosocial Adjustment: Life Change
Anxiety
Aggression Control
Anxiety Control
Coping
Decreased Intracranial Adaptive Capacity
Electrolyte and Acid-Base Balance
Fluid Balance
Neurologic Status: Autonomic
Neurologic Status: Cranial
    Sensory/Motor Function

Neurologic Status: Spinal
    Sensory/Motor Function
Ineffective Coping
Aggression Control
Coping
Decision-Making
Impulse Control
Role Performance
Ineffective Health Maintenance
Knowledge: Health Behaviors
Knowledge: Treatment Regimen
Treatment Behavior: Illness
Risk for Disturbed Thought Processes
Cognitive Ability
Cognitive Orientation
Decision-Making

Risk for Ineffective Tissue Perfusion: Cerebral
Cognitive Ability
Neurologic Status
Neurologic Status: Central Motor
    Control
Neurologic Status: Consciousness
Tissue Perfusion: Cerebral
Risk for Injury
Safety Status: Falls Occurrence
Safety Status: Physical Injury
Symptom Control
Risk for Spiritual Distress
Anxiety Control
Coping
Grief Resolution
Hope
Quality of Life
Spiritual Well-Being

Seizures are classified as *genetic, acquired,* or *idiopathic.*[43] What is not well understood is how these three factors may cause the seizure threshold to be lowered, thereby increasing the possibility of seizures. For example, with idiopathic seizures, what is the offending agent? Is it structural, neurochemical, or a combination of several factors?

Idiopathic epilepsy most often begins before the age of 20 years and rarely begins after age 30. Seizures beginning in newborns and infants are often caused by congenital brain defects, birth injuries, or metabolic problems such as anoxia, hypoglycemia, or hypocalcemia. Although the underlying cause may be perinatal, seizures may not begin for many years, often with onset during puberty. Other than in children younger than age 5 years, the highest incidence of new-onset epilepsy is in people older than 65. In this group, the increased risk is attributed to the increase in conditions that cause neurologic changes in this group. These include cerebrovascular disease, tumor, delirium, Alzheimer's disease, infection, accumulated trauma, and chronic alcoholism, as well as the aging process itself.[21,26,28,45,49,51]

When the cause of seizures is known, the disorder is called *secondary epilepsy.* After age 20 years, generalized seizures usually have an identifiable cause. These causes include traumatic brain injury, brain tumor, and infection. Approximately two thirds of cases of epilepsy are idiopathic; the remainder are caused by secondary causes.

Pathophysiology

When the integrity of the neuronal cell membrane is altered, the cell begins firing with increased frequency and amplitude.[21,51,53] When the intensity of the discharges reaches a threshold, the neuronal firing spreads to adja-cent normal neurons. Discharges in the brain stem cause muscle contraction and possibly loss of consciousness. The excitation of the cells can spread to the spinal cord.

Normally, excitatory messages from a single hypersensitive neuron in the cerebral cortex are modulated by deeper structures (e.g., thalamus and brain stem) (Figure 71-1). In epilepsy, these bursts of electrical activity from the cortex are not controlled or modulated. These discharges block normal inhibition and perpetuate a feedback loop. Eventually, inhibitory neurons in the cortex, anterior thalamus, and basal ganglia slow the neuronal firing. This inhibition interrupts the seizure and produces an intermittent contraction-relaxation phase. Once the epileptogenic neurons are exhausted and inhibitory processes build, the seizure stops. These later events depress CNS action and impair consciousness. This period of impaired consciousness after a seizure, called a *postictal state,* may be manifested as sleep, confusion, or fatigue.

Seizure activity increases the need for adenosine triphosphate (ATP) and for cerebral oxygen consumption. Supplies of oxygen and glucose are rapidly consumed. To meet these demands, the cerebral blood flow increases during a seizure. If the seizure is ongoing (as in status epilepticus), severe hypoxia and lactic acidosis occur and may result in brain tissue destruction.[21,37,50]

Clinical Manifestations

Epilepsy has been classified according to the age at onset, cause, area of origin, abnormalities on the electroencephalogram (EEG), and clinical type of seizure. The International Classification of Epileptic Seizures, used here, is based on the clinical seizure type and on EEG findings during seizures (the ictal period) and between

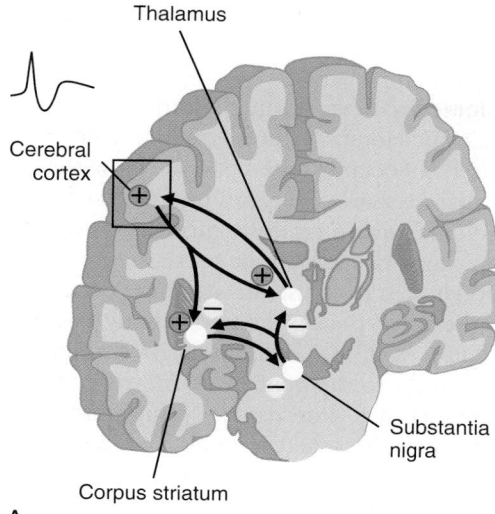

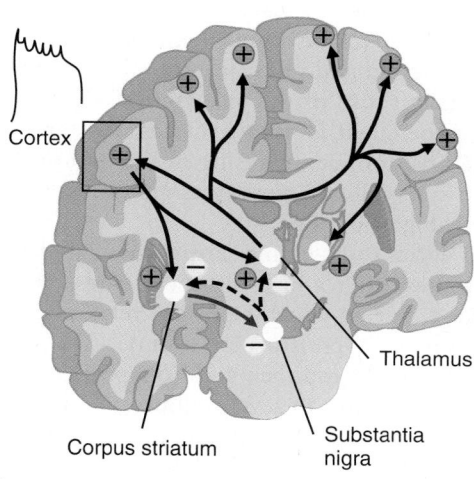

FIGURE 71-1 **A,** Normally, excitatory messages from the cerebral cortex are modulated by deeper structures. **B,** In clients with epilepsy, bursts of activity from the cortex are not modulated and these bursts spread. (From Devinsky, O. [1994]. Seizure disorders. *Clinical Symposia, 46*[1], 1-54. Modified from an original illustration in *Clinical Symposia,* illustrated by John Craig, M.D., copyright by Ciba-Geigy Corporation.)

seizures (the interictal period). According to this classification, there are two major categories of seizures. The neurologic abnormality may be limited to a specific part or focus of the brain, hence the term *partial seizures*. Additionally, the seizure may involve the entire cortical surface, to produce a generalized seizure exist.[46]

Partial (Focal, Local) Seizures with No Loss of Consciousness

Partial seizures are the most common type of epilepsy. The first clinical and electroencephalographic changes indicate initial activation of neurons in one part of the cerebral hemisphere. They are further classified according to whether or not consciousness is impaired. There are four types of simple partial seizures that do not impair consciousness. These include seizures with motor manifestations, those with somatosensory or "special senses" manifestations, those with autonomic manifestations, and psychic manifestations.[46]

Motor Manifestations. Partial seizures with motor manifestations arise from a focus in the region of the brain's motor cortex. The resulting motor activity (seizure) occurs in the part of the body innervated by motor neurons originating in the affected region of the cortex. Because the hand and fingers have the largest cortical representation, many focal motor seizures begin with convulsive movement in an upper extremity. Involuntary movements may spread centrally and involve the entire limb, and even the same side of the face and lower extremity. This progression or spread is known as the "Jacksonian march." The client also may exhibit changes in posture or spoken utterances.[46]

Somatosensory or Special Senses Manifestations. If the epileptogenic focus is in the parietal region, the client experiences sensory phenomena such as numbness and tingling in the affected area. If the focus is in the occipital region, the client may experience bright, flashing lights in the field of vision opposite the side of the focus. Likewise, the client can have changes in speech or taste. Involvement of the posterior temporal area of the dominant hemisphere (usually the left) causes difficulty with speaking, or aphasia.[46]

Autonomic Manifestations. Stimulation of the autonomic system produces epigastric sensations, pallor, sweating, flushing, piloerection (goose flesh), pupillary dilation, tachycardia, and tachypnea.[46]

Psychic Manifestations. Seizures arising in the anterior temporal lobe can begin with psychic manifestations. These seizures frequently begin with an aura, a subjective sensation that helps localize the focus. An aura may be a strange smell, noise, or sensation preceding a seizure, or a sense of "rising" or "welling up" in the epigastric region. Visual distortions and feelings such as déjà vu are common.[46]

Complex Partial Seizures

There are two types of complex partial seizures: complex partial seizures with automatisms and partial seizures evolving into generalized seizures.

Complex Partial Seizures with Automatisms. The most characteristic features of a complex partial seizure are the accompanying *automatisms*. These automatic behaviors include purposeless repetitive activities such as lip-smacking, chewing, patting a part of the body, or picking at clothes while in a dreamy state. Inappropriate or antisocial behavior may also automatically occur during the seizure. This unusual behavior may cause the client to be viewed as psychotic or otherwise mentally disturbed. However, some abnormalities are subtle and may not be detected by an untrained observer.

Temporal lobe seizures usually last 2 to 3 minutes but may last up to 15 minutes. The client is usually unaware of any activity during the seizure and may be confused or drowsy postictally. Attempts to restrain the client during a seizure may induce combative and uncooperative behavior.[46]

Partial Seizures Evolving to Secondary Generalized Seizures. These seizures start from a particular focus, and then the electrical discharges spread throughout the brain. Clinically, the client first shows focal manifestations; for example, one side of the face moves, and then the whole body becomes involved. Consciousness is lost if the discharges spread throughout the brain.[46]

Generalized Seizures

Generalized seizures lead to a loss of consciousness. They can be convulsive or nonconvulsive. Generalized seizures begin with manifestations involving both hemispheres. Consciousness may be impaired, which may be the first clinical manifestation. About one third of seizures are generalized. Types of generalized seizures are absence, myoclonic, clonic, tonic, tonic-clonic, and atonic.[46]

Absence Seizures. Absence seizures occur in childhood and early adolescence. "Grand mal" or partial seizures may develop at any time in clients who have had absence seizures.[46]

Myoclonic Seizures. Myoclonic seizures involve sudden uncontrollable jerking movements of either a single muscle group or multiple groups, sometimes causing the client to fall. The client loses consciousness for a moment and then is confused postictally. These seizures often occur in the morning, and clients often report that they spill their coffee with their fall.[46]

Clonic Seizures. The clinical manifestations of clonic seizures include rhythmic muscular contraction and relaxation lasting several minutes. Distinct phases of clonic seizures are not easily observed.[46]

Tonic Seizures. Tonic seizures include an abrupt increase in muscular tone and muscular contraction. In addition, with tonic seizures there is a loss of consciousness and the presence of autonomic manifestations.

Tonic seizures may last from 30 seconds to several minutes.[46]

Tonic-Clonic Seizures. Formerly known as "grand mal" seizures, tonic-clonic seizures are the type of seizures most closely associated with epilepsy. However, this type of generalized seizure comprises only 10% of all seizures. A tonic-clonic seizure typically proceeds as follows:

1. Aura may or may not be present.
2. Sudden loss of consciousness may occur.
3. In the tonic phase, the entire body becomes rigid (Figure 71-2, *A*). If standing or sitting, the client falls stiffly to the floor. A cry may be uttered. Respirations are interrupted temporarily, and the client may become cyanotic. The jaw is fixed and the hands are clenched. The eyes may be opened wide; the pupils are dilated and fixed. The tonic phase lasts 30 to 60 seconds. At the end of this phase the client breathes deeply.
4. The clonic phase begins next, with rhythmic, jerky contraction and relaxation of all body muscles, especially those of the extremities (see Figure 71-2, *B*). The client is usually incontinent and may bite the lips, tongue, or inside of the mouth. Excessive saliva is blown from the mouth, which creates frothing at the lips.
5. An entire tonic-clonic seizure may last from 2 to 5 minutes, after which the client enters the postictal phase, during which he or she relaxes and remains totally unresponsive for a time. The client may rouse briefly and then go into a postictal sleep lasting 30 minutes to several hours. This sleep may be followed by general fatigue, depression, confusion, or headache, all of which gradually resolve. The client has complete amnesia for the seizure episode and may feel nauseated, stiff, and sore. Bruising may occur as the result of falls. Petechial hemorrhages may develop on the face and chest due to the vasovagal responses. Falling during the seizure may cause other injury.

Tonic-clonic seizures vary in frequency from many times daily to once or twice a year. Tonic-only and clonic-only seizures may also occur.[21,46,50]

Atonic Seizures. Atonic seizures are associated with a total loss of muscle tone. They may be mild, with the client briefly nodding the head, or the client may fall to the floor. Consciousness is impaired only briefly.[46]

Diagnostic Tests

The major diagnostic tool for assessment of clients suspected of having epilepsy is the EEG (see Chapter 69). This test assists in (1) locating the focus of abnormal electrical discharges, if present, (2) establishing a diagnosis of epilepsy, and (3) identifying the specific type of

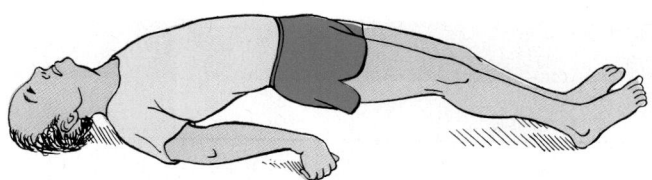

A Tonic phase

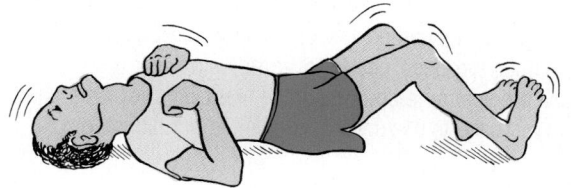

B Clonic phase

FIGURE 71-2 **A,** The tonic phase of a seizure is marked by loss of consciousness, falling, crying, and generalized stiffness. There may be incontinence. **B,** During the clonic phase, there is jerking of the limbs and salivary frothing.

seizures. The EEG records only the electrical activity of the cerebral cortex. With this limitation, a normal EEG tracing does not always exclude a diagnosis of epilepsy, and EEG abnormalities do not always confirm the diagnosis. During a seizure, EEG abnormalities involve all parts of the cortex. Between seizures, clients with epilepsy may show EEG abnormalities not characteristic of seizure disorders. An ambulatory EEG study can be used to clarify suspected seizures that occur frequently. The monitor used is similar to a Holter monitor. Long-term video EEG monitoring may also be used to rule out pseudoseizures.

Occasionally, diagnostic tests such as skull radiography, computed tomography (CT), and magnetic resonance imaging (MRI) are used to rule out brain lesions that can trigger seizures. Positron emission tomography (PET) and single-photon emission computed tomography (SPECT) may be helpful to measure cerebral blood flow in clients undergoing surgery for epilepsy. As important as the EEG and other diagnostic studies are, a complete seizure profile and history must be established. The seizure profile includes a baseline neurologic examination and description of the seizure activity, as well as laboratory studies.[21,52]

Outcome Management
■ Medical Management

The goals of management of clients with seizures and epilepsy are to prevent injury during seizures, to eliminate factors that precipitate seizures, to diagnose and treat the cause of the seizure, and to control seizures to allow a desired lifestyle.

Prevent Injury During a Seizure. During a seizure, the major goals are to maintain the airway, to prevent injury

to the client, to observe the seizure activity, and to administer appropriate anticonvulsant medications. Currently, "seizure precautions" as identified in a hospital setting refers to the availability of an oral airway and suction equipment. In the home or the community, turning the person to his or her side displaces the tongue and usually results in an open airway once the tonic phase has ceased. Any tight clothing around the person's neck is loosened.

The person experiencing a seizure usually requires protection from the environment. For example, objects should be moved out of the way so that the client does not strike his or her head or extremities. Put a pillow or folded blanket under the affected person's head, but do not flex the neck sharply or close the airway.

Observers' descriptions of a seizure can be helpful in making a diagnosis, especially if the descriptions include details such as the sequence in which phenomena occurred. Instruct the family and unlicensed assistive personnel to make the following observations:
- How long did the seizure last?
- Where in the body did the seizure begin and how did it progress?
- Did the client's eyes or head deviate?
- Were the respirations labored or frothy?
- Was the client incontinent?
- Did the client lose consciousness?
- What were the types of movements and what body parts moved?

Eliminate Factors That Precipitate Seizures. For decades, the main antiepileptic drugs (AEDs) were phenytoin (Dilantin), phenobarbital, carbamazepine (Tegretol), and valproate sodium (Depakote). Since the 1990s, other AEDs have been approved and show promising effectiveness. Currently available antiepileptic drugs appear to act primarily by blocking the initiation or spread of seizures. (See the Integrating Pharmacology feature on Antiseizure Drugs on p. 2078.)

Phenytoin, fosphenytoin sodium (Cerebyx), carbamazepine, valproic acid, and lamotrigine inhibit sodium-dependent action potentials, blocking the burst and firing neurons in a seizure focus. Phenytoin also appears to suppress seizure spread through inhibition of specific voltage-gated calcium channels.

Benzodiazepines and barbiturates augment inhibition by distinct interactions with gamma-aminobutyric acid (GABA) receptors (see the Unit 16 Anatomy and Physiology Review). Valproic acid elevates the concentration of GABA in the brain, perhaps through interaction with enzymes involved in the synthesis (glutamic acid decarboxylase) and catabolism (GABA transaminase) of GABA. Gabapentin, which is a structural analog of GABA, appears to increase GABA levels by enhancing GABA synthesis and release and may also cause a decrease in glutamate synthesis. The two most effective drugs for absence

INTEGRATING PHARMACOLOGY

Antiseizure Drugs

Many seizure disorders are controlled by various types of anti-seizure drugs (sometimes called anticonvulsants). As well, different types of seizures require different medications. Epilepsy medication may be prescribed alone or in combination. If a client has more than one type of seizure, he or she may have to take more than one type of drug to gain control. More than 20 different antiepileptic drugs are available, all with different benefits and side effects. The choice of which drug to prescribe, and at what dosage, depends on many different factors, including the type of seizures, the person's lifestyle and age, how frequently the seizures occur, and, for a woman, the likelihood that she will become pregnant. People with epilepsy should follow their physician's advice and share any concerns they may have regarding their medication.

The first line of drug therapy is often carbamazepine, valproate, or phenytoin, unless the epilepsy is a type that is known to require a different kind of treatment. For absence seizures, ethosuximide is often the primary treatment. For the client with stereotyped recurrent severe seizures that can be easily recognized by the person's family, the drug diazepam is available as a gel that can be administered rectally by a family member. This method of drug delivery may stop prolonged seizures before they develop into status epilepticus.

Most side effects of antiepileptic drugs are relatively minor, such as fatigue, dizziness, or weight gain. However, severe and life-threatening side effects such as allergic reactions can occur. Epilepsy medication also may predispose people to developing depression or psychoses. Clients with epilepsy should consult a physician immediately if they develop any kind of rash while on medication, or if they find themselves depressed or otherwise unable to think in a rational manner. Other danger signs that should be discussed with a physician immediately are extreme fatigue, staggering or other movement problems, and slurring of words. Clients with epilepsy should be aware that their epilepsy medication can interact with many other drugs in potentially harmful ways. For this reason, people with epilepsy should always tell their treating physicians which medications they are taking. Women also should know that some antiepileptic drugs can interfere with the effectiveness of oral contraceptives, and they should discuss this possibility with their physicians.

Because older adults are more sensitive to medications, blood levels of medication are checked occasionally to determine whether the dose needs to be adjusted. The effects of a particular medication also sometimes wear off over time, leading to an increase in seizures if the dose is not adjusted.

Discontinuing Medication

Some physicians advise clients with epilepsy to discontinue their antiepileptic drugs after 2 years have passed without a seizure. Others believe it is better to wait for 4 to 5 years. Discontinuing medication should only be done with a physician's advice and supervision. It is very important to continue taking epilepsy medication for as long as it is prescribed. Clients should ask their physician or pharmacist ahead of time what they should do if they miss a dose. Discontinuing medication without a physician's advice is one of the major reasons people who have been seizure-free begin having new seizures. Seizures that result from suddenly stopping medication can be serious and can lead to status epilepticus. Furthermore, there is some evidence that uncontrolled seizures trigger changes in neurons that can make it more difficult to treat the seizures in the future.

The chance that a client will eventually be able to discontinue medication depends on the person's age and his or her type of epilepsy. More than half of children who go into remission with medication can eventually stop their medication without having new seizures. One study showed that 68% of adults who had been seizure-free for 2 years before stopping medication were able to do so without having more seizures and that 75% could successfully discontinue medication if they had been seizure-free for 3 years. However, the odds of successfully stopping medication are not as good for clients with a family history of epilepsy, those who need multiple medications, those with partial seizures, or those who continue to have abnormal EEG results while on medication.

seizures, ethosuximide and valproic acid, probably act by reducing calcium conduction in thalamic neurons.

In contrast to the relatively large number of antiepileptic drugs that can attenuate seizure activity, there are no drugs known to prevent the formation of a seizure focus after CNS injury in humans. The eventual development of such "antiepileptogenic" drugs will provide an important means of preventing the emergence of epilepsy after injuries such as head trauma, stroke, and CNS infection.

The use of AEDs is not without adverse effects. Although myriad adverse effects can occur, for the most part they can be grouped into three categories: idiosyncratic, dose-related, and allergic reactions. It is the responsibility of the nurse, as well as of other health care team members, to instruct the client about the action, dosing, and possible side effects of the various AEDs. Developing a program of correctly prescribed anticonvulsants requires weeks of medication adjustment by trial and error. (See the Integrating Pharmacology feature on Antiseizure Drugs, above.) The desired outcome of pharmacologic management is monotherapy (use of one anticonvulsant medication).[20,46] Large doses of a single anticonvulsant are often more helpful than smaller doses of several drugs. Ideally, initial treatment begins

COMPLEMENTARY AND ALTERNATIVE THERAPY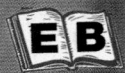

Low Carbohydrate or Ketogenic Diet for Seizures

The ketogenic diet (KD) is actually a non-drug therapy for epileptic seizures. It was developed in the 1920s and was based on the clinical observation that fasting suppresses seizures, probably through the induction of ketosis. Interestingly, the high-fat, low-carbohydrate KD tends to mimic the ketogenic effects of fasting and places the body into a constant state of ketosis. KD suppresses many different types of seizures, including those that do not respond to the conventional anticonvulsant drugs. The KD is given only after drug therapy has failed to provide adequate seizure control. KD is effective for tonic-clonic, absence, complex partial, and the multiple types of intractable seizures associated with the Lennox-Gastaut syndrome.

Reference
Likhodii, S., et al. (2003). Anticonvulsant properties of acetone, a brain ketone elevated by the ketogenic diet. *Annals of Neurology, 54,* 219-226.

CLIENT EDUCATION GUIDE
Epilepsy

- Take prescribed dosages of medications to maintain your blood levels.
- Consult your physician if you are unable to take medication because of illness.
- Observe for side effects of anticonvulsant drugs. Do not stop taking medications because of annoying side effects; this is very dangerous. Consult your physician first.
- Notify the physician if seizure activity is not being controlled. Provide specific descriptions of the seizure activity.
- Do not take any over-the-counter medications without consulting your physician.
- Obtain a medical alert identification card (or bracelet or tag) with the name of the drug, dosage, and frequency, and your physician's name and phone number. Carry this identification with you at all times.

with a single drug (primary anticonvulsant) until either seizure control is attained or unacceptable side effects appear. If side effects become intolerable before seizures are controlled, another drug is added. Combining medications does carry the potential risk of drug-drug interactions, which decrease effectiveness. For more information on non-drug therapies, see the Complementary and Alternative Therapy feature on Low Carbohydrate or Ketogenic Diet for Seizures, above.

■ Nursing Management of the Medical Client

The management of epilepsy does not usually involve hospitalization. However, a client may initially be hospitalized for assessment, diagnosis, and education immediately after a first seizure (i.e., in a person with previously undiagnosed epilepsy). Hospitalization may also be required if seizures become uncontrolled or if status epilepticus develops. Nurses have a role in assessing for Ineffective Health Maintenance related to knowledge deficit or other barriers, anticipating risk of injury, and providing support for clients and their families who experience life changes related to seizure disorders.

Assessment

Assessment of clients not actively experiencing seizures includes the following:
- History, including prenatal, birth, and developmental history; family history; age at seizure onset; history of all illnesses and trauma; previous brain sur-

gery or stroke; complete description of seizures, including precipitating factors; and presence of an aura
- Medication use and postictal (period of time following a seizure) manifestations
- Psychosocial assessment, including mental status examination
- Complete physical examination, focusing on neurologic manifestations (usually physical findings between seizures are normal)

Diagnosis, Outcomes, Interventions

Diagnosis: Ineffective Health Maintenance. *Ineffective Health Maintenance* is the nursing diagnosis appropriate for clients who are having difficulty adjusting their life to their epileptic condition.

Outcomes. The client will have improved health maintenance related to knowledge deficit, as evidenced by maintaining routine dosing, consulting a physician whenever there is a problem, and wearing a medical alert identification tag or bracelet.

Interventions. Provide the client with verbal information and written reinforcement about (1) how anticonvulsants prevent seizures, (2) the importance of taking prescribed medication regularly, and (3) care during seizures. Consult with the client to plan ways to make taking medication part of daily activities (e.g., keeping medication by the toothbrush). Also, help the client to identify factors that precipitate seizures and ways of avoiding these factors. Such factors include increased stress, lack of sleep, emotional upset, and alcohol use. See the Client Education Guide feature on Epilepsy above for other important teaching information.

Evaluation

The short-term outcomes for the client who is experiencing a seizure are usually met within hours. An example is that the seizure stops and the client returns to the previous level of functioning. Nursing care of clients with confirmed epilepsy should focus on the long-term outcomes with self-care.

■ Modifications for Older Clients

With the increasing frequency of epilepsy in the older population, nurses need to be more aware of the changes in pharmacokinetics in this age group. Concurrent disease, foods, and drug-drug interactions affect absorption of anticonvulsant medication. A decrease in albumin, as is commonly seen in the older adult, can increase the free plasma level of these drugs. Decreased metabolism can increase the half-life of these drugs, and decreased elimination can result in higher plasma levels.

Enteral feedings inhibit the absorption of phenytoin (Dilantin). Therefore the feeding should be turned off 2 hours before and after administration of phenytoin, or the dose should be altered on the basis of plasma levels. Altered vitamin D metabolism with phenytoin increases the risk of osteoporosis. Carbamazepine (Tegretol) carries an increased risk of slowed cardiac conduction and heart failure; hyponatremia secondary to increased secretion of antidiuretic hormone, especially if the client is on a low-sodium diet; and altered cholesterol metabolism in the older population. Valproate (Depakene) carries an increased risk of causing hyperammonemia in older clients, leading to hepatic dysfunction, decrease in platelets, and toxicity related to its longer half-life in this population.[21,26,45,51-53]

■ Surgical Management

For approximately 75% of clients with seizures, medical management with AEDs and follow-up evaluation suffices. The remaining 25% continue to have seizures. For about 5% of people with epilepsy, surgery is recommended to control the disease.

The safest and most effective surgical treatment is cortical resection of the anterior temporal lobe for complex partial seizures.[10,16] Criteria for resection include (1) failure of the medical approach and (2) localization and identification of a focus of abnormal discharge that is easily accessible surgically and is located in the "dispensable" areas of the cerebral cortex. Dispensable areas are those for which there is a duplicative area in the cortex.

Thorough assessment is necessary before surgery. This is usually done in three phases:

- *Phase 1* involves using video EEG, SPECT, or PET to locate the epileptogenic focus.[41] Intelligence quotient (IQ) testing and psychological assessments are usually performed.[50,68]

- *Phase 2* is used when surface EEG electrodes are not sensitive enough to locate the seizure focus exactly. Depth electrodes are placed in the temporal and frontal lobes of the brain or in the subdural space. These techniques allow detailed maps of the brain for surgery.[18]

- *Phase 3* involves cerebral angiography with *Wada's test* to determine hemispheric dominance and location of the speech center. The functional supremacy of one cerebral hemisphere is crucial to language function. Wada's test is a method of determining which side of the brain is dominant for speech production. An injection of amobarbital sodium (Amytal Sodium) is introduced into the left internal carotid artery. If the left hemisphere is dominant, speech is arrested for 1 or 2 minutes, followed by misnaming and misreading for 8 to 9 minutes altogether. After 30 minutes, the process is repeated in the right internal carotid artery. The physician looks for changes in sensation, abstract thought, and coordination. Postprocedural care is the same as for cerebral angiography (see Chapter 69).[54]

Cortical Resection/Corpus Callosotomy. Corpus callosal resection is considered palliative surgery designed to make the seizures more tolerable. It involves the excision of one section of cortex to reduce the spread of epileptic discharges (Figure 71-3, *A*). One complication, called *disconnection syndrome,* results when the pathways responsible for communication from one hemisphere to another are severed. Clinical manifestations range from motor apraxias and mutism to minimal losses detected only on neuropsychological testing. Staged resections are performed to reduce the risk of disconnection syndrome.[49,67]

Temporal Lobectomy. This form of curative surgery for epilepsy is performed to remove the area in which the seizures begin without causing neurologic or cognitive deficits (see Figure 71-3, *B*). If the dominant hemisphere is removed, the client experiences some language defects for a few weeks. Visual defects from loss of visual projection fibers are compensated for quickly.[49,67]

Hemispherectomy. Removal of most of the cortex of one hemisphere is done in children with intractable seizures to control those that are injurious, not to stop all seizures (see Figure 71-3, *C*).[49,67]

Vagal Nerve Stimulator Implantation. The implantation of a vagal nerve stimulator (VNS) offers clients another treatment modality. Although the underlying mechanism is not fully understood, the VNS is believed to provide a stimulus that desynchronizes the abnormal uncontrolled electrical discharge of the brain activity

Corpus callosotomy

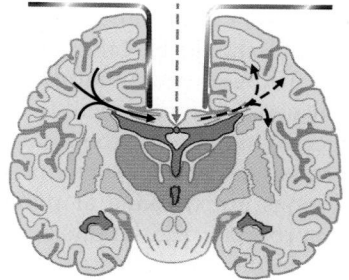

A

Division of the corpus callosum disrupts the interhemispheric pathway for secondary generalization of partial seizures (unilateral seizure focus)

Temporal lobectomy

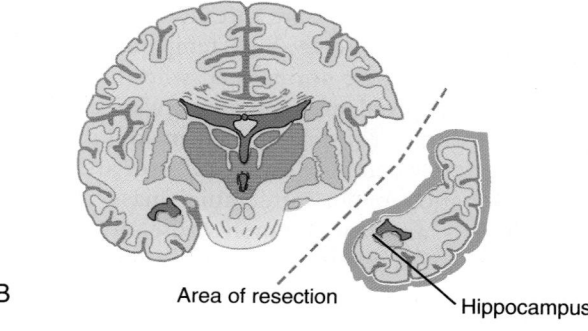

B   Area of resection   Hippocampus

Hemispherectomy

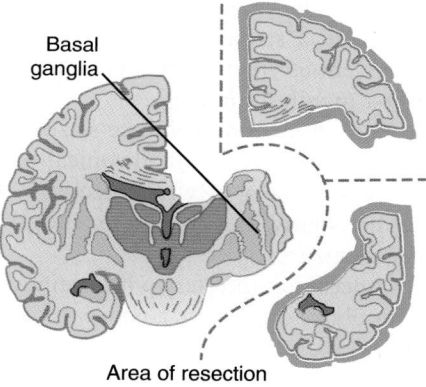

Basal ganglia

C   Area of resection

FIGURE 71-3 Surgery for epilepsy can consist of corpus callosotomy (**A**), temporal lobectomy (**B**), or hemispherectomy (**C**). (From Devinsky, O. [1994]. Seizure disorders. *Clinical Symposia, 46*[1], 1-54. Modified from an original illustration in *Clinical Symposia,* illustrated by John Craig, M.D., copyright by Ciba-Geigy Corporation.)

during a seizure. One study has reported that the benefit from VNS increases over time. For example, 40% to 45% of clients continue to experience a decrease in the frequency of seizures at 18 months after implantation of the VNS.[40,50,57,65]

■ Nursing Management of the Surgical Client

Preoperative Care

The role of the nurse during the evaluation phase before surgery is to provide support and education. Clients who have epilepsy have been trying to control their seizures for most of their lives. Now, as part of the preoperative assessment, the health care team needs to observe the client during seizure activity. Therefore AEDs are tapered and discontinued. This withdrawal of effective medication is often confusing and frightening. In addition, some clients are far from family and may be rethinking their decision to undergo surgery. Memory impairments are common because of both the side effects of medications and postictal states. Be certain to provide written material and reinforce education often.[28,50]

Postoperative Care

Postoperative nursing care is the same as for any client undergoing a craniotomy (see later discussion). The client is often placed in an intensive care unit (ICU) to facilitate frequent assessment. Anticonvulsant medications are resumed immediately after surgery as well as after leaving the hospital.[35,48]

■ Self-Care

It is important for the client with epilepsy to live as normal a life as possible. The client and family members must learn to accept the condition and not exaggerate it or overprotect the client. Although certain dangerous activities should be avoided or performed with special safeguards (e.g., swimming or horseback riding), a wide range of activities can still be enjoyed. Driving motor vehicles depends on state laws and the client's medical control of seizures. There is a wide range of time during which the client must be seizure-free before driving. Times can range from 3 months to 2 years. This restriction on driving can be emotionally and economically devastating for clients of all ages and socioeconomic backgrounds.

A regular pattern of adequate diet, fluid intake, sleep, and moderate recreation and exercise is helpful. Many clients find that skipping meals or not getting enough sleep lowers the threshold for seizures. Alcoholic beverages are contraindicated for two reasons. First, alcohol lowers the seizure threshold; second, alcohol is detoxified by the liver. Most anticonvulsant drugs are also metabolized by the liver. Consuming alcohol while taking an anticonvulsant places an increased strain on the metabolizing functions of the liver.

For some clients, the psychosocial impact of epilepsy is overwhelming. Because most seizures occur without warning, many clients spend their lives anticipating inappropriate behavior, embarrassment, and self-injury.

Clients with epilepsy often have a poor self-image, feelings of inferiority, self-consciousness, guilt, anger, depression, and other emotional problems. Education and support groups can help clients deal with the emotional impact of epilepsy.

The client and family members should be taught that epilepsy is a chronic disorder that requires long-term management. Even though the client may have been seizure-free for some time, it is important to take medication as prescribed. Phenytoin, a common anticonvulsant, leads to excessive gingival (gum tissue) growth. Brushing two to three times daily helps retard gingival growth. Some clients have excess gingival tissue excised every 6 to 12 months. Medications may also cause diplopia, ataxia, sedation, and bone marrow depression. Most anticonvulsant drugs require periodic monitoring of serum drug levels, liver function, and complete blood counts. Clients with epilepsy should always wear or carry identification stating that they have epilepsy and providing the name and telephone number of their physician.

If the client is able to recognize that certain activities trigger the seizure, the activities can be avoided, or the client can be desensitized in some cases. For example, flickering lights can trigger seizures. Fluorescent lights and flickering shadows from trees on the road while driving during the late afternoon are common precipitants of seizures. If the client experiences an aura, precautions should be taken immediately to prevent self-injury from the impending seizure—for example, lying down on the ground or floor or, if driving a vehicle, pulling over to the side of the road and lying on the seat. Instruct clients to carry a large pillow in the vehicle or to use the arms to protect the head.

Some clients with epilepsy cannot find employment if they admit to having seizures. However, falsifying job applications can result in dismissal from employment. These factors contribute to a higher incidence of depression among clients with epilepsy. Nurses can educate the public regarding epilepsy and help to dissipate prejudices. When discussing the long-term impact of epilepsy with the client, be empathetic but realistic. It is hoped the client can accept the lifestyle limitations of the disorder and not be overwhelmed by them.[5]

The client's family needs to know what to do in the event of a seizure. The affected person should be protected from self-injury. Clothing should be loosened, the head protected from impact, and sharp objects in the environment removed. The person should not be forcibly restrained during a seizure but protected from self-injury. Hard objects or fingers should not be inserted into the mouth. People experiencing a seizure do not swallow the tongue—a common misconception. However, the tongue can occlude the airway, and positioning the head is important to protect the airway. After the head is protected from injury, the person should be placed in a side-lying position to displace the tongue and allow oral secretions to drain from the airway. Someone should stay with the person until full consciousness has returned. An ambulance should be called if the seizure lasts for longer than 10 minutes, if another seizure occurs before consciousness returns, if there is respiratory difficulty on evidence of injury, or if the person is pregnant. Sleepiness is common in the postictal period.

Various organizations are working at public education, introducing appropriate legislation, and assisting people with epilepsy. In the United States, these include the Epilepsy Foundation of America and Epilepsy Services. Similar organizations exist in other countries.

SEIZURES

Not all seizures are epileptic. Not only do clients differ in their susceptibility to experiencing a seizure, but they also have variations in seizure thresholds. For example, seizures may be induced by high temperatures in children who are otherwise normal and who never develop other neurologic problems, including epilepsy.

The cause of seizures varies widely in adults. Brain tumors are the most common cause. Seizures are often the first manifestation of an intracranial mass. Traumatic brain injury is another common cause of seizures in young adults. With severe closed head injuries, seizures occur in a small percentage of clients. However, with open head injuries in which the skull and dura are penetrated, the incidence of seizures increases markedly.

Cerebrovascular disease is the most common cause of seizures in clients older than age 50 years. These seizures usually accompany a stroke. In other vascular lesions, such as arteriovenous malformations (AVMs), seizures may be the first manifestation.[45]

CNS infections frequently produce seizures, either in the acute phase of infection or chronically thereafter. Seizures can be a sequela of viral infections, brain abscesses, and meningitis. Postinfectious encephalitis can cause persistent seizures.

Toxic substances that interfere with brain metabolism or with the supply of oxygen or glucose to the brain can cause seizures. Alcohol is one of the most frequently ingested toxins and can cause seizures either during ingestion or during withdrawal. Chronic substance abuse, especially of barbiturates, can lead to seizures when the drug is withdrawn (see Chapter 26).

Simulated convulsive episodes may occur in clients with psychiatric disorders. These are called "pseudoseizures." One key to differentiating between pseudoseizures and actual seizures is to look for stereotypical movements and a paroxysmal nature of the episodes. Clients with recurrent seizures exhibit the same stereotypic movements with each seizure. Clients exhibiting pseudoseizure make different movements with each seizure.[35,52]

Management of the client who is experiencing a single seizure focuses on protecting the client during the seizure and then identifying and correcting the underlying problem. Care of clients during a seizure is as discussed earlier.

Controversy exists over the best pharmacologic approach to seizure management. Many authorities recommend a single antiepileptic drug therapy approach, which decreases the risk of drug interactions and adverse effects, makes monitoring easier, and increases client compliance.

STATUS EPILEPTICUS

Status epilepticus, a medical emergency, is a state in which a client has continuous seizures or seizures in rapid succession, without regaining consciousness, lasting at least 30 minutes. The most common cause of status epilepticus is the sudden withdrawal of anticonvulsant medication. During a seizure, the brain's metabolic needs increase dramatically. If these heightened requirements continue without opportunity for the body to recover, the supply of glucose and oxygen to the brain becomes inadequate, and permanent brain damage may occur.

Outcome Management

The major goals in managing a client with status epilepticus are to establish and protect the airway, to control the seizure, and to monitor for cessation or other outcomes.

The airway is maintained and aspiration prevented by placing the client in a side-lying position, suctioning the airway, and providing oxygen. Oxygen offers nothing to a client who is apneic; therefore intubation may be necessary to ventilate and oxygenate the client.

Anticonvulsant medications are given to terminate seizures and to prevent exhaustion. Intravenous (IV) infusion is begun immediately and maintained during treatment. Status epilepticus is treated with diazepam in doses of 5 to 10 mg (0.2 mg/kg) given every 10 to 20 minutes, for a total dose of up to 30 mg in an 8-hour period. Lorazepam (0.1 mg/kg) can also be given in 4-mg doses given over 2 to 5 minutes, repeated every 10 to 15 minutes to a maximum of 8 mg (0.2 mg/kg). In addition, phenytoin can be given to a total dose of 15 to 18 mg/kg by slow IV push (no more than 50 mg/min). Assess the client for bradycardia and heart block while phenytoin is given. If this agent is not effective, diazepam or lorazepam can be used. Because all of these medications can depress respiration, emergency ventilation equipment should be readily available.

If diazepam or lorazepam is not effective, pentobarbital can be used to bring on a barbiturate coma and suppress brain activity. Inducing coma is used only after the anticonvulsant treatments have been tried and have not been successful. The client in barbiturate coma is ventilator-dependent and requires nursing care in an ICU.

A last resort involves the use of general anesthesia. If a general anesthetic agent or a neuromuscular blocking agent such as vecuronium bromide (Norcuron) is required, the client requires mechanical ventilation, continuous EEG monitoring, and hemodynamic monitoring.

The client's neurologic status is assessed frequently. Even when the status epilepticus has been controlled, the client may be unresponsive for a period of time. Absence of manifestations of seizure does not mean the seizure has stopped. The manifestations may not be evident. Semiconscious clients thought to be in a postictal state have been found to be still experiencing seizure. After the seizures have been controlled, maintenance anticonvulsants are prescribed.

Clients experiencing status epilepticus are especially difficult for significant others to watch. They need support and assessment. Always explain to family members the treatment being given.[21,26,35,48-50]

BRAIN TUMORS

Brain tumors are identified as primary or secondary lesions. Tumors arising from the brain or its supporting structures are called *primary* brain tumors; those metastasizing from other areas in the body are *secondary* tumors. Brain tumors may also be referred to as *intra-axial* or *extra-axial*. Intra-axial tumors are those originating from the glial cells (cells supporting the neurons) and arise from within the cerebrum, cerebellum, or brain stem. Extra-axial tumors have their origin in the skull, meninges, cranial nerves, or pituitary gland.

The Central Brain Tumor Registry for the United States (CBTRUS) estimated that 190,600 brain tumors would be diagnosed in the United States in 2003. Of that total, 40,600 were estimated to be primary brain tumors and 150,000 to be secondary or metastatic. The overall incidence for primary brain and CNS tumors is 14 cases per 100,000 person years. The incidence of brain tumors appears to be increasing but may reflect improved and earlier diagnosis.[2,13,55,56] CBTRUS notes that, as of 2000, approximately 359,000 people in the United States were living with a primary brain tumor, with 75% having benign tumors and 23% having malignant tumors.

Etiology

A clear etiologic factor has not been established for any of the primary brain tumors. Although the type of cell that gives rise to the tumor can often be identified, the mechanism causing the cells to act abnormally remains unknown. Most primary brain tumors do not metastasize out of the brain to other areas. Neuroscience researchers are searching for the answers. Familial tendencies, immunosuppression, and environmental factors are being considered.[2,13,16,55,56]

Pathophysiology

Space-Occupying Lesions

Brain tumors are described as "space-occupying lesions." This phrase explains that the tumor displaces normal tissue or occupies normal tissue spaces. When normal brain tissue is compressed, blood flow is altered and ischemia leading to necrosis may occur, destroying major functions.

Increased Intracranial Pressure

Not only are the tumors space-occupying lesions, but they also often produce considerable cerebral edema. The skull is a rigid, box-like structure, containing little room for expansion of any of the intracranial contents. Brain tumors cause progressively increased intracranial pressure (ICP), which leads to displacement of brain structures with herniation of the brain (see Chapter 75).

Intracranial Tumors

Intracranial tumors may arise from neurons (neuromas) or from the support cells, the neuroglial cells (gliomas). Brain tumors can be encapsulated, nonencapsulated, or invasive. Much confusion exists with regard to the pathologic and histologic nomenclature. Historically, staging or grading scales identified tumors as grade I (benign) through grade IV or V (malignant). The World Health Organization (WHO) classifies tumors using a three-tiered or four-tiered scale. The grading scales are determined according to the maturity of the tumor cells—for example, "mature cells, benign," or "immature cells, malignant"[28,33,49,67] (Box 71-1).

BOX 71-1	*Schema for Classifying Brain Tumors**
Astrocytoma	Increased number of astrocytes; mature astrocytes; normally developed astrocytes
Anaplastic astrocytoma	Increased number of less mature astrocytes; possibility of mitotic figures (mitotic figures represent increased cellular division and malignant changes)
Glioblastoma multiforme	Increased number of astrocyte cells; immature astrocytes; presence of mitotic figures; hemorrhage, necrosis, swelling, and obscure tumor margins

*This schema of astrocytoma, anaplastic tumor, and glioblastoma multiforme is also used for the astrocytoma, ependymoma, and oligodendroglioma.

Glial Tumors. Gliomas are tumors of the neuroglia (supporting brain tissue). Astrocytomas are the most common type of glial cell tumor and can be found throughout the brain or spinal cord. These tumors occur in adults and children. Depending on the exact location, clinical manifestations may result in increased ICP or focal compression.[49,67]

Oligodendrogliomas. Oligodendroglial cells are found in the CNS and produce myelin. Oligodendrogliomas are tumors of the white matter of the brain. They tend to develop in the cortex of the frontal and parietal lobes. This tumor is fairly slow-growing and calcifies, which makes it recognizable on x-ray studies. The calcification may contribute to the development of seizures as a presenting clinical manifestation. Oligodendrogliomas peak in clients between the ages of 30 and 50 years. Clinical manifestations in addition to seizures are headache, personality changes, and papilledema.[49,67]

Ependymomas. The ependymal cells line the ventricles and form the inner lining of the spinal cord. Ependymomas may be found anywhere within the CNS; however, there is an increased incidence in the fourth ventricle and intramedullary (within the spinal cord tissue). This tumor affects all age groups. Manifestations are caused by ventricular obstruction and include headache, vomiting, diplopia, dizziness, ataxia, vision changes, and motor and sensory abnormalities.[49,67]

Pituitary Tumors. Pituitary tumors are usually slow-growing tumors that involve only the anterior lobe of the pituitary gland or extend into the floor of the third ventricle. Most of these are benign, small, and encapsulated. Manifestations can be related to hypofunctioning of the gland and include visual field defects, irregular or absent menstrual cycles, infertility, decreased libido, impotence, decreased body hair, and decreased production of pituitary-stimulating hormones; this decrease results in decreased thyroid and adrenal function. Hypersecretion can also occur and is related to the hormones that are in excess. Combinations of hyposecretion and hypersecretion can also be seen. Manifestations of pituitary tumors are often overlooked for months because they are so diverse. Clients are usually diagnosed by testing blood for the presence of pituitary-stimulating hormones.[12,15,49,62,67]

Tumors of Supporting Structures. These tumors include meningiomas and acoustic neuromas.

Meningiomas. Meningiomas are common benign tumors that may involve all meningeal layers; however, these tumors are believed to originate in the arachnoid cells (Figure 71-4). Most meningiomas are benign, but some tumors may become malignant.[14] Meningiomas may be found in the brain or spinal cord. They are slow-growing and occur at any age, most commonly at midlife and in women. Manifestations depend on location of the tumor and can be diverse. Outcomes are related to the site of the tumor. Recurrence is a concern.[35,49,67]

Acoustic Neuromas. Acoustic neuromas are tumors of the Schwann cells of the eighth cranial nerve, the acoustic nerve. Manifestations are tinnitus, dizziness, and unilateral hearing loss. If the tumor is allowed to grow, it can displace the other cranial nerves—especially cranial nerves IV to X—and the brain stem. An excellent outcome can be expected with surgical resection and preservation of the remaining cranial nerves. However, most clients experience at least temporary tinnitus, balance problems, and facial weakness after surgery.[25,49,67]

Metastatic Brain Tumors

Metastatic brain tumors are those with primary sites outside of the brain. Cancers of the lung, breast, and kidney and malignant melanoma are the major sources

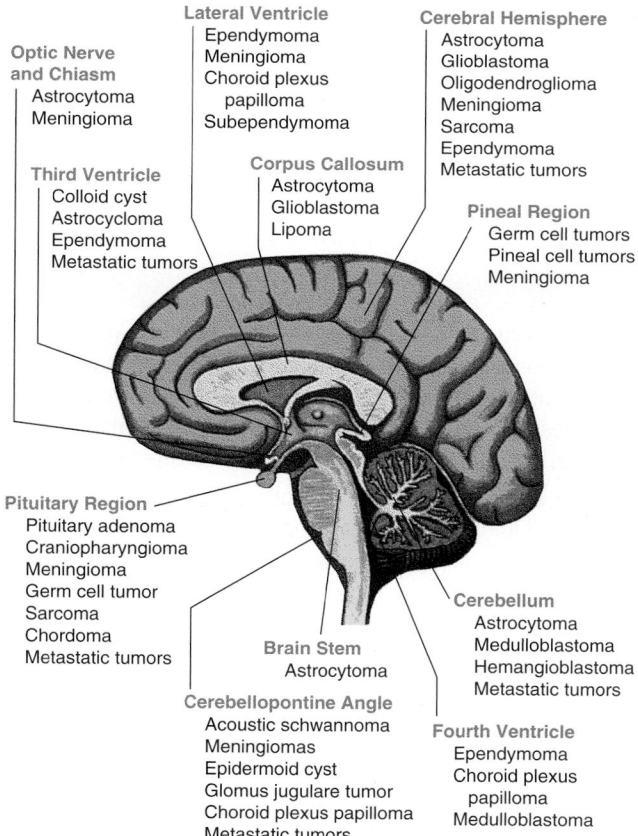

FIGURE 71-4 Common intracranial tumors and their usual locations. (Modified from Murphy, G.P., Lawrence, W., & Lenhard, R.E. [1995]. *American Cancer Society textbook of clinical oncology* [2nd ed., p. 381]. Atlanta: American Cancer Society.)

of metastatic brain cancers. The tumor location may also be within the brain or on the arachnoid. The common locations of brain tumors are shown in Figure 71-4.

Clinical Manifestations

General clinical manifestations are caused by changes in cerebral function resulting from edema and increased ICP. The classic triad of clinical manifestations for increased ICP is headache, nausea, and vomiting. Papilledema, a hallmark of increased ICP, is a clinical manifestation and is often added to the triad.

Mental Status Changes

As in any neurologic or neurosurgical disorder, a change in the level of consciousness (LOC) or sensorium is often noted. Mental and emotional status changes such as lethargy and drowsiness, confusion, disorientation, and personality changes may be found.

Headaches

Headaches may be localized or generalized and are most severe in the frontal or occipital region. They are usually intermittent, are of increasing duration, and may be intensified by a change in posture or straining. Recurrent, severe headaches in a client who was previously free of headaches, or recurrent headaches in the morning, increasing in frequency and severity, may indicate an intracranial tumor and indicate the need for further assessment.

Nausea and Vomiting

Classically, the clinical manifestations of nausea and vomiting are believed to occur because of pressure on the medulla, where the vomiting center is found. The occurrence of these manifestations may be related to generalized swelling, cerebral edema, increasing headache, and stimulation of the chemoemetic trigger zone (CETZ). The CETZ has numerous neural connections from areas within the cerebral hemispheres that transmit or synapse with the vomiting center in the medulla. In a frequent clinical scenario, the client complains of a severe headache after lying flat in bed. As the headache increases in severity, the client may also experience nausea related to the involvement of the CETZ. With increasing signaling to the vomiting center, the client then vomits. During the episode of emesis, the client may hyperventilate and after the episode may note that the headache is less severe.

Papilledema

Compression of the second cranial nerve, the optic nerve, may result in papilledema. The underlying pathophysiologic mechanism of papilledema is not clearly understood. The cause may be increased pressure in the central retinal vein as a result of obstructed venous return from the eye. Papilledema, also known as "choked disc," is common in clients with intracranial tumors and may be the first manifestation. Early papilledema does not cause visual acuity changes and can be detected only through an ophthalmologic examination. Prolonged papilledema causes optic atrophy and severely diminished visual acuity.

Seizures

Seizures, focal or generalized, are common in clients with intracranial tumors, especially cerebral hemisphere tumors (see earlier discussion).

Localized Manifestations

Localized clinical manifestations are caused by destruction, irritation, or compression of the part of the brain in or near the tumor. Blood supply to the affected area is also impaired. Localized manifestations include the following:

- Focal weaknesses (e.g., hemiparesis)
- Sensory disturbances, including absence of feeling (anesthesia) or abnormal sensation (paresthesia)
- Language disturbances
- Coordination disturbances (e.g., staggering gait)
- Visual disturbance such as diplopia (double vision) or visual field deficit (monopia)

As with other cranial disorders, the clinical manifestations associated with a brain tumor correlate with the area of the brain involved. Table 71-1 lists specific clinical manifestations based on tumor location. As an intracranial tumor enlarges, it shifts intracranial structures, which may lead to herniation.

Despite the availability of extremely sensitive and sophisticated equipment, brain tumor diagnosis is often delayed because of difficulty recognizing early manifestations. No two adults with the diagnosis of brain tumor present with the same clinical manifestations. Older clients especially fail to report such problems during regular examinations because they forget or think that the manifestations are "just part of growing old."

Diagnostic Findings

If an intracranial tumor is suspected, noninvasive studies such as CT, MRI, and x-ray examination are performed (Figure 71-5). Other disorders may be ruled out with EEG, radionuclide scans, angiogram, or lumbar puncture. A stereotactic biopsy may confirm the diagnosis of a brain tumor and help in planning chemotherapy and radiation therapy. Three-dimensional thresholding techniques help visualize the tumor's location in the brain and can assist with plans for resection. PET scans can also be used to study the biochemical and physiologic effects of the tumor.

TABLE 71-1	*Clinical Manifestations of Brain Tumors by Location*
Location	**Clinical Manifestations**
Frontal lobe	Disturbed mental state, apathy, inappropriate behavior, dementia, depression, emotional lability, inattentiveness, inability to concentrate, indifference, loss of self-restraint and social behavior, impaired long-term memory, difficulty with abstraction, quiet but flat affect, dominant hemisphere expressive speech disturbance, impaired sphincter control with bowel and bladder incontinence, motor disorders, gait disturbances, paralysis, "frontal release signs," seizures
Temporal lobe	Receptive aphasia, generalized psychomotor seizures, visual field changes, personality changes, ataxia, headache, manifestations of increased ICP, tinnitus, recent memory impairment
Parietal lobe	Sensory deficits, motor and sensory focal seizures, agnosias, hypoesthesias, paresthesias, dyslexia, visual field cut, diminished appreciation of side opposite the tumor, headache, apraxia, tactile inattention, right/left disorientation
Occipital lobe	Headache, manifestations of increased ICP, visual impairment (homonymous hemianopsia), visual agnosia, cortical blindness, hallucinations, seizures
Cerebellar	Unsteady gait, falling, ataxia, incoordination, tremors, head tilt, nystagmus, CSF obstruction/hydrocephalus, truncal ataxia if vermis is tumor site
Brain stem	Vertigo, dizziness, vomiting, CN III-XII palsies/dysfunction, nystagmus, decreased corneal reflex, headache, vomiting, gait disturbance, motor and sensory deficits, deafness, intranuclear ophthalmoplegia, sudden death from cardiac and respiratory failure
Pituitary and hypothalamus	Visual deficits, headache, hormonal dysfunction, sleep disturbances, water imbalance, temperature fluctuations, imbalance in fat and carbohydrate metabolism, Cushing's syndrome
Ventricle	Obstruction of CSF circulation, hydrocephalus, rapid increase in ICP, postural headache

CN, Cranial nerve; *CSF,* cerebrospinal fluid; *ICP,* intracranial pressure.

Outcome Management
■ Medical Management

For the adult client with a brain tumor, there are many options for treatment. Regardless of which treatment modality is selected, there are several goals. First and foremost, the initial goal is to remove or reduce as much of the tumor burden as possible; therefore surgical management is discussed first. Additional goals include managing increased ICP, controlling or preventing seizures, and monitoring for motor or sensory deficits and cranial nerve deficits.

Intervention depends on the type and location of the intracranial tumor and the client's medical condition. Management is always interdisciplinary, with several members forming a clinical team to support the client through care.

■ Surgical Management

Surgical intervention may range from biopsy to total removal of the brain tumor by way of a craniotomy. The primary goal of surgery, whether biopsy or resection, is to arrive at the histologic or pathologic diagnosis. Surgical resection decreases the tumor bulk or burden, making other treatments and adjunctive therapeutic treatments more effective. With only a few exceptions, all clients with brain tumors require a craniotomy for surgical intervention.

Craniotomy. The term *craniotomy* means to surgically create an opening into the skull. A craniectomy (removal of a portion of the cranium) may be performed for decompression. There are many methods of removing the tumor, regardless of the type of tumor and the extent of tumor removed (Table 71-2).

Intraoperatively the client may be positioned in various ways to facilitate exposure and visualization. Such positions and head-supporting frames have the potential to cause skin pressure on the head, edema of the face, and muscle soreness, especially in the neck. Preoperatively or postoperatively, a ventriculostomy—in which a catheter is inserted through a burr hole into the ventricle—may be needed to drain cerebrospinal fluid (CSF) or blood. Drains may be used if a large area of dead space remains after the removal of the tumor.

■ Nursing Management of the Surgical Candidate

Preoperative Care

More than at any other time, the role of the nurse caring for the client with the diagnosis of a brain tumor is diverse. The nurse in the neurosurgeon's office begins preoperative teaching. The nurse is usually the first person the client sees when being admitted for diagnostic procedures. During the perioperative and the postoperative periods, the nurse prepares the client for various transitions in the continuum of care.

Preoperative assessment includes the routine assessment data (see Chapter 4). In addition, a detailed history and physical examination provides a baseline for comparison of neurologic data. The nurse will obtain and record data on the following:

- Vital signs, level of consciousness, orientation to person, place, and time; ability to follow instructions; pupil equality, size, reactivity, accommodation, and reaction to light; extraocular eye movements; and cranial nerve function
- Limb strength and movement—note limited or exaggerated movements, pronator drift, hand grip, dorsiflexion/plantiflexion, any paresis or paralysis, or sensory abnormalities
- Manifestations of increased ICP, such as changes in Glasgow Coma Scale score, difficulties in problem-solving, limited memory, changes in pupil response, or loss of limb strength or movement

Preoperative interventions are similar to those for the care of other clients before surgery (see Chapter 16). In addition, the client undergoing a craniotomy requires hair removal at the surgical site. If the operation is for treatment of cancer, the client and family members may have anxiety over the potential outcome. Offer explanations and clarification as needed. Be certain not to offer empty promises about recovery.

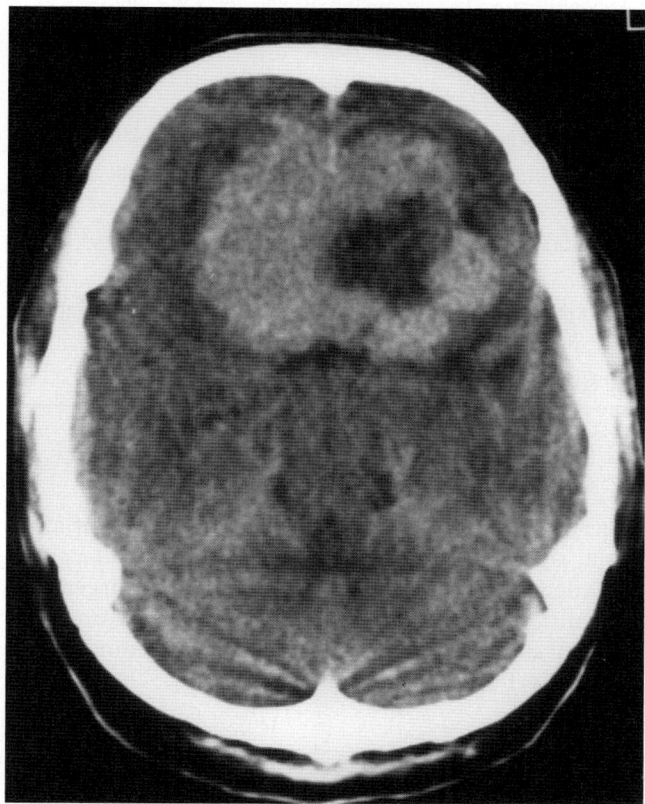

FIGURE 71-5 Magnetic resonance image revealing a midline frontal meningioma.

TABLE 71-2	*Surgical Options for Brain Tumor Diagnosis and Excision*
Procedure	**Description**

Preoperative Procedures to Locate and Map the Tumor and Nearby Structures

Procedure	Description
Brain-mapping technique	Uses viewing wand to precisely identify location of specific anatomical functions (i.e., motor, sensory, and/or speech); methods developed include localizing tumors with ultrasound techniques and various wand-like devices
Cortical mapping	Intraoperative cortical EEG recording and monitoring, facilitating areas for greater accuracy of resection without loss of eloquent motor and/or sensory functions
Direct cortical stimulation	Electrical current is directed to a specific area in the brain, causing a visible movement of the corresponding body part
Frameless stereotactic localization systems	External devices are placed preoperatively and the client's body is scanned using CT or MRI; scanning data are transferred to the operating room, allowing determination of the boundaries of the lesion by means of a surgical "wand"
Intraoperative ultrasonography	Utilizes a hand-held device to differentiate tumors with a cystic component; ultrasound techniques allow identification of tumor margins
Somatosensory evoked potentials (SSEPs)	Measurement of electrical response of specific areas (e.g., visual, auditory, brain stem); after the function of such critical areas has been determined, these areas can be avoided during surgical manipulation

Surgical Techniques Used for Precise Location of the Tumor

Procedure	Description
Intraoperative imaging techniques	Real-time CT or MRI for improved visualization
Photodynamic therapy	Combination of a sensitizing agent and laser surgery; goal is for the "sensitizing" agent to make the tumor more visible or "fluorescent" when the laser is used
Stereotactic surgery	Localization of a specific target within a three-dimensional space; with the client stabilized in a head frame, the tumor is imaged using either CT or MRI; data from the scans are analyzed by a computer and a trajectory location is identified; stereotactic procedures may be used for biopsy or craniotomy

Treatment Options for Tumor Excision

Procedure	Description
Embolization	Decreases blood supply to the tumor; may be used in conjunction with surgical procedures
Laser surgery	Destroys tumor tissue using the heat from the laser without causing adjacent edema or damage
Neuro-endoscopic techniques	For treatment of third and/or lateral ventricle lesions; provides access to lesions in areas otherwise difficult to locate
Polymer wafer implants	Chemotherapeutic wafers are placed in the tumor bed; carmustine is currently available, and other agents are being tested
Ultrasonic aspirator	Suction-like device used in removing solid tumors

CT, Computed tomography; *EEG,* electroencephalography; *MRI,* magnetic resonance imaging.

After any brain surgery, the client is closely assessed for injury to and edema of the brain. Specific complications from intracranial surgery depend on the area of surgery and the procedure being performed. Examples include increased ICP, motor or sensory deficits and cranial deficits, seizures, CSF leak, wound infection, and CNS infections. If there is loss of significant functions, these problems can be psychosocially and physically devastating. Some postoperative complications gradually resolve, but others are permanent.

General postoperative complications after intracranial surgery do not differ from those after other forms of surgery. Complications may occur as the result of anesthesia, opioids, or immobility. Ecchymosis and periorbital edema may be present after intracranial surgery but are transient. These changes affecting the appearance of the eyes and the face overall can be frightening to the client as well as to the family members.

Postoperative Care

Postoperative care of the client after craniotomy is shown in the accompanying Care Plan feature on The Client Who Has Undergone Craniotomy on pp. 2089 to 2091.

CARE PLAN

The Client Who Has Undergone Craniotomy

Nursing Diagnosis: Risk for Ineffective Tissue Perfusion: Cerebral related to edema or bleeding after craniotomy.

Outcomes. The client will have intracranial pressure (ICP) less than 15 mm Hg, mean arterial pressure (MAP) greater than 70 mm Hg, cerebral perfusion pressure (CPP) greater than 50 mm Hg, neurologic assessments and vital signs at baseline values or improved, no clinical manifestations of increased ICP and/or herniation, and body temperature less than 38.5° C.

Interventions	Rationales
1. Assess neurologic status and vital signs frequently and compare with baseline values.	1. A change in level of consciousness is the first sign of increasing intracranial pressure (ICP).
2. Elevated head of bed to 30 degrees.	2. Elevation facilitates venous drainage and reduces edema.
3. Maintain head and neck in neutral alignment.	3. This facilitates venous drainage and reduces edema.
4. Change position slowly.	4. Rapid changes in position increase cerebral blood flow and pressure.
5. Avoid a Valsalva maneuver.	5. Straining during coughing, movement in bed, or moving bowels increases ICP.
6. Monitor intake and output frequently.	6. Excess fluids can promote edema; dehydration can decrease cerebral arterial flow.
7. Monitor pulse oximetry and arterial blood gases.	7. The cerebrum is sensitive to lack of oxygen, and damage can occur within minutes after onset of hypoxia.
8. Suction airway as needed.	8. Routine suctioning not advised because it stimulates cough and increases ICP; however, sputum plugs cause retention of carbon dioxide and need to be removed because carbon dioxide increases cerebral blood flow and pressure.
9. Administer steroids as ordered.	9. Steroids reduce cerebral edema.
10. Administer antiepileptic drugs as ordered.	10. Seizures are a common sequelae of brain surgery.

Evaluation. Depending on the etiology of edema or amount of bleeding, it may require hours to days to control ICP.

Nursing Diagnosis. Ineffective Coping related to fear of changes in body image, role performance, or life expectancy.

Outcomes. The client will have improved individual coping, as evidenced by statements indicating feelings of self-worth, behaviors demonstrating self-worth, and less use of dependent behaviors.

Interventions	Rationales
1. Encourage family members/significant others to assist in meeting need for close contact.	1. Family members may also fear that they will injure the client.
2. Anticipate needs.	2. Anxiety increases feelings of loneliness.
3. Offer praise and encouragement during ongoing assessment of client's readiness to move toward more competent coping.	3. Positive reinforcement helps to guide future steps toward independence.
4. Reduce environmental stress by minimizing interruptions and stimuli.	4. Noise and frequent interruptions may decrease needed sleep and alter ability to cope.
5. Provide opportunities for expression and ventilation of feelings.	5. Problem-solving coping styles are initiated by talking about feelings and issues.
6. Utilize consistent personnel.	6. A therapeutic relationship is easier to maintain than to build.
7. Establish trust relationship; follow through on promises.	7. Feelings of fear and anxiety are reduced.

Continued

CARE PLAN

The Client Who Has Undergone Craniotomy—cont'd

Evaluation. Coping skills will wax and wane over time. Expect periods of coping and periods of failure to cope with changes in prognosis.

Nursing Diagnosis. Anxiety related to uncertain future and prognosis.

Outcomes. The client will have decreased anxiety and express fears and concerns openly.

Interventions	Rationales
1. Repeat information; provide information in different forms; encourage the client and/or significant other to write down questions and/or concerns.	1. Depending on the type of tumor, the location of the tumor, and/or motor or sensory deficits, the client may be faced with the loss of specific functions and the possibility of having a malignancy. Appropriate interventions may help the client better understand the prescribed plan of care.
2. Encourage open communication between the client, significant others, and members of the health care team.	2. Having a diagnosis of brain cancer may immobilize all of the normal coping mechanisms of the client and significant others.
3. Involve the client's clergy or hospital chaplain if desired.	3. Spiritual support is crucial at times of serious illness for the client, family members, and significant others. The client need not be "religious" to gain support from clergy.

Evaluation. Anxiety should be controllable in a short time. However, changes in response to therapy or other outcomes will increase anxiety.

Nursing Diagnosis. Risk for Disturbed Thought Processes related to neurologic changes from edema or surgical excision of sections of brain or tumor.

Outcomes. The client will make decisions and process information at expected levels, express and identify anger, exercise control over own behavior, make appropriate choices, and/or cease hostile behavior.

Interventions	Rationales
1. Allow client to verbalize concerns, and channel these concerns to the appropriate person.	1. Problem-solving coping begins with verbalization of concerns.
2. Offer reasonable choices to client.	2. Feelings of control can be reestablished by offering choices to client. All options must be safe and implementable for the client.
3. Assist client to recognize alternatives and the implications of choices.	3. This measure helps client with problem-solving abilities.
4. Report client's status to client, and allow for opportunity to make decisions about treatment or no treatment.	4. Do not keep facts from the client. The client has the right to know his or her diagnosis and to be a part of decisions about care.
5. Inform family about physiologic reasons for behavior, and teach them how to respond to client.	5. The family needs to be informed about any abnormal behavior and how best to respond to it.
6. Use a consistent approach to inappropriate behavior; establish contracts if needed.	6. Consistent approaches help the client relearn acceptable ways of personal expression.
7. Maintain nonjudgmental behavior.	7. The nurse realizes that the client's outbursts are not personal attacks but are due to the disease or feelings of loss of control.

Evaluation. Expect restoration of thought and behavior control to take weeks or months. Long-term coping by the family is important.

CARE PLAN

Nursing Diagnosis. Anticipatory Grieving related to potential loss of function, previous abilities, or life from brain cancer or surgery.

Outcomes. The client will have resolution of grief or progression through stages of grief, as evidenced by expressing feelings, maintaining hope, identifying problems with changes in body function, seeking help with anticipated problems, or developing realistic plans for the future.

Interventions	Rationales
1. Acknowledge reality, but do not force its acceptance.	1. Denial is a powerful defense mechanism; clients will examine reality when they are ready.
2. Establish regular time to spend with client, family members, and/or significant others for the exclusive purpose of discussing feelings and concerns.	2. Discussions about feelings can be difficult; giving the client time to plan and prepare facilitates the discussion.
3. If denial is beneficial, respond by listening with and reflecting statements by client.	3. It is important to understand that not all clients reach acceptance of their disease; some remain in complete denial.
4. Accept emotions and assist client, family members, and/or significant others to clarify them.	4. This measure reinforces the ideas that emotional response is normal and that family members should be accepting of the client at all stages of grief.
5. Assess perceptions about realistic goals and the future.	5. Inaccurate perceptions about the future can prevent or stall planning.
6. Have the client list those activities he or she wants to perform/resume.	6. Plans for the future can be uplifting.

Evaluation. Expect each client and family to cope differently with grief over losses or impending death. Clients may go through the "typical" stages in order or go back and forth between them.

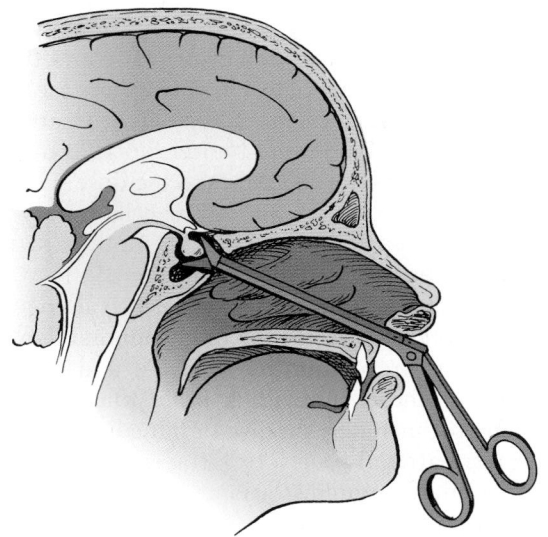

FIGURE 71-6 Transsphenoidal hypophysectomy for the excision of pituitary tumors.

See also the information on care of clients with increased ICP in Chapter 75.

Transsphenoidal Hypophysectomy. Clients with tumors of the pituitary gland have surgical options for the excision of the tumor. Historically, the procedure has been the transsphenoidal hypophysectomy, to remove small tumors housed in the sella turcica (bony structure housing the pituitary gland). For this procedure, the incision is made horizontally at the junction of the inner aspect of the upper lip and gingival, extending bilaterally to the canine teeth. From this incision, a surgical area is created beneath the nasal cartilage extending superiorly through and up to the floor of the sella turcica. At this location, the area of the floor of the sella turcica is accessed and the tumor is removed (Figure 71-6). Fat or muscle grafts, using tissue from the abdomen or upper thigh, are implanted at the surgical site to assist in healing of the hypophysectomy operative wound. Nasal packing may or may not be used.

Recently, the endoscopic endonasal approach has been used. This procedure provides a minimally invasive approach for the resection of pituitary tumors. The procedure involves passing a rigid endoscope into the nostril to provide illumination and visualization. No incision is made, nor is it necessary to break or fracture the nose. The sphenoid sinus and pituitary fossa are then entered using microsurgical instruments and the tumor is excised.[12,15,67]

Postoperative Care Following Pituitary Surgery

Postoperative care after pituitary surgery using a transsphenoidal approach includes prohibition of the use of straws for drinking any fluid to prevent trauma to the oral/gingival incision site. Frequent oral hygiene is provided, and a cool vaporizer mist may be used to keep oral mucous membranes moist. The nasal drip pad ("moustache" dressing) is assessed frequently for blood or clear fluid (CSF). The donor site and dressings are also assessed, and dressings are changed as needed. For the client undergoing the endoscopic endonasal procedure, a nasal drip pad is used as well.

A fairly common effect of pituitary surgery is the development of diabetes insipidus (DI). In most clients, the DI is temporary; however in clients in whom the stalk of the pituitary is removed, DI is permanent. DI results from a decreased secretion of antidiuretic hormone (ADH). The main clinical manifestations of DI are polyuria (large urine volumes) and polydipsia (increased thirst). Clients with DI produce large volumes (2 to 15 L/day) of dilute urine with a specific gravity of 1.005 or less. These clients require laboratory assessment of serum and urine levels of sodium and serum osmolalities. Aside from the inconvenience of polyuria, the client often suffers no serious effects from DI unless deprived of oral or IV fluids. When this happens, circulatory collapse (hypovolemic shock) and hypertonic encephalopathy occur as a result of fluid shifts in the brain. Usual treatment is with IV vasopressin (Pitressin) or inhalation desmopressin (DDAVP). Long-acting forms of these agents can be used to treat chronic DI.

■ Medical Management

Surgical excision is completed initially to reduce the bulk of the brain tumor or to excise it completely. After surgery, when an exact histologic diagnosis has been obtained, the client is given adjuvant therapy or medical management, including radiation therapy and chemotherapy. These modes of cancer treatment are discussed in Chapters 18 and 19; this material is also applicable to the care of clients with brain cancer.

Radiation Therapy. Conventional radiotherapy uses two different machines to deliver radiation: the linear accelerator and the cobalt machine. Both of these machines are used in treating brain tumors. In radiotherapy, the standard dose for primary brain tumors is approximately 6000 Gy given four to five times a week for 4 to 6 weeks. For clients with metastatic tumors, a standard dose of ra-

diation is approximately 3000 Gy. The exact dose depends on tumor characteristics, volume of tissue to be irradiated, and the goals of radiation therapy. Radiation treatments are usually given over shorter periods of time to allow for protection of normal surrounding tissues. The cancer cells in CNS tumors tend to be more slowly dividing; therefore the tumor response often takes longer. This concept is important for clients to understand, because they may be disappointed when they do not see effects during or immediately following irradiation.

As in many areas of medicine, new methods of treatment and improved delivery devices are helping clients daily. This is also the case with radiation therapy. Newer methods of delivery and more sophisticated machines are available. Table 71-3 lists examples of advances made in the area of radiotherapy for clients with brain tumors.[2] Additional forms of radiation therapy, although not considered conventional and, more important, not readily available, are heavy particle radiation therapy, fast neutron radiotherapy, photodynamic therapy, and boron neutron capture therapy.[2] Despite its wide use, radiation therapy is not without consequences. Effects may be acute, early, delayed, or late delayed; see Chapter 19. Work is progressing with the use of an inflatable balloon-filled catheter with radioactive iodine-125 placed in the tumor bed (GliaSite Radiation Therapy System).[60]

Chemotherapy. In addition to surgery and radiotherapy, chemotherapy is used in the management of brain tumors. As part of a multimodality approach, chemotherapy may be given before, during, or after other therapies. The goal of chemotherapy is to match the appropriate agent with the appropriate cell cycle phase and then attack the rapidly dividing cells. However, there are several challenges in the use of chemotherapy in the treatment of brain tumors: the blood-brain barrier blocks transportation, there are few data to guide specific dose schedules, and the mitotic cycle of brain tumor cells is very long. There does not appear to be one chemotherapy agent that can overcome all of the challenges.

The nitrosoureas are the most frequently used and effective chemotherapy agent for brain tumors. Examples of these drugs are carmustine (BCNU) and lomustine (CCNU). For the client with a brain tumor, the chemotherapy regimen may involve oral medication; IV solutions; intra-arterial routes; or intraventricular, intratumor, or epidural administration; or the use of other implanted devices, such as the Ommaya reservoir[8] (see Chapter 19, Figure 19-3).

Some progress has been made in delivery of chemotherapy across the blood-brain barrier. Of recent interest is the use of substances to open up the blood-brain barrier. In opening or unlocking the blood-brain barrier, certain agents may enter and directly bind with the CSF or have a direct effect on the tumor. The osmotic diuretic mannitol may be used to disrupt the blood-brain barrier,

TABLE 71-3	*Radiation Therapy Modalities for Treatment of Brain Tumors*
Procedure	**Description**
Interstitial radiation (also called brachytherapy, tumor implants, tumor seeding, or radioactive pellets)	Temporary or permanent placement of radioactive substances in the tumor bed Advantages: minimal effects to the surrounding tissue Generally not advised in large tumors because of secondary swelling and edema Disadvantages: implantation requires a surgical procedure; because of the radioactive substances, the client must be protected and isolated to prevent exposure to family members and health care personnel
Stereotactic radiosurgery, stereotactic radiotherapy	Allows for a high dose of radiation beams to be directed precisely to a small brain tumor in a single session by localizing the specific tumor site three dimensionally Gamma knife, linear accelerator, or cyclotron is used to deliver the radiation Best used on small, round, well-defined tumors The Peacock technique incorporates stereotaxis, radiosurgery, and computers to deliver radiation exactly to the tumor, skipping over vital areas that may be embedded in the tumor such as nerves or blood vessels
Hyperthermia	Application of heat into the tumor; electrodes with small catheters/antennae are placed through burr holes in the skull into the tumor bed; using computer-assisted stereotactic methods, the heat is delivered into the tumor Several features of brain tumors make tumor cells more susceptible to the increased temperature: poor blood supply, hypoxic areas, and increased acidity; these factors alone allow the increased temperature to kill the tumor cells Nerve cells in the brain can tolerate temperatures up to 40° C before cellular death occurs Hyperthermia uses heat from radiofrequency or microwave sources
Radiation sensitizing therapy	Use of various pharmacologic agents as "sensitizers" to make the tumor more responsive to radiation therapy and other therapies
Intraoperative radiation	Direct irradiation of the tumor while exposed in surgery; bypasses normal tissues
Conformal radiation	High or higher dose of external radiation "conformed" to match tumor's shape; the goal is to deliver a uniform amount of radiation to the entire tumor
Radioactive monoclonal antibodies	Antibodies that are cloned or mated to kill tumor cells

allowing for greater drug concentration. There are also newer chemotherapeutic agents that cross the blood-brain barrier.[2,5,28] As with the treatment of any cancer invading the body and especially the brain, the hope lies in future research. Biologic response modifiers and modulation of the immune system are two of the keys that scientists hope may hold the answers.

The care of the client with a brain tumor is a challenging task for all involved. The client should not feel abandoned or uninformed during any portion of the care or treatment. To assist the client, family members, significant others, and the health care team, the American Cancer Society and the American Brain Tumor Association are valuable resources.

HEMORRHAGIC CEREBROVASCULAR DISORDERS

There are two types of hemorrhagic cerebrovascular disorders (CVDs): (1) intracerebral hemorrhage (ICH) (see Chapter 72) and (2) subarachnoid hemorrhage (SAH).

The following section discusses SAH resulting from bleeding due to intracranial aneurysms and AVMs.

SUBARACHNOID HEMORRHAGE

SAH is bleeding into the subarachnoid space. SAH most often develops from traumatic brain injury (TBI) (see Chapter 75), intracranial aneurysms, and AVMs. Other potential causes of SAH include brain tumors (see earlier discussion), blood dyscrasias, and anticoagulant therapy.

Etiology

An SAH can occur when any of the aforementioned conditions weakens the artery, causing either a leaking or rupturing of the artery. Trauma is the leading cause of SAH, and intracranial aneurysms are the second leading cause of SAH. Most intracranial aneurysms are either congenital or developmental.

Aneurysms

An intracranial aneurysm is from a weakness in the tunica media, the middle layer of the blood vessel. The most common type of intracranial aneurysm is the saccular or berry aneurysm. These congenital aneurysms are present from birth and begin to weaken over time. The muscular walls of the artery weaken and lead to formation of a sac-like or berry-like structure.

Conditions that hasten the development of this type of aneurysm are hypertension, atherosclerosis, the aging process, and stress.[49,67] Greater than 25% of all clients with intracranial aneurysms present with multiple intracranial aneurysms. Statistically, SAH is more common in females than in males.[49,67]

Intracranial aneurysms are found more often in the anterior cerebral circulation (internal carotid artery and its branches—the anterior cerebral artery [ACA], the middle cerebral artery [MCA], and the posterior cerebral artery [PCA])—than in the posterior cerebral circulation, including the vertebral and basilar arteries. Intracranial aneurysms are found in locations where normal anatomic weaknesses occur—that is, in bifurcations and trifurcations.

Pathophysiology

Saccular aneurysms occur at the bifurcations of the large arteries at the base of the brain and rupture into the subarachnoid space in the basal cisterns. Approximately 85% of aneurysms occur in the anterior circulation, mostly in the circle of Willis. The common sites include the junction of the anterior communicating artery with the ACA, the junction of the PCA with the internal carotid artery, and the bifurcation of the MCA. The top of the basilar artery, the junction of the basilar artery and the superior cerebellar artery or the anterior inferior cerebellar artery, and the junction of the vertebral artery and the posterior inferior cerebellar artery comprise most of the remainder.

As an aneurysm develops, it often forms a neck with a dome. The arterial internal elastic lamina disappears at the base of the neck. The media thins, and connective tissue replaces smooth muscle cells. At the site of rupture (most often the dome), the wall thins, and the tear that allows bleeding is often no more than 0.5 mm long. It is not possible to predict which aneurysms are likely to rupture, but limited data suggest that most ruptured aneurysms are large, averaging 7 mm in diameter.

Vasospasm is defined as the constriction or narrowing of the cerebral vessels. Narrowing of the arteries at the base of the brain regularly occurs after SAH. This vasospasm causes ischemia and infarction. Vasospasm is a serious consequence and is the major cause of delayed morbidity or death. Although the precise mechanism of delayed vasospasm is uncertain, it seems related to direct effects of clotted blood and its breakdown products on the artery. In general, the more blood there is surrounding the arteries, the more likely there will be symptomatic vasospasm.

Clinical Manifestations

Aneurysms are found during incidental assessment, such as a work-up for headache, or they may be detected because of a mass effect, when the accumulated blood pushes on other structures. Occasionally, mild premonitory manifestations are present, such as mild headache, confusion, fainting, or vertigo. However, the onset of the hemorrhage is usually sudden. The client experiences a sudden, severe headache, often accompanied by vomiting. The headache is often described as "the worst headache I have ever had."

The client may lose consciousness immediately or may become confused and lethargic and gradually become comatose within hours, or the client may remain conscious and coherent. Generalized seizures may occur. Manifestations of meningeal irritation (e.g., nuchal rigidity, photophobia, back pain) are often present, caused by blood in the subarachnoid space. Depending on the location and size of the aneurysm and the SAH, focal clinical manifestations may be noted (e.g., motor or sensory deficits, speech and cranial nerve deficits). Retinal hemorrhages may be present. Various grading scales have been developed. Table 71-4 presents criteria for the Hunt-Hess scale and the Fisher scale.

Manifestations of vasospasm vary according to the specific arterial territories involved. However, collateral blood flow may prevent the appearance of some expected manifestations. Spasm of the MCA typically causes contralateral hemiparesis and dysphasia (domi-

TABLE 71-4	*Grading Scales for Subarachnoid Hemorrhage*
Grade	**Clinical Criteria**

Hunt-Hess Clinical Grading Scale for Clients with Aneurysmal Subarachnoid Hemorrhage

I	Alert, minimal headache
II	Alert, moderate to severe headache (cranial nerve palsy allowed)
III	Lethargic or confused or mild focal deficit
IV	Stuporous, moderate to severe hemiparesis, possibly early decerebrate rigidity
V	Deep coma, decerebrate rigidity, moribund appearance

Fisher Scale for CT Grading of Clients with Suspected Aneurysmal Subarachnoid Hemorrhage

1	No SAH on CT scan
2	Thin SAH (<1 mm)
3	Thick SAH (>1 mm)
4	Intracerebral or intraventricular hemorrhage, with no or thin SAH (<1 mm)

CT, Computed tomography; *SAH,* subarachnoid hemorrhage.

nant hemisphere). Proximal ACA vasospasm causes abulia (faulty problem-solving) and incontinence, whereas severe vasospasm of the PCA causes hemianopia. Severe spasm of the basilar or vertebral arteries occasionally produces focal brain stem ischemia. All of these focal neurologic manifestations may develop over a few days, fluctuate, or present abruptly.

Manifestations of ischemia appear 4 to 14 days after the hemorrhage, most frequently at about 7 days. The severity and distribution of vasospasm determine whether infarction occurs subsequently.

Diagnosis of SAH is usually based on history and physical examination. The hallmark of aneurysmal rupture is presence of blood in the CSF. In about 80% of affected clients, enough blood is present to be visualized on a noncontrast CT scan obtained within 72 hours. A small hemorrhage may not be seen on CT scan. If the scan neither establishes the diagnosis of SAH nor demonstrates a mass lesion or obstructive hydrocephalus, a lumbar puncture is performed to establish the presence of subarachnoid blood. Lumbar puncture is contraindicated when pressure is high in the cerebrum.

CT scan may identify blood in the subarachnoid space, intracerebral clots, and large clots surrounding an aneurysm. However, cerebral angiography is the definitive diagnostic test. A four-vessel study provides adequate visualization of the carotid and vertebrobasilar circulation. An angiogram usually provides information about the aneurysm location and type, vessels supplying the aneurysm, presence of an intracerebral blood clot, and presence of cerebral vasospasm.[49,67] Depending on the client's condition, angiography may be performed immediately or when the client's condition stabilizes. (See Chapter 4 regarding angiography.) Transcranial Doppler can be used to diagnose vasospasm. This test measures blood flow through major cerebral vessels.

Outcome Management
■ Medical Management

The client with an SAH resulting from an intracranial aneurysm presents a challenge to all members of the interdisciplinary health care team. Until the 1980s it was not unusual to place a client on bed rest, imposing severe physical and environmental limitations (complete bed rest for 10 to 14 days, dimming lights, feeding the client, keeping the room quiet, and minimizing visitors). This management approach was believed to lessen the effects of the SAH, allowing for better visualization during surgery and decreasing swelling and cerebral edema. Many innovations have developed over the intervening years to cause a paradigm shift not only in the treatment interventions but also in the medical and nursing management.[49,67] Currently, treatment is often instituted within 24 hours of onset of the headache, and the client typically makes a full recovery.

The goals for the management of a client with SAH include maintaining cerebral perfusion pressure, controlling ICP, minimizing effects of vasospasm, managing hydrocephalus, managing cardiac dysrhythmias, and preventing bleeding (or rebleeding).

Ongoing neurologic assessment is essential regardless of the setting in which care is provided. For the first 24 to 72 hours, the nurse examines the serial data to note trends in the neurologic assessments that suggest changes or deterioration. The client with an intracranial aneurysm is at great risk for the development of increased ICP. The LOC is the most sensitive and early indicator of neurologic change, usually evident before pupillary changes, new hemiparesis, or changes in respiratory patterns are noted. The onset of lethargy or restlessness may be the first clinical manifestation of increased ICP, hydrocephalus, or vasospasm.

Cardiac and respiratory function is also closely monitored, particularly because of the direct role in providing adequate cerebral perfusion pressure (CPP) and oxygen supply to the brain. Because cardiovascular disease is common in people with aneurysms, continuous electrocardiographic monitoring is necessary to identify life-threatening dysrhythmias. Pulse oximetry is imperative to monitor peripheral oxygen saturation. In the ICU setting, most clients have a central IV line or a pulmonary artery catheter in place to monitor hemodynamic status for prescription of fluids and vasoactive medications. The pulmonary capillary wedge pressure is often used for targeted therapy to manage fluid administration.[11,22,49,59,61,68]

Reduce Vasospasm. To reduce the damaging effects of vasospasm, hypervolemic therapy is the treatment of choice (often referred to as the "triple-H" therapy—for hypertension, hypervolemia, and hemodilution). Various therapies are used. For example, calcium channel blockers, vasopressor agents, and hyperosmotic diuretics may be indicated. The treatment of vasospasm in these clients necessitates consideration of a delicate balance between benefit and risk. With the major goal of improving and increasing cerebral blood flow, as well as CPP, many measures used have the potential to precipitate a cardiopulmonary crisis. Simply stated, if the client cannot tolerate an increase in fluid status or an increase in blood pressure, how can the vasospasm be relieved? Table 71-5 is a guide to various clinical interventions. The goal of such therapies is to increase cerebral blood flow and CPP without producing cerebral infarction or cardiopulmonary compromise.[11,59]

Maintain Cerebral Perfusion Pressure. Medical and nursing management focuses on maintaining blood pressure to facilitate CPP. The blood pressure must be maintained to keep the systemic pressure at a level high enough to provide adequate CPP, yet not so high as to

TABLE 71-5 *Example Treatment Protocol for Vasospasm*	
Interventions	**Rationales**
1. Glasgow Coma Scale and other neurologic assessments q 1 hr. Compare findings to baseline, and report changes.	1. Hourly observations allow early intervention when change occurs.
2. Maintain patent airway with Po_2 values greater than 85 mm Hg and Pco_2 between 25 and 30 mm Hg.	2. Prevent cerebral hypoxia; hypercapnia increases cerebral blood flow.
3. Continuous hemodynamic monitoring of RAP, PAP, and PAWP. Perform CO/CI assessments as ordered. Titrate medications and fluids to maintain desired ranges. Usual ranges are as follows: RAP: 1-7 mm Hg PAWP (no congestion): 6-12 mm Hg CI: >2.5 L/m. Target hematocrit is 33%-38%. Hypertensive goals are a minimally hypertensive state (10 mm Hg above baseline), with SBP 110-160 mm Hg.	3. Hypervolemic, hemodilution, and hypertensive therapies are used to improve perfusion through the cerebral vessels. Fluid balance must be monitored closely to prevent fluid volume overload.
4. Nimodipine (Nimotop) 60 mg q 4 hr for at least 3 weeks.	4. Calcium channel blocker; promotes relaxation of blood vessels, decreasing vasospasm.
5. Morphine as required.	5. Sedative effect; allows for continuous monitoring.
6. Accurate I & O q 1 hr.	6. Fluid balance is crucial to maintaining CPP.

BP, Blood pressure; *CI,* cardiac index; *CO,* cardiac output; *CPP,* cerebral perfusion pressure; *I & O,* (fluid) input and output; *MAP,* mean arterial pressure; *PAP,* pulmonary artery pressure; *PAWP,* pulmonary artery wedge pressure; *RAP,* right atrial pressure; *SBP,* systolic blood pressure.

cause rebleeding. Various medications and infusions are used to maintain the blood pressure approximately 10% above the client's normal pressure. In addition to medications supporting the blood pressure, blood products and albumin are used when indicated. When the blood pressure exceeds the acceptable range, antihypertensive and diuretic agents are used to decrease the blood pressure slowly. Any sudden decrease in blood pressure has a dramatic effect on the cerebral blood flow as well as on the CPP, and may increase the risk of cerebral infarction.[63]

■ Surgical Management

To successfully treat the aneurysm requires either a surgical procedure or endovascular intervention (Figure 71-7). If surgery is the chosen treatment, many different procedures may be used; however, the one most commonly used is clipping of the intracranial aneurysm. Aneurysms not anatomically suited to clipping can be wrapped in a surgical gauze material and coated with an acrylic material.[49,67]

Aneurysm Clipping. Surgical obliteration of the aneurysm with a metal clip eliminates the risk of rebleeding. A craniotomy incision is used, and the aneurysm is isolated. A metal clip is placed over the neck of the aneurysm. The timing of surgery is based on the clinical status and the grade of the aneurysm. Clients with grade I or II aneurysms are operated on within 3 days of the SAH event. Clients with lesions of grades III to V undergo clipping later on, between 10 and 14 days afterward. Surgery is delayed while vasospasm is present. Operating on vessels in spasm increases mortality and morbidity. For clients with high-grade aneurysms, the risk of rebleeding is less than that for morbidity and mortality of early surgery. Medical instability, delay in transfer from one hospital to another, and client or family reluctance to consent to surgery may also delay prompt intervention.

Postoperatively, the client's neurologic status is carefully monitored. The usual postoperative care is given, including cardiac monitoring. As with any neurologic disorder, the physician must be promptly notified about any neurologic changes.

Endovascular Therapy and Embolization. An embolization procedure involves clotting of the aneurysm by means of platinum coils, wires, or embolic substances or liquid substances. An interventional radiologist performs the procedure in an angiography suite. A cerebral angiogram is first performed to facilitate advancing a catheter to the selected vessel in the brain. Once the neck of the aneurysm is visualized, a small platinum wire is guided carefully into the aneurysm. Each coil is advanced until it curls into a ball shape inside the aneurysm, not allowing arterial blood to flow into the aneurysmal sac. As each coil is fitted into the sac, a small current of electricity is deployed that breaks the solder

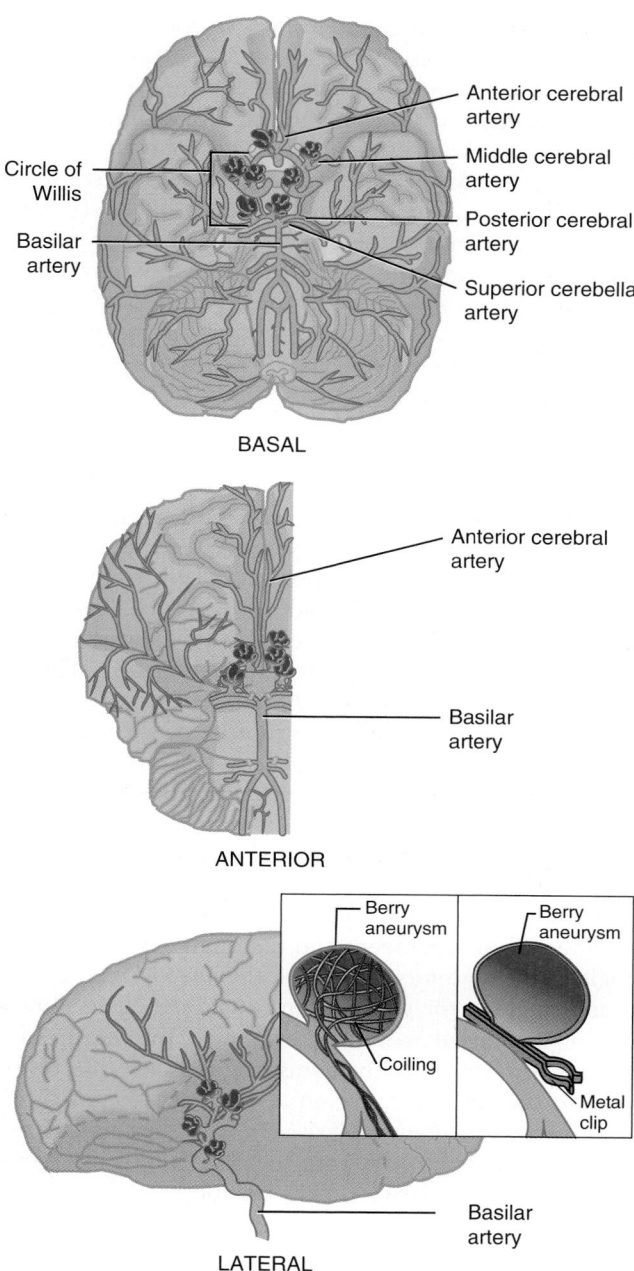

BASAL

Circle of Willis

Basilar artery

Anterior cerebral artery

Middle cerebral artery

Posterior cerebral artery

Superior cerebellar artery

ANTERIOR

Anterior cerebral artery

Basilar artery

LATERAL

Berry aneurysm

Coiling

Berry aneurysm

Metal clip

Basilar artery

FIGURE 71-7 Common locations of cerebral aneurysms. Surgical resection of aneurysms includes clipping the neck of the aneurysm or inserting a heated coil into the sac to destroy the tissue.

and leaves the coils in the aneurysm. When the aneurysm becomes embolized, thrombosing begins. To complete the procedure, an angiogram is performed.

After embolization, the client is admitted to the ICU. The client may receive heparin for 12 to 24 hours after the procedure. The catheter sheath (from the angiogram site) remains in the femoral/groin area with a saline infusion to maintain patency of the artery. Care of the femoral/groin site includes assessing the puncture site for

bleeding and hematoma formation, as well as frequent checking of peripheral pulses of the legs. The client is instructed to remain flat in bed and to avoid bending the leg at the groin. Nursing measures to maintain comfort are provided. Ongoing and frequent assessment of neurologic status is required.

Complications. Minimal complications result from the embolization procedure. If the aneurysm has not bled, there is a risk of bleeding at the time of embolization. Other problems may be related to the cerebral angiogram (see Chapter 69). Regardless of the treatment used, one factor of importance not only in selection of the treatment protocol but also in the clinical course is whether or not the aneurysm has ruptured or bled.[41,59,63] If the SAH aneurysm ruptures, the client experiences a hemorrhagic stroke (see Chapter 72).

ARTERIOVENOUS MALFORMATIONS

Etiology and Pathophysiology

AVMs are vascular lesions in which there is a congenital lack of capillaries and a tangled array of arteries and veins form. Because of the lack of a capillary bed, the blood is shunted directly from the artery to the vein. At the core or center of the AVM is the major artery, referred to as the *nidus*. From the nidus are multiple feeding vessels. Some AVMs have been associated with traumatic brain injuries, wherein the blood is shunted around a hematoma.[67] AVMs range in size from small to those encompassing an entire hemisphere.

AVMs may be found in the brain or spinal cord. Intracranially, the majority of AVMs are found in the cerebral hemispheres. In the spinal cord, AVMs predominantly occur on the posterior aspect of the cord. Depending on the size of the malformation, the number of feeders, and the magnitude of circulatory steal, the AVM can bleed or undergo thrombosis, resulting in transient to permanent spinal cord damage.

Clinical Manifestations

The onset of clinical manifestations may be seen at any age; however, increased incidence is noted in clients younger than 40 years of age. Manifestations are related to the anatomy of the malformation and the vessels involved, and occur as the result of the weakening of the vessels and of the shunting of blood in the tortuous mass. Manifestations may also be due to increasing size of the AVM. As the AVM expands, the anomalous vessels dilate and require more blood. The process of acquiring more blood flow is referred to as circulatory "steal." In this phenomenon, blood is diverted (stolen) from normal areas to maintain flow through the anomalous vessels. Consequently, localized hypoperfusion and hypoxia occur in the tissue adjacent to the AVM.

When the AVM bleeds, the client may present with any of the following: complaints of headache, seizures, SAH, or infracerebral hemorrhage. Once an AVM has bled, there is a 25% chance of rebleeding.

Outcome Management

The management of AVMs is similar to that of intracranial aneurysm. Nursing goals are comparable to those for aneurysm management, with limitation of activity, seizure control, and blood pressure management. The goals of AVM treatment are complete and permanent obliteration of the lesion. This goal may be accomplished with surgery, endovascular embolizations, or radiosurgery. The client's condition and the characteristics of the AVM determine the course of treatment. For example, in a client who has had a large SAH, vasospasm may develop. In this case, treatment is delayed until the vasospasm is decreased or resolved. With an improvement in the clinical status of the client, a treatment plan can then be developed.[49,67]

Clients commonly require a combination of treatments. Surgical resection may be the preferred treatment. Depending on the size and location of the aneurysm, the client may undergo serial embolizations, and surgery is the final form of treatment. For the serial embolizations, a thrombosing agent, histoacryl glue may be used. The goal of the embolization is to place the glue as close to the nidus of the AVM as possible.

Another treatment option for cerebral AVMs is radiosurgery. This approach may constitute the main treatment or may be used in combination with other therapies. Radiosurgery consists of direction of a focused beam of radiation toward the nidus of the AVM. The dose delivered is determined by the size of the AVM. The use of radiotherapy is recommended with small AVMs.

The treatment and management of hemorrhagic cerebral disorders is an area of active research. For example, "liquid coils" (coils that take the shape within the vascular lesion) and new coatings on currently used coils are being studied.[49,67]

▌INFECTIONS
BACTERIAL MENINGITIS

Bacterial meningitis is characterized by inflammation of all the meninges; however, the organisms predominantly involve the arachnoid and subarachnoid spaces. The infection spreads throughout the subarachnoid space via the CSF around the brain and spinal cord and usually involves the ventricles.

Etiology

Almost any bacteria entering the body can cause meningitis. The most common are meningococci (*Neisseria*

meningitidis), pneumococci (*Streptococcus pneumoniae*), and *Haemophilus influenzae*. These organisms are often present in the nasopharynx. It is not known how they enter the bloodstream and the subarachnoid space. *S. pneumoniae* and *N. meningitidis* are found most often in adults. Factors predisposing to bacterial meningitis include traumatic brain injury, systemic infection, postsurgical infection, meningeal infection, anatomic defects, and other systemic illnesses. Toxins such as intrathecal drugs or tumor cytokines may directly trigger meningeal irritation.

Pathophysiology

The route of entry into the intact CNS is uncertain. Invasion may occur through the choroid plexus (across the blood-brain barrier) or within monocytes as a component of normal cellular movement. Little change occurs in brain structure in the early stages of meningitis. Later in bacterial meningitis, inflammation leads to formation of exudate. The arachnoid and pia tissues become thickened, and adhesions form, especially in areas where there normally is an increased amount of CSF. The arteries supplying the subarachnoid space, may be engorged with blood, leading to rupture or thrombosis of these vessels.

Clinical Manifestations

The classic manifestations of meningitis are nuchal rigidity (rigidity of the neck), Brudzinski's sign and Kernig's sign, and photophobia. To assess for *Kernig's sign,* begin with the client recumbent and the thigh flexed at a right angle to the abdomen, and with the knee flexed at a 90-degree angle to the thigh. Then extend the client's lower leg. In meningeal irritation, extending the leg upward causes pain, spasm of the hamstring muscles, and resistance to further leg extension at the knee (Figure 71-8, *A*). To assess for *Brudzinski's sign,* with the client supine lift the head rapidly up from the bed. If meningeal irritation is present, forward neck flexion produces flexion of both thighs at the hips and flexure movements of the ankles and knees (see Figure 71-8, *B*).

Other general manifestations related to infection are also present, such as fever, tachycardia, headache, prostration, chills, fever, nausea, and vomiting. The client may be irritable at first, but, as the infection progresses, the client appears acutely ill and confused, stuporous, or semicomatose. Seizures may occur. A petechial or hemorrhagic rash may develop. CSF is cloudy. Gram stain of the CSF reveals organisms in 70% to 80% of cases.[39] When the organism cannot be identified, bacterial antigens can be determined. *H. influenzae* is frequently detected with this technique. Clients with bacterial pneumomeningitis demonstrate the following:

- Moderately elevated CSF pressures
- Elevated CSF protein (normal, 15 to 45 mg/dl)

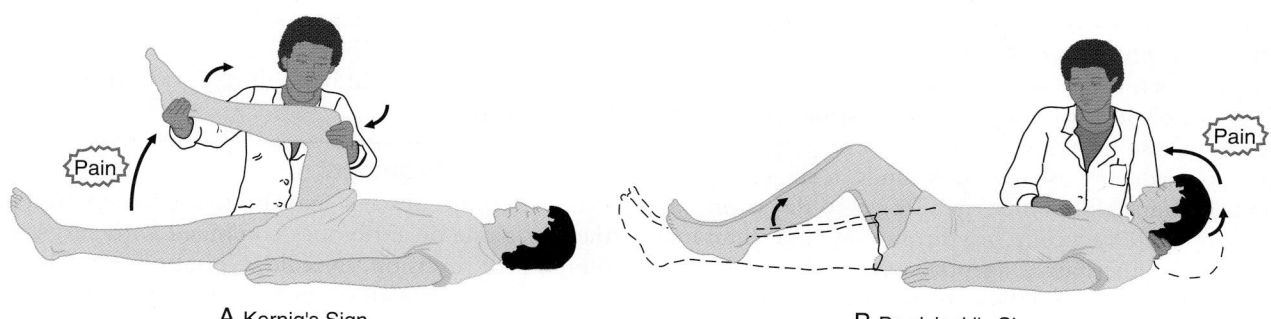

A Kernig's Sign   **B** Brudzinski's Sign

FIGURE 71-8 Assessment of meningeal irritation. Stretching the inflamed meninges by flexing the neck or legs causes pain. **A,** Kernig's sign. **B,** Brudzinski's sign.

- Decreased CSF glucose (normal 60 to 80 mg/dl, or two thirds of the serum glucose value)
- Elevated white blood cell count, usually increased (100 to 10,000/cm³), with predominantly polymorphonuclear leukocytes

Outcome Management

Bacterial meningitis constitutes a medical emergency. If untreated, it can be fatal within hours to days. Medical diagnosis is made by assessment of clinical manifestations and is confirmed by isolating the causative organism from the CSF. The use of antibiotics has reduced the mortality rate for all types of bacterial meningitis. Prognosis varies according to the causative organism. The mortality rate is less than 5%.[32] Deaths most often occur in newborn infants and in older adults. Complications are rare but may include septic shock, vasomotor collapse, seizures, and increased ICP due to hydrocephalus, brain swelling, and fluid overload. Residual neurologic deficits are rare in adults.[32]

Intervention depends on the causative microorganism and the source of the infection. Empirical therapy in bacterial meningitis includes cephalosporins, rifampin, and vancomycin. The empirical use of penicillin or ampicillin in the treatment of CNS infections is avoided because of the beta-lactamase–producing *H. influenzae* and *N. meningitidis*. It is believed that the cephalosporins are more potent against the beta-lactamase organisms. Chloramphenicol and trimethoprim-sulfamethoxazole are recommended for clients allergic to penicillin. Once the organism is known, antibiotics with greater sensitivity may be used. High doses of the appropriate antibiotic are usually prescribed for at least 10 days. If the primary focus of infection is located in the frontal area, such as the parasinuses, or if cranial osteomyelitis is present, surgery may be indicated after the acute phases of meningitis have subsided.

A unique problem in treating CNS infection is that an intact blood-brain barrier prevents complete penetration of the antibiotic. However, inflammation inhibits the blood-brain barrier, so for a short time antibiotics penetrate the CNS. Antibiotics are given intravenously; the blood-brain barrier recovers as inflammation subsides, and high doses are required to reach the CSF.

Adequate fluid and electrolyte balance must be maintained. Frequent assessment of the neurologic status is indicated to detect early manifestations of increasing ICP and seizures. Anticonvulsants may be prescribed for seizure prevention.

Outbreaks of meningitis can be a major health problem in the community, especially when they occur in schools. Refer to your facility's isolation protocols.

BACTERIAL TOXINS

Toxins produced by several pathogenic bacteria have a special affinity for the nervous system. They cause conditions such as tetanus, diphtheria, and botulism. Tetanus, a preventable disease, is caused by the anaerobic spore-forming rod *Clostridium tetani*. Tetanus may be found in people with some form of trauma and no history of tetanus immunization. Bacteria enter the CNS from a wound in which the spores were introduced and produced a toxin. The toxin enters the bloodstream from the wound and travels to the central and peripheral nervous systems. It is important to note that with wounds that are closer to the head, the neurotoxin causes tetanus more quickly.

Clinical Manifestations

Clinical manifestations may be limited to painful muscular spasms and contractions in the affected extremity. However, generalized tetanus is more common, with painful, involuntary muscular contractions involving the neck and facial muscles, especially cheek muscles, the jaw becomes locked closed (trismus), resulting in a grotesque grinning expression (risus sardonicus). The involuntary muscular contractions may further involve the pharyngeal and respiratory muscles, neck, trunk, and limbs. The affected muscles become rigid, with occurrence of painful paroxysms of tonic contractions in response to even the slightest external stimuli. The client may also exhibit seizures as a result of airway problems or hypoxia.

Outcome Management

Interventions for the acute care of the client with tetanus include the respiratory support with possible mechanical ventilation, use of neuromuscular blocking agents, surgery to debride any associated wounds, a single dose of tetanus immune globulin (Hyper-Tet), a 10-day course of penicillin G (tetracycline, erythromycin, and chloramphenicol are alternative agents), enteral feedings, and prophylactic anticoagulation to prevent thrombus. The overall mortality rate for tetanus is 25% to 50%, even in modern facilities with extensive resources. Tetanus is best prevented by immunization and regular booster doses of the toxoid.

BRAIN ABSCESS

A brain abscess is a collection of either encapsulated or free pus within brain tissue arising from a primary focus elsewhere (e.g., ear, mastoid sinuses, nasal sinuses, heart, distal bones, lungs, or primary bacteremia). The frontal lobe is the most common site of a brain abscess, which varies in size. A large abscess may involve most of one cerebral hemisphere. Other abscesses are microscopic. Brain abscesses are relatively rare; when they do occur, they are most common in persons younger than age 30 years. Morbidity and mortality increase greatly with multiple brain abscesses.

A brain abscess may occur after penetrating traumatic brain injuries or intracranial surgery. Staphylococci are the most common organisms in trauma-related cases; however, many organisms may be implicated. *Toxoplasma* is the usual agent found in clients with human immunodeficiency virus (HIV) infection.

In its early stages, the abscess produces inflammation, necrotic tissue, and surrounding edema. Within several days, the center of the abscess is purulent, and a wall of granulation tissue forms, encapsulating the abscess. Infection may spread through thin places in the wall of the capsule, resulting in development of additional abscesses.

Clinical Manifestations

Clinical manifestations of a brain abscess are essentially the same as those seen with any space-occupying brain lesion. Headache and lethargy are the most common manifestations. Manifestations of infection (e.g., fever, chills) are present about half the time. The client may experience drowsiness, confusion, and a depressed mental status as a result of the cerebral edema, increasing ICP, and intracranial effects of the brain abscess. Transient focal neurologic disorders (e.g., weakness on one side, loss of speech) occur when the abscess is located in a specific area such as the motor or speech area. Early manifestations may subside, and then within a few days or weeks, indications of increasing ICP may develop (e.g.,

recurrent headaches, changes in LOC, focal or generalized seizures).

Medical diagnosis of brain abscess is made by CT and MRI.

Outcome Management

Pyogenic brain abscess may be treated with antibiotic therapy alone or antibiotics combined with surgical aspiration or excision. Needle aspiration may be performed stereotactically (guided by CT imaging) with the use of local anesthesia. Corticosteroids may also be given to reduce cerebral edema. Penicillin is the antibiotic of choice for this type of infection. When antibiotics are used to treat the abscess, follow-up CT scans are used to monitor progress.[6,32]

OTHER SOURCES OF CNS INFECTIONS

Viruses, fungi, and parasites can also lead to CNS infections. They are discussed in Table 71-6.

HEADACHE

Headache, the most common of pains, may occur either in the absence of organic disease or as a manifestation of serious disease. Most headaches are transient and of only moderate or slight severity. However, a few types are chronic, intense, and recurrent over a period of months or years. Headache is a manifestation of an underlying disorder, rather than a disease itself. The cause of headache must be identified so that appropriate treatment can be given.

Clients often self-treat headaches with over-the-counter medications. Most headaches do not indicate serious disease. However, some headaches and headache patterns require more complete assessment (see the Critical Monitoring feature on Headache on p. 2102). Serious disorders that typically produce headache include intracranial tumors and hemorrhage, CNS infections, acute systemic infections, TBI, cerebral hypoxia, severe hypertension, and acute or chronic diseases of the eye, ear, nose, or throat.

Assessment of headaches may include detailed history, psychosocial assessment, and physical examination. Neurologic assessment is particularly important. Possible neurologic diagnostic tests include skull x-ray studies, CT, EEG, and lumbar puncture with CSF examination.[31]

History should determine (1) location of the pain, intensity, and paths of radiation, (2) character of the headache (e.g., sharp, dull, throbbing), (3) mode of headache onset, duration, and frequency, (4) methods used to treat the headache, (5) presence of localized tenderness, (6) associated phenomena or precipitating factors, and (7) familial incidence.

TABLE 71-6 *Central Nervous System Infections*

Type of Infection	Organism	Clinical Manifestations	Management
Viral Infections			
Viral meningitis Aseptic meningitis	Mumps virus Picornaviruses Enteroviruses (coxsackievirus, echovirus)	Drowsiness, headache, weakness, photophobia Nuchal rigidity (Brudzinski's sign) Spine stiffness with flexion (Kernig's sign) Blood in CSF Clinical manifestations usually resolve in 2 weeks Seizures may be present	Symptomatic management to reduce headache, control fever, and increase general comfort Anticonvulsants for seizure Isolation
	Arthropod-borne virus (arbovirus)	Unpredictable course of illness Acute fever, malaise, sore throat, vomiting, listlessness, photophobia Later, mental deterioration, personality changes, hemiparesis May develop coma or seizures Arbovirus encephalitis often leads to severe residual disabilities including mental retardation, seizures, blindness, deafness, speech disorders, and hemiplegia	Symptomatic management with close assessment for neurologic deterioration If antiviral medications, close monitoring of vital signs, lungs, airway, fluid balance, and serum electrolytes
	Herpes simplex 1	Similar to above, plus headache, fever, vomiting, and seizures Permanent neurologic and mental disabilities are common If not aggressively treated, will lead to brain herniation, coma, and brain death	Infectious agent confirmed with biopsy Symptomatic management with close assessment for neurologic deterioration Acyclovir given early in the course
Fungal Infections			
Granulomatous meningitis	*Cryptococcus*	Concurrent diseases that reduce the immune response Drowsiness, headache, weakness, photophobia, fever Nuchal rigidity Spine stiffness with flexion Cryptococci in the CSF	IV antifungal medications, such as amphotericin B, flucytosine, and fluconazole
Parasitic Infections			
Neurocysticercus	Cysticercus	Consumption of raw or undercooked pork by history May be asymptomatic unless near a vital portion of the brain, which leads to local manifestations CT or MRI reveal cysts	Praziquantel Surgical excision of the cyst if medication is ineffective
Toxoplasmosis	*Toxoplasma gondii*	Most common opportunistic infection in clients with AIDS Confusion, headache, lethargy, low-grade fever Focal manifestations of weakness, ataxia, speech problems, apraxia, seizures, and sensory changes (depending on location of mass) Multiple brain abscesses	Pyrimethamine, sulfadiazine, leucovorin, or clindamycin Symptomatic treatments

AIDS, Acquired immunodeficiency syndrome; *CSF,* cerebrospinal fluid; *CT,* computed tomography; *IV,* Intravenous; *MRI,* magnetic resonance imaging.

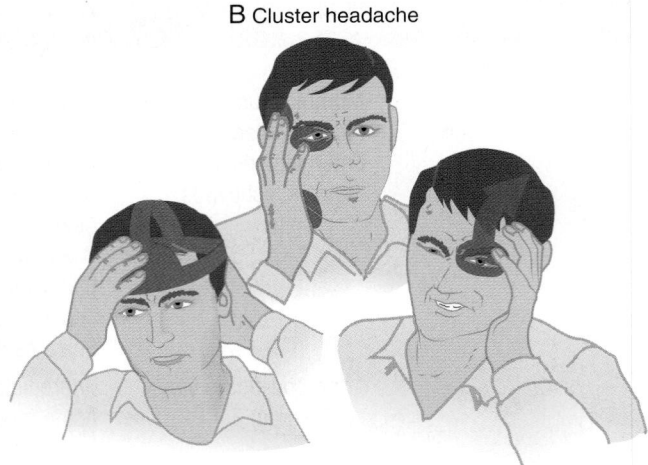

FIGURE 71-9 Types of headaches. The red areas show the regions of greatest pain. **A,** Muscle contraction headache. **B,** Cluster headache. **C,** Migraine headache.

CRITICAL MONITORING

Headache

Headaches are the most common form of pain and most headaches are due to primary causes, such as migraines or tension. However, headache requires further evaluation when:

- There is a significant change in the progression or pattern of the pain
- The pain recurs in one particular area, such as over the eye or in the temple
- The pain is described as "the worst headache" the client has ever had
- The pain is severe and begins abruptly, waking the client from sleep
- The client also has neck stiffness or fever
- The client had a recent injury to the head
- The client has neurologic changes lasting more than 1 hour, or loss of consciousness
- There is a change in vision, such as light waves in the line of vision
- The headache is present in clients with cancer, immuno-suppression, or pregnancy
- The headache is triggered by physical exertion, sexual activity, or the Valsalva maneuver

Classification and Etiology

Tension Headaches

Tension headaches result from muscle contraction (Figure 71-9, *A*). This type of headache is described as a tight band-like discomfort that is unrelenting, with few headache-free intervals. The pain typically builds slowly, fluctuates in severity, and may persist more or less continuously for many days. Triggers include fatigue and stress. The diagnosis of tension headache is confirmed when the headaches occur more often than 15 days a month. Clients may report that the head feels as if it is in a vise or that the posterior neck muscles are tight. In some clients, anxiety or depression coexists with tension headache.[31]

Cluster Headaches

Cluster headaches are sometimes classified as a form of migraine (see Figure 71-9, *B*). These headaches have a cyclical pattern of one to three short-lived attacks of periorbital pain lasting from 4 to 8 weeks, with an increased incidence in spring and fall. These headaches also have quiescent periods lasting months to years. Cluster headaches occur more often in men.

The headache lasts between 15 minutes and 3 hours. It may occur one to four times each day and may awaken the client from sleep. The pain is described as deep, boring, intense pain of such severity that the client has difficulty remaining still. The client may also develop Horner's syndrome with constricted pupils, injected conjunctiva, unilateral lacrimation, and rhinorrhea during the headaches. Cluster headaches are triggered by consumption of alcohol.

Propranolol and amitriptyline are largely ineffective. Lithium is beneficial for cluster headache and ineffective in migraine. The most satisfactory treatment is the administration of drugs to prevent cluster attacks until the bout is over. Effective prophylactic drugs are prednisone, lithium, methysergide, ergotamine, and verapamil. Lithium appears to be particularly useful for the chronic form of the disorder. A 10-day course of prednisone, followed by a rapid taper, may interrupt the pain bout for many clients.[31]

For the attacks themselves, oxygen inhalation (9 L/min via a loose mask) is the most effective modality; inhalation of 100% oxygen for 15 minutes is often necessary. The self-administration of intranasal lidocaine, either 4% topical or 2% viscous, to the most caudal aspect of the inferior nasal turbinate, can produce a ganglionic block that is usually remarkably effective in terminating an attack.

Migraine Headaches

Migraine headache is often considered to be a "vascular" headache, with vasospasm and ischemia of intracranial vessels being the cause of the pain (see Figure 71-9, *C*). These headaches usually begin in puberty and are more common in women, often associated with hormonal changes following the menstrual cycle. About 66% of cases of migraine are familial.

CLIENT EDUCATION GUIDE
Migraine Headache

- Many things can trigger a migraine headache. Find out what things trigger your headaches and avoid those triggers. If this is not possible, consult your physician about adjusting the dosage of your medication.
- If menstruation and ovulation are triggers, consult your physician for adjustments to your medication dosage.
- Alcohol temporarily increases the diameter of your blood vessels (a process called vasodilation), which may trigger migraines.
- Some foods, such as chocolate, cheese, citrus fruits, coffee, pork, and dairy products, contain substances that may trigger migraines.
- Low food intake may lead to a low blood glucose (sugar) level (hypoglycemia), which can trigger migraines. Eat small, frequent meals to decrease this risk.
- Stress management is essential. Adjust your lifestyle to reduce fatigue and exposure to bright sunlight, heat, or humidity. Get enough sleep. If you are having trouble managing the stresses in your life, seek expert guidance.

COMPLEMENTARY AND ALTERNATIVE THERAPY

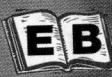

High-Dose Vitamin B₂ (Riboflavin) for Headaches

Because of the high cost and side effects of current migraine drug treatments, there is ongoing interest in alternative and cheaper options. For example, in a controlled trial, 55 clients were randomized to 3 months of vitamin B_2 (riboflavin) 400 mg once a day or placebo for 3 months. Clients were included who experienced 2 to 8 migraines a month. Responders were defined as those having a 50% reduction in manifestations. The two groups were similar in terms of age, co-morbidities, and severity of migraine at baseline. After 3 months of treatment, the number of migraines per month for clients taking riboflavin was reduced from 3.83 to less than 2 ($P = .0001$), with parallel reductions in the number of days ($P = .0001$) and the duration of migraines ($P = .018$). There were no changes in the placebo group. These changes were moderate but were also significant. Headache severity and medication use during headache did not change. Side effects were minimal; only one riboflavin recipient left the study, complaining of diarrhea after 2 weeks. Health professionals should keep in mind that riboflavin may work more slowly than other agents (taking 2 to 3 months to reach full effect). High doses of other B vitamins such as B_6 (pyridoxine) may cause peripheral neuropathy. Clients should be warned about the potential of this vitamin to create a fluorescent yellow urine, as well as not attempting to obtain the 400 mg of B_2 with a multivitamin, which contains other toxic vitamins in excess. Thus clients should take B_2 as a separate individual supplement.

Reference

Schoenen, J., Jacquy, J., & Lenaerts, M. (1998). Effectiveness of high-dose riboflavin in migraine prophylaxis: A randomized controlled trial. *Neurology, 50,* 466-470.

Migraine headaches last between 4 and 72 hours, with headache-free intervals between attacks. The headache is most often unilateral, but pain may occur on alternate sides with different attacks. Pain is described as throbbing and pulsatile. Photophobia, phonophobia, anorexia, nausea, vomiting, and focal neurologic manifestations are often present. Some clients have a visual aura that precedes the headache by 10 to 60 minutes (usually 20 minutes). The client sees a jagged edge of light in the visual fields. Other premonitory manifestations occur 12 to 24 hours before an attack and may include euphoria, fatigue, yawning, and craving for sweets. Migraine headache can be triggered by relief of intense stress, missing meals, or tyramine-rich foods.[31] See the Client Education Guide feature on Migraine Headache, above.

Typically, the client finds pain reduction in a quiet, dark environment. When aspirin and acetaminophen alone fail, the addition of butalbital, caffeine, ibuprofen (600 to 800 mg), and naproxen (375 to 750 mg) is often useful. Isometheptene compound, one to two capsules, is effective for mild to moderate "common migraine." When these measures fail, more aggressive therapy should be considered. Drug absorption is impaired during migrainous attacks because of reduced gastrointestinal motility. Delayed absorption occurs in the absence of nausea and is related to the severity of the attack and not its duration. Therefore when oral agents fail to cure, alternative therapies, including rectal ergotamine, subcutaneous sumatriptan, parenteral dihydroergotamine, and IV chlorpromazine and prochlorperazine, should be tried. For more information, see the Complementary and Alternative Therapy feature on High-Dose Vitamin B_2 (Riboflavin) for Headaches, above.

A number of drugs have the capacity to stabilize migraine. They must be taken daily. The decision to use daily medication as a prophylactic measure depends on the frequency of attacks and on how well acute treatment is working. The occurrence of at least two or three attacks per month may be an indication for this approach. There is usually a lag of 2 weeks before an effect is seen. The major drugs are propranolol, amitriptyline, valproate, verapamil, phenelzine, and methysergide.

Lumbar Puncture Headaches

Loss of CSF volume with lumbar puncture decreases the brain's supportive cushion. Headache after lumbar puncture usually begins within 48 hours but may be delayed for up to 12 days. Head pain is dramatically positional; it begins when the client sits or stands upright, and reduction is obtained upon reclining or with abdominal compression. The longer the client is upright, the longer the latency before head pain subsides. It is worsened by head shaking and jugular vein compression. The pain is usually a dull ache but may be throbbing; its location is occipitofrontal. Nausea and stiff neck often accompany headache, and occasionally blurred vision, photophobia, tinnitus, and vertigo are reported. The pain usually resolves over a few days but may sometimes persist for weeks to months.

Treatment with IV caffeine sodium benzoate promptly terminates headache in most clients. An epidural blood patch accomplished by injection of 15 ml of autologous whole blood rarely fails for those who do **EB** not respond to caffeine. The mechanism for these treatment effects is not certain. The blood patch has an immediate effect, making it unlikely that sealing off a dural hole with blood clot is its mechanism of action.

Postconcussion Headaches and Syndrome

After seemingly trivial head injuries and particularly after rear-end motor vehicle collisions, many clients report varying combinations of headache, dizziness, vertigo, **EB** and impaired memory. Anxiety, irritability, and difficulty with concentration are other hallmarks of *postconcussion syndrome*. Manifestations may remit after several weeks or persist for months and even years after the injury.

Postconcussion headaches may occur whether or not a client was rendered unconscious by head trauma. Typically, findings on neurologic examination are normal, with the exception of the behavioral abnormalities. Chronic subdural hematoma may on occasion mimic this disorder. Although the cause of postconcussive headache disorder is not known, it should not in general be viewed as a primary psychological disturbance. It often persists long after the settlement of pending lawsuits.

Treatment is symptomatic support. Repeated encouragement that the syndrome eventually remits is important.

Other Causes of Headache

Head pain may also develop from disorders of the eyes, ears, teeth, and paranasal structures. Headaches may result from errors of refraction, glaucoma (with increased intraocular pressure), inflammation, and ocular muscle disturbances (see Chapter 67). Pain associated with sinus infection is usually caused by irritation and inflammation of sinus openings. Sinus walls are less sensitive. The pain of a sinus headache may be reduced or eliminated by decongestants and analgesics. Sometimes antibiotics are needed. Surgery to drain the sinuses may also be required (see Chapter 62).[31]

CONCLUSIONS

Because of the complexity of brain disorders and the emotional reactions of the client and family members to these problems, neurologic nursing is one of the most challenging areas of nursing practice. Common nursing problems center on cerebral perfusion and cognition as well as on those related to functional rehabilitation. Prevention and early intervention are key to optimal client outcome.

THINKING CRITICALLY *evolve*

1. A client suffered a temporal lobe contusion from a motor vehicle accident 3 days ago. He is disoriented to time and place and has short-term memory deficits. During your assessment of the client, he stops answering questions and begins tonic movements of his extremities.

Factors to Consider. What are the highest priorities for this client? What are the interventions related to these priorities? What interventions come next? What significance does the site of injury have?

2. A client with a history of headaches, dizziness, and vertigo experienced a first-time seizure at age 27 years. Immediately after this episode, he noted the onset of blurred vision. Subsequent studies revealed the presence of a brain tumor, and cranial surgery was scheduled. Two days after surgery, the client is transferred to the regular unit. What are your responsibilities regarding monitoring for an increase in intracranial pressure? What are the general interventions for the client after craniotomy?

Factors to Consider. What is the major complication following intracranial surgery? How do the general interventions prevent complications associated with this type of surgery?

3. You are caring for a client who had a malignant brain tumor resected 72 hours ago. During previous assessments, she was alert and oriented; her pupils were equal, round, reactive to light, and accommodative (PERRLA); her eyes opened spontaneously; and she was moving all four extremities equally and on command. Her Glasgow Coma Scale score was 15. Now, however, she is slow to respond although still oriented to person, place, and time. Her right pupil is equal in size to the left but exhibits a sluggish reaction to direct light. Her left pupil responds normally. She still responds to verbal commands appropriately, has equal motor strength, and opens her eyes spontaneously. Thus her score on the Glasgow Coma Scale is still 15. You decide to notify the physician. Why?

Factors to Consider. How sensitive is the Glasgow Coma Scale? What abnormality may be indicated by the decreased response time and the change in pupil reaction?

4. A 33-year-old woman, Miss Brown, arrives in the emergency department with a severe headache. She has vomited twice. She states, "This is the worst headache I have ever had." The headache has lasted for about 6 hours, and two doses of acetaminophen have given no relief. Miss Brown cannot lift her head off of the pillow or position herself for comfort. Her pupils are equal, and there is no diaphoresis. What further nursing history and assessments should be done? How soon can medication to alleviate the headache be administered?

Factors to Consider. How crucial is a thorough pain assessment? How can a migraine headache mimic manifestations of a cerebral disorder? Would it be advisable to delay giving an analgesic? Why? Why not?

Discussions for these questions can be found on the website and the CD-ROM.

BIBLIOGRAPHY

1. American Association of Neuroscience Nursing. (1978). *Core curriculum for neurosurgical nurses.* Chicago: Author.
2. American Brain Tumor Association. (2000). *A primer of brain tumors* (7th ed.). Chicago: Author.
3. Anderson, S.I., et al. (1999). Mood disorders in patients after treatment for primary intracranial tumors. *British Journal of Neurosurgery, 13*(5), 480-485.
4. Angelle, D. (2002). Brain attack. *Leading Medicine, 1*(Spring), 8-12.
5. Barad, M.B. (1999). Functional assessment for transitions in patient acuity. *Nursing Clinics of North America, 34*(3), 607-620.
6. Bauman, C.K. (1997). Multiple bilateral cerebral abscesses with hemorrhage. *Journal of Neuroscience Nursing, 29*(1), 4-14.
7. Bauman, G.S., et al. (1998). Bihemispheric malignant glioma: One size does not fit all. *Journal of Neuro-oncology, 28,* 83-89.
8. Berweiler, U., et al. (1998). Reservoir systems for intraventricular chemotherapy. *Journal of Neuro-oncology, 38,* 141-143.
9. Billings, C.V. (1980). Emotional first aid. *American Journal of Nursing, 80*(11), 2006-2009.
10. Breslau, N., et al. (2000). Headache and major depression. *Neurology, 54*(2), 308-313.
11. Brisman, M.H., & Bederson, J.B. (1997). Surgical management of subarachnoid hemorrhage. *New Horizons, 5*(4), 376-386.
12. Buffalo Neurosurgery Group. (2003). *Endoscopic endonasal removal of pituitary tumors.* Available: http://buffaloneuro.com/pittumo.
13. Byock, I. (2000). Completing the continuum of care: Integrating life-prolongation and palliation. *CA: A Cancer Journal for Clinicians, 50*(2), 123-132.
14. Coke, C.B., et al. (1998). Atypical and malignant meningiomas: An outcome report of 17 cases. *Journal of Neuro-oncology, 39,* 65-70.
15. Columbia-Presbyterian Department of Neurological Surgery. (2003). Endoscopic neurosurgery. Available: http://cpmcnet.columbia.edu/dept/nsg.
16. Davis, F., & Preston-Martin, S. (1998). The epidemiology of brain tumors. In Bigner D., et al. (Eds.), *Russell and Rubinstein's pathology of tumors of the nervous system* (6th ed.). London: Edward Arnold.
17. Dawson, H., & Segal, M.B. (1996). *Physiology of the CSF and blood-brain barriers.* New York: CRC Press.
18. Dewar, S., et al. (1996). Intracranial electrode monitoring for seizure location: Indications, methods and the prevention of complications. *Journal of Neuroscience Nursing, 28*(5), 280-292.
19. Doolittle, N., et al. (1998). Blood-brain barrier disruption for the treatment of malignant brain tumors: The national program. *Journal of Neuroscience Nursing, 30*(2), 81-90.
20. Engle, G. (1964). Grief and grieving. *American Journal of Nursing, 64*(9), 93-98.
21. Engle, J., & Pedley, T.A. (Eds.). (1998). *Epilepsy—a comprehensive textbook* (Vols. I, II, and III). Philadelphia: Lippincott-Raven.
22. Faylor, C.R. (1999). Using transcranial Doppler to augment the neurological examination after aneurysmal subarachnoid hemorrhage. *Journal of Neuroscience Nursing, 31*(5), 285-293.
23. Fisher, C.M., et al. (1980). Relation of cerebrovasospasm to subarachnoid hemorrhage visualized by computerized tomographic scanning. *Neurosurgery, 6*(1), 1-9.
24. Gahart, B., & Nazareno, A. (2004). *Intravenous medications* (20th ed., pp. 362-365). St. Louis: Mosby.
25. Gormely, W.B., et al. (1997). Acoustic neuromas: Results of current surgical management. *Neurosurgery, 41*(1), 50-60.
26. Gumnit, R. (1997). *Living well with epilepsy* (2nd ed.). Minneapolis: Demos Vermande.
27. Gurney, J., et al. (1999). The contribution of nonmalignant tumors to CNS tumor incidence rates among children in the United States. *Cancer Causes and Control, 10*(2), 101-105.
28. Hickey, J.V. (1997). *The clinical practice of neurological and neurosurgical nursing.* Philadelphia: Lippincott-Raven.
29. Hunt, W.E., & Hess, R.M. (1968). Surgical risks as related to time of intervention in the repair of intracranial aneurysms. *Journal of Neurosurgery, 28,* 14-20.
30. Kajs-Wylie, M. (1999). Antihypertensive therapy for the neurological patient: A nursing challenge. *Journal of Neuroscience Nursing, 31*(3), 142-151.

31. Kaniecki, R. (2003). Headache assessment and management. *Journal of the American Medical Association 289*(11), 1430-1433.

32. King, D. (1999). Central nervous system infection. *Nursing Clinics of North America, 34*(3), 761-771.

33. Kleihues, P., et al. (1993). The new WHO classification of brain tumors. *Brain Pathology, 3,* 225-268.

 34. Laino, C. (2003). Changes in brain function associated with recovery identifiable two weeks after stroke. *Neurology Today,* September, 45-46.

35. Long, L., & Reeves, A. (1997). The practical aspects of epilepsy: Critical components of comprehensive patient care. *Journal of Neuroscience Nursing, 29*(4), 249-254.

36. Mayo Clinic. (2003). *Treatment options for brain tumors.* Available: http://mayoclinic.org/braintumors.

 37. McCarthy, B., et al. (1998). Factors associated with survival in patients with meningioma. *Journal of Neurosurgery, 88,* 831- 839.

38. Minton, M. (1999). Primer of neuroanatomy and neurophysiology. *Nursing Clinics of North America, 34*(3), 555-572.

39. Moloney, M.F., et al. (2000). Caring for the woman with migraine headaches. *Nurse Practitioner, 25*(2), 17-41.

40. Morris, G.L., et al. (1999). Long-term treatment with vagus nerve stimulation in patients with refractory epilepsy. *Neurology, 53*(7), 1731-1735.

 41. Morrison, S.R. (1997). Guglielmi detachable coils: An alternative therapy for surgically high-risk aneurysms. *Journal of Neuroscience Nursing, 29*(4), 232-237.

42. Noebels, J. (1998). Genetics and epilepsy. In Ozuna, J., et al. (Eds.), *Clinical nursing practice in epilepsy* (Vol. 2, pp. 4-7). Secaucus, NJ: Churchill Communications.

43. *Radiation therapy and you: A guide to self-help during treatment.* NIH Publication No. 97-2227, Revised October 1993; reprinted January 1997. Bethesda, MD: National Institutes of Health, National Cancer Institute.

44. Raskin, N.H. (1996). Approach to the patient with migraine. *Hospital Practice, 31*(2), 93-106.

45. Rowan, JA, & Tuchman, L. (2003) Management of seizures in the elderly. *Profiles in Seizure Management, 2*(4), 4-9.

46. Santillli, N., & Sierzant, T. (1987). Advances in the treatment of epilepsy. *Journal of Neuroscience Nursing, 19,*143-144.

 47. Sargent, J., et al. (1995). Oral sumatriptan is effective and well tolerated for the acute treatment of migraine. *Neurology, 45*(Suppl. 7), S10-S14.

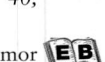 48. Schiller, Y., et al. (2000). Discontinuation of antiepileptic drugs after successful epilepsy surgery. *Neurology, 54*(2), 346-349.

49. Schmidek, H.H., & Sweet, W.H. (1995). *Operative neurosurgical techniques* (3rd ed., Vols. I and II). Philadelphia: W. B. Saunders.

50. Shafer, P.O. (1999). Epilepsy and seizures—advances in seizure assessment, treatment and self-management. *Nursing Clinics of North America, 34*(3), 743-759.

51. Shafer, P.O. (1999). New therapies in the management of acute or cluster seizures and seizure emergencies. *Journal of Neuroscience Nursing, 31*(4), 224-230.

52. Shah, S.M., & Kelly, K.M. (1999). *Emergency, neurology—principles and practices.* Cambridge: Cambridge University Press.

53. Spencer, D.C., et al. (2000). The role of intracarotid amobarbital procedure in evaluation of patients for epilepsy. *Surgery, 42*(3), 302-325.

54. Surawiez, T.S., et al. (1998). Brain tumor survival: Results from the National Cancer Data Base. *Journal of Neuro-Oncology, 40,* 151-160.

55. Surawiez, T.S., et al. (1999). Results from the central brain tumor registry of the United States, 1990-1994. *Neuro-oncology 1*(1), 14-25.

56. Surveillance, Epidemiology, and End Results (SEER). (1998). *Cancer statistics review, 1973-1995 U.S. populations.* Bethesda, MD: National Cancer Institute.

57. Snively, C., et al. (1998). Vagal nerve stimulator as a treatment for intractable epilepsy. *Journal of Neuroscience Nursing, 30*(5), 286-289.

58. Solomon, G. (1997). Diagnosis of primary headache disorders: Validity of the International Headache Society criteria in clinical practice. *Neurology Clinics, 15* (1), 15-26.

59. Tamargo, R.J., et al. (1997). Aneurysmal subarachnoid hemorrhage: prognostic features and outcomes. *New Horizons, 5*(4), 364-374.

60. Tatter, S.B., et al. (2003). An inflatable balloon catheter and liquid ^{125}I radiation source (GliaSite Radiation Therapy System) for treatment of recurrent malignant glioma: multicenter safety and feasibility trial. *Journal of Neurosurgery, 99*(2), 297-303.

61. Vale, F.L., et al. (1997). The relationship of subarachnoid hemorrhage and the need for postoperative shunting. *Journal of Neurosurgery, 86,* 462-466.

62. Vannemreddy, P.S.S.V., et al. (2000). Glioblastoma multiforme in a case of acquired immunodeficiency syndrome: Investigating a possible oncogenic influence of human immunodeficiency virus on glial cells. *Journal of Neurosurgery, 92,* 161-164.

63. Vinuela, F., et al. (1997). Guglielmi detachable coil embolization of acute intracranial aneurysm: Perioperative anatomical and clinical outcome in 403 patients. *Journal of Neurosurgery, 86,* 475-482.

64. Vitners, H.V. (1998). *Diagnostic neuropathology.* New York: Marcel Dekker.

65. Vonck, K., et al. (1999). Long-term results of vagus nerve stimulation in refractory epilepsy. *Seizure, 8,* 328-334.

66. Walters, P. (1990). Chemo: A nurse's guide to action, administration, and side effects. *RN, 53*(2), 52-67.

67. Youmans, J.R. (Ed.). (1996). *Neurological surgery: A comprehensive reference guide to the diagnosis and management of neurosurgical problems.* Philadelphia: W. B. Saunders.

68. Yundt, K.D., et al. (1996). Hospital resource utilization in the treatment of cerebral aneurysms. *Journal of Neurosurgery, 85,* 403-409.

Chapter 72

Management of Clients with Stroke

Lisa Bowman

---

evolve

Web Enhancements

http://evolve.elsevier.com/Black/medsurg/

Case Management
Stroke
Case Study
Meningioma, Fractured Hip, and Possible Stroke
Client Education Guide
Transfer from Bed to Wheelchair by a Hemiplegic Client
(Spanish Translation)

Clinical Pathway
Stroke
Appendix C
Laboratory Values of Clinical Importance in Medical-Surgical
Nursing

STROKE: SCOPE OF THE PROBLEM

Stroke is a term used to describe neurologic changes caused by an interruption in the blood supply to a part of the brain. The two major types of stroke are *ischemic* and *hemorrhagic*. Ischemic stroke is caused by a thrombotic or embolic blockage of blood flow to the brain. Bleeding into the brain tissue or the subarachnoid space causes a hemorrhagic stroke. Ischemic strokes account for about 83% of all strokes. The remaining 17% of strokes are hemorrhagic.

Cerebrovascular disorders are the third leading cause of death in the United States and account for about 164,000 mortalities annually.[25] An estimated 550,000 people experience a stroke each year.[2] When second strokes are considered in the estimates, the incidence increases to 700,000 per year in the United States alone. Stroke is a leading cause of adult disability and a leading primary diagnosis for long-term care. More than four million stroke survivors are living with varying degrees of disability in the United States.[2] Along with a high mortality rate, strokes produce significant morbidity in people who survive them. Of stroke survivors, 31% require assistance with self-care, 20% require assistance with ambulation, 71% have some impairment in vocational ability up to 7 years following the stroke, and 16% are institutionalized.[33]

The advent of thrombolytic therapy for the treatment of acute ischemic stroke has revolutionized the care of the client following a stroke. Before 1995 health care professionals could offer only supportive measures and rehabilitation to stroke survivors. New therapies can now prevent or limit the extent of damage to brain tissue caused by acute ischemic stroke. Thrombolytic therapy must be administered as soon as possible after onset of the stroke; a treatment window of 3 hours from the onset of manifestations has been established. To convey this sense of urgency regarding the evaluation and treatment of stroke, health care professionals now refer to stroke as a *brain attack*. Public education is focused on prevention, recognition of manifestations, and early treatment of brain attack.[39]

Etiology and Risk Factors

Ischemia

Ischemia occurs when the blood supply to a part of the brain is interrupted or totally occluded. Ultimate survival of ischemic brain tissue depends on the length of time it is deprived plus the degree of altered brain metabolism. Ischemia is commonly due to thrombosis or embolism (Figure 72-1). Thrombotic strokes are more common than embolic strokes.

---

evolve *Be sure to check out the bonus material on the Evolve website and the CD-ROM, including free self-assessment exercises.*

http://evolve.elsevier.com/Black/medsurg/

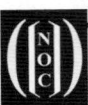

Nursing Outcomes Classification (NOC)
for Nursing Diagnoses—Clients with Stroke

Disturbed Sensory Perception: Visual
 Vision Compensation Behavior
 Risk Control: Visual Impairment
Disturbed Thought Processes
 Cognitive Ability
 Cognitive Orientation
 Information Processing
 Memory
Imbalanced Nutrition: Less Than Body Requirements
 Nutritional Status: Food and Fluid
  Intake
 Nutritional Status: Biochemical
  Measures
 Nutritional Status: Body Mass
Impaired Physical Mobility
 Ambulation: Walking
 Ambulation: Wheelchair
 Body Positioning: Self-Initiated
 Joint Movement: Active

Mobility Level
 Transfer Performance
Impaired Verbal Communication
 Communication: Expressive Ability
 Communication: Receptive Ability
 Muscle Function
Ineffective Coping
 Coping
 Role Performance
 Social Support
 Caregiver-Patient Relationship
Ineffective Tissue Perfusion
 Risk for Aspiration
 Neurologic Status
 Swallowing Status
Ineffective Tissue Perfusion: Cerebral
 Neurologic Status: Consciousness
 Tissue Perfusion: Cerebral
Risk for Aspiration
 Aspiration Control
 Swallowing Status

Risk for Hyperthermia
 Thermoregulation
Risk for Impaired Skin Integrity
 Immobility Consequences: Physiologic
 Tissue Integrity: Skin and Mucous
  Membranes
Risk for Injury
 Neurologic Status
 Safety Behavior: Fall Prevention
 Safety Behavior: Home Physical
  Environment
 Safety Status: Falls Occurrence
 Safety Status: Physical Injury
Self-Care Deficit
 Self-Care: Activities of Daily Living
 Self-Care: Eating
 Self-Care: Dressing
 Self-Care: Bathing
 Self-Care: Hygiene
Unilateral Neglect
 Self-Care: Activities of Daily Living

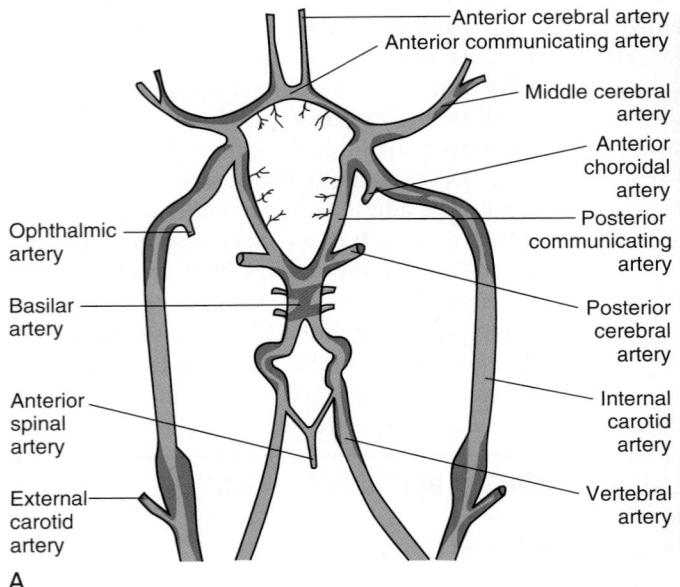

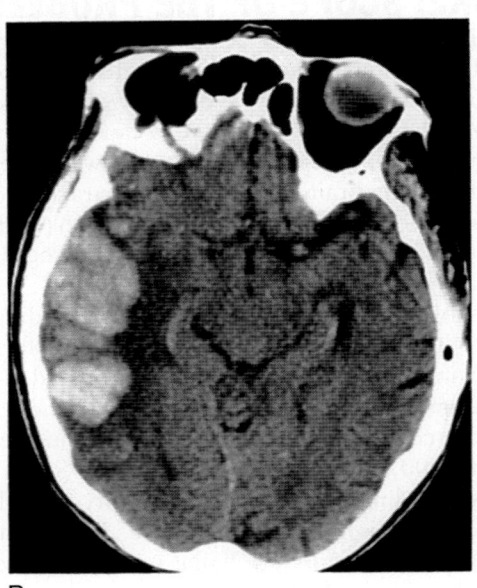

FIGURE 72-1 A, Events causing stroke. **B,** Magnetic resonance image showing a hemorrhagic stroke in the left cerebrum.

Strokes can also be "large vessel" and "small vessel." Large vessel strokes are caused by blockage of a major cerebral artery, such as the internal carotid, anterior cerebral, middle cerebral, posterior cerebral, vertebral, and basilar arteries. Small vessel strokes affect smaller vessels that branch off the larger vessels to penetrate deep into the brain.

Thrombosis

A thrombus starts with damage to the endothelial lining of the vessel. Atherosclerosis is the primary culprit. Atherosclerosis causes fatty material to deposit and form plaques on vessel walls. These plaques continue to enlarge and cause stenosis of the artery. Stenosis alters the usual smooth flow of blood through the artery. Blood swirls around the irregular surface of the plaques, causing platelets to adhere to the plaque. Eventually the vessel lumen becomes obstructed. Rarely occlusion is due to inflammation of the arteries, called *arteritis* or *vasculitis*.

A thrombus can develop anywhere along a carotid artery or its branches. A common site is at the bifurcation of the common carotid into the internal and external carotid arteries. Thrombotic stroke is the most common type of stroke in people with diabetes.

Lacunar strokes are small vessel strokes. The endothelium of smaller vessels is affected primarily by hypertension, which causes a thickening of the vessel wall and stenosis. Lacunar infarctions are also common in people with diabetes mellitus.

Embolism

The occlusion of a cerebral artery by an embolus causes an embolic stroke. An embolus forms outside the brain, detaches, and travels through the cerebral circulation until it lodges in and occludes a cerebral artery. A common embolus is plaque. A thrombus can detach from the internal carotid artery at the site of an ulcerated plaque and travel into the cerebral circulation. Chronic atrial fibrillation is associated with a high incidence of embolic stroke. Blood then pools in the poorly emptying atria. Tiny clots form in the left atrium and move through the heart and into the cerebral circulation. Mechanical prosthetic heart valves have a rougher surface than the normal endocardium and can cause an increased risk of clots. Both bacterial and nonbacterial endocarditis can be sources of emboli. Other sources of emboli include tumor, fat, bacteria, and air. Any cerebrovascular territory may be affected. The incidence of cerebral embolism increases with age.

Hemorrhage

Intracerebral hemorrhage results from rupture of a cerebral vessel, which causes bleeding into brain tissue. Intracerebral hemorrhage is most often secondary to hypertension and is most common after age 50 years. These hemorrhages usually produce extensive residual functional loss and have the slowest recovery of all types of stroke. The overall mortality of intracerebral hemorrhage varies between 25% and 60%.[18] The volume of the hemorrhage is the single most important predictor of client outcome.[17,18] Bleeding may also occur from rupture of an aneurysm or a vascular malformation. The effects of these hemorrhages depend on the site and the extent of the bleeding.

Other Causes

Cerebral arterial spasm, caused by irritation, reduces blood flow to the area of the brain supplied by the constricted vessel. Spasm of short duration does not necessarily cause permanent brain damage.

Hypercoagulable states, including protein C and protein S deficiencies and disorders of the clotting cascade, can cause thrombosis and ischemic stroke. Compression of cerebral vessels may result from a tumor, large blood clot, swollen brain tissue, brain abscess, or other disorders. These causes are fairly rare.

Risk Factors

The incidence of stroke and stroke mortalities has gradually declined in many industrialized countries in recent years as a result of increased recognition and treatment of risk factors. Modifiable risk factors can be reduced or eliminated through lifestyle changes. Hypertension is the most important modifiable risk factor for both ischemic and hemorrhagic stroke. Adequate blood pressure control is associated with a 38% reduction in stroke incidence.[6]

Cardiovascular disease and atrial fibrillation are also associated with an increased risk of stroke (see the Complementary and Alternative Therapy feature on Elevated Homocysteine Levels and Stroke, below). Diabetes mellitus increases the risk of stroke and morbidity and mor-

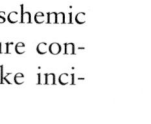

COMPLEMENTARY AND ALTERNATIVE THERAPY

Elevated Homocysteine Levels and Stroke

A recent meta-analysis of studies from 1966 to 1999 was conducted to evaluate the ability of homocysteine to predict heart disease or stroke. A total of 30 studies were found (12 prospective and 18 retrospective) that met the inclusion criteria. Researchers found that lower plasma homocysteine levels were associated with a modest reduction in cardiovascular disease (CVD) risk, but a true causal association cannot be concluded. No studies reviewed adjusted for the presence of renal impairment, a condition known to increase both plasma homocysteine and risk for CVD. Also, genetic studies and large intervention trials are required to establish causation. Interestingly, plasma homocysteine can be lowered in most clients using 1 mg/day oral folic acid, with or without vitamins B_{12} and B_6. Some researchers suggest that until ongoing primary and secondary prevention trials of homocysteine reduction and CVD are completed, the measurement of homocysteine should be done only in those with unexplained premature CVD.

Reference

The Homocysteine Studies Collaboration. (2002). Homocysteine and risk of ischemic heart disease and stroke: A meta-analysis. *Journal of the American Medical Association, 288,* 2015-2022.

tality after stroke. The mechanism is related to macrovascular changes in people with diabetes mellitus. Prior stroke, carotid stenosis, and a history of transient ischemic attacks (TIAs) are considered modifiable risk factors for stroke. Reduction in the risk factors for initial stroke may prevent stroke recurrence.[41] Early recognition and treatment of carotid stenosis and treatment of TIAs with antiplatelet agents reduce the risk of stroke.

Other modifiable risk factors for stroke include hyperlipidemia, cigarette smoking, heavy alcohol consumption, cocaine use, and obesity. Current research suggests that although heavy alcohol consumption increases one's risk of a stroke, light or moderate alcohol consumption may protect against ischemic stroke.[32] Stroke is uncommon in women of childbearing age; however, high-dose estrogen oral contraceptives combined with hypertension, cigarette smoking, migraine headaches, and increasing age increase the risk of stroke in women.[14] (See the Complementary and Alternative Therapy feature on Vitamin E and Stroke, below.)

Client education is aimed at stroke prevention. *Primary* prevention of stroke includes the following:

- Maintaining an ideal body weight
- Maintaining safe cholesterol levels
- Stopping smoking
- Using low-dose estrogen contraceptives only in the absence of other risk factors
- Reducing heavy alcohol consumption
- Eliminating illicit drug use

Secondary prevention includes the following:

- Adequate blood pressure control
- Care of diabetes mellitus
- Treatment of cardiovascular disease, TIA, and atrial fibrillation

Nonmodifiable risk factors cannot be prevented or treated. Advancing age is one of the most significant risk factors for stroke. The incidence of stroke in men is slightly higher than that in women. Stroke is also more prevalent in African Americans than in whites or Hispanics.[20] This difference is probably related to the increased incidence of hypertension and diabetes mellitus in this group.[8] Family history of stroke increases one's risk for stroke.

Pathophysiology

The brain is very sensitive to a loss of blood supply. Unlike other body tissues, such as muscle, the brain cannot resort to anaerobic metabolism in the absence of oxygen and glucose. The brain is perfused at the expense of other less vital organs to preserve cerebral metabolism. Hypoxia can cause cerebral ischemia. Short-term ischemia leads to temporary neurologic deficits or a TIA. If blood flow is not restored, brain tissue sustains irreversible damage or infarction within minutes. The extent of infarction depends on the location and size of the occluded artery and the adequacy of collateral circulation to the area it supplies.

Ischemia quickly alters cerebral metabolism. Cell death and permanent changes can occur within 3 to 10 minutes. The client's baseline oxygen level and ability to compensate determine how quickly irreversible changes occur. Blood flow can be altered by localized perfusion problems, such as stroke, or by generalized perfusion problems, such as hypotension or cardiac arrest. Cerebral perfusion pressure must fall to two thirds of normal (a mean arterial pressure of 50 mm Hg or below) before the brain does not receive adequate blood flow. These numbers assume a normal baseline of blood flow. A client who has lost compensatory autoregulation experiences manifestations of neurologic deficit sooner.

Decreased cerebral perfusion is usually caused by occlusion of a cerebral artery or intracerebral hemorrhage. Occlusion produces ischemia in the brain tissue supplied by the affected artery and edema in the surrounding tissue. Cells in the center of the stroke area, or the core, die almost immediately after stroke onset; this is referred to as *primary neuronal injury*. A zone of hypoperfusion also exists around the infarcted core; this zone is called the *penumbra*.[16] The size of this zone depends on the amount of collateral circulation present. Collateral cir-

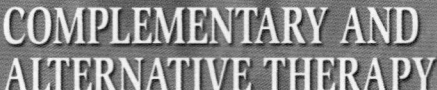

COMPLEMENTARY AND ALTERNATIVE THERAPY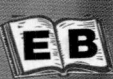

Vitamin E and Stroke

In a randomized, controlled clinical trial of 29,133 Finnish male smokers, the overall net stroke morbidity and mortality with alpha-tocopherol (vitamin E) and beta-carotene was not significantly different from placebo; however, a trend toward higher rates of subarachnoid hemorrhages was found (relative risk [RR] = 1.5, number needed to harm = 833), but the cerebral infarction rate was decreased (RR = 0.86, number needed to treat = 239).[2] The Italian GISSI* study of 11,324 clients with a recent myocardial infarction showed no effect of vitamin E on the combined outcomes of death, myocardial infarction, and stroke.[1] Therefore recommending vitamin E supplements for cardiovascular disease reduction cannot be advocated at this time.

References

1. GISSI investigators. (1999). Dietary supplementation with n-3 polyunsaturated fatty acids and vitamin E after myocardial infarction: Results of the GISSI Prevenzione Trial. *Lancet, 354,* 447-455.
2. Leppala, J., et al. (2000). Controlled trial of alpha-tocopherol and beta-carotene supplements on stroke incidence and mortality in male smokers. *Arteriosclerosis, Thrombosis, and Vascular Biology, 20,* 230-235.

*Gruppo Italiano per lo Studio della Streptochinasi Nell'Infarto Miocardico (Italian Group for the Study of Streptokinase in Myocardial Infarction).

culation describes the vessels that augment the major circulatory vessels of the brain. Differences in the size and number of collateral vessels help to explain variations in the severity of manifestations experienced by clients with strokes in the same anatomic area.

A cascade of biochemical processes occurs within minutes of cerebral ischemia. Neurotoxins, including oxygen free radicals, nitric oxide, and glutamate, are released. Local acidosis develops. Membrane depolarization occurs. This results in an influx of calcium and sodium. Cytotoxic edema and cell death are a result; this is secondary neuronal injury. Penumbral neurons are highly susceptible to the effects of the ischemic cascade. The area of edema after ischemia may lead to temporary neurologic deficits. Edema may subside in a few hours or sometimes in several days, and the client may regain some function.

EB Most intracerebral hemorrhages are caused by the rupture of arteriosclerotic and hypertensive vessels. Most intracerebral hemorrhages are very large. Therefore it is not surprising that hemorrhage into the brain causes the most fatalities of all strokes. Aneurysms are weakened outpouchings in a vessel wall. Although cerebral aneurysms are usually small (2 to 6 mm in diameter), they can rupture. An estimated 6% of all strokes are caused by aneurysm rupture. A stroke secondary to bleeding often produces spasm of cerebral vessels and cerebral ischemia because the blood outside of the vessels acts as an irritant to the tissues.

Clinical Manifestations

General findings of stroke unrelated to specific vessel sites include headache, vomiting, seizures, changes in mental status, fever, and changes on the electrocardiogram (ECG). ECG changes include T-wave changes, shortened PR interval, prolonged QT interval, premature ventricular contractions, sinus bradycardia, and ventricular and supraventricular tachycardias.[9]

Early Warnings

Manifestations of impending ischemic stroke include transient hemiparesis, loss of speech, and hemisensory loss. Manifestations of a thrombotic stroke develop over minutes to hours to days. The slow onset is related to the increasing size of the thrombus, with partial and then complete occlusion of the affected vessel. In contrast, manifestations of embolic strokes occur suddenly and without warning.

Hemorrhagic stroke occurs rapidly, with manifestations developing over minutes to hours. Common manifestations include severe occipital or nuchal headaches, vertigo or syncope, paresthesias, transient paralysis, epistaxis, and retinal hemorrhages.

Manifestations of deficit must persist longer than 24 hours to be diagnostic of stroke. TIAs are focal neurologic deficits lasting less than 24 hours.

Specific Deficits After Stroke

Stroke manifestations can be correlated with the cause (Table 72-1) and with the area of the brain in which perfusion is impaired (Table 72-2). The middle cerebral artery is the most common site of ischemic stroke. The client's deficit also varies according to whether the dominant or the nondominant side of the brain is affected. The degree of deficit can also vary from little impairment to serious functional loss.

Hemiparesis and Hemiplegia. *Hemiparesis* (weakness) or *hemiplegia* (paralysis) of one side of the body may occur after a stroke. These deficits are usually caused by a stroke in the anterior or middle cerebral artery, leading to an infarction in the motor strip of the frontal cortex. Complete hemiplegia involves half of the face and tongue as well as the arm and leg of the ipsilateral side of the body. Infarction in the right side of the brain causes left-sided hemiplegia and vice versa because nerve fibers cross over in the pyramidal tract as they pass from the brain to the spinal cord. Strokes causing hemiparesis or hemiplegia usually affect other cortical areas in addi-

TABLE 72-1	*Clinical Manifestations of the Various Causes of Stroke*
Cause	**Clinical Manifestations**
Thrombosis	Tends to develop during sleep or within 1 hour of arising
	Ischemia is produced gradually; therefore the clinical manifestations develop more slowly than those caused by hemorrhage or emboli
	Relative preservation of consciousness
	Hypertension
Embolism	No discernible time pattern, unrelated to activity
	Clinical manifestations occur rapidly, within 10-30 seconds, and often without warning
	May have rapid improvement
	Relative preservation of consciousness
	Normotension
Hemorrhage	Typically occurs during active, waking hours
	Severe headache and nuchal rigidity occur (if client is able to report manifestations)
	Rapid onset of complete hemiplegia, occurs over minutes to 1 hour
	Usually results in extensive, permanent loss of function with slower, less complete recovery
	Rapid progression into coma

TABLE 72-2	*Clinical Manifestations of Stroke Associated with Area of Brain Affected*		
Location	**Middle Cerebral Artery**	**Anterior Cerebral Artery**	**Posterior Cerebral Artery**
Motor changes	Contralateral hemiparesis or hemiplegia, face and arm deficits greater than leg	Contralateral hemiparesis, foot and leg deficits greater than arm, foot-drop, gait disturbances	Mild contralateral hemiparesis (with thalamic or subthalamic involvement) Intention tremor
Sensory changes	Contralateral hemisensory alterations Neglect of involved extremities	Contralateral hemisensory alterations	Diffuse sensory loss (thalamic)
Visual or ocular changes	Homonymous hemianopia Inability to turn eyes toward affected side	Deviation of eyes toward affected side	Pupillary dysfunction (brain stem) Loss of conjugate gaze, nystagmus Loss of depth perception Cortical blindness Homonymous hemianopia
Speech changes	Dyslexia, dysgraphia, aphasia	Expressive aphasia	Perseveration Dyslexia
Mental changes	Memory deficits	Confusion, amnesia Flat affect, apathy Shortened attention span Loss of mental acuity	Memory deficits
Other changes	Vomiting may occur	Apraxia (inability to carry out purposeful movements in nonaffected areas) Incontinence	Visual hallucinations

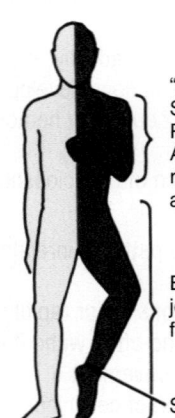

"Frozen" shoulder
Subluxation of the shoulder
Painful shoulder-hand dystrophy
Adduction of arm with internal rotation; flexion of elbow, wrist and fingers

External rotation of leg at hip joint; flexion at knee; and plantar flexion and supination at ankle

Shortened heel cord

FIGURE 72-2 Hemiplegic contractures. The elbow is bent, the wrist is flexed, and the fingers are curled into palmar flexion; the knee is bent and the heel cord is shortened.

tion to the motor strip. As a result, hemiparesis and hemiplegia are often accompanied by other manifestations of stroke, including hemisensory loss, hemianopia, apraxia, agnosia, and aphasia. Muscles of the thorax and abdomen are usually not affected because they are innervated from both cerebral hemispheres.

When voluntary muscle control is lost, strong flexor muscles overbalance the extensors. This imbalance can cause serious contractures. For example, a hemiplegic client's affected arm tends to rotate internally and to adduct because adductor muscles are stronger than abductors. The elbow, wrist, and fingers also tend to flex. The affected leg tends to rotate externally at the hip joint, flex at the knee and plantar flex, and supinate at the ankle joint (Figure 72-2).

Aphasia. *Aphasia* is a deficit in the ability to communicate. Aphasia may involve any or all aspects of communication, including speaking, reading, writing, and understanding spoken language. The primary language center is usually located in the left cerebral hemisphere and is affected by stroke in the left middle cerebral artery. Several different types of aphasia exist; the most common are described here.

Wernicke's (sensory or *receptive) aphasia* affects speech comprehension as a result of an infarction in the temporal lobe of the brain. *Broca's (expressive* or *motor) aphasia* affects speech production as a result of an infarction in the frontal lobe of the brain. Branches of the middle cerebral artery supply both areas. *Global aphasia* affects both speech comprehension and speech production.

Internal Carotid Artery	Vertebrobasilar System	Anteroinferior Cerebellar (Lateral Pontine)	Posteroinferior Cerebellar
Contralateral hemiparesis with facial asymmetry	Alternating motor weaknesses Ataxic gait, dysmetria (uncoordinated actions)	Ipsilateral ataxia Facial paralysis	Ataxia Paralysis of larynx and soft palate
Contralateral sensory alterations	Contralateral hemisensory impairments	Ipsilateral loss of sensation in face, sensation changes on trunk and limbs	Ipsilateral loss of sensation in face, contralateral on body
Homonymous hemianopia Ipsilateral periods of blindness (amaurosis fugax)	Double vision Homonymous hemianopia Nystagmus, conjugate gaze paralysis	Nystagmus	Nystagmus
Aphasia if dominant hemisphere is involved	Dysarthria Memory loss Disorientation		Dysarthria
Mild Horner's syndrome Carotid bruits	Drop attacks Tinnitus, hearing loss Vertigo Dysphagia Coma or locked-in syndrome	Horner's syndrome Tinnitus, hearing loss	Horner's syndrome Hiccups and coughing Vertigo Nausea, vomiting

Other methods of classifying aphasia are by fluency or by the degree of difficulty in articulation. Clients with fluent aphasia (Wernicke's) have speech that is well articulated and grammatically correct but lacks content. Clients with nonfluent aphasia (Broca's) have varying degrees of difficulty in producing speech, and what words are spoken are uttered slowly, with great effort and poor articulation. Clients with global aphasia typically repeat the same sounds they hear and have poor comprehension.

Sensory or fluent aphasias involve loss of the ability to comprehend written, printed, or spoken words. A client with acoustic aphasia can hear the sounds of speech, but the parts of the brain that give meaning to these sounds are damaged. Clients have difficulty understanding what is being said. They hear sound but cannot make sense of it because they cannot understand the symbolic communication associated with the sound. Visual aphasia is similar. Affected clients cannot read words but can see them. They cannot understand the symbolic content of printed or written symbols.

Motor or nonfluent aphasias include aphasias in which the ability to write, make signs, or speak is lost. For example, with motor aphasia, words may be recalled but the client cannot combine speech sounds into words and syllables. Pure motor or pure sensory aphasias are rare. Most aphasias are mixed, affecting both expressive and receptive elements.

Most aphasias are partial rather than complete. The severity of aphasia varies with the area involved and the extent of cerebral damage. Severe damage may deprive the client of any meaningful relationship with the environment and family. Global aphasia can be so extensive that neither expressive nor receptive language abilities are retained. Early determination of the client's yes-no reliability facilitates communication. Verbal skills are often the best. Reading and writing are usually more impaired. The use of gestures can aid in communication.

Aphasia is frequently associated with hemiplegia involving the dominant hemisphere. The speech center for a right-handed client is usually located in the left cerebral hemisphere; the speech center for a left-handed client may be in the brain's right or left side. Thus a right-handed client with right-sided hemiplegia usually has aphasia because the speech center is in the damaged left hemisphere. Most people have left-sided speech dominance.

Dysarthria. *Dysarthria* is imperfect articulation that causes difficulty in speaking. It is important to differentiate between dysarthria and aphasia. With dysarthria the client understands language but has difficulty pronouncing words and may slur them, enunciating poorly. No disturbance is evident in grammar or in sentence construction. A dysarthric client can understand verbal speech and can read and write (unless the dominant hand is paralyzed, absent, or injured).

Dysarthria is caused by cranial nerve (CN) dysfunction from a stroke in the vertebrobasilar artery or its branches. It may result from weakness or paralysis of the muscles of the lips, tongue, and larynx or from a loss of sensation. In addition to speaking problems, clients with dysarthria often have difficulty chewing and swallowing because of poor muscle control.

Dysphagia. Swallowing is a complex process that requires the function of several cranial nerves. The mouth must open (CN V), the lips must close (CN VII), and the tongue must move (CN XII). The mouth must sense the quantity and quality of the food bolus (CN V and VII) and must send messages to the swallowing center (CN V and IX). During swallowing, the tongue moves the food bolus toward the oropharynx. The pharynx elevates and the glottis closes. Contraction of the pharyngeal muscles transports food from the pharynx to the esophagus. Peristalsis moves food to the stomach. A stroke in the territory of the vertebrobasilar system causes dysphagia.

Apraxia. *Apraxia* is a condition that affects complex motor integration and therefore can result from a stroke in several areas in the brain. In apraxia the client cannot carry out a skilled act such as dressing in the absence of paralysis. A client with apraxia may be able to conceive or conceptualize the content of messages to send to muscles. The motor patterns or schema necessary to convey the impulse message cannot be reconstructed, however. Thus accurate "instructions" do not reach the limb from the brain, and the desired action or movement does not happen. Apraxia ranges from relatively simple to highly complex disorders. For example, a client may have less difficulty writing than speaking or vice versa.

Visual Changes. Vision is a complex process controlled by several areas in the brain. Parietal and temporal lobe strokes may interrupt visual fibers of the optic tract en route to the occipital cortex and impair visual acuity. Depth perception and visual perception of horizontal and vertical planes may also be impaired. In clients with hemiplegia, this causes motor performance problems in gait and posture (Figure 72-3). Clients may or may not be aware of a perceptual difficulty, but it may cause them to be accident prone, and their behavior may appear bizarre. Visual disorders can interfere with a client's ability to relearn motor skills. Infarcts affecting the function of CN III, IV, and VI may produce CN palsies and result in diplopia.

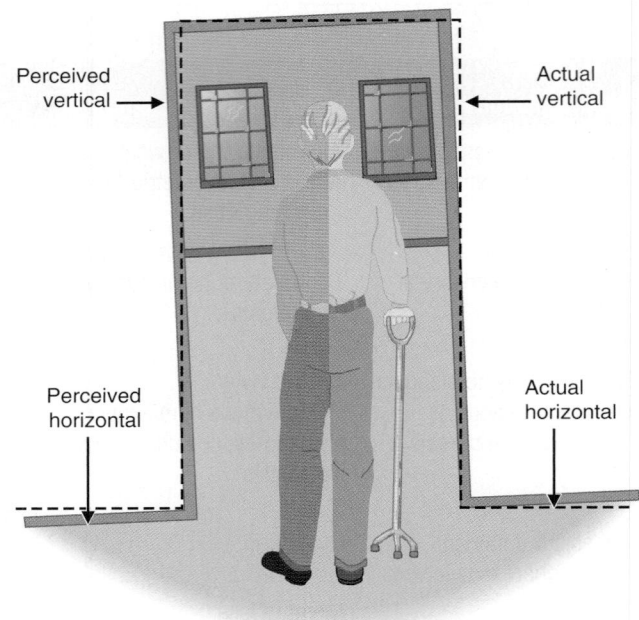

FIGURE 72-3 Perceptual disturbances in left sided hemiplegia. Such disturbances can be both unpleasant and unsafe.

Homonymous Hemianopia. *Homonymous hemianopia* (Figure 72-4) is a visual loss in the same half of the visual field of each eye, so the client has only half of normal vision. For example, the client may see clearly on one side of the midline but see nothing on the other side. Clients with homonymous hemianopia cannot see past the midline without turning the head toward that side.

Horner's Syndrome. *Horner's syndrome* is paralysis of the sympathetic nerves to the eye, causing sinking of the eyeball, ptosis of the upper eyelid, slight elevation of the lower lid, constriction of the pupil, and lack of tearing in the eye.

Agnosia. *Agnosia* is a disturbance in the ability to recognize familiar objects through the senses. The most common types are visual and auditory. Agnosia may result from an occlusion of the middle or posterior cerebral arteries supplying the temporal or occipital lobes.

A client with visual agnosia sees objects but is unable to recognize or attach meaning to them. Disorientation occurs because of an inability to recognize environmental cues, familiar faces, or symbols. Such a client may examine objects curiously but might be unable to determine their function. This can cause considerable self-care deficit when common, necessary objects, such as silverware, clothing, or toilet articles, are unfamiliar. Visual agnosia greatly increases the risk for injury because the client cannot recognize danger or symbols that warn of danger. Extensive visual agnosia can produce

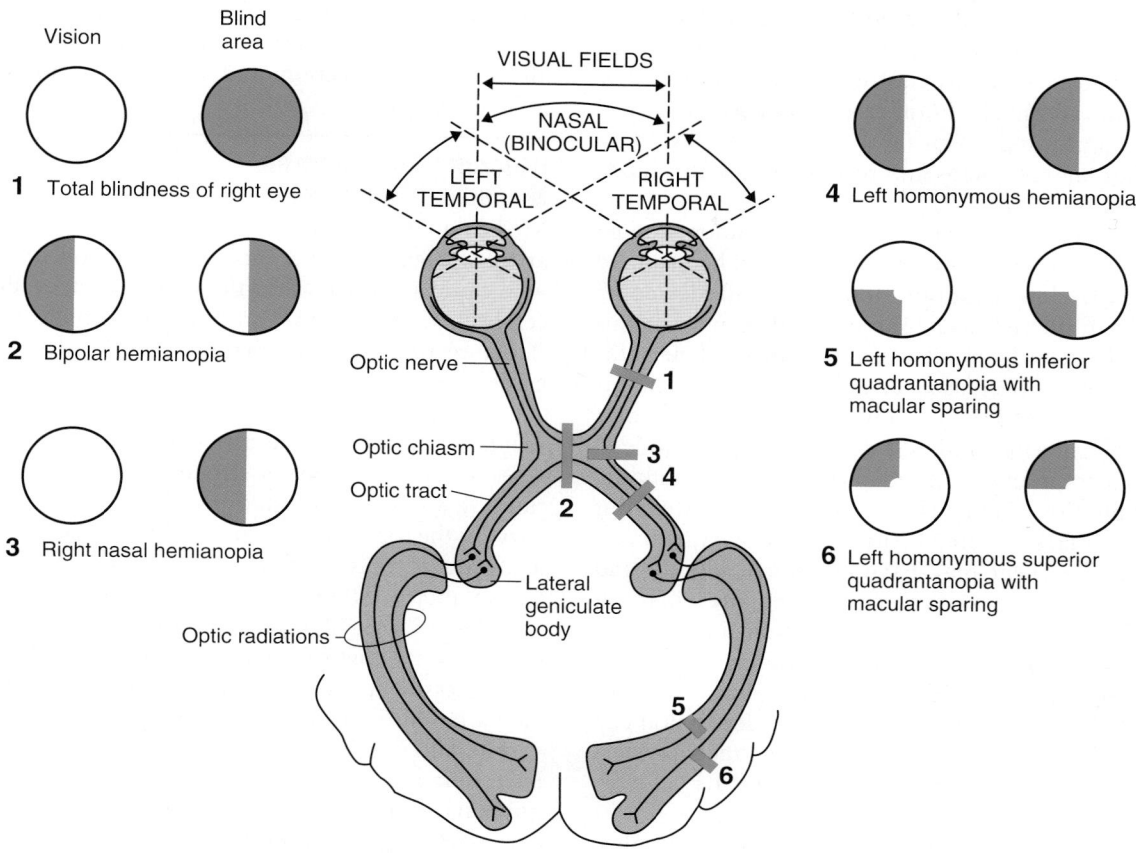

FIGURE 72-4 Visual-field defects associated with optic nerve lesions.

such extreme behavioral effects that the client's condition may be inaccurately diagnosed as diffuse dementia.

A client with auditory agnosia cannot attach meaning to sounds in the absence of hearing loss or decreased level of consciousness. Some degree of aphasia is almost always present. Often these people are initially considered hysterical or psychotic.

Unilateral Neglect. *Unilateral neglect* is the inability of a person to respond to stimulus on the contralateral side of a cerebral infarction. Clients with injury to the temporoparietal lobe, inferior parietal lobe, lateral frontal lobe, cingulate gyrus, thalamus, and striatum as a result of a middle cerebral artery occlusion most commonly develop neglect. Because of the dominance of the right hemisphere in directing attention, neglect is most commonly seen in clients with right hemisphere damage.

Clinical manifestations of unilateral neglect include failure to (1) attend to one side of the body, (2) report or respond to stimuli on one side of the body, (3) use one extremity, and (4) orient the head and eyes to one side. Unilateral neglect may be accompanied by inaccurate beliefs about the position of a limb in space or its existence or ownership. For example, a man with unilateral neglect may not believe that his arm is part of his body, he may be unaware of his arm's position, or he may deny that a limb is paralyzed when it is.

Sensory Deficits. Several types of sensory changes can result from a stroke in the sensory strip of the parietal lobe supplied by the anterior or middle cerebral artery. The deficit is on the contralateral side of the body and is frequently accompanied by hemiplegia or hemiparesis. *Hemisensory loss* (a loss of sensation on one side of the body) is generally incomplete and may not be noticed by the client. The superficial sensations of pain, touch, pressure, and temperature are affected in varying degrees. *Paresthesia* is described as persistent, burning pain; feelings of heaviness, numbness, tingling, or prickling; or heightened sensitivity. *Proprioception* (the ability to perceive the relationship of body parts to the external environment) and postural sense disturbances may occur with loss of muscle-joint sense. This may seriously interfere with the client's ability to ambulate because of a lack of balance control and inappropriate movements. The risk of falling is high because of the tendency to misposition the feet when walking.

Behavioral Changes. Various portions of the brain assist with control of behavior and emotions. The cerebral cortex interprets stimuli. The temporal and limbic areas modulate emotional responses to stimuli. The hypothalamus and pituitary glands coordinate the motor cortex and language areas. The brain can be seen as a modulator of emotions, and when the brain is not fully functional, emotional reactions and responses lack this modulation.

Behavioral changes after a stroke are common. People with stroke in the left cerebral, or dominant, hemisphere are frequently slow, cautious, and disorganized. People with stroke in the right cerebral, or nondominant, hemisphere are frequently impulsive, overestimate their abilities, and have a decreased attention span, which increases their risk of injury. Frontal lobe infarcts from a stroke in the anterior or middle cerebral arteries can lead to disturbances in memory, judgment, abstract thinking, insight, inhibition, and emotion.[39] The client may exhibit a flat affect, a lack of spontaneity, distractibility, and forgetfulness. The client may have emotional lability and burst into tears or, less commonly, laughter without provocation. There is little or no relationship between the emotion and what is occurring in the person's environment. Significant clinical depression occurs in 25% to 60% of clients with strokes.[15] Because depression can interfere with rehabilitation and functional recovery, it is important to identify it and initiate treatment.[29]

Incontinence. Stroke may cause bowel and bladder dysfunction. One type of neurogenic bladder, an uninhibited bladder, sometimes occurs after stroke. Nerves send the message of bladder filling to the brain, but the brain does not correctly interpret the message and does not transmit the message not to urinate to the bladder. This results in frequency, urgency, and incontinence. Sometimes clients with a type of neurogenic bowel seem fixated on having a bowel movement. Other causes of incontinence may be memory lapses, inattention, emotional factors, inability to communicate, impaired physical mobility, and infection. The duration and severity of the dysfunction depend on the extent and location of the infarct.[34]

Diagnostic Findings

With the advent of thrombolytic therapy in the treatment of acute ischemic stroke, accurate brain imaging plays an important role in the diagnosis and treatment of stroke.[12] A noncontrast head computed tomography (CT) scan is performed to rule out hemorrhagic stroke as a cause of acute neurologic deficits. Cellular changes that are diagnostic of stroke do not appear on the head CT scan acutely.[31] Standard magnetic resonance imaging (MRI) has limited value in diagnosing acute ischemic stroke because the infarct is usually not apparent until 8 to 12 hours after the onset of symptoms.[12] New MRI techniques—diffusion-weighted imaging (DWI) and perfusion imaging (PI)—may improve the diagnosis and

treatment of acute stroke. These techniques have greater sensitivity and anatomic resolution and the potential to allow earlier detection and characterization of acute ischemic stroke.[30]

Outcome Management
■ Medical Management

Medical management of the client with stroke is directed at early diagnosis and early identification of the client who can benefit from thrombolytic treatment. Preserving cerebral oxygenation, preventing complications and stroke recurrence, and rehabilitating the client are other goals.

Identify Stroke Early. A critical factor in the early intervention and treatment of stroke is the proper identification of stroke manifestations. Because manifestations vary by the location and size of the infarct, standardized assessment tools, including the Acute Stroke Quick Screen and the National Institutes of Health Stroke Scale (NIHSS) (Table 72-3), can be used to identify rapidly which clients might benefit from thrombolytic therapy.[31] The assessment must be complete and accurate to provide a baseline for ongoing assessments.

The initial assessment of the client who is thought to have had a stroke includes the level of consciousness, pupillary response to light, visual fields, movement of extremities, speech, sensation, reflexes, ataxia, and vital signs. These data are often recorded and scored on the Glasgow Coma Scale (GCS). In addition, if intracranial pressure monitors are in place, baseline pressure values and waveforms should be noted.

A complete history of the presenting problem as well as past medical and social history can provide data about the cause of the stroke. This information also guides stroke treatment. The time of onset of manifestations must be determined because thrombolytic therapy must be administered within 3 hours of the onset of manifestations. A history of hypertension or cardiac valve disorders is commonly associated with stroke.

Maintain Cerebral Oxygenation. Emergency care of the client with stroke includes maintaining a patent airway. The client should be turned on the affected side if he or she is unconscious to promote drainage of saliva from the airway. The collar of the shirt should be loosened to facilitate venous return. The head should be elevated, but the neck should not be flexed. The client should be kept quiet, and emergency help should be contacted.

Once the client is in the emergency department (ED), a patent airway is maintained and oxygen is supplied. If the client demonstrates poor ventilatory effort, intubation and mechanical ventilation may be required to prevent hypoxia and increased cerebral ischemia. An ECG is performed to assess for cardiac disorders, such as atrial fibrillation, that increase the

TABLE 72-3 · *National Institutes of Health (NIH) Stroke Scale*

Administer stroke scale items in the order listed. Scores should reflect what the patient does, not what the clinician thinks the patient can do. Except where indicated, the patient should not be coached (i.e., repeated requests to patient to make a special effort).

Instruction	Scale Definition
1a. Level of Consciousness The investigator must choose a response, even if a full evaluation is prevented by such obstacles as an endotracheal tube, language barrier, or orotracheal trauma or bandages. A **3** is scored only if the patient makes no movement (other than reflexive posturing) in response to noxious stimulation.	0 = Alert, keenly responsive 1 = Not alert, but arousable by minor stimulation to obey, answer, or respond 2 = Not alert, requires repeated stimulation or painful stimulation to make movements (not stereotyped) 3 = Responds only with reflex motor or autonomic effects, or totally unresponsive, flaccid, areflexic
1b. LOC Questions The patient is asked the month and his or her age. The answer must be correct—there is no partial credit for being close. Aphasic and stuporous patients who do not comprehend the questions will score **2**. Patients unable to speak because of endotracheal intubation, orotracheal trauma, severe dysarthria from any cause, language barrier, or any other problem not secondary to aphasia are given a **1**. It is important that only the initial answer be graded and that the examiner not "help" the patient with verbal or nonverbal cues.	0 = Answers both questions correctly 1 = Answers one question correctly 2 = Answers neither question correctly
1c. LOC Commands The patient is asked to open and close the eyes and then to grip and release the nonparetic hand. Substitute another one-step command if the hands cannot be used. Credit is given if an unequivocal attempt is made but not completed due to weakness. If patients do not respond to command, the task should be demonstrated to them (pantomime) and score the result (i.e., follows none, one, or two commands). Patients with trauma, amputation, or other physical impediments should be given suitable one-step commands. Only the first attempt is scored.	0 = Performs both tasks correctly 1 = Performs one task correctly 2 = Performs neither task correctly
2. Best Gaze Only horizontal eye movements will be tested. Voluntary or reflexive (oculocephalic) eye movements will be scored, but caloric testing is not done. If the patient has a conjugate deviation of the eyes that can be overcome by voluntary or reflexive activity, the score will be **1**. If a patient has an isolated peripheral nerve paresis (CN III, IV, or VI), score a **1**. Gaze is testable in all aphasic patients. Patients with ocular trauma, bandages, pre-existing blindness, or other disorder of visual acuity or fields should be tested with reflexive movements, and a choice made by the investigator. Establishing eye contact and then moving about the patient from side to side will occasionally clarify the presence of a gaze palsy.	0 = Normal 1 = Partial gaze palsy; this score is given when gaze is abnormal in one or both eyes, but where forced deviation or total gaze paresis is not present 2 = Forced deviation or total gaze paresis not overcome by the oculocephalic maneuver
3. Visual Visual fields (upper and lower quadrants) are tested by confrontation, using finger counting or visual threat as appropriate. Patient must be encouraged, but if he or she looks at the side of the moving fingers appropriately, this can be scored as normal. If there is unilateral blindness or enucleation, visual fields in the remaining eye are scored. Score **1** only if a clear-cut asymmetry, including quadrantanopia, is found. If patient is blind from any cause, score **3**. Double simultaneous stimulation is performed at this point. If there is extinction, patient receives a **1** and the results are used to answer question 11.	0 = No visual loss 1 = Partial hemianopia 2 = Complete hemianopia 3 = Bilateral hemianopia (blind, including cortical blindness)

Modified from National Institutes of Health, Bethesda, MD.
CN, Cranial nerve; *LOC,* level of consciousness.

Continued

TABLE 72-3	*National Institutes of Health (NIH) Stroke Scale—cont'd*
Instruction	**Scale Definition**

4. Facial Palsy

Ask or use pantomime to encourage the patient to show teeth or smile and close eyes. Score symmetry of grimace in response to noxious stimuli in the poorly responsive or noncomprehending patient. If facial trauma or bandages, orotracheal tube, tape, or other physical barrier obscures the face, these should be removed to the extent possible.

0 = Normal symmetrical movement
1 = Minor paralysis (flattened nasolabial fold, asymmetry on smiling)
2 = partial paralysis (total or near total paralysis of lower face)
3 = Complete paralysis (absence of facial movement in the upper and lower face)

5 and 6. Motor Arm and Leg

The limb is placed in the appropriate position: extend the arms 90 degrees (if sitting) or 45 degrees (if supine) and the leg 30 degrees (always tested supine). Drift is scored if the arm falls before 10 seconds or the leg before 5 seconds. The aphasic patient is encouraged using urgency in the voice and pantomime but not noxious stimulation. Each limb is tested in turn, beginning with the nonparetic arm. Only in the case of amputation or joint fusion at the shoulder or hip may the score be **9,** and the examiner must clearly write the explanation for scoring as a **9.**

0 = No drift; limb holds 90 degrees (or 45 degrees) for full 10 seconds
1 = Drift; limb holds 90 degrees (or 45 degrees) but drifts down before full 10 seconds; does not hit bed or other support
2 = Some effort against gravity; limb cannot get to or maintain (if cued) 90 degrees (or 45 degrees); drifts down to bed but has some effort against gravity
3 = No effort against gravity; limb falls
4 = No movement
9 = Amputation, joint fusion; explain:
5a = Left arm
5b = Right arm

0 = No drift; leg holds 30 degrees for full 5 seconds
1 = Drift; leg falls by the end of the 5-second period but does not hit bed
2 = Some effort against gravity; leg falls to bed by 5 seconds but has some effort against gravity
3 = No effort against gravity; leg falls to bed immediately
4 = No movement
9 = Amputation, joint fusion; explain:
6a = Left leg
6b = Right leg

7. Limb Ataxia

This item is aimed at finding evidence of a unilateral cerebellar lesion. Test with eyes open. In case of visual defect, ensure testing is done in intact visual field. The finger-nose-finger and heel-shin tests are performed on both sides, and ataxia is scored only if present out of proportion to weakness. Ataxia is absent in the patient who cannot understand or is hemiplegic, only in the case of amputation or joint fusion may the item be scored **9,** and the examiner must clearly write the explanation for not scoring. In case of blindness, test by touching nose from extended arm position.

0 = Absent
1 = Present in one limb
2 = Present in two limbs
If present, is ataxia in
  Right arm: 1 = yes   2 = No
    9 = Amputation or joint fusion; explain:
  Left arm: 1 = yes   2 = No
    9 = Amputation or joint fusion; explain:
  Right leg: 1 = yes   2 = No
    9 = Amputation or joint fusion; explain:
  Left leg: 1 = Yes   2 = No
    9 = Amputation or joint fusion; explain:

Modified from National Institutes of Health, Bethesda, MD.
CN, Cranial nerve; *LOC,* level of consciousness.

TABLE 72-3	*National Institutes of Health (NIH) Stroke Scale—cont'd*
Instruction	**Scale Definition**

8. Sensory

Sensation or grimace to pinprick when tested or withdrawal from noxious stimulus in the obtunded or aphasic patient. Only sensory loss attributed to stroke is scored as abnormal, and the examiner should test as many body areas (arms [not hands], legs, trunk, face) as needed to accurately check for hemisensory loss. A score of **2,** "severe or total," should only be given when a severe or total loss of sensation can be clearly demonstrated. Stuporous and aphasic patients will therefore probably score **1** or **0.** The patient with brain stem stroke who has bilateral loss of sensation is scored **2.** If the patient does not respond and is quadriplegic, score **2.** patients in coma (question 1a =3) are arbitrarily given a **2** on this item.

0 = Normal; no sensory loss
1 = Mild to moderate sensory loss; patient feels pinprick is less sharp or is dull on the affected side, or there is a loss of superficial pain with pinprick but patient is aware he or she is being touched
2 = Severe to total sensory loss; patient is not aware of being touched

9. Best Language

A great deal of information about comprehension will be obtained during the preceding sections of the examination. The patient is asked to describe what is happening in the attached picture, to name the items on the attached naming sheet, and to read from the attached list of sentences. Comprehension is judged from responses here as well as to all of the commands in the preceding general neurologic examination. If visual loss interferes with the tests, ask the patient to identify objects placed in the hand, repeat, and produce speech. The intubated patient should be asked to write a sentence. The patient in coma (question 1a = 3) will arbitrarily score **3** on this item. The examiner must choose a score in the patient with stupor or limited cooperation, but a score of **3** should be used only if the patient is mute and follows no one-step commands.

0 = No aphasia; normal
1 = Mild to moderate aphasia; some obvious loss of fluency or facility of comprehension, without significant limitation on ideas expressed or form of expression. Reduction of speech and/or comprehension, however, makes conversation about provided material difficult or impossible. For example, in conversation about provided materials examiner can identify picture or naming card from patient's response.
2 = Severe aphasia; all communication is through fragmentary expression; great need for inference, questioning, and guessing by the listener. Range of information that can be exchanged is limited; listener carries burden of communication. Examiner cannot identify materials provided from patient response.
3 = Mute, global aphasia; no usable speech or auditory comprehension

10. Dysarthria

If the patient is thought to be normal, an adequate sample of speech must be obtained by asking patient to read or repeat words from the attached list. If the patient has severe aphasia, the clarity of articulation of spontaneous speech can be rated. Only if the patient is intubated or has other physical barriers to producing speech may the item be scored **9,** and the examiner must clearly write an explanation for not scoring. Do not tell the patient why he or she is being tested.

0 = Normal
1 = Mild to moderate; patient slurs at least some words and, at worst, can be understood with some difficulty
2 = Severe; patient's speech is so slurred as to be unintelligible in the absence of or out of proportion to any dysphasia, or is mute/anarthric
9 = Intubated or other physical barrier; explain:

11. Extinction and Inattention (formerly Neglect)

Sufficient information to identify neglect may be obtained during the prior testing. If the patient has severe visual loss preventing visual double simultaneous stimulation, and the cutaneous stimuli are normal, the score is normal. If the patient has aphasia but does appear to attend to both sides, the score is normal. The presence of visual spatial neglect or anosognosia may also be taken as evidence of neglect. Because neglect is scored only if present, the item is never untestable.

0 = No abnormality
1 = Visual, tactile, auditory, spatial, or personal inattention or extinction to bilateral simultaneous stimulation in one of the sensory modalities
2 = Profound hemi-inattention or hemi-inattention to more than one modality; does not recognize own hand or orients to only one side of space

Continued

TABLE 72-3	*National Institutes of Health (NIH) Stroke Scale—cont'd*
Instruction	**Scale Definition**

Additional item, not part of the NIH Stroke Scale score.

12. Distal Motor Function
The patient's hand is held up at the forearm by the examiner, and patient is asked to extend his or her fingers as much as possible. If the patient cannot or does not extend the fingers, the examiner places the fingers in full extension and observes for any flexion movement for 5 seconds. The patient's first attempts only are scored. Repetition of the instructions or of the testing is prohibited.

0 = Normal (no flexion after 5 seconds)
1 = At least some extension after 5 seconds but not fully extended; any movement of the fingers that is not a command is not scored
2 = No voluntary extension after 5 seconds; movement of the fingers at another time is not scored
 a. Left arm
 b. Right arm

Modified from National Institutes of Health, Bethesda, MD.
CN, Cranial nerve; *LOC,* level of consciousness.

risk for embolic stroke. Blood pressure is also evaluated, and hypertension may be reduced with vasodilators. Caution is exercised when treating blood pressure because lowering the blood pressure too far may lower cerebral perfusion pressure and increase cerebral ischemia.[16,31] Laboratory tests for hematology, chemistry, and coagulation are obtained to rule out stroke-mimicking conditions and to detect bleeding disorders that would increase the risk of bleeding during thrombolytic therapy.

Restore Cerebral Blood Flow. The client is evaluated as a candidate for thrombolytic therapy once an intracerebral hemorrhage is ruled out. The goal of thrombolytic therapy is recanalization of the occluded vessel and reperfusion of ischemic brain tissue.[11,21] Thrombolytic agents are exogenous plasminogen activators, which dissolve the thrombus or embolus blocking the cerebral blood flow. Clients who receive recombinant tissue plasminogen activator (rt-PA) within 3 hours of the onset of stroke are 30% more likely to have minimal or no disability from acute ischemic stroke without an increase in mortality.[24] Several contraindications to thrombolytic therapy are shown in Box 72-1.

Treatment should begin immediately after the client is deemed to be a candidate for rt-PA. The dose of rt-PA for acute ischemic stroke is 0.9 mg/kg administered intravenously over 1 hour. Ten percent of the total dose is given as a bolus over 1 minute before initiation of the intravenous dose.[26,31] The pharmacologic half-life of rt-PA is approximately 5 to 7 minutes. After thrombolytic therapy, the client is sent to the intensive care unit (ICU) for careful monitoring of blood pressure, neurologic status, and bleeding.

The risk-benefit ratio for the use of thrombolytic therapy must be considered in certain client populations. The choice of whether to pursue aggressive treatment focuses on several factors, such as the client's age, his or her preference (if known), the presence and severity of

---

BOX 72-1	*Exclusion Criteria for Intravenous rt-PA Therapy for Acute Ischemic Stroke*

- Current use of oral anticoagulants or prothrombin time >15 seconds
- Use of heparin in previous 48 hours and a prolonged partial thromboplastin time
- Platelet count <100,000/mm³
- Another stroke or serious head injury in previous 3 months
- Major surgery within preceding 14 days
- Pretreatment systolic BP >185 mm Hg or diastolic BP >110 mm Hg
- Rapidly improving neurologic signs
- Isolated, mild neurologic deficits, such as ataxia alone, sensory loss alone, dysarthria alone, or minimal weakness
- Prior intracranial hemorrhage
- Blood glucose <50 mg/dl or >400 mg/dl
- Seizure at onset of stroke
- Gastrointestinal or urinary bleeding within preceding 21 days
- Recent myocardial infarction

From Urden, L.D., Stacy, K.M., & Lough, M.E. (2002). *Thelan's critical care nursing: Diagnosis and management* (4th ed.). St. Louis: Mosby.

other disorders, the severity of the stroke, and how much time has elapsed since the infarction. The risk of intracerebral hemorrhage after rt-PA is greater in clients with early signs of a major infarct on CT scan.[36,38] Clients who have severe neurologic deficits at presentation (NIHSS >22) are at increased risk for intracerebral hemorrhage and poor outcome.[31,38]

At present the treatment for most clients with large areas of infarction or large intracerebral hemorrhage is supportive care. It is hoped that future research can improve the treatment outcomes for these clients.

Prevent Complications

Bleeding. After administration of rt-PA, the client is monitored for potential complications of rt-PA, which may include intracranial hemorrhage and systemic bleeding.[3] In the initial studies of rt-PA in acute ischemic stroke, symptomatic intracranial hemorrhage occurred in 6.4% of clients within the first 36 hours after treatment.[24] Intracranial hemorrhage carries a mortality rate greater than 50%.[21] All fatal intracranial hemorrhages occurred within the first 24 hours of treatment.[3] The expanding clot of an intracranial hemorrhage destroys brain tissue. The pressure of the clot also disrupts blood flow and causes additional ischemia. Increased intracranial pressure (ICP) results from the space-occupying clot and surrounding edema of ischemic tissue and can lead to midline shift of intracranial contents, possible brain stem herniation, and death. To decrease the risk of intracranial or systemic bleeding, administration of anticoagulants and antiplatelet medications are not recommended until 24 hours after administration of rt-PA.[7]

Stringent blood pressure management is the single most important measure to prevent intracranial hemorrhage after thrombolysis.[3] Frequent vital signs and neurologic checks are necessary to prevent hypertension and detect manifestations of intracranial hemorrhage. Hypertension frequently accompanies acute ischemic stroke. Therefore blood pressure is usually not treated unless it increases to 185 mm Hg systolic or 105 mm Hg diastolic.[3] In addition, the mean arterial pressure should be lowered by no more than 10% and in gradual increments.[33] This is less likely to lead to hypoperfusion and worsening cerebral ischemia.

An intracranial hemorrhage should be suspected if the client has new complaints of headache, nausea and vomiting, or sudden change in level of consciousness. An intracranial hemorrhage should be assumed with any acute worsening of neurologic function until it can be ruled out by CT scan. If the rt-PA is still infusing, the infusion should be stopped. A complete blood count, coagulation studies, and type and cross are done. If a head CT scan reveals intracranial hemorrhage, fresh frozen plasma with fibrinogen or cryoprecipitate is administered to correct coagulopathies.

Systemic bleeding may also occur as a complication of rt-PA. Clinical manifestations include change in level of consciousness (LOC), tachycardia, hypotension, and cool, clammy, and pale skin. Thrombolytic therapy may be stopped depending on the site and severity of the bleeding.[16]

Cerebral Edema. Increased ICP is a potential complication of large ischemic strokes.[22] Increased ICP is also a potential complication of intracerebral hemorrhage, either primary or secondary to thrombolytic therapy. Manifestations of increased ICP include change in LOC, reflex hypertension, and worsening neurologic status. Invasive monitoring of ICP is done for clients with decreased LOC who are at high risk for increased ICP. All clients are placed on bed rest with the head of the bed elevated to 30 degrees to decrease ICP and to facilitate venous drainage. Ideally the degree of head elevation is based on the response of the client's ICP for those clients on ICP monitoring.[23]

External *ventriculostomy* drainage is sometimes used to reduce pressure from cerebrospinal fluid (CSF) accumulation. A burr hole is placed through the skull, and a catheter is passed into the lateral ventricle to allow for controlled drainage of CSF. Blood pressure is closely monitored. The goal is to maintain blood pressure low enough to prevent another stroke or hemorrhage without decreasing cerebral perfusion. The client may require continuous mechanical ventilation and hyperventilation to decrease ICP. Mannitol, an osmotic diuretic, helps in lowering increased ICP. Surgical evacuation of the intracerebral hematoma may be performed. Increasing ICP, central herniation, and brain stem hemorrhage can lead to death from depression of the vital centers in the medulla, that is, brain stem failure.

Stroke Recurrence. The incidence of stroke recurrence in the first 4 weeks after acute ischemic stroke ranges from 0.6% to 2.2% per week.[37] The risks of anticoagulation include intracranial hemorrhage, systemic bleeding, and death. Therefore the general use of heparin in all clients with acute ischemic stroke is no longer recommended. Heparin is indicated to prevent stroke recurrence in clients at risk for cardiogenic emboli. Initially unfractionated heparin is administered intravenously, and then warfarin is administered orally. Intravenous heparin is delivered with an infusion pump for accurate and safe delivery. Monitoring of clotting times is important to detect over-anticoagulation, which increases the risk of bleeding. Activated partial thromboplastin time (aPTT) should be at 1.5 to 2.5 times control for anticoagulation to be effective.

After a therapeutic anticoagulant level has been achieved with heparin therapy, warfarin is begun. Because warfarin has a long half-life, the physician initiates the warfarin therapy while the client is still receiving intravenous heparin. Once the client has a therapeutic response to warfarin, in about 24 to 48 hours, the physician discontinues the heparin and continues the warfarin therapy. The therapeutic International Normalized Ratio (INR) for prophylaxis against cardiogenic embolization is 2.0 to 3.0.[33] Clients receiving anticoagulation therapy should be assessed for bruising, hematuria, blood in feces, bleeding from mucous membranes, and new-onset or worsening headaches.

The long-term risk for stroke recurrence is 4% to 14% per year.[3] Antiplatelet agents, including aspirin, ticlopidine, extended-release dipyridamole plus aspirin, and clopidogrel, decrease the risk for secondary stroke.[9,41] Antiplatelet agents inhibit platelet function to decrease the risk of thrombus formation. The selection of the specific antiplatelet agent is individualized according to the client's medical history.

Aspiration. Clients with stroke are at high risk for aspiration pneumonia, which is the direct cause of death in 6% of clients following stroke.[4] Aspiration is most common in the early period and is related to loss of pharyngeal sensation, loss of oropharyngeal motor control, and decreased LOC. Oral food and fluids are generally withheld for 24 to 48 hours. If the client cannot eat or drink after 48 hours, alternate feeding routes are used, such as tube feeding or hyperalimentation. When the swallowing mechanism has returned, the client can be fed orally. Progressive feeding programs for dysphagia are based on the degree of swallowing ability.

Other Potential Complications. Other complications of stroke depend primarily on the location of the lesion or infarcted tissue. If the brain stem is affected, blood pressure fluctuations, altered respiratory patterns, and cardiac dysrhythmias are all possible. Physical injury related to the client's inability to realize his or her limitations can occur. Complications of immobility can also occur.

Coma can follow strokes of various causes. The blood supply to the brain stem or reticular activating system, which controls consciousness, may have been directly occluded. Similarly, the deep structures of the thalamus that relay information to the cerebral cortex may be involved. Vascular occlusion of the internal carotid artery or one of its major branches may also decrease LOC. Sometimes the cerebral edema that follows stroke may produce midline shifts, resulting in coma.

Hyperthermia is treated immediately with antipyretics. Temperature elevations lead to increased cerebral metabolic needs, which in turn cause cerebral edema and increased risk for cerebral ischemia. In addition, a hypothermia blanket or ice packs may be required to reduce body temperature. Causing the client to shiver should be avoided, however, because shivering increases oxygen consumption and ICP. If seizures develop, phenytoin (Dilantin) or phenobarbital may be used. Hyperglycemia is common after a stroke and has been associated with poor outcomes in clients with a stroke.[40] Glucose monitoring should be performed, and normoglycemia should be maintained.[40]

Strokes caused by occlusive disease (e.g., thrombus, embolus) rarely cause sudden death. When stroke is fatal, death may occur within 3 to 12 hours, but it occurs more often between 1 and 14 days after the original episode. Typically, with any type of fatal stroke, a rise in temperature, heart rate, and respiratory rate occurs along with deepening coma several hours or days before death. These result from damage to the vasomotor and heat-regulating centers. See the Case Study feature on Meningioma, Fractured Hip, and Possible Stroke, below.

Rehabilitation After Stroke. From the onset of stroke, interventions are aimed at maximizing the client's physical and cognitive recovery.[13] Early pre-mobilization efforts are aimed at preventing the complications of neurologic deficit and immobility. After the first few days of the acute event, cerebral edema has usually subsided and the residual deficits of stroke can be identified. Clients with stroke and their families face difficult adjustments as the acute stages pass and residual disabilities become obvious.

Previously it was thought that damage to the central nervous system (CNS) was irreversible. Now it has been shown that even in adults with significant brain injury, relearning can take place. It is extremely important that relearning take place as soon as possible after the injury. Early rehabilitation makes this relearning possible. The severity of a client's stroke will impact the length of time it may take to recover their function.

An interdisciplinary rehabilitation team is necessary to assist and support clients and their families during this time. Assessing the functional abilities of the client and setting realistic goals are part of this approach. To optimize recovery, all clinicians should use the Clinical Practice Guidelines developed by the Agency for Health Care Policy and Research (AHCPR) on post-stroke rehabilitation to guide the care of a client suffering from a stroke.[29]

Because stroke is a common health care problem, many facilities have developed clinical pathways to guide care. (See the CareMap of the Clinical Pathway feature on Stroke on the website.)

The recommended plan of care includes using interdisciplinary services to do the following:

- Document the client's condition and course fully, including deficits, status of other diseases, compli-

---

CASE STUDY *evolve*

Meningioma, Fractured Hip, and Possible Stroke

Mrs. Olsen is a 72-year-old white woman who resides at Shady Oaks Care Center. She fell today and could not get up again because of the pain. An x-ray examination obtained at the nursing home showed a proximal femoral fracture near the right hip joint. She has been transferred to your hospital for a preoperative medical evaluation in preparation for possible surgical repair of her right hip fracture later today. . . . *Case Study continued on the website and the CD-ROM with discussions, multiple-choice questions, and a nursing care plan.* *evolve*

cations, changes in status, and functional status before stroke

- Begin physical activity as soon as the client's medical condition is stable; use caution with early mobilization in clients with progressing neurologic deficit, subarachnoid or intracerebral hemorrhage, severe orthostatic hypotension, acute myocardial infarction, or acute deep vein thrombosis
- Assist in managing general health functions throughout all stages of treatment, such as managing dysphagia, nutrition, hydration, bladder and bowel function, sleep and rest, co-morbid conditions, and acute illnesses
- Prevent complications, including deep vein thrombosis and pulmonary embolism, aspiration, skin breakdown, urinary tract infections, falls, spasticity and contractures, shoulder injury, and seizures
- Prevent recurrent strokes through control of modifiable risk factors, oral anticoagulation, antiplatelet therapy, or surgical intervention
- Assess throughout acute and rehabilitation stages
- Use reliable standardized instruments for evaluation
- Evaluate for formal rehabilitation during the acute stage
- Choose an individual or interdisciplinary program based on the client's and family's needs; success of the program requires full support and active participation of the client and family; families must be involved at the outset
- Choose the local rehabilitation program that best meets the client's and family's needs

Interdisciplinary Management. Several other disciplines join to facilitate recovery of the client following a stroke. It is the coordinated effort of the entire team that best serves the client and family.

Physical Therapy. Physical therapists work with the client to build strength and preserve range of motion (ROM) and tone in noninvolved muscles. Physical therapy also builds ROM and tone and retrains muscles affected by the stroke. The client also works on balance and proprioception skills. This may enable the client, with continued improvement, to sit on the edge of the bed and eventually to ambulate. Exercise and bed mobility skills are taught at the client's bedside, as are wheelchair mobility and transfers. Clients who would benefit from the use of an orthosis are identified and instructed on how to apply and remove it. A hemiplegic client is usually able to ambulate using a quad cane following gait training.

Occupational Therapy. Occupational therapists work with the client to relearn activities of daily living (ADL) and to use assistive devices that promote independence. For example, a client with hemiplegia may be able to dress if the clothing can be closed with self-fastening tape (Velcro) fasteners rather than buttons.

Many clients experience severe pain in the affected shoulder and hand after a stroke. This pain can be so severe that it results in lack of balance and loss of ROM, which further restricts mobility and self-care. Overstretching from turns and transfers can aggravate the problem. Some clients have experienced partial dislocation or subluxation of the shoulder both from having the shoulder pulled on and from the weight of the arm pulling it. Chronic subluxation results in shoulder-hand syndrome, characterized by a painful or frozen shoulder and hand edema. Occupational therapists assist in treating this problem and in instructing the client and caregivers in proper transfer and positioning techniques to prevent further injury.

Speech Therapy. Speech pathologists work with the client to foster the maximum amount of speech recovery possible through relearning, accentuation of speech sounds, or use of alternative communication devices. The speech pathologist also assesses the client's swallowing mechanism and makes recommendations for initiation and progression of foods and fluids to decrease the risk of aspiration.

Case Management. Case managers are often assigned to clients following stroke. Their role is to facilitate all care providers and to advocate for the client and family. (See Case Management feature on Stroke on the website.)

■ Nursing Management of the Medical Client
Assessment

Ongoing assessments of all body systems are needed. The use of a standardized neurologic assessment tool such as the GCS assists the nurse in documenting changes in the client's status and in monitoring progress. In addition to the neurologic assessment, the client's heart sounds, heart rate and rhythm, respiratory rate and rhythm, temperature, levels of nutrition, ability to swallow, bladder and bowel elimination, communication, and sexuality need to be assessed. The client's and family's psychosocial and learning needs should be assessed daily.

Diagnosis, Outcomes, Interventions

Diagnosis: Ineffective Tissue Perfusion: Cerebral Perfusion of the cerebrum is critical for survival and long-term outcome. Therefore it should be the first priority in the care of clients with acute stroke. Decreased cerebral blood flow may be secondary to thrombus, embolus, hemorrhage, edema, or spasm. Ongoing assessment and intervention are required beyond the critical stage. Data indicating that the risk for altered perfusion has become an actual problem are shown in Box 72-2.

Outcomes. The client will have improved cerebral tissue perfusion as evidenced by ICP less than 15 mm Hg, cerebral perfusion pressure (CPP) greater than 65 mm Hg, no type A waves (when using intracranial monitors), no reports of headache, no decreases in LOC, and stable or improving GCS score.

Interventions. Serial assessments of these data may be required as often as every 15 minutes for unstable clients to every 2 to 4 hours for stable clients. Analyze data for trends, and if the client is deteriorating neurologically, notify the physician. Manifestations of progressive deterioration include decreasing LOC, changes in motor or sensory function, pupillary changes, respiratory difficulty, and development of visual or perceptual defects or aphasia.

Maintain the client's blood pressure within the range prescribed by the physician to maintain perfusion without promoting cerebral edema. Maintain normothermia to reduce cerebral glucose and oxygen consumption. Cluster nursing interventions to reduce unneeded movement and stimulation. Elevate the head of the bed 30 degrees to reduce cerebral edema. Maintain the client's head in a neutral position to improve venous drainage.

Administer medications to improve cerebral tissue perfusion as prescribed. The drugs prescribed to decrease risk for further thrombus formation include anticoagulants or antiplatelet agents. Nimodipine, a calcium-channel blocker, is used to treat vasospasm secondary to subarachnoid hemorrhage.[19]

BOX 72-2 *Manifestations Indicating an Acute Change in Cerebral Perfusion*

- Intracranial pressure greater than 15 mm Hg sustained for 15 to 30 seconds or longer
- Cerebral perfusion pressure less than 70 mm Hg
- Decrease in Glasgow Coma Scale score of two or more points from baseline
- Decreasing levels of consciousness
- Mean arterial pressure of less than 80 mm Hg or systolic blood pressure less than 100 mm Hg
- Bradycardia
- Altered pattern of breathing
- Loss of response to painful stimuli
- Change in pupil size or response to light
- Headache
- Vomiting
- Abnormal flexion or extension posturing

Delirium and restlessness should be controlled, with sedatives if necessary. Be certain, however, that restlessness is not the result of treatable causes, such as hypoxia, full bladder, bowel impaction, or pain. Restraints should be avoided because they often increase agitation and ICP.

Straining at stool or with excessive coughing, vomiting, lifting, or use of the arms to change position should be avoided, because the Valsalva maneuver increases ICP. Mild laxatives and stool softeners are often prescribed.

Collaborative Problem: Hemorrhage. Because of the increased risk for systemic bleeding secondary to the use of thrombolytic therapy or anticoagulation, monitoring for bleeding is an important collaborative problem. Write the collaborative problem as *Risk for prolonged bleeding times related to use of thrombolytic agents or anticoagulation.*

Outcomes. The nurse will monitor for hemorrhage and, if present, will control bleeding and notify the physician.

Interventions. For the client who is receiving thrombolytic therapy, certain interventions can prevent systemic bleeding. These include no arterial punctures or insertions of nasogastric tubes for 24 hours after the infusion; monitor all puncture sites and body fluids for manifestations of bleeding for 24 hours; and maintain bed rest for 24 hours after completion of the infusion. Gingival bleeding and oozing from intravenous sites have been associated with intracranial hemorrhage.[3] Pressure may be applied to any compressible bleeding sites.

For the client who is receiving anticoagulation, monitor the aPPT and INR and adjust the client's dosage based on the physician's orders. Report any manifestations of bleeding to the physician immediately.

Diagnosis: Risk for Aspiration. The nursing diagnosis *Increased Risk for Aspiration* is listed here because of its importance in maintaining airway and oxygenation. Not all clients are at risk for aspiration after stroke, and their risk depends on the time since injury and area of infarction. When considering this nursing diagnosis, use the following causes of aspiration to guide your problem-solving: impaired swallowing, depressed cough and gag reflexes, and decreased LOC.

Outcomes. The client will have a reduced risk of aspiration as evidenced by easily managing saliva, no choking or coughing while eating, no fever, and no crackles or rhonchi.

Interventions. Assess the client for clinical manifestations of aspiration, such as fever, dyspnea, crackles and rhonchi, confusion, and decreased PaO$_2$ in arterial blood gases. Use caution in feeding the client, either orally or enterally. If the client is receiving enteral feedings, add food coloring to the tube feeding to assist with identifying aspiration via suctioned aspirate. Monitor chest x-ray results, and report findings of pulmonary infiltrate.

Diagnosis: Impaired Physical Mobility.

Almost all clients have some degree of immobility after a stroke. In the early phases of stroke recovery, the client may be completely immobile and need assistance just to turn over in bed. Later in recovery, mobility may be hampered in one extremity only. Various causes can be used to individualize this diagnosis. These include (1) loss of muscle tone secondary to flaccid paralysis or spasticity and (2) reluctance to move because of the fear of self-injury or prolonged disuse.

Outcomes.
The client will achieve maximal physical mobility within the limitations imposed by the stroke as evidenced by more normal movement of the affected extremity, improved muscle strength, and effective use of adaptive devices.

Interventions.
Assess the client's degree of muscle strength to use as a baseline value and for determining and evaluating outcomes. A comprehensive assessment by a physical therapist helps to determine appropriate activity levels.

Encourage Bed Exercises. Encouraging clients with hemiplegia to exercise while at bed rest not only prepares them for later activities but also offers hope and a sense of optimism about recovery. A hemiplegic client can learn to move the weak leg by sliding the unaffected leg under it to lift and move the weak leg. The client can also use the unaffected arm to move the affected arm and hand. Keep in mind that clients may have difficulty crossing the midline.

Frequent gluteal and quadriceps muscle setting exercises during the day help to prepare the client for later ambulation. Begin with five repetitions, and increase gradually to 20 repetitions each time. Instruct the client as follows:

1. *Gluteal setting:* "Pinch" or contract the buttocks together and count to five. Then relax and count to five. Repeat.
2. *Quadriceps setting:* Contract the quadriceps muscles on the anterior portion of the thigh while raising the heel and trying to squash a rolled towel placed under the popliteal fossa against the mattress. While keeping the muscle contracted, count to five. Then relax and count to five. Repeat. Perform on both legs if possible. Start quadriceps setting exercise as soon as the client is conscious. The quadriceps muscle is the most important in giving knee joint stability in walking.

Help the Client Sit Up. Help the client out of bed as soon as the client's condition is medically stable. Remember, however, that hemiplegia can severely affect balance. Assistance is needed to provide security and safety. Raise the head of the bed slowly to reduce orthostatic hypotension.

When the client first sits up, support the affected side, especially the back and the head. Gradually the client will learn to sit alone with the head of the bed elevated and then to sit on the edge of the bed with the feet on a firm surface. Help the client maintain balance by extending the affected arm and placing the palm flat on the bed. Be patient and encouraging as the client regains balance. When the client is sitting in a chair, support the weak side with pillows.

Eventually the client will learn to raise the weak leg with the unaffected leg and to swing both legs laterally over the side of the bed onto the floor. It is safest to have the client pivot on the unaffected leg. Therefore position the chair at a right angle to the unaffected side.

Teach the Client How to Use a Wheelchair. A hemiplegic client needs to learn safe transfers from the bed to the chair, commode, or wheelchair. The Client Education Guide feature on Transfer from Bed to Wheelchair by a Hemiplegic Client on p. 2126 shows one method. The client with hemiplegia can propel a wheelchair with the unaffected arm and leg; one-arm-drive wheelchairs also are available. Once the client is in a wheelchair, his or her level of independence increases greatly. Deficits in spatial relations, decreased awareness, and unilateral neglect can result in problems such as falling and running into doors. Clients must not be allowed to perform wheelchair self-transfers until they have demonstrated competence.

Promote Walking. A tilt table may be used in physical therapy to help the client assume a standing position if difficulty with balance is a problem. The client can begin standing as soon as the quadriceps muscles on the unaffected side have normal strength. Have the client seated on the edge of the bed. Encourage the client to rise by using the muscle power of the unaffected leg. The client may tend to swing around toward the affected side. Gradually the client will learn to take increasing amounts of weight onto the weaker side.

Despite weakness in the affected limb, a hemiplegic client often develops an extensor reflex, which facilitates standing. Position yourself on the weaker side when helping the client to stand. To avoid pulling on the affected arm and increasing the risk for shoulder injury, provide support with ambulation by using a gait belt. A quad cane should be used on the unaffected side to allow walking with a three-point gait.

Most hemiplegic clients can be taught to walk. Remind them to keep the body weight forward over the feet. Practice is important for learning to walk correctly.

CLIENT EDUCATION GUIDE

Transfer from Bed to Wheelchair by a Hemiplegic Client

- Lock the wheelchair for safety, and keep it beside the bed on your unaffected side.
- Use your unaffected arm and leg **(A, B)** to move your affected arm and leg.
- As your legs drop over the edge of the bed, swing your torso up to a sitting position **(C)**.

- Push yourself up to a standing position **(D)** by using your unaffected arm and leg.
- Reach across the wheelchair **(E)** to grasp the far arm of the chair, and turn to seat yourself.
- Shading on the right side of the client indicates the affected side.

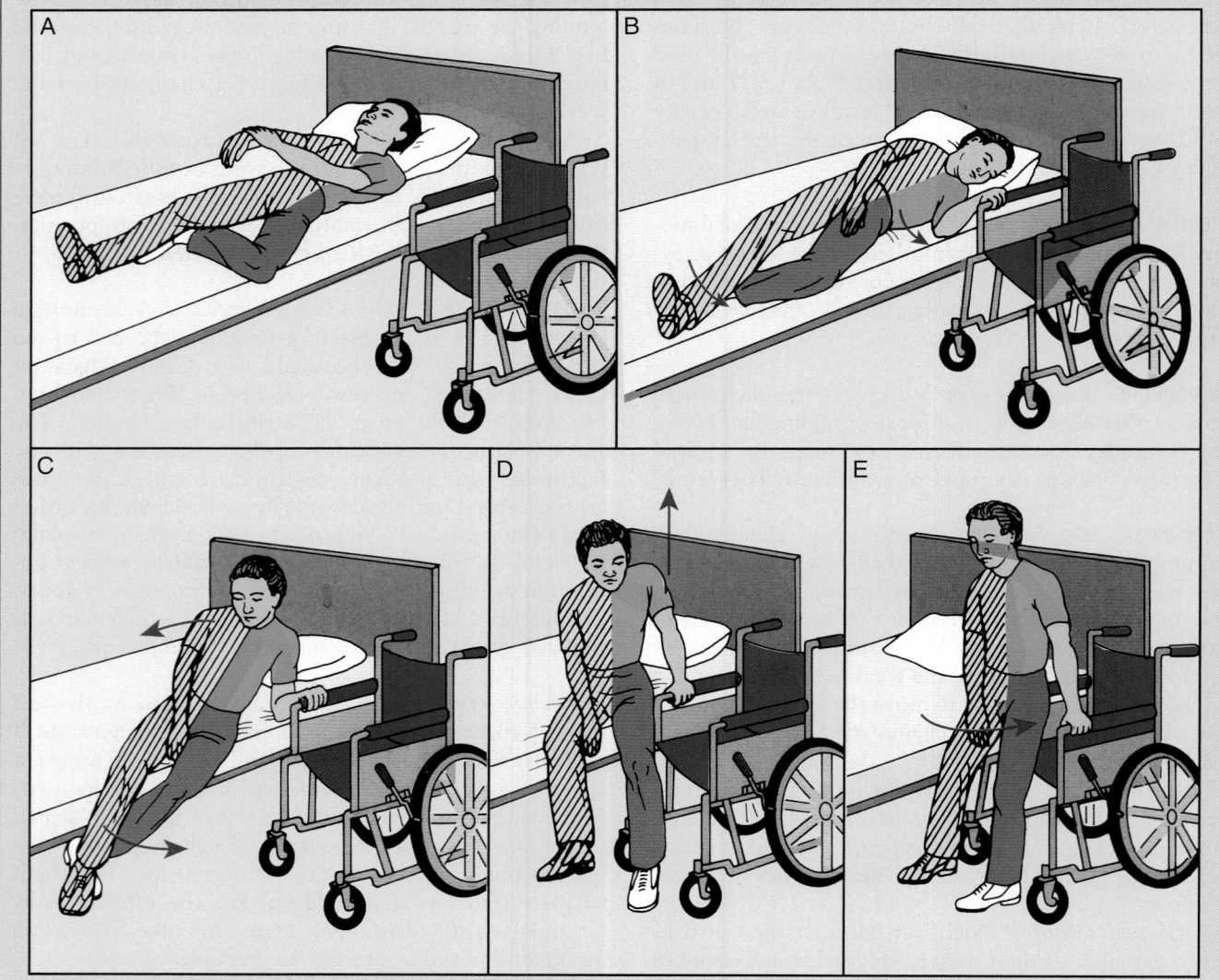

Incorrect habits, once developed, may be difficult to overcome later. Supervise clients carefully until they can safely walk alone without fear of falling. When walking, the client should not show circumduction or toe scraping or stoop forward. Heel-toe walking with a reciprocal gait pattern is the goal of ambulation.

Teach Bracing. If bracing is used, teach the client and family how to apply and remove the brace, to observe skin for breakdown, to give proper skin care, and to care for the brace itself.

Diagnosis: Risk for Hyperthermia. Bleeding or edema of the hypothalamus can lead to ischemia of the thermoregulatory center of the brain.

Outcomes. The client will have a reduced risk of hyperthermia or will have a normal temperature.

Interventions. Treat fever with antipyretics. A hypothermia blanket may be used to bring down a high temperature quickly. When hypothermia blankets are used, assess the skin frequently for pressure points and cold injury. Shivering must be avoided because the muscle activity increases body temperature. Keeping the feet warm with blankets may decrease shivering. Phenothiazine agents may be used to help stabilize neuronal membranes if fever is related to damaged brain structures.

Diagnosis: Risk for Impaired Skin Integrity.

The loss of protective sensation and decreased ability to move increases the risk for injury to the skin. In addition, skin damage may develop from friction and shearing or increased skin fragility from inadequate nutritional status or edema.

Outcomes. The client's skin will remain intact as evidenced by an absence of stage I pressure ulcer development and an absence of manifestations of redness from friction or shearing.

Interventions. Assess the skin every 2 hours. Change the position of a client with hemiplegia or decreased LOC every 2 hours. Develop a written turning schedule for other health care providers and family members to follow. When positioning the client on the affected side, make sure that body weight does not harm affected limbs. Support the affected arm and leg when turning and positioning a hemiplegic client. Complete shoulder and hip dislocation can occur if the flaccid extremity is not supported properly. Place a pillow between the client's legs to provide support. The client may be able to tolerate lying only for 30 minutes on the affected side because of the impaired circulation or pain.

Collaborative Problem: Risk for Contracture.

One of the normal activities of the brain is to inhibit spastic muscle contraction. Early in stroke recovery, flaccidity is usually present because of a loss of cerebral connections for afferent sensory and efferent motor nerves. During recovery affected muscles may be spastic because the injured brain cannot inhibit spastic muscle contraction. Therefore the collaborative problem *Risk for Contracture* is due to flaccid paralysis or spasticity.

Outcomes. The nurse will monitor for the development of contractures as evidenced by no muscle shortening and by maintaining normal ROM.

Interventions. Assess the client's ROM in both the involved and noninvolved joints. These findings can be used as a baseline and as an expected outcome.

Perform passive ROM exercises two times daily after the first 24 hours following a stroke unless otherwise prescribed. Motor impulses usually begin to return between 2 and 14 days after a stroke. The affected part

(initially flaccid) becomes spastic as the spinal cord motor systems establish their autonomy and the potential for contractures increases. Passive ROM exercises are more difficult to perform once affected muscles begin to tighten.

Do not force extremities beyond the point of initiating pain or continuous spasm. Always support the joint you are exercising, and move the extremity smoothly, without jerking movements. Frequent passive ROM exercises (1) prevent joint immobility, tendon contractures, and muscle atrophy; (2) stimulate circulation; and (3) help reestablish neuromuscular pathways. Performing these exercises before dressing and undressing the client may facilitate self-care.

Teach the client to use the unaffected hand to lift the weak arm and to put it through ROM exercises. Exercise each finger separately. While the client is in bed, teach him or her (1) to exercise the affected arm by grasping it at the wrist with the unaffected hand and raising it above the head and (2) to stretch and rub the fingers of the affected hand several times each day. Active ROM to the unaffected extremities assists in maintaining or increasing muscle strength.

Once some voluntary movement returns, encourage the client with assisted movements. As motor strength increases, resisted movements may strengthen weakened muscles and help restore muscle bulk. Shoulder slings are not recommended because they may increase the risk of contractures.

Several interventions are used to reduce the risk for joint contracture:

1. Allow the client to sit upright for short periods only; sitting can contribute to hip and knee flexion deformities.
2. When the client is on one side, do not flex the hip acutely.
3. Do not place a pillow under the affected knee when the client is supine; this encourages flexion deformity and impedes circulation.
4. If the client's knees tend to hyperextend, place a folded towel under the knee for short periods while the client is lying supine.

If the client can tolerate the prone position, place the client in this position for 15 to 30 minutes several times a day, with a small pillow placed under the pelvis (from the umbilicus to the upper third of the thigh) to hyperextend the hip joints.

Prevent foot drop, heel cord shortening, and plantiflexion by (1) avoiding pressure on the feet, (2) performing frequent passive ROM exercises, and (3) having the client sit in a chair as soon as possible with the feet flat on the floor. While the client is in bed, keep the foot flexed at 90 degrees by using high-top tennis shoes or orthotics.

A trochanter roll, extending from the crest of the ilium to midthigh, prevents external hip rotation by wedging under the projection of the greater trochanter and stopping the femur from rolling. Because trochanter rolls increase the risk of skin impairment, assess the skin beneath the roll often.

When the client is in bed, prevent adduction of the affected shoulder by placing a pillow in the axilla, between the upper arm and the chest wall, to keep the arm abducted about 60 degrees. Keep the arm slightly flexed in a neutral position. Place the forearm on another pillow with the elbow above the shoulder and the wrist above the elbow. This position stretches the shoulder's internal rotators. Elevating the arm also helps to prevent edema and resultant fibrosis.

Place the affected hand in a position of function (i.e., slightly supinated with fingers slightly flexed and the thumb in opposition). Frequent passive ROM exercises are important. The use of splints to prevent flexion contractures is more effective if the splints are designed individually by occupational therapists and scheduled for on-and-off periods to allow for skin assessment and ROM. Squeezing a rubber ball is not recommended because it promotes flexion when extension is desired.

The weight of an immobile arm may cause pain and movement limitation (frozen shoulder) or subluxation of the shoulder joint. Prevent these by supporting a completely flaccid arm with a pillow when the client is in bed or seated in a chair.

Diagnosis: Self-Care Deficit.

Self-care deficits may range from not being able to reach with a weak arm to full dependence on others. This diagnosis is applicable if an achievable outcome can be obtained. Clients with complete paralysis and cognitive deficits may not be able to perform self-care. Other nursing diagnoses may be more applicable, such as *Impaired Physical Mobility* and *Impaired Skin Integrity*. Several nursing diagnoses can be used to describe *Self-Care Deficit*, including *Impaired Physical Mobility, Disturbed Sensory Perception (Visual), Unilateral Neglect,* or *Disturbed Thought Processes.*

Outcomes. The client will perform as many ADLs as possible within limitations as evidenced by use of adaptive devices and techniques.

Interventions. Initially a client who has had a stroke may need considerable help with all self-care activities, including washing, eating, and grooming. Encourage clients to perform as many self-care activities as possible and to use the affected arm to avoid the tendency to do everything with the unaffected arm. This activity helps to preserve independent self-care, prevents complications of immobility, and enhances self-esteem.

Remember that stroke clients are easily frustrated and may need a lot of encouragement. Self-care activities provide an excellent opportunity for family teaching. Family members find it difficult to watch a loved one struggle with a task, and they often perform the task for the client. Explain how it benefits the client to be as independent as possible.

In clients with diplopia, an eye patch over one eye removes the second image and promotes better vision. Alternating the patch daily helps to maintain the function and strength of the extraocular muscles in both eyes. Provide mouth care at least three or four times a day, giving special attention to the affected side of the tongue and mouth. Focus rehabilitation plans on self-care deficits and ADL.

Diagnosis: Risk for Injury.

The *Risk for Injury* and trauma continues throughout recovery from stroke. It may also extend into the home environment, where clients attempt to perform former activities, such as cooking or driving. Factors that increase the risk for injury include decreased LOC, weakness, flaccidity, spasticity, impulsive behavior, altered thought processes, and motor, visual, and spatial-perceptual impairments.

Outcomes. The client will remain free from injury as evidenced by an absence of abrasions, burns, or falls. The client will also seek needed help to perform tasks that are beyond his or her capabilities.

Interventions. Keep the side rails of the bed raised for clients with recent hemiplegia to protect them from rolling out of bed. As recovery proceeds, the client may pull against side rails when sitting up or turning. Once the client can get out of bed unassisted, half side rails may be more useful. Full side rails hinder ambulation.

A client with impaired sensation is especially prone to injury. Frequent skin inspections for manifestations of injury are essential. Visual disturbances may also increase a hemiplegic client's potential for injury. Weakness on one side makes clients susceptible to falls. Remind clients to walk slowly, rest adequately between intervals of walking, use effective lighting, and look where they are going. Be especially alert during toileting. Make sure that support staff and family members know not to leave these clients alone in the bathroom.

Diagnosis: Imbalanced Nutrition: Less Than Body Requirements.

Use the nursing diagnosis *Imbalanced Nutrition: Less Than Body Requirements* if your client has an inability to swallow secondary to stroke. Support the diagnosis with data on intake and output, ability to swallow, caloric intake and weight change over the past 3 days, hemoglobin, hematocrit, albumin, prealbumin, and lymphocyte count over the past 3 days.

Outcomes. The client will demonstrate manifestations of adequate nutrition as evidenced by (1) maintenance of stable weight; (2) consumption of adequate calories for age, height, and weight; (3) intake equaling output; (4) hemoglobin and hematocrit levels within normal limits for age and gender; (5) lymphocyte count, prealbumin, and albumin levels within normal limits; and (6) healing of incisions and wounds within 12 to 14 days, as applicable.

Interventions. Carefully assess the client's diet to ensure adequate nutrition. Assess total intake. Feeding clients with partial paralysis of the tongue, mouth, and throat requires patience and care for prevention of choking and aspiration. Clients often fear choking and are embarrassed and frustrated by eating difficulties. Consequently, they may avoid eating and may not obtain adequate nutrition. Give supplemental meals as necessary. If the client cannot swallow at all, tube feeding may be used. With help and encouragement, hemiplegic clients can usually learn to feed themselves. Many helpful orthotic devices are available through consultation with an occupational therapist. These might include utensils with built-up handles or scoop plates. Make mealtimes pleasant and unhurried. Serve food attractively and at an appropriate temperature.

Feeding can be very frustrating for a dysphagic client, especially if the caregiver is not familiar with the client's **EB** specific disabilities. Support personnel and family members need to be taught basic feeding techniques and also to be informed of each client's individual needs and limitations. To facilitate feeding, assess the following and intervene as necessary. The speech pathologist can recommend additional feeding techniques based on the client's specific deficits and needs.

Promote Head Control. If the client has limited or no voluntary head control, placing a hand on the forehead may help. The caregiver approaches the client from the midline rather than from the side so that the client does not have to turn the head to be fed. Remind the client not to throw the head back to propel food because this can lead to aspiration. The head should be midline and flexed slightly forward.

Assist in Positioning. Have the client in an upright position, as close to 90 degrees as possible, either in bed or in a chair. Support the client's head to counteract hyperextension.

Promote Mouth Opening. If the client does not open the **EB** mouth, lightly touch both lips with the tip of a spoon. If this does not work, apply light pressure with a finger to the chin just below the lower lip. Ask the client to open at the same time. Stroking the muscle under the chin (digastric muscle), without crossing the midline, also stimulates mouth opening.

Stimulate Mouth Closing. If a client does not close the **EB** lips, swallowing is more difficult. Stimulate lip closure by stroking the lips with a finger or ice or by applying gentle pressure just above the upper lip with your thumb or forefinger.

Help the Client with Swallowing. A dysphagic client must concentrate on swallowing. A quiet environment, free from distractions, is helpful. Feed the client slowly and offer small amounts. Begin feeding the client with foods that require no chewing and are easy to swallow (Table 72-4). Gradually progress to foods that require more chewing and swallowing effort as tolerated. Alternate liquids with solids whenever possible to prevent food from being left in the mouth. Avoid unthickened liquids. Place food in the unaffected side of the mouth. Encourage the client to chew each bite thoroughly. After clients have swallowed, teach them to check for food on the paralyzed side by turning the head to the unaffected side and sweeping the mouth with the tongue.

Diagnosis: Impaired Verbal Communication. The inability to speak is frustrating for clients. Early recognition of this problem decreases some of the frustration in meeting everyday needs. Loss of verbal communication is usually caused by ischemia of the dominant cerebral hemisphere, leading to loss of the function of muscles that produce speech.

Outcomes. The client will be able to communicate effectively, the client's needs will be understood and met, and the client will indicate understanding of the communication of others.

Interventions. Communication involves the dual processes of sending and receiving language. Although either can be affected, the expressive deficit is usually greater than the receptive deficit after initial recovery. Clients may understand more than they can respond to clearly.

Most aphasic clients regain some speech through spontaneous recovery or speech therapy. Speech therapy should be started early. Occasionally residual brain function is not adequate for an aphasic client to relearn the complicated processes of communication. A picture board may be helpful.

Assessment of dysarthria usually includes examination of the peripheral muscles of speech, tests for specific speech skills, and assessment of the client's functional ability based on the clarity of speech in conversation. Speech therapy is beneficial for many dysarthric clients.

Reinforce the lessons that a speech therapist has initiated. Remember, the client may have a short attention span. Use every encounter to encourage and support communication, and yet be careful not to cause frustration and fatigue. In general, when working with an aphasic client, speak at a slower rate and give the client time to respond. Listen and watch carefully when an aphasic client attempts to communicate. Try hard to un-

TABLE 72-4	*Progressive Feeding Program for Clients with Dysphagia*			
	Stage I	**Stage II**	**Stage III**	**Stage IV**
Description	Severe swallowing difficulty	Chewing and swallowing difficulty with various textures	Less difficulty swallowing, beginning to control foods better in mouth, able to tolerate various food textures and consistencies	Able to swallow most foods very well
Meats	Puréed meat with gravy, baby food, egg yolks	Junior baby food meats with gravy; scrambled, soft, or poached eggs; cottage cheese	Ground meat with gravy, soft meats (tuna) in casseroles, macaroni and cheese, fish without bones, chopped meats	Soft diet
Starch	Mashed potatoes with gravy	Muffins (no seeds), pancakes, French toast, cooked cereal (thick)	Toast (no seeds), rice, soft baked potato	Soft foods
Vegetables	Puréed	Junior vegetables	Peas, squash, cooked carrots; avoid stringy foods (celery, spinach)	Soft foods
Fruits	Puréed	Cooked fruit, ripe banana, soft canned fruit	Grapefruit and orange sections; peeled ripe peaches, pears, and nectarines	Soft foods
Dessert	Custard, pudding	Cakes (no seeds, nuts)	Pies, cakes, sherbet, ice cream	Soft foods
Liquids	None	None	Thick liquids, nectars, strained cream soups, eggnog, liquid caloric supplements, milk shakes	May be able to have thickened liquids

derstand. This reduces the client's frustration. Anticipate an aphasic client's needs to reduce feelings of communication helplessness.

When a client *cannot identify objects by name,* give the client practice in receiving word images. For example, point to an object and clearly state its name. Then ask the client to repeat the word.

When a client *cannot understand spoken words or has receptive difficulty,* repeat simple directions until they are understood. Do not shout; the client can hear. Speak slowly and clearly. Talk without pressing for a response. Use nonverbal methods of communication to reinforce your words. Stand within 6 feet, and face the client directly. Gradually shift topics of conversation, and tell the client when you are going to change the topic.

When a client has *difficulty with verbal expression,* give the client practice in repeating words after you. Begin with simple words and then progress to simple sentences.

Help the family to communicate with the aphasic client. Act as a role model for such communication by being calm, patient, and gentle. Explain how damaging it can be to the client's self-image if others appear to be embarrassed or amused by the client's attempts to communicate. Likewise, the family should not do all of the speaking for the client.

Always try to put aphasic clients at ease. Reduce the feelings of panic that may occur when they first realize that they cannot communicate as before. The fact that others understand the problem is helpful. Offer calm reassurance. Demonstrate the use of the call light and allow the client to practice. Use gestures and one-step commands.

Collaborative Problem: Risk for Corneal Abrasion.
Following stroke, clients may lose their ability to blink. Without a blink reflex, the cornea will dry and become abraded. The collaborative problem is *Risk for Corneal Abrasion.*

Outcomes. Monitor the client for risk factors for the development of corneal abrasion, including the absence of eye closure or blinking and lack of eye moisture.

Interventions. Protect the eye with an eye patch if no blinking is noted. Instill prescribed artificial tears or consult the physician for a prescription if none exists.

Diagnosis: Disturbed Thought Processes. Sometimes it is difficult to make a nursing diagnosis of *Disturbed Thought Processes* unless you spend time with the client. Asking simple or common questions may get fixed, yet correct, answers. Often, after spending a morning with a client, you may note difficulty with thought processing that was not evident on first assessment. Changes in behavior may be caused by alterations in body image, sensation, vision, mobility, and perception. Cerebral edema may also increase confusion.

Outcomes. The client will have improved thought processing as evidenced by recall of information, improved Mini-Mental State examination scores, decreased agitation, cooperation with interventions, and appropriate responses to questions about recent and past events.

Interventions. Try to prevent disorientation by reorienting the client as LOC improves. Continually reorient a confused client. Glasses and hearing aids assist the client in maintaining awareness of the environment and thus improve thought processes. Activity such as sitting up in a chair for meals or at scheduled times throughout the day also improves LOC and orientation. Position a calendar and a clock where the client can see them. Stroke contributes to altered behavioral patterns, including confusion, memory loss, and emotional lability. To decrease agitation, explain all nursing activities before initiating them. Avoid sensory overload.

Diagnosis: Disturbed Sensory Perception: Visual. Ischemia of visual pathways can lead to altered vision. The client may not notice you when you approach from one side or may not eat food from one side of the food tray. A thorough assessment of visual fields is usually needed for this diagnosis.

Outcomes. The client will successfully compensate for altered visual perceptions as evidenced by safely performing ADLs and safely compensating for visual deficit through scanning or other techniques.

Interventions. Approach the client from the side that is not visually impaired. Position the call light and telephone on that side. If possible, position the bed so that the client's side that is not visually impaired is toward the center of the room. Teach clients to position the head to increase the visual field. Warn hemiplegic clients to be careful when crossing streets because they may not see traffic approaching from the affected side. An eye patch over one eye in clients with diplopia removes the second image and assists vision.

A client with perceptual deficits benefits from simplicity. A busy or noisy environment is difficult to interpret and may increase confusion. Reduce complexity and the need for decision-making. The following are examples:

1. Obtain clothing that is simply designed and easy to put on.
2. Give brief, simple directions.
3. Prepare food trays with a minimum number of utensils, dishes, and foods.

Diagnosis: Unilateral Neglect. *Unilateral Neglect* is a pattern of lack of awareness of one side of the body. The client behaves as if that part is simply not there. He or she does not look for the paralyzed limb when moving about. It is caused by damage to portions of the non-dominant cerebral hemisphere. Unilateral neglect creates an increased risk of injury. It is possible to relearn to look for and to move the limb.

Outcomes. The client will be able to compensate for unilateral neglect as evidenced by being free from injury and demonstrating an increased awareness of the neglected body side.

Interventions. Initially adapt the environment to the deficit by focusing on the client's unaffected side. Greet the client as you enter the room, especially if the entrance is toward the neglected side. Keep personal care items and a bedside chair and commode on the unaffected side. Set up the client's food tray toward the unaffected side. Position the client's extremities in correct alignment. Gradually begin to focus the client's attention to the affected side. Move the personal items, bedside chair, and commode to the affected side. Assist the client from the affected side. Have the client groom the affected side first. Cue the client to scan the entire environment and remind the client to keep track of the affected extremities.

Diagnosis: Ineffective Coping. Coping strategies are quite varied among people. Any major illness or change in the body challenges a client's or family's coping skills. This process is particularly true after a stroke because of the physiologic changes and frustrations associated with the resulting deficits. The term *coping* refers to the use of all forms of coping strategies: emotional, cognitive, support systems, and risk appraisal.

Outcomes. The client will develop effective coping strategies as evidenced by appropriate lifestyle modifications, use of the assistance of others, and appropriate social interactions.

Interventions. After a stroke, the client may experience grief over lost mobility, inability to communicate, alterations in sensation and vision, and loss of roles within society. Stroke clients express feelings of profound suffering related to the sudden, devastating changes that accompany stroke.[28] Be understanding and kind. Supportive statements are often helpful, such as "I am sure it's hard for you not to be able to dress alone." The client needs to feel listened to and cared about.

Loss of independence is of particular concern for the stroke client.[35] Care for clients in a way that encourages their independence. Arrange the environment and anticipate needs to reduce frustration. Praise all successes, however small. Break a long-term goal into several short-term goals so that the client can experience successes along the way. For example, a long-term goal may be to walk independently, but short-term goals such as sitting on the side of the bed and ambulating with a quad cane will allow the client to have successes and the long-term goal will seem more attainable. Inappropriate behavior may occur. When necessary, point out the behavior in a matter-of-fact manner and ask the client to stop. Significant others often need help to understand that these behaviors may be caused by damage to the inhibitory centers in the brain or they may be a part of the normal grief response. Provide support by helping the client and family understand this.

Aphasic clients often express their emotional state by irritability and "moodiness." These frustrated clients are often anxious, bewildered, and depressed. Emotional lability may also be present. Accept such behavior in a matter-of-fact but kind manner, without embarrassment. Help families by encouraging short visits by one or two people. If children are allowed to visit, ensure that they are adequately supervised.

Psychosocial Nursing Diagnoses. Various psychosocial nursing diagnoses may be appropriate for clients experiencing stroke, depending on the client and the circumstances. These include *Interrupted Family Processes. Deficient Diversional Activity, Anxiety, Fear, Powerlessness, Situational Low Self-Esteem,* and *Social Isolation.* Shift in spousal roles often occurs. The ways a couple copes will determine how satisfying their lives are after a stroke.[35] Include significant others in the plan of care; let them help care for the client if they wish. Provide them with the information they need to understand the client's condition. Many clients with strokes are in ICUs during the acute phase. The complexity of equipment and activity within an ICU may be frightening to the client and to significant others. Explain carefully what is happening, and provide opportunities for questions and discussion. Give frequent reassurance and support.

Evaluation

Evaluate the degree of outcome attainment on an ongoing basis. After a stroke, some outcomes, such as cerebral perfusion, are achieved early; others, such as self-care deficit, may require long-term rehabilitation. Monitor progress toward outcomes, working with both the client and the family.

■ Surgical Management

Several criteria are used to identify candidates for rapid evacuation of the hematoma in hemorrhagic stroke. The clients most likely to benefit from surgery are those who are younger than 70 years of age, can open their eyes and follow commands, have elevated ICP (>30 mm Hg), or are rapidly deteriorating neurologically. Clients who have large blood clots removed often can recover a substantial portion of speech. Surgery is usually not performed in clients with bleeding in deep cerebral structures such as the basal ganglia or thalamus.

Most therapies are aimed at reducing increased ICP.[18] Surgery is also performed on some intracranial aneurysms and on the carotid arteries to reduce the risk for stroke.

■ Modifications for Older Clients

Because stroke affects older people more than it affects others, the nursing care discussed here does not have to be significantly altered for older clients. Older people often have multiple medical problems that must be monitored and treated simultaneously.

■ Self-Care

Clients who have experienced a stroke often are transferred to a rehabilitation unit after they are medically stable. The client is evaluated for rehabilitation potential, and plans are made for ongoing therapy. The plan of care established during acute care can continue. The major nursing diagnoses and collaborative problems include *Impaired Physical Mobility, Self-Care Deficit, Impaired Verbal Communication, Risk for Contracture, Imbalanced Nutrition: Less Than Body Requirements,* and *Ineffective Coping.*

The following are adjuncts to discharge from rehabilitation settings to home:

- Self-medication
- Use of therapeutic passes
- Rehabilitation home visits

Self-medication means that clients can manage their own medications. Goals are to help the client learn about the medications, including dosage, action, and side effects. Provide a supervised trial to evaluate the client's knowledge and compliance and to enable clients to develop increased responsibility for their own care. A clear and accurate medication chart is helpful.

Therapeutic passes allow the client to return to home or family for short stays. They facilitate discharge planning and improve the transition into the community. Passes help the stroke survivor adjust to the home environment and to practice self-care activities at home and help the family adjust to living with the stroke survivor and to any alterations in physical, cognitive, and emotional functioning. Clients and family members can practice problem-solving and can perform some physical care skills needed after discharge from the facility. Much effort goes into planning for the passes and preparing the client and family. Passes are usually for 8 hours at first and then are increased to a weekend. When the client returns to the facility, the client and family discuss any difficulties they had during the pass interval. Team members intervene with information, retraining, or procurement of needed supplies.

For the *rehabilitation home visit,* team members, including the nurse, social worker, and physical and occupational therapists, visit the client's home. The purpose is to evaluate the accessibility of the home and the safety of the home environment based on the client's level of functioning, specifically, the client's ability (1) to get in and out of the house; (2) to perform specific tasks in each room; (3) to transfer onto and off of the toilet, bed, and chair; and (4) to move about from room to room. The client's ability to use the telephone and various appliances safely is also evaluated. On the basis of findings from the visit, the team recommends home modifications, further teaching, or adaptive equipment.

The family needs a clear understanding of the client's residual deficits. If spatial or perceptual deficits or unilateral neglect is present, emphasize the need for assistance with ADLs and the need for adherence to safety precautions to prevent injury. Writing lists of tasks or activities may help clients with impaired memory. Reinforce measures to improve mobility and the ability to perform ADLs. The client should have a plan for exercises. Equally important, the family and client need to have realistic expectations about the client's abilities so that they can encourage independence when and where the client is able.

Provide written documentation of any anticoagulant schedule as well as a list of warning signs of bleeding. Reinforce the need for caution when the client is using sharp instruments and tools. If appropriate, contact sports must be curtailed while the client is receiving anticoagulants. The INR is closely monitored, and medications are adjusted as needed. The client should be taught to carry Medic-Alert identification.

Provide information about community resources that can assist the client and family with home management and adjustments to residual deficits. These resources include Meals-on-Wheels, the American Stroke Association (a division of the American Heart Association), the National Stroke Association, stroke support groups, social services, local service groups to assist with the purchase of equipment, and individual and family counselors.

At times the stroke client may not be able to tolerate the intensive therapy of a rehabilitation setting, and placement in an extended care facility may be necessary. This is usually very stressful for the client and family, particularly an older spouse. In some cases, care by nurses and allied health professionals in the home may prevent placement in an extended care facility. If both partners are older or in poor health, placement in an extended care facility may be the only option, which can create feelings of guilt and abandonment. Emotional support must be provided to both the client and family members. Education in how to choose a facility and how to monitor care can be helpful.

TRANSIENT ISCHEMIC ATTACKS

Transient ischemic attacks (TIAs) are sudden, brief episodes of neurologic dysfunction caused by temporary, focal cerebral ischemia. Recovery is complete. By definition, a TIA lasts less than 24 hours, and most TIAs last only 5 to 20 minutes. TIAs that last longer than 1 hour are often caused by small infarcts.[6] TIAs often serve as warning signs of an impending stroke. In fact, one third of people with untreated TIAs experience a stroke within 5 years.[6]

Etiology and Risk Factors

During a TIA, a transient decrease in blood supply to a focal area of the cerebrum or brain stem occurs. Many factors can cause this ischemia. Thromboembolism from ulcerated plaque on the carotid arteries is the most common cause of TIAs, accounting for 80% of cases. Thromboemboli may originate in the vertebrobasilar system. Other sources of emboli include blood clots forming on diseased or prosthetic heart valves, atrial fibrillation, or breakdown of plaque.

Pathophysiology

The pathophysiology of a TIA is similar to that of a stroke. The major differences are the short duration of ischemia and the lack of permanent deficits.

Clinical Manifestations

Manifestations of TIAs vary, depending on which area of the brain is affected. Common manifestations of a TIA in the carotid artery circulation include a rapid onset of weakness or numbness in an arm or leg, aphasia, and visual-field cuts. Manifestations of a TIA in the vertebrobasilar circulation include two or more of the following: vertigo, diplopia, dysphagia, dysarthria, and ataxia.

Transient ischemic attacks are often recurrent; however, some clients have only one or two episodes before having a complete stroke. TIAs may occur for 1 to 6 years before cerebral infarction, or clusters of TIAs may first appear only a few hours or days before a cerebral infarction. Between episodes, neurologic assessment findings are normal.

The diagnosis of TIA is confirmed by the client's reported clinical manifestations. The causes of the TIA and the potential risk for stroke are diagnosed by the following examinations:

1. Auscultation for a carotid bruit
2. CT to rule out stroke or other causes of neurologic deficit

3. Doppler, computed tomographic angiography (CTA), or magnetic resonance angiography (MRA) studies of the carotid arteries
4. Cerebral angiogram
5. ECG to assess for atrial fibrillation
6. Transthoracic or transesophageal echocardiography (TTE and TEE, respectively) to rule out mural thrombosis and valvular disorders

The results of the noninvasive carotid artery studies, which include the Doppler, CTA, and MRA, determine whether the more invasive cerebral angiogram is performed. The TTE is often performed before the TEE because it is less invasive; however, the TEE may better visualize prosthetic valves and the left atrium.

Conditions that mimic a TIA include intracranial hemorrhage, seizures, hypoglycemia, migraine, and inner ear disorders.

Outcome Management
■ Medical Management

Preventing the progression of a TIA to a stroke is the goal of medical management. Every effort is made to determine the cause of the TIAs. Another important medical intervention is to identify and decrease the client's modifiable risk factors for stroke.[9] Antihypertensives or antiplatelet drugs may be prescribed. Warfarin may be administered for emboli of cardiac origin.

Teach the client and family about the manifestations of stroke, risk factors for stroke, and emergency care if a stroke occurs at home. If the client is hospitalized, assess neurologic status frequently for progressive ischemia.

Clients experiencing TIAs are often afraid that they are having a stroke. They need emotional support and education during this stressful time. The diagnostic work-up as well as the manifestations themselves can produce anxiety. Thorough, simple explanations of upcoming events can help. Stress the importance of completing the work-up. Baseline neurologic status must be recorded for postoperative comparison.

■ Surgical Management

Clients who are considered for surgery are those who have a low risk for postoperative morbidity and mortality and one of the following: (1) asymptomatic carotid artery disease with 60% or greater stenosis or (2) symptomatic carotid artery disease with 70% or greater stenosis.[1,5] In these clients, the incidence of stroke with surgical management is significantly reduced compared with those with medical management. Clients considered at increased risk for postoperative morbidity and mortality include those with coronary artery disease, pulmonary disease, and moderate to severe stroke on the ipsilateral side.[1,5] Surgery is usually performed only on stenotic arteries, not on those that are totally occluded. A client may require bilateral endarterectomy. The inter-

val between surgeries is determined by the client's tolerance of the procedure and the likelihood of symptom progression from the remaining stenotic vessel.

Surgeons may perform cerebral angiography before carotid artery surgery to quantitate accurately the degree of carotid stenosis.[1] The risk for stroke from cerebral angiography is 1% to 3%.[1] Because of the vast improvements in the technology of noninvasive carotid artery studies (carotid ultrasound, carotid duplex, and MRA), these studies may also be used to evaluate stenosis and guide the planning for surgery.[1,5] Preoperative aspirin is often administered to decrease the formation of embolism at the carotid suture line. If the client is receiving heparin, it is usually stopped on arrival to the operating room.

Carotid Endarterectomy. Carotid endarterectomy is useful in preventing stroke. Carotid endarterectomy is the opening of the carotid artery to remove obstructing and embolizing plaque (Figure 72-5). After coronary artery bypass, it is the second most common vascular surgical procedure. An incision is made on the anterior border of the sternocleidomastoid muscle. The vessel is clamped, and the plaque or atheroma is removed. The potential for cerebral perfusion during the operation is reduced because the artery must be clamped during the procedure. Some surgeons use intraoperative electroencephalogram (EEG) and transcranial Doppler monitor-

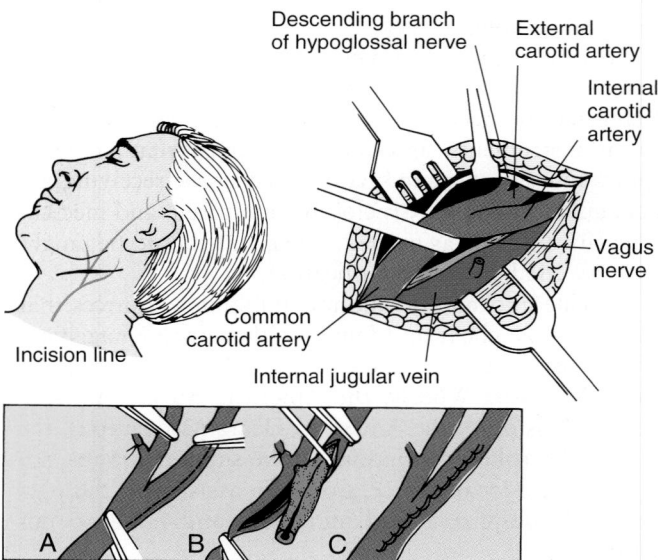

FIGURE 72-5 Carotid endarterectomy. **A,** The common carotid artery is clamped, and an incision is made along the carotid bifurcation. **B,** Plaque is removed. Sometimes portions of the artery are also removed and reconstructed with vein grafts or polyester, such as Dacron. **C,** The artery is sutured closed, and the clamps are removed.

ing to detect decreased cerebral perfusion while the carotid artery is clamped. In addition, some surgeons shunt blood from below the targeted carotid artery incision to above it to provide a temporary blood supply to the brain. The client is admitted to the ICU for monitoring of neurologic and vital signs and is usually discharged the following day.

Prognosis. Follow-up Doppler studies are performed at 3 months postoperatively to assess for artery patency and again at 6 months to 1 year to detect restenosis on the operated side and disease on the nonoperated side. Restenosis may occur in about 1% to 37% of clients after carotid endarterectomy.[1]

Complications. Neurologic complications of carotid endarterectomy include the following:
- Embolization during surgery, causing cerebral vessel occlusion and ischemia
- Thrombosis of the artery at the endarterectomy site, causing cerebral ischemia
- Inadequate cerebral perfusion from intolerance of the temporary artery clamping during surgery

Other Techniques. Recent advances in microcatheter and microballoon technology have lead to the investigational use of interventional neurovascular procedures to treat and prevent cerebrovascular disorders. Results of studies of the use of carotid angioplasty and stenting have been promising. The less invasive procedures would treat severe carotid stenosis in a less invasive way than traditional surgery.[10]

Cerebral angioplasty is similar to coronary angioplasty. A balloon catheter is threaded through the arterial system via the femoral artery to the area of carotid stenosis. A small balloon is inflated to dilate the lesion. A stent catheter can also be used to further open the area of stenosis. The U.S. Food and Drug Administration (FDA) views both these procedures to be experimental. The complications and complication rate are comparable to those of carotid endarterectomy.

■ Nursing Management of the Surgical Client

Postoperative care after carotid endarterectomy includes neurologic assessments every 1 to 2 hours. Immediately report indications of deterioration of neurologic status. In addition, several CNs are close to the operative site. The function of the following CNs is assessed: facial (VII), vagus (X), spinal accessory (XI), and hypoglossal (XII). CN dysfunction is usually temporary but may last for months. The most common CN damage causes vocal cord paralysis, difficulty managing saliva, or tongue deviation.

Keep the client's head aligned in a straight position to help maintain airway patency and to minimize stress on

the operative site. Antiplatelet agents are often administered. The client can lie supine or on the side so long as the neck is not flexed.

Elevate the head of the bed when vital signs are stable. Local applications of cold to the operative site may be prescribed.

Frequently assess the client's breathing pattern, pulse, and blood pressure. Maintain the client's blood pressure within 20 mm Hg of the preoperative normal values. Hypertension or hypotension may lead to hemorrhage, ischemia, or occlusion of the anastomosis. Labile blood pressure is a common postsurgical problem. Baroreceptors located in the lining of the carotid sinus are one of the primary mechanisms of maintaining normotension. Manipulation of the baroreceptors during surgery causes a short-term disruption in blood pressure regulation.

Observe the operative site. Airway obstruction can occur from excessive swelling of the neck or hematoma formation. Bleeding and hemorrhage are a concern because anticoagulation from intraoperative heparin is not yet reversed. Risk factor modification is essential to the long-term success of the surgery and the general health of the client.[1,5]

CLIENT AND PUBLIC EDUCATION

The general public has limited knowledge of the manifestations of stroke. In one study, only slightly more than half of the respondents could name at least one stroke manifestation.[35] In addition, only 68% could name a risk factor for stroke.[35] A public education campaign is under way to promote awareness of the manifestations of a stroke. In this campaign, stroke is referred to as a "brain attack" to indicate the need for emergency care with the same intensity as a heart attack (Box 72-3). Prompt recognition allows for early treatment of a stroke, which may lessen residual deficits and decrease disability. Recognition and modification of risk factors for stroke are the most important preventions available.

BOX 72-3	*I Am A Stroke*

Learn to recognize a stroke and act quickly:
- Sudden numbness or weakness of the face, arm, or leg, especially on one side of the body
- Sudden confusion, trouble speaking or understanding
- Sudden trouble seeing in one or both eyes
- Sudden trouble walking, dizziness, loss of balance or coordination
- Sudden, severe headache with no known cause

Call 9-1-1 immediately if you experience symptoms! Time lost is brain lost!

From the National Stroke Association, Englewood, CO. Retrieved February 2004 from http://www.stroke.org.

CONCLUSIONS

Stroke is being managed today as a treatable problem if recognized early; however, because of the limited knowledge of the public about early warning signs, many clients still suffer the consequences of stroke. Treatment of the client with stroke is aimed at maximizing function and preventing disability.

THINKING CRITICALLY *evolve*

1. A 70-year-old man had a left-sided stroke 2 days ago. While obtaining his assessment, you note that his blood pressure is elevated at 200 mm Hg systolic; his usual systolic blood pressure is 140 to 160 mm Hg. He is receiving oxygen at 5 L, but his oxygen saturation has dropped from 95% to 88% in the last hour. The client was oriented to person, place, and time an hour ago but has become increasingly restless and slightly confused. The confusion has led him to pull out the nasogastric tube that had been placed for nutritional maintenance. What other neurologic assessments should you do? What is the first priority? Is the suddenness of this change significant?

Factors to Consider. How has the client's assessment changed from baseline values? Is there any relationship between the increased blood pressure and the hypoxia? Is the removal of the nasogastric tube an immediate problem?

2. A 78-year-old woman with a history of hypertension has a stroke. Her family reports that she has felt good and has refused to take her antihypertensive medication. She now has hemiparesis and is able to respond verbally. She does not recognize people or objects in her line of vision on the left side. Three days after her stroke, she is able to move her fingers and wiggle her toes on the affected side, and she is transferred to the rehabilitation unit. What are the most likely rehabilitation goals for this client? How should you proceed with teaching about the complications, motivation to comply with the prescribed therapies, and the importance of antihypertensive medications?

Factors to Consider. What types of rehabilitation will she require? How soon can teaching begin? How will you teach the client and family to provide her care after discharge?

3. A client is seen in the emergency department at 9 AM on Monday morning. His chief complaint is a severe headache. He states, "I am having the worst headache of my life. The pain awakened me around 5 AM and has gotten worse and worse." On examination, the client scores 15 on the Glasgow Coma Scale, complains of nausea, and has a stiff neck. The left-hand grip is slightly weaker than the right-hand grip, and there is a slight pronator drift of the left arm. In addition, there is flattening of the left nasolabial fold. A computed tomography scan of the brain reveals moderate hemorrhage on the right side with increased blood present in the right sylvian fissure. What tests would you expect to be ordered? What complications are important to assess for in this client?

Factors to Consider. What problem is probably in progress? Is the client a surgical candidate, either at present or later on?

Discussions for these questions can be found on the website and the CD-ROM.

BIBLIOGRAPHY

1. Ailawadi, G., et al. (2002). Carotid stenosis: Medical and surgical aspects. *Cardiology Clinics, 20*(4), 599-609.
2. American Heart Association. (2002). *Heart disease and stroke statistics—2003 update.* American Heart Association; Dallas, TX.
3. Barch, C., et al., and the NINDS rt-PA Stroke Study Group. (1997). Nursing management of acute complications following rt-PA in acute ischemic stroke. *Journal of Neuroscience Nursing, 29*(6), 367-372.
4. Bernardine, G.L., & Mayer, S.A. (1999). Cardiac and pulmonary complications of cerebrovascular disease. *The Neurologist 5*(1), 24-32.
5. Biller, J., et al. (1998). Guidelines for carotid endarterectomy, a statement for healthcare professionals from a special writing group of the stroke council, American Heart Association. *Circulation, 97*, 501-509.
6. Biller, J., & Love, B.B. (2000). Ischemic cerebrovascular disease. In W.G. Bradley (Ed.), *Neurology in clinical practice: Principles of diagnosis and management* (3rd ed.). Boston: Butterworth-Heinemann.
7. Braimah, J., et al., and the NINDS rt-PA Stroke Study Group. (1997). Nursing care of acute stroke patients after receiving rt-PA therapy. *Journal of Neuroscience Nursing, 29*(6), 373-383.
8. Broderick, J., et al. (1998). The greater Cincinnati/northern Kentucky stroke study: Preliminary first-ever and total incidence rates of stroke among blacks. *Stroke, 29*(2), 415-421.
9. Caplan, L.R. (1998). 10 most commonly asked questions about stroke. *The Neurologist, 4*(4), 227-231.
10. Cates, C. (2000). 10 most commonly asked questions about carotid angioplasty and stenting. *The Neurologist, 6*(1), 58-62.

evolve *Did you remember to check out the bonus material on the Evolve website and the CD-ROM, including free self-assessment exercises?*

http://evolve.elsevier.com/Black/medsurg/

11. Deibert, E., & Diringer, M.N. (1999). The intensive care management of acute ischemic stroke. *The Neurologist, 5*(6), 313-325.

12. Fisher, M., & Albers, G. W. (1999). Applications of diffusion-perfusion magnetic resonance imaging in acute ischemic stroke. *Neurology, 52,* 1750-1756.

13. Gelber, D.A., & Callahan, G.D. (1999). Neurorehabilitation. *The Neurologist, 5*(5), 271-278.

14. Hershey, L. (1999). 10 most commonly asked questions about stroke in women. *The Neurologist, 5*(3), 166-168.

15. Hinkle, J.L. (1998). Biological and behavioral correlates of stroke and depression. *Journal of Neuroscience Nursing, 30*(1), 25-31.

16. Hock, N. (1998). Neuroprotective and thrombolytic agents: Advances in stroke treatment. *Journal of Neuroscience Nursing, 30*(3), 175-184.

17. Jeffrey, S. (1998). Managing the "dynamic process" of hemorrhagic stroke. *Neurology Reviews, 6*(1), 28-29.

18. Kase, C.S. (2000). Intracerebral hemorrhage. In W.G. Bradley (Ed.), *Neurology in clinical practice: Principles of diagnosis and management* (3rd ed.). Boston: Butterworth-Heinemann.

19. Kasner, S.E. (2000). Stroke treatment-specific considerations. *Neurologic Clinics, 8*(2), 399-417.

20. Liskay, A.M. (1999). Stroke: Are you at risk? *The Neurologist, 5*(1), 53-54.

21. Lyden, P.D., et al. (1997). Intravenous thrombolysis for acute stroke. *Neurology, 49,* 14-29.

 22. Manno, E.M., et al. (1999). The effects of mannitol on cerebral edema after large hemispheric cerebral infarct. *Neurology, 52,* 583-587.

23. Mayer, S.A., & Dennis, L.J. (1998). Management of increased intracranial pressure. *The Neurologist, 4*(1), 2-12.

24. Mayo, N.E., et al. (2000). There's no place like home: An evaluation of early supported discharge for stroke. *Stroke, 31*(5), 1016-1023.

 25. National Center for Health Statistics, Center for Disease Control. (2001). Fast stats A to Z, stroke. Retrieved February 2004 from http://www.cdc.gov/nchs/fastats/stroke.htm.

26. National Institute of Neurological Disorders and Stroke rt-PA Stroke Study Group. (1995). Tissue plasminogen activator for acute ischemic stroke. *New England Journal of Medicine, 333*(24), 1581-1587.

27. Pancioli, A., et al. (1998). Public perception of stroke warning signs and knowledge of potential risk factors. *Journal of the American Medical Association, 279*(16), 1288-1292.

28. Pilkington, F.B. (1999). A qualitative study of life after stroke. *Journal of Neuroscience Nursing, 31*(6), 336-347.

29. Post-stroke Rehabilitation Guideline Panel. (1995). *Post-stroke re-* *habilitation: Assessment, referral and patient management. Quick reference guide for clinicians.* No. 16. Rockville, MD: U.S. Department of Health and Human Services, Agency for Health Care Policy and Research Publication No. 95-0663.

30. Prichard, J.W., & Grossman, R.I. (1999). New reasons for early use of MRI in stroke. *Neurology, 52,* 1733-1736.

31. Rapp, K., et al., and the NINDS rt-PA Stroke Study Group. (1997). Code stroke: Rapid transport, triage and treatment using rt-PA therapy. *Journal of Neuroscience Nursing, 29*(6), 361-366.

32. Reynolds, K., et al. (2003). Alcohol Consumption and risk of stroke. A meta-analysis. *Journal of the American Medical Association, 289*(5), 579-588.

33. Shepard, T.J., & Fox, S.W. (1996). Assessment and management of hypertension in the acute ischemic stroke patient. *Journal of Neuroscience Nursing, 28*(1), 5-12.

34. Siroky, M.B. (2003). Neurological disorders, cerebrovascular disease and parkinsonism. *Urologic Clinics of North America, 30*(1), 27-47.

35. Smith, G.R., & Mahoney, C. (1995). Coping and marital equilibrium after stroke. *Journal of Neuroscience Nursing, 27*(2), 83-89.

36. Suarez, J.L., et al. (1999). Predictors of clinical improvement, angiographic recanalization, and intracranial hemorrhage after intra-arterial thrombolysis for acute ischemic stroke. *Stroke, 30,* 2094-2100.

37. Swanson, R.A. (1999). Intravenous heparin for acute stroke: What can we learn from the megatrials? *Neurology, 52,* 1746-1750.

38. Tanne, D., et al. (2002). Markers of increased risk of intracerebral hemorrhage after intravenous recombinant tissue plasminogen activator therapy for acute ischemic stroke in clinical practice, the multicenter rt-PA acute stroke survey. *Circulation, 105,* 1679-1685.

39. Testani-Dufour, L., & Marano Morrison, C.A. (1997). Brain attack: Correlative anatomy. *Journal of Neuroscience Nursing, 29*(4), 213-222.

40. Williams, L.S., et al. (2002). Effects of admission hyperglycemia on mortality and costs in acute ischemic stroke. *Neurology, 59,* 67-71.

41. Wolf, P.A., et al. (1999). Preventing ischemic stroke in patients with prior stroke and transient ischemic attack, a statement for healthcare professionals from the stroke council of the American Heart Association. *Stroke, 30,* 1991-1994.

Management of Clients with Peripheral Nervous System Disorders

Sharon R. Redding

The peripheral nervous system is that portion of the nervous system that exists outside of the brain and spinal cord itself. This chapter addresses problems with the spine and cranial nerves.

LOWER BACK PAIN

The spine is a mechanical organ that has been described as a crane with the ability to support weight, maintain balance, and counter numerous daily strains during normal work and recreational activities. Although it has tremendous ability to withstand most mechanical stresses, it can be stressed beyond its limits. Forces that exceed the capacity of the tissues to stretch can lead to injury and pain. Lower back pain is the second most common reason for visits to health care providers (the most common reason being respiratory problems) and results in more health care costs due to treatment and lost work hours than any other medical condition.

The problem of lower back pain is a source of fascination, frustration, and often confusion by clinicians and scientists who attempt to study and treat clients with this problem. The spine is the only organ that consists of bones, joints, ligaments, fatty tissue, multiple layers of muscles, peripheral nerves, sensory ganglia, autonomic ganglia, and the spinal cord. These structures are in turn fed by an intricate system of arteries and veins. Furthermore, the movement of the spine is complex and injury to the spine and other structures leads to unique patterns of pain.

Etiology

The origin of back pain is not well known and has never been fully described. Many groups have given up trying to describe the cause of lower back pain and instead have listed several *red flag* conditions that are associated with the problem. Three groups of problems lead to back pain:

1. *Biomechanical and destructive* origins include compression of the disks, herniation of the disk, torsion injury, and vibration. These problems are seen when clients have occupations that require strenuous or repetitive lifting in a stooped position or jobs that require operating vibrating machinery.
2. *Destructive origins* include infection, tumors, and rheumatoid disorders. These conditions can place

Nursing Outcomes Classification (NOC)
for Nursing Diagnoses—Clients with Peripheral Nervous System Disorders

Activity Intolerance
  Ambulation: Walking
  Activity Tolerance
  Pain: Disruptive Effects
Acute Pain
  Comfort Level
  Pain Level
Anxiety
  Psychosocial Adjustment: Life Change
  Symptom Control
Chronic Pain
  Body Image
  Hope

Role Performance
  Self-Esteem
  Social Interaction Skills
Deficient Knowledge
  Knowledge: Disease Process
  Knowledge: Treatment Regimen
Disturbed Body Image
  Acceptance: Health Status
  Self-Esteem
Fear
  Coping

Impaired Physical Mobility
  Mobility Level
  Pain Level
Impaired Urinary Elimination
  Urinary Continence
  Urinary Elimination
Ineffective Role Performance
  Role Performance
  Psychosocial Adjustment: Life Change
Ineffective Tissue Perfusion: Peripheral
  Sensory Function: Cutaneous
  Tissue Perfusion: Peripheral

pressure on the spinal roots or cord, or alter the structure of the vertebrae.

3. *Degenerative* problems include osteoporosis and spinal stenosis. Osteoporosis can cause collapse of the vertebrae and lead to compression of the nerve roots. The spinal canal can narrow and compress the nerves, a condition called *spinal stenosis,* usually occurring in older people. The severity ranges from entrapment of one nerve root to compression of the entire cord.

Other disorders include those that have no clear physiologic cause, yet lead to loss of income and pain. There is a growing body of data that show strong psychological influences on the response of clients to lower back pain. The primary determining factors for disability from lower back pain appear to be based on whether the client is depressed, unhappy in a work setting, or involved in litigation. These psychosocial issues do not negate the presence of real pain. The manner in which the brain processes pain may by implicated. The psychosocial aspects may suppress the serotonergic pathways and limit the secretion of endorphins.

Back Strain

Back strain is an acute injury leading to lower back pain. Back strain occurs when the client flexes the back without bending the knees or makes rotating movements, creating significant stress on the intervertebral disk and muscles of the lower back.

Disk Herniation

An intervertebral disk is a pad that rests between the centers of two adjacent vertebrae. Disks provide cushions for spinal movement. The intervertebral disk is composed of three parts:

1. Cartilaginous plates act as the superior and inferior limits of the disk. These are composed of hyaline

cartilage and cover the top and bottom of the vertebrae.
2. The annulus fibrosus is a ring of tissue that gives size and shape to the disk and holds the nucleus pulposus in place.
3. The nucleus pulposus is a semigelatinous material that forms the center of the disk and provides the cushioning effect.

Strenuous activity or degeneration of the disk or vertebrae can permit movement of the disk from its normal location. With aging, changes in disk cartilage and elasticity of the disk may cause the disk to prolapse. Displacement of intervertebral disk material may be referred to as *prolapse, herniation, rupture,* or *extrusion.* Ruptured intervertebral disks may occur at any level of the spine. Lumbar disks are more likely to rupture than cervical disks, due to the force of gravity, continual movement in this region, and improper movements of the spine as with lifting or turning. As in spinal cord injury, thoracic disk disorders are the least common.

More than half of the people with clinical manifestations of a herniated disk give a history of a previous back injury. Heavy physical labor, strenuous exercise, and weak abdominal and back muscles all increase the risk of herniated disk. Repeated stress progressively weakens the disk, resulting in bulging and herniation.

Lordosis

Lordosis is an excessive backward concavity in the lumbar spine. It is commonly associated with sagging shoulders, medial rotation of the legs, and an exaggerated pelvic angle. Excessive lordosis may result in swayback and kyphosis. Back pain is common.

Spondylolisthesis

Spondylolisthesis is the forward slipping of one vertebra. It commonly occurs at L4–5, where the upper vertebra

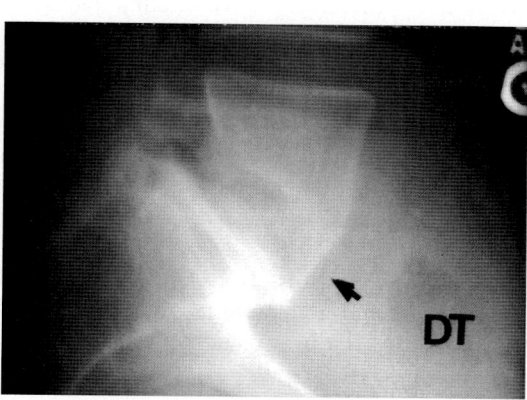

FIGURE 73-1 Preoperative radiograph of spondylolisthesis. Note the slippage of the vertebrae. (Courtesy of James Manz, M.D., Mayo Clinic, Eau Claire, WI).

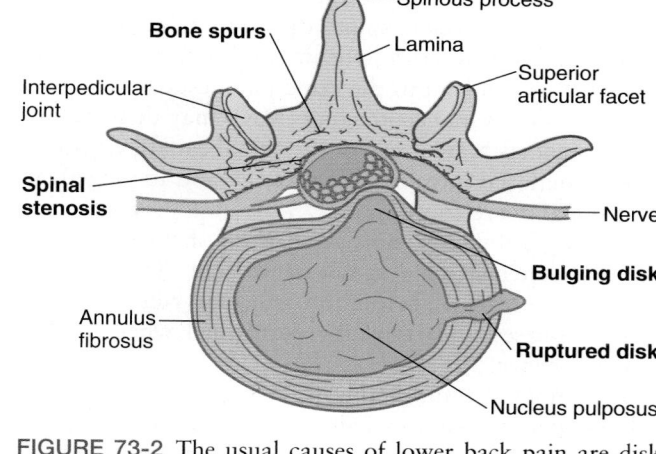

FIGURE 73-2 The usual causes of lower back pain are disk herniation and spinal stenosis.

slips forward out of alignment. Spondylolisthesis is graded from 1 to 4. Grades 1 and 2 are managed conservatively. Grades 3 and 4 usually require surgery for stabilization (Figure 73-1).

Spondylolysis

Spondylolysis is a structural defect in the lamina or neural arch of the spine. The vertebral arch slips forward. The lumbar spine is most commonly involved.

Spinal Stenosis

Spinal stenosis is due to ligamentous infolding and hypertrophy of the bone (Figure 73-2). It produces pressure on the entire spinal cord. If compression remains untreated, weakness or paralysis of the innervated muscle groups may result.

Pathophysiology

Compressive loads have different effects on the intervertebral disk, body of the vertebrae, facets, and spinal ligaments. Under compressive loads, the annular fibers of the disks are stretched. The vertebrae are also compressed and may fracture at the end plates. Spinal ligaments tend to buckle easily and the facet joints offer little resistance to compression.

The result is that the disk can herniate. When the disk only bulges, the annulus remains intact. With herniation, the annulus is usually torn, allowing extrusion of the nucleus pulposus (see Figure 71-3). Compression of spinal nerve roots may result from herniation of the disk. The disks that separate and pad the vertebrae are innervated with fine nerve endings. When the disk impinges on the sciatic nerve, the condition and resulting pain is called *sciatica*. Sciatica is a severe, usually constant pain in the

leg that occurs along the course of the sciatic nerve and its branches.

Clinical Manifestations

Rupture or herniation of a lumbar disk leads to lower back pain that radiates down the sciatic nerve into the posterior thigh as a result of compression of the spinal nerve roots. Typically, the pain of sciatica begins in the buttocks and extends down the back of the thigh and leg to the ankle. Disk herniation can result in groin pain. The client frequently has muscle spasms and hyperesthesia (numbness and tingling) in the area of distribution of affected nerve roots. The pain is aggravated by straining (coughing, sneezing, defecation, bending, lifting, and straight-leg raising) or prolonged sitting and is reduced by side-lying with the knees flexed. Any movement of the lower extremities that stretches the nerve causes pain and involuntary resistance. Straight-leg raising on the affected side is limited. Complete extension of the leg is not possible when the thigh is flexed on the abdomen (Lasègue sign). There may be depression of deep tendon reflexes.

Manifestations of spinal stenosis usually begin slowly and are due to pressure placed on nerve roots as they exit the vertebrae. The most common manifestations are aching pain with standing and walking, paresthesias, and heaviness in the legs that progressively worsens with walking. There is rapid improvement in manifestations with trunk flexion, stooping, or sitting. The manifestations of spinal stenosis must be differentiated from claudication.

Diagnostic Findings

X-ray studies may show spinal degenerative changes (at any level) that may indicate disk problems but usually do not show a ruptured disk. Osteophytes and narrowed disk interspaces are degenerative changes visible on radiographs. Also, other spinal disorders (e.g., spinal tumors, vertebral fracture, rheumatoid arthritis, and osteoarthritis) can lead to the same manifestations.

Magnetic resonance imaging (MRI) may demonstrate spinal stenosis (narrowing of the spinal canal), extrusion of disk material into the spinal canal, and impingement of a spinal nerve root (Figure 73-3).

Myelography may show narrowing of the disk space and impingement of a spinal nerve root. This test can identify the level of herniation and may rule out other spinal diseases. It is typically performed when MRI is not conclusive.

A computed tomography (CT) scan is usually done following a myelogram. This sequence allows better imaging with only one administration of contrast material. CT scanning may demonstrate spinal stenosis or other changes associated with degenerative disk disease. CT scans are more useful at the thoracic or lumbar level than at the cervical level.

Diskography is the injection of a water-soluble imaging material into the nucleus pulposus. It is used to determine internal changes in the disk. During the injection, information is recorded about the amount of dye accepted and the pressure needed to inject the material. Clients can have allergic responses to the dye and disk space infections can develop from the injection. Electromyography of the peripheral nerves may also be used to localize the site of the ruptured disk. Paraspinal mapping and somatosensory evoked potentials may also be used for diagnosis.

Outcome Management
■ Medical Management

Goals of medical care include reducing pain and spasms, improving mobility, and repairing any structural problems in the spine or disks.

Initial assessment of the client with lower back pain helps pinpoint the cause. The client's medical history is obtained to help determine whether a serious underlying condition is responsible for the pain, such as a fracture, tumor, or infection. The client's psychological and socioeconomic history is obtained, because these problems can complicate both assessment and management. The client is also asked to rate the pain. Physical examination determines whether lumbar nerve roots are involved by testing for reflexes, muscle strength, and the presence of neurologic deficits (Figure 73-4).

Control Pain and Spasms. Initial care of acute lower back pain is directed at managing the client's pain and directing activities. Pain is usually managed with non-

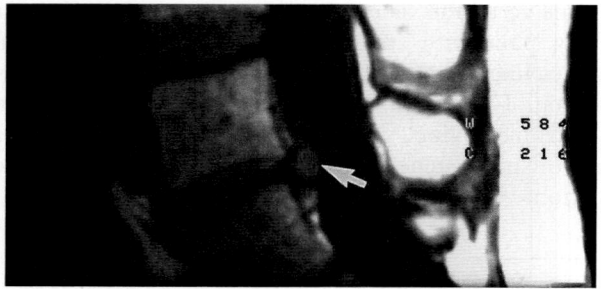

FIGURE 73-3 Magnetic resonance imaging of the lumbar spine showing herniation of the disk between L5 and S1.

Nerve root	L4	L5	S1
Pain	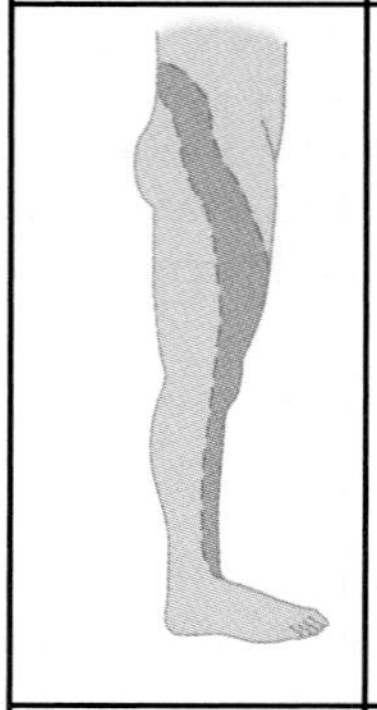	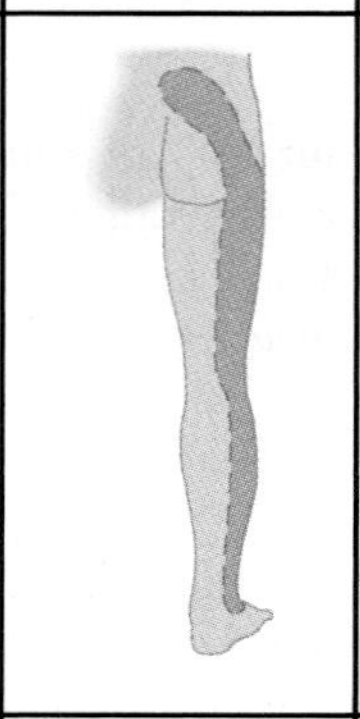	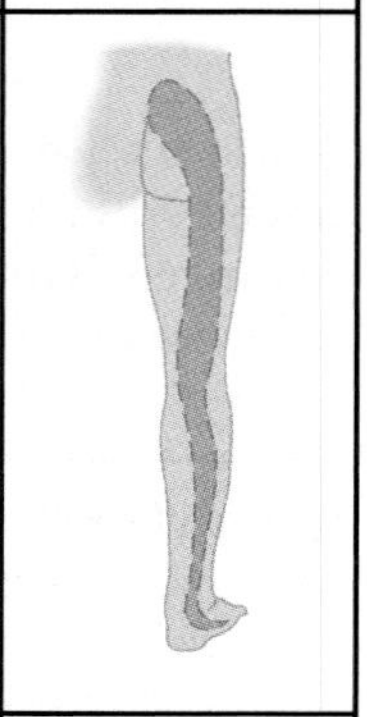
Numbness	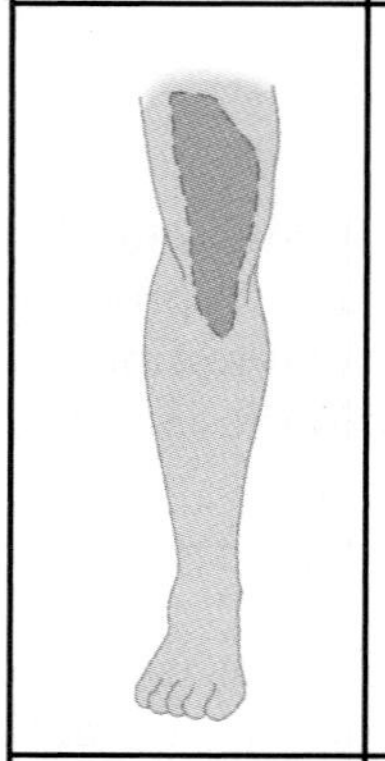	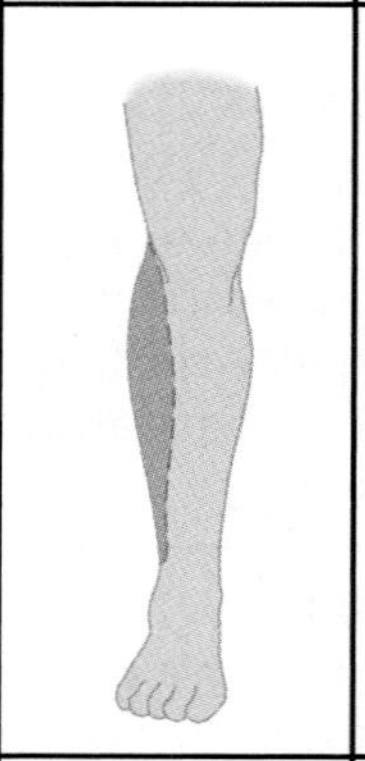	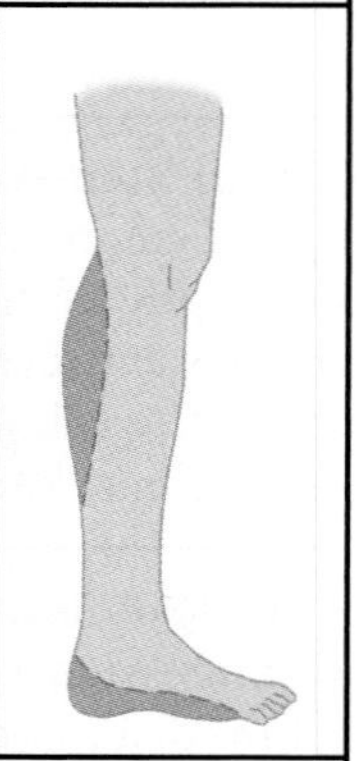
Motor weakness	Extension of quadriceps	Dorsiflexion of great toe and foot	Plantar flexion of great toe and foot
Screening Exam	Squat and rise	Heel walking	Walking on toes
Reflexes	Knee jerk diminished	None reliable	Ankle jerk diminished

FIGURE 73-4 Assessment of lumbar nerve root compromise includes testing for motor weakness and reflexes, and eliciting pain (screening examination). (Redrawn from Agency for Health Care Policy and Research. [1994]. *Acute low back problems in adults: Assessment and treatment. Quick reference guide for clinicians,* No. 14. Rockville, MD: Author.)

steroidal anti-inflammatory agents (NSAIDs), COX-2 inhibitors, muscle relaxants, and short-term opioids. Ice may be used to reduce pain with acute disk herniation for the first 48 hours. After that, heat is usually a better analgesic. A semi-sitting position (in a recliner chair) is usually comfortable and promotes forward lumbar spine flexion, thus reducing back strain. Other positions of comfort include (1) the supine position with pillows under the knees or legs or (2) the lateral position, in which the client lies on the unaffected side with a thin pillow between the knees and with the painful leg flexed to reduce tension on the sciatic nerve. Lying in a prone position and sleeping with thick pillows under the head should be avoided. Physical therapists may be able to reduce pain and spasm with stretching exercises, massage, ultrasonic heat treatments, or transcutaneous electrical nerve stimulation (TENS). Work space or environmental modifications may also be necessary. Complementary alternative therapies such as the use of acupuncture may be of therapeutic benefit.

For the client with nonspecific lower back pain, manipulation may be used by a physical therapist or chiropractor. *Spinal manipulation* is the use of the hands on the spine to stretch, mobilize, or manipulate the spine and paravertebral tissues. It is usually performed for clients with manifestations of more than 1 month's duration. These is no evidence that spinal traction with weights is effective in reducing lower back pain. Although unproven, deep ultrasonic heat treatment and moist local heat applications may help reduce pain.

Progressive muscle relaxation exercises and other stress reduction techniques can be helpful. Muscle stretching has also been effective for fascial pain.

For severe lumbar disk problems with leg pain, conservative intervention involves 2 to 4 days of bed rest on a firm mattress. Bed rest reduces back pain by relieving the back muscles and vertebrae of the stresses. The forces of gravity (e.g., weight of the head with cervical problems) and motion can increase back pain during activity.

Improve Mobility. Activity modifications are prescribed to reduce back irritation and prevent debilitation from inactivity. Most clients do not require bed rest; in fact, more than 4 days of bed rest can be debilitating and slow recovery. The client is taught to minimize the stress of lifting by using good body mechanics, keeping objects close to the body, and to avoid twisting when lifting. Sitting may aggravate leg pain and clients who sit at work should change positions often. Aerobic activities should be prescribed to help avoid debilitation.

Walking, stationary bicycling, and even light jogging can be performed. Exercise should begin within the first 2 weeks after injury and each activity should be performed for 20 to 30 minutes, two or three times a week, for best aerobic conditioning.

Work activities need to be individualized for each client based on his or her job requirements. See the Client Education Guide feature on Lower Back Care on the website.

A back brace or corset is often prescribed for a client with a ruptured lumbar disk. Back supports are usually not recommended once clinical manifestations are relieved, because restricted back motion progressively weakens muscles and causes further degeneration of spinal structures. Strengthening the back and abdominal muscles helps prevent further problems when the exercises are done daily throughout life.

Nursing Care of the Medical Client

Nursing care focuses on assisting the client to adjust his or her lifestyle to reduce the risk of further back injuries. Many clients are frustrated with the lack of cure of their back pain. Clients have become accustomed to having a well-defined cause of a problem and a well-researched approach for management. Many clients with lower back pain have pain for years without relief. This level of chronic pain can lead to depression and personality changes or relationship difficulties. Nurses should remain sensitive to the exasperation felt by the clients as well as the health care team.

Nurses teach the client safe methods to lift and bend, how to lie down and rise up from bed to avoid twisting, and how to take NSAIDs correctly to reduce the risk of gastric ulceration. If the client requires opioids for pain, instruct the client to eat high-fiber foods to reduce constipation, to avoid alcohol, and to not operate machinery or drive. The Client Education Guide on Lower Back Care is a useful tool in client teaching.

Surgical Management

Surgery is indicated for spinal disk problems when (1) sciatica is severe and disabling, (2) manifestations of sciatica persist without improvement or worsen, and (3) physiologic evidence of specific nerve root dysfunction is present. Surgery is also used to stabilize spinal fractures and correct scoliosis and kyphoscoliosis. Some surgeons use other criteria. Chemonucleolysis, which involves injecting chymopapain into the disk, is a practice that has been abandoned because of the frequency of immediate and delayed allergic responses.

Percutaneous Diskectomy. Herniated disk material can be removed using a trocar to remove the center of the disk. This procedure may also involve using laser to destroy the damaged disk.

Microdiskectomy. Microdiskectomy is the use of microsurgical instruments to remove the herniated fragment of disk. Use of this technique results in less trauma to the surgical site than standard diskectomy and more tissue integrity is preserved. Advantages of microsurgery in-

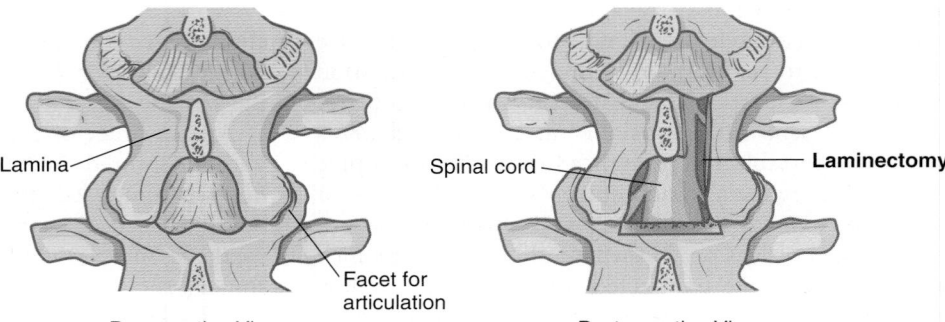

FIGURE 73-5 Laminectomy for the interlaminal removal of a herniated disk.

Lamina

Facet for articulation

Preoperative View

Spinal cord

Laminectomy

Postoperative View

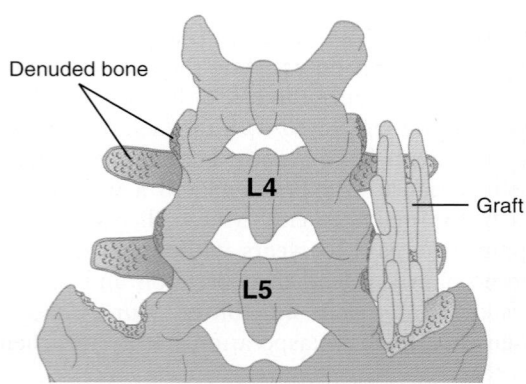

Denuded bone

L4

Graft

L5

FIGURE 73-6 Lumbar interbody spinal fusion. Bone grafts are taken from the iliac crest and inserted between the vertebrae. In this illustration, the "bed" of raw bone is shown on the left, and the graft material is shown in place on the right.

clude (1) minimal nerve root retraction, (2) preservation of an intact joint capsule (no bone is removed), (3) improved hemostasis, and (4) minimal stripping of the muscle and fascia from the spine.

Decompressive Laminectomy. The term *laminectomy* is confusing and is used loosely. The term *laminectomy* means complete removal of the bone between the spinous process and the facet. This is seldom necessary. The more correct term for what is done is *laminotomy,* which is the creation of a hole in the lamina.

Decompressive laminectomy is surgical removal of the posterior arch of a vertebra, exposing the spinal cord (Figure 73-5). This gives access to the spinal canal for (1) removing a spinal cord tumor, (2) removing portions of the facets, or (3) decompressing bony infringement on the spinal cord. Sometimes foraminotomy is performed to enlarge the intervertebral foramen if it is narrowed and osteophytic processes (overgrowth of bone) entrap the nerve root and impinge on neural structures

Artificial Disk Replacement. Recent advances in research have developed replacement disks to provide spinal motion rather than fusion. Postoperative care is similar to other spinal surgery except that clients are am-

bulated sooner. Outcomes of ambulation and recreation are positive.[18]

Spinal Fusion/Arthrodesis. Spinal fusion is the placement of bone grafts (bone chips) between vertebrae (Figure 73-6). The new bone that grows fuses the two vertebrae and immobilizes them to reduce the pain. Usually no more than five vertebrae are fused; fusing more than five vertebrae causes considerable loss of movement in the spine. Bone grafts may be obtained from a bone bank or the anterosuperior iliac crest. During healing, the graft gradually grows onto the vertebrae and forms a bony union. This union causes permanent stiffness in the area. After a while, the stiffness is hardly noticed in the lumbar area but is noticeable in the cervical area. The client cannot be guaranteed that back pain will be relieved permanently or that further surgery will not be required.

Spinal Fusion with Instrumentation. Metal rods may be used to straighten and fuse the spine in disorders such as scoliosis or multiple vertebral fractures. Other devices can also be used to provide additional support while the bones heal in a fused manner (see Figure 29-4).

Complications. General potential complications following spinal disk surgery at any level include infection and inflammation, injury to nerve roots, dural tears, cauda equina syndrome, and hematoma. Non-union of the surgical area is also a risk and is associated with smoking. Some surgeons assess serum or salivary nicotine levels before surgery to reduce the risk of non-union and validate statements of smoking cessation.

Prognosis. The Agency for Health Care Policy and Research (AHCPR) reviewed outcomes of surgery for lower back problems.[2] In general, lumbar diskectomy often relieved manifestations of pain in persons with severe and disabling leg pain faster than continued medical management. However, in individuals with no leg pain, there appeared to be little difference in outcome between diskectomy and conservative care. Most clients who had chymopapain injections required eventual diskectomy for permanent pain relief. More study is needed to determine who is best served by the various techniques; client preference also plays a big role in the technique chosen.

■ Nursing Management of the Surgical Client

Preoperative Care
Assessment

A baseline neurologic assessment is obtained for comparison after surgery. Assessment should include motor and sensory function of extremities and psychological readiness for surgery.

Diagnosis, Outcomes, Interventions

Diagnosis: Deficient Knowledge.
Perioperative care of a client having spinal surgery includes providing knowledge about the preoperative, operative, and postoperative phases. It also includes evaluating the client and family's understanding of the experience. A common nursing diagnosis in this circumstance is *Deficient Knowledge*.

Outcomes. The client and family will be able to explain the surgical procedure, preoperative preparations, and the postoperative precautions and needs. The client will demonstrate safe mobility, including logrolling, and transfer to and from the bed.

Interventions. The family is included in preoperative education. Explain to the client that frequent turning follows surgery and that correct turning protects the back and helps the recovery process. Explain the logrolling method of turning, the necessity for limitations on activity to prevent damage (flexion, extension, or twisting) to the surgical site, and the importance of not straining. Advise the client to ask for help rather than stretching to reach for objects. Stool softeners are given daily while the client is in the hospital to minimize straining with bowel movements. Clients with a recent injury may not be permitted to ambulate before surgery. For these clients, explain and demonstrate the various interventions to be used.

EB Encourage clients who smoke to stop smoking. Smoking increases cardiovascular complications and increases the risk of poor wound healing and non-union if a fusion is performed.

When a fusion is to be done, clients need to be evaluated for autologous blood donations. Two or three units should be donated, the last one at least a week before the surgery. Older clients may require more time for blood donation. A fusion also necessitates informing the client about the bone autograft donor site and about the additional pain associated with this site.

The client may also require changes in the home environment. These changes should be considered and dis-

cussed before surgery. Topics include bathroom facilities, devices needed for ambulation, the ability to use a shower and toilet, and the need for seat risers and grab bars in strategic locations such as near the toilet or shower.

Diagnosis: Fear and Anxiety.
Many people fear postoperative problems such as paralysis and chronic pain. *Fear* and *Anxiety* are common nursing diagnoses in this situation.

Outcomes. The client will express a low level of fear or anxiety related to the upcoming surgery and will use positive coping strategies to decrease his or her fear or anxiety.

Interventions. Encourage the client and family to express their concerns and fears about the spinal surgery. Concerns and fears should be allayed whenever possible. For example, clients need to be aware that some edema is expected at the surgical site and therefore some of the preoperative deficit may still exist after surgery, but the client's condition should improve as the edema lessens.

Evaluation

Preoperative education should allay some of the concerns of the client and family. Do not expect all anxiety to be relieved; in fact, some new areas of concern may arise. If questions arise about the operation, ask the surgeon to answer them. Do not attempt to provide information outside of your area of expertise.

Postoperative Care
Assessment

Following spinal surgery, assessment is similar to that performed for other surgical clients. A head-to-toe assessment is done. Dressings and drains are checked, including those at the donor site. Evaluate the level of pain and the response to analgesia. Assess neurologic function by asking the client to move his or her legs and comparing the results with those of the baseline evaluation. Question the client about the presence of numbness or tingling and changes in sensation or pain. These paresthesias may be a consequence of the edema from the surgery and should improve. If progressive weakness or paralysis of the lower extremities, loss of sphincter control, anal numbness, or urinary retention (called the *cauda equina syndrome*) occurs, notify the physician immediately. Emergency surgical decompression may be required.

Clients who have had fusions are on bed rest longer and thus are at greater risk for deep vein thrombosis (DVT). Compression devices on the legs may be used to improve venous return. Observe for and report any manifestations of DVT: positive Homans' sign, redness or swelling in the one leg, or sudden chest pain or dyspnea. Assess the wound for bulging or clear drainage, which may indicate cerebrospinal fluid (CSF) leakage. If the client had an anterior approach for surgery, usual care following abdominal surgery is required (e.g., assessment for ileus).

Disk problems often create fears and concerns related to pain, treatments, sexual activity, possible length of illness, and possible lifestyle changes. Provide psychosocial support to the client and family. Impaired mobility and altered urinary or bowel elimination are also common problems experienced after disk surgery. Considerations about employment and finances should be referred to a social worker.

Diagnosis, Outcomes, Interventions

Diagnosis: Acute Pain. Pain secondary to incisional trauma and edema is an expected response after spinal surgery. Write this common postoperative nursing diagnosis as *Acute Pain related to tissue trauma secondary to back (and/or abdominal) incision.*

Outcomes. The client will express comfort, for example, a low level of pain, such as a 3 on a pain scale of 0 to 10.

Interventions. Although acute incisional pain is present, often the pain in an extremity is significantly less after herniated disk surgery. In addition, many surgeons inject long-acting local anesthetics into disk spaces during surgery. This gives the client immediate relief from pain and promotes a positive attitude toward the outcome of surgery. Often the pain recurs on the second postoperative day. This is due to both the increase in swelling and the fact that the local anesthetic is wearing off.

Acute postoperative pain can be managed by using a basal (continuous) dose of an opioid per intravenous (IV) pump or by mouth in combination with a patient-controlled analgesia (PCA) dose for pain peaks (breakthrough pain) not controlled by the continuous dose. Another method of providing basal (continuous) pain medication is by epidural catheter. If the client is on an as-needed (prn) pain management, teach the client to keep pain levels tolerable by asking for opioids before the pain is too great. Ice may also be applied to the incision using an abdominal wrap that holds sheets of ice along the lumbar area and reduces the risk of ice burns. Ice may also be applied to the bone graft donor site.

Diagnosis: Impaired Physical Mobility. Clients who have spinal surgery will have varying degrees of mobility limitations. The nursing diagnosis can be written as *Impaired Physical Mobility related to pain, leg weakness,* *prolonged immobility, or fear of pain and spasms.* Choose the etiology that best fits your client.

Outcomes. The client will resume a maximal level of progressive activity, starting with logrolling on the day of surgery, progressing to independent movement from the bed to a standing position, followed by independent ambulation before discharge.

Interventions. When the client is being transferred to bed initially from surgery, ample people should assist. Transfer devices such as a sliding board may be used with adequate help. Transfer the client gently and smoothly, with the spine supported and properly aligned at all times.

Immediately following lumbar diskectomy, the client typically is not turned for an hour or so but remains flat to aid hemostasis. Begin side-to-side logrolling and repeat every 2 hours. If a dural tear was repaired, the surgeon may order the client to remain flat longer to minimize the risk of CSF leak or a tear in the dural sutures.

After lumbar fusion, the bed is generally kept flat. The client logrolls from side to side, usually beginning about 4 hours after surgery and then every 2 to 4 hours thereafter. Twisting the client's spine or twisting at the hips must be avoided. Ensure safety during turning to prevent straining of the spine or rolling off the bed. It is beneficial to have extra help in turning a client the first few times after spinal surgery. Spinal bone grafts are delicate and heal slowly. Eventually, turning is permitted without help, while keeping the spine rigid.

It is common for the client to have spasms and pain with turning, and analgesics should be administered before moving. If the client is receiving medication by PCA, administer the medication about 10 minutes before moving the client. The advanced dose reduces pain without the immediate nausea and flushing that may occur. Once the client is turned, tilt the client back onto pillows to reduce pressure on the iliac crest. Back strain may then be reduced by (1) keeping the client's spine straight, (2) flexing the upper leg and placing a pillow between the legs, and (3) placing a pillow to support the upper arm and prevent the upper shoulder from sagging. If the iliac crest was used as a donor site, the client may not be able to turn onto that side because of pain. Abdominal incisions should be splinted to reduce pain.

Follow the surgeon's orders on how high the head can be elevated. Use a pressure-reduction mattress to reduce the risk of pressure ulcers when the client had spinal surgery for fracture stabilization or when the client will be in bed for an extended period. Use of a trapeze over the bed is contraindicated because it promotes twisting. The call light and PCA control are placed so the client can access them without straining or twisting. Once the client is allowed to reach for things, the objects needed should be placed conveniently.

Encourage the client to move his or her legs and feet while on bed rest to promote venous return. In addition, alternating or continuous compression stockings may be used to promote venous return. Keep the bed linens loose at the foot of the bed to promote independent movement. If the client requires assistance to turn, or when turning to place a bedpan, turn the client in the logrolling manner. A fracture bedpan is used to reduce back arching and strain.

If a client is supine following spinal surgery (e.g., using a bedpan), the lower back muscles may be relaxed somewhat if pillows are placed under the entire length of the legs. This may also prevent thrombophlebitis in the femoral vessels. Do not flex the client's knees by placing anything under the popliteal space; this is hazardous because it increases the risk of DVT. A sign is placed on the bed describing the prescribed position for the bed. Instruct the client clearly about contraindicated activities and positions.

To assist the client into a chair, keep the bed flat and teach the client to roll onto his or her side (Figure 73-7), then push the torso from the bed with the arms to rise from the bed. This technique has often been used by clients with long-standing back pain and may be familiar to the client. If the client has had long-standing back pain, review the client's technique for rising from the bed. Usually the client is assisted to a chair the morning following surgery. Be sure to follow the physician's activity prescriptions.

After spinal surgery, a brace or corset may be required temporarily to support the spine. Clients who have lumbar or thoracic spinal fusions wear a fiberglass brace, which resembles a shell. Initially, back braces or corsets may be worn constantly, whether the client is in or out of bed. As the client's muscles strengthen, the use of braces or corsets is usually decreased. Again, follow the physician's activity prescriptions. Casts may be used for a while following any thoracic spinal surgery for clients with unstable thoracic spines (e.g., thoracic spinal cord trauma).

Diagnosis: Impaired Urinary Elimination. After spinal surgery, urinary retention may occur, most commonly because of pain and spasms when resting supine and as a side effect of opioids. Urinary retention also occurs when the cauda equina is affected. Write the nursing diagnosis as *Risk for Impaired Urinary Elimination related to pain and spasms with movement, inability to void in a supine position, and side effects from opioids.*

Outcomes. The client will resume normal bladder emptying by the time he or she is ambulating.

Interventions. Assess for bladder distention and pain 8 hours after surgery. If the client's bladder is distended and painful on palpation, noninvasive measures should be tried first. The client is commonly catheterized with an in-and-out catheter (straight catheterization) twice, after which an indwelling catheter is placed if the client still

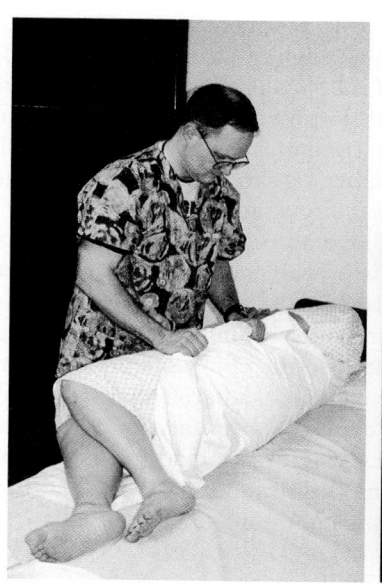 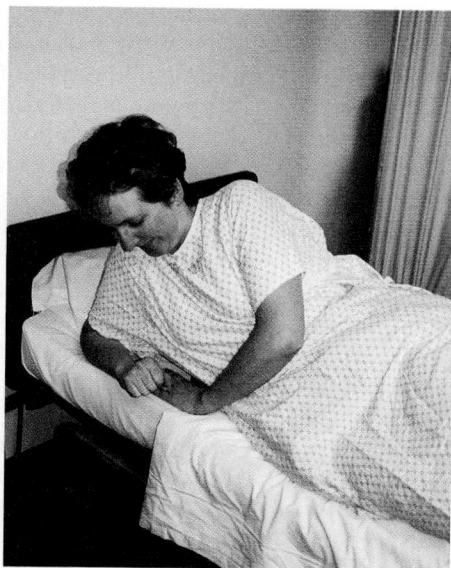 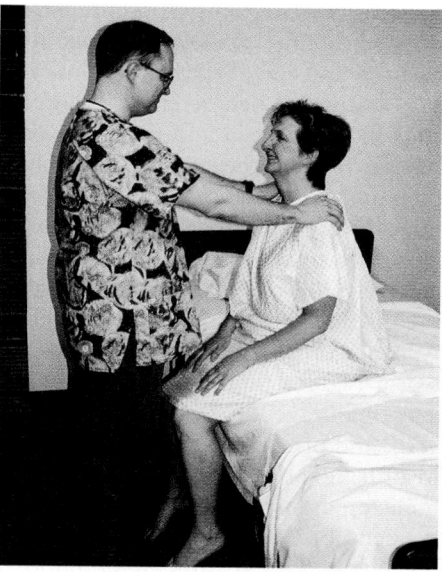

A   B   C

FIGURE 73-7 Helping the client stand after lumbar fusion. **A,** Logroll the client to the edge of the bed using a turning sheet if needed. Leave the bed in that position. **B,** The client pushes off the bed with the hand and the other elbow to sit up without twisting. The client drops his or her legs off the side of the bed at the same time. **C,** With the client seated on the edge of the bed, the nurse assesses for orthostatic hypotension. The client stands from the bed without flexing the back.

does not void spontaneously. Indwelling catheters may be used for the first few days until the client is ambulating and using less pain medication. When the catheter is removed, generally clients can urinate when sitting or standing rather than lying supine. If the bladder is full or cannot be emptied completely, the physician may order straight catheterization to check for residual urine.

Collaborative Problem: Risk for Paralytic Ileus.
The most common bowel problem after laminectomy and spinal fusion is paralytic ileus. This loss of bowel sounds and abdominal distention is due to lack of peristalsis from a sudden loss of parasympathetic function innervating the bowels and manipulation of the intestines in anterior approaches to spinal surgery.

Outcomes. The nurse will assess the client for return of normal bowel function, including normal bowel sound patterns, and evacuation without straining, by the time he or she is ambulating. This problem is expressed as a collaborative problem, therefore the outcome is written in terms of the nurse's actions. The nurse's actions cannot independently alter the outcome, as occurs with nursing diagnoses.

Interventions. Assessment findings with paralytic ileus include nausea, vomiting, a hard and possibly distended or tympanic abdomen, and absence of bowel sounds. The client is assessed every 4 hours postoperatively for bowel distention.

If the client has paralytic ileus or is expected to develop ileus due to extensive manipulation during surgery, a nasogastric tube connected to low intermittent suction is inserted and the client has no fluid or food by mouth (NPO status). When a client's gag reflex and bowel sounds have returned and the client passes gas or has a bowel movement, the nasogastric tube is removed and a clear liquid diet is prescribed. The client progresses to a regular diet as tolerated.

Bowel dysfunction may occur for several days postoperatively. Inactivity and the use of opioid analgesia often cause problems with bowel elimination. Bowel movements are documented. Fluids are forced as ordered; a regular time for bowel movements and bowel care is encouraged; fiber is provided in the diet (when allowed), and prescribed medications (e.g., stool softeners, mild bulk laxatives, or a suppository) and enemas are administered. Instruct the client not to strain for a bowel movement, because this increases pain and CSF pressure. Often clients find it difficult or impossible to defecate when lying flat. A bowel movement may not occur until sitting up is possible.

Evaluation

Expect pain to be controlled with mild to moderate opioid analgesics, bowel and bladder function to be intact,

the client to be able to walk steadily for several yards, and the client to be able to eat before discharge.

■ Self-Care

Approximately 80% of the population experience lower back pain at some point in their lives. It is estimated that 10% of those who seek medical attention for back pain have herniated disks. Because of the frequency of herniated disk problems, health promotion is an essential activity for health care providers. The Client Education Guide provides suggestions for lower back care.

CERVICAL DISK DISORDERS

Disks may become entrapped in the cervical spine. The process is much like that with herniated lumbar disks. Manifestations include arm pain, neck pain and spasms, and loss of function (grip strength) and changes in sensation in the hands.

Outcome Management

Initial treatment is with NSAIDs, muscle stretching, and teaching proper body mechanics. Opinions differ concerning the advisability of performing head and neck range-of-motion exercises in the presence of significant cervical disease. Tell the client to avoid activities that increase cervical disk pain. To prevent neck extension when in bed, only one flat pillow (to prevent neck flexion) is recommended. The neck should not be hyperextended. Intermittent traction may be applied for cervical disk herniation (5- to 8-lb weight) to reduce pain. The head of the bed may be slightly elevated with cervical traction. Otherwise, it is best kept flat when cervical pain is present. A review of posture at work is important for clients who work at computer terminals. Keyboards, screens, and written materials should be kept at a height that reduces strain on the neck and shoulders.

A soft cervical collar may be prescribed for mild to moderate cervical disk problems to keep the head slightly flexed. After fracture of a cervical vertebra, cervical disk rupture, or whiplash injury, the client may wear a neck brace (fitted so the chin rests on a cup and the neck is kept hyperextended), a hard collar (which extends up under the chin and prevents flexion of the neck), or a soft collar. Neck braces tend to limit vision, because people wearing them cannot look down at their feet. Safety awareness is important to prevent falls.

■ Surgical Management

Sometimes conservative treatment does not work and clients require surgery. Surgery to stabilize bone fragments is necessary when a neck injury involves a bone fracture. Cervical fusion is most commonly performed through an anterior approach (Figure 73-8). Immediately after a posterior cervical diskectomy, a cervical collar is worn (Figure 73-9). A hard cervical collar is usu-

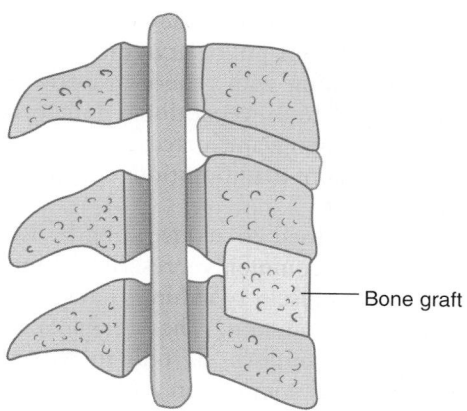

FIGURE 73-8 Anterior cervical fusion. A trough has been cut into the anterior cervical spine for insertion of an iliac graft as a splint. The intervertebral spaces have been filled with bone chips.

ally prescribed following fusion. Complications after posterior cervical surgery include soft tissue hematoma, air embolism, and subcutaneous wound dehiscence. Complications following anterior cervical surgeries include laryngeal nerve damage and injury to neck structures such as the carotid arteries, trachea, esophagus, and soft tissue.

After microdiskectomy, the client may have the head of the bed elevated to whatever position is comfortable. Following cervical spine fusion, the surgeon indicates the degree of head elevation for comfort and to reduce edema. Make sure the spine is in anatomic alignment. The client's head may be elevated and a folded small towel, bath blanket, or small pillow is placed under the head to maintain spinal alignment while the client lies supine or on the side.

Assess and document the client's neurologic status frequently. The development or worsening of a neurologic deficit must be promptly reported to the surgeon. During the first 24 hours after an anterior cervical diskectomy, assess the client's ability to breathe, check the operative site for excessive swelling, and look for shifting of the trachea and changes in the client's voice. Laryngeal nerve damage during surgery may cause permanent vocal impairment, such as hoarseness. If a spinal fusion was performed with the anterior cervical diskectomy, the surgeon is notified if radicular pain suddenly recurs. This could mean that the bone graft has moved out of place and surgery needs to be repeated. Also assess the client for indications of postoperative improvement such as absence of paresthesias.

After surgery on the cervical spine, watch for indications of respiratory paralysis resulting from spinal cord edema. Emergency tracheostomy equipment is kept at hand.

Tell the client that it is not unusual for preoperative manifestations to persist for a few days secondary to

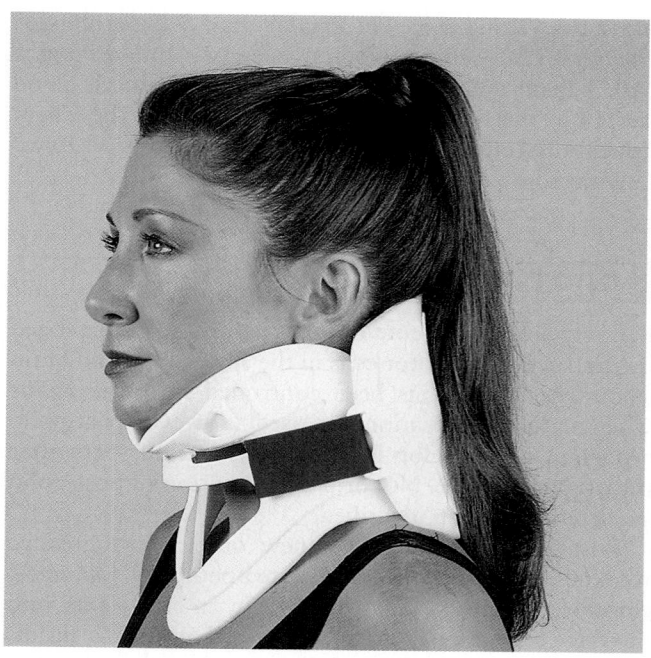

FIGURE 73-9 A cervical collar with a chin piece. This orthosis provides additional support for the head and some restriction of cervical spine motion. (Courtesy of Zimmer, Inc., Dover, OH.)

edema at the operative site, although these manifestations are usually less uncomfortable. Difficulty swallowing and throat discomfort are usually present for several days and are commonly due to local irritation from the endotracheal tube. A soft diet, throat lozenges, a viscous lidocaine (Xylocaine) solution, humidified air, minimal talking, and other comfort measures lessen the discomfort.

A wound drain may be present and is usually removed by the surgeon on the second postoperative day, after drainage has decreased. Bladder and bowel management are the same as for clients after lumbar surgery. Cervical surgery may affect the parasympathetic chain, causing urinary retention.

■ Self-Care

With shorter postoperative hospital stays, most clients are discharged before suture or staple removal. Instruction for care of the incision includes keeping the sutures or staples clean and dry and noting any increased redness or drainage from the wound. Clients need clear instructions on walking, lifting, driving, and returning to work. Most clients can resume regular activity 6 weeks after surgery. Specific physician instructions need to be followed.

Prolonged sitting or standing in one position strains the healing back. Contraindicated activities vary. The client is instructed to ask the surgeon when it will be safe to perform activities that could damage the back (climbing stairs, lifting a weight greater than 5 lb, prolonged travel, sexual activity, sports, exercise, and driving a car). Clients must not smoke. Smoking reduces blood supply to the tissues and delays healing. See the Client Education Guide feature on Home Care After Cervical Laminectomy or Fusion on the website.

POST-POLIO SYNDROME

Poliomyelitis is an acute form of paralysis characterized by destruction of motor cells in the spinal cord and brain stem. The disease has been controlled since the 1950s when mass immunization was used. However, post-polio syndrome can develop in polio survivors 30 years after the original disease. No form of prevention of post-polio syndrome has been identified.

Post-polio syndrome is a new onset of progressive weakness, fatigue, decreased temperature tolerance, emotional distress, dysphagia, pain in the joints and muscles, and respiratory problems. The onset is insidious, and weakness occasionally extends to muscles that were not involved during the initial illness. The prognosis is generally good; progression to further weakness is usually slow, with plateau periods that range from 1 to 10 years. The syndrome is thought to be due to progressive dysfunction and loss of motor neurons that compensated for the neurons lost during the original infection and not to persistent or reactivated poliovirus infection.

Management of post-polio syndrome has three components: energy conservation and lifestyle modification, medications, and measures to promote quality of life. Energy conservation includes pacing of activities, making the environment more ergonomic, sitting rather than standing, and use of electric mobility. Assistive devices to correct and minimize postural and gait abnormalities (e.g., canes, crutches, walkers) and braces designed to provide support to weakened muscles and joints can reduce pain, improve safety and enhance energy conservation, help clients reduce fatigue, avoid overuse, and recover faster after activity. Occupational therapists can help clients assess their lifestyles and design appropriate changes. Despite the benefits of assistive devices, many polio survivors are reluctant to use them. They remember the intense rehabilitation efforts during their childhood and how they were encouraged to become independent and "like everyone else" again. It is important for a knowledgeable orthotist to fully explain the advantages of assistive devices and discuss the newer designs and materials.

Polio survivors may have also been taught to give up exercise to avoid activity-induced muscle pain to "save" what they have. This advice results in declining strength as a result of muscle deconditioning and increased long-term risk of cardiac deconditioning. Currently, several studies have demonstrated both the safety and efficacy of nonfatiguing exercise for polio survivors. Progressive resistive strength training with reduced repetitive motion (e.g., three sets of 4 to 10 repetitions) done every other day demonstrated significant increases in static and dynamic strength without manifestations of injury or worsening manifestations.

Medications are used to reduce fatigue. Pyridostigmine (Mestinon) is commonly prescribed, but side effects of increased muscle twitching, nausea, diarrhea, and frequency are common. The weakness is treated with strengthening exercises, steroids to reduce inflammation, and electrical stimulation. Other manifestations are treated symptomatically also.

Symptomatic treatment of pain is important for optimizing both functional ability and quality of life. Polio survivors with pain can benefit from a multidisciplinary approach to pain management, which may include medication. The cause of the pain determines the choice of drug used to treat it.

Primary post-polio muscle pain may have features of neuropathic pain. Additionally, primary neuropathic pain from nerve compression may be present. Neuropathic pain responds to NSAIDs, topical capsaicin, lidocaine (Xylocaine) preparations, and membrane-stabilizing agents.

Biomechanical pain can be treated with steroids (oral or injectable), NSAIDs, or muscle relaxants, as well as with rehabilitation techniques, topical cold or heat, TENS, and relaxation/biofeedback. Overuse pain and cramps should not be casually medicated, because they are signs that changes in lifestyle and body mechanics are overdue.

Quality of life can be affected when post-polio syndrome develops in clients who have successfully adapted to their disease and disability. Respiratory distress may bring back memories of the initial infection and treatment in an iron lung (a very early form of a respirator in which the client's entire body was placed in a large metal cylinder).

Perceived barriers to health that furthered disablement in polio survivors have included fatigue, lack of money and time, lack of convenient resources, and lack of supportive health care providers. Additional restrictions are difficult to accept. Emotional support is vital. Teach the client to balance rest and activity.

SPINAL CORD DISORDERS
SYRINGOMYELIA

Syringomyelia is often associated with the Arnold-Chiari malformation (an abnormal protrusion of the medulla into the spinal canal) or spina bifida. Syringomyelia consists of abnormal cavities filled with dense, glue-like tissue in the spinal cord substance, especially the cervical cord. Scar tissue surrounds the cysts. Syringomyelia is characterized by (1) muscular weakness and wasting, (2) sensory defects, and (3) indications of injury to the long tracts of the spinal cord, such as hyperreflexia.

Early manifestations of cervical syringomyelia often include the following:

1. Atrophy, weakness, and fibrillations of the small muscles of the hands
2. Loss of pain sensation in the fingers or forearms
3. Weakness and atrophy of the shoulder girdle muscles
4. Horner's syndrome, which is characterized by ptosis of the upper eyelid, constriction of the pupil, anhidrosis (absence of sweating), and flushing of the affected side of the face
5. Nystagmus
6. Vasomotor and trophic disturbances of the upper extremities

Although there is segmental loss or impairment of pain and temperature sensation, sensation for light touch remains. Segments of sensory loss may be separated by zones of normal sensation. Spasticity, ataxia, or paralysis of the lower extremities may occur, as may disturbed bladder control, if the lumbosacral region of the spinal cord is involved.

Cranial nerve involvement may produce additional problems such as impairment of facial pain and temperature sensation, loss of the corneal reflex (necessitating protection of the eye), dysphagia, dysarthria, laryngeal stridor (possibly necessitating tracheostomy), nystagmus, and atrophy and fibrillation of the tongue muscles.

Syringomyelia may progress rapidly at first and then become quiescent for many years. Some clients live 40 years after onset. Others become incapacitated (from paralysis or sensory defects) or die within a few years.

Treatment includes relieving increased pressure on the cord from the fluid content of the cavities within the spinal canal. The fluid buildup can be removed and CSF outflow restored by direct surgical drainage or by shunt placement.

VASCULAR SPINAL CORD LESIONS

As with stroke, spinal cord vascular lesions may be caused by rupture, thrombosis, or embolism. Trauma is the usual cause of hemorrhage into the spinal cord. Thrombosis of the spinal vessels is usually secondary to meningitis or to compression of the vessels by tumors, granulomas, or abscesses in the epidural space.

MYELOMALACIA

Myelomalacia is softening or infarction of the spinal cord from spinal artery occlusion. Prognosis is poor because there is little or no return of normal function to the involved areas. Myelomalacia is suspected when indications of transverse myelitis develop suddenly. Clinical manifestations depend on the level of the lesion in the

cord. There is always motor paralysis and dissociated sensory loss below the level of the lesion, accompanied by paralysis of bladder and bowel sphincters. Paralysis is usually bilateral but rarely complete. Initially, the limbs are flaccid and no deep tendon or superficial reflexes are elicited, as in spinal shock. After several weeks, spasticity, hyperreflexia, and clonus develop. Intervention focuses on maintaining body functions, preventing complications of immobility, and providing pain relief. The person usually begins intensive rehabilitation 12 to 14 hours after onset of manifestations.

HEMATOMYELIA

Hematomyelia is hemorrhage into the substance of the spinal cord. It almost always follows trauma but may be caused by vascular malformation or a bleeding disorder. Clinical manifestations of hematomyelia usually develop suddenly, immediately after spinal injury, and depend on the size of the hemorrhage. Following trauma, it is important to differentiate between hematomyelia and a vertebral fracture dislocation. Immediate surgery to relieve cord compression is indicated if fracture dislocation is evident on x-ray film. Spinal angiography, spinal CT scans, and MRI enable visualization of vascular lesions. Some of these lesions are treated by ligating their feeding vessels, others by excising the entire malformation. Management is the same as for myelomalacia. If surgery is needed, postoperative care is like that given to clients with other forms of spinal surgery.

NEUROSYPHILIS

Neurosyphilis is a chronic or late stage of syphilis involving infection of the brain or spinal cord. The oculomotor nerves may be affected, leading to an inability of the pupil to react to light, called an Argyll Robertson pupil. The posterior columns and nerve roots of the spinal cord may be affected, which is called *tabes dorsalis*. Because these are sensory nerves, the most common manifestation is pain. The pain can occur almost anywhere in the body, although abdominal pain is most common. The pain is severe enough to be confused with gastric ulcers and gallbladder disease. In addition to pain, areas of paresthesias may be noted. A common finding in tabes dorsalis is the loss of position sense in the feet and legs. As a result, clients walk with a slapping step. They are at increased risk of falls when walking in the dark because they must rely on visual cues for placement of their feet with each step. In addition, because the gait is abnormal, bone alignment with walking is altered. Eventually the foot is abnormally shaped (called *Charcot's joint*). This alteration in foot structure can lead to foot ulcerations, because the client bears the body weight on abnormal areas. The brain can also be involved in later stages of syphilis. A general deterioration of mental status can develop.

With improved case finding and the use of penicillin to treat syphilis in its early stages, the management of syphilis is improving. However, with development of resistant strains of organisms and a recent increase in the incidence of sexually transmitted diseases, problems may recur in the future.

UPPER MOTOR NEURON LESIONS

Upper motor neurons are long nerve cells that originate in the brain and travel in tracts through the spinal cord. These pathways constitute the upper motor neurons (UMNs). The UMNs originate in the motor strip of the cerebral cortex and in multiple brain stem nuclei. From the cortex, these axons pass through the internal capsule; most of them cross over in the medulla and descend in the spinal cord through the corticospinal tracts. A few do not cross in the brain but cross later in the spinal cord. The corticospinal tracts are primarily responsible for precise, fine, voluntary motor movements. However, they also assist in modulating muscle tone and reflexes to some degree. Any injury to these nerves cuts off contact with brain control. Reflex activity is still intact, however, resulting in spasticity.

Any lesion that destroys the UMNs initially results in contralateral paralysis, such as is seen with stroke. Initially, the involved area is flaccid and hyporeflexic. The flaccidity gradually recedes, and the reflex arc becomes hyperactive due to the lack of inhibition by the UMNs. Muscle tone is hypertonic and the extremity becomes spastic. Despite the spasms, the muscle becomes atrophied from disuse. The atrophy seen with UMN lesions occurs later than that seen with lower motor neuron (LMN) problems. The Babinski reflex is present.

LOWER MOTOR NEURON LESIONS

LMNs consist of the anterior horn cells located in the anterior gray matter of the spinal cord. They are also located in the motor cranial nuclei of the brain stem. Each anterior horn cell has a long axon that leaves the cord via the anterior spinal root and extends out the peripheral nerve, eventually synapsing at the motor end-plate of a neuromuscular junction. These structures form a motor unit that controls skeletal muscle activity, both voluntary and reflex activity. They are the last cells to carry information from the nervous system out to the muscles.

When a lesion develops in these structures, the client develops flaccid muscle weakness or paralysis, loss of reflexes, loss of muscle tone, and atrophy of the involved muscles. The degree to which these clinical manifestations develop depends on the extent of the lesion. Each anterior horn cell innervates several separate muscle fibers, and because several anterior horn cells exist at each spinal level, a lesion confined to one spinal segment may not damage all of the anterior horn cells innervating an entire muscle. This type of lesion would cause muscle weakness rather than paralysis. Paralysis occurs when a lesion involves the column or anterior horn cells in several spinal segments. When all the peripheral motor nerves are involved, the entire muscle becomes flac-

cid. The muscles atrophy early due to lack of innervation. LMN lesions are often associated with spinal cord injury or tumors and surgery on the aorta, which alters blood flow to the spinal cord.

SPINAL TUMORS

Spinal tumors are similar in nature and origin to intracranial tumors but occur much less often. They are most common in young or middle-aged adults and most often involve the thoracic region. Spinal tumors may occur outside of the spinal cord such as in the meninges, nerve roots, or vertebrae (extramedullary) or within the substance of the spinal cord (intramedullary). Neurofibromas and meningiomas are the most common spinal cord tumors. Both are benign and operable and may not produce permanent damage if removed early.

Clinical manifestations of spinal tumors vary according to their location. Extramedullary tumors cause manifestations by compressing the spinal cord or some of its nerve roots or by occluding blood vessels supplying the cord. Early characteristics of spinal cord compression include pain, sensory loss, muscle weakness, and muscle wasting. Progressive cord compression is manifested by spastic weakness below the level of the lesion, decreased sensation, and increased reflexes. Severe cord compression at the cervical level destroys cord function and produces quadriplegia; compression at the thoracic or lumbar level results in paraplegia.

Intramedullary tumors produce more variable clinical manifestations. High cervical cord involvement causes spastic quadriplegia and sensory changes. Tumors in descending areas of the spinal cord produce motor and sensory changes appropriate to functions at that level.

Medical diagnosis is made after a complete general neurologic examination. Diagnostic testing includes a spinal radiograph, CT scan, MRI scan, and a myelogram, individually or serially.

Intervention for spinal tumors is usually surgery, radiation therapy, or both. Immediate surgery is indicated if compression of the cord or nerve roots is evident. Often, surgery results in marked improvement or even complete restoration of function, especially when the tumor is benign and encapsulated (e.g., meningioma or lipoma). However, functional improvement is less common when cord necrosis has developed. Complete surgical removal of an intramedullary tumor is rare. However, partial resection followed by radiation may improve the client's condition. Usually the course of the condition is gradually progressive.

DISORDERS OF THE CRANIAL NERVES

Cranial nerves can be affected in many ways by various nervous system disorders. For example, they may be secondarily affected by compression resulting from increased intracranial pressure or they may be directly damaged as a result of head injuries. In this section, only the two most common disorders specific to the cranial nerves, not those associated with other disorders, are discussed. Other cranial nerve disorders do exist. Regeneration of the cranial nerves can occur except for the first (olfactory) or second (optic) cranial nerve, because these nerves are actually part of the central nervous system (CNS).

TRIGEMINAL NEURALGIA

Chronic irritation of the fifth cranial nerve results in trigeminal neuralgia, also called *tic douloureux*. Although most commonly occurring in 50- to 70-year-old persons, trigeminal neuralgia can occur in adults of any age. Approximately 60% of clients are women. The trigeminal nerve has three divisions: the ophthalmic, maxillary, and mandibular (Figure 73-10). Trigeminal neuralgia may occur in any one or more of these divisions.

Causes of trigeminal neuralgia can be divided into intrinsic and extrinsic lesions within the nerve itself, such as gross abnormalities of the axon or myelin, as may occur with multiple sclerosis. Extrinsic lesions are outside the trigeminal root and include mechanical compression by tumors, vascular anomalies, dental abscesses, or jaw malformation.

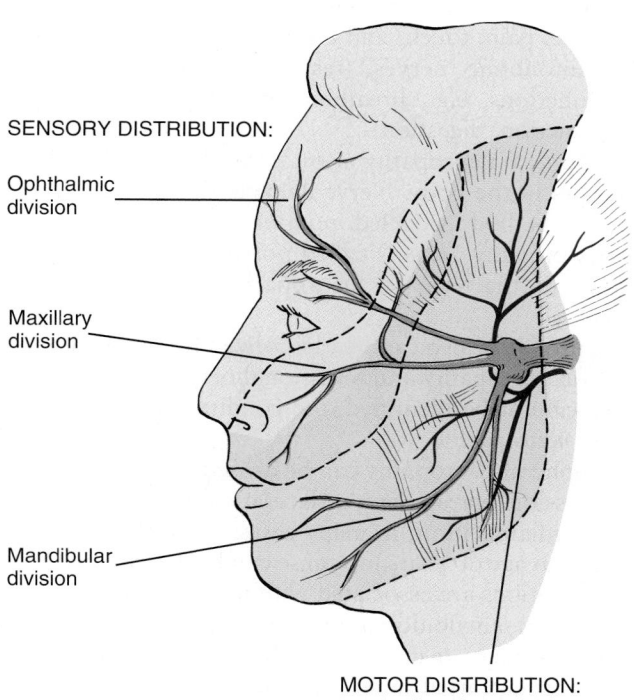

SENSORY DISTRIBUTION:

Ophthalmic division

Maxillary division

Mandibular division

MOTOR DISTRIBUTION:
to muscles of mastication

FIGURE 73-10 Distribution of the trigeminal nerve. Trigeminal neuralgia develops along the course of this nerve.

Trigeminal neuralgia is characterized by intermittent episodes of intense pain of sudden onset. The pain is rarely relieved by analgesics. Tactile stimulation, such as touch and facial hygiene, and even talking, may trigger an attack. Trigeminal neuralgia is more prevalent in the maxillary and mandibular distributions and on the right side of the face. Bilateral trigeminal neuralgia is rare but does occur. The pain from trigeminal neuralgia can become so intense that the client ponders suicide.

None of the current diagnostic studies identify trigeminal neuralgia. Angiography, CT scan, and MRI can identify a causative lesion. The actual diagnosis is made on the basis of an in-depth history with attention paid to triggering stimuli and the nature and site of the pain.

A careful history is obtained from the client regarding stimuli that trigger an attack. This information is used to plan care so as to minimize triggering events. The client's dental hygiene and nutritional intake are evaluated. These clients often do not eat enough to meet their daily nutritional needs and neglect their teeth because of the pain.

Outcome Management

Anticonvulsants such as carbamazepine (Tegretol) are often prescribed as the initial treatment of trigeminal neuralgia. These drugs may dampen the reactivity of the neurons within the trigeminal nerve. For some clients, these medications are all the treatment that is ever needed. Liver impairment may result from administration of both carbamazepine and phenytoin. Liver enzymes must be monitored before and during therapy. If the client cannot tolerate the dose needed for pain control, phenytoin can be used. These medications should be used cautiously in clients with a history of alcohol abuse. Baclofen (Lioresal) is an antispasmodic that may be used alone or in conjunction with anticonvulsants. Opioids are not particularly effective in relieving trigeminal neuralgia pain.

Help clients use and improve any pain control strategies they have developed. Clients with trigeminal neuralgia need emotional support to help them deal with pain that has often been present for a long time.

Surgery includes nerve blocks with alcohol and glycerol, peripheral neurectomy, and percutaneous radiofrequency wave forms that create lesions that alter pain transmission. The relief obtained with these procedures is not always permanent. Complications include development of facial paresthesias and muscular weakness. These procedures, being less invasive, are often better tolerated by older or debilitated clients.

More invasive techniques include major surgical procedures. Microvascular decompression involves removing the vessel from the posterior trigeminal root. A rhizotomy is the resection of the root of the nerve. These procedures require a craniotomy to allow access to the nerve.

Complications include those of any surgical procedure, as well as facial weakness and paresthesias. If facial anesthesia is present following surgery, clients must learn to test the temperature of food before putting it into their mouth. They should chew on the unaffected side and inspect mucous membranes for irritation. Assess for aspiration and advance the diet slowly. Teach clients to use a water jet device instead of a toothbrush for dental hygiene and advise them to visit their dentist as soon as possible after surgery.

If the corneal reflex has been impaired, the client should be taught eye care. During the acute postoperative period, apply eye drops and a protective shield. The client assumes these tasks with supervision and then independently.

BELL'S PALSY

Bell's palsy affects the motor aspects of the facial nerve, the seventh cranial nerve (Figure 73-11). Bell's palsy is the most common type of peripheral facial paralysis. It affects both women and men in all age-groups. However, it occurs most commonly between ages 20 and 40 years.

Bell's palsy results in a unilateral paralysis of the facial muscles of expression. There is no evidence of a pathologic cause. Facial paralysis may be central or peripheral in origin. Central facial palsy is an upper motor neuron paralysis or paresis. Sometimes it produces dissociation of motor function. In this situation, the client cannot voluntarily show his or her teeth on the paralyzed side, but can show them with emotional stimulation such as that causing smiles or laughter. This phenomenon is called *voluntary emotional dissociation.*

Typical clinical manifestations include (1) upward movement of the eyeball on closing the eye (Bell's phenomenon), (2) drooping of the mouth, (3) flattening of the nasolabial fold, (4) widening of the palpebral fissure, and (5) a slight lag in closing the eye. Eating may be difficult.

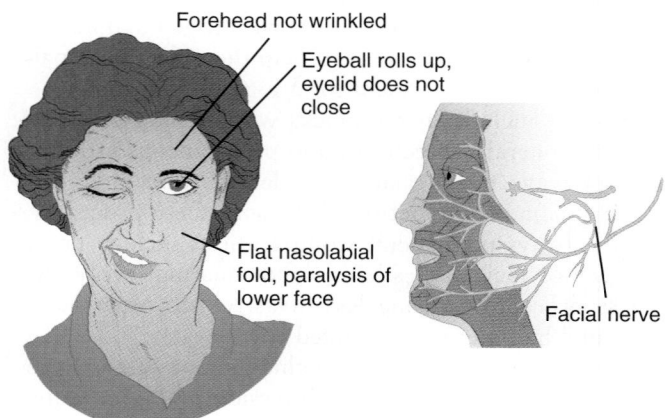

Forehead not wrinkled

Eyeball rolls up, eyelid does not close

Flat nasolabial fold, paralysis of lower face

Facial nerve

FIGURE 73-11 Bell's palsy is paralysis of the facial muscles innervated by the seventh cranial nerve.

There is no known cure for Bell's palsy. Care is palliative and includes analgesics if discomfort occurs from herpetic lesions, corticosteroids to decrease nerve tissue edema, physical therapy with moist heat, gentle massage, and stimulation of the facial nerve with faradic current. The cornea is protected with artificial tears, sunglasses, an eye patch at night, and periodic gentle closure of the eye.

Clients experiencing Bell's palsy often think they have had a stroke. Reassure the client that this is not the case. Most clients recover from Bell's palsy within a few weeks without residual manifestations. If permanent complete facial paralysis occurs, surgery may be necessary. Anastomosis of the peripheral end of the facial nerve with the spinal accessory or hypoglossal nerve allows closure of the eye during sleep and restores tone to the facial musculature.

DISORDERS OF THE PERIPHERAL NERVES

Peripheral neuropathy is a general term referring to disorders of peripheral nerves. Peripheral neuropathy can be associated with poor nutrition, a large number of diseases, and pressure or trauma. Many people suffer from the disorder without ever identifying the cause.

Peripheral neuropathy can be broadly categorized by the type of nerve that has been damaged. The peripheral nervous system is made up of three types of nerves:

- Motor nerves (responsible for voluntary movement)
- Sensory nerves (responsible for sensing temperature, pain, touch, and limb positioning)
- Autonomic nerves (responsible for involuntary functions, e.g., breathing, blood pressure, sexual function, digestion)

Peripheral neuropathy also can be classified by where it occurs in the body. Nerve damage that occurs in one area of the body is called *mononeuropathy;* that which occurs in many areas is called *polyneuropathy.* Radiculopathy is the term for neuropathy that affects nerve roots.

Neuropathy also can be categorized by cause, such as diabetic neuropathy and nutritional neuropathy. When a cause cannot be identified, the condition is called *idiopathic neuropathy.*

Peripheral neuropathy can be caused by disease; nerve compression, entrapment, or laceration; exposure to toxins; or inflammation. In many cases, especially in clients older than age 60 years, no cause can be determined. Several conditions are associated with neuropathy, including alcoholism, amyloidosis (metabolic disorder), autoimmune disorders (e.g., Guillain-Barré syndrome), Bell's palsy, cancer, carpal tunnel syndrome, renal failure, connective tissue diseases (rheumatoid arthritis), diabetes, Lyme disease, and vitamin deficiencies.

Clinical manifestations depend on the type of nerve affected (motor, sensory, autonomic) and where the nerve is located in the body. One or more types of nerve may be damaged.

Muscle weakness, cramps, and spasms are associated with motor nerve damage. In some cases, there may be loss of balance and coordination.

Sensory nerve damage can produce tingling, numbness, and pain. Pain associated with sensory nerve damage is variably described in the following manner:

- Sensation of wearing an invisible "glove" or "sock"
- Burning, freezing, or electric-like
- Extreme sensitivity to touch

If the autonomic nerves are damaged, involuntary functions may be affected. Orthostatic hypotension, bradycardia, reduced ability to perspire, constipation, bladder dysfunction, and sexual dysfunction may occur.

Because analgesics (e.g., aspirin, ibuprofen) are usually ineffective against pain caused by neuropathy, treatment often involves medications that target nerve cells. Anticonvulsants and antidepressants such as gabapentin (Neurontin) and amitriptyline (Elavil) are usually the first medications prescribed. Topical treatment with capsaicin cream (Zostrix) may be prescribed for focal neuropathy. The area surrounding the affected nerves may also be injected with lidocaine (Xylocaine) to temporarily reduce pain. Vitamin supplements may be used to treat nutritional neuropathy.

Physical therapy (e.g., exercise, massage, heat) and acupuncture may be used to reduce manifestations.

CUMULATIVE TRAUMA DISORDERS

Cumulative trauma disorders (CTDs) include a group of overuse syndromes that predominately affect the wrist and hand. They are also called *repetitive strain injuries* because some repetitive work activities seem to cause or exacerbate the manifestations. There are several forms (Table 73-1). The client often describes fatigue in the extremity, and aching and tiredness during the activity. Rest generally relieves the manifestations in the first clinical stage. As the disorder progresses, manifestations persist despite rest. Finally, chronic aching, fatigue in the extremity, and weakness develop despite rest. To minimize the incidence and effects of CTDs, health specialists in business and industry have modified work tasks, work stations, work environment, tools, and equipment.

CARPAL TUNNEL SYNDROME

Carpal tunnel syndrome (CTS) is an entrapment neuropathy that occurs when the median nerve is compressed as it passes through the wrist along a pathway to the hand. The tunnel, called the *carpal tunnel,* is bordered by the flexor retinaculum, which is a band of fibrous tissue that prevents the wrist tendons from bowing when the wrist is flexed. Compression causes sensory and motor changes in the thumb, the index and middle finger,

and the radial aspect of the ring finger. CTS also leads to atrophy of the radial half of the thenar eminence.

CTS may develop spontaneously without a known cause or may result from disease or injury. The most commonly reported cause of CTS is repetitive motion of the wrist, with the wrist in constant flexion. A higher incidence of CTS is reported among homemakers, factory workers, bricklayers, cashiers, musicians, secretaries, and computer operators. Pregnancy, hypothyroidism, gout, and rheumatoid arthritis are other conditions associated with CTS.

Initially, the client may be awakened at night by pain and paresthesia. Although these initial manifestations are temporary and relieved by shaking the hand, later stages may be accompanied by motor loss (e.g., progressive weakness, inability to perform fine motor activities, and burning or numbness in the thumb, index finger, or middle finger) and daytime pain.

Assessment of the client begins with a thorough history, including occupational tasks. Diagnostic assessment for CTS includes assessing for Tinel's and Phalen's signs (Figure 73-12, *A* and *B*). Tinel's sign is the development of tingling in the hands and fingers when the wrist is tapped. Phalen's test is assessing for the development of numbness and tingling following forceful flexion of the wrists for 20 to 30 seconds (see Figure 73-12, *B*). Finally, the wrist compression test is done. The wrist compression test is manual application of 30 seconds of pressure over the flexor retinaculum (see Figure 73-12, *C*). If paresthesias develop after compression, the result is positive. The wrist compression test has been demonstrated to be 87% accurate in diagnosing CTS. Electromyography may also be used in differential diagnosis to rule out other possible causes.

Management

Initially the wrist is splinted in a neutral position to prevent mechanical irritation of the nerve. Injection of steroids into the flexor tendons is done less frequently than in the past because of reported problems with scarring, median nerve damage, and infection. In addition to rest, pyridoxine hydrochloride (vitamin B_6) has been reported to be helpful. For some clients, pain can be relieved by gently squeezing the distal metacarpal heads together with the affected hand palm up; in some instances, stretch of digits III and IV is also required. This maneuver may also help in the clinical diagnosis of CTS.

Surgery is indicated with (1) severe manifestations of long duration, (2) muscle atrophy, or (3) progressive sensory loss in the fingers and hand. Carpal tunnel release can be performed by opening the wrist or through an endoscope. General or regional anesthesia can be used. During the surgery, the transverse carpal ligament is divided to relieve pressure.

After surgery, blood flow is assessed hourly by checking the color, capillary refill, and warmth of the finger-

TABLE 73-1 *Repetitive Motion Injuries*

Condition	Manifestations	People/Occupations at Risk	Usual Treatment
Neck			
Tension neck syndrome	Stiff, aching neck; headache	Typists, keypunch operators, cashiers, and others who must maintain a restricted posture	Prevention is key: (1) pause frequently when typing or keying to stretch about 30 sec every 30 min; (2) place screen directly in front of typist, avoid twisting; (3) place material to be typed at eye level if possible; avoid having materials to be typed consistently on one side of typist; conservative*
Cervical syndrome	Pain on flexion or extension of the neck with radiation down the arm	Common in people who assume awkward positions for a long time, such as painters, dentists	Conservative,* cervical collar, surgery
Shoulder			
Thoracic outlet syndrome	Numbness, pain, ischemia, and weakened pulse in upper extremity with hyperextension of the shoulder	Overhead assembly workers, automobile, repair mechanics, letter carriers	Conservative,* transcutaneous nerve stimulation, surgery
Supraspinatus tendinitis	Pain on elevating arm above 70 degrees at the shoulder	People who must maintain abduction with elbow extended-painters, construction workers	Conservative,* physical therapy, steroid injections
Bicipital tendinitis	Pain over the bicipital tendon in bicipital groove	Window washers, construction workers, shipping clerks	Conservative,* physical therapy, steroid injections
Elbow, Hand, and Wrist			
Lateral or medial epicondylitis (tennis elbow)	Local pain and pain on resisted hand motion	Repeated and forceful rotation of the forearm with the wrist bent; can be seen in bowlers, tennis players, and pitchers	Conservative,* steroid injections, surgery
de Quervain's tenosynovitis (inflammation of the extensor pollicis brevis tendons)	Gradual onset of pain, and sometimes swelling of the radial styloid; popping sensation on extension of the thumb	Middle-aged women and those subject to repetitive stress of the thumb	Conservative,* steroid injections, surgery
Carpal tunnel syndrome	Pain and paresthesias on percussion over the median nerve at the wrist (Tinel's sign) or with flexed wrists pressed together (positive Phalen's maneuver); night pain after 3-4 hr of sleep, morning stiffness, daytime numbness	Repetitive forced hand movements, keypunch operators, cashiers, typists, people with degenerative joint disease	Prevention is key: (1) while typing pause frequently at least 30 sec every 30 min; (2) adjust keyboard so the elbows are at 90-degree angle and wrists are straight; (3) do not rest wrists on a hard surface or restpad; wrists should "float" above keyboard; (4) use a light touch when striking the keys; conservative,* steroid injections, surgery
Ulnar nerve entrapment	Pain and paresthesias on percussion of the ulnar nerve over the epicondyle (Tinel's sign); local swelling and tissue hypertrophy around elbow	Rheumatoid arthritis clients, occupational stress on elbow	Conservative,* surgery

*Conservative treatment consists of restriction of the harmful motion, splinting (if appropriate and only for short periods of time or at night), application of ice or heat, mild analgesics, and nonsteroidal anti-inflammatory drugs, and gentle stretching exercises.

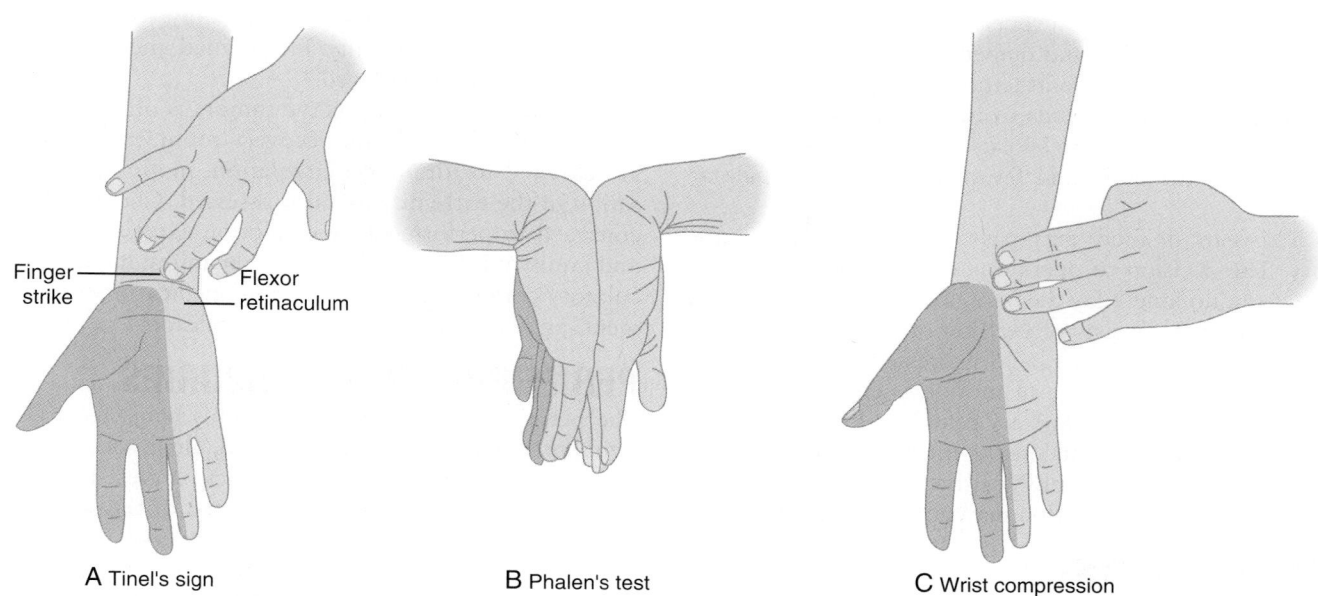

Finger strike
Flexor retinaculum

A Tinel's sign   B Phalen's test   C Wrist compression

FIGURE 73-12 Clinical examination for carpal tunnel syndrome includes tests for (**A**) Tinel's sign, (**B**) Phalen's sign, and (**C**) wrist compression. Each of these maneuvers elicits numbness and pain in the thumb, the index and middle fingers, and the radial aspect of the ring finger when carpal tunnel syndrome is present.

tips. When the anesthetic has worn off, assess the fingers for sensation.

Initially, postoperative care centers on wrist immobilization using bulky dressings and a wrist splint. The arm is elevated on pillows to reduce edema. Encourage the client to try to move the fingers, even though they are splinted. Heavy gripping and pinching should be avoided for up to 6 weeks. These actions need to be avoided to keep the tendons from pushing out against the healing transverse ligament. After 6 weeks, the client should be safe to resume gripping and pinching without irritating the wrist. The client often returns to the same type of work, so recovery of strength and flexibility are imperative. Work site analysis should also be completed to avoid reinjury.

The client and family are the care providers beyond the immediate postoperative period. Because this surgery is usually performed on an outpatient basis, provide detailed instructions on home care. See the Client Education Guide feature on Home Care After Carpal Tunnel Release on the website.

CUBITAL TUNNEL SYNDROME

Cubital tunnel syndrome results from a combination of local pressure and stretching of the ulnar nerve at the elbow as it passes behind the medial epicondyle. The problem may arise following local trauma, but most often is spontaneous, with elbow position during sleep being the largest contributing factor. Problems include pain, numbness, altered sensation, and weakness, and may be permanent if nerve damage has occurred. Electrical nerve testing may be helpful in assessing nerve damage, but may be

normal even in clients with symptomatic nerve compression. Nerve irritation at the neck may produce similar manifestations and may coexist with this problem. Most mild cases can be treated with a splint or elbow pad and avoidance of flexion and direct pressure on the nerve. More advanced cases require surgery to decompress and transpose the nerve out of the cubital tunnel.

TARSAL TUNNEL SYNDROME

Tarsal tunnel syndrome is the counterpart of the CTS in the lower extremity. In this syndrome, the posterior tibial nerve is trapped beneath the flexor retinaculum and deep fascia along the foot's medial border. Entrapment compresses the nerve, causing pain, burning, and tingling on the sole of the foot; it usually worsens as the day progresses. This pain can usually be reduced by rest, elevation, or massage.

Conservative treatment, such as arch supports and wider shoes, may successfully relieve the discomfort of tarsal tunnel syndrome. If inflammation of the nerve is causing the compression, NSAIDs may be prescribed. Steroid injections may also be effective. If the problem is caused by flat feet, custom orthotics can help restore the foot's natural arch.

Surgery to release the laciniate ligament may be required to provide room for expansion of the nerve. If a cyst is impinging on the nerve, it can be removed.

DUPUYTREN'S CONTRACTURE

Dupuytren's contracture is permanent flexor contracture of the fourth and fifth fingers. Dupuytren's contracture is inherited as an autosomal dominant trait and is common in people of Northern European descent. It is also more common in alcoholic and diabetic clients.

In severe forms of contracture, a longitudinal fibrous cord forms, which extends from the fingers to the palm and pulls the fingers into a locked position. Milder forms have less contracture and fewer nodules in the palmar fascia.

Ten years or more may pass before surgery is necessary. The decision to operate is usually made when the client can no longer lay the hand outstretched on a table. The operation consists of excision of part of the palmar fascia. After surgery, the hand is dressed in a large compression dressing. Range of motion is encouraged. Frequent assessments of capillary refill and finger color are needed. Splints are often used at night to promote extension. Many months of physical therapy may be needed, and even then, full function may not be achievable.

GANGLION CYST

A ganglion can be described simply as a fluid-filled sac arising from an adjacent joint capsule or tendon sheath. A ganglion can form from almost any joint or tendon sheath in the wrist and hand. Trauma or degenerative changes in the fibrous joint capsule are thought to contribute to development of ganglia.

Ganglions may limit motion in the adjacent joints, or produce discomfort from compression or distention of local soft tissues. Particularly large ganglions can be cosmetically unpleasant. Ganglion cysts of the distal interphalangeal (DIP) joint may produce deformities of the fingernail. Ganglion cysts arising from the flexor tendon sheath at the base of the finger may produce pain when grasping. On rare occasions, ganglion cysts (particularly those associated with the wrist) may cause changes in the bone. Ganglion cysts can frequently be diagnosed simply by their location and shape. They are usually not adherent to the overlying skin and are firmly attached to the underlying joint or tendon sheath. Large ganglions may permit the passage of light through their substance (transillumination). X-ray studies are sometimes helpful in diagnosing ganglion cysts, particularly about the DIP joint where associated degenerative arthritis is often found.

To relieve pain or numbness, the ganglion may be aspirated or surgically excised. The area may then be injected with a corticosteroid before a pressure dressing and splint are applied. NSAIDs are commonly used for pain. Wrist ganglions may recur in up to 30% of clients.

PERIPHERAL NERVE TUMORS

Although solitary tumors (generally neurofibromas) may develop on any peripheral nerve, multiple tumors most often occur and are part of a syndrome known as *neurofibromatosis* (von Recklinghausen's disease). This hereditary disorder is characterized by multiple tumors of the spinal and cranial nerves along with involvement of many other systems. The disease is usually not life-threatening, and lesions are excised only when they interfere with normal activity. Intracranial and intraspinal tumors are usually removed.

Surgery for peripheral nerve tumors is often done on an outpatient basis. In the recovery room, the dressings are checked for drainage; circulation, motion, and sensation in the extremity are also assessed. Clients are encouraged to perform range-of-motion exercises. Clients and family members are taught the manifestations of circulatory compromise and infection, medication management, and care of the dressing and incision.

PERIPHERAL NERVE INJURIES

The peripheral nerves most commonly subjected to external pressure are the median, radial, ulnar, sciatic, common peroneal, tibial, and long thoracic nerves. The common peroneal nerve (a terminal branch of the sciatic) is injured more frequently than any other nerve. Because of its course and distribution, the sciatic nerve is exposed to internal and external trauma and inflammation more than any other nerve. The median nerve is most often injured by constriction from fascial bands. The axillary nerve may be injured as the result of an allergic reaction to serum injections or secondary to improper crutch walking. The sciatic nerve may be injured directly during medication injections. Any peripheral nerve can be injured by bone fractures or perforating wounds. Nerves can be injured in common household accidents (cut on glass) or in severe motor vehicle accidents.

Assessment includes a full examination of the injured area. Assessment findings with nerve damage depend on the type of nerve injured and the extent of damage. Damaged motor nerves cause clinical manifestations such as flaccid paralysis, muscle wasting, and reflex loss in the muscle innervated by the injured nerve. Damaged mixed nerves or sensory nerves cause vasomotor and trophic disturbances following either partial or complete interruption of the nerve. Following partial injury or incomplete division of a nerve, the person may experience stabbing pains, paresthesias (pins-and-needles sensation) and, occasionally, the burning pains of causalgia. Damaged sensory nerves cause loss of sensation in the nerves' area of anatomic distribution. If the hand is injured, the client's occupation and documentation of the dominant hand is included in the assessment.

Conservative management may include splinting, ice, elevation of the limb, administration of anti-inflammatory and analgesic agents, or a combination of these. If a peripheral nerve is traumatically severed, the ends should be surgically anastomosed to enable healing. The nearer the site of injury occurs to the CNS, the less chance of regeneration. When nerves are only slightly damaged, mild edema occurs at the injury site. This may cause temporary manifestations that recede in a few days or possibly weeks.

Postoperative care of clients having nerve repair or grafting includes elevation of the extremity. Elevation is critical to reduce edema and improve venous return. The procedure is usually performed with local anesthesia, so assessment of neurovascular status is not conclusive until the anesthesia has worn off. Color, warmth, movement, sensation, capillary refill, and strength are assessed. Some of these assessments can be hampered by dressings, but as many as possible should be performed. Monitor the fingertips for blood flow with Doppler laser or standard Doppler ultrasonography and temperature probes. The temperature of the hand is usually less than the core temperature and the surgeon indicates acceptable ranges of temperature. Physical therapy begins within a few days to promote movement after severe injuries.

If the injury is severe, the client may have recurring dreams about the accident and his or her injury. These dreams are generally normal, but if they are bothersome to the client, a psychiatric consultant may be helpful.

CONCLUSIONS

The physical and psychological impairments vary with the degree of damage as well as the client's response and ability to cope with the body changes. The coping response is not always related to the degree of physiologic damage. A client can have facial paralysis or trigeminal neuralgia and be more compromised psychologically than a client with spinal cord injury who has strong coping skills. It is imperative that nurses comprehend the severity of the client's dysfunction as it relates to quality of life, as well as the impact it has on family dynamics.

THINKING CRITICALLY *evolve*

1. The client, a 34-year-old woman, had a lumbar laminectomy done earlier today. An earlier assessment showed that movement and sensation of both lower extremities were intact. During the current postoperative assessment, she states that her right toes feel numb, and the dorsiflexion and plantar flexion of the right foot are a little weaker than earlier. She has requested an analgesic because she is starting to get a headache. What are the priorities for her care? What assessments and interventions might be used?

Factors to Consider. What assessment methods can be used to determine the extent of vascular insufficiency? What type of neurologic checks should be done?

A discussion for this question can be found on the website and the CD-ROM.

BIBLIOGRAPHY

1. Aflatoon, K., & Carboone, J. (2002). Cauda equina syndrome with acute lumbar burst fracture. *Topics in Spinal Cord Injury and Rehabilitation*, 8(2), 1-8.
2. Agency for Health Care Policy and Research (AHCPR). (1994). *Acute low back problems in adults: Assessment and treatment.* No. 95-0642. Rockville, MD: U.S. Department of Health and Human Services, Public Health Service, Agency for Health Care Policy and Research.
3. Becker, F.C. (2001). Acute low back pain: Diagnostics and treatment. *Clinical Excellence for Nurse Practitioners* 5(2), 80-84.
4. Chem, T.Y. (2000). The clinical presentation of uppermost cervical disc protrusion. *Spine* 25(4), 439-442.
5. Currie, H. (2001). A critical analysis of the evidence for chiropractic management of low back pain. *Journal of Orthopaedic Nursing* 21(91), 139-144.
6. Freidman, R.A. (2000). The surgical management of Bell's palsy: A review. *American Journal of Otolaryngology* 21(1) 139-144.
7. Galloway, G. (2003). An update on carpal tunnel syndrome. *Patient Care for the Nurse Practitioner*, Feb 9.
8. Hall, F. (2003). Use of exercise in the management of nonmalignant chronic pain. *Professional Nurse* 18(7), 412-414.
9. Kling, C., et al. (2000). The health-related quality of life of patients suffering from the late effects of polio (post-polio). *Journal of Advanced Nursing* 32(1), 164-173.
10. Kuklo, T.R., & Lenke, L.G. (2000). Thorascopic spine surgery: Current indications and techniques. *Orthopaedic Nursing* 19(6), 15-22.
11. Massy-Westropp, N., Grimmer, K., Bain, G. (2000). A systematic review of the clinical diagnostic tests for carpal tunnel syndrome. *Journal of Hand Surgery* 25(1), 120-127.
12. North American Spine Society. (2000). Herniated disc. La Grange, IL: North American Spine Society (NASS). National Clearinghouse Available: http://www.guideline.gov.
13. North American Spine Society. (2000). Spondylolysis, lytic spondylolisthesis and degenerative spondylolisthesis. La Grange, IL: North American Spine Society (NASS). National Clearinghouse Available: http://www.guideline.gov.
14. Pinnock, D. (2002). Pain management. Effective services for the care of patients with back pain. *Professional Nurse* 17(7), 422-444.
15. Schoen, D.C. (2002). Upper extremity nerve entrapments. *Orthopaedic Nursing* 21(2), 15-33.
16. Washington State Department of Labor and Industries. (2001). Guidelines for lumbar fusion (arthrodesis). Olympia, WA: Washington State Department of Labor and Industries National Clearinghouse Available: http://www.guideline.gov.
17. Yuras, S. (2000). Syringomyelia: An expanding problem. *Journal of the American Academy of Nurse Practitioners* 35(91), 61-85.
18. Zigler, J.E, et al. (2003). Lumbar spine arthroplasty. *Journal of Spinal Disorders*, 16(4), 352-361.

evolve Did you remember to check out the bonus material on the Evolve website and the CD-ROM, including free self-assessment exercises?
http://evolve.elsevier.com/Black/medsurg/

Chapter 74

Management of Clients with Degenerative Neurologic Disorders

Joyce M. Black

Degenerative neurologic disorders pose a great challenge to the client, the family, and the caregiver, whether it is a nurse, a family member, or a significant other. By their very nature, these disorders cause progressive decline in neurologic function (see the Critical Monitoring feature on Manifestations of Changes in Neurologic Status on p. 2059). Some progress relatively quickly (over months to 1 or 2 years), whereas others progress more gradually, sometimes over decades. Common nursing diagnoses for clients with these disorders are *Altered Thought Processes, Memory Deficit, Visual-Perceptual Alteration, Impaired Physical Mobility, Incontinence, Self-Care Deficit,* and *Impaired Individual and Family Coping.* A major goal of intervention is to help the client achieve an optimal level of functioning in light of chronic neurologic deficits. The family should also be taught what to expect, such as the usual areas of decline, how to provide care and support to the client, and how to manage stress and cope with the progressive nature of the disorder.

The diagnosis of degenerative neurologic disease is most often made in an outpatient setting; however, hospital admission may be necessary when acute relapses or life-threatening events occur. Many clients return to their homes and have regular follow-up in outpatient clinics; however, some may require rehabilitation, in either inpatient or outpatient settings, for newly acquired deficits. Other clients may require transfer to long-term care facilities because of a significant decline in their ability to provide self-care. Still other clients may not survive their acute illness.

ALZHEIMER'S DISEASE AND RELATED DEMENTIAS

The term *dementia* refers to the loss of memory, reasoning, judgment, and language to such an extent that it interferes with everyday life. The changes may occur gradually or quickly, and how they come about is key to determining whether the condition causing dementia is temporary.

Cognition is the act or process of thinking, perceiving, and learning. Cognitive activities that become impaired in dementia include decision-making, judgment, memory

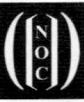

Nursing Outcomes Classification (NOC)
for Nursing Diagnoses—Clients with Degenerative Neurologic Disorders

Activity Intolerance
  Activity Tolerance
  Energy Conservation
  Self-Care: Activities of Daily Living
    (ADLs)
Caregiver Role Strain
  Caregiver Emotional Health
  Caregiver Performance: Direct Care
  Caregiver Performance: Indirect Care
  Caregiver Physical Health
  Caregiver Stressors
  Caregiver Well-Being
  Depression Control
  Knowledge: Health Resources
Chronic Low Self-Esteem and Situational Low Self-Esteem
  Self-Esteem
  Body Image
  Social Support

Constipation
  Bowel Elimination
  Hydration
Deficient Knowledge
  Knowledge: Disease Process
  Knowledge: Health Resources
  Knowledge: Medication
Disturbed Thought Processes
  Cognitive Ability
  Cognitive Orientation
  Information Processing
  Memory
Impaired Physical Mobility
  Body Positioning: Self-Initiated
  Joint Movement: Active
  Mobility Level
Impaired Urinary Elimination
  Urinary Continence
  Urinary Elimination
Impaired Verbal Communication
  Communication Ability

Communication: Expressive Ability
Communication: Receptive Ability
Cognitive Orientation
Distorted Thought Control
Risk for Injury
  Neurological Status
  Risk Detection
  Safety Behavior: Fall Prevention
  Safety Behavior: Home Physical
    Environment
  Safety Status: Falls Occurrence
Risk for Self-Care Deficit
  Self-Care: Activities of Daily Living
  Mobility Level
Self-Care Deficit
  Self-Care: Activities of Daily Living
Urge Urinary Incontinence
  Tissue Integrity: Skin and Mucous
    Membranes
  Urinary Continence
  Urinary Elimination

---

spatial orientation, thinking, reasoning, and verbal communication. A client with dementia may undergo behavioral and personality changes as well, depending on the area(s) of the brain affected.

Types of Dementia

Alzheimer's disease (AD) is the most common form of dementia among people 65 years of age and older. Dementia is intellectual deterioration severe enough to interfere with occupational or social performance. It involves progressive decline in two or more areas of cognition, usually memory and language, calculation, visuospatial perception, constructional praxis, judgment, abstraction, or personality. AD constitutes at least half of all dementias.

Multi-infarct (multiple stroke) disease is the second most common cause of irreversible dementia. Blood clots block small blood vessels in the brain and destroy brain tissue. Typically multiple infarct dementia occurs in men over 50 years old. The effect of multiple infarcts (strokes) over time leads to the progressive decline in cognition.

Lewy body dementia is similar to Alzheimer's disease but may progress more rapidly. Abnormal brain cells called cortical Lewy bodies occur throughout the brain and produce manifestations. Lewy bodies are also associated with Parkinson's and Alzheimer's diseases, but it is not clear whether dementia with Lewy bodies is a distinct clinical entity or perhaps a variant of Alzheimer's or Parkinson's disease.

Pick's disease also is a form of dementia but differs from AD in several ways. First, the two diseases produce different abnormalities in the cells of the brain. Pick's dis-

BOX 74-1 *Causes of Dementia*

- Alzheimer's disease
- Multi-infarct dementia (arteriosclerotic dementia)
- Parkinson's disease
- Lewy body disease
- Alcoholic dementia
- Binswanger's disease
- Creutzfeldt-Jakob disease
- Huntington's chorea
- AIDS-related dementia
- Normal pressure hydrocephalus
- Genetic or metabolic disease (e.g., thyroid)
- Toxic or traumatic injury
- Malignant disease; primary, metastatic, or iatrogenic from the treatment

ease is marked by "Pick bodies," rounded, microscopic structures found within affected cells. Neurons swell, taking on a "ballooned" appearance. Neither of these changes appears in Alzheimer's disease, and the pathology of Alzheimer's disease (plaques and tangles) is not found in Pick's disease. Second, Pick's disease is usually sharply confined to the front parts of the brain, particularly the frontal and anterior temporal lobes. This contrasts with Alzheimer's disease, which is more widely distributed.

There are many causes of dementia. Because the brain is quickly injured from hypoxia, reduced blood flow or drugs, the causes are numerous (Box 74-1).

GENETICS LINKS

Examples of Neurodegenerative Genetic Disorders

Disorder	Features	Inheritance	Gene defect	Genetic Testing Available?
Huntington's disease (HD)	Progressive disorder of motor, cognitive, and psychiatric disturbance; onset 35-44 yr; median survival 15-18 yr after onset	AD	HD	Yes
Early-onset familial Alzheimer's disease (EOFAD)	Early onset of progressive impairment of memory, judgment, decision making, and language; mean onset under age 65 yr; comprise <2% of all AD cases	AD	PSEN1 APP PSEN2	Yes No Yes
Late-onset Alzheimer's (AD2)	Multiple affected family members, with onset of dementia after age 60-65 yr; estimated to account for ~25% of Alzheimer's disease	Complex trait; one or more susceptibility genes	APOE	Yes*
Parkinson's disease (familial PD)	Progressive disorder characterized by resting tremor, akinesia, and rigidity; rare occurrence	AD	PARK1 PARK2 PARK3 PARK4 UCH-L1 PARK6 PARK7 PARK8	Yes No No No No No No No
Spinocerebellar ataxias, 21 types	Poor coordination of movement and a wide-based uncoordinated, unsteady gait; poor coordination of limbs and speech often present; onset, frequency, and features vary and overlap	AD AR XL	SCA1 SCA2 SCA3 SCA6 SCA7 SCA8 SCA10 SCA12 SCA17	Yes Yes Yes Yes Yes Yes Yes Yes Yes
Friedreich's ataxia	Slowly progressive ataxia; onset <age 25 yr; depressed tendon reflexes	AR	FRDA	Yes
Early onset primary dystonia (DYT1)	Onset <age 21 yr; involuntary sustained muscle contractions that cause posturing of limbs	AD	DYT1	Yes

AR, Autosomal recessive; *AD*, autosomal dominant; *XL*, X-linked.
*Presymptomatic testing is not routinely performed.

Alzheimer's disease affects about four million Americans. Slightly more than half of these people receive care at home, and the remainder receive institutional nursing care. The prevalence of AD doubles every 5 years after the age of 65. In fact, some estimates indicate that nearly half of all people over age 85 years have AD.

Etiology and Risk Factors

The cause of AD has not been found, although several risk factors have been identified. Increasing age is a risk factor. Genetic factors are also linked to AD. At least five chromosomes (1, 12, 14, 19, 21) are involved in some forms of familial AD. Four genetic loci have also been identified as contributing to AD, including the amyloid precursor gene, the presenilin 1 gene, the presenilin 2 gene, and the apolipoprotein E gene. Research has also shown that the age of AD development is also genetic. See the Genetic Links feature on Examples of Neurodegenerative Genetic Disorders, above.

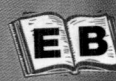

COMPLEMENTARY AND ALTERNATIVE THERAPY

Omega-3 Fatty Acids from Fish and a Lower Risk of Alzheimer's Disease

A prospective study conducted from 1993 to 2000 followed 815 individuals (aged 65 to 94 years) in a community in the United States for an average of 3.9 years. These individuals completed a dietary questionnaire on average 2.3 years before clinical evaluation. A total of 131 individuals developed Alzheimer's disease in this study. Individuals who consumed fish once per week or more had 60% less risk of developing Alzheimer's disease compared with those who rarely or never ate fish.

Reference

Morris, M., et al. (2003). Consumption of fish and Omega-3 fatty acids and risk of incident Alzheimer Disease. *Archives of Neurology, 60,* 940-946.

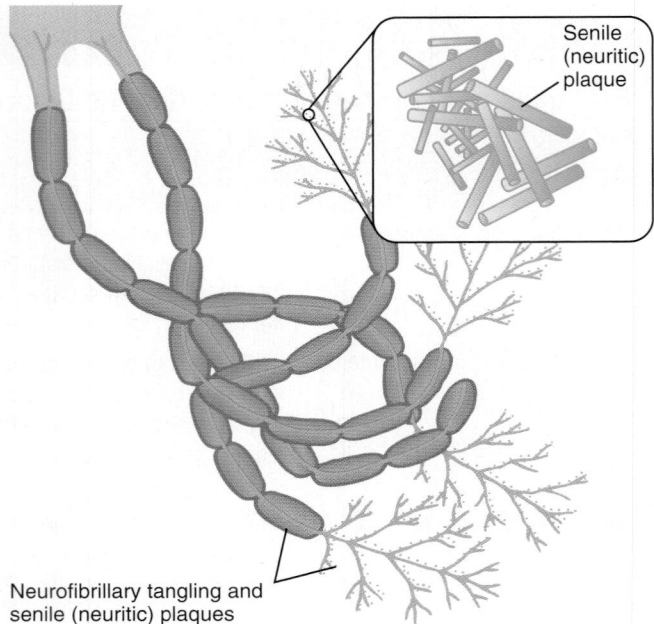

Neurofibrillary tangling and senile (neuritic) plaques

FIGURE 74-1 Neurofibrillary tangles. In clients with Alzheimer's disease and some other neurologic disorders, these tangles replace the normal neuronal cytoplasm. The tangles are often seen with senile plaques and appear throughout the cortex, hippocampus, and amygdala. The number of plaques and tangles correlates roughly with the severity of the dementia.

Clinical situations associated with AD development include elevated homocysteine, a risk factor for heart disease, inflammation, stroke, and oxidative damage from free radicals (see the Complementary and Alternative Therapy feature on Omega-3 Fatty Acids from Fish and a Lower Risk for Alzheimer's Disease, above). Research is active in these areas to find the pathophysiologic connections and prevent them.

Pathophysiology

Alzheimer's disease disrupts the three processes that keep neurons healthy: communication, metabolism, and repair. Alois Alzheimer first described presenile dementia in 1907. He used a new staining technique of human brain tissue to demonstrate the pathologic changes. The changes he noted are now termed *beta-amyloid plaques* and *neurofibrillary tangles* (Figure 74-1). *Plaque* is a cluster of beta-amyloid, a protein fragment snipped from a larger protein, called *amyloid precursor protein.* Plaques have been described as dense, mostly insoluble deposits of protein and cellular material outside and around the neuron. Plaques develop in the hippocampus, an area of the brain that helps encode memories. Degenerating nerve terminals, both dendritic and axonal, contain amyloid protein. Healthy neurons have an internal support structure, called *microtubules.* These tubules serve as tracts to guide nutrients to the end of the axon and back. The tubule is stable due to a protein called tau. In AD, the tau is changed chemically and becomes tangled. Once tangled, the tubules degenerate and so do the cells they support. The destruction leads to memory failure, personality changes, and problems carrying out activities of daily living (ADL).

Acetylcholine (ACh) is also decreased in clients with AD. This neurotransmitter is commonly used in the hippocampus and the cerebral cortex.

Gross brain changes evident in clients with AD include thickening of the leptomeninges, shrunken gyri, widened sulci, enlarged ventricles, hippocampal shrinkage, and generalized atrophy (Figure 74-2). In addition to structural changes, neurotransmitter changes are evident in the brain of clients with AD. A decline in cholinergic neurons in the basal nucleus leads to loss of choline acetyltransferase in the neocortex and hippocampus.

Clinical Manifestations

Clinically, AD is characterized by a relentless impairment of decision-making that generally begins insidiously and can progress for a decade or so. Manifestations can vary depending on the portion of the brain involved and on genetic predisposition. The onset of AD typically occurs in late middle age (age 65 years and older), although some familial cases occur in a person's 40s and 50s.

Preclinical Alzheimer's Disease

Alzheimer's disease begins near the hippocampus, a structure essential to the formation of both short- and

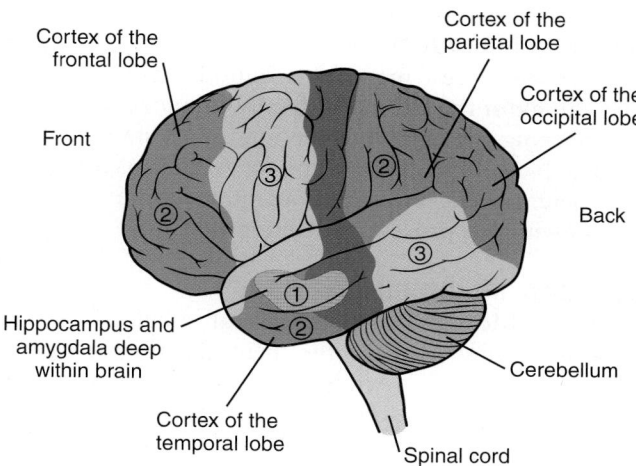

FIGURE 74-2 Alzheimer's disease affects many portions of the brain, especially those required for memory and thought.

long-term memories. Affected regions begin to shrink and in time (10 to 20 years perhaps) lead to memory loss.

Mild Alzheimer's Disease

As the cerebral cortex begins to shrink, other cognitive losses become apparent. *Memory disturbance* is usually noticed by family members or co-workers before the client does. The client may demonstrate poor judgment and problem-solving skills and become careless in work habits and household chores. Clients may become confused about where they are and they begin to get lost easily. Routine activities such as bill paying and other daily tasks take longer. The client may do well in familiar surroundings and may be able to follow well-established routines but lacks the ability to adapt to new challenges. The person may become irritable, suspicious, or indifferent. Agitation, apathy, dysphoria, and aberrant motor behavior are associated with cognitive impairments.

Moderate Alzheimer's Disease

The client may demonstrate *language disturbance*, characterized by impaired word-finding and *circumlocution* (talking around a subject rather than about it directly). Later, spontaneous speech becomes increasingly empty, and *paraphasias* (words used in the wrong context) are used. Clients may repeat words and phrases just spoken by themselves *(palilalia)* or by others *(echolalia)*. Motor disturbance *(apraxia)* is characterized by difficulty in using everyday objects such as a toothbrush, comb, razor, and utensils. Apraxia combined with forgetfulness can create serious safety problems. The person may leave a stove burner on in the kitchen or forget to extinguish a cigarette. Indifference worsens, and restlessness with frequent pacing appears. *Hyperorality* (the desire to take everything into the mouth to suck, chew, or taste) may develop. Swallowing may become difficult.

Depression and irritability may worsen, and delusions and psychosis may appear. The person fears personal harm, theft of property, or infidelity of the spouse. Clients may see bugs crawling on the bed or throughout the house. Wandering at night is common. Occasional incontinence may occur.

Severe Alzheimer's Disease

In the final stage, plaques and tangles are widespread throughout the brain. Clients cannot recognize family or friends and do not communicate in any way. Voluntary movement is minimal, and the limbs become rigid with flexor posturing. Urinary and fecal incontinence is frequent. Aspiration and aspiration pneumonia are frequent.

Diagnostic Findings

Because there is no definitive test for AD, the diagnosis is made by exclusion of known causes of dementia (e.g., toxic or metabolic alterations, drug side effects, cerebrovascular disease, neoplasm, infection). The diagnosis is confirmed with (1) the presence of dementia involving two or more areas of cognition, (2) insidious onset and steady progression, and (3) loss of normal alertness.

Computed tomography (CT) scan can be used to identify ventricular dilation and sulcal enlargement and cerebral atrophy of the portions of the brain most affected. Magnetic resonance imaging (MRI), single-positron emission computed tomography (SPECT), and positron emission tomography (PET) are also used to detect changes in brain function.

Finally, laboratory studies are performed to rule out metabolic and drug-related causes of dementia. These studies include urinalysis, complete blood count (CBC), erythrocyte sedimentation rate (ESR), electrolytes, blood urea nitrogen (BUN) and creatinine values, thyroid and liver function tests, calcium, serum B_{12} levels, syphilis serology, and human immunodeficiency virus (HIV) testing.

Manifestations of Other Dementias

Manifestations of multi-infarct dementia (MID) often develop in a stepwise manner and include confusion, problems with recent memory, wandering or getting lost in familiar places, incontinence, emotional lability such as laughing or crying inappropriately, difficulty following instructions, and problems handling money. Usually the damage is so slight that the change is noticeable only as a series of small steps. Over time, however, as more small vessels are blocked, gradual mental decline occurs. MID, which typically begins between the ages of 60 and 75, affects men more often than women.

Manifestations of Lewy body dementia can range from traditional parkinsonian effects, such as loss of spontaneous movement *(bradykinesia)*, rigidity (muscles feel stiff and resist movement), tremor, and shuffling gait, to effects similar to those of AD, such as acute confusion, loss of memory, and loss of or fluctuating cognition. Visual hallucinations may be one of the first manifestations noted, and clients may suffer from other psychiatric disturbances such as delusions and depression.

COMPLEMENTARY AND ALTERNATIVE THERAPY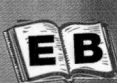

Vitamin E Supplements for Clients with Alzheimer's Disease

The only agent that has been shown to slow the progression of Alzheimer's disease in a prospective study (in clients diagnosed with this condition) is vitamin E supplements. A multi-institutional, double-blind, placebo-controlled prospective study included 341 moderately impaired clients (Clinical Dementia Rating score of 2). Clients were randomly assigned to receive 2000 international units of vitamin E, 10 mg of selegiline, vitamin E and selegiline, or placebo for 2 years. The primary end-point was the time to progression to any of the following endpoints: institutionalization, loss of any two of three basic activities of daily living (eating, dressing, and toileting), a rating of 3 on the Clinical Dementia Rating Scale, or death. Using an intention-to-treat analysis and after adjusting for differences among the groups in the baseline Mini-Mental State Examination score, the researchers observed a significant delay in the primary outcome among the treatment groups. There was an increase in median survival of 230 days for clients taking vitamin E alone, 215 days for clients taking selegiline, and 145 days for clients taking vitamin E and selegiline compared with clients on placebo.[2] The interpretation of this trial was somewhat controversial because of the need to include the baseline Mini-Mental State Examination score as a covariant in order to reveal a statistically significant difference between the treatment and placebo groups. Regardless, the American Academy of Neurology now recommends 2000 international units of vitamin E daily (1000 international units twice daily) as a standard care for the treatment of clients with Alzheimer's disease.[1]

References
1. Doody, R., et al. (2001). Practice parameter: management of dementia (an evidence-based review). Report of the Quality Standards Subcommittee of the American Academy of Neurology. *Neurology, 56,* 1154-1166.
2. Sano, M., et al. (1997). A controlled trial of selegiline, alpha-tocopherol, or both as treatment for Alzheimer's disease. The Alzheimer's Disease Cooperative Study. *New England Journal of Medicine, 336,* 1216-1222.

Outcome Management

A diagnosis is best made by a multidisciplinary group that can assist the client and family to understand what is happening and what interventions or assistance will be needed. No cure has been found for AD. Management of the client centers on helping maintain mental function and slowing the process of deterioration.

■ Medical Management

Maintain Mental Function. Several medications are used to retain ACh in the neurojunctions. Tacrine (Cognex), donepezil (Aricept), galanthamine (Reminyl), and rivastigmine (Exelon) are approved by the U.S. Food and Drug Administration (FDA) for use in AD. These drugs can have small but noticeable effects, depending on the stage of disease, differences in the way the drugs act in different clients, and other factors. At least tem-

COMPLEMENTARY AND ALTERNATIVE THERAPY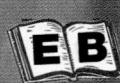

Ginkgo Biloba in Healthy Individuals for Memory Enhancement

Extracts or compounds from ginkgo have shown some initial promise in enhancing memory in demented older individuals.[1] However, researchers wanted to test the potential claims of some manufacturers that ginkgo could, in general, enhance mental focus and improve memory and concentration. Community-dwelling, functionally independent individuals older than 60 years volunteered for this study of memory.[2] Participants were excluded if they scored less than 27 out of a possible 30 points on the Mini-Mental Status Examination at baseline. Highly educated or intelligent participants with mild dementia may have been included in this study. Participants in this randomized controlled trial received 40 mg of ginkgo biloba three times daily (dose recommended by many manufacturers) or placebo for 6 weeks. This duration was 2 weeks longer than the manufacturer's suggested onset of action. A total of 230 participants were included. No statistically significant differences were observed between ginkgo and placebo on any of the scales measured. No significant changes from baseline to post-treatment and no adverse effects were noted of the groups. In other words, ginkgo, in standard doses for 6 weeks, was ineffective in improving memory, intelligence, and concentration in older clients without dementia.

References
1. Le Bars, P., et al. (2002). Influence of the severity of cognitive impairment on the effect of the ginkgo biloba extract Egb 761 in Alzheimer's disease. *Neuropsychobiology,45,* 19-26.
2. Solomon, P., et al. (2002). Ginkgo for memory enhancement: A randomized controlled trial. *Journal of the American Medical Association, 288,* 835-840.

porarily, many clients taking these drugs experience improvements in their thinking abilities and are less likely to demonstrate common manifestations of advanced AD, such as wandering, agitation, and socially inappropriate behaviors. None of these drugs prevents AD from worsening over time.

In an effort to combat the effect of oxygen free radicals, alpha-tocopherol (vitamin E) and selegiline have been studied. Both agents have been reported to delay the development of the later stages of AD and show some improvement in levels of independent and behavioral manifestations (see the Complementary and Alternative Therapy features on Vitamin E Supplements for Clients with Alzheimer's Disease and on Ginkgo Biloba in Healthy Individuals for Memory Enhancement on p. 2166). An extract of ginkgo biloba may improve cognitive function for 6 to 12 months.[10] Propentofylline has been effective in the management of AD. See the Complementary and Alternative Therapy feature on Use It or Lose It: Reducing the Risk of Dementia on the website.

Over the short term, other medicines can somewhat relieve anxiety, agitation, depression, and psychotic or inappropriate behavior. Anxiolytics for anxiety and agitation, neuroleptics for unusual or troublesome behavior, and antidepressants or mood stabilizers for mood disorders and specific problems like spells of anger or rage. No specific drugs or dosages address the wide range of problems that clients with AD experience. Medications like risperidone (Risperdal), olanzapine (Zyprexa), quetiapine (Seroquel), sertraline (Zoloft), or citalopram (Celexa) should be used as seldom as possible and at the lowest effective doses. This will help minimize side effects in frail older clients. The use of these medications to "control behavior problems" is avoided; rather, the behavior should be considered an attempt to communicate a specific need.

■ Nursing Management of the Medical Client
Assessment

When AD is suspected, a complete history should be taken to assess for other causes of dementia. Data should be obtained from the client, family, and co-workers (if possible). Secondary sources are used because the client is often unaware of a problem with thought processing and minimizes it. Ask specific questions about difficulties with ADL, increasing forgetfulness, and changes in personality. Assess past medical history for previous head injury or surgery, recent falls, headache, and a family history of AD. A Mini-Mental State examination may provide objective data for ongoing evaluation of the client (see Chapter 69). AD has a profound impact on psychosocial behaviors. Ask about the client's reactions to changes in routine or in the environment. It is not uncommon for a client with AD to become very agitated

over small changes, and apathy, social isolation, and irritability may be noted. As the brain continues to atrophy and the limbic system becomes dysfunctional, the client may become paranoid, use abusive language, and become suspicious of others.

Alzheimer's disease has a profound impact on the family. Assess the family for strengths and weaknesses, their ability to provide care for the client, and their financial concerns. In large centers, assessment of the client and family is performed through a team approach. The Client Education Guide feature on Caring for Family Members with Alzheimer's Disease on the website provides instructions and resources for caregivers of people with AD.

Diagnosis, Outcomes, Interventions

Diagnosis: Impaired Verbal Communication. Use the nursing diagnosis *Impaired Verbal Communication related to neuronal degeneration* to describe the client with AD.

Outcomes. The client's needs will be communicated effectively as evidenced by making his or her needs known and interacting meaningfully with others. This outcome is often possible only in the early stages. In later stages, a more appropriate outcome might be expressed as the client's needs are interpreted appropriately.

Interventions. In the initial stage of AD, the client's receptive and expressive language skills are relatively intact. The nurse must be prepared to adapt to the communication level of the client. If the client speaks only single words or short phrases, the nurse should do likewise. It is best to speak slowly and simply, with a firm volume and low pitch. The tone of voice should always be calm and reassuring and project control of the situation. When language becomes impaired in the second stage of the illness, be prepared to apply new techniques for communicating with the client.

Nonverbal behavior can provide clues about specific needs. Clients with AD often avert their eyes, look down, back away, and increase hand gesturing when they do not understand. If they are frustrated, angry, or hostile, they may increase motor activity by pacing, rattling doorknobs, waving their arms or shaking their fists, frowning, raising their voice volume and pitch, or tightening their facial muscles. These behaviors should signal staff to increase their alertness, search for the cause of the distress, and prepare to intervene.

Interventions can include the following:
- Decreasing environmental stimuli
- Approaching the client calmly and with assurance
- Taking care not to place any demands on the client
- Gently distracting the client
- Making sure that all verbal and nonverbal communication cues are concordant

- Using multiple sensory modalities (visual, auditory, and tactile) to send the message but do not use all forms at the same time

The client's memory loss can be an advantage in distracting him or her from the stressful situation. If removed from the situation and provided with a calm, non-threatening environment, clients may forget why they are upset. Elicit listening behavior by reaching out and touching, holding a hand, putting an arm around the waist, or in some way maintaining physical contact with the client. Dementia sufferers can perceive nonverbal behavior of others and can become agitated or upset if they sense negative nonverbal behavior from them. Having activities or interest, exercise periods, and opportunities to wander in a safe environment can do much to reduce anxiety and stress.

The identification of pain or discomfort in clients with advanced AD is also difficult. Behavioral indicators of discomfort include noisy breathing, negative vocalization (constant muttering, making sounds with a negative quality), a sad or frightened facial expression, frowning, tense body language, and fidgeting.

Diagnosis: Disturbed Thought Processes.
Neuronal degeneration also affects thought processing. State this nursing diagnosis as *Disturbed Thought Processes related to neuronal degeneration.*

Outcomes. The client will have appropriate thought processing as evidenced by retention of information to maximal capacity, maintaining orientation to maximal capacity, and sharing meaningful life experiences.

Interventions. Because memory deficit occurs in all stages of AD, you must continually apply interventions to enhance memory. Reorient the client as necessary by placing a calendar and clock in obvious places. Because the client's long-term memory is retained longer than short-term memory, allow clients to reminisce. Become aware of a client's past experiences so that they can be shared meaningfully. Repetition is useful for ensuring maximal retention of information by the client.

Diagnosis: Risk for Injury.
Altered thought processes lead to impaired judgment and forgetfulness. These changes increase risk for injury. State this common nursing diagnosis as *Risk for Injury related to impaired judgment, forgetfulness, and motor impairments* (specify).

Outcomes. The client's physical and environmental safety will be maintained as evidenced by the absence of physical injury and the existence of a safe living environment.

Interventions. Impaired judgment, forgetfulness, and motor impairment can make any environment unsafe for the client with AD. In the home, electrical devices, toxic substances, loose rugs, hot tap water, inadequate lighting, and unlocked doors can be sources of injury. Teach family members how to eliminate these safety hazards. In the inpatient setting, ensure that clients cannot leave the premises without being noticed, that they wear an identification badge in case they become lost, and that doors and windows are secured. Dangerous objects should be kept out of reach, and potentially dangerous activities, such as cooking, should be supervised. The client's driving skill should be evaluated at regular intervals. See the Bridge to Home Health Care feature on Safety Solutions for People with Alzheimer's Disease on p. 2169.

Diagnosis: Self-Care Deficit.
State the nursing diagnosis of self-care problems as *Self-Care Deficit related to loss of memory and motor impairments.*

Outcomes. Clients will maintain self-care ability as evidenced by completing the tasks they are capable of performing and receiving assistance with ADL they are incapable of performing.

Interventions. Encourage the client with AD to do as much as possible, as long as it is safe and appropriate. Carefully balance helping the client with maintaining his or her autonomy; this can boost the client's confidence and self-respect, which can be very fragile during the early and middle stages of the disease. Give the client plenty of time to complete a task. Constantly encouraging, urging, and reminding the client in a step-by-step approach are necessary.

Diagnosis: Urge Urinary Incontinence.
Clients with AD develop urge incontinence as cortical neurons degenerate and no longer provide inhibition of the micturition and defecation responses. State this nursing diagnosis as *Urge Urinary Incontinence related to neuronal degeneration and forgetfulness.*

Outcomes. The client will have optimal continence of bladder and bowel as evidenced by having clean, dry clothing and bedding as much as possible; having intact skin; and voiding appropriately in the bathroom.

Interventions. Anticipation of elimination needs and scheduled voiding and defecation times can help in the initial stages. The client may show nonverbal signs of needing to void or defecate, like restlessness, grasping the genital area, or picking at clothing. Sometimes the client forgets where the bathroom is located. Having clear, bright signs indicating where the bathroom is and frequently taking the client there may help control incontinence. Fluid intake after the dinner meal can be restricted to help maintain continence during the night.

BRIDGE TO HOME HEALTH CARE

Safety Solutions for People with Alzheimer's Disease

To live with damaged thinking and judgment is to live at risk. People with Alzheimer's disease cannot take responsibility for their own safety. They are unable to evaluate the potential consequences of their actions and they forget quickly. Verbal reminders and written notes have little value, but there are many other ways to promote safety.

Older people love to live surrounded by their treasures. Although a neat home is always safer than a cluttered one, anticipate that only small changes can be made. Suggest moving knickknacks so that the edges of surfaces can be used for balance. Retain the existing furniture arrangements but consider removing or altering furniture with sharp corners, rocking chairs that tip easily, coffee tables, and fragile antiques. Block off unsafe areas by placing a sturdy chair in front of them. Eliminate hazards such as trailing wires, extension cords, or telephone cords. Caution caregivers to watch for paper or wooden objects that are tossed into gas fireplaces.

Most accidents happen in the kitchen and the bathroom. Therefore it is important to thoroughly assess how the person with Alzheimer's disease uses those areas. Disable stoves by removing knobs, installing a special switch behind the stove, removing a fuse, or turning the stove off at the breaker. Because people may retain overlearned food preparation skills, they may be able to use sharp utensils and hot surfaces safely but do need to be supervised. Encourage them to participate in meal preparation by doing single steps of a task, such as tearing lettuce for a salad or putting plates on the table.

Remove rugs and runners that tend to slide, especially those in the bathroom. Install grab bars to help prevent falls during transfers into or out of the tub or shower. Bars should be attached to structural supports rather than drywall or plaster. Consider using a raised toilet seat if rising is difficult and a bedside commode at night if urgency is a problem. Bath benches with nonskid feet are best, and hand-held showers minimize the need for the person to move about. Lower the temperature on the water heater to 120° F so that the water cannot become hot enough to scald anyone. If hot pipes are exposed, cover them with insulation.

While walking is good exercise and can reduce stress, wandering can become a safety issue. If the environment is secured with a fence, camouflaged doors, or locks, people with dementia may move freely within a relatively safe area, reducing the stress of caregivers who are afraid to let them out of sight. It is important to balance freedom, safety, and client rights. If wandering away from home is a potential hazard, the Alzheimer's Association has an excellent program called "safe return." More information about this low-cost program is available by calling 1-800-272-3900.

Try to arrange a bowel program to coincide with the client's usual pattern. In the later stages of AD, clients may need to wear incontinence briefs during the day and external urinary drainage devices at night. Indwelling catheters should be avoided because of the risk of infection and injury. Several varieties of disposable and extra absorbent washable underwear, bed pads, and mattress covers are available. If the client is male, choose undergarments that allow him to urinate through an opened fly.

Diagnosis: Caregiver Role Strain.
Family members and especially caregivers (usually a spouse or adult child) of clients with AD face a great deal of emotional and physical burden. State this nursing diagnosis as *Caregiver Role Strain related to grieving the loss of a family member to AD, change in social role, and intense demands for time commitment and provision of care.*

Outcomes. The family will demonstrate decreased role strain as evidenced by voicing their emotional concerns, seeking appropriate assistance, and providing adequate care for the client.

Interventions. Family members grieve the loss of the person they used to know. Each decline in cognitive function becomes another source of grief. Two stages of grief in the family have been described.

The process of grief begins during the caregiving stage and continues after the client's death. Normal family routines are lost, and the relationship between the family member and the dementia sufferer changes. Factors that have the most profound effect on the emotional well-being of caregivers include incontinence, overly demanding behavior, and the need for constant supervision.

Wives tend to experience a higher degree of emotional burden as caregivers than husbands do. Paradoxically, the closer the emotional bond between caregiver and dementia sufferer, the less the strain for the caregiver. Conversely, a low past level of intimacy is associated with an increased level of both perceived strain and depression in the spouse caregiver. Caregivers are most likely to be depressed if they feel a loss of control over their spouse's behavior, if they feel unable to cope with the impact of caregiving, and if they perceive the situation to be stable and to affect everything.

Studies have not determined that formal support of the caregiver (home visits by special practitioners, chore workers, and day care workers) relieves the caregiver's burden more than informal support (family member visits and support groups). The Alzheimer's Disease and Related Disorders Association has local chapters that offer support groups in many major cities in the United States (Phone: 1-800-272-3900).

Interview family members to determine their understanding of the diagnosis and prognosis of AD and to allow them to discuss their concerns about caring for the client:

- Do they know about community resources?
- Do they have someone to call when they can no longer cope with caregiving?

The home environment should be evaluated for safety before the client is sent home from the hospital:

- Is the home on a busy street?
- Can doors be secured so that the client cannot leave without supervision?
- Are potentially dangerous appliances out of reach?

A variety of options are available to caregivers. Chore service workers can help with household chores and relieve the caregiver of these duties. Other paid help can provide in-home respite care by observing the dementia sufferer while the caregiver tends to business outside the home, seeks social interaction, or meets recreational needs.

Adult day care provides time away from home for the dementia sufferer. Day care usually offers a lunchtime meal as well as several hours of scheduled activities that are tailored to the client's abilities. These activities may include games, crafts, music, and exercise.

Respite care involves admission to an extended care facility for a few days to a few weeks to allow the caregiver time to recover from the demands of providing 24-hour care (see the Bridge to Home Health Care on Respite Care for Caregivers of People with Alzheimer's Disease on the website).

Assisted living facilities with dementia units can also be used. These settings are home like and can provide needed supervision as long as the client is ambulatory.

Nursing home care is usually the final and most difficult and trying option for a caregiver. This decision creates guilt, self-doubt, and anxiety; however, it may be the only option when the caregiver suffers burnout and becomes unable to provide adequate care. Table 74-1 lists nursing guidelines for meeting family needs.

When the person with AD reaches the terminal stage of illness, the following questions about end-of-life treatments arise:

- Should a feeding tube be used to provide nourishment?
- Should antibiotics be used to treat pneumonias or other infections?
- Should cardiopulmonary resuscitation be used?

Ideally, decisions about these questions are raised and discussed with the client and family members before the person loses the capacity to make decisions.

Two forms of *advance directives* (means of expressing one's wishes about life-sustaining treatment after losing the mental capacity to make informed decisions) are available. One is the *living will,* a written document signed by the individual (while he or she is still mentally capable of making informed decisions) in the presence of a witness. The living will lists conditions under which the person wishes life-sustaining treatments to be withheld or withdrawn. The other advance directive is a *durable power of attorney for health care.* This is a legal document in which the person (while still mentally capable) assigns someone to act on his or her behalf in matters of health care decisions if the person loses decisional capacity (e.g., becomes demented). The family needs to be advised early to seek legal assistance to set up trusts, power of attorney documents for finances and for health care, and a living will.

Evaluation

Continually evaluate the degree of expected outcome attainment. You should expect progress toward outcomes to be slow. If the client is transferred to a new center (e.g., hospital), some regression can be expected. Family evaluation should be completed on regular intervals.

PARKINSON'S DISEASE

Parkinson's disease (PD) is a chronic, progressive, neurologic disorder that results from the loss of the neurotransmitter dopamine in a group of brain structures that control movements. Its major manifestations are variable but can include hand tremor, slowness of movements, limb stiffness, and difficulties with gait and balance. For the vast majority of individuals, PD is not thought to be an inherited disease. Even when a second person within a family is diagnosed with PD, this is thought to be more of a coincidence than an emerging genetic pattern because PD is a fairly common disorder among the older population.

Parkinsonian manifestations may also develop from other problems, such as long-term use of phenothiazines; poisoning from carbon monoxide, mercury, or manganese; or traumatic injury to the midbrain.

When PD occurs, degenerative changes are found in an area of the brain known as the *substantia nigra,* which produces *dopamine,* a chemical substance that enables people to move normally and smoothly. Once cell loss in the substantia nigra reaches 80%, manifestations appear. The cause of nigral cell degeneration is not known. PD is characterized by a severe shortage of dopamine in relation to ACh in the basal ganglia, which leads to the clinical characteristics of PD.

Clinical Manifestations

Parkinson's disease develops most often in people in their 60s, although it can strike much younger people as

TABLE 74-1	*Nursing Guidelines for Meeting the Needs of the Family of the Client with Dementia of the Alzheimer's Type*
Goals	**Selected Interventions**

Physical

Monitor chronic health problems or physical limitations of family caregiver.

Identify development of new health problems.

Obtain health history of family caregiver to identify past and new health problems.
Support family in following through with routine health examinations.
Refer family members to physician when health problems are observed.
Assess family's understanding of medical management of own health problems.
Teach family members to preserve own health in order to continue caring for patient with Alzheimer's disease.

Identify cues for stress.

Examine somatic health problems.

Emphasize family's need for adequate nutrition, hydration, exercise, and rest.

Help family members to be alert to signs of caregiver stress.

Psychosocial

Assist family in coping positively with stress.

Instruct family to get respite regularly for rest and relaxation.
Teach stress management techniques (i.e., relaxation, supportive relationships, goal setting, time management, diversion).

Identify destructive methods of coping (i.e., alcohol, drugs, tobacco, overeating or undereating, physical abuse of patient).

Refer family to physician, therapist when stress remains unmanageable even with social or psychological resources.

Assess family dynamics.

Assist family members in dealing with role change and conflict.

Refer signs of physical abuse to adult protective services.

Recognize the family's role, discuss capacity to provide care, and give reinforcement for care provided.
Counsel family in dealing with role conflicts, unmet expectations, or interpersonal conflicts.
Teach family the need to maintain roles and social activities outside caregiving experience.
Administer burden interview.
Reinforce family's attempt to cope.
Acknowledge family fears of being unable to continue with caregiving.

If need for support identified, direct family members to sources.

Refer family to a support group to share with others in similar situations.
Refer family to nearest office on aging or Alzheimer's Disease and Related Disorders Association, Inc. (ADRDA) to identify benefits in community available to Alzheimer's disease clients.

Identify family's mixed emotions (i.e., depression, anger, resentment, pity, embarrassment, guilt).

Listen to family and facilitate sharing of emotions and feelings in supportive, empathic environment.

Identify alternative plans for care if family members or social support systems become unable to provide care or are ineffective.

Counsel and support family if patient placed in care of others (i.e., day care, respite service, home care, nursing home); allay feelings of guilt.
Facilitate family meeting to identify time for socialization.

Identify financial limitations.

Encourage family to be specific about financial limitations.
Offer family referrals (legal, financial, or social service) for information on eligibility for private, county, state, or federal financial support for home services; advise and counsel regarding power of attorney or guardianship, trust or estate planning.

Assess family's ability to make funeral plans.

Help family anticipate and cope with grief process.
Assist family in making prefuneral arrangements.
Address family's fear regarding the possible role of heredity in development of Alzheimer's disease, and assist in making decision regarding autopsy.

Modified from Stevenson, J.P. (1990). Family stress to home care of Alzheimer's disease patients and implications for support. *Journal of Neuroscience Nursing, 22*(3), 185.

Continued

TABLE 74-1	*Nursing Guidelines for Meeting the Needs of the Family of the Client with Dementia of the Alzheimer's Type—cont'd*	
Goals	**Selected Interventions**	

Environmental

Identify compatibility of environment with family and client.	Conduct a family meeting to discuss relationship of family, patient, and environment.
Assess learning needs regarding client care tasks.	Teach management of concurrent physical health problems of the client with Alzheimer's disease.
	Include family in development of patient care plan.
	Teach family to encourage the client to continue daily habits to extent possible.
	Complete behavior problems checklist.
	Anticipate likely problems and tech how to manage them.
	Teach environmental modification (consistent, simple, calm routines) to maximize family endurance and enhance safety.
	Teach family to relate to patient with creative connectedness (touch, humor, flexibility, reminiscence, music, planned activities).
Assess family need and desire for information about Alzheimer's disease and how it affects the client's behavior.	Assist family in understanding symptoms related to memory loss, nature of the illness, symptoms, stages of disease progression, and behavior manifestations.
	Provide written material to reinforce education and understanding (i.e., *The 36-Hour Day, Coping and Caring: Living with Alzheimer's Disease;* literature from local, state, or national ADRDA chapters).
	Supply ADRDA 24-hour hotline number: 1-800-272-3900; website: http://www.alz.org.

Modified from Stevenson, J.P. (1990). Family stress to home care of Alzheimer's disease patients and implications for support. *Journal of Neuroscience Nursing, 22*(3), 185.

---

well. It occurs worldwide. About 1% of people over age 50 have PD. The disease has six cardinal features: (1) tremor at rest; (2) rigidity; (3) bradykinesia (slow movement); (4) flexed posture of the neck, trunk, and limbs; (5) loss of postural reflexes; and (6) freezing movement.

Early in the disease, the client may notice a slight slowing in the ability to perform ADL *(bradykinesia).* A general feeling of stiffness *(rigidity)* may be noticed, along with mild, diffuse muscular pain. *Tremor* is a common early manifestation that usually occurs in one of the upper limbs. It occurs at rest and involves a coarse "pill-rolling" movement of the thumb against the fingers that can vary in intensity and distribution. Voluntary movement stops or reduces the tremor in some people; however, others may have tremor during voluntary movement *(intention tremor)* as well.

Bradykinesia makes voluntary movements difficult to execute. When manifestations are severe, total lack of movement *(akinesia)* may occur and the client is literally frozen in one spot. Bradykinesia also affects gait. Initially there may be a slight stiffness of one leg while walking, and the ipsilateral arm may be held flexed at the elbow and abducted at the shoulder. The person may catch or drag one foot. Later, when both sides of the body are involved, the typical shuffling gait with short steps may develop. There is lack of associated swinging of the arms while walking. In advanced PD, the client stands with head, shoulders, and spine flexed forward, giving the appearance of a stooped posture (Figure 74-3).

The face of someone with advanced PD appears stiff, mask-like, and without expression. Speech is low in volume, monotonous in tone, and slow. Words are poorly articulated *(dysarthria).* Saliva may flow involuntarily from the mouth because of the lack of spontaneous swallowing.

Usually PD does not affect intellectual ability; however, a dementia similar to that of AD develops in 15% to 20% of clients with PD. Mood disturbance can occur, and emotional stress may intensify clinical manifestations.

The course of the disease is slowly progressive. The person becomes more rigid and more disabled, eventually requiring full assistance with ADL.

Outcome Management

The manifestations of PD can be relieved by providing dopamine to the basal ganglia. The purpose of anticholinergic drugs is to block release of ACh, thereby creating a better balance between ACh and dopamine. The most common levodopa drug is carbidopa-levodopa (Sinemet). Levodopa is a synthetic metabolic precursor of dopamine.

The benefit of the drug seems to decline with prolonged use. The therapy is more effective in treating bradykinesia and rigidity than tremor. The dosage of

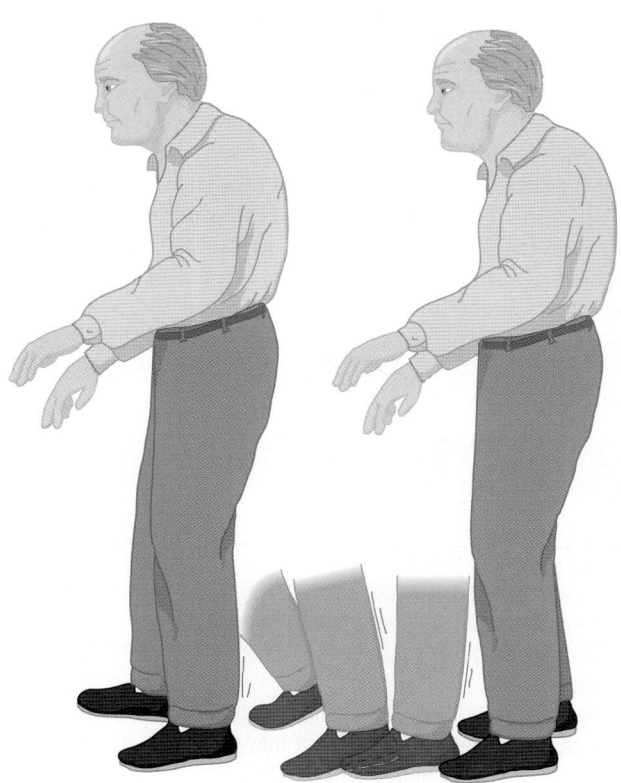

FIGURE 74-3 Gait changes seen in Parkinson's disease. Some of the clinical manifestations of Parkinson's disease are stooped posture, bradykinesia, and a festinant gait.

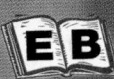

COMPLEMENTARY AND ALTERNATIVE THERAPY

Coenzyme Q10 Supplements and Parkinson's Disease

Parkinson's disease is a neurological disorder that currently has no treatment that has demonstrated a reduction in the progression of this disease. Researchers conducted a multicenter, randomized, parallel-group, placebo-controlled, double-blind, dosing-ranging trial. The participants in this trial were 80 individuals with early Parkinson's disease that did not require treatment for their condition. Clients were randomly assigned to placebo or coenzyme Q10 at dosages of 300, 600, or 1200 mg/day. Clients were followed for 16 months or until disability requiring treatment with levodopa had developed. Researchers found that coenzyme Q10 supplements were safe and well tolerated at dosages of up to 1200 mg/day. Less overall disability developed in clients assigned to coenzyme Q10 than in those assigned to placebo, and the benefit was greatest in the clients consuming the highest dose. Coenzyme Q10 seemed to slow the progressive deterioration of function in Parkinson's disease. Clients taking the highest dosage (1200 mg/day) had deterioration slowed by 44%. The greatest benefit was observed for daily activities such as feeding, dressing, bathing, and walking. By the eighth month, clients taking the highest dose scored significantly better than the placebo group.

Reference

Shults, C., et al. (2002). Effects of coenzyme Q10 in early Parkinson Disease: Evidence of slowing of the functional decline. *Archives of Neurology, 59,* 1541-1550.

levodopa is gradually increased until the optimal therapeutic response is achieved. This process may take several months. When the daily dose of levodopa approaches the desired level, the client often has involuntary *dyskinesias* (jerky, writhing movements), especially of the face, mouth, and tongue. Some clients prefer this stage to being severely bradykinetic because at least they can be mobile and perform voluntary movements more easily.

A relatively new class of drugs for PD is the catechol O-methyltransferase (COMT) inhibitors. COMT inhibitors are given with levodopa-carbidopa to increase the available dopamine in the brain.

See the Complementary and Alternative Therapy feature on Coenzyme Q10 Supplements and Parkinson's Disease on p. 2173.

■ Medical Management

Manage the Parkinsonian Crisis. Occasionally clients with PD experience a parkinsonian crisis as a result of emotional trauma or sudden or inadvertent withdrawal of anti-parkinsonian medication. Severe exacerbation of tremor, rigidity, and bradykinesia, accompanied by acute anxiety, sweating, tachycardia, and hyperpnea, occur. Intervention for parkinsonian crisis includes respiratory and cardiac support. The client should be placed in a quiet room with subdued lighting. Barbiturates may be prescribed in addition to anti-parkinsonian drugs.

Manage the On/Off Response. An *on/off response* (rapid fluctuation of clinical manifestations) may occur in clients with PD; the client may be mobile and active ("on") one moment and akinetic and rigid ("off") the next. This transition may happen quickly, within 1 to 2 minutes. Initially the off periods tend to occur 3 to 4 hours after a dose of anti-parkinsonian medication. Later the transition may happen anytime and may be unrelated to medication ingestion. Apparently off periods are due to dopamine deficit, but this factor is not clear. A person experiencing on/off response may be temporarily helped by shortening the interval between medication doses or by gradually increasing the total dosage.

Medications such as ropinirole may be given in addition to other PD medications to help smooth out the fluctuations.

■ Nursing Management of the Medical Client

Nursing care of the PD client includes health assessment, medication instruction and monitoring, liaison with other members of the health care team, and client and family education. Case managers are often used to guide transitions from one facility to the next (see Chapter 3 and the Chapter 63 Case Management feature on The *evolve* Older Adult on the website).

Advise the client to maintain fluid intake of 2L every 24 hours and to increase the intake of dietary fiber. Stool softeners and mild laxatives can be used. A regular time for bowel movements should be established, usually a half-hour after the morning or evening meal.

Teach the client various techniques to enhance voluntary movement. Clients often need to try different strategies on their own to find what helps most. Some clients grasp coins in their pocket to reduce embarrassing hand tremor. Others grip the arms of a chair. Mental thoughts, such as walking over imaginary lines, can aid ambulation. One client finds that tossing small scraps of paper

---

CLIENT EDUCATION GUIDE

Parkinson's Disease

Make sure that you understand how to take your medications, the importance of following the correct diet, and what side effects you can expect from your medications.

To avoid rigidity and the development of contractures:
- Exercise and stretch regularly.
- Perform the exercises recommended in your self-help booklets.
- Exercise first thing in the morning, when your energy levels are highest.
- Exercise in bed if getting to the floor is difficult.
- Get out of a chair by bending over slowly so that your head is over your toes; avoid soft, deep chairs.

If your health care provider has told you that you have bradykinesia (slow movements):
- Rock back and forth to get going.
- Imagine that you are stepping over an imaginary line when you walk.
- Throw small objects (e.g., small scraps of paper) in front of you to practice fine motor movements.
- Count to yourself while walking.
- Visualize your intended movement.

If you have a tremor:
- Hold change in your pocket or squeeze a small rubber ball.
- Use both hands to accomplish tasks.
- Lie face down on the floor and relax your entire body.
- Sleep on the side that has the tremor.

If you have trouble getting dressed:
- Dress and undress in front of a mirror.
- Use adaptive devices such as long-handled shoehorns and button fasteners.
- Buy clothes with self-fasteners (e.g., Velcro) and slide-locking buckles.

To ensure safety:
- Wear good, sturdy shoes.

- Use a cane or walker.
- Concentrate on standing upright.
- Consciously pick up your feet to take steps.
- Remove all throw rugs, electrical cords, and clutter from the floor.
- Make sure that you have adequate lighting.
- Arrange essential items so that they are within easy reach.
- Use a bath chair and a hand-held shower nozzle.
- Have grab bars installed in the bathroom.
- Have a raised toilet seat installed.

To ensure good communication:
- Pause between every few words.
- Exaggerate the pronunciation of words.
- Finish saying the final consonant of a word before starting to say the next word.
- Express ideas in short, concise phrases.
- Plan what to say.
- Face the listener.

To ensure adequate swallowing and prevent aspiration:
- Think through the steps of swallowing:
    Keep your lips closed.
    Keep your teeth together.
    Put food on your tongue.
    Lift your tongue up and back.
    Swallow.
- Eat slowly, taking small bites.
- Chew hard and move food around with your tongue.
- Finish one bite before taking another.

To keep saliva from building up in your mouth:
- Make a conscious effort to swallow saliva often.
- Keep your head in an upright position so saliva will collect in the back of your throat and stimulate automatic swallowing.
- Swallow excess saliva before attempting to speak.

in front of him aids his walking; another finds that rocking back and forth helps initiate movement. Encourage daily range-of-motion exercises to avoid rigidity and contractures. Remind the client to maintain good posture and to avoid flexion of the neck and shoulders. The client should sleep on a firm mattress. When resting, the client should avoid using a pillow to prevent flexion of the spine. Periodically lying prone also helps.

Because self-care activities are performed more slowly by the client with PD, extra time should be allowed for completion of tasks such as dressing, bathing, and eating. Warming trays can keep food hot. Recommend rest periods during meals to avoid aspiration.

As PD progresses, clients become rigid and unresponsive to verbal stimuli. During these stages, continue to treat clients with dignity, speaking to the clients rather than ignoring them.

Teach the client about home safety. Loose carpeting should be removed. Grab bars should be placed in the bathroom. An elevated toilet seat should be installed. Clients with severe tremor should avoid carrying hot liquids. Walking aids such as a cane or walker can provide added stability (see the Client Education Guide feature on Parkinson's Disease on p. 2174).

The client and family need emotional support. Support groups are available in most major cities. Refer the client and family to the American Parkinson Disease Association.

■ Surgical Management

Surgical interventions are used for PD. Intractable tremor *(dyskinetic movement)* may be ameliorated by pallidotomy. Fetal tissue transplantation and genetically engineered cells that produce dopamine are in experimental stages. Deep brain stimulation is also used to treat uncontrollable movement. Electrodes implanted in the thalamus or globus pallidus can be connected to a pacemaker-like device that the client can control.

CREUTZFELDT-JAKOB DISEASE

Creutzfeldt-Jakob disease (CJD) is a rare, fatal brain disease that produces progressive dementia, myoclonus, and distinctive electroencephalographic (EEG) changes. CJD is a unique disease that apparently can arise from two separate mechanisms: genetic and infectious. People with the genetic form have a mutated gene. The infectious form does not develop from a known virus or other pathogen; therefore words such as *virion, slow virus,* and *prion* are sometimes used to describe the etiologic agent. Several reports document human-to-human spread of CJD from transplanted tissue from a person with CJD. Incubation periods have ranged from 4 to 21 years, which indicates the enormous difficulty of tracing the infection. In 1996, CJD was associated with ingestion of infected beef. This led to the popular term *mad cow disease.*

Clinical Manifestations

Manifestations include vague psychiatric or behavior changes suggesting a personality change. About one third of clients report weight loss, anorexia, insomnia, malaise, and dizziness for a period of weeks to months. In the early stages, there is progressive memory loss, visual impairment, and dysphagia. Within a few weeks or months, a relentlessly progressive dementia develops and marked deterioration is noted from week to week. *Myoclonus* (twitching) is usually present. Deterioration is rapid, with 90% of clients dying within 1 year.

A definitive diagnosis attempts to differentiate CJD from AD, which has a more protracted course and no myoclonus or EEG changes. Lithium toxicity can mimic the manifestations, but they clear within about 2 weeks after discontinuation of the drug. Brain biopsy during hospitalization or on autopsy is the usual method of establishing a definitive diagnosis.

Outcome Management

No effective treatment is available, and CJD appears to be uniformly fatal. Nursing care is directed at supportive care, preventing skin breakdown, furnishing nutrition, and providing emotional support to the client and family. Families require much support, care, and concern as they try to cope with the sudden onset of this debilitating disease and with managing the day-to-day care of the client.

Although CJD can be transmitted, the risk to health care workers and others having contact with the client is no more than that to the general population. Isolation of clients is not indicated, but personnel should wear gloves when handling tissues, blood, and spinal fluid. Accidental skin contact with possibly infected material should be followed by washing in 10% normal sodium hydroxide or a solution of 5% household chlorine bleach. The agent can be inactivated on surfaces by using a 10% bleach solution for 1 hour. Surgical and pathologic instruments should be steam-autoclaved for 1 hour at 132° C. No organs, tissue, or tissue products from clients with CJD or any other ill-defined neurologic disorders should be used for transplantation or replacement therapy.

HUNTINGTON'S DISEASE

Huntington's disease (HD), also known as *Huntington's chorea,* is a genetically transmitted degenerative neurologic disease. It is characterized by abnormal movements *(chorea),* intellectual decline, and emotional disturbance. Clinical manifestations usually begin in the 30s and 40s, although occasionally they begin in young adulthood or even in children. Women and men are equally affected. The disease is relentlessly progressive, leading to disability and death within 15 to 20 years. Death usually results from respiratory complications caused by aspiration.

The disease is autosomal dominant; offspring of an affected person have a 50% chance of inheriting the disease. Because HD does not skip generations, offspring who have not inherited the disease will not pass it on to their offspring. The abnormal gene has been isolated on chromosome 4.

Pathophysiology

The pathologic changes of HD involve degeneration of the striatum (caudate and putamen) in the basal ganglia. Other subtle changes occur in the cortex and cerebellum, namely, loss of neurons and an increased number of glial cells (gliosis). The degeneration of the caudate nucleus leads to a reduction in several neurotransmitters, including gamma-aminobutyric acid, ACh, substance P, and metenkephalin, and their synthetic enzymes. This change leaves relatively higher concentrations of the other neurotransmitters, dopamine and norepinephrine. The relative excess of dopamine in HD, a disorder of excessive movement, can be contrasted to the lack of dopamine in Parkinson's disease (PD), a disorder of lack of movement.

Clinical Manifestations

Emotional disturbances and mental deterioration may precede the abnormal movements. The person may become negative, suspicious, and irritable. This condition may progress to depression and psychosis. Temper outbursts and sexual promiscuity may also occur. Severe mood swings are common. Cognitive decline progresses, and eventually the person becomes demented, incontinent, and completely unable to care for himself or herself.

The abnormal movements in HD are subtle at first. The person may appear restless or fidgety. The person may be aware of these movements and try to mask them by making them seem to be parts of intentional movements, such as head scratching or leg crossing. As the disease progresses, the rapid, jerky choreiform movements become more pronounced and involve all muscles. The person is constantly in motion. Stress, emotional situations, and attempts to perform voluntary movement can aggravate the abnormal movements. During sleep the movements diminish or disappear.

The diagnosis of HD is made on the basis of clinical manifestations and family history because there is no specific diagnostic test for the disease itself. CT or MRI imaging of the brain may show atrophy of the head of the caudate, but this factor alone is not diagnostic of HD.

Outcome Management

There is no known treatment to cure or alter the course of HD. Haloperidol, a dopamine blocker, can control the abnormal movements and some behavioral manifestations. Diazepam can be used to lower anxiety, thereby aiding in control of movements. Antidepressants can help depression.

■ Medical Management

Late-Stage Dysphagia. One of the most common and dangerous problems in the middle to late stages is dysphagia. Several interventions should be tried. Medications need to be evaluated for their anticholinergic and sedative effects, which may impair swallowing. Mealtimes should be free of stress and clutter and have an unhurried atmosphere. Use of adaptive eating utensils can encourage and extend independence in eating. The diet should include foods that are easy to swallow and form a bolus in the mouth (e.g., canned peaches, chopped meat in gravy and mashed potatoes, custards). Many clients with HD require high caloric intake because of excessive movements and should try eating frequent, small meals containing high-calorie foods. Clients should sit upright when eating. While swallowing, they should keep the chin down toward the chest. They can be trained to hold their breath before swallowing and cough after each mouthful is swallowed to clear the throat of any residual food.

■ Nursing Management

If the client continues to have difficulty eating and loses weight despite dietary and environmental modifications, a feeding tube may become necessary; however, artificial feeding methods often frighten families, and they pose ethical dilemmas about prolonging life. Nurses can help clients and their families make these difficult decisions by clarifying the issues and providing information on the types, risks, benefits, and long-term effects of artificial feeding methods.

Poor control of oral and respiratory muscles can make communication difficult. The nurse can assist the family in developing signals such as raising a hand or keeping the eyes open or closed for yes and no responses. If physical signals are not an option, cards with printed words may be helpful. Keep communication simple and unstrained. Repeat words that are understood to let the client know that communication has been successful.

Excessive movements and falls may cause physical injury and can restrict independence. Pads on wheelchairs and beds, shin guards, and walking belts can prevent injury. Aids for ambulation (e.g., walking behind a wheelchair) can extend independence. Clothing should be light and simple to don and doff.

Huntington's disease has a major impact on the family, not only because of the burden of caregiving but also because of the risk to offspring of inheriting the disease. Many ethical dilemmas surrounding the issue of privacy can surface in cases of HD. Whether test results are positive or negative, the results are of interest to the spouse, other family members, employers, and insurers; however, principles of confidentiality forbid disclosure of medical information to anyone without the client's consents. Be sensitive to the client's desire for confidentiality, but use this opportunity to teach the client about the effect the disease may have on other family members. Because a blood test is now available to check for the presence of the abnormal gene, family members face difficult choices about whether to find out if they have the Huntington gene.

MULTIPLE SCLEROSIS

Multiple sclerosis (MS) is a chronic demyelinating disease that affects the myelin sheath of neurons in the central nervous system (CNS). The myelin sheath is essential for normal conduction of nerve impulses. Patches of myelin deteriorate at irregular intervals along the nerve axon, causing slowing of nerve conduction. Axonal destruction also occurs in MS.

The onset of MS usually occurs between 20 and 40 years of age, and it affects women twice as often as men. Whites are affected more often than Hispanics, blacks, or Asians. The disease is most prevalent in the colder climates of North America and Europe. If someone is born in an area of high risk for MS and moves to an area of low risk after age 15, the person carries the risk of the area of origin.

Etiology and Risk Factors

The exact cause of MS is unknown. Most theories suggest that MS is an immunogenetic-viral disease, that is, an immune-mediated demyelination triggered by a viral infection, probably with the Epstein-Barr virus. A genetic susceptibility apparently alters the body's immune response to viral infection. Multiple genes are probably involved; however, the only consistently identified disease locus is on the human leukocyte antigen (HLA) gene complex on chromosome 6.

A variety of precipitating factors can precede the onset or an exacerbation of MS, such as infection, physical injury, emotional stress, pregnancy, and fatigue. Most pregnancy-related exacerbations occur 3 months postpartum and may relate more to the stress of labor and fatigue during the puerperium than to the pregnancy itself.

Pathophysiology

Myelin is a highly conductive fatty material that surrounds the axon and speeds conduction of nerve impulses along the axon. In MS, plaques form along the myelin sheath, causing inflammation, edema, and eventually scarring and destruction (Figure 74-4). Plaques are characterized by primary demyelination and death of oligodendrocytes in the center of the lesion. Initially perivascular inflammatory cells (autoreactive T cells) invade the myelin-covered axons in the CNS. This is followed by extensive gliosis or scarring by astrocytes and aberrant attempts at remyelination, with oligodendro-

cytes proliferating at the edges of the plaque. When edema and inflammation subside, some remyelination occurs but is often incomplete.

Although plaques may occur anywhere in the white matter of the CNS, the areas most commonly involved are the optic nerves, cerebrum, and cervical spinal cord.

Clinical Manifestations

The wide variety of manifestations possible with MS and the unpredictable nature of the disease pose many challenges to the client and family. The course of illness **EB** varies from person to person. Four clinical patterns have been identified (Figure 74-5). The most common initial pattern is *relapsing-remitting* MS. Clients experience manifestations that eventually remit with little or no progression of disability.

The random distribution of MS plaques leads to several clinical manifestations:

- Weakness or tingling sensations (paresthesias) of one or more extremities caused by involvement of the cerebrum or spinal cord
- Vision loss from optic neuritis
- Incoordination that is due to cerebellar involvement
- Bowel and bladder dysfunction as a result of spinal cord involvement

Bladder dysfunction can take several forms, depending on which neural pathways are affected. Dysfunction may involve hesitancy, frequency, loss of sensation,

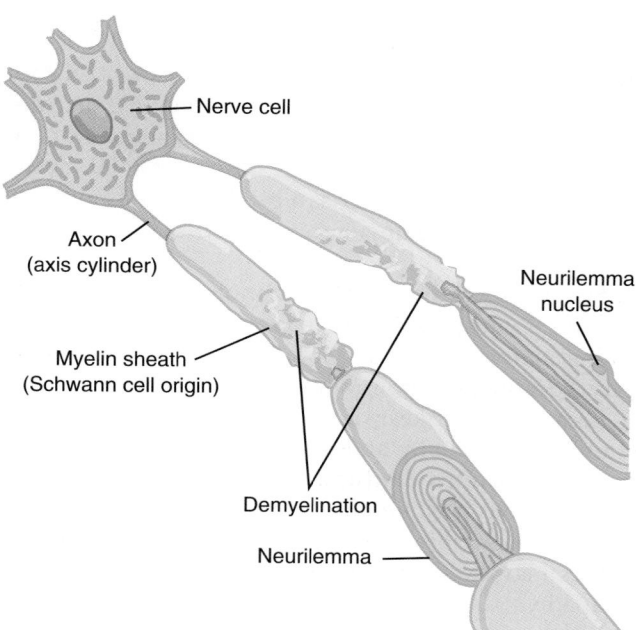

FIGURE 74-4 Changes in the nerve sheath, as seen in multiple sclerosis. Myelin is made by the oligodendrocyte and coats peripheral nerves, facilitating nervous impulse. In clients with multiple sclerosis, the myelin degenerates in patches, causing nerve transmission to become erratic.

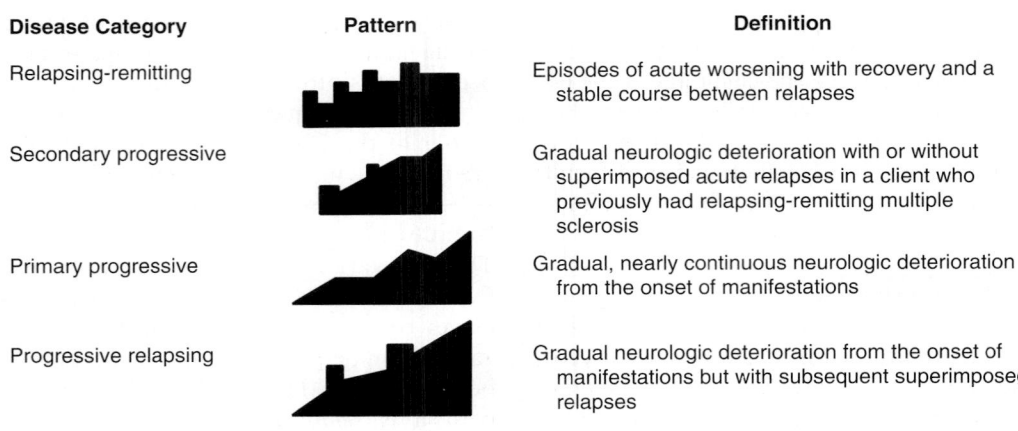

Disease Category	Pattern	Definition
Relapsing-remitting		Episodes of acute worsening with recovery and a stable course between relapses
Secondary progressive		Gradual neurologic deterioration with or without superimposed acute relapses in a client who previously had relapsing-remitting multiple sclerosis
Primary progressive		Gradual, nearly continuous neurologic deterioration from the onset of manifestations
Progressive relapsing		Gradual neurologic deterioration from the onset of manifestations but with subsequent superimposed relapses

FIGURE 74-5 Clinical patterns of multiple sclerosis. (Modified from Lublin, F. D., & Reingold, S.C. [1996]. Defining the clinical course of multiple sclerosis: Results of an international survey. *Neurology, 46,* 907-911.)

incontinence, and retention. Increased or decreased detrusor, bladder neck, external sphincter tone, or a combination of these problems may occur. The ultimate bladder dysfunction, however, is usually hyperreflexia in association with sphincter dyssynergia (sphincter contraction during detrusor contraction).[3] Proper diagnosis of the type of bladder dysfunction requires a thorough history, laboratory assessment of kidney function, and identification of possible infection. If bladder emptying is defective, further investigation with urography, cystoscopy, and urodynamic studies should be performed.

Constipation is commonly experienced by clients with MS. Dysfunction can result from one or more of the following factors: spinal cord lesion, immobility, dehydration, medications, and nutritional deficiencies. Stool incontinence, although rarer, is also possible. Sexual dysfunction can also occur as a result of lesions in the ascending or descending autonomic and sensory fibers in the spinal cord.

 Fatigue is a common manifestation of MS and usually one of the most disabling. Spasticity can reduce energy, inhibit motor control, and interfere with self-care, sexuality, vocational responsibilities, and recreation.

Because MS strikes young adults during their years of establishing a family and an occupation, the impact of the disease can be devastating. Depression often occurs in clients, but it is not clear whether depression is a reaction to disability or a function of the disease itself. Others may experience euphoria, emotional instability, or apathy.

Because there is no definitive test for MS, clinicians rely on a detailed history, clinical findings, and a variety of diagnostic tests. The history often reveals several episodes of neurologic dysfunction, separated by time and by different locations in the CNS. Current research looking at clients who experience only one manifesta-

tion, such as optic neuritis, is changing the way clinicians diagnose MS.

Diagnostic tests include the following:
- Cerebrospinal fluid (CSF) evaluation for the presence of oligoclonal banding
- Evoked potentials of the optic pathways and auditory system to assess the presence of slowed nerve conduction
- MRI of the brain and spinal cord to determine the presence of MS plaques

Outcome Management
■ Medical Management
Treatment generally falls into one of three categories: (1) treatment of acute relapses, (2) treatment aimed at disease management, and (3) symptomatic treatment.

Treat Acute Relapses. Treatment of acute relapses usually involves the use of intravenous (IV) or oral corticosteroids, which have both anti-inflammatory and immunosuppressive properties. They are often used to enhance recovery from an exacerbation. Methylprednisolone is standard therapy for acute exacerbations sometimes followed by an oral prednisone taper. Azathioprine (Imuran) and cyclophosphamide (Cytoxan), other immunosuppressive agents, may be used for more severe exacerbations or progressive MS.

Treat Exacerbations. Interferon β_{1b} (Betaseron) is used for ambulatory clients with relapsing-remitting MS. Interferon β_{1b} is a genetically engineered complex protein with both antiviral and immunoregulatory properties that can reduce the number of MS exacerbations. The drug is injected subcutaneously every other day. Interferon β_{1a} (Avonex) is also available for the treatment of relapsing forms of MS. In addition to reducing the number and severity of relapses, interferon β_{1a} has provided a delay in disability in placebo-controlled studies.

The third disease-modifying agent available for use in the United States is glatiramer acetate (Copaxone), a synthetic polypeptide approved for use in relapsing-remitting MS. It is not an interferon but is believed to work by mimicking myelin basic protein and interrupting the inflammatory cascade to prevent damage to myelin.

Side effects of the interferons include fever, fatigue, and flu-like manifestations. Clients on interferon β_{1a} have also reported increased depression and injection site reactions. Copaxone does not produce the interferon-type side effects of fever and flu-like manifestations, but rare episodes of face flushing, chest tightness, and shortness of breath lasting less than 15 minutes have been reported. Numerous other therapeutic agents are undergoing clinical trials.

Symptomatic Treatment. Several strategies are available for symptomatic management in MS. Pharmacologic interventions can be used for bladder dysfunction (oxybutynin, propantheline); constipation (psyllium hydrophilic mucilloid, bisacodyl pills or suppositories), fatigue (amantadine, modafinil), spasticity (baclofen, diazepam, dantrolene), tremor (propranolol, phenobarbital, clonazepam), and dysesthesias and trigeminal neuralgia (carbamazepine, phenytoin, amitriptyline).

Transcutaneous electrical nerve stimulation (TENS) is also helpful for dysesthesias. Areas of numbness should be inspected regularly to prevent injury and development of pressure ulcers. Skin should be kept dry and free of urine and feces. A seat cushion that distributes pressure should be used for wheelchair-bound clients with insensate buttock skin. Blindness or severely impaired vision may occur. In this case, refer the client to Services for the Blind for rehabilitation. Cognitive and perceptual impairment necessitates psychometric and functional testing for accurate assessment and rehabilitation services.

■ Nursing Management of the Medical Client
Assessment

If the client is being assessed for possible MS, you should assess the client for clinical manifestations of the disorder. Ocular manifestations are very common. As a result of the fluctuations of clinical manifestations, the client may report a past history of similar findings that went away.

If the client is being hospitalized for an exacerbation of MS, focus on the client's ability to perform ADL as well as other areas that require fine motor movements. Gross motor activities, such as walking, may also be impaired and may lead to problems with bowel and bladder continence.

Diagnosis, Outcomes, Interventions

Diagnosis: Impaired Urinary Elimination.
Demyelination of the nerves supplying the bladder may result in altered bladder function. This nursing diagnosis is stated as *Impaired Urinary Elimination related to bladder dysfunction.*

Outcomes. The client will maintain urinary continence and normal bladder filling as evidenced by residual volumes of less than 100 ml, application of appropriate bladder elimination procedures, and verbalization of personal satisfaction with urinary elimination status.

Interventions. The following interventions are for neurogenic bladder, the most common type of bladder dysfunction in MS.

Fluid intake should be maintained at 2000 ml/24 hr, ideally, 400 to 500 ml with each meal and 200 ml at midmorning, midafternoon, and late afternoon. Avoiding fluid intake after the evening meal reduces the need for emptying the bladder during the night.

Voiding should be attempted every 3 hours during waking hours. If voiding is not successful, a catheter should be inserted into the bladder and then removed once emptying is complete. This is called *intermittent catheterization.* If the volume of catheterized urine exceeds 500 ml, catheterization may need to be scheduled more frequently.

Instruct the client on how to do self-catheterization if he or she is capable. A clean red rubber catheter can be reused for up to 1 week so long as it is washed thoroughly with soap and water and placed in a clean, tightly sealed plastic bag after every catheterization. Sterile equipment is not required for ongoing self-catheterization in the hospital or at home for these clients.

Diagnosis: Constipation.
Immobility and demyelination lead to constipation. State this common nursing diagnosis as *Constipation related to immobility and demyelination.*

Outcomes. The client will have bowel movements of normal consistency and frequency.

Interventions. A high-fiber diet, bulk formers, and stool softeners are useful for maintaining stool consistency. Adequate fluid intake also assists bowel elimination; 2000 ml should be taken. Explain that laxatives and enemas should be avoided because they lead to dependence. A bowel program should be performed every other day, approximately 45 minutes after the largest meal, to take advantage of the gastrocolic reflex. Rectal evacuation may be augmented by the use of glycerin or bisacodyl suppositories or digital stimulation.

Diagnosis: Activity Intolerance. State this common nursing diagnosis as *Activity Intolerance related to fatigue and muscle weakness.*

Outcomes. The client will demonstrate improved activity tolerance as evidenced by (1) maintaining a balance between work, rest, and exercise and recreation; (2) performing ADL without excessive fatigue; (3) using energy-saving devices and techniques; (4) avoiding elevations in environmental and body temperatures; and (5) consuming a diet adequate in calories and protein for body size, frame, and age.

Interventions. Because fatigue can be precipitated by warm temperatures, the environment should be kept cool. If air-conditioning is unavailable, cool baths and ice packs may help lower body temperature.

Assist the client in planning activities at his or her peak energy level, which is usually in the morning. This schedule promotes optimal synchrony between circadian rhythms and the client's physical demands. The client should plan for periods of rest throughout the day. Collaboration with the physical and occupational therapist can reveal methods to reduce energy consumption with repeated tasks and apply adaptive devices for ambulation and toileting. The drugs amantadine (Symmetrel) and modafinil (Provigil) may alleviate fatigue in some clients.

Diagnosis: Impaired Physical Mobility. Several problems lead to difficulties with mobility. State this nursing diagnosis as *Impaired Physical Mobility related to weakness, contractures, spasticity, and ataxia.*

Outcomes. The client will achieve optimal physical mobility as evidenced by improved or maintained range of motion in all joints, optimal control of spasticity, and effective use of adaptive aids.

Interventions. Although some clients are bothered by painful muscle spasms, others may rely on spasticity to stabilize weak limbs during transfers and ambulation. Spastic muscles must be stretched at least twice daily through their full range of motion. The drug baclofen (Lioresal) provides synaptic inhibition of spinal reflexes, which can reduce spasticity, although it may increase weakness and fatigue in some clients. Diazepam (Valium), tizanidine (Zanaflex), and dantrolene (Dantrium) are other anti-spasmodic drugs. Surgical intervention or nerve blocks may be necessary if contractures develop. Monitor the effect of medications on spasticity, promote activity to decrease spasms, and use spasms for muscle strength when transferring.

Advise that strengthening exercises for muscle weakness *(paresis)* must be done with caution because they can exacerbate paresis by causing muscle fatigue; however, selective strengthening of unaffected or less affected muscles can enhance physical function and well-being. Range-of-motion exercises should be performed at least twice daily. Active movement is preferable to passive movement. Correct body alignment should be maintained to reduce the risk of contractures. Splints may help maintain position and provide support for weak hands and ankles. Ataxia and tremor of the extremities can be lessened by the use of small weights applied to the distal extremities or the use of weighted utensils. Weakness and fatigue can worsen ataxia. Ambulation aids such as a cane or a walker may be necessary.

Diagnosis: Risk for Self-Care Deficit. Clients with MS may experience a decline in self-care abilities. State this nursing diagnosis as *Risk for Self-Care Deficit related to muscle weakness.*

Outcomes. The client will reduce the risk for self-care deficits by using ADL aids.

Interventions. Clients may require aids, such as wheelchairs or canes, to perform ADLs and ambulate. The performance of ADLs may be enhanced if counters and tabletops are adjusted to a comfortable working height. Work in combination with the physical therapist, occupational therapist, social worker, and home health nurse to identify, purchase, and teach the client how to use ADL aids.

Diagnosis: Deficient Knowledge. The client with a new diagnosis of MS often lacks knowledge about MS, its unpredictable course, and the role of stress in MS. State this nursing diagnosis as *Deficient Knowledge related to new diagnosis of MS.*

Outcomes. The client will have more knowledge about MS as evidenced by stating facts about the course of MS and the role of stress in MS.

Interventions. The client with MS needs to have a clear understanding of the unpredictability of this disorder. The client may be free of manifestations for many weeks to months, even years, and then experience them. If the client can identify stressors that exacerbate the clinical manifestations, sometimes these stressors can be avoided. The National Multiple Sclerosis Society can be an excellent resource for education and support. For clients on one of the three disease-modifying agents, each company has a support program to offer education, financial information, and support for people with MS and their families.

Diagnosis: Situational Low Self-Esteem. Because of the client's age, loss of independence and fear of disability can be devastating. Psychosocial diagnosis is important in providing holistic care. State this nursing diagnosis as *Situational Low Self-Esteem related to loss of independence and fear of disability.*

Outcomes. The client will achieve improved self-esteem as evidenced by verbalizing awareness that personal goals and body image will need to be adjusted, willingness to maintain appropriate independence, and positive thoughts and statements about self.

Interventions. Regardless of the cause of disturbance in self-esteem, carefully assess the individual and family history for the presence and type of depressive episodes and the clinical manifestations. Identify previous treatment for depression, including psychotherapy and drug therapy. By assessing the client's problem-solving strategies, you can identify coping behavior strengths and defense mechanisms such as denial, avoidance, or intellectualization that the client may use to mask depression.

Evaluate the client's social support system, which contributes to a sense of well-being. Grieving the loss of function in MS can lead to a reactive depression and require provision of support group therapy for both the client and family. Some clients may not benefit from this

type of therapy, however, because they may see people whose condition is much worse than their own and fear developing that level of disability. On-line computer services for MS clients can provide a means of social support.

Evaluation

The degree of expected outcome attainment should be evaluated on an ongoing basis. Most outcomes are long-term and may require weeks to months to attain.

PARALYTIC DISEASES

Paralysis, the lost of both motor and sensory function, can occur from virus-like poliomyelitis or Guillain-Barré syndrome. Unfortunately, it can also develop from botulism in the form of terrorism (see the Terrorism Alert feature on Botulism, below).

GUILLAIN-BARRÉ SYNDROME

Guillain-Barré syndrome (GBS) is an inflammatory disease of unknown origin that involves degeneration of the myelin sheath of peripheral nerves. GBS is seen worldwide and affects people of all ages and races. Since the

---

TERRORISM ALERT

Botulism

Botulism is a serious paralytic illness caused by a nerve toxin that is produced by the bacterium *Clostridium botulinum.* Botulinum is the most poisonous substance known. Two types of botulinum toxin are of concern in bioterrorism: foodborne and inhalational forms. Foodborne botulism can be especially dangerous because many people can be poisoned by eating a contaminated food. Foodborne botulism can occur from contaminated low-acid foods such as asparagus, green beans, beets, and corn. Outbreaks of botulism have been reported from chopped garlic in oil, chile peppers, tomatoes, improperly handled baked potatoes wrapped in aluminum foil, and home-canned or fermented fish. Inhalational botulism has been released intentionally via weapons.

The classic clinical manifestations of botulinum toxin exposure depend on the amount of toxin absorbed into the circulation. Manifestations include double vision, blurred vision, drooping eyelids, slurred speech, difficulty swallowing, dry mouth, and muscle weakness. All manifestations are due to muscle paralysis caused by the bacterial toxin. If untreated, these manifestations may progress to cause paralysis of the arms, legs, trunk, and respiratory muscles. In foodborne botulism, symptoms generally begin 18 to 36 hours after eating a contaminated food, but they can occur as early as 6 hours or as late as 10 days. The most direct way to confirm the diagnosis is to detect the botulinum toxin in the serum or stool.

The respiratory failure and paralysis that occur with severe botulism may require mechanical ventilation for weeks. After several weeks, the paralysis slowly improves. If diagnosed early, foodborne and wound botulism can be treated with an antitoxin that blocks the action of the toxin. Contaminated food still in the gut can be partially removed by inducing vomiting or by using enemas. Wounds should be treated, usually surgically, to remove the source of the toxin-producing bacteria. After exposure to suspected botulism, clothing and skin should be washed with soap and water. Contaminated surfaces should be cleaned with 0.1% hypochlorite solution.

Botulism in a rare disease. Intentional exposure should be considered if a large number of clients are seen with flaccid paralysis, if unusual types are found that are not seen in food poisoning, or if outbreaks are occurring in unusual settings (e.g., airports). Suspected outbreaks of botulism are quickly investigated. If they involve a commercial product, the appropriate control measures are coordinated among public health and regulatory agencies. Physicians should report suspected cases of botulism to a state health department.

Reference

Arnon, S., et al. (2001). Botulinum toxin as a biological weapon. *Journal of the American Medical Association, 285* 1059-1070.

virtual elimination of poliomyelitis, GBS has become the most common cause of acute generalized paralysis, with an annual incidence of 0.75 to 2 per 100,000 population. In one half to two thirds of cases, an upper respiratory or gastrointestinal infection precedes the onset of the syndrome by 1 to 4 weeks.

Although many organisms have been suspected, including *Cytomegalovirus* and Epstein-Barr virus, *Campylobacter jejuni* is the organism most often implicated. This gram-negative rod is found in poultry, pets, raw milk, and contaminated water. *C. jejuni* targets the myelin sheath. Macrophages penetrate the basal lamina surrounding the axon, displace the Schwann cell from the myelin sheath, and phagocytose the myelin lamellae. An association between HIV and GBS has also been reported, and clients with GBS should be tested for HIV.

Clinical Manifestations

A characteristic feature is ascending weakness, usually beginning in the lower extremities and spreading, sometimes rapidly, to the trunk, upper extremities, and even the face. The weakness evolves over hours to days, with maximal deficit by 4 weeks in 90% of cases. Deep-tendon reflexes are lost. Paresthesias (tingling sensation) in the limbs may occur early in the course of the illness.

This *initial phase* is usually followed by a *plateau phase* during which the disease no longer seems to progress, but the client does not recover functions initially lost. Deep, aching muscle pain in the shoulder girdle and thighs is common. The two most dangerous features of the disease are respiratory muscle weakness and autonomic neuropathy involving both the sympathetic and parasympathetic systems. The latter feature can involve orthostatic hypotension, hypertension, pupillary disturbances, sweating dysfunction, cardiac dysrhythmias, paralytic ileus, and urinary retention.

The third phase of the disease is the *recovery phase.* Improvement and recovery occur with remyelination. If nerve axons are damaged, however, some residual deficits may remain. Remyelination occurs in a descending pattern; the functions lost last are thus the first to be regained. Recovery is usually maximal at 6 months, although severe cases may take up to 2 years for maximal recovery. Fortunately, 85% to 90% of clients with GBS recover completely.

Diagnosis of GBS is based on history and physical examination, CSF examination, and electrophysiologic studies. The CSF contains increased protein, with few or no white blood cells. Nerve-conduction velocity is slowed, although it may be normal in the early stage of the illness. *Conduction block,* a diminution in amplitude or an absence of elicited muscle action potentials from stimulation of a peripheral nerve, also occurs.

Outcome Management

The focus of therapy is supportive care. Monitor respiratory or cardiovascular status carefully: vital signs, se-

rial measurement of vital capacity, peripheral oxygen saturation, and electrocardiography. When vital capacity falls to 15 ml/kg of body weight, intubation and artificial ventilation are usually necessary. Early treatment with plasmapheresis may accelerate recovery, although the exact mechanism for this effect is not known. Hypotheses include the removal of circulating antibodies or other humoral myelinotoxic or immunopathogenic factors. IV immunoglobulin G (IVIG) therapy may prove to be the treatment of choice because it can be administered easily and can be given with other drugs simultaneously (plasmapheresis removes co-medication jointly with adverse disease factors).

During the first several days after hospital admission, it is crucial to assess the client's respiratory, swallowing, and autonomic function (see the Critical Monitoring feature on Respiratory Distress with Guillain-Barré Syndrome on p. 2183). Assess the following at least every 4 hours: vital signs, forced vital capacity, swallowing, strength in the extremities, and intake and output balance. If ascending weakness is noted, increase the frequency of assessment to every 2 hours or even more often. Cardiac monitoring and supplemental oxygen are often needed. Common complications include bladder infection, deep vein thrombosis, pulmonary emboli, pneumonia, and syndrome of inappropriate antidiuretic hormone (SIADH).

Interventions to control infection and prevent complications of immobility are vital. Proper body alignment should be maintained to prevent deformities and injury to paralyzed limbs. Once the client's condition is stabilized, rehabilitative interventions can be implemented.

Assist the client in coping with the progressive nature of GBS. During the early stages, clients are frightened because their paralysis can ascend rapidly. They are often admitted to an acute care agency with progressive weakness and within days are completely paralyzed. Clients fear they will never recover. Help clients in verbalizing their fears, and offer support and encouragement that although the disorder is progressive, most clients gain full recovery. Encouragement is not hollow, however. The client is not taught to expect immediate resolution but is assisted to realize the usual time frames for recovery.

MYASTHENIA GRAVIS

Myasthenia gravis (MG) is an autoimmune disease that presents as muscular weakness and fatigue that worsens with exercise and improves with rest. The manifestations result from a loss of ACh receptors in the postsynaptic neurons of the neuromuscular junction. The cause of MG is unknown, but 80% of people with the generalized form of the disease have elevated titers of antibodies to the ACh receptor in their serum. MG may appear at any age, although there are two peaks of onset. In early-onset MG, at age 20 to 30 years, women are more often affected than men. In late-onset MG, after age 50, men are more often affected. The overall incidence of

CRITICAL MONITORING

Respiratory Distress with Guillain-Barré Syndrome

Monitor the client for:
- Complaints of headache
- Myoclonic jerks
- Drowsiness
- Confusion
- Restlessness
- Reduced cough
- Decreased ability to move pulmonary secretions

Assess pulmonary function studies for:
- Decreased forced vital capacity (<15 ml/kg)
- Decreased tidal volume (<3-4 ml/kg)
- Decreased maximum inspiratory pressure (<10-20 cm H_2O)
- Decreased maximum expiratory pressure (<40 cm H_2O)

Assess arterial blood gases for:
- Decreased Pao_2 (<80 mm Hg on 50% Fio_2 with normal Pco_2)
- Alveolar-arterial gradient >300 on 50% Fio_2
- $Paco_2$ >50 mm Hg
- V_D/V_T >0.6

Fio₂, Fraction of inspired oxygen; *Paco₂*, partial pressure of arterial carbon dioxide; *Pao₂*, partial pressure of arterial oxygen; *V_D/V_T*, ratio of dead space volume to tidal volume.

MG is 0.4 per 100,000 and the prevalence is 0.5 to 5 per 100,000.

Clinical Manifestations

The primary feature of MG is increasing weakness with sustained muscle contraction. For instance, if the person is asked to hold the arms up, the power of muscle contraction diminishes and the arms gradually drift downward. After a period of rest, the muscles regain their strength. Muscle weakness is greatest after exertion or at the end of the day.

Ocular manifestations are most common, with *ptosis* (drooping of the upper eyelid) or *diplopia* (double vision) occurring in many clients. Ptosis is due to weakness of the levator palpebrae muscles of the eye. If not present at the examination, ptosis can be elicited by prolonged upward gaze, which creates fatigue of the muscle.

Diplopia is a result of weakness or fatigue of the extraocular muscles. Other manifestations are weakness of the orbicularis oculi muscles (which help close the eye), the facial muscles, the muscles of chewing and swallowing, and the limbs. Weakness of the facial and levator palpebrae muscles produces an expressionless face, with droopy eyelids, smoothed features, and a tendency for the mouth to hang open.

An attempt to smile often turns into a snarl because of the weakness. A person may hold a hand under the jaw to keep it closed. Dysphagia and a nasal quality to speech occur when the muscles of chewing and swallowing are involved. In severe cases, respiratory muscle weakness may occur, which may necessitate intubation and mechanical ventilation (see Myasthenic Crisis).

The course of MG varies, and remissions and exacerbations may occur. Clinical manifestations may progress quickly or slowly and may fluctuate from day to day. The severity of the disease varies greatly from person to person.

Diagnostic Findings

The diagnosis of MG is based on the clinical presentation and can be confirmed by testing the client's response to anticholinesterase drugs. These drugs inhibit cholinesterase, an enzyme that breaks down ACh in the neuromuscular junction, thereby allowing more ACh to bind to the remaining ACh receptors. Edrophonium (Tensilon) is a short-acting drug that is given intravenously *(Tensilon test)*. A test dose of 2 mg (for adults) is injected first. If no untoward reaction occurs (such as increased weakness, change in heart rate or rhythm, nausea, or abdominal cramps), the remaining 8 mg is injected. The client is then observed for objective manifestations of improvement in muscle strength. The effect is transitory, wearing off after 3 to 5 minutes. Another drug, neostigmine methylsulfate (Prostigmin), may be used because of its longer duration of effect on muscle strength (1 to 2 hours), which allows better analysis of its effect.

When either drug is used, IV atropine sulfate should be available to inject as an antidote. This medication counteracts any severe cholinergic reactions (cardiac dysrhythmias or abdominal cramping). Electromyography (EMG) helps confirm the diagnosis. Repetitive stimulation of the nerve with recording from the involved muscle shows a characteristic decrementing response of the muscle action potential.

Outcome Management

No cure for MG exists as yet. Pharmacologic intervention consists of two groups of medications: (1) short-acting anticholinesterase compounds and (2) corticosteroids. The most effective anticholinesterase drugs are pyridostigmine (Mestinon) and neostigmine (Prostigmin). Dosages are highly individualized, based on physiologic response to the medication. The goal is to achieve the maximum benefit (muscle strength and endurance) with the fewest side effects (excessive salivation, sweating, nausea, diarrhea, abdominal cramps, or tachycardia). Corticosteroids (usually prednisone) are directed toward reducing the levels of serum ACh receptor antibodies. Corticosteroids may temporarily worsen manifestations; however, this is followed by gradual improvement in muscle strength.

After a peak of improvement is reached and maintained for several weeks, the dosage of both prednisone and anticholinesterase medication may be gradually decreased. A low maintenance dose of alternate-day prednisone may be effective for many months or years. Precautions with any steroid therapy are important, including potassium supplements if indicated and liberal use of antacids.

Potential complications of steroid use are cataracts, hypertension, diabetes, fluid retention, delayed wound healing, insomnia, and osteoporosis. Other treatments include azathioprine (Imuran) and cyclosporine (Sandimmune), which reduce the level of circulating ACh receptor antibodies, and plasmapheresis and IVIG.

Plasmapheresis

Plasmapheresis is an adjunctive therapy for clients with refractory MG. It is a process by which plasma is separated from formed elements of blood. The plasma is discarded and the packed red blood cells are joined with albumin, normal saline, and electrolytes and returned to the client. The purpose is to remove plasma proteins containing antibodies that are believed to cause MG. Plasmapheresis may produce transient improvement in clients who have actual or pending respiratory failure.

Usually, three to five treatments given once daily over 5 to 7 days are required. Potential complications include myasthenic or cholinergic crisis and, rarely, hypovolemia. Muscle strength should be assessed before and after the procedure, with particular attention paid to vital capacity, swallowing ability, diplopia, and ptosis to evaluate the effectiveness of the treatment.

Complications

Two major complications of MG may occur: *myasthenic crisis* and *cholinergic crisis* (see the Critical Monitoring feature on Myasthenic and Cholinergic Crises in Clients with Myasthenia Gravis at right).

Myasthenic Crisis. Clients with moderate or severe generalized MG, especially those who have difficulty swallowing or breathing, may experience a sudden worsening of their condition. This is usually precipitated by an intercurrent infection or sudden withdrawal of anticholinesterase drugs, but it may occur spontaneously. If an increase in the dosage of the anticholinesterase drug does not improve the weakness, endotracheal intubation and mechanical ventilation may be required. In many instances, drug responsiveness returns in 24 to 48 hours, and weaning from the respirator can proceed.

Cholinergic Crisis. Cholinergic crisis occurs as a result of overmedication. The muscarinic effect of a toxic level of anticholinesterase medication causes abdominal

---

CRITICAL MONITORING
Myasthenic and Cholinergic Crises in Clients with Myasthenia Gravis

Myasthenic Crisis Is Caused by Undermedication

Clinical Manifestations

Sudden marked rise in blood pressure due to hypoxia

Increased heart rate

Severe respiratory distress and cyanosis

Absent cough and swallow reflex

Increased secretions, increased diaphoresis, and increased lacrimation

Restlessness, dysarthria

Bowel and bladder incontinence

Intervention

Increased doses of cholinergic drugs as long as the client responds positively to edrophonium treatment

Possible mechanical ventilation if respiratory muscle paralysis is acute

Cholinergic Crisis Is Caused by Depolarization Block Resulting from Excessive Medications

Clinical Manifestations

Weakness with difficulty swallowing, chewing, speaking, and breathing

Apprehension, nausea, and vomiting

Abdominal cramps and diarrhea

Increased secretions and saliva

Sweating, lacrimation, fasciculations, and blurred vision

Intervention

Discontinue all cholinergic drugs until cholinergic effects decrease

Provide adequate ventilatory support

1 mg intravenous atropine may be necessary to counteract severe cholinergic reactions

---

cramps, diarrhea, and excessive pulmonary secretions. The nicotinic effect paradoxically worsens weakness and can cause bronchial spasm. If respiratory status is compromised, the client may need intubation and mechanical ventilation.

■ Nursing Management of the Medical Client

Clients with MG are usually managed in an outpatient setting. When clients are hospitalized for diagnosis or during a crisis, the following nursing management procedure may be pertinent.

Because MG may involve the muscles of respiration, the client may experience dyspnea and ineffective cough and swallow mechanisms, which may lead to aspiration and pneumonia. Encourage deep breathing and coughing. Have suction equipment available at the bedside, and instruct the client on how to use it. Instruct the client to sit upright when eating, to swallow only when the chin is tipped downward toward the chest, and never to speak while food is in the mouth. Oxygen and, in severe cases, mechanical ventilation may be required.

In MG, weakness is usually greatest following exertion and at the end of the day. Activities should be carefully planned to include rest periods so that energy is conserved and the muscles have a chance to regain their strength. Rearrangement of the home environment may help prevent unnecessary energy expenditure. Vocational retraining may be indicated for those who can no longer meet the physical demands of their jobs. Clients with severe disease or an acute exacerbation will be totally dependent on nursing care for ADL. This level of care requires that complications of immobility be avoided.

Provide the client and family with information about MG and its treatment. They should be aware of adverse reactions of both anticholinesterase drugs and steroids. Explain how to recognize myasthenic and cholinergic crises and how to have a plan to seek medical intervention, if necessary.

■ Surgical Management

Thymectomy can be used for treatment. The thymus gland, located in the superior mediastinum, is important during fetal growth for development of the immune system. It is usually atrophied and nonfunctioning in adulthood. The effect of thymectomy is not fully understood. It may alter some immunologic control mechanism that affects the production of antibodies to the ACh receptor, or it may eliminate a trigger to antibody production. Thymectomy is indicated for clients with thymoma, selected clients with generalized MG without thymoma, and selected clients with disabling ocular MG.[14] The procedure is recommended early in the course of the disease. Nursing management is similar to care following thoracic surgery.

EATON-LAMBERT (MYASTHENIC) SYNDROME

Eaton-Lambert syndrome (also called *myasthenic syndrome*) is a myasthenia-like condition in which weakness is noted in the limbs. It is characterized by defective release of ACh, possibly caused by autoantibodies (IgG). Eaton-Lambert syndrome is found almost exclusively in people with oat cell carcinoma of the lung and has been noted less often in people with cancers of the prostate, stomach, rectum, and breast.

The onset is insidious, and clinical manifestations are progressive. Compared with MG, diplopia is less common and there is proximal weakness of the legs, arms, and pelvic girdle. Muscle action potential is reduced when muscle is stimulated, but repetitive stimulation augments muscle action. Weakness tends to develop with exertion, although some clients have a temporary increase in power when muscles are repeatedly stimulated. Autonomic dysfunction is common, presenting as dry mouth, impotence, and peripheral paresthesias.

Treatment is directed at the primary cancer. Guanidine HCl may improve manifestations by increasing ACh release. Plasmapheresis and immunotherapy have also been used. Calcium-channel blockers can worsen the transmission defect. Because MG can precede the development of cancer by many years, clients with Eaton-Lambert syndrome should be assessed yearly for the development of cancer.

AMYOTROPHIC LATERAL SCLEROSIS

Amyotrophic lateral sclerosis (ALS) is the most common of the motor neuron diseases. It is an age-dependent, fatal paralytic disorder also known as *Charcot's disease* and *Lou Gehrig's disease*. Onset is usually in middle age. Men are affected more often than women. The overall incidence of ALS is 0.4 to 1.8 per 100,000, and the prevalence is 4 to 6 per 100,000.

Clinical Manifestations

Amyotrophic lateral sclerosis involves degeneration of both the anterior horn cells and the corticospinal tracts. Consequently, both upper and lower motor neuron clinical manifestations are seen. Lower motor neuron clinical manifestations include weakness, atrophy, cramps, and fasciculations (irregular twitchings of muscle fibers or bundles). Upper motor neuron manifestations include spasticity and hyperreflexia. Involvement of the corticobulbar tracts causes dysphagia (difficulty swallowing) and dysarthria (slurred speech). The sensory system is not involved, and cognition is not affected. The client remains alert and mentally intact throughout the course of the disease.

The course of the disease is relentlessly progressive. Death usually results from pneumonia caused by respiratory compromise within 2 to 5 years.

Weakness typically begins in the upper extremities and progressively involves the upper arms and shoulders and then the muscles of the neck and throat. The trunk and lower extremities are usually not affected until late in the disease. When the intercostal muscles and diaphragm become involved, respirations are shallow and coughing is ineffective. Cognition, as well as bowel and bladder sphincters, remains intact, even when the client is totally debilitated. In some cases, weakness begins in the brain stem, causing problems with speech and swallowing. This is called *bulbar ALS*.

Diagnosis of ALS is made by the clinical presentation and EMG. The EMG criteria for the diagnosis of ALS include the presence of widespread anterior horn cell dysfunction with fibrillations, positive waves, fasciculations, and chronic neurogenic motor unit potential changes in multiple nerve root distribution in at least three limbs and the paraspinal muscles in the presence of normal sensory responses.

Outcome Management

Supportive therapy was the only intervention for ALS until riluzole (Rilutek) was approved in 1996. Its mechanism of action is unknown, but it is thought to have a neuroprotective effect. The drug extends the life of ALS clients by a few months. Clients with ALS are usually admitted to health care facilities only twice in their illness, first for diagnosis and later in the final stage of debilitation.

The antibiotic minocycline is being studied for ALS. Laboratory studies have linked inducible nitric oxide and caspase enzyme activation to motor nerve cell death in ALS. Minocycline is in the tetracycline group of antibiotics that penetrates barriers around the CNS when taken orally and helps to inhibit caspase enzymes, which are involved in cell death pathways. Genetic treatments are also being researched.

 Supportive nursing care is an important aspect of managing the ALS client. In the outpatient arena, the nurse can provide ongoing assessment of daily living needs and make suggestions for modifications in activity level, clothing, and diet. Often just allowing the client or family to talk about problems reduces anxiety and helps them find solutions to problems.[19] Interventions should be aimed at conserving energy. Activities should be spaced during the day. Muscle stress, strenuous activity, and extremes of hot and cold should be avoided. Leg braces, canes, and walkers can prolong independence in ambulation. Hand braces, special utensils, and adaptive devices such as buttonhooks can help with dressing and self-feeding. Pressure ulcers are not usually a problem because the sensory system remains intact and the client can feel when pressure on a body part is too great.

In the acute care setting, gather information from the client and family about communication needs and which positions are best for respiration, handling secretions, eating, and turning routines.

Encourage fluid intake regularly, when the client is not fatigued. Proper positioning is imperative. Providing a cup with a spout may prevent liquid from running out of the corners of the mouth. Give liquids by using a large syringe with short tubing on the tip. The tube is placed on the anterior portion of the tongue, and gentle force is used to deliver small amounts of liquid.

Encourage small, frequent, high-nutrient feedings. Tell the client to sit upright, with the head slightly flexed forward while eating. Papase tablets placed under the tongue 10 minutes before meals can make thick saliva less sticky. Plenty of time should be allowed for eating, and the client should not attempt to speak while food is in the mouth. Have suction equipment available during meals to reduce the risk of aspiration of food and secretions that become lodged in the mouth and pharynx. The

head may need to be stabilized with a soft cervical collar. Consult the dietitian for special diet recommendations.

Although speech remains intelligible, the client can be trained to slow the rate of speech and exaggerate articulation. As manifestations progress, the client may need to repeat words or have an interpreter (usually the spouse). At this stage, it is important to eliminate extraneous noise, face the client when he or she is talking, and maintain eye contact. When the client's speech contains only one-word phrases or is no longer possible, writing can be an effective means of communicating and should be encouraged. When writing is no longer possible, a speech pathologist can provide communication devices such as alphabet boards and portable memo writers.[9]

If the client is a smoker, encourage him or her to stop. Exposure to people with respiratory infections should be avoided. Remind the client to use good posture. Pulmonary function tests should be performed regularly to assess ventilatory status. Clients generally experience respiratory fatigue when vital capacity is less than 1.5 L. Some clients can be taught to use their abdominal muscles to enhance respirations when the intercostal muscles and diaphragm become weak. A manifestation of pending respiratory insufficiency is shortness of breath while eating.

Encourage the client and family to talk about the losses they are experiencing and the feelings associated with them. Family members should be encouraged to take time for rest and activities away from the client. Refer the client and family to an ALS support group.

Eventually clients face the difficult choice of deciding whether they will accept artificial ventilation. Encourage them to discuss this with family and friends and to seek input from ALS support groups. Encourage clients to complete advance directives to indicate whether they desire life-sustaining treatments such as cardiopulmonary resuscitation, but this should be reassessed at regular intervals. Clients may change their minds on the basis of their experience with their illness, changes in their subjective appreciation of their quality of life, or changes in their evaluation of the benefits and burdens of life-sustaining measures as they come to terms with the imminence of death.[21]

CONCLUSIONS

Degenerative neurologic disorders have many causes, including viruses, autoimmune responses, and heredity. Some have no known cause. In general, they are relentlessly progressive, slowly taking away both physical and mental ability. Nurses should focus care on the management of clinical manifestations and prevention of complications. Family support throughout the process of care is essential.

THINKING CRITICALLY *evolve*

1. A 52-year-old man with multiple sclerosis is wheelchair-bound and has a neurogenic bladder. He complains of a sudden onset of generalized weakness, fever, and chills and is admitted to the hospital. What priorities should be set for his care?

Factors to Consider. What do generalized weakness, fever, and chills suggest in *any* client? If your client has not been following good bladder management, how can you intervene?

2. A 70-year-old man with Parkinson's disease is admitted to the hospital after experiencing severe nightmares and periods of confusion. During lucid periods, he is very disturbed by these manifestations. At other times, he believes that his wife is participating in a conspiracy to harm him. What assessments and interventions should you consider?

Factors to Consider. Are hallucinations and paranoia typical manifestations of Parkinson's disease? Might the client's manifestations be related to treatment or to some cause other than Parkinson's disease?

3. A 41-year-old woman with myasthenia gravis is taking pyridostigmine and prednisone. She is complaining of increased fatigue and weakness and has difficulty breathing. What concerns should you have?

Factors to Consider. Might the client's difficulty breathing be related to her fatigue and weakness? Could these manifestations be related to myasthenia gravis or its treatment?

Discussions for these questions can be found on the website and the CD-ROM.

BIBLIOGRAPHY

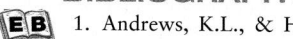 1. Andrews, K.L., & Husmann, D.A. (1997). Bladder dysfunction and management in multiple sclerosis. *Mayo Clinic Proceedings, 74*, 1176-1183.

2. Brown, P. (1997). The risk of bovine spongiform encephalopathy ('mad cow disease') to human health. *Journal of the American Medical Association, 278*(12), 1008-1011.

3. Friedlander, R. (2003). Apoptosis and caspases in neurodegenerative diseases. *New England Journal of Medicine, 348*(14), 1365-1375.

4. Gwyther, L.P. (2000). Family issues in dementia: finding a new normal. *Neurology Clinics, 18*(4), 993-1010.

5. Halper, J., et al. (2003). Rethinking cognitive function in multiple sclerosis: A nursing perspective. *Journal of Neuroscience Nursing, 35*(2), 70-81.

6. Hecht, M.J., et al. (2003). Burden of care in amyotrophic lateral sclerosis. *Palliative Medicine, 17*(4), 327-333.

7. Hogancamp, W.E., Rodriguez, M., & Weinshenker, B.G. (1997). The epidemiology of multiple sclerosis. *Mayo Clinic Proceedings, 74*, 871-878.

8. Jones, P.S., & Martinson, I.M. (1992). The experience of bereavement in care givers of family members with Alzheimer's disease. *Image—The Journal of Nursing Scholarship, 24*(3), 174-176.

9. Lang, A.E., & Lozano, A.M. (1998). Parkinson's disease. *New England Journal of Medicine, 339*(16), 1130-1143.

10. Le Bars, P.L., et al. (1997). A placebo-controlled, double-blind, randomized trial of an extract of ginkgo biloba for dementia. *Journal of the American Medical Association, 278*(16), 1327-1332.

11. Levin, L.I., Munger, K., Ruberton, M., et al. (2003). Multiple sclerosis and Epstein Barr virus. *Journal of the American Medical Association, 289*(12), 1533-1536.

12. Lucchinetti, C.F., & Rodriguez, M. (1997). The controversy surrounding pathogenesis of the multiple sclerosis lesion. *Mayo Clinic Proceedings, 74*, 665-678.

13. Mayo Foundation for Medical Education and Research. (1996, October). Alzheimer's disease: Living with a 'long goodbye.' *Mayo Clinic Health Letter* (Suppl), 1-8.

14. Mezey, M., et al. (1996). Life-sustaining treatment decisions by spouses of patients with Alzheimer's disease. *Journal of the American Geriatrics Society, 44*(2), 144-150.

15. Nowotny, M.L. (1998). My journey with amyotrophic lateral sclerosis. *Journal of Neuroscience Nursing, 30*(1), 68-70.

16. Perry, J. (2002). Wives giving care to husband's with Alzheimer's disease: a process of interpretive caring. *Research in Nursing and Health, 25* (4), 307-316.

17. Post, S.G., et al. (1997). The clinical introduction of genetic testing for Alzheimer disease: An ethical perspective. *Journal of the American Medical Association, 277*(10), 832-836.

18. Prusiner, S. (2001). Neurodegenerative diseases and prions. *New England Journal of Medicine, 344*(20), 1516-1524.

19. Robinson, L. (2003). The importance of touch for the patient with dementia. *Home HealthCare Nurse, 21*(1), 16-19.

20. Robinson, B.E. (1997). Guideline for initial evaluation of the patient with memory loss. *Geriatrics, 52*(12), 30-39.

21. Rodriguez, M. (1997). Multiple sclerosis: Insights into molecular pathogenesis and therapy. *Mayo Clinic Proceedings, 74*, 663-664.

22. Rudick, R.A., et al. (1997). Management of multiple sclerosis. *New England Journal of Medicine, 337*(22), 1604-1611.

23. Vrabec, N.J. (1997). Literature review of social support and caregiver burden, 1980 to 1995. *Image—The Journal of Nursing Scholarship, 29*(4), 383-388.

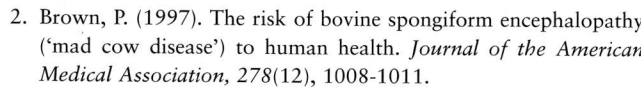 *evolve* Did you remember to check out the bonus material on the Evolve website and the CD-ROM, including free self-assessment exercises?

Chapter 75

Management of Clients with Neurologic Trauma

Norma D. McNair
Judi L. Kuric

evolve

Web Enhancements

http://evolve.elsevier.com/Black/medsurg/

Case Study
  Spinal Cord Injury
Client Education Guide
  Monitoring Family Members After Head Injury (English Version
    and Spanish Translation)
  Use of a Halo Vest (English Version and Spanish Translation)

Ethical Issues in Nursing
  What Is the Government's Obligation to Put Care for Its
    Citizens Above Care for Noncitizens, Given Scarce
    Resources?
Figure
  A Neurologic Observation Chart
Appendix C
  Laboratory Values of Clinical Importance in Medical-Surgical
    Nursing

The complexity of the central nervous system (CNS) allows the human organism to evaluate information about the outside world. Failure of the brain or the spinal cord to process information accurately prevents the affected person from accurately performing tasks and may impair interactions with others as well as self-appraisal.

Admission of a client with CNS trauma to the emergency department requires rapid mobilization of a trauma team. The team provides initial assessment and resuscitation of the trauma victim and performs triage to the appropriate radiologic studies and surgical service. Ultimately the management of a client with a head injury, spinal cord injury, or a combination of neurologic injuries is directed by the neurosurgical service. This chapter examines the needs of clients with CNS trauma, including head and spinal cord injuries.

INCREASED INTRACRANIAL PRESSURE

The skull is a hard, bony vault filled with brain tissue, blood, and cerebrospinal fluid (CSF). A balance between these three components maintains the pressure within the cranium. The modified *Munro-Kellie hypothesis,* a theory for understanding intracranial pressure (ICP), states that because the bony skull cannot expand, when one of the three components expands, the other two must compensate by decreasing in volume for the total brain volume and pressure to remain constant.

Intracranial pressure is the pressure exerted in the cranium by its contents: the brain, blood, and CSF (Figure 75-1). ICP is measured with a monitor in the ventricle, the brain parenchyma, or the subarachnoid space. The normal ICP is 5 to 15 mm Hg. Pressures greater than 20 mm Hg are considered to represent *increased ICP,* which seriously impairs cerebral perfusion. Recognition of increased ICP is one of the most important assessments made by nurses caring for clients with neurologic disorders.

Cerebral perfusion pressure (CPP) is the amount of blood flow from the systemic circulation required to provide adequate oxygen and glucose for brain metabolism. *Mean arterial pressure* (MAP) represents the average pressure during the cardiac cycle. It is calculated by adding the systolic pressure to twice the diastolic pres-

Nursing Outcomes Classification (NOC)
for Nursing Diagnoses—Clients with Neurologic Trauma

Anticipatory Grieving
Adaptive Coping
Psychosocial Adjustment: Life Change
Bowel Incontinence
Bowel Elimination
Self-Care: Toileting
Chronic Pain
Comfort Level
Depression Control
Lifestyle Adaptation
Constipation
Bowel Elimination
Hydration
Disabled Family Coping
Readiness for Enhanced Family Coping
Effective Family Therapeutic Regimen
   Management
Family Coping
Disturbed Thought Processes
Intact Short-Term Memory
Effective Problem-Solving
Cognitive Ability
Neurologic Status: Consciousness
Imbalanced Nutrition: Less Than Body
Requirements
Nutritional Status: Food and Fluid
   Intake
Impaired Gas Exchange
Respiratory Status: Ventilation
Vital Signs Status
Impaired Oral Mucous Membrane
Oral Health
Tissue Integrity: Skin and Mucous
   Membrane

Impaired Physical Mobility
Independent Walking
Independent Wheelchair Mobility
Independent Transfer Ability
Independent Bed Mobility
Activity Tolerance
Impaired Spontaneous Ventilation
Neurologic Status: Central Motor
   Control
Vital Signs Status
Ineffective Airway Clearance
Spontaneous Ventilation
Airway Patency
Ineffective Coping
Effective Therapeutic Regimen
   Management
Adjustment
Social Support
Ineffective Health Maintenance
Risk Detection
Social Support
Ineffective Therapeutic Regimen
Management
Compliance Behavior
Knowledge: Treatment Regimen
Treatment Behavior: Illness or Injury
Ineffective Thermoregulation
Thermoregulation
Ineffective Tissue Perfusion: Cerebral
Intracranial Adaptive Capacity
Interrupted Family Processes
Family Coping
Caregiver Role Performance
Role Performance

Social Support
Adjustment
Post-Trauma Syndrome
Adaptive Coping
Risk for Aspiration
Cognitive Ability
Functional Swallowing
Neurologic Status
Respiratory Status: Ventilation
Risk for Impaired Skin Integrity
Immobility Consequences: Physiologic
Tissue Integrity: Skin and Mucous
   Membranes
Risk for Injury
Neurologic Status
Risk Control
Self-Care Deficit
Self-Care: Activities of Daily Living
Self-Care: Feeding
Self-Care: Hygiene
Self-Care: Toileting
Direction of Self-Care
Sexual Dysfunction
Sexual Functioning
Role Performance
Total Urinary Incontinence
Urinary Elimination
Self-Care

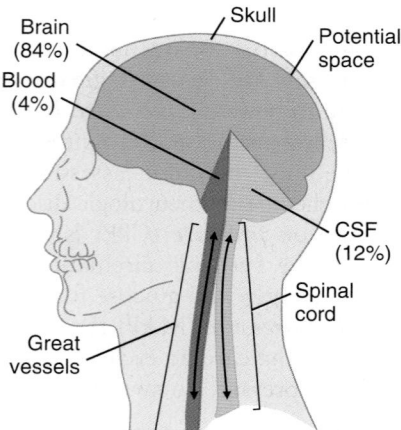

FIGURE 75-1 Components of the intracranial vault. A balance between these three compartments maintains normal intracranial pressure.

sure and dividing by 3. (Diastole is twice as long as systole.) The formula for calculating CPP is as follows:

$$CPP = MAP - ICP$$

When MAP and ICP are equal, there is no CPP and brain perfusion ceases. Therefore it is crucial to maintain control of ICP and MAP.

Etiology and Risk Factors
Increased ICP is most often associated with a space-occupying lesion, a cerebral infarction, an obstruction to the outflow of CSF, an abscess, an ingested or accumulated toxin, impaired blood flow to or from the brain, vasodilation from increased carbon dioxide ($PaCO_2$) or decreased partial pressure of oxygen (PaO_2), systemic hypertension, or increased intrathoracic pressure. Risk factors include head injury, brain tumors, cerebral bleeding, hydrocephalus, and edema from surgery or injury.

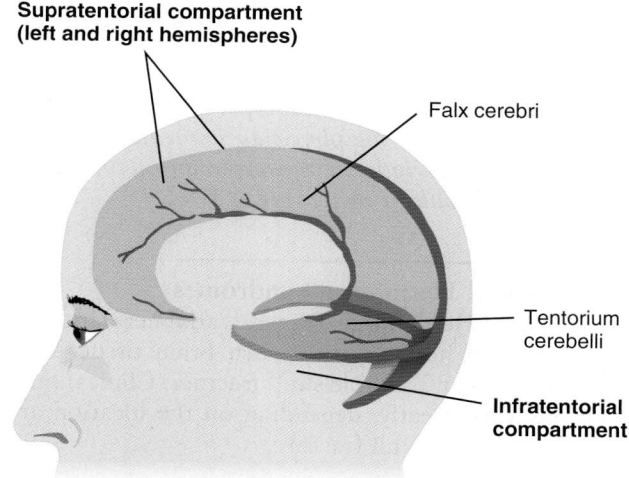

Supratentorial compartment (left and right hemispheres)

Falx cerebri

Tentorium cerebelli

Infratentorial compartment

FIGURE 75-2 The intracranial compartments are divided by inelastic fibers to provide support.

Pathophysiology

As an intracranial mass enlarges, initial compensation occurs through *displacement of CSF* into the spinal canal. The ability of the brain to adapt to increasing pressure without increasing ICP is called *compliance*. The movement of CSF out of the cranium is the first and major compensatory mechanism, but the cranial vault can accommodate increasing intracranial volume only to a point. When the compliance of the brain is exceeded, the ICP rises, clinical manifestations develop, and other compensatory efforts to reduce pressure begin.

The second form of compensation is *reduction of blood volume* in the brain. When blood flow is reduced by 40%, cerebral tissue becomes acidotic. When 60% of blood flow is lost, the electroencephalogram (EEG) begins to change. This stage of compensation alters cerebral metabolism, eventually leading to brain tissue hypoxia and areas of brain tissue ischemia.

The last stage of compensation and the most lethal is *displacement of brain tissue* across the tentorium, under the falx cerebri, or through the foramen magnum into the spinal canal. This process is called *herniation* and often results in death from brain stem compression. The brain is supported within various intracranial compartments (Figure 75-2). The supratentorial compartment contains all the brain tissue from the top of the midbrain upward. This section is divided into right and left chambers by the tough, inelastic fibers of the falx cerebri. The supratentorial compartment is separated from the infratentorial compartment (containing the brain stem and cerebellum) by the tentorium cerebelli. The brain is capable of some movement within these compartments. Pressure increases in one compartment affect surrounding areas of lower pressure.

With regard to ICP maintenance, *autoregulation* is the occurrence of compensatory changes in the diameter of intracranial blood vessels designed to maintain a constant blood flow during changes in CPP. Autoregulation is lost with increasing ICP. Small increases in brain volume can then cause dramatic increases in ICP, with a longer time required to return to baseline level. When ICP approaches systemic blood pressure, cerebral perfusion decreases and the brain suffers severe hypoxia and acidosis.

Cerebral Edema

The terms *cerebral edema, brain swelling,* and *increased ICP* are sometimes used interchangeably, but they are not the same. Cerebral edema and brain swelling are causes of increased ICP. An increase in brain bulk caused by an increase in cerebral blood volume is called *brain swelling. Brain edema,* in contrast, is an increase in the fluid content surrounding the tissues of the brain, such as in the extracellular spaces or the white matter, or within the cells themselves. The distinction between these two conditions is important because the interventions differ.

After head injury, edema develops because of a disruption of the blood-brain barrier. This type of edema is similar to other forms of edema, such as that seen in a sprained ankle. The fluid contains electrolytes, proteins, and blood. Edema reaches its maximum within 48 to 72 hours after brain surgery or injury. The fluid returns to the systemic circulation via the CSF or the venous system. This form of edema is usually treated with osmotic diuretics.

Brain swelling is also caused by increased blood volume resulting from dilated cerebral blood vessels. Brain swelling appears to be the major mechanism responsible for increasing ICP and for decreasing the size of the ventricles when compensation occurs. This form of swelling may be treated with therapeutic hyperventilation using mechanical ventilation to cause vasoconstriction.

Clinical Manifestations

Manifestations of increased ICP are caused by traction on the cerebral blood vessels from swelling tissues and by pressure on the pain-sensitive dura mater and various structures within the brain. The pathologic process of increased ICP actually comprises several entities that occur at the same time. No single set of clinical manifestations occurs in all clients. Indications of increased ICP relate to the location and cause of the raised pressure and to the speed and extent of its development.

Manifestations of increased ICP are subtle, and diligent observation for changes in the client's condition is necessary. Clinical manifestations include *any* alteration in level of consciousness (e.g., restlessness, irritability, confusion) and may include a decrease in the Glasgow Coma Scale (GCS) score. In addition, the client may have changes in speech, pupillary reactivity, motor or sensory ability, or cardiac rate and rhythm. Headache, nausea, vomiting, or blurred or double vision (diplopia) may be reported. The optic nerve is an extension of the brain, and increased tension in the skull is transmitted to the optic nerve to cause papilledema. *Papilledema* is swelling and hyperemia of the optic disc and can be observed only through an ophthalmoscope. Early detection (i.e., before clinical manifestations develop) by means of periodic ophthalmologic examination and ICP monitoring in the critical care unit can greatly improve a client's outcome.

Cushing's triad—increased systolic blood pressure with widened pulse pressure and bradycardia—is a late response and indicates severe increased ICP with failure of autoregulation. Respiratory patterns progress from Cheyne-Stokes respiration to central neurogenic hyperventilation to apneustic breathing and ataxic breathing as ICP increases (see Chapter 70). Hyperthermia is typically present when the hypothalamus is first affected by the increase in pressure, followed by hypothermia as ICP increases (Figure 75-3).

Common diagnostic studies performed to determine the source of increased ICP include skull radiography, computed tomography (CT) scanning, and magnetic resonance imaging (MRI). A lumbar puncture is not usually performed because of the risk of causing herniation of the brain stem when the pressure of the CSF in the spinal cord is lower than in the cranium. In addition, the CSF pressure at the lumbar level is not always an accurate reflection of the intracranial CSF pressure.

Herniation Syndromes

Herniation syndromes have been classified into five types (Figure 75-4). These conditions occur late in the course

of increased ICP and represent the body's last attempt to restore normal brain volume and pressure through displacement of blood, brain tissue, or CSF.

Herniation, regardless of the type, always constitutes an emergency. *Notify the physician immediately of any manifestations that indicate a worsening of the client's condition as a result of increasing ICP.*

Supratentorial Herniation Syndromes

Transcalvarial Herniation. Transcalvarial herniation occurs with open head injuries when brain tissue is extruded through an unstable skull fracture. Clinical manifestations vary greatly, depending on the location and extent of the open skull fracture.

Central Transtentorial Herniation. Central transtentorial herniation is the result of the downward displacement of the diencephalon through the tentorial notch. It is caused by injuries or masses located in the cerebral cortex or on the outward perimeter of the cerebrum. An early indication of central transtentorial herniation is a rapid change in the level of consciousness. As the pressure increases, changes in respiratory patterns are seen: first, Cheyne-Stokes respirations and then central neurogenic hyperventilation; later, apneustic breathing and also ataxic breathing (Biot's respiration); and, fi-

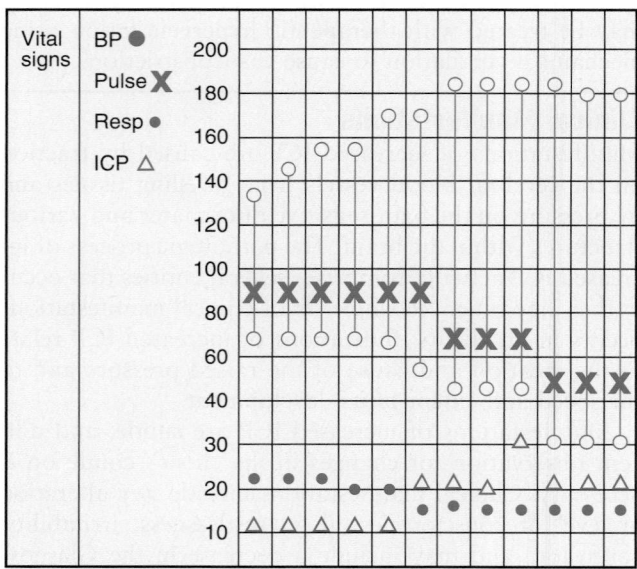

FIGURE 75-3 A late response to increased intracranial pressure is Cushing's triad (also called Cushing's response): bradycardia, systolic hypertension, and a wide pulse pressure, which result from pressure on the medulla. These manifestations can occur with intracranial hypertension or herniation. Alterations in the respiratory pattern also accompany Cushing's triad.

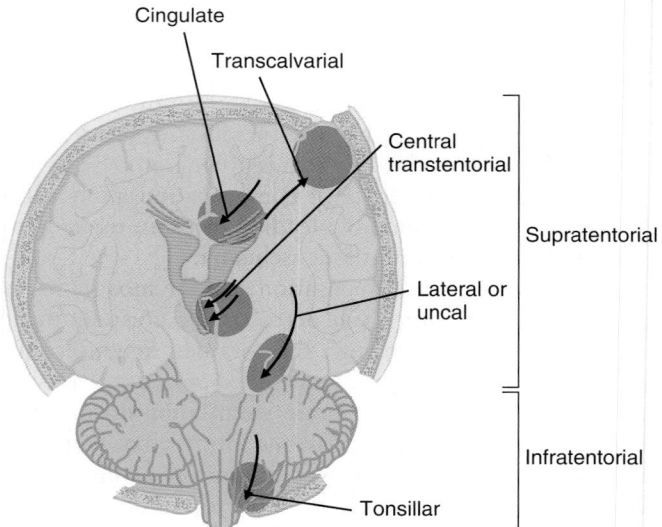

FIGURE 75-4 Types of intracranial herniation. In *transcalvarial* herniation, edematous brain tissue is extruded through the skull. In *central* transtentorial herniation, the lesion is located centrally or superiorly in the cranium, and compression of central and midbrain structures may result. In *lateral*, or *uncal*, herniation the lesion is located laterally within the cranium and can cause pressure on the midbrain. *Cingulate* herniation occurs between the two frontal lobes; the brain is pressed under the falx cerebri. In *tonsillar* herniation, the cerebellar tonsils are driven between the posterior arch of the atlas and the medulla and may be compressed.

nally, apnea (see Chapter 70). Pupils become small but at first remain reactive, with progression to a dilated and fixed state. Pathologic reflexes begin with Babinski's sign (see Chapter 69) and then progress from abnormal flexion to abnormal extensor posturing. Doll's eye reflex and a positive response to caloric testing are noted when brain stem function is still intact but are absent if the brain stem dies (see Chapter 70). The Critical Monitoring feature Manifestations of Changes in Neurologic Status on p. 2194 lists the specific areas of brain involvement that are correlated with pathologic manifestation.

Lateral Transtentorial Herniation. Lateral transtentorial herniation occurs from displacement by masses in or along the temporal lobe. It is also called *uncal herniation* because as the temporal lobe is compressed, the *uncus* (the anteromedial portion of the hippocampus) or the hippocampal gyrus shifts from the middle fossa through the tentorial notch into the posterior fossa. As the herniation progresses, the pupils first become sluggish in response to light and then become unresponsive; lack of response is seen first in the ipsilateral pupil and then in the contralateral pupil, secondary to third cranial nerve compression at the midbrain level. Other progressive clinical manifestations include a decreasing level of consciousness (stupor to coma), Cheyne-Stokes respirations followed by central neurogenic hyperventilation, and abnormal flexor posturing that progresses to abnormal extensor posturing.

Cingulate Herniation. Cingulate herniation occurs when the frontal lobes of the cerebrum are compressed, resulting in compression of the cingulate gyrus (an arch-shaped convolution situated just above the corpus callosum) under the falx cerebri. Manifestations are related to cerebral artery compression resulting in ischemia and congestion, edema, and increasing ICP.

Infratentorial (Tonsillar) Herniation Syndrome

Tonsillar herniation, also known as *cerebellar herniation,* occurs when the cerebellar tonsil shifts through the foramen magnum, compressing the medulla and upper portion of the spinal cord. Increasing pressure in the posterior fossa, often secondary to cerebellar bleeding, is the usual underlying problem. Manifestations often progress rapidly and include erratic changes in blood pressure, pulse rate, and breathing; decreased level of consciousness; an arched, stiff neck; and quadriparesis.

Outcome Management of Herniation Syndromes

Hyperventilation has been the standard treatment for herniation for many years. Based on the reduction in cerebral blood flow by vasoconstriction by "blow-ing off carbon dioxide," CPP is reduced in the brain. The tradeoff, however, is a serious reduction in arterial blood flow to the brain; therefore the routine practice of hyperventilation is questioned because the lack of arterial blood flow causes secondary brain injury. Today hyperventilation is used as a temporary measure for clients who exhibit manifestations of herniation.[9]

Outcome Management
■ Medical Management

The goals of medical management are to maintain cerebral oxygenation, to decrease ICP, to maintain optimal neurologic function, and to ready the client for rehabilitation.

Maintain Cerebral Oxygenation. The swollen or bruised brain has an increased need for oxygen and glucose because of an increased metabolic rate. The PaO_2 must be kept between 90 and 100 mm Hg. Hypoxemia (apnea, cyanosis, oxygen saturation below 90%) is corrected immediately by opening the airway or intubating the client. Routine prophylactic hyperventilation is avoided unless the client shows evidence of cerebral herniation (see later discussion).

Steroids have been prescribed for decades to control cerebral edema, and their use was shown to improve outcomes over 30 years ago. Recent studies, however, have not shown improve outcomes with steroids, and so the use of steroids remains unclear.[9]

Decrease Intracranial Pressure. Emergency care of the client at high risk for development of increased ICP focuses on maintaining the airway, improving breathing, and promoting circulation. Hypoxemia and hypotension are often associated with poor outcomes in head injuries. Immediate interventions may include intubation followed by hyperventilation, osmotic diuretics, and elevation of the head to promote venous drainage.

Cerebral Perfusion. Intravenous (IV) fluids are administered to avoid or limit hypotension and to prevent secondary brain injury. Vasoactive medication, given either to raise or lower blood pressure, may be required to maintain CPP at a normal level. CPP is a result of the relationship between blood pressure and ICP. If the physician has not left orders to treat blood pressure changes, notification must occur if the blood pressure range is below 100 or above 150 mm Hg systolic. Several clinical studies suggest that a CPP of 70 to 80 mm Hg is the critical threshold. Often physician orders specify titration of medication to maintain the CPP at greater than 70 mm Hg. General reduction measures include elevating the head of the bed, preventing obstruction of the jugular veins, controlling body temperature, preventing seizures, and sedation.

CRITICAL MONITORING

Manifestations of Changes in Neurologic Status

"Change" is the key word. Notify the physician whenever there is a change in the client's neurologic status. The following manifestations are listed in the order that indicates a *worsening* in the client's condition. Remember, a client may display a "transient" deterioration in neurologic responses that does not warrant calling a physician. For example, after you have just performed suctioning of the client's airway or have turned the client, you would anticipate a possible change in neurologic status. If you hyperoxygenate the client and ensure proper positioning for venous return from the jugular veins and airway maintenance, however, any manifestations of increased deficit should last only a few seconds or no more than 4 or 5 minutes. Worsening deficit that lasts longer than this increases the risk for irreversible brain injury and requires immediate attention.

Normal

Alert, oriented to person, place, time
Responds appropriately to verbal commands
Eyes open spontaneously with any stimulus, unless in a deep sleep

Abnormal; Changes Due to Altered Perfusion of the Cerebral Cortex

Altered level of consciousness
Altered perception of time, then place, and lastly person
Motor deficits (e.g., hemiparesis, hemiplegia)
Speech deficits (e.g., expressive or receptive speech or both)
Memory deficits (e.g., recent, intermediate, remote)
Hyperreflexia
Babinski's sign
Seizures
Decorticate rigidity
Emotional lability
Altered sensory interpretation
Cheyne-Stokes respiration
Headache, nausea, vomiting, papilledema

Abnormal; Changes Due to Altered Perfusion Just Inferior to the Cortex

Pupillary changes: asymmetry of size, shape, or time-responsiveness
Loss of reaction to direct light
Visual field changes (e.g., homonymous hemianopsia; see Chapter 72)

Abnormal; Changes Due to Altered Perfusion of the Diencephalon

Altered temperature; first high fevers, then hypothermia
Cheyne-Stokes respiration

Abnormal; Changes Due to Altered Perfusion of the Posterior Pituitary Gland

Diabetes insipidus (decreased antidiuretic hormone)

Abnormal; Changes Due to Altered Perfusion of the Midbrain

Dysfunction of CN III (loss of reaction to indirect or consensual light, dysconjugate eye movement)
Dysfunction of CN IV (dysconjugate eye movement)
Central neurogenic hyperventilation

Abnormal; Changes Due to Altered Perfusion of the Upper Pons

Dysfunction of CN V (altered sensory function to cornea, nasal membranes, face, oral cavity, tongue, teeth, or altered mastication)
Dysfunction of CN VI (altered lateral eye movement)
Dysfunction of CN VII (altered facial expression, taste, and salivation)
Central neurogenic hyperventilation
Abnormal extension posture
Pinpoint pupils

Abnormal; Changes Due to Altered Perfusion of the Lower Pons

Apneustic breathing
Flaccidity

Abnormal; Changes Due to Altered Perfusion of the Medulla

Dysfunction of CN VIII (altered equilibrium and hearing)
Dysfunction of CN IX (altered taste, pharyngeal sensations, and cough and swallowing)
Dysfunction of CN X (altered sensations in pharynx, larynx, external ear, and altered cough and swallowing; altered parasympathetic nervous system functions in thoracic and abdominal viscera)
Dysfunction of CN XI (altered neck and shoulder movement)
Dysfunction of CN XII (altered tongue movement)
Projectile vomiting
Cushing's triad (increased systolic blood pressure, wide pulse pressure, bradycardia)
Ataxic (Biot's respiration)

CN, Cranial nerve.

Hyperventilation. Hyperventilation had been recommended as the primary treatment of head-injured clients because carbon dioxide causes cerebral blood vessels to dilate. By manually hyperventilating or increasing the ventilator settings to cause hyperventilation, a hypocarbic (low carbon dioxide) blood level is created. A partial pressure of CO_2 ($PaCO_2$) level between 30 and 35 mm Hg results in vasoconstriction of the cerebral blood vessels, leading to decreased blood flow and thus decreased ICP. In traumatic brain injury, however, cerebral blood flow is reduced by as much as two thirds of normal and hyperventilation can seriously compromise cerebral perfusion. Therefore routine hyperventilation is no longer recommended unless the client is manifesting herniation. If the client has extensor posturing or pupillary asymmetry or nonreactivity, the client should be hyperventilated at a rate of 20 breaths/min until blood gas analyses can provide guidelines for ventilation rates.[9]

Mannitol. Mannitol, a hyperosmotic agent, is used to expand immediately the volume of plasma that increases cerebral blood flow and oxygen delivery. Mannitol has a delayed effect of creating an osmotic gradient and pulls fluid out of the cells, creating diuresis over the following hours. Mannitol may accumulate in the brain over time; so to reduce this risk, it is usually given in bolus doses rather than by continuous infusion. Renal function, electrolytes, and serum osmolality need to be monitored when the client is receiving mannitol. Diuresis is expected, and the client may become hypotensive and dehydrated with the excessive use of mannitol. Dehydration is manifested by increased serum sodium and osmolality values.[9]

Prevent Complications. Many complications are associated with head injury (Box 75-1). Antibiotics may be prescribed, especially with an open head injury, the placement of an ICP monitor, or an infection in another body system. Infections increase metabolism and thus raise ICP.

Anti-seizure medications (e.g., phenytoin, carbamazepine) are given prophylactically to reduce the risk of seizures. Seizures significantly increase metabolic requirements and cerebral blood flow and volume and thus increase ICP. Chapter 71 describes the care of the client with seizures.

Intravenous fluids are given by IV infusion pump to help monitor the amount of fluids given. The client is maintained in a state of euvolemia. Hypotonic IV solutions are avoided because of the risk of promoting cerebral edema.

Temperature reduction decreases metabolism and cerebral blood flow and thus ICP. Antipyretics should be the first intervention to reset the hypothalamic thermostat. Other cooling measures include hypothermic blankets, bathing with tepid water, or placement of ice packs. Muscle relaxants are given to prevent shivering.

BOX 75-1 *Complications of Head Injury*

- Cerebral edema
- Stress ulcers
- Seizures
- Infections
- Acute hydrocephalus
- Diabetes insipidus
- Syndrome of inappropriate secretion of antidiuretic hormone
- Cardiac dysrhythmias
- Neurogenic pulmonary edema
- Subarachnoid hemorrhage/aneurysms
- Altered behavior
- Post-trauma response

Malnutrition, with wasting of lean muscle mass, can develop quickly because of the metabolic response to severe head injury. Hypoglycemia must be avoided; glucose is the primary fuel for the brain. Hypoglycemia should be avoided by close monitoring. Furthermore, severe hypoglycemia can also result in seizures and coma. Nutritional support is provided with jejunal feeding to reduce the risk of gastric regurgitation and aspiration. Recommended calorie intake is 140% of resting metabolic expenditures in nonparalyzed clients and 100% of resting metabolic expenditures in paralyzed clients with 15% of caloric intake as protein. Nutritional support should begin by the seventh day after injury.[9]

Monitor Intracranial Pressure. Continuous ICP monitoring is used for clients experiencing conditions associated with potentially elevated ICP (e.g., head trauma with GCS scores of 8 and lower), preoperative and postoperative aneurysms, tumors, and posterior fossa lesions). ICP monitoring aids in earlier detection of intracranial mass lesions; it can limit the use of indiscriminate therapies to control ICP, which themselves can be harmful; it can reduce ICP by draining CSF and thus improve cerebral perfusion; it helps to determine prognosis; and it may improve outcomes.

Several methods of ICP monitoring are available. The most common types measure CSF pressure in the ventri- cles, brain parenchyma, or subarachnoid space. Intraventricular catheters provide the most accurate results. All monitoring devices are invasive and carry a risk of infection/colonization, hemorrhage, and obstruction, especially when the device is left in place for over 5 days.[9] Most surgeons prescribe antibiotics, limit the length of time for which the ICP monitor remains in place, and monitor CSF samples on a regular basis. The Bridge to Critical Care feature on Intracranial Pressure Monitoring on pp. 2196 and 2197 describes the nurse's role in caring for clients with these devices.

Monitoring ICP also allows the measurement of intracranial compliance. Introducing a known volume of

BRIDGE TO CRITICAL CARE

Intracranial Pressure Monitoring

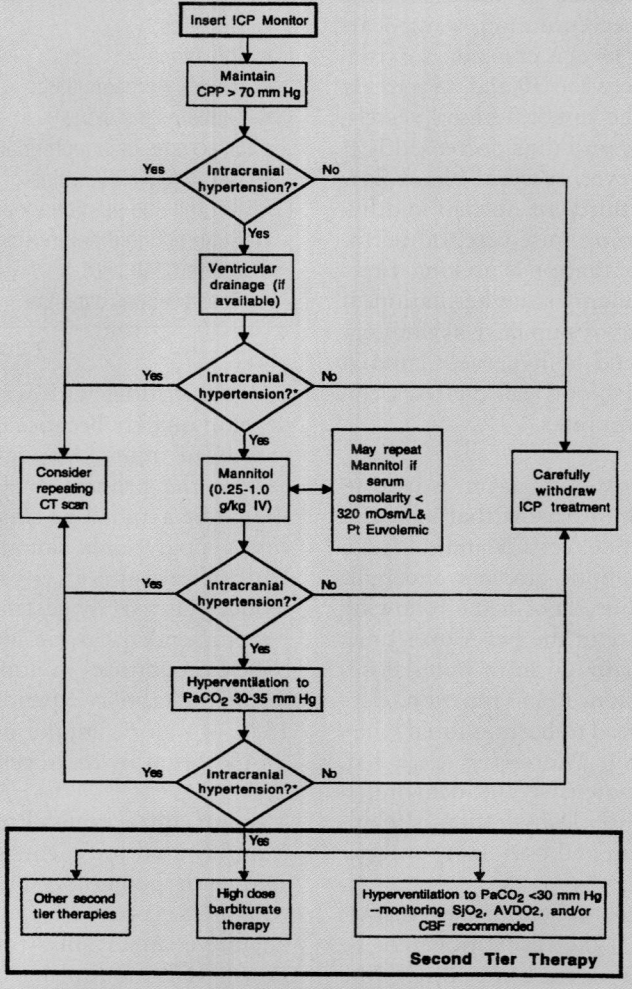

Intracranial Pressure Waveforms

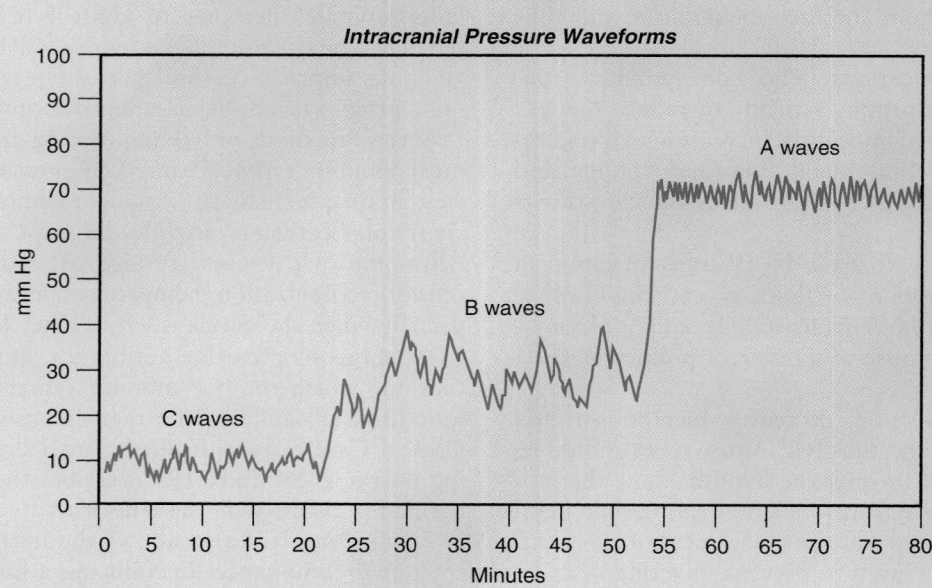

BRIDGE TO CRITICAL CARE

Intracranial Pressure Monitoring—cont'd

The shape of the waves is influenced by cardiac pulsations and respirations as well as by intracranial pressure (ICP).

C waves occur 4 to 8 times per minute and reflect fluctuations in arterial pressure. C waves are not considered significant.

B waves occur at intervals of 30 seconds to 2 minutes and represent increases in ICP to 50 mm Hg. They may be precursors to A waves.

A waves are most pronounced when the amount of cranial contents is increased. Also called *plateau waves*, A waves represent recurrent ICP elevations to 100 mm Hg. An A wave may be caused by coughing or straining but, if recurrent or sustained, may indicate a reduced ability of the brain to compensate. The client may also show other manifestations of increasing ICP.

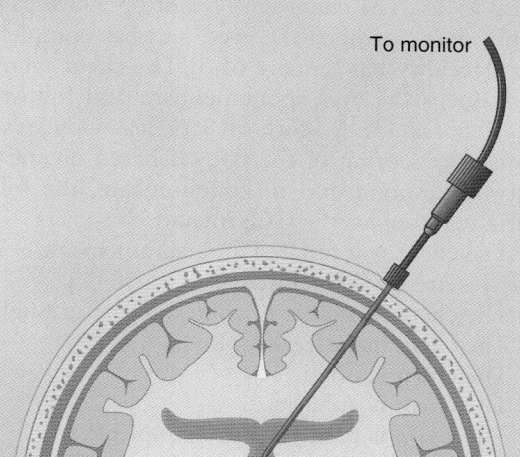

Ventricular catheter (ventriculostomy)

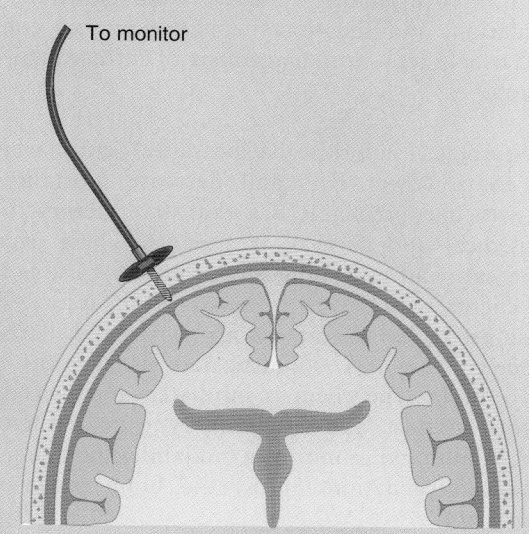

Subarachnoid screw (bolt)

General Interventions for Monitoring Intracranial Pressure

- Ensure that the tubing is long enough to allow the client to be moved in bed but that it is no longer than 14 feet. Use of tubing longer than 14 feet may cause inaccurate readings.
- Be careful to prevent kinks in the tubing.
- Place the catheter at the preset level of the transducer to take a reading.
- Use sterile technique when setting up the device.
- Monitor for manifestations of infection.
- Notify the physician if the readings show damping (lessening of amplitude) of the waves. The catheter may need to be flushed by the physician.
- If inaccurate readings occur, check for the following:
    Leaks in the system
    Differences in the height of the transducer and the device
    Kinks in the tubing
    Client activity or behavior involving performance of the Valsalva maneuver
    Obstruction in the system

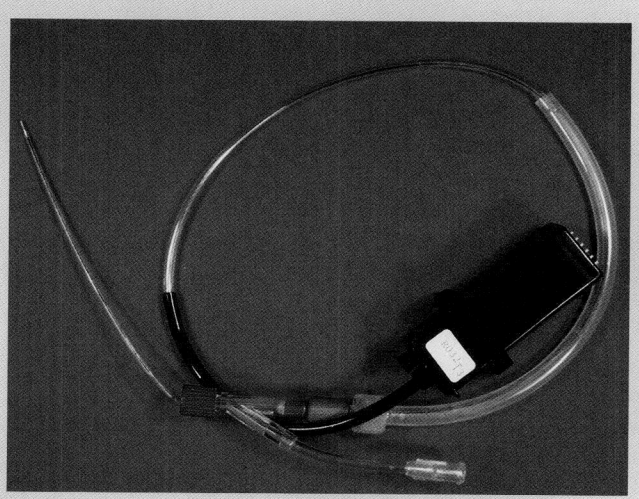

fluid into the ventricle and measuring its effect on ICP tests compliance. Detecting a change in the critical relationship between volume and pressure allows early treatment before the onset of clinical manifestations or sustained elevated ICP. Measurements of CPP can be made with ICP monitors. Ideally, CPP should be maintained at greater than 70 mm Hg.

Prevent Intracranial Hypertension. Intracranial hypertension is defined as an ICP greater than 20 to 25 mm Hg and can lead to a fatal herniation of the brain. When the herniation occurs at the level of the medulla, death is imminent. CSF drainage, mannitol administration, hyperventilation, and sedation/chemical paralysis constitute the usual steps in management of intracranial hypertension.

Barbiturates. High-dose barbiturates (pentobarbital) induce coma, lower ICP, and decrease mortality in clients with uncontrollable ICP that is refractory to all other medical and surgical treatments. These agents, however, can lead to hypotension, and their use is limited to clients with severe traumatic brain injury. Prophylactic use of barbiturates is not warranted. Barbiturate therapy requires sophisticated monitoring and special training. The client is intubated and placed on ventilatory support, and a pulmonary artery catheter is inserted. Additional monitoring modalities include jugular venous oxygenation ($SjvO_2$) and brain tissue oxygenation (tbO_2).[9]

Monitor serum drug levels daily; the dose should be reduced if serum levels exceed 5 mg/dl or if the burst suppression pattern on the EEG lasts longer than 10 seconds. Monitor temperature because barbiturates reduce metabolism, thereby cooling the body. If the temperature falls below 36° C, active warming is indicated.

Continue pupillary assessment. Even when a client is in a coma, the pupils dilate if the brain stem becomes compressed. Notify the physician of this change. Barbiturate therapy eliminates the client's normal protective functions. The client is completely dependent on nursing care for all basic needs (see Chapter 70). Wean clients slowly from barbiturate therapy to prevent rebound intracranial hypertension.

Neuromuscular Blocking Agents. Nondepolarizing neuromuscular blocking agents are sometimes used to induce skeletal muscle relaxation and to promote synchronous breathing during mechanical ventilation. Decreasing muscle activity may be necessary to control ICP. Nurses use a peripheral nerve stimulator to monitor for adequacy of drug dosage as well as for the risk of overdose (see Chapter 65). Pentobarbital and neuromuscular blocking agents usually are not given concomitantly. If the client is receiving a neuromuscular blocking agent, sedation and analgesia must be given because the neuro-

muscular blocking agents do not provide it. Other complications may result and are described in Box 75-1.

■ Nursing Management
Assessment

The Glasgow Coma Scale (GCS) is the most commonly used neurologic assessment tool in clinical care (Box 75-2). This scale provides objective measurement of three essential components of the neurologic examination: spontaneity of eye opening, best verbal response, and best motor response. The three scores can range from 3 to 15. The client who is unresponsive to painful stimuli, does not open the eyes, and has complete muscular flaccidity has a score of 3. The client who is oriented, opens the eyes spontaneously, and follows commands scores 15. A score of 8 or less indicates coma. Because the scoring of the GCS is based on the client's ability to respond and to communicate, the following criteria may render the GCS invalid:

- The client is intubated and cannot speak.
- Eyes are swollen closed.
- The client is unable to communicate in English.
- The client has a hearing loss.
- The client is blind.
- The client is aphasic.
- The client is paralyzed or hemiplegic.

The first GCS score recorded for the client becomes the baseline score. Subsequent scores allow assessment of trends or changes in neurologic status and provide a significant and reliable indicator of the severity of head injury. A single measurement cannot predict outcome; however a decrease of two points in the GCS with a score of nine or lower indicates serious injury. The use of consistent criteria for client assessment is more important than the specific tool used. Specific behaviors dictating a given score should be indicated. If variations occur in scoring criteria, the value of the scale is lost, and serious changes in the client's condition can be overlooked or treated unnecessarily (see the neurologic observation chart on the website). More detailed neurologic assessments are conducted to identify specific trends in responses.

Level of Consciousness. The first change in a client who presents with altered cerebral tissue perfusion is a change in the level of consciousness (LOC). When decreased LOC is noted, serial and detailed assessments are required until the client has achieved maximum recovery. To eliminate the subjectivity associated with use of terms such as *lethargy, obtundation, semi-coma,* or *coma,* the GCS both objectifies the client's LOC and assists in identifying very subtle changes.

Pupil Response. A pupil check includes assessing pupil appearance and physiologic response. The affected pupil

BOX 75-2   *Assessment of Clients Using the Glasgow Coma Scale*

The Glasgow Coma Scale (GCS) is a numeric expression of cognition, behavior, and neurologic function. It is the most commonly used scale and was designed to measure level of consciousness and severity of injury through eye opening, verbal responsiveness, and motor response. The total of the three scores ranges from 3 to 15, with 3 being the most severe and 15 being normal. Assessments of abstract thought and problem solving should be combined with the GCS to give a more complete picture of neurologic status.

Documentation should contain specific descriptive terms. For example, instead of just indicating that the client is "stuporous," record the evidence of stupor that you observe: "no response to verbal commands, responded only to tracheal suctioning with abnormal flexor posturing." Words such as "lethargic," "stuporous," or "comatose" or open to individual interpretation, and a clear description of behavior is less likely to be misunderstood.

Scale Components
Eye Opening
Observe eye opening without speaking to the client. Does the client open the eyes and look around? If the eyes are closed, call the client's name. If no response is noted, raise your voice. If there is still no response, use a mildly painful stimulus, given in the central part of the body, such as squeezing the trapezius muscle or rubbing the sternum.

Avoid supraorbital pressure, as it can cause damage to the eyes. Pinching of the body can cause severe bruising and is unnecessary in a neurologic examination.

Motor Response
Asking the client to follow specific commands such as "Raise your right arm" or "Wiggle your toes" assesses motor responses. Do not ask the client to squeeze your hand, because grasp is a reflexive response that can occur with head injury. If agency protocol lists grasp as a neurologic assessment component, ask the client to "let go" after grasping to measure cognitive ability to control movement.

In a client who is unable to follow commands, observe the response to a painful stimulus. Responses may include (1) localizing (trying to remove the stimulus), (2) withdrawing, and (3) posturing. In addition, a response may not be elicited and the client may remain motionless.

Compare the right and left sides and the upper and lower extremities. Record the best response while also recording any abnormality that indicates decreased movement in a particular extremity.

Motor Activity
Motor activity assessment is the measure of strength of voluntary movement of the arms and legs. If a client cannot cooperate with testing, paralysis may be difficult to detect. Observe the client carefully. If a client is restless, paralysis may become ob-

vious because the paralyzed part does not move as other body parts move. Additional information may be obtained by:
1. Comparing the tone of one side of the body with that of the other.
2. Lifting the arms or legs on both sides, releasing them, and watching them drop to the bed.
3. Observing the position of the limbs at rest.

If a client can cooperate, assessing "drift" may demonstrate subtle tone and strength alterations. For this assessment, have the client hold both arms up in front of the body with the palms upward and the eyes closed. Muscles are weak if one arm "drifts" (gradually moves) downward or if the hand pronates (turns over). This maneuver is often referred to as the *pronator drift test*.

Posturing
Review posturing in Chapter 70. As the client's intracranial pressure increases at the cortical level, abnormal flexor posturing occurs. As pressure reaches the pons level, abnormal extensor posturing occurs. When the pressure reaches further to the medullary level, flaccidity is noted, or a response is totally lacking—the gravest of all signs.

Verbal Response
Verbal responses assess the client's orientation to self, environment, and time. Ask appropriate questions such as the following: "What is your name? Where are you? What is the month, year, season, nearest holiday?" Avoid asking questions about the date or day of the week.

Being hospitalized can alter the accuracy of that response even in a person with normal cognitive function. Structure the conversation to elicit information that can be verified by family members, such as home address or employer's name. In many cases, a slight degree of confusion is not noticeable until some time is spent with the client. An apparently oriented client may ask the same question a few minutes after it was originally asked and answered, or the client may have "learned" the answers to common questions such as "What is your name?" and "What hospital are you in?" Therefore it is helpful to reassess the client regularly to check memory or to challenge cognitive integrity with various questions. If addition, observing the course of a normal conversation may give evidence of confusion or disorientation.

Scoring
After obtaining the data for all three parts of the GCS, total the points for each part and compare the score obtained with the client's baseline score. If a decrease in the score of even 1 point occurs, complete a detailed neurologic assessment, including pupillary responses, and notify the physician.

is usually on the same *(ipsilateral)* side as the brain lesion, whereas the motor and sensory deficits are usually on the opposite *(contralateral)* side. Be careful not to mistake a prosthetic eye for a fixed pupil.

Pupil Equality. Document pupil equality, noting the relative size of each pupil.

Pupil Size. Estimate the size of each pupil in millimeters (mm) before and after light stimulation. A penlight provides more accurate data than obtainable with a flashlight owing to the smaller size of the light and the ability to focus the beam directly at the pupil.

Pupil Position. Note whether the pupil is positioned in the midline or deviated from midline.

Pupil Reaction to Light. Bring the penlight from the lateral aspect of the client's head toward the eye. Observe for constriction in that eye as well as in the opposite eye. Then test the opposite eye in the same way. The detection of subtle change may require four approaches with the penlight. Brisk and equal constriction of the pupils to direct and indirect light is a normal response. Sluggish or unequal direct or indirect *(consensual)* response is abnormal. *Anisocoria,* or unequal pupils, occurs normally in about 17% of the population, with one pupil being about 1 mm larger. It is important to ascertain information about pupil inequality from the client or family members so that an unnecessary procedure is not performed.

Pupil Shape. Normally, pupils are round. Describe abnormal shapes with a drawing. Pupils may be oddly shaped as the result of previous eye surgery. A pupil that looks oval may be early evidence of increasing ICP.

Pupil Accommodation. Normally, the size of the pupil and the lens (which is not visible to the naked eye) accommodates (adjusts) to varying focal lengths. Having the client focus on a distant object and then quickly focus on a close object tests accommodation. Pupils should become smaller as the object is brought nearer the eye and should dilate when the object is moved away from the eye. Accommodation is often not tested in the acute care setting because of the client's inability to cooperate.

The acronym PERRLA is often used in practice and indicates that the *p*upils are *e*qual, *r*ound, and *r*eactive to *l*ight and *a*ccommodation. Notify the physician immediately if any change occurs in the pupillary response.

Eye Movement. Document any changes in eye movement. Observe the position of the eyes when assessing the pupils. The eyes should move together. If *dysconjugate* (not together) movement is noted, the physician should be notified.

Vital Signs. Initially vital signs should be assessed every 15 minutes until they are stable. Body temperature should be monitored every 2 hours. If hypothermia or hyperthermia occurs, temperature should be monitored continuously. Trends in vital signs and respiratory patterns should be analyzed. As ICP increases and herniation occurs at the level of the medulla, Cushing's response occurs (see Figure 75-3).

Vital sign changes are *late* changes. See the following discussion of altered cerebral tissue perfusion for care of a client with increasing ICP. Once the vital signs begin to deteriorate, many other changes have already occurred, such as a decrease in LOC. Ongoing monitoring for such changes is imperative; do not wait for vital signs to change because the delay may prove fatal for the client. Any changes in neurologic status may be significant and must be reported to the physician, no matter how minor they may seem.

Other assessments can also be made of the cranial nerves. Extraocular movements are tested on clients who are awake enough to follow directions. Ask the clients to follow your fingers with their eyes without moving the head. Move your fingers in a figure H, and observe both eyes as they move across, up, and down. Conjugate eye movements occur when both eyes move in a parallel motion. Dysconjugate eye movements occur when the eyes do not move in a lateral direction together (one eye may move laterally while the other is fixed or moves in another direction). Tracking occurs when the client is consciously following someone's or something's movement around the room.

The *blink reflex* can be tested by lightly stroking the eyelashes. When the eyelids are closed, they will flutter slightly if the reflex is present. Observe for blinking in the conscious and alert client. The *gag reflex* is tested by asking the alert client to cough or swallow. If the client is unable or unconscious, stroke the back of the client's throat with a long cotton-tipped swab. Gag reflex should be swift.

Note the symmetry of the facial muscles. Note the ability of the eyelids to open spontaneously and equally. Ask the client to close the eyes as tightly as possible. Ask the client to smile, and note the corners of the mouth to identify symmetrical patterns. Ask the client to frown/wrinkle the forehead. Finally, note whether speech is clear, slurred, rambling, or aphasic.

Diagnosis, Outcomes, Interventions

Diagnosis: Ineffective Tissue Perfusion: Cerebral.

If your patient is in a coma because of increased ICP, use this diagnosis to reflect the risk to cerebral tissue perfusion. Write the diagnosis as *Ineffective Tissue Perfusion: Cerebral related to increased ICP.* The term *patient* is used to refer to a person in a coma. The *client* in this case is the patient's family, who serves as his or her advocate.

Outcomes. The patient will maintain normal cerebral perfusion as evidenced by (1) stable or improving levels of consciousness; (2) stable or improving GCS score; (3) ICP of 15 mm Hg or less; (4) no restlessness, irritability, or headache; and (5) no pupillary changes, no seizures, no widening pulse pressure, no respiratory irregularity, and no hypertension or bradycardia.

Interventions. Administer the medications ordered to reduce cerebral edema (e.g., osmotic diuretics) and to decrease the risk of seizure (e.g., anticonvulsants), and monitor the patient's response to these medications. If the patient's baseline manifestations of increased ICP are not improving, if the patient's status deteriorates, or if seizures develop, notify the physician. Also, consult the physician for medication to promote bowel evacuation without straining because straining increases ICP. Disimpaction is not advised because of the vasovagal response that occurs.

Position the Patient. Place the patient supine with the head elevated 30 degrees unless contraindicated (e.g., with some spinal injuries, some aneurysms). Keep the patient's head in a neutral position to facilitate venous **EB** drainage from the brain. Avoid extreme rotation and flexion of the neck because these positions compress the jugular veins and increase ICP. Also avoid extreme hip flexion because this position increases intra-abdominal and intrathoracic pressure, which increase ICP. As the coma lightens, the patient may become disoriented and combative, making it difficult to maintain proper positioning. If restraints must be used, remember that they often increase agitation, which increases ICP.

Maintain a Patent Airway. Patients need to maintain a patent airway even in the presence of increased ICP. Suctioning assists in preventing buildup of secretions and **EB** CO_2 and a resultant elevation of ICP. Adequately oxygenate intubated patients before initiating suctioning, between suctioning efforts, and after suctioning. Try to limit suctioning to three passes, and limit each pass to 10 seconds. Nasal drainage may indicate a dural tear; therefore suctioning of the nares is contraindicated because of the risk of meningitis.

Balance Fluid Levels. In the past, only small amounts of fluids were administered to clients with head injury, in **EB** an effort to decrease cerebral edema. Current data indicate that fluid restriction may actually reduce blood volume and decrease cerebral circulation. The lack of volume causes the blood to be thick and sluggish and may decrease the mobilization of nutrition and toxins into and out of the circulation. Patients should be maintained in a euvolemic state rather than a fluid-restricted state. Fluid restriction may be appropriate for certain conditions (such as syndrome of inappropriate secretion of an-

tidiuretic hormone [SIADH]) but otherwise is contraindicated. Strict intake and output measurement is necessary to assess fluid balance.

Control Body Temperature. Hyperthermia increases ICP because of the increased metabolic demand. Therefore notify the physician immediately if hyperthermia occurs. If a patient's ICP is being managed with a hypothermia blanket, notify the physician if the patient's response is not within the prescribed parameters. Observe for shiv- ering because this phenomenon also increases metabolism and ICP. Assess for skin breakdown if cooling blankets are used for extended periods, especially in patients who are thin.

Monitor Intracranial Pressure. The ICP reading should be less than 15 mm Hg, the MAP reading 80 mm Hg or above, and the CPP reading above 70 mm Hg.

Plateau waves (A waves) are noted when ICP goes above 50 mm Hg and can be sustained for longer than 5 minutes. Whenever these sustained pressures are present, assess for contributing factors and intervene appropriately. For example, neck flexion, excessive hip flexion, airway secretions, excess water in the ventilator tubing, taping the endotracheal tube tightly over the jugular veins, and discussing the patient's condition at the bedside all have been known to increase ICP. Spacing and planning of nonessential nursing interventions (e.g., turning the patient) for when the patient's ICP is not elevated help to prevent plateau waves. Plateau waves may not be obvious on the ICP monitor screen; a printout generated at a slow rate may be required for accurate observation of these waves. Whenever ICP is over 20 mm Hg, interventions to decrease ICP should begin.

Assessing the ICP monitor site for infection and leakage, using sterile technique for dressing and drainage bag changes, and maintaining a closed system are helpful in preventing infection or in promoting early intervention if infection occurs. If CSF drainage is required, most systems have a stopcock for attaching the tubing and drainage bag that maintains the closed system, decreasing the likelihood of infection. The system is opened only to change the drainage bag. The drainage bag is changed using strict sterile technique.

Evaluation

Evaluate the client's response to treatment as often as every 15 minutes, progressing to hourly, then every 2 to 4 hours, and every 8 hours as the client improves. Once the physician has determined that the client's clinical condition has been optimized, the frequency and extent of evaluation can diminish even further. In the immediate and acute stages, anticipate ongoing modification in the care plan to help the client reach maximum recovery.

■ Surgical Management

Various surgical techniques are used to treat increased ICP. Optimally, the cause of increased ICP is located and removed. Other techniques include surgical placement of a ventriculoperitoneal shunt to allow drainage if CSF circulation is blocked (Figure 75-5) and decompressive surgery. The latter is done by removing some brain tissue (e.g., part of the temporal lobe) to give the remaining structures room to expand. If compliance is low during surgery, the bone flap removed to gain access to the brain is not replaced, or the dura may not be closed. Subsequent surgery is then required to repair the defect. Postoperative care is the same as that required after craniotomy (see Chapter 71). If the bone flap remains out, special care is required to keep the patient off the side of the defect and a helmet may be required until the bone flap is replaced.

TRAUMATIC BRAIN INJURY

Traumatic brain injury is an insult to the brain that is capable of producing physical, intellectual, emotional, social, and vocational changes. In the United States, a head injury is experienced approximately every 15 seconds. Head injuries occur in about seven million Americans every year. Among these head-injured people, more than 500,000 are hospitalized, 100,000 experience chronic disability, and about 2000 are left in a persistent vegetative state.[8,24]

In more than 30% of cases, because of the seriousness of the injury, head injuries are fatal before the injured person arrives at the hospital. An additional 20% die later because of secondary brain injury. Secondary brain events include ischemia from hypoxia and hypotension, secondary hemorrhage, and cerebral edema.[75]

Clients with traumatic head injuries often have other major injuries, including injury to the facial structures, lungs, heart, cervical spine, abdomen, and bones. Facial fractures and lung injuries may contribute to respiratory insufficiency. Airway obstruction and decreased ability to breathe (e.g., from pulmonary contusion, flail chest, pneumothorax) contribute to respiratory insufficiency and poor oxygenation of the brain and other tissues. Ischemia of brain tissue may result.

Hemorrhagic shock in clients with multiple trauma is rarely caused by head injury alone. Frequently shock is due to ruptured abdominal organs or musculoskeletal injuries (e.g., fractured femur and pelvis). Circulation may be further compromised by cardiac contusion and associated dysrhythmias.

Etiology and Risk Factors

Motor vehicle accidents are the leading cause of head injuries. Of clients admitted to the emergency room, most are males younger than 30 years of age and 50% have evidence of ingestion of alcohol or other substances of abuse. Alcohol slows the reflexes and alters cognitive processes and perception. These physiologic changes increase the chances of being involved in an accident or altercation. A second risk factor is driving without seat belts. Peak occurrence is during evenings, nights, and weekends. Other causes are assaults, falls, and sports-related injuries.

Mechanisms of Injury

Head injuries are caused by a sudden impact force to the head or inertial forces within the skull (Figure 75-6). The results are complex. Three mechanisms contribute to head trauma.

Primary injuries occur on impact and are the direct result of the impact resulting in injury to the area of the brain beneath the contact site. Skull fractures commonly occur (Figure 75-6, *A*). Diffuse injuries occur when a blow is received that does not result in fracture but causes the brain to move enough to shear or tear some of the veins going from the cortical surface of the brain to the skull. (Figure 75-6, *B*). Because the brain is able to move within the skull, movement of the brain can result in injuries at different locations. As the brain moves, it scrapes over the skull's irregular inner prominences, which bruise and lacerate brain tissue. Disruption of the brain's small surface blood vessels may occur. Changes in capillary integrity lead to fluid shifts and petechial hemorrhages. Cranial nerves, nerve tracts, larger blood vessels, and other structures may be stretched, twisted,

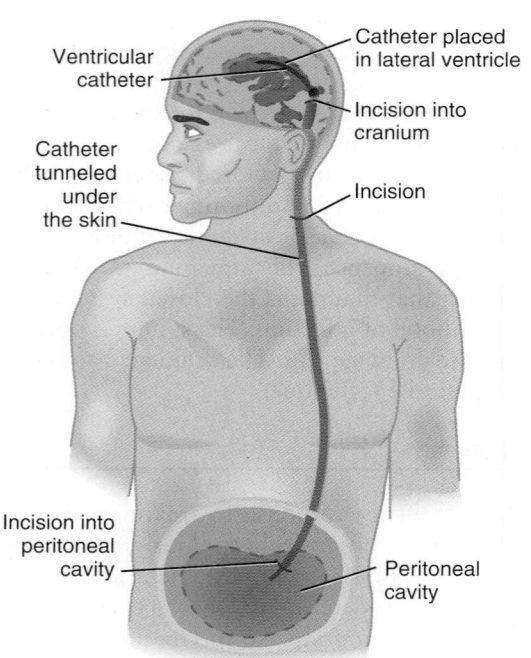

FIGURE 75-5 Ventriculoperitoneal shunt placed for chronic hydrocephalus.

or rotated, and their functions disrupted. An example is an automobile accident in which the head hits the steering wheel.

Coup-Contrecoup Injuries. A unique term can be used for this complex head injury: *coup-contrecoup injury.* From the French word *coup,* which means "blow," this diagnosis indicates that the client has sustained a combined injury at the point of impact and an injury on the side of the brain opposite from the movement of the brain within the skull. That is, a contrecoup injury (see Figure 75-6, C) from the French for "counterblow" (see also Figure 75-7).

Penetrating Trauma. *Penetrating injuries* are a form of primary injury and include head wounds made by foreign bodies (e.g., knives or bullets) or those made by bone fragments from a skull fracture. The damage caused by a penetrating injury often relates to the velocity with which a penetrating object pierces the skull and brain. Bone fragments from a skull fracture may cause local brain injury by lacerating brain tissue and damaging other structures (e.g., nerves, blood vessels). If a major blood vessel is severed or ruptured, a large clot *(hematoma)* may form, with resultant damage to adjacent or remote structures (e.g., brain compression as in a herniation syndrome). Thus a hematoma itself can cause extensive brain tissue damage.

High-velocity objects (e.g., bullets) produce shock waves in the skull and brain. The shock waves may significantly damage brain structures beyond those in the object's path. Frequently penetrating wounds create an open communication between the external environment

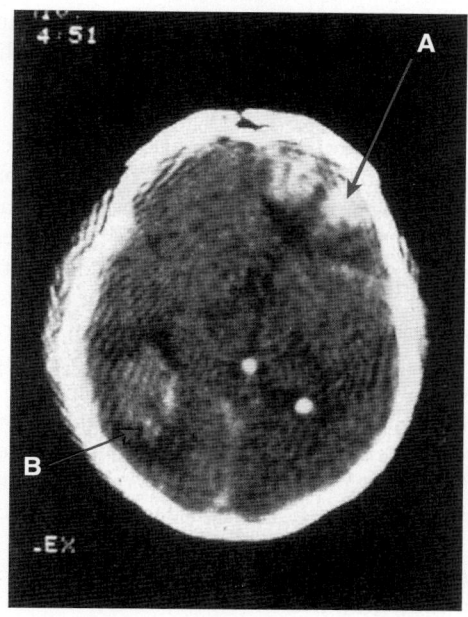

FIGURE 75-7 A magnetic resonance imaging scan showing coup (**A**) contrecoup (**B**) injury after head injury.

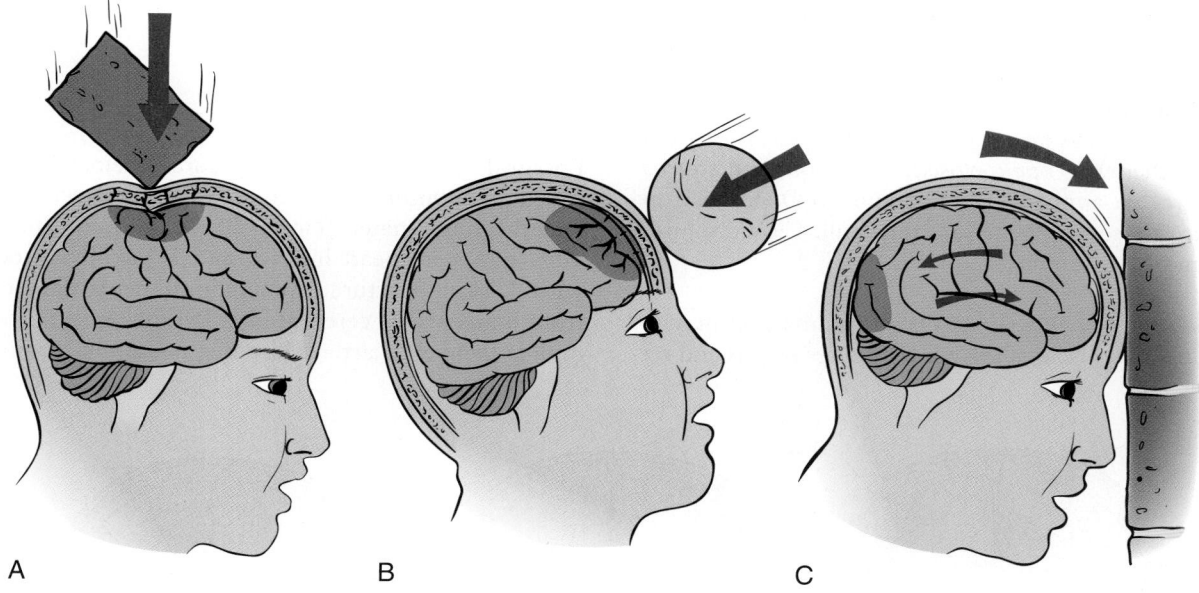

FIGURE 75-6 Some mechanisms of head injury. **A,** Penetrating injury may fracture the skull. **B,** Diffuse injuries such as a blow to the skull do not result in fracture; they may cause the brain to move enough to tear some of the veins going from the cortical surface to the dura. Subdural hematoma may then develop. Note the areas of cerebral contusion (dark brown). **C,** Rebound of the cranial contents may result in an area of injury opposite the point of impact. Such an injury is called a *contrecoup* injury. In addition to the direct damage sustained in the three injuries depicted, additional brain damage may occur.

and the cranial cavity, and infection is thus a possible complication.[8]

Scalp Injuries. Scalp injuries can cause lacerations, hematomas, and contusions or abrasions to the skin. These injuries may be unsightly and may bleed profusely. Clients with minor scalp injuries not accompanied by damage to other areas do not require hospitalization. The care of these injuries is discussed in Chapter 84.

Skull Fractures. Skull fractures are often caused by a force sufficient to fracture the skull and cause brain injury. The fractures themselves do not signal that brain injury is also present; however, skull fractures often cause serious brain damage. Depressed skull fractures injure the brain by bruising it (resulting in a contusion) or by driving bone fragments into it (causing lacerations). The site of a fracture and the extent of brain injury may not correlate.

The three types of skull fractures are as follows:
- *Linear skull fractures* appear as thin lines radiographically and do not require treatment; they are important only if there is significant underlying brain damage.
- *Depressed skull fractures* may be palpated and are seen radiographically.
- *Basilar skull fractures* occur in bones over the base of the frontal and temporal lobes. These are not observable on plain radiographs but may be manifested as ecchymosis around the eyes or behind the ears or by blood or CSF leakage from the ear.

Brain Injuries
A single classification of brain injuries does not exist; however, the terms *open, closed, contusion,* and *concussion* are often applied to brain injuries. Open head injuries are those that penetrate the skull. Closed injuries are from blunt trauma.

Concussions. A *concussion* is head trauma that may result in loss of consciousness for 5 minutes or less and retrograde amnesia. There is no break in the skull or dura, and no visible damage on a CT or MRI scans.

Contusions. Contusions are associated with more extensive damage than that from concussions. With contusions the brain itself is damaged, often with multiple areas of petechial and punctate hemorrhage and bruised areas in brain tissue. Diffuse axonal injury resulting in anatomic disruption of the white matter may result from serious contusions. Microscopic nerve fiber lesions also occur. Abnormalities may be located primarily in one area of the brain, but other areas may also be injured. This is particularly true of brain stem contusions, which are a very serious type of lesion.

Diffuse Axonal Injury. Diffuse axonal injury is the most severe form of head injury because there is no focal lesion to remove. The injury involves the tissue of the entire brain and occurs at the microscopic level. Diffuse axonal injury is classified as mild, moderate, or severe. With *mild diffuse axonal injury,* loss of consciousness lasting 6 to 24 hours is characteristic, and short-term disability may be associated with it. With *moderate diffuse axonal injury,* coma lasting less than 24 hours is the predominant clinical feature, with incomplete recovery on awakening. *Severe diffuse axonal injury* involves primary injury to the brain stem. The patient may present with abnormal posturing and in coma, but there may not be evidence of cerebral edema or increased ICP. Diffuse axonal injury begins with immediate loss of consciousness, prolonged coma, abnormal flexion or extensor posturing, hypertension, and fever.

Focal Injuries
Epidural Hematoma. An epidural hematoma, also called an *extradural hematoma,* forms between the skull and the dura mater (Figure 75-8). It occurs in about 10% of severe head injuries and is usually associated with a skull fracture. An epidural hematoma occurs from injury to the cerebral blood vessels, most often the middle meningeal artery. Bleeding is usually continuous,

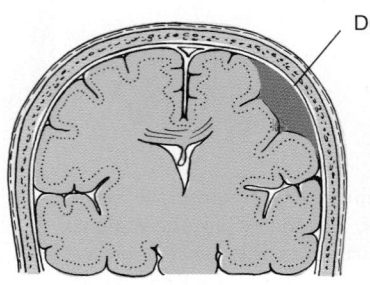
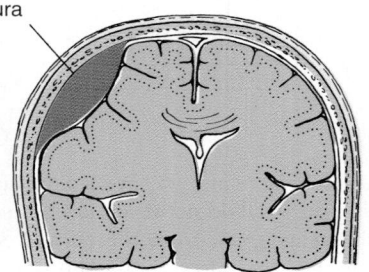
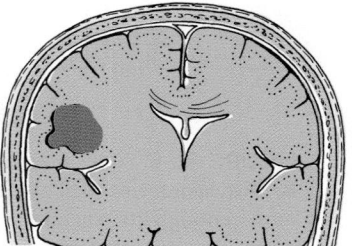

A. Subdural hematoma   B. Epidural hematoma   C. Intracerebral hematoma

FIGURE 75-8 Formation of a hematoma after head injury. Note movement of the brain structures.

and a large clot forms, which separates the dura from the skull.

Manifestations are usually acute in onset because the bleeding is often arterial. With an epidural hematoma, the following sequence of events may occur:

1. The client is unconscious immediately after head trauma.
2. The client awakens and is quite lucid.
3. Loss of consciousness occurs and pupil dilation response rapidly deteriorates, with onset of eye movement paralysis, on the same side as that of the hematoma.
4. The client lapses into a coma.

Although these manifestations are often described as "classic" for an epidural hematoma, few clients present with such classic manifestations, and astute assessment is necessary to prevent death.

Computed tomography scanning confirms the diagnosis. Rapid diagnosis and prompt intervention are essential with an epidural hematoma. Careful, ongoing assessment of neurologic status is also necessary.

Subdural Hematoma. Subdural hematoma is a collection of blood in the subdural space (i.e., between the dura mater and arachnoid mater). Tearing of the bridging veins over the brain causes most subdural hematomas.

Subdural hematomas may be classified as acute, subacute, or chronic, depending on how rapidly clinical manifestations develop. Another classification recognizes only acute and chronic, combining the acute and subacute categories.

Acute and Subacute Subdural Hematoma. Acute subdural hematoma usually results from brain or blood vessel laceration. Acute subdural hematomas are a serious complication requiring prompt treatment because they compress and distort an already damaged, edematous brain. Acute subdural hematoma is symptomatic within 24 to 48 hours of injury and is seen in about 24% of clients with severe head injuries.

Clinical manifestations of acute subdural hematoma are similar to those of acute epidural hematoma. The onset and development of the clinical manifestations may be somewhat slower because the bleeding is more often venous rather than arterial. Recognition of clinical manifestations may be difficult because subdural hematoma is often associated with moderate or severe brain injury. A patient who develops an acute subdural hematoma may remain unconscious after injury or may have a variable LOC (depending on the extent of injury). A conscious client usually has a headache. The client may become irritable and confused and lapse into a coma or show a fluctuating LOC. Manifestations of increasing ICP appear. Subtle changes in LOC and development of lateralizing changes (i.e., on one side) such as hemipare-

sis, pupillary dilation, or extraocular eye movement paralysis may be the only findings.

Chronic Subdural Hematoma. Chronic subdural hematoma is most common in older and alcoholic clients (Figure 75-9). These clients experience atrophy of the brain, which results in stretching of the bridging veins and an increase in the size of the subdural space. These stretched veins are easily ruptured in a fall, even if the fall does not result in other injuries. It develops several weeks or even months after injury because of a slow accumulation of fluid in a larger-than-normal space. Older or alcoholic clients may not even recall the mechanism of injury. The initial injury may have been relatively minor, and the client may not associate current clinical manifestations with the past injury. In addition, family members may not recognize the subtle neurologic changes or may not give credence to them because of the client's age or alcohol use.

Gradually the enlarging blood clot creates pressure on the brain. There is an interval during which the client appears to be recovering or seems completely recovered. Later, manifestations of neurologic deterioration develop. The client may become drowsy, inattentive, and incoherent and display personality changes. Headaches are another prominent symptom. These indications of chronic subdural hematoma may be overlooked until focal or lateralizing signs appear (e.g., hemiparesis, pupil signs). Changes in LOC continue, and LOC may fluctuate widely. Clinical assessment with subdural hematoma

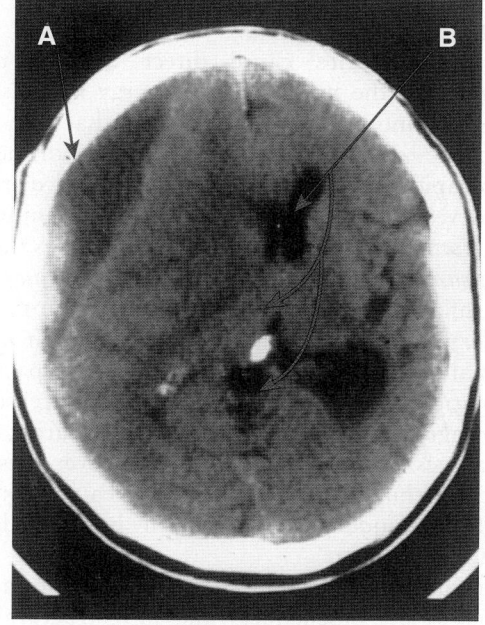

FIGURE 75-9 A, Magnetic resonance image of a chronic subdural hematoma with an area of acute bleeding. **B,** Severe midline shift results.

is similar to that with epidural hematomas. Surgical intervention usually consists of placing several burr holes or performing a craniotomy to remove the hematoma. Treatment results depend on the client's condition before surgery and the degree of primary brain tissue damage.

A client who has undergone evacuation of a chronic subdural hematoma usually has a drain placed in the cavity to prevent reaccumulation of the fluid and blood. These clients are typically kept flat during the immediate postoperative period, which allows the brain to reexpand to fill the cranial cavity.

Intracerebral Hematoma. Intracerebral hematomas occur less often than epidural or subdural hematomas. They are caused by bleeding directly into brain tissue and may occur at the area of injury, some distance away, or deep within the brain. These hematomas cause problems with increased ICP. Surgical resection may cause as much damage as the clot itself and is usually not performed unless the clot is easily accessible. Clinical manifestations are similar to those that occur with epidural or subdural hematomas, although hemiplegia is more common than hemiparesis. Many assessment findings relate to the lesion's mass effect. Various other clinical manifestations may also be present, depending on the location of the intracerebral hematoma. A diagnosis is established as with other types of hematomas. One form of hematoma, called *delayed traumatic intracerebral hematoma*, occurs after a few days. It is most common in persons with disseminated intravascular coagulation, hypertension, a history of alcohol abuse, or hypoxia. It carries a poor prognosis.

Pathophysiology

Major head injuries cause direct damage to the parenchyma of the brain. Kinetic energy is transmitted to the brain, and bruising analogous to that seen in soft tissue injuries results. A blow to the surface of the brain leads to rapid brain tissue displacement and disruption of blood vessels, leading to bleeding, tissue injury, and edema. Damage to the brain and skull includes the blow itself *(primary injury)* and continuing injury from edema, inflammation, and hemorrhage within the brain *(secondary injury)*. Secondary injury can result in more severe manifestations than those due to the impact itself. Inflammation leads to cerebral edema and increased ICP. Hemorrhage may be diffuse if it is due to tearing of several small vessels within the brain. Whenever pressure is increased within the brain, the brain can become hypoxic. The secondary problems occur hours to days after the initial impact.

A concussion usually causes injury to the brain that is 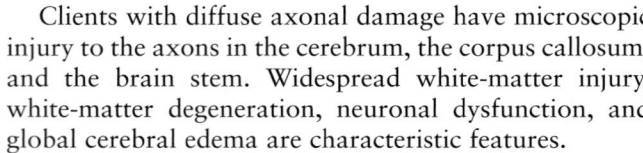 reversible. Some biochemical and ultrastructural damage, such as depletion in mitochondrial adenosine triphosphate and changes in vascular permeability, also can occur.

Clients with diffuse axonal damage have microscopic injury to the axons in the cerebrum, the corpus callosum, and the brain stem. Widespread white-matter injury, white-matter degeneration, neuronal dysfunction, and global cerebral edema are characteristic features.

Studies have noted a significantly increased mortality rate in the client who experiences hypotension, especially early in the post-injury period. When autoregulation is disrupted, as in head injury, cerebral hypoperfusion leads to brain tissue ischemia. Hypoxia has a lesser effect on mortality so long as cerebral perfusion is adequate because the brain can extract extra oxygen for short periods. The combination of arterial hypotension and hypoxemia is significant in the progression of secondary injury. Other causes of secondary brain injury include increased ICP, respiratory problems, electrolyte imbalance, and infection.

Reperfusion injury occurs when ischemia is reversed and blood flow is reestablished; it also leads to secondary injury. Reperfusion injury is probably caused by oxygen free radicals, which are normal by-products of aerobic metabolism that usually break down into oxygen and water. In cell injury, breakdown of these radicals is impaired so that they accumulate, causing destruction of nucleic acids, proteins, carbohydrates, and lipids and, eventually, cell membranes in the brain tissue. Currently research is targeted at developing neuroprotective agents that prevent delayed injury progression.[61]

Clinical Manifestations

Skull Fractures

Other than a history of skull fracture, clients may not have clear manifestations of the injury. Therefore they need careful ongoing assessment. They may develop other clinical signs, including the following:

- CSF or other fluid draining from the ear or nose
- Evidence of various cranial nerve injuries
- Blood behind the tympanic membrane
- Periorbital ecchymoses (bruises around the eyes)
- Later, a bruise over the mastoid process (Battle's sign)

Indications of cranial nerve and inner ear damage may be noted at the time of the initial injury or may not appear until later. They include the following:

- Vision changes from optic nerve damage
- Hearing loss from auditory nerve damage
- Loss of the sense of smell from olfactory nerve damage
- Squint or fixed, dilated pupil and loss of some eye movements from oculomotor nerve damage
- Facial paresis or paralysis (unilateral) from facial nerve damage
- Vertigo caused by damage from otoliths in the inner ear
- Nystagmus from damage to the vestibular system

Basilar skull fractures, depressed fractures, and other open (compound) fractures allow communication between the external environment and the brain. Infection is therefore a possible complication. See Chapter 71 for a discussion of brain abscess and meningitis. Increasing ICP with basilar skull fractures can be difficult to assess because the pressure is not exerted on the motor strip of the frontal lobes, which means that there will be no weakness in the contralateral extremities. Assess for subtle changes in vital signs, especially heart rate and rhythm and breathing patterns. Headache may be present if there is bleeding at the site of injury.

Concussions

After concussion, observers report loss of consciousness for 5 minutes or less. Retrograde amnesia, posttraumatic amnesia, or both may be present. The duration of amnesia may directly correlate with the severity of the concussion. The client usually has a headache and dizziness and may complain of nausea and vomiting. There is no break in the skull or dura, and no visible damage is seen on CT or MRI scans.

Contusions

The clinical manifestations of contusions are varied, partly because any area of the brain can suffer contusion. Contusions are often associated with other serious injuries, including cervical fractures. Secondary effects (e.g., brain swelling and edema) accompany serious contusions. Increased ICP and herniation syndromes may result. Contusions may be divided into cerebral contusions and brain stem contusions.

Cerebral Contusions. Manifestations of cerebral contusions vary, depending on which areas of the cerebral hemispheres are damaged. An agitated, confused head-injured client who remains alert may have a temporal lobe contusion. Hemiparesis in an alert head-injured client may indicate a frontal contusion. An aphasic head-injured client may have a frontotemporal contusion. Other findings indicate contusions in other areas. Although these findings correlate with cerebral contusion, they do not rule out other abnormalities, such as a developing mass lesion. Adverse changes in the client's condition require immediate medical attention. If treated early, these complications may be reversible.

Brain Stem Contusions. Brain stem contusions render a client immediately unresponsive or partially comatose because of significant brain stem disruption. Typically an altered LOC continues for at least several hours and usually days or weeks. The client may regain partial consciousness within hours or remain in a coma.

Damage to the reticular activating system may render the client permanently comatose. Other neurologic abnormalities are present and are usually symmetrical (i.e., evenly distributed on both sides of the body). Some may be lateralized (asymmetrical, or on one side of the body only), indicating development of a secondary event, such as a hematoma.

In addition to the altered LOC that is always present with brain stem contusion, respiratory, pupillary, eye movement, and motor abnormalities may occur.

- Respirations may be normal, periodic, very rapid, or ataxic.
- Pupils are usually small, equal, and reactive. Damage to the upper brain stem (third cranial nerve) may cause pupillary abnormalities.
- Loss of normal eye movements may occur because pathways controlling eye movements traverse the midbrain and pons.
- The client may respond to light or noxious stimuli by purposeful movements, such as pushing the stimulus away, or the client may have no response to stimuli (i.e., may be in a flaccid state). In the presence of profound alteration in LOC, flexor or extensor posturing may be elicited with or without noxious stimuli (see Chapter 70).

Brain stem contusions do not usually injure the brain stem alone. Localized swelling or direct injury to the hypothalamus may produce autonomic nervous system effects. The client may have a high temperature and a rapid pulse and respirations and may perspire profusely. These effects may wax and wane but, if sustained, can lead to serious complications.

These clinical manifestations often vary from one observation to another, whereas findings with a developing hematoma are more consistent. Careful documentation of assessment findings to identify patterns or trends in the client's condition is important.

Diagnostic assessments such as CT or MRI scanning may reveal fractures and areas of bleeding or brain shift (see Figure 75-9). Lumbar puncture can also be used to assess for bleeding within the subarachnoid space if any possibility of increased ICP has been ruled out. Currently CT scans can identify blood in the subarachnoid space, and lumbar punctures are rarely done for this purpose.[65]

Outcome Management

Major goals in the care of severely head-injured clients are as follows:

- Prompt recognition and treatment of hypoxia and acid-base disorders that can contribute to cerebral edema
- Control of increasing ICP resulting from factors such as cerebral edema or expanding hematoma
- Stabilization of other conditions

■ Medical Management

The medical management of severely head-injured clients focuses on supporting all organ systems while recovery from the injuries takes place. This involves (1) ventilatory support, (2) management of fluid balance and elimination, and (3) management of nutrition and gastrointestinal function. Head trauma affects all systems of the body, and managing its effects requires a holistic perspective. Also see the Evidence-Based Practice in Action feature on Management of Fever in Clients with Head Injury, below. Clinical manifestations may be the result of the initial head injury or may arise from a complicating process.

Initial Management. The initial management of clients with head injury is the same as for any other injured client: airway, breathing, and circulation. There is a high association of cervical fracture with head injury; therefore the client must be immobilized at the scene of the injury. Lateral cervical spine x-ray films are obtained before the client's head is moved, or the immobilization devices are removed. The client with head injury is pro-

---

EB EVIDENCE-BASED PRACTICE IN ACTION

Management of Fever in Clients with Head Injury

Fever is defined as a core temperature greater than 38° C or 100.4° F. Other definitions of fever include two or more consecutive elevations greater than 38.3° C or 101° F.[5,6] Fever (hyperpyrexia) implies that the thermoregulatory response is intact but that the body temperature is maintained at a higher level. In the presence of fever, compensatory cooling responses occur. Hyperthermia is the loss of thermoregulatory ability, which can occur with injury to the hypothalamus or in malignant hyperthermia. Hyperthermia requires aggressive treatment to prevent cellular damage as the temperature approaches 40° C.

The management of fever in the head-injured patient can be complex because the etiology of fever is not always clear. Assessment of the fever is the first step in management. The nurse needs to evaluate the diagnosis of the patient, the disease processes that might be occurring in conjunction with the fever, and the pattern of the fever that the patient is experiencing. In addition, the presence of intravenous lines or other invasive devices (e.g., ICP monitor or indwelling bladder catheter) needs to be evaluated.

Infectious causes of fever include nosocomial pneumonia, bacteremia from central lines, drug fever from antimicrobials, diuretics, or other medications. Noninfections fever can occur as a result of neurologic events (stroke, head injury, seizure or hemorrhage), malignancies, or acute myocardial infarction.

Whereas the literature suggests that fever can enhance the host defense by activating the body's physiologic adaptive response, in certain vulnerable populations (neurologic, cardiac, immune compromised, and older clients), evidence shows that fever is maladaptive and needs aggressive management.[2,3,7]

Once the patient is assessed for fever, the physician is notified, and appropriate cultures are obtained, the patient should be given an antipyretic as the first line of therapy for temperatures greater than 38.5° C. Acetaminophen, aspirin or nonsteroidal anti-inflammatory drugs are given to "re-set" the thermoregulatory mechanism or "thermostat."[5,6]

Which cooling measures to use and when to use them has not been answered in the literature in scientifically rigorous studies. Cooling measures should be directed toward increasing heat loss. Examples of this include placing ice packs at the groin or axilla or sponging with alcohol and tepid water. It is important to observe the patient for shivering, which should be avoided because of the increase in metabolic activity and the potential to increase rather than decrease the fever. Cooling measures that allow evaporation may be more effective than the use of cooling blankets.[1,4]

The use of cooling blankets should be reserved for patients whose core temperatures rise to 39 to 40° C (>103.5° F). The cooling blanket should be set at 23.9° C to prevent shivering episodes and patients should not be cooled at greater than 0.5° C every 30 minutes. The cooling blanket should be turned off once the patient temperature reaches a desirable level (<38° C).[1]

References
1. Caruso, C.C., et al. (1992). Cooling effects and comfort of four cooling blanket temperatures in humans with fever. *Nursing Research, 41*(2), 68-72.
2. Henker, R. (1999). Evidence-based practice: Fever-related interventions. *American Journal of Critical Care, 8*(1), 481-489.
3. Kluger, M.J. (1986). Is fever beneficial? *Yale Journal of Biological Medicine, 58*, 89-95.
4. O'Donnell, J., et al. (1997). Use and effectiveness of hypothermia blankets for febrile patients in the intensive care unit. *Clinical Infectious Diseases, 24,* 1208-1213.
5. UCLA Nursing Practice Research Council. (n.d.).Research-based practice guideline for blood cultures. Retrieved July 10, 2003, from http://www.mednet.ucla.edu/nursing.
6. UCLA Nursing Practice Research Council. (n.d.).Research-based practice guidelines for fever and cooling measures. Retrieved July 10, 2003, from http://www.mednet.ucla.edu/nursing.
7. Vaughn, L.K., Veale, W.L., & Cooper, K.E. (1980). Antipyresis: Its effect on mortality rate of bacterially infected rabbits. *Brain Research Bulletin, 5*, 69-73.

tected from possible complications of cord injury by immobilizing the head and neck immediately, using a cervical collar or sandbags until a collar can be obtained.

 If intubation is necessary, a jaw thrust maneuver must be used. A baseline assessment of the client's motor and sensory function is obtained at the scene of the accident. Interventions include achieving oxygenation and lowering the ICP with hyperventilation by mechanical ventilation or by manually ventilating the client with a bag-valve-mask device if the client has evidence of herniation.[9]

An IV line is placed and fluids are given to stabilize the blood pressure to systolic pressures over 90 mm Hg. Head injury alone does not cause major loss of blood. If substantial blood loss is suspected, look for other injuries (e.g., fractures, abdominal injury, severe scalp laceration).

A complete history, including the mechanism of injury, is important. These data allow the physician to determine the probable extent of injury and allow emergency department personnel to prepare for the client's arrival. Open head wounds should be covered and pressure applied to control bleeding unless there appears to be an underlying depressed or compound skull fracture.

Do not attempt to remove foreign objects or any penetrating objects from the wound. Uncomplicated scalp wounds (that do not lie over depressed or compound skull fractures) are anesthetized with a local anesthetic agent, cleansed, and sutured. In the emergency department, primary and secondary surveys of the client's injuries are performed. Resuscitation continues with fluid administration.

Laboratory studies are performed, as are necessary radiologic studies. If any identified injuries require emergency surgery, the client is taken directly to the operating room (OR) before admission to the intensive care unit (ICU). Once the client is stabilized enough for transfer to the ICU, the neurosurgical and trauma teams and the nursing staff maintain ongoing care.

Ongoing Management. Ongoing care to maintain cerebral perfusion and reduce ICP is the focus of critical care. The cerebral metabolic rate is reduced with sedatives, paralytic agents, antipyretics, barbiturates, and hypothermia. Morphine is a commonly used opioid for the head-injured client. It reduces pain and can be given intravenously. Respiratory depression is controlled in the client who is intubated and ventilated. Paralytic agents may be used to promote adequate ventilation and should be administered in conjunction with a sedative and an analgesic because paralytic agents have no sedative or analgesic effect.

Prognosis. Not many clients die instantly from head injury; however, many head-injured clients die within the first few minutes after injury from shock or impaired respiration. Early death may also result from brain stem damage. According to the results of several studies, coma duration is the best predictor of damage severity because it correlates highly with the probability of death, intellectual deficit, and social skill impairment. These studies classified a *mild* head injury as loss of consciousness for 20 minutes or less, a *moderate* head injury as 21 to 59 minutes of unconsciousness, and *severe* head injury as coma for 1 hour or longer.

■ Nursing Management
Assessment

A description of the mechanism of injury is helpful in understanding the nature of a head injury. Whenever there are witnesses to the accident, information obtained can be valuable in determining the extent of the injury. Information about the client's activity and LOC before and after the injury is also helpful. Also important is whether the client was conscious at all or unconscious after injury.

As soon as possible after head injury, assess and document the client's vital signs and neurologic status. This initial assessment and the data obtained from witnesses at the accident scene establish a baseline for later observations. Carefully document all assessment findings. Assessment data collection is described earlier in this chapter.

The physician should be notified promptly of any findings that indicate the possible development of complications. It is particularly difficult to assess the condition of a head-injured client who has ingested large amounts of alcohol or other drugs before injury because the effects of these substances may obscure significant clinical abnormalities.

Diagnosis, Outcomes, Interventions

Many nursing and collaborative problems are present in the client with a head injury, such as risk for *Ineffective Airway Clearance, Ineffective Tissue Perfusion,* seizures, paralysis, infection, diabetes insipidus, and *Post-trauma Syndrome.* Other problems that a client with a head injury may experience include the following:

- Risk for contractures
- Impaired skin integrity
- Impaired oral mucous membranes
- Imbalanced nutrition
- Risk for imbalanced fluid volume
- Risk for falls
- Risk for increased ICP
- Disturbed thought processes
- Interrupted family processes

Nursing diagnoses for these problems are discussed in Chapters 70 and 71. Investigation of the underlying cause of these problems and the interventions for them must be individualized according to the client's needs.

Diagnosis: Risk for Ineffective Airway Clearance.
The client with traumatic brain injury may have an altered state of consciousness and may not be able to expectorate secretions. The client is also at increased risk for aspiration.

Outcomes. The client will have effective airway clearance. The upper airway should be free of secretions. Respirations should be of a regular rate (16 to 22 breaths/min), rhythm, and depth. Breath sounds should be clear in both lungs, and the chest should have symmetrical movement. The trachea should be in a midline position, and no dyspnea or accessory muscle use should be noted. Aspiration should be prevented. The PaO_2 should be maintained greater than 90 mm Hg and $PaCO_2$ between 30 and 35 mm Hg initially. The chest film should be clear.

Interventions. Nursing actions aimed at maintaining adequate airway clearance include clearing the mouth and oral pharynx of foreign bodies (e.g., broken teeth) and suctioning the oropharynx and trachea every 1 or 2 hours and as needed. Avoid suctioning the nasopharynx until after a basilar fracture or meningeal tear is ruled out. A semiprone lateral position may facilitate drainage of secretions and prevent aspiration but is contraindicated with increased ICP or a cervical fracture. Humidified oxygen, endotracheal intubation, mechanical ventilation, or a tracheostomy may be required to maintain the client's PaO_2 and $PaCO_2$ within set parameters.

Diagnosis: Ineffective Tissue Perfusion: Cerebral.
In clients who suffer from traumatic brain injuries, another appropriate nursing diagnosis is *Risk for Ineffective Tissue Perfusion: Cerebral secondary to hypotension, hypertension, intracranial hemorrhage, hematoma, or other injuries.*

Outcomes. The client will have adequate cerebral tissue perfusion. The client will have a stable or improving LOC with a stable GCS score and an ICP of less than 15 mm Hg. Temperature will be maintained at less than 38.5° C. The client's blood pressure will be maintained within established parameters. Urine output will be at a minimum of 0.5 ml/kg/hr and not greater than 200 ml/hr. Laboratory values will remain within normal limits.

Interventions. Although anticipatory, prudent monitoring is key to early detection of ineffective cerebral tissue perfusion; nursing interventions can actually prevent, delay, or minimize ineffective cerebral perfusion. These interventions are discussed earlier in this chapter. Briefly they include maintaining all physiologic parameters within normal limits, positioning the client for optimal venous return, and monitoring extracerebral systems for complications. Communicating a client's neurologic status accurately and completely through verbal reporting and documentation is essential to early identification of change and early intervention. ICP monitoring may be required (see earlier discussion).

■ Surgical Management
Conditions that may require surgery include subdural and epidural hematomas, depressed skull fractures, and penetrating foreign bodies. An epidural clot may be surgically evacuated through burr holes (Figure 75-10) or a craniotomy. During surgery the wound may be drained and bleeding vessels ligated. After surgery nursing care is the same as for any client recovering from a craniotomy. Simple skull depressions are treated electively by surgically elevating the depressed bone tissue, removing fragments, and repairing lacerated dura. Compound depressed skull fractures are immediately treated surgically. The scalp, skull, and devitalized brain are debrided, and the wound is cleaned thoroughly. Unless all foreign material is removed, a brain abscess or seizures may develop. Debridement of a penetrating wound or depressed skull fracture frequently leaves a cranial defect that is cosmetically unsightly. The defect may be surgically corrected by cranioplasty later.[72]

Before surgery ICP is reduced as much as possible. Baseline neurologic data are documented. Informed consent needs to be obtained from the family if the patient is unconscious or confused. After surgery, provide nursing care for the client following the guidelines for craniotomy (see Chapter 71).

■ Self-Care
Clients with possible head injury or mild head injury were previously hospitalized for observation for a minimum of 6 hours (ideally for 48 hours) because of the risk of extradural hemorrhage. If the client is sent home, give clear instructions to help the client's caregiver assess for

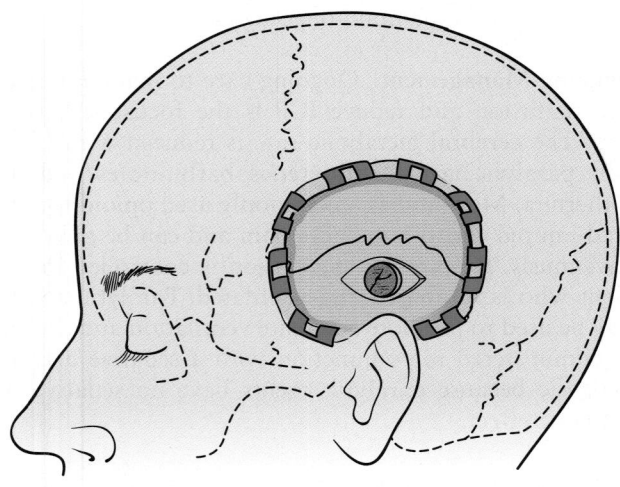

FIGURE 75-10 Placement of burr holes in the skull.

complications (see the Client Education Guide feature on Monitoring Family Members After Head Injury on *evolve* the website).

■ Rehabilitation

Most clients hospitalized for more than 48 hours because of a head injury ultimately require some rehabilitation. Clients with mild head injury may be overlooked in the population of people who need follow-up care. Mild head injuries can cause headache, memory difficulties, difficulty performing simple tasks, and irritability. These clinical manifestations may persist for a month or longer.[10,24]

Rehabilitation may take place in an inpatient or outpatient setting, depending on the client's condition. Rehabilitation may include physical, occupational, speech, and cognitive therapy and is essential in returning the client to maximal function. Nurses play a major role in the rehabilitation of the head-injured client and in the education of significant others.

More severely injured clients may be sent to rehabilitation facilities with feeding tubes or tracheostomy tubes in place. Clients and families need assistance in choosing a new health care facility that can deliver the level of care needed. If recovery is unlikely, the client may need to be transferred to an extended-care facility. Because many head-injured clients are young, previously healthy people, placement in a nursing home may be a very difficult reality for family members to accept. Teaching and support can greatly improve coping. Involvement of disciplines such as social services, pastoral care, or discharge planning can increase the family members' understanding of the next phase of care.[32]

The rehabilitation of clients with brain injuries is challenging. In some cases, community reintegration is unsuccessful. Studies have reported improvement in the client's ability to lead a productive life with the use of interdisciplinary techniques that include rehabilitation in cognition, compensatory techniques, social skills, emotional adjustment, leisure skills, physical fitness, and health maintenance. Most clients require at least 6 months in a rehabilitation program.

■ Modifications for Older Clients

Although most head injuries do not occur in the older population, diagnosis is often more difficult in older adults because of an atypical presentation. These clients also experience more complications. An older client may be less able to tolerate respiratory problems or cardiac dysrhythmias. The presence of chronic diseases such as chronic obstructive pulmonary disease or heart failure can make managing ventilation and fluid balance more difficult. If any type of mental impairment was present before the injury, recovery to full independence is less likely. Poor stamina and medical complications may impede rehabilitation.[56]

SPINAL CORD INJURY

Injury to the spinal cord can range in severity from mild flexion-extension "whiplash" injuries to complete transection of the cord with permanent quadriplegia. Trauma to the cord can occur at any level but most commonly occurs in the cervical and lower thoracic–upper lumbar vertebrae. This finding is due in part to the support given by the ribs to the thoracic spine and the flexibility of the cervical and lumbar spinal segments.

Although this discussion focuses on nursing management of *acute* spinal cord injury (SCI), it should be appreciated that about 200,000 people with spinal cord injury are living in the United States.

Etiology and Risk Factors

Trauma is the most common cause of SCI. Each year about 10,000 people sustain such injury. Most are males between the ages of 16 and 30 years. Nine percent of injuries occur in people over the age of 60. Traumatic SCI is most often caused by automobile or motorcycle accidents, gunshot or knife wounds, falls, and sports mishaps. More than half of all SCIs involve the cervical spine, and the rest occur in the thoracic, lumbar, and sacral spinal segments.

The feeling of immortality often experienced by adolescents and young adults contributes strongly to their risk of SCI. Young people may believe they can engage in dangerous behavior without being injured. The use of alcohol and illicit drugs can reinforce this belief in immortality. A young person who has experienced the devastation of SCI may best deliver the message of primary prevention. In several nationwide programs, head-injured and spinal cord–injured people are available to speak at school-sponsored educational programs.

Nontraumatic disorders may also result in SCI. These problems include the following:

- Cervical spondylosis with myelopathy (spinal canal narrowing with progressive injury to the cord and roots)
- Myelitis (infective or noninfective)
- Osteoporosis causing vertebral compression fractures
- Syringomyelia (central cavitation of the cord)
- Tumors, both infiltrative and compressive
- Vascular diseases, usually infarction or hemorrhage

Whatever the cause, SCI produces distinctive and debilitating damage. Nowhere else in the body can a local insult produce such devastation in proportion to the extent of tissue involved.

Flexion-Rotation, Dislocation, and Fracture-Dislocation Injuries

By far the most common SCI is flexion injury. When a person strikes the head against the steering wheel or windshield, the spine is forced into acute hyperflexion

(Figure 75-11, *A*). Rupture of the posterior ligaments results in forward dislocation of the vertebrae. Blood vessels may be damaged, leading to ischemia of the spinal cord. The cervical spine, usually at the C5-6 level, is most commonly affected by a flexion injury. In the thoracic-lumbar spine, this type of injury is most frequently seen at the T12-L1 level.

Hyperextension Injuries

Hyperextension injuries result after a fall in which the chin hits an object and the head is thrown back (see Figure 75-11, *B*). The anterior ligament is ruptured, with fracture of the posterior elements of the vertebral body. Hyperextension of the spinal cord against the ligamen-

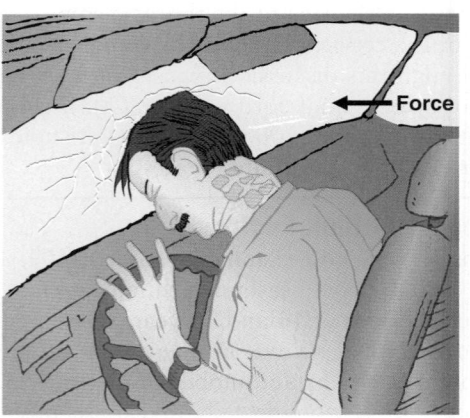

A Hyperflexion

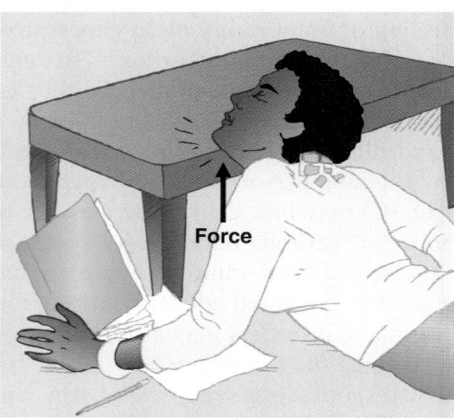

B Hyperextension

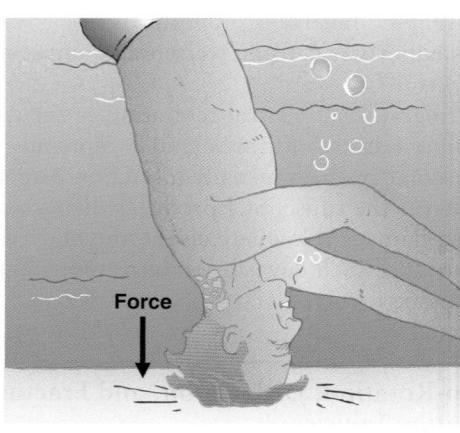

C Compression

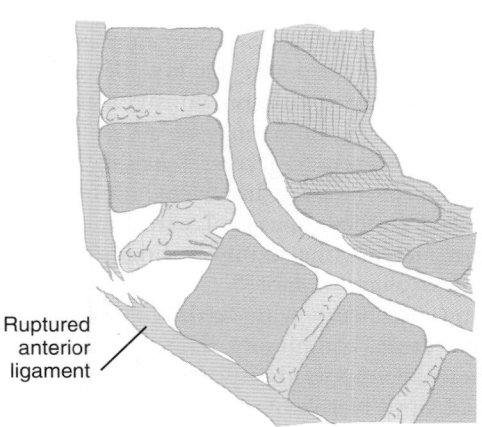

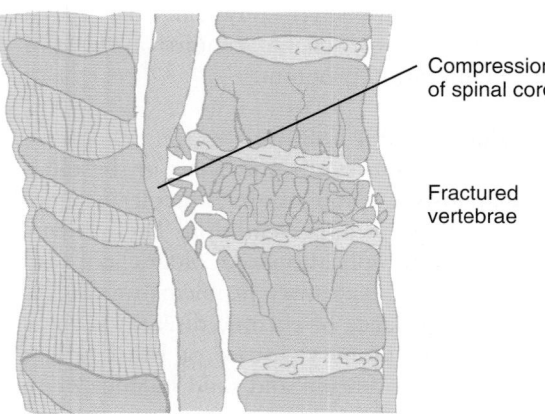

FIGURE 75-11 Patterns of cervical spine injury. **A,** Hyperflexion injury of the cervical spine ruptures the posterior ligaments. **B,** Hyperextension injury of the cervical spine ruptures the anterior ligaments. **C,** Compression fractures crush the vertebrae and force bony fragments into the spinal canal.

tum flavum can lead to dorsal column contusion and posterior dislocation of the vertebrae. Complete transection of the cord can follow a hyperextension injury, although transection of the cord is rare. Clients who have complete lesions of the spinal cord do not necessarily have transection of the cord. Complete lesions of the cord result in loss of all voluntary movement and sensation below the lesion and loss of reflex function in isolated segments of the cord.

Compression Injuries

Compression injuries are often caused by falls or jumps in which the person lands directly on the head, sacrum, or feet (see Figure 75-11, C). The force of impact fractures the vertebrae, and the fragments compress the cord. Disk and bone fragments may be propelled into the spinal cord on impact. The lumbar and the lower thoracic vertebrae are the most commonly injured regions after a compression impact when the person lands on the feet. If the person lands on the head (as in diving into shallow water), the injury is to the cervical spine. About 50% of these injuries result in incomplete lesions. Incomplete lesions occur when some of the spinal tracts remain intact.

Unique Cervical Injuries

Three types of fractures are unique to the cervical spine (Figure 75-12):
1. *Fractures of the odontoid process* (the odontoid process is the superior projection of the bone on C2) may be intact, with no detectable movement, or may be displaced, with movement and entrapment of the spinal cord.

2. A *hangman's fracture* is a bilateral fracture through the pedicles of C2, separating the posterior elements from the body of the vertebra.
3. The *Jefferson fracture* involves bursting of the ring of C1. The spinal canal usually widens.

These injuries are usually associated with other spinal injuries. Clients with these cervical fractures either die of the injury immediately or are stable and may walk into the emergency department reporting only neck pain.

Pathophysiology

Most often SCIs occur as a result of injury to the vertebrae. The most common sites of injury are at the C1-2, C4-6, and T11-L2 vertebrae. These segments of the spine are the most mobile and therefore the most easily injured.

The cord is injured as the result of acceleration, deceleration, or another force (e.g., impact) applied to the spine. The forces injure the spinal cord by compressing, pulling, or tearing the tissues. Microscopic bleeding occurs immediately after injury, primarily in the gray matter of the cord. Within the first hour, edema develops and often spreads along segments of the spinal cord. Arachidonic acid and its metabolites (prostaglandins, thromboxanes, and leukotrienes) cause edema. Cord edema peaks within 2 to 3 days and subsides within the first 7 days after injury. Although the site of the initial injury has the most edema and bleeding, some edema and bleeding extend at least for two cord segments on either side of the injury. The edema of the cord leads to temporary loss of sensation and function. Spinal cord tissue injury is related to the initial insult, biochemical changes, and hemodynamic instability. Therefore immediately after injury, it is not easy to determine the ultimate degree of permanent impairment.

Further changes include fragmentation of the axonal covering and loss of myelin. Phagocytic cells can injure surviving axons as they scavenge cellular debris. Chemotactic and inflammatory mediators further extend tissue necrosis. Macrophages engulf the spinal cord tissue and may cause a central cavity (called *post-traumatic syringomyelia*) to develop as early as 9 days after injury.

In addition, the oligodendroglial cells that support the cord are lost. Injury to the cord leads to rapid loss of axonal conduction from ion changes, such as very rapid increases in extracellular potassium and influx of calcium into the cell. Finally, free radicals are produced. Free radicals are normally found in the body but are quickly controlled by antioxidant enzyme systems. When the antioxidant systems are overwhelmed, the free radicals damage tissues.

The physiologic response to SCI extends beyond changes within the spinal cord. For example, the sympathetic nervous system stress response results in reduced perfusion of the gastrointestinal tract and reduced production of gastric mucus to protect the lining. Ulceration and bleeding may develop.

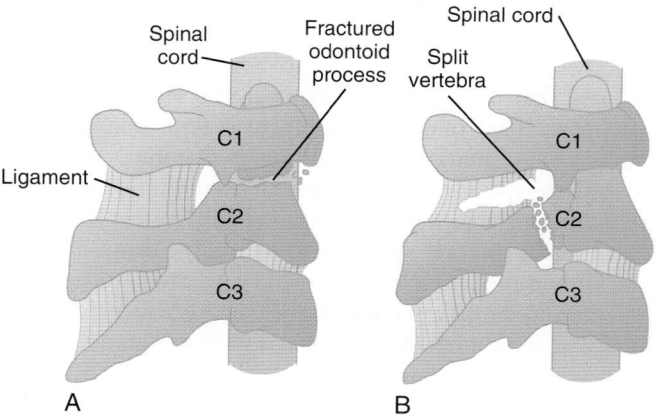

FIGURE 75-12 Fractures of the cervical spine. **A,** Odontoid fractures are fractures of the superior projection of C2 that normally projects into C1. **B,** Hangman's fractures are of the pedicle of C2. The vertebra is split in half.

Spasticity is the increased tone or contraction of muscles, producing stiff movements. Various CNS injuries or diseases such as SCI, strokes, and cerebral palsy may result in spasticity. After SCI, the brain can no longer influence reflex movements through the spinal cord. Eventually the lower part of the cord, using spinal reflex arcs, begins to work automatically. Spinal reflex activities include the flexor withdrawal reflex and reflex emptying of the bladder and bowel. These primitive spinal mechanisms, normally kept inactive by higher centers, are "released" when the normal inhibitions of the higher centers are destroyed. As recovery progresses, flexor responses are interspersed with extensor spasms. These movements ultimately develop into predominantly extensor activity. The client's limbs spasm into extension with movement. Spasticity may remain indefinitely or gradually decrease over time.

Clinical Manifestations

Level of Injury

The initial clinical manifestations of acute SCI depend on the level and extent of injury to the cord. Below the level of injury or lesion, the following functions are lost:

- Voluntary movement
- Sensation of pain, temperature, pressure, and *proprioception* (the ability to know where the body is in space)
- Bowel and bladder function
- Spinal and autonomic reflexes

The level of injury may be described in terms of (1) skeletal injury and (2) neurologic level of injury. Skeletal injury refers to the vertebral damage demonstrated by x-ray study. The criterion of the American Spinal Injury Association (ASIA)[3] is useful in describing the level of spinal cord involvement: *The neurologic level of injury is the lowest segment of the spinal cord with bilateral intact sensory and motor function.* Assess sensory function according to dermatomes to identify the areas of skin with normal sensation. Motor function is measured by testing myotomes to identify muscles with active movement and full range of motion (ROM) against gravity. The ASIA Impairment Scale is as follows:

- Normal with sensory and motor function preserved
- Incomplete with the majority of motor function preserved
- Incomplete with nonfunctional motor function preserved
- Incomplete with only sensation preserved
- Complete with loss of sensation and motor function

Injury to the cervical cord produces quadriplegia. Injuries above the C4 level may be fatal because of loss of innervation to the diaphragm and intercostal muscles. Without immediate rescue breathing after the accident, the injured person will die of respiratory failure. Today, with the general public's knowledge of cardiopulmonary

resuscitation, many people survive this injury to the cervical spine. Injuries to the remainder of the cervical spine create specific patterns of motor loss. Note that a person with a C7 injury is able to lift the shoulders, elbows, and wrists and has some hand function, but below C7 no motor function or sensation remains.

Injuries to the thoracic or lumbar spinal segment produce paraplegia. People with such injuries have function in their upper extremities and can be mobile in a wheelchair or with crutches and braces. People with L5 injury can extend the great toe and dorsiflex the ankle. They have no sensation in the perianal area, calf, heel, or small toe.

Changes in Reflexes

Reflexes, which normally cross the spinal cord and return to the stimulated limb, are absent in early SCI because of spinal shock. Blood pressure and temperature in denervated (without nervous function or innervation) areas fall markedly and respond poorly to reflex stimuli.

After spinal shock subsides, some body functions may return by reflex (e.g., control of the urinary bladder), but they lack integration with other visceral activities. Visceral activities may be initiated by atypical stimuli. For example, scratching the skin may cause vasodilation, sweating, and urination. Nervous system lesions may produce a type of defective urinary bladder function known as *neurogenic bladder*. For example, stimulation of the skin on the lower abdomen or thighs may cause reflex urination. This form of cord bladder is called a *reflex bladder*. Such stimulation may also cause reflex ejaculation and priapism (persistent abnormal penile erection without sexual desire) in paralyzed men.

Muscle Spasms

Intense and painful muscular spasms of the lower extremities occur following a traumatic complete transverse spinal cord lesion. In assisting the client and the family members to understand these movements, it should be explained that these muscle spasms are involuntary and do not mean that voluntary movement is returning. This information, although disappointing, is essential.

Muscle spasms range in intensity from mild muscular twitching to vigorous mass reflexogenic states. Extreme, involuntary muscle spasms can actually throw a client out of bed or wheelchair. Bed side rails are kept up, and restraining straps are comfortably secured over the client lying on a stretcher. Muscle spasms, often aggravated by cold weather, prolonged periods of sitting, infections, or emotionally upsetting events, may become intolerable. Reflex spasms may be triggered by extrinsic or visceral stimuli, such as a distended bladder.

Emotion (e.g., anxiety, crying, anger, laughing) or cutaneous stimulation (e.g., tickling, stroking, pinching) may initiate spastic movements. By learning to recognize events that trigger such reflex spasms, the client may use these potentially annoying movements to achieve functional activities such as urination.

Autonomic Dysreflexia

Autonomic dysreflexia, also known as *autonomic hyperreflexia,* is a life-threatening syndrome. It is a cluster of clinical manifestations that results when multiple spinal cord autonomic responses discharge simultaneously. This syndrome, observed in as many as 85% of clients with cord injury above the T6 level, can occur anytime after spinal shock has resolved. Dysreflexia often lessens as time after injury passes, but it may recur. The manifestations of autonomic dysreflexia result from an exaggerated sympathetic response to a noxious stimulus below the level of the cord lesion. Common stimuli are bladder and bowel distention but may also include pressure ulcers, spasms, pain, pressure on the penis, excessive rectal stimulation, bladder stones, ingrown toenails, abdominal abnormalities, or uterine contractions.

Exaggerated sympathetic responses cause the blood vessels below the level of injury to constrict. As a result, the client develops hypertension (readings of 20 mm Hg above baseline is considered hypertensive), a pounding headache, flushing above the level of the lesion, nasal stuffiness, diaphoresis, piloerection ("gooseflesh"), dilated pupils with blurred vision, bradycardia (30 to 40 beats/min), restlessness, and nausea. The manifestations are a result of compensatory efforts to overcome the severe hypertension. Initially baroreceptors sense the hypertensive stimuli and stimulate the parasympathetic nervous system, which results in vasodilation above the level of cord injury (headache, flushing) and bradycardia. The problem is that the visceral and peripheral vessels do not dilate because the efferent impulses cannot pass through the damaged cord. Thus the overall effect is one of extreme hypertension (with pressures possibly as high as 300 mm Hg). Seizures and cerebral hemorrhage occur in about 10% to 15% of cases. See the later discussion on Risk for Autonomic Dysreflexia for interventions.

Clinical Syndromes Causing Partial Paralysis

Five spinal cord syndromes cause partial paralysis (Figure 75-13): central cord syndrome, anterior cord syndrome, Brown-Séquard syndrome, conus medullaris syndrome, and cauda equina syndrome. Each has distinctive neurologic features.

Central Cord Syndrome. Central cord syndrome (most common with hyperextension-hyperflexion injuries) produces more weakness in the upper extremities than in the lower extremities. This type of injury occurs most often in the older adult who has a pre-existing spinal stenosis. This injury may also occur in a person who lands on the head such as when diving into shallow water and hitting the bottom. The common mechanism of injury is a fall forward. The weakness is caused by edema and hemorrhage in the central area of the cord, which is predominantly occupied by nerve tracts to the hands and arms.

Anterior Cord Syndrome. A lesion in the anterior spinal cord causes anterior cord syndrome, with complete motor function loss and decreased pain sensation. Deep pressure, position sense, and two-point discrimination sensations remain intact. Often the anterior spinal artery is affected, causing an infarction of spinal cord tissue. Cervical cord concussion may produce various degrees of motor and sensory deficit, which completely resolve within hours. Occasionally cervical cord trauma produces only root injuries, which may paralyze isolated muscles or muscle groups in the arms and shoulders. These deficits are usually permanent.

Brown-Séquard Syndrome. Brown-Séquard syndrome is caused by lateral hemisection of the cord (i.e., when half the cord is cut or otherwise damaged) as a bullet wound or knife wound. This injury results in ipsilateral (same side) motor paralysis, loss of vibratory and position sense, and contralateral (opposite side) loss of pain and temperature sensation.

Conus Medullaris Syndrome. *Conus medullaris syndrome* follows damage to the lumbar nerve roots and the conus medullaris in the spinal cord. The client usually has bowel and bladder areflexia and flaccid lower extremities. The bulbocavernosus penile (erection) and micturition reflexes may be preserved when damage is limited to the upper sacral segments of the spinal cord.

Cauda Equina Syndrome. Injury to the lumbosacral nerve roots below the conus medullaris results in the cauda equina syndrome. The client experiences areflexia of the bowel, bladder, and lower extremities.

Spinal Shock

The immediate response to cord transection is called *spinal shock.* The client with SCI experiences a complete loss of skeletal muscle function, bowel and bladder tone, sexual function, and autonomic reflexes. Loss of venous return and hypotension also occur. The hypothalamus cannot control temperature by vasoconstriction and increased metabolism; therefore the client's body assumes the environmental temperature. Spinal shock is most severe in clients with higher levels of SCI. Clients with thoracic or lumbar injuries are often unaffected because the sympathetic nervous system is spared with these levels of injury.

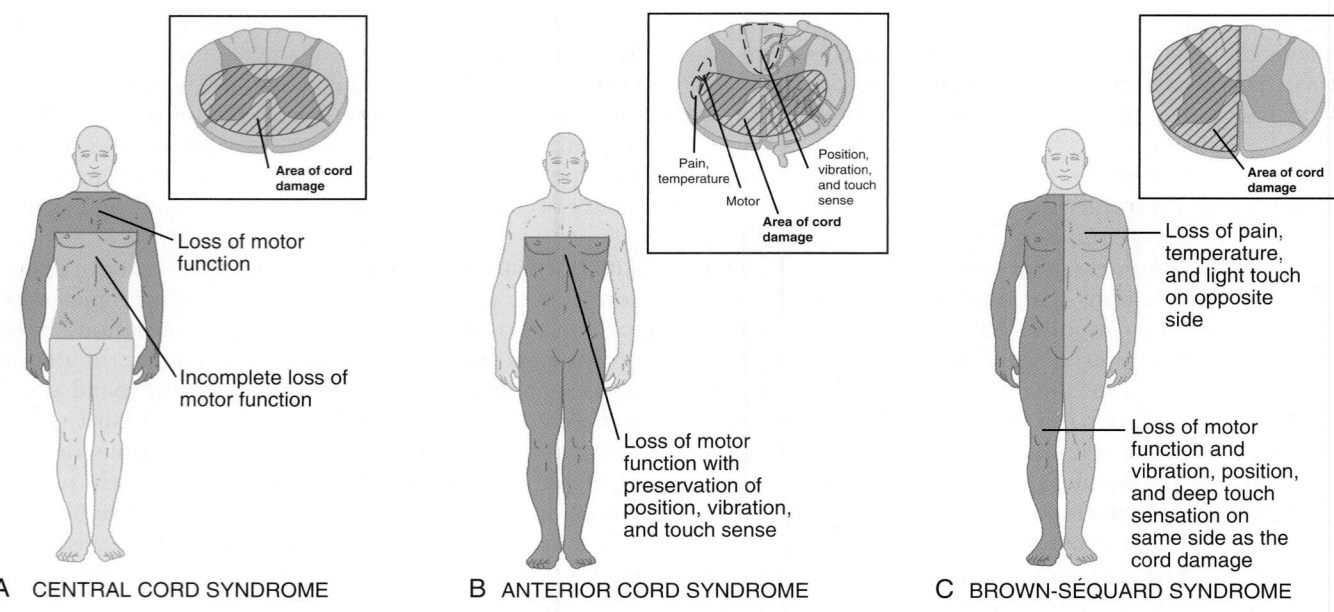

A CENTRAL CORD SYNDROME

Loss of motor function

Incomplete loss of motor function

Area of cord damage

B ANTERIOR CORD SYNDROME

Pain, temperature

Motor

Position, vibration, and touch sense

Area of cord damage

Loss of motor function with preservation of position, vibration, and touch sense

C BROWN-SÉQUARD SYNDROME

Area of cord damage

Loss of pain, temperature, and light touch on opposite side

Loss of motor function and vibration, position, and deep touch sensation on same side as the cord damage

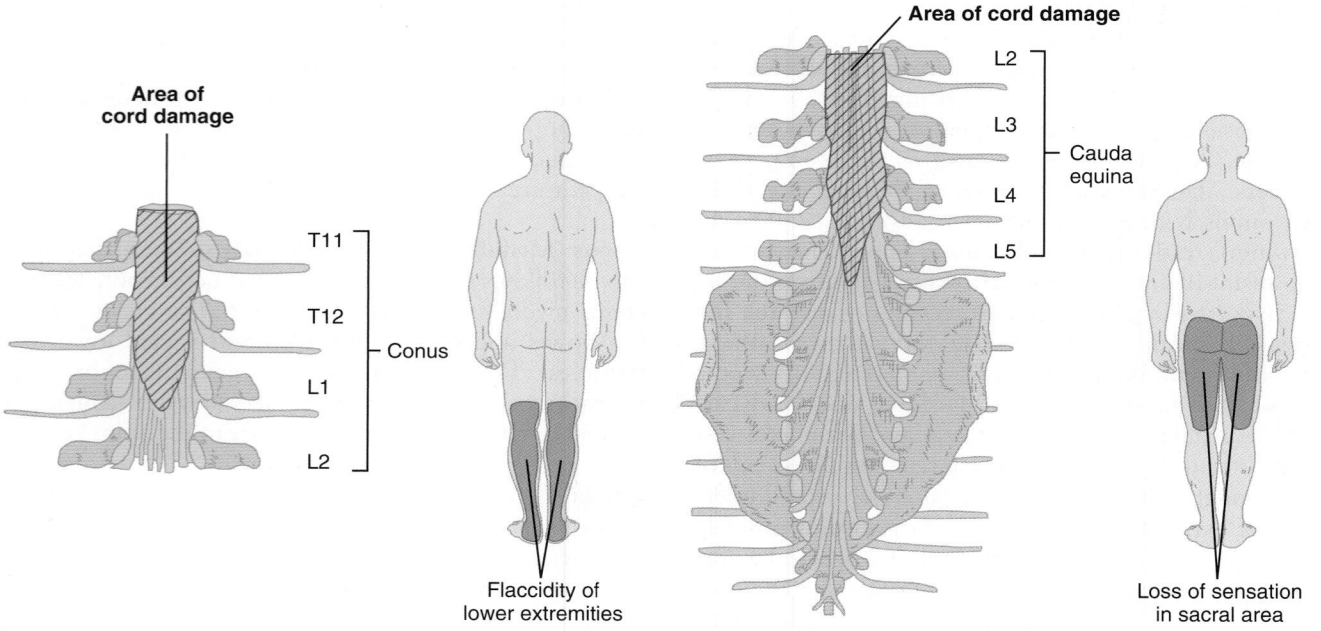

D CONUS MEDULLARIS SYNDROME

Area of cord damage

T11

T12

L1

L2

Conus

Flaccidity of lower extremities

E CAUDA EQUINA SYNDROME

Area of cord damage

L2

L3

L4

L5

Cauda equina

Loss of sensation in sacral area

FIGURE 75-13 Patterns of injury leading to partial paralysis. **A,** Central cord syndrome. **B,** Anterior cord syndrome. **C,** Brown-Séquard syndrome. **D,** Conus medullaris syndrome. **E,** Cauda equina syndrome.

Spinal shock may last for 1 to 6 weeks. Indications that spinal shock is resolving include return of reflexes, development of hyperreflexia rather than flaccidity, and return of reflex emptying of the bladder. The earliest reflexes recovered are the flexor reflexes evoked by noxious cutaneous stimulation. The return of the bulbocavernosus reflex in male patients is also an early indicator of recovery from spinal shock. Babinski's reflex (dorsi-flexion of the great toe with fanning of the other toes when the sole of the foot is stroked) is an early returning reflex.

Diagnostic Findings

Initially, full spinal x-ray films are obtained. If a high-level cervical lesion is suspected, films of the odontoid bone viewed through the open mouth may be required. CT scans may be obtained after the client has achieved hemodynamic and ventilatory stabilization. These studies provide more information regarding the nature of fractures and the status of the spinal cord. They are also useful when a fracture is not seen on x-ray films but neurologic deficit is present. MRI may also be used to locate the level of the lesion. Although controversial, myelography may be used if SCI is suspected and the degree of deficit is increasing.

Outcome Management

Both initial (especially during the first hour after injury) and long-term interventions provided for a client who has sustained an SCI significantly influence the following:

- The extent of the injury and associated deficits
- How well the person survives the acute phase of injury
- The success of recovery and rehabilitation

People with SCI can lead productive and, in many cases, independent lives. As with head injury, information obtained from witnesses to the accident can assist in diagnosis and treatment. Information from witnesses or the client should include the mechanism of injury, the presence and duration of loss of consciousness, and impairment of motor function. It is also important to diagnose SCI correctly. Delays in diagnosis can be attributed to alcohol intoxication, concomitant head injury, or other multiple injuries.

Initial Care

At the scene of the accident, the injured person should be moved only when adequate numbers of people are present to accomplish this with immobilization of the spine. The neck should be stabilized in a neutral position without flexion or extension until a fixed immobilizing device can be applied. Cervical traction should not be applied. Without x-ray films to guide movements, the spinal cord can be injured. The simplest method of immobilizing the spine is to place the affected person on a spine board and to secure the spine with a hard collar around the neck and self-fastening ties across the torso and legs. Transparent stiff collars have become popular because they allow visualization of the carotid arteries and trachea. Excellent on-the-scene care has increased the number of persons who are neurologically intact despite vertebral column fractures. Accurate reporting of the person's baseline deficits is essential to help the physician plan the aggressiveness of treatment interventions.

Spinal trauma is often associated with other injuries, such as head injury, chest trauma, extremity fractures, and abdominal injury. Anyone who has sustained multiple trauma should be handled as though spinal injuries are present until assessment proves otherwise. In handling a client in whom cervical spine injury is present, the spine is kept in neutral alignment and flexion is prevented.

When turning is required, a *logrolling* maneuver is used. The client is placed in a supine position on a firm surface. The head is supported in alignment with the body and is immobilized with a firm, padded cervical collar. Some physicians use halter traction immediately to keep the cervical spine aligned and prevent movement. Clothing is cut off rather than removed. The client is transported on a flat, firm stretcher with the neck immobilized. SCI-trained personnel should remain with the client while x-ray studies are taken to ensure that the cervical spine is not moved.

Cervical spine injury may produce respiratory distress. When breathing difficulty is noted, immediate action is taken to maintain a patent airway and to provide adequate oxygenation. It is important that the client's neck not be hyperextended during intubation; therefore the jaw-thrust technique is used. Suctioning is performed as necessary to maintain a patent airway. Mechanically assisted ventilation is required when definite loss or impairment of respiratory muscle function occurs. Respiratory parameters can be used to guide the decision of whether to ventilate the client mechanically. Serial decreases in vital capacity, along with an increase in partial pressure of arterial carbon dioxide ($PaCO_2$), constitute a good predictor of impending pulmonary failure. A vital capacity of less than 15 ml/kg is cause for serious concern.

In the emergency department, a client who has sustained a severe cervical injury should be placed immediately in skeletal traction to immobilize the cervical spine and reduce the fracture and dislocation. Gardner-Wells tongs are inserted through the outer table of the skull (Figure 75-14). Traction is applied to the tongs via rope, pulleys, and weights. Traction weight is begun with 10 to 20 pounds (4.5 to 9.1 kg) and is gradually increased to accomplish bone reduction. When proper alignment is obtained and verified by x-ray examination, the traction weight may be lessened to maintain the reduction. Traction is not used to stabilize and immobilize thoracic or lumbar spinal fractures or fracture-dislocations because there is no effective way to provide it. Therefore the spine is kept in alignment, and logrolling is used as needed, until surgical stabilization can be performed.

A cross-table lateral x-ray film of the cervical spine is obtained before transport of the injured person. Lateral and anteroposterior x-ray studies are not usually sufficient. To visualize lower cervical fractures, it is necessary either to apply downward traction to the arms or have the arms in the swimmer's position during x-ray examination. If a high-level cervical lesion is suspected, a view of the odontoid bone through the open mouth may be required. A brief but thorough neurologic examination is made to assess the extent of injury and to establish a baseline of function and involvement for later comparison.

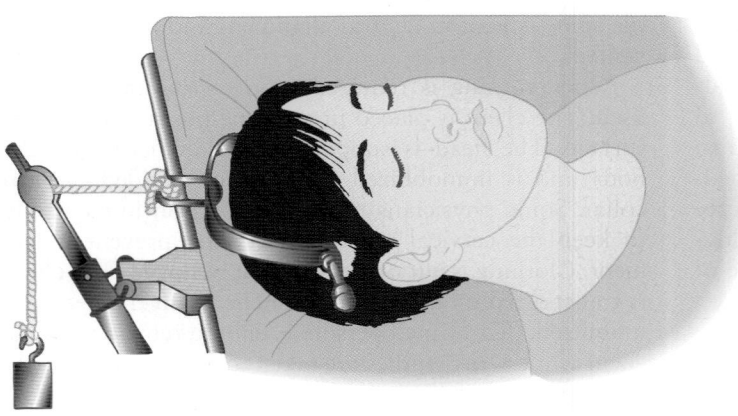

FIGURE 75-14 Gardner-Wells tongs are used to provide skeletal traction on the cervical spine before operative stabilization.

Common emergency interventions include insertion of an IV line and infusion of normal saline, insertion of an indwelling catheter, administration of high-dose steroids, administration of vasoactive medications to maintain systolic blood pressure, insertion of a nasogastric tube, and provision of oxygen if oxygen saturation is low.

Once orthopedic and medical stabilization of the fracture has been achieved, the client is transferred to an ICU or to an SCI center. It is important that the client be appropriately immobilized before transport.

■ Medical Management

Once the client's spine and emergency medical conditions have been stabilized, a complete neurologic assessment is performed. Several associated injuries are commonly seen with SCI. These include orthopedic injury to the spine, head injury, chest injury, abdominal injury, and genitourinary injury. Some of these injuries may not be immediately evident in the emergency department, and ongoing assessments are made until the problem is ruled out.

The client is monitored for spinal shock and the effects of hypotension, bradycardia, and decreased cardiac output. Respiratory compromise may occur if the client develops diaphragmatic fatigue; mechanical ventilation may be needed. Arterial blood gases are monitored closely. The client may be transferred to a kinetic treatment bed to reduce the risk of pressure ulcer development, improve pulmonary function, and minimize complications of immobility. These beds are shown in Figure 70-2.

Potential complications include atelectasis, pneumonia, bradycardia, hypotension, deep vein thrombosis (DVT), gastrointestinal bleeding, pressure ulcers, joint contractures, and psychological dysfunction such as denial and depression.

Vasoactive agents are commonly used to support blood pressure immediately after injury. Short-term high-dose methylprednisolone therapy is started in people with SCI less than 8 hours old. A bolus dose of 30 mg/kg infused over 1 hour followed by 5.4 mg/kg infused over 23 hours is usual. Other therapies may include the use of neuropeptides and thyrotropin-releasing hormone, which may induce some reversal of lesions by decreasing post-traumatic ischemia. Histamine-2 (H_2) receptor-blocking agents are often given to reduce the risk of gastric and intestinal bleeding. Long-term pharmacologic management may include urinary antiseptics, anticoagulants, laxatives, and antispasmodics.

Respiratory impairment, position, emotional status, or gastrointestinal function may compromise nutritional intake. Intubation eliminates the possibility of oral intake, whereas a tracheostomy does not. Clients with a tracheostomy require time to adjust to swallowing with the tube in place and must be carefully monitored to prevent aspiration.

Aspiration is also a risk for clients who must remain flat while in tongs and traction. Although these clients may be capable of swallowing, it is unlikely that they will be able to consume safely enough food to meet their metabolic needs. Clients wearing a halo jacket (Figure 75-15) often experience difficulty eating because the halo jacket immobilizes the head. They should be encouraged to take small bites, eat slowly, and concentrate on swallowing.

Depression is a common reaction to SCI and may be associated with inhibition of the appetite. Choosing when and what to eat may be one of the few areas of control left to the person with SCI. As much free choice of dietary intake as is feasible should be encouraged.

Any of these conditions can severely limit a spinal injury client's oral intake at a time when a high-calorie, high-protein diet is needed. Enteral feeding or total parenteral hyperalimentation is often prescribed until oral intake is sufficient to meet the body's needs.

■ Initial Nursing Management of the Client with Spinal Cord Injury
Assessment

A holistic assessment approach is essential in planning for nursing care of clients with SCI. Every system of the body is affected with these injuries. A complete baseline

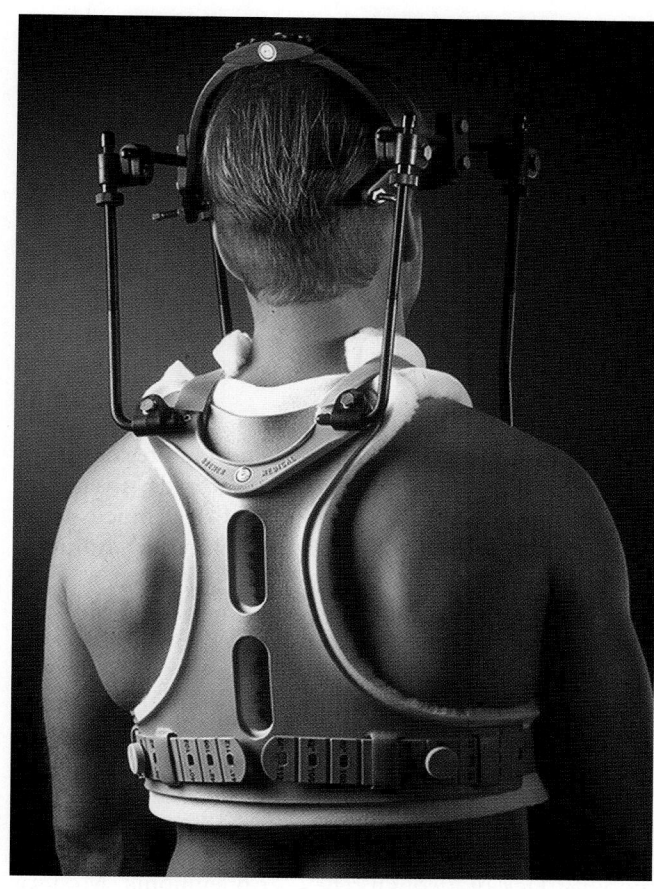

FIGURE 75-15 Halo traction. This form of traction immobilizes the cervical spine so that the client can move without risk of further injury. (Courtesy of DePuy Spine, A Johnson & Johnson Company, Raynham, MA.)

TABLE 75-1	*Motor Assessment After Spinal Cord Injury*
Spinal Nerve(s)	**Assessment Technique**
C4-5	Shoulders are shrugged against downward pressure of examiner's hands
C5-6	Arm is pulled up from resting position against resistance
C7	From the flexed position, arm is straightened out against resistance
C7	Index finger is held firmly to thumb against resistance to pull it away
C8	Hand grasp strength if evaluated
L2-4	Leg is lifted from the bed against resistance
L2-4	From flexed position, knee is extended against resistance
L5-S1	Knee is flexed against resistance
L5	Foot is pulled up toward nose against resistance
S1	Foot is pushed down (as in stepping on automobile gas pedal) against resistance

assessment is obtained initially. The results of subsequent assessments are then compared with the baseline results. Specific components in the assessment of the client with an SCI depend on the client's phase of treatment. Therefore assessment is addressed within the following sections.

Careful monitoring of hemodynamic parameters is essential. Heart rate, blood pressure, temperature, respirations, fluid balance, and peripheral oxygen saturation (as determined by pulse oximetry) should be monitored continuously.

If the client is conscious, ask whether there is any pain. Determining whether the client can feel a touch or a pinprick in the feet, legs, trunk, hands, and arms tests sensation. Levels of sensation are documented according to dermatomes. To assess motor function, ask the client to wiggle toes, move ankles, flex knees, and move hands and arms. The location, symmetry, and strength of muscle movement are documented (Table 75-1). The major reflexes—that is, the Achilles, patellar, biceps, and triceps tendon reflexes—are briefly tested. Assessment for intact sensation in areas such as the perineum is also nec-

essary. If the patient is unresponsive, assessment is more limited. Assess respiratory status by observing for spontaneous movement and thorax expansion. Sensation and movement of extremities are assessed by watching the client for a few moments or by applying a painful stimulus (nail bed pressure) and observing for withdrawal.

Usually the client is awake and may be concerned about obtaining pain relief, the chances of survival, and the safety of any other people in the accident. Once these issues are addressed, the client may begin to appraise the severity of his or her own injury.

Rehabilitation begins when the client is admitted to the acute health care facility. During the acute stage, nursing and medical attention is appropriately focused on immediate needs. It is also imperative to remember that the client probably will have severe residual disabilities and must make major lifestyle changes. Care provided in the acute period can significantly affect the client's later life. Prevention of complications such as infection, pressure sores, and contractures facilitates rehabilitation and reduces suffering, disability, and expense. Challenges in caring for clients with SCI are presented in the Case Study feature on Spinal Cord Injury on p. 2220.

Diagnosis, Outcomes, Interventions

Collaborative Problem: Risk for Hypotension. Clients suffering from SCI are at risk for the development of hypotension. The collaborative problem of *Risk for Hypotension* is related to vasodilation and the inability to vasoconstrict rather than to volume depletion.

CASE STUDY *evolve*

Spinal Cord Injury

Ben Brown is a 21-year-old college junior who was admitted to the intensive care unit (ICU) via the emergency department for evaluation and treatment of a spinal cord injury (SCI) sustained in a diving accident. Consider the type of fracture most typical from this type of accident. He is accompanied by his fiancée and his parents. . . . *Case Study continued on the website and the CD-ROM with discussions, multiple-choice questions, and a nursing care plan.* *evolve*

Outcomes. Expected outcomes for collaborative problems address actions of the nurse, rather than client outcomes. Management of the problem is within the physician's domain; therefore nurses monitor for it.

State the goal as follows: The nurse will monitor for hypotension and pulmonary fluid overload as evidenced by systolic blood pressure greater than 90 mm Hg, heart rate more than 60 beats/min, and the client alert and oriented with an adequate urine output.

Interventions. Hypotension associated with spinal shock is initially treated with IV fluid. It is important to remember that fluid depletion is not the cause of hypotension; rather, lack of reflexes is the cause. Therefore fluid resuscitation should be carefully monitored to avoid fluid overload, which can lead to pulmonary edema. Vasopressor agents are often given in the acute phase of SCI to maintain blood pressure.

Diagnosis: Impaired Spontaneous Ventilation, Ineffective Airway Clearance, Impaired Gas Exchange.

Cervical-level SCI carries a high risk of respiratory compromise. Any or all three of these nursing diagnoses may be appropriate.

Outcomes. The client will show no manifestations of respiratory compromise as evidenced by clear lung sounds; PaO_2, PcO_2, pH, and oxygen saturation values within normal limits; unlabored respirations; and normal vital capacity.

Interventions. Chest physical therapy can help mobilize secretions and prevent pneumonia, as can suctioning and assisted coughing. When spinal cord edema has temporarily impaired respiratory function, mechanical ventilation is used to support respiration. Intubation and ventilation can be frightening to a person who has been able to breathe independently. Provide reassurance that mechanical ventilation will probably not be permanent. Clients may also be placed on a kinetic bed to maximize pulmonary function. Sedation is administered as needed after intubation.

For extended airway management, a tracheostomy may be required to allow for long-term controlled ventilation, to facilitate the removal of tracheobronchial secretions, and to seal off the esophagus from the trachea for the prevention of aspiration. An abdominal binder is often used to provide abdominal support, to facilitate diaphragmatic breathing, and to increase venous return.

Diagnosis: Risk for Aspiration.
Clients without a tracheostomy or with ineffective airway clearance or in whom the gag reflex is absent are at higher risk for aspiration. Aspiration is a common cause of morbidity in SCI clients.

Outcomes. The client will exhibit no manifestations of aspiration as evidenced by clear lung sounds; absence of stridor and fever; minimal amounts of clear mucus upon suctioning; and PaO_2, $PaCO_2$, pH, and oxygen saturation values within normal limits.

Interventions. Suctioning equipment should be kept available and breath sounds assessed every 1 or 2 hours in acutely ill clients. The results of arterial blood gas analysis and pulse oximetry are monitored to determine the degree of oxygenation provided with mechanical ventilation or supplemental oxygen administration. Tracheobronchial suctioning is performed frequently to prevent or reduce the accumulation of secretions from immobility, lack of a cough reflex, or pneumonia. Monitor the electrocardiogram for dysrhythmias (e.g., premature ventricular contractions) resulting from hypoxia during suctioning.

Diagnosis: Ineffective Thermoregulation.
Thermoregulation may be altered because of loss of hypothalamic control of the sympathetic nervous system in clients with SCI above the T6 level.

Outcomes. The client will maintain normothermic status.

Interventions. Rectal or core temperature is monitored every 4 hours during the first 72 hours after injury. Skin surfaces are palpated for areas of warmth, coolness, and moisture. Control the environmental temperature by using bed linens as needed to warm the client, eliminating drafts in the room, and using hypothermia blankets cautiously.

Evaluation

The problems identified in the early period of SCI care may resolve within 72 hours, especially if no other serious injuries or medical problems are present. If the client remains in an ICU for a prolonged time, implement other aspects of SCI care as discussed later.

■ Surgical Management

Surgical intervention for progressive neurologic deficit is indicated for any of the following:

- Compound fractures and penetrating wounds of the spine
- Presence of bone fragments in the spinal canal
- Syndrome of acute anterior spinal cord trauma

There are various surgical approaches for spinal stabilization. Decompressive laminectomy can be used for complete SCIs in which the laminae of the vertebrae are removed to minimize pressure on the spinal cord. Stabilization by surgical fusion can be done by insertion of metal plates and screws or the use of bone grafts alone or in combination.

Cervical fractures can also be allowed to heal with stabilization of bone fragments achieved by immobilization in a brace or halo jacket (see Figure 75-15). The halo jacket has a ring that is fixed to the skull with pins. This ring is then attached to the jacket by rods. This system provides the traction required to maintain cervical alignment. A halo jacket allows early mobilization and rehabilitation. The wrench that comes with the brace should always be taped to the front of the jacket to allow quick removal in case of emergency. If the client has some mobility remaining, always assist during the client's first attempt at any activity. The halo jacket changes the client's center of gravity, making falls a constant risk. Never grasp the rods to help reposition the client. Perform pin site care around the pin insertion sites daily. Refer to your agency's policy manual for guidelines.

Burst fractures of the thoracic and lumbar spinal segments can be treated with body casts, Harrington rods, or other devices for spine stabilization. Spine stabilization devices are commonly inserted through a posterior incision (Figure 75-16). After the operation, perform the usual postoperative assessments, including an assessment of the neurovascular status of the legs. Chest tubes and nasogastric tubes are inserted during surgery. The client is logrolled to facilitate maintenance of respiration and skin perfusion. Pain is managed with continuous-infusion or injected opioids. The client usually is fitted for a body brace, and mobilization begins on the fourth day.

Complications of surgery include infection and poor wound healing as well as those related to anesthesia. Both infection and impaired wound healing are more likely to occur in a malnourished client.

■ Spinal Cord Injury Rehabilitation

In 1970 the United States Rehabilitation Service Administration adopted a model system for rehabilitation of people with SCI. The key to the system is the use of multidisciplinary teams of physicians, nurses, and allied health care providers (physical therapists, occupational therapists, speech and language pathologists) to reduce morbidity, maximize functional recovery, and promote independence.

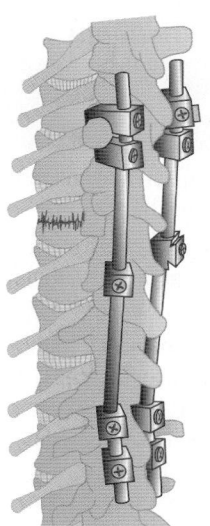

FIGURE 75-16 Fractures of the spine are often stabilized with internal fixation devices.

Establish Functional Goals. Prediction of functional ability after SCI can generally be guided by the degree of residual muscle function (Table 75-2). Clients with all levels of injury and of all ages benefit from rehabilitation. The client and family are involved in all phases. The client delegates needed skills to another caregiver so that care can be provided at home. The skills learned in a rehabilitation setting must be adapted to the home environment and community setting before hospital discharge. This process can be accomplished by the use of therapeutic weekend passes and participation in community activities as a part of the rehabilitation process.

In all phases of rehabilitation, it is imperative that a motivated client be given the opportunity to perform any skill, even if the nurse or the physician can accomplish it more quickly. Allowing the client to attempt a complex skill demonstrates support of the client's self-care abilities. A description of functional outcomes for rehabilitation is provided in Table 75-2. It is intended to be a guide and might not represent ability in all clients with various levels of injury.

Promote Mobility. Wheelchairs provide mobility, and having the proper wheelchair is crucial. The wheelchair design must provide the client with the ability to propel the chair and prevent development of spinal deformities and pressure ulcers. A high back and head support are needed for clients without arm function (Figure 75-17). For clients who can use their arms, the back of the wheelchair should be at the level of the scapula and the wheelchair should be lower than normal to facilitate transfers. Cushions help reduce pressure and the risk of pressure ulcers. Cushions, however, do not prevent pressure ulcers, and weight shifts are still needed every 10 to

TABLE 75-2 *Functional Goals in Rehabilitation After Spinal Cord Injury*

Spinal Cord Level	Muscle Function/Sensory Impairment	Functional Goals
C1-2	No phrenic nerve function; no sensation below neck	Respirations managed with phrenic pacemaker
C3-4	Neck control; scapular elevators; diaphragm function may be weak or absent	Manipulate electric wheelchair with breath control, chin control, or voice activation
C5	Fair to good shoulder control; functional deltoids/biceps; elbow flexion No sensation below clavicles	Dress upper trunk; turn self in bed with or without arm slings Propel wheelchair with hand splints or after tenodesis Assist in getting into and out of bed May learn to write or type
C6	Ability to lift shoulders, elbows, and wrists (partial) Sensation as in C5 but more in arms and thumbs	Dress upper trunk; sometimes dress lower trunk Propel wheelchair with hand rim projections Self-feeding with hand splints Transfer from wheelchair to bed with or without minimal assistance (e.g., sliding board) Assist in getting to and from bedside commode; self-catheterization
C7	Ability to lift shoulders, elbows, wrists, and hands (partial) Sensation as in C6 level, with more in arms and middle fingers	Independent in transfer to bed, car, and toilet Total dressing independence Propel wheelchair with standard hand rims Self-feeding with no assistive devices
C8	Ability to lift shoulders, elbows, wrists, and hands (partial) Sensation as in C7 level, with more in arms and little fingers	Independent in transfer to bed, car, and toilet Total dressing independence Propel wheelchair with standard hand rims Self-feeding with no assistive devices
T1-4	Ability to use arms and hands normally No sensation below nipple line No trunk control	Independent in transfer to bed, car, and toilet Total dressing independence Propel wheelchair with standard hand rims Self-feeding with no assistive devices Transfer from wheelchair to floor and return Propel wheelchair up and down curb Transfer from wheelchair to tub and return
T5-L2	Partial to good trunk stability Able to use intercostal muscles No sensation below level of injury	Total wheelchair independence Limited ambulation with bilateral long leg braces and crutches (injury at T12 or below)
L3-4	All trunk-pelvic stabilizers intact; hip flexors, adductors, quadriceps	Ambulation with short leg braces with or without crutches depending on level of injury
L5-S3	Hip extensors, abductors; knee flexors; ankle control No sensation below midanterior thigh or in perianal area	No equipment needed if plantiflexion is strong enough for push-off at end of stance

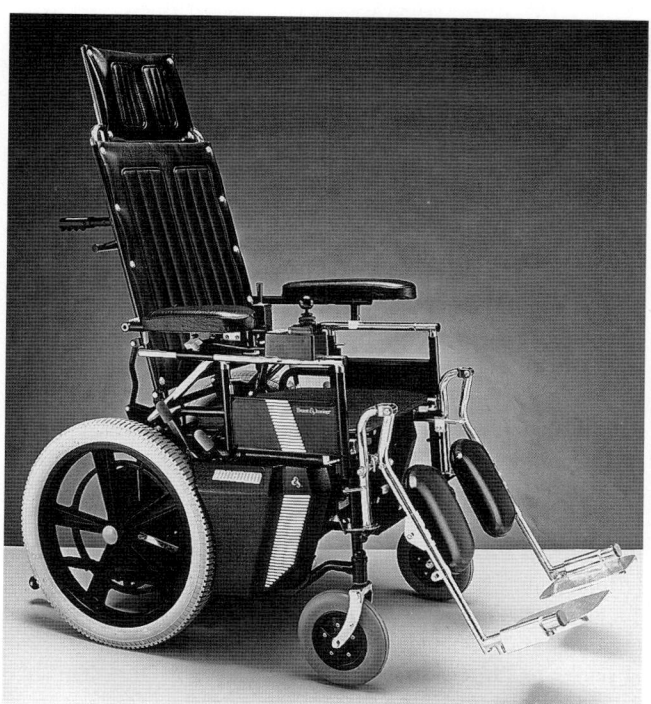

FIGURE 75-17 A wheelchair with power hand controls for clients with C1-3 cervical spine injury. A respirator can be attached to the wheelchair. (Courtesy of Everett and Jennings, St. Louis, MO.)

15 minutes of time spent in the wheelchair. Physical therapists work with the client to teach how to transfer from bed to a wheelchair, from a wheelchair into and out of a car, and from the wheelchair onto a toilet.

Current emphasis is on strengthening muscles rather than using braces; however, back braces may be prescribed after lumbar spinal injury or for intervertebral disk problems. More frequently, a thoracolumbosacral orthosis is used. This device is a custom-made plastic brace with front and back pieces that attach together with self-fastening straps. This brace provides stability for the healing spine. The nurse is responsible for supervising the unlicensed professional whenever he or she is assisting with positioning transfers for a client with a spinal abnormality.

Reduce Spasticity. Spasticity often interferes with positioning and functional activities. Spasticity does serve to maintain muscle bulk, facilitate venous return, prevent DVT, and it can aid in transfers. Treatment includes ROM exercises and oral antispasmodic medications such as baclofen, dantrolene sodium, and clonidine. Medications for the treatment of spasms are given only when the spasms cause discomfort or safety concerns. An implanted pump designed to deliver baclofen through a catheter into the intrathecal space can be used to increase the efficacy of the baclofen and decreasing dosages.

Improve Bladder and Bowel Control. The term *neurogenic bladder* is used to describe bladder control changes that occur with both upper and lower motor neuron disorders. Upper motor neuron disorders produce a spastic or reflex bladder. Lower motor neuron disorders produce a flaccid bladder. The bladder can be managed in many ways, and treatment options must be tailored to fit the client's preferences and lifestyle as well as his or her functional abilities.

Intermittent urinary catheterization is begun when the urine output drops to less than 600 ml in 4 to 6 hours. This reduces the risk of infection and bladder stone formation caused by indwelling catheters. Clients with injuries at the C6 level and lower can perform self-catheterization, although the technique requires adequate hand function and the ability to manage lower extremity clothing. External catheters are used for men who void between catheterizations or for those who leak urine during bladder spasms. Clients with arm function are taught to facilitate the emptying of their bladder using the Credé maneuver over the bladder to relax the sphincter and express urine (see Promote Bladder Retraining in the later nursing management section).

Suprapubic catheters seem to offer the advantages of less infection and urethral injury over indwelling catheters. Indwelling catheters are not ideal from a medical standpoint but are preferred by many clients because of the ease of management. Complications include infection, bladder stones, urethral damage, and a reported increased incidence of bladder cancer. A neurogenic bladder may also be managed pharmacologically with medications such as bethanechol (Urecholine) to stimulate bladder contraction or oxybutynin (Ditropan) to reduce bladder contraction. Urine-acidifying agents may also be prescribed to reduce the risk of infection.

A neurogenic bowel is similar to a neurogenic bladder in that the client cannot control defecation. The goal is to develop a bowel elimination method that is convenient, effective, and least expensive for the client. Sufficient fluid and fiber intake is essential. Consistent timing and position are important to a successful program. When fiber is added to or increased in the diet, it must be done slowly to avoid cramping and diarrhea. Stool softeners and bulk laxatives may also be used.

Bowel movements of clients with upper motor neuron damage are generally regulated with suppositories or digital stimulation every day or every other day to reduce the risk of autonomic dysreflexia. A lower motor neuron neurogenic bowel is more difficult to regulate, and often the client requires manual removal of impacted material.

Prevent Pressure Ulcers. Numb skin is associated with an increased frequency of pressure ulcers. During the acute care period, the risk of pressure ulcer development is related to the level of injury, completeness of the injury, and duration of immobilization. Once the client is seated in a wheelchair, pressure ulcers can develop on the ischia as a result of prolonged sitting. Clients should be turned every 2 hours when in bed. Once the client is seated, he or she should be taught to perform a daily systematic skin inspection using a long-handled mirror to see the buttocks when going to bed. Clothing should not be worn that has seams, pockets, or rivets because these items cause unusual pressure points. Prevention of pressure ulcers should include use of pressure-relieving devices (such as gel cushions in the chair or specialty water bed or mattress overlay). Pressure relief in wheel chairs is usually done by pushing off the arms of the wheelchair or leaning forward every 15 to 30 minutes.

Reduce Respiratory Dysfunction. Respiratory dysfunction is a significant cause of morbidity and mortality after SCI. Clients with injury to C3 have paralyzed diaphragms and will need phrenic pacing once they are weaned from a ventilator. In injuries lower than C3, the diaphragm may be the only functional muscle that is active in respiration because the intercostal and abdominal muscles are often paralyzed. Vital capacity and inspiratory reserve volume are markedly diminished. The client should be taught to use incentive spirometry and diaphragmatic breathing to enhance vital capacity. Glossopharyngeal breathing uses the tongue and muscles of the pharynx to force air into the lungs. This technique enhances vital capacity and promotes chest expansion.

Promote Expression of Sexuality. Sexual function in spinal cord–injured men depends on the location of the lesion (Box 75-3). Reflex erection is possible in some clients with upper motor neuron lesions and also with some lower motor neuron lesions. Ejaculation is possible with lower motor neuron lesions and if the lesion is more caudal. Fertility after SCI remains low but has been improved by electroejaculation, artificial insemination, and in vitro fertilization. Sexual dysfunction is approached from two avenues: psychological counseling and education about technological advances in the facilitation of sexual activity. Erection can be restored with external aids, an implantable penile prosthesis, or medications.

Female clients retain fertility after SCI. Problems with sexual function generally relate to positioning and the lack of vaginal lubrication. These problems can usually be addressed through client education.

Control Pain. Long-term pain occurs frequently in spinal cord–injured clients with intact sensation. Dysesthetic pain, which is distal to the site of injury, is extremely disabling. It is similar to the phantom pain experienced after amputation. It is described as cutting, burning, piercing, radiating, or tightening. The usual treatment is with non-opioid analgesics and transcutaneous nerve stimulators. An "as-needed" approach to pain management is not recommended for chronic pain;

BOX 75-3 *Sexual Function in Clients with Spinal Cord Injury*

Females

Lesions at C1-3: Reflex lubrication is probable; erogenous areas may develop above injury; libido is intact

Lesions at C4-6: Psychogenic lubrication is unlikely; nongenital orgasm may be experienced

Lesions at C7: Able to use hands for holding and caressing

Lesions at T12-L5: Psychogenic stimulation of the clitoris, lubrication, labial swelling, and skin flush are possible but unlikely

Males

Lesions at C1-3: Reflex erection is caused by genital stimulation; psychogenic erection is not possible; erogenous zones above injury site may develop; libido is intact

Lesions at C4-6: Reflex erection is possible; nongenital orgasm may be experienced; no ejaculation; oral sex is possible; libido is intact

Lesions at C7: Able to use hands for holding

Lesions at T12-L6: Psychogenic stimulation and erection are possible; no reflex erection

Lesions at S2-4: Reflex erection is possible; ejaculation is possible but may be retrograde

---

however, routine analgesics may need to be supplemented with other pain-relieving medications given as needed during a client's pain peaks. Gabapentin (Neurontin) has been used successfully for patients with neuropathic pain.

Reduce Abnormal Bone Growth. Heterotopic ossification is the formation of bone in abnormal locations, occurring most often around the hips and knees after SCI. The client may develop swelling in the joint or loss of ROM. Heterotopic ossification is diagnosed by x-ray study or bone scan. Treatment includes the use of etidronate disodium (Didronel) and ROM exercises of the affected joints. Sometimes the bone is removed surgically.

Promote Psychological Adjustment. Psychological counseling is ongoing. Commonly, spinal cord–injured clients participate in peer group counseling sessions in which experiences and solutions are shared to help newly injured clients to cope better with their losses. Vocational rehabilitation may help clients reach their maximum rehabilitation potential.

■ Ongoing Nursing Management of the Client with Spinal Cord Injury
Assessment

The client usually is transferred from the ICU after becoming hemodynamically stable. Clients with high cervical injuries may remain on ventilators. The care of the ventilator-dependent client is discussed in Chapter 65. Some of the nursing diagnoses that applied in the critical care unit may still apply after transfer. The client remains at risk for skin impairment and may still have difficulty swallowing, with attendant risk for aspiration. A baseline assessment should be completed at transfer.

Diagnosis, Outcomes, Interventions

Diagnosis: Impaired Physical Mobility.

Spinal cord injury that causes permanent impaired physical mobility produces problems with ambulation and potential complications arising from immobility. The relevant nursing diagnosis is *Impaired Physical Mobility related to inability to move upper and/or lower extremities secondary to paralysis.*

Outcomes.

The client will have maximal physical mobility as evidenced by absence of tendon contractures, joint ankylosis, and muscle shortening and will demonstrate effective use of adaptive devices.

Interventions.

Throughout the acute and rehabilitative phases of nursing care, make every effort to maximize functional abilities and independence by encouraging the client to perform independently any activities of daily living (ADL) for which capability remains.

Provide Positioning and Adaptive Equipment. Improper positioning of the client in the bed or chair and lack of joint movements (e.g., related to spasticity or immobility) lead to tendon contractures, joint ankylosis, and muscle shortening. Interventions to prevent such problems include the following:

- Frequent position changes
- Proper positioning of joints
- Use of splints and removable casts
- Intermittent turning to a prone position
- Positioning of upper extremities away from the body
- Draping of bed linen over frames to keep pressure off the feet
- Keeping knee joints flexed 15 degrees when the client is supine
- Use of active and passive conditioning exercises (see Risk for Contractures)

Wristdrop and footdrop are inevitable sequelae in paralyzed extremities unless specific preventive measures are used. Footdrop may be prevented by keeping the client's feet firmly supported in dorsiflexion at right angles to the hips to counteract the force of gravity on weakened muscles. Many devices are available to prevent footdrop. Skin must be frequently assessed to prevent associated skin breakdown. Support a paralyzed arm in a sling when the client is out of bed and in a cockup splint when the client is in bed. Usually the hand end

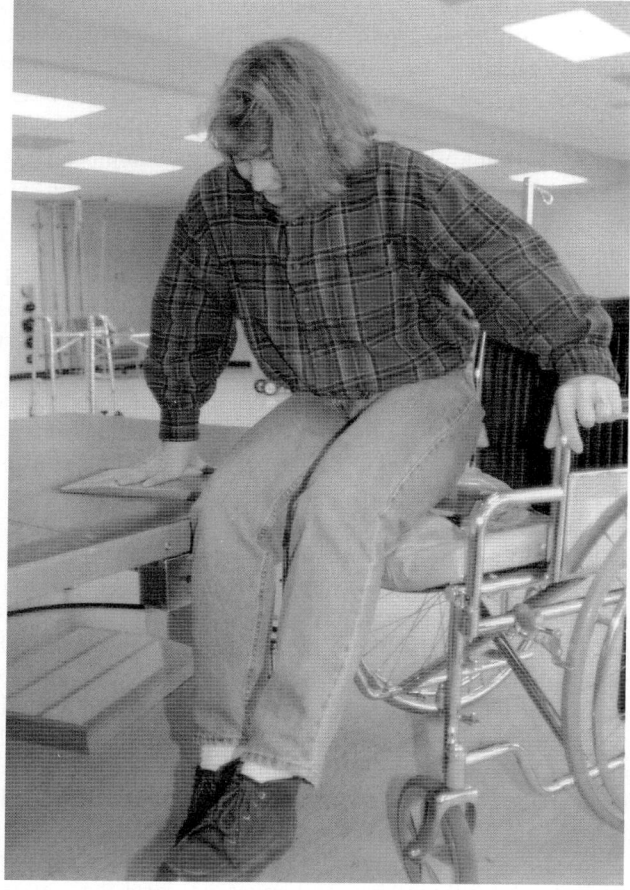

FIGURE 75-18 Bed-to-wheelchair lateral transfer using a sliding board.

of the splint is elevated 2 inches to support the wrist, and the fingers are maintained in a position of function. Posterior molded casts may be used instead of splints to support a paralyzed wrist while the client is in bed. For some clients, pillows and a hand roll are adequate.

Assist with Transfers and Ambulation. Rehabilitative programs often require strength and endurance. To prepare a client for ambulation, the unaffected parts of the body must be strengthened and suitable exercises started early. Tolerance for activity gradually increases. Take care not to fatigue the client. Periods of planned rest and recreation are important.

Physical therapy is essential for all clients with SCI. Paraplegic clients need to learn various transfers to become self-sufficient. One transfer method is illustrated in Figure 75-18. Learning to sit up precedes learning to transfer. Many paralyzed clients become mobile by using a wheelchair. Many types of wheelchairs are available, and selection needs to be made carefully, according to individual needs.

The brace or corset should be applied before the client is assisted to get out of bed. A thin, knitted undershirt is worn under the brace or corset to protect the skin and to keep the appliance clean. To apply the brace or corset, turn the client to one side, place the appliance against the back, and then roll the client back into it. The brace or corset is secured while the client lies supine. As recovery and rehabilitation progress, many clients learn to apply their own brace or corset while in bed. Others continue to need help. The degree of arm and hand function determines the client's ability to apply a brace.

Weight-bearing begins as early as possible after SCI. Weight-bearing stimulates osteoblastic activity and thus decreases demineralization of bone (osteoporosis) that develops with prolonged immobilization. Use of a standing board or tilt table assists the client to tolerate gradually a standing position. Having the client assume a standing position periodically each day also helps prevent contractures (e.g., hip contractures resulting from long periods of sitting).

Take care in helping clients to stand or sit in a chair for the first time. Because of the effects of loss of muscular activity on the peripheral venous system, these clients are prone to orthostatic hypotension. Always check blood pressure before and after transfers. Syncope during a wheelchair transfer may be avoided in the quadriplegic client by using an abdominal binder, thigh-high support hose, and slowly elevating the head of the bed to 90 degrees. Using a recliner or a wheelchair with an adjustable back will help achieve gradual elevations.

Clients easily lose balance when wearing braces, particularly the halo brace, and must be careful to avoid falling. See the Client Education Guide feature on Use of a Halo Vest on the website. A brace feels surprisingly heavy at first, especially if the client is weak. For safety, shoes rather than slippers or just stockings or socks should be worn during ambulation. Shoes should tie or have self-fastening straps for firm support and have a low heel. High-top athletic shoes give added support. Slick soles, high or narrow heels, and stocking feet are hazardous. Wearing shoes also helps prevent footdrop when the client lies down.

The fit, comfort, and appearance of braces, corsets, and shoes are important to the client. Try to accommodate the preferences of clients who want to be as stylish as possible as well as benefit from therapeutic garments. Disabled clients are helped by being encouraged to express their feelings concerning their self-image and by having their desires taken into consideration when being fitted for therapeutic garments. Some garments can be painful when first worn. The pain worsens if the garments do not fit properly. The client's skin should be inspected frequently, especially at first, because pressure sores can develop very quickly.

Diagnosis: Ineffective Airway Clearance.

Airway clearance may be impaired because of paralysis of the abdominal and intercostal muscles. The relevant nursing diagnosis is *Ineffective Airway Clearance related to inability to cough.*

Outcomes. The client has adequate airway clearance as evidenced by participating in "quad-assisted" coughing, remaining afebrile, and having normal blood gas or pulse oximetry values and clear sputum.

Interventions. Use the "quad-assisted" cough maneuver to promote airway clearance. Quad-assisted coughing is accomplished by placing a fist or heel of the hand between the umbilicus and the xiphoid process. Press inward and upward during the client's cough (Figure 75-19). Other interventions, such as turning, hydration, and chest physical therapy, may also be used.

Collaborative Problem: Risk for Contractures.

Active ROM is severely limited or nonexistent in the upper extremities and nonexistent in the lower extremities in a client with cervical cord damage; it is also nonexistent in the lower extremities in a client with thoracic or lumbar cord damage. This deficit increases the risk for contractures. The collaborative problem is *Risk for Contractures related to inability to move purposefully.*

Outcomes. The client will have reduced risk of contractures as evidenced by maintaining ROM compared with the degree of ROM before injury.

Interventions. Monitor the degree of ROM in all involved joints. Passive exercises prevent contractures and painful reflex dystrophies of the hand and shoulder. Such exercises may be prescribed as soon as 48 to 72 hours after injury. Active exercises, massage, and electrical stim-

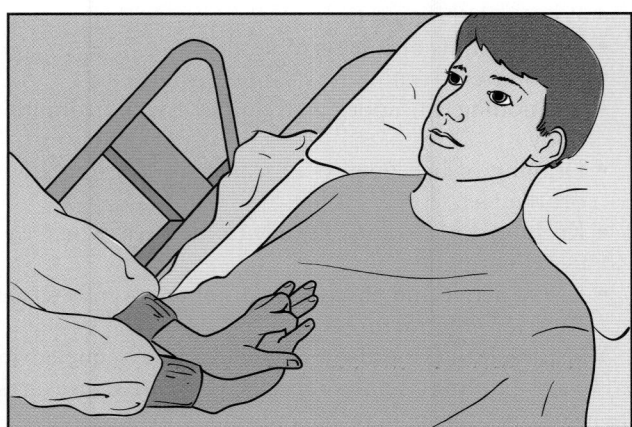

FIGURE 75-19 Cough assistance. A hand or both hands are placed over upper diaphragm. After the client inhales, pressure is directed inward and upward as the client attempts to cough. (From Urden, L.D., Stacy, K.M., & Lough, M.E. (2002). *Thelan's critical care nursing diagnosis and management* (4th ed.) St. Louis: Mosby.)

ulation may also be prescribed. Begin shoulder and arm exercises early. Strength in these areas and in the chest and back is essential for effective self-transfers and ambulation. Clients may find that the prone position is helpful to prevent hip flexure contracture.

Diagnosis: Self-Care Deficit.
The client who has suffered an SCI is often unable to perform many self-care activities.

Outcomes. The client will have a satisfactory level of self care as evidenced by independently performing as many ADL tasks as possible. If unable to perform an activity independently, the client will be able to direct a caregiver's performance. These goals will be evaluated by observing successful performance of ADL by the client or under the client's direction.

Interventions. Self-care deficit can lead to a feeling of powerlessness. Assisting the client to maximize independence can lessen this feeling. The client is assisted with muscle-strengthening exercises and the use of adaptive devices. Clients with high cervical injuries are able to perform few activities independently. Allow them adequate time to accomplish whatever tasks they can. If help with ADL is needed, adapt nursing care to the client's routine. In collaborating to maintain intact oral mucous membranes, a schedule is established for brushing the teeth at least twice daily and cleaning the tongue, roof of the mouth, and gums with agents that do not contain lemon or alcohol.

Diagnosis: Risk for Imbalanced Nutrition: Less Than Body Requirements.
After traumatic injury metabolic demand increases because of the response to stress and the body's requirements for healing. The relevant nursing diagnosis is written *Risk for Imbalanced Nutrition: Less Than Body Requirements related to increased metabolic demand and inability to access nutrients.* Anorexia related to depression may be another etiologic factor.

Outcomes. The client will have balanced nutrition as evidenced by maintaining a reasonable weight for height.

Interventions. The client should be weighed on admission to obtain a baseline measurement. Compare current weight to ideal body weight. Whereas weight loss is not encouraged during the healing phase of injury, once the client is stable, excess weight should be shed to promote activity and transferring. For clients below ideal body weight, nutrient supplementation should begin by 72 hours after injury if the client is not eating. Enteral feeding can be used if the client has bowel sounds. If the client still has paralytic ileus, hyperalimentation is commonly used. Weigh the client at least once a week to monitor progress. Laboratory values for albumin and prealbumin should also be monitored.

Diagnosis: Total Urinary Incontinence.
Observe the client carefully for indications of faulty bladder control and infection, including incontinence, retention, urgency, dribbling, frequency, enuresis, and precipitate micturition. Document such observations and inform the physician. The relevant nursing diagnosis is written *Total Urinary Incontinence related to paralysis.*

Outcomes. The client will have improved bladder control as evidenced by no infection and emptying of the bladder every 4 to 6 hours.

Interventions. Nursing intervention is planned to prevent urinary tract infection, to preserve existing bladder capacity and muscle tone, and to establish and maintain a routine pattern of elimination requiring minimal artificial assistance.

Urinary bladder *atony* (absence of tone) may last several weeks or months after SCI. In clients with upper motor neuron lesions, when spinal shock subsides and the reflexes return, a reflex contraction may empty the bladder. It is important to check a postvoid residual or to use an ultrasound to measure bladder volume to ensure near complete bladder emptying. During the period of atony, a retention catheter may be inserted to prevent bladder distention and keep the client dry and comfortable. Bladder overdistention causes stretching and fissure formation—a predisposing factor for infection—and may result in bladder rupture. When sensory pathways are damaged, the client does not feel the discomfort of bladder distention; however, prolonged catheter use also predisposes to infection. Therefore catheterization every 4 to 6 hours to keep urine volumes less than 600 ml is preferred over a retention catheter.

Urinary complications may be avoided by periodically examining the client for bladder distention, accurately documenting fluid intake and output, using aseptic technique when handling urinary catheters, and observing for manifestations of bladder infection. Encourage the client to drink water to keep the urine diluted, which lessens the possibility of infection. Urine acidifiers may be prescribed.

Urinary complications occur because of incomplete emptying of the bladder, necessitating catheterization. Catheterization may predispose the client to infection and vesicoureteral reflux, which may lead to kidney complications. Renal calculi, pyelonephritis, and hydronephrosis are major causes of considerable disability and even death in paralyzed clients.

To prevent development of renal calculi, encourage the client to drink about 3000 ml of fluid per day, unless contraindicated by other medical conditions. This is sufficient to maintain a minimal urine output of 2000 ml/day. Drinking this much fluid may increase incontinence but is necessary to prevent renal calculi.

Diagnosis: Bowel Incontinence or Constipation.

Bowel dysfunction is a common but manageable problem in a client with SCI. This common nursing diagnosis is written as *Constipation related to paralysis.*

Outcomes. The client will have reduced risk of bowel incontinence or constipation as evidenced by a bowel movement every 1 to 2 days, no manifestations of fecal impaction, no incontinence, and no manifestations of hyperreflexia.

Interventions. Nursing intervention is planned to prevent constipation, distention, and impaction; to detect and treat these conditions if they occur; and to reestablish habitual, controlled bowel movements by conditioned reflex activity. Paralytic ileus is common after SCI. By frequently assessing bowel sounds and documenting the passage of stool, return of peristalsis can be determined and the client can resume oral intake. The client is observed carefully for indications of constipation, diarrhea, or *tenesmus* (straining at stool). If the bowel becomes impacted, a cleansing enema may be prescribed to initially empty the lower bowel. Enemas should be avoided for long-term bowel management, however. A paraplegic or quadriplegic client cannot retain an enema solution, nor can the degree of intestinal distention be felt. Therefore enemas must be administered carefully to avoid overdistending the intestine with excessive fluid; 500 ml or less is usually given.

Document the client's intake of fluid and food and elimination patterns. A bowel program should be established early. The program should occur at the same time every day (or every other day), after a meal or large snack with the patient as upright as possible. The use of water-based suppositories or digital stimulation provides a signal to the body for reflex evacuation.

A daily fluid intake of 3000 ml/day is important for proper bowel function as well as bladder function. Also, the diet must be high in bulk and roughage, such as bran, whole grains, fresh and dried fruits, and leafy green and raw vegetables. A stool softener such as docusate sodium (Colace) may be taken daily, but laxatives should be carefully administered. Bulk-forming medications (e.g., psyllium hydrophilic mucilloid [Metamucil]) are effective for spinal cord–injured clients so long as adequate hydration is maintained.

Diagnosis: Risk for Impaired Skin Integrity.

Clients with SCI are at higher risk of impairment of skin integrity because of immobility and loss of protective functions.

Outcomes. The client will have intact skin as evidenced by no reddened areas over bony prominences and no areas or manifestations of skin irritation or dryness.

Interventions. The spinal cord–injured client cannot respond to the sensory cues to local tissue hypoxia resulting from being in one position for an extended period. Impaired skin sensation occurring with quadriplegia and paraplegia predisposes the client to the development of pressure ulcers and other injuries. Spinal cord–injured clients should be placed on pressure-reducing beds or mattresses. Use of these special beds does not, however, eliminate the need to assess the skin every 2 to 4 hours and does not eliminate the risk of pressure ulcers. In addition, the client's nutritional needs must be met to reduce the risk of pressure ulcers.

A client with spinal fractures may be placed on an oscillating or rotating bed (see Figure 70-2). It is equipped with supportive packs and straps that keep the body in neutral alignment while it continuously oscillates from side to side. If rotation is greater than 35 degrees, the continuous motion helps to prevent skin breakdown, reduce urinary stasis, and promote lung aeration. Skin inspection must be performed closely on the sacrum for signs of shearing. Unfortunately the constant movement may also stimulate peristalsis, resulting in severe diarrhea. Some clients also experience disorientation from the constant movement and have reported fear of falling. Staff members should remain with the client initially to provide emotional support and reassurance. Also, it is important to pull window curtains at night because a client in a rotating bed who can see himself or herself "floating" in the window reflection can become disoriented or frightened.

Wheelchairs need to be fitted with pressure reduction seating cushions that allow movement for transfers as well as pressure reduction. Because ischial pressure ulcers can develop quickly, clients should be taught to inspect their own skin with a long handled mirror or have their caregiver do so daily. Once an ulcer forms, complete bed rest may be needed to heal the ulcer; so prevention and early detection are crucial.

Diagnosis: Chronic Pain.

Clients with SCI may experience pain at the level of the injury and radiating along spinal nerves originating in the area. Phantom pain may also be experienced. The onset of pain is usually later than for muscle spasms. Some paraplegic and quadriplegic clients experience both pain and spasm. Pain most often occurs in the lower extremities.

Outcomes. The client will experience adequate pain relief as evidenced by verbalization of improvement in comfort, ability to rest without interruption by pain, and ability to participate in therapies without hindrance by pain.

Interventions. Analgesics such as aspirin and nonsteroidal anti-inflammatory drugs (NSAIDs) may be prescribed. Opioids are seldom used after the initial injury and are contraindicated in clients with high cervical-level injuries because of the risk of respiratory depression.

Clients with thoracic pulmonary injuries tend to breathe more shallowly to avoid pain. Inadequate depth of respirations can lead to complications. Give prescribed pain medication and encourage deep breathing and coughing to aerate the lungs and remove secretions from the respiratory tract.

Antispasmodics, NSAIDs, and non-opioid analgesics are prescribed for pain associated with spasticity. Surgery (e.g., neurectomy, chordotomy) is sometimes required for pain relief.

Collaborative Problem: Risk for Autonomic Dysreflexia.

Autonomic dysreflexia/hyperreflexia is a serious complication of SCI when injury is above the T6 level. This collaborative problem is documented as *Risk for Autonomic Dysreflexia related to spinal cord injury.*

Outcomes.

The nurse will monitor for clinical manifestations of autonomic dysreflexia and respond to them quickly.

Interventions.

Assess the client for sudden onset of severe hypertension, severe throbbing headache, profuse diaphoresis, flushing of the skin above the level of the lesion, nasal stuffiness, pilomotor spasm, blurred vision, nausea, and bradycardia. (See the Critical Monitoring feature on Features of Autonomic Dysreflexia, below.)

Educate the client about early warning signs and symptoms of autonomic dysreflexia and the importance of calling for a nurse immediately if any occur. Adaptive call lights are available to facilitate calling for assistance. If autonomic dysreflexia does occur, institute the following measures:

1. Elevate the head of the bed to a sitting position immediately.
2. Check blood pressure.
3. Check for possible sources of irritation (e.g., kinked or clogged catheter or distended bladder or lower bowel).

4. Remove the stimulus if it can be done quickly. Once the source of irritation is removed, manifestations of autonomic dysreflexia usually subside.
5. If blood pressure remains elevated, antihypertensive medication (nitrates, hydralazine, guanethidine, or diazoxide) may be administered according to prescription or procedural policy (intravenously, intranasally, or sublingually).
6. If there is no order or policy or if these measures do not correct the problem, notify the physician.

Once manifestations have subsided, observe the client's vital signs and neurologic status closely for 3 to 4 hours. If an antihypertensive medication has been given, the client may become hypotensive after the stimulus is removed. Autonomic dysreflexia may recur if the stimulus is not completely removed. If the identified source is bladder distention, use caution when emptying the bladder. Remove 500 ml every 5 to 15 minutes. If the identified source of irritation is bowel distention, be careful when removing the impacted material from the bowel. An anesthetic lubricant is used, and another nurse must monitor the client's blood pressure every few minutes. The stimulation of trying to remove the impacted material can increase the severity of the autonomic response. When a quadriplegic client complains of a headache, *do not automatically give analgesics without first checking the blood pressure.*

Diagnosis: Risk for Injury.

In clients with SCI, another appropriate nursing diagnosis is *Risk for Injury related to abnormal reflexes, spasms, and corneal drying.* Corneal abrasions may result unless proper interventions are instituted.

Outcomes.

The client will sustain no injuries from spasms as evidenced by no abrasions or bruising. Corneal abrasions will not occur.

Interventions.

Injections should be avoided whenever possible. Medications should be given orally or intravenously if needed. When injections are unavoidable, give above the level of the cord lesion whenever possible. Absorption may be compromised in denervated areas of the body with impaired capillary and precapillary circulation. Moisten the cornea with natural tears every 4 hours for a client with altered blinking reflexes.

Clients can also be injured from involuntary spasms. Avoid unnecessary stimulation of areas that elicit reflex spinal automatisms. When such reactions do occur, an unembarrassed, accepting response helps relieve the client's anxiety and embarrassment. Gentle, slow hyperextension of a limb in spasm can often override the trigger points and interrupt the spasm. Abnormal spinal reflexes make people respond to stimuli in ways that may be puzzling to them and others unless the origin of such responses is explained. For example, stimulation of the

---

CRITICAL MONITORING
Features of Autonomic Dysreflexia

- Severe hypertension (up to 300 mm Hg)
- Pounding headache
- Flushing (above the level of the lesion)
- Piloerection
- Diaphoresis
- Dilated pupils, blurred vision
- Nasal stuffiness
- Bradycardia (pulse <60 beats/min)
- Restlessness
- Nausea

limbs (perhaps toe flexion while the person's foot is being dried) may cause mass flexion of the upper and lower extremities. Mass flexion reactions may be accompanied by massive contractions of the abdominal wall, evacuation of the urinary bladder and bowel, and automatic response such as sweating, flushing, penile erection, or pilomotor reactions below the level of the lesion.

Collaborative Problem: Risk for Thrombophlebitis.
Muscular activity is a major factor in venous circulation. A paralyzed client experiences slowed venous return and pooling of blood in dependent limbs. These phenomena constitute the basis for the collaborative problem *Risk for Thrombophlebitis.*

Outcomes. The nurse will monitor for thrombophlebitis as evidenced by unilateral leg edema, erythema, and warmth.

Interventions. In the acute phase of SCI, antiembolism stockings, sequential compression devices, and subcutaneous heparin may be used prophylactically.

Education is vital to preventing vascular complications and minimizing their impact. Teach the client the importance of all preventive activities. During assessment of the legs for manifestations of clot formation (i.e., redness and unilateral swelling and warmth), explain the components of assessment and emphasize the importance of incorporating this activity into daily routines. Measuring calf diameter on both legs daily to detect any changes is a more objective way of assessing swelling. Clients also learn not to cross their legs while sitting in a wheelchair.

Diagnosis: Ineffective Coping.
When the reality of the injury and the permanence of deficit are understood, coping skills may need to be taught. The nursing diagnosis can be written as *Ineffective Coping related to paralysis.*

Outcomes. The client will use adaptive coping strategies and resources appropriately.

Interventions. Clients need to find appropriate methods for coping with new approaches to performing ADL and managing bodily functions. The learning needs of spinal cord–injured clients and their family members are complex and ongoing. In the acute phase, education about spinal anatomy and physiology is needed. This teaching begins in the acute phase of hospitalization and should be incorporated into all aspects of care. Successful learning in this stage affects the client's entire life. Over time many SCI clients develop unique and resourceful adaptations to their living and work environments to facilitate independence.

Diagnosis: Anticipatory Grieving.
Clients with SCI experience many changes (e.g., functional ability, role def-

inition, body image, financial security). Grief is a normal response to these losses. Write the nursing diagnosis as *Anticipatory Grieving related to multiple losses.*

Outcomes. The client will progress through the grieving process and develop adaptive coping strategies as evidenced by verbalizing his or her feelings about the injury and the future, participating in community activities, and expressing positive thoughts about the future.

Interventions. Adjusting to paralysis is difficult physically and psychosocially for the client and family. Family members may experience the same reactions as those experienced by the disabled client and may need the same type of help. Sudden paralysis in a previously healthy, active person can be devastating. Typically the sudden lifestyle changes brought about by serious SCI produce a grief reaction. The reaction may involve initial shock and denial, leading to depression and anger. Crying and talking about the injury may be helpful. Social services or pastoral care may also be of assistance during this time of grief.

It takes time to adjust to disability and to develop ways of coping. Psychological adjustment occurs when the client can function appropriately in the real world.

A client may use psychological defense mechanisms in adjusting to paralysis. When caring for such a client, assess the possible reasons for observed behavior. Hostility, depression, anger, or withdrawal may be upsetting to staff and family. These emotions and behaviors represent coping mechanisms and should not be taken personally.

Paralysis may cause complex changes in self-concept and body image. In the acute phase, immobilization can contribute to sensory deprivation and its consequences (e.g., hallucinations). Providing visual, auditory, and tactile stimulation as desired by the client may minimize the experience of deprivation.

Paralyzed clients are often helped initially by being with others who are experiencing similar problems. Clients should be allowed to wear their own clothing as soon as possible and encouraged to be out of bed and out of the hospital room. Planned social activities may reduce feelings of social isolation and may help clients regain self-confidence. Peer counseling, in which newly disabled clients are provided opportunities to talk with others who have adjusted to similar disabilities, may be helpful.

A sense of security is particularly important for a newly paralyzed client adjusting to enforced dependency. A paralyzed client should always have a means of summoning help and yet needs to learn that it is safe to be alone at times. Blow lights, minimal-pressure call lights, pads, and voice-activated call lights are now available in many settings.

Gradually the client develops trust in his or her abilities and resources and relinquishes some reliance on others. These feelings and attitudes develop slowly as the client experiences genuinely trustworthy relationships.

To avoid unnecessary frustrations, try to keep the client's environment comfortable, with necessary items conveniently placed. It is difficult and depressing for the client to have to ask for help repeatedly. Although recent advances have been made in the rehabilitation prognosis of paraplegic and quadriplegic clients, it is important to be realistic as well as optimistic. Nurses need to understand the tremendous lifestyle changes disabled clients must make. Some people can be rehabilitated to a level of near-independence: walking (perhaps with braces or other appliances), driving a car, and coping with full-time employment outside the home. Quadriplegic clients usually rely on a wheelchair and other devices and appliances.

Most paralyzed clients can become productive and happy. One well-known SCI victim, actor Christopher Reeve, has been serving as a positive role model regarding *abilities* that remain after SCI. Even if some clients are unable to be "productive," all disabled clients have a right to a satisfying, happy life. Although many paralyzed clients achieve complete rehabilitation, others lead lives that are difficult, frustrating, and psychophysiologically complex. At times severe mental depression develops. Depression is assessed, and professional counseling is offered as indicated. Unfortunately, ideations of suicide are frequent.

Diagnosis: Disabled Family Coping.

A family is a unit. A trauma as devastating as SCI to one of the members of the family unit affects the entire family. The relevant nursing diagnosis can be written *Disabled Family Coping: related to multiple changes in the family roles.*

Outcomes.

The client and family members will use adaptive coping by identifying areas of significant or potential loss and changes in family roles, working together to overcome obstacles, seeking appropriate support services, and being able to restore a supportive family structure.

Interventions.

The injury affects not only physical functioning but also the psychological, vocational, educational, and social aspects of life. An organized team approach is vital to helping the injured client and family cope with lifestyle changes. Nurses are often the first health care professionals to assess client and family coping. An open, empathetic manner can allow the people involved to express their grief and uncertainty and to ask questions. Educate the family about the normal grief response. Also carefully probe into persistent denial of grief or lack of progression through grieving. Encouraging as much optimism as possible while remaining truthful and realistic may help SCI survivors to face the future.

Assess the previous roles of the client and other family members and how they have handled stressful situations or losses. Identify the family's sources of strength. Assess patterns of interaction between family members; their spiritual, social, and economic status; and their lifestyle. Cultural or ethnic influences should also be noted. These variables often influence how the family responds to grief. Sometimes the nurse can play a valuable role simply by giving family members permission to have a day off from visiting.

Diagnosis: Ineffective Therapeutic Regimen Management.

Clients with SCI have bladder function changes. Bladder emptying has to be learned using a different approach, and bowel retraining is often necessary. A common nursing diagnosis in this circumstance is *Ineffective Therapeutic Regimen Management.*

Outcomes.

The client will be able to manage his or her bowel and bladder or instruct others how to do so.

Interventions.

One of the most common stimuli for autonomic dysreflexia, a life-threatening complication in people with SCI, is bladder distention. Therefore intervention leading to bladder management is crucial.

Promote Bladder Retraining. When the initial indwelling catheter is removed, a program of intermittent catheterization is commonly prescribed to empty the bladder regularly every 4 to 6 hours for several weeks. During this time, the client may be taught methods of emptying the bladder without catheterization. Such methods promote urination by increasing intra-abdominal pressure on the bladder. For some clients with SCI, urinary flow can be initiated by using the Credé maneuver, the Valsalva maneuver, or the rectal stretch.

The *Credé maneuver* involves placing the fist or fingers directly over the bladder and pressing down toward the pubic bone with a kneading motion. This motion is continued until the bladder is empty.

The *Valsalva maneuver* involves inhaling deeply, holding the breath, and bearing down as hard as possible, as if for a bowel movement.

The *rectal stretch* involves inserting a lubricated, gloved finger into the rectum. When the anal sphincter is relaxed, the client maintains the relaxation by gently pulling on the sphincter. This relaxes the perineal floor. The Valsalva maneuver is performed at the same time.

Urination may also be prompted by reflex stimulation. The following stimuli may be successful: tapping the suprapubic area; stroking the glans penis, thigh, or vulva; tugging pubic hairs; or flexing the toes. The client or caregiver may apply the stimulation. As training continues, less stimulation is needed to initiate urination.

Catheterization may be required at home. Teach the client and caregiver clean, rather than sterile, technique.

This technique has the same infection rate as for sterile insertion methods used for home catheterization. Suprapubic catheters may be inserted for long-term bladder management.

Occasionally a surgical procedure such as sphincterotomy is necessary. The bladder then empties continuously. An external, condom-type catheter connected to a closed drainage bag may be used to collect urine in men. External appliances for females are not consistently effective.

The Mitrofanoff procedure is a surgical option that creates an opening from the bladder to the umbilicus. It allows for catheterization of the stoma and bladder emptying with less hand function and disrobing needed.

Teach Bowel Retraining. Bowel retraining is possible for most paraplegic and quadriplegic clients. It involves developing controlled bowel movements by conditioned reflex activity. Begin bowel retraining as soon as feasible. Ensure privacy during the daily bowel routine, and if possible, have the client sitting upright. When possible, include appropriate family members in the bowel retraining program because they may be involved in this aspect of long-term management. Always assess the family members' willingness to participate in such care. If the sexual partner is also responsible for hygiene and personal care, problems in role separation and intimacy may result. These issues should be openly discussed between partners.

With an effective bowel program, a client has a bowel movement once a day or every other day and is not incontinent at other times. Attaining continence may influence a paralyzed client's vocational future and positively affect ability to have satisfying social relationships. It can also give the client the confidence to cope with other problems.

Diagnosis: Sexual Dysfunction.

Spinal cord–injured clients are often concerned about sexuality and their ability to achieve sexual fulfillment. They often worry about such concerns long before they express them to others. Nurses are often asked about sexuality issues before other professionals are approached, perhaps because nurses provide intimate care. Such care can promote a high degree of trust.

Outcomes. The client will develop personally satisfying and socially acceptable means of expressing sexuality as evidenced by interacting appropriately in social situations, verbalizing the effects of the injury on sexual function, discussing sexual issues with a health care team member, verbalizing methods of sexual expression, and verbalizing understanding of contraceptive implications.

Interventions. Some clients discuss their own sexual potential directly. Others refer to it subtly or appear crude in the way they introduce the topic, such as making inappropriate sexual comments or gestures. Such behaviors are attempts to acknowledge sexuality. Try to look beyond the behavior to the underlying emotional concerns. Acknowledge the client's concerns and offer to open a discussion, by saying, for example, "You seem concerned about your sexuality, James. This is a common concern that others with spinal cord injury have had. Sometimes talking about it helps. If you like, we can talk about how this has affected you, and when you are ready, I can share with you interventions that have helped others who have had similar problems."

To be helpful, nurses need to be able to talk about sexuality without embarrassment. They also need accurate information about "normal" sexuality and how physiologic changes that occur because of the injury affect sexual function.

The client can be referred to another person or an agency if appropriate. Referral should not be made too hastily, however. If a client talks with a nurse about this subject, it is probably because the client feels most comfortable speaking with that nurse at that time. Allow the client to lead the conversation, which may be difficult. Professionals must be aware that they do not always know what a client needs and wants and should listen carefully to the client's voiced concerns.

In general, a physiologic sexual response requires an intact nervous system. For example, psychogenic erection requires an intact spinal cord with preservation of S2-4 nerve roots and spinal reflexes; ejaculation is a function of skeletal muscle controlled by the somatic center in the pudendal nerve originating in the S2-4 roots; and orgasm involves contraction of both smooth and skeletal muscle. It should be remembered, however, that there is more involved in sexual expression than physiologic response.

To some extent, sexual function can be predicted by the level of the spinal cord lesion (see Box 75-3). For example, psychogenic erection is often difficult or impossible after SCI. Although physical limitations certainly exist, every person is different. Many men do have reflex erections after SCI. Many disabled people enjoy *paraorgasm* (phantom orgasm) by developing alternative erogenous zones. The genitals are not the only body areas where sexual stimulation is possible, and intercourse is not the only means of sexual expression.

Some people find it disappointing, perhaps devastating, that they can no longer function sexually as they did before the injury; however, they can be helped to learn new ways of giving and receiving sexual pleasure. Sex and relationship counseling is sometimes helpful. Some form of sexual expression is possible for anyone, regardless of disability. Before making specific suggestions for alternative expressions of sexuality, discussion with the client should occur to identify past sexual behavior and cultural taboos. Some clients may find some methods of giving and receiving sexual pleasure unacceptable. Lack of a sexual partner may be a deterrent but should not preclude discussion of sexuality. Society as a whole is becoming progressively more open about sexuality.

Increasingly, the parenting potential of disabled people is receiving societal attention. Physical assessment is needed to determine a client's ability to reproduce. Male infertility is a frequent complication of SCI because of testicular atrophy, decreased sperm formation, and infrequent ejaculation. Most men are unable to ejaculate after SCI. Women usually remain fertile and can conceive and deliver a child. Adoption is a viable option, and conception by artificial insemination is possible.

Disabled people may have contraception concerns. Little is known about the effects of various kinds of contraceptives on disabled people. Oral contraceptives may be contraindicated. Paralyzed women often have slowed circulation, increasing the potential circulatory complications of oral contraceptives. To use an intrauterine device, a woman must have feeling in her pelvis to be able to recognize early manifestations of pelvic inflammatory disease. Many paralyzed women do not have such sensation. Barrier devices, such as a diaphragm, a condom, or foam, may be used if at least one partner has enough manual dexterity to insert the diaphragm or foam or put on the condom.

Diagnosis: Risk for Injury.
Sensory loss poses serious problems for paralyzed clients because they cannot feel the pain or pressure that normally warns of tissue damage.

Outcomes. The client will be free of injury as evidenced by absence of abrasions, reddened areas, ulcerations, or burns.

Interventions. Spinal cord–injured clients should not wear tight, restrictive clothing or ill-fitting shoes or braces. They need to develop the habit of preventive thinking to avoid potential danger. Dangerous situations include getting too close to heaters, radiators, and fireplaces and using heating pads or hot-water bottles and rubbing against shoes or parts of the wheelchair. Burns can be a serious problem because impaired circulation delays healing. External heat should not be applied if there is a loss of sensation, and the bath water should not be too hot.

Regular foot and nail care is required to prevent overgrown nails from rubbing or cutting the skin and to prevent ingrown nails. Instruct the client not to cut corns or calluses; cutting too deep is easy to do and may lead to a foot infection. Cocoa butter or oils without alcohol may be used to soften calluses and reduce cracking.

Diagnosis: Ineffective Health Maintenance.
Spinal cord injuries result in many alterations in physiologic functioning that place the client at risk for maintaining normal health status. A possible nursing diagnosis is *Ineffective Health Maintenance.*

Outcomes. The client and family members will be able to meet the client's needs as evidenced by intact skin, bowel and bladder continence, ability to transfer into and out of a wheelchair, absence of infection, maintenance of appropriate weight, and satisfaction with personal relationships.

Interventions. Teaching should be conducted in short sessions, using easily understood terms. For example, teach the caregiver the importance of providing good skin care on the hands and skin folds to prevent *Candida* overgrowth. Complex tasks should be taught in steps, with return demonstrations provided by the client or caregiver.

Most spinal cord–injured people are transferred from an acute care hospital to a rehabilitation facility. After functional capabilities have been maximized, the person is then discharged from the rehabilitation facility. The Bridge to Home Health Care feature on Managing the Immobile Client in Chapter 29 provides suggestions for helping caregivers support the client with SCI who lives at home.

Evaluation

Spinal cord–injured clients are hospitalized for a long time. Therefore certain functions important to expected outcomes need to be evaluated frequently, such as respiratory and cardiac function. Other expected outcomes will not be achieved for months, such as independence in performing ADL. The plan of care must reflect these individual needs of the client.

■ Modifications for Older Clients

For older adults with SCI, the most important modification of the nursing care plan is increased vigilance. Older people are more prone to the complications of immobility. A person with heart failure may have difficulty breathing when lying flat. Before initiation of halo traction in this age group, some neurosurgeons perform a temporary prophylactic tracheostomy because the older client has difficulty swallowing oral secretions and eating. Older people are also more susceptible to sensory deprivation. The nurse must make sure the client has his or her eyeglasses and hearing aid. If a window or clock is not within the range of vision, the client should be reoriented as needed. Discharge plans for older clients may be complicated if the caregiver is also an older adult. The spouse of an older spinal cord–injured person may not have the physical strength to provide the needed care. Learning to provide home care may also be problematic.

■ Self-Care

Paraplegic clients can usually live independently. Most quadriplegic clients need assistance with ADL. Depending on the amount of assistance needed and the specific situation, this care may be provided by family members or by a part-time or full-time paid attendant. By using a wheelchair, clients may become completely independent in ADL, with minimal help of social services personnel, a home health aide, or family members. Many clients drive and hold outside jobs.

Ventilator-dependent people who cannot obtain in-home care and others who do not have the personal or financial resources for in-home care may have no option except institutional living. The problem of limited government resources for all clients requiring rehabilitative care remains an important ethical issue in nursing. Group living situations, especially for young adults, are becoming more available, however.

CONCLUSIONS

Disorders of the spinal cord and peripheral nervous system range from life-threatening SCIs to temporary peripheral nerve compressions. The physical and psychological impairments vary with the degree of damage as well as the client's response to and ability to cope with the body changes. The coping response is not always related to the degree of physiologic damage. A client who has facial paralysis or trigeminal neuralgia can be more compromised psychologically than a client with SCI who has developed strong coping skills. It is imperative that nurses comprehend the severity of the client's dysfunction as it relates to quality of life as well as the impact it has on family dynamics.

Management of the client with SCI is complex and multidisciplinary. Successful rehabilitation provides the client with the opportunity to be productive in society in spite of severe neurologic deficit.

THINKING CRITICALLY *evolve*

1. A 23-year-old man was admitted from the emergency department (ED) following a car accident in which he sustained a concussion and thoracic injuries with thoracic spinal cord involvement. The client's baseline data included loss of consciousness for 15 minutes, headache, nausea, and an inability to move or feel any sensation from his thorax down. One hour after this man arrived in the intensive care unit (ICU), additional assessment changes included an inability to move his fingers and hands and to flex or extend his arms. Shoulder movement was still intact. He was fully conscious, and his vital signs were stable. What critical interventions initiated in the ED need to be continued in the ICU? What do these changes in data indicate? What nursing interventions are appropriate both initially and as precautions?

Factors to Consider. What are the implications when a high thoracic injury occurs? What changes indicate ascending cord dysfunction?

2. A 22-year-old man was admitted 4 hours after sustaining a C6 spinal cord compression injury. No neurologic deficits were found, but his blood alcohol level was very high on admission. Initially, he kept falling asleep after you completed your assessments. Gardner-Wells tongs with 10 pounds of traction were placed. Now that the client is more awake, he has begun thrashing his arms and attempting to roll over in bed. What are the priorities for his care? What nursing interventions should be used?

Factors to Consider. What is the purpose of the Gardner-Wells tongs? How would edema and microscopic bleeding compromise recovery in this client?

Discussions for these questions can be found on the website and on the CD-ROM.

BIBLIOGRAPHY

1. Aito, S., Cariaggi, B., & Perazza, S. (2002).The use of high-dose methylprednisolone in acute spinal cord injuries: NASCIS review. National Acute Spinal Cord Injury Study. *Europa Medicophysica*, 38(2): 89-95.
2. American Association of Neuroscience Nurses. (1997). *Clinical guideline series: Intracranial pressure monitoring.* Chicago: Author.
3. American Spinal Injury Association (ASIA). (2002). *International standards for neurological classification of SCI.* Chicago: Author.
4. Bader, M.K., & Palmer, S. (2000). Keeping the brain in the zone. *Critical Care Nursing Clinics of North America, 12(4),* 413-427.
5. Barker, E., & Saulino, M.F. (2002) First-ever guidelines for spinal cord injuries. *RN, 65(10),* 32-37.
6. Bauman, W.A., & Spungen, A.M. (2000). Metabolic changes in persons after spinal cord injury. *Physical Medicine and Rehabilitation Clinics of North America, 11(1),* 109-140.
7. Bell, G.B. (1999). Spinal cord injury, pressure ulcers, support surfaces. *Ostomy and Wound Management, 45(6),* 48-50, 52-53.
8. Blank-Reid, C., & Reid, P.C. (2000). Penetrating trauma to the head. *Critical Care Nursing Clinics of North America, 12(4),* 477-487.
9. Brain Trauma Foundation. (2000). *Management and prognosis of severe traumatic brain injury.* New York: Author.

 evolve **Did you remember to check out the bonus material on the Evolve website and the CD-ROM, including free self-assessment exercises?**

http://evolve.elsevier.com/Black/medsurg/

10. Brewer, T., & Therrien, B. (2000). Minor brain injury: New insights for early nursing care. *Journal of Neuroscience Nursing, 32*(6): 311-317.

 11. Bryce, T.N., & Ragnarsson, K.T. (2000). Pain after spinal cord injury. *Physical Medicine and Rehabilitation Clinics of North America, 11*(1), 157-168.

12. Buckley, D.A., & Guanci, M.M. (1999). Spinal cord trauma. *Nursing Clinics of North America, 34* (3), 661-687.

13. Cantella, D. (1999). Sports-related spinal cord injuries. *Critical Care Nursing Quarterly, 22*(2), 14-19.

 14. Caruso, C.C., et al. (1992). Cooling effects and comfort of four cooling blanket temperatures in humans with fever. *Nursing Research, 41*(2), 68-72.

15. Chaviano, A.H., et al. (2000). Mitrofanoff continent catheterizable stoma for pediatric patients with spinal cord injury. *Topics in Spinal Cord Injury Rehabilitation, Summer Suppl*(6), 30-35.

16. Chen, D., & Nussbaum, S.B. (2000). The gastrointestinal system and bowel management following spinal cord injury. *Physical Medicine and Rehabilitation Clinics of North America, 11*(1), 45-56, viii.

17. Christensen, M.A., Janson, S., & Seago, J.A. (2001). Alcohol, head injury and pulmonary complications. *Journal of Neuroscience Nursing, 33*(4), 184-189.

18. Clear, D., & Chadwick, D.W. (2000). Seizures provoked by blows to the head. *Epilepsia, 41*(2), 243-244.

19. Consortium for Spinal Cord Medicine. (2001). *Autonomic dysreflexia in individuals with spinal cord injury presenting to health care facilities.* (2nd ed.). Washington, D.C.: Paralyzed Veterans of America.

20. Consortium for Spinal Cord Medicine. (1999). *Neurogenic bowel management in adults with spinal cord injury.* Washington, D.C.: Paralyzed Veterans of America.

 21. Consortium for Spinal Cord Medicine. (1999). *Outcomes following traumatic spinal cord injury.* Washington, D.C.: Paralyzed Veterans of America.

 22. Consortium for Spinal Cord Medicine. (2000). *Pressure ulcer prevention and treatment following spinal cord injury.* Washington, D.C.: Paralyzed Veterans of America

 23. Consortium for Spinal Cord Medicine. (1999). *Prevention of thromboembolism in spinal cord injury.* Washington, D.C.: Paralyzed Veterans of America.

24. Davis, A.E. (2000). Cognitive impairments following traumatic brain injury. *Critical Care Nursing Clinics of North America, 12*(4): 447-456.

25. Davis, A.E. (2000). Mechanisms of traumatic brain injury: Biomechanical, structural and cellular considerations. *Critical Care Nursing Quarterly, 23*(3), 1-13.

26. Domeier, R.M., et al. (2002). Multicenter prospective validation of prehospital clinical spinal clearance criteria. *Journal of Trauma: Injury, Infection, and Critical Care, 53*(4), 744-750.

27. Dubendorf, P. (1999). Spinal cord injury pathophysiology. *Critical Care Nursing Quarterly, 22*(2), 31-35.

28. Flannery, J., & Land, K. (2001). Teaching acute care nurses cognitive assessment using LOCFAS: What's the best method? *Journal of Neuroscience Nursing, 33*(1), 50-56.

29. Franzen, M.D. (2000). Neuropsychological assessment in traumatic brain injury. *Critical Care Nursing Quarterly, 23*(3), 58-64.

30. Goldstein, B. (2000). Musculoskeletal conditions after spinal cord injury. *Physical Medicine and Rehabilitation Clinics of North America, 11*(1), 91-108, viii-ix.

31. Guerra, W.K.W., Piek, J., & Gaab, M.R. (1999). Decompressive craniectomy to treat intracranial hypertension in head injured patients. *Intensive and Critical Care Medicine, 25*(11), 1327-1329.

32. Hauber, R.P., & Testani-Dufour, L. (2000). Living in limbo: The low-level brain-injured patient and the patient's family. *Journal of Neuroscience Nursing, 32*(1), 22-26.

33. Henker, R. (1999). Evidence-based practice: Fever-related interventions. *American Journal of Critical Care, 8*(1), 481-489.

34. Henker, R. (2000). Use of blood cultures in the critically ill. *Critical Care Nurse, 20*(1), 45-50.

35. Hickey, J.V. (2003). Craniocerebral trauma. In J.V. Hickey (Ed.), *The clinical practice of neurological and neurosurgical nursing* (5th ed., pp. 373-406). Philadelphia: J.B. Lippincott.

36. Hickey, J.V. (2003). Intracranial hypertension: Theory and management of increased intracranial pressure. In J.V. Hickey (Ed.), *The clinical practice of neurological and neurosurgical nursing* (5th ed., pp. 285-318). Philadelphia: J.B. Lippincott.

37. Hickey, J.V. (2003). Vertebral and spinal cord injuries. In J.V. Hickey (Ed.). *The clinical practice of neurological and neurosurgical nursing* (5th ed., pp. 407-450). Philadelphia: J.B. Lippincott.

38. Iacono, L.A. (2000). Exploring the guidelines for the management of severe head injury. *Journal of Neuroscience Nursing, 32*(1), 54-60.

39. Jean-Bay, E. (2000). The biobehavioral correlates of post-traumatic brain injury depression. *Journal of Neuroscience Nursing, 32*(3), 169-176.

40. Karlet, M.C. (2001). Acute management of the patient with spinal cord injury. *International Journal of Trauma Nursing, 7*(2), 43-48.

41. Kavchak-Keyes, M.A. (2000). Autonomic hyperreflexia. *Rehabilitation Nursing, 25*(1), 31-35.

42. Kemp, B., & Thompson, L. (2002). Aging and spinal cord injury: Medical, functional, and psychosocial changes. *SCI Nursing, 19*(2), 51-60.

42a. Kluger, M.J. (1986). Is fever beneficial? *Yale Journal of Biological Medicine, 59*, 89-95.

43. Kirshblum, S. (1999). Treatment alternatives for spinal cord injury related spasticity. *Journal of Spinal Cord Medicine, 22*(3), 199-217.

43a. Kirshblum, S.C., & O'Connor, K.C. (2000). Levels of spinal cord injury and predictors for neurologic recovery. *Physical Medicine and Rehabilitation Clinics of North America, 11*(1), 1-27, vii.

44. Lanig, I.S., & Peterson, W.P. (2000). The respiratory system in spinal cord injury. *Physical Medicine and Rehabilitation Clinics of North America, 11*(1), 29-43, vii.

44a. LeJeune, G., & Howard-Fain, T. (2002). Nursing assessment and management of patients with head injuries. *Dimensions of Critical Care Nursing, 27*(6), 226-229.

45. Linsenmeyer, T.A. (2000). Sexual function and infertility following spinal cord injury. *Physical Medicine and Rehabilitation Clinics of North America 11*(1), 141-156, ix.

46. Little, J.W., et al. (2000). Neurologic recovery and neurologic decline after spinal cord injury. *Physical Medicine and Rehabilitation Clinics of North America, 11*(1), 73-89.

46a. Lohne, V. (2001). Hope in patients with spinal cord injury: A literature review related to nursing. *Journal of Neuroscience Nursing, 82*(2), 173-187.

47. Lovasik, D. (1999). The older patient with a spinal cord injury. *Critical Care Nursing Quarterly, 22*(2), 20-30.

48. March, K. (2000). Intracranial pressure monitoring and assessing intracranial compliance in brain injury. *Critical Care Nursing Clinics of North America, 12*(4), 429-435.

49. Marion, D.W., & Speigel, T.P. (2000). Changes in the management of severe traumatic brain injury: 1991-1997. *Critical Care Medicine, 28*(1), 16-18.

50. Marion, D.W., et al. (1993). The use of moderate therapeutic hypothermia for patients with severe head injuries: A preliminary report. *Journal of Neurosurgery, 79,* 354-362.

51. McIlvoy, L., et al. (2001). Successful incorporation of the severe head injury guidelines into a phased-outcome clinical pathway. *Journal of Neuroscience Nursing, 33*(2), 72-78.

52. McNair, N.D. (1999). Traumatic brain injury. *Nursing Clinics of North America, 34*(3), 637-659.

53. Mitcho, K., & Yanko, J.R. (1999). Acute care management of spinal cord injuries. *Critical Care Nursing Quarterly, 22*(2), 60-79.

54. Morgan, S.P. (1990). A comparison of three methods of managing fever in the neurologic patient. *Journal of Neuroscience Nursing, 22*(1), 19-24.

55. Neatherlin, J.S. (1999). Foundation for practice: Neuroassessment for neuroscience nurses. *Nursing Clinics of North America, 34*(3), 573-592.

56. Neatherlin, J. (2000). Head trauma in the older adult population. *Critical Care Nursing Quarterly, 23*(3), 49-57.

57. O'Donnell, J., et al. (1997). Use and effectiveness of hypothermia blankets for febrile patients in the intensive care unit. *Clinical Infectious Diseases, 24,* 1208-1213.

58. Quint, D.J. (2000). Indications for emergent MRI of the central nervous system. *Journal of the American Medical Association, 283*(7), 853-855.

59. Proctor, M.R. (2002). Spinal cord injury. *Critical Care Medicine, 30*(11) Suppl, S489-S499.

60. Quint, D.J. (2000). Indications for emergent MRI of the central nervous system. *Journal of the American Medical Association, 283*(7), 853-855.

61. Roth, P., & Farls, K. (2000). Pathophysiology of traumatic brain injury. *Critical Care Nursing Quarterly, 23*(3), 14-25.

62. Rovlias, A., & Kotson, S. (2000). The influence of hyperglycemia on neurologic outcome in patients with severe head injury. *Neurosurgery, 46*(2), 335-342.

63. Segatore, M. (1999). Corticosteroids and traumatic brain injury: Status at the end of the decade of the brain. *Journal of Neuroscience Nursing, 31*(4), 239-250.

64. Seidl, E.C. (1999). Promising pharmacological agents in the management of acute spinal cord injury. *Critical Care Nursing Quarterly, 22*(2), 44-50.

65. Shpritz, D.W. (1999). Neurodiagnostic studies. *Nursing Clinics of North America, 34*(3), 593-606.

66. Stempien, L., & Tsai, T. (2000). Intrathecal baclofen pump use for spasticity: a clinical survey. *American Journal of Physical Medicine & Rehabilitation, 79*(6), 536-541, 547-550, 564.

67. Sullivan, J. (2000). Positioning of patients with severe traumatic brain injury: Research based practice. *Journal of Neuroscience Nursing, 32*(4), 204-209.

68. Thurman, D.J., et al. (1999). Traumatic brain injury in the United States: A public health perspective. *Journal of Head Trauma Rehabilitation, 14*(6), 602-615.

69. UCLA Nursing Practice Research Council. (n.d.).Research-based practice guideline for blood cultures. Retrieved July 10, 2003, from http://www.mednet.ucla.edu/nursing.

70. UCLA Nursing Practice Research Council. (n.d.).Research-based practice guidelines for fever and cooling measures. Retrieved July 10, 2003, from http://www.mednet.ucla.edu/nursing.

71. Vaughn, L.K., Veale, W.L., & Cooper, K.E. (1980). Antipyresis: Its effect on mortality rate of bacterially infected rabbits. *Brain Research Bulletin, 5,* 69-73.

72. Wick, J., et al. (1999). Use of decompressive craniectomy after severe head trauma. *AORN Journal, 69*(3), 517-529.

73. Winemuller, M.K., et al. (1999). Prevention of venous thromboembolism in patients with spinal cord injury: Effects of sequential pneumatic compression and heparin. *Journal of Spinal Cord Medicine, 23*(3), 182-191.

74. Winkelman, C. (2000). Effect of backrest position on intracranial and cerebral perfusion pressures in traumatically brain-injured adults. *American Journal of Critical Care, 9*(6), 373-380.

75. Wong, F.W.H. (2000). Prevention of secondary brain injury. *Critical Care Nurse, 20* (5), 18-27.

76. Zuccarelli, L.A. (2000). Altered cellular anatomy of acute brain injury and spinal cord injury. *Critical Care Nursing Clinics of North America, 12*(4), 403-411.

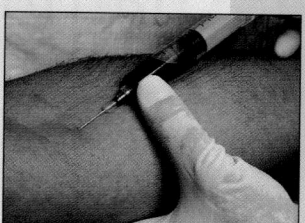

Unit 17

Protective Disorders

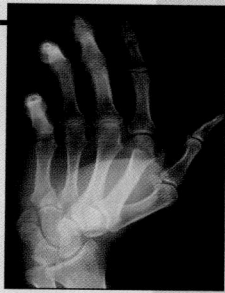

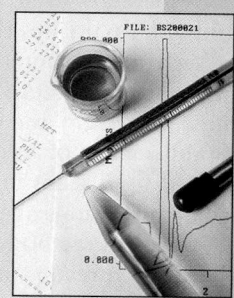

Anatomy and Physiology Review

The Hematopoietic System

Robert G. Carroll

Survival depends on maintaining a barrier separating the inside of the body from pathogens outside of the body and on employing effective defense mechanisms against those pathogens that break that barrier. The epithelium of the skin, gastrointestinal (GI), respiratory, urinary and reproductive tracts, provide the barrier. The body defends itself against attack by viruses, bacteria, and other parasites that enter the body by using two sets of separate but interrelated functions: (1) innate immunity and (2) adaptive immunity. Both of these systems must be present and operating properly in order to block establishment of infectious agents, to minimize damage caused by disease in progress, and to expel, destroy, or isolate infectious agents that gain access to inner tissues.

Together, the body is protected using both *surveillance* ("inside" threats) and *defense* ("outside" threats) functions. The importance of these mechanisms to our health and well-being becomes apparent when the defenses of a healthy body are compromised by infection or suppressed by medication or chemotherapy. Parts of the defense system in a healthy body may function inappropriately to reject organ and tissue transplants and may produce autoimmune disease or hypersensitivity states that cause pathologic changes and sometimes death.

RESISTANCE: A FORM OF NONSPECIFIC DEFENSE

The first line of defense in the body is the aspect of resistance that stops a threatening agent or condition. Defenses provide a form of resistance against disease by combating anything not recognized as *self*. Resistance components are usually the first to encounter infectious agents or parasites. Many of these functions operate independently of the immune system but, as shown later, some of the components and features participate in or amplify acquired immune responses.

SURFACE DEFENSES

Intact skin and mucous membranes, combined with surface-clearing mechanisms, are sufficient to provide barriers that prevent penetration to underlying tissues by many pathogens. Lysozyme in tears and bile in the gut inhibit gram-positive bacteria; hydrochloric acid in the stomach is lethal to many pathogens; and fatty acids help protect the skin from infectious agents.

The *reticuloendothelial system* (RES) includes mononuclear phagocytic cells (macrophages). Fixed (attached) macrophages in the sinusoids of the liver, spleen, and bone marrow monitor the circulating blood and remove all foreign particulates and any moribund self cells. Resident mobile macrophages in lymph nodes remove foreign particulate matter. Macrophages in the alveolar spaces are the most active of the RES cells and help remove inspired particulates that reach the lower recesses of the lung.

ORGANS OF THE IMMUNE AND HEMATOLOGIC SYSTEMS

The organs of the immune and hematologic systems are shown in Figure U17-1. There are both the peripheral sites for the production of the molecules and cells that serve as effector units of the immune response, and the central organs that prepare antigens for recognition.

Lymph Nodes

Lymph nodes are mostly small organs (many are less than 5 mm in diameter) that are present throughout the body interconnected by means of lymph vessels. Their structure is fairly complex and provides both RES and immune functions. The lymph node receives fluids, particulates, and solutes that are taken up by lymphatic capillaries from distal tissue sites. Resident macrophages within the node monitor the lymph fluid passing through for the presence of foreign particulates and remove them by phagocytic action. Antigenic substances, either particulates or solutes, are taken up by the macrophages or dendritic cells serving as antigen-presenting cells (APCs). Immunocompetent cells in the lymph node can give rise to either a humoral immune response or a cell-mediated immune response.

Lymph nodes are found in large numbers in the thoracic and abdominal cavities. Those lying close to the body surface are called *superficial nodes*. Cervical nodes

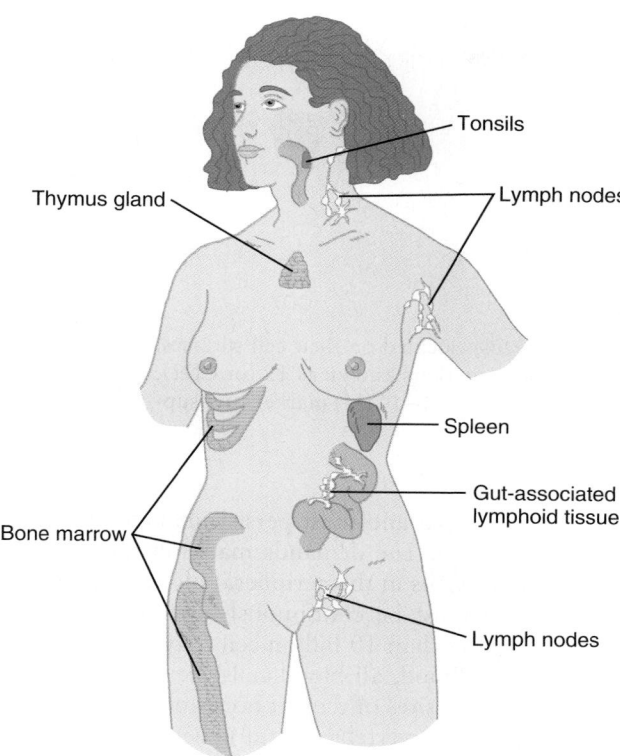

FIGURE U17-1 Organs of the immune system. The bone marrow, spleen, lymph nodes, tonsils, and gut-associated lymphoid tissue (GALT) function in both specific and nonspecific immunity, whereas the thymus functions primarily in specific immunity.

lie alongside the neck, axillary nodes in the armpit, and inguinal nodes in the crease between the upper thigh and the trunk. When inflamed, these nodes become swollen and may be palpated, serving as diagnostic signs.

Lymph Nodules

The structure of the lymph nodules is much less organized than that of the lymph nodes. The nodules occur in the mucosal epithelium lining the respiratory, GI, and urogenital tracts. Antigenic materials are translocated across the epithelium through a special cell (M cell). The translocated material is deposited directly into the nodule structure where it is taken up by APCs. Immunocompetent B cells in lymph nodules produce either immunoglobulin E (IgE) or A (IgA). These immunoglobulins provide for the development either of allergy of the immediate hypersensitivity type or, for IgA, of a mucosal immune response.

Spleen

The spleen is the largest lymphoid organ in the body. Its defensive functions include the blood-clearing process via fixed macrophages in sinusoids as well as serving as a major site of humoral immune responses to blood-borne antigens. The splenic pulp is divided into red

zones and white zones. The white zones are accumulations of lymphocytes and APCs. Loss of the spleen or diminished function due to injury or infection greatly increases the risk of infection with extracellular bacteria.

Other functions of the spleen include (1) assisting in recycling iron by capturing hemoglobin released from destroyed red blood cells (RBCs) and (2) performing pitting (removal of particles from RBCs without destroying the cell itself).

Thymus

The thymus is located in the mediastinum, and reaches peak development during childhood. After puberty, it begins to atrophy but remnants persist into old age. The thymus is an endocrine organ that secretes hormones that contribute to the maintenance and function of peripheral T-cell populations.

A fundamental paradigm in immunology is the rearrangement of germ line genes during differentiation of lymphocytes in the central lymphoid tissues, leading to the production of molecules for the recognition of antigen. In both cell types, the antigen recognition unit is inserted into the membrane with the antigen-reactive ends extending out into the extracellular environment. The T cell uses the T-cell antigen receptor, and the B cell has a tetrapeptide monomer called *surface immunoglobulin* (SIg). The individual cells each have a unique receptor capable of reacting only with a single antigenic determinant (Figure U17-2). Each specifically reacting cell is called a *clonotype;* when properly stimulated by antigen, the clonotype produces effector units (either antibody molecules or specially reactive cells) and a memory cell clone, both of which have the identical specificity of the original clonotype.

The positive and negative selection processes acting on cells in the thymus make it possible for the mechanism to discriminate between *self* and *non-self* in immune function. This distinction is accomplished by making antigen recognition absolutely dependent on the variable but individually unique composition of the transcription products of gene loci located in the major histocompatibility region of the genome.

Class I major histocompatibility complex (MHC) molecules are found on nearly all nucleated cells in the body and represent a major antigenic distinction between individuals of a given species with different genotypes. This molecule is necessary for antigen recognition by T cells with CD8 surface markers. Class II MHC molecules are found on some APCs, on all B cells, and on antigen-activated T cells. This molecule is necessary for antigen recognition by T cells with CD4 surface markers. MHC antigens in humans were initially discovered on leukocyte membranes and are thus called *human leukocyte antigens* (HLAs). It is this recognition system that forms the basis for the rejection of foreign or transplanted tissue. The cells in the recipient's immune system

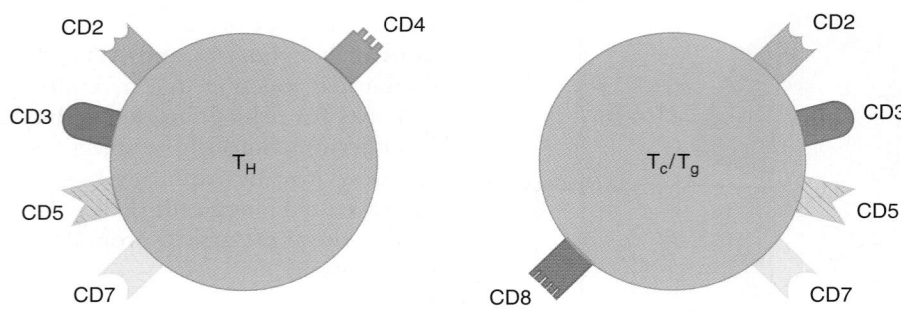

FIGURE U17-2 T cells can be distinguished by distinctive molecules located on their cell surfaces. They are called cluster designations (CDs). All mature T cells carry markers known as T2 (or CD2), T3 (or CD3), T5 (or CD5), and T7 (or CD7). T helper (T_H) cells carry a T4 (CD4) marker, and suppressor and cytotoxic T (T_c/T_g) cells carry a T8 (CD8) marker.

recognize the surface HLA proteins of the donor's tissue as being non-self.

Bone Marrow

Bone marrow constitutes one of the largest organs in the body, with an aggregate weight in adults of about 3000 g (comparable in mass to the liver). Based on visual appearance, the marrow mass was originally described as being either red or yellow. *Red marrow* consists of a mass of supporting cells surrounding aggregates of hematopoietic cells and interspaced with sinusoidal capillaries. *Yellow marrow,* is less active in hematopoiesis, with the light color resulting from adipose cells.

Function of Bone Marrow

Bone marrow provides for the following:

- Maintenance of a self-renewing pluripotent stem cell population from which all blood cells are derived
- An environment for the differentiation and maturation of blood cells
- A storage site for large numbers of neutrophils and erythrocytes
- Transformation of undifferentiated lymphocytes into mature B cells
- A site of antibody production in a secondary immune response to thymic-dependent antigens administered intravenously

Sinusoids bearing fixed macrophages serve an RES function in blood clearing. This is a defensive action based on the phagocytic activity of the macrophages attached to the luminal side of the marrow sinuses. These phagocytes, part of the RES or mononuclear phagocytic system, monitor the blood for the presence of foreign particulate matter, remove it, and destroy it.

Formation of Blood Cells

Hematopoiesis, the process of formation and development of blood cells, begins early in the development of the human embryo and must persist unabated throughout one's lifetime. The demands made on this function are enormous. Cells in the peripheral blood have a finite life span and must be continuously renewed at a rate probably greater than 10 billion cells/day.

During childhood, all blood cells are essentially produced in marrow sites of the flat bones of the skull, clavicle, sternum, ribs, vertebrae, and pelvis. After puberty, hematopoiesis becomes localized within the flat bones of the sternum, ilium, ribs, and vertebrae, sometimes occurring in the proximal ends of long bones (humerus and femur).

Blood

Blood is a complex fluid in which a variety of cells RBCs, white blood cells (WBCs), and platelets are suspended in plasma. Blood circulates continuously through the heart and vascular system. Circulating blood performs many functions, including the following:

- Supplying cells with oxygen from the lungs and absorbed nutrients from the GI tract
- Removing waste products from tissues to the kidney, skin, and lungs for excretion
- Transporting hormones from their origin in the endocrine glands to their targets in other parts of the body
- Protecting the body from dangerous microorganisms
- Promoting *hemostasis* (the arrest of bleeding)
- Regulating body temperature by heat transfer

Composition

About 8% of our total body weight is blood; for example, a healthy young female has 4 to 5 L and a male has about 5 to 6 L. Blood volume also varies by age and body composition. The less body fat, the more blood per kilogram of body weight is present.

Arterial blood is bright red because of the oxygen bound to the hemoglobin within RBCs. Venous blood is dark red because of the lower amount of oxygenated hemoglobin. Pulse oxymetry uses this change in color to estimate the oxygen saturation in tissues. Blood is three to four times more viscous (thick) than water. Specific gravity is 1.048 to 1.066. Blood normally has a pH of 7.35 to 7.45.

Plasma

Plasma, the liquid portion of the blood, is one of the three major body fluids (along with interstitial and intracellular fluids). A straw-colored, watery substance, plasma is composed of 92% water, 7% proteins, and less than 1% nutrients, metabolic wastes, respiratory gases, enzymes, hormones, clotting factors, and inorganic salts. Serum albumin and gamma globulin contribute to colloidal osmotic pressure (see Chapter 13). Gamma globulin also contains the antibody immunoglobulins IgM, IgG, IgA, IgD, and IgE, which are essential in the body's defense against microorganisms.

Plasma makes up about 55% of the blood, and solid suspended particles (blood cells and platelets) compose the other 45%. If a tube of blood is allowed to stand or is spun in a centrifuge, the cells separate. The term *packed cell volume* or *hematocrit* is used to express the volume or percent of the RBCs in the sample. Normal hematocrit levels are 35% to 45%. Hematocrit can be increased from loss of plasma (e.g., dehydration) or increased production of RBCs (polycythemia). Low hematocrit levels are seen in overhydration and low numbers of RBCs (Figure U17-3). The WBCs and platelets make up less than 1% of the blood volume. These cells form a buffy coat or white layer and are seen at the interface of the RBCs and plasma.

Hematopoiesis

Stem cells are poorly characterized, undifferentiated cells that exist within the red marrow. These totipotent, or pluripotent, stem cells are self-replicating and maintain a small population throughout the lifetime of the individual. Following stimulation by one or more signal molecules called *poietins*, the stem cells can undergo differentiation into erythrocytes (RBCs), megakaryocytes, and leukocytes. The steps of hematopoiesis and the divisions of each cell, once it takes a committed path, are shown in Figure U17-4.

Control of Hematopoiesis. Growth factors *(cytokines)* control blood cell growth, proliferation, and differentiation. Growth factors are usually identified by using acronyms that are a legacy from original studies of colony-forming cells. The suffix "-CSF" (colony-stimulating factor) describes the growth factor that stimulates or regulates the development of the corresponding cell type identified by the prefix "CFU-." For example, G-CSF is the growth factor for CFU-G (colony-forming unit–granulocytic series), and M-CSF is the growth factor regulating the development of monocytes (CFU-M). Other growth factors, interleukins (ILs), are given numbers to distinguish between different molecules.

Red Blood Cells

RBCs (erythrocytes) carry oxygen to the cells and help transport carbon dioxide back to the lungs. RBCs also assist with acid-base balance. They contain carbonic anhydrase, an enzyme that joins carbon dioxide to water to form carbonic acid. The acid dissociates to form bicarbonate and hydrogen ions, which diffuse out of the RBC.

The mature RBC has no nucleus and is only 7.5 mm in diameter. Each RBC has a depression on the flat surface that provides a thin center and thicker edges. The unique structure of the RBC supplies a large surface area relative to its volume (to facilitate exchange by diffusion) and allows the cell to change shape passively as it is transported through capillaries that are smaller than 7.5 mm in diameter. The average RBC count is 5,500,000 cells/mm³ of blood.

Packed within each RBC are about 200 to 300 million molecules of hemoglobin. Each hemoglobin molecule is composed of four protein chains (globin). The globin is bound to a heme group that contains one iron atom. In healthy men, 100 ml of blood contains 14 to 16 g of hemoglobin. Women have slightly less, about 12 to 14 g. Anemia is present when hemoglobin levels decrease to less than 10 g per 100 ml of blood.

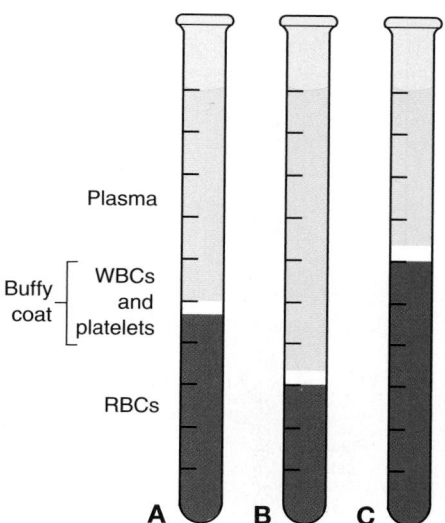

Plasma

Buffy coat — WBCs and platelets

RBCs

A **B** **C**

FIGURE U17-3 Tubes showing hematocrit levels of normal blood, anemia, and polycythemia. Note the buffy coat located between the packed red blood cells (RBCs) and the plasma. **A,** A normal percentage of RBCs (45%). **B,** Anemia (a low percentage of RBCs, 30%). **C,** Polycythemia (a high percentage of RBCs, 60%). *WBCs,* White blood cells. (Modified from Thibodeau, G., & Patton, K. [2003]. *Anatomy and physiology* [5th ed., p. 532]. St. Louis: Mosby.)

CELLS SEEN
IN BONE MARROW

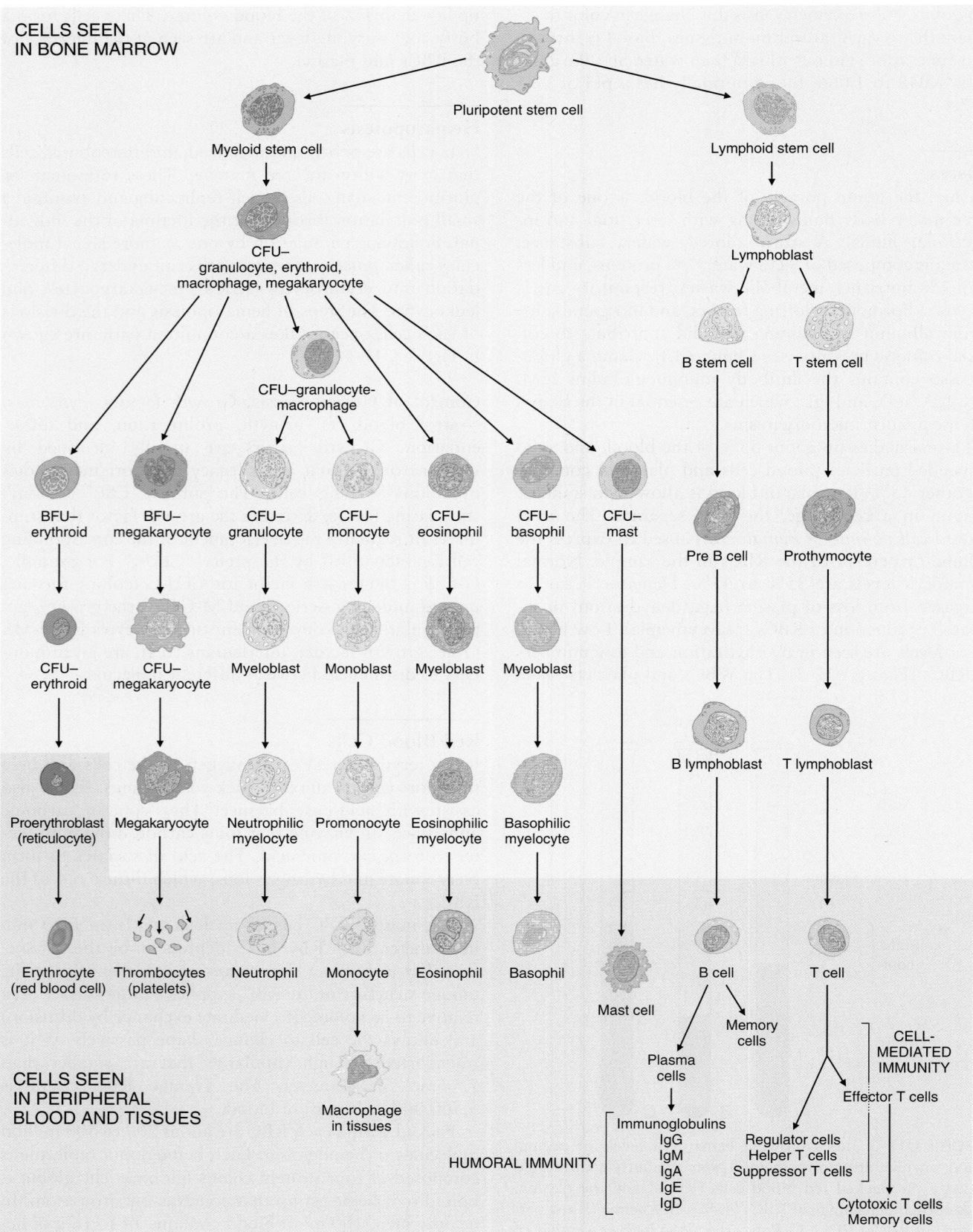

CELLS SEEN
IN PERIPHERAL
BLOOD AND TISSUES

FIGURE U17-4 Hematopoietic cascade. The pluripotent stem cell is the origin of all cells. Once a pathway is chosen, the cell is committed to the final cell type.

Erythrocyte Production. The production of erythrocytes is termed *erythropoiesis.* Normally, more than 100 million RBCs, or about 1% of the body's total, are formed to replace an equal number of destroyed cells. Erythropoietin increases the rate of RBC production when oxygen levels decrease or during pregnancy. Healthy bone marrow has the capacity to increase its production of erythrocytes six to eight times over the normal rate and is thus able to keep pace with increased destruction or loss of RBCs. This response mechanism leads to a remarkably constant number of erythrocytes.

Erythrocytes are produced in the red bone marrow. Required for this process are (1) precursor cells, (2) a proper microenvironment, and (3) adequate supplies of iron, vitamin B$_{12}$, folic acid, protein, pyridoxine, and traces of copper. If any of these factors is missing, the resultant erythrocytes are fragile, misshapen, abnormally large or small, deficient in hemoglobin, or too few in number. Erythrocytes arise from nucleated cells called *hematopoietic stem cells. Stem cells* can maintain a constant population of newly differentiating cells. Differentiation takes about 7 days and involves about six stages (see Figure U17-4).

Immature erythrocytes leave the bone marrow via veins in the marrow and enter the general circulation as nucleated reticulocytes. After their release from the marrow sites, the reticulocytes travel to the spleen, where they undergo conditioning and evolve into mature erythrocytes before being released into the general circulation.

The life span of RBCs is about 105 to 120 days. As erythrocytes age, they become increasingly fragile and eventually rupture. The released hemoglobin and the empty membranes ("ghost cells") are taken up by macrophages within the liver, spleen, lymph nodes, and bone marrow. The hemoglobin is broken down into heme (iron and porphyrin) and globin (polypeptide chain) fractions. The iron of the heme fraction is returned to the liver, spleen, and bone marrow to be reused in making hemoglobin. The liver converts the porphyrin of the heme fraction into bilirubin, an orange pigment, and secretes it into the bile to be excreted from the body in the feces and urine (Figure U17-5). During periods of increased RBC destruction (e.g., in hemolytic anemia), excessive amounts of bilirubin are formed and may accumulate in the body's tissues.

Nutritional Influences on Red Blood Cell Production. Vitamin B$_{12}$ and folic acid are essential for normal RBC maturation and nervous system functions. Because it is not synthesized in the body, vitamin B$_{12}$ must be a component of the daily diet. Animal products such as meat and dairy products are primary sources of this vitamin. When released from food during digestion, vitamin B$_{12}$ binds with *intrinsic factor,* and the complex is absorbed in the distal ileum. Folic acid, a B-group vitamin synthe-

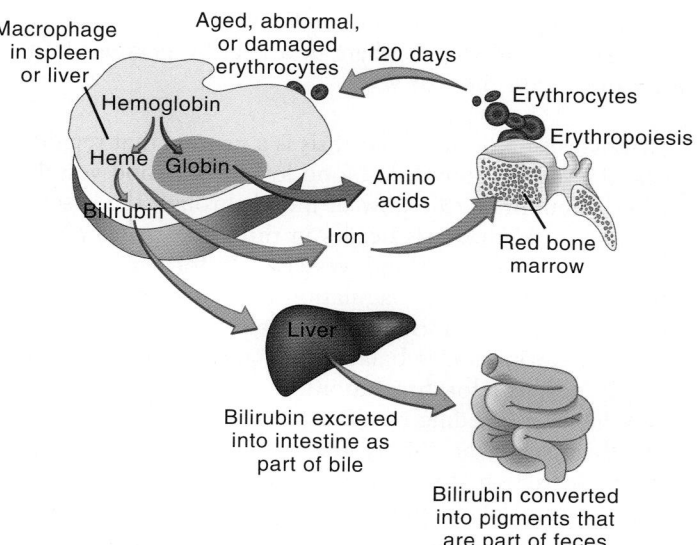

FIGURE U17-5 Destruction of red blood cells. (From Thibodeau, G., & Patton, K. [2003]. *Anatomy and physiology* [5th ed., p. 537]. St. Louis: Mosby.)

sized by many plants and bacteria, is also necessary for RBC formation and maturation.

Iron is essential to hemoglobin production. The adult human body contains about 50 mg of iron per 100 ml of blood. Total body iron ranges between 2 and 6 g, depending on the size of the person and the amount of hemoglobin sequestered within the cellular compartment. Hemoglobin accounts for about two thirds of the total iron (called *essential iron*). The other one third resides in the bone marrow, spleen, liver, and muscle. When an iron deficiency develops, the latter iron stores are depleted first, followed by a gradual loss of the iron contained in hemoglobin.

Megakaryocytes and Platelets

Platelets *(thrombocytes)* have two essential roles in hemostasis: (1) occlusion of small openings in blood vessels (a hemostatic function) and (2) provision of chemical components in the molecular cascade leading to coagulation (a thromboplastic function).

Individual platelets are produced by a fragmentation process from giant multinucleated cells in the red bone marrow called *megakaryocytes* (see Figure U17-4). The time required for the formation of human platelets is about 5 days. Cytoplasmic extensions from megakaryoblasts are extruded into sinusoids, and platelets are formed by fragmentation at the terminal ends of the filaments. Normal human marrow may have up to 6 million megakaryocytes per kilogram of body weight, with each megakaryocyte being able to give rise to 1000 or more individual platelets. Platelet production in a normal person appears to be under tight control by the hepatic hormone *thrombopoietin* and is remarkably consistent, with the numbers in a healthy person often remaining constant for years.

Hemostasis. Normal hemostasis is a process that repairs vascular breaks to reduce blood loss from blood vessels while maintaining the flow of blood through the vascular system. Hemostasis occurs in three stages: (1) *vasoconstriction* of the blood vessels, (2) formation of a platelet plug, and (3) coagulation or formation of a fibrin clot. Once the fibrin clot has served its purpose, further clot formation is balanced by anticoagulation and by *fibrinolysis* (clot dissolution).

Whenever bleeding results from injury or disease, the blood vessels that supply the damaged site constrict. Vasoconstriction slows the flow of blood to the injured area, decreasing blood loss. Vasoconstriction results from muscular tissue and reflex nervous system reactions. *Thromboxane A₂*, a potent local vasoconstrictor, is secreted by platelets and promotes constriction of small blood vessels following injury.

Adequate numbers of platelets (150,000 to 400,000/mm³) are required in the peripheral blood for hemostasis. When platelets come into contact with an alteration of the endothelial cell lining of a blood vessel, they become sticky and adhere to one another, thus sealing the surface of the vessel lining. These platelet constituents can activate additional platelets that aggregate to form a *thrombus*.

Platelets control hemostasis unless large blood vessels have been damaged. If bleeding is severe, coagulation factors must join with platelets to form a permanent clot. The coagulation system consists of a series of interactions that result in the formation of a fibrin clot. The system consists of clotting proteins, most of which circulate in the plasma in an inactive state.

The formation of a fibrin clot can result from activation of one of two pathways: *intrinsic* or *extrinsic* (Figure U17-6). Various factors are needed by these two pathways for completion of a final common pathway that results in a fibrin clot. The *extrinsic pathway* is initiated when tissue injury occurs outside the vessels, such as a burn. The *intrinsic pathway* involves the blood itself (i.e., antigen-antibody reactions and endotoxins) or damage to the blood vessels. Blood in normal vessels that is stagnant for a long period of time can form clots.

Activated factor X is responsible for the conversion of prothrombin to thrombin and of soluble fibrinogen to an insoluble fibrin clot. The protein fibrin forms dense interlacing threads that entrap erythrocytes and platelets. The platelets then release a contractile protein, which causes shrinkage and retraction of the clot into a firm, insoluble fibrin mass. The process of retraction squeezes out the clear yellow serum. Serum differs from plasma, in that it does not contain clotting factors.

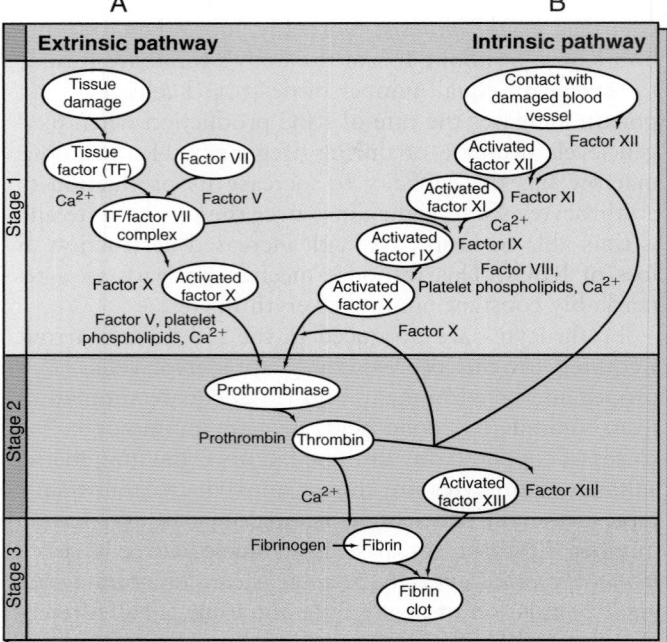

FIGURE U17-6 Clot formation. **A,** Extrinsic clotting pathway. *Stage I:* Damaged tissue releases tissue factor (TF), which with factor VII and calcium ions activate factor X. Activated factor X, factor V, phospholipids, and calcium ions form prothrombinase. *Stage 2:* Prothrombin is converted to thrombin by prothrombinase. *Stage 3:* Fibrinogen is converted to fibrin by thrombin. Fibrin forms a clot. **B,** Intrinsic clotting pathway. *Stage 1:* Damaged vessels cause activation of factor XII. Activated factor XII activates factor XI, which activates factor IX. Factor IX, along with factor VIII and platelet phospholipids, activates factor X. Activated factor X, factor V, phospholipids, and calcium ions form prothrombinase. *Stages 2* and *3* take the same course as in the extrinsic clotting pathway. (From Thibodeau, G., & Patton, K. [2003]. *Anatomy and physiology* [5th ed., p. 547]. St. Louis: Mosby.)

In some cases, formation of a fibrin clot is unnecessary because hemostasis occurs at an early stage. Temporary clots are sometimes insufficient. For example, bleeding from a small pinprick can normally be ended by a platelet plug, whereas more serious cuts require the interaction of the various coagulation factors.

Fibrinolysis and Anticoagulants. The coagulation system is controlled by several mechanisms to maintain a flow of blood through the vascular space. The blood carries natural anticoagulants (e.g., heparin, antithrombin, antithromboplastin) that act continuously to inhibit coagulation. The liver and RES also aid in controlling coagulation by removing activated clotting factors and fibrin.

In fibrinolysis, the fibrin clot is dissolved. The fibrinolytic mechanism activates in less than a day after clot formation. Formation of plasmin by *tissue plasminogen activator* is the major mechanism for dissolving a clot. Plasmin, a proteolytic enzyme, can dissolve such protein material as fibrin, fibrinogen, and factors V and VIII. Plasminogen, a serum globulin, is the inactive precursor of plasmin. Lysis of the clot produces formation of fibrin split products (or fibrin degradation products), which also act as anticoagulants.

Blood vessels break and are repaired continuously in the body. The multiple and complex interactions between clot formation, clot lysis, and anticoagulation allows normal vessel repair without precipitating a massive clot throughout the vascular system. Clots formed in the venous system often break free (embolus) and are transported to the lung capillaries, which have enhanced clot lysis properties. In contrast, emboli formed on the arterial system travel progressively through the arteriolar tree, until they occlude an arteriole and block blood flow to areas distal to the occlusion.

Roles of the Liver and Spleen

The spleen and liver both have important roles in the hematopoietic system. The spleen, lung, and liver sequester some of the peripheral blood erythrocytes, providing a ready reserve supply whenever the RBC count decreases significantly. The liver is also important in the blood-clearing process. Fixed macrophages *(Kupffer cells)* remove inanimate particulates and bacterial cells that appear in the peripheral blood. The roles of the liver in hematopoiesis are mostly indirect, related to the synthesis of plasma proteins and clotting factors, the decomposition of hemoglobin into bilirubin, and the storage of iron in the form of *ferritin*

White Blood Cells (Leukocytes)

There are five types of WBCs, or *leukocytes,* classified according to the presence or absence of granules and the staining characteristics of their cytoplasm. As a group, the leukocytes appear brightly colored when stained. *Granulocytes* are derived from a myeloid stem cell that differentiates (see Figure U17-4). Granulocytes include three types of WBCs that have large granules in their cytoplasm. Their names are derived from the staining properties: (1) *neutrophils,* (2) *eosinophils,* and (3) *basophils.* There are two types of agranulocytes (WBCs without cytoplasmic granules): (1) *monocytes* and (2) *lymphocytes.*

Granulocytes

Neutrophils. Neutrophils stain very light pink-purple with neutral dyes. The granules in their cytoplasm make them appear "coarse," and they have nuclei with many lobes. Because of the appearance of their nuclei, they are also called polymorphonuclear leukocytes ("polys").

The neutrophil is the primary cell to respond during an acute inflammatory response (see Figure U17-4). About 90% of mature neutrophils remain in the bone marrow, a storage arrangement that enables the body to quickly release large numbers of these cells when inflammation occurs in perimeter tissues. The remaining 10% of neutrophils in the peripheral blood are subdivided, about half and half, into a circulating cell group and a cell group that adheres to endothelial linings in small blood vessels.

Thus a complete blood count (CBC) for a healthy person accounts for only about 5% of the total number of mature neutrophils actually present in the body at that time. The increases seen in peripheral WBC counts during episodes of inflammation are the result of large numbers of neutrophils being released from the bone marrow reserve. If the inflamed state is prolonged, the supply of mature cells with lobed nuclei becomes exhausted, and immature neutrophils with a banded nucleus appear in the circulating blood. The life span of the neutrophil is hours to 3 days.

Eosinophils. Eosinophils contain numerous large granules that stain orange. Under normal circumstances, mature eosinophils do not remain long in the marrow; they are present only in small numbers in the peripheral blood (less than 3% of the total WBC count in a healthy person). These cells exit the peripheral blood compartment and accumulate in extravascular sites near epithelial surfaces. From there, they can be recruited to protect against parasitic infections and to modulate IgE-mediated allergic responses. Their life span is hours to 3 days.

Basophils. The basophil stains purple and has large granules. Details of its normal role in body homeostasis are lacking. The intracytoplasmic granules (storage vesicles) include heparin, histamine, and a chemotactic factor for eosinophils. There is disagreement as to whether this cell is a precursor to a similar cell found in solid tissues: the mast cell. Vesicular contents in the mast cell are similar to those found in the basophil, and the human mast cell is known to bind IgE and to be a primary participant in the induction of IgE-mediated allergic cascades.

Agranulocytes

Monocytes. The monocyte is derived from a precursor cell that is indistinguishable from a myeloblast. Subsequent differentiation, however, leads to a cell structure that is markedly different from that of the granulocyte. The monocyte released from the bone marrow into the circulation is a hypoactive phagocytic cell. After becoming attached to sinusoidal endothelium in the spleen, bone marrow, and liver, or after emigrating from the blood into lung, connective, or lymphoid tissue, this cell becomes transformed into a *macrophage* with full phagocytic function. These cells constitute the RES and are responsible for removing all foreign particulate material that enters the body.

The macrophage is attracted secondarily to acute inflamed sites and is the characteristic cell in chronic and in many secretory T-cell–orchestrated inflammatory lesions. Some macrophages also have immune functions by serving as antigen-processing cells and APCs.

Lymphocytes. In their mature form, lymphocytes are assigned to one of three groups according to the presence of characteristic surface markers and cell function (see Figure U17-2): (1) Some lymphocytes are programmed in the thymus to become *T cells;* (2) others are programmed in the bone marrow become *B cells;* (3) some lymphocytes, not identifiable as either T cells or B cells, are *natural killer (NK) cells. B cells* function in antibody-mediated immune responses helping to defend the body against invasive types of bacteria, bacterial toxins, and some viruses. *T cells* are the basis of cell-mediated immune functions that defend against facultative and obligate intracellular pathogens, fungi, and viruses. *NK cells* make up about 5% to 10% of the circulating lymphocytes. They are involved in killing some tumor cells and some virally infected cells. Their cytotoxicity can be enhanced by exposure to cytokines, which convert a naive NK cell into a lymphokine-activated cell. After binding to a target cell, the NK cell secretes *perforins,* which cause holes to form in the target cell membrane in a manner analogous to the membrane attack complex (MAC) of complement. Interestingly, people who have normal T-cell and B-cell populations but who are deficient in NK cells experience repetitive life-threatening infections by viruses such as varicella and cytomegalovirus.

Inflammation

Inflammation is a complex response to sublethal injury to a tissue, having both local and systemic consequences. The process can be initiated by products released from damaged cells, by components from microbial cells, and by the interaction of effector units and antigen. Within the injured tissue site, the first indication is a transient constriction followed by a sustained dilation of small blood vessels. Swelling at the site is caused by increased capillary permeability and the escape of plasma (with its solutes: complement, fibrinogen, immunoglobulins). At about the same time that the vessels are responding, WBCs begin to stick to the vascular endothelium, a process called *margination.* Neutrophils are the first to escape from the vessels *(diapedesis)* and, in response to a chemotactic gradient, accumulate at the site of injury.

After a few hours, monocytes from the local circulation and macrophages present in local connective tissues begin to infiltrate the site of injury. In a limited type of injury, the healing and resolution begin shortly afterward (see Chapter 20). Some cytokines produced by stimulated macrophages act locally to stimulate vascular changes and to activate fibroblasts and other cells. The same or other cytokines are distributed systemically and help to initiate the *acute phase response.* This systemic response accompanies a strong local inflammatory response. Many aspects of the acute phase response are initiated by the action of cytokines produced by stimulated macrophages. These stimulatory molecules include IL-1, tumor necrosis factor (TNF), and IL-6. The systemic responses of the host include (1) elevation of serum cortisol, (2) induction of fever, (3) leukocytosis, (4) the *de novo* appearance of C-reactive protein, an opsonizing protein that aids in phagocytosis, (5) increased production of complement components, and (6) increased production of siderophores (iron-binding proteins).

▌IMMUNITY

We can become immunized following *direct* (active) exposure to an antigen and generation of our own effector units or following *indirect* (passive) receipt of effector units produced by an animal, by another human, or by gene-engineering procedures. Indirect natural immunity occurs in utero via colostrum (topologic protection in humans) and across the placenta (systemic protection in humans). Artificial indirect immunity is produced through pooled gamma (immune)-globulin, $RH_0(D)$ immunoglobulin (RhoGAM), and genetically engineered human antibody.

ACQUIRED IMMUNITY

Four types (or compartments) of active immunity are identified based on the type and body location of the effector units:

1. *Humoral immunity.* The effector units are immunoglobulins (IgM, IgG, and IgA) present in the peripheral blood.
2. *Mucosal immunity.* The effector unit is an immunoglobulin (secretory IgA) present in mucous secretions of the respiratory tract, GI tract, and urogenital tract.
3. *Cell-mediated immunity.* The effector units are cytotoxic T cells that circulate in peripheral blood and are present in peripheral lymphoid tissues.
4. *Atopic hypersensitivity (type I hypersensitivity).* The effector unit is IgE, which is attached to surface receptors on mast cells found in connective tissues and subsurface tissues of the respiratory and GI tract.

THE PRIMARY IMMUNE RESPONSE AND THE IMMUNE CASCADE

A primary immune response arguably occurs only once (Figure U17-7). The quality and quantity of the primary immune response depend on many factors, some of which are host-related whereas others depend on the composition of the antigen and how it is presented to the recipient. The primary immune response can be divided into three stages (the immune cascade).

Phase I: Afferent Phase

Application or Exposure to the Antigen

Topical (skin) exposure is successful only with certain materials called *proantigens*. Examples of these substances include plant secretions (poison oak, poison ivy), salts of nickel and chromium, and formaldehyde. Mucosal exposure, through epithelia in the respiratory, GI, or urogenital tract, is triggered by foods (strawberries, peanuts), drugs (aspirin), pollens, or house dust. Parenteral (subcutaneous, intradermal, intravenous) exposure is via vaccines or allergens for testing.

Transport of Antigen

Lymph nodules lie immediately under modified mucosal epithelium (M cells in the gut). No transport of antigen is required. Antigen deposited into solid tissues gains access to draining lymphatics and is then carried to the nearest regional lymph node. Antigen introduced intravenously localizes in the white pulp of the spleen. Proantigens applied to the skin are absorbed and, in conjunction with Langerhans cells in the subepithelial tissues, are coupled with an autogenous protein. The resultant complex is transported to a regional lymph node.

Arrival of Antigen

Arrival of antigen in peripheral lymphoid tissue is followed by its uptake by APCs.

Any exogenous molecule or any cell that does not have the self-markers of the recipient can serve as an antigen. Antigens may be natural, artificial, or synthetic.

Natural antigens include unmodified bacteria, fungi, viruses, parasites, foreign tissue cells, and large individual molecules such as proteins.

Artificial antigens are natural antigens that have been altered, usually to produce a vaccine: killed or attenuated bacteria, inactivated viruses, and toxoids.

Synthetic antigens are not found in nature but are produced in the laboratory (e.g., molecules genetically engineered to improve current or proposed immunization protocols).

The reactive sites of antigens are called determinant sites (or *epitopes*) and consist of three to five monosaccharide or amino acid residues that act together as a unit. The determinant sites are complementary to the reactive sites of the T-cell antigen receptor (on T cells) and the serum immunoglobulin (on B cells). Each natural antigen has many different epitopes, each of which is capable of stimulating a specific B-cell or T-cell clonotype (Figure U17-8).

Phase 2: Central Phase

In phase 2, the central phase, antigen is taken up by or becomes affiliated with processing and presenting cells. Protein antigens are processed intracellularly by the APCs into peptide fragments. The fragments, in association with the major histocompatibility molecules, are placed on the surface of the APCs for presentation to T cells. B cells can react to antigen in solute form, or the antigen can be adsorbed to the surfaces of follicular

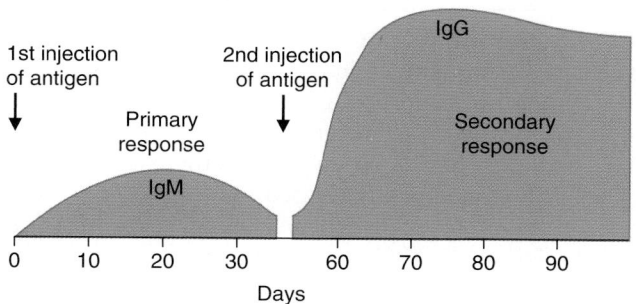

FIGURE U17-7 Primary and secondary antibody response. The second exposure of an antigen to the host causes a more rapid, stronger, and longer-acting response than the first exposure, owing to the presence of memory cells. Immunoglobulin M (IgM) is most often produced in the primary response, whereas IgG is more likely to be produced predominantly in the secondary response.

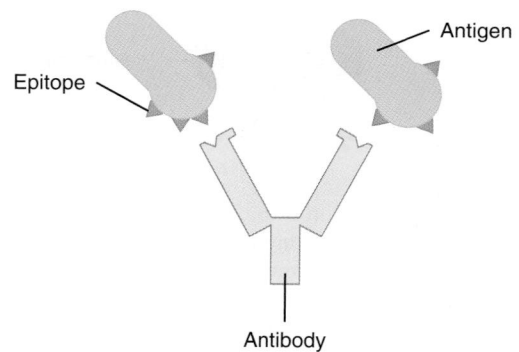

FIGURE U17-8 Epitopes protrude from the surface of an antigen and combine with the appropriate receptor of an antibody, much as a key fits into a lock.

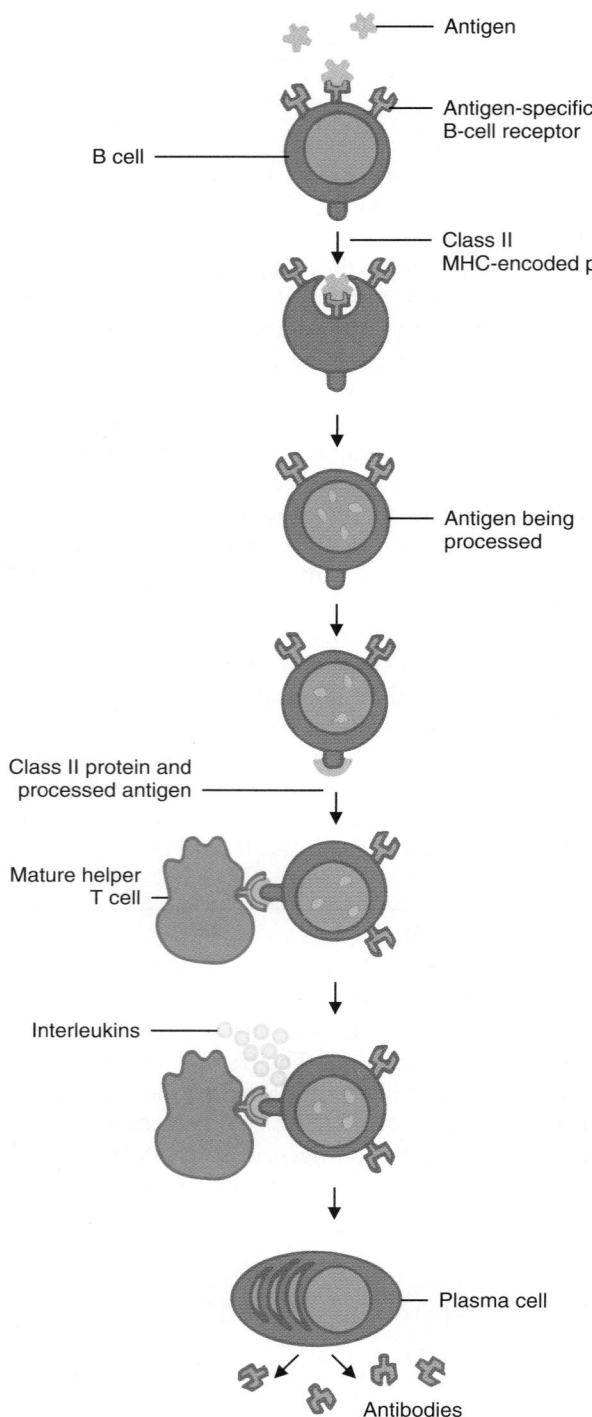

- Antigen
- Antigen-specific B-cell receptor
- B cell
- Class II MHC-encoded protein
- Antigen being processed
- Class II protein and processed antigen
- Mature helper T cell
- Interleukins
- Plasma cell
- Antibodies

FIGURE U17-9 Activation of B cells to make antibody. The B cell uses its receptor to bind matching antigen, which it engulfs and processes. The B cell then presents a piece of antigen, bound to class II protein, on its surface. The complex binds to the mature T helper cell, which releases interleukins that transform the B cell into an antibody-secreting plasma cell. (Redrawn from Schindler, L.W. [1991]. *Understanding the immune system.* Washington, DC: National Institutes of Health.)

dendritic cells. T and B lymphocytes become activated and produce effector units and memory clonotypes.

Phase 3: Efferent Phase

Effector units and memory clonotypes are exported to all body sites. If residual antigen remains in the tissues, effector units may combine with it, causing manifestations until the antigen is neutralized or removed. Residual antigen is most often seen with obligate or facultative intracellular parasites or pathogens. This condition is not likely to occur with an extracellular pathogen.

THE SECONDARY IMMUNE RESPONSE

The secondary immune response occurs when a person who has been previously immunized with an antigen is rechallenged later with the same substance. In this second (and any subsequent) response, effector units are generally produced in greater quantity for a longer period of time, and antibody molecules may exhibit a higher affinity for antigen (see Figure U17-7).

Antigen Processing and Presentation

T-cell recognition of antigen is limited to peptide fragments presented by an APC in conjunction with an MHC molecule. The recognition process is assisted by CD4 or CD8 molecules on the T-cell surface. Class I MHC molecules are used to present peptides to CD8 cells, and class II molecules present peptides to CD4 cells. This recognition process is said to be self-MHC–restricted; that is, the APC and the T cell both must have the same MHC molecules (each must recognize the other as self). The cells that can function as APCs in peripheral lymphoid tissue sites are B cells, dendritic cells, and some macrophages. Other locations include endothelial cells in peripheral vasculature (in humans) and Langerhans cells in the skin.

B Cells and the Antibody Response

B cells recognize antigen in one of two forms:

1. When free, unprocessed antigen (characteristically carbohydrate) is encountered, the response is limited; only IgM is produced, and there are no memory B clonotypes developed.
2. When proteins or protein conjugates are used as antigens, the APCs must first process the molecules to produce peptide fragments, which are combined with MHC molecules and then presented to T helper cells (Figure U17-9).

The activated T cells secrete cytokines, which assist the B cell in responding to its own set of determinant sites present on the protein antigen. The cytokines stimulate growth and maturation in B cells, induce isotype switching, and make possible the development of memory clonotypes in both T and B cell lines.

After being activated by antigen and stimulated by cytokines, the B cell is transformed morphologically and physiologically into a distinct cell type: the *plasma cell.* Plasma cells are highly differentiated and specialized cells that are capable of producing large quantities of secreted immunoglobulin.

Immunoglobulins

Antibodies, or immunoglobulins (Ig), are a family of glycoprotein molecules that are present in the body as solutes in body fluids (plasma and mucous secretions) and attached to a group of cells in solid tissues. Once attached, they inactivate and bind to antigens to facilitate phagocytosis and initiate inflammation by activating the complement cascade (Figure U17-10). The terminal amino acid residues react with receptors on the surface of macrophages, neutrophils, B cells, and mast cells. There are five types (Table U17-1).

IgG. IgG is available to react either by opsonizing antigens for accelerated uptake by RES cells or by activating complement via the classic pathway. When inflammation occurs in extravascular tissues, IgG is carried out of the vascular compartment to the septic site. There are four subclasses of IgG based on variation in amino acid composition in the heavy chain.

IgA. IgA is the predominant immunoglobulin in saliva, tears, colostrum, breast milk, and intestinal and bronchial secretions. The secretory (or mucosal) form of IgA prevents the adherence of microorganisms to mucosal epithelium and thus supplements resistance mechanisms against local infections in the respiratory, GI, and urogenital tracts.

IgM. IgM is normally present as a pentamer stabilized by a peptide J chain. It is the largest of the immunoglobulin molecules and is the class identified by the designation "natural." It is produced in response to challenge by bacteria in the normal gut flora and not only acts against these and similar bacteria that may infect tissue sites but also is the main immunoglobulin composing the isoagglutinins reacting with blood group antigens.

IgM is more effective than IgG in activating complement, because only a single pentameric molecule bound to a cell is sufficient to initiate the cascade sequence (IgG

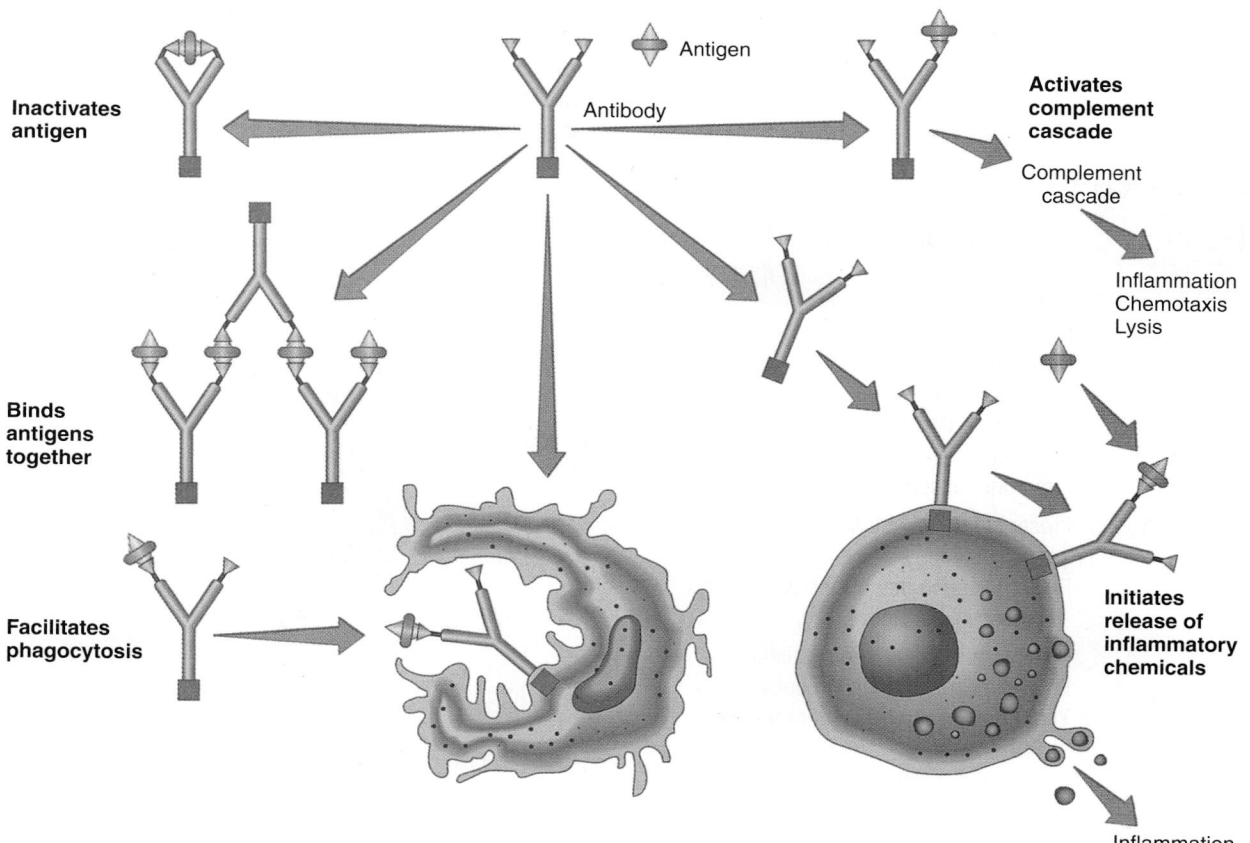

FIGURE U17-10 Actions of antibodies. Antibodies act on antigens by inactivating and binding them together to facilitate phagocytosis and by initiating inflammation and activating the complement cascade. (From Thibodeau, G., & Patton, K. [2003]. *Anatomy and physiology* [5th ed., p. 654]. St. Louis: Mosby.)

requires the presence of two adjacent molecules bound to the cell surface). IgM is the early antibody seen in response to a thymic-dependent antigen and is the sole antibody produced against a thymic-independent antigen.

IgE. In most people, IgE is normally present only in trace amounts within the blood. Exceptions occur in people who have active atopic allergies or who are infected with parasitic worms. In humans, IgE is normally bound to a surface receptor on mast cells, where, following antigen binding, it triggers the release of chemical mediators such as histamine, which helps initiate the cascade of events leading to the expression of atopic allergy.

IgD. The physiologic function of IgD is unknown. It is present in large numbers on the cell membrane of naive B lymphocytes, and its only role is thought to be for antigen recognition.

MONOCLONAL ANTIBODIES

Monoclonal antibodies are immunoglobulins that can be synthesized by fusing a normal plasma cell (for antibody) with a myeloma cell (for longevity). The products of such a hybrid cell are immunoglobulins with an identical specificity. Current technology enables large quantities of immunoglobulins with almost any specificity to be produced at reasonable cost. Because they have a single specificity, they are widely used in research and for diagnostic and therapeutic regimens. Some of the applications include leukocyte identification, parasite and pathogen identification, quantitative estimation of peptide hormones, antitumor therapy, immunosuppression, and fertility control.

COMPLEMENT AND AMPLIFICATION OF ANTIBODY FUNCTION

Complement refers to a group of dissolved plasma proteins. When activated, the various components react in a cascade fashion. Complement activated by antibodies forms holes in the plasma membrane of the bacterium. Sodium and water diffuse into the cell and cause it to swell and burst (Figure U17-11). Plasma complement can be activated by either of two methods: (1) a classic pathway requiring the participation of antibody and (2) an alternative pathway that is independent of antibody.

Activation of complement by the classic pathway must be preceded by the interaction of antigen with antibody (either IgG or IgM). The advantage of this pathway is that complement can be recruited to assist in the removal of any solute or of any cell against which antibody can be produced. The alternative pathway helps defend against pathogens. Surface molecules of many bacterial species can initiate the complement cascade, leading to the destruction of the bacterial cell either indirectly by opsonization or by direct cell lysis.

TABLE U17-1		*Classes and Characteristics of Immunoglobulins (Ig)*
Class	**% of Total**	**Characteristics**
IgG	75	Present in circulation and tissue spaces Opsonizes antigen Activates complement Transferred transplacentally The first Ig synthesized in secondary immune response
IgA	15	Present in the circulation and seromucous secretions Prevents adherence of microorganisms to mucosal surface
IgM	10	Present primarily in the circulation Powerful agglutinating antibody The first Ig of the primary immune response Activates complement
IgE	<1.0	Mediates hypersensitivity reactions Binds to mast cells and triggers mediator release
IgD	<1.0	Lymphocyte differentiation Full function unknown

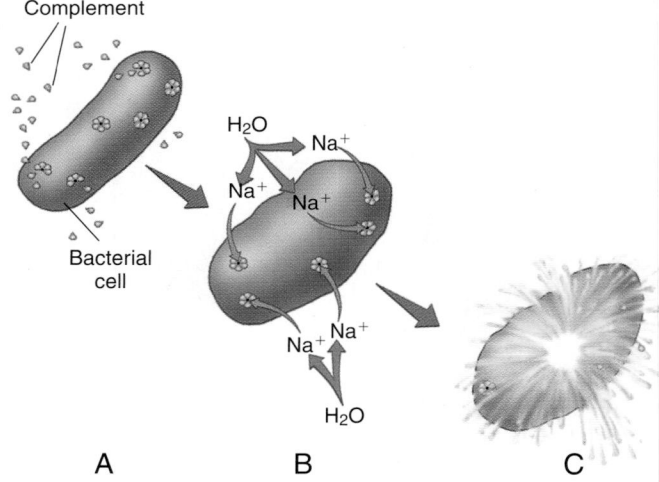

FIGURE U17-11 Complement fixation. **A,** Complement molecules activated by antibodies form doughnut-shaped complexes in a bacterium's plasma membrane. **B,** Holes in the complement complex allow sodium (Na^+) and then water (H_2O) to diffuse into the bacterium. **C,** After enough water has entered, the swollen bacterium bursts. (From Thibodeau, G., & Patton, K. [2003]. *Anatomy and physiology* [5th ed., p. 655]. St. Louis: Mosby.)

T LYMPHOCYTES AND CELL-MEDIATED IMMUNITY

Cell-mediated immunity (CMI) includes immune responses in which antibodies are not involved. CMI is vital in protecting the body against infection by viruses, slow-growing bacteria, and fungal infections. It also has a major role in immunosurveillance, reacting to abnormal clones of self cells, some of which are malignant. Such altered self cells can be destroyed in early stages by cytotoxic T cells or by NK cells, preventing them from becoming established tumors. Other CMI functions include primary rejection of allografts and development of delayed hypersensitivity reactions such as contact dermatitis (poison oak) and hypersensitivity to products of the tubercle bacillus. Many of the biologic actions of T lymphocytes are mediated through the secretion of factors called *lymphokines* (cytokines). Although humoral

and cell-mediated responses are often discussed separately, these two arms of the immune system work together (Figure U17-12), sometimes inseparably, and failure or malfunction in one part of the system frequently alter the effectiveness of the other.

The T lymphocytes that play a predominant role in CMI belong to a variety of T-cell subsets. Some have a regulatory function and are designated as *T helper cells* or *T suppressor cells*; others act as effector cells. Cytokines from antigen-activated T helper cells assist B cells to mature and produce antibody and also modulate the maturation and function of cytotoxic T cells (see Figure U17-12). The importance of T helper cell function is reflected by the severe consequences seen when it is suppressed by physical or chemical means or depleted during infection with human immunodeficiency virus (HIV); the T helper cell is a primary target of HIV. The decline of T helper cells in infected people is almost inevitably

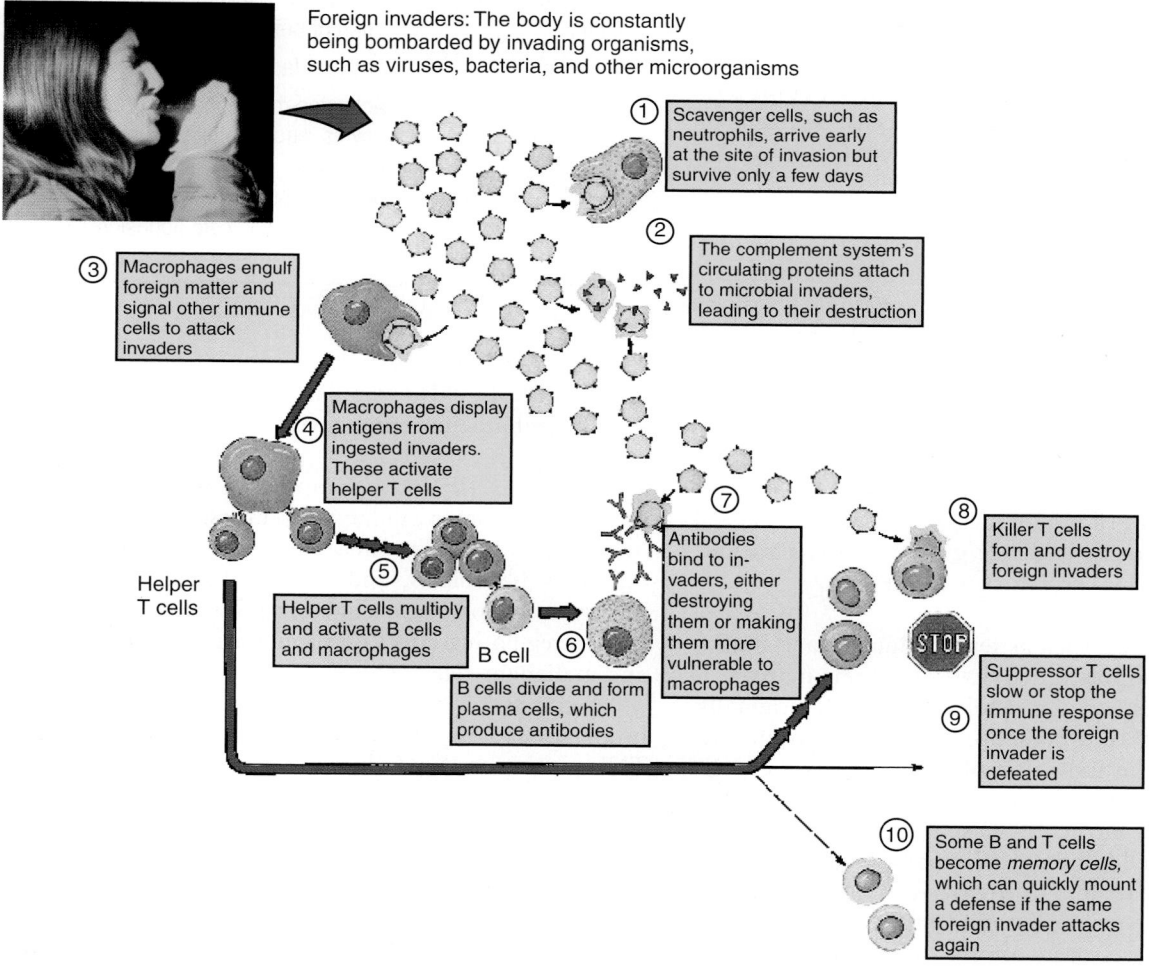

FIGURE U17-12 The protective systems include both arms of defense. Sneezing decreases exposure to the virus. Humoral immunity is shown in steps *1* and *2*, cell-mediated immunity in steps *3* and *10*. (From Thibodeau, G., & Patton, K. [2003]. *Anatomy and physiology* [5th ed., p. 659]. St. Louis: Mosby.)

followed by recurrent episodes of opportunistic infections and the development of malignancy in people with acquired immunodeficiency syndrome (AIDS).

The homeostatic reduction or suppression of B- and T-cell responses to antigen is no longer considered to be restricted to a single suppressor cell population (once thought to be a subset of T cells bearing the CD8 marker). It is currently hypothesized that this type of negative regulation may be a function of essentially all T cells. Whether a given cell will act to produce a positive immune response (produce effector units) or will mediate a negative response (tolerance) may be a function of the mechanism by which an individual T cell is activated by antigen.

The cytotoxic T lymphocyte reacts individually with target cells to establish a contact boundary that is required for target cell destruction. The intimate contact between the target cell and the cytotoxic T lymphocyte is mediated by an antigen-specific process and allows the cytotoxic T lymphocyte to release lytic molecules *(porins)* directly into the membrane of the target cell. Cytokines produced and released by the cytotoxic T lymphocyte during the cell contact phase enhance the action of porins. The cytotoxic T-lymphocyte function is to kill viral-infected host cells, malignant cells, and cells in allograft transplants.

CYTOKINES

The *cytokine* is a general term for cell-derived factors that mediate interactions between cells. Cytokines produced by lymphocytes are called *lymphokines;* those produced by monocyte-macrophage cells are called *monokines.* Some of these factors are called interleukins, indicating service as regulatory signals between various leukocytes (Table U17-2).

Cytokines are a diverse group of proteins with four areas of function:

1. Enhancement of mononuclear phagocytes
2. Regulation of lymphocyte growth, differentiation, maturation, and secretory activities
3. Inflammation
4. Systemic effects such as fever induction and induction of hemopoietic activity in the bone marrow

One of the best known cytokines is *IL-1*, originally described in the early 1960s. Produced by macrophages, IL-1 plays a role in induction of fever, acts as a coactivator of T cells, assists in activation of B cells and NK cells, and initiates the acute-phase response.

IL-2 is also well known from its first identification as a T-cell growth factor. The growth-enhancing function was crucial in the original studies of some of the retroviruses. Current research efforts are directed toward finding an application for IL-2 for treatment of malignant conditions.

IL-3 and *IL-4* are necessary for inducing antigen-stimulated B cells to undergo isotype switching to

TABLE U17-2	*Major Cytokines*
Cytokine	**Principal Effects**
Interleukin-1 (IL-1)	Lymphocyte activation
	Macrophage and neutrophil stimulation
	Stimulation of acute phase proteins
	Fever and sleep
	Pituitary hormone regulation
Interleukin-2 (IL-2)	Enhances T cell growth and function
Interleukin-3 (IL-3)	Stimulates differentiation of hematopoietic cells (colony-stimulating factor)
Interleukin-4 (IL-4)	B cell growth factor
Interleukin-5 (IL-5)	B cell growth and differentiation
Interleukin-6 (IL-6)	B cell growth and differentiation
	Stimulates the acute phase response
Colony-stimulating factor	Stimulates division and differentiation of bone marrow stem cells
Interferon	Antiviral factor
Tumor necrosis factor	Activates macrophages, granulocytes, and cytotoxic cells
	Cachexia
	Mediates septic shock
	Increases leukocyte adhesion
	Enhances antigen presentation

change from synthesis and secretion of IgM to IgG (or IgA or IgE). IL-3 also stimulates bone marrow stem cells to differentiate into monocytic and granulocytic precursors.

Interferons (IFNs) are another group of molecules that serve as intercellular messengers. There are three major types: IFN-α, produced by many cells, IFN-β, produced by fibroblasts, and IFN-γ, produced by T lymphocytes. All interferons have antiviral activity and have a downregulating effect on proliferation of both normal and malignant cells.

Tumor necrosis factor acts as a growth factor for fibroblasts and has a necrotizing effect on tumor cells. TNF participates in inducing the acute-phase response and is apparently one of the major factors in inducing endotoxic shock (sometimes seen in infections with gram-negative bacteria). This cytokine is thought to be a major cause of infection-related cachexia.

BLOOD GROUPS AND BLOOD TYPING

Human RBCs display antigens that are either glycoproteins or glycolipids on the surface of the membrane. Together the various blood group systems contribute more than 400 characterized antigens. Antigens are inherited from the parents. Fewer than a dozen of these blood group antigens attract frequent clinical notice, and of these only the ABO and rhesus (Rh) systems are major determinants of compatibility testing.

The ABO Blood Group System

The ABO blood type is inherited as an autosomal trait. The four major blood types of clinical importance in this genetic system are A, B, AB, and O. Blood is typed according to the antigens found on the RBC and the antibodies found in the serum.

The two major antigens within the blood group system are antigens A and B. For the antibodies to be formed, usually there must be exposure to foreign or homologous RBC antigens through pregnancy or transfusion. The major exceptions are the A and B antigens, for which there are structurally similar proteins in the environment, resulting in antibody formation against the missing A or B, or both antigens by the age of 3 months. Table U17-3 shows the antigen and antibody combinations for the different blood groups.

The Rh System

The Rh blood groups are nearly equal in clinical importance to the ABO groups. Although Rh serology involves more than 20 different antigens, the D antigen has the most clinical significance because of the high risk of formation of an anti-D in an Rh-negative recipient. The term *Rh-positive* means that the client has the D antigen; the *Rh-negative* client has no D antigen.

The most striking difference between the ABO and Rh systems is that, in the ABO system, there is spontaneous development of antibodies directed against A and B antigens not present on the RBC. In the Rh system, antibody formation is never spontaneous. Instead, a client must first be exposed to the Rh antigen, for example, through a blood transfusion or pregnancy. Thus clients with Rh-negative blood, transfused for the first time with Rh-positive blood, do not experience a reaction because their blood does not yet contain anti-Rh antibodies (anti-D). About 50% of people, however, develop sensitivity and form antibodies against the D antigen as a result of exposure to it from transfusion or pregnancy. If a sensitized client receives a second transfusion or has a second pregnancy with exposure to the D antigen, some degree of RBC destruction will occur. However, it is usually possible to prevent sensitization from occurring the first time by administering a single dose of anti-

TABLE U17-3 *The ABO Blood Group System*

Blood Type	Agglutinogens on RBCs	Agglutinins in Plasma	Frequency in United States
A	A	Anti-B	41%
B	B	Anti-A	10%
AB	A and B	None	4%
O	None	Anti-A and anti-B	45%

RBCs, Red blood cells.

Rh antibodies in the form of $Rh_0(D)$ immune globulin (RhoGAM) immediately following exposure to the D antigen.

THE HLA SYSTEM

HLAs are also called *histocompatibility antigens* because the antigens (glycoproteins) are found on the surface of most cells in the body except RBCs (including circulating and tissue cells). The HLA system is a series of closely linked genes located on the short arm of chromosome 6. The major function of the HLA antigen is regulation of the immune response, distinguishing self from non-self. This plays a major role in the rejection of transplanted tissues when donor and recipient HLA antigens do not match. There also is an association between HLA antigens and some diseases. For example, in ankylosing spondylitis, the association with HLA factor is so strong that HLA typing can be used diagnostically.

CONCLUSIONS

The immune system is extremely complex. It has evolved through the years to become a pervasive and highly structured group of complex functions that defend the body against pathogens and parasites from the outside and that are able to detect and attack altered self cells that pose threats to an individual's homeostasis.

BIBLIOGRAPHY

1. Goldsby, R.A., et al. (2000). *Kuby immunology* (4th ed.). Philadelphia: W. H. Freeman.
2. Thibodeau, G., & Patton, K. (1999). *Anatomy and physiology* (4th ed.). St. Louis: Mosby.
3. Travers, P., Walport, M., & Shlomchik, M. (2001). *Immunobiology* (5th ed.). New York: Garland.

Chapter 76

Assessment of the Hematopoietic System

Mary A. Allen

evolve

Web Enhancements

Assessment Terms
English and Spanish
Appendix A
Religious Beliefs and Practices Affecting Health Care

http://evolve.elsevier.com/Black/medsurg/

Appendix B
A Health History Format That Integrates the Assessment of Functional Health Patterns
Appendix C
Laboratory Values of Clinical Importance in Medical-Surgical Nursing

HISTORY

The nature of the presenting problem determines the focus of the health history for the hematopoietic system. Clients may present with manifestations that suggest a hematologic or immunologic problem.

Biographical and Demographic Data

When assessing the hematopoietic system, note the client's age, gender, race, ethnicity, and family health history. The immune response is diminished in both very young and older people. Some hematologic and immunologic disorders occur more frequently at certain ages, in women or men, and in those of a particular race or ethnic background. In addition, the normal values of some hematologic tests have age-specific and gender-specific norms. For example, hemoglobin and hematocrit levels are lower in women, particularly during the menstrual years, than in men. Hemoglobin values in African Americans are about 0.5 g/dl lower than in whites.

Collect family health history data because several hematologic and immunologic disorders are inherited. Note occupations, housing, and hobbies to identify possible exposure to chemicals, radiation, and allergens. Inquire about residence and work locations to determine environmental triggers of allergic responses.

Current Health

Chief Complaint

Disorders of the hematopoietic system often affect all organs and tissues of the body, resulting in widespread pathophysiologic manifestations. Manifestations may be vague and nonspecific, such as fatigue, malaise, fever, anorexia, weight loss, and chronic diarrhea. In general, anemias often manifest with fatigue, paleness, and weakness; bleeding disorders with bruising, petechiae, epistaxis, and bleeding gums; and immunodeficiencies with recurrent infections, fever, and chronic diarrhea. Allergic manifestations range from mild to severe and can be systemic or organ specific, such as integumentary, respiratory, gastrointestinal, or cardiovascular reactions. Conduct a symptom analysis (see Chapter 4). The review of systems outlines the body systems, their common hematopoietic findings, and the possible pathophysiologic bases.

---

evolve *Be sure to check out the bonus material on the Evolve website and the CD-ROM, including free self-assessment exercises.*
http://evolve.elsevier.com/Black/medsurg/

Symptom Analysis

Timing. Ask the client when the manifestations began and whether the onset was abrupt or gradual. Manifestations of anemias and immunodeficiencies can develop over time. Bleeding disorders may be present since childhood or may be of recent onset. Some allergic manifestations begin in childhood, whereas others develop later in life. Ask which allergens trigger a response and whether allergies are seasonal in appearance. Determine how long the allergic manifestations last and whether they are relieved or persist once the allergen is removed.

Quality and Quantity. How long do bleeding episodes last, and how severe are they? Does blood ooze from a site, or does sudden, massive bleeding occur? (Sudden bleeding is less common than prolonged, slow hemorrhage.) How often do bleeding episodes occur, and how long do they last? What does the client do to stop them? Ask about injury or physical trauma resulting in a break in the skin's integrity. Does the client report associated manifestations, such as lymph node swelling, edema, fever, pain, tenderness, pruritus, redness, or drainage?

Note allergic manifestations such as rhinitis, sneezing, nasal stuffiness, postnasal drip, sore throat, voice changes, hoarseness, wheezing, persistent cough, dyspnea, malaise, fatigue, tearing, or altered hearing acuity. Manifestations vary, depending on the nature of the allergen and individual sensitivity patterns. A symptom analysis for each reported manifestation assists in identifying the allergen.

Severity and Location. Fatigue is the most common manifestation of anemia. Is more than usual rest needed? Is endurance affected? Ask the client to compare how activities and activity tolerance have changed over time (in the past month compared with a year ago).

Attempt to quantify the severity of bleeding tendency. Does the client bruise easily? Has bleeding into the joints occurred? For menstruating women, ask whether the number and saturation of sanitary products used during a recent cycle have increased from the usual pattern.

Do allergic manifestations present as simple skin rashes, nasal stuffiness, and cough, or are they more severe, such as wheezing and respiratory distress? Do different allergens trigger different responses? Has the client ever experienced an anaphylactic reaction?

Precipitating Factors. Hepatic, splenic, or renal diseases may manifest as hematologic or hemorrhagic problems. Anticoagulant medications can precipitate bleeding episodes. Bone marrow suppression can lead to anemia, leukopenia, and thrombocytopenia. Causative agents include antineoplastic drugs, some antibiotics, and radiation. Other hematologic effects from certain drugs include hemolysis and disruption of platelet aggregation.

Has the client recently been exposed to infectious agents? Does the client take corticosteroids or other immunosuppressive drugs, thus increasing the risk of infection? Systemic and local infections can result from broken skin integrity, ingrown nails, or puncture wounds. Altered lymph vessel structure (from surgical disruption, trauma, neoplasm, or scarring from radiation) can lead to edema, particularly in an extremity.

The major types of allergic triggers include (1) inhalants (pollens, molds, spores, dust mites, trees, grasses, animal dander), (2) contact agents (dyes in clothing, fibers, cosmetics, metals in jewelry, plant oils and secretions, topical drugs, numerous chemicals), (3) ingested agents (foods, food additives, drugs), and (4) injectable agents (drugs, vaccines, insect venom).

Aggravating and Relieving Factors. Medications containing salicylates, including many over-the-counter (OTC) drugs, can aggravate bleeding tendencies (see later discussion). Is the client's edema aggravated by dependent positioning or tight, restrictive clothing? Does elevation of the affected body part reduce or relieve swelling? Are elastic support garments worn to reduce or prevent edema?

What relieves allergic manifestations (antihistamines, antipruritic agents)? What does the client use for relief from a rash? Is an inhaled medication needed for respiratory manifestations?

Past Health History

Assess for hematologic disorders by asking whether there is a history of anemia; concurrent disorders, such as renal, liver, or autoimmune disease; cancer; or organ transplantation.

Assess for bleeding disorders. Ask whether the disorder might be related to genetic factors, exposure to toxins, or liver disease. Cirrhosis, hepatitis, and other liver diseases can result in reduced production of clotting factors as well as reduced clearance of factors that inhibit clotting or promote fibrinolysis.

When assessing the client with a bleeding disorder, ask the following: How long has there been a bleeding problem? Was it present in childhood, or did it appear recently? Do any family members have a history of bleeding disorders? Is the bleeding linked to any specific event or procedure? For example, does severe bleeding occur with menses or following minor trauma, a tooth extraction, minor surgery (including circumcision), shaving, or participation in contact sports? Does the client have frequent nosebleeds (epistaxis)? Is there a history of bleeding into the joints or cavities? Does the client bruise easily or report petechiae? How severe are bleeding episodes, and how long do they last? Is bleeding slow and prolonged or sudden and massive?

Immunodeficiencies may be present at birth or may develop later in life, and they may be *iatrogenic* (a result of treatment with cytotoxic agents, corticosteroids or other immunosuppressants, or radiation). Immunodeficiencies may also result from protein-deficiency malnutrition, protein-losing enteropathy, nephrotic syndrome, or hypercatabolic states (major trauma, severe thermal injury). Immunodeficiencies may be related to loss of anatomic integrity from instrumentation (catheters), impaired dermatologic barrier function (burns, psoriasis, atopic dermatitis), mucosal inflammation (atopic diseases, irritants such as cigarette smoke), or mucociliary elevator dysfunction (cystic fibrosis or the immotile cilia syndrome).

Ask the client about indications of a possible immunodeficiency: poor or delayed wound healing; chronic diarrhea; unusually frequent bacterial infections; unusually severe viral infections; development of an infection with an unusual microorganism (fungus or protozoa); exposure to human immunodeficiency virus (HIV) through sexual activity, injection drug use, transfusion of blood or blood products, or other source; or family history of recurrent infection.

When assessing lymphatic problems, inquire about trauma or other injury, especially to an extremity. Has the client had a recent infection or neoplasm? Edema may be related to altered anatomy or disorders affecting the vascular system, such as heart failure, deep vein thrombosis, or renal disease.

Ask whether allergic manifestations have been present since childhood. Can the client identify triggers? Is there a seasonal pattern associated with the manifestations? Has hospitalization or emergency treatment been necessary for a severe allergic reaction? Was desensitization therapy (allergy shots) undertaken, and if so was it effective?

Childhood and Infectious Diseases

Did the client experience an unusually severe course of measles, mumps, or other infectious diseases of childhood? Were there severe reactions to vaccinations, especially immunizations with live virus vaccines such as measles and mumps? Are vaccinations current? (See Chapter 4.)

Major Illnesses and Hospitalizations

Ask about major illnesses and hospitalizations. Has the client received a blood or blood product transfusion, and for what reason? Have there been retroperitoneal, intracranial, or paratracheal hemorrhages? Were there problems or reactions to the blood or blood products? Does the client know his or her blood type, including Rh factor? This information is important for the pregnant client who is Rh negative (see Chapter 39).

Has the client recently donated blood or blood components? Donating whole blood, erythrocytes, leuko-cytes, platelets, or plasma can affect laboratory values for days or weeks.

Ask the client about the occurrence of any major illnesses, including (1) cancer, (2) lymphoproliferative diseases (lymphoma, leukemia, multiple myeloma), (3) infection (HIV-1, HIV-2, rubella, cytomegalovirus, influenza, varicella zoster), (4) systemic inflammatory diseases (rheumatoid arthritis, systemic lupus erythematosus, sarcoidosis, vasculitis), (5) diabetes mellitus, (6) renal or liver disease, and (7) sickle cell disease.

Is there a history of diseases involving the terminal ileum, Crohn disease, tropical sprue, ulcers, or severe atrophic gastritis? Ask the client to describe the disorder and its treatment.

Operations

Surgical procedures can influence the development of hematologic disorders or immunodeficiency. For example, cardiac valve replacement may cause erythrocyte hemolysis and subsequent anemia. Anemia may also occur following partial or total gastrectomy or removal of the terminal portion of the ileum because of the consequent reduction in absorption of vitamin B_{12}. Surgical removal of duodenal tissue can decrease iron absorption and thus produce iron deficiency anemia. Splenectomy increases the risk of overwhelming infections with encapsulated bacteria such as *Streptococcus pneumoniae*. Surgical instrumentation and loss of anatomic integrity increase the risk of infection.

Medications

Note the client's past and current use of both prescription and OTC drugs as well as herbal or complementary remedies and alcohol intake. Many medications can prolong bleeding; cause hemolysis of red blood cells; or, through selective or general bone marrow suppression, produce anemia, thrombocytopenia, or leukopenia. Medications can also inhibit folic acid absorption from the intestine, leading to folic acid deficiency and anemia.

Inquire whether the client takes medications that can cause hemolysis: (1) hypoglycemic (antidiabetic) agents, such as chlorpropamide, glyburide, and tolbutamide; (2) cardiovascular medications, such as mefenamic acid, methyldopa, and procainamide; and (3) antibiotics, including sulfonamides and penicillins.

Ask about current or recent anticoagulant therapy or thrombolytic treatment. The anticoagulants heparin and warfarin prolong bleeding, and heparin may also cause immune-mediated thrombocytopenia. The thrombolytic agents streptokinase, tissue plasminogen activator (t-PA), and urokinase also prolong bleeding.

A wide range of medications can affect platelet function or cause thrombocytopenia. Ask about OTC medications that contain aspirin or other nonsteroidal anti-inflammatory drugs (NSAIDs) that can interfere with platelet aggregation and prolong bleeding.

Has the client taken corticosteroids, cytotoxic agents (cyclophosphamide, chlorambucil, cisplatin, etoposide), other immunosuppressants (gold salts, NSAIDs), or therapies (irradiation) for the treatment of cancer or autoimmune diseases? These agents may suppress bone marrow production of blood cells or the immune response. Effects may continue long after the medications have been stopped. Treatment with cytotoxic agents or high doses of corticosteroids can mask fever and other manifestations until an infection is serious and widespread.

Has the client received other medications for which myelosuppression is an adverse effect? These include chloramphenicol, cephalosporins, clindamycin, penicillin, tetracycline, sulfonamides, D-penicillamine, amphotericin B, antimalarials, captopril, phenothiazines, antithyroid drugs, zidovudine, and ganciclovir.

Determine whether the client has received intravenous immune globulin (IGIV) or intramuscular immune globulin (IMIG) to treat an immunoglobulin deficiency or other condition.

Ask the client about herbal preparations and nutritional supplements including comfrey *(Symphytum officinale)*, echinacea *(Echinacea angustifolia, E. pallida, E. purpura)*, evening primrose *(Oenothera biennis)*, ginseng *(Panax ginseng, P. quinquefolius, Eleutherococcus senticosus)*, goldenseal *(Hydrastis canadensis)*, licorice *(Glycyrrhiza glabra, G. uralensis)*, maitake *(Grifola frondosa)*, St. John's wort *(Hypericum perforatum)*, and stinging nettle *(Urtica dioica)*. Topical comfrey acts as an anti-inflammatory on wounds. Herbs used to boost the immune system include echinacea, evening primrose, ginseng, goldenseal, and maitake. St. John's wort has antiviral actions. Licorice is used to reduce inflammation, fight viruses and bacteria, and reduce asthma and allergy manifestations. Stinging nettle is used as a hay fever remedy. Nutritional supplements associated with anticancer properties include vitamins E and C, beta-carotene, selenium, garlic *(Allium sativum)*, and green tea. Folic acid (vitamin B_6) and cobalamin (vitamin B_{12}) are necessary to prevent pernicious anemia.

Assess the client for potential interactions of herbal preparations with prescription medications. Ephedra *(Ma-huang, Ephedra sinica)*, a sympathomimetic, might reduce the effect of prednisone. St. John's wort can reduce warfarin levels. There is some limited anecdotal evidence that gingko, garlic, fish oil, and the Chinese herbs danshen and dong quai may exert an anticoagulant effect. Hence the use of these products may need to be avoided in people with bleeding disorders or on anticoagulant therapy.

Allergies

If the client has a history of transfusions with blood or blood products, ask about complications. Reactions to blood products include fever, chills, back or flank pain, wheezing, headache, vomiting, urticaria (hives), and shock.

Ask the client about past episodes of allergic reactions. Is there a seasonal pattern to the episodes? What manifestations developed? What treatment was given, and was it effective? Inquire about food and drug allergies or sensitivities. Has the client ever had an anaphylactic reaction or been hospitalized for an allergic reaction? Has the client had desensitization treatment with allergy injections. If so, was it effective?

Has the client undergone procedures requiring administration of radiopaque contrast medium, or is this likely in the future? Clients with a history of allergies or asthma may be at higher risk of a reaction to these media and may be candidates for low-ionic contrast media or pretreatment with medications to reduce the risk of serious reaction. Previously clients often were asked about allergies to shellfish or iodine before the administration of radiopaque contrast media because it was thought that iodine-based cross-reactions could occur. Seafood allergies, however, are immunoglobulin E (IgE)–mediated reactions to the muscle protein tropomyosin that is present in shellfish and mollusks and do not involve reactions to iodine. Conversely, most reactions to radiopaque contrast media do not appear to be IgE mediated and are unrelated to allergies to tropomyosin or iodine.

Family Health History

Explore the family history for (1) anemia; (2) thrombocytopenia; (3) bleeding disorders, such as hemophilia or von Willebrand's disease; (4) congenital blood disorders, such as sickle cell anemia; (5) jaundice; (6) infections that are unusually frequent, unusually severe, or caused by an unusual organism; (7) delayed healing; (8) cancer; or (9) autoimmune disease. A family history of neonatal jaundice or early cholecystectomy (gallbladder removal) may indicate a genetic hematologic disorder.

Ask the client to identify allergies and sensitivities in family members, particularly atopic reactions. Hay fever tends to occur among family members.

Psychosocial History

Hematopoietic disorders can result in physiologic changes that affect the client's psychosocial status and ability to perform activities of daily living (ADL). Assess for work-related problems, sexual dysfunction, and fatigue that may interfere with role performance. Encourage the client to discuss current levels of stress and whether they seem to relate to the appearance of allergic manifestations. How does the client react to allergic manifestations? For example, some people break out in hives when under emotional stress. Their appearance triggers more emotional distress and can lead to further outbreaks. A cycle may develop that is difficult to interrupt.

Occupation

Ask about occupational exposure to agents that might predispose the client to the development of hematopoietic disorders: radiation, aromatic hydrocarbons 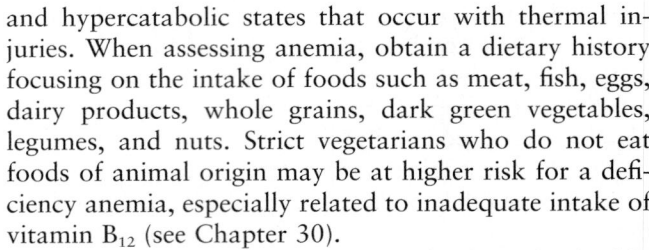 (kerosene, gasoline), benzene (used in the manufacture of pharmaceuticals, rubber, leather, and explosives), inorganic arsenics, trinitrotoluene, insecticides, weed killers, lead, and phenylbutazone. Exposure to toxic chemicals and ionizing radiation may occur in several industries (chemicals, plastics, ceramics, steel, metal refinery); in the manufacturing of rubber tires, shoes, incandescent lamps, vacuum tubes, glue, and varnish; in nuclear reactors, uranium mines, research laboratories, hospital radiology, or sterile supplies; and in farming and horticulture.

Does the client have sufficient energy to perform normal activities and occupational tasks? Do fatigue, dyspnea, or other manifestations interfere with a productive lifestyle? Has the client missed time from work or school, resulting in financial loss or other economic concerns, such as health or life insurance eligibility?

Exposure to allergens at work may trigger reactions. Ask about the heating and cooling systems if airborne allergens are suspected.

Geographical Location and Environment

Geographical location may be associated with exposure to possible health hazards. Living at altitudes above 10,000 feet may result in increased hemoglobin levels and other physiologic adaptations. Immunologic disorders may be more prevalent in certain geographical areas. High levels of air pollution can increase the incidence of allergy-related respiratory problems. Ask about home and work environments. Are pets, houseplants, or fresh-cut flowers present? What type of vegetation is in the immediate vicinity?

Nutrition

The hematopoietic system depends on the adequate intake of protein, calories, vitamins (A, B_{12}, folic acid), minerals, and trace elements such as iron and zinc. Inadequate intake of any of these substances can lead to anemia or immunodeficiency. Assess for conditions that increase nutritional needs, such as pregnancy, lactation, and hypercatabolic states that occur with thermal injuries. When assessing anemia, obtain a dietary history focusing on the intake of foods such as meat, fish, eggs, dairy products, whole grains, dark green vegetables, legumes, and nuts. Strict vegetarians who do not eat foods of animal origin may be at higher risk for a deficiency anemia, especially related to inadequate intake of vitamin B_{12} (see Chapter 30).

Does the client have allergies to foods or food additives? Do these allergies limit the intake of specific nutrients as previously identified? A food diary (see Chapter 30) is useful to help identify food-related allergic reactions. See Chapter 78 for further discussion of food allergy.

Habits

Assess the client's current and past use of tobacco (including exposure to second-hand smoke that can aggravate allergies), alcohol, and illicit drugs. Excessive use of alcohol in particular often results in poor nutrition, folic acid deficiency, and decreased immunity as well as acute or chronic loss of blood from gastritis and esophageal varices. Many substances, most notably alcohol, damage the structure and function of liver cells, decreasing the production of clotting factors and reducing the clearance of factors that promote clot dissolution; the result is a bleeding tendency.

Review of Systems

General manifestations of hematopoietic disorders include fatigue, malaise, weakness, and fever. Specific manifestations can vary if the disorder is related to anemia, bleeding, or immunodeficiency. Allergic manifestations can be general or specific.

Anemia is characterized by pallor, weakness, and lightheadedness; severe anemia manifests with chronic severe fatigue, exertional dyspnea, headache, or vertigo. Clients with bleeding disorders manifest petechiae, purpura, and ecchymoses (bruises); spontaneous bleeding from the nose, gingiva, vagina, and rectum; oozing of blood from cuts and venipuncture sites; jaundice; conjunctival or retinal hemorrhage; hemoptysis, hematemesis, hematuria, and back and flank pain.

Clients with hemophilia and other congenital coagulation disorders have a history of lifelong bleeding tendencies, such as (1) excessive or prolonged bleeding after circumcision or dental extraction; (2) repeated episodes of spontaneous bleeding into joints (hemarthrosis), and (3) life-threatening hemorrhages (retroperitoneal, intracranial, paratracheal).

Clients with immunodeficiencies have a history of recurrent infections, especially of mucous membranes (oral cavity, anorectal area, genitourinary tract, respiratory tract); poor wound healing; diarrhea; and manifestations of systemic activation of the inflammatory response (fever, malaise, fatigue, anorexia, unexplained weight loss, headache, and irritability). Clients with allergies may have rhinitis, sinusitis, urticaria, and pruritus.

Skin

Integumentary manifestations may be pallor (anemia); pruritus and ruddy skin (polycythemia vera); jaundice (bile pigment accumulation from hemolytic anemia), dry skin, dry hair, brittle nails, and spoon-shaped concave nails with longitudinal ridges (iron deficiency anemia); petechiae, especially of the lower legs and hard palate (thrombocytopenia), purpura, and ecchymoses (thrombocytopenia and bleeding disorders); delayed wound healing, lymphadenopathy, and severe acne or acne scars (immunodeficiency); and rashes, urticaria, pruritus, dryness, and scaling (allergies).

Assess for local inflammation (redness, heat, swelling, pain). Clients with severe neutropenia or immunosuppression may be unable to mount the inflammatory response of fever, redness, and pus formation.

Eyes

Ocular manifestations include visual disturbances (anemia, polycythemia), blindness (retinal hemorrhage related to thrombocytopenia or bleeding disorder), scleral jaundice (hemolytic anemia) and conjunctivitis, tearing, eye rubbing, styes, and dark circles or "allergic shiners," or "raccoon eyes" (allergies).

Ears

Aural manifestations are vertigo or tinnitus (severe anemia). Bleeding disorders may manifest as blood in the external auditory canal or as a bluish tympanic membrane, suggesting blood in the middle ear. Immunodeficiencies can manifest as chronic otitis media, mastoiditis, and hearing impairment related to chronic infections (eardrum rupture, scarring, perforated tympanic membrane) or treatment with ototoxic drugs.

Nose

Nasal manifestations include epistaxis (thrombocytopenia and bleeding disorders); crusting around nares, sinopulmonary drainage, and indications of chronic sinusitis (immunodeficiency); and sneezing, sniffling, rhinitis, nasal polyps, nasal voice quality, a crease across the bridge of the nose from chronic rubbing, and stuffiness (allergies).

Mouth

Oral manifestations include a smooth, glossy, bright red, and sore tongue (pernicious anemia, iron deficiency ane-

mia); gingival bleeding (thrombocytopenia, bleeding disorders); and oral ulcers (aphthous, herpetic), candidiasis, gingivitis, periodontitis, dental caries, and tooth loss (immunodeficiencies). The tonsils may be absent without a history of tonsillectomy, or they may be enlarged, inflamed, or pustular. Lip and tongue swelling, frequent throat clearing from postnasal drip, sore throat, itching of the palate, throat, or neck, and hoarseness can occur (allergies).

Lungs

Respiratory manifestations include dyspnea and orthopnea (anemia, sickle cell crisis), wheezing, frequent cough, ineffective cough, and respiratory arrest (allergies).

Cardiovascular System

Cardiovascular manifestations include tachycardia, palpitations (compensatory mechanism to increase cardiac output secondary to anemia), murmurs, particularly systolic (increased volume and velocity of blood through valves related to anemia), and angina (decreased oxygen supply to the heart related to rapid-onset anemia).

Gastrointestinal Tract

The gastrointestinal system may be affected by dysphagia (mucous membrane atrophy related to iron deficiency anemia), abdominal pain (sickle cell disease, retroperitoneal bleeding, acute hemolysis), hepatomegaly, splenomegaly (hemolytic anemia resulting in increased need for removal of erythrocytes), hematemesis and melena (thrombocytopenia and bleeding disorders), vomiting, cramping, and diarrhea (allergies).

Genitourinary Tract

Urinary manifestations include hematuria (hemolysis and bleeding disorders). Reproductive manifestations are amenorrhea and menorrhagia (iron deficiency and bleeding disorders) and decreased fertility (severe anemia).

Musculoskeletal System

Musculoskeletal manifestations are back pain *(hemolysis)*, sternal tenderness and excruciating bone pain (sickle cell crises), and joint pain (hemarthroses or bleeding into joints, often related to hemophilia).

Nervous System

Neurologic manifestations are headache and confusion (anemia, polycythemia); brain hemorrhage (thrombocytopenia or a bleeding disorder); and peripheral neuropathy, paresthesias, and loss of balance (pernicious anemia). The client may experience mental depression (hematopoietic disorders that cause fatigue, discomfort, and acute and chronic problems related to a disease process) or coping difficulties related to a diagnosis of life-threatening illness.

PHYSICAL EXAMINATION

The physical examination of the hematopoietic system can entail both a complete head-to-toe examination and examinations of specific systems, depending on the nature of the client's problem. For example, anemia or fever can cause tachycardia and systolic ejection murmur; immunodeficiency manifested by repeated episodes of pulmonary infections may result in adventitious breath sounds. (See Chapters 56 and 61 for discussions of cardiac and respiratory assessment, respectively.) The Physical Assessment Findings in the Healthy Adult feature on The Hematopoietic System below outlines expected findings.

The portions of the lymphatic system accessible for a physical examination are the superficial lymph nodes, liver, and spleen (see Chapter 44). Note the presence of a surgical splenectomy scar. Assess the superficial lymph nodes using inspection and palpation. Supplement the findings from the history and physical examination with results from laboratory tests and specific diagnostic studies.

Inspection

Inspect surfaces overlying the lymph nodes for masses, scars, swelling, and redness. Note extremity swelling or edema. Look for symmetry and compare with the contralateral side.

Palpation

Use a methodical approach to examine the lymph nodes; do not overlook single nodes or chains of nodes. Palpate nodes for location, size, shape, consistency, symmetry, discreteness, mobility, tenderness, temperature, overlying edema, or red streaks. Avoid excessive pressure to discern small, yet palpable nodes. Chapter 4 describes the palpation technique.

Lymph nodes are generally nonpalpable; however, small (1 cm in diameter), single, round, soft, mobile, nontender nodes are common, particularly in the head, neck, and inguinal areas, and are usually not significant. Nodes that are inflamed, tender, large (>1 cm in diameter), hard, matted together, or fixed to underlying structures are abnormal. Describe their characteristics thoroughly. If you see a mass, palpate the area and compare with the contralateral side. The supraclavicular area is a frequent site of metastatic disease; investigate palpable nodes in this site.

The nodes of the head and neck and the clavicular and epitrochlear areas are most easily palpated while the client is sitting. Palpate the inguinal and popliteal nodes when the client is lying down. Axillary nodes may be palpated with the client sitting or lying. Specific guidelines for palpating the lymph nodes are presented in Table 76-1. Palpation techniques are shown in Chapter 4.

DIAGNOSTIC TESTS

Diagnosis of hematologic, bleeding, or immunologic disorders depends primarily on laboratory analysis. No particular preprocedure or postprocedure care is associated with the simple blood tests involved in most hematopoietic assessments.

Although dozens of specific tests are used to diagnose individual disorders, all cases generally call for (1) a complete blood count (CBC) to determine the number of leukocytes, erythrocytes, and platelets; (2) a white blood cell (WBC) differential count to indicate the relative percentages of the different leukocytes; (3) coagulation studies such as prothrombin time (PT), partial thromboplastin time (PTT), and bleeding time; and (4) a peripheral blood smear for red blood cell (RBC) morphology to differentiate various anemias and blood dyscrasias.

The diagnosis of deficiency anemias may require measuring serum levels of iron, total iron-binding capacity (TIBC), transferrin saturation, ferritin, folic acid, and vitamin B_{12} (Table 76-2). Bone marrow aspiration and biopsy are performed to determine both the cellularity of the bone marrow and the morphology of the cells present. The diagnosis of particular hematologic disorders requires specialized blood tests, such as the Schilling test, hemoglobin electrophoresis, and measure-

---

PHYSICAL ASSESSMENT FINDINGS IN THE HEALTHY ADULT

The Hematopoietic System

Inspection

Alert and oriented; afebrile. Skin color even, without pallor, flushing, jaundice, bruises, or petechiae. Lumps or masses absent; no draining lesions. Sclerae white. Lingual papillae visible; oral lesions absent. Eupneic. Joints not swollen; full range of motion

Palpation

Lumps, masses absent. Lymph nodes, liver, and spleen nonpalpable and nontender. Joints nontender. Several round, small (<0.5 cm), discrete, soft, mobile nodes palpable in submandibular area

Auscultation

Heart sounds regular, without murmurs or palpitations

TABLE 76-1	*Sequence and Palpation Technique for Lymph Nodes*	
Nodes	**Location**	**Palpation Technique**
Occipital	Posterior at base of skull and lateral to cervical spine	Flex the client's neck forward slightly to relax the trapezius. Palpate right and left node centers simultaneously.
Posterior auricular (mastoid)	Behind auricle of ear, over outer surface of mastoid process	Palpate over both mastoid processes simultaneously.
Preauricular (anterior auricular)	In front of tragus of ear	Palpate right and left sides simultaneously, anterior to the tragus and posterior to the temporomandibular joint.
Retropharyngeal (tonsillar)	Near angle of jaw at jaw margin	Flex the client's neck slightly in the midline. Palpate behind both jaw angles simultaneously.
Submandibular (submaxillary)	Along medial border of mandible, between angle of jaw and chin	Palpate along the medial borders of the mandible from the angle of the jaw toward the chin. Palpate right and left node centers simultaneously.
Submental	At the midline, posterior to tip of mandible under chin	Palpate with one hand under the client's chin just behind the tip of the mandible. Steady the client's head with the free hand if necessary.
Anterior superficial cervical chain	Along and over (anterior to) sternocleidomastoid, in anterior triangle	Flex the client's neck forward to relax the sternocleidomastoid. Palpate one side at a time. Palpate slowly against the sternocleidomastoid, progressing from the clavicle toward the jaw.
Posterior superficial cervical chain	Along anterior edge of trapezius, in posterior triangle	Flex the client's neck to relax the trapezius muscles. Palpate slowly against the trapezius muscles, progressing from the mastoid processes toward the clavicles.
Deep cervical chain	Under sternocleidomastoid	Flex the client's neck laterally toward the side being examined to relax the muscles and soft tissue. Palpate one side at a time. Hook the thumb (on one side) and fingers (on the other side) around the sternocleidomastoid muscle to feel deep to the muscle. Progress from the jaw toward the sternum.
	Along anterior edge of sternocleidomastoid, in anterior triangle	With the client's neck still flexed laterally, palpate along the anterior edge of the sternocleidomastoid from the sternum to the jaw angle. Repeat on the opposite side of the neck.
Supraclavicular (scalene)	Above clavicle, in angle formed by clavicle and sternocleidomastoid	Flex the client's neck sharply with one hand and encourage the client to relax the shoulders so the clavicles drop. Palpate one side at a time with the fingers over the client's right clavicle lateral to the sternocleidomastoid. Ask the client to inhale deeply while pressing in and behind the clavicle. Repeat using the right hand to palpate the client's left node centers.
Infraclavicular	Below the clavicle, in midclavicular area	Palpate the right and left sides simultaneously, pushing in and up, under the clavicles.
Axillary (anterior pectoral, midaxillary, and posterior subscapular)	In the axilla (performed during breast examination)	Palpate one side at a time anteriorly, centrally, and posteriorly. If the client is sitting, support the client's right forearm with your right hand and use the finger tips of your left hand to palpate—starting low in the anterior axilla, advancing higher to the central nodes, and then to the posterior nodes. If nodes are palpable, try to slide fingers beneath to evaluate. Repeat on the other side (see Chapter 39).
Epitrochlear (cubital)	Medial surface of upper arm in groove between the biceps and triceps muscles (included in breast examination)	Flex the client's elbow about 90 degrees; support the elbow with one hand and palpate with the other. Feel for nodes in the fossa, about 3 cm proximal to the medial epicondyle of the humerus (see Chapter 39).
Inguinal	Superior (horizontal) chain, just below inguinal ligament Inferior (vertical) chain: close to upper portion of great saphenous vein	Have the client lie supine with the knee slightly flexed. Palpate one side at a time, rolling fingers along the inguinal ligament.
Popliteal	In popliteal fossae on lateral aspect of the knee	Have the client lie supine with the knee slightly flexed. Palpate one side at a time.

TABLE 76-2	*Laboratory Tests Used in the Diagnosis of Anemia*
Test	**Normal Value**
Iron	50-150 μg/dl
Total iron-binding capacity (TIBC)	250-350 μg/dl
Transferrin	250-430 mg/dl
Transferrin saturation	20%-55%
Ferritin	Men: 15-200 μg/ml
	Women: 11-200 μg/ml
Folate	7-20 μg/ml
Vitamin B$_{12}$	200-800 pg/ml
Schilling test (vitamin B$_{12}$ absorption)	8.5%-28% excretion in 24-48 hr

dl, Deciliter; *ml*, milliliter; *μg*, microgram; *pg*, picogram.

TABLE 76-3	*Normal Values for Complete Blood Counts in Adults*
Measure	**Value***
Erythrocytes	
RBC count (number of cells/ mm³ of blood)	Women: 4.2-5.4 million/mm³
	Men: 4.7-6.1 million/mm³
Hemoglobin (oxygen-carrying pigment of RBC)	Women: 12-16.0 g/dl
	Men: 13.5-18.0 g/dl
Hematocrit (% volume of RBCs in whole blood)	Women: 37%-47% (pregnancy >33%)
	Men: 42%-52%
Reticulocytes	0.5%-2% of total erythrocytes
Leukocytes	
WBC count (number of cells/ mm³ of blood)	4000-9000/mm³
WBC differential	
Granulocytes	
Neutrophils	55%-70%
Eosinophils	1%-4%
Basophils	0.5%-1.0%
Agranulocytes	
Lymphocytes	20%-40%
Monocytes	2%-8%
Platelets	
Platelet (thrombocyte) count (number of cells/mm³ of blood)	150,000-450,000/mm³

g/dl, Grams per deciliter; *mm³*, cubic millimeter; *RBC*, red blood cell; *WBC*, white blood cell.
*Normal values may differ significantly among laboratories.

ment of levels of specific clotting factors. These specialized tests are discussed in Chapter 77.

Hematologic Tests

Complete Blood Count

The CBC includes the RBC count, hemoglobin, hematocrit, RBC indices, WBC count with or without differential, and platelet count. Table 76-3 presents reference values for the CBC. Table 76-4 reviews the effects of diseases, disorders, and conditions on the CBC and the RBC indices.

Red Blood Cell Count. The RBC count measures the number of RBCs per cubic millimeter (mm³) of blood. This value is useful in verifying findings from other hematopoietic tests for diagnosis of anemia and polycythemia. Normal values vary with age and gender.

Hemoglobin Level. A hemoglobin determination is used to evaluate the hemoglobin content (and thus the iron status and oxygen-carrying capacity) of erythrocytes by measuring the number of grams of hemoglobin per deciliter (100 ml) of blood. This measurement helps to indicate anemias and polycythemia. Normal hemoglobin levels vary with age and gender.

Hematocrit Level. Often used in place of the RBC count, the hematocrit is a measure of the volume of RBCs in whole blood expressed as a percentage. This test is useful in the diagnosis of anemia, polycythemia, and abnormal hydration states. The hematocrit value is roughly three times the hemoglobin concentration. Normal values vary with age and gender.

Red Blood Cell Indices. The RBC indices are measures of erythrocyte size and hemoglobin content. These val-

ues derive from the RBC count and hemoglobin level. Table 76-5 describes the three RBC indices: mean corpuscular volume, mean corpuscular hemoglobin, and mean corpuscular hemoglobin concentration. The indices are helpful in assessing the various anemias.

Platelet Count. The platelet count measures the number of platelets (thrombocytes) per cubic millimeter (mm³) of blood. Platelets have a key role in blood clotting. The count is valuable in assessing the severity of thrombocytopenia (abnormally low platelet count), which can result in spontaneous bleeding, as well as thrombocytosis (abnormally high platelet count).

White Blood Cell Count. The WBC count measures the number of WBCs in a cubic millimeter of blood. It is used to detect infection or inflammation and to monitor a client's response to or adverse effects of chemotherapy or radiation therapy.

TABLE 76-4	*Diseases, Disorders, and Conditions Affecting the Complete Blood Count (CBC), and Red Blood Cell (RBC) Indices*	
CBC, RBC Index	**Increased by**	**Decreased by**
RBC count	Polycythemia vera, cardiac and pulmonary disorders characterized by cyanosis, dehydration, acute poisoning	Anemia, fluid overload, recent hemorrhage, leukemia
Reticulocyte count	Hemolytic anemia, hemorrhage, following effective treatment for pernicious anemia	Bone marrow failure, pernicious anemia
Hemoglobin	Hemoconcentration from polycythemia or dehydration	Hemodilution (fluid overload), anemia, recent hemorrhage
Hematocrit	Hemoconcentration from loss of fluid, dehydration, polycythemia	Hemodilution, anemia, acute massive blood loss
Mean corpuscular volume	Pernicious anemia, macrocytic anemia, folic acid or vitamin B_{12} deficiency anemias	Microcytic anemia, iron deficiency anemia, hypochromic anemia, thalassemia, lead poisoning
Mean corpuscular hemoglobin	Macrocytic anemia	Microcytic anemia
Mean corpuscular hemoglobin concentration	Spherocytosis	Microcytic anemia, hypochromic anemia, thalassemia, iron deficiency anemia
WBC count	Infection, leukemia, tissue necrosis	Bone marrow depression
Neutrophils	Inflammatory disease or response, tissue necrosis (burns, myocardial infarction), granulocytic leukemia and other malignancies, acute stress response, bacterial infection	Bone marrow depression, viral diseases, drugs (chemotherapy, some antibiotics, psychotropics)
Eosinophils	Allergic reactions, parasitic infections, skin diseases, neoplasms, pernicious anemia	Stress response, Cushing's syndrome
Basophils	Leukemia, some hemolytic anemias, polycythemia vera	Corticosteroids, allergic reactions, acute infections (*Note:* decline is unlikely to be detected because normal count is 0%-2%)
Lymphocytes	Infectious mononucleosis, chronic bacterial infections, tuberculosis, pertussis, lymphocytic leukemia	AIDS, corticosteroids, immunosuppressive drugs
Monocytes	Infections (tuberculosis, malaria, Rocky Mountain spotted fever), collagen-vascular diseases, monocytic leukemia	Drug therapy, prednisone
Platelet count	Malignancies, polycythemia vera, splenectomy (rebound thrombocytosis)	Idiopathic thrombocytopenia purpura, aplastic anemia, hemolytic disorders, chemotherapeutic drugs or radiation, hypersplenism or splenomegaly, infiltrative bone marrow disease, disseminated intravascular coagulation, viral infections, AIDS

RBC, Red blood cell; *WBC,* white blood cell; *AIDS,* acquired immunodeficiency syndrome.

White Blood Cell Differential. The WBC differential determines the proportion of each of the five types of WBCs in a sample of 100 WBCs. To determine the actual (absolute) count of a specific WBC type, multiply the total WBC count by the cell percentage reported in the differential. The differential helps in evaluating the body's capacity to resist and overcome infections, in detecting and classifying leukemias and other disorders, and in detecting allergies and helminthic infections.

Peripheral Blood Smear

A peripheral blood smear is obtained to determine variations and abnormalities in erythrocytes, leukocytes, and platelets. Cells of normal size and shape are termed *normocytes;* cells of normal color are *normochromic.* Abnormalities of erythrocyte size, shape, and color usually indicate some form of anemia (Table 76-6).

TABLE 76-5	Red Blood Cell Indices	
Mean Corpuscular Volume (MCV)	**Mean Corpuscular Hemoglobin (MCH)**	**Mean Corpuscular Hemoglobin Concentration (MCHC)**
Measures average size or volume of individual RBC; differentiates anemias into microcytic, normocytic, and macrocytic	Measures hemoglobin content within one RBC of average size	Measures average hemoglobin concentration within 100 ml (1 dl) of packed RBCs
Formula: $\dfrac{Hct}{RBC}$	Formula: $\dfrac{Hb}{RBC}$	Formula: $\dfrac{Hb}{Hct}$
Normal value: 80-95 μm	Normal value: 27-31 pg	Normal value: 32-36 g/dl of packed RBCs
MCV <80 μm means abnormally small (*microcytic*) RBCs	MCH <27 pg indicates hemoglobin deficiency, hypochromic RBCs	MCHC <32 g/dl indicates hemoglobin deficiency
MCV >94 μm means abnormally large (*macrocytic*) RBCs	MCH >32 pg indicates macrocytic cells with abnormally large volume of hemoglobin	MCHC remains normal when MCH >32 g/dl because cells are oversized (fewer cells can be packed together within 1 dl)
	MCH >35.5 pg suggests spherocytosis	

Hb, Hemoglobin; *Hct,* hematocrit; *RBC,* red blood cell; μm, micrometer; *pg,* picogram; *g/dl,* grams per deciliter.

TABLE 76-6	Abnormalities of the Erythrocyte	
Abnormality	**Characteristics of Abnormal Cell**	**Conditions Characterized by Abnormality**
Anisocytes	Vary from normal in size	Any of the anemias
Poikilocytes	Abnormally shaped (tear- or club-shaped)	Any of the anemias; most bizarre shapes seen in the severe anemias
Microcytes	Abnormally small (<6 mm)	Microcytic anemias (iron deficiency anemia, thalassemia major)
Macrocytes	Abnormally large (>9 mm)	Macrocytic anemias (pernicious anemia, folic acid deficiency anemia)
Hypochromic cells	Pale appearance because of abnormally low hemoglobin content	Any of the anemias
Spherocytes	Relatively small and round rather than biconcave	Hereditary spherocytosis, warm antibody-induced immunohemolytic disease
Schistocytes	Fragmented, with bizarre shapes (triangles, spirals)	Hemolytic anemia, thrombotic thrombocytopenic purpura
Sickle cells	Crescent- or sickle-shaped from presence of abnormal hemoglobin (Hb S)	Sickle cell anemia
Target cells	Thin, with small amount of hemoglobin in center	Hemoglobin C diseases, thalassemia major, sickle cell anemia
Metarubricytes	Nucleated	Severe anemia

Reticulocyte Count

A reflection of RBC production, the reticulocyte count measures the responsiveness of the bone marrow to a diminished number of circulating erythrocytes. Specifically, this test measures the number of reticulocytes released from the bone marrow into the blood. An increased reticulocyte count indicates increased erythrocyte production, probably because of excessive RBC destruction (hemolytic anemia) or loss (hemorrhage). A decrease in the reticulocyte count may indicate bone marrow failure or pernicious anemia. The reticulocyte count is also used to evaluate the effectiveness of treatment of pernicious anemia and bone marrow failure.

Antiglobulin Tests

The *direct* antiglobulin test (Coombs' test) is used to (1) detect certain antigen-antibody reactions between serum antibodies and RBC antigens, (2) differentiate between various forms of hemolytic anemia, (3) determine unusual blood types, and (4) identify hemolytic disease in newborns. This test examines erythrocytes for the presence of antibodies (agglutinins) that damage erythrocytes without causing clumping or hemolysis. It is used to crossmatch blood for blood transfusions, test umbilical cord blood for erythroblastosis fetalis, and diagnose acquired hemolytic anemia.

The *indirect* antiglobulin test identifies antibodies to erythrocyte antigens in the serum of clients who have a greater than normal chance of developing transfusion reactions. Both the direct and the indirect tests are agglutination procedures that use a suspension of RBCs.

Coagulation Screening Tests

Laboratory studies are the most crucial for pinpointing the type and cause of bleeding disorders (Table 76-7). Initially, four basic laboratory tests are performed to discern whether the bleeding problem is related to a platelet, coagulation, or vascular defect: (1) platelet count, (2) PT, (3) PTT, and (4) bleeding time. Most bleeding disorders are diagnosed by the PT and PTT.

Because the normal and therapeutic ranges for PT vary according to the type of reagent used in the assay, the PT is standardized by conversion to the International Normalized Ratio (INR). For most clinical conditions that necessitate anticoagulation, the recommended INR is 2 to 3.5. Clients with mechanical prosthetic valves or recurrent systemic embolism need higher INR levels. PT may be performed with a finger-stick sample at the point of care via a portable laser photodetector.

Additional coagulation screening tests are (1) the D-dimer, which confirms diagnosis of disseminated intravascular coagulation (DIC); (2) the fibrinogen level, which is low in DIC; and (3) fibrin degradation products (FDP), which are elevated in DIC.

Bone Marrow Aspiration and Biopsy

Bone marrow aspiration and biopsy are used to assess and identify most blood dyscrasias (aplastic anemia, leukemias, pernicious anemia, thrombocytopenia). Examination of the bone marrow reveals the number, size, and shape of the RBCs, WBCs, and platelet precursors. Hematologists examine marrow cells for various maturational abnormalities. Bone marrow aspiration and biopsy may be performed by a physician or a specially trained nurse. The practitioner may elect to perform the biopsy first and the aspiration second. Bone marrow samples are most commonly taken from the poste-

rior iliac crests. An alternative site for specimens is the sternum.

Preprocedure Care

Prepare the client for the test. Explain the purpose of the procedure and what to expect. Advise the client that there will be pain during the procedure. Verify that the client has signed an informed consent form. Provide sedation as prescribed. Some protocols use conscious sedation or anesthesia (see Chapter 16).

Procedure

Help the client assume the lateral decubitus position, with the side from where the biopsy will be taken uppermost. Clean the client's skin with an antiseptic solution such as povidone-iodine. A local anesthetic is administered to numb the skin and subcutaneous tissue to the level of the periosteum. Applying ice to the contralateral side reduces pain.

Bone Marrow Aspiration. The skin is incised with a scalpel. The bone marrow aspiration needle containing an obturator is inserted through the incision to the bone cortex and into the marrow space. Once the needle is in place, the obturator is removed. A syringe is then attached to the needle, and about 1 ml of marrow is withdrawn. Because the marrow space itself cannot be anesthetized, removal of the marrow usually produces moderate to severe pain of short duration. The pain usually stops as soon as suction on the marrow space is stopped. The marrow is ejected onto labeled slides. The needle is withdrawn. Specimens should be sent to the laboratory immediately.

Bone Marrow Biopsy. The bone marrow biopsy needle is advanced through the soft tissue to the periosteum of the biopsy site. The obturator is removed, and the biopsy needle is advanced into the cortex. After the cortex is penetrated, the biopsy needle is advanced another 2 to 3 cm through the bony trabeculae. The needle is rotated several times in a circular back-and-forth motion to cut the core sample and then is withdrawn. A small probe is used to remove the core sample from the end of the biopsy needle, and the sample is placed in formalin. Specimens are labeled and sent to the laboratory immediately.

Postprocedure Care

After the procedure, apply pressure until bleeding stops. Most clients require only a small bandage over the site because bleeding is usually minimal; however, many clients who require bone marrow aspiration are thrombocytopenic and may need a longer period of pressure to

TABLE 76-7 — Laboratory Tests Used in the Diagnosis of Hemorrhagic Disorders

Name of Test	Purpose	Normal Values	Interpretation of Findings
Platelet count	Measures number of circulating platelets in venous or arterial blood	150,000-450,000/mm³	Low count results in prolonged bleeding time and impaired clot retraction; diagnostic of thrombocytopenia
Prothrombin time (PT)	Determines activity and interaction of factors V, VII, and X, prothrombin, and fibrinogen; determines dosages of oral anticoagulant drugs	11-15 sec (one-stage) INR: 2-3.5	Prolonged PT is seen in clients receiving anticoagulant therapy; with low levels or deficiencies of fibrinogen, clotting factors II, V, VII, and X; impaired prothrombin activity; in the presence of circulating anticoagulants as seen in SLE
Partial thromboplastin time (PTT, aPTT)	Complex method for testing the normalcy of intrinsic coagulation process; used to identify deficiencies of coagulation factors, prothrombin, and fibrinogen; used to monitor heparin therapy	25-38 sec	Prolongation of time indicates coagulation disorder that is related to deficiency of a coagulation factor; not diagnostic for platelet disorders
Thrombin time	Measures functional fibrinogen available, as shown by the time needed to form fibrin clot after thrombin is added	10-15 sec	Prolonged time indicates DIC or hypofibrinogenemia; presence in blood of excess heparin or other anticoagulants
Thromboplastin generation test (TGT)	Measures generation of thromboplastin; if result abnormal, second stage is done to identify missing coagulation factor	<12 sec (100%)	Abnormal values found in hemophilia
Fibrinogen level	Measures level of fibrinogen	200-400 mg/dl	Abnormally low values may indicate DIC, liver disease, congenital or acquired afibrinogenemia
Fibrin split products (FSPs), fibrin degradation products (FDPs) test	Measures products that result from breakdown of fibrin	Less than 10 μg/ml	Abnormally high levels are seen in DIC; helpful in monitoring fibrinolytic therapy
D-dimer	Measures a specific product resulting from breakdown of fibrin	Less than 0.5 μg/ml	Abnormally high levels confirm the diagnosis of DIC; screen for abruptio placentae (placental abruption)
Activated clotting time	Crude measure of coagulation process in venous blood; used to control heparin therapy; commonly used during cardiovascular surgery and in the ICU	7-120 sec (depends on type of activator used)	Prolonged time occurs in severe coagulation problems and therapeutic administration of heparin
Bleeding time	Measures ability to stop bleeding after a small puncture wound	3-8 min in adults (varies with test method)	Prolonged bleeding time occurs in vascular maladies and after aspirin ingestion
Capillary fragility test (tourniquet test, Rumpel-Leede test)	Crude test of vascular resistance and platelet number and function; a BP cuff is placed on the arm and inflated to a pressure midway between systolic and diastolic BP for 5 min; petechiae in area are counted	No petechiae	Petechiae (five or more) are seen in thrombocytopenia and vascular purpura
Clot retraction	Indicates function and number of platelets; measures time needed for contraction of an undisturbed clot	50%-100% in 24 hr	Clot retraction is retarded in thrombocytopenia; clot is small and soft in thrombasthenia (functional disturbance of platelets)

BP, Blood pressure; DIC, disseminated intravascular coagulation; ICU, intensive care unit; INR, International Normalized Ratio; SLE, systemic lupus erythematosis.

TABLE 76-8	*Lymphocyte Immunophenotyping*			
Cell	**Total Lymphocyte Count (%)**	**Absolute Count**	**Decreased**	**Increased**
CD3 (mature T cells)	56%-77%	860-1880/mm³	AIDS, chronic lymphocytic leukemia, SCID, immuno-suppressive therapy	Acute lymphocytic leukemia, infectious mononucleosis, multiple myeloma
CD19 (total B cells)	7%-17%	140-370/mm³	Acute lymphocytic leukemia, SCID	Chronic lymphocytic leukemia, multiple myeloma, SLE
CD4 (T helper cells)	32%-54%	530-1190/mm³	AIDS	—
CD8 (T killer/suppressor cells)	24%-37%	430-1060/mm³	AIDS	—

AIDS, Acquired immunodeficiency syndrome; *SLE*, systemic lupus erythematosus; *SCID*, severe combined immunodeficiency disease.

stop bleeding. A pressure dressing and sandbag may be applied in these cases. Instruct the family to observe the site frequently on the day of the procedure and for several days thereafter for clients with an increased risk for bleeding. Clients may experience some discomfort or pain and may require a mild analgesic.

Immunologic Status Tests

Most immunodeficiencies can be identified through three blood tests that require no preprocedure or postprocedure care: (1) WBC and differential, (2) immunoglobulin levels, and (3) total serum complement. Additional immunodeficiencies can be determined through more complex tests, including lymphocyte immunophenotyping, measures of immunoglobulin subclasses, complement assays, and the presence of specific antibodies (after immunizations or exposure to antigens as with communicable diseases).

Lymphocyte Immunophenotyping

Lymphocyte subpopulation analysis by flow cytometry measures total numbers and percentages of B lymphocytes, T lymphocytes, and T lymphocyte subsets (CD4, CD8) in a peripheral blood sample. Table 76-8 lists normal levels of T and B lymphocytes and conditions in which abnormal levels of T cells and B cells occur.

Advanced lymphocyte assays (not detailed here) include the following:

- Mixed lymphocyte culture reaction with the client as stimulator and the client as responder
- Lymphoproliferation assays using chemicals such as phytohemagglutinin (PHA) or concanavalin A (ConA) to stimulate T cells and pokeweed mitogen to stimulate B cells
- Tests of natural killer cell activity
- Tests for deficiencies of adenosine deaminase and purine nucleoside phosphorylase

TABLE 76-9	*Immunoglobulin (Ig) Isotypes*
Immunoglobulin	**Normal Range (mg/dl)**
IgG	550-1990
IgG1	280-1020
IgG2	60-790
IgG3	14-240
IgG4	11-330
IgM	45-145
IgA	70-310
IgE	0.01-0.04
IgD	0-8

Immunoglobulin Isotypes

The immunoglobulin isotype examination measures the serum level of the various immunoglobulins: IgG, IgA, IgM, IgD, and IgE (Table 76-9). Subclasses of IgG may also be measured (IgG1, IgG2, IgG3, IgG4).

Complement Assays

Immunodeficiencies or disorders that are related to a lack of normal levels of complement components may be detected by the level of the total serum complement (CH50) or may require measuring levels of specific complement components such as C3 and C4. In rare cases functional complement assays are required to diagnose complement disorders. Table 76-10 provides normal complement levels.

Radiography

Congenital absence of thymic tissue (diagnostic of certain immunodeficiencies) or tumor of the thymus gland (associated with myasthenia gravis) can be detected by a chest radiograph (see Chapter 4).

TABLE 76-10	*Complement Assays*	
Test	**Normal Range**
Total serum complement (CH50)	75-160 units/ml
C3	55-177 mg/dl
C4	15-50 mg/dl

Other radiographic procedures may be performed to assist the diagnosis of allergy-related disorders. X-ray films and computed tomography (CT) may be ordered to assess the integrity of the sinuses (see Chapter 4).

Lymphangiography allows visualization of the lymphatic system to assess malignancy, metastases, or obstruction. After the administration of local anesthesia, blue dye is injected into the dorsa of the feet and is taken up by the lymphatics. When a lymphatic channel is located, a surgical incision into the channel allows insertion of a catheter. An oil-based dye is injected, and its progress through the lymphatic system is monitored with x-rays taken over 1 to 2 days.

Postprocedure care and complications are similar to those for angiography (see Chapter 4). Explain that the dye colors the urine blue until it is completely excreted. The dorsa may also remain blue for months.

Skin Tests

Skin tests confirm sensitivity to a specific allergen. A known antigen is placed on or directly beneath the skin to detect the presence of antibodies. Antigens are applied by one of three methods:

1. *Patch tests* (see Chapter 50)
2. *Scratch tests* (also known as *tine tests* or *prick tests*) (see Chapter 78)
3. Delayed-type hypersensitivity skin testing (see the following section)

Delayed-Type Hypersensitivity Skin Testing

Delayed-type hypersensitivity (DTH) skin tests may be administered in an *anergy panel* to evaluate cell-mediated immune response, or it may be administered to aid in the diagnosis of certain infectious diseases. To assess cell-mediated immunity, antigens to which people have been immunized (mumps, tetanus) or to which they commonly have been exposed *(Candida albicans)* are injected intradermally into the ventral forearm. After 24 to 72 hours, people with normal T-cell immunity exhibit an area of hard, reddened swelling *(induration)* at the injection site. The localized thickening and redness indicate accumulation of sensitized T lymphocytes at the site of antigen administration. An absence of induration may indicate *anergy* (a state of immunologic hyporesponsiveness) and an inability to react to common antigens. Anergy is associated with congenital T-cell immunodefi-

ciency, malnutrition, cancer, HIV infection, immunosuppressant therapy (including treatment with cytotoxic agents, corticosteroids, or radiation), and, in older clients, aging of the immune system. A negative result may also occur if the antigen was deposited too deeply into the skin (subcutaneously rather than intradermally). Conversely, induration and erythema occurring only 4 to 6 hours after test administration may represent an *Arthrus reaction* that is antibody based and not a measure of cellular immunity.

The DTH antigens for anergy testing are most accurately administered by separate intradermal injections of mumps antigen, *C. albicans* antigen, and tetanus toxoid fluid (1:5 dilution). Other antigens such as streptokinase, streptodornase, or trichophytin may be used but may be less reliable in assessment of T-cell immunity.

In addition, DTH skin tests are a component of diagnostic testing for certain infectious diseases such as tuberculosis and coccidioidomycosis. Disease antigens such as purified protein derivative (PPD) for tuberculosis or coccidioidin for coccidioidomycosis are injected intradermally. The presence at the injection site of induration and erythema of a specified size and at a specified time ranging from 24 to 72 hours indicates past or present infection with the microorganism on which the antigen is based. (See Chapter 64 for discussion of PPD testing for tuberculosis.)

Nurses often administer DTH skin tests and interpret test results. Take a thorough client history of allergies, and explain the purpose of the test and the procedure. Verify the specific antigens prescribed by the physician for testing, and ensure the availability of emergency resuscitation equipment in the event of an anaphylactic reaction. For consistency, it is best if the same person administers and reads the skin test.

Procedure

Use a 1-ml syringe with a 0.5-inch 26- to 27-gauge needle to administer the antigen. Select a site on the ventral surface of the forearm, avoiding veins or bruises. Clean the skin with alcohol and allow it to dry. Stretch the skin taut. Inject 0.1 ml of the antigen intradermally, producing a wheal 6 to 10 mm in diameter. Circle the area with a marking pen. If more than one antigen is administered, administer each antigen 5 cm (2 inches) apart. Document the site of administration of each antigen using a schematic drawing.

Postprocedure Care

Assess the injection site at the specified interval for the type of testing being performed. For anergy testing, palpate the site for induration after 48 hours. DTH responses begin to resolve after 48 hours; hence, if the anergy skin test is read at 72 hours, a borderline positive reaction may appear negative. Use a flexible ruler to measure the area of induration; redness alone is not significant. Induration of 5 mm or more with erythema indicates a positive response to the antigen and probable intact cell-mediated immunity. Record the results.

Problems following DTH skin testing range from minor itching and discomfort at the injection site (common) to anaphylaxis (rare). Relieve itching and minor discomfort by applying cool compresses and topical corticosteroids. If ulceration of the injection site occurs, keep the area clean and dry. Anaphylaxis is potentially lethal. Clients who have known anaphylactic reactions to specific antigens should never be tested for allergy to that substance. Anaphylaxis is treated by administering oxygen and subcutaneous epinephrine and by establishing intravenous access for administration of corticosteroids, antihistamines, and other medications, such as bronchodilators.

CONCLUSIONS

The hematopoietic system is extremely complex. Understanding the structure, function, and assessment of the hematopoietic system will help you care for clients with any of the wide variety of disorders that affect this highly complex system.

BIBLIOGRAPHY

1. Abbott, M.B., & Levin, R.H. (2001). Anaphylactoid reactions to radiocontrast agents. *Pediatric Revue, 22*(10), 356.
2. Ahya, S., et al. (Eds.). (2001). *The Washington manual of medical therapeutics* (30th ed.). Philadelphia: Lippincott Williams & Wilkins.
3. Anderson, K.N. (Ed.). (2002). *Mosby's medical, nursing, & allied health dictionary* (6th ed.). St. Louis: Mosby.
4. Bickley, L.S., & Szilagyi, P.G. (2003). *Bates' guide to physical examination & history taking* (8th ed.). Philadelphia: Lippincott Williams & Wilkins.
5. Braunwald, E., et al. (Eds.). (2001). *Harrison's principles of internal medicine* (15th ed.). New York: McGraw Hill.
6. Cavanaugh, B.M. (2003). *Nurse's manual of laboratory and diagnostic tests* (4th ed.). Philadelphia: F.A. Davis.
7. Chernecky, C.C., & Berger, B.J. (Eds.). (2001). *Laboratory tests and diagnostic procedures* (3rd ed.). Philadelphia: W.B. Saunders.
8. Corbett, J.V. (2000). *Laboratory tests and diagnostic procedures with nursing diagnoses* (5th ed.). Upper Saddle River, NJ: Prentice Hall.
9. Fishbach, F.T. (2000). *A manual of laboratory and diagnostic tests* (6th ed.). Philadelphia: Lippincott Williams & Wilkins.
10. Goldman, L., & Bennett, C. (Eds.). (2001). *Cecil's textbook of medicine* (21st ed.). Philadelphia: W.B. Saunders.
11. Guyton, A.C., & Hall, J.E. (2000). *Textbook of medical physiology* (10th ed.). Philadelphia: W.B. Saunders.
12. Harmening, D. (Ed.). (2001). *Clinical hematology and fundamentals of hemostasis* (4th ed.). Philadelphia: F.A. Davis.
13. Hash, R.B. (1999). Intravascular radiographic contrast media: Issues for family physicians. *Journal of American Family Practice, 12*(1), 32-42.
14. Henry, J.B., & Davey, F.R. (Eds.). (2001). *Clinical diagnosis and management by laboratory methods* (20th ed.). Philadelphia: W.B. Saunders.
15. Jacobs, D.S., et al. (Eds.). (2001). *Laboratory test handbook* (5th ed.). Cleveland: Lexi Comp.
16. Jarvis, C. (2000). *Physical examination and health assessment* (3rd ed.). Philadelphia: W.B. Saunders.
17. Kee, J.L. (2002). *Laboratory and diagnostic tests with nursing implications* (6th ed.). Upper Saddle River, NJ: Prentice Hall.
18. Mandell, G.L., et al. (Eds.). (2000). *Mandell, Douglas, and Bennett's principles & practice of infectious diseases* (5th ed.). Philadelphia: Churchill Livingstone.
19. Miller, B.F. (Ed.). (2003). *Encyclopedia & dictionary of medicine, nursing, & allied health* (7th ed.). Philadelphia: W.B. Saunders.
20. Pagana, K.D., & Pagana, T.J. (2001). *Mosby's diagnostic and laboratory test reference* (5th ed.). St. Louis: Mosby.
21. Seidel, H.M., et al. (Eds.). (2002). *Mosby's guide to physical examination* (5th ed.). St. Louis: Mosby.
22. Skidmore-Roth, L. (2001). *Mosby's handbook of herbs & natural supplements*. St. Louis: Mosby.
23. Tierney, L.M., & Whooley, M. (Eds.). (2002). *Current medical diagnosis and treatment* (42nd ed.). New York: McGraw-Hill.
24. Turgeon, M.L. (1999). *Clinical hematology: Theory and procedures* (3rd ed.). Philadelphia: Lippincott Williams & Wilkins.
25. Wallach, J. (2000). *Interpretation of diagnostic tests* (7th ed.). Philadelphia: Lippincott Williams & Wilkins.

evolve *Did you remember to check out the bonus material on the Evolve website and the CD-ROM, including free self-assessment exercises?*

http://evolve.elsevier.com/Black/medsurg/

Management of Clients with Hematologic Disorders

Tricia C. Corbett
Patricia C. Buchsel

This chapter discusses disorders that affect red blood cells *(erythrocytes)*, white blood cells *(leukocytes)*, the spleen, platelets, and clotting factors. Priorities of nursing care center around the lack of oxygenated blood flow and risk of hemorrhage. Leukemia and lymphoma are discussed in Chapter 81.

DISORDERS AFFECTING RED BLOOD CELLS

THE ANEMIAS

Anemia is a clinical condition that results from an insufficient supply of healthy red blood cells (RBCs) to oxygenate the body's tissues adequately; hypoxia results. Not a disease in itself, anemia reflects a number of underlying pathologic processes leading to an abnormality in RBC number, structure, or function. Those at risk for developing anemia differ with the various etiologies. Because the prevalence of anemia increases with age, adults 65 and older are at particular risk; the estimated prevalence in this group is 20%. Aging cannot be assumed to be the cause of anemia, however, without excluding other reversible causes.

Etiology, Risk Factors, and Classification

The anemias are classified by either the etiology or the morphology of the specific anemia. Anemia is caused in one of three ways: (1) decreased production of healthy RBCs, (2) increased RBC destruction *(hemolysis)*, or (3) loss of blood. A number of underlying problems lead to these conditions. Etiologic categories are listed in Table 77-1.

The production of RBCs *(erythropoiesis)* takes place in the bone marrow. The requirements for healthy RBCs include precursor cells *(reticulocytes)* and adequate supplies of iron, vitamin B_{12}, folic acid, protein, pyridoxine, and traces of copper. If any of these factors is missing, the RBCs will be fragile, misshapen, of abnormal size, lacking hemoglobin, or too few. Such complications in production may be inherited or nutritional.

Increased destruction of RBCs can be due to extrinsic causes such as physical trauma from prosthetic heart valves and thrombotic thrombocytopenic purpura, antibodies triggering isoimmune and autoimmune reactions, and infectious agents and toxins such as malaria. Intrinsic causes may include defective hemoglobin (HbS) as seen in sickle cell disease or membrane abnor-

Nursing Outcomes Classification (NOC)
for Nursing Diagnoses—Clients with Hematologic Disorders

Activity Intolerance
Activity Tolerance
Circulation Status
Endurance
Pain: Disruptive Effects
Acute Pain and Chronic Pain
Comfort Level
Pain Control
Pain: Disruptive Effects
Pain Level
Symptom Control
Symptom Severity

Fatigue
Activity Tolerance
Comfort Level
Energy Conservation
Rest
Quality of Life
Imbalanced Nutrition: Less than Body Requirements
Nutritional Status: Food and Fluid
Intake
Nutrient Intake
Ineffective Protection
Coagulation Status

Infection Status
Ineffective Tissue Perfusion
Tissue Perfusion: Skin and Mucous
Membranes
Tissue Perfusion: Peripheral
Readiness for Enhanced Therapeutic Regimen Management
Health-Promoting Behavior
Health-Seeking Behavior
Knowledge: Health Promotion, Illness
Care, Prescribed Activity, Treatment
Regimen

TABLE 77-1 *Etiologic Categories of Anemia*

Genetic	Drugs and chemicals
Hemoglobinopathies	Chemotherapeutic agents
Thalassemias	Anticonvulsants
Enzyme abnormalities of the glycolytic pathways	Antimetabolites
Defects of the red blood cell cytoskeleton	Certain oral contraceptives
Hereditary spherocytosis	Toxic chemicals
Fanconi anemia	Thrombotic thrombocytopenic purpura and hemolytic uremic
Nutritional	syndrome
Iron deficiency	Physical effects
Cobalamin/vitamin B_{12} deficiency	Trauma
Folate deficiency	Burns
Alcoholism, generalized malnutrition, and starvation	Prosthetic valves and surfaces
Hemorrhage	Snake venom
Immunologic: Antibody-mediated abnormalities	Chronic diseases and malignancies
Infections	Renal disease
Viral: Hepatitis, infectious mononucleosis, cytomegalovirus,	Hepatic disease
Epstein-Barr virus, parvovirus	Chronic infections
Bacterial: Clostridia, gram-negative sepsis	Neoplasia
Protozoal: Malaria, leishmaniasis, toxoplasmosis	Collagen vascular disease

 malities resulting in osmotic injury to the cell. Exposure to certain drugs and chemicals and conditions such as hypersplenism or neoplasms are additional causes of hemolysis.

Anemia may also be due to acute blood loss, most commonly seen in trauma or vessel rupture, or chronic loss, such as gastrointestinal (GI) tract hemorrhaging and menses.

Morphologic classification is based on erythrocyte size, shape, and color. Normal RBCs are shown in Figure 77-1, *A*. Morphologic categories include normocytic/normochromic (normal size and color), macrocytic/normochromic (large size, normal color), and microcytic/hypochromic (small size, pale color). Normocytic/normochromic morphology is caused by acute blood loss, hemolysis, chronic renal disease, cancers, sideroblastic anemia, refractory anemia, diseases of en-

docrine dysfunction, aplastic anemia, and pregnancy. Macrocytic/normochromic morphology is a result of cobalamin (vitamin B_{12}) deficiency, folic acid deficiency, liver disorders (including alcoholism), and splenectomy. Microcytic/hypochromic morphology is present in iron-deficiency anemia, thalassemia, and lead poisoning.

Some anemias are named for the abnormal shape of the RBCs. For instance, normal RBCs have a biconcave shape, and *sickle cell anemia* has sickle-shaped RBCs (Figure 77-1, *B*); spherocytosis, a hereditary disorder leading to hemolytic anemia, has spherical-shaped RBCs. (See Table 76-4 for other abnormalities of erythrocytes and their associated conditions.) Although the morphologic system is the most accurate means of classifying anemias, the etiologic system provides a better basis for identifying clinical and nursing management requirements.

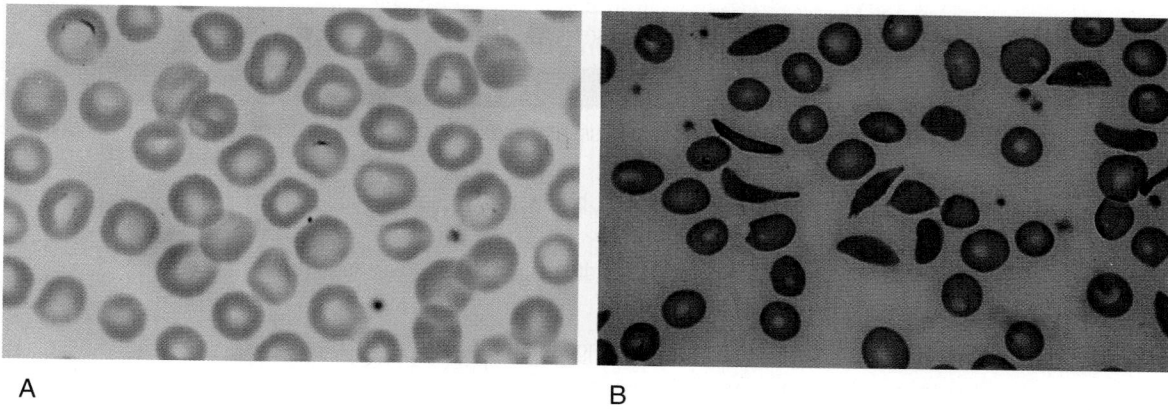

FIGURE 77-1 **A,** Normal red blood cells. **B,** Sickle cell anemia. (Magnification ×875.) Note the elongated and sickle-shaped cells. (From Rodak, B. [2002]. *Hematology: Clinical principles and applications* [2nd ed.]. Philadelphia: W.B. Saunders.)

Pathophysiology

Transport of oxygen (O_2) is impaired with anemia. Hemoglobin is lacking or the number of RBCs is too low to carry adequate O_2 to tissues, and hypoxia develops. The body attempts to compensate for tissue hypoxia in four major ways: (1) a shift in oxygen-hemoglobin dissociation curve to the right to facilitate the removal of more O_2 by the tissues at the same partial pressure of O_2, (2) redistribution of blood from tissues of low O_2 needs to tissues of high O_2 needs, (3) increased cardiac output achieved by increased heart rate or increased stroke volume to meet O_2 demands of the tissues, and (4) increased rate of RBC production resulting from erythropoietin synthesis by the kidneys in response to tissue hypoxia.

Clinical Manifestations

Manifestations accompanying anemia are due primarily to the body's response to hypoxia. The manifestations differ depending on the severity and speed of blood loss, the chronicity of the anemia, the client's age, and the presence of other disorders. Hb levels are used to determine the severity of anemia. Clients with mild anemia (Hb 10 to 12 g/dl) are usually asymptomatic. If manifestations do occur, they typically follow strenuous exertion. Clients with moderate anemia (Hb 6 to 10 g/dl) may suffer from *dyspnea* (shortness of breath), palpitations, *diaphoresis* (profuse perspiration) with exertion, and chronic fatigue. Some clients with severe anemia (Hb <6 g/dl), such as those with chronic renal failure, may be asymptomatic because their anemia develops gradually; others may have significant clinical manifestations involving multiple body systems. Additional manifestations are due to the underlying etiology; a careful work-up can provide clues to the etiology. Table 77-2 lists typical manifestations of anemia by body system (see the Evidence-Based Practice in Action feature on Fatigue and Quality of Life on p. 2275).

Hereditary anemias have several cultural and ethnic considerations. The prevalence of sickle cell disease and thalassemia is high in African Americans. Thalassemia is also high in people of Mediterranean origin. Pernicious anemia rates are high in Scandinavians and African Americans.

Assessment of clients with manifestations of anemia was detailed in Chapter 76. Clients often appear pale, particularly of palm lines, nail beds, conjunctivae, and circumoral area. Because of tissue hypoxia, clients are fatigued. Other manifestations may include shortness of breath, dyspnea on exertion, or palpitations. Hypotension is common, especially if the client has lost blood. If the client has GI bleeding, tarry stools may be present. If heart failure develops, orthopnea, angina, tachycardia, dependent edema, bruits, and tachypnea may occur.

The RBC count, hemoglobin level, and hematocrit confirm the presence of anemia. A bone marrow specimen may be required to confirm the type of anemia. A peripheral blood smear (RBC indices) is needed to determine the size of the RBC. Table 76-4 identifies laboratory study findings in various anemias.

Outcome Management
Medical Management

The goals of care for clients with anemia include (1) alleviating or controlling the causes, (2) relieving the manifestations, and (3) preventing complications. Treatment varies in intensity and duration because some anemias resolve after blood transfusion, others resolve within a few weeks or months, and still other forms require lifelong intervention.

Alleviate and Control the Causes. Depending on the etiology of the anemia, interventions may include (1) supplemental iron therapy, (2) nutritional therapy, (3) surgery to repair sites of hemorrhage, (4) splenectomy, (5)

TABLE 77-2	*Clinical Manifestations of Severe Anemia (Hb <6 g/dl)*
Area	**Clinical Manifestations**
General	Pallor, severe fatigue, malaise, weakness, light-headedness, fever, exertional dyspnea, headache, vertigo, sensitivity to cold, weight loss.
Skin (Integumentary)	Pallor (anemia); jaundice (HA); dry skin, brittle nails, spoon-shaped concave nails with longitudinal ridges (IDA)
Eyes	Blurred vision (anemia, PV); sclera jaundice and retinal hemorrhage (HA)
Ears	Vertigo, tinnitus
Mouth	Smooth, glossy, bright red, and sore tongue (PA, IDA)
Lungs	Dyspnea, orthopnea (anemia, HbS crisis)
Cardiovascular	Tachycardia, palpitations, murmurs (particularly systolic), angina, hypertension, cardiomegaly, intermittent claudication, heart failure, MI
Gastrointestinal	Anorexia; dysphagia (IDA); abdominal pain (Hb S, HA); hematemesis (vomiting blood), tarry stools (HA); hepatomegaly, splenomegaly
Genitourinary	Amenorrhea and menorrhagia (IDA); decreased fertility (anemia); hematuria (HA)
Musculoskeletal	Back pain (HA); sternal tenderness and severe bone and joint pain (Hb S)
Nervous System	Headache, confusion (anemia); peripheral neuropathy, paresthesias, and loss of balance (PA); mental depression, anxiety, coping difficulties (especially life-threatening conditions)

AP, Aplastic anemia; *HA,* hemolytic anemia; *HbS,* sickle cell anemia; *IDA,* iron-deficiency anemia; *MI,* myocardial infarction; *PA,* pernicious anemia; *PV,* polycythemia vera.

removal of toxic agents that cause aplasia, (6) stem cell or bone marrow transplantation, (7) corticosteroid therapy, and (8) immunosuppressive therapy.

Relieve Manifestations

Oxygen Therapy. Oxygen therapy may be prescribed for clients with severe anemia because their blood has a reduced capacity for oxygen. Oxygen helps to prevent tissue hypoxia and lessens the workload of the heart as it struggles to compensate for the lower Hb levels.

Erythropoietin. Subcutaneous injections of erythropoietin can be given to treat anemias of chronic disease because this drug increases the production of RBCs. For this drug to be effective, the client must have bone marrow capable of producing RBCs and sufficient nutrients for the production of RBCs.

Iron Replacement. Iron can be given to augment oral intake in cases where the need for iron is immediate or the demands are beyond dietary measures (e.g., pregnancy). The oral form of iron should be used because it is inexpensive and convenient. It is usually given for mild forms of anemia. The medications of choice are ferrous sulfate (Feosol) or ferrous gluconate (Fergon), 200 to 325 mg orally in three or four doses a day, with or after meals. Taking iron with vitamin C or orange juice aids in the absorption of iron. Clients usually receive iron supplements for at least 6 months for repletion of the body stores. Side effects may include nausea, vomiting, constipation or diarrhea, and blackened stools.

Few indications exist for the use of parenteral therapy. It is usually given only if the client has malabsorption syndrome, has an intolerance to oral iron, continues to suffer blood losses, habitually forgets to take oral preparations, or if a rapid response is needed. Iron dextran (Imferon), 100 to 250 mg intramuscularly (IM) or intravenously (IV), or iron-sorbitol-citrate complex, IM only, may be given. However, because IM administration is painful, stains the skin, and results in less of the iron being absorbed, IV administration is preferable. IV iron should be infused at a rate no greater than 1 ml/min. Side effects of this form of iron may include flushing, hives, arthralgia, fever, lymphadenopathy, phlebitis, and anaphylaxis. Peak reticulocytosis occurs at about day 10. RBC indices and Hb level gradually return to normal. Because of the high risk of allergic reaction, if iron is to be given IV, the client must be closely monitored during the administration of the first dose (see the Integrating Pharmacology feature on Oral and Parenteral Iron Replacement Therapy on p. 2278).

Blood Transfusions: Homologous. For a general overview of blood component transfusion, including composition, compatibility, special considerations and outcomes, see Table 77-3.

Blood transfusions are valuable in treating anemia resulting from acute blood loss; it also may benefit clients with severe chronic anemia (Hb <6 g/dl) who have responded poorly to other forms of therapy. Packed RBCs may be given to clients who have lost blood in surgery or due to trauma; however, several issues related to

📖 EVIDENCE-BASED PRACTICE IN ACTION

Fatigue and Quality of Life

One of the most debilitating manifestations of anemia is profound fatigue that significantly affects the client's quality of life. A growing body of literature documents that not only is fatigue often overlooked and undertreated but often is considered an inevitable sequela of disease and treatment to be endured. Most of the research in fatigue and its management has occurred in the cancer model; however, manifestations accompanying fatigue in the ill client are endemic to all client populations. For example, clients with anemia experience classic clinical manifestations of profound fatigue, dyspnea, shortness of breath, pallor, weakness, and below normal Hb serum blood levels.[1]

Only recently have researchers found that fatigue is so far reaching that it is known to decrease the quality of life in the four domains of living: physical, psychological, social, and spiritual well-being.[1,2] The correlation between fatigue and physical well-being is well known but not always well understood. Clients most often report that they cannot keep pace with their normal activities of functioning as a parent, work at their jobs, exercise, or have energy for pleasurable activities such as going to the movies or visiting friends.

The psychological well-being domain address is impacted by emotional distress, fears of the unknown, the inability to concentrate, forgetfulness, and the notion that their disease is worsening. Cognitive dysfunction secondary to cancer treatment is only beginning to be explored. Studies suggest that women with cancer who have been treated with adjuvant therapy show cognitive dysfunction 2 years after treatment.[3] The cognitive functions that appear to be affected by chemotherapy include verbal and short-term memory, verbal fluency, and concentration.[3] A recent randomized study on the impact of the use of epoetin alfa on cognitive function, fatigue, and quality of life in women with breast cancer who had received adjuvant or neoadjuvant chemotherapy found that fatigue and quality of life as measured by standardized tests showed that fatigue and quality of life was seen in a lesser extend in the epoetin alfa arm than in the placebo arm during chemotherapy.[4]

Social well-being affected by fatigue is manifested in the client's reluctance to attend support groups or attend community activities because of their profound fatigue. Clients find themselves becoming isolated and often depressed because they must conserve their energy for the basic tasks of daily living.[1]

Finally, the spiritual well-being domain encompasses the client's concern for his or her mortality and often causes a shift in life priorities from the need to accumulate tangible goals (e.g., promotions at work, gaining more financial security) to focus on the small but joyous events of even one day (e.g., the change of seasons, gardening, or return to a religion that might have abandoned for some years).

More research is required to understand fully the manifestation of fatigue and its enormous consequences in the client and his or her family. Although the impact of fatigue is well documented in its physical consequences, psychological, social, and spiritual consequences are only beginning to be researched.

Similar to shifts in understanding and treating the manifestation of pain in a humanistic and nonjudgmental fashion, fatigue is emerging as an important manifestation to be managed by health care clinicians.

Nursing research is emerging to document that all the domains of fatigue can be diminished by teaching clients and their families to practice certain behaviors.[5-7]

1. Treating anemia with erythropoietin colony stimulating factors or RBC transfusion when appropriate
2. Promoting sleep and rest
   a. Taking short naps instead of long ones
3. Providing optimal nutritional support
   a. Eat low-fat, high-fiber meals
4. Alternative therapies
   a. Relaxation techniques, biofeedback, massage therapy
5. Energy conservation and body mechanics
   a. Wash hair in the shower, not in the tub or over a sink
   b. Use a terry-cloth robe instead of a towel to dry off
   c. Use a hand-held shower while sitting in the tub
   d. Install a handrail
6. Exercise
   a. Exercise moderately
   b. Take walks
7. Cognitive dysfunction
   a. Do crossword puzzles
   b. Do jigsaw puzzles

References

1. Yoder, L. (2001). Management of clients with hematologic disorders. In Black J.M., Hawks, J.H., & Keene, A.M. (Eds.). Medical surgical nursing: Clinical management for positive outcomes (6th ed., pp. 2103-2128). Philadelphia: W.B. Saunders.
2. Ferrell, B.R., et al. (1996). "Bone tired": The experience of fatigue and impact on quality of life. *Oncology Nursing Forum, 23,* 1539-1547.
3. Schagen, S.B, et al. (1998). Impairment of cognitive function in women receiving adjuvant treatment for high-risk breast cancer; high dose versus standard-dose chemotherapy. Journal of the National Cancer Institute *90,* 210-218.
4. O'Shaughnessy, J., et al (2002). Impact of epoetin alfa on cognitive function, asthenia, and quality of life in women with breast cancer receiving adjuvant or neoadjuvant chemotherapy: Analysis of a 6-month follow-up data. Presented at the 25th Annual San Antonio Breast Cancer Symposium, December 11-14, San Antonio.
5. Crimpton, B. (1995). Symptom management: Loss of concentration. *Seminars in Oncology Nursing, 11,* 279-288.
6. Swartz, A. (1998). Patterns of exercise and fatigue in physically active cancer survivors. *Oncology Nursing Forum, 25*(3), 1-12.
7. Mock, V., et al. (1997). Effects of exercise on fatigue, physical function, and emotional distress during radiation therapy for breast cancer. *Oncology Nursing Forum,* 23, 991-1000.

TABLE 77-3	*Blood Components*		
Whole Blood	**Red Blood Cells**	**Platelet Concentrates**	**Fresh Frozen Plasma**
Composition RBC, plasma, plasma proteins (globulins, antibodies), 63 ml of anticoagulant-preservative	RBC with CPDA-1 solution (anticoagulant-preservative only), final hematocrit no higher than 80% (80% RBC, 20% plasma) RBC with 100 ml additive solution, final hematocrit about 55%-60%	Single-unit platelets contain a minimum of 5.5×10^{10} (1 unit) platelets in 50-70 ml of plasma obtained by separating platelet-rich plasma from 1 unit of fresh whole blood; 6-10 units may be pooled for 1 transfusion Single-donor platelets contain a minimum of 3.0×10^{11} platelets (6 units) obtained from single donor by use of automated cell separator during apheresis; recipient exposed to fewer donors, which decreases complications	91% water, 7% protein (globulin, antibodies, clotting factors), and 2% carbohydrates Freezing within 8 hr of collection preserves all clotting factors
Volume 500 ml/unit	250-350 ml/unit 350-400 ml/unit	50-70 ml/unit 200-400 ml/unit	200-250 ml
ABO/Rh Compatibility The ABO type of the donor should be identical with the recipient's Rh− blood can be given to an Rh− or Rh+ recipient	A can match with A or 0; B can match with B or 0; 0 can match only with 0; AB can match with A, B, or 0 Rh− blood can be given to either Rh+ or Rh− recipient	Whereas platelets have no ABO or Rh antigens, they are suspended in 200-400 ml of plasma containing donor antibodies and a small number of RBC ABO and Rh compatibility is recommended	A can match with A or AB; B can match with B or AB; AB can match only with AB; 0 can match with A, B, AB, or 0 Rh− and Rh+ blood can be given to either Rh+ or Rh− recipient
Special Considerations Whole blood transfusion is rarely indicated Treatment with specific blood components is usually recommended	RBC may be viscous, thus 0.9% saline may be added to achieve optimal flow rates For some clients, a leukocyte depletion filter may be used to prevent complications	Because platelet concentrates contain few RBC, crossmatch testing is not required Plasma ABO and Rh compatibility is recommended, especially when the total volume of the transfusion exceeds 150-200 ml Only filters specially designed for platelet transfusion should be used	Plasma carries same risk of disease transmission as does whole blood If only volume expansion is required, products of choice are crystalloid or colloid solutions, such as saline or albumin Plasma contains no RBC, and Rh compatibility and crossmatching are not required ABO compatibility must be confirmed before administration

CPDA-1, Citrate-phosphate-dextrose-adenine; *FFP,* fresh-frozen plasma; *HIV,* human immunodeficiency virus; *IV,* intravenous; *PPF,* plasma protein fraction; *PT,* prothrombin time; *PTT,* partial thromboplastin time; *RBC,* red blood cells; *vWF,* von Willebrand's factor; *WBC,* white blood cells.

Cryoprecipitate	Granulocyte Concentrates	Plasma Derivatives	Coagulation Factor Concentrates
Each unit contains 50% of antihemophilic factor VIII (80-120 units) and 20%-30% of factor XIII originally present in a unit of whole blood, as well as vWF and 250 mg of fibrinogen suspended in 10-20 ml of plasma	Unit obtained by granulocytaphresis contains a minimum of 1×10^{10} granulocytes, variable amounts of lymphocytes (usually <10%), 30-50 ml of RBC and 100-400 ml of plasma, and 6-10 units of platelets; the platelets can be separated from the unit if the granulocyte recipient is not thrombocytopenic	*Albumin:* 96% albumin, 4% globulin and other proteins extracted from plasma; available as a 5% solution, oncotically equivalent to plasma, and also a concentrated 25% solution *Plasma protein fraction:* 83% albumin and 17% globulins extracted from plasma; less pure than albumin and has higher degree of contamination with other plasma proteins; in 5% solution only	*Factor VIII:* Lyophilized concentrate containing large quantities of factor VIII; prepared from large pools of donor plasma, but heat treatment during fractionation process significantly reduces risk of transmitting viral disease *Factor IX:* Lyophilized concentrate containing large quantities of factor IX; also contains factors II, VII, and X; product prepared from large pools of donor plasma, but heat treatment during fractionation process significantly reduces risk of transmitting viral disease
5-10 ml/unit	200-400 ml with platelets 100-200 ml without platelets	Albumin: 250 and 500 ml (5%); 50 and 100 ml (25%)	Multiple-dose vial
Cryoprecipitate contains no RBC and a small volume of plasma ABO crossmatching not needed, and plasma compatibility preferred but not required	Granulocytes contain a significant number of RBC and plasma; therefore ABO of donor should be identical with recipient's Rh− components may be transfused to an Rh+ recipient	Antibodies destroyed during processing; therefore compatibility not a factor	Antibodies destroyed during processing, so compatibility not a factor
Single units of cryoprecipitate may be pooled into 1 container by the blood collection center If individual bags are issued, 0.9% saline may need to be added to rinse residual cryoprecipitate from bags and tubing	Granulocytes have short survival (<24 hr); infuse as soon as possible Granulocyte concentrates contain a significant number of RBC; pretransfusion testing recommended Increased incidence of febrile, nonhemolytic reactions with granulocyte transfusions; infuse slowly, observe client closely; premedication with an antihistamine, acetaminophen, steroids advised Do *not* administer amphotericin B within 4 hr of granulocyte transfusion to avoid pulmonary insufficiency	PPF and albumin cannot transmit hepatitis or HIV infection; the pasteurization process used to prepare the products destroys such viruses Hypotension has been associated with rapid infusion of PPF; 25% albumin can cause a significantly increased blood pressure because of its ability to draw fluid into the intravascular space	Factor VIII and factor IX assays should be performed at appropriate intervals to assess response Factor VIII concentration lacks vWF and should not be used in treatment of von Willebrand's disease

Continued

TABLE 77-3	*Blood Components—cont'd*		
Whole Blood	**Red Blood Cells**	**Platelet Concentrates**	**Fresh Frozen Plasma**
Outcomes			
Prevention or resolution of hypovolemic shock and anemia In a nonbleeding adult, 1 unit of whole blood should increase hematocrit by 3% and hemoglobin by 1 g/dl	Resolution of manifestations of anemia In a nonbleeding adult, 1 unit of RBC should increase hematocrit by 3% and hemoglobin by 1 g/dl	Prevention or resolution of bleeding due to thrombocytopenia or platelet dysfunction 1 unit should raise peripheral platelet count 5000-10,000/mm³ if underlying cause is resolved or controlled Efficacy of platelet transfusion can be determined by obtaining platelet counts at 1 hr and 18-24 hr after infusion	Treatment effectiveness is assessed by monitoring coagulation function (specifically PT and PTT) or by specific factor assays

CPDA-1, Citrate-phosphate-dextrose-adenine; *FFP*, fresh-frozen plasma; *HIV*, human immunodeficiency virus; *IV*, intravenous; *PPF*, plasma protein fraction; *PT*, prothrombin time; *PTT*, partial thromboplastin time; *RBC*, red blood cells; *vWF*, von Willebrand's factor; *WBC*, white blood cells.

INTEGRATING PHARMACOLOGY

Oral and Parenteral Iron Replacement Therapy

Iron-deficiency anemia is often treated with oral ferrous sulfate and, more recently, with parenteral iron administration. Although oral iron is an over-the-counter medication, its frequent side effects often cause the client to discontinue the medication. Nurses can teach clients the nature of the side effects and how to manage them. You may teach your client to drink ginger tea or suck on ginger candy to avoid or minimize nausea and vomiting. Stool softeners to avoid constipation are also important. Conversely, IV iron replacements, long discouraged because of the dangers of anaphylactic shock, are being replaced by newer preparations with fewer adverse effects. Because of the history of adverse events, fears of administering the IV iron agent warrants discussion of this new preparation.

Functional iron deficiency may develop in clients with normal ferritin levels but low transferrin saturation (<20%) due to the inability of the client to mobilize iron stores rapidly enough to support increased erythropoiesis. Some factors that influence the absorption of iron include the dose, iron stores, the degree of erythropoiesis, diet, and the route of administration. In iron-deficiency clients, the amount of iron absorbed can be 10% to 30% and as high as 60%. In healthy clients, about 5% to 10% of dietary iron is absorbed. In clients with iron deficiencies such as iron-deficient anemia, oral or IV iron replacement may be needed.

Oral iron supplementation therapy is preferred, provided the client can adequately absorb iron and can tolerate oral therapy. If no blood is lost, the usual adult daily dose of elemental iron is in the range of 180 to 200 mg daily in divided doses preferably taken on an empty stomach. Oral iron supplementation is available as ferrous sulfate, ferrous gluconate, or ferrous fumarate. These iron salts are absorbed equally; however, they differ in the amount of elemental iron they contain. Ferrous gluconate, ferrous sulfate, and ferrous fumarate provide about 11%, 20%, and 33% of elemental iron, respectively. All three iron salts are known to be associated with GI side effects such a nausea and vomiting, constipation, diarrhea, or dark coloration of feces.

Some clients may inadequately respond to oral iron supplementation because of poor absorption, noncompliance, or intolerance of therapy.

Parenteral iron therapy does not induce GI side effects, thereby reducing client noncompliance, and it is convenient to take; however, parenteral iron preparations are also known to be associated with hypersensitivity reactions, including anaphylactic reactions and local adverse reactions. Three different IV iron preparations are currently available for iron-deficiency anemia: (1) iron dextran, (2) sodium ferric gluconate, and (3) iron sucrose. All iron dextran products are indicated for use as a second line therapy only after clients fail oral iron therapy.

Cryoprecipitate	Granulocyte Concentrates	Plasma Derivatives	Coagulation Factor Concentrates
Correction of factor VIII, vWF, factor XIII, and fibrinogen deficiency; cessation of bleeding in uremic clients Laboratory values required to assess effectiveness of treatment	Improvement in or resolution of infection Increase in peripheral WBC count not usually seen after granulocyte transfusion in adults, although increase may be seen in children An improvement in clinical condition because of resolving infection is the only measure of treatment effectiveness	The client will acquire and maintain adequate blood pressure and volume support	The client will develop hemostasis because of increased levels of factor VIII and factor IX activity

transfusion warrant judicial use. Transfusion should not be used as a substitute for a specific therapy. A transfusion can have significant risks for the client. These risks include hemolytic transfusion reactions and the possibility of contracting infectious diseases such as human immunodeficiency virus (HIV)/acquired immunodeficiency syndrome (AIDS), hepatitis B or C, graft-versus-host disease (GVHD), cytomegalovirus (CMV), Epstein-Barr virus (EBV), and West Nile virus. Transfusions should be avoided in clients who might be candidates for BMT (e.g., those with aplastic disorders or sickle cell disease) because transfusion decreases the probability of cure. In addition, clients who may have multiple antibodies against RBCs and those with autoimmune antibodies are at a higher risk for complications due to the complexities of obtaining cross-matched donor blood.

Considering the potential risks, alternative interventions should be taken when possible to reduce the need for transfusion. The Joint Commission on Accreditation of Healthcare Organizations (JCAHO) requires that all blood transfusions be evaluated to confirm that clear medical indications for the transfusion exist and that the client responds as expected. The physician's order for transfusion should specify blood component, volume, and rate of infusion. Table 77-3 describes blood components.

Because of the risks associated with blood transfusion, a client's informed consent is required. Blood is administered only after informed consent is obtained. Consent includes an explanation to the client or family member, if necessary, of medical indications for homologous transfusion and its benefits, risks, and alternatives. Documentation of informed consent may consist of a form in the medical record stating that this information was presented in a manner understandable to the client or family member. (e.g., the risks of and alternatives to blood transfusion were explained, and the client consented). If no family member is available or time does not allow, place a note to this effect in the chart.

An option to random donors is for transfusion recipients to designate their own donors; however, directed donations have not decreased the risk of contracting HIV infection. Directed donors also appear to have a higher incidence of hepatitis. Despite this evidence, clients frequently feel more comfortable identifying their donors. Discuss all the options and risks with the client in sufficient time to permit donation and blood testing.

Pretransfusion Testing. Current blood donation procedures initiated to increase the safety of the blood supply have significantly reduced the risk of contracting HIV and hepatitis B and C. A thorough donor history with an emphasis on lifestyle and other known risks for contracting HIV and hepatitis is obtained, and many diagnostic tests for serologic and infectious diseases are routinely performed on the donor's blood.

When a need for blood is identified, several tests are done to confirm that the client's blood is compatible with that of the donor. First, the recipient's ABO and Rh type are identified through routine serologic studies. Routine serologic testing requires a 10-ml clotted sample and a 7-ml citrated sample. About 1 hour is required for testing. In the event of a medical emergency, O-negative RBCs and AB plasma can be safely administered to most clients without serologic testing.

Second, to determine the presence of antibodies other than anti-A or anti-B, an antibody screen (the "indirect" antiglobulin test) is performed. More than 400 minor RBC antigens have been identified in RBCs, each of which can stimulate the production of an antibody; however, only a few (i.e., about 30) that are of sufficiently potent antigenicity to be clinically significant are included in the routine antibody screen.

The third test, crossmatching, is another test for compatibility of blood products. It requires identifying antibodies and obtaining blood from donors who do not possess the corresponding antigens. This testing procedure is complicated, lengthens the time required for blood preparation, and is costly. The test adds little to the safety of transfusion (0.01% to 0.1%) if a negative antibody screen is initially obtained. However, crossmatching is important for clients who may have multiple antibodies against RBCs, such as those who are chronically transfused or are known to have autoimmune antibodies. Some clients with autoimmune hemolytic anemia cannot be crossmatched in vitro. These clients require in vivo tests in which incompatible blood is transfused slowly and the client is continually monitored for developing hemoglobinemia. This method should be used only in clients with significant hypoxia or evidence of coronary insufficiency.

Finally, although not a test, failure to label correctly the samples used for blood bank testing can lead to fatal errors. Several precautionary measures should be taken to reduce this risk. Label the sample at the bedside after asking the client to state his or her name and comparing it with the name on the identification bracelet. If the client cannot state his or her name, identity should be confirmed by a family member or other person familiar with the client whenever possible. The date and initials of the phlebotomist must be written on the sample label. To ensure correct labeling, many institutions have adopted a secondary identification system.

Transfusion Complications. Complications can be acute or delayed, occurring days to years after a transfusion. Acute reactions may be immunogenic or nonimmunogenic. Immunogenic reactions include allergic, acute hemolytic, and anaphylactic reactions, and fever; nonimmunogenic reactions include circulatory overload and septicemia. See Table 77-4 for details on acute transfusion reactions.

Delayed reactions may include a delayed hemolytic reaction, hepatitis B, hepatitis C, HIV, GVHD, iron overload, and other infections and agents such as CMV, EBV, human T-cell leukemia virus type 1 (HTLV-1), the organism that causes malaria, and West Nile virus. Table 77-5 provides details on delayed transfusion reactions.

Blood Transfusion: Autologous. *Autologous* blood transfusion is the alternative to *homologous* (random) transfusion and should be considered. Clients who do not have leukemia or bacteremia should be offered the option of donating their own blood before a scheduled surgical procedure when there is a reasonable expectation that blood will be required. Although the risk-benefit ratio should be evaluated, experience to date indicates that even clients with heart disease and other high-risk conditions tolerate donating blood well. The elimination of disease transmission, alloimmunization, and other potential transfusion complications makes this a reasonable option for many surgical clients.

Autologous donations can be made every 3 days if the donor's Hb remains at or above 11 g/dl. For the blood to be maintained in a liquid state, donations should begin within 5 weeks of the transfusion date. RBCs can be stored frozen for 10 years, but the expense involved and time required for final preparation limit this practice to clients who have extremely rare blood types. Donations should cease at least 3 days before the date of transfusion.

Another commonly used method of autologous blood collection is intraoperative, postoperative, or posttraumatic blood salvage. Blood is suctioned from body cavities, joint spaces, and other closed operative or trauma sites. Tissue debris and other sterile contaminants may necessitate special processing, such as washing. Salvaged blood must be reinfused within 6 hours of collection.

■ Nursing Management
Assessment

The general nursing care of clients with anemia includes adequate assessment by the nurse to help identify the cause of the anemia and client education deficits relating to the illness. You can help in the diagnosis by taking a complete health history focusing on the elements outlined in Chapter 76. Client and family teaching is extremely important in treating the anemias because most of the care takes place in an outpatient clinic or in the client's home. Help the client and family to become knowledgeable about self-care in both preventing and treating anemia.

Diagnosis, Outcomes, Interventions

Diagnosis: Activity Intolerance and/or Fatigue. Write the nursing diagnosis as *Activity Intolerance and/or fatigue related to decreased blood supply or low hemoglobin levels as evidenced by complaints of fatigue and lack of energy, dyspnea, pallor, tachycardia, and cognitive dysfunction.*

Outcomes. The client will tolerate activity as evidenced by being able to sit up without fatigue; dyspnea, pallor, or tachycardia; walking increasing distances; and participating in activities of daily living (ADL), such as bathing, dressing, grooming, feeding, to the greatest extent possible.

TABLE 77-4	*Acute Transfusion Reactions*			
Reaction	**Cause**	**Clinical Manifestations**	**Management**	**Prevention**
Immunogenic				
Allergic Incidence: 1%	Sensitivity to foreign proteins in plasma	Urticaria, flushing, itching (no fever)	Administer antihistamines as directed If manifestations mild and transient, transfusion may resume	Treat prophylactically with antihistamines
Febrile, nonhemolytic Incidence: 0.5%-1%	Sensitization to donor white blood cells, platelets, or plasma proteins	Fever and/or pulmonary symptoms Sudden chills and fever (rise in temperature >1° C [1.8° F]), headache, flushing, anxiety, muscle pain	If fever and/or pulmonary manifestations occur, *do not* resume transfusion Give antipyretics as prescribed; avoid aspirin thrombocytopenic clients Treat shock	Consider leukocyte-poor blood products (filtered, washed, or frozen) if fever occurs more than once
Acute hemolytic Incidence: 1:25,000 Fatal: $2:1 \times 10^6$	Infusion of ABO-incompatible red blood cells	Chills, fever, low back pain, flushing, tachycardia, tachypnea, hemoglobinuria, hemoglobinemia, hypotension, vascular collapse, bleeding, acute renal failure, shock, cardiac arrest, death	Send blood samples for serologic testing, and send urine samples to lab Maintain blood pressure Give diuretics as prescribed to maintain urine flow Insert indwelling catheter or measure hourly output Dialysis may be needed	Meticulously verify recipient from sample collection to transfusion
Anaphylactic Incidence: 1:150,000	Infusion of IgA proteins to IgA-deficient recipient who has developed anti-IgA antibodies	Anxiety, urticaria, wheezing progressing to cyanosis, shock, and possible cardiac arrest	Do not transfuse additional RBC Initiate CPR if indicated Have epinephrine ready for injection (0.4 ml of a 1:1000 solution SC)	Give blood components from IgA-deficient donors or remove *all* plasma by washing
Nonimmunogenic				
Circulatory overload Estimated Incidence: 1:10,000 (not usually reported to blood bank)	Infusion of blood at a rate too rapid for size, cardiac status, or clinical condition of recipient	Cough, dyspnea, pulmonary congestion (rales), headache, hypertension, tachycardia, distended neck veins	Place client in upright position with feet in dependent position Administer diuretics, oxygen, and morphine as prescribed Phlebotomy may be required	Adjust transfusion volume and flow rate on basis of client size and clinical status If slow transfusion will exceed 4 hr, request that unit be aliquoted into smaller volumes
Septicemia Incidence: very rare	Transfusion of component contaminated with microorganism	Rapid onset of chills, high fever, vomiting, diarrhea, marked hypotension, and shock	Treat manifestations and administer antibiotics, IV fluids, vasopressors, and steroids as directed Obtain culture of client and blood containers	Collect, process, store, and transfuse blood according to industry standards Infuse within 4 hr of starting time

CPR, Cardiopulmonary resuscitation; *IG*, immunoglobulin; *IV*, intravenous; *RBC*, red blood cells; *SC*, subcutaneously.

Interventions. Plan alternate periods of activity and rest so as not to tire the client. Assist the client with ADL as needed. Place objects within client's reach to conserve energy. Limit demands on the client (e.g., visitors, phone calls, noise, interruptions by hospital staff). Monitor vital signs, hematocrit, and Hb as a guide for activity tolerance. If needed, provide a unit of packed RBCs to improve overall blood volume or increase hematocrit (see earlier description of blood transfusion).

Transfusion Procedures

Obtain Venous Access. The gauge of the needle used for transfusion varies with the product being infused. When packed RBCs weighing less than 300 g are infused, a 20-gauge or larger needle is needed to achieve the maximal flow rate. If a smaller-gauge needle must be used, the RBCs can be diluted with 0.9% saline. To prevent hemolysis, add no solution other than normal saline to blood components.

TABLE 77-5	*Delayed Transfusion Reactions*
Reaction	**Clinical Manifestations**
Delayed hemolytic	Fever, mild jaundice, decreased hemoglobin and hematocrit. Occurs as early as 3 days or as late as several months but usually 7 to 14 days posttransfusion as the result of destruction of transfused RBCs by alloantibodies not detected during crossmatch. Generally, no acute treatment is required, but hemolysis may be severe enough to warrant further transfusions. Although uncommon, severe complications such as renal failure and DIC have been reported.
Hepatitis B*	Elevated liver enzymes (AST and ALT), anorexia, malaise, nausea and vomiting, fever, dark urine, jaundice. Incubation period is about 8-12 wk, although it may extend to 6 mo or longer. Usually resolves spontaneously within 4-6 wk. Chronic carrier state can develop and can result in permanent liver damage. Treat symptomatically.
Hepatitis C*	Similar to hepatitis B, but manifestations are usually less severe. Approximately 20% of acute infections resolve. Chronic liver disease and cirrhosis may develop. Before introduction of anti-HCV test, accounted for 90%-95% of all posttransfusion hepatitis. Treat symptomatically.
Human immunodeficiency virus (HIV)	Can be asymptomatic for up to several years or may develop flulike manifestations within 2-4 wk. Later manifestations include weight loss, diarrhea, fever, lymphadenopathy, thrush, *Pneumocystis* pneumonia.
Iron overload	Heart failure, dysrhythmias, impaired thyroid and gonadal function, diabetes, arthritis, cirrhosis. Excess iron is deposited in the heart, liver, pancreas, and joints, causing dysfunction. Commonly occurs in clients receiving >100 units for chronic anemia over a period of time. Prevented by iron chelation therapy [Deferoxamine (Desferal)], which chelates and removes accumulated iron via the kidneys, may be administered IV or SC. Treat clinical manifestations.
Graft-versus-host disease	Fever, rash, diarrhea, nausea, jaundice, hepatitis. Result of replication of donor lymphocytes (graft) in the transfusion recipient (host). Onset 3-30 days posttransfusion. No effective therapy available. To prevent, irradiate blood products before transfusion in at-risk recipient. Some believe that irradiated blood products are indicated for first-degree family members' donations also.
Other	Other infectious diseases and agents may be transmitted via transfusion, including cytomegalovirus, HTLV-1, and those causing malaria.

 Data from National Blood Resource Education Program's Transfusion Therapy Guidelines for Nurses (NIH Publication no. 90-2668). Washington, D.C.: U.S. Government Printing Office; Blaney, K.D., & Howard, P.R. (2000). *Basic & applied concepts of immunohematology.* St. Louis: Mosby; and Hillyer, C.D., et al. (2003). *Blood banking and transfusion medicine: Basic principles and practice.* Philadelphia: Churchill Livingstone.
ALT, Alanine aminotransferase; *AST,* aspartate aminotransferase; *HTLV-1,* human T cell leukemia virus, type 1; *IV,* intravenous; *RBCs,* red blood cells; *SC,* subcutaneous.
*New cases of transfusion-related hepatitis B and C are not common.

Components that contain a significant volume of plasma or other diluent can be safely infused at a rapid rate through smaller-gauge needles or catheters. A central venous catheter is an acceptable access option for blood transfusion; however, a large volume of refrigerated blood infused rapidly into the ventricle of the heart may cause cardiac dysrhythmias. Warming the blood can reduce the risk of this complication.

Another issue of concern is the use of multilumen catheters, which may allow blood to mix with incompatible solutions and medications as they exit the catheter tips. Experience indicates that the circulation achieved through a blood vessel that is suitable for central line placement results in rapid mixing of fluids. As a result no harmful effects have been reported.

Request Blood Release. Blood-bank regulations state that refrigerated components may not be returned to inventory if they have been warmed to more than 10° C (50° F). To meet this requirement, most transfusion medicine services consider 30 minutes to be the maximal allowable time out of monitored storage. To avoid wasting a scarce commodity, certain procedures should be performed before blood is requested: (1) An IV catheter appropriate for transfusing the requested component should be functional, flushed with normal saline, and maintained at a keep-vein-open (KVO) rate. (2) Vital signs should then be taken and recorded. (3) The existence of a fever may be a reason for delaying the transfusion. In addition to masking a possible manifestation of an acute transfusion reaction, fever can also compromise the efficacy of platelet transfusions. (4) Premedication also may be required if the client has a history of adverse reactions. In many cases, febrile reactions can be prevented by administering acetaminophen. A history of allergic reactions may warrant prophylactic administration of antihistamines (e.g., diphenhydramine HCl). To ensure effectiveness, administer oral medication 30 minutes before the transfusion is started. IV medication may be given immediately before the transfusion is initiated.

The name and identification number of the recipient must be provided, and a permanent record of this information must be maintained in the blood bank. To avoid delivery to the wrong client, blood should be transported to only one client at a time.

Confirm Blood Acceptability. The most crucial phase of transfusion is confirming product compatibility and verifying the client's identity. An estimated 80% of transfusion reactions are due to labeling errors. Before going to the client's bedside, verify ABO and Rh compatibility, usually by comparing the bag label with the medical record and forms issued from the blood bank. Also check the bag label to ensure that the correct component has been issued, and check for the expiration date. Components expire at midnight of the day marked on the bag unless otherwise specified.

Inspect the unit for leaks, abnormal color, clots, excessive air, and bubbles. Check carefully for important labels (e.g., "autologous" or "directed") or instructions (e.g., "use a leukocyte-depleting filter"). Cellular components (whole blood, RBCs, and platelets) for an immunosuppressed client should be clearly marked "irradiated." Clients with Hodgkin's or non-Hodgkin's lymphoma, acute leukemia, or congenital immunodeficiency disorders and BMT recipients may develop post-transfusion GVHD if lymphocytes contaminating cellular components engraft and divide. Transfusions from first-degree family members may also cause fatal GVHD. A small dose of radiation delivered to the component before release from the blood bank renders the lymphocytes incapable of mitotic action.

At the bedside compare the name and number on the identification bracelet with the tag on the blood bag. If applicable, check the secondary identification system. The American Association of Blood Banks recommends that two qualified people perform this critical step.

Infuse Blood. Most blood products should be infused through administration sets designed specifically for this use. The set usually contains a 170-mm filter designed to trap fibrin clots and other debris that accumulates during blood storage. Most standard filters can filter 4 units of blood.

Tubing is available in two basic configurations: straight or Y-type. The use of Y-type tubing simplifies the process of adding normal saline to RBCs and provides ready access to a saline flush if the transfusion must be interrupted. Straight tubing usually has a medication injection site a few inches from the needle. If an adverse reaction develops, a KVO saline drip initiated at this site maintains patency of the IV line but avoids exposure to the 30 to 50 ml of blood remaining in the tubing and filter. To reduce the risk of septicemia, change the administration set every 4 to 6 hours or according to institution policy.

Several types of infusion devices are available to regulate and monitor the flow of IV solutions. There are basically two types of infusion devices:

- Infusion controllers, which regulate flow by gravity
- Infusion pumps, which deliver solutions under pressure

Infusion controllers may be used with all blood products if they are designed to function with opaque solutions; however, the negative pressure exerted by the peristaltic or syringe-like cassette action of infusion pumps may cause RBC hemolysis. If the transfusion product contains a significant number of RBCs, consult the manufacturer before a pump designed for crystalloid and colloid solutions is used.

If manual pressure cuffs are used to increase RBC flow rate, the pressure should not exceed 300 mm Hg.

Do not use standard sphygmomanometers for this purpose because they do not exert uniform pressure against all parts of the bag.

Blood warmers may be used to prevent hypothermia, which can be induced by rapid infusion of large volumes of refrigerated blood. Neonatal exchange transfusion, plasma exchange, surgery, and trauma are all clinical situations that might require the use of a blood warmer. Other clients of concern are those with cold agglutinin disease. These clients have antibodies that react at temperatures below 37° C (98.6° F). Systemic circulatory cooling can cause intravascular agglutination. This condition may be detected during serologic testing. Once this client has been identified, the transfusion service may recommend the use of a blood warmer for all transfusions.

Two types of devices are approved by blood-bank regulatory agencies for warming blood. For dry heating a bag is placed between two aluminum heating plates or a disposable cuff-style bag is wrapped around a cylindrical aluminum heating element. A second type uses warm water to increase the temperature of the blood. Water baths containing water warmed to 37° C (98.6° F) may be used only if they have been specifically designed for warming blood. The blood bag should never be fully immersed in water.

Monitor During the Transfusion. The first 10 to 15 minutes of any transfusion are the most critical. If a major ABO incompatibility exists or a severe allergic reaction such as anaphylaxis occurs, it is usually evident within the first 50 ml of the transfusion. Therefore it is recommended that the transfusion begin slowly and that the client be closely monitored. If no evidence of a reaction is noted within the first 15 minutes, flow can be increased to the prescribed rate.

Before leaving the client unattended, instruct the client to report anything unusual immediately. Take and record vital signs before the transfusion begins, after the first 15 minutes, and every hour until 1 hour after the transfusion has been discontinued. Check vital signs immediately if the client displays any untoward manifestations.

The recommended rate of infusion varies with the blood component being transfused. Components such as platelets, plasma, and cryoprecipitate may be infused rapidly, but you must take care to avoid circulatory overload, especially with geriatric clients and clients with cardiac disease. To avoid the risk of septicemia, infusions should not exceed 4 hours. If the client's size or medical condition does not allow infusion within 4 hours, the unit may be split into smaller aliquots in the blood bank.

 Regulatory agencies require complete documentation of the transfusion, including identification of personnel starting and ending the transfusion, unique product number, and outcome (e.g., "no reaction noted"). If an adverse reaction does occur, document the manifestations, actions taken, and future recommendations in the client's record.

Watch for Transfusion Reaction. Exposure to foreign blood elements may mediate immunologic and nonimmunologic reactions affecting all major body systems. Consider any unusual manifestation that occurs during or immediately after a transfusion a potential reaction. Monitor unconscious clients closely because manifestations of a reaction may be inhibited in the unconscious state. The acute reactions most frequently seen are described in Table 77-4.

Whereas treatment may vary depending on the manifestations, follow certain standard procedures when a reaction is suspected. In all cases, stop the transfusion and keep the IV line open with normal saline. Treat life-threatening manifestations such as respiratory or circulatory failure immediately. Contact the client's physician and the blood bank. In accordance with institutional policy, obtain appropriate laboratory samples. Samples used to evaluate a reaction include blood and urine. Free Hb found in either indicates that RBCs have hemolyzed, which is the most serious serologic finding.

To avoid clouding the diagnostic picture by venous trauma, obtain blood samples from a large peripheral vein using at least a 19-gauge needle. The blood sample is also used to repeat ABO and Rh typing, antibody screening, and direct antiglobulin testing. A discrepancy in results between initial and repeat testing may indicate that incompatible blood was transfused. When future transfusions are required, special processing (e.g., washing) may then be performed in the blood bank to reduce the risks of another adverse reaction.

Diagnosis: Ineffective Tissue Perfusion. The lack of circulating blood volume can create tissue hypoxia. State this nursing diagnosis as *Ineffective Tissue Perfusion related to loss of blood volume.*

Outcomes. The client will have adequate tissue perfusion as evidenced by normotension, warm extremities, heart rate between 60 and 100 beats/min, the ability to perform ADLs, or walk without dyspnea or tachycardia.

Interventions. Monitor vital signs and peripheral pulses, peripheral skin temperature, and activity tolerance. Monitor for manifestations of hypoxia such as dyspnea, a decrease in O_2 saturation, an increase in $PaCO_2$, and cyanosis so that early intervention can be initiated. Administer O_2 and transfuse with blood products as ordered. Clients should receive adequate food and fluids to assist with blood volume and provide protein for Hb manufacturing. Keep the client warm, adding blankets to the feet for additional comfort.

Diagnosis: Imbalanced Nutrition: Less Than Body Requirements.

Write the nursing diagnosis as *Imbalanced Nutrition: Less Than Body Requirements related to disease, treatment, or lack of knowledge of adequate nutrition.*

Outcomes. The client will have nutritional deficiencies corrected and optimal nutrition will be achieved, as evidenced by blood test results reaching normal range, improved tolerance for activity, and anemia resolved.

Interventions. Teach the basics of good nutrition, and encourage a diet high in protein, iron, and vitamins. Encourage foods cooked in iron pots and ingestion of foods such as liver (the richest source), oysters, lean meats, kidney beans, whole wheat bread, kale, spinach, egg yolks, turnip tops, beet greens, carrots, apricots, and raisins. Encourage the use of a food diary to increase the client's awareness of actual intake. Suggest eating small, frequent meals throughout the day. Document the client's weight. Encourage good oral hygiene.

Diagnosis: Readiness for Effective Therapeutic Regimen Management or Risk for Ineffective Therapeutic Regimen Management.

This nursing diagnosis is *Readiness for Effective Therapeutic Regiment Management or Risk for Ineffective Therapeutic Regimen Management* related to the client's lack of knowledge about the condition, self-care ability, lifestyle adjustments, appropriate nutrition, and the ability to take iron preparations.

Outcomes. The client will verbalize correct dosage of, route of, and indications for iron preparations as evidenced by correct administration of iron medications and an absence of complications.

Interventions. Teach the client about the condition, self-care activities, lifestyle changes, nutritional needs, and medication information necessary to achieve compliance. Inform the client that iron salts are gastric irritants and should always be taken with or after meals. Liquid iron preparations should be well diluted and taken through a straw (undiluted liquid iron stains teeth). The client can avoid constipation, commonly seen during iron therapy, by eating a high-fiber diet and the use of stool softeners or laxatives as required. Avoid consumption of coffee and tea with iron; absorption is hampered by the tannates. To administer parenteral iron medications, use Z-track methods (see fundamentals textbooks for a review).

Evaluation

Resolution of anemia requires time. When packed RBCs are used, anemia will be corrected immediately. When oral iron preparations are used, it takes weeks for anemia to resolve; the client will thus need assessments at intervals to monitor the progress of therapy. Ultimate prognosis depends on how well the underlying disease is resolved or controlled; progress in this regard should also be monitored.

■ Modifications for Older Clients

Older adults have an especially high prevalence of anemia primarily attributable to poor nutrition with a decreased intestinal absorption of iron, often resulting from debilitation or depression or both. Anemia in older clients is often asymptomatic or mistakenly diagnosed as normal aging changes. Such manifestations include fatigue, confusion, angina, ataxia, and heart failure. Special care should be taken to provide a thorough work-up of these clients to determine whether an etiology exists that might be reversible and thus treatable.

ANEMIA CAUSED BY DECREASED ERYTHROCYTE PRODUCTION

Normally the production and destruction of erythrocytes are in equilibrium in the body. In situations where the production of erythrocytes is decreased, anemia results. Decreased production may be due to (1) decreased synthesis of normal hemoglobin, as seen in iron deficiency anemia, thalassemia, and sideroblastic anemia; (2) defective DNA synthesis, as seen in megaloblastic anemia resulting from cobalamin (vitamin B_{12}) and folate deficiency; or (3) reduced availability of erythrocyte precursors as seen in aplastic anemia and anemia of chronic disease.

IRON-DEFICIENCY ANEMIA

Iron-deficiency anemia (IDA) is a chronic, hypochromic, microcytic anemia resulting from an insufficient supply of iron in the body. Without iron, hemoglobin concentration in the RBCs is reduced and the cells are unable to oxygenate the body's tissues adequately, resulting in anemia.

Etiology and Risk Factors

The National Academy of Sciences recommends an iron intake of 15 mg daily for women and 10 mg daily for men. An average diet supplies the body with about 12 to 15 mg/day of iron, of which only 5% to 10% (0.6 to 1.5 mg) is absorbed. IDA is associated with either inadequate absorption or excessive loss of iron. Major risk factors for IDA include (1) insufficient dietary intake of iron, (2) blood loss, (3) impaired absorption of iron, and (4) excessive demands for RBC production as a result of hemolysis. It is important to know the population groups that have a higher association with these risk factors.

Populations in poor countries and people whose diets lack meat are at particular risk for iron-deficiency anemia from insufficient dietary intake of iron, the most prevalent hematologic disorder worldwide. About 30% of the world's population has this anemia. It is an important international economic concern for two reasons: (1) the diminished capacity of individuals to perform physical labor and (2) the impact on the growth, development and learning of infants and children. Alcoholics are also at increased risk because of poor diets.

Other populations may have increased requirements for iron intake at particular times in their lives. The amount of iron normally absorbed daily is sufficient for meeting the needs of healthy men and women past childbearing age, but it does not meet the additional needs of menstruating and pregnant women, infants, children, adolescent females, older adults (>65 years), regular blood donors, and those on strict vegetarian diets. These groups are at a sufficiently high risk to warrant consideration of prophylactic iron therapy. In the United States women have twice the prevalence of IDA as men (8% versus 4%) because of the excess needs of women of childbearing age. An estimated 4% to 8% of premenopausal women are iron deficient. The most common etiologies of IDA for women are menstruation and pregnancy. Normal iron excretion is less than 1 mg daily. Iron is excreted in urine, sweat, bile, and feces and from the skin in desquamated cells. The average woman loses another 15 mg monthly during menses. About 500 mg of iron is lost during a normal pregnancy.

Infants, children, and female adolescents are also at higher risk for IDA and should be monitored carefully because of associated problems such as failure to thrive, delayed growth and development, and learning difficulties. Infants are born with adequate stores of iron (250 mg) from their mothers; however, once breast-feeding ends, a 25% drop in iron levels occurs. Infants on cows' milk have a higher incidence rate because calcium competes with iron for absorption. Growing children deficient in iron tend to have lower IQs than their nonanemic peers and often exhibit behavioral disturbances frequently manifested as attention deficit disorder (ADA). Malnutrition and lead poisoning should also be considered possible etiologies in this age group.

Older adults are a population at risk for IDA. An estimated 20% of adults over 65 years of age suffer from this condition. Economic constraints, poor dentition, lack of interest in food preparation, malnutrition, and increased rates of chronic disease and cancers, particularly of the GI tract, contribute to a higher prevalence rate in older adults.

Blood loss is the most common etiologic factor in men; and the GI tract is the most common site. Hemorrhage may result from peptic ulcers, hiatal hernia, gastritis, GERD, cancer, hemorrhoids, diverticula, Crohn's disease, ulcerative colitis, or salicylate poisoning. It may also be related to gastritis from the use of aspirin, steroids, or nonsteroidal anti-inflammatory drugs (NSAIDs). Bleeding from the GI tract is usually chronic and occult (too small to be seen). A chronic blood loss of as little as 2 to 4 ml daily can result in iron deficiency anemia because every 2 ml of blood contains 1 mg of iron. The body can compensate for such losses to some degree by excreting less than 0.5 mg of iron daily rather than the normal 1 mg.

Malabsorption of iron may result from alterations in the mucosa of the duodenum and proximal jejunum (as in chronic diarrhea, malabsorption syndromes such as sprue and celiac disease, gastrectomy, and removal of the proximal small bowel) resulting in IDA. Tannates (in tea and coffee), carbonates, the chelating agent ethylenediaminetetraacetic acid (EDTA), and the medicinal antacid magnesium trisilicate all hinder non-heme iron absorption. Eating starch and clay, which occurs in some cultures, also leads to malabsorption.

Pathophysiology

Iron is used in the bone marrow to form iron compounds called *heme*, which are required to synthesize Hb, the key molecule responsible for the transport of oxygen in RBCs. Heme accounts for two thirds of the body's iron. Iron is also vital for the metabolic processes of DNA synthesis and electron transport. Iron concentration in the body is regulated by the absorptive cells in the proximal small intestine; these cells alter iron absorption to match body losses or iron. Errors in this balance also lead to anemia. Fortunately the GI tract can increase its absorption of iron from 10% daily to about 20% to 30% daily. In this way, the body often compensates for diminishing iron stores resulting from inadequate iron intake or excessive iron loss. The other one third of the body's iron (non-heme) is stored in the form of ferritin, an iron-phosphorus-protein complex that contains about 23% iron. It is formed in the intestinal mucosa when ferric iron joins with the protein apoferritin. Ferritin is stored in the tissues, primarily in the reticuloendothelial cells of the liver, spleen, and bone marrow. Iron storage problems can also lead to IDA.

Clinical Manifestations

In mild cases of iron deficiency anemia, the client is asymptomatic; in more severe cases, assessment reveals the general manifestations of anemia, including fatigue, headache, dyspnea, palpitations, pallor in the face, palm of the hand, nail bed, and mucous membranes of the mouth and conjunctiva; *angular stomatitis* (inflammation of the mucosa of the mouth), *glossitis* (inflammation of the tongue), and *cheilitis* (inflammation of the lips); and brittle nails. Laboratory results (Table 77-6) show the following:

- Peripheral blood smears that reveal microcytic and pale (hypochromic) RBCs
- Hb level decreased to as low as 6 to 9 g/dl
- Moderately reduced total RBC count, rarely dropping below 3 million cells/mm^3

TABLE 77-6 Laboratory Study Findings in Erythrocytic Disorders

	Iron Deficiency	Thalassemia Major	Cobalamin B$_{12}$	Folic Acid Deficiency	Aplastic Anemia	Hemolytic Anemia	Sickle Cell Anemia	Polycythemia Vera	Hemachromatosis
RBC Count	−	N to −	−	−	−	−	−	+	+
Hb/HcT	−	− (beta trait +)	−	−	−	−	−	+	+
RBC morphology	Mic/H	Mic/H Target cells	Mac/N Hypersegmented polymorphonuclear leukocytes	Mac/N Hypersegmented polymorphonuclear leukocytes	N/N	N/N Fragmented Bizarre shape	Sickle cell Target cell	Few cells N/N	
Reticulocyte	N or −	+	−	−	−	+	+	+	
Platelets	N or −		+	+	−		+	+	
MCV	−	−	+	+	N			−	
MCH	−	−	− to N	− to N	N				
MCHC	−	−	+	+	N	+ with spherocytosis >36			
Serum iron	−	+	− with malabsorption			N or +	N or +	−	+
TIBC	+	+				−	N or −	−	+
Serum ferritin	−	+							+
Bilirubin	N or −	+				N or + − Indirect bilirubinemia	+		
Marrow aspirate	Absence of hemosiderin		Megaloblasts	Megaloblasts	− Aplastic: remaining cells normal Myelodysplastic: remaining cells abnormal			Hyperplastic	
Other	− Transferrin saturation	Hb electrophoresis Amniocentesis	− Serum vitamin B$_{12}$ + Schilling	− Serum folate	− WBC	− Folate	+ Hb S on Hb electrophoresis − Haptoglobin + Fibrinogen + Urobilinogen + Stercobilinogen Amniocentesis	− Serum erythropoietin + Serum B$_{12}$ + Fibrinogen + WBC (neutrophils)	+ Transferrin saturation Liver biopsy: + iron stores Genetic test to detect HFE gene mutation

+, Increase or positive; −, decrease or negative; *Hb*, hemoglobin; *Hb/Hct*, hemoglobin/hematocrit; *Hb S*, sickle hemoglobin; *HFE*, hemachromatosis gene symbol; *Mac/N*, macrocytic/normochromic; *MCB*, mean corpuscular volume; *MCH*, mean corpuscular hemoglobin; *MCHC*, mean corpuscular hemoglobin concentration; *Mic/H*, microcytic/hypochromic; *N*, normal; *N/N*, normocytic/normochromic; *RBC*, red blood cell; *TIBC*, total iron-binding capacity; *WBC*, white blood cell.

- Reduced mean corpuscular volume (MCV), mean corpuscular hemoglobin (MCH), and mean corpuscular hemoglobin concentration (MCHC)
- Serum iron level (normally 50 to 150 mg/dl) decreased to 10 mg/dl
- Total iron-binding capacity elevated to 350 to 500 mg/dl (normally 250 to 350 mg/dl)
- Complete absence of hemosiderin (an insoluble form of storage iron) from bone marrow
- Immunoradiometric serum ferritin level below normal

Outcome Management

Management of IDA focuses on (1) diagnosis of and correction of the underlying cause and (2) treatment through diet and supplemental iron preparations. Once the diagnosis of iron deficiency anemia is confirmed, studies are conducted to find the cause. Radiographic studies (GI tract series), stool examination for occult blood, esophagoscopy, gastroscopy, and sigmoidoscopy are commonly done to identify the site of blood loss. Correction of the underlying problem (malnutrition, alcoholism, hemorrhage) must follow so that the deficiency does not recur.

Supplemental iron is administered to increase iron available in the blood. Oral and injectable forms of iron are available (see discussion earlier in this chapter). Monitoring the client to ensure compliance is important. An increase in reticulocytes 5-10 days after initiation of iron therapy can document a positive response. Clients with increased daily needs should be given supplemental iron prophylactically (during pregnancy) (see the Integrating Pharmacology feature on Oral and Parenteral Iron Replacement Therapy on p. 2278).

Diets high in iron should be planned with the client and his or her family. The nurse plays a key role in this intervention. Clients and families may need to be taught the elements of high-iron diets, both in terms of the food to be consumed (Table 77-7) and how it should be prepared to increase (cooking in iron skillets) or prevent the loss of dietary iron. Older clients should be informed that tannins in coffee and tea reduce the absorption of iron. These clients can be put in contact with community services (e.g., Meals on Wheels) that will provide at least one nutritious meal daily.

THALASSEMIA (MAJOR)

Thalassemia is a group of genetic disorders that result in inadequate normal Hb production. Whereas IDA affects heme synthesis, thalassemia disrupts the synthesis of globin. These disorders include alpha-thalassemia, a relatively benign and asymptomatic condition; beta-thalassemia minor, a mild to moderate form of microcytic anemia; and beta-thalassemia major, a severe, microcytic, hypochromic anemia that may be fatal. These disorders also cause hemolysis. All are chronic conditions.

Etiology and Risk Factors

The genes for thalassemia are frequently found in people of Mediterranean, African, and Southeast Asian origin. The condition is thought to be a response to endemic malaria. Prevalence rates are as high as 10% in these geographical areas. Individuals who inherit an alpha-gene(s) have alpha-thalassemia, the most common of the thalassemias; the alpha-trait (*heterozygous* state) is asymptomatic in about 30% of African Americans. Those who inherit just one beta-gene *(heterozygotes)* have thalassemia minor, also called *thalassemia trait*, the carrier state of thalassemia major. Those who inherit both beta-genes *(homozygotes)* have thalassemia major, which results in a profound and life-threatening anemia.

Pathophysiology

Thalassemias are autosomal-recessive genetic disorders associated with mutations in the globin genes. The globin protein, vital for the synthesis of hemoglobin, is

TABLE 77-7	*Food High in Iron, Vitamin B$_{12}$, and Folic Acid*

Excellent Source of Iron

Almonds, asparagus, bran, beans, Boston brown bread, carrots, cauliflower, celery, chard, dandelions, egg yolk, graham bread, kale, kidney, lettuce, liver, oatmeal, oysters, soybeans, spinach, and whole wheat. (Cook foods in iron pans.)

Good Source of Iron

Apricots, beef, beets, cabbage, cornmeal, cucumbers, currants, dates, duck, goose, greens, lamb, molasses, mushrooms, oranges, parsnips, peanuts, peas, peppers, potatoes, prunes, radishes, raisins, rhubarb, pineapple, tomatoes, and turnips.

Vitamin B$_{12}$

Red meats, especially liver, dairy products, and eggs

Folic Acid

Asparagus, broccoli, spinach, lettuce, lemons, bananas, melons, green leafy vegetables, fish, legumes, whole grains, liver, organ meats, mushrooms, strawberries, milk, eggs, yeast, wheat germ, kidney beans, beef, potatoes, dried peas and beans, and nuts. (Foods should not be cooked with excessive heat or large amounts of water.)

composed of two alpha- and two beta-polypeptide chains known as alpha-globin and beta-globin. In alpha-thalassemia, there is a mutation in the alpha-globin gene(s). In thalassemia minor, one beta-globin gene is mutated, leading to minor disruptions in beta-globin synthesis. In thalassemia major, a mutation exists in both beta-genes, resulting in significant impairment of beta-globin synthesis, marked reduction in hemoglobin production, and profound anemia.

Hemolysis results from an imbalance in the alpha- and beta-globin chains, which are normally paired. The excess unpaired alpha- or beta-globin chains aggregate and form a precipitate that damages RBC membranes, leading to intravascular hemolysis.

Clinical Manifestations

Individuals with alpha thalassemia may have very mild anemia and are typically asymptomatic. Those with thalassemia minor have clinical manifestations of mild to moderate anemia. These disorders may go undiagnosed for several years.

Individuals with thalassemia major are diagnosed early in life because the lack of Hb becomes quickly apparent. Affected children appear normal at birth because fetal Hb contains no beta-globin; however, in the first few months of life, as Hb synthesis switches from fetal to adult form, manifestations of severe anemia begin to appear. The children also have pain, failure to thrive, frequent infections, diarrhea, splenomegaly, hepatomegaly, jaundice from RBC hemolysis, and bone marrow hyperplasia.

Fetal diagnosis for a specific type of thalassemia can be made through amniocentesis. Molecular diagnostic tests can determine whether a mutation(s) is present after 8 weeks of gestation.

Outcome Management

Thalassemia minor usually does not require treatment. For thalassemia major, the treatment goals are to provide adequate normal Hb for erythropoiesis and to alleviate the effects of iron overload. Chronic transfusions are administered to correct the anemia with the targeted Hb at 9 to 10 g/dl. Iron chelation with deferoxamine is necessary to prevent iron overload. Iron supplementation should not be used. Splenectomy may be undertaken to decrease transfusion requirements. Allogenic hematopoietic transplantation may be curative for some clients. Experimental gene strategies are under development. Dietary interventions include increased tea consumption to help reduce iron absorption in the intestinal tract and increased use of vitamin C to improve iron excretion in those receiving chelation therapy. Genetic counseling and testing for families should be encouraged.

MEGALOBLASTIC ANEMIA

Megaloblastic anemias are a group of disorders caused by impaired DNA synthesis resulting in defective RBCs.

These anemias share the morphology of megaloblasts (large, abnormal, and premature RBCs) in the blood and bone marrow. They are caused by deficiencies of vitamin B_{12} (cobalamin) and folic acid. Common features include the following:

- *Leukopenia*, a decreased number of white blood cells (WBCs)
- *Thrombocytopenia*, a decreased number of platelets
- Oral, GI, and neurologic manifestations
- A favorable response to injections of either vitamin B_{12} or folic acid

COBALAMIN/B_{12} DEFICIENCY (PERNICIOUS ANEMIA)

Pernicious anemia is an autoimmune disorder characterized by the absence of intrinsic factor (IF) in gastric secretions, leading to malabsorption of cobalamin (vitamin B_{12}).

Etiology and Risk Factors

Pernicious anemia (PA) is a type of megaloblastic or macrocytic anemia caused by failure of absorption of vitamin B_{12} (cobalamin). It is the most prevalent form of vitamin B_{12} deficiency in the United States and Canada (Table 77-8). It is associated with gastric atrophy and loss of IF as well as a rare genetic autosomal-recessive disorder (congenital pernicious anemia) in which IF is lacking without gastric atrophy. Ninety percent of people with PA have antibodies that react specifically against the parietal gastric cells where IF is produced;

TABLE 77-8	*Causes of Cobalamin and Folate Deficiencies*

- Insufficient dietary intake: Rare with cobalamin (Cbl) but common with folate
- Drugs that impede absorption in the stomach: Purine analogs (azathioprine), pyrimidine analogs (5-FU), ribonucleotide reductase inhibitors (hydroxyurea), anticonvulsants (phenytoin), and oral contraceptives
- Drugs that impair uptake in the ileum: Nitrous oxide, cholestyramine, para-aminosalicylic acid, neomycin, metformin, phenformin, and colchicine
- Genetic disorders causing defects in the ileal receptors of intrinsic factor (IF) (Imerslünd-Grasbeck syndrome), hereditary transcobalamin II (TCII) deficiency
- Impaired absorption resulting from medications, neoplasms, gastrointestinal (GI) diseases, or surgical resection of the terminal ileum
- GI disorders: Gastric atrophy, gastrectomy, gastric stapling, bypass for pancreatic insufficiency of protease, which releases Cbl from r binders so that Cbl can bind with IF
- Zollinger-Ellison syndrome

60% have anti-IF antibodies. It occurs more often in families of PA clients and is associated with human leukocyte antigen (HLA) types A-2, A-3, and B-7 and in type A blood groups. PA typically arises in people between 40 and 70 years of age with peak incidence around 70 years of age. It is more prevalent in people of Celtic and Scandinavian ancestry.

Pathophysiology

Cobalamin (B_{12}) and folate deficiency are believed to lead to attenuated production of DNA. In normal metabolism cobalamin (extrinsic factor) is released from its ingested protein-bound state by gastric acid. It is bound to IF, a glucoprotein produced by parietal cells of the gastric lining and absorbed in the terminal ileum. It is then bound to the protein transcobalamin II (TCII) and transported to storage sites in the liver. Problems with any of these steps can lead to deficiency. Without cobalamin, DNA synthesis and cell replication are impaired. RBC precursors (erythrocytes/reticulocytes) do not divide normally, and large, poorly functioning RBCs are created. Production of myelin on nerves is greatly affected, also resulting in neurologic deterioration.

Clinical Manifestations

The major manifestations of PA are low Hb, hematocrit, and RBC levels. The diagnosis is based on the presence of anemia, GI manifestations (weight loss, appetite loss, nausea, vomiting, abdominal distension, diarrhea, constipation, steatorrhea) and neurologic disorders (paresthesias of feet and hands, poor gate, memory loss, cognitive problems, depression). Laboratory studies include a complete blood count (CBC), peripheral smear, reticulocyte count, Hb and hematocrit levels, serum iron, total iron-binding capacity, and serum ferritin levels (see Table 77-6). In addition the Schilling test is the definitive test for PA and is used to diagnose and determine the cobalamin deficiency. The Schilling test measures the absorption of orally administered radioactive vitamin B_{12} (tagged with cobalt 60) before and after parenteral administration of intrinsic factor. Gastric secretion analysis to check for the presence of free HCl is another important test. Most clients with pernicious anemia have low-volume gastric secretions with high pH and free hydrochloric acid levels. These findings do not change, even after the administration of histamine, which normally stimulates gastric secretion.

Outcome Management
■ Medical Management

Cobalamin/Vitamin B_{12} Therapy. Clients with PA need both immediate treatment and lifelong therapy with maintenance vitamin B_{12}. The standard treatment is parenteral administration of cobalamin (cyanocobalamin or hydroxocobalamin) at 1000 μg daily for 2 weeks and then weekly until the hematocrit returns to normal.

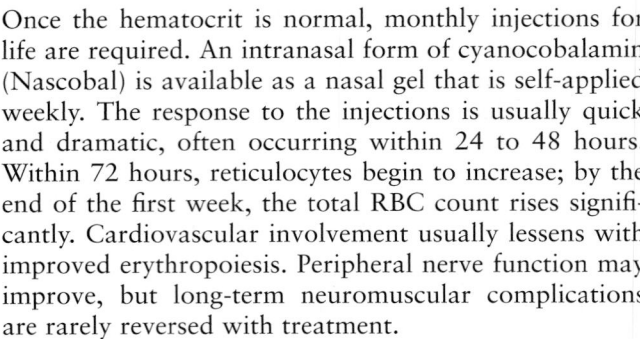

Once the hematocrit is normal, monthly injections for life are required. An intranasal form of cyanocobalamin (Nascobal) is available as a nasal gel that is self-applied weekly. The response to the injections is usually quick and dramatic, often occurring within 24 to 48 hours. Within 72 hours, reticulocytes begin to increase; by the end of the first week, the total RBC count rises significantly. Cardiovascular involvement usually lessens with improved erythropoiesis. Peripheral nerve function may improve, but long-term neuromuscular complications are rarely reversed with treatment.

Iron Supplements. Additionally the client may need oral or IV iron supplementation if the Hg level fails to rise in proportion to an increased RBC count. Iron deficiency may be an etiologic factor in pernicious anemia and must be corrected if it is present. Iron-deficiency anemia can also develop during treatment of pernicious anemia. Injections of vitamin B_{12} may cause a rapid regeneration of RBCs that depletes iron. As a result the Hg level remains low, although the total RBC count rises. Once the acute stage of the illness is past, the client with pernicious anemia must undertake a lifelong program of maintenance therapy. Monthly injections of vitamin B_{12} are needed to avoid relapse. Encourage the client to eat a diet high in folic acid and iron (see Table 77-7) to supplement the medication used to treat the anemia. If the cause involves altered absorption of vitamin B_{12}, nutritional supplements are useless. If the disease is related to decreased intake of the vitamin, a diet high in vitamin B_{12} is encouraged.

Folic Acid. Folic acid is sometimes given to clients with a history of poor nutrition. Folic acid can be dangerous, however, because it does not address neurologic problems that will continue unchecked in the absence of vitamin B_{12}. Therefore a therapeutic trial of folate should never be given before PA is either diagnosed or ruled out.

Digestants. Digestants may be given to enhance the metabolism of vitamins such as HCl diluted in water and given with meals during the first few weeks of vitamin B_{12} therapy.

Treat Neurologic Complications. Multidrug combinations of high doses of folate, cobalamin, and pyridoxine have been proposed to help prevent neurologic complications.

■ Nursing Management

Because clients with PA must receive weekly or monthly treatment for life, the nurse plays an important role in monitoring client progress. Response to treatment should be carefully monitored with blood counts and clinical blood chemistry tests. The client must be educated about the importance of adherence to the treatment regimen on a lifelong basis if the anemia is to be controlled and about the life-threatening consequences of not doing so. The progress of neurologic complications should be continually assessed. Clients with existing neurologic problems should be monitored for and educated about the possibility of injuries attributable to diminished sensitivity to heat and pain from nerve damage. Because gastric carcinoma is commonly associated with PA, clients should be evaluated frequently for the presence of this neoplasm.

FOLIC ACID DEFICIENCY ANEMIA

Etiology and Risk Factors

Anemia associated with folic acid deficiency is common. There are many causes, most of which are the same as those of vitamin B_{12} deficiency. Usually folic acid deficiency results from a diet lacking in such foods as green leafy vegetables, liver, citrus fruits, nuts, grains, and yeast. Clients with chronic alcoholism or eating disorders, such as anorexia, because of their typically inadequate diets, are particularly at risk. High levels of alcohol in the blood also partially block the response of the bone marrow to folic acid, which thereby interferes with erythropoiesis.

Folic acid deficiency, like vitamin B_{12} deficiency, can develop with malabsorption syndromes (e.g., sprue, celiac disease, steatorrhea). Certain medications can also impede folic acid absorption and utilization. For example, a serious anemia may develop under the following conditions:

- Long-term use of anticonvulsant medications (e.g., primidone, phenytoin, phenobarbital)
- Administration of antimetabolites (e.g., folic acid antagonists, purine, pyrimidine analogs) to clients with cancer and leukemia
- Use of certain oral contraceptives

Finally, folic acid deficiency may occur with increased demands for folate, such as during pregnancy and the growth spurts of childhood and adolescence.

Clinical Manifestations

Folic acid, like vitamin B_{12}, is necessary for DNA synthesis; unlike PA, however, folic acid deficiency does not cause neurologic manifestations. The presence of neurologic problems generally rules out folic acid deficiency as the etiology. Anemia resulting from folic acid deficiency has a slow and insidious onset. The client, often thin and emaciated, usually appears quite ill. The client's malnourished and debilitated state frequently leads to other deficiencies, for example, of iron, protein, minerals, and other vitamins. Some clients may also have an electrolyte imbalance, and neurologic manifestations may develop as a result of thiamine, calcium, or magnesium deficiency (commonly linked with alcoholism). Cirrhosis of the liver and bleeding varices further complicate anemia for the alcoholic client.

The megaloblastic anemia caused by folic acid deficiency is the same as that seen in pernicious anemia (see Table 77-6). The diagnosis is confirmed by blood smear and bone marrow examinations. With folic acid deficiency, the serum folate level is less than 4 ng/ml (normal, 7 to 20 ng/ml); the Schilling test finding is normal. HCl is probably present in the gastric juice. Neurologic manifestations are absent; and the client responds favorably to a therapeutic trial of 50 to 100 mg of folic acid administered IM daily for 10 days.

Outcome Management

For correction of anemia caused by folate deficiency, the client receives oral doses of folic acid 0.1 to 5 mg daily until the blood profile improves or the cause of intestinal malabsorption is corrected. Clients with malabsorption syndromes may need parenteral folic acid initially, followed by maintenance therapy with oral doses. Folic acid is administered IM in the form of folinic acid (leucovorin calcium injection). Additionally, vitamin C is sometimes prescribed because it increases the role of folic acid in promoting erythropoiesis. Diets with foods rich in folic acid (see Table 77-7) and food preparation methods that ensure that folate is not destroyed are important. Lifelong monthly doses of folate may be necessary for clients with partial or total gastrectomies. Multivitamins with folate are often prescribed for older clients. Nursing interventions are similar to those discussed for the client with PA.

APLASTIC ANEMIA

Aplastic anemia is caused by a failure of the bone marrow, leading to insufficient production of peripheral blood elements. The marrow failure is due to primary defects in, or damage to, the stem cell or marrow microenvironment. The disorder is characterized by a severely hypoplastic (underdeveloped) fatty marrow that is devoid of all three hematopoietic cell lines (erythroid, myeloid, and megakaryocytic). The stem cell and early progenitor populations are reduced significantly and are unresponsive to hematopoietic growth factors. Hypoplastic bone marrow results in anemia, leukopenia, and thrombocytopenia, collectively known as *pancytopenia*.

Etiology and Risk Factors

The incidence of aplastic anemia is approximately 2 per million population in the United States and Europe. Rates are higher in Asia than in the West (Thailand is 4 per million; Japan is 14 per million); environmental exposure is considered the likely cause. It affects people of all ages, and both genders are equally susceptible; however, idiopathic cases are most common in adolescents and young adults.

Aplastic anemia may be either hereditary or acquired (Table 77-9). In the hereditary forms, anemia typically ap-

TABLE 77-9	*Causes of Aplastic Anemias*

Hereditary

Fanconi syndrome
Dyskeratosis congenita
Shwachman-Diamond syndrome
Pearson syndrome
Diamond-Blackfan syndrome
Amegakaryocytic thrombocytopenia (absent radius [TAR] syndrome)

Acquired

High-dose radiation and chemotherapy drugs (e.g., antimetabolites, alkylating agents)
Toxic chemicals: hair and aniline dyes, herbicides and insecticides (e.g., DDT); and benzene and its derivatives (gasoline, mothballs, paint and varnish removers, dry-cleaning solutions, and household cleaners
Certain drugs: chloramphenicol, sulfonamides, quinacrine, phenylbutazone, the anticonvulsants phenytoin and mephenytoin, gold compounds, streptomycin, tripelennamine, meprobamate, carbon tetrachloride, arsenic
Autoimmune disorders such as systemic lupus erythematosus
Infectious agents: hepatitis, Epstein-Barr virus, human immunodeficiency virus, parvovirus, miliary tuberculosis, and mycobacterial infections
Diseases of the bone marrow (leukemia, graft-versus-host disease, eosinophilic fasciitis, and fulminant hepatitis)
Pregnancy (rare, likely autoimmune)
Idiopathic (an environmental etiology is rarely identified)

pears in childhood. The acquired forms account for nearly 80% of aplastic anemia and appear to result from an autoimmune mechanism. Immunity is controlled genetically and can be influenced by the environment. A number of environmental causes have been associated with aplastic anemia, and yet an estimated 40% to 70% of acquired cases are *idiopathic* (no known cause). Agents that cause destruction of bone marrow are termed *myelotoxins*.

Pathophysiology

The onset of aplastic anemia may be insidious or rapid. In idiopathic or hereditary cases, the onset is usually gradual. Inherited marrow failure syndromes are associated with physical stigmata such as skin pigmentation, short stature, microcephaly, hypogonadism, mental retardation, and skeletal anomalies. When bone marrow failure results from a myelotoxin, however, the onset may be explosive and manifestations developing quickly. If the condition does not reverse itself when the offending agent is removed, it can be fatal.

Clinical Manifestations

Clinical manifestations include fatigue, weakness, headache, dyspnea, rapid heart rate, pallor, frequent infections, unexplained bruising, easy bruising, nose-

bleeds, bleeding gums, heavy menses, blood in the stool, prolonged bleeding from cuts, skin rash, bone pain, foot swelling, and fever.

Manifestations of pancytopenia are particularly severe. The RBC count and leukocyte and platelet counts all decline. The three conditions then develop: (1) normocytic anemia, (2) neutropenia, and (3) thrombocytopenia. The RBC count is usually below 1 million/mm^3, and the reticulocyte count is low. The leukocyte count may be less than 1000/mm^3 (normal range, 5000 to 10,000/mm^3). Neutropenia manifests as overt infection or mouth and pharyngeal ulcerations. If the absolute neutrophil count drops below 500/mm^3, a fulminating bacterial infection may develop, often from the client's own normal flora. The platelet count may fall below 30,000 to 15,000/mm^3 (normal range, 150,000 to 450,000/mm^3). Thrombocytopenia presents as mucosal or gingival bleeding or petechial rashes, purpura, or ecchymoses. Retinal and intracranial hemorrhages may also occur. If the platelet count is severely reduced, spontaneous hemorrhage may also be seen. Some clients show evidence of hepatitis.

Aplastic anemia can be confused with myelodysplastic syndrome because the clinical manifestations are generally the same. A bone marrow biopsy is required to differentiate the two. Aplastic anemia marrow is hypoplastic; that is, the blood cells are reduced, but those that remain are normal. In myelodysplastic syndrome the marrow is hyperplastic; that is, the blood cells are markedly increased and abnormal.

In clients suspected to have aplastic anemia, take a history to elicit the possible etiology, including a work history with a focus on solvent and radiation exposure and family, environmental, travel, and medical histories that include information about recent infectious diseases, cancer therapy, and pregnancy. The diagnosis of aplastic anemia (*pancytopenia*) is based on the client's manifestations, verification of a hereditary disorder, history of exposure to a suspected myelotoxin, a differential blood count, and a bone marrow examination.

Outcome Management

The client with pancytopenia is often critically ill. The major causes of morbidity and mortality are infections and bleeding. Prompt medical attention and skillful nursing care are necessary.

■ Medical Management

Withdrawal of Offending Agent. The first step in halting the process of aplastic anemia is immediate withdrawal of the offending agent if exposure to a causal agent is determined. Any client undergoing radiotherapy or receiving a medication that is a suspected myelotoxin should be monitored by frequent CBCs. A significant drop in the RBC, leukocyte, or platelet count signals the need to stop the drug. Usually stopping a suspected agent is followed by a rise in the CBC. Unfortunately, marrow failure due to chloramphenicol may progress despite discontinuation of the drug.

Transfusion Therapy. If aplastic anemia develops from a suspected myelotoxic agent, blood transfusions are the mainstay of therapy until bone marrow activity signals recovery. If, however, the client is a candidate for a marrow transplant, transfusion should be used judiciously because clients with minimal transfusions have better therapeutic outcomes. Avoid transfusions from family members because sensitization against non-HLA tissue antigens may occur. Because the marrow of the aplastic client is severely depressed, cellular blood components should undergo leukocyte-poor reduction if possible to prevent alloimmunization and be irradiated before transfusion to prevent transfusion-associated GVHD (see Chapter 81). If the marrow does not recover and long-term RBC support is required, the client should be monitored for iron overload. Iron-chelating therapy should be instituted if iron overload occurs. Before iron chelating therapy became available, this complication was a leading cause of death.

Treatment of Infection. Infection is a major cause of mortality for clients with aplastic anemia. Fungal infections, particularly *Aspergillus,* are a major risk. Clients should be treated with a broad-based antibiotic with gram-negative and staphylococcal coverage. For clients with febrile neutropenia, antipseudomonal therapy should be initiated. Antifungal agents should be considered for those with persistent fever.

Bone Marrow Transplantation. Bone marrow transplantation is now the treatment of choice for clients with aplastic anemia who are less than 60 years of age when (1) an autoimmune phenomenon is suspected or (2) the bone marrow fails to regenerate after discontinuation of myelotoxic agents. Currently transplantation can take place only if the client has a HLA–matched donor, usually a sibling. Unrelated donors should be used only if immunosuppressive therapy is unsuccessful. Comparison of the results of clients treated by BMT with conventional therapy of steroids and androgens reveals a 2-year survival rate of 60% to 80% with BMT versus 25% for those treated conventionally. Successful transplantation occurs in about 80% of younger clients and 40% to 70% of older recipients.

Immunosuppressive Therapy. Immunosuppressive therapy should be undertaken if a matched donor cannot be found or if the client is over 60 years of age. Combination therapy is used and usually includes cyclosporine (Neoral, Sandimmune), ATG (antithymocyte globulin), ALG (antilymphocyte globulin), cyclosporine A, and methylprednisolone, with or without cytokine support. The response rate is good, although the initial response (usually 4 to 12 weeks) and continued improvement are slow. Relapse is common. Most clients who receive this therapy become transfusion independent. Preliminary data show that high-dose cyclophosphamide may result in remissions, but this approach has a high risk for fungal infections. Because a central venous catheter is re- quired for immunosuppressive therapy, clients should be carefully monitored for the development of infection.

Diet Adjustments. For clients who are neutropenic or are on immunosuppressive therapy, foods that are likely to harbor bacteria, fungi, or mold (e.g., raw meat, dairy products, certain fruits and vegetables) should be avoided.

Experimental Treatments. Clinical trials are currently under way to determine whether the various hematopoi- etic growth factors can increase the production of blood cells by the bone marrow. The male hormone androgen, which is known to stimulate blood cell production, is also being studied.

Client Education. The client and family should be educated about the causes and treatment of the illness, measures to prevent infection and bleeding (using an electric razor, a humidifier to avoid drying out the mucous membranes), the importance of meticulous oral and perianal hygiene, and adequate rest. The client should be advised to avoid any activity that increases the risk of trauma during periods of thrombocytopenia and unnecessary exposure to the community during periods of neutropenia.

ANEMIAS CAUSED BY INCREASED ERYTHROCYTE DESTRUCTION

HEMOLYTIC ANEMIA

Hemolytic anemia is an end result of many conditions that lead to hemolysis. Hemolysis, the premature destruction of erythrocytes, can result from physical damage, intrinsic membrane defects, abnormal Hb, erythrocytic enzymatic defects, immune destruction of RBCs by macrophages, or hypersplenism. Anemia occurs when the bone marrow fails to replace RBCs at the rate they are destroyed.

Etiology and Risk Factors

Hemolytic anemias constitute about 5% of all anemias. More than 200 causes of hemolytic anemia have been identified.

Hemolysis can result from hereditary disorders or acquired hemolytic conditions. All hereditary disorders are due to intracorpuscular defects. Hereditary disorders that lead to erythrocytic membrane and enzyme defects and Hb abnormalities include spherocytosis (most common of the hereditary disorders) and the hereditary hemoglobinopathies (glucose-6-phosphate dehydrogenase deficiency [G-6-PD], thalassemia, and sickle-cell anemia).

Hereditary spherocytosis is a condition characterized by the spherical shape of the erythrocyte and an abnormal osmotic fragility in vitro. It is caused by an intrinsic genetic defect that leads to defects in membrane proteins. G-6-PD deficiency is an X-linked genetic disorder that causes an erythrocytic enzyme abnormality. The G-6-PD enzyme is the catalyst for glycolysis in the RBC and protects the cell from oxidative agents. A deficiency in this enzyme leads to damage in older cells that undergo rapid hemolysis. G-6-PD confers protection against malaria.

Most cases of acquired hemolytic anemia are due to extracorpuscular abnormalities. Immune reactions, toxic chemicals and drugs, infections, and physical damage can cause acquired hemolytic conditions. Immune reactions may be isoimmune or autoimmune hemolytic anemia (AIHA). Isoimmune reactions occur when host antibodies develop against donor antigens; this is most commonly seen with blood transfusions. Autoimmune reactions occur when antibodies are developed against the body's own erythrocytes. Such reactions may be secondary to lymphomas, leukemias such as chronic lymphocytic (CLL), or systemic lupus erythematosus (SLE). Other examples include acquired immunohemolytic anemia, disseminated intravascular coagulation (DIC), hemolytic uremic syndrome (HUS), and idiopathic (immune) thrombocytopenic purpura (ITP).

Chemicals known to induce hemolytic anemias include arsenic, lead, copper, and certain snake venoms. Drugs that can cause immune hemolysis include penicillin, cephalothin, ampicillin, methicillin, phenylbutazone, phenacetin, quinine, quinidine, and L-dopa. Oxidants (acetanilide, furazolidone, isobutyl nitrite, nalidixic acid, naphthalene, niridazole) can lead to hemolysis in clients with G-6-PD deficiency. Fava beans can induce hemolysis in individuals with the Mediterranean variant of G-6-PD deficiency. The drug-induced hemolytic anemias are clinically indistinguishable from AIHA and usually are classified with this disorder.

Hemolysis may also result from certain parasitic disease that disrupt the RBC membrane (malaria, *Clostridium welchii*) and stress from infections (particularly in those with G-6-PD). Physical damage to the erythrocyte membrane due to hemodialysis, heart-lung machines, and prosthetic cardiac valves also leads to hemolysis.

Intravascular hemolysis occurs in such conditions as G-6-PD deficiency, thrombotic thrombocytopenic purpura (TTP), and DIC. Extravascular hemolysis, which takes place in the spleen and other reticuloendothelial organs, is seen in AIHA and hereditary spherocytosis.

Clinical Manifestations

The clinical manifestations of hemolytic anemia are numerous and diverse and are due primarily to anemia, the extent of compensation, previous treatment, and the underlying cause. The client with hemolytic anemia may suffer from all the general manifestations of anemia discussed earlier (lassitude, fatigue). Manifestations of specific disorders may be present, such as *hemochromatosis* (bronze skin tone and diabetes), *hemoglobinuria* (dark urine), intravascular hemolysis, TTP (fever, neurologic signs, petechiae), thalassemia, and sickle cell anemia. Renal failure, caused by an increased load of RBC degradation products, may be a complication of severe hemolysis. Jaundice, leg ulcers, hepatosplenomegaly, folate deficiency, hemosiderosis, and gallstones may be seen. Clients may also exhibit clinical manifestations that suggest CLL, some lymphomas, and SLE.

Because of the large number of causes for hemolytic anemia, numerous laboratory tests are conducted to determine or rule out known etiologies. These include a CBC, peripheral smear and morphologic examination, RBC indices, increased red blood cell distribution width (RDW), reticulocyte count, lactic acid dehydrogenase, serum haptoglobin, indirect bilirubin, and other studies suggested by the history or physical examination (see Table 77-6). Typically seen are increased RBC fragility, shortened erythrocyte life span, increased fecal and urinary urobilinogen, and hemoglobinemia in cases of massive intravascular hemolysis.

Outcome Management

Interventions are undertaken to counter the complications of the hemolysis and to treat the underlying disorder. Removal of the offending agent, if it is known, is key. Transfusion therapy may be necessary (packed RBCs should be administered slowly to avoid cardiac arrest). Adequate fluids are given to flush the kidneys. In addition, sodium bicarbonate or sodium lactate is administered to alkalize the urine, which decreases the likelihood of precipitation in the renal tubules. Folate acid may be given to offset the consumption of folate that results from active hemolysis. Corticosteroids (prednisone) are indicated for those with AIHA. Iron replacement therapy may be needed for those with severe intravascular hemolysis to counter persistent hemoglobinuria. Splenectomy is the treatment of choice for hereditary spherocytosis. Erythropoietin is given for anemia that has resulted from renal failure. Finally, clients should be educated to recognize the manifestations of hemolysis and to seek immediate medical attention if they occur.

SICKLE CELL ANEMIA

Sickle cell disease (SCD) is a group of inherited disorders of mutant hemoglobin (HbS) that causes the characteristic sickling of RBCs. Sickling occurs only under conditions of low oxygenation. The abnormally shaped RBCs become trapped in capillaries, causing organ damage from infarcts and tissue hypoxia, or are damaged in transit, leading to severe anemia. The most common variant, *sickle cell anemia,* is an autosomal-recessive disorder in which the person is homozygous for HbS. The heterozygous form, known as *sickle cell trait,* is a much milder form of the disease and the carrier state of HbS. SCD is a lifelong condition that manifests in the first year of life and persists throughout one's life span.

Etiology and Risk Factors

Sickle cell disease is found in races of people from areas of the world where malaria is endemic, including Africa, the Mediterranean, the Middle East, and India. The heterozygous form (trait) appears to be a selective advantage for the survival of malaria because the parasite infected cells sickle and are removed.

It is the most common form of anemia worldwide. The highest prevalence rate is in West Africa, where the HbS mutation is thought to have arisen. In the United States, about 75,000 people have SCD; 1 in 500 African-American infants is affected; and 8% of African Americans (about two million) carry the sickle cell gene. It is also found, although rarely, in people of Mediterranean, Middle East, or East Indian descent. The prevalence rate is less than the incidence rate because of high early mortality. Whether an individual will have sickle cell anemia, sickle cell trait, or will be free of the disorder depends on the Hb genes inherited from each parent. Figure 77-2 shows the distribution of the sickle cell gene and the inheritance pattern for the gene. Life expectancy is currently 42 years for males and 48 years for females. The leading cause of death is *acute chest syndrome.*

Pathophysiology

The genetics, molecular biology, and pathophysiology of SCD are well understood. SCD arises from an autosomal-recessive mutation in the allele that codes for the beta-chain of Hb. The mutation causes a substitution of the amino acid valine for glutamic acid at six positions in the chain. The defective hemoglobin (HbS), when exposed to a decrease in oxygen, becomes viscous, has decreased solubility, and forms a gel-like substance containing hemoglobin crystals within the affected RBCs. These crystals clump together into long chains that form a parallel array of filaments, which disrupt the membrane, and the cell assumes a crescent or classic sickle shape (see Figure 77-1, *B*). The sickled cells become rigid, sticky, and fragile. These cells agglutinate and impede circulation in the capillaries, causing microinfarcts, tissue hypoxia, and further sickling. These responses to HbS lead to the profound clinical manifestations of sickling disorders: hemolytic anemia, painful sickle cell crisis, and multiple organ system damage.

Sickle cell crisis is an acute, episodic exacerbation of the disorder brought on by reduced oxygen levels and associated crises. Exposure to low oxygen levels (low oxygen tension) triggers the process of sickling, such as high altitudes, flying in planes that are not pressurized, exercising strenuously (including military boot camp), respiratory infections, or undergoing anesthesia without receiving adequate oxygenation. A sickle cell crisis is most typically the result of vaso-occlusion in tissues and organs *(vaso-occlusive crisis).* This crisis is the most common reason for seeking medical care. It may be induced by stress, exposure to cold water or temperature, hypoxia, or infection; most occur with no obvious cause. Sickled cells have increased immunoglobulin G on the cell surface, which may partially explain why infection often triggers vaso-occlusive crisis.

Organ-damage syndromes are also a hallmark of SCD. Organ damage is due to increased fibrinogen levels and plasma-clotting factors (products of hemolysis) that contribute to the formation of microthrombi and the resultant microinfarcts and tissue necrosis of vital organs. The organs most vulnerable to infarction and necrosis are the brain, heart, lung, and kidneys because of their constant demand for oxygen and the bone marrow and spleen because of increased demands on these organs to replace damaged erythrocytes.

Clinical Manifestations

The typical clinical picture of SCD is associated with profound manifestations of chronic hemolytic anemia, painful sickle cell (vaso-occlusive) crisis, and manifesta-

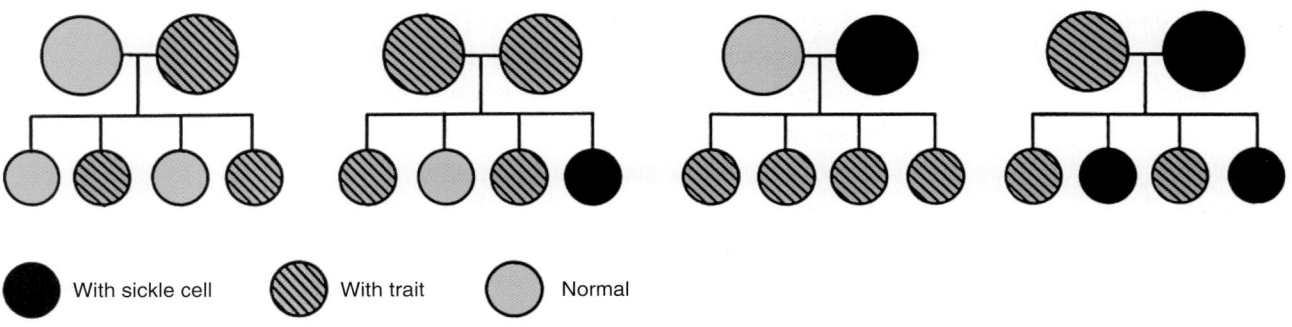

○ With sickle cell   ◩ With trait   ○ Normal

FIGURE 77-2 Inheritance pattern of sickle cell gene. (Redrawn from Page, J., et al. [1981]. *Blood: The river of life.* Washington, DC: Torstar Books.)

tions of the various associated organ-damage syndromes. SCD usually manifests after a child is 6 months of age, when fetal Hb is no longer present. For infants certain factors are predictive of SCD: a Hb lower than 7 g/dl, leukocytosis in the absence of infection, and dactylitis (*hand-foot syndrome)* before the age of 1 year. Young children and adolescents typically exhibit growth retardation and delayed sexual maturity and tend to be underweight. Occasionally clinical manifestations do not appear until adulthood. Many people with SCD are in good health and asymptomatic, except for the occasional but painful periods of vaso-occlusive crisis, the most common manifestation of SCD in adulthood.

Chronic hemolytic anemia is universally present but usually well tolerated. Clients often present with the classic manifestations of chronic anemia such as pallor of the mucosa, fatigue, and low tolerance for exercise. Jaundice is a common side effect of chronic hemolysis. Folate deficiency with resulting megaloblastic changes is also common because of increased demands for folate required for the replacement of destroyed cells.

Sickle cell crisis is predominately a *vaso-occlusive crisis* (sometimes referred to as *pain crisis*), a serious manifestation that requires immediate medical attention. It has a sudden onset and results in severe pain in the long bones, joints, the chest, the back, and the abdomen (resembling acute abdomen); the face may also be involved. Because of the abdominal pain, acute abdomen must be ruled out. Fever, malaise, and leukocytosis may be seen. The duration of crises is extremely variable from client to client and may range from six or more per year, to relatively few over a lifetime, to none. Individual clients appear to have established frequency patterns. About 50% of individuals with homozygous HbS have vaso-occlusive crises.

Aplastic, hemolytic, and sequestration crises are seen much less frequently but also require immediate medical attention. *Aplastic crisis* is a serious complication caused by infection with the parvovirus B-19. This virus infects red cell progenitors in the bone marrow, leading to cessation of erythropoiesis. Hb levels drop precipitously; however, this condition is self-limiting because bone marrow usually recovers in 7 to 10 days. Pain may be a presenting manifestation of this condition. *Hemolytic crisis,* due to the abnormal destruction of RBCs, also may be seen. This condition presents with manifestations of severe hemolytic anemia. The client is usually febrile. *Sequestration crisis* occurs when there is a sudden and massive trapping of destroyed RBC components by visceral organs; splenic sequestration is a common and painful complication.

Acute chest syndrome is the current most common cause of SCD-related mortality followed by cerebrovascular, cardiac, and pulmonary infarcts. This syndrome presents with chest pain, fever, cough, tachypnea, leukocytosis, and pulmonary infiltrates. Fat emboli resulting from bone marrow infarction are thought to be the major etiology of this syndrome. It is a medical emergency and, if not treated immediately, can result in acute respiratory distress and death.

The involvement of multiple organ systems, due primarily to microinfarcts and resulting tissue necrosis, is the basis for the complications most commonly seen in SCD. Nearly every major organ system is affected (Table 77-10). Cerebrovascular, myocardial, and pulmonary infarctions are serious complications. Central nervous systems (CNS) involvement is most prevalent in childhood and adolescence and can have devastating consequences. The most severe manifestation is stroke, typically of thrombotic origin. It is a life-threatening condition and often leads to brain-related deficits (e.g., sensory, motor, cognitive, affective) and paralysis. Heart involvement, due to ischemia from chronic anemia and microinfarcts, usually includes hemosiderin deposits in the myo-

TABLE 77-10	*Organ System Manifestations in Sickle Cell Anemia*
Organ Systems	**Clinical Manifestations**
Central nervous system	Thrombosis- or hemorrhage-related paralysis, cerebral deficits, or death
Cardiac	Systolic murmur, cardiomegaly, heart failure
Pulmonary	Acute chest syndrome, hypertension, infiltrates, pneumonia, heart failure
Renal	Hematuria, renal failure
Spleen	Splenomegaly, splenic atrophy (autosplenectomy)
Hepatic	Hepatomegaly, gallstones
Skeletal	Hand-foot syndrome, osteonecrotic skeletal deformities, osteomyelitis, osteoporosis
Genital	Penal priapism
Optic	Hemorrhage, retinal detachment, retinopathy, blindness
Dermis	Stasis ulcers of the extremities

cardium, systolic murmur, and dilation of the ventricles and left atrium, leading to heart failure. Pulmonary infarcts lead to pulmonary hypertension, heart failure, and eventually cor pulmonale.

Splenomegaly is evident by the latter part of the first year and may present as a sudden and painful splenic sequestration crisis. Impaired function follows, and eventually the spleen shrinks *(autosplenectomy)*. As a result immune deficiency develops, and infections are commonly seen, particularly with encapsulated microorganisms such as *Streptococcus pneumonia*. Hepatomegaly- and infarction-related hepatopathy are often present, as are bile stones, as a result of chronic hemolysis with hyperbilirubinemia. Renal medullary ischemia may be present, resulting in a diminished capacity to concentrate urine; nephritic syndrome, although uncommon, may occur.

Hyperactivity of the bone marrow can lead to spindly legs, a short trunk, and a tower-shaped skull. Skeletal manifestations of aseptic necrosis, especially on the heads of weight-bearing long bones, are due to repeated infarction of the bone, joints, and growth plates, and may lead to osteomyelitis, osteoporosis, and osteosclerosis. Related pain in the joints and long bones is common and usually severe. Necrotic bone marrow with associated development of infection is often seen. Skeletal and joint involvements are associated with chronic pain and disability and may require changes in lifestyle and employment. This is the single most important economic effect of the disease.

Impaired circulation leads to edema of the hands and feet and often results in leg and feet ulcers because of delayed healing and opportunistic infections. Leg ulcers are a chronic painful problem and are found in about 75% of older children and adults with the disease. Ophthalmologic manifestations may include ptosis from paraorbital infarction, retinal vascular changes, and proliferative retinitis, which may result in a loss of vision. The major genitourinary complication is *priapism* (persistent abnormal erection), which tends to occur repeatedly; if prolonged, it may lead to impotence.

Diagnosis of HbS disease is suggested by findings of chronic hemolytic anemia and vaso-occlusive crisis and is confirmed by the existence of homozygous HbS. Typical laboratory study findings are shown in Table 77-6.

Four specific laboratory procedures demonstrate the presence of HbS in either homozygous or heterozygous clients. A stained blood smear is examined for the presence of sickle cells. A sickle slide preparation is used to detect the sickling phenomenon after deoxygenation of the blood. This test is accurate but time consuming. The sickle-turbidity tube test is an excellent mass screening test to detect HbS. After a finger prick, blood is mixed with Sickledex solution in a test tube. Five minutes later, the specimen is observed for cloudiness, which indicates the presence of HbS. Solutions mixed with normal Hb

will remain clear. If the test demonstrates HbS, it does not differentiate SCD from sickle cell trait and other variants. The final study, Hb electrophoresis, is the diagnostic test for HbS and also differentiates SCD from sickle cell trait. The various types of Hb within a blood specimen are separated by means of an applied electric field. If a blood specimen contains both HbS and HbA, the client is heterozygous and has sickle cell trait. If HbS is 75% to 100% of the total and the rest HbF or HbA_2, the client is homozygous and has sickle cell anemia. If the specimen contains 50% HbS and 50% HbC, the client has the HbC variant. If only HbS is found, but HbA_2 is elevated on other tests, Hb S-beta O thalassemia is indicated. Hb S-beta + thalassemia specimens have levels of HbA between 10% and 30%.

Imaging studies are also frequently used. Skeletal x-rays may show deformities and flattening of the bones and joints and areas of infarction. Magnetic resonance imaging (MRI) can demonstrate areas of avascular necrosis and distinguish between osteomyelitis and bony infarction. An abdominal sonogram can document spleen size and the presence of bile stones. Transcranial Doppler ultrasonography can identify clients at risk for stroke.

Many African Americans are unaware that they carry the sickle cell trait and that they can transmit this trait to their offspring. Consequently researchers are perfecting mass screening tests for the detection of HbS among the black population. Clients who have only the sickle cell trait may never be detected unless they are exposed to extremely low oxygen tension, strenuous work or exercise, or pregnancy. When exposed to extreme stressors, the client with the trait may experience manifestations of SCD.

Outcome Management
■ Medical Management

No safe, effective treatment is currently available. Treatment strategies are aimed at control of manifestations and management of disease complications and include management of the following: (1) vaso-occlusive crisis; (2) acute and chronic pain; (3) chronic hemolytic anemia; (4) complications particularly acute chest syndrome and organ-damage syndromes; and (5) infections. Vaso-occlusive crisis is treated with hydration and analgesics. Intravenous fluids (normal saline or 5% dextrose in saline) are administered to correct dehydration and to replace continuing loss.

Reduce Pain. Acute pain control is best accomplished by the administration of opioids, and morphine sulfate is the drug of choice. The drug is given IV, hourly at first, until an effective dose is established; then the dose is tapered off once pain control is achieved usually in 24 to 48 hours. When the client is discharged, sustained-release morphine is given with the dose gradually reduced over several days. Morphine elixir is most commonly used for breakthrough pain. Chronic pain control is achieved with acetaminophen and NSAIDs. The NSAIDs are best for treating deep bone pain, although the use of opioids may be required. If so, codeine and hydrocodone should be tried first; morphine should be used only for more severe cases. Tricyclic antidepressants may reduce the dose of opioids because of their ability to interfere with pain perception. Many clients are depressed, and lifting depression may have a positive effect on the pain. Nonpharmacologic measures, such as physical therapy, heat and cold applications, transcutaneous nerve stimulation (TENS), hypnosis, and acupuncture may also be used.

Bone Marrow Transplantation. Allogenic BMT is the only known cure, but the risks of this procedure may outweigh the benefits. In addition, a matched donor may not be available. Current advances in cord blood stem cell transplantation and immunoablative conditioning regimens may improve the odds of an SCD cure in the not too distant future.

Pharmacologic Agents. Hydroxyurea is the only drug currently approved by the Food and Drug Administrative (FDA) for the treatment of SCD. Hydroxyurea increases the production of HbF, which retards sickling, the Hb level increases, and vaso-occlusive crises become less frequent and less severe or totally eliminated. A decrease in chronic pain and a lowering of reticulocytes also occur; however, hydroxyurea has been identified as a potential leukemogenic and carcinogenic agent. Data on long-term use are currently not available. Candidates for this therapy should include only those who have frequent, painful crises (>6/year), uncontrolled pain using conservative treatment, acute chest syndrome, or a history of or high risk for stroke. For clients receiving hydroxyurea, frequent blood tests to monitor for leucopenia or thrombocytopenia are necessary.

Sodium cromoglycate has shown promising results in significantly reducing the percentage of sickle cells in venous blood. This effect appears to be retained when the blood is deoxygenated. The drug is given by inhalation or the nasal route.

Folic acid supplementation is required because all clients have a folate deficiency. Iron supplementation may also be required for menstruating women.

Blood Transfusion. Blood transfusion is indicated only for special situations such as acute chest syndrome, stroke, aplastic crisis, pregnancy, and general anesthesia. The goal of the transfusion is to reduce the concentration of HbS to 30% or less. Those receiving repeated transfusions should be given iron-chelating agents.

Acute chest syndrome is treated with analgesics, oxygen, antibiotics, and transfusion. The goal of treatment is to reduce the level of HbS to 30% or less. If the hematocrit is 30% or higher, an exchange transfusion is required. This entails removing 1 unit of blood, transfusing 1 unit, and repeating the process or using a continuous-flow phoresis machine.

Prevent Infection. Prevention of infection greatly improves survival. In the past infection was the leading cause of mortality. Penicillin prophylaxis, beginning in infancy, and pneumococcal vaccination at 2 years with a booster at 5 years, controls infections of pneumoniae origin. All infections must be treated promptly with broad-spectrum antibiotics until the causative organism is identified and appropriate antibiotic therapy instituted.

Leg ulcers require debridement and antibiotics. A zinc oxide occlusive dressing (Unna boot) and leg elevation are used. Skin grafting may also be necessary.

■ Nursing Management
Assessment

Assess the client for the pattern of data that may indicate sickle cell crisis. Assess for the ability of the family and client to cope with the disorder and their understanding of the disease and the triggers of crisis.

Diagnosis, Outcomes, Interventions

Diagnosis: Acute Pain. Because of the long bone pain, joint swelling, and abdominal pain secondary to sickling crisis, one nursing diagnosis is *Acute Pain related to sickle cell crisis.*

Outcomes. The client will experience diminished pain as evidenced by verbalization of pain reduction and reliance on fewer opiates for control of pain.

Interventions. Assess for the earliest manifestations of vaso-occlusive crisis and initiate analgesics as needed and ordered. Monitor for the effectiveness of analgesia. Apply heat to joints as ordered. Provide rest periods. Administer fluids to prevent dehydration and recurrence of pain crisis. Increase oral fluid intake, and monitor intake and output.

Diagnosis: Chronic Pain. Because of long-term chronic pain experienced by clients with SCD, another nursing diagnosis is *Chronic Pain related to manifestations of sickle cell anemia.*

Outcomes. The client will experience diminished pain as evidenced by verbalization of pain reduction and will undertake self-management of analgesics for control of pain.

Interventions. Initiate a plan for outpatient use of either acetaminophen or long-acting NSAIDs (a weak opioid such as codeine or hydrocodone may be needed) for chronic pain control as ordered. Monitor the effectiveness of pain reduction during scheduled outpatient visits, and adjust medications as ordered.

Diagnosis: Readiness for Enhanced Therapeutic Regimen Management.

Another nursing diagnosis is *Readiness for Enhanced Therapeutic Regimen Management related to disease, treatment, and prevention of crises.*

Outcomes. The client and family will understand the disease, treatment, and prevention of crises as evidenced by the client's and his or her family's statements and the absence or lessened frequency of crises.

Interventions. When educating clients about sickle cell anemia or sickle cell trait, remember the following:

1. Explain the nature of the disease and answer any related questions the client or family may have.
2. Explain that because SCD is a lifelong condition, adherence to therapy and follow-up visits is critical for effective control of the disease.
3. Encourage African-American parents to have themselves and their children tested for the presence of HbS. Advise parents-to-be that sickle cell screening procedures for the fetus and newborn are available, as is genetic counseling.
4. Advise the client and family to have routine medical examinations that include an RBC count.
5. Encourage young adults who carry HbS to ask their physician for genetic counseling before marrying or having children.
6. Alert young women with sickle cell anemia that pregnancy carries a high risk for them.
7. Explain that multiple organ system complications, particularly pulmonary, cerebrovascular, cardiovascular or renal complications, may develop. The client and family should be taught the manifestations of these complications and advised to seek prompt medical attention if any arise.
8. Explain how to prevent crises, such as (a) avoiding lower oxygen tension and (b) taking caution against becoming dehydrated. Instruct the client and family to call a physician if vomiting, diarrhea, high fever, or any other cause of water loss develops.

The nurse plays an important role in the lifelong management of this disease. The nurse should be aware that the risk for failure to maintain the treatment regimen might be high. Many clients may be of lower socioeconomic and education levels and without adequate health insurance coverage. These factors often lead to noncompliance with treatment regimens.

Evaluation

An appropriate outcome for the client with SCD is that the disease will remain in remission as long as possible. It is impossible to prevent every crisis; however, with education and an effort by the client and family, the number of attacks can be reduced and the severity lessened.

POLYCYTHEMIA VERA

Polycythemia vera (PV), the excessive production of erythrocytes, leukocytes, and platelets is caused by excessive activation of pluripotent stem cells in the bone marrow. It is a chronic, life-shortening, pan-hyperplastic, malignant, and neoplastic marrow disorder. The inordinate mass production of these three cell lines results in (1) an increase in blood viscosity; (2) an increase in the total blood volume, which may be twice or even three times greater than normal; and (3) severe blood congestion of all tissues and organs. Because of these problems, the client suffers many manifestations, including an increased risk of clot formation.

Etiology and Risk Factors

In the United States, PV is relatively rare; its prevalence is 0.6 to 1.6 per million population. Although it occurs in persons of every age-group, its peak incidence is in the group 50 to 70 years of age. All ethnic groups are affected, and predilection of people of Jewish descent may exist. No cure is currently available. With the advent of new therapeutic regimens for management of PV, survival is now between 10 and 20 years. The most common causes of mortality are thrombosis, particularly pulmonary emboli (up to 40%), and hemorrhage complications, especially for those with myelofibrosis or pancytopenia (up to 30%).

Pathophysiology

Polycythemia vera is due to the excessive production of a single line of clonal stems cells present in the bone marrow. These cells interfere with or stimulate normal stem cell growth and maturation. Unregulated neoplastic proliferation is thought to be the etiology. The origin of the abnormal clonal cells is currently unknown; however, these cells have an increased sensitivity to growth factors for maturation, indicating the presence of a defect in the signal pathway (likely in the transmission of the signal) common to different growth factors. Clonal and cytogenic studies are currently under way in an attempt to determine the molecular basis of PV.

Clinical Manifestations

In its early stages polycythemia usually remains asymptomatic (an increased hematocrit level may be an incidental finding). Presenting manifestations are usually related to hypoxia from impairment of the microcirculation caused by blood hyperviscosity secondary to hypervolemia. Manifestations include dizziness, headache, vertigo, tinnitus, visual disturbances, and angina pectoris. Other manifestations can appear depending on the body system that is affected. The client may also have a ruddy complexion (plethora) and dusky, red mucosa; cardiovascular hypertension (with dizziness, headache, and a sense of fullness in the head) and heart failure (shortness of breath, orthopnea); increased clotting leading to stroke, myocardial infarction, or peripheral gangrene; and bleeding (hemorrhage in capillaries, venules, and arterioles), which causes rupture of vessels; GI peptic ulcers, enlargement of liver and spleen; and skeletal gout (painful swollen joints, usually the big toe) characterized by an increased uric acid level.

Diagnostic findings (see Table 77-6) include (1) an RBC count as high as 8 to 12 million/mm³; (2) Hb level of 18 to 25 g/dl; (3) hematocrit greater than 54% in men and 49% in women; (4) platelet count usually increased; (5) normal arterial blood gases (ABG) values; (6) hyperplastic bone marrow; and (7) a serum uric acid level three to four times normal.

Outcome Management

A permanent cure for PV is currently unavailable, but remission of many years can be achieved. The goals of care in PV are 2-fold: reduction of (1) blood volume and viscosity and (2) myeloproliferative activity. These decreases are accomplished through phlebotomy, administration of myelosuppressive agents, and radiation therapy. Emergency phlebotomy can be used to normalize red cell mass as quickly as possible (removal of 500 to 2000 ml of blood until the hematocrit reaches 45%). Clients with hematocrits of less than 70% may be bled twice a week. Clients who are older or who have cardiovascular compromise or cerebrovascular complications should receive volume replacement with saline solution to avoid postural hypotension. If platelet counts are elevated, a myelosuppressive agent should be used in combination with aspirin (300 mg three times a day) to avoid thrombotic or hemorrhagic complications. Women of childbearing age should be treated only with phlebotomy. Once normal hematocrit levels are reached, subsequent phlebotomies should be carried out as frequently (monthly) as necessary to maintain the hematocrit at about 45%. Iron deficiency will likely result, but as it supervenes RBC production will be retarded so that clients managed by phlebotomy alone may require as few as two or three phlebotomies a year.

The myelosuppressive agent hydroxyurea is commonly used in clients over 50 years of age. Radioactive phosphorus, chlorambucil, busulfan (Myleran), and melphalan (Alkeran) have also been tried but are not indicated for long-term use because of the increased incidence of acute leukemia (17%) after 15 years. Radioactive phosphorus, however, may be used for clients older than 80 years or for those with co-morbid conditions in which life expectancy is shorter than 5 to 10 years. Anagrelide may be used in younger clients (50 to 70 years of age) if hydroxyurea is contraindicated. In young males, myelosuppressive therapy can lead to aspermia; use of

this treatment should be carefully evaluated for these clients.

Hyperuricemia is treated with allopurinol (100 to 300 mg/day) until remission is attained; acute gouty attacks are treated with colchicine or other anti-inflammatory agents.

HEMOCHROMATOSIS

Hemochromatosis (HH), also called *iron overload disease,* is the most common genetic disorder in the United States. It is an inherited metabolic disorder that causes increased absorption of iron that is deposited in the body tissues and organs, particularly the liver, heart, and pancreas. As iron levels increase, toxicity results and leads to damage of vital organs.

Etiology and Risk Factors

Hemochromatosis is associated with a defect in the gene called *HFE,* which helps regulate the amount of iron absorbed from food. The body's normal iron concentration level is 2 to 6 g. Individuals with HH accumulate between 0.5 and 10 g/yr and eventually may have in excess of 50 g. Individuals who inherit a defective gene from each parent *(homozygous)* may develop the disease. Those with only one defective gene from each parent *(heterozygous)* are carriers and rarely develop the disease. HH is present at birth, but manifestations seldom manifest before adulthood.

Most often HH affects Caucasians of Northern European heritage. About 0.5% (5 in 1000) of the American Caucasian population is homozygous for the disorder. About 1 person in 10 is a carrier. Men and women are equally at risk for HH, but men are five times more likely to be diagnosed than women and to have manifestations at a much younger age. Women seldom have manifestations before menopause.

Clinical Manifestations

Joint pain is the most common manifestation of HH. Other manifestations include fatigue, lack of energy, irritability, depression, loss of body hair, abdominal pain, loss of sex drive, and heart problems. Early diagnosis and treatment are critical to a positive outcome in HH. If the disease is not detected early and treated before the accumulation of iron in the body tissues, serious disorders such as arthritis, liver disease, pancreatic disease, heart complications, impotence, bronzing of the skin, and other problems can arise.

Hemochromatosis is one of the most underdiagnosed disorders. Certain blood tests can determine whether iron stores in the body are higher than normal. The transferring saturation test (TS) can calculate how much iron is bound to the protein that carries iron in the blood. The serum ferritin test shows the level of iron in the liver. If HH is suspected, a special blood test to detect the *HFE* mutation can be ordered as a definitive diagnosis. A liver biopsy is sometimes undertaken to determine how much damage the liver has sustained (see Table 77-6).

Outcome Management

Treatment is simple, inexpensive, and safe. The major goal of treatment is to rid the body of excess iron, which is accomplished with phlebotomy. Depending on the severity of iron overload, 500 ml of blood can be drawn each week for up to 2 or 3 years until iron levels return to normal limits. Then maintenance phlebotomy, usually once every 2 to 4 months for life, is initiated. Clients with HH should not take iron supplements, and dietary intake of iron may be limited. Those with liver damage should avoid alcoholic beverages. If tissue damage has occurred, specialists in the organ system involved usually treat the resulting organ system complications.

DISORDERS AFFECTING WHITE BLOOD CELLS

White blood cells (WBCs), also called *leukocytes,* are divided into two groups:

- *Granulocytes* (polymorphonuclear leukocytes)
- *Agranulocytes* (mononuclear cells)

Granulocytes, in turn, are divided into three groups: (1) neutrophils, (2) basophils, and (3) eosinophils. The names denote affinity for the dyes used in staining. Agranulocytes include lymphocytes (B and T) and monocytes.

Plasmacytes (plasma cells) are derived from B lymphocytes. Plasmacytes are formed within the bone marrow and lymph nodes and are active in producing immunoglobulins (antibodies). Leukemia and lymphoma are discussed in Chapter 81.

AGRANULOCYTOSIS

Agranulocytosis (granulocytopenia, malignant neutropenia) is an acute, potentially fatal blood dyscrasia characterized by profound *neutropenia* (a reduced number of circulating neutrophils). Because neutrophils make up roughly 93% of all granulocytes, the terms *neutropenia* and *agranulocytosis* are often used interchangeably. This condition is also known as *Schultz's disease.*

Etiology and Risk Factors

Agranulocytosis is a fairly rare condition. For unknown reasons, females are much more susceptible to this condition than males, although even among females, agranulocytosis is relatively rare.

Agranulocytosis results from either inadequate neutrophil production or excessive destruction of neutrophils, The most common cause of agranulocytosis is drug or chemical toxicity or hypersensitivity. Any drug or chemical that leads to aplasia can also cause agranu-

locytosis. More than 75 drugs have been associated with development of agranulocytosis. Agents that also produce neutropenia, when given in sufficiently large does over time, include many cancer chemotherapeutic agents, ionizing radiation, and benzene. Agents that frequently produce neutropenia (usually only in clients sensitive to the drug) include tranquilizers (phenothiazine, chlorpromazine), antithyroid agents (thiouracil, propylthiouracil), anticonvulsants (phenytoin), antibiotics (chloramphenicol, sulfonamides), and analgesics (aminopyrine, phenylbutazone). Some of these agents (including valproic acid, carbamazepine, and beta-lactam antibiotics) inhibit myelopoiesis, whereas others induce the formation of antibodies that destroy granulocytes (antithyroid drugs, gold aminopyrine).

Additional causes include (1) anemias related to diminished erythropoiesis (aplastic and megaloblastic anemias); (2) certain diseases such as uremia, tuberculosis, typhoid fever, malaria, yellow fever, EBV, hepatitis B, CMV, and influenza; (3) ionizing radiation exposure; (4) autoimmune diseases such as lupus erythematosus and rheumatoid arthritis; and (5) genetic aberrations, which may be suspected if a family history of recurrent infections beginning in childhood exists.

Pathophysiology

The exact mechanisms of neutropenia are not clearly understood. Bone marrow and the peripheral blood are the organ systems most affected in neutropenia. Neutrophils are the first blood cells to respond to an injury and constitute a swift and powerful defense against invading microorganisms through normal surveillance and phagocytosis. Failure to produce adequate numbers of neutrophils leads to a greater susceptibility to bacterial invasion, especially when the absolute neutrophil count (ANC) drops below 500/mm^3. In profound neutropenia (<100/mm^3), infection occurs in nearly 100% of cases.

Clinical Manifestations

The manifestations of agranulocytosis are a result of neutropenia. Typically the onset of this acute disease is rapid. For the first 2 or 3 days, severe fatigue and weakness occur, followed by a sore throat, ulcerations of the pharyngeal and buccal mucosa, dysphagia, high fever, weak and rapid pulse, and severe chills. The mucous membranes of the throat and mouth are particularly vulnerable. Without prompt antibiotic treatment, the disorder usually causes septicemia and death within a week.

The diagnosis of agranulocytosis rests on the following:

- Leukopenia, evidenced by WBC counts of 500 to 3000/mm^3 with extreme reduction in polymorphonuclear cells (0 to 2%)
- Bone marrow examination revealing an absence of granulocytes, a maturational arrest of young developing cells, or an increased number of myeloid pre-

cursors (signifying peripheral granulocyte destruction)
- Cultures of urine, blood, and ulcerative lesions in the throat and mouth that are positive for bacteria, usually gram-positive cocci (anaerobic and fungal infections are also frequently seen)
- A test for antineutrophil antibodies
- A history of exposure to an offending agent

Outcome Management

Treatment of clients with agranulocytosis involves eliminating potentially toxic agents that may be responsible for marrow suppression. Agranulocytosis caused by toxic substances is usually reversed within 2 to 3 weeks after their elimination. An allogenic BMT may be required for survival if agranulocytosis is not reversed when the cause is removed.

Surveillance cultures of blood, throat, sputum, urine, and stool should be taken at frequent intervals to monitor the status of infections. Broad-spectrum antibiotics are usually administered until the offending organism is identified and appropriate antibiotic therapy, along with rehydration, is initiated to treat the infection. Control of oral and gingival pain is performed with saline rinses and local anesthetic gels and gargles. Diet needs include soft or liquid foods until mouth and gum sores are diminished. Also all raw foods should be thoroughly cooked to avoid bacteria commonly found on these items.

Treatment of agranulocytosis includes various *colony-stimulating factors*, such as granulocyte colony-stimulating factor (G-CSF), granulocyte macrophage colony-stimulating factor (GM-CSF), and erythropoietin (EPO). These factors are given after the offending agent has been eliminated. Recent use of the recombinant neutrophil cytokine filgrastim (Neupogen) is showing good results. If given before a serious infection sets in, the duration of the infection is shortened and recovery hastened. Granulocyte transfusions are currently in disfavor because of the many associated complications.

MULTIPLE MYELOMA

Multiple myeloma is a malignancy of the plasma B cell characterized by infiltration of the cells into the bone marrow, which leads to destruction of other marrow cells, destruction of the bone cortex, and the secretion by the cells of the monoclonal paraprotein (Bence-Jones).

Etiology and Risk Factors

The etiology of multiple myeloma is a neoplastic proliferation of the plasma B cells. Risk factors include an increased incidence in some families, ionizing radiation, and occupational chemical exposures. The incidence rate is 4 per 100,000 people. Men are affected twice as often as women and blacks twice as often as whites. It usually develops after the age of 40 and peaks in the sixth decade. It accounts for 1% of all malignancies and 10% of hematologic malignancies.

Pathophysiology

Multiple myeloma is characterized by an abnormal proliferation of plasma B cells. These cells infiltrate the bone marrow and produce abnormal and excessive amounts of immunoglobulin *(myeloma protein)*. Accumulation of these cells in the marrow disrupts RBC, leukocyte, and platelet production, which lead to anemia, increased vulnerability to infection, and bleeding tendencies, respectively. In addition abnormal and excessive amounts of cytokine are produced, which plays an important role in bone destruction (lytic lesions and osteoporosis). Cell destruction leads to hypercalcemia, which can cause renal problems and failure (polyuria, hyperuricemia), GI problems (nausea, anorexia), and neurologic manifestations (confusion). Further complications include hematopoietic suppression, immunosuppression, chronic infections, proteinuria, and soft tissue masses.

Clinical Manifestations

Once manifestations appear, they typically involve the skeletal system, particularly the pelvis, spine, and ribs. The most common presenting complaint is bone pain (70%). The most common cause of the pain is pathologic fractures and bone lesions, which occur in 93% of clients over the course of the illness. Diffuse osteoporosis is common and manifests as multiple osteolytic lesions of the skull, sternum, rib cage, and spine (10% to 20% have spinal cord compression). Thirty percent of clients present with manifestations of hypercalcemia (confusion, somnolence, bone pain, constipation, nausea, and thirst); renal stones may be seen with this condition. Hyperuricemia is usually present and manifests as renal impairment or renal failure attributable to renal tubule obstruction and interstitial nephritis. Infections resulting from leukopenia, hyperviscosity caused by the high volume of monoclonal proteins, bleeding attributable to thrombocytopenia, and carpal tunnel syndrome may also be present.

Diagnosis of multiple myeloma rests on radiographic studies, bone marrow biopsy, and blood and urine examination. Radiographic studies reveal diffuse lesions in the bone, widespread demineralization, and osteoporosis. The CBC shows anemia, leucopenia, and thrombocytopenia. The bone marrow contains large numbers of immature plasma cells, which usually constitute 5% of the bone marrow cell population. Because of the abnormal number of plasma cells producing immunoglobulins, peripheral blood samples sent for plasma electrophoresis reveal a large amount of abnormal immunoglobulins. Another diagnostic manifestation of multiple myeloma is the appearance of Bence-Jones paraprotein in a 24-hour urine. A beta-2 microglobulin test is an important test because it is an overall marker of the total body tumor burden and (along with the level of renal damage) is a strong prognosticator of outcome. Median survival is 3 years.

Outcome Management

Currently no cure for multiple myeloma exists. Management is aimed at early recognition and treatment of complications of the disease. Clients may require hospitalization for pain management and treatment of bone-related complications. Not all clients with multiple myeloma should be treated initially. Clients who are asymptomatic are often carefully monitored until the disease progresses and then are treated with chemotherapy.

■ Medical Management

Suppress the Bone Marrow. If overt manifestations are present, chemotherapy is the preferred initial treatment. Some controversy exists over which chemotherapy regimen is most effective. The most commonly used regimen is melphalan and prednisone (M and P) given orally for 4 to 7 days and repeated at 4- to 6-week intervals. It is well tolerated and has a 50% to 60% response rate. Other combinations of alkylating agents, such as melphalan cyclophosphamide carmustine (BCNU), and chlorambucil can also be effective. The VAD regimen of vincristine (Oncovin), doxorubicin (Adriamycin), and dexamethasone (Decadron) is used for clients who do not respond to alkylating agents and is well tolerated. Thalidomide has recently been shown to have positive results, with a 30% response rate. (Melphalan should not be used for clients who are candidates for transplantation). Leukocyte and platelet counts are monitored regularly and doses are adjusted until modest cytopenia occurs. Chemotherapy may continue for 1 to 2 years, but almost all cases recur when chemotherapy is discontinued. Interferon-alfa appears to be beneficial in prolonging the duration of remission.

Autologous bone marrow and peripheral blood stem cell transplantation in combination with high-dose chemotherapy has had a significantly higher response rate (80% versus 57%) and better 5-year event-free survival (28% versus 10%) than those treated with chemotherapy alone. Allogeneic transplant may be used but carries a much higher risk for complications.

Reduce Serum Calcium Levels. Corticosteroids and hydration are used to reduce serum calcium levels. A new group of corticosteroid agents now exists for treating hypercalcemia. The most effective agent to date is pamidronate sodium (Aredia); etidronate disodium (Didronel) or gallium nitrate (Ganite) are also effective. Medications such as furosemide (Lasix), steroids, and plicamycin, etidronate, gallium, or pamidronate are used to increase calcium excretion and to decrease calcium loss from bone. If the client

is able, encourage activity that places stress on the long bones to increase calcium absorption.

Administer IV fluids in amounts adequate to maintain an output of 1.5 to 2 L daily. Clients with multiple myeloma usually require about 3 L of fluid per day. The client needs sufficient fluid not only to dilute the calcium overload but also to prevent protein from precipitating in the renal tubules.

Treat Complications. Nursing care is focused primarily on management of the various complications caused by dissemination of the disease. Bone pain management can be obtained with palliative radiotherapy of localized myeloma lesions (appropriate skin care techniques must be used) and with NSAIDs, acetaminophen, or an acetaminophen-opioid combination.

Antiemetics may be required for relief of nausea and vomiting. Small, frequent feedings may be better tolerated, and stool softeners may be routinely required. Closely monitor intake, output, and blood studies to determine the effectiveness of treatment. Weigh the client daily so that any significant loss can be noted and corrected. Measure the client's calcium level at regular intervals (outpatient) for assessment of the development of hypercalcemia.

Because of skeletal complications, care should be taken when moving the client. Closely monitor the client's mental status. If disorientation or confusion occurs, remove sharp objects and other potentially hazardous items from the environment. The side rails should be raised, and light restraints may be required.

Teach the client and family about the manifestations of hypercalcemia and instruct them to report any manifestations immediately to the physician. Instruct family members or significant others on how to institute safety measures to prevent falls and injuries. The client may need some assistive devices at home, such as a toilet riser and handhold bars in the bathroom. Counseling may be needed for the client and family to deal with the eventual fatal outcome of multiple myeloma.

INFECTIOUS MONONUCLEOSIS

Infectious mononucleosis is an acute disorder that is self-limiting and usually is benign. It is also known as the *glandular disease* or the *kissing disease*.

Etiology and Risk Factors

The cause of 85% of infectious mononucleosis-like cases is the EBV, a herpes virus. The mode of transmission is through the saliva during close contact such as kissing. The epithelial cells of the oropharynx, nasopharynx, and salivary glands are infected first before spreading to the lymphoid tissue via infected B lymphocytes. It is characterized by painful enlargement of the lymph nodes, numerous large lymphoblasts, lymphocytosis, sore throat, and fever. CMV, adenovirus, and *Toxoplasma gondii* cause similar clinical manifestations.

Primarily a disease of the young, it usually strikes children between the ages of 3 and 5 years and young adults between the ages of 15 and 25 years. The greatest incidence occurs among college students, medical students, and nurses.

Clinical Manifestations

The onset of infectious mononucleosis follows an incubation period of 2 to 6 weeks. Before frank clinical manifestations occur, the person may experience fatigue, headaches, malaise, and myalgias. Subsequently, assessment reveals temperatures up to 39° C (102.2° F), pharyngitis, and lymphadenopathy that is more pronounced in the cervical regions. In 10% to 15% of affected people, a maculopapular rash develops that closely resembles the rash of rubella. Splenic enlargement causes left upper quadrant pain. In rare cases, liver involvement may develop into a hepatitis-like syndrome. When infectious mononucleosis is severe, two complications may develop: (1) splenic rupture resulting from the infiltration of the spleen by massive numbers of lymphocytes and (2) streptococcal pharyngitis (Vincent's angina) secondary to bacterial invasion of the throat.

The diagnosis of infectious mononucleosis is based on three criteria: (1) physical assessment, (2) laboratory tests, and (3) the tests specific for EBV antibodies (mono spot test and the Paul-Bunnel test). The WBC count usually ranges from 12,000 to 20,000/mm^3, of which 50% are lymphocytes and monocytes and 10% to 20% are large, atypical lymphoblasts. The *mono spot test* is also performed with a throat swab. It detects EBV antibodies and is positive in 50% of cases within the first week and 90% of cases in the fourth week. The Paul-Bunnel test is a more specific test and can detect antibodies after 1 week of infection. It is used if the mono spot test is negative.

Outcome Management

No specific intervention either mitigates or shortens the disease process. Because infectious mononucleosis must simply run its course, treatments are directed at control of manifestations. Bed rest is recommended until fever is resolved. NSAIDs are used to treat fever, headache, sore throat, and myalgias. Cool sponge baths and a large fluid intake help control fever. Warm saline throat irrigation may relieve the sore throat. Aspirin is avoided because of the risk of Reye's syndrome. Contact sports must be avoided to reduce the risk of splenic rupture. A 5-day course of corticosteroids has been used to reduce swelling and has been reported to decrease the severity and length of the illness.

Although complications sometimes develop, the prognosis for clients with infectious mononucleosis is generally excellent. The febrile phase of this disorder typically lasts 2 to 4 weeks. During the long convalescence, the client slowly regains strength and energy.

SPLENIC RUPTURE AND HYPERSPLENISM

Rupture of the spleen, complicated by severe hemorrhage, is the most frequent indication for splenectomy. Hypersplenism is the second most important indication for splenectomy.

Etiology and Risk Factors

Causes of splenic rupture include the following:
- Trauma (e.g., automobile accidents, bullet or knife wounds, severe blows to the spleen)
- Accidental tearing of the splenic capsule during surgery on neighboring organs
- Disease of the spleen that causes softening or damage (e.g., infectious mononucleosis and malaria)

In hypersplenism the spleen destroys, in excessive numbers, one of the blood cell types (i.e., erythrocytes, leukocytes, or platelets). Primary hypersplenism occurs in idiopathic thrombocytopenic purpura and congenital spherocytosis. Some etiologic factors associated with secondary hypersplenism include lymphomas (including Hodgkin's disease), leukemia, PV, acute infections (including infectious mononucleosis), chronic infections, malaria, syphilis, hemoglobinopathy, and cirrhosis of the liver.

Clinical Manifestations

Manifestations of hypersplenism include moderate to massive splenomegaly, anemia, leukopenia, or thrombocytopenia and a compensatory increase in the production of the affected cell line by the bone marrow. Overactivity of the spleen develops either as a primary condition of unknown origin or as a condition secondary to another disease.

Laboratory indications for splenectomy include granulocytopenia of less than 500/mm^3 and thrombocytopenia of less than 20,000/mm^3.

Outcome Management

Primary hypersplenism can be alleviated by splenectomy. Splenectomy is palliative only for clients with secondary hypersplenism because the surgery has little or no effect on the course of the primary illness. When the diagnosis is confirmed, it is important to teach the client to prevent complications associated with the specific cytopenia.

The spleen has an important role in the phagocytosis of circulating opsonized organisms. After splenectomy, young children are at high risk for fulminant infections caused by *Streptococcus pneumoniae, Haemophilus influenzae, Neisseria meningitidis,* and other encapsulated organisms. Continuous prophylactic antibiotics may be advisable during the early years or indefinitely. Adults are also at increased risk for infection, especially during the first 3 years after surgery. The splenectomized client should be advised to seek medical treatment at the earliest manifestations of infection.

The unique functions performed by the spleen are eventually taken over by other organs; however, loss of the spleen because of the cessation of function or splenectomy does require the client to be monitored for potentially serious complications. Nursing care of the client undergoing splenectomy is generally the same as that discussed in Chapter 16 for any client undergoing surgery.

lems underlying hemorrhagic (bleeding) disorders are as follows:

- Weak, damaged vessels that rupture easily or spontaneously
- Platelet deficiency (*thrombocytopenia*) due to hypoproliferation, excessive pooling of platelets in the spleen, or excessive platelet destruction

DISORDERS OF PLATELETS AND CLOTTING FACTORS

Disorders of hemostasis that affect platelets and clotting factors include (1) purpura and (2) coagulation disorders (Box 77-1). They are classified with the hemorrhagic disorders. (See the Terrorism Alert feature on Hemorrhagic Fever Viruses below for a discussion of viruses that result in hemorrhage.)

HEMORRHAGIC DISORDERS

Normal clot formation and lysis depend on (1) intact blood vessels, (2) an adequate number of functioning platelets, (3) sufficient amounts of the 12 clotting factors (I-XIII; VI is no longer used), and (4) a well-controlled fibrinolytic system. Consequently, the four basic prob-

---

BOX 77-1 *Classification of Disorders of Hemostasis*

Purpura
Vascular defect purpura
 Familial hemorrhagic telangiectasia
 Anaphylactoid purpura (allergic purpura)
 Toxic purpura
Platelet disorder purpura
 Idiopathic thrombocytopenic purpura
 Secondary thrombocytopenias

Coagulation Disorders
Hemophilia
Hypoprothrombinemia
Disseminated intravascular coagulation (DIC)

TERRORISM ALERT

Hemorrhagic Fever Viruses

Historically, hemorrhagic fever viruses (HFVs) refer to a clinical illness associated with fever and a bleeding disorder caused by a virus belonging to one of four distinct families: Filoviridae, Arenaviridae, Bunyaviridae, and Flaviviridae. Ebola and Marburg are in the Filoviridae family; Lassa and New World Arenaviridae are in the Arenaviridae family; Rift Valley fever is in the Bunyaviridae family; and Dengue, Omsk hemorrhagic fever, Kyasanur Forest Disease, and yellow fever are in the Flaviviridae family.

The HFVs are transmitted to humans via contact with infected animal reservoirs or arthropod vectors, although the reservoirs and vectors for Marburg and Ebola viruses are unknown. The Working Group on Civilian Biodefense previously established nine features that characterize biologic agents that pose serious risks if used as biologic weapons against civilian populations. Several HFVs exhibit a number of these features and pose serious risk as biologic weapons, including Ebola and Marburg viruses, Lassa fever and New World arenaviruses, Rift Valley fever, yellow fever, Omsk hemorrhage fever, and Kyasanur Forest disease. These viruses can be spread through unannounced aerosol attacks. The overall incubation period is 2 to 21 days.

A variety of clinical manifestations follow infection with HFVs, including fever, headache, hypotension, abdominal pain, diarrhea, myalgias, skin rash, encephalitis, and eventually manifestations of progressive hemorrhaging such as conjunctival hem-

orrhage, petechiae, hematuria, hematemesis, and melena. DIC and circulatory shock may ensue. Therefore in the event of a bioterrorist attack with one of these agents, infected clients may have a variety of clinical presentations, complicating early detection and management.

The mainstay of treatment of HFV is supportive, with careful maintenance of fluid and electrolyte balance, circulatory volume, and blood pressure. Vasopressor support is with hemodynamic monitoring as well as mechanical ventilation and renal dialysis. IM injections, aspirin, NSAIDs, and anticoagulant therapies are contraindicated. Steroids are not indicated. No antiviral drugs have been approved by the U.S. FDA for treatment of HFVs. Ribavirin (used for treatment of chronic hepatitis C) has some in vitro and in vivo activity against Arenaviridae and Bunyaviridae but no utility against Filoviridae or Flaviviridae.

Protective measures against nosocomial transmission of HFVs include double gloves, impermeable gowns, strict hand hygiene, N-95 masks or powered air-purifying respirators, a negative isolation room with 6 to 12 air changes per hour, leg and shoe coverings, face shields, goggles for eye protection, restricted access of nonessential staff and visitors, environmental disinfection with 1:100 dilution of household bleach, and placing all clients with HFVs in the same part of the hospital to minimize exposures to other clients and health care workers.

Data from Borio, L, et al. (2002). Hemorrhagic fever viruses as biological weapons: Medical and public health management. *Journal of the American Medical Association, 287*(18), 2391-2405.

- Deficiency or total lack of one of the clotting factors
- Excessive or insufficient fibrinolysis

The diagnosis of a hemorrhagic disorder is based on a complete health and family history, physical examination, and laboratory tests for platelet and clotting defects. The history usually offers numerous clues to the type of bleeding problem and its cause. *Petechiae* (tiny hemorrhagic spots caused by intradermal or submucosal bleeding) are usually present in vascular and thrombocytopenic purpuras. The presence of *ecchymoses* (large, blotchy subcutaneous hemorrhagic areas), *hematomas* (subdermal hemorrhage), and *hemarthrosis* (blood within the joints) points to *hemophilia*; however, ecchymoses may develop in any hemorrhagic disorder. Clients who hemorrhage severely from several areas during childbirth or a major surgical procedure may have a fibrinogen deficiency. In addition to any evidence of bleeding, search for manifestations of hepatic cirrhosis (e.g., hepatomegaly, jaundice) and splenomegaly. Laboratory studies provide the most crucial evidence for pinpointing the type and cause of a bleeding disorder.

Clients with hemorrhagic disorders need to understand (1) why they are at risk for bleeding, (2) the manifestations of bleeding, and (3) preventive measures to avoid bleeding. Those who can be managed by home health care should be referred to appropriate health care agencies. Clients with bleeding disorders should carry an identification card at all times that indicates their diagnosis, name of their physician or health care agency, and blood type.

IDIOPATHIC THROMBOCYTOPENIC PURPURA

Idiopathic thrombocytopenic purpura is the most common thrombocytopenic disorder. It is a hemorrhagic autoimmune disease that results in the destruction of platelets.

Etiology and Risk Factors

Idiopathic thrombocytopenic purpura is an acquired disorder in which circulating platelets are destroyed because of autoantibodies that bind with antigens on the platelet membrane. Although the platelets perform normally in the bloodstream, they are recognized as foreign and are destroyed by the macrophages when they reach the spleen and liver. The decrease in the number of platelets results in bruising and spontaneous bleeding into the skin and mucous membranes (purpura). Platelets normally survive 8 to 10 days within the circulation; with ITP, however, platelet survival is as brief as 1 to 3 days or less. ITP may be acute or chronic; in most cases, the course is one of remissions and exacerbations that, if untreated, may continue for years.

Clinical Manifestations

Clinical manifestations include petechiae, ecchymosis, epistaxis, bleeding from the gums, and easy bruising.

Women may have extremely heavy menses or bleeding between periods.

Diagnostic findings that confirm the presence of ITP include the following:
- A platelet count below 100,000/mm^3
- Prolonged bleeding time with normal coagulation time (all coagulation factors are present and normal)
- Increased capillary fragility as demonstrated by the tourniquet test
- Positive platelet antibody screening
- Bone marrow aspirate containing normal or increased numbers of megakaryocytes

Complications of ITP include (1) spontaneous cerebral hemorrhage, which proves fatal in 1% to 5% of clients with ITP; (2) severe hemorrhages from the nose, GI tract, and urinary system; (3) bleeding into the diaphragm, which can result in pulmonary complications; and (4) nerve pain, extremity anesthesia, or paralysis resulting from the pressure of hematomas on nerves or brain tissues.

Outcome Management

Idiopathic thrombocytopenic purpura is treated with high-dose corticosteroids to inhibit the macrophage ingestion of the antibody-coated platelets. Plasmapheresis is sometimes used as short-term therapy until the steroid therapy takes effect. If the client is actively bleeding or requires surgery, IV gamma globulin can be used to increase the platelet count.

If the client does not have a sustained remission, splenectomy may be needed (see discussion earlier in this chapter). In 60% to 80% of cases, removal of the spleen results in complete and permanent remission. Danazol (Danocrine) has been used with success in some clients. Immunosuppressive therapy used in refractory cases includes vincristine, vinblastine (Velban), azathioprine (Imuran), and cyclophosphamide.

Nursing care of clients at high risk for bleeding is discussed in Chapter 81.

COAGULATION DISORDERS

Coagulation disorders stem from a defect in the clotting mechanisms. One or more of the clotting factors (I-XIII) is depleted or absent. The important coagulation disorders discussed here are (1) hypoprothrombinemia, (2) DIC, and (3) the hemophilias. See Figure U17-6 for an explanation of the coagulation cascade.

HYPOPROTHROMBINEMIA

Hypoprothrombinemia is a congenital or acquired deficiency of the clotting factor II (prothrombin), a protein produced in the liver and normally found in the blood.

Etiology and Risk Factors

Hypoprothrombinemia may develop from a vitamin K deficiency, a severe liver disorder, or from an overdose of anticoagulants (aspirin, coumarin, or coumarin-derivatives such as warfarin) that antagonizes the action of vitamin K. Dicumarol is an effective anticoagulant, interfering with vitamin K in prothrombin synthesis. In excessive doses, prothrombin time (PT) is prolonged. If the PT is too long, the danger of bleeding or spontaneous hemorrhage increases.

Vitamin K deficiency is seen in newborns who arrive with a limited supply and a largely sterile digestive tract. It is also seen in clients with GI tract disorders that interfere with the absorption of vitamin K such as (1) malabsorption syndrome and jaundice due to bile duct obstruction; (2) liver damage so extensive that liver cells cannot produce bile or synthesize prothrombin; and (3) prolonged sulfonamide or antibiotic administration that sterilizes the bowel, thereby halting vitamin K manufactured by GI tract bacteria.

Pathophysiology

For prothrombin synthesis to take place, vitamin K (a fat-soluble vitamin) must be present in the liver to act as a catalyst. Bacteria in the small intestine synthesize vitamin K, but it can also be supplemented through the diet. Currently no standard dietary daily allowance for this vitamin has been established. Because vitamin K is fat soluble, it depends on the presence of bile for absorption. Once absorbed, vitamin K catalyzes prothrombin synthesis within the liver cells.

Clinical Manifestations

The major manifestations of hypoprothrombinemia are ecchymosis after minimal trauma, epistaxis, postoperative hemorrhage from the incision, hematuria, GI tract bleeding, and prolonged bleeding from a venipuncture. The outstanding laboratory finding is a prolonged PT.

Outcome Management

Treatment of hypoprothrombinemia is aimed at providing prothrombin and addressing the underlying cause. The infusion of fresh frozen plasma may be given to boost the level of prothrombin. Vitamin K deficiency resulting from malabsorption is corrected through IM or IV administration of vitamin K, such as phytonadione (AquaMEPHYTON) or menadione (Synkayvite). If overdosage with a coumarin anticoagulant is the underlying problem, anticoagulant therapy is stopped. To normalize the PT, phytonadione is administered orally for minor bleeding problems or IV for hemorrhage. Finally, if prothrombin deficiency results from liver disease, concentrates of prothrombin or of prothrombin and factors VII, IX, and X may be transfused.

DISSEMINATED INTRAVASCULAR COAGULATION

Disseminated intravascular coagulation is a complex syndrome of activated coagulation that results in bleeding and thrombosis. It is basically a loss of balance between the clotting and lysing systems in the body caused by the simultaneous presence of thrombin and plasmin. Too much thrombin tips the balance toward the prothrombic state, resulting in thrombosis; too much plasmin triggers excessive clot lysis (fibrinolysis), in which clotting factors are consumed to such an extent that generalized bleeding occurs. This concept is referred to as consumptive coagulopathy. In DIC these seemingly contradictory states of excessive thrombosis and excessive lysis occur simultaneously.

Etiology and Risk Factors

The causes of DIC are many. Four categories of causative factors are (1) infection, (2) introduction of tissue coagulation factors into the circulation, (3) damage to vascular endothelium, and (4) stagnant blood flow. Infection is the leading cause (e.g., gram-negative septicemia, typhoid fever, Rocky Mountain spotted fever, viremia, parasites). Conditions that may lead to DIC are listed in Box 77-2.

Pathophysiology

Excessive clotting can be precipitated through extrinsic or intrinsic coagulation pathways (Figure U17-6). The extrinsic pathway is a response to massive tissue damage (e.g., burns or trauma); the intrinsic pathway is a response to damaged blood vessels (endothelium). Both release thromboplastic substances that activate thrombin, which in turn activates fibrinogen. This results in deposition of fibrin throughout the microcirculation. The formation of fibrin is triggered by increased production of thrombin, the suppression of anticoagulation mechanisms, and delayed removal of fibrin due to impaired fibrinolysis).

Platelet aggregation or adhesiveness is increased enabling fibrin clots and microthrombi to form in the brain, kidneys, heart, and other organs; microinfarcts and tissue necrosis ensue. RBCs become trapped in the fibrin strands and are destroyed (hemolysis). The resultant sluggish circulation of blood reduces the flow of nutrients and oxygen to the cells. Platelets, prothrombin, and other clotting factors are consumed in the process, which compromises coagulation and predisposes to bleeding.

Excessive clotting activates the fibrinolytic mechanism, which causes the production of fibrin degradation products. Fibrin degradation products act to inhibit platelet clotting functions, which causes further bleeding. Ultimately, with lysis of clots and depletion of clotting factors, the blood loses its ability to clot (see the Concept Map feature on Understanding DIC and Its Treatment on p. 2309).

Clinical Manifestations

Clinically, DIC is termed acute, subacute, or chronic. *Acute* DIC usually presents as a hemorrhagic condition associated with excess plasmin formation. The onset is usually within days to hours after an initial assault to the

BOX 77-2	*Conditions That May Precipitate Disseminated Intravascular Coagulation*

Shock
Cirrhosis
Purpura fulminans
Glomerulonephritis
Acute fulminant hepatitis
Acute bacterial and viral infections (septicemia)
Conditions that may cause the release of platelet factor III:
• Fat emboli
• Snakebites

Hemolytic processes caused by:
• Infection
• Transfusion reactions
• Immunologic disorders

Tissue damage caused by:
• Trauma
• Heatstroke
• Extensive burns
• Transplant rejections
• Surgery—particularly if extracorporeal circulation was used
• Glomerulonephritis
• Acute anoxia
• Prosthetic devices

Conditions that may cause the release of thromboplastin from tissues:
• Neoplastic growths
  • Adenocarcinomas
  • Acute leukemias
  • Prostatic cancer
  • Bronchogenic cancer
  • Giant cavernous hemangioma
• Obstetric conditions
  • Abruptio placentae (placental abruption)
  • Retained dead fetus
  • Amniotic fluid embolism
  • Septic abortion
  • Eclampsia

TABLE 77-11	*Laboratory Tests Used in Diagnosis of Disseminated Intravascular Coagulation*

Test	Results
Prothrombin time	Prolonged (75%)
Partial thromboplastin time	Usually prolonged
Thrombin time	Usually prolonged
Fibrinogen level	Usually depressed
Platelet count	Usually depressed
Fibrin degradation products	Elevated (75%-100%)
D-Dimer (cross-linked fibrin fragments)*	Positive
Protamine sulfate test	Strongly positive
Antithrombin III	Reduced (90%)
Factor assays II, V, VII, VIII, X, XIII	Reduced

*Important diagnostic test. Identifies presence of both thrombin and plasmin. More reliable than fibrin split products (FSP).

hemorrhage during surgery or childbirth; (4) excessive bleeding from gums and the nose; (5) intracerebral and GI bleeding; (6) renal hematuria; (7) tachycardia and hypotension; and (8) dyspnea, hemoptysis, and respiratory congestion. Manifestations of microvascular thrombosis include oliguria and acute renal failure; pulmonary emboli and acute respiratory distress; delirium, convulsions and coma; hemorrhagic necrosis, and ischemia of the peripheral tissue (acral cyanosis) with the risk of gangrene.

The prognosis for clients with DIC varies. Associated mortality is quite high, primarily because of the underlying illness. Hemorrhage, organ damage (especially adult [acute] respiratory distress syndrome [ARDS]), or even death may occur within a matter of hours if associated with gram-negative sepsis. In severe cases the mortality rate reaches 80%. Morbidity is usually due to vascular thrombosis, acral cyanosis, and limb ischemia. Some cases are self-limiting.

Diagnostic tests include screening assays and confirmatory assays. Findings of the screening assays show prolonged PT and activated partial thromboplastin time (PTT), a very low (and falling) platelet count (<100,000/mm³), reduced fibrinogen, and prolonged clotting times. Confirmatory tests such as fibrinogen degradation product (FDP), D-dimer, and factor assays identify the presence of products of DIC pathology. Table 77-11 lists the laboratory tests used in the diagnosis of DIC.

Outcome Management
■ Medical Management
The treatment of DIC is controversial, and efforts are under way to determine the most suitable regimen for managing this syndrome. Goals of treatment include (1) identification and correction of the precipitating cause or

body system. *Subacute* DIC may not be apparent initially but may become fulminant as the clinical course progresses. *Chronic* cases of DIC are typically seen in clients with cancer or in women carrying a dead fetus. Subacute and chronic cases usually present as thrombosis attributable to excessive formation of thrombin.

Manifestations of acute DIC (hemorrhagic) include (1) purpura, petechiae, and ecchymoses on the skin, mucous membranes, heart lining, and lungs; (2) prolonged bleeding from venipuncture; (3) severe, uncontrolled

CONCEPT MAP

Understanding DIC and Its Treatment

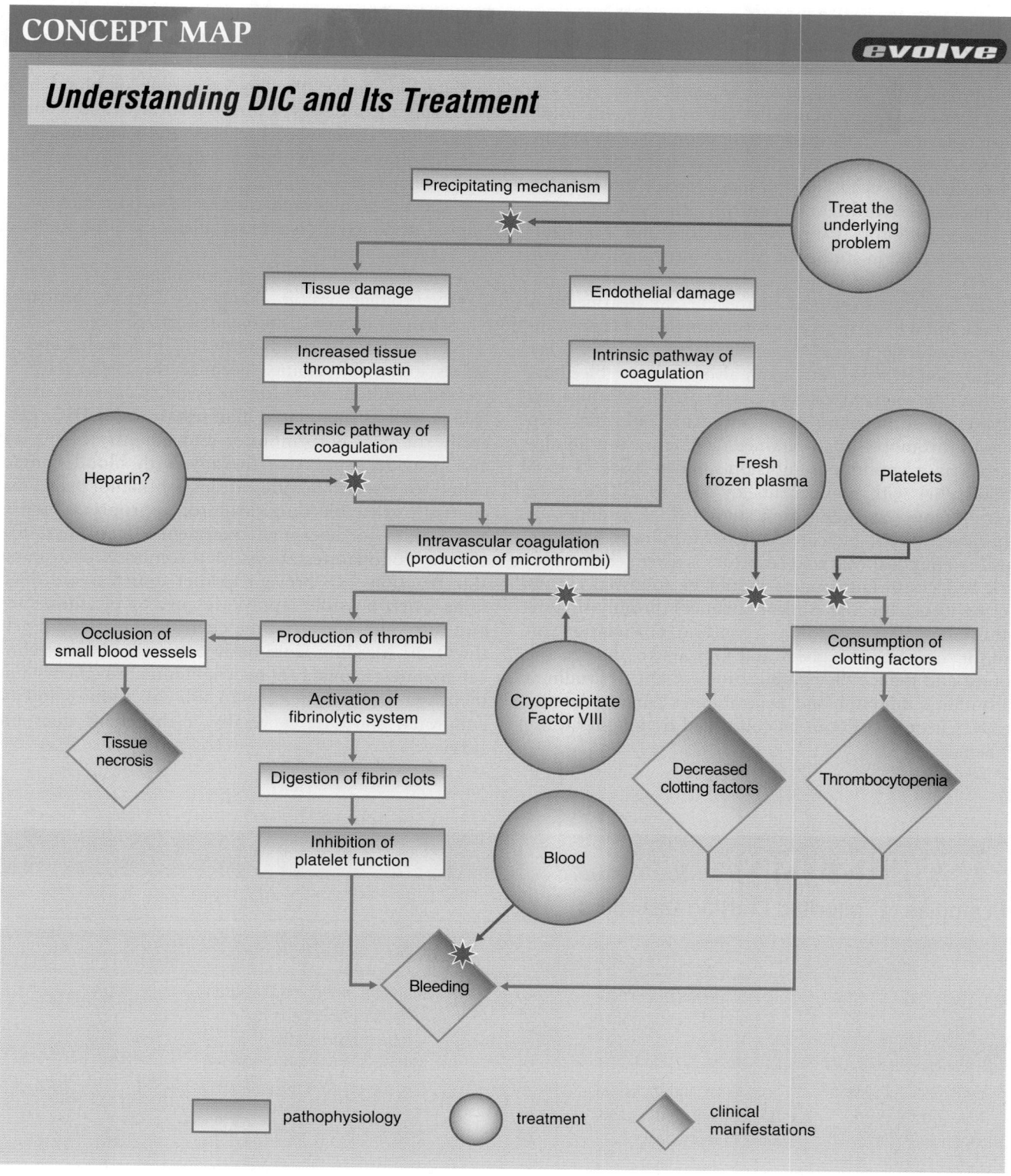

problem (e.g., infection, delivery of a fetus, surgery, or irradiation for cancer); (2) reinstitution of hemostasis by replacing missing blood components; and (3) provision of supportive therapy to control manifestations of hemorrhage and thrombosis.

Appropriate treatment is determined when (and if) the underlying cause is identified; for instance, antibiotic

therapy to control infections or surgery to control severe obstetric complications. In the meantime, manifestations of hemorrhage and thrombosis must be addressed. Replacement of missing blood components is an important first step, particularly if bleeding is present. Washed packed RBCs can be administered to replace blood volume lost through hemorrhage without introducing anticoagulant substances, The specific blood product to be transfused is determined by the deficiency. Platelets are given for thrombocytopenia. If fibrinogen levels are below 100 mg/dl, transfusions of cryoprecipitate is given until levels can be maintained at 100 to 150 mg/dl. Fresh frozen plasma is transfused if coagulation factors are decreased. Concerns that this may reaccelerate coagulation are unfounded because the plasma protease inhibitors in the plasma are sufficient to control such a reaction. The protease inhibitors gabexate and aprotinin (Trasylol) have been used in studies to control bleeding with some success.

The most controversial of the current treatments is the use of IV heparin to control thrombosis. Heparin inhibits the production of thrombin, factor Xa, and other coagulation enzymes, but it can also accelerate bleeding. It should be reserved for clients with digital ischemia and acral cyanosis, purpura fulminans, acute leukemia, deep venous thrombosis, or a retained dead fetus. It is administered as a continuous infusion at low doses (3 to 5 units/kg/hr) with adjustments by 100 to 200 units/hr every 4 hours as monitoring studies (FDP, D-dimer, or fibrinogen levels) indicate. If heparin induces bleeding, epsilon aminocaproic acid (Amicar) is given; cardiac, renal, and electrolyte studies should be followed closely during its use because Amicar enhances thrombosis. Antithrombin III (desirudin), a natural coagulation inhibitor, may also be given and appears to shorten the course and reduce the complications of DIC. Hirudin, a thrombotic inhibitor and neutralizer is currently under study. Chronic DIC can be controlled by long-term use of heparin.

■ Nursing Management

Assess all body systems for the effects of DIC, including the following:

- Integumentary bleeding or oozing of blood from venipuncture sites or mucosal surfaces and wounds, pallor, petechiae, ecchymoses, and hematomas
- Respiratory tachypnea, hemoptysis, orthopnea, and basilar rales
- Cardiovascular tachycardia and hypotension
- GI abdominal distention, guaiac-positive stools or gastric contents
- Genitourinary hematuria and oliguria
- Neurologic vision changes, dizziness, headache, changes in mental status, and irritability

Nursing care of clients with DIC is complex and requires extreme vigilance because the client must be treated simultaneously for the primary causative problem as well as the related manifestations of DIC. Generally the goal is to monitor and quantify blood loss and provide supportive therapy with blood components to resolve manifestations of hemorrhage and control further bleeding. Monitor appropriate laboratory values to determine treatment effectiveness and observe for manifestations of thrombosis or transfusion reactions. To prevent further injury, avoid injections when possible, apply pressure to bleeding sites, and turn and reposition the client frequently and gently. Overt bleeding from body orifices and other clinical manifestations can be frightening to clients and their significant others, who all will require intense emotional support, especially if the client does not survive.

GENETICS LINKS

Examples of Inherited Clotting Disorders

Disorder	Features	Inheritance	Metabolic/Gene Defect	Genetic Testing Available?
von Willebrand disease	Mucocutaneous bleeding; prolonged bleeding time	AD	Mutation in the von Willebrand factor (VWF) gene on chromosome 12	Yes
Hemophilia A (factor VIII deficiency; classic hemophilia)	Easy bruising and hemorrhage into joints and muscles due to deficient clotting ability	XR	Mutation in the factor VIII (F8) gene on chromosome X	Yes
Hemophilia B (factor IX deficiency; Christmas disease)	Similar to Hemophilia A	XR	Mutation in the factor IX (F9) gene on chromosome X	Yes
Hemophilia C (factor XI deficiency)	Mild to moderate bleeding; mucocutaneous bleeding	AR	Mutation in the factor XI (FXI) gene on chromosome 4; deficiency of plasma thromboplastin antecedent (PTA)	Yes

AD, Autosomal dominant; XR, X-linked recessive; AR, autosomal recessive.

HEMOPHILIA

Hemophilia is an X-linked genetic disorder that results in a deficiency of coagulation factors. Two major forms are hemophilia A (HA), the classic form, which is due to a deficiency of factor VIII, and hemophilia B (HB), also known as Christmas disease, which is due to a deficiency of factor IX. See the Genetic Links feature on Examples of Inherited Clotting Disorders on p. 2310.

Etiology and Risk Factors

Factor VIII and factor IX deficiencies result in an insufficient production of thrombin through the intrinsic pathway of the coagulation cascade, which creates a profound tendency for spontaneous bleeding. Both are usually found only in males. Factor VIII deficiency also may be caused by a congenitally acquired molecular defect in the FVIII binding domain of von Willebrand factor (vWF). FVIII circulates in the blood bound to vWF. This disorder, von Willebrand disease, is the most common congenital bleeding disorder and may affect both genders. A comparison of the three forms of hemophilia appears in the Table 77-12. Because HA makes up 80% of all hemophilia, the discussion of manifestations and treatment refers only to this form.

Hemophilia is classified as severe (<1% normal factor level), moderate (1% to 5% of normal factor level), or mild (5% to 40% of normal factor level). The prevalence of HA in the United States is 20.6 cases per 100,000 males, with 60% having severe disease; the HB rate is 5.3 cases per 100,000 males, with 40% having severe disease.

Clinical Manifestations

All manifestations are related to bleeding. Severe hemophilia often presents at circumcision or at the beginning of ambulation or primary dentition. The hallmark of this disorder is *hemarthrosis* (bleeding into the joints) in the knees, ankles, elbows, wrists, fingers, hips, and shoulders. Hemarthrosis is painful and leads to deterioration of the joints, which may become deformed and permanently crippled. Synovial hypertrophy, hemosiderin deposition, fibrosis, damage to the cartilage, and subchondral cyst formation are seen with this condition.

HA typically manifests in the following ways:
- Slow, persistent bleeding from cuts, scratches, and other minor traumas
- Delayed hemorrhage that follows minor injuries; bleeding may not start from a site until hours or even days after the traumatic event
- Severe hemorrhaging from the gums after dental extraction or even brushing the teeth with a hard toothbrush
- Severe, sometimes fatal, epistaxis after injury to the nose
- Overwhelming gastric hemorrhage, which may be linked to gastric disorders such as ulcers or gastritis
- Recurrent hematoma formation in the deep subcutaneous tissue in the intramuscular tissues (muscular atrophy sometimes results), and around the peripheral nerves causing compression which can result in severe pain, anesthesia of the innervated part, nerve damage, and paralysis
- Hematuria from genitourinary trauma
- Splenic rupture from falls or abdominal trauma
- Intracranial bleeding, which is the leading cause of hemorrhagic death

Life expectancy dramatically increased with the advent in the 1960s of antihemophilic factor (AHF) replacement therapy and prophylactic therapy with lyophilized concentrates that eliminate bleeding. Before this time, the life expectancy for clients with severe HA was 5 to 11 years; today it is 50 to 60 years. By 1983 more than 50% of clients were infected with HIV be-

TABLE 77-12	*Comparison of the Three Forms of Hemophilia*		
Form of Hemophilia	**Etiology**	**Transmission**	**Major Laboratory Findings**
Hemophilia A (classic hemophilia)	Inherited factor VIII (antihemophilic globulin) deficiency	Transmitted as sex-linked *recessive* trait; transmitted by females; occurs in males and, rarely, homozygous females	Coagulation time prolonged but bleeding time normal; factor VIII missing from plasma
Hemophilia B (Christmas disease)	Inherited factor IX (plasma thromboplastin component) deficiency	Transmitted as sex-linked *recessive* trait; transmitted by females; occurs in males and, rarely, homozygous females	Laboratory findings and symptoms same as in hemophilia A; factor IX missing
von Willebrand's disease	Inherited factor VIII deficiency and defective platelet dysfunction	Transmitted as autosomal *dominant* trait to both sexes; occurs in both males and females	Both coagulation time and bleeding time prolonged; low factor VIII levels; platelet adhesiveness decreased

cause of contamination of the blood supply; AIDS accounted for 55% of hemophiliac deaths. Mortality rates jumped from 0.4 per million population to 2.1. Fortunately, subsequent measures taken to ensure a safe supply of blood products has virtually eliminated this threat and greatly reduced the mortality rate in recent years. Intracranial hemorrhages currently account for about a third of HA-related deaths.

Platelet function, platelet count, bleeding time, and prothrombin time are normal. The activated partial thromboplastin time (aPTT) is prolonged. Quantitative assays for factor VIII determine the severity of the disease.

Outcome Management

The goals of care for clients with hemophilia are as follows:

- Stop topical bleeding as quickly as possible
- Supply the missing factor causing hemorrhage
- Prevent complications leading to and caused by bleeding

The nurse can control topical bleeding quickly by applying pressure or ice to the injured site, packing the area with fibrin foam, and applying topical hemostatic agents such as thrombin.

Primary factor replacement therapy should be initiated as ordered. This typically is the immediate transfusion of factor VIII (or IX) concentrate supplied as a lyophilized powder. One unit per kilogram of concentrate increases the plasma level of FVIII by 2%, with a reaction half-time of 8 to 12 hours. Because the procoagulant activity AHF disappears rapidly, clients need transfusions every 12 hours until bleeding stops. For mild hemorrhage, an FVIII level of 30% should be maintained; for major hemorrhage, the level should be maintained at 50%; life-threatening bleeds require a level of 80% to 90%. Plasma levels must be maintained at higher than 50% for a minimum of 7 to 10 days. Prophylactic administration of FVIII to a level 50% above normal is recommended in cases of minor injury, surgery, and dental extractions. Transfusion of packed RBCs or WBCs is used only to replace blood volume when there has been severe loss.

 With repeated transfusions and AHF therapy, some clients become sensitized to AHF and develop alloantibody inhibitors that can neutralize FVIII and complicate replacement therapy. These antibodies are seen in about 30% of clients with severe cases by the age of 10. In case of major and life-threatening hemorrhages, these clients are treated with massive doses of factor VIII from animal sources (bovine and porcine), inactivated prothrombin complex concentrates (Konyne 80, Proplex T), or activated prothrombin complex concentrates (Feiba VH Immuno, Autoplex T). Recent treatment with FVIIa for hemarthrosis has been effective for these clients. Clinicians are using various experimental

treatments such as immunosuppressive therapy to combat this problem.

Hemarthrosis may be controlled if the client receives AHF in the early stages of bleeding. Joint immobilization and local chilling (such as packing ice around the joint) may bring relief. If pain is severe, it may be necessary to aspirate blood from the joint. Once bleeding stops and swelling subsides, the client should perform active range-of-motion exercises without weight-bearing to prevent further complications such as deformity and muscle atrophy.

Prophylactic home infusion of AHF can greatly reduce bleeding episodes and related complications. Training programs with strict guidelines for this regimen have been developed. As a result, clients with hemophilia lose less time from work or school and need fewer visits to the emergency department.

Analgesics (acetaminophen, oxycodone, propoxyphene, pentazocine) and corticosteroids often reduce joint pain and swelling and the pain of chronic arthritis. Avoid all aspirin products. In mild hemophilia, the use of IV desmopressin may eliminate the need for AHF. Desmopressin acts by causing an increase in plasma factor VIII activity.

Although most clients with hemophilia are successfully maintained with home health care, they may be seen in the hospital during acute bleeding episodes or for unrelated treatments. If even a minor invasive procedure is planned, it is crucial to assess the factor VIII level and to administer a sufficient quantity of factor concentrate before the procedure. During routine medical examinations, these clients should be assessed for the frequency of bleeding episodes and the effectiveness of home therapy. Examine joints for manifestations of bleeding and related atrophy.

Teach the client and family to recognize early manifestations of bleeding and why it is critical to intervene with treatment immediately. Effective and prompt administration of factors to reduce the incidence of bleeding episodes and resultant complications is a priority. The client and family will need to learn IV infusion administration techniques to control the bleeding. Discuss situations that require medical consultation. Discuss the need to curtail physical activities such as contact sports, minor invasive procedures, falls, and cuts that may precipitate a bleeding episode. If a client has HIV seroconversion, arrange for a referral for appropriate care.

CONCLUSIONS

Hematologic diseases are complex disorders that require the nurse to understand the hematopoietic system. The nurse is often involved in the administration of blood and blood products for treatment of these various disorders. Many of the blood disorders are life-threatening; others are easily controlled with proper nutrition or regular medication.

Because blood and blood product transfusions are widely used in the treatment of hematologic disorders, it is vital that you understand these procedures, the implications of these procedures, and the proper techniques of administration so the client will receive safe and effective care.

THINKING CRITICALLY *evolve*

1. A 62-year-old client underwent a gastric resection for peptic ulcer disease 3 months ago at a hospital in another state. She comes to the nursing clinic complaining of shortness of breath and fatigue with minimal physical exertion. She currently takes ranitidine (Zantac). What assessments should you make now?
Factors to Consider. What is the significance of the history of gastric resection? How might this contribute to the client's lethargy? What might be causing the shortness of breath and fatigue? What laboratory results would be appropriate to evaluate? What teaching should you consider with this client?

2. A 40-year-old client has recently been told that she has multiple myeloma. She has been admitted to the oncology inpatient unit for initial evaluation and treatment. On her fourth day after admission, she becomes confused and difficult to arouse. Bowel sounds are diminished, and she begins to vomit. What priority assessment should you make now?
Factors to Consider. What might predispose the client to this change in her level of consciousness? What additional assessments would you need to make? What interventions should you anticipate at this time?

Discussions for these questions can be found on the website and the CD-ROM.

BIBLIOGRAPHY

1. Agaliotis, D. (2003). Hemophilia overview. *EMedicine.* Available: http://www.eMedicine.com/med/topic 3528.htm.
2. Alyea, E., & Anderson, K. (2000). Allogenic bone marrow transplantation in the treatment of multiple myeloma. *PPU Updates, 14,* 1-10.
3. Bakshi, S., Baynes, R., & Abella, E. (2003). Aplastic anemia. *EMedicine.* Available: http://www.eMedicine.com/med/topic 162. htm.
4. Ballas, S. (1999). Complications of sickle cell anemia in adults: Guidelines for effective management. *Cleveland Clinics Journal of Medicine, 66*(1), 48-58.
5. Besa, E., & Woermann, U. (2003). Polycythemia vera. *eMedicine.* Available: http://www.emedicine.com/med/topicXXX.htm.
6. Borio, L., et al. (2002). Hemorrhagic fever viruses as biological weapons: Medical and public health management. *Journal of the American Medical Association, 287*(18), 2391-2405.
7. Boyland, L., & Gleeson, C. (1999). Clinical management: The management of anemia. *European Journal of Palliative Care, 6*(5), 145-148.
8. Busch, M., Kleinman, S., & Nemo, G. (2003). Current and emerging infectious risks of blood transfusions. *Journal of the American Medical Association, 289*(8), 959-961.
9. Castro, O. (1999). Management of sickle cell disease: Recent advances and controversies. *British Journal of Haematology, 107*(1), 2-11.
10. Cella, D., & Bron, D. (1999). The effect of epoetin alfa on quality of life in anemia cancer patients. *Cancer Practice, 7*(4), 177-182.
11. Conrad, M. (2003). Anemia. *EMedicine.* Available: http://www.emedicine.com/med/topic 132.htm.cce.
12. Conrad, M. (2003). Iron deficiency anemia. *EMedicine.* Available: http://www.emedicine.com/med/topic 1188.htm.
13. Conrad, M. (2003). Pernicious anemia. *EMedicine.* Available: http://www.emedicine.com/med/topic132.htm.
14. Distenfeld, A., & Woermann, U. (2003). Sickle cell anemia. *EMedicine.* http://www.emedicine.com/med/topic 12126.htm.
15. Distenfeld, A. (2003). Agranulocytosis. *EMedicine.* Available: http://www.emedicine.com/med/topic 82.htm.
16. Gaines, K. (2003). Aminocaproic acid (Amicar): Potent antifibrolytic agent for treating hematuria. *Urologic Nursing, 23*(2), 156-158.
17. Gobel, B.H. (1999). Disseminated intravascular coagulation. *Seminars in Oncology Nursing, 15*(3), 174-182.
18. Gonzalez, G., & Eichner, E. (2003). Spherocytosis, hereditary. *EMedicine.* Available: http://www.emedicine.com/med/topic 82. htm.
19. Grethlein, S. (2003). Multiple myeloma. *EMedicine.* Available: http://www.emedicine.com/med/topic 1521.htm.
20. Hawkins, R. (1999). Disseminated intravascular coagulation. *Clinical Journal of Oncology Nursing, 3*(3), 127, 131.
21. Hebert, P., et al. (2003). Clinical outcomes following institution of the Canadian universal leukoreduction program for red blood cell transfusions. *Journal of the American Medical Association, 289*(15), 1941-1949.
22. Horowitz, M. (2000). Current status of allogenic bone marrow transplantation in acquired aplastic anemia. *Seminars of Hematology, 37*(1), 30-42.
23. Levi, M., & Cate, H.T. (1999). Disseminated intravascular coagulation. *New England Journal of Medicine, 341*(8), 586-592.
24. Miller, S., Sleeper, L., & Pegelow, C. (2000). Prediction of adverse outcomes in children with sickle cell disease. *New England Journal of Medicine, 342*(2), 83-89.
25. National Institute of Diabetes, Digestive, and Kidney Diseases. (2003). Hemochromatosis. National digestive diseases information clearinghouse. Available: http://www.niddk.nih.gov/health/digest/pubs/hemochrom/hemochromatosis.htm.
26. Overturf, G. (1999). Infections and immunizations of children with sickle cell disease. *Advances in Pediatric Infectious Disease, 14,* 191-218.

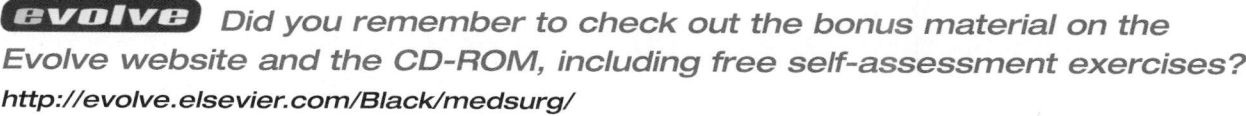

evolve *Did you remember to check out the bonus material on the Evolve website and the CD-ROM, including free self-assessment exercises?*
http://evolve.elsevier.com/Black/medsurg/

27. Quinn, C., & Buchanan, G. (1999). The acute chest syndrome of sickle cell disease. *Journal of Pediatrics, 135*(4), 416-422.

28. Rajkumar, S., et al. (2002). Current therapy for multiple myeloma. *Mayo Clinic Proceedings, 77,* 813-822.

29. Reed, W., & Vichinsky, E. (1999). Transfusion practice for patients with sickle cell disease. *Current Opinions in Hematology, 6*(6), 432-436.

 30. Rosenfeld, S., et al. (2003). Antithymocyte globulin and cyclosporine for severe aplastic anemia: Association between hematologic response and long-term outcome. *Journal of the American Medical Association, 289*(9), 1130-1135.

31. Schick, P. (2003). Hemolytic anemia. *eMedicine.* Available: http://www.emedicine.com/med/topic 979.htm.

32. Schick, P. (2003). Megaloblastic anemia. *eMedicine.* Available: http://www.emedicine.com/med/topic 1420.htm.

33. Schmaier, A. (2003). Disseminated intravascular coagulation. *eMedicine,* http://www.emedicine.com/med/topic 557.htm.

34. Steinberg, M., et al. (2003). Effect of hydroxyurea on mortality and morbidity in adult sickle cell anemia: Risks and benefits up to 9 years of treatment. *Journal of the American Medical Association, 289*(13), 1645-1651.

35. Stephan, F., et al. (1999). Thrombocytopenia in a surgical ICU. *Chest, 115*(5), 1363-1370.

36. Takeshita, K. (2003). Thalassemia beta. *EMedicine.* Available: http://www.emedicine.com/med/topic 2260.htm.

37. Weiner, D., & Brugnara, C. (2003). Hydroxyurea and sickle cell disease: A chance for every patient. *Journal of the American Medical Association, 289*(13), 1692-1695.

38. Worrall, L.M., Thompkins, C.A., & Rust, D.M. (1999). Recognizing and managing anemia. *Clinical Journal of Oncology Nursing, 3*(4), 153-160, 180-182.

Chapter 78

Management of Clients with Immune Disorders

Linda M. Scott

evolve

Web Enhancements

http://evolve.elsevier.com/Black/medsurg/

Bridge to Home Health Care
Managing Immunosuppression and Nutrition

Appendix C
Laboratory Values of Clinical Importance in Medical-Surgical Nursing

The immune system constitutes the body's defense system against invading foreign substances. A functioning immune system must protect the body from potential pathogens. An immune system that is malfunctioning predisposes an individual to the development of a wide variety of diseases ranging from severe infection to autoimmune disease and the resultant tissue injury. The Unit 17 Anatomy and Physiology Review describes the normally functioning immune system; this chapter looks at alterations in the immune system and how these changes affect the human organism.

HYPERSENSITIVITY DISORDERS

As health care providers, nurses deal with allergic conditions far more often than might be suspected. Allergic rhinitis, asthma, and dermatitis are a few examples of these immunologic diseases.

The tendency to develop allergies for which there is a genetic predisposition and that involve immunoglobulin E (IgE) antibody formation is known as *atopy*. The terms *atopic, allergic,* and *hypersensitive* are frequently used interchangeably. *Allergy* (or, more appropriately, hypersensitivity) describes the increased immune response to the presence of an allergen, also known as an *antigen*.

Between 20% and 30% of the population have allergies. We cannot predict who will have allergies; however, there is a higher incidence of allergies among children of allergic parents.

People must progress through a two-step process to become allergic. Step 1 starts with *sensitization*. Sensitization occurs when one develops IgE antibodies against a substance that is inhaled, ingested, or injected. Newly formed IgE antibodies stick to basophils and mast cells, which are found in the skin's mucosal surfaces and in the respiratory and gastrointestinal (GI) tracts. Hypersensitivity can be claimed only after IgE antibodies against a certain foreign substance have formed and are bound to the surface of tissue mast cells and circulating basophils.

Hypersensitivity does not produce any of the manifestations typically associated with allergic disease. It is not until step 2, *reexposure to the allergen*, that allergic manifestations such as sneezing, asthma, and anaphylaxis occur. Although the cellular events for all immediate allergic reactions tend to be similar, differences are found in the clinical sequelae that occur, based on the state of the individual's host defenses, the nature of the allergen, the concentration of the allergen, the route by which the allergen enters, the amount of allergen exposure received, and which organ is affected.

evolve *Be sure to check out the bonus material on the Evolve website and the CD-ROM, including free self-assessment exercises.*

http://evolve.elsevier.com/Black/medsurg/

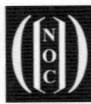

Nursing Outcomes Classification (NOC)
for Nursing Diagnoses—Clients with Immune Disorders

Health-Seeking Behaviors
  Health Belief: Perceived Resources
  Health-Promoting Behavior
  Health-Seeking Behavior
  Knowledge: Health Behaviors
  Knowledge: Health Promotion
  Knowledge: Health Resources
  Knowledge: Treatment Regimen
  Participation: Health Care Decisions
  Psychosocial Adjustment: Life Change

Risk Detection
  Self-Direction of Care
  Social Support
  Treatment Behavior: Illness or Injury
Latex Allergy Response
  Immune Hypersensitivity Control
  Symptom Severity
  Tissue Integrity: Skin and Mucous
    Membranes

Risk for Latex Allergy Response
  Immune Hypersensitivity Control
  Knowledge: Health Behaviors
  Risk Control
  Risk Detection
  Tissue Integrity: Skin and Mucous
    Membranes

Etiology and Risk Factors

Host Defenses

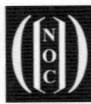 Some people are more susceptible to hypersensitivity than others for reasons that are unclear (see the Complementary and Alternative Therapy feature on Allergies, below). The increasing prevalence of allergic disease suggests that environmental factors acting either before or after birth contribute to the regulation of the development of Th_2 cells or their function. Th_2 cells play a triggering role in the activation and recruitment of IgE antibody–producing B cells, mast cells, and eosinophils, the cellular triad involved in allergy. The decrease in the number or reported childhood infectious diseases that has resulted from vast vaccination programs, antimicrobial therapy, and changing lifestyles are important influences on an individual's outcome in the Th response to an allergen. Specific IgE formation can be influenced by vital infections, especially those caused by cytomegalovirus (CMV) and mononucleosis. Factors such as air pollution, gender, age, and exposure to second-hand smoke can influence the manifestations of allergies.

Nature of the Allergen

Allergens are proteins that are capable of inducing IgE antibody, thus triggering an allergic response. Molecules that combine with proteins to produce antibodies are called *haptens*. Haptens, along with other environmental allergens, are carried on vectors that may become airborne (e.g., pollen, molds, dust particles, animal dander). Contact with these allergens causes sensitization and atopy and evokes the acute manifestations of allergy. Some haptens (e.g., penicillin) are highly antigenic.

Concentration of the Allergen

Higher concentrations usually result in hypersensitivity responses of greater intensity. Lower concentrations of the allergen may then cause severe manifestations when reexposure occurs.

Route of Entrance into the Body

Routes by which allergens enter the body include inhalation, injection, ingestion, and direct contact. Most allergens are inhaled.

Exposure to the Allergen

Sensitization to allergens is necessary for hypersensitivity to occur. A few factors that influence the likelihood of development of allergy are a person's age at the time of exposure (exposure early in life), the type of allergen

---

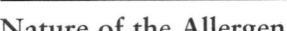

COMPLEMENTARY AND ALTERNATIVE THERAPY

Allergies

Several studies have found a number of environmental factors that may be associated with a lower incidence of allergic disease. For example, taking oral supplements of a probiotic supplement such as *Lactobacillus ruminus*,[2] having a dog or other pet in the home,[3] and attending a day care or having siblings in the home[1] have all been found to decrease the incidence of allergic disease.

References
1. Celedon, J., et al. (2002). Day care attendance, respiratory tract illnesses, wheezing, asthma, and total serum IgE level in early childhood. *Archives of Pediatric Adolescent Medicine, 156,* 241-245.
2. Kalliomaki, M., et al. (2001). Probiotics in primary prevention of atopic disease: A randomised placebo-controlled trial. *Lancet, 357,* 1076-1079.
3. Reijonen, T., et al. (2000). Predictors of asthma three years after hospitalization admission for wheezing in infancy. *Pediatrics 106,* 1406-1412.

(house dust mite, cockroach, various medications, and pollen), the allergen load (lower levels are capable of inducing specific IgE production), and the month of a person's birth (a greater affinity for allergies is seen in those born in the spring and fall).

Pathophysiology

The key intermediate in allergic disease is the IgE antibody. The production of IgE in response to an allergen renders an individual allergic. The two general categories of hypersensitivity reactions are (1) *immediate* (humoral or antigen-antibody) and (2) *delayed* (cell-mediated).

Immediate Reaction

The immediate (antigen-antibody) reaction occurs within minutes after exposure to the allergen. The resultant IgE production mediates the immediate response by activating mast cells and basophils, causing them to degranulate and release mediators such as histamine, leukotrienes from basophils and prostaglandins, and platelet-activating factor from eosinophils.

The mediators, whether preformed or newly formed after activation, are able to increase vascular permeability, dilate vessels, cause bronchospasm, contract smooth muscle, and ignite other inflammatory cells. Table 78-1 describes chemical mediators of the allergic reaction, their action, and the associated manifestations.

Manifestations of mediator release vary, depending on the organ where the mediators' receptors are found. For example, histamine is a preformed mast cell mediator that has receptors in various organs, including skin, oral and nasal mucosa, lungs, and the smooth muscle in the GI tract. Once histamine binds to its receptor, it can cause many reactions. Vasodilation causes edema; smooth muscle contraction results in dangerous airway narrowing; and glandular stimulation leads to increased mucus secretion in the nose, lungs, and GI tract.

TABLE 78-1	*Chemical Mediators of the Allergic Reaction*	
Mediator	**Action**	**Manifestations**
Histamine	Dilates blood vessels and increases vascular permeability	Erythema, tissue swelling, and shock
	Constricts smooth muscles in the bronchial airways	Shortness of breath and wheezing
	Stimulates nerve endings	Itching and painful skin
	Increases mucus production in the airways and GI tract	Congestion, gastric reflux, and heartburn
Platelet-activating factor	Dilates the blood vessels and constricts the bronchial airways	Same as for histamine
	Aids in the secretion and aggregation of platelets	Same as for histamine
Eosinophil chemotactic factor of anaphylaxis (ECF-A)	Increases eosinophil migration	Inflamed airways
Neutrophil chemotactic factor	Increases neutrophil migration	Inflamed airways
Heparin	Anticoagulation	Increased bleeding and bruising
Bradykinin	Slows smooth muscle contraction	Mucus plugging
	Increases vascular permeability	Swelling
	Increases mucus production	Congestion
Lipid Mediators or SRS-A		
Leukotrienes	Increase vascular permeability	Same as for histamine
	Increase smooth muscle contraction	
Prostaglandin D	Constricts bronchial airways	Wheezing, shortness of breath, and cough
	Vasodilation	Flushing and swelling
Cytokines (IL-4, IL-5, TNF-α)	Allow cells to influence the activity and development of other unrelated cells	Inflammation, edema, and fibrosis
	Aid in eosinophil production	
	Increase vascular permeability	

GI, Gastrointestinal; *IL,* interleukin; *SRS,* slow-reacting substance of anaphylaxis; *TNF,* tumor necrosis factor.

Newly formed mediators, including lipid mediators and cytokines, are made after the mast cell has been activated and have similar actions to those of histamine, but their effects tend to last much longer. Once released into the blood and after binding to their receptors, these mediators cause more bronchial smooth muscle contraction, vasodilation in the skin, nasal congestion, and edema.

Delayed Reaction

The delayed (cell-mediated or late-phase) reaction is seen when there is a prolonged response to the initial allergen. T cells govern the delayed inflammatory response that occurs about 2 to 8 hours after mast cells have been activated by the initial allergen exposure.

Hypersensitivity reactions are divided into four main types (Table 78-2):
- Type 1, immediate or anaphylactic
- Type 2, cytolytic or cytotoxic
- Type 3, immune complex
- Type 4, cell-mediated or delayed

Type 1 (Anaphylactic) Hypersensitivity. The anaphylactic response (described previously) is a rapidly occurring reaction that is mediated by IgE antibodies. The allergen binds to IgE antibodies, which are attracted to the surface of mast cells and basophils, causing the release of mediators (see Table 78-1). Examples of type 1 hypersensitivity reactions include anaphylaxis, allergic rhinitis, asthma, and acute allergic drug reactions.

Type 2 (Cytolytic or Cytotoxic) Hypersensitivity. Cytolytic or cytotoxic reactions are complement dependent and thus involve IgG or IgM antibodies. The antigen-antibody binding results in activation of the complement system and destroys the cell on which the antigen is bound, usually a circulating blood cell, thus causing tissue injury. Examples of tissue injury caused by type 2 hypersensitivity include hemolytic anemia, Rh hemolytic disease in newborns, autoimmune hyperthyroidism, myasthenia gravis, and blood transfusion reactions.

During a blood transfusion, blood group incompatibility causes cell lysis, which results in a transfusion reaction. The antigen responsible for initiating the reaction is a part of the donor red blood cell membrane. Manifestations of a transfusion reaction result from intravascular hemolysis of red blood cells and include headache and back pain (flank), chest pain similar to angina, nausea and vomiting, tachycardia and hypotension, hematuria, and urticaria.

Transfusions of more than 100 ml of incompatible blood can result in severe, permanent renal damage, circulatory shock, and death. Therefore if manifestations develop, stop the transfusion at once, maintain an open intravenous (IV) line, check the client's vital signs, and notify the physician immediately. For detailed nursing interventions related to transfusion reactions, see Chapter 77.

Type 3 (Immune Complex) Hypersensitivity. Immune complex reactions result when antigens bind to antibodies, leading to tissue injury. The molecular size of the antigen-antibody complexes is an important feature in eliciting immune complex reactions. Larger complexes are rapidly cleared by phagocytic cells. The smaller complexes formed in antigen excess persist longer in the circulation because they are not so easily captured by

TABLE 78-2	*Types of Hypersensitivity Reactions*			
	Type	**Causative Component**	**Pathologic Process**	**Reaction**
I	Immediate/anaphylactic	IgE	Mast cell degranulation ↓ Histamine and leukotriene release	Anaphylaxis Atopic diseases Skin reactions
II	Cytolytic/cytotoxic	IgG IgM Complement	Complement fixation ↓ Cell lysis	ABO incompatibility Drug-induced hemolytic anemia
III	Immune complex	Antigen-antibody complexes	Deposition in vessels and tissue walls ↓ Inflammation	Arthus reaction Serum sickness Systemic lupus erythematosus Acute glomerulonephritis
IV	Cell-mediated/delayed	Sensitized T cells	Lymphokine release	Tuberculosis Contact dermatitis Transplant rejection

Ig, Immunoglobulin.

phagocytic cells in the spleen and liver. Inflammation results and leads to acute or chronic disease of the organ system in which the immune complexes were deposited.

Immune complex–mediated inflammation is produced by IgG or IgM antibodies, antigen, and complement. The mediators of inflammatory injury include the complement cleavage peptides, which can activate mast cells, neutrophils, monocytes, and other cells. The release of lysosomal granules from white blood cells and macrophages causes further tissue injury.

The antigen may be tissue fixed or released locally, as in Goodpasture's syndrome, in which circulating antibodies react with autologous antigens in the glomerular basement membranes of the kidneys, causing inflammation of the glomerulus.

Antigen-antibody complexes are formed in the bloodstream and get trapped in capillaries or deposited in vessel walls, causing urticaria, arthritis, arteritis, or glomerulonephritis.

Alternatively, antigen-antibody complexes may form in the joint space, with resultant synovitis, as in rheumatoid arthritis and systemic lupus erythematous.

The Arthus reaction is a localized area of tissue necrosis that results from immune complex hypersensitivity.

The antigen may also be circulating, as in serum sickness. Serum sickness develops 6 to 14 days after injection with a foreign serum. Deposition of complexes on vessel walls causes complement activation, with resultant edema, fever, inflammation of blood vessels and joints, and urticaria. Classic serum sickness is rare because large doses of heterologous sera (e.g., horse antisera to human lymphocytes) are seldom used.

A serum sickness–like reaction may occur, however, after administration of such medications as penicillin, sulfonamides, streptomycin, thiouracils, and hydantoin compounds. Rather than being dominated by cutaneous vasculitis, these reactions more often manifest with fever, arthralgias, lymphadenopathy, and urticaria. The illness is usually benign and self-limiting, and it resolves after discontinuation of the offending medication.

Nursing care of the client with serum sickness depends on the severity of the reaction. For a mild reaction, care includes control of fever and pain with aspirin and antihistamines. For a severe reaction, care may require steroids.

Serum sickness can be prevented by avoiding allergen exposure. Obtain an allergy history and information about any previous reactions to drugs or vaccines. Document findings in the client's chart, care plan, and medication record so that the risk of subsequent exposure is minimized.

Type 4 (Cell-Mediated, Late-Phase, or Delayed) Hypersensitivity. In cell-mediated hypersensitivity, sensitized T cells respond to antigens by releasing lymphokines, some of which direct phagocytic cell activity. This reaction occurs 24 to 72 hours after exposure to an allergen. Delayed hypersensitivity is induced by chronic infection (e.g., tuberculosis) or by contact sensitivities, as in contact dermatitis.

Type 4 reactions occur after the intradermal injection of tuberculosis antigen or purified protein derivative (PPD). If the client has been sensitized to tuberculosis, sensitized T cells react with the antigen at the injection site. The reaction leads to edema and fibrin deposits, which result in the induration characteristic of a positive tuberculosis reaction.

Graft-versus-host disease (GVHD) and transplant rejection are also type 4 reactions. In GVHD, immunocompetent donor bone marrow cells (the graft) react against various antigens in the bone marrow recipient (the host). Various clinical manifestations result, including skin, GI, and hepatic lesions. Transplant rejection is discussed in Chapter 82, and GVHD is discussed in Chapter 81.

Contact dermatitis is another type 4 reaction that occurs after sensitization to an allergen, commonly a cosmetic, adhesive, topical medication, drug additive (such as lanolin added to lotions), or plant toxin (such as poison ivy). With the first exposure, no reaction occurs, but antigens are formed. On subsequent exposures, hypersensitivity reactions are triggered, which lead to itching, erythema, and vesicular lesions.

Clinical Manifestations

During an allergic response, mast cell activation and the release of chemical mediators result in increased vascular permeability, edema, dilation of blood vessels, smooth muscle contraction, bronchospasm, and increased mucus secretion in the nose, lungs, and GI tract.

The diagnosis of an allergic disease is based on the client's history, manifestations experienced during or after allergen exposure, and the results from commonly used allergy tests. Common allergy tests include (1) skin testing; (2) radioallergosorbent test (RAST) or fluoroenzyme immunoassay test (ImmunoCAP FEIA), which are used to measure IgE levels to certain allergens in vitro; (3) pulmonary function tests (PFTs) to diagnose asthma; and (4) blood assays for IgE levels.

Skin Testing

The health care practitioner introduces a small quantity of allergen into the skin by quickly pricking, scratching, or puncturing it or by using intradermal injection. A wheal and flare reaction usually occurs soon after the allergen is introduced into the skin if the client is allergic. Skin testing is generally considered safe, but it always carries a risk of causing a systemic reaction such as anaphylaxis.

Intradermal testing or injecting the known allergen directly below the skin is the most accurate skin test but is linked to a higher incidence of severe allergic reactions. Therefore it should be used with extreme caution and under close supervision. A patch test can be used to evaluate contact allergies; the allergen is applied directly to the skin and then covered with a gauze dressing.

Nurses often administer skin tests and interpret test results. An *immediate* reaction (i.e., appearing within 10 to 20 minutes after the injection), marked by erythema and wheal formation greater than 3 mm of the positive control (usually histamine), denotes a positive reaction. *Positive* reactions indicate antibody response to previous exposure to this antigen and suggest that the client is allergic to the particular substance that causes the reaction. *Negative* reactions may be inconclusive, requiring further assessment. Negative results may indicate the following: (1) antibodies have not formed to this antigen, (2) the antigen was deposited too deeply into the skin (e.g., subcutaneously), (3) the client is immunosuppressed from disease or therapies (e.g., steroids, chemotherapy, radiation therapy), or (4) the client has taken antihistamines within the past 72 hours.

Problems that arise from skin testing range from minor itching to anaphylaxis. Itching and discomfort at the injection site are common and can be relieved by the application of cool compresses, topical steroid or antihistamine creams, and oral antihistamines such as diphenhydramine (Benadryl). Ulceration of the injection site is best treated by keeping the area clean and dry. Anaphylactic shock is a rare but potentially lethal complication of skin testing. A client with a history of an anaphylactic reaction to a substance should never undergo skin testing for an allergy to that substance. This is especially true of allergens such as penicillin, which can produce lethal anaphylaxis in susceptible clients.

Radioallergosorbent Test

The RAST uses the principle of immunoabsorption and reveals elevated levels of allergen-specific IgE associated with atopy. The allergen of interest is first bound to some solid surface, usually a paper disk. The client's blood is then incubated with the disk. If the client has antibodies specific to the allergen being tested, they bind to that allergen. The unbound antibodies are washed away, and the level of antigen-specific IgE can be measured. This test is somewhat less sensitive than skin testing and is more time consuming and costly.

ImmunoCAP FEIA (Fluoroenzyme Immunoassay Test)

This method uses as the solid phase a flexible, hydrophobic cellulosic disk to which an allergen has been linked. The advantage of this system compared to RAST testing is that it has a very high antigen binding capacity and has minimal nonspecific binding with high total IgE

output. This test is more readily used worldwide based on its increased sensitivity and equal specificity.

Pulmonary Function Test

The PFTs are done to confirm the diagnosis or to evaluate the respiratory status in asthmatic disease, to assess the severity of lung obstruction, and to guide the medical treatment of asthma. The principal abnormality associated with asthma is reversible airway obstruction, reflected by a reduction in the forced expiratory volume measured in 1 second (FEV_1). Reversibility is noted if an increase of more than 15% in the FEV_1 is noted after giving a bronchodilator such as albuterol (Ventolin).

Blood Assays

Immunometric blood assays measure the total amount of IgE normally present in the circulation. Most studies have shown that blood concentrations of IgE are increased in the presence of allergic disease; however, a normal or even decreased level may occur in IgE-mediated sensitivities. Elevated serum eosinophil levels also may suggest hypersensitivities.

Outcome Management
■ Medical Management

Allergies are among the most common disorders seen in the medical community. The client often requires a combination of treatments, ranging from avoidance of known allergens to environmental control, immunotherapy, and follow-up.

Identify Allergen. It is imperative to obtain a detailed history that identifies any previous allergic problems in the client and also the presence of allergy in close family members, to perform a thorough assessment and examination, and to ensure that appropriate diagnostic tests are performed. The clinician must know the times of the year during which manifestations occur to determine a correct diagnosis on the basis of the offending allergen. If year-round manifestations are present, find out whether they are worse at any time. A careful search for environmental factors should be undertaken. The client should be questioned in detail regarding the home environment: location, type of heating, insulation, humidity, nature of the bedding, presence of carpeting, method of house cleaning, and so on.

Avoid Allergen. Avoidance of the allergen is often the easiest, cheapest, and safest way of dealing with allergies; however, identification of the specific allergen is sometimes difficult, especially if the client refuses, cannot afford, or cannot locate allergen-testing services. Even if the allergen can be identified, complete avoidance may not be possible, as with pollens and food additives.

Control Environment. Environmental control sometimes helps to eliminate airborne allergens. Figure 78-1 illustrates ways to desensitize a room. These environmental controls, combined with air filters that remove small particles from the air, can help to eliminate many allergens.

Administer Medications. Atopic clients benefit greatly from selected prescriptions and over-the-counter medications. Usually, clients self-administer these agents, although in some settings the nurse or a family member administers them. See the Integrating Pharmacology feature on Medications for Allergies on p. 2322.

Promote Desensitization. Immunotherapy ("desensitization therapy") is designed for the treatment of type 1, IgE-mediated hypersensitivity reactions. Precise doses of allergens are injected at intervals over a prolonged period with the goal of altering the immune system's response to an allergen, thus reducing manifestations of rhinitis,

sneezing, and generalized pruritus triggered by subsequent exposures. The doses are increased gradually over time, or infections may be given several times a day in increasing doses in "rush" protocols. Immunotherapy increases IgG antibody levels and may increase suppressor T-cell function. Specific IgG interferes with IgE binding to allergens and thus mitigates the hypersensitivity response. Immunotherapy is widely used in the treatment of allergic rhinitis (hay fever), for which its greatest success has been achieved because immunotherapy blunts the seasonal rise in specific immunoglobulin IgE antibody levels. It also is used for Hymenoptera sensitivity (bee, yellow jacket, wasp, and hornet stings) with reportable success. There is some controversy regarding the efficacy of this treatment in the management of asthma.

Nurses often administer these injections and assess and treat side effects. Clients are asked to wait at least 30 to 40 minutes after receiving the injections so that immediate reactions can be treated. Side effects are similar to those seen in skin testing.

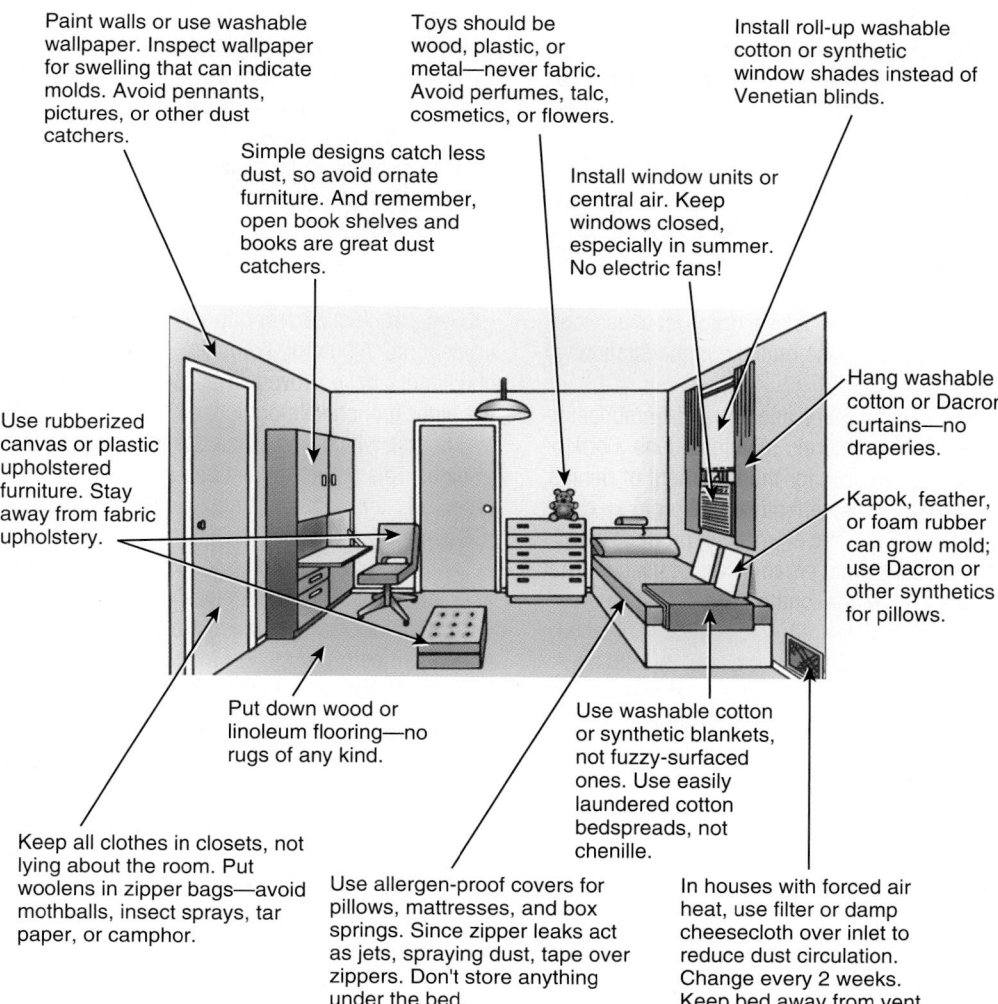

Paint walls or use washable wallpaper. Inspect wallpaper for swelling that can indicate molds. Avoid pennants, pictures, or other dust catchers.

Toys should be wood, plastic, or metal—never fabric. Avoid perfumes, talc, cosmetics, or flowers.

Install roll-up washable cotton or synthetic window shades instead of Venetian blinds.

Simple designs catch less dust, so avoid ornate furniture. And remember, open book shelves and books are great dust catchers.

Install window units or central air. Keep windows closed, especially in summer. No electric fans!

Use rubberized canvas or plastic upholstered furniture. Stay away from fabric upholstery.

Hang washable cotton or Dacron curtains—no draperies.

Kapok, feather, or foam rubber can grow mold; use Dacron or other synthetics for pillows.

Put down wood or linoleum flooring—no rugs of any kind.

Use washable cotton or synthetic blankets, not fuzzy-surfaced ones. Use easily laundered cotton bedspreads, not chenille.

Keep all clothes in closets, not lying about the room. Put woolens in zipper bags—avoid mothballs, insect sprays, tar paper, or camphor.

Use allergen-proof covers for pillows, mattresses, and box springs. Since zipper leaks act as jets, spraying dust, tape over zippers. Don't store anything under the bed.

In houses with forced air heat, use filter or damp cheesecloth over inlet to reduce dust circulation. Change every 2 weeks. Keep bed away from vent.

FIGURE 78-1 Controlling the environment of a room. Dacron is a trade name for polyester. (Courtesy of A.H. Robins Company, Richmond, VA.)

INTEGRATING PHARMACOLOGY

Medications for Allergies

In addition to avoiding the allergen, several medications are available to minimize manifestations and decrease the inflammatory process.

Antihistamines are the major group of prescription and over-the-counter drugs used to alleviate the early phase allergic manifestations. These medications relieve sneezing, rhinitis, itching, and other manifestations of allergic rhinitis. They bind to the H_1 receptor. Traditional antihistamines such as diphenhydramine (Benadryl) pass the blood-brain barrier and can produce significant drowsiness. Because newer agents (cetirizine [Zyrtec], fexofenadine [Allegra], and loratadine [Claritin]) do not cross the blood-brain barrier (or do so poorly), they do not cause the drowsiness that limits the use of older medications.

Decongestants (oral sympathomimetics) such as pseudoephedrine and phenylephrine help relieve nasal congestion by stimulating the alpha-adrenergic receptors that control the capillary sphincters at the entrance to the venous plexuses of the turbinates. Nasal decongestants such as oxymetazoline, hydrochloride, and phenylephedrine sprays act primarily on turbinate swelling and are more effective and rapid in onset when used topically rather than orally. Because the prolonged use of topical nasal sprays can cause rhinitis medicamentosa (recurrence of congestion), however, it is advisable to limit their use to no more than 3 to 5 days. Practitioners are cautioned against the use of oral agents by clients with heart disease, hypertension, thyroid disease, diabetes, and urinary difficulties resulting from prostatic hypertrophy. These drugs can be combined with antihistamines to treat the multiple manifestations of allergy.

Corticosteroids, anti-inflammatory agents, and immunosuppressants can be used to treat allergic manifestations. Corticosteroids are the most effective drug for the treatment of rhinitis. Oral steroids are in general more effective and rapid in onset than topical forms, but their systemic effects can produce a myriad of complications. Topical steroid creams can be used to treat dermatitis. Beclomethasone dipropionate (Beconase), triamcinolone (Nasacort), flunisolide (Nasarel), budesonide (Rhinocort), and fluticasone (Flonase) are nasal sprays useful in treating allergic rhinitis, and they evoke few systemic side effects.

Cromolyn sodium is a topical or aerosol medication used to treat allergic rhinitis (Nasalcrom) and asthma (Intal). Its mechanism of action is not completely understood, but it helps prevent the release of chemical mediators (e.g., histamine and leukotrienes) by stabilizing mast cells during both immediate and late-phase reactions. Cromolyn sodium should be administered before allergen exposure. It should be started a week before allergy season to be most effective in the treatment of seasonal allergic rhinitis. It must be used on a regular basis and, unfortunately, dosing is required four to six times a day. Nasal steroids such as Flonase and Rhinocort are the mainstay of therapy for allergic rhinitis.

Inhaled steroids are fundamental to the treatment of asthma. New inhaled steroids with a greater topical potency ratio and fewer systemic effects allow greater control in asthma management. Fluticasone (Flovent), fluticasone and Serevent (Advair), triamcinolone (Azmacort), and beclomethasone (Vanceril) are examples of inhaled steroids.

Anticholinergics are used primarily to treat allergic rhinitis and rhinorrhea caused by the common cold. Ipratropium (Atrovent) was a major advance in the therapeutic regimen for asthma. It does not cross the blood-brain barrier and is relatively free of side effects. Anticholinergics inhibit the effects of acetylcholine by blocking its binding to receptors at neurotransmitter sites on glandular tissue, thereby decreasing the amount of watery discharge in clients with rhinitis. Anticholinergics are also available in oral forms in combination with antihistamines and decongestant preparations (Dura-Vent DA, Extendryl SR).

$Beta_2$ agonists are commonly used to control bronchospasm in asthma. Albuterol (Ventolin) and other short-acting bronchodilators have proved to be well tolerated. The drawback of the older bronchodilators is their short duration of action (only 4 to 6 hours), which limits their use for manifestations experienced at night. This problem has been addressed with the new generation of long-acting $beta_2$ agonists such as salmeterol (Serevent).

Anti-leukotrienes are used to treat manifestations of asthma and anaphylaxis. They block the synthesis or action of leukotriene mediators, which are known to contribute to airway edema, smooth muscle contraction, and the process of inflammation. These drugs include zafirlukast (Accolate), zileuton (Zyflo), and montelukast (Singulair).

■ Nursing Management of the Medical Client
Assessment

As a nurse, you play a crucial role in obtaining a detailed medical history of the client and ensuring that appropriate diagnostic tests are performed. The most important part of evaluating the allergic client is the history. The history should elicit all the client's current manifestations. It is important for clinicians to know whether the manifestations are always present or what times of the year they worsen.

Indoor allergens are causing increasing amounts of distress. House dust mites and cockroach and animal allergens are problematic and are present year-round in many homes. Assess whether animals are present in the home and, if so, how many. Is the house filled with plants that could harbor mold spores? Is the client exposed to moist rooms, such as a basement, that is constantly damp?

Environmental factors such as smoke can exacerbate manifestations. Determining where these manifestations present is very important. Many occupations involve exposure to certain allergens such as smoke, latex, chemicals, and animals. Manifestations may be reported as worse during the workweek compared with the weekend. Inquiries such as these help to narrow down possible causes of manifestations.

Diagnosis, Outcomes, Interventions

Diagnosis: Health-Seeking Behaviors.

The key nursing diagnosis for the client with hypersensitivity disorders is *Health-Seeking Behaviors related to the desire to learn about the disease process, treatment regimen, and risk control methods.*

Outcomes.

The client will follow a mutually agreed on health maintenance plan that includes stated understanding of the disease process, treatment regimen, and control of risk factors.

Interventions

Provide Teaching. Although clients usually self-administer medications, as described under the medical management section, you are responsible for instructing clients and their significant others about these medications. The client needs to learn what the medication is, why it is being prescribed, how to take it, when to take it, and what the possible side effects might be. In addition, the client needs to know what to do during an anaphylactic reaction (see Anaphylaxis, Insect Sting Allergy, and Latex Allergy).

If an inhaler is prescribed, the client must be taught how to use it correctly (see Chapter 63). A spacer (an attachment added to the inhaler that holds the medication in the additional chamber or space until the client inhales) may be recommended to help the client obtain the maximal effect. Some clients are taught to perform desensitization injections themselves. In this case, teach clients the proper injection technique and the manifestations of any untoward reactions to the medications, such as shortness of breath, hoarseness, urticaria, and generalized flushing.

Clients may need to carry medications for anaphylaxis with them at all times. In such instances, clients should also wear a medical-alert bracelet. Other nursing interventions are described in the following sections under specific disorders.

Evaluation

It is expected that the client will obtain relief from allergic manifestations when the treatment regimen is followed. The client will be able to avoid or control risk factors for allergic manifestations. Ideally, the client will be able to avoid anaphylactic events and obtain treatment before serious problems develop.

ALLERGIC DISORDERS
FOOD ALLERGY

Adverse food reactions can be classified in one of two ways: (1) *food allergies,* which occur by a specific IgE-mediated response to the offending food, such as food-induced anaphylaxis from peanuts; and (2) *food intolerances,* which do not result from an IgE-mediated response but cause manifestations such as diarrhea and vomiting. The prevalence of food intolerances is much higher than that of food allergies. Although food allergies can occur at any age, the condition is more common among infants and very young children, affecting about 8% of those under age 3.

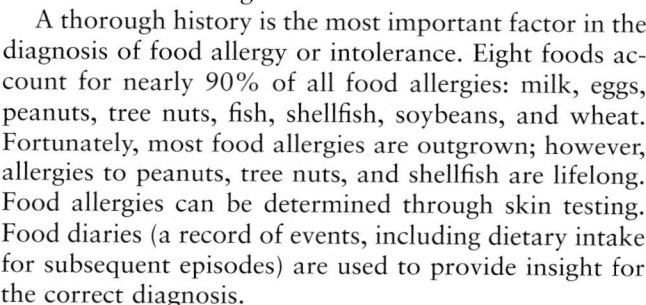

A thorough history is the most important factor in the diagnosis of food allergy or intolerance. Eight foods account for nearly 90% of all food allergies: milk, eggs, peanuts, tree nuts, fish, shellfish, soybeans, and wheat. Fortunately, most food allergies are outgrown; however, allergies to peanuts, tree nuts, and shellfish are lifelong. Food allergies can be determined through skin testing. Food diaries (a record of events, including dietary intake for subsequent episodes) are used to provide insight for the correct diagnosis.

The standard of diagnosis in food allergy is the double-blind, placebo-controlled food challenge. The suspected food is eliminated from the diet for 10 to 14 days. Antihistamines are not to be taken for at least 24 hours before the challenge, and a fasting state should be maintained for 12 to 18 hours before testing. The challenge starts with the introduction of a very low dose of the suspected food, and the dose is gradually increased every 20 to 30 minutes until a reaction is noted or the amount of food present in a normal feeding is reached. *Elimination diets* are also used and consist of removing one food at a time until the adverse manifestations are relieved.

Measuring serum blood tryptase levels can also prove helpful because elevations in tryptase occur and are detectable in the blood for up to 2 hours after a severe systemic reaction. Negative results do not, however, rule out a positive reaction.

See the Bridge to Home Health Care on Managing Immunosuppression and Nutrition on the website.

ATOPIC DERMATITIS

Atopic dermatitis occurs in about 10% of the population. Clients typically have a history of or complaints about itchy skin, in addition to a history of rashes in the area of skin creases. Other common complaints are of generally dry skin initially experienced in children younger than 2 years of age, accompanied by manifestations of asthma, hay fever, or dermatitis. Lesions of atopic dermatitis are red and pruritic, contain exudates, and are maculopapular in younger clients, becoming drier and thicker as clients age. The lesions are typically found on the cheeks, scalp, and forehead; in later years, they may occur on the trunk and extremities.

■ Medical Management

Treatment is aimed at controlling and reducing the manifestations because there is no true cure. Antihistamines 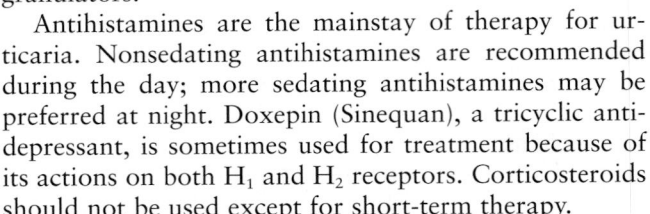 are used with good results to help alleviate the itch-scratch cycle that is common to atopic dermatitis. The mainstay of therapy is topical corticosteroids, which control the inflammation in the skin lesions. Gels penetrate more effectively but are drying. Ointments should be used in more severe cases because they promote hydration; however, some clients prefer not to use them because they are oily and become messy in the heat. Creams and lotions are the least penetrating but are preferred by most clients. They are absorbed quickly and promote comfort. Antibiotics may be needed to treat superficial skin infections caused by intense pruritus and scratching.

■ Nursing Management of the Medical Client

Teach clients the importance of environmental control. A key strategy is to minimize allergen exposure and physical stimuli that provoke pruritus. Explain that the client can reduce itching by avoiding severe changes in temperature, wearing loose cotton clothing, using gentle detergents, and rinsing clothing completely. Advise clients to avoid chemical irritants, emotional stress, aeroallergens such as dust and animal dander, and dietary allergens. Teach the client general skin care measures, such as how to perform the following:

1. Maintain good skin hydration by bathing in lukewarm water
2. Use gentle soaps (e.g., Basis, Dove)
3. Apply a lubricant like Alpha Keri, petroleum jelly, Eucerin, or Aquaphor to the skin immediately after bathing
4. Avoid scratching
5. Keep fingernails trimmed to avoid infection

URTICARIA

Urticaria (or hives) is a cutaneous reaction associated with several different causes. It occurs in as many as 25% of all people at some time. Hives that are present daily or intermittently over a period of less than 6 weeks are termed *acute* urticaria. Hives present for more than 6 weeks are referred to as *chronic* urticaria.

Lesions of urticaria tend to be papules or plaques that fade within 24 hours. They do not leave areas of hyperpigmentation. Hives are round or oval and range in size from a few millimeters to several centimeters. Numerous

agents can trigger the onset of urticaria: cold, heat, the sun, vibrations, rubbing, or pressure. Urticaria can also be caused by medications, foods, and infections.

Mast cells and their mediators may play a key role in urticaria, causing intense pruritus and vascular changes. A lesional skin biopsy to identify which types of inflammatory cells are present in the lesion is useful in structuring treatment. Some known provoking stimuli of urticaria are medications, foreign substances, foods and food additives, infections, insect bites and stings, contact irritants, inhalants, heat, cold, light, and pressure.

■ Medical Management

Although management focuses on identifying and eliminating any known causative factors, in about 80% of chronic cases no cause of urticaria is found. All clients with urticaria should be cautioned about aspirin and nonsteroidal anti-inflammatory drugs (NSAIDs), which may exacerbate existing hives. Opiates should be used cautiously as well because they are typically mast cell degranulators.

Antihistamines are the mainstay of therapy for urticaria. Nonsedating antihistamines are recommended during the day; more sedating antihistamines may be preferred at night. Doxepin (Sinequan), a tricyclic antidepressant, is sometimes used for treatment because of its actions on both H_1 and H_2 receptors. Corticosteroids should not be used except for short-term therapy.

■ Nursing Management of the Medical Client

Urticaria tends to evoke anxiety and frustration in both clients and clinicians. The most effective treatment is to eliminate any triggers. Help the client identify factors that may be suspect, and suggest elimination diets and challenges if foods or food additives are thought to provoke manifestations. Encourage clients to avoid initiating physical factors, such as pressure from tight clothing, heat, vibration, sunlight, and rubbing of the skin. Good skin hydration is mandatory; counsel the client to avoid harsh soaps and irritants and to apply moisturizing lotions after bathing while the skin is still damp.

ANAPHYLAXIS, INSECT STING ALLERGY, AND LATEX ALLERGY

The most common causes of anaphylaxis are drugs, foods, latex exposure, and insect bites and stings. Common food offenders in adults are peanuts, tree nuts, and shellfish (Table 78-3). Insect stings cause many deaths in the United States every year. The incidence of anaphylaxis related to latex exposure, especially in health care workers, has dramatically increased since the 1990s with the increased use of latex gloves.

Anaphylactic events commonly present with hives and angioedema and often with dyspnea, wheezing, syncope, hypotension, nausea, vomiting, diarrhea, abdomi-

TABLE 78-3	*Common Agents Causing Anaphylaxis*

Drugs

Penicillins (most common)	Vancomycin
Cephalosporins	Amphotericin B
Tetracyclines	Polymyxin
Streptomycin	Bacitracin
Kanamycin	Aspirin, other anti-
Neomycin	inflammatory agents
Heparin	Colchicine
Protamine	Tranquilizers

Foods

Peanuts	Milk
Seafood	Citrus fruits
Eggs	Strawberries
Nuts	Legumes

Insect Venoms

Hymenoptera (honeybees, wasps, yellow jackets, hornets, fire ants)

Biologicals

Heterologous antisera (especially equine)
Enzymes
Hormones
Vaccines (especially egg-cultured types)

Blood Products

Plasma	Whole blood
Cryoprecipitate	Gamma globulin

Allergen Extracts

Skin-testing agents
Desensitization

Diagnostic Agents

Sulfobromophthalein
Iodinated contrast media

---

nal pain, flushing, headache, rhinitis, substernal pain, and itching. Cardiovascular collapse, shock, and respiratory obstruction, which can occur immediately and without other manifestations, are the primary cause of death from anaphylaxis. Although manifestations usually begin 5 to 30 minutes after the offending trigger has been encountered, there can be a delay of an hour or more. The more rapid the onset, the more severe the episode.

The incidence of anaphylaxis related to insect stings ranges from 0.3% to 3% in the general population. The sting insects are members of the order Hymenoptera. People may be allergic to one or all of the stinging insects, but the sting of the yellow jacket is the most common cause of allergy. Common reactions to an insect sting include pain, swelling, and redness that may be lo-

calized or may extend over a large area. The swelling usually peaks in 24 to 48 hours and may last for 7 to 10 days. There are no factors that identify those at potential risk for anaphylaxis from an insect sting other than a prior history. Those who have had severe anaphylaxis have an 80% chance of another reaction.

Health care workers are at particular risk for latex allergy. About 700,000 health care workers are affected. Workers with allergies to latex also have a high incidence of reactions to certain foods, such as chestnuts, bananas, kiwi, avocado, apricot, and papaya. Manifestations range from simple dermatitis to generalized itching, urticaria, sneezing, coughing, wheezing, hypotension, and shock on exposure. The diagnosis of type 1 hypersensitivity to latex is confirmed by in vivo skin testing with raw latex extracts or in vitro blood assays that measure specific IgE responses to latex.

■ Medical Management

Anaphylaxis is treated by (1) subcutaneous epinephrine injection, (2) removing or discontinuing the causative agent, (3) administering emergency oxygen, (4) maintaining an open airway, (5) placing the client in the Trendelenburg position, and (6) giving supportive IV fluids, such as 0.9% normal saline or lactated Ringer's solution as necessary.

■ Nursing Management of the Medical Client

Nursing Diagnoses *Risk for Latex Allergy and Latex Allergy Response* are more specific nursing diagnoses for latex allergy reactions. Most of the interventions for these diagnoses have been described under the nursing diagnosis *Health-Seeking Behaviors*. In addition, the incidence and severity of anaphylactic reactions are decreased by both general and specific measures. Take a thorough history for drug, food, insect, pollen, and animal allergies from every client. Counsel all clients with a history of anaphylaxis or anaphylactic-like reactions to carry epinephrine with them at all times in the form of an Epi-Pen or Ana-Kit for self-injection. Recommend that they carry a medical-alert bracelet or necklace and an identification card in their wallet or purse and that they register with the proper authorities.

ALLERGIC RHINITIS

Manifestations of allergic rhinitis are persistent and show seasonal variation. Nasal manifestations are often accompanied by eye irritation, which causes pruritus, erythema, and excessive tearing. Numerous allergens may cause these manifestations, such as tree pollens (most common in the spring), grasses (summer), ragweed (fall), or dust mites and animal dander (year-round).

When the nasal mucosa is exposed to an allergen, a series of events is set in motion. Allergen exposure increases the production of IgE, which binds to the receptors on mast cells and basophils and eventually causes a release of mediators. The mediator release leads to increased swelling and blockage of the nose, watery discharge, sneezing, and nasal itching.

■ Medical Management

Nasal glucocorticoid sprays are used with good results for the treatment of allergic rhinitis. The newer, nonsedating antihistamines are beneficial in maintaining control over allergic rhinitis and are a crucial component of therapy.

■ Nursing Management of the Medical Client

Educating the client is the most important component of therapy. Teach clients to avoid allergens and to use air filters and air conditioning. Emphasize that compliance with medication is essential. Explain the reasoning behind daily medication use as well as how to adjust the medication to control minor flare-ups and to prevent progression of the disease.

ASTHMA

Because the diagnosis and treatment of asthma account for a substantial number of outpatient visits in allergy clinics, a heightened awareness and thorough understanding of the disease are warranted. See Chapter 63 for a thorough discussion of asthma management.

CONCLUSIONS

The immune system is a complex, interrelated system that affects the whole body. As a nurse, you must understand immune responses to provide clients with complete and individualized care. Because the care of these clients requires multifaceted interventions, you must be able to develop and implement complex care plans to meet their needs.

THINKING CRITICALLY *evolve*

1. L.S. is a 41-year-old woman admitted for surgery. After surgery, she was to receive prophylactic IV cephalosporin but received a dose of penicillin by mistake. She has a known allergy to penicillin. With a history of allergy to penicillin, what type of hypersensitivity reaction is L.S. most likely to experience? Using the concepts of hypersensitivity, explain this process.

Factors to Consider. What reactions might the nurse expect? What should be the nurse's first actions? What medications might the nurse expect the physician to pre-scribe to treat this reaction? How can such a reaction be prevented from occurring in the future?

2. A.W. is a 21-year-old college student admitted with an asthmatic attack that has not responded to his usual treatments. He is admitted for a course of IV medications and respiratory treatments. When you enter the room to start the IV line, his wheezing is audible. He is also anxious and gasping for air. What actions should you implement? What problems might you experience when you start the IV line?

Factors to Consider. After the acute phase is over, what might the nurse assess to determine the cause of the asthma attack and why the typical interventions were unsuccessful? What additional teaching might be required?

3. R.H. is a newly graduated registered nurse on an oncology unit. She has been wearing gloves more than ever during the past 2 weeks following orientation. A rash develops on her hands, and she complains of itching all over her body. What type of allergic reaction might be occurring? What actions to assess the allergy should be taken?

Factors to Consider. Can R.H. expect to continue in her new job? Does the organization have a responsibility to keep her employed?

Discussions for these questions can be found on the website and the CD-ROM.

BIBLIOGRAPHY

1. Alfonso, L., & Hogan, D. (1999). Contact dermatitis for primary care providers. *Nurse Practitioner Forum, 10*(2), 67-73.
2. Becker, H. (2000). An analysis of the epidemiology of latex allergy: Implications for primary prevention. *MEDSURG Nursing, 9*(3), 135-143.
3. Bunn, B. (1999). Itch, scratch, sweat and wheeze: Managing allergic reactions. *Emergency Medical Services, 28*(7), 75-77.
4. Burt, S. (1999). What you need to know about latex allergy. *Nursing Management, 30*(8), 18-26.
5. Casale, T., et al. (2001). Effect of omalizumab on symptoms of seasonal allergic rhinitis: A randomized controlled trial. *Journal of the American Medical Association, 286*(23), 2956-2968.
6. Cohen, S. (2001). About latex allergy. *Nursing, 31*(2), 76.
7. Craig, T.J. (2002) Allergic rhinitis remains an important disease. *Journal of the American Osteopathic Association, 102*(6 Suppl 2), S1-S2.
8. Doutre, M. (1999). Physiopathology of urticaria. *European Journal of Dermatology, 9*(8), 601-605.
9. Gehring, L.L. (2000). Latex allergy: Creating a safe environment. *Dermatological Nursing, 12*(3), 197-201.

evolve *Did you remember to check out the bonus material on the Evolve website and the CD-ROM, including free self-assessment exercises?*
http://evolve.elsevier.com/Black/medsurg/

10. Jones, T. (2001). Allergic rhinitis. In M. Groer (Ed.), *Advanced pathophysiology: Application to clinical practice* (pp. 118-137). Philadelphia: J.B. Lippincott.

EB 11. Parronchi, P., et al. (2000). Genetic and environmental factors contributing to the onset of allergic disorders. *International Archives of Allergy and Immunology,121*(1), 2-9.

12. Phelps, D., & Groer, M. (2001). Asthma and other allergic disorders. In M. Groer (Ed.), *Advanced pathophysiology: Application to clinical practice* (pp. 138-152). Philadelphia: J.B. Lippincott.

13. Putman, H. (2002). Food allergies: Keeping kids safe. *RN, 65*(6), 26-30.

14. Putman, H. (2001). Relief for patients with severe allergies. *RN, 64*(6), 26-31.

15. Solomon, W. (2003). Atopic dermatitis and urticaria. In S. Price & L. Wilson (Eds.), *Pathophysiology: Clinical concepts of disease processes* (6th ed., pp. 149-153). St. Louis: Mosby.

16. Solomon, W. (2003). Bronchial asthma: Allergic and otherwise. In S. Price & L. Wilson (Eds.), *Pathophysiology: Clinical concepts of disease processes* (6th ed., pp. 139-148). St. Louis: Mosby.

17. Solomon, W. (2003). Familiar (IgE-mediated) allergic disorders: Anaphylaxis and the atopic diseases. In S. Price & L. Wilson (Eds.), *Pathophysiology: Clinical concepts of disease processes* (6th ed., pp. 129-138). St. Louis: Mosby.

18. Sommers, M. (2003). Alterations in immunocompetence. In V. Carrieri-Kohlman, A. Lindsay, & C. West (Eds.), *Pathophysiological phenomena in nursing: Human responses to illness* (3rd ed., pp. 297-317). Philadelphia: W.B. Saunders.

19. Willsie, S.K. (2002). Improved strategies and new treatment options for allergic rhinitis. *Journal of the American Osteopathic Association, 102*(6 Suppl 2), S7-S14.

Chapter 79

Management of Clients with Rheumatic Disorders

Patricia A. MacDonald

The United Nations, the World Health Organization, and 37 countries have proclaimed the years 2000 to 2010 as the "Bone and Joint Decade." This global initiative is intended to improve the lives of people with musculoskeletal disorders, such as arthritis, and to advance understanding and treatment of musculoskeletal disorders through prevention, education and research.

By 2035, more than 20% of the United States population will be 65 years of age or older. The term *arthritis* literally means "inflammation of a joint," but arthritis is actually a collection of more than 100 related, but distinct conditions. Approximately 49% of all Americans older than age 65 years think they have arthritis. The disease touches one in every seven Americans, that is, one in every three families. Arthritis is the primary reason for work-related disability and is the leading cause of disability among people 65 years of age or older.[3] The Centers for Disease Control and Prevention (CDC) reports that 70 million Americans suffer from arthritis. In 1999, a consortium of national organizations produced "The National Arthritis Action Plan: A Public Health Strategy," which is a comprehensive and ambitious plan for addressing the increasing concerns regarding arthritis.[12]

Rheumatic disorders are comprised of autoimmune and inflammatory disorders, which have been called "the primary crippling diseases" of the developed world. They are the most prevalent chronic condition in the United States and a leading cause of disability. Rheumatic disorders encompass more than 100 diseases and conditions, including osteoarthritis (OA) (discussed in Chapter 28), rheumatoid arthritis (RA), psoriatic arthritis (PsA), systemic lupus erythematosus (SLE), fibromyalgia (FMS), scleroderma (SSc), ankylosing spondylitis (AS), reactive arthritis (Reiter's syndrome), idiopathic inflammatory myopathies, polymyositis (PM), dermatomyositis (DM), gout, and bursitis. Less common disorders include rheumatic syndromes associated with infectious agents, metabolic and endocrine diseases associated with rheumatic states, connective tissue neoplasms, extra-articular disorders, and miscellaneous disorders associated with joint manifestations.

Although the conditions have different clinical patterns, pain and impaired mobility are common problems with these disorders. Chronic pain and progressive physical impairment of joints and soft tissues characterize rheumatic disorders. The ultimate goals of the health care team are to reduce pain and other physical

evolve *Be sure to check out the bonus material on the Evolve website and the CD-ROM, including free self-assessment exercises.*

http://evolve.elsevier.com/Black/medsurg/

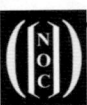

Nursing Outcomes Classification (NOC)
for Nursing Diagnoses—Clients with Rheumatic Disorders

Activity Intolerance
Self-Care: Activities of Daily Living
Endurance
Activity Tolerance
Energy Conservation
Chronic Pain
Comfort Level
Depression Control
Pain Control
Pain: Psychological Response
Effective Therapeutic Regimen Management/Risk for Ineffective Therapeutic Regimen Management
Health Promoting Behavior

Knowledge: Health Promotion
Knowledge: Treatment Regimen
Participation: Health Care Decisions
Social Support
Fatigue
Activity Tolerance
Endurance
Energy Conservation
Impaired Physical Mobility
Ambulation: Walking
Mobility
Self-Care: Activities of Daily Living
Impaired Social Interaction
Role Performance

Social Involvement
Ineffective Role Performance
Coping
Depression Control
Psychosocial Adjustment: Life Change
Role Performance
Ineffective Tissue Perfusion: Peripheral
Tissue Perfusion: Peripheral
Sensory Function: Cutaneous
Sleep Deprivation
Rest
Sleep
Symptom Severity

 manifestations, assuage psychological distress, improve physical function, and generally aid in the well-being of the client. Equally important are interventions to prevent and ameliorate socioeconomic problems. A majority of the costs, both economic and social, are due to lost function rather than direct medical costs. Until cures for the many types of rheumatic disorders and arthritis are found or until more effective therapies to prevent joint damage and physical disability are developed, clients will continue to suffer severe, premature economic and social dislocations that seriously affect their lives. As the population ages, society can expect that these impacts will mushroom.[13]

As the incidence of autoimmune and inflammatory disorders continues to increase, research efforts focus on the role of overuse, injury, obesity, gene defects, infection, immunosuppression, amino acids, interleukin, and environmental agents in both the development and treatment of these life-altering diseases. In addition, autoimmunity was named a major priority in women's health issues by the Office of Research on Women's Health, a unit of the National Institutes of Health, because these disorders occur in women three times more often than in men.

Clinical trials and their results are used to support evidence-based practice. The American College of Rheumatology (ACR) has set the standard for what is an acceptable indicator of disease improvement. The *ACR 20* and the *Sharp Score,* outcome variables, are the most consistent measures used. The ACR 20 is defined as a 20% improvement in tender and swollen joint counts and a 20% improvement in three of the five remaining core data (Table 79-1). The Sharp Score, named after its originator John Sharp, is a standardized means of scoring the damage done to the joints, joint space narrowing, and erosions.[10] In early studies there were no radiographic results. It was not until the early 1990s that x-ray studies were done in clinical trials; reported data

were inconsistent and the results difficult to interpret. These same problems are still being addressed. Joint space narrowing and erosions are seen in 67% of clients within the first 2 years of disease. Radiographic progression occurs early and continues over the client's lifetime.[10]

The difficulty in evaluating the results of these clinical trials is due to design differences (e.g., single agent versus combination, active comparator versus placebo, no prior methotrexate [MTX] versus MTX failures) and differences in client populations (early versus late disease, rheumatoid factor [RF]-positive versus RF-negative). The radiographic results show that there is slowing of radiographic progression with the use of disease-modifying antirheumatic drugs (DMARDs) and biologic response modifiers (BRMs). None of the studies were read for "healing." The lower the Sharp Score, the less damage from erosions and joint space narrowing. Clients treated with MTX alone have less damage than those given placebo. The addition of the newer medications should limit further damage—as much as 70% less. MTX and leflunomide are effective DMARDs, with etanercept, infliximab, adalimumab, and anakinra being effective BRMs. Combined usage with MTX appears to lead to greater efficacy. In the early rheumatoid arthritis (ERA) trial, etanercept stopped progression in 63% of clients and 72% of clients achieved a 20% improvement in manifestations with an ACR score of 20 (results at 2 years). See the Evidence-Based Practice in Action feature on Rheumatoid Arthritis Treatment on p. 2331.

AUTOIMMUNITY

Relationships between altered immune function and rheumatic disease are better understood as a result of continued research efforts. Autoimmune diseases are defined as conditions in which immunologic self-tolerance

TABLE 79-1	1987 Revised Criteria of the American Rheumatism Association for the Classification of Rheumatoid Arthritis*
Criterion	**Description**
1	Morning stiffness in and around joints lasting at least 1 hr before maximal improvement
2	Soft tissue swelling (arthritis) of three or more joint areas (including the right and left PIP, MCP, wrist, elbow, knee, ankle, and MTP joints)
3	Swelling of at least one wrist, MCP, or PIP joint
4	Simultaneous symmetrical swelling in joints listed in criterion 2
5	Subcutaneous rheumatoid nodules
6	Presence of rheumatoid factor
7	Radiographic erosions or periarticular osteopenia in hand or wrist joints

Data from Arnett, F.C., et al. (1988). The American Rheumatism Association 1987 revised criteria for the classification of rheumatoid arthritis. *Arthritis and Rheumatism, 31,* 315-324.

MCP, Metacarpophalangeal; *MTP,* metatarsophalangeal; *PIP,* proximal interphalangeal.

*NOTE: Rheumatoid arthritis is defined by the presence of four or more criteria. Criteria 1 through 4 must have been present for at least 6 weeks. The American Rheumatism Association 1987 revised criteria for the classification of rheumatoid arthritis.

EB EVIDENCE-BASED PRACTICE IN ACTION

Rheumatoid Arthritis Treatment

Have new pharmacologic treatments made a difference in treatment outcomes for rheumatoid arthritis (RA)? RA is a chronic, systemic autoimmune disorder whose major distinctive feature is exhibited primarily by chronic, symmetrical, and erosive inflammation of the synovial tissue of joints. Pharmacologic treatment of this disorder is one of the most thoroughly researched areas in the treatment of rheumatic disorders. (Many new medications, approved by the Food and Drug Administration following thorough research studies, are discussed in the Integrating Pharmacology feature on Medications Used in the Treatment of Rheumatoid Arthritis on pp. 2342 to 2344.) However, this has not always been true. Many of the early treatments were based on anecdotal reports written by health care providers about clients treated within their own practice.

Careful review of the literature relating to new therapies as well as new evidence about older treatment standards is necessary. Four selected studies that address the use of biologic response modifiers (BRMs) in addition to the more traditional disease-modifying antirheumatic agents (DMARDs) have been reviewed.[1-4] As a result of these studies, much more is known about RA, its progression, and the damage that occurs to joints without overt clinical manifestations.

All four studies used double-blind, controlled methods to evaluate the medications studied by measuring ACR 20 and Sharp Scores as recommended by the American College of Rheumatology.[1-4] Study sizes ranged from 148 participants in the Tugwell study[4] to 999 in the Emery study.[2] Methotrexate and placebo were found to be less effective than methotrexate and cyclosporine combined.[4] Leflunomide and methotrexate were both found to be effective when compared, but methotrexate had more side effects while showing some clinical benefit qualities.[2] Leflunomide, methotrexate, and sulfasalazine all resulted in statistically significantly less radiographic progression of RA compared with placebo.[3] Etanercept provided better and more rapid improvement than methotrexate while also resulting in fewer adverse effects and infections for clients on the etanercept regimen.[1] The use of more than one drug provided better outcomes according to ACR 20 and Sharp Scores than did single use of a drug.

Implications

As more pharmacologic agents are introduced for treatment of RA, the nurse will need to monitor results of studies according to ACR 20 and Sharp Scores. All of these agents have potential toxic side effects that need to be monitored closely by the nurse and the client. Additional research is needed to determine whether continued long-term use of multiple agents will result in less progression of RA over time while also limiting adverse side effects.

References

1. Bathon, J., et al. (2000). A comparison of etanercept and methotrexate in patients with early rheumatoid arthritis. *The New England Journal of Medicine, 343,* 1586-1593.
2. Emery, P., et al. (2000). A comparison of the efficacy and safety of leflunomide and methotrexate for the treatment of rheumatoid arthritis. *Rheumatology, 39,* 655-665.
3. Sharp, J., et al. (2000). Treatment with leflunomide slows radiographic progression of rheumatoid arthritis: Results from three randomized controlled trials of leflunomide in patients with active rheumatoid arthritis. Leflunomide Rheumatoid Arthritis Investigators Group. *Arthritis and Rheumatism, 43,* 495-505.
4. Tugwell, P. (1995). Combination therapy with cyclosporine and methotrexate in severe rheumatoid arthritis. The Methotrexate-Cyclosporine Combination Study Group. *The New England Journal of Medicine, 333,* 137-141.

has been disrupted, with resultant damage to body tissues or cells normally recognized as self. Autoimmune disorders with muscle and joint involvement include SLE, RA, dermatomyositis, scleroderma, Sjögren's syndrome, and mixed connective tissue disease.

To understand systemic, arthritic autoimmune diseases, it is important to briefly review key components of the immune system. The immune system consists of immune cells (primarily B lymphocytes, T lymphocytes, and macrophages) and central and peripheral lymphoid structures. Immune cells are primarily produced in the central immune organs of the bone marrow and thymus. These cells interact with antigens (i.e., substances perceived as foreign to the body) in the peripheral lymphoid structures of the lymph nodes, spleen, tonsils, and other areas where lymphoid tissue is located. As the B lymphocytes and T lymphocytes travel throughout the body, they selectively seek out and destroy foreign antigens while sparing cells identified as self.

The ability of the immune system to distinguish self from non-self depends in large part on cell-surface antigens. These antigens (which are unique to every person) are encoded by a large cluster of genes called the *major histocompatibility complex* (MHC) located on the short end of chromosome 6. Histocompatibility antigens are also more typically referred to as *human leukocyte antigens* (HLAs) because they were first discovered on leukocytes. Seven closely related gene loci have been identified: HLA-A, HLA-B, HLA-C, HLA-D, HLA-DR, HLA-DQ, and HLA-DP. Each of these gene loci is occupied by multiple alleles (alternate genes) that code the development of each surface antigen. At least 23 gene products are associated with the HLA-A group, and 47 are associated with the HLA-B group.

HLAs have been categorized into two groups. Found on the surface of nucleated cells, class I antigens include HLA-A, HLA-B, and HLA-C antigens. Class II antigens (D, DR, DQ, and DP) are found on macrophage and B cells, among others.[4]

As a result of aberrations in HLA activity genetic coding, the body may lose some of its ability to recognize and differentiate self from non-self, resulting in autoimmune disorders. In other words, the body has decreased self-tolerance. Abnormalities of the HLA system, however, are but one key to the development of autoimmunity. Others involve abnormal T- or B-cell reactivity, resulting in altered recognition of foreign antigens and self by the immune system. For example, altered T-cell function has been implicated in the pathogenesis of arthritic diseases, such as RA. Research has begun to identify the specific roles of various T cells in these disease processes. For example, CD4$^+$ T cells have been shown to have a crucial role in the pathogenesis of arthritis, and CD8$^+$ T cells may play an immunoregulatory role. In addition, research suggests that B cells in the synovial membrane of joints expand as a result of local antigen stimulation.

It is also likely that the immune system can be altered by interactions with chemical, environmental, viral, and bacterial agents.

Another important aspect of autoimmune disease is familial aggregation (or clustering), which suggests that there is a genetic predisposition to the development of specific disorders. This possibility is not surprising because an individual's HLA type is inherited. Indeed, some HLA types appear more frequently in certain disease conditions. For example, in Caucasians HLA-B27 appears in 80% to 90% of persons with ankylosing spondylitis but in only 7% to 10% of persons in the general population.

RHEUMATOID ARTHRITIS

RA is a chronic, systemic autoimmune disorder whose major distinctive feature is chronic, symmetrical, and erosive inflammation of the synovial tissue of joints. The severity of the joint disease may fluctuate over time, but progressive development of various degrees of joint destruction, deformity, and disability are the most common outcomes of established disease. Associated nonarticular manifestations may include subcutaneous nodules, vasculitis, pulmonary nodules or interstitial fibrosis, and pericarditis.

Table 79-1 illustrates the seven criteria for the 1987-revised classification of RA.[2] The criteria highlight the symmetrical involvement of inflamed joints of the wrist, the metacarpophalangeal (MCP) joints, and the proximal interphalangeal (PIP) joints. The distal interphalangeal (DIP) joints are rarely involved in RA and are more commonly affected in osteoarthritis. Four or more of the seven criteria must be met before the disease is classified as RA. In addition, the first four criteria relating to stiffness and swelling must be present for at least 6 weeks, and criteria 2 through 5 (swelling and subcutaneous nodules) must be observed by a physician. These criteria remain the hallmark for classification of RA.

The prevalence of RA is estimated to range from 0.5% to 1.5% of the population. After age 55 years, the prevalence rates for men and women are estimated to be 2% and 5%, respectively. Prevalence rates for African Americans are similar to those for Caucasian Americans. RA appears to be a relatively "recent" disease. It was first described in the mid-18th century and has not been found in skeletal remains from ancient European or Asian civilizations. However, erosive polyarthritis has been documented in the skeletons of prehistoric (3000 to 5000 years ago) Native Americans, which might indicate an infectious agent confined to a small geographic area before the 18th century.[19]

Rheumatoid arthritis occurs worldwide and affects all racial and ethnic groups. It can occur at any time of life, but its incidence tends to increase with age, peaking between the fourth and sixth decades. Women are affected two to three times more often than men. Clients with RA have a substantially reduced life expectancy, and mortality can be predicted, in most instances, by more severe clinical status.[4] Overall, the disease is characterized by cycles of exacerbation and remission, the duration of which adds to the feelings of powerlessness and uncertainty that clients with RA often experience. A small percentage of clients have a severely progressive disease that does not respond to aggressive therapy.[4]

Etiology and Risk Factors

RA is characterized by the presence of RF, an autoantibody directed against immunoglobulin G (IgG) in more than 80% of clients with the disease.[19] In addition to RF, antibodies against collagen, Epstein-Barr virus, encoded nuclear antigen, and certain other antigens have been identified in clients with RA. The role of autoantibodies in RA is still unclear, but research has focused attention on pre-illness immunologic status in the pathogenesis of RA. Antikeratin antibody (AKA) and anti-perinuclear factor (APF) appear to be markers that predict the development of RA in RF-positive clients. However, RA develops in only a proportion of cases. Other immunogenetic markers may aid in the identification of clients with early RA with more severe disease. RA may be mild and relapsing, involving a few joints for a brief period, or markedly progressive, with the development of deformities and severe systemic disease.

Genetic factors are important in the epidemiology of the disease. A genetic predisposition for RA is seen with a higher concordance rate of 32% in identical twins rather than the 9% rate observed in fraternal twins. Other research suggests that the reason for consistent reports by female RA clients that joint pain and swelling disappear during pregnancy is because of the genetic differences between mother and fetus. Although these data are speculative, this is an exciting area for continuing research. The strongest genetic evidence, however, is seen in the association of RA with HLA-DR4, a genetically determined allele of the MHC on the short arm of chromosome 6.

Pathophysiology

The histologic changes in RA are not disease specific but rather largely depend on the organ involved. The primary joint lesion involves the synovium. RF antibodies develop there against IgG, the largest of the five classes of immunoglobulins, to form immune complexes. IgG is a natural human antibody. It is not clear, however, why the body produces an antibody (RF) against its own antibody (IgG) and, in effect, transforms IgG to an antigen or foreign protein that must be destroyed. The products of macrophages and lymphocytes are thought to have critical roles in the pathogenesis of RA as part of the immune response to an unidentified antigen. Moreover,

it is the formation of these antibody-antigen immune complexes that leads to the activation of the complement system and the release of lysosomal enzymes from leukocytes. Both of these reactions cause inflammation. Initial research has demonstrated that interleukin-8, known as neutrophil-activating peptide 1 (NAP-1), has a definite role in the inflammatory process of RA and that circulating autoantibodies may provide a clinically useful marker for RA severity. With the initial formation of immune complexes, synovitis develops as the synovial membrane becomes swollen, irritated, and inflamed. See the Concept Map feature on Understanding Rheumatoid Arthritis and Its Treatment on p. 2334.

As the immune complexes are deposited onto the synovial membrane or the superficial layers of the articular cartilage, they are phagocytized by polymorphonuclear (PMN) leukocytes, monocytes, and lymphocytes. Phagocytosis deactivates the immune complexes and simultaneously produces additional enzymes (oxygen radicals, arachidonic acid) that lead to hyperemia, edema, swelling, and thickening of the synovial lining. The hypertrophied synovium invades the surrounding tissue, including cartilage, ligaments, joint capsule, and tendons. Eventually, granulation tissue forms to cover the entire articular cartilage, leading to the formation of *pannus*, a highly vascularized fibrous scar tissue composed of lymphocytes, macrophages, histiocytes, fibroblasts, and mast cells. Pannus, which is the most destructive element in RA, can erode and destroy articular cartilage, eventually resulting in subchondral bone erosions, bone cysts, fissures, and development of bone spurs and osteophytes. Research has identified tumor necrosis factor (TNF), which is produced by cells at the cartilage-pannus junction and which may lead to cartilage destruction. Pannus can also scar and shorten tendons and ligaments, conditions that in turn lead to ligamentous laxity, subluxation, and contractures. See the Concept Map feature on Understanding Rheumatoid Arthritis and Its Treatment on p. 2334.

The course of RA is variable and unpredictable.[21] Some people experience flares and remissions and others a progressive course. Over the years, structural damage may occur, often leading to articular deformities and functional impairment. Thanks to increased awareness, research, and more aggressive treatment, clients with RA can expect a less ominous future than that described by Yellin in 1987, which predicted that most persons with RA would be unable to work 10 years after the initial diagnosis.[3]

Clinical Manifestations

Clinical manifestations of RA vary not only from one client to another but also in individual clients over the course of their disease. Explosive acute polyarticular onset evolving over several days also can occur. Rheumatoid arthritis usually begins gradually, over a period of

CONCEPT MAP   *evolve*

Understanding Rheumatoid Arthritis and Its Treatment

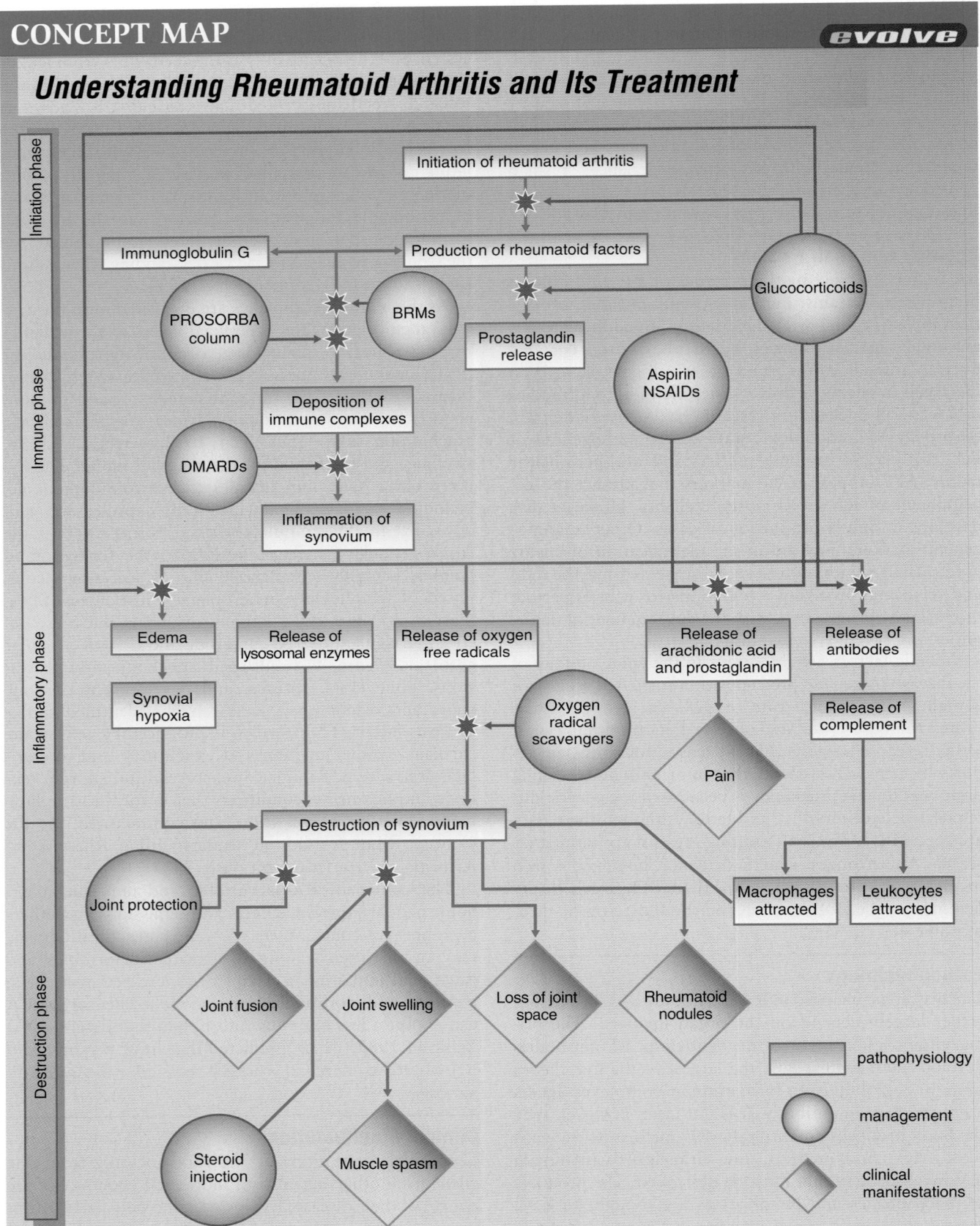

several weeks to months; accompanied by systemic manifestations, such as anorexia, weight loss, fatigue, muscle aching, and stiffness. Joint pain and swelling are associated with morning stiffness that can last several hours. Joint involvement is usually polyarticular and symmetrical, with the most frequently affected joints being those in the fingers, hands, wrists, knees, and feet.

Bilateral symmetrical involvement of the hands (wrists, MCP joints, and PIP joints) is characteristic of RA. Inflammation of the PIP joints contributes to the spindle-shaped appearance of the fingers. Tenosynovitis of the flexor tendons of the fingers is common, along with swelling and tenderness of the ulnar styloid process. Decreased dorsiflexion of the wrist occurs early in the disease and can be more painful than changes in the finger joints. With time, progressive synovial damage leads to characteristic deformities of the hands: ulnar deviation of the MCP joints of the fingers and medial deviation of the wrist. Figure 79-1 depicts three types of hand deformities characteristic of RA. A swan-neck deformity (hyperextension of the PIP joint with flexion of the MCP and DIP joints) results from contractures of the intrinsic muscles and tendons. The boutonnière deformity (flexion of the PIP and hyperextension of the DIP joints) is due to rupture of the extensor tendons over the fingers. Carpal tunnel syndrome, the compression of the median nerve as a result of tenosynovitis on the volar aspect of the wrist, is fairly common in RA. All of these changes lead to decreased hand strength and the ability to maintain a tight pinch.

The shoulders, elbows, and spine are also affected. Shoulder arthritis is seen with late disease, whereas the elbows can become flexed and contracted with early disease. Spinal involvement is usually limited to the cervical area. Atlantoaxial subluxation can lead to tenderness, muscle spasm, persistent head tilt, and occipital headache.

In the lower extremities, RA frequently affects the feet and knees. Cock-up toes result from plantar subluxation of the metatarsal heads. Walking can be difficult because of limited flexion and extension of the ankle. Active synovitis is often seen in swelling over the medial and lateral aspects of the patella. Popliteal cysts (Baker's cysts) can develop behind the knee joint.

As a systemic disease, RA can affect almost every body system. Extra-articular manifestations of RA are summarized in Table 79-2. Three of them, however, are more frequently seen in RA. These include rheumatoid nodules (Figure 79-2), Sjögren's syndrome, and Felty's syndrome. Rheumatoid nodules, granuloma-type lesions that develop around small blood vessels, can develop in up to 50% of clients with RA. Usually, those affected have high titers of RF.[19] Generally firm, mobile, and painless, rheumatoid nodules appear over the extensor surfaces of joints, such as elbows and fingers, but may be found anywhere in the body, even in the lungs. These can

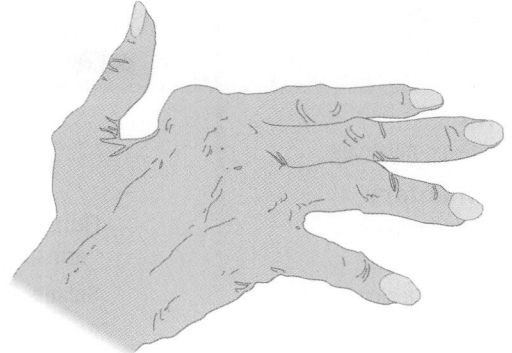

Ulnar drift

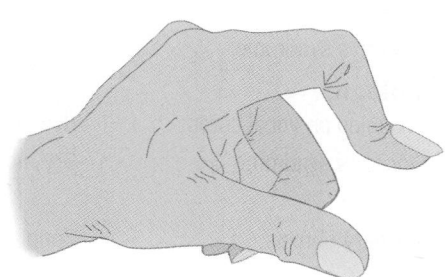

Boutonnière deformity

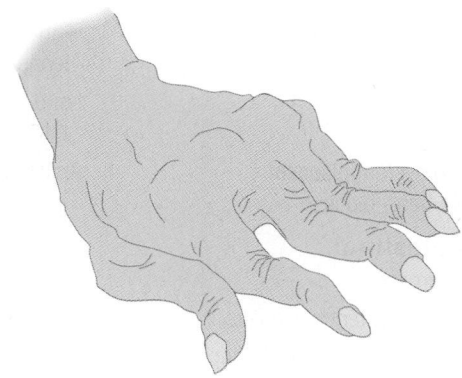

Swan-neck deformity

FIGURE 79-1 Three types of hand deformity characteristic of clients with rheumatoid arthritis.

easily break down or become infected. What part these nodules play in RA is unknown.

Secondary Sjögren's syndrome, keratoconjunctivitis sicca, is seen in about 10% to 15% of clients with RA. It may also occur as a disorder by itself or with other connective tissue disease, such as SLE or polymyositis. Clients with Sjögren's syndrome have diminished lacrimal and salivary gland secretion. They may complain of gritty, burning, or sandy eyes, with decreased tearing, itching, and photosensitivity.[8]

TABLE 79-2	*Extra-Articular Manifestations of Rheumatoid Arthritis*
Feature	**Assessment Parameter**
General	
Fatigue, fever, myalgias	
Integumentary	
Rheumatoid nodules	Firm, mobile, nontender subcutaneous nodes on the extensor surface of the fore-arms, legs, occiput, sacrum. May occur wherever there is pressure.
Vasculitic skin lesions	Splinter hemorrhages on nails.
Purpura	Ecchymosis, bruises, or ischemic involvement, especially on lower extremities.
Ocular	
Episcleritis	Pain and visual discomfort.
Scleritis	Pain and visual impairment; raised nodules on superior sclerae.
Secondary Sjögren's syndrome	Dry eyes, burning, itching, photophobia, decreased tearing.
Otolaryngologic	
Rheumatoid nodules on vocal cords	Hoarseness.
Secondary Sjögren's syndrome	Dry mouth, decreased saliva.
Pulmonary	
Pleuritis, pulmonary fibrosis, pleural effusions	Cough, dyspnea, crackles (fine rales), decreased thoracic expansion.
Pulmonary nodules, with or without cavitation	As described for pleuritis.
Cardiac	
Pericarditis, myocarditis	High-pitched, scratchy pericardial friction rubs. May increase in intensity when client leans forward and exhales.
Mitral valve disease	Loud, high-pitched blowing murmur characteristic of mitral regurgitation. May have third heart sound (S_3).
Conduction system disease: complete heart block	Apical pulse, usually 25 to 45 beats/min.
Gastrointestinal	
Felty's syndrome	Enlarged spleen.
Bowel and mesenteric vasculitis	Pain after meals; epigastric bruit.
Malabsorption due to amyloid deposits	Frequent loose, watery stools; abdominal distention.
Renal	
Proteinuria	Urinalysis.
Neurologic	
Myelopathy (C1–2 vertebral subluxation)	History of transient ischemic attacks (dizziness, numbness, paresthesias, temporary loss of vision).
Carpal tunnel syndrome	Decreased grip strength, thenar atrophy, positive Phalen's test, Tinel's sign.
Posterior tibial nerve entrapment	Decreased sensation in first dorsal web space. Eliciting numbness and paresthesias after tapping the tarsal tunnel at the ankle joint medial to the dorsalis pedis.
Hematologic	
Anemia	Hypochromic, microcytic anemia with low serum ferritin and low or normal iron-binding capacity.
Felty's syndrome	Combination of splenomegaly, leukopenia, lymphadenopathy, thrombocytopenia, HLA-DR4 haplotype, and leg ulcers.

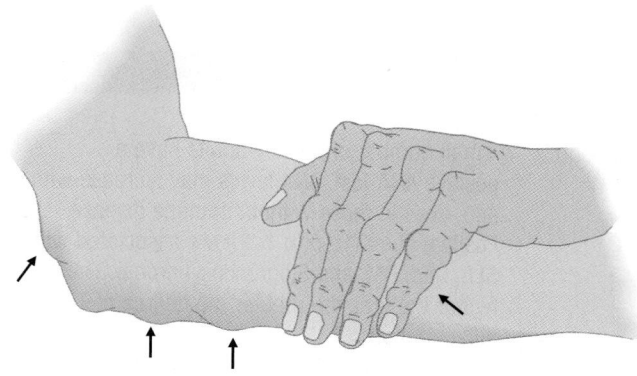

FIGURE 79-2 Rheumatoid nodules.

Felty's syndrome was originally described as the combination of RA, splenomegaly, leukopenia, and leg ulcers. Subsequent observations have shown an association with lymphadenopathy, thrombocytopenia, and the HLA-DR4 haplotype occurring most commonly in clients with severe, nodule-forming RA. Other extra-articular problems seen in RA include inflammatory eye disorders, infection, pulmonary disease, vasculitis, and cardiac abnormalities.[19]

The 1987 revised criteria for the classification of RA (see Table 79-1) serve as a framework for the clinical diagnosis.[2] The classification system, however, is not intended to explicitly define diagnostic criteria. Other findings, including the results of laboratory tests, radiologic examination, and synovial fluid analysis, help to confirm the diagnosis.

Laboratory Testing

The laboratory evaluation of clients with rheumatic disease is often informative but rarely definitive. Laboratory testing is important in the diagnosis of RA, even though no single set of chemical, serologic, or hematologic tests confirms the diagnosis. Table 79-3 lists laboratory tests commonly used in the diagnosis of RA and other rheumatic diseases. Serum and urine chemistries are usually normal in RA. Occasionally, proteinuria and microscopic hematuria are seen as a result of amyloid deposits in the kidney. Elevated erythrocyte sedimentation rates (ESRs) and C-reactive protein (CRP) levels are typical of active disease, with the CRP being a more definitive indicator of inflammation. Hematologic studies often indicate a mild normocytic, hypochromic anemia along with thrombocytosis. An underlying iron anemia is usually present if the hemoglobin is less than 10 g/ml and ferritin levels are low. Low eosinophil counts occur with increased disease activity, and granulocytopenia may indicate Felty's syndrome.

Serologic tests used to confirm the diagnosis of RA include antinuclear antibodies (ANAs) and RF. ANA titers

are seen in 15% to 20% of clients; of these, more half have Felty's syndrome. RF, an autoantibody directed against IgM, is positive in only 80% of clients. Higher titers are seen in active disease. The presence of IgM RF, however, is not specific for RA. Increased levels can be seen in older adults or after infections or immunizations. RF titers are also present in other rheumatic disorders, including SLE, dermatomyositis, and SSc, and in liver and pulmonary disease. The absence of a positive RF test does not exclude the diagnosis of RA in a client with typical clinical characteristics. Clients can convert from negative to positive with an exacerbation in their manifestations. Clients with seronegative RA, however, have better outcomes and rarely have extra-articular involvement. Recent evidence points to recognition that seronegative and seropositive polyarthritis are separate entities.

Radiologic Studies

Radiologic findings help to confirm disease activity and monitor treatment results. In the early stages, soft tissue swelling is indicated by increased shadowing around the affected joint (Figure 79-3). Massive tissue swelling of the entire joint often precedes further destructive changes, such as periarticular osteoporosis. Subchondral cysts may develop from the invasion of granulation tissue. As the disease progresses, subchondral bone erosions develop, ultimately causing a narrowing of the joint space. In mild disease, erosions may not develop for 6 to 12 months. Initially occurring at the joint margins where the capsule is attached, erosions are first seen in the small joints of the hands and feet, where the bone is less dense. Subluxation and malalignment of the joints can be seen on x-ray study, reflecting the destructive changes seen on physical examination. With advanced disease, subchondral bone destruction and diffuse osteoporosis appear.[10]

Other Procedures

Synovial fluid analysis indicates a change from the normal transparent color to a milky, cloudy, or dark yellow fluid. Arthroscopic examinations typically show pale, thick, edematous synovial villi, cartilage destruction, and fibrous scar formation (pannus). Bone and joint scans can be used to detect early joint changes and more readily confirm the diagnosis.

Outcome Management

There has been considerable effort devoted to the development of outcome measures in RA. A proposed set of core RA measures includes pain measurement, disability, physician and client global assessment, number of tender and swollen joints, and acute-phase reactants. In addition, the ACR developed a statistically powerful

TABLE 79-3	*Common Diagnostic Studies Used in Rheumatic Diseases*	
Test and Purpose	**Normal Value**	**Significance**
Antinuclear antibody (ANA) ANAs are gamma globulins that react to specific antigens. ANA titer indicates the presence of antibodies that are produced in response to the nuclear part of the white blood cell. Positive ANA should be interpreted in light of titer and specific autoantibody profile.	Titer >1:32 (lab dependent) Patterns: Peripheral Diffuse Speckled Nucleolar	A small number of healthy adults have a positive ANA test. ANA levels may increase with age, even in those without immune disease. Positive titers (1:10 to 1:30) are associated with SLE, SSc, DM, and Sjögren's syndrome. The higher the titer, the greater the degree of inflammation.
ANA subsets: anti-Ro antibody and CH50.	Positive	When SLE is suspected and the ANA is negative.
Anti-Sm and anti-dsDNA.	Positive	Highly specific for SLE but not highly sensitive and subject to variability by laboratory and assay used.
Antineutrophilic cytoplasmic antibodies (ANCAs): ANCAs are directed against several antigens—c-ANCA cytoplasmic staining and p-ANCA peripheral staining.	Positive	c-ANCA 80% sensitive for active diffuse Wegener's granulomatosis, and for crescentic or necrotizing glomerulonephritis, P-ANCA drug-induced lupus, and SLE.
C4 Complement Method to determine serum hemolytic complement activity. Complement is a protein that binds antigen-antibody complexes for purposes of lysis. Activation of the entire complement system leads to an inflammatory response that destroys or damages cells. When the number of antigen-antibody complexes increases markedly, complement is used for lysis, thus decreasing its availability.	Men: 12 to 72 mg/dl Women: 14 to 75 mg/dl	Increased in active inflammatory disease and in autoimmune disorders (rheumatoid spondylitis, JRA). May be decreased in RA and SLE.
C-Reactive protein (CRP) Indicates presence of abnormal plasma protein (glycoprotein) that appears as a nonspecific response to a variety of inflammatory stimuli.	Trace to 6 mg/ml	CRP is a nonspecific antigen-antibody reaction test to help determine the extent or severity of a disease process. Elevated measurements indicate active inflammation, both infectious and noninfectious. Elevated in RA, bacterial and viral infections, disseminated lupus erythematosus. In RA, test becomes negative with successful therapy, indicating that the inflammatory reaction has disappeared, although the ESR may continue to be elevated.
Erythrocyte sedimentation rate (ESR) Measures the rate at which RBCs settle out of unclotted blood in 1 hr.	*Wintrobe* Men: 0 to 7 mm/hr Women: 0 to 25 mm/hr *Westergren* Men: 0 to 20 mm/hr Women: 0 to 30 mm/hr Higher elevations are seen in both men and women older than age 50 years.	Increased rate seen in inflammation and necrotic processes. An increase is often seen in any inflammatory connective tissue disease, often indicating increased inflammation and resulting in clustering of RBCs, which makes them heavier than normal. The higher the sedimentation rate, the greater the inflammatory activity. ESR is particularly useful as a guide to the management of the client with RA. ESR is decreased in salicylate toxicity. ESR is falsely elevated with excessive exercise, anxiety, pain, or dehydration.

DM, *Diabetes mellitus;* ESR, *erythrocyte sedimentation rate;* SLE, *systemic lupus erythematosus;* SSc, *systemic sclerosis (scleroderma);* JRA, *juvenile rheumatoid arthritis;* RA, *rheumatoid arthritis;* RBCs, *red blood cells;* AS, *ankylosing spondylitis.*

TABLE 79-3 *Common Diagnostic Studies Used in Rheumatic Diseases—cont'd*		
Test and Purpose	**Normal Value**	**Significance**
HLA-B27 antigen Measures the presence of HLA-B27, which is used for tissue typing/tissue recognition. Five series have been designated for HLA (i.e., A, B, C, D, DR), each with 10 to 20 distinct antigens	Titer 1:32	Primary use is to predict the compatibility of donor/recipient tissues and platelets. HLA-B27 is found in 80% to 90% of those with AS and Reiter's syndrome. It is also found in persons with the pauciarticular subgroup of JRA. The presence of HLA-B27 does not always signify disease, in that HLA-B27 is also seen in 8% of general population.
Immunoglobulin electrophoresis Measures the values of immunoglobulins, serum antibodies produced by the plasma cells of the B lymphocytes. Five classes: IgA—protects mucous membranes from viruses and bacteria IgM—first responder to appear after antigens enter body; produces antibody against rheumatoid factor IgG—produces antibodies against bacteria, viruses, toxins IgD—less active IgE—less active	*IgA:* 85 to 385 mg/dl *IgG:* 565 to 1700 mg/dl *IgM:* 55 to 370 mg/dl *IgD:* trace *IgE:* trace	Basic function of immunoglobulins is to neutralize toxic substances (antigens) to allow phagocytosis. Unique because of their genetic coding: each immunoglobulin interacts with other molecules. The recognition mechanism of the immunoglobulin forms the basis of the immune response. Increased levels are found in autoimmune diseases, specifically IgM (lupus, RA) and IgG (RA).
Radioallergosorbent test (RAST) Measures the quantity and increase of the antigen IgE present in the serum after exposure to a specific antigen.	0.01 to 0.04 mg/dl	Elevated with allergic reactions: asthma, hay fever, dermatitis. May be used to evaluate suspected allergic responses in clients on gold therapy.
RBC count Measures the number of circulating erythrocytes per cubic millimeter of blood.	Men: 4.7 to 6.1 million (mn)/mm³ Women: 4.2 to 5.4 mn/mm³	Normal values vary according to age. When the value is >10% below the normal value, the client is considered to be anemic. Decreased in SLE, RA, chronic inflammation.
Rheumatoid factor (RF) Determines the measurement for RF, a macroglobulin (antibody) directed toward a gamma globulin (IgG). Two tests are used: latex fixation and sheep red cell agglutination	≥1:160 considered significant in latex fixation Greater than 1:16 considered significant for agglutination titer (lab dependent)	Positive RF present in 70% to 90% of persons with RA. Negative RF found in 10% to 30% of clients with clinical diagnosis of RA. Positive RF may also suggest SLE or mixed connective tissue disease. The higher the titer (the number to the right of the colon), the greater the degree of inflammation. Titer is normally increased in older persons and in those who have had multiple vaccinations or blood transfusions.

definition of improvement in RA: 20% improvement in tender and swollen joint counts and 20% improvement in three of the five remaining ACR core set measures of client and physician global assessments, pain, disability, and an acute-phase reactant. These research advances continue to clarify effective and appropriate management strategies for RA clients. The plan of care for clients with manifestations suggestive of RA should (1) establish a diagnosis of RA as early as possible, (2) determine the stage of disease (joint destruction) and disease activity (inflammation), (3) define relevant factors that affect prognosis, (4) establish a plan for treatment as early as possible, (5) monitor disease activity and response to treatment, and (6) modify the treatment when client response is absent or inadequate.

■ Medical Management

Effective management of RA involves a combination of medications, rest, exercise, and methods of joint protection to achieve the primary goals of providing pain reduction, reducing joint inflammation, protecting articular surfaces to prevent bone and cartilage destruction,

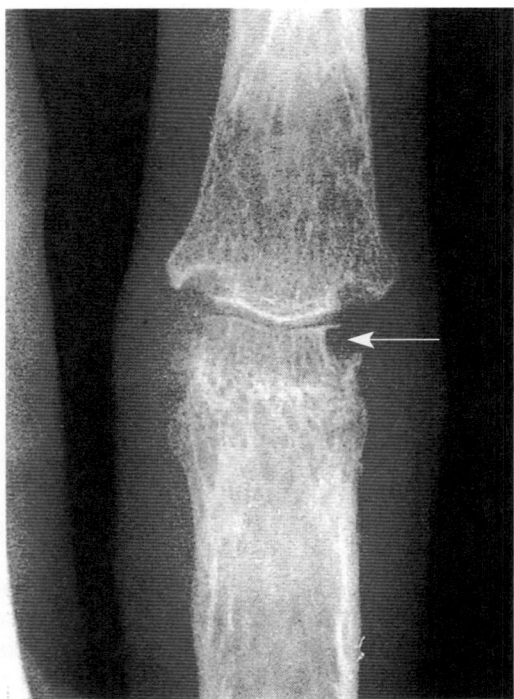

FIGURE 79-3 Radiograph of an interphalangeal joint affected by rheumatoid arthritis. Pocket erosion is shown with the arrow. Pocket erosions can spread into trabecular bone and weaken the bone surface. There is also joint space narrowing and soft tissue swelling. (From Resnick, D., Berthiaume, M.J., & Sartoris, D. [1993]: Imaging. In Kelley, W.N., et al. [Eds.], *Textbook of rheumatology* [4th ed., p. 600]. Philadelphia: W. B. Saunders.)

maintaining or restoring joint function, and controlling systemic involvement. The treatment paradigms for severe RA have changed significantly since 1998 and the advent of the immunomodulator leflunomide (Arava); the BRMs, such as etanercept (Enbrel), infliximab (Remicade), and adalimumab (Humira); and a medical device known as the PROSORBA column.

The treatment and management of RA depend on successful collaboration between the client and the entire health care team—physician, nurse, and physical or occupational therapist. Other team members—orthopedic surgeon, nutritionist, social worker, and orthotist—may be required as the client's needs change. The totally dependent RA client is uncommon today, in large part due to advances in joint replacement surgery and the advent of new therapies.

Education is the foundation of the successful treatment of RA. Many of the major content areas, such as fatigue, energy conservation, exercise, and stress management, require considerable follow-up, monitoring, and reinforcement over time. Families must also be educated about the disease process and its impact on the family unit. Families must be helped to become partners with the client to effectively manage the disease and enable the client to function at the highest level of his or her abilities.

Collaboration between health care providers is necessary for teaching and reinforcing the unpredictable nature of the disease. Clients need to understand that the disease is chronic, characterized by remission and exacerbation in most of those affected, and therefore it is somewhat unpredictable. This unpredictability can affect, on a daily basis, the client's ability to do simple tasks. The lack of certainty with which the client and

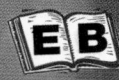

COMPLEMENTARY AND ALTERNATIVE THERAPY

Can Writing Heal?

In a unique study, clients with asthma or rheumatoid arthritis were told to either (1) write about the most stressful event of their lives for 20 minutes a day (for 3 consecutive days a week) or (2) write about nonstressful things (e.g., grocery lists). The group that wrote about stressful events actually had a decrease in their asthma (within 2 weeks) or rheumatoid arthritis manifestations (within 4 months), whereas the other group did not experience this benefit.

Reference
Hurewitz, A., et al. (1999). Effects of writing about stressful experiences on symptom reduction in patients with asthma or rheumatoid arthritis: a randomized trial, *Journal of the American Medical Association, 281,* 1304-1309.

family can plan ahead for outings and special activities can be frustrating for all parties. Individual and family stress can escalate to the point where family counseling is required. Reinforcing positive coping strategies and recommending stress management techniques, however, can help clients avoid feelings of powerlessness and helplessness.

For more information on alternative therapy, see the Complementary and Alternative Therapy feature on Can Writing Heal? on p. 2340.

Reduce Pain and Inflammation. Reduction of pain and inflammation is most often achieved with pharmacologic management, which usually combines a nonsteroidal anti-inflammatory (NSAID), a DMARD/BRM, and short intermittent courses of oral corticosteroids. Medications are changed in response to lack of efficacy or if the initial improvement fades. The use of single-drug therapy has been shown to be of limited benefit in the treatment of RA. Most clients who are prescribed a single agent are no longer taking that agent 3 years later. Combination therapy is most effective if introduced within the first 2 years after diagnosis of RA. MTX in combination with the BRMs has a synergistic effect, as does MTX and the immunomodulator leflunomide. See the Integrating Pharmacology feature on Medications Used in the Treatment of Rheumatoid Arthritis on pp. 2342 to 2344. These medications reduce pain and inflammation as well as control systemic involvement.

Whole-body rest can decrease joint inflammation. Many clients with RA find that an afternoon nap reduces fatigue and helps them cope with the rest of the day.

PROSORBA Column. PROSORBA column, a medical device used in conjunction with apheresis, employs approximately 200 mg of protein A covalently bound to an inert silica matrix that is contained within a 300-ml polycarbonate housing. Each column contains 123 *plus or minus* 2 g of this matrix. Protein A is a component of certain strains of the *Staphylococcus* bacterium and it has the propensity to bind IgG with IgG bound to an antigen, that is, circulating immune complex. The PROSORBA column is indicated for use in the therapeutic reduction of the manifestations of severe RA in adult clients with long-standing disease that has failed or who are intolerant of DMARDs. The procedure requires 12 weekly apheresis procedures. A plasma volume of 1250 plus or minus 250 ml is passed through the column. Clients must have good intravenous access. The therapeutic effect is usually not noticed until completion of the 12 weeks.

Protect Articular Surfaces. One important interrelated area of content concerns principles of joint protection and work simplification. In a multidisciplinary setting, principles of joint protection and work simplification can be taught by the occupational therapist and rein-

forced by the nurse. Education in these areas can have a positive effect on increased energy levels and decreased fatigue, thereby improving the client's coping abilities and sense of control.

Specific suggestions or anticipatory guidance about self-care can be beneficial. For example, clients should select easy-to-grip combs and brushes with large handles. These devices are readily available at almost all department stores. Using a long-handled bath brush to reach the feet and back during bathing is much less stressful on the joints. Selecting attractive, adaptable clothing is easier now that many department stores and mail-order catalogs have included a home care section. Jogging suits with pull-on pants and large, easily zippered tops are comfortable and attractive. Adaptive equipment for dressing includes long-handled shoehorns, zipper pulls, and buttoners. Involvement of the feet, the metatarsophalangeals (MTPs), can seriously affect the ability to ambulate and enjoy life. Referral to an orthotist for proper supportive shoes and or the use of orthotics is essential to reduce pain and prevent further joint damage. Table 79-4 discusses principles of joint protection and associated work simplification strategies.

Maintain Function. Therapeutic exercise is another important modality in the initial and ongoing treatment of RA. Three types of exercises are typically used: range of motion (ROM), strengthening, and endurance. The purpose of ROM exercises is to improve joint motion. ROM exercises can be passive, assisted, or active. Carried out by the therapist without any client effort, passive exercises are most often done when the client is totally unable to move the joint because of the lack of strength or voluntary control. The purpose of passive ROM is to ensure joint movement when there is a risk of developing contractures. Recent research has begun to identify a safe role for progressive resistance exercise training in selected clients with well-controlled RA that leads to significant improvements in strength, pain, and fatigue without exacerbating disease activity or joint pain.

When joint inflammation and flares have diminished, the client performs active ROM exercises as prescribed by the therapist. Although clients may be able to enjoy other therapeutic and recreational exercises, they need to understand that engaging in other activities or activities of daily living (ADL) is not a substitute for the ROM program.

Strengthening exercises are done to preserve or improve the muscle's ability to perform work. Two types of strengthening exercises are commonly used, isometric and isotonic. With isometric exercises, the muscle is contracted for 5 to 6 seconds, but the joint is not permitted to move. Common isometric techniques include gluteal folds and quadriceps-setting exercises. Isotonic exercises are used carefully in clients with RA because they require

INTEGRATING PHARMACOLOGY

Medications Used in the Treatment of Rheumatoid Arthritis

Nonselective NSAIDs

Nonsteroidal anti-inflammatory drugs (NSAIDs) are used to treat inflammation and swelling. NSAIDs suppress inflammation by interfering with the body's production of substances called prostaglandins. Prostaglandins play a major role in the process of inflammation and NSAIDs act by inhibiting their synthesis. The most common side effects of NSAID therapy occur in the gastrointestinal tract and include nausea and dyspepsia. More importantly, NSAIDs may cause gastric and duodenal ulcers. Studies have shown that 10% to 25% of arthritis clients who are on regular treatment with these drugs are found to have NSAID-related ulcers upon endoscopy. The primary serious complications from NSAID-induced ulcers are upper gastrointestinal perforation, obstruction, and hemorrhage. Serious complications develop in 2% to 4% of all clients.[1]

Selective NSAIDs

Cyclooxygenase-2 (COX-2) inhibitors, a group of drugs known as selective NSAIDs, block the key enzyme involved in the production of prostaglandin—cyclooxygenase. There are two forms of this enzyme, cyclooxygenase-1 (COX-1) and COX-2. COX-1 is present in all cells at all times and its purpose is to produce prostaglandins that regulate normal cellular processes; drugs that inhibit this enzyme are called nonselective NSAIDs. COX-2 is expressed almost completely in response to inflammation. COX-2 produces prostaglandins in the joints and synovium. Evidence suggests that the gastrointestinal side effects of NSAIDs are related to their ability to inhibit COX-1, whereas the beneficial anti-inflammatory effects are primarily the result of inhibition of COX-2.[1] Three selective NSAIDs that inhibit COX-2 have been developed. They are celecoxib (Celebrex), valdecoxib (Bextra), and rofecoxib (Vioxx). Efficacy is comparable between the COX-1 and COX-2 medications with the COX-2 drugs causing less gastrointestinal toxicity. In studies of 1 to 6 months' duration (although most were 3 months long), 0.04% of clients (2 of 5825) receiving celecoxib experienced significant upper gastrointestinal bleeding.[3] Twelve-month data showed no statistical difference between selective and nonselective NSAIDs.

Disease-Modifying Rheumatic Agents

When NSAIDs do not alter the course of RA, disease-modifying rheumatic agents (DMARDs) are usually considered when the client does not show an appropriate clinical response (i.e., decreases in pain, swelling, and stiffness) or when x-ray study shows evidence of bony erosions within the first 30 to 60 days of onset. DMARDs include the antimalarial agents hydroxychloroquine (HCQ), gold salts, penicillamine, methotrexate (MTX), azathioprine, sulfasalazine, and cyclosporine. Added to this array are the immunomodulatory drug leflunomide (Arava) and the biologic response modifiers (BRMs), etanercept (Enbrel), adalimumab (Humira) and infliximab (Remicade).

The antimalarial drug HCQ is widely used and has an acceptable toxicity profile and can be safely combined with other DMARDs. Maculopathy occurs almost exclusively at higher than recommended doses (6 mg/kg/day), although eye examinations are recommended every 6 months during therapy. HCQ is particularly effective in the early treatment of clients with mild to moderate or seronegative RA. Gold preparations have been used successfully to treat RA since the 1920s, although they are rarely used currently because of the length of onset of action. Recent 3-month to 6-month and long-term studies have demonstrated little clinical efficacy and continued disease progression.

After 20 years of research, MTX was approved in 1988 for the treatment of RA unresponsive to other agents. MTX was the first agent to demonstrate early onset of action and superior efficacy and tolerability compared to gold, HCQ, and sulfasalazine. Clinical benefit may be seen as early as 3 weeks after initiating treatment, and the maximal improvement is generally achieved by 6 months. Low-dose MTX administered once a week as a single dose (7.5 to 12.5 mg) has been reported to be effective with little toxicity. Adverse effects have been reported with both low-dose and parenteral administration, but they do not generally require discontinuing the drug. The most common side effect is gastrointestinal intolerance (anorexia, nausea, vomiting, diarrhea, weight loss). Other reactions are stomatitis, alopecia, and central nervous system effects, such as headache, dizziness, and depression. When bone marrow depression occurs, it is usually associated with renal impairment, folic acid depletion, and the use of trimethoprim-sulfamethoxazole. Opportunistic infections (e.g., *Pneumocystis carinii* infection) also occur in RA clients treated with MTX. It is uncertain whether preexisting lung disease predisposes RA clients to MTX pneumonitis. It appears that the most vulnerable time for developing infection during MTX therapy is in the first year of treatment. Literature also suggests that more MTX-associated infections occur in severe RA than in moderate RA. Drug toxicity, as opposed to lack of response to the medication, is the primary factor limiting the client's continued treatment. The probability of developing toxic effects (e.g., hepatotoxicity) when taking MTX is significant, especially during the first year of therapy. However, research has shown that folic acid supplementation decreases toxicity without compromising efficacy. The probability of continuing MTX up to 6 years after it was initiated, however, was nearly 50% in one study. These results were far superior to the less than 20%, 5-year retention rate of clients on sulfasalazine, penicillamine, or gold salts. MTX has become the accepted means of treatment for early RA. In addition, MTX in combination with cyclosporine has been shown to be more effective than cyclosporine alone and in combination with the BRMs. Folic acid, 1 mg/day, should be given because MTX inhibits folic acid reductase, leading to inhibition of DNA synthesis and inhibition of cellular replications.

INTEGRATING PHARMACOLOGY

Medications Used in the Treatment of Rheumatoid Arthritis—cont'd

Although numerous studies have shown penicillamine to be safe and effective in low doses (250 mg/day), it is not routinely used to treat RA. Penicillamine has a slow onset of action and a high frequency of side effects such as leukopenia and autoimmune disorders.

Another slow-acting agent, azathioprine, is metabolized in the body to 6-mercaptopurine, the active form of the drug. Azathioprine inhibits DNA synthesis and both humoral and cell-mediated immune responses. Consequently, B and T lymphocytes are reduced so that antibody production is limited. The clinical response to azathioprine is not evident for 3 to 4 months. When azathioprine is used in low doses of 1 to 2.5 mg/kg/day, most side effects are troublesome but short term; these include stomatitis, nausea, and vomiting. Bone marrow toxicity can occur, however, so complete blood counts are mandatory to screen for leukopenia. Oncogenesis is a major concern with the long-term use of azathioprine. Transplant clients who receive high doses of azathioprine have a higher incidence of lymphomas and neoplasms. It is not known, however, whether tumor development will occur in RA clients, who typically receive much lower doses of the drug.

Despite many studies demonstrating the clinical effectiveness of cyclosporine, its cost and potential for irreversible toxicity, even at low doses (2.5 to 5 mg/kg/day), have limited its use to severe, progressive RA refractory to all other DMARDs. A multicenter short-term study comparing RA clients treated with MTX alone to those receiving both cyclosporine and MTX demonstrated a clinically important (20%) improvement in disease activity, without substantial differences in side effects.

The alkylating agent cyclophosphamide is a highly effective agent for treating RA. However, this drug has been abandoned for routine use because of its high toxicity profile (i.e., oncogenicity, bladder hemorrhage, bone marrow toxicity, infertility). Cyclophosphamide is the drug of choice in RA vasculitis unresponsive to corticosteroids.

Leflunomide (Arava), a de novo blocker of purine synthesis, has been found to be effective in the treatment of RA. Leflunomide reversibly blocks the enzyme DHODH, which is active in the autoimmune process that leads to RA; blocking this enzyme relieves the manifestations of inflammation and blocks the structural damage caused by the inflammatory response to the autoimmune process.

Biologic Response Modifiers

BRMs that target specific cells or cytokines involved in the inflammatory response hold great promise for RA therapy because of their improved efficacy and limited toxicity. The first BRM to be approved by the Food and Drug Administration was etanercept. Etanercept binds specifically to tumor necrosis factor (TNF) and blocks its interaction with cell surface TNF receptors. TNF is a naturally occurring cytokine that is involved in normal inflammatory and immune responses. Etanercept is genetically engineered (TNF) receptors from Chinese hamster ovary cells that keep the inflammatory response to autoimmune disease in check by reacting with and deactivating free-floating TNF released by active leucocytes. Etanercept is currently indicated for reducing manifestations and delaying structural damage in clients with moderately to severely active RA.[4] Etanercept is a twice-weekly subcutaneous injection of 25 mg. Clients and their families have been very receptive to this form of treatment.

Infliximab (Remicade), in combination with MTX, is currently indicated for the reduction in manifestations of RA in clients who have had an inadequate response. Infliximab is a monoclonal antibody to TNF-alpha. It may be given alone or in combination with MTX. This is an intravenous infusion of 3 mg/kg over 2 hours. It is given initially, at 2 weeks, at 6 weeks, and then every 8 weeks.

Adalimumab is a recombinant fully human monoclonal anti-TNF-alpha antibody for the treatment of RA. The antibody is specific for TNF-alpha and does not bind to other cytokines. It does not possess nonhuman or artificially fused human sequences, suggesting a low propensity for immunogenicity.

Anakinra is a recombinant form of human interleukin-1 receptor antagonist. A subcutaneous injection of 100 mg/day is recommended for clients with RA. Anakinra was associated with an increased incidence of serious infections in clinical trials (2% versus less than 1% in placebo groups). Anakinra therapy should not be initiated in clients with active infections or neutropenia. Clients with asthma had higher rates of serious infection (5%) and concomitant treatment with etanercept was associated with higher rates of serious infections (7%) and neutropenia (3%). Injection site reactions are common (71%). Anakinra is indicated for adult clients with moderately to severely active RA who have failed at least one DMARD. It may be used as monotherapy or in combination with other DMARDs other than TNF-blocking agents. Candidates for this therapy must have good intravenous access. The therapeutic effect is usually not noticed until completion of the 12 weeks.

Corticosteroids

Corticosteroids produce an immediate and profound anti-inflammatory response in clients with RA. At low doses, corticosteroids demonstrate characteristics that are primarily anti-inflammatory rather than immunosuppressive. At higher doses, these agents are immunosuppressive by appearing to exert the greatest suppressive effect on T helper cells. In the 1940s and 1950s, cortisone was almost universally prescribed for the treatment of RA. Its use was quickly modulated by the many adverse effects associated with long-term administration and its lack of effectiveness in preventing disabling deformities.

Low-dose prednisone is used as a bridge, to carry clients from unsuccessful NSAID therapy until they experience the benefits of the slow-acting, disease-modifying agents. This time interval has

Continued

Medications Used in the Treatment of Rheumatoid Arthritis—cont'd

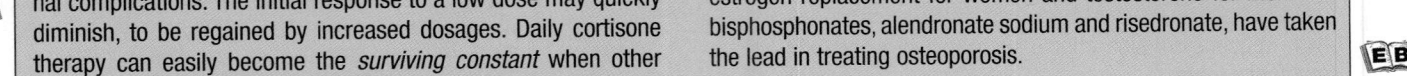

shortened considerably with the advent of the BRMs. More recent research found low-dose long-term prednisone use of less than 5 mg/day to be correlated with the development of adverse effects, specifically serious infections, fractures, and gastrointestinal complications. The initial response to a low dose may quickly diminish, to be regained by increased dosages. Daily cortisone therapy can easily become the *surviving constant* when other agents are discontinued because of toxicity or lack of effectiveness. Clearly, this therapy must be carefully monitored.

Determining whether a surgical client is steroid dependent has important implications for those undergoing surgery. Taking a drug history of the client with RA requires exploration of the use of steroids: when they were initiated, dosage history, and date they were discontinued. Steroid-dependent clients are those currently taking corticosteroids as well as those weaned from chronic corticosteroid therapy within the last year. Other clients at risk of steroid dependency include those who received regular intra-articular injections of steroids, psoriasis clients who routinely used topical steroids on large areas of the skin, and clients with inflammatory bowel disease who routinely used steroid enemas.[2] Steroid-dependent clients who undergo general anesthesia must receive stress doses of corticosteroids to prevent intraoperative shock. Three doses of intravenous hydrocortisone (100 mg each) are usually given before, during, and immediately after the surgical procedures. Corticosteroids have several unfortunate effects on bone metabolism: decreased calcium absorption, increased urinary calcium excretion, decreased bone formation, and bone resorption that may remain normal or increase. Treatment guide-lines have been published for treatment of steroid-induced osteoporosis. The defect in calcium absorption is treated with daily doses of 1500-mg calcium supplements and 800 international units of vitamin D. Treatment of low gonadotropin levels includes estrogen replacement for women and testosterone for men. The bisphosphonates, alendronate sodium and risedronate, have taken the lead in treating osteoporosis.

Investigational Agents

Research is currently being conducting using, IL-1RA, vaccines, CTLA 4 blockers of CD28, blockers of $CD4^+$, and inhibitors of IL-1β–converting enzyme (ICE). Research is focusing on the pathogenesis of disease and in halting disease progression.

References

1. Graham, D., et al. (2002). Ulcer prevention in long-term users of nonsteroidal anti-inflammatory drugs. *Archives of Internal Medicine, 162,* 169-175.
2. Mayes, M., et al. (2003). Prevalence, incidence, survival, and disease characteristics of systemic sclerosis in a large U.S. population. *Arthritis and Rheumatology, 48*(8), 2246-2255.
3. Simon, L., et al. (2002). Controversies on COX-2 selective inhibition. Consensus Conference Report. *Journal of Rheumatology, 29*(7), 1501-1510.
4. Weinblatt, M., et al. (1999). A trial of etanercept, a recombinant tumor necrosis factor receptor: Fc fusion protein, in clients with rheumatoid arthritis receiving methotrexate. *New England Journal of Medicine, 340,* 253-259.

TABLE 79-4	*Principles of Joint Protection and Associated Work Simplification Strategies*
Joint Protection Principles	**Strategies to Simplify Work**
1. Respect pain (fear of pain can lead to inactivity; ignoring pain can lead to joint damage).	Carry out activities and exercise only to the point of fatigue or discomfort. Reduce the time spent in doing painful activities. Avoid doing activities (other than gentle ROM) when joints are inflamed.
2. Balance work and rest.	Rest 5 to 10 min periodically when doing tasks that take more time. Get sufficient sleep. Take a 30-min rest during the afternoon.
3. Reduce effort to joints.	Slide objects rather than lift them. Store items at appropriate heights. Avoid stooping, bending, or overreaching. Sit to work whenever possible.
4. Avoid positions of stress on joints.	Avoid tight pinch or grip, for example, by using built-up handles and holders for such objects as toothbrushes and pens. Avoid turning fingers toward the little finger: turn fingers toward the thumb. Avoid wrist flexion and rotation during stirring, for example, by using a spoon like a dagger. Use two hands to lift or carry objects. Always consider adaptive devices (jar opener, reachers, built-up keys) to protect joints from deformities.
5. Use larger/stronger joints.	Lift with palm and forearm instead of fingers. Use a backpack, waist pack, or shoulder bag instead of a handbag.
6. Use joints in most stable positions.	Avoid or minimize excessive stretch of joint ligaments, for example, by rising rise from a chair symmetrically and not leaning to either side. Maintain good posture.
7. Avoid remaining in one position.	Change position (or stretch) every 20 min. Balance sitting tasks with those that require moving around.
8. Avoid activities that cannot be stopped.	Break activities into defined parts.

repetitive joint motion. After joint pain and inflammation have been controlled, however, and the client has achieved increased isometric strength, dynamic, low-resistance exercises are appropriate. Appropriate low-resistance exercises (Figure 79-4) for the client with RA include bike riding, swimming, golf, ping-pong, swimming, and dancing.

Other physical therapy modalities are also useful. For severely inflamed joints, splints appear to help resolve inflammation more quickly than does leaving the joint unsplinted. Heat and cold therapy are important adjuncts to an exercise and rehabilitation program. Superficial heat therapy can be given with hot packs, hydrotherapy, or paraffin baths. Deep heat is achieved through the use of diathermy or ultrasound. Superficial heat appears to cool joints by increasing the local blood flow, but deep heat actually raises the intra-articular joint temperature. As a result, superficial heat is generally preferred to deep heat. Heat seems to be more beneficial in the treatment of chronic conditions characterized by minimal swelling and inflammation. It also permits more effective stretching exercises.

Many persons prefer cold therapy because it appears to provide greater reduction of pain and stiffness than does heat. Cold packs, however, should not be used in clients with Raynaud's phenomenon, cold sensitivity, or cryoglobulinemia or in anyone who finds it uncomfortable. The Arthritis Foundation has developed a wide selection of literature about RA regarding support groups, self-help classes, and water-based and land-based exercises. To obtain this information from the Arthritis Foundation, call 1-800-283-7800. Requests for information can also be mailed to The Arthritis Foundation, 1414 Spring Street, NW, Atlanta, GA 30309 or visit their website at http://www.arthritis.org.

■ Nursing Management of the Medical Client

The goal of nursing care for clients with RA is to promote a healthy, positive life with adaptation to the chronicity of the disease. To achieve this goal, the nurse focuses on comfort, self-care, control, and coping. Adapting to a chronic illness is a complex process that is physically, emotionally, and socially demanding. The energy required to achieve this adaptation can be easily exhausted, especially in the early stages of RA. Achieving normalcy, regulation, or adjustment can become a life-long process, consuming increasing amounts of energy, unless clients learn to participate actively in modulating their responses to the illness. By working together with the client, the nurse helps the client master adaptive strategies so that physical, psychological, and social energy are renewed.

The nurse's role is to assess, educate, and coordinate treatments, facilitate adaptations in the home, reevaluate periodically, and serve as client advocate. Providing information to help the client deal with chronic pain, comply with treatment, and cope with a chronic disease are some of the challenges faced in managing clients with RA. The nurse provides information and encourages the client's self-management by allowing choices about when to exercise, which adaptive equipment to use, and what other self-care techniques to use. Clients with RA appreciate caring and empathy by nurses. See the Bridge to Home Health Care feature on Increasing Independent Living with Rheumatoid Arthritis on the website. **evolve**

Assessment

Nursing assessment begins by identifying the client's concerns and needs. The history should include information about the duration of clinical manifestations and ways the client has been managing those manifestations, particularly pain. It is important to identify other conditions the client may have. The client's current understanding of RA and the coping strategies used for dealing with pain and fatigue are important. Determine the methods that the client is now using to reduce pain (and the amount of pain the client considers tolerable). Find out what methods the client is using for joint protection.

Evaluate the amount of swelling and pain in each joint and the number of affected joints (to obtain a "joint count"). Determine physiologic measures of function such as a timed walk, measures of grip strength, and results of self-reported instruments that evaluate flexion

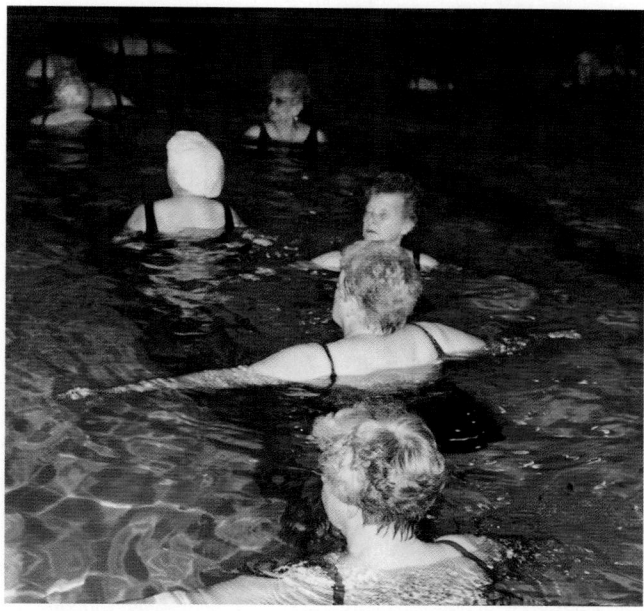

FIGURE 79-4 A community water exercise program. Many clients with rheumatoid arthritis find that water exercise helps to control pain and disability and improves exercise tolerance. The people in this class demonstrate the importance of keeping the shoulders submerged to allow the buoyancy of the water to protect their joints.

and extension. Assess for clinical manifestations in the client's eyes, heart, lungs, and peripheral nerves. It is important to note new manifestations and marked changes in previous clinical manifestations. Also evaluate the client's perception of his or her quality of life, usual role in the family, and social involvement. Physical changes in the body can lead to lower self-esteem. Western society values beauty and youth. Clients may find it psychologically difficult to be seen in public and deal with stares brought on by a hand deformity and other changes. As the client grieves the loss of a healthy, youthful body, thoughts of suicide can occur. Be sensitive to these issues and bring them into the discussion if the client or family hints of suicidal thoughts. The medical treatment available today has reduced the crippling affects of RA and made it possible for many clients to maintain a healthy, productive, active lifestyle.

Diagnosis, Outcomes, Interventions

Diagnosis: Chronic Pain.
The primary nursing diagnosis of clients with RA is *Chronic Pain related to inflammation and swelling, pressure on surrounding tissues, joint deformity, and joint destruction.* The amount of pain that these clients experience permeates all aspects of their life.

Outcomes.
The client's pain will be controlled at a level that permits the client to perform ADL.

Interventions.
Modulating the client's response to the experience of joint pain is another key principle of pain management. The uncertainty and unpredictability of the disease, with its concomitant impact on comfort, have been well documented. Four interventions to help clients with the pain of RA include (1) making them comfortable, according to what has worked for them in the past, (2) listening to and learning from clients, (3) reducing anxiety, and (4) enlisting family and community support. Not all clients with RA have the same pain or the same experience with pain, so it is critical to understand the phenomenon from the individual client's perspective.

Achieving a reasonable degree of comfort is a continuous challenge. Pain can be so pervasive and encompassing that it becomes a veil over daily activities, only to lift at unpredictable moments. Clients frequently use military terms, such as "struggle," "battle," "siege," "in the trenches," "attack," "fight," and "surrender," to describe their experiences with pain and discomfort. The importance of hiding the pain and keeping up with activities as a means of rejecting or disengaging from the disease has been emphasized. In fact, achieving some degree of comfort is the primary predictor of psychological well-being.

Numerous strategies can be used to help clients achieve pain reduction. Teaching clients about their medications and monitoring their response are im-

portant nursing responsibilities (see the Integrating Pharmacology feature on Medications Used in the Treatment of Rheumatoid Arthritis on pp. 2342 to 2344). Providing medication instruction is another significant aspect of RA client education programs. Clients should receive information about the purpose, dose, frequency, and anticipated side effects of each medication they take. Clients need to understand clearly when they are to report adverse clinical manifestations to the health care team and what to do if they miss a dose. Some of the new therapies are self-injectable medications requiring that clients and their families be taught injection and preparation techniques. Preprinted or written instructions are essential to help clients recall the information. Appropriate educational materials on a variety of pharmacologic agents are available from the Arthritis Foundation and the pharmaceutical manufacturers. See the Client Education Guide feature on Using Topical Agents to Reduce Pain, below.

Nurses play an important role in teaching clients to participate in their care by keeping a medication history. Clients can use a notebook or flow sheet to record essential medication information useful to themselves and other health care providers, such as dentists, other medical specialists, or acute care nurses. It is most helpful for information to be recorded about the medication name, date started, dosage, date discontinued, and reason for discontinuing the drug.

CLIENT EDUCATION GUIDE
Using Topical Agents to Reduce Pain

Topical pain reducers work in several ways depending on their ingredients. Some, which contain salicylates (the substance found in aspirin) may penetrate through the skin to the joint and reduce pain. Other pain relievers contain ingredients such as menthol or camphor that irritate the skin and distract attention from the actual pain. Still others contain capsaicin, a substance found in hot peppers, which reduces the pain signal to the brain.

Regardless of the mechanism of action of the pain reducer, the Arthritis Foundation recommends that topical pain reducers be only one part of a comprehensive treatment program that includes medication, exercise, rest, joint protection and, in severe cases, surgery.

Convey these additional instructions to the client as follows:
- Read and follow the directions of the package.
- Wash your hands after every application.
- Keep topical pain relievers away from your eyes, mucous membranes, cuts, or irritated skin.
- If you are allergic to aspirin or are taking an anticoagulant ("blood thinner"), talk with your physician before using any rubs, creams, or sprays that contain salicylates.
- Keep all topical pain reducers out of the reach of children.

Positioning the client, ensuring that the limbs are correctly supported, and reinforcing the use of heat and cold, however, are all important measures for promoting comfort. Some clients find that flannel nightwear, sleeping blankets, and thermal underwear are helpful means of retaining warmth while reducing pain and stiffness.

Other nonpharmacologic pain management strategies can be useful. They not only help reduce pain but also decrease anxiety and thus enhance overall comfort and a sense of control. A variety of relaxation techniques, including imagery, self-hypnosis, and controlled, rhythmic breathing, have been suggested. Progressive muscle relaxation techniques should be used with caution in clients with RA, however, because there is a danger that muscles could be tensed too tightly, thus exacerbating joint and muscle pain.

Other comfort-promoting activities include the management of stiffness and the promotion of adequate sleep. If these areas are addressed through the nurse-client partnership, fatigue can also be significantly reduced. Clients need to be taught to distinguish between pain and stiffness and understand why the nurse is interested in differentiating between the two manifestations. As one of the most important diagnostic criteria of RA (as well as several other arthritic diseases), *morning stiffness* can vary in duration or quality depending on disease activity. Typically, clients with morning stiffness wake up feeling comfortable until they begin to move. If the morning stiffness lasts longer than 1 hour or does not show evidence of decreasing, they may require additional rest and sleep plus changes in their medical regimen.

Occasionally, if stiffness is severe, family members may need to provide early morning assistance so the client is prepared for the day ahead. Another option is for clients to begin (or organize) as many tasks as possible the night before so they have enough time to complete ADL without rushing or anxiety. Clients might also be able to rearrange schedules so chores normally performed in the morning, when stiffness is most pronounced, are deferred until later in the day. Daytime stiffness can occur, but frequent position changes and pacing or alternating the types of activities usually alleviates it.

One unusual aspect of stiffness is that it is a disabling phenomenon that is not readily understood by other family members. Initially, family and co-workers may wonder whether the client is feigning his or her inability to move rapidly or perform optimally in the morning. Helping the client and family understand the need for additional time to complete activities is an important measure in decreasing the family's frustration and the client's anxiety about moving slowly.

Diagnosis: Fatigue/Sleep Deprivation.
Two nursing diagnoses that are related are sleep deprivation and fatigue. Fatigue is a complex physiologic process involving the muscles, heart, lungs, and immune system. Clients with RA often experience fatigue, in part because of their chronic inflammatory process, pain, and depression. In addition, pain and stiffness may prevent them from getting a good night's sleep. When pain prevents sleep and causes fatigue, the experience of pain may be further increased because of the sleep deprivation and fatigue. The nursing diagnoses may be *Fatigue and Sleep Deprivation related to joint pain, stiffness, generalized musculoskeletal aching, anxiety, chronic inflammation, and/or depression.*

Outcomes. The client will develop methods to balance rest and activity and will express satisfaction with his or her current amount of sleep and level of activity and energy.

Interventions. Help the client explore reasonable options for gaining enough sleep and finding time during the day to rest or nap. This may require changes in job performance or working relationships (if others need to do the client's work while he or she rests). Be sensitive to these concerns, and ask whether your suggestions are reasonable in the client's personal setting. Practitioners can find it easy to say "be sure to rest now" without determining the feasibility of this protocol. For example, if your client is a young mother, she may need to send her young children to a neighbor for an hour or two each afternoon, or nap while the children nap.

With RA, sleep is often interrupted because of joint pain, excessive fatigue, stiffness, or generalized musculoskeletal aching. Other important causes are anxiety and poor sleep hygiene. Before specific interventions are suggested, the nurse needs to determine how the sleep has been disturbed—for example, difficulty falling asleep, frequent periods of waking up during the night, or early morning awakening. Often the nurse's first interventions are to reinforce good sleep habits, such as maintaining a regular sleep schedule, avoiding caffeine or alcohol before bed, or engaging in soothing activities before retiring. Other strategies address specific causes of impaired sleep in persons with RA. For example, warming the bed or taking a bath before bedtime can ease painful joints. Taking the prescribed NSAID (with a light snack of milk and crackers) half an hour before retiring can also promote sleep by reducing joint pain. If clients are awakened during the night because of pain or stiffness, they may need to use a smaller pillow, bed boards, or even lighter weight blankets. Those clients who have difficulty falling asleep because of worries or diffuse anxiety may benefit from using relaxation-imagery exercises.

Diagnosis: Impaired Physical Mobility.
Another common nursing diagnosis is *Impaired Physical Mobility related to pain, stiffness, and joint deformity.*

Outcomes. The client will maintain mobility at the highest possible level to carry out desired activities.

Interventions. Encourage the client to stay active. In cooperation with a physical therapist or trained exercise physiologist, help the client develop an exercise program to preserve ROM while protecting joints. Maintaining function and mobility are necessary for the client to manage self-care activities.

Exercise can decrease morning stiffness, pain, and fatigue while enhancing the client's self-esteem. Participating in group exercise programs such as community water exercise programs (see Figure 79-4) provides social support and strengthens coping. Seek programs led by arthritis-certified instructors who monitor movement for adequate joint protection. Each session should include a warm-up period, full ROM exercises, endurance exercises, muscle-strengthening exercises, and cool-down exercises. Clients may use pain medication before exercise to permit increased freedom of movement. If a joint becomes painful during the exercise and if the pain persists for 2 hours or more after the exercise, the activity should be modified.

Diagnosis: Chronic Low Self-Esteem, Disturbed Body Image, Hopelessness, Ineffective Role Performance, Powerlessness.

Several psychosocial nursing diagnoses may apply to the client with RA. Choose the one that best fits the client. All of these nursing diagnoses may be related to chronic pain, the need for others to perform previous roles, feelings of helplessness, powerlessness, hopelessness, and embarrassment.

Outcomes. Although the actual outcomes statement depends on the client's particular diagnosis, most outcomes focus on the client's being able to express improved satisfaction with the problem. The problems identified by the three psychosocial nursing diagnoses are usually closely related and improvement in one area can lead to improvement in others.

Interventions. RA and side effects of some of the medications used to treat RA alter appearance and may alter self-esteem and body image. As the disease progresses, disfiguring joint changes or systemic alterations, such as rheumatoid nodules, may contribute to clients' sensitivity about their appearance and attractiveness. Coping with changes in body image may take months to accept. Be sensitive to negative self-talk by the client and express acceptance of the client's appearance. Suggest clothing options that may minimize visible changes.

Successful coping strategies help the client with RA to integrate the disease into the demands of daily living. Coping strategies can be viewed as either approach (positive or healthy) or avoidance strategies. Healthy approach strategies include seeking out information and assistance, finding strength through spiritual support, verbalizing feelings and concerns, setting goals, expressing positive thoughts, and maintaining realistic independence. The less adaptive, avoidance strategies include denial, excessive sleeping, other passive behaviors, and depression. Research findings indicate that depression is associated with increased levels of pain and functional impairment and increased use of health care services. In addition, the relationship between depression and pain may be influenced by the use of adaptive or maladaptive coping strategies and by clients' beliefs about their abilities to control their pain. Therefore the nurse's goal is clearly to help the client realize the benefits of the healthier approach strategies. Healthy coping strategies and the reframing of negative behaviors can be discussed, modeled, and safely tried out in nurse-led client support groups.

If changes occur in the performance of occupational, family, or social roles, self-esteem can be significantly affected. The client and family need time to plan for and accept the changes in the client's ability to perform previous tasks. Initially, it may seem easy to fill the role of two people in the home, and clients and their families may seem wary of efforts to encourage them to think about this change over the years that follow. Clients may also think initially that they will be able to go back to work full-time and that joint inflammation is only temporary. Be sensitive to this type of denial and work with the family "where they are." Gradually as the client's disease progresses, clients and families may need additional help as they try to come to terms with the long-term implications of the disease.

In general, clients with RA have a difficult time learning to live in partnership with the disease. RA clients may experience the fears of becoming crippled, being perceived as being old and nonproductive, and not being understood by loved ones. As with any chronic illness, clients need to maintain some degree of physical and psychologic control over the disabling effects of their manifestations. For some clients, however, the need to exercise control is so great that they can experience extreme powerlessness and helplessness during exacerbations of the illness. Clients who can view their relationship with RA as an evolving partnership have better outcomes, both physically and psychosocially, than clients who perceive the disease to be the "enemy." This sense of partnership helps the client let go (i.e., rest and take care of himself or herself) during exacerbations of the disease yet respond actively by agreeing to engage in health-promoting, self-care practices. It can also help clients not to waste precious energy with anxiety, anger, and unresolved grief or guilt.

Exercising healthy control over the disease may include formulating causes of the illness. In one study, clients who reported causes for their arthritis (such as fate, personal habits, heredity, or the environment) were

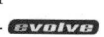

less anxious, depressed, and hostile than were those who did not report any cause. Most likely, clients who continue to ask "Why me?" and are unable to identify a specific cause of the illness have a more difficult time feeling in control.

Powerlessness can have physically and mentally detrimental effects on the client and can lead to anxiety, depression, and hopelessness. The key intervention for powerlessness is to increase the client's active participation in decision-making by allowing him or her as many choices as possible, for example, when to take medications or how to perform required ADL. Helping clients to reframe their relationship with the disease to one of active partnership, as previously mentioned, can also increase the sense of control.

Two other areas are important to the client's perception of control: client education and hope. Arthritis education provides information that clients can use to make informed decisions about their care. Knowledge about the disease, its course, the appropriate treatment, and what clients can do to promote their well-being increases their mastery of the unknown. Client education in the safe environment of a support group can also decrease the uncertainties of the disease and thus enhance control.

Having a sense of hopefulness about the future is a powerful ally against powerlessness. Everything clients do can be based on some level of hope. Nursing interventions to promote hope include avoiding false reassurance, helping clients to set realistic goals, praising them for all accomplishments (no matter how small), and active listening. Being sensitive to changes in mood and affect is important, particularly for clients on corticosteroid therapy. When clients are on steroids, views about the future often change from hopeful and positive to depressed, despairing expressions about their lives. If medication changes are not possible or if dosage adjustments do not relieve the depression, the nurse should consult the physician about the need for a psychiatric evaluation.

Diagnosis: Effective Therapeutic Regimen Management or Risk for Ineffective Therapeutic Regimen Management.

A final nursing diagnosis for the medically managed client with RA is *Effective Therapeutic Regimen Management or Risk for Ineffective Therapeutic Regiment Management related to complex medication schedules, high risk of side effects from medications, health maintenance, and self-care.* The management of RA as a chronic disorder is complex. Clients often have to take several types of medications with many undesirable side effects. They must plan for exercise and rest and cope with daily pain and stiffness.

Outcomes.

The client will make informed decisions about the management of RA that will lead to a satisfactory quality of life despite the disease.

Interventions.

Education focuses on coping skills, alternative methods of managing pain, joint protection, exercise, and adaptations for retaining functional independence and self-care. Inadequate knowledge may contribute to noncompliance with treatment regimens. Also, because of the pattern of remissions and exacerbations characteristic of RA, people tend to become discouraged with their prescribed treatments. Likewise, the medications used in the treatment of RA may provide only moderate pain reduction, and many are slow-acting. Clients with RA therefore are susceptible to "quack" cures and unproven remedies (see the box on Unproven Remedies for Arthritis on the website). Unproven arthritis remedies are treatments that in scientific studies have not been shown to work and to be safe. Proven treatments for arthritis must show in repeated, controlled scientific clinical trials that they are safe and provide benefit in one or more of the following areas:

- Reduction of pain
- Reduction of inflammation
- Safe joint mobility
- Avoidance of stress damage to joints

Self-care includes all of those practices that clients undertake to promote their health and well-being despite having a chronic illness. Interestingly, in one study of older clients with arthritic joint pain, the most common self-care practice reported was the administration of prescription or nonprescription medications. Other modalities, such as heat, exercise, rest, positioning, or joint protection, were reported occasionally or seldom. Although taking medication is an important aspect of the plan of care for a client with RA, the results of this study emphasize that other beneficial self-care practices must be taught and reinforced so the client does not develop self-care deficits.

Nutrition is an important aspect of self-care that is often misunderstood by the client with RA. This misunderstanding can occur because the popular press has promoted nutrition and unique diet therapies as instant cures for arthritis. Clients with RA may become overweight (because of decreased activity or mobility) or underweight (because of the anorexia of a chronic illness, the side effects of medications, or alterations in oral mucous membranes). In addition, diets may not provide sufficient iron to restore the deficit that results from the anemia of a chronic illness.

Clients need to understand that it is just as important to consume nutritionally sound diets as it is to achieve a reasonable body weight. Strategies to promote nutrition in anorexic clients include good oral hygiene before and after meals, small, frequent feedings, and high-calorie snacks. Clients with a dry mouth (xerostomia) benefit from moister foods and extra fluids with meals. Eliminating spicy or acidic foods, sitting upright to eat, and taking all medications with food and a full glass of water can ameliorate gastrointestinal distress. Clients with stiffness or hand deformities need assistive devices to feed themselves or help with opening cartons or packages.

Despite the many problems that people with RA face daily, many of these people courageously overcome these problems to maintain active, productive lives. Clients or health care providers can access arthritis news on America On-Line and World Wide Web browsers can go to http://www.arthritis.org for more information.

Evaluation

RA is progressive, and improvement can be slow. It takes several weeks to months for the expected outcomes to be met. When joints are already severely damaged and pain is uncontrollable, joint replacement may become an option. These and other surgical therapies are discussed under Surgical Management.

■ Surgical Management

Surgical procedures may be helpful for clients with arthritis. Surgery may be used to reduce pain, improve function, and correct deformities. Previously, surgery was considered only late in the course of arthritis, often after severe joint destruction or deformity had developed. Now, however, early surgery is used to prevent deformities during the early phases or active stages of the disease.

Tendon Transfer and Osteotomy. Tendon transfers can prevent progressive deformity. During these procedures, nodules or benign bony tumors (*exostoses*) may be surgically removed and flexion contractures surgically relieved. *Osteotomies* (excising or cutting through bone) may improve the function of deformed joints or limbs. For example, a femoral head osteotomy may give symptomatic relief by changing the position of the head of the femur when it is being subjected to the stress of impact against the acetabulum. Postoperative care varies, depending on the joint treated. Postoperative physical therapy is critical.

Synovectomy. Synovectomy (surgical removal of synovia, as in the elbows, wrists, fingers, or knees) may be used in clients with RA to help maintain joint function. With RA, joint destruction begins in the synovial tissue and then proceeds to involve bone, cartilage, and other structures. Short-term immobilization and physical therapy is needed after surgery.

Arthrodesis. Arthrodesis is a surgical procedure to produce bony fusion of a joint and is used for clients with bone loss after joint infection, tumors, musculoskeletal trauma, and paralysis. Arthrodesis may also help certain clients with RA or degenerative arthritis to regain some mobility. Although arthrodesis immobilizes the joint, the procedure may eliminate some of the discomfort of the arthritic process and improve functional mobility. The ankle is the joint most commonly treated with arthrodesis, usually to relieve post-traumatic arthritis. Arthrodesis often results in stiffness in adjacent joints and increases the energy required for ambulation. After surgery, the limb is put in a cast. Nursing care is the same as for clients with casts (see Chapter 29).

Joint Replacement. Arthroplasty (joint replacement) is the surgical replacement of natural diseased joints or joint components with artificial joints or joint components. The operation restores motion to a joint and function to the muscles, ligaments, and other soft tissue structures that control a joint. Joint prostheses are a combination of a metal surface articulating with a polyethylene surface. The metal surfaces are made of strong, lightweight alloys such as cobalt-chromium and titanium-aluminum-vanadium. Both surfaces of an arthritic joint are replaced. Arthroplasty of the shoulder, elbow, and fingers is discussed next; hip and knee replacement is described in Chapter 28 following discussion of osteoarthritis.

Shoulder Arthroplasty. Disorders of the shoulder that require arthroplasty are much less common than those problems in weight-bearing joints. Although the shoulder is classified as a ball-and-socket joint, it permits more mobility than any other joint in the body. The large head of the humerus articulates against, not inside, the small glenoid cavity. The shoulder relies on soft tissue and ligaments for stability, particularly the rotator cuff muscle-tendon unit. The rotator cuff muscle-tendon unit is composed of four muscles and their tendons, which allows the normal shoulder to move through three planes: flexion and extension, abduction and adduction, and internal rotation and external rotation.

Shoulder arthroplasty is the replacement of the humeral head and glenoid articulating surface with a metal and polyethylene prosthesis (Figure 79-5). The primary indication for total shoulder replacement is pain and secondarily it is improvement in function and ROM. Contraindications include infection and inability to comply with rehabilitation, such as clients with physiologic (e.g., neuropathy) or psychological problems. Complications include brachial nerve palsy, prosthetic loosening, joint dislocation or subluxation, and impingement syndrome. See the Critical Monitoring feature on Postoperative Brachial Plexus Compromise on p. 2351.

Postoperative Care

Nursing assessment includes neurovascular examination of the operative arm at least every 4 hours. A possible complication is development of impingement syndrome

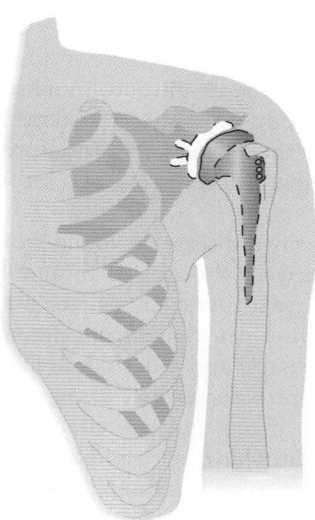

FIGURE 79-5 Total shoulder arthroplasty.

because of the proximity of the brachial plexus. Hemovac drainage should be less than 100 ml during the first 12 hours. Elevate the head of the bed 30 degrees to reduce swelling and improve comfort. Aggressive pain management is needed; the shoulder arthroplasty usually causes more pain during the first 24 hours than the other joint replacements. Patient-controlled analgesia (PCA) works well when supplemented with non-opioid anti-inflammatory agents. Ice is applied to the shoulder and the shoulder is positioned for comfort. Shoulder rehabilitation begins quickly after surgery and continues for about 6 weeks. For no other joint is rehabilitation as important as for the shoulder. The shoulder is placed through progressive external and internal ROM, hyperextension, and finally exercises with resistance once the rotator cuff has healed (about 6 weeks). Usually, the client can be taught how to use the nonoperative arm to move the operative arm through ROM.

Elbow Arthroplasty. Elbow arthroplasty uses hinge joints made from metal and polyethylene. This metal and plastic joint allows for some medial to lateral and rotational movements. A nonhinged elbow joint contains a metal and polyethylene component. Indications for elbow arthroplasty are pain, mechanical instability, and bilateral elbow arthrodesis (fusion of the elbow). A resection arthroplasty is done to reduce pain in the elbow by resecting the olecranon. Severe RA is the most common indication for total elbow arthroplasty.

Postoperative Care

Postoperative care includes elevating the arm above the shoulder for 4 to 5 days. Assess the client every 4 hours for ulnar nerve entrapment. Check the client's hand

CRITICAL MONITORING
Postoperative Brachial Plexus Compromise

- To assess median nerve status, have the client grasp your hand. Note the strength of the first and second fingers. A weak grip may indicate compromise of the median nerve.
- To assess radial nerve status, note the movement of the client's thumb toward the palm and then back to neutral. Problems with this motion may indicate compromise of the radial nerve.
- To assess ulnar nerve status, have the client spread all the fingers wide and resist pressure. Weakness against pressure may indicate compromise of the ulnar nerve.
- To assess cutaneous nerve status, assess for flexion of the biceps by having the client raise the forearm. Poor biceps flexion may indicate compromise of the cutaneous nerve.
- To assess axillary nerve status, have the client push the elbow outward against pressure. Hold the arm still while you palpate the deltoid for contraction. Weak contraction may indicate compromise of the axillary nerve.

strength; especially assess the thumb and index finger's ability to pinch and ability to adduct the fourth and fifth fingers. The ulnar nerve lies close to the posteromedial surface of the elbow. This nerve is called the "funny bone" because of the uncomfortable sensation that occurs in the arm and fingers when it is hit.

Assess for radial and ulnar pulses and capillary refill. Some institutions use pulse oximetry to continuously assess tissue perfusion. Pain is managed with PCA opioids. Elbow flexion and extension are allowed as tolerated. Personal items should be placed within easy reach of the nonoperative arm.

An occupational therapist should guide the client on how to modify ADL. Clients should not lift more than 5 pounds or begin triceps and biceps strengthening exercises for 3 months. The client will never be able to lift heavy items or play sports with the operative arm.

Hand Arthroplasty. Various hand deformities develop from synovitis. Synovitis stretches the central portion of the extensor tendon, causing it to shift. Eventually, the tendons become shortened and fixed. Ulnar drift occurs when the imbalance of damaged extensor tendons and intact flexor tendons cause subluxation of the MCP joint. Other hand deformities develop from synovitis of the PIP joint: boutonnière deformity and swan-neck deformity. A boutonnière deformity is flexion of the PIP joint and hyperextension of the DIP joint. There is no loss of MCP joint mobility. In the swan-neck deformity, the DIP joint is flexed and the PIP joint is hyperextended. Surgery includes tendon transfers to improve pinch grasp and arthrodesis for strength and position of the thumb for opposition. Hinge implants are placed to restore function to the fingers.

Postoperative Care

After surgery, neurovascular assessments are performed every hour for several hours. If the client has regional block anesthesia, the hand may be numb. The hand is elevated off the bed to prevent ulnar pressure. The hand is usually placed in a stockinette and suspended from the bed. An opening is made to assess the fingers. Encourage the client to exercise the fingers 10 times every hour, attempting full extension and flexion. Finger exercises reduce edema and pain. Place the client's personal items within easy reach of the nonoperative arm. If the opposite hand is equally deformed from RA, the client is often helpless and requires assistance with most components of ADL.

Encourage the client to use the nonoperative arm as much as possible. Some clients may express great concern about being dependent. Promote independence, and praise actions that foster self-care.

Rehabilitation is a long process. Most clients are fitted with outrigger splints with rubber bands that allow exercise with resistance after 1 week. Therapy continues for several weeks to assist the client to regain strength and control.

■ Modifications for Older Clients

Older clients may have adapted to RA very well but often find any further dependency needed after surgery difficult to handle. They tend to be slower in their recovery from total joint replacement. They may require prolonged hospitalization in an extended care facility or subacute care setting until they regain adequate mobility to function independently or with some assistance and safety.

CONNECTIVE TISSUE DISORDERS
SYSTEMIC LUPUS ERYTHEMATOSUS

The use of the term *lupus,* Latin for "wolf," to describe various disfiguring cutaneous disorders dates to medieval times. The first clinical description of rashes that continue to be recognized as lupus was by Biett in 1833. Credit is usually given to Kaposi for describing the systemic nature of the disease, including fever, weight loss, lymphadenopathy, and mental disturbances. Insights into the pathogenesis of systemic lupus erythematosus (SLE) were enhanced by the discovery of the lupus erythematosus (LE) cell phenomenon and the antinuclear factor.

SLE is a multisystem, inflammatory disorder associated with abnormalities of the immune system. It is a chronic condition characterized by various degrees of increased disease activity that are generally followed by a less active, remitting course. So many classic immunologic abnormalities can be present in SLE that it is considered the prototype of an autoimmune disease. Typically, multiple body organs and systems are affected at different times, thus producing widespread damage to connective tissues, blood vessels, and serous and mucous membranes.

SLE is primarily a disease of young women. Peak incidence occurs between the ages of 15 and 40 years during the childbearing years, with a female-to-male ratio of 5:1.[4] However, the onset can range from infancy to advanced age; in both pediatric and older onset clients, the female-to-male ratio approximates 2:1. In the general outpatient population, SLE affects approximately 1 in 2000 individuals. Incidence rates have increased over the past 40 years, most likely owing to an increased availability of serologic tests and increased awareness of the disease. The disease has a predilection for women in their childbearing years, with young black women being the majority group affected. The prevalence of SLE varies with race, ethnicity, and socioeconomic status. SLE has been estimated to be as high as 50.8 cases per 100,000, with an overall prevalence of 500,000 persons in the United States. The female-to-male prevalence ratio is 10:1 for women in the childbearing years. However, men and African-American females have been found to have a worse renal outcome than Caucasian women who have SLE.[14]

Once considered a fatal disease in young women, SLE now has improved outcomes. More than 85% of persons with the disorder live longer than 15 years after diagnosis. Increased mortality, however, has been noted in African Americans, Asians, Puerto Ricans, and persons of Hispanic descent living in the southwest United States. Poor survival has been associated with high serum creatinine, low hematocrit, and proteinuria. The most common causes of death in SLE are active lupus nephritis, vascular events, and infections.[14]

The 1982 revised criteria for the classification of SLE are listed in Table 79-5. The diagnosis of SLE is confirmed if a person has any 4 of the 11 criteria present, either serially or simultaneously, during any observation period.[18]

Etiology and Risk Factors

An underlying hormonal change may explain why the disease affects so many more women. Genetic factors may also be involved. Familial aggregation occurs in 10% of persons having a first-degree relative with SLE, including its occurrence in identical twins. Acute lupus-like reactions have been reported after taking drugs, such as hydralazine, procainamide, isoniazid, and chlorpromazine (Box 79-1).

Pathophysiology

The pathologic findings of SLE occur throughout the body and are manifested by inflammation, blood vessel abnormalities that encompass both bland vasculopathy

TABLE 79-5	1982 Revised Criteria for the Classification of Systemic Lupus Erythematosus
Criterion	**Definition**
Malar rash	Fixed erythema, flat or raised, over the malar eminences, tending to spare the nasolabial folds
Discoid rash	Erythematous raised patches with adherent keratotic scaling and follicular plugging; atrophic scarring may occur in older lesions
Photosensitivity	Skin rash as a result of unusual reaction to sunlight, by client history or physician observation
Oral ulcers	Oral or nasopharyngeal ulceration, usually painless, observed by a physician
Arthritis	Nonerosive arthritis involving two or more peripheral joints, characterized by tenderness, swelling, or effusion
Serositis	Pleuritis—convincing history of pleuritic pain or rub heard by a physician or evidence of pleural effusion *or* Pericarditis—documented by electrocardiogram or rub or evidence of pericardial effusion
Renal disorder	Persistent proteinuria greater than 0.5 g/day or greater than 3 g if quantification not performed *or* Cellular casts—may be red cell, hemoglobin, granular, tubular, or mixed
Neurologic disorder	Seizures—in the absence of offending drugs or known metabolic derangements, e.g., uremia, ketoacidosis, or electrolyte imbalance *or* Psychosis—in the absence of offending drugs or known metabolic derangements, e.g., uremia, ketoacidosis, or electrolyte imbalance
Hematologic disorder	Hemolytic anemia—with reticulocytosis *or* Leukopenia—less than 4000/mm^3 total on two or more occasions *or* Lymphopenia—less than 1500/mm^3 on two or more occasions *or* Thrombocytopenia—less than 100,000/mm^3 in the absence of the offending drugs
Immunologic disorder	Positive lupus erythematosus cell preparation *or* Anti-DNA—antibody to native DNA in abnormal titer *or* Anti-Sm—presence of antibody to Sm nuclear antigen *or* False-positive serologic test for syphilis known to be positive for at least 6 months and confirmed by *Treponema pallidum* immobilization or fluorescent treponemal antibody absorption test
Antinuclear antibody	An abnormal titer of antinuclear antibody by immunofluorescence or an equivalent assay at any point in time and in the absence of drugs known to be associated with "drug-induced lupus" syndrome

Data from Tan, E., et al. (1982). The 1982 revised criteria for the classification of systemic lupus erythematosus (SLE). *Arthritis and Rheumatism, 25,* 1271-1277.

and vasculitis, and immune complex deposition. SLE results from an abnormal reaction of the body against its own tissues, cells, and serum proteins. In other words, as an autoimmune disease, SLE is characterized by a decreased self-tolerance. In the North American white population, there is a positive association between SLE and two HLA antigens (DR2 and DR3) that are coded by the MHC. Persons with SLE have increased numbers of both self and non-self antigens, suggesting hyperactivity of the B cells. Interleukin-6 may have a role in B-cell hyperac-

tivity. Table 79-6 summarizes the changes in organ systems that occur in SLE. Another antibody, anti–double-stranded DNA (anti-dsDNA) of the IgG type, may be responsible for the development of the engulfed LE bodies in the LE cells. The relationship between the serum LE factor and the pathologic changes that occur with SLE is not clear. The absence of the LE factor, however, is a strong indication that the disease is not present. Increased levels of anti-dsDNA antibodies are associated with increased disease activity in clients with SLE.

Clinical Manifestations

The clinical manifestations vary considerably, from general complaints of fever, fatigue, and malaise to painful, swollen joints, to the psychologic distress of a variety of skin lesions. The latter can include the classic butterfly rash over the bridge of the nose and cheeks, erythematous discoid lesions (which can result in permanent scars on the scalp, ears, face, or neck), the temporary loss of hair on the scalp, painless mouth ulcers, and cutaneous vascular lesions. Photosensitivity can be especially problematic for some clients with SLE. Sunlight may trigger a local dermatitis or more severe disease activity.

Other systemic manifestations include the following:

- Raynaud's phenomenon secondary to peripheral vascular vasospasm
- SLE glomerulonephritis, which may progress to chronic renal failure

- Pericarditis
- Pleural effusion
- Hepatomegaly
- Lymphadenopathy
- Psychosis and convulsions
- Serum, immunologic, and antibody abnormalities
- Thrombocytopenic purpura
- Severe hemolytic anemia

SLE can be differentiated by the presence or development of glomerulonephritis, photosensitivity, characteristic skin rashes, central nervous system disease, and various cytopenias such as the Coombs' positive hemolytic anemia, leukopenia, and thrombocytopenia.

The *most specific tests* for SLE are antibodies to dsDNA, antibodies to Sm, and ribosomal P proteins, which are seen exclusively in SLE. Measuring C-reactive protein can sometimes be a useful test for distinguishing between a lupus flare and infection. It usually remains normal in a flare but is elevated with an infection.

The *most sensitive test* for SLE is the relatively nonspecific fluorescent ANA assay. Almost all clients with SLE have ANAs, but they also occur in many other situations, such as infections, advanced age, and RA, and with certain drug therapy regimens. Complements C3, C4, and CD 50 are useful measures of disease activity.

Outcome Management
■ Medical Management

Management of SLE is based on the organ systems involved. It is critical in the management of these clients to be aware of and to aggressively treat the co-morbid conditions that commonly occur in SLE such as hypertension, infections, seizures, hyperlipidemia, and osteoporosis. The goals of care focus on maintaining skin integrity, promoting a healthy lifestyle, reducing stress, maintaining proper nutrition, promoting comfort, increasing independence, and maintaining emotional well-being.

BOX 79-1	*Medications Associated with Lupus-Like Syndrome*

Definite
Hydralazine
Procainamide

Possible
Chlorpromazine
Ethosuximide
Hydantoin
Isoniazid
Methyldopa
D-Penicillamine
Oral contraceptives
Quinidine

TABLE 79-6	*Systems Changes with the Pathogenesis of Systemic Lupus Erythematosus*
System	**Pathogenesis with Systemic Lupus Erythematosus**
Integumentary	Immune complex deposition, inflammation of dermal-epidermal junctions, vasculitis
Gastrointestinal	Collagen degeneration and vasculitis leading to mucous membrane ulcers; vasculitis leading to organ infarction and necrosis
Musculoskeletal	Increased fibrin deposits at synovial surfaces; inflammation of arterioles, venules, and tendon sheaths; eventual necrosis, degeneration, and fibrosis of muscle tissue
Pulmonary	Pleural inflammation; intestinal vasculitis
Cardiovascular	Diffuse vasculitis; inflammation and scarring of atrioventricular and sinoatrial nodes; inflammation of pericardial sac
Renal	Deposition of immune complexes in the glomerular basement membranes
Neurologic	Immune complex deposition; antineuronal antibody activity leading to cerebritis, seizures, organic brain syndrome, and peripheral neuropathies

The primary management of SLE involves the use of drugs that suppress end-organ inflammation or interfere with immune function. Very few drug therapies have been subjected to randomized clinical trials. Treatment of acute SLE is based on the use of steroids, immunosuppressive agents, and experimental therapies.[9]

In general, the clinical pattern and prognosis of SLE are variable. The illness may develop rapidly with an acute fulminant course. More commonly, it develops insidiously and becomes chronic, with remissions and exacerbations. The course of the disorder is more severe when onset occurs at a young age. The survival rate has improved dramatically in recent years, although the disease is still potentially fatal. More than 95% of clients are alive 5 years after diagnosis. Improvements in treatments mean that clients can now live for many years.

Reduce Inflammation and Minimize Complications.
NSAIDs are given to reduce musculoskeletal manifestations, mild serositis, and constitutional manifestations such as fever. Care must be taken when using NSAIDs in clients with SLE. NSAIDs inhibit prostaglandin synthesis within the kidney and impair renal blood flow. Clients with lupus nephritis are particularly susceptible because of a heightened dependency on prostaglandins to maintain renal function compromised by glomerular inflammation. Clients should be questioned about their nonprescription use of NSAIDs. Renal abnormalities produced by NSAIDs, particularly impaired renal function, are generally promptly reversible.

Corticosteroids are required to control serious complications, such as thrombocytopenic purpura, hemolytic anemia, myocarditis, pericarditis, seizures, and nephritis. Prednisone is usually given orally in low doses (up to 15 mg/day), moderate doses (16 to 40 mg/day), or high doses (up to 120 mg/day). Divided doses are generally administered to ensure more sustained antiinflammatory action and greater lupus-suppressing activity than the same amount of drug given as a single morning dose. Once the disease is under control, however, gradual reduction (tapering) is essential. Clients on a regimen in which the daily dose is divided into several doses throughout the day must first be converted to a single morning dose before attempting to reduce the actual drug dose. The length of time the client has been on the drug directly affects the length of drug taper. Many methods have been used, with the most common being to decrease the dose by 10 mg in weekly increments.

An alternative to the use of high-dose oral corticosteroids is bolus intravenous steroid pulse therapy. Usually 1 to 1.5 g of methylprednisolone is given daily for 3 days to persons with severe disease, such as active nephritis, fulminating central nervous system disease, and hematologic crises. Generally, oral steroids (up to 60 mg/day of prednisone) are also given following this treatment period. Dysrhythmias and seizures have been associated with sudden death after administration of pulse therapy.

The antimalarial drug hydroxychloroquine (HCQ) is useful in managing cutaneous manifestations of lupus and in treating musculoskeletal and constitutional manifestations. Improvements in cutaneous manifestations, including discoid, subacute cutaneous, and erythematous inflammatory lesions, can be remarkably rapid, often evident within days. Discontinuation is associated with an increased risk of lupus flares, including major exacerbations such as vasculitis, transverse myelitis, and nephropathy. As a consequence, there is reluctance to discontinue HCQ in clients in stable condition who have clearly benefited from the drug. Low doses (200 to 400 mg/day) are well tolerated and rarely associated with side effects. Ophthalmologic examinations are required before starting this drug and every 6 to 12 months thereafter, although the risk of retinal toxicity is extremely small.

The use of immunosuppressive agents has gradually become an accepted therapy for SLE. MTX in low doses (7.5 to 15 mg/week) appears to be useful in managing arthritis, skin rashes, serositis, and constitutional manifestations. Treatment regimens, including azathioprine (Imuran) or cyclophosphamide (Cytoxan), have been able to halt the progression of glomerulonephritis or result in significantly less renal deterioration. Azathioprine and intravenous cyclophosphamide can be given.

Danazol, the attenuated androgen, has been shown to be useful in managing lupus thrombocytopenia. The mechanism of action has not been defined, but it is thought to involve endocrine influences such as the suppression of pituitary follicle-stimulating hormone and luteinizing hormone on immune or reticuloendothelial functions.

Intravenous immunoglobulin has been shown to be useful in managing severe lupus thrombocytopenia. The platelet count increases rapidly within hours of administration, occasionally peaking with extraordinarily high counts in which thrombotic events become a clinical concern. The rate of relapse following treatment is high. The primary role is to control acute bleeding associated with lupus thrombocytopenia or to rapidly increase the platelet count to allow for splenectomy or other surgery.

Dapsone has been used to manage cutaneous manifestation of lupus, including discoid, subacute cutaneous lupus, bullous, and lupus profundus lesions. Hematologic side effects are common and require close monitoring.

Drugs in clinical trials for the treatment of lupus nephritis include mycophenolate mofetil (CellCept) and tolerogens that arrest the production of dsDNA antibodies. A placebo-controlled trial of dehydroepiandrosterone (DHEA) has reported benefits in clients with mild to moderate lupus activity. Experimental research has shown that zileuton (a selective 5-lipoxygenase inhibitor) may be beneficial in treating mild SLE.

Hypertension is aggressively managed with medications because it commonly leads to renal failure and death. Advise the client to reduce salt, fat, and cholesterol intake and to stop smoking to reduce the risk of hypertension and coronary artery disease.

Cases of end-stage lupus nephropathy are managed with dialysis or kidney transplantation. There is a tendency for decreased clinical and serologic lupus activity following the onset of end-stage renal disease. Survival of lupus clients and other end-stage renal clients is comparable. Most studies note an increased incidence of infections among SLE clients on dialysis. Kidney transplantation during an acute exacerbation of SLE is controversial and may increase the risk of poor outcome. Recurrence of lupus nephritis in transplanted allografts, often with the same histopathology as in the native kidney, develops in 2% to 4% of transplanted kidneys.

Provide Supportive Therapy. Although drug therapy and the use of experimental treatments play a significant part in the management of SLE, perhaps the more important aspects of treatment are the supportive therapies of physical and emotional rest, diet and nutrition, and skin protection. Clients should receive the pneumococcal pneumonia vaccine and yearly influenza vaccines. Teach clients to report any manifestations of infection quickly.

■ Nursing Management of the Medical Client

The nursing history of persons with confirmed or suspected SLE must be sufficiently thorough to capture the range of possible manifestations that accompany an autoimmune disease. Clients need to be asked about general problems, such as fever, weight loss, and fatigue, and about changes in energy levels. A detailed medication history is essential in identifying the need for additional client teaching as well as in determining that the condition has not been drug induced. Clients should be asked about the names of their current medications, dosage, purpose, side effects, and length of time that they have been taking these drugs. Approximately 25 drugs have been implicated as causing a lupus-like syndrome, but only a few (hydralazine, procainamide, isoniazid) cause the disorder with any great frequency.

Questions about changes in skin should be elicited. The presence, location, and nature of rashes should be explored as should whether the rashes are associated with exposure to sunlight or even fluorescent lighting. Clients should be asked about changes in their nails and nailbeds, loss of hair on the scalp, and mouth or nasal sores.

Because SLE is occasionally characterized by generalized cerebritis, careful attention should be paid to the neuropsychiatric system. If seizure activity occurs, it is usually the generalized tonic-clonic type. The client should be asked about visual disturbances, vertigo, facial weakness, and presence of headaches. Changes in emotional status, including anxiety, insomnia, disorientation, and mood swings, are fairly common due to the disease and steroid therapy. The client may also complain of impaired cognition, such as mental dullness or a slow reaction time.

The nursing assessment should begin with an examination of the integumentary and musculoskeletal systems because clients with SLE have a high percentage of physical changes involving the skin, muscles, and joints. Inspect the entire body carefully, noting the location, nature, and size of cutaneous and vascular lesions. Transient rashes can appear in any location, particularly after exposure to sunlight. The classic butterfly rash over the bridge of the nose and cheeks affects fewer than half of those with SLE. Discoid lesions, characterized by annular erythematous plaques, can appear as atrophied, scaling areas on the face, neck, and arms. Severe scarring is also possible. Fingers can be affected by erythema under the nailbeds or by digital gangrene. Mild to moderate loss of scalp hair can occur when the disease is active. Vascular lesions can include petechiae, purpuric lesions, and Raynaud's phenomenon.

Joint manifestations, with or without active synovitis, occur in more than 90% of those affected. Along with Raynaud's phenomenon, these findings are often the earliest features of the disease. Therefore the musculoskeletal examination should focus on a full assessment of the ROM of all joints, noting the location and presence of synovitis, diffuse swelling, joint and muscle pain, and stiffness. Joint involvement is symmetrical in SLE, but deformities are usually the result of soft tissue stresses rather than erosive changes. One of the more common deformities is Jaccoud's arthropathy, a rheumatoid-like deformity of the hands present in about 10% of clients with SLE. In this condition, the MCP joints are subluxed, ulnar deviation develops, and hyperextension of the PIP joints can be observed.

Nurses have an important role in teaching clients how to manage the daily stress of coping with a chronic illness. The nursing care of clients with SLE can be challenging and demanding. During exacerbations, clients may become acutely and seriously ill. Infectious complications can develop in about one half of the clients with SLE, especially bacterial infections of the skin, respiratory tract, and urinary tract. Nursing care during this time is directed toward the assessment and management of acute confusional states, the prevention of seizures, the maintenance of skin integrity, the prevention of additional infection, the assessment of renal function, and the management of impaired gas exchange associated with lung disease and infection.

During this acute phase, increased fatigue, joint pain, and stiffness are often present as a result of inflammation and increased disease activity. Nursing activities to manage these acute flares are similar to those used during exacerbations of RA. Self-care deficits are often exacerbated because of the increased disease activity. It is important to help clients maintain as much independence as possible during periods of acute flares, so both self-esteem and physical functions are enhanced. Clients may require considerably more time to complete even one task, so nursing interventions may need to help the client focus on conserving energy and prioritizing self-care actions.

Caring for a client with acutely impaired thought processes can be perplexing. Several factors can contribute to the cause of this nursing diagnosis, including increased inflammation of the central nervous system and psychosis from high doses of steroids. Clients typically have severe throbbing headaches that are sometimes accompanied by generalized tonic-clonic seizures. They may display impaired judgment, inappropriate speech and behavior, difficulty concentrating or comprehending simple instructions, or short-term memory deficits. As the disease progresses, they may have personality changes, with a decreased ability to carry out purposeful activity. Clients with impaired thought processes should be cared for in a quiet environment, particularly when headaches are severe. Clocks and calendars should be provided to help with orientation. Communication must be caring but clear and concise to decrease ambiguity and anxiety.

If clients are susceptible to seizures, they should be observed carefully for auras or specific activities that might trigger the seizure. During the seizure, the client should be protected from injury by removing dangerous objects, by providing padding and blankets, and by turning him or her to the side after muscle activity has stopped to prevent aspiration. Restraints should never be applied during the seizure because the intense muscular activity beneath the restraint could lead to fractures (see Chapter 71 for information regarding management of seizures).

Another focus of nursing care during exacerbations of the disease is the management of excess fluid volume typically seen in peripheral edema. The goal is to maintain optimal renal function by assessing urine output and specific gravity every 2 to 4 hours, monitoring fluid intake and electrolyte levels, and assessing changes in the level of consciousness. The skin of a steroid-dependent client with SLE is characteristically tissue thin and fragile, so clients with peripheral edema must be moved and handled gently. The excess osmotic pressure beneath the skin surface can stress it easily so that minimal shearing forces can quickly denude the dermal layers.

During the chronic phase of the illness, clients can experience intense frustration because they often do not appear ill. The extreme weakness and fatigue they encounter during exacerbations of the disease, however, can lead to feelings of powerlessness and helplessness, ineffective coping, and a disturbance in self-concept.[15] Helping clients with SLE develop a traditional support group is difficult. Lupus clients are often homebound because of extreme fatigue, impaired mobility, and commitment to their roles of spouse and parent. In these situations, the use of telephone support networks or Internet support networks for clients with SLE can be a powerful nursing strategy. At the same time that these networks provide social support and counseling for the homebound, they also encourage personal growth and development among other clients with SLE who have developed positive coping skills. Nurses can play an important role in helping to establish this type of network through the education and support of peer counselors.

During remissions, clients often wonder about whether they can safely have children. This is a natural concern because most clients are women of childbearing age. Because fertility in clients with SLE is comparable to that in the general population, initiating and responding to clients' requests for health information are important functions of the nurse. Relapses of SLE can occur at any time during pregnancy but have not shown an increase in the risk of fetal loss. The incidence of relapses during pregnancy varies from 22% to 58%. However, most disease exacerbations can be reasonably well controlled with increasing doses of prednisone. Oral contraceptives containing low doses of estrogen are safe with mild lupus but should be used with caution by clients with severe lupus, because they can cause a flare. In addition, most studies report good neonatal outcomes in infants born to women with SLE, although a high incidence of prematurity has been observed.

SYSTEMIC SCLEROSIS (SCLERODERMA)

Systemic sclerosis (SSc) or scleroderma, literally "hard" (scleros) "skin" (derma) encompasses both a disease restricted to the skin (localized scleroderma) and disease with internal organ involvement (diffuse scleroderma or systemic sclerosis). One of the earliest definite descriptions of scleroderma in a child was published by W. D. Chowne (1842, London) and in an adult by James Startin (1846, London). Maurice Raynaud (1862, Paris) described the vasospastic phenomenon that bears his name.[11]

SSc is one of the least well understood of the rheumatic disorders.[11] It occurs as a multisystem inflammatory disease characterized by skin thickening (scleroderma) and deposition of excessive quantities of connective tissue (particularly collagen), which eventually results in severe fibrosis. The skin, blood vessels, synovium, and skeletal muscles are affected along with the microvasculature of internal organs, such as the heart, lung, kidney, and gastrointestinal tract. Widespread vascular involvement, perhaps the earliest and most significant pathologic change, is also a prominent feature of SSc.

SSc is considered one of the eight types of scleroderma, the classification of which depends on the degree and extent of skin thickening. The term *scleroderma* was first introduced in the mid-19th century to describe skin induration. Later, others used the term *progressive systemic sclerosis* to reflect its often generalized multisystem course. Currently, the term *systemic sclerosis* is preferred because many clients have limited skin and organ involvement.

Etiology and Risk Factors

SSc is seen worldwide. The incidence for women is more than three times that for men, especially for those between the ages of 14 and 40 years. The prevalence has been calculated at 10 per 100,000 population,[4] with a total estimate of 250,000 to 300,000 cases in the United States. Several risk factors have been associated with SSc. Overproduction of collagen and fibrous skin thickening have been associated with environmental factors (working with plastics, coal, or silica dust) and a high alcohol intake. Scleroderma-like conditions can also be present as a result of genetic factors (phenylketonuria), metabolic disorders (Hashimoto's thyroiditis), malignancies, postinfectious disorders, and neurologic conditions.[11]

Pathophysiology

SSc is the result of an excessive production of collagen by fibroblasts. It seems likely that lymphocytes accumulate in the lower dermis. These cells, almost entirely T lymphocytes, generate lymphokines, which in turn stimulate fibroblasts to produce excessive amounts of procollagen. After the procollagen is secreted from the cell, it undergoes cross-linking in the extracellular environment to produce mature, relatively insoluble collagen. The skin undergoes fibrotic changes, leading to loss of elasticity and movement.

Vascular changes are also important in the development of SSc. When the vascular endothelium is injured, damaged blood vessels release vasoactive substances, which are stimulated to overproduce collagen and mucopolysaccharides. Proliferation of the subintimal connective tissue results, along with fibrous thickening and narrowing of the lumina, thus leading to tissue ischemia. In a small number of clients with CREST syndrome (calcinosis, Raynaud's phenomenon, esophageal hardening, sclerodactyly, telangiectasias), pulmonary hypertension and intestinal malabsorption develop; these are the leading causes of death for these clients.

Clinical Manifestations

The two major types of SSc are classified according to the degree of their skin and systemic involvement. The first type, characterized by diffuse, cutaneous scleroderma, begins with symmetrical, widespread thickening of the skin on the extremities, the face, and the trunk. In the early stages of the disease, bilateral symmetrical swelling of the fingers, face, and feet can be seen, and the skin has a tense, wrinkle-free appearance (Figure 79-6). As the disease progresses, the skin becomes more thickened, hidebound, and shiny. Changes in pigmentation (both hypopigmentation and hyperpigmentation) are associated with the loss of normal skin folds. Distal thickening is always more severe than proximal thickening, so the extremities may show more changes than the face. Eventually, the face can become mask-like. The mouth is

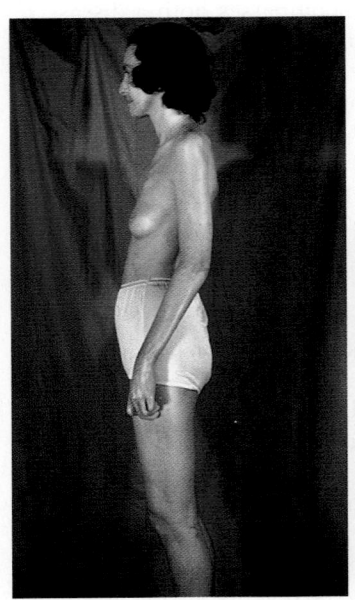

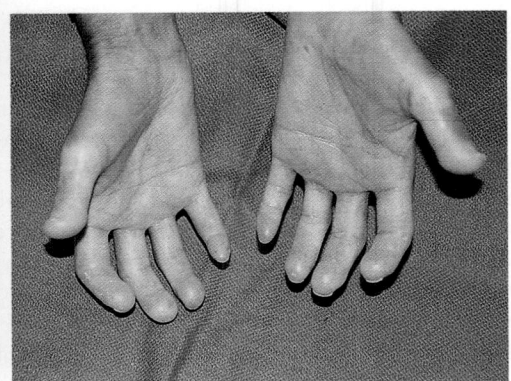

FIGURE 79-6 A, Long-term scleroderma. Note wrinkle-free appearance and shinyness of the skin. **B,** Appearance of the hands in a client with scleroderma. Note thickening of the skin and swelling of the fingers.

A   B

rigid, and the overall expression is blunted or immobile. Persons with this diffuse type have a tendency to develop early problems in the gastrointestinal tract, heart, lungs, and kidneys. The esophagus is particularly affected. Because of the early development of visceral changes, the pace, progression, and complications can be rapid.

The second type, limited cutaneous scleroderma, is characterized by skin changes that are usually confined to the fingers and distal portions of the extremities and face. In general, skin changes progress much more slowly than they do in the diffuse type of SSc. Truncal scleroderma is absent. Visceral changes (e.g., severe pulmonary arterial hypertension and biliary cirrhosis), if they do appear, are rare and are seen late in the course of the disease. CREST syndrome often develops in persons with the limited scleroderma:

- *Calcinosis*—Calcium (small white deposits) in the tissues
- *Raynaud's phenomenon*—Intermittent vasospasm of the fingertips often brought on by cold or stress
- *Esophageal hardening*—Sclerosis of the esophagus
- *Sclerodactyly*—Scleroderma of the digits
- *Telangiectasias*—Capillary dilations that form vascular lesions on the face, lips, and fingers

The presence of the CREST manifestations is a poor prognostic indicator. The 10-year survival rate after diagnosis is approximately 65%.

Raynaud's phenomenon, a generally bilateral vasospastic condition, can be an especially important predictor of SSc. Tricolor changes affecting the fingers in Raynaud's disease consist of pallor (white) accompanying vasoconstriction, followed by cyanosis (blue), as capillary blood is desaturated of oxygen and hyperemia secondary to vasodilatation. Clients with the CREST syndrome often develop painful ulcers on the fingertips or in the areas of calcinosis because of chronic vascular insufficiency. Although not identified in the acronym CREST, there is evidence of pulmonary involvement in most clients. Pulmonary artery hypertension occasionally develops in the client with limited cutaneous scleroderma.

Laboratory findings are relatively normal in persons with scleroderma. Mild hemolytic anemia is often present because of mechanical damage to red cells from diseased small vessels. Mild hypergammaglobulinemia (IgG) and RF are found in 30% of those affected. Slight elevation of the ESR is also common. Proteinuria is common with renal involvement. Most clients have positive titers for ANA. Anticentromere and anticentriole antibodies seem to be relatively specific for scleroderma. Clients with the serum anticentromere antibody have a more favorable prognosis. SCL-70, an antibody to topoisomerase, is found in about 35% of persons with diffuse SSc but is rarely seen in persons with limited cutaneous involvement and the CREST syndrome. The anticentromere ANA is seen in 80% of clients with limited

cutaneous involvement and in only 5% of those with diffuse cutaneous involvement.

A definite diagnosis of SSc requires the presence of one major or two minor criteria. The major criterion is proximal scleroderma with skin thickening and tightening of areas proximal to the MCP joints. These changes can affect the entire extremity, face, neck, thorax, and abdomen. The three minor criteria are (1) sclerodactyly (in which the skin changes are limited to the fingers), (2) digital pitting scars, with depressed areas at the tips of the fingers or loss of finger pad tissue, and (3) bibasilar pulmonary fibrosis.

Outcome Management
■ Medical Management

The treatment of SSc involves the shared management of a chronic illness and pharmacologic support.[1] Members of the health care team should educate the client about the nature, course, and treatment of SSc, the importance of avoiding cold, stress management techniques as a means to control Raynaud's phenomenon, the prevention of hand contractures and facial rigidity, the nutritional management of constipation and diarrhea and ideal body weight, and the prevention of injury. Protecting digits by using gloves or wearing warm socks, avoiding cold temperatures, and not smoking are important self-care measures that may require behavior modification so the client believes that he or she can have some control over the illness.

Reduce Inflammation, Sclerosis, and Vasospasm. Many medications are used in SSc, but no single agent has been proved convincingly effective. Symptomatic treatment and prevention of complications are the current goals of therapy. Three types of therapeutic agents have been used to treat SSc: (1) vasoactive agents, (2) anti-inflammatory medications, and (3) immunosuppressive drugs. In Raynaud's disease, calcium channel blockers have become widely prescribed. Nifedipine, 10 to 20 mg three times a day, was effective for Raynaud's disease in a controlled, double blind trial. Digital ulcer and digital infarcts have been successfully treated with digital sympathectomies. Corticosteroids are the major anti-inflam- matory agent used in SSc when clients have significant joint and muscle involvement or extensive skin disease. Low-dose steroid therapy (prednisone, 10 mg/day or every other day) is preferred.

Overall, immunosuppressive agents (azathioprine, cyclophosphamide, cyclosporine and MTX) have not consistently been proved effective in the treatment of SSc. Cyclophosphamide is often used in clients with progressive lung fibrosis.

Penicillamine, an immunomodulating agent that also interferes with the cross-linking of collagen, is a widely used drug in treating scleroderma. A large retrospective study showed significant improvement in skin thickening after 2 years of therapy and improved 5-year survival in clients taking penicillamine compared with untreated clients. Not all clinicians, however, accept penicillamine as established therapy for SSc. Initial doses should be low (125 mg/day), and the dose should increase gradually. Reduction of skin thickness requires long-term therapy, so clients need considerable support and monitoring while they are taking penicillamine. In addition, numerous toxic side effects can occur, including lupus-like syndrome, myasthenia gravis, glomerulonephritis, pemphigus, excessive skin wrinkling, and blood and liver dyscrasias. Clients on penicillamine must be carefully instructed to report skin rashes, burning, bleeding, sore throats, or fevers that might indicate serious side effects. The nurse and physician must explain the importance of periodic laboratory follow-up of liver and renal function to the client.

Various other agents are used to treat specific system problems. Minocycline has been effective in the treatment of diarrhea associated with malabsorption syndrome. This drug may reduce inflammation by blocking metalloproteases. A proton pump inhibitor should be administered to reduce the acidity of gastric reflux.

Renal crisis and associated hypertension was the most feared complication of systemic sclerosis. The introduction of angiotensin-converting enzyme (ACE) inhibitors, which are capable of reversing underlying hyperreninemia and controlling hypertension, has improved the outcome of renal crisis. Clients with renal manifestations who are taking ACE inhibitors have an 80% rate of 1-year survival and a 60% rate of 5-year survival in contrast to a 15% rate of 1-year survival without the use of ACE inhibitors.

No single drug or combination of drugs has proved successful as the standard treatment in controlled research studies. Etanercept in an initial small (10 client), open-label pilot study was encouraging, as was the long-term extension, but further research is necessary.[5] Ongoing clinical trials are rare in this orphan disease.

■ Nursing Management of the Medical Client

Clients should be interviewed with great sensitivity because of their possible fears about the disease and the changes in body image. The first manifestation of SSc is often puffiness of the fingers and toes and, in limited scleroderma, Raynaud's phenomenon. Question clients carefully about their experiences. Ask them whether they have had the sequence of blanching, cyanosis, and erythema that is associated with periodic vasospasm of the peripheral blood vessels. Ask which parts of the body have been affected. Although Raynaud's phenomenon is commonly seen in the hands and toes, it can affect the earlobes, nose, and tongue. It is also important to ask clients under what circumstances (i.e., cold or stress) they have experienced Raynaud's phenomenon.

Clients should be asked about changes in the texture, color, consistency, and moisture of their skin. Because skin changes can be widespread, it is usually helpful to tell clients you would like to review changes according to body location. Clients should be asked about subcutaneous nodules that they may have noticed under their fingertips. Other systemic changes to be explored include those associated with the gastrointestinal tract. Clients should be asked about the ease with which they swallow food and the types of food they have had difficulty swallowing. The presence of diarrhea (related to bacterial overgrowth), which can create malabsorption, constipation (related to colonic hypomotility), nausea, vomiting, and abdominal distention, should be explored within the framework of onset, severity, duration, aggravating factors, and relieving factors. The respiratory system can be affected, secondary to interstitial pulmonary fibrosis. Therefore ask clients whether they have had any cough, shortness of breath, or dyspnea with activity. Clients should be asked questions about their musculoskeletal health. The presence of bilateral symmetric joint pain and swelling should be elicited. Changes in endurance and muscle strength, as indicated by the ability to perform ADL, should be explored.

A careful assessment is required of the entire integumentary system, including the skin on the feet, trunk, and abdomen. The face and lips (as well as fingers, palms, and fingernails) may have telangiectasias. They are macular dilatations of superficial blood vessels that collapse after firm palpation. The hands are inspected and palpated for edema, thickened or hardened skin, loss of skin folds, or absence of wrinkles (see Figure 79-6). Fingers are also inspected and palpated for subcutaneous calcific nodules and dilated capillary loops or venules or ulcers on the tips of the fingernails. Nailbeds are inspected for pitting, changes in contour, and the appearance of suppurative cuticles.

Changes in skin over the forearms, face, legs, and trunk can occur in diffuse cutaneous scleroderma. Therefore each area should be carefully assessed for edema, thickening, or tightening. The face should be inspected for mobility of expression and ability to open the mouth. Persons with SSc are often unable to open the mouth fully as the disease progresses. Skin thickening is often accompanied by areas of hypopigmentation and hyperpigmentation, so these changes are most commonly observed on the extremities and chest.

The musculoskeletal assessment includes a thorough evaluation of ROM because reduced joint mobility and polyarthritis characterize SSc. Flexor and extensor tendons should be palpated for the presence of friction rubs. Often, coarse crepitus caused by fibrin deposits can be heard with tendon motion—a manifestation that is often considered specific for SSc. Eliciting Tinel's sign to rule out or confirm carpal tunnel syndrome is useful. Muscle strength should be assessed and graded because SSc may have a polymyositis-type myopathy affecting the proximal muscles.

Other body systems should be assessed to provide baseline data or to determine possible organ involvement. The respiratory system should be assessed for the ease and extent of thoracic excursion, presence of dyspnea, and presence of adventitious lung sounds. The heart is examined for changes in rhythm or manifestations of heart failure. Blood pressure must be monitored closely because sudden malignant hypertension associated with renal disease can occur in SSc.

Most clients with SSc have significant muscle and joint involvement, including arthralgias, myalgia, and fibrosis of the tendons. When contractures develop, they are often due to the fibrotic changes in the skin. These muscle and joint changes lead to problems often encountered in clients with RA—joint pain, stiffness, fatigue, self-care deficits, and impaired physical mobility.

From the client's perspective, coping with an altered body image that accompanies extensive skin changes can be an overwhelming task. Nurses can help clients understand that successful coping often means assuming responsibility for self-care and the prevention of complications. Nursing interventions, therefore are targeted at maintaining a full ROM of the mouth and hands as well as suggesting creative use of clothing and make-up to enhance the appearance.

Changes in skin integrity require meticulous nursing care. For the acutely ill client, all digits and extremities must be handled carefully and gently. If possible, the client should try to move or reposition himself or herself so minimal discomfort occurs. Debilitated or steroid-dependent clients or those undergoing orthopedic surgery should be placed on pressure-reducing beds or air mattresses to prevent the development of skin breakdown over bony prominences. Dressings must be removed carefully so that additional trauma does not occur. Although moist dressings are applied to injured areas, they should be dampened with sterile saline if they do not come off easily. Tape should be used only when absolutely essential, for example, to stabilize an intravenous catheter needle. Otherwise, all dressings should be secured with stretchable gauze.

Whenever possible, the administration of injections and intravenous therapy should be in sites free of fibrosis and sclerosis. Areas of tough, thickened skin and sclerotic veins cannot be easily punctured. It is possible, also, to cause additional damage (and a portal for infection) if needle punctures are not made successfully.

Client education is the cornerstone to effective nursing care of the client with Raynaud's phenomenon. Clients must be assisted to modify their dress and health practices so all controllable sources of vasospasm are eliminated. Newly diagnosed clients may need anticipatory guidance about how to dress protectively in cold weather and in air conditioning. They may readily recognize the need for gloves but not realize the importance of protecting the head, ears, nose, lips, and feet. Keeping a pair of gloves in a tote bag or pocket is helpful when in air-conditioned stores or when taking frozen items out of the grocery freezer. Clients must maintain their core temperature, always dressing warmly. Clients must often be helped to change their health practices, so they eliminate the use of vasoconstrictive substances, such as alcohol and caffeine. Learning biofeedback or other stress management skills is indicated when clients identify stress as a cause of altered tissue perfusion.

Clients with SSc often have difficulty maintaining their weight because of esophageal changes leading to dysphagia, esophagitis, and decreased intestinal motility. Consultation with the dietitian can help the nurse provide appropriate, easy-to-swallow, high-calorie snacks. The dietitian can plan meals to avoid foods contributing to esophagitis and gastric reflux. Remaining upright for 1 to 2 hours after eating also helps to prevent esophageal reflux. Avoiding heavy snacks close to retiring, using a large wedge pillow to elevate the head and shoulders, or elevating the head of the bed on shock blocks can prevent bedtime reflux. The client's ability to chew and swallow dry, compact foods, such as meat and bread, should be carefully evaluated. Often, these foods cause severe choking spells. Moistening them with gravies, sauces, or jellies helps them to be more easily tolerated. The achievement of nutritional goals is often affected by dental hygiene practices. Because of sclerotic skin changes, clients may have a difficult time completely opening the mouth. Mucous membranes may become inflamed or ulcerated owing to lack of moisture or inadequate brushing and rinsing. Using a small angled toothbrush or WaterPik can help prevent these problems. Reinforcing the need to perform facial exercises to prevent rigidity of the face and mouth is a priority nursing intervention.

Chronic constipation and diarrhea are two other problems that are usually amenable to nursing intervention. Chronic constipation is associated with the decreased motility of the gastrointestinal tract that accompanies SSc. Nursing interventions include eating easy-to-swallow, high-fiber foods along with increased fluids and exercise. The use of bulk stool softeners and suppositories may be needed as part of the bowel program. Diarrhea is associated with the malabsorption syndrome. Foods known to precipitate diarrhea should be eliminated from the diet, and natural antidiarrheal agents can be added to meals. When infectious organisms are present, antibiotic agents (often tetracycline) are prescribed.

Nursing care is also directed toward the monitoring and detecting of potential problems. The potential for impaired gas exchange exists when interstitial fibrosis of the lungs occurs. The presence of dyspnea, changes in activity tolerance, and an increased rate and depth of respirations may be noted. Auscultation of lung sounds may indicate fine crackles. Oxygen is usually administered as supportive therapy, and clients are educated about factors (pollen, smoking, humidity) that exacerbate the pulmonary condition.

SPONDYLOARTHROPATHIES

The *spondyloarthropathies* are a group of interrelated disorders that include psoriatic arthritis (PsA), reactive arthritis, arthritis-associated inflammatory bowel disease, and ankylosing spondylitis (AS). Spondyloarthropathies are distinguished from RA by three characteristics: (1) a negative test for RF, (2) the absence of rheumatoid nodules, and (3) an inflammatory peripheral arthritis that is typically asymmetrical. Three other features of the spondyloarthropathies have been noted. First, inflammation occurs where the ligament inserts into the bone (enthesis) rather than at the synovium. Extraskeletal changes can occur in the eye, skin, lung parenchyma, or aortic valve. Second, there is considerable overlap between the various spondyloarthropathies. For example, a person with PsA can develop the classic sacroiliitis seen in AS. Finally, there is a tendency toward familial aggregation in the development of the disease, with genes other than B27 probably playing a role.

ANKYLOSING SPONDYLITIS

Literally, *ankylosing spondylitis* refers to fusion (ankylosis) of inflamed vertebrae (spondylitis) (Figure 79-7). The disease typically begins in the spine of young men in their late teens or early twenties. Most clients have bilateral sacroiliitis that causes pain and some degree of restricted motion in the lumbar spine. Peripheral arthritis of the large joints, usually the hips and shoulders and more rarely the knees, occurs in 20% to 30% of persons with AS. Small joint involvement is not usually seen. Chest expansion can also be decreased owing to an associated costovertebral arthritis. By the time the client is 50 or 60 years old, the fusion of the lumbar spine has proceeded to the cervical region. If AS is not treated, the disease tends to progress with remissions and exacerbations to a final stage of rigid lumbar and thoracic kyphosis that leaves the neck in a flexed position. AS is associated with a shortening of the life span.

Etiology and Risk Factors

The average annual age-adjusted incidence rate of AS has been reported to be 6.6 per 100,000 population, with men being affected three times as frequently as women. Although the usual age of onset is set between 15 and 35 years of age, the age group with the highest

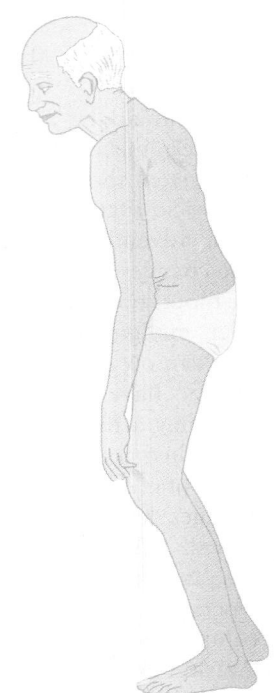

FIGURE 79-7 Ankylosing spondylitis.

incidence rate is the 25- to 34-year-old group. The overall prevalence rate is estimated to be 129 per 100,000 population. Thus the overall prevalence rate for the entire U.S. population is between 1 and 2 per 1000 population.

Risk factors associated with AS include gender (with a 3:1 to 4:1 predominance of males over females), the young adult years of adolescence through adulthood (15 to 35 years old), and a genetic predisposition. A strong tendency toward familial aggregation has been seen and a sex-linked hormone may be important. The presence of HLA-B27 may also be a risk factor, in that it appears frequently in the high-risk Native American population but is almost nonexistent in the low-risk U.S. African-American population. Although the disease is generally seen in men in the third decade of life, the condition may go undetected in women because of its milder course and because fewer pelvic x-ray examinations are done in women of childbearing age.

Clinical Manifestations

Initially, morning backache and stiffness begin during adolescence or young adulthood. The back pain and stiffness subside with movement but often return with inactivity. Back pain throughout the spinal column, difficulty sleeping, fever, and neurologic changes such as bowel and bladder incontinence, paresthesias, and numbness may also occur. Several other systemic manifestations of AS can be seen: uveitis, pulmonary fibrosis, inflammatory bowel disease, and aortic insufficiency.

Uveitis occurs in up to 25% of all clients with AS, especially in HLA-B27–positive clients with peripheral joint disease, but its incidence seems to be unrelated to the severity of the spondylitis. Upper lobe pulmonary fibrosis is rare, but it has been reported. Intestinal inflammation is frequent in clients with spondyloarthropathy, and one fourth of clients have early features of Crohn's disease. Aortic insufficiency, accompanied by a typical diastolic murmur, occurs in 5% of clients with AS, and this problem frequently leads to the need for an aortic valve replacement. Cardiac problems, however, do not usually appear for several years.

The diagnosis of AS is based on the results of the history, physical examination, and radiologic findings. Positive physical examination findings include the presence of sacroiliitis, spinal muscle spasms, and decreased hip mobility. Decreased chest expansion is seen later in the disease. Along with symptomatic sacroiliitis, radiologic confirmation of sacroiliac joint changes is probably the most important finding early in the disease. Radiographs may show no abnormalities, but later, the typical changes of sacroiliitis develop, with patchy sclerosis at the joint margins. Early changes in AS include a squaring off of the anterior lumbar vertebral surfaces. This squaring is caused by erosion of the upper and lower margins of the vertebrae at the site of insertion of the annulus fibrosus. The intervertebral ligaments involved in the inflammatory process heal by ossification, leading to the formation of syndesmophytes in the outer layers of the annulus fibrosus. Eventually, the disk space becomes bridged by these bony syndesmophytes. In the end stage of the disease, complete spinal fusion (bamboo spine) and fusion of the sacroiliac joints occur along with ossification of all of the ligamentous structures.

In general, laboratory studies are not helpful in diagnosing AS. Although the HLA-B27 antigen is seen in 90% of clients with AS, it is found in up to 10% of those without the disease, thus limiting its specificity in diagnosis. An elevated ESR is seen in most clients, but it may be normal in those with severe disease. Other findings may include an elevated creatine kinase (CK) and alkaline phosphatase level, but these are not confirming diagnostic tests.

Outcome Management
■ Medical Management
The treatment goals for AS are to maintain mobility, decrease inflammation, and control pain.[7] As with other chronic conditions, treatment is more successful when clients are engaged in and assume responsibility for health promotion and other self-care activities.

Maintain Mobility. Instructing the client to perform appropriate exercises and engage in ADL is critical if he or she is to maintain mobility with minimal spinal curvature. Good posture must be encouraged through exercises that promote stretching and extension of the spine. Swimming is an excellent general conditioner as well as an activity that promotes spinal extension without increased pain. The nurse may need to help the client solve problems about awkward furniture or equipment that reinforces spinal flexion. For example, the client who has a desk job may need to invest in a tilting artist's table so the neck and head are not forced into flexion with constant activity. Selecting ergonomic chairs or ensuring the correct placement of a computer workstation can also be beneficial for the client's comfort. Appropriate sleep posture must be reinforced, particularly in those with mild cervical flexion who are accustomed to sleeping with two pillows. Spinal extension is maximized during sleep if clients lie on a firm mattress, preferably with bed boards underneath, in a supine position, without a pillow. If the client insists on using a pillow, it should be as flat as possible.

Reduce Pain and Inflammation. As with many other chronic arthritic conditions, successful pain management depends on reducing inflammation and stiffness. NSAIDs are used to reduce inflammation, and the application of heat (or a warm shower or bath) helps reduce morning pain and stiffness. Sulfasalazine is somewhat effective in the treatment of active spondyloarthropathy. MTX has also shown beneficial effects in the treatment of severe AS but is not considered standard drug therapy. In randomized clinical trials, infliximab has been shown to be effective.

■ Nursing Management of the Medical Client
Questions should focus on the typical manifestations of pain, stiffness, and fatigue and on their effects on performing ADL, as well as screening for extra-articular involvement. Question clients about the nature, onset, location, duration, and quality of their pain. Ask what self-care measures (e.g., use of heat or cold, showers or baths) they have tried to cope with the pain-stiffness-fatigue cycle and which measures have been effective.

Determine whether the pain is in the lower back, thorax, or cervical area and whether other large peripheral joints, such as the knees, hips, or shoulders, cause discomfort. During the early phase of AS, clients complain of lumbosacral pain that radiates to the buttocks and thighs. Sleep for clients with AS is different from normal sleep. Therefore an assessment of sleep patterns should be completed. Ask clients whether the pain is worse on rising, whether it is associated with morning stiffness, and whether it decreases with activity. Also determine the length of time that the client has been affected with back pain. These points are important because five features strongly suggest inflammatory spinal disease: (1) insidious onset of discomfort, (2) being younger than 40 years of age, (3) persistence of discomfort for more than 3 months, (4) association with morning stiffness, and (5) improvement with exercise.

Clients should also be questioned about fatigue, weight loss, and the presence of a low-grade fever. With advanced disease, cord compression can occur as a result of spinal fractures, so it is important to elicit information about neurologic changes, such as decreased motor activity, paresthesias, numbness, and bowel and bladder incontinence. Because of the possibility of extra-articular disease, it is important to ask clients about their eyes, respiratory status, and heart. Suggested screening parameters for each system are listed:

- *Eyes*—Presence of blurred vision, decreased vision, pain, excessive tearing, photophobia
- *Respiratory*—Presence and quality of cough, sputum production, dyspnea, shortness of breath, smoking history
- *Cardiovascular*—History of murmurs, tachycardia, and extra heart sounds

The spinal assessment is often normal early in the disease, or there can be tenderness with deep palpation of the sacroiliac joints. As the disease progresses into the upper spinal segments, loss of the normal lumbar lordosis occurs, followed by decreased flexion, extension, and lateral movement. Asking the client to flex at the waist and observing the flattening of the lumbar spine can assess loss of lumbar lordosis. Tenderness along vertebral structures and marked paravertebral spasm can also be present with decreased lumbar lordosis.

A useful measure of lumbar flexion is the Schober test. With the client standing erect, the nurse makes a mark at the L5-S1 area and another 10 cm above it. When the client bends forward in maximal flexion, the distance between the two marks normally should increase to 15 cm. In AS, however, this measurement does not significantly increase. The Schober test is most useful in evaluating young persons because spinal flexion generally decreases with age. An alternative technique to screen for AS is to measure the distance from fingers to floor when the client attempts to touch the toes. Persons with decreased flexion have a greater distance between their fingers and the floor. The tendency to develop a kyphotic posture in AS is reflected in diminished thoracic expansion. To assess chest expansion, place the tape line at the nipples and then note the chest measurement with full lung expansion. A distance of less than 3 cm, along with other physical manifestations, is highly suggestive of AS.

As the disease progresses, loss of ROM in the neck leads to a fixed kyphosis that can seriously impair visual function. The serial tracking of measurements of the distance from the client's head to the wall can be used to detect the progression of cervical kyphosis. Positioning the client with the heels against the wall and instructing him or her to extend the neck fully can obtain consistent results.

Clients with AS should also be assessed for two other musculoskeletal changes. The first change is the development of an inflammatory peripheral joint involvement, particularly of the hips, knees, and shoulders. Assess these joints bilaterally for changes in ROM, pain, tenderness, and synovitis. Also observe for manifestations of enthesitis, a problem commonly seen in juvenile AS and occasionally present in adults. Enthesitis can involve the plantar aspect of the foot (plantar fasciitis), the heel (Achilles tendinitis), and the knee. Other sites include the greater trochanters, superior anterior iliac crests, and ischial tuberosities. Attachment sites may or may not be swollen, but typically they are extremely painful to palpation. Because of the potential for developing extra skeletal problems with the eyes, lungs, and heart, these systems should be carefully assessed during the baseline screening.

The nurse plays a key role in educating the client about health promotion activities, exercise, and the management of pain. One of the most critical areas for skillful nursing intervention involves being attentive to and providing positive, unconditional regard for those persons with changing appearances. If the disease progresses rapidly or if the client has not sought help until skeletal changes are noticeable, he or she may be quite self-conscious and even depressed about his or her appearance. Businessmen may have found it increasingly more difficult to find clothing that fits. Some men have been known to avoid buying suits because of their embarrassment about being seen by salespersons or tailors. The client may be so concerned about appearance that he or she avoids social interaction outside of the job.

Helping clients who have an altered body image or who are socially isolated is a significant challenge and an opportunity to establish a meaningful therapeutic relationship. Although specific nursing interventions can be implemented that encourage group participation and interaction, it is often the nurse's positive, unconditional regard that helps the client work toward reintegration of the self. Approximately one third of clients experience depression, and women report more depression than men.

Another important area for nursing intervention, especially as the disease progresses, is the maintenance of effective breathing patterns and adequate oxygenation. Ongoing assessment of chest wall expansion, instructions in deep-breathing exercises, and the avoidance of smoking and respiratory depressants can help the client to maintain optimal breathing. If dyspnea becomes a problem, instruct the client in pursed-lip breathing and the pacing of activities. For those clients with cervical involvement who become acutely ill or require surgery, notify the anesthesia department. AS in the cervical area frequently causes problems with intubation.

REACTIVE ARTHRITIS (REITER'S SYNDROME)

Reactive arthritis and Reiter's syndrome are both designations for a form of peripheral arthritis, often accompanied by one or more extra-articular manifestations, which appear shortly after certain infections of the genitourinary or gastrointestinal tracts. Most affected individuals, usually young men, have inherited the human leukocyte antigen HLA-B27. Reiter's syndrome originally referred to the clinical triad of nongonococcal urethritis, conjunctivitis, and arthritis. Because of many overlapping clinical, epidemiologic, and genetic features, reactive arthritis is classified as a seronegative spondyloarthropathy. Approximately 80% of clients experience chronic problems marked by periods of remission and exacerbation.[16]

Etiology and Risk Factors

Reactive arthritis occurs following exposure to a bacterial gastrointestinal or genitourinary infection. Although the exact mechanism remains unclear, certain infective agents and a specific genetic background (HLA-B27) are associated with reactive arthritis. Epidemic reactive arthritis has occurred in association with dysentery. Endemic or postvenereal reactive arthritis is the more common type found in the United States.

Endemic reactive arthritis occurs more frequently in young men (9:1) and is linked to the greater prevalence of HLA-B27 antigen in this population. Cases following food-borne enteric infections affect both genders equally. Whites are affected more commonly than African Americans or other racial groups who have a lower frequency of HLA-B27. Reactive arthritis is difficult to diagnose and probably occurs more frequently than is reported.

Clinical Manifestations

Reactive arthritis demonstrates features in almost every system of the body; the most common of which are polyarthritis and urethritis or cervicitis and conjunctivitis. There is a link between the genitourinary system and reactive arthritis. Urethritis can occur with clinical manifestations (discharge, slight burning on urination) or can be asymptomatic, which is a component in the difficulty in establishing a diagnosis. Reactive arthritis has been reported frequently in clients with human immunodeficiency virus (HIV) infection. There is a high incidence of prostatitis and acquired immunodeficiency syndrome (AIDS). The role of AIDS in the pathogenesis of reactive arthritis is still being investigated. Urethral infection is commonly accompanied by stomatitis, balanitis, and keratoderma blennorrhagicum. The keratodermal lesions are similar to psoriatic lesions and can appear on the soles of the feet, glans penis, and toes.

Conjunctivitis, considered a classic manifestation, is typically a transient, mild phenomenon. If a sterile discharge is present, it subsides within a few days. Uveitis can become a more significant clinical problem in this disorder.

Reactive arthritis is characteristically additive, asymmetrical, and oligoarticular, affecting an average of four joints. The arthritic process generally affects weight-bearing joints, especially of the knees and ankles. Large effusions can accompany it.

Diagnostic work-up includes radiography and laboratory examinations. Early in the disease, there are no radiographic changes. With disease progression, joint space narrowing and erosive changes can be seen. In advanced disease, the individual may develop sacroiliitis, as found in AS. Laboratory findings may show an elevated ESR, but the ESR may be normal despite active joint involvement. Mild hypochromic or normochromic anemia may be present. Routine typing for HLA-B27 is considered unnecessary.

Outcome Management
■ Medical Management

Reactive arthritis usually runs a self-limited course of from 3 to 12 months in most clients; however, some studies suggest that many clients continue to be plagued by minor musculoskeletal manifestations. Management of the client targets client education and management of clinical manifestations.

Pharmacologic management is similar to that used for AS. The attacks tend to be self-limiting, lasting 2 to 4 months, with a recurrence rate of 15% per year. The use of antibiotic therapy in the prevention or management of reactive arthritis remains controversial. For clients with ocular manifestations, steroid eyedrops or subconjunctival preparations may be needed. Severe uveitis is relatively common and is a difficult clinical management problem. Small numbers (less than 12 clients) have limited clinical trials in determining the management of reactive arthritis. Larger randomized, controlled trials are needed.

Joint pain and dysfunction are managed with a regimen of physical therapy. Splinting for joint protection along with a managed exercise and activity program are indicated.

There is a general recognition that reactive arthritis has a greater propensity for chronicity than previously appreciated, which should temper an overly optimistic prognosis. One study reported that at 1 year, 40% of clients with post-genitourinary-acquired reactive arthritis and 20% of post-gastrointestinal-acquired reactive arthritis still had active disease, but almost all had recovered at 2-year follow-up.

■ Nursing Management of the Medical Client

While collecting the nursing history, the nurse should examine the pattern of orthopedic pain. Joint pain, back pain, heel pain, and a tendinitis-type pain can manifest in reactive arthritis. Clients with a nonspecific arthritis should be questioned about the presence of genitourinary and ocular manifestations. Ask the client if he or she has noted any atypical urethral discharge or slight pain or burning on urination for even a few days. An examination of past history of sexually transmitted diseases is important, as is the sexual history in relation to number and frequency of sexual partners. Interview for the presence of eye disease. Has the client experienced recent eye irritation and perhaps attributed it to smog or other chemical irritants? The client may have noted dermatologic lesions. Ask the client about any lesions for which he or she may have used a corticosteroid cream. Has the client noticed any other vesicle-type lesions? Physical examination targets the involved joints and inspects for dermatologic lesions and the presence of localized infections.

As with any chronic disease, client education plays a crucial role in helping the individual understand and manage the disease. Similar to RA (see prior discussion), clients and their families need information about the disease process and management. Because of the link to genitourinary pathology, education must target safe sexual practices. There is some evidence that use of a condom protects the client from postvenereal exacerbation of reactive arthritis. Clients are advised to avoid multiple sexual partners.

PSORIATIC ARTHRITIS

Psoriasis is a common skin disorder characterized by stippled nails, pruritus, and silvery scales on bright red plaques, usually on the elbows, knees, and scalp. It is a genetically determined disease associated with several histocompatibility antigens, including HLA-B14, HLA-Bw17, and HLA-Cw6. About 5% to 10% of those with psoriasis develop a distinctive inflammatory arthritis, i.e., PsA.

Three to five types of PsA have been proposed. In asymmetrical oligoarthropathy, there is asymmetrical involvement of both large and small joints, and sausage-shaped joints are common. With this type of arthritis, the asymmetrical pattern involves the interphalangeal and MTP joints of the feet and the DIP joints of the fingers. The second type, symmetrical polyarthropathy, closely resembles RA. Arthritis mutilans, a severe form of destructive arthritis, is characterized by telescoping digits, also known as the "opera-glass hand." Psoriatic spondylitis is characterized by the sacroiliitis of AS. Clients with this last type, characterized by DIP involvement, often have nail changes, such as pitting, transverse depressions, and subungual hyperkeratosis, along with DIP joint disease.

The overall prevalence of PsA is approximately 0.1% in the United States. Arthritis occurs in approximately 5% to 7% of clients with psoriasis, but it may affect 40% of hospitalized clients with extensive skin involvement. Two percent of white North Americans and Europeans are believed to be affected with psoriasis, but it is relatively uncommon in Asians. The male-to-female ratio is equal but varies in subsets of this disease. In contrast to psoriasis in which the peak age is between 5 and 15 years, the peak age of PsA is between 30 and 55 years, which is similar to that for RA.[4]

Etiology and Risk Factors

The cause of psoriatic arthritis appears to be a complex combination of immunologic, genetic, and environmental factors. Immunologic changes seen in some clients include elevated titers of IgG and IgA and the presence of immune complexes. There is an increased prevalence of the disease among family members who have PsA. Possible environmental factors include group A streptococci and trauma.

Clinical Manifestations

The diagnosis of PsA is usually confirmed after a positive history of psoriasis and specific x-ray findings. It is important; however, to realize that, in some clients, particularly children, joint changes precede skin changes. Nevertheless, most rheumatologists agree that the diagnosis cannot be made without evidence of psoriatic skin or nail changes.

Some changes that appear on x-ray film are suggestive of PsA. In early cases, soft tissue swelling can be seen in clients with psoriasis similar to that observed in RA. Periarticular demineralization of the bone, however, is less common in PsA. Radiologic findings indicative of the disease include erosions of the DIP joints (both hands and feet), which can lead to a whittled, "pencil-in-cup" appearance. Clients with spinal involvement have radiologic evidence of sacroiliitis, but the distribution of the joint changes is less predictable than it is in AS.

Laboratory tests often reveal a slightly elevated sedimentation rate and hypochromic anemia. Many clients have mild hyperuricemia, a confusing finding that could initially lead to the diagnosis of gout. Tests for RF are negative in 75% of clients; among the 25% with positive tests, many have coexisting psoriasis and RA.

Outcome Management
■ Medical Management

Although clients with PsA can have an explosive onset of polyarticular or monoarticular joint pain, erythema, and swelling, treatment goals are directed to the management of a chronic illness. Clients can be confused or discouraged when they first realize their diagnosis. They may perceive themselves as having not just one but two chronic diseases and thus feel increasingly powerless or helpless about their illness. Nurses and physicians, therefore, must work collaboratively to educate clients about the cause of the disease and the expected course of treatment. As with all other arthritic diseases, engaging the client's interest and partnership in actively managing the disease is essential for the best outcomes.

Nurses work with physicians to educate clients about key treatment strategies, many of which are similar to those implemented in RA and AS. During exacerbations of the disease, clients must avoid stressing inflamed joints, participate in active assistive ROM exercises to prevent joint contractures, and alternate periods of rest with activity. Those with foot and toenail involvement must be instructed to select appropriate footwear to protect swollen digits and keratotic nailbeds.

Reduce Inflammation. The initial treatment for stable plaque psoriasis is topical. However topical therapy may be impractical for clients with extensive psoriasis (more than 20% involvement) and systemic therapy may be indicated at the outset. Topical treatment includes emollients and keratolytic agents alone or in combination with anthralin, corticosteroids, and vitamin D derivatives. Stress and certain drugs (beta-adrenergic blockers, ACE inhibitors, lithium, and antimalarial drugs) may exacerbate psoriasis and should be used with caution.

In general, PsA is managed following the same principles used to treat RA or spondylitis.[7] Treatment depends on the type of joint disease (axial versus peripheral) and the severity of the joint and skin involvement. Simultaneous joint and skin disease activity has been observed in up to one third of clients, particularly those with non-spondylitis disease. The medical management of PsA begins with the administration of NSAIDs. If the response to NSAIDs is inadequate or if the disease is progressive, erosive, or polyarticular, DMARDs should be initiated **EB** as early as possible. MTX is effective for both the skin disease and peripheral arthritis. Dosage and monitoring is the same as for RA. Sulfasalazine (2 to 3 g/day) is helpful for both axial and peripheral arthritis. Sulfasalazine has no significant effect on the skin disease. Almost all of the DMARDs have been studied in small, open-label, uncontrolled studies and have shown some efficacy. Etanercept (Enbrel) significantly improves the arthritis **EB** and the skin disease and is approved for the treatment of PsA.

For clients with intractable pain or loss of joint function, surgery may be indicated. Although several reports have raised concerns about a higher risk of infections, recurrent contracture or stiffness, or excessive bone formation after surgery, most of these fears seem ill founded and surgery should not be withheld.

■ Nursing Management of the Medical Client

The focus of the nursing history for persons with psoriatic arthritis is similar to that for persons with RA. Asymmetric pauciarticular arthritis, however, often occurs in PsA, so clients should be questioned about the nature, onset, and location of any acutely occurring painful, swollen joints. Questions about back pain and stiffness can help identify psoriatic spondylitis. In addition, clients should be asked about their psoriasis-associated skin changes—location, size, color, and degree of scaling of the plaques—as well as changes in the nailbeds of the fingers and the toes. Because the disease seems to be caused by several other factors, ask clients whether there is a family history of arthritis, PsA, or psoriasis.

Determine whether they have had a history of severe infection before or after developing manifestations of the disease or any episodes of local trauma to the hands, feet, or spine.

Assessment of the client with PsA begins with a thorough assessment of the skin for evidence of psoriatic plaques or nailbed changes. Such completeness is essential because the disease cannot be confirmed, even with characteristic radiologic changes, unless there is evidence of psoriasis. Usually located on extensor surfaces, psoriatic skin lesions are either macular or papular round scales that tend to bleed when they are removed. If clients deny that they have any skin involvement, examine all areas carefully, particularly the scalp, axillae, and umbilicus. Look carefully for pitting nails, which often precede skin rashes and are highly suggestive of psoriasis.

Defer the assessment of the musculoskeletal system until the examination of the integument is complete so subtle changes in either system are not overlooked. Because the range of joint involvement in PsA is extensive (e.g., asymmetrical or symmetrical, small or large, pauciarticular or monoarticular), each joint must be assessed for swelling, bogginess, and erythema. Pay particular attention to the small joints of the hands and feet, watching for swollen, sausage-shaped digits, which result from tenosynovitis of the flexor tendon sheath. Note whether any of the digits have assumed a spindle or telescopic shape.

Nursing interventions are especially important for the client with PsA experiencing impaired skin integrity and body image disturbance. Clients with psoriatic arthritis may need basic instruction about how to care for their skin. If skin changes are severe, the client should be referred to a dermatologist, or the nurse (and physician) should collaborate with the dermatologist if the client has previously sought care from this specialist. The nurse should review skin care principles, such as the purpose and application techniques of emollients to keep the skin soft, patting the skin dry after bathing instead of vigorous towel drying, and the correct application of topical ointments with a thin layer, sparingly applied. If the client is hospitalized, it is important that he or she assume responsibility for skin care as soon as it is feasible.

Because of the changes in both the skin and the joints, it is likely that the client has experienced a significant body image disturbance. Being sensitive to clients' expressions can help assess the degree of integrity they perceive they have. It is not unusual for persons to be so affected by their appearance that they wear long-sleeved shirts on the hottest days and buy only clothes with pockets to hide their altered fingers. The communication of positive unconditional regard by the nurse—and all members of the health care team—can be a powerful tool to help clients begin to feel comfortable exploring their feelings.

FIBROMYALGIA SYNDROME

Not all people complaining of musculoskeletal pain have arthritis. Fibromyalgia syndrome is an increasingly recognized chronic musculoskeletal pain disorder of unknown cause. It occurs in about 2% to 5% of the general population, predominately in girls and young women. Active research is being conducted to find the cause. Clinical manifestations include fatigue, morning stiffness, nonrefreshing sleep due to lack of stage 4 sleep, and postexertional muscle pain. About one third of clients have associated problems such as irritable bowel syndrome, tension headaches, premenstrual syndrome, numbness and tingling, and Raynaud's phenomenon. Fatigue is the most common clinical manifestation, and the most common cause of the fatigue is chronic depression.[14]

Outcome Management

Management involves reducing clinical manifestations and includes L-tryptophan to increase sleep, tricyclic antidepressants to inhibit serotonin uptake, benzodiazepines for the treatment of anxiety associated with depression, and corticosteroids and NSAIDs for pain control. Low-intensity exercise is also important and helps decrease pain. Biofeedback, acupuncture, and hypnotherapy have also been used to help manage nonmuscular problems such as functional diarrhea, tension headache, and fatigue. The efficacy of these treatments is yet to be fully ascertained.

Many clients with fibromyalgia perceive themselves to be significantly disabled and have a reduced quality of life that rivals conditions such as RA and terminal emphysema. Clients with fibromyalgia have difficulty coping with "daily hassles" and this, in turn, increases the psychological stress. Cognitive behavioral therapy is often effective in providing these clients with a sense of control over their lives.

IDIOPATHIC INFLAMMATORY MYOPATHY (POLYMYOSITIS AND DERMATOMYOSITIS)

Inflammatory diseases of muscle are a heterogeneous group of disorders characterized by proximal muscle weakness and nonsuppurative inflammation of skeletal muscle. Traditionally, the terms *polymyositis* and *dermatomyositis* have been used to represent these diseases. It is currently more appropriate to use the term *idiopathic inflammatory myopathy* to describe the entire group and reserve the terms polymyositis (PM) and dermatomyositis (DM) for more specific conditions or subsets.

Etiology

The idiopathic myopathies are relatively rare diseases. Accurate estimates of their prevalence are difficult to obtain because the diseases are uncommon and lack uni-versally accepted specific diagnostic criteria. Estimates of incidence range from 0.5 to 8.4 cases per million. The incidence appears to be increasing, although this may simply reflect increased awareness and more accurate diagnosis. Although PM and DM affect all age groups, there is a bimodal distribution of the age of onset with peaks at ages 10 and 15 years in children and between 45 and 60 years in adults. As with other rheumatic diseases, there is a 2:1 female-to-male predominance in PM-DM, with the exception of inclusion body myositis, which affects men twice as often. Racial differences are apparent. In adults, the lowest rates are reported in the Japanese and the highest in African Americans. Although no direct relationships have been established between an inflammatory myopathy and a specific genetic marker, several associations have been recognized. The strongest associations are for HLA-B8, HLA-DR3, and DRW52 phenotypes with PM and DM in all age groups.

Muscle weakness with an underlying malignancy develops in a subset of clients with inflammatory myopathies. Malignancy may precede or follow the onset of muscle weakness. The association is rare in children, but has occurred in clients of all ages in all subsets of disease, although associated malignancy may be more common with DM. Subsequent studies seem to indicate that the types of tumors found roughly paralleled those found in the general population with the exception of ovarian cancer, which is overrepresented in women with DM.

Increased mortality has been associated with DM rather than PM. Mortality in PM is predicted by more extensive clinical involvement and is considerably higher in blacks than in whites.

Pathophysiology

The results of muscle biopsies, usually of the deltoid or quadriceps muscles, have provided useful information about the pathology of the disease. Several changes have been noted, including focal or extensive degeneration of muscle fibers caused by inflammatory infiltrates of lymphocytes and macrophages. In some cases, necrosis of parts or entire groups of muscle fibers can occur. Fibers, however, can also show evidence of regeneration.

The idiopathic myopathies are believed to be immune-mediated processes that are triggered by environmental factors in genetically susceptible individuals. This is supported by two observations: (1) there is a recognized association with other autoimmune and connective tissue diseases and (2) there is a high prevalence of circulating autoantibodies. The autoantibodies associated with PM-DM include the myositis specific autoantibodies (MSAs) found almost exclusively in these diseases. The triggering event of PM-DM is unknown, but viruses have been strongly implicated. The seasonal variation in the onset of disease is direct evidence that infectious agents play a role and there is further such evidence found in animal models. Genetic factors play an important role. Individuals with HLA-DR3 are at increased risk for development of inflammatory muscle disease including PM and juvenile DM. All clients with the anti-Jo-1 antibodies have the HLA antigen DR52, and white clients also have a high prevalence of HLA-B8, HLA-DR3, and DR6. Inclusion body myositis is more likely associated with HLA-DR1, DR6, and DQ1.

Clinical Manifestations

The most frequently occurring idiopathic myopathies in adults—PM and DM—are diffuse, systemic, inflammatory connective tissue diseases. Although these disorders can have an acute onset and progress rapidly, more typically there is a slower progression. Clients gradually develop significant weight loss, fatigue, and weakness over a period of months, sometimes not even being aware of when the changes began. Both diseases cause symmetrical progressive weakness of the proximal or limb-girdle muscles and occasionally atrophy of the muscles of the limbs, neck, and pharynx. Decreased muscle strength occurs in the pelvic girdle first, followed by weakness of the legs and shoulders and arms. Weakness of the flexor muscles of the neck occurs in about half of those affected with PM-DM. In acute disease, muscles can be tender or swollen and doughy. When classic skin changes are associated with PM, the disease is classified as *dermatomyositis*. The classification of idiopathic inflammatory myopathies, to which PM and DM belong, includes seven groups: (1) PM, (2) DM, (3) amyopathic DM, (4) juvenile DM, (5) myositis associated with neoplasia, (6) myositis associated with collagen vascular disease, and (7) inclusion body myositis.[22]

The criteria developed in 1975 for the diagnosis of PM and DM continue to be used: (1) proximal, symmetrical muscle weakness, with or without dysphagia or respiratory muscle weakness, (2) elevation of serum muscle enzymes, (3) characteristic electromyographic (EMG) changes, (4) muscle biopsy evidence of myositis, and (5) the typical skin rash of DM. In addition, the diagnosis is confirmed after excluding other neuromuscular diseases, such as myasthenia gravis, amyotrophic lateral sclerosis, polymyalgia rheumatica, and Guillain-Barré syndrome. Research continues to refine the diagnostic criteria for PM-DM, and four additional criteria may become standard in the future.

The most important laboratory test is the measurement of the muscle enzyme CK (formerly creatine phosphokinase). An elevated CK level indicates muscle injury, but it is not specific to PM-DM. Elevated CK levels can be seen after intramuscular injections, muscle biopsies, or exercise, for example. The level of CK changes according to the activity of the disease. Other muscle enzymes are also elevated, in most cases including aldolase, SGOT, SGPT, and LDH. The sedimentation rate is normal in 50% of clients.

EMG results often show bizarre, high-frequency discharges with spontaneous fibrillations and positive spikes at rest. Muscle biopsies are done if there is doubt about the diagnosis. The muscle chosen should be affected by the disease but not atrophied. The site should not be one where a previous EMG needle has been introduced. When biopsies are performed under general anesthesia, a permanent scar usually forms, and the area is sore for several weeks. For these reasons, physicians may prefer not to perform the biopsy unless it is essential to making the diagnosis. Muscle biopsy results, as previously mentioned, show changes associated with necrosis and degeneration as well as evidence of regeneration. Fibrosis may be seen.

Outcome Management
■ Medical Management

Treatment of PM-DM usually begins with the daily administration of high doses of oral corticosteroids. Prednisone (1 to 2 mg/kg/day) is given until elevated muscle enzymes begin to decrease toward normal and clients show improvement in their ability to perform ADL. In severe cases, the daily dose can be divided or intravenous methylprednisolone may be used. Reduction in steroid dosages to alternate-day therapy may not be possible for several months. Some clients require long-term treatment with maintenance doses of steroids because the disease can recur when the steroids are withdrawn. Clients who do not respond to steroids or who cannot tolerate the high steroid doses usually require the addition of an immunosuppressive agent, such as daily azathioprine (50 to 150 mg/day) or weekly MTX therapy (7.5 mg/week orally or 0.5 to 0.8 mg/kg/week intravenously). Other immunosuppressive agents have been used in steroid-resistant clients. Cyclophosphamide, 6-mercaptopurine, chlorambucil, total-body (or total-nodal) irradiation, and intravenous immunoglobulins have also been used. HCQ can be used to treat the cutaneous lesions of DM, although it has no recognized effect on the myositis.

■ Nursing Management of the Medical Client

Eliciting the history of a person with PM-DM begins with the client's perspective. He or she seeks health care because of the nonspecific changes, usually occurring over several months, of increasing fatigue, weight loss, and malaise. When questioned about the nature of the fatigue and how it affects his or her ability to carry out ADL, clients usually describe difficulty performing tasks because of muscle weakness. Good screening questions include queries about the changes in ability to perform ADL that require the use of large muscle groups. Questions about the onset, duration, location, and quality of muscle pain should be asked. Muscle pain or tenderness may or may not be present in the early phases of the disease. Ask the client whether he or she has had difficulty brushing hair, reaching overhead for objects on a shelf or putting on clothes, or performing repetitive chores, such as mowing the lawn, hanging up laundry, or putting away groceries.

For a history of pelvic limb weakness, determine whether the client has had difficulty rising from an armless chair, getting out of a car, climbing steps, or riding a bike. Ask whether the client has had difficulties in raising the neck off the bed or pillow. Question the client about associated joint pains because arthritis and arthralgia occur in many persons who are in overlap group V (i.e., they have both PM and DM and evidence of another collagen vascular disease, such as RA or SSc). Some clients may report a tendency to fall that is unrelated to balance, so explore changes in gait patterns with them. Because muscle weakness in the face and larynx is seen in PM-DM, determine whether there has been any difficulty in chewing or swallowing, facial swelling, or hoarseness.

Because PM-DM is a systemic disease, questions must also be included about the integumentary, pulmonary, and cardiovascular systems. Determine whether the client has experienced any skin or nail changes—rash, reddened areas, scaling—typical of those seen in DM. Common respiratory complications of PM-DM include aspiration pneumonia (because of a weakened cough, slow protective movements with vomiting, and pharyngeal muscle weakness) and interstitial lung disease. Questions about whether clients had previous respiratory diseases, particularly pneumonia and influenza-like illnesses, and about how they recovered give important information to surgical nurses for preoperative and postoperative pulmonary care. The client's cardiac history should be assessed via questions about dysrhythmias and whether the person has a prolapsed mitral valve.

The physical examination of the client with PM-DM requires a meticulous assessment of the skin and nailbeds for the presence of erythema, macular-papular rashes, plaques, scaling, and nodules. Skin changes can help direct this examination. To confirm the presence of a heliotrope rash on the client's face, hold the neck and head securely while it is lowered off the examination table or the side of the bed. This maneuver elicits increased suffusion to bring out the distinctive color of the bluish red hue of the rash.

Initially test for muscle weakness by asking the client to walk, get up from a chair without arms, raise the neck off the bed or table, or lift a heavy book. Loss of hand strength is less noticeable, but it can be detected by a test of grip strength. Asking the client to shrug the shoulders upward against the nurse's hands can test proximal weakness of the shoulder girdle. Weakness of the masseter muscles (which can be seen in clients who have difficulty chewing) is assessed by palpating their strength when the client clenches the teeth. All muscle groups should be palpated for symmetry, atrophy, pain or tenderness, and the presence of contractures. Atrophy generally appears late in the disease, but contractures develop early if muscle weakness has been severe. As muscles are being assessed, large and small joints should be inspected for erythema, pain, presence of synovitis, and limitations in ROM.

Although the focus of the examination is on the integumentary and musculoskeletal systems, thorough assessment of the cardiopulmonary system is required because of the systemic nature of the disease. The bilateral assessment of chest expansion (diaphragmatic excursion) helps the nurse know how compliant the muscles of respiration are. The quality of the breathing, the presence of dyspnea with simple activities, and the presence of a cough can indicate an acute or chronic respiratory problem with muscle disease. The quality of the lung sounds should be carefully assessed for fine rales (crackles) because aspiration pneumonia is a frequent complication of advanced PM-DM.

The education of clients on high-dose steroid therapy focuses on teaching them about the potential side effects of long-term prednisone (see the Integrating Pharmacology feature on pp. 2342 to 2344). Clients should be aware that they have an increased risk of infection, so they should monitor and report any manifestations, such as low-grade fevers, chills, or joint pain, to their primary caregivers. Other long-term effects include facial edema, increased appetite, and the development of diabetes mellitus, osteoporosis, and avascular necrosis. Clients should also be instructed to wear a MedicAlert identification tag as long as they are on prednisone therapy. Clients must clearly understand that they should never change a dose of prednisone. Steroids must be tapered slowly after high-dose or long-term use because the body cannot respond quickly to changes in cortisol levels. During the period in which high doses of steroids have been administered, the hypothalamus-pituitary-adrenocortical axis has been suppressed, thus leading to negative feedback for the natural production of cortisol. Steroid-dependent clients who abruptly discontinue their therapy can experience an addisonian crisis (characterized by circulatory collapse, vomiting, and severe weakness) with minimal stress.

Clients with involvement of the pharyngeal and respiratory muscles must be carefully monitored for the prevention of aspiration pneumonia. Helping clients maintain or regain effective swallowing can significantly reduce aspiration. Resting before meals, eating easily swallowed foods (such as those of a smooth, slippery consistency), and sitting upright during meals are measures that can enhance the client's ability to swallow.

Clients with PM-DM are also at risk of falling because of muscle weakness, gait changes, and the possibility of osteoporosis from high-dose prednisone therapy. Balancing a muscle-strengthening program with the use of assistive devices and instructions about safe ambulation helps to keep the client injury free.

BURSITIS

Bursitis is a painful inflammation of the bursae, those closed, minimally fluid-filled sacs that are lined with a synovium similar to the lining of joint spaces. The purpose of bursae is to reduce friction between adjacent tissues—tendon and bones or tendons and ligaments—by lubricating these enclosed structures with synovial fluid from the bursal sac. Approximately 150 bursae are found in the human body. They typically cover bony prominences, such as the olecranon, trochanter, and patella, or they provide protection between the skin and other structures, such as the calcaneal bursa. Bursae are usually thin, but with repeated stress, they can become thickened and fluid-filled secondary to inflammation. Bursitis can be either an acute or a chronic condition.

Approximately 3% of the adult population has been estimated to have painful, symptomatic bursitis. The problem peaks between the ages of 40 and 50, presumably as active adults first experience the beginning of degenerative changes in the joints. The shoulder joint is the most commonly affected, followed by the elbow, knee, and hip. When bursitis involves the upper extremities, the dominant arm is usually affected.

Risk factors associated with the development of bursitis include acute or chronic trauma, typically through participation in mechanical, highly repetitive activities. Other causes include such arthritic conditions as RA, gout, tumors, and degenerative changes associated with increasing age. Bursitis is considered a true inflammatory condition with the classic manifestations of inflammation, local redness, warmth, and swelling.

Typically, the client with acute bursitis complains of exquisite localized pain in the target area. Clients may experience point tenderness; that is, they can point specifically to the spot of greatest discomfort. They may also have diffuse soreness radiating to the tendons at the site. Depending on the location of the bursitis, clients may complain of interrupted sleep (e.g., with subacromial bursitis, calcaneal bursitis), difficulty walking (trochanteric bursitis, calcaneal bursitis), or difficulty performing ADL (subacromial or olecranon bursitis).

Occupational or avocational activities can also provide insight into the nature of the pain, for example, a woodcarver who has developed acute subacromial bursitis or a businesswoman who walks long distances in medium to high heels and develops retrocalcaneal bursitis.

The diagnosis of bursitis is generally based on the results of the history and physical examination. Radiographs of the affected joint are usually normal in acute bursitis, whereas in chronic conditions, calcium deposits may be present. Results of laboratory tests and synovial fluid analysis are normal unless the bursa has become infected.

Outcome Management

Acute bursitis is treated with rest and immobilization of the affected joint, non-opioid analgesics, and ROM exercises. In general, the pain of acute bursitis is controlled with NSAIDs. Client education focuses on the causes of bursitis, the prevention of additional attacks (by avoiding activities that cause constant friction or pressure),

the correct application of moist heat, and medication and exercise instruction.

Appropriate nursing diagnoses for clients with bursitis include acute or chronic pain, impaired physical mobility, and temporary self-care deficits. Helping clients obtain reduction of pain is the primary focus of nursing interventions. Without pain reduction, joint mobility is impaired through guarding, protective measures. Nurses must instruct clients about the purpose of anti-inflammatory medications, the appropriate dose, and the untoward side effects. Pain reduction is also achieved by resting or immobilizing the joint or by elevating or compressing the involved area to control edema. Teaching clients about the correct application of ice and heat is important so they receive maximum pain reduction. If clients receive intra-articular injections of cortisone, they should be informed about the possibility of a postinjection flare. They should also be reassured that the pain responds quickly to the application of ice packs.

Self-care deficits are usually temporary in acute bursitis. If the condition becomes chronic, clients may experience more difficulties, particularly if the shoulder or elbow is involved. Dressing is easier when oversized garments are worn, especially those with long sleeves or wide pant legs. Shirts and tops that button in the front are also helpful. Clients can be taught to minimize shoulder or elbow pain by putting clothing on the affected arm first and by taking it off the affected arm last.

VASCULITIS

Vasculitis comprises a group of disorders leading to inflammation and necrosis of blood vessel walls. Soluble immune complexes are deposited in blood vessel walls in areas where capillaries have increased permeability. After deposition, the immune system is activated and the complex is destroyed along with the blood vessel wall. These disorders include polyarteritis nodosa, systemic necrotizing vasculitis, and allergic granulomatous angiitis. Inflammation and damage to large and small vessels result in end-stage organ damage.

Specific manifestations vary, depending on the organs affected. Steroids are the treatment of choice for these disorders.

POLYMYALGIA RHEUMATICA

Polymyalgia rheumatica is a clinical syndrome occurring more commonly in women than in men. It is a disease of aging, rarely occurring before age 60 years. It is characterized by pain and stiffness in the neck, shoulder, back, and pelvic girdle, especially in the morning. Headaches or painful areas on the head may be present. The client also may have a low-grade fever or temporal arteritis. Laboratory findings include an elevated ESR, mild anemia, and possible elevation of immunoglobulins. Steroids usually produce symptomatic relief within days.

GIANT CELL ARTERITIS

Giant cell arteritis, also known as temporal or cranial arteritis, is also a disease of older people. The client often has manifestations of polymyalgia rheumatica for months, then suddenly experiences the severe headaches associated with temporal arteritis. The onset of this disorder is usually sudden, with severe pain often appearing in the temporal area. The pain also may be felt in the occipital area, face, jaw, or side of the neck. It is usually associated with hyperesthesia, which makes any touch exquisitely painful. The client may experience visual changes, including sudden onset of blindness in one or both eyes.

It is important to diagnose and treat this disorder before blindness occurs. Because older women are often affected, their complaints of decreased vision and headaches are sometimes ignored as normal aging. Treatment is with corticosteroids, which are highly effective in controlling this disorder.

MIXED CONNECTIVE TISSUE DISEASE

Mixed connective tissue disease is a combination of several connective tissue diseases. Clients have manifestations that are not typical of any one disorder. Frequent combinations are SLE and SSc and RA. Mixed connective tissue diseases are managed according to their manifestations.

LYME DISEASE

Lyme disease is one form of rheumatic joint disease with a known cause. It is included as a connective tissue disorder because the skin, joints, nervous system, and heart are involved. This complex multisystem disease is caused by the tick-borne spirochete *Borrelia burgdorferi.* Clinical manifestations found from 3 to 32 days after the bite may include a red flat rash that clears in the center, severe headache, stiff neck, fever, chills, myalgias, joint pain, severe malaise, and fatigue.

The disease can be treated with a course of antibiotic therapy. Doxycycline is the most common antibiotic used. Neurologic abnormalities may occur if treatment is ineffective. Intra-articular steroids and NSAIDs may be used to reduce joint inflammation and pain. Long-term effects include fatigue and arthralgia for many years after the initial infection.

CONCLUSIONS

Nursing clients with rheumatic disorders prove to be challenging. Clients can experience acute exacerbations or crises with almost all of these diseases. Systemic manifestations can be as devastating as the musculoskeletal manifestations. The unpredictable nature of these disorders results in considerable uncertainty, which in turn leads to a cycle of ineffective coping, disturbed self-esteem, helplessness, and powerlessness. In many respects, the psychological and social problems that are associated with these chronic illnesses are more disabling than the physical complaints.

Physiologically, clients with autoimmune disorders, spondyloarthropathies, or inflammatory joint diseases experience many common problems. The triad of pain, fatigue, and stiffness must be controlled so that function is enhanced or maintained. If this triad, which represents a runaway inflammatory response, is not held in check, essential self-care deficits develop. Difficulty with self-care is usually accompanied by sleep disturbances, altered nutrition, and impaired mobility. All of these problems can adversely affect the individual's self-concept and self-esteem and so lead to social isolation.

Because of the chronicity of these disorders, clients need skilled, knowledgeable nursing care that draws on the disciplines of rehabilitation, counseling, and self-care. The unique role of the nurse for these clients is one that assumes accountability and responsibility for guiding and directing the client through the health care maze. Clients with chronic, usually systemic illnesses require multiple therapies and follow-up appointments for pharmacologic management, nutritional counseling, lifestyle assessment, physical and occupational therapy, and psychological support, to name just a few. The personal and financial cost demanded by the arthritic disorder can exhaust the client's enthusiasm, job security, support systems, and sense of purpose in life. The nurse can provide a sense of consistency, hope, and reassurance that the client can learn to cope with, and positively adapt to, the demands of a chronic illness. Clients with arthritis need the nurse's expertise to teach them how to explore new self-care strategies so successful adaptation to the disease is a reality. Nurses help clients learn to become partners with the entire health care team as well as with themselves. When clients assume the role of partner, they exhibit greater control, greater accountability, and increased self-esteem as they learn self-management skills. This is nowhere more self-evident than in the clients giving themselves their bi-weekly or daily injections.

THINKING CRITICALLY *evolve*

1. You are working in an outpatient clinic and receive a call from a 66-year-old woman who is experiencing a

flare-up of rheumatoid arthritis. She was seen 2 days ago in the clinic and was given a high dose of prednisone. Now she reports epigastric abdominal pain. She reports that her pain has a burning quality, is worse between meals, is relieved by food, and is aggravated by coffee. She has taken some over-the-counter ibuprofen for the pain but states, "It didn't help." What other information do you need to collect? What interventions would you advise?

Factors to Consider. Consider the side effects of corticosteroids and NSAIDs.

2. A 55-year-old woman with a history of joint pain is scheduled for shoulder arthroplasty. She has experienced increasing pain while working as a waitress and handling orders that must be carried to tables of restaurant guests. She hopes to be able to work pain-free so she can resume her job as a waitress. What nursing assessments are pertinent to this type of condition and proposed surgery? How realistic is the client's desire to return to work as a waitress?

Factors to Consider. How will assessments help in the prevention of postoperative complications? Are clients able to return to an improved level of functioning after joint replacement surgery?

Discussions for these questions can be found on the website and the CD-ROM.

BIBLIOGRAPHY

1. Acorn, J., Joachim, G., & Wachs, J. (2003). Scleroderma: Living with unpredictability. *AAOHN Journal, 51*(8), 358-359.
2. Arnett, F.C., et al. (1988). The American Rheumatism Association 1987 revised criteria for the classification of rheumatoid arthritis. *Arthritis and Rheumatism, 31,* 315-324.
3. Callahan, L., & Yelin, E. (2001). The social and economic consequences of rheumatic disease. In Klippel, J.H. (Ed.), *Primer on the rheumatic disease* (12th ed., pp. 1-4). Atlanta: Arthritis Foundation.
4. Cooper, G., & Stroehla, B. (2003). The epidemiology of autoimmune diseases. *Autoimmune Review, 2*(3), 119-125.
5. Ellman, M.H., MacDonald, P.A., & Hayes, F.A. (2000). Etanercept as treatment for diffuse scleroderma: A pilot study. *Arthritis and Rheumatism, 43,* S392.
6. Graham, D., et al. (2002). Ulcer prevention in long-term users of nonsteroidal anti-inflammatory drugs. *Archives of Internal Medicine, 162,* 169-175.
7. Guidelines for the management of rheumatic diseases. (2001). In Klippel, J.H. (Ed.), *Primer on the rheumatic disease* (12th ed., pp. 649-650). Atlanta: Arthritis Foundation.
8. Hansen, A., Lipsky, P., & Dorner, T. (2003). New concepts in the pathogenesis of Sjögren's syndrome: Many questions, fewer answers. *Current Opinions in Rheumatology, 15*(5), 563-570.
9. Manzi, S. (2001). Systemic lupus erythematosus: Treatment. In Klippel, J.H. (Ed.), *Primer on the rheumatic diseases* (12th ed., pp. 346-352). Atlanta: Arthritis Foundation.
10. Marchesoni, A., et al. (2003). Radiographic progression in early rheumatoid arthritis: A 12-month randomized controlled study comparing the combination of cyclosporine and methotrexate with methotrexate alone. *Rheumatology, 42,* 1-5.
11. Mayes, M., et al. (2003). Prevalence, incidence, survival, and disease characteristics of systemic sclerosis in a large U.S. population. *Arthritis and Rheumatology, 48*(8), 2246-2255.
12. Meenan, R., Callahan, L., & Helmich, C. (1999). The Arthritis Action Plan: A public health strategy for a looming epidemic. *Arthritis Care and Research, 12,* 79-81.
13. National Center for Chronic Disease Prevention and Health Promotion. (1999). *National Arthritis Action Plan: A public health strategy.* Atlanta: Centers for Disease Control and Prevention.
14. Neumann, L., & Buskila, D. (2003). Epidemiology of fibromyalgia. *Current Pain and Headache Reports, 7*(5), 362-368.
15. Pisetsky, D.S. (2001). Systemic lupus erythematosus: Epidemiology, pathology and pathogenesis. In Klippel, J.H. (Ed.), *Primer on the rheumatic diseases* (12th ed., pp. 329-335). Atlanta: Arthritis Foundation.
16. Schneider, J., Matthews, J., & Graham, B. (2003). Reiter's syndrome. *Cutis, 71*(3), 198-200.
17. Simon, L., et al. (2002). Controversies on COX-2 selective inhibition. Consensus Conference Report. *Journal of Rheumatology, 29*(7), 1501-1510
18. Tan, E., et al. (1982). The 1982 revised criteria for the classification of systemic lupus erythematosus (SLE). *Arthritis and Rheumatism, 25,* 1271-1277.
19. Turesson, C., O'Fallon, W., & Crowson, C. (2003). Extra-articular disease manifestations in rheumatoid arthritis: Incidence, trends and risk factors over 46 years. *Annals of Rheumatic Diseases, 62*(8), 722-727.
20. Weinblatt, M., et al. (1999). A trial of etanercept, a recombinant tumor necrosis factor receptor: Fc fusion protein, in clients with rheumatoid arthritis receiving methotrexate. *New England Journal of Medicine, 340,* 253-259.
21. Wolfe, F., et al. (2003). Predicting mortality in patients with rheumatoid arthritis. *Arthritis and Rheumatology, 48*(6), 1530-1542.
22. Wortmann, R. (2001). Inflammatory and metabolic disease of muscle. In Klippel, J.H. (Ed.), *Primer on the rheumatic diseases* (12th ed., pp. 369-376). Atlanta: Arthritis Foundation.

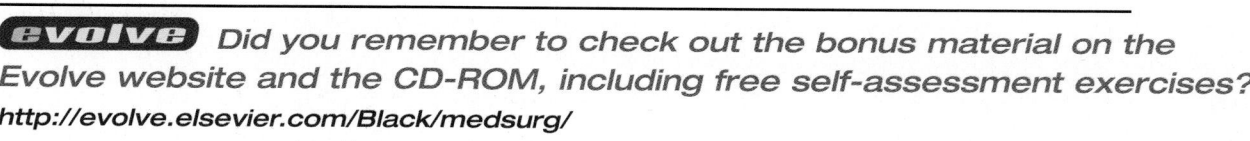

evolve *Did you remember to check out the bonus material on the Evolve website and the CD-ROM, including free self-assessment exercises?*
http://evolve.elsevier.com/Black/medsurg/

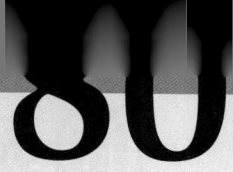

Management of Clients with Acquired Immunodeficiency Syndrome

Meg Blair

The human immunodeficiency virus (HIV) infects people worldwide and results in destruction of the body's host defenses and immune system. By 2002, HIV infected more than 42 million people throughout the world, with an estimated five million people newly infected each year. The Centers for Disease Control and Prevention (CDC) has reported an overall increase in new diagnoses of HIV from 1999 to 2002. The incidence of HIV increased 55% in blacks and 26% in Hispanics. There were no significant changes in incidence for Asian-Americans or Native Americans. New diagnoses increased 17% in homosexual and bisexual men. HIV kills more people than any other infectious disease and ranks fourth among the leading causes of death worldwide.

For many years, because of our lack of understanding and effective treatment, HIV was considered a rapidly progressing fatal disease. Today HIV infection is viewed more optimistically as a chronic disease that can be controlled with appropriate health care. The cost of such health care (~$12,000 yearly per person), however, limits its accessibility to developed, industrialized nations such as the United States. Because many parts of the world, such as Africa and Asia, lack adequate economic resources to treat this disease, HIV infection continues to be a rapidly progressing fatal illness in these areas.

From both a medical and nursing perspective, clinical management parallels the HIV illness trajectory. Once infected with HIV, a person who receives appropriate treatment can live for many years and continue to function without major problems. In the latter stages of disease, for a variety of reasons to be discussed, the illness progresses, wearing out the immune system. The person is then given the diagnosis acquired immunodeficiency syndrome (AIDS). Because of this dual clinical picture, the material presented in this chapter is divided into (1) caring for the person with HIV disease and (2) caring for the person with AIDS.

Etiology and Risk Factors

Etiology

The etiologic agent associated with AIDS was first isolated by French scientists in 1983 and named the *lymphadenopathy-associated virus*. One year later, an Ameri-

Nursing Outcomes Classification (NOC)
for Nursing Diagnoses—Clients with HIV/AIDS

Acute Pain or Chronic Pain
  Comfort Level
  Pain Control
  Pain: Disruptive Effects
  Pain Level
Effective Therapeutic Regimen Management
  Adherence Behavior
  Compliance Behavior
  Family Participation in Professional Care

  Knowledge: Treatment Regimen
  Participation: Health Care Decisions
  Risk Control
  Symptom Control
Fatigue
  Activity Intolerance
  Endurance
  Energy Conservation
  Nutritional Status: Energy
  Psychomotor Energy

Hyperthermia
  Immune Status
  Thermoregulation
Imbalanced Nutrition: Less Than Body Requirements
  Nutritional Status
  Nutritional Status: Food and Fluid Intake
  Nutritional Status: Nutrient Intake

can scientist claimed the discovery of the etiologic agent and named it the *human T-cell lymphotropic virus type III*. Although both scientists actually identified the same virus, much confusion took place. In 1986 the International Society on the Taxonomy of Viruses renamed the virus, calling it the *human immunodeficiency virus*. In that same year, to everyone's surprise, a second and distinctly different strain of the virus was discovered in Africa. Therefore since 1986, the scientific names to distinguish between the two viruses are HIV-1 and HIV-2.

This was a major—and alarming—discovery because it was the first clue that HIV could change its appearance, or mutate, rapidly. This capability is called *genetic promiscuity*, and it has become the hallmark of the virus, creating a monumental challenge for scientists and researchers alike. HIV-1 is distributed worldwide, but it is most prevalent in Europe and the United States. HIV-2 predominates in west African nations but has been isolated in other parts of the world. By 1999 approximately 79 cases of HIV-2 had been identified in the United States; most of the infected people had been born in Africa. Most worldwide infections are HIV-1.

By 1996 scientists discovered that HIV-1 had also mutated several times. It has two major subtypes, which are designated as (1) HIV-1 major (group M) viruses, and (2) HIV-1 outlier (group O) viruses.

HIV-1 Group M. Group M viruses are assigned to 10 genetic subtypes, designated HIV-1, group M, subtype A, B, C, D, E, F, G, H, I, and J, according to the phylogenetic analysis of their genes. The distribution of subtypes varies worldwide. For example, subtype B predominates in North America and Europe, and subtypes A, B, C, and E have been identified in India. There is concern that subtypes other than B will invade the United States because American service personnel assigned to overseas duty

who have become infected with HIV-1 have been found to be infected with subtypes A, D, and E.

It is important to mention these complexities to illustrate the rapidly changing nature of HIV. The virus poses a considerable challenge to researchers investigating new drugs to treat the disease or developing vaccines because their work is usually limited to one specific subtype of HIV-1. Indeed, vaccine trials have shown that a vaccine for one subtype may not work for other subtypes.

HIV-1 Group O. The designation O was deliberate because this mutation was an outlier and differed from the others in that it cannot be detected with the routine HIV antibody tests used in the United States. Group O was identified primarily in west and central Africa, with a few isolated cases found through special tests in France and the United States.

Risk Factors

Modes of transmission have remained constant throughout the course of the HIV pandemic. The virus is spread through certain sexual practices, through exposure to blood, and through perinatal (vertical) transmission. The patterns in the spread of HIV changed considerably during the first 19 years of the epidemic in the United States. Comparing the 1980s with the 1990s, significant increases have been noted in intravenous (IV) drug users, women, and heterosexuals. Although most Americans infected with HIV continue to be men who have sex with men, the overall number has decreased considerably. This decline, however, has been limited to white men; the number of new HIV infections among racial and ethnic minority men who have sex with men continues to increase, as outlined in the Diversity in Health Care feature on HIV and AIDS in Minority Populations on the website. In young adults (19 to 29 years of age), the number of new infections has been increasing, especially in the South and Midwest. HIV infection and AIDS are

The authors would like to thank Peter J. Ungvarski for his contribution to this chapter in the sixth edition of *Medical-Surgical Nursing*.

the second leading causes of death among adults 25 to 44 years of age.

Perhaps the most overlooked population in the HIV epidemic is adults over 50 years of age. By 1999 about 11% of the nation's total number of reported AIDS cases were in this age group; current estimates are as much as 20% to 30% of new cases. People over 50 years of age may not be tested promptly for HIV because they and their health care providers may not perceive them to be at risk for this disease. Women over 50 years of age acquire HIV infection primarily through heterosexual contact. Although the largest numbers of AIDS and HIV cases have been reported in large cities, such as New York and San Francisco, a shift has occurred of newly diagnosed infections to small cities and rural areas, especially in the South and Midwest.

The principal mode of transmission of HIV throughout the world has been through sexual exposure. Except in Australia, Europe, and the United States, most HIV transmission has been through heterosexual activity. One important lesson health care professionals have learned from this epidemic is that sexual *practices,* not sexual *preferences,* place people at risk for sexually transmitted diseases (STDs). Homosexual men who do not engage in unprotected sex or expose themselves to another person's body fluids are no more at risk for acquiring HIV infection than anyone else; similarly, heterosexual or homosexual couples in long-term, monogamous relationships are at low risk. Unsafe sexual encounters outside of these relationships do, however, pose a risk.

Sexual practices that are *completely safe* include (1) autosexual activities (such as masturbation), (2) mutually monogamous relationships between noninfected partners, and (3) abstinence. *Very safe* sexual practices include noninsertive activity. Insertive practices with a condom are considered *probably safe* so long as the condom does not break and no contact with body fluids occurs. Everything else is considered risky. Other cofactors, such as engaging in sexual activities while under the influence of drugs or alcohol, having multiple sex partners, and the presence of sores in the genital area, increase the risk of acquiring HIV. Although the number of reported cases is small, oral sexual practices, whether performed on a man or a woman, have been implicated as a possible transmission activity.

Transmission by exposure to blood is a broad category encompassing numerous possible routes. The most obvious are through the administration of blood or blood products, transplantation of donated tissue or organs, and implantation of semen contaminated with HIV. Prevention of HIV infection by any of these means is possible by donor exclusion (excluding persons from high-risk groups), routine serologic testing of donated tissues or fluids for HIV antibodies, and heat inactivation of certain blood products, such as factor VIII con-

centrate. Other means of preventing HIV infection related to blood products are *autologous* (self-donated) blood programs and limiting the administration of any blood product to situations in which it is absolutely necessary.

Use of injected drugs accounts for the largest number of HIV infections through exposure to contaminated blood. The only *absolutely safe* injecting drug use behavior is not to inject. *Very safe* practice is to use sterilized injection paraphernalia and never share needles and syringes. A *probably safe* practice is to clean injection paraphernalia with full-strength bleach before injecting, although disposable needles and syringes are difficult to clean. Anything else is considered risky. Other cofactors that increase the chances of acquiring HIV by drug injection include the seroprevalence of HIV in the geographical area of the drug user, the social setting of the drug use (e.g., "shooting galleries," where injection paraphernalia is shared), and the frequency of injection.

Needle exchange programs provide sterile injection equipment, latex condoms, counseling, and access to social and health programs, including drug treatment. Numerous studies have shown that needle exchange programs decrease the spread of HIV and hepatitis B and C and do not increase or promote injection drug use. Despite the proven success of this approach to disease prevention, state and federal legislators have been reluctant to appropriate funds to support this model of care. In the United States, because of existing attitudes about IV drug use, needle exchange programs may operate as legal, illegal but tolerated, or illegal or underground programs. In Europe, where the approach to preventing disease has received more favorable support, governments providing national health care services for their citizens have found that needle exchange programs not only reduce the incidence of disease but also have significantly reduced health care spending for diseases associated with IV drug injection.

Occupational exposure to blood is a potential problem not only for health care workers but also for members of other occupations, such as police and corrections officers. The state of Connecticut legalized the sale of sterile needles and syringes in certain drugstores and found they not only reduced the incidence of needle sharing in IV drug users but also resulted in a significant decrease in the number of occupationally acquired needle-stick injuries of police officers.

The problem of HIV transmission to health care workers by clients is an ongoing concern of workers, employers, and public health officials. In the United States, by January 1999, the cumulative total number of health care workers with documented, occupationally acquired HIV or AIDS was 54. The number with possible (less clear evidence) transmission was 134. Although most health care workers occupationally infected with HIV acquired the virus after percutaneous exposure, other modes of transmission included mucocutaneous exposure and direct exposure to HIV in the laboratory setting. The actual average risk to a health care worker for exposure to HIV is extremely low (0.3% after a needle-stick or sharp instrument injury and 0.09% after a mucous membrane exposure). The risk, when an exposure occurs, is increased in situations in which a deep injury occurs, when there is visible blood on the device causing the injury, when the device involved was previously placed in a client's artery or vein, and when AIDS was diagnosed in the source client who died within 60 days after the health care worker's exposure (presumably because concentrations of HIV in the blood are very high at this time).

Accidental needle-stick exposure poses the greatest hazard to health care workers. As health care workers, nurses should learn and follow Standard Precautions when handling blood and body fluids and when performing procedures that could lead to exposure to blood and body fluids. When any incident reflects potential exposure to blood-borne pathogens, seek medical treatment immediately. The U.S. Public Health Service has issued guidelines for evaluating and treating exposures to HIV. In the case of high-risk exposures, they recommend that combination antiretroviral therapy be given for at least 4 weeks for after-exposure prophylaxis.

In the United States, only one case of HIV transmission from a health care worker to clients has been documented. It was reported in 1990 and involved a Florida dentist. Six clients reportedly became infected with HIV after receiving dental care. The circumstances of this case implied inadequate disinfection and sterilization of instruments in the dental office. Since this incident, *retrospective* (look-back) studies of possible HIV transmis- sion from infected health care workers to clients have not identified any other cases in the United States. In 1999 one additional case of HIV transmission from a health care worker to a client was reported in France. An HIV-positive physician who was injured during orthopedic surgery transmitted HIV to the client. The surgeon acquired HIV in 1983 when he sustained an injury while operating on an HIV-infected client.

Perinatal HIV exposure can occur during pregnancy, during vaginal delivery, and post-partum through breast-feeding. Of all infants born to HIV-infected women worldwide, about 23% are infected. The risk of transmission from mother to child increases if viral activity is high and the CD4$^+$ titer is low, which is usually the case in later stages of HIV disease, when the diagnosis is AIDS. Administration of zidovudine to pregnant women has been shown to reduce the rate of vertical HIV infection from 23% to 8%. The CDC has published guide- lines for the use of zidovudine and other antiretroviral therapies for pregnant women and their newborn infants.

The only absolute method of preventing perinatal exposure is to avoid pregnancy. All health care workers should discuss HIV infection as part of routine prenatal care with all clients because many mothers may be unaware that they are infected with HIV. Infected women who carry to term should be advised against breast-feeding because this has been implicated as a mode of HIV transmission.

Primary prevention of HIV infection for exposed individuals is an emerging concept being applied not only to health care workers but also to the treatment of other accidental exposures. Post-exposure prophylaxis is being used as a health maintenance strategy by some clinicians for people who do the following:

- Have unprotected anal or vaginal intercourse
- Have receptive oral intercourse with ejaculation
- Share needles with an infected partner
- Have a single-event exposure, such as a rape
- Intend to stop high-risk behaviors

Considerable controversy surrounds the use of post-exposure prophylaxis except in cases of rape, and the ethical aspects of providing such treatment continue to be discussed.

Vaccine research has been ongoing since 1987. Vaccines are being developed to prevent HIV infection (*preventive vaccine*) and to treat people infected with HIV (*therapeutic vaccine*). Currently there are 11 classes of vaccine, with more in development, and 22 phase I or phase I/II vaccine trials ongoing. One major drawback to soliciting volunteers for these trials is the possibility that they will have a false-positive result for HIV after receiving the vaccine because their bodies have developed antibodies to the virus. This may pose a problem for these people when HIV testing is required, such as when they are seeking employment or applying for insurance.

Pathophysiology

HIV-1 is a member of the lentivirus subfamily of human retroviruses. Diseases caused by lentiviruses are characterized by an insidious onset with progressive involvement of the central nervous system (CNS) and may result in disorders of the immune system. HIV-1 is one of five viruses in the lentivirus family (Figure 80-1). The others are HIV-2 and human T-lymphotropic virus (HTLV) types I, II, and IV.

A retrovirus belongs to the family Retroviridae and possesses ribonucleic acid (RNA)-dependent deoxyribonucleic acid (DNA) polymerase (reverse transcriptase). HIV infects T helper cells (T4 lymphocytes), macrophages, and B cells. HIV does not directly affect the CNS or peripheral neurons, astrocytes, or oligodendrocytes. HIV infection in the CNS is indirectly caused by neurotoxins produced by infected macrophages or chemical substances produced by the dysregulation of cytokines and chemokines.

T helper cells are infected more readily than are other cells. The depletion of T helper cells occurs in the following steps:

1. Once inside the host, HIV attaches to the target cell membrane by way of its receptor molecule, CD4$^+$.

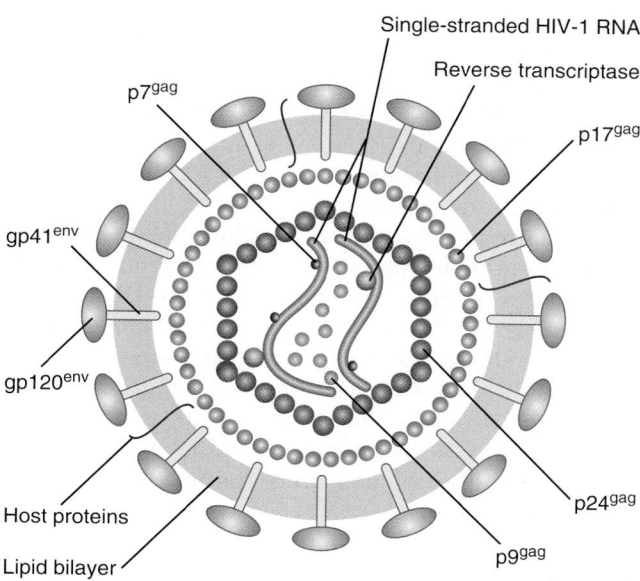

FIGURE 80-1 Schematic diagram of the human immunodeficiency virus-1 (HIV-1) virion. RNA, ribonucleic acid. (Redrawn from Sande, M., & Volberding, P. [1999]. *The medical management of AIDS* [6th ed.]. Philadelphia: W.B. Saunders.)

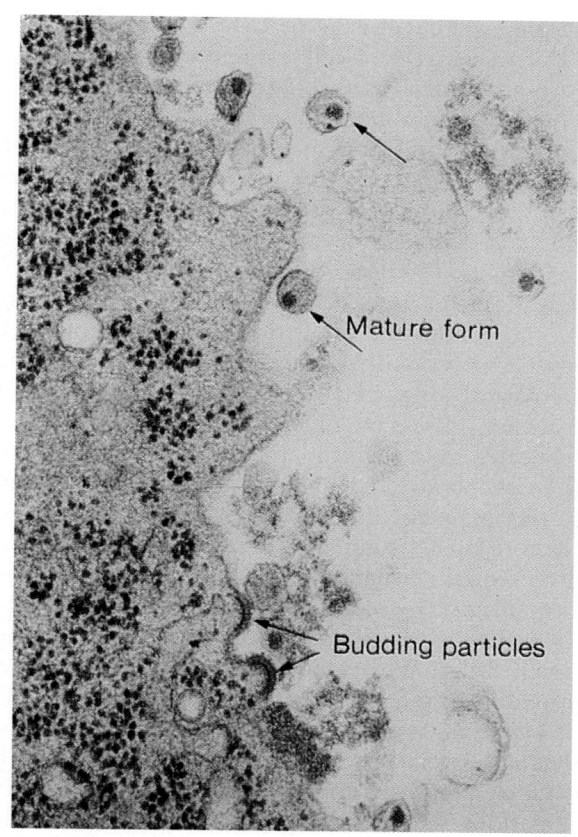

FIGURE 80-2 Human immunodeficiency virus. Electron micrograph of the virus budding from a T lymphocyte. (From Friedman-Kien, A., & Cockerell, C. [1996]. *Color atlas of AIDS* [2nd ed.]. Philadelphia: W.B. Saunders, p. 11.)

2. The virus is uncoated, and the RNA enters the cell.
3. The enzyme known as reverse transcriptase is released, and viral RNA is transcribed into DNA.
4. This newly created DNA moves into the nucleus and the DNA of the cell.
5. A provirus is created when the viral DNA integrates itself into the cellular DNA or genome of the cell.
6. Once the provirus is in place, its genetic material is no longer pure cell but is part virus.
7. The cell may function abnormally.
8. The host cell dies, and viral budding occurs (Figure 80-2). The new virus now infects other cells.

The main target for HIV is the T4 helper cell; however, the "glue" to which HIV is attracted is the CD4$^+$ molecule, which acts as the receptor for HIV on the T4 helper cell. Even though the CD4$^+$ molecule is also found on other cells, such as macrophages and monocytes, clinicians usually refer to T4 helper cells as CD4$^+$ cells. Therefore in articles, research papers, or laboratory reports about HIV, the labels *T4, T4 helper, CF4$^+$,* and *CD4$^+$ T helper cell* are used synonymously. Another substance, *chemokines,* acts as a messenger to facilitate HIV entry into cells. In 1996 scientists discovered that certain people have a genetic defect in a gene related to chemokines and, despite repeated exposure to HIV, never become infected.

The CD4$^+$ T helper cells are the regulating cells in the immune system. They interact with monocytes, macrophages, cytotoxic T cells, natural killer cells, and B cells. In the analogy of an orchestra and a conductor, the T cells are the "conductor" of the immune system,

directing all the activity ("music") produced by the other immune cells ("orchestra"). Therefore the loss of the CD4$^+$ T helper cells results in chaos. The body loses its ability to maintain a consistent state of health. With significant losses of these regulatory cells, the HIV-infected person becomes highly susceptible to acquired infection. Pathogens that previously caused disease may reactivate and also cause infection. An example is the varicella zoster virus, which may have caused chickenpox when an HIV-infected person was a child and may reappear as shingles when the CD4$^+$ T-cell count drops to low levels.

The average laboratory range for the CD4$^+$ T-cell count is 500 to 1600 mm^3. A gradual physiologic decline occurs in these cells over the life of an individual. In fact, CD4$^+$ T-cell counts in newborns are almost double those of an adult. In the adult, CD4$^+$ cell counts below 200/mm^3 are considered dangerously low and infection is likely to develop. Other laboratory changes that indicate immune dysfunction include the following:

- An overall decline in the total numbers of white blood cells
- Decreases in both the total number and percentage of lymphocytes

- Significant changes in the CD4$^+$/CD8$^+$ ratio
- Decreased CD4$^+$ T-cell test findings
- Absent or decreased skin test reactivity *(anergy)*
- Increased immunoglobulin levels

The cause of all this damage to the immune system is the extensive amount of HIV activity that takes place in the body of an infected person from the time of infection. HIV replicates at a rapid rate. In fact, it may produce 10 million new *virions* (viral particles) daily. Although a person with HIV may be asymptomatic and CD4$^+$ cell counts may be within the normal range, insidious destruction of the immune system is taking place. Antiretroviral drugs play a key role in interrupting the HIV disease process by inhibiting the ability of the virus to replicate, thus reducing the amount of circulating virus in the body and halting its destructive activity. Once this happens, the immune system begins to heal and restore itself, as noted by rising CD4$^+$ cell counts.

Sustaining the beneficial effects of antiretroviral therapy entails many challenges. The greatest problem is HIV's ability to mutate and become resistant to antiretroviral drugs. When this *drug failure* occurs, plasma viral load rises and the CD4$^+$ cell count decreases. The treatment regimen must then be changed. Because two to three drugs are usually used at the same time and the list of available approved drugs is still small, the number of combinations that can be prescribed is limited. Additionally, although the drugs can contain the disease in plasma, the virus can hide in many other cells in the body. Finally, because most antiretroviral agents do not cross the blood-brain barrier in the CNS, treatment of CNS problems caused by HIV infection can be very difficult.

The course of HIV illness varies from person to person. Several cofactors may accelerate immunodeficiency, including malnutrition, continued substance abuse, allergic conditions, genetics, age, pregnancy, gender, and presence of infections. Research has clearly implicated some of these cofactors as contributing to a more rapid decline in CD4$^+$ cell levels; for others, the evidence is less clear. Factors that have been linked to increased mortality and morbidity include lower socioeconomic status, lack of access to adequate care, receiving care in a hospital with limited AIDS experience, and being treated by a physician with little experience in AIDS care.

Overall, survival among clients with AIDS has been dramatic since the advent of *Highly Active Antiretroviral Therapy* (HAART), which uses varying combinations of drugs from three different classes of antiretroviral medications. Combined with prophylactic treatment for commonly occurring opportunistic infections, HAART has led to HIV disease changing from a rapidly fatal disease to a chronic, mostly manageable condition (Figure 80-3).

To illustrate further the differences observed in HIV-infected people, scientists have reported that about 5%

are perfectly healthy after many years and show no manifestations of disease progression. These *long-term non-progressors* have the following:

- Documented evidence of HIV infection for more than 10 years
- Lack of manifestations
- Normal, stable immune profiles
- Never required any treatment for HIV disease

Long-term non-progressors appear to produce vigorous amounts of serum antibodies that keep HIV activity at extremely low levels, thus preventing damage to the immune system. Do not confuse a long-term non-progressor with a *long-term survivor,* defined as someone who has lived for more than 8 years after an AIDS diagnosis, who shows all clinical and laboratory manifestations of disease, and who continuously requires treatment.

Although the principal target of HIV is the immune system, considerable damage occurs to other parts of the body as a direct result of HIV in body tissues. A few examples of clinical conditions that can be directly attributed to HIV include cranial and peripheral neuropathies, uveitis, cardiomyopathy, pneumonitis, malabsorption in the small intestine, nephritis, cervicitis, arthritis, psoriasis, gonad dysfunction, and adrenalitis. Additionally, damage to the hematologic system, which is due in part to impaired blood cell production, commonly results in anemia, granulocytopenia, and thrombocytopenia throughout the course of disease.

In addition to managing HIV disease, clinicians are challenged with addressing those illnesses that existed before the person acquired HIV infection. These not only require continuing treatment and attention but also may complicate the course of illness. Frequently encountered pre-existing and co-morbid conditions seen in HIV-infected clients include, but are not limited to, alcoholism, drug dependence, liver disease, kidney disease, psychiatric illness, and a history of STDs. As therapy improves and people with HIV disease live longer, they will also require treatment for such illnesses as cancer, coronary artery disease, chronic obstructive lung disease, hypertension, and diabetes, all of which may occur in the aging population not infected with HIV.

Clinical Manifestations

As knowledge has evolved regarding the HIV disease process, the CDC has developed and revised numerous classification systems (see the box on HIV and AIDS Classification System for Adolescents and Adults on the website). The most recent classification system for HIV disease in adults and adolescents is based on two monitoring parameters used to follow a client: (1) laboratory data (CD4$^+$ cell counts) and (2) clinical presentation (the person's clinical manifestations of diseases). The period in which a person becomes infected is referred to as *primary infection.* If HIV is detected at the

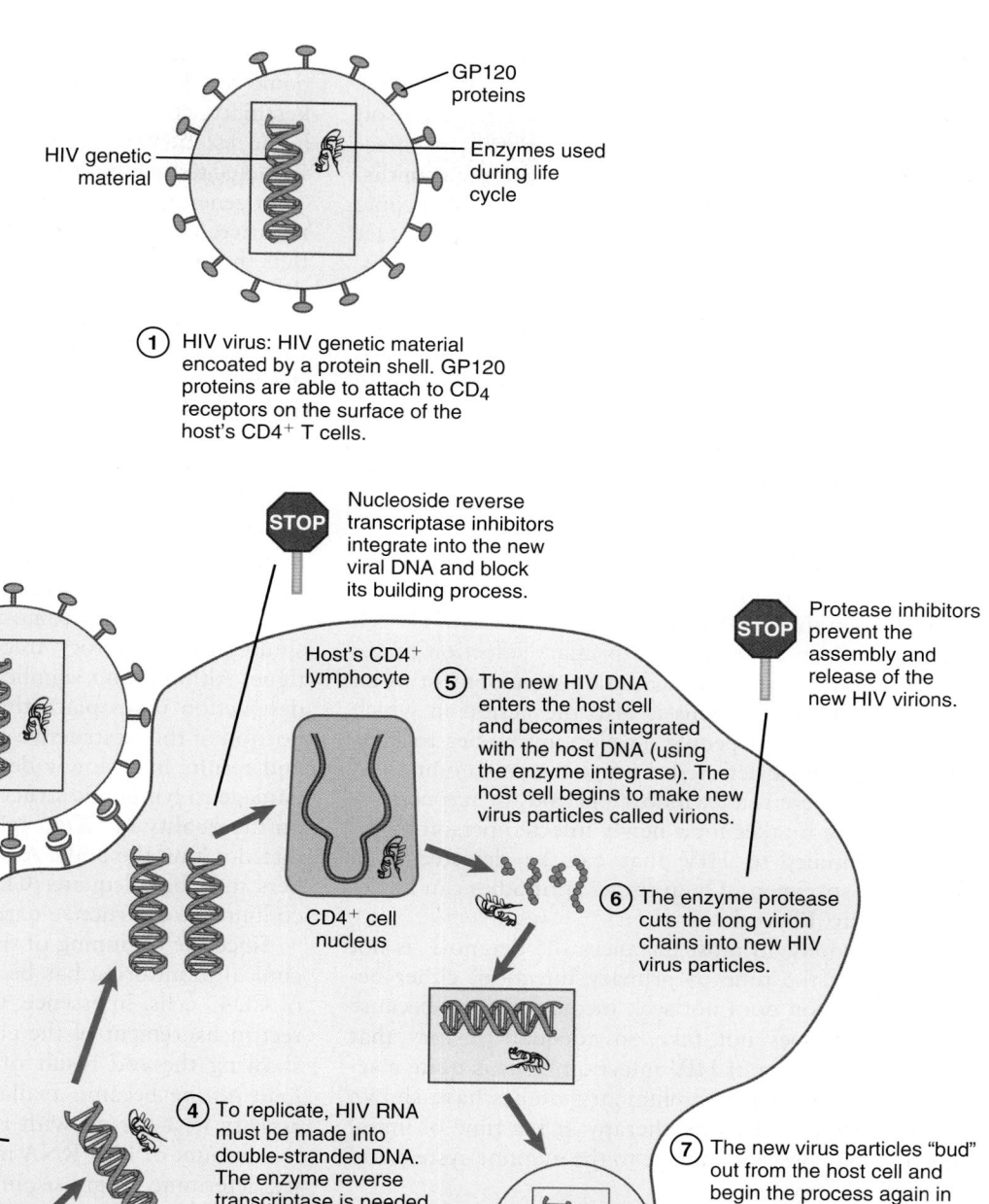

FIGURE 80-3 The steps in the life cycle of the HIV virus with correlation to medications.

time of initial infection, the client is considered to be in category A.

Primary infection is the initial period after a person has acquired HIV. The length of time the primary infection lasts varies from several weeks to a few months. During primary infection, 50% to 70% of people become sick. Many clinicians are unaware of this fact and tend to think that primary infection is silent. In addition to systemic manifestations (fever, fatigue, lymphadenopathy, nausea, vomiting), the infected person may experience headache; truncal (torso and arms) rash; ulcers of the mouth, genitals, or both; thrush; pharyngitis; diarrhea; hepatomegaly; myalgia; arthralgia; anemia; thrombocytopenia; and leukopenia. In some people, the manifestations are mild and similar to mononucleosis. Other people have severe manifestations requiring hospitalization.

During primary infection, a sudden and intense burst of HIV activity results in a high viral load and a dramatic drop in the $CD4^+$ cell count. In fact, the $CD4^+$ cell count may drop at the time of primary infection to below 100 mm³, with the concomitant development of an AIDS-defining illness. This is also the period in which most newly infected people develop antibodies to HIV, which can then be detected through enzyme immunoassay testing. There is a "window" period for *seroconversion* (the time it takes for a newly infected person to develop antibodies to HIV that can be detected in a laboratory specimen). On average, antibodies can be detected in 4 to 12 weeks.

 Unfortunately, in most instances the diagnosis is not confirmed at the time of primary infection, either because the person does not seek medical care or because the clinician does not take an adequate history that raises the suspicion of HIV infection. This is quite a serious situation because preliminary studies have shown that starting antiretroviral therapy at the time of initial infection may prevent damage to the immune system and to other body systems.

Except in certain instances, such as when seeking a federal job or when testing infant umbilical cord blood, the decision to seek an enzyme immunoassay test for HIV antibodies is left up to the individual. Testing also involves pretest and post-test counseling. Laws that govern the reporting of HIV antibody test results vary from state to state, and testing may be performed either anonymously or confidentially. If the enzyme immunoassay result is positive, a second test, the Western blot, is performed to confirm a positive HIV status.

If testing is performed too early in the initial infection period, a false-negative result may occur. A few cases of outliers also did not test positive for up to 3 years after becoming infected. False-positive results are extremely rare but may occur in clients with autoimmune disorders, such as lupus erythematosus, or in clients who have taken part in HIV vaccine studies.

Other methods for detecting HIV infection include home test kits, salivary tests, and urine tests. The marketability, cost, and popularity have limited the use of home test kits thus far. Saliva test results are as accurate as serologic testing, but the urine test is slightly less accurate.

In general, test results are reported as (1) positive, (2) negative, or (3) indeterminate. A *positive* result means that the person is HIV-infected, but it does not predict the future course of disease. A *negative* result means that HIV antibodies were not detected. Indeterminate results usually mean that the enzyme immunoassay test was positive, but the Western blot test did not confirm the findings. Repeated testing later is commonly recommended as a means of validating initial test results.

The period following primary infection is one in which the person usually remains asymptomatic for many years. Therefore clients with HIV disease are commonly categorized in group A for extended periods. Although the clients have no obvious major manifestations, they may start to notice recurrent infections of the sinuses or respiratory tract or may feel increasing fatigue. Although no significant disease is apparent, viral destruction takes place throughout the body. A major portion of this destructive activity occurs in lymph tissue and results in a slowly declining $CD4^+$ cell count. The damage to lymphatic structures also has a negative effect on the quality of $CD4^+$ cells that are continuously produced within the body. After a while, although the numbers may be adequate, $CD4^+$ cells lose their ability to contain the destructive nature of HIV.

Since the beginning of the HIV epidemic, the focus of clinical monitoring has been on evaluating the quantity of $CD4^+$ cells. In essence, $CD4^+$ cell counts are an indirect measurement of the clinical course of HIV disease, showing the end result of HIV activity. In 1996 *viral load testing* became available to measure directly viral activity in a person with HIV. Viral load tests measure the amount of HIV RNA in plasma, quantify HIV activity, determine prognosis, indicate the need for treatment, evaluate the biologic response to treatment, and detect treatment failure. $CD4^+$ cell counts should not be a substitute for viral load testing because the correlation between the two is weak. High viral loads may not always correlate with clinical manifestations and a low $CD4^+$ cell count and vice versa. Viral load results may be reported in copies per milliliter (e.g., 10,000 copies/ml). The actual numbers may be reported as follows:
- Decimal numbers, as in 10,000 copies
- Exponents, as in 10^4, where the exponent 4 indicates the number of zeros after the 1
- A logarithm, in this case 4, which indicates 10^4 or 10,000

Thus a report that sets viral activity at 5 logs would be interpreted as 10^5 or 100,000 copies/ml.

As the disease progresses, manifestations such as thrush or vulvovaginal candidiasis usually appear, which are distinct manifestations of an underlying immunodeficiency. This development is what commonly causes people to seek HIV antibody testing. Those who have symptomatic illness are then classified into group B (see the box on HIV and AIDS Classification System for Adolescents and Adults on the website). Eventually a client with HIV infection develops one or more AIDS-defining diseases and is finally classified into group C. Once again, this may be the first time that HIV infection is discovered.

Outcome Management for HIV Infection
■ Medical Management of the Client with HIV Infection

The outcomes for medical and nursing management of the client infected with HIV are to maintain the person's health, initiate and maintain an effective antiretroviral regimen, and prevent infectious complications. This requires health care follow-up at specified intervals and an understanding that to achieve these outcomes the client has to make lifestyle changes.

Maintain Health. Initiating a plan of care for any client infected with HIV requires a detailed laboratory and clinical assessment not only for the initial evaluation but also on an ongoing basis. Initial and follow-up laboratory testing provides invaluable information on disease progression, serves as a guide for treatment decisions, and determines the efficacy of treatment prescribed. A complete blood count is needed to identify anemia, thrombocytopenia, leukopenia, and developing infections. Multichannel chemistry panels and urinalysis reveal renal, liver, metabolic, or nutritional disease. Both tests are repeated at 6- to 12-month intervals to detect any abnormalities resulting from disease progression or prescribed drugs. These results are also needed to modify dosages of antiretroviral drugs for clients with impaired kidney or liver function.

An annual tuberculin skin test detects mycobacterial disease, and a chest x-ray identifies pulmonary problems. For women a pregnancy test and Papanicolaou (Pap) smear are usually performed. Pap smears are performed twice during the first year after a diagnosis of HIV infection and then at least annually. Screening for STDs includes testing for syphilis, gonorrhea, and *Chlamydia*. These are repeated annually if the client is sexually active. Hepatitis antibody testing is performed to identify acute or prior infection and to determine the need for immunization. There is a high incidence of hepatitis C in people infected with HIV.

Testing for pathogens known to cause opportunistic infections in people infected with HIV includes serologic tests intended to detect previous exposure to toxoplasmosis, histoplasmosis, cryptococcosis, and cytomegalovirus. For seronegative clients, repeated testing may reveal a primary exposure. For seropositive clients,

rising titers of antibodies to these pathogens indicate the need for prophylactic therapy.

Finally, CD4+ cell counts, ratios, and percentages are performed to determine the degree of immunodeficiency, and viral load testing is ordered to calculate the amount of viral activity. Viral load test result interpretations are as follows:

- 10,000 copies/ml: poses a low risk for AIDS
- 10,000 to 100,000 copies/ml: doubles risk for AIDS
- >100,000 copies/ml: poses a high risk for AIDS

The initial test, without any treatment, may reveal viral loads of 80,000 to one million copies per milliliter or even higher. These same tests are repeated at intervals determined by the presence or absence of manifestations or disease in the client through the course of illness. Because several viral load tests have been approved for use, clinicians are advised to use the same viral load test when performing serial measurements to control variations in test results. Diseases such as influenza, herpes, or pneumonia, as well as testing immediately after the influenza vaccine is administered, can cause a temporary rise in test results. Therefore testing should be deferred in any of these situations.

Initiate and Maintain Antiretroviral Therapy. The decision to treat HIV disease should involve both the primary care provider and the client. Many clients, because of personal experience or preference, may refuse recommended antiretroviral therapy. Clinicians should, in a noncoercive manner, provide as much objective information as possible so that the person with HIV can make an informed choice about taking these drugs. Most clinicians recommend starting an antiretroviral combination therapy regimen early in the course of disease; however, this has become somewhat controversial (see the Evidence-Based Practice in Action feature on Adherence to HAART on pp. 2384 and 2385).

Current guidelines from the U.S. Department of Health and Human Services are as follows:

- Symptomatic clients: Treat
- Asymptomatic clients with a CD4+ count <200: Treat
- Asymptomatic clients with CD4+ counts 200-350: Therapy should generally be offered
- Asymptomatic clients with CD4+ counts >350: Defer or consider therapy if viral load is high

The following classes of antiretroviral agents are most commonly used:

- Nucleoside/nucleotide reverse transcriptase inhibitors (NRTIs)
- Protease inhibitors (PIs)
- Non-nucleoside reverse transcriptase inhibitors (NNRTIs)
- Entry inhibitors

Also called nucleoside/nucleotide analogs, NRTIs block HIV replication by protecting noninfected cells.

📖 EVIDENCE-BASED PRACTICE IN ACTION

Adherence to HAART

Adherence to prescribed medication is known to be problematic. Clients have difficulty fully complying with therapy, whether it is of short duration for an acute episode (for instance, antibiotics), or of long duration, as in the case of chronic illness. It is well documented that adherence declines as the urgency of treating the disease declines and as the duration of therapy lengthens.

The literature shows that overall medication adherence rates vary from 40% to 80%. Unfortunately HIV presents a unique challenge. Among individuals taking HAART (highly active anti-retroviral therapy), only 40% to 60% are 90% adherent. Non-adherence to therapy allows the viral load to increase as immune functioning decreases and is the major contributing factor to the development of resistant strains of HIV, which can be transmitted to others. Compliance with anti-HIV medication must occur at an incredible 95% to prevent these sequelae.

Persons living with HIV (PLWH) undergoing treatment face a daunting challenge in remaining adherent to their regimen. HAART requires that the person take multiple medications, at precise dosing intervals, and with specific restrictions regarding timing the medications with food and fluid. In addition, there may be particular dietary or storage requirements. A client may be taking a medication that needs to be accompanied by a low-fat meal at the same time another medication requires a high-fat meal. PLWH may also be taking several drugs to combat or prevent opportunistic infections, nutritional supplements, drugs to counteract unpleasant side effects, and, as the population of PLWH ages, medications to control other chronic conditions.

Many research studies have attempted to shed light on this topic by investigating factors leading to non-adherence as well as factors promoting adherence to therapy. Non-adherence can be because of personal factors or systems-level factors. Personal factors include such things as "forgot", being unwilling to suffer side effects, lack of knowledge, large pill burden, social support, or changes to lifestyle required by the treatment regimen. Systems-level factors include client-health care provider relationship; having multiple services available at one location; ease of obtaining refills; and simplicity of arranging follow-up care, especially in light of new manifestations or side effects. Ongoing substance abuse and psychiatric conditions also are important considerations.

Medication non-adherence seems to be a multifactorial and unique experience to each client. It is incumbent on the nurse to assess this topic gently at every opportunity, attempting to learn, from the client's point of view, what barriers he or she is facing in remaining adherent to the medical regimen.

Implications

Several strategies to improving medication adherence seem to be beneficial. First and foremost is education. PLWH need detailed information about their medications and knowledge regarding the consequences of non-adherence. They also need ongoing information regarding their viral load and CD4+ counts, which can be correlated with medication use. Motivate the client by including him or her in all decisions regarding drug treatment. Give the client information regarding dosing schedule, food and storage requirements, and side effects; then let the client decide whether that treatment is feasible. Some clinics let the PLWH "practice" the regimen with candy or jelly beans for several weeks before the client is asked to commit to the regimen.

Simplify the regimen as much as possible and use drugs that require the least amount of change in the client's lifestyle. Help the client schedule taking medications along with other daily routines. Anticipate unpleasant side effects and be prepared to deal with them promptly. Several "adherence-promoting devices" are available, including simple pill boxes, beepers and alarms, and computer-generated telephone reminder calls. PLWH may need specific skills-building sessions or assistance with problem-solving barriers to taking medications.

Clients with active substance abuse or untreated and under-treated psychiatric conditions (depression, anxiety) may not be able to adhere until these issues are under control. Likewise, a person must fulfill "survival needs" before managing a complex condition such as HIV. If a client is homeless, finding shelter will be a much higher priority than adhering to medications. For these types of clients, it probably is best to delay the start of therapy until these conditions have been stabilized.

Adherence to HIV medication regimen is demanding, complex, and requires vigilance on the part of the client in maintaining his or her treatment schedule. It also requires the nurse to be vigilant, sensitive, creative, and a partner with the PLWH to design strategies to improve adherence. Adherence to therapy is the most significant determinant of its success. Nurses must be in the forefront to help their clients combat this disease.

Bibliography

Bartlett, J.A. (2002). Addressing the challenges of adherence. *Journal of Acquired Immune Deficiency Syndromes and Human Retrovirology, 29*(Suppl 1), S2-S10.

Brook, MG., et al. (2001). Adherence to highly active antiretroviral therapy in the real world: Experience of twelve English HIV units. *AIDS Patient Care and STDs, 15*(9), 491-494.

Jones, S.G. (2002). The other side of the pill bottle: The lived experience of HIV-positive nurses on HIV combination drug therapy. *Journal of the Association of Nurses in AIDS Care, 13*(3), 22-36.

Kalichman, S.C., et al. (2001). HIV treatment adherence in women living with HIV/AIDS: Research based on the Information-Motivation-Behavioral Skills Model of Health Behavior. *Journal of the Association of Nurses in AIDS Care, 12*(4), 58-67.

Kemppainen, J.K., et al. (2001). HAART adherence in culturally diverse patients with HIV/AIDS: A study of male patients from

EVIDENCE-BASED PRACTICE IN ACTION

Adherence to HAART—cont'd

a Veteran's Administration hospital in northern California. *AIDS Patient Care and STDs, 15*(3), 117-127.

Malone, S.B., & Osborne, J.J. (2002). Improving treatment adherence in drug abusers who are HIV-positive. *Lippincott's Case Management, 5*(6), 236-247.

Simoni, J.M., et al. (2002). Mediators of social support and antiretroviral adherence among an indigent population in New York City. *AIDS Patient Care and STDs, 16*(9), 431-439.

Van Servellen, G., et al. (2002). Individual and system level factors associated with treatment nonadherence in human immunodeficiency virus-infected men and women. *AIDS Patient Care and STDs, 16*(6), 269-281.

Winland-Brown, J.E., & Valiante, J. (2000). Effectiveness of different medication management approaches on elders' medication adherence. *Outcomes Management for Nursing Practice, 4*(4), 172-176.

PIs render HIV particles noninfectious in cells already infected with HIV. NNRTIs work in a manner similar to that of NRTIs. Entry inhibitors, the newest class of drugs for treatment of HIV, prevent HIV from entering healthy T cells in the body (see Figure 80-3 and the Integrating Pharmacology feature on Understanding HAART on p. 2386). Use of entry inhibitors is reserved for HIV-positive clients who have become resistant to PIs, NRTIs, and NNRTIs. Combination pills are available that greatly decrease the number of pills needed daily and facilitate adherence to treatment (see the Evidence-Based Practice in Action feature on Adherence to HAART on p. 2384 and above). In HAART, a combination of three drugs from two of the first three drug classes (NRTIs, PIs, NNRTIs) is used. Clinicians and clients strive to find combinations that are the least toxic and that produce the largest and most long-lasting viral response (lowest viral load) and the best immune response (highest CD4$^+$ cell counts). The goals of therapy are to inhibit the replication of HIV, reduce the viral load to undetectable levels, and stabilize the disease.

The first NRTI, approved in March 1987, was zidovudine (Retrovir, AZT). The original dosage was 1200 mg/day taken at specified intervals. The most profound side effect was myelosuppression, resulting in anemia and leukopenia, which often required repeated transfusions. Many people currently infected with HIV remember the difficult experience of a friend or loved one and consequently may be reluctant to try antiretroviral therapy. By 1990 research demonstrated that 600 mg/day of zidovudine (half the original dose) was sufficient to achieve the desired effects. Eager anticipation preceded the approval of PIs, a new class of drugs, because large numbers of clients developed resistance to NRTIs.

Perhaps the greatest challenge in treating HIV infection has been the genetic promiscuity of this virus. As stated earlier, HIV mutates rapidly. In the presence of an antiretroviral drug, it can develop resistance to the drug and continue to grow in the presence of the drug. Three types of drug resistance are of concern:

- *Genotype resistance,* in which the virus mutates
- *Phenotype resistance,* in which the virus shows a decrease in sensitivity to the drug
- *Cross-resistance,* in which the virus, having developed resistance to one drug, becomes resistant to other drugs in that class

Monotherapy (prescription of one antiretroviral agent at a time) is more likely to result in drug resistance than is combination therapy. *Subtherapeutic* levels of a drug also lead to drug resistance. Subtherapeutic levels can occur when the client does not take the prescribed dosage, does not take doses at specified intervals, or both and can also occur when other prescribed drugs interact with the antiretroviral drug and cause lower blood levels.

In an attempt to prevent drug resistance, clinicians order combination therapy, believing that combinations of drugs "confuse" the virus, thus interfering with its ability to develop resistance. Unfortunately, preliminary data show that even in combinations of three drugs at once, resistance develops to one or more of the agents being taken. Evaluation of the efficacy of antiretroviral therapy is based on the client's clinical manifestations and on laboratory tests of viral load and CD4$^+$ cell counts. The most reliable objective determinant is viral load testing, which is performed 3 to 4 weeks after initiating or changing therapy. If the decrease in viral load is not at least three times the original laboratory reports, or decreased by at least 0.5 log, the therapy is usually changed. Repeated testing is usually performed at 3- to 4-month intervals.

Drug failure, in which the ordered combination is no longer effective, can occur after trying several standard combinations of anti-retrovirals. The challenge to the clinician at that point is to try combinations of four to six drugs in an effort to suppress HIV activity once again. This approach to therapeutic intervention is commonly called *salvage therapy.* In many instances, salvage therapy fails because the HIV-infected person has developed drug resistance to most of the available drugs.

Studies are also being conducted to identify other chemotherapeutic strategies to control HIV infection. Sci-

INTEGRATING PHARMACOLOGY

Understanding HAART

Compared with the early days of the epidemic, many drugs now exist to treat HIV/AIDS and more are being developed. Treating HIV with monotherapy (using one drug) leads to rapid drug resistance. Combination therapy (HAART, or highly active antiretroviral therapy) consists of the simultaneous administration of drugs that have different mechanisms of action and without similar toxicities. HAART drug combinations attack the HIV virus at different points necessary for its replication. Utilizing multiple drugs decreases the chance of developing resistance.

Since the advent of HAART, dramatic declines in AIDS morbidity and mortality have occurred. Inhibiting viral replication allows for "reconstitution" (rebuilding) of the immune system and reducing clinical progression and the risk of death. Drugs to treat HIV/AIDS fall into categories based on which part of the viral replication cycle they are effective against.

Reverse Transcriptase Inhibitors

To replicate, HIV's viral RNA must be converted into double-stranded DNA. The enzyme *reverse transcriptase* is responsible for this activity. The first drugs approved to treat HIV/AIDS were reverse transcriptase inhibitors, which prevent the enzyme from changing viral RNA into DNA.

Non-Nucleoside Reverse Transcriptase Inhibitors

Non-nucleoside reverse transcriptase inhibitors (NNRTIs) bind directly to the enzyme and prevent the conversion of RNA to DNA. Examples include the following:
- Rescriptor (delavirdine, DLV)
- Sustiva (efavirenz, EFV)
- Viramune (nevirapine, NVP)

Nucleoside/Nucleotide Reverse Transcriptase Inhibitors

Nucleoside/nucleotide reverse transcriptase inhibitors (NRTIs) incorporate themselves into viral DNA and cause its construction to be terminated. Examples include the following:
- Combivir (zidovudine/lamivudine, AZT + 3TC)
- Epivir (lamivudine, 3TC)
- Hivid (zalcitabine, ddC)
- Retrovir (zidovudine: ZDV or AZT)
- Zerit (stavudine or d4T)
- Ziagen (abacavir or ABC)
- Videx, Videx EC (didanosine, ddI)
- Viread (tenofovir disoproxil fumarate, DF)
- Trizivir (abacavir/lamivudine/zidovudine, ABC + AZT + 3TC)

Protease Inhibitors

These drugs work by preventing the successful assembly and release of new virus particles (virions). Problems with this class include intolerance, high "pill burden", and poor adherence to treatment. Examples include the following:
- Agenerase (amprenavir, APV)
- Crixivan (indinavir, IDV)
- Fortovase (saquinavir soft gels, SQV-SGC)
- Invirase (saquinavir capsules, SQV-HGC)
- Kaletra (lopinavir/ritonavir, LPV)
- Norvir (ritonavir, RTV)
- Viracept (nelfinavir, NFV)

The optimal time to start therapy has not been definitively determined by research studies. Most clinicians favor the "hit early and hard" approach; however, recent guidelines from the U.S. Department of Health and Human Services and the International AIDS Society—USA Panel delineate several factors to consider prior to initiating therapy: CD4$^+$ count, viral load, presence of manifestations or opportunistic infections, and the client's willingness to adhere to the regimen. Client willingness is key: nonadherence to this complex regime leads to drug resistance (see the Evidence-Based Practice in Action feature on Adherence to HAART on pp. 2384 and 2385). Other considerations include drug toxicity profile, "pill burden," dosing/storage/food requirements, and interactions with other drugs the client is taking.

There is no specific prescription for HAART. Recommended combinations include the following:
- 2 NRTIs plus either 1 NNRTI or 1 PI or 2 PIs
- 3 NRTIs

Entry Inhibitors

Entry inhibitors work by preventing HIV from entering healthy T cells. They work differently from the approved anti-HIV drugs described earlier that are active against HIV after it has infected a T cell. These drugs are reserved for use in people who have become resistant to PIs, NRTIs, and NNRTIs. Entry inhibitors include fusion inhibitors such as enfuvirtide (Fuzeon, ENF). Fuzeon binds to the gp41 protein on the HIV's surface so that it cannot bind with T cells, thus preventing the virus from infecting healthy cells. Administration is more difficult because enfuvirtide cannot be taken by mouth and must be given as an injection twice a day every 12 hours. Other entry inhibitors are currently under investigation.

Other drugs that work to inhibit different phases of the HIV life cycle are currently being studied. Supervised drug interruptions are also being investigated as a way to boost the client's immune system and decrease the financial and emotional burden of such complex therapy.

entists are looking at the use of HIV vaccines as a therapeutic strategy to stimulate host responses and control viral replication. Research continues to investigate the development of *immunomodulators,* drugs designed to modulate or reconstitute the immune system. Other novel approaches to therapy include entry inhibitor agents, nonpeptidic protease inhibitors, second-generation NNRTIs, integrase inhibitors, and chemokine antagonists.

Prevent Infection. By 1986 surveillance data indicated that in more than 80% of people with HIV disease, *Pneumocystis carinii* pneumonia occurred at least once before death. Studies eventually showed that morbidity and mortality rates could be reduced significantly by giv-ing a drug prophylactically for *P. carinii* pneumonia. Since 1989 the U.S. Public Health Service has recommended that all HIV-infected clients with a CD4$^+$ cell count below 200 mm^3 receive prophylaxis for *P. carinii* pneumonia. Drugs include trimethoprim-sulfamethoxazole (TMP-SMX); dapsone; dapsone, pyrimethamine, and folinic acid; aerosolized, intravenous, or intramuscular pentamidine; or atovaquone. TMP-SMX and dapsone also provide protection against toxoplasmosis.

Although surveillance data alone do not reflect the true incidence of infection with *Mycobacterium avium-intracellulare* complex, postmortem examinations revealed that more than 60% of HIV-infected people had an active infection. Since 1993 the U.S. Public Health Ser-vice has recommended that all HIV-infected clients with a CD4$^+$ cell count below 50 mm^3 receive prophylaxis for *M. avium-intracellulare* complex. Recommended drugs include clarithromycin, azithromycin, and rifabutin. However, these drugs may interact with anti-retrovirals.

All HIV-infected clients with a positive result to a tuberculin skin test that have no evidence of active tuberculosis should receive 9 months of preventive therapy with isoniazid. Pyridoxine should be added to reduce the potential for peripheral neuropathy. An alternative regimen is rifabutin and pyrazinamide for 2 months; however, these drugs may interact with anti-retrovirals.

Other recommended prophylactic measures include prevention of respiratory infections by using pneumococcal vaccine and influenza vaccine and prevention of traveler's diarrhea when traveling to countries where diarrhea is common by using antimicrobials such as ciprofloxacin. Finally, prophylactic medication may be ordered to prevent cytomegalovirus infection, recurrent candidiasis, cryptococcosis, or histoplasmosis.

■ Nursing Management of the Client with HIV Infection
Assessment

To help a client with health maintenance behaviors, nurses should not restrict assessment to the client's immediate clinical status. Instead, focus on potential prob-

lems the client may encounter during the illness. For example, it is of no value to tell people they need regular health care follow-up if they have no insurance and no money to pay for it. Social work intervention is needed to find an alternative source of health care services, such as the federally funded AIDS Drug Assistance Program, which provides more than just drugs. If the client lives alone and has no one willing to assist, he or she may need to be placed in an institution when the illness progresses. As a coordinator of care, have information readily available to identify problems and plan ahead.

Before performing any teaching, evaluate the client's existing level of knowledge about HIV infection. Some clients may know little, whereas others may be knowledgeable. Try to assess exactly what the client does or does not know about transmission and health-promoting behaviors instead of making any assumptions.

The psychological burden of HIV disease can be overwhelming. Crisis points at which the nurse can anticipate anxiety, fear, or depression include the following:
- Time of the initial HIV-positive diagnosis
- Time of the initial AIDS diagnosis
- Changes in treatment
- Development of new manifestations
- Recurrence of problems or relapse
- Terminal illness

Psychological conflicts that clients commonly experience include fear of transmitting HIV to others, constant worry about developing an infection, guilt about a previous lifestyle, and changes in personal relationships. Social stressors may include disclosure of one's HIV status, stigma related to that status, insecurity about employment and insurance, and loneliness and social isolation.

Diagnosis, Outcomes, Interventions

Diagnosis: Effective Therapeutic Regimen Management. The primary nursing diagnosis encountered with newly diagnosed HIV infection is *Effective Therapeutic Regimen Management related to behaviors that will improve the level of health and prevent complications.* Although some clients may know about HIV disease, it is unlikely that they know all that can be done to improve their health.

Outcomes. The client will know about HIV disease, how to prevent transmission, how to manage the disease, and how to prevent complications.

Interventions
Provide Education. Health teaching should be ongoing and repeated at frequent intervals. An HIV-infected person can adopt several behaviors that not only improve immune function but also increase a sense of well-being. The content outline for teaching health maintenance includes stress management, exercise, safer sex practices,

pregnancy and HIV infection, nutrition (emphasizing a high-protein, high-calorie, low-fat diet), food and water safety, skin and care, routine mouth care, proper hand-washing, environmental cleaning and safety, pet care, limiting alcohol consumption, use of injected drugs, travel safety and avoiding exposure to infectious pathogens, importance of health care follow-up, and understanding and interpreting viral load tests and CD4$^+$ cell counts.

Carefully explain viral load test results because many people misunderstand the results. When successful therapy begins, the viral load drops from high levels, such as 750,000 copies/ml, down to what are called "undetectable" levels; however, most laboratory personnel can detect HIV copies down to only 400 copies/ml. Because anything lower cannot be measured, the laboratory report reads "undetectable levels." Although this is great news and indicates the success of the prescribed regimen, it does not mean that the person no longer has HIV infection. Some clients with HIV infection leave their primary care provider thinking that they are disease free and no longer at risk of spreading HIV. This must be clarified whenever you report laboratory results to a client; emphasize that the client must still practice safer sex, avoid sharing needles, and so on.

Encourage clients to tell their health care providers about any self-prescribed therapies they are taking because these therapies might have a positive or negative influence on the outcomes of care. Keep track of over-the-counter medications because they may interact with prescribed therapies. Some clients may also obtain drugs through buyers' clubs or underground pharmacies. This may not only be detrimental to the effectiveness of prescribed treatments but may also have an adverse effect on observations made during a drug trial.

Some clients may opt to try alternative or complementary treatments, including (1) spiritual or psychological interventions (e.g., guided imagery, meditation, faith healing), (2) nutritional alternatives (e.g., a macrobiotic diet), (3) drug and biologic therapies, (e.g., homeopathy, oxygen, ozone therapy), and (4) physical forces (e.g., acupuncture, acupressure, massage therapy). In most cases, these choices can have a positive effect on the person's emotional well-being but may also have a negative effect. For example, a macrobiotic diet can lead to vitamin and mineral deficiencies as well as weight loss. Herbal remedies may cause nausea, vomiting, diarrhea, or CNS depression. Despite these effects, some clients will continue to use these methods.

Initiate and Maintain Antiretroviral Therapy. One of the most important aspects of providing nursing care to the HIV-infected client is helping with the antiretroviral regimen. Studies suggest that clients with chronic diseases such as hypertension and diabetes take their prescribed drugs about 50% of the time. In contrast, to sustain the

durability and efficacy of antiretroviral therapy, clients must maintain about a 95% compliance rate. This places high expectations on both the HIV-infected client and the physicians and nurses. Because therapy may last for many years, it is vital that the client understand the potential benefits and drawbacks of any regimen and the potential consequences of not adhering to therapy. Potential benefits of anti-retroviral therapy include the following:

- Control of HIV replication and mutation, with reduction in viral load
- Prevention of destruction of the immune system and loss of CD4$^+$ T helper cells
- Delayed progression to AIDS-defining illnesses
- Decreased risk for development of HIV resistance to drugs
- Decreased risk of drug toxicity (drugs are started when the client is healthier)
- Increased survival with HIV disease (the most important benefit)

Potential risks include the following:

- Reduced quality of life from adverse drug effects and the inconvenience of a complex regimen
- Earlier development of drug resistance
- A limited number of drugs available to respond to drug resistance
- Unknown long-term toxicity of antiretroviral therapy
- Unknown duration of the effectiveness of current antiretroviral therapies

The decision of whether to take anti-retrovirals is ultimately up to the client. The regimens ordered are commonly complex and require the client to take large numbers of pills daily (as many as 30 to 40), often at exactly spaced intervals and with differing requirements as to timing the pills related to food. Liquid preparations often taste horrible, and the client must try various strategies to mask the taste. All the drugs have side effects to which the person must learn to adjust and control, and they also interact with numerous other drugs. These drug-drug interactions are usually not life-threatening, but they may interfere with anti-retroviral blood levels, causing subtherapeutic effects, drug resistance, and drug failure. Instruct all clients taking anti-retrovirals as follows:

- Take the drug at specified intervals.
- Do not skip a dose.
- Do not increase or decrease the number of pills you take.
- Follow meal and fluid requirements.
- If side effects occur, tell your physician or nurse. If side effects are significant, ask your primary care provider for information or medication to help manage them.
- Store all drugs as instructed.
- If you do not want to take the drugs, tell your primary care provider.

- If you take the drugs only periodically, it would be better not to take them at all. Discuss this with your physician or nurse.
- Remember, the treatment plan is yours. If you do not agree with it, discuss it with your physician or nurse.

Because of concern over the development of drug resistance and drug failure, several studies have been started on methods to help people infected with HIV adhere to their drug regimens. Several strategies have proved very helpful, especially when used together. See the Evidence-Based Practice in Action feature on Adherence to HAART on pp. 2384 to 2385. Primary care providers also need to incorporate cultural and religious beliefs when addressing drug adherence behaviors. Meal planning because of fat content requirements or dietary restrictions or preferences as well as the need to abstain from food and water on certain days because of religious practices may be necessary.

Prevent Infection. Nursing strategies to prevent infection include health teaching and helping the client take drugs properly to prevent opportunistic infections. Health teaching focuses on safer sex practices not only to prevent HIV transmission but also to keep clients from acquiring STDs. Practicing food and water safety can prevent such diseases as salmonellosis, cryptosporidiosis, and toxoplasmosis. Maintaining skin and mucous membrane integrity with good skin and mouth hygiene can reduce the incidence of candidiasis.

Evaluation

Evaluation includes the client's understanding of teaching that has been provided and the choices that are available. If a client chooses not to adopt a recommended behavior, it does not mean that the client is noncompliant. People with HIV who smoke may find that their stress level rises too high when they try to quit, even when using a nicotine patch or gum. Such clients may choose to continue to smoke. Health care providers can have a difficult time evaluating the outcomes of teaching and weighing them against the client's free choice. Remember that the ultimate decision about following a health care provider's advice belongs to the client. The client's decisions do not reflect failure on the part of the health care professional.

Evaluation of a client's ability to adhere to a prescribed drug regimen includes both subjective and objective techniques. *Subjective* evaluation is by self-report; clients and their care partner describe the client's ability to take all prescribed medications. *Objective* analysis of the success of the plan of care is by laboratory evaluation of CD4$^+$ cell counts and viral load. Avoid "pill counting" to evaluate whether a client is taking drugs as prescribed. This should be performed only if the client

wants this intervention and participates. Pill counts have been used for many years by nurses as a sort of policing activity when they find a client is not following a drug regimen properly. Today pill counts are considered by many nurse experts to be a waste of time because clients often simply discard leftover pills if they know that a nurse will be performing a pill count.

A totally different situation exists when minimal learning takes place because of cognitive impairment. It is well documented that problems with thinking or memory may exist and go unidentified if they are not obvious. This is more likely to occur in clients with less than a 12th grade education and in clients over 50 years of age. In such a situation, a care partner should be designated who receives all information when it is provided to the client. Whenever the care partner cannot make a clinic or office visit, provide telephone teaching and document that you accomplished this.

Outcome Management for AIDS

As both the quantity and quality of CD4$^+$ cells diminish, "AIDS-indicator" diseases occur. The categories of AIDS-defining illnesses include opportunistic infections, cancers, and other conditions specific to HIV disease. The four main types of opportunistic infections are (1) bacterial, (2) fungal, (3) protozoal, and (4) viral. Bacterial infections are the easiest to treat, and viruses are the most difficult. Neoplasms associated with AIDS include Kaposi's sarcoma (KS), non-Hodgkin's lymphoma, and invasive cervical cancer. Two other conditions that are unique to AIDS are (1) HIV encephalopathy and (2) HIV wasting syndrome. Hepatitis C is now considered an AIDS-indicator disease. Since the introduction of HAART in 1996, the onset of AIDS-defining illness has been delayed and treating these diseases has become easier.

■ Medical Management of the Client with AIDS

Prevent and Treat Opportunistic Infections. Most of the pathogens responsible for opportunistic infections are ubiquitous; that is, they are all around us. *P. carinii* is in the air we breathe. Most people do not become sick from this organism because their immune systems are intact. Once the regulators of the immune system (CD4$^+$ cells) are destroyed by HIV, however, infection can occur. Most opportunistic infections result from secondary reactivation of previously acquired pathogens rather than from a new or primary infection. For example, most people are infected with *P. carinii* in the early preschool years, when it causes respiratory manifestations and is probably dismissed as a common cold. The child's intact immune system brings the infection under control; however, the organism remains dormant in the person's body. The potential then exists for the organism to reactivate, causing disease again in an immunocompromised person. This concept applies to any person with an immunodeficiency, regardless of the cause. For example, clients with cancer who receive chemotherapy and become immunodeficient may also develop infection from *P. carinii.*

Single opportunistic infections are rare, and clients may have multiple infections. Many of these opportunistic infections are not curable. Because the immune system no longer has the strength to contain the infection, it becomes chronic and requires lifetime suppressive therapy. Helping the client comply with the antibiotic regimen to keep opportunistic infections under control is an essential part of the care planning process. Because the client must take antibiotics for extended periods, drug resistance may develop, and both physicians and nurses must constantly observe the client for recurrence of the infection.

Bacterial Infections

Mycobacterium tuberculosis Infection. Co-infection with *M. tuberculosis* (TB) and HIV is common, especially in large metropolitan areas. Because the bacterium is airborne, the presence of an immunodeficiency makes the person with HIV very susceptible to TB. All HIV-infected people should be tested annually to detect infection. Nosocomial spread of TB among clients hospitalized on AIDS units has been a problem. Manifestations of active infection are categorized as constitutional, pulmonary, or extrapulmonary. Constitutional manifestations include fever, chills, weight loss, night sweats, lymphadenopathy, and fatigue. Pulmonary manifestations may include cough, dyspnea, chest pain, and hemoptysis. Extrapulmonary presentation may involve bones, joints, liver, spleen, CNS, skin, gastrointestinal tract, mass lesions, urine, and blood.

 The recommended therapy includes a combination of drugs that may include isoniazid, rifampin, pyrazinamide, and either ethambutol or streptomycin. Drug selection is based on culture and sensitivity reports and potential drug-drug interactions with anti-retrovirals already being taken.

 Multi-drug–resistant TB was identified as an emerging problem in the United States around 1987. By 1990 significant numbers of cases were identified, especially among people with HIV infection. Studies attributed the development of multi-drug–resistant TB to physicians prescribing insufficient numbers of drugs to treat new cases of TB. Based on drug sensitivity reports, second-line therapy for multi-drug–resistant TB includes ciprofloxacin, ofloxacin, kanamycin, amikacin, capreomycin, ethionamide, cycloserine, aminosalicylic acid, or clofazimine as single-drug or combination therapy. Rifampin is contraindicated in the client taking some PIs and NNRTIs.

In institutional settings, clients are placed in respiratory isolation until sputum tests reveal that they are no longer infectious. In many cases of multi-drug–resistant TB, despite therapy, it is not uncommon to have clients remain in respiratory isolation until discharge. TB is a reportable communicable disease, and health care professionals are required to report new cases to local health authorities.

Follow-up care focuses on management of clinical manifestations. Monitoring drug compliance is essential to ensure effective treatment and to prevent recurrent active disease. In cities where multi-drug–resistant TB has become a significant problem, local health departments have established monitoring programs (known as *directly observed therapy*), in which health care workers travel to client locations and watch them take their medications. Psychological stressors for the client include coping with the stigma of both HIV and TB.

Mycobacterium avium Complex. *M. avium* complex is also sometimes called *M. avium-intracellulare.* The organism exists in soil, water, animals, eggs, and unpasteurized dairy products. Not all members of the *Mycobacterium* family of bacteria are communicable. *M. avium* complex is referred to as an atypical, noncommunicable mycobacterial disease. Because most people with HIV develop active disease and the risk of infection increases with CD4$^+$ cell counts below 50 mm^3, prophylaxis to prevent infection is recommended. Additionally, *M. avium* complex infection is much easier to prevent than to treat.

The clinical presentation of *M. avium* complex infection includes fever, night sweats, fatigue, anorexia, weight loss, abdominal pain, and diarrhea. Because the disease is difficult to treat and side effects of the medications are numerous, the decision of whether to treat *M. avium* complex infection depends on the severity of manifestations and the presence of renal or hepatic disease. Two to six drugs may be used at one time, including some combination of azithromycin, clarithromycin, ethambutol, ciprofloxacin, rifabutin, and amikacin.

Follow-up care focuses on managing clinical manifestations because they may persist despite drug therapy. It is important to evaluate the client's ability to comply with the prescribed therapy because some clients may decrease the dosage of prescribed pills on their own to minimize side effects. Both clients and their care providers need to be taught that this is not a communicable disease.

Salmonellosis. *Salmonella* infection can be prevented by teaching the client about food and water safety and proper food handling. Infection occurs after ingestion of contaminated food, including (1) beef, pork, poultry, and eggs; (2) drinking contaminated water; (3) ingesting contaminated drugs or diagnostic agents; (4) directly handling contaminated feces; or (5) sexual activity involving oral-anal contact. Food handlers may be asymptomatic carriers, and pets, especially turtles, may be a source of exposure. Presenting clinical manifestations include fever, night sweats, fatigue, anorexia, weight loss, abdominal pain, and diarrhea. Treatment includes ampicillin, chloramphenicol, TMP-SMX, ciprofloxacin, or norfloxacin. Follow-up care focuses on management of manifestations, including preventing and managing skin breakdown in the perianal region.

Bacterial Pneumonia. Recurrent bacterial pneumonia is common among IV drug users. Predisposing factors include needle sharing, environmental exposure, heavy alcohol use, smoking, and inadequate nutrition. Pathogens most often associated with bacterial pneumonia, seen in people infected with HIV, are *Streptococcus pneumoniae* and *Haemophilus influenzae.* The risk of bacterial pneumonia increases when the CD4$^+$ cell count is below 200 mm^3. Antibiotic treatment is based on culture and sensitivity reports. Follow-up care includes focusing on behavioral changes that decrease the possibility of recurrence.

Pneumococcal vaccination should be given at 5-year intervals. Prophylactic therapy prescribed to prevent *P. carinii* pneumonia or *M. avium* complex may provide some protection against recurrent bacterial pneumonia.

Fungal Infections

Candidiasis. *Candida albicans* not only is ubiquitous (in soil and food, on fomites) but is also normally found on the skin and in the mouth, vagina, and large intestine. Most infections are *endogenous;* that is, the person's own organism is the source of the infection. *Nosocomial* spread in hospitals and nursing homes can also occur. Human-to-human transmission can occur from mother to infant during vaginal delivery and between sexual partners. Clinical presentation is related to the site of infection: dysphagia with esophagitis, oral lesions with thrush, cutaneous lesions with intertrigo, vulvovaginal irritation and discharge with vaginitis, and constitutional manifestations with disseminated disease. Treatment is also site dependent:

- For *oral/esophageal candidiasis,* clotrimazole troches, nystatin suspension, fluconazole: For esophagitis, fluconazole, itraconazole, ketoconazole, or amphotericin B
- For *intertrigo* and *vaginitis,* clotrimazole, miconazole, ketoconazole, fluconazole, and itraconazole (for nail infection)
- For *disseminated disease,* amphotericin B, with or without flucytosine

Follow-up care includes teaching routine skin and mouth care. Encourage the client to eat 8 ounces of yogurt made from live cultures (*Lactobacillus acidophilus*) to help control recurrent infection with *Candida.* For recurrent, frequent episodes or after a severe episode, prophylactic therapy with fluconazole, ketoconazole, or itraconazole may be ordered.

Cryptococcosis. *Cryptococcus neoformans* is ubiquitous and is found in pigeon droppings, nesting places, soil, fruit, and unpasteurized fruit juices. The organism is aerosolized and inhaled. As an AIDS-indicator disease,

it causes lung and brain infection. HIV-infected smokers are more prone to development of cryptococcosis. Clinical manifestations primarily involve the CNS but can also include the lungs, skin, and mouth.

The CNS manifestations include low-grade fever, fatigue, headaches, nausea, vomiting, and altered mental status. Pulmonary manifestations include cough, dyspnea, and pleuritic chest pain. Cutaneous and oral manifestations include painless lesions that may mimic KS or molluscum contagiosum. Treatment includes amphotericin B, with or without flucytosine, fluconazole, or itraconazole. Maintenance lifetime suppressive therapy is required with fluconazole, itraconazole, or amphotericin B, and follow-up care focuses on assisting with medication compliance and monitoring for recurrence of manifestations that indicate resistance to maintenance drug therapy.

Histoplasmosis. *Histoplasma capsulatum,* a fungus endemic to certain regions of the United States, is most prevalent in the middle, central, and south central states and Puerto Rico. Therefore people with HIV disease and living in these areas are susceptible to the disease. When diagnosed in other parts of the country (e.g., New York, California), the disease usually appears in a client who either grew up in or traveled to the endemic regions. Manifestations include fever; weight loss; enlarged lymph nodes, liver, and spleen; abdominal pain; oral and skin lesions; anemia; leukopenia; and thrombocytopenia.

Treatment includes amphotericin B, itraconazole, or fluconazole. Maintenance lifetime suppressive therapy (itraconazole or amphotericin B) is required. Follow-up care focuses on helping with drug compliance and monitoring for recurrence of manifestations that indicate resistance to maintenance drug therapy.

Coccidioidomycosis. *Coccidioides immitis* is a fungus endemic to the southwestern United States. It was originally discovered in the San Joaquin Valley in southern California and is also referred to as *valley fever.* As an AIDS-defining diagnosis, it is commonly seen in people infected with HIV residing in Arizona, California, Nevada, New Mexico, Texas, and Utah. When diagnosed in other parts of the United States, the disease usually appears in a client who either grew up in or traveled to the endemic regions. Clinical presentation includes fever, dyspnea, fatigue, weight loss, and cough.

Treatment includes amphotericin B, ketoconazole, itraconazole, or fluconazole. Maintenance lifetime suppressive therapy is required using fluconazole, itraconazole, or amphotericin B. Follow-up care focuses on helping with drug compliance and monitoring for recurrence of manifestations that indicate resistance to maintenance drug therapy.

Protozoal Infections

Pneumocystosis. *P. carinii* is a ubiquitous organism that is airborne and can be found in the lungs of humans and animals. Most healthy people have had a primary infection by 4 years of age. Although most of the literature suggests that *P. carinii* infection in people with HIV is a secondary appearance of a previously acquired pathogen (reactivation), more recent information has revealed that some clients have different strains of the organism, which may indicate that reinfection is possible through airborne transmission.

Clinical presentation can be elusive, and about 7% of clients with the infection are asymptomatic. With *P. carinii* pneumonia, coughing is a frequent first manifestation. The pneumonia begins with a nonproductive cough and progresses to a productive cough. Eventually the client has fever and dyspnea on exertion, then dyspnea at rest. Extrapulmonary *P. carinii* infection can occur in the eyes, ears, lymph nodes, heart, spleen, liver, pleural space, and on the skin.

Clients who are receiving prophylaxis for *P. carinii* pneumonia sometimes also go on to have infection because of poor drug compliance, unusual or erratic pharmacokinetics, or development of drug resistance. Treatment may be with TMP-SMX, pentamidine, atovaquone, TMP-dapsone, clindamycin-primaquine, or trimetrexate. Maintenance lifetime suppressive therapy is required with TMP-SMX, pentamidine aerosol, atovaquone, dapsone, or clindamycin-primaquine. Follow-up care focuses on helping with drug compliance and monitoring for recurrence of manifestations that indicate resistance to maintenance drug therapy.

Toxoplasmosis. Toxoplasma gondii is ubiquitous in nature and is acquired through ingestion of contaminated meat (lamb and pork), vegetables, eggs, and unpasteurized dairy products. Human-to-human transmission can occur from mother to fetus if the mother acquires primary infection during pregnancy. Toxoplasmosis can also be acquired through direct handling of contaminated cat feces; however, fewer than 1% of domestic cats are infected with *T. gondii*. A veterinarian can perform a simple blood test to determine whether a cat is infected. Studies of cat owners infected with HIV have not shown any increased risk for the development of toxoplasmosis. The potential for the development of toxoplasmosis increases when the CD4$^+$ cell count is below 100 mm³. If TMP-SMX or dapsone is prescribed for *P. carinii* pneumonia prophylaxis, the drug would provide prophylaxis against toxoplasmosis as well.

Clinical manifestations of CNS infection include headache, impaired cognition, hemiparesis, aphasia, ataxia, vision loss, cranial nerve palsies, motor problems, and seizures. Infection can also involve the heart, lungs, skin, stomach, abdomen, and testes. Treatment includes pyrimethamine plus sulfadiazine, leucovorin, clindamycin plus pyrimethamine, clarithromycin, or azithromycin. Maintenance lifetime suppressive therapy calls for pyrimethamine plus sulfadiazine plus leucovorin. Follow-up care focuses on helping with drug com-

pliance and monitoring for recurrence of manifestations that indicate resistance to maintenance drug therapy.

Cryptosporidiosis. Cryptosporidium is found in mammals, birds, reptiles, and fish. The primary mode of transmission in people infected with HIV is through the ingestion of contaminated food or water. Water-borne transmission can occur when drinking supplies become contaminated, including municipal water supplies, because chlorine does not destroy the organism. Boiling water for 1 minute destroys this organism.

Cryptosporidial disease can also be acquired from contaminated swimming pools, from handling infected animals, and through anal-oral sexual contact with an infected person. When cryptosporidiosis occurs in immunocompetent people, the disease is self-limiting. In an immunodeficient person with HIV, the disease is chronic and causes malabsorption, dehydration, and malnutrition. It can lead to death. Clinical presentation includes profuse diarrhea, steatorrhea (1 to 25 L/day), flatulence, abdominal cramping and pain, anorexia, nausea, vomiting, profound weight loss, fever, fatigue, myalgia, and electrolyte imbalance.

No effective treatment for cryptosporidiosis has been found. Drugs that may be tried include paromomycin, azithromycin, clarithromycin, nitazoxanide, thalidomide, and symptomatic therapy to decrease peristalsis and control pain. Spontaneous remission has occurred once combination anti-retroviral therapy was started, presumably because the immune system restores itself and controls the disease. Special attention is also needed to manage skin breakdown in the perianal region. Clients with cryptosporidiosis are vulnerable to depression and social isolation.

Isosporiasis. Isospora belli is a parasite that is transmitted through contact with infected animals or humans or contaminated water. The disease is often seen in immigrants from Mexico, Haiti, and Central America. Clinical manifestations of the disease include diarrhea, anorexia, nausea, vomiting, weight loss, abdominal pain, and fever. Drug therapy includes TMP-SMX or pyrimethamine plus folinic acid. Treatment is usually successful, and lifetime suppressive therapy is not usually required.

Viral Infections

Cytomegalovirus Disease. Cytomegalovirus (CMV) is ubiquitous in humans throughout the world. Almost everyone eventually becomes infected with CMV, which is transmitted through direct contact with infected secretions, including saliva, cervical fluid, urine, semen, breast milk, feces, and blood. In people infected with HIV, CMV infection can be asymptomatic or can cause chorioretinitis, pneumonitis, encephalitis, adrenalitis, colitis, esophagitis, hepatitis, or cholangitis.

Drugs used to treat CMV infection systemically include ganciclovir, foscarnet, and cidofovir plus probenecid.

Treatment also may involve intraocular ganciclovir implants or intravitreal injection of ganciclovir, foscarnet, or cidofovir. Maintenance lifetime suppressive therapy is required using any of these drugs. Follow-up care focuses on helping with drug compliance and monitoring for recurrence of manifestations that indicate resistance to maintenance drug therapy.

Herpes Simplex. Herpes simplex virus (HSV) is ubiquitous and is spread by direct contact with infected secretions. HSV-1 is present in oral secretions, and HSV-2 is present in genital secretions. Transmission also takes place with "symptom-free excreters" (people previously infected with HSV and with no apparent lesions). Clinical presentation includes painful vesicular lesions that coalesce and rupture. Lesions usually occur in the oral, genital, or perianal region. HSV can also cause encephalitis, esophagitis, bronchitis, keratitis, pericarditis, and hand infection.

Treatment includes acyclovir, foscarnet, or famciclovir. Topical acyclovir also reduces pain and itching associated with skin lesions. Follow-up care focuses on monitoring the client for recurrent disease. Chronic disease requires lifetime suppressive therapy with acyclovir.

Progressive Multifocal Leukoencephalopathy. Progressive multifocal leukoencephalopathy is caused by the JC virus (initials of the first client in whom it was discovered). The JC virus is ubiquitous in nature and appears to infect most middle-aged people. Active disease in people infected with HIV results in limb weakness, ataxia, cognitive impairment, vision loss, speech impairment, and headache. In the latter stages of illness, it progresses to dementia, blindness, paralysis, and death.

No effective therapy has been found, but drugs that may be used include acyclovir, foscarnet, adenine arabinoside, cytosine arabinoside, and interferon alfa. There have been reports of spontaneous remission of this disease once combination antiretroviral therapy is started, presumably because the immune system restores itself and controls the disease. Follow-up care focuses on palliative therapy, safety measures, and preventing complications from immobility.

Hepatitis. The leading cause of death among AIDS clients is now hepatic failure secondary to hepatitis B. See Chapter 49 for a discussion of hepatitis.

Treat Neoplasms

Kaposi's Sarcoma. Four types of KS may be encountered in clinical practice: (1) classic KS, which tends to occur in older men who are black, of Mediterranean descent, or from certain Jewish populations; (2) African KS, seen in Africa; (3) Transplant KS, seen in people who receive organ transplants; and (4) HIV-related KS, which differs from the others in that it runs a fulminant course, is disseminated throughout the body, and results in shorter survival.

The only form associated with HIV disease is HIV-related KS sarcoma. It has been diagnosed predominantly in men who have sex with men and is thought to be associated with a sexually transmitted pathogen that then predisposes the person to development. Researchers think it is caused by either human herpesvirus type 8 (HHV-8) or KS-associated herpes virus (KSHV). KS differs from most AIDS-defining diseases in that it is unrelated to low CD4+ cell counts and can occur early in HIV infection.

Clinical presentation typically starts with an initial "patch" that is flat and pink, looks like a bruise, and is symmetrical on both sides of the body. Later, it turns into dark violet or black plaques. Clinical presentation of the lesions can include the mouth, skin, mucous membranes, head, neck, torso, limbs (soles of feet), genitals, lung, brain, intestines, testes, liver, spleen, pancreas, adrenal gland, and lymph nodes. They can be painful.

Treatment depends on the extent of tumors (tumor burden), CD4+ cell count, associated manifestations and diseases, and the client's functional ability. Local therapy includes radiation, localized chemotherapy, and cryotherapy. Systemic therapy includes doxorubicin, alpha interferon, bleomycin, paclitaxel, and daunorubicin. Experimental therapies under investigation include possible treatment of the underlying viral cause of KS with foscarnet or ganciclovir. Initially several therapies may be tried, which may be effective in suppressing the course of KS; eventually, however, the clinical decline in the client's condition makes continued treatment impossible.

Non-Hodgkin's Lymphoma. Non-Hodgkin's lymphoma tends to occur late in the course of HIV disease and is related to low CD4+ cell counts. The primary sites of occurrence are the brain, gastrointestinal tract, bone marrow, and liver. The initial clinical presentation may be nonspecific and include fever, night sweats, and weight loss, all of which are associated with *M. avium* complex infection, TB, and CMV infection.

Treatment includes methotrexate, bleomycin, doxorubicin, cyclophosphamide, and vincristine. Despite aggressive treatment, the prognosis is poor except in clients on combination anti-retroviral therapy, who tend to survive longer.

Invasive Cervical Cancer. Cervical intraepithelial neoplasia (CIN), the precursor to cervical cancer, occurs at a high rate in women infected with HIV, progresses more rapidly, is less responsive to therapy, and is related to low CD4+ cell counts. In early stages of disease, the client is asymptomatic. Cervical dysplasia is usually detected by Pap smear. Early clinical manifestations include postcoital bleeding, metrorrhagia, and a blood-tinged vaginal discharge. Manifestations of more extensive disease include back, pelvic, and leg pain; weight loss; vaginal bleeding; anemia; lymphadenopathy; and edema of the legs.

Treatment of CIN can include conization, laser therapy, cryosurgery, electrocautery, or hysterectomy. For invasive cancer, treatment may involve surgery, radiation, and chemotherapy with cisplatin, vincristine, bleomycin, or mitomycin. Follow-up care focuses on recurrent disease and control of manifestations and metastasis.

Treat Conditions Specific to AIDS

AIDS Dementia. HIV encephalopathy, also referred to as *AIDS dementia complex,* appears to affect the very young and older HIV-infected clients and clients with anemia and weight loss. In addition, HIV-infected people with less than a 12th grade education may be more likely to show clinical manifestations. Manifestations include cognitive dysfunction, motor problems, and behavioral changes. Cognitive manifestations include an inability to concentrate, decreased memory, impaired judgment, and slowed thinking. Motor impairment may be manifested as leg weakness, ataxia, and clumsiness. Behavioral changes can range from apathy, reduced spontaneity, and social withdrawal to irritability, hyperactivity, anxiety, mania, and delirium.

The staging system for AIDS dementia complex is as follows:

- Stage 1: Minimal manifestations, mild neurologic manifestations, no impairment of work or ability to perform activities of daily living (ADL)
- Stage 2: Obvious intellectual or motor impairment, still able to do all but the most demanding ADL
- Stage 3: Cannot work or perform demanding ADL, still capable of basic self-care, ambulatory but may need a single assistive device
- Stage 4: Major intellectual disability, cannot walk without assistance
- Stage 5: Nearly vegetative, paraplegic or quadriplegic, only rudimentary cognition remains

Some studies have shown a favorable response to combination anti-retroviral therapy. Psychotropic drugs may be tried in small doses, but benzodiazepines, drugs with strong anticholinergic properties, and amitriptyline should be used with caution. Follow-up monitoring focuses on detecting the progression of AIDS dementia complex and on evaluating the client's ability to safely maintain independent living and comply with prescribed therapies.

HIV Wasting Syndrome. Weight loss occurs at some point in more than 90% of people with HIV infection. *HIV wasting* is defined as profound involuntary weight loss (>10% of total body baseline weight) with either chronic diarrhea or chronic weakness and fever. The primary causes of HIV wasting syndrome are reduced food intake, malabsorption of nutrients, and altered metabolism of nutrients. The evaluation of a client with HIV wasting syndrome includes determining and treating the cause. Treating the underlying cause usually alleviates the progressive weight loss. In men with HIV, low testosterone levels lead to weight loss and can be reversed with testosterone replacement.

Once wasting has begun, treatment usually results in only partial recovery. The goal of drug therapy is to stimulate appetite, produce weight gain, and increase lean muscle mass. Weight gain that results in increased body fat is of little benefit. Identified conditions that contribute to wasting should be treated first. Drugs used to treat HIV wasting syndrome include megestrol acetate, and dronabinol (the major psychoactive component of marijuana). The drug used most successfully to treat wasting is human growth hormone. Follow-up therapy includes constant assessment for factors that may interfere with the plan of care.

■ Nursing Management of the Client with AIDS

In advanced HIV disease, the goal of nursing care is to diagnose and treat human responses to actual or potential health problems related to the development of clinical manifestations and the diagnosis of AIDS. All efforts are directed at controlling manifestations. Actual or potential problems seen in people with AIDS include fever, fatigue, weight loss, nausea, diarrhea, dry and painful mouth, dry skin, skin lesions, pain, dyspnea, cough, impaired cognition, impaired vision, insomnia, and sexual dysfunction. Common nursing diagnoses associated with the diagnosis of AIDS are presented in the box on Common Nursing Diagnoses for Clients with HIV and AIDS on the website. Four problems that affect most AIDS *evolve* clients are described here. Also see the Case Study feature on Human Immunodeficiency Virus below and the Bridge to Home Health Care feature on Living with HIV/AIDS on the website. *evolve*

Assessment

Assessment of clinical manifestations should include both subjective and objective data. All clinical manifes-

---

CASE STUDY *evolve*

Human Immunodeficiency Virus

Edith Jones is a white woman, age 50 years, who presents to an outpatient clinic with complaints of fever, fatigue, "swollen glands," and a sore throat. She is an elementary school teacher and states that she believes she has been exposed to some virus in her classroom. She is concerned because the manifestations have not resolved as quickly as they usually do when she catches a "classroom bug" . . . . *Case Study continued on the website and the CD-ROM with discussions, multiple-choice questions, and a nursing care plan.* *evolve*

tations should be quantified. The easiest way to measure the severity of a clinical manifestation is by asking the client to rate it on a scale from 0 to 10, with 0 being no problem at all and 10 being the worst possible. This method works well for most manifestations, such as fatigue and pain. Fever assessment can be made easy if the client is willing to keep a fever diary (writing down his or her temperature whenever he or she takes it). For clients who have no scale at home, the nurse will have to rely on client self-report to detect trends in weight.

Pain is a subjective experience. The single most reliable indicator of the existence and intensity of acute pain and any related discomfort or distress is the client's self-report. Neither behavior nor vital signs can substitute for that self-report. A client may be in excruciating pain even while smiling or laughing to cope with it. Trying to figure out whether a client has pain when the client is actually reporting pain is a waste of time.

Diagnosis, Outcomes, Interventions

Diagnosis: Hyperthermia.
An important nursing diagnosis for a client with AIDS is *Hyperthermia related to chronic HIV infection, secondary opportunistic infection, malignancy, autoimmune disorders, diarrhea, dehydration, allergic response to medications, or infection at IV sites, catheters, drains, and incisions.*

Outcomes.
After discussing the finding of assessment and the nursing diagnosis, select interventions in concert with the client, care partner, or both to control fever and replace fluid loss.

Interventions.
Because of the underlying immunodeficiency and impaired inflammatory response, clinical manifestations of infection, including fever, may be greatly muted. Nonpharmacologic interventions include keeping the client in a warm room to avoid shivering and applying a sheet and a loosely woven blanket. Avoid fanning the bed covers, exposing skin, or rapidly removing clothing that might cause chilling.

Avoid counterproductive treatments, such as tepid water sponge bathing, which causes defensive vasoconstriction and has not been shown to be an effective coolant in fever. Indeed sponge baths can cause shivering and can be distressing. Avoid alcohol sponging as well, which also causes vasoconstriction, shivering, and toxic fumes. The alcohol also can be absorbed cutaneously, causing hypoglycemia.

Increase caloric and fluid intake by providing a plan for six feedings distributed over 24 hours and high-protein, high-calorie nutritional supplements, especially if the client has anorexia. Provide 2 to 2.5 L of fluid to drink daily.

Maintain comfort and safety by providing dry clothes and bed linens made out of cotton rather than synthet-

ics. Use emollient creams for dry skin. Monitor mental status frequently, especially when the client has a fever. Evaluate the client's need for assistance with all ADL. Teach the client how to manage chronic recurrent night fever and night sweats by doing the following:
- Take the antipyretic agent of choice before going to sleep
- Have a change of bedclothes nearby in case a change is necessary
- Keep a plastic cover on the pillow
- Place a towel over the pillow in case of profuse diaphoresis
- Keep liquids at the bedside to drink

Pharmacologic treatment can include aspirin, nonsteroidal anti-inflammatory drugs (NSAIDs), or acetaminophen. Follow-up should include comparing patterns of use of these agents with laboratory evaluation of hepatic and hematologic abnormalities as well as interactions with other agents.

Diagnosis: Fatigue.
Another common nursing diagnosis is *Fatigue related to chronic HIV infection, anemia, secondary opportunistic infection, malnutrition, dehydration, prolonged immobility, and psychological and situational factors.* Fatigue is the most common complaint of clients with AIDS and of their caregivers.

Outcomes.
After discussing and validating the findings of assessment and nursing diagnosis, select interventions in concert with the client, care partner, or both to increase self-awareness of fatigue, associated clinical manifestations, environmental factors affecting fatigue, and activity tolerance. Identify interventions to highlight the importance of resting when needed and accepting assistance when needed. Develop a plan for a lifestyle that keeps the client independent, socially active, and involved in activities of daily living.

Interventions.
Promote self-care and self-awareness by having the client keep a daily fatigue diary for at least 1 week to identify sources of fatigue and appropriate interventions as well as patterns of peak fitness. Advise the client to avoid coffee, tobacco, and alcohol, any of which may increase fatigue. Promote adequate sleep by increasing the amount of sleep each day. Reduce the amount of sleep-cycle interruptions by preparing for sleep and keeping needed items at the bedside.

Promote rest and activity by developing a written 24-hour schedule of daily activities that alternates short activities with rest periods. Identify activity priorities, such as eating breakfast and then resting before bathing in the morning, as opposed to the reverse. Evaluate the client's needs and point out ways to conserve energy, such as sitting down while dressing, shaving, or preparing food; sitting on a shower chair while bathing; or using disposable items for eating so that no cleanup is needed. Help the client write a plan for rest and activities that progresses from daily to weekly. Encourage the client to always plan activities ahead of time.

Prepare an exercise schedule (immobilization may lead to decreased endurance and increased fatigue) and plan exercises at peak energy times (after a rest period). Follow the exercises with rest. Aerobic exercise, which increases endurance, can reduce fatigue. Additional natural techniques that may be of benefit include progressive muscle relaxation, acupressure, massage, reflexology, imagery and visualization, autogenic relaxation, reframing and positive affirmations, therapeutic touch, and social support and support groups.

Diagnosis: Imbalanced Nutrition: Less Than Body Requirements.

A frequently encountered nursing diagnosis is *Imbalanced Nutrition: Less Than Body Requirements related to increased nutrient requirements, decreased food intake secondary to side effects of medications and infection such as an anorexia, nausea, vomiting, altered taste, or impaired swallowing or chewing, diarrhea, fatigue, depression, or impaired cognition.*

Outcomes. After discussing and validating the findings of assessment and the nursing diagnosis, select interventions in concert with the client, care partner, or both to increase food intake, preserve lean body mass, and provide adequate levels of all nutrients.

Interventions

Minimize Anorexia. Minimize factors contributing to anorexia. For *hyperosmia* (increased sense of smell), avoid cooking odors by keeping windows open and the home well aerated. Encourage meals that include cold foods. For *hyposmia* (decreased sense of smell), use spices such as basil, oregano, rosemary, thyme, cloves, mint, cinnamon, or lemon juice to enhance the aroma. For alterations in sense of taste (especially related to distaste for red meat), marinate meat in a commercial marinade, wine, or vinegar before cooking it, and use substitutes for red meat, such as eggs, peanut butter, tofu, cheeses, poultry, and fish.

Prevent Weight Loss. Weight loss can be a significant problem for clients who live alone or who have fatigue or depression. Interventions include the following:

- Eating small meals frequently throughout the day
- Eating high-calorie snacks or commercially prepared supplements (liquids or bars)
- Indulging in favorite foods
- Consuming more nutrient-dense foods and beverages rather than filling up on low-calorie items
- Drinking liquids 30 minutes before eating instead of with meals
- Preparing meals (such as soups or casseroles) ahead of time so they can be divided into individual servings and frozen until ready to use

- Keeping easy-to-prepare foods on hand, such as frozen dinners, canned foods, and eggs
- Encouraging the client to dine with friends or family
- Getting family members and friends involved in meal preparation; the pleasant atmosphere they can provide may stimulate the client's appetite

Many communities have home food delivery service for people with AIDS as well.

Improve Food Intake. Minimize factors related to difficulty in chewing, dysphagia (difficulty in swallowing), or odynophagia (painful swallowing) by advising clients to avoid rough foods, such as (1) raw fruits and vegetables; spicy, acidic, or salty foods; (2) alcohol or tobacco; (3) excessively hot or cold foods; and (4) sticky foods, such as peanut butter; and (5) slippery foods, such as gelatin, bologna, and elbow macaroni. Encourage the client to do the following:

- Eat foods at room temperature
- Choose mild foods and drinks, such as apple juice rather than orange juice
- Eat dry grain foods (such as breads, crackers, and cookies) after softening them in milk, tea, or another mild beverage
- Eat nonabrasive foods that are easy to swallow, such as ice cream, pudding, well-cooked eggs, noodle dishes, baked fish, and soft cheese
- Eat Popsicles (frozen dessert) to numb pain
- Use a straw when drinking
- Tilt the head forward or back to make swallowing easier

Increase the Availability of Food. Minimize factors related to the client's inability to obtain food by evaluating his or her financial resources and the need for referral for Medicaid, food stamps, or other services. Evaluate the client's home and ability to prepare and obtain food. Look for problems such as an absence of cooking facilities and the need for alternative housing arrangements. Explore community resources that provide free meals.

Teach Nutritional Requirements. If the client has no metabolic condition that requires a special diet, the prescribed diet for people with HIV disease should include high-protein, high-calorie, low-fat foods. Help the client plan a 24-hour menu, and review the essential elements of a low-microbe diet and food safety and preparation. Nutritional teaching should, as much as possible, follow the client's usual pattern of food intake rather than expect the client to follow a totally new, unfamiliar prescription for meal planning.

Diagnosis: Acute Pain or Chronic Pain.

A common nursing diagnosis is *Acute Pain or Chronic Pain related to arthralgia, myalgia, or neuropathy associated with HIV disease, mass lesions associated with opportunistic infection(s) or cancer, side effects of medications, co-morbid disease such as diabetic neuropathy, or interventions such as surgery.*

Outcomes. After discussing and validating the findings of assessment, select interventions in concert with the client, care partner, or both to reduce the incidence and severity of pain, communicate effectively about pain experiences, and enhance comfort and satisfaction.

Interventions

Provide Comfort Measures. Non-drug interventions include identifying ADL that increase the intensity and severity of pain. Provide additional comfort measures, such as using a pressure-relieving mattress, positioning and supporting limbs comfortably when in bed or a chair, and using a "pull sheet" to move clients or help them change positions. For institutionalized clients, encourage family members or significant others to bring in familiar objects, such as pillows and blankets, favorite photographs, religious articles, personal clothing, cologne, make-up, face powder, and other cosmetics.

Provide Physical Therapy. Physical therapy can be very helpful in managing pain. The physical therapist can provide the following:

- Exercise to maintain or increase physical activity levels and endurance
- Ultrasound and physical treatments, such as application of heat or cold, to reduce musculoskeletal pain
- Therapeutic massage
- Instruction and supervision in using a transcutaneous electrical nerve stimulation (TENS) device, commonly called a *TENS unit*

Administer Pain Medications. Pharmacologic treatments usually include *non-opioid analgesics,* such as aspirin and acetaminophen for mild pain; (2) *weak opioids,* such as codeine and oxycodone for moderate pain; and (3) *strong opioids,* such as morphine for severe pain. For neuropathic pain (such as HIV-associated polyneuropathy, acute and postherpetic neuralgia, and nucleoside toxicity with didanosine, zalcitabine, and stavudine), adjuvants such as ibuprofen may be used as well as amitriptyline, desipramine, nortriptyline, doxepin, carbamazepine, divalproex, phenytoin, gabapentin, or mexiletine.

Primary care providers should anticipate several changes in prescriptions for analgesics when starting the client with a pain-control regimen. A major error in initial pain management occurs when a clinician prescribes a 2-week supply of an analgesic, assumes that the prescription works, and has no further contact until the client returns 2 weeks later for follow-up. On the contrary, during the initial phase of pain control, the clinician should have daily contact with the client, even if by telephone, and should anticipate schedule changes. Dosage frequency should be adjusted to prevent pain from recurring once the duration of analgesic action is determined. Similarly, it is a waste of money to prescribe large amounts of an analgesic, such as a 30-day supply, knowing that the orders will change. Orders for opioid analgesics should include "rescue" doses for breakthrough pain when regularly scheduled doses are insufficient.

Orders for analgesics as needed result in delays in administration and intervals of inadequate pain control. Tell clients and their care partners that the client may sleep for extended periods and may appear very drowsy during the first few days of a pain control regimen. Although this may result in part from the initial effects of the drug, it probably also reflects exhaustion and the need for rest as a result of sleep deprivation caused by pain. This situation usually reverses itself within a few days after a scheduled pain management regimen is begun.

Clients may refuse an analgesic if they are not in pain or may forgo it when they are asleep. Explain that this decision may lower blood analgesia levels and cause a resurgence of pain and failure of the pain control plan. Although the anti-inflammatory effects of aspirin are highly effective as an analgesic adjuvant, because aspirin inhibits platelet function, it may be contraindicated if the client has a low platelet count.

Helpful guidelines for managing pain in the injecting drug user include (1) having a single practitioner prescribe medications, (2) refusing to refill lost prescriptions, (3) carefully rationing opioid prescriptions, and (4) limiting rescue doses of opioid analgesics on a monthly basis. Clients who are in recovery for opioid addiction and are being treated with methadone maintenance still experience pain and in most instances require higher and more frequent doses of analgesia than a opioid-naive client would. Some anti-retroviral drugs, such as nevirapine and ritonavir, interfere with the half-life of methadone and may decrease its blood levels. The client will experience mild withdrawal manifestations. Increasing the daily dose of methadone usually resolves the problem.

Because diarrhea is common in clients with HIV disease, especially when protease inhibitors are prescribed, the constipating effects of analgesics may actually be beneficial. Evaluate each client's response to therapy instead of automatically using stool softeners when initiating the pain control plan.

Encourage Complementary Therapies. Complementary therapies that may be used include cognitive-behavioral interventions, such as education and instruction in pain control, relaxation exercises, imagery, music distraction, biofeedback, and therapeutic touch.

Evaluation

It is expected that the client will maintain or increase weight. It is expected that the client, care partner, or both will (1) identify factors related to anorexia, diffi-

culty in chewing, dysphagia, or odynophagia; (2) identify sufficient resources to obtain and prepare food or
make use of social work interventions employed to obtain food stamps or public assistance; (3) identify ways
to increase protein and calorie intake; (4) identify key
concepts in planning a low-microbial diet; and (5) select
a balanced 24-hour menu. The client's weight will fluctuate during the course of HIV disease related to new
disease processes and the side effects of prescribed medications.

It is expected that the client, care partner, or both will
be able to (1) identify appropriate measures to take for
a fever, (2) initiate and maintain adequate hydration
and nutrition, and (3) demonstrate the ability to take
and record the client's temperature accurately. Although
infection-related fever can be controlled with appropriate antibiotic therapy, this problem can be expected to
recur throughout the illness.

It is expected that the client, care partner, or both will
be able to (1) identify causative factors that increase fatigue, (2) plan a schedule of paced activity for a 24-hour
period, (3) demonstrate the ability to participate in a
program of exercise, and (4) verbalize a decrease in the
client's fatigue for a 24-hour period. Fatigue is a manifestation that can be expected to recur throughout HIV
disease, especially because it is a side effect of some antiretroviral medications.

It is expected that the client, care partner, or both will
(1) identify aggravating factors or precipitating factors
related to the pain experienced, (2) identify measures to
control pain, and (3) verbalize a decrease in the amount
and type of pain experienced over 24 hours. Pain may be
either chronic or acute, depending on the cause. In most
instances, it can be managed effectively, as with any
client with another diagnosis.

CONCLUSIONS

Human immunodeficiency virus continues to be a major
threat to human health worldwide. At one time or another, you will care for a person with HIV infection or
AIDS. To provide adequate care for a person with HIV infection, you must understand the illness trajectory and the
therapeutic interventions needed to maintain health. Always seek expert guidance when starting to care for a
client with HIV infection or AIDS. The nature of care is
very complex, and the client's clinical needs are numerous.

THINKING CRITICALLY *evolve*

1. A 30-year-old woman presents with fever, fatigue,
   lymphadenopathy, thrush, diarrhea, and pain in her
   muscles and joints. She has a rash on her torso and
   arms. What questions would you ask to determine her
   possible exposure to HIV? How will the client be
   evaluated and treated?

   Factors to Consider. What tests confirm the diagnosis of
   AIDS? How is the CD4+ cell count used? What is the
   purpose of the viral load test? What treatment should be
   used?

2. You are working in a homeless shelter and are scheduled to present a 20-minute program on AIDS prevention. A small class of four men and three women
   has gathered. They are all known to you, and you suspect that one couple may be infected with HIV. What
   should you plan to teach?

   Factors to Consider. What main areas of HIV education
   should be addressed? What is an effective method of
   communicating this information?

3. Your HIV-infected female client leaves the physician's
   office and comes over to you and says, "I don't have
   HIV anymore. The doctor just told me that my viral
   load was undetectable." How would you respond?

   Factors to Consider. What does an undetectable viral load
   test result mean? What would you tell this client about
   safer sex practices and becoming pregnant?

4. Your 40-year-old male client with AIDS and *P. carinii*
   pneumonia is about to be discharged from the hospital. His CD4+ cell count is 35. He asks you what he
   should do now. What teaching would you provide?

   Factors to Consider. When does a person with HIV infection get an AIDS diagnosis? Does this client need any
   medication for his pneumonia? Given the fact that the
   CD4+ cell count is 35, does he need any medication to
   prevent any other opportunistic infections?

*Discussions for these questions can be found on the
website and the CD-ROM.*

BIBLIOGRAPHY

1. (2002). New drugs, new data hold promise for next decade of HIV
   treatment. *AIDS Alert, 17*(5), 53, 55-57.

evolve **Did you remember to check out the bonus material on the
Evolve website and the CD-ROM, including free self-assessment exercises?**
http://evolve.elsevier.com/Black/medsurg/

2. (2002). STI may work in some patients. *AIDS Patient Care and STDs, 16*(2), 97.

 3. Abbaticiola, M.M. (2000). A team approach to the treatment of AIDS wasting. *Journal of the Association of Nurses in AIDS Care, 11*(1), 45-56.

 4. American Dietetic Association. (1994). Position of the American Dietetic Association and the Canadian Dietetic Association: Nutrition intervention in the care of persons with human immunodeficiency virus infection. *Journal of the American Dietetic Association, 94*, 1042-1045.

5. Barroso, J. (2002). HIV-related fatigue. *American Journal of Nursing, 102*(5), 83-86.

6. Bartlett, J. (2002). Addressing the challenges of adherence. *Journal of Acquired Immune Deficiency Syndromes and Human Retrovirology, 29*(Suppl 1), S2-S10.

 7. Centers for Disease Control. (1992). 1993 Revised classification system for HIV infection and expanded surveillance case definition for AIDS among adolescents and adults. *Morbidity and Mortality Weekly Report, 41* (RR-17), 1-19.

 8. Centers for Disease Control and Prevention. (1998). *HIV/AIDS Surveillance Report, 10*(2), 1-39.

 9. Centers for Disease Control and Prevention. (1999). *1999 USPHS/IDSA guidelines for the prevention of opportunistic infections in persons infected with human immunodeficiency virus.* Atlanta: Author.

10. Centers for Disease Control and Prevention. (1999). *Guidelines for the use of antiretroviral agents in HIV-infected adults and adolescents.* Atlanta: Author.

11. Daugherty, L.M., Bankston, J.B., & Deshotels, J.M. (2002). Keeping trouble at bay. *RN, 65*(2), 31-36.

12. Demmer, C. (2001). Dealing with AIDS-related loss and grief in a time of treatment advances. *American Journal of Hospice & Palliative Care, 18*(1), 35-41.

13. Jones, S.G. (2001). How to support patient with HIV/AIDS. *Nursing 2001, 31*(12), 36-42.

14. Laurence, J. (2002). Bullet points: New topics in HIV/AIDS. *AIDS Patient Care and STDs, 16*(1), 1-4.

15. Keiser, P. (2002). Roles of sequencing in therapy selection. *Journal of Acquired Immune Deficiency Syndromes and Human Retrovirology, 29*(Suppl. 1), S19-S27.

16. Kirton, C.A., Talotta, D., & Zwolski, K. (2001). *Handbook of HIV/AIDS Nursing.* St. Louis: Mosby.

17. Powderly, W.G. (2002). Long-term exposure to lifelong therapies. *Journal of Acquired Immune Deficiency and Human Retrovirology, 29*(Suppl 1), S28-S40.

18. Ress, B. (2001). Caring for patients with HIV disease in the new millennium. *Critical Care Nurse, 21*(1), 69-77.

19. Tsasis, P. (2001). Adherence assessment to highly active antiretroviral therapy. *AIDS Patient Care and STDs, 15*(3), 109-115.

20. Weller, V.D., & Williams, I.G. (2001). ABC of AIDS: Antiretroviral drugs. *British Journal of Medicine, 322*, 1410-1412.

21. World Health Organization. (2002). AIDS epidemic update. Available at: http://www.unaids.org/worldaidsday/2002/press/update/epiupdate2002_en.doc

Chapter 81

Management of Clients with Leukemia and Lymphoma

Susan Newton

evolve

Web Enhancements

http://evolve.elsevier.com/Black/medsurg/

Appendix C
Laboratory Values of Clinical Importance in Medical-Surgical Nursing

Cancers of the hematopoietic system are disorders that result from the proliferation of malignant cells originating in the bone marrow, thymus, and lymphatic tissue. Blood cells that originate in bone marrow are called *hematopoietic cells;* cells that originate in the lymph are called *lymphoid cells. Leukemia* is cancer of the bone marrow, and *lymphoma* is cancer of the lymphoid tissue.

LEUKEMIA

Leukemia is a malignant disease of the blood-forming organs. The American Cancer Society estimated that in 2003 about 30,600 new cases of leukemia would be diagnosed, and about 21,900 deaths would be attributed to the disease.[2] Leukemia is the most common malignancy in children and young adults. Half of all leukemias are classified as *acute,* with rapid onset and progression of disease resulting in 100% mortality within days to months without appropriate therapy. The remaining leukemias, classified as *chronic,* have a more indolent course. In children 80% of leukemias are lymphocytic and 20% are nonlymphocytic. In adults the percentages are reversed, with 80% nonlymphocytic.

Etiology and Risk Factors

Although the cause of leukemia is unknown, several risk factors are associated with leukemia, including (1) genetic factors, (2) exposure to ionizing radiation and chemicals, (3) congenital abnormalities (e.g., Down syndrome), and (4) the presence of primary immunodeficiency and infection with the human T-cell leukemia virus type 1 (HTLV-1). Genetic factors increase the risk of leukemia. A high incidence of acute leukemias and *chronic lymphocytic leukemia* (CLL) is reported in certain families. Hereditary abnormalities associated with an increased incidence of leukemia are Down syndrome, Fanconi aplastic anemia, Bloom's syndrome, ataxia telangiectasia, trisomy 13 (Patau's syndrome), Wiskott-Aldrich syndrome, and congenital X-linked agammaglobulinemia. Identical twins, fraternal twins, and siblings of children with leukemia are also at increased risk. In *chronic myelogenous leukemia* (CML), more than 90% of clients have the Philadelphia chromosome, an abnormal chromosome (see Chronic Leukemia later in this chapter).

Overexposure to ionizing radiation is a major risk factor for development of leukemia, with the disease developing years after the initial exposure. Alkylating

Nursing Outcomes Classification (NOC)
for Nursing Diagnoses—Clients with Leukemia and Lymphoma

Acute Pain or Chronic Pain
  Comfort Level
  Pain Control
  Pain Level
  Symptom Control
  Well-Being
Anticipatory Grieving
  Coping
  Family Coping
  Grief Resolution
  Sleep
Death Anxiety
  Dignified Dying
  Fear Control
  Depression Level
Disturbed Body Image
  Acceptance: Health Status
  Body Image
  Self-Esteem
Dysfunctional Grieving
  Coping
  Family Coping
  Grief Resolution
  Role Performance
Fatigue
  Activity Tolerance
  Endurance
  Energy Conservation

  Nutritional Status: Energy
  Psychomotor Energy
Imbalanced Nutrition: Less Than Body Requirements
  Nutritional Status
  Nutritional Status: Food and Fluids
  Nutritional Status: Nutrient Intake
  Sensory Function: Taste and Smell
Impaired Oral Mucous Membrane
  Immune Status
  Infection Status
  Oral Health
  Self-Care: Oral Hygiene
  Pain Level
  Swallowing Status
  Tissue Integrity: Skin and Mucous
    Membranes
Ineffective Protection
  Coagulation Status
  Coping
  Immune Status
  Infection Status
  Nutritional Status
Nausea
  Comfort Level
  Hydration
  Nutritional Status: Food and Fluid
    Intake

  Symptom Severity
Risk for Ineffective Therapeutic Regimen Management/ Risk for Ineffective Family Therapeutic Regimen Management
  Knowledge: Therapeutic Regimen
Risk for Infection
  Immune Status
  Nutritional Status
Risk for Injury
  Fall Prevention Behavior
  Immune Status
  Personal Safety Behavior
  Risk Control
  Safe Home Environment
Risk for Sexual Dysfunction
  Acceptance
  Sexual Functioning
Spiritual Distress
  Anxiety Control
  Coping
  Dignified Dying
  Hope
  Quality of Life
  Spiritual Well-Being
  Well-Being

agents used to treat other cancers, especially in combination with radiation therapy, increase a person's risk of leukemia. Workers exposed to chemical agents, such as benzene, an aromatic hydrocarbon, are at a much higher risk.

Causal risk factors acting together with a genetic predisposition can alter nuclear deoxyribonucleic acid (DNA). The leukemic cell is then unable to mature and respond to normal regulatory mechanisms. Abnormal chromosomes are reported in 40% to 50% of clients with acute leukemia, and certain chromosomes are repeatedly more involved than others. A mutation in a single cell appears to give rise to some leukemias.

Pathophysiology

In normal bone marrow, efficient regulation ensures that cell proliferation and maturation are adequate to meet a person's needs. Pluripotent stem cells commit to differentiate along the myeloid, erythroid, or lymphoid path-

way in the presence of growth factors. In leukemia control is missing or abnormal. Leukemia is an uncontrolled proliferation of leukocytes. This lack of control causes normal bone marrow to be replaced by immature and undifferentiated leukocytes, or *blast cells* (Figure 81-1). Abnormal, immature leukocytes then circulate in the blood and infiltrate the blood-forming organs (liver, spleen, lymph nodes) and other sites throughout the body.

The French-American-British (FAB) Cooperative Group developed a classification system that is universally accepted. Under this system, acute leukemias are classified on the basis of morphologic characteristics and histochemical staining of blast cells, which indicates the percentage of immature cells in the bone marrow (Table 81-1).

Acute Leukemia

Acute leukemia is caused by a block in the differentiation of cells in the hematopoietic cell line. The result is a massive accumulation of immature, nonfunctional cells or blasts in the bone marrow or in other organs. *Acute lymphoblastic leukemia* (ALL) is most common in children

The authors would like to thank Linda Yoder for her contribution to this chapter in the sixth edition of *Medical-Surgical Nursing*.

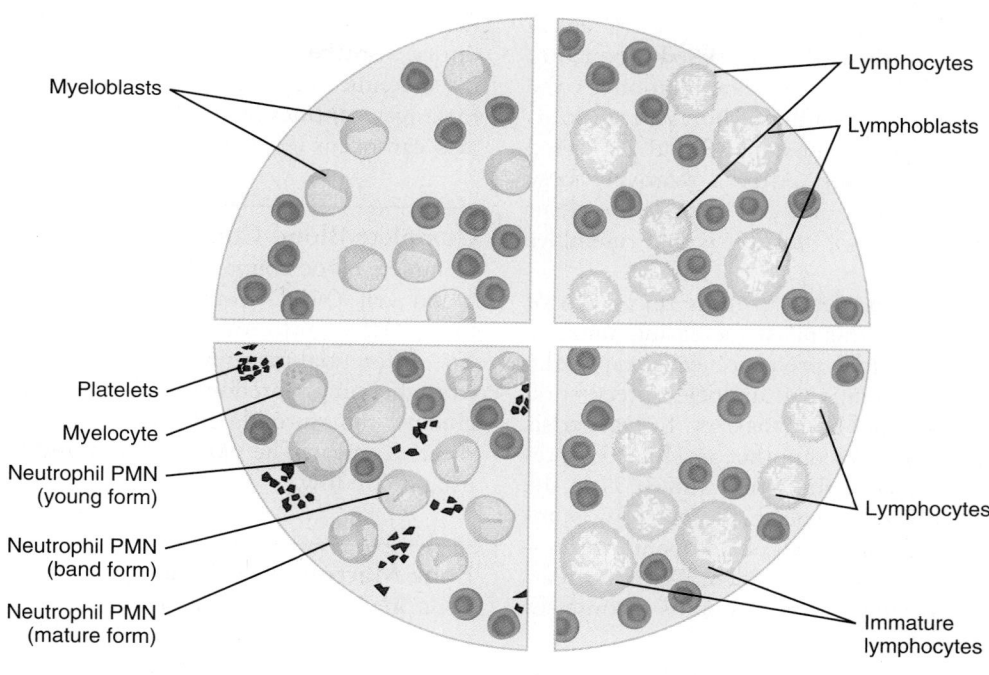

A Acute nonlymphocytic leukemia (ANLL)

Myeloblasts

B Acute lymphocytic leukemia (ALL)

Lymphocytes

Lymphoblasts

Platelets

Myelocyte

Neutrophil PMN
(young form)

Neutrophil PMN
(band form)

Neutrophil PMN
(mature form)

Lymphocytes

Immature
lymphocytes

C Chronic myelogenous leukemia (CML)

D Chronic lymphocytic leukemia (CLL)

FIGURE 81-1 Comparison of types of leukemia.

(median age, 10 years). *Acute nonlymphocytic leukemia* (ANLL), also referred to as *acute myeloid leukemia* (AML) is more common in adults (median age, 65 years). Leukemias are considered clonal disorders in that a single cell undergoes transformation, and leukemic cells then proliferate. An interesting paradox is that leukemic cells apparently divide more slowly and take longer to synthesize DNA than do other blood precursors. Acute leukemia is not caused by rapid cellular proliferation but instead is caused by the blocking of blood cell precursors. Leukemic cells accumulate relentlessly in most affected individuals, and they compete with normal cellular proliferation. Acute leukemia has also been termed an *accumulation disorder* and *proliferation disorder.*

The development of leukemia occurs in the most primitive blood precursors, pluripotent stem cells, which give rise to all other blood cells (see the Unit 17 Anatomy and Physiology Review). The leukemia blasts, or precursor cells, literally "crowd out" the marrow and cause cellular proliferation of the other cell lines to cease. Normal granulocytic, monocytic, lymphocytic, erythrocytic, and megakaryocytic stem cells cease to function, causing *pancytopenia* (a reduction in all cellular components of the blood). Transformation also may occur, most often in the granulocyte-monocyte series, but transformation could also occur in the erythrocyte series.

TABLE 81-1	*French-American-British (FAB) Classification of Acute Leukemia*

Acute lymphocytic leukemia
  L1   Common childhood leukemia
  L2   Adult acute lymphocytic leukemia
  L3   Rare subtype, blasts resembling those in Burkitt's lymphoma

Acute myeloblastic leukemia
  Granulocytic
    M1   Myeloblastic leukemia without maturation
    M2   Myeloblastic leukemia with maturation
    M3   Hypergranular promyelocytic leukemia
  Monocytic
    M4   Myelomonocytic leukemia
    M5   Monocytic
  Erythroid
    M6   Erythroleukemia

Chronic Leukemia

Chronic leukemias are caused by unregulated proliferation of hematopoietic cells or disordered cell death (*apoptosis*). Chronic leukemia is classified as CML or

CLL. CML originates in the pluripotent stem cell. Initially the marrow is hypercellular with most cells normal. Typically the peripheral blood smear reveals leukocytosis and thrombocytosis with an increased production of granulocytes. In 90% of cases examination of the bone marrow cells during metaphase shows a translocation of the long arms of chromosomes 9 and 22, called the *Philadelphia chromosome*. After a relatively slow course for a median period of 3 to 4 years, the client with CML invariably enters a *blast crisis* that resembles acute leukemia.

Blast crisis results in the death of more than 70% of clients with CML. During this phase increasing numbers of *blasts* (immature myeloid precursor cells, especially *myeloblasts*, the most primitive granulocyte precursors) proliferate in the blood and bone marrow. In blast crisis the blasts and *promyelocytes* (another myeloid cell precursor type) exceed 20% in the blood and 30% in the marrow. Increased fibrotic tissue in the marrow is another manifestation of blast crisis. Leukopenia, thrombocytopenia, and anemia also are evident. Without treatment death usually occurs within 6 months of onset of the blast crisis.

Chronic lymphocytic leukemia, which is characterized by the proliferation of early B lymphocytes, is an indolent leukemia that is seen most often in men older than 50 years of age. It is usually discovered when the complete blood count (CBC) is performed as part of a routine physical examination. A peripheral blood smear reveals increased numbers of mature and slightly immature lymphocytes. As the disease progresses, lymphocytes infiltrate the lymph nodes, liver, spleen, and ultimately the bone marrow. A staging system is based on the extent of lymphocyte infiltration. Progression of the disease may take up to 15 years, during which the client may not require therapy.

Clinical Manifestations

The manifestations of all types of leukemia are similar. The clinical history usually reveals anemia, thrombocytopenia, and leukopenia.

Clinical manifestations of bone marrow depression include fatigue caused by anemia, bleeding resulting from thrombocytopenia (reduced numbers of circulating platelets), fever caused by infection, anorexia, headaches, and papilledema. Bleeding can occur in the skin, gums, mucous membranes, and gastrointestinal (GI) and genitourinary tracts. Bleeding also is the underlying cause of petechiae and *ecchymosis* (discoloration visible through the skin).

Anorexia is associated with weight loss, diminished sensitivity to sour and sweet tastes, wasting away of muscle, and difficulty swallowing. Liver, spleen, and lymph node enlargement are more common in ALL than in ANLL. Splenomegaly and hepatomegaly usually occur together. The client with leukemia commonly experiences abdominal pain with tenderness and breast tenderness.

Headache, vomiting, and papilledema are associated with central nervous system (CNS) involvement. Facial nerve involvement causes facial palsy. Blurred vision, auditory disturbances, and meningeal irritation can occur if leukemic cells infiltrate the cerebral or spinal meninges. Intracranial hemorrhage and compression also can occur (Figure 81-2).

Complete Blood Count

Complete blood count values vary greatly. The total white blood cell (WBC) count may be normal, abnormally low (<1000/mm³), or extremely high (>200,000/mm³). The differential may reveal that one type of leukocyte is overwhelmingly predominant. Abnormal leukocytes, including immature blast forms, may be noted on the peripheral smear. The platelet count and hemoglobin level usually are low.

Bone Marrow Aspiration

Bone marrow aspiration or biopsy is a key diagnostic tool for confirming the diagnosis and identifying the malignant cell type. Typical findings in the bone marrow aspirate and biopsy are an overall increase in the number of marrow cells and an increase in the proportion of earlier forms, suggesting immature cells.

Other Findings

Lumbar puncture determines the presence of blast cells in the CNS; 5% of clients have this abnormality at diagnosis. Lumbar puncture is rarely if ever performed during the acute phase of leukemia secondary to an increased risk of iatrogenic introduction of blast cells into the CNS. It is usually performed post induction, especially in clients with ALL. Radiography of the chest and skeleton and magnetic resonance imaging (MRI) and computed tomography (CT) scans of the head and body detect lesions and sites of infection. Lymphangiography or lymph node biopsy may be performed to locate malignant lesions and classify the disease accurately.

Outcome Management

The treatment goals of all classifications of leukemia are targeted at destroying neoplastic cells and maintaining a sustained remission. During each phase of therapy, the medical treatment may vary, but the basic nursing principles are the same.

■ Medical Management

Acute Leukemia

The treatment plan for acute leukemia is determined by disease classification, the presence or absence of prognostic factors, and disease progression. The goal of treat-

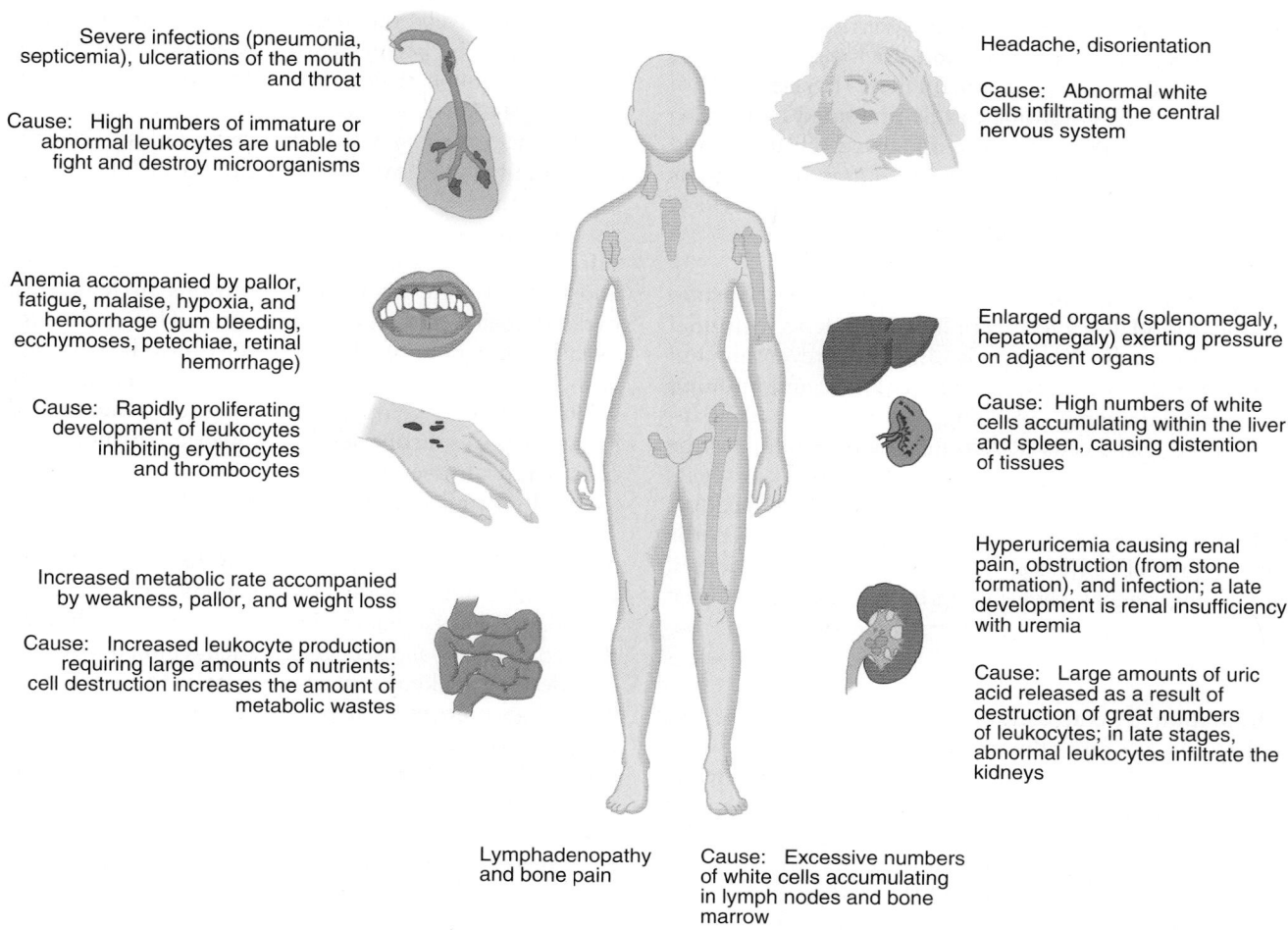

Severe infections (pneumonia, septicemia), ulcerations of the mouth and throat

Cause: High numbers of immature or abnormal leukocytes are unable to fight and destroy microorganisms

Anemia accompanied by pallor, fatigue, malaise, hypoxia, and hemorrhage (gum bleeding, ecchymoses, petechiae, retinal hemorrhage)

Cause: Rapidly proliferating development of leukocytes inhibiting erythrocytes and thrombocytes

Increased metabolic rate accompanied by weakness, pallor, and weight loss

Cause: Increased leukocyte production requiring large amounts of nutrients; cell destruction increases the amount of metabolic wastes

Headache, disorientation

Cause: Abnormal white cells infiltrating the central nervous system

Enlarged organs (splenomegaly, hepatomegaly) exerting pressure on adjacent organs

Cause: High numbers of white cells accumulating within the liver and spleen, causing distention of tissues

Hyperuricemia causing renal pain, obstruction (from stone formation), and infection; a late development is renal insufficiency with uremia

Cause: Large amounts of uric acid released as a result of destruction of great numbers of leukocytes; in late stages, abnormal leukocytes infiltrate the kidneys

Lymphadenopathy and bone pain

Cause: Excessive numbers of white cells accumulating in lymph nodes and bone marrow

FIGURE 81-2 Clinical manifestations and pathophysiologic bases of leukemia.

ment is complete remission with restoration of normal bone marrow function; this means a level of blast cells in the marrow less than 5%. About 70% to 80% of adults with ALL achieve complete remission, with 35% to 45% surviving 2 years. The cure rate remains low without bone marrow transplantation (BMT); however, of adults with ANLL, 60% to 70% achieve complete remission, and about 25% surviving 5 years or longer.

Destruction of Neoplastic Cells

Chemotherapy. Chemotherapy is given to destroy the malignant cells of the bone marrow. The treatment protocol for acute leukemia may involve up to three phases: the induction phase, consolidation phase, and maintenance phase. Maintenance phase is usually only used in adult ALL. The three phases of the treatment protocol are as follows:

1. *Induction phase.* The client receives an intensive course of chemotherapy designed to induce complete remission. The usual criteria for complete remission are blast cells less than 5% of the bone marrow cells and normal peripheral blood counts. Both conditions must be sustained for at least 1

month. Once remission is achieved, the consolidation phase begins.
2. *Consolidation phase.* Modified courses of intensive chemotherapy are given to eradicate any remaining disease. Usually a higher dose of one or more chemotherapeutic agents is administered.
3. *Maintenance phase.* Small doses of different combinations of chemotherapeutic agents are given every 3 to 4 weeks. This phase may continue for a year or longer and is structured to allow the client to live as normal a life as possible. This phase is used more commonly with ALL.

Tumor Lysis Syndrome. A potentially fatal complication resulting from the treatment of acute leukemia, *tumor lysis syndrome* is a group of metabolic complications associated with the rapid destruction of a large number of WBCs. If the WBC count is high when chemotherapy is initiated, rapid cell lysis can lead to (1) increased serum uric acid, phosphate, and potassium levels; and (2) decreased serum calcium levels. Manifestations include confusion, weakness, numbness, bradycardia, electrocardiographic (ECG) changes, and dysrhythmias (hyperkalemia);

numbness, tingling, muscle cramps, seizures, tetany, and ECG changes (hypocalcemia); and uric acid crystalluria, renal obstruction, and acute renal failure (hyperuricemia). Acute tumor lysis syndrome can be prevented by increasing intravenous (IV) hydration, alkalizing the urine, and administering allopurinol (Zyloprim). Often hemodialysis is necessary to decrease creatinine levels or leukapheresis is necessary to reduce the WBC count.

Replacing Cells and Controlling Infection. Current treatment modalities for acute leukemia destroy normal and aberrant cells. Therapy is aimed at preventing and resolving the complications of acquired and induced pancytopenia: anemia, bleeding, and infection. Transfusions of red blood cells (RBCs) may be required until the marrow produces mature cells. All blood products should be human leukocyte antigen (HLA) matched, cytomegalovirus (CMV) negative, and irradiated. If the client requires IV infusions of RBCs and amphotericin B, an antifungal agent, they should be separated by at least 1 hour so that adverse (e.g., allergic) reactions can be detected.

Radiation Therapy. Radiation therapy may be administered as an adjunct to chemotherapy when leukemic cells infiltrate the CNS, skin, rectum, and testes or when a large mediastinal mass is noted at diagnosis (as may occur in ALL).

Targeted Therapy. When AML relapses, treatment options are limited because of the associated toxicities and the health status of the client. Targeted therapies affect only the tumor cells and spare normal cells, hence decreasing the associated toxicities. Gemtuzumab ozofamicin (Mylotarg) is an anti-CD 33 monoclonal antibody linked to calicheamicin, which is a potent cytotoxic agent. CD33 antigens are found on the surface of leukemic blast cells and myeloid precursors. This agent is approved for the treatment of CD33-positive AML in clients with first relapse who are 60 years of age or older and who are not candidates for cytotoxic chemotherapy.

Chronic Myelogenous Leukemia
Treatment of CML is usually divided into four areas: (1) stem cell transplantation (discussed later in this chapter), (2) interferon alfa therapy with or without chemotherapy, (3) single-agent chemotherapy (hydroxyurea), or (4) the use of specific tyrosine kinase inhibitors.

The goal of therapy in the chronic phase of CML is to control leukocytosis and thrombocytosis. When unwanted cells accumulate, apheresis is a method of blood collection in which blood is withdrawn. The unwanted component is separated, and the remainder of the blood is returned to the client. *Apheresis* is usually performed with use of automated blood cell separators designed to

remove selectively the desired blood element. *Leukapheresis* may be performed to lower an extremely high peripheral leukocyte count quickly and to prevent acute tumor lysis syndrome (Figure 81-3). Leukapheresis is rarely performed in CML, however, unless peripheral blast count rises above 300,000 and the client is exhibiting abnormal clinical manifestations such as leukostasis. Leukapheresis can lower WBC counts rapidly and safely in clients with WBC counts greater than 300,000 and can alleviate acute manifestations of leukostasis, hyperviscosity, and tissue infiltration. This reduction is usually only temporary and often must be combined with chemotherapy for more lasting effects. If painful splenomegaly develops, irradiating or removing the spleen may be recommended; however, splenectomy is considered an avenue of last resort secondary to high surgical mortality in this population.

The most widely used medications are interferon alfa administered IV or subcutaneously (SC) and hydroxyurea administered orally (PO). Clients with a blast crisis (Figure 81-4) require intensive chemotherapy with the same agents as used in acute leukemia. These drugs can destroy leukemic blast cells, transform them into normal granulocytes, or prevent leukemic cells from inhibiting formation of normal granulocytes. Unfortunately, drugs are usually ineffective in achieving long-term remission.

Targeted Therapy. STI571 or imatinib mesylate (Gleevec) inhibits proliferation and induces apoptosis by

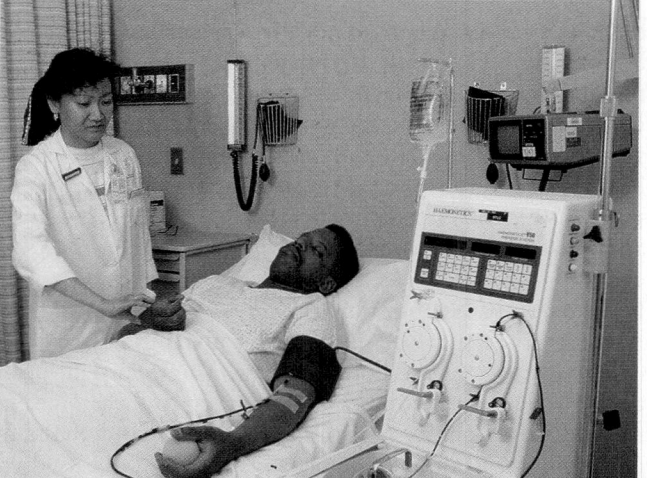

FIGURE 81-3 The white blood cell (WBC) level can be temporarily lowered by leukapheresis. Several automated blood cell separators effectively remove large numbers of WBCs and return red blood cells and plasma to the client. The Haemonetics V50 cell separator is commonly used to perform this procedure.

inhibiting tyrosine kinase activity in cells positive for *bcr-abl*. This agent also targets new leukemic cells in CML that are positive for the Philadelphia chromosome. This drug was approved rapidly by the U.S. Food and Drug Administration (FDA) because data demonstrate that Gleevec can induce hematologic response in 52% to 82% of clients. The results were sustained for at least 4 weeks in 31% to 64% of the clients. Complete response is lower at 7% to 34%.

Chronic Lymphocytic Leukemia

The goal of therapy in CLL is palliation or control of undesired manifestations. Local radiation to the spleen may be given as a palliative treatment to reduce complications. Two complications seen during the later stages are hemolytic anemia resulting from autoimmune disorder and hypogammaglobulinemia, which further increases susceptibility to infection. Antibiotics, transfusions of RBCs, and injections of gamma-globulin concentrates may be required for these clients. Leukapheresis is performed when the WBCs are enough to cause vascular thrombosis or embolism, especially in clients who are unresponsive to chemotherapy.

Chemotherapy. Chlorambucil (Leukeran) or cyclophosphamide (Cytoxan) may be given orally to reduce the manifestations of CLL. Chemotherapy generally is given for 2 weeks of every month. When anemia (stage III) and thrombocytopenia (stage IV) develop, daily oral prednisone is given as an adjunct to the alkylating agents. Prednisone has a marked lymphocytolytic effect and may stimulate the production of RBCs and platelets.

Fludarabine is a newer chemotherapeutic agent that appears effective in treating CLL.

Targeted Therapy. Targeted therapies are now being used in the treatment of CLL. Alemtuzumab (Campath) is a monoclonal antibody approved by the FDA for the treatment of CLL in clients who have been treated with alkylating agents and for whom fludarabine therapy has not been successful. This agent is directed at the CD52 receptor of the lymphocytes, which slows their proliferation. Rituximab (Rituxan) also is effective as a second-line or third-line treatment and may have a prominent role in the future.

■ Nursing Management of the Medical Client
Assessment

Obtain a thorough health history from the client and family members to aid in diagnosis and treatment. The initial history and physical examination provide baseline data to facilitate assessment of complications of ablative chemotherapy and radiation therapy. The severity and longevity of the manifestations of leukemia are important facts to obtain and document.

Ask the client about risk factors and causative factors. Age is important to note because the incidence of leukemia increases with age. The client's occupational history and hobbies may also give hints about environmental exposures. Previous illnesses and medical history may indicate risk factors.

Because leukemia increases the risk of infection resulting from loss of WBC function, ask about the frequency and severity of infections, such as colds, pneu-

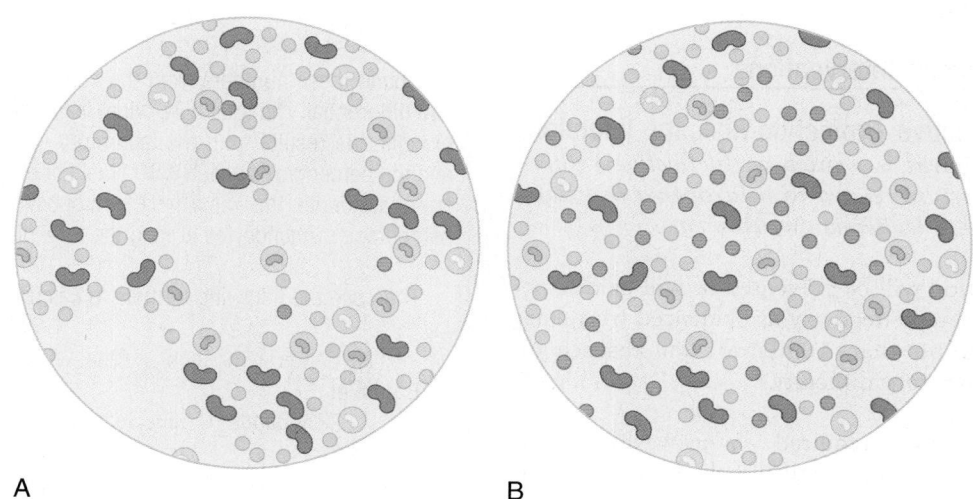

FIGURE 81-4 **A,** Microscopic view of a normal bone marrow specimen showing a normal distribution of blood cell types and fatty spaces. Blast cells appear as round, dark gray circles. **B,** During blast crisis the number of blast cells increases and fatty spaces shrink.

monia, bronchitis, and unexplained fever during the past 6 months. Leukemia reduces the production of RBCs. The client may report activity intolerance, headache resulting from cerebral hypoxia, increased sleepiness, decreased attention span, anorexia, and weight loss.

The loss of platelet function increases the risk of bleeding. The client may report a tendency to bleed or bruise easily (e.g., nosebleeds), an inability to stop bleeding from small nicks, bleeding in saliva when brushing teeth, increased menstrual flow, or blood in the stool or urine.

Physical examination findings may include the manifestations shown in Figure 81-2. A complete head-to-toe assessment is performed. Clients with leukemia or blast crisis may have tachycardia, hypotension, tachypnea, murmurs or bruits, and increased capillary fill time resulting from low RBC counts. Skin and mucous membranes may show evidence of bruising and bleeding. *Petechiae* (small, raised red spots) may be present. Lymph node enlargement may be present. If the leukemic cells have infiltrated the spleen or liver, abdominal tenderness may be noted. If the leukemic cells have infiltrated the brain, the client may be confused, have seizures, or become comatose.

The therapeutic relationship initiated during assessment is used to support the psychosocial needs of clients and their families. Leukemia is a life-threatening illness, and working with the client and family as a team is beneficial. Educating the client is an ongoing process to increase understanding of the disease and may help in obtaining compliance with treatment.

The nursing role during the acute phases of leukemia is extremely challenging because the client has many physical and psychosocial needs. Modern therapies offer hope for remission and possibly cure for some clients, but leukemia is still a diagnosis equated with pain, expensive long-term therapy, and potential death.

Diagnosis, Outcomes, Interventions

Diagnosis: Ineffective Protection/Risk for Infection.
The nursing diagnosis is written as *Ineffective Protection/Risk for Infection related to neutropenia or leukocytosis secondary to leukemia or treatment.*

Outcomes. Infection will be prevented or will be discovered early and treated effectively as evidenced by a neutrophil count greater than 1000/mm³, an absence of fever, and no respiratory difficulty.

Interventions. Institute required hand-washing for everyone coming in contact with the client. The client's risk for infection is estimated by calculating the absolute neutrophil count (ANC) (Box 81-1). The client should be in protective isolation if the ANC count is below 500/mm³. Visitors with possible communicable diseases

should be screened for the presence of infection, and visitors or staff with colds or respiratory infections should not be allowed near the client. Avoid all live plants and flowers in the client's room.

The client should be on a low-bacteria diet that excludes raw fruits and vegetables. Assist the client with a daily bath using antimicrobial soap. Encourage the client to perform meticulous oral hygiene several times a day. Female clients should not douche and should avoid the use of tampons. Daily stool softeners are ordered to reduce the risk of anal fissures. Perineal cleansing should occur after every bowel movement. Avoid insertion of rectal suppositories and rectal thermometers. Oral, axillary, or tympanic temperature should be taken every 4

BOX 81-1   *Determining the Absolute Neutrophil Count*

A leading complication in oncology clients is infection. To recognize this risk, the absolute neutrophil count (ANC) is calculated daily. The ANC (or granulocyte count) provides a numeric estimate of the client's immune status, risk for bacterial infection, and need for reverse isolation. For example, a client with leukemia may have a high white blood cell (WBC) count or a normal count. On calculating the ANC, however, you may find that he or she is at high risk for infection. For example, if a client has a WBC count of 9000 mm³, composed of 10% segmented neutrophils (segs), 60% blast cells, and 30% other WBCs, he or she would have an increased risk of infection because the functional neutrophils are only 900.

Three numbers are required:
- Banded neutrophil count
- Segmented neutrophil count
- Total WBC

Obtain these numbers from the complete blood cell count and differential. The total WBC count is composed of five types of cells; the results from the laboratory show the total count and the percentage of each WBC type. For example, on the differential counts, the value next to monocytes represents the percentage of monocytes among the total number of WBCs.

Then use the following formula to calculate the ANC:

(% Bands + % Segs) × Total WBC count = ANC
Example:
(2% Bands + 55% Segs) × 1600 = 912

When the ANC is less than 1000, the client is at risk for bacterial infection.
When the ANC count is less than 500, the client is at high risk for bacterial infection.

hours, and the physician should be notified if a temperature is higher than 38° C (100.5° to 101° F) or lower than 36° C (97° to 97.5° F). Fever may be the only manifestation in a neutropenic client. Assess the cause of fever before initiation of therapy by obtaining specimens of blood, sputum, urine, central line sites, and other potential sources of infection for culture.

Administer antibiotics as ordered. Therapy usually consists of multiple IV broad-spectrum antibiotics administered on alternating schedules. Administer analgesics as ordered for the relief of discomfort, avoiding aspirin if the client is thrombocytopenic. Aspirin, aspirin-containing products, and acetaminophen should be avoided because they may mask fever.

Invasive procedures should be avoided if possible. Provide meticulous skin decontamination before venipunctures. Maintain sterile occlusion of central venous catheters and perform routine dressing care according to institutional policy. Change IV tubing according to agency policy.

Monitor the client closely for manifestations of fungal or viral infections (i.e., increased respirations, rales, dyspnea, changed oral mucosa). Monitor the respiratory rate and auscultate breath sounds regularly. Viral and fungal pneumonia are common causes of death in the neutropenic client.

Diagnosis: Ineffective Protection/Risk for Hemorrhage.
The client eventually becomes thrombocytopenic because of the progression of the disease or because of chemotherapy treatment, leading to the nursing diagnosis of *Ineffective Protection/Risk for Hemorrhage related to thrombocytopenia secondary to either leukemia or treatment.*

Outcomes. Bleeding as a result of injuries, such as falls, punctures, cuts, or other environmental hazards, will be prevented or will be diagnosed and treated successfully as evidenced by absence of bleeding and a platelet count greater than 20,000/mm³.

Interventions. Institute bleeding precautions as follows:

EB
- Provide oral sponges or a soft toothbrush for oral hygiene; avoid flossing, hard toothbrushes, and commercial mouthwashes containing alcohol.
- Instruct the client to avoid blowing or picking the nose, straining at bowel movements, douching or using tampons, or using razors. Men and women should use only electric razors to shave with during the neutropenic phase.
- Do not give any intramuscular (IM) or SC injections.
- Do not insert rectal suppositories.
- Do not give medications containing aspirin, and instruct the client to avoid aspirin-containing medications.

- Avoid urinary catheters whenever possible. If a catheter must be inserted, use the smallest size possible, lubricate it well, and insert it gently.
- Avoid mucosal trauma during suctioning.
- Remove all potential hazards and sharp objects from the environment. Sharp corners or edges on furniture should be padded.
- Use a pressure-reducing mattress, and turn the client frequently to prevent pressure sores. Use bed cradles to protect extremities.
- Avoid overinflation of the blood pressure cuff, and rotate the cuff to different sites. Avoid prolonged use of tourniquets.
- Use only paper tape, and avoid strong adhesives that may cause skin adhesions.

Teach the client and significant others or family members to institute bleeding precautions during periods of thrombocytopenia. Monitor the client at least every 4 hours for manifestations of bleeding, such as ecchymosis, petechiae, epistaxis, gingival bleeding, hematuria, occult blood in stools, enlarged abdominal girth, disorientation, confusion, and changes in level of consciousness. All urine, stools, and emesis should be tested for blood. Take and record vital signs routinely, noting manifestations of altered tissue perfusion related to anemia (increased respirations and pulse, decreased blood pressure).

Check the platelet count, hemoglobin level, and hematocrit daily. Report a hemoglobin level of less than 10 g/dl and a platelet count of less than 20,000/mm³. Administer packed RBCs and platelets as ordered. Keep a current blood sample in the laboratory for cross-matching if needed in an emergency.

Diagnosis: Fatigue.
Fatigue is a common complaint by clients. It may be cumulative, a gradually worsening response to treatments for cancer, low hematocrit, low hemoglobin, altered blood glucose levels, decreased oxygen saturation levels, abnormal electrolyte levels, or unintentional weight loss. Fatigue is the greatest about 2 to 3 days after IV chemotherapy. The nursing diagnosis is written *Fatigue related to side effects of treatments, low hemoglobin levels, pain, lack of sleep, or other causes* as made evident by the client. A scale to rate fatigue numerically may be used, such as the Piper Fatigue Scale or, more simply, a 0 to 10 numeric scale (see Chapter 24).

Outcomes. The client will report less fatigue, plan adequate rest periods, and be able to do an increasing amount of usual activities with decreasing assistance from others.

Interventions. Assess for anemia and for the physical, psychological, and treatment-related causes of fatigue. Encourage exercise to maintain strength. Ask a physical therapist to assist with bed and strengthening exercises. An occupational therapist may be able to offer suggestions or devices to conserve energy. If the client has thrombocytopenia or fever or has just received chemotherapy (past 24 hours), exercise is not encouraged to avoid injury. Advocate for adequate pain reduction, minimizing interruptions, and reducing visitors when rest is needed.

Diagnosis: Imbalanced Nutrition: Less Than Body Requirements.

The client usually experiences decreased appetite and decreased nutritional intake as a result of the effects of radiation therapy and chemotherapy on the GI tract. Write the nursing diagnosis as *Imbalanced Nutrition: Less Than Body Requirements related to anorexia, pain or fatigue.*

Outcomes. The client will maintain adequate nutrition, maintain body weight as evidenced by stable weight, adequate caloric intake, and maintenance of fluid and electrolyte balance.

Interventions. Administer antiemetics, as ordered, around the clock as necessary to prevent nausea and vomiting. Premedicate the client with sufficient antiemetics before meals to encourage food and fluid intake. Administer local and IV analgesics, as ordered, to reduce pain caused by mucositis.

Discuss daily dietary requirements with the client and provide high-carbohydrate meals and oral supplements. Allow the client to make food selections. Cold foods, shakes, and sandwiches are tolerated better than hot or spicy foods. Small, frequent feedings may be tolerated better than three large meals a day. Monitor weight daily. If the client cannot tolerate food for an extended period, begin total parenteral nutrition (TPN), as ordered, and monitor intake. The client's own digestive system should be used as long as possible, with TPN used as a last resort. Coordinate and plan rest periods and activities of daily living in increments as needed to minimize fatigue.

Diagnosis: Disturbed Body Image.

Most clients experience body image disturbance. The nursing diagnosis is written as *Disturbed Body Image due to alopecia, weight loss, and fatigue.*

Outcomes. The client will be able to demonstrate and discuss understanding of the disease condition and the temporary nature of changes in body image and energy.

Interventions. Before treatment, inform the client about the potential for hair loss over the entire body. Encourage the use of scarves, hats, or wigs as desired. Explain the temporary nature of alopecia, although the hair may have a different color or texture when it returns. Alope-

cia may be permanent with whole-brain radiation therapy (WBXRT).

Encourage the client to balance rest with exercise and activities to maintain muscle tone without developing severe fatigue. Discuss daily dietary requirements with the client, and provide high-carbohydrate meals and oral supplements in an attempt to help clients maintain their body weight and an appearance that is acceptable to them.

Diagnosis: Risk for Sexual Dysfunction.

Many clients experience reproductive or sexual dysfunction. The nursing diagnosis is written *Risk for Sexual Dysfunction related to the effects of chemotherapy or radiation therapy on reproductive organs.*

Outcomes. The client will be able to discuss the potential for sterility and decreased libido that may result from therapy.

Interventions. Describe the normal cellular destruction that might lead to temporary or permanent destruction of reproductive function in the client. Inform the client that sexual libido may be altered during and after the acute phase of the illness because of fatigue or other side effects of therapy. Provide the client with emotional support and references to support groups. Provide manuals for alternative sexual positioning and techniques. In appropriate cases, inform the client of reproductive alternatives, such as sperm banking, artificial insemination, and egg harvesting.

Diagnosis: Risk for Ineffective Therapeutic Regimen Management and Risk for Ineffective Family Therapeutic Regimen Management.

Because hospital lengths of stay have become shorter and many oncology clients receive their care in outpatient settings, there is *Risk for Ineffective Therapeutic Regimen Management and Risk for Ineffective Family Therapeutic Regimen Management* related to the chronic nature of the disease process and the risk for complications.

Outcomes. The client and family will manage the therapeutic regimen as evidenced by effective medication administration, an absence of infections, no hemorrhage, and the client's ability to remain independent at home.

Interventions. After the induction phase of therapy is completed successfully, the client frequently returns home to recover and to await subsequent courses of therapy that may be given on an outpatient basis if no serious complications arise. It is common for clients to return home with anemia and thrombocytopenia. They also may suffer from the residual effects of chemotherapy or radiation therapy, such as loss of appetite, nausea, and mucositis. Some clients find it difficult to leave the security of the hospital setting because of significantly altered body image, fatigue, and fear.

Teach the client and his or her significant others how to recognize manifestations of complications as well as appropriate actions to take. Inform them of measures to ensure safety and to reduce risks of bleeding and infection. Provide clients with phone numbers of nursing personnel to call with questions and for suggestions for interventions. The client and family should be referred to an oncology clinical nurse specialist or case manager as soon as possible after diagnosis. These nurses often assist the client and family about the disease process, the planned treatment, and strategies for successful transition from the hospital to home and outpatient care.

Evaluation

The desired outcome for the client with leukemia is that the disease will become a chronic condition that the client and family can cope with in a positive manner. If acute leukemia does not respond to therapy, the client's life expectancy is short.

■ Surgical Management

Bone Marrow Transplantation. To achieve cure with acute leukemia, BMT is the most common current recommended treatment. Allogeneic BMT presents a treatment option for clients younger than 60 or 70 years of age, depending on the client's performance status, who have a suitable HLA-matched donor. Transplantation performed during the first remission has a higher success rate than transplantation performed during repeated remissions or in the blast phase of chronic leukemia. BMT is discussed later in this chapter.

■ Modifications for Older Clients

Older clients are at greater risk for chronic leukemia. The treatment of chronic leukemia in older clients is less vigorous. BMT is an option in older clients if they are otherwise fit and if their organ systems can endure the stress of the procedure. Some older adults with excellent physical and psychological functioning have done quite well with BMT.

▌LYMPHOMAS

Primary tumors originating from the lymphatic system were identified in 1932. Lymphoma is the most common tumor of the lymphoid system, with about 61,000 new cases diagnosed in 2003 and an estimated 24,700 deaths.[2] About 53,400 new cases of lymphoma will be non-Hodgkin's lymphoma (NHL) and about 7600 Hodgkin's lymphoma (Hodgkin's disease [HD]). *Lymphomas* are tumors of primary lymphoid tissue (thymus and bone marrow) or secondary tissue (lymph nodes, spleen, tonsils, and intestinal lymphoid tissue). Most lymphomas are neoplasms of secondary lymphoid tissue and involve mostly lymph nodes, the spleen, or both. Malignant lymphoid cells sometimes are found in circulating blood, indicating bone marrow involvement. The major subdivisions of malignant lymphomas are HD and NHL. Bone marrow involvement occurs more often in NHL than in HD.

HODGKIN'S DISEASE

In 1832 Hodgkin reported observations from autopsies showing unusually enlarged lymph nodes and biopsy tissue that showed a distinctive, large cell. Sixty years later Sternberg and Reed described the giant cells, which are called Reed-Sternberg cells of Hodgkin's lymphoma. Today the disease is called *Hodgkin's disease* and is known to be cancer of the lymph, or a lymphoma. Incidence rates differ with respect to age, gender, geographic locations, and socioeconomic class. In 2003 the American Cancer Society estimated the diagnosis of 7600 new cases of HD with 1300 related deaths in the United States.[2]

In economically advantaged countries, the incidence of HD is bimodal, with the first peak occurring in the mid-20s and the second peak occurring after age 50. In economically underdeveloped countries, the overall incidence of HD is lower than in developed countries but the incidence of HD before age 15 is higher, with only a modest increase into young adulthood. The incidence in people older than age 60 is declining, probably because of improved diagnostic techniques that classify NHL more accurately.

Etiology and Risk Factors

The exact cause of HD is unknown, although indirect evidence indicates a viral cause. The Epstein-Barr virus (EBV) is believed to be a causative agent. EBV-associated lymphomas are well documented in clients who have received organ transplants or who have an immunodeficiency disease. A 2-fold to 3-fold increase in HD is seen among clients who have a history of mononucleosis, a disease caused by EBV. Researchers have shown that 30% to 50% of HD specimens contained EBV genome fragments in the diagnostic Reed-Sternberg cells.

Some studies indicate a genetic predisposition for HD. The disease occurs more frequently in Jews and among first-degree relatives. Siblings were shown to have a 2- fold to 5-fold increased risk, and same-sex siblings have a 9-fold increased risk. An increased risk was found among parent-child pairs but not among spouses, suggesting a genetic rather than an infectious cause. Research continues in an attempt to identify the genetic role in the development of HD.

Pathophysiology

Cancerous transformation occurs from a particular site in the lymph node. With continuing growth the entire node becomes replaced, with zones of necrosis obscuring the normal nodular pattern. The mechanism of growth and spread of HD remains unknown. Some have suggested that the disease progresses by extension to adjacent structures. It also may disseminate by the lymphatics because lymphoreticular cells inhabit all tissues of the body except the CNS. Hematologic spread also may occur, possibly by means of direct infiltration of blood vessels.

Clinical Manifestations

Clients often are asymptomatic and may have painless lymphadenopathy. Enlarged lymph nodes most commonly are found in the supraclavicular, cervical, and mediastinal regions (Figure 81-5). Local manifestations produced by lymphadenopathy usually are caused by pressure or obstruction. Involvement of the extremities can be manifested by pain, nerve irritation, and obliteration of the pulse. Clients may experience a nonproductive cough, with the chest radiograph revealing a mediastinal mass, which is present in about 50% of clients.

Pericardial involvement can occur by direct invasion from mediastinal lymph nodes. This involvement can cause pericardial friction rub, pericardial effusion, and engorgement of neck veins. Other manifestations arise when enlarged lymph nodes obstruct or compress an adjacent structure (e.g., edema of the face, neck, and right arm secondary to superior vena cava compression or renal failure secondary to urethral obstruction).

If the tumor infiltrates the spine and presses on the spinal cord, manifestations of spinal cord compression can develop. Manifestations range from early back pain with motor weakness and sensory loss to loss of motor function, urinary retention, constipation, and other manifestations of compression of the cord late in the disease.

Associated clinical manifestations of unexplained weight loss of more than 10% of body weight in 6 months, frequent drenching night sweats, and fever above 38° C also may be present. Pruritus is a systemic manifestation that can be significant if it is recurrent. These additional

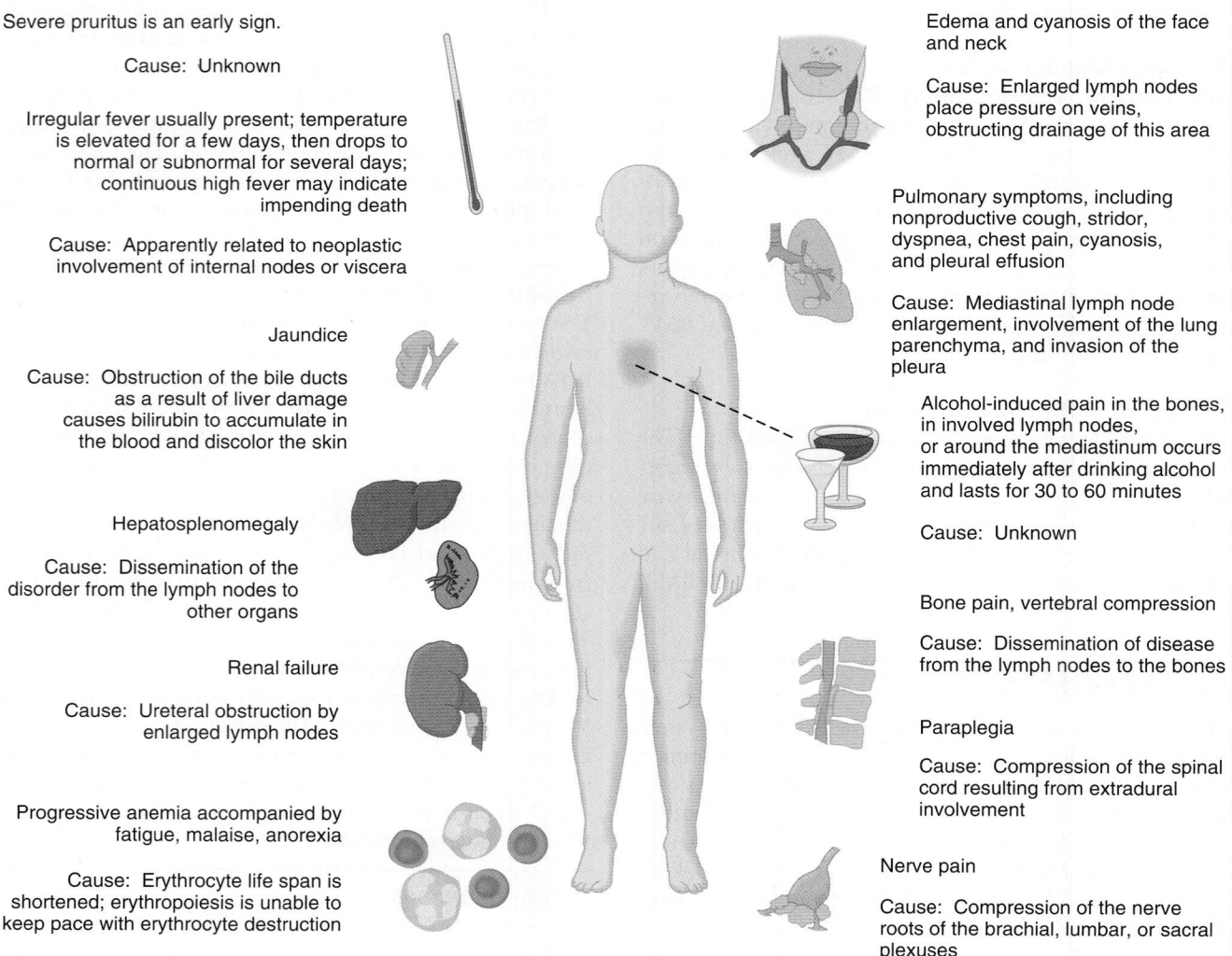

Severe pruritus is an early sign.

Cause: Unknown

Irregular fever usually present; temperature is elevated for a few days, then drops to normal or subnormal for several days; continuous high fever may indicate impending death

Cause: Apparently related to neoplastic involvement of internal nodes or viscera

Jaundice

Cause: Obstruction of the bile ducts as a result of liver damage causes bilirubin to accumulate in the blood and discolor the skin

Hepatosplenomegaly

Cause: Dissemination of the disorder from the lymph nodes to other organs

Renal failure

Cause: Ureteral obstruction by enlarged lymph nodes

Progressive anemia accompanied by fatigue, malaise, anorexia

Cause: Erythrocyte life span is shortened; erythropoiesis is unable to keep pace with erythrocyte destruction

Edema and cyanosis of the face and neck

Cause: Enlarged lymph nodes place pressure on veins, obstructing drainage of this area

Pulmonary symptoms, including nonproductive cough, stridor, dyspnea, chest pain, cyanosis, and pleural effusion

Cause: Mediastinal lymph node enlargement, involvement of the lung parenchyma, and invasion of the pleura

Alcohol-induced pain in the bones, in involved lymph nodes, or around the mediastinum occurs immediately after drinking alcohol and lasts for 30 to 60 minutes

Cause: Unknown

Bone pain, vertebral compression

Cause: Dissemination of disease from the lymph nodes to the bones

Paraplegia

Cause: Compression of the spinal cord resulting from extradural involvement

Nerve pain

Cause: Compression of the nerve roots of the brachial, lumbar, or sacral plexuses

FIGURE 81-5 Clinical manifestations and pathophysiologic bases of Hodgkin's disease.

manifestations are known as *B symptoms* for staging purposes; they occur in greater frequency in older clients and are negatively related to the prognosis.

The diagnosis is confirmed by lymph node and bone marrow biopsy. A chest radiograph to evaluate complaints of persistent cough or dyspnea may identify mediastinal involvement. The extent of disease is determined by CT scans of the thoracic, abdominal, and pelvic areas as well as gallium scan of mediastinal or hilar lymph nodes and lymphangiography of the lower extremities. If the extent of the disease cannot be determined by these diagnostic tests and confirmation of abdominal disease is necessary for determining treatment choice, a staging laparotomy may be performed.

Staging

Hodgkin's disease is divided into categories, or stages, according to the microscopic appearance of the involved

TABLE 81-2	*Cotswold Staging Classification for Hodgkin's Disease*
Stage I	Involvement of a single lymph node region or a lymphoid structure (e.g., spleen, thymus, Waldeyer's ring)
Stage II	Involvement of two or more lymph node regions on the same side of the diaphragm (i.e., the mediastinum is a single site, hilar lymph nodes are lateralized). The number of anatomic sites should be indicated by a subscript (e.g., II$_2$)
Stage III	Involvement of lymph node regions or structures on both sides of the diaphragm: III$_1$: With or without involvement of splenic, hilar, celiac, or portal nodes III$_2$: With involvement of para-aortic, iliac, or mesenteric nodes
Stage IV	Involvement of extranodal site(s) beyond that designated as E.

Designation Applicable to Any Disease Stage

A	No manifestations
B	Fever, drenching sweats, weight loss (B symptoms)
X	Bulky disease: >⅓ the width of the mediastinum <10 cm maximal dimension of nodal mass
E	Involvement of a single extranodal site, contiguous or proximal to a known nodal site
CS	Clinical stage
PS	Pathologic stage

Data from Goldman, L., Krevans, J., & Ausiello, D. (2004). *Cecil textbook of medicine* (22nd ed.). Philadelphia: W.B. Saunders.

lymph nodes, the extent and severity of the disorder, and the prognosis. Accurate staging of HD is important for determining treatment options. Table 81-2 shows the Cotswold staging classification, which modified the Ann Arbor classification system, primarily to incorporate the newer diagnostic tests and the evidence that bulky disease is an important prognostic indicator.

Outcome Management
■ Medical Management

Since the advent of combination chemotherapy, adult HD has become one of the most curable malignancies, resulting in a long-term survival rate of about 70%. The goal of therapy for clients with stage I and II disease is to achieve long-term disease-free survival with minimal acute and long-term complications that affect quality of life. Treatment consists of radiation therapy alone or combined with chemotherapy.

Eradication of Tumor Cells

Radiation. Radiation treatment for HD involves three locations: the mantle, the para-aortic region, and the pelvis (Figure 81-6). The mantle field encompasses the submandibular, cervical, infraclavicular, axillary, mediastinal, subcarinal, and hilar lymph nodes. In clinical stage I and II disease, combined chemotherapy and radiation therapy are recommended for clients with unfavorable prognostic indicators. Most cancer centers classify B symptoms (fever, night sweats, and unexplained weight loss), high erythrocyte sedimentation rate (ESR), or large mediastinal adenopathy as poor prognostic factors. Some centers include large numbers of site involvement and older age as poor prognostic indicators.

Chemotherapy. Chemotherapy has become the primary treatment strategy, with or without radiation therapy, in stage I and II disease with poor prognostic indicators and in clients with advanced HD. Numerous chemotherapy regimens are available for HD. For years, MOPP (mechlorethamine, vincristine [Oncovin], procarbazine, prednisone) was the gold standard of therapy; however, ABVD (doxorubicin [Adriamycin], bleomycin, vinblastine, and dacarbazine) has emerged as the best alternative to MOPP. The primary advantages of ABVD are its ease of delivery in full doses, fewer side effects, and less risk of subsequent development of leukemia. With proper treatment, the 20-year disease-free survival rate of HD is 70% to 80%, and the overall survival rate, with salvage chemotherapy for clients who relapse, is 80% to 95%.

Research has shown that clients with advanced disease (stage II and IV) may achieve better treatment results with MOPP plus ABVD than with MOPP alone. Other studies showed that ABVD alone could achieve results similar to MOPP plus ABVD. Many physicians recommend that ABVD alone be given for as many cycles

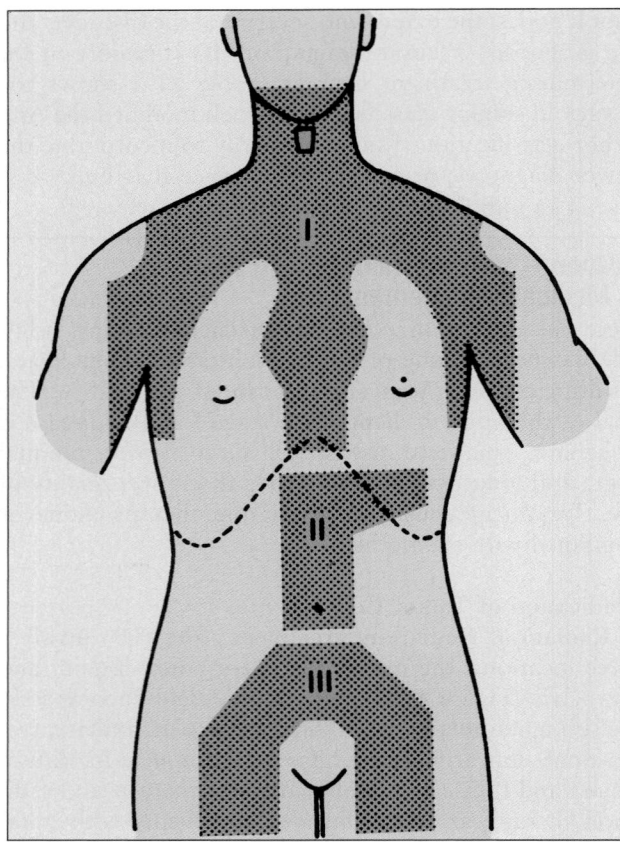

FIGURE 81-6 Radiation fields in therapy for Hodgkin's disease. *Shaded areas* represent the three treatment fields. The *mantle field* is the uppermost field (I). Lungs and vocal cords are protected by lead blocks; the heart and thyroid gland are within the field. The *para-aortic field,* or middle field (II), extends from the diaphragm to just above the bifurcation of the aorta. When the spleen has not been removed, this field is extended to include the entire spleen and splenic hilum. The *pelvic* or *inverted Y field* is the lowest field (III). It encompasses the pelvic and inguinal nodes and includes a large area of bone marrow. (Modified from Murphy, G.P., Lawrence, W., & Lenhard, R.E. [1995]. *American Cancer Society textbook of clinical oncology* [2nd ed.]. Atlanta: American Cancer Society.)

as required to achieve a complete remission plus two consolidation cycles (usually six cycles total). The use of radiation therapy in advanced disease is individualized to the client, especially those with local-regional disease problems.

Clients who relapse after definitive HD therapy generally require some type of systemic therapy, which depends on the type of initial therapy used. Therapies range from chemotherapy and wide-field radiation to high-dose chemotherapy with autologous or allogeneic stem cell transplant. Of clients with stages I to II HD, 20% to 30% relapse within 5 years after radiation therapy. In these cases, the use of combination chemotherapy produces a 57% to 62% disease-free survival at 10

TABLE 81-3	*Complications of Hodgkin's Disease*
Problem	**Cause**
Thyroid dysfunction Thymic hyperplasia	Underlying disease, therapy, or both
Hypothyroidism Thyroid cancer	Direct or indirect radiation exposure
Sexual dysfunction Male impotence Male and female infertility Female dyspareunia	Underlying disease, therapy, or both
Herpes zoster or varicella	Underlying disease, therapy, or both
Pulmonary dysfunction Pneumonitis (acute, chronic, or both)	Direct or indirect radiation exposure, bleomycin, nitrosoureas, radiation recall
Cardiac dysfunction Cardiomyopathy	Mediastinal radiation therapy, pericarditis (acute), doxorubicin, radiation recall
Pericarditis (chronic)	Mediastinal radiation therapy
Dental caries	Salivary changes related to radiation therapy
Myelodysplastic syndrome	Therapy, especially if age >40 yr or lymphocytic leukemia
Non-Hodgkin's lymphoma	Therapy
Solid tumors	Direct or indirect radiation exposure

years. At the National Cancer Institute, a 93% second complete remission rate was seen in clients with initial remissions longer than 12 months after chemotherapy. The positive results of several studies investigating the use of stem cell transplant have provided the basis for recommending BMT and stem cell transplantation for all HD clients who relapsed or did not respond to any primary chemotherapy, regardless of the length of the initial remission.

Complications

The complications related to HD are numerous because they are a result of the disease itself or of radiation therapy, chemotherapy, or a combination of several of these factors (Table 81-3).

■ Nursing Management of the Medical Client

Obtain a thorough health history from the client and family members. The severity and longevity of the manifestations of the disease are important facts to obtain and document. Nurses play an essential role in symptom management associated with therapy. Because of the side effects of chemotherapy, clients may ask for a reduction of the dosage or may want to stop therapy completely. Provide clients with information about the effect of reducing or stopping therapy on long-term survival.

NON-HODGKIN'S LYMPHOMA

Non-Hodgkin's lymphoma comprises a group of malignancies with a common origin in the lymphoid cells. They are heterogeneous in cellular origin, morphologic appearance, and clinical behavior. For 2003 the American Cancer Society estimated that in the United States about 53,400 new cases of NHL were diagnosed, with 23,400 related deaths.[2]

Between 1973 and 1991, the incidence of NHL increased by about 73%. Part of this increase was attributed to acquired immunodeficiency syndrome (AIDS). NHL is about 60 times more common in people with AIDS than in the general population of the United States. NHL is the fifth (male) and sixth (female) most common cause of cancer-related deaths in the United States. Men are affected more often than women, and the incidence is higher in whites than other races. NHL can occur in any age group, but an increase in incidence occurs in the 50s and 60s. Because the average age at diagnosis is in the 50s, the number of years of life lost to these malignancies ranks NHL fourth in economic impact among cancers in the United States.

Etiology and Risk Factors

No hereditary, ethnic, or dietary risk factors have been associated with NHL. An increased risk is associated with immunodeficiency states, autoimmune disorders, and infectious physical and chemical agents. As with HD, a viral or bacterial cause has been implicated (EBV, HTLV-1, human herpes virus 8, *Helicobacter pylori*). A greater than expected incidence of NHL is reported in people with ataxia-telangiectasia, Wiskott-Aldrich syndrome, and Chédiak-Higashi syndrome.

Classifications

Terminology describing NHL is complex, inconsistent, and ambiguous, and several classifications exist. Rappaport's widely used classification, developed in 1956, distinguishes two major histopathologic patterns: nodular and diffuse (Table 81-4). These two patterns in NHL illustrate two different pathologic states. The nodular (and diffuse, well-differentiated lymphocytic) pattern involves nodal and extranodal sites. The diffuse pattern does not show the cell aggregates that are evident in the nodular pattern.

Based on expanding knowledge of the lymphatic system physiology, six distinct classification systems emerged worldwide in the 1970s. To standardize terminology, the Revised European-American Lymphoma (REAL) classification system was proposed in 1994. This classification includes all lymphoma types as well as

TABLE 81-4	*Rappaport Staging Classification*	
Grade	**Characteristics**
Low grade	Diffuse, lymphocytic, well differentiated
	Nodular, lymphocytic, poorly differentiated
	Nodular, mixed, lymphocytic, and histiocytic
Intermediate grade	Nodular, histiocytic
	Diffuse, lymphocytic
	Diffuse, mixed, lymphocytic, and histiocytic
High grade	Diffuse, histiocytic
	Diffuse, lymphoblastic
	Diffuse, undifferentiated

the extranodal lymphomas not included in the other classification systems.

Pathophysiology

In clients with NHL, an abnormal proliferation of neoplastic lymphocytes occurs. The cells remain fixed at one phase of development and continue to proliferate. Both T and B lymphocytes mature in the lymph nodes. Clinical manifestations are due to mechanical obstruction of the enlarged lymph nodes. Lymphocytic infiltration of the abdomen or oropharynx also can occur.

Clinical Manifestations

Clients with NHL show localized or generalized lymphadenopathy. The cervical, axillary, inguinal, and femoral chains are the most frequent sites of lymph node enlargement. The swelling is generally painless, and the nodes have enlarged and transformed over months or years. Extranodal sites of involvement are the nasopharynx, GI tract, bone, thyroid, testes, and soft tissue. Some clients have retroperitoneal and abdominal masses with abdominal fullness, back pain, ascites (fluid in the peritoneal cavity), and leg swelling.

Several sites of involvement in NHL are not common in HD, such as Waldeyer's ring (lymphoid tissue that encircles the tonsils), the stomach, the small and large bowel, mesenteric lymph nodes, the thyroid, the skin, the pancreas, the kidneys, and the CNS. With diffuse NHL, clinical manifestations are variable and generally involve more systemic findings. Clients also may experience systemic B symptoms, including night sweats, fever, and weight loss. About one third of clients have hepatomegaly or splenomegaly.

Certain other clinical conditions mimic the malignant lymphomas, including tuberculosis, syphilis, systemic lupus erythematosus, lung cancer, and bone cancer. A thorough diagnostic evaluation is required.

Blood work includes a CBC, ESR, and peripheral smear to rule out other causes of lymphadenopathy, such as mononucleosis. Blood cultures and other serologic studies for viral and autoimmune diseases provide important differential information. Elevated lactate dehydrogenase (LDH) levels may be seen in advanced NHL.

A lymph node biopsy is an important diagnostic tool. The following are indications for biopsy:

- Adenopathy for longer than 3 weeks, which progresses in size or spreads to other areas
- B symptoms that cannot be attributed to other causes
- Abnormal blood test results indicative of lymphoma
- Radiographs that suggest possible extranodal involvement

Because of the aggressive nature of AIDS-related NHL, any symptomatic client at increased risk or known to be positive for human immunodeficiency virus (HIV) should have a biopsy to rule out high-grade lymphoma.

Just as in HD, once the diagnosis of NHL is made, disease staging should take place. Noninvasive imaging techniques, such as CT and MRI, are useful tools in the initial staging of NHL. Renal and liver function tests are performed to determine the presence of extranodal involvement. Bilateral bone marrow biopsies are important because metastasis to the bone marrow is common, especially in low-grade disease.

Outcome Management
■ Medical Management

Eradication of Tumor Cells. Many classification systems are used to differentiate NHL according to histologic type and cytologic characteristics. Treatment varies based on the histology and stage of the tumor. The treatment of a low-grade lymphoma is different from that for high-grade disease. Low-grade tumors tend to progress slowly and often are asymptomatic for long periods; the natural course of the disease may fluctuate considerably over 5 to 10 years, with or without treatment. Low-grade cells eventually transform into a more aggressive disease process, however, and may quickly cause the death of the client. Because of this process, indolent NHL is believed to be incurable, and many controversies exist concerning treatment standards, especially for clients who have disseminated disease.

Radiation and Chemotherapy. The progression of intermediate-grade and high-grade lymphomas is similar to that of other cancers. Because of their higher growth fraction, however, these tumors tend to be more sensitive to chemotherapy and radiation therapy; the response rate is higher when these tumors are treated. Combination chemotherapy is used to produce tumor shrinkage

and remission. Cyclophosphamide and doxorubicin are active against lymphoma. Various combination drug regimens that include these two drugs are used in the treatment of NHL. Controversy regarding first-line standard of care therapy is ongoing. Studies comparing various treatment protocols affirmed the practice of using CHOP (cyclophosphamide, hydroxydaunorubicin [doxorubicin], vincristine [Oncovin], and prednisone) as first-line therapy in many academic and community settings.

For clients with low-grade NHL in stage I to II, radiation therapy alone may be curative, although there are reports of recurrence past 10 years. Depending on whether the disease is supradiaphragmatic or subdiaphragmatic, single-mode therapy includes mantle and inverted Y field irradiation (see Figure 81-6).

Clients with stage III to IV intermediate-grade lymphoma require combination chemotherapy as an immediate intervention. Clients who are older than 60 years of age and have elevated LDH levels, poor performance status, and stage III to IV intermediate disease are at higher risk and should be offered aggressive regimens that provide higher-dose intensities.

The diagnosis of a high-grade NHL warrants immediate and aggressive treatment. Clients may present with rapidly growing disease that has the potential to double in bulk in days or hours. Treatment includes dose-intense chemotherapy, with or without radiation therapy, and prophylactic CNS therapy. It is necessary to provide prophylaxis for the CNS because the blood-brain barrier prevents most chemotherapy drugs from getting into CNS spaces. Without such treatment, lymphoma cells may look for "sanctuary" in the CNS (CNS metastasis). High-grade NHL clients also are excellent candidates for BMT or stem cell transplantation because the tumors respond dramatically to high-dose chemotherapy, which is part of the preparative regimen of transplant.

Monoclonal Antibodies. Rituximab (Rituxan) is an unconjugated chimeric monoclonal antibody that binds to the CD20 antigen found on the surface of most B-cell lymphomas. This surface antigen is present in about 90% of B-cell lymphomas. This IV drug is FDA approved as a single agent in the treatment of relapsed low-grade follicular NHL, and it is also under investigation for use in combination regimens for mantle cell and diffuse aggressive NHL. Rituxan was the first monoclonal antibody to gain FDA approval for the treatment of cancer.

Targeted Therapy. Targeted therapy utilizing radiolabeled monoclonal antibodies is also available for the treatment of NHL. These radiolabeled agents recognize and react with specific antigens to target and kill specific tumor cells. Greater amounts of radiation are delivered to tumor cells than to normal cells, and critical organs are spared that do not express the specific antigen. The only FDA-approved agent in this class of drugs for the treatment on clients with NHL is ibritumomab tiuxetan (Zevalin), and it is labeled with yttrium-90. Another agent that utilizes iodine-131 is under investigation.

Other Therapies. Experimental therapies are emerging in the treatment of NHL. Such therapies include vaccines, high-dose radioimmunotherapy and stem cell transplantation, and antisense antiangiogenesis agents. These therapies are currently being investigated in clinical trials.

■ Nursing Management of the Medical Client
Assessment

Although the appearance of an enlarged lymph node in the absence of infection may cause worry, 56% of healthy adults may experience cervical adenopathy; however, any enlargement of lymph nodes warrants further evaluation.

The work-up for NHL begins with a thorough history and physical examination. On examination, lymph nodes involved in infectious processes may be tender or painful, whereas lymphomatous nodes tend to be firm and "rubbery" and are found in generalized patterns. Carcinomatous nodes often are hard and sometimes matted to one another or fixed to underlying structures in contiguous or regional patterns. Other hallmarks of lymphoma, such as systemic B symptoms (fever, night sweats, unexplained weight loss), are seen in 20% to 30% of clients, but these manifestations also may be seen in other disease states, such as certain infections and connective tissue diseases.

The heterogeneous nature of NHL challenges nurses to meet a variety of physical and psychosocial needs for both clients and their families. The client and family members are confronted with managing a demanding diagnosis and treatment and the effects of the disease on daily routines. Health care professionals often assume that clients with supportive families manage well, but family members share the strain of the illness, are deeply affected (psychologically, financially, and perhaps physically), and need ongoing support. It is crucial that nurses adapt their plans of care for these clients along the disease trajectory, which can wax and wane for many years.

Diagnosis, Outcomes, Interventions

The nursing diagnosis, outcomes, and interventions for HD and NHL are the same as those for the client with leukemia.

Nursing Diagnoses. These clients may have *Ineffective Protection/Risk for Infection* (related to neutropenia or the result of chemotherapy and radiation therapy), *Inef-*

fective Protection/Risk for Hemorrhage (as a result of thrombocytopenia secondary to treatment), *Fatigue, Risk for Sexual Dysfunction, Imbalanced Nutrition: Less than Body Requirements, Disturbed Body Image,* and *Risk for Ineffective Therapeutic Regimen Management* (Individuals and Families).

Outcomes. The desired outcome for the client with lymphoma is that the disease will become a chronic condition that the client and family can cope with in a positive manner. If the disease becomes terminal, the outcome should include a death with dignity, in which comfort measures and psychological support are emphasized.

Interventions. Interventions for these problems were discussed previously for clients with leukemia.

Evaluation

Physiologic problems may resolve quickly with medication. Psychological diagnosis will require prolonged intervention.

■ BONE MARROW TRANSPLANTATION

Since the 1970s BMT has progressed from a treatment of last resort to a viable therapeutic modality for a variety of hematologic, malignant, and nonmalignant disorders. Peripheral stem cell transplantation and autologous transplants have further revolutionized the field. The status of the disease to be treated by BMT is an important determinant of the outcome for the client. When BMT is performed in clients with acute leukemia in full relapse, the disease-free survival rates approximate 15%, whereas BMT mortality falls dramatically in clients with chemotherapy-induced remission.

INDICATIONS

Bone marrow transplant may be considered as a treatment for clients with the following:
- Aplastic anemia
- Malignant disorders, specifically myelodysplastic syndromes, leukemia (certain types of acute leukemic, chronic leukemic, and preleukemic states), lymphoma, multiple myeloma, neuroblastoma, and selected solid tumors (breast cancer, ovarian cancer, testicular cancer, poor-risk germ cell tumors)
- Nonmalignant hematologic disorders, such as Fanconi anemia, thalassemia, and sickle cell anemia
- Immunodeficiency disorders, such as severe combined immunodeficiency disease and Wiskott-Aldrich syndrome

BONE MARROW HARVESTING

Sources of Bone Marrow

The three types of bone marrow donors are (1) allogeneic, (2) syngeneic, and (3) autologous.

Allogeneic Bone Marrow

Allogeneic bone marrow is obtained from a relative or unrelated donor having a closely matched HLA type. This was the most common type of marrow transplant, but it carried the highest rate of morbidity and mortality because of complications of incompatibility such as graft-versus-host disease (GVHD). The rate of allogeneic transplants has dropped with the drop in the birth rate and the increased use of autologous and peripheral stem cell transplants.

Syngeneic Bone Marrow

Syngeneic marrow is donated by an identical twin. Although syngeneic marrow is a perfect HLA match, which eliminates the risks of marrow rejection, the incidence of leukemic relapse is higher than when an allogeneic donor is used because GVHD is considered to have an antileukemic effect.

Autologous Bone Marrow

Autologous marrow is removed from the intended recipient during the remission phase to allow another course of ablative therapy to be given if a relapse occurs. Although autologous marrow eliminates the risk of adverse immunologic responses, such as GVHD and graft rejection, relapse after autologous BMT is a frequent occurrence. This relapse may be due to contamination of the harvested bone marrow by malignant cells or to failure of pre-transplant chemotherapy to eradicate completely the tumor cells from the body.

Histocompatibility Testing for Allogeneic and Syngeneic Transplantation

Immunologic recognition of the differences in HLA antigens is the first step in host transplant rejection. The HLA system antigens are a complex set of protein structures found on the surface membrane of all human nucleated cells, solid tissues, and circulating blood cells except RBCs. This genetically inherited mixture of antigens is considered representative of the tissue type of each person.

Siblings have a one in four chance of having identical sets of HLA antigens. This situation would provide the optimally matched allogeneic bone marrow donor. Because of the complexity of the HLA system, unrelated clients have less than a 1 in 5000 chance of having identical HLA types. The establishment of the National Bone Marrow Donor Program (NMDP) in 1986 has given hope to many clients who do not have a compatible relative donor. As of June 2000, about one million donors are listed in the NMDP's registry, with about 25,000 new volunteer donors added to the registry every month. This has increased the availability of unrelated donors for allogeneic transplants.

ALLOGENEIC DONOR PREPARATION

An extensive work-up is performed for ensuring compatibility and the mental and physical well-being of the prospective donor. This evaluation includes histocompatibility testing, medical history, physical examination, chest film, ECG, laboratory evaluation (CBC, chemistry profile, viral testing, rapid plasma reagin test [syphilis], ABO and Rh blood typing, coagulation studies), and psychological testing (may include psychiatric consultation).

Before marrow harvest, an informed consent, including potential donor complications (pain, fever, hematoma), must be obtained. In rare instances, the donor may experience serious adverse effects from general anesthesia. Spinal anesthesia is sometimes used instead of general anesthesia during the harvest. Because of the potential for significant blood loss during the harvesting process, syngeneic and allogeneic donors are required to donate autologous blood for reinfusion before the procedure.

Newborns are currently being used as potential donors through the use of their cord blood, which is rich in stem cells. Some parents are being encouraged to freeze their newborn's cord blood for potential future use, especially if there is a history of cancer in the family.

Marrow Collection

When collecting marrow, the client or donor is given general or spinal anesthesia in the operating room. The marrow is obtained in 5- to 10-ml aliquots from the marrow spaces of the posterior and occasionally the anterior iliac crest and sternum. Numerous skin punctures may be required; the aspiration needle is redirected to various marrow spaces without being withdrawn. A total of 500 to 1000 ml of marrow usually is obtained. The blood is placed in heparinized tissue culture media and filtered for removal of fat and bone particles. Marrow can be infused immediately or frozen in a solution containing dimethyl sulfoxide (DMSO), which preserves stem cells in the frozen state.

Peripheral Stem Cell Collection

Peripheral stem (progenitor) cells are harvested by apheresis or leukapheresis, a process that removes blood through a large-bore catheter and runs it through a machine that removes the stem cells before returning the blood to the client. Because stem cell concentration is much lower in peripheral blood compared with bone marrow, a process to increase the concentration in the peripheral blood must be initiated first. To increase the number of circulating stem cells, a stimulus, such as a granulocyte colony-stimulating factor (GCSF), interleukins (ILs), fusion molecules (made from a combination of a CSF and IL-3), or some chemotherapeutic agents, may be given to the donor before the stem cell harvest. As mentioned earlier, the umbilical cord of newborns also is rich in stem cells.

Once the stem cells are harvested, they are preserved in the same manner as bone marrow. The engraftment of stem cells occurs at about the same rate as or slightly faster than with BMT.

ALLOGENEIC TRANSPLANT

Recipient Preparation

The physical and psychological evaluation of the recipient is similar to that of the donor. Additional testing may be required to stage existing disease accurately. The recipient must undergo a preparative regimen before transplantation. Such a regimen serves three purposes:

1. Malignant cells are destroyed.
2. The immune system is inactivated, which reduces the risk of GVHD in allogeneic transplant clients.
3. The marrow cavities are emptied to provide space for implantation of the transfused stem cells.

 Common protocols combine total body irradiation and high doses of a single chemotherapeutic agent (cyclophosphamide is one of the most common agents used) or fractionated/high doses of multiple agents. A multilumen central venous catheter is inserted to provide suitable access for marrow infusion as well as for antibiotics, blood products, hyperalimentation, and frequent blood sampling.

Bone Marrow Infusion

The infusion of the marrow is commonly anticlimactic after the client has undergone the rigorous preparatory chemotherapy and radiation therapy (often referred to as the *conditioning regimen*). The marrow is usually administered immediately after the conditioning regimen is complete. Marrow is administered from a large blood infusion bag by a multilumen catheter, using an infusion pump, or small volumes may be prefiltered and given by IV push by a physician.

The BMT client remains pancytopenic until the transplanted stem cells make their way to the medullary cavities, where subsequent growth and reconstitution of the marrow are confirmed. Indications of successful engraft- ment are an increase in platelets and RBCs in the peripheral blood count. This change may occur 14 days after marrow infusion. Each day that recovery is delayed places the client at added risk. Graft rejection is evident if the bone marrow fails to produce peripheral blood cells after several weeks.

■ Nursing Management

Nursing management of BMT clients follows the plan of care for any completely immunosuppressed client. Clients receiving allogeneic transplants must be observed closely for manifestations of GVHD. Potential immediate adverse reactions are allergic (urticaria, chills, fever), volume overload, and pulmonary complications secondary to fat emboli. Renal damage may occur from too many erythrocytes. The period immediately after transplant is crucial. Multisystem failure related to ablative therapy is common, as are immune reactions caused by the transplanted cells.

■ GRAFT-VERSUS-HOST DISEASE

The most common and potentially disastrous complication of allogeneic BMT is GVHD, which may occur 7 to 30 days after infusion of viable lymphocytes. The donor T lymphocytes form an immunologic reaction against the host cells. The clients at highest risk for development of GVHD are those who have had allogeneic BMT. Of those clients, risk is greatest when the donor mismatched two to three antigens and when the client is older than 30 years. A moderate risk (35% to 50% incidence) remains for clients who have HLA-identical donors.

ACUTE GRAFT-VERSUS-HOST DISEASE

Acute GVHD is staged according to the organ system affected (Table 81-5). It usually affects the gut, skin, lungs, or liver. *Stage I* GVHD occurs in many allogeneic transplant clients. Skin manifestations may resolve without treatment. Systemic complications may be treated with immunosuppressive drug therapy.

Therapy for GVHD includes high doses of methylprednisolone, antithymocyte globulin, antilymphocyte globulin, cyclosporine, and anti–T-cell immunotoxins. These also leave the client immunosuppressed and vulnerable to infection. The prognosis and treatment depend on the severity of the syndrome. Acute GVHD that does not respond to treatment greatly increases the morbidity and mortality of BMT.

Nursing management is shown in the Care Plan feature on The Client with Stage I Graft-Versus-Host Disease on p. 2420.

CHRONIC GRAFT-VERSUS-HOST DISEASE

Chronic GVHD, a long-term form of the disease with less acute manifestations, may occur even if the client has not experienced acute GVHD. Chronic GVHD appears about 100 days after transplantation; it may affect the liver, GI system, oral mucosa, and lungs as well as

Stage	Skin Manifestations	Liver Manifestations	Gastrointestinal Manifestations
TABLE 81-5	*Stages of Acute Graft-Versus-Host Disease*		
1	Maculopapular rash >25% of body surface area	Bilirubin 2-3 mg/dl	Diarrhea 500-1000 ml/day
2	Maculopapular rash 25%-50% of body surface area	Bilirubin 3-6 mg/dl	Diarrhea 1000-1500 ml/day
3	Generalized erythroderma	Bilirubin 6-15 mg/dl	Diarrhea >1500 ml/day
4	Desquamation and bullae	Bilirubin >15 mg/dl	Abdominal pain or ileus

CARE PLAN

The Client with Stage I Graft-Versus-Host Disease

Nursing Diagnosis. Risk for Injury related to graft-versus-host disease (GVHD).

Outcome. Client exhibits resolution of early GVHD as evidenced by healing of skin, return of liver functions to normal, resolution of diarrhea and abdominal cramping, normal serum electrolytes, and control of pain.

Interventions	Rationales
1. Assess client's or significant others' knowledge of GVHD.	1. The client or significant others also can monitor for clinical manifestations and by reporting them early enhance treatment.

2. Teach client or significant others about the early manifestations of GVHD and to report them:
  a. Erythematous rash on palms, soles, ears, and trunk
  b. Anorexia, abdominal cramping, diarrhea, nausea, vomiting
	2. Client is ambulatory and may not recognize the need to report these data to the nurse.

3. Determine baseline status or skin condition, liver function (alkaline phosphatase, bilirubin), and gastrointestinal function before donor marrow infusion.	3. Baseline data guide assessments of further data.
4. Assess for manifestations of GVHD at day 25 post-transplant.	4. The median onset time of GVHD is 25 days after bone marrow transplant.
5. Administer prescribed preventive agents.	5. Medications such as methotrexate and cyclosporine are used to suppress response.
6. Monitor magnesium levels daily.	6. Cyclosporine can induce seizures in hypomagnesemic clients.
7. Monitor renal function daily.	7. Bilirubin levels rise in GVHD.
8. Irradiate all blood products before infusing.	8. Irradiation prevents the infusion of immunocompetent T lymphocytes.
9. Bathe daily in warm saline or warm Hibiclens solution diluted to 1:8 with sterile water. Pat skin dry.	9. Skin care is important to reduce the risk of infection and avoid injury to the skin.
10. Apply prescribed lotions to the moist skin after bathing.	10. Keeping the skin moist reduces the risk of cracks, which increase the risk of infection.
11. Monitor characteristics of stools. If diarrhea develops, keep the client on NPO (nothing by mouth). Administer antidiarrheal agents, and test all stools for blood.	11. Diarrhea is a manifestation of GVHD. Blood loss through stool may require transfusion for replacement.
12. Monitor intake and output strictly, and record daily weights.	12. GVHD can lead to dehydration. Clients receiving chemotherapeutic agents need ample fluids during administration to prevent renal damage.

Evaluation. If the client develops GVHD, treatment with methotrexate and cyclosporine will result in resolution of skin impairment and diarrhea as well as relief of pain and a return of serum electrolyte and liver function laboratory values to normal limits.

the skin. Chronic GVHD resembles autoimmune collagen-vascular disorders, such as systemic lupus erythematosus. It is characterized by scleroderma-like skin fibrosis and Sjögren's syndrome, in which the mucosa and lacrimal ducts are abnormally dry.

Diagnosis of chronic GVHD is confirmed by skin and oral mucosal biopsy. Although severe GVHD usually is fatal, researchers believe that a complete absence of this immune reaction increases the risk of leukemic relapse. This situation may be due to a beneficial graft-versus-leukemic reaction that mild GVHD stimulates. In allogeneic BMT recipients with GVHD stages II through IV, the relapse rate is 2.5 times lower than in syngeneic recipients or allogeneic recipients without GVHD.

CONCLUSIONS

Leukemia and lymphoma are complex diseases affecting physiologic and psychological aspects of the client and the family. Nursing care focuses on protecting the client from infection resulting from loss of WBC function, protection from hemorrhage resulting from loss of platelet function, and protection from hypoxia resulting from loss of RBC function.

THINKING CRITICALLY *evolve*

1. A 68-year-old woman is admitted with acute nonlymphocytic leukemia (ANLL). She is receiving chemotherapy. Her WBC is 1000; 3% are banded neutrophils, and 54% are segmented neutrophils. What, if any, precautions are needed?

Factors to Consider. How is her risk of sepsis determined? Why does body temperature serve as one marker of infection? What precautions are followed?

2. A 34-year-old man with acute myelogenous leukemia comes to the outpatient oncology facility for his second round of chemotherapy. Three days later the client calls the clinic nurse and is complaining of bleeding gums. What is the priority problem you should address? What instructions should you give the client at this time?

Factors to Consider. What pathologic process underlies the client's manifestations? Are there laboratory results you would want to check? What other precautions should you institute based on the client's other manifestations and the laboratory data? What other data are significant to collect at this time?

Discussions for these questions can be found on the website and the CD-ROM.

BIBLIOGRAPHY

1. Abraham, J., & Allegra, C. (2001). Bethesda handbook of clinical oncology. Philadelphia: Lippincott Williams & Wilkins.
2. American Cancer Society. (2003). *Cancer facts and figures.* Atlanta, GA: Author.
3. Bush, S. (2002). Monoclonal antibodies conjugated with radioisotopes for the treatment of non-Hodgkin's lymphoma. *Seminars in Oncology Nursing,* 18(1 Suppl 1), 16-21.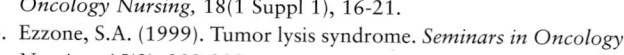
4. Ezzone, S.A. (1999). Tumor lysis syndrome. *Seminars in Oncology Nursing,* 15(3), 202-208.
5. Accessed January 19, 2004 from http://seer.cancer.gov/faststats/html/inc-leuks.html.
6. Kosits, C., & Callaghan, M. (2000). Rituximab: A new monoclonal antibody therapy for non-Hodgkin's lymphoma. *Oncology Nursing Forum,* 27(1), 51-59.
7. Leukemia and Lymphoma Society. Accessed January 19, 2004 from http://www.leukemia-lymphoma.org.
8. O'Brien, T. (2002). Current therapeutic approaches in the treatment of non-Hodgkin's lymphoma. *Seminars in Oncology Nursing,* 18(1 Suppl 1), 3-9.
9. Seeley, K.M., & DeMeyer, E. (2002). Nursing care of patients receiving Campath. *Clinical Journal of Oncology Nursing,* 6(3), 138-43.
10. Shannon-Dorcy, K. (2002). Nursing implications of Mylotarg: A novel antibody-targeted chemotherapy for CD33+ acute myeloid leukemia in first relapse. *Oncology Nursing Forum,* 29(4), E52-9.
11. Stolar, K. (1999). A graft versus host disease prevention and management tool: A mechanism for improving continuity of care. *Oncology Nursing Forum,* 26(6), 977-978.
12. Vogelsang, G.B. (2000). Advances in the treatment of graft-versus-host disease. *Leukemia (England),* 14(3), 509-510.
13. Yeager, K.A., et al. (2000). Implementation of an oral care standard for leukemia and transplantation patients. *Cancer Nursing,* 23(1), 40-47.

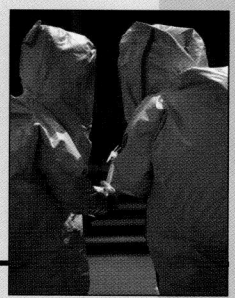

Unit 18

Multisystem Disorders

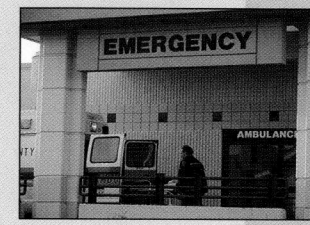

Management of Clients Requiring Transplantation

Connie White-Williams

The field of organ transplantation has evolved from the early beginnings of experimental kidney transplantation to the current practice of multiple organ transplantation. The advances made have been due largely to the increased knowledge in the areas of immunology and organ preservation, recipient and donor selection, and management of postoperative complications.

Organ transplantation is needed when an organ is irreversibly diseased or injured, leading to end-stage organ failure. Transplantation offers people with end-stage organ failure a chance to live longer and to overcome conditions that were once considered hopeless. Thus nurses have an increasing opportunity to care for clients with end-stage disease who are awaiting transplantation or who have undergone organ transplantation. In addition, nurses may also play a vital role in identification of potential donors and their management during the donor maintenance period.

HISTORICAL PERSPECTIVE

Transplantation had its beginnings in the 17th century with blood transfusions; however, the era of modern transplantation originated with a tooth replacement by John Hunter in the 18th century.[16] In 1912, Alexis Carrel developed the techniques for surgical suturing and vascular anastomosis that opened the pathway to solid organ transplantation.[15] Much of the work during the succeeding years focused on immunology, the importance of ABO and Rh blood group compatibility, and, later, the development of histocompatibility testing, all of which are crucial to organ transplantation today.[15,25] In 1945, Medawar[33] described the immune response of acute rejection, and by 1970 the relationship between donor and recipient histocompatibility in the role of acute rejection was recognized.[16]

Although many attempts at kidney transplantation were made in the early 1900s, it was not until 1954 that

evolve Be sure to check out the bonus material on the Evolve website and the CD-ROM, including free self-assessment exercises.
http://evolve.elsevier.com/Black/medsurg/

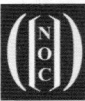

Nursing Outcomes Classification (NOC)
for Nursing Diagnoses—Clients Requiring Transplantation

Effective Therapeutic Regimen Management/Deficient Knowledge Adherence Behavior Compliance Behavior Knowledge: Transplant Treatment Regimen Knowledge: Infection Control Knowledge: Illness Care	**Participation: Health Care Decisions** Risk Control **Ineffective Protection/Risk for Infection** Immune Status Infection Status Knowledge: Infection Control Risk Control	**Risk for Imbalanced Nutrition: More or Less Than Body Requirements** Nutritional Status Nutritional Status: Food and Fluid Intake Nutritional Status: Nutrient Intake Weight Control

Merrell and Murray performed the first successful kidney transplantation between identical twin brothers.[16] Experimental heart transplantation took place in the early 1900s. Hardy transplanted a chimpanzee heart (xenograft) into a 68-year-old man in 1964. In 1967, Barnard performed the first human-to-human heart transplantation.[5,16,22] The first lung transplantation was performed by Hardy in 1963.[16] Experimental liver transplantation began in the 1950s. The first human liver transplant was performed in 1963 by Starzl.[36] For a summary of the number of transplantation procedures reported by the United Network of Organ Sharing (UNOS), visit *evolve* http://www.optn.org/data/annualReport.asp.[40]

With current success and survival statistics, these procedures are no longer deemed experimental. Organ transplantation is clearly an option for clients with end-stage organ disease. Much of the success is due to the availability of new immunosuppressive therapies, advances in organ preservation, improved surgical techniques, and the recognition of risk factors that affect survival after transplantation. Because transplant recipients now live longer, however, numerous social, economic, ethical, and quality of life (QOL) issues have arisen.

RELATED ISSUES

Cost

Average costs for the surgical procedure plus 5-year post-transplantation expenses are approximately $196,000 for kidney transplantation, $434,000 for heart transplantation, $361,000 for lung transplantation, and $394,000 for liver transplantation.[40] The Social Security Act was amended in 1972 to cover the cost of dialysis and transplantation for end-stage renal disease. Although coverage by private insurance companies, health maintenance organizations, (HMOs), preferred provider organizations (PPOs), and Medicare/Medicaid has increased, the high cost remains a factor for clients who wish to undergo transplantation. In 1996, Medicare extended the coverage of immunosuppressive medications to 3 years after transplantation, which was a positive step toward helping clients financially.

Shortage of Organ Donors

The shortage of organ donors is the most significant limitation to transplantation. There are simply not enough organs for the thousands of clients waiting for transplantation. As of September 2003, the number of clients with end-stage disease waiting for an organ were as follows: 55,644 for a kidney, 3688 for a heart, 3893 for a lung, 17,325 for a liver, and 1441 for a pancreas.[40,41] (Because this information changes hourly, see http://www.unos.org/data/ for the most current data.[41]) Required request/referral and presumed consent programs are being implemented to increase organ donation. Also, the transplant community is investigating methods to increase donor organ supply. For example, redefining brain death to include cerebral death and anencephaly, use of xenotransplantation (transplanting organs from one species to another), and expanding the donor criteria to include older donors and living extrarenal donors (as in lobar transplantation of lung or liver) all are methods that increase donor organ supply.

Ethical Considerations

Many moral and ethical issues surround transplantation. Religious and cultural customs and beliefs related to death and organ donation and transplantation create challenges for health care professionals (see the table on Religious and Cultural Customs and Beliefs Related to Death and Organ Donation/Transplantation on the website).[32] As ways to increase the organ donor pool are explored, additional ethical dilemmas may be encountered. The future trends for transplantation include more living-related donation and new experimentation such as cell transplantation. It is important for nurses to be knowledgeable about these issues and to communicate and discuss dilemmas with peers and professionals.

Definition of Death

Debate continues regarding the definition of *death*. The Uniform Determination of Death Act states that "an individual is considered dead if sustaining either (1) irreversible cessation of circulatory and respiratory function or (2) irreversible cessation of all functions of the entire brain, including the brain stem."[38] Different criteria are recognized for children and infants. In clients in chronic vegetative states or in anencephalic infants, brain stem function is intact but body and mental functions are not. Should death be redefined to include these people as donors? In transplantation, there will always be the dilemma of too few organs available in the face of the need to respect the life of people in a vegetative state who may be potential donors.

Buying and Selling of Organs

The National Organ Transplant Act of 1984 prohibits the sale of human organs and tissues. In addition, the Uniform Anatomical Gift Act of 1968 prohibits the sale or purchase of body parts or organs.[38] The conflict arises with respect to property rights. Supporters of organ sales believe that people own their bodies and have the right to do what they wish with their bodies—including the sale of their organs. The legal sale of blood plasma and sperm, which are body fluids, fuels the debate. The sale of organs in the United States is unlawful. A change in the law would alter the existing practice of free, altruistic donation.[21]

Prisoners as Donors or Recipients

A number of concerns arise in exploring solutions to the organ donor shortage. Once again, payment for organs enters the picture. Should prisoners be allowed to donate a kidney or bone marrow for a reduced sentence? This practice would not comply with current altruistic donation. In the same context, should a convicted criminal be allowed to be a transplant recipient? Some authorities believe that being a convicted criminal should not be an exclusion criterion, whereas others argue that it should be an exclusion criterion because of the prisoner's limited life expectancy outside prison.[21] Criminals may continue a life of crime outside of prison (drugs, guns, robberies), and therefore their chances of early death are greater.

Non–Heart-Beating Donors

Other potential organ donors are people who have experienced a respiratory or circulatory death. The hearts of these potential donors stop beating at the time of organ recovery. Ethical issues here involve the definition of brain death and determining when death occurs after asystole.

Xenotransplantation

Xenotransplantation, the transplantation of organs, tissues, or cells from one species to another (e.g., transplantation of a baboon heart into a human body), has been proposed as one answer to the organ donor shortage. There are still many medical and ethical issues to consider with this concept. Medical issues include organ rejection, new modes of infection transmission, and incompatible immune system responses. Ethical considerations include informed consent, the use of animals as donors, potential benefits versus risks, and public health issues.[21]

OUTCOME MANAGEMENT

Clients with End-Stage Organ Disease

Referral and Recipient Selection

A primary responsibility of the transplant team is to transplant organs into clients who have the best chance for a long-term successful outcome. It is expected that the transplant recipient will experience an improvement in functional status, maintain long-term graft function, and enjoy improved QOL. This result is accomplished by the selection of an appropriate candidate. The transplant evaluation is a complex, multidisciplinary process that is usually initiated after a referral by the primary physician. The evaluation begins with an initial assessment of medical records and an examination of the client by the transplant team. On the basis of findings from the client's history and physical examination, the transplant team determines whether the client should undergo further evaluation for transplantation. Figure 82-1 shows the referral and evaluation process.

The goals of the evaluation process are to determine the following:
- The medical necessity for transplantation
- The surgical feasibility of the procedure
- Risk factors and the proper timing of transplantation
- Psychosocial suitability
- Immunologic status

The evaluation can be performed on either an inpatient or outpatient basis and usually takes 3 to 5 days. During this period, extensive testing is completed, client education is provided, and the client and family members meet the members of the transplant team. Tests and procedures performed during the evaluation are listed in Table 82-1. These tests provide the transplant team with information regarding the status of all organ systems, infections, coexisting medical conditions, organ matching, and psychosocial issues that may affect the client and family. Psychosocial factors include neurocognitive status, coping skills, compliance history, availability of support systems, financial status, and extent of resources (Table 82-2). (See the website for an example of an evaluation summary sheet to be completed for transplantation candidates.)

The details of the evaluation process may vary between transplant centers and with the organs being evaluated. It is important for you to understand the evalua-

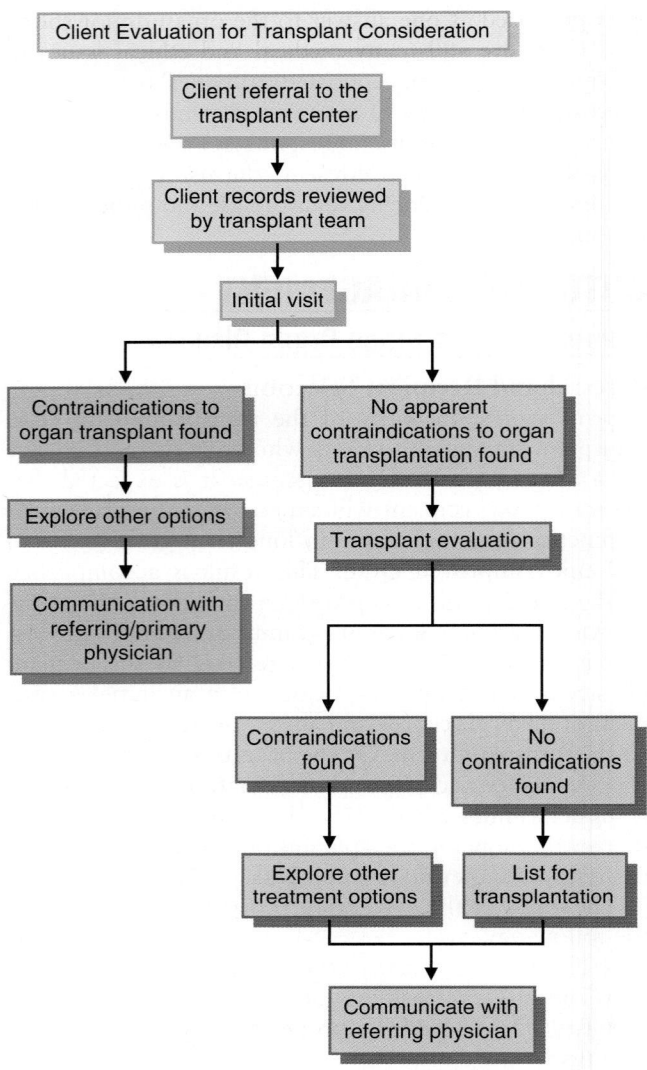

FIGURE 82-1 Client evaluation for transplantation.

tion process and to know the indications for and contraindications to transplantation. In addition, preoperative education is an important responsibility of the nurse. The goal of education of the potential organ recipient is to provide the client and family with factual information regarding the waiting time for an organ, the surgical procedure, and the post-transplantation regimens, including diet, exercise, medication, routine follow-up, complications, and return to "normal" life expectations (return to work). Many centers provide this education using several teaching skills, such as one-to-one teaching, group classes, and written information. The client uses this information to make an informed decision whether to undergo transplantation.

If contraindications are found during the transplant evaluation (Box 82-1), the transplant team reviews treatment options with the client and family. If no contraindications are found, the client can then be listed on

the national waiting list according to criteria established by UNOS, a nationwide system dedicated to the equitable sharing and distribution of donor organs.

Listing for Transplantation and Waiting for a Donor Organ

The criteria for listing a client for transplantation are governed by UNOS and vary according to the organ to be transplanted. These criteria include urgency, blood type, and recipient weight and height.

Stable clients wait at home or near the transplant center. Many clients choose local housing, such as an apartment. A few centers provide hospital-owned housing dedicated to use by pre- and post-transplant clients and their families. Cellular telephones or beeper systems must be available to allow the transplant team to contact the client at any time. Usually, a client who lives at a distance from the transplant center requiring more than 2 hours' travel time must relocate or arrange air transportation to arrive at the center within an acceptable time.

Clients whose condition is unstable wait in the hospital, often in an intensive care unit. Some clients, particularly those awaiting heart transplantation, may live outside the hospital with continuous inotropic support. Intermittent hospitalization may be needed throughout the waiting period. Heart transplantation candidates who become hemodynamically unstable may need an intra-aortic balloon pump or a ventricular-assist device. Clients waiting for renal transplantation may be receiving dialysis, and those waiting for lung transplantation may require ventilator assistance. In liver transplantation candidates, mechanical assistance devices are not used during the wait for the transplant. Cardiac or pulmonary rehabilitation before transplantation is beneficial to optimize the client's strength and aerobic capacity.

Waiting for transplantation is perhaps the most stressful time for clients and families as they cope with terminal illness, altered lifestyles, financial strain, and impending surgery. Both the client and family members may experience feelings of anxiety, depression, and helplessness.[11,13] An often forgotten but important component of transplantation nursing is the care of clients with end-stage organ disease who are waiting for transplantation. The transplant nurse may care for clients while they wait in the hospital for a donor organ, in the clinic setting, or in the home. This wait may be days, months, or even years, and it is natural for the nurse to develop strong personal and professional relationships with these clients.

Along with the intense nursing that is involved in keeping the client alive during the waiting period, emotional stress may develop in nurses caring for these clients. It is important for nurses to have periodic meetings to discuss their feelings and difficult cases and to de-

TABLE 82-1 | *Evaluation for Organ Transplantation*

General

Complete medical history and physical examination
Psychiatric and social evaluation
Laboratory studies
    Electrolyte and metabolic profile
    Liver function tests
    Hematologic profile
    Fasting cholesterol/lipid profile
    Arterial blood gas analysis
    Urinalysis, urine specific gravity determination
    Creatinine clearance determination
    ABO blood typing
    Antibody screen
    Human leukocyte antigen (HLA) tissue typing
    Lymphocyte cytotoxicity screen (assay for preformed reactive antibodies)
Virologic and microbiologic profile testing for the following:
    Cytomegalovirus (CMV)
    Toxoplasmosis
    Human immunodeficiency virus (HIV)
Hepatitis B surface antigen (HBsAg)
    Hepatitis C antibody
    Epstein-Barr virus (EBV)
    Syphilis: Venereal Disease Research Laboratory (VDRL) assay
    Tuberculosis: Purified protein derivative (PPD) testing with controls

Kidney

Laboratory studies
Glomerular filtration rate determination
Radiographic and radionuclide scanning studies
    Renal ultrasound examination
    Kidney-urethra-bladder radiographic series
    Renal radionuclide scanning
    Renal angiography

    Magnetic resonance imaging
    Renal biopsy
    Cystourethrography

Heart

Radiographic and radionuclide scanning studies
    Posteroanterior (PA) and lateral chest radiographs
    Sinus and panoramic films
    Resting radionuclide angiography
    Pulmonary function tests
    Ventilation-perfusion lung scan
    Nuclear magnetic resonance imaging when indicated
    CT studies when indicated
    Resting and exercise gas exchange studies
Cardiac catheterization
Two-dimensional echocardiography
Electrocardiography

Liver

Laboratory studies: additional blood work for diagnosis of specific liver disease may be indicated
Radiographic and radionuclide scanning studies
    Ultrasound examination of liver and biliary tree
    CT scan of head
    CT scan of abdomen with liver volumes
    Endoscopic retrograde cholangiopancreatography
    Percutaneous transhepatic cholangiogram
    Pulmonary and cardiac evaluation

Lung

Radiographic and radionuclide scanning studies
    CT scan of chest
    Ventilation-perfusion scan
    Pulmonary function tests
    Cardiac evaluation

CT, Computed tomography.

velop plans of care for the clients. More than 20 million people in the United States have chronic renal disease, whereas 400,000 have chronic kidney failure and receive dialysis each year.[34a] Approximately 1.1 million Americans are expected to experience a new or recurrent heart failure by year 2010.[1] Cirrhosis is the fourth leading cause of death, accounting for 25,000 deaths yearly.[2] It is important for transplant nurses to understand that, although there may be many happy moments when an organ becomes available for the clients, there will also be tragedies when death occurs before an organ is located. Working with transplant clients can be both emotionally draining and frustrating during the waiting period for organ availability. Nurses can strive to provide excellent care for the client but they have little control over the availability of organs. It is important that emotional support be provided not only for transplant clients and their families but also for health care staff members and their families. Many centers have established support groups vital to the emotional well-being of the people involved.

During the waiting time, the nurse, as part of the transplant team, and the client with end-stage organ disease begin to establish a trusting relationship, participate in the client's education, and work together to grasp the realities of life after transplantation. Many clients and their families unrealistically expect that transplantation will cure all life's problems. The problems of end-stage organ disease may be resolved, but new problems associated with transplantation, including medication side effects, rejection, infections, and financial limitations,

TABLE 82-2	*Considerations in the Psychosocial Evaluation for Transplantation*

Demographics Age Marital status Support systems	Compliance with medication regimen Compliance with clinical appointments
Financial Insurance Savings	**Transportation** Ability to get to clinic or hospital Travel time to transplantation center
Social Habits Smoking Drinking Illicit drugs Coping skills	**Home Environment** Telephone Running water Trailer/home (e.g., Financial? Steps? Cleanliness?) Heating and air-conditioning
Health Maintenance Oxygen requirements Dialysis	

BOX 82-1 *General Contraindications to Organ Transplantation*

- Presence of active systemic infection (bacteremia, fungemia, viremia)
- Malignant disease (except skin cancer and some primary tumors of the diseased organ)
- Active peptic ulcer disease
- Active abuse of alcohol or other substances
- Severe damage to organ system(s) other than that to be transplanted (such as severe cardiovascular dysfunction in the potential liver transplant recipient)
- Severe psychiatric disease
- Demonstration of past or current inability to comply with a prescribed medical regimen
- Lack of a functional social support system
- Lack of sufficient financial resources to pay for surgery, hospitalization, medication, and follow-up care

---

are frequently encountered. Help the client understand the post-transplantation regimen, and explain what to expect once the client is discharged from the hospital.

Organ Donation and Recovery

The gifts of organ and tissue by donation are a vital part of transplantation. Without the gracious decision of the donor or donor family to give the "gift of life" by donation, there would be no post-transplantation miracles.

If the potential donor is a living relative, careful physical and psychosocial assessment is necessary. Potential donors must be psychologically evaluated as to their real desire to donate an organ, usually a kidney, and the ability to make a lifelong adjustment to having one kidney. To avoid conflict of interest, evaluation of the donor is commonly done by a team different from that caring for the recipient. Discussions with the donor should be held in strict confidence; if the potential donor decides not to donate, the medical team frequently cites a physical contraindication in order to allow continued acceptance of that person by the other family members.

Several legislative initiatives have advanced issues of donation and transplantation. In 1968, the Uniform Anatomical Gift Act, aimed at increasing volunteer organ donation, became law. Included in this law were the specifications for notifying legal next of kin of donation wishes, uniform donor cards, and designation of donation preference on the driver's license.[16] The National Transplant Act of 1984 addressed medical, legal, ethical, and social issues of donation such as requiring national scientific registries for assessment by the federal government and declaring it illegal to buy and sell human organs.[38] Also, the Organ Procurement and Transplant Network (OPTN) was established to create a national client registry and to coordinate organ allocation and distribution. UNOS is under contract from the U.S. Department of Health and Human Services to operate OPTN.[16]

The Omnibus Budget Reconciliation Act (OBRA) of 1986 requires hospitals to have written policies and procedures for identification and referral of potential donors. Under the 1987 Organ Donation Request Act, consideration of the donor's religious beliefs is mandated, and guidelines are set forth to guide the health care team's approach to next of kin for donor consent, attainment of consent, and notification of the organ procurement organization (OPO).

OBRA also requires transplant centers and OPOs to be members of OPTN. OPOs are nonprofit organ recovery services in the United States that constitute an integral link in the identification, acceptance, and management of the potential organ donor. In addition to the coordination of organ recovery, transplant procurement coordinators within the OPO provide professional and public education, assist hospitals during donor evaluation, and offer family counseling. Other responsibilities of the procurement coordinators are assisting in donor management, arranging transportation to and from the donor hospital, and assisting surgical personnel in the operating room. The procurement coordinator provides information to the clinical transplantation coordinator and the transplantation surgeon throughout the recovery process.[11,16]

OPOs are either hospital-based or independent. They must meet criteria mandated by the Health Care Finance Administration (HCFA), which includes (1) arranging for appropriate tissue typing, (2) demonstrating a working relationship with 75% of hospitals within the OPO area, (3) discussing accounting procedures, (4) providing a method of transport of donated organs, (5) submitting center-specific data, (6) cooperating with local tissue banks, and (7) having a governing board of directors.

Role of the Nurse in Organ Donation

The nurse plays an important role in organ donation and recovery with early identification of potential donors, making referrals to the OPO, and assisting in the medical management of the organ donor.[11] The nurse may act as a liaison with donor families or may be involved in the clinical management of the donor. This nursing role can be a very emotional experience. A nurse involved in this process must acknowledge the personal loss incurred when faced with the brain death of a donor client. The nurse then begins to focus on managing that client's vital systems until donation is completed.

The nurse's identification of a potential organ donor is a vital link to transplantation. To be a donor, a person must meet certain criteria, including sustaining an injury resulting in brain death. According to the Uniform Determination of Death Act, "An individual is dead if he has sustained either irreversible cessation of circulatory and respiratory functions or irreversible cessation of all functions of the brain, including the brain stem, as determined in accordance with accepted medical standards."[38]

The nurse may be the first to recognize the manifestations of brain death, including lack of responsiveness; absence of cough, gag, or corneal reflexes; and lack of response to painful stimuli. These findings should be reported to the physician. Refer all clients who meet brain death criteria to the local OPO.[8] It is most often a nurse who notifies the OPO of the potential donor. Notification should occur when brain death is imminent, to allow the procurement coordinator to become familiar with the potential donor's case. Figure 82-2 depicts the organ donor referral and triage procedure.

The first step in the donation process is awareness of potential organ donors. Organ donors are people who have suffered an injury leading to brain death. The most common causes of injury are head trauma, strokes, subarachnoid hemorrhage, and primary brain tumors. Once a potential donor is identified, the organ procurement agency should be notified. The next steps are documentation of brain death and family consent of donation.

Next, medical management of the potential donor begins. The goal of donor management is to maintain optimal conditions ensuring functional and infection-free organs for transplantation. This goal is accomplished by the diligent management of hydration and tissue perfusion, oxygenation, infection control, diuresis, and temperature regulation. Guidelines that have been helpful in maintaining organ viability include the "rules of 100's,"

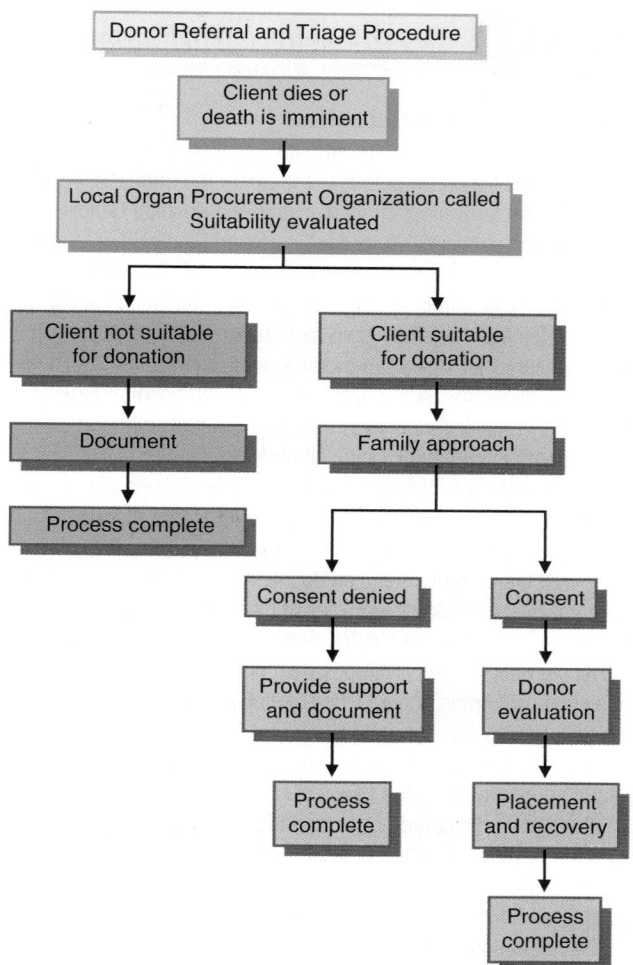

FIGURE 82-2 Organ recovery process.

in which (1) systolic blood pressure is maintained at 100 mm Hg, (2) urine output at 100 ml/hr, (3) heart rate at 100 beats/min, and (4) PaO$_2$ at 100 mm Hg.[8] Common problems encountered in management of the potential donor are hypotension, shock, electrolyte imbalances, disseminated intravascular coagulation (DIC), and loss of thermoregulation. The ideal organ donor is a person whose fatal injury resulted in brain death but who was otherwise healthy and infection-free. Criteria for organ donation are listed in Table 82-3.

Initiation of the organ donor process should proceed according to hospital policy. Organ recovery occurs in the operating room only after (1) identifying a potential donor, (2) notifying an OPO, (3) diagnosing brain death, (4) obtaining family consent, and (5) managing the donor until organ removal is complete.

Organ Recovery

Multiple organ procurement, or recovery of more than one type of organ from a single donor, is standard practice. As

TABLE 82-3	*Conditions of Participation for Organ Donation*

Conditions of Participation

The Department of Health and Human Services (HHS), in an attempt to optimize donor potential and abate the critical shortage of organs for transplantation, issued the Hospital Conditions of Participation (COP) for Medicare and Medicaid on June 22, 1998. This rule took effect on August 21, 1998, and requires all U.S. hospitals to adopt a "routine notification" policy or mandates that hospitals have and implement written protocols to ensure that the organ procurement organization (OPO) is notified of all deaths. According to the COP, the hospital must, "in a timely fashion," notify the OPO of individuals who die or whose death is imminent," thus eliminating the need for hospital staff to identify a potential donor.* All patients who die should be considered a potential organ and/or tissue donor.

Routine notification ensures that an individual who is most familiar with the current criteria on donation, specifically the OPO, evaluates every individual who dies to determine suitability for donation. If the policy were consistently followed, routine notification would make it virtually impossible for the hospital not to refer all potential organ donors. Thus routine notification places the decision making and determination of medical suitability for a person to be a donor in the hands of the procurement and transplant community, not in the hands of hospital staff.

This rule is designed not to exclude hospital professionals from the process but, rather, to ensure that the procurement professionals are included.

Five stipulations are contained in the COP:

- A hospital must have an agreement with an OPO and must contact the OPO in a timely manner about all individuals who die or whose death is imminent. The OPO will then determine medical suitability for donation.
- Every hospital must have an agreement with a designated eye and tissue bank to cooperate in the recovery of eyes and tissues.
- Every hospital must ensure that the family of every potential donor is offered the option to donate organs and/or tissues or not to donate.
- Every hospital must work in collaboration with the OPO and tissue or eye bank in educating their staff, participating in death records to identify potential donors and maintain potential donors during the donor management period while necessary testing and the placement of organs and tissues take place.
- Every hospital must provide organ-transplant–related data, as requested by the national Organ Procurement and Transplantation Network and the U.S. Scientific Registry of Transplant Recipients and the OPOs.†

Source: United Network for Organ Sharing.
*Final Rule: *Federal Register,* Vol. 63, No. 119, June 22, 1998. 42 CFR Part 482.4.5. Department of Health and Human Services: Health Care Financing Administration. Medicare and Medicaid Programs; Hospital Conditions of Participation; Identification of Potential Organ, Tissue and Eye Donors and Transplant Hospitals, Provision of Transplant Related Data.
†From Chabalewski, F.L. et al. *Donation and transplantation: Into the new millennium.* Available: www.medscape.com, October 5, 2000.

many as four separate surgical teams may be present in the operating room, each focusing on recovery of one organ. Usually, a separate surgical team prepares the recipient for the new organ. After a midline incision is made, dissection of organs occurs. Once cross-clamping of the aorta is done and cardioplegia is begun, the heart is removed. Then lungs, liver, and finally kidneys are procured.

The organs are preserved in a cold storage solution selected by the transplant center. Examples of such solutions are University of Wisconsin solution (UW solution), Euro-Collins solution, Belzer's solution, and other, institution-specific solutions. Organs are preserved in a sterile storage solution, packed in ice, and transported to the recipient in a cooler.

Viability times for donated organs vary. Standard periods after organ recovery are as follows: for kidney, 48 to 72 hours; for heart, 4 to 5 hours; for lung, 4 to 6 hours; for liver, 24 to 30 hours; and for pancreas, 24 hours. For successful transplantation, the timing of organ removal, transport, and preparation of the recipient is essential. Surgical transplantation procedures for specific organs are discussed in their respective chapters.

Preparation of Recipient

While the procurement coordinator manages and coordinates the donor process, the clinical transplant coordinator manages and coordinates the preparation of the potential recipient. The potential recipient (or recipients—in many cases a second client is also told to come to the hospital in case the transplant team encounters a problem with use of the donated organ in the primary potential recipient) is admitted to the hospital and immediately prepared for surgery. Preparation involves obtaining blood work, administering preoperative medications, and performing other standard preoperative interventions such as shaving and skin preparation. Preparation of the recipient may become a race against the clock as the transplant team works within the time constraints of organ viability.

Postoperative Transplant Clients

Management of the post-transplant client involves an intensive collaborative effort of the various members of the transplant team. The transplant team consists of transplant surgeons and other physicians, nurse coordinators, social workers, pharmacists, psychologists, nurse practitioners, nutritionists, members of the clergy, staff nurses, and consultants. Depending on which organ is transplanted, usually the same team members provide care to clients from initial referral throughout the client's lifetime. In many cases, kidney or liver transplant recipients return to their referring physicians for long-term care. Nursing care should be designed to recognize life-threatening clinical problems, to prevent complications, and to promote the client's return to normal activities with improved QOL.

Basic Immunology Related to Transplantation

To effectively care for the transplant client, you must understand basic immunology concepts related to transplantation (see Chapters 76 and 78). The immune response elicits mechanisms that direct the body to recognize transplanted organs as foreign (non-self). Although this immune response is normal, it is the goal of immunosuppressive agents to alter this immune response in transplanted clients.

The innate or nonspecific immune responses consist of natural mechanisms for the protection of the client against foreign antigens. These natural defenses are present at birth, lack memory, and do not need prior exposure for antigens to develop. Innate immunity mechanisms include physical barriers, chemical barriers, and leukocyte reactions, all of which play a role in the body's immune response.

Acquired or specific immunity involves mechanisms elicited by the lymphoid system. Lymphoid cells include plasma cells and lymphocytes. Lymphocytes constitute 30% of the white blood cells (WBCs) and are responsible for the recognition of antigens. These lymphocyte defense mechanisms recognize foreign antigens and can elicit rejection of transplanted organs. Two types of lymphocytes can elicit a response: B lymphocytes, which mediate a humoral immune response through the production of antibodies, and T lymphocytes, which are derived from maturing stems cells in the thymus and act to defend the body by interaction with an antigen with a sensitized T lymphocyte.[22,24,35,37,42] There are regulator (T helper and T suppressor) and effector (cytotoxic and memory) T lymphocytes.

In humans, the genetic factor used to determine specific antigen recognition is called the major histocompatibility complex (MHC). The MHC is the human leukocyte antigen (HLA) gene complex, located on chromosome 6. Antigens of the HLA complex are divided into two classes: class I comprises HLA types A, B, and C; class II consists of HLA types DR, DQ, and DP. Histocompatibility testing is used to minimize specific immune responses to the transplanted organ. The type of histocompatibility testing varies according to the organ transplanted and with time limitations. Before transplantation, the potential recipient undergoes ABO typing, Rh typing, and HLA tissue typing. An assay for preformed reactive antibodies (PRAs) determines the presence of preformed antibodies to HLA antigens. Results range from 0% to 100%. If a potential recipient is found to have antibodies against specific HLA antigens, a donor organ with those antigens is not suitable for transplantation.

Several types of cross-matching procedures can be performed to identify the presence of antibodies in the potential recipient to antigens located on the lymphocytes of the potential donor. A positive result on cross-matching means that antibodies are present, and transplantation is usually inadvisable because of the associated higher risk of rejection. A negative result on cross-matching means that no antibodies are present, with a reduced risk of rejection.

Immunosuppression

The goal of immunosuppressive therapy involves the delicate balance of adequately suppressing the immune response to prevent organ rejection without developing complications from the therapy itself. This intricate balance of the immunosuppressive medication regimen is individualized for each client. The transplant team aims to keep the dose of each drug within the therapeutic range. Management of the immunosuppressive regimen is crucial to long-term outcomes in post-transplant clients; for example, excessive immunosuppression may lead to increased risk of infection, liver or kidney insufficiency, joint necrosis, cataracts, or malignancies, whereas inadequate immunosuppression may lead to rejection of the transplanted organ. Although in many cases long-term graft acceptance can be maintained with less drug as time goes by, most clients require immunosuppression for life to prevent rejection of the transplanted organ.[7,22]

Immunosuppressive agents are used in the post-transplant population in three categories of use: induction, maintenance, and antirejection. Specific agents and dosages vary according to category of use. Protocols are dependent on the type of organs transplanted, transplant center–specific practices, and the client's history and current health status. See the Integrating Pharmacology feature on Immunosuppressive Agents Used in Transplantation on p. 2434. Most transplant centers use multiple-drug regimens containing agents that act on various functions of the immune system as well as minimize side effects. Many new immunosuppressant medications are being developed and tested in the United States and Europe.

Complications

Rejection. Transplantation of allografts (organs transplanted between genetically different individuals in the same species) elicits an immune response in which the antigens in tissue of the transplanted organ are recognized as foreign; hence a series of events occur, resulting in rejection of the organ. Rejection is classified into three types: (1) hyperacute, (2) acute, and (3) chronic (Figure 82-3).[39]

Hyperacute Rejection. Hyperacute rejection can occur within minutes to hours of implantation of the organ. It is caused by the presence of antibodies. Usually, a destructive humoral or B-cell reaction to antigens on the vascular endothelium results in organ necrosis. Most hyperacute rejection episodes can be prevented by previous PRA assay, histocompatibility testing, and cross-matching. If hyperacute rejection occurs, treatment options are

INTEGRATING PHARMACOLOGY

Immunosuppressive Agents Used in Transplantation

Following transplantation, clients require continuous immunosuppression to prevent rejection of the transplanted organ unless it is received from an identical twin. These immunosuppressive agents are often given in a combination of two to three agents that may vary from one transplant center to another. There are three classifications of immunosuppressive agents: (1) cytokine inhibitors, (2) antiproliferatives, and (3) antibodies.

Cytokine inhibitors are used to prevent and treat organ rejection and include agents such as cyclosporine (Sandimmune, Neoral, Gengraf), corticosteroids, tacrolimus (Prograf), and sirolimus (Rapamune). These drugs inhibit production of T lymphocytes, suppress T lymphocytes activity, and inhibit production of interleukin-2 (IL-2).

Antiproliferative agents are used to prevent organ rejection and include azathioprine (Imuran), mycophenolate mofetil (CellCept), methotrexate and cyclophosphamide (Cytoxan). These drugs inhibit proliferation of T and B lymphocytes, and interfere with DNA and RNA synthesis.

Antibodies are divided into monoclonal antibodies (muromonab-CD3 [Orthoclone OKT3], daclizumab [Zenapax], basiliximab [Simulect]) or polyclonal antibodies (Thymoglobulin, antithymocyte globulin [ATG]). These drugs inhibit T lymphocyte function, decrease the number of circulating lymphocytes, or block IL-2, which inhibits the activation of lymphocytes. They are used to prevent and treat organ rejection.

Because the client on immunosuppressive agents is at increased risk of infection, the clients must be taught to recognize the clinical manifestations of infection as well as rejection. Many of the medications may cause serious side effects such as hypertension, fatigue, tremor, diabetes, renal dysfunction, cataracts, obesity, and various gastrointestinal manifestations such as nausea, vomiting, bleeding, and diarrhea. These problems may also require medical or surgical management.

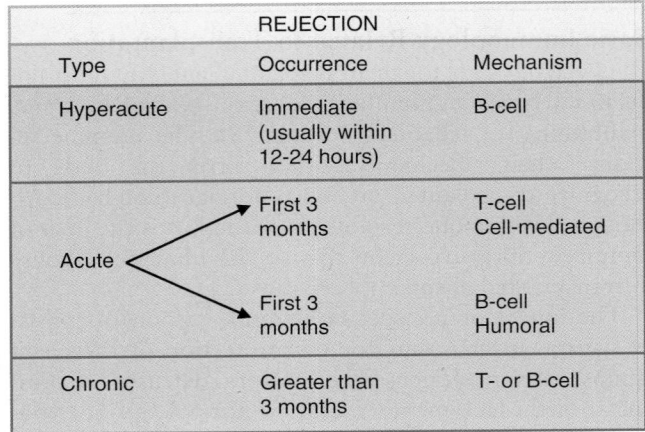

REJECTION		
Type	Occurrence	Mechanism
Hyperacute	Immediate (usually within 12-24 hours)	B-cell
Acute	First 3 months	T-cell Cell-mediated
	First 3 months	B-cell Humoral
Chronic	Greater than 3 months	T- or B-cell

FIGURE 82-3 Transplant rejection.

BOX 82-2 · Clinical Manifestations of Graft Rejection

- Fever
- Graft tenderness
- Fatigue
- Heart: shortness of breath, irregular heart beat
- Lung: shortness of breath
- Abnormal laboratory test results
  Kidney: ↑ serum creatinine, blood urea nitrogen levels
  Liver: ↑ total bilirubin, liver enzyme levels
  Pancreas: ↑ urine amylase

ical manifestations, laboratory data, or results of tests such as organ biopsy. Clinical manifestations of rejection are listed in Box 82-2.

Treatment usually consists of high-dose steroids; if recurrent episodes occur, muromonab-CD3 (Orthoclone OKT3) may be administered.

Chronic Rejection. Chronic rejection evolves gradually, usually after the first 3 months after transplantation. It may be the result of frequent episodes of acute rejection, increased ischemic time, or cytomegalovirus (CMV) infection. Chronic rejection results in progressive loss of graft function. The transplanted organ develops a persistent, perivascular inflammation associated with focal myocyte necrosis. Chronic rejection is treated in similar fashion to test for acute rejection; however, retransplantation may be required as a result of the progressive deterioration of organ function.

Infection. Infection is the leading cause of morbidity and mortality after transplantation. Many factors contribute to the potential risk of infection, including the client's age, nutritional status, medical condition before transplantation, infection history and exposure, and the im-

limited. Clients who have received kidney or kidney-pancreas transplants may need to return to dialysis. Clients who have received other organ transplants may receive plasmapheresis, a procedure that removes circulating antibodies from the blood. If this measure fails, retransplantation is indicated.

Acute Rejection. Acute rejection usually occurs in the first 3 months after transplantation; however, it can occur at any time, particularly if the immunosuppression regimen is altered or if an infection develops. Acute rejection can be a purely cellular immune response mediated by T cells or an antibody-mediated response, or a combination of the two.[22,24,39] Diagnosis is based on clin-

TABLE 82-4	*Common Infections After Transplantation*	
Infecting Organism	**Site(s) Affected**	**Therapeutic Agent of Choice**
Bacteria		
Gram-negative bacilli		Ticarcillin-
Klebsiella	Lung	clavulanate
Pseudomonas	Blood	(Timentin)
Escherichia coli	CNS	Gentamicin
Legionella	Lung	
Enterobacter		
Gram-positive cocci		Vancomycin
Enterococci		
Staphylococci		
Streptococci		
Viruses		
Cytomegalovirus	Lung	Ganciclovir
	Blood	
	GI tract	
Varicella-zoster virus	Skin	Acyclovir
	Blood	
Protozoa		
Toxoplasma gondii	Transplanted	Pyrimethamine
	organ	Sulfadiazine
	Lung	Folinic acid
	Liver	
Pneumocystis	Lung	Trimethoprim-
		sulfamethoxazole
Fungi		
Aspergillus	Lung	Amphotericin B
	CNS	
Candida	Oral mucosa	Nystatin
		Fluconazole
		Amphotericin B

CNS, Central nervous system; *GI*, gastrointestinal.

munosuppressive regimen. Infections seen in transplant recipients are usually the result of immunosuppression or altered immune defenses.[24,35,42] During the first month after transplantation, nosocomial infections are common; then, between 1 and 6 months after transplantation, opportunistic infections such as *Pneumocystis carinii* pneumonia, candidiasis, and CMV infection occur.[35,42] The lungs are the most common site for infection, followed by blood, urine, and the gastrointestinal tract. Common infections seen in transplant recipients are listed in Table 82-4. Infection is the most common indication for hospital readmission after transplantation.[20,42]

Malignancy. The development of post-transplantation malignancies caused by the immunodeficient state is well

documented.[35,42] Types of malignancies seen in the post-transplantation population include basal cell and squamous cell carcinomas of the skin and lip, seen most commonly, followed by the lymphoproliferative disorders and cancers of the vulva, perineum, and lungs. Reduction in the level of immunosuppression, surgical resection, chemotherapy, and radiation therapy are treatment options.

All clients should be screened for development of cancer after transplantation. Routine gynecologic examinations, including mammography and cervical smear in women, annual prostate-specific antigen (PSA) testing in men, and regular physical examination of neck and groin lymph nodes should be performed to detect any problems. Report any unusual lesions to the transplant team. In addition, monitor clients who are seronegative for Epstein-Barr virus for conversion to seropositivity, which may place them at higher risk for lymphoproliferative disease after transplantation. Clients need to be educated to use sunscreen products with a sun protection factor (SPF) of 15 or greater and to wear protective clothing to help prevent skin malignancies. (See the Bridge to Critical Care feature on Solid Organ Transplantation on p. 2436.)

Clients Receiving a Specific Organ Transplant

Renal Transplantation

The potential renal transplant recipient has end-stage renal disease, most commonly the result of hypertension, diabetic nephropathy, or a hereditary or congenital disorder.[34] In most cases, the renal transplant candidate is anemic and fatigued and has been maintained on chronic hemodialysis (see Chapter 38). Contraindications to renal transplantation include seropositivity for the human immunodeficiency virus (HIV), active infection, severe coronary artery disease with left ventricular dysfunction, malignancy, severe peripheral vascular disease, severe carotid artery disease, and chronic active hepatitis.

Unlike the heart, lung, liver, or pancreas transplant candidate, the kidney transplant candidate has several potential donors: living related, living nonrelated, and cadaver. Eighty-five percent of all renal transplants are from cadaveric donors.

Extensive histocompatibility testing is completed for renal transplantation, because evidence indicates that six antigen matches are necessary for long-term graft survival. Six-antigen-matching means that six antigens recognized on recipient HLA tissue typing match six antigens found on donor HLA tissue typing. A negative result on cross-matching is required for transplantation to occur.

Nursing Care. Nursing care of the renal transplant recipient is focused on the recognition and prevention of

BRIDGE TO CRITICAL CARE

Solid Organ Transplantation

Core Body Temperature Changes

The client arrives at the intensive care unit directly from the operating room with the anesthetic agents unreversed. Postoperative hypothermia prolongs clearance of the anesthetic agents and can lead to other complications such as cardiac dysrhythmias, altered platelet function, and decreased oxygen delivery to the tissues. Nursing measures in the early postoperative phase are directed toward supporting and assisting the client while the core body temperature returns to normal. Warming blankets, heat lamps, commercially available rewarming devices, and head covers are important measures to expedite rewarming of the client. Frequent monitoring of arterial blood pressure, cardiac rhythm, central venous pressure, pulmonary artery pressures, and core body temperature is essential during this phase. Arterial blood pressure, systemic vascular resistance, and cardiac output are expected to decrease as core body temperature rises and vasodilation occurs; thus additional support measures often are required during this time of instability.

Early Graft Dysfunction

The intensive care nurse must be aware of the manifestations of early graft dysfunction. During the first 24 hours, serologic laboratory findings, physical assessments, and objective hemodynamic measurements must be critically evaluated frequently for indications of graft function.

Organ	Indicators of Adequate Early Graft Function
Kidney	High volume urine output Decreasing BUN and creatinine Normal serum potassium level Normal serum glucose Nontender over graft (avoiding incision)
Heart	Normal cardiac output and cardiac index Decreasing to normal CVP Decreasing to normal PAP and PCWP Normal SVR Normal sinus rhythm with a ventricular rate of 90-100 beats/min Normal LVEF ($>$55%) by echocardiogram Normal S_1, S_2 heart sounds (pericardial rub may be present) Decreasing mediastinal drainage ($<$200 ml/hr in first 4 hours)
Lung	Normal Pao_2 Normal CO_2 Normal oxygen saturation Breath sounds clear and present in all allograft lung fields Decreasing pleural drainage Chest radiograph clear and well expanded
Liver	Adequate bile output Decreasing AST and ALT Increasing serum protein levels Normal to slightly elevated serum glucose

ALT, alanine aminotransferase; AST, aspartate aminotransferase; CVP, central venous pressure; LVEF, left ventricular ejection fraction; PAP, pulmonary artery pressure; PCWP, pulmonary capillary wedge pressure; SVR, systemic vascular resistance.

complications. Ongoing assessment of renal function—by determination of blood urea nitrogen (BUN), serum creatinine, glomerular filtration rate (GFR), fluid intake and output, weight, and serum electrolytes—is routine in these clients. If indicated, a renal scan or ultrasound study may be used to detect complications. Renal biopsy may be performed to make a definitive diagnosis, in that rejection, acute tubular necrosis (ATN), and obstructive complications have similar manifestations.

Goals are to maintain hydration, promote diuresis, avoid fluid overload, and prevent infection. Complications after renal transplantation include fluid and electrolyte imbalances, ATN, obstructive or vascular complications, rejection, and infection. Clinical manifestations of potential complications in the renal transplant client are decreased urine output, graft tenderness or pain, increasing serum creatinine level, fever, and weight gain.

Pancreas and Pancreas-Kidney Transplantation

Pancreas transplantation is indicated for the client with type 1 diabetes mellitus to restore normal glucose metabolism.[17] Pancreas-kidney transplantation is performed in the diabetic client with end-stage renal disease (see Chapter 47).[12] Contraindications are the same as in renal transplantation.

Nursing Care. Nursing care includes monitoring for fluid and electrolyte imbalances, especially BUN, serum creatinine, bicarbonate, and CO_2. Urine amylase is also monitored to assess pancreatic function. Clinical manifestations of graft thrombosis are a sudden increase in blood glucose, severe graft pain, and increased serum creatinine with combined kidney-pancreas transplantation.

Heart Transplantation

Potential candidates for heart transplantation are usually New York Heart Association class III or IV clients who are younger than 65 years of age and have a life expectancy of less than 12 months. The most common diseases treated by heart transplantation are coronary artery disease and cardiomyopathy.[20,23] Contraindications to heart transplantation include malignancy, active infection, autoimmune disorders, irreversible kidney, lung, or liver disease, and severely elevated pulmonary vascular resistance. Relative contraindications, which vary between transplant centers, are peptic ulcer disease, stroke, peripheral vascular disease, diabetes mellitus, and obesity.[23]

When listed for transplantation, candidates are evaluated periodically, usually every 4 to 6 weeks, to monitor their overall condition. Clients whose condition is stable wait at home or near the hospital, and clients whose condition is hemodynamically unstable wait at the hospital. Clients who become critically ill may need continuous inotropic infusions or ventricular-assist devices.

Cardiac Transplantation Physiology Alterations. Unique to the cardiac transplant recipient is cardiac transplant denervation. Denervation occurs after orthotopic transplantation, in which the vagus nerve is severed. The resultant lack of vagal nerve stimulation results in (1) a higher resting heart rate, (2) a gradual increase in heart rate with exercise and delayed return to baseline, (3) absence of angina, and (4) enhanced response to certain drugs (e.g., adrenaline, adenosine) and decreased re-

sponse to other drugs (e.g., atropine, digoxin).[6,23] Finally, two P waves may be detected on the electrocardiogram resulting from the presence of both donor and recipient heart sinoatrial (SA) nodes. It is important to note that only the donor heart SA node regulates the electrical conduction of the heart.

Nursing Care. The nursing assessment is a vital component in the care of the cardiac transplant recipient. The physical assessment should include auscultation of heart and breath sounds and assessment of pedal pulses and of the jugular vein for distention. Ongoing assessment of renal and liver function and monitoring of immunosuppressant drug levels and the complete blood count (CBC) are important in the overall care of the client. Complications seen after heart transplantation include organ dysfunction, rejection, infection, coronary vasculopathy, and malignancy.[6,23] Chest radiography is used to monitor possible lung infection, whereas echocardiography and endomyocardial biopsy are used to detect rejection. Clinical manifestations of rejection include fever, shortness of breath, fatigue, presence of S_3 or S_4 heart sound, decreased blood pressure, decreased ejection fraction, and jugular vein distention.

Liver Transplantation

Indications for liver transplantation include chronic irreversible liver disease due to a number of underlying disorders. In adults, the most common indications are cirrhosis secondary to chronic hepatitis, cryptogenic cirrhosis, primary biliary cirrhosis, and primary sclerosing cholangitis (see Chapter 49).[28,29] Contraindications to liver transplantation are center-specific and may include portal vein thrombosis, active alcoholism, active infection, malignancy outside the hepatobiliary system, and advanced cardiopulmonary disease. The client evaluation takes into account technical feasibility and optimal timing of surgery in addition to the usual physical and psychosocial indications.

Nursing Care. The postoperative care of the liver transplant client is complex. Nursing care focuses on monitoring graft function, managing fluid and electrolyte imbalances, preventing problems with other organ systems, and assessing for manifestations of rejection or infection. Clinical manifestations of rejection include fever, elevation of liver enzymes, and change in color, amount, and consistency of bile drainage through the T tube.

Diagnosis of rejection is confirmed by liver biopsy. In addition, a sudden increase in the International Normalized Ratio (INR) (a system for reporting prothrombin values), serum bilirubin, or liver enzymes may indicate a complication such as hepatic artery thrombosis or biliary obstruction. If neurologic status is affected, serum ammonia levels may be monitored. Finally, as in all organ transplantation procedures, renal function, immunosuppressant drug levels, and white blood cell (WBC) count should be closely monitored.

Lung Transplantation

The lung transplantation candidate has end-stage pulmonary disease (1) is generally younger than 65 years of age for single-lung transplantation, 60 years for two-lung transplantation, or 55 years for heart-lung transplantation and (2) is able to participate in pulmonary rehabilitation (i.e., is not wheelchair-dependent).[4,6,44] The decision whether to perform a single-lung or double-lung procedure varies among transplant centers but is based on the likelihood of achieving the best outcome and most improvement in QOL.

Contraindications to lung transplantation are active malignancy, positive results on hepatitis B antigen assay, hepatitis C infection, autoimmune disorders, and dysfunction of organs other than the lungs. Risk factors that affect eligibility include symptomatic osteoporosis, the need for steroid therapy in doses greater than 20 mg/day, severe musculoskeletal disease, impaired nutritional status (malnutrition or obesity), the need for mechanical ventilation, and colonization with fungi or atypical mycobacteria.

Lung Transplantation Physiology Alterations. Removal of native lung and lung replacement entail denervation of the transplanted lung. Denervation interferes with autonomic nervous system communication, resulting in dysfunctional ciliary movement, loss of cough reflex, and changes in mucus production, which lead to ineffective clearance of airway secretions. Health maintenance interventions to maintain patent airways are chest vibropercussion, postural drainage, and use of an incentive spirometer.

Nursing Care. The postoperative care of the lung transplant recipient is gratifying. It is a pleasure to watch a pretransplantation oxygen-dependent client gasping for breath become an active person requiring no oxygen after transplantation. Immunosuppressant drug levels, electrolyte determinations, liver function tests, CBC, chest radiography, and pulmonary function tests are important monitoring tests in this population.

Complications include surgical side effects, graft dysfunction, rejection, infection, and bronchiolitis obliterans or obliterating bronchiolitis (OB).[4,6,44] OB is the greatest limiting factor to long-term survival after lung

---

BOX 82-3 *Client and Family Education After Transplantation*

Members of transplantation team
When to call the transplant coordinator
Immunosuppression
- Administration of medications
- Side effects of medications

Rejection
- Definition, manifestations, diagnosis, treatment

Infection
- Definition, manifestations, diagnosis, treatment

Routine care
- Temperature
- Weight
- Skin care
- Incision care
- Fluid intake and output
- Pedal pulses
- Incentive spirometry
- Clinic schedule

Diet after transplantation
Activities after transplantation
- Precautions
- Exercise
- Physical therapy

Self-care
- Blood pressure
- Blood glucose levels
- Medical identification bracelet and card
- Sun exposure
- Sexual activity
- Sending specimens for laboratory monitoring tests
- Vacations
- Over-the-counter medicines to be avoided
- Driving
- Birth control

Psychosocial issues
- Physical appearance
- Family participation and support
- Writing to the donor family
- Cost of transplantation

Health maintenance
- Dental care
- Ophthalmologic examinations
- Gynecologic examinations
- Yearly evaluations of transplant

transplantation. OB is progressive in nature, resulting in severe shortness of breath, and must be treated aggressively. Usual medical management may include administration of intravenous steroids, cytolytic therapy (with OKT3), administration of Thymoglobulin, photopheresis, and retransplantation. Goals in nursing management are to prevent and recognize complications and to promote return to a functional lifestyle.

SELF-CARE

Before discharge from the hospital, pertinent information is discussed with the client and family members. Postoperative education after transplantation can be challenging, because many clients are discharged between 1 and 2 weeks after surgery. Many institutions provide client education booklets. Information discussed with the client and family is presented in Box 82-3.

Of special importance are knowledge of the clinical manifestations of rejection and infection and indications for contacting the transplant team. A schedule of return appointments is usually given at discharge. Most clients reside close to the transplant center for 2 to 8 weeks before going home. This proximity allows for frequent medical visits, ongoing education, and familiarization of the client with the postoperative regimen. It also allows the client to become more independent and resume self-care responsibilities. Often it is the nurse who is best able to monitor compliance with the medical regimen and to identify difficulty coping with the post-transplantation regimen. Once the client returns home, it may be necessary for a home health nurse to provide wound care, perform intravenous infusions, or perform other nursing care measures. Findings on home visits are communicated to the transplant coordinator. Box 82-4 lists

nursing diagnoses related to care of the post-transplant client.

Meticulous follow-up evaluation (assessing for manifestations of rejection, infection, or other complications) is essential to the long-term well-being of the post-transplant client. Long-term care of the transplant recipient requires communication between the client and transplant team. Each client should be assessed for infection, rejection, malignancy, organ dysfunction, and adverse manifestations of immunosuppression such as diabetes, hypertension, abnormalities on liver function testing, and gastrointestinal distress.

Psychosocial issues that should be investigated are financial status, family dynamics, and return to work. The social worker at the transplant center can assist the client with insurance questions, medication assistance programs, and ways of dealing with the financial stresses of transplantation. QOL may also be an issue that the transplant client must cope with. See the Evidence-Based Practice in Action feature on Quality of Life After Transplantation on pp. 2440 and 2441.

Health maintenance areas to evaluate are screening by mammography and Papanicolaou (Pap) smears in women, colon cancer screening, and immunizations such as with the influenza vaccine and pneumococcal vaccine (Pneumovax). Routine dental and ophthalmologic examinations should be scheduled. Communication with the referring physician or the primary health care provider is also important. Constant relaying of information including laboratory findings, clinic visit results, and follow-up plans should occur between the transplant center and the client's primary health care provider.

CONCLUSIONS

Nursing care of the transplant client is both challenging and rewarding. With thorough understanding of the end-stage disease process and its manifestations, the organ donation and recovery process, and postoperative management, the nurse has the unique ability to work as a member of the interdisciplinary team caring for this group of clients. The nurse may serve as primary care provider, client advocate, and liaison with other team members. To maximize QOL, caring for the client and family must focus on both the physical and psychosocial aspects of transplantation, including not only medical treatments but also nursing interventions that address the client's specific QOL issues. If psychosocial issues are not fully explored, the client is likely to experience poorer satisfaction with the post-transplantation outcome. Meticulous medical care, long-term follow-up, and addressing physical and psychosocial QOL issues all are important components of management to improve both survival and QOL in the population of clients who have undergone organ transplantation.

BOX 82-4	*Nursing Diagnoses for the Post-Transplant Client*

- *Risk for Imbalanced Nutrition: More Than Body Requirements* related to side effects of immunosuppressant agents/*Less Than Body Requirements* related to increased caloric needs after transplantation
- *Ineffective Protection and Risk for Infection* related to immunosuppression required after organ transplantation
- *Effective Therapeutic Regimen Management/Deficient Knowledge* related to post-transplantation regimen
- *Pain* related to transplantation surgery
- *Risk for Ineffective Coping* after transplantation related to increased stress, anxiety, fear, and lifestyle changes
- *Risk for Injury:* rejection of transplanted organ related to impaired immunocompetence; malignancy/diabetes/hypertension related to immunosuppression

EB EVIDENCE-BASED PRACTICE IN ACTION

Quality of Life After Transplantation

Quality of life (QOL) before and after transplantation, as well as how the client functions, copes, and lives after transplantation, is being investigated by nurses.[1-14] Research studies may evaluate QOL at a specific period either before or after transplantation.[2,4] Differences in the effects of drug treatment, device intervention, or medical therapy on QOL may be examined also.[8] The diabetic client who is no longer insulin-dependent or the client who had end-stage renal disease who no longer requires dialysis has experienced a major change in lifestyle. Although there are challenges related to immunosuppressive therapy, most clients who undergo successful transplantation report improved QOL.[2] Dew and colleagues reviewed 218 published studies using almost 15,000 total subjects from 1972 through 1996 and evaluated QOL in three areas: physical functioning, mental/cognitive health, and social functioning. Physical functioning was improved in all studies involving pancreas/kidney, pancreas, lung, and heart/lung clients.[2] Mental/cognitive and social improvement were reported in less than 80% of studies reviewed.[2] Of the studies reviewed by Dew and colleagues, few compared QOL ratings by transplant clients to QOL ratings by healthy people.[2]

Hathaway and colleagues and Johnson and colleagues reported improved QOL in renal transplant recipients regardless of race or gender of the client.[6,10] Hathaway and colleagues also completed a longitudinal study of 91 kidney transplant recipients who underwent QOL testing before transplantation and at 6 and 12 months after transplantation. The Sickness Impact Profile, the Adult Self-Image Scale, and the Personal Resource Questionnaire were used for this study. Variables that predicted posttransplantation QOL were employment status, the number of transplantation-related hospitalizations, and available social support.[7] White-Williams and colleagues found that males reported better QOL than females, both before heart transplantation and at 6 months after transplantation.[14]

Grady and colleagues reported on compliance at 1 year and at 2 years after heart transplantation in 120 recipients. Compliance was measured with the Heart Transplant Compliance Instrument developed for this study. The heart transplant recipients had no difficulty following medication regimens but did have difficulty with diet, exercise, and taking their vital signs.[5] De Geest and associates also examined compliance with taking medications in heart transplant recipients. They found that compliance with immunosuppressive medication was high; however, clients who were considered "moderate noncompliers" had a higher incidence of late acute rejection episodes. The findings in this study suggest that client compliance plays a pivotal role in long-term outcome after transplantation.[1]

Limbos and colleagues studied QOL in women before and after lung transplantation. Overall QOL improved after transplantation; however, the women reported impairments with sexuality and body satisfaction.[11] Manzetti reported that a health maintenance program of education and exercise improved QOL in clients awaiting lung transplantation.[13] Similarly, LoBiondo-Wood and colleagues reported improved QOL over time in 41 liver transplant recipients.[12]

Implications

QOL findings may vary from one type of transplant procedure to another requiring nurses to be familiar with the QOL data for the type of transplant they work with most frequently. Nurses working with a particular population of transplant clients may also share data about QOL that may be useful for transplant clients and families. It is important to remember that rating one's QOL may be relative because the experience of having a life-threatening illness changes how one thinks about life in general and about one's own particular life. Studies that compare QOL ratings by transplant recipients to QOL ratings by clients who have experienced near-death experiences, life-altering accidents, or medical treatment for severe illness should also be explored. Many studies were short term or asked clients about QOL only once or twice. This suggests that longitudinal studies of QOL are needed to enable nurses to understand and appreciate the impact of chronic illnesses and transplantation on clients and families.

References

1. De Geest, S., et al. (1998). Late acute rejection and subclinical noncompliance with cyclosporine therapy in heart transplant recipients. *Journal of Heart and Lung Transplantation, 17,* 854-863.
2. Dew, M., et al. (1997). Does transplantation produce quality of life benefits? A quantitative analysis. *Transplantation, 64,* 1261-1273.
3. Forsberg, A. (2002). Liver transplant recipient's experienced meaning of health and quality of life one year after transplantation. *Theoria Journal of Nursing Theory, 11*(3), 4-14.
4. Grady, K., Jalowiec, A., & White-Williams, C. (1995). Predictors of quality of life in patients with advanced heart failure awaiting transplantation. *Journal of Heart and Lung Transplantation, 14,* 2-10.
5. Grady, K., et al. (1998). Patient compliance at one year and two years after heart transplantation. *Journal of Heart and Lung Transplantation, 17,* 383-394.
6. Hathaway, D., et al. (1996). Racial and gender differences in quality of life prior to and following kidney transplantation. *Proceedings of the Tenth Annual Southern Nursing Research Society Conference.* February 29, 2006, Miami, FL.
7. Hathaway, D., et al. (1998). Post kidney transplantation quality of life prediction models. *Clinical Transplantation, 12,* 168-174.
8. Hilbrands, L., et al. (1995). The effect of immunosuppressive drugs on quality of life after renal transplantation. *Transplantation, 59,* 1263-1270.
9. Houle, N., et al. (2002). Health promoting behaviors, quality

EB EVIDENCE-BASED PRACTICE IN ACTION

Quality of Life After Transplantation—cont'd

of life, and hospital resource utilization of patients receiving kidney transplants, *Nephrology Nursing Journal, 29,* 35-40.

10. Johnson, C., et al. (1998). Racial and gender differences in quality of life following kidney transplantation. *Image: Journal of Nursing Scholarship, 30,* 125-130.

11. Limbos, M., Chan, C., & Kesten, S. (1997). Quality of life in female lung transplant candidates and recipients. *Chest, 112,* 1165-1174.

12. LoBiondo-Wood, G., et al. (1997). Impact of liver transplantation on quality of life: A longitudinal perspective. *Applied Nursing Research, 10*(1), 27-32.

13. Manzetti, J., et al. (1994). Exercise, education and quality of

life in lung transplant candidates. *Journal of Heart and Lung Transplantation, 13,* 297-305.

14. White-Williams, C., Jalowic, A., & Grady, K. (1997). Gender differences in quality of life outcomes before and 6 months after heart transplantation. *Journal of Heart and Lung Transplantation, 16,* 100.

THINKING CRITICALLY *evolve*

1. A client has been receiving dialysis for several years awaiting kidney transplantation. She is notified that a kidney donor has been found and that she should proceed to the hospital. What teaching will be completed before she goes to surgery? What psychosocial care should be offered?

Factors to Consider. What teaching and support will the family require? What are the ramifications if the donor kidney is found to be an unsuitable match for the client?

2. A client has recently undergone heart transplantation and is to be discharged from the hospital in 2 days. What client education should be completed? What education should be completed for the family?

Factors to Consider. What living arrangements are required for the client after discharge? What are the long-term concerns related to financial factors, quality of life issues, and long-term immunosuppressive therapy?

3. At a pretransplantation support group, a client makes the following statement: "I think I may need to buy my new organ." How should the nurse react to this statement? What ethical issues are raised by this statement?

Factors to Consider. Of what other ethical considerations regarding organ donation should the transplant nurse be aware?

Discussions for these questions can be found on the website and the CD-ROM.

BIBLIOGRAPHY

1. American Heart Association. Retrieved January 31, 2004, from http://www. americanheart.org.

2. American Liver Foundation. Retrieved January 31, 2004, from http://www.liverfoundation. org.

3. American Lung Association. Retrieved January 31, 2004, from http://www.lungusa.org.

4. Banner, N., Polak, J., & Yacoub, M. (2003). *Lung transplantation.* Cambridge: Cambridge University Press.

5. Barnard, C.N. (1967). A human cardiac transplant. *South African Medical Journal, 41,* 1271-1274.

6. Baumgartner, W. (2002). *Heart and lung transplantation* (2nd ed.). Philadelphia: W. B. Saunders.

7. Beniaminovitz, S., et al. (1999). Use of daclizumab decreases the EB frequency of early allograft rejection: De novo heart transplant recipients. *Journal of Heart and Lung Transplantation, 18,* 47.

8. Bogan, L., Rosson, M., & Peterson, F. (2000). Organ procurement and the donor family. *Critical Care Clinics of North America, 12,* 23-33.

9. Costanzo, M., et al., & The Cardiac Transplant Research Database Group. (1996). Heart transplant coronary artery disease detected by angiography: A multi-institutional study. *Journal of Heart and Lung Transplantation, 15,* S39.

10. De Geest, S., et al. (1998). Late acute rejection and subclinical EB noncompliance with cyclosporine therapy in heart transplant recipients. *Journal of Heart and Lung Transplantation, 17,* 854-863.

11. Ehrle, R., Shafer, T., & Nelson, K. (1999). Referral, request, and consent for organ donation: Best practice—a blueprint for success. *Critical Care Nurse, 19*(2), 21-33.

12. Freise, C, et al. (1999). Simultaneous pancreas-kidney transplantation: An overview of indications, complications and outcomes. *Western Journal of Medicine, 170,* 11-18.

13. Grady, K., Jalowiec, A., & White-Williams, C. (1995). Predictors of EB quality of life in patients with advanced heart failure awaiting transplantation. *Journal of Heart and Lung Transplantation, 14,* 2-10.

---

evolve **Did you remember to check out the bonus material on the Evolve website and the CD-ROM, including free self-assessment exercises?**

http://evolve.elsevier.com/Black/medsurg/

14. Grady, K., et al. (1998). Patient compliance at one year and two years after heart transplantation. *Journal of Heart and Lung Transplantation, 17,* 383-394

15. Guthrie, C. (Ed.). (1912). Applications of blood vessel surgery. In *Blood vessel surgery.* New York: Longmans, Green.

16. Hakim, N., & Papalois, V. (2003). *History of organ and cell transplantation* . River Edge, NJ: Imperial College Press.

17. Hakim, N., Stratta, R., & Gray, D. (2002). *Pancreas and islet transplantation.* New York: Oxford University Press.

 18. Hathaway, D., et al. (1996). Racial and gender differences in quality of life prior to and following kidney transplantation. *Proceedings of the Tenth Annual Southern Nursing Research Society Conference.* February 29, Miami, FL.

19. Hathaway, D., et al. (1998). Post kidney transplantation quality of life prediction models. *Clinical Transplantation, 12,* 168-174.

20. International Society for Heart and Lung Transplantation. (2003). *Twenty-third Annual Meeting and Scientific Sessions: April 9-12, 2003, Vienna, Austria.*

21. Kaserman, D., & Barneett, A. (2002). *The U.S. organ procurement system: A prescription for reform.* Washington, DC: AEI Press.

22. Kirklin, J., & George, J. (2002) Immunosuppressive modalities. In J. Kirklin, J. Young, & D. McGiffin (Eds.), *Heart transplantation* (pp. 390-463). New York: Churchill Livingstone.

23. Kirklin, J., Young, J., McGiffin, D. (2002). *Heart transplantation.* New York: Churchill Livingstone.

24. Kuo, P., Schroeder, R., & Johnson, L. (2001). *Clinical management of the transplant patient.* New York: Arnold.

25. Landsteiner, K. (1928). Cell antigens and individual specificity. *Journal of Immunology, 15,* 589-600.

26. Limbos, M., Chan, C., & Kesten, S. (1997). Quality of life in female lung transplant candidates and recipients. *Chest, 112,* 1165-1174.

27. LoBiondo-Wood, G., et al. (1997). Impact of liver transplantation on quality of life: A longitudinal perspective. *Applied Nursing Research, 10*(1), 27-32.

28. Lucey, M., Neuberger, J., & Shaked, A. (2003). *Liver transplantation.* Georgetown, TX: Landes Bioscience.

29. Maddrey, W., Schiff, E., & Sorrell, M. (2001). *Transplantation of the liver* (3rd ed.). Philadelphia: Lippincott Williams & Wilkins.

30. Manzetti, J., et al. (1994). Exercise, education and quality of life in lung transplant candidates. *Journal of Heart and Lung Transplantation, 13,* 297-305.

31. Maurer, J., et al. (1998). International guidelines for the selection of lung transplant candidates. *Journal of Heart and Lung Transplantation, 17,* 703-709.

32. McCoy, J. & Argue, P. (1999). The role of the nurse in the donation process: A case study. *Critical Care Nurse, 2*(9), 48-52.

33. Medawar, P.B. (1945). A second study of the behavior and fate of skin homografts in rabbits: A report to the War Wounds Committee of the Medical Research Council. *Journal of Anatomy, 69,* 157-176.

34. Morris, P. (2001). *Kidney transplantation: Principles and practice* (5th ed.). Philadelphia: W. B. Saunders.

34a. National Kidney Foundation. Retrieved January 31, 2004, from http://www.kidney.org.

35. Norman, D., & Turka, L. (2001). *Primer on transplantation* (2nd ed.). Mt. Laurel, NJ: American Society of Transplantation.

36. Starzl, T.E., et al. (1963). Homotransplantation of the liver in humans. *Surgery, Gynecology and Obstetrics, 117,* 659-676.

37. Smith, S. (2002). Immunosuppressive therapies in organ transplantation. In S. Smith (Ed.). Available: http://www.medscape.com.viewarticle/437182.

38. Task Force on Organ Transplantation. (1986). *Organ transplantation: Issues and recommendations.* (HRP-0906976.) Rockville, MD: Health Resources and Services Administration.

39. Thiru, S., & Waldmann, H. (2001). *Pathology and immunology of transplantation and rejection.* Malden, MA: Blackwell Science.

40. United Network of Organ Sharing (UNOS). (September 14, 2003). *Annual report of the U.S. Scientific Registry for Transplant Recipients and Organ Procurement and Transplantation Network— Transplant data.* Richmond, VA: Author. Retrieved September 14, 2003, from http://www.optn.org/data/annualReport.asp

41. United Network of Organ Sharing (UNOS) OPTN and Scientific Registry Data. (2003). Retrieved September 14, 2003, from http://www.unos.org/data/.

42. Urden, L., Stacy, K., & Lough, M. (2002). Transplantation. In L. Urden, K. Stacey, & M. Lough (Eds.), *Thelan's critical care nursing: Diagnosis and management* (4th ed., pp 993-1026). St. Louis: Mosby.

43. White-Williams, C., Jalowic, A., & Grady, K. (1997). Gender differences in quality of life outcomes before and 6 months after heart transplantation. *Journal of Heart and Lung Transplantation, 16,* 100.

44. White-Williams, C. (2002). Lung transplantation. In S. Smith (Ed.) *Organ transplantation: Concepts, issues, practice, and outcomes.* Available: http://www.medscape.com/viewpublication704.

Management of Clients with Shock and Multisystem Disorders

Louise Nelson LaFramboise

evolve

Web Enhancements

http://evolve.elsevier.com/Black/medsurg/

Client Education Guide
Shock (Spanish Translation)
Concept Map
Understanding Septic Shock and Its Treatment

Ethical Issues in Nursing
Is There a Moral Difference Between Withholding and Withdrawing Treatments?
Appendix C
Laboratory Values of Clinical Importance in Medical-Surgical Nursing

SHOCK

Shock is a complex clinical syndrome that may occur at any time and in any place. It is a life-threatening condition often requiring team action by many health care providers, including nurses, physicians, laboratory technicians, pharmacists, and respiratory therapists. Shock causes thousands of deaths and unknown numbers of permanent injuries each year. The economic impact of shock is staggering, with annual health care costs for treatment of shock in the billions of dollars. Because shock is potentially lethal, debilitating, and costly, it is essential that nurses identify clients at risk for shock, recognize the early assessment findings indicating shock, and initiate appropriate interventions before shock ensues.

Shock is defined as failure of the circulatory system to maintain adequate perfusion of vital organs. Disorders leading to inadequate tissue perfusion result in decreased oxygenation at the cellular level. Inadequate oxygenation results in anaerobic cellular metabolism and accumulated waste products in cells. If this condition is untreated, cell and organ death occur.

Shock is commonly divided into three major classifications:

- Hypovolemic
- Cardiogenic
- Distributive

Hypovolemic shock is due to inadequate circulating blood volume resulting from hemorrhage with actual blood loss, burns with a loss of plasma proteins and fluid shifts, or dehydration with a loss of fluid volume. It is the most common type of shock and develops when the intravascular volume decreases to the point where compensatory mechanisms are unable to maintain organ and tissue perfusion.

Cardiogenic shock is due to inadequate pumping action of the heart because of primary cardiac muscle dysfunction or mechanical obstruction of blood flow caused by myocardial infarction (MI), valvular insufficiency caused by disease or trauma, cardiac dysrhythmias, or an obstructive condition, such as pericardial tamponade or pulmonary embolus. Cardiogenic shock occurs in 10% to 15% of all clients after MI and carries an associated mortality rate of up to 80%. Cardiogenic shock after an MI usually occurs when 40% or more of the myocardium has been damaged.

The term *obstructive shock* is sometimes used to include conditions that lead to a sudden obstruction of blood flow (i.e., cardiac tamponade, tension pneumo-

---

evolve *Be sure to check out the bonus material on the Evolve website and the CD-ROM, including free self-assessment exercises.*
http://evolve.elsevier.com/Black/medsurg/

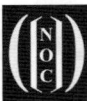

Nursing Outcomes Classification (NOC)
for Nursing Diagnoses—Clients in Shock

Ineffective Tissue Perfusion: Cerebral, Cardiopulmonary, Renal, Gastrointestinal, Peripheral
Bowel Elimination
Circulation Status
Cognitive Ability
Electrolyte and Acid-Base Balance
Fluid Balance
Hydration
Neurologic Status

Neurologic Status: Consciousness
Neurologic Status: Central Motor
  Control
Pain Level
Sensory Function: Cutaneous
Swallowing Status
Tissue Integrity: Skin and Mucous
  Membrane
Tissue Perfusion: Cerebral
Tissue Perfusion: Pulmonary

Tissue Perfusion: Cardiac
Tissue Perfusion: Abdominal Organ
Tissue Perfusion: Peripheral
Urinary Elimination
Vital Signs Status
Interrupted Family Processes
Caregiver Emotional Health
Depression Control
Family Coping
Family Normalization

---

thorax, pulmonary embolism). Obstructive causes are discussed under the topic of cardiogenic shock because the ability of the heart to pump effectively is the primary problem.

Distributive shock (also called *vasogenic shock*) is due to changes in blood vessel tone that increase the size of the vascular space without an increase in the circulating blood volume. The result is a relative hypovolemia (total fluid volume remains the same but is redistributed). Distributive shock is further divided into three types:

- *Anaphylactic shock,* a severe hypersensitivity reaction resulting in massive systemic vasodilation
- *Neurogenic shock,* or interference with nervous system control of the blood vessels, such as with spinal cord injury (especially cervical spine injury), spinal anesthesia, or severe vasovagal reactions caused by pain or psychic trauma
- *Septic shock,* caused by a release of vasoactive substances

Some amount of neurogenic shock is seen with all spinal cord injuries. More dramatic cases of neurogenic shock are seen with cervical spine injuries. The duration of neurogenic shock is usually 1 to 6 weeks, as long as there is no irreparable cord injury. The incidence of septic and anaphylactic shock is variable. Clients who are at risk for either type of shock should be monitored closely.

Etiology and Risk Factors
All causes of shock focus on some component of blood distribution throughout the body. There can be an insufficient quantity of blood (hypovolemic shock), an incompetent pump (cardiogenic shock), or an ineffective delivery of blood (distributive shock).

Hypovolemic Shock
The primary event precipitating hypovolemic shock is a large reduction in the circulating blood volume so that the body's metabolic needs cannot be met. Hypovolemic shock may be due to a loss of plasma or blood. Condi-

tions that may cause a reduction in the circulating volume include hemorrhage, burns, and dehydration.

Health promotion activities to prevent hypovolemic shock include client education to avoid injuries that would put someone at risk for hypovolemic shock (see Client Education Guide on Shock on p. 2473). Health maintenance activities are the use of oxygen and maintenance of fluid and electrolyte balance. To restore health, monitor the client with telemetry and hemodynamic monitoring, and give vasoactive medications and blood and fluid replacements as ordered.

Hemorrhage. Hemorrhage is the loss of blood. Clinical manifestations may begin to appear with a blood volume deficit of 15% to 25%, or about 500 to 1500 ml in an adult with a normal circulating volume. Shock fully develops if a previously healthy client loses about one third of the normal circulating blood volume of 5 L.

The loss of smaller amounts of blood may cause shock in clients less able to compensate rapidly (e.g., older people with decreased vascular tone and impaired cardiac function). The extent to which shock develops after blood loss also depends on the length of time over which the blood loss occurs. Clients experiencing slow blood loss over a period of days or weeks tolerate their blood loss better than clients whose blood loss occurs rapidly over minutes or hours. Hypovolemic shock following trauma is typically the result of hemorrhage. The classes of hemorrhage and the associated assessment findings are listed in Table 83-1.

Burns. Hypovolemic shock produced by burns occurs most often in people with large partial-thickness or full-thickness burns. It is caused primarily by a shift of plasma from the vascular space into the interstitial space. In addition to these fluid losses or shifts, the client may have cardiac dysfunction that is due to the presence of *myocardial depressant factor* (MDF), a polypeptide (see later). MDF affects the contractility of cardiac muscle by depressing myocardial muscle function. The result is impaired cardiac output, even in the presence of a nor-

TABLE 83-1	*Assessment Findings and Classifications of Acute Hemorrhage**			
Assessment Finding	**Class I**	**Class II**	**Class III**	**Class IV**
Blood loss (%)	<15	15-30	30-40	>40
Blood loss (ml)	<750	750-1500	1500-2000	>2000
Pulse rate/min	<100	>100	>120	>140
Respiratory rate/min	Normal (14-20)	20-30	30-40	>35
Blood pressure	Normal	Normal	Decreased	Decreased
Pulse pressure	Normal or increased	Decreased	Decreased	Decreased
Central nervous system/ mental status	Slightly anxious	Mildly anxious	Anxious, confused	Confused, lethargic
Urine output (ml/hr)	>30	20-30	5-15	Negligible
Intravenous fluid replacement	Crystalloid at 3 ml/ 1 ml of blood loss	Crystalloid at 3 ml/ 1 ml of blood loss	Crystalloid plus blood at 3 ml/1 ml of blood loss	Crystalloid plus blood at 3 ml/1 ml of blood loss

Data from American College of Surgeons Committee on Trauma. (1997). *Advanced trauma life support student manual* (p. 98). Chicago: Author.
*Assumes a normal 70-kg man.

mal circulating volume. Shock related to burns is discussed in Chapter 52.

Other causes of hypovolemic shock that may produce fluid shifts similar to those in burns include nephrotic syndrome, severe crush injuries, starvation, surgery, and conditions causing plasma fluids to accumulate in the abdominal cavity (e.g., cirrhosis of the liver, pancreatitis, bowel obstruction).

Dehydration. Shock may also occur from either reduced oral fluid intake or significant fluid losses (e.g., rigorous exercise causing fluid loss from sweating and insensible fluid loss through the respiratory tract and hot environments). Loss of fluid, leading to dehydration-induced hypovolemic shock, may occur in people with excessive urine output or prolonged vomiting or diarrhea. Clients with chronic illnesses, especially older people, may be at increased risk because of impaired recognition of thirst or an inability to obtain fluids, inadequate maintenance of chronic conditions (i.e., increased blood glucose levels with diabetes), or inadequate monitoring of therapeutic regimens (i.e., diuretic-induced dehydration). With prolonged fluid deficit, all compartments—intravascular, interstitial, and intracellular—are depleted.

Cardiogenic Shock

Cardiogenic shock results primarily from an inability of heart muscle to function adequately or mechanical obstructions of blood flow to or from the heart. As with other causes of shock, the lack of blood flow decreases tissue and organ perfusion.

Myocardial Infarction. Impaired heart muscle action is most often caused by MI (see Chapter 60). The area of dead or dying tissue that occurs with infarction impairs contractility of the myocardium, and the cardiac output decreases. Impaired myocardial contractility may also occur with blunt cardiac trauma, cardiomyopathy, and heart failure.

Prevention of cardiogenic shock related to MI begins with health promotion activities directed at client education for decreasing the risk factors associated with coronary artery disease (e.g., increasing exercise and modifying dietary intake). Supportive oxygenation and administration of inotropic agents and vasodilators are health maintenance activities. An intra-aortic balloon pump (IABP) (see Chapter 58) may be needed for health restoration.

Clients in cardiogenic shock may also develop some degree of hypovolemic shock. This is most often due to the therapeutic use of diuretics or to edema in the extremities or other dependent areas (caused by inadequate cardiac pumping activity and venous congestion).

Obstructive Conditions. Several types of mechanical obstructions to blood flow may cause cardiogenic shock:

1. *Large pulmonary embolism.* An *embolus* is usually the result of a blood clot that breaks loose in a person with deep vein thrombosis (DVT). This embolus travels through the venous system to the right side of the heart and into the pulmonary artery. The size of the embolus determines at what point it lodges in the pulmonary artery. A large embolus can inhibit perfusion of a major portion of the lung field, resulting in an increased workload for the right ventricle.
2. *Pericardial tamponade* is an accumulation of blood or fluid in the pericardial space that compresses the myocardium and interferes with the ability of the myocardium to expand.
3. A *tension pneumothorax* is a significant amount of air in the pleural space compressing the heart and great vessels, thus interfering with venous return to the heart.

Other Causes of Cardiogenic Shock. Additional causes of cardiogenic shock include (1) cardiac valvular insufficiency from trauma or disease, (2) myocardial aneurysms (usually due to previous MI or congenital abnormalities), (3) rupture of a valvular papillary muscle, (4) ventricle rupture, (5) aortic stenosis, (6) mitral regurgitation, and (7) cardiac dysrhythmias.

Clients with hypovolemic shock are also at risk for cardiogenic shock. The myocardium normally receives its blood supply during diastole. When the heart rate increases to compensate for the decreased volume and to increase cardiac output, diastole is shortened, leading to insufficient time for the coronary arteries to fill with blood. Because these arteries supply blood to the myocardium, the myocardial oxygen supply is impaired. The increased heart rate also increases the need of the myocardium for oxygen, predisposing the myocardium to injury because of the decreased blood flow and resultant decreased oxygen supply. In addition, the decreased venous return associated with hypovolemia results in decreased coronary artery perfusion and inadequate oxygenation of the myocardium.

Finally, shock results in the release of MDF and lactic acid, which depresses myocardial function.

Distributive (Vasogenic) Shock

Distributive shock results from inadequate vascular tone. Blood volume remains normal, but the size of the vascular space increases dramatically because of massive vasodilation. The result is maldistribution of the blood because of decreased blood pressure (BP) and lack of blood returning to the heart, which is why it is often referred to as "relative" hypovolemia. The volume of blood remains constant, but the blood has pooled because of increased capacity of the vascular system.

After extensive vasodilation, the BP, return of venous blood to the heart, and cardiac output are decreased. As with other forms of shock, tissue anoxia and cell destruction result. The massive vasodilation present with distributive shock has several major causes.

Acute Allergic Reaction (Anaphylactic Shock). Anaphylactic shock occurs as a result of an acute allergic reaction from exposure to a substance to which the client has been sensitized. Common sensitizing agents are penicillin, penicillin derivatives, bee stings, chocolate, strawberries, peanuts, snake venom, iodine-based contrast for x-ray studies, foods, and nonsteroidal anti-inflammatory drugs (NSAIDs).

Re-exposure to the foreign substance results in the offending antigen binding to previously made immunoglobulins (i.e., IgE) located on the mast cell. This binding causes the release of several chemical mediators from the cell, such as histamine, platelet-activating factor, leukotrienes, and prostaglandins (see Chapter 78). Manifestations include massive vasodilation, urticaria (hives), laryngeal edema, and bronchial constriction. Without prompt treatment, a person with anaphylactic shock will die of cardiovascular collapse and respiratory failure.

To help prevent the onset of anaphylactic shock, teach clients to avoid precipitators and to use an epinephrine injection (e.g., EpiPen). Encouraging clients to wear medical alert bracelets and to seek allergy desensitization also decreases their potential for anaphylactic shock.

Spinal Cord Injury (Neurogenic Shock). With injury to the cervical spine, the autonomic nervous system is affected. Below the level of injury, there is blocking of sympathetic nervous stimulation and the parasympathetic system goes unopposed. This unopposed stimulation causes vasodilation, decreased venous return, decreased cardiac output, and decreased tissue perfusion. Teaching clients safety measures may help prevent spinal cord injury and neurogenic shock.

Health maintenance actions are to protect the client's spine, maintain the client's airway and breathing, provide circulatory support, and provide for thermoregulation. Health restoration involves rehabilitation when the client is stable.

Infection (Septic Shock). *Sepsis* is the systemic response to infection. The process begins with the growth of various microorganisms at the site of infection. Organisms may invade the bloodstream directly (leading to positive blood cultures) or may remain in one area. The organisms release various substances into the bloodstream. These substances include structural parts of the organism, such as endotoxins and elements synthesized by them called *exotoxins*. Once these substances are released into the body, they activate the complement cascade, and a complex shock picture occurs. Septic shock is lethal. With a mortality rate of up to 50%, it is the 11th leading cause of death in the United States.

Encouraging clients to treat infections immediately and completely may help reduce the incidence of septic shock. Older and immunocompromised clients should be monitored closely for infection, and treatment should begin immediately when infection is diagnosed. Shock is a serious development. Identify high-risk clients, and implement measures to prevent shock whenever possible.

Pathophysiology

Adequate circulating volume is dependent on three interrelated components of the cardiovascular system: (1) the heart, (2) vascular tone, and (3) blood volume. A minor impairment in one component is compensated for by the other two. Prolonged or severe impairments lead to shock. Some of the problems with decreased organ and tissue perfusion in shock are due to failure of the normal mechanisms (see the Concept Map on Understanding Septic Shock and Its Treatment on p. 2447).

Blood flows throughout the body because of its driving pressure as it leaves the left ventricle (LV). Nowhere else in the cardiovascular system is blood under as high a pressure as it is in the LV. About 100 ml of blood (called *stroke volume*) leaves the LV at systolic BP about 80 times

CONCEPT MAP

Understanding Septic Shock and Its Treatment

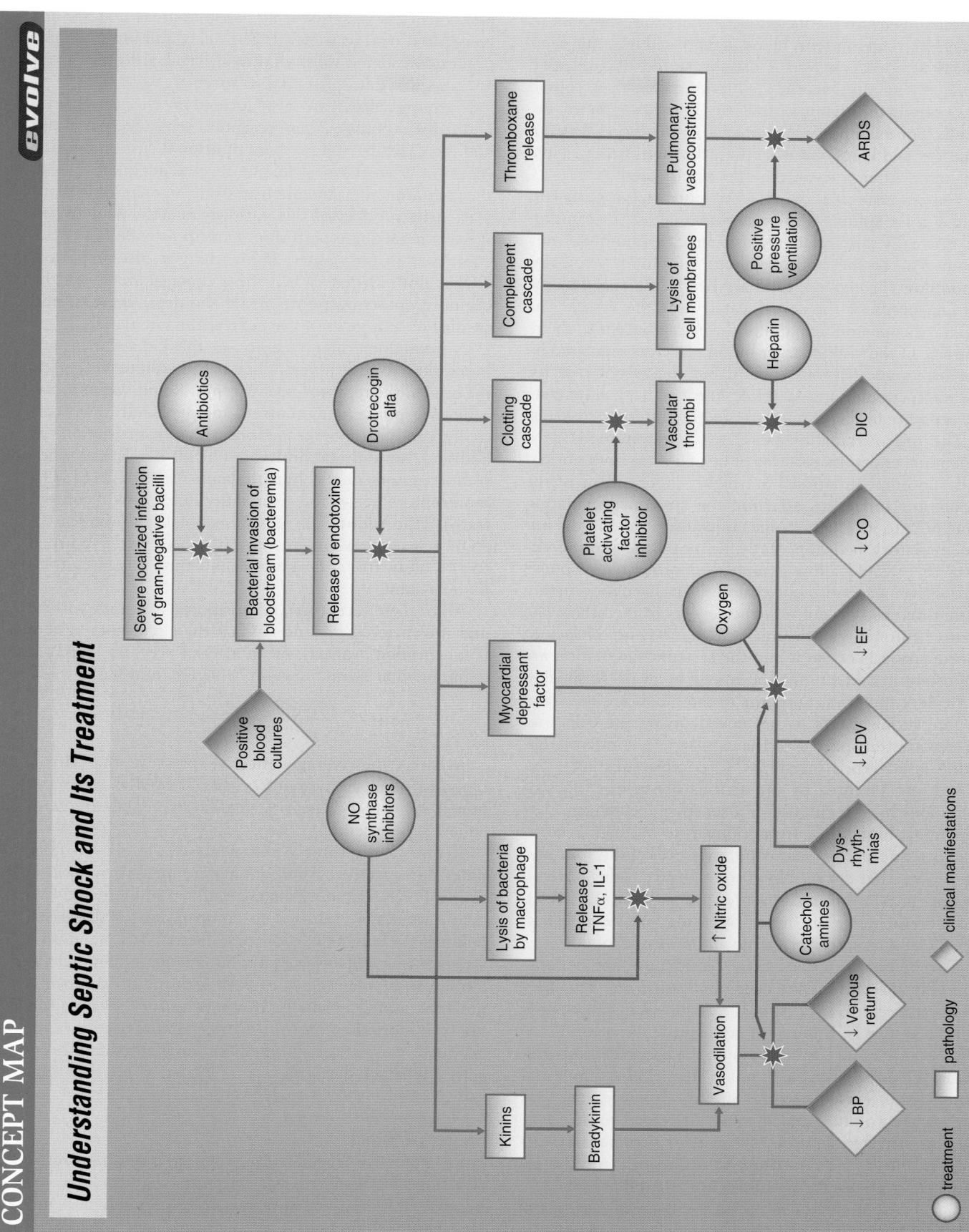

ARDS, Adult (acute) respiratory distress syndrome; BP, blood pressure; CO, cardiac output; DIC, disseminated intravascular coagulation; EDV, end diastolic volume; EF, ejection fraction; IL-1, interleukin 1; NO, nitric oxide; TNF, tumor necrosis factor.

a minute. Because the metabolic demands are continuous rather than intermittent, blood is delivered into muscular walled arterioles, where it can be stored and released more consistently into the capillaries. From there, blood flows slowly through the capillaries that have greatest demand. (For example, when you run, more blood flows to your legs and lungs and less flows to your gastrointestinal [GI] tract. After you eat, the opposite is true.)

The microcirculation has the potential capacity to hold a great volume of blood. Nonetheless, the capillaries normally are relatively ischemic, containing only about 5% of the body's volume of blood. Typically, blood flow through the capillary bed is influenced by the varying needs of the cells located near the vessel. The capillaries open on demand of the cells adjacent to them. The size of the body's larger blood vessels is regulated by the autonomic nervous system, but this is not true for the microcirculation. Arteriole and capillary sphincters are separate mechanisms governed by different controls.

The microcirculation is relatively autonomous as a functional entity. Its patterns of behavior (in both normal and abnormal situations) are highly independent of the vasomotor influences affecting the systemic circulation lying next to it. The systemic circulatory bed and the microcirculatory bed apparently do not have sensing devices that would allow a unified, coordinated response throughout the entire circulation. Thus events occurring within one bed do not influence events in the other. The relative autonomy of the microcirculation and the lack of coordination between it and the systemic circulation are important in determining the course of events in shock.

In the capillaries, nutrients in the blood are delivered to interstitial spaces to be picked up by the cells and wastes are transported to the capillary. The microcirculation is governed locally by vasoactive substances released into the area by the actions of various types of cells. This local regulation is a sensitive mechanism that can adjust blood flow from moment to moment according to tissue needs. The capillaries eventually join and meet veins that deliver blood to the heart. Veins have no muscle and are very low-pressure systems in which blood returns to the heart by using one-way valves. Veins can also store very large amounts of blood.

Two major receptors sense blood flow and volume and help the body make needed adjustments. The *arterial baroreceptor,* located in the aortic arch, senses how full the system is. If pressure in the muscular arterioles is low because of increased demand, the baroreceptor stimulates the sympathetic nervous system. This stimulation results in increased cardiac output, by increasing rate and stroke volume, and through increased muscle tension on the arteriole walls (*systemic* or *peripheral vascular resistance*). If BP was low to begin with, there is insufficient pressure for perfusion at the capillary end.

On the right side of the heart is the *atrial baroreceptor,* which measures the fluid volume returning to the heart. It also stimulates the sympathetic nervous system

and constricts vessels storing blood in areas that are not considered vital to survival. The heart and brain are the organs considered most vital to survival. All other areas are considered less essential to survival.

Chemoreceptors are also located in the aortic arch and carotid bodies. These receptors sense decreased pH and increased partial pressure of arterial carbon dioxide ($PaCO_2$). When tissues do not receive adequate blood, they maintain their metabolism using an anaerobic pathway. A by-product of this pathway is lactic acid. When there is inadequate perfusion, carbon dioxide (CO_2) accumulates in the tissues. If breathing is also impaired, CO_2 is not exhaled. When these changes are sensed by chemoreceptors, respiratory rate and depth increase and cardiac output increases to correct the imbalance.

A juxtaglomerular receptor in the kidney measures blood flow to the kidney. When blood volume decreases, the cells in the receptor release renin. Renin begins a cascade of response (angiotensin I, angiotensin II) that eventually produces potent peripheral vasoconstriction. In addition, antidiuretic hormone (ADH) is released when osmoreceptors in the hypothalamus are triggered. Osmoreceptors sense the osmolality (i.e., how "concentrated" the blood is). When osmolality is increased, ADH release prevents diuresis, increases water returned to the body from the kidney, and thus increases total blood volume.

All of these receptors and hormones maintain volume and thus arterial pressure. When the circulatory system is functioning properly, mean arterial pressure (MAP) is maintained at normal levels (70 to 105 mm Hg):

$$MAP = \frac{(Systolic + [2 \times Diastolic])}{3}$$

MAP is the average effective pressure that drives blood through the systemic organs. If MAP is not maintained at normal or near-normal levels, tissues are inadequately perfused.

If one of the three components of circulation fails, other parts of the system initiate compensatory mechanisms. For example, vasoconstriction and increased cardiac output may be used to compensate for decreased volume. As long as two of these factors can maintain a satisfactory compensatory action, adequate blood circulation can be maintained even though the third factor is not functioning normally. If compensatory mechanisms fail or if more than one of the three factors necessary for adequate circulation malfunction, circulatory failure results and shock develops.

Stages of Shock

Nonprogressive Stage. During the initial or nonprogressive stage of shock, cardiac output is slightly decreased because of loss of actual or relative blood volume. During this stage, the body's compensatory mechanisms can maintain BP within a normal to low-normal range and can maintain tissue perfusion to the vital organs. During the compensatory phase, the systemic circulation and microcirculation work together. Both undergo a major readjustment in which their activities are coordinated to preserve the entire system. Figure 83-1 illustrates these readjustments.

Progressive Stage. If shock and the compensatory vasoconstriction persist, shock progresses as the body begins to decompensate and the systemic circulation and microcirculation no longer work in unison. As vasoconstriction continues, the supply of oxygenated blood to the tissues is reduced. This results in anaerobic metabolism and lactic acidosis. Acidosis and the increasing PaCO$_2$ cause the microcirculation to dilate. This dilation causes decreased venous return and decreased circulation of reoxygenated blood.

Lactic acidosis also causes increased capillary permeability and relaxation of the capillary sphincters. Relaxation of the sphincters allows increased blood in the capillaries and increased capillary pressure. This increased pressure along with the increased capillary permeability allows fluid to move out of the vascular space and back into the tissues. In doing so, the microcirculation has reversed its pattern and is trying to secure for itself (and the tissue it supplies) more of the limited supply of available blood. Thus the blood supply is progressively retained in the capillary bed and blood pools in the microcirculation. Because the cells demand greater perfusion time, many or most of the capillaries remain open at any one time, increasing the vascular space in the microcirculation.

Increased vascular capacity, decreased blood volume, or decreased heart action reduces the MAP. In turn, the pressure gradient for the venous return of blood decreases. This also contributes to venous pooling of blood, decreased venous return to the heart, and decreased cardiac output.

Because there are no feedback systems within the body to change this pattern, the cycle of events becomes progressively more severe. Eventually, the circulation is totally disrupted. Once the vascular space enlarges (because of vasodilation of the microcirculation), even a normal blood volume cannot fill all these small vessels and the larger ones as well. The result is a low central venous pressure (CVP), except in cardiogenic shock, and inadequate venous return to the right side of the heart, with a further decrease in cardiac output.

This resultant decrease in circulating volume and capillary flow does not allow adequate perfusion and oxygenation of the vital organs. With the prolonged decrease in capillary blood flow, the tissues become hypoxic. This cycle of events is illustrated in Figure 83-2.

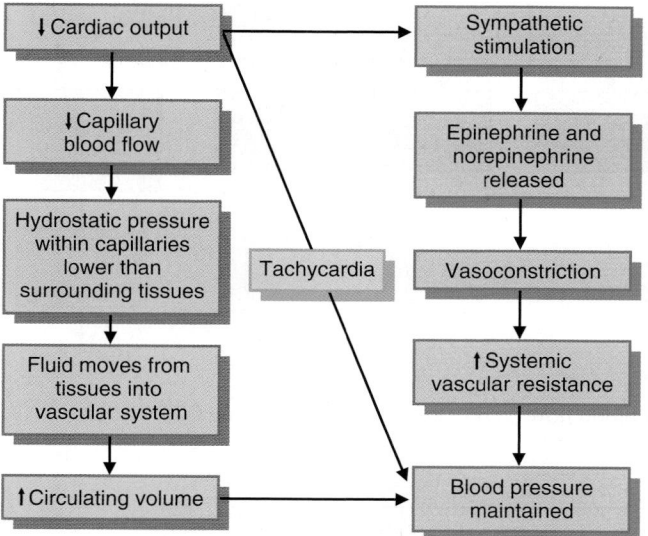

FIGURE 83-1 Nonprogressive stage of shock. Regardless of the cause, a decreased cardiac output is generally the stimulus that precipitates the body's response to compensate for the hypovolemia (relative or actual) to maintain blood pressure.

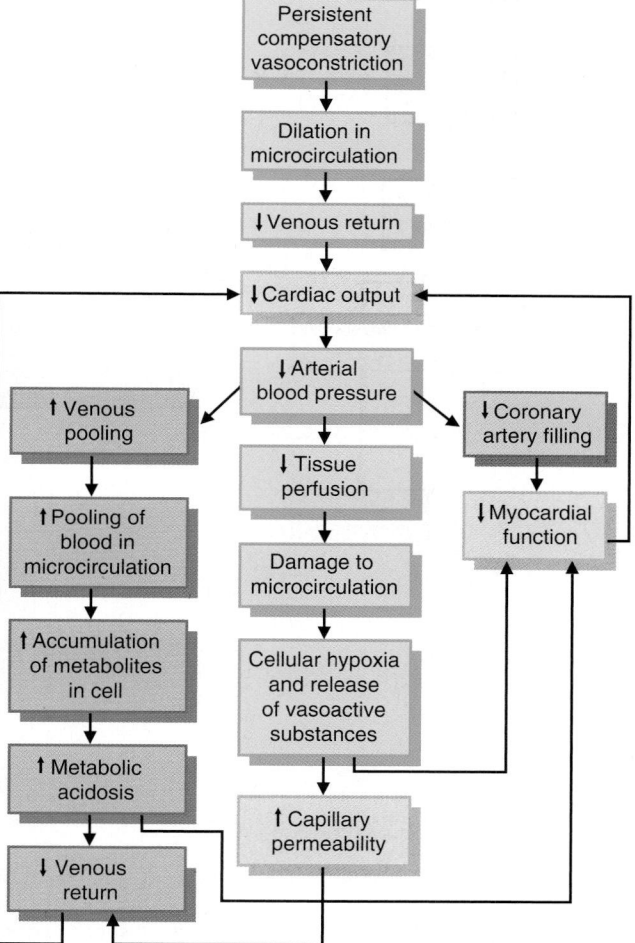

FIGURE 83-2 Vicious cycle of events occurring in the progressive stage of shock. The shock syndrome can be initiated anywhere in the cycle, depending on the precipitating cause (e.g., impaired myocardial function due to myocardial infarction, blood loss due to trauma, or the release of vasoactive toxins due to sepsis). Hypovolemic shock resulting from blood loss, for example, results in decreased arterial blood pressure, setting in motion a cascade of events that worsen the shock state.

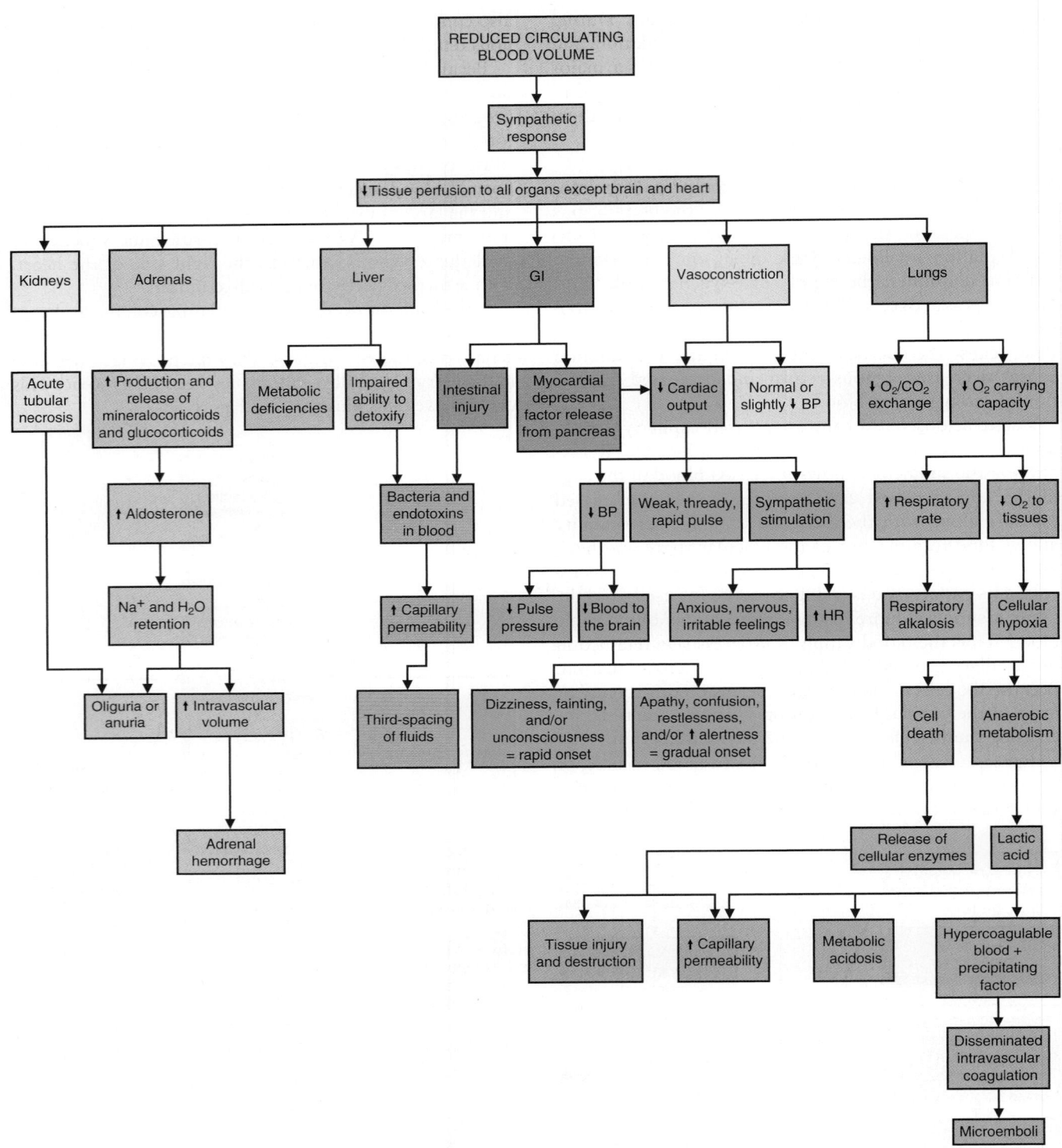

FIGURE 83-3 Systemic effects of shock. The lack of blood flow is compensated by constricting flow to nonessential organs (all organs except the brain and heart).

Irreversible Stage. The irreversible stage of shock occurs if the cycle of inadequate tissue perfusion is not interrupted. The shock state becomes progressively more severe, even though the initial cause of the shock is not itself becoming more severe. Cellular ischemia and necrosis lead to organ failure and death.

Systemic Effects of Shock
Shock affects every system within the body. Equally important to understanding the cellular level of shock is understanding what happens to the various organs (Figure 83-3).

Respiratory System. Getting oxygen in (*ventilation*) and delivering oxygenated blood to the tissues (*perfusion*) are crucial for survival. Shock produces prolonged circulatory insufficiency. This leads to variable and inadequate perfusion of certain organs and tissues, particularly at the microcirculation level. Such circulatory deprivation results in tissue hypoxia and anoxia. Hypoxia and anoxia can be tolerated for a short time. As the time lengthens, the chances of recovery diminish. A lack of oxygen appears to initiate the irreversible stage of shock. The greater the difference between the amount of oxygen available and the amount needed, the more rapidly irreversible shock develops. If sufficient oxygen is available to the cells to meet the body's needs, irreversible shock is less likely to occur.

Respiratory failure continues to be a major cause of death in shock, despite many advances in shock prevention, early recognition, and management. The magnitude of this problem surfaced during the Vietnam War era when soldiers sustaining massive injuries and profound blood loss were successfully resuscitated only to die several days later of adult (acute) respiratory distress syndrome (ARDS) (see Chapter 65). Although ARDS remains the greatest contributing factor to respiratory failure, other causes of respiratory failure during shock include aspiration and loss of neurologic control of breathing.

Acid-Base Balance. To function properly, cells depend on adequate circulation to receive nutrients, electrolytes, and oxygen and to remove waste products. Oxygen and nutrients are essential to life because they make possible chemical transformations resulting in the synthesis of adenosine triphosphate (ATP). ATP is the ultimate source of energy for life processes.

When oxygen is not present, ATP is produced through a different set of reactions called *anaerobic metabolism*. Although production of ATP in this manner is a useful emergency measure, it is inefficient compared with the normal process of *aerobic* (oxidative) *metabolism*. Anaerobic metabolism produces anaerobic metabolites, such as lactic acid (which causes intracellular acidity with consequent cellular damage) and substrates of the adenylic acid system (which depress the heart) (Figure 83-4).

In response to the chemoreceptors sensing decreased pH, the rate and depth of respirations are increased to "blow off" (exhale) CO_2 to compensate for the metabolic acidosis. This results in respiratory alkalosis. However, the cellular hypoxia is caused not by inadequate ventilation but rather by inadequate tissue perfusion. Therefore the increased respiratory effort does little to correct the problem.

Because lactic acid is not exhaled, it accumulates in tissue fluids, which thus become increasingly acidic. Eventually, metabolic acidosis is produced. During metabolic acidosis, blood pH and bicarbonate levels decrease.

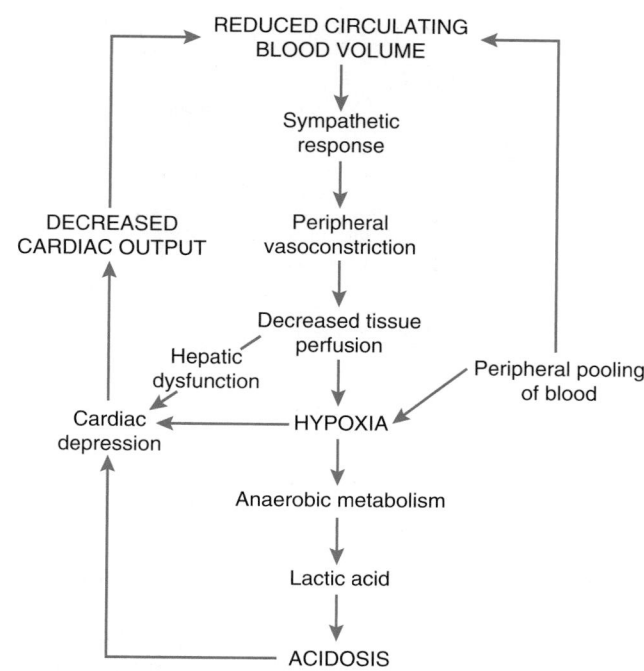

FIGURE 83-4 Shock leads to tissue hypoxia, with blockage of normal aerobic metabolism. Lactic acid accumulates, resulting in tissue acidosis. (Modified from Condon, R.E., & Nyhus, L.M. [1978]. *Manual of surgical therapeutics* [4th ed.]. Boston: Little, Brown.)

Pyruvate, lactate, phosphate, and sulfate levels increase. Unless circulation is restored, the acidotic reaction resulting from metabolic acidosis ultimately kills the cells. The buildup of lactic acid causes such a severe local acidosis that cellular enzymes are inactivated. As a result, the cells soon die.

Respiratory alkalosis or *respiratory acidosis* (induced by pulmonary ventilatory or diffusion changes) may be superimposed on the metabolic acidosis. As perfusion and oxygen delivery to the tissues decrease, cellular energy production decreases. To compensate, cells increase anaerobic metabolism, which results in the buildup of lactic acid in the cell. As the pH of the cells decreases, lysosomes within the cell explode, releasing powerful, destructive enzymes. These enzymes destroy the cellular membrane and digest the cell contents. Once this process begins, the cellular changes are irreversible. The final result is cellular death (Figure 83-5).

Lysosomal Enzymes. Lysosomal enzymes are released from dead cells undergoing autolysis. They are also released just before cell death produced by cellular anoxia or some other form of injury. For example, these enzymes may be liberated as a result of trauma and endotoxins. During shock, the disruption of lysosomes and the release of their enzymes seem to occur in the liver. This is one mechanism of cell destruction resulting from

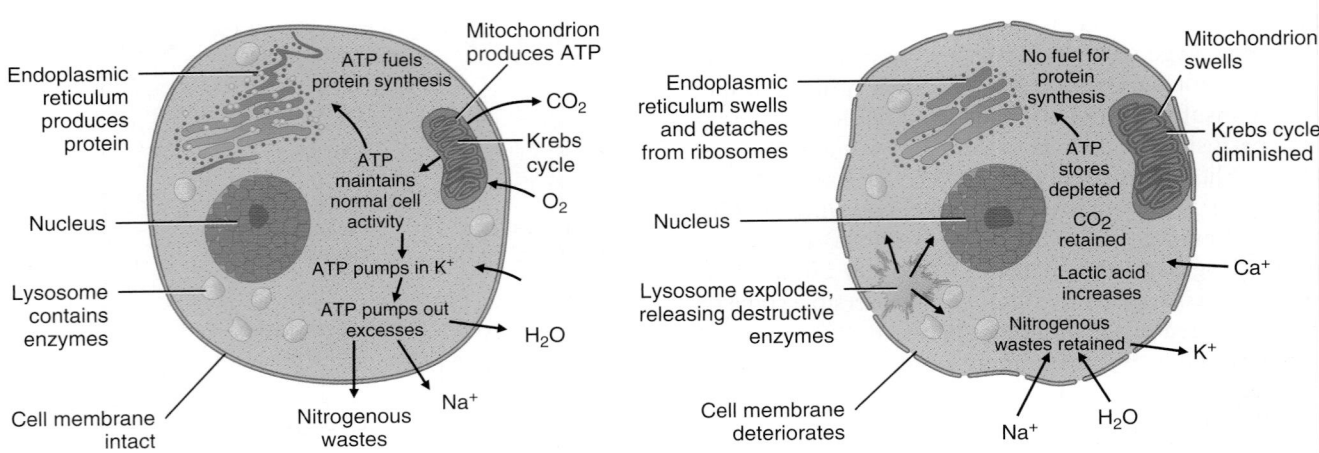

FIGURE 83-5 *Left,* Normal cell. *Right,* Alterations in cell function during late shock. *ATP,* Adenosine triphosphate; Ca^+, calcium; CO_2, carbon dioxide; H_2O, water; Na^+, sodium; O_2, oxygen.

prolonged shock. The presence of hepatic lysosomal active enzymes in the bloodstream, along with blocking of the *reticuloendothelial system* (RES), may contribute to death from shock. Blockade of the RES drastically reduces its capacity to clear bacteria from the bloodstream.

Lysosomal enzymes become most active in an acid pH range. Thus as long as normal acid-base balance is maintained within the body, these enzymes are repressed within normal cells. During shock, however, the accompanying metabolic acidosis accelerates the activation of these enzymes in hypoxic tissues. The activation of lysosomal hydrolases within the cells and their release into the circulation markedly exacerbate the tissue injury that occurs during shock. The release of active lysosomal proteases and other enzymes from damaged tissue into the bloodstream and their action on extracellular and intracellular structures probably contribute to the progression of injury from cell to cell.

Cardiovascular System

Myocardial Deterioration. As shock progresses, the heart deteriorates. Cardiac deterioration is one of the major causes of death in shock. Although the exact cause of myocardial depression is unclear, much attention has been directed at MDF. MDF, a polypeptide with vasoactive properties, is released in response to ischemia of the GI tract. It causes a significant reduction in cardiac output, even in the presence of a normal circulating volume of blood. Another factor contributing to cardiac deterioration may be myocardial zonal lesions, which appear in the myocardium after ischemia or infarction. Cells in these areas do not fully repolarize and thus interfere with the usual efficient electrical conduction in the heart, which results in impaired contraction and possibly cardiac failure.

Cardiac depression is often compensated for by the large cardiac reserve of a normal person. Because of this reserve, the heart can deteriorate to less than one third

(sometimes less than one fifth) of its normal pumping strength without measurable evidence of cardiac failure.

Disseminated Intravascular Coagulation. During shock, tissue hypoxia results from the sluggish movement of blood in the capillaries. Anaerobic metabolism begins, increasing the production of lactic acid. The slow-moving acidic blood is hypercoagulable; however, it does not coagulate unless a clot-initiating factor is present. Such factors include bacterial endotoxins and thromboplastin of red blood cells (liberated by hemolysis). Hemolysis (destruction of red blood cells with the liberation of hemoglobin) accompanies trauma, especially when massive crushing injury occurs. When any of these factors is present, along with the stagnant, acidic blood of shock, widespread intravascular clotting may occur in the vessels. This disorder is called *disseminated intravascular coagulation* (DIC) (see Chapter 77).

DIC is associated with multiple thrombi or emboli that are deposited in the microvascular circulation, with resultant organ obstruction and increased tissue ischemia. As blood attempts to flow through partially obstructed vessels, widespread hemolysis may occur. When red blood cells are destroyed, again hemoglobin is liberated. Anemia occurs because the liberated hemoglobin is excreted by the kidneys.

Because of the inappropriate clotting that occurs with DIC, the body attempts to reverse the process by breaking down clots. However, clots are destroyed throughout the body, not just the inappropriately formed clots. This results in bleeding in areas previously sealed by clots (i.e., venipuncture sites, vascular leaks in the brain). As DIC progresses, clotting factors are depleted, causing an inability for normal clot formation in the presence of bleeding.

Treatment of the precipitating cause, anticoagulant therapy, and replacement of clotting factors must be started as soon as possible for maximal effectiveness.

DIC is a serious complication that occurs in almost 40% of clients in septic shock and is often fatal.

Vasoconstriction. Sluggish circulation also results in decreased removal of CO_2 from the tissues. Increased CO_2 dilates arterioles located in active tissues and constricts those in nonactive tissues. Because of the heart's increased activity, excessive CO_2 is produced in the myocardium. Increased CO_2 directly dilates the coronary arteries leading to the myocardium, which allows the myocardium to receive more arterial blood. CO_2 is also a powerful stimulant of the vasoconstrictor center in the sympathetic nervous system. With vasoconstriction of nonactive tissues, blood is shunted to the more active tissues, which have a greater immediate need.

Vasoactive Substances. Vasoactive substances are highly variable in promoting vasoconstriction or vasodilation in a person experiencing shock. The influence they exert may be altered by factors such as pH, the specific tissue (e.g., heart, lung), the presence of drugs or other substances, serum electrolyte levels, and the sensitivity of the end organ.

Catecholamines. Catecholamines, such as epinephrine and norepinephrine, are present early in shock and are related to the fight-or-flight response. Their general effects are to increase blood flow to the brain, heart, and striated (skeletal) muscle and to decrease blood flow to the skin, kidneys, and splanchnic bed. Although the initial effect of vasoconstriction in the skin, kidneys, and splanchnic bed (GI tract) increases the intravascular volume, sustained vasoconstriction contributes to stagnant hypoxia and cellular death.

Histamine. Histamine causes vasodilation, increased capillary permeability, bronchoconstriction, coronary vasodilation, and cutaneous reactions (flares, wheals). The effects of histamine are especially obvious in anaphylactic and septic shock.

Vasoactive Polypeptides. Among the more important vasoactive polypeptides that appear to play significant roles in shock are the following:

1. *Bradykinin.* A kinin peptide, bradykinin produces vasodilation, increased capillary permeability, smooth muscle relaxation, pain, and infiltration of an area with leukocytes. Kinins appear to be most active in late shock. They may be a factor in the development of pulmonary insufficiency associated with shock.
2. *Angiotensin.* Angiotensin results from the action of renal renin on angiotensinogen. This potent substance causes vasoconstriction and increased vascular resistance. Although similar to norepinephrine in effect, angiotensin may produce fewer negative effects. Its role in sodium and water retention (through the stimulation of aldosterone secretion) is discussed under Adrenal Response.
3. *MDF.* MDF is a vasoactive polypeptide that contributes to cardiac failure in clients in shock by depressing cardiac muscle contraction.

Neuroendocrine System

General Adaptation Syndrome Response. Neuroendocrine responses during shock are defensive reactions that occur during the body's stage of resistance in the general adaptation syndrome (GAS). Because the length of the stage of resistance varies among people and is determined by a body's ability to compensate for its deficiencies, one person may be able to combat shock longer than another. For example, a previously healthy person may have a longer stage of resistance against shock compared than a client who is debilitated before shock develops.

Adrenal Response. Basic features of the neuroendocrine responses include (1) the release of epinephrine and norepinephrine from the adrenal medulla (which re- sults in increased respiratory and heart rates, increased BP, increased blood flow to organs, decreased blood flow to peripheral tissues) and (2) the release of mineralocorticoids (which control fluid and electrolyte balance) and glucocorticoids (which affect energy and tissue resistance) from the adrenal cortex.

Increased production of adrenocortical mineralocorticoid hormones occurs. The main mineralocorticoids—aldosterone and desoxycorticosterone—help increase intravascular fluid volume by stimulating the kidneys to retain sodium and water. The renal tubular conservation of sodium occurs with any type of fluid loss or blood volume depletion. Aldosterone is essential to conservation of sodium. Because water is retained in the body along with sodium, urine excretion is diminished during shock. This fluid is retained in the bloodstream to increase blood volume. Increasing the volume of blood in this way is aimed at increasing venous return, cardiac output, and BP.

Pituitary Response. Of major importance in regulating water and sodium balance are aldosterone and ADH, also called *vasopressin.* ADH is produced by the posterior pituitary gland. The osmolality (osmotic concentration) of blood increases with dehydration. This stimulates osmoreceptors in the hypothalamus to release ADH from the posterior pituitary gland. Via the blood, the ADH is carried to the kidneys where it causes the body to retain water.

Various components of the sympathoadrenal (sympathetic part of the autonomic nervous system and adrenal medulla) response to a major stressor are shown in Figure 83-6.

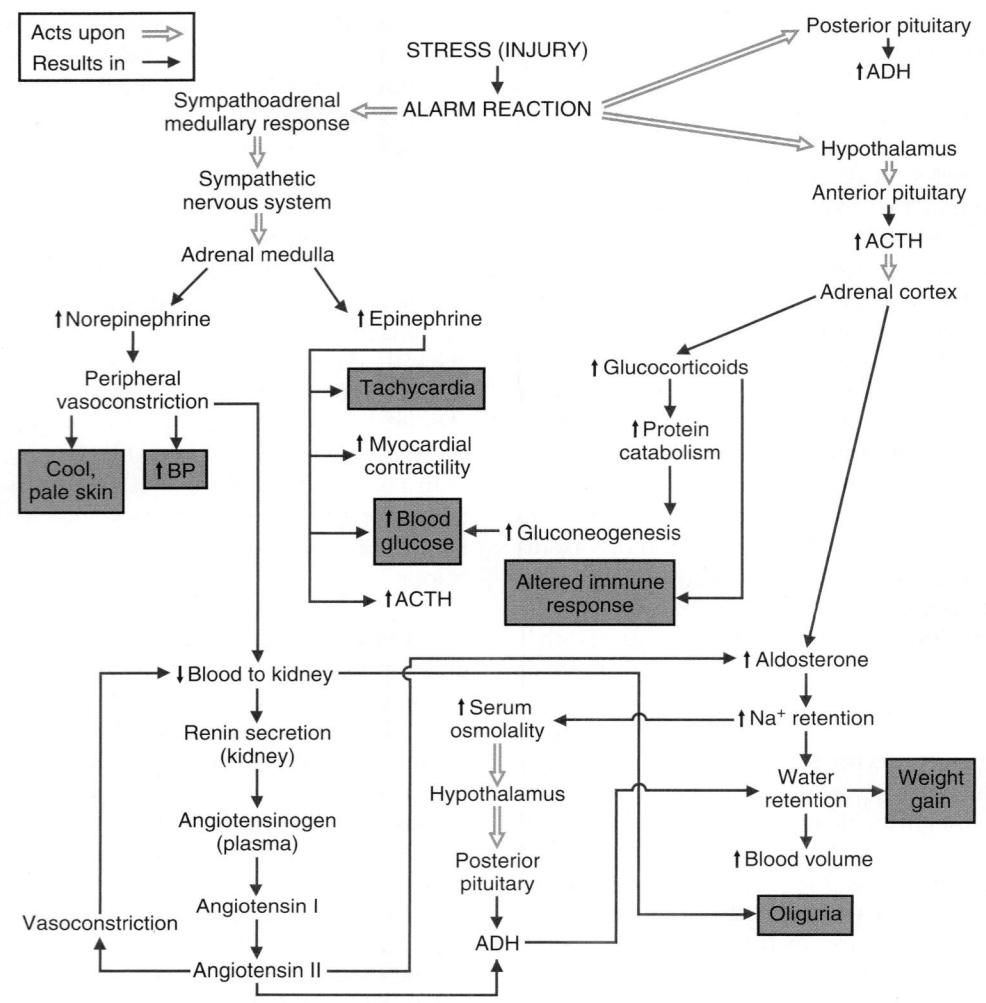

FIGURE 83-6 Components of the neuroendocrine response to a major stressor. Readily observed clinical manifestations as well as laboratory values are indicated by the boxes. *ACTH,* Adrenocorticotropic hormone; *ADH,* antidiuretic hormone; *BP,* blood pressure.

Metabolic Response. Generally, the hormonal response to stress rapidly provides fuel for the body's various tissues, organs, and systems. These fuels (e.g., amino acids, fatty acids, glucose) are produced by the breakdown of food. These substances are then chemically converted into energy, resulting in the formation of ATP. ATP is the main source of energy produced and used inside the body's cells.

The glucocorticoids, particularly hydrocortisone, mobilize energy stores. During the initial phase of shock, the body's small stores of available carbohydrate are rapidly depleted. It then becomes necessary to mobilize protein and fat stores to meet the body's energy requirements. Protein catabolism and negative nitrogen balance occur as part of the metabolic response, because of gluconeogenesis (resulting from glucocorticoid action) and starvation.

Neurologic Response. With shock, cerebral blood flow and cerebral metabolism may become insufficient

to maintain normal mental functioning and level of consciousness. Brain cells are highly sensitive to a shortage of oxygen and glucose and to fluid imbalances. When the brain becomes hypoxic, the cerebral vessels dilate to restore blood flow. Likewise, blood is diverted to the brain from the other, less vital organs.

Immune System. All forms of shock severely depress macrophages, which are located in both the blood and tissues. The capacity of macrophages to remove bacteria and the constantly formed endotoxins from the bloodstream is greatly reduced. Alterations in the blood itself are partially due to tissue hypoxia and impairment of monitoring activities of the macrophage. The stasis, sludging, tendency for venular thrombosis, impaired capillary permeability, and subnormal vascular reactivity that occur during shock can all be traced to macrophage dysfunction.

The impaired ability of macrophages to ward off toxic agents is critical. Reduced blood flow through the intestines during shock extensively impairs the integrity of intestinal tissue. This results in the movement of normal GI flora across the impaired intestinal tissue into the bloodstream, leading to a possible bacteremic state. The person in a state of shock is more susceptible than normal to bacterial products, particularly bacterial endotoxins, because of alterations in macrophage function.

Gastrointestinal System. Under sympathetic stimulation, vagal stimulation to the GI tract slows or stops, resulting in ileus with an absence of peristalsis. A lack of nutrient blood supply to the intestines increases the risk of tissue necrosis and sepsis.

GI changes appear to have a more important role in the progression of shock than was previously thought. The submucosa of the intestine becomes ischemic early in shock. If ischemia is prolonged, actual tissue necrosis of intestinal mucosa occurs. The intestinal arterioles and venules seem highly susceptible to the extensive vasoconstriction that occurs during shock. The massive amount of tissue destruction within the intestines that results from vasoconstriction and tissue anoxia is sufficient to cause death even if bacteria are not present. Bacteria and their toxins contribute to shock by escaping into the systemic circulation following destruction of the intestinal mucosa barrier.

Shock causes serious changes in the functions of the liver, the major organ of detoxification. The liver also suffers from this impaired circulation and appears to be a source of toxic materials. Normally, the liver protectively traps and disposes of toxic materials (released from the bowel contents) that are products of bacterial enzyme actions. During shock, the anoxic liver develops metabolic deficiencies, has an impaired ability to detoxify, and may release vasoactive substances. In addition, enhanced bacterial invasion of the liver from the intestine apparently occurs.

Finally, during shock, pooling of blood occurs in the viscera. Pooling of blood in the liver and portal bed may result from masses of agglutinated (clotted) blood plugging numerous small hepatic vessels, sinusoids, and intrahepatic radicles of the portal vein and hepatic artery.

Renal System. The rate of urinary production reflects visceral blood flow and body fluid balance. Thus urine output indicates the status of circulation through the vital organs. Adequate urine output indicates adequate circulation even if the arterial BP is below normal.

Altered Capillary Blood Pressure and Glomerular Filtration. Glomerular filtration within the kidneys depends on the pressure at which the blood is circulating through the glomerular capillaries. Usually, the average capillary pressure of blood is much higher in the glomeruli than in other capillaries. Under usual circumstances, the kidneys can maintain this heightened capillary pressure in the glomeruli even though there are changes in systemic BP. Afferent arterioles supplying the glomeruli dilate as the BP declines and constrict as it increases. However, eventually this adaptive mechanism cannot protect the kidneys against damage from a decreasing systemic BP.

During shock, when blood volume and BP decline steadily, glomerular filtration is progressively reduced, which leads to an inability of the kidneys to excrete sodium and water. To compensate, the body excretes some sodium and water through the sweat glands. Damaged kidneys also lose their crucial ability to regulate electrolyte and acid-base balance.

Inadequate perfusion of renal capillaries is believed to be the cause of early prerenal failure in shock. The afferent and efferent arterioles constrict, shunting blood away from the glomeruli. Later, if shock persists, actual renal shutdown occurs from focal tubular necrosis. Vasoconstriction in the kidneys may continue for a prolonged period of time after the systemic BP is restored to normal levels.

Renal Ischemia. During shock, the kidneys may experience renal ischemia. Because the kidneys have a high rate of metabolism, they are highly susceptible to injury of the tubule cells when the blood supply is deficient. When injury to the kidneys is extensive and renal failure ensues, acute tubular necrosis (ATN) occurs. With appropriate intervention, including careful fluid administration, the kidneys can heal. Normal kidney function usually returns after 10 to 14 days.

Clinical Manifestations

Systemic Manifestations of Shock

Because shock affects every system within the body, there are numerous clinical manifestations. The body is made up of many cells, which may function or malfunction at different stages of metabolic impairment. Subjective complaints are usually nonspecific and may not be particularly helpful to the clinician attempting to diagnose shock and treat the client. The client may report feeling sick, weak, cold, hot, nauseated, dizzy, confused, frightened, thirsty, or short of breath. Observable and measurable manifestations are often conflicting (Figure 83-7). BP, cardiac output, and urine output are usually decreased. Respiratory rate is usually increased. Variable indicators of shock include alterations in heart rate, core body temperature, skin temperature, systemic vascular resistance, and skin color. Dyspnea, altered sensorium, and diaphoresis may be present. The manifestations discussed in the sections that follow are usually present in people with shock of any type.

Respiratory System. Rapid, shallow respirations (tachypnea) typically occur during shock because of decreased tissue perfusion. The respiratory rate increases as the oxygen-carrying capacity of the blood decreases.

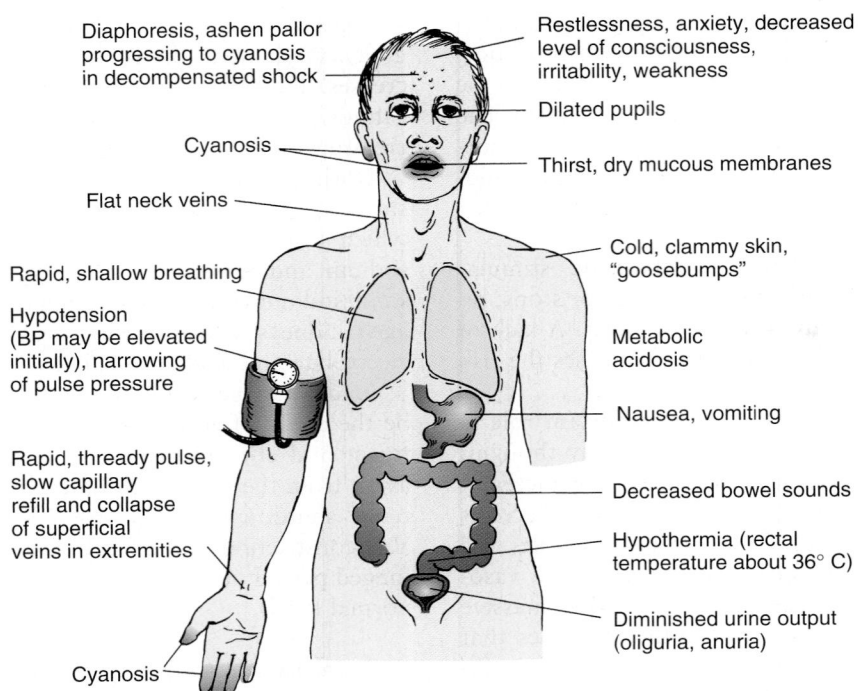

Diaphoresis, ashen pallor progressing to cyanosis in decompensated shock

Restlessness, anxiety, decreased level of consciousness, irritability, weakness

Cyanosis

Dilated pupils

Flat neck veins

Thirst, dry mucous membranes

Rapid, shallow breathing

Cold, clammy skin, "goosebumps"

Hypotension (BP may be elevated initially), narrowing of pulse pressure

Metabolic acidosis

Rapid, thready pulse, slow capillary refill and collapse of superficial veins in extremities

Nausea, vomiting

Decreased bowel sounds

Hypothermia (rectal temperature about 36° C)

Cyanosis

Diminished urine output (oliguria, anuria)

FIGURE 83-7 Clinical manifestations of the client with hypovolemic shock.

These changes may signal the development of hypoxemia and respiratory alkalosis.

Cardiovascular System

Tachycardia. During shock, the pulse rate usually increases as a result of increased sympathetic stimulation. Tachycardia (rapid heartbeat) occurs in an attempt to maintain adequate cardiac output and MAP when the blood's circulating volume is declining. With increased rate, the pulse becomes typically weak and thready. At the onset of shock, the pulse rate does not relate as directly to the severity of shock as does BP, because, in the early stage of shock, worry, excitement, and fear may influence the heart rate out of proportion to the underlying conditions. However, when emotional factors are no longer significant, serial observations of the pulse rate over a period of time are highly useful to assess the client's condition and the direction of the shock state and to evaluate the effectiveness of intervention.

Older clients (with and without various degrees of heart block) and clients taking beta-blocking medications, however, may show little change in heart rate despite the presence of conditions causing circulatory failure (e.g., hemorrhage). The pulse rate may become extremely slow in the terminal stages of shock and is usually slow in neurogenic shock.

Hypotension. The systolic BP indicates the integrity of the heart, arteries, and arterioles. The diastolic BP indicates the resistance (*systemic vascular resistance* [SVR] or *vasoconstriction*) of blood vessels. For example, an increasing diastolic BP indicates increasing systemic blood vessel resistance. Conversely, a declining diastolic BP indicates decreasing SVR. When the diastolic BP decreases significantly, vasoconstriction is being lost as a compensatory mechanism. When vasoconstriction is replaced by marked vasodilation, there is no resistance to blood flow and an adequate BP is difficult to maintain.

Usually, the BP begins to decrease when total blood volume is decreased by about 15% to 20%, although some people may lose as much as 25% of the total blood volume without having a decline in BP. This is especially true in young adults; therefore in young adults, declining BP is a *very* late manifestation of shock.

Typically, as shock progresses, both the systolic and diastolic BPs drop, with the systolic pressure dropping more than the diastolic. The pulse pressure narrows because it is equal to the difference between the systolic and diastolic BPs.

During shock, pulse pressure is actually more significant than BP because it tends to parallel cardiac stroke volume. Pulse pressure is affected by stroke volume (amount of blood ejected by the LV during contraction) and by peripheral resistance. If stroke volume is decreased from a decreased circulating blood volume, pulse pressure decreases. In shock, pulse pressure may decrease even in the presence of an acceptable systolic BP. This may provide a clue to worsening shock. In shock, pulse pressure is often less than 20 mm Hg (see the Critical Monitoring feature on Worsening Shock on p. 2457).

CRITICAL MONITORING

Worsening Shock

- Systolic blood pressure decreased more than 20 mm Hg with heart rate increased more than 20 beats indicates actual or relative hypovolemia requiring immediate assessment of need for fluid replacement and support of cardiovascular status.
- Decreased oxygen saturation or any manifestations of respiratory distress require immediate intervention. Interventions may range from administration of supplemental oxygen via a nasal cannula to endotracheal intubation with mechanical ventilation. Other interventions to support respiratory status (e.g., decreasing anxiety, positioning to support optimum respiratory functioning) are also important.

To maintain coronary circulation, a minimal systolic BP of 60 to 70 mm Hg is necessary. In interpreting BP readings, it is important to know what the client's BP has been. A systolic BP of 100 mm Hg or less is significant for clients whose systolic BP usually ranges from 110 to 140 mm Hg. When a client is supine, a decline in BP may be a late finding. Hypotension by itself is not shock. Healthy clients often have BP readings lower than textbook normal values.

Additional problems need to be considered in assessment of BP that make BP an unreliable criterion for assessing the presence and severity of shock. In the early, nonprogressive stage of shock, BP changes are generally unreliable because the arterial pressure may actually be normal or slightly elevated even though shock is present. In fact, blood volume deficits of 1 L or more may occur even though arterial and venous pressures are normal or elevated. When severe vasoconstriction is present, BP may be normal even though the circulation is actually highly inadequate. Conversely, the blood flow may be adequate even though BP is decreased (e.g., because of mechanisms such as vasodilation).

Valuable information about the level of arterial pressure in clients with vasoconstriction can be gained by assessing the strength of the femoral pulses. Doppler study may also be appropriate to obtain an accurate peripheral BP. With displaced or depleted blood volume, it is important to consider adequate venous filling. Hypovolemia, whether actual or relative, causes superficial veins to flatten. This change may hamper attempts to insert intravenous (IV) catheters for fluid replacement.

Neuroendocrine System. Early in shock, hyperactivity of the sympathetic nervous system with increased secretion of epinephrine usually causes the client to feel anxious, nervous, and irritable. Anxiety and worry are seen in the client's facial expressions.

Assessment findings associated with lack of blood to the brain are determined by the suddenness with which the shock develops and by its severity. With sudden, severe shock, the body may not have time to initiate its compensatory adjustment mechanisms. Consequently, the brain is deprived of its blood supply. The client may feel dizzy and faint on sitting up from a horizontal position because of postural hypotension. Fainting and unconsciousness may occur. If shock develops gradually over a period of hours, early assessment findings may include apathy and confusion or the opposite, restlessness and unusual alertness.

The systolic BP is important in maintaining blood flow to the brain. A cerebral perfusion pressure (CPP) of at least 50 mm Hg is required to deliver blood to the brain.

$$CPP = MAP - ICP$$

Usually, a decrease in systolic BP is accompanied by a reduced flow of blood to the brain. The vessels of the brain, like those of the heart, however, are not constricted by the vasoconstrictor center in the medulla oblongata. Thus blood from the peripheral vessels can be shifted to the brain as an emergency compensatory measure.

A client's level of consciousness decreases as circulation to brain tissue becomes increasingly impaired. Confusion, agitation, and restlessness may occur. In trauma situations, restlessness can be mistaken for pain. If opioids are given, the client's situation may be worsened or it may be difficult to detect worsening hypoxia. Drowsiness and stupor are more likely in shock related to severe infection than in shock caused by trauma and hemorrhage. As compensatory mechanisms fail, apathy may ensue. Ultimately, a comatose condition may be reached.

Renal System. A decrease in urinary volume, often the earliest manifestation of developing shock, may occur even while arterial BP and pulse remain stable. Although urine output is one of the most sensitive indices in shock, any form of shock that develops rapidly shows other manifestations before decreased urine output is noticed.

Urine output should be kept greater than 0.5 ml/kg/hr. If the hourly output diminishes significantly, treatment must be instituted to prevent renal failure. Urinary flow of less than 0.5 ml/kg/hr can cause ATN from inadequate renal circulation.

Clinical Manifestations of Specific Types of Shock

Hypovolemic Shock. Initially, urine osmolality and specific gravity increase because of sodium and water reabsorption, which attempts to support circulating volume. As altered tissue perfusion and the hypovolemic shock progress, urine osmolality and specific gravity decrease because of the inability of the kidneys to reabsorb sodium and water.

Sympathetic nervous system stimulation of the skin leads to marked diaphoresis. Clients sweat profusely, which increases insensible fluid loss, leading to further hypovolemia and temperature instability. Sympathetic stimulation also results in increased pulse and respirations and decreased tissue perfusion to the skin, causing the skin to feel cool and clammy and to appear pale.

Cyanosis may indicate either decreased tissue perfusion or decreased oxygenation or both. Cyanosis is a late manifestation of decreased oxygenation.

Cardiogenic Shock. Because of the impaired muscle action or mechanical obstruction that caused the cardiogenic shock, blood is inadequately pumped through the heart. This results in a back-up of blood. When the shock is due to right-sided heart failure, this back-up is evidenced as jugular venous distention and increased CVP. (See Chapters 58 and 65 for discussions of cardiac tamponade and tension pneumothorax.) When the shock is due to left-sided failure, blood backs up into the pulmonary circulation, resulting in pulmonary edema, crackles in the lungs, and increased pulmonary capillary wedge pressure (PCWP). As in hypovolemic shock, there is stimulation of the sympathetic nervous system because of decreased cardiac output and decreased BP and all of the resultant clinical manifestations.

Distributive Shock

Anaphylactic Shock. Initially, the client may complain of a vague feeling of uneasiness or a feeling of impending doom. The massive vasodilation that occurs with anaphylaxis may cause complaints of headache as well. This may be followed by severe anxiety, dizziness, disorientation, and loss of consciousness.

Respiratory involvement may be apparent through a variety of manifestations. The initial complaint may be a feeling of a lump in the throat, which is due to laryngeal edema and is followed by hoarseness, coughing, dyspnea, and stridor. Diffuse wheezes and a prolonged expiratory phase are heard on auscultation. If a pulse oximeter is in use, there may be a rapid decline in oxygen saturation.

Additional complaints may include pruritus and urticaria. Direct observation may also demonstrate edema of the eyelids, lips, or tongue (angioedema).

Neurogenic Shock. In neurogenic shock, abnormal distribution of fluid volume occurs from interruption or loss of innervation. Exceptions to the usual clinical manifestations are bradycardia and hypotension (which cannot be corrected because of loss of the ability of vasoconstriction). Below the level of injury, skin temperature takes on the same temperature as the room (poikilothermia). Skin is dry to the touch because of an inability to sweat.

Septic Shock. In the early stages of septic shock, the body experiences massive vasodilation. Warm, dry, flushed skin is apparent during this hyperdynamic stage of septic shock. The compensatory increase in cardiac output and resultant increased perfusion of the skin give this stage the name "warm shock." During later stages, when compensatory mechanisms fail, the release of MDF and decreased venous return result in decreased perfusion and "cold shock," or the hypodynamic stage. At this point, the skin becomes pale, cold, clammy, and mottled. Body temperature decreases to subnormal levels. Auscultation of the lungs reveals crackles and wheezes, which develop secondary to pulmonary congestion as ARDS ensues. In addition to the clinical manifestations seen with shock in general, changes in the level of consciousness may include drowsiness and stupor progressing to coma. See the Concept Map on Understanding Septic Shock and Its Treatment on p. 2447.

Diagnostic Assessment

Diagnostic assessments of clients in shock should include oxygenation, organ perfusion, and fluid balance. Assessment of respiratory status can be accomplished to some degree by noninvasive procedures such as spirometry, pulse oximeter, or arterial blood gas (ABG) analysis.

ABG analysis may also be done to determine whether the metabolic acidosis that occurs with shock is being effectively combated by hyperventilation. A low $PaCO_2$, along with low pH and bicarbonate levels (metabolic acidosis), indicates that hyperventilation is trying to compensate. However, an increasing $PaCO_2$ in the presence of a persistently low pH indicates that respiratory assistance is needed. It is also important to monitor PaO_2 levels to determine whether the client is being adequately oxygenated (see the Critical Monitoring feature on Worsening Shock on p. 2457 and Chapter 65 for discussions of respiratory interventions).

CVP measurement is one of the first invasive assessments made in the presence of shock to estimate fluid loss. A pulmonary artery or Swan-Ganz catheter may also be inserted to assist with assessments of fluid status, cardiac function, and tissue oxygen consumption (see Chapter 56).

Other noninvasive assessment and monitoring tools are the cardiac monitor and the 12-lead electrocardiogram (ECG). Laboratory studies include a complete blood count, blood chemistry, and blood and body fluid cultures for certain clients.

Outcome Management

Treatment should generally be instituted for shock whenever at least two of the following three conditions occur: systolic BP of 80 mm Hg or less, pulse pressure of 20 mm Hg or less, and pulse rate of 120 or more. Pulse pressure is calculated by subtracting diastolic BP from systolic BP and is normally between 30 and 50 mm Hg.

The therapeutic management of shock has changed markedly over recent years. Lowering the head, raising the feet, and administering potent vasoconstrictor drugs were once the foundation of treatment for a client in shock. Now, emphasis is placed on maintaining adequate circulating volume, positions that do not interfere with pulmonary ventilation, and the use of medications having both vasoconstrictor and vasodilator effects.

■ Medical Management

Correct the Causative Factor. Assessment and an accurate differential medical diagnosis, which establish the specific cause of the shock state, form the basis for treatment. The differential medical diagnosis is usually readily made unless the shock is in an advanced stage, at which point several specific forms of shock may exist at the same time. Some forms of shock more easily recognized are hypovolemic shock that is due to extensive burns or trauma and cardiogenic shock with severe chest pain and acute MI. Septic shock is probably the most difficult shock state to diagnose because of its insidious onset and complex manifestations.

Improve Oxygenation. Maintaining the client's airway is vital to the treatment of shock. In all types of shock, supplemental oxygen is administered to protect against hypoxemia. Oxygen can be delivered via a nasal cannula, a mask, a high-flow non-rebreathing mask, an endotracheal tube, or a tracheostomy tube.

Endotracheal intubation, or tracheostomy, may be performed to rest an exhausted client during severe or prolonged shock and to correct respiratory failure. By increasing the rate of pulmonary ventilation (through spontaneous or mechanical hyperventilation), it is possible to compensate for minor degrees of metabolic acidosis. This increased "blowing off" of carbon dioxide with hyperventilation begins to compensate for acid-base imbalance. Positive end-expiratory pressure may be added when the client is being mechanically ventilated. This assists in preventing atelectasis and may provide a higher PaO_2 for the client at a lower oxygen concentration setting. The goal of therapy is to maintain a PaO_2 greater than 50 mm Hg and an SaO_2 greater than 90% to avoid anaerobic metabolism. If the chest is congested, chest physical therapy, including vibration, percussion, and postural drainage, may be required.

EB Sometimes the interventions discussed cannot establish optimal tissue oxygenation. In these instances, hyperbaric oxygenation (HBO) or extracorporeal membrane oxygenation may be used. HBO involves the administration of 100% oxygen under 2 to 3 atmospheres of pressure. This raises tissue oxygen tension to normal or above-normal levels. HBO requires the use of special chambers, which usually are available only in highly specialized institutions.

Extracorporeal membrane oxygenation is most commonly used in adults as a temporary intervention for refractory ARDS. Arterial and venous catheters are inserted, and some of the client's blood is diverted through them into a machine that artificially oxygenates the blood. This is a relatively expensive form of therapy and is usually done only in large medical centers.

Restore and Maintain Adequate Perfusion. The primary aim in treating shock is to maintain an adequate circulating blood volume. Unless this is accomplished early, subsequent therapeutic measures are of no avail, and death can be anticipated. In addition, other treatment adjuncts are necessary, which are discussed in the sections that follow. The adjuncts facilitate the distribution of blood to the body and enhance perfusion and oxygenation of the tissues with the circulating blood.

Administer Vasoactive Medications. Please refer to the Integrating Pharmacology feature on Vasoactive Medications for Shock Management, below, for a discussion of vasoactive medications commonly used to treat shock.

Vasoconstrictors. Vasoconstrictors elevate the systemic BP by constricting peripheral arterioles. Vasoconstrictor agents may be used briefly in shock if compen-

INTEGRATING PHARMACOLOGY

Vasoactive Medications for Shock Management

It may seem contradictory to use medications that vasoconstrict and medications that vasodilate in caring for individuals in shock. However, both actions are needed at times during shock and many of the medications used have actions that are beneficial during each stage.

In the nonprogressive stage of shock, when the body is experiencing significant vasodilation, vasoconstrictors, such as high-dose dopamine, norepinephrine, and phenylephrine, help maintain blood pressure (BP). Adding medications that increase cardiac contractility, such as amrinone and dobutamine, further support BP by increasing cardiac output. As shock progresses and vasoconstriction ensues, these same drugs, with some changes in dosing, are still effective in supporting the client's hemodynamic stability. Low-dose dopamine causes vasodilation of the renal and mesenteric blood vessels, helping to support perfusion of the kidneys and gut. Amrinone and dobutamine contribute to vasodilation of blood vessels in the heart and skeletal muscle, ensuring adequate oxygenation to those organs and tissues. If significant systemic vasoconstriction continues, relaxation of the vascular smooth muscle may be necessary with drugs such as nitroglycerin and nitroprusside.

Titration and changing of medications is continued until the client's shock is clearly reversed. If the client progresses to the irreversible stage of shock despite the health care teams best efforts, these drugs will have little, if any, effectiveness.

satory vasoconstriction is unable to maintain blood flow to vital organs. They may also be used to correct hypotension secondary to vasoconstrictor nerve paralysis, as in spinal anesthesia or conditions associated with massive vasodilation. However, vasoconstrictors should not be used exclusively but should be given concomitantly with IV fluids to restore adequate circulation and perfusion.

Perfusion of vital organs with blood is impossible when systolic BP is less than 50 mm Hg. Usually, the goal of using vasoconstrictors is to achieve and maintain a mean BP of 70 to 80 mm Hg, which is sufficient to perfuse tissues. Generally, attempts to increase the BP beyond this level are not advisable because vasoconstrictors increase the oxygen demand of the heart and may cause fatal dysrhythmias. Vasoconstrictors are used with extreme caution in cardiogenic shock. Other major adverse effects of vasoconstrictors include decreased renal and splanchnic blood flow, excessive or sudden increase in arterial BP (which may precipitate heart failure), pulmonary edema or LV decompensation, and gangrene of the fingers and toes from prolonged vasoconstriction.

Although the use of vasoconstrictors during shock is being critically evaluated, they do favorably increase blood flow to the brain and heart in severely hypotensive clients. Reduced tissue perfusion when systolic pressures are less than 60 to 70 mm Hg may precipitate an MI or a stroke.

Vasodilators. Agents that induce vasodilation or inhibit vasoconstriction may promote recovery from shock in which intensive vasoconstriction is contributing to the problem. These include adrenergic blocking agents, ganglionic blocking agents, and direct-acting peripheral vasodilators.

Adrenergic blockade prevents harmful effects of prolonged vasoconstriction such as increased pressure in capillaries, promoting fluid loss from the vascular to the interstitial compartment, and altered blood flow, especially in the splanchnic area. Prolonged vasoconstriction also impairs cellular nutrition and allows accumulation of waste products. Adrenergic blockade prevents these changes in circulation and may also induce opposite beneficial changes.

Vasodilators may be helpful during shock when vasoconstriction is severe and persists even though fluids have been infused in what should be adequate amounts for fluid replacement. Vasodilators may be administered to inhibit vasoconstriction of peripheral blood vessels (the result of norepinephrine from sympathetic stimulation) so that blood can be redistributed to enhance tissue perfusion and increase vascular volume.

When shock is caused by hypovolemia, rapid and adequate fluid replacement is essential before vasodilators are used. Vasodilators are dangerous because they lower arterial BP if they are given while circulating blood volume is deficient. When the circulating blood volume is inadequate, the body depends on vasoconstriction to maintain arterial pressure. However, when the vascular space is full and cardiac venous return is adequate, vasodilation should open arterioles in the lungs and elsewhere. This lets blood circulate, increasing cardiac output and capillary perfusion without lowering systemic BP. In fact, a vasodilator may produce a dramatic, sustained increase in the systemic arterial pressure.

Keep clients who are receiving vasodilators lying relatively flat. Elevation of the head can produce dangerous orthostatic hypotension. Older clients may have sclerotic blood vessels and may not tolerate the hypotension that may accompany administration of vasodilators. In this situation, a cardiotonic drug (such as dobutamine) may be given with the vasodilator to increase cardiac output.

Vasoconstrictor medications are sometimes given in combination with vasodilator medications to offset the profound effects that may occur with some vasoconstrictors and to provide the benefits both types of drugs have to offer.

Characteristically, impaired tissue perfusion is correctable during early shock. However, it may be fatal if treatment is not received or is inadequate. In the later stages of shock, impaired tissue perfusion becomes irreversible, leading to death despite treatment. However, treatment for irreversible shock is never abandoned while the client remains alive. Before a client's shock state is viewed as probably irreversible, identification and treatment of occult bleeding and restoration of circulating volume, correction of any factors interfering with cardiopulmonary function, and treatment of overwhelming infection must be attempted.

During shock intervention, all of the basic pathophysiologic changes associated with the development of shock must be corrected. Some problems that must often be treated are (1) the vascular problem of vasoconstriction with the diminished tissue perfusion it causes, (2) the intravascular problem of coagulation and sludging of blood cells, and (3) the extravascular problem of extravasation of fluid into the extravascular space.

Assist Circulation. Mechanical devices that assist circulation or decrease the workload of the heart may be used as temporary measures in managing clients in shock. Examples of these include the military or medical antishock trousers (MAST), IABP, and external counterpulsation device. (See Chapter 60 for more information.)

MAST Garment. MAST, also called pneumatic antishock garment (Figure 83-8), encases the lower part of the body in a one-piece, three-chambered (one abdominal and two leg chambers) suit from the lower costal margin to the ankles. The external pressure provided by the MAST garment causes increased vascular resistance and reduces the diameter of blood vessels in the abdomen and legs. This results in impedance of blood flow and may decrease leakage into the tissues, resulting in increased perfusion of vital organs. Cardiac output and arterial BP increase.

MAST garments are most often used in trauma situations occurring outside the hospital setting for management of massive blood loss with no obtainable BP, fluid loss other than hemorrhage, and cardiac arrest caused by severe fluid or blood loss. They also help further reduce bleeding in areas being compressed, immobilize fractures of the femur and pelvis, and facilitate insertion of the IV line by increasing upper extremity cardiac output and vein filling. The use of MAST garments continues to be controversial because the decreased perfusion in the lower extremities leads to acidosis in the compressed tissues and compression of the tissues may lead to compartment syndrome. MAST garments may be contraindicated in cardiogenic shock.

Intra-Aortic Balloon Pump. An IABP is used primarily in clients with cardiogenic shock and after open heart surgery. The ability of the heart to adequately pump blood is augmented by a balloon-tipped catheter placed in the descending thoracic aorta. The catheter is attached to a unit that inflates during diastole and deflates just before systole. This counterpulsation displaces blood back into the aorta and improves coronary artery circulation. In cardiogenic shock, use of the IABP re-

duces preload, allowing the heart to more efficiently empty, thereby increasing cardiac output. Details of the IABP are found in the Bridge to Critical Care feature on Intra-Aortic Balloon Pumping in Chapter 60.

External Counterpulsation Device. This device uses the same general principles as an IABP but is applied externally to the legs. The legs are encased in air- or water-filled tubular bags connected to a pumping unit. Pressure is applied to the legs during diastole and is released in systole. A form of external counterpulsation is also being used in the cardiac setting with clients experiencing chronic angina, because it has been shown in some client groups to decrease their episodes of angina.

Modified Trendelenburg Position. A client in shock is usually placed in a modified Trendelenburg position with the lower extremities elevated 30 to 45 degrees, the knees straight, the trunk horizontal or very slightly raised, and the neck comfortably positioned with the head level with the chest or slightly higher (Figure 83-9). This position promotes increased venous return from the lower extremities without compressing the abdominal organs against the diaphragm.

Elevating the legs mobilizes blood that has pooled in the lower extremities. As a result of gravity, the additional circulating blood increases venous return to the heart, thus improving cardiac output. The position is of temporary value in moderate hypovolemia. However, it does not help in severe hypovolemia, because the extremities have very little blood in them in such a state. Generally, the modified shock position is not used with cardiogenic shock, when there is already circulatory overload.

The traditional Trendelenburg position (head down, with legs elevated at least 30 degrees above the head) was once the classic shock position but is no longer used for shock management because it compresses the abdominal contents against the diaphragm, interfering with pulmonary excursion, and promotes congestion of blood in the brain, possibly contributing to cerebral edema.

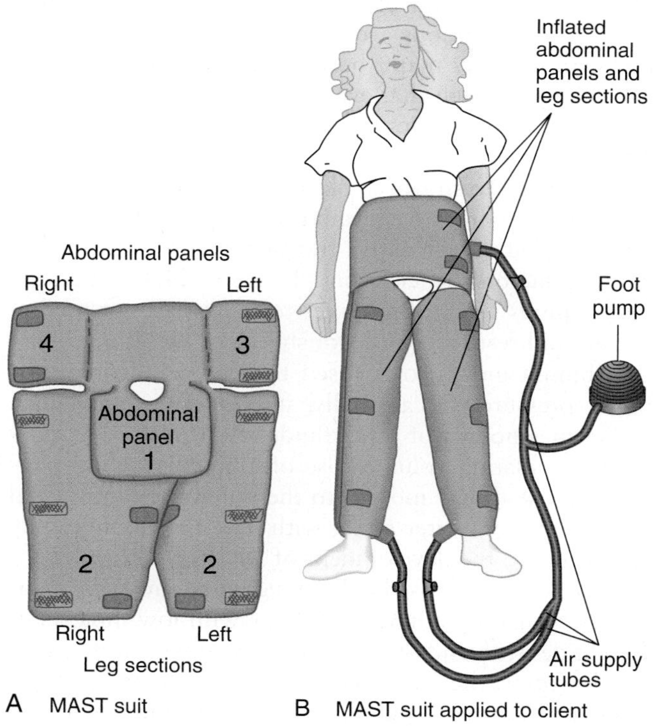

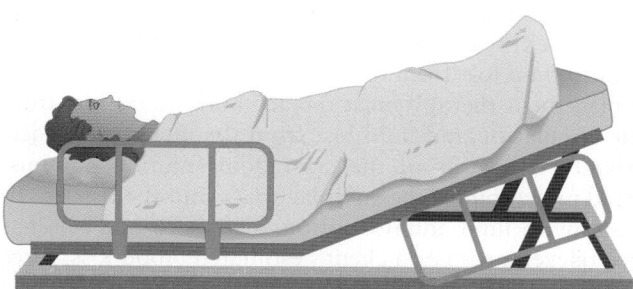

FIGURE 83-8 MAST suit, or pneumatic antishock garment. **A,** The suit is composed of two leg compartments and an abdominal compartment. **B,** MAST suit in place. Abdominal and leg compartments are attached to air tubes and a foot pump for inflation. *MAST, Military antishock trousers.*

FIGURE 83-9 Positioning of the person in shock. This position is a modification of Trendelenburg position and includes elevating the legs, leaving the trunk flat, and elevating the head and shoulders slightly.

Replace Fluid Volume. The mainstay of hypovolemic shock therapy is expansion of circulating blood volume by IV administration of blood or other appropriate fluids. Fluid replacement should be administered through large-bore peripheral lines, central venous lines, or both.

Various fluids are given to correct specific problems, such as electrolyte or protein deficiencies or other defects of the blood, including acidosis and hyponatremia. However, in treating hypovolemic shock, the immediate results of therapy seem to depend less on the type of fluid administered for fluid replacement than on the amount of fluid administered. In general, enough fluid is given to exceed the normal blood volume. In part, this "extra" fluid is required because the vascular space is expanded as a result of dilation of the microcirculation. Additional fluid is also administered to replace intracellular fluid that was mobilized into the circulation as an early response to the hypovolemia.

In replacing fluids, enough volume must be administered to fill the capillaries and run through into the veins. Such fluid replacement maintains CVP and provides an adequate venous return to the heart. This promotes additional cardiac output. In addition, adequate fluid replacement decreases the blood catecholamine level and thus produces a vasodilation that promotes capillary flow. Adequate flow of fluids in the capillaries in turn perfuses tissues and prevents sludging and coagulation of blood within the vessels. Carefully monitor IV fluid replacement therapy to prevent circulatory overload. Hypervolemia can be lethal; thus aggressive fluid replacement should be tapered off when urine output is at least 0.5 ml/kg/hr, systolic BP is greater than 100 mm Hg, or the heart rate is 60 to 100 beats/min.

IV fluids used in shock management may include warmed crystalloids or balanced salt solutions, colloids, and blood. Dextrose and water should not be used to resuscitate a client; once the dextrose is metabolized, only hypotonic water remains, which leads to greater fluid shifts.

Crystalloid or Balanced Salt Solutions. During hypovolemic shock, the loss of circulating blood volume is also associated with redistribution of extravascular fluid. A sizable amount of fluid (about 4 L in moderately severe shock) leaves the interstitial space. This is in addition to fluid lost from the circulating volume. Thus fluid replacement therapy must replace both blood lost from the circulation and fluid lost from the interstitial space. About two thirds of the crystalloid solution administered moves out of the vascular space into the tissues. To assist with fluid administration, a three-to-one rule has been developed. For a client's estimated blood loss, three times as much crystalloid solution must be administered for adequate volume resuscitation. Crystalloid solutions that may be administered include normal saline, Ringer's lactate, or half-normal saline.

Electrolyte solutions such as Ringer's lactate help expand extracellular volume, reduce viscosity, and prevent sludging. In a client with impaired liver function, a solution containing lactate could further compound the problem of lactic acidosis. In a normally functioning liver, lactate is converted to bicarbonate and does not accumulate. Because the liver is not an organ of primary perfusion during times of stress for the body and may not be functioning normally, other solutions should be considered before Ringer's lactate.

Abnormalities of electrolyte and acid-base balance are corrected with the specific substance needed rather than with a solution that administers multiple electrolytes and acid-base components. Therapy is gauged by serial ABG and electrolyte determinations.

Colloid Solutions. Colloid solutions contain proteins normally too large to exit at the capillary; thus they remain in the vascular compartment and increase osmotic pressure of the capillaries. This increased osmotic pressure helps retain fluid in the vascular compartment and maintain circulating volume. These solutions may be used in conjunction with crystalloid solutions in treating hypovolemic shock to maintain an adequate circulating volume. The most commonly used colloid solutions include plasma and its components, plasma substitutes (e.g., dextran), oxygen-carrying solutions other than blood (e.g., perfluorochemicals), and hetastarch. (See discussions of blood and blood transfusions, Chapter 77.) Colloid solutions are often not used in initial fluid resuscitation after major burn injury. The capillary leakage is large enough that even the proteins escape.

Plasma is sometimes used in treating clients with low serum protein levels to control fluid escape from the vascular system. Fresh frozen plasma (FFP) is the form commonly used to improve serum protein levels. FFP may be administered after massive transfusions to restore some clotting factors deficient in "banked" blood. Because FFP requires 15 to 30 minutes to thaw, it is not used in initial fluid resuscitation with shock.

Albumin may also be used to achieve adequate osmotic pressure. Occasionally, it is administered when sufficient amounts of other fluids fail to restore an adequate circulating volume. Use of albumin is controversial because it may move into the pulmonary interstitial space, drawing water along with it. Thus albumin may contribute to the development of ARDS.

Dextran may be used in both high- and low-molecular-weight forms. By initiating therapy with low-molecular-weight dextran and then progressing to high-molecular-weight forms, the incidence of hypersensitivity reactions to dextran can be lowered. The advantage in using dextran is that it contains large molecules that should effectively and rapidly expand the intravascular volume. Dextran can interfere with blood type and crossmatch procedures and with clotting factors. It should therefore be used only after type and crossmatch have been done and until blood is available for transfusion.

Although the administration of crystalloids, albumin, and blood has been the standard treatment of hypovolemic shock for many years, several new substances have been introduced for shock management. Perfluorochemicals (e.g., Fluosol, Oxygent) are non-blood, oxygen-carrying solutions that remain in the circulation for about 12 to 24 hours. Major limitations associated with the use of perfluorochemicals relate to limited immediate availability (the product must be stored frozen), administration of 80% to 100% O_2 for the solution to be effective, and accumulation of the chemicals in the body. Advantages include the high solubility of perfluorochemicals, making them readily available to the tissues, and their acceptability to clients whose religious beliefs prohibit the use of blood products. Perfluorochemicals have been researched since the 1970s and are still in various stages of experimentation.

Hemoglobin-based oxygen carriers (e.g., PolyHeme, Hemopure, Hemolink) are made from hemoglobin that has been extracted from red blood cells and have been developed from bovine, recombinant, and human sources. Advantages are that no type and crossmatch is required for administration, so oxygen-carrying solutions are more readily available for situations in which major traumas occur or during periods of diminished blood availability. Concerns that still exist relate to the toxicity of the solutions, their short half-life, and their relatively high colloid oncotic pressure.

Hetastarch, a glycogen-like synthetic colloid, has been used to treat hypovolemic shock and may provide alternatives to blood administration.

Blood. When hemorrhage is the primary cause of shock, the rapid administration of large volumes of packed cells or whole blood may be necessary. Type-specific, crossmatched blood is the most desirable form of blood replacement. However, if the client is hemorrhaging, it may be necessary to administer type-specific, un-crossmatched blood: O-negative blood or O-positive, low antibody titer blood. Women should receive Rh-negative blood.

When shock resulting from hemorrhage is treated, a crystalloid is usually given as an initial emergency treatment to sustain BP. Later, the acute anemia resulting from hemorrhage must be corrected by administration of packed cells for the prevention of hypoxemia.

During fluid replacement, a normal red blood cell mass should be maintained. Fluids given in excess of normal volume should be fluids other than blood so that they can be easily removed from the circulation by the kidneys once the shock is corrected. If the normal red blood cell mass is exceeded, it is difficult for the body to eliminate the excess red blood cells after the vascular volume contracts to normal (after adequate perfusion of tissues with blood is achieved). Because dangers also are involved in blood transfusions, blood should not be used if another fluid can satisfactorily maintain an adequate oxygen-carrying capacity and can sufficiently increase blood volume. Blood can become so dilute that there are relatively few blood cells as the result of up to 8 to 12 L of fluid being administered in only a few hours.

Autotransfusion. Autotransfusion involves collecting and retransfusing blood into the same client. Autotransfusion is used to prevent or treat hypovolemic shock caused by hemorrhage. It is common in the treatment of chest injuries.

Evaluate Fluid Replacement. Often, fluid replacement is the only treatment required for shock. However, it is difficult to evaluate whether fluid replacement is adequate. Internal losses of circulating fluid volume, including whole blood, into areas of traumatized tissue, infection, and so forth are difficult to estimate. If a vasoconstrictor drug has been administered or if prolonged vasoconstriction occurs, an additional considerable loss of circulating volume may also occur because of vasoconstriction. Large volumes of IV fluid may be administered either until systemic BP, urinary volume, and lactate levels become relatively normal or until central venous or pulmonary artery pressures, or both, stabilize or become elevated.

Infusion of blood or other fluids usually continues only as long as the CVP is low, that is, less than 4 cm H_2O or 2 mm Hg. When the CVP is higher than normal (e.g., greater than 15 cm H_2O or 11 mm Hg), benefit cannot be expected from the continued infusion of fluids or blood beyond maintenance amounts. When the CVP is low and the lungs are clear, with no indications of heart failure, fluids are administered to improve the return of blood to the heart. However, some clients have a normal or low CVP despite faulty LV function. They readily develop heart failure or pulmonary edema. Thus a low or normal CVP does not always mean that fluid administration is advisable.

IV fluid administration should be stopped before extremely high elevations of pulmonary artery pressures occur if there is an adequate systemic response. An adequate volume of circulating fluid causes an ample venous return to the right side of the heart and increases the right-sided output. Pulmonary artery hypertension may develop if continued pulmonary obstruction is present because of coagulation in the microcirculation or vasoconstriction. This appears as increased pulmonary artery pressure. In the presence of right-sided heart failure, this increased pressure may back up through the right side of the heart, causing an abnormal elevation in CVP. Vasodilators may help open this partially blocked pulmonary microcirculation.

Prevent Complications

Prevent Renal Impairment. Impaired kidney function and ATN may result from inadequate renal tissue perfusion, as discussed earlier. To prevent acute renal damage, the urine output is monitored with an indwelling catheter, and diuretics (e.g., furosemide) may be given. Correcting metabolic acidosis (see Chapter 15) and using other measures to increase blood volume and improve cardiac output also benefit the kidney as well as other tissues. If tubular necrosis is present, peritoneal dialysis or hemodialysis may be needed until regeneration of functioning renal tubular epithelium occurs. (See also Chapter 38.)

During shock, urine output should be measured and compared with normal urinary production. The normal rate of urinary excretion from the kidneys is 1 ml/min or 60 ml/hr. A client who becomes acutely hypovolemic or is experiencing a redistribution of circulating volume cannot maintain an hourly output of 40 to 60 ml of urine. Decreased urine output (oliguria) typically occurs in shock. Often during shock, the urine output may stop completely (anuria). When this occurs, the client is said to be in renal shutdown or renal failure.

Oliguria does not contraindicate the administration of large volumes of fluid in the treatment of shock. In fact, restoring renal capillary perfusion along with that of other vital capillaries restores urine volume production as long as tubular necrosis is not already present. Fluid administration may prevent ATN in the kidneys.

A large amount of tissue damage (e.g., crush injuries) may cause a release of myoglobin from muscle tissue. Because the myoglobin molecule is large, a type of mechanical renal failure may result from attempts to excrete large amounts of myoglobin. Fluid administration is again important to decrease damage to the tubules.

Prevent Gastrointestinal Bleeding. An early physiologic response to shock is a decrease in splanchnic circulation. This reduces the blood supply to the stomach and bowel, causing inadequate GI tissue perfusion and delayed gastric emptying; thus vomiting with aspiration of gastric contents into the lung may occur. For this reason and for diagnostic purposes, nasogastric (NG) suction is often used during treatment of shock. A double-lumen, 16-French NG tube is usually used in adults.

Assess gastric aspirate periodically for blood. Guaiac solution or Hemoccult tablets and reagent can be used to check for blood; litmus paper checks the pH to determine the acidity of the stomach. Promptly report new findings of blood or increases in the amount of blood. Histamine blockers and proton pump inhibitors are used to reduce gastric acid in the stomach. Antacids

TABLE 83-2	*Summary of the Management of Hypovolemic Shock*	
Etiology	**Clinical Situation**	**Intervention***
Blood loss	Massive trauma Gastrointestinal bleeding Ruptured aortic aneurysm Surgery Erosion of vessel from lesion, tubes, or other devices DIC	Stop external bleeding with direct pressure, pressure dressing, tourniquet (as last resort) Reduce intra-abdominal or retroperitoneal bleeding by applying MAST garment or prepare for emergency surgery Administer lactated Ringer's solution or normal saline Transfuse with fresh whole blood, packed cells, fresh frozen plasma, platelets, or other clotting factors, if significant improvement does not occur with crystalloid administration Use non-blood plasma expanders (albumin , hetastarch, dextran) until blood is available Conduct autotransfusion if appropriate
Plasma loss	Burns Accumulation of intra-abdominal fluid Malnutrition Severe dermatitis DIC	Administer low-dose cardiotonics (dopamine, dobutamine) Administer lactated Ringer's solution or normal saline Administer albumin, fresh frozen plasma, hetastarch, or dextran if cardiac output is still low
Crystalloid loss	Dehydration (e.g., diabetic ketoacidosis, heat exhaustion) Protracted vomiting, diarrhea Nasogastric suction	Administer isotonic or hypotonic saline with electrolytes as needed to maintain normal circulating volume and electrolyte balance

DIC, Disseminated intravascular coagulation; *MAST*, military or medical antishock trousers.
*Assumes that airway management and cardiac monitoring are ongoing.

may also be instilled through the tube when the pH is acidic.

When shock is caused by GI bleeding, other NG tubes may be used. If the suspected cause of bleeding is a gastric ulcer, a 36-French Ewald tube may be used. The many large holes in this tube facilitate saline lavage and removal of blood clots. If esophageal varices are suspected or present, a Sengstaken-Blakemore tube may be used. This triple-lumen tube exerts pressure on the lower portion of the esophagus and the upper portion of the stomach where varices are most prominent. Pressure is created by esophageal and gastric balloons inflated with air. Gentle traction is applied to keep the balloons in proper position (see Chapter 33).

Tables 83-2, 83-3, and 83-4 give specific interventions for hypovolemic, cardiogenic, and distributive shock, respectively.

Provide Pharmacologic Management

Antibiotics. Antibiotics are essential when shock is due to infection. If septic shock is suspected, a blood specimen for culture and sensitivity is taken at once, and broad-spectrum antibiotics are started even though the specific infectious organism has not yet been identified. When the blood sample is drawn, samples of urine, sputum, and fluid from draining wounds, sinuses, and so forth are also obtained for culture. The antibiotic selected depends on the cause of the infection and should not be initiated until after all cultures have been obtained. However, once cultures have been obtained, treatment with empirical broad-spectrum antibiotics should be initiated. Cephalosporins, gentamicin, and aminoglycosides may be used in combination until specific culture and sensitivity information is available. Antibiotics may also be administered along with appropri-

TABLE 83-3	*Summary of the Management of Cardiogenic Shock*	
Etiology	**Clinical Situation**	**Intervention***
Myocardial disease or injury	Acute myocardial infarction Myocardial contusion Cardiomyopathies	Fluid-challenge with up to 300 ml of normal saline solution or Ringer's lactate to rule out hypovolemia, unless heart failure or pulmonary edema is present Insert CVP or pulmonary artery catheter; monitor cardiac output, pulmonary artery pressure, and PCWP; administer IV fluids to maintain left ventricular filling pressure of 15-20 mm Hg Administer inotropics (e.g., dopamine or dobutamine) Vasodilators (e.g., sodium nitroprusside, nitroglycerin, calcium-channel blockers, morphine) Diuretics (e.g., mannitol or furosemide) Cardiotonics (e.g., digitalis) Beta-blockers (propranolol) Glucocorticosteroids† Intra-aortic balloon pump or external counterpulsation device if unresponsive to other therapies
Valvular disease or injury	Ruptured aortic cusp Ruptured papillary muscle Ball thrombus	Same as above: if rapid response does not occur, prepare for prompt cardiac surgery
External pressure on the heart interferes with heart filling or emptying	Pericardial tamponade due to trauma, aneurysm, cardiac surgery, pericarditis Massive pulmonary embolus Tension pneumothorax Ascites Hemoperitoneum Mechanical ventilation	Relieve tamponade with ECG-assisted pericardiocentesis; repair surgically if it recurs Thrombolytic (streptokinase) or anticoagulant (heparin) therapy; surgery for removal of clot Relieve air accumulation with needle thoracostomy or chest tube insertion Relieve fluid accumulation with paracentesis Reduce inspiratory pressure
Cardiac dysrhythmias	Tachydysrhythmias Bradydysrhythmias Pulseless electrical activity	Treat dysrhythmias; be prepared to initiate CPR, cardiac pacing

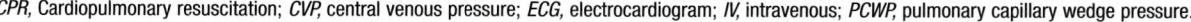

CPR, Cardiopulmonary resuscitation; *CVP,* central venous pressure; *ECG,* electrocardiogram; *IV,* intravenous; *PCWP,* pulmonary capillary wedge pressure.
*Assumes that airway management and cardiac monitoring are ongoing.
†Controversial.

TABLE 83-4	*Summary of the Management of Distributive Shock*	
Etiology	**Clinical Situation**	**Intervention***
Anaphylactic shock	Allergy to food, medicines, dyes, insect bites, stings, or latex	Prepare for surgical management of the airway Decrease further absorption of antigen (e.g., stop IV fluid, place tourniquet between injection or sting site and heart if feasible) Epinephrine (1:100) 2 inhalations every 3 hours, *or* Epinephrine (1:1000) 0.2-0.5 ml every 5-15 min given subcutaneously, *or* Epinephrine (1:10,000) 0.5-1.0 ml every 5-15 min given at a rate of 1 mg/min IV fluid resuscitation with isotonic solution Diphenhydramine HCl or H_1-receptor antagonist IV Theophylline IV drip for bronchospasm Steroids IV Vasopressors (e.g., norepinephrine, metaraminol bitartrate, high-dosage dopamine) Gastric lavage for ingested antigen Ice pack to injection or sting site Meat tenderizer paste to sting site
Septic shock	Often gram-negative septicemia but also caused by other organisms in debilitated, immunodeficient, or chronically ill clients	Identify origin of sepsis; culture all suspected sources Vigorous IV fluid resuscitation with normal saline Empirical antibiotic therapy until sensitivities are reported If suspected organism is gram-positive, vancomycin is used; if suspected organism is gram-negative, give expanded-spectrum penicillin or a cephalosporin and aminoglycoside Administer cardiotonic agents (e.g., dopamine or dobutamine, norepinephrine, isoproterenol, digitalis, calcium) Naloxone (narcotic antagonist) Prostaglandins Monoclonal antibodies Temperature control (both hypothermia and hyperthermia are noted) Heparin, clotting factors, blood products if DIC develops
Neurogenic (spinal) shock	Spinal anesthesia Spinal cord injury	Normal saline to restore volume Treat bradycardia with atropine Vasopressors (e.g., norepinephrine, metaraminol bitartrate, high-dosage dopamine, and phenylephrine) may be given Place client in modified Trendelenburg position
Vasovagal reaction	Severe pain Severe emotional stress	Place client in a head-down or recumbent position Give atropine if bradycardia and profound hypotension; eliminate pain

DIC, Disseminated intravascular coagulation; *IV*, intravenous.
*Assumes airway management and cardiac monitoring are ongoing.

ate surgical management to clients with open or potentially contaminated wounds who are experiencing hypovolemic shock.

Monoclonal Technology. Multiple therapies that specifically target the mediators of septic shock are being researched. Monoclonal antiendotoxin (e.g., HA-1A and E5) neutralizes the endotoxin or toxicity of the offending pathogen or the immune response itself. Interleukin-1 receptor agonists, anti-tumor necrosing factor antibodies, and platelet-activating factor inhibitors are also in research trials for their effectiveness in reducing the morbidity and mortality from septic shock. Research results to date on these therapies are mixed, but researchers continue to search for the solution in preventing the significant negative outcomes of septic shock.

Drotrecogin Alfa. Drotrecogin alfa (Xigris) is a new drug that is expected to help diminish the negative outcomes of severe sepsis. Septic shock does not develop simply because an infection is present. Rather, a person with severe sepsis develops the hypotension, coagulation disorders, and multisystem organ dysfunction of septic shock due, in part, to a dysregulated expression of the body's mediators of inflammation. The relationship between the outcomes of sepsis and the inflammatory response has led to a multitude of research. Drotrecogin alfa is a recombinant form of human activated protein C and has the ability to inhibit inflammation, inhibit coagulation, and promote fibrinolysis. It is expected that this drug will diminish the negative outcomes and mortality associated with septic shock. Preliminary studies have indicated that use of drotrecogin alfa can decrease septic shock–related mortality by 6% to 11%.

Heparin. The anticoagulant effect of heparin may help prevent complications or treat DIC. The dosage is usually adjusted according to clotting studies. Heparin is also used because of the prolonged immobility often associated with shock. Immobility predisposes clients to venous thrombosis and pulmonary emboli. The treatment of DIC may include heparin administration to minimize consumption of clotting factors. Heparin also may be appropriate for clients with ARDS if the primary cause of the respiratory insufficiency is suspected to be DIC or massive microembolism.

Steroids. Steroids have several effects that may assist the client in neurogenic shock after spinal cord injury. They are given to reduce edema in the cord and have been shown to improve recovery. They assist in treatment by stabilizing lysosomal membrane and preventing intracellular release of enzymes. Complications from high-dose steroid therapy include acute GI bleeding, aggravation of diabetes, and immunosuppression. In the past, steroids were given to treat septic shock, but mortality was not reduced and the practice was abandoned.

Naloxone. Naloxone (Narcan), an opiate antagonist, is commonly used to treat opioid and synthetic opioid overdosages. During stress, opiate-like substances known as *enkephalins* and *endorphins* are released from the brain. Although the mechanisms of action are not clear, endorphins may play a role in capillary bed vasodilation found in all forms of shock. Studies indicate that when naloxone is administered to animals not in shock, no significant cardiovascular effects are noted. However, when administered during shock, naloxone reverses the hypotension and decreases cardiac contractility. It is believed that naloxone blocks the effects of endorphins and enkephalins.

Epinephrine. Epinephrine is the drug of choice for emergency treatment of allergic reactions (anaphylaxis). Epinephrine inhibits histamine release and antagonizes 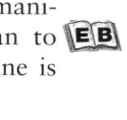 its effects on end organs, resulting in reversal of the bronchial constriction, increased capillary permeability, and vasodilation that occur with acute anaphylactic reactions. The overall effect is improved respiratory status and cardiovascular stability.

Diphenhydramine. Anaphylaxis can also be treated with antihistamines, like diphenhydramine (Benadryl). This medication acts primarily to relieve clinical manifestations associated with anaphylaxis rather than to stop the release of histamine. Therefore epinephrine is always administered first in treating anaphylaxis.

Histamine H$_2$-Receptor Antagonists. Histamine H$_2$-receptor antagonists, which inhibit gastric acid secretion, may be administered intravenously to a client experiencing shock to prevent stress ulcers. They may be prescribed in combination with oral antacids. Stress ulcers are often lethal complications of severe illness or injury produced by continuous shunting of blood from the GI tract from extended sympathetic nervous system stimulation.

Opioids. The need for pain reduction may be obvious in clients experiencing different types of shock. However, the use of opioids for pain management may be dangerous. Opioids interfere with vasoconstriction, and vasoconstriction may be the mechanism by which the client's BP is maintained. Morphine sulfate, however, causes pooling of blood in the extremities and contributes to a decrease in anxiety. These effects may prove useful for the client in cardiogenic shock.

Cardiotonic Medications. Medications that improve myocardial contraction are basic in treating those forms of shock that decrease cardiac output (e.g., hypovolemic shock and cardiogenic shock):

- Digitalis is often used if there is evidence of cardiac failure. By strengthening and slowing the heartbeat, digitalis supports a weakened heart and may reduce the heart rate to a more normal level.
- Amiodarone, lidocaine, bretylium, quinidine, and procainamide may treat dysrhythmias that tend to reduce cardiac efficiency. However, these medications reduce myocardial contractility.
- Atropine may treat bradycardia, which predisposes clients to cardiogenic shock.

Calcium. Calcium is needed for normal functioning of the nervous and cardiovascular systems and for blood clotting. The value and dosages of calcium in treating shock are not clear. However, calcium may be administered if impaired cardiac function is evident. Calcium

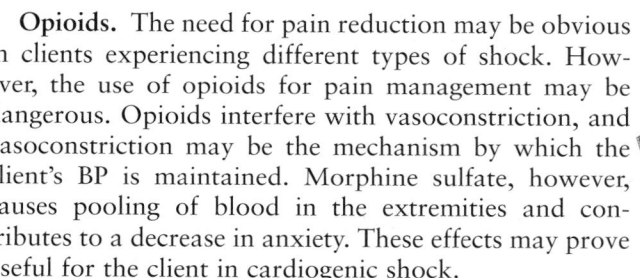

may precipitate toxic effects in a person who has received digitalis. It is given only with extreme caution to such a person. Monitor for evidence of digitalis toxicity (e.g., bradydysrhythmias or tachydysrhythmias, ST-segment depression).

Calcium chloride should be given intravenously only. Calcium gluconate may be given intramuscularly but is irritating to tissues. Although calcium chloride and calcium gluconate are both available as 10% solutions, they are not identical in concentration. Do not substitute one for the other. Indications of hypocalcemia may be subtle. Careful assessment is essential. (See discussions of calcium in Chapter 14.)

■ Nursing Management of the Medical Client

Nursing outcomes are similar to medical outcomes in that the overall goals of care are to correct the causative factor if possible, improve oxygenation, restore and maintain adequate tissue perfusion, and prevent complications. However, most of the interventions provided for clients in shock require a physician's order and are not independent nursing actions. The nurse's major responsibilities in shock include assessment of the client's condition and timely and accurate performance of dependent interventions.

Assessment

Because a client's condition can change rapidly in shock, frequent nursing assessment is essential. Documentation of the progress and response to interventions needs to be concise, yet convey the client's status minute by minute.

Initiate a flow sheet containing all pertinent data in an easily read format. This flow sheet must contain the assessments essential in treating shock. Blood chemistries, blood gases, oxygen saturations, and electrolytes need to be determined frequently and reported promptly so therapy can be adjusted to the client's rapidly changing physiologic status.

The first step in assessing a person in shock is a general overview, giving attention to airway, breathing, and circulation (ABC). Once the airway is patent, air exchange is adequate, a pulse is present, and the cervical spine is immobilized (if it is a trauma situation), perform a rapid, cursory initial head-to-toe physical assessment. The initial assessment goal is to identify major problems and gross abnormalities. Give further detailed attention to specific injuries or problems after shock is stabilized.

Improve Oxygenation. Several assessments should be performed to determine that no airway or breathing problems exist. To determine airway patency, assess for the presence of noisy respirations and check for obstructions. Listen to lung sounds to determine adequate air movement. Assess the respiratory rate and effort to evaluate the adequacy of breathing. Evaluate chest wall ex-

pansion and assess for chest wall bulges or defects. Monitor for tracheal deviation, which could indicate tension pneumothorax.

When caring for clients experiencing shock, carefully differentiate nursing diagnoses concerning pain and impaired gas exchange. Restlessness is an assessment finding common to both and can thus be easily misinterpreted. Too often clients who are restless, especially trauma victims, are given opioids because their behavior is incorrectly interpreted as resulting from pain. However, the restlessness frequently is actually due to hypoxia, and opioids worsen the problem. The decision to administer opioids is often a nursing decision. It is important to assess the need for these medications carefully. Attention to positioning, splinting of injured areas, breathing techniques, and comfort measures may provide safer and more effective pain reduction than opioids. (Pain is discussed in detail in Chapter 22.)

Restore and Maintain Adequate Perfusion. To complete the critical assessment of ABCs, circulation must be evaluated. Assess the client's pulse, BP, skin color, temperature, heart sounds, peripheral pulses, state of hydration, and skin perfusion (e.g., capillary refill time less than 3 seconds). Check the condition of the mucous membranes, sclera, and conjunctivae; the presence of pallor or cyanosis; and fullness of the neck veins (jugular venous distention, which may suggest right heart failure and cardiogenic shock).

It is imperative that the adequacy of blood volume be determined before administration of opioids to a client suffering from acute, multiple trauma. Opioid administration causes vasodilation, which results in severe hypotension or shock. If a opioid is administered intramuscularly to a client in shock, it also may not be completely absorbed because of the vasoconstriction that is present. Because the client experiences little or no pain reduction, a second injection may be given. Once fluid resuscitation is complete and the circulating volume is restored, the client may absorb both doses of the opioid. No one in shock should be given intramuscular medications when rapid onset of action of the drug is needed.

When opioids are appropriate for a client in shock, they are most effective if administered intravenously in small doses. When caring for trauma victims, especially those with massive injury, the extent of the injury does not necessarily coincide with the amount of pain being experienced. Careful assessment is necessary once opioid administration seems safe (in terms of the client's hemodynamic status). Assess the client's BP more closely after IV administration of opioids to watch for hypotension.

Even though a person in shock may feel cold and may be hypothermic, do not apply heat to the skin. Heat application dilates peripheral blood vessels and draws blood away from the vital organs (where it is life-sustaining) into the vessels of the skin. This interferes with the body's initial compensatory mechanism of peripheral vasoconstriction. Heat also increases the body's metabolism. In turn, this increases the need for oxygen and puts an added strain on the heart.

This does not mean that the person is kept in a cold environment. The environment is kept warm because it is important that the person not become chilled. Chilling and shivering require energy expenditure needed to maintain vital functions. Chilling also contributes to sludging of blood in the microcirculation. Hypothermia slows the heart, increases the likelihood of ventricular fibrillation, and inhibits the body's reparative processes.

After potentially life-threatening problems are treated, obtain complete vital signs, with BP taken in both arms to rule out other causes of hypovolemic shock (i.e., thoracic dissection, aneurysm). It is important to take postural vital signs if applicable and if it is safe to do so. Do not take postural vital signs (1) if the client has multiple traumatic injuries, (2) if there is evidence of vertebral, pelvic, or femoral fracture, or (3) if hypotension already exists. Clients with postural hypotension should not be sent to the x-ray department for upright films until they are adequately volume-resuscitated. If x-ray studies must be obtained, clients require constant attendance by a nurse who monitors vital signs, administers IV fluids, and provides guidance to x-ray department personnel regarding movement, positioning, and timing of studies.

Measurement of postural vital signs is done when there is a history or presence of significant blood loss, unexplained tachycardia, a history of fluid loss (e.g., diarrhea, vomiting, diuretic therapy, or third-space loss), unexplained syncope, blunt chest or abdominal trauma, or abdominal pain.

Alternative Methods of Blood Pressure Monitoring.
 Often when a client is in shock, it is difficult to auscultate BP with a standard stethoscope. Two commonly used techniques to obtain BP measurements are palpation of the radial or brachial pulse during deflation of the BP cuff and use of a Doppler instrument. When palpation is used, the first palpable pulse noted during deflation of the cuff is the systolic BP. Document the BP as such (e.g., 90/palp). A Doppler instrument amplifies arterial and venous pulsations by ultrasonography. Various Doppler probes are available and are used instead of a stethoscope to measure BP. Systolic BP is easily heard by placing the probe over the brachial artery after applying transmission gel. The diastolic BP is not obtainable when the Doppler is used.

For clarity and accuracy, document the method by which BP readings are taken (in addition to the readings themselves) and whether palpation or a Doppler monitor is used. This is important because these readings may be higher or lower than those obtained in the standard way with a cuff and stethoscope. Likewise, document

whether readings are obtained by automatic BP machines even though readings from these machines may not differ from those taken in the standard way.

Direct measurement of arterial BP by use of an arterial line often is done during shock. Discussion of arterial lines is found in Chapter 56.

Temperature Monitoring. An accurate core temperature measurement is important in assessing a client in shock. Sometimes an indwelling flexible rectal probe connected to a continuous display monitor is more accurate and less traumatic than intermittent rectal temperature measurements with a standard thermometer. Core temperature can also be measured with an indwelling urinary catheter that contains a thermometer. Tympanic temperatures are commonly used in critical care settings and provide core temperature measurements. Core temperature can also be obtained if the client has a thermodilution (Swan-Ganz) catheter in place.

Oral temperature measurement is neither accurate nor safe. During shock, the buccal mucosa is poorly perfused, and the client should be receiving oxygen by mask or nasal prongs. (Because clients in shock are hypoxemic, the procedure of removing the oxygen long enough to obtain an oral temperature is not routinely recommended.)

Cardiac Monitoring. For assessment and evaluation purposes, the electrical activity of the heart needs to be continuously monitored in all clients in shock, regardless of age. Nurses caring for clients experiencing shock need to be able to initiate cardiac monitoring, recognize cardiac dysrhythmias, and initiate treatment for any potentially lethal dysrhythmias that occur (see Chapter 56).

During the initial resuscitation period, it may be more appropriate to place the ECG monitor electrodes on the client's shoulders than on the chest. This placement does not interfere with chest film findings. It also allows better access to the chest for thoracic procedures such as insertion of chest tubes, pericardiocentesis, and CVP line placement. Once the client's condition is stabilized, the electrodes may be moved to the chest.

Hemodynamic Monitoring. Measurement of CVP is one hemodynamic technique that may be used in initial shock management, especially with hypovolemic shock. However, because CVP only provides information regarding preload, peripheral intra-arterial lines or a pulmonary artery catheter is inserted as soon as possible. Blood volume needs to be expanded as the vascular space enlarges, and CVP measurements are used to determine the amount of fluid needed to fill the enlarging vascular space. The rate of fluid replacement is adjusted to maintain the desired CVP. It is serious if the CVP continues to decrease despite fluid replacement. This means that the rate and volume of fluid replacement are not sufficient to meet the client's physiologic needs.

Peripheral arterial catheters are commonly used in shock to measure arterial BP and MAP and to obtain blood samples for chemical and blood gas analysis. These catheters are usually placed in the radial artery but may also be placed in the femoral or brachial arteries. Pulmonary artery and PCWP measurements are monitored to assess left-sided heart function and to guide fluid administration. These pressures are measured through a Swan-Ganz catheter. The PCWP corresponds to the LV end-diastolic pressure. This is the pressure in the LV just before contraction. An increase in this pressure in a client with cardiogenic shock may indicate left-sided heart failure. A low value in a client with hypovolemic shock may indicate that volume replacement is needed. In a client with septic shock, lower values would be expected during the warm phase and higher values during the cold phase.

Depending on the type of Swan-Ganz catheter used, additional measurements may be obtained. Some catheters have a fiberoptic tip that allows measurement of oxygen saturation of hemoglobin in the venous blood (SvO_2). SvO_2 is measured in the pulmonary artery, just before reoxygenation of the blood in the lungs. This reading gives an average of the tissue uptake or use of oxygen in the body. The normal range for SvO_2 is 60% to 80%. When the SvO_2 goes below 60%, it may indicate either decreased arterial oxygenation or increased tissue oxygen demand. If the SvO_2 is greater than 80%, the indication, in relation to shock, is that the oxygen is unable either to reach the tissues or to be extracted by the tissues.

Most Swan-Ganz catheters also have a thermistor bead just proximal to the balloon. This may be used to determine cardiac output by a thermodilution technique. A fourth lumen opens at the level of the right atrium, and CVP measurements (preload) can be obtained through this lumen.

Cardiac Output Monitoring. Cardiac output, measured in liters per minute, is the amount of blood pumped by the LV into the aorta each minute. During shock, cardiac output may be decreased because of myocardial damage resulting from an MI or, in hypovolemic shock, from inadequate volume replacement.

Because of the widespread use of Swan-Ganz catheters and the ease of obtaining measurements, cardiac output monitoring is used in managing all types of shock. These measurements assess overall cardiac function and the function of the LV. Factors that may alter cardiac output include heart rate, SVR, age, body size, exercise, and (in persons with cardiac problems) decreased filling or emptying of the LV.

Cardiac index is the cardiac output divided by the body surface area. Cardiac output as a separate reading does not take into account the amount of tissue that needs to be perfused. By figuring body size into the calculation, a more accurate assessment is obtained.

SVR can be determined by using the cardiac output and the MAP. SVR measures afterload and provides information regarding vasoconstriction or vasodilation. Decreased SVR indicates systemic vasodilation and may indicate the need for administration of vasoconstrictors. Increased SVR indicates systemic vasoconstriction and the potential need for vasodilators. Arterial BP and cardiac function should always be taken into consideration before administering vasoconstrictors or vasodilators.

Prevent Complications. Although it is important to begin assessments and interventions with the ABCs, additional assessments are necessary to evaluate the client's overall condition and prevent complications. Additional assessments important in preventing complications include evaluation of the following:

- Level of consciousness and orientation $\times$ 3 (i.e., person, place, time)
- Ability to move extremities
- Sensation in all extremities
- Hand grasps
- Response to verbal and painful stimuli
- Pupil size and reaction to light
- Presence of abnormal posturing; presence, location, intensity, and duration of pain and what reduces the pain
- Bowel sounds
- Abdominal distention or rigidity
- Circumference of abdomen or extremities
- Presence of lacerations, contusions, ecchymoses, petechiae, and purpura (also check for bruising over flank area)
- Bone deformities
- Presence of medical alert tags or bracelets

Prevent Renal Impairment. An indwelling urinary catheter is a simple means of monitoring a client during shock. Continuously measuring urinary flow provides important information about peripheral blood flow and kidney function. Because the amount of urine excreted during shock is often small, it is important to have an accurate, calibrated urine collector. In some settings, the catheter may be attached to a urinometer collector or to a more complex electric urinometer.

Urinary volume changes can be highly important as an index of the success or failure of therapy. Minimal (less than 0.5 ml/kg/hr) or absent urine output indicates treatment is not successful. Increasing urine output is a favorable sign. Assess the client's urine output routinely and record it at least every hour.

Diagnosis, Outcomes, Interventions

Diagnosis: Ineffective Tissue Perfusion. The nursing diagnosis *Ineffective Tissue Perfusion* can be used to describe the reduced tissue perfusion and inadequate effective circulating intravascular blood volume. This diagnosis does not describe the oxygen-carrying capacity of the blood, but rather the volume of circulating blood and its ability to reach the tissues. The nursing diagnosis can be written *Ineffective Tissue Perfusion (specify type) related to actual or relative (specify type) hypovolemia secondary to shock (specify type)*. Other potential nursing diagnoses for the client in shock are listed in Box 83-1.

Outcomes. Nursing care of the client with shock is complex. Specific nursing and medical interventions vary according to individual needs and the setting in which care is delivered (e.g., emergency department versus intensive care unit). However, two major physiologic outcomes of care are desired:

1. Adequate blood flow (tissue perfusion) and cellular oxygenation are achieved to maintain the integrity of the tissue or organ.
2. The metabolic needs of the tissue or organ are reduced or maintained.

Interventions. Provide continuous assessment of the client. Cardiovascular and respiratory changes can occur

---

BOX 83-1   *Potential Nursing Diagnoses for the Client in Shock*

Activity Intolerance
Acute Pain
Anticipatory Grieving
Anxiety
Bathing/Hygiene, Dressing/Grooming, Toileting Self-Care
    Deficit
Compromised Family Coping
Constipation
Decreased Cardiac Output
Deficient Fluid Volume
Disturbed Body Image
Disturbed Personal Identity
Disturbed Sleep Pattern
Disturbed Sensory Perception: Visual, Auditory, Kinesthetic,
    Gustatory, Tactile, Olfactory
Fear
Imbalanced Nutrition: Less than Body Requirements
Impaired Gas Exchange
Impaired Physical Mobility
Impaired or Risk for Impaired Skin Integrity
Impaired Tissue Integrity
Impaired Verbal Communication
Ineffective Airway Clearance
Ineffective Breathing Pattern
Ineffective Protection
Ineffective Tissue Perfusion: Cerebral, Cardiopulmonary, Gastrointestinal, Renal, Peripheral
Interrupted Family Processes
Spiritual Distress

---

rapidly, and interventions must be adjusted promptly. Document observations clearly and concisely.

Help decrease tissue oxygen demand. Because shock states can double the body's O_2 consumption, promote factors that decrease tissue oxygen need. Interventions aimed at decreasing total body work, pain, anxiety, and temperature decrease tissue oxygen demand.

Keep equipment and supplies (e.g., suction, emergency drugs) available and in working order. Implement appropriate, planned nursing interventions to prevent complications that can develop from enforced immobilization. Provide adequate pain reduction, because pain intensifies shock. Base this intervention on careful assessment.

Diagnosis: Interrupted Family Processes. Sudden changes in the family's communication and ability to problem solve without the client and concerns about the cause of illness, or worry about the outcome create a situational crisis. The appropriate nursing diagnosis is *Interrupted Family Processes*.

Outcomes. The goal is that the usual processes of coping for the family remain intact or that a new process be adopted to facilitate problem solving. Outcomes may include that the family members remain supportive of each other, cope reasonably well with the crisis, and participate in problem solving or decision making with the health care team. Another goal might be that the client and significant others understand the cause of the problem and modify their lifestyle to minimize or eliminate the causative factor.

Interventions. Facilitate expression of concerns and questions by the client and family. For example, try to reduce the client's fears and anxieties about what is happening and about the equipment being used.

A client in shock is extremely ill and may die. In addition, the stress of the situation is compounded by emergency medical treatment, with all the people, equipment, and movement this entails. During shock management, nurses attend to numerous delegated medical care activities. However, there must be sufficient nursing resources to provide psychosocial care (e.g., reassurance, emotional support) to the client and family. All of the people involved may be frightened, anxious, confused, and dependent (see the Evidence-Based Practice in Action feature on Helping Family Members Deal with Life-Threatening Illnesses on p. 2472).

Keep the client's family informed of what is happening. They need information on which to base decisions. Because of the family's anxiety, the nurse may need to calmly repeat information several times. See the Client Education Guide feature on Shock on p. 2473 for information to be conveyed. Remember that the client and significant others may be experiencing "psychological shock." They often need (and greatly appreciate) oppor-

EB EVIDENCE-BASED PRACTICE IN ACTION

Helping Family Members Deal with Life-Threatening Illnesses

The etiologies leading to the various types of shock usually have a sudden onset. Families and significant others have little warning or preparation for the life-threatening nature of their loved one's illness and few have had experience with a family member being critically ill. The illness trajectory is often characterized by periods of stability and instability, and the critically ill client may move back and forth between the two states. All of this leads to a great deal of uncertainty for the families of individuals with shock.

Uncertainty as a concept has been described as having four components: (1) ambiguity concerning the state of the illness, (2) complexity concerning treatment and the system of care, (3) lack of information regarding diagnosis and the severity of illness, and (4) unpredictability of the course of illness and outcome.[2] All four of these components may be experienced by families of an individual in shock.

Three studies were reviewed to determine the factors that lead to uncertainty and to identify those interventions most effective in alleviating the uncertainty for families of critically ill clients.

Uncertainty may stem from the tension between the capabilities of modern medicine (i.e., high-tech interventions) to maintain life and the philosophical perspective held by some of death with dignity and the obligation to honor their loved one's wishes related to extraordinary measures to sustain life. Contributors to uncertainty include (1) the client's current health status, (2) treatments necessary to save the loved one's life and the decisions families make about those treatments, (3) lack of information overall, (4) unfamiliarity with the setting, and (5) the need to be with and to be vigilant for their loved one. The experiences families have described resemble a vortex in which there is a downward spiral of prognoses, difficult decisions, feelings of inadequacy, potential for loss despite best efforts, and the possibility that the loved one may remain unconscious and die with no opportunity to say goodbye.

Despite the best efforts of the health care team, sometimes critically ill clients die. However, there are many opportunities during the care of a critically ill client to diminish the family's feelings of uncertainty. Families describe "living it one day at a time" and often need "just in time" information rather than the entire trajectory of information laid out before them. Family members may feel positive about what they have to offer their loved one if they are allowed to participate in the loved one's care.

Families remain vigilant for their loved one. It is unhelpful to provide false hope, but it is equally unhelpful to paint a bleak picture if the outcomes for the client are not yet certain. Families have also described "drawing on God's strength" as something that helps them cope with the uncertainty. Family members may find comfort in talking with someone from pastoral care if that service is available.

Implications for practice include allowing open visitation so that families can spend as much time as they need with their loved one. Families also need to have access to the physicians, nurses, and other health care providers who will listen to their concerns, provide information, and correct any misperceptions they may have. Contact pastoral care or other hospital personnel who can help families find comfort if the family requests it.

Implications for research include exploring the interventions most helpful to families of clients in shock. How much information can families take in at one time? How can the overwhelming nature of the technology be made more manageable for families? Considering the time constraints of health care professionals, how can families' questions and concerns be addressed in a timely manner?

References

1. Kirchhoff, K.T., et al. (2002). The vortex: Families' experiences with death in the intensive care unit. *American Journal of Critical Care, 11*(3), 200-209.
2. Mishel, M.H. (1981). The measurement of uncertainty. *Nursing Research, 30,* 258-263.
3. Pelletier-Hibbert, M., & Sohi, P. (2001). Sources of uncertainty and coping strategies used by family members of individuals living with end stage renal disease. *Nephrology Nursing Journal, 28*(4), 411-419.
4. Plowfield, L.A. (1999). Living a nightmare: Family experiences of waiting following neurological crisis. *Journal of Neuroscience Nursing, 31*(4), 231-238.

tunities to discuss with care providers their important concerns.

EB Help the client (and family) feel physically and emotionally comfortable. Do not keep loved ones away from the client unnecessarily. Because of limited space, there may be times when they must wait in another room for a period of time. However, they should not be kept away long and should be given a reasonable explanation of why it is necessary to leave their loved one.

A client experiencing shock requires emotional support. When caught up in the sudden drama of an emergency or critical care, health professionals sometimes forget that the experience and setting are often new and very frightening for the client. Unfortunately, "dehumanization" of the client may occasionally occur during the rush of emergency treatment. Whether a client appears to be conscious or not, always explain what is happening. Keep the atmosphere as quiet and orderly as possible. Eliminate

CLIENT EDUCATION GUIDE
Shock

- It is difficult to prevent the occurrence of shock because the causes are often unpredictable. If your family member is in shock, obtain precise, consistent information about his or her current status and prognosis.
- Learn about the monitoring equipment in use.
- Learn how to communicate with the client who is intubated or unconscious.
- Learn how to demonstrate love and caring to someone surrounded by equipment.
- Participate in your family member's care during the hospital stay; this increases your ability to provide care at home.
- Learn how to prevent recurrence if the cause was avoidable.

unnecessary chatter. Commonly, recovered clients remember hearing what was said and were aware of what happened to them even though they appeared to be unconscious.

Provide care to the family. Among a nurse's greatest responsibilities are providing support, comfort, and advocacy to clients receiving care and to their significant others. This is very important for nursing clients who are critically ill and are experiencing shock.

Evaluation

It is expected that the client will achieve adequate tissue perfusion and make a full recovery without complications from the type of shock being experienced, be transferred to a medical unit, and eventually be dismissed to home. Recovery from the cause of the shock may be delayed because of the complications created from the shock episode (e.g., wound healing).

■ Surgical Management

Although surgical interventions that can help in shock states are limited, they may be very useful in trauma situations. In hypovolemic shock caused by trauma, surgery can be performed to control sources of bleeding. Once bleeding is controlled, interventions aimed at restoring adequate fluid volume are more effective.

■ Self-Care

Shock must be fully resolved before a client is transferred or discharged (unless the client is being transported for the treatment of shock). Clients who survive shock find that recovery from the precipitating problem is delayed. They may also experience some feelings of confusion, depression, or grief when they realize that they lived through a very critical illness.

MULTIPLE ORGAN DYSFUNCTION SYNDROME

Single organ failure (e.g., heart failure, renal failure) has long been recognized as a cause of morbidity and mortality in critically ill clients. In trauma centers in the late 1960s, a new form of organ failure was recognized, that of sequential failure of the lungs, liver, and kidneys usually followed by death. By the 1970s, the syndrome of sequential organ failure was well described. Today, this problem is named *multiple organ dysfunction syndrome* (MODS), *multiple organ system failure*, or *multiorgan system failure* and is considered to be present when two or more organs fail. More recently, the precursor to MODS has been labeled as *systemic inflammatory response syndrome* (SIRS). Twenty percent to 60% of clients in septic shock develop SIRS, and up to 90% of clients who go on to develop MODS die.

Etiology and Risk Factors

Causes of MODS include dead tissue, injured tissue, infection, perfusion deficits, and persistent sources of inflammation such as pancreatitis or pneumonitis. Acute lung injury is usually present in some form. People known to be at high risk for developing MODS include those with impaired immune responses such as older adults, clients with chronic illnesses, clients with malnutrition, and clients with cancer. In addition, clients with prolonged or exaggerated inflammatory responses are at risk, including victims of severe trauma and clients with sepsis.

Prevention is a primary direction of current therapy. Source control is a major emphasis. When possible, the potential source of sepsis or inflammation is excised or removed (e.g., full-thickness burn wound). In many cases, however, the source cannot be removed, such as pneumonia, pancreatitis, soft tissue injury, and hematoma. When the source cannot be removed, empirical antimicrobial agents are used to reduce risk.

It would be helpful to clinicians to be able to predict which clients are at the highest risk, but accurate prediction remains elusive. The most predictive variables appear to be the ratio of arterial oxygen tension (PaO_2) to the fraction of inspired oxygen (FiO_2) on day 1; the plasma lactate on day 2; the serum bilirubin on day 6; and the serum creatinine on day 12 after injury. When nurses note these predictors, increased surveillance should begin.

Pathophysiology

In the healthy person, the normal integrated inflammatory immune response (IIR) protects tissue from microbial invasion and rids the body of cellular debris and foreign material. The IIR is a continual process of responses until the insult slows and the client's condition stabilizes. The IIR stops once it is no longer needed. SIRS is a case of unchecked inflammatory responses. MODS is the end result of the prolonged response.

Most inciting events start with a local injury from trauma, infection, or lack of perfusion. Bacteria introduced into the wound or allowed to grow in necrotic tissues because of a decreased immune response activate the systemic inflammatory responses. Bacteria release toxins that activate systemic mediators of inflammation. Activation of the systemic response is an effort to "recruit help" to battle the invasion of microorganisms.

Once the inflammatory response becomes systemic, it is controlled by chemical mediators of inflammation. Mediators include bradykinin, complement, histamine, interleukin-1, prekallikrein, prostaglandins, and tumor necrosis factor. These powerful mediators of inflammation induce a systemic response. Endothelial cells are a common target for some mediators. The endothelium is destroyed and blood flow is reduced to the tissues. Endothelial damage is produced by endotoxins from bacteria, tumor necrosis factor, interleukin-1, platelet activating factors, and many others. When this inflammatory response is unchecked, it produces damage to organs and tissues by altering perfusion, disturbing oxygen supply or demand, or changing metabolic dysfunctions. Metabolism increases under the direction of mediators such as cortisol and the catecholamines.

Many organs are affected by MODS. The lungs are usually the first to malfunction, because of the large surface area of pulmonary epithelium combined with the presence of bacterial contamination from systemic blood return. The GI tract is generally the second system to malfunction, and it propagates conditions for further deterioration of other organs. Once the GI tract is malfunctioning, bacteria quickly relocate from the GI tract to other organs. Additionally, the hypermetabolic state increases gastric acid production, increasing the risk of ulceration and bleeding. The most serious metabolic problem is hypermetabolism. The hypermetabolic state is continued by cell-to-cell communication and the sympathetic nervous system responds with its usual "fight-or-flight" response.

Classification

There are two types of MODS. *Primary* MODS results directly from "a well-defined insult in which organ dysfunction occurs early and is directly attributed to the insult itself."[1] The direct insult initially causes a localized inflammatory response that may or may not progress to SIRS. An example of primary MODS is a primary pulmonary injury, such as aspiration. Only a small percentage of clients develop primary MODS.

Secondary MODS is a consequence of widespread systemic inflammation, which develops after a variety of insults, and results in dysfunction of organs not involved in the initial insult.[1] The client enters a hypermetabolic state that lasts for 14 to 21 days. During this time, the body engages in autocatabolism, which causes profound changes in the body's metabolic processes. Unless the process can be stopped, the outcome for the client is death. Secondary MODS occurs with conditions such as septic shock and ARDS.

Clinical Manifestations

There is usually a precipitating event to MODS, including aspiration, ruptured aneurysm, or septic shock, which is associated with resultant hypotension. The client is resuscitated; the cause is treated; and the client appears to do well for a few days. The following possible sequence of events often develops.

The client experiences SIRS before MODS develops. Within a few days, there is an insidious onset of a low-grade fever, tachycardia, increased numbers of banded and segmented neutrophils on the differential count (called a left shift), and dyspnea with the appearance of diffuse patchy infiltrates on the chest x-ray film. The client often has some deterioration in mental status, with reasonably normal renal and hepatic laboratory results. Dyspnea progresses, and intubation and mechanical ventilation are required. Some evidence of consumptive coagulopathy (DIC) is usually present. The client is usually stable hemodynamically and has relative polyuria, an increased cardiac index (greater than 4.5 L/min), and systemic vascular resistance of less than 600 dynes cm^{-5}. Clients often have increased blood glucose levels in the absence of diabetes. Some physicians use the criteria presented in Table 83-5 to make the diagnosis of MODS.

Between 7 and 10 days, the bilirubin level increases and continues to increase, followed by an increase in serum creatinine. Blood glucose and lactate levels continue to increase because of the hypermetabolic state. Other progressive changes include excretion of urinary nitrogen and protein combined with decreased levels of serum albumin, prealbumin, and retinol binding protein. Bacteremia with enteric organisms is also common. In addition, infections from *Candida* and viruses such as herpes and cytomegalovirus are common. Surgical wounds fail to heal, and pressure ulcers may develop. During this time, the client needs increasing amounts of fluids and inotropic medications to keep blood volume and cardiac preload near normal and to replace fluids lost through polyuria.

Between day 14 and day 21, the client is unstable and appears close to death. The client may lose consciousness. Renal failure worsens to the point of considering dialysis. Edema may be present because of low serum protein levels. Mixed venous oxygen levels may increase because of problems with tissue uptake of oxygen caused by mitochondrial dysfunction. Lactic acidosis worsens, liver enzymes continue to increase, and coagulation disorders become impossible to correct.

TABLE 83-5	*Modified Apache II Criteria for Diagnosis of Multiple Organ Dysfunction Syndrome*

Cardiovascular Failure (Presence of One or More of the Following)

Heart rate <54 beats/min

Mean arterial pressure ≤49 mm Hg (systolic pressure ≤60 mm Hg)

Occurrence of ventricular tachycardia or ventricular fibrillation

Serum pH ≤7.24 with a $Paco_2$ of ≤40 mm Hg

Respiratory Failure (Presence of One or More of the Following)

Respiratory rate ≤5 breaths/min or ≥49 breaths/min $Paco_2$ ≥50 mm Hg

Alveolar-arterial oxygen difference ≥350 mm Hg (calculate as follows, at sea level: [713 × % oxygen in inspired gas] − $Paco_2$ − Pao_2)

Dependent on ventilator or CPAP on the second day

Renal Failure (Presence of One or More of the Following)

Urine output ≤479 ml/24 hr or ≤159 ml/8 hr

Serum BUN ≥100 mg/dl (35.7 mmol/L)

Serum creatinine ≥3.5 mg/dl (309 μmol/L)

Hematologic Failure (Presence of One or More of the Following)

WBC count ≤1000/μl (1 × 10^9/L)

Platelets ≤20,000/μl (20 × 10^9/L)

Hematocrit ≤20%

Neurologic Failure

Glasgow Coma Scale score ≤6 (in absence of sedation)

Hepatic Failure (Presence of Both of the Following)

Serum bilirubin ≥6 mg%

Prothrombin time ≥4 sec over control in the absence of systemic anticoagulation

From Knaus, W. A., & Wagner, D. P. (1989). Multiple systems organ failure: Epidemiology and prognosis. *Critical Care Clinics, 5*(2), 221.
CPAP, Continuous positive airway pressure; *BUN,* blood urea nitrogen; *WBC,* white blood cell.

Prognosis

 If the process of MODS is not reversed by day 21, it is usually evident that the client will die. Death usually occurs between days 21 and 28 after the injury or precipitating event. Not all clients with MODS die; however, MODS remains the leading cause of death in the intensive care unit, with mortality rates from 50% to 90% despite the development of better antibiotics, better resuscitation, and more sophisticated means of organ support. For those clients who survive, the average duration of intensive care unit stay is about 21 days. The rehabilitation, which is directed at recovery of muscle mass and neuromuscular function, lasts about 10 months.

Outcome Management
■ Medical Management

Restrain the Activators. Manifestations of potential infection must be quickly treated to restrain the activators of MODS. If the agent is known, antibiotics to which the organism is sensitive should be administered. If the organism is not known, broad-spectrum antibiotics are given. Antibiotics are sometimes directed at the probable organism (an empirical treatment). Early aggressive management of sources of infection should be carried out. For example, the client may need to have a large infected wound incised and drained or necrotic tissue excised. Extreme caution must be taken to avoid infecting the client. These clients have many invasive monitors and may have open wounds. Unfortunately, clients in critical care units exist in a paradox. The ICU is the only environment with sophisticated equipment and health care professionals to provide safe care, yet it is an environment where the risk of infection is higher. In addition, there is a high prevalence of multiresistant organisms, such as vancomycin-resistant *enterococci* (VRE) and methicillin-resistant *Staphylococcus aureus* (MRSA).

If the severity of the sepsis is identified early and drotrecogin alfa (Xigris) (see earlier discussion) is administered, progression to MODS may be prevented. However, if there is progression, the lungs are often the first organs to fail and so require special attention. Aggressive pulmonary care is needed in all clients who are at risk of MODS. Interventions may be as simple as coughing and deep breathing or ambulation. The client's oxygen saturation should be monitored as well.

Because malnutrition develops from the hypermetab-olism and the GI tract often seeds other areas with bacteria, some clinicians require the client to be fed enterally. They believe that feeding enhances perfusion and decreases the bacterial load and the effects of endotoxins. Nutrient intake is usually 30 to 35 kcal/kg/day of carbohydrates. Fats are restricted to 0.5 to 1 g/kg/day. Proteins are given to the client via modified amino acids. Some practitioners administer protein until an increase in plasma transferrin or prealbumin is noted. Increases in these values indicate hepatic protein synthesis rather than a breakdown of body stores. Decontamination of the GI tract and pharynx decreases infection but has shown no effect on the death rate from MODS.

Control the Mediators. Controlling the mediators of inflammation is directed at (1) general levels of care and (2) specific treatments targeted at the problem cells. Maintenance of a positive nitrogen balance via nutrition, promotion of sleep and rest, and management of pain are important general care areas. Specific treatments include monoclonal antibodies to control mediators such as interleukin-1, endotoxins, and tumor necrosis factors. These therapies are shown in Table 83-6. Outcomes from research in these treatments are conflicting, and it appears that there is no "magic bullet" to cure the problem. Development of more specific monoclonal antibodies is ongoing.

Protect the Affected Organs. Care is directed toward maintaining the function of organs that fail with MODS. The client is intubated and mechanically ventilated to maintain adequate oxygenation. Oxygen is given to the client until blood levels of lactate decrease toward normal. Elevated serum lactate levels indicate the use of anaerobic metabolism. Nurses must recognize that certain clinical problems further increase the need for oxygen. Problems such as fever, seizures, and shivering increase oxygen demands. These problems should be controlled with medications or environmental changes (e.g., warming).

TABLE 83-6	Summary of Potentially Useful Therapies for Multiple Organ Dysfunction Syndrome
Rationale	**Therapy**
Treatment of infection	Monoclonal antibodies Passive antibody protection Gut decontamination regimens
Support of gut function	Mucosal trophic agents: e.g., glutamine, bombesin, ketone bodies Early enteral feeding Regulation of gut microbial flora
Improved resuscitation	Hypertonic saline In-line sensors Tissue-specific sensors Noninvasive monitoring
Endothelial cell protection	PAF inhibitors WBC adherence inhibition Antioxidant therapy Eicosanoid modulation
Modulation of macrophage function	n3 polyunsaturated fatty acids Signal transduction modulation
Stimulation of lymphocyte function	Arginine w3 polyunsaturated fatty acids

From Lekander, B. J., & Cerra, F. B. (1990). The syndrome of multiple organ failure. *Critical Care Clinics of North America 2*(2), 338.
PAF, Platelet activating factor; *WBC,* white blood cell.

Fluids and inotropic drugs are used to support hemodynamic parameters. The client often becomes more unstable and needs continuous monitoring. Nutritional support is also critical to reduce the catabolism that accompanies hypermetabolism. Dialysis is often used to reduce azotemia from renal failure.

■ Nursing Management of the Medical Client

Care of the client with MODS is multifaceted, balancing the needs of one system against the needs of another while trying to maintain optimal functioning of each system. Nursing diagnoses appropriate for the client with MODS are determined by the system involved and the clinical manifestations identified.

The number of independent nursing interventions for the client with MODS is limited. The overall goal for nursing is effective client and family coping. This complex disorder taxes the client and family. Nurses must remain sensitive to the needs of the family. Caring for the family of critically ill clients is a challenge in that understanding, predicting, and intervening with families in crisis is less exact than the calculation of oxygen needs. There are no easy formulas to use to provide hope, courage, coping, and caring. Nurses must remain alert to the needs of the family as well as the client during this stressful time.

CONCLUSIONS

This chapter discusses shock under three major classifications: hypovolemic, cardiogenic, and distributive. The pathophysiology, clinical manifestations, and medical and nursing management are presented. Shock is a critical condition with a high mortality rate. Early diagnosis and intervention are necessary for the best possible outcomes. Multiple organ dysfunction syndrome is a syndrome of multiple organs progressively failing because of prolonged inflammatory responses.

THINKING CRITICALLY *evolve*

1. The client is a 20-year-old man with a gunshot wound to the right chest and massive hemorrhage. His systolic BP is 60 mm Hg (palpated), heart rate is 130 beats/min, and respiratory rate is 36 breaths/min. The skin is pale, cold, and clammy; capillary refill is greater than 3 seconds; pulses are weak and thready. What priority assessments should be done? What interventions might be performed?

Factors to Consider. What do his vital signs tell you? What injuries might have occurred with a major chest trauma? How can his need for fluid and blood replacement best be met?

2. A 69-year-old man was brought to the emergency department by a rescue squad. He had undergone a

colon resection 2 weeks ago. His wife said that he was having increased difficulty breathing, and he could feel his heart beating in his chest. He also has seemed "slower" to her. He is not moving as fast as usual and gets very dizzy when he stands up. He almost passed out, which is why she called the rescue squad. What priority assessments should be done? What interventions might be performed?

Factors to Consider. What might be happening that could lead to all of the problems with breathing, dizziness, and confusion? What risk might be present as a result of the surgery?

3. A 65-year-old man in the coronary care unit had an acute MI 3 days ago. The monitor alarms and assessments reveal that his BP is 76/50 mm Hg, and his respiratory rate is 20 breaths/min. His pulse is rapid (128 beats/min) and thready. His skin is cool and diaphoretic, with a slight ashen color; the capillary refill is greater than 3 seconds. The client is restless and confused. What priority assessments should be done? What interventions might be performed?

Factors to Consider. What form of shock can quickly develop in a client after an MI? Does he need fluid resuscitation to increase his blood pressure? Why or why not? What medications are commonly used to support a heart in distress? Are special forms of monitoring needed while these medications are used?

Discussions for the questions can be found on the website and the CD-ROM.

BIBLIOGRAPHY

1. Alia, I., et al. (1999). A randomized and controlled trial of the effect of treatment aimed at maximizing oxygen delivery in patients with severe sepsis or septic shock. *Chest, 115*(2), 453-461.
2. American College of Chest Physicians/Society of Critical Care Medicine Consensus Conference Committee. (1992). Definitions for sepsis and organ failure and guidelines for the use of innovative therapies in sepsis. *Critical Care Medicine, 20*(6), 864-874.
3. Bernard, G.R., et al. (2001). Efficacy and safety of recombinant human activated protein C for severe sepsis. *New England Journal of Medicine, 344,* 699-709.
4. Brealey, D., et al. (2002). Association between mitochondrial dysfunction and severity and outcome of septic shock. *Lancet, 360*(9328), 219-223.
5. Coopersmith, C.M., et al. (2002). Inhibition of intestinal epithelial apoptosis and survival in a murine model of pneumonia-induced sepsis. *Journal of the American Medical Association, 287*(13), 1716-1721.
6. Crowther, M.A., & Marshall, J.C. (2001). Continuing challenges of sepsis research. *Journal of the American Medical Association, 286*(15), 1894-1896.
7. Eli Lilly and Company. (2001). Xigris. Drotrecogin alfa (activated). Indianapolis, IN: Author.
8. Fahey, M. (2002). Spinal shock: A nurse's perspective. *Journal of Orthopaedic Nursing, 6*(1), 18-22.
9. Fitch, S.J., & Gossage, J.R. (2002). Optimal management of septic shock. *Postgraduate Medicine, 111*(3), 53-60.
10. Hollenberg, S.M., Kavinsky, C.J., & Parrillow, J.E. (1999). Cardiogenic shock. *Annals of Internal Medicine, 131,* 47-59.
11. Hynes-Gay, P. (2002). Understanding sepsis: From SIRS to septic shock. *Dynamics, 13*(1), 17-18, 20, 22-26.
12. Jindal, N., Hollenberg, S.M., & Dellinger, R.P. (2000). Pharmacologic issues in the management of septic shock. *Critical Care Clinics, 16*(2), 233-249.
13. Khalaf, S., & DeBlieux, P.M.C. (2001). Managing shock: The role of vasoactive agents, Part 1: Making the best choices for patients with septic or cardiogenic shock. *Journal of Critical Illness, 16*(6), 281-284.
14. Kirchhoff, K.T., et al. (2002). The vortex: Families' experiences with death in the intensive care unit. *American Journal of Critical Care, 11*(3), 200-209.
15. Koide, T., et al. (2002). Systemic mastocytosis and recurrent anaphylactic shock. *Lancet, 359*(9323), 2084.
16. Larson, A.M. (2002). Xigris: Reducing mortality in adult patients with severe sepsis. *Urologic Nursing, 22*(3), 200-201.
17. Lent, M. (2001). Systemic toxins: Signs, symptoms, and management of patients in septic shock. *Journal of Emergency Medical Services, 26*(12), 54-56, 58-67.
18. Mayers, I., & Johnson, D. (2000). Septic shock: Treating more than just blood pressure. *Canadian Medical Association Journal, 162*(3), 369-370.
19. Mira, J., et al. (1999). Association of TNF2, a TNF-α promoter polymorphism, with septic shock susceptibility and mortality. *Journal of the American Medical Association, 282*(6), 561-568.
20. Mishel, M.H. (1981). The measurement of uncertainty. *Nursing Research, 30,* 258-263.
21. Mora Santiago, M.R., et al. (1999). Treatment of anaphylactic shock. *Farmacia Hospitalaria, 23,* 131-133.
22. Natanson, C. (2002). Early goal-directed therapy reduced mortality and multiorgan dysfunction in severe sepsis or septic shock. *ACP Journal Club, 136*(3), 90.
23. Pelletier-Hibbert, M., & Sohi, P. (2001). Sources of uncertainty and coping strategies used by family members of individuals living with end stage renal disease. *Nephrology Nursing Journal, 28*(4), 411-419.
24. Plowfield, L.A. (1999). Living a nightmare: Family experiences of waiting following neurological crisis. *Journal of Neuroscience Nursing, 31*(4), 231-238.
25. Przybelski, R.J., et al. (1999). A safety assessment of diaspirin cross-linked hemoglobin (DCLHb) in the treatment of hemorrhagic, hypovolemic shock. *Prehospital Disaster Medicine, 14*(4), 251-264.
26. Rivers, E., et al. (2001). Early goal-directed therapy in the treatment of severe sepsis and septic shock. *The New England Journal of Medicine, 345*(19), 1368-1377.

evolve Did you remember to check out the bonus material on the Evolve website and the CD-ROM, including free self-assessment exercises?

http://evolve.elsevier.com/Black/medsurg/

27. Sanborn, T.A., et al. (2000). Impact of thrombolysis, intra-aortic balloon pump counterpulsation, and their combination in cardiogenic shock complicating acute myocardial infarction: A report from the SHOCK trial registry. *Journal of the American College of Cardiology, 36*(3),1123-1129.

28. Sloan, E.P., et al. (1999). Diaspirin cross-linked hemoglobin (DCLHb) in the treatment of severe traumatic hemorrhagic shock. *Journal of the American Medical Association, 282*(19), 1857-1864.

29. Smith, C., et al. (2001). An extracorporeal membrane oxygenation-based approach to cardiogenic shock in an older population. *Annals of Thoracic Surgery, 71,* 1421-1427.

30. Snooks, H., Moore, F., & Palmer, Y. (2000). Snapshot audit. Care of patients with anaphylactic shock. *Pre-hospital Immediate Care, 4*(1), 51.

31. Stoll, E.H. (2001). Clinical focus: Sepsis and septic shock. *Clinical Journal of Oncology Nursing, 5*(2), 71-72.

32. Walters, M.I., & Norell, M.S. (1999). Cardiogenic shock after myocardial infarction: What should we do? *Care of the Critically Ill, 15*(3), 105-108.

33. Warren, B.L., et al. (2001). High-dose antithrombin III in severe sepsis. *Journal of the American Medical Association, 286*(15), 1869-1878.

34. Wynne, A.L., Woo, T.M., & Millard, M. (2002). *Pharmacotherapeutics for nurse practitioner prescribers.* Philadelphia: F. A. Davis Company.

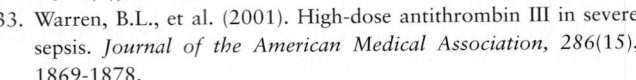
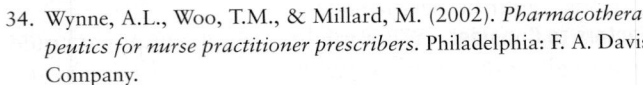

Chapter 84

Management of Clients in the Emergency Department

Judy Selfridge-Thomas

evolve

Web Enhancements

Ethical Issues in Nursing
Are Emergency Personnel Obliged to Honor Clients' Advance Directives?

Appendix A
Religious Beliefs and Practices Affecting Health Care

http://evolve.elsevier.com/Black/medsurg/

Appendix C
Laboratory Values of Clinical Importance in Medical-Surgical Nursing

---

During the mid-1960s, the need for specialization of emergency services throughout the United States was identified as a national priority to reduce the associated morbidity and mortality resulting from catastrophic illness or injury. Since then, the specialties of emergency medicine, emergency nursing, and prehospital care services have grown. In the United States, more than 100 million clients use emergency departments (EDs) for health care services each year.[23,51,76] The number of EDs throughout the United States has not increased over the past decade; in fact they have decreased, but the average daily client census has increased by 35,000 clients per day since 1992.[23] Adults older than 75 years of age are responsible for the highest annual rate of ED visits: 63 visits per 100 people.[23] There were 1154 trauma centers in the United States in 2002.[49]

The scope of services provided in an ED range from treatment of acute conditions that threaten the loss of life, limb, or vision to management of non-urgent, chronic conditions. Current statistics indicate that one third of ED visits are injury related.[23] The most frequent types of client complaints for which clients seek treatments are related to stomach, chest, or abdominal pain, and fever.[23] Problems related to drugs or complications of medical care resulted in 1.4 million ED visits per year in 1999.[23]

EMERGENCY MEDICAL SERVICES

The Emergency Medical Services (EMS) system encompasses all aspects of emergency care. Federal, state, and county EMS systems are designed to complement each other. The systems are responsible for establishing, regulating, coordinating, and monitoring the components involved in the provision of emergency care. These components include entities such as 911 telephone access systems, Emergency Medical Technician (EMT) and paramedical personnel scopes of practice, ground and air ambulance services, dispatch communication between points of incident and responding personnel, and telecommunications between paramedical personnel and specialty-designated EDs known as *base station hospitals*. EMS systems are also instrumental in the coordination of activities for management of disaster situations.

Two goals of the EMS system are (1) to provide emergency care to a client as quickly as possible and (2) to assure that the "right client arrives at the right hospital in the least amount of time." Consequently, EMS systems are involved with specialty-designated hospital departments and EDs such as local or state trauma centers, burn centers, and pediatric care centers.

---

evolve Be sure to check out the bonus material on the Evolve website and the CD-ROM, including free self-assessment exercises.
http://evolve.elsevier.com/Black/medsurg/

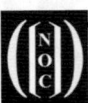

Nursing Outcomes Classification (NOC)
for Nursing Diagnoses—Clients in the Emergency Department

Acute Pain or Chronic Pain
  Comfort Level
  Pain Control
  Pain: Disruptive Effects
  Pain Level
Acute Confusion
  Cognitive Ability
  Distorted Thought Control
  Information Processing
  Memory
  Neurologic Status: Consciousness
  Sleep
Decreased Cardiac Output
  Cardiac Pump Effectiveness
  Circulation Status
  Tissue Perfusion: Abdominal Organs
  Tissue Perfusion: Peripheral
  Vital Signs Status
Deficient Fluid Volume
  Electrolyte and Acid-Base Balance
  Fluid Balance
  Hydration
  Nutritional Status: Food and Fluid
    Intake
Disturbed Sensory Perception
  Anxiety Control
  Body Image
  Cognitive Ability
  Cognitive Orientation
  Distorted Thought Process
  Energy Conservation
  Hearing Compensation Behavior
  Vision Compensation Behavior
Excess Fluid Volume
  Electrolyte and Acid-Base Balance

Fluid Balance
  Hydration
Hypothermia
  Thermoregulation
Hyperthermia
  Thermoregulation
Impaired Gas Exchange
  Electrolyte and Acid-Base Balance
  Respiratory Status: Gas Exchange
  Respiratory Status: Ventilation
  Tissue Perfusion: Pulmonary
  Vital Signs Status
Impaired Physical Mobility
  Ambulation: Walking
  Ambulation: Wheelchair
  Body Positioning: Self-Initiated
  Joint Movement: Active
  Mobility Level
  Sensory Function: Proprioception
  Transfer Performance
Impaired Skin Integrity
  Tissue Integrity: Skin and Mucous
    Membranes
  Wound Healing: Primary Intention
  Wound Healing: Secondary Intention
Ineffective Airway Clearance
  Aspiration Control
  Respiratory Status: Airway Patency
  Respiratory Status: Gas Exchange
  Respiratory Status: Ventilation
Ineffective Breathing Pattern
  Respiratory Status: Airway Patency
  Respiratory Status: Ventilation
  Vital Signs Status

Ineffective Coping
  Aggression Control
  Coping
  Decision Making
  Impulse Control
  Information Processing
  Role Performance
  Social Support
Risk for Infection
  Dialysis Access Integrity
  Immobility Consequences: Physiologic
  Immune Status
  Immunization Behavior
  Knowledge: Infection Control
  Nutritional Status
  Risk Control
  Risk Control: Sexually Transmitted
    Diseases (STDs)
  Risk Detection
  Tissue Integrity: Skin and Mucous
    Membranes
  Treatment Behavior: Illness or Injury
  Wound Healing: Primary Intention
  Wound Healing: Secondary Intention
Risk for Poisoning
  Knowledge: Medicine
  Medication Response
  Risk Control
  Risk Control: Drug Use
  Risk Detection
  Safety Behavior: Home Physical
    Environment
  Self-Care: Nonparenteral Education
  Self-Care: Parenteral Medication
  Suicide: Self-Restraint

EMERGENCY NURSING

Emergency nursing was officially recognized as a specialty in 1970. The national association representing these nurses is the Emergency Nurses Association (ENA). Its current membership comprises more than 25,000 nurses who have chosen this area of professional nursing. The ENA is recognized internationally and by 1999 had approximately 400 members from 35 different countries. Emergency nurses throughout the world have realized both their similarities and differences through use of the World Wide Web and increasing international globalization.

According to the ENA, the definition of emergency nursing involves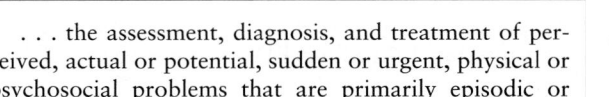

> . . . the assessment, diagnosis, and treatment of perceived, actual or potential, sudden or urgent, physical or psychosocial problems that are primarily episodic or acute. These may require minimal care or life-support measures, education of client and significant others, appropriate referral and knowledge of legal implications.[40]

The ED of the future is being formulated today.[51] Not only is technology changing, but the day-to-day processes that support the ED infrastructure are being challenged and redesigned. These include concepts such as incorporating multiple triage stations and bedside or back-end client registration; using computerized protocols, guidelines, and electronic medical records; integrating nontraditional health care modalities; initiating wireless communication technology; and creating "virtual" EDs.[51]

In addition to the provision of direct client care, other multifaceted roles exist within emergency nursing. The emergency nurse is involved in the initial triaging of clients according to illness severity, may perform as a mobile intensive care nurse (MICN) by directing prehospital care personnel via telecommunication, and frequently provides client care in the prehospital environment. Community clinics use ED nurses, and many emergency nurses have become active in injury prevention programs at both national and local levels. Advanced practice roles such as clinical nurse specialists and nurse practitioners are integrated into many EDs throughout the United States. Nurses in these advanced practice roles often have a master's degree level of education or higher in addition to specialty certification.

Nurses working in an ED must be prepared to provide care to clients of all age-groups who have a myriad of possible illnesses or injuries. It is often cited that emergency nurses must have an understanding of almost all disease processes specific to any age-group. However, ED nursing is not usually addressed in depth in generic nursing programs. The education of ED nurses frequently occurs through hospital orientation programs, post-employment internship courses, and continuing education programs. ED nurses can obtain national specialty certification through an examination process. A certified ED nurse can use the credential of Certified Emergency Nurse (CEN).

▮ LEGAL ISSUES

Nurses deal with a variety of legal issues in whatever specialty area they practice. The ED is no exception; however, certain issues are of paramount importance in this setting.

Federal Legislation

Past federal legislation has mandated that any client who presents to an ED seeking treatment must be rendered aid regardless of financial ability to pay for services. Since the mid-1980s, additional specific legislation has been enacted requiring ED personnel to stabilize the condition of any client considered medically unstable before transfer to another health care facility—the Consolidated Omnibus Budget Reconciliation Act (COBRA) of 1986 and the Omnibus Budget Reconciliation Act (OBRA) of 1990. This stabilization must occur regardless of the client's financial ability to pay for services. ED personnel who transfer clients to another institution

without first providing this initial stabilization can incur substantial fines and penalties, as can the hospital administration.

Clients have continued to seek health care services in the ED, even with the proliferation of managed health care plans and gatekeeping policies. The financial integrity of the ED has been challenged over the years due to the legal obligations of the ED to provide service. Retrospectively, financial reimbursement for rendered services has been denied to EDs from managed health care plans following a determination that the client's problem did not constitute a true emergency. Additional legislation was enacted (Emergency Medical Treatment and Active Labor Act [EMTALA] in 1988, 1989, 1990, and 1994) requiring that a medical screening examination be performed on all ED clients before solicitation of information about ability to pay.[3] This medical screening examination must be inclusive enough to determine whether the client is experiencing an emergency medical condition requiring treatment or, in the case of a pregnant woman, is experiencing labor contractions. An emergency medical condition includes drug abuse, hemodynamic instability, psychiatric illness, intoxication, severe pain, and labor. If a client has an emergency medical condition, stabilization must be rendered. Stabilization is interpreted to mean that deterioration of the client is unlikely during possible transfer or discharge of the client. Continued interpretations of this act have expanded the facilities that come under EMTALA. These include not only EDs, but also hospital-owned urgent care centers, anywhere unscheduled clients appear for medical care, and off-site locations that are within a 250-yard zone of a main hospital that is covered under the 2001 outpatient prospective payment system.[26,27,45,67] Violations of this legislation can again result in fines and penalties. Each congressional year, new legislation and interpretations of existing law are proposed for providing appropriate emergency medical treatment to the public while continuing to acknowledge cost-containment issues.

Consent to Treat

Most adult clients seeking treatment in the ED give voluntary consent to the standard and usual treatment performed in this setting. In some instances, however, a client is deemed unable to give consent for treatment.[73] This inability may be due to the critical nature of the client's illness or injury or to other conditions, such as an altered level of consciousness. In these instances, emergency care may be rendered to the client under the implied emergency doctrine This doctrine assumes that the client would consent to treatment to prevent death or disability if the client were so able.

Children younger than the age of legal majority must have the consent of their parent or legal guardian for medical care to be rendered. Exceptions include (1) emancipated minors, (2) minors seeking treatment for communicable diseases, including sexually transmitted diseases, injuries from abuse, and alcohol or drug rehabilitation, and (3) minor-aged females requesting treatment for pregnancy or pregnancy-related concerns. Some states also allow the adult caregiver with whom the child resides to give treatment authorization even though that caregiver may not be the parent.

The issue of informed consent in the ED is the same as in any other health care setting. Adult clients must be informed about the necessity of required treatments, expected outcomes, and potential complications. Clients must also be mentally competent and understand the information being explained. As in any other setting, a mentally competent adult client always maintains the right to refuse treatment or withdraw previously given consent.

Restraints

Restraining a client while he or she is in the ED may at times be necessary. The need for restraints usually arises because the client is becoming agitated or potentially violent.[44] Hard leather or chemical restraints are used in the ED if the client is in danger of injuring self or others and when nonphysical methods of controlling the client are not viable. Restraints may not be used to control a client solely for convenience or because of staffing issues. When restraints are required, departmental and hospital guidelines that are in compliance with Joint Commission and the Centers for Medicare & Medicaid Services (formerly the Health Care Financing Administration) must be followed.[31] A physician's order for applying restraints as well as the client's behavior mandating the use of restraints must be documented. The client must be periodically reevaluated both for the continued need for restraints and the integrity of distal circulation, motor movement, and sensory level of the restrained extremities. The findings must be documented. Offering water to the client and providing opportunities to urinate or relieve other body needs are required, as is documentation of this nursing care. No client may be kept in restraints against his or her will unless the client's behavior indicates the existence of safety issues. Behavior modification techniques used in an attempt to release the client from restraints must also be documented. The ED staff must receive appropriate education pertaining to dealing with clients requiring physical restraint.[31]

Clients in the ED who have psychological conditions that render them a danger to themselves or to others, or who are unable to provide food or shelter for themselves, can be placed and held on a legal psychiatric restraining order. This order mandates that such clients be placed in a locked psychiatric facility for their protection for a maximum of 72 hours. Within that 72-hour period, the client must be evaluated by a psychiatrist to determine whether the legal hold needs to be extended or whether the client can be released.

Mandatory Reporting

Every state has mandatory reporting regulations that affect emergency nurses. Incidents and conditions may need to be reported to federal, state, or local authorities or to the Department of Public Health, Department of Motor Vehicles, coroner's offices, or animal control agencies. The types of incidents requiring reporting are suspected child, sexual, domestic, and elder abuse; assaults; motor vehicle crashes; communicable diseases such as hepatitis, sexually transmitted diseases, chicken pox, measles, mumps, meningitis, tuberculosis, and food poisoning; first time or recurrent seizure activity; death; and animal bites. Every ED has written policies regarding these mandatory reports.

Evidence Collection and Preservation

Recognition of unusual circumstances surrounding a client's injury or death is an important aspect of ED nursing because of the associated legal implications. Not only must the legal authorities be notified, but also, in many instances, the ED nurse may be required to collect and preserve evidence taken from the client. This evidence can include bullets, weapons, clothing, and body fluid specimens.

All collected evidence must be identified by the client's name, hospital identification number, date and time of evidence collection, type of evidence and source (e.g., venipuncture, hematoma, aspiration vomitus, swab), and the initials or signature of the person collecting the evidence. Once the evidence has been collected, its preservation and the maintenance of the "chain of custody" are extremely important. Table 84-1 and Boxes 84-1 and 84-2 relate to evidence collection.

Violence

Violence directed against ED personnel has become an issue of concern throughout the late 1990s and into the 21st century.[1,29,93] The environment inherent in the ED, the emotional circumstances often surrounding the illness or injury that affect both clients and family members, and the increasingly violent trends in the United States all play a role in this phenomenon.[46,47] Administrative changes have been made in some EDs to enhance both public and health care worker safety. These measures have included the installation of items such as metal detectors, "panic buttons," bullet-proof glass, and lockdown doors at public entrances; increasing the visibility of security guards; using patrol guard dogs; and instituting visitor control policies. Changing the perception of the ED from one of fear and isolation for both clients and family members is also occurring. Instituting family-centered practices that recognize the importance of family participation and addressing the emotional needs of clients and families is a trend in ED management.[4,21] However, education of ED personnel in violence preven-

TABLE 84-1	*Evidence Collection in the Emergency Department*
Evidence	**Collection/Container**
Glass fragments, bullets, broken fingernails, paint chips, loose hair follicles, fibers, or trace evidence such as soil	Place each item in a paper envelope or specimen container.
Head or pubic hair samples	Collected samples from combings and cuttings are each placed in a paper envelope.
Blood (from both venipuncture and possible hematoma evacuation), urine, gastric washings, or vomitus	A 20- to 30-ml sample placed in a sealed container.
Swabs from wounds, membranes, or orifices	Air-dry before placing in a collection container or paper envelope.

From Selfridge-Thomas, J. (1995). *Manual of emergency nursing* (p. 382). Philadelphia: W.B. Saunders.

tion is also of paramount importance in reducing the toll of violence. The following areas are crucial to address[93]:

- Recognizing potentially violent clients and situations
- Identifying verbally and physically abusive signs from clients, family members, or friends
- Understanding the importance of instinct or "gut reactions"
- Using simple communication strategies to defuse potentially problematic situations
- Requiring clients to completely undress before physical examination
- Minimizing the presence of "potential weapons" in client care areas such as scalpels, needles, excess tubing attached to oxygen flow meters, scissors, stethoscopes worn around the neck, and personal jewelry
- Restraining clients, when necessary, using a team approach
- Avoiding becoming a hostage in a volatile situation
- Having safety committee track all reported assaults on clients and employees
- Ensuring Occupational Safety and Health Administration violence guidelines are followed
- Encouraging employees to report both verbal and physical assaults

Once a violent situation has erupted, the protection of ED personnel and others in the department is of utmost concern. Any means necessary to ensure their safety must be undertaken.

BOX 84-1	*Tips for Preserving Evidence in the Emergency Department*

1. Minimally handle the body of a deceased person.
2. Place paper bags on the hands and feet and possibly over the head of a deceased person to protect trace evidence or residue.
3. Place wet clothing in individual paper bags. Do not use plastic bags, as wet clothes can "sweat," thereby destroying evidence.
4. Photograph inflicted wounds or injury before cleansing or repair.
5. Do not insert invasive tubes through pre-existing wounds or holes (e.g., do not place chest tubes through chest wounds or intravenous catheters through needle track marks).
6. Do not cut clothing through evidence holes such as stab wounds or bullet wounds.
7. Collect the client's personal items such as written notes, drugs or medications, and items from clothing pockets.
8. Do not allow family members, significant others, or friends to be alone with the client.

From Selfridge-Thomas, J. (1995). *Manual of emergency nursing* (p. 382). Philadelphia: W.B. Saunders.

BOX 84-2	*Maintaining "Chain of Custody" of Evidence in the Emergency Department*

1. Label all collected evidence with client information data.
2. Document all collected evidence with the date and time and the initials of the person collecting evidence.
3. Document all transfers of evidence from one person to another, and include the reason for transfer of evidence.
4. Obtain signatures of the person releasing evidence and of the person receiving evidence.
5. *Never* leave collected evidence unattended.

From Selfridge-Thomas, J. (1995). *Manual of emergency nursing* (p. 383). Philadelphia: W.B. Saunders.

ETHICAL ISSUES

The ethical issues confronting ED nurses usually deal with end-of-life concerns. Initial resuscitation and stabilization of clients in critical condition constitute universal standard practice in the ED. At times, however, the desired outcome of client survivability is not achievable.

Unexpected Death

When death occurs in the ED setting, it is usually sudden and unexpected, even if the client has had a prolonged illness. The unexpected nature of the death, or impending death, can present ethical dilemmas for both the family survivors and the ED personnel.[87] One such issue deals with the length to which resuscitation is performed. This is usually a physician's decision; however, family members may at times have input. Allowing family members or significant others to be present during client resuscitation is becoming more common. This practice is not necessarily disruptive to the resuscitation process, and it can be of comfort to the survivors and the involved ED personnel.[22,52]

When death does occur, the ED nurse and the ED physician have important roles in informing the family:

- Inform the family of the client's death, and refer to the deceased client by name.
- Provide the family with an explanation of the course of events related to the death; use simple explanations.
- Offer the family an opportunity to view the body. If a child has died, allow the parent to hold the child. Providing the parent with a lock of the child's hair may be comforting.
- Help the family to focus on decisions requiring immediate attention such as taking possession of the deceased person's valuables, arranging postmortem examination if desired or required, identifying possible organ or tissue donation, and selecting a funeral home.
- Inform family members when they can leave the ED setting.
- Provide community agency referral as needed.

Advance Directives

In 1991, Congress enacted the Patient Self-Determination Act (PSDA), which allows a client, or the client's health care proxy, to make determinations related to end-of-life measures. Emergency care personnel are obligated to abide by the client's advance directive decisions, if that information is available and provided in writing. When this written information is not available, ED personnel have a responsibility to stabilize or resuscitate any client according to standard treatment guidelines regardless of a family member's expressed wishes.

Organ and Tissue Donation

Issues related to potential organ or tissue donation often arise in the ED setting. Once a potential donor is identified, the surviving family members need to be approached. A team approach involving a physician, a nurse, and possibly an organ procurement coordinator is optimal. Utmost dignity and professionalism must be maintained. (Chapter 82 reviews religious and cultural customs and beliefs related to death and organ transplantation. Also see the WebLinks icon for Chapter 82, which includes links to various agencies, organizations, and the latest medical information.) Whatever decision the family makes regarding organ or tissue donation, that decision must be supported by health care personnel.

Child Abandonment

States are beginning to pass child abandonment laws in response to the number of newborn infants being abandoned following birth. In general, the law allows mothers to bring their newborn child to the ED and abandon the child in the care of the ED personnel. The mother bears no criminal responsibility. Local Departments of Social Services are then contacted so the child can be placed in their custody.

COMPONENTS OF EMERGENCY CARE

Even though treatment decisions in the ED may at first appear to occur in a chaotic fashion, there is an inherent order in the timing and choice of interventions performed throughout a client's stay. The organizational flow of events involves client triage (prioritizing), in-depth nursing assessment of the client, diagnostic testing, formulation of diagnoses, outcome management, evaluation, disposition, and documentation.

Triage

Whether clients arrive in the ED via ambulance or are ambulatory, they are triaged at some point by either an ED physician or an ED nurse. The purpose of this triage process is to expediently determine the severity of a client's problem or condition. The acuity level of the presenting problem is rated according to predetermined categories; the most frequently used ratings are *emergent*, *urgent*, and *non-urgent*. Box 84-3 provides a definition for each of these categories. Newer systems using a five-level rating approach are being incorporated into client triage. See the Evidence-Based Practice in Action feature on Emergency Department Triage Priority Rating Systems on p. 2485. These five-level rating systems are one of two types. In one type, the previous *urgent* and *non-urgent* categories may be further subdivided into unstable and stable clients.[84] Another five-level rating system is the Emergency Severity Index (ESI).[94] This system is

---

BOX 84-3 | *Three-Category Triage Rating in the Emergency Department*

Emergent category: Client must be treated immediately; otherwise, life/limb/vision is threatened.

Urgent category: Client requires treatment, but life/limb/vision is not threatened if care cannot be provided within 1 to 2 hours.

Nonurgent category: Client requires evaluation and possible treatment, but time is not a critical factor.

based on the triage nurse identifying the critical clients and then predetermining the number of department resources most likely required to treat the non-urgent client. Figure 84-1 displays this algometric approach. Once an initial determination is made about the severity of the client's condition, a more in-depth nursing and medical assessment is completed. Appropriate diagnostic testing and specific interventions are performed using a team approach as emergency physicians and nurses work collaboratively to provide appropriate and expeditious management of the client's problem.

Nursing Assessment

The nursing assessment process for any client entering the ED is divided into *primary* and *secondary* assessments (Figure 84-2).

The purpose of the *primary assessment* is to immediately identify any client problem that poses a threat, immediate or potential, to life, limb, or vision. Information is gathered primarily through objective data.[85] If any abnormalities are found during the primary assessment, immediate interventions such as cardiopulmonary resuscitation (CPR) and Advanced Life Support (ALS) must be instituted to aid in preserving the client's life, limb, or vision. The primary assessment uses the *ABC* mnemonic:

- *A* Airway patency
- *B* Breathing effectiveness
- *C* Circulation (both peripheral and organ-specific)

For any client arriving in the ED who has been involved in a major traumatic injury, the primary assessment must also include an evaluation of the cervical spine area for any potential injury.

Once it is determined that a client's ABC status is satisfactory, the *secondary assessment* is performed to identify any other non–life-threatening problems the client may be experiencing.[85] Both subjective information and objective data are obtained. The secondary assessment includes the following elements.

Neurologic Assessment

Determine the client's (1) level of consciousness; (2) orientation to person, place, time, and event; (3) Glasgow Coma Scale (GCS) score (Table 84-2); (4) pupillary size, equality, and reaction to light and accommodation; and (5) motor movement and strength of hand grips and pedal pushes. In children, a brief neurologic assessment can be determined using the *AVPU* mnemonic: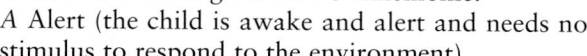

- *A* Alert (the child is awake and alert and needs no stimulus to respond to the environment)
- *V* Verbal (the child requires a verbal stimulus to elicit a response)
- *P* Pain (the child requires a painful stimulus to evoke a response)
- *U* Unresponsive (the child is unresponsive to any applied stimulus)

EB EVIDENCE-BASED PRACTICE IN ACTION

Emergency Department Triage Priority Rating Systems

Accurate triage is an essential component of ED nursing. Determining appropriate client assessments and priority ratings enhances both client care and client flow. The current three-tiered priority rating system of classifying client acuity according to emergent, urgent, and non-urgent categories has recently been challenged in terms of reliability and interrater agreement.[5] Under the three-tiered system, reliability in the ranking of client acuity has been shown to be poor among experienced emergency nurses.[1] The five-tiered systems that are standard in Australia and Canada have been shown to be superior in terms of reliability. The five-tiered systems provide a more discriminating rating of clients, using categories of emergent, high urgent, urgent, low urgent, and non-urgent.[2-4]

Various five-tiered systems have been explored to incorporate as the national standard for triage rating systems within the United States. One such system, the Emergency Severity Index (ESI), is a flowchart-style algorithm incorporating both client acuity and resource allotment in determining client illness severity. Use of the ESI and other five-tiered systems has consistently shown a decrease in undertriaging of clients as well as more accuracy among less experienced triage nurses.[4,5]

Implications

Incorporating a five-tiered acuity rating system at triage may become the national standard for performing triage in the ED. Nurses in the ED triage nurse role may have greater flexibility in determining client illness or injury severity, and better opportunity to more accurately reflect the urgency of the client's complaint.

References

1. Beveridge, R., et al. (1999). Reliability of the Canadian ED triage and acuity scale: inter-rater agreement. *Annals of Emergency Medicine, 34,* 155-159.
2. Fernandez, C., et al. (1999). How reliable is emergency department triage? *Annals of Emergency Medicine, 34,* 41-7.
3. McMahon, M. (2003). ED triage. *American Journal of Nursing, 103*(3), 61-63.
4. Travers, D., et al. (2002). Five-level triage system more effective than three-level in tertiary emergency department. *Journal of Emergency Nursing, 28*(5), 395-400.
5. Zimmerman, P. (2001). The case of a universal, valid, reliable 5-tier triage acuity scale of US emergency departments. *Journal of Emergency Nursing, 27*(3), 246-254.

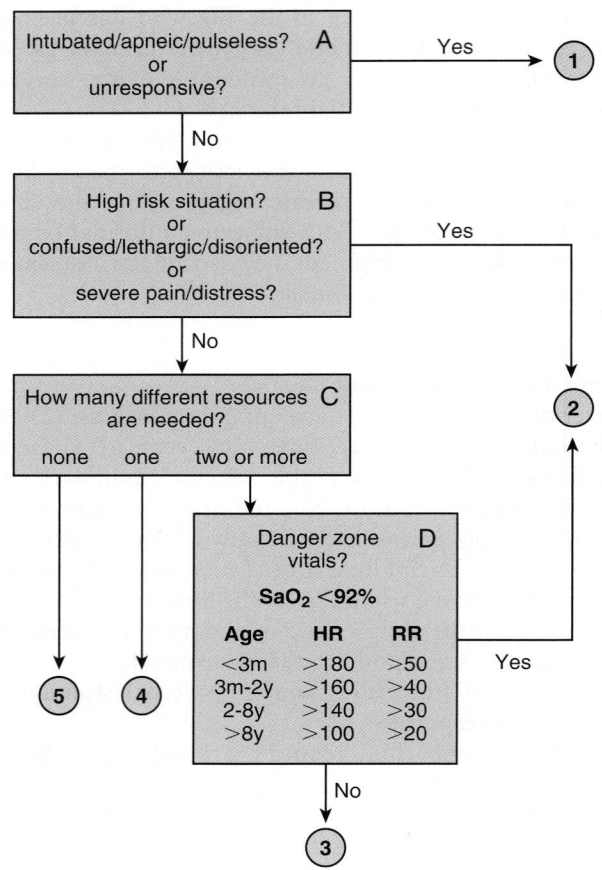

FIGURE 84-1 Emergency Severity Index triage algorithm. (From Wuerz, R.C., et al. (2001). Implementation and refinement of the emergency severity index. *Academic Emergency Medicine 8*, 170-176.

History

Elicit the nature of the client's chief complaint, duration of the problem, mechanism of injury from blunt or penetrating forces (Box 84-4), associated manifestations related to the primary problem, past pertinent medical history, current medications and compliance, use of over-the-counter (OTC) medications or herbs, routine use of alcohol or illicit drugs, known medication allergies, and immunization history. Women of childbearing age may need to be questioned about the date of the last normal menstrual period (LNMP), number of pregnancies and outcomes, and

TABLE 84-2	*Glasgow Coma Scale*	
Eye-opening response	Spontaneous	4
	To voice	3
	To pain	2
	None	1
Best verbal response	Oriented	5
	Confused	4
	Inappropriate words	3
	Incomprehensible sounds	2
	None	1
Best motor response	Obeys command	6
	Localizes pain	5
	Withdraws (to painful stimulus)	4
	Flexion (to painful stimulus)	3
	Extension (to painful stimulus)	2
	None	1
Total		3-15

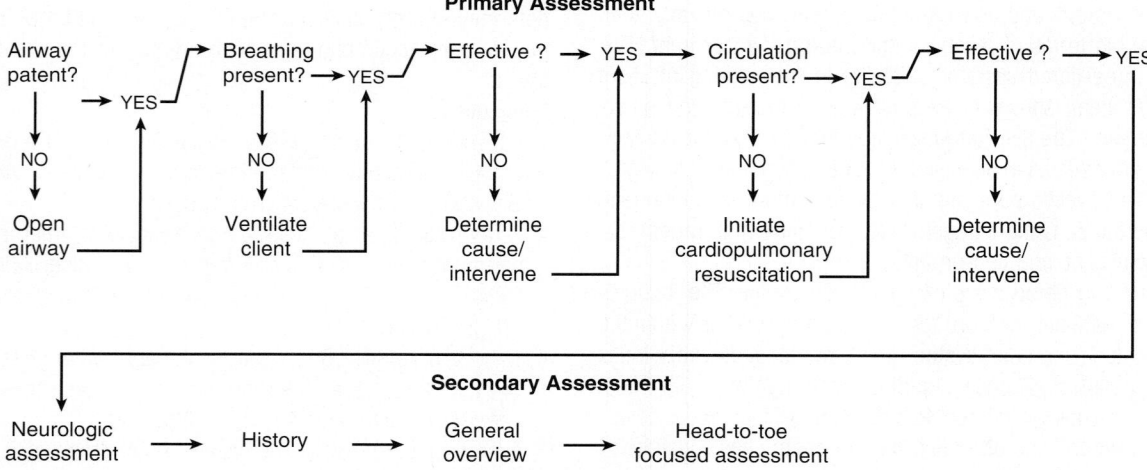

FIGURE 84-2 Primary and secondary assessment process.

age at onset or at end of menstruation. Questions related to potential or actual child, sexual, domestic, or elder abuse situations also must be addressed.

Pain

The most frequent complaint for which clients seek emergency care is related to both acute and chronic pain. Obtaining specific information regarding pain patterns

---

BOX 84-4 · *History Questions Related to Injury*

Motor Vehicle Crashes
- Were you the driver or passenger?
- Were you wearing a seat belt or shoulder harness (or both) correctly?
- Did the airbag deploy?
- Did you hit the steering wheel or the dashboard? If so, with what part of your body?
- Did you lose consciousness? If so, for how long?
- How fast was the vehicle going?
- What did the vehicle hit?
- Did the vehicle hit a moving object or a nonmoving object? (Paramedical personnel may provide information describing the condition of the car.)
- Where is your pain?
- How far were you thrown from the car?
- What is the condition of the other passengers?

Blunt Injury from Falls
- How far did you fall?
- What precipitated the fall?
- What did you land on?
- Where is your pain?
- Did you lose consciousness?

Gunshot Wounds
- How long ago did the incident occur?
- How many shots did you hear?
- What type of gun was it?
- From what direction do you think the bullet entered your body?
- How far away was the assailant?
- Where is your pain?

Penetrating Wounds or Stab Wounds
- How long ago did the injury occur?
- How many times were you stabbed?
- How long was the knife or sharp object?
- How far in did the sharp object go?
- From what direction were you stabbed?
- Where is your pain?

From Kitt S., et al. (Eds.). (1995). *Emergency nursing: A physiologic and clinical perspective* (2nd ed.). Philadelphia: W.B. Saunders.

---

can be extremely helpful. Asking questions according to the *PQRST* mnemonic often provides useful information: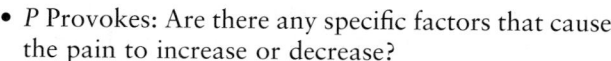

- *P* Provokes: Are there any specific factors that cause the pain to increase or decrease?
- *Q* Quality: What descriptive terminology identifies the type of pain—dull, sharp, colicky, pressure?
- *R* Region/Radiation: Where is the pain located? Does it move to other areas?
- *S* Severity: Use a rating scale of 1 to 10, visual analogs, or word descriptors to describe pain severity.
- *T* Timing: How long has the pain been present? Are there cycles related to when the pain is present or absent?

Both adult and pediatric clients who rate their pain at a level of 7 or above, or use descriptive words denoting "severe" pain need to be considered high risk. They require a more thorough evaluation by the ED physician, which should be performed as expediently as possible.[48] Clients have a right to have their pain treated appropriately, in a timely manner, and effectively, without exception.[74,82]

General Overview

Note the client's overall health condition, skin color, gait, posture, unusual skin markings or body odors, and mood and affect. Measurements of blood pressure, pulse rate, respiratory rate, pulse oximetry values, and temperature are important.

Head-to-Toe (Focused) Assessment

Remove the client's clothing and examine the areas where the chief complaint and any other associated complaints are focused. The techniques of inspection, auscultation, percussion, and palpation are used to determine additional normal or abnormal findings.

Diagnosis

Upon completion of the medical and nursing assessment process, diagnostic tests (radiographic, cardiology, laboratory, special studies) may be initiated. Once all pertinent information has been collected, a working diagnosis is formulated. The physician provides a medical diagnosis; in addition, the ED nurse may incorporate a variety of nursing diagnoses. These diagnoses provide a framework on which to build a plan of appropriate client care and against which to measure outcomes.

Outcome Management

Client care interventions may be initiated by the ED nurse, the ED physician, or other health care providers. There is frequent collaboration among all health care providers involved, and interventions are assigned priority according to the severity of the client's condition.

Evaluation

The desired goal in client care is to achieve positive client outcomes after medical and nursing management. This is an integral component of ED nursing care. If the client's condition does not improve with initial interventions, the plan of care must be reexamined and additional interventions may be required.

Client Disposition

All clients entering the ED are eventually discharged from the ED. They may be transferred to another health care facility, admitted to the hospital, or released to home or another facility. Most clients are released to home following treatment. Before being discharged from the ED, a client or family members must be given both oral and written instructions concerning follow-up care. These instructions should identify the client's diagnosed problem, explain necessary continued treatments, describe potential complications, and specify time frames for rechecks and the name of the physician to whom the client is being referred. These instructions should be presented in both oral and written form in the client's primary language. At times, a hospital or family interpreter may be required to accomplish this outcome.

Nursing Documentation

Because ED nurses frequently are responsible for an assigned area, zone, or "pod" within the department and because clients enter and exit those areas on a continual basis, nursing documentation is of paramount importance. Documentation must include the recording of all assessment findings, diagnostic tests, interventions and management, responses to treatment, achieved outcomes, and client education. Documentation needs to be complete but concise, providing an ongoing record of the client's condition and responses. The format may be a flow sheet, narrative, computer-generated design, or a combination of these.

▍EMERGENCY CONDITIONS
INEFFECTIVE AIRWAY CLEARANCE

A compromised or ineffective airway may be due to either complete or partial airway obstruction. Common causes of airway compromise include the presence of a foreign object in the airway, airway edema, airway infection, facial or airway injury, and tongue obstruction.

Clinical Manifestations

The clinical manifestations of airway compromise include absence of respirations, drooling, stridor, intercostal or substernal retractions, cyanosis, and agitation. A decreased level of consciousness may lead to airway compromise as a result of obstruction of the posterior pharynx by the relaxed tongue.

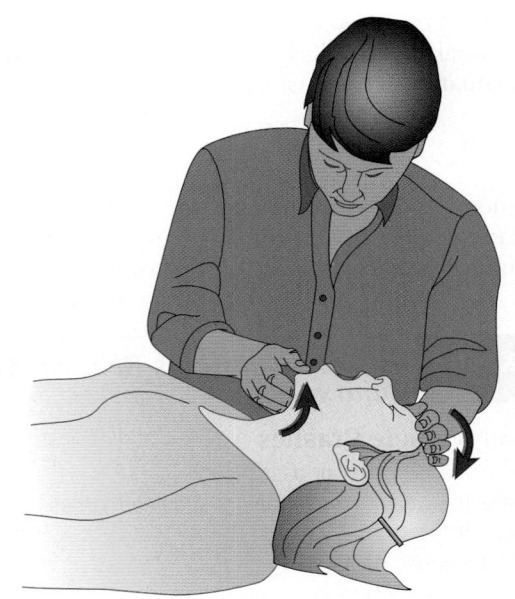

FIGURE 84-3 Chin lift maneuver to open the airway.

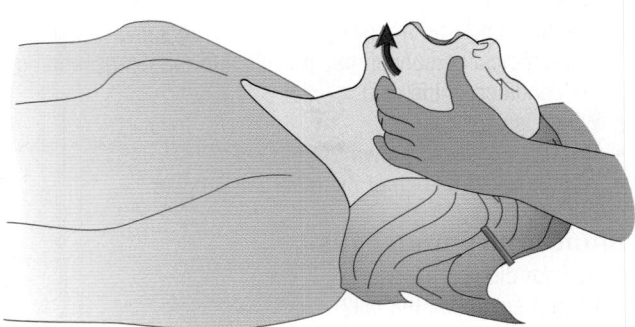

FIGURE 84-4 The jaw thrust maneuver to open the airway is the preferred method for use in clients with head or cervical neck injury.

Outcome Management

Remove Obstruction. If an obstruction is present, the airway should be opened by a chin lift or jaw thrust maneuver (Figures 84-3 and 84-4). If either of these maneuvers opens the client's airway, patency is maintained via the insertion of a nasopharyngeal or oral airway device. If these maneuvers fail to relieve the obstruction, more aggressive interventions must be instituted, such as (1) performing abdominal or chest thrusts if an aspirated foreign object is the suspected cause (Figure 84-5), (2) suctioning the oral cavity to remove secretions or visible foreign objects, (3) intubating via the nasal or oral route, (4) using a laryngeal mask airway (LMA), or (5) assisting with creating a surgical airway via a cricothyroidotomy (Figure 84-6).

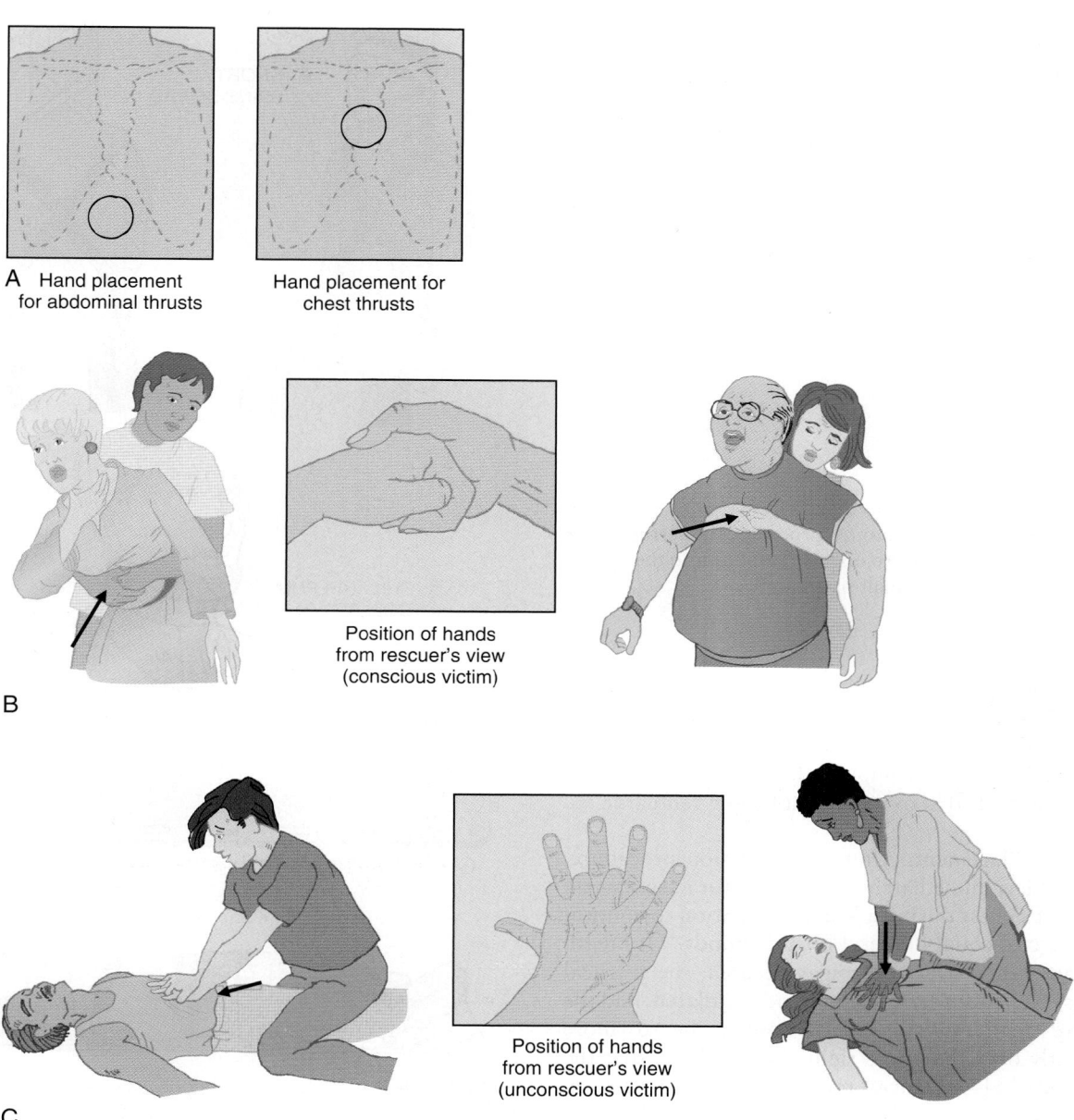

A Hand placement for abdominal thrusts

Hand placement for chest thrusts

Position of hands from rescuer's view (conscious victim)

B

Position of hands from rescuer's view (unconscious victim)

C

FIGURE 84-5 Heimlich maneuver, used for removal of foreign bodies blocking the upper airway. Vigorous upward chest or abdominal thrusts produce a rush of air that expels the foreign body. The abdominal thrust is the original Heimlich maneuver. The chest thrust is an adaptation that is useful for obese or pregnant victims. Use four quick thrusts in the positions shown. **A,** Hand placement. **B,** Maneuver for conscious victims. **C,** Maneuver for unconscious victims.

Intubate. In some cases, oral or nasal intubation may require the use of *rapid-sequence induction* (RSI). This procedure is used in awake clients who require intubation either to maintain the airway or as a mechanism to provide adequate ventilation. RSI is most frequently used in clients who have sustained a head or spinal injury and in clients who are rapidly tiring from the effort of maintaining respirations. RSI involves (1) establishing venous access, (2) hyperventilating the client with 100% oxygen, (3) administering intravenous (IV) lidocaine 1 mg/kg to blunt any transient increase in intracranial

pressure from the actual intubation procedure, and (4) administering an IV general barbiturate or anesthetic medication such as thiopental 3 to 5 mg/kg, fentanyl (Sublimaze) 3 to 15 μg/kg, ketamine (Ketalar) 1 to 2 mg/kg, etomidate (Amidate) 0.3 mg/kg, propofol (Diprivan) 2 mg/kg, or midazolam (Versed) 0.1 mg/kg followed immediately by the administration of an IV muscle-paralyzing agent such as succinylcholine (Anectine) 1.5 to 2 mg/kg, pancuronium (Pavulon) 0.04 to 0.1 mg/kg, or vecuronium (Norcuron) 0.08 to 0.1 mg/kg. [95] Once the client loses consciousness and adequate muscle

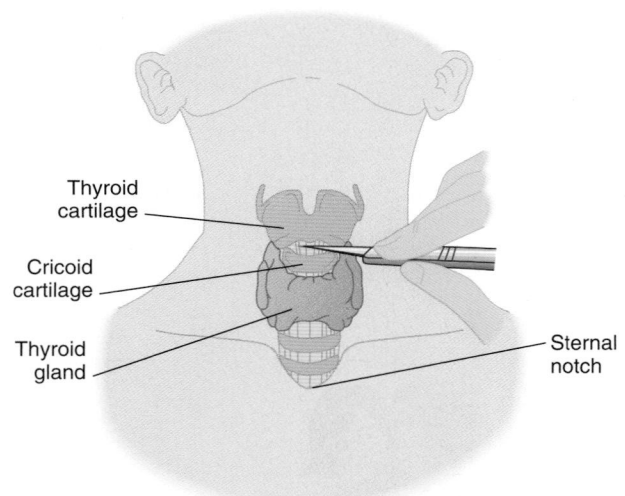

FIGURE 84-6 A cricothyrotomy procedure is performed to create a temporary airway. An opening is made into the trachea and is maintained with a small plastic tube.

relaxation and paralysis have been obtained, intubation using equipment such as an intubating laryngeal mask airway, intubating fiberoptic bronchoscope, or nasal/endotracheal tubes is accomplished.[5,57,96] The client is then ventilated using 100% oxygen via a bag or ventilator.

Verify Tube Placement. After an intubation procedure, the ED nurse is immediately responsible for auscultation of the client's chest during assisted ventilation to confirm the presence of equal bilateral breath sounds.[97] If breath sounds are heard over the epigastric area, the tracheal tube must be removed, the client hyperventilated, and the procedure reattempted. Breath sounds heard more prominently over the upper right chest indicate that the tracheal tube has advanced too far into the right main bronchus. The tube needs to be pulled back and breath sounds reassessed. Once the presence of equal and bilateral breath sounds is confirmed, the tube is secured in place and a chest film is obtained to document correct tube placement. An end-tidal CO_2 monitoring device may be attached to the end of the tracheal tube to aid in confirming correct tube placement.[97]

Securing and maintaining a patent airway constitutes the first priority in any ED client. Other treatments directed at the cause of airway compromise are then instituted. These measures may include administration of IV medications if infection or local edema of the airway is present.

Immobilize the Spine. If the client with an actual or potential airway problem has also sustained a traumatic injury, simultaneous stabilization of the client's cervical, thoracic, and lumbar spine must be instituted and maintained to prevent any further possible spinal injury. Stabilization is accomplished using a team approach and in-

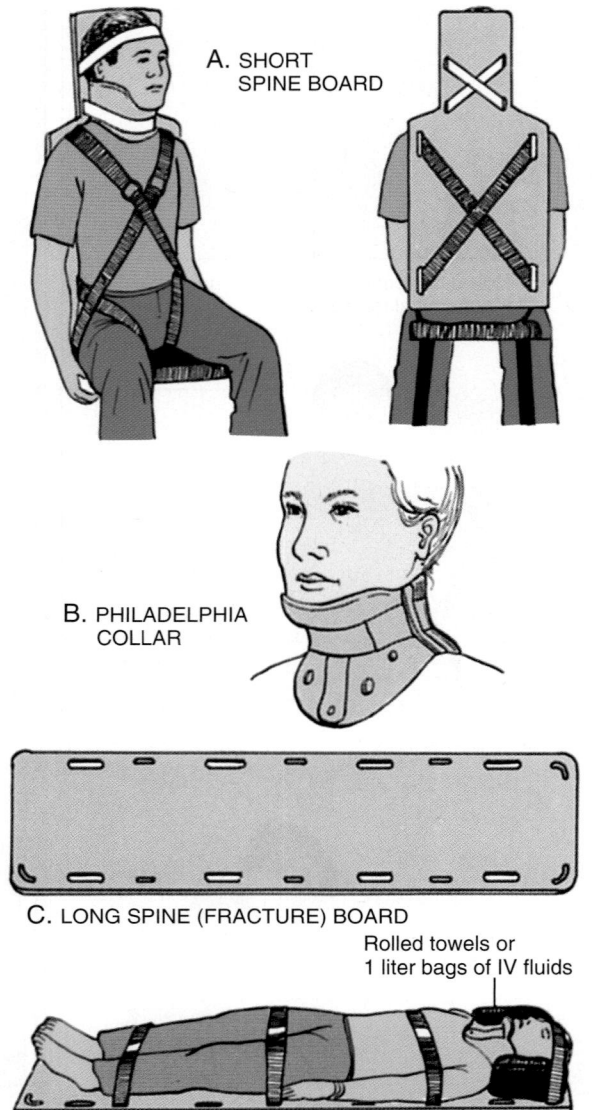

FIGURE 84-7 Spine-immobilizing devices. **A,** The short spine board is applied to a client who is seated (e.g., in an automobile) and is applied along with a cervical collar before extrication of the person from the vehicle. **B,** The Philadelphia collar, a two-piece, hard, molded plastic device, can be applied without manipulating the neck and provides good immobilization of the cervical spine. **C,** The long spine (fracture) board is made of wood and contains cut-out sections along the sides for securing restraining straps and for lifting the injured client.

volves the following steps: (1) manually stabilizing the client's head and cervical spine, (2) applying a hard cervical collar around the client's nuchal area, (3) placing the client on a long, rigid backboard, (4) securing the client to the backboard, (5) placing immobilization devices, such as rolled towels, at the side of the client's head and neck, and (6) placing a strip of adhesive tape across the client's forehead and immobilization devices and then onto the backboard (Figure 84-7).

INEFFECTIVE BREATHING PATTERN

Breathing patterns are affected if a client is either hyperventilating or hypoventilating. The normal respiratory rate for an adult is between 12 and 20 breaths/min; infant respiratory rates are between 30 and 40 breaths/min; and children sustain respiratory rates between 25 and 30 breaths/min until approximately the age of 10 years.

HYPERVENTILATION

Clinical Manifestations

Respiratory rates faster than normal constitute tachypnea and, in many cases, hyperventilation. Common causes for hyperventilation include anxiety reactions, pulmonary infections, and metabolic deviations. With excessive and prolonged hyperventilation, carbon dioxide levels decrease and respiratory alkalosis can result. The client may report numbness and tingling sensations in the distal extremities or around the lips, along with carpal or pedal spasms. A sensation of chest pain may also be present. Frequently this condition is caused by client anxiety, but it is important to also investigate other possible causes, such as pain, aspirin toxicity, diabetic ketoacidosis, fluid loss, central nervous system (CNS) lesions, and pulmonary embolism.

Outcome Management

The goals of treatment are to return the client's breathing pattern and rate to normal and to restore normal gas exchange. If anxiety is the cause of the hyperventilation, the client needs to be instructed to take slow, deep breaths through the nose and slowly exhale through the mouth. Having clients breathe into a paper bag and rebreathe their own carbon dioxide may be helpful. If another cause is identified as the reason for the client's altered breathing pattern, specific treatments such as administration of oxygen and inhaled, intravenous, or oral medications are initiated to reverse the process.

HYPOVENTILATION

Clinical Manifestations

Hypoventilation occurs when an adult client's respiratory rate falls below 12 breaths/min or in the case of a child the respiratory rate is below what is normal for the age-group. At these rates, not enough oxygen is available to maintain adequate tissue oxygenation. Clinical manifestations may include a decrease in the client's level of consciousness, pallor, cyanosis, and pulse oximetry readings of less than 96%. Carbon dioxide is retained, and respiratory acidosis develops. Causes of hypoventilation include brain stem lesions, head injury, drug-induced depression of the respiratory center, impaired respiratory muscle innervation from spinal cord injury, and the presence of neuromuscular diseases such as muscular dystrophy or Guillain-Barré syndrome.

TABLE 84-3	*Respiratory Sounds Associated with Illness*
Illness	**Lung Sounds**
Asthma	Wheezes
COPD	Rales, rhonchi, wheezes
Bronchitis	Rhonchi
Pneumonia	Rhonchi, abnormal bronchial sounds
Tuberculosis	Rhonchi, abnormal bronchial sounds
Bronchiolitis	Wheezes

COPD, Chronic obstructive pulmonary disease.

Outcome Management

Administering high-flow oxygen via a bag-valve-mask device is often required to reduce the systemic hypoxemia and to return oxygen levels to between 80 and 100 mm Hg. Recommendations for ventilating infants include using a pediatric size bag-valve-mask instead of an infant bag.[2]

IMPAIRED GAS EXCHANGE

Etiology

Obstructions, infections, and injury within the pulmonary system can lead to the development of gas exchange abnormalities. Common causative disorders include asthma, other reactive airway diseases, chronic obstructive pulmonary disease, pulmonary embolism, bronchitis, pneumonia, tuberculosis, pneumothorax, and chest injuries such as a flail chest.[38,53]

A less common cause of a gas exchange problem is noncardiac pulmonary edema, which results from acute damage to the alveolocapillary membrane. This damage can occur from inhalation injury, near-drowning, sepsis, trauma, and opioid overdose. As the alveolocapillary membrane permeability increases, fluid collects in the interstitial space, surfactant levels decrease, and the alveoli eventually collapse.

Clinical Manifestations

With constriction of the bronchi, accumulation of fluid, or lung consolidation, abnormal lung sounds such as wheezes, rales, or rhonchi (Table 84-3) are often heard throughout the client's lung fields. With pulmonary infections, the client may have concurrent fever. If a pneumothorax is present, breath sounds are diminished or absent on the side of the pneumothorax. Asymmetrical chest wall movement with respirations, especially if the client has sustained a blunt force traumatic injury, should raise suspicion of a possible flail chest. In such cases, a chest film provides valuable diagnostic information about the cause of the client's problem. A D-dimer assay, ventilation-perfusion ($\dot{V}/\dot{Q}$) scan, or spiral computed tomography (CT) aid in the diagnosis of pulmonary embolism.[91]

Outcome Management

Administer Oxygen. Oxygen therapy with a flow rate of between 2 and 10 L/min via nasal cannula or face mask is the priority intervention for clients with an obstructive or infectious cause of ineffective gas exchange. Biphasic positive airway pressure (BiPAP) or continuous positive airway pressure (CPAP) are noninvasive ventilation masks used to provide high-flow oxygen.

Administer Medications to Open Lower Airways. Oxygen administration is frequently followed by administering aerosolized bronchodilator medications such as metaproterenol (Alupent) or albuterol (Ventolin) to open constricted upper or lower bronchi.[33] Subcutaneous epinephrine 1:1000 may be administered to relax constricted bronchi and to reduce the degree of airway or bronchial edema. Administration of steroid medications, either intravenously or orally, is also frequently used as first-line therapy.[33,60] A client with a suspected pulmonary embolus may be given IV fibrinolytic medications, such as tissue-type plasminogen activator (t-PA [Activase]), to lyse the offending embolus and heparin to prevent the formation of new emboli. Low-molecular-weight heparin (enoxaparin) is being used to treat deep venous thrombus to prevent pulmonary emboli development.[9,36]

Minimize Spread of Infection. Infectious diseases that are the cause of impaired gas exchange are treated with IV or oral antibiotic medications.[13,34] A client thought to have a highly contagious pulmonary disease such as tuberculosis must be isolated from the general ED client population. The use of a high-efficiency particulate air (HEPA) filter mask placed over the nose and mouth is indicated to prevent spreading of aerosol droplets. ED personnel caring for the client may also need to wear this type of mask to decrease exposure risks.

TRAUMATIC PNEUMOTHORAX

A pneumothorax can be classified as a simple pneumothorax, open pneumothorax, or tension pneumothorax (Figure 84-8). In a *simple pneumothorax,* air from the bronchus, bronchioles, or alveoli escapes into the pleural space and diminishes lung expansion capacity. With an *open pneumothorax,* a traumatically created opening in the client's chest wall allows air to move freely into and out of the thoracic cavity during inspiration and exhalation. A tension pneumothorax occurs when air continues to become trapped in the pleural cavity with no mechanism of escape during the exhalation process. This type of pneumothorax is an emergent condition.

Clinical Manifestations

A simple pneumothorax can occur spontaneously but is frequently associated with penetrating injury forces delivered to the chest or with blunt forces causing a rib fracture. Pain with respirations is present, as is the auscultative finding of unequal breath sounds. Pulse oximetry readings are less than 94%.

An obvious chest wound is present with an open pneumothorax, because this type of pneumothorax is most commonly caused by penetrating injury forces. As air moves into and out of the wound, a sucking sound is heard. The client is in pain and tachypnea is present. Breath sounds are diminished or absent on the side of the injury.

A tension pneumothorax produces the clinical manifestations of extreme respiratory distress, distended jugular neck veins, and a mediastinal shift of the heart, trachea, esophagus, and great vessels to the side away from the tension pneumothorax. Hypotension and decreased cardiac output are other findings. Pneumothorax is diagnosed by a chest radiograph.

Outcome Management

Administer Oxygen. High-flow oxygen delivered via a face mask is the priority treatment for a client who has 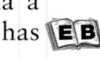 sustained a pneumothorax.

Apply Occlusive Dressing. Any open chest wall wound should be covered with an occlusive gauze dressing, but this intervention may convert an open pneumothorax into the more dangerous tension pneumothorax because the gauze covering blocks the trapped air's escape route. If manifestations of a tension pneumothorax appear, the occlusive dressing must be immediately removed.

Release Trapped Air. If a tension pneumothorax is thought to be the cause of respiratory distress and if it has not been iatrogenically produced by covering an open chest wound, a 14- to 16-gauge catheter needle is immediately inserted into the client's anterior chest wall on the affected side at the second midclavicular intercostal space. This life-saving intervention allows the immediate release of trapped air and decompresses the pleural cavity.

Place Chest Tube. The simple, open, and tension varieties of pneumothorax are definitively treated with the insertion of a chest tube that is attached to a suction/collection device. This measure aids in reexpansion of the lung, leading to improvement in the client's gas exchange.

FLAIL CHEST

A flail chest involves serious rib fractures. It occurs when two or more ribs are fractured in two or more places on the same chest wall side or when the sternum is detached from the ribs. The fractured segment has no connection with the remaining rib cage. This segment then moves in a direction opposite that of the rest of the chest wall during the processes of inhalation and exhalation—so-called

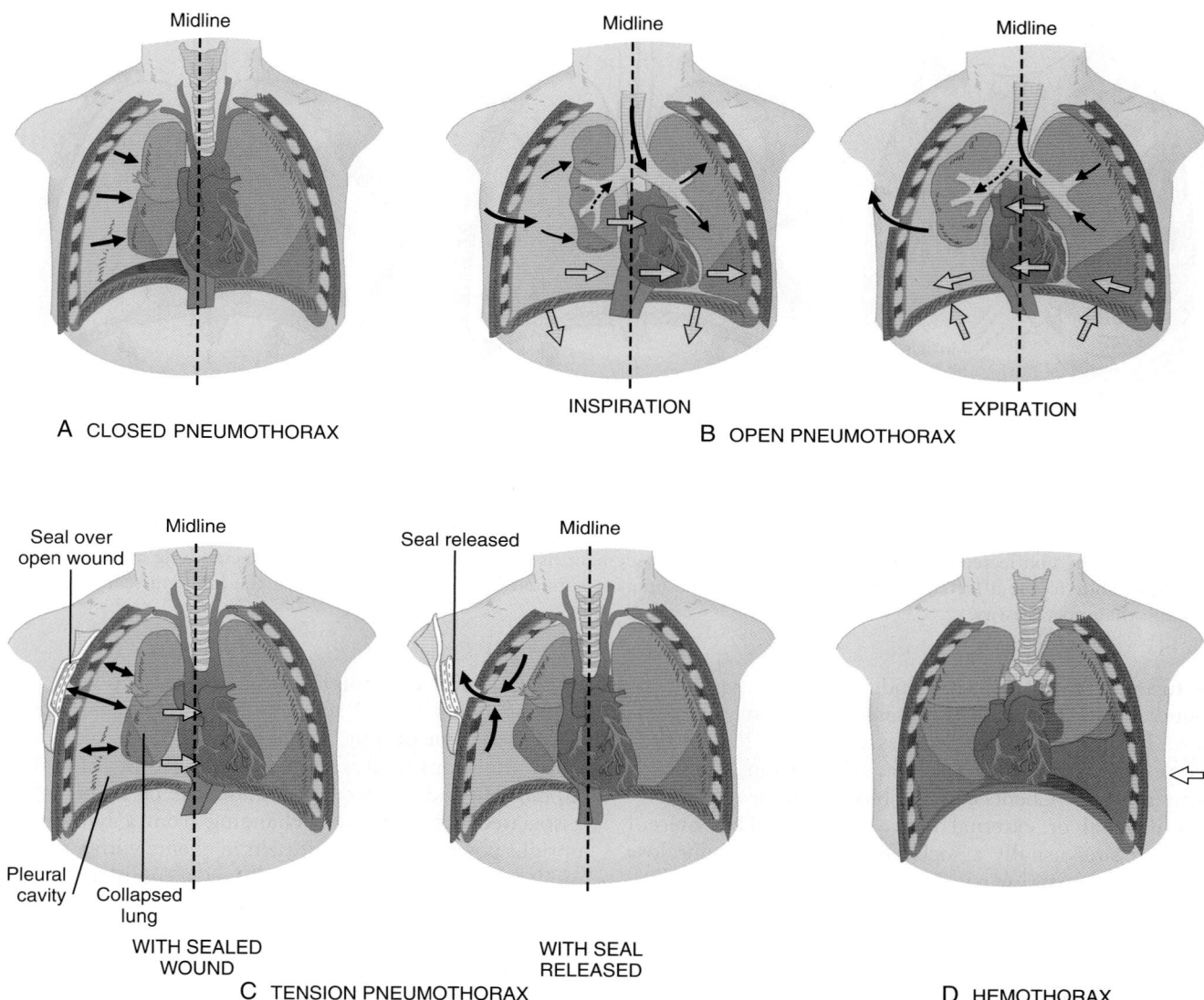

FIGURE 84-8 Pneumothorax. **A,** Closed pneumothorax. The lung collapses as air gathers in the pleural space. **B,** Open pneumothorax (sucking chest wound). *Solid arrows* indicate air movement; *open arrows,* structural movement. A chest wall wound connects the pleural space with atmospheric air. During inspiration, atmospheric air is sucked into the pleural space through the chest wall wound. Positive pressure in the pleural space collapses the lung on the affected side and pushes the mediastinal contents toward the unaffected side. This reduces the volume of air in the unaffected side considerably. During expiration, air escapes through the chest wall wound, lessening positive pressure in the affected side and allowing the mediastinal contents to swing back toward the affected side. Movement of mediastinal structures from side to side is called *mediastinal flutter.* **C,** Tension pneumothorax. *Left,* If an open pneumothorax is covered (e.g., with a dressing), it forms a seal, and tension pneumothorax with a mediastinal shift develops. A tear in lung structure continues to allow air into the pleural space. As positive pressure builds in the pleural space, the affected lung collapses, and the mediastinal contents shift to the unaffected side. *Right,* Tension pneumothorax is corrected by removing the seal (e.g., dressing), allowing air trapped in the pleural space to escape. **D,** Hemothorax. Massive hemothorax *(arrow)* below the left lung causes collapse of lung tissue.

paradoxical chest wall movement (Figure 84-9). Respiratory distress is present, as are skin pallor and cyanosis.

Treatment involves nasal or tracheal intubation and mechanical ventilation with positive end-expiratory pressure (PEEP). Pulmonary contusions are commonly present in conjunction with a flail chest, and within 24 to 48 hours, noncardiac pulmonary edema or adult (acute) respiratory distress syndrome (ARDS) may develop.

DEFICIENT FLUID VOLUME

A decrease in circulating blood volume leads to a deficit in fluid volume and, subsequently, to decreased tissue

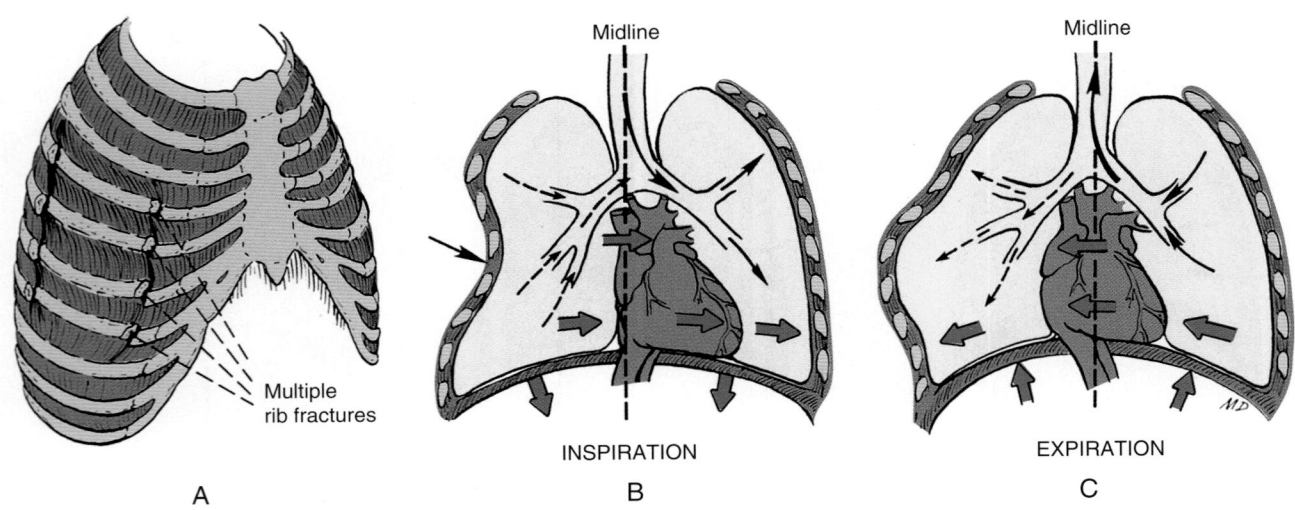

A

B INSPIRATION

C EXPIRATION

Multiple rib fractures

Midline

Midline

FIGURE 84-9 Flail chest. *Dashed arrows* indicate air movement; *solid arrows,* structural movement. **A,** A flail chest consists of fractured rib segments that are unattached (free-floating) to the rest of the chest wall. **B,** On inspiration, the flail segment of ribs is sucked inward. The affected lung and mediastinal structures shift to the unaffected side. This compromises the amount of inspired air in the unaffected lung. **C,** On expiration, the flail segment of ribs bellows outward. The affected lung and mediastinal structures shift to the affected side. Some air within the lungs is shunted back and forth between the lungs instead of passing through the upper airway.

perfusion. Therefore any condition producing a profound volume deficit necessitates immediate intervention. The more common causes of volume loss include shock due to acute hypovolemia, dehydration, and major burn injuries.[35] Clients can lose blood volume through either internal or external active bleeding. The internal bleeding sites usually associated with large volume loss include the posterior nasal passages, aortic vessel injury or dissecting aneurysm,[30] pulmonary vasculature, stomach, liver, spleen, uterus, or fallopian tube, and fractures of the pelvis and femur. Illness leading to prolonged vomiting or diarrhea can also produce large fluid losses. "Third-spacing" volume loss or interstitial volume sequestering associated with major burn injury occurs approximately 12 hours after injury (see Chapter 52).

As volume loss occurs, various compensatory mechanisms produce vasoconstriction of the vasculature, retain fluid via the renal tubules, and increase cardiac output. These compensatory mechanisms—such as stimulation of the sympathetic nervous system; the release of renin, angiotensin, aldosterone, and antidiuretic hormones; and fluid shifts—continue in an effort to restore tissue perfusion, thus ensuring cell survival. However, these mechanisms are limited in scope, and if the lost volume is not restored, eventually cellular structures incur irreversible damage from the oxygen debt, and death ensues.

Clinical Manifestations

The client often provides a history of recent injury or illness with associated volume loss. Clinical manifestations may include agitation or decreasing level of conscious-

ness, pale and diaphoretic skin, delayed capillary refill time of longer than 2 seconds, tachycardia, tachypnea, decreased urine output, and hypotension. Positive orthostatic vital signs (a decrease in systolic blood pressure by 20 mm Hg and an increase in pulse rate by 20 beats/min associated with the client changing from a lying to an upright position) may be present in clients with a mild to moderate volume loss. If blood has accumulated in the thoracic cavity (hemothorax) or abdominal cavity, percussion over the area elicits a dull sound. A collection of blood under the thoracic diaphragm or in the peritoneal cavity can produce Kehr's sign (referred shoulder pain unrelated to injury) or a rigid, hard abdomen with increased rebound tenderness upon palpation.

Diagnostic testing is directed at locating the source of any internal bleeding. Tests may include radiography, ultrasonography, and CT scans of the chest, pelvis, extremities, or abdomen. The laboratory tests of blood typing, complete blood count (CBC), hemoglobin concentration and hematocrit, and electrolyte panel are performed on collected blood samples. A urine specimen should be tested for specific gravity and the presence of blood and leukocytes and, in females, for pregnancy. If gastrointestinal bleeding is suspected, a nasogastric tube is passed and the aspirate tested for the presence of blood. Stool is tested for blood.

A diagnostic peritoneal lavage (DPL) procedure is occasionally performed in unstable clients who have sustained abdominal injury. A peritoneal catheter is inserted into the client's peritoneal cavity, and 1 L of normal saline is infused. The fluid is then drained, via gravity, from the peritoneal cavity back into the emptied fluid bag. The fluid is

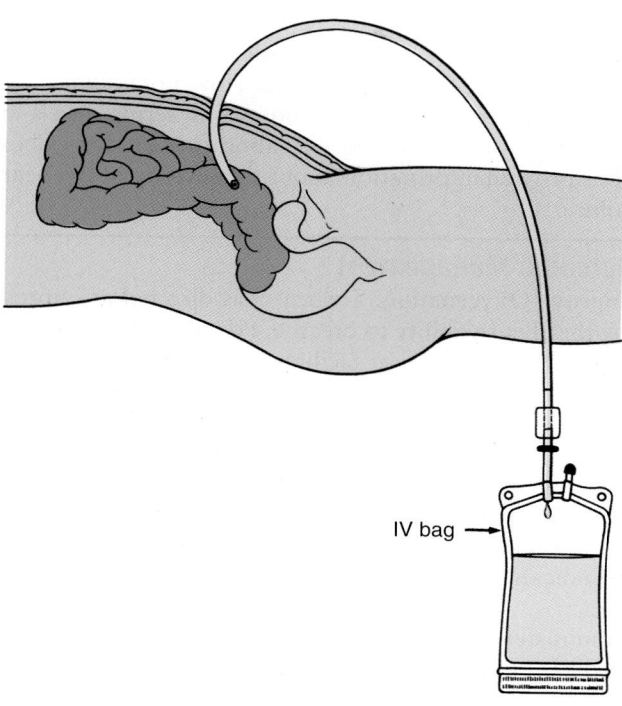

INTERPRETATION OF RESULTS

Positive result	Free-flowing blood on aspiration
	Grossly bloody lavage return
	>100,000 RBC/mm³
	>500 WBC/mm³
	Exit of lavage fluid from urinary or thoracic catheters
Equivocal result	50,000-100,000 RBC/mm³
	100-500 WBC/mm³
Negative result	<50,000 RBC/mm³
	<100 WBC/mm³

FIGURE 84-10 Diagnostic peritoneal lavage.

examined for the presence of blood, bile, feces, amylase, and white blood cells to determine whether organs within the peritoneal cavity have been injured (Figure 84-10).

Diagnostic testing not only helps in identifying the source and severity of volume loss but also aids in determining whether the client requires immediate surgery or hospital admission.

Outcome Management

Treatment is directed at preventing further volume loss and replacing fluid volume.

Maintain Blood Flow to Vital Organs. High-flow oxygen is delivered via face mask to provide additional oxygen to tissues. Positioning the client in a supine position with the legs elevated is appropriate.

Stop or Decrease Bleeding. If external bleeding is present, direct pressure should be applied to control further blood loss. The application of tourniquets and clamping

of exposed vessels should be avoided if possible. If the bleeding source is the posterior nasal passages, the client needs to be seated and leaning forward in a high Fowler position. Nasal packing is required.

Replace Fluids. Venous access must be obtained using a large-bore catheter (14 to 16 gauge). Usually two IV sites are required for fluid replacement. At the time of vein cannulation, blood samples should also be obtained for laboratory testing. If peripheral venous access is not possible, an intraosseous procedure may be performed. This involves inserting an intraosseous needle into the proximal anterior tibia. Fluids, blood, and medications can then be infused into the bone marrow. This is a temporary lifeline and is removed once peripheral venous access can be obtained. The procedure is usually performed by a physician, but it may also be performed by educated personnel such as paramedics and ED nurses. In the past, this procedure was performed only on children younger than age 3 years, but this has recently been expanded so that the procedure can be performed on individuals of any age.

Crystalloids. Crystalloid fluids (normal saline, lactated Ringer's solution) are the replacement fluids of choice. They should be warmed and administered at a ratio of 3:1 (3 L of solution for every 1 L of volume loss) in an adult. In children, the infusion rate is 20 ml/kg administered as a bolus. This bolus may need to be repeated.

Colloids. Colloid fluids (e.g., blood, hetastarch, albumin) may also be given for fluid resuscitation. These fluids contain proteins and are infused at a 1:1 ratio (1 unit of solution for every 1 unit of blood loss). Blood can be administered as whole blood or as packed red blood cells. It is best if the client's blood has been typed or, optimally, typed and cross-matched with the donor's blood, but universal type O Rh-negative blood can be used if speed is a vital consideration. All administered blood must be warmed and can be infused quickly in an adult using a rapid infuser machine. In children, blood is infused at a rate of 40 ml/kg bolus.

Autotransfusion. Following chest trauma, if a large amount of blood due to a hemothorax (see Figure 84-8) is sequestered in the thoracic cavity, the procedure of autotransfusion can be life-saving. With this procedure, a large chest tube is inserted into the client's thoracic cavity and into the hemothorax. The blood is collected into an autotransfuser drainage system and then reinfused into the client through an IV catheter.

Open Thoracotomy. It may be necessary to perform an emergency open thoracotomy on a client who has sustained major chest trauma and is near death. The client's ribs are cut and spread to expose the internal thoracic cavity. Any bleeding sites may then be identified and potentially repaired.

Replace Fluids for Burns. Clients who have sustained major partial or full-thickness burn injuries are at risk for associated fluid loss. Fluid replacement is calculated according to the client's weight in kilograms and the total body surface area (TBSA) involved, as determined by the *rule of 9*s (see Chapter 52). The usual formula is 2 to 4 ml of fluid × body weight in kilograms × TBSA. The calculated amount of fluid is used as the total fluid replacement volume required over the 24-hour period from the time of injury. One half of the total fluid amount is infused in the first 8-hour period, one fourth of the fluid amount in the second 8-hour period, and the remaining one fourth amount in the last 8-hour period.

Institute Other Measures. Once fluid resuscitation is begun, other interventions can be instituted. A nasogastric tube is passed to prevent vomiting and possible aspiration. In clients with gastrointestinal bleeding, gastric lavage is performed, instilling room-temperature normal saline, then, using a large syringe, the fluid is aspirated through the nasogastric tube. This procedure is repeated until there is a clearing of the bloody fluid aspirate. An indwelling urinary catheter is inserted to measure urine output. The client with volume loss is susceptible to the development of mild hypothermia. Keeping the client warm with blankets, warming lights, and infusion of warmed fluids aids in maintaining a normal body temperature. Continual monitoring of cardiac rate and rhythm, blood pressure, pulse oximetry readings, respiratory rate, level of consciousness, and temperature is indicated.[15]

EXCESS FLUID VOLUME

Clients who have an excess of fluid volume can concurrently have pulmonary congestion, leading to respiratory distress. Although clients with renal failure experience fluid volume excess, the disorder most commonly associated with fluid overload in the ED is heart failure. Heart failure results in fluid excess because of the inability of the cardiac muscle to function effectively. Ejection fraction decreases, pressure in the left ventricle increases, and eventually pressure increases affect the left atrium and right ventricle and atrium.

Clinical Manifestations

The clinical manifestations of heart failure include agitation or restlessness, tachypnea and increased respiratory effort, respiratory rales, distended jugular neck veins, tachycardia, skin pallor, diaphoresis, ascites, and pitting-dependent edema.[92] Pulse oximetry readings are less than 94%, and the client may also cough up excessive, frothy sputum. Cardiac dysrhythmias, such as atrial fibrillation, may be noted with cardiac monitoring.

Because these clients often have a chronic history of heart failure, their daily medication regimen usually includes digoxin, furosemide (Lasix), and potassium. Electrolyte imbalances are common, and serum levels of digoxin must be assessed via laboratory studies. Chest films provide information about the severity of the heart failure.

Outcome Management

Improve Oxygenation. Treatment is directed at improving the client's ability to breathe. Positioning the client in a high Fowler position facilitates the ability to breathe. Oxygen is administered at a high flow rate via face mask, although this intervention may be difficult for the client to tolerate. Noninvasive ventilatory assistance via BiPAP may be required. However, if respiratory fatigue develops, the client must be intubated to provide adequate ventilation. The use of RSI before intubation may be indicated.

Administer Medications. Establishing venous access for medication administration is necessary. The most current therapy involves administering recombinate human B-type natriuretic peptide nesiritide (Natrecor).[14] This naturally occurring protein is secreted by the ventricles during exacerbations of heart failure. However, the amount secreted is insufficient in terms of being therapeutic. This medication is replacing the use of nitroglycerin and nitroprusside. The recommended dose is 2 μg/kg IV followed by an infusion of 0.01 μg/kg/min. The actions of the medication increase salt and water excretion in addition to producing vasodilation. The client must be monitored for urine output, hypotension, and respiratory improvement. If Natrecor is not administered, the more common medications include nitroglycerin 5 to 10 μg/min IV infusion, furosemide (Lasix) 40 to 100 mg IV, and morphine sulfate 2 to 10 mg IV. If serum digoxin levels are subtherapeutic and the client is not hypokalemic, then digoxin may be administered 0.6 to 1 mg IV. Dobutamine, angiotensin-converting enzyme (ACE) inhibitor, and beta-blocker medications may be administered cautiously in some settings to reduce cardiac preload and to produce inotropic effects.

Monitor Response to Treatment. Continual monitoring of the client's response to treatment is of paramount importance. Assessments should include level of consciousness, cardiac status, blood pressure, respiratory rate and effort, pulse oximetry, and urine output.

DECREASED CARDIAC OUTPUT

Any illness or injury that has a direct effect on the heart can produce a decrease in cardiac output. Such disorders include cardiac dysrhythmias, acute myocardial infarction, cardiac injury, cardiac tamponade, and cardiac infection or myopathy.[19,56]

When cardiac output decreases, tissue perfusion is adversely affected. Cardiac output (CO) is determined by stroke volume (SV) and heart rate (HR):

$$CO = SV \times HR$$

Therefore any disease process that produces a reduction in stroke volume or an alteration in heart rate has a direct effect on cardiac output. Entities such as cardiac dysrhythmias and acute myocardial infarction have a direct affect on heart rate. Acute myocardial infarction also reduces stroke volume as a result of the death of cardiac muscle. Cardiac tamponade results in compression of the cardiac muscle by the collection of blood or fluid in the pericardial sac. This effect produces a decrease in stroke volume. Infection and cardiac myopathy also affect the cardiac muscle structures, thereby reducing stroke volume.

Clinical Manifestations

Depending on the cause of the reduced cardiac output, clients may present with differing clinical manifestations.[59] Dysrhythmias are self-evident on cardiac monitoring. The most prominent manifestations associated with a decrease in cardiac output include chest pain, skin pallor, diaphoresis, hypotension, nausea, and agitation or a decrease in level of consciousness.[70] External chest wall injury may be evident with cardiac contusions. Cardiac tamponade produces the additional findings of distended jugular neck veins and muffled heart sounds. Fever may be present with cardiac infections.

Diagnostic tests include cardiac monitoring, electrocardiography (ECG), chest radiography, ultrasonography, laboratory studies, noninvasive stress testing, two-dimensional echocardiography, myocardial perfusion imaging, CT scans, and invasive coronary angiography. Levels of the cardiac enzymes creatine kinase (CK) and the CK-MB fraction and of the cardiac markers myoglobin and troponin T (cTnT) and troponin I (cTnI) are especially important in diagnosing the occurrences of a myocardial infarction.

Outcome Management

Improve Cardiac Output. The goal of treatment is to improve cardiac output. High-flow oxygen should be administered via face mask, and venous access should be secured for the administration of medications. Supraventricular tachycardic dysrhythmias are frequently treated with the IV adenosine (Adenocar) 6 mg, whereas bradycardic rhythms may be treated with IV atropine 0.5 to 2 mg or with the insertion of a cardiac pacemaker. Amiodarone 150 mg IV[6] or lidocaine 1 mg/kg is administered to clients with premature ventricular contractions, as long as they are not associated with a bradycardic rhythm. Clients who have sustained a cardiac contusion from traumatic injury may also develop cardiac dys-

rhythmias. For further discussion of dysrhythmia treatment, see Chapter 59.

Increase Coronary Artery Blood Flow. An acute myocardial infarction is often caused by an embolus or thrombus that occludes a coronary artery. Initially, nitroglycerin, administered sublingually or intravenously, and morphine sulfate are given to reduce pain and to produce vasodilation of the coronary arteries. Treatment may then involve the administration of oral aspirin, fibrinolytic medications IV, heparin IV, glycoprotein (GP) IIb/IIIa inhibitors IV, or the more invasive procedure of percutaneous transluminal coronary angioplasty (PTCA).[36,54,68,75,88] Beta-blocker therapy is also instituted in clients who do not have concurrent heart failure or cardiogenic shock.[68] Clients who are diagnosed with non–Q-wave myocardial infarctions are treated with oxygen, low-molecular-weight heparin subcutaneously or IV heparin, beta-blocker medications IV or orally, and GP IIb/IIIa receptor inhibitors IV.[36]

Clients who have received fibrinolytic medications must be continuously monitored for the presence of active bleeding. Other monitoring parameters include pain reduction, cardiac rate and rhythm, ST segment patterns, blood pressure, pulse oximetry readings, and respiratory rate.

Remove Pericardial Fluid. Blunt or penetrating force injury to the left chest can cause cardiac tamponade. If this injury is suspected or diagnosed, treatment involves pericardiocentesis (Figure 84-11). A long spinal needle attached to a 60-ml syringe is inserted beneath the xiphoid process and into the pericardial sac. The accumulated blood is removed, compression of the ventricles is relieved, and cardiac output is restored.[66]

Treat Infectious Causes. Infections of the heart structures, such as pericarditis or endocarditis, may be treated with pain-reducing medications or antibiotics. Pericarditis is frequently caused by a viral organism, whereas endocarditis is of bacterial origin and requires antibiotic therapy.

ACUTE PAIN OR CHRONIC PAIN

Pain is the most common complaint of clients seeking emergency care.[62,82] Pain can be caused by almost any entity; therefore identifying the source of pain is of paramount importance. The sensation of pain may be the only complaint, or pain may be associated with other clinical evidence of illness or injury. Pain is assessed as described earlier in the chapter.

Outcome Management

Promote Comfort. Pain reduction is the goal of treatment and may be provided by administering oral, intramuscular (IM), or IV analgesic or opioid medications. With isolated orthopedic injuries, such as digit injuries,

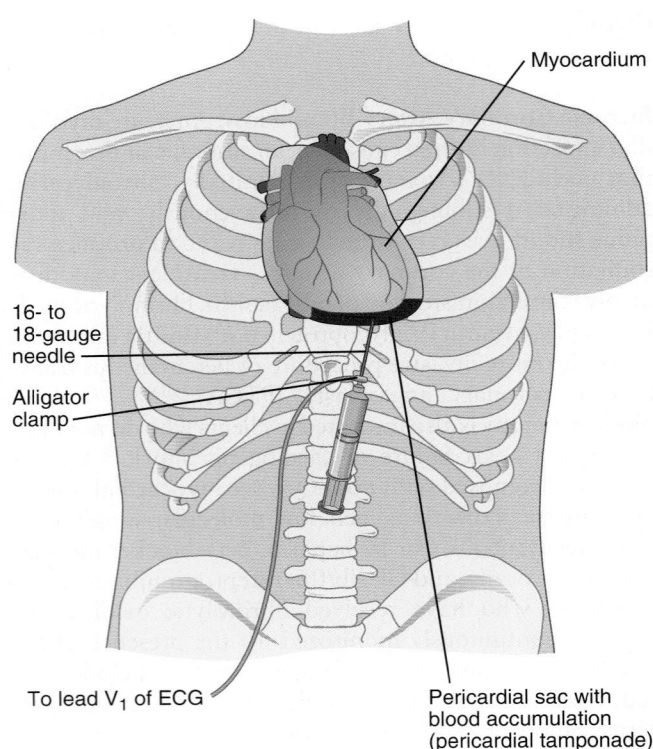
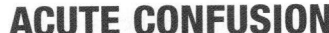

Myocardium

16- to
18-gauge
needle

Alligator
clamp

To lead V₁ of ECG

Pericardial sac with
blood accumulation
(pericardial tamponade)

FIGURE 84-11 Pericardiocentesis procedure. (Modified from Kosmos, C.A. [1995]. In Kitt, S., et al. [Eds.], *Emergency nursing: A physiologic and clinical perspective* [2nd ed., p. 66]. Philadelphia: W. B. Saunders.)

pain reduction may be obtained by injecting affected nerves with anesthetizing medications.[25] Client comfort measures should also be instituted.[71] Measures may include client positioning to ease stress on painful areas, elevating injured extremities, applying ice or cool compresses to injured areas, and attempting to make the room environment comfortable for the client.

Induce Conscious Sedation. Instituting conscious sedation is a routine practice in many EDs. This procedure involves controlled pharmacologic depression of the level of consciousness that nevertheless allows maintenance of the client's reflexes to protect the airway as well as maintain spontaneous ventilation. Conscious sedation is most commonly induced with medications such as midazolam (Versed), ketamine (Ketalar), or fentanyl (Sublimaze).[42] Dose and route of administration vary with the agent used. The most common routes are IM, IV, and nasal. The ED nurse's responsibility is to continually monitor the client for airway patency, oxygen saturation levels, cardiac activity, and response to physical or verbal stimulation until recovery from the anesthesia has occurred.[42] The duration of sedation may be from 30 to 60 minutes. The only two absolute contraindications to conscious sedation are (1) hemodynamic instability and (2) refusal by a competent client or a parent.

ACUTE CONFUSION

Clients can have an altered level of consciousness from many causes. Underlying disorders such as stroke, metabolic abnormalities, seizure, intoxication, hemorrhage, or injury need to be considered.[63,69,81] A helpful guide to use in attempting to determine the cause is the "vowels-TIPS" mnemonic: *A,* alcohol; *E,* epilepsy, encephalopathy, endocrine; *I,* insulin; *O,* overdose; *U,* underdose or uremia; *T,* trauma; *I,* infection; *P,* psychogenic; *S,* stroke or shock.

The normal state of wakefulness and consciousness is controlled by the reticular activating system (RAS) and the brain's cerebral hemispheres. Various factors can produce a decreased state of wakefulness. These include impairment of the central nervous system (CNS) from lesions, infection, or hemorrhage; a decreased supply of oxygen, blood, or glucose to cerebral tissues; and exposure to, ingestion of, or withdrawal from substances toxic to cerebral tissue.

Family members or prehospital personnel may be the only sources for obtaining historical information concerning the client's state of consciousness. It is extremely important to determine any known illnesses of the client, current medications, recent injury, known alcohol or drug use, and duration of the client's altered mental state.

Clinical Manifestations

Clinical manifestations vary according to the cause of the client's illness or injury. The Glasgow Coma Scale score is less than 15 and, in children, either a verbal or painful stimulus is required to elicit a response, or the child is unresponsive. Pupil size and equality may be altered. Unequal pupil size and reaction may indicate compression of the third cranial nerve caused by increased intracranial pressure. Small, pinpoint pupils may signify opiate overdose, pontine hemorrhage, cholinesterase poisoning, or recent use of miotic eye drops. Cranial nerve abnormalities and unilateral decreased muscle strength may be present with a recent stroke. Tongue lacerations can indicate recent seizure activity. Pale, cool, clammy skin can occur with shock or hypoglycemia. Fresh needle marks on the skin indicate recent IV drug use. A petechial rash on the skin can be an indication of a lethal bacterial meningitis. Bruising of the face, eyes (raccoon eyes), or mastoid process (Battle's sign) or a bluish hue to the tympanic membrane can indicate recent head injury and an associated basilar skull fracture.[58,81]

Diagnostic testing involves first obtaining a bedside blood glucose level. Other laboratory studies may be indicated, including serum levels of specific medications, serum and urine toxicology screening tests, CBC, blood cultures, electrolyte panel, arterial blood gas analysis, and urinalysis.[81] Urine specimens should also be tested for the presence of myoglobin, because clients who have been comatose for a prolonged time can develop rhabdomyolysis, resulting from ischemia and damage to large muscle groups. Other diagnostic studies include ECG, chest film, and brain CT scan. Occasionally a lumbar puncture may need to be performed.

Outcome Management

Establish and Maintain Airway. The first treatment priority in a client with an altered level of consciousness is establishing and maintaining the airway. If required, oral or nasal airway devices should be inserted, or preparations for intubation should be undertaken. During interventions directed at maintaining airway patency, spinal immobilization should also be considered if there is any suspicion that a traumatic injury may have occurred. High-flow oxygen via a face mask must be administered to provide supplemental oxygen to brain tissue.

Establish Vascular Access for Appropriate Medications. Venous access must be secured for possible IV fluid or medication administration. If a bedside glucose level reading is less than 45 mg/dl, 50% dextrose (D_{50}) is administered IV. If the bedside glucose level reading indicates a high level of glucose, therapy should be instituted for treatment of diabetic ketoacidosis or hyperglycemic hyperosmolar nonketotic coma (see Chapter 47).

Naloxone (Narcan) 2 to 4 mg IV may also be administered. If the cause of the alteration in consciousness is an opiate overdose, naloxone reverses the process.

If a stroke is considered to be the cause of the client's altered level of consciousness, treatment may involve administering the IV fibrinolytic medication of t-Pa. The window of time for administration of this medication has recently been expanded from 3 to 6 hours from the time of symptom onset.[10,18] The fibrinolytic medication is administered only after a brain CT scan has been obtained and interpreted by a radiologist to rule out a hemorrhage cause of the stroke. Research is currently being conducted on the early administration of brain-protective medications for the treatment of a stroke.[18]

If tonic-clonic seizure activity begins, the client is medicated with diazepam (Valium) 5 to 10 mg IV or lorazepam (Ativan) 0.05 to 0.1 mg/kg IV to terminate the seizure. This intervention may need to be followed by IV administration of phenytoin (Dilantin). Phenytoin must be diluted in normal saline solution and infused at a rate of less than 50 mg/min.

IV antibiotic medications are administered in any client with known or suspected bacterial infection within the brain tissue or cerebrospinal fluid. In clients with bacterial meningitis, this can be a life-saving intervention.

Monitor Intoxicated Clients and Treat Toxicity States. Intoxicated clients with an altered level of consciousness must be monitored in the ED for a minimum of 4 to 6

TABLE 84-4	Classification of Concussion
Grade	**Clinical Manifestations**
I	No loss of consciousness; transient confusion (lasting a few minutes); rapid return to normal functioning; no amnesia
II	Brief loss of consciousness; mild confusion; some amnesia, usually anterograde
III	Loss of consciousness for less than 6 hours; profound confusion; anterograde and retrograde amnesia
IV	Loss of consciousness for more than 6 hours; confusion; anterograde and retrograde amnesia

hours. Treatment involves IV fluid support and nutritional supplementation with thiamine, multivitamins, and occasionally folic acid. If level of consciousness does not improve within 4 to 6 hours, a brain CT scan should be obtained. It is not unusual for clients to have suffered minor head trauma during their intoxicated state, with subsequent development of a subdural hematoma.

Monitor Clients with Head Trauma and Treat the Injuries. Neurologic trauma can result in minor disturbances such as a concussion[7] (Table 84-4). The majority of minor head-injury clients are released to home without any definitive treatment. Before leaving the ED, the client or family members must be given instructions on manifestations that indicate worsening of the client's condition.

Other types of neurologic trauma, such as skull fractures, cerebral edema, subdural hematomas, epidural hematomas, and cerebral contusions, may require operative intervention.[77] The client must be closely monitored in the ED for any manifestations of increasing intracranial pressure. Diuretic medications such as mannitol and corticosteroid medications may be administered IV to prevent or diminish cerebral edema.

Prevent Injury. Safety is an important issue in a client with an altered level of consciousness. The client may need to be positioned on the left side, and frequent oral suctioning may be necessary. If in place, spinal immobilization must be maintained. Bed side rails must be up and locked in position at all times. Clients are monitored for changes in level of consciousness along with cardiac rate and rhythm, blood pressure, pulse oximetry, and respiratory rates.

DISTURBED SENSORY PERCEPTION

Sensory perceptions may be disturbed in any of the sensory organs, but an alteration in vision is one of the more common client complaints associated with sensory perceptual changes. Such alterations can be caused by infection, inflammation, or trauma.[16]

Clinical Manifestations

The client may be able to provide information related to the visual changes and the circumstances surrounding the onset of the changes. The affected eye should be assessed for discharge from the eye, excessive tearing, redness of the conjunctiva, presence of a ciliary flush (a ring of inflammation surrounding the corneal-scleral junction), periorbital cellulitis, obvious foreign objects, presence of a cloudy cornea, extruded globe contents, and obvious ecchymosis, laceration, or trauma to the eye and surrounding structures.[24] A baseline visual acuity test must be performed on all clients with a complaint related to the eye.

Changes in vision can be present with non-urgent conditions such as conjunctivitis. This infection of the conjunctival tissue is highly contagious. Foreign objects or chemicals in the eye, corneal abrasions, and deep structure infections or injury are more significant problems, and the client usually presents with a complaint of pain as well as visual changes.

Outcome Management

Anesthetizing ophthalmic drops can be placed in the affected eye to diminish pain and allow for a more thorough examination of the eye. Superficial conjunctival infections are treated with topical ophthalmic antibiotic drops or ointments. Small superficial foreign objects are removed by the ED physician. For exposure to harmful chemicals, the eye must be irrigated with a minimum of 1 L of normal saline. After irrigation, the pH of the eye is checked; if it has not returned to a normal pH of 6 to 7, irrigation may need to be continued. If corneal abrasions are present, the client is given oral pain reduction medications and topical ophthalmic antibiotic medication. Patching of the affected eye is not recommended.

More serious problems associated with the eye necessitate an immediate consultation with or referral to an ophthalmologist. These problems include complaints of sudden changes in or loss of vision with or without pain, impaled foreign objects, extensive injury or infection, and globe rupture. Any client who receives treatment from the ED physician for an eye problem should be instructed to be rechecked within 24 hours by his or her primary physician or an ophthalmologist.

RISK FOR INFECTION

Clients frequently present to the ED because of an infectious process. The infection may be caused by either viral or bacterial organisms. The source of the infection may be localized, or the infection may have spread to surrounding tissues or be systemic. It also may be contagious. Hospital employees are frequently treated in the ED for needle-stick injury and prophylactically for hepatitis B and human immunodeficiency virus exposure.

Clinical Manifestations

Clinical manifestations depend on the organism causing the infection, the extent of the infection, and the location of the infection. Bacterial infections usually produce more obvious and severe manifestations than those seen in viral infections. With bacterial infections, the client may have a fever. However, older adults and neonates frequently have subnormal temperatures with an infectious process. The client may complain of pain at the site of the infection, such as in the ear, eye, throat, abdomen, genitourinary tract, or an area of skin. It is important to consider that airway, pharyngeal, and mouth infections can be associated with airway compromise. Meningeal infections can produce headache, vomiting, neck pain, and occasionally petechiae. Pulmonary infections are frequently accompanied by productive cough and sputum. Erythema, edema, lymphadenopathy, and observable discharge or pus may be present with ear, throat, or skin infections. A skin rash or abscess may also be the presenting problem of an underlying infection.[61] Abdominal infections often present with pain and palpable abdominal tenderness. A systemic infectious process can lead to septic shock, in which endotoxins from bacterial organisms are released into the circulation. The client is acutely ill and may have clinical manifestations of fever, tachycardia, hypotension, and decreased urine output. In later stages of sepsis, the client may become hypothermic, the skin may have a mottled appearance, and the level of consciousness becomes diminished. These findings are usually associated with a high mortality rate.[15]

A primary decision must be made about whether the infection is considered contagious to other clients in the ED. If the infection is thought to be contagious, the client must be isolated as quickly as possible from other clients. It then becomes important to identify the primary source of the infection. The ears, eyes, throat, lungs, skin, and genital and pelvic areas must be assessed for evidence of infection. A chest film is obtained, in addition to possible abdominal and pelvic ultrasound studies. Laboratory studies include a urinalysis, CBC, and culture of discharge and blood specimens. If the source of the infection is not identified, a lumbar puncture may be required.

Outcome Management

When dealing with clients with known or potential infections, it is important that the ED nurse be cognizant of the hospital-wide infection control policies. Wearing gloves, using proper hand-washing techniques, and protecting oneself against contamination of infected body fluids must be a high priority.

Administer Medications. Treatment involves administering antibiotic or antiviral medications selected according to the identified or probable source of the infection.

These agents may be administered orally, IM, or IV. The antipyretic medications acetaminophen (Tylenol) and ibuprofen can be administered orally to reduce temperature. Other treatments to reduce temperature involve undressing the client and allowing heat to dissipate into the environment. Cooling the client using tepid bath water is not routinely performed. Abscesses due to skin infections may need to be incised, drained, and packed.

Hepatitis B prophylaxis treatment for unvaccinated employees exposed to a needle-stick consists of administering HBIG (hepatitis B immunoglobulin) and beginning the series of hepatitis B vaccinations. There is a risk of exposure to hepatitis C from needle-sticks, but to date there is no prophylactic treatment.[39,64]

Monitor and Treat Sepsis. If sepsis is suspected, it is important to also administer high-flow oxygen to the client, infuse IV fluids of normal saline, and insert a nasogastric tube and an indwelling urinary catheter. Additional infused medications, after antibiotic administration, may include dopamine and corticosteroids.[17,35] The client must be closely monitored for changes in blood pressure, heart rate, respiratory rate, oxygen saturation, cardiac rhythm, urine output, level of conscious changes, and prolonged bleeding times. These clients are at risk for developing disseminated intravascular coagulopathy (DIC).

IMPAIRED PHYSICAL MOBILITY

Any injury to the musculoskeletal system can lead to a decrease in the client's mobility. Other causes of impaired mobility are injuries to the vertebral bodies and possibly the spinal cord. Sprains of ligaments, fractures to bones, dislocated joints, muscle strains, and amputated extremities or digits are the majority of problems for which clients seek emergency care related to mobility deficits.

Spinal cord injury can involve edema of the cord, with transitory or minimal deficits, or other cord injury, or the cord can actually be severed. With marked edema or cord severance, deficits are usually devastating and permanent. Neurogenic shock can develop with loss of the sympathetic component of the autonomic nervous system. With only the parasympathetic nervous system functioning, massive vasodilation occurs, and tissue perfusion is decreased.[32]

Clinical Manifestations

Clinical manifestations in most musculoskeletal injuries include swelling around the injured area, presence of ecchymosis, obvious deformity of the area, palpable tenderness, and limited movement of the area.[90] Amputations are self-evident, and depending upon whether a complete or partial amputation has occurred, active bleeding may be minimal or profuse. With a complete amputation, active bleeding is minimal as a result of constriction of the severed vessels. It is important that the

ED nurse assess the effectiveness of circulation, motor movement, and presence and degree of sensation distal to any musculoskeletal injury.

An injury to the spinal cord produces a motor or sensory deficit, or both, below the level of injury. If the injury is in the upper thoracic or cervical area, the diaphragm and thoracic intercostal muscles can be affected, leading to respiratory compromise.[32] A client with neurogenic shock has warm, dry skin caused by the massive vasodilation, hypotension, and bradycardia, with no movement or sensation below the level of injury.

Radiographic films of the injured area are obtained to aid in identifying fractures. Depending on the extent of the injury, additional laboratory tests or other diagnostic studies may be performed.

Outcome Management

Treat Sprains, Strains, and Fractures. Treatment of extremity sprains and fractures consists of immediately elevating the extremity above the level of the client's heart, applying ice to the area, and immobilizing the extremity with pillows or cardboard splints.[8] Oral, IM, or IV pain-reducing medication may also need to be administered. More definitive immobilization of the area with the application of splints, molds, or immobilizers is accomplished before the client leaves the ED. Lower extremity injuries may require the client to use crutches. Detailed crutch-walking instructions must be provided (Box 84-5), and the client should be able to demonstrate adequate use of the crutches to the ED nurse before his or her discharge from the department.

Pain-reducing medication is also administered to clients with muscle strains. Once clients achieve reduction

---

BOX 84-5 *Crutch-Walking Instructions*

1. Measure for correct size of crutches. With client standing, measure from 3.75-5.0 cm below the axillary fold to a point on the floor 10 cm in front of the client and 15 cm lateral to the small toe.
2. With client standing, shoulders and back are straight, elbows flexed at 30 degrees, wrists extended, and hands dorsiflexed. Do not bear weight on axilla.
3. Three-point gait sequence involves movement of the weaker leg with both crutches simultaneously.
4. To go down stairs, place crutches on affected side, place weight on unaffected leg, place crutches on next lower step, and bring unaffected leg down to share the work of lowering the body with the support of the crutches.
5. To walk up stairs, place crutches on affected side a half-step width from the lowest step, place weight on hands, and lift the stronger leg to the step.

From Kitt S., et al. (Eds.). (1995). *Emergency nursing: A physiologic and clinical perspective* (2nd ed.). Philadelphia: W.B. Saunders.

of pain, they are usually discharged to home with instructions to rest and to apply alternating ice and heat to the injured area for the next 24 hours.

Reduce Dislocations. A joint dislocation requires reduction in the ED.[86] This procedure is performed by the ED physician. Pain-reducing and muscle-relaxant medications may need to be administered before the reduction procedure. Once joint reduction has been achieved, a post-reduction radiographic film must be obtained. After successful reduction, the joint is immobilized with the required orthopedic device.

Treat Amputation. The goal in the management of a client who has sustained an amputation is to attempt to salvage the part so that possible replantation can occur.[90] Any profuse bleeding from the stump should be controlled with direct pressure. The use of tourniquets and clamps is discouraged, because these measures can further damage the injured tissue. If the client has sustained significant blood loss, high-flow oxygen is administered, venous access is established, and replacement fluids are given.

The stump is then gently cleansed with normal saline. The amputated part is wrapped in sterile gauze moistened with normal saline. It is then placed in a plastic bag or container, and the plastic bag or container is placed on ice. The amputated part should *never* be placed directly on ice, because the resultant freezing of the tissues makes replantation impossible. The client is given pain-reducing medications, antibiotic medications, and possible tetanus prophylaxis with tetanus and diphtheria toxoids (Td) 0.5 ml if more than 5 years have elapsed since the last tetanus immunization.

Treat Spinal Cord Injury. Clients with a spinal cord injury must be maintained in complete spinal immobilization. At a minimum, a cross-table lateral cervical spine radiograph is required, and this study may be followed by more extensive spinal films or a CT scan. When a high thoracic or cervical injury is present, the client may become fatigued with the effort of maintaining respirations. The need for nasal intubation and assisted ventilation must be considered. IV fluids are necessary to maintain perfusion. Administration of high-dose IV steroids such as methylprednisolone (Solu-Medrol), 30 mg/kg over 15 minutes and then 5.4 mg/kg by infusion over the following 23 to 48 hours, may be considered to reduce cord edema.[35,89] IV administration of high-dose dopamine to counteract parasympathetic nervous system effects is another treatment consideration. This therapy, however, must be instituted cautiously, because the vasoconstrictive effect of dopamine may decrease perfusion to the injured cord. A nasogastric tube and indwelling urinary catheter are inserted.

The client must be kept warm with blankets and heating lights as necessary, because often the ability to regulate internal body temperature has been lost. Stabilization of cervical fractures may involve applying Gardner-Wells tongs with traction or a halo traction device. Monitoring of body temperature, cardiac rate and rhythm, blood pressure, respiratory rate and effort, pulse oximetry, urine output, and changes in sensory and motor movement is vital.

IMPAIRED SKIN INTEGRITY

Skin and soft tissue injury is a common problem encountered in ED clients. Injury to the skin and surrounding soft tissue can occur from sharp objects, blunt force injury, scraping mechanisms, or bites resulting in lacerations, contusions, abrasions, avulsions, or puncture wounds.[20]

Clinical Manifestations

Once the skin barrier is interrupted, the potential for infection is increased. Skin flora and other bacteria then have access to the underlying structures. After injury to the skin, natural or secondary healing processes occur, resulting in skin closure and scarring. Primary closure, or suturing, of skin wounds also closes the skin and reduces the amount of scarring. Wounds caused by forces in which bacteria were deeply embedded in the tissues, or that are older than approximately 12 hours, are not routinely managed by primary closure because of the risk for developing infection. Diagnostic tests may involve radiographic films of the wound area. Such studies are important when a foreign object is suspected to be embedded in the wound or when gas in the wound may have developed.

Outcome Management

Skin and soft tissue wounds can occur anywhere on the body. Scalp and facial lacerations often bleed profusely because of the high vascularity of these areas. Direct pressure over the wound is usually sufficient to control bleeding.

Cleanse the Wound. Cleansing of wounds is best achieved using high-pressure irrigation and normal saline solution. Directing the stream flow from a 20- to 30-ml syringe directly into the wound adequately cleanses most wounds.[20] A minimum of 100 ml of solution should be used. Shaving an area around a wound to remove hair is controversial. In most instances, shaving is not necessary and should *never* be performed on a wound located in a client's eyebrow.

Open wounds often need to be anesthetized before cleansing and must be anesthetized before primary repair is attempted. A cotton ball can be saturated with a topical solution of tetracaine-adrenaline-cocaine (TAC) or lidocaine-epinephrine-tetracaine (LET) and then applied directly to a face or scalp wound, as long as it is not used near mucous membranes. Other anesthetic agents

TABLE 84-5	*Suture Material*
Suture Size	**Indicated Use: Body Area(s)**
2-0, 3-0	Tissue subjected to strong tensile forces (e.g., knees, elbows, over joints)
3-0, 4-0	Epidermal and dermal layers, except for face
5-0, 6-0	Facial area

TABLE 84-6	*Tetanus Prophylaxis in Wound Management*			

Immunization History (No. of Doses)	Clean Minor Wounds		All Other Wounds	
	Td*	TIG†	Td	TIG
Uncertain	Yes	No	Yes	Yes
0-2	Yes	No	Yes	Yes
3 or more	No (Yes, if >10 yr since last dose)	No	No (Yes, if >5 yr since last dose)	No

Modified from Centers for Disease Control and Prevention: *MMWR Morbidity and Mortality Weekly Report,* 1999.
*Td, tetanus and diphtheria toxoids: used for persons 7 years of age or older. For children younger than 7 years, diphtheria-pertussis-tetanus (DPT).
†TIG, tetanus immune globulin (Hyper-Tet).

include lidocaine 1% or 2%, with or without epinephrine, and bupivacaine (Marcaine) 0.25% or 0.5%, with or without epinephrine. Anesthetic agents with epinephrine should never be injected into wounds located on the fingers, toes, ears, nose, or penis because of the vasoconstricting effects of epinephrine. Bupivacaine provides a longer anesthetic effect than that obtained with lidocaine. Sodium bicarbonate at a 1:10 ratio may be added to lidocaine or bupivacaine to reduce pain when the medication is injected into the wound.[55]

Close the Wound. Small, superficial wounds may be closed with adhesive paper strips or Dermabond glue. It is important to evert and bring the wound edges close together and then apply the paper strips or glue.

Larger wounds that are gaping, that involve injury to deeper structures, that occur over joints, or that are located in high-tension areas need to be sutured for optimal healing. The type of suture material required varies depending on the size and location of the open wound (Table 84-5).

Abrasion injuries are not sutured. Abrasion injuries need to be thoroughly cleansed in order to remove any particles or debris left in the wound. If particles remain in the wound, a tattooing effect results with the healing process. Human and animal bites are not routinely sutured because of the highly contaminated nature of the wound. The wound is thoroughly irrigated, and prophylactic antibiotic medications are frequently administered. Animal bites should be reported to the local animal control authorities.

Apply a Dressing. Protective dressings must be applied to wounds before the client leaves the ED. Most dressings involve first applying a thin layer of antibacterial ointment or gauze impregnated with petrolatum (Vaseline) or other occlusive substance. Then dry, sterile gauze is applied for padding, followed by a wrap of woven gauze (Kling or Kerlix). Adhesive tape is used to hold the dressing in place.

Administer Tetanus and Rabies Prophylaxis. Clients must be questioned about their tetanus immunization status. Table 84-6 presents current recommendations for tetanus prophylaxis. Td 0.5 ml is the preferred agent for active

immunization in adults. When passive immunization is necessary, human tetanus immune globulin (TIG) 250 units is administered. If both preparations must be administered, separate sites for injection should be selected.

Rabies prophylaxis should be considered in clients who have been bitten by dogs, cats, skunks, raccoons, bats, squirrels, or opossums, even though the incidence of rabies is low in the United States. Prophylaxis is especially important if the animal cannot be located and placed under quarantine for an observation period. The dose of human rabies immune globulin (RIG) for passive immunization is 20 units/kg, with as much medication as possible injected into and around the wound site and the remainder of the dose injected intramuscularly in the buttocks.[43] For active immunization with human diploid cell vaccine (HDCV), the dose is 1 ml initially and again on days 3, 7, 14, and 28 following the bite incident.

Instruct on Wound Care. Instructions related to the care of the wound are given to the client or family members before they leave the ED. These instructions should identify the manifestations of infection and explain care of the wound. Timing for a follow-up appointment with the appropriate physician for a recheck of the wound and suture removal must also be included in the instructions.

RISK FOR POISONING

ACCIDENTAL AND INTENTIONAL POISONINGS

Poisonings are either accidental or intentional. Accidental poisonings occur more commonly in the pediatric age-group, whereas intentional poisonings are more frequent in the adolescent and adult population. Poisoning can also occur from injected venom, such as snake or insect bites.

Obtaining accurate information about the offending substance, amount, and time of ingestion or exposure can be difficult. Details may be available from family or friends. Other important information to obtain is whether the client has vomited since the exposure, whether the client has been depressed or had any previous episodes of intentional poisoning, and any other associated details.[50]

Clinical Manifestations

Assessment must be directed toward the intactness of the client's ABCs (airway, breathing, and circulation). There may be few outward clinical manifestations that aid in determining the substance that was ingested, inhaled, or injected.

Diagnostic tests may include electrocardiography and continual cardiac monitoring. Blood and urine specimens need to be obtained for toxicology screening and testing. In many cases, the results of these tests are not rapidly available. Chest films may aid in diagnosing possible aspiration. If envenomation is the source of poisoning, bleeding and coagulation studies must be performed.

Outcome Management

Maintain Airway. If the client demonstrates a decrease in level of consciousness, initial interventions include establishing and maintaining a patent airway, possibly with airway adjunct devices. Oxygen should be administered, and venous access should be obtained.

Remove Offending Substance. Treatment is directed at removing or absorbing the offending substance. If the substance was injected, naloxone 2 to 4 mg IV may be administered. If the client's level of consciousness is decreased, a large nasogastric (Ewald) tube is passed either nasally or orally and gastric lavage performed if the ingestion was recent, potentially toxic, or considered significant. This procedure involves instilling approximately 250 to 500 ml normal saline solution through the tube and then removing the solution either with a syringe or gravity drainage into a collection bag. This process is repeated until the returned contents are clear of pill fragments. Then liquid-activated charcoal and a cathartic are instilled through the Ewald tube and allowed to remain in the stomach. The charcoal aids in adsorbing any other remaining particles of the toxic substance.

Awake and alert clients are given liquid-activated charcoal to drink. This medication provides the greatest benefit of adsorption if administered within 1 hour of the ingestion. Occasionally, the charcoal slurry may cause the client to vomit, and an additional dose of the charcoal may be required. The purpose of activated charcoal is again to quickly adsorb the ingested toxic substance to minimize its harmful effects. Syrup of ipecac is not routinely administered. It is not effective in

TABLE 84-7	*Poisonings and Antidotes*
Toxic Substance	**Treatment**
Beta-blocker medications	Treat hypotension initially with fluids; if unsuccessful, administer glucagons 100-150 µg/kg IV followed by 2-5 mg/hr by infusion
Calcium channel blocker medications	Calcium chloride 5-10 ml IV, or calcium gluconate 10-20 ml IV
Carbon monoxide	100% oxygen; possibly use of hyperbaric chamber
Iron	Deferoxamine (Desferal) 80 mg/kg IV or IM and repeated q 8 hr
Isoniazid (INH)	Pyridoxine (vitamin B_6) IV in a dose equivalent to amount ingested (gram for gram); if ingested amount is unknown, administer 5 g IV over 3-5 min, then repeat q 3-5 min until seizures are controlled
Methanol, ethylene glycol	50% ethanol 0.7 g/kg, or 7 ml/kg of 10% ethanol IV; continuous IV infusion of 0.07 to 0.1 g/kg/hr to maintain blood ethanol concentration between 100 and 200 mg/dl
Phenothiazine medications	Diphenhydramine (Benadryl) 0.5-1 mg/kg IV or benztropine (Cogentin) 1-2 mg IM

removing the toxic substance, unless the ingestion occurred within the previous 30 minutes. Its emetic effect prolongs the time until activated charcoal can be administered. Clients who have ingested an alkaline-based substance are not given syrup of ipecac, charcoal, or any substance that can cause emesis.

If a specific toxic substance exposure is known and an antidote is available, the antidote is administered. Table 84-7 provides a list of the more common poisoning substances and antidotes.

Dry chemicals that may be present on the client's skin or external surfaces must first be brushed off. Then the contaminated area is copiously irrigated with water or normal saline.

Provide Psychiatric Evaluation as Needed. Any client who is in the ED because of an intentional poisoning must have a psychiatric evaluation before discharge and release from the ED. Many communities have psychiatric evaluation teams (PETs) that provide this service.[65]

SNAKE BITE

Snake antivenin is available for clients who have been envenomated by a pit viper (a poisonous snake).[12] The area of the envenomation may be swollen and ecchymotic, and pain may be present at the site. Pit viper venom produces both proteolytic and hemotoxic effects. Massive swelling producing a compartment syndrome may develop, and a coagulation disorder such as DIC may result. The wound area should be gently cleansed. Ice should not be applied to reduce swelling. Antivenin is administered intravenously, but skin or conjunctival testing must be performed before administering the antivenin.

HYPERTHERMIA

Hyperthermic emergencies are usually the result of environmental exposure. The pediatric and geriatric populations are at the greatest risk for developing hyperthermia. The types of hyperthermic problems are heat cramps, heat exhaustion, and heat stroke.[72] Heat stroke is the most severe.

Clinical Manifestations

Muscle spasms of the arms and legs are evident with heat cramps. Often there is a depletion of sodium because the client has been perspiring excessively. Excessive sweating can lead to dehydration and heat exhaustion. The client may complain of headache, dizziness, nausea, and weakness. Mild hypotension can be present, and the skin is frequently cool and clammy to the touch.

Heat stroke is an emergent condition. The client is often comatose. Other clinical manifestations include hypotension, tachycardia, hot and flushed-appearing skin, and a core temperature of greater than 105° F (40.5° C).

Outcome Management

Administer Fluids and Electrolytes. For the client with mild heat cramps, administering oral fluids with electrolytes and removal from the hot environment are usually the only necessary treatments. Treatment of a client with heat exhaustion also involves removal from the hot environment and administering either oral or IV fluids to correct the problem.

Resolve Heat Stroke. Heat stroke treatment involves establishing and maintaining a patent airway, administering high-flow oxygen, and establishing venous access. IV normal saline is administered to restore fluid volume. Cooling measures must be instituted quickly. These measures include removing all clothing from the client; spraying tepid mist over the client's body and using a fan to increase air flow; placing ice packs on the scalp and neck and in the axillae and groin; and using a cooling blanket. Gastric lavage with cool saline and peritoneal dialysis may be necessary. Cooling measures

TABLE 84-8	*Stages of Hypothermia*
Stage	**Clinical Manifestations**
Mild: 93° to 95° F (34.0°-35° C)	Person is conscious and alert but may have lethargy and confusion Shivering Bradycardia or tachycardia
Moderate: 86° to 93° F (30°-34° C)	Decreased level of consciousness or coma Hypoventilation Bradycardia Atrial fibrillation Hypovolemia Cessation of shivering Possible hyperglycemia due to underutilization of glucose
Severe: <86° F (<30° C)	Coma Fixed and dilated pupils Bradycardia Apnea Hypotension Ventricular fibrillation Asystole

should continue until the client's body temperature is 101° F (38.4° C).[72] As the temperature decreases, administering chlorpromazine (Thorazine) or diazepam (Valium) may be required to reduce shivering.

A nasogastric tube and indwelling urinary catheter must be inserted. Continual cardiac, pulse oximetry, blood pressure, respiratory rate, level of consciousness, and temperature monitoring are performed.

HYPOTHERMIA

Clinical Manifestations

A body temperature less than 94° F (34.4° C) indicates the condition of hypothermia. The development of hypothermia is usually unintentional and involves accidental and prolonged exposure to cold temperatures.

Hypothermia severity can be divided into stages depending on the client's core temperature. Different clinical manifestations are present with each stage (Table 84-8).

Outcome Management

Rewarm the Client. After the establishment and maintenance of a patent airway, heated high-flow oxygen administration, and venous access with warmed fluid replacement, treatment is then directed at rewarming the client. Rewarming must be done slowly, because the hypothermic client is especially susceptible to the development of ventricular fibrillation and cardiovascular collapse if warmed blood is returned too rapidly to a cold heart. Rewarming methods include the following[72]:

1. *Passive warming*
   a. Removing wet clothing
   b. Covering the client with warm blankets
   c. Placing the client in a warm room
2. *Active warming*
   a. Immersing the client in a warm bath (104° F [40° C])
   b. Placing the client on a warming blanket
   c. Placing radiant lamps over the client
3. *Active core warming*
   a. Infusing warmed IV fluids
   b. Providing heated, humidified supplemental oxygen
   c. Performing warm fluid lavage (peritoneal, gastric, bladder, or colonic lavage)
   d. Performing continuous arteriovenous rewarming (CAVR), hemodialysis, or cardiopulmonary bypass

Insertion of a nasogastric tube and indwelling urinary catheter is an additional component of care. Continual cardiac, pulse oximetry, blood pressure, respiratory rate, level of consciousness, and temperature monitoring must be instituted.

FROSTBITE

Hypothermia to the extremities can lead to frostbite injury. The feet, hands, nose, ears, and cheeks are most commonly affected.[72] Damage to the tissues occurs, and peripheral blood flow is reduced. The area may appear red and swollen or may be pale in color. Formation of blisters containing either clear or purple bloody fluid may be seen. Rewarming of the frostbitten area should begin once the client is removed from the cold environment. The frostbitten part should be immersed in heated water at 105° to 115° F (40.6° to 46.1° C). The frostbitten area needs to be handled gently so that blood-filled blisters remain intact. Loose, sterile, bulky dressings are then applied and changed daily. The rewarming process is painful; therefore pain-reducing medications must be administered.

INEFFECTIVE COPING

Clients present to the ED not only with medical and traumatically induced problems but with psychological issues as well. Psychological disorders can range from mild anxiety to psychosis to deep depression. It is important that clients with psychological problems be taken as seriously as clients seeking treatment for medical problems.[65]

A brief mental status examination needs to be conducted to assess the client's behavior, speech patterns, mood and affect, thought processes, and judgment and insight.[11] Has the client recently experienced a crisis-producing situation? Is the client experiencing auditory or visual hallucinations? A physical examination must be performed to identify any concurrent medical condition or injury that may be compounding the problem.

It is important to communicate with the client in a calm, nonjudgmental, and accepting manner. Focusing the client on reality and explaining expected behaviors constitute part of the therapeutic communication process. In some cases, involuntary psychiatric hospitalization may be required. If the client is discharged from the ED, providing outside agency assistance and referral can be helpful.

DISASTER PLANNING/BIOTERRORISM

The ED has always been involved in both community and internal disaster planning.[28,41] When a disaster strikes, the ED is the portal through which injured clients are admitted to the hospital. In the aftermath of the 9/11/01 tragedy, disaster planning also involves vigilance on the part of ED personnel in recognizing clients exposed to outbreaks caused by weapons of mass destruction.[37,80] These weapons include nuclear radiation attacks and biochemical agent exposure. Not only must the ED be able to function as a triaging station and treatment area in a disaster scenario, but it must also have special decontamination areas to prevent the spread of these agents.[78-80] See the Terrorism Alert features on Disaster and Weapons of Mass Destruction, on Sarin, and on Being Alert to Patterns of Illness below and on pp. 2508 and 2509.

TERRORISM ALERT
Disaster and Weapons of Mass Destruction

Disaster planning is not only a hospital-wide requirement, but also an integral component of the ED. The term *disaster* is used whenever an event occurs that is of such magnitude that the normal operations of the ED are disrupted. During a disaster episode, the ED is the hospital port of entry for incoming wounded clients. A disaster triage area is established adjacent to the ED and is frequently staffed by an emergency physician and nurse. Their purpose is to identify clients whose condition is critical with a chance of survival, clients whose condition is critical or close to death with minimal chance of survival, clients requiring hospital admission, clients with minor and treatable injuries, and clients with psychological injury. Clients are then sent to the appropriate area for stabilization or treatment, or to the makeshift morgue.

TERRORISM ALERT

Disaster and Weapons of Mass Destruction—cont'd

In the past, most disasters in the United States have involved transportation accidents, such as airplane, train, or motor vehicle crashes with multiple injured patients, or natural disasters, such as tornados, earthquakes, fires, hurricanes, floods, or falling buildings, again with multitudes of injured clients. Plans have been instituted within the hospital communities, cities, counties, states, and federal government to provide support and medical treatment to the victims and survivors of a disaster.

Since September 11, 2001, disaster planning has taken on different responsibilities. Terrorist activities have prompted concern regarding transportation accidents that may involve scores of clients as well as use of weapons of mass destruction. It is likely that, in cases of use of biochemical weapons, the ED personnel may be the first to identify that a terrorist activity has occurred. For example, following a terrorist attack using biochemical weapons, clusters of otherwise healthy individuals may begin appearing at EDs requesting treatment for unknown illnesses. These illnesses may be caused by the release of substances such as radiation, bacterial agents, toxic agents such as anthrax, nerve gas, or viral agents into the atmosphere, food supply, or other medium.

It is imperative that ED nurses understand how to respond quickly when a disaster occurs. This involves knowing *who* needs to know and both *how* and *what* to do.[2] A core set of competencies for emergency preparedness has been developed at the request of the Centers for Disease Control and Prevention (CDC).[2] These competencies include (1) understanding the necessary roles involved in responding to a disaster, (2) initiating and following the chain of command, and (3) activating the response plan.[2]

Clinical Manifestations

Each disaster situation is unique in terms of the clients involved and the type of disaster that has occurred. Victims may have traumatic injuries, psychological manifestations, or a constellation of clinical manifestations indicating a bioterrorist attack.

Radiation Manifestations

The type and severity of clinical manifestations that clients demonstrate will be a direct result of the blast itself and the type and dose of the thermal radiation. The effects may occur within hours of exposure up to months afterward. Clinical manifestations include nausea, diarrhea, malaise, development of immunocompromised infections, bleeding, shock, and death.[3,7]

Biological and Chemical Agents

The bacterial agents *Bacillus anthracis* (anthrax) and *Yersinia pestis* (plague) may enter the body through inhalation, ingestion, or openings in the skin. Clinical manifestations involve the appearance of skin lesions, abdominal pain, bloody diarrhea, nausea, hematemesis, fever, respiratory distress, lymphadenopathy, shock, and death.[5] Incubation periods last from 1 to 40 days depending on the agent and the degree of exposure.

Clostridium botulinum can be ingested or inhaled. Clinical manifestations include paralysis, visual disturbances, ptosis, dysphagia, and dysphonia, which begin to occur from 2 hours to 10 days after exposure.[6]

Airborne viral agents such as variola (smallpox) produce manifestations of malaise, fever, vomiting, and characteristic lesions. These lesions begin primarily on the face and extremities with scattered lesions on the trunk of the body. Clinical manifestations begin to appear approximately 12 days after exposure.[7]

Nerve gas agents use inhalation, skin contact, or ingestion as their portal of entry. Clinical manifestations may begin to appear as soon as 20 to 30 minutes after exposure. These include respiratory arrest due to muscle paralysis, excessive salivation, diaphoresis, dyspnea, vomiting, incontinence, muscle weakness, and miosis.[1,8]

Outcome Management

Depending on the agent used to expose the population to biochemical agents, client decontamination may or may not be required. If decontamination is necessary, specialized rooms and equipment must be used to prevent the spread of the agent to other clients or health care workers.

Medications used in treating biochemical exposure include antibiotics, vaccines, atropine, and antitoxins. The U.S. Federal Government has stockpiled these medications in case they are needed.

Managing a terrorist biochemical incident involves being able to recognize its occurrence and reacting quickly. In the effort to detect the occurrence of possible terrorist activities, emergency nurses must use epidemiologic clues to identify biochemical incidents, such as identifying (1) small or large outbreaks of a disease, (2) an increase in deaths of hospitalized clients within 72 hours of admission, (3) clusters of clients from a single location with the same illness, (4) childhood diseases in adults, (5) healthy people dying of flu, (6) unexplained blood disorders, and (7) unusual increases in complaints of fever, pulmonary, or gastrointestinal manifestations.[4]

References

1. Armstrong, J. (2002). Chemical warfare. *RN, 65*(4), 32-39.
2. Gebbie, K., & Qureshi, K. (2002). Emergency and disaster preparedness: Core competencies for nurses. *American Journal of Nursing, 102*(1), 46-51.
3. Fell-Carlson, D. (2003). Terrorist danger. *Nurseweek California, 16*(2), 19-21.
4. Howard-Ruben, J. (2001). Disarm bioterrorism with knowledge and vigilance. *Nursing Spectrum Metro Edition, 2*(12), 26W-27W.
5. Stilp, R. (2002). Biological weapons & emergency preparedness, Part I. *Nursing Spectrum Metro Edition, 3*(1), 30-34.
6. Stilp, R. (2002). Biological weapons & emergency preparedness, Part II. *Nursing Spectrum Metro Edition, 3*(2), 30-34.
7. Veenema, T. & Karam, P. (2003). Emergency: Radiation. *American Journal of Nursing, 103*(5), 32-50.
8. Yergler, M. (2002). Nerve gas attack. *American Journal of Nursing, 102*(7), 57-60.

TERRORISM ALERT

Sarin

Sarin is one of the dangerous chemical weapons called nerve agents or nerve gases that have dominated chemical warfare since World War II. These gases are the most toxic and rapidly acting of the known chemical warfare agents. Sarin, a colorless and odorless gas, has a lethal dose of 0.5 mg for an adult and is 26 times more deadly than cyanide gas and 20 times more lethal than potassium cyanide. Just 0.01 mg/kg can kill a human. The vapor is slightly heavier than air, so it hovers close to the ground when released. Under cool, wet, and humid weather conditions, sarin degrades swiftly, but as the temperature increases, the lethal duration of the chemical increases despite high levels of humidity. Food and water may also be contaminated with sarin.

Nerve agents (e.g., sarin, tabun, soman, and VX) are potent acetylcholinesterase inhibitors. These agents alter cholinergic synaptic transmission at neuroeffector junctions (muscarinic effects), at skeletal myoneural junctions and autonomic ganglia (nicotinic effects), and in the central nervous system.

Exposure

Following sarin gas release into air, people can be exposed through skin or eye contact or by breathing air that contains sarin. Small containers of sarin gas or liquid can be easily carried and released for an immediate, short-lived attack. Sarin mixes easily with water and can be used to poison water or food. Touching or drinking water that contains sarin or eating food contaminated with sarin may cause clinical manifestations such as those seen with sarin gas exposure.

Protection

Chemical warfare suits that include body (skin and eye) and respiratory (mask) protection are available but are very hot when worn and are rarely available outside military or emergency rescue situations.

If exposure occurs without protection, persons should leave the area where sarin was released and get into fresh air immediately, remove clothing, rapidly wash their entire body with soap and water, rinse eyes with plain water, and seek medical attention immediately. Contaminated clothing must be disposed of carefully with placement in plastic bags. Sarin is easily decontaminated with basic solutions.

Clinical Manifestations

Exposure to large doses of sarin by any route results in loss of consciousness, convulsions, paralysis, and respiratory failure leading to death within seconds and minutes of the exposure if treatment is not initiated immediately. Other clinical manifestations are described below.

Exposure to small doses results in the following clinical manifestations within seconds to hours of exposure:

Muscarinic Effects
- Small, pinpoint pupils
- Blurred vision and eye pain
- Hypersecretion of salivary (drooling), lacrimal (watery eyes), sweat (diaphoresis), and bronchial (coughing) glands
- Runny nose
- Nausea and vomiting
- Diarrhea and abdominal cramps
- Urinary and fecal incontinence
- Slow heart rate

Nicotinic Effects
- Skeletal muscle twitching and weakness
- Convulsions
- Rapid heart rate and high blood pressure (which can mask muscarinic effects)

Treatment

Treatment consists of removing sarin from the body as soon as possible and providing supportive medical care. Emergency respondents must be trained and appropriately attired (skin and respiratory protection) before treating clients. Before transport to a hospital, all casualties must be decontaminated (clothing, skin, eyes). A patent airway must be ensured and administration of antidotes, such as 2 mg atropine IM and 600 mg pralidoxime chloride (2-PAM Cl) IV, given as soon as possible. These antidotes may be repeated at 5- to 10-minute intervals during transport and upon arrival to an ED. Emesis should not be induced if the client is alert and able to swallow a slurry of activated charcoal. Diazepam may be required to control convulsions. ALS guidelines are followed for clients with cardiac dysrhythmias or hypotension.

Data from CDC Fact Sheet on Chemical Emergencies, Department of Health and Human Services, Centers for Disease Control and Prevention. Retrieved October 21, 2003, from http://www.bt.cdc.gov/agent/sarin/basics/facts.asp and CDC Medical Management Guidelines (MMG): Nerve agents. Retrieved October 21, 2003, from atsdr.cdc.gov/MHMI.mmgd4.pdf.

TERRORISM ALERT
Being Alert to Patterns of Illness

All health care providers must remain alert for unusual illness patterns and clinical manifestations that might indicate an unusual infectious disease outbreak associated with intentional release of a biologic agent. The covert release of a biologic agent may not have an immediate impact because of the delay between exposure and illness onset, and outbreaks associated with intentional releases might closely resemble naturally occurring outbreaks. Indications of intentional release of a biologic agent include (1) an unusual temporal or geographic clustering of illness (e.g., persons who attended the same public event or gathering or development of a disease at an airport) or clients presenting with clinical manifestations that suggest an infectious disease outbreak (e.g., more than two clients presenting with an unexplained febrile illness associated with sepsis, pneumonia, respiratory failure, or rash or a botulism-like syndrome with flaccid muscle paralysis, especially if occurring in otherwise healthy persons); (2) an unusual age distribution for common diseases (e.g., an increase in what appears to be a chickenpox-like illness among adults, but which might be smallpox); and (3) a large number of cases of acute flaccid paralysis with prominent bulbar palsies, suggestive of a release of *botulinum* toxin.

CONCLUSIONS

Providing care to clients in the ED setting can be challenging and rewarding. An understanding of the principles of emergency care is the cornerstone of the specialty of emergency nursing. Most clients present to the ED without a working diagnosis but only a cadre of clinical manifestations. Therefore assessing each client using an organized approach is paramount for the ED nurse in order to be able to establish care priorities and institute appropriate interventions. The nursing process from assessment to evaluation is continually used. The scope of ED nursing is constantly changing and expanding beyond the hospital walls into the areas of community practice and community education.

THINKING CRITICALLY *evolve*

1. A 23-year-old man walks into the emergency department. He tells you that he was in a motor vehicle accident about 4 hours ago. The police were at the scene, but he refused to be transported to the emergency department because he felt fine; he went home. At home, however, the client started to experience worsening shoulder and posterior neck pain. His mother urged him to come to the emergency department. He tells you that he has "numbness" in his fingers and a "tingling" feeling in his right elbow. If you were the triage nurse, what potential problems would you consider that this client might have? Would you classify the client as emergent, urgent, or non-urgent? What measures should you take to ensure the client's safety?

Factors to Consider. What injuries sustained in a motor vehicle accident might account for the client's clinical manifestations?

2. A 35-year-old man is brought into the emergency department by the city police, who were arresting him for drunk and disorderly conduct. He had been involved in a barroom brawl, during which he acquired several small lacerations about the face and arms from broken glass, a hit to the head, and kicks to his ribs. He is conscious, verbally abusive, and threatening to fight his way out of the emergency department because he wants "to go home and be left alone." He has twice threatened you with bodily harm if you persist in preventing him from leaving. How would you proceed with this case?

Factors to Consider. Whom should you call? Would it be appropriate to sedate this client? What should you do if the client actually harms you physically?

3. A 60-year-old man has arrived at the emergency department with a complaint of headache. He states that he never had headaches until about 2 weeks ago, when he began awakening in the mornings with head pain. The headache would go away each day after he had been up and around for a few hours and had taken aspirin. In the last few days, however, neither aspirin nor acetaminophen has helped, and the headache has become nearly continuous. His wife states that his speech and balance have been "off" a little. He wonders whether there can be any connection between his headaches and a recent fall or a recent elevation in blood pressure. Describe how you would proceed with an evaluation of this client. What further information should you elicit from him? What is your assessment priority? What triage classification would be best for this client? What interventions should you anticipate?

evolve Did you remember to check out the bonus material on the Evolve website and the CD-ROM, including free self-assessment exercises?

http://evolve.elsevier.com/Black/medsurg/

Factors to Consider. What diagnostic assessments should you anticipate? What should you include in your physical examination and nursing history?

4. The client, a 70-year-old man, has been brought to the emergency department by ambulance. His wife states that he has become increasingly confused over the past few months. Within the past few days, he has become worse, is difficult to awaken in the morning, and is "sleepy" all day. This situation progressed until today, when the client's wife could not keep him awake at all; she called an ambulance and had him brought in. The client has a long history of hypertension, coronary artery disease, diabetes mellitus, and depression. Ambulance records show evidence that the client is difficult to arouse, but upon aggressive stimulation he "wakes up" and can follow basic commands. His vital signs are stable, but his pulse is slow and irregular. Blood pressure is lower than his "norm." His wife has brought his medications with her in a large paper bag. What is your priority assessment? What should you include in your physical assessment? What interventions should you anticipate?

Factors to Consider. What body systems should you assess? What diagnostic studies should you anticipate?

Discussions for these questions can be found on the website and the CD-ROM.

BIBLIOGRAPHY

1. Alexander, M. (2001). Violence in the emergency department: A first hand account. *Journal of Emergency Nursing, 27*(3), 279-285.
2. American Health Consultants. (2001). Don't use outdated approaches for critically ill infants and children. *ED Nursing, 4*(4), 45-50.

3. American Health Consultants. (2002). EMTALA compliance. *ED Nursing, 5*(6), 78-81.
4. American Health Consultants. (2002). Make your ED stand out—trend grows toward family-centered practices. *ED Nursing, 5*(4), 45-48.
5. American Health Consultants. (1999). Cutting-edge concepts for airway management. *ED Nursing, 2*(8), 110-112.
6. American Health Consultants. (2000). Become familiar with these new cardiac drugs. *ED Nursing, 4*(1), 13-14.
7. Anthony, M. (2000). Loss of consciousness after a minor injury. *Clinical Reviews, 10*(9), 80-84.
8. Barry, M. (2001). Ankle sprains. *American Journal of Nursing, 101*(10), 40-42.
9. Benton, L. (2000). DVT Prevention. *American Journal of Nursing, 100*(2), 84.
10. Blank, F., Keyes, M. (2000). Thrombolytic therapy for patients with acute stroke in the ED setting. *Journal of Emergency Nursing, 26*(1), 24-39.
11. Book, S., Kates, M., & Strauss G. (1999). A form-free psychiatric evaluation. *Patient Care for the Nurse Practitioner, 2*(8), 17-33.
12. Caywood, M. (2000). Near-fatal rattlesnake envenomation. *Journal of Emergency Nursing, 26*(2), 113-116.

13. Chan-Tack, K.,& Schaffner, W. (2001). CAP: Advice from the new guidelines. *Patient Care for the Nurse Practitioner, 4*(12), 42-52
14. Colucci, W., et. al. (2000). Intravenous nesiritide, a natriuretic peptide, in the treatment of decompensated congestive heart failure. *New England Journal of Medicine, 343,* 246-253.
15. Cryer, H., et al. (1999). Multiple organ failure: By the time you predict it, it's already there. *Journal of Trauma, 46,* 597-606.
16. Cuculino, G. (2002). Common ophthalmologic emergencies: A systematic approach to evaluation and management. *Emergency Medicine Reports, 23*(13), 163-178.
17. Curran, C., Martin, G., & Bernard, G. (2001). Sepsis: What you can do to improve the odds for your patient. *Consultant, 41*(1), 63-69.
18. Dashe, J. (2000). Acute stroke: Evaluation and treatment. *The Clinical Advisor, January,* 40-53.
19. Dunn, J. (2002). Missed MI: Costly, deadly, and sometimes unpreventable. *ED Legal Letter, 13*(7), 73-84.
20. Durham, C. (2001). Laceration assessment and management. *Patient Care for the Nurse Practitioner, 4*(6), 17-23.
21. Eckle, N., & MacLean, S. (2001). Assessment of family-centered care policies and practices for pediatric patients in nine U.S. emergency departments. *Journal of Emergency Nursing, 27,* 238-245.
22. Eichhorn, D., et al. (2001). Family presence during invasive procedures and resuscitation: Hearing the voice of the patient. *American Journal of Nursing, 101*(5), 48-55.
23. Emergency Department Overload: A Growing Crisis. The Results of the American Hospital Association Survey of Emergency Department (ED) and Hospital Capacity, April 2002.
24. Epifanio, P. (2000). Ocular emergencies. In K. Jordan (Ed.), *Emergency nursing core curriculum* (5th ed.). Philadelphia: W. B. Saunders.
25. Flarity-Reed, K. (2002). Methods of digital block. *Journal of Emergency Nursing, 28*(4), 351-354.
26. Frank, G. (2000). "I was born a rambling law": Complying with EMTALA when "coming to the emergency department" may not mean actually coming to the emergency department. *Journal of Emergency Nursing, 26*(4), 360-362.
27. Frank, G. (2001). EMTALA: An expert tells us what it's all about. *Journal of Emergency Nursing, 27*(1), 65-67.
28. Gebbie, K., & Qureshi, K. (2002). Emergency and disaster preparedness: Core competencies for nurses. *American Journal of Nursing, 102*(1), 46-51.
29. Gilmore-Hall, A. (2001). Violence in the workplace. *American Journal of Nursing, 101*(7), 55-56.
30. Goldsmith, C. (2001). Aortic aneurysms. *Nurseweek California, 14*(17), 19-20.
31. Gurney, D. (2002). Behavioral and medical-surgical restraints: New protocols, forms, and competencies that comply with all regulatory mandates. *Journal of Emergency Nursing, 28*(4), 313-322.
32. Habel, M. (2002). Spinal cord injury: The acute phase. *Nurseweek California, 15*(15), 22-23.
33. Henderson, D. (2000). Coping with asthma: The National Institutes of Health Asthma Guidelines. *Journal of Emergency Nursing, 26*(1), 70-75.
34. Hines, S. (2001). Treating respiratory tract infection in the age of resistance. *Patient Care for the Nurse Practitioner Supplement, 4*(9), 1-13.
35. Horvath, C. (2000). Shock emergencies. In K. Jordan (Ed.), *Emergency nursing core curriculum* (5th ed.). Philadelphia: W. B. Saunders.

36. Hovanessian, H. (1999). New-generation anticoagulants: The low molecular weight heparins. *Annals of Emergency Medicine, 34,* 768-779.

37. Howard-Ruben J. (2001). Disarm bioterrorism with knowledge and vigilance. *Nursing Spectrum Metro, 2*(12), 26w-27w.

38. James, C. (2000). Respiratory emergencies. In K. Jordan (Ed.), *Emergency nursing core curriculum* (5th ed.). Philadelphia: W. B. Saunders.

39. Kallenborn, J., et al. (1999). Occupational exposure: Organizing ED care to determine rapid postexposure prophylaxis within hours instead of days. *Journal of Emergency Nursing, 25*(6), 505-508.

 40. Killian, M. (Ed). (1999). *Standards of emergency nursing practice* (4th ed.). Park Ridge, IL: Emergency Nurses Association.

41. Klein, J. (2000). Disaster preparedness/disaster management. In K., Jordan (Ed.), *Emergency nursing core curriculum* (5th ed.). Philadelphia: W. B. Saunders.

42. Knight, S., & Proehl, J. (1999). Conscious sedation. In J. Proehl (Ed.), *Emergency nursing procedures* (2nd ed.). Philadelphia: W. B. Saunders.

43. Le, T., & Dire, D. (2002). Managing human and animal bites. *The Clinical Advisor, April,* 27-40.

44. Lee, G. (2002). The legal use of restraints. *Journal of Emergency Nursing, 28*(4), 335-337.

45. Lee, G. (2000). Update of EMTALA. *American Journal of Nursing, 100*(9), 57-59.

 46. May, D., & Grubs, L. (2002). The extent, nature, and precipitating factors of nurse assault among three groups of registered nurses in a regional medical center. *Journal of Emergency Nursing, 28*(1), 11-17.

 47. Mayer, B., Smith, F., & King, C. (1999). Factors associated with victimization of personnel in emergency departments. *Journal of Emergency Nursing, 25*(5), 361-366.

48. Mayer, D., et al. (2001). Speaking the language of pain. *American Journal of Nursing, 101*(2), 42-49.

 49. MacKenzie, E., et al. (2003). National inventory of hospital trauma centers. *Journal of the American Medical Association, 289*(12), 1515-1522.

50. McDeed-Breault, C. (2000). Toxicological emergencies. In K. Jordan (Ed.), *Emergency nursing core curriculum* (5th ed.). Philadelphia: W. B. Saunders.

51. McKay, J. (1999). The emergency department of the future—The challenge is in changing how we operate! *Journal of Emergency Nursing, 25*(6), 480-488.

52. Meyers, T., et al. (2000). Family presence during invasive procedures and resuscitation: The experience of family members, nurses, and physicians. *American Journal of Nursing, 100*(2), 32-42.

53. Moody, L., & Galanowsky, K. (2002). TB or not TB: A continuing challenge. *Nursing Spectrum Metro, 3*(3), 14-19.

54. Moore, J., & Wilson, M. (2000). Treatment of acute myocardial infarction emergencies in a community hospital setting. *American Journal of Nursing, 100*(9, Supplement), 15-19.

55. Moy, R., & Pfenninger, J. (2000). Taking the sting out of local anesthesia. *Patient Care for the Nurse Practitioner, 3*(3), 49-57.

56. Ng, S., et al. (2001). Ninety-minute accelerated critical pathway for chest pain evaluation. *American Journal of Cardiology, 88,* 611-617.

57. Odell C. (1999). Combitube airway. In J. Proehl (Ed.), *Emergency nursing procedures* (2nd ed.). Philadelphia: W. B. Saunders.

58. O'Hanlon-Nichols, T. (1999). Neurologic assessment. *American Journal of Nursing, 99*(6), 44-50.

59. Ornato, J. (2001). Evaluating the patient with chest pain. *Patient Care for the Nurse Practitioner, 4*(3), 28-43.

60. Owen, C. (1999). New directions in asthma management. *American Journal of Nursing, 99*(3), 26-33.

61. Parhizgar, B. (2001). Skin signs of systemic disease. *The Clinical Advisor, July/August,* 33-40.

62. Pasero, C. (2002). Pain assessment in infants and young children: Neonates. *American Journal of Nursing, 102*(8), 61-65.

63. Peabody, S.P. (2000). General medical emergencies: Part I. In K. Jordan (Ed.), *Emergency nursing core curriculum* (5th ed.). Philadelphia: W. B. Saunders.

64. Philie, P. (2001). Management of bloodborne fluid exposures with a rapid treatment prophylactic caremap: One hospital's 4-year experience. *Journal of Emergency Nursing, 27*(5), 440-449.

65. Polli, G., & Lazear, S. (2000). Mental health emergencies. In K. Jordan (Ed.), *Emergency nursing core curriculum* (5th ed.). Philadelphia: W. B. Saunders.

66. Rembacz, J., & Abel, C. (2000). Pericardial tamponade. *American Journal of Nursing, 100*(9, Supplement), 10-14.

67. Robinson, K. (2001). HCFA's 250-year rule for patients requiring assistance outside: EMS' or the hospital's responsibility? *Journal of Emergency Nursing, 27*(3), 264-266.

68. Roettiz, M., & Tanabe, P. (2000). Emergency management of acute coronary syndromes. *Journal of Emergency Nursing, 26*(6), S1-S42.

69. Ruckenstein, M. (2001). The dizzy patient: How can you help. *Consultant, 41*(1), 29-34.

70. Sams, R. (2001). Chest pain: Eight steps to definitive diagnosis. *ADVANCE for Nurse Practitioners, 9*(12), 22-26.

71. Selman, J. (2000). Contemporary diagnosis and management of headache. *The Clinical Advisor, June,* 37-46.

72. Semonin-Holleran, R. (2000). Environmental emergencies. In K. Jordan (Ed.), *Emergency nursing core curriculum* (5th ed.). Philadelphia: W. B. Saunders.

73. Sheehy, S., & George, J. (1999). Emergency consent: How would you act? *Journal of Emergency Nursing, 25*(5), 401-402.

74. Slaughter, A., Pasero, C., & Manworren, R. (2002). Unacceptable pain levels. *American Journal of Nursing, 102*(5): 75-77.

 75. Smith, A. (1999). New MI treatment guidelines reflect current findings. *Clinical Reviews, 9*(10), 79-84.

76. Stephens, N. (2000). One emergency department's responses to the increasingly complex challenges of patient care at century's change. *Journal of Emergency Nursing, 26*(4), 318-328.

77. Stillwell, S. (2000). When you suspect epidural hematoma. *American Journal of Nursing, 100*(9), 68-76.

78. Stilp, R. (2002). Biological weapons & emergency preparedness, Part I. *Nursing Spectrum Metro, 3*(1), 30-34.

79. Stilp, R. (2002). Biological weapons & emergency preparedness, Part II. *Nursing Spectrum Metro, 3*(2), 30-34.

80. Stopford, B. (2001). Responding to the threat of bioterrorism: Practical resources and references, and the importance of preparation. *Journal of Emergency Nursing, 27*(5), 471-475.

81. Snyder, J. (2000). Neurological emergencies. In K. Jordan (Ed.), *Emergency nursing core curriculum* (5th ed.). Philadelphia: W. B. Saunders.

 82. Tanabe, P., & Buschmann, M. (1999). A prospective study of ED pain management practices and the patient's perspective. *Journal of Emergency Nursing, 25*(3), 171-177.

 83. Tanabe, P., et al. (2002). The effect of standard care, ibuprofen, and distraction of pain relief and patient satisfaction in children with musculoskeletal trauma. *Journal of Emergency Nursing, 28*(2), 118-125.

84. Travers, D., et al. (2000). Comparison of three-level and five-level triage acuity systems. *Journal of Emergency Nursing, 26,* 411.

85. Twedell, D. (2000). Nursing process: Assessment and priority setting. In K. Jordan (Ed.), *Emergency nursing core curriculum* (5th ed.). Philadelphia: W. B. Saunders.

86. Urquhart, B. (2001). Anterior shoulder dislocation. *American Journal of Nursing, 101*(2), 33-35.

87. Valentino, R. (2001). Recognizing and responding to grief. *ADVANCE for Nurse Practitioners, 9*(1), 52-55.

88. van Vlaanderen, D. (2001). Revised guidelines for acute MI. *The Clinical Advisor, March,* 31-34.

89. Walker, J., & Criddle, L. (2001). Methylprednisolone in acute spinal cord injury: Fact or fantasy? *Journal of Emergency Nursing, 27*(4), 401-403.

90. Walker, J. (2000). Orthopedic emergencies. In K. Jordan (Ed.), *Emergency nursing core curriculum* (5th ed.). Philadelphia: W. B. Saunders.

91. Wells, J., & Salyer, S. (2001). Diagnosing pulmonary embolism. *Clinical Reviews, 11*(2), 67-78.

92. Welsh, J., et al. (2002). Characteristics and treatment of patients with heart failure in the emergency department. *Journal of Emergency Nursing, 28*(2), 126-131.

93. Worthington, K. (2000). Violence in the health care workplace. *American Journal of Nursing, 100*(11), 69-70.

94. Wuerz, R., et al. (2001). Implementation and refinement of the emergency severity index. *Academy of Emergency Medicine, 8,* 170-176.

95. York, D. (1999). Rapid sequence induction for intubation. In J. Proehl (Ed.), *Emergency nursing procedures* (2nd ed.). Philadelphia: W. B. Saunders.

96. York, D. (1999). Laryngeal mask airway. In J. Proehl (Ed.), *Emergency nursing procedures* (2nd ed.). Philadelphia: W. B. Saunders.

97. York, D. (1999). General principles of endotracheal intubation. In J. Proehl (Ed.), *Emergency nursing procedures* (2nd ed.). Philadelphia: W. B. Saunders.

Additional Online Content

THE FOLLOWING LEARNING TOOLS AND KEY REFERENCE CONTENT CAN BE FOUND ON THE EVOLVE WEBSITE AT http://evolve.elsevier.com/Black/medsurg/

Audio Pronunciations for more than 250 words

Audio Clips, Animations, and Video Clips for physical examination and health assessment

Health Assessment Images on normal and abnormal findings

Fluid & Electrolyte Module

Concept Map Creator

List of Nursing Interventions Classification (NIC) Labels

List of Nursing Outcomes Classification (NOC) Labels

List of NANDA International Approved Nursing Diagnoses

APPENDIX A
Religious Beliefs and Practices Affecting Health Care

APPENDIX B
A Health History Format That Integrates the Assessment of Functional Health Patterns

APPENDIX C
Laboratory Values of Clinical Importance in Medical-Surgical Nursing

Index

A

AAACN. *See* American Academy of Ambulatory Care Nursing
ABC mnemonic, 2485
ABCDE mnemonic
   for angina management, 1705
   in preoperative assessment, 265
Abdomen
   assessing, 680-682
   auscultation of, 682
   endoscopy of, 783-784
   inspection of, 682
   palpation of, 682
   percussion of, 681, 1162
   physical examination of, 779-780
      in elimination assessment, 793-794
   quadrants and anatomic regions of, 681f
   radiography of, 683-684, 783
   rebound tenderness of, 780
   trauma to, 852-853
   ultrasonography of, 783
Abdominal angina, intestinal obstruction due
      to, 844
Abdominal aortic aneurysm, 1528-1532
   resection of, acute renal failure and, 947
   rupture of, 1532
Abdominal bruits, assessing for, 779f
Abdominal cancer, 843-844
Abdominal films, plain, 99
Abdominal pain, 780
   in appendicitis, 812-813
   assessment of, 672, 673t, 776
   in endocrine disorders, 1158, 1158f
Abdominal reflex, normal, 2034t
Abdominal trauma, pancreatic injury in, 1301
Abdominal-perineal resection for colorectal cancer,
      835, 835f
Abdominoplasty, 1426
Abducens nerve, function of, 2012
ABI. *See* Ankle-brachial index
ABO blood group system, 2253, 2253t
ABO blood group typing for transplantation, 2433
Abortion
   federal funding for, 122
   spontaneous, herpes simplex infection and, 1136
   spontaneous/planned, 989
   threatened, treatment of, 978
Abscess
   anorectal, 851
   brain, manifestations/management of, 2100
   crypt, in ulcerative colitis, 817
   liver, 1363-1364
   lung, manifestations/management of, 1843-1844
   pancreatic, 1295
   in pelvic inflammatory disease, 1064-1065
   pericholecystic, 1303
   peritonsillar, manifestations/management of, 1800
   renal/perinephric, manifestations, diagnosis,
      treatment, 921t
   subdiaphragmatic, 1874

b indicates numbered box material, *f* indicates illustrations, and *t* indicates tables.

Absence seizures, 2076
Absolute neutrophil count, 366
   determining, 2408b
Absolute refractory period, 2009
Absorptiometry, dual-energy x-ray, of
      musculoskeletal system, 576
Absorption
   facilitators of, 665
   and intestinal ion/water balance, 666
   of vitamins, 666
   of water and electrolytes, 666
Abstinence, defined, 540t
Abuse. *See also* Child abuse; Domestic violence;
      Elder abuse; Sexual abuse
   domestic, 40
   elder, 56
   mandatory reporting of, 2482
A1C testing, 1251, 1265
Acaia senegal, adverse GI effects of, 777
Acalculous cholecystitis, 1312
   acute, 1313
Accidents
   alcohol-related, 37
   coma due to, 2052
   prevention of, 36
   screening/preventive measures for, 14t
Accommodation
   assessing, 2028
   defined, 1912
   pupil, with increased intracranial pressure, 2200
Accreditation Association for Ambulatory Health
      Care, functions of, 144
Accreditation in ambulatory nursing care, 144
ACE. *See* Angiotensin-converting enzyme
Acetaminophen
   analgesic effects of, 437
   with codeine, 60t
   liver damage from, 1339t
   for osteoarthritis, 583
Acetate, daily requirement for, 706t
Acetazolamide (Diamox)
   increased urinary oxalate levels and, 882
   for metabolic alkalosis, 256
   for reducing intraocular pressure, 1953
Acetic acid, indications/wound healing effects
      of, 409t
Acetylcholine
   in Alzheimer's disease, 2164
   in muscle movement, 563
   nerve fibers secreting, 2012
Acetylcysteine supplements for preventing renal
      deterioration, 937
Achalasia, 659, 727-731
   medical management of, 727-728
   nursing management of, 728-729
   pathophysiology/manifestations, 727
   surgical management of, 729-731
Achilles reflex
   normal, 2034t
   testing, 1178
Achlorhydria, defined, 1194
Acid perfusion test, 686
Acid phosphatase, reference values/conditions with
      altered levels, 357t

Acid-base balance, 247-261
   arterial blood gas analysis in, 252
   compensation in, 251-252, 252b
   correction in, 252
   disorders of, 252-260
      metabolic acidosis, 256-260
      metabolic alkalosis, 255-256
      mixed, 257-260
      respiratory acidosis, 254-255
      respiratory alkalosis, 253-254
      triple, 257
   in metabolic coma, 2057
   regulation of, 247-249
      buffer systems in, 247-248
      interactions of systems involved in, 251-252
      kidneys in, 249-251, 249f
      lungs in, 248-249, 248f, 249f
      pulmonary, 1741
   renal mechanisms of, 771-772
   in shock, 2451
Acid-base map, 257, 257f
Acidemia
   defined, 253
   in metabolic acidosis, 256
   in respiratory acidosis, 254
Acidosis, 666. *See also* Metabolic acidosis;
      Respiratory acidosis
   defined, 253
   high anion gap, 256
   non-anion gap, 256
   overcorrection of, 255
Acids
   exogenous
      for acid-base imbalances, 260
      for metabolic alkalosis, 256
   fixed, kidney regulation of, 249-251, 249f, 250f
   volatile, pulmonary regulation of, 248-249,
      248f, 249f
ACL. *See* Anterior cruciate ligament
Acne, topical medications for, 1392t
Acne rosacea, characteristics/management of,
      1401-1402
Acne vulgaris, 1401
Acoustic nerve, assessing, 2029
Acoustic neuroma, 2085
   hearing loss due to, 1972
   tumor removal in, 1980
   unilateral tinnitus and, 1974
Acquired immunodeficiency syndrome. *See* AIDS
Acral-lentiginous melanoma, characteristics
      of, 1416t
Acromegaly, 1155, 1233, 1234f
   in hyperpituitarism, characteristics and
      management of, 1236t
   symptoms of, 1155
ACTH. *See* Adrenocorticotropic hormone
ACTH syndrome, ectopic, therapies for, 1228t
ACTH test, plasma, in Cushing's syndrome, 1223
ACTH-reducing agents, 1229
Actinic keratosis, 1374
   characteristics/management of, 1411-1413
Action potentials, 563, 2009
Activated clotting time, purpose, normal values,
      interpretations, 2266t

I-1

Antineutrophilic cytoplasmic antibodies, normal value/significance, 2338t
Antinuclear antibody
 normal value/significance, 2338t
 in systemic lupus erythematosus, 2353t
Antinuclear antibody tests for musculoskeletal conditions, 578t
Antinuclear factor in systemic lupus erythematosus, 2352
Antioxidant vitamins for reducing cardiovascular disease, 1517
Antioxidants
 for acute respiratory distress syndrome, 1897
 mechanism of, 20
 sources of, 20
Anti-perinuclear factor in rheumatoid arthritis, 2333
Antiplatelet agents
 for angina, 1705
 for coronary heart disease, 1637
Antiretroviral agents
 classes of, 2383
 correlation to HIV life cycle, 2381f
 failure of, 2385
 for HIV infection, 2383-2387
 HIV resistance to, 2385
 initiating/maintaining, 2388-2389
 mechanism of action of, 2380
 resistance to, 2389
Antirheumatic drugs, disease-modifying, studies of, 2330, 2331
Antiseizure drugs. *See* Antiepileptic drugs
Antiseptic solutions for wounds, 409t
Antispasmotics
 effect on urination, 791t
 for irritable bowel syndrome, 848
 for neurogenic bladder, 904
Antithyroglobulin antibody, normal value/test description, 1166t-1167t
Antithyroid antibody tests, 1164
Antithyroid medications for Graves' disease, 1200-1201
Antivertigo agents, 1991
Antiviral agents. *See also* Antiretroviral agents
 for STDs, 1129
Antixoidants, appropriate use of term, 114
Antrectomy for peptic ulcer disease, 757
Anuria
 defined, 785, 942
 versus urinary retention, 893
Anus
 inspection of, 682
 palpation of, 682
 physical examination of, 780-781
 structure and function of, 774
Anxiety
 about amputation, 1523
 about anesthesia, 286
 in acute pancreatitis, 1295
 after craniotomy, 2090
 AMI-related, 1723
 with cholecystectomy, 1309
 in chronic renal failure, 967
 client, in renal trauma, 932-933
 in COPD, 1825
 in dying client, 491-492
 interventions for decreasing, 526b
 manifestations of, 525t
 mechanical ventilation-related, 1890-1891
 medications for, 492t
 pain response and, 453
 preoperative, 278
 risk for, in heart failure, 1667
 spinal fusion and, 2145
 tracheostomy-related, 1785

Anxiety (*Continued*)
 as universal phenomenon, 525
 in viral hepatitis, 1331
Anxiety disorders
 outcome management/interventions, 528-530
 referrals for, 529-530
Anxiolytic abuse, 549
 health consequences of, 550t-551t
Anxiolytic withdrawal, symptoms of, 544t
Anxiolytics
 in Alzheimer's disease, 2167
 effects of, 542t
Anzemet. *See* Dolasetron (Anzemet)
Aorta, disorders of, impotence and, 1476
Aortic aneurysm
 abdominal, resection of, acute renal failure and, 947
 dissecting
  differential assessment of, 1564t-1565t
  hypertension due to, 1495b
 palpation for, 1482, 1483f
Aortic dissection, 1532-1533
Aortic regurgitation
 clinical manifestations of, 1603-1604
 etiology/risk factors, 1603
 management of, 1604
 manifestations of, 1602-1603
 pathophysiology of, 1603
Aortic stenosis
 clinical manifestations of, 1603
 etiology/risk factors, 1603
 management of, 1604
 manifestations of, 1602
 pathophysiology of, 1603
Aortic valve disease, 1602-1604
Aortic valve stenosis/regurgitation, manifestations of, 1600t
Aortoiliac stenosis, 1511, 1511f
Aphasia
 Broca's, 1998, 2112-2113
 defined, 2112
 in epilepsy, 2075
 global, 2112
 with hemiplegia, 2113
 motor/nonfluent, 2113
 sensory/fluent, 2113
 stroke-induced, 2112-2113
 Wernicke's, 2112-2113
Apheresis for chronic myelogenous leukemia, 2406
Aphthasol. *See* Amlexanox (Aphthasol)
Aphthous stomatitis, 719, 719f
Aplastic anemia
 agranulocytosis and, 2301
 hereditary *versus* acquired, 2291-2292, 2292t
 lab findings in, 2287t
 manifestations/management of, 2291-2293
Aplastic crisis in sickle cell anemia, 2296
Apley's scratch test, purpose, techniques, findings, 573t
Apnea
 respiratory pattern in, 1751f
 sleep. *See* Sleep apnea
Apocrine glands
 structure and function of, 1371
 sympathetic/parasympathetic stimulation of, 2014t
Apolipoprotein E in Alzheimer's disease, 324
Apomorphine (Uprima) for erectile dysfunction, 1047
Apoptosis
 definition and role in cell death, 345, 345f
 in heart failure, 1651
 in metastasis, 344-345
Appearance, assessing, 88
Appendectomy, 813

Appendicitis, 812-814, 812f
 clinical manifestations of, 812f, 812-813
 etiology, risk factors, pathophysiology, 812
 outcome management of, 813-814
Appendicular skeleton, 558
Appetite
 changes in, assessment of, 672-673
 interventions for increasing, 696-697
 loss of. *See also* Anorexia nervosa
  in gastrointestinal disorders, 743
Applanation tonometry, 1912
Apraxia
 assessing, 2031
 stroke-related, 2114
Aqueous flow, promoting, in glaucoma, 1945-1946
Aqueous humor
 composition of, 1912
 normal flow of, 1944f
Arachnoid, structure and function of, 2004
Arava. *See* Leflunomide (Arava)
Arcus senilis, 1914
 assessing for, 1923
  in cardiovascular exam, 1571
ARDS. *See* Acute respiratory distress syndrome; Adult respiratory distress syndrome
Aredia. *See* Pamidronate (Aredia)
ARF. *See* Acute renal failure
L-Arginine supplements for erectile dysfunction, 1048
Argyll Robertson pupil in neurosyphilis, 2151
Arimidex. *See* Anastrozole (Arimidex)
Arm exercises after breast cancer surgery, 1109-1110
Arnica for skin disorders, 1378
Aromatase inhibitor in cancer treatment, 367b
Aromatherapy, 110
 description of, 116t
Arousal
 early morning, in hospital, 517
 physiology of, 438, 508-510, 509f
Arousal disorders, 514
Arrhythmias. *See* Dysrhythmias; specific dysrhythmias
ARS. *See* Artificial rectal sphincter
Art therapy, description of, 116t
Arterial baroreceptors in shock, 2448
Arterial blood gases
 analysis of, 252, 252b, 1764-1765
 in complex acid-base disorders, 257, 258
 in metabolic acidosis, 256
 in metabolic alkalosis, 255
 minimizing sampling errors in, 259, 259t
 in respiratory alkalosis, 253
Arterial blood sampling, 97
Arterial bypass surgery
 for peripheral vascular disease, 1517f, 1517-1518
 postoperative care for, 1519-1521
Arterial disorders. *See also* Peripheral vascular disease
 clinical manifestations of, 1476
 in lower extremities, 1477t
Arterial embolism, 1526-1527, 1527f
 versus arterial thrombosis, 1527
Arterial flow, promoting, in peripheral vascular disease, 1513, 1514
Arterial insufficiency
 manifestations of, 1476, 1477-1478
 objective/subjective data in, 1511, 1512t
Arterial occlusion
 acute, 1526-1528
 six Ps of, 1528b
Arterial oxygen, partial pressure of, in acute respiratory failure, 1877

Cutaneous stimulation, pain management with, 476
Cutaneous T-cell lymphoma, characteristics and management of, 1417-1418
CVP. *See* Central venous pressure
CVVH. *See* Continuous venovenous hemofiltration
CWHD. *See* Continuous venovenous hemodialysis
CWHDF. *See* Continuous venovenous hemodiafiltration
Cyanosis, assessing, 91, 1383, 1567
  in cardiovascular exam, 1571-1572
Cyclic adenosine monophosphate, 1151
Cyclodestructive procedures for glaucoma, 1948
Cyclophosphamide (Cytoxan)
  for bladder cancer, 870
  for breast cancer, 1114
  for preventing/treating organ rejection, 2434
  for prostate cancer, 1032
  for rheumatoid arthritis, 2343
  and risk of bladder cancer, 867
Cyclospora infection, intestinal infections due to, 810-811
Cyclosporine
  for psoriasis vulgaris, 1401
  for rheumatoid arthritis, 2342, 2343
    studies of, 2331
Cylert. *See* Pemoline (Cylert)
Cymatic therapy, description of, 117t
Cyproheptadine (Periactin) for ACTH hypersecretion, 1229
Cystadenocarcinoma, pancreatic, 1301
Cystectomy. *See also* Urinary diversion
  partial, for bladder cancer, 872
  radical
    for bladder cancer, 872
    sexual dysfunction after, 880-881
Cystic disease, adult-onset medullary, 937
Cystic fibrosis
  genetic error and symptoms in, 320
  manifestations/management of, 1869-1870
  pancreatic effects of, 1301-1302
Cystic fibrosis transmembrane conductance regulator, 1297
Cystine, urinary, normal values/causes of abnormal values, 798t
Cystine stones, 884
  medications for, 885
Cystitis, 857-863. *See also* Urinary tract infections
  clinical manifestations, 859-860
  defined, 857
  etiology/risk factors, 858-859
  interstitial, 789, 864-866
    caffeine and, 792, 792t
    etiology/risk factors, 864
    outcome management of, 865-866
    pathophysiology/clinical manifestations of, 865
  medical management of, 860-862
  nursing management of, 862-863
  pathophysiology of, 859
  surgical management of, 863
Cystocele
  assessing for, 996
  characteristics of, 1076-1077, 1077f
  urinary retention and, 891
  vaginal, 795
Cystograms, 800
Cystolitholapaxy, 888
Cystolithotomy, 889
Cystometry, 803-804
Cystoscopy for assessing prostate/urologic problems, 1011
Cystotomy, suprapubic, for urinary retention, 894
Cystourethrogram, voiding, 800
  in urinary elimination assessment, 805
Cystourethroscopy, 801

Cysts
  characteristics of, 1381f
  chocolate, 1067
  of ear, otalgia due to, 1983
  ganglion, manifestations/management of, 2158
  ovarian, 1079
  pilonidal, 852
  sebaceous, 1374
Cytadren. *See* Aminoglutethimide (Cytadren)
Cytogenetics, 319
Cytokine inhibitors for preventing/treating organ rejection, 2434
Cytokines, 2251
  defined, 334t
  functions of, 2241, 2252, 2252t
  in inflammatory response, 401
  in mediation of allergic reactions, 2317t
  secretion of, 401
Cytologic specimens in cancer diagnosis, 359
Cytologic studies, 105-106
Cytology, urine, 797
Cytomegalovirus infection
  opportunistic, with HIV infection, 2392-2393
  renal, 916
Cytomegalovirus retinitis, opportunistic, 1965-1966
Cytometry, flow, 797
Cytoplasm, organelles of, description and function of, 198t
Cytoskeleton, description and function of, 198t
Cytotec. *See* Misoprostol (Cytotec)
Cytotoxic agents, bone marrow production and, 2257
Cytoxan. *See* Cyclophosphamide (Cytoxan)

D

Dacryocystitis, definition, manifestations, management, 1963t
Dactylitis in sickle cell anemia, 2296
Dakin's solution, indications/wound healing effects of, 409t
Dalfopristin (Synercid), microbial resistance to, 425
Dalmane. *See* Flurazepam (Dalmane)
Danazol (Danocrine)
  for endometriosis, 1067
  for systemic lupus erythematosus, 2355
Dance therapy, description of, 116t
Danocrine. *See* Danazol (Danocrine)
Dapsone for systemic lupus erythematosus, 2355
DASH diet, 1499, 1500t, 1570
Dawn phenomenon, 1278
DCA. *See* Directional coronary atherectomy
DCIS. *See* Ductal carcinoma in situ
D-dimer, purpose, normal values, interpretations, 2266t
D-dimer blood test, 1537
De Quervain's tenosynovitis, manifestations, occupations at risk, treatment, 2156t
Dead space in deep wounds, 411
Deafness. *See also* Hearing impairment; Hearing loss
  central, 1972
  versus hearing impairment, 1974
Death/dying
  in America, 488
  and care for caregivers, 500
  communication and, 500
  definition of, 2426-2427
  imminent, indicators of, 499-500, 500t
  informing family of, 2484
  Kübler-Ross's stages of, 487-488, 488t
  leading causes of, 20b, 489-490
  and support of grieving family, 14-16, 15t, 210t
  unexpected, in emergency department, 2483-2484

Debridement
  autolytic, 412
  of burn injuries, 1451-1452
  enzymatic, 411-412
  of necrotic tissue, 411
  types of, for pressure ulcers, 1404-1405
  wound, 406, 407-408
Decisional conflict
  in COPD, 1828
Decision-making, client involvement in, in CAM, 110
Decompression
  by gastrointestinal intubation, 744
  tubes for, 745
Decompressive laminectomy for herniated disk removal, 2144, 2144f
Decongestants for allergic reactions, 2322
Decortication for pleural effusions, 1873
Decubitus ulcers. *See* Pressure ulcers
Deep tendon reflexes, 2035
  assessing, 2036b
Deep venous thrombosis
  chronic venous insufficiency and, 1540
  conditions associated with, 1535b
  fracture-related, 630, 635, 640
  Homans' sign and, 1483
  preventing, after total hip arthroplasty, 586
  risk for, after hip arthroplasty, 591-592
Deep-breathing exerciser, postoperative use of, 305, 305f
Deep-breathing exercises. *See* Breathing exercises
Defecation, 774
Defense mechanisms
  antioxidants as, 20
  immune/hematologic systems as, 2238-2246
  resistance as, 2238-2246
  surface, 2238
Deformities
  musculoskeletal, 566
  varus *versus* valgus, 570
Dehiscence, wound, 414
Dehydration. *See also* Fluid imbalances, extracellular deficit; Fluid volume deficit
  in acute hyperglycemia, 1270z
  cellular, manifestations of, 208
  delirium due to, interventions for, 496t
  in diabetic ketoacidosis, 1259
  in dying client, 495
  in HHNS, 1273
  hypovolemic shock due to, 2445
  morbidity/mortality due to, 205
  pathophysiology of, 207
Dehydration tests, 1177-1178
Dehydroepiandrosterone (DHEA)
  availability of, 113
  for systemic lupus erythematosus, 2355
Deinfibulation, 1088
Delayed-type hypersensitivity skin tests, 2268-2269
Delegation, rights of, 122
Delirium
  classification of, 2065-2066
  versus dementia, 57
  DSM-IV-TR criteria for, 494
  of dying client, 494-495
  features of, 2065
  in older adults, 57, 58t
  reversible causes of, 494, 496t
Deltoid muscles, assessing, 570t
Delusions in brain disorders, 2066
Demeclocycline for hyponatremia in SIADH, 227
Dementia. *See also* Alzheimer's disease
  causes of, 2162b
  classification of, 2066
  versus delirium, 57
  features of, 2066

Infective endocarditis (*Continued*)
　etiology/risk factors, 1617
　manifestations of, 1618
　medical management of, 1618
　nosocomial, 1617
　nursing management of, 1618-1620
　pathophysiology of, 1617-1618
　prevalence of, 1616-1617
　prophylaxis of, during dental procedures,
　　1620b1618-1620
Infertility
　chlamydial infection and, 1131
　education about, 1043
　in endometriosis, 1066
　male, 1041-1043
　preventing, 1043
　radiation-related, 365
　STDs and, 1126
Infibulation, 1087
Inflammation
　acute, 402-406
　chemical mediators of, 449
　chronic, 406
　mechanism and function of, 2246
　pain due to, 449
　purpose of, 399
　wound-related, 398-401
　　reducing, 404
Inflammation modulator imidazoles for
　　inflammatory bowel disease, 819
Inflammatory bowel disease, 815-829
　clinical manifestations of, 817-818
　etiology/risk factors, 815
　versus irritable bowel syndrome, 776
　medical management of, 818-819
　medications for, 819
　nursing management of, 819-821, 824-829
　pathophysiology of, 815, 817
　prognosis for, 818
　quality of life with, 822
　surgical management of, 821-829
Inflammatory disorders, intestinal, 808-829
Inflammatory responses
　coronary artery disease and, 1631
　in SIRS and MODS, 2473-2474
Infliximab (Remicade) with MTX for rheumatoid
　　arthritis, 2343
Influenza
　manifestations/management of, 1838-1839
　vaccination against, 427-428, 1746
　　in health care workers, 429-430
　　recommendations for, 427t
Influenza A, agent, infection site, reservoir,
　　transmission of, 420t
Informed consent
　in emergency departments, 2482
　for genetic testing, 328b
　by surgical client, 280-282, 281f
　for transfusion, 2279
Infusion devices, intravenous, client education
　　about, 280
Ingestive disorders, 717-742. *See also* Digestive
　　disorders
　dental disorders, 717-718
　of esophagus, 726-740
　nursing outcomes classification for, 718
　oral, 718-725
　　candidiasis, 720-721
　　stomatitis, 718-720
　　tumors, 721-725
　of salivary glands, 725-726
　vascular, 740
Inguinal canal, physical exam of, 1010
Inguinal hernia, 838-841
　assessing for, 779
　direct, 840

Inguinal hernia (*Continued*)
　etiology/risk factors, 839
　indirect, 840
　medical management of, 840
　nursing management of, 841
　pathophysiology of, 839-840
　surgical management of, 841
Inhalant abuse, health consequences of, 550t-551t
Inhalant withdrawal, symptoms of, 544t
Inhalants, 548
　effects of, 541t
Inhalation anesthesia, 287
　action, side effects, nursing implications, 288t
Inhalation injuries, 1434
　pulmonary effects of, 1437
Inhalations
　flow-triggered, 1885
　negative pressure, 1885
　time-triggered, 1885
　volume-triggered, 1885
Inhalers
　instructions for, 1816
　metered-dose, 1746
Inheritance. *See also* Genetic conditions; Genetic
　　factors
　autosomal dominant, 321-322
　autosomal recessive, 320-321
　mendelian, 320
　multifactorial, 323-325
　X-linked, 322-323, 323f
Initial Pain Assessment Tool, 454, 456f
Injuries. *See also* Trauma
　aging and, 19
　alcohol-related, 37
　history questions related to, 2487b
　laryngeal, manifestations/management of, 1803
　to nervous system, 2012-2013
　preventing, 36-37
　　in prostatectomy, 1031
　　during seizures, 2077
　　in surgical client, 294-295
　pulmonary response to, 1741-1742
　remobilization after, 654-655
　risk for, 77
　　in acute hypothyroidism, 1197-1198
　　in Addisonian crisis, 1220
　　from adrenalectomy, 1234
　　after adrenalectomy, 1226-1227
　　after axillary node dissection, 1108
　　after hip arthroplasty, 590
　　after nephrectomy, 924
　　after spinal cord injury, 2229-2230, 2232
　　after stroke, 2128
　　in altered states of consciousness, 2499
　　in Alzheimer's disease, 2168
　　in bladder cancer client, 871
　　from chemotherapy, 368
　　with chest tubes, 730
　　from cholecystectomy, 1309-1310
　　in comatose patient, 2064
　　with colostomy, 836
　　in confusional disorders, 2068
　　in Cushing's syndrome, 1226
　　from endourologic procedures, 889-890
　　in esophageal cancer surgery, 739-740
　　with gallstones, 1306
　　from gastric surgery, 760
　　in heart failure, 1661-1662
　　in hemodialysis, 967
　　in hepatic disorders, 1340-1341
　　in hepatic encephalopathy, 1358
　　in hyperparathyroidism, 1211, 1213
　　in hyperthryoidism, 1202
　　hypokalemia and, 234
　　in hypoparathyroidism, 1215
　　in pheochromocytoma surgery, 1232-1233

Injuries (*Continued*)
　　from prostate surgery, 1024-1025
　　from stoma formation, 825
　　from thyroidectomy, 1203, 1205
Innovar. *See* Fentanyl citrate-droperidol
　　(Innovar)
Inotropic agents
　assessing response to, 1660t
　for heart failure, 1657-1658
Inotropic state, function of, 1649t
Inpatient Rehabilitation Facility-Patient
　　Assessment Instrument, 191
Insect sting allergy, manifestations/management of,
　　2324-2325
Insect venom, anaphylaxis due to, 2325t
Insight, assessing, 74-75, 2026
Insomnia, 510-511
　interventions for, 511
　psychophysiologic, 510
Inspection, 80, 83
Inspiration
　muscles of, 1737-1738
　normal, 1736f
Inspiratory capacity, defined, 1735, 1762t
Inspiratory pressure, maximal, defined, 1762t
Inspiratory reserve volume, 1735, 1735f
　defined, 1762t
Inspiratory-to-expiratory ratio, assessing, 1748,
　　1751f
Institute of Medicine
　dietary recommendations of, 30t
　studies of, 181
Instruments, 82f, 83
　preparation of, 86
Insulin
　administration of
　　by client, 1261-1262
　　in diabetic ketoacidosis, 1271-1272
　　instructions for, 1262-1265
　in chronic renal failure, 954
　function of, 1149, 1150
　hormones counteracting, 1244
　needle-free technology for, 1265
　prefilled syringes for, 1264
　preparation and injection of, 1264
　for preventing hypoglycemia, 1253
　renal metabolism of, 914
　role in growth, 1149
　secretion of, 1146
　self-injection of, 1263-1265, 1264f
　sick day management of, in diabetes, 1286
　storage of, 1263-1264
　syringes for injecting, 1263, 1263f
Insulin pumps, 1255-1256, 1256f
Insulin resistance, 1247
　insulin secretion and, 1247f
　type 2 diabetes and, 1280
Insulin shock, 1262
Insulin therapy, 1253-1257
　in chronic pancreatitis, 1298
　combination, 1256-1257
　dosage of, 1255, 1255f
　for HHNS, 1273
　intensive, 1256-1257
　overdose of, 1273
　for preventing hypoglycemia, 1275
　with pumps, 1255-1256, 1256f
　rapid-acting, 1254-1255, 1254t
　sources of, 1253-1255
　types of, 1254t
Insulin-like growth factors, 1144
Insulin:proinsulin ratio, 1247
Insurance. *See* Health insurance
Intake and output, measurement of, fluid loss and,
　　207-208
Intal. *See* Cromolyn (Nasalcrom, Intal)

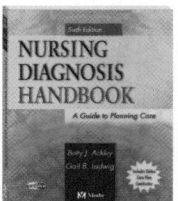
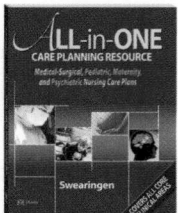
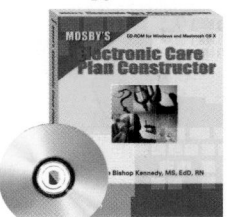
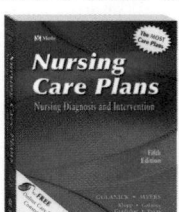
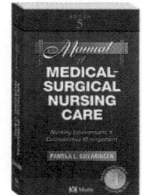
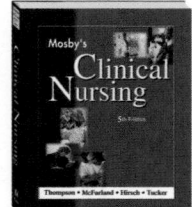
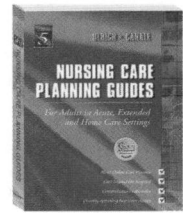
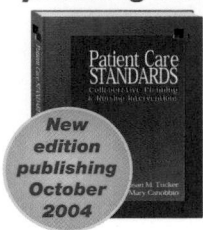

SPECIAL FEATURES—cont'd

Health & Physical
Assessment

Health & Physical Assessment

VIOLET H. BARKAUSKAS,
PhD, RN, CNM, FAAN
Associate Professor
Associate Dean for Administration
School of Nursing
The University of Michigan
Ann Arbor, Michigan

KATHRYN STOLTENBERG-ALLEN,
MSN, RN
Formerly Assistant Professor
Department of Public Health Nursing
College Nursing
University of Illinois at the Medical Center
Chicago, Illinois

LINDA CIOFU BAUMANN,
PhD, RN
Associate Professor
School of Nursing
University of Wisconsin—Madison
Madison, Wisconsin

CYNTHIA DARLING-FISHER,
PhD, RN
Assistant Professor
School of Nursing
The University of Michigan
Ann Arbor, Michigan

with 900 illustrations

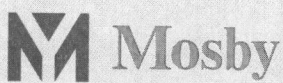

St. Louis Baltimore Boston Chicago London Madrid Philadelphia Sydney Toronto

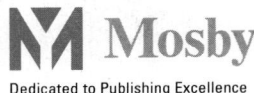

Mosby

Dedicated to Publishing Excellence

Editor: Sally Schrefer
Developmental Editor: Janet Livingston
Project Manager: Karen Edwards
Production Editor: Richard Barber
Designer: Elizabeth Fett
Manufacturing Supervisor: Betty Richmond

Printed in the United States of America
Composition by Graphic World, Inc.
Printing/binding by Von Hoffmann Press, Inc.

Mosby−Year Book, Inc.
11830 Westline Industrial Drive
St. Louis, Missouri 63146

International Standard Book Number 0-8016-7663-0

94 95 96 97 98 / 9 8 7 6 5 4 3 2 1

Beverly A. Priefer, PhD, RN
Geriatrics Research, Education, and Clinical Center
William S. Middleton Memorial Veterans Hospital;
Assistant Clinical Professor
School of Nursing
University of Wisconsin-Madison
Madison, Wisconsin
Chapter 25: Aging Clients

Donna R. Seibels, MS, RD
Adjunct Professor
Department of Family and Consumer Education
Samford University
Birmingham, Alabama
Chapter 4: Nutritional Assessment

Michele Soest, MSN, RN
Director of Health Technologies
BiLevel Nursing Program
Jefferson College
Hillsboro, Missouri
*Chapters 3-5, 8-26: Clinical Applications in Nursing
   Diagnosis—The Next Step*

Debbie Gemoules Wolf, BSN, RN
Coronary Care Unit
St. Louis University Medical Center
St. Louis, Missouri
*Chapters 3-5, 8-26: Defining Characteristics and Related
   Factors in Nursing Diagnosis—The Next Step*

REVIEWERS

Cheryl Anderson, PhD, RN
Department of Obstetrics
University of Texas at Arlington
Arlington, Texas

Eileen K. Baldwin, MSN, RN
Allentown College of St. Francis de Sales
Department of Nursing
Center Valley, Pennsylvania

Donna H. Bedsole, EdD, RN
Troy State University
School of Nursing
Montgomery, Alabama

Charlotte Breithaupt, MN, RN
School of Nursing
Baylor University
Dallas, Texas

Mary Ann Broda, PhD, RN, CPNP
Assistant Professor, Parent-Child Nursing
University of Michigan
Ann Arbor, Michigan

Pamela S. Brown, MS, RN
Blessing-Rieman College of Nursing
Quincy, Illinois

Brenda Leigh Cameron, MScN, RN
Assistant Professor
Faculty of Nursing
University of Alberta
Edmonton, Alberta

Linda S. Dillion, MS, RN
Baylor University School of Nursing
Dallas, Texas

Marty Downey, BSN, RN, CCRN
Boise, Idaho

Linda A. Eastham, MSN, RN, FNP
Charlottesville, Virginia

Helen Hansen, MS, RN
Instructor
College of Nursing
University of Tulsa
Tulsa, Oklahoma

Janice Hausauer, MS, RN, CCRN
Adjunct Assistant Professor
Department of Nursing
Montana State University
Bozeman, Montana

Anne Hummer, PhD, RN
University of Detroit
Detroit, Michigan

Mary C. Kavoosi, PhD, RN
Clarion University
Oil City, Pennsylvania

Nancy Lospinoso, MS, RN, ONC
Orange, New Jersey

Meredith A. McCord, MS, RN
Assistant Professor
Adult Health and Illness Nursing
Oregon Health Sciences University
Portland, Oregon

Graham McDougall, PhD, RN, CS
Assistant Professor
Gerontological Nursing
Frances Payne Bolton School of Nursing
Case Western Reserve University
Cleveland, Ohio

Joan C. Murphy, MS, RN
Director, College of Nursing
Utica College
Utica, New York

Yvonne G. Newberry, MSN, RN, FNP
Department of Obstetrics and Gynecology
University of Virginia Health Sciences Center;
Clinical Faculty, School of Nursing
University of Virginia
Charlottesville, Virginia;
Clinical Faculty
Medical College of Virginia-Virginia Commonwealth
  University
Richmond, Virginia

Marybeth Paradowski, MPH, MSN, RN
Assistant Professor, Nursing
Allentown College of St. Francis de Sales
Center Valley, Pennsylvania

Charlene Pope, MPH, RN, CNM
Clinical Associate Faculty
Women's Health Care/School of Nursing
University of Rochester
Rochester, New York

Patricia K. Reed, MA, RN, CNAA
Albany Medical Center
Project Learn
Albany, New York

Susan D. Schaffer, MS, RN, CFNP
Assistant Professor of Nursing
Old Dominion University
Norfolk, Virginia

Anita Singleton, MSN, EdS, RN
Assistant Professor
Missouri Southern State College
School of Nursing
Joplin, Missouri

Elaine Steinke, PhD, RN
Wichita State University
Department of Nursing
Wichita, Kansas

Health and Physical Assessment reflects recent changes in the practice of health assessment by nurses, including assessment in relationship to nursing diagnoses. This new textbook represents our beliefs in holistic health assessment as the basis for nursing intervention and practice. Health assessment is presented as the systematic collection of data that health professionals can use to make decisions about how they will intervene to promote, maintain, or restore health. Our goal for this new text is to provide an innovative product that reflects and anticipates the ways in which nursing practice and health care are changing.

Health and Physical Assessment is designed for students and beginning practitioners. It contains the theory and skills necessary to collect a comprehensive health history and to perform a complete physical examination. These skills can be most effectively mastered when the text is used within a structured learning environment, which includes supervised student practice in skills laboratories or clinical settings. Because *Health and Physical Assessment* contains a great deal of substantive detail on examination techniques and findings, the student is not expected to outgrow the text but to continue to use it as a valuable reference in clinical practice.

Throughout this text, the consumer of health care is referred to as the *client* because the term implies the ability of a person, whether well or sick, to contract for health care as a responsible participant, along with the providers, in the health-care process. Health care providers cannot expect consumers to accept assessment or intervention unless they have been actively included in the process.

ORGANIZATION

The content in *Health and Physical Assessment* is organized in five units. Unit One, *Taking the Health History*, consists of thorough discussions of the art and science of effectively taking and recording a comprehensive health history for purposes of health or illness assessment and management. Unit Two, *Holistic Assessment*, assists the reader to understand and assess a client holistically with chapters on developmental, nutritional, and sleep assessment and cultural considerations in health assessment.

Unit Three, *Physical Assessment*, follows the traditional body-system approach and contains detailed, richly illustrated discussions of the physical examination of body systems or regions. The chapters in Unit Three are consistently organized and include the following headings and content:

Anatomy and Physiology
Health History
Preparation for the Examination: Client and Environment
Technique for Examination and Normal Findings
Variations from Health

Although this book focuses on the general care of the healthy adult client, no comprehensive text on health assessment can ignore the special assessment techniques required by clients of other age groups and with special health needs. Thus, Unit Four, *Assessing Special Populations*, includes chapters that present assessment techniques unique to pregnant women, children, older adults, and individuals with functional limitations. These client groups are frequently served by nurse practitioners.

Unit Five, *The Complete Health and Physical Assessment*, assists the reader to bring together all physical assessment components into a logical system for performing the comprehensive physical examination. The concluding chapter of the text assists the reader to make the linkages from health assessment to subsequent steps of the client care process—diagnosis, care planning, and implementation.

FEATURES

Color photographs of physical examination techniques are extensively used to enhance learning, and carefully crafted illustrations clarify significant aspects of the discussion, especially anatomy and physiology.

Other special features of *Health and Physical Assessment* include the following:

- **Helpful Hints** boxes provide tips for performing a thorough and accurate assessment.
- **Preparation for the Examination: Client and Environment** boxes quickly present needed equipment and special considerations for preparing the client and setting for an examination.
- **Examination Step-by-Step** outlines provide a quick overview of the physical examination discussed in a chapter.
- **Sample Documentation** boxes highlight the importance of documenting assessment findings

and can be used as models for students' own documentation in the clinical setting.

- **Teaching Self-Assessment** is included in all applicable chapters and provides information on health maintenance.
- **Nursing Diagnosis—The Next Step** boxes present critical-thinking content and demonstrate the progression from assessment to formulating nursing diagnoses.
- **Glossary** with every chapter provides definitions of key terms, which are discussed and in bold-face type when they first appear in the text.

ANCILLARIES

A copy of *Quick Reference to Cultural Assessment* is included with every copy of the text. This quick reference is a compilation of boxes and tables that the student will find useful. The information in the quick reference will enable the reader to become familiar with culturally influenced variables that should be taken into account during a health assessment.

An *Instructor's Manual and Test Bank to accompany Health and Physical Assessment* is available. The *Instructor's Manual* includes, for every chapter in the text, learning objectives, detailed lecture outlines, and learning activities. The *Test Bank* has approximately 700 questions with answers and cross references to the text page where the answer can be found.

ACKNOWLEDGMENTS

It is our pleasure to express gratitude to a number of individuals who helped us prepare this publication. Without their support and assistance it would not have been possible. The beautiful color photographs are the products of Don Price, Tim Ford, Joe Welch, and Lin Goings of BMC Photographics, University of Michigan. Illustrations were prepared by Holly Fischer and Valorie Loomis of Biomedical Communications, University of Michigan. Youngshook Han, of the University of Wisconsin-Madison, greatly facilitated the library research for Dr. Baumann. Jean Gittings, medical librarian at Trinity Medical Center in Rock Island/Moline, Illinois, helped Ms. Stoltenberg-Allen with computer searches.

The authors wish to especially acknowledge the guidance and mentoring of two very talented Mosby editors—Terry Van Schaik and Janet Livingston. Terry was especially skillful in negotiating the resources needed for this book. We appreciated her tenacity and her wisdom throughout its creation and missed her guidance when she was transferred to another Mosby division. Janet has been a positive mentor and an effective conscience, very skilled in keeping us focused, bringing out the best in us, and helping us solve the multitude of problems along the way. We thank them for making this hard work an enjoyable and rewarding experience.

Violet H. Barkauskas
Kathryn Stoltenberg-Allen
Linda Ciofu Baumann
Cynthia Darling-Fisher

. . .

DEDICATIONS

To family, friends, colleagues, and students who have extended their love, support, wisdom, encouragement, and perspective during our professional lives and during the development of this book, especially:

Sally Dymek and Sally Ann Dymek
V.H.B.

Lawrence, Laurel, Douglas, and Matthew Allen
James and Sadye Stoltenberg
John and Kathy Stoltenberg
Joan, Art, and Katy Kiehn
Carolyn Piatek, Jane Martin, Suzanne Auman, Melanie Landa,
Diane Otte, Sue Ickes,and Naomi Nelson
K. S-A.

Alice Simonds, mentor and teacher
L.C.B.

Daniel C., Cara, and Noah Fisher
Elaine C. and R. Clement Darling
Clem and Julie Darling
Wendy and Doug Nickerson
Elisabeth and Michael Botelho
C. D-F.

DETAILED CONTENTS

UNIT ONE
Taking the Health History

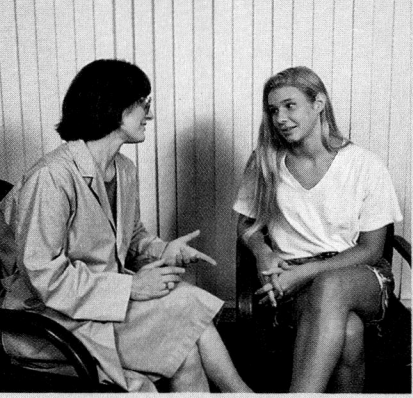

UNIT TWO
Holistic Assessment

UNIT THREE
Physical Assessment

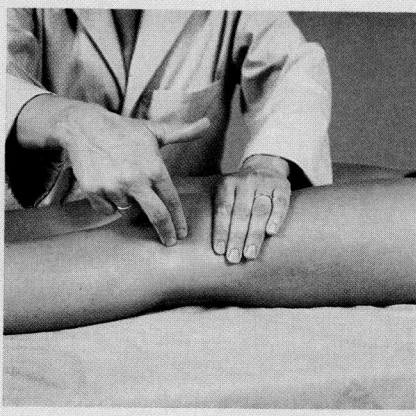

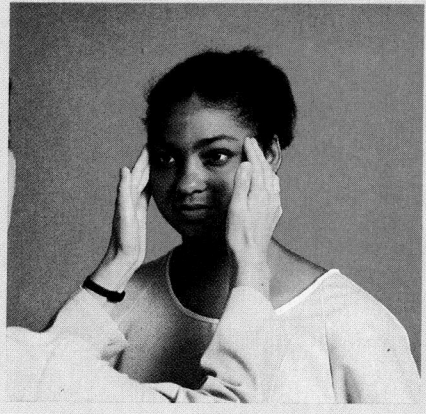

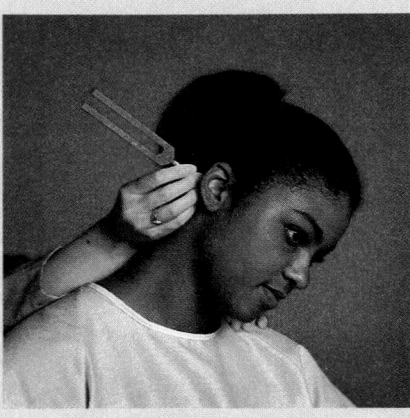

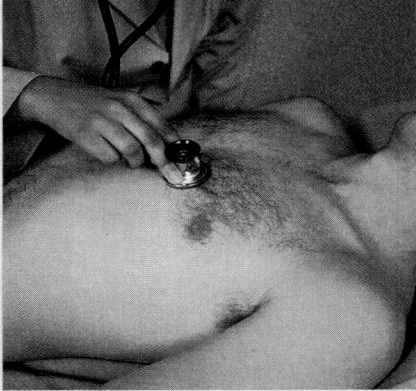

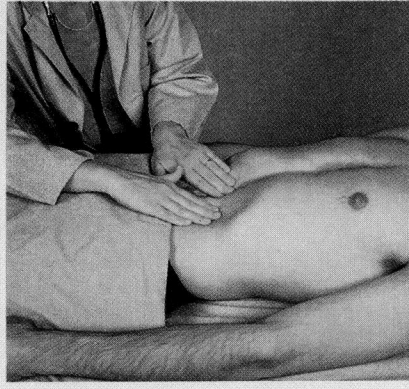

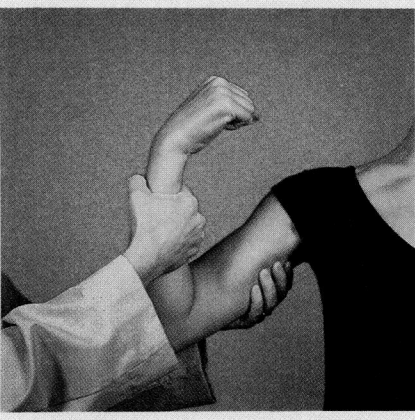

UNIT FOUR
Assessing Special Populations

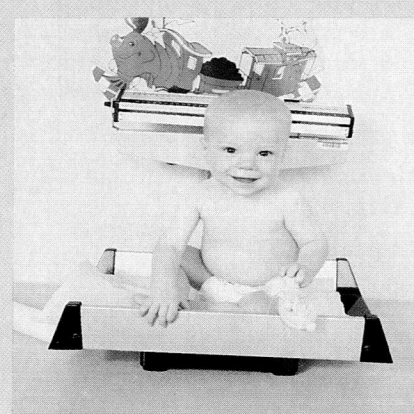

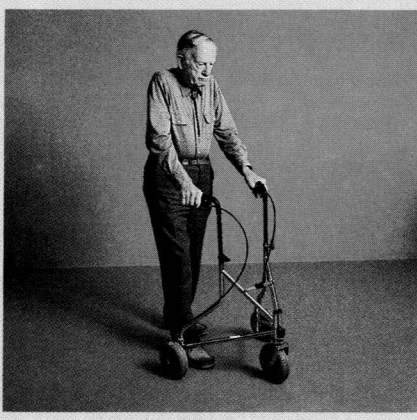

UNIT FIVE
The Complete Health and Physical Assessment

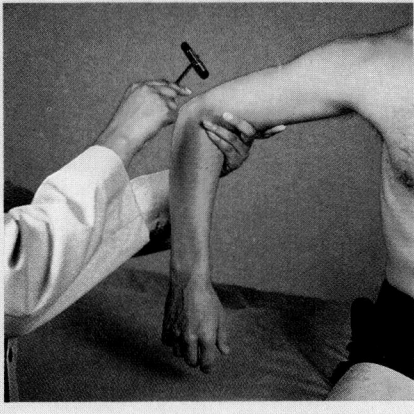
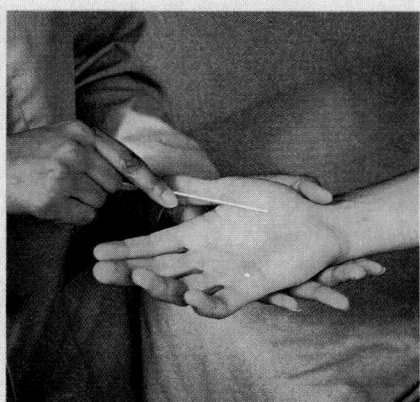

*U*nit I, Taking the Health
History, focuses on interviewing
skills for the health history and the
content of the health history.
Chapter 1, Interviewing Skills and
Techniques, is a discussion of the
interviewing skills needed to take a
health history. Chapter 2, The
Health History, provides the outline
for and content of the health history
for both well clients and clients with
health problems.

Taking the Health History

Outline

Interviewing Skills and Techniques

PURPOSE OF THE INTERVIEW

Developing Relationships

The major purpose of interviewing a client before performing the physical examination is to obtain a health history. Practitioners must be skillful in communication techniques to enable a client to fully share life experiences relevant to his or her health status. When the initial interview is problem-focused, the practitioner also asks about the signs and symptoms associated with the client's problems or concerns.

Beginning with introductions, the practitioner observes and analyzes the client's reactions to the interview. The examiner must establish a climate of trust to promote interaction necessary for a **therapeutic relationship,** or an interaction that maintains a focus on the client's needs. As a practitioner, you can create a climate of trust by the way you introduce yourself, how you conduct the interview, and the environment you arrange for the interview. To create a respectful and warm environment, introduce yourself, including your full name and your role in the agency, describe your

3

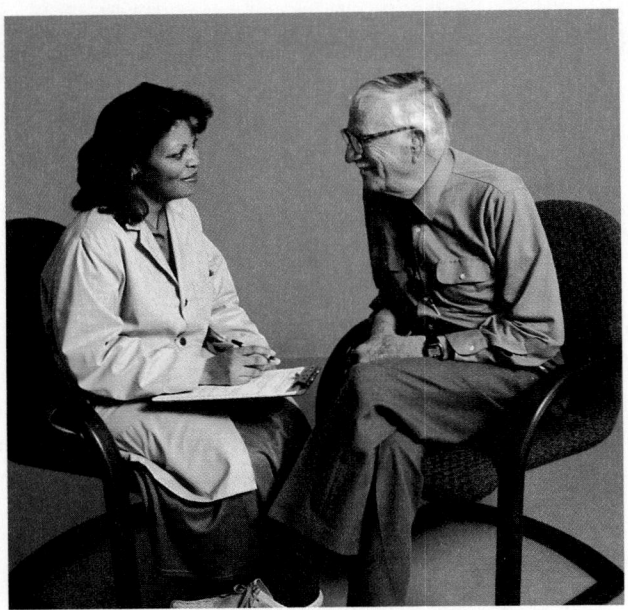

FIGURE 1-1 Establishing a climate that is comfortable and respectful to the client promotes communication.

understanding of the purpose of the interview, and address the client by his or her full name or surname (Figure 1-1).

Another way to promote trust and acknowledge the client as an active participant in the interview is to ask about the client's primary concerns and goals for the visit. Use communication skills that create a climate in which the client feels free to talk about his or her health condition. These strategies are necessary for obtaining the most reliable data about both the client's physical and mental status (see Chapter 19).

Contracting

The initial interview is the basis for establishing a client-provider contract. **Contracting** is an agreement between the provider and client that makes explicit the expectations of each party. For example, the provider might state that in order for the client to receive appropriate preventive care, the client will agree to make an appointment at least yearly. The client is then encouraged to respond to this. It is not necessary to label this a "contract," but it is important for the client and provider to agree on the plan and modify it as needed.

Sometimes contracts are written, but most often they are verbal agreements. Written contracts are often useful when using behavior modification techniques for dealing with behavior changes such as smoking cessation or medication taking.

Timing is important when the examiner introduces discussion of a contract. Allow enough time so that you and the client have exchanged introductions and you

have some awareness of the client's needs and purpose of the visit. However, it is important not to wait until the very end of the visit to discuss a plan of care or treatment. Adequate time should be available for negotiating any modifications to the course of action or plan based on the client's response.

Modifications in the Interview

The interview will be modified by the age of the client, the reason for the visit, and the existing relationship between you and the client. A young child will be accompanied by a parent or adult who will be the major source of information. It is important to remember that although the adult may be providing the verbal information, the child needs to feel included in the interview. Introduce yourself to the child, ask the child questions, and let the child touch equipment. Adults may also prefer to have a family member or significant other with them during a health visit. Confirm with the client that he or she chooses to have another person present and acknowledge the presence and concerns of the family member or significant other (Figure 1-2).

On the first visit with a client who is being seen for a general health assessment, allocate a considerable amount of time for the interview and history. This allows you to obtain baseline data and develop a relationship with the client. When you see a client who has an acute problem, less time is focused on past history and greater emphasis is placed on understanding the immediate problem. An established practitioner who has known a client and/or the family members over many years may be quite familiar with many aspects of the client's health status and may need a shorter amount of time for a visit. However, a provider in this situation will need to periodically and systematically update history information.

Guide for Focusing the Physical Examination

Always ask for basic information such as the client's reason for seeking care, his or her current health status, information about allergies, medications taken, and levels of stress and support available to cope with health concerns (see Chapter 2). The focus and types of questions you ask will vary according to the client's presenting problem or concerns. Chapters 9 through 26 include history questions related to a specific body system or to the health concerns of special populations (such as children, the elderly, and the functionally limited).

From information obtained in the history you will determine what to explore in more depth during the physical examination. For example, if a client's major reason for a visit is a cough, nasal congestion, and fullness in the head, focus on examining the head, eyes,

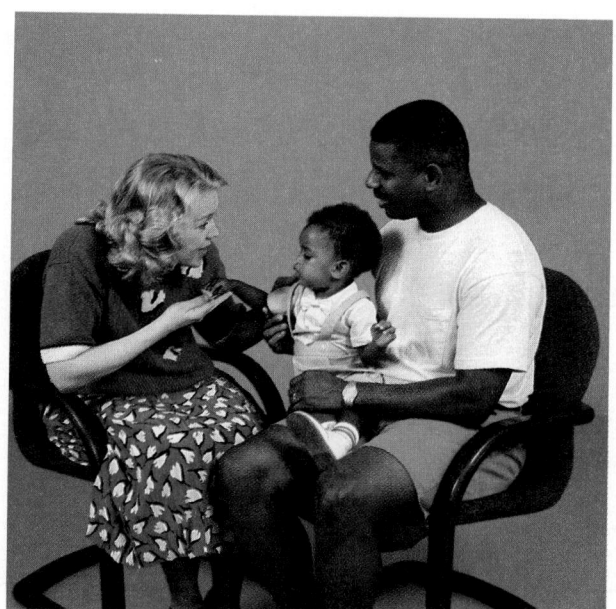

FIGURE 1-2 The practitioner modifies the interview by the client's age and the presence of other family members.

ears, nose, and throat (HEENT) as well as the lungs. A neurological or musculoskeletal examination, for example, may not be necessary during that visit.

> **Helpful Hint:** *A self-administered history form helps the practitioner to focus the interview and can save time. (See Figure 1-3.)*

Therapeutic Use of Self

Therapeutic use of self is a term that describes how certain personal qualities of the interviewer can be used to support the client's perspective or feelings. For example, an interviewer might say, "As a woman I have also experienced . . ." or "As a mother I can understand how difficult this can be . . ." This technique can be especially helpful when the client's background, such as ethnicity, race, or socioeconomic status, appears to be very different from the examiner's background. It helps to find a common connection that can facilitate communication.

CONDUCTING THE INTERVIEW

Health History

Begin by finding out the client's **chief complaint** or major reason for seeking care. It is also important to find out why the client came at this point in time. It

may be that it was simply a convenient time or an acute problem started to get worse and the client felt the need for treatment. Other underlying concerns related to a chief complaint may exist. An individual may have had a "blue-black" mole for a number of years and now wants it evaluated "immediately." By asking what triggered the visit now, you may find that a friend or relative recently died of malignant melanoma and the client is now concerned about having cancer. Because you are aware of the concern, you can provide the appropriate evaluation and also reassure (if appropriate) the client and educate him or her about the warning signs of melanoma.

A client may also have a specific agenda that is not obvious from the stated reason for a visit. By asking a question such as "How did you hope I could help you today?" toward the end of the visit, you can identify the client's underlying concerns as well as address the health issues obvious to a clinician (Molde, 1986).

You may also obtain data from secondary sources such as parents, guardians, family members, significant others, written records, and interpreters. The use of interpreters will be discussed in more detail later in this chapter under "Cultural Variation."

Client explanatory models. You can ask the client a series of questions to uncover his or her explanatory model (Kleinman, Eisenberg, and Good, 1978). Answers to these questions provide a meaningful explanation of the events surrounding an illness and suggest the appropriate course of action. These questions also help to uncover the client's level of understanding about a health problem. These questions include:
What do you think caused your problem?
Why do you think it started when it did?
What do you think your illness does to you?
What are the symptoms?
How long do you think it will last?
Based on information you obtain, you can develop a plan that will be sensitive to the client's needs and level of understanding.

Dimensions of a symptom. Symptoms are the perceived change in body sensations or functions. During an interview, obtain a thorough understanding of the dimensions of a symptom. This understanding will help guide the focus of the physical examination. Seven criteria can be used to describe a symptom: location, quality, quantity, timing, setting in which it occurs, aggravating or alleviating factors, and associated symptoms.

Dimensions of a symptom	Questions to ask
1. Location	"Where do you feel it? Does it move around? Does it radiate? Show me where it hurts."

I.D. #: _____

NAME: _____

PHONE: _____

GYNECOLOGY CLINIC
Confidential To be completed by patient

ELIGIBILITY: E   P   F   O   M   C
                                    O

DATE: _____

Reason for Visit

First Day of Last
Menstrual Period

Drug Allergies

Present Medications

REPRODUCTIVE HISTORY: Age at 1st period _____   Date of Last Pap _____

Number of: Live births _____   Pregnancies _____   Abortions _____   Miscarriages _____

Have you ever had: Breast _____   Uterus/Tube _____   Sexually _____   Abnormal Pap _____
                     Abnormality   Infection   Transmitted
                                                                Disease

Other OB/Gyn Problems: _____

Did your mother take DES (a hormone) while pregnant with you?   ❑ Yes   ❑ No   ❑ Unsure

Do you have: **Flow:** ❑ excessively heavy   ❑ missed periods
                          ❑ excessively light

❑ painful periods
❑ spotting between periods
❑ unusual discharge/infection
❑ sexual concerns

Are you sexually active?   ❑ Yes   ❑ No

Current contraception? (Specify) _____

List any problems you are experiencing: _____

FAMILY HISTORY:

Have any members of your immediate family i.e., Grandparent(s) Parent(s) Sibling(s) ever had

❑ high blood pressure   ❑ heart attack or stroke
❑ diabetes   ❑ cancer, type _____

MEDICAL HISTORY: please check any condition(s) that applies to you

❑ heart disease   ❑ anemia   ❑ gallbladder disease   ❑ kidney or bladder infections
❑ high blood pressure   ❑ asthma   ❑ cancer   ❑ thyroid disease
❑ migraine headaches   ❑ epilepsy   ❑ high cholesterol   ❑ liver disease/jaundice
❑ blood clots (leg or lungs) ❑ diabetes   ❑ sickle cell disease   ❑ surgery, type _____
❑ eating disorder   ❑ depression   ❑ other _____

HEALTH BEHAVIORS: (Please refer to pamphlet (p) or video (v) for more information)

Do you: **(Please check all that apply to you)**

❑ smoke (p)   ❑ eat a well balanced diet (p)
❑ have a weight problem (p)   ❑ exercise regularly (p)
❑ have a history of alcohol or other drug use (p) ❑ perform monthly self breast examinations (p) (v)
❑ more than 2 sexual partners in the past six months (p) (v)   ❑ have Rubella immunization (p)

FIGURE 1-3 Self-administered history form.

Dimensions of a symptom	Questions to ask
2. Quality or character	"What does it feel like?"
3. Quantity or severity	"On a scale of 1 to 10, with 10 being the worst pain you could have, how would you rate the discomfort you have now?"
	"How does this interfere with your usual activities?"
	"How bad is it?"
4. Timing	"When did you first notice it? How long does it last? How often does it happen?"
5. Setting	"Does this occur in a particular place or under certain circumstances? Is it associated with any specific activity?"
6. Aggravating or alleviating factors	"What makes it better? What makes it worse?"
7. Associated symptoms	"Have you noticed other changes that occur with this symptom?"

Preparation for the Interview: Client and the Environment

A comfortable, private, and quiet environment is essential for conducting an interview. Meet the client before he or she has undressed for the physical examination. In some clinics, clients are asked to undress before they meet the clinician. If you are in such a situation, try to at least introduce yourself before the client undresses. Address the client using his or her full name or surname. Identify yourself using your full name and title. This greeting respectfully acknowledges the client and conveys your personal accountability as part of the health care team.

You and the client should both be comfortably seated during the interview. To put the client at ease, directly state that the information you obtain will be confidential, recorded in the medical record, and shared only with those individuals directly involved in the care and treatment plan.

During the interview you will need to take some notes regarding dates, events, or short phrases related to specific aspects of the history. It is not desirable to complete the final report during the interview because it will likely divert attention from the client. You will need to practice to determine what relevant information you must document during the interview and what data can be later written or dictated into the permanent record. History forms that are partially completed by the client before the interview and flow sheets are useful devices for facilitating documentation of history information (see Figure 1-3).

Preparation for the Interview

Equipment

Item	Purpose
Pencil and paper	To write brief notes during the interview
Health record/referral information	To refer to for validating events

Techniques for Conducting the Interview

Start with the concerns the client stated in the chief complaint. Be aware of the pace of your questions and the tone of your voice. You do not want to appear rushed or abrupt.

Types of questions

Open-ended questions. Open the interview with a broad opening statement such as "Tell me about your problem." You can prompt the client to explain details using minimal verbal activity. For example, you might say "You feel . . . . ?"

The aim of an open-ended question is to elicit a response that is more than one or two words. A client will answer this type of question by describing signs or symptoms in his or her own words and at his or her own pace. Examples of open-ended questions are "Can you tell me a little about yourself?" or "How have you been feeling since your last visit?" A risk of asking an open-ended question is when a client is unable to focus on the topic being asked or takes an excessive amount of time to tell his or her story. In cases like these, you will need to focus the interview.

Closed-ended questions. A closed-ended question requires a response of one or two words such as "yes" or "no," or briefly stating marital status, age, or a list of medications one may be taking. An examiner asks closed-ended questions when specific information is required, such as age, presence of a specific health risk such as smoking, or when the client has a limited ability to respond. The client might be limited in his or her responses by anxiety, lack of verbal skill, or physical discomfort. If a practitioner is rushed, he or she may ask more closed-ended questions to speed up the process of obtaining a history of the problem. A word of caution: Failure to allow clients to express in their own words the nature of their problem may lead to inaccurate conclusions and in the long run will waste time.

Directive questions. Directive questions lead the client to focus on one set of thoughts. This type of question is most often used in reviewing systems or in evaluating functional status. Allow the client time for **reflection**, at least 5 to 10 seconds, before answering or before you ask the next question. For example, you might ask "Have you experienced any problems with urination in the past, such as infections or unusual frequency, urgency, or difficulty urinating?"

Permission-giving questions. Frequently you will need to ask clients questions about sensitive areas or concerns. One way to deal with such questions is to ask clients in a way that lets them know that it is alright to speak of such things to you. For example, you might tell a male client, "Many young men I see have questions or concerns about sexually transmitted diseases; what questions do you have?"

Use of silence. Periods of silence during the interview can be helpful for both you and the client. Short periods of silence allow the client to organize his or her thoughts. During silent periods, you can observe the client's emotional state and note nonverbal cues. Silence may also indicate that either you or the client may need time to reflect upon what was just said.

Validating information from the interview

Clarification. Use clarification to obtain more information about conflicting, vague, or ambiguous statements. By asking the client to elaborate, or clarify, on the thoughts and feelings he or she has expressed, you will communicate understanding. An example of clarification is "You say you feel depressed. Tell me what you mean."

Restatement. Restatement involves repeating what the client has said using different words. It is a way to acknowledge that you are listening to the client and to validate your interpretation of what the client has said. An example is "I'd like to review the timing of your symptoms with you. You said that first you experienced a headache; then nausea and vomiting followed an hour later. Is that correct?"

Reflection. **Reflection** is repeating a phrase or sentence the client just said. This suggests to the client that you are still interested in the topic being discussed and you would like further elaboration on the facts or feelings involved. An example of reflection follows:
Client: I love my children but sometimes they are so misbehaved that I am afraid I'll hurt them.
Interviewer: You are afraid you might hurt them?
Use reflection to describe nonverbal behavior and ask the client what it means. For example, "I notice that you haven't taken your sunglasses off. Is there a reason?" Verbalizing that you perceive what the client feels communicates empathy. For example, "I see you

have tears in your eyes. You must feel quite sad about this."

Confrontation. In confrontation, you make the client aware that what you observe is not consistent with what he or she said. An example: "You are telling me how depressed you feel but I notice you are smiling a lot." Another example: "You said you were so sick this morning you stayed home from work, yet you show no distress now. Can you help me understand what is going on?"

Interpretation. During **interpretation**, you share with the client the conclusion you have drawn from the information you obtained in the interview. Sharing your interpretation or the meaning of the facts provides the client with an opportunity to confirm, deny, or offer an alternative interpretation to the facts.

Summary. Summary is a technique that orders and condenses the information obtained during an interview to help clarify the situation being discussed. This is particularly useful when you obtain information from a client who rambles and has difficulty conveying the sequence of events.

When you terminate the interview, it may be helpful to summarize the information you obtained to highlight the main areas discussed. A summary also allows the client to assess whether information pertinent to his or her health problem was completely obtained and can help demonstrate to both the client and examiner what was accomplished during the interview.

Focusing/refocusing. Focusing or refocusing involves guiding the direction of the interview. During focusing or refocusing, you will attempt to help the client expand on a particular topic of concern. It is particularly useful if the client comes in for an acute complaint but has multiple health problems. It is also useful if the client begins to ramble or tries to avoid a particular topic. When attempting to focus the interview, acknowledge the value of the information being given but redirect the discussion to the problem at hand. An example is: "I would like to hear about your past history shortly; for the moment I need more information about your headaches."

Nonverbal communication

Body posture. **Body language** is the conveyance of messages by movements or gestures of the body or limbs, facial expressions, and eye contact. Body posture may convey anxiety, boredom, attention, or indifference. Both the examiner and the client communicate nonverbally. In a closed-body posture one holds limbs in a defensive position, close to the body as though hugging oneself. This often conveys mistrust or anxiety. An open-body posture is one that is more relaxed with arms extended or hanging loosely at sides. An examiner who remains standing during an interview conveys a message of time urgency. An examiner who is seated comfortably during the interview conveys to the client that they will take some time to conduct the interview.

Facial expressions such as frowns or smiles may represent an effort to avoid saying something unpleasant. These expressions are also indicators of emotional states such as anxiety, fear, surprise, or joy.

> **Helpful Hint:** *Appropriate nonverbal behavior is subject to considerable cultural variation. In the United States dominant culture, it is important to look directly at the person with whom you are speaking. In other cultures (Asian, Native American, Indochinese, Arab, Appalachian), looking directly at another person may be a sign of disrespect or aggression. In many cultures it is not acceptable for a younger person or woman to have direct eye contact with a male. In many Asian cultures it is considered inappropriate to express openly pain or sadness to a stranger.*

Eye contact. Use eye contact and eye movement to engage or remove oneself from a situation. You may convey the message that the interview is over by looking at a watch or clock. A client who looks around the room while answering questions or talking and avoids eye contact with an examiner may have anxiety about the situation being discussed. Prolonged direct gaze into an examiner's eyes or an excess or absence of blinking might be cues to the client's mental status.

Mirroring activity. **Mirroring** involves awareness of nonverbal aspects of the client's communication to you, such as speed and volume of speech and body position. Imitate or mirror these characteristics in an unobtrusive way. For example, if a client is sitting forward with her arms folded across her chest, you can also fold your arms across your chest and lean forward in the client's direction. This is an action that individuals who are engrossed in a conversation frequently do without thinking. Mirroring has been shown to increase the client's comfort level and sense of rapport. It is also a nonverbal way to evaluate how comfortable the client is with the discussion. If in the course of the interview, the client suddenly changes from an open-body posture that had been similar to your own posture to a closed-body posture, the discussion may have raised a sensitive topic or the client may have lost interest in the discussion.

Interpersonal distance. **Interpersonal distance** is the distance between two individuals interacting. This may vary by the nature of the relationship or cultural practices. The distance most acceptable in the United States dominant culture is to be close enough to be able to extend one's arm to shake hands, to hear a moderate to low volume voice, and to clearly observe the client. Trust is best developed from this distance.

Cultural variation. If you work with a particular cultural group, it is necessary to obtain some understanding of the group's health beliefs and practices as well as some language skills to facilitate communication. The use of interpreters may be critical. A useful guide for overcoming barriers in cross-cultural communication is the LEARN model (Berlin and Fowkes, 1983).

L Listen with sympathy and understanding to the client's perception of the problem
E Explain your perceptions of the problem
A Acknowledge and discuss the differences and similarities
R Recommend a course of action
N Negotiate an agreement

Given current projections about the number of cultural groups who will receive health care in the United States in the next 50 years, it is unrealistic to assume that health providers can have in-depth knowledge of the health practices and beliefs of multiple cultural groups. In addition, it is unwise to assume that because a client is a member of a particular cultural or ethnic group, he or she holds a certain belief. Beliefs *within* one cultural or ethnic group vary as much as they do among different groups.

Therefore, the process of uncovering health care beliefs in each client is an essential skill for any health provider. Questions to elicit a client's explanatory model of an illness (Kleinman, and others, 1978) is one approach to gathering this information.

Listening. Listening is probably the most effective communication technique available. **Active listening** is concentrating on what the client is saying so that subtle cues may be detected. Active listening gives the client the nonverbal message that he or she is "a person of worth" whose opinions, ideas, and concerns are valued. Active listening involves blocking out environmental noise and distractions as well as intrusive thoughts you may have about what to do next.

Providing support

Acceptance. Never discount what the person says. **Acceptance** is recognition of what is said without necessarily agreeing. An example is: "You say you fear this pain could mean that you have cancer."

GUIDELINES FOR THE USE OF INTERPRETERS

1. Unless you are fluent in the client's language, use an interpreter.
2. Allow extra time when using an interpreter. The interview becomes a discussion among people.
3. Avoid using family members as interpreters. They may respond to your questions based on their own knowledge without asking the client.
4. Make sure the interpreter has a basic understanding of medical terminology. Become familiar with the meaning of special words or phrases that connote practices or traditions of a particular cultural group.
5. Make sure the interpreter understands the confidential nature of the information obtained in the interview.
6. Direct questions to the client. The client may then direct responses to you directly or to the interpreter.
7. Some cultures are unfamiliar with direct questions. If necessary, adjust the type and tone of your questions to a style that is more conversational. Use short questions with minimal jargon.
8. Validate information you heard using repetition; summarize what you heard at the end of the interview.
9. Instructions to the client may need to be in writing in the client's language to ensure clear understanding.
10. Get feedback from the interpreter about the client's emotional state and comprehension.

Touch. The art of touching is one of the most intimate forms of nonverbal communication. It precedes speech in every person's life. Cultural traditions prescribe the ritual of touch or define the taboos. For example, in North American middle-class culture, touch (when used by health care providers) conveys a message of closeness, encouragement, and caring. A warm handshake can be a familiar comfort to a client who is concerned about a health problem and who is fearful of unfamiliar surroundings. Clients may also express appreciation and trust in the health provider by hugging or initiating touch. Other cultural groups see touch as an invasion of privacy.

Many Asian cultures believe that the head is the most sacred part of the body. The clinician should therefore obtain permission before touching an Asian client's head. Many Asians believe that feet are the lowest part of the body, and it is therefore disrespectful to show the bottom of your shoe to the client or point your toe at him or her.

Openness to more information. It is important not to appear too rushed or impatient because the client may hesitate to share concerns that could be crucial to identifying and treating a problem. Before concluding an interview ask, "Do you have any additional concerns you want to discuss?" This question encourages a client to bring up important issues, which may save a great deal of time in the long run.

COMMON ERRORS IN INTERVIEWING

Giving Advice

By giving advice or telling clients what to do, you communicate that they may not be capable of handling the problem. You also accept responsibility for the outcomes. A health provider should provide sufficient information about risks, side effects, and benefits of available treatment and management options so clients can decide what is right for themselves.

Changing the Subject

Changing the subject introduces a new topic inappropriately. A client may be expressing concern about the discomfort of the examination and the practitioner asks what medication he is taking. Practitioners may do this unintentionally when feeling, for example, both pressured for time and anxious about ensuring that they obtain specific information.

Social Versus Therapeutic Response

A social response focuses attention on the practitioner instead of the client. An example is a client stating that she just returned from a trip to South America and the practitioner responds by talking about her own vacation. The sharing of this story by the practitioner becomes the focus of the interchange. This exchange would be a therapeutic response by focusing on the client. An example is after the client states that she just returned from a trip to South America the practitioner responds with "Tell me about your trip."

False Reassurance

In an attempt to reassure the client, statements may be made that are not true such as "it will be all right," "you'll be just fine," "you'll get over it."

Overloading or Underloading Client with Questions

Overloading is continuing to ask a client questions before he has a chance to answer the first one. Underloading is failing to answer when a client asks a question or failing to respond to cues. An example might be:

Client: "This is going to hurt." Client is wincing, teeth clenched.

Nurse: Smiles and walks away.

Jumping to Conclusions

The following is an example of jumping to conclusions, or making assumptions without verifying information: A client who is sexually active states that she does not use a birth control method and the practitioner responds, "How long have you been trying to get pregnant?" The client might lack knowledge of birth control methods or be in a homosexual relationship where pregnancy is not a risk.

The Halo Effect

Because of the "halo effect," the practitioner may neglect to ask about potential problem areas because the client appears to be happy, prosperous, and coping well. In fact, the client may have serious financial or psychosocial problems that she does not feel comfortable discussing. For example, although the practitioner might say, "Oh, I never asked Mrs. Smith about her alcohol intake; she seems like such a happy, well-adjusted person and has such a nice family," Mrs. Smith may in fact have a serious problem with drinking.

Biased Questions

Biased questions make assumptions about the client's feelings or behavior and may lead the examiner to make false conclusions. For example, "You practice safe sex, don't you?" This question not only assumes that the client is sexually active and knows what "safe sex" means, but also conveys a certain negative judgment on the part of the practitioner toward someone who does not practice safe sex.

INTERVIEW VIGNETTES

An example of an appropriate sequence of questions (Can you identify the techniques of interviewing used in the example that follows?)

Provider: Hello, Mr. Chang, my name is Linda Jones, the nurse practitioner at the clinic. What brings you here today?

Mr. Chang: I'm worried about my heart.

Ms. Jones: Worried?

Mr. Chang: Yes. I was gardening last week and noticed that it became very hard for me to catch my breath after raking only 10 or 15 minutes. I know this is a sign of a heart problem.

Ms. Jones: Yes, shortness of breath can be a sign of a heart problem. But there can be other reasons someone becomes short of breath. I need to get more information from you before coming to any conclusions. I'm going to ask you some questions about the symptoms you experience that cause you concern . . .

An example of an inappropriate sequence of questions (Can you identify the common errors discussed in the chapter in the exchange that follows?)

Provider: Hello, my name is Linda, I'm a special kind of a nurse. What's your name?

Mr. Chang: George Chang

Provider: Well, George, what's wrong with you today?

Mr. Chang: I'm not sure. But I'm worried about my heart.

Provider: Oh at your age it's unlikely you have a heart problem. And anyway, it's my job to diagnose the problem. I just need for you to tell me what your symptoms are. Do you have chest pain?

Mr. Chang: No.

Provider: Do you have trouble breathing?

Mr. Chang: Well, yes, as a matter of fact that was my biggest worry

Provider: (Interrupts.) You don't look like you're having trouble breathing to me. By the way, exactly how old are you?

GLOSSARY

acceptance Recognition of what is said without necessarily agreeing.

active listening A communication technique that involves concentration on what is said by blocking out environmental noise, distractions, and intrusive thoughts. Active listening conveys a nonverbal message to the speaker that what is being said is valued.

body language The conveyance of messages by movements or gestures of the body or limbs, facial expressions, and eye contact. Body posture may convey a variety of emotions, including anger, anxiety, boredom, attention, or indifference.

chief complaint The major reason for seeking care stated in the client's own words.

contracting A contract is an oral or written agreement between the provider and client that makes explicit the expectations of each party.

interpersonal distance The distance between two individuals interacting that will vary by the nature of the relationship or cultural practices.

interpretation Sharing the meaning of the facts provided so that the client has an opportunity to confirm, deny, or offer an alternative explanation.

mirroring Awareness of and imitation or mirroring of characteristics of nonverbal aspects of the client's communication, such as speed and volume of speech and body position.

reflection Repeating a phrase or sentence the client has said. Allow a period of silence lasting at least 5 to 10 seconds to allow a client to think before answering a question or responding to a suggestion; after 10 seconds without a response the interviewer will need to initiate another question or suggestion.

therapeutic relationship A relationship in which the focus of exchange is on the client and the client's needs.

therapeutic use of self A communication technique in which the use of personal qualities of the interviewer supports the client's perspective or feelings by finding a common connection. This technique can be especially helpful when the client's ethnicity, race, or socioeconomic status appear to be very different from that of the interviewer's.

BIBLIOGRAPHY

Berlin EA, Fowkes WC: A teaching framework for cross-cultural health care, *Western J of Med* 139:934-938, 1983.

Long L: *Understanding/responding: a communication manual for nurses,* ed 2, Boston, 1992, Jones and Bartlett.

Kleinman A, Eisenberg L, Good B: Culture, illness, and care, *Ann Intern Med* 88:251-258, 1978.

Molde S: Understanding patient agendas, *Image* 18:145-147, 1986.

Putsch RW: Cross-cultural communication, *JAMA* 254: 3344-3348, 1985.

Stuart GW and Sundeen SJ: *Principles and practice of psychiatric nursing,* ed 4, St. Louis, 1991, Mosby—Year Book.

Sundeen SJ and others: *Nurse-client interaction,* St. Louis, 1989, Mosby—Year Book.

The Health History

PURPOSE

The **health history** is an extremely important part of the health assessment. It serves as the primary vehicle by which the practitioner establishes rapport with the client. The history-taking interview helps the practitioner assess and diagnose the client's health needs and problems and obtain knowledge of these matters within the context of that particular client's life. The health history not only documents the client's needs and problems but also provides a picture of the client as a whole person, in relation to his or her social and physical environment. Thus it registers both the deficits and abnormalities and the strengths that will support health interventions and care.

Other important components of the history database are the client's perceptions regarding health, illness, therapies, and experiences with health care providers and delivery systems. Understanding these beliefs, perceptions, and responses is necessary to providing future care that is relevant and, consequently, effective.

The practitioner implements the health history in two phases: (1) the client interview phase, which elicits the information, and (2) the documentation of data phase. The sequence for obtaining a history, as presented in this chapter, follows a systematic method for recording the history. The client interview itself may not proceed in the same sequence because of the nature of the client's health need or problem, the condition of the client, or other contextual variables. The interviewer needs to understand the essential components of a health history fully, develop a personal scheme for taking a health history, and be ready to alter the sequence and nature of data obtained according to the conditions of a particular encounter.

The health history usually is done in the examiner's office or the client's home or hospital room. If the interview takes place in the examiner's space, the examiner can control the environment to facilitate privacy, comfort, and quiet. However, if the interview is done in the client's space, the examiner must assess the environment and, in some instances, alter it to facilitate an adequate interview. For example, closing the curtains in a multibed hospital room or requesting that the television be turned off in the home will make the environment more conducive to the interview situation.

Whether the examiner or the client initiates the encounter, the client will have certain ideas about its purpose and content. Clarification of the client's purpose and expectations and orientation of the client to the examiner's goals and methods early in the encounter will minimize the potential for misunderstanding and frustration. Often the client's priorities are different from those of the examiner, or the examiner may have an inaccurate perception of the client's goals. The interviewer must clarify any discrepancies and negotiate priorities if the encounter is to be productive.

The various types of health histories include the following:

1. A complete health history, as described in this chapter, is taken on the initial visit to a health care facility when the health care providers within that facility will be providing comprehensive and/or continuous care.
2. An interval health history is used to collect information during visits subsequent to the one in which the initial database was collected. Depending on the time since the last entry to the history and the purpose of the encounter, selected information about current needs and problems and updates of health history information are obtained.
3. A problem-focused or chief complaint–focused health history is used to collect data about a specific problem system or region. Examples of such health histories are included in the systems and region examination chapters in this book.

The interviewer should strive for balance between allowing clients to talk freely and tell their story in their own way and using time efficiently. Clients must be able to provide information that they consider relevant. However, the examiner must probe, clarify, and quantify client information in structured ways. Because the examiner is the "expert" in history taking, he or she must take the lead in managing the interview to obtain appropriate information as efficiently as possible. Also, time is not an unlimited resource. Often other clients are waiting for services, and the examiner must control the costs of encounters.

Because it is usually not possible to write the entire health history during the interview, the interviewer takes notes. Forms are useful in structuring note taking and are appropriate for many data components. The interviewer records as much of the health history as possible during the interview, and the remainder is added as soon as possible after the interview has been completed.

PREPARATION: CLIENT AND ENVIRONMENT

Organize the environment for the history in a manner that will increase the physical and psychological comfort of the client (see box below). At the first encounter, introduce yourself to the client with a formal greeting and use the client's full name. In a clinic setting, seat yourself facing the client. Allow the client to remain in street clothes until the history portion of the assessment has been completed.

Make sure that you and the client understand each other's expectations for the encounter. Brief the client about the purposes and structure of a health history, and ask the client about his or her expectations early in the interaction.

PREPARATION FOR THE HEALTH HISTORY

Establish an environment that is conducive to effective communication—private, comfortable, and quiet.

Introduce yourself to the client.

Address the client formally with his or her full name.

If children or others are in attendance, determine the client's wishes about the presence of the additional person(s) during the interview and examination.

Allow the client to state the problems and his or her expectations for the encounter.

Orient the client to the purposes, structure, and components of the health history.

If this is not the client's first encounter with the health system and a record exists of past data and care for the client, review this record with the client.

Make some judgment early in the interview about the priorities for the encounter, given your and the client's constraints. Communicate and negotiate priorities with the client.

FORMAT

The health history described in this chapter is extremely detailed and complete. In many actual client care situations, it may not be possible, or even appropriate, to obtain the complete history at the first encounter or at all. For clients who are receiving continuous care, the history can be done in portions during several encounters. For clients who require episodic care, decisions regarding the data that are essential for immediate therapy will guide the content of the history.

The beginning health historian should practice obtaining the complete health history to develop skill in interviewing and in recording data and to establish priorities for focused interviews (see box below). During this practice process the learner will gain an appreciation for the information obtained from each portion of the health history.

The recommended format for the complete health history is as follows:

A. Biographical information
B. Client's reason for seeking care (chief complaint)
C. Present health and present illness status
D. Past health history
E. Current health information
F. Family health history
G. Review of systems
    1. Physical systems
    2. Functional status
    3. Sociological system
    4. Psychological system
H. Developmental data
I. Nutritional data

Biographical Information

At the beginning of any health record, list commonly used, and sometimes critical, biographical information. Obtain this information early during the client's first visit or at admission. Otherwise, the information may be omitted and later needed in an emergency or at a time when the client is unavailable or unable to respond.

Record the information listed in the box on p. 16 in the introductory biographical section of the history. Sometimes this information is recorded by an assistant in the health care setting, or it may be on the record from a previous encounter. If the information is already recorded, review it with the client to verify that it is complete, accurate, and up to date.

SUGGESTED SCRIPT FOR INTRODUCING COMPONENTS OF THE HEALTH HISTORY

Biographical information

"I will start the history by asking you some general questions about yourself. First, could you please give me the correct spelling of your full name?"

Client's reason for seeking care

"Please tell me why you came to see me today."

Past health history

"Because some of the health problems you had in the past may have some implications for what we do today, I will now be asking you about your past illnesses, health problems, and immunizations."

Current health information

"Because my advice must take into account your current health habits and practices, I will now ask you various questions about your current habits and medications."

Family health history

For ill client: "Because others in your family may have health problems that relate to your problems or affect your treatment, I will ask you some questions about their health."

For well client: "Because others in your family may have health problems that relate to your current health risks and future health, I will ask you some questions about their health."

Review of systems
Physical systems

"Up to now in the interview, we have concentrated on certain parts of your body. To have a complete picture of your physical health, I will now ask you a number of questions about the other parts of your body."

Sociological systems and psychological systems

"Because I want to know more about you as a total person, I will now ask you some questions about you, your family, and your relationships with others."

Developmental data

[Usually the interview up to this point in the history will provide information for this section.]

Nutritional data

"Because nutrition is important to health, I will next ask you some questions about your diet."

CLIENT BIOGRAPHICAL INFORMATION

A. Full name
B. Address and telephone numbers
 1. Client's permanent
 2. Contact of client (person to contact in case of emergency)
C. Birthdate
D. Sex
E. Race
F. Religion
G. Marital status
H. Social Security number
I. Occupation
 1. Usual
 2. Present
J. Birthplace
K. Source of referral
L. Usual source of health care
M. Source and reliability of information
N. Date of interview

First, record the client's name. Since persons who live in an ethnically homogenous geographical area often have similar names, it is important that this key information be exact. Precise identification, including first, middle, and last names, assists in ensuring accurate information retrieval and coordination. If additional identifying information is needed, record the parents' names, including the mother's maiden name.

Next, record the client's full mailing address and telephone numbers. Also include the name, address, and telephone number of one of the client's friends or relatives. This person should be someone with whom the client is in frequent contact and who would be willing and able to relay a message to the client in an emergency or if the client cannot be located.

The birthdate, sex, race, religion, marital status, and birthplace entries are self-explanatory. Many health problems and needs are related to age, sex, race, or social situation. This information provides initial insight into the client as a unique person and can be correlated with the client's needs and problems discovered later in the history.

Justifiable reasons for recording the client's Social Security number include the precise identification of each client and potential access to a large pool of health-related information. The potential for violation of client confidentiality is a disadvantage.

A significant difference may exist between the client's current and usual occupations. The nature of the difference may indicate the severity of the client's health problems and the level of disability resulting from them.

In addition, knowledge of past occupations might provide clues to past or present environmental hazards contributing to the present illness. A mine worker with a respiratory system complaint is an example.

Knowledge of the client's birthplace provides geographical information associated with the origin of problems and cultural implications for therapy and health maintenance.

If the current caregiver is not the usual and primary source of the client's care, record the name and address of the individual or institution so identified by the client. In addition, document the reason that the client is entering a new health care system. The client may be in crisis, may be dissatisfied with past care, or may be "shopping." If the past source of care possesses significant data about the client's health and if the client intends to continue in the current health care system, ask the client to sign a permission for the transfer of information. Later in the health history, you will have the opportunity to record, in some detail, past patterns of health care.

The source of client payment for care is usually included on administrative records. However, noting this information in the health history might be useful in guiding choices of interventions.

Next, make a statement about the source of the information to follow. In most instances the source is the client, but do not assume that this is so unless the source is specifically identified. If the information is given by someone other than the client, describe the nature of the informant's contact with the client. For example, in the case of a child, a history given by a grandmother who resides with the child should be viewed differently from one given by a grandmother who visits the child once a week.

Along with the statement of the informant, give an evaluation of that person's reliability. For example, you could describe the informant as "inconsistent," "unclear about recent events," "evasive," or "cooperative and

Helpful Hints for Effective Interviewing: Make judgments about the balance between allowing the client to talk in an unstructured way and the need to control the interview.
Avoid questions that can be answered with "yes" or "no" if details are needed.
Clarify the client's diagnostic statements and conclusions.
Be alert to concerns that the client is having difficulty in presenting.
Do not formulate premature conclusions about the nature of the client's problem.

reliable." Such statements serve as simple criteria by which the remainder of the information in the history is judged by other health care providers. In addition, this type of information may indicate a need to retake or supplement the history at a future date or to consult with other informants to verify the data.

It is important to date the history. In a situation in which the client's condition changes rapidly, events can be correlated only if their temporal relationships are known.

For suggestions about how to conduct an effective health history interview, see the box on p. 16.

Client's Reason for Seeking Care (Chief Complaint)

Record the reason for seeking care as a short statement in the client's own words and in quotation marks, indicating the client's purpose for requesting health care at this time. In the case of a well client, the statement of the reason for seeking care may be the client's request for a health examination for health screening or health promotion.

With an ill client, the statement is sometimes called a chief complaint (CC), defined as the **acute** or chronic problem that is the client's priority for treatment. Whenever relevant, include a notation of the duration of the problem. The duration stated by the client may not be the actual time span of the symptoms. However, it indicates the time during which the complaint was important enough to motivate the client to seek help.

Keep in mind that the reason for seeking care is not a diagnostic statement. In fact, formulating this statement in diagnostic terms can be hazardous. For example, a client who has frequent asthmatic attacks may appear for treatment with respiratory system complaints and state that he or she is having an "asthmatic attack." However, this may not be the actual situation. In this early portion of the history, care must be taken to avoid client and interviewer bias. Otherwise the interview and the problem solving may be set in one potentially incorrect direction.

The following are examples of good statements of reasons for seeking care:

Chest pain for 3 days.
Swollen ankles for 2 weeks.
Fever and headache for 24 hours.
Pap smear needed. Last Pap 9/8/90.
Physical examination needed for camp.

In contrast, these are examples of inadequately stated chief complaints:

Thinks she might be pregnant.
Sick.
Nausea and vomiting.
Hypertension.

The client's reason for seeking care may seem superfluous, especially since the next section of the history involves a description of the health need or problem in detail. However, this entry is one of the few places in the recorded histories of encounters with the health care system where clients are given the opportunity to have their needs recorded in their own words. Too often, practitioners lose sight of the clients' priorities for care. The consistent documentation of clients' reasons for seeking care assists in keeping the system responsive to their perceived needs.

In some instances a client presents several complaints. However, do not state more than three in this portion of the history, and note the client's priorities as stated. All the client's problems can be addressed in the present health/present illness (PH/PI) portion of the health history.

Be alert to the possibility that some clients may be reluctant to state their priority for seeking health care and may provide the interviewer with a reason perceived to be more acceptable than the actual reason. Watch for clues to any underlying and unstated concerns throughout the interview.

Present Health/Present Illness Status

general information

The present health/present illness section describes the information relevant to the client's reasons for seeking care. For a well client, the interviewer commonly describes the client's usual health and briefly summarizes his or her health maintenance needs and activities.

When the client has a health problem, this portion of the health history challenges the practitioner's interviewing, clinical knowledge, and written communication skills. The practitioner must learn the minute details of the chief complaint and its associated phenomena. First, the information must be comprehensive. Second, it must be recorded logically and concisely. Third, it must provide the practitioner with enough information to initiate additional assessment and the intervention measures.

The interviewing and recording for the present illness portion of the health history is especially difficult for beginning practitioners because the processes involved require both skill in interviewing and history taking and clinical knowledge. Outlining the progression of the present illness before writing the narrative discussion is sometimes helpful. Although the student who is learning health assessment has probably not yet studied client care management, the student may find that the use of clinical management references for the system(s) discussed with the client will often provide valuable learning by highlighting important omissions, which can be incorporated in future interviews.

The following are the components of the present health/present illness section of the health history:

A. Introduction
   1. Client summary
   2. Usual health
B. Investigation of symptoms: chronological story
   1. Onset
      a. Date
      b. Manner (gradual or sudden)
      c. Duration
      d. Precipitating factors
   2. Course since onset
      a. Incidence (frequency)
      b. Manner
      c. Duration (longest, shortest, and average times)
      d. Patterns of remissions and exacerbations
   3. Location
   4. Quality
   5. Quantity
   6. Setting
   7. Associated phenomena
   8. Alleviating or aggravating factors
C. Negative information
D. Relevant family information
E. Disability assessment

Introduction. The introduction to the present illness section should be succinct. Its major purpose is to provide the reader with a general orientation to the client.

State the client's previous visits or admissions, if any, to the institution or service. Next, briefly summarize the client's biographical data (usually age, race, marital status, employment status, and occupation). If the client is being hospitalized and also has been hospitalized in the past, note the client's total number of hospitalizations and the number of hospitalizations for complaints related to the present illness.

Next, describe the client's usual health and record any significant past diagnoses and past and current health problems.

Investigation of symptoms: chronological story
Initiate the exploration of symptoms by saying to the client: "Tell me about it [the problem mentioned in the chief complaint statement]," or "How did it [the problem] start, and what has happened since it started?" The client usually will respond to this inquiry with a long but diagnostically incomplete discourse about health problems and needs. Exercise skill in determining when to interrupt the client—specifically, when to direct the responses by asking additional clarifying questions and when to allow the client to continue the narration of events perceived as significant by that individual.

Create a mental or written list of the areas of **symp-**

tom investigation to be explored as an aid in attaining comprehensive information. Regardless of the nature of the problem, each of the areas of investigation is relevant, and any health problem analysis would be incomplete without the description of all areas.

Determine the chronological sequence of the client's problem. The client is apt to remember best the most recent episode of illness. When a prolonged illness is being discussed, the client will need direction in tracing the problem to its first symptomatic event. Once this first event has been identified, investigate it in detail and specify its date, manner of onset, duration, and precipitating factors.

Describe each symptom's course since onset. Determine its frequency as a specific time interval. Clients may state vaguely that they have a symptom "all the time." Such a statement may mean once a month to one client or 10 times a day to another. To obtain specific information, ask: "How many times a day [or a week or a month] does it occur?" Although suggesting answers with questions is to be avoided, occasionally it may be necessary to pursue the issue of frequency by asking leading questions, for example, "Does it occur more often than five times a day?"

Determine the usual manner of onset for the illness episodes. Note specifically any change in onset. When many episodes have occurred, specify the longest, shortest, and average durations of the episodes. If there have been only several episodes, identify the length of each one.

For prolonged illnesses, describe the patterns of remission and exacerbation according to their duration and frequency. Be watchful for environmental or other clues that might be precipitating factors for the illness events.

For recording the symptoms, several methods can be used to assist readers in identifying temporal relationships easily. Describe the initial event first, then the subsequent events. A chronological story can be indexed in the left-hand column of the history sheet, with prior to admission (PTA) or visit (PTV) used as a reference. For example, the chronological index can be listed as follows: "6 years PTA," "3 years PTA," "6 months PTA," or "1 day PTA," with the corresponding narrative alongside it and continuing below the temporal index heading.

One method of demonstrating the progression of an illness is to use a diagram illustrating the disease process (Figure 2-1). This type of diagram is especially helpful with multisymptomatic illnesses.

As the chronological story evolves, integrate the other areas of symptom investigation into the text of the narrative. Whenever appropriate, describe the sign's or symptom's location, quality, quantity, setting, associated phenomena, and alleviating and aggravating factors, especially when a change in pattern occurs.

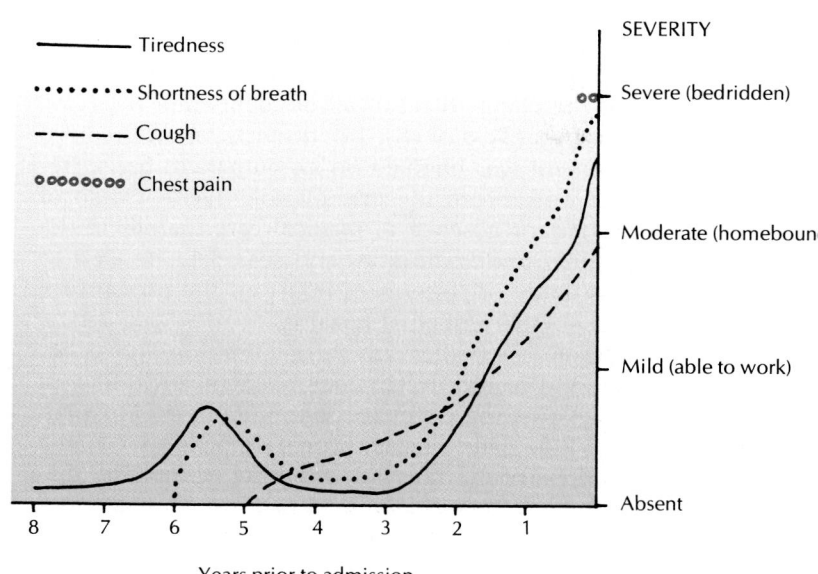

——— Tiredness

•••••••• Shortness of breath

– – – – – Cough

ooooooo Chest pain

SEVERITY

Severe (bedridden)

Moderate (homebound)

Mild (able to work)

Absent

8 7 6 5 4 3 2 1

Years prior to admission

FIGURE 2-1 Example of a graph to illustrate symptomatic progress of an illness.

Determine the exact site of the sign or symptom. Subjective events, such as pain, pose certain problems. Having a client point to the exact location of pain and trace its radiation with a finger assists in determining the site. In recording the location, use body hemispheres and anatomical landmarks.

Quality refers to the unique properties of the complaint. Signs such as discharge are described according to their color, texture, composition, appearance, and odor. Sound and temperature may be descriptive attributes of other phenomena. Subjective events such as pain challenge the descriptive skills of the practitioner. The quality of pain is frequently characterized as dull, aching, sharp, nagging, throbbing, stabbing, or squeezing. Whenever appropriate, use the client's descriptions with quotation marks.

Quantity refers to the size, extent, number, or amount (e.g., of pain, rash, discharge, or lesion). With objective signs, use common measurements, such as centimeters, cups, or tablespoons. In describing subjective events, for example, pain, remember that evaluations such as "a little" or "a lot" have different meanings for different persons. The quality of subjective phenomena can be more accurately conveyed by describing the client's response to the symptom. For example, when the pain occurs, does the client stop and sit or continue with activities?

Whenever illness occurs, the client is in a particular environment, either with someone or alone. It may be useful to ask about the setting in which certain symptoms occur because, physically or psychologically, the setting may have an effect on the client. This information can provide the practitioner with clues to the cause of the problem and implications for treatment.

Associated phenomena are those symptoms, such as nausea and vomiting, that occur with the chief complaint. They may be related to the chief complaint or may be a part of a totally different syndrome. Often the client will spontaneously identify these events. Always ask if there is anything else occurring with the chief complaint, or inquire about the presence or absence of certain specific events. Review the implicated problem system or systems. Record the client's positive responses and completely describe all reported symptoms. Document the negative responses in the negative information section.

When an illness occurs, initially the affected person often adapts to it or attempts self-treatment. The individual may decrease activity, eat more or less, wait, or actively medicate and treat himself or herself. Often cultural responses to illness and treatment influence this self-care. The client's actions in response to the problem and the effect of these actions should be addressed in a nonjudgmental way. If there has been professional intervention, the nature, source, and effect of each intervention need to be recorded. The client, through treatment or accommodation, may have discovered something that alleviates the symptom. Therefore the client should be asked what makes the situation better. The client's solution may provide valuable therapeutic data and may reflect the individual's adaptation to illness.

Ask the client about what makes the chief complaint worse. Usually the client has noticed aggravating factors but may need assistance in recalling them. Inquire about the effect of movement, positioning, or eating, for example. Again, this information may offer valuable therapeutic data.

Negative information. In the analysis of a problem, negative information is as significant as positive information for determining the diagnosis. Thoroughly review each system implicated in the present illness section. Record the client's positive replies in the text of the chronological story. Document all negative information in this separate category of the present illness section.

Relevant family history. Ask the client whether any problem similar to the chief complaint is known to exist among blood relatives. Record positive replies, specifically identifying the relative and the problem. Document negative replies in general terms, for example: "None of the client's blood relatives has diabetes." In the case of a client who is adopted, the family history of the biological family (if known) must be differentiated from that of the adoptive family, in which bloodlines are not shared.

Disability assessment. The purpose of the disability assessment is to determine the extent to which the symptoms identified in the present illness section have affected the client's total life. Note physiological effects as well as sociological, psychological, and financial consequences of the problem.

Past Health History

The purpose of the past health history (PH) section of the health history is to identify all the client's major past health problems. Past illnesses may have some effect on the client's current health needs and problems. In addition, information about the management of and response to past problems provides some indication of the client's possible response to current and future health issues.

The following information is obtained and recorded in the present history section of the health history:
A. Past general health
B. Childhood illnesses
C. Accidents and disabling injuries
D. Hospitalizations
E. Operations
F. Major acute and chronic illnesses
G. Immunizations
H. Medications and transfusions
I. Allergies

Ask about the client's usual health status. Try to elicit a sense of the client's perception of his or her health and feelings about usual health status.

The recording of childhood illnesses is probably more relevant to, and more easily obtained for, a child's history than an adult's. At minimum, however, ask all adults if they have had rheumatic fever. Whenever a positive reply is given, determine the age of the client

at occurrence, the fact or absence of a medically confirmed diagnosis, and the short-term and long-term effects of the disease.

Ask the client to recall all accidents and disabling injuries, regardless of whether hospitalization occurred or treatment was handled on an outpatient basis. Determine and record the precipitating event, extent of injury, fact or absence of medical care, names of the practitioner and institution, and sequelae. Be alert to the possibility of patterns of injury or the presence of consistent environmental hazards.

Determine whether any hospitalizations have occurred, and record descriptions of them, including all the times that the client was admitted to an inpatient unit. Include dates of stay, primary practitioner, name and address of the hospital, admitting complaint, discharge diagnosis, and follow-up care and sequelae. Record any obstetrical hospitalizations in this section or in the review of systems portion of the health history (review of female genital system).

Record all operations together, under the specific operations category. Include a description of the nature of the repair or removal, making it as complete as possible. Frequently, clients are unaware of the exact nature of their operations. It may be necessary to consult past records for accurate and complete information.

If the client has had major acute illnesses or chronic illnesses that have not required hospitalization, note the course of treatment, the person making the diagnosis, and the follow-up care and sequelae.

Information under the categories of hospitalizations, operations, and other major illnesses may, in some instances, be redundant. Do not record detailed information more than once. Instead, state the presence of a past problem, and refer the reader to the section where the original notation was made.

Information regarding medications currently being taken is covered in the next section of the health history. At this point, ask about previous medications that may have been taken for a long time and/or those that might have an effect on the current health need or problem. Given current concerns about blood transfusions and AIDS, be sure to record information about blood transfusions in this section.

Record all immunizations according to type and date. Accurate immunization records are commonly kept for children but not usually for adults. For adults, obtain the exact (or at least approximate) date of the last tetanus immunization.

Current Health Information

The purpose of the current health information section is to record major current health-related information. A recommended outline for the information is as follows:

A. Allergies
   1. Environmental
   2. Ingestion
   3. Drug
   4. Other
B. Habits
   1. Alcohol
   2. Tobacco
   3. Drugs
   4. Caffeine
C. Medications taken regularly (names, dosages, frequency, intended effect, and compliance)
   1. By health care provider prescription
   2. By self-prescription
D. Exercise patterns
E. Sleep patterns

Ask specifically about allergies to food, environmental factors, animals, and drugs. If the client reports an allergy, obtain specific information about the causative factor, reaction, diagnosis of causative factor, therapy, and sequelae. Exercise caution in assessing drug allergies. A drug reaction may not always be an allergic response. It may be an interaction with a concurrently administered drug, a misdose, a side effect, or an adverse effect.

Habits relevant to the health of an individual are excessive alcohol or caffeine ingestion, smoking, and the addictive use of legal or illegal mood-altering substances. In recording habits, note the number of cigarettes, ounces, or tablets per day along with the duration of the habit. Determine and record both past and current use of these substances.

If therapy is to be planned by informed practitioners logically, all medications currently being used by the client must be known and recorded. Clients usually admit to vague patterns, such as taking "a white pill once a day for water," but they may forget to tell the practitioner about the aspirin or antacid they take several times a day unless they are specifically asked about nonprescription items. This situation presents the opportunity to educate clients about the names, doses, and uses of their medications and the necessity of knowing such information.

Explore the pattern of physical and sedentary activities in the client's usual routine. Include a weekly or daily profile of the individual's usual activities.

Describe the client's sleep pattern. Record the daily routine for a typical week. Determine the client's assessment of the adequacy of his or her sleep and satisfaction with the pattern.

Family Health History

The purpose of the family health history (FH) section is to learn about the general health of the client's blood relatives, spouse, and children and to identify any ill-nesses of a genetic, familial, or environmental nature that might have implications for the client's current or future health problems and needs or their solution or resolution. Genetic problems are those that are directly inherited through the genes. Familial problems are ones that have not yet been demonstrated to be genetic exclusively but appear more often in family clusters for various reasons. An example of a familial problem is alcoholism. Environmental problems, for example, exposure to toxic substances, may be shared by families.

The health status of the client's family is significant for several reasons. First, the client's health status affects and is affected by health conditions in other family members. Communicable disease is an example of this situation. Second, heredity and constitutional factors are associated with the causation of many diseases. A strong family history of certain problems might offer important clues in assessment and diagnosis.

Inquire about the health of the client's blood relatives, including maternal and paternal grandparents, parents, siblings, aunts, uncles, spouse, and children. In certain situations information regarding roommates, sexual partners, and significant others might be relevant to a family history. Information also needs to be obtained about the current health status of, presence of disease in, and current age or age at death of each family member. If a member is deceased, record the cause of death.

If the nature of the client's established or possible illnesses have known or suspected familial tendencies, question the client again about similar problems of family members.

Inquire about the presence of the following diseases because of their genetic, familial, or environmental tendencies: alcoholism, allergies, epilepsy, diabetes, hematological disorders (e.g., hemophilia, sickle cell anemia, thalassemia, hemolytic jaundice, and severe anemia), Huntington's chorea, cancer, hypertension, arteriosclerosis, gout, obesity, coronary artery disease, tuberculosis, and kidney disease. Often printed history forms list these diseases. Check whether or not the client or a family member has the diagnosis. Inquire about selected additional health problems because of the client's family history, occupation, socioeconomic status, ethnic origins, or environment.

The information in the family history section can be outlined in the record or put in the form of a family tree chart. Figure 2-2 is an example of such a chart. This type of chart is especially useful in situations in which genetically transmitted diseases are present or suspected or if the understanding of family composition is an important factor in management. The traditionally used symbols for genogram notations are included in the box on p. 22. For an adopted individual, two genograms may be useful if the information is available. The

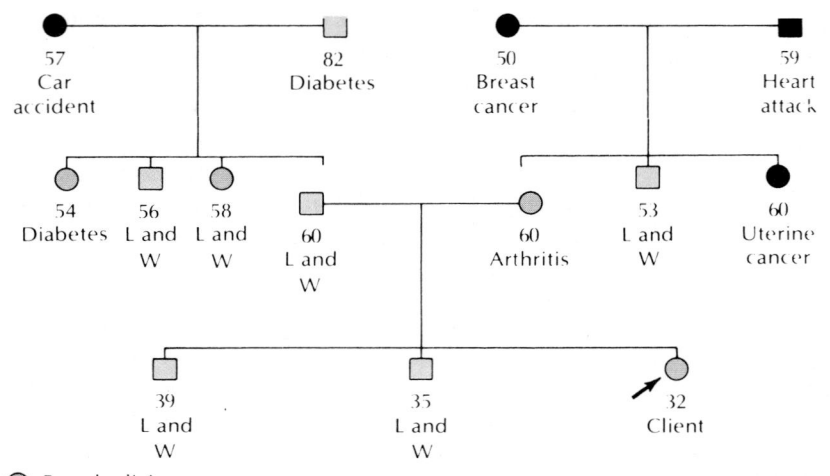

FIGURE 2-2 Example of a family tree to illustrate family health.

genogram for the biological family would indicate genetic health issues and familial ones that may be genetically linked. The genogram for the adoptive family would include familial health issues and those affected by environment.

Review of Systems

The review of systems (ROS) portion of the history includes a collection of data about the past and present health of each of the client's systems. This review of the client's physical, functional, sociological, and psychological health status may identify problems not uncovered previously in the history. It also provides an opportunity to indicate the client's strengths and weaknesses.

Generally, this portion of the history is organized from a **cephalad** to **caudad** body direction and from physical to psychosocial factors. The client is told that he or she will be asked a number of questions. For both beginning and experienced interviewers, a checklist or written reminder of the routine is useful.

Physical systems. In the review of physical systems section, ask a question about the client's symptoms. Then pause to allow the client to think and respond. If the client responds positively, analyze the symptoms according to the characteristics of symptoms discussed in the present health/present illness section of the history. Ask questions quickly enough to be efficient, yet slowly enough to allow the client time to think. In general, emphasize the presence of past or current com-

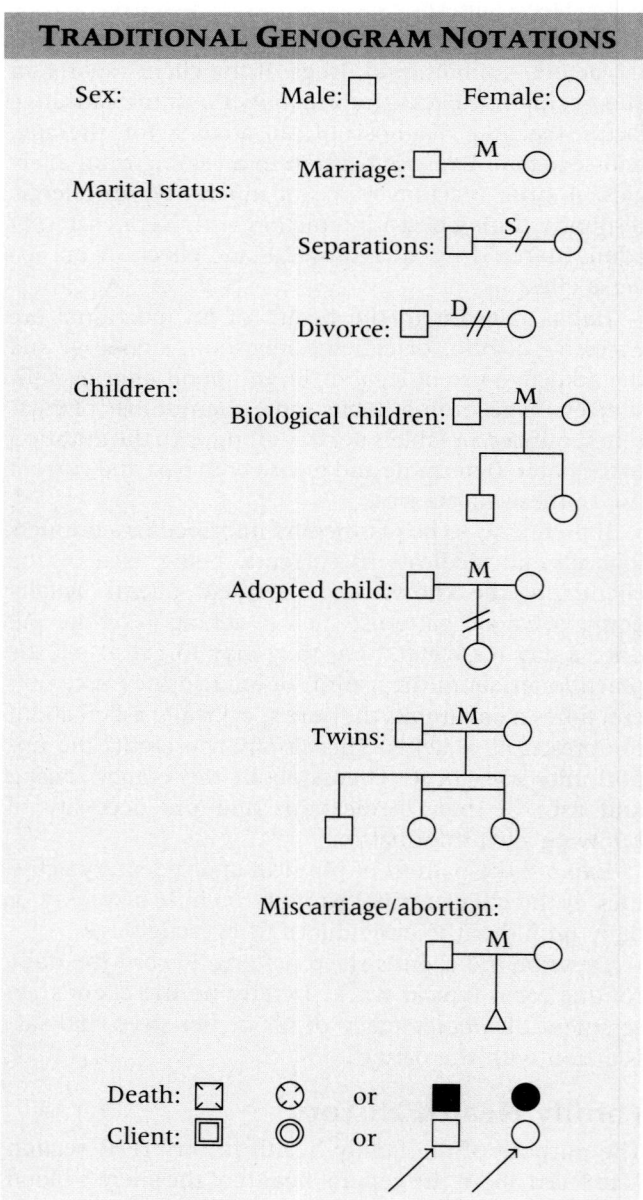

mon anatomical or functional problems of the system and the health functioning and maintenance of the system.

It is important to translate the signs and symptoms into questions and terms that the client can understand. For example, questions concerning a symptom such as **intermittent claudication** need to be presented in descriptive lay terms. Examples of questions related to intermittent claudication follow:

"Do you ever have any **cramp**like pains in your legs?"

"When do these cramps occur?"

"What happens to the pain if you rest your legs?"

In documenting the health history, record the presence or absence of all signs or symptoms included in the inquiry. Using the general term "negative" for a total system is meaningless. If such a broad notation is made, the reader will not know which questions were asked and consequently will not understand the context of "negative." If the reader is also the recorder, he or she probably will not, at a later time, remember which specific questions were asked. An exception might exist in a health care system where the review of physical systems section is routinized and where "negative" indicates an inquiry into and a negative response to predetermined, universally known, and always reviewed items of exploration.

In the present health/present illness section of the health history, a body region or system may have already been reviewed along with the exploration of a health problem. In this situation, in the review of physical systems section, a notation is made that refers the reader to the present health/present illness section for information about that system.

Systems and body regions to review and areas of exploration about the health status, functional and anatomical problems, and health maintenance of those systems are presented in the following list.

GENERAL
Usual state of health
Episodes of chills
Episodes of weakness or **malaise**
Fatigue

FEVER
Recent and significant gain or loss of weight (if present, amount, time interval, and possible causes are recorded)
Sweats
Usual, maximum, and minimum weight

SKIN
Usual condition
Care habits
Previously diagnosed and treated disease
Color changes

Dryness
Ecchymosis
Lesions
Masses
Odors
Petechiae
Pruritus
Temperature changes
Texture changes

HAIR
Usual state of health
Alopecia or hair loss
Excessive growth or change in distribution
Texture changes
Use of dyes

NAILS
Usual state of health
Changes in appearance
Texture changes

HEAD AND FACE
Usual state of health
Dizziness
History of trauma
Injuries
Pain
Syncope
Unusual or frequent headaches

EYES
Usual state of health
Pattern of eye examinations
Visual acuity, without and with corrective lenses, if applicable
Date of last ophthalmological examination and results
Cataracts
Changes in visual fields or vision
Diplopia
Excessive tearing
Glaucoma
Infections
Pain
Photophobia
Pruritus
Redness
Unusual discharge or sensations
Visual disturbances, such as "rainbows" around lights, flashing lights, or blind spots

EARS
Usual state of health
Care habits, especially cleaning
Use of prosthetic devices
Discharge
Hearing ability

Infections
Otalgia
Presence of excessive environmental noise
Tinnitus, buzzing, or ringing
Vertigo (subjective or objective)

NOSE AND SINUSES
Usual state of health
Olfactory ability
Discharge (seasonal associations)
Epistaxis
Frequency of colds
Obstruction
Pain in infraorbital or sinus areas
Postnasal drip
Sinus infection
Sneezing (frequent or prolonged)

MOUTH AND THROAT
Usual state of health
Pattern of dental care
Pattern of dental hygiene
Use of prosthetic devices
Abscesses
Bleeding or swelling of gums
Change in taste
Dysphagia
Dryness
Excessive salivation
Hoarseness
Lesions
Odors
Pain
Sore throats
Voice changes

NECK AND NODES
Usual state of health
Masses
Node enlargement
Pain with movement or palpation
Swelling
Tenderness

BREASTS
Usual state of health
Self-examination pattern
Dimpling
Discharge
Masses
Pain
Tenderness

RESPIRATORY AND CARDIOVASCULAR SYSTEMS
Usual state of health
Past diagnosis of respiratory or cardiovascular system
  disease

Date of last roentgenogram and electrocardiogram
  and results
Cough
Cyanosis
Dyspnea (if present, amount of exertion precipitating
  it is recorded)
Edema
Hemoptysis
High blood pressure
Orthopnea (number of pillows needed to sleep
  comfortably is recorded)
Pain (exact location, radiation, and effect of respira-
  tion are recorded)
Palpitations
Paroxysmal nocturnal dyspnea
Sputum (if present, amount and characteristics are
  described)
Stridor
Wheezing

GASTROINTESTINAL SYSTEM
Usual state of health
Previous roentgenograms and results
Abdominal pain
Appetite
Ascites
Bowel habits
Change in stool color
Constipation
Diarrhea
Dyschezia
Dyspepsia
Dysphagia
Flatulence
Food idiosyncrasies
Hematemesis
Hemorrhoids
Hernia
Indigestion
Infections
Jaundice
Nausea
Previously diagnosed problems
Pyrosis
Recent changes in habits
Rectal bleeding
Rectal discomfort
Thirst
Vomiting

URINARY SYSTEM
Usual state of health
Past diagnosed problems
Usual pattern of urination
Anuria
Change in stream

Dysuria
Enuresis
Flank pain
Frequency
Hematuria
Hesitancy of stream
Incontinence
Nocturia
Oliguria
Polyuria
Pyuria
Retention
Stress incontinence
Suprapubic pain
Urgency
Urine color change
Urine odor change

GENITAL SYSTEM
MALE
Usual state of health
Impotence
Lesions
Masses
Pain
Prostate problems
Swelling
Urethral discharge

FEMALE
Usual state of health
Frequency of Pap smear and results
Care habits
Diagnosed problems
Dyspareunia
Lesions
Menstrual history
  Age at menarche
  Amenorrhea
  Amount of flow
  Date of last normal menstrual period (LNMP)
  Duration of flow
  Dysmenorrhea
  Frequency of menses
  Menorrhagia
  Metrorrhagia
  Polymenorrhea
Pruritus
Vaginal discharge
Obstetrical history (for each pregnancy)
  Complications of pregnancy
  Condition, sex, and weight of baby
  Date of delivery
  Description of labor
  Duration of pregnancy
  Place of prenatal care and hospitalization

Postpartum course
Prenatal course
Type of delivery (vaginal, cesarean section)

SEXUAL HISTORY (BOTH SEXES)
Ability to perform and enjoy satisfactory sexual inter-
  course
  Age at onset
Infertility
Number of sexual partners and number of sexual
  partners with multiple partners
Problems with sexual function or sexuality
Satisfaction with sexual activity
Sexual activity
Sexual preference
Sexually transmitted diseases
Sterility
Use of contraceptives

EXTREMITIES AND MUSCULOSKELETAL SYSTEM
Usual state of health
Past diagnosis of disease
Extremities
  Coldness
  Deformities
  Discoloration
  Edema
  Intermittent claudication
  Pain
  Thrombophlebitis
Muscles
  Cramping
  Pain
  Weakness
Bones and joints
  Back pain
  Deformities
  Fractures
  Heat
  Limitation of movement
  Pain
  Redness
  Stiffness
  Swelling

CENTRAL NERVOUS SYSTEM
Usual state of health
Past diagnosis of disease
Anxiety
General **behavior** change
Loss of consciousness
Mood change
Nervousness
Seizures
Speech
  Aphasia

Dysarthria
Cognitive ability
  Changes in memory
  Disorientation
  Hallucinations
Motor
  Ataxia
  Imbalance
  Paralysis
  Paresis
  Tic
  Tremor
  Spasm
Sensory
  Pain
  Paresthesia (hyperesthesia, anesthesia)

ENDOCRINE SYSTEM
History of physical growth and development
Adult changes in size of head, hands, or feet
Diagnosis of diabetes or thyroid disease
Dryness of skin or hair
Exophthalmos
Goiter
Hair distribution
Hormone therapy
Hypoglycemia
Intolerance of heat or cold
Polydipsia
Polyphagia
Polyuria
Postural hypotension
Presence of secondary sex characteristics
Weakness

HEMATOPOIETIC SYSTEM
Past diagnosis of **hematopoietic** disease
Anemia
Bleeding tendencies
Blood transfusion
Blood type
Bruising
Exposure to radiation
Lymphadenopathy

Functional status. If the client has functional limitations, measure the extent of abilities. Chapter 26 contains approaches and tools for the specific assessment of functional abilities. If this area of assessment is included, choose tools appropriate to the client group being assessed.

Sociological system. Diagnosis and treatment cannot be effectively done by knowing the client's physical status only. Since the client is a unique and whole person, diagnosis and treatment must be addressed within the context of that person. Therefore it is necessary to gather, in some organized way, information about the client's sociological, psychological, developmental, and nutritional status.

The following is a suggested organization of sociological data:
A. Relationships with family and significant others
  1. Client's position in the family
  2. Persons with whom client lives
  3. Persons with whom client relates
  4. Recent family **crisis** or changes
B. Environment
  1. Home
  2. Community
  3. Work
  4. Recent changes in environment
C. Occupational history
  1. Jobs held
  2. Satisfaction with present and past employment
  3. Current place of employment
D. Economic status and resources
  1. Source of income
  2. **Perception** of adequacy or inadequacy of income
  3. Effect of illness on economic status
E. Educational level
  1. Highest degree or grade attained
  2. Judgment of intellect relative to age
F. Daily profile
  1. Rest-activity patterns
  2. Social activities
  3. Special weekend activities
  4. Recent changes in daily activities
G. Patterns of health care
  1. Private and public primary care agencies
  2. Dental care
  3. Preventive care
  4. Emergency care

This outline is useful for gathering the sociological data for the majority of adult clients; however, it may be necessary to make adaptations for some individuals. Many clients may be unaccustomed to extensive questioning about nonphysical matters during the taking of a health history. Therefore the use of such data may need to be explained to the client, by stating, for example, "To treat you most effectively, it is important that I know something about you as a person."

First, ask about the client's role or roles in the family and household. A member may have a societally assigned role relating to birth, for example, that of son, father, or grandfather. In addition, the client may have a circumstantially defined role, for example, that of provider, "black sheep," or child. Identify all roles if possible.

Next, inquire about the people whom the client lives with and relates to on a regular basis. This information can be useful in hypothesizing, for example, the effect that a long illness of the care provider may have on the family. Also, identify strengths by the presence of strong family or friend relationships. Ask the client about the closeness and compatibility of these relationships. Sometimes unsatisfactory social relationships produce stress, which can be a factor in exacerbating or causing illness.

Ask the client if any recent event has had a significant impact on his or her health. Resultant positive data might provide clues of causation or implications for prevention of illness.

Physical and psychological environments can have a profound effect on an individual's health status and potential. Ask about the client's satisfaction with the appearance and general comfort of house, community, and work situations. Also, inquire whether the client considers the environment healthy or unhealthy. The pursuit of "why" in the case of negative responses will provide some insight into the client's value system, possible information regarding significant health hazards, clues to the cause of the present illness, and a validation of the negative responses. Again, ask about recent change or loss. Record positive responses.

Occupational history information can be used to specify past environmental hazards, determine the fit between personal ability and productivity, and plan rehabilitation. Inquire about jobs held, satisfaction with those jobs, and place of current employment.

Although it is usually not necessary to know the client's exact annual income, find out the source of that income and his or her assessment of its adequacy. Identify clients whose resources are insufficient to enable them to follow therapy, and make appropriate referral for financial assistance. For a probable prolonged illness, discuss and record financial reserves. If the client is covered by any health insurance, note the type of insurance, name of the insurer, and policy number.

Determine the educational level of the client, and record the highest degree or grade completed. In addition, make a judgment about the client's intellectual ability relative to age. Interviewing up to this point in the history has provided the opportunity for extensive observation of the client's understanding, response, and judgment.

Knowing the client's daily pattern helps in understanding the client as a person, with habits that encourage or impede health. Ask the client to describe a typical 24-hour day and to indicate weekend differences. Specifically, identify work, activity, sleep, rest, and recreational pursuits in the recording.

Part of the client's past social interaction has been with the health care system, and past responses may predict future patterns. Ask about health agencies used for acute, preventive, and maintenance health care. Determine whether the client is a health facility "shopper" or whether his or her care has had continuity.

Psychological system. The following information needs to be obtained during the psychological assessment of the client:

A. Cognitive abilities
1. Comprehension
2. Learning patterns
3. Memory
B. Responses to illness and health
1. Reaction to illness
2. Coping patterns
3. Value of health
C. Response to care
1. Perceptions of the caregivers
2. Compliance
D. Cultural implications for care
1. Patterns of therapy
2. Patterns of illness response

In assessing cognitive abilities, determine the client's comprehension ability. Usually comprehension can be assessed well indirectly rather than directly. Up to this point in the history-taking process, the client has demonstrated the ability to respond to rather complex questions. With this background in mind, record your judgment summary regarding the client's general comprehension ability.

Because education should be an essential component of all therapy, determine the client's health-learning patterns. Some clients need personal instructions. Others learn best through reading or group discussion. Knowing the client's preference can enable efficient use of provider effort and also involve the client in decision making concerning the process of therapy.

Discuss the client's behavior in past illnesses and in health to help predict future responses. Ask questions such as: "What does health mean to you, and what do you do to keep yourself healthy?" "How do you feel, and what do you do when you become slightly ill? When you become very ill?" "Who do you go to for help if you are ill?" Most clients will be able to answer these questions easily. Record a concise summary of the client's responses. This information can indicate the client's strengths and weaknesses and possible problems in therapy.

Skill may be required in learning the client's real responses to care since people are often placed in a position of subjugation by the health care system. Ask the client how comfortable he or she feels in asking questions of health care providers and whether he or she feels like a partner in care with them. You may record answers verbatim or summarize them.

Ask about the client's degree of compliance with past courses of therapy. If compliance has been minimal, determine the reasons for noncompliance. Problems resulting from lack of understanding and financial constraints are more easily solved than problems relating to distrust, indifference, or denial.

If the client is of a cultural group that is different from yours and that of the majority of the care providers, ask the client what he or she expects of care and therapy and if his or her culture has particular traditions regarding persons with similar needs. If the chief complaint is an illness, ask about the feelings and responses of the client and significant others to the fact of the illness. The responses may help to guide the care provider in a more efficient direction and to avoid unacceptable routes of intervention. (For more information on the collection of culturally relevant information, see Chapter 6.)

Developmental Data

A detailed description of the developmental assessment is presented in Chapter 3. At minimum, the recording of these data includes a summary of the client's development to date and a statement of current developmental functioning.

Nutritional Data

A detailed description of nutritional assessment is presented in Chapter 4. The recording of data minimally includes a description of an average day's food intake; an assessment of adequacy, inadequacy, or excess of the components of the basic four food groups; and the presence of any past nutritional problems.

ORGANIZATION BY FUNCTIONAL HEALTH PATTERNS

The format for the health history presented in this chapter is based on the traditional approaches in health care delivery systems. Within nursing, alternate systems of health assessment are being developed around the organizing framework of functional health patterns (Gordon, 1987 and 1993). Functional health patterns are defined as sequences of health behavior across time. Following is the currently used taxonomy of functional health patterns. Listed under each pattern are areas of specific assessment relevant to that health pattern.

Health Perception–Health Management Pattern

This category describes the client's perceived pattern of health and well-being and how health is managed. It includes the relevance of health perception to current activities and future planning. Also included is the individual's health risk management and general health care behavior, such as adherence to mental and physical health promotion activities, medical or nursing prescriptions, and follow-up care (Gordon, 1993).

Reason for seeking health care
Current and usual health status
Perception of individual's own health
Health management and adherence behavior
Risk factors—family, health habits, environment
Preventive health screening activities

Nutritional-Metabolic Pattern

This area describes the pattern of food and fluid consumption relative to metabolic need and pattern indicators of local nutrient supply. It includes daily eating times, types and quantity of food and fluids consumed, particular food preferences, and use of nutrient or vitamin supplements. This area also describes breast-feeding and infant feeding patterns. It includes reports of any skin lesions and general ability to heal. The condition of skin, hair, nails, mucous membranes, and teeth and measurements of body temperature, height, and weight are included (Gordon, 1993).

General information—height, weight, appetite
Food and fluid intake
Weight patterns
Activity level
Psychosocial/cultural/personal influences
Nutrition information
Pertinent physiological alterations
Drug history
Skin and dental problems

Elimination Pattern

This class describes the patterns of excretory function (bowel, bladder, and skin). It includes the individual's perceived regularity of excretory function, use of routines or laxatives for bowel elimination, and any changes or disturbances in time pattern, mode of excretion, quality, or quantity. Also included are any devices used to control excretion (Gordon, 1993).

Bladder elimination
    Usual pattern of voiding
    Self-care practices
    Symptoms of altered bladder elimination
    Pertinent physiological alterations
Bowel elimination
    Usual pattern of defecation
    Self-care practices
    Symptoms of altered bowel elimination
    Pertinent physiological alterations
Skin problems

Activity-Exercise Pattern

This area describes the pattern of exercise, activity, leisure, and recreation. It includes activities of daily living requiring energy expenditure, such as hygiene, cooking, shopping, eating, working, and home maintenance. Also included are the type, quantity, and quality of exercise, including sports, that describe the typical pattern for the individual. Factors that interfere with the desired or expected pattern for the individual (e.g., neuromuscular deficits and compensations, dyspnea, angina, or muscle cramping on exertion, and cardiac/pulmonary classification, if appropriate) are noted. Leisure patterns are also included and describe the activities that the individual undertakes as recreation either with a group or as an individual. Emphasis is on the activities of high importance or significance to the individual (Gordon, 1993).

Usual activities
Self-care activities
Adequacy of energy for requirements
Symptoms related to activity and exercise
Pertinent physiological alterations
Functional status

Sleep-Rest Pattern

This category describes the patterns of sleep, rest, and relaxation during the 24-hour day. It includes the individual's perception of the quality and quantity of sleep and rest and perception of energy level. Also noted are aids to sleep such as medications or nighttime routines that the individual employs (Gordon, 1993).

Usual sleep pattern
Sleep/bedtime rituals
Sleep environment
Sleep position
Psychophysiological influences
Sleep-pattern disturbance symptoms

Cognitive-Perceptual Pattern

This class describes the sensory-perceptual and cognitive pattern. It includes the adequacy of sensory modes, such as vision, hearing, taste, touch, or smell, and the compensation or prosthetics used for disturbances. Reports of pain perception and how pain is managed are also noted when appropriate. In addition, the cognitive functional abilities, such as language, memory, and decision making, are included (Gordon, 1993).

Special senses
  Eyes and vision
  Ears and hearing
Other special senses
Symptoms of neurological dysfunction
Pertinent physiological alterations and medications
Learning styles
Comfort

Self-Perception-Self-Concept Pattern

This area describes the self-concept pattern and the perceptions of self. It includes the individual's attitudes about himself or herself, perception of abilities (cognitive, affective, or physical), body image, identity, general sense of worth, and general emotional pattern. Pattern of body posture and movement, eye contact, voice, and speech pattern are noted (Gordon, 1993).

Social identity
Personal identity
Physical self
Self-esteem
Self-concept threats

Role-Relationship Pattern

This class describes the pattern of role engagements and relationships. It includes the individual's perception of the major roles and responsibilities in current life situations. Satisfaction or disturbances in family, work, or social relationships and responsibilities related to these roles are noted (Gordon, 1993).

Roles
Family relationships
Family problems
Family functioning
Work environment
Neighborhood environment

Sexuality-Reproductive Pattern

This category describes the patterns of satisfaction or dissatisfaction with sexuality and delineates the reproductive pattern. It includes the individual's perceived satisfaction or disturbances in his or her sexuality. The female's reproductive stage, premenopausal or postmenopausal, and any perceived problems are also noted (Gordon, 1993).

Sex roles and gender identification
Knowledge about sexuality and reproduction
Concerns about sexual performance and satisfaction
Reproductive history
Use of contraception

Coping-Stress Tolerance Pattern

This area describes the general coping pattern and the effectiveness of the pattern in terms of stress tolerance. It includes the individual's reserve or capacity to resist challenge to self-integrity, modes of handling stress, family or other support systems, and perceived ability to control and manange situations (Gordon, 1993).

Nature of stresses
Perception of stresses/roles
Coping strategies
Resolution of stress

Value-Belief Pattern

This class describes the pattern of values, goals, or beliefs (including spiritual) that guide choices or decisions. It includes what is perceived as important in life, quality of life, and any perceived conflicts in values, beliefs, or expectations that are health related (Gordon, 1993).

    Culture
    Spirituality
    Values

COMPUTER-ASSISTED HISTORY

Computer science is an important and permanent component of health care technology, and the computer can be an important tool in obtaining the client health history. Studies have demonstrated that the use of the computer in history taking can save the practitioner time and yield a reliable, comprehensive, and readable printout. In addition, this approach is acceptable to clients. In situations where personnel is in short supply and time allocated to history taking is routinely inadequate, the computer-assisted history can be superior to a verbal history.

Computer systems for history taking can be either client- or practitioner-interactive. The client-interactive systems are more commonly used because they can save the practitioner time. A number of client-interactive, computerized history-taking systems are available. Self-administered histories involve the client's either completing a paper-and-pencil questionnaire or interacting with a computer. With the paper-and-pencil questionnaire, the client's responses are computerized in a variety of ways, and the practitioner receives a printout of those responses. In the client-interactive systems, the client responds to inquiries from a computer terminal. In general, clients have viewed computer-assisted interviews favorably, and printouts from such systems have been complete, accurate, and legible.

In any client self-administered system, the practitioner's time is needed to review the client's history. Usually this review involves only a small amount of time. However, the amount of time spent by the client in the history-taking process is not shortened by the computer-assisted methods. The client's age, the number of client problems, and the time required by the client to complete the instructional portion of the computer program are positively correlated with the overall time needed to complete a computer-assisted history. The number of the client's years of formal education is negatively correlated with the overall time.

The computer-assisted history is more appropriate for the ambulatory client than for the hospitalized client. The ambulatory client can be scheduled for a computer interview or can complete a form for computerization that will yield a printout for the practitioner within several days. For hospitalized clients, information is generally needed immediately, and client access to terminals becomes problematic. Also, the hospitalized client often is too ill to complete a questionnaire or to use a computer terminal.

Practitioner-based computer systems for history taking involve either the practitioner's direct interaction with a computer, which is programmed for questions related to the history and into which answers are placed, or the practitioner's completion of a form that is computer-processed at a later time. The practitioner-interactive systems require a terminal for each practitioner, a situation that may not be cost-effective in ambulatory care situations. A more common approach is to perform computer processing of questionnaires. The advantage of this method is that it produces a legible printout, an improvement over most handwritten documents.

The computer-assisted history can be as effective as the verbal history. In fact, it may be more effective because remembering items for review is not a problem. Any question that can be asked verbally can be programmed into a computer system, and computer technology allows for additional branching questions if the client gives certain significant responses. Before additional assessment is done and therapy is begun, it is important for the practitioner to discuss, review, and verify the information to determine the validity of significant responses. The client may have misunderstood instructions, or mechanical errors may be reflected in the information.

As computers become more prevalent in health care systems, especially microcomputers, the use of computer-assisted histories is likely to increase. However, there will always exist situations in which the computer-assisted history is not feasible and a verbal history is necessary. Therefore skill in history taking is, and will continue to be, an important ability of the health care practitioner.

WRITTEN RECORD

The written record is the permanent, legal, and working documentation of what the practitioner sees, hears, and feels during the examination. It serves as the baseline for evaluation of subsequent changes and decisions related to therapy. This record is commonly used by a reader who does not have access to the recorder and is consequently subject to interpretation.

The recorded history must be as objective, clear, complete, and concise as possible. It should be free of recorder bias. In particular, the history is not the place for the recorder to include his or her opinions of possible diagnoses. Other portions of a client's record allow for the recorder to elaborate on hypotheses and plans.

Text continued on p. 41.

EXAMPLE OF HEALTH HISTORY DOCUMENTATION: ILL CLIENT

Client: John Donald Doe

Address: 9037 N. Sheridan St.
           St. Louis, MO 63125

Telephone: 735-1946

Contact: Mrs. Clara Doe (mother)

Address: Same address as above; client will move in with mother after discharge from hospital

Telephone: Same telephone number as above

Birthdate: March 3, 1960   **Sex:** Male   **Race:** White

Religion: Presbyterian (inactive)   **Marital status:** Separated

Social Security number: 097-32-7259

Usual occupation: Offset printer

Present occupation: None; on disability for 1 year

Birthplace: New York, N.Y.

Source of referral: Self

Usual source of health care: Dr. Christopher Ryan
                              1346 W. North Ave.
                              St. Louis, MO 63122

Source and reliability of information: Client; attempted to be cooperative; however, was frequently vague about the nature and time of events

Date of interview: Jan. 9, 1992

Chief complaint

"Pain in the left side of stomach for 2 days."

Present illness
Usual health

This is the fifth Healer's Hospital admission for this 31-year-old white, separated, unemployed male who has been drinking an average of 2 to 3 fifths of hard liquor daily. Total past admissions number 8; one of these has been for gastrointestinal complaints: hemorrhoidectomy. Client is presently on disability income as a result of a diagnosis of tuberculosis (11/90). Also has a history of drug abuse and gastric ulcer.

Chronological story

14 years PTA*	Began drinking heavily and regularly.
7 years PTA	Diagnosed as having a gastric ulcer by Dr. Ryan. Treated by him on an outpatient basis with Maalox and Valium prn. Had x-rays at that time. Has complained of slight to moderate gastric discomfort and food intolerance intermittently since then. Unable to relate the specific frequency or specific characteristics of episodes of illness. States that they are usually accompanied by "hangovers." Generally experiences left upper quadrant (LUQ) discomfort, feelings of hunger, nausea, and vomiting of mucous material 6 to 8 hours after drinking heavily. Drinks heavily 3 to 4 days a week and states symptoms occur approximately 2 times a week. Appetite generally has been good. Meal patterns are erratic. Takes Valium for sleep each night. Drinks 2 to 3 8-oz bottles of Maalox per week. No pattern of follow-up care with Dr. Ryan. Symptoms relieved somewhat with Maalox. Bowel movements have been regular, formed, and brown.
1 day PTA	Had not been drinking the night before. Awoke at approximately 7:00 AM and took several alcoholic drinks (amount approximately 1 cup). An hour after an attempt to drink orange juice experienced nausea and vomiting.
	At 10:00 AM walked to his mother's home (2 blocks). On arriving, experienced a sharp, continuous, nonradiating pain in his upper left abdominal area. Indicates LUQ. The intensity required him to lie down. Position changes provided no relief. A whole bottle of Maalox did not affect the pain, which built in intensity over the next 2 hours. After 2 hours the pain remained constant but was more nagging than sharp. Tried to take some soup and orange juice but immediately vomited it. At 2:00 PM vomited again, and this time there were red streaks in the vomitus, which was a green, thick material. (Exact amount of vomitus or blood streaks unknown.)

*PTA, prior to admission.

Continued.

EXAMPLE OF A RECORDED HEALTH HISTORY: ILL CLIENT—cont'd

Throughout the remainder of the afternoon and early evening, took 5 mg Valium for a total of 4 times. Obtained no relief; pain remained nagging and continuous. Was able to walk with no increase in discomfort but felt most comfortable lying down.

At bedtime took a sleeping pill but states it did not really help him sleep. Spent a fitful night, and the pain persisted with increased intensity. States he took his temperature at midnight and had a fever of 102° F.

Date of admission   Rose at 9:00 AM and was driven to Dr. Ryan's office but found it closed. Then came directly to Healer's outpatient clinic, where he was seen and admitted.

Negative information   Important to "rlo"

Denies unusual weakness, chills, or fever before the onset of symptoms. Denies injury to the abdomen, unusual activity or exercise, pain in other locations, diarrhea, constipation, change in stools, jaundice, ascites, flatulence, hemorrhoids, rectal bleeding, or dysphagia.

Relevant family history

The only significant family history (hx) for a serious, persistent gastrointestinal disorder was a maternal uncle who was a heavy drinker and who died of stomach cancer at age 40.

Disability assessment

Client states that he has not felt really well in the past 7 years. Has not spent a great deal of time in bed but has not worked regularly and has been either drinking or "hung over" most of the time. Was diagnosed as having tuberculosis, 11/90, and was placed on a disability income plan at that time. This insurance will cover medical expenses.

Past health history
Childhood illnesses

Exact illnesses or dates unknown. Assumes he had all childhood illnesses, for example, measles, mumps, chickenpox; denies hx of rheumatic fever.

Injuries

Client unable to provide exact dates for any of the following:
1. Age 9 (1969). Hit in the eye by rock. States has had a permanent decrease in vision in that eye. No medical care.
2. Age 14 (1974). In an automobile accident. Was hospitalized in Lakeside Hospital, Chicago, for 1 week. Physician unknown. Discharged from hospital with no follow-up required.
3. Age 15 or 16 (1975 or 1976). Fractured right ankle while playing football. Cast applied at Johnson Hospital, Chicago, and was followed in their orthopedic clinic. Apparently healed.
4. Age 18 (1978). Head injury from blow with blunt object, which was thrown. Was unconscious for approximately 30 minutes. Head sutured in emergency room (ER) of Healer's Hospital, St. Louis. No follow-up except for removal of sutures. No sequelae.
5. Age 21 (1981). Stab wound in left shoulder; was attacked and robbed. Sutured in ER of Lakeside Hospital, Chicago. No follow-up except for removal of sutures. No sequelae.

how many? what kind? age group

Hospitalizations

1. Age 10 (1970). Hernia repair at Lakeside Hospital, Chicago. Dates and events of hospitalization unclear.
2. Age 14 (1974). Automobile accident. See item 2 under Injuries.
3. Age 20 (1980). Pneumonia. Under the care of Dr. Warner at St. Peter's Hospital, Chicago. Hospitalized for 2 weeks during December. No follow-up.
4. Age 23 (1983). Surgery for priapism at Lakeside Hospital. Under the care of Dr. Meyer. Follow-up for 1 year after surgery because was unable to obtain an erection. No other complications or current disability.
5. Age 24 (1984). Drug overdose. Under the care of Dr. Ryan, Healer's Hospital, St. Louis. Hospitalized for 2 weeks; was to start methadone maintenance; did not. Dates of stay not known.
6. Age 26 (1986). Drug overdose. Under the care of Dr. Ryan, Healer's Hospital. In the hospital for 1 week. Discharged against medical advice.
7. Age 28 (1988). Drug overdose. Under the care of Dr. Ryan. Hospitalized at Healer's Hospital for 2 weeks (1/83). Discharged on methadone maintenance.

EXAMPLE OF A RECORDED HEALTH HISTORY: ILL CLIENT—cont'd

8. Age 28 (1988). Hemorrhoidectomy. Under the care of Dr. Ryan and Dr. Jones, Healer's Hospital. Hospitalized 1 week. No complications; 1 follow-up visit.

Operations

See Hospitalizations for details.
1. Age 10 (1970). Hernia repair.
2. Age 23 (1983). Correction of priapism.
3. Age 28 (1988). Hemorrhoidectomy.

Other major illnesses

1. Age 23 (1983). Diagnosed as having gastric ulcer by Dr. Ryan after an outpatient evaluation including x-rays. See Present Illness section for follow-up and sequelae.
2. Age 30 (1990). Tuberculosis diagnosed and treated by staff of the St. Louis Health Department as an outpatient. Medications for 1 year. Off medications for the past 3 months. Followed with yearly x-rays and evaluation.

Current health information

Allergies

None known. Denies allergies to penicillin, other drugs, foods, or environmental components; has had at least 3 courses of penicillin.

Immunizations

Unknown.

Habits

Cigarettes—smokes 1 pack a day. Habit regular since age 12.
Hard drugs—all types, including heroin. 1984-1988 had a "$90-a-day-habit." No recent history.
Alcohol—started to drink heavily at age 16. Drinking decreased during period of drug addiction. Has been drinking 2 to 3 fifths of hard liquor a day for the past 2 years.
Coffee—drinks 6 to 7 cups a day.

Medications

Maalox—for ulcer prn with varied dosage since 1983. Prescribed by Dr. Ryan. Client states he uses 2 to 3 8-oz bottles a week.
Valium—10 mg prn for ulcer and nervousness since 1983. Client states he uses at least 1 to 2 tablets a day.
Methadone—40 mg daily for 6 months, 1988. Given through drug abuse program.
Streptomycin—IM daily, dose? For TB, 11/90 to 9/91.
INH—tid for TB, 11/90 to 9/91.
Salve—name unknown, a nonprescription drug; topically every day for scaling skin on soles of feet; since approximately 8/89.
Magnesium citrate—for constipation approximately once (× 1) monthly or less frequently; prescribed by self. Uses 1 tbsp prn.
Sleeping pill—prn. Name and dose unknown. Prescribed by Dr. Ryan; 1 every night.

Exercise patterns

Largely sedentary due to life-style and low energy. No regularly scheduled exercise.

Sleep patterns

Sleeps about 7 to 8 hours during a 24-hour period. Often patterns are irregular because of alcohol consumption.

Family health history

Maternal and paternal grandparents deceased. Ages at death and causes of death unknown. Denies family hx of diabetes, blood disorders, arteriosclerosis, gout, obesity, coronary artery disease, tuberculosis, cancer, hypertension, epilepsy, kidney disease, or allergic disorders. Uncertain about health history of aunts and uncles.
  Mother—age 52; alive and well.
  Father—deceased, age 50, 1975; cause unknown.
  Siblings—no maternal miscarriages.

Continued.

EXAMPLE OF A RECORDED HEALTH HISTORY: ILL CLIENT—cont'd

    1. ♀ Age 27; alive and well.
    2. ♂ Age 20; deceased 1988; drug overdose.
    3. ♀ Age 21; alive and well.
    4. ♂ Age 19; alive and well.
Children
    1. ♂ Age 10; alive and well.
    2. ♂ Age 7; alive and well.
Wife—age 31; obese, otherwise well.

Review of physical systems
General

Chronically ill, white male adult; usual wt about 176 lb. Reports approximately 10-lb wt loss over the past 3- to 4-month period. Feels this is a result of not eating when drinking heavily. States he has felt a generalized fatigue and malaise for over 1 year, since onset of TB, but denies requiring daily naps or extra sleep. States he cannot exercise due to fatigue. Denies chills (other than those associated with present illness), sweats, and seizures.

Skin, hair, and nails

Denies lesions, color changes, ecchymoses, petechiae, texture changes, unusual odors, or infections. Pruritus; soles of feet dry and scaling for 6 months; condition stable (using nonprescription salve, name unknown). States he has had small cracks at corners of mouth for 1 month. Denies cold sores. States hair breaks off and falls out but denies patchy alopeica. Denies brittle, cracking, or peeling nails. States bites nails. Has 1 birthmark on upper back but is not aware of any change in size or color.

Head and face

Denies pain, headache, dizziness, or vertigo. Hx of injury with blow to forehead. Reports frequent losses of consciousness after drinking; duration unknown, probably 1 to 8 hours.

Eyes

Has worn corrective lenses since 1970, age 10. States rt eye 20/20, lt eye 20/50. Hx of 1 eye injury, age 9. States visual acuity decreased after injury. Denies pain, infection, watery or itching eyes, diplopia, blurred vision, glaucoma, cataracts, decreased peripheral vision. Last ophthalmological examination 2 years ago.

Ears

Denies hearing loss. Denies discharge, pain, irritation, or ringing in ears. States he was "cut in a fight" on rt auricle. Cleans ears with a toothpick.

Nose and sinuses

Denies sinus pain, postnasal drip, discharge, epistaxis, soreness, excessive sneezing, or obstructed breathing. Denies injuries. States he has approximately 2 colds a year. Olfaction not good; attributes this to smoking.

Oral cavity

Complains of frequent dryness in mouth and cracking of lips and tongue. No false teeth. Gums bleed frequently. Denies hoarseness, pain, odor, frequent sore throats, voice change. Dental care infrequent. Brushes teeth "occasionally."

Neck

Denies pain, stiffness, or limitation of range of motion. Denies masses.

Nodes

Denies enlarged or tender nodes in neck, axillary, or inguinal area.

Breasts

Denies surgery, pain, masses, or discharge.

EXAMPLE OF A RECORDED HEALTH HISTORY: ILL CLIENT—cont'd

Chest and respiratory system

Denies pain, wheezing, asthma, or bronchitis. Hx of pneumonia, age 20 (see Hospitalizations). Denies shortness of breath or dyspnea. Sleeps on 2 pillows but is not dependent on them for breathing. Hx of TB, 1990-1991. Last chest x-ray on present admission, negative. States he had 1 episode of hemoptysis, 1983, associated with his ulcer. Details of this unclear. States he has "smoker's cough" (dry cough in the morning) but denies sputum.

Cardiovascular system

Denies chest pain, coronary artery disease, rheumatic fever, or heart murmur. Denies hypertension, palpitations, cyanosis, or diagnosis of cardiac disorder. States he has occasional slight edema in rt ankle.

Gastrointestinal system

See PI. Also see Hospitalizations re: hemorrhoidectomy. Appetite good. Denies melena, clay-colored stools, or diarrhea. Takes laxative, magnesium citrate, approximately × 1 monthly or less for constipation. Denies jaundice. Reports decreased appetite with alcohol intake but denies specific intolerance to any food.

Genitourinary system

Denies bladder or kidney infections, urgency, frequency, hesitancy, painful micturition, incontinence, nocturia, or polyuria, hx of VD. Denies testicular pain. Hx of surgery for priapism with inability to have erection for 1 year following (p) surgery. No dysfunction at present. States sex life is "fair." Alcohol decreases "urge." Heterosexual. No homosexual encounters.

Extremities

Hx of fractured rt ankle, age 15 or 16. Reports swelling of ankle without pain. Denies varicose veins, thrombophlebitis, joint pain, stiffness, swelling, gout, arthritis, limitation of movement, or color changes.

Back

Denies pain, stiffness, limitation of movement, or disk disease.

Central nervous system

Reports loss of consciousness (1978) following blow to head; duration approximately 30 minutes. Denies clumsiness of movement, weakness, paralysis, tremor, neuralgia, or paresthesia. States he is a "nervous" person but denies hx of nervous breakdown. Hx of drug and alcohol abuse. States he will periodically (every 2 to 3 weeks) have spontaneous jerky movement of legs during rest. There are 4 to 5 movements in each episode. This has never occurred while legs were bearing weight. Denies disorientation or memory disorders. Denies seizures or epilepsy. "Passes out" frequently after heavy alcohol ingestion and sleeps for 5 to 6 hours. Wakes with headache and nausea.

Hematopoietic system

Denies bleeding, bruising, blood transfusion, or exposure to x-rays or toxic agents.

Endocrine system

Denies diabetes, thyroid disease, or intolerance to heat or cold. Growth has been within normal range.

Review of sociological system
Family relationships

Has been separated from wife for 6 to 7 months and is in the process of being divorced. States his marital problems do not interfere with seeing his children. Plans to move to his mother's home when discharged from hospital. States relationships with his family of origin are good.

Occupational history

Offset printer since 1986. Presently unemployed. Was advised not to work for 6 months when tuberculosis was diagnosed and has not been "able to get back to work." States he liked that occupation but expresses no urgency to return to work.

Economic status

On disability income because of tuberculosis and need to rest. States he does not have trouble making ends meet on present income. Expresses no concern for financial status of wife and children who are on "welfare" and being assisted by wife's family.

Continued.

EXAMPLE OF A RECORDED HEALTH HISTORY: ILL CLIENT—cont'd

Daily profile

Lives alone in a room. States he spends time during the day at home or with friends, drinking. Has no special hobbies or activities to occupy time. Has habit of heavy daily drinking. States "I just hang around all day." Does do some spur-of-the-moment traveling. Weekdays are no different than weekends. States he dropped out of college because of disinterest.

Educational level

States he is "smart enough." Dropped out of college after 2 years because of disinterest. States he has no aspiration except to "get by in life."

Patterns of health care

Has maintained relationship with same physician for the episodic care for the last 10 years. Does return for periodic examinations and follow-up when symptoms "scare him."

Environmental data

Birthplace—New York, N.Y. No travel outside of USA; no armed forces duty.
Home—Plans to move to his mother's home. Will share the 5-bedroom residence with his mother and 2 siblings. Neighborhood is residential; describes it as "beautiful."

Review of psychological system
Cognitive abilities

Oriented to present events. Has fairly adequate vocabulary. Has a fair to poor memory. Cannot recall details of some important events. No history of psychiatric treatment.

Response to illness

States he "quit" drinking when he entered the hospital and plans to abstain in the future. Verbalizes that his health problems are his own fault and that he will die soon if he does not resolve them. States illness does not bother him except when "it gets out of control." Definition of health entails being able to play baseball again.

Response to care

States he has sometimes not followed medical advice because of fear or because drugs or alcohol did not allow him to think "straight." "People have been nice to me." States all care has been "OK."

Cultural implications

Inactive Presbyterian at present but is concerned about conflict with religious beliefs and life-style. Fourth-generation American.

Developmental data

Adult male who has had problems with interpersonal relationships in his marriage. Has demonstrated drug and alcohol abuse since entering adulthood. Does not express concern regarding his inability to work; has abandoned his college attendance. Immediate plans for the future involve moving in with his mother and trying to stop drinking. Speaks of his children as playmates; expresses few fathering needs or activities.

Nutritional data

States he does not eat or has erratic meal patterns when drinking heavily and must build his tolerance to food by taking liquids such as soup or juices after drinking. States he does eat 3 complete meals daily when not drinking. Includes foods from the four basic food groups.

EXAMPLE OF HEALTH HISTORY DOCUMENTATION: WELL CLIENT

Client: Mary Rose Doe

Address: 1056 N. East St.
St. Louis, MO 63047

Telephone: 278-9274

Contact: Mrs. Elsa Smith (mother)

Address: 3496 Oak St.
St. Louis, MO 63047

Telephone: 926-8711

Birthdate: Feb. 6, 1959   **Sex:** Female   **Race:** Black

Religion: Methodist (active)   **Marital status:** Married

Social Security number: 396-47-8911

Usual occupation: Grade school teacher

Present occupation: Same—Greenwich School

Birthplace: Greenwood, Mississippi

Source of referral: Self

Usual source of health care: St. Louis Health Maintenance Organization
4693 C. Division St.
St. Louis, MO 63044

Source and reliability of information: Client; cooperative, apparently reliable

Date of interview: Dec. 12, 1992

Reason for visit

Annual physical examination; last exam, 11/91

Present health status
Usual health

This is the third St. Louis Health Maintenance Organization (HMO) visit for this 33-year-old black, married, female school teacher who has been in good health for all of her life. Client has been hospitalized twice for the purposes of normal childbirth only. Has no major chronic diseases.

Summary

Client is presently well and requests a physical examination for health maintenance and screening purposes. Is concerned about a strong family history of hypertension and believes that monitoring of her blood pressure status is important.

Also requests a Pap smear and evaluation for continuance of oral contraceptives. Has been taking Ortho-Novum 1 + 50 since the birth of her last child in 1983. Client enrolled in the health plan a year ago.

Past health history
Childhood illnesses

Had rubella, chickenpox—not diagnosed by a physician. Has not had rheumatic fever.

Injuries

None.

Hospitalizations

See obstetrical data in Review of Physical Systems.
1. Age 20 (1979). Childbirth.
2. Age 24 (1983). Childbirth.

Operations

None.

Major illnesses

None.

Continued.

EXAMPLE OF A RECORDED HEALTH HISTORY: WELL CLIENT—cont'd

Current health information

Allergies

None known. Denies allergy to penicillin, other drugs, foods, or environmental components. Has had a course of penicillin (10 d, oral).

Immunizations

Had full series of diphtheria-pertussis-tetanus (DPT) when a preschooler. Had oral polio when an adolescent. No others.

Habits

Cigarettes—smoked 15 cigarettes a day for 5 years (age 20-25).
Hard drugs—none.
Alcohol—drinks 3 to 4 mixed drinks a weekend.
Coffee, tea—drinks approximately 10 cups of coffee a day. Drinks tea rarely.

Medications

Ortho-Novum 1 + 50 oral contraceptive since 1983.
Aspirin (ASA) for headache—takes approximately × 10 gr twice a month.
Milk of magnesia for constipation—takes 1 tablespoon about once a month.
One-a-Day multiple vitamins—takes 1 a day.

Exercise patterns

Attends aerobics classes 2 to 3 times a week during the winter. In summer, walks 3 to 4 times a week.

Sleep patterns

Sleeps 7 to 8 hours a night regularly with occasional naps on weekends.

Family health history

Denies family history of diabetes, blood disorder, gout, obesity, tuberculosis, epilepsy, kidney disease, or gastrointestinal disease.

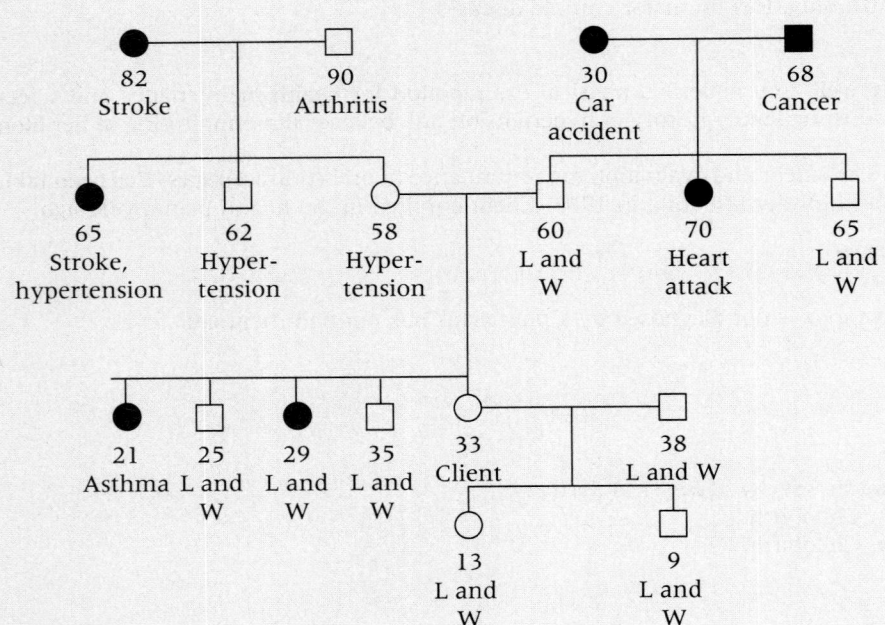

EXAMPLE OF A RECORDED HEALTH HISTORY: WELL CLIENT—cont'd

Review of physical systems

General

Usually well. Usual-minimum-maximum weight: 135-125-160 lb. No recent increase or decrease in weight. Denies fatigue, malaise, chills, sweats, fever, seizures, or fainting. Reports height as 5 ft 6 in.

Skin, hair, and nails

Denies lesions, color change, ecchymoses, masses, petechiae, texture changes, pruritus, sweating, or unusual odors. No alopecia or brittle hair. Denies brittle, cracking, or peeling nails. No birthmarks. Washes hair once a week; does not use dyes.

Head and face

Denies pain, dizziness, vertigo, or history of injury or loss of consciousness.

Eyes

Has worn corrective lenses since age 7; currently wears contact lenses all day. Denies recent change in visual acuity, pain, infection, watery or itching eyes, diplopia, blurred vision, glaucoma, cataracts, or decreased peripheral vision. Last ophthalmoscopic examination, 2 years ago.

Ears

Denies hearing loss, discharge, pain, irritation, or ringing in ears. Cleans ears with cotton-tipped applicator.

Nose and sinuses

States she has sinus pain, congestion, and subsequent nasal discharge several times each winter. Takes Contac prn (approximately 1 q 12 hours × 3 d) for each episode of rhinitis; gets relief. Denies epistaxis, soreness, excessive sneezing, obstructed breathing, or injuries. States olfaction is good.

Oral cavity

Visits a dentist every 6 months for cleaning and examination. Brushes teeth twice a day. Denies toothache, lesions, soreness, bleeding of gums, coated tongue, disturbance of taste, hoarseness, or frequent sore throat.

Neck

Denies pain, stiffness, limitation of movement, or masses.

Nodes

Denies enlarged or tender nodes in neck, axillary, or inguinal area.

Breasts

Denies masses, pain, tenderness, or discharge. Examines breasts monthly, right after menses.

Chest and respiratory system

Denies pain, wheezing, shortness of breath, dyspnea, hemoptysis, or cough. Denies hx of asthma, pneumonia, or bronchitis. Has yearly chest x-ray, required for work in the schools.

Cardiovascular system

Denies precordial pain, palpitations, cyanosis, edema, or intermittent claudication. Frequently bicycles in summer and downhill skis in winter. Walks 2 miles a day. Denies diagnosis of heart murmur, hypertension, coronary artery disease, or rheumatic fever.

Gastrointestinal system

Denies history of gastrointestinal (GI) disease. Appetite good. Bowels active daily, stools are always brown. Denies pain, constipation, diarrhea, flatulence, vomiting, hemorrhoids, hernias, jaundice, pyrosis, or bleeding. Has never had GI x-rays.

Continued.

EXAMPLE OF A RECORDED HEALTH HISTORY: WELL CLIENT—cont'd

Genitourinary system

Denies hx of bladder or kidney infections, hematuria, urgency, frequency, dysuria, incontinence, nocturia, polyuria, or VD. Menses—onset 13 years; frequency, every 26 to 30 days; duration, 5 days; flow, heavy for 3 days, light for 2 days; last menstrual period (LMP), 12/1/92. Denies dysmenorrhea, menorrhagia, metrorrhagic discharge, or pruritus. Last Pap smear, 12/91.

Obstetrical history

1. Sept. 12, 1979. Girl, 6 lb, 8 oz. Vaginal delivery at St. Francis Hospital, St. Louis. Prenatal, intrapartum, and postpartum course normal for mother and baby.
2. Oct. 9, 1983. Boy 7 lb, 2 oz. Vaginal delivery at St. Francis Hospital, St. Louis. Prenatal, intrapartum, and postpartum course normal for mother and baby.

Sexual history

Age at first intercourse was 17 years. Enjoys intercourse with husband—no dyspareunia and able to achieve satisfactory orgasm most of the time. Using oral birth control medication. Not sure yet if she will have another child. Will consider sterilization when family is complete.

Extremities

No past problems. Denies deformities, varicose veins, thrombophlebitis, joint pain, stiffness, swelling, gout, arthritis, limitation of movement, color changes, or temperature changes.

Back

No past problems. Denies pain, stiffness, or limitation of movement; no history of disk disease.

Central nervous system

No past problems. Denies loss of consciousness, clumsiness of movement, difficulty with balance, weakness, paralysis, tremor, neuraligia, paresthesia, history of emotional disorders, drug or alcohol dependency, disorientation, memory lapses, or seizures. Speech articulate.

Hematopoietic system

No past problems. Denies excessive bleeding and bruising, blood transfusions, or excessive exposure to x-rays or toxic agents. Blood type A, Rh positive.

Endocrine system

Denies history of diabetes or thyroid disease, polyuria, polydipsia, polydysplasia, intolerance to heat or cold, or hirsutism.

Review of sociological system
Family relationships

Lives in own home with husband and 2 children. Husband is a school teacher also; couple shares finances, child-rearing, and housekeeping responsibilities. Client's parents live ½ mile away, and relationships are described as "good." Couple has several close friends; also, siblings are in frequent contact. No recent family crisis or change.

Occupational history

Has been a grade school teacher for 5 years. No other jobs. Holds bachelor's and master's degrees and feels secure that she can retain her job as long as she wants it. Enjoys children and states job is very satisfying.

Economic status

Client and husband achieve a combined gross income of over $60,000 a year. Feels this is very adequate. Has hospitalization insurance.

Daily profile

During the week, works 8 AM to 3 PM. Returns home around 3:30 and works until 5 PM on school work. Then cooks dinner and interacts with family. Has meetings 1 or 2 evenings a week. Weekends, client and husband usually have 1 evening out with friends, to movie or concert. Family attends church each Sunday. Client is involved with photography as a hobby.

EXAMPLE OF A RECORDED HEALTH HISTORY: WELL CLIENT—cont'd

Educational level

Highest degree attained is the master's degree. Obtains most of health knowledge by reading.

Patterns of health care

Has always had a primary care provider. Cared for by Dr. Richard Smith, a family practitioner until first pregnancy. Then seen regularly by Dr. Janice Lawson for obstetric and gynecologic care. Family enrolled in HMO a year ago; all family members are being seen here. Dental care regular and at the HMO.

Environmental data

Birthplace—Greenwood, Miss. Grew up in Trenton, N.J.
Home—family lives in their own 8-room home in a residential St. Louis neighborhood. Client describes home as comfortable. Has lived there for 10 years.
Community—community is middle income, integrated, consisting primarily of young professional families.
Work—teaches fourth grade in a community school. States that the work situation is fairly good. School is in good condition, and classes are small. A recent stress is a new assistant principal with whom client does not get along. May consider transfer to another school.

Review of psychological system
Cognitive abilities

Oriented to time, place, and person ($\times$ 3). Is articulate, asks questions, has a good memory. Able to understand directions.

Response to illness

States she has never been seriously ill, so does not know what personal response would be. Feels she is "too busy" to be ill for any length of time. Uses the resources of HMO for preventive and therapeutic needs of self and family.

Response to care

States she enjoys encounters with health care providers. States she usually follows through on the advice that is given. Feels that the services of the HMO are adequate to meet her family care needs and she has been very satisfied with the care to date.

Cultural implications

Client states she and her family are involved in a racially integrated community. She grew up in a predominantly black northern community. Cannot identify any way in which her black culture would especially affect her response to illness or therapy in the case of illness. Active Methodist; believes that religious concerns would influence her response to illness and treatment.

Developmental data

Adult female; wife, mother, and career teacher.

Nutritional data

Diet adequate; high in fats and carbohydrates. Has no food intolerances.
Usual breakfast—toast with butter, fried egg, orange juice and coffee with cream.
Usual lunch—eats with school children; consists of meat, 1 vegetable, 1 carbohydrate, dessert, and beverage.
Dinner—meat (beef, chicken, or pork), salad, 1 vegetable, potato or bread, dessert, and coffee with cream.
Snacks—may have cheese and crackers or peanuts in the evening.

In addition, the practitioner should integrate the client's responses in an accurate but objective way. This can be accomplished in one of two ways: (1) by paraphrasing the client, using statements such as "States he had the same symptoms 4 years ago" or "Denies chest pain," or (2) by quoting the client directly, for example, "The pain was so severe, I fell back into the chair I had just gotten up from."

Because most health histories are read by many health care providers over time, the clarity of the presentation is important. A clear presentation is often difficult for the beginning health historian to achieve, but feedback about written histories from colleagues and instructors can assist in identifying strengths and deficits in this area. Most beginners must pay specific attention to chronology and the quality and quantity of symptoms.

The written record should be a complete history of the practitioner-client encounter. It should be specific enough for the reader to determine clearly what questions were asked, what areas of examination were covered, and the results of the interview and examination. An entry such as "Eyes—negative" or "Eyes—normal" does not supply any information regarding what questions were asked about the eyes. The range of "normal" is wide, and any change in condition, even within the range of normal, may be significant for an individual client.

Although the written record must be complete, it should also be concise. A reader should be able to locate and read regional entries easily. A verbose and disorganized record may be even less effective than an incomplete one because its appearance may frustrate the busy reader, who simply will not read it. The record does not need to be composed of complete sentences. In fact, the use of clear phrases can save both time and space.

Two examples of documented health histories are presented on pp. 31-41. One is an example of a history taken from an ill client being admitted to a hospital. The other is an example of a history taken from a well client. An example of a documented physical examination is included in Chapter 27.

GLOSSARY

acute Characterized by sharpness and severity; usually involves rapid onset and short duration.

amenorrhea Absence of menstruation.

anesthesia State characterized by loss of sensation.

anuria Absence of excretion of urine.

anxiety Motor tension, autonomic hyperactivity, apprehension, or hyperattentiveness.

ascites Abnormal intraperitoneal accumulation of fluid containing large amounts of protein and electrolytes.

behavior Any observable, recordable, and measurable move, response, or act (verbal or nonverbal) of an individual.

caudad Toward the tail or end of the body; away from the head.

cephalad Toward the head; away from the tail or end.

cognitive Pertaining to mental processes of knowing, thinking, learning, and judging.

constipation Infrequent or difficult evacuation of feces; often associated with drying and hardening of the stool.

cramp Involuntary, painful skeletal muscle contraction.

crisis Sudden change in the course of a disease.

cyanosis Bluish discoloration of the skin and mucous membranes caused by an excess of deoxygenated hemoglobin in the blood or a structural defect in the hemoglobin molecule.

diarrhea Increased frequency and liquid content of fecal evacuation.

diplopia Double vision.

disease Abnormality of structure or function that has a single pathogenic mechanism and a predictable course.

dysarthria Difficult, poorly articulated speech.

dyschezia Painful defecation.

dysmenorrhea Pain associated with menstruation.

dyspareunia An abnormal condition in women in which sexual intercourse is accompanied by pain.

dyspepsia Impairment of the ability to digest food, especially discomfort after eating a meal.

dysphagia Difficult or painful swallowing.

dysuria Difficult or painful urination.

ecchymosis Discoloration of an area of the skin or mucous membranes caused by the extravasation of blood into the subcutaneous tissues as a result of trauma to the underlying blood vessels or fragility of the vessel walls.

edema Abnormal increase in the quantity of interstitial fluid.

enuresis Involuntary urination.

epistaxis Bleeding or hemorrhage from the nose.

exophthalmos Abnormal condition characterized by a marked protrusion of the eyeballs.

fever Elevation of the body temperature above normal for a given individual. Also called **pyrexia.**

flatulence Excessive amount of gas in the gastrointestinal tract.

goiter Increase in size of the thyroid gland.

health history Comprehensive body of information obtained from the client and other select sources. Includes information on the client as a whole, health/illness status (past and present), social and physical environment, and past interactions with health care systems.

hematemesis Vomiting of blood.

hematopoietic Relating to the formation and development of blood cells in the bone marrow.

hematuria Presence of blood in the urine.

hemoptysis Spitting or coughing up of blood from the respiratory tract.

hyperesthesia Abnormally increased sensitivity of the skin or another sense organ.

hypertension Persistent elevation of blood pressure.

incontinence Failure of control of excretory functions.

intermittent claudication *Claudication* is a weakness of the legs accompanied by cramplike pains in the calves caused by poor circulation to the leg muscles. *Intermittent claudication* is a form of this disorder that is manifested only at certain times, usually after an extended period of walking, and is relieved by a period of rest.

jaundice Accumulation of bilirubin-to-serum concentration greater than 2 mg/dl; produces yellow-green to bronze color of skin and itching.

lymphadenopathy Any disorder of the lymph nodes or lymph vessels.

malaise Feeling of general discomfort or uneasiness.

menorrhagia Abnormally heavy or long menstrual periods.

metrorrhagia Uterine bleeding other than that caused by menstruation.

nausea Feeling that vomiting is impending.

nocturia Excessive urination at night.

oliguria Abnormally decreased urine secretion (less than 400 ml/24 hr).

orthopnea Shortness of breath that is relieved by sitting upright.

otalgia Earache.

palpitation Forcible pulsation of the heart and arteries that is perceptible to the client.

paresis Slight or incomplete paralysis; weakness.

paresthesia Abnormal or perverted sensation; may include burning, itching, pain, or a feeling of electric shock.

perception Awareness of objects and relations that follows stimulation of peripheral sense organs.

petechiae Tiny purple or red spots that appear on the skin as a result of minute hemorrhages within the dermal or submucosal layers.

phobia Persistent and exaggerated fear of a particular object or situation.

photophobia Abnormal intolerance of light.

polydipsia Excessive thirst.

polymenorrhea Abnormally frequent menstruation.

polyphagia Excessive ingestion of food.

polyuria Excessive urinary excretion.

pruritus Itching.

pyrexia Fever; elevation of the body temperature above normal for a given individual.

pyrosis Heartburn.

pyuria Presence of pus in the urine.

sign Objective evidence of disease that is perceptible to the examiner.

sinus Hollow in a bone or other tissue.

spasm Involuntary sudden contraction of a muscle or a group of muscles accompanied by pain and interference with function.

stress incontinence Involuntary urination incurred by straining, coughing, or lifting.

stridor Abnormal, high-pitched respiratory sound caused by an obstruction in the trachea or larynx.

symptom Alteration of bodily or mental function as subjectively perceived by the client from basal conditions.

syncope Fainting; temporary unconsciousness.

temporal Of or limited by time.

thrombophlebitis Inflammation of a vein, often accompanied by formation of a clot.

tinnitus Sensation of noise in the ear caused by abnormal stimulation of the auditory apparatus or its afferent pathways; may be described as ringing, buzzing, swishing, roaring, blowing, or whistling.

tremor Involuntary, somewhat rhythmic oscillatory quivering of muscles caused by alternate contraction of opposing groups of muscles. *Cerebellar tremor:* occurs during intentional movement, becoming more pronounced near end of the movement; associated with lesions of the dentate nucleus. *Coarse tremor:* slow rate and high-amplitude movements. *Essential (familial) tremor:* usually begins around age 50 with fine tremors of the hands; aggravated by intentional movement; commonly affects head, jaws, lips, or voice. *Fine tremor:* rapid rate (10 to 20 oscillations/sec) and low-amplitude movements, usually in the fingers and hands. *Moderate tremor:* medium rate and medium-amplitude movements. *Passive tremor:* present at rest; may improve during intentional movement, for example, pill-rolling tremor or Parkinson's disease. *Physiological tremor:* experienced by healthy people in fatigue, cold, and stress. *Toxic tremor:* caused by endogenous (thyrotoxicosis, uremia) or exogenous toxins (alcohol, drugs).

vertigo Illusion of movement, with imagined rotation of oneself (subjective vertigo) or one's surroundings (objective vertigo).

BIBLIOGRAPHY

Bernstein L, Bernstein RS: *Interviewing: a guide for health professionals,* ed 4, Norwalk, Conn, 1985, Appleton-Century-Crofts.

Billings JA, Stoeckle JD: *The clinical encounter: a guide to the medical interview and case presentation,* Chicago, 1989, Mosby–Year Book.

Cohen-Cole SA: *The medical interview: the three function approach,* St Louis, 1991, Mosby–Year Book.

Crouch MA, Thiedke CC: Documentation of family health history in the outpatient medical record, *J Fam Pract* 22:169-174, 1986.

Fuller J, Schaller-Ayers J: *Health assessment: a nursing approach,* Philadelphia, 1990, JB Lippincott.

Gordon M: *Manual of nursing diagnosis: 1993-1994,* St Louis, 1993, Mosby–Year Book.

Gordon M: *Nursing diagnosis: process and application,* ed 2, New York, 1987, McGraw-Hill.

Kraytman M: *The complete patient history,* ed 2, New York, 1991, McGraw-Hill.

Mosby's medical, nursing, and allied health dictionary, ed 3, St Louis, 1990, Mosby–Year Book.

Pagana KD, Pagana TJ: *Mosby's diagnostic and laboratory test reference,* St Louis, 1992, Mosby–Year Book.

Roter DL, Hall JA: Physicians' interviewing styles and medical information obtained from patients, *J Gen Intern Med* 2:325-329, 1987.

Sherwood MJ, and others: *Determining nursing diagnosis through assessment,* Baltimore, 1988, Williams & Wilkins.

US Preventive Services Task Force: *Guide to clinical preventive services: an assessment of the effectiveness of 169 interventions,* Baltimore, 1989, Williams & Wilkins.

U nit II, Holistic Assessment, provides in-depth discussions of aspects of assessment that will assist the reader to assess the individuality of clients in the context of life-styles and cultures and to identify strengths and assets to support interventions. Chapter 3, Developmental Assessment Across the Lifespan, focuses on the assessment and understanding of the client in the context of his/her life roles and relationships. Chapter 4, Nutritional Assessment, provides tools for the efficient measurement of nutritional habits and health. The discussion on Sleep Assessment in Chapter 5 provides a framework for assessing sleep and rest patterns of clients. Chapter 6, Cultural Considerations in Health Assessment, provides an appreciation for the impact of culture on responses to health and illness, physical and psychosocial findings, and responses to health care providers, health care systems, and interventions.

Holistic Assessment

Outline

Developmental Assessment Across the Life Span

PURPOSE OF DEVELOPMENTAL ASSESSMENT

Birth is the first of numerous developmental stages over the life span. From infancy through old age, individuals continue to develop some aspect of who they are. Each person is unique, but his or her individuality occurs within some broadly shared patterns.

The family is a powerful influence on human development. How each person develops through each phase of life and how he or she comes to view the world and interact with the people in it are largely learned within the family. While the focus of this chapter is on the individual, it is always with the acknowledgment that all individuals are part of family units, or substitutes for family units, for at least some significant portion of their lives.

Humans are dynamic, complex, changing beings. They interact continuously with the environment, and their responses to life are highly individualized. Personal growth and development patterns along with social, cultural, economic, and historical forces affect each person's responses to life.

While you are learning to obtain a health history and perform a physical examination, you are focused on assimilating new skills, handling new tools, performing new techniques, remembering lists of questions for the health history, and performing the many components of the physical examination. However, from the onset of this learning process, you need to remember to include a perspective on the individual client as a whole person. The whole person includes the mind, body, and spirit. You cannot assess parts of the person in isolation from each other or from the whole. You must take into account the client's life developmental processes and the phases of growth and maturation through which that person is progressing. Take time to observe the client as a person and to discuss and discover the client's world—her or his interaction and growth within the self, with significant others, and with society at large.

Discussing developmental phases, stages, or crises with the client can provide both of you with a perspective of greater breadth and depth on the client's life situation and its relationship to health or illness. As a health care practitioner, you are in a position to help individuals and families look at the developmental aspects of their lives. Your openness in discussing the life tasks of individuals can help them appreciate the appropriateness and normalcy of their own or their children's growth patterns, changes, behaviors, and feelings. With anticipatory guidance parents can gain a greater appreciation of ways to support their child's development. Your guidance may also assist those who are blocked in their growth to understand and deal with the problem area more effectively. Help clients review their past, compare it with the present, look at progressive phases and intervals, and plan for the future in whatever ways are appropriate and necessary.

You should not expect to learn everything about a client's developmental accomplishments in one or even several interviews. It is a personal story that requires time and trust. Determining the presence of a developmental deficit is sometimes difficult in a busy clinical setting. You may need additional time to focus attention on assessing development, or you may need to seek the assistance of others who specialize in the field.

You can perform some developmental assessment during each encounter with a client of any age. With children, have a parent or primary caregiver present, as this person will be the main source of information. This person's descriptions are essential because limited opportunities exist to observe a child's behavior and responses in the clinical setting. In addition, keep in mind that the behavior demonstrated may not be typical because of stress from the unfamiliar environment or the particular problems related to the child's illness.

Record developmental assessment data in the health history.

For further information on the developmental changes of children and older adults, see Chapter 24: Pediatric Clients and Chapter 25: Aging Clients.

STAGES OF DEVELOPMENT

Developmental stages and categories are used for purposes of organization. In life, such stages are not totally distinct or exclusive. During particular phases, certain aspects of growth may be more prominent, but many overlap. Some of the early work done on the development of children by Jean Piaget and of children and adults by Erik Erikson was based on a "stage" approach. One stage and its accomplishments was followed by another, and moving from one to the other was premised on the completion of tasks at the earlier level. Piaget asserted that biological growth combines with children's interaction with the environment to take them up a development staircase, step by step, with each step signaling an increase in complexity of the child's thinking. He believed that changes in memory, perceptual skills, learning ability, and other aspects of mental development all occurred in this fashion. More recently it has been argued that more variations in children's growth can be observed and that some children develop in one area much more quickly than in others. See the box on page 49 for general characteristics of growth and development.

SOME GENERAL CHARACTERISTICS OF GROWTH AND DEVELOPMENT

1. Growth and development are cyclical. Children tend to grow in spurts, then level off for periods. Adolescents tend to have cycles of outward activity and then inner reflection. Adults also experience periods of greater outward involvement and inner orientation.
2. Growth and development continue throughout the life cycle. From birth until death, some aspect of the complex human being is changing. This process of growth and development is both universal and unique and includes physical, emotional, psychological, social, and cognitive components. It ranges from changes that are slow, subtle, and often elusive to those that occur with astonishing rapidity.
3. All aspects of the growth and development of an individual are interrelated. The physical, mental, social, emotional, sexual, moral, and spiritual components of the self are all a part of the complex matrix that is the whole person.
4. There are periods of readiness for certain developmental tasks. During these periods a necessary degree of maturation is present for the behavior to occur. If the appropriate environment or stimulus is not present, the behavior may not develop, may be delayed, or may occur in a defective way.

SELECTED THEORIES OF HUMAN DEVELOPMENT

The developmental aspect of infancy and childhood has received much attention and study since the late 1800s. A considerable amount of literature has surfaced on these phases, although much still remains to be studied and understood. Of more recent vintage are the studies and theories about adolescence and old age. The most recent literature on human development is material on the age span between youth and old age, middle adulthood.

The theories of development briefly described here include:

Psychosocial development: Erik Erikson
Intellectual development: Jean Piaget
Development of sexuality: Sigmund Freud
The work of Carl Jung and Carol Gilligan is also briefly discussed.

TABLE 3-1

Erikson's Eight Stages of Development

Stage	Task	Threat
Infant	Trust	Mistrust
Toddler	Autonomy	Shame and doubt
Preschooler	Initiative	Guilt
School age	Industry	Inferiority
Adolescent	Identity	Identity diffusion
Early adulthood	Intimacy	Isolation
Middle adulthood	Generativity	Self-absorption
Late adulthood	Integrity	Despair

Erik Erikson—Psychosocial Development

Erikson is one of the theorists who suggested a developmental framework for the entire life span (1963). His framework is outlined here and is incorporated into the discussion at the various stages of growth used in this chapter. Erikson suggested eight developmental stages and for each stage identified a central task and a threat to the accomplishment of that task. These central tasks are called developmental "crises," not in the sense of an emergency but rather to designate a necessary turning point when development must move one way or another. Each crisis is marked by a pair of opposite qualities that the person must resolve and integrate in order to proceed with ego development. Dealing with each task at a particular stage of development provides the basis for progress to the next stage. As a person faces each challenge, she or he assumes both increased vulnerability and increased potential. A new strength emerges that contributes to further development. These stages and tasks are shown in Table 3-1.

Jean Piaget—Intellectual Development

Piaget's theory concerns intellectual, or cognitive, development. He noted certain signposts of development that indicate maturation and growth. The newborn perceives the world as a vague mass, but gradually integrates the various sensory inputs from sight, sound, touch, taste, and smell. The young child does not understand that objects continue to exist though they cannot be seen, but gradually learns that objects have constancy—they are there even when they cannot be seen. The use of symbols and language to represent reality is another developmental milestone in childhood. A young schoolchild gains the cognitive ability to focus on more than one aspect of a situation and to realize that although things may change superficially, they remain the same. Piaget described four major stages of intellectual development. These stages are listed in the box on page 50.

PIAGET'S STAGES OF COGNITIVE DEVELOPMENT

1. Sensorimotor stage: age 0 to 2, primary concern is learning about physical objects.
2. Preoperational stage: age 2 to 7, primary concern is with symbols in language, dreams, and fantasy.
3. Concrete operational stage: age 7 to 11, primary concern is with the abstract world, mastering numbers and relationships and how to reason about them.
4. Formal operational stage: age 11 to 15, primary concern is logical thought, thinking about one's own thoughts as well as those of others.

Sigmund Freud—Development of Sexuality

The sex of a child is genetically determined, but the development of human sexuality is influenced by many aspects of life: physical, mental, emotional, and sociocultural. Sexuality is a large dimension of life related to many aspects of total personality functioning. It is

FREUD'S STAGES OF SEXUAL DEVELOPMENT

1. Oral stage: infancy through 18 months. During this period, the oral region (the sensory area of the mouth, lips, and tongue) provides the greatest sensual satisfaction. Sucking and swallowing reduce tension and provide pleasure.
2. Anal stage: age 18 months to 3 years. During this period, the greatest amount of sensual pleasure is obtained from the anal and urethral areas. Toilet training is a source of tension between child and parent.
3. Phallic stage: age 3 to 5 years. The region of greatest sensual pleasure is the genital region. The Oedipal/Electra complex occurs in the later part of the phallic stage. During this stage the child "loves" the parent of the opposite sex. The parent of the same sex is considered a rival.
4. Latency stage: age 6 to 12 years. At the beginning of the latency stage the child is resolving the Oedipal/Electra conflict, so this is a phase of sexual latency. During this period, children form close relationships with others of their own age and sex. They direct energy to physical and intellectual quests.
5. Genital stage: puberty to adulthood. Increased hormones stimulate sexual development. Sexual urges reawaken but are now directed outside the family.

expressed through cultural beliefs, attitudes, stereotypes, feelings, self-image, and body image.

Freud thought that sexual feelings were present from infancy, changing from one form to another into adulthood. Freud's four stages of psychosexual development center on the early years of life. At each stage, instinctual sexual energy (libido) is invested in different areas of the body. This determines how the individual interacts with other people. The box on the lower left lists Freud's stages of sexual development.

Freud's theory has had a strong and lasting impact in the field of psychology. Many now feel, however, that while his focus on the sexual aspect of development was important, it was also narrow and limited and that human psychological and sexual development need to be considered in the broader context of the whole person.

Carl Jung

Jung focused his extensive psychoanalytic work on the adult years of life. Jung's first developmental stage, extending from about 18 to 35 or 40, was called "youth." He saw this stage as marked by individual development, involvement in the outside world, and investment in a family. During this period the individual's task is to give up the world of childhood while broadening one's horizons and engaging in the task-oriented and achievement-oriented work of the world. Jung saw the second half of life beginning at age 35 or 40, with the change in orientation occurring slowly, developing largely through the unconscious. During this time individuals become increasingly oriented to the inner life through introversion and self-reflection. Throughout life there is a drive toward individuation of the self and an effort to develop those aspects of the personality that have been underdeveloped, such as the qualities of extroversion, introversion, intuition, or thinking.

Carol Gilligan

Recent studies focusing on men's or women's development across the life span have provoked controversy over the applicability of previous theories to both sexes. Many of the theories on human growth and development were developed based on research or observations of males only, or with only a small sample of females. In her study of the psychosocial processes by which women develop, Carol Gilligan takes the position that women's development does not match men's development because women's identity formation takes place in a context of an ongoing relationship with the mother rather than separation from the mother. The female child experiences attachment to the mother that does not require separation for self and sexual identity that the male child requires. Masculine identity becomes defined through separation and is threatened by intimacy, while feminine identity is defined through attachment and is threatened by separation. This leads to life experiences where males tend to have greater difficulty with relationships, while females have greater difficulty with individuation. Gilligan notes that when maturity is equated with personal autonomy, a focus on relationships appears to be a weakness rather than a human strength, and she suggests that both forces must be in balance as the person moves toward maturity.

This chapter organizes developmental assessment around eight major life phases based on age:

Infancy: Birth to 12 months

Toddler years: 1 to 3 years

Preschooler: 3 to 6 years

School age: 6 to 12 years

Adolescence: approximately 12 to 20 years

Young adulthood: approximately 20 to 30-35 years

Middle adulthood: approximately 30-35 to 65-70 years

Late adulthood: approximately 65-70 to 95+ years

Characteristics of each stage are described. The length of the chronological divisions increases with each division, ranging from months for infants to decades for adults.

For infants through the school age child, developmental characteristics in the categories of physical, cognitive, and psychosocial development are discussed. For adolescence through late adulthood, the developmental tasks are added to the other three categories.

TOOLS FOR DEVELOPMENTAL ASSESSMENT

Numerous tools are available to assess child development and a few to assess certain aspects of adult development. Some of the more commonly used ones are presented here. These tools assess various components including gross motor skills, fine motor skills, personal-social behaviors, and language abilities. As a health care practitioner, you will not be administering intelligence tests. Special training in the administration of each tool and careful adherence to standardized procedures are necessary to obtain valid results.

For adolescents through adults you can accomplish much assessment by talking with the client in an accepting, unrushed manner. Use nonthreatening questions about thoughts, feelings, work, family, and other activities, accompanied by an attitude of active listening to encourage clients to share significant information about themselves regarding their own development tasks and accomplishments.

Screening Tools Used with Infants and Children

Screening tools assist in determining an infant's or child's progress in accomplishing age-appropriate developmental tasks. For further information on childhood assessment tools, see Chapter 24.

The Denver II (1989 revision of the Denver Developmental Screening Test [DDST]) (Figure 3-1). The Denver II is a screening tool commonly used to assess developmental level from 1 month to 6 years of age. It is easy to administer, useful for determining developmental level, and helpful in providing guidance to parents. A series of developmental tasks are used to determine whether a child's development is within the normal range. The Denver II provides a developmental profile of the individual child in four areas: personal-social, fine motor-adaptive, language, and gross motor skills. If development in any of these four areas is questionable when compared with normal standards, refer the child for an in-depth evaluation. Children who have questionable or abnormal scores on the Denver II are at risk for developing later problems in school regardless of their intelligence. The Denver II is a *screening* tool; it is *not* a *diagnostic* tool, nor is it an intelligence test.

Denver Prescreening Developmental Questionnaire (PDQ). The PDQ (box on pp. 54-55) is a brief test answered by the parent. It identifies those children who will need a more thorough screening with the Denver II (or the DDST). It assesses the same four categories as the Denver II, and it can be administered quickly and easily. The questionnaire consists of 97 questions, divided according to the child's age. The parent is asked to answer the questions from the appropriate age grouping.

Denver Articulation Screening Examination (DASE). The DASE (box on pp. 56-57) is used to detect articulation disorders in children age 2 ½ to 7 years. It assesses a child's ability to imitate word sounds, which provides information on a child's speech development. The child is asked to repeat 30 different sound elements: the tester listens for errors in articulation.*

Goodenough-Harris Drawing Test. This test is used to screen children between 3 and 12 years. Children are requested to make three drawings: a man, a woman, and a representation of the self. The interpretation is

*Further information on the Denver II, PDQ, DASE, and other developmental screening and training materials can be obtained from Denver Developmental Materials, Inc.
P. O. Box 6919
Denver, CO 80206-0919
(303) 355-4729

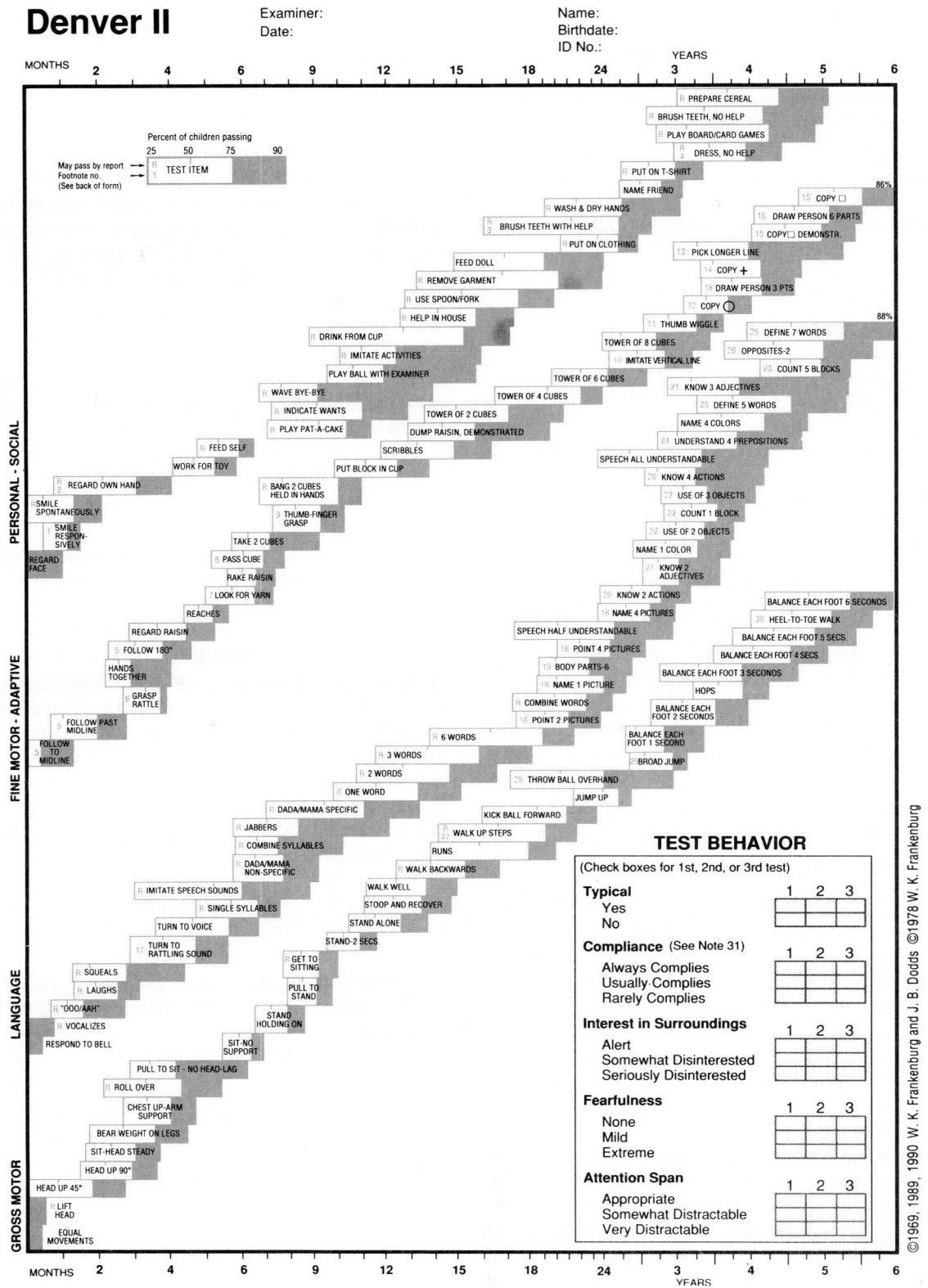

FIGURE 3-1 The Denver II Developmental Screening Test.

DIRECTIONS FOR ADMINISTRATION

1. Try to get child to smile by smiling, talking or waving. Do not touch him/her.
2. Child must stare at hand several seconds.
3. Parent may help guide toothbrush and put toothpaste on brush.
4. Child does not have to be able to tie shoes or button/zip in the back.
5. Move yarn slowly in an arc from one side to the other, about 8" above child's face.
6. Pass if child grasps rattle when it is touched to the backs or tips of fingers.
7. Pass if child tries to see where yarn went. Yarn should be dropped quickly from sight from tester's hand without arm movement.
8. Child must transfer cube from hand to hand without help of body, mouth, or table.
9. Pass if child picks up raisin with any part of thumb and finger.
10. Line can vary only 30 degrees or less from tester's line.
11. Make a fist with thumb pointing upward and wiggle only the thumb. Pass if child imitates and does not move any fingers other than the thumb.

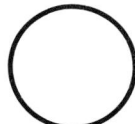      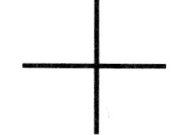   

12. Pass any enclosed form. Fail continuous round motions.

13. Which line is longer? (Not bigger.) Turn paper upside down and repeat. (pass 3 of 3 or 5 of 6)

14. Pass any lines crossing near midpoint.

15. Have child copy first. If failed, demonstrate.

When giving items 12, 14, and 15, do not name the forms. Do not demonstrate 12 and 14.

16. When scoring, each pair (2 arms, 2 legs, etc.) counts as one part.
17. Place one cube in cup and shake gently near child's ear, but out of sight. Repeat for other ear.
18. Point to picture and have child name it. (No credit is given for sounds only.)
    If less than 4 pictures are named correctly, have child point to picture as each is named by tester.

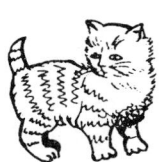   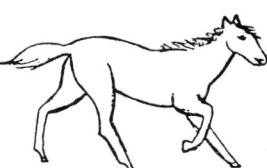   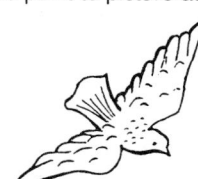   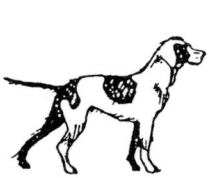   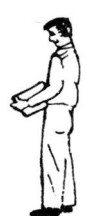

19. Using doll, tell child: Show me the nose, eyes, ears, mouth, hands, feet, tummy, hair. Pass 6 of 8.
20. Using pictures, ask child: Which one flies?… says meow?… talks?… barks?… gallops? Pass 2 of 5, 4 of 5.
21. Ask child: What do you do when you are cold?… tired?… hungry? Pass 2 of 3, 3 of 3.
22. Ask child: What do you do with a cup? What is a chair used for? What is a pencil used for?
    Action words must be included in answers.
23. Pass if child correctly places <u>and</u> says how many blocks are on paper. (1, 5).
24. Tell child: Put block **on** table; **under** table; **in front of** me, **behind** me. Pass 4 of 4.
    (Do not help child by pointing, moving head or eyes.)
25. Ask child: What is a ball?… lake?… desk?… house?… banana?… curtain?… fence?… ceiling? Pass if defined in terms of use, shape, what it is made of, or general category (such as banana is fruit, not just yellow). Pass 5 of 8, 7 of 8.
26. Ask child: If a horse is big, a mouse is __? If fire is hot, ice is __? If the sun shines during the day, the moon shines during the __? Pass 2 of 3.
27. Child may use wall or rail only, not person. May not crawl.
28. Child must throw ball overhand 3 feet to within arm's reach of tester.
29. Child must perform standing broad jump over width of test sheet (8 1/2 inches).
30. Tell child to walk forward, ⚬⚬⚬⚬⚬⚬➔ heel within 1 inch of toe. Tester may demonstrate.
    Child must walk 4 consecutive steps.
31. In the second year, half of normal children are non-compliant.

OBSERVATIONS:

FIGURE 3-1, cont'd.

REVISED DENVER PRESCREENING DEVELOPMENTAL QUESTIONNAIRE

0-9 MONTHS (R-PDQ)

Child's Name _____

Person Completing R-PDQ: _____

Relation to Child: _____

For Office Use		
Today's Date:	___ yr	___ mo	___ day
Child's Birthdate:	___ yr	___ mo	___ day
Subtract to get Child's Exact Age:	___ yr	___ mo	___ day
R-PDQ Age:	(___ yr ___ mo)	___ completed wks)

CONTINUE ANSWERING UNTIL 3 "NOs" ARE CIRCLED

1. Equal Movements
When your baby is lying on his/her back, can (s)he move each of his/her arms as easily as the other and each of the legs as easily as the other? Answer **No** if your child makes jerky or uncoordinated movements with one or both of his/her arms or legs.

Yes   No   (0)   FMA

2. Stomach Lifts Head
When your baby is on his/her stomach on a flat surface, can (s)he lift his/her head off the surface?

Yes   No   (0-3)   GM

3. Regards Face
When your baby is lying on his/her back, can (s)he look at you and watch your face?

Yes   No   (1)   PS

4. Follows To Midline
When your child is on his/her back, can (s)he follow your movement by turning his/her head from one side to facing directly forward?

Yes   No   (1-1)   FMA

5. Responds To Bell
Does your child respond with eye movements, change in breathing or other change in activity to a bell or rattle sounded outside his/her line of vision?

Yes   No   (1-2)   L

6. Vocalizes Not Crying
Does your child make sounds other than crying, such as gurgling, cooing, or babbling?

Yes   No   (1-3)   L

7. Smiles Responsively
When you smile and talk to your baby, does (s)he smile back at you?

Yes   No   (1-3)   PS

8. Follows Past Midline
When your child is on his/her back, does (s)he follow your movement by turning his/her head from one side *almost all the way to the other side?*

Yes   No   (2-2)   FMA

9. Stomach, Head Up 45°
When your baby is on his/her stomach on a flat surface, can (s)he lift his/her head 45°?

Yes   No   (2-2)   GM

10. Stomach, Head Up 90°
When your baby is on his/her stomach on a flat surface, can (s)he lift his/her head 90°?

Yes   No   (3)   GM

11. Laughs
Does your baby laugh out loud without being tickled or touched?

Yes   No   (3-1)   L

12. Hands Together
Does your baby play with his/her hands by touching them together?

Yes   No   (3-3)   FMA

13. Follows 180°
When your child is on his/her back, does (s)he follow your movement from one side *all the way* to the other side?

Yes   No   (4)   FMA

14. Grasps Rattle
It is important that you follow instructions carefully. Do *not* place the pencil in the palm of your child's hand. When you touch the pencil to the back or tips of your baby's fingers, does your baby grasp the pencil for a few seconds?

Yes   No   (4)   FMA

TRY THIS   NOT THIS

(Please turn page)

© Wm. K. Frankenburg, M.D., 1975, 1986

Side #2

	For Office Use	

23. Sits, Looks For Yarn
Please follow directions carefully. Get your baby's attention with a scarf, handkerchief, or a tissue and then drop it *out of sight.* Did your baby try to find it? For example, did (s)he look for it under the table or continue to watch where it disappeared?   **Yes   No**   (7-2) FMA

24. Passes Cube Hand To Hand
Can your baby pass something, such as a small block or a small cookie, from one hand to the other? Long objects like a spoon or rattle do not count.   **Yes   No**   (7-2) FMA

25. Sits, Takes 2 Cubes
Can your baby pick up 2 things, such as toys or cookies, and hold one in each hand at the same time?   **Yes   No**   (7-2) FMA

26. Bears Some Weight On Legs
When you hold your baby under his/her arms, can (s)he bear some weight on his/her legs? Answer **Yes** only if (s)he tries to stand on his/her feet and supports some of his/her own weight.   **Yes   No**   (7-3) GM

27. Rakes Raisin, Attains
Can your baby pick up small objects, such as raisins or pieces of food with his/her hand using a raking or grabbing motion?   **Yes   No**   (7-3) FMA

28. Sits Without Support
Without being propped by pillows, a chair, or wall, can your child sit by himself/herself for 60 seconds?   **Yes   No**   (7-3) GM

29. Feed Self Crackers
Can your baby feed himself/herself a cracker or cookie? Answer **No** if (s)he has never been given one.   **Yes   No**   (8) PS

30. Turns To Voice
When your child is playing and you come up *quietly* behind him/her, does (s)he sometimes turn his/her head as though (s)he heard you? *Loud sounds do not count.*   **Yes   No**   (8-1) L

© Wm. K. Frankenburg, M.D., 1975, 1986

0-9 MONTHS (R-PDQ)

CONTINUE ANSWERING UNTIL 3 "NOs" ARE CIRCLED

	For Office Use

15. Sits, Head Steady
When sitting, can your child hold his/her head upright and steady? Answer **No** if his/her head falls to either side or upon his/her chest.   **Yes   No**   (4) GM

16. Stomach Chest Up-Arm Support
When your baby is on his/her stomach on a flat surface, can (s)he lift his/her chest using his/her arms for support?   **Yes   No**   (4-1) GM

17. Squeals
Does your baby make happy high-pitched squealing sounds which are not crying?   **Yes   No**   (4-2) L

18. Rolls Over
Has your baby rolled over at least 2 times, from stomach to back, or back to stomach?   **Yes   No**   (4-3) GM

19. Regards Raisin
Can your child focus his/her eyes on small objects the size of a pea, a raisin, or a penny?   **Yes   No**   (5) FMA

20. Reaches For Object
Can your child pick up a toy if it is placed within his/her reach?   **Yes   No**   (5) FMA

21. Smiles Spontaneously
Does your child smile at crib toys, pictures, or pets when (s)he is playing by himself/herself?   **Yes   No**   (5) PS

22. Pull To Sit, No Headlag
With your baby on his/her back, gently pull him/her up to a sitting position by his/her wrists. Does your baby hold his/her neck stiffly like the baby in the picture below left? Answer **No** if his/her head falls back like the baby in the picture below right.   **Yes   No**   (6-1) GM

Yes   No

DENVER ARTICULATION SCREENING EXAMINATION (DASE)

Denver Articulation Screening Examination

NAME

HOSPITAL NO.

(For children 2.5 to 6 years of age)

ADDRESS

Instructions: Have child repeat each word after you. Circle the underlined sounds that he or she pronounces correctly. Total number of correct sounds is the raw score. Use charts below to score results.

Date: _____ Child's age: _____ Examiner: _____ Raw score: _____

Percentile: _____ Intelligibility: _____ Result: _____

1. table	6. zipper	11. sock	16. wagon	21. leaf
2. shirt	7. grapes	12. vacuum	17. gum	22. carrot
3. door	8. flag	13. yarn	18. house	
4. trunk	9. thumb	14. mother	19. pencil	
5. jumping	10. toothbrush	15. twinkle	20. fish	

Intelligibility (circle one): 1. Easy to understand   3. Not understandable
                               2. Understandable half of the time   4. Cannot evaluate

Comments:

DENVER ARTICULATION SCREENING EXAMINATION (DASE)—CONTINUED

To score DASE words: Note raw score for child's performance. Match raw score line (extreme left of chart) with column representing child's age (to the closest *previous* age group). Where raw score line and age column meet denotes percentile rank of child's performance when compared with other children that age. Percentiles above heavy line are *abnormal*, below heavy line are *normal*.

Percentile rank

Raw score	2.5 yr	3.0 yr	3.5 yr	4.0 yr	4.5 yr	5.0 yr	5.5 yr	6 yr
2	1							
3	2							
4	5							
5	9							
6	16							
7	23							
8	31	2						
9	37	4	1					
10	42	6	2					
11	48	7	4					
12	54	9	6	1	1			
13	58	12	9	2	3	1	1	
14	62	17	11	5	4	2	2	
15	68	23	15	9	5	3	2	
16	75	31	19	12	5	4	3	
17	79	38	25	15	6	6	4	
18	83	46	31	19	8	7	4	
19	86	51	38	24	10	9	5	1
20	89	58	45	30	12	11	7	3
21	92	65	52	36	15	15	9	4
22	94	72	58	43	18	19	12	5
23	96	77	63	50	22	24	15	7
24	97	82	70	58	29	29	20	15
25	99	87	78	66	36	34	26	17
26	99	91	84	75	46	43	34	24
27		94	89	82	57	54	44	34
28		96	94	88	70	68	59	47
29		98	98	94	84	84	77	68
30		100	100	100	100	100	100	100

To score intelligibility:

	NORMAL	ABNORMAL
2.5 years	Understandable half of the time or easy to understand	Not understandable
3 years and older	Easy to understand	Understandable half of the time or not understandable

Test result: 1. Normal on DASE and intelligibility = *normal*
2. Abnormal on DASE or intelligibility = *abnormal**

*If abnormal on initial screening, rescreen within 2 weeks. If abnormal again, child should be referred for complete speech evaluation.

based on gradually increasing complexity of the figures as the child becomes older.

Adult Assessment Tools

Although few tools are available to assess life changes and their effects on adults, two that have been developed are the Recent Life Changes Questionnaire and the Life Experiences Survey. Both attempt to assess life stresses and to indicate a possible relationship between life stresses and susceptibility to physical and psychological problems or illnesses.

Recent Life Changes Questionnaire. The Recent Life Changes Questionnaire (Rahe, 1975) is a self-administered questionnaire containing a list of events that subjects respond to by checking those events that they have experienced in the previous 6 months to 1 year. (Table 3-2). To determine the scores for these events, the researchers had a large group of subjects rate each of the items with regard to the amount of social readjustment each event required. Mean values for each item were taken to represent the average amount of social readjustment required. The values, called Life Change Units, were added to yield a life stress score. Studies using this tool have shown correlations between high recent life change scores and the development of health problems. This tool combines a life stress score based on both desirable and undesirable events; health care professionals should take these differences into account in assessing an individual's life change and its impact on health. They also should consider the client's own assessment of both the intensity of the life changes and the strength of his or her coping abilities.

Life Experiences Survey. The Life Experiences Survey (Sarason, Johnson, and Siegel, 1978) is a self-report tool that allows respondents to indicate events they have experienced over the past year. (Table 3-3). It includes events that occur fairly frequently and allows respondents to weigh the desirability or undesirability of events. Ratings are on a seven-point scale from extremely negative (-3) to extremely positive ($+3$). A positive change score is obtained by adding those events rated as positive, the negative change score is obtained by adding the negatively rated events, and a total change score is obtained by adding those two values.

As the integrated nature of the human organism becomes more fully understood, we will likely gain better understanding of the relationship between life changes and problems of a psychological nature. The cause-effect relationship is often unclear between life changes and health status, and the effect of life changes or stresses differs from person to person depending on unique characteristics, including the degree of perceived control over events and the degree of psychosocial assets.

TABLE 3-2

Recent Life Changes Questionnaire

Life Change Unit (LCU) Weights for Life Change Events

Health
Within the time periods listed, have you experienced:

	1. An illness or injury that:
42	(a) Kept you in bed a week or more, or took you to the hospital?
25	(b) Was less serious than described above?
29	2. A major change in eating habits?
31	3. A major change in sleeping habits?
30	4. A change in your usual type or amount of recreation?
40	5. Major dental work?

Work
Within the time periods listed, have you:

38	6. Changed to a new type of work?
33	7. Changed your work hours or conditions?
	8. Had a change in your responsibilities at work:
31	(a) More responsibilities?
29	(b) Less responsibilities?
31	(c) Promotion?
51	(d) Demotion?
38	(e) Transfer?
	9. Experienced troubles at work:
39	(a) With your boss?
35	(b) With co-workers?
30	(c) With persons under your supervision?
31	(d) Other work troubles?
38	10. Experienced a major business readjustment?
49	11. Retired?
	12. Experienced being:
64	(a) Fired from work?
57	(b) Laid off from work?
29	13. Taken courses by mail or studied at home to help you in your work?

Home and family
Within the time periods listed, have you experienced:

	14. A change in residence:
28	(a) A move within the same town or city?
38	(b) A move to a different town, city, or state?
26	15. A change in family "get-togethers"?
52	16. A major change in the health or behavior of a family member (illness, accidents, drug, or disciplinary problems, etc.)?
39	17. Major change in your living conditions (home improvements or a decline in your home or neighborhood)?

From Rahe RH: Epidemiological studies of life change and illness, Int J Psychiatry Med 6(1-2):133-146, 1975. © Baywood Publishing Co, Inc.

TABLE 3-2—cont'd

Recent Life Changes Questionnaire

Life Change Unit (LCU) Weights for Life Change Events	
105	18. The death of a spouse?
	19. The death of a:
105	(a) Child?
64	(b) Brother or sister?
66	(c) Parent?
	(d) Other close family member?
46	20. The death of a close friend?
	21. A change in marital status of your parents:
38	(a) Divorce?
33	(b) Remarriage?
50	22. Marriage?
	(NOTE: Questions 23-33 concern marriage. For persons never married go to item 34.)
34	23. A change in arguments with your spouse?
29	24. In-law problems?
	25. A separation from spouse:
49	(a) Due to work?
56	(b) Due to marital problems?
45	26. A reconciliation with spouse?
62	27. A divorce?
	28. A gain of a new family member?
49	(a) Birth of a child?
45	(b) Adoption of a child?
57	(c) A relative moving in with you?
37	37. Wife beginning or ceasing work outside the home?
60	30. Wife becoming pregnant?
29	31. A child leaving home:
28	(a) Due to marriage?
30	(b) To attend college?
29	(c) For other reasons?
53	32. Wife having a miscarriage or abortion?
31	33. Birth of a grandchild?

Personal and social
Within the time periods listed, have you experienced:

33	34. A major personal achievement?
31	35. A change in your personal habits (your dress, friends, life-style, etc.)?
49	36. Sexual difficulties?
32	37. Beginning or ceasing school or college?
28	38. A change of school or college?
29	39. A vacation?
29	40. A change in your religious beliefs?
28	41. A change in your social activities (clubs, movies, visiting)?
32	42. A minor violation of the law?
57	43. Legal troubles resulting in your being held in jail?
25	44. A change in your political beliefs?

TABLE 3-2—cont'd

Recent Life Changes Questionnaire

Life Change Unit (LCU) Weights for Life Change Events	
32	45. A new, close, personal relationship?
39	46. An engagement to marry?
35	47. A "falling out" of a close personal relationship?
30	48. Girlfriend (or boyfriend) problems?
40	49. A loss or damage of personal property?
44	50. An accident?
45	51. A major decision regarding your immediate future?

Financial
Within the time periods listed, have you:

26	52. Taken on a moderate purchase, such as a television, car, freezer, etc.?
39	53. Taken on a major purchase or a mortgage loan, such as a home, business, property, etc.?
57	54. Experienced a foreclosure on a mortgage or loan?
	55. Experienced a major change in finances:
27	(a) Increased income?
60	(b) Decreased income?
43	(c) Credit rating difficulties?

Subjective life change unit (SLCU) instructions
Instructions for scoring your adjustment to your recent life changes

Persons adapt to their recent life changes in different ways. Some people find the adjustment to a residential move, for example, to be enormous, while others find very little life adjustment necessary. You are now requested to "score" each of the recent life changes that you marked with an "X" as to the amount of adjustment you needed to handle the event.

Your scores can range from 1 to 100 "points." If, for example, you experienced a recent residential move but felt it required very little life adjustment, you would choose a low number and place it in the blank to the right of the question boxes. On the other hand, if you recently changed residence and felt it required a near maximal life adjustment, you would place a high number, toward 100, in the blank to the right of that question's boxes. For immediate life adjustment scores you would choose intermediate numbers between 1 and 100.

Please go back through your questionnaire and for each recent life change you indicated with an "X," choose your personal life adjustment score (between 1 and 100) which reflects what you saw to be the amount of life adjustment necessary to cope with or handle the event. Use both your estimates of the intensity of the life change and its duration to arrive at your scores.

TABLE 3-3

The Life Experiences Survey

Listed below are a number of events which sometimes bring about change in the lives of those who experience them and which necessitate social readjustment. *Please check those events which you have experienced in the recent past and indicate the time period during which you have experienced each event.* Be sure that all check marks are directly across from the items they correspond to.

Also, for each item checked below, *please indicate the extent to which you viewed the event as having either a positive or negative impact on your life* at the time the event occurred. That is, *indicate the type and extent of impact that the event had.* A rating of − 3 would indicate an extremely negative impact. A rating of 0 suggests no impact either positive or negative. A rating + 3 would indicate an extremely positive impact.

	0 to 6 mo	7 mo to 1 yr	Extremely negative	Moderately negative	Somewhat negative	No impact	Slightly positive	Moderately positive	Extremely positive
1. Marriage			− 3	− 2	− 1	0	+ 1	+ 2	+ 3
2. Detention in jail or comparable institution			− 3	− 2	− 1	0	+ 1	+ 2	+ 3
3. Death of spouse			− 3	− 2	− 1	0	+ 1	+ 2	+ 3
4. Major change in sleeping habits (much more or much less sleep)			− 3	− 2	− 1	0	+ 1	+ 2	+ 3
5. Death of close family member:									
a. Mother			− 3	− 2	− 1	0	+ 1	+ 2	+ 3
b. Father			− 3	− 2	− 1	0	+ 1	+ 2	+ 3
c. Brother			− 3	− 2	− 1	0	+ 1	+ 2	+ 3
d. Sister			− 3	− 2	− 1	0	+ 1	+ 2	+ 3
e. Grandmother			− 3	− 2	− 1	0	+ 1	+ 2	+ 3
f. Grandfather			− 3	− 2	− 1	0	+ 1	+ 2	+ 3
g. Other (specify)			− 3	− 2	− 1	0	+ 1	+ 2	+ 3
6. Major change in eating habits (much more or much less food intake)			− 3	− 2	− 1	0	+ 1	+ 2	+ 3
7. Foreclosure on mortgage or loan			− 3	− 2	− 1	0	+ 1	+ 2	+ 3
8. Death of close friend			− 3	− 2	− 1	0	+ 1	+ 2	+ 3
9. Outstanding personal achievement			− 3	− 2	− 1	0	+ 1	+ 2	+ 3
10. Minor law violations (traffic tickets, disturbing the peace, etc.)			− 3	− 2	− 1	0	+ 1	+ 2	+ 3
11. *Male:* Wife/girlfriend's pregnancy			− 3	− 2	− 1	0	+ 1	+ 2	+ 3
12. *Female:* Pregnancy			− 3	− 2	− 1	0	+ 1	+ 2	+ 3
13. Changed work situation (different work responsibility, major change in working conditions, working hours, etc.)			− 3	− 2	− 1	0	+ 1	+ 2	+ 3
14. New job			− 3	− 2	− 1	0	+ 1	+ 2	+ 3
15. Serious illness or injury of close family member:									
a. Father			− 3	− 2	− 1	0	+ 1	+ 2	+ 3
b. Mother			− 3	− 2	− 1	0	+ 1	+ 2	+ 3
c. Sister			− 3	− 2	− 1	0	+ 1	+ 2	+ 3
d. Brother			− 3	− 2	− 1	0	+ 1	+ 2	+ 3
e. Grandmother			− 3	− 2	− 1	0	+ 1	+ 2	+ 3
f. Grandfather			− 3	− 2	− 1	0	+ 1	+ 2	+ 3
g. Spouse			− 3	− 2	− 1	0	+ 1	+ 2	+ 3
h. Other (specify)			− 3	− 2	− 1	0	+ 1	+ 2	+ 3

From Sarason IG, Johnson JH, Siegal JM: Assessing the impact of life changes: development of life experiences survey, *J Consult Clin Psychol* 46(5):932-946, 1978.

TABLE 3-3—cont'd

The Life Experiences Survey

	0 to 6 mo	7 mo to 1 yr	Extremely negative	Moderately negative	Somewhat negative	No impact	Slightly positive	Moderately positive	Extremely positive
16. Sexual difficulties			−3	−2	−1	0	+1	+2	+3
17. Trouble with employer (in danger of losing job, being suspended, demoted, etc.)			−3	−2	−1	0	+1	+2	+3
18. Trouble with in-laws			−3	−2	−1	0	+1	+2	+3
19. Major change in financial status (a lot better off or a lot worse off)			−3	−2	−1	0	+1	+2	+3
20. Major change in closeness of family members (increased or decreased closeness)			−3	−2	−1	0	+1	+2	+3
21. Gaining a new family member (through birth, adoption, family member moving in, etc.)			−3	−2	−1	0	+1	+2	+3
22. Change of residence			−3	−2	−1	0	+1	+2	+3
23. Marital separation from mate (due to conflict)			−3	−2	−1	0	+1	+2	+3
24. Major change in church activities (increased or decreased attendance)			−3	−2	−1	0	+1	+2	+3
25. Marital reconciliation with mate			−3	−2	−1	0	+1	+2	+3
26. Major change in number of arguments with spouse (a lot more or a lot less arguments)			−3	−2	−1	0	+1	+2	+3
27. *Married male:* Change in wife's work outside the home (beginning work, ceasing work, changing to a new job, etc.)			−3	−2	−1	0	+1	+2	+3
28. *Married female:* Change in husband's work (loss of job, beginning new job, retirement, etc.)			−3	−2	−1	0	+1	+2	+3
29. Major change in usual type and/or amount of recreation			−3	−2	−1	0	+1	+2	+3
30. Borrowing more than $10,000 (buying home, business, etc.)			−3	−2	−1	0	+1	+2	+3
31. Borrowing less than $10,000 (buying car, TV, getting school loan, etc.)			−3	−2	−1	0	+1	+2	+3
32. Being fired from job			−3	−2	−1	0	+1	+2	+3
33. *Male:* Wife/girlfriend having abortion			−3	−2	−1	0	+1	+2	+3
34. *Female:* Having abortion			−3	−2	−1	0	+1	+2	+3
35. Major personal illness or injury			−3	−2	−1	0	+1	+2	+3
36. Major change in social activities, e.g., parties, movies, visiting (increased or decreased participation)			−3	−2	−1	0	+1	+2	+3
37. Major change in living conditions of family (building new home, remodeling, deterioration of home, neighborhood, etc.)			−3	−2	−1	0	+1	+2	+3

Continued.

TABLE 3-3—cont'd

The Life Experiences Survey

	0 to 6 mo	7 mo to 1 yr	Extremely negative	Moderately negative	Somewhat negative	No impact	Slightly positive	Moderately positive	Extremely positive
38. Divorce			−3	−2	−1	0	+1	+2	+3
39. Serious injury or illness of close friend			−3	−2	−1	0	+1	+2	+3
40. Retirement from work			−3	−2	−1	0	+1	+2	+3
41. Son or daughter leaving home (due to marriage, college, etc.)			−3	−2	−1	0	+1	+2	+3
42. Ending of formal schooling			−3	−2	−1	0	+1	+2	+3
43. Separation from spouse (due to work, travel, etc.)			−3	−2	−1	0	+1	+2	+3
44. Engagement			−3	−2	−1	0	+1	+2	+3
45. Breaking up with boyfriend/ girlfriend			−3	−2	−1	0	+1	+2	+3
46. Leaving home for the first time			−3	−2	−1	0	+1	+2	+3
47. Reconciliation with boyfriend/ girlfriend			−3	−2	−1	0	+1	+2	+3
Other recent experiences that have had an impact on your life. List and rate.									
48. _____			−3	−2	−1	0	+1	+2	+3
49. _____			−3	−2	−1	0	+1	+2	+3
50. _____			−3	−2	−1	0	+1	+2	+3

THE INFANT: BIRTH TO 12 MONTHS

More dramatic changes occur within the brief period of infancy than during any other time of life. During the period from birth to 12 months, the child develops from a dependent, helpless newborn to a busy little person who is mobile and communicative and relates to people in terms of their importance in her or his life. Infants enter the world with all sensory systems functioning in at least a rudimentary fashion. They begin to interact with and influence their environment from the moment of birth. As the neuromuscular system becomes more integrated, they are intent on taking in everything in the environment within their reach. Soon they can display a wide range of primary, unselfconscious emotions: interest, distress, disgust, joy, anger, surprise, sadness, and fear. They are responsive to the caregivers' mood: sadness or happiness affects their behavior.

The boxed material on page 63, "Child Development from 1 Month to 5 Years," summarizes child development using the categories of motor development, language development, and personal–social-adaptive development. (These categories are slightly different from but complementary to the categories used in the text.)

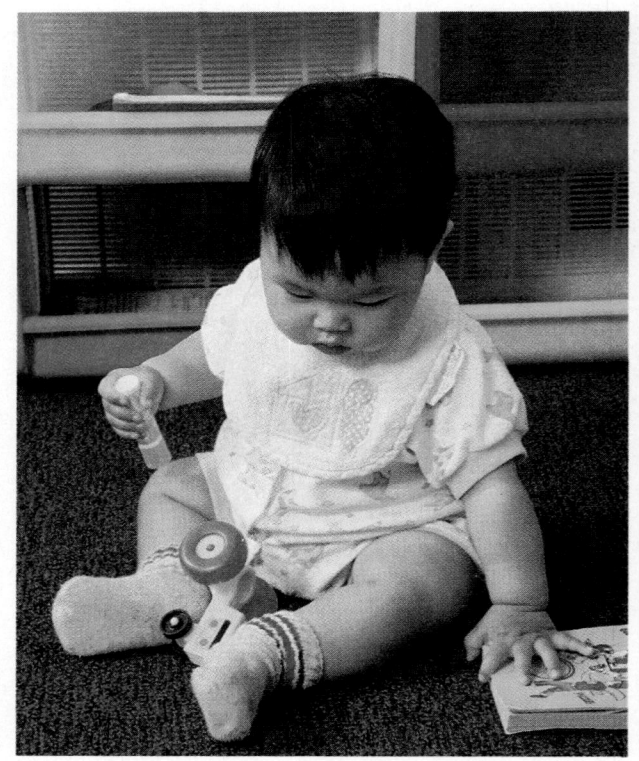

CHILD DEVELOPMENT FROM 1 MONTH TO 5 YEARS

1 Month
Motor

1. Moro reflex present.
2. Vigorous sucking reflex present.
3. Lying prone (face down): lifts head briefly so chin is off table.
4. Lying prone: makes crawling movements with legs.
5. Held in sitting position: back is rounded, head held up momentarily only.
6. Hands tightly fisted.
7. Reflex grasp of object with palm.

Language

8. Startled by sound; quieted by voice.
9. Small throaty noises or vocalizations.

Personal-social-adaptive

10. Ringing bell produces decrease of activity.
11. May follow dangling object with eyes to midline.
12. Lying on back: will briefly look at examiner or change activity.
13. Reacts with generalized body movements when tissue paper is placed on face.

2 Months
Motor

1. Kicks vigorously.
2. Energetic arm movements.
3. Vigorous head turning.
4. Held in ventral suspension (prone): no head droop.
5. Lying prone: lifts head so face makes an approximate 45° angle with table.
6. Held in sitting position: head erect but bobs.
7. Hand goes to mouth.
8. Hands often open (not clenched).

Language

9. Is cooing.
10. Vocalizes single vowel sounds, such as: ah-eh-uh.

Personal-social-adaptive

11. Head and eyes search for sound.
12. Listens to bell ringing.
13. Follows dangling object past midline.
14. Alert expression.
15. Follows moving person with eyes.
16. Smiles back when talked to.

3 Months
Motor

1. Lying prone: lifts head to 90° angle.
2. Lifts head when lying on back (supine).
3. Moro reflex begins to disappear.
4. Grasp reflex nearly gone.
5. Rolls side to back (3-4 months).

Language

6. Chuckling, squealing, grunting, especially when talked to.
7. Listens to music.
8. Vocalizes with two different syllables, such as: a-a, la-la (not distinct), oo-oo.

Personal-social-adaptive

9. Reaches for but misses objects.
10. Holds toy with active grasp when put into hand.
11. Sucks and inspects fingers.
12. Pulls at clothes.
13. Follows object (toy) side to side (and 180°).
14. Looks predominately at examiner.
15. Glances at toy when put into hand.
16. Recognizes mother and bottle.
17. Smiles spontaneously.

4 Months
Motor

1. Sits when well supported.
2. No head lag when pulled to sitting position.
3. Turns head at sound of voice.
4. Lifts head (in supine position) in effort to sit.
5. Lifts head and chest when prone, using hands and forearms.
6. Held erect: pushes feet against table.

Language

7. Laughs aloud (4-5 months).
8. Uses sounds, such as: m-p-b.
9. Repeats series of same sounds.

Personal-social-adaptive

10. Grasps rattle.
11. Plays with own fingers.
12. Reaches for object in front with both hands.
13. Transfers object from hand to hand.
14. Pulls dress over face.
15. Smiles spontaneously at people.
16. Regards raisin (or pellet).

5 Months
Motor

1. Moro reflex gone.
2. Rolls side to side.
3. Rolls back to front.
4. Full head control when pulled to or held in sitting position.
5. Briefly supports most of weight on legs.
6. Scratches on tabletop.

Language

7. Squeals with high voice.
8. Recognizes familiar voices.
9. Coos or stops crying on hearing music.

Reprinted by permission of Walter M. Block, MD, Child Evaluation Clinic of Cedar Rapids, Iowa © Copyright 1972.

Continued.

CHILD DEVELOPMENT FROM 1 MONTH TO 5 YEARS—cont'd

Personal-social-adaptive

10. Grasps dangling object.
11. Reaches for toy with both hands.
12. Smiles at mirror image.
13. Turns head deliberately to bell.
14. Obviously enjoys being played with.

6 Months
Motor

1. Supine: lifts head spontaneously.
2. Bounces on feet when held standing.
3. Sits briefly (tripod fashion).
4. Rolls front to back (6-7 months).
5. Grasps foot and plays with toes.
6. Grasps cube with palms.

Language

7. Vocalizes at mirror image.
8. Makes four or more different sounds.
9. Localizes source of sound (bell, voice).
10. Vague, formless babble (especially with family members).

Personal-social-adaptive

11. Holds one cube in each hand.
12. Puts cube into mouth.
13. Resecures dropped cube.
14. Transfers cube from hand to hand.
15. Conscious of strange sights and persons.
16. Consistent regard of object or person (6-7 months).
17. Uses raking movement to secure raisin or pellet.
18. Resists having toy taken away.
19. Stretches out arms to be taken up (6-8 months).

8 Months
Motor

1. Sits alone (6-8 months).
2. Early stepping movements.
3. Tries to crawl.
4. Stands few seconds, holding on to object.
5. Leans forward to get an object.
6. Held in sitting position: head erect but bobs.

Language

6. Two-syllable babble, such as a-la, ba-ba, oo-goo, a-ma, mama, dada (8-10 months).
7. Listens to conversation (8-10 months).
8. "Shouts" for attention (8-10 months).

Personal-social-adaptive

9. Works to get toy out of reach.
10. Scoops pellet.
11. Rings bell purposely (8-10 months).
12. Drinks from cup.
13. Plays peek-a-boo.
14. Looks for dropped object.
15. Bites and chews toys.

16. Pats mirror image.
17. Bangs spoon on table.
18. Manipulates paper or string.
19. Secures ring by pulling on the string.
20. Feeds self crackers.

10 Months
Motor

1. Gets self into sitting position.
2. Sits steadily (long time).
3. Pulls self to standing positon (on bed railing).
4. Crawls on hands and knees.
5. Walks when held or around furniture.
6. Turns around when left on floor.

Language

7. Imitates speech sounds.
8. Shakes head for "no."
9. Waves "bye-bye."
10. Responds to name.
11. Vocalizes in varied jargon-patterns (10-12 months).

Personal-social-adaptive

12. Plays "pat-a-cake."
13. Picks up pellet with finger and thumb.
14. Bangs toys together.
15. Extends toy to a person.
16. Holds own bottle.
17. Removes cube from cup.
18. Drops one cube to get another.
19. Uses handle to lift cup.
20. Initially shy with strangers.

1 Year
Motor

1. Walks with one hand held.
2. Stands alone (or with support).
3. Secures small object with good pincer grasp.
4. Pivots in sitting position.
5. Grasps two cubes in one hand.

Language

6. Uses "mama" or "dada" with specific meaning.
7. "Talks" to toys and people, using fairly long verbal patterns.
8. Has vocabulary of two words besides "mama" and "dada."
9. Babbles to self when alone.
10. Obeys simple requests, such as: "Give me the cup."
11. Reacts to music.

Personal-social-adaptive

12. Cooperates with dressing.
13. Plays with cup, spoon, saucer.
14. Points with index finger.

CHILD DEVELOPMENT FROM 1 MONTH TO 5 YEARS—cont'd

15. Pokes finger (into stethoscope) to explore.
16. Releases toy into your hand.
17. Tries to take cube out of box.
18. Upwraps a cube.
19. Holds cup to drink.
20. Holds crayon.
21. Tries to imitate scribble.
22. Imitates beating two cubes together.
23. Gives affection.

15 Months
Motor

1. Stands alone.
2. Creeps upstairs.
3. Kneels on floor or chair.
4. Gets off floor and walks alone with good balance.
5. Bends over to pick up toy without holding on to furniture.

Language

6. May speak four to six words (15-18 months).
7. Uses jargon.
8. Indicates wants by vocalizing.
9. Knows own name.
10. Enjoys rhymes or jingles.

Personal-social-adaptive

11. Tilts cup to drinks.
12. Uses spoon but spills.
13. Builds tower of two cubes.
14. Drops cubes into cup.
15. Helps turn page in book, pats picture.
16. Shows or offers toy.
17. Helps pull off clothes.
18. Puts pellet into bottle without demonstration.
19. Opens lid of box.
20. Likes to push wheeled toys.

18 Months
Motor

1. Runs (stiffly).
2. Walks upstairs—one hand held.
3. Walks backwards.
4. Climbs into chair.
5. Hurls ball.

Language

6. May say six to ten words (18-21 months).
7. Points to at least one body part.
8. Can say "hello" and "thank you".
9. Carries out two directions (one at a time), for instance: "Get ball from table."—"Give ball to mother."
10. Identifies two objects by pointing (or picking up), such as: cup, spoon, dog, car, chair.

Personal-social-adaptive

11. Turns pages.
12. Builds tower of three to four cubes.
13. Puts 10 cubes into cup.
14. Carries or hugs a doll.
15. Takes off shoes and socks.
16. Pulls string toy.
17. Scribbles spontaneously.
18. Dumps raisin from bottle after demonstration.
19. Uses spoon with little spilling.

21 Months
Motor

1. Runs well.
2. Walks downstairs—one hand held.
3. Walks upstairs alone or holding on to rail.
4. Kicks large ball (when demonstrated).

Language

5. May speak fifteen to twenty words (21-24 months).
6. May combine two to three words.
7. Asks for food, drink.
8. Echoes two or more words.
9. Takes three directions (one at a time), for instance: "Take ball from table."—"Give ball to Mommy."—"Put ball on floor."
10. Points to three or more body parts.

Personal-social-adaptive

11. Builds tower of five to six cubes.
12. Folds paper once when shown.
13. Helps with simple household tasks (21-24 months).
14. Removes some clothing purposefully (besides hat or socks).
15. Pulls person to show something.

2 Years
Motor

1. Runs without falling.
2. Walks up and down stairs.
3. Kicks large ball (without demonstration).
4. Throws ball overhand.
5. Claps hands.
6. Opens door.
7. Turns pages in book, singly.

Language

8. Says simple phrases.
9. Says at least one sentence or phrase of four or more syllables.
10. Can repeat four to five syllables.
11. May reproduce about five or six consonant sounds. (Typically: m-p-b-h-w).
12. Points to four parts of body on command.
13. Asks for things at table by name.
14. Refers to self by name.
15. May use personal pronouns, such as: I-me-you (2-2½ years).

Continued.

CHILD DEVELOPMENT FROM 1 MONTH TO 5 YEARS—cont'd

Personal-social-adaptive

16. Builds five- to seven-cube tower.
17. May cut with scissors.
18. Spontaneously dumps raisin from bottle (without demonstration).
19. Throws ball into box.
20. Imitates drawing vertical line from demonstration.
21. Parallel play predominant.

2½ Years
Motor

1. Jumps in place with both feet.
2. Tries standing on one foot (may not be successful).
3. Holds crayon by fingers.
4. Imitates walking on tiptoe.

Language

5. Refers to self by pronoun (rather than name).
6. Names common objects when asked (key, penny, shoe, box, book).
7. Repeats two digits (one of three trials).
8. Answers simple questions, such as: "What is this?"—"What does the kitty say?"

Personal-social-adaptive

9. Builds tower of eight cubes.
10. Pushes toy with good steering.
11. Helps put things away.
12. Can carry breakable objects.
13. Puts on clothing.
14. Washes and dries hands.
15. Eats with fork.
16. Imitates drawing a horizontal line from demonstration.
17. May imitate drawing a circle from demonstration.

3 Years
Motor

1. Stands on one foot for at least 1 second.
2. Jumps from bottom stair.
3. Alternates feet going upstairs.
4. Pours from a pitcher.
5. Can undo two buttons.
6. Pedals a tricycle.

Language

7. Repeats six syllables, for instance: "I have a little dog."
8. Names three or more objects in a picture.
9. Gives sex. ("Are you a boy or a girl?")

10. Gives full name.
11. Repeats three digits (one of three trials).
12. Knows a few rhymes.
13. Gives appropriate answers to: "What: swims-flies-shoots-boils-bites-melts?"
14. Uses plurals.
15. Knows at least one color.
16. Can reply to questions in at least three-word sentences.
17. May have vocabulary of 750 to 1,000 words (3-3½ years).

Personal-social-adaptive

18. Understands taking turns.
19. Copies a circle (from model, without demonstration).
20. Builds three-block pyramid.
21. Dresses with supervision.
22. Puts 10 pellets into bottle in 30 seconds.
23. Separates easily from mother.
24. Feeds self well.
25. Plays interactive games, such as "tag."

4 Years
Motor

1. Stands on one foot for at least 5 seconds (two of three trials).
2. Hops at least twice on one foot.
3. Can walk heel-to-toe four or more steps (with heel 1 inch or less in front of toe).
4. Can button coat or dress; may lace shoes.

Language

5. Repeats ten-word sentences without errors.
6. Counts three objects, pointing correctly.
7. Repeats three to four digits (4-5 years).
8. Comprehends: "What do you do if: you are hungry, sleepy, cold?"
9. Spontaneous sentences, four to five words long.
10. Likes to ask questions.
11. Understands prepositions, such as: on-under-behind, etc. ("Put the block *on* the table.")
12. Can point to three out of four colors (red, blue, green, yellow).
13. Speech is now an effective communication tool.

Personal-social-adaptive

14. Copies cross (+) without demonstration.
15. Imitates oblique cross (×).
16. Draws a man with four parts.
17. Cooperates with other children in play.
18. Dresses and undresses self (mostly without supervision).

CHILD DEVELOPMENT FROM 1 MONTH TO 5 YEARS—cont'd

19. Brushes teeth, washes face.
20. Compares lines: "Which is longer?"
21. Folds paper two to three times.
22. Can select heavier from lighter object.
23. Cares for self at toilet.

5 Years
Motor

1. Balances on one foot for 8 to 10 seconds.
2. Skips, using feet alternately.
3. May be able to tie a knot.
4. Catches bounced ball with hands (not arms) in two of three trials.

Language

5. Knows age ("How old are you?")
6. Performs three tasks (with one command), for instance: "Put pen on table—close door—bring me the ball."
7. Knows four colors.

8. Defines use for: fork-horse-key-pencil, etc.
9. Identifies by name: nickel-dime-penny.
10. Asks meaning of words.
11. Asks many "why" questions.
12. Relatively few speech errors remain—90% of consonant sounds are made correctly.
13. Counts number of fingers correctly.
14. Counts by rote to 10.
15. Comments on pictures (descriptions and interpretations).

Personal-social-adaptive

16. Copies a square.
17. Copies oblique cross (×) without demonstration.
18. May print a few letters (5-5½ years).
19. Draws man with at least six identifiable parts.
20. Builds a six-block pyramid from demonstration.
21. Transports things in a wagon.
22. Plays with coloring set, construction toys, puzzles.
23. Participates well in group play.

Physical Development

The rate of growth during the first few months and years of life is greater than at any other time. The average full-term infant weighs about 7 to 7 ½ pounds (3.4 Kg) and is about 20 inches (50 cm) long. An infant typically loses up to 10% of that weight during the first few days, then regains it within 10 days and continues to gain steadily. Although infants vary, most double their birth weight by 4 to 6 months and triple it by 1 year. Length increases by about 50% during the first year.

Marked changes occur in body contour during infancy. The head grows at a rapid rate during the first year, and the head circumference is greater than the chest circumference. Growth in head circumference reflects brain growth, most of which occurs during the first 2 years of life. The thickness of the subcutaneous fat increases during the first year, reaching a peak around 9 months, then decreasing during the second year. Teeth begin to erupt, and the infant advances from a liquid diet to table food.

The newborn makes many rapid adjustments necessary to sustain life outside the uterus, which are actually a continuum of the development during fetal life. At birth, respirations are initiated and changes in the circulatory system occur, the digestive system begins to assimilate the food obtained from an external source, body wastes are excreted, and maintenance of body heat depends on the infant's own resources. Behavior includes many reflex actions that reflect the immaturity of the newborn's nervous system but also assist in adaptation with the new environment. One of the most striking physiological changes is the continuing maturation and increasing function of the nervous system. **Myelination** continues at a rapid rate during the first months of life but is not completed for several years. The functional development of various body structures probably corresponds to the order of myelination and occurs in a cephalocaudal direction, from head to foot. The development of head control precedes sitting, standing, and walking. As the brain and central nervous system continue to develop, an increasingly sophisticated range of cognitive and behavioral skills follows.

The first 3 months of life can be called a period of adjustment. Reflexes become more regulated during the first month, and the infant learns how to search, to suck, and to let needs be known. Sleeping and feeding patterns become more regular. The **tonic neck reflex** becomes more prominent at the end of the first month. (The tonic neck reflex is a normal response in newborns. It consists of extending the arm and the leg on the side of the body to which the head is quickly turned while the infant is supine and flexing the limbs of the opposite side.) During the second and third months, new behaviors appear that are not reflexes. The infant begins to follow objects with the eyes, allowing exploration of the environment. There is coordination of movement of hand and mouth, such as sucking the thumb at will. The **grasp reflex** gradually lessens as more purposeful movements begin. The infant begins to prolong interesting events that occur more or less by accident. The little wails that precede crying may be continued for their own sake. The squeals of the 2- to 3-month-old baby are loud, repeated, and joyful. The infant begins to smile in response to environmental stimuli and to vocalize. Most responses are generalized and frequently involve movements of the whole body. The infant during this period has social responses but does not discriminate; any person who can satisfy their needs is accepted.

By 3 months of age the baby becomes more discriminating and begins to differentiate his or her mother from others and produces special types of smiles and crying for her. This is the beginning of attachment behavior and the development of awareness of the self as separate from her. Between 3 and 6 months, or even earlier, the infant repeats some actions that are interesting as well as prolonging those that occur accidentally, such as repeated hitting of suspended toys to produce movement. There is more imitation of facial movements and beginning imitation of sounds. The infant attempts somewhat of a search for a displaced object, but not a true search. Infantile reflexes are replaced by purposeful movements, especially those seen in the development of eye-hand coordination. The infant begins to reach for and grasp objects with a raking motion. The tonic neck reflex and **Moro reflex** disappear during the fifth or sixth month. (The Moro reflex is a normal mass reflex in a young infant elicited by a sudden loud noise resulting in flexion of the legs, an embracing posture of the arms, and usually a brief cry.) At 3 months the infant, while prone, can raise the head and chest from a surface with arms extended, and at 4 months the head can be held steadily while the infant is supported in the sitting position. At 6 to 7 months the infant can sit without support. Crawling typically begins at about 9 months. At about the same time, the baby will begin to pull up to a standing position while holding onto something for support. At 10 to 11 months, the child starts to "cruise," walking while holding onto the furniture. Walking alone usually begins at about 12 months, though it may be several months earlier or later.

Fine motor skill development includes using the hands and fingers for grasping. The infant is born with a grasp reflex, which disappears by about 3 months. At 4 months, the infant seems to discover his or her hands and inspects them. By 5 months, the baby is able to grasp with two hands. By 10 months, the **pincer grasp,** with the index finger in apposition to the thumb, is present. The child can pick up finger foods and small toys.

Cognitive Development

Piaget defined the infancy stage of cognitive development as the **sensorimotor period.** Mental development during this period begins with reflexes and ends with the early appearance of language and other symbolic ways of representing the world. The infant is egocentric, and sensorimotor learning is related to the self. The infant changes from response through reflexes (crying, grasping, rooting, and sucking) to organization of sensorimotor activities in relation to the environment. Even the very young infant is a cognitive being capable of rather sophisticated mental operations. For example, infants are more responsive to a new stimulus than to one that has been repeated several times, showing discrimination known as habituation. They are also able to imitate certain facial gestures, such as sticking out the tongue or opening the mouth, which are indications of early cognitive abilities and integrative function.

During the first 7 to 9 months of life, the infant's learning is focused on bodily actions. Around 8 to 9 months the concept Piaget called "object permanence" can be observed. The infant learns that objects and people continue to exist even when she or he cannot see them. The 5-month-old infant will not reach for an object after it is hidden, but the 8-month-old infant will. Through this sequence of mental and physical actions and the gradual development of memory, the child begins to have a sense of self as separate from and yet a part of the environment. It is the beginning of the child's construction of reality.

The first mode of communication is crying. Although all the cries may sound the same initially, by about 1 month of age, the parents are usually able to differentiate the meaning of cries of varying pitch and intensity. For example, the infant has different cries for discomfort and hunger. Vocalization during this period changes from babbling and cooing to the use of several words that can be understood. Generally, the baby laughs at about 3 months, babbles at about 4 months, and by 9 or 10 months can imitate the sounds of others. By 12 months several words besides "mama" and "dada" are acquired.

Psychosocial Development

During the first year of life, great strides in behavioral development occur. The infant develops social skills that bond the baby with others in the environment. Socially, the infant progresses from staring at faces and crying to smiling, demanding company, vocalizing, and actively participating in games.

The period between 6 and 12 months is dominated by the social modality of "taking and holding on" as described by Erikson. It is a period of attachment behavior. The infant at 8 to 9 months of age has a beginning permanence concept and becomes fearful that the mother or other primary caregiver will disappear. The infant actively initiates contact with the caregiver and seeks to maintain that contact. There is true searching for a vanished object, although the search may be in several inappropriate places. Behavior becomes more complex and aggressive. The infant coordinates earlier repetitive actions into behaviors with a purposeful aim. Now the child explores objects more fully by rubbing, banging, and chewing and by discovering the correct procedures for manipulating them. Motor development is dramatic as coordination increases. The pincer grasp, using thumb and forefinger, develops.

Erikson described this first stage of ego development as one of **trust versus mistrust.** During this critical period of personality development, the child develops a sense of trust based on consistent nurturing in terms of food, warmth, comfort, and the presence of the mother. Successful growth during this period means that the child comes to trust both the self and the people in the environment. The threat at this stage is mistrust of the environment and self. According to Erikson (1963), a sense of trust develops when there is a mutual regulation of the baby's pattern of accepting things and the mother's way of giving them that changes as the baby develops. The social modality of the baby's development during the first 6 months is to satisfy needs by getting, receiving, and accepting. This is not passive behavior, since the infant influences people in the environment from birth. The first reflexive behaviors of looking, rooting, sucking, and crying elicit responses in the mother or other caretaking adults that cause them to act in ways that will meet the infant's needs. Parental bonding is influenced by these behaviors. The infant's social modality during the second half of the first year is taking and holding on, which begins with the eruption of teeth and the ability to sit upright and voluntarily reach out. The infant begins to be aware of being separate from the mother. The infant may become more demanding of the mother and is faced with the frustrations that result when the pleasure experienced in biting or grasping and holding on to things is met with interference. The infant displays helpless rage when strong desires are thwarted. When this behavior is understood and the infant continues to receive loving attention, trust in self and others can be maintained and strengthened. Some of the infant's early emotional expressions, such as timidity and shyness or boldness and sociability, may indicate enduring personality characteristics. Temperament, or basic behavioral style, is inborn. Aspects of temperament include activity level, regularity in biological functioning (hunger, sleep, elimination), readiness to accept new people and situations, adaptability to change, sensitivity to noise, light, and other sensory stimuli, mood (cheerfulness or unhappiness), intensity of responses, distractibility, and persistence. Infants vary in these characteristics from birth and have a tendency to continue in one style, although parental handling and experiences may cause change.

Freud described infancy as the oral stage. The pleasure zone is the mouth; the child seeks to take in everything for sensory exploration and takes great pleasure in sucking and eating. Weaning and teething are challenges at this stage.

THE TODDLER: 1 TO 3 YEARS

The child enters the toddler years well equipped to continue learning about the self and the world. Autonomy blossoms as the child begins to recognize self as separate from others. Toddlers have a sense of hope and trust and are developing intellectual and motor skills. A basic competence develops with the expansion of language, memory, and self-control. The toddler years are characterized by energetic exploration and intense inquisitiveness, and also by some obstinate and ritualistic behaviors. Ego growth is rapid during the second and third years of life as the child learns about people and objects in the environment and gradually gains increasing mastery over impulses and bodily functions.

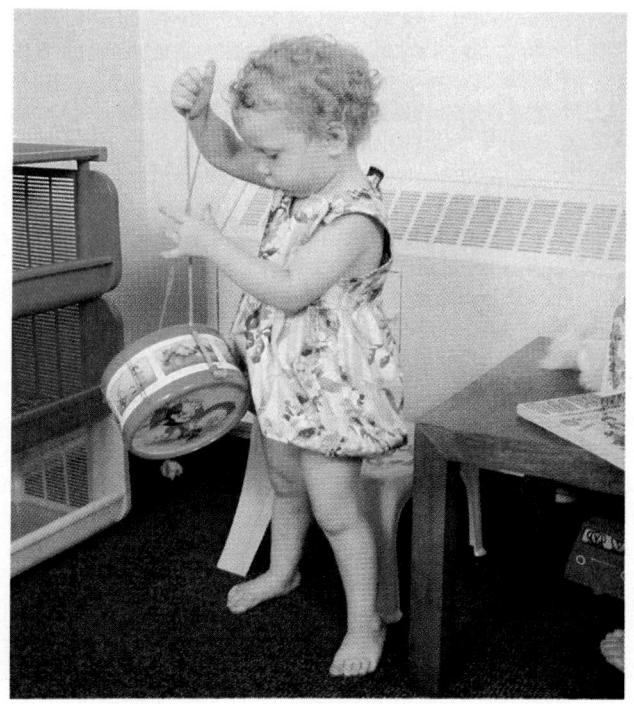

Physical Development

The rate of growth in height and weight decreases during the second year of life. The toddler gains an average of 5 ½ pounds (2.5 kg) in weight and 4 to 5 inches (10 to 13 cm) in height. The child's adult height will be roughly twice what it is at age 2. As the growth rate in height and weight decreases, it becomes less consistent month by month.

The changes in the child's physical appearance are dramatic. The toddler who is beginning to walk looks top-heavy, with short legs and a potbelly. Fat pads fill the arch of the foot, and most young children appear to be flat-footed until 3 or 4 years of age. There is also a tendency for the legs to bow outward and for lordosis to be apparent. Gradually the child becomes less chubby, the abdomen becomes flatter, and the face loses its baby look. The posture and body proportions change as the chest becomes larger in proportion to the head and abdomen. After 2 years of age, the extremities continue to grow faster than the trunk, and the jaw and lower face grow more rapidly than the cranium. The subcutaneous fat decreases rapidly in thickness during the second year.

Visual acuity improves: at 2 years it is about 20/40. The brain reaches 75% of its adult weight by 3 years. Myelination in the spinal cord is almost complete by age 2. The skin changes after the first year, becoming firmer with less water content. The primary teeth continue to erupt, and the child will have the full complement of 20 primary teeth early during the third year, when the second molars erupt.

Gross and fine motor skills increase during the toddler years due to the myelination of nerve fibers. Neuromuscular maturation contributes to gross motor abilities such as sitting, crawling, standing, and walking and to fine motor skills such as scribbling and using a pincer grasp. The child usually walks by about 12 months, though it may be as early as 9 months or as late as 18 months. By age 2, the toddler can run and can walk up and down stairs. Toilet training, a major developmental milestone, is also dependent on neuromuscular maturation and generally occurs around age 3.

As the toddler learns to perform self-care skills such as drinking, eating, dressing, toothbrushing, and bathing, her or his sense of independence and competence is enhanced. Initially, the child's efforts are clumsy and incomplete, but by about 3 years, the child displays a fair degree of competence in these areas. Competence increases with physical maturation and is enhanced by parents who give their child the opportunity to practice these skills.

On the average, during the toddler years, girls' development tends to be a bit ahead of boys'. Girls talk, walk, and are toilet trained a month or two earlier than boys.

Cognitive Development

During the second year of life, the child is in the sensorimotor stage as described by Piaget. The toddler, increasingly ready for independence, experiments with new ways to achieve a goal. During the last half of the second year, the child reaches a cognitive milestone: he or she becomes capable of the mental representation of external events. The toddler can think through plans to achieve a goal, rather than performing and watching what happens. The concept of object permanence is developed: the toddler searches for an object even when it is not visible.

Language skills increase dramatically during the toddler years. The use of language reflects the child's cognitive development. Speech enables the child to become more independent as well as to better make needs known. Most children begin to use a few words at about 14 months, though some do not begin until around age 2. By age 2 most children have an effective vocabulary (words that can be spoken and/or understood) of 250 to 300 words. The first words a child learns are nouns of one syllable; subsequently the noun is connected with an action verb. During the second year, the child moves from having personal, nonverbal mental images of objects and events and the use of words and gestures invested with personal meaning, to having the capacity for thought and communicative language. A burst of vocabulary occurs toward the end of the second year. This is a period of symbolic thought, a time when the toddler can use mental symbols and words to refer to objects and people, seen and unseen, and to anticipate future events. Language develops sequentially, with adjectives and adverbs following the use of nouns and verbs. The toddler gradually learns other grammatical components of the language from 18 months on. By the third birthday, the child has an effective vocabulary of about 900 words. The greater the child's vocabulary and comprehension, the more the cognitive processes can advance. As children share speech and communication with adults, they also learn ideas, attitudes, and values.

The toddler's thinking is characterized by centering, which means that only one aspect of an object or event is perceived by the child, and by egocentrism, the notion that there is only one point of view—the child's own. Toddlers are unaware of how other people think.

Psychosocial Development

Autonomy and independence are major goals for a toddler. The core task for this stage of ego development as described by Erikson is **autonomy versus shame.** Each child is developing a sense of individuality and separateness from other people. The toddler experiences autonomy in many ways, including the ability to gain a new level of control over motor abilities, bodily functions, and self-care skills; making and acting on decisions; coping with problems or getting the necessary help; and giving generously or holding on. Neuromuscular and cognitive development make it possible for the toddler to explore and experiment, which lead to a sense of autonomy. Failure to establish autonomy results in a sense of shame and of doubt in one's ability to function effectively.

Freud described the period from 18 months to 3 years as the anal stage of psychosexual development. The focus of this stage is on the buildup and release of tension at the orifices. The child experiences pleasure from expelling urine and feces. However, the parents begin to insist that these actions occur only at the proper time and in the proper location. Toilet training is part of socializing the child. Self-control and delayed gratification are necessary skills for socialized behavior. Freud believed that the parent's approach to toilet training and the child's response greatly influence the personality of the individual.

Socialization is an important aspect of the child's development during the toddler years. Socialization is the process by which an individual becomes a member of a social group by acquiring the group's values and behaviors. In our society, socialization during this period focuses on numerous issues including bowel and bladder habits, cleanliness, control of anger and aggressive behaviors, acquisition of language skills, and control of excessive motor activities, egocentric behavior, and antisocial behavior.

During infancy, the child had few restrictions or responsibilities. The toddler must develop new roles and relationships with the world and the people in it. The rules for acceptable behavior are changing, and the growing child must adapt.

Social relationships during this period continue to revolve mainly around the parents or other primary caregivers, but the toddler is increasingly equipped to expand her or his social world to include siblings, other children, relatives, and neighbors. Through social relationships the toddler learns about socially approved behaviors such as cooperation, sharing, waiting one's turn, and respecting the feelings and possessions of others.

Socialization as a male or female begins during infancy. From age 1 to 3 the child has a beginning awareness of sexual differences and sexual roles. Children begin exploring their own bodies and those of others. This is normal and is an important means for the toddler to learn about physical differences between males and females. Parents generally interact differently with boys and girls and have different expectations regarding behaviors and attitudes such as dependence/independence, achievement, vigor, cooperation/competition, and assertiveness. The attributes that are affirmed or negated by the parents greatly influence the child's sex

role development. Observation and imitation of the same-sex parent also contribute to gender identity.

The toddler is uninhibited in the pursuit of personal goals. She or he wants to explore everything in the environment. Since the toddler has not yet acquired any sense of judgment or discrimination, parents are constantly balancing the child's drive to explore and experience with the need to protect the child from situations that could be harmful or are beyond the child's ability level. This leads to conflict with the parents when the child encounters restrictions that the parent must set to protect the child, or help her or him adapt to socially acceptable behaviors. Displays of the toddler's temper are common, especially when the child is also fatigued. While temper tantrums are expressions of frustration, they are fear-provoking for the child because he or she also wants to please the parent and desires the parent's love and approval. An environment that is safe for exploration and allows the child to make choices is beneficial. It is also important for the parents to maintain control of their own emotions in situations where the toddler is not yet prepared to do so. As the toddler matures and gains greater control over self and environment, many situations become less stressful.

Play is important developmental work for the toddler. It is a process of exploration and discovery. Gradually, as the child begins to form mental images, play becomes more imaginative and imitative. The child thoroughly enjoys newly acquired abilities and manipulates objects with persistence and enthusiasm. Play provides practice for newly acquired motor skills. The toddler exhibits repetitive play and enjoys putting things in and out of containers. Children who are given the freedom to explore and make reasonable choices develop a sense of self-assurance and spontaneity. If the toddler is not allowed to play in a safe and interesting environment or if play activities are stopped by constant limit setting, the child may begin to doubt his or her ability to accomplish tasks or to meet new challenges.

Young toddlers engage in parallel play, where they play beside, but not with, each other. Initially, they treat other children like objects; toddlers may push, pinch, bite, or poke others because they have no inner sense that this may hurt. Gradually the toddler moves into interactive play with peers.

The toddler gradually becomes able to play alone for longer periods of time, but attachment behavior continues. Periodically, the toddler seeks out the parent or caregiver, particularly if there is a problem or perceived threat. When faced with a new person or situation, most toddlers face it with more assurance if the parent is present, and return to the parent quickly if things become too difficult.

The toddler is sensitive to changes in the environment. If one alteration occurs in the toddler's world, it is as if everything changes and becomes strange and unmanageable. Consistent routines for daily activities are helpful. They allow the child to anticipate what will happen, learn the behaviors that are expected, and gain a sense of control. Routines, habits, or rituals may be particularly important around mealtime or at bedtime when the child must deal with separation and darkness. If parents do everything the same way each night, the child feels reassurance that the world will not change while he or she sleeps.

During the toddler years, the child learns to cope with separation from the parents or caregivers. Fear of separation begins at about 7 months. Between the age of 1 and 3 years, long separations are not well tolerated and may damage the child emotionally. Although unable to express or understand the feelings, the child is able to sense loss. Learning to tolerate brief separations is an important developmental task. As children learn that parents return, they become more accepting and adaptable.

Closely related to separation anxiety are the fears and fantasies commonly expressed by toddlers. The child may experience nightmares or behavioral changes, such as anxiety about taking a bath or about flushing the toilet for fear of disappearing. The toddler's feeling of power may contribute to these fears because the child believes that by wishing something, it can be made to happen. For example, the child fears that by wishing harm toward someone, it may occur. Imaginary beings and animals, some of them ferocious, are common in the imaginations of toddlers. Some of the child's own aggressive feelings may be projected onto the imaginary being. Sympathetic understanding of these fears and fantasies by the parents helps them deal with the child's concern about separation.

Emotional feelings and reactions vary in toddlers depending on age and temperament and on how others in their environment react to them. A toddler cannot express or explain personal emotions, so they are expressed in behaviors. These behaviors may include showing affection, sharing, playing cooperatively, timidity, contrariness, selfish or aggressive behavior, temper tantrums, or dawdling. A degree of self-awareness, and emotions such as pride, sympathy, jealousy, guilt, and shame begin to emerge during the second year. Parents need to be sensitive to the acting out of the toddler's emotions, and the need to be supportive and loving in helping the toddler as he or she learns to deal with various emotions.

The word "no" is spoken with increasing frequency during the toddler years. This is often labeled "negativism," but it is essential to the child's efforts to gain self-control and a sense of mastery over the environment. The child may be saying "no" and at the same time complying with the parent's request.

Children begin to develop a self-concept at a very young age. By the time a child enters the toddler years, and certainly during these years, the child has positive or negative perceptions of the self and a personal sense of worth. Adults in the child's world are very influential in determining the direction of the child's inner sense of self. Supportive reinforcement of positive feelings is essential for nurturing an emotionally healthy human being.

THE PRESCHOOLER: 3 TO 6 YEARS

The preschool years are marked by physical, social, emotional, and intellectual development. While the child still has many dependent needs and behaviors, she or he is also beginning to exhibit more independence in action and thoughts. The child is developing a sense of self as a social person in relation to other people and is also learning a great deal about the physical world. Preschool children are emerging from their toddler years and becoming social beings. Expanded language and gross motor skills enable them to explore further in the environment. Preschoolers are involved in increasing independence, developing basic motor and language skills, and adding to their social skills.

Physical Development

Physical growth continues at a slow rate. On the average, the preschooler gains about 1.5 to 2.5 kg (3 to 5 pounds) in weight, and 5 to 7 cm (2 to 2 ¾ inches) per year. The face and body become more slender as

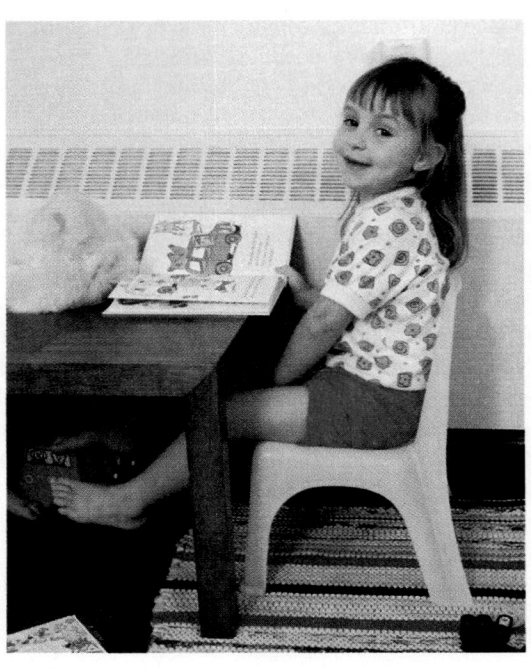

the baby fat disappears. The musculoskeletal system continues to develop with muscles growing and cartilage changing to bone. Most of the bone growth is in the long bones. At about age 5, the child begins to lose the first set of teeth. Visual acuity reaches 20/20 between 4 and 5 years.

Preschoolers have an increased sense of balance and enjoy both gross and fine motor skills. Their ability to run, jump, hop, swim, skate, and ride tricycles and bicycles demonstrates their increasing gross motor abilities. Their use of building toys and art materials exhibits their increase in coordination and fine motor skills.

The preschooler is dependent on parents and other caregivers for nutritious foods and good eating habits. Family food preferences, culture, and life-style also influence food selections. Appetite fluctuates, and many preschoolers go for several months without gaining weight. However, for some preschoolers excessive eating may be a problem and is a cause for concern as lifetime habits are beginning during these years. During the preschool years, the child learns to eat with the family and to enjoy many of the foods that the family eats. The child should be able to feed himself or herself early in the preschool years, and should be using eating utensils with little difficulty toward the end of the preschool years.

The preschooler shows increasing skills in dressing and other personal care skills. Toilet training is usually completed before or during the early preschool years.

Cognitive Development

Piaget described the child from 2 to 7 years as being in the **preoperational stage** of cognitive functioning. The child is increasingly able to use mental symbols to represent people, objects, and events. This means that the child is able to think about people, for example, without seeing or hearing them. This is liberating for the child, making it possible to act out thoughts during play. The preschooler's thinking is still limited by the inability to focus on more than one aspect of a situation at a time. At times, preschoolers will group unrelated characteristics of a person or event together into a confusing whole. A major characteristic of this period is egocentric thinking: children in this stage cannot see another's point of view and assume that their own viewpoint is shared by everyone. This affects the preschooler's language, thought, and reasoning. The older preschooler begins to be able to consider more aspects of a situation, another person's viewpoint, and the intent and outcome of behavior. Cognitive growth of the preschooler includes increasing memory ability.

Language development includes use of an increasing number of words, improved articulation, use of correct grammatical structure, and a growing ability to categorize objects in the environment using words. The early preschooler uses both communicative and non-communicative speech. When using communicative speech, the child tries to communicate a message to a listener. Noncommunicative speech consists of monologues during which the child converses out loud to herself or himself, though others may be present. The child may repeat and elaborate on statements made by parents and other adults. These monologues are often a source of great amusement to other people.

Interactions with parents, siblings, relatives, other adults, and peers all contribute to the child's educational process. In addition, many preschoolers begin structured educational programs such as Headstart, nursery school, or preschool, when they are 3 or 4 years of age. An environment at home or away from home that stimulates and affirms discovery and learning is necessary for the child to practice new skills and extend earlier experiences.

Psychosocial Development

The child identifies with the parents and is motivated to try to be what they want and to be like them. The child becomes more socially responsive and able to give love and affection. The development of initiative is characterized by the wish to "become," in which the child wants to find out what kind of person he or she can be. During the earlier years, the child undergoes a growth of the sense of self as a separate person with some power to influence the environment and to control impulses and her or his own body. These accomplishments make it possible to approach new tasks with feelings of confidence and an abundance of energy. The child becomes intrusive in a desire to attack new situations. Preschool children are noisy, active, and on the move. They thrust themselves into each situation, driven by curiosity and imagination. Erikson described this stage of ego development, particularly around 4 to 5 years, as one of **initiative versus guilt.** The child now has adequate energy, motor skills, and mental ability to attack new tasks with gusto and determination. When the parent provides encouragement and enthusiasm, while also protecting the child from harm, the child learns self-sufficiency, direction, and purpose. If the parent prevents the child from doing tasks she or he is capable of trying, or ridicules or punishes the child, the child learns guilt and shame and a sense of inadequacy. The child may then experience these negative feelings when he or she tries to do the same thing, or even when the child thinks about trying it again. This can have long-term effects on the child's psychological makeup.

Love and admiration for the parents and other significant adults intensify during the preschool years, although they may be mixed with defiance at times; identification with the parents increases. Sexual identification began at an earlier age when the child learned that he was a boy or that she was a girl, but during the preschool years it is heightened. It becomes evident as the child begins to imitate the parent of the same sex, learns more of a sex role identity, and becomes acutely aware of sexual differences. The interest in the parent of the opposite sex is somewhat romantic, which results in conflict when the child learns that he or she cannot replace the parent of the same sex, whom the child also loves. These feelings of intense love and the wish to be rid of one parent can cause anxiety, guilt, and fear because the child believes that wishes are as real as the actual deed. Because the child cannot compete with this larger and more powerful rival, she or he resolves the tension by identifying with the parent of the same sex. Freud called this the Oedipal complex for boys and the Elektra complex for girls, named after characters in Greek mythology. Parents and other significant adults influence early sex role development.

Sexuality Patterns

The preschooler is very interested in his or her own body and its intactness and how it compares with other children. This sexual curiosity is an important developmental phase and helps the child gain an understanding of sexual identity. The child's curiosity may be manifested in direct questions to parents about sex. Such questions are an attempt to understand how the body functions and why girls and boys are different. Curiosity may also be evident in overt behaviors such as actual visual exploration of oneself or of the opposite sex. The sexual development of the preschooler also centers around resolution of the Oedipal complex for boys and the Electra complex for girls. According to Freud's psychoanalytical theory, a boy wishes to possess his mother solely and thus competes with his father to win affections from his mother. The child imitates the behaviors of the same-sex parent closely in an attempt to replace the opposite-sex parent, thus taking on characteristics of masculinity or femininity and resolving the complex. By the end of the preschool period, the child begins to realize that such a sexual relationship is not possible and instead expresses interest in the same-sex peer group. Nevertheless, child-rearing practices and imitation of the same-sex parent influence the specific sex typing of the child. One activity related to sexuality that tends to confuse or disturb parents is the preschooler's interest in masturbation, or self-stimulation of the genitals. If this behavior is not excessive, it is both normal and healthy, since it is part of a child's bodily exploration and helps satisfy sexual curiosity.

When assessing sex and sexuality, it is important to also determine the parents' perceptions of sex roles for both male and female, their understanding of sexual development in the preschooler, and any biases they may have due to certain attitudes or beliefs.

The preschooler's social environment increasingly extends beyond the family and other primary caregivers to include other adult and peer encounters. The child learns to interact more easily with unfamiliar people. Temperament enables some children to do this with great ease; other children require more encouragement. Experiencing a variety of interactions with people of all ages is important for preschoolers to help them develop a range of personal-social behaviors.

The preschooler is able to experience many feelings, including happiness, joy, affection, excitement, wonder, anger, frustration, jealousy, sadness, loneliness, and fear, all which are normal emotions. Emotional feelings and reactions are determined by both innate temperament and by the pattern of emotional expression of adults around the child. Children need to be able to express the range of their emotions in a supportive and loving environment, and to begin to name and understand their own emotional reactions. Preschool children who experience a death, loss, separation, significant change in life-style, or illness require support and help in dealing with their feelings. Preschoolers may express their feelings through physical symptoms such as headaches or stomachaches, or they may become irritable or withdrawn. The finality of death is not well understood by a child at this age. She or he may ask many questions and continue to search for the lost person. The most important aspect of dealing with a loss or death is for the parents to be honest with the child.

The behaviors of a preschool child are a composite of many interacting factors including heredity, culture, the environment, and developmental level. The child continually experiments with old and new behaviors. As the child's experience moves beyond the home, she or he encounters a vast number of experiences that affect behavior. As the behavioral repertoire enlarges, the preschooler tries many new behaviors. Many of these are useful and help the child develop. However, some are negative, harmful, or dangerous and must be curtailed. Some of the common negative behaviors of the preschooler include: negative use of language, negative facial gestures, aggressive or hostile behavior, excessively dependent behavior, and noncompliance. If the parent or other caregiver does not intervene when the child displays negative behaviors, behavioral problems may develop. Some discipline is necessary, but it must be delivered within the context of love and concern for the child's present and future well-being. The preschooler is developing concepts of "good" and "bad." If a child behaves in an unacceptable manner and is told repeatedly that he or she is "bad," this affects self-image. The situation is similar with a child who is repeatedly told that he or she is "good," and then becomes limited in self-expression and self-development to someone else's definition of "good." Adults should identify the behavior, rather than label the child. Children become restricted by labels and may find it difficult to move beyond them to enlarge their field of experience.

Play during the preschool years becomes increasingly more social, imaginative, and complex. While playing together, children develop concepts, imagination, neuromuscular coordination, and language. "Let's pretend" is a favorite phrase and activity. Through imaginative play the child tries out the roles of different people in a variety of situations. In play the child can take on any role and master fears. The child can have feelings of strength and adequacy instead of smallness and vulnerability.

Imaginary playmates are important to some preschoolers. They may include these "playmates" in dreams, fantasies, and certain daily rituals, such as eating, as well as including them in their play. Rituals continue to be a significant part of the preschooler's daily pattern.

By internalizing the parents' standards and ideals, the child gradually develops a sense of moral responsibility and a conscience, which makes resisting temptation possible even though the parents are not present. The child can feel guilt for misbehavior, and at about 5 years of age he or she even has some feelings of guilt for wanting to misbehave. This early conscience is modified through the years of childhood as intellectual abilities increase and the ability to identify reasons for moral action becomes more mature.

THE SCHOOL AGE CHILD: 6-12

During the middle years of childhood, from age 6 to 10, the child moves from the close ties of family and home to the larger world of peers, school, and neighborhood. The family "romance" is less intense, and the child is able to go out into the world. This is the period of latency during which the child is free from earlier concentration on sexuality and strong basic drives. The child can now direct energy toward learning the skills and competencies of the mind and body that lead to practical achievements and accomplishment in the world. Tremendous intellectual growth occurs during this lull before the "storm" of adolescence, and the child is introduced to experiences that help in learning the fundamentals of society and culture.

Physical Development

Physical growth during the middle years of childhood is relatively slow and smooth. The most pronounced period of growth usually comes toward the end of this stage, at 10 to 12 years. Some children begin the growth spurt as early as age 8 or 9. The increments in weight are less regular than those in the young infant and child, and weight may remain stationary for weeks at a time.

The approximate annual increase in weight is about 5 to 7 pounds. The average annual increase in height is approximately 2 to 3 inches. Boys on the average are taller and heavier than girls until the adolescent growth spurt, which occurs earlier in girls.

The physical changes that occur make school-age children more agile and graceful. They become slimmer, with longer legs and a lower center of gravity than the younger child. They are stronger and better coordinated and are able to fit into the adult physical environment more easily. The size of the cranium increases only slightly because nearly 90% of the growth of the brain is accomplished by age 7. The lower parts of the face continue to grow, giving the child a more mature appearance and making room for the larger teeth to erupt. The first permanent teeth, which usually erupt at 6 to 6½ years of age, are usually the mandibular central incisors. The eruption of the large permanent teeth contributes to the temporarily less attractive appearance of the school-age child.

The eyeball continues to grow until 10 or 12 years of age. Visual acuity is usually 20/20 to 20/30 between 4 and 5 years of age, but depth perception is not very accurate until 6 to 7 years of age. Hearing is well-established at a much earlier age. Growth of lymphoid tissue increases steadily until puberty and then decreases. This accounts for the abundance of lymphoid tissues such as adenoids and tonsils. The skeleton continues to ossify, with cartilage being replaced by bone. The child acquires the basic neuromuscular mechanisms by age 6 or 7 and spends the school years refining physical skills, resulting in an increase in motor skills and coordination. Thus, the school-age child engages in repetitive practice in all areas of neuromuscular activities from the fine motor skills of writing, drawing, and playing instruments, to the large motor skills used in baseball, biking, running, and swimming, depending on individual interests.

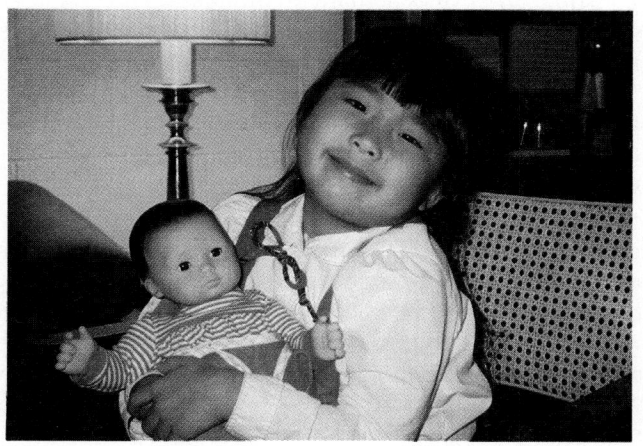

The appetite fluctuates, and nutritious eating may become a problem. Problems with excessive weight may also begin to occur. Although taste preferences continue to influence what the child eats, the ongoing establishment of good eating habits is important.

Cognitive Development

The cognitive development of the school-age child, according to Piaget, is characterized by the ability to begin to do mentally what the child would have had to do with real action at an earlier age. Piaget termed this the **stage of concrete operations,** meaning that the child can now use mental representations or symbols of objects and events. What had to be done physically before, the child can now experience mentally. This enables the child to use numbers, read, order objects on an increasing or decreasing scale, and classify objects by a common characteristic. The stage of concrete operations begins at about age 8. The school-age child also begins to see the multiple characteristics of objects rather than centering on any one aspect. Piaget also found that during these years the child masters the concept of conservation. Piaget's classic test illustrating the principle of conservation is to give the child two jars of equal size containing equal amounts of liquid. The contents of one jar are then poured into two smaller containers of equal size, and the child is asked whether the amount of liquid poured into the two smaller jars is still the same as that remaining in the other container. Younger children cannot comprehend that the liquid has been conserved when placed in smaller containers. The older child comprehends that the quantity remains the same. She or he is beginning to distinguish the difference between how things seem and how they really are.

Throughout the school years, memory and language skills increase. This enhances the child's ability to share experiences and observations and to articulate questions and new understandings. Older children can think more logically because they can now make mental comparisons rather than actually manipulating objects, can see the whole as well as the parts, and have mastered the concept of conservation.

As school-age children develop, thinking gradually becomes more logical. Egocentric thinking and behavior progressively diminish and are replaced by a larger view of self and others. Children begin to realize that their own is not the only point of view and that others see things differently. This new ability to reason and to carry out mental operations in solving problems is limited in an important respect. They cannot yet differentiate clearly between their own assumptions and the facts. In other words, they treat their own hypotheses as if they were facts and reject facts that do not agree with that position.

Creativity continues to develop in the young school-age child. Frequently, however, children appear more reluctant to express creativity while they are in school, perhaps due to the responses of adults who are more interested in the "right" answers. This attitude can suppress the child's creative impulses, because adult approval is so important.

As children internalize the standards and ideals of the significant adults around them, they begin to develop a conscience and sense of moral behavior. They have greater knowledge of what is right and wrong, though they may break the rules made by adults. They begin to have feelings of guilt about misbehavior. The younger child may follow certain rules somewhat rigidly and be quick to condemn the supposed wrongs of others. This early sense of morality is expanded and modified during the years of middle childhood as intellectual skills increase and the ability to understand reasons for moral thought and action matures. Parents can enhance their child's moral growth by modeling their own values, such as honesty and fairness, at every opportunity, and by helping the child understand punishment as the result of a deed and not as a judgment of the child's worth.

School is an exciting adventure, and most children anticipate it eagerly. Mixed in with the excitement are often some fears and anxieties. The child needs to separate from home and parents, adjust to new authority figures, accept restrictions on previously acceptable activities, learn new routines, and participate in large groups. These situations can create tension within the child. This transition can be facilitated by parents and teachers who express understanding and encouragement.

Certain characteristics are indicators of readiness to enter the world of school. Of course, one child is unlikely to possess all these. Some of these characteristics include the ability to communicate, ability to participate in social interactions, capacity to make friends, attainment of a basic body of knowledge, and independence in basic self-care activities.

Psychosocial Development

Erikson described the ego development stage of middle childhood as a period focused on industry versus inferiority. This is a stage when ideally the child develops a sense of industriousness and accomplishment rather than a sense of inadequacy. During this period the child leaves home for school where the views, esteem, and approval of people outside the family become important. The child becomes a worker, one who is required to develop intellectual, physical, and social skills that contribute to a sense of adequacy. The child's attainments in cognitive, interpersonal, and social develop-

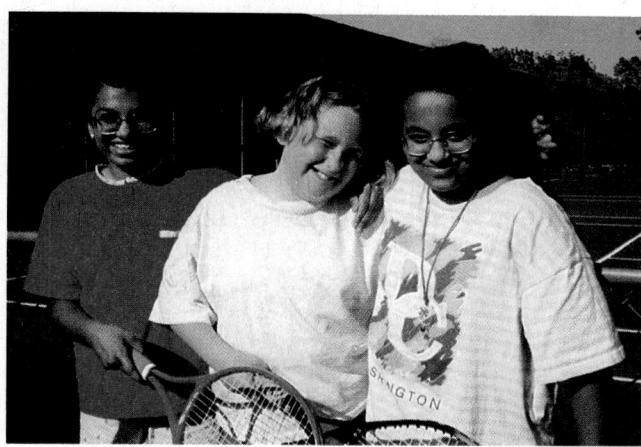

ment are significant. The child is now able to see a higher organization of behavior in which to participate. The child wants to operate in socially accepted ways of thinking and behaving, can understand another person's point of view, and is able to take what she or he hears and sees and compare it with what is already known of reality. The child learns to reason and act according to rules, which allows for benefit from the school experience and for participation in organized sports or other activities. Participation in activities that develop skills both in cooperation and competition is beneficial.

Achievement at this stage enhances feelings of competence, confidence, and industry. The child who achieves in some areas begins to feel rewarded both from outside sources, such as teachers and parents, and from within, by feelings of satisfaction. The child who does not achieve in some way begins to develop feelings of inferiority, low self-esteem, loss of confidence, and a sense of incompetence. These feelings may haunt the developing individual for many years, even when success and achievement come later. Children experience success during this stage of industry as they participate in many productive activities. School-age children's great desire to win at games and willingness to work to achieve a variety of skills demonstrate their need to be adequate in their own eyes as well as in the eyes of others. Parents, teachers, and other adult figures should encourage school-age children even when performance is incomplete or imperfect. And adults must realize that success comes sooner for some children than for others.

Freud described the period of relative sexual quiet as a time of latency. In terms of sexual development, middle childhood is a span of time between the sexual struggles and resolutions of earlier childhood, and the sexual turbulence of adolescence. Awareness of sexuality is not absent; curiosity, questions, and jokes remain a part of the child's growing sexual identity.

By 6 years of age the child's personality has become structured. Through accomplishment of earlier developmental tasks, the child has achieved a concept of the self, acquired a sense of trust, developed autonomy with some power over impulses and the environment, and incorporated standards of the culture as interpreted by the parents.

During these school years, the peer group becomes increasingly important, and the child needs to find a place in a group of peers. The child is ready to be involved in the private world of children, where adults are not always welcome. At age 6 and 7, peers are partners in play, with boys and girls participating together much of the time. During ages 8 and 9, the child usually selects a best friend and moves toward group activities with friends of the same sex. Feelings of group solidarity and belonging are promoted by secret languages, codes, and clubs, as well as a common culture. Together children explore ideas and values, learn fair play, practice leadership roles, and experience cooperation and compromise. Children who show difficulty with peer relationships may have problems in developing future relationships.

As these children move into the larger world of school and peers, they continue to need their parent(s). Demands for conformity are placed on them by people outside the family, such as teachers, scout leaders, and peers. The family should be children's source of strength and support. They continue to need the approval of parents, teachers, and other important adults for their uniqueness and any special talents. As children approach adolescence, they view their parents in a more critical light. This puts a strain on the parent-child relationship and can lead to tension and arguments. Parents need to understand the changing viewpoint of the child, and reassure him or her of their continuing love, even when this is difficult. Parents also need to allow greater independence and responsibility for the child in appropriate areas. This reinforces the child's sense of self and prepares the child for future developmental stages.

ADOLESCENCE: 11-13 TO 20

Adolescence is the period of life beginning with puberty and extending for 8 or 10 years to the onset of adulthood. The age boundaries of adolescence vary but range from 11-13 to 19-22, and sometimes longer. Adolescence generally extends to the time when the person is physically and psychologically mature, ready to assume adult responsibilities, and to be self-sufficient. Throughout the adolescent years the individual struggles with the transition from the role of a child to the role of an adult and struggles to develop a personal identity. The adolescent moves toward greater independence and personal freedom to make decisions.

Developmental Tasks of Adolescence

The adolescent faces the following developmental tasks:

1. Searching for self-identity and a sense of self-worth
2. Achieving a gradual independence from parents
3. Establishing relationships with peers
4. Developing academic and vocational skills
5. Adjusting to rapid physical and sexual changes
6. Developing an internalized set of values
7. Considering choices for a career

According to Erikson, the task of adolescence is the development of ego identity versus role confusion. The formation of a self-identity separate from others is a process that begins in infancy and continues throughout adulthood, but it has a very distinct focus during adolescence. Without the emerging understanding of self-identity as expressed through interests, preferences, and personality temperament, individuals feel confused about who they are in comparison with the group. Part of the need to identify the self as a separate person is the need to establish independence from the parents.

The word *conflict* is often associated with the words *teenager* and *adolescent,* and adolescence is truly a stage of conflict and turmoil, as well as one of high growth potential in the physical, sexual, and social areas. The adolescent must learn to cope with increasingly intense impulses, developing sexuality, and an altering body form. Spurts of growth occur, along with increased muscular energy and strength. The reproductive system matures; the individual develops secondary sexual characteristics and becomes capable of reproduction. The social world broadens in adolescence, and the individual develops a growing sensitivity to the perceived judgments of others.

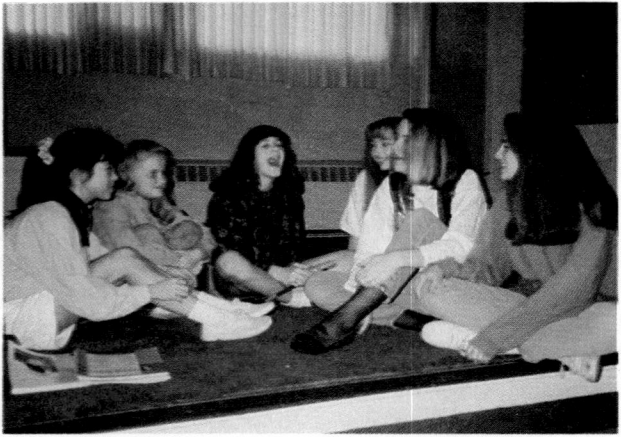

Stages of Adolescence

Adolescence may be divided into four phases or stages:

Preadolescence
Early adolescence
Middle adolescence
Late adolescence

Preadolescence is a stage covering the years of 10 through 12 for girls and 10 to 11 through 13 for boys. It is characterized by increases in physical activity, energy, and restlessness. Running is more natural than walking, and sitting still even for a short time may be nearly impossible. Muscular strength, skill, and agility are very important to the individual and among peers. Adolescents may have quiet moments during which they seem to be simply staring into space. They may have fears, worries, and concerns but are generally not interested in talking about them. Signs of earlier childhood problems such as nervous habits, childish antics, or bed-wetting may reappear temporarily.

Preadolescence is a continuation of the change in primary affiliation with parents and their codes to primary affiliation with peers. These years are often trying times for parents because the parent-child bonds appear to be loosening and breaking. Although preadolescents love and feel loyalty toward their parents, they may frequently treat them with surprising suspicion, distrust, and irritability. They are easily offended and respond to seemingly minor incidents with the ready accusation that adults do not understand them and treat them unfairly. Other adults in the neighborhood may receive more admiration than the parents receive. Parental recommendations regarding use of language and matters of appearance and cleanliness are often met with indignation and conflict. Preadolescents are increasingly sensitive about having a parent see their bodies and about public displays of affection toward parents. They are often seemingly unaware of the effect of their own inconsiderations on the feelings of others and appear surprised when it is pointed out to them that their behavior has caused some hurt.

At this stage, boys and girls typically have little to do with each other socially. Girls may move through this phase more quickly than boys. Clique and secret club formation is a prominent characteristic. If peer codes do not meet with parental approval, they are all the more desirable. The changes of preadolescence are not easy for the parents, nor are they easy for the preadolescent. Conflicting and painful situations are common, but the preadolescent must experience these to move on in establishing an individual identity.

Early adolescence begins with **puberty** and lasts for several years (11 to 12 through 13 to 14 for females and 12 to 14 through 15 to 16 for males). The growth spurt focuses attention on the self and on the task of

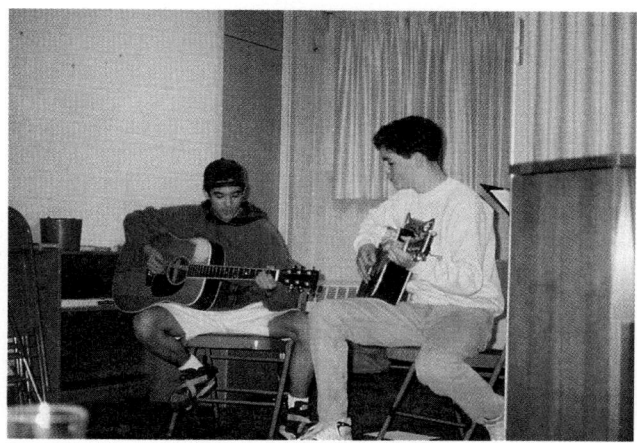

becoming comfortable with body changes and appearance. The teen tries to separate from the parents; the dependency-independency struggle is apparent by less involvement in family activities, criticism of parents, and rebellion against parental and other adult discipline and authority. Conformity to and acceptance of peer group standards and peer friendships gain importance. The peer group usually consists of same-sex friends; however, the early adolescent shows an increased interest in the opposite sex. Early adolescence usually coincides with menarche in females and active spermatogenesis in males.

Middle adolescence begins when physical growth is completed and usually extends from age 13 to 14 through 16 for females and 14 to 16 through 18 to 20 for males. The major tasks during this period are an increased sense of ego identity, attainment of greater independence, interest in the future and career possibilities, and establishment of heterosexual relationships. The individual is working to overcome feelings of insecurity and inadequacy and to move toward self-assurance and independence. Peer group allegiance, at a peak in 15- to 16-year-olds, is manifested by clothing, food, and other fads, musical preference, and common jargon. Most teenagers relate increasingly with the opposite sex, while some begin to be aware of their homosexual orientation. The middle adolescent gradually becomes more self-assured and able to make some independent decisions. For these reasons the youth at this stage has particular difficulty in adjusting to controlling or confining situations. Some societal privileges and responsibilities increase during middle adolescence such as driving a car. Experimentation with adult-like behavior and risk taking is common in an attempt to prove oneself to peers. Sexual experimentation often begins now as a result of social exploration and physical maturation. Family relationships and communication may be disrupted as the adolescent's activity outside the

home is increased. Changes in cognitive functioning may first be evident in that the adolescent moves to abstract thinking, returning to more concrete thinking during times of stress.

Late adolescence may occur from about age 17 to 18 until 20 to 25 years of age. The person has usually finished adolescent rebellion, formed some significant views, and established a fairly stable sense of self. Many youths are not yet committed to one occupation, and they often question relationships to existing social, vocational, and emotional roles and life-styles. He or she may be a student or an apprentice. Lack of economic freedom may be a concern and can lead to prolonged dependence on parents. Continued dependence may lead to delayed maturity. The late adolescent is clarifying his or her value system and examining issues of philosophy, religion, life and death, and ethical decisions. The peer group has lost its primary importance, and a relationship with a particular person may become the focal point for social activity. There is more individual dating and fewer group activities with friends; often the first emotionally intimate relationship develops. The late adolescent may take a major step in establishing independence from parents by moving away from home. Activities with family members tend to decrease and more adult-like friendships begin between late adolescents and their parents as the earlier family turbulence subsides. At that point, the person is developmentally a young adult, having made the transition from adolescence. He or she is more realistically aware of strengths and self-limitations and the limitations of others. Thought processes become more logical and the ability to utilize abstract ideas increases. The end of late adolescence is marked by planning for the future in the form of higher education, occupation, and committed relationships.

Some fluctuation in this progression may continue to some degree for several years in the direction of greater maturation. The tasks of finding an acceptable career that is personally satisfying and potentially economically adequate assumes a more central position during the later high school years and subsequent period of college, vocational training, or apprenticeship. This is a time of becoming ready to leave the parents' home both physically and emotionally.

At age 18 people may marry without parental consent and may vote, and males become subject to the military draft in times of national need. In most states alcoholic beverages are prohibited at this age. At age 21 individuals attain most adult privileges and responsibilities conferred by society. At this time an individual is allowed to drink all alcoholic beverages, sign a binding financial document, and accept full legal penalties for crimes.

The end of adolescence is more difficult to define than the beginning. Our society observes no specific ritual of passage into adulthood. The adolescent may remain dependent on the parents because of economic need or educational endeavors. In general, the adolescent moves into adulthood when she or he can prepare realistic plans for the future, including plans for education, occupation, and a shared or single life-style. The status of young adulthood is reached when the adolescent begins to adjust to societal responsibilities and moves toward achieving personal life goals.

Physical Development

Puberty marks the beginning of adolescence. It is characterized by dramatic physical and physiological changes, including the beginning of the ability to reproduce. There is a spurt of rapid growth in height, weight, and muscular development. Secondary sex characteristics appear and the reproductive organs mature. In girls, puberty lasts about 3 years, from age 10-11 to 14. **Menarche,** the onset of menses, usually occurs at 12 to 13 years, though it may begin about a year earlier or several years later. It often begins just after the peak of the physical growth spurt. In boys, puberty lasts about 4 years, from age 12 to 16.

Girls between the ages of 10 to 12 experience a spurt in height; by age 14 to 15 their growth is nearly complete. During these years, females grow 2.5 to 5 inches (6 to 12.5 cm) and gain 8 to 10 pounds (3.5 to 4.5 kg). Boys have their rapid growth spurt at age 12 to 14. By age 16, their growth is nearly complete. Males average 3 to 6 inches (7.5 to 15 cm) and gain 12 to 14 pounds (5.5 to 6.5 kg). An adolescent's self-concept is continually readjusting as the body changes.

Sexual development and sexuality. Adolescents struggle with notions of body image and what is normal growth and development. At this stage, teenagers begin to develop curiosity and interest in sexual relationships. They are very aware of the development of secondary sex characteristics and continually compare how their body looks with that of their peers and to some ideal standard of attractiveness.

Frequently, formerly supportive adults are confused or uncomfortable with the teenager's sexual curiosity. The changing roles of males and females leave many teenagers with little idea of what is expected from them.

Females. As previously mentioned, menarche may occur anywhere between 10 and 16 years of age. This onset of menstruation marks puberty in the female. In the United States, the average age of onset is at about 12½ years of age. Ovulation usually begins 12 to 24 months after menarche. The onset of menarche varies among population groups and is influenced by heredity,

nutrition, health care, and other enivronmental factors. Most adolescent females view the menarche as a normal developmental milestone separating them from childhood. They may view it with curiosity or pride. Others view the onset of menstruation with fear or anxiety. A wide variety of attitudes exists among different groups in society. The presence of physical discomfort during and/or around the time of menstruation may also lead to a negative reaction, with some females experiencing headaches, backaches, cramps, and abdominal pain. They may also experience mood changes before menstruation such as depression, irritability, anxiety, and a sense of low self-esteem.

Secondary sex characteristics in the female begin to develop before puberty and may take 2 to 8 years for completion. Breast development, often the earliest sign of puberty in girls, occurs between the ages of 8 and 18. Pubic hair develops between years 11 to 14.

Males. **Spermatogenesis** (sperm production) and seminal emissions mark puberty and sexual maturity in the male. The first ejaculate of seminal fluid occurs about 1 year after the penis has begun its adolescent growth, and nocturnal emissions, loss of seminal fluid during sleep, occur at about age 14. Just as the onset of menstruation produces a new set of feelings in girls, nocturnal emissions may produce new feelings including pride, fear, or shame. Erotic dreams may accompany the nocturnal emissions.

Secondary sex characteristics in the male also begin before puberty and may take 2 to 5 years for completion. Changes in body shape, growth of body hair, and muscle development may continue until 19 or 20, or even until the late twenties. Testicular enlargement is usually the first pubescent change, starting between 10 and 13 and ending between 13 and 17. The penis and scrotum enlarge; the scrotum reddens and scrotal skin changes texture. Hair grows at the axilla and pubic area between 12 and 16 years. The growth of facial and chest hair usually occurs somewhat later, around age 16. The voice begins to deepen at age 13 to 14.

Sexual role development. Maturation of an individual's sexual identity involves more than development of primary and secondary sexual characteristics and strong sexual impulses. It also involves the ability and desire to give and receive love, respect, and affection. The development of a sexual identity begins very early in life, but it is particularly strong during adolescence because of the physical changes and the search for self-identity. Conflict with parents over issues of sexual identity and behaviors is common. This conflict is due in part to the changes between childhood and adolescence in what parents find acceptable, such as kissing others, and in part because of the differences between what different generations believe is acceptable.

Intellectual curiosity about sexuality and the act of sexual intercourse is a major component in adolescent sexual development. Frustration at this age results from a general lack of sufficient information about sex in a culture where sexual innuendos are associated with almost every facet of daily adult life.

Traditional attitudes and values regarding sexuality are changing. Because of the dichotomy of American values relating to sexual behavior and rules for sexual identity, present-day adolescents are left to search for their own sexual identity and moral code with very few parental or societal guidelines. Understandably, many teenagers have difficulty establishing a consistent sexual identity.

Adolescent pregnancy. Teen pregnancies occur within all cultural and socioeconomic groups. Teenagers may find it difficult to deal with the tension between their emotional needs and their developing sexuality. During this time of sexual development and exploration of a sexual role, pregnancy may occur. Babies born to teen mothers are at risk for low birth weight and related problems. If both parents are not committed to caring for the child, this complicates the already difficult situation. Frequently, the teen mother is left with little support to take on an enormous burden of raising a child while she is still developing herself.

Educating adolescents about sexuality, birth control, and the realities of parenting is very important in avoiding unwanted pregnancy and helping teens learn about the responsibilities of parenthood.

Skin. Skin texture changes during adolescence. Sebaceous glands become more active and increase in size. Acne may develop. The sweat glands are fully developed and begin to secrete in response to emotional stimuli.

Health risks. Physical health is generally good. Risks to the health of adolescents include poor judgment resulting in accidents, drug or alcohol abuse, unwanted pregnancy, or sexually transmitted diseases. Emotional stress due to unmet or unrealistic expectations may show up as depression, anorexia nervosa, or suicide attempts. Accidents and suicide are the leading causes of death in the adolescent population.

Cognitive Development

During adolescence, the mind has a great ability to acquire and utilize knowledge. The thought process of the adolescent becomes more logical and the ability to utilize abstract ideas increases. The adolescent is working on the beginning structure of a philosophy of life. This process requires the use of abstract thinking. Piaget described this level of cognitive process as the **period of formal operations.** This thinking moves beyond the concrete into the area of abstract thought where reasoning occurs and symbolic and logical processes are used. Abstract thinking is a new and more aware level of consciousness. It allows for greater creativity and inner awareness. The individual can contemplate the past and future, as well as the present, can develop theories, and can consider scientific hypotheses. Abstract thinking liberates the person for mental processes of greater depth and breadth. This can be a period of academic achievement for the adolescent.

The conscious development of a personal value system also occurs during this period. This is another component of the search for self-identity. Part of the questioning of the values of parents and institutions is the process of developing a set of values that works for the person. The adolescent becomes more aware of inconsistencies, hypocrisy, and injustices.

Adolescents are subject to many stresses placed on them by their families, schools, peer groups, and society at large. Adolescents are vulnerable to stress as they have not yet developed a strong identity with sufficient coping mechanisms to deal with negative stress. Problems such as teen pregnancy, drug abuse, conflict with parents, dropping out of school, or delinquency may result. As our sociey grows in complexity, there is an increase in potential stress factors to which adolescents are subject. An individual teenager's response to stress may result in growth in personal identity and self-confidence, or in vulnerability to less healthy coping patterns.

Psychosocial Development

According to Erikson, the task of adolescence is the development of **ego identity versus the danger of role diffusion.** Adolescents become increasingly sensitive to how they think others perceive them as compared to how they perceive themselves. Finding one's own identity is stressful and difficult work. In many ways, it is a life-long task. If the adolescent can emerge with a reasonably strong sense of his or her own identity, he or she has successfully experienced this stage. If an adolescent does not develop a personal sense of identity, she or he feels an ongoing personal sense of confusion, anxiety, alienation, and incompleteness. The person may then look to a group outside the family for a sense of identity. The peer group becomes an important place for experimentation with various roles outside the family, and the adolescent often feels intense pressure to join one.

Adolescents may also follow or identify with popular entertainers and wear personal apparel or use speech patterns that mark them as part of a group. Because of the vulnerability of young teenagers, the pressures of peer group conformity may be harmful. Individual judgment may often be forfeited to the desires of the group as a whole, creating great stress and anxiety in some adolescents. It is the rare adolescent who has developed enough ego strength to stand alone against the crowd. Teenagers, however, perceive their behavior as highly individualistic or original because it is different from that of adults, even though it may conform to group codes.

During preadolescence, close friendships are important to identity development. During the later teen years, relationships with the opposite sex usually develop. They may take the form of group activties or couple dating. Adolescents begin to experience the possibilities for trust and intimacy with others. Some individuals become aware that they may have a homosexual orientation.

Another important characteristic is the relationship between the parent of an adolescent and his or her peer group of friends. Frequently, values and beliefs of parents are dramatically different from those of the adolescent's friends. This can result in friction between these two influential factions and can be a source of stress, especially if the teenager feels that he or she must make a choice between loved family members and friends.

The emotional life of an adolescent ranges from exhilarating peaks to depressing lows. Much energy goes into this effort to understand the meanings of this shifting complex of feelings. Outwardly these emotional expressions may be the source of tension and conflict. Gradually the emotions even out to some extent, and a sense of balance develops.

YOUNG ADULTHOOD: 20 to 30-35

Leaving adolescence and entering young adulthood means separation from the family and its financial support as well as greater freedom to choose experiences and friends. It is also a time of taking greater responsibility for one's own life. During the first several years of early adulthood, some of the major tasks are to achieve relative independence from parental figures, to establish an independent life-style, and to develop a sense of emotional, social, and economic responsibility for one's own life. The young adult faces many complex issues that affect personal and professional growth. Coping mechanisms that were developing during childhood and adolescence are challenged and expanded during the young adult years when choices and responsibilities increase. The young adult must balance the desire to explore options with the need for some stability. During the later years of young adulthood the individual may establish a career commitment, form significant relationships, and even take on parenthood.

During the middle years of young adulthood, there is often a period of questioning and reflection. Questions the individual reflects upon may include: "Why am I doing this, and not something else?", "Where am I going with my life, my career?", or "What other alternatives should I consider?" This is probably the first period of conscious self-examination. Sometimes this search reaffirms the direction a person's life is taking; sometimes change seems desirable. Depending on the set of circumstances, the person may decide to get married, change jobs, get divorced, have children, develop a career as a parent, or return to work.

This period of questioning and transition is often followed by a period of settling in with the choices that have been made. The individual can use energy to develop the chosen life-style and find a special place or role in a family and in society. People at this stage invest in home, career, and family.

Developmental Tasks

The major developmental tasks of early adulthood include:

1. Becoming independent from parents
2. Establishing a household
3. Choosing and beginning to establish a career or vocation
4. Developing a personal style of living, including shared living or single living
5. Establishing an intimate relationship
6. Establishing friendships and a social network
7. Choosing activities in social and community organizations
8. Developing parenting behaviors for biological offspring or in the broader framework of social parenting
9. Implementing personal values in home, employment, and community settings

Physical Development

Physical growth reaches its peak during early adulthood. The body is operating efficiently with good muscle tone, strength, and coordination, and a high energy level. The young adult has the physical strength and stamina for many activities that influence life patterns.

Sexual development is a part of this period of peak physical development. Exploration with sexuality and various sexual roles occurs at this time. During young adulthood, the individual establishes a sense of identity with his or her sexual role. This is also the time for decisions on childbearing.

Nutritional needs are no longer for growth, but for maintenance and repair. Weight control becomes a problem for many adults, especially for those who continue to consume food as they did during adolescence, but whose energy expenditure is less than it was during those years.

Cognitive Development

The young adult years are a time of optimal cognitive functioning. The individual is engaged in the mastery of new skills and new knowledge, and the intellect is stimulated by these exciting and challenging events. Cognitive functioning at the level of formal operations, the capacity for abstract thinking, emerged during adolescence. The young adult expands on this base by becoming less egocentric and more realistic and objective. The young adult has an excellent ability to acquire and use knowledge, and to engage in problem-solving and creative endeavors.

For many, education continues during the early years of young adulthood. College, graduate school, on-the-job training, and/or continuing education classes prepare the young adult to enter some field of work. Depending on the career path chosen, educational preparation may continue well into the 20s.

Psychosocial Development

Erikson's sixth stage, intimacy versus isolation, focuses on one of the tasks of young adulthood: forming an intimate relationship. After establishing self-identity, the individual can enter a relationship with another without losing self-identity. Because neither the development of self-identity nor readiness for an intimate relationship are clearly defined, young adults often experience some fear that they will experience a loss of personal identity when entering a relationship. Intimacy involves more than physical contact: it is the ability to share personal identity with another without losing one's own unique identity. The desired outcome is mutual satisfaction and support.

Although Erikson focused on the heterosexual marriage relationship, intimate bonds are also formed within a homosexual relationship. Erikson suggested that affiliation or intimacy was expressed as mutuality with a loved partner with whom one is willing and able to share the cycles of work, family life, and recreation. This bond involves the capacity to enter a committed relationship and to stand by it through difficult times.

The danger of this stage is isolation or an avoidance of those persons and settings that promote and provide intimacy. A young adult whose identity work is not well underway may settle for sets of stereotyped interpersonal relationships that lead to a deep sense of isolation. This false "intimacy" is not a love relationship; it bypasses the accomplishment of improved understanding of one's own inner resources and those of others. The person feels isolated, lonely, and withdrawn.

Another of Erikson's stages of ego development, which is important during young adulthood, as well as during middle and late adulthood, is the stage of generativity versus stagnation. Generativity refers to a productive life: productivity within personal relationships (family and friends), a chosen career, and in the community.

Establishing independence. Young adults may move out of the parental home or establish a more equal role with their parents if they stay in it. During difficult economic times, when jobs for high school and college graduates are hard to find, many young adults continue to live in their parents' home until they are able to establish themselves financially. Whether the young adult remains temporarily in the parents' home or moves out to establish an independent living situation, the young adult should work toward emotional, social, and economic independence.

Marriage or singlehood. Marriage is increasingly viewed today in our society as a loving, sharing relationship between two people, rather than as a social institution for creating and rearing a family. Most marriages are heterosexual; however, there are also homosexual unions. While many young adults still choose marriage, singlehood is another viable option. Remaining single may meet the needs of those not ready for the complex interdependent relationship of marriage, or those who by temperament are not suited to the roles of spouse and parent. Single persons may experience pressure from the family. Even people who remain single by choice may have difficulty with feelings of aloneness and lack of companionship. Singlehood, however, may increase the opportunities for career advancement, creative expression, and community service.

Divorce. The expectations for marriage as a close, loving and sharing relationship where both individuals benefit from the union are often unmet. Divorce is a common result in our society. Divorce may be a freeing experience, but initially, it may be quite traumatic as each person deals with feelings of anger, disappointment, grief, and disillusionment. They must develop new roles. Financial strain is a frequent problem, most commonly for the woman.

The development of adult maturity includes the quest for independence, willingness to assume responsibility, the ability to deal constructively with frustration and to maintain self-control, sensitivity to others, and the ability to communicate effectively.

Parenting. Parenting tasks may be initiated by bearing children, adopting, becoming a foster parent, or reaching out in other ways, such as coaching children's teams or participating in child development organizations. The decision to raise children involves a major change in a couple's relationship. The arrival of a child is usually a happy event in the life of a couple, yet it can also bring

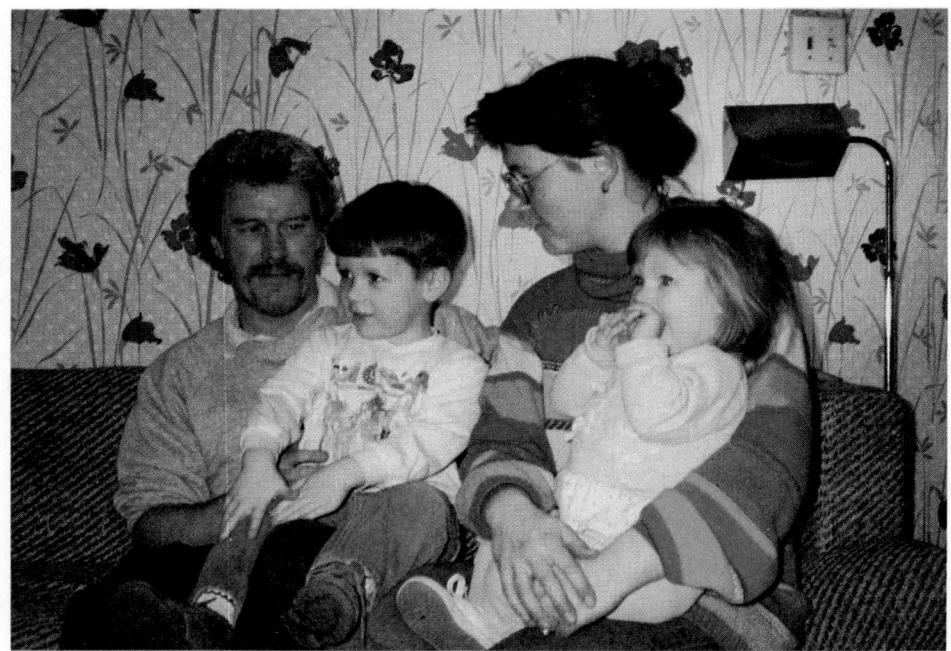

great stress to the marriage. The role of parent is very demanding and requires changes in roles, relationships, and in time commitments within and outside the home. For those who choose to develop work roles at home and in a career outside the home, the stress can be significant.

Many individuals raise children as single parents. This may be a deliberate choice to remain single, or may occur as a result of divorce or the death of a spouse. When divorce and remarriage occur in families with children, the difficult roles of stepparent and stepchild must be worked through and established.

Career, work, and occupation. The young adult also chooses a career or a vocation and may begin to consider how beliefs about self and society affect that choice. During these years, work is closely tied with identity. A young adult who feels satisfied with her or his work feels challenged, fulfilled, and rewarded. Frustration with work can lead to boredom and apathy. Work satisfaction is important for maturation and mental health. It can provide prestige and social recognition, a sense of self-worth, opportunities for service, creative self-expression, varied interactions, and a means of self-support. The individual is in a position to stand on his or her own, take risks, and accept consequences for personal actions. This can produce both excitement and fear and holds great potential for personal growth.

Organizational participation. During young adulthood, many individuals begin to establish connections with various organizations in the community. These affiliations may be related to commitment to a cause or belief system, development of friendship networks, physical exercise, or social purposes. Group membership serves the important purpose of providing an outlet for self-expression. However, groups may be problematic if they become a substitute for development of the individual. Maintaining a healthy balance within various group memberships and time for self-orientation is important for young adults. Self-direction, or the knowledge of one's own goals, and recognition of what membership with certain adult groups means to those goals are necessary if an individual is to achieve appropriate group affiliation.

MIDDLE ADULTHOOD: 30-35 TO 65-70

Middle adulthood is a stage of life when growth is strongest in the areas of personal, social, and emotional development. By this time, individuals have generally chosen a life-style, a family or single pattern of living, and an occupation. The span of time considered to cover the middle adulthood years is variable; some consider ages 40 to 65, and others use ages 30 to 70. Stevenson (1977) uses the term *middlescence* to describe this age span of 30 to 70 years. She further subdivides it into two categories: middlescence I from 30 to 50 and middlescence II fom 50 to 70. The boundaries of this stage of life must be considered tentative and flexible. Regardless of the parameters used, this is likely to be the longest stage of a person's life.

Developmental Tasks

The categories of early middle age and late middle age are used here to describe major developmental tasks.

The major development tasks for people in early middle age, between 30-35 and 50-55, include:

1. Adjusting to the physical changes of aging
2. Continuing to learn in the areas of personal and career interests
3. Reviewing, evaluating, and refining career goals (orientation) in light of a personal value system
4. Reaching desired level of achievement in career
5. Working on a maturing relationship with spouse or significant other
6. Choosing organizational and civic activities in which to participate
7. Helping younger persons develop as they search for their own identity
8. Coping with the "empty nest" as children leave home
9. Assisting aging parents, or planning for the time when that will be necessary
10. Developing hobby and leisure activities for current enjoyment and for long-range retirement planning
11. Planning for the financial, personal, and social aspects of retirement

The major developmental tasks for people in late middle age, between 50-55 to 65-70, include:

1. Developing supportive, interdependent relationships with grown children, their families, and other members of the younger generation
2. Enhancing the relationship with spouse or most significant other person
3. Adjusting to the loss of a spouse or significant other person, if necessary
4. Maintaining an affiliation with some civic, political, professional, religious, and/or social organization(s)
5. Maintaining an interest in current scientific, political, and cultural changes
6. Helping aged parents or other relatives cope with changes in their lives
7. Developing satisfying leisure time activities
8. Preparing for or adapting to retirement, which may include another career, a move, a change in financial status, and numerous other changes
9. Adapting to changes accompanying the aging processes

Physical Changes (also see Chapter 25)

During the years of early middle age, physical changes are generally gradual. During the years of late middle age, they become more marked. In our society, aging changes are often the focus of humor, denial, and

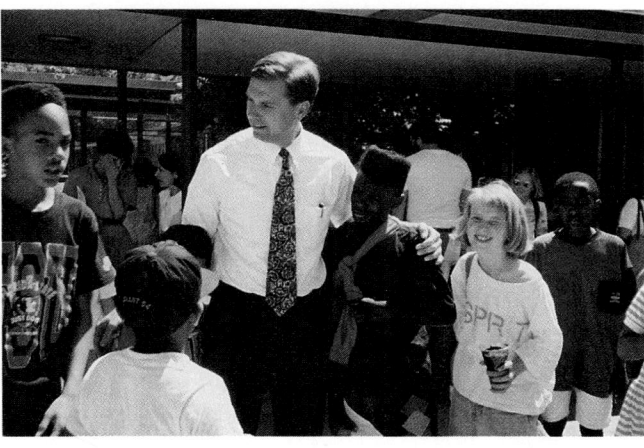

depression. However, many adults accept the physical changes of aging with grace. Aging changes may begin over a wide span of time. For some people they begin in the early 30s; for others, changes do not occur until well into the 40s. The skin loses some of its elasticity: wrinkles gradually begin to form around the eyes and mouth and on the forehead. The skin sags a bit under the eyes and around the chin and jaw. The hair begins to lose pigment and turns grey or white. It may thin somewhat, and in men the hairline often recedes. Because of decreased muscular tone, the abdominal muscles are no longer as firm. Frequently weight gain occurs, especially when activity level decreases but caloric intake does not. Sensory function remains generally intact except for decreased accommodation for near vision (presbyopia). Internal organ function remains fairly constant in the healthy adult, although some decrease may occur in respiratory and cardiac function. If the individual actively pursues physical fitness, these changes may not occur until later.

During the late 40s or early 50s, women experience menopause. The menstrual cycle becomes irregular in frequency and flow pattern. Periods of heavy bleeding alternate with amenorrhea for 1 to 2 years and finally cease altogether. The decrease in the hormones estrogen and progesterone produces symptoms that may include vasomotor changes (hot flashes and sweating) and mood changes.

Men do not experience such an abrupt halt to their reproductive ability. During the late 50s or during the 60s, testosterone production decreases somewhat, leading to decreased sperm production, longer erection time, and less intense orgasms.

During middle adulthood many individuals experience for the first time the diagnosis of a chronic health problem such as hypertension, diabetes, or arthritis. A history of smoking may lead to cardiovascular or respiratory problems, which are evident for the first time during middle age.

As the individual moves through late middle adulthood and toward late adulthood in the late 60s and into the 70s, many develop more chronic health status changes. While none of them may be life-threatening, together they do take a toll on the energy level and sense of well-being.

Cognitive Development

Cognitive processes in adulthood include learning, problem solving, memory, and creativity.

Learning continues in adulthood. Much of it comes from life experiences that are integrated by thought and reflection. Adult learning is enhanced by interest, motivation, self-confidence, a sense of humor, and flexibility. The middle-aged adult is interested in how knowledge is applied to living and improving life. The growth in continuing education and outreach programs makes ongoing, life-long learning available to interested adults. These programs enable persons to update their knowledge for their profession or occupation and to develop new personal interest areas. Some adults use middle age as the opportunity to enroll in college for the first time, and others return to earn an advanced degree. Reaction time or speed of intellectual performance is individual and generally stays the same or diminishes during late middle age. Most adults experience no decrease in the ability to learn, though they may need a longer learning period.

Problem-solving abilities remain fairly constant throughout adulthood. The levels of education and intelligence, and the accumulation of life experiences influence the ability to solve problems at this age, as they do at any age. People of various ages will perceive problems and situations differently. Early formative experiences differ somewhat with each generation and affect how people view problems and how they seek resolution. The older the person is, the greater the store of past experiences used to evaluate current situations. Moving through the middle adult years, individuals have the opportunity to broaden their perspectives and deepen their insights.

Memory generally remains intact during the middle adulthood years. Some decrease in recent memory may occur during the late middle years. Memory is aided by the presentation of well-organized material.

Creativity continues and may increase during middle adulthood. The insight needed for many creative thoughts, acts, and productions depends on the range of life experiences accumulated over the years.

Psychosocial Development

Generativity versus stagnation. Erikson believed that the important task for personality development at this stage of life is resolution of generativity versus stagnation. Adults need to contribute to the next generation either by raising children or producing something that can be passed on. The latter may involve creative, socially useful work. The motivation is to create and/or nurture those who will follow and to leave a mark on the world. Generativity means sharing, giving, and contributing to the growth of others as well as passing something on to the next generation. For some this means parenthood; for others this means generativity through creative acts of expression in the arts or through community involvement. Stagnation means experiencing boredom and a sense of emptiness in life, which leads to being inactive, self-absorbed, and self-indulgent.

Between the ages of 30 and 50, major life goals and activities concentrate on the areas of self-development, career development, assistance to both the younger and older generations, and organizational endeavors. Individuals feel a need to come to terms with both their own values and society's values. Personal values undergo a major change or numerous minor changes during these years when patterns are beginning to seem set but may not feel comfortable. Individuals move into various roles in a number of settings: in the family, at work, in religious organizations, and in community and civic affairs. In Western society, much of the implementation of the goals of major institutions, such as business, industry, government, education, religion, and charitable agencies, is done by the middle-aged population.

Work/career. Work is a major activity and motivating force during middle age. For some the work itself is rewarding and gratifying; for others, the only rewards are a paycheck and fringe benefits. Success in a line of work enhances the self-image; lack of success can damage that image. As the person advances through middle age, she or he becomes more aware of the years remaining before retirement. The person reflects on whether he or she is on schedule with the career goals,

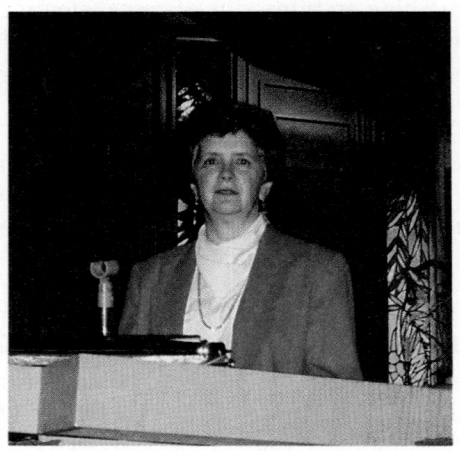

and whether this is the desired career path for the remaining years of employment. Middle-aged individuals may realize that they have expended time and energy in doing what their family and society felt they "should" do. They may begin to feel too restricted by the career and personal choices made earlier. They may find that other aspects of themselves are struggling to surface and find expression. This reflection may involve an uprooting of the life that seemed well grounded and striking out after a new vision. During the 40s and early 50s individuals may be enjoying success and promotions at work or may harbor a concern that this is the last chance to "make it." Some experience tension from a fear of being passed by and are sensitive to any indications that peers or superiors are losing confidence. While much energy is going into the work setting, the home setting may suffer.

For the working woman, involvement in a career may be a source of strength, since work brings its own rewards and sense of personal accomplishment. A mother benefits from having an identity outside her family role. However, it may also be a source of stress, since demands from both work and family may be high. Women in the work world who may already have experienced some discrimination can find promotions increasingly rare and even when they occur, they may be resented by a husband who has not been similarly recognized.

Family roles and relationships. New roles emerge as the middle-aged adult deals with growing children and aging parents. The adult may feel sandwiched between the concurrent needs of the older and younger generations. As the children grow through their own life stages, the parents must switch from a role of great involvement during young childhood, to lesser involvement with continued support as the offspring move through their adolescent years. When the children reach young adulthood, it is healthy for the relationship if the roles of children and parents become more equal. With aging parents, a role change for the middle-aged adult depends to a great extent on the health and dependency needs of the parents. If they become weak and frail, requiring more health care and a change in housing arrangements, middle-aged adults often feel as if their roles with their parents have switched; they are now increasingly in charge. When a parent dies, the middle-aged adult may feel lonely, vulnerable, and aware of the limited time to live one's life.

Caring for children. A major family task facing the middle-aged adult with children is to help the child(ren) live up to their potential and to assist them in their search for personal identity. The parent must adjust to the increasing desire of a child to be independent. As adolescence evolves, the child becomes less involved in family activities and desires increased responsibility and freedom. Some parents nurture the independence and delight in the developing individual. Others tend to be overprotective and controlling. Parents may believe they are protecting their children from the same mistakes they made as youths, but children usually resent overly protective efforts. When the last child moves out of the family home, the middle-aged adult again needs to reconsider her or his role in the family and in the community. For some parents this event leaves a void; for others it presents a new opportunity for growth. A woman who has devoted years to home and family may be eager to get involved in the outside world of school, business, or community activities.

If two parents remain in the home, they need to face one another as a couple again. This opportunity can bring the positive experience of increased closeness and more time and freedom for shared activities. Or the couple may realize that their relationship was based on the children, and that apart from the children, they have little in common. A reconsideration of the marriage may occur. Changes also occur for the parent in a single-parent household. The single parent may experience loneliness, but this time may also be an opportunity for new relationships or career goals. During late middle adulthood the role of grandparent may be realized.

Mid-life transition. The phrase "mid-life crisis" has become popular in recent decades, but because the term *crisis* often has a negative connotation, the term *transition* is used here. Also, many middle-aged individuals are aware of the changes and challenges they must confront but see it more as a period of reassessment and reevaluation than as a period of crisis. This phase may begin in the early 40s, although it may be some years earlier or later. People look at the realities of life and at the goals and dreams they have been carrying. Some of these have or can be met; others must be set aside. It is a time of taking stock, readjusting, and emerging with a new understanding. Questions frequently asked include: "What have I done with my life?," "Is this what I want out of life?," or "Have I set aside my own deepest dreams and desires for practicalities that are not satisfying?" Individuals may move their lives onto a different track or they may accept the one they are on, adjusting to it with greater understanding.

There may be gender differences in mid-life perception of the mid-life transition. Men still tend to be more involved in career assessment because their traditional role has been focused on becoming established in the career world. Many women, including those who are employed, still tend to see the family as the central issue. This difference does not mean that family is not important to men, nor that career issues are not important to women. Many women have experienced the situation of children growing in independence and leaving home. This affects the women's identity. They feel that they are no longer needed in the same way. Some women see this as liberating, because they can now focus on their own needs with greater energy.

Sheehy believes that women enter the mid-life transition earlier than men, at age 35 (1974). This is the age at which the average woman sees her youngest child enter school, at which the average married woman reenters the work force, and at which the biological boundary of childbearing is now in sight. (It must be noted, however, that with the recent developments in fertility technology, it is increasingly possible for women to become pregnant at a later age.) Aging and biology force women to review options that were set aside and that will be closed off in the now foreseeable future. Women with or without children face this review.

Whatever the central issue, all those in mid-life transition explore the meaning of their career, their family, and their personal identity. An individual who has spent some years searching for power and responsiblity now may crave more inner growth and meaning. Childless couples reconsider having children, while those who have spent a number of years raising young children may move toward involvement outside the home. Single people may reconsider the choice of career over marriage. The mid-life transition may mean a diminishing acceptance of stereotyped roles and acknowledgment that few answers are absolute. The years 35 to 45 are a time of reevaluating choices, purposes, and the expenditure of resources. It is a period of uncertainty and opportunity, a chance to restructure a narrower, earlier identity.

The mid-life transition is variable; some may never sense a transition at all, while others experience profound searches and changes.

Development of interests outside of work. At some point in middle age, the attitude toward work may change from one of total involvement to one of lesser involvement, with a growing interest in focusing on home and family and/or developing skill in a sport or hobby. Work may become more acceptable and be viewed more in terms of its responsiblities than in terms of power. The meaningfulness of activities is a frequent theme, as individuals rethink daily routines at work and home and reevaluate beliefs in religion, politics, and relationships. This situation offers potential for psychological growth and a reintegration and stabilization of identity. During these years, aspects of the personality and talents that have been latent may begin to emerge.

Coping with physical changes. Part of self-knowledge and self-acceptance is an acknowledgment of the changes at the physical, emotional, and intellectual levels that accompany the aging process. Physical changes may be difficult to accept in a culture where the signs of youthfulness are highly acclaimed. Middle-age adults ideally find some balance between accepting the inevitable changes in appearance while striving to maintain a high level of health with positive approaches toward exercise, diet, and the socioemotional environment. They may also appreciate the changes of added years in terms of the emotional and intellectual benefits that accumulate.

Weight may become an eminent concern; a battle against weight gain may also be a battle against aging and the loss of physical attractiveness, and all that this implies in our culture. Difficulties in this area may well depend on the amount of self-esteem that a person previously derived from physical attractiveness. Gray hair is yet another manifestation of a physical change accompanying aging. The adult may perceive it as a source of distress or as a sign of hard-won wisdom.

Menopause. Menopause, which normally occurs during the 40s or early 50s, involves both physiological and psychological changes. The hormonal changes may result in episodes of rapid mood shifts, nervousness, irritability, insomnia, hot flashes, diaphoresis, and fatigue. These changes cause some women to experience confusion or depression. Other women experience relatively minor physical and psychological distress. In some cultures, menopause is recognized as a time of a woman's greater wisdom, creativity, and participation in the life of the community. Menopause may be followed by increased enjoyment of sex as concerns about pregnancy are now absent.

Loss of peers. Many middle-aged adults are suddenly made aware of the relatively brief and fragile nature of life because of the death of peers. Most deaths that occur during the middle years of adulthood are due to cardiovascular disease and cancer. These events are also cause for reflection and stocktaking on the meaning and direction of one's own life.

Personal inner growth. Individuals examine and reexamine many issues during these years of middle adulthood: issues of personal qualities, relationships, commitments, career choices, and organizational affiliations. All the choices and reflections concerning those choices provide an opportunity for personal growth.

Maintaining interest in current affairs. People in this age group, as in any age group, are confronted with rapid changes in technology and in the social environment. However, they often prefer to advise some caution and restraint in the type and rate of change. Life experiences have brought some sense of wisdom and judgment to the middle-aged; although some younger people may view them as overly cautious and nonprogressive, the balance between the two views is important. At the same time, openness and flexibility continue to be important characteristics to health and well-being. Those who stay current with ideas and trends have a more positive approach to life and less need to maintain a defensive posture. They will probably also be able to communicate more effectively with younger individuals.

Retirement. Preparation for retirement is an important task, both for people who have been employed outside the home, and for those who have maintained the household. For a married couple, both must readjust to more shared time. Single individuals need to adjust to more time alone. Preparation through adult education or development of new skills can pave the way for a refocusing of talents and interests. Preparation for retirement is actually lifelong. People bring to retirement all that they have become during their lifetime. During the entire span of middle age, the activities an individual chooses to participate in are worthy of thoughtful consideration. A person should not delay specific planning for retirement until retirement is imminent but should integrate it throughout the adult years.

Special characteristics of late middle age. While many of the issues and characteristics described above continue to affect the years of late middle adulthood, some changes and special characteristics may become more prominent during the 50s and 60s. These individuals have an opportunity to define and integrate the emotional and intellectual growth of the earlier adulthood years. It may be a time of changes outside the family, thus giving the individual time and energy to develop new areas of interest. In the work world, although advancement is still possible, many have attained much or most of what they can. In certain areas, such as in law, business, government, religion, and community service, this period may include the prime years of activity. People in the late middle years occupy many of the highest positions in these areas. Within the family setting, spouses may be back to the couple stage, or fast approaching it, and must readjust to the contracted nuclear family or to life alone if a spouse should die. Grandparenting is a new role often acquired during this stage. Parents must reassess their relationships with their children and move from the adult-child type of interactions to adult-adult interactions. Men may become more aware of, less fearful of, and more accepting of their tendencies to provide care and nurturance, while women may accept and develop more fully their assertiveness through an interest in business, politics, or other organizations and activities outside the home.

The aging parents of 50- to 70-year-olds often require a great deal of emotional, physical, and/or financial assistance.

LATE ADULTHOOD: 65-70 to 95+

As is the case with other stages of adulthood, the parameters of late adulthood and old age are not easy to determine. Some people seem old at 40, while others seem young at 65. Some gerontologists have attempted to deal with this situation by setting apart the years from 60 to 75 as early old age and the years after age 75 as late old age.

Later adulthood has become a subject of increasing interest because of longer life spans and declining death rates in Western society. The elderly are now the fastest growing portion of the population. The larger numbers of the elderly and the changes that come with aging have created numerous challenges for individuals and for society as a whole. Institutional forms of care have been developed but have often proved unsatisfactory; major pieces of legislation have been passed on behalf of the elderly, but often this has not eased the passage of time and the financial, social, and emotional problems that develop. The emphasis in our society on youth and their culture, behavior, and attitudes is accompanied by a negative attitude toward those on the other end of the age continuum. This prejudice is known as "ageism," a negative attitude toward aging and discrimination based on age. This attitude characterizes the elderly as burdensome, sick, and senile. It is an indication of much anxiety about aging. This attitude is changing somewhat because the ever increasing numbers of elderly are commanding more attention to the process of aging. It is often said that in this culture, everyone wants to live long but no one wishes to grow old. This is in marked contrast to other cultures, where old age is respected and even revered. Older adults are not a homogenenous group. Most people become more individualized as their years increase. Each individual's story, responses, and needs are unique.

Developmental Tasks

Late adulthood is similar to all other developmental stages in that individuals must be able to make certain adaptations and achieve certain developmental tasks. These developmental tasks are different from earlier ones in that these are the final ones in life. Among the most significant developmental tasks in late adulthood are:

1. Maintaining and developing activities that enhance self-image, contribute to a sense of worth in society, and help to retain functional capacity

2. Developing new family roles as in-laws and grandparents
3. Accepting retirement and adjusting to reduced income
4. Adapting to changes in physical status and health
5. Adjusting to satisfactory living arrangements
6. Adapting to losses of spouse, other family members, friends
7. Working on a life review
8. Preparing for one's own death

Physical Changes

Individuals age at different rates. How people age depends on a number of factors including:

Personal attitude toward aging and life
Level of physical activity
Nutrition
Personal habits
Presence or absence of illness

Even in the absence of illness, some decline in physical function comes with advancing years. Usually this occurs gradually. Reaction times slow and eyesight and hearing may diminish. In addition, older adults experience an increased incidence of chronic disease, less resistance to acute illnesses, and a slower recovery period. These physical changes produce an increase in use of the health care system.

Some older persons adjust to these changes with an attitude of acceptance and humor. Others become preoccupied with their discomforts and ailments.

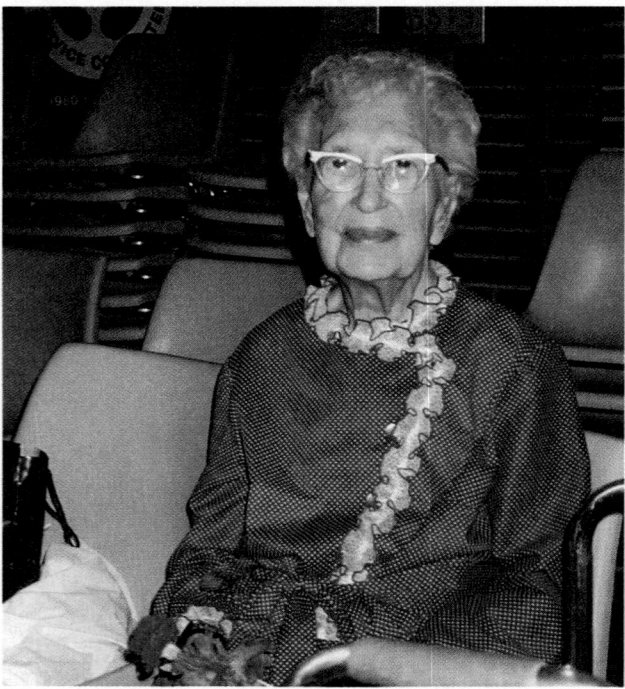

Cognitive Changes

There are few predictable changes in intellectual function that accompany aging. No decrease in general knowledge occurs, and an increase in wisdom may come with advancing years. Speed in mental performance and in complex decision making may slow. Maintenance of mental function is affected by many factors including:

Personal motivation
Interest in the subject
Sensory function, especially vision and hearing
Educational accomplishments
Recency of learning
Personal value on intellectual activity

Psychosocial Development

During the early part of late adulthood, the major life commitments to job and family are nearing completion. Ideally, planning for the next phase of life has been going on for many years. Most older adults have time and energy during the retirement years to further develop interests in many areas. The person may pursue development in the areas of learning, sports, hobbies, travel, or community service. The older adult has an opportunity to develop a new balance with others and society. It can be a time for creative endeavors.

Retirement. As both demands from work and family and living arrangements change somewhat with the onset of retirement, the time to do other things becomes more available. As mentioned previously, advance planning for postretirement activities that enhance self-respect is crucial. Failure to plan can make the change come as a shock, and the hours may seem empty, heavy, or endless. If adults prepare, they can use the time to advantage in the development of new careers, hobbies, sporting skills, or community activities. This productive use should enhance self-worth, a sense of usefulness, and functional capacity. Educational opportunities for adults of all ages are increasing. For the older adult, continuing education can provide an opportunity to learn again simply for the pleasure of learning or to develop another set of skills or an avocation. Both physical and mental well-being depend on continuing involvement in and contribution to society.

If one or both elderly spouses have been employed, the marriage relationship is affected by retirement. They must adjust to having more shared time and to weaving their lives together effectively. A spouse may have, at least initially, a sense of the other person being more "underfoot" and of losing privacy. Couples can develop a more equal relationship with regard to household and leisure activities.

How a person reacts to retirement is related to the meaning and satisfaction the job held. Feelings of relief and release may be present if the job lacked personal meaning and satisfaction. If the job held much meaning and gave a person satisfaction and authority, the loss is more deeply felt and may lead to depression. In addition to the loss of a job, the retiree also feels the loss of work associates, and the social network and friendships they may have provided.

Retirement usually involves a financial change, typically a decrease in income. This change is difficult because it affects the person's life-style in the areas of daily living, home ownership and maintenance, socializing, entertainment, and travel.

New roles. New roles emerge for older adults as their children marry and have children of their own. Acceptance of their children's spouses into the family network is instrumental in the ongoing interaction of the family. Interaction with grandchildren can be a pleasant aspect of aging if it does not become too time-consuming or burdensome. Grandparents can provide a sense of family and history. Another role that may begin in an earlier phase of late adulthood is the caring for elderly parents who may be ill or dependent. One needs to reevaluate personal identity in light of these new roles.

Living arrangements. The older adult may need to change living arrangements for many reasons, including physical status and finances. This may mean giving up a home of many years, with all the comfort and memories that it holds. Some individuals are able to find more suitable arrangements in single homes; others may move in with adult children or to a retirement or nursing home. In our society, the extended family is no longer expected to take care of the elders in their own homes, so a move to a facility may be seen as necessary but not desirable. Such a move usually involves giving up some or many personal belongings and some loss of privacy. These moves can, however, also involve the positive aspects of more efficient accommodations and an increase in socialization with peers.

Losses. Many of the numerous changes that occur in late adulthood are felt as losses. These include employment status, income, deaths of significant people, and changes in physical strength and sensory acuity.

The loss of a job after many years of employment may be one of the greatest developmental and situational crises in an individual's life. As retirement incomes become relatively smaller in an inflationary era, lowered income becomes more of a loss. Homes, entertainment styles, and lifelong travel plans may have to be given up or diminished in scope to meet the costs of food, housing, and health care.

Other losses may include the deaths of friends, a spouse, or other family members. These losses are among the most difficult aspects of later adulthood. Coping with bereavement for the person with whom one has shared life experiences, memories, and plans leaves a great personal void. Ideally the older adult experiences the profound emotions that accompany the loss and then goes on living and fostering the development of new relationships. This process requires time and patience. Serious illnesses and deaths of people who have been close during life are also a reminder that there is an unknown but limited amount of time left to live.

Older adults may also feel physical changes as losses. Physical strength, energy, and sensory acuity of eyes and ears typically decline gradually over the years. By age 60, most people are aware of some physical decline, and most have at least one illness or limiting condition. The occurrence of one or more chronic health conditions may affect strength, energy, and self-image. The ability to live independently may change, leading to more assistance in the home or to a move to the home of an adult child or to a nursing or retirement home. The older adult faces challenges in accepting physical changes and limitations and in using energy most effectively.

Life review. The process of performing a life review is an important developmental task of later adulthood. The goal is to achieve a sense of integrity, acceptance, and wholeness in looking back on the life one has lived. Most older persons do spend some time reflecting on their accomplishments and failures, satisfactions, and disappointments in an effort to integrate and evaluate the diverse elements of their life so they can reach a reasonably positive view of their life's worth. Failure to accomplish this task may lead to serious psychological problems. The life review process is far more than useless reminiscence. It allows for some gratification and also for the revision in understanding and clarification of experiences that a person may have poorly understood or accepted when they occurred. It is an inventory that helps put past successes and failures into some perspective. If considered with others, particularly with the younger generation, this review can be mutually beneficial; it gives the older person a sense of usefulness and some credit for age and wisdom and can provide the younger person with a sense of family and history. Today's older Americans have lived through more changes than any other single group in human history.

This developmental task is well described by Erikson as the last ego stage: ego integrity versus despair. Successful consideration leads to the acceptance of one's life as the way it had to be, given the person, the choices, and the circumstances. The inability to come to terms with the life one lived can lead to negative feelings such as despair, anger, resentment, and hopelessness. Life for most people is complex, so the life review is unlikely to be entirely "good" or "bad." For most, it involves some satisfactions, some disappointments. Some hopes and dreams are realized, some remain unfulfilled. The task is to accept what happened and to accept oneself.

Preparation for death. Preparation for one's own death, views on death, and the possibility of an afterlife are likely to evolve from the life review process. For many, considering the issue of their own death is important and they want to prepare for it in terms of

finishing their business or setting their affairs in order. This preparation takes many forms: finalizing a will, achieving some goal, resolving some or many interpersonal relationships, and saying farewell to significant family members and friends. If the dying process is prolonged because of some chronic illness, the individual goes through several phases of dealing with eventual death. To die in a way as close as possible to what the individual desires may be thought of as life's final developmental task.

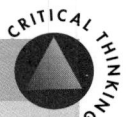

Nursing Diagnosis—*THE NEXT STEP*

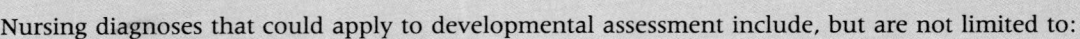

Nursing diagnoses that could apply to developmental assessment include, but are not limited to:

ALTERED GROWTH AND DEVELOPMENT The state in which an individual demonstrates deviations in norms from his/her age-group.

Defining Characteristics

- Delay or difficulty in performing skills (motor, social, or expressive) typical of age group
- Altered physical growth
- Inability to perform self-care or self-control activities appropriate for age
- Flat effect
- Listlessness, decreased responses

Related Factors

- Inadequate caretaking: indifference, inconsistent responsiveness, multiple caretakers
- Separation from significant others
- Environmental and stimulation deficiencies
- Effects of physical disability
- Prescribed dependence

PERSONAL IDENTITY DISTURBANCE Inability to distinguish between self and nonself.

Defining Characteristics

- Inability to distinguish self from others or objects
- Verbalization of "not knowing who I am"

Related Factors

- Refusal to look into mirror
- Increasing dependence on others
- Self-destructive behavior (alcohol, smoking, drug abuse)

ALTERED ROLE PERFORMANCE Disruption in the way one perceives one's role performance.

Defining Characteristics

- Denial of role
- Conflict in roles
- Change in self-perception of role
- Change in others' perception of role
- Change in physical capacity to resume role
- Lack of knowledge of role
- Change in usual patterns of responsibilities

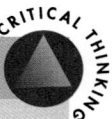

Nursing Diagnosis—*THE NEXT STEP—cont'd*

Related Factors

- Change in employment
- Change in financial status
- Change in health status
- Cultural transition
- Developmental crisis
- Ineffective coping mechanisms
- Role loss

SOCIAL ISOLATION Aloneness experienced by an individual and perceived as imposed by others and as a negative or threatened state.

Defining Characteristics

- Apathy
- Verbalization of isolation from others
- Low contact with peers
- Absent or limited contact with community
- Lack of contact with or absence of significant others
- Seclusion
- Expresses feelings of aloneness imposed by others, rejection, or feelings of difference from others
- Expresses values acceptable to subculture but unacceptable to dominant cultural group
- Perceived inadequacy of significant purpose in life or absence of purpose in life
- Perceived inability to meet expectations of others or insecurity in public
- Observed or expressed interests/activities inappropriate to the developmental age/stage
- Shows behavior unaccepted by dominant cultural group
- Seeks to be alone or to exist in a subculture
- Sad, dull affect
- Uncommunicative, withdrawn, no eye contact
- Preoccupation with own thoughts, repetitive meaningless actions
- Absence of supportive significant other(s): family, friends, group

Related Factors

- Impaired mobility
- Therapeutic isolation
- Sociocultural dissonance
- Insufficient community resources
- Body image disturbance
- Fear (environmental hazards, violence)
- Immature interests
- Unacceptable social behaviors or values
- Inability to engage in satisfying personal relationships
- Alteration in mental status
- Altered state of wellness
- Developmental delay
- Immature interests

Clinical Application

Susan M., age 16, was admitted to the stress unit following an overdose attempt. Her brother found her at home, barely arousable, following ingestion of an unknown quantity of her mother's tranquilizers. Susan's parents describe behavior changes over the last 6 months. She shows lack of interest in her own care or her surroundings. She appears unkempt and takes no interest in her physical upkeep. Her family describes her as being withdrawn and isolated, with increasing mood

Continued.

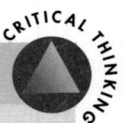

Nursing Diagnosis—*THE NEXT STEP*—*cont'd*

swings and emotional outbursts. Her grades in school have dropped and she has no close friends nor does she participate in social activities.

Interviewing Susan upon her admission to the unit 1 day post-intensive care, the nurse identifies the following information. Susan states, "I can't do anything right, that's what my parents always say." She has difficulty identifying any positive qualities and/or strengths and describes herself as "stupid and a failure." Susan describes her relationship with her parents as "okay, but my mother and father always seem to find things wrong with me and compare me to my older brother." She describes communication problems with her parents. "My parents don't listen to me. They just holler and say that until I'm old enough to live on my own I need to listen to them, and follow their rules. So, I just don't talk to them. They don't understand. Nobody understands. I feel so alone."

All through her interview, Susan maintains very little eye contact and stares down at the floor.

SUBJECTIVE DATA:
Client states:
I can't do anything right
I am stupid and a failure
No one listens to me
I feel alone

OBJECTIVE DATA:
Lack of interest in her physical upkeep
Lack of interest in her surroundings
Withdrawal and isolation of self
Increasing mood swings and emotional outbursts
Grades have dropped
No friends
No social activities
Maintains little or no eye contact when talking with others

NURSING DIAGNOSIS

Personal identity disturbance related to self-destructive behavior (overdose on tranquilizer).

Defining Characteristics
- Poor image of physical self
- Frequent self-criticism
- Inability to describe positive aspects/strengths about self
- Maintains little or no eye contact with others

Altered role performance related to developmental crisis.

Defining Characteristics
- Conflict in role self-perception versus parents' perception
- Self-imposed withdrawal from peers and family
- Dysfunctional parent-child communication

Social isolation related to body image disturbances.

Defining Characteristics
- Poor image of self
- Frequent self-criticism
- Inability to describe positive strengths about self
- Self-imposed withdrawal from peers and family
- No friends
- No social activities

GLOSSARY

adolescence The stage of life beginning at puberty and extending to adulthood.

diagnostic Pertaining to the identification of a disease or condition by a scientific evaluation of physical signs, symptoms, history, laboratory tests, and procedures.

grasp reflex Normal reflex in young infants elicited by stroking the infant's palms; the examiner's fingers are grasped so firmly that the child can be lifted into the air. (In older individuals, the tonic grasp reflex is pathological, occurring in diseases of the premotor cortex.)

menarche The first menstruation and the commencment of cyclic menstrual function.

menopause The gradual cessation of the menses, usually occurring between 45 and 60 years of age.

middlescence A term for the years of middle adulthood.

Moro reflex A normal mass reflex in a young infant elicited by a sudden loud noise resulting in flexion of the legs, an embracing posture of the arms, and usually a brief cry. Also called startle reflex.

myelination Development of the myelin sheath around a nerve fiber.

pincer grasp The index finger in apposition to the thumb.

puberty The period of life at which the ability to reproduce begins.

screening A preliminary procedure, such as a test or examination, to detect the most characteristic sign or signs of a disorder that may require further investigation.

spermatogenesis The process of development of spermatozoa, the male germ cells.

tonic neck reflex A normal response in newborns to extend the arm and the leg on the side of the body to which the head is quickly turned while the infant is supine and to flex the limbs of the opposite side. The reflex prevents the infant from rolling over until adequate neurological and motor development occurs and disappears by 3 to 4 months of age. At this time the reflex is replaced by symmetric positioning of both sides of the body.

BIBLIOGRAPHY

Berk LE: *Child development*, ed 2, Boston, 1991, Allyn and Bacon.

Blair KA: Aging: physiological aspects and clinical implications, *Nurse Pract* 15:2, 14-28, 1990.

Comfort A: *A good old age*, New York, 1976, Crown.

Duvall E, Miller B: *Marriage and family development*, ed 6, New York, 1984, Harper & Row.

Elkind D: *The hurried child: growing up too fast too soon*, New York, 1981, Addison-Wesley.

Erikson EH: *Childhood and society*, ed 2, New York, 1963, WW Norton.

Erikson EH: *Identity: youth and crisis*, New York, 1968, WW Norton.

Erikson EH: *Adulthood*, New York, 1978, WW Norton.

Foster RLR, and others: *Family-centered nursing care of children*, Philadelphia, 1989, WB Saunders.

Frankenburg WK, Camp BW, editors: *Pediatric screening tests*, Springfield, Ill, 1975, Charles C. Thomas.

Frankenburg WK, Dodds JB: The Denver Developmental Screening Test, *J Pediatr* 71:181-191, 1967.

Gordon M: *Manual of Nursing Diagnosis 1993-1994*, St. Louis, 1993, Mosby.

Gilligan C: *In a different voice, psychological theory and women's development*, Cambridge, Mass, 1982, Harvard University Press.

Hall CS, Nordby VJ: *A primer of Jungian psychology*, New York, 1973, New American Library.

Havinghurst R: *Human development and education*, St. Louis, 1953, Warren H. Green, Inc.

Holmes TH, Rahe RH: The social readjustment rating scale, *J Psychosom Res* 11:213-218, 1967.

Jones DA, and others: *Health assessment across the life span*, New York, 1984, McGraw-Hill.

Kimmel DC: *Adulthood and aging: An interdisciplinary development view*, ed 3, New York, 1989, John Wiley.

Levinson DJ, and others: *The seasons of a man's life*, New York, 1978, Ballantine.

Marlow DR, Redding BA: *Textbook of pediatric nursing*, ed 6, Philadelphia, 1988, WB Saunders.

McElmurry BJ, LiBrizzi SJ: The health of older women, *Nurs Clin North Am*, 21:1, 161-171, 1986.

Murray RB, Zentner JP: *Nursing assessment & health promotion strategies through the life span*, ed 4, Norwalk, Conn, 1989, Appleton & Lange.

Piaget J: *The construction of reality in the child*, New York, 1975, Ballantine.

Rahe RH: Epidemiological studies of life changes and illness, *Int J Psychiatry Med* 6(1-2):133-146, 1975.

Sarason IG, Johnson JH, Siegel JM: Assessing the impact of life changes: development of the life experiences survey, *J Consult Clin Psychol* 46:932-946, 1978.

Sheehy G: *Passages*, New York, 1974, EP Dutton.

Sheehy G: *The silent passage: menopause*, New York, 1991, Random House.

Stein M: *In midlife: a Jungian perspective*, Dallas, 1983, Spring Publications.

Stevenson JS: *Issues and crises during middlescence*, New York, 1977, Appleton-Century-Crofts.

Turner JS, Helms DB: *Lifespan development*, ed 3, New York, 1987, Rinehart and Winston.

Wadsworth B: *Piaget's theory of cognitive and affective development*, ed 3, White Plains, NY, 1988, Longman.

Whaley LF, Wong DL: *Nursing care of infants and children*, ed 4, St. Louis, 1991, Mosby—Year Book.

Whitborn SK, editor: *Adult development*, ed 2, New York, 1986, Praeger.

Nutritional Assessment

Nutrition plays a major role in the way an individual looks, feels, and behaves. The body's ability to maintain health and fight disease and the effectiveness of any type of therapy in illness greatly depend on the individual's nutritional status.

A patient with optimum or normal nutritional status has more **nutrient** reserves and is better able to withstand the stress of disease or illness. A patient with mild nutritional deficiencies that occur before clinical signs of **malnutrition** appear cannot fully combat the stress placed on the body during illness. These deficiencies slow down or halt patient recovery time and increase hospital cost (Hirsch, Jensen, 1981).

Nutritional assessment has become an integral component of health care in terms of preserving patient health and decreasing length and cost of patient hospitalization. Nutritional assessment involves collecting information about a client to assess nutritional status, identify nutritional needs, and develop a plan of action to meet those needs. This plan is known as a nutritional care plan. In ideal circumstances where optimum staff is available a registered dietitian most often develops this plan.

GOALS OF NUTRITIONAL ASSESSMENT

Three major goals in the assessment of nutritional status include:

1. Identification of malnutrition and its effects on an individual's health status.
2. Identification of patterns of overconsumption and their link with the development of obesity, diabetes, hypertension, cardiovascular disease, and cancer.
3. Identification of nutritional parameters for optimal health and fitness.

When assessing the nutritional status of a client and developing a nutritional care plan, the examiner should consider the needs of the whole client as they relate to nutrition. Components to assess in a holistic approach to nutrition and wellness include cultural food habits, food consumption, levels of physical activity, and standard of living.

Knowledge of the parameters for optimal health and fitness allows the health care professional to assess an individual's health and fitness status. Assessment of current status and identification of existing patterns are the first steps in helping an individual to make any necessary changes toward optimal health and fitness. As recommendations for optimal nutrient intake and physical activity are modified based on ongoing research and study of population groups, health care professionals have a major responsibility to educate individuals on how to attain a healthier life-style.

NUTRITIONAL ASSESSMENT: A TEAM APPROACH

The team approach to nutrition assessment involves the nurse, the physician, and the dietitian. A nurse most often performs an initial nutritional assessment or screen as part of a routine admission to a hospital or clinic. Nurses are in an ideal position for initial nutritional assessments. Much of the information readily available to the nurse through the medical chart can be evaluated with nutrition in mind (Henneman, 1981). If after an initial screen the nurse determines with a given set of criteria (usually determined by each clinic or hospital) that the client is at risk, he or she can make an appropriate referral to the physician or registered dietitian.

The level of nutritional assessment by the nurse depends on the size and availability of personnel in each clinical setting. The dietitian in most cases carries the major responsibility for the nutritional care of clients but may not be available to visit each client personally. Early detection of possible nutritional problems by the nurse and quick referral to the dietitian or physician can have a positive impact on the well-being and care of the client (Henneman, 1981).

COMPONENTS OF NUTRITIONAL ASSESSMENT

Anthropometric measurements, biochemical measurements, clinical examination, and dietary history are techniques for assessing nutritional status. Depending on the level of nutritional assessment necessary, all techniques may not be used on all clients and all may not be performed by a nurse only.

Anthropometric Measurement

Anthropometric measurement is the measurement of size, weight, and proportions of the human body.

The purpose of anthropometric measurements is to evaluate growth and assess nutritional status and body energy stores. These measurements are also used in the clinical setting to establish a client's initial baseline nutritional status. If initial nutritional status is recorded, health care professionals can quickly assess changes in nutritional health during illness or treatment.

The most common measurements taken include height, weight, skinfold thickness, and circumference of various body parts, including the head, chest, and arm. Measurements are compared with appropriate reference standards based on the individual or population being assessed. Standardization of equipment and procedure is essential, so that results are accurate and can be interpreted meaningfully. Results that deviate from standards may indicate malnutrition or overconsumption of various nutrients.

The nurse should inform the client before the physical assessment what areas of the body will be measured, and for what purpose.

COMPONENTS OF NUTRITIONAL ASSESSMENT

Nutritional assessment of an individual involves various parameters:
- Anthropometric measurement
- Biochemical measurement
- Clinical examination
- Dietary analysis

TABLE 4-1

Anthropometric Measurement

Anthropometric measurement	Equipment needed
Weight	Scale, accurate in measuring pounds or kilograms, as well as fractions of these units of measure
Height	Wall scale or rigid freestanding measuring device with a right-angle headboard, or wooden length board, accurate in measuring centimeters or inches, as well as fractions of these units of measure
Midpoint of arm and mid-arm circumference	Nonstretchable cloth tape measure marked in centimeters or special tape designed for use in nutritional assessment that has been developed by companies supplying nutritional products (Insertape, Ross Laboratories)
Skinfold thickness	Skinfold calipers

Height. In adults and older children measure height by having the client stand erect, without shoes, against a flat vertical measuring surface with a right-angle headboard (Table 4-1). Measure height on the line where the crown of the head intersects the height scale (Figure 4-1). For small children, measure height using a wooden length board with the child lying flat on the back (Figure 4-2).

Have one person (often a caregiver) hold the infant's head against the headboard while the nurse holds the leg straight and completes the measurement. Graph these measurements on a chart using recumbent length. For the nonambulatory elderly and elderly persons who are not able to stand erect due to spinal curvature, specific recumbent measurements have been developed to determine stature. Some of these include sitting height or crown-rump length and knee height (Zeman and Ney, 1988). The most accurate of these is knee height, which will be discussed later in this chapter.

Height may be recorded in centimeters or in inches. Standards for height exist for children and adolescents and will be discussed in depth in the part of this chapter dealing with pediatric assessment. For adults, the only standard for comparison of measured height is the Mean Height and Weight Table, from the Recommended Dietary Allowances, revised 1989, Food and Nutrition Board (Table 4-2).

Weight. Several types of instruments are commonly used for measuring weight, but the preferred instrument appears to be a balance beam scale with nondetachable

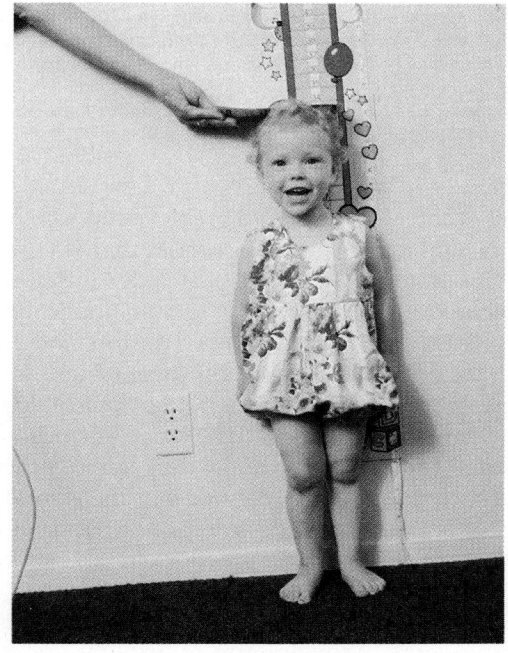

FIGURE 4-1 Measurement of standing height.

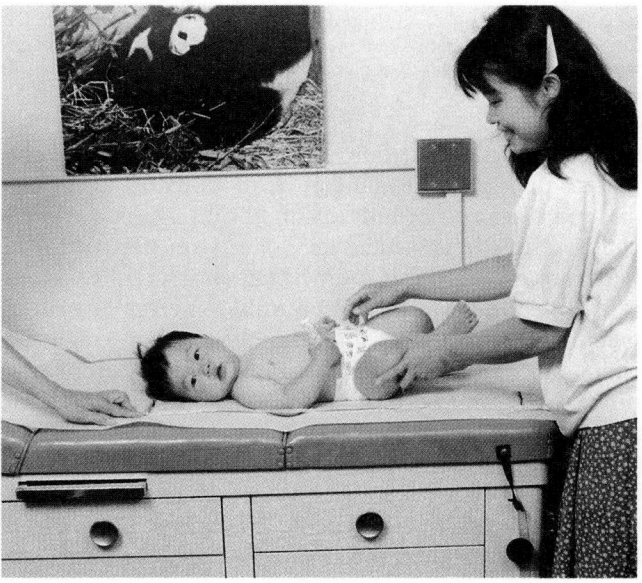

FIGURE 4-2 Measurement of recumbent length.

TABLE 4-2

Mean Heights and Weights and Recommended Energy Intake

Category	Age (years) or Condition	Weight (kg)	Weight (lb)	Height (cm)	Height (in)	REE[a] (Recommended Energy Expenditure) (kcal/day)	Multiples of REE	Average energy allowance (kcal)[b] Per kg	Average energy allowance (kcal)[b] Per day[c]
Infants	0.0-0.5	6	13	60	24	320		108	650
	0.5-1.0	9	20	71	28	500		98	850
Children	1-3	13	29	90	35	740		102	1,300
	4-6	20	44	112	44	950		90	1,800
	7-10	28	62	132	52	1,130		70	2,000
Males	11-14	45	99	157	62	1,440	1.70	55	2,500
	15-18	66	145	176	69	1,760	1.67	45	3,000
	19-24	72	160	177	70	1,780	1.67	40	2,900
	25-50	79	174	176	70	1,800	1.60	37	2,900
	51+	77	170	173	68	1,530	1.50	30	2,300
Females	11-14	46	101	157	62	1,310	1.67	47	2,200
	15-18	55	120	163	64	1,370	1.60	40	2,200
	19-24	58	128	164	65	1,350	1.60	38	2,200
	25-50	63	138	163	64	1,380	1.55	36	2,200
	51+	65	143	160	63	1,280	1.50	30	1,900
Pregnant	1st trimester								+0
	2nd trimester								+300
	3rd trimester								+300
Lactating	1st 6 months								+500
	2nd 6 months								+500

[a]Calculation based on FAO equations (Table 3-1), then rounded.
[b]In the range of light to moderate activity, the coefficient of variation is ±20%.
[c]Figure is rounded.

From Recommended Dietary Allowances, revised 1989, Food and Nutrition Board, Academy of Sciences—National Research Council, Washington, DC. The data in this table have been assembled from the observed median heights and weights of children, together with desirable weights for adults for heights of men (70 in) and women (64 in) between the ages of 18 and 34 years as surveyed in the U.S. population (DHEW/NCHS data). Energy allowances for the young adults are for men and women doing light work. The allowances for the two older groups represent mean energy needs over these age spans, allowing for a 2% decrease in basal (resting) metabolic rate per decade and a reduction in activity of 200 kcal per day for men and women between 51 and 75 years; 500 kcal for men over 75 years; and 400 kcal for women over 75. The customary range of daily energy output is shown for adults in the range column and is based on a variation in energy needs of ±400 kcal at any one age, emphasizing the wide range of energy intakes appropriate for any group of people.
Energy allowances for children through age 18 are based on median energy intakes of children of these ages followed in longitudinal growth studies. Ranges are the 10th and 90th percentiles of energy intake, to indicate range of energy consumption among children of these ages.

weights. Digital electronic platform scales have become increasingly popular and can be modified to weigh individuals in a compromised condition (e.g., in a wheelchair). The client stands, lies, or sits on the platform, with minimal clothing and without shoes, while weight is recorded in kilograms or pounds. When taking serial weights, the examiner should make sure to weigh the client on the same scale, at approximately the same time of day, and with the same amount of clothing for accurate comparison.

Several standards for comparison of weight to normal exist, and the examiner must use the proper standard for the individual being measured. The Mean Height and Weight Table (see Table 4-2) is one standard. Another standard used is the Metropolitan Height and Weight Tables, published first in 1959 and revised

in 1983 (Table 4-3). The 1983 tables reflect higher desirable weight ranges for all categories than do the 1959 tables. The National Institutes of Health Consensus Development Conference on the Health Implications of Obesity, held in February 1985 (Burton and Foster, 1985), suggested less reliance on these tables alone for a variety of reasons: They may not be applicable to the entire population, particularly lower socioeconomic groups and some ethnic groups; they ignore other risk factors, such as smoking; they do not measure degree of obesity or regional distribution of fat; and, in addition, they have relied on an ill-defined concept of "frame size."

The measurement of waist/hip circumferences is a valid assessment of the amount of body fat and its potential for health risk. With an increased waist to hip

TABLE 4-3

1983 Metropolitan Life Table*

Men					Women				
Height		Small frame	Medium frame	Large frame	Height		Small frame	Medium frame	Large frame
Feet	Inches				Feet	Inches			
5	2	128-134	131-141	138-150	4	10	102-111	109-121	118-131
5	3	130-136	133-143	140-153	4	11	103-113	111-123	120-134
5	4	132-138	135-145	142-156	5	0	104-115	113-126	122-137
5	5	134-140	137-148	144-160	5	1	106-118	115-129	125-140
5	6	136-142	139-151	146-164	5	2	108-121	118-132	128-143
5	7	138-145	142-154	149-168	5	3	111-124	121-135	131-147
5	8	140-148	145-157	152-172	5	4	114-127	124-138	134-151
5	9	142-151	148-160	155-176	5	5	117-130	127-141	137-155
5	10	144-154	151-163	158-180	5	6	120-133	130-144	140-159
5	11	146-157	154-166	161-184	5	7	123-136	133-147	143-163
6	0	149-160	157-170	164-188	5	8	126-139	133-150	146-167
6	1	152-164	160-174	168-192	5	9	129-142	139-153	149-170
6	2	155-168	164-178	172-197	5	10	132-145	142-156	152-173
6	3	158-172	167-182	176-202	5	11	135-148	145-159	155-176
6	4	162-176	171-187	181-207	6	0	138-151	148-162	158-179

From Society of Actuaries, Build Study, 1979, Chicago, 1980, Society of Actuaries and Association of Life Insurance Medical Directors of America, Metropolitan Life Insurance Co., New York, 1983. Courtesy Statistical Bulletin, Metropolitan Life Insurance, New York.
*Weight in pounds at ages 29 to 59 years according to build. In shoes and 3 lb of indoor clothing for women and 5 lb for men.

circumference ratio or an increased accumulation of upper body fat, the client's risk of complications from obesity increases. The examiner should measure the waist at the smallest part with the client lying down, and the hips at the largest part with the client standing with feet together (Jensen, 1992). A waist/hip circumference ratio of greater than .85 in women and 1.0 in men is indicative of increased risk of health complications associated with obesity (Jensen, 1989, 1992).

Body mass index (BMI) is an indicator of body fat that is useful in almost every situation. BMI shows a direct and continuous relationship to morbidity and mortality in studies of large populations. The regional distribution of body fat (abdomen in contrast with hips and thighs) was described repeatedly as an important predictor of the health hazards of obesity.

BMI is calculated according to the following formula (Burton and Foster, 1985):

$$BMI = \frac{\text{Weight in kilograms}}{(\text{Height in meters})^2}$$

Nomograms, or graphic representations of the variables used to calculate BMI, were developed to aid in calculation and interpretation of BMI. One nomogram is given, based on the 1983 Metropolitan Life Insurance Company Tables (Figure 4-3). The values provided by the nomogram indicate (1) desirable weight, (2) the 20% overweight level, and (3) the 40% overweight level for an individual (Burton and Foster, 1985). The

implications of degree of obesity are discussed later in this chapter. From the nomogram, weight values less than desirable are also evident.

Daily weight measurement can be beneficial in assessing fluid balance in some clients. Weight gain of more than 1 pound in 24 hours would indicate the client is accumulating fluid over new tissue (Jensen, 1981).

Measured weight can also be compared with reference norms listed by percentile, specific for height, sex, and age (Tables 4-4 and 4-5). A formula for calculating desirable body weight, which takes into account frame size, is given in Table 4-6.

To determine frame size, measure wrist circumference or elbow breadth. See Figure 4-4 and the box on page 105.

When calculating an individual's desirable weight, consider the individual's personal weight goal as well as any numbers calculated from a formula. Looking at the person's past weight pattern and ascertaining his idea of a comfortable weight is important in establishing a realistic goal.

Measured weight can be compared with desirable weight according to the following (Blackburn and others, 1977):

$$\% \text{ Ideal body weight} = \frac{\text{Actual weight}}{\text{Ideal body weight}} \times 100$$

Weight equal to or greater than 20% above or equal to

TABLE 4-4

Weight (lb) for Height (in), Males

Height (in)	Percentile	Age group in years					
		18-24	25-34	35-44	45-54	55-64	65-74
62	50	130	141	143	147	143	143
	15	102	109	115	118	113	116
	5	85	91	98	100	96	100
63	50	135	145	148	152	147	147
	15	107	113	120	123	117	120
	5	90	95	103	105	100	104
64	50	140	150	153	156	153	151
	15	112	118	125	127	123	124
	5	95	100	108	109	106	108
65	50	145	156	158	160	158	156
	15	117	124	130	131	128	129
	5	100	106	113	113	111	113
66	50	150	160	163	164	163	160
	15	122	128	135	135	133	133
	5	105	110	118	117	116	117
67	50	154	165	169	169	168	164
	15	126	133	141	140	138	137
	5	109	115	124	122	121	121
68	50	159	170	174	173	173	169
	15	131	138	146	144	143	142
	5	114	120	129	126	126	126
69	50	164	174	179	177	178	173
	15	136	142	151	148	148	146
	5	119	124	134	130	131	130
70	50	168	179	184	182	183	177
	15	140	147	156	153	153	150
	5	123	129	139	135	136	134
71	50	173	184	190	187	189	182
	15	145	152	162	158	159	155
	5	128	134	145	140	142	139
72	50	178	189	194	191	193	186
	15	150	157	166	162	163	159
	5	133	139	149	144	146	143
73	50	183	194	200	196	197	190
	15	155	162	172	167	167	163
	5	138	144	155	149	150	147
74	50	188	199	205	200	203	194
	15	160	167	177	171	173	167
	5	143	149	160	153	156	151

From Abraham S, Johnson CL, Najjar MF: Weight by height and age of adults 18-74 years; United States, 1971-74, *Advancedata* 14:7-8, 1977. Reprinted with permission of Ross Laboratories, Columbus, OH 43216, from Nutritional Assessment Summary Sheet G636, © 1987, Ross Laboratories.
15th Percentile values computed from reference 1 data by Ross Laboratories.

or more than 10% below ideal warrants further investigation.

Determining the percentage of weight change a client has experienced over a specific recent period is important in evaluating nutritional status. The following formula may be used (Blackburn and others, 1977):

% Weight change

$$= \frac{\text{Usual weight} - \text{Actual weight}}{\text{Usual weight}} \times 100$$

A change in weight of greater than 10% over 6 months is significant and warrants further investigation.

Circumstances that make the measurement of weight alone an unreliable measure of nutritional status include the body's degree of hydration and increases in muscle mass. For instance, a person who is retaining fluid may appear to be at an appropriate weight for height but may actually have decreased fat stores and muscle mass. The excess water hides this fact when

TABLE 4-5

Weight (lb) for Height (in), Females

Height (in)	Percentile	Age group in years					
		18-24	25-34	35-44	45-54	55-64	65-74
57	50	114	118	125	129	132	130
	15	85	85	89	94	97	100
	5	68	65	67	73	77	82
58	50	117	121	129	133	136	134
	15	88	88	93	98	101	104
	5	71	68	71	77	81	86
59	50	120	125	133	136	140	137
	15	91	92	97	101	105	107
	5	74	72	75	80	85	89
60	50	123	128	137	140	143	140
	15	94	95	101	105	108	110
	5	77	75	79	84	88	92
61	50	126	132	141	143	147	144
	15	97	99	105	108	112	114
	5	80	79	83	87	92	96
62	50	129	136	144	147	150	147
	15	100	103	108	112	115	117
	5	83	83	86	91	95	99
63	50	132	139	148	150	153	151
	15	103	106	112	115	118	121
	5	86	86	90	94	98	103
64	50	135	142	152	154	157	154
	15	106	109	116	119	122	124
	5	89	89	94	98	102	106
65	50	138	146	156	158	160	158
	15	109	113	120	123	125	128
	5	92	93	98	102	105	110
66	50	141	150	159	161	164	161
	15	112	117	123	126	129	131
	5	95	97	101	105	109	113
67	50	144	153	163	165	167	165
	15	115	120	127	130	132	135
	5	98	100	105	109	112	117
68	50	147	157	167	168	171	169
	15	118	124	131	133	136	139
	5	101	104	109	112	116	121

From Abraham S, Johnson CL, Najjar MF: Weight by height and age of adults 18-74 years: United States, 1971-74, *Advancedata* 14:7-8, 1977. Reprinted with permission of Ross Laboratories, Columbus, OH 43216, from Nutritional Assessment Summary Sheet G636, © 1987, Ross Laboratories.
15th Percentile values computed from reference 1 data by Ross Laboratories.

other way a weight measurement may be interpreted incorrectly is in an athlete, whose increased muscle mass is reflected in greater total body weight, yet whose fat stores may be low.

Weight standards for children are based on the National Center for Health Statistics Growth Charts, published by Ross Laboratories (see sample on pp. 102-103) and will be discussed in the portion of this chapter dealing with pediatric assessment. Children at either extreme of the scale may require further assessment.

Skinfold thickness. Measuring skinfold thickness is one method of determining body fat. Skinfold measurements indicate subcutaneous fat, muscle mass, and caloric status. Their accuracy and usefulness are greater in assessing clients who are malnourished, normal, or moderately fat as opposed to those who are extremely obese (Kamath, 1986).

Skinfold thickness can be measured at a variety of body sites. The tricep skinfold measurement (TSF) is commonly used for evaluation. Some adults, however, carry a higher percentage of body fat than is considered

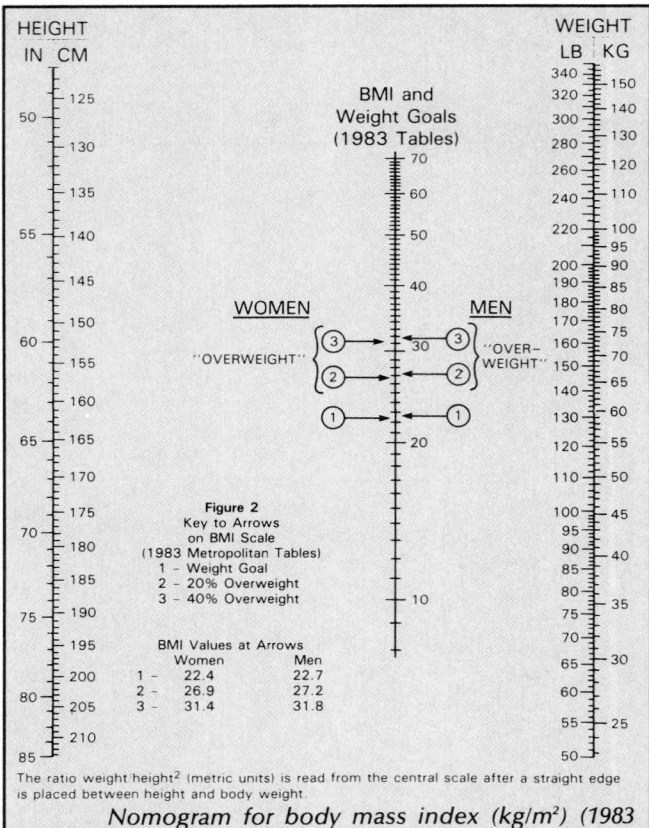

The ratio weight/height² (metric units) is read from the central scale after a straight edge is placed between height and body weight.

Nomogram for body mass index (kg/m²) (1983 Metropolitan Life Insurance Co. tables. Weights and heights are without clothing. With clothes, add 5 lb (2.3 kg) for men or 3 lb for women, and 1 in. (2.5 cm) in height for shoes.

FIGURE 4-3 Nomogram for body mass index (kg/m²) 1983 Metropolitan Life Insurance Co. tables. Weights and heights are without clothing. With clothes add 5 lb (2.3 kg) for men or 3 lb (1.4 kg) for women and 1 in (2.5 cm) in height for shoes. (From Burton BT, Foster WR: Health implications of obesity: an NIH consensus development conference, *J Am Diet Assoc* 85(9):1117-1121, 1985.)

normal in their upper arms. In this case, and when assessment of total body fat is desired, other skinfold measurements such as subscapular and suprailiac can be useful. Electrical impedance and underwater weighing are two other methods that have been used to measure total body fat (see Figures 4-5 and 4-6).

For triceps skinfold measurement, have the client expose the arm (see Table 4-1). Make sure clothing permits easy access to the shoulder area as well as to the upper arm. If taking other skinfold measurements, ensure that clothing permits easy access to the particular area while covering private parts of the body to avoid embarrassment. Take measurements on the bare skin. Client privacy and assurance of confidentiality are important.

TABLE 4-6

Calculating Desirable Body Weight

Frame size	Adult females	Adult males
Medium	Count 100 lb for the first 5 ft of height, plus 5 lb for each additional inch over 5 ft	Count 106 lb for the first 5 ft of height, plus 6 lb for each additional inch over 5 ft
Small	Subtract 10%	Subtract 10%
Large	Add 10%	Add 10%

TABLE 4-7

Triceps Skinfold (mm), Males

	Percentile		
Age (yr)	50th	15th	5th
18-19	8.5	6.0	4.5
20-24	10.0	6.0	4.0
25-34	12.0	6.0	4.5
35-44	12.0	7.0	5.0
45-54	11.0	7.0	5.0
55-64	11.0	6.5	5.0
65-74	11.0	6.5	4.5

Basic data on anthropometric measurements and angular measurements of the hip and knee joints for selected age groups 1-74 years of age, United States, 1971-1975. National Health Survey, Vital and Health Statistics Series No. 219, US Dept of Health and Human Services, Public Health Service, 1981, pp 20, 26. Reprinted with permission of Ross Laboratories, Columbus, OH 43216, from Nutritional Assessment Summary Sheet G636, © 1987, Ross Laboratories.

TABLE 4-8

Triceps Skinfold (mm), Females

	Percentile		
Age (yr)	50th	15th	5th
18-19	17.5	12.0	9.0
20-24	18.0	12.0	10.0
25-34	21.0	13.5	10.5
35-44	23.0	16.0	12.0
45-54	25.0	17.0	13.0
55-64	25.0	16.0	11.0
65-74	23.0	16.0	11.5

Basic data on anthropometric measurements and angular measurements of the hip and knee joints for selected age groups 1-74 years of age, United States, 1971-1975. National Health Survey, Vital and Health Statistics Series No. 219, US Dept of Health and Human Services, Public Health Service, 1981, pp 20, 26. Reprinted with permission of Ross Laboratories, Columbus, OH 43216, from Nutritional Assessment Summary Sheet G636, © 1987, Ross Laboratories.

FORMULA FOR CALCULATING ELBOW BREADTH

Method 1*

Record height without shoes on.

Measure wrist circumference just distal to the styloid process at the wrist crease on the right arm using a tape measure.

Use the following formula:

$$r = \frac{\text{Height (cm)}}{\text{Wrist circumference (cm)}}$$

Determine frame size as follows:

	Males	Females
Small	r > 10.4	r > 11.0
Medium	r = 9.6-10.4	r = 10.1-11.0
Large	r < 9.6	r < 10.1

Method 2†

Have the patient extend the right arm forward perpendicular to the body, with the arm bent so the angle at the elbow forms 90° with the fingers pointing up and the palm turned away from the body. Measure the greatest breadth across the elbow joint with a sliding caliper along the axis of the upper arm, on the two prominent bones on either side of the elbow. If a sliding caliper is not available, place the thumb and index finger on the two prominent bones. Measure the distance between the fingers and compare with the table below. Record this as the elbow breadth. The following data give the elbow breadth measurements for medium-framed men and women of various heights. Measurements lower than those listed indicate a small frame size; higher measurements indicate a large frame size.

	Height in 1" heels	Elbow breadth
Men	5 ft 2 in-5 ft 3 in	2½ in-2⅞ in
	5 ft 4 in-5 ft 7 in	2⅝ in-2⅞ in
	5 ft 8 in-5 ft 11 in	2¾ in-3 in
	6 ft 0 in-6 ft 3 in	2¾ in-3⅛ in
	6 ft 4 in	2⅞ in-3¼ in
Women	4 ft 10 in-4 ft 11 in	2¼ in-2½ in
	5 ft 0 in-5 ft 3 in	2¼ in-2½ in
	5 ft 4 in-5 ft 7 in	2⅜ in-2⅝ in
	5 ft 8 in-5 ft 11 in	2⅜ in-2⅝ in
	6 ft 0 in	2½ in-2¾ in

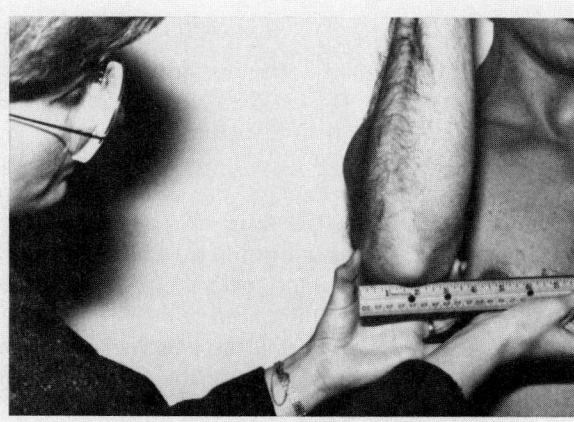

*Data from Grant JP: *Handbook of total parenteral nutrition,* Philadelphia, 1980, WB Saunders Co.

†Data from the Metropolitan Life Insurance Co., New York, 1983.

FIGURE 4-4 Measurement of wrist circumference. Measure the wrist just distal (toward the hand) to the styloid process at the wrist crease of the right hand.

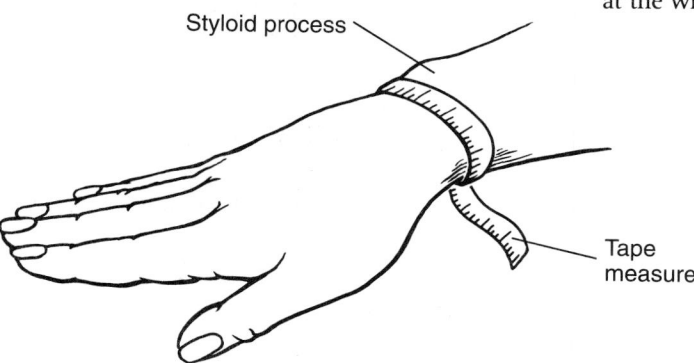

Styloid process

Tape measure

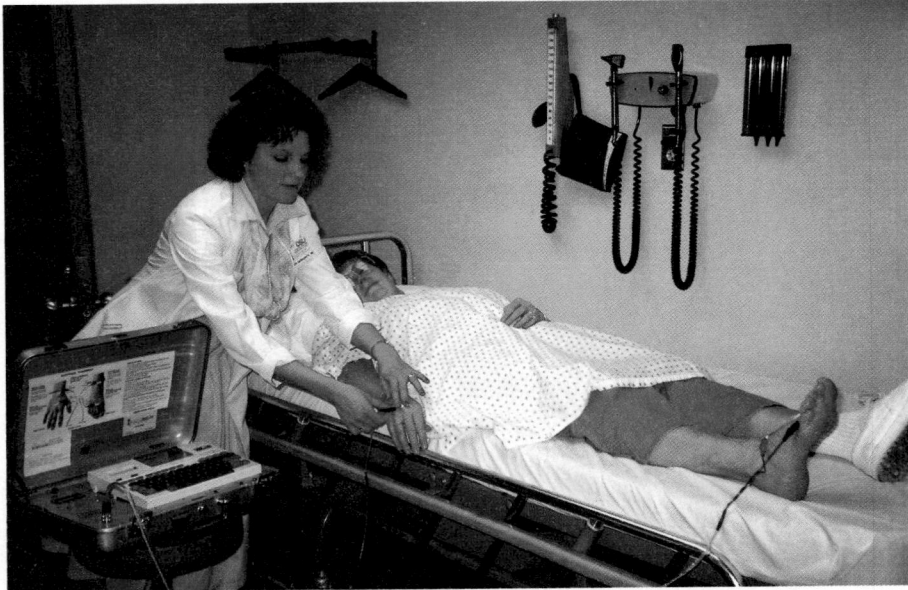

FIGURE 4-5 Bioelectrical impedance. This method can accurately be used to estimate total body fat in less than 5 minutes. (From Wardlaw GM, Insel PM: *Perspectives in nutrition,* St. Louis, 1990, Mosby–Year Book.)

In measuring the TSF, the nondominant arm is preferred. Measure the TSF on the back of the arm midway between the acromion and olecranon process (Figure 4-7). After assessing the midpoint, with the arm relaxed, firmly grasp a fold of bare skin above the midpoint and parallel to the long axis between your left thumb and forefinger and pull it away from underlying muscle. Place the contact surfaces of the **caliper** on either side of the skinfold directly at the midpoint (Figure 4-8). When the initial movement of the caliper stops, read the measurement to the nearest 0.5 mm.

Repeat the measurement one or two times for reliability. Measurements should be within 1 to 2 mm of each other. If trials yield similar values, record the last value. Tables 4-7 and 4-8 present TSF norms for comparison.

When determining total body fat in assessment of physical fitness, measure various sites on the body, add the sum of the skinfold thickness, and compare with norms based on age and sex. Determining the percentage of body fat gives a better perspective on overall fitness as opposed to weight alone. A discussion of optimal body fat is presented in the portion of this chapter dealing with obesity.

Circumference. Common circumferences measured are the head, chest, mid-arm, and mid-arm muscle. Chest and head circumference are used in assessing

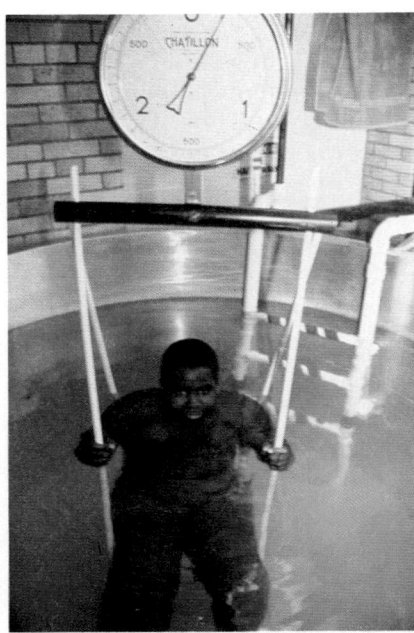

FIGURE 4-6 Underwater weighing. (From Wardlaw GM, Insel PM: *Perspectives in nutrition,* St. Louis, 1990, Mosby–Year Book.)

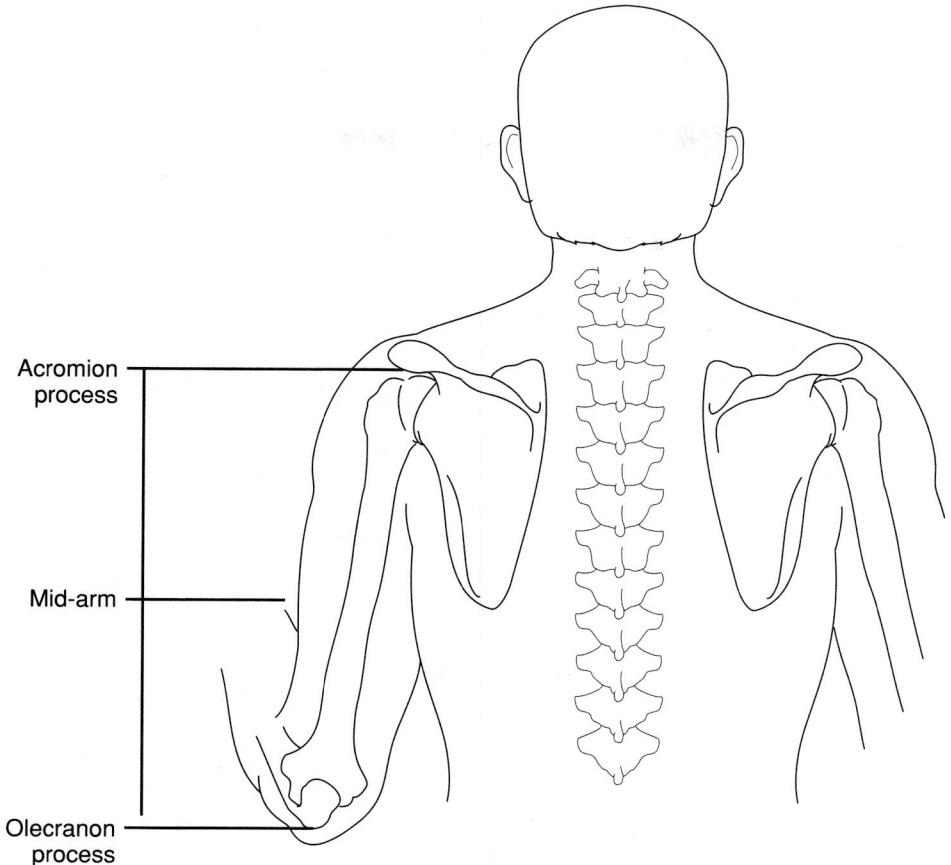

FIGURE 4-7 Assessing mid-point of upper arm.

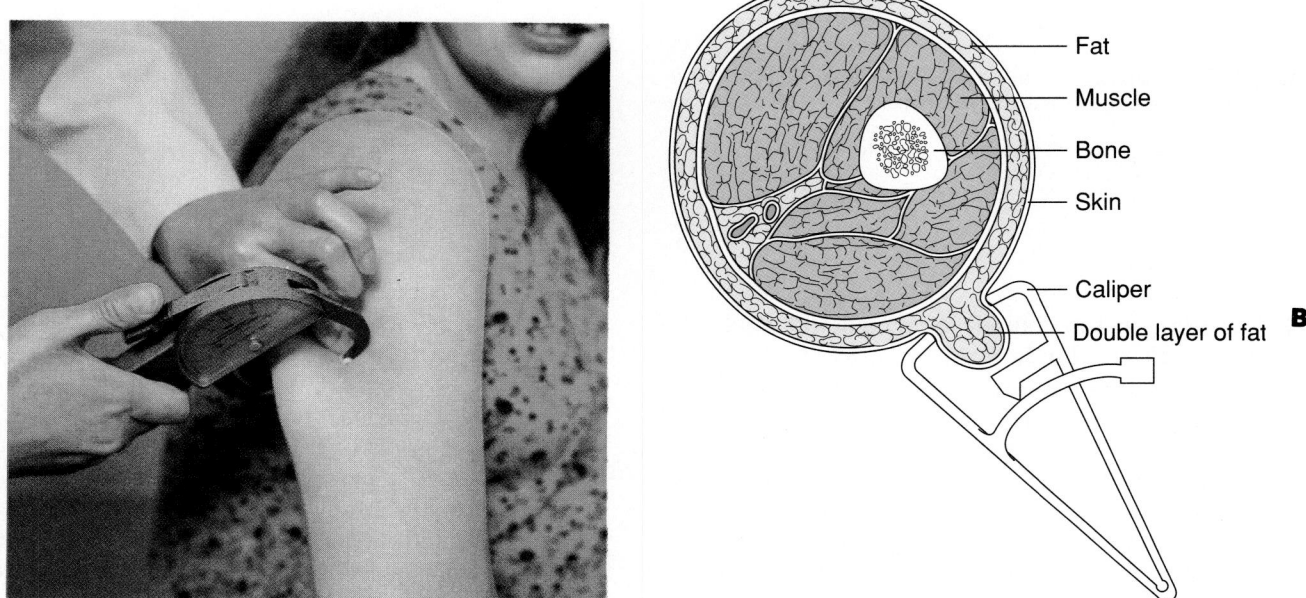

FIGURE 4-8 A, Measuring triceps skinfold with calipers. **B,** Cross-section of arm.

TABLE 4-9

Mid-Arm Circumference (cm), Males

Age (yr)	Percentile		
	50th	15th	5th
18-19	30.1	27.4	25.3
20-24	31.0	27.7	26.1
25-34	32.0	28.9	27.0
35-44	32.7	29.6	27.8
45-54	32.1	28.9	26.7
55-64	31.7	28.1	25.6
65-74	30.7	27.3	25.3

Basic data on anthropometric measurements and angular measurements of the hip and knee joints for selected age groups 1-74 years of age, United States, 1971-1975. National Health Survey, Vital and Health Statistics Series No. 219, US Dept of Health and Human Services, Public Health Service, 1981, pp 20, 26. Reprinted with permission of Ross Laboratories, Columbus, OH 43216, from Nutritional Assessment Summary Sheet G636, © 1987, Ross Laboratories.

TABLE 4-10

Mid-Arm Circumference (cm), Females

Age (yr)	Percentile		
	50th	15th	5th
18-19	26.2	23.2	22.1
20-24	26.5	23.6	22.2
25-34	27.8	24.8	23.3
35-44	29.2	25.8	24.1
45-54	30.3	26.6	24.3
55-64	30.2	26.1	23.9
65-74	29.9	26.2	23.8

Basic data on anthropometric measurements and angular measurements of the hip and knee joints for selected age groups 1-74 years of age, United States, 1971-1975. National Health Survey, Vital and Health Statistics Series No. 219, US Dept of Health and Human Services, Public Health Service, 1981, pp 20, 26. Reprinted with permission of Ross Laboratories, Columbus, OH 43216, from Nutritional Assessment Summary Sheet G636, © 1987, Ross Laboratories.

TABLE 4-11

Mid-Arm Muscle Circumference (cm), Males*

Age (yr)	Percentile		
	50th	15th	5th
18-19	27.4	25.5	23.9
20-24	27.9	25.8	24.8
25-34	28.2	27.0	25.6
35-44	28.9	27.4	26.2
45-54	28.7	26.7	25.1
55-64	28.3	26.2	24.0
65-74	27.2	25.3	23.9

Reprinted with permission of Ross Laboratories, Columbus, OH 43216, from Nutritional Assessment Summary Sheet G636, © 1987, Ross Laboratories.
*Values computed using MAMC (cm) = MAC (cm) − [3.14 × TSF (cm)] from data in Tables 3-8 and 3-10.

TABLE 4-12

Mid-Arm Muscle Circumference (cm), Females*

Age (yr)	Percentile		
	50th	15th	5th
18-19	20.7	19.4	19.3
20-24	20.8	19.8	19.1
25-34	21.2	20.6	20.0
35-44	22.0	20.8	20.3
45-54	22.5	21.3	20.2
55-64	22.4	21.1	20.5
65-74	22.7	21.2	20.2

Reprinted with permission of Ross Laboratories, Columbus, OH 43216, from Nutritional Assessment Summary Sheet G636, © 1987, Ross Laboratories.
*Values computed using MAMC (cm) = MAC (cm) − [3.14 × TSF (cm)] from data in Tables 3-9 and 3-11.

infants' growth and brain development and will be discussed in the section on pediatric assessment.

Mid-arm and mid-arm muscle circumference (MAC and MAMC, respectively) are useful in evaluating somatic protein stores and are most commonly used in assessing malnutrition. Measure the MAC in centimeters using a cloth tape around the midpoint of the nondominant arm (Figure 4-9). Calculate the MAMC from the following formula (Blackburn and others, 1977):

$$MAMC_{(cm)} = MAC_{(cm)} - [3.14 \times TSF_{(cm)}]$$

Compare values for both the MAC and MAMC with norms listed in Tables 4-9 through 4-12.

• • •

Anthropometry is of great value as a part of overall assessment, but standardization of instruments and consistency in technique are critical for reliable measurements. In interpreting anthropometric data, the examiner must consider all parameters together for accurate assessment and take serial measurements to document *changes* in anthropometric status. Measurements

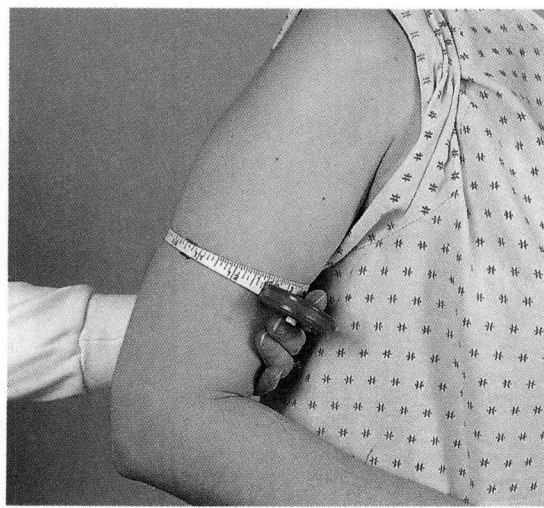

FIGURE 4-9 Measurement of mid upper arm circumference. (From Seidel HM and others: Mosby's guide to physical examination, ed 2, St. Louis, 1991, Mosby—Year Book.)

at either extreme above or below the 50th percentile warrant further investigation. Measurements significantly lower than the 50th percentile are evidence of depletion; measurements significantly above the 50th percentile, particularly weight and TSF, may be associated with increased risk of obesity.

Examiners should use caution in interpreting the results of skinfold measurements, especially in the critically ill client. Skinfold measurements are most useful in population surveys, not for determining small changes in muscle mass due to malnutrition over a short period of time; the techniques and equipment used to measure skinfold thickness can cause measurements to vary from one assessor to another and one instrument to another (Jensen, 1992). Use of anthropometric measurements to assess nutritional status should include more than one measurement parameter. Using skinfold alone or height/weight alone often does not truly represent the client's nutritional status. Analysis should include other body components such as **adipose tissue,** skeletal muscle protein, and **visceral protein,** which will give a more accurate analysis of body composition than weight alone (Jensen, 1981).

Biochemical Measurement

In nutritional assessment, commonly used biochemical values include total lymphocyte count (TLC), serum albumin, total iron binding capacity (TIBC), serum transferrin, creatinine height index (CHI), hemoglobin, hematocrit, nitrogen balance, and skin antigen tests. These values, taken with anthropometric measurements, give a good overall picture of an individual's skeletal and visceral protein status as well as fat reserves and immunologic response.

Total lymphocyte count. Both TLC and antigen skin testing are measures of immune function or the body's ability to fight disease. TLC is derived from the total white blood cell (WBC) and differential count, which gives the percentage in the blood of each of the five types of red blood cells. Lymphocyte count of below 1500 cells/mm³ may indicate depletion. TLC is expressed in cells/mm³ and Table 4-13 lists normal values for this parameter. The measured value is expressed as percentage of standard, with 60% to 90% of standard indicating moderate depletion and less than 60% of standard indicating severe depletion.

A lowered TLC can reflect a protein deficiency related to malnutrition such as **kwashiorkor.** However, the examiner should use caution in interpeting this value or using this test as a means of assessing the course of nutritional recovery because many other conditions and diseases affect both the TLC and WBC daily (Weinseir, 1989).

Conditions that may alter the accuracy and meaningfulness of TLC measurement include conditions where **leukocytosis** is present, such as bacterial infection, severe sepsis, tuberculosis, and chronic leukemia.

A depressed WBC and therefore a lower TLC can be caused by viral infections or induced by certain medications even if the nutritional status is normal.

Leukopenia may also distort the reliability of TLC in evaluation of malnutrition. Leukopenia may be associated with aberrations in white blood cells; it may be induced by certain medications or be a manifestation of viral infection. TLC is not a valid indicator of nutritional status in clients with acquired immunodeficiency syndrome (AIDS).

Skin antigen tests. Protein malnutrition is associated with impaired cell-mediated immunity, as manifested by skin antigen testing. Failure of a delayed cutaneous response is called **anergy** and is a well-documented feature of malnutrition (Jensen and others, 1981).

Anergy has been shown to be a risk factor for sepsis, infection, and mortality in the elderly and in hospitalized clients.

Four antigens are commonly used together in skin testing:
- Mumps
- *Candida albicans*
- Streptokinase/streptodornase
- Purified protein derivative (PPD)

The antigens are injected intradermally, and the area of induration is read after 24 hours and 48 hours. A client with a response over 15 mm on any *one* test is considered immune competent. The following values

TABLE 4-13

Selected Normal Values for Adults

Hematocrit (vol % red cells)
 Male 40%-54%
 Female 37%-47%
Hemoglobin
 Male 14-17 g/dl
 Female 12-15 g/dl
Lymphocytes, total count 1500-3000/mm³
Albumin, serum 4.0-5.5 g/dl
Iron-binding capacity
 Total, serum 250-410 µg/dl
 Percent saturation 20%-50%
Transferrin 170-250 mg/dl
Creatinine 1.0-1.5 g/24 hr

From Lagua RT, Claudio VS, Thiele VF: Nutrition and diet therapy reference dictionary, ed 2, St Louis, 1974, The CV Mosby Co. Reprinted with permission of Ross Laboratories, Columbus, OH 43216, from Nutritional Assessment Summary Sheet G636, © 1987, Ross Laboratories.

TABLE 4-14

Ideal Urinary Creatinine Value (mg), Adults

Male*		Female**	
Height (cm)	Ideal creatinine (mg)	Height (cm)	Ideal creatinine (mg)
157.5	1288	147.3	830
160.0	1325	149.9	851
162.6	1359	152.4	875
165.1	1386	154.9	900
167.6	1426	157.5	925
170.2	1467	160.0	949
172.7	1513	162.6	977
175.3	1555	165.1	1006
177.8	1596	167.6	1044
180.3	1642	170.2	1076
182.9	1691	172.7	1109
185.4	1739	175.3	1141
188.0	1785	177.8	1174
190.5	1831	180.3	1206
193.0	1891	182.9	1240

From Bistrian BR, Blackburn GL, Sherman M, Scrimshaw NS: Therapeutic index of nutritional depletion in hospitalized patients, *Surg Gynecol Obstet* 141:512-516, 1975. Reprinted with permission of Ross Laboratories, Columbus, OH 43216, from Nutritional Assessment Summary Sheet G636, © 1987, Ross Laboratories.
*Creatinine coefficient (males) = 23 mg/kg of ideal body weight.
**Creatinine coefficient (females) = 18 mg/kg of ideal body weight.

indicate a deficit in immune response (Kaminski and Winborn, 1978):

Severe	Moderate	Mild
<5-0 mm	<10-5 mm	<15-10 mm

Surgery or severe thermal injury will obliterate the immune response; therefore, antigen testing should probably not be done during the first 48 hours following such stresses. Immune response is also diminished in iron-deficiency states but is usually restored once the deficiency is corrected (Jensen and others, 1981).

Results of antigen testing, as with TLC, may be affected by other conditions such as infections, renal and hepatic disease, and treatments such as radiation and drug therapy, which may interfere with immune response. Skin antigen testing is not valid in clients with AIDS.

Serum albumin. Serum albumin is an important indicator of nutritional status and protein synthesis. A drop in serum albumin levels often occurs in conjunction with severe stress such as infection, injury or disease affecting the liver, kidney, or gastrointestinal tract.

Table 4-13 lists normal values for serum albumin. A concentration under 3.4 g/dl warrants further investigation and a concentration under 2.5 g/dl is associated with severe protein depletion (Jensen and others, 1981). The degree of hydration may have a significant effect on the reliability of serum albumin values.

Total iron binding capacity and serum transferrin. Serum transferrin concentration is another parameter useful in assessing visceral protein status. Serum

transferrin is calculated using TIBC according to the following formula (Blackburn and others, 1977):

$$\text{Serum transferrin} = (.8 \times \text{TIBC}) - 43$$

It is assessed in milligrams per deciliter. Normal values are represented in Table 4-13, with results expressed as percentage of standard; values between 60% and 90% of standard indicate moderate depletion, and values under 60% of standard indicate severe depletion.

Creatinine height index. CHI is a measure of urinary creatinine excretion. Creatinine is protein that is released from skeletal muscle at a fairly constant rate. For this reason, urinary creatinine levels are proportional to muscle mass and can give an assessment of the skeletal muscle mass in a client.

Creatinine height index is calculated from a 24-hour urine sample using the following equation:

$$\% \text{ CHI} = \frac{\text{Actual 24 hr creatinine excretion}}{\text{Expected 24 hr creatinine excretion}} \times 100$$

Table 4-14 gives standard urinary creatinine values.

A CHI of 60% to 90% of standard indicates moderate depletion; under 60% of standard indicates severe depletion. CHI values may be invalid in some cases of renal disease, amputations, fever, and with certain drug therapy. Accurate collection of urine is crucial in the reliability of this test.

Nitrogen balance. Nitrogen balance studies are useful in determining a client's level of body protein breakdown. In normal conditions the body takes in through food and excretes in urine the same amount of protein each day. In cases where the body is **catabolizing** more protein than it takes in through food each day, the body is in negative nitrogen balance. This disorder occurs in cases of severe stress, injury, or disease. If negative nitrogen balance continues, the patient is at risk for developing protein malnutrition. A positive nitrogen balance occurs during periods of growth such as in infancy, childhood, adolescence, pregnancy, and during wound healing.

Nitrogen balance studies involve calculating protein intake through dietary or intravenous means as well as measuring urine losses. The formula

$$N_2 \text{ balance} = \frac{\text{Protein intake}}{6.25}$$
$$- (\text{Urinary urea nitrogen} + 4)$$

is used, indicating either a positive or negative value (Blackburn and others, 1977). The degree to which the number is either negative or positive may document the severity of catabolism or the benefit of therapy, respectively.

Nitrogen balance calculated by this formula is unreliable in patients with renal disease and in those in whom urine collection is impaired and may underestimate nitrogen excretion in those patients with burns, diarrhea, vomiting, fistula drainage, and other abnormal nitrogen losses (Jensen and others, 1981).

Hemoglobin and hematocrit. Hemoglobin and hematocrit are measurements that may indicate many nutritional deficiencies. With severe protein malnutrition, the hemoglobin level may reflect protein status. Hemoglobin is expressed in grams per deciliter; hematocrit is expressed as a percentage (see Table 4-13 for normal values). Decreased values may occur (1) in iron, B_{12}, folate, and pyridoxine (B_6) deficiencies, (2) with chronic blood loss, (3) with overhydration, and (4) with genetic defects. Increased values may occur in (1) dehydration, (2) chronic anoxia, (3) polycythemia, and (4) the presence of some tumors.

Serum lipids. One of the primary risk factors in the development of coronary heart disease (CHD) is elevated blood lipid levels. The National Institutes of Health in 1984 made recommendations regarding serum cholesterol levels and relative risk of coronary heart disease (Table 4-15).

TABLE 4-15

Cholesterol Recommendations

Age	Blood cholesterol levels (mg/dl)		
	Recommended	Moderate risk	High risk
20-29	under 180	200-220	220+
30-39	under 200	220-240	240+
40+	under 200	240-260	260+

From National Institutes of Health: *Cholesterol counts*, Bethesda Md, 1985, Public Health Service, US Department of Health and Human Services.

Beyond measuring serum cholesterol value, measurement of the **high-density lipoprotein (HDL)** fraction and the low-density fraction of the cholesterol molecule gives more insight into the relative risk of heart disease, particularly after age 50. The HDL fraction appears to act as a scavenger molecule in the bloodstream, facilitating removal of cholesterol from the body. Elevated **low-density lipoprotein (LDL)** cholesterol is associated with increased CHD risk (American Heart Association, 1980). An optimal LDL:HDL ratio appears to be less than 3:1, with total LDL cholesterol less than 130 mg/dl. An HDL level lower than 35 mg/dl indicates some degree of CHD risk. Diet, exercise, and drug therapy can lower unacceptable lipid levels to more desirable levels.

Normal serum **triglyceride** levels range from 40 to 150 mg/dl. An elevated serum triglyceride level may also be associated with increased risk of CHD, particularly in individuals with other characteristics of increased risk. Individuals with an elevated serum triglyceride level should also be assessed for levels of total cholesterol, HDL, and blood glucose; degree of obesity; alcohol intake; and estrogen-containing medication (American Heart Association, 1980).

Serum glucose. Hyperglycemia is associated with diabetes mellitus, obesity, hypertriglyceridemia, hypertension, and elevated LDL and depressed HDL levels. All are associated with increased risk of CHD. A normal fasting serum glucose value is 80 to 120 mg/dl, but it may vary by 10 mg on either end of the range based on the specific laboratory used for testing.

Clinical Examination

Clinical examination of a client involves close physical evaluation and may reveal signs suggesting malnutrition or overconsumption of nutrients. Although clinical examination alone does not permit definitive diagnosis of a nutritional problem, the examiner should not overlook it in nutritional assessment. Table 4-16 lists physical signs suggesting malnutrition.

TABLE 4-16

Physical Signs Suggesting Malnutrition

Body area	Signs associated with malnutrition	Possible causes
Hair	Lack of natural shine; hair dull, dry, thin, and sparse; color changes (flag sign); can be easily plucked	Protein-calorie (P-C) deficiency; may be deficiency of other nutrients
Face	Skin color loss; skin dark over cheeks and eyes	P-C deficiency; deficiency of B complex vitamins
	Moon face; enlarged parotid glands	P-C deficiency
	Scaling of skin around nostrils	Niacin, riboflavin, pyridoxine deficiency
Eyes	Small, yellowish lumps around eyes (xanthelasma); white rings around both eyes (corneal arcus)	Hyperlipidemia
	Eye membranes pale (pale conjunctivae)	Vitamin B_{12}, folic acid, or iron-deficiency anemia
	Xerophthalmia: (1) night blindness, (2) dryness of eye membranes (conjunctival xerosis), and (3) dull-appearing or soft cornea (corneal xerosis)	Vitamin A deficiency
	Redness of membranes (conjunctival injection); ring of fine blood vessels around cornea (circumcorneal injection); Bitot's spots	General poor nutrition
	Redness and fissuring of eyelid corners (angular palpebritis)	Niacin and riboflavin deficiency
Lips	Redness and swelling of mouth or lips (cheilosis), especially corners of mouth (angular fissures and scars)	Niacin, riboflavin, iron, or vitamin B_6 deficiency
Tongue	Swelling; scarlet and raw tongue; smooth tongue; swollen sores; hyperemic and hypertrophic papillae; atrophic papillae	Folic acid, niacin, riboflavin, vitamin B_{12}, pyridoxine, iron, or zinc deficiency
	Magenta (purplish) tongue	Riboflavin deficiency
Gums	Spongy and bleeding	Vitamin C deficiency
Teeth	Teeth may be missing or erupting abnormally	General poor nutrition
	Caries	Excessive intake of highly refined carbohydrates; general poor nutrition
	Gray or white spots (fluorosis)	Excessive fluoride intake
Glands	Thyroid enlargement	Iodine deficiency or toxicity
	Parotid enlargement (cheeks become swollen)	General poor nutrition
	Hypogonadism	Zinc deficiency
Skin	Small or large tumors around joints of hands, legs, or skin (xanthoma)	Hyperlipidemia
	Dryness of skin (xerosis); sandpaper feel of skin (follicular hyperkeratosis); flakiness of skin	Vitamin A deficiency or excess; essential fatty acid deficiency; P-C deficiency
	Black and blue marks due to skin bleeding (petechiae)	Vitamin C or K deficiency
	Skin swollen and dark; red swollen pigmentation of exposed areas (pellagrous dermatosis)	Niacin deficiency
	Lack of fat under skin	P-C deficiency
	Yellow skin	Carotene toxicity
	Hyperpigmentation	Multiple vitamin deficiencies
	Cutaneous flushing	Niacin toxicity
Nails	Nails spoon shaped (koilonychial)	Iron deficiency
Cardiovascular system	Tachycardia (heart beat greater than 100); enlarged heart	Thiamine deficiency
	Elevated blood pressure	Excessive sodium intake
	CHD	Excessive cholesterol, fat, or caloric intake

From Roberts SLW: *Nutrition assessment manual,* Iowa City, 1977, University of Iowa Hospitals and Clinics. Reprinted with permission.

TABLE 4-16—cont'd

Physical Signs Suggesting Malnutrition

Body area	Signs associated with malnutrition	Possible causes
Nervous system	Listlessness	P-C deficiency
	Loss of position and vibratory sense; decrease and loss of ankle and knee reflexes	Vitamin B_{12} and thiamine deficiency
Muscular and skeletal systems	Muscle weakness	Phosphorus deficiency
	Muscles have "wasted" appearance	P-C deficiency
	Baby's skull bones are thin and soft; round swelling of front and side of head (frontal and parietal bossing); baby's soft spot on head does not harden (persistently open anterior fontanelle); small bumps on both sides of chest wall (ribs); bowed legs; swelling of ends of bones (epiphyseal swelling)	Vitamin D and calcium deficiency
	Musculoskeletal hemorrhages	Vitamin C deficiency
	Pseudoparalysis	
	Calf tenderness	Thiamine deficiency
	Bilateral edema of lower extremities	Protein deficiency
	Demineralization of bone (osteoporosis)	Calcium deficiency
Gastrointestinal system	Liver enlargement	Protein deficiency
	Liver and spleen enlargement	Hyperlipidemia
	Gastritis	Niacin toxicity
	Anorexia, nausea	Magnesium deficiency
	Nausea and vomiting	Vitamin A toxicity
General	Growth failure	P-C or zinc deficiency

Dietary Analysis

Assessment of dietary intake and patterns involves eliciting information regarding usual foods consumed and habits of food purchasing, preparation, and consumption. Individuals rely on foods for much more than physical nourishment. Food may represent cultural and ethnic background and socioeconomic status and have many emotional or psychological meanings. Gaining as much background information into daily food habits as possible aids in client assessment and identification of any nutritional problems, therapy, and education.

Diet history. In assessing actual food intake, consider using a 24-hour recall. Ask the client to recall everything consumed within the past 24 hours including all foods, fluids, and any vitamins, minerals, or other supplements. Be careful not to bias the client's response to questions based on personal habits or knowledge of recommended food consumption.

Another method of ascertaining food intake involves the client's keeping food records for 1 to 3 days. Asking open-ended questions that elicit a more detailed answer from the client, other than a yes or no, is best. Clients often tend to underreport amounts eaten when using the 24-hour recall, and day-to-day variations are also common (Wynder, 1992). For these reasons a food diary in which the client records food intake for 1 to 4 days is often useful. A detailed food record sheet, an example of which is given in the box on p. 114, supplies a wide variety of information regarding habits of consumption and behaviors linked with food consumption. Because an individual's weekends or days away from work or school may differ from the usual "routine," clients should include at least one weekend day in their records.

Using food records as above, the examiner can use one of the many popular computer programs to analyze the client's actual intake according to the **Recommended Dietary Allowances (RDAs)** based on age and sex (Table 4-17). Intakes of two thirds or greater of the RDA are considered adequate, although individuals may require greater amounts of a specific nutrient in particular situations.

Without computer analysis, the examiner can quickly assess the records using the "Guide to Good Eating," developed by the National Dairy Council, as shown in Table 4-18. A more detailed but very time-consuming analysis is possible using food analysis reference books.

The box on p. 116 can help elicit further information in a detailed dietary history.

Rephrasing a question or statement in various ways

TABLE 4-17

Recommended Dietary Allowances

Food and Nutrition Board, National Academy of Sciences

National Research Council
Recommended Dietary Allowances, Revised 1989

Category	Age (years) or Condition	Weight[b] (kg)	Weight[b] (lb)	Height[b] (cm)	Height[b] (in)	Protein (g)	Fat-soluble vitamins Vita-min A (μg RE)[c]	Vita-min D (μg)[d]	Vita-min E (mg α-TE)[e]	Vita-min K (μg)	Vita-min C (mg)
Infants	0.0-0.5	6	13	60	24	13	375	7.5	3	5	30
	0.5-1.0	9	20	71	28	14	375	10	4	10	35
Children	1-3	13	29	90	35	16	400	10	6	15	40
	4-6	20	44	112	44	24	500	10	7	20	45
	7-10	28	62	132	52	28	700	10	7	30	45
Males	11-14	45	99	157	62	45	1,000	10	10	45	50
	15-18	66	145	176	69	59	1,000	10	10	65	60
	19-24	72	160	177	70	58	1,000	10	10	70	60
	25-50	79	174	176	70	63	1,000	5	10	80	60
	51 +	77	170	173	68	63	1,000	5	10	80	60
Females	11-14	46	101	157	62	46	800	10	8	45	50
	15-18	55	120	163	64	44	800	10	8	55	60
	19-24	58	128	164	65	46	800	10	8	60	60
	25-50	63	138	163	64	50	800	5	8	65	60
	51 +	65	143	160	63	50	800	5	8	65	60
Pregnant						60	800	10	10	65	70
Lactating	1st 6 months					65	1,300	10	12	65	95
	2nd 6 months					62	1,200	10	11	65	90

[b]Weights and heights of Reference Adults are actual medians for the U.S. population of the designated age, as reported by NHANES II. The use of these figures does not imply that the height-to-weight ratios are ideal.
[c]Retinol equivalents. 1 retinol equivalent = 1 μg retinol or 6 μg β-carotene.
[d]As cholecalciferol. 10 μg cholecalciferol = 400 IU of vitamin D.
[e]α-Tocopherol equivalents. 1 mg d-α tocopherol = 1 α TE.
[f]NE (niacin equivalent) is equal to 1 mg of niacin or 60 mg of dietary tryptophan.

SAMPLE FOOD RECORD SHEET

Name: Height:
Date: Weight:
Age: Sex:

Foods and fluids consumed	Amount	Time of day	Place	Alone or with whom	Mood while eating
Note: Include water and any vitamins, minerals, and nutritional supplements. Specify brand name whenever possible.	*Be as specific as possible: oz., cups, etc.*				

Designed for the maintenance of good nutrition of practically all healthy people in the United States

Water-Soluble Vitamins						Minerals						
Thia-mine (mg)	Ribo-flavin (mg)	Niacin (mg NE)ᶠ	Vita-min B₆ (mg)	Fo-late (µg)	Vita-min B₁₂ (µg)	Cal-cium (mg)	Phos-phorus (mg)	Mag-nesium (mg)	Iron (mg)	Zinc (mg)	Iodine (µg)	Sele-nium (µg)
0.3	0.4	5	0.3	25	0.3	400	300	40	6	5	40	10
0.4	0.5	6	0.6	35	0.5	600	500	60	10	5	50	15
0.7	0.8	9	1.0	50	0.7	800	800	80	10	10	70	20
0.9	1.1	12	1.1	75	1.0	800	800	120	10	10	90	20
1.0	1.2	13	1.4	100	1.4	800	800	170	10	10	120	30
1.3	1.5	17	1.7	150	2.0	1,200	1,200	270	12	15	150	40
1.5	1.8	20	2.0	200	2.0	1,200	1,200	400	12	15	150	50
1.5	1.7	19	2.0	200	2.0	1,200	1,200	350	10	15	150	70
1.5	1.7	19	2.0	200	2.0	800	800	350	10	15	150	70
1.2	1.4	15	2.0	200	2.0	800	800	350	10	15	150	70
1.1	1.3	15	1.4	150	2.0	1,200	1,200	280	15	12	150	45
1.1	1.3	15	1.5	180	2.0	1,200	1,200	300	15	12	150	50
1.1	1.3	15	1.6	180	2.0	1,200	1,200	280	15	12	150	55
1.1	1.3	15	1.6	180	2.0	800	800	280	15	12	150	55
1.0	1.2	13	1.6	180	2.0	800	800	280	10	12	150	55
1.5	1.6	17	2.2	400	2.2	1,200	1,200	320	30	15	175	65
1.6	1.8	20	2.1	280	2.6	1,200	1,200	355	15	19	200	75
1.6	1.7	20	2.1	260	2.6	1,200	1,200	340	15	16	200	75

From Recommended Dietary Allowances, Revised 1989, Food and Nutrition Board, National Academy of Sciences–National Research Council, Washington, DC.

*The allowances are intended to provide for individual variations among most normal persons as they live in the United States under usual environmental stresses. Diets should be based on a variety of common foods to provide other nutrients for which human requirements have been less well defined.

†Retinol equivalents: 1 retinol equivalent = 1 µg retinol or 6 µg β-carotene.

‡As cholecalciferol: 10 µg cholecalciferol = 400 IU of vitamin D.

§α-tocopherol equivalents: 1 mg d-α-tocopherol = 1 α TE.

‖1 NE (niacin equivalent) = 1 mg niacin or 60 mg dietary tryptophan.

¶The folacin allowances refer to dietary sources as determined by *Lactobacillus casei* assay after treatment with enzymes ("conjugases") to make poly-glutamyl forms of the vitamin available to the test organism.

#The RDA for vitamin B₁₂ in infants is based on average concentration of the vitamin in human milk. The allowances after weaning are based on energy intake (as recommended by the American Academy of Pediatrics) and consideration of other factors, such as intestinal absorption.

**The increased requirement during pregnancy cannot be met by the iron content of habitual American diets nor by the existing iron stores of many women; therefore, the use of 30-60 mg of supplemental iron is recommended. Iron needs during lactation are not substantially different from those of nonpregnant women, but continued supplementation of the mother for 2-3 months after parturition is advisable to replenish stores depleted by pregnancy.

during an interview may be necessary to ascertain the reliability of information given.

A detailed dietary history can often point out a client's nutritional risk and may indicate the need for further evaluation or referral.

Estimated caloric needs. Table 4-2 lists mean heights and weights and mean values as well as ranges for recommended caloric intake. An individual's needs may vary considerably due to present nutritional status, activity, or compromising medical conditions.

Table 4-19 on p. 117 gives formulas for calculating estimated caloric expenditure in various types of injury or trauma.

Estimated protein needs. Table 4-18 lists suggested daily protein intakes for maintaining good health. As with caloric needs, an individual's protein needs may vary due to present nutritional status, activity, or compromising medical condition.

NUTRITIONAL ASSESSMENT EVALUATION

After gathering information in the four parameters of nutritional assessment—anthropometric measurement, biochemical measurement, clinical examination, and dietary analysis—the examiner should try to thoroughly integrate it to present a detailed, clear analysis

TIPS FOR ELICITING FURTHER INFORMATION FOR THE DIETARY HISTORY

1. Do you eat away from home?
2. What type of restaurants do you frequent?
3. Who cooks at home?
4. What methods of food preparation are normally used—e.g., baking, broiling, frying?
5. What are your particular food likes and dislikes?
6. What are your food allergies or intolerances?
7. What medications do you take, including vitamins, minerals, or other nutritional supplements?
8. Do you have drug allergies?
9. What are your significant medical problems, past and present?
10. Have you any difficulty chewing or swallowing?
11. Have you any problems with nausea, vomiting, diarrhea, or constipation?
12. What is your occupation? (Note the amount of time sedentary vs physically active.)
13. What are your hobbies or relaxation activities?
14. Do you exercise—type, frequency, intensity, and duration?
15. What is your target weight, if different than current weight?
16. What is your pattern of weight throughout life?
17. Have you had any significant change in weight within the last 6 months?
18. Have you ever followed dietary restrictions?
19. Have you ever received nutritional counseling? By whom?
20. Have you any episodes of food bingeing and purging?
21. Have you consumed nonfood substances (pica)?
22. Are there any religious restrictions regarding your food preparation or consumption?
23. Do you participate in special food programs?
24. How many people are in your household?

of the client's current state of health and well-being. A sample nutritional assessment form is given on pp. 18-19.

Collecting detailed information, however, is often not practical or economical in terms of time and cost. Many institutions screen clients for potential nutrition-related problems as they enter the hospital or clinic. A basic nutritional screen that would be applicable to all clients includes a review of:

Client's diet history and medical history. See page 116 (sample questions and 24-hour recall).

Client's present weight and weight change over 6 months, BMI, current lab reports such as serum albumin, TLC, hemoglobin, and hematocrit

Results of physical examination. See Table 4-18 (physical signs).

If the nurse has concerns over the results of this review he or she can then communicate them to the registered dietitian or physician.

After documenting malnutrition and beginning therapy, a suggested protocol (Blackburn and others, 1977) for evaluating therapy and the client's nutritional status involves the following:

1. Daily—body weight
2. Twice weekly—nitrogen balance
3. Weekly—TLC
4. Every three weeks—anthropometrics, serum transferrin, skin tests

DIET-RELATED CONDITIONS

Malnutrition

Malnutrition has long been recognized and well documented in developing countries. Television commercials and magazine advertisements portraying malnourished children in developing countries describe pictorially its devastating effect on human growth and development. However, malnutrition in affluent countries, such as the United States, has been identified and revealed in a variety of settings and population groups only within the past 20 years. *Subclinical* nutrient deficiencies more often occur in developed countries, but overt malnutrition also exists in affluent societies.

The problem of malnutrition in hospitalized patients was brought into focus in the early 1970s (Butterworth, 1974). Another study of hospital patients in a major midwestern city in the mid-1980s revealed a large percentage of patients who had subnormal values for the nutritional assessment parameters studied, and a large number of patients were considered to be at nutritional risk (Kamath and others, 1986).

Malnutrition is most basically defined as a lack of essential nutrients at the cellular level resulting from psychological, personal, social, educational, economic, cultural, or political factors in the individual's environment.

Malnutrition may be classified as a primary deficiency or a secondary deficiency. A *primary deficiency* occurs when a specific essential nutrient is lacking in the diet. A *secondary deficiency* can result from the body's inability to digest, absorb, metabolize, or use a specific nutrient properly or because the body has an increased requirement for or increased excretion of a specific nutrient. Malnutrition may be *acute,* a result of temporary conditions and reversible without long-term side effects, or it may be chronic, existing over a long period with possible irreversible consequences (Williams, 1985). Although the effects of various forms of malnutrition

TABLE 4-18

Guide to good eating: A Recommended Daily Pattern

The recommended daily pattern provides the foundation for a nutritious, healthful diet.
The recommended servings from the four food groups for adults supply about 1200 calories. The chart below gives recommendations for the number and size of servings for several categories of people.

Food group	Child	Teen-ager	Adult	Pregnant woman	Lactating woman	Food group	Child	Teen-ager	Adult	Pregnant woman	Lactating woman
Milk						**Fruit-vegetable**	4	4	4	4	4
1 cup milk, yogurt, OR	3	4	2	4	4	½ cup cooked or juice					
						1 cup raw					
Calcium equivalent:						Portion commonly served such as a medium-size apple or banana					
1½ slices (1½ oz) cheddar cheese*											
1 cup pudding						**Grain,** whole grain, fortified enriched	4	4	4	4	4
1¾ cups ice cream						1 slice bread					
2 cups cottage cheese*						1 cup ready-to-eat cereal					
						½ cup cooked cereal, pasta, grits					
Meat	2	2	2	3	2						
2 ounces cooked, lean meat, fish, poultry, OR											
Protein equivalent:											
2 eggs											
2 slices (2 oz) cheddar cheese*											
½ cup cottage cheese*											
1 cup dried beans, peas											
4 tbsp peanut butter											

*Count cheese as serving of milk OR meat, not both simultaneously.
"Others" complement but do not replace foods from the four food groups. Amounts should be determined by individual caloric needs.
Adapted from National Dairy Council, 1992.

TABLE 4-19

Estimated Caloric Expenditure (ECE)

$ECE\ (men) = (66.47 + 13.75W + 5.0H - 6.76A) \times (activity\ factor) \times (injury\ factor)$

$ECE\ (women) = (655.10 + 9.56W + 1.85H - 4.68A) \times (activity\ factor) \times (injury\ factor)$

W = weight in kg
H = height in cm
A = age in yrs

Activity factor
Confined to bed, use 1.20
Out of bed, use 1.30

Injury factor
Surgery: Minor, use 1.10
   Major, use 1.20
Infection: Mild, use 1.20
   Moderate, use 1.40
   Severe, use 1.80

Trauma: Skeletal, use 1.35
   Head injury with steroid therapy, use 1.60
   Blunt, use 1.35

Burns: Body Surface Area (BSA)
   40% BSA, use 1.50
   100% BSA, use 1.95

From Long CL, Schaffel N, Geiger JW, and others: Metabolic response to injury and illness: Estimation of energy and protein needs from indirect calorimetry and nitrogen balance, *JPEN* 3:452-456, 1979, and Long CL: Energy and protein requirements in stress and trauma. In *Critical Care Nursing Currents*, vol 2, no 2, Columbus, OH, 1984, Ross Laboratories, pp. 7-12. Reprinted with permission of Ross Laboratories, Columbus, OH 43216, from Nutritional Assessment Summary Sheet G636, © 1987, Ross Laboratories.

NUTRITIONAL ASSESSMENT

Name: _____ Age: _____ Gender: _____

Date: _____

Address: _____

Telephone: _____

Present Health Condition or Health Problem: _____

Parameter	Value	Percentile	Degree of depletion or elevation
0 + Weight/height	_____ kg/_____ cm	_____	_____
0 + Usual weight	_____ kg	_____	_____
0 + % Weight change	_____ %	NVA*	NVA*
0 + Desirable weight	_____ kg	NVA*	NVA*
0 + Triceps skinfold	_____ mm	_____	_____
+ Mid-arm circumference	_____ cm	_____	_____
+ Mid-arm muscle circumference	_____ cm	_____	_____
0 Body fat	_____ %	NVA*	_____

Parameter	Value	% Of standard	Degree of depletion or elevation
+ Total lymphocyte count	_____ mm³	_____	_____
0 + Serum albumin	_____ g/dl	_____	_____
+ Total iron binding capacity	_____ μg/dl	NVA*	NVA*
+ Serum transferrin	_____ mg/dl	_____	_____
+ Urinary creatinine	_____ mg	NVA*	NVA*
+ Creatinine height index	_____ %	_____	_____
0 + Hemoglobin	_____ mg/dl	NVA*	_____
0 + Hematocrit	_____ %	NVA*	_____
0 Serum cholesterol	_____ mg/dl	NVA*	_____
0 LDL:HDL ratio	_____	NVA*	_____
0 Serum triglyceride	_____ mg/dl	NVA*	_____
+ Nitrogen balance	_____ pos. or neg. number	NVA*	_____
+ Cellular immunity	_____ pos. or neg.	NVA*	_____
0 Serum glucose	_____ mg/dl	NVA*	_____

Clinical: Unusual physical signs _____

_____

_____

_____

+ indicates parameters which may be used to assess malnutrition.
0 indicates parameters which may be used to assess physical fitness or determine existence or risk of various chronic diseases, such as CHD, diabetes, and so on.
*NVA means no value appropriate.

NUTRITIONAL ASSESSMENT—cont'd

Dietary:

Approximate number of calories consumed per 24 hours _____

Approximate grams of protein consumed per 24 hours _____

Estimated caloric needs per 24 hours _____

Estimated protein needs per 24 hours _____

Adequacy of basic food groups _____

Nutrient deficiencies _____

_____

Nutrient excesses _____

_____

Daily fluid intake _____

Other dietary information pertinent to current health status _____

_____

_____

Problem identification: _____

_____

Action plan: _____

_____

_____

_____

_____

_____

_____

_____

_____

may be manifested in similar ways, isolating the cause is important for successful treatment.

Several steps occur in the development of malnutrition. A primary or secondary nutrient deficiency appears, as noted above. In an attempt to maintain necessary nutrients at the cellular level, the body mobilizes tissue reserves, leading to measurably reduced levels of the nutrients in the tissues. As tissue reserves are depleted and cellular supplies of essential nutrients decrease, biochemical alterations appear, as measured by enzyme and metabolite levels. With further progression, clinical symptoms are manifested. Malnutrition can be identified at any of these stages (Figure 4-10).

Malnutrition resulting from a deficiency of protein, calories, or both, is referred to as protein energy malnutrition or PEM. PEM can be classified as kwashiorkor or **marasmus.**

Kwashiorkor is caused by protein deficiency. Symptoms include retarded growth and development, muscle wasting, depigmentation of the hair and skin, and edema. The edema and presence of existing fat stores can give this client the appearance of being well-nourished (Williams, 1993).

In marasmus the client is deficient in both protein and calories. It is a chronic condition that produces gradual wasting of the body. Characteristics of marasmus include atrophy of muscle mass and fat stores with little edema. Clients with marasmus appear to have stunted growth and look emaciated (Williams, 1989).

These conditions occur mainly in children from poverty stricken areas, although marginal to chronic deficiencies of these types may occur in conditions such as liver disease, hypermetabolic disease, AIDS, cancer, chronic obstructive pulmonary disease, cystic fibrosis, and any prolonged illness, especially in the elderly. When body protein is depleted, specific body functions

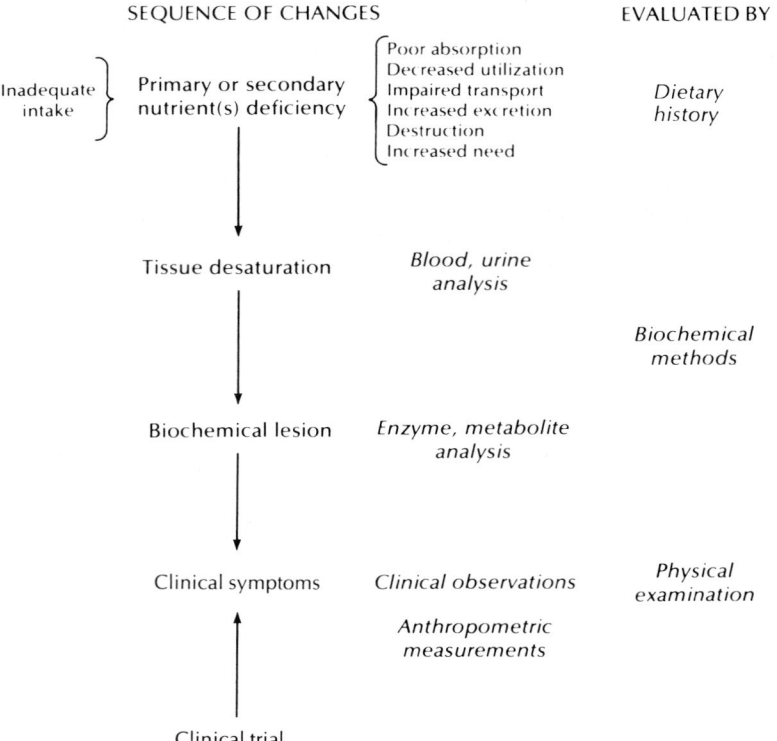

SEQUENCE OF CHANGES   EVALUATED BY

Inadequate intake } Primary or secondary nutrient(s) deficiency { Poor absorption / Decreased utilization / Impaired transport / Increased excretion / Destruction / Increased need   *Dietary history*

Tissue desaturation   *Blood, urine analysis*

Biochemical methods

Biochemical lesion   *Enzyme, metabolite analysis*

Clinical symptoms   *Clinical observations*   *Physical examination*

Anthropometric measurements

Clinical trial

FIGURE 4-10 Sequence of body changes in the development of malnutrition.

can be lost or minimized. Some of these functions include skeletal muscle function necessary to a client's mobility, respiratory function, and protein synthesis in the liver and other organs including the production of antibodies and tissue repair (Windsor, 1991).

Specific nutrient deficiencies may be present in an individual due to lack of adequate intake of the nutrients, or may be associated with various disease states or induced through the use of certain medications, particularly if dietary intake of essential nutrients is marginal. The health care practitioner should use a drug-nutrient interaction handbook to determine possible drug-nutrient interactions a client may be experiencing.

Obesity

Obesity is defined as body weight 20% above the recommended weight listed in insurance tables. It can also be defined as having a BMI above 27.8 for men and above 27.3 for women. Obesity must be distinguished from being overweight as a result of extra muscle development that occurs in certain types of athletes. Determining percentage of body fat can be helpful in some clients to determine the level of body fat. Techniques such as biochemical impedance (see Figure 4-5), underwater weighing (see Figure 4-6), and skinfold measurements are useful in determining total body fat. The

examiner can determine total body fat by comparing measured values to tables based on age and sex. Normal body fat percentages are 10 to 20% for men and 20 to 30% for healthy adult women.

Obesity may result from a complexity of factors, and several theories regarding the development of obesity exist. In terms of psychological aspects of obesity, the use of food to handle other problems in life results in overconsumption, weight gain, and possibly other health risks. The obese individual often knows *what* to eat, but the control of eating behavior is elusive. An overweight individual may consume much less than a thin individual in terms of total calories, but a decreased metabolic rate, often due to repeated strict dieting and low activity levels, may aid the body's storage of fat. Being overweight may be a predisposing factor in some cases of **anorexia nervosa;** adolescent obesity may be a predisposing factor in the development of **bulimia nervosa** in adult life. Important in planning a holistic therapy program is a detailed diet history, including

1. Weight history
2. History and patterns of dieting
3. Present food consumption
4. Eating behavior patterns
5. Exercise habits
6. Feelings about food—psychological meanings

Obesity threatens health as follows:

1. Obesity may aggravate existing health conditions such as high blood pressure, cardiovascular problems, liver disorders, and arthritis and may pose increased risk for development of these diseases.
2. Obesity often occurs with diabetes, particularly type II.
3. Obesity can increase the risk of developing gallbladder disease.
4. Obesity can increase surgical risks.
5. Obesity restricts mobility, which can lower one's general level of fitness.
6. Obesity can decrease life expectancy. The morbidly obese have the highest rate of premature death.

In addition, obese individuals often suffer emotional and psychological difficulties (National Dairy Council, 1985).

Assessment of the obese individual involves a close look at

1. Current height and weight
2. BMI—degree of overweight
3. Percentage of body fat (may not be reliable with the severely obese client)
4. Abnormalities that may be present in blood pressure, serum lipids, and serum glucose
5. Food consumption habits
6. Physical activity patterns

The examiner can determine height, weight, BMI, and degree of obesity by methods previously described in this chapter.

Weight reduction is recommended in the following circumstances:

1. Excess body weight of 20% or more. This corresponds to a BMI above 27.8 for men and 27.3 for women.
2. Family history or risk factors for maturity-onset (type II) diabetes.
3. High blood pressure.
4. Hypertriglyceridemia or hypercholesterolemia.
5. CHD (or atherosclerosis).
6. Gout.
7. Functional impairment due to heart disease, chronic obstructive pulmonary disease, or osteoarthritis of the spine, hips, and knees (which bear weight).
8. History of childhood obesity (Burton and Foster, 1985).

A team approach is suggested in the diagnosis and treatment of obesity. In many cases, when elevations of blood sugar, blood pressure, or serum lipids coexist with obesity, a loss of body fat and achievement of desirable weight will reduce these elevations. Psychological factors important in assessing and treating obesity are discussed in the section on assessment of eating disorders later in this chapter.

Diabetes

Diabetes, although not caused by diet or activity level alone, may be aggravated by obesity, poor food choices, and a sedentary life-style. The diabetic client is at increased risk of developing microvascular complications. In assessing the diabetic client, the practitioner must pay close attention to the following:

1. Current height and weight versus desirable weight for height
2. Regularity of physical activity patterns
3. Daily food consumption patterns:
   a. Calories consumed
   b. Percentages of carbohydrate, protein, and fat in the diet
   c. Types of dietary fat consumed
   d. Amount of dietary fiber consumed
   e. Regularity of meal schedule and coordination with insulin action
   f. Methods of food preparation
4. Diet tolerance
5. Monitoring of blood and/or urine glucose

Dietary and activity recommendations should be based on maintaining desirable weight, controlling blood sugar and serum lipid levels, and promoting a general state of fitness.

Hypertension

Predisposing factors that increase a person's risk of developing hypertension include heredity, sex, age, race, obesity, calcium intake, and sensitivity to sodium. Related factors that appear to have some effect on hypertension include heavy alcohol consumption, use of oral contraceptives, and a sedentary life-style (American Heart Association, 1986). Nutritional assessment of the client with hypertension or of the client who is at increased risk for developing hypertension involves assessing weight and dietary factors, with particular attention to the amount of sodium, calcium, and calories consumed as well as the overall balance of nutrients in the diet. Assessing physical activity patterns is important. BMI has been related to hypertension, and an estimated 25% to 35% of hypertensive individuals are overweight. Moderate weight loss can produce decreases in blood pressure similar to those produced with initial doses of diuretics (Elmer, 1985).

The practitioner should assess the client's needs based on

1. Achieving and maintaining desirable weight
2. Reducing sodium intake, if elevated, to suggested levels based on the severity of hypertension and the client's past response to diet or drug modifications

3. Ensuring a balance of all essential nutrients in the diet
4. Promoting regular physical activity according to individual tolerance
5. Evaluating the effect of antihypertensive drugs and diuretic therapy on dietary intake

Coronary Heart Disease

The three major risk factors in the development of CHD are high blood cholesterol, hypertension, and cigarette smoking. Other risk factors in the development of CHD include

- Emotional stress
- Sedentary life-style
- Overweight
- Diabetes
- Heart abnormalities
- Family history of heart disease
- Age
- Sex
- Race

The American Heart Association's (1991) current recommendations for healthy adult Americans include the following:

1. Total fat intake should be less than 30% of calories.
2. **Saturated fat** intake should be less than 10% of calories.
3. **Polyunsaturated fat** should be less than 10% of calories.
4. **Monounsaturated fat** should be less than 10% of calories.
5. Cholesterol intake should be less than 100 mg/1000 calories, not to exceed 300 mg daily.
6. Protein intake should be approximately 15% of calories.
7. Carbohydrate intake should make up 50% to 55% or more of calories, with emphasis on increasing sources of complex carbohydrates.
8. Sodium intake should be reduced to approximately 1 g/1000 calories, not to exceed 3 g daily.
9. If alcoholic beverages are consumed, the limit should be 15% of total calories, not to exceed 50 ml of ethanol daily.
10. Total calories should be sufficient to maintain the individual's body weight (see Table 4-3).
11. A wide variety of foods should be consumed.

Modification of the diet in individuals whose lipid levels are elevated involves individualization. HDL levels may be positively affected by regular physical activity and by modifying specific types of fat consumed. LDL levels may be lowered by modifying dietary saturated fat and cholesterol intake and by regulating body weight combined with exercise training.

Cancer

Scientific research has demonstrated an association between the amount of dietary fat consumed and the incidence of cancer, especially of the breast, large bowel, and prostate. Certain nutrients and other food constituents, such as vitamins A, C, and E, selenium, and dietary fiber, may be potential anticancer substances when consumed at levels found in a balanced diet.

For dietary fiber some investigators recommend intakes of approximately 25 grams/day (Wynder, 1992).

The American Institute for Cancer Research has produced the following dietary guidelines to lower cancer risk:

1. Reduce daily intake of dietary fat—both saturated and unsaturated—to 30% of total calories.
2. Increase consumption of fruits, vegetables, and whole grain cereals.
3. Consume salt-cured, salt-pickled, smoked, and charcoal-broiled foods in moderation.
4. Drink alcoholic beverages in moderation if at all.

In certain countries, eating large amounts of salt-cured, salt-pickled, and smoked foods has increased the incidence of stomach and esophageal cancer. Ingesting large amounts of charred foods, such as those cooked over an open flame, may also lead to cancer. In the United States this guideline is only intended for those who consume these foods in excess; most Americans do not fall into this category. In addition, although alcoholic beverages are low in most nutrients, they are high in calories. A high intake of such "empty" calories reduces the intake of other nutrient-rich foods needed in a balanced diet. When excessive alcohol consumption is combined with cigarette smoking, cancers of the mouth, esophagus, and larynx are increased. Also, excessive alcohol consumption may be a factor in the development of liver cancer (The American Institute for Cancer Research, 1990).

These guidelines to lower cancer risks are consistent with and extend the *Dietary Guidelines for Americans* published by the U.S. Departments of Agriculture and Health and Human Services (The American Institute for Cancer Research, 1990). Nutritional assessment involves dietary analysis with the above guidelines in mind.

SPECIALTY POPULATIONS AND CONCERNS

Pediatric Assessment

Pediatric assessment involves evaluating growth and activity patterns as well as foods consumed and eating behavior.

Nutritional needs per kilogram body weight are higher during infancy than in any other stage of the life cycle. Nutritional monitoring is an essential part of the health assessment in order to monitor growth and development. During puberty a second large growth spurt occurs and along with hormonal changes can greatly change nutritional needs (Williams, 1993).

The examiner can evaluate height, weight, head circumference, and growth pattern using the National Center for Health Statistics growth charts. Table 4-20 lists standards for height and weight for children 4 to 18 years of age. The examiner should pay specific attention to *individuality* and *consistency* in the growth pattern, recognizing that trends and variations may occur. Height indicates long-term nutritional status, while weight signals a change in nutritional status (Satter, 1991). Measurements in children and adolescents below the 15th percentile may indicate some type of disorder and warrant closer investigation of the condition. Children and adolescents whose weight is at the 85th percentile or greater may warrant closer investigation of food habits and activity patterns, especially with rapid changes. Eating disorders can develop in early childhood, and early intervention is critical if the individual is to mature with a healthy view of food and the eating experience.

The assessment of food intake and eating behavior begins with the infant. The information contained under Nutritional Data in Chapter 24, Assessment of the Pediatric Client, details important aspects of infant feeding to include in pediatric assessment. Determining the appropriateness of the formula used, if the child is not breast-fed, is important, along with ensuring that the child is growing at a consistent rate. Assess developmental patterns and the introduction of solid foods according to the schedules shown in Tables 4-21 through 4-24. The child who is growing normally will experience changes in appetite and food intake as growth trends occur. Refer to Tables 4-18 and 4-24 for recommended daily servings from the four basic food groups for children and teens.

Along with the basics, an evaluation of types of foods consumed, method of preparation (e.g., fresh, convenience, fried, baked), and snacking habits will indicate other aspects of nutritional quality such as the level of fat, sodium, sugar, and fiber.

Evaluating a child's or adolescent's intake of iron, calcium, and vitamins A and C may indicate a less than desirable intake. The RDAs for these nutrients, along with other essential nutrients, are found in Table 4-17. Inclusion of recommended servings from the basic food groups every day ensures that the average healthy child's nutrient needs will be met.

Nutritional assessment of the pediatric client also involves assessment of family attitudes toward food, family knowledge of proper nutrition, and family food budget.

Maternal Assessment

In the best of circumstances assessment of maternal nutrition begins before conception. In reality, because the majority of women are seen for evaluation once conception has occurred, the pregnant woman should be assessed early in the pregnancy.

A health evaluation including assessment of the woman's current height and weight status, dietary intake, and any preexisting health concerns allows the health care practitioner to determine if the client is in optimal health or if changes in health habits (e.g., diet and exercise) would serve to make pregnancy healthier and safer for the mother and baby.

Prepregnancy weight and maternal weight gain have both been positively associated with infant birth weight (Committee on Maternal Nutrition, 1970). Other factors associated with gestational weight gain and low birth weight include maternal prepregnancy weight for height, prepregnant weight, race, marital status, educational level, age, parity, cigarette smoking, socioeconomic status, and energy intake (Institute of Medicine, 1990). Table 4-25 gives values for optimum weight gain during pregnancy, based on weight for height, BMI.

Poor gestational weight gain or less than recommended for the client's prepregnancy height/weight are associated with an increased risk of giving birth to a growth-retarded infant (Institute of Medicine, 1990).

TABLE 4-20

Body Composition of Reference Children

Age	Length (cm) Males	Length (cm) Fem.	Weight (kg) Males	Weight (kg) Fem.	Fat 1% Males	Fat 1% Fem.
Birth	51.6	50.5	3.545	3.325	13.7	14.9
3 mo.	61.5	59.6	6.435	5.743	23.2	23.8
6 mo.	67.6	65.8	8.030	7.250	25.4	26.4
12 mo.	76.1	74.3	10.15	9.18	22.5	23.7
18 mo.	82.4	80.2	11.47	10.78	20.8	21.8
24 mo.	87.2	85.5	12.59	11.91	19.5	20.4
3 yr.	95.3	94.1	14.675	14.10	17.5	18.5
4 yr.	102.9	101.6	16.69	15.96	15.9	17.3
5 yr.	109.9	108.4	18.67	17.66	14.6	16.7
6 yr.	116.1	114.6	20.69	19.52	13.5	16.4
7 yr.	121.7	120.6	22.85	21.84	12.8	16.8
8 yr.	127	126.4	25.30	24.84	13	17.4
9 yr.	132	132.2	28.13	28.46	13.2	18.3
10 yr.	137.5	138.3	31.44	32.55	13.7	19.4

Adapted from Foman SJ, Haschke F, Zeigler EE, Nelson SE: Body composition of reference children from birth to age i0 years, *Am J Clin Nutr* 35:1171, 1982.

TABLE 4-21

Developmental Patterns and Feeding Style in the First 6 Months

	Birth	1 mo	2 mo	3 mo	4 mo	5 mo	6 mo
Mouth pattern	Sucking, "extrusion" pattern.				Beginning swallow pattern; can transfer food from front of tongue to back. Beginning of drooling		
Hand coordination	Random motion of hands				Hands beginning to go to mouth		Palmar grasp
Body control	Prone on back: can raise head when on stomach				Sits supported; loses balance when reaches		Sits unsupported; can balance while manipulating with hands
Digestive ability	Can digest appropriate milk				Intestinal amylase begins to increase to allow starch digestion		
Homeostatic ability	Low; needs carefully adapted formula						
Nutritional requirements	Relatively high nutrient requirement for rapid growth		Iron stores depleted in premature infants				Iron stores begin to be depleted in term babies
Feeding style	Nipple-feeding by breast or bottle						Beginning spoon feeding
Food selection	Breast milk or formula						Beginning solids: iron source

From Satter E: *Child of mine—feeding with love and good sense,* Palo Alto, Calif, Bull Publishing 1991. Reprinted with permission.

Current anthropometric methods for assessing gestational weight gain are BMI and rate of weight gain.

The pattern of weight gain is important, with about 4.4 to 8.8 kg (2 to 4 lb) as an average gain during the first trimester and an average weight gain of about 2.2 kg (1 lb) per week during the second and third trimesters for the normal weight woman.

For underweight women the rate of weight gain should be .5 kg per week or 1.1 lb. In the overweight woman the pattern should be .3 kg per week or .66 lb (Institute of Medicine, 1990). Weight should be assessed at each prenatal visit. If weight gain is less than .5 kg (1 lb) per month for overweight women and 1 kg (2.2 lb) per month for normal weight women further assessment and planning are recommended (Institute of Medicine, 1990).

The recommended number of servings from the basic food groups for pregnant and lactating women can be found in Table 4-18. Intakes of less than the RDA (Recommended Dietary Allowances) have been seen most often for vitamins B_6, D, E and folate and for the minerals iron, zinc, calcium, and magnesium (Institute of Medicine, 1990).

Recommendations vary but, supplementation of the pregnant woman's diet with 30 to 60 mg of iron daily during the second and third trimesters, as well as a daily

TABLE 4-22

Development Patterns and Feeding Recommendations

	6 mo	7 mo	8 mo	9 mo	10 mo	11 mo	12 mo	13 mo	14 mo	15 mo	16 mo
Mouth pattern	Beginning swallow pattern; can transfer food from front of tongue to back		Beginning chewing pattern; side-to-side motion of tongue and mashing food with jaws				Continuing maturation of biting, chewing, swallowing				
Hand coordination	Palmar grasp	Pincer grasp beginning	Grabs spoon		Can get spoon in mouth but generally turns it over		Beginning mastery of spoon—still spilling most times			Spoon to mouth—with load intact	
	Urge to put anything in mouth continues until about three; increased risk for poisoning throughout this time										
Body control	Sits unsupported; can balance while manipulating with hands		Continuing improvement in balance while sitting								
			Begins to stand; can pull self to feet and move around				Beginning and increasing mastery of walking				
Digestive			Gastric acid volume begins to increase		Can handle balanced amounts of all reasonably soft, moderately seasoned family food						
Homeostatic ability		Increasing ability to maintain hydration and chemical balance									
Nutritional requirements	Iron stores begin to be depleted in term babies		Gradually increasing proportion of adequate diet offered by foods other than milk feeding							All daily nutritional requirements provided by a mixed table food diet: primary source of nutrients and calories in table food and cup	
Feeding style	Spoon feeding	Introduce cup at meals		Begin self-feeding with cup; beginning proficiency with spoon						Reasonably adept with spoon and cup. Can feed self with spoon, drink from cup. Weaned from bottle. Continuance of breast-feeding up to baby and parents	
Food selection	Semisolid foods	Increase texture, stiffness of solids			Pieces of soft, cooked foods						

From Satter E: *Child of mine—feeding with love and good sense,* Palo Alto, Calif, 1983, 1986, Bull Publishing. Reprinted with permission. Ages overlap and are given as ranges because of variations in rate of infant development.

TABLE 4-23

Feeding Schedule: Six to Twelve Months

	4-7 months	6-8 months	7-10 months	10-12 months
Milk feeding	Breast milk or formula	Breast milk or formula	Breast milk or formula	Breast milk or formula Evaporated milk diluted 1:1 with water Whole pasteurized milk or combination
Cereal and bread	Begin iron-fortified baby cereal mixed with milk feeding	Continue baby cereal; begin other breads and cereals	Continue baby cereal Other breads and cereals from table	Continue baby cereal until 18 months Total of four servings bread and cereal from table
Fruit and vegetables (including juice)	None	Begin juice from cup: 3 oz vitamin C source Begin fork-mashed, soft fruits and vegetables	3 oz juice Pieces of soft and cooked fruits and vegetables from table	Table-food diet to allow 4 servings a day, including juice
Meat and other protein sources	None	None	Gradually begin milled or finely cut meat Casseroles, ground beef, eggs, fish, peanut butter, legumes, cheese	Two servings daily; one ounce total, meat or equivalent

From Satter E: *Child of mine—feeding with love and good sense,* Palo Alto, Calif, 1991, Bull Publishing. Reprinted with permission. Ages overlap and are given as ranges because of variations in rate of infant development.

supplement of 0.2 to 0.4 mg of folate, is commonly advised. Other nutritional considerations involve the mother's use of caffeine, artificial sweeteners, and alcohol during pregnancy. The safest strategy, in terms of protecting the baby from possible side effects, is to abstain from using these substances in the diet. Amounts of these substances consumed by the pregnant woman must be evaluated. Assessment of the mother's intake of dietary fiber, found in whole grains, fruits and vegetables (especially raw), and legumes, as well as assessment of fluid intake is helpful in preventing constipation.

Assessment of the mother's diet while breastfeeding is important, following the recommendations listed in Table 4-21, as well as ensuring that the mother is drinking enough fluids to support milk production. It is important during this time that the mother not omit basic foods—and thus essential nutrients—from her diet in an attempt to lose weight rapidly. Alcohol, caffeine, and artificial sweeteners should be used with caution if at all, as in the pregnant woman.

Geriatric Assessment

Assessment of the older adult requires recognition of nutritional risk factors that are associated with the normal aging process as well as prevention or control of chronic diseases that are known to occur in over 85% of the older adult population (Nutrition Screening Initiative, 1991). Poor nutritional status in the aging can significantly increase hospital stay and recovery time in cases of disease or chronic illness.

TABLE 4-24

A Feeding Guide for Children

This is a guide to a basic diet. Fats, desserts, and sauces will contribute additional kilocalories to meet the needs of the growing child.

Food	1 year old		2-3 years old		4-6 years old		7 years to puberty		Comments
	Portion sizes	No. of servings	Portion sizes	No. of servings	Portion sizes	No. of servings	Portion sizes	No. of servings	
Milk	½ cup	4-5	¼-¾ cup	4-5	½-¾ cup	3-4	1 cup	3	The following may be substituted for one-half cup of liquid milk: ½-¾ oz cheese ¼-½ cup yogurt 2½ tbsp non-fat dry milk powder
Meat and meat equivalents	¼-1 oz 2-4 tbsp	1	1-2 oz	2	1-2 oz	2	2-3 oz	3	The following may be substituted for one ounce of meat, fish, poultry: 4-5 tbsp cooked legumes 1 egg 2 tbsp peanut butter
Fruit and vegetables		4-5		4-5		4-5		4-5	Include one green leafy or yellow vegetable, e.g., spinach, broccoli, carrots, winter squash
Vegetables									
Cooked	1-2 tbsp		2-3 tbsp		3-4 tbsp		½ cup		
Raw	1-2 tbsp		Few pieces		Few pieces		½ cup		
Fruit									
Canned	2-4 tbsp		2-4 tbsp		4-6 tbsp		½ cup		Include one vitamin C–rich fruit or juice per day
Raw	2-4 tbsp (chopped)		½-1 small		½-1 small				
Juice	2-4 oz		3-4 oz		4 oz		4 oz		
Grains and grain products	½ slice	3	¼-1 slice	3	1 slice	4	1 slice	6	The following may be substituted for one slice of bread: ½ cup cooked cereal ½ cup spaghetti or other pasta ½ cup rice 5 saltines Whole grain products provide additional bulk to the diet

Adapted from Lowenberg ME: *The development of food patterns in young children.* In Pipes P: *Nutrition in infancy and childhood,* ed 3, St Louis, 1985, Mosby–Year Book.

TABLE 4-25

*Recommended Total Weight Gain Ranges
for Pregnant Women,^a by Prepregnancy
Body Mass Index (BMI)^b*

Weight-for-height category	Recommended total gain	
	kg	lb
Low (BMI < 19.8)	12.5-18	28-40
Normal (BMI of 19.8 to 26.0)	11.5-16	25-35
High^c (BMI > 26.0 to 29.0)	7-11.5	15-25

^aYoung adolescents and black women should strive for gains at the upper end of the recommended range. Short women (<157 cm, or 62 in.) should strive for gains at the lower end of the range.
^bBMI is calculated using metric units.
^cThe recommended target weight gain for obese women (BMI > 29.0) is at least 6.0 kg (15 lb).

In the process of aging, some lean body mass is lost as the weight of vital organs decreases, while increased fat deposition occurs, mainly around internal organs and to a lesser degree in the blood.

There is a slight decrease in total body water. A decrease in bone mass is experienced, more so in women than in men that can lead to osteoporosis.

Because of bodily changes that occur during aging and the difficulty of obtaining certain measurements, anthropometric measurements routinely used in assessing nutritional status are not entirely appropriate for the geriatric population. The particular measurements that may be difficult to obtain in some elderly clients include height, weight, skinfold thickness, and MAC. Various recumbent measurements can be used to assess nutritional status when standard methods are not possible.

Reference data have been established for anthropometric assessment of the elderly (Chumlea and others, 1987). Estimation of height may be necessary as curvature of the spine and other problems may be present. Chumlea and associates have formulated an equation for the estimation of height based on knee height:

Men: 64.19 × (0.04 × age) + (2.02 × knee height)
Women: 84.88 − (0.24 × age) + (1.83 × knee height)

Knee height should be measured from the bottom of the foot to the anterior of the knee.

The appropriate data must be used for accurate assessment and interpretation of nutritional status. Taking into account a decrease in basal metabolic rate and generally decreasing physical activity with aging, recommended energy intake decreases with age, as listed in Table 4-2.

BMI for the aging should ideally fall between 24 and 27. Levels below 24 may indicate poor nutritional status. Levels at 28 or above indicate increased risk for the medical complication of obesity (Nutrition Screening Initiative, 1991).

Physiological changes occurring during aging may interfere with the body's ability to digest, absorb, and use food consumed. In addition, many elderly persons are taking one or more drugs, which may interfere with the body's absorption and metabolism of nutrients consumed.

With a decrease in calorie level and difficulties with digestion and absorption it is more difficult to plan a diet that meets all nutrient needs. A diet that is high in nutrient density is recommended, which is a diet with maximum nutritional benefit for the minimum amount of calories.

Other common characteristics in the geriatric client that are important in nutritional assessment include (1) tooth loss, (2) loss of perception of taste and smell, (3) changes in vision, (4) specific physical and psychological disorders, (5) social isolation and depression, and (6) poverty.

All these factors affect the food choices a person might make. Causes and any possible corrections should be evaluated thoroughly so that the feeding environment is as pleasant and as positive an experience as possible, ensuring consumption of a nutritious diet. Alterations in the composition and consistency of the diet and the timing and size of meals and snacks may be necessary. An evaluation of activity habits is important, considering that moderate activity is thought to have a positive effect on health and well-being and to prevent the premature loss of muscle mass and calcium.

The following laboratory values may be altered in the elderly:

May be increased	*May be decreased*
Serum glucose	Hemoglobin
Serum cholesterol	Hematocrit
Serum triglycerides	Serum albumin
Blood urea nitrogen	Creatinine clearance
	Adrenocorticotropic hormone

In addition, reduced levels of serum folate, vitamin C, B12, and zinc are also seen.

Assessment of the Physically Active

Assessment of the physically active client involves evaluating physical status, including such factors as body composition, flexibility, muscular strength, and cardiovascular endurance. For a healthy individual, suggested laboratory analysis could include serum cholesterol, serum glucose, hemoglobin, and hematocrit determinations. The measurement of blood pressure is of further value in assessing health status.

Nutritional assessment involves a close look at energy expended during various activities as well as evaluation of the client's current dietary patterns regarding calories consumed; percentages of carbohydrate, protein, and fat in the diet; balance and variety of food consumption; appropriate amounts of vitamins and minerals in the diet; and fluid consumption.

Table 4-26 lists caloric expenditure for various recreational activities based on body weight. Endurance athletes may require as many as 5000 to 6000 calories daily to supply sufficient energy for performance. *Where* these calories are obtained, in terms of food sources, can have a tremendous impact on the athlete's health and performance.

Table 4-18 is used as a guideline for consumption by physically active individuals. Although endurance athletes appear to require slightly more protein than nonathletic and moderately active adults (1.2 g of protein/kg body weight daily vs 0.8 g of protein/kg body weight daily, respectively) these needs are usually met without any problem if the endurance athlete consumes 15% of total calories daily in the form of protein. The recommended amounts of carbohydrate, protein, and fat in the diet of the nontraining adult are as follows:

- 55% to 60% of calories in the form of carbohydrate
- 12% to 15% of calories in the form of protein
- Up to 30% of calories in the form of fat

Endurance training athletes are advised to increase the carbohydrate content of their diet slightly, up to about 65% of total calories, to increase muscle **glycogen** stores and ensure available energy to the body during the training process. The food groups that supply the major amounts of carbohydrate in the diet are the grain group and the fruit and vegetable group. Foods in the milk group also supply some carbohydrate but may supply unwanted fat if not chosen carefully.

It is important to assess if an individual is consuming adequate fluid to meet metabolic needs. A sedentary

TABLE 4-26

Energy Expenditure/Hour During Various Activities

Light activities (120-150 kcal/hr)	Light to moderate activities (150-300 kcal/hr)	Moderate activities (300-420 kcal/hr)	Heavy activities (420-600 kcal/hr)
Personal care	**Domestic work**	**Yard work**	**Yard work**
Dressing	Making beds	Digging	Chopping wood
Washing	Sweeping floors	Mowing lawn (not motorized)	Digging holes
Shaving	Ironing	Pulling weeds	Shoveling snow
	Washing clothes		
Sitting		**Walking**	**Walking**
Rocking	**Yard work**	3½ to 4 mph on level surface	5 mph
Typing	Light gardening	Up and down small hills	Up stairs
Writing	Mowing lawn (power mower)		Up hills
Playing cards		**Recreation**	Climbing
Peeling potatoes	**Light work**	Badminton	
Sewing	Auto repair	Calisthenics	**Recreation**
Playing piano	Painting	Ballet exercises	Bicycling 11 to 12 mph or up
	Shoe repair	Canoeing 4 mph	and down hills
Standing or slowly moving around	Store clerk	Dancing (waltz, square)	Cross-country skiing
	Washing car	Golf (no cart)	Jogging 5 mph
Billiards		Ping-Pong	Swimming
	Walking	Tennis (doubles)	Tennis (singles)
	2 to 3 mph on level surface or down stairs	Volleyball	Water-skiing
	Recreation		
	Archery		
	Bicycling 5½ mph on level surface		
	Bowling		
	Canoeing 2½ to 3 mph		

*Energy expenditure will depend on the physical fitness (that is, amount of lean body mass) of the individual and continuity of exercise. Note that some of these activities can be used as aerobic activities to promote cardiovascular fitness.
From Williams, SR: *Nutrition and diet therapy,* ed 6, St. Louis, 1989, Mosby–Year Book.

individual needs approximately 1 liter of water daily per 1000 calories consumed (O'Neil and others, 1986) and large, very active athletes may require two or three times this amount. Inadequate fluid intake hampers performance and can cause serious heat-related problems.

Specific concerns related to nutritional health of athletes involve the misuse of dietary supplements (vitamins, minerals, protein, and steroids) and the development of eating disorders in an attempt to achieve an unrealistic body size or shape. Although athletes require a few vitamins and minerals in increased amounts, these needs can be easily met through a diet that is varied and balanced and that supplies enough calories to meet energy needs. The athlete who consumes megadoses of vitamins, minerals, or protein in an attempt to increase muscle mass or improve performance may cause serious **toxicities** or risk developing such problems as renal disease from long-term overload of protein. According to O'Neil and others (1986), "Athletes at high risk for developing iron deficiency include male and female long-distance runners, menstruating girls and women, children, vegetarians, and other individuals who do not meet iron needs through diet."

Although athletes do not generally require more calcium than nonathletes, the athlete's diet should be assessed for adequate calcium consumption, providing at least the RDA. The amenorrheic athlete's calcium needs may be increased, resembling the needs of postmenopausal women (O'Neil and others, 1986).

Athletes, because they may be told to lose a few pounds to make weight, wish to be a certain body size or shape for a specific sport, or are striving toward perfectionism, may be prone to consume inadequate diets to meet nutritional needs as well as to develop eating disorders. Assessment of eating disorders is discussed in the next section.

Because of the positive effects of regular physical activity in controlling weight, increasing cardiovascular fitness, reducing stress, and contributing to an overall sense of health and well-being, an assessment of current activity patterns is important in determining health status and providing recommendations to the client.

ASSESSMENT OF EATING DISORDERS

An eating disorder is an aberration of the function and process of eating, indicating a complexity of psychological, emotional, and social problems or maladaptation. Assessment of eating disorders involves identification of

1. The signs and symptoms associated with particular disorders

2. Medical, psychological, and social complications or consequences resulting from particular disorders

3. A client's present nutritional status, dietary habits, activity patterns, and psychological background

Two major categories of eating disorders will be discussed, anorexia nervosa and bulimia nervosa.

Anorexia Nervosa

Anorexia nervosa is "characterized by persistent, intentional loss of weight and maintenance of weight at an abnormally low level" (Huse and Lucas, 1983). Discriminating features in identifying the disorder include those listed in the box below, left.

Onset of the disorder typically occurs in early to late adolescence but may range from prepubescence to, rarely, the early thirties. Anorexia nervosa occurs predominantly in females.

MEDICAL COMPLICATIONS OF ANOREXIA NERVOSA

Metabolic complications

Yellowing of skin
Impaired taste
Hypoglycemia

Gastrointestinal complications

Altered gastric emptying
Salivary gland swelling
Superior mesenteric artery syndrome
Gastric dilatation
Constipation

Cardiovascular complications

Bradycardia
Arrhythmias
Pericardial effusion
Edema
Heart failure

Renal complications

Water concentration defect
Kaliopenic nephropathy

Fluid and electrolyte complications

Dehydration
Weakness
Tetany

Hematologic complications

Bleeding diathesis
Anemia

Dental problems

Decalcification
Caries

Endocrine complications

Amenorrhea
Lack of sexual interest
Impotence

General complications

Weakness
Hypothermia

From Brownell KD and Foreyt JP, editors: *Handbook of eating disorders: physiology, psychology, and treatment of obesity, anorexia, and bulimia,* New York, 1986, Basic Books.

DISCRIMINATING FEATURES IN IDENTIFYING ANOREXIA NERVOSA

1. Self-inflicted weight loss accompanied thereafter by a sustained avoidance of mature body shape, which cannot be directly ascribed to other identifiable psychiatric causes, **cachexia**-inducing diseases, or externally imposed demands for reduced food intake.
2. A morbid and persistent dread of fat.
3. The manipulation of body weight through dietary restraint, self-induced vomiting, abuse of purgatives, or excessive exercise.
4. Disturbances in body image manifest in the misrepresentation of actual body dimensions or extreme loathing of bodily functions.
5. Amenorrhea and the development of other behavioral physiological sequelae of starvation.

From Brownell KD and Foreyt JP, editors: *Handbook of eating disorders: physiology, psychology, and treatment of obesity, anorexia, and bulimia*, New York, 1986, Basic Books.

TABLE 4-27

Symptoms and Signs of Anorexia Nervosa

Symptoms	Prevalence of symptoms (%)	Signs	Prevalence of signs (%)
Amenorrhea	100	Hypotension	20-85
Constipation	20	Hypothermia	15-85
Bloating	30	Dry skin	25-85
Abdominal pain	20	Bradycardia	25-90
Cold intolerance	20	Lanugo	20-80
Lethargy	20	Edema	20-25
Excess energy	35	Petechiae	10

From Brownell KD and Foreyt JP, editors: *Handbook of eating disorders: physiology, psychology, and treatment of obesity, anorexia, and bulimia*, New York, 1986, Basic Books.

Ten percent of females are thought to be affected. Most anorexics include excessive strenuous exercise in their daily activities. Many are also involved in school athletic programs (Rees, 1991).

The symptoms and signs associated with anorexia nervosa are listed in Table 4-27. Clinical features of anorexia nervosa include those listed in Table 4-28. Medical complications resulting from anorexia nervosa involve various organ systems (see the box on p. 130). Nutritional assessment involves the following:

1. Anthropometric measurement to assess current physical status
2. Biochemical evaluation for nutrient deficiencies
3. Clinical examination

4. Detailed dietary history, determining
   a. Development of the disorder
   b. Current food consumption—calories, protein, other nutrients
   c. *Patterns* of food intake and eating behavior
   d. Feelings about and preoccupation with food
   e. Psychological and social influences on eating behavior
   f. Use of any drugs, including vitamins, minerals, laxatives, and diuretics
   g. Exercise habits

Treatment of anorexia nervosa is usually long term and requires a team effort. In addition to nutritional assessment data, medical and psychological evaluation and assessment are needed before a treatment plan can be initiated. Treatment plans involve not only the client but the client's family as well.

Early recognition of symptoms is important and can be accomplished through education of those in frequent contact with adolescents such as teachers, coaches, friends, and health personnel. The consequences of long-term self-starvation can be severe.

TABLE 4-28

Clinical Features of Anorexia Nervosa

Feature	Anorexia nervosa
Intense drive for thinness	Marked
Self-imposed starvation	Marked (due to fear of body size)
Disturbance in body image	Present (lack of awareness of change in body size and lack of satisfaction or pleasure in the body)
Appetite	Maintained (but with fear of giving in to impulse)
Satiety	Usually bloating, nausea, early satiety
Avoidance of specific foods	Present (for carbohydrates or foods presumed to be high in "calories")
Bulimia	Present in 30% to 50%
Vomiting	Present (to prevent weight gain)
Laxative abuse	Present (to prevent weight gain)
Activity level	Increased
Amenorrhea	Present

From Garfinkel PE, and others. *Can Med Assoc* 129:940, 1983. Reprinted from, by permission of the publisher, CMAJ Vol. 129, November 1, 1983.

Bulimia Nervosa

Bulimia nervosa is typically characterized by episodes of binge eating, or rapid consumption of large amounts of food within a given time, alternating with episodes of vomiting, use of laxatives or diuretics, strict dieting, or exercise to prevent weight gain. Bulimia nervosa usually begins during adolescence or early adulthood and occurs predominantly in females. The disorder occurs in individuals of normal weight as well as in obese persons and persons with anorexic behavior (Kirkley, 1986). The condition can also occur during pregnancy (Rees, 1992).

Diagnostic criteria for bulimia nervosa are outlined in the box below.

Laboratory and medical complications can be extensive and, as with anorexia nervosa, involve various organ systems (see box in right column).

The bulimic individual may show no outward signs of the disorder. Physical complaints may bring the client in for medical treatment and may include dental erosion, throat irritation, and inflammation of the esophagus.

Bulimic behavior is secretive, and, as with anorexics, denial may exist.

Dietary analysis should detail the following:
1. Weight history
2. Dieting history and behavior
3. History of the bulimic behavior
4. Patterns of bingeing and purging
5. Foods consumed during a binge—"trigger" foods
6. Food likes and dislikes
7. Eating behavior and pattern when not bingeing
8. Feelings regarding food and self
9. Exercise habits

As with anorexia nervosa, a team approach to treatment is essential. Psychological assessment by a qualified professional is critical for treatment to be individualized and successful.

DIAGNOSTIC CRITERIA FOR BULIMIA NERVOSA

1. Recurrent episodes of binge eating (rapid consumption of a large amount of food in a discrete time).
2. A feeling of lack of control over eating behavior during the eating binges.
3. The person regularly engages in either self-induced vomiting, use of laxatives or diuretics, strict dieting or fasting, or vigorous exercise to prevent weight gain.
4. A minimum average of two binge eating episodes a week for at least 3 months.
5. Persistent overconcern with body shape and weight.

From the *Diagnostic and Statistical Manual of Mental Disorders*, ed 3, rev., Washington DC, 1987, American Psychiatric Association. Reprinted with permission.

THE REGISTERED DIETITIAN

The registered dietitian is the health care professional best qualified to work as a member of the health care team in assessing an individual's nutritional needs, planning appropriate nutritional intervention, and educating the individual on a healthy life-style. Registered dietitians can be found in a variety of settings, including hospitals and clinics, community health care, extended care facilities, private practice, business and industry, the armed forces, and educational settings. A client with a suspected or diagnosed nutritional problem or concern can be referred to the registered dietitian for further assessment, counseling, and follow-up regarding the problem or concern. As people strive for high-level wellness, registered dietitians do preventive counseling in the area of health and fitness. National, state, and local dietetic associations exist for the public and act as a resource to the community and other professionals.

LABORATORY ABNORMALITIES AND MEDICAL COMPLICATIONS OF BULIMIA

Renal complications
Dehydration
Hypokalemic nephropathy

Gastrointestinal complications
Gastric dilatation
Sialodenosis
Amylase elevations
Pancreatitis

Electrolyte abnormalities
Hyperuricemia
Hypokalemia
Alkalosis
Acidosis

Laxative abuse complications
Hyperuremia
Hypocalcemia
Tetany
Osteomalacia
Clubbing
Skin pigmentation
Hypomagnesemia
Fluid retention
Malabsorption syndromes
Protein-losing enteropathy
Cathartic colon

Hematologic abnormalities
Bleeding tendency

Neurologic abnormalities
Electroencephalogram abnormalities

Endocrine abnormalities
Blunted thyroid-stimulating hormone response to thyroid-releasing hormone
Pathologic growth hormone response to thyroid-releasing hormone glucose
Prolactin elevations
Dexamethasone suppression test nonsuppression

Dental problems
Caries
Enamel erosion

From Brownell KD and Foreyt JP, editors: *Handbook of eating disorders: physiology, psychology, and treatment of obesity, anorexia, and bulimia*, New York, 1986, Basic Books.

SUMMARY

Assessment of nutritional status is an essential component of health assessment. The parameters of nutritional assessment, including

- *A*nthropometric measurement
- *B*iochemical measurement
- *C*linical examination
- *D*ietary analysis

can be applied to any client, noting particular features that may be of value in assessing a specific condition or disorder. Integration of all these components, along with other health assessment data obtained, is important in evaluating health status accurately and in recommending any treatment or client education.

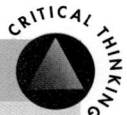

Nursing Diagnosis *THE NEXT STEP*

Nursing diagnoses that could apply to nutritional assessment include, but are not limited to:

ALTERED NUTRITION: HIGH RISK FOR MORE THAN BODY REQUIREMENTS The state in which an individual is at risk of experiencing an intake of nutrients that exceeds metabolic needs.

Defining Characteristics (Risk Factors)

- Hereditary factors
- Excessive intake relative to energy expenditure during late gestational life, early infancy, and adolescence
- Dysfunctional eating patterns (e.g., pairing food with other activities, concentrating food intake at the end of the day, eating in response to external cues such as time of day or social situation, and eating in response to internal cues such as anxiety and depression)
- Sedentary activity level
- Use of food as a reward or comfort measure
- Frequent, closely spaced pregnancies
- Limited financial resources

ALTERED NUTRITION: MORE THAN BODY REQUIREMENTS The state in which an individual is experiencing an intake of nutrients that exceeds metabolic needs.

Defining Characteristics

- Weight 10%-20% over ideal for height and frame
- Triceps skinfold greater than 15 mm in men and 25 mm in women
- Sedentary activity level

Related Factors

- Food intake-energy expenditure imbalance
- Dysfunctional eating patterns

ALTERED NUTRITION: LESS THAN BODY REQUIREMENTS The state in which an individual experiences an intake of nutrients insufficient to meet metabolic needs.

Defining Characteristics

- Weight 20% under ideal body weight
- Weight loss (with or without adequate intake)
- Reported or observed inadequate food intake relative to minimum daily requirements
- Excessive hair loss
- Poor muscle tone
- Pale conjunctiva and mucous membranes
- Fatigue
- Decreased serum albumin
- Capillary fragility

Continued.

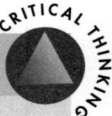

Nursing Diagnosis *THE NEXT STEP—cont'd*

Defining Characteristics—cont'd
- Diarrhea and/or steatorrhea
- Hyperactive bowel sounds; abdominal cramping, pain

Related Factors
- Inability to prepare/procure food
- Knowledge deficit (daily requirements)
- Financial limitations
- Edentulous
- Social isolation
- Anorexia
- Early satiety
- Chemical dependency
- Emotional stress
- Dieting practices
- Muscle weakness (mastication, swallowing)

Clinical Application

Mr. F. is a 42-year-old black male, who has come to the clinic for complaint of intermittent severe headaches, nausea, and dizzy spells. Weight 250 lbs; height 5'll"; oral temperature 98.6° F, pulse 100, respirations 20, blood pressure 180/94. Mr. F. is a bus driver who works the 0600 to 1400 shift in a large metropolitan area. He reports "it's a very stressful job." He sits 8 hours/day and his meals during the day are usually "fast food." When questioned he reports that he does not exercise regularly and relaxes mostly by watching television and playing video games. He has not been to a health care provider in 12 years. He is very concerned about his health at the present time.

SUBJECTIVE DATA: Patient complains of:
Intermittent headaches
Job being very stressful
Job sedentary
Fast food diet
No regular exercise
Hobbies are sedentary activities

OBJECTIVE DATA:
BP 180/94
Pulse 100
Respirations 20
Temperature 98.6° F
Weight 250 lbs
Height 5' 11"
Triceps skin fold 18 mm
Serum lipids 200 mg/dL
Serum cholesterol 250 mg/dL HDL 35 mg/dL LDL 150 mg/dL
(PERRLA)
Neurological checks for strength—hand grips equal and strong; push/pulls equal and strong

NURSING DIAGNOSIS

Altered nutrition: more than body requirements related to food intake energy expenditure imbalance.

Defining Characteristics
- Weight 20% over ideal for height and frame
- Sedentary activity level

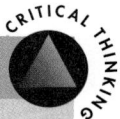

Nursing Diagnosis *THE NEXT STEP—cont'd*

Altered health maintenance related to failure to seek help to maintain health.

Defining Characteristics
- History of lack of health seeking behaviors
- Expression of interest in improving health behaviors

Knowledge deficit related to lack of interest or motivation to learn.

Defining Characteristics
- Inadequate understanding of nutrition
- Inadequate understanding of obesity and its effect on other body systems
- Inadequate knowledge of the relationship between sedentary activity and weight gain.

Activity intolerance related to obesity

Defining Characteristics
- Sedentary life style
- Abnormal response to activity
- Complains of shortness of breath when walking—Level III

GLOSSARY

adipose tissue Composed of fat cells arranged in lobules.

anergy An immunodeficient condition characterized by a lack of or diminished reaction to an antigen or group of antigens.

anorexia nervosa A psychoneurotic disorder characterized by a prolonged refusal to eat, resulting in emaciation, amenorrhea, emotional disturbance concerning body image, and an abnormal fear of becoming obese.

anoxia An abnormal condition characterized by a lack of oxygen.

anthropometry The science of measuring the human body as to height, weight, and size of component parts, including measurement of skinfolds.

body mass index An index for estimating obesity. The weight in kilograms is divided by the height in meters squared.

bulimia nervosa An insatiable craving for food, often resulting in episodes of continuous eating followed by periods of depression and self-deprivation.

cachexia General ill health and malnutrition, marked by weakness and emaciation.

caliper An instrument with two hinged, adjustable, curved legs, used to measure the thickness or the diameter of a convex body or solid.

catabolism A complex, metabolic process in which energy is liberated for use in work, energy storage, or heat production by the destruction of complex substances by living cells to form simple compounds.

glycogen A polysaccharide that is the major carbohydrate stored in animal cells.

high-density lipoprotein (HDL) A plasma protein containing about 50% protein with cholesterol and triglycerides.

hyperglycemia A greater than normal amount of glucose in the blood.

kwashiorkor A malnutrition disease, primarily of children, caused by severe protein deficiency, usually occurring when the child is weaned from the breast.

leukocytosis An abnormal increase in the number of circulating white blood cells.

leukopenia An abnormal decrease in the number of white blood cells to fewer than 5000 cells per cubic millimeter.

low-density lipoprotein (LDL) A plasma protein containing relatively more cholesterol and triglycerides than protein.

malnutrition Any disorder concerning nutrition. It may result from an unbalanced, insufficient, or excessive diet or the impaired absorption, assimilation, or use of foods.

marasmus A condition of extreme malnutrition and emaciation, occurring chiefly in young children, that is characterized by progressive wasting of subcutaneous tissue and muscle.

monounsaturated fat Has only one double or triple bond per molecule and is found in such foods as fowl, almonds, pecans, cashew nuts, and olive oil.

nutrient A substance that provides nourishment and affects the nutritive and metabolic processes of the body.

nutrition The sum of the processes involved in the taking in of nutrients and in their assimilation and use for proper body functioning and maintenance of health.

polycythemia An abnormal increase in the number of erythrocytes in the blood.

polyunsaturated fat Has more than one double or triple bond per molecule and is found in fish, corn, walnuts, sunflower seeds, soybeans, cottonseeds, and safflower oil.

recommended dietary allowance (RDA) The amount of nutrients, particularly vitamins, recommended as a necessary part of one's daily food intake to maintain normal health.

satiety The satisfied feeling of being full after eating.

saturated fat Any number of glyceryl esters of certain organic acids in which all the atoms are joined by single-valence bonds. These fats are chiefly of animal origin.

toxicity A condition that results from exposure to a toxin or to toxic amounts of a substance that does not cause adverse effects in smaller amounts.

triglyceride A compound consisting of a fatty acid (oleic, palmitic, or stearic) and glycerol. Triglycerides make up most animal and vegetable fats.

visceral protein Protein that is contained in the internal organs.

BIBLIOGRAPHY

Ardell DB: *Fourteen days to a wellness lifestyle,* San Rafael, Calif, 1982, Whatever Publishing.

American Dietetic Association: *Handbook of clinical dietetics,* New Haven, Conn, 1981, Yale University Press.

American Heart Association: *About high blood pressure,* Dallas, 1986, American Heart Association.

American Heart Association: *Dietary guidelines for healthy American adults,* Dallas, 1986, American Heart Association.

American Heart Association: *Risk factors and coronary disease: a statement for physicians,* Dallas, 1980, American Heart Association.

The American Institute for Cancer Research: *Dietary guidelines to lower cancer risk,* Washington, DC, 1990, The American Institute for Cancer Research.

Blackburn GL, and others: Nutritional and metabolic assessment of the hospitalized patient, *JPEN* 1:11–22, 1977.

Burton BT, Foster WR: Health implications of obesity: an NIH consensus development conference, *J Am Diet Assoc* 85:1117–1121, 1985.

Butterworth CE Jr: The skeleton in the hospital closet, *Nutrition Today* 9:4–8, 1974.

Chumlea WC, Roche AF, and Mukherjee, D: *Nutritional assessment of the elderly through anthropometry,* Columbus, Ohio, 1987, Ross Laboratories.

Committee on Maternal Nutrition, Food and Nutrition Board, National Research Council, National Academy of Sciences: *Maternal nutrition and the course of pregnancy: summer report,* Bethesda, Md, 1970, Department of Health and Human Services.

Elmer PJ: *Dietary intervention in hypertension: current status, weight and sodium, and new directions,* Iowa City, 1985, Presented at Diet Therapy USA.

Huse DM, Lucas AR: Dietary treatment of anorexia nervosa, *J Am Diet Assoc* 83:687–690, 1983.

Jensen TG, Englert DM, Dudrick SJ: Interpretation of nutritional assessment data, *Nutr Support Serv* 1:14–20, 1981.

Kamath SK, and others: Hospital malnutrition: a 33-hospital screening study. *J Am Diet Assoc* 86:203–206, 1986.

Kaminski MV Jr, Winborn AL: Nutritional assessment guide, Chicago, 1978, Midwest Nutrition, Education, and Research Foundation.

Kirkley BG: Bulimia: clinical characteristics, development, and etiology, *J Am Diet Assoc* 86:468–472, 1986.

National Dairy Council: LIFESTEPS®, Rosemont, Ill, 1985, The Council.

O'Neil FT, Hynak-Hankinson MT, Gorman J: Research and application of current topics in sports nutrition, *J Am Diet Assoc* 86:1007–1012, 1986.

Satter E: *Child of mine—feeding with love and good sense,* Palo Alto, Calif, 1991, Bull Publishing.

National Institutes of Health: *Cholesterol counts,* Bethesda, Md, 1985, Public Health Service, U.S. Department of Health and Human Services.

Williams SR: Nutrition and diet therapy, ed 7, St Louis, 1993, Mosby-Year Book.

ADDITIONAL REFERENCES

American Heart Association: *The American Heart Association diet: an eating plan for healthy Americans,* Dallas, 1991, American Heart Association.

Henneman A, and others: Teaching nutritional assessment to nursing students, *J Am Diet Assoc,* 78:498–500, 1981.

Hirsch S, and others: Nutritional status of surgical patients and the relationship of nutrition to postoperative outcome, *J Am Coll Nutr* 11(1):21–24, 1992.

Institute of Medicine (U.S.) Subcommittee on Nutritional Status and Weight Gain During Pregnancy, Washington, DC, 1990, National Academy of Sciences, National Academy Press.

Jensen M: Research techniques for body composition assessment, *J Am Diet Assoc* 92:454–460, 1992.

Jensen MD, and others: Influence of body fat distribution on free fatty acid metabolism in obesity, *J Clin Invest* 83:1168–1173, 1989.

Jensen T, Dudrick S: Implementation of a multidisciplinary nutritional assessment program, *J Am Diet Assoc* 79:258–266, 1981.

Nutrition Screening Initiative: *Nutrition screening manual for professionals caring for older Americans. A project of Am Academy of Family Physicians, Am Diet Assoc and National Council on the Aging,* 1991, Nutritional Screening Initiative, 2626 Pennsylvania Ave, Washington, DC.

Rees JM: *Nutrition in adolescence.* In Williams SR, Worthington-Roberts, BS, editors: *Nutrition throughout the life cycle,* ed 2, St. Louis, 1992, Mosby–Year Book.

Weinseir RL: *Handbook of clinical nutrition,* ed 2, St. Louis, 1989, Mosby–Year Book.

Williams SR: *Nutrition and diet therapy,* ed 6, St. Louis, 1989, Mosby–Year Book.

Williams SR, Worthington-Roberts B: *Nutrition throughout the life cycle,* ed 3, St. Louis, 1992, Mosby–Year Book.

Windsor JA, Hill GL: Nutritional assessment: a pending renaissance, *Nutrition* 7:377–379, 1991.

Wynder EL, Weisburger JH, Nq SK: Nutrition: the need to define "optimal" intake as a basis for public policy decisions, *Am J Public Health* 82:346–350, 1992.

Zeman F, Ney P: *Applications of clinical nutrition,* Englewood Cliffs, NJ, 1988, Prentice Hall.

Sleep Assessment

PURPOSE OF THE EXAMINATION

Sleep is a basic human need. It has a restorative function, both physically and psychologically. Adequate sleep is essential to a sense of well-being. **Circadian rhythms** are those physiological functions that occur within a period of approximately 24 hours. The sleep-wakefulness pattern is a part of this rhythm. During sleep, the brain goes through a series of stages: stages 1 through 4 of **nonrapid eye movement (nonREM) sleep** and **rapid eye movement sleep (REM)**, which includes dreaming. People who are sleep-deprived usually have less ability to cope with psychological stressors. During illness, the sleep state can be difficult to attain and can be a frustrating accompaniment to the illness.

Shakespeare described sleep as a natural healer when he wrote:

"Sleep that knits up the ravel'd sleave of care,
The death of each day's life, sore labor's bath,
Balm of hurt minds, great nature's second course,
Chief nourisher in life's feast."

—Macbeth, Act II, Scene II
William Shakespeare

137

The purpose of assessing the client's sleep-rest pattern is to incorporate that aspect of the client's daily pattern into your holistic assessment of her or his life, health, and abilities to function and cope. A client's sense of adequate sleep and rest can affect that individual's sense of physical and psychological well-being.

PHYSIOLOGY

Sleep Neurophysiology

We do not yet fully understand the neurophysiology of sleep. We know that certain brain structures are involved, including the suprachiasmatic nuclei of the anterior hypothalamus, the reticular activating system, the cerebral hemispheres, and the sleep-producing areas located in the lower brainstem. Neurotransmitters involved in sleep processes include serotonin, norepinephrine, dopamine, and acetylcholine. Researchers continue to study the exact way in which they influence sleep and wakefulness.

Soon after sleep begins, bone marrow and skin cell division reach a peak. During sleep stages 3 and 4, hormones associated with growth and development are secreted in greater amounts. If the individual is awakened during these sleep stages, growth hormone secretion is interrupted. Strenuous exercise during the day is associated with increased stage 3 and 4 sleep periods. Cerebral blood flow usually increases during REM sleep. This increased blood flow may be necessary to meet internal metabolic demands, which may be higher in children, who usually spend a proportionately longer time in rapid eye movement sleep. During REM sleep, increased protein synthesis occurs. Rapid eye movement sleep is associated with memory storage and learning.

Categories, Stages, and Cycles of Sleep

Categories of sleep. As mentioned, sleep is divided into two major categories:
- nonrapid eye movement (nonREM) sleep, which consists of 4 stages
- rapid eye movement (REM) sleep during which dreaming occurs

The brain is active and produces electrical patterns during wakefulness and sleep. These electrical patterns can be traced by electroencephalogram (EEG) recordings. Other monitoring devices that are used to differentiate stages of sleep and wakefulness include the electro-oculogram (EOG), which records eye movements, and the electromyelogram (EMG), which monitors muscle tone and activity.

Stages of sleep. Wakefulness is characterized by rapid eye movements and high muscle tone. People are awake when they are alert and aware of their surroundings.

Stage 1 nonREM sleep. Stage 1 occurs as a person falls asleep. It is the transition between wakefulness and sleep and may last only 5 minutes. There is a sensation of drowsiness, drifting, or relaxation. A person may be easily awakened from stage 1 sleep by noise or other stimuli and may state that he or she has not yet fallen asleep. This stage is characterized by:
- absence of rapid eye movements (the eyes roll slowly from side to side)
- decreasing heart and respiratory rates, relatively high muscle tone, and jerks or sudden twitching in the face or extremities

Stage 2 nonREM sleep. Stage 2 lasts from 10 to 15 minutes and is a deeper sleep state. Awakening a person from this stage is more difficult. There is little eye movement, and body temperature and metabolic rates decrease somewhat.

Stage 3 nonREM sleep. Stage 3 is deeper and more restful sleep. It is dominated by parasympathetic nervous system activity with decreased blood pressure, and lowered heart and respiratory rates. Awakening the person is difficult.

Stage 4 nonREM sleep. Stage 4 sleep is the deepest sleep, and awakening the person during this stage is difficult. The sleeper enters it anywhere from 15 to 30 minutes after he or she falls asleep. The eyes remain still. Muscle tone is relaxed, respiratory rate, heart rate, and blood pressure are lowered. Restorative physiological processes occur during stage 4, including increased protein synthesis and secretion of growth hormone. Sleep quality is often judged by the amount of time spent in stage 4 sleep. People who report that they have not slept well, although the actual time spent sleeping may have been adequate, may not have obtained sufficient stage 4 sleep.

REM sleep. REM sleep differs from nonREM sleep in that it is a relatively active sleep state. It shows bursts of increased sympathetic nervous system activity. This activity is exhibited by muscle twitches and variability in pulse, blood pressure, and respiratory rates. Gastric secretion may increase, and steroid hormones are released. Penile erections may occur in males of all ages during this stage. Paradoxically, during this stage the muscles are relaxed, and deep tendon reflexes are reduced. Thus, during REM sleep, some characteristics associated with wakefulness and others associated with deep sleep are present. Episodic bursts of rapid eye movements associated with dreaming are present.

These movements are visible even though the person's eyes are closed. REM sleep varies in duration. People who do not have adequate REM sleep also feel they have had too little sleep.

Sleep cycles. The sleep stages occur in a cyclical fashion. During an average 8-hour sleep period, an individual may experience four to six sleep cycles. An average cycle is 90 minutes long, and each cycle has varying amounts of REM and nonREM sleep. For example, during early sleep, nonREM sleep is longer, lasting from 70 to 100 minutes, and REM sleep is shorter. During a later part of the sleep period, REM sleep lengthens. The normal sequence varies with age, environment, and the effect of daily activities.

The first sleep cycle generally follows the most orderly progression through each of the sleep stages. The stages proceed 1 through 4 and then on to REM sleep. During a subsequent cycle, stage 1 may be absent, and the stages may proceed in a different order, such as stage 4 to stage 2 to REM sleep. At all ages, stage 2 accounts for 50% or more of total sleep time, and REM sleep usually arises from stage 2. The number of REM periods varies between four and six nightly, accounting for about 20% to 25% of the total sleep time. During a sleep cycle, the length of each stage can be influenced by physical and mental states and by medication. As an individual ages, there is a gradual decrease in stages 3 and 4 of sleep. The elderly have little or no stage 4 sleep. During REM sleep, there is general relaxation of skeletal muscles, including pharyngeal muscles. This may play a role in the development of upper airway obstruction during sleep.

As people age, the sleep cycle changes (Figure 5-1). The newborn spends 50% of sleep time in REM sleep, and the sleep cycles are 45 to 60 minutes long. Total sleep time for the newborn is 14 to 18 hours a day. By age 1, REM sleep is only 20% to 30%. Stage 4 sleep is greater in duration during childhood, As the child matures, the sleep cycle increases in length and the total sleep time decreases. Sleep patterns of 8 to 10 hours develop during childhood. Many adolescents go through stages of needing increased amounts of sleep. Most healthy adults spend 7 to 9 hours sleeping each day, although many require less than 6 hours or more than 9 hours of sleep. Of this time, about 25% of sleep is in REM sleep, 50% in stage 2 sleep, and 5% to 10% in stage 1 sleep. The remaining 15% to 20% is a combination of stage 3 and 4. Older adults have a decrease in total sleep time and in stage 4 sleep. The elderly may experience more frequent awakenings during the night; some need to compensate for this with rest periods during the day. Some elderly clients view their pattern of diminished sleep with frustration, while others accept it as an opportunity to have more time for other activities.

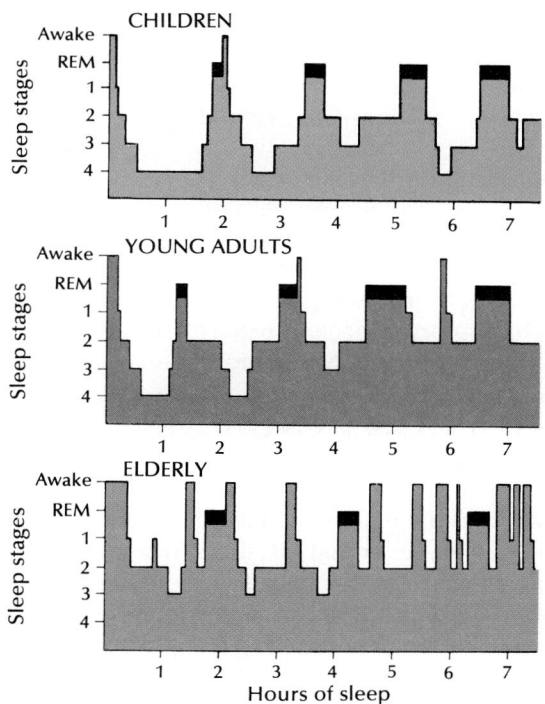

FIGURE 5-1 Sleep cycles of normal subjects. The sleep of children and young adults shows early preponderance of stages 3 and 4, progressive lengthening of the first three REM periods, and infrequent awakenings. In elderly adults there is little or no stage 4 sleep, REM periods are fairly uniform in length, and awakenings are frequent and often lengthy. (From Kales A, et al: *Ann Intern Med* 68:1078, 1968.)

EXAMINATION

Health History

Find out how the client perceives the effectiveness of sleep and relaxation. Most people take sleep for granted until they have a problem with it. Use open-ended questions to elicit descriptions in the client's own words. Assess effectiveness of waking and sleeping patterns from the client's perspective. If possible, obtain some sleep history, such as information on snoring or apneic periods, from the client's bed partner.

Client's usual or desired waking and sleep-rest pattern. This describes the client's pattern of activities, sleep, rest, and relaxation in a 24-hour period. Request the following information:
- Typical daytime activities, including any naps
- Usual bedtime activities or rituals, including all efforts to enhance sleep

—reading
—beverage
—music
—restful position
—other environmental aids
—medications, prescription and nonprescription
- Change(s) in sleep pattern
  —Difficulty falling asleep, staying asleep, or awakening too early
  —Time it takes client to fall asleep
  —When client awakens during sleep period
  —Time when client awakens at end of sleep cycle
  —Duration of change in pattern
  —What client thinks prevents sleep or causes the awakenings
- The sleep environment
  —sleeping arrangement
  —comfort level
  —noise
  —light
  —temperature
- Feelings at time of awakening
  —rested, refreshed, ready for the day
  —fatigued, anxious
- Effects of inadequate sleep on the individual
  —fatigue
  —irritability
  —inability to think and/or speak clearly
  —inability to stay awake during the day
  —excessive napping during the day
  —decreased attention span
  —memory changes
- Pertinent psychological influences
  —current life situation, including situations for which sleep is providing escape, relief
  —relationships
  —role of work
  —sense of meaning, purpose in life
  —coping skills, ability to deal with stress, anxiety, unresolved feelings
- Pertinent physiological factors
  —pain
  —nocturia
  —shortness of breath
- Personal beliefs about the value of sleep, rest, dreams

Information from bed partner

- snoring
- apneic periods
- restless movements during sleep period

Family sleep-rest pattern

- family beliefs and practices regarding sleep and rest
- general family pattern

- sufficient space and quiet
- family relaxation habits

Technique for Examination and Normal Findings

Use the technique of observation to help assess the sleep/rest status of the client. Physical findings are grossly normal in most clients.
- Observe:
  —client's mental alertness status, thought patterns, speech patterns, facial appearance, gross motor movements, and posture
- Measure:
  —blood pressure
  —body weight
- Inspect:
  —nose: nasal septum may be deviated
  —neck: clients with sleep apnea syndrome may have a short, thick neck
  —throat: look for narrow pharyngeal space; bulky, elevated base of the tongue; and a long or edematous uvula; tonsils and adenoids may be enlarged

Screening Tests and Procedures

With a suspected sleep disorder, an EEG may be appropriate. A more comprehensive study is **polysomnography,** which is an overnight sleep study. This study includes:
  —observation of sleep stages
  —EEG (electroencephalogram)
  —EOG (electrooculogram)
  —EMG (electromyelogram)
  —ECG (electrocardiogram)
  —Respiratory effort and pattern analysis
  —Arterial hemoglobin saturation analysis

VARIATIONS FROM HEALTH

Insomnia

Insomnia is the inability to fall asleep or to stay asleep for an adequate period of time. Insomnia may be chronic or may last for only a brief period in an individual's life. It can result from a variety of causes. Insomnia may be due to the sleep interruptions involving the needs of a newborn child. Stressful situations caused by loss, grief, or unresolved emotional pain, and environmental factors, such as uncomfortable temperatures or a change in work schedule, may contribute to insomnia. The noise level in a hospital, and the need to awaken patients for treatments or medications may cause insomnia. Drugs such as amphetamines or caffeine, which remain active in the bloodstream for up to 12 hours, may also cause insomnia. Some people who believe they have insomnia may actually be sleeping, but do not feel rested or refreshed by their sleep. Insomnia may be a symptom of depression.

Insomnia may occur during any part of the sleep cycle: early, midway, or late. Most people fall asleep within 5 to 15 minutes of the time they lie down to go to sleep. People with initial insomnia need 30 or more minutes to fall asleep. This is the most common sleep disorder in young adults. Autonomic nervous system activity is higher in these clients; stress and anxiety also play a role.

Intermittent insomnia is the most common form of insomnia in all age groups. It occurs when sleep is interrupted midcycle. The person may or may not be aware of a sleep pattern disturbance if she or he falls asleep easily again. Factors causing intermittent insomnia may be environmental, such as a baby crying. They may be physiological, such as pain or the need to void. Or it may be an aspect of the sleep state itself, such as nightmares. Some people return to sleep if they stay in bed; others find getting up for a while to engage in some activity helps them return to sleep more easily.

Insomnia that occurs toward the end of the sleep cycle becomes more common as people age. This type of insomnia is characterized by early awakenings with an inability to return to sleep. The person may report final awakening as early as 3 or 4 AM. End cycle insomnia may be associated with daytime napping or an early bedtime. It may also be an important sign of depression or other change in emotional state.

The finding of insomnia indicates a need to carefully assess the overall sleep pattern, current life stresses, coping abilities, and self-concept. Individuals experiencing insomnia may interpret it very differently: some find it upsetting while others see it as extra time to accomplish their goals.

Sleep Apnea Syndrome (SAS)

Apnea is the temporary cessation of airflow at the level of the nostrils and mouth for at least 10 seconds.

Apnea occurring during sleep may be categorized as:
1. Obstructive sleep apnea (OSA)
2. Central sleep apnea (CSA)
3. Mixed sleep apnea

Obstructive sleep apnea (OSA) is the most common form of **sleep apnea,** accounting for about 95% of sleep apneas. OSA is caused by a physical blockage to the flow of air. It results when the flow of air is obstructed as the soft palate and the tongue move backward against the posterior pharyngeal wall and partially or completely obstruct the pharynx.

Obesity is a risk factor, especially if the neck is short and thick. However, persons of normal weight with normal neck features can also have OSA. Enlarged tonsils, a large tongue, or a narrowed pharyngeal passageway can be causative factors.

In OSA, the neural stimulus is present, so a persistent effort to breathe continues even during the occlusive phase of the cycle. Thus, an observer can see thoracic and abdominal movements.

The individual with obstructive sleep apnea exhibits a cyclical breathing pattern in which periods of apnea alternate with arousal and breathing. Sometime after the individual falls asleep, a loss of upper airway muscle tone occurs, creating an airway occlusion. The apneic period ranges from 20 to 120 seconds and results in hypoxemia, which stimulates the respiratory drive. The person arouses to a lighter stage of sleep or may awaken, and the upper airway muscles are activated, resulting in the return of airflow. The individual returns to sleep and the cycle starts again. The duration of the apneic periods and the degree of hypoxemia increase gradually as the disease progresses, resulting in a higher degree of hypoxemia necessary to stimulate arousal. The increasing stimulus necessary to create arousal may also be a result of the fragmented sleep caused by the disease process.

Central sleep apnea (CSA) is the least common form of SAS. It is characterized by cessation of airflow caused by decreased respiratory center output. The neural signal to breathe is interrupted, so that both respiratory effort and airflow are absent. The absence of rib cage and abdominal movement is characteristic. Individuals with central sleep apnea syndrome are usually of normal weight or underweight. Their reported difficulty tends to be disrupted sleep rather than excessive daytime sleepiness. Clients with CSA generally fall asleep easily and rapidly but subsequently wake up several times during the night with a choking sensation.

Mixed sleep apnea occurs when a person experiences both disorders. It starts as central apnea and is followed by upper airway obstruction. Mixed apneas are less common than obstructive apnea but more frequent than central apnea.

Persons with SAS may experience several to hundreds of apneic periods each night, with each period lasting from 10 seconds to 2 minutes. Sleep disruption and sleep deprivation result. Men over age 50 are most frequently affected.

Characteristics of sleep apnea syndrome. The primary symptoms of sleep apnea are nighttime snoring and daytime sleepiness, often referred to as nocturnal snoring and daytime **hypersomnolence.** Other symptoms include abnormal physical movements during sleep, morning headache, hallucinations, personality changes, deterioration of intellectual capacity, sexual problems, and altered cardiac function.

Nocturnal snoring. The family or sleeping partner may be a better source of information than the client, as the client may not be aware of alterations that occur during the sleep period. The family or partner may report the following about the individual's snoring and other sleep period symptoms:

- snores loudly and sometimes irregularly
- has multiple apneic periods while sleeping, each lasting more than 10 seconds
- may or may not make respiratory efforts during the apneic period
- awakens or partially awakens coughing and/or choking on secretions in the throat
- makes grunting or gurgling noises during sleep
- flails about in bed

The incidence of these events increases if the individual consumes alcohol, takes a depressant drug, or has a change in his or her sleeping pattern.

Daytime hypersomnolence. This is often the symptom that makes an individual seek help, because it interferes with his or her life-style. The person experiences excessive drowsiness and a strong urge to sleep at various and often inappropriate times during the day. The client may be resisting the urge to sleep, or may be taking short naps, though they are often not restful and may be accompanied by headaches and a sense of fogginess or confusion. These changes may lead to difficulty with work and relationships. These difficulties may lead to depression or other emotional changes. Excessive daytime sleepiness can lead to serious accidents if the individual is operating a car or other machinery. The life of the client and of others in the environment may be endangered.

Abnormal physical movements. Abnormal movements during sleep are usually reported by the sleeping partner or show up on polysomnographic tests. Agitation is evidenced by movement of the extremities or of the whole body. These movements, in addition to the snoring, may be so disruptive to the bed partner that she or he will sleep in a different bed or different room. Other abnormal sleep behaviors may include sleeptalking and sleepwalking. The person may suddenly sit upright in bed gasping for breath. These movements may or may not awaken the client.

Morning headache. Recurrent morning headache is a complaint of many clients with sleep apnea syndrome. The headache is usually frontal but is occasionally diffuse. It usually diminishes several hours after the patient awakens, but may recur if there are episodes of sleep during the day. The headache may be accompanied by some confusion.

Hallucinations. Hallucinatory images may appear during the waking state when the urge to sleep arises.

Though they usually persist for only a short time, the individual may react to the image before recognizing its hallucinatory nature. For example, if the client visualizes a tree while driving, he or she may swerve or brake to avoid hitting it. Obviously, hallucinatory images pose a threat to the safety of the client and others.

Personality changes. Irritability is an early personality change reported by persons with SAS. Other changes can develop such as paranoia, confusion, depression, aggressiveness, jealousy, suspicion, and hostility. Emotional and/or psychological assessment is appropriate.

Deterioration of intellectual capacity. Diminished intellectual function, decreased memory retention, poor judgment, and difficulty concentrating may seriously affect job performance and personal life activities.

Sexual problems. Many clients with sleep apnea report a progressive decrease in sexual drive and, for men, difficulty in obtaining erection and ejaculation.

Altered cardiac function. During the apneic period, the client experiences hypoxemia (decreased Pao_2), hypercapnia (increased $Paco_2$), and acidosis. The hypoxemia may lead to serious cardiac dysrhythmias. Clients with sleep apnea, as a rule, have normal sinus rhythm while awake, but during sleep the EKG shows progressive sinus bradycardia during apnea and sinus acceleration when breathing resumes. Electrocardiographic abnormalities may include left anterior hemiblock, ST-T wave abnormalities, marked sinus arrhythmias, sinus bradycardia, asystole, second-degree AV block, atrial tachycardia, atrial fibrillation, premature ventricular contractions, and ventricular tachycardia. The asphyxia experienced by the individual may result in pulmonary and systemic vasoconstriction. The vasoconstriction may lead to pulmonary hypertension, right-sided heart failure, and systemic hypertension.

Narcolepsy

Narcolepsy is a disorder of excessive sleep. It is characterized by the following:

- Sudden, irresistable attacks of sleep during the day, which may last anywhere from a few minutes to several hours
- **Cataplexy**—a sudden loss of motor tone that may lead to falls or other accidents because the person cannot move or speak
- Sleep paralysis of the skeletal muscles, which occurs during the transition from wakefulness to stage 1
- Nightmares, usually as the person falls asleep

Involuntary daytime sleep attacks may begin in adolescence or young adulthood. People with this problem may have symptoms for years before the disorder is diagnosed. Not all persons with the disorder experience all four symptoms.

Parasomnias

Parasomnias are other events that occur during sleep.

Somnambulism (sleepwalking) occurs most often in children; boys are affected more often than girls. Sleepwalking occurs most often in the first third of the sleep period during stage 3 or 4 nonREM sleep. The episode lasts from several minutes to a half hour. The person usually cannot remember the sleepwalking episode. It is more likely to occur if the individual is fatigued or under stress or has taken a sedative or hypnotic medication at bedtime. Other predisposing factors include seizure disorders, central nervous system infections, and trauma.

Sleep terror disorder, or night terrors, most often affect children and are more common in boys than in girls. After a few hours of sleep, the child bolts up in bed, may or may not awaken, shakes, screams, and appears terrified. There is intense anxiety, confusion, agitation, disorientation, and unresponsiveness. Children usually do not remember these episodes. Night terrors occur predominantly in stages 3 and 4 of nonREM sleep. The episodes are extremely variable in frequency. They are more likely to occur if the individual is fatigued, is under stress, or has been given a tricyclic antidepressant at bedtime.

Nocturnal enuresis (bed-wetting) is primarily a childhood disorder, occurring more frequently in boys. It may be either primary or secondary. Primary enuresis may persist from birth to age 6 or older. In secondary enuresis, bed-wetting occurs because of psychological factors. Urination usually occurs just before entering REM sleep. The child may wake up due to the wet clothing and bed linens. When assessing enuresis, the practitioner should interview both the parent(s) and the child.

Bruxism (teeth grinding) during sleep may be a symptom of tension and may cause the teeth to become chipped. The individual with bruxism may not be aware of it, but it can be quite irritating to the bed partner. It usually occurs during stage 2 nonREM sleep.

DOCUMENTATION

Sample Documentation

56-year-old male reports disrupted sleep during past 10 years. He is able to fall asleep fairly easily, but wakes up repeatedly during the night, often because of phone calls due to his occupation; but he sometimes wakes up for no apparent reason. Once awake, he may or may not fall asleep again right away. Also, he occasionally wakes up at 4 or 5 AM and is not able to fall asleep again. He has noticed increased daytime sleepiness, with strong urges to "just get away and take a nap," though this is not interfering with his work. His spouse states that she has noted an increase in episodes of apnea during sleep over the past 5 to 6 months. She reports that he stops breathing for 10 to 30 seconds several times during the night, and after several such periods will wake up coughing. He snores occasionally. These symptoms are causing her to lose sleep.

Examination:
Appears healthy, not overweight
Height: 6'
Weight: 175 lb.
Neck: normal size, not short or thick
ENT: nasal septum deviated to right; tonsils not enlarged; tongue normal size, tongue strength good

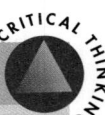

Nursing diagnoses that could apply to alterations in the client's sleep pattern include, but are not limited to, the following:

SLEEP PATTERN DISTURBANCE Disruption of sleep time causes discomfort or interferes with desired life-style.

Defining Characteristics

- Verbal complaints of difficulty falling asleep (sleep onset)
- Early awakening
- Interrupted sleep
- Sleep pattern reversal
- Reduction in performance (work, school, home)
- Increasing irritability
- Restlessness
- Disorientation (progressive)
- Lethargy
- Listlessness
- Mild, fleeting nystagmus
- Slight hand tremor
- Ptosis of eyelids
- Expressionless face
- Thick speech with mispronunciation and incorrect words
- Dark circles under eyes
- Frequent yawning
- Changes in posture
- Fatigue upon awakening or during the day
- Frequent dozing
- Light-headedness

Related Factors

- Physical discomfort (specify)
- Personal stress
- Family stress
- Environmental or habit changes
- Daytime boredom, inactivity
- Fear (specify)

FATIGUE An overwhelming sense of exhaustion and decreased capacity for physical and mental work regardless of adequate sleep.

Defining Characteristics

- Verbalization of an unremitting and overwhelming lack of energy
- Inability to maintain usual routines
- Perceived need for additional energy to accomplish routine tasks
- Increase in physical complaints
- Emotionally labile or irritable
- Impaired ability to concentrate: lethargic or listless
- Decreased performance; accident-prone
- Disinterest in surroundings/introspection
- Decreased libido
- Heart palpitations
- Poor memory
- Decreased appetite

Related Factors

- Overwhelming psychological/emotional demands
- Increased energy requirements to perform activities of daily living

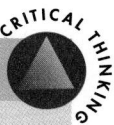

Related Factors—cont'd

- Excessive social and/or role demands
- Discomfort
- Altered body chemistry (for example, medications, drug withdrawal, chemotherapy); decreased/increased metabolic energy production

ANTICIPATORY GRIEVING The state in which an individual grieves before an actual loss.

Defining Characteristics

- Potential loss of significant object
- Verbal expression of distress at potential (anticipated) loss
- Anger
- Sadness, sorrow, crying
- Crying at frequent intervals, choked feeling
- Alteration in sleep or dream patterns
- Alteration in activity level
- Altered libido
- Idealization of anticipated loss
- Alteration in concentration or pursuit of tasks
- Verbalized feeling of numbness

Related Factors

- Expected loss/change (specify)

DYSFUNCTIONAL GRIEVING The state in which actual or perceived object loss (object loss is used in the broadest sense) exists. Objects include people, possessions, a job, status, home, ideals, parts and processes of the body, etc.

Defining Characteristics

- Verbal expression of distress at loss or denial of loss
- Anger
- Sadness
- Crying
- Difficulty in expressing meaning of loss
- Alterations in eating habits
- Alterations of sleep or dream pattern
- Alteration in activity level, work, or socialization
- Altered libido
- Reliving past experiences
- Labile affect
- Alteration in concentration and/or pursuits of tasks
- Continued indicators of grieving beyond expected time for cultural group

Related Factors

- Loss of perceived loss/change (specify)
- Unavailable support systems

INEFFECTIVE INDIVIDUAL COPING Impairment of adaptive behaviors and problem-solving abilities of a person in meeting life's demands and roles.

Defining Characteristics

- Verbalization of inability to cope
- Inability to ask for help
- Anxiety, fear, anger, irritability, tension
- Presence of life stress
- Inability to meet role expectations

Continued.

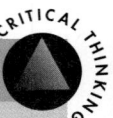

Nursing Diagnosis   *THE NEXT STEP—cont'd*

Defining Characteristics—cont'd

- Inability to meet basic needs
- Destructive behavior toward self and others
- High rate of accidents
- Verbal manipulation
- Excess food intake, alcohol consumption; smoking
- Digestive, bowel, appetite disturbance; chronic fatigue or sleep pattern disturbance

Related Factors

- Situational crises (specify type)
- Maturational crises (specify type)
- Personal vulnerability
- Knowledge deficit (specify)
- Problem-solving skills deficit

Clinical Application

Mrs. K. is a 34-year-old R.N. who has worked the night shift for the past 7 years. She has been admitted to the hospital and had an appendectomy. She has frequently been observed walking in the hallways at night, yawning, and taking frequent short naps during the day. Her meal trays are not touched, and she complains of no appetite and feeling nauseated off and on. She states, "I feel tired all the time. Look at me! I have circles under my eyes. I walk around half asleep day and night and I can't relax or sleep here."

SUBJECTIVE DATA:
Daytime and nighttime fatigue.
Dark circles under eyes.
Cannot sleep or relax in the hospital.
Nauseated off and on.

OBJECTIVE DATA:
Yawning.
Frequent short naps during the day.
Walking the halls at night.
No appetite—does not eat from tray.
Dark circles under eyes.

NURSING DIAGNOSES

Sleep pattern disturbance related to environmental and habit changes.

Defining Characteristics

- Sleep pattern reversal
- Verbal complaints of not feeling rested
- Restlessness
- Dark circles under eyes
- Expressionless face
- Frequent yawning
- Changes in posture
- Fatigue upon awakening or during the day
- Frequent dozing.

Fatigue related to altered body chemistry (circadian rhythm change).

Defining Characteristics

- Verbalization of an unremitting and overwhelming lack of energy
- Inability to maintain usual routine

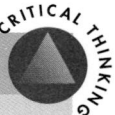

Nursing Diagnosis *THE NEXT STEP—cont'd*

Defining Characteristics—cont'd
- Disinterest in surrounding and introspection
- Decreased appetite

Ineffective individual coping related to situational crises (emergency hospitalization).

Defining Characteristics
- Verbalization of inability to cope
- Presence of life stress
- Appetite disturbance
- Sleep pattern disturbance

GLOSSARY

apnea Cessation of airflow lasting 10 seconds or longer

bruxism The compulsive, unconscious grinding of the teeth, especially during sleep

cataplexy A condition characterized by sudden muscular weakness and hypotonia, caused by emotions, as anger, fear, or surprise; often associated with narcolepsy

central sleep apnea A form of sleep apnea resulting from a decreased respiratory center output. Characterized by cessation of both airflow and respiratory movements

circadian rhythm A cyclical pattern based on a 24-hour cycle, especially the repetition of certain physiological phenomena, such as sleeping and waking

hypersomnia 1. sleep of excessive depth or abnormal duration. 2. extreme drowsiness, often associated with lethargy. 3. a condition characterized by periods of deep, long sleep

insomnia Chronic inability to sleep or to remain asleep throughout the night: wakefulness; sleeplessness

mixed sleep apnea A condition marked by signs and symptoms of both central sleep apnea and obstructive sleep apnea

narcolepsy A syndrome characterized by sudden sleep attacks, cataplexy, sleep paralysis, and visual or auditory hallucination at the onset of sleep

nocturnal enuresis Urinary voiding during sleep

obstructive sleep apnea A form of sleep apnea involving a physical obstruction of the upper airway

polysomnography A multicomponent sleep study that monitors arterial oxygen saturation, brain waves (electroencephalogram—EEG), eye movements (electrooculogram—EOG), muscle tone and movements (electromyelogram—EMG), intraesophageal pressure, inspiratory flow, and rib cage and abdominal circumference changes. The length of time slept, the total number of apneic periods, the number of apneic periods per hour, the percentage of apneic time, the mean duration of apneas, and the cumulative Sao_2 are calculated for each individual

REM sleep Rapid eye movement sleep characterized by episodic bursts of rapid eye movements on the electrooculogram and by low-voltage, high-frequency waves on the electroencephalogram

sleep A state marked by reduced consciousness, diminished activity of the skeletal muscles, and depressed metabolism. People normally experience sleep in patterns that follow four observable, progressive stages

sleep apnea Periodic cessation of breathing during sleep

sleep apnea syndrome (SAS) A sleep disorder characterized by multiple episodes of cessation of breathing during sleep

sleep terror disorder A condition occurring during stages 3 or 4 of nonrapid eye movement (nonREM) sleep that is characterized by repeated episodes of abrupt awakening, usually with a panicky scream, accompanied by intense anxiety, confusion, agitation, disorientation, unresponsiveness, marked motor movements, and amnesia concerning the event

somnambulism Sleepwalking; a condition occurring during stages 3 or 4 of nonrapid eye movement (nonREM) sleep that is characterized by complex motor activity, usually culminating in leaving the bed and walking about, with no recall of the episode on awakening

BIBLIOGRAPHY

Feinsilver SH: Recognizing and treating the sleep apnea syndromes, *Emergency Medicine* 19(11):147-159, 1987.

Fletcher EC, and others: Undiagnosed sleep apnea in patients with essential hypertension, *Annals of Internal Medicine* 103:190-195, 1985.

Goothe B: Recognizing sleep apnea syndrome, *Respiratory Management* 17(1):27-30, 1987.

Gordon M: *Manual of nursing diagnosis, 1991-1992,* St. Louis, 1991, Mosby—Year Book.

Jaquis J: Obstructive sleep apnea syndrome, *Nurse Pract* 12(6):50-56, 1987.

Mishoe SC: The diagnosis and treatment of sleep apnea syndrome, *Respiratory Care* 32(3):183-201, 1987.

Riley TL, editor: *Clinical aspects of sleep and sleep disturbance,* Boston, 1985, Butterworth Publishers.

Cultural Considerations in Health Assessment

The information in this book enables nurses to perform a comprehensive assessment for virtually all clients whom they are likely to encounter. In addition to a comprehensive approach to the physical examination, this book presents special considerations and techniques appropriate for clients of all age groups and some frequently encountered special populations. Along the way, the text emphasizes documentation of the client's health history, psychosocial issues related to systems and groups, and an awareness of the family and environmental considerations affecting both health and illness. That is the meaning of holistic health assessment, an approach that is a predominant focus of nursing. A truly holistic assessment, however, cannot ignore the critical cultural considerations that are an essential dimension of every client.

The first section of this chapter presents the rationale for cultural considerations as part of the health assessment. Then terms related to culture are briefly defined. Emphasis is then placed on certain broad variables likely to be encountered when performing health assessments on members of various cultural groups. Finally, specific characteristics of the prevalent cultural groups in North America that may influence health care needs are reviewed.

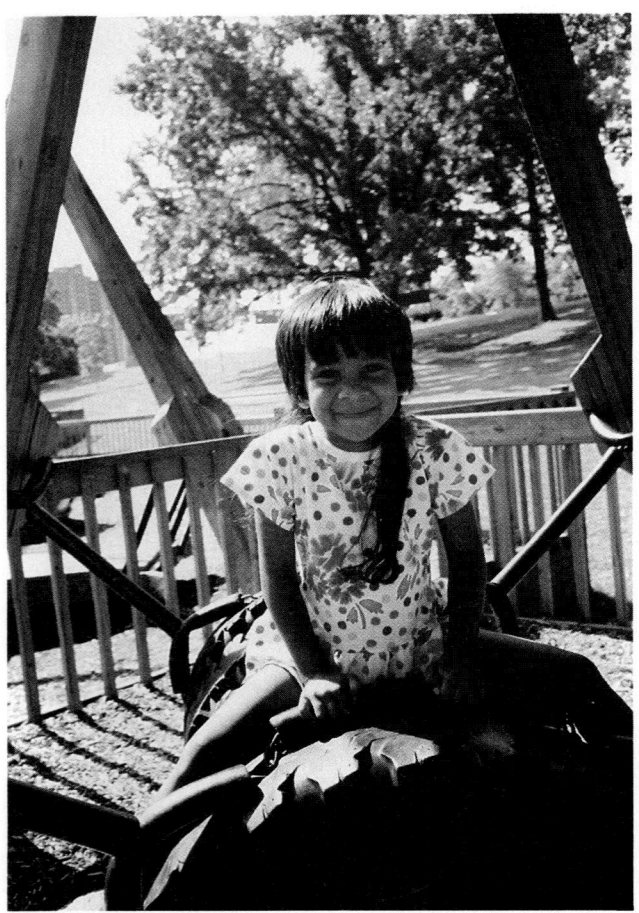

NURSING AND CULTURE

Cultural beliefs and personal characteristics determine health behavior in individuals and families. More than half of all health problems are the result of behavior and life-style. If nursing's goal is to promote health while respecting individual value systems and life-styles, culture-based health behavior must be understood.

Nurses as a group reflect society's cultural mix. In North America, the majority of nurses hold values, beliefs, and attitudes typical of the dominant middle class. In addition, nurses belong to a separate culture as members of the health care team. When two people of differing cultural backgrounds interact, significant communication barriers may arise unless at least one of the persons is willing and able to recognize and adapt to the other's values. To care for others, nurses must be able to accept a wide diversity of beliefs, practices, and ideas about health and illness, including many that differ from their own.

Acceptance of alternate beliefs about health and illness can be more difficult for nurses than might be initially assumed. As health care professionals educated in and exposed to the established health care system, nurses share certain values, attitudes, and beliefs about health and illness that they may not consciously think about. These ways of thinking have been shaped by more than 2000 years of Western thought broadly known as Hippocratic medicine. Modern health care is based on rational, scientific, biomedical principles directed toward solving human health problems. As part of the dominant culture, the health care culture is interwoven with established social, religious, political, and economic systems. Certain aspects of the health care culture, such as nurse-physician relationships and provider-patient relationships, are governed by a broadly shared set of customs and protocols.

The cultural beliefs of some clients may conflict with the cultural beliefs many nurses share. Nurses cannot hope to plan meaningful health care for their clients without at least understanding their health beliefs. That is why performing a sensitive cultural assessment is necessary. A thorough assessment of the cultural aspects of a client's life-style, health beliefs, and health practices enhances decision making and clinical judgment during care.

TERMINOLOGY ASSOCIATED WITH CULTURAL CONSIDERATIONS

Culture is a complex, integrated system that includes knowledge, beliefs, skills, art, morals, law, customs, and any other *acquired* habits and capabilities of a group of people. Culture is characterized by being learned, shared with others, and adapted to the environment. It is stable but subject to and capable of change. As a learned set of traits, culture is transmitted from one generation to the next by both formal education and imitation.

Subculture is a group of persons within a culture with one or more shared traits. These include age, socioeconomic status, race, ethnic origin, education, and occupation. Literally thousands of subcultures exist within a culture, and everyone is a member of several. Although subcultures have an identity uniquely their own, they are also related to the overall culture in certain ways. Major subcultural groups in the United States include African Americans (12.1%), Hispanic Americans (9%), Asian Americans (2.9%), and Native Americans (0.8%). In Canada, major subcultures include French Canadians (27%) and Natives (2%).

Race refers to the classification of human beings on the basis of physical characteristics such as skin pigmentation, head form, or stature that are transmitted through generations. The recognized races are Caucasian, Negroid, and Mongoloid.

Ethnic groups share traits such as a common national or regional origin and linguistic, ancestral, and physical characteristics. Within the major North American subcultures, distinct ethnic groups include African, Haitian, or Dominican (Black); Mexican, Cuban, or Puerto Rican (Hispanic); Japanese, Chinese, Filipino, Korean, Vietnamese, Guamian, or Samoan (Asian); many European ethnic subcultures (German, Italian, Polish, Slavic, Scandinavian, Swiss, French, Dutch,

Russian, English, Irish, Scottish); and Native American and Alaska Native subcultures.

Minority group is a frequently misunderstood term. More normative than descriptive, it refers to any group that receives different and unequal treatment from others in the larger group or society and whose members see themselves as victims of discrimination. This concept is important for caregivers to understand, since many people in our society are discriminated against, and discrimination takes place in the health care system. However, an individual's membership in a minority group is not necessarily related to the individual's cultural affiliations, and this distinction has an important bearing on cultural assessment.

Customs refer to the learned behaviors shared by and associated with a particular cultural group. They include dietary practices, communication patterns, family and kinship relations, religious practices, and health behaviors.

Rituals are highly structured patterns of behavior characteristic of cultural groups. They are prescribed ways to define basic human activities within a cultural context. Rituals may govern a group's approach to communication, traditions, taboos, religion, healing and care for the sick, trade, means of travel, sexual activities, or recreation.

Values and norms are judgments that cultural groups apply to behavior. Values are universal to all cultures and define the desirable or undesirable state of affairs within a culture. Norms provide direction for applying values and are the rules that govern human behavior. Cultural norms set limits. Members of a culture are rewarded or punished as they conform or de-

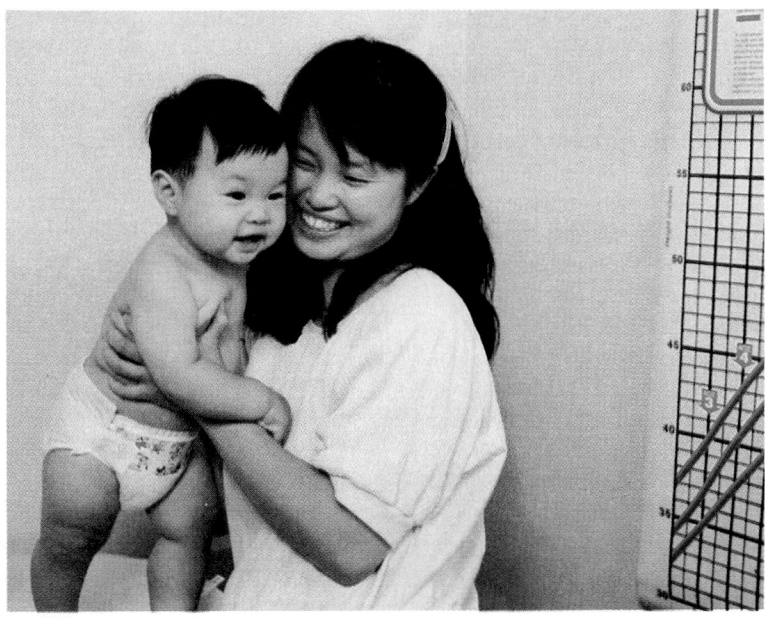

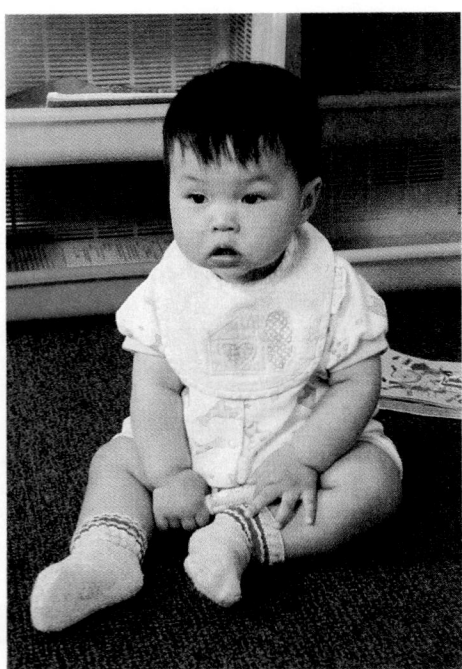

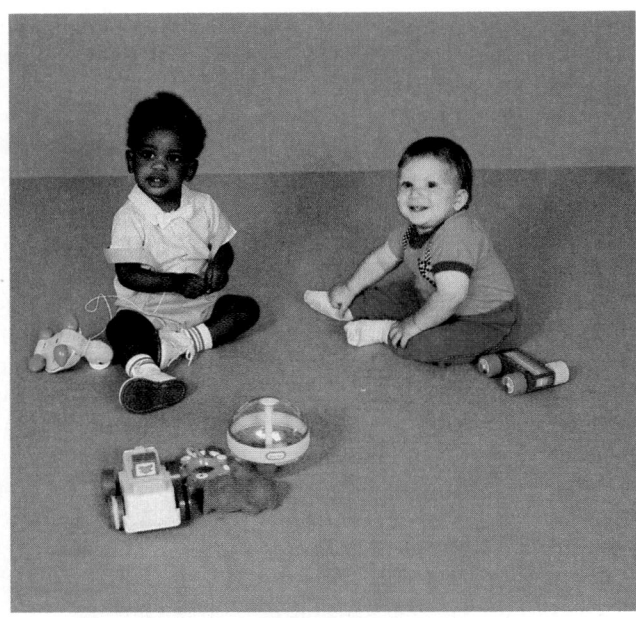

viate from them. Norms perform a number of important functions. They influence a person's perception of others. They direct a person's responses to situations and to others. They provide a basis for self-evaluation. They provide a foundation for forming opinions. They motivate behavior, and they give meaning to life and self-esteem. Values and norms exert a powerful influence over an individual's beliefs, attitudes, and practices. You must explore the client's value system to gain an appreciation for health-related behavior.

Cultural paradigms encompass abstract explanations used by groups to account for major life events. The term is synonymous with the idea of world view. The three dominant cultural paradigms are magico-religious, holistic, and scientific. This concept is crucial to health care professionals because all beliefs and values regarding health are derived from a person's basic world view. Aspects of all three world views are identifiable in most cultures, but one view usually predominates. The magico-religious paradigm offers a mystical cause-and-effect relationship between health and illness. The holistic paradigm provides the basis for a sense of balance and harmony between humans and the larger environment. The scientific view defines health as the absence of disease symptoms.

Enculturation is the process of acquiring one's cultural identity as it is transmitted by the previous generation. The *degree* of enculturation is important to assess before planning care, especially if you anticipate that the client will obtain health benefits by modifying

some culturally based aspect of health beliefs, attitudes, or practices. You can also act as an advocate or "culture broker" for the client by educating teachers, other health care workers, or representatives of social agencies about specific cultural beliefs and practices that may influence the client's and his or her family's behaviors or response to recommendations (DeSantis and Thomas, 1992).

Acculturation refers to the process of adapting to a culture different from the one in which a person was enculturated. Because North America is a continent of immigrants, you will frequently encounter clients undergoing acculturation. Culture is a learned group of traits, so it is possible for an individual to acquire a new cultural identity. Again, you must assess the *degree* of acculturation to predict the client's inclination to comply with a desirable modification in health care beliefs, attitudes, or practices. The degree of acculturation has been shown to be related to a variety of health concerns such as mental health (Rogler and others, 1991), psychosocial distress (Krause and Goldenhar, 1992), and childrearing attitudes (Raugh and others, 1990). When a client is undergoing acculturation, you can play a significant role in teaching the sort of acquired health behavior the client is already attempting to learn.

Cultural determinism is simply a term for conveying the notion that a person's behavior is *determined* by cultural beliefs. The concept is central to cultural assessment because one must understand it to formulate client goals. A goal is something the client, not the

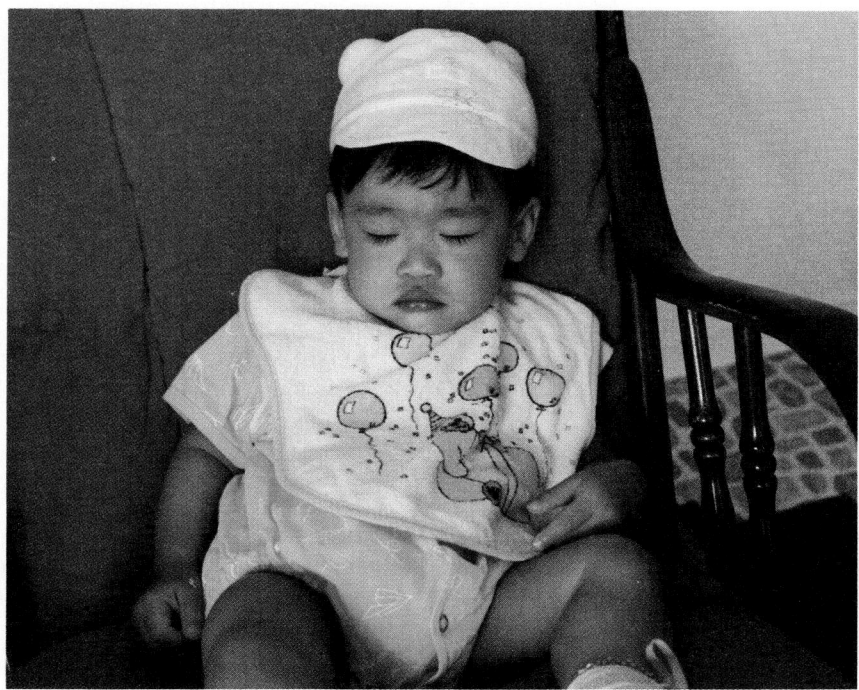

nurse, wants to achieve. A goal therefore must take into account the client's culturally determined behavior; otherwise, you cannot expect client compliance.

Ethnocentrism is the tendency to view people unconsciously by using one's group and one's own customs as the standard for all judgments. A nurse with this tendency will gather data only selectively in accordance with personal standards, values, and judgments and will not be able to see what the patient has to offer or the different ways in which the patient views the world. This bias will limit the data a nurse gathers and will distort interpretation.

Cultural relativity refers to the attempt to view or interpret behavior of culturally different individuals within the context of those individuals' culture. This perspective acknowledges that behavior that is appropriate in one culture may not be so defined in another culture. Providing nursing care from a perspective of cultural relativity involves viewing behaviors within the context of the client's culture. This approach may provide meaning to behaviors that caregivers might otherwise consider negative or confusing.

Ethnoscience refers to a systematic study of the way of life of a designated cultural group to obtain an accurate account of the people's behavior and how they perceive and interpret their universe. An ethnoscience approach includes the various ethnic groups' views on health and illness. This chapter takes an ethnoscience approach to cultural assessment because it presents the beliefs of cultural groups as they relate to health and illness. Research by Morse and others (1991) examines the differences between Cree Indian methods of treating a chronic skin disease (psoriasis) and the Western health care system approach. Using an ethnographic approach, they were able to identify conflicts between the two types of health care and reasons for client dissatisfaction with the Western approach.

Disease, illness, and sickness are similar terms that are frequently used and misused. The distinctions among them are important to cultural assessment. **Disease** is a medical term, arising from the dominant, scientifically based health care subculture. It refers to a pathologic process within human structure and function. **Illness** is a subjective term clients may use to describe the symptoms of discomfort. **Sickness,** on the other hand, is a personal state of illness with distinct social dimensions. Depending on the norms within any given culture, role behaviors are modified when a person becomes sick. These modified role behaviors are an important aspect of cultural assessment.

MAJOR VARIABLES IN CULTURAL ASSESSMENT

Trip-Reimer (1992) describes an anthropological model of cultural strata that is useful for examining the variables in cultural assessment (Figure 6-1). As is shown

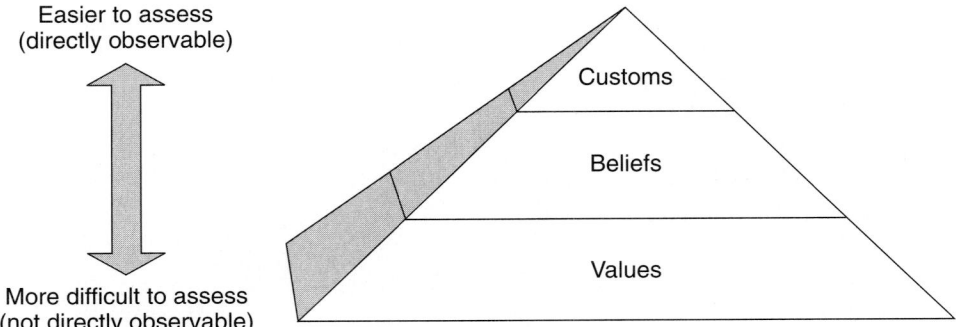

FIGURE 6-1 Model of cultural strata. Modified from Tripp-Reimer, T: *Cultural assessment.* (Redrawn from J Bellack and B Edlund, editors: Nursing assessment and diagnosis, Boston, 1992, Jones and Bartlett.)

in the model, customs (or behaviors) are based on beliefs, and beliefs are rooted in values. A nurse may observe and describe customs and therefore they are the easiest to assess. People, however, frequently learn values through an unconscious process of socialization; values are the most difficult to assess.

Values

Values provide the foundation for beliefs, attitudes, and behaviors. Often people are unaware of their values even though they are able to describe their beliefs and customs. They acquire values through socialization early in childhood, and these values guide the individual's goals, aspirations, and behaviors. Kluckhohn (1976) describes values common to all cultural groups. Table 6-1 compares five major value orientations among different groups. Kluckhohn proposes that variation in value orientation is one of the most important differences among cultures.

Recognizing the underlying value orientation of the culture of the health care system, and the impact it may have on interactions with clients is particularly helpful for nurses. The health care culture tends to have the following value orientations:
1. Time orientation–have a future orientation, which means an expectation for promptness and keeping scheduled appointments.
2. Activity orientation–value individuals for their accomplishments (a "doing" orientation), which may include getting healthy or taking medications as prescribed.
3. Human-nature orientation–view humans as having mastery over nature and value the omnipotence of technology.
4. Relational orientation–should be individualistic in its focus, emphasizing autonomy and putting the needs of the individual over the needs of the family.

Be aware of your own values in these areas so that when conflicts with clients arise, you can have an understanding that your expectations (based on the above values) may be contributing to the difficulty.

Beliefs

Beliefs include opinions, knowledge, and faith about various aspects of the world. Beliefs of particular concern to nurses are those related to illness causation, preferred method of treatment, expected outcomes, and fears about the illness. How the individual defines illness is based on his or her belief system and is largely determined by his or her culture. Tripp-Reimer (1992) notes that an individual with obvious pathology may not consult the "scientific" health care professional because the condition may be ignored, undetected, or attributed to a nonscientific cause.

Many chronic illnesses like hypertension and renal problems may go undetected because they do not exhibit symptoms obvious to a lay person. Illnesses attributed to nonscientific causes are referred to as "folk illnesses." A client usually seeks treatment for folk illnesses from a folk practitioner. Health professionals, such as physicians and nurses, are usually not seen as knowledgeable in these areas, and the client may not mention folk remedies or treatments unless you specifically ask. Tripp-Reimer (1992) divides folk illnesses into two major categories: naturalistic illness and personalistic illness.

Naturalistic illnesses are caused by impersonal factors that have no regard for the individual. These illnesses usually involve the concept of equilibrium. Problems develop when the balance is disturbed. One of the most common imbalances is between "hot" and "cold." These beliefs exist in Hispanic, Chinese, Filipino, and Arab cultures. In traditional Chinese health beliefs, the forces are called yin (cold) and yang (hot). Treatments

TABLE 6-1

Comparison of Value Orientations Among Eastern Asians, Hispanics, Native Americans, Blacks, and the Dominant American Culture

Value orientation	Cultural group
Time orientation	
Present oriented: accepts each day as it comes; little regard for the past; future unpredictable	Hispanic, Black, Native American
Past oriented: maintains traditions that were meaningful in the past; worships ancestors	Eastern Asian
Future oriented: anticipates "bigger and better" future; high value on change	Dominant American
Activity orientation	
"Doing" orientation: emphasizes accomplishments that are measurable by external standards	Dominant American
"Being" orientation: spontaneous expression of self	Hispanic, Black, Native American
"Being-in-becoming": emphasizes self-development of all aspects of self as an integrated whole	Eastern Asian
Human nature orientation	
Human being basically evil but with perfectable nature; constant self-control and discipline necessary	Dominant American, Hispanic, Black
Human being as neutral, neither good nor evil	Eastern Asian, Native American
Human-nature orientation	
Human being subject to environment with very little control over own destiny	Hispanic, Black
Human being in harmony with nature	Eastern Asian, Native American
Human being master over nature	Dominant American
Relational orientation	
Individualistic: encourages individualism: impersonal relationships occur more with outsiders and less with family	Dominant American
Lineal: group goals dominant over individual goals; ordered positional succession (father to son)	Eastern Asian
Collateral: group goals dominant over individual goals: more emphasis on relationship with others on one's own level	Hispanic, Black, Native American

Adapted from Kluckhohn F: Dominant and variant value orientation. In Brink P, editor: *Transcultural nursing: a book of readings,* Englewood Cliffs, NJ, 1976, Prentice-Hall.

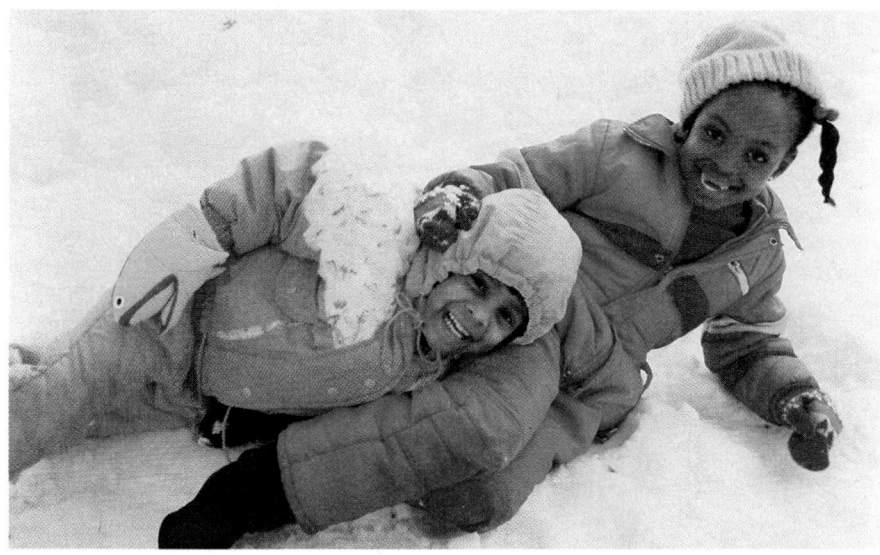

usually involve restoring balance by applying opposing forces, for example, application of the appropriate "hot" remedy to treat a "cold" illness and vice versa. Hot-cold classifications for treatments and illnesses are culturally determined and have nothing to do with actual temperature. The box below gives examples of hot-cold

---

HOT-COLD CONDITIONS AND THEIR CORRESPONDING TREATMENT

Hot conditions	Cold conditions
Fever	Cancer
Infections	Pneumonia
Diarrhea	Malaria
Kidney problems	Joint pain
Rashes	Menstrual period
Skin ailments	Teething
Sore throat	Earache
Liver problems	Rheumatism
Ulcers	Tuberculosis
Constipation	Colds
	Headache
	Paralysis
	Stomach cramps

Hot foods	Cold foods
Chocolate	Fresh vegetables
Cheese	Tropical fruits
Temperate-zone fruits	Dairy products
Eggs	Meats such as goat, fish, chicken
Peas	Honey
Onions	Cod
Aromatic beverages	Raisins
Hard liquor	Bottled milk
Oils	Barley water
Meats such as beef, waterfowl, mutton	
Goat's milk	
Cereal grains	
Chili peppers	

Hot medicines and herbs	Cold medicines and herbs
Penicillin	Orange flower water
Tobacco	Linden
Ginger root	Sage
Garlic	Milk of magnesia
Cinnamon	Bicarbonate of soda
Anise	
Vitamins	
Iron preparations	
Cod-liver oil	
Castor oil	
Aspirin	

Adapted from Wilson H, Kneisl C: *Psychiatric nursing,* Reading Mass, 1988. Addison-Wesley.

---

classifications. Understanding this belief system may help explain a client's desire for or rejection of a specific medical treatment. For example, the client may insist on penicillin (a "hot" medicine) or an x-ray (a "hot" treatment) for a viral respiratory infection (a "cold" condition) and may not be satisfied with his care without receiving what he believes to be an appropriate treatment.

Personalistic illnesses result from aggression directed at or punishment of the individual. The "evil eye" and witchcraft are two examples of personalistic folk beliefs. The "evil eye" is a concept known throughout Mediterranean (for example, Greek and Italian cultures) and Spanish-speaking cultures. It is usually caused unintentionally and is related to envy and admiration. Complimenting another person's child may be considered a way to "cast the evil eye," and the symptoms may be interpreted as related to this. Usually some general methods can protect against the evil eye. Children may wear protective amulets, beads, or gold crosses, for example. Respect these cultural beliefs and help the client determine ways to resolve the situation along with appropriate medical interventions, if they are required.

Belief in witchcraft as a cause of illness is prevalent in many cultures. Snow (1978) noted evidence of this belief in Puerto Ricans, Haitians, and black Americans. He estimated that one third of black clients treated in psychiatric centers in the southern United States felt they were victims of witchcraft. The common theme he noted was that someone had done something to cause another person's injury, illness, or death.

Clients usually seek out a folk healer for treatment of these conditions. For many clients, the practitioner can be most helpful by working in a collaborative and cooperative manner with the folk healer to provide holistic care to the client. An example of this approach is the effort of the Indian Health Service to involve traditional healers in the client's care and make the services of traditional healers accessible to clients even when they are hospitalized (Giger and Davidson, 1991). Table 6-2 describes some folk illnesses in Spanish-speaking and African American cultures.

While health practitioners may assess health beliefs in a variety of ways, an assessment model proposed by Kleinman, Eisenberg, and Good (1978) is very useful. These authors suggest the following set of questions to elicit the client's explanatory model:

1. What do you think caused your problem?
2. Why do you think it started when it did?
3. What does your sickness do to you? How does it work?
4. How severe is your sickness? Will it have a long or a short duration?
5. What kind of treatment do you think you should receive?

TABLE 6-2

Folk Illnesses in Spanish-Speaking and African-American Cultures

Culture	Folk illness	Etiology	Behaviors	Practitioner	Treatment
Hispanic	*Susto* (fright)	An individual experiences a stressful event at some time prior to the onset of symptoms. The stressor may vary from death of a significant person to a child's nightmare to inability to adequately fulfill social-role responsibility. Children are more susceptible to *susto*. It is believed that the soul or spirit leaves the body.	Restlessness during sleep Anorexia Depression Listlessness Disinterest in personal appearance	*Curandero* or *Espiritualista (Espiritista)*	A ceremony is performed using branches from a sweet pepper tree and a candle. Motions by the ill person and the curer are performed that form a cross. Three Ave Marias or credos (Apostles' Creed) are said.
	Empacho	Bolus of undigested food adheres to the stomach or wall of intestine. The cause may be the food itself, or it may be due to eating when one is not hungry or when one is stressed.	Stomach pain Diarrhea Vomiting Anorexia	Family member *Sabador* *Curandero*	Massage of the stomach or back until a popping sound is heard. A laxative may be given.
	Caida de la Mollera (fallen fontanel)	Trauma—a fall or blow to the head or the rapid dislodging of a nipple from an infant's mouth causes the fontanel to be sucked into the palate.	Inability to suckle Irritability Vomiting Diarrhea Sunken fontanel	Family member *Curandero*	One or more of these practitioners insert a finger into the child's mouth and push the palate back into place. Hold the child by the ankles with the top of the head just touching a pan of tepid water for a minute or two. Apply a poultice of soap shavings to the fontanel. Administer herb tea.
	Mal de ojo (evil eye)	A disease of magical origin cast by a person who is jealous or envious of another person or something the person owns. The evil eye is cast by the envious person's vision upon the subject thereby heating the blood and producing symptoms. Usually a beautiful child is envied or admired but is not touched by the admirer and the evil eye can be inflicted. The admirer may not be aware of the damage done. If the child is admired and then touched by that person the evil eye is not inflicted.	Fever Diarrhea Vomiting Crying without apparent cause	*Curandero* *Brujo*	Passing an unbroken egg over the body or rubbing the body with the egg to draw the heat (fever) from the body. Prayers such as the Our Father or Hail Mary may be said simultaneously with the passing of the egg. The egg is then broken in a bowl, placed under the head of the bed and left there all night. By morning if the egg is almost cooked from the heat of the body, this is a sign that the sick person had *mal de ojo*.

Continued.

TABLE 6-2—cont'd

Folk Illnesses in Spanish-Speaking and African-American Cultures

Culture	Folk illness	Etiology	Behaviors	Practitioner	Treatment
	Mal Puesto (evil)	Illness caused by a hex put on by a *brujo,* witch, or *curandero,* or other person knowledgeable about witchcraft.	Vary considerably Strange behavioral changes Labile emotions Convulsions	*Curandero* *Brujo*	Varies, depending on the hex.
African American	High blood (too much blood)	Diet very high in red meat and rich food. Belief that high blood causes stroke.	Weakness, paralysis, vertigo, or other behaviors related to stroke	Family member or friend of Spiritualist or self (the latter does this after referring to a Zodiac almanac)	Take internally lemon juice, vinegar, epsom salts, or other astringent food to sweat out the excess blood. Treatment varies depending on what is appropriate for each person according to the Zodiac almanac.
	Low blood (not enough blood)	Too many astringent foods, too harsh a treatment for high blood. Remaining on high blood-pressure medication for too long.	Fatigue Weakness	Same as for high blood	Eat rich red meat, raw beets. Stop taking treatment for high blood. Consult the Zodiac almanac.
	Thin blood (predisposition to illness)	Occurs in women, children, or old people. Blood is very thin until puberty and again in old age.	Greater susceptibility to illness	Individual	Individual should exercise caution in cold weather by wearing warm clothing or by staying indoors.
	Rash appearing on a child after birth (no specific disease name—the concept is that of body defilement)	Impurities within the body coming out. The body is being defiled and will therefore produce skin rashes.	Rash anywhere on the body; may be accompanied by fever	Family member	Catnip tea as a laxative or other commercial laxative. The quantity and kind depend on the age of the individual.
	Diseases of witchcraft, hex, or conjuring	Envy and sexual conflict are the most frequent causes of having someone hex another person.	Unusual behavior not normal for the person Sudden death Symptoms related to poisoning (i.e., foul taste, fall off [weight loss], nausea, vomiting) A crawling sensation on the skin or in the stomach Psychotic behavior	Voodoo Priest(ess) Spiritualist	*Conja* is the help given to the conjured person. Treatment varies depending on the spell cast.

From Hautman, MA: Folk health and illness beliefs, *Nurse Pract* 4(4):27, 1979.

6. What are the most important results you hope to receive from this treatment?
7. What are the chief problems your sickness has caused you?
8. What do you fear most about your sickness?

Customs

Customs are learned behaviors that you can easily assess through observation and direct questioning. However, problems and misunderstandings can arise if you do not assess customs or if you do not validate the meaning of observed behaviors. Customs include dietary practices, communication patterns, family and kinship relations, religious practices, and health behaviors. Tables 6-3 through 6-5 and the box on p. 179 summarize characteristic behaviors related to the health care of different cultural groups.

Diet and nutrition. Anthropologists have shown that cultural groups differ in their dietary beliefs and practices, but this is obvious to anyone who associates particular foods with specific ethnic groups. The development of national cuisines is a complex process related to the availability of certain kinds of food, the price, the efficiency of its distribution, the subjective preferences of taste and spices, and patterns of trade and commerce. Hotter, spicier food is preferred by groups living relatively closer to the equator, where the climate is warmer, while groups living in higher latitudes in more temperate climates prefer relatively less spicy food. The variety of foods available in industrialized countries is greater than that in Third World countries. Moreover, apart from its nutritional value, food carries a range of symbolic meanings. Food that is popular in one society may be rigorously forbidden in an-

TABLE 6-3

Characteristic Food Choices for Six Groups

Vegetables	Fruits	Meats and alternatives	Grain products	Others
African American				
Broccoli, corn, greens (mustard, collard, kale, turnips, beets, etc.), lima beans, okra, peas, pumpkin	Grapefruit, grapes, nectarine, plums, watermelon	Sausage, pig's feet, ears, etc., bacon, luncheon meat, organ meats, turkey, catfish, perch, red snapper, tuna, salmon, sardines, shrimp, kidney beans, red beans, blackeyed peas, peanuts and peanut butter	Corn bread, hominy grits, biscuits, muffins, cooked cereal, crackers	Chitterlings, salt pork, gravies, buttermilk
Hispanic-American				
Avocado, chilies, corn, lettuce, onion, peas, potato, prickly pear (cactus leaf called *nopales*), zucchini	Guava, lemon, mango, melons, prickly pear (cactus fruit called *tuna*), zapote (or sapote)	Lamb, tripe, sausage *(chorizo)*, bologna, bacon, pinto beans, pink beans, garbanzo beans, lentils, peanuts and peanut butter	Tortillas, corn flour, oatmeal, sweet bread *(pan dulce)*	Salsa (tomato, pepper, onion relish), chili sauce, guacamole, lard *(manteca)*, pork cracklings
Japanese				
Bamboo shoots, broccoli, burdock root, cauliflower, celery, cucumbers, eggplant, gourd *(Kampyo)*, mushrooms, napa cabbage, peas, peppers, radishes (daikon or pickles called *takuwan*), snow peas, squash, sweet potato, turnips, water chestnuts, yamaimo	Apricot, cherries, grapefruit, grapes, lemon, lime, melons, persimmon, pineapple, pomegranate, plums (dried pickled *umeboshi*), strawberries	Turkey, raw tuna or sea bass *(sashimi)*, mackerel, sardines *(mezashi)*, shrimp, abalone, squid, octopus, soybean curd *(tofu)*, soybean paste *(miso)*, soybeans, red beans *(azuki)*, lima beans, peanuts, almonds, cashews	Rice crackers, noodles (whole wheat noodle called *soba* or *udon*), oatmeal	Soy sauce, Nori paste (used to season rice), bean thread *(konyaku)*, ginger *(shoga:* dried form called *denishoga)*

Continued.

TABLE 6-3—cont'd

Characteristic Food Choices for Six Groups

Vegetables	Fruits	Meats and alternatives	Grain products	Others
Chinese				
Bamboo shoots, bean sprouts, bok choy, broccoli, celery, Chinese cabbage, corn, cucumbers, eggplant, greens (collard, Chinese, broccoli, mustard, kale), leeks, lettuce, mushrooms, peppers, scallions, snow peas, taro, water chestnuts, white turnips, white radishes, winter melon	Figs, grapes, kumquats, loquats, mango, melons, persimmon, pineapple, plums, pomegranate	Organ meats, duck, white fish, shrimp, lobster, oyster, sardines, soybeans, soybean curd *(tofu)*, black beans, chestnuts *(kuri)*	Barley, millet	Soy sauce, sweet and sour sauce, mustard sauce, ginger root, plum sauce, red bean paste
Vietnamese*				
Bamboo shoots, bean sprouts, cabbage, carrots, cucumbers, greens, lettuce, mushrooms, onions, peas, spinach, yams	Apple, banana, eggfruit *(o-ma)*, grapefruit, jackfruit, lychee, mandarin, mango, orange, papaya, pineapple, tangerine, watermelon	Beef, blood, brain, chicken, duck, eggs, fish, goat, kidney, lamb, liver, pork, shellfish, soybeans	French bread, rice, rice noodles, wheat noodles	Fish sauce, fresh herbs, garlic, ginger, lard, MSG, peanut oil, sesame seeds, sesame seed oil, vegetable oil
Indian (East)				
Cauliflower, carrots, cucumber, corn-gourds, leeks, eggplant, beets, radishes, hot pepper, bell pepper, peas, French beans, okra, pumpkin, red and white cabbage, mung sprouts, bean sprouts, potatoes, tapioca root, sweet potatoes	Oranges, limes, grapes, watermelon, mango, guava, honeydew, chiku, cantaloupe, pineapple, green, yellow, and red bananas, berries, custard apples	Lamb, beef, duck, chicken, shrimp, catfish, buffalo, sunfish, sardines, fresh crab, lobster, peanuts, cashews, almonds, chickpeas, split peas, black-eyed peas, dry mung beans	Rice pancakes, wheat chapati, puri, mixed grain flour bread	Fresh coconut juice, curries, tomato sauce, tamarind sauce, dried grain curries *(pulses)*, yogurt-curry garnished with coriander (fresh leaves)

From Endres JB, and Rockwell RE: *Food, nutrition, and the young child*, St. Louis, 1980, Mosby–Year Book, pp. 182-183. Modified from Nutrition during pregnancy and lactation, California Department of Public Health, revised 1975.

NOTE: Foods common to all ethnic groups have been omitted.

*Information supplied by Hanh-Trang Tran-Viet, Carbondale, Ill.

other. Food, and the social aspects of eating it, play a central role in daily life. Consequently, the practitioner should appreciate that dietary beliefs and practices are notoriously difficult to change, even if they interfere with adequate nutrition.

Try to understand the ways in which various cultures view their food, and the ways food is classified, before attempting to change nutrition practices. Food is usually classified into definitions of (1) what is edible and what is not, (2) what is sacred and what is profane, (3) the ways food is grouped, (4) food as medicine, and (5) social food. Rancid butter is not normally considered edible in North American culture, yet it is a standard condiment in tea in many central Asian regions. By the same token, food commonly eaten in North America, such as pork rinds, would be considered repulsive in some other cultures. Snails and eel, for instance, are considered delicacies by some people but inedible by others. Table 6-3 summarizes characteristic food choices for six cultural groups.

In the United States and Canada, industrialized countries with many immigrants, few foods are generally considered profane. But among specific religious groups, some examples of sacred and profane foods are familiar. Many Jews will not eat pork, whereas strict Catholics will not eat meat on Fridays (although this has become a less common practice). Apart from religious-based sanctions, many people are vegetarians, while other groups eschew highly processed foods.

In American culture, food is classified into four main groups—dairy, grains, meat, and fruits and vegetables. Many people regard food in terms of its use by the body—protein, fat, and starch and carbohydrates. We live in a culture strongly influenced by science, and the biochemistry of food is part of our general fund of knowledge. The staples in the diets of a great many North Americans are meat and potatoes, something sweet for dessert, salads, soups, and fruit juices, all reflecting the conception of a healthy diet as one containing a balance of the food groups widely recognized and accepted as healthy. In other cultures, standard dishes might include pastas or rice, sausage, or bread.

Medicinal qualities are ascribed to various foods, rightly or wrongly, across the world. North Americans have their own widely shared beliefs associating food with medicine. Apples keep doctors away. Honey and lemon help reduce congestion. Fish is brain food. Citrus fruits provide protection from colds. Oats unclog arteries.

Finally, all cultures tend to associate foods with social occasions unique to their cultures. Some occasions seem to demand wine and others seem to demand hot chocolate. Certain foods are consumed at baseball games, while other foods are eaten as family traditions on various holidays.

Other cultures are no different from the dominant culture in these broad aspects of food. Only the foods that carry strong cultural preferences or taboos vary from one culture to another.

Communication patterns. Communication patterns are closely intertwined with culture and may be the source of misunderstandings between you and your client. Communication patterns include both verbal and

Text continued on p. 174.

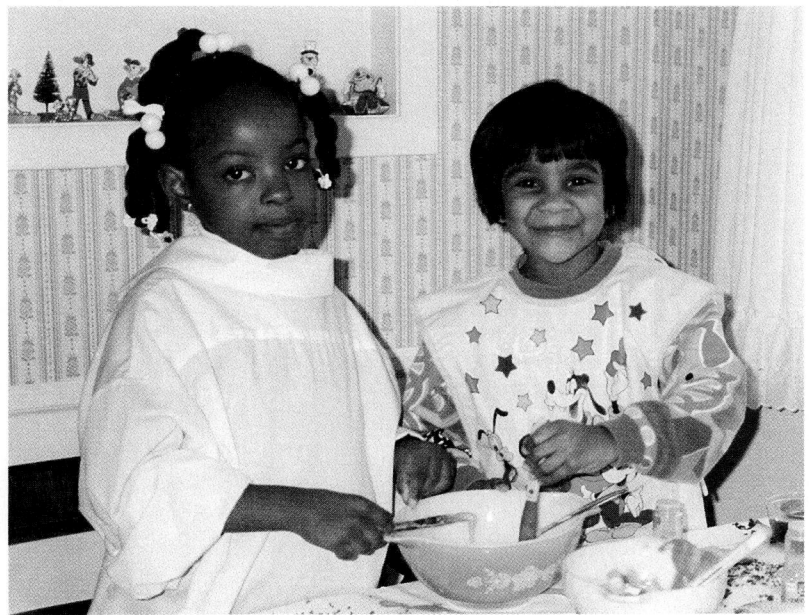

TABLE 6-4

Religious Beliefs that Affect Nursing Care

Religion	Beliefs about birth and death	Beliefs about diet and food practices
Adventist (Seventh Day Adventist; Church of God)	*Birth:* Opposed to infant baptism Baptism in adulthood	Meat prohibited in some groups No alcohol, coffee, or tea
Baptist (27 groups)	*Birth:* Opposed to infant baptism Believers baptize by immersion as adults *Death:* Counsel and prayer with clergy, family, patient	Some groups discourage coffee, tea, and alcohol
Black Muslim	*Birth:* No baptism *Death:* Carefully prescribed procedure for washing and shrouding dead	Prohibit alcohol, pork and meat of dead animals, or foods traditional among American blacks, e.g., corn bread, collard greens
Buddhist Churches of America	*Birth:* No infant baptism Infant presentation *Death:* Last rite chanting often practiced at bedside soon after death Priest should be contacted	No requirements or restrictions Some sects are strictly vegetarian Discourage use of alcohol and drugs
Church of Christ Scientist (Christian Science)	*Birth:* No baptism *Death:* No last rites	No requirements or restrictions
Church of Jesus Christ of Latter Day Saints (Mormon)	*Birth:* No baptism at birth Infant is "blessed" by church official at first opportunity after birth (in church) Baptism by immersion at 8 years *Death:* No special rites	Prohibit tea, coffee, alcohol Encourage sparing use of meats Fasting for 24 hours on first Sunday each month (from after evening meal Saturday until evening meal Sunday)
Eastern Orthodox (Turkey, Egypt, Syria, Rumania, Bulgaria, Cyprus, Albania, etc.)	*Birth:* Most believe in infant baptism by immersion 8 to 40 days after birth *Death:* Last rites obligatory for impending death	Restrictions depend on specific sect
Episcopal (Anglican)	*Birth:* Infant baptism mandatory; urgent if poor prognosis *Death:* Last rites available but not mandatory	Abstain from meat on fast days May fast on Wednesday, Friday, during Lent, and before Christmas Some fast for 6 hours before receiving Holy Communion
Friends (Quakers)	*Birth:* No baptism Infant's name recorded in official book	No requirements or restrictions Most practice moderation Avoid alcohol and illicit drugs

Beliefs regarding medical care	Comments
Some believe in divine healing and practice anointing with oil and use of prayer	Sabbath: Saturday for many
May desire communion or baptism when ill	Accept Bible literally
Believe in man's choice and God's sovereignty	
Some oppose hypnosis as therapy	
"Laying on of hands" (some)	Fundamentalist and conservative groups accept Bible as inspired word of God
May encounter some resistance to some therapies, such as abortion	
Believe God functions through physician	
Some believe in predestination; may respond passively to care	
Faith healing unacceptable	General adherence to Moslem tenets overlaid, in many instances, by antagonism to whites especially Christians and Jews
Always maintain personal habits of cleanliness	Do not indulge in activities (such as sleeping) more than is necessary to health
Illness believed to be a trial to aid development of soul; illness due to Karmic causes	Optimistic outlook; teach ways to overcome fears, anxieties, apprehension
May be reluctant to have surgery or certain treatments on holy days	
Cleanliness believed to be of great importance	
Family may request Buddhist priest for counseling	
Deny the existence of health crisis; see sickness and sin as errors of mind that can be altered by prayer	Many desire services of Practitioner or Reader; will sometimes refuse even emergency treatment until they have consulted a Reader
Oppose human intervention with drugs or other therapies; however, accept legally required immunizations	Unlikely to donate organs for transplant
Many adhere to belief that disease is a human mental concept that can be dispelled by "spiritual truth" to extent that they refuse all medical treatment	
Devout adherents believe in divine healing through anointment with oil and "laying on of hands" by church officials (elders)	Married adults wear special undergarments
Medical therapy not prohibited	May request Sacrament on Sunday while in hospital
	Financial support for sick available through well-funded welfare system
	Discourage cremation
	Discourage use of tobacco
Anointment of the sick	Discourage cremation
No conflict with medical science	
Some believe in spiritual healing	Religious icons very important
Rite for anointing sick available but not mandatory	Communion four times yearly: Christmas, Easter, June 30, and August 15; may be mandatory for some
No special rites or restrictions	Believe in plain speech and dress
	Pacifists

Continued.

TABLE 6-4 — cont'd

Religious Beliefs that Affect Nursing Care

Religion	Beliefs about birth and death	Beliefs about diet and food practices
Greek Orthodox	*Birth:* Baptism considered important Performed 40 days after birth If not possible to baptize by sprinkling or immersion, Church allows child baptism "in the air" by moving the child in the form of a cross as appropriate words are said *Death:* Last rites, administration of Sacrament of Holy Communion Should be performed while dying person is still conscious	Church prescribed fast periods — usually occur on Wednesday, Friday, and during Lent; consist of avoiding meat and (in some cases) dairy products If health compromised, priest may be contacted to convince family to forego fasting
Hindu	*Birth:* No ritual *Death:* Special prescribed rites Priest pours water into the mouth of dead child, ties a thread around neck or wrist to signify blessing (should not be removed) Family washes body and is particular about who touches body	Many dietary restrictions Beef and veal not eaten Some strict vegetarians
Islam (Muslim/Moslem)	*Birth:* No baptism *Death:* Patient must confess sins and beg forgiveness before death; family should be present Family washes and prepares body, then turns it to face Mecca Only relatives and friends may touch body	Prohibit all pork products Daylight fasting practiced during ninth month of Mohammedan year (Ramadan) Strict Muslims do not use alcohol
Jehovah's Witness	*Birth:* No baptism *Death:* No last rites	Eat nothing to which blood has been added; can eat animal flesh that has been drained
Judaism (Orthodox and Conservative)	*Birth:* No baptism Ritual circumcision of male infants on eighth day; performed by Mohel (ritual circumciser familiar with Jewish law and aseptic technique) Reform Jews favor ritual circumcision, but not as a religious imperative *Death:* Remains are ritually washed by members of the Ritual Burial Society Burial should take place as soon as possible	Numerous dietary kosher laws exist that may be influenced by local practices and family and cultural tradition Allowed only meat from animals that are vegetable eaters, are cloven hoofed, chew their cud, and are ritually slaughtered; fish that have scales and fins Prohibit any combination of meat and milk; milk products served first can be followed by meat in a few minutes but milk may not be consumed for several hours after eating meat. Fasting for 24 hours is part of Yom Kippur observance Matzo replaces leavened bread during Passover week

Beliefs regarding medical care	Comments
Each health crisis handled by ordained priest; deacon may also serve in some cases Holy Communion administered in hospital Some may desire Sacrament of the Holy Unction performed by priest	Oppose euthanasia Believe every reasonable effort should be made to preserve life until termination by God Discourage autopsies that may cause dismemberment Prefer burial to cremation
Illness or injury believed to represent sins committed in previous life Accept most modern medical practices	Cremation preferred
Faith healing not acceptable unless psychologic condition of patient is deteriorating; performed for morale Ritual washing after prayer; prayer takes place five times daily (upon rising, midday, afternoon, early evening, and before bed); during prayer, face Mecca and kneel on prayer rug	Older Muslims often have a fatalistic view that may interfere with compliance to therapy May oppose autopsy
Adherents are generally absolutely opposed to blood transfusions, including banking of own blood; individuals can sometimes be persuaded in emergencies May be opposed to use of albumin, globulin, factor replacement (hemophilia), vaccines	Often possible to obtain a court order appointing a hospital official as temporary guardian to consent to a child's transfusion when parents refuse consent Autopsy approved only as required by law
May resist surgical procedures during Sabbath, which extends from sundown Friday until sundown Saturday Seriously ill and pregnant women are exempt from fasting Illness is grounds for violating dietary laws, e.g., patient with congestive heart failure does not have to use kosher meats, which are high in sodium	Oppose all forms of mutilation, including autopsy; body parts not donated or removed; amputated limbs, organs, or surgically removed tissues should be made available to family for burial Donation or transplantation of organs requires rabbinical consent May oppose prolongation of life after irreversible brain damage

Continued.

TABLE 6-4—cont'd

Religious Beliefs that Affect Nursing Care

Religion	Beliefs about birth and death	Beliefs about diet and food practices
Lutheran	*Birth:* Baptize only living infants shortly after birth *Death:* Last rites optional	No requirements or restrictions
Mennonite (similar to Amish)	*Birth:* No baptism in infancy Baptism during early or middle teens	No requirements or restrictions
Methodist	*Birth:* No baptism at birth; performed on children or adults *Death:* No ritual	No requirements or restrictions
Nazarene	*Birth:* Baptism optional *Death:* No last rites	No requirements or restrictions Alcohol prohibited
Pentecostal (Assembly of God, Four-square)	*Birth:* No baptism at birth Baptism by complete immersion after age of accountability *Death:* No last rites	Abstain from alcohol, eating blood, strangled animals, or anything to which blood has been added Some individuals may resist pork
Orthodox Presbyterian	*Birth:* Infant baptism by sprinkling *Death:* Last rites not a sacramental procedure; scripture reading and prayer	No requirements or restrictions
Roman Catholic	*Birth:* Infant baptism mandatory; especially urgent in poor prognosis, when it may be performed by anyone *Death:* Rite for Anointing of the sick is mandatory Family or patient may request anointing if prognosis is grave	Fasting or abstaining from meat mandatory on Ash Wednesday and Good Friday; fasting optional during Lent; no meat on Fridays during Lent as general rule Most hospital patients exempt from fasting Some older Catholics may adhere to older rule of eating fish on Friday
Russian Orthodox	*Birth:* Baptism by priest only *Death:* Traditionally after death arms are crossed, fingers set in a cross	No meat or dairy products on Wednesday, Friday, and during Lent
Unitarian Universalist	*Birth:* Some practice infant baptism; most consider it unnecessary *Death:* No ritual	No requirements or restrictions

From Whaley LF and Wong DL: *Nursing care of infants and children*, ed 4, St. Louis, 1991, Mosby—Year Book.
Data from Recognizing your patients' spiritual needs, *Nursing* 77 7(12):64-68, 1977; Beliefs that can affect therapy, *Pediatr Nurs* 5(3):40-43, 1979; Carpenito, LJ: Nursing diagnosis: application to clinical practice, ed 3, Philadelphia, 1989, JB Lippincott; Kozier, B and Erb, G: *Fundamentals of nursing*, ed 3, Menlo Park, Calif., 1987, Addison-Wesley Publishing; Spector, RE: *Cultural diversity in health and illness*, ed 2, New York, 1985, Appleton Century-Crofts: personal communications.

Beliefs regarding medical care	Comments
If grave prognosis, family may request anointing and blessing of sick or visit by church official	Accept scientific developments
No illness rituals	
Deep concern for dignity and self-determination of individual that would conflict with shock treatment or medical treatment affecting personality or will	
Communion may be requested before surgery or similar crisis	Encourage donation of body or body parts to medical science
Church official administers communion and laying on of hands	Cremation permitted
Adherents believe in divine healing but not exclusive of medical treatment	
No restrictions regarding medical care	Some insist illness is divine punishment; most consider it an intrusion of Satan
Deliverance from sickness is provided for in atonement; may pray for divine intervention in health matters and seek God in prayer for themselves and others when ill	Practice glossolalia (speaking in tongues)
Communion administered when appropriate and convenient	Full forgiveness granted for any illness connected with a sin
Blood transfusion accepted when advisable	
Pastor or elder should be called for ill person	
Believe science should be used for relief of suffering	
Encourage anointing of sick, although this may be interpreted by older members of church as equivalent to the old terminology "extreme unction" or "last rites"; they may require a careful explanation if their reluctance is associated with fear of imminent death	Family may request that major amputated limb be buried in consecrated ground
	Transplant accepted as long as loss of organ does not deprive donor of life or functional integrity of body
Traditional church teaching does not approve of contraceptives or abortion; however, some clergy advocate more liberal views on these issues	Autopsy acceptable
	Religious articles important
Cross necklace is important and should be removed only when necessary and replaced as soon as possible	Opposed to autopsy, embalming, or cremation
Adherents believe in divine healing, but not exclusive of medical treatment	
Believe God helps those who help themselves	Cremation preferred to burial
Some may prefer not to have clergy visit them in hospital	

TABLE 6-5

Cultural Characteristics Related to Health Care

Cultural group	Health beliefs	Health and diet practices
Asian Americans **Chinese**	A healthy body viewed as gift from parents and ancestors and must be cared for Health is one of the results of balance between the forces of *yin* (cold) and *yang* (hot), energy forces that rule the world Illness caused by imbalance Believe blood is source of life and is not regenerated *Chi* is innate energy Lack of *chi* and blood results in deficiency that produces fatigue, poor constitution, and long illness	Goal of therapy is to restore balance of *yin* and *yang* Acupuncturist applies needles to appropriate meridians identified in terms of *yin* and *yang* Acupressure and *tai chi* replacing acupuncture in some areas Moxibustion is application of heat to skin over specific meridians Wide use of medicinal herbs procured and applied in prescribed ways Folk healers are herbalist, spiritual healer, temple healer, fortune healer Meals may or may not be planned to balance hot and cold Milk intolerance relatively common Use of condiments, e.g., monosodium glutamate and soy sauce, may create difficulty with some diet regimens, e.g., low-salt diets

Japanese	Three major belief systems:
	  Shinto religious influence
	    Humans inherently good
	    Evil caused by outside spirits
	    Illness caused by contact with polluting agents, e.g., blood, corpses, skin diseases
	  Chinese and Korean influence
	    Health achieved through harmony and balance between self and society
	    Disease caused by disharmony with society and not caring for body
	  Portuguese influence
	  Upholds germ theory of disease
		Believe evil removed by purification
		Energy restored by means of acupuncture, acupressure, massage, and moxibustion along affected meridians
		Kampō medicine — use of natural herbs
		Believe in removal of diseased parts
		Trend is to use both Western and Oriental healing methods
		Care for disabled viewed as family's responsibility
		Take pride in child's good health
		Seek preventive care, medical care for illness
		Older persons avoid some food combinations (e.g., milk and cherries, watermelon and crab) and believe pickled plums to have special properties

Vietnamese	Good health considered to be balance between *yin* (cold) and *yang* (hot) Believe person's life has been predisposed toward certain phenomena by cosmic forces Health believed to be result of harmony with existing universal order, harmony attained by pleasing good spirits and avoiding evil ones Belief in *am duc*, the amount of good deeds accumulated by ancestors Many use rituals to prevent illness Practice some restrictions to prevent incurring wrath of evil spirits	Family uses all means possible before using outside agencies for health care Fortune-tellers determine event that caused disturbance May visit temple to procure divine instruction Use astrologer to calculate cyclical changes and forces Regard health as family responsibility; outside aid sought when resources run out Certain illnesses considered only temporary (such as pustules, open wounds) and ignored Seek generalist health healers May use special diets to prevent illness and promote health Lactose intolerance prevalent

*Most Asian cultures consider the child 1 year old at the time of birth. Traditional Chinese custom adds 1 year on January 1 regardless of the birthday — a child born in December is 2 years old the next January.

Family relationships	Communication	Comments
Extended family pattern common Strong concept of loyalty of young to old Respect for elders taught at early age — acceptance without questioning or talking back Children's behavior a reflection on family Family and individual honor and "face" important Self-reliance and self-restraint highly valued; self-expression repressed Males valued more highly than females; women submissive to men in family	Open expression of emotions unacceptable Often smile when do not comprehend	Do not react well to painful diagnostic workup; are especially upset by drawing of blood Deep respect for their bodies and believe it best to die with bodies intact; therefore may refuse surgery Believe in reincarnation Older members fear hospitals; often believe hospital is a place to go to die Children sometimes breast-fed for up to 4 or 5 years*

Close intergenerational relationships
Family provides anchor
Family tends to keep problems to self
Value self-control and self-sufficiency
Concept of *haji* (shame) imposes strong control; unacceptable behavior of children reflects on family
Many adopt practices of contemporary middle class
Concern for child's missing school may result in sending to school before fully recovered from illness
	Issei — born in Japan; usually speak Japanese only
	Nisei, Sansei, and *Yonsei* have few language difficulties
	New immigrants able to read and write English better than to speak or understand it
	Make significant use of nonverbal communication with subtle gestures and facial expression
	Tend to suppress emotions
	Will often wait silently
		Generational categories:
		  Issei — 1st generation to live in U.S.
		  Nisei — 2nd generation
		  Sansei — 3rd generation
		  Yonsei — 4th generation
		Issei and *Nisei* — tolerant and permissive childrearing until 5 or 6, then emphasis on emotional reserve and control
		Cleanliness highly valued
		Time considered valuable and used wisely
		Tendency to practice emotional control may make assessment of pain more difficult

Family is revered institution Multigenerational families Family is chief social network Children highly valued Individual needs and interests are subordinate to those of family group Father is main decision maker Women taught submission to men Parents expect respect and obedience from children	Many immigrants are not proficient in speaking and understanding English May hesitate to ask questions Questioning authority is sign of disrespect; asking questions considered impolite Use indirectness rather than forthrightness in expressing disagreement May avoid eye contact with health professionals as a sign of respect	Consider status more important than money Children taught emotional control Time concept more relaxed — consider punctuality less significant than other values, i.e., propriety Place high value on social harmony

Continued.

TABLE 6-5 — cont'd

Cultural Characteristics Related to Health Care

Cultural group	Health beliefs	Health and diet practices
Filipino	Believe God's will and supernatural forces govern universe Illness, accidents, and other misfortunes are God's punishment for violations of His will Widely accept "hot" and "cold" balance and imbalance as cause of health and illness	Some use amulets as a shield from witchcraft or as good luck pieces Catholics substitute religious medals and other items
African American	Illness classified as: 　Natural — affected by forces of nature without adequate protection, e.g., cold air, pollution, food, and water 　Unnatural — evil influences, e.g., witchcraft, voodoo, hoodoo, hex, fix, rootwork; symptoms often associated with eating Believe serious illness sent by God as punishment, e.g., parents punished by illness or death of child Believe serious illness can be avoided May resist health care because illness is "will of God"	Self-care and folk medicine very prevalent Folk therapies usually religious in origin Attempt home remedies first; poorer people do not seek help until illness serious Usually seek help from: 　"Old lady" — woman in community with a common knowledge of herbs; consults regarding pediatric care 　Spiritualist — has received gift from God for healing incurable diseases or solving personal problems; strongly based in Christianity 　Priest (voodoo priest/priestess) — most powerful healer 　Root doctor — meets need for herbs, oils, candles, and ointments Prayer is common means for prevention and treatment
Haitian	Illnesses have supernatural or natural origin Supernatural illnesses are caused by angry voodoo spirits, enemies, or the dead, especially deceased ancestors Natural illnesses are based on conceptions of natural causation: 　Irregularities of blood volume, flow, purity, viscosity, color and/or temperature (hot/cold) 　Gas (*gaz*) 　Movement and consistency of mother's milk 　Hot/cold imbalance in the body 　Bone displacement 　Movement of diseases Health is maintained by good dietary and hygienic habits	Health is a personal responsibility Foods have properties of "hot"/"cold" and "light"/"heavy" and must be in harmony with one's life cycle and bodily states Natural illnesses are treated by home remedies first Supernatural illness treated by healers: voodoo priest *(houngan)* or priestess *(mambo)*, midwife *(fam saj)*, and herbalist or leaf doctor *(dokte fey)* Amulets and prayer used to protect against illness due to curses or willed by evil people
Hispanic American 　**Mexican-American (Latino, Chicano, Raza-Latino)**	Health beliefs have strong religious association Believe in body imbalance as a cause of illness, especially imbalance between *caliente* (hot) and *frio* (cold) or "wet" and "dry" Some maintain good health is a result of "good luck" — a reward for good behavior	Seek help from *curandero* or *curandera* especially in rural areas Curandero(a) receives his/her position by birth, apprenticeship, or a "calling" via dream or vision Treatments involve use of herbs, rituals, and religious artifacts Practice for severe illness — make promises, visit shrines, offer medals and candles, offer prayers

Family relationships	Communication	Comments
Family is highly valued with strong family ties	Immigrants and older persons may not be able to speak or understand English	Tend to have a fatalistic outlook on life
Multigenerational family structure common, often with collateral members as well		Believe time and providence will solve all
Personal interests are subordinated to family interests and needs		
Members avoid any behavior that would bring shame on the family		
Strong kinship bonds in extended family; members come to aid of others in crisis	Alert to any evidence of discrimination	High level of caution and distrust of majority group
Less likely to view illness as a burden	Place importance on nonverbal behavior	Social anxiety related to tradition of humiliation, oppression, and loss of dignity
Augmented families common (unrelated persons living in same household)	May use nonstandard English or "black English"	Will elect to retain dignity rather than seek care if values are compromised
Place strong emphasis on work and ambition	Use "testing" behaviors to assess personnel in health care situations before seeking active care	Strong sense of peoplehood
Sex-role sharing among parents	Best to use simple, direct, but caring approach	High incidence of poverty
		African American minister a strong influence in black community
		Visits by family minister are sought, expected, and valued in helping to cope with illness and suffering
Maintenance of family reputation is paramount	Recent immigrants and older persons may speak only Haitian creole	Will use biomedical and ethnomedical (folk) systems simultaneously
Lineal authority supreme; children in a subordinate position in family hierarchy	May prefer family/friends to act as translators and confidants	Resistant to dietary and work restrictions
Children valued for parental social security in old age and expected to contribute to family welfare at an early age	Often smile and nod in agreement when do not understand	Adherence to prescribed treatments directly related to perceived severity of illness
Children viewed as "gifts from god" and treated with indulgence and affection	Quiet and gentle communication style and lack of assertiveness lead health care providers to falsely believe they comprehend health teaching and are compliant	
	Will not ask questions if health care provider is busy or rushed	
Traditionally men considered breadwinners, women homemakers	May use nonstandard English	High degree of modesty — often a deterrent to seeking medical care
Males are considered big and strong (*macho*)	Most bilingual; many only speak Spanish	Youngsters often reluctant to share communal showers in schools
Strong kinship; extended families include *compadres* (godparents) established by ritual kinship	May have a strong preference for native language and revert to it in times of stress	Relaxed concept of time — may be late for appointments
Children valued highly and desired, taken everywhere with family		Magicoreligious practices common
		May view hospital as place to go to die

Continued.

TABLE 6-5 — cont'd

Cultural Characteristics Related to Health Care

Cultural group	Health beliefs	Health and diet practices
Hispanic American Mexican-American — cont'd	Illness prevented by performing properly, eating proper foods, and working proper amount of time; accomplished through prayer, wearing religious medals or amulets, and sleeping with relics at home Illness is a punishment from God for wrongdoing, forces of nature, and the supernatural	prayers Adhere to "hot" and "cold" food prescriptions and prohibitions for prevention and treatment of illness
Puerto Rican	Subscribe to the "hot-cold" theory of causation of illness Believe some illness caused by evil spirits and forces	Infrequent use of health care systems Seek folk healers — use of herbs, rituals Consult spiritualist medium for mental disorders *Santeria* is system and practitioners are called *santeros* Treatments classified as "hot" or "cold"
Cuban-American	Prevention and good nutrition are related to good health	Diligent users of the medical model, in part because of aggressive public health practices on the island prior to and after the revolution Eclectic health-seeking practices, including preventive measures, extensive use of the medical model, and, in some instances, folk medicine of both religious and nonreligious origins; home remedies; in many instances seek assistance of *santeros* (Afro-Cuban healers) and spiritualists to complement medical treatment Nutrition is important; parents show overconcern with eating habits of their children and spend a considerable part of the budget on food; traditional Cuban diet is rich in meat and starch; consumption of fresh vegetables added in U.S.

Native American (numerous tribes)	Believe health is state of harmony with nature and universe
	Respect of bodies through proper management
	All disorders believed to have aspects of supernatural
	Violation of a restriction or prohibition thought to cause illness
	Fear of witchcraft
	May carry objects believed to guard against witchcraft
	Theology and medicine strongly interwoven
		Medicine persons:
		  Altruistic persons who must use powers in purely positive ways
		  Persons capable of both good and evil — perform negative acts against enemies
		  Diviner-diagnosticians — diagnose but do not have powers or skill to implement medical treatment
		  Specialists — use herbs and curative but nonsacred medical procedures
		  Medicine persons — use herbs and ritual
		  Singers — cure by the power of their song obtained from supernatural beings, effect cures by laying on of hands

From Whaley LF and Wong DL: *Nursing care of infants and children,* ed 4, St. Louis, 1991, Mosby—Year Book.

Family relationships	Communication	Comments
Many homes contain shrines with statues and pictures of saints		
Family usually large and home centered — the core of existence Father has complete authority in family — family provider and decision-maker Wife and children subordinate to father Children valued — seen as a gift from God Children taught to obey and respect parents; corporal punishment to ensure obedience	May use nonstandard English Spanish speaking or bilingual Strong sense of family privacy — may view questions regarding family as impudent	Relaxed sense of time Pay little attention to *exact* time of day Suspicious and fearful of hospitals
Strong family ties with mother and father kinships Children supported and assisted by parents long after becoming adults Elderly cared for at home	Most are bilingual (English/Spanish) except for segments of the senior population	In less than 30 years Cubans have been able to obtain a higher standard of living than other Hispanic groups in U.S. Have been able to retain many of their former social institutions: bilingual and private schools, clinics, social clubs, the family as an extended network of support, etc. Many do not feel discriminated against nor harbor feelings of inferiority with respect to Anglo-Americans or "mainstream" population
Extended family structure — usually includes relatives from both sides of family Elder members assume leadership roles	Most continue to speak their Indian language as well as English Nonverbal communication	Time orientation — present Respect for age Going to hospital associated with illness or disease; therefore may not seek prenatal care since pregnancy viewed as natural process

Sources: Bloch, 1983; Chen-Louie, 1983; Chow, 1976; Char, 1981; Ehling, 1981; Greathouse and Miller, 1981; Hashizume and Takano, 1983; Holland and Sweeney, 1985; Hollingsworth, Brown, and Brooten, 1980; Jacques, 1976; Lacay, 1981; Monrroy, 1983; Orque, 1983a, 1983b; Sodetaini-Shebata, 1981.

nonverbal behaviors. Verbal behaviors include language, vocabulary, grammatical structure, voice qualities, intonation, speed, pronunciation, and silence. Nonverbal behaviors include touch, facial expression, eye movement, posture, personal space, and distance.

Determining what language is spoken at home is an important part of a cultural assessment. Find out how well the client understands written and spoken English, since this is important for both verbal interactions and for giving the client written information such as health education pamphlets. Even when the client speaks English, colloquialisms may be confusing. For example, "bad" may have a negative connotation for one group and a more positive connotation for another group. Certain groups may use lay terms such as "high blood" for hypertension and "low blood" for anemia. These may vary among different ethnic groups, so confirm your understanding of the term with the client.

Also be aware of cultural norms related to the way you address clients, for example, whether you address them by their first name or use more formal titles. Proper forms of address may vary according to ethnic or regional groups.

Nonverbal communication may also have different meanings in different cultures. In North American middle-class culture looking directly at the person with whom you are speaking is important. However, in many cultures (Asian, Native American, Indochinese, Arab, Appalachian) looking directly at another person may be a sign of disrespect or aggression. Touch also has many different interpretations by different cultural groups. Some groups, such as those of Mediterranean descent, use touch to communicate feelings, while other groups see touch as an invasion of privacy. Many Asian groups believe that the head is the most sacred part of the body; therefore, obtain permission before touching the client's head. The feet are the lowest part of the body so showing the bottom of your shoe or pointing your toe at the client is disrespectful.

Family relationships. Attitudes toward family structure and family roles and relationships have been traditionally mediated by cultural considerations. However, over the past 20 years, cultural differences related to families, once a defining characteristic of different cultural groups, are rapidly changing. Our society has become highly mobile and more integrated, tearing down barriers that previously kept family norms intact within subcultures. The media have focused our attention on alternate family arrangements and practices, making them more familiar and thus acceptable.

As of 25 years ago, the concept of the nuclear family was predominant. Typically, young men and women married someone who was raised within 25 miles of them. People married people with whom they shared cultural or group affiliations. Couples tended to share the same race, religion, and socioeconomic status. They had children, and the mother provided child care while the father earned the income. They tended to stay married for life and they tried to transmit these values to their children. Because of mass communication, easy access to cheap and fast transportation, and economic changes promoting urbanization, today's young people often move far away from their parents. More young people attend college and use this opportunity to migrate elsewhere. Far from the daily influences of their families, new group affiliations develop based on common interests, education, and jobs. There has been an increased incidence and acceptance of divorce, dual-income families, single-parent families, teenage parents, and involvement of fathers in child care. The nuclear family is not nearly as prevalent now, and neither are culturally mediated family practices that used to distinguish one cultural group from another.

This is not to say that cultural differences in attitudes toward family structure and role no longer exist. Rather, they cannot be taken for granted. Therefore, avoid making any assumptions about the relationship between family and culture and take a value-free approach to assessing family dimensions, which can be so important to health and well-being.

A neutral starting point in assessing the client's family is to determine the family structure. Use a simple family tree or family diagram, sometimes called a **genogram,** to establish who the members of the family are and how the client fits in. Particularly with individuals who live far from their natural families, extend the gen-

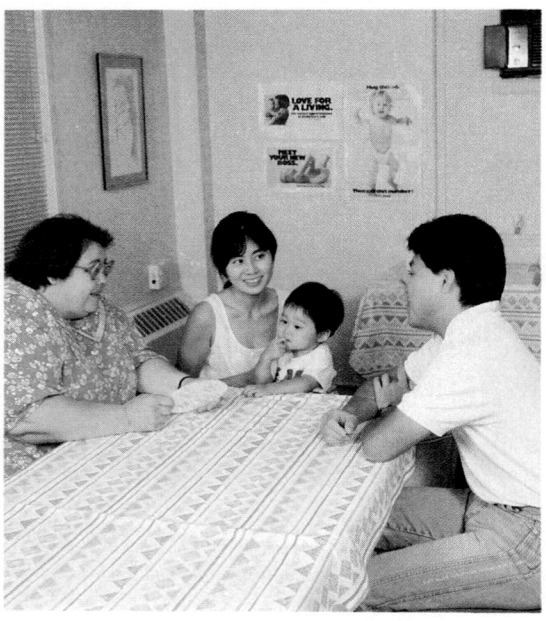

ogram concept to a broader tool known as an **ecogram.** This tool maps the network of the client's significant others, including friends, neighbors, peers, and associates who may be more important to the client's health and well-being than are actual family members.

Once the structure is clear, explore roles and relationships to determine whom the client is attached to and how the dynamics of various relationships work. Relationships, both within families and in broader associations, can be close or distant, dependent or hostile. In each relationship, the sharing of power and decision making, as well as approaches to problem solving, can vary widely. Assess communication patterns and willingness to express feelings and offer support. Individuality may be submerged or fostered. Many tools exist to provide for an orderly assessment of these roles and functions. A familiar one that assesses the person's satisfaction with relationships in the immediate family (and is both reliable and valid and clinically useful) is the Family APGAR (see box below).

Keep in mind that despite the rapid change in family structure and function associated with distinct cultural groups, cultural considerations remain very important for many individuals.

Religious practices. Religion has an influence on the life-styles of most cultures and may affect health care practices. Most religions have rituals or ceremonies that mark life cycle stages such as birth, entrance into adulthood, marriage, and death. Religions may have certain dietary restrictions such as prohibitions against eating pork (Jewish and Muslim religions) or abstaining from specific foods on certain days (Roman Catholic). Religions may prohibit certain types of health care interventions such as the administration of blood (Jehovah's Witnesses) or use of medications containing caffeine or made from pork products. Table 6-4 describes a variety of religious beliefs that may affect nursing care. Remember that the strictness of adherence to these rules will vary with individuals and subgroups within the religion.

Religious beliefs may influence a client's perception

FAMILY APGAR

Definition

Adaptation is the use of intrafamilial and extrafamilial resources for problem-solving when family equilibrium is stressed during a crisis.

Partnership is the sharing of decision-making and nurturing responsibilities by family members.

Growth is the physical and emotional maturation and self-fulfillment that is achieved by family members through mutual support and guidance.

Affection is the caring or loving relationship that exists among family members.

Resolve is the commitment to devote time to other members of the family for physical and emotional nurturing. It also usually involves a decision to share wealth and space.

Functions measured by the Family APGAR

How resources are shared, or the degree to which a member is satisfied with the assistance received when family resources are needed.

How decisions are shared, or the member's satisfaction with mutuality in family communication and problem-solving.

How nurturing is shared, or the member's satisfaction with the freedom available within the family to change roles and attain physical and emotional growth or maturation.

How emotional experiences are shared, or the member's satisfaction with the intimacy and emotional interaction that exists in the family.

How time (and space and money) is shared, or the member's satisfaction with the time commitment that has been made to the family by its members.

Relevant open-ended questions

How have family members aided each other in time of need?

In what way have family members received help or assistance from friends and community agencies?

How do family members communicate with each other about such matters as vacations, finances, medical care, large purchases, and personal problems?

How have family members changed during the past years?

How has this change been accepted by family members?

In what ways have family members aided each other in growing or developing independent life-styles?

How have family members reacted to your desires for change?

How have members of your family responded to emotional expressions such as affection, love, sorrow, or anger?

How do members of your family share time, space, and money?

Modified from Smilkstein G: The Family APGAR: a proposal for a family function test and its use by physicians, *J Fam Pract* 6:1231-1239, 1978.

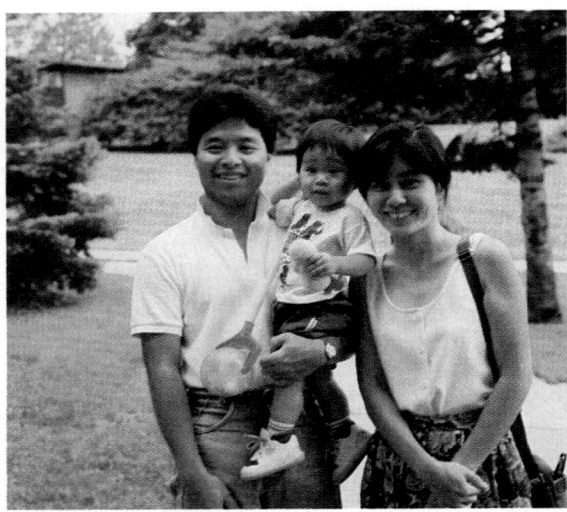

of the cause of an illness, its severity, and the type of healer required. The religion and religiosity of the individual determine the role that religious faith plays in the recovery process. In many instances religiosity also affects the response to a specific treatment and the process of healing. Although cultural heritage and religion may be interrelated, do not assume that membership in a particular ethnic or cultural group is equated with membership in a specific religion. For example, although many Mexican Americans are Catholic, do not assume that your Mexican American client is Catholic and in a time of crisis offer to contact a priest for support. This approach, although well-intentioned, may add to the client's stress and sense of frustration. Gathering initial information about the client's religious affiliation and the role that religious beliefs and practices play in health and illness helps avoid mistaken assumptions and provides information that is important to the client's care.

Health and illness behaviors. Cultures also influence the client's attitudes toward health, response to illness, and even experience of symptoms such as pain. Individuals learn about health behaviors through socialization in their families. Beliefs about illness and alternative types of health providers have been discussed in the section on beliefs. Specific illness behaviors also are culturally determined. Zola (1966) examined the differences in symptoms that caused clients to seek health care by a physician. In his comparison of diagnostically matched clients from different ethnic groups, he found that the definition of an illness and the pattern of response to symptoms varied according to ethnic group. The experience of pain is another symptom that is strongly influenced by culture.

Pain. Pain is among the most common symptoms in clinical practice, yet it is not purely a neurophysiological response. Pain is influenced by social, psychological, and cultural factors.

Culture influences both pain intensity and pain tolerance. Culture determines a person's attitudes toward pain and beliefs about it. Emotions associated with the context in which pain is experienced can have a powerful effect on how pain is felt. Sometimes soldiers are wounded in battle and do not realize it until afterward. In some cultures, meditation or religious trances dissipate the sensation of pain, as in the firewalkers of Sri Lanka, who are apparently oblivious to the expected intensity of the pain they experience. Other cultures value the ability to withstand pain without complaint or physical manifestations, as in the case of certain American Indian and African tribes, who demonstrate their adulthood by withstanding painful stimuli.

It is difficult to separate culturally determined pain from pain that is mediated by neurological mechanisms. Nurses often encounter the so-called "placebo effect," in which an inactive drug relieves suffering. A simple *belief* in the effectiveness of the placebo can release endorphins in the brain, actually providing physiological pain relief.

Culture also determines when pain is abnormal, requiring medical attention and treatment. The extent to which pain is considered a normal part of life also affects a person's willingness to withstand it. Studies show, for instance, that Polish women are far more able to accept the pain associated with childbirth than their American counterparts, who have greater access to anesthesia during labor.

Each culture has its own language of distress, which includes facial expressions, changes in activity, sounds, and words describing feeling. These norms determine acceptable ways clients express pain to others. For example, Zbrowski (1952) in a classic study found that Italian-Americans tended to dramatize their pain as a means of allaying anxiety and dissipating the pain. Irish-Americans, by contrast, were more reticent about their bodily complaints. Villarruel and Ortiz de Montellano (1992) identified themes related to the cultural meanings of pain and pain-related behaviors in Mesoamerican cultures (with particular reference to Mexican-Americans).

Pain is a subjective sensation that has physiological, cultural, and emotional components. The actual cause or intensity of pain is difficult to assess. In treating pain remember that it is the client's experience of pain, as the client feels it, that determines how you treat it. Carefully assess, however, cultural considerations that affect a client's ability or willingness to report pain as a sign of illness, as well as inclination to seek treatment, because of these implications for ascertaining the person's actual degree of illness.

TABLE 6-6

Distribution of Selected Genetic Traits and Disorders by Population or Ethnic Group

Ethnic or population group	Genetic or multifactorial disorder present in relatively high frequency	Ethnic or population group	Genetic or multifactorial disorder present in relatively high frequency
Åland Islanders	Ocular albinism (Forsius-Erikkson type)	Gypsies (Czech)	Congenital glaucoma
		Hopi Indians	Tyrosinase positive albinism
Amish	Limb-girdle muscular dystrophy (IN—Adams, Allen counties)	Iceland	Phenylketonuria
	Ellis-van Creveld (PA—Lancaster county)	Irish	Phenylketonuria Neural tube defects
	Pyruvate kinase deficiency (OH—Mifflin county)	Japanese	Acatalasemia Cleft lip/palate Oguchi's disease
	Hemophilia B (PA—Holmes county)		
Armenians	Familial Mediterranean fever Familial paroxysmal polyserositis	Jews *Ashkenazi*	Tay-Sachs disease (infantile) Niemann-Pick disease (infantile) Gaucher's disease (adult type) Familial dysautonomia (Riley-Day syndrome) Bloom's syndrome Torsion dystonia Factor XI (PTA) deficiency
Blacks (African)	Sickle cell disease Hemoglobin C disease Hereditary persistence of hemoglobin F G-6-PD deficiency, African type Lactase deficiency, adult β-Thalassemia	*Sephardi*	Familial Mediterranean fever Ataxia-telangiectasia (Morocco) Cystinuria (Libya) Glycogen storage disease III (Morocco)
Burmese	Hemoglobin E disease	Lapps	Congenital dislocation of hip
Chinese	Alpha thalassemia G-6-PD deficiency, Chinese type Lactase deficiency, adult	Lebanese	Dyggve-Melchoir-Clausen syndrome
Costa Rican	Malignant osteopetrosis	Mediterranean people (Italians, Greeks)	G-6-PD deficiency, Mediterranean type β-Thalassemia Familial Mediterranean fever
Druze	Alkaptonuria		
English	Cystic fibrosis Hereditary amyloidosis, type III		
Eskimos	Congenital adrenal hyperplasia Pseudocholinesterase deficiency Methemoglobinemia	Navaho Indians	Ear anomalies
		Nova Scotia Acadians	Niemann-Pick disease, type D
Finns	Congenital nephrosis Generalized amyloidosis syndrome, V Polycystic liver disease Retinoschisis Aspartylglycosaminuria Diastrophic dwarfism	Oriental	Dubin-Johnson syndrome (Iran) Ichthyosis vulgaris (Iraq, India) Werdnig-Hoffmann disease (Karaite Jews) G-6-PD deficiency, Mediterranean type
French Canadians (Quebec)	Tyrosinemia Morquio's syndrome		

From Whaley LD and Wong DL: Nursing care of infants and children, ed. 4, St. Louis, 1991, Mosby—Year Book.
Data from Cohen FL: Clinical genetics in nursing practice, Philadelphia, 1984, JB Lippincott Co., pp. 23-24; Damon A: Race, ethnic group and disease, Soc Biol 16:69, 1969; Der Kaloustian VM, Maffah J, and Loiselet J: Genetic diseases in Lebanon, Am J Med Genet 7:187, 1980; Goodman RM: Genetic disorders among the Jewish people, Baltimore, 1979, Johns Hopkins University Press; McKusick V: Mendelian inheritance in man, ed. 8, Baltimore, 1988, Johns Hopkins University Press; Tamot B: Genetic polymorphisms and diseases in man, New York, 1974, Academic Press, Inc.; Stanbury JB: The metabolic basis of inherited disease, New York, 1983, McGraw-Hill, Inc.; Ferak V, Gencik A, and Gencikova A: Population genetical aspects of primary congenital glaucoma, Hum Genet 61:193, 1982.

Continued.

TABLE 6-6—cont'd

Distribution of Selected Genetic Traits and Disorders by Population or Ethnic Group

Ethnic or population group	Genetic or multifactorial disorder present in relatively high frequency	Ethnic or population group	Genetic or multifactorial disorder present in relatively high frequency
	Phenylketonuria (Yemen) Metachromatic leukodystrophy (Habbanite Jews, Saudi Arabia)	Scots	Phenylketonuria Cystic fibrosis Hereditary amyloidosis, type III
Polish	Phenylketonuria	Thai	Lactase deficiency, adult Hemoglobin E disease
Polynesians	Clubfoot	Zuni Indians	Tyrosinase positive albinism
Portugese	Joseph's disease		
Scandinavians (Norwegians, Swedes, Danes)	Cholestasis-lymphedema (Norwegians) Sjögren's syndrome (Swedes) Krabbe's disease Phenylketonuria		

Other Variables to Consider

Heredity. Information concerning ethnic, cultural, or racial heritage is also important for assessing the client's susceptibility to specific genetic disorders. Because of intermarriage within a relatively narrow range of ethnic, geographic, or religious groups, certain traits are passed on that place members of those groups at risk for genetic disorders. Table 6-6 provides an overview of disorders and genetic traits for a variety of population or ethnic groups. Knowledge of these susceptibilities is important for screening clients for problems, providing interventions to avoid complications related to problems, and counseling clients who are considering having children and are concerned about the risks of passing on such traits.

Socioeconomic status. Virtually all cultures are stratified. That is, they contain the range of socioeconomic classes. When members of a cultural group can be called a minority group (defined as a group receiving unequal treatment from the dominant group), socioeconomic characteristics can have implications for health and health care.

Public health research shows that people in lower socioeconomic groups have the highest rates of death and disease resulting from virtually every health problem. Thus, although speaking of "a culture of poverty" is incorrect, socioeconomic status is an important predictor of health and disease. Because of the way health care systems are structured, particularly in the United

States, people in poverty make less use of the health care system; their choice of providers, as well as their criterion for seeking health care, is different from the frequency and criterion associated with more affluent citizens. Therefore, an awareness of a client's economic status has implications for care.

Health care in North America. North Americans place a high premium on their health. They pay a large percentage of their national wealth for health care, and in recent years they have devoted more energy and resources to preventive health care through proper diet, more exercise, and the avoidance of health hazards. Canadians spend about 9% of their gross national product on health care, and Americans spend about 12%. The United States has a highly stratified free-enterprise approach to health care. Consequently, affluent people buy a great deal of health care, while those in the lower socioeconomic groups have far more restricted access to quality health care. Canada offers all its citizens comprehensive health insurance that allows clients access to the same quality of care regardless of income level.

Two common measures of national health are infant mortality and longevity. Although both countries rank very high in longevity (life expectancy for American men is 72 and women is 79, life expectancy for Canadian men is 73 and women 80), there is considerable difference in infant mortality rates. Canada has an infant mortality rate of 7.2/1000 while the United States has an infant mortality rate of 10.3/1000 (U.S. Bureau of the Census, World Population Profile, 1991). This ranks Canada in 6th place while the United States ranks 22nd among the nations of the world in infant mortality (National Center for Health Statistics, 1989). Although both countries have made progress in relation to birth control, spread of infectious diseases, and better nutrition, Canada's national health care program provides all citizens with access to care. The United States, however, suffers from restricted access to wellness-oriented health care and inconsistent prenatal care. This lack of access to health care results in a much higher prevalence of very low birth weight infants, accounting for the higher infant mortality in the United States.

ASSESSMENT CONSIDERATIONS FOR MAJOR CULTURAL GROUPS IN NORTH AMERICA

Tables 6-3 through 6-6 describe characteristics of different cultural groups related to health care. Note that these are generalizations and are meant as guidelines only. Cultural traits are not uniform and static. How important cultural influences are to health care concerns varies according to the degree of enculturation and acculturation, the type of problem, and the con-

---

CULTURAL ASSESSMENT GUIDE

Health beliefs and practices

How does the client define health and illness?

Are there particular methods used to help maintain health, such as hygiene and self-care practices?

Are there particular methods being used by the client for treatment of illness?

What is the attitude toward preventive health measures such as immunizations?

Are there health topics that the client may be particularly sensitive to or that are considered taboo?

What are the attitudes toward mental illness, pain, handicapping conditions, chronic disease, death, and dying?

Is there a person in the family responsible for various health-related decisions, such as where to go, whom to see, and what advice to follow?

Religious influences and special rituals

Is there a religion that the client adheres to?

Is there a significant person that the client looks to for guidance and support?

Are there any special religious practices or beliefs that may affect health care when the client is ill or dying?

What events, rituals, and ceremonies are considered important within the life cycle, such as birth, baptism, puberty, marriage, and death?

Language and communication

What language is spoken in the home?

How well does the client understand English, both spoken or written?

Are there special signs of demonstrating respect or disrespect?

Is touch involved in communication?

Are there culturally appropriate ways to enter and leave situations, including greetings, farewells, and convenient times to make a home visit?

Parenting styles and role of family

Who makes the decisions in the family?

What is the composition of the family, how many generations are considered to be a single family, and which relatives comprise the family unit?

When the marriage custom is practiced, what is the attitude about separation and divorce?

What is the role of and attitude toward children in the family?

When do children need to be disciplined or punished, and how is this done (if physical means are used, in what way)?

Do the parents demonstrate physical affection toward their children and each other?

What major events are important to the family, and how are they celebrated?

Are there special beliefs and practices surrounding conception, pregnancy, childbirth, lactation, and child rearing?

Dietary practices

What does the family like to eat, and does everyone in the family have similar tastes in food?

Who is responsible for food preparation?

Are any foods forbidden by the culture, or are some foods a cultural requirement in observance of a rite or ceremony?

How is food prepared and consumed?

Are there specific beliefs or preferences concerning food, such as those believed to cause or to cure an illness?

From Stulc DM: The family as bearer of culture. In Cookfair JN: *Nursing process and practice in the community*, St. Louis, 1990, Mosby–Year Book.

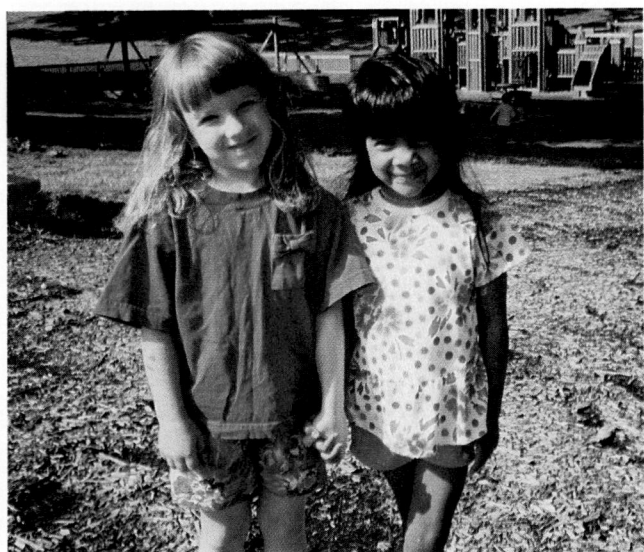

gruence with the health care culture. Knowledge of cultural factors provides a context for understanding behaviors and designing care to meet the client's (or family's) needs. A cultural assessment does not require exhaustive information on every element of the culture. Make sure to identify major values, beliefs, and behaviors related to particular health concerns. Tailor actual assessments and interventions to the individual client and family. Also avoid making assumptions about cultural beliefs and behaviors without receiving validation from the client. This assessment involves a shared negotiation between you and the client in which each person is equal in bringing important and relevant information to the interview. The box on p. 179 provides guidelines for material to cover in a cultural assessment.

GLOSSARY

acculturation Process of adapting to a culture different from the one a person was encultured in

culture Complex, integrated system that includes knowledge, beliefs, skills, art, morals, law, customs, and any other acquired habits and capabilities of a group of people

ecogram Diagram that maps the network of significant others, including friends, neighbors, peers, and associates

enculturation Process of acquiring one's cultural identity as it is transmitted by the previous generation

ethnic group Group of persons with shared traits such as common national or regional origin and linguistic, ancestral, and physical characteristics

ethnocentrism Tendency to view people unconsciously by using one's group and one's own customs as the standard for all judgments

genogram Diagram that depicts family relationships over at least three generations

minority group Any group that receives different and unequal treatment from others in the larger group or society and whose members see themselves as victims of discrimination

race Classification of human beings on the basis of physical characteristics such as skin pigmentation, head form, or stature that are transmitted through generations

subculture Group of persons within a culture with one or more shared traits

BIBLIOGRAPHY

AAN expert panel on culturally competent nursing care: AAN expert panel report: culturally competent health care, *Nurs Outlook,* 40:277-283, 1992.

American Nurses Association: *Cultural diversity in the nursing curriculum: a guide for implementation* (ANA #G-171:11), Kansas City, 1986, American Nurses Association.

Boyle JS, Andrews MM: *Transcultural concepts in nursing care,* Boston, 1989, Little, Brown.

DeSantis L, Thomas JT: Health education and the immigrant Haitian mother: cultural insights for community health nurses, *Public Health Nurs* 9:87-96, 1992.

Fuchs VR, Hahn JS: How does Canada do it? A comparison of expenditures for physicians' services in the United States and Canada, *N Engl J Med* 323:884-890, 1990.

Giger JN, Davidhizar RE: Transcultural nursing: assessment and intervention, St. Louis, 1991, Mosby—Year Book.

Hartog J, Hartog EA: Cultural aspects of health and illness behavior in hospitals, *West J Med* 139:911-916, 1983.

Hautman MA: Folk health and illness beliefs, *Nurse Pract* 4:4, 1979.

Health Resources and Service Administration: *Health status of minorities and low income groups,* DHHS pub. no. HRS-P-DV 85-1, Washington, DC, 1985, US Government Printing Office.

Helman C: *Culture, health and illness,* ed 2, London, 1990, John Wright and Sons.

Henderson G, Primeaux M: *Transcultural health care,* Menlo Park, Calif, 1981, Addison-Wesley.

Kleinman A, Eisenberg L, Good B: Culture, illness and care: clinical lessons from anthropologic and cross-cultural research, *Ann Intern Med* 88:251-258, 1978.

Kluckhohn F: Dominant and variant value orientations. In Brink PJ, editor: *Transcultural nursing: a book of readings,* Englewood Cliffs, NJ, 1976, Prentice-Hall.

Krause N, Goldenhar LM: Acculturation and psychological distress in three groups of elderly Hispanics, *J Gerontol* 47:S279-S288, 1992.

Leininger MM: *Transcultural nursing: concepts, theories and practices,* New York, 1978, John Wiley & Sons.

Martin MM, Henry M: Cultural relativity and poverty, *Public Health Nurs* 6:28-34, 1989.

Morse JM, Young DE, Swartz L: Cree Indian healing practices and western health care: a comparative analysis. *Social Science and Medicine* 32:1361-1366, 1991.

National Center for Health Statistics, *Prevention profile, Health United States,* 1991, Hyattsville, Md., 1992, Public Health Service.

Olness K: Cultural issues in primary pediatric care. In Hoekelman R, and others: *Primary pediatric care,* ed 2, St Louis, 1992, Mosby—Year Book.

Overfield T: Biological variation: concepts from physical anthropology. In Henderson G, Primeaux M, editors: *Transcultural health care,* Menlo Park, Calif, 1981, Addison-Wesley.

Raugh VA, Wasserman GA, Brunelli SA: *J Am Acad Child Adolesc Psychiatry* 29:375-381, 1990.

Rogler LH, Cortes DE, Malgady RG: Acculturation and mental health status among hispanics, *Am Psychol* 46:585-605, 1991.

Smith LS: Ethnic differences in knowledge of sexually transmitted diseases in North American Black and Mexican-American migrant farmworkers, *Res Nurs Health* 11:51-58, 1988.

Snow LF: Folk medical beliefs and their implications for the care of patients: a review based on studies of black Americans. In Henderson G, Primeaux M, editors: *Transcultural health care,* Menlo Park, Calif, 1981, Addison-Wesley.

Snow LF, Johnson SM: Folklore, food, female reproductive cycle, *Ecol Food Nut* 7:41-49, 1978.

Spector R: *Cultural diversity in health and illness,* ed 3, Norwalk, Conn, 1991, Appleton-Lange.

Stulc DM: The family as bearer of culture. In Cookfair JN, editor: *Nursing process and practice in the community,* St Louis, 1990, Mosby—Year Book.

Syme SL: Social determinants of disease, *Ann Clin Res* 19:44-52, 1987.

Thierderman SB: Ethnocentrism: a barrier to effective health care, *Nurse Pract* 11:53-59, 1986.

Tripp-Reimer T: Cultural assessment. In Bellack J, Edlund B, editors: *Nursing assessment and diagnosis,* Boston, 1992, Jones and Bartlett.

Tripp-Reimer T, Brink PJ, Saunders JM: Cultural assessment: content and process, *Nurs Outlook* 32:78-82, 1984.

US Bureau of the Census: *Statistical abstract of the United States: 1992,* ed 112, Washington, DC, US Government Printing Office.

US Department of Health and Human Services. Public Health Service. *Healthy people 2000: National health promotion and disease prevention objectives,* 1990, DHHS Publication No. 91-50213, Washington, DC.

van der Horst M: Canada's health care system provides lessons for NPs: 1992, *Nurse Pract* 17:44-60, 1992.

Villarruel AM, Ortiz de Montellano B: Culture and pain: a Meso-american perspective, *Adv Nurs Sci* 15:21-32, 1992.

Whaley LF, Wong DL: *Nursing care of infants and children,* ed 4, St Louis, 1991, Mosby—Year Book.

Zbrowski M: *People in pain,* San Francisco, 1969, Jossey-Bass.

Zbrowoski: Cultural components in response to pain, *Sociol Issues* 8:16-30, 1952.

Zola IK: Culture and symptoms: an analysis of patients presenting complaints, *Am Sociol Rev* 31:615-630, 1966.

*U*nit III, Physical Assessment, contains 16 chapters that present detailed orientations to physical assessment techniques and tools for assessment of body systems and regions. All physical areas of the body are covered in detail and all chapters contain information about regional health histories for the system or region as well as examples of recording the history and physical findings for the system or body region.

Physical Assessment

CHAPTER 7

Assessment Techniques

PURPOSE OF EXAMINATION

The overall goal of the physical examination is to identify variations from the normal state. This information will then become a part of the client's database. The health assessment database consists of both subjective and objective information. Subjective information is the client's verbalized **perceptions** and interpretations. In the interview the history and review of systems provide subjective information. This information alerts the nurse to areas to be focused on during the examination. The nurse obtains objective information through the physical examination by observation or measurement of data with all the senses. This information is used to support the subjective information given by the client during the interview.

CONDUCTING THE EXAMINATION

Basic Principles

The examiner's goal is to conduct an efficient and complete examination that involves as little trauma and fatigue to the client as possible. Accomplishing this goal requires a consistent, systematic pattern of performing the examination. Following such a pattern will prevent omitting a step and possibly vital information. The nurse examiner must be thorough and exacting in the examination routine. With experience, he or she will develop an individual examination technique and sequence. However, the following six general principles will help to ensure that the examiner conducts a comprehensive examination in a logical order.

First, explain the procedures to the client at the beginning of the evaluation and restate them as the examination proceeds. Assist the client in appropriate positioning and warn the client of any uncomfortable maneuvers.

Second, use a head-to-toe approach. The head and face are examined before the genitals or feet because this sequence is generally more acceptable to the adult client.

Third, move from external to internal. Begin with observation, and then use instruments or perform digital examinations. Initial observations are general impressions such as the client's appearance. Later observations might involve using an instrument such as an otoscope to identify anatomical landmarks of the eardrum or **tympanic membrane**.

Fourth, examine normal or unaffected areas before observing abnormal areas or parts of the body where the client describes **symptoms**. The regions that are to be examined must be exposed completely to ensure an accurate finding. The examiner must be sensitive to a client's **anxiety** and possible embarrassment when certain areas of the body are exposed.

Fifth, observe for body **symmetry,** comparing one side to the other. Although minor asymmetry may be a normal finding, right to left differences in leg circumference or joint movement may be the first clue to other problems.

Sixth, perform the physical examination while standing on the client's right. This consistency of examiner position will help to locate anatomical landmarks while the examination is being performed.

Safety

Health care providers must be increasingly aware of the need to protect themselves and their clients from the risk of infection. They must be aware that whenever they come in close physical contact with clients, infection can be transmitted. Hand washing is one of the most effective methods of reducing the transmission of infection and must be done before and after any

---

SAFETY FIRST

The goal of **universal precautions** is that the health care provider avoid contact with all the client's body fluids. This approach involves wearing latex gloves whenever examining an area of the client's body (e.g., mouth, genitals) or obtaining a specimen (e.g., blood, sputum) when there is potential for contact with body fluids. Disposable specula and tongue blades must be available. Protective eyewear should be worn when dealing with secretions that can be passed through the air and might come in contact with the examiner's eye (for example, during suctioning). Protective clothing, such as a fully buttoned lab coat, a disposable gown, or a uniform, should be worn to reduce the risk of transmission of infectious organisms.

Risk of transmission of infection to the practitioner and to housekeeping and maintenance personnel can be reduced by proper disposal of any equipment that has come in contact with the client's body fluids. Needles should not be recapped. Needles and other sharp objects should be disposed of in a "sharps" container to avoid accidental puncture or incision wounds.

---

physical contact with a client during an examination (see box on the bottom of the left column).

Equipment Preparation for Health Assessment

Equipment needed in a comprehensive health assessment is shown in Figure 7-1. The examiner should keep all equipment within easy reach and place it out on a table before beginning the examination. In addition to the equipment shown in the figure, the examiner may use a thermometer and a visual acuity chart during a screening examination. The purpose of each piece of equipment will be discussed in detail in the various assessment chapters.

Examination Techniques

The four assessment techniques used in the physical examination are **inspection**, **percussion**, **palpation**, and **auscultation**. Positioning of the client is sometimes used as a fifth assessment technique. The examiner uses these techniques as an organizing framework for bringing the senses of sight, hearing, touch, and smell into focus. These techniques are explained further in the chapters that deal with their application to specific organs and systems.

Inspection. During inspection the examiner concentrates attention on a thorough and unhurried visualization of the client. Inspection also involves listening to any sounds coming from the client and being aware of any odors that may be present. The inexperienced examiner often moves too quickly to a "hands on" technique and may miss information that can be obtained only through careful observation. Up to 80% of diagnoses are based on data obtained from a history and inspection.

Lighting must be adequate for inspection. Either daylight or artificial light is suitable. **Tangential lighting** is a method of directing light from an adjustable lamp at a right angle to the area being observed. This technique produces shadows that are useful in assessing movements, such as abdominal pulsations or **precordial** movement.

Percussion. Percussion involves tapping on the surface of the skin. This tapping creates a vibration of underlying organs that produces sound. **Immediate or direct percussion** is the striking of a finger or hand directly against the body.

In **mediate (indirect) percussion** the middle finger of the dominant hand (plexor) is used to strike against the middle finger (pleximeter) of the other hand. Only the distal portion of the middle finger of the pleximeter hand is placed firmly against the skin. The middle finger is used to strike at, or immediately distal to, the

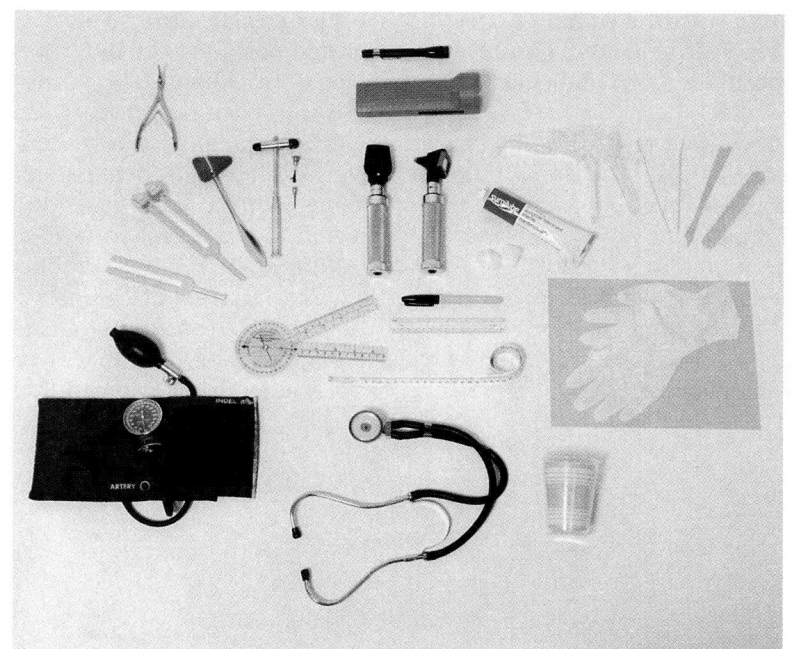

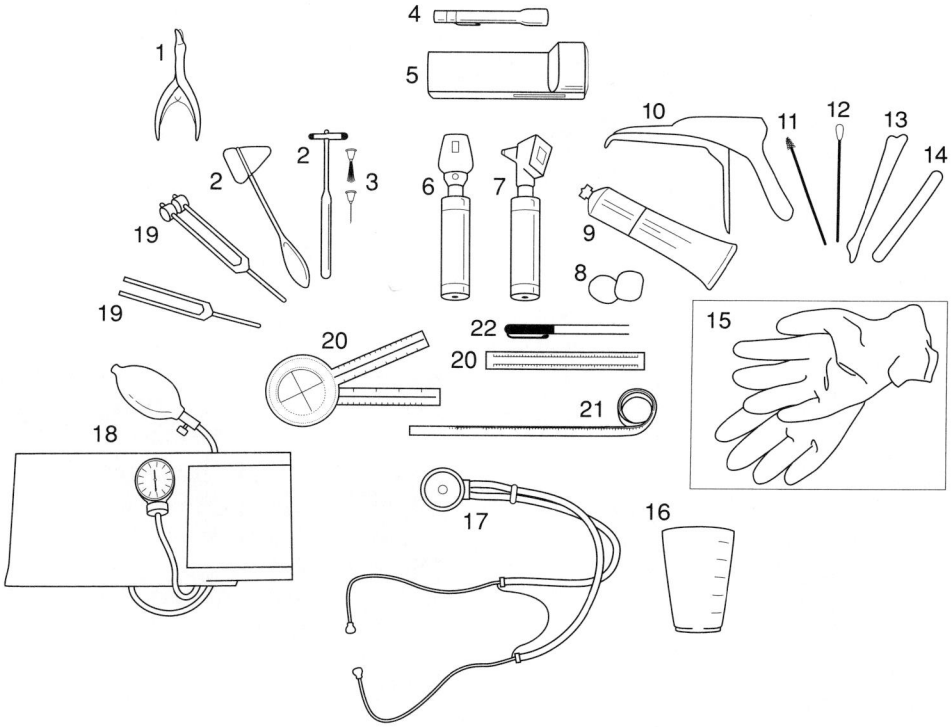

FIGURE 7-1 Equipment used during the physical examination (clockwise from upper left): 1. Nasal speculum, 2. reflex hammer (2 types shown), 3. sharp and dull end objects (for sensory exam), 4. penlight, 5. flashlight, 6. ophthalmoscope, 7. otoscope, 8. cotton balls, 9. lubricant, 10. disposable vaginal speculum, 11. cervical brush, 12. cotton-tip applicator, 13. cervical spatula, 14. tongue depressor, 15. disposable gloves, 16. specimen cup, 17. stethoscope, 18. sphygmomanometer, 19. tuning fork (2 types shown) and (*center*): 20. centimeter rulers (2 types shown), 21. tape measure, and 22. marking pen.

distal interphalangeal joint with the middle finger of the plexor hand. The blow is delivered crisply and sharply with the plexor positioned perpendicular to the pleximeter.

Wrist action controls the speed and force of a blow. The hand is flexed backward on the forearm and brought forward with a quick, snapping motion that follows a fast strike and rapid removal of the plexor to avoiding dampening the vibration (Figure 7-2). The fingernails of the plexor finger must be kept short to avoid cutting the skin of the pleximeter. The vibration produced through percussion involves only the tissue adjacent (3 to 5 cm) to the pleximeter.

Fist percussion involves striking with the hand in a fisted position. The blow is delivered with the lateral aspect of the hand. The purpose of this type of percussion is to elicit sensation by the vibration of the tissue, which stimulates pain or tenderness of organs (e.g., liver, kidneys). Fist percussion may be direct or indirect. When indirect fist percussion is used, the blow is delivered to the dorsal surface of the opposite hand.

Vibrating structures produce sound. The vibrations generate a series of compression waves in a medium that is capable of sound transmission. For example, solids, liquids, and gases that are sufficiently elastic to convert energy to motion can transmit sound. The exam-

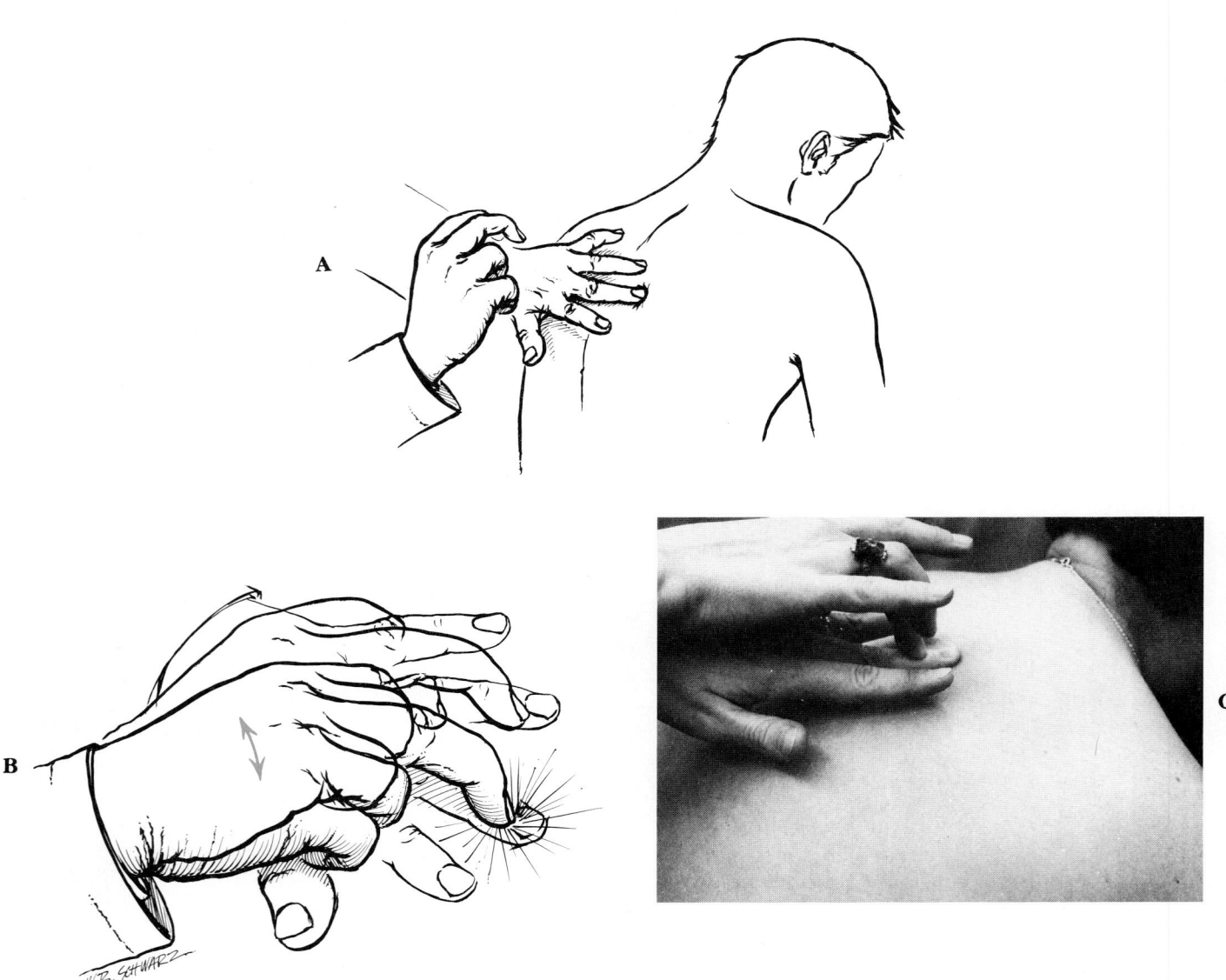

FIGURE 7-2 A, Positioning of the hands. **B,** Hand movement. **C,** Percussion of the posterior thorax.

TABLE 7-1

Sounds Produced by Percussion

Record of finding	Intensity	Pitch	Quality	Example of where sounds may be heard
Tympany	Loud	High	Drumlike	Gastric air bubble
Hyperresonance	Very loud	Very low	Booming	Air-filled lungs (e.g., in emphysema)
Resonance	Loud	Low	Hollow	Normal lung
Dullness	Moderate	Moderate	Thudlike	Liver
Flatness	Soft	High	Flat	Muscle

iner evaluates the following characteristics of percussion sounds: intensity, pitch, and quality (Table 7-1).

Intensity. **Intensity** refers to the loudness of sound. As a sound wave travels, air molecules are compressed and then expanded in the wake of the compression wave. The difference between maximum pressure and minimum pressure is the amplitude of the sound wave. The greater the displacement of air, the more movement will occur during vibration of the tympanic membrane and the louder the perception of sound will be. Loudness is a subjective quality. The perception of loudness is affected by the attentiveness of the individual or selectively competing sounds in the environment.

Pitch. Pitch is related to the frequency of sound. It is the number of vibrations of the sound source per second. The waveform of a sound of single frequency is sinusoidal:

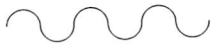

with perfectly matched peaks and valleys. The distance from one peak to the next is one cycle. The recording of frequency is done in cycles per second (cps) or **hertz** (Hz). The human ear can detect sounds in the frequency range of 20 to 20,000 Hz. With advancing age, the human ear becomes progressively less sensitive to the higher sound frequencies. The sounds of speech and music (300 to 3000 Hz) are most frequently lost in elderly persons.

Quality. Harmonic refers to the physical property of sound that causes the effect called quality or **timbre.** A sound of single frequency produces a pure tone. The examiner records the quality in descriptive terms, such as humming, buzzing, or roaring. A musical sound is one in which the mix of intensity and pitch is pleasing to the ear. **Noise** refers to a sound that produces an unpleasant sensation. Most sounds heard in the course of the physical examination are perceived as noise.

The more air that the tissue contains (i.e., the less dense the tissue), the deeper and louder the sound will be. The denser the tissue, the higher and fainter the sound will be. The examiner records sounds elicited in percussion in relation to the density of the tissue being vibrated. The least dense tissues produce **tympany.** Successively denser tissue results in hyperresonance, resonance, dullness, and flatness.

The change from **resonance** (less density) to **dullness** (greater density) is more easily perceived than the change from dullness to resonance. Thus percussion should be done from more resonant to less resonant areas.

Palpation. In performing palpation, the examiner uses his or her hands to augment the data gathered through inspection. The skilled examiner uses the most sensitive parts of the hand for each type of palpation (Table 7-2). The examiner's hands should be warm and have well-trimmed nails. Rubber gloves should be worn for any examination of mucous membranes or any area where contact with body fluids or drainage is likely. Touch is used to determine the extent of tenderness and to note any **tremor** or **spasm** of muscle tissues. It is also used to elicit **crepitus**, or crackling, in bones and joints.

> **Helpful Hint:** *Always palpate areas of tenderness last.*

The examiner may palpate individual structures within body cavities, particularly the abdomen, for position, size, shape, consistency, and mobility. The examining hand can be used to detect masses. Palpation may also serve as a means of evaluating abnormal collections of fluid. Both light and deep palpation are used in the examination. Light palpation involves applying slight pressure to the area being examined to assess skin, tenderness, or pulsations. Deep palpation is done to assess the size or contour of organs, such as the liver or kidney. Light palpation should always be performed first because it is less likely to create discomfort for the client. Touch is used to examine the skin and hair for moisture and texture.

TABLE 7-2

Discriminating Areas of the Hands Used in Palpation

Discriminating sense	Sensitive regions
Fine tactile discrimination	Fingertips
Skin texture	General differences: fingertips
	Fine discrimination: back of hands and fingers
Position, consistency, and form of a structure or mass	Fingertips using grasping fingers
Vibration	Palmar aspects of metacarpophalangeal joints (ball of hand)
	Alternative method: ulnar side of hand
Temperature	Dorsal side of hands or fingers (back of hand)

From Talbot L, Meyers-Marquardt M: *Pocket guide to critical care assessment.* St Louis, 1989, Mosby—Year Book.

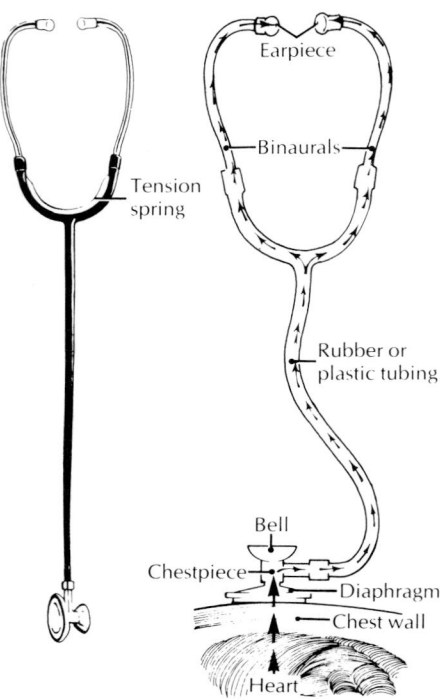

FIGURE 7-3 Acoustic stethoscope. (Modified from Patient Care, March 15, 1974. Copyright 1974, Miller & Fink Corp., Darien, Conn. All rights reserved.)

Auscultation. Auscultation is the process of listening for the sounds that the human body produces. The particularly important sounds are those produced by (1) the thoracic or abdominal viscera and (2) the movement of blood in the cardiovascular system. Direct auscultation involves listening with the unassisted ear, that is, without any amplifying device. However, auscultation is routinely done with a stethoscope, an instrument developed by René Laënnec in 1816. The purpose of the stethoscope is to exclude environmental sound and to augment internal sound.

The **acoustic stethoscope** is the type currently used (Figure 7-3). Essentially, it is a closed cylinder that inhibits the dissipation of sound waves produced by the sound source. The diaphragm of the stethoscope screens out low-frequency sounds and is therefore most effective in assessing high-frequency sounds such as breath and bowel sounds. The diaphragm is applied firmly to the skin so that it creates a seal between the skin surface and the diaphragm.

Helpful Hint: *A water-soluble jelly applied to the diaphragm will improve the transmission of sound.*

The bell-type head of the stethoscope is most effective in detecting low-frequency sounds such as vascular sounds or blood pressure. It is important to avoid pressing the bell too firmly on the skin surface because stretching the skin inhibits vibration by actually con-

verting the tissue to a diaphragm. The bell chestpiece should be wide enough to span an intercostal space in an adult and deep enough so that it will not fill with tissue.

Several sizes of earpieces are supplied with better stethoscopes. The examiner should determine which size fits his or her external **meatus** most snugly. The

STEP-BY-STEP

Examination Step-by-Step

Using the techniques of examination in combination for assessment of the lungs would include the following steps:

1. Inspecting the anterior and posterior thorax to observe symmetry of movement.
2. Using direct percussion over the posterior thorax to assess intensity, pitch, and quality of sound.
3. Palpating the posterior and anterior thorax to assess tenderness and vibrations produced by underlying tissues.
4. Auscultating over the anterior and posterior thorax to assess for breath sounds.
5. Positioning the client in a sitting position with the shoulders rounded to expose maximum lung tissue when examining the posterior thorax.

TABLE 7-3

Positions for Examination

Position	Areas assessed	Rationale	Limitations
Sitting	Head and neck, back, posterior thorax and lungs, anterior thorax and lungs, breasts, axillae, heart, vital signs, and upper extremities	Sitting upright provides full expansion of lungs and provides better visualization of symmetry of upper body parts.	Physically weakened client may be unable to sit. Use supine position with head of bed elevated instead.
Supine	Head and neck, anterior thorax and lungs, breasts, axillae, heart, abdomen, extremities, pulses	This is most normally relaxed position. It prevents contracture of abdominal muscles and provides easy access to pulse sites.	If client becomes short of breath easily, examiner may need to raise head of bed.
Dorsal recumbent	Head and neck, anterior thorax and lungs, breasts, axillae, heart	Clients with painful disorders are more comfortable with knees flexed.	Position is not used for abdominal assessment because it promotes contracture of abdominal muscles.
Lithotomy	Female genitalia and genital tract	This position provides maximal exposure of genitalia and facilitates insertion of vaginal speculum.	Lithotomy position is embarrassing and uncomfortable, so minimize time client spends in it. Keep client well draped. Client with severe arthritis or other joint deformity may be unable to assume this position.
Sims'	Rectum and vagina	Flexion of hip and knee improves exposure of rectal area.	Joint deformities may hinder client's ability to bend hip and knee.
Prone	Musculoskeletal system	This position is used only to assess extension of the hip joint.	This position is intolerable for client with respiratory difficulties.
Knee-chest	Rectum	This position provides maximal exposure of rectal area.	This position is embarrassing and uncomfortable. Clients with arthritis or other joint deformities may be unable to assume this postion.

From Potter PA, Perry AG: *Basic nursing: theory and practice,* ed 2, St Louis, 1991, Mosby–Year Book.

earpiece should occlude the meatus, thus blocking extraneous sound. However, the earpiece should not cause the examiner pain. The binaurals (metal tubing) are angled slightly toward the nose of the wearer to project the sound onto the tympanic membrane. The direction of the angle may be adjusted by the tension spring. The tubing should not be longer than 30 to 35 cm to minimize sound distortion. Longer tubing increases the chance of diminishing the sound.

Special maneuvers—positioning. Positioning the client can help in using the four modalities described here. For example, positioning the client in a right side-lying position will aid in palpating the spleen. Positioning also makes certain body areas more accessible to the examiner. Table 7-3 summarizes the positions used for assessing different body parts. The inability of a client to assume a position may be an important objective finding. For example, the inability to lie flat may be a sign of a cardiovascular problem.

DOCUMENTATION

Sample Documentation

An example of recording the assessment data obtained by using the four examination techniques and positioning is given for the spleen:

With the client in a supine position, inspection revealed a flat abdomen with smooth contours and without bulging or visible pulsation. No friction rubs were detected on auscultation. With the client in a right side-lying position, percussion done just posterior to the left midaxillary line between the level of the 5th and 9th rib revealed an area of dullness. Light palpation of the left anterior costal margin elicited tenderness but suggested no enlargement of the spleen.

GLOSSARY

acoustic stethoscope An instrument used in mediate auscultation consisting of two earpieces connected by means of flexible tubing to a diaphragm, which is placed on the client's skin.

anxiety Motor tension, autonomic hyperactivity, apprehension, or hyperattentiveness.

auscultation Examination technique done by listening, usually through a stethoscope.

crepitus A dry, crackling sound in (1) the lung, when air passes through abnormally accumulated moisture; (2) the joints, when dry synovial surfaces rub together; and (3) the skin, when air is present subdermally.

dullness Decreased resonance on percussion, such as percussion sound produced over the liver.

fist percussion Striking the body with the lateral aspect of the hand to elicit pain or tenderness.

hertz (Hz) Unit of frequency of a periodic process equal to one cycle per second.

immediate (direct) percussion Use of the finger or hand to strike the body to evaluate the sound waves produced.

inspection Visual evaluation of the body that incorporates the senses of sight, smell, and hearing.

intensity Loudness of sound.

meatus Passage or opening of a canal.

mediate (indirect) percussion Technique in which the middle finger of one hand strikes the middle finger of the other hand to emit a sound or vibration.

noise Sound that produces an unpleasant auditory sensation.

palpation Examination technique that involves feeling or touching the object to be evaluated.

perception Awareness of objects and relations that follows stimulation of the peripheral sense organs.

percussion Examination technique that involves listening to reverberation of tissue after striking the surface with short, sharp blows.

pitch Quality of a tone or sound that is dependent on the relative rapidity of the vibrations by which it is produced.

precordial Related to the part of the chest that overlies the heart and lower thorax.

resonance Low-pitched, hollow sound produced over normal lung tissue when the chest is percussed.

spasm Involuntary sudden contraction of a muscle or group of muscles accompanied by pain and interference with function.

symmetry Similarity in size, shape, and position to the corresponding body part on the opposite side.

symptom Client's subjective perception of an alteration of bodily or mental function from basal conditions; change perceived by the individual.

tangential lighting Use of light shining from the side to create shadows over the area being examined; accentuates subtle differences in contour and movement.

timbre The quality of a sound that distinguishes it from other sounds of the same pitch and volume

tympany Resonant sound obtained by percussion

tremor Involuntary, somewhat rhythmic oscillatory quivering of muscles caused by alternate contraction of opposing groups of muscles. *Cerebellar tremor:* occurs during intentional movement, becoming more pronounced near end of the movement; associated with lesions of the dentate nucleus. *Coarse tremor:* slow rate and large-amplitude movements. *Essential (familial) tremor:* usually begins at approximately age 50 with fine tremors of the hands; aggravated by intentional movement; commonly affects head, jaws, lips, or voice. *Fine tremor:* rapid (10 to 20 oscillations/sec) and low amplitude movements, usually in the fingers and hands. *Passive tremor:* present at rest, may improve during intentional movement; for example, pill-rolling tremor or Parkinson's disease. *Physiological tremor:* experienced by healthy people in fatigue, cold, and stress. *Toxic tremor:* caused by endogenous (thyrotoxicosis, uremia) or exogenous toxins (alcohol, drugs).

tympanic membrane (eardrum) Membranous structure separating the external ear from the middle ear.

universal precautions Constellation of safeguards for handling materials, tissues, and fluids that may contain human pathogens; exposure to blood and body fluids is minimized by using removable and disposable barriers (e.g., latex and vinyl gloves, protective eyewear, masks and gowns, and "sharps" containers).

BIBLIOGRAPHY

American College of Physicians, Medical Practice Committee: Periodic health examination: a guide for designing individualized preventive health care in asymptomatic patients, *Ann Intern Med* 95:729, 1981.

Breslow L, Somers AR: The lifetime health monitoring program: a practical approach to preventive medicine, *N Engl J Med* 296:601, 1977.

Canadian Task Force: Report on the periodic health examination, *Can Med Assoc J* 121:1193, 1979.

Canadian Task Force: The periodic health examination, II, 1987 update, *Can Med Assoc J* 138:618, 1988.

Hayward RSA, and others: Preventive care guidelines: 1991, *Ann Intern Med* 114:758, 1991.

King C: Refining your assessment techniques, *RN* 46:42-47, 1983.

Kozier B, Erb G, Olivieri R: *Fundamentals of nursing: concepts, process and practice*, Menlo Park, Calif, 1991, Addison-Wesley.

Leavell HR, Clark EG: Preventive medicine for the doctor in his community, ed 3, New York, 1965, McGraw-Hill.

Talbot L, Marquardt M: Pocket guide to critical care assessment, St Louis, 1989, Mosby–Year Book.

US Preventive Services Task Force: *Guide to clinical preventive services: an assessment of the effectiveness of 169 interventions*, Baltimore, 1989, William & Wilkins.

General Assessment, Including Vital Signs

Outline

PURPOSE OF THE EXAMINATION

After obtaining subjective data from the client using methods of interviewing and history taking discussed in previous chapters, the examiner proceeds to the physical examination. Techniques of the physical examination provide the *objective* measurements of health assessment. The client's and examiner's coordinated efforts lead to the recognition and identification of abnormal phenomena.

Symptoms are elicited in the interview. The examiner gains valuable insights from the client's description and presentation into whether a pathological condition exists. Furthermore, the examiner may obtain indications of the client's cooperation, motivation, and objectives.

The examiner's observations and measurements are essential in verifying the client's descriptions and in identifying *signs* or objective findings. The tools of physical assessment also allow the examiner to explore facets not usually available to the client. Conclusions about an individual's health are drawn from synthesizing information from the client's description and the physical assessment.

GENERAL INSPECTION

General inspection begins with observing the client entering the room, during introductions, and as he or she follows instructions before the interview begins. General observation is the overall impression given by the client's general state of health and outstanding characteristics.

The survey proceeds from head to toe. The examiner observes thoroughly and discerningly. Many professionals experience some difficulty in gazing at the client without doing some task simultaneously. Nevertheless, one must be totally absorbed in the process of looking and perceiving.

Inspection is a more detailed observation that includes smell, hearing, and touch as well as visual inspection. Make observations only in good light, particularly when assessing skin color.

Make every attempt to concentrate on the person being examined. With practice and by carefully guarding against distractions, either from the environment or unrelated thoughts, you will learn to become completely absorbed with the client. Total and focused concentration on the client allows the examiner to process information using all sensory modalities.

The general observations continue throughout the interview. In some cases, the initial impression sets the focus of the interview and of the physical examination. For instance, some feature of the client's appearance

---

may point immediately to the problem. Slow speech and a hoarse voice, for example, may indicate the need to look further for the dry skin and sluggish movements of hypothyroidism.

Helpful Hint: *Give the client total attention. Do not allow yourself to be interrupted to take phone calls or to be distracted by other responsibilities. Consider the time with the client as precious.*

Although the initial inspection is a scanning procedure, the astute practitioner gathers information that may be used as the basis for planning portions of the examination that deserve special attention.

ASSESSMENT OF BODY MORPHOLOGY AND GAIT

Normal Body Types

Although body **morphology**, or the size and physical shape of a person, is to some degree genetically determined, the environment plays a significant role in altering body type. Several normal variations in body types are shown in Figure 8-1.

Mesomorphic type. The mesophorphic body type is characterized by average height, well-developed musculature, wide shoulders with a subcostal angle that is approximately a right angle, and a flat abdomen.

Ectomorphic type. The ectomorphic body build is often described as tall and willowy. The musculature

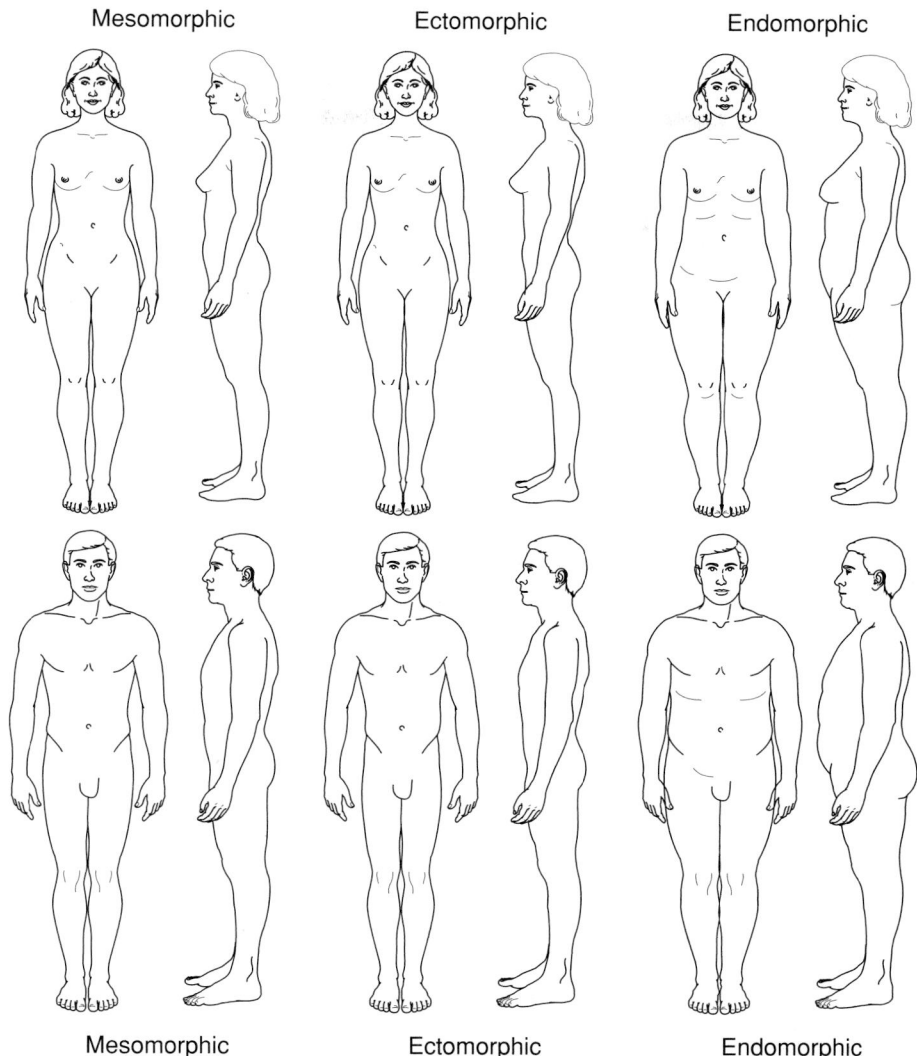

FIGURE 8-1 Body types (Redrawn from Manual of Orthopaedic Surgery Chicago, *Am Orthop Assoc*, 1953).

and subcutaneous fat are poorly developed. The extremity bones are long and thin. The clavicles, ribs, and spinous processes protrude because of the deficient subcutaneous fat. The chest is long and narrow. Because abdominal muscles are not as well developed, the abdominal wall may sag outward. The stomach is lower in the abdomen and more vertical in position. The neck is long.

Endomorphic type. The endomorphic body build is short, stocky, and the most likely of the body types to be obese. The neck is short and thick. The extremities are large and sturdy. Compared to the mesomorphic and ectomorphic types, the chest is shorter and broader and the costal margin is a wider angle (obtuse). The

heart is likely to lie in a transverse position. The abdomen is long and of great capacity. The stomach is higher in the abdomen than it is in the other two body types and more or less in a transverse position.

Symmetry

The arrangement of most structures of the human body is symmetrical; that is, size and shape of parts correspond. If inspection reveals obvious areas of lack of symmetry, note this and investigate it later.

Posture

Posture is a part of **body image**. Good body alignment is a sign of good health. Correct posture is the position in which minimum stress will be applied to each joint.

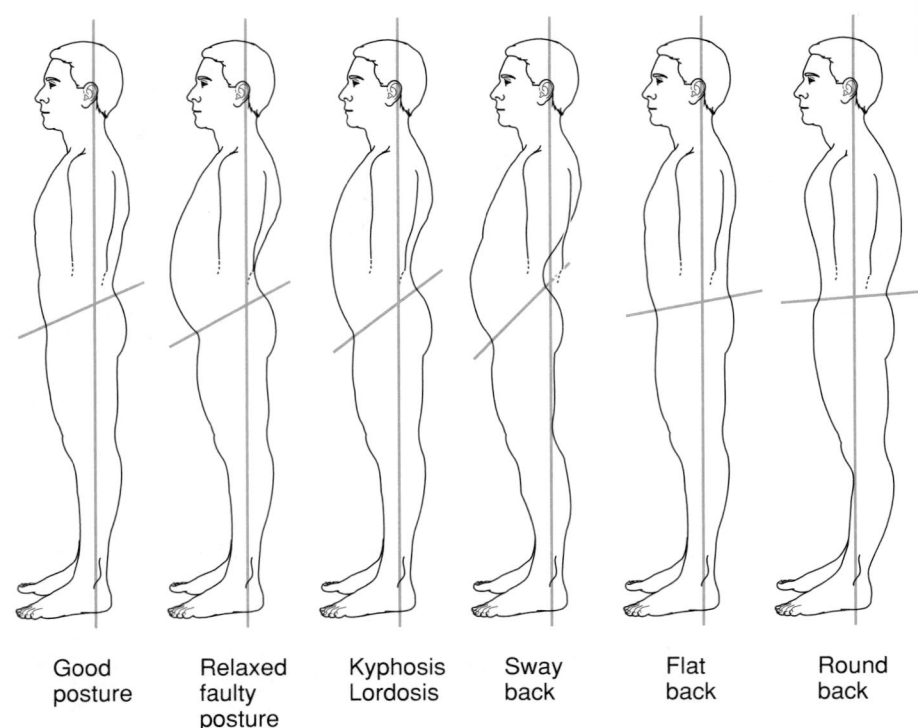

| Good posture | Relaxed faulty posture | Kyphosis Lordosis | Sway back | Flat back | Round back |

FIGURE 8-2 Types of faulty posture. (Redrawn from McMorris RO: *Pediatr Clin North Am* 8:217, 1961).

Minimum muscular effort is required to maintain an upright posture, which is achieved when the line of the center of gravity bisects the principal weight-bearing joints and is the same distance from each foot. Frequent changes of posture are necessary for comfort. Good posture depends on a normal sense of balance and muscular coordination. Faulty posture is any position that increases stress to joints (Figure 8-2).

Aging and posture. Bone and joint changes contribute to the bent posture often seen in the elderly. Joint degeneration and **osteoporosis** occur with aging. Aging changes, such as widening and flattening of the third cervical vertebrae and drying of the intervertebral disks, may result in a decrease from baseline adult height of as much as 2 to 3 cm.

CULTURAL INFLUENCES

Some evidence points to appropriate exercise as an aid to maintaining erect posture. Chinese shadow-boxing exercises are purported to maintain body awareness and erect posture despite advancing years.

Although all muscles decline in girth and strength with aging, the muscles of the trunk are particularly affected. Weakness of the abdominal muscles also contributes to the slumped posture of the elderly.

Gait

The phases of normal **gait** are stance and swing (Figure 8-3). The stance phase occurs when the foot is on the ground and bearing weight. The lower leg supports the body weight and the body advances over the supporting limb. The five components of stance are: (1) initial contact (heel strike), (2) load response, (3) midstance, (4) terminal stance, and (5) preswing.

The normal heel strike is quiet and smoothly coordinated with the knee extended. The load response, the movement to full contact of the foot with the floor, should be complete and proceed smoothly. The midstance of the foot is the shift of weight onto the foot. The weight should be supported evenly by all aspects of the foot and the knee is slightly flexed. In the terminal stance, the metatarsal pushoff is a smoothly coordinated lift off the floor. The swing phase occurs when the foot is nonweight bearing and moving forward. The swing phase allows the toes to clear the floor and the swing leg to advance forward.

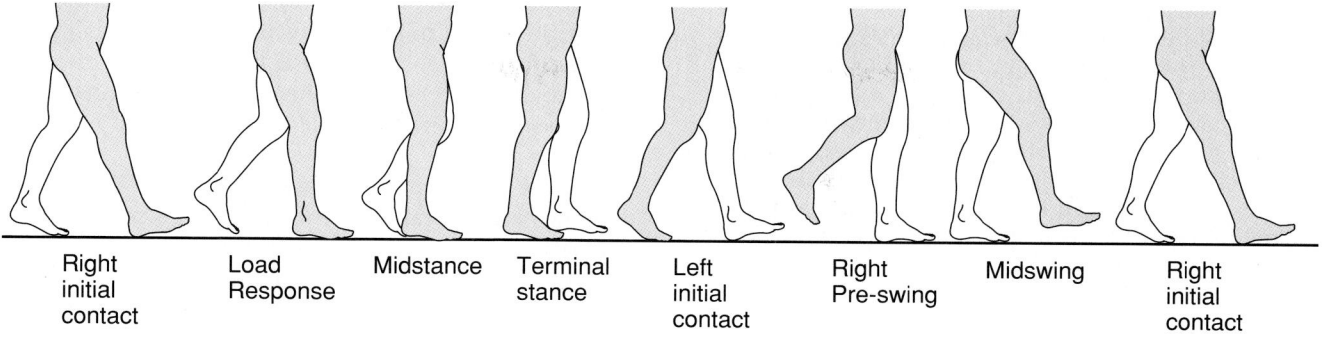

| Right initial contact | Load Response | Midstance | Terminal stance | Left initial contact | Right Pre-swing | Midswing | Right initial contact |

FIGURE 8-3 Stance and swing phase of gait. (Modified from Magee DJ: *Orthopedic physical assessment*, Philadelphia, 1987, WB Saunders and Inman VT, et al: *Human walking*, Baltimore, 1981, Williams & Wilkins.)

Technique for Examination of Posture and Gait

Develop a protocol for accurately observing the main postures of the body in all its common acts. Beginning observations are made by watching the client come into the room and sit down and by observing while the client lies on the examining table. It is important to note whether the client sits tensely or slumps in the chair.

The characteristics of the client's walk provide clues to the client's problems. Ask the client to walk a straight line and observe the client walking a short distance both toward and away from you. Note the speed of step as well as the smoothness and style of movement.

ASSESSMENT OF GENERAL APPEARANCE

Weight

Weight is sometimes considered a vital sign because unexplained weight loss frequently is one of the early signs of illness. With aging, weight tends to increase, and a more sedentary life-style may also contribute to weight gain. Body fat distribution changes with age; abdominal and truncal fat increases and the extremities thin.

Adipose deposition varies by gender. Women have fat deposits over the shoulders, breasts, buttocks or lateral aspect of the thighs, and pubic symphysis. The fat deposits in men are more evenly dispersed throughout the body.

An essential part of the assessment of children or anyone who has not completed the growth cycle is the accurate, serial measurement of height and weight. Growth charts (see Chapter 24), which are assembled from data gathered from large populations, allow the examiner to compare an individual client's pattern of growth to national standards.

Hair Growth Patterns

Hair growth is influenced by hereditary and racial factors. Excessive hairiness is thought to be a dominant hereditary trait related to the presence of androgens, whereas thinning or absent hair is a recessive trait.

Hair grows at various rates. The most rapid rate of growth is that of the beard, followed by that of the scalp, axillae, thighs, and eyebrows. The rate of hair growth is affected by environmental temperature and by the general state of health. Extremely cold temperatures impede hair growth, whereas hot climates appear to promote increased length.

Axillary and pubic hair growth is initiated by adrenal hormones, ovarian hormones, and testicular hormones. True sexual hair grows on the face, chest, abdomen, back, and extremities. The hair may be classified by the types of hormonal influences the growth receives:

1. Hair dependent on growth hormone (GH) is that which grows on the head, including eyelashes and eyebrows; midphalangeal area; distal portions of limbs; and, to some extent, on the lumbosacral area.
2. Hair dependent on female hormones is that which grows on the pubic area, axillae, limbs, and hypogastric area. The male pubic hair configuration is that of a diamond, with its superior angle at the umbilicus. The female pubic hair pattern is triangular, with the base over the mons pubis.
3. Hair dependent on male hormones is that of the beard, mustache, nasal tip, ear, and body hair (particularly on the back).

CULTURAL VARIATIONS

Caucasian persons have more abundant and coarser body hair than Asians. Facial **hirsutism,** or excessive hair growth, occurs in more than 40% of Caucasian women. Japanese women, on the other hand, do not develop excessive facial hair growth, and Japanese men have sparser beards than Caucasian men. Blacks have kinky hair, whereas Caucasians have straight or wavy to curly hair. American Indians have straight hair.

A heavier distribution of hair is correlated with darker skin pigmentation; that is, the brunette individual is more likely to have more hair than the blonde person.

Some male hair growth characteristics may be normal for women of certain ethnic or familial groups and could include sideburns, hair growth on the upper lip, abdomen, and lower limbs, and hair growth around the areola of the breasts.

Alopecia (balding) is more frequently noted in individuals with abundant coarse-hair growth on the body. Alopecia is thought to be related to androgen production. Male pattern baldness is recession of the hairline and baldness of the crown. As a rule, women do not bald unless androgens are present in relatively increased amounts or if the baldness occurs as a result of disease or chemotherapy.

Technique for Examination of General Appearance and Normal Findings

Weight. Weigh the client and measure his or her height. Compare the client's parameters with actuarial tables of average weights and heights, which are prepared by insurance companies. Record weight in kilograms or pounds and height in centimeters or inches, depending on the requirements of the particular setting.

> **Helpful Hint:** *Weigh the client with or without clothes; however, note whether or not the client was clothed. The client should not wear shoes when height is measured.*

Hair. Inspect for hair growth on the following body regions: scalp, beard, mustache, ears, hypogastric area, thoracic area, lower limbs, genital area, lumbosacral area, upper back, midphalangeal area, pubis, and axillae. Observe hair for growth characteristics, distribution, density of growth, appearance, and hygiene.

Nails. The nails may indicate the level of concern and care the client has for appearance. Inspect the nails for length, cleanliness, neatness of filing, and the presence and condition of polish. Inspection of the actual nail is obscured in females who use artificial nails that are glued to the nail bed. Note the texture, recording thickness and ridging when present.

Personal hygiene. General cleanliness of the body is an important indication of the individual's **self-esteem** and access to necessary supplies to maintain good body care. Standards of cleanliness are a sociocultural value. Deodorants are not used in all cultures. Although shaving the legs is normal in some groups of women in the United States, it is not practiced by all women. However, although norms may vary, poor personal hygiene can indicate serious mental or physical illness.

Odors. Note odor of the body and breath. The smell of alcohol on the client's breath should alert one to look for other effects of alcohol, a central nervous system (CNS) depressant. Foul breath points to the possibility of an oral or pulmonary infection or may simply be the result of poor oral hygiene. The odor of ammonia may be detectable in the patient with uremia. Body odor may be related to the activities of the sweat and **sebaceous** glands and to the general cleanliness of the body.

The odors emanating from the client may provide clues helpful in defining the client's condition. Some diseases are characterized by particular odors emanat-

TABLE 8-1

Association of Breath Odors to Disease

Breath odor	Description	Associated condition
Halitosis, foul	Odor of necrotic tissue	Pyorrhea
		Poor dental hygiene
		Tonsilitis
		Sinusitis
		Lung abcess
		Bronchiectasis
Feculent	Odor of feces	Bowel obstruction
Fetor hepaticus	"Fishy" odor	Hepatic failure
Acid	Acrid, acid smell	Peptic disease
Uriniferous, ammoniacal	Odor of urine	Renal failure
Acetone	Odor of acetone, "fruity"	Diabetic ketoacidosis
Bitter almonds	Odor of almonds	Cyanide poisoning

ing from the mouth. The odors known to have diagnostic importance are listed in Table 8-1.

Manner of dress. Note the fit of the clothing as well as its appropriateness to season or room temperature. General cleanliness and neatness of clothing may provide further clues to the client's cultural or socioeconomic status as well as ego strength and self-image. If a client is unshaven or unwashed, these may be signs of self-neglect or neglect by relatives or others on whom the client is dependent. Carefully note such signs of neglect.

ASSESSMENT OF VITAL SIGNS

The most frequent clinical measurements made by the health practitioner are temperature, *pulse*, respiratory rate, and blood pressure. These measures provide valuable data on the client's state of health. Because of the importance of these indicators in predicting normal body function, they have been termed the **vital** or **cardinal** signs. Obtain vital signs at the beginning of any examination.

Variations from the client's baseline values or from the previous measurement are clinically significant. The client's baseline measures are important because there is considerable variability among individuals. The examiner assesses vital signs to establish a database; data obtained on future occasions may then be compared to baseline values.

Bear in mind that your manner of approach to the client may alter the client's vital signs, especially if the client reacts emotionally to your actions. For instance, a curt, impatient, rude interaction or awkward handling of the instruments may upset the client, increasing pulse rate, respiration, blood pressure, and even temperature if the interaction is prolonged.

Temperature

For most individuals, the optimum temperature for metabolic function of all cells of the human body is 37° C (98.6° F). The core temperature of the body is maintained within very narrow limits. The normal ranges for temperature are 36.1° to 37.6° C (97° to 99.6° F). Factors that influence temperature are described in the boxed material above.

Temperature regulation. Body temperature is an excellent example of both *homeostasis* and biological rhythms. The hypothalamus serves as the body's thermostat. Two hypothalamic centers trigger heat-dissipating or heat-conserving mechanisms. The delivery of overwarmed blood to thermoreceptors in the anterior hypothalamus results in sweating and redistribution of blood, which dilates surface capillaries and causes flush-

FACTORS INFLUENCING TEMPERATURE

Biological rhythms are reflected in temperature assessment (Figure 8-4). Diurnal variations of up to 1.0° C are observed; the trough occurs in the hours before waking; the peak occurs in the late afternoon or early evening.

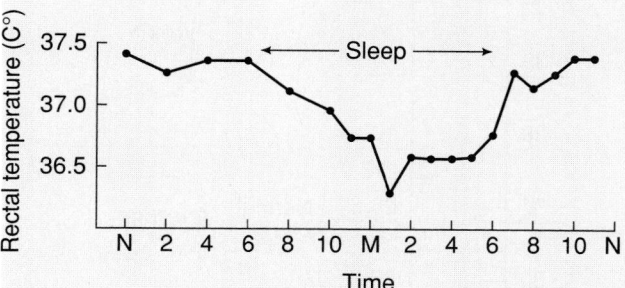

FIGURE 8-4 Biological rhythms for temperature in a 24-hour cycle. (From Mountcastle VB: *Medical physiology*, vol 2, ed 14, St. Louis, 1980, Mosby–Year Book.)

Hormones can increase temperature. Increased secretion of thyroid hormone increases body temperature. Progesterone secretion at the time of ovulation correlates with temperature increases of 0.5° C, which continue until the menses.

Environment affects temperature. Although body temperature may be altered little by seasonal changes in temperature, hot and cold baths are known to produce temporary changes in temperature.

Exercise increases body temperature because of the physiological changes incurred.

Eating food is associated with a rise in temperature. This rise in temperature is a result of the specific dynamic action (SDA) of the food.

Age is a factor in temperature assessment. Because heat control mechanisms are not as well established in the child as in the adult, considerable variation in a child's temperature may occur. Normal body temperature declines with age, from 37.2°C in young children, to 37°C in adults, and 36°C in older adults.

ing. Temperature loss from the skin occurs when blood flow to the skin increases and sweat evaporates. This heat loss is related to the temperature difference between the skin and external environment.

Conduction, convection, radiation, and evaporation are the physical phenomena involved in temperature regulation. Heat loss from the object of higher temperature to the object of lower temperature is **conduction.** **Convection** is the loss of heat to the molecules of air.

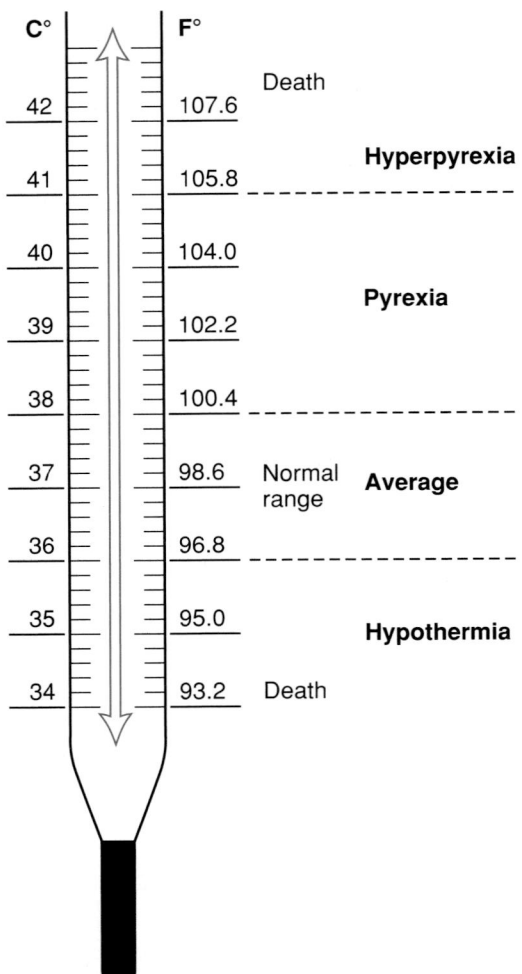

FIGURE 8-5 Comparison of Celsius and Fahrenheit oral temperatures in the range compatible with survival in humans. (Redrawn from Kozier B, Erb, G, Olivieri R: *Fundamentals of nursing: concepts, process and practice,* ed 4, Redwood City, Calif., 1991, Addison-Wesley.)

Conduction and convection occur only when the ambient temperature is lower than the body temperature.

Radiation is the loss of heat by electromagnetic infrared waves. The radiation does not heat the air through which it passes. **Evaporation** is the conversion of liquid (sweat) to gaseous form. Vaporization of perspiration depends on ambient humidity and does not occur when air is very humid.

Heat-conserving mechanisms are activated when overcooled blood is delivered to thermoreceptors in the posterior hypothalamus. These mechanisms include reducing blood flow to the distal extremities and constricting peripheral capillary beds (blanching). Com-

pensatory heat production is enhanced both at the metabolic level (nonshivering thermogenesis) and through voluntary muscle contraction and shivering. Shivering occurs when vasoconstriction is ineffective in preventing heat loss.

Temperature acclimatization. Clients who have spent a good deal of time in very cold climates show an increased ability to tolerate cold. These individuals show (1) increased metabolic rate with increased rates of secretion of thyroid hormones, (2) reduction in shivering, and (3) growth of hair.

Adaptation to heat changes the secretion of sweat. The amount of sweat produced declines from the profuse, dripping, early response to a quantity that will evaporate upon reaching the air.

Temperature recording. Record body temperature in degrees Celsius (°C) or in degrees Fahrenheit (°F), according to the protocol of the practice setting. The metric system is generally the preferred system in health care. Each scale may be readily converted through the use of the following formulas:

$$°C = 5/9 \ (°F - 32)$$
$$°F = 9/5 \ (°C + 32)$$

Figure 8-5 equates Fahrenheit and Celsius temperatures in the compatible range for human survival.

Techniques for Temperature Measurement

For accurate temperature measurement, insert the glass or electronic thermometer properly and leave in place for the recommended length of time. Explain to the client what is being done. The box on p. 203 describes steps in taking a temperature with a glass thermometer.

Oral temperature. The oral temperature is the most convenient method for registering body temperature in the alert, adult client. Normal oral temperature in adults is 37° C. Wait 15 minutes before taking a temperature if the client has smoked or ingested hot or iced liquids. For a glass mercury thermometer, placement in the mouth for 3 to 5 minutes is recommended although the oral thermometer may take as long as 7 minutes to reach maximum registration. Other measurements may be obtained at this time.

Rectal temperature. The rectal site for temperature registration is preferable for the confused or comatose client, the client who is unable to close his or her mouth, or the client who is receiving oxygen. The normal rectal temperature in adults is 37.5° C. The lubricated thermometer placed in the rectum will register within 2 minutes.

STEPS IN TAKING A TEMPERATURE WITH A GLASS THERMOMETER

Oral temperature

1. Explain to client what you will be doing.
2. Hold the thermometer at the end opposite the bulb and rinse in cold water.
3. Wipe from your fingers to the bulb with clean paper or gauze.
4. Holding the thermometer horizontal at eye level, rotate it until the scale is visible and read the mercury.
5. Grasp the end opposite the bulb and shake the thermometer downward with a brisk flick of the wrist.
6. Ask the client to open his or her mouth with the tip of the tongue against the upper teeth.
7. Insert thermometer tip gently under the tongue between the frenulum and lower gum; leave in place at least 3 minutes.
8. Hold the distal tip and ask client to open his or her mouth to remove the thermometer.
9. Wipe the thermometer clean from the distal end to the bulb.
10. Read the temperature indicated by the mercury column and record.

Rectal temperature

Same steps as 1-5 above.
6. Apply a lubricant to the bulb end.
7. Assist the client to a lateral position with upper leg flexed.
8. Separate the buttocks to view the anus, while instructing the client to breathe deeply; insert the thermometer 2.5 to 3.5 cm for an adult and 1 to 2 cm for an infant.
9. Leave thermometer in place for at least 2 minutes and then remove gently.

Axillary temperature

Same steps as 1-5 above.
6. Insert thermometer into the center of the axilla and lower the client's arm over the thermometer.
7. Fold the client's arm across his or her chest to keep thermometer in place.
8. Leave thermometer in place at least 5 minutes in children and somewhat longer in adults.

Axillary temperature. The axillary method is safe and accurate for infants and small children and is not often used with adult clients unless oral and rectal routes are not accessible. The normal axillary temperature in adults is 36.5° C. It can take up to 10 minutes for the full registration of axillary temperature in adults and about 5 minutes for children.

Tympanic temperature. Tympanic thermography is a noninvasive technique for assessment of body temperature. It uses an infrared sensor to detect the temperature of blood flowing through the eardrum. It records an even more reliable temperature than do oral or rectal thermometers. The tympanic thermometer registers an electronic display within 2 seconds (Figure 8-6).

Respiration

The assessment of respiratory pattern is discussed in Chapter 14, Assessment of the Respiratory System.

Pulses

The detailed assessment of pulses is discussed in Chapter 16. General assessment usually includes assessment of

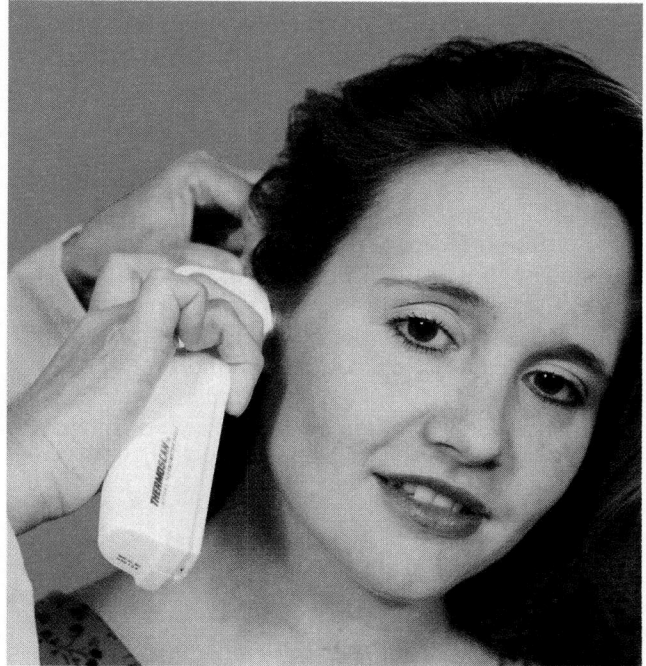

FIGURE 8-6 Tympanic temperature measurement.

TABLE 8-2

Normal Age Variations in Pulse Rate

Age	Pulse rate (beats/min)
Birth	70-170
Neonate	120-140
1 year	80-140
2 years	80-130
3 years	80-120
4 years	70-115
Adult	60-100
Conditioned athlete	≅ 50

the peripheral (radial) or apical pulse for rate, rhythm, and volume. The peripheral arterial pulse is a pressure wave transmitted from the left ventricle to the aorta to the peripheral vessels. The nature of the peripheral pulse gives an indication of cardiac function and perfusion of the peripheral tissues.

Pulse rate. Normal heart rate is between 50 and 100 beats per minute. Table 8-2 shows normal variations of pulse rate by age. When obtaining baseline data, count the pulse rate for 1 full minute to accurately evaluate rate, rhythm, and volume. Normal rhythm is an even tempo. For subsequent measures, count 15 to 30 seconds for pulses that are regular. Auscultate the apical pulse for 1 minute if irregularities are felt. Because of diurnal rhythm, pulse rate is lowest in the early morning hours and most rapid in the late afternoon and evening.

Pulse volume. Pulse volume represents the strength of left ventricular contraction or stroke volume. Estimate pulse volume from the feel of the vessel as blood flows through it with each heartbeat. **Bounding** is the descriptive term used to describe the full pulse that is difficult to depress with the fingertips. The normal pulse is easily palpable, does not fade in and out, and is not easily obliterated. Weak, feeble, and thready are descriptive words for the pulse of a vessel with low volume. The artery with low volume is readily compressed.

Technique for Examination of Vital Signs

The techniques used to assess vital signs include inspection, palpation, auscultation, and the use of instruments to obtain specific measures of physiological functioning.

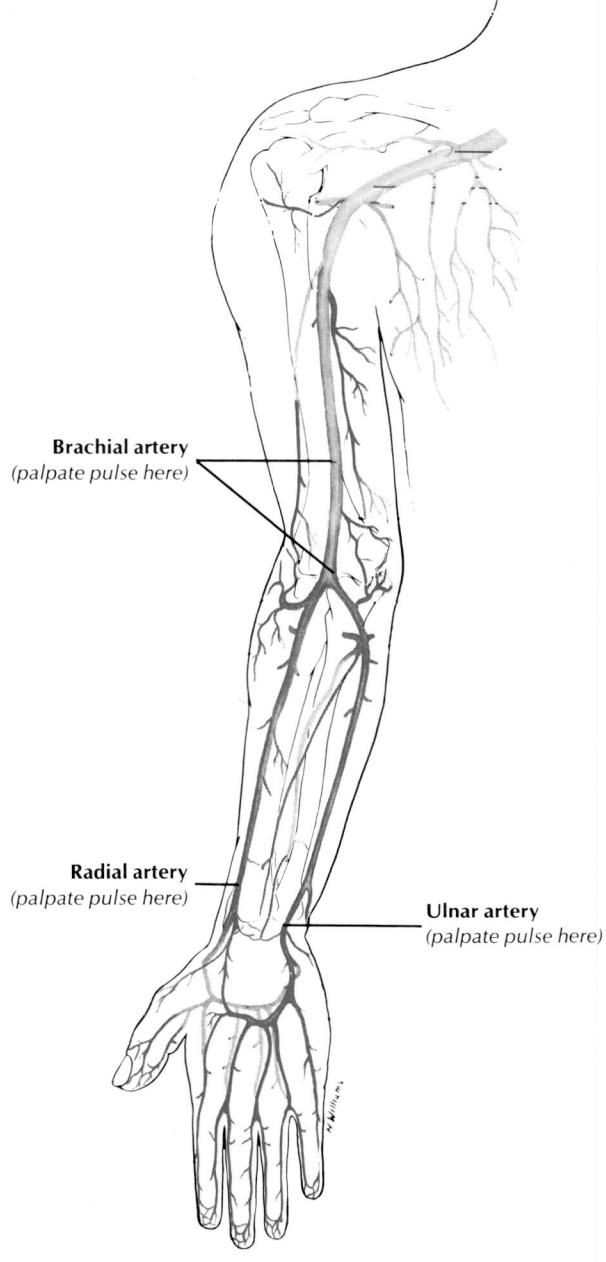

FIGURE 8-7 Arteries of the upper extremity. (Adapted from Francis CC, Martin AH: *Introduction to human anatomy*, ed 7, St Louis, 1975, Mosby–Year Book.)

Inspection. Inspect for changes in color such as the flush of **fever**, the pallor in response to cold, or the dusky blueness of **cyanosis**.

Palpation

Palpation to assess body temperature. Palpate to determine temperature using the dorsal aspect of your hand or fingers, which are more sensitive to temperature variation. Palpation may reveal moisture and texture variations as well as the vibration of shivering.

Palpation to assess arterial pulses. The pulse is best palpated over arteries that are close to the surface of the body and that lie over a bony surface.

RADIAL PULSE. The radial pulse is the pulse that clinicians most frequently use to initially assess the rate and rhythm of pulsation, the pattern of pulsation, and the shape (consistency) of the arterial wall. The examiner has easy access to this pulse, and its evaluation causes little inconvenience to the client. Other pulses in the upper extremity that are easy to evaluate are the ulnar and brachial pulses (Figure 8-7).

Evaluate the radial pulse by placing the pads of your first and second fingers on the palmar surface of the client's relaxed and slightly flexed wrist medial to the radial styloid process (Figure 8-8). Occasionally the arteries run in a deeper and more lateral course. Feel both radial pulses simultaneously to assess symmetry. Exert sufficient pressure to occlude the artery during diastole yet allow the vessel to return to normal *contour* during systole.

BRACHIAL PULSE. The brachial pulse is palpated and auscultated as part of the blood pressure evaluation.

Palpate the pulse over the upper half of the antecubital fossa at the midline (anterior surface of the elbow joint), because halfway through the fossa, it bifurcates into the radial and ulnar arteries. The brachial artery is medial to the biceps tendon.

Assessment of other pulses are discussed in Chapter 16.

Blood Pressure

Anatomy and physiology. Blood pressure is the result of the interaction of cardiac output and peripheral resistance and is dependent on the velocity of the arterial blood, the intravascular volume, and the elasticity of the arterial walls. **Arterial pressure** is the force exerted by the blood against the wall of the artery as the heart contracts and relaxes. **Systolic** (systole) arterial blood pressure is the force exerted against the wall of the artery when the ventricles are contracted, and **diastolic** (diastole) arterial blood pressure is the force when the heart is in the filling or relaxed phase. **Pulse pressure** is the difference between the systolic and diastolic blood pressures. The usual pulse pressure is between 30 and 40 mm Hg.

The examiner may assess the systemic arterial blood pressure by direct or indirect methods. The direct method requires cannulation of the artery and is not

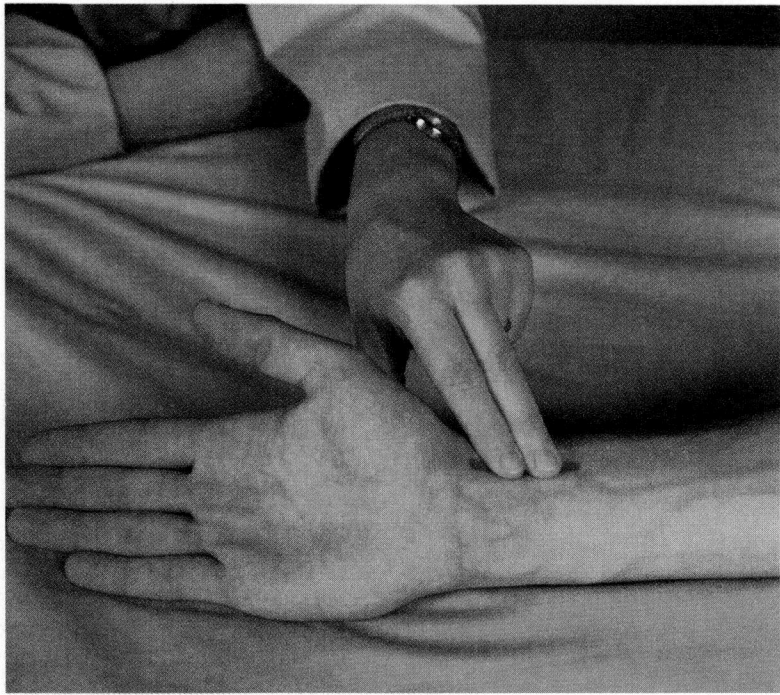

FIGURE 8-8 Palpation of the radial pulse. The site for palpation of the ulnar artery is also marked.

NORMAL VARIATIONS IN BLOOD PRESSURE

The blood pressure in a normal individual varies continually with respiration, autonomic state, emotional levels, and biological rhythms. Furthermore, successive readings of indirect measures of blood pressure by the same or different observers may differ by as much as 10 mm Hg.

In the normal individual, the change from a supine to an erect position causes a slight decrease in systolic blood pressure (less than 15 mm Hg) and a slight rise in diastolic pressure (less than 5 mm Hg).

The blood pressure also shows a **circadian pattern**; it is higher in the afternoon and evening hours and lower in the late hours of sleep.

Because blood pressure is readily altered by stressful events, an effort should be made to relax the client as much as possible before taking the blood pressure.

The blood pressure in the arm increases when the arm is lower than the level of the heart and, conversely, raising the arm above the level of the heart lowers the blood pressure. If you are measuring a standing blood pressure, rest the elbow of the client's arm in your hand, with the weight of his or her forearm on your arm.

done routinely. Indirect blood pressure measurement can be made without opening the artery. The valid methods of indirect measurement are those that are closest in values to those made from direct techniques. Direct blood pressure standards are used to calibrate indirect pressure instruments.

Indirect measurement of blood pressure. Indirect methods of blood pressure measurement take into account the following three physiological facts: (1) the arterial wall may be occluded by direct pressure, resulting in obliteration of the pulse distal to the compression; (2) oscillations that vary directly with the amount of applied pressure may be measured from the compressed artery; and (3) the normal extremity blanches (pales) when its arterial blood supply is occluded by pressure, and there is flushing or return of color when the pressure is removed.

The most commonly used method of indirect assessment of blood pressure is the auscultatory technique. The proper application of the auscultatory method yields values that are within 4 ± 5 mm Hg of the results of the direct method of measurement.

The two types of sphygmomanometers that clinicians commonly use to assess arterial blood pressure are the mercury gravity and the aneroid instruments. Each in-

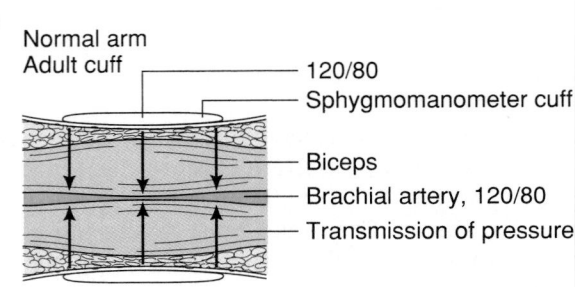

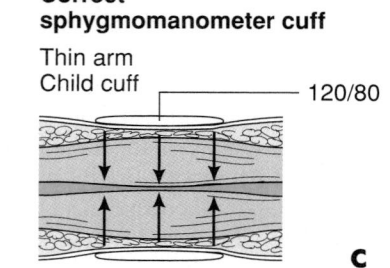

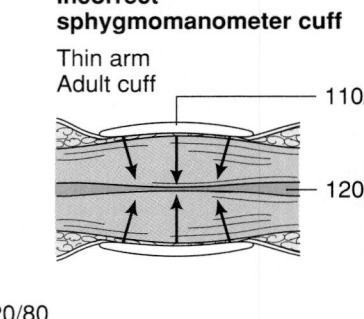

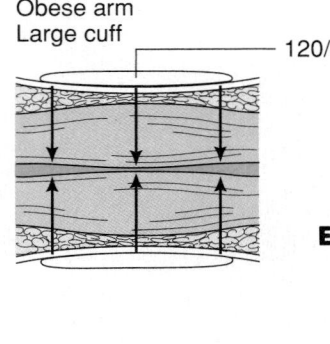

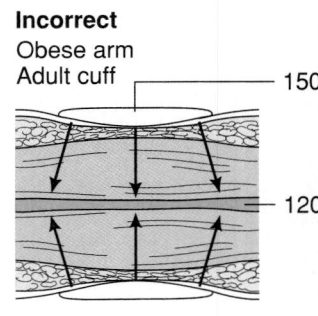

FIGURE 8-9 Longitudinal sections of arms of different diameters to which sphygmomanometer cuffs have been applied. **A,** Normal arm. **B,** Thin arm, correct application. **C,** Thin arm, incorrect application. **D,** Obese arm, correct application using large arm cuff. **E,** Obese arm, incorrect application using adult cuff. (Redrawn from American Heart Association, Wisconsin Affiliate: *Blood pressure measurement training program: nurse instructor manual,* 1980, The Association.)

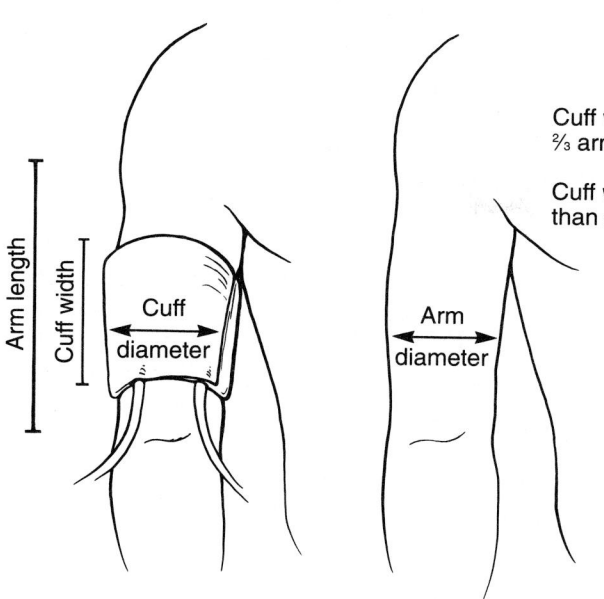

Cuff width =
⅔ arm length

Cuff width = 20% more
than arm diameter

FIGURE 8-10 Guidelines for determining proper cuff size. (Modified from American Heart Association, Wisconsin Affiliate: *Blood pressure measurement training program, nurse instructor manual*, 1980, The Association.)

BLOOD PRESSURE EQUIPMENT

A stethoscope equipped with a bell type diaphragm is used to listen to sounds produced by each type of the blood pressure measurement devices described below.

The mercury gravity manometer (Figure 8-12) is a straight glass tube connected to a reservoir of mercury. The reservoir in turn is connected to the pressure bulb so that pressure created on the bulb causes the mercury to rise in the tube. Because the weight of mercury depends on gravity, a given amount of pressure will always support a column of mercury of the same height if the tube is straight and of uniform diameter. The mercury manometer does not need further calibration after the initial setting.

The aneroid sphygmomanometer (Figure 8-13) is made up of a metal bellows connected to the compression cuff. Changes in pressure within the apparatus cause the bellows to expand and collapse. The movement of the bellows rotates a gear that moves a pointer across the calibrated dial. The aneroid sphygmomanometer is calibrated against a mercury manometer because the more complex mechanisms have been shown to need routine and frequent adjustment. This is simply done by using a connecting Y tube between the manometers.

Electronic devices are available for blood pressure measurement and are used for continuous blood pressure monitoring as well as for self-monitoring of the client's blood pressure at home. The electronic units determine blood pressure by analyzing the sounds of blood flow or measuring oscillations. A cuff is automatically inflated to occlude the artery. Battery operated units produce a digital readout of the systolic and diastolic measures after the cuff is manually inflated.

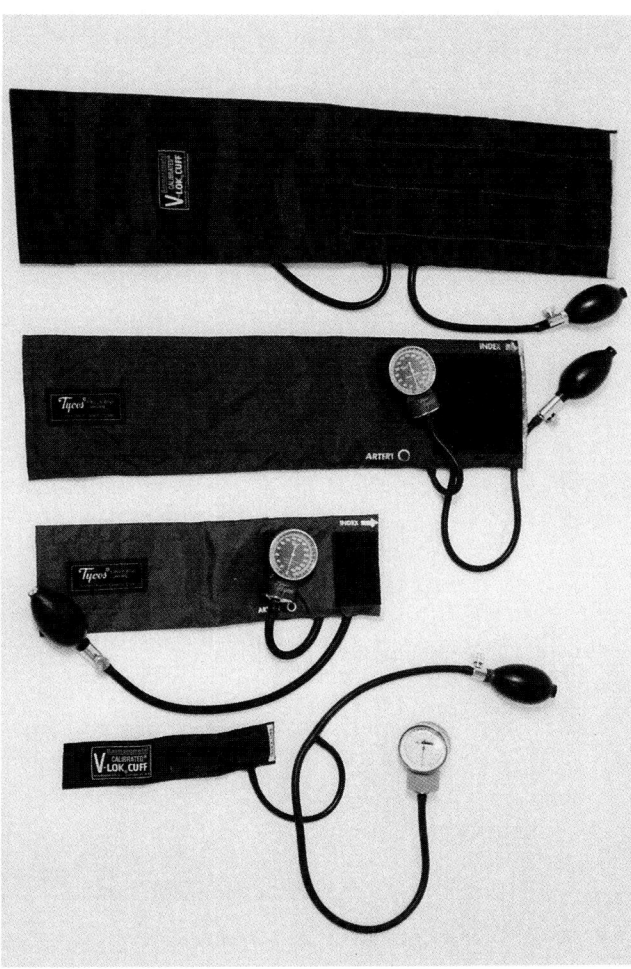

FIGURE 8-11 Blood pressure cuff sizes, *top to bottom*: thigh, large adult, adult, and child cuffs.

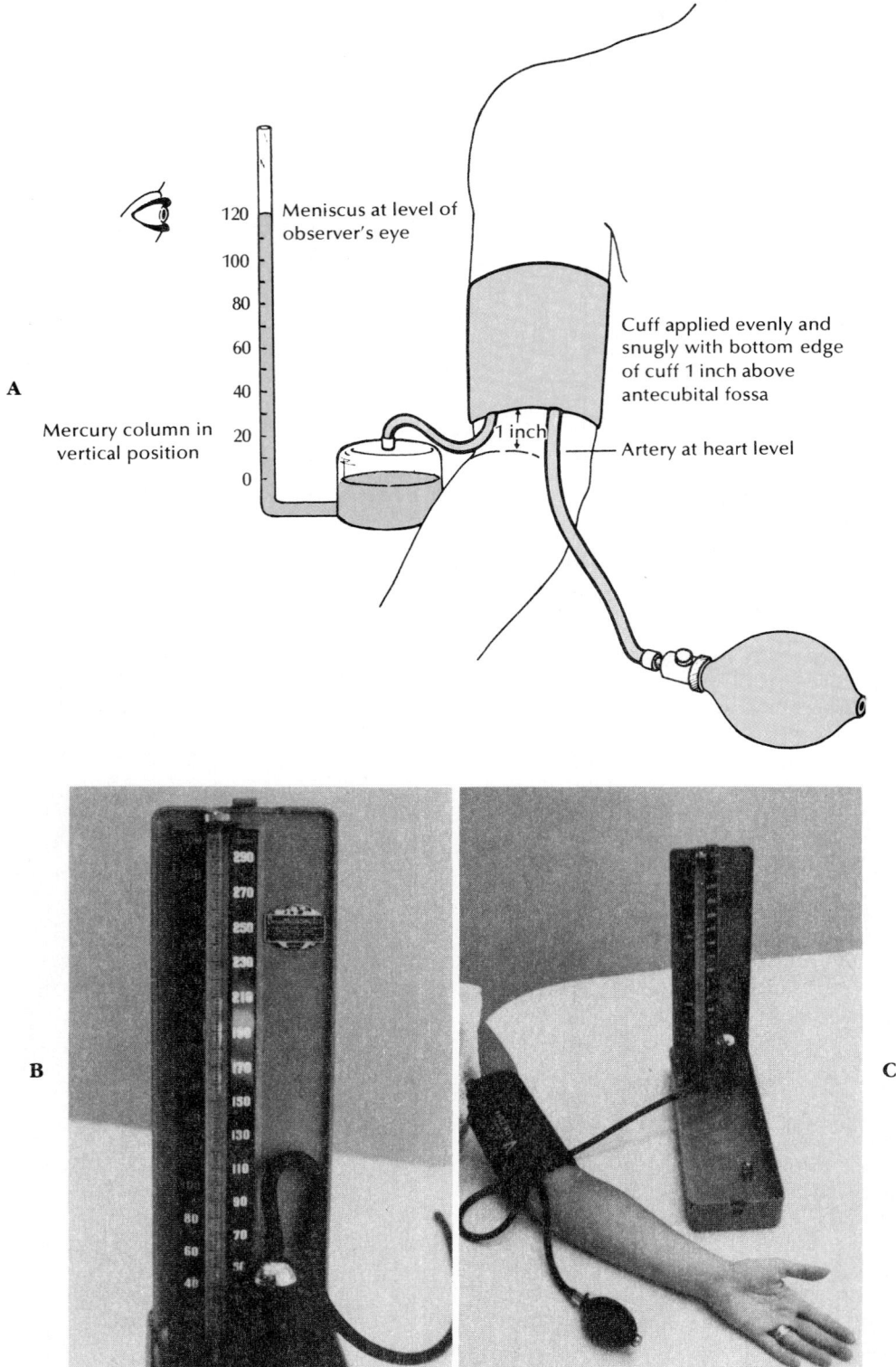

FIGURE 8-12 A, Mercury gravity manometer (diagrammatic). **B,** Mercury manometer. **C,** Mercury sphygmomanometer applied to client. (**A** from Burch GE, DePasquale NP: *Primer of clinical measurement of blood pressure,* St Louis, 1962, Mosby–Year Book. **B** and **C** reproduced with permission from Chicago Heart Association: *Blood pressure measurement: a handbook for instructors,* 1979, The Association.)

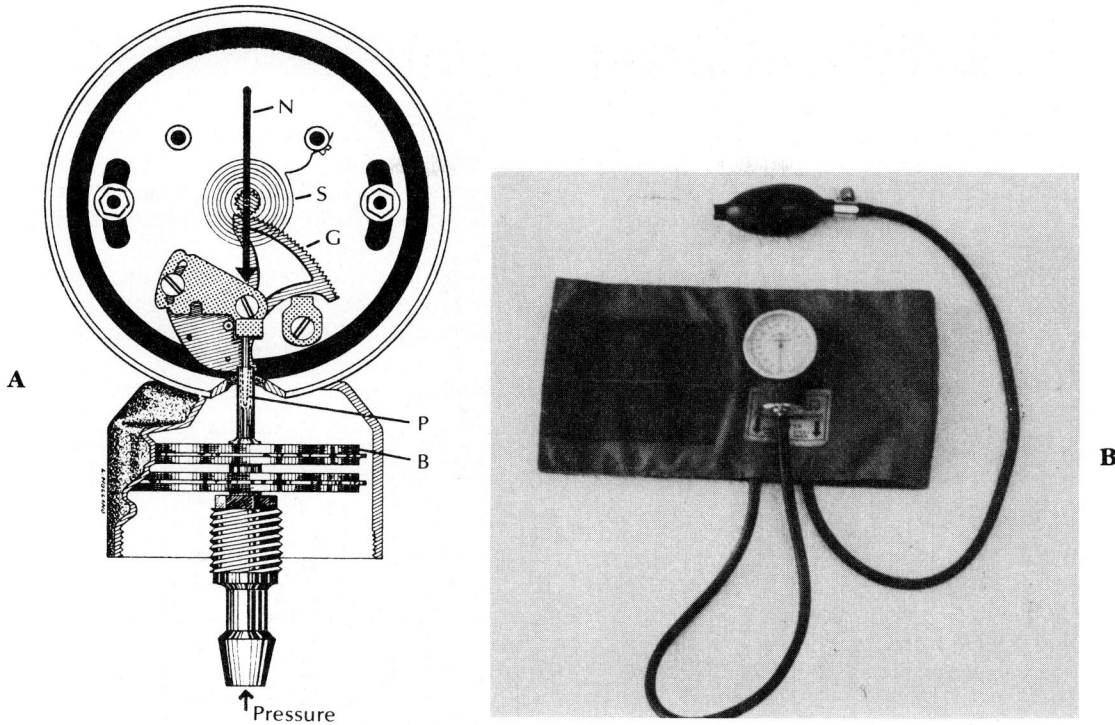

FIGURE 8-13 A, Aneroid sphygmomanometer (diagrammatic). Variations within the bellow *(B)* activate a pin *(P)*, which sets a gear *(G)* into motion. The gear, in turn, operates the spring *(S)*, which causes the needle *(N)* to move across the face of a calibrated dial. **B,** Aneroid sphygmomanometer. (**A** from Burch GE, DePasquale NP: *Primer of clinical measurement of blood pressure*, St Louis, 1962, Mosby–Year Book. **B** reproduced with permission from Chicago Heart Association: *Blood pressure measurement: a handbook for instructors*, 1979, The Association.)

strument includes a pressure manometer, an inflatable rubber bladder used to occlude an artery encased in a cloth cuff, and a rubber hand bulb with a pressure control valve. The mercury sphygmomanometer is considered to be the most accurate and reliable measure when properly used.

Cuff size. If the cuff is too narrow, the blood pressure reading will be erroneously high. Using a cuff that is too small is a common pitfall in blood pressure measurement. A wide cuff increases the risk of an erroneously low reading. (See Figure 8-9.) The sphygmomanometer cuff should be 20% wider than the diameter of the arm. The cuff should cover two thirds of the upper arm (Figure 8-10). Cuffs may be obtained in several sizes as shown in Figure 8-11.

Auscultatory method of arterial blood pressure assessment. When the cuff is properly placed on the client's limb, the arterial blood can flow past the cuff

only when **arterial pressure** exceeds that in the cuff. Partial obstruction of arterial blood flow disturbs the **laminar flow** pattern, creating turbulence. This turbulence produces sounds called **Korotkoff sounds**, which can be heard over arteries distal to the cuff through a stethoscope (Figure 8-14).

Record the **systolic blood pressure** at the point when you initially hear Korotkoff sounds. This is also the beginning of *phase I*, which starts with faint, clear, and rhythmic tapping noises that gradually increase in intensity. At this point the intraluminal pressure is the same as the cuff pressure, but it is not great enough to produce a radial pulse.

Phase II is characterized by a **murmur** or swishing sound that is heard as the vessel distends with blood. *Phase III* is the period when the sounds are crisper and more intense. In phase III the vessel remains open in systole but obliterated in diastole.

The muffling of the Korotkoff sounds is the beginning of *phase IV,* and the pressure at this point is the closest

---

TAKING A BLOOD PRESSURE STEP-BY-STEP

1. Situate the client in a comfortable sitting position, with the arm resting on a flat surface at heart level and the palm turned upward. Expose the upper arm fully. Have the person rest 5 minutes before taking the blood pressure. Wait 30 minutes if the client has smoked or ingested caffeine.
2. Palpate the brachial artery. Center the bladder of the cuff over the brachial artery with the bottom edge of the cuff 2.5 cm (1 in) above the antecubital space. Do not rely on cuff markings; find the center by folding the bladder in half.
3. If you do not know the client's usual blood pressure, estimate the systolic pressure first by applying the cuff, palpating the radial pulse, and inflating the cuff until the pulse disappears. The point when the pulse disappears is the estimated systolic pressure. Deflate the cuff completely and wait 30 seconds before measuring the blood pressure.
4. Be sure the cuff is fully deflated. Wrap the cuff evenly and snugly around the upper arm. Place the manometer at eye level.
5. Place the bell of the stethoscope over the brachial artery. Apply light pressure to ensure good skin contact. Heavy pressure may distort sounds. The bell of the stethoscope is more effective than the diaphragm in transmitting the low-frequency Korotkoff sounds.
6. Close the valve of the pressure bulb clockwise until tight.
7. Rapidly and steadily inflate the cuff to 30 mm Hg above the client's normal or estimated systolic level.
8. Slowly release the valve, allowing the mercury to fall at a rate of 2 to 3 mm Hg per second.
9. Note the point on the manometer at which the first clear sound is heard (phase I). This is the systolic pressure. Continue to deflate the cuff, noting the point at which sound is muffled (phase IV) and when sound disappears (phase V). In children, record Phase IV and Phase V for the diastolic pressure. In adults, Phase V is recorded.
10. Listen 10 to 20 mm Hg below the last sound, then deflate the cuff rapidly and remove it from the client's arm. If repeating the procedure, wait 1 to 2 minutes.

When initially evaluating a client, take blood pressure measures in both sitting and lying positions on each arm. In the normal client there may be a slight decrease in blood pressure, less than 10 mm Hg, from supine to sitting.

---

to the diastolic arterial pressure measured by a direct method. Phase IV is frequently called the first diastolic pressure.

Cessation of sound is *phase V* or the second diastolic pressure. During the entire phase V, the vessel remains open.

For children, the muffling of sound (phase IV) is regarded as the true diastolic pressure, whereas for adults, true diastolic pressure is the disappearance of sound (phase V). An example of a blood pressure recorded for a child might be 96/54/46.

Normal systolic and diastolic pressure. In adults, a normal systolic blood pressure is below 140 mm Hg. Normal diastolic pressure is below 90 mm Hg. A client with a systolic blood pressure less than 55 mm Hg may be considered **hypotensive**. Hypotension in the absence of other signs and symptoms is generally innocent although the blood pressure must be high enough to perfuse blood to the kidneys, brain, and other tissues.

Blood pressure gradually increases until late adolescence, when adult blood pressure levels are reached. To get the best estimate of a person's usual blood pressure, take two or three readings and average them. A single blood pressure reading can be a very unreliable measure.

Technique for Examination and Normal Findings
Measurement of blood pressure in the leg

Measure blood pressure in the leg with the client lying prone, if possible. Apply a large cuff (thigh) to the lower third of the thigh. Center the bladder of the cuff over the popliteal artery. Auscultate in the popliteal fossa. The systolic blood pressure is normally 20 to 30 mm Hg higher in the leg than the arm.

Auscultatory gap

Occasionally, as the cuff is deflating, the Korotkoff sounds disappear and then are heard 10 to 15 mm Hg later. This is called auscultatory gap. When this happens, the examiner may seriously underestimate the systolic pressure or overestimate the diastolic pressure. Auscultatory gap occurs in about 5% of adults and is prevalent in individuals with hypertension. The auscultatory gap will not be a cause for error if the examiner palpates the pulse for disappearance while the cuff is

---

Helpful Hint: *Place the bell lightly over the skin. The bell of the stethoscope transmits low frequency sounds better than the diaphragm.*

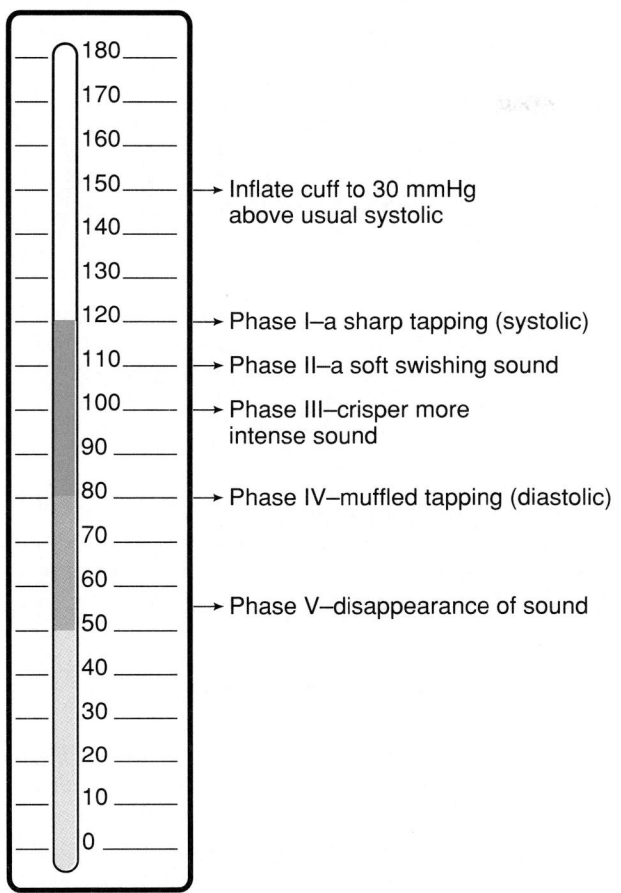

FIGURE 8-14 Phases of Korotkoff sounds that would be recorded as a blood pressure of 120/80/50 mmHg.

Inflate cuff to 30 mmHg above usual systolic

Phase I–a sharp tapping (systolic)

Phase II–a soft swishing sound

Phase III–crisper more intense sound

Phase IV–muffled tapping (diastolic)

Phase V–disappearance of sound

inflated to 30 mm Hg above the point at which the artery is occluded.

> **Helpful Hint:** *If you have not inflated the cuff 30 mm Hg above the systolic pressure (obliteration of the pulse) and begin to listen during Phase II, the sounds may be too soft to hear.*

Absent Phase V

In some individuals, the Korotkoff sounds do not disappear but are heard until the manometer falls to 0 mm Hg. This is especially common in children. In this situation, phase IV, or the change in Korotkoff sounds, is a more reliable estimate of the diastolic pressure than phase V. The blood pressure would be recorded as 140/80/0.

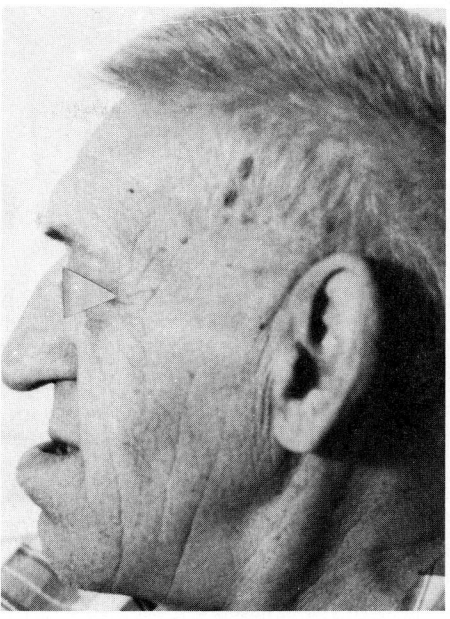

FIGURE 8-15 Acromegaly. Note the prominent jaw and forehead, the large zygomatic arches and supraorbital ridges, enlarged nose, and coarse and oily skin. (Reprinted by permission of Elsevier Science Publishing Co., Inc. From Mazzaferri EL: Endocrinology case studies, ed 2, Flushing NY, 1975, Medical Examination Publishing Co.)

VARIATIONS FROM HEALTH

General Inspection

Be aware of signs of distress in the client. If you detect distress, you may need to deal with the underlying problem immediately and postpone the full interview and physical examination to a later time. Some of the signs that may indicate a need for immediate intervention are (1) anxiety, indicated by a clenched jaw; fidgety movements; cold, moist palms, and an apparent inability to process questions normally; (2) pain, indicated by moaning, writhing, facial grimacing, or guarding of the painful part; (3) cardiopulmonary distress, signaled by labored breathing, coughing, cyanosis, and/or pallor; (4) alteration in consciousness; or (5) observable hemorrhage.

Facial expression. Individuals with **Parkinson's disease** tend to have motionless faces because of limited movement of the musculature. In addition, their blinking rate is slowed so that the client appears to stare.

The facial changes that occur with **acromegaly**, caused by excessive growth hormone production, include a prominent supraorbital ridge, jutting jaw, and enlarged nose and lips (Figure 8-15).

In **myxedema** (hypothyroidism) the features are flattened because they are swollen from fluid retention

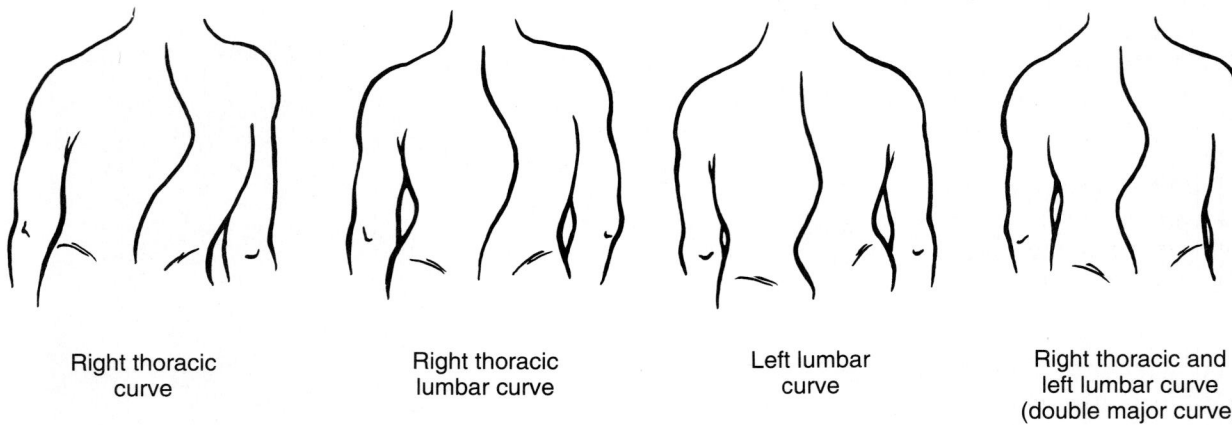

| Right thoracic curve | Right thoracic lumbar curve | Left lumbar curve | Right thoracic and left lumbar curve (double major curve) |

FIGURE 8-16 Examples of scoliosis curve patterns. (Redrawn from Magee DJ: *Orthopedic physical assessment*, Philadelphia, 1987, WB Saunders.)

that is caused by the accumulation of mucopolysaccharides. The face appears heavy and coarse.

The individual with **Bell's palsy** has paralysis of muscles that are innervated by the facial nerve and is unable to close the eye on the affected side; the face appears flaccid, and the mouth droops on the affected side.

Posture. Faulty posture is most likely to result from postural or structural problems. Postural problems result from poor posture habits, muscle imbalance, or pain. Examples are the deviation of the spine toward the affected side in **sciatica** (irritation to the sciatic nerve) and the maintenance of a position that elevates the clavicles, such as leaning forward on extended arms, by the client with chronic obstructive lung disease. Children may have poor postural habits because they do not want to appear taller than their peers.

Occupations that require positions that deviate from normal alignment may result in chronic pain or deformity. Examples include bent shoulders in mine workers and painful shoulders in sewing machine operators.

Structural factors, especially spinal deformities, can also cause faulty posture. Disordered body alignment may lead to changes of the surrounding soft tissue. An example of this is the change in lung volume and ventilation, as well as in circulation, that occurs with **scoliosis** or lateral curvature of the spine (Figure 8-16).

Weight. Anorexia nervosa is a psychological disorder in which the person has a distorted body image and perceives that he or she needs to lose weight. To lose weight the person with anorexia nervosa severely restricts his or her food intake. Bulimia nervosa includes cycles of bingeing and purging by vomiting or using laxatives. Anorexia nervosa and bulimia occur mostly in adolescent females and is associated with amenorrhea. Anorexia nervosa is present if the client is at or

below 85% of his or her expected weight (Figure 8-17). Although over 40% of clients recover from anorexia nervosa, it is associated with a fivefold increase in mortality compared to the general population of the same age and sex.

Obesity is defined as having a body weight that is 20% greater than ideal weight for height.

Endocrine disorders. When hypothyroidism begins in infancy it is called **cretinism** and is characterized by retarded bone maturation and multiple abnormal areas of epiphyseal ossification. Juvenile myxedema is also a cause of retarded growth. In adults, hypothyroidism is identified by the presence of generalized signs and symptoms such as fatigue, modest weight gain, dry

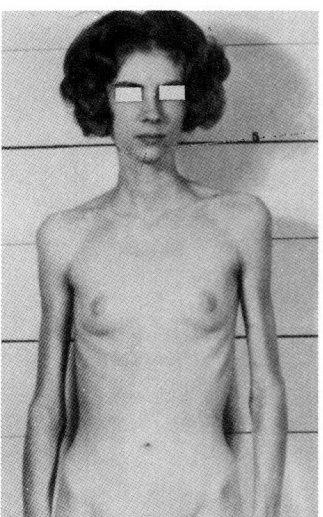

FIGURE 8-17 Young female with anorexia nervosa. (From Ezrin D, Godden JO, Volpe R: Systematic endocrinology, ed 2, New York, 1979, Harper & Row.)

skin, cold intolerance, constipation, slowed pulse, and periorbital swelling.

Gigantism is caused by excess growth hormone (GH) before puberty and before the ossification of the epiphyseal plates. The excess results in the overgrowth of the long bones.

Pituitary dwarfism is the result of hyposecretion of GH. Mental development is usually normal. Men are affected twice as often as women.

Acromegaly is a disease caused by hypersecretion of GH secondary to pituitary tumor; it is usually detected in the fourth or fifth decade of life. In most instances, growth of the acral (small) parts proceeds so slowly that it is not noticed until the changes are well advanced. Bony changes in the skull are most apparent. The mandible is increased in length and width. There is little increase in height because the epiphyseal plates have closed. The features are exaggerated as a result of the expansion of the facial, molar, and frontal bones. The skull itself, as well as the **sinuses**, may be markedly enlarged. **Arthralgia** and **arthritis** are commonly present in acromegaly.

Cushing's syndrome is a disease caused by an excess of endogenous cortisol or exogenous glucocorticoids. The fat distribution that is characteristic of Cushing's syndrome (hyperadrenalism) or administration of the glucocorticoid hormone is in the facial, *nuchal* (neck), truncal, and girdle areas. Cushing's syndrome (Figure 8-18) is characterized by thin skin, purplish **striae, plethora** (red cheeks), muscle weakness, evidence of osteoporosis, redistribution of fat deposits, truncal obesity, *"buffalo hump"* (cervicodorsal fat), "moon facies" (fat cheeks), and thin extremities.

Hair. In starvation, general protein production is inhibited, which leads to reduced hair growth, dullness in appearance, and loss of color. In some ethnic groups, especially those with black or dark brown hair, this loss of hair pigment results in a reddish-brown hair color.

Chemotherapeutic drugs inhibit cell division and thereby inhibit hair growth.

X-ray radiation causes **atrophy** of perifollicular structures, resulting in hair loss.

Increased hair growth in normal sites has been associated with adrenal tumors.

Hirsutism, the appearance of excessive hair in normal and abnormal sites caused by increased androgens, has been observed in the following pathophysiological conditions: bilateral polycystic ovary, Cushing's syndrome, and ovarian tumor. Hirsutism can be most disturbing to the affected female client. The degree of overgrowth need not be marked to pose a threat to the client's feelings of femininity. When the examiner notes hirsutism in a female client, he or she should also be alerted to the presence of other virilizing signs, which

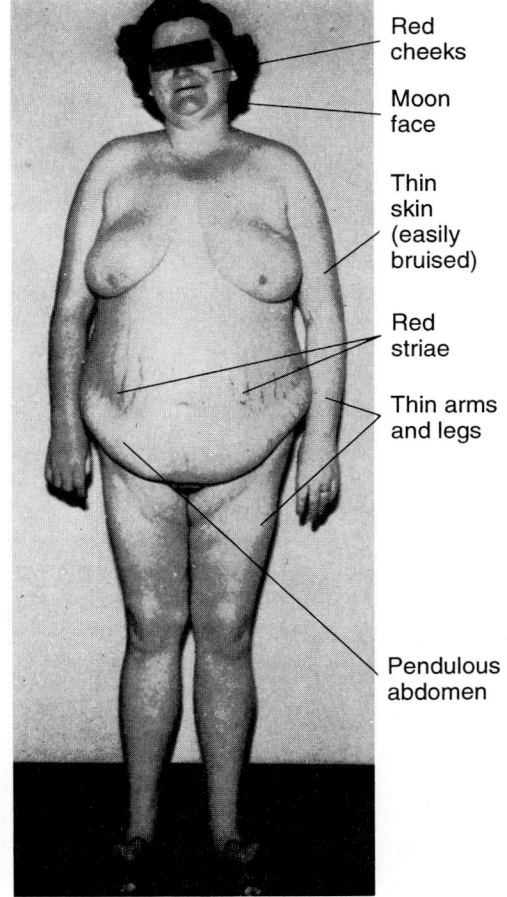

Red cheeks

Moon face

Thin skin (easily bruised)

Red striae

Thin arms and legs

Pendulous abdomen

FIGURE 8-18 Physical characteristics of Cushings syndrome. Prominent features include moon facies, red cheeks, thin skin, bruisability, red striae, poor wound healing. Fat distribution is in trunk with thin arms and legs.
(Modified from Prior JA and others: *Physical diagnosis: the history and examination* of the patient, ed 6, St. Louis, 1981, Mosby–Year Book.)

include a deepening of the voice, clitoral enlargement, and changes in fat distribution. Because of the identity confusion that may exist in the presence of hirsutism, approach the problem with sensitivity.

Fungal infections (tinea capitis) may cause hair loss. The fungal contamination is frequently acquired from pets and contaminated cosmetics.

Chemical, thermal, and physically abusive treatment of the hair causes damage to the surface characterized by breaking and splitting.

Symmetry. Defects of the thoracic cage might change the nature of respiration. Some defects are **pectus carinatum**, in which the sternum is markedly protuberant (as in a bird); funnel chest, or **pectus excavatum**, in

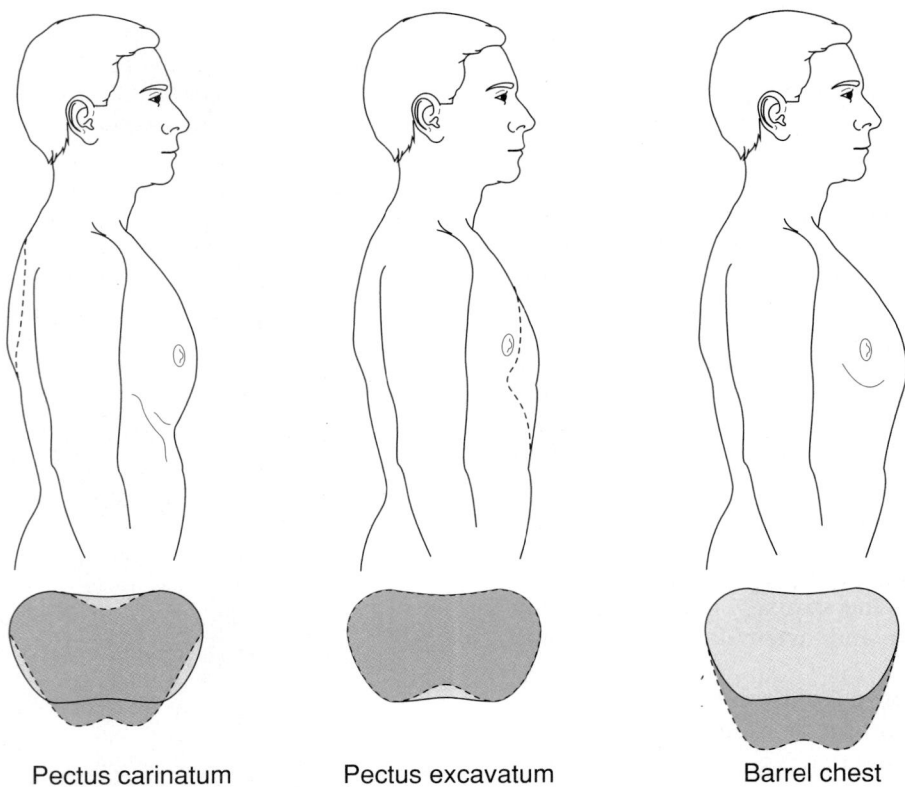

Pectus carinatum   Pectus excavatum   Barrel chest

FIGURE 8-19 Chest deformities. Lower vertical views show change in chest wall contours with deformity. (Modified from Magee DJ: *Orthopedic physical assessment,* Philadelphia, 1987, WB Saunders.)

which the sternum is retracted; and barrel chest (Figure 8-19).

Fever

Fever, or **pyrexia,** is the elevation of body temperature above normal limits compared with a given individual's basal data. For example, a temperature of 37° C (98.6° F) in a client whose normal temperature is 36.1° C (97° F) would be considered a fever. Fever is described in three stages: cold, hot, and **defervescence** (decline).

Cold stage. The cold stage is the period of a developing increase in core temperature and is characterized by heat conservation reactions. Cutaneous circulation is decreased and the skin looks blanched and feels cold. Heat production produces shivering and piloerection ("goose pimples"). Chills and **rigor** are the extremes of shivering and produce rapid increases in temperature.

Hot stage. The hot stage is the period after the fever has peaked (regulated at the new set point). During this stage blood flow to the periphery is increased. The body radiates excess heat, feels hot, and is flushed.

Defervescence. The stage of defervescence is the period of fever **abatement** and is characterized by heat-loss mechanisms, particularly vasodilation and sweating. Diaphoresis is diffuse perspiration, which may accompany fever abatement.

Irregularities in Pulse

Tachycardia. Rates that are persistently over 100 beats per minute **(tachycardia)** suggest some abnormality. Heart rates are increased during fever, anemia, hypoxia, and low volume states (shock). However, tachycardia can also be the result of exercise, anger, anxiety, or fear.

Bradycardia. **Bradycardia** is a slow heart rate of less than 50 beats per minute. A slow rate may indicate stimulation of the parasympathetic system or failure in the electrical conduction system of the heart. Bradycardia may be caused by overdoses of digitalis. Bradycardia occurs normally in the well-trained athlete. This is due to heart muscle increasing in strength with development of skeletal muscle. This increased strength results in greater stroke volume, which in turn requires fewer beats per minute to maintain cardiac output.

Irregular rhythm. An irregular rhythm of the pulse is caused by cardiac **arrhythmia**. Some arrhythmias are caused by atrial **fibrillation**; atrial flutter with block; second degree heart block resulting in dropped beats; and irregular sinus depolarization.

Bigeminal pulse. Bigeminal pulse is a pulse that alternates in amplitude from beat to beat. This alteration may be produced by a small, premature ventricular beat after a strong beat, resulting from normal electrical cardiac conduction. The strong pulse occurs after a long diastolic filling phase following the premature beat. The pulse is irregular. Identify the bigeminal pulse by simultaneously palpating the radial pulse and listening at the precordium.

Pulsus alternans. Pulsus alternans is a pulse that alternates between strong and weak beats while the rhythm is regular. When the variation is marked, the alternation from weak to strong beats is palpable.

Palpitations. Palpitation is a term used when the client describes feeling his or her heartbeat. Common terms used by clients to describe this phenomenon are "pounding," "thudding," "fluttering," "flopping," and "skipping." Palpitation is more common just before falling asleep or during sleep.

Palpitations may be experienced by the normal individual following strenuous exercise or when that person is aroused emotionally or sexually. In this case, the cardiac contraction is of a greater rate and amplitude. A common feature of the anxiety state (arousal) is palpitations caused by the increased adrenergic activity. The relationship between anxiety and palpitations creates some problem for the examiner; because the presence of palpitations frequently creates anxiety, ask questions carefully so as not to cause further anxiety.

Palpitations are also associated with anemia, fever, hypoglycemia, and thyrotoxicosis. Irregularities in cardiac rhythm have also been associated with palpitations, particularly extra systoles and ectopic tachycardia.

Variations in Blood Pressure

Differences in blood pressure indicating disease. On initial examination, measure blood pressures in both the client's arms. Differences in blood pressure between the two arms may be caused by congenital aortic obstruction **(coarctation),** acquired conditions such as aortic dissection, or obstruction of the arteries of the upper arm.

Marked drops in pressure (greater than 30 mm Hg) incurred when the client stands may indicate a vasopressor defect or hypovolemia.

Sudden changes in blood pressure may produce changes in body function, and sudden drops in normal blood pressure may result in fainting. Fainting is observed in **orthostatic hypotension**, defined as a blood pressure decrease of 30 mm Hg and a 10 to 20 beats per minute increased pulse from a lying to a standing position. In orthostatic hypotension, the blood pressure may be normal when an individual is reclining but drops when he or she rises to a sitting or standing position, particularly when the position change is rapid. Faintness and dizziness from orthostatic hypotension is common in individuals on antihypertensive medications, or individuals who are elderly or confined to bed.

Hypertension. The screening examination is especially important for recognizing the client who has **hypertension** (persistently elevated blood pressure). Because hypertension may be present without symptoms, it is known as the silent disease. A client who does not feel ill does not usually come to a clinic or hospital for health care. Thus, the screening examination may be instrumental in prompting the hypertensive client to begin early treatment to prevent some of the complications of untreated hypertension.

In their 1988 report, the Joint National Committee on Detection, Evaluation and Treatment of High Blood Pressure Guidelines defines hypertension as being at least two blood pressure readings that average greater than 140/90 mm Hg or as a blood pressure below 140/

TABLE 8-3

Follow-Up Criteria for Initial Blood Pressure Measurement for Adults Age 18 Years or Older

Range, mm Hg	Recommended follow-up*
Diastolic	
<85	Recheck within 2 years
85-89	Recheck within 1 year
90-104	Confirm within 2 months
105-114	Evaluate or refer promptly to source of care within 2 weeks
≥115	Evaluate or refer immediately to source of care
Systolic, when diastolic blood pressure is <90	
<140	Recheck within 2 years
140-199	Confirm within 2 months
≥200	Evaluate or refer promptly to source of care within 2 weeks

*If recommendations for follow-up of diastolic and systolic blood pressure are different, the shorter recommended time for recheck and referral should take precedence.
From Joint National Committee on Detection, Evaluation, and Treatment of High Blood Pressure: The 1988 report of the Joint National Committee on Detection, Evaluation, and Treatment of High Blood Pressure, *Arch Intern Med* 148:1023, May 1988.

90 in an individual who is currently using antihypertensive medication. Elevation of either systolic or diastolic blood pressure above 140/90 needs further evaluation. Hypertension should not be diagnosed on the basis of a single reading but on the average of two or three blood pressure readings. The timing of subsequent readings should be based on the initial blood pressure level. Table 8-3 presents follow-up criteria for ranges of systolic and diastolic readings.

The prevalence of hypertension in the United States is considerably greater in blacks than in whites. Ninety percent of adults have **essential** or **idiopathic hypertension.** In essential hypertension, no physiological cause is identified for the elevated blood pressure level.

Obtain a blood pressure measurement with well-child visits beginning at age 3. The screening examination may yield an incidence of hypertension in less than 3% of children 4 to 15 years of age. Early detection of the hypertensive children may mean that diagnosis and treatment may be initiated in time to prevent the sequelae of the underlying disease process.

TEACHING SELF-ASSESSMENT

Maintaining a normal weight reduces the risk of hypertension. Weight loss often results in a substantial decrease in blood pressure even when ideal weight is not achieved. Restriction of daily dietary sodium to 2 g is also recommended. Alcohol consumption should not exceed 1 ounce per day (i.e., 8 ounces of wine or 24 ounces of beer). Other risk-reducing behaviors include avoiding tobacco use, following a regular program of exercise, and using behavior modification therapies such as relaxation and biofeedback.

A client can identify his or her maximal heart rate to measure the amount of exertion in physical exercise. To do this, he or she subtracts his or her age from 220. To exercise aerobically, the pulse must reach 80% of an individual's maximal heart rate. The client should obtain a radial or carotid baseline pulse before exercising by feeling the pulse, counting for 10 seconds, and then multiplying that count by 6. The count should be repeated immediately after exercise to obtain the maximal heart rate and 2 minutes later to assess recovery to baseline. If after 2 minutes the pulse has not returned to near baseline, the exercise involved too much exertion.

DOCUMENTATION

Sample Documentation

Certain characteristics of the total person are noted when recording general appearance from head to toe: apparent age; sex; race; body type and symmetry; weight and nutritional status; posture and motor activity; mental status; speech; general skin condition; apparent state of health and signs of distress. An example of the record of the general survey might read as follows:

Mr. A. is an alert, talkative 25-year-old Asian male who appears younger than his stated age and exhibits no acute distress.

A description of the client's bodily proportions should be included in the written record of the general survey. For example:
Mr. R. is a tall, thin male with an erect posture.

An example of obtaining and recording general appearance information, based on brief history data follows:
Past health history:
Ms. C is a white 45-year-old married female. She has no history of hospital admissions. Her chief complaint is that she has not slept well in weeks and feels fatigued.
Physical examination:
General appearance: Ms. C is a well-dressed, well-nourished female of average body type in no apparent distress. Skin color appears slightly pale. She has symmetrical, coordinated but slow body movements and a slumped posture. Hair and nails appear clean, and dress and grooming is appropriate. She is alert and oriented and answers questions but does not initiate conversation.
Vital signs:
Height 173 cm, Weight 68.2 Kg
Oral temperature 37.1° C, radial pulse 78, regular and strong, respirations 12, unlabored, blood pressure 130/80 mmHg right arm sitting and 124/84 mmHg left arm sitting.

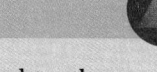

Nursing Diagnosis *THE NEXT STEP*

Nursing diagnoses that could apply to the general assessment include, but are not limited to, the following:

HIGH RISK FOR ALTERED BODY TEMPERATURE The state in which an individual is at risk for failure to maintain body temperature within normal range.

Defining Characteristics (risk factors)
- Extremes of age or weight
- Exposure to cold or hot environments
- Dehydration
- Inactivity or vigorous activity
- Medications causing vasoconstriction/vasodilation
- Altered metabolic rate
- Sedation
- Inappropriate clothing for environmental temperature
- Illness or trauma affecting temperature regulation

INEFFECTIVE THERMOREGULATION The state in which an individual's temperature fluctuates between hypothermia nad hyperthermia.

Defining Characteristics
- Fluctuations in body temperature above or below the normal range

Related Factors
- Trauma or illness
- Immaturity
- Aging
- Fluctuating environmental temperature

HYPERTHERMIA The state in which an individual's body temperature is elevated above his/her normal range.

Defining Characteristics
- Increase in body temperature above normal range
- Flushed skin, warm to touch
- Increased respiratory rate
- Tachycardia
- Seizures/convulsions

Related Factors
- Dehydration
- Exposure to hot environment
- Vigorous activity
- Medication/anesthesia
- Inappropriate clothing
- Increased metabolic rate
- Illness or trauma
- Dehydration
- Inability/decreased ability to perspire

Continued.

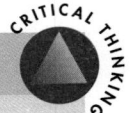

Nursing Diagnosis—*cont'd*

HYPOTHERMIA The state in which an individual's body temperature is reduced below his/her normal range but not below 35.6° C (rectal)/36.4° C (rectal, newborn).

Defining Characteristics

- Decrease in body temperature below normal range
- Shivering (mild)
- Slow capillary refill
- Cyanotic nail beds
- Tachycardia
- Cool skin, pallor

Related Factors

- Exposure to cold or cold environment
- Illness or trauma
- Inability/decreased ability to shiver
- Malnutrition
- Decreased metabolic rate
- Aging
- Vasodilation
- Damage to the hypothalmus

DECREASED CARDIAC OUTPUT The state in which the blood pumped by an individual's heart is sufficiently reduced to the extent that it is inadequate to meet the needs of the body's tissues.

Defining Characteristics

- Variations in blood pressure readings
- Jugular vein distention
- Decreased peripheral pulses
- Arrhythmias
- Fatigue
- Oliguria
- Dyspnea
- Orthopnea
- Restlessness
- Changes in mental status
- Syncope/vertigo
- Edema
- Cough/frothy sputum
- Weakness
- Rapid pulse
- Cyanosis
- Angina
- Rales
- Gallop rhythm
- Cold/clammy skin

Related Factors

- Reduced stroke volume as a result of electrophysiologic problems
- Hypovolemia
- Mechanical or structural problems

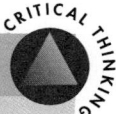

Nursing Diagnosis—*cont'd*

ACTIVITY INTOLERANCE The state in which an individual has insufficient physiological or psychological energy to endure or complete required or desired daily activities.

Defining Characteristics

- Verbal report of fatigue or weakness
- External discomfort or dyspnea
- Abnormal responses to activity (heart rate, blood pressure, or EKG changes reflecting ischemia or arrhythmias)
- Weakness
- Confusion and vertigo

Levels of Activity Intolerance:

Level I:
  Walk, regular pace, on level indefinitely; one flight or more but more short of breath than normally.

Level II:
  Walk one city block 500 feet on level; climb one flight slowly without stopping.

Level III:
  Walk no more than 50 feet on level without stopping; unable to climb one flight of stairs without stopping.

Level IV:
  Dyspnea and fatigue at rest.

Related Factors

- Bed rest
- Immobility
- Sedentary life-style
- Imbalance between oxygen supply and demand
- Generalized weakness

FATIGUE An overwhelming sense of exhaustion and decreased capacity for physical and mental work regardless of adequate sleep.

Defining Characteristics

- Inability to maintain casual routines
- Decreased performance, accident prone
- Verbalization of an unremitting and overwhelming lack of energy
- Perceived need for additional energy to accomplish routine tasks
- Increased physical complaints
- Emotionally labile or irritable
- Impaired ability to concentrate; lethargic/listless
- Decreased libido
- Disinterest in surroundings/introspection

Related Factors

- Overwhelming psychological/emotional demands
- Increased energy requirements to perform activities of daily living
- Excessive social and/or role demands
- Discomfort
- Altered body chemistry (e.g., medications, drug withdrawal, chemotherapy)
- Decreased/increased metabolic energy production

Continued.

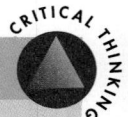

Nursing Diagnosis—*cont'd*

SELF-CARE DEFICIT, BATHING/HYGIENE The state in which one experiences an impaired ability to perform or complete bathing/hygiene activities for oneself.

Defining Characteristics

- Inability to wash body or body parts
- Inability to obtain or get to water source
- Inability to regulate temperature or flow

Levels of Self-Bathing Hygiene Deficit:

Level I:
  Requires use of equipment or devices
Level II:
  Requires help from another person(s): assistance, supervision, teaching
Level III:
  Requires help from another person(s) and equipment or device
Level IV:
  Is dependent and does not participate in self-bathing/hygiene

Related Factors

- Intolerance to activity
- Pain
- Uncompensated perceptual-cognitive, musculoskeletal, or neuromuscular impairment
- Depression
- Anxiety

SELF-CARE DEFICIT, DRESSING/GROOMING The state in which one experiences an impaired ability to perform or complete dressing and grooming activities for oneself.

Defining Characteristics

- Impaired ability to put on or take off necessary items of clothing
- Impaired ability to obtain or replace articles of clothing
- Impaired ability to fasten clothing
- Inability to maintain appearance at a satisfactory level

Levels of Self-Dressing—Grooming Deficit:

Level I:
  Requires use of equipment or devices
Level II:
  Requires help from another person(s): assistance, supervision, teaching
Level III:
  Requires help from another person(s) and equipment or device
Level IV:
  Is dependent and does not participate in self-dressing/grooming

Related Factors

- Intolerance to activity
- Pain
- Uncompensated perceptual-cognitive, musculoskeletal, or neuromuscular impairment
- Depression
- Anxiety

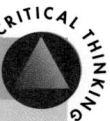

Nursing Diagnosis—*cont'd*

PAIN The state in which an individual experiences and reports the presence of severe discomfort or an uncomfortable sensation.

Defining Characteristics

- Communication of pain descriptors
- Guarding behavior
- Self-focusing
- Narrowed focus (altered time perception, withdrawal from social contact, impaired thought processes)
- Distraction behavior (moaning, crying, pacing, seeking out other people and/or activities, restless)
- Facial mask of pain (eyes lack luster, "beaten look," fixed or scattered movement, grimace)
- Alteration in muscle tone (from listless to rigid)
- Autonomic responses (diaphoresis, blood pressure and pulse rate changes, pupillary dilation, increased or decreased respiratory rate)

Related Factors

- Deficit (pain management techniques)
- Injuring agents (biological, chemical, physical, psychological)

CHRONIC PAIN The state in which an individual experiences pain that continues for more than 6 months.

Defining Characteristics

- Verbal report or observed evidence of pain experienced for more than 6 months
- Facial masks (of pain)
- Guarded movement
- Fear of reinjury
- Physical and social withdrawal
- Altered ability to continue previous activities
- Anorexia
- Weight changes
- Changes in sleep patterns

Related Factors

- Chronic physical/psychological disability.

SELF-ESTEEM DISTURBANCE Negative self-evaluation/feelings about self or self-capabilities, which may be directly or indirectly expressed.

Defining Characteristics

- Self-negating verbalizations
- Lack of eye contact
- Expression of shame/guilt
- Rationalization/rejection of positive feedback
- Exaggerations of negative feedback about self
- Hesitation to try new things/situations
- Denial of problems obvious to others
- Rationalization of personal failures
- Hypersensitivity to criticism
- Grandiosity
- Projection of blame/responsibility for problems
- Evaluations of self as unable to deal with events

Continued.

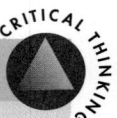

Nursing Diagnosis—*cont'd*

Related Factors

- Self-negating verbalizations
- Lack of eye contact
- Expressions of shame/guilt
- Evaluations of self as unable to deal with events
- Rationalizations/rejections of positive feedback
- Exaggerations of negative feedback about self
- Hesitation to try new things/situations
- Denial of problems obvious to others
- Projection of blame/responsibility for problems
- Rationalization of personal failures
- Hypersensitivity to criticism
- Grandiosity

BODY IMAGE DISTURBANCE Disruption in the way one perceives one's body image.

Defining Characteristics

- Verbalized actual or perceived change in structure and/or function of body or body part
- Verbalized change in life-style because of negative feelings or perception of body
- Verbalized fear of rejections by others
- Repeated verbalizations focusing on past strengths, function, or appearance
- Verbalized negative feelings about body (dirty, big, small, unsightly)
- Verbalized feelings of helplessness, hopelessness, powerlessness in relation to the body
- Preoccupation with change in body or loss of part
- Personalization of part or loss by name
- Guilt, shame
- Refusal to verify actual change in body or body part
- Hiding or overexposing body part
- Not touching/looking at body part
- Change in social involvement or social relationships
- Emphasis on remaining strengths or heightened achievement

Related Factors

- Nonintegration of change in body characteristics, function, or limits
- Perceived developmental imperfections

Clinical Application

It is the middle of summer; the temperature is 102° F with a heat index of over 110° F. Mrs. H., an 84-year-old female, is brought into the emergency room by ambulance. Her daughter found her in a chair where she had been sitting all night, after she didn't answer the phone several times. The room was very hot and the windows were closed. Mrs. H. did not know who her daughter was nor who she was. She could not get out of the chair. Upon admission, Mrs. H. complained of black spots floating in front of her eyes, a severe headache, weakness, and nausea. Vital signs were as follows: rectal temperature 40° C (104° F); apical pulse rate 120 beats/min; respirations 32 and slightly labored; blood pressure 100/50 mm Hg. Her skin is flushed with her lower extremities beginning to mottle. Her arms and legs are cool to touch, while skin on her trunk feels very warm and dry. She is just beginning to shiver. Her peripheral pulses are weak. Mrs. H. is diagnosed with hyperthermia.

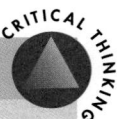

Nursing Diagnosis—*cont'd*

SUBJECTIVE DATA: Client complains of:
Black spots in front of eyes
A severe headache
Nausea

OBJECTIVE DATA:
Confused
PERRLA
Rectal temperature 40° C
Pulse 120
Respirations: 32 labored, fast and shallow
Blood pressure 100/50 mm Hg
Skin flushed all over
Lower extremities with weak peripheral pulses and mottled skin
Skin on trunk flushed, warm, and very dry
Extremities starting to shake slightly (shiver)

NURSING DIAGNOSES

Hyperthermia related to exposure to hot environment.

Defining Characteristics

- Increase in body temperature above normal range
- Flushed skin, warm to touch
- Increased respiratory rate
- Tachycardia

Activity intolerance related to generalized weakness

Defining Characteristics

- Verbal report of weakness
- Dyspnea
- Confusion

Decreased cardiac output related to alterations in rhythm

Defining Characteristics

- Decreased peripheral pulses
- Fatigue
- Dyspnea
- Changes in mental status
- Weakness
- Rapid pulse
- Cold peripheral skin

GLOSSARY

abatement Decrease in intensity of a pain or other symptom.

acromegaly Chronic disease caused by hypersecretion of growth hormone; it occurs in middle-age and is characterized by overgrowth of the small skeletal parts.

alopecia Loss of hair to baldness.

anorexia Loss of appetite.

Anorexia nervosa A psychological disorder, occurring mostly in adolescent females, in which the person has a distorted body image and perceives that he or she needs to lose weight by severely restricting food intake. Anorexia is present if the client is at or below 85% of his or her expected weight. Bulimia nervosa includes cycles of bingeing and purging by vomiting or using laxatives.

arrhythmia Any deviation from the normal pace of the heart.

arterial pressure The force exerted by the blood against the arterial walls. Blood pressure is measured in millimeters of mercury above sea level. The contraction of the heart results in a pulsatile ejection of the blood, resulting in variation of the pressure from a systolic peak of about 120 mm Hg at maximum left ventricular stroke output and a minimum diastolic pressure of about 80 mm Hg. The pulse pressure is equal to the difference between systolic and diastolic pressure.

arthralgia Any pain that affects a joint.

arthritis Inflammation of a joint.

atrophy Wasting; decrease in the size of a cell, tissue, organ, or body part.

Bell's palsy A lower motor neuron lesion that affects both the upper and lower facial motor function.

bigeminal, bigeminy A pattern of arrhythmia consisting of coupled or paired ventricular beats; alternating QRS complexes are ventricular premature depolarizations.

body image A person's subjective concept of his or her physical appearance.

bounding pulse A pulse that, on palpation, feels full and springlike because of an increased thrust of cardiac contraction or an increased volume of circulating blood within the elastic structures of the vascular system.

bradycardia Slower than normal heart rate (<50 beats per minute).

buffalo hump An accumulation of fat on the back of the neck associated with the prolonged use of large doses of glucocorticoids or the hypersecretion of cortisol caused by Cushing's syndrome.

circadian pattern A cyclic pattern or period of 24 hours.

coarctation A tightening or compression of the walls of a vessel, producing a narrowed lumen.

conduction A process in which heat is transferred from one substance to another because of a difference in temperature.

contour Surface outline or shape of the part being described.

convection The transfer of heat through a gas or liquid by the circulation of heated particles

cretinism Disease caused by congenital lack of thyroid hormone; characterized by retarded physical and mental development, deafness, dystrophy of bones and soft tissue, and abnormally low concentrations of thyroid hormones.

Cushing's syndrome Hypersecretion of the glucocorticoids of the adrenal cortex, characterized by fragility of the skin, poor wound healing, truncal fat deposition, and thin extremities.

cyanosis Dusky blue skin color, seen especially in the lips and nail beds, when the hemoglobin saturation is less than 75% to 85% or PaO_2 is less than 50 mm Hg.

defervescence The diminishing or disappearance of a fever.

diastolic (diastole) The force of blood against the arterial wall during the filling phase of the cardiac cycle.

dysplasia Disorder in the size, shape, or organization of adult cells.

ectomorph A person whose physique is characterized by slenderness, fragility, and predominance of structures derived from the ectoderm.

endomorph A person whose body build is characterized by a soft, round physique with a large trunk and thighs, tapering extremities, an accumulation of fat throughout the body, and a predominance of structures derived from the endoderm.

essential hypertension An elevated arterial pressure for which no cause can be found and that is often the only significant clinical finding.

evaporation The change of a substance from a solid or liquid state to a gaseous state. The process of evaporation is hastened by an increase in temperature and a decrease in atmospheric pressure.

fever Pyrexia; elevation of the body temperature above normal for a given individual.

fibrillation Fine, continuous twitching caused by irregular, random contraction of a single muscle or group of fibers. Atrial fibrillation usually benign; ventricular fibrillation can be life-threatening.

gait The manner of progression in walking. *Ataxic gait:* foot raised high with sole striking down suddenly.

gigantism Excessive growth of the body or its parts; may be the result of hypersecretion of growth hormone in childhood.

hirsutism Excessive hairiness, especially in females.

homeostasis A relative constancy in the internal environment of the body, naturally maintained by adaptive responses that promote healthy survival.

hypertension Persistent elevation of blood pressure above 140 mmHg systolic or 90 mmHg diastolic.

hypotension An abnormal condition in which the blood pressure is not adequate for normal perfusion and oxygenation of the tissues.

idiopathic Without a known cause.

Korotkoff sounds Turbulent sounds heard when auscultating the blood pressure.

laminar flow An airflow that is concentrated into a narrow pathway.

mesomorph A person whose physique is characterized by a predominance of muscle, bone, and connective tissue, structures that develop from the mesodermal layer of the embryo.

morphology The study of the physical shape and size of a specimen, plant, or animal.

murmur Blowing sound caused by turbulence of blood flow, heard through the stethoscope over the heart; when heard in the great vessels the sound is called a bruit.

myxedema Hypothyroidism. Hypometabolism is present, and nonpitting edema results from the presence of hydrated mucopolysaccharides in connective tissue.

nuchal Pertaining to the nape of the neck.

obesity A condition in which the amount of fat in the body is excessive in relation to total body weight; exceeding 20% of ideal body weight.

orthostatic (postural) hypotension Lower blood pressure of greater than 30 mm Hg that occurs on rising from a lying or sitting to an erect position.

osteoporosis A disorder characterized by loss of bone density, occurring most frequently in postmenopausal women, in sedentary or immobilized individuals, and in persons on long-term steroid therapy.

palpitation Client's sensation of a pounding or racing of the heart, associated with normal emotional responses or with certain heart disorders.

Parkinson's disease A progressive disorder of the basal ganglia, characterized by tremor, difficulty in initiating voluntary movements, muscle weakness and rigidity, and a peculiar gait.

pectus carinatum Structural deformity of the thoracic cage where the sternum is displaced anteriorly, increasing the anteroposterior diameter. The costal cartilages adjacent to the sternum are depressed.

pectus excavatum Structural deformity of the thoracic cage where the lower sternum is depressed. Compression of the heart and great vessels may cause murmurs.

pituitary dwarfism A condition of being abnormally small, especially small of stature due to a deficiency of growth hormone.

plethora Pertaining to a red, florid complexion.

pulse Palpable, rhythmic expansion of the artery.

pulse pressure The difference between the systolic and diastolic blood pressure.

pulsus alternans A pulse characterized by a regular alternation of weak and strong beats without changes in the length of the cycle.

pyrexia Fever; elevation of the body temperature above normal for a given individual.

radiation The emission of energy, rays, or waves.

rigor Common term for shivering accompanying a chill or for muscle rigidity accompanying depletion of adenosine triphosphate, as in death (rigor mortis).

sciatica Pain, weakness, or paresthesias associated with inflammation or pressure on the sciatic nerve; posterior aspect of the thigh, posterolateral and anterolateral aspects of the leg into the foot.

scoliosis Lateral deviation of the spine.

sebaceous Pertaining to or secreting sebum, an oily secretion composed of fat and epithelial debris.

self-esteem The degree of worth and competence one attributes to oneself.

sign Objective evidence of disease that is perceptible to the examiner.

sinus A hollow cavity in a bone or other tissue.

stria, *pl.* **striae (lineae albicantes)** Atrophic line or streak that differs in texture and color from the surrounding skin because of disrupted elastic fibers of the reticular layer of the cutis.

symptom A client's subjective perception of an alteration of bodily or mental function.

systolic (systole) The force of blood against the arterial wall during the ejection phase of the cardiac cycle.

tachycardia Rapid heart rate (≥ 100 beats per minute). *Atrial flutter:* rapid, regular, uniform atrial contraction caused by AV block; ventricular rhythm varies with the degree of AV block. *Atrial tachycardia:* arrhythmia caused by the atria; rapid, regular beat of the entire heart. *Ventricular tachycardia:* arrhythmia caused by the ventricles; rapid, relatively regular heartbeat.

vital or cardinal signs Indicators of bodily function such as blood pressure, temperature, pulse, and respiration.

BIBLIOGRAPHY

American Heart Association: *Recommendations for human blood pressure determination by sphygmomanometers,* Dallas, 1987, The Association.

American Heart Association, Wisconsin Affiliate: *Blood pressure measurement education program,* Nurse instructor manual, 1980, The Association.

Centers for Disease Control: *Recommendations for prevention of HIV transmission in health-care settings,* MMWR (suppl 36):SS, August, 1987.

Carnoni-Huntley, LaCroix AZ, Havlik RJ: Race and sex differentials in the impact of hypertension in the United States, *Arch Intern Med* 149:780, 1989.

Edelman CL, Mandle CL: *Health promotion throughout the lifespan,* ed 2, St Louis, 1990, Mosby–Year Book.

Fever and tympanic thermometry: a symposium, *Clin Pediatr* (suppl) 30, 1991.

Fontana SA: Update on high blood pressure. Highlights from the 1988 national report, *Nurse Pract* 13:8, 1988.

Gordon M: *Manual of nursing diagnosis* 1993-1994, St. Louis, 1993, Mosby–Year Book.

Guyton AC: *Textbook of medical physiology,* ed 8, Philadelphia, 1991, WB Saunders.

Hill MN, Grim CM: How to take a precise blood pressure, *Am J Nurs* 91:38, 1991.

Joint National Committee on Detection, Evaluation, and Treatment of High Blood Pressure: The 1988 report of the Joint National Committee on Detection, Evaluation and Treatment of High Blood Pressure, *Arch Intern Med* 148:1023, May 1988.

Magee DJ: *Orthopedic physical assessment,* Philadelphia, 1987, WB Saunders Co.

Mountcastle VB: *Medical physiology,* vol 2, ed 14, St Louis, 1980, Mosby–Year Book.

Rook RK, Petersdorf RC: Alteration in body temperature. In Wilson JD, and others, editors: *Harrison's principles of internal medicine,* ed 12, New York, 1991, McGraw-Hill.

Shafer RC: *Clinical biomechanics. Musculoskeletal actions and reactions,* Baltimore, 1983, Williams & Wilkins.

Sparks SM, Taylor CM: *Nursing diagnosis reference manual. An indispensable guide to better patient care.* Pennsylvania, 1991, Springhouse Corporation.

Summers S: Axillary, tympanic and esophageal temperature measurement. Descriptive comparisons in postanesthesia patients, *J Post Anesth Nurs* 6:420, 1991.

Task Force on Blood Pressure Control in Children: Report of Second Task Force on Blood Pressure Control in Children—1987, *Pediatrics* 79:1-15, 1987.

Thibodeau GA: *Anatomy and physiology,* St Louis, 1987, Mosby–Year Book.

Timby BK, Lewis LW: *Fundamental skills and concepts in patient care,* ed 5, New York, 1992, JB Lippincott.

U.S. Department of Health and Human Services: *Working group report on management of patients with hypertension and high blood cholesterol,* August, 1990.

Whaley LF, Wong DL: *Nursing care of infants and children,* ed 4, St Louis, 1991, Mosby–Year Book.

CHAPTER 9

Skin, Hair, and Nails

Outline

PURPOSE OF THE EXAMINATION

The skin, or integumentary system, is an organ system readily accessible to examination. It provides a membrane barrier between the individual and the external environment. The skin responds to changes in the external environment. It also reflects changes in the internal environment. A careful examination of the skin may yield valuable information about the client's general health. It can provide specific information needed to identify a systemic disease or a skin problem. A description of the skin of the healthy client, as well as a description of the client with a skin problem, is important. The examiner should pay special attention to any deviation from normal.

Examination of the skin requires some understanding of the structure and function of the system and familiarity with the appearance of the skin, hair, nails, and mucous membranes in health and disease. This chapter includes a brief discussion of the anatomy and function of the skin, hair, and nails; methods for conducting a health history; and the systematic examination of the skin, hair, and nails. (The examination of the sclera and conjunctiva is discussed in Chapter 11, and the examination of the oral mucosa is discussed in Chapter 12.)

ANATOMY AND PHYSIOLOGY

The skin combined with its appendages (the hair, nails, sebaceous glands and eccrine and apocrine sweat glands), is the largest organ of the body. It has many important functions: (1) provides a barrier to loss of water and electrolytes; (2) provides protection from external agents injurious to the internal structures; (3)

regulates body temperature and blood pressure; (4) acts as sense organ for touch, pressure, temperature, and pain; (5) maintains body surface integrity by ongoing cell replacement and increased regeneration for wound repair; (6) maintains a buffered protective skin film by eccrine and sebaceous glands to protect against microbial and fungal agents; (7) participates in production of vitamin D; (8) delays hypersensitivity reactions to foreign substances; and (9) indicates emotion through color change.

Skin

The skin is composed of three distinct layers: the epidermis, the dermis, and the subcutaneous tissue (Figure 9-1).

Epidermis. The epidermis is the outermost layer of the skin and varies from about 0.3 mm to 1.5 mm thick. It is an avascular, cornified cellular structure that depends on the underlying dermis for its nutrition. The epidermis is continuous with the mucous membranes and the lining of the ear canals. It is stratified into several layers and is composed chiefly of keratinocytes, cells that produce keratin. Keratin makes up much of the horny material in the outermost epidermal layer, the stratum corneum, and is the principal constituent of the harder, keratinized structures of nails and hair. The innermost layer of the epidermis contains melanocytes, the source of melanin, which is the pigment that gives color to the skin and hair. The outermost or horny layer is made up of stratified layers of dead keratinized cells. This outer layer is constantly shed in an inconspicuous way and replenished by mitosis of the underlying cells, so there is almost a complete turnover every 3 to 4 weeks.

Epidermal appendages include the hair, nails, eccrine sweat glands, apocrine sweat glands, and sebaceous glands. These appendages are formed by invagination of the epidermis into the underlying dermis. The eccrine, sebaceous, and apocrine appendages are glandular.

Dermis. The dermis underlying the epidermis constitutes the bulk of the skin. It is often referred to as the "true skin." It is a tough connective tissue that contains lymphatics and nerves and is highly vascular. The dermis consists of predominantly collagen fibers. It supports and nourishes the epidermis.

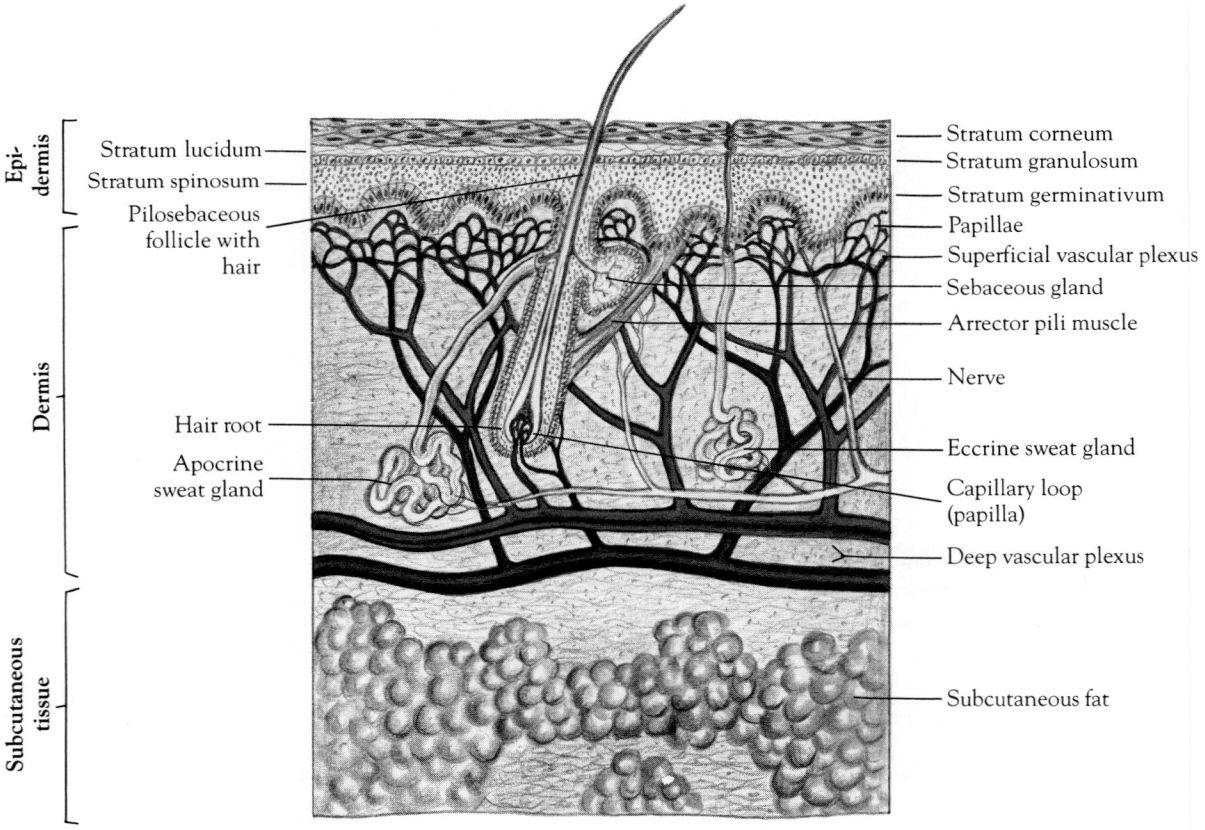

FIGURE 9-1 Structures of the skin. (From Thompson JM and others: *Mosby's manual of clinical nursing,* ed 3, St. Louis, 1993, Mosby–Year Book.)

Subcutaneous tissue. The subcutaneous layer immediately under the dermis is composed of adipose tissue. It stores fat for energy and is important in temperature insulation.

Sebaceous glands. The sebaceous glands usually arise from the hair follicles and produce sebum, which has a lubricating effect on the horny outer layer of the epidermis. Sebaceous glands are on all parts of the body except the palms and soles. They are most abundant on the forehead, face, chin, and scalp. Excessive production of sebum is called seborrhea.

Sweat glands. The eccrine sweat glands open onto the surface of the skin and produce a dilute saline solution, or sweat. They are widely distributed and in great density on the palms and other parts of the hands. They have an important function in the dissipation of body heat as sweat is produced and evaporates. The apocrine sweat glands are found in the axillary and genital areas. They usually open into the hair follicles and produce a milky, viscid fluid or sweat. The sweat produced by the apocrine glands decomposes when contaminated by bacteria, resulting in the characteristic body odor. The apocrine glands do not function until puberty.

Hair

Hair is formed by invagination of epidermal cells into the dermal layers. Hair consists of a root, shaft, and hair follicle. Hair follicles are formed in utero and continue functioning through old age. No new follicles are formed after birth. Hair follicles produce the keratin of mature hair. Adults have two types of hairs: vellus hairs, which are short, fine, nonpigmented hairs; and terminal hairs, which are thick, coarse, and pigmented. Terminal hairs are found most extensively on the scalp, brows, and extremities.

Each hair goes through cyclic growth phases: a growing (anagen) phase, a transition (catogen) phase lasting only a few days, and a resting (telogen) phase. Ninety percent of normal scalp hairs are in the growing (anagen) phase and 10% are in the resting stage. Hairs in the resting stage are subsequently expelled by the regenerating new hair. Hair growth is different depending on its location. Axillary, pubic, beard, and body hair is influenced by hormones. Hair on the scalp, eyelashes, and extremities does not require hormonal stimulus. Hair loss may be related to factors such as destruction of the hair matrix, slowing of hair growth due to medications or metabolic disorders, and genetic characteristics.

Nails

The nails are keratinized appendages of the epidermis. The nails consist of (1) the nail matrix (root), wherein the nail plate is developed; (2) the nail plate; (3) the nail bed, which is attached to the nail plate; and (4) the periungual tissue, including the eponychium and the perionychium (Figure 9-2).

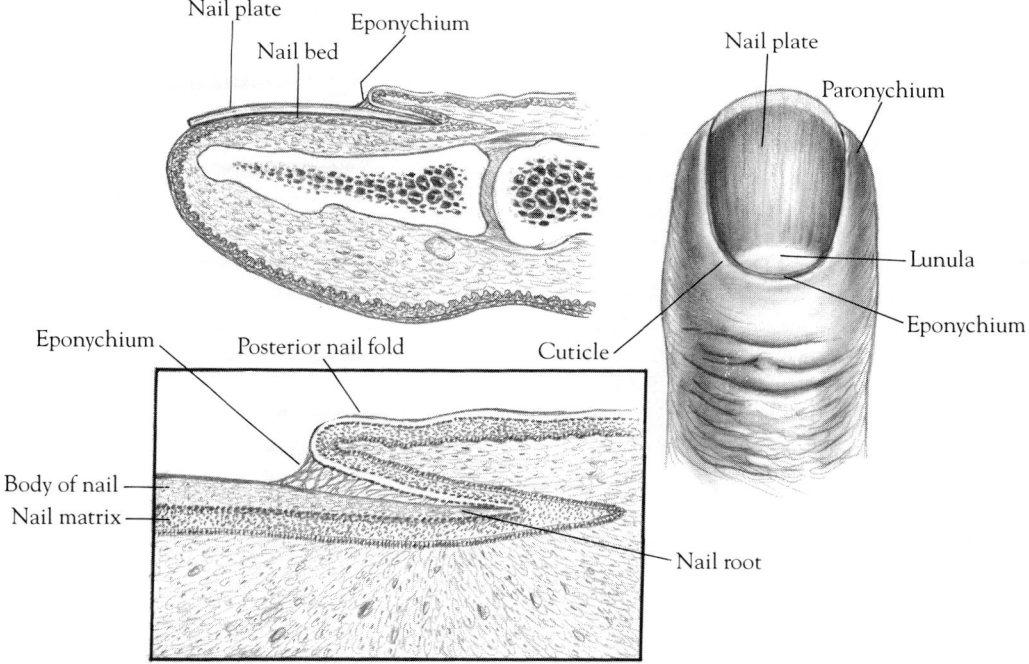

FIGURE 9-2 Structures of nail. (From Thompson JM and others: *Mosby's manual of clinical nursing*, ed 3, St. Louis, 1993, Mosby–Year Book.)

The nail matrix is not visible. The lunula, located at the base of the visible nail, has the shape of a half moon. It marks the end of the nail matrix, the site of nail growth. A bluish hue is visible in the nails of more darkly pigmented individuals. The size of the lunula is variable; it may not be visible in older individuals. The nail plate is a horny, semitransparent structure with a dorsal convexity. The nail bed lies distal to the lunula and is not known to participate in nail formation. The visible nail has a roughly rectangular shape. Normal thickness of the nail is 0.3 to 0.65 mm. It is somewhat thicker in men. The free edge of the nail fold is continuous with the cuticle, which is an extension of the stratum corneum of the dorsum of the finger. The eponychium lies below this and is the anterior extension of the roof of the nail fold on the nail plate. The hyponychium is the portion of the fingertip underlying the free portion of the nail. The perionychium is the epidermis bordering the nail.

The nail plate is formed continuously and uniformly at all points in the matrix. Reports of the fingernail growth rate in the normal adult vary from 0.1 to 1 mm per day. The rate varies with nutrition, age, and activity level. Nail growth also has a circadian and seasonal rhythm. It is greater in the morning, lessening progressively in the afternoon and the night. Nail growth is greater in warm seasons than in cold, and accelerated growth has been observed in warm climates. The growth rate slows with aging. The total time required for reaching the free margin of the nail from the lunula is called the migration time and is normally 130 days. The time required for complete renewal of the fingernail (regeneration time) is 170 days, while that of the toenail is 1 to 1 1/2 years.

EXAMINATION

Health History

A. Present health status
   1. Chief complaint
   2. Allergies: medications, foods, pollens, seasonal
   3. Exposures: travel, environmental or occupational hazards or irritants, frequent sun exposure, use of tanning salons, frequent handwashing or immersion in water, family members or close contacts with skin problems
   4. Medications: prescribed or over-the-counter, topical or systemic, new or previously taken
   5. Skin care habits: cleansing patterns, skin care products used (soaps, oils, astringents, alcohol, facials, etc.), use of sunscreens, recent changes in skin care habits or products
   6. Nail care habits: difficulty cutting or clipping toenails and/or fingernails, type of instruments used, nail biting, use of adhesives for false fingernails

   7. Hair care habits: cleansing routines, recent changes in routine or products used, use of dyes, hair straighteners, permanents or other chemical treatments, hair styles that put tension on the hair
   8. Diet: any recent dietary changes, liquid protein diet, new foods
   9. Recent life changes, losses, or psychological or physiological stress
B. Specific Problems
   1. Skin
      a. Changes in usual state of health, rashes, sores, lumps, *pruritus*, pigmentation changes, texture, dryness, odor, changes in or new presentation of wart or mole, lesion that is repeatedly irritated or that is slow to heal.
      b. Onset: sudden or gradual, date of onset
      c. Duration: how long has problem persisted
      d. Frequency: previous occurrence or progressive problem
      e. Location: extensor or flexor surfaces, skinfolds, generalized or localized, any progression of rash or pattern
      f. Precipitating factors: change in skin care products, tried new perfumes, detergents or other products that come in contact with the skin, diet changes, exposures (travel, other family members or close contacts with a similar problem, new pet), stress-related reactions.
      g. Alleviating factors: medications, relaxation, not using certain products or avoiding contact with allergens, etc.
      h. Associated symptoms: recent viral illness, high fever, systemic diseases, relationship to leisure activities or stress
      i. Efforts to treat: medications or home remedies, response to treatment
   2. Hair
      a. Changes in usual state of health, thinning, hair loss, excess hair, distribution of hair, color
      b. Onset: sudden or gradual, asymmetrical or symmetrical pattern
      c. Duration: how long has problem persisted
      d. Frequency: recurrence or progressive problem
      e. Precipitating factors: dietary changes, dieting (particularly liquid protein diet), malnutrition, hair care products/chemicals
      f. Alleviating factors: not using particular products, diet, specific actions
      g. Associated symptoms: any other health problems, skin disorders, hormonal changes (medications or menarche, pregnancy, menopause), thyroid disease

h. Efforts to treat: medications or other preparations used, response to treatment

3. Nails
   a. Changes in usual state of health, splitting, breaking, biting, thickening, discoloration, separation from nail bed, inflammation
   b. Onset: sudden or gradual, related to illness or trauma
   c. Duration: how long has problem persisted
   d. Frequency: recurrent or intermittent, how often
   e. Precipitating factors: exposure to drugs, chemicals, immersion in water, nail care products
   f. Alleviating factors: diet, stopping specific behaviors
   g. Associated symptoms: any other health problems such as cardiac or respiratory disease, psoriasis, hypothyroidism
   h. Efforts to treat: medications or other remedies used, response to treatment

C. Past health history
   1. Previous occurrences of the problem and their resolution
   2. Previous skin problems, history of allergies, eczema, lesions, and their response to treatment
   3. Previous hair problems: loss, unusual growth or distribution, thinning, breakage, response to treatment
   4. Previous nail problems: injury, infections (fungal, bacterial, viral), allergic reactions (to nail care products), response to treatment
   5. Systemic health problems: Severe cardiac, endocrine, respiratory, liver, hematologic, or other systemic diseases.

D. Family health history
   1. History of allergic diseases such as asthma, hay fever, or other sensitivities.
   2. Dermatologic disorders: skin cancer; melanoma; psoriasis; eczema; infestations (lice, scabies); fungal, bacterial, or viral infections
   3. Familial patterns of hair loss, coloration, or distribution

RISK FACTORS: MALIGNANT MELANOMA

Malignant melanoma is the most rapidly increasing form of cancer in the United States. Detection and surgical treatment of early stages are usually curative, while treatment of later stages has a poor prognosis. Those at high risk for melanoma have one or more of the following (The NIH Consensus Development Panel on Melanoma, 1992):
1. Large number of typical moles
2. Presence of atypical moles
3. Family history of melanoma
4. Prior melanoma
5. History of repeated severe sunburns, ease of burning, freckling, or inability to tan

The NIH Consensus Development Panel on Melanoma (1992) recommends that individuals be taught self-examination of the skin, know the warning signs of melanoma, and contact their health care provider if such signs appear. Warning signs include these ABCD's of melanoma (Figure 9-3):

Asymmetry: Early melanoma is asymmetric. Most typical or common moles are symmetrical.

Border: Melanomas may have notching, scalloping, or poorly defined borders. Most common moles have very clear-cut borders.

Color: Melanomas are usually variegated. They may have shades of brown, tan, red, white, blue/black, or combinations thereof. Common moles tend to be uniform in color.

Diameter: Melanomas are frequently larger than 6 mm in diameter, although they may be diagnosed at a smaller size. Most common moles are less than 6 mm in diameter (about the size of a pencil eraser).

RISK FACTORS TO CONSIDER

Skin cancer

Over age 50
Male
Family history of skin cancer
Light-colored hair or eyes
Precancerous skin lesions (dysplastic nevi, certain congenital nevi)
Extended periods of exposure to sunlight (occupational or recreational)
Tendency to burn easily
Geographic location: high altitudes or near equator
Exposure to radium, isotopes, x-rays
Exposure to coal, tar, creosote, and/or petroleum products
Repeated skin trauma or irritation

PREPARATION FOR THE EXAMINATION: CLIENT AND THE ENVIRONMENT

The examination of the skin is important in the assessment of the client's overall health and as a screening method for skin cancer. A complete examination of the skin needs to be a part of every complete physical exam. This requires that you take a brief but careful view of the entire body and then examine specific areas in more detail. Provide a warm exam room with sufficient privacy. Have the client remove clothing so you can fully

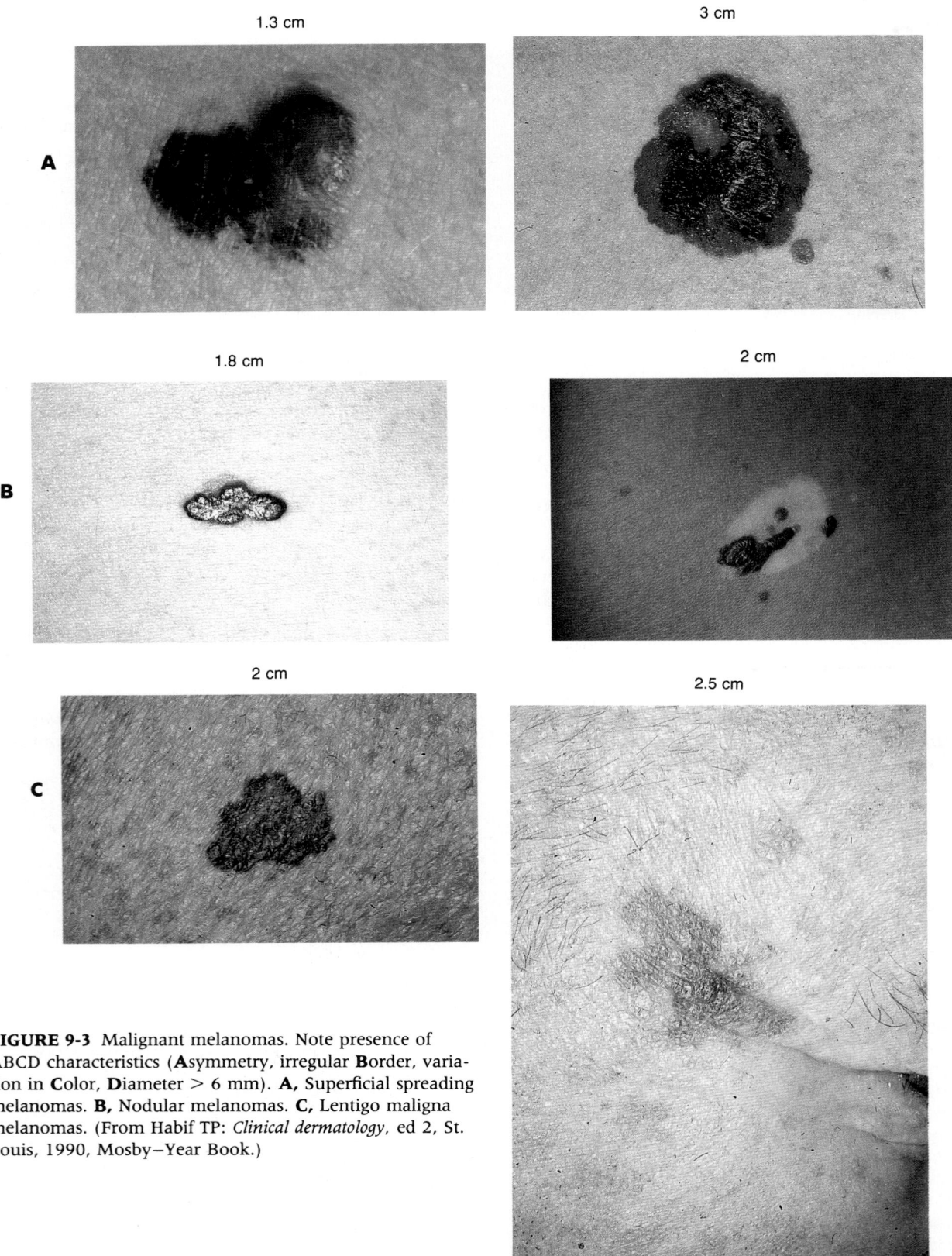

FIGURE 9-3 Malignant melanomas. Note presence of ABCD characteristics (**A**symmetry, irregular **B**order, variation in **C**olor, **D**iameter > 6 mm). **A,** Superficial spreading melanomas. **B,** Nodular melanomas. **C,** Lentigo maligna melanomas. (From Habif TP: *Clinical dermatology,* ed 2, St. Louis, 1990, Mosby–Year Book.)

Preparation for the Examination

Equipment

Item	Purpose
Metric ruler	To measure lesions
Flashlight	To illuminate lesions
Magnifying glass (optional)	To aid in evaluation of lesions
Disposable latex gloves	To protect the examiner when examining lesions
For special procedures:	
Wood's lamp (filtered ultraviolet light)	To assess for tinea capitis
Glass slides and 20% KOH solution	To assess for fungal infection

Client and the environment

Provide a warm room with adequate lighting
Protect the client's modesty while exposing areas to be examined as fully as possible
Explain examination before beginning
Use short, clear instructions

view each section of the body. Protect client modesty by draping areas you are not examining.

TECHNIQUE FOR EXAMINATION AND NORMAL FINDINGS

The examination of the skin and appendages needs to include a general inspection of the entire body, followed by a detailed regional examination. A good source of illumination is necessary; indirect natural daylight is preferred. Consider using a small magnifying glass to aid in examining individual lesions of the skin. Use a clear, flexible measure to assess the size of the lesions. Always wear gloves when examining lesions.

When doing a complete physical examination, you may want to begin the skin examination with areas the client is more used to having exposed (hair, face, hands, and arms). This technique may be less threatening to the client. Then inspect and palpate the skin, mucous membranes, and epidermal appendages of each body part as you examine it. Examine the entire body (with client disrobed) at the end of the exam when the client is standing. For example, assess the skin on the back, buttocks, and legs before or after the examination of the spine.

If the client's main reason for being examined is to evaluate a skin problem, do a full body inspection first to get an idea of the distribution pattern and extent of any lesions. Follow this with a detailed examination of the specific areas affected. To protect client modesty, drape the client's front as you are examining the back and vice versa.

Compare symmetric anatomic areas throughout the examination. Also compare sun-exposed to non–sun-exposed areas. Examine **intertriginous** areas (those with skin folds), which are dark, warm, and moist, such as large breasts, the groin, the obese abdomen, for signs of irritation and/or infection. Make sure to have the client remove the socks and examine the feet, between the toes, and toenails.

Skin

Inspection. Inspect the skin for color and vascularity and for evidence of perspiration, edema, injuries, or skin lesions. During the examination, think about the underlying structures and the particular kind of exposure of a body part. Note those changes in the skin that indicate past injuries and habits, such as calluses, stains, scars, needle marks, and insect bites. Also note the grooming of hair and nails. See the Helpful Hints box on p. 234 for tips on assessing dark skin.

Color. Skin color varies from person to person and from one part of the body to another. Normally it is a whitish pink or a brown shade, depending on race. The exposed areas of the body, including the face, ears, back of neck, and backs of hands and arms, are noticeably different from the unexposed areas and may be more damaged after long exposure to the sun and weather. The vascular flush areas are the cheeks, the bridge of the nose, the neck, the upper chest, the flexor surfaces of the extremities, and the genital area. These areas may be involved in a vascular disturbance or may demonstrate increased color caused by blushing or temperature elevation. Compare them with areas of less vascularity.

The pigment labile areas are the face, the backs of the hands, the flexor of the wrists, the axillae, the mammary areolae, the midline of the abdomen, and the genital area. These areas may demonstrate normal systemic pigmentary changes, such as during pregnancy (see Helpful Hints box below).

Helpful Hints for Evaluating Skin Color Changes:
If you notice a color change in the client's skin, consider:

> *The lighting in the examination room*
> *The position of the client or the client's extremity*
> *The room temperature*
> *The client's emotional condition*
> *The cleanliness of the skin*
> *The presence of edema*

Helpful Hints for Assessing Dark Skin

1. *Skin color should be observed in the sclera, conjunctiva, buccal mucosa, tongue, lips, nail beds, palms, and soles.*
2. *Inspection should be accompanied by palpation, especially if inflammation or edema is suspected.*
3. *Findings should always be correlated with the patient's history to arrive at a nursing diagnosis.*
4. *Pallor in brown-skinned patients may present as a yellowish-brown tinge to the skin. In a black-skinned patient the skin will appear "ashen-gray." It can be difficult to determine. Pallor in dark-skinned individuals is characterized by absence of the underlying red tones in the skin.*
5. *Jaundice may be observed in the sclera but should not be confused with the normal yellow pigmentation of the dark-skinned black patient. The best place to inspect is in that portion of the sclera that is observable when the eye is open. If jaundice is suspected, the posterior portion of the hard palate should also be observed for a yellowish cast. This is most effective when done in bright daylight.*
6. *The oral mucosa of dark-skinned individuals may have a normal freckling of pigmentation that may also be evident in the gums, the borders of the tongue, and the lining of the cheeks.*
7. *The gingiva normally may have a dark blue color that may appear blotchy or be evenly distributed.*
8. *Petechiae are best observed over areas of lighter pigmentation—the abdomen, gluteal areas, and volar aspect of the forearm. They may also be seen in the palpebral conjunctiva and buccal mucosa.*
9. *To differentiate petechiae and ecchymosis from erythema, remember that pressure over the area will cause erythema to blanch but will not affect either petechiae or ecchymosis.*
10. *Erythema usually is associated with increased skin temperature, so palpation should also be used if an inflammatory condition is suspected.*
11. *Edema may reduce the intensity of the color of an area of skin because of the increased distance between the external epithelium and the pigmented layers. Therefore, darker skin would appear lighter. On palpation the skin may feel "tight."*
12. *Cyanosis can often be difficult to determine in dark-skinned individuals. Familiarity with the precyanotic color is often helpful. However, if this is not possible, close inspection of the nail beds, lips, palpebral conjunctiva, palms, and soles should show evidence of cyanosis.*
13. *Skin rashes may be assessed by palpating for changes in skin texture.*

From Roach B: Color changes in dark skin, *Nursing '77*, January, 1977.

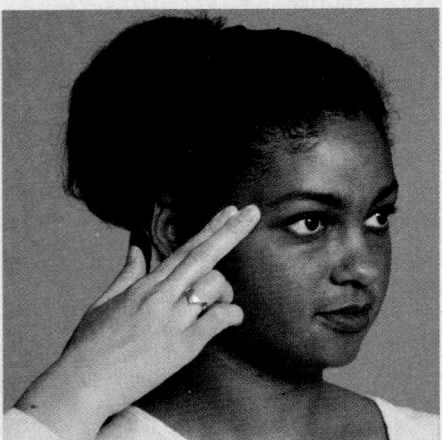

Other changes in skin color may provide evidence of systemic disease.

These changes include the following:

1. Cyanosis, a dusky blue color, may be visible in the nail beds and in the lips and the oral mucosa. It results from decreased oxyhemoglobin binding, or decreased oxygenation of the blood, and can be caused by pulmonary or heart disease, by abnormalities of hemoglobin, or by cold.
2. Jaundice, a yellow or green hue, occurs when tissue bilirubin is increased and may be visible first in the sclerae and then in the mucous membranes and the skin.
3. Pallor, or decreased color in the skin, results from decreased blood flow to the superficial vessels or from decreased amounts of hemoglobin in the blood. Pallor is most evident in the face, the palpebral conjunctiva, the mouth, and the nail beds.
4. **Erythema,** or an intense redness of the skin, may be generalized or localized. Generalized redness of the skin may be caused by fever, whereas defined areas of redness may be the result of a localized infection or sunburn.
5. Pigmentation changes or alterations in the normal pattern of pigmentation result from changes in the distribution of melanin or in the

function of the melanocytes in the epidermis. Either hyperpigmentation or depigmentation can occur. The **nevus,** or birthmark, is an example of a defined area of hyperpigmentation that may be an innocent manifestation, such as the mongolian spots found on infants, or it may be a more serious finding, such as the numerous cafe au lait spots of neurofibromatosis. Depigmentation of the skin, which occurs in vitiligo, may involve only one or few areas or may be more generalized. Common sites of vitiligo are the face, neck, axillae, groin, anogenital area, eyelids, hands, and wrists. Table 9-1 lists other conditions causing variations in pigmentation.

It is important to be aware that expression of the above skin color changes will vary depending on the client's racial group. Table 9-2 summarizes the differences in assessment of color changes in light-skinned and dark-skinned individuals.

Other localized changes in color may indicate a problem such as edema, which tends to blanch skin color.

Palpation. Palpate the skin to augment your findings on inspection. In general, perform palpation simultaneously as you examine each body part. Note changes in temperature, moisture, texture, and turgor.

Temperature. Skin temperature increases when blood flow through the dermis increases. Localized elevations in skin temperature occur with a burn or a localized infection. Generalized increase in skin temperature may occur with a fever, which may be due to a localized infection or systemic disease. Temperature of the skin is reduced when blood flow through the dermis decreases. Generalized skin coolness occurs when the client is in shock. Localized hypothermia occurs in conditions such as arteriosclerosis. Always check for bilateral symmetry. Inequality in temperature may indicate circulatory problems or infection.

Moisture. Moisture on the skin varies from one body area to another. The soles of the feet, the palms of the hands, and the intertriginous areas (where two surfaces are close together) contain more moisture than other parts. The amount of moisture found over the entire integument also varies with changes in the environmental temperature, muscular activity, and body temperature. The skin regulates body temperature by producing perspiration that evaporates, thus cooling the body when the temperature increases. The skin is normally drier during the winter months, when environmental temperatures and humidity are lower and as the individual ages. Abnormal dryness of the skin occurs with dehydration. In this instance, the skin feels dry

TABLE 9-1

Variation in Pigmentation

Condition	Characteristic color	Location
Diffuse hyperpigmentation		
Addison's disease, ACTH-producing tumors*	Tan to brown, "bronzing"	Generalized, more marked on exposed areas, flexures, mucous membrane of mouth
Arsenic toxicity	Dusky, diffuse, paler spots	Trunk, extremities
Chloasma (mask of pregnancy), phenytoin ingestion	Tan to brown	Forehead—adjacent to hair line, malar prominence, upper lip, chin
Hemochromatosis	Bronze to grayish brown, deposits of hemosiderin	Generalized
Ichthyosis	Tan, fine to coarse scales	Generalized
Malabsorption syndrome (sprue)	Tan to brown patches	Any area of body
Scleroderma	Yellow to tan (may also have depigmentation)	Generalized
Uremia (chronic renal failure)	Yellow-brown, retention of urinary chromogens	Generalized
Lack of pigmentation		
Vitiligo	Circumscribed lack of pigmentation	
Albinism—hereditary	Complete or partial lack of melanin	Generalized (universal albinism), skin, hair, eyes

*ACTH, adrenocorticotropic hormone.

TABLE 9-2

Differences in Color Changes of Racial Groups

Color change	Light skin	Dark skin
Cyanosis	Blue tinge, especially in palpebral conjunctiva (lower eyelid), nail bed, earlobes, lips, oral membranes, soles, and palms	Ashen-gray lips and tongue
Pallor	Loss of rosy glow in skin, especially face	Ashen-gray appearance in black skin More yellowish-brown color in brown skin
Erythema	Redness easily seen anywhere on body	Much more difficult to assess; rely on palpation for warmth or edema
Ecchymoses	Purple to yellowish-green areas; may be seen anywhere on skin	Very difficult to see unless in mouth or conjunctiva
Petechiae	Purple pinpoints most easily seen on buttocks, abdomen, and inner surfaces of the arms or legs	Usually invisible except in oral mucosa, conjunctiva of eyelids, and conjunctiva covering eyeball
Jaundice	Yellow staining seen in sclera of eyes, skin, fingernails, soles, palms, and oral mucosa	Most reliably assessed in sclera, hard palate, palms, and soles

From Whaley LF, Wong DL: *Nursing care of infants and children*, ed 4, St Louis, 1991, Mosby–Year Book.

even when the temperature increases. Dryness of the skin also occurs in conditions such as myxedema and chronic nephritis.

Texture. Texture refers to the fineness or coarseness of the skin. Changes in skin texture may indicate local irritation or trauma to defined skin areas or may be associated with problems of other systems. The skin becomes soft and smooth in hyperthyroidism and rough and dry in hypothyroidism.

Turgor. Turgor refers to the elasticity of the skin. You can most easily determine turgor by picking up a fold of skin over the abdomen and observing how quickly it returns to its normal shape (Figure 9-4). A

loss of turgor is associated with dehydration. The skin demonstrates a laxness and a loss of normal mobility, returning to place slowly. Loss of turgor is also associated with aging; the skin becomes wrinkled and lax. Increased turgor is associated with an increase in tension, which causes the skin to return to place quickly when pinched. Increased turgor occurs in progressive systemic sclerosis (PSS), a connective tissue disorder.

Lesions. Perform the initial examination of any skin lesion at a distance of 3 feet or more to determine the

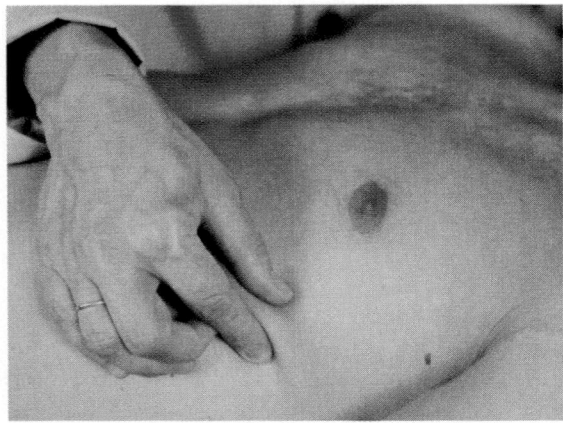

FIGURE 9-4 Testing skin turgor.

Helpful Hints for Assessing Skin Lesions: *If a lesion is present, consider:*

Are there any associated symptoms, for example, pruritus?

What is the chronology of the appearance of these lesions?

Are they changing in morphology? Are they disappearing?

Are there associated variables or precipitants such as:

Environmental exposures
Injury
Infection
Use of medications (prescribed or self-treatment)
Diet
Clothing
Emotional factors
Personal care items such as soaps and cosmetics

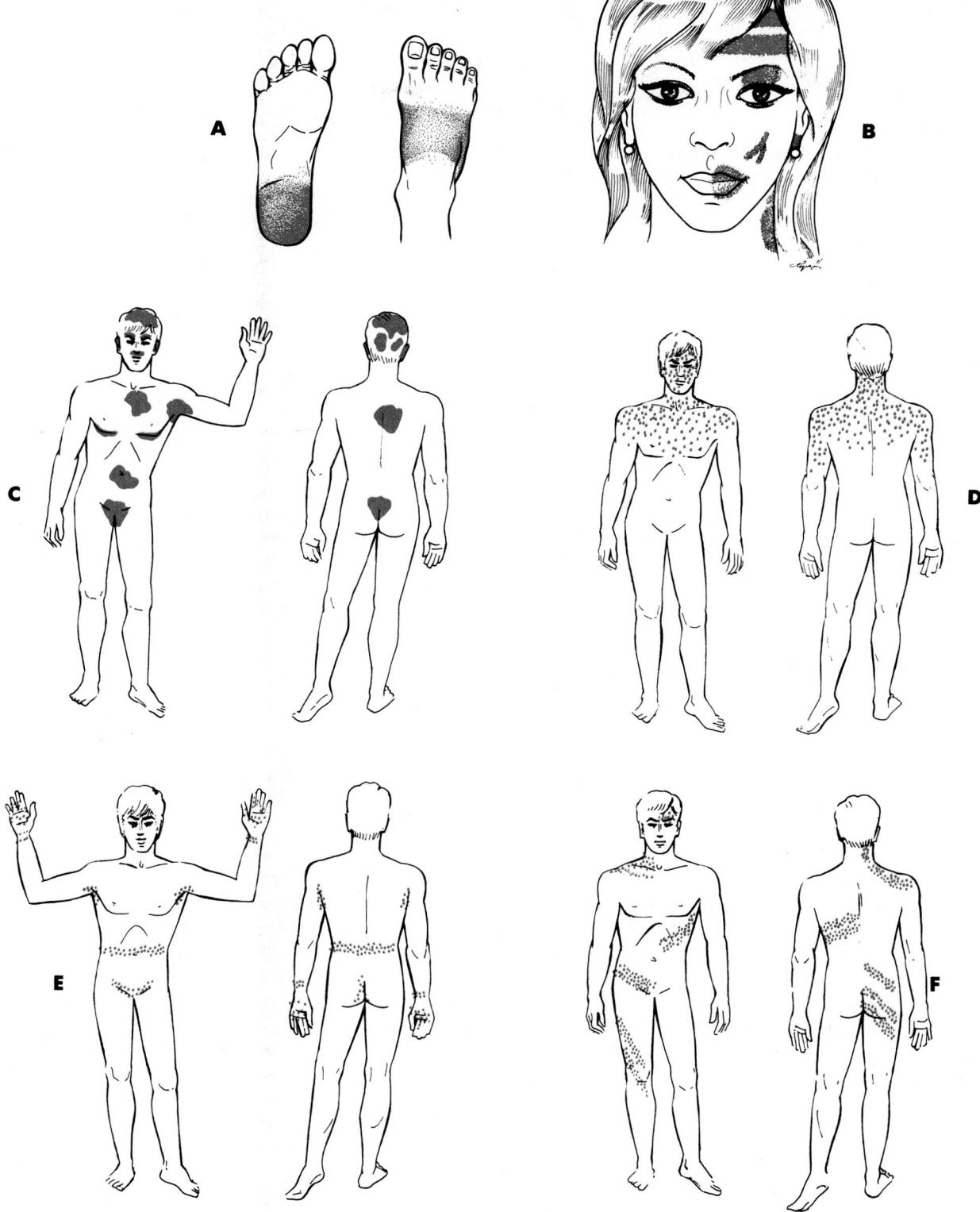

FIGURE 9-5 Distribution of lesions in selected problems of the skin. **A,** Contact dermatitis (shoes). **B,** Contact dermatitis (cosmetics, perfumes, earrings). **C,** Seborrheic dermatitis. **D,** Acne. **E,** Scabies. **F,** Herpes zoster.

general characteristics of the eruption. This first observation provides the opportunity to determine the location, distribution, and configuration of the lesions. Next, carry out a closer examination to determine the color, size, shape, texture, firmness, and morphological characteristics of the individual lesions (see Helpful Hints Box on p. 236).

1. Distribution—Describe the distribution of skin lesions according to the location or body region affected and the symmetry or asymmetry of findings in comparable body parts. Keep in mind the characteristic patterns that provide the major clue in the diagnosis of a specific skin problem. Figure 9-5 illustrates a few distribution patterns observed in specific problems.

2. Configuration—Note the configuration of skin lesions, which is equally important in defining the problem. Configuration refers to the arrangement or position of several lesions in relation to each other. For example, the skin lesions of tinea corporis, which is ringworm of the body, have an annular configuration that is circular. Use the following terms to describe the configuration of skin lesions, as appropriate:

Grouped	Lesions clustered together
Herpetiform or zosteriform	Multiple groups of vesicles erupting unilaterally following the course of cutaneous nerves
Linear	Lesions arranged in a line
Annular	Lesions arranged in a circle, ring-shaped
Polycyclic	Multiple annular arrangements of lesions
Arciform	Lesions arranged in an arc, bow-shaped
Reticular	Lesions meshed in the form of a network
Confluent	Lesions become merged together, not discrete

Figure 9-6 illustrates some configurations.

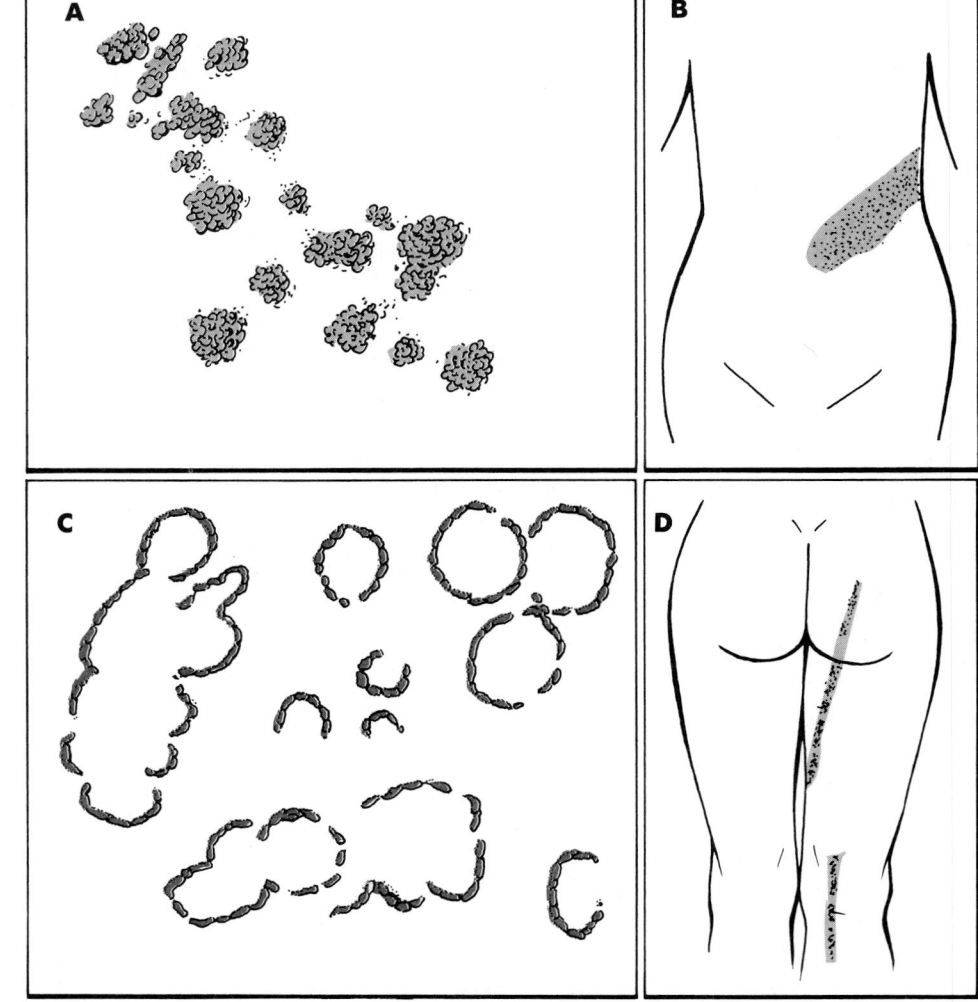

FIGURE 9-6 Examples of different configurations of skins lesions. **A,** Grouped. **B,** Zosteriform. **C,** Annular (*circular*) and arciform (*arc*). **D,** Linear.

3. Type of Lesion. The morphologic classification of skin lesions organizes lesions in terms of their structure. It is based on the size, shape, elevation, or depression of the lesions. Determining the morphological structure of the individual lesion (macule, papule, vesicle, etc.) helps identify the specific problem. Table 9-3 provides detailed parameters for classification of skin lesions. Figures 9-7, 9-8, and 9-9 illustrate descriptions and characteristics of lesions.

Classify lesions as primary, secondary, or vascular. Primary lesions are those that appear initially in response to some change in the external or internal environment of the skin. Secondary lesions do not appear initially but result from modifications such as trauma, chronicity, or infection in the primary lesion. For instance, the primary lesion may be a vesicle, which is a small, circumscribed, elevated lesion containing clear fluid. The vesicle will rupture, leaving a small moist area, which is classified as a secondary lesion called an erosion. Figures 9-7 and 9-8 illustrate some of the primary and secondary lesions. Table 9-4 describes types of skin lesions that characterize stages of dermatitis. Primary and secondary lesions may occur at the same time.

Vascular lesions usually appear as red pigmented lesions. They may be indicative of problems such as bleeding (petechiae and ecchymoses) or liver disease (spider angioma), or they may be due to benign conditions such as telangiectasia. Determining whether or not the lesion blanches will help identify the type of lesion. Place a glass slide over the lesion and apply pressure. If the lesion loses color or fades, it blanches. Vascular lesions are described in Figure 9-9.

Measure the lesion with a small, clear, and flexible ruler. Report sizes in centimeters (inches may also be used but are less desirable). Measure all the dimensions possible (length, width, height/depth). If possible, draw a diagram with location and dimensions included. This

---

TABLE 9-3

Identification of Skin Lesions

	Name of lesion	**Description**	**<1 cm**	**>1 cm**
Type of lesion:				
Primary	Macule—patch	Flat, circumscribed discoloration	Macule	Patch
	Papule—plaque	Solid, elevated lesion	Papule	Plaque
	Nodule—tumor	Solid, elevated lesion also has depth	Nodule	Tumor
	Vesicle—bulla	Fluid filled, superficial, elevated	Vesicle	Bulla
Primary of	Pustule	Vesicle or bulla containing pus		
varying	Wheal	Lesion caused by cutaneous edema irregular in shape, elevated, transient		
size	Telangiectasia	Dilated capillary, fine red line(s)		
Secondary	Scale	Accumulation of loose surface epithelium		
	Crust	Dried surface fluids: serum or pus		
	Excoriation	Scratch mark		
	Erosion	Superficial denuded lesion		
	Scar	First red, then pale smooth hyaline wound repair; may be flat, depressed, elevated, or hypertrophic (keloid)		
	Ulcer	Loss of tissue from a surface caused by destruction of a superficial lesion		
	Atrophy	Thinning of skin, loss of hair and sweat glands		
	Fissure	Linear crack in skin that extends to dermis		
	Lichenification	Thickening of skin caused by chronic scratching		

Number of lesions: ☐ Single ☐ Numerous ☐ Actual count
Size of lesion: (Measure)
Shape of lesion: ☐ Round ☐ Oval ☐ Umbilicated ☐ Irregular
Color of lesion: ☐ Red ☐ Brown ☐ Black ☐ Gray-blue ☐ White ☐ Purple ☐ Orange ☐ Yellow
 ☐ Circumscribed? ☐ Diffuse? ☐ Change with diascopy*?
Configuration: ☐ Single ☐ Grouped: ☐ Herpetiform ☐ Linear ☐ Annular ☐ Arciform ☐ Reticular ☐ Scattered
Distribution: ☐ Localized ☐ Generalized ☐ Symmetrical
 Site of predilection _____

*Diascopy consists of the application of firm pressure against a microscope slide or clear plastic placed over a skin lesion, allowing identification of capillary dilatation and thus differentiating telangiectasia from purpura. The technique also makes lymphoma, sarcoidosis, and tuberculosis of the skin appear yellow-brown.

Macule—flat; nonpalpable; circumscribed; less than 1 cm in diameter; brown, red, purple, white, or tan in color
Examples: Freckles; flat moles; rubella; rubeola

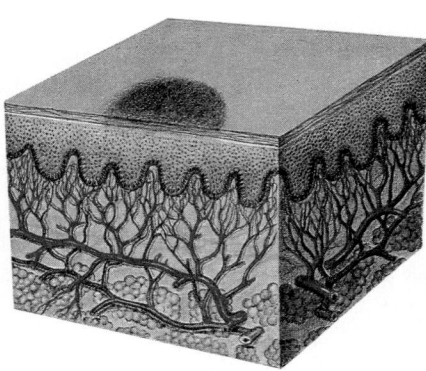

Plaque—elevated; flat topped; firm; rough; superficial papule greater than 1 cm in diameter; may be coalesced papules
Examples: Psoriasis; seborrheic and actinic keratoses

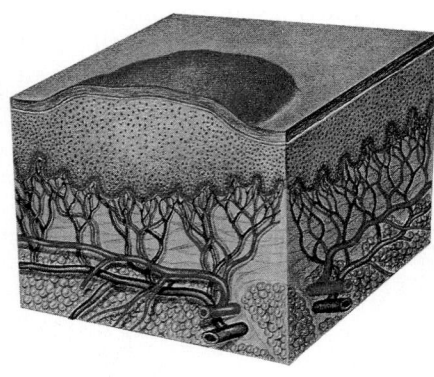

Wheal—elevated, irregular-shaped area of cutaneous edema; solid, transient, changing, variable diameter; pale pink with lighter center
Examples: Urticaria; insect bites

Patch—flat; nonpalpable; irregular in shape; macule that is greater than 1 cm in diameter
Examples: Vitiligo; port-wine marks

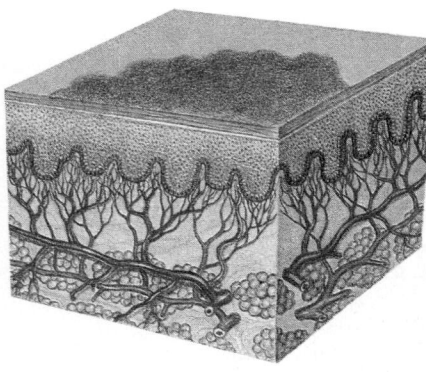

Nodule—elevated; firm; circumscribed; palpable; deeper in dermis than papule; 1 to 2 cm in diameter
Examples: Erythema nodosum; lipomas

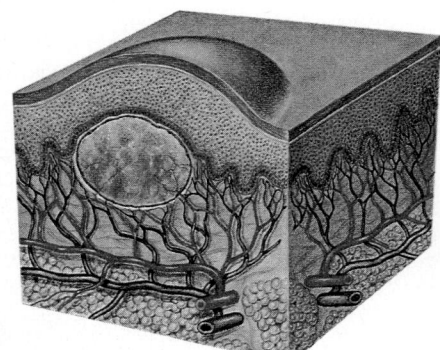

Papule—elevated; palpable; firm; circumscribed; less than 1 cm in diameter; brown, red, pink, tan, or bluish red in color
Examples: Warts; drug-related eruptions; pigmented nevi

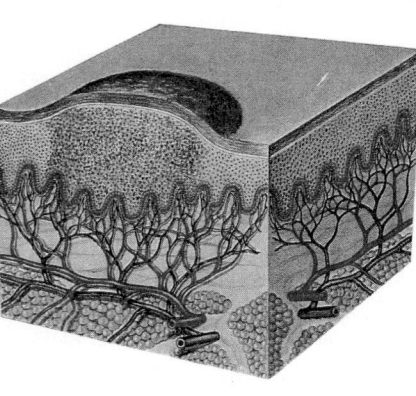

FIGURE 9-7 Descriptions and characteristics of primary skin lesions. (From Thompson JM and others: *Mosby's manual of clinical nursing,* ed 3, St. Louis, 1993, Mosby–Year Book.)

Tumor—elevated; solid; may or may not be clearly demarcated; greater than 2 cm in diameter; may or may not vary from skin color
Example: Neoplasms

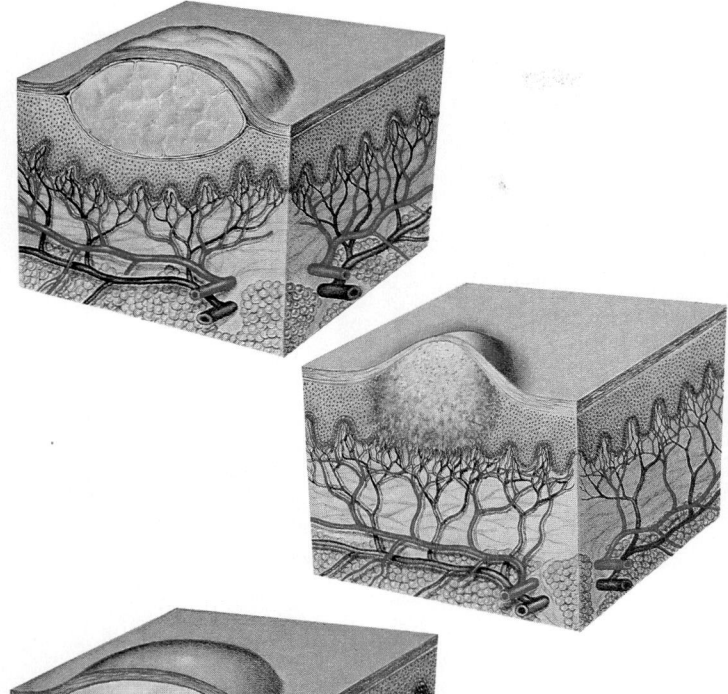

Pustule—elevated; superficial; similar to vesicle but filled with purulent fluid
Examples: Impetigo; acne; variola

Vesicle—elevated; circumscribed; superficial; filled with serous fluid; less than 1 cm in diameter
Examples: Blister; varicella

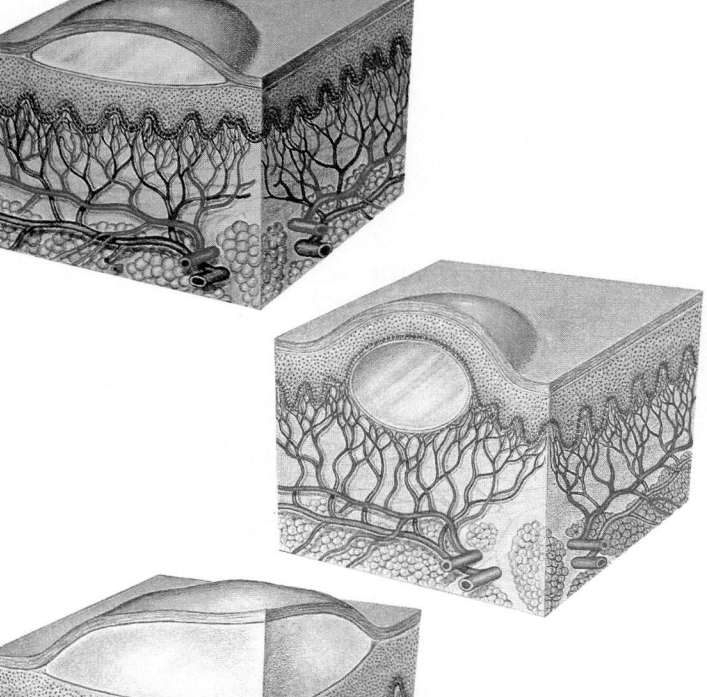

Cyst—elevated; circumscribed; palpable; encapsulated; filled with liquid or semi-solid material
Example: Sebaceous cyst

Bulla—vesicle greater than 1 cm in diameter
Examples: Blister; pemphigus vulgaris

Scale—heaped-up keratinized cells; flaky exfoliation; irregular; thick or thin; dry or oily; varied size; silver, white, or tan in color
Examples: Psoriasis; exfoliative dermatitis

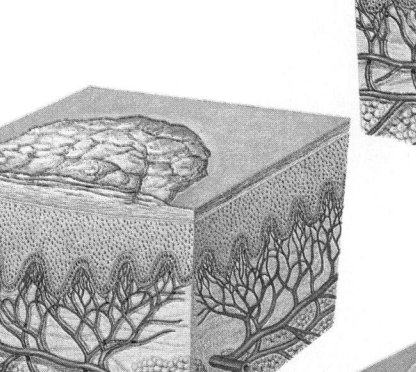

Scar—thin to thick fibrous tissue replacing injured dermis; irregular; pink, red, or white in color; may be atrophic or hypertrophic
Example: Healed wound or surgical incision

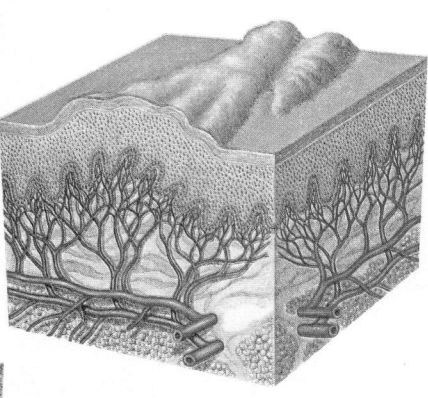

Keloid—irregularly shaped, elevated, progressively enlarging scar; grows beyond boundaries of wound; caused by excessive collagen formation during healing
Example: Keloid from ear piercing or burn scar

Crust—dried serum, blood, or purulent exudate; slightly elevated; size varies; brown, red, black, tan, or straw in color
Examples: Scab on abrasion; eczema

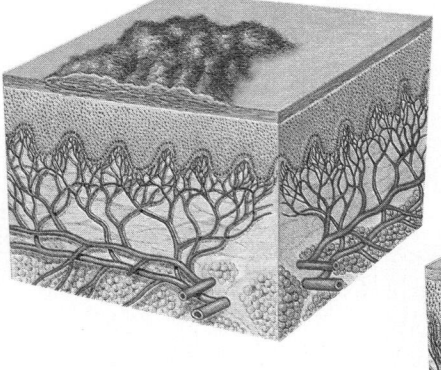

Excoriation—loss of epidermis; linear or hollowed-out crusted area; dermis exposed
Examples: Abrasion; scratch

Lichenification—rough, thickened epidermis; accentuated skin markings caused by rubbing or irritation; often involves flexor aspect of extremity
Example: Chronic dermatitis

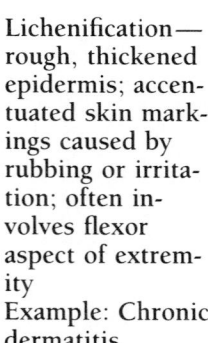

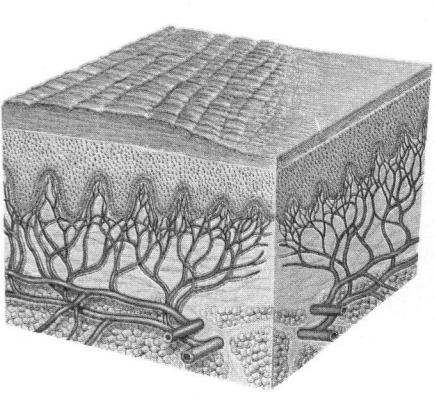

FIGURE 9-8 Description and characteristics of secondary skin lesions. (From Thompson JM and others: *Mosby's manual of clinical nursing,* ed 3, St. Louis, 1993, Mosby–Year Book.)

Fissure—linear crack or
break from epidermis to
dermis; small; deep; red
Examples: Athlete's foot;
cheilois

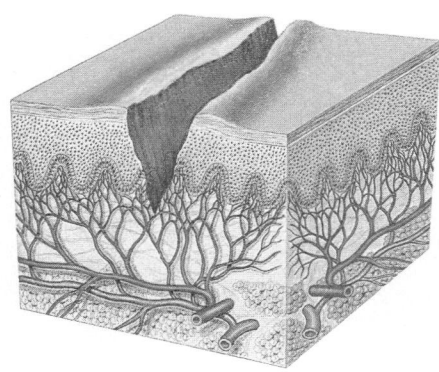

Erosion—loss of all or
part of epidermis;
depressed; moist;
glistening; follows rupture
of vesicle or bulla; larger
than fissure
Examples: Varicella;
variola following rupture

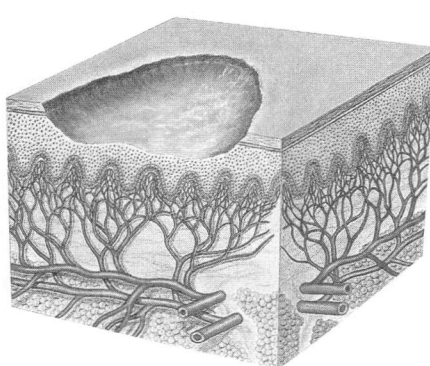

Ulcer—loss of epidermis
and dermis; concave;
varies in size; exudative;
red or reddish blue
Examples: Decubiti; stasis
ulcers

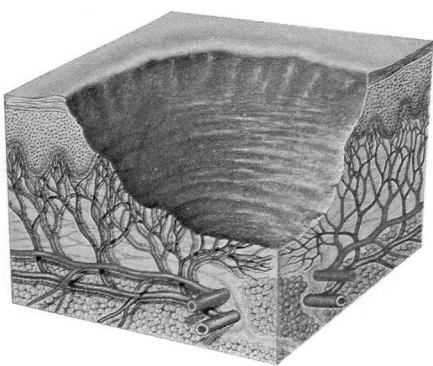
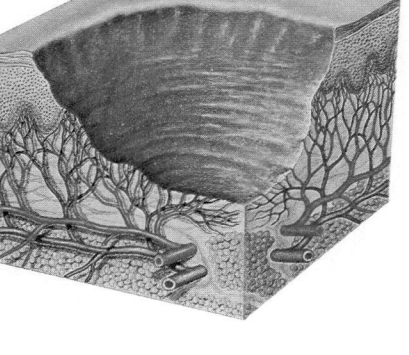

Atrophy—thinning of
skin surface and loss of
skin markings; skin
translucent and paperlike
Examples: Striae; aged
skin

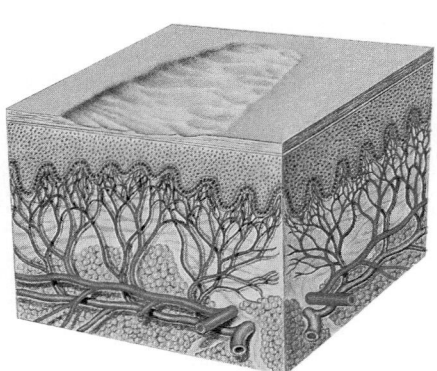

Purpura—red-purple nonblanchable discoloration greater than 0.5 cm diameter. Cause: Intravascular defects, infection

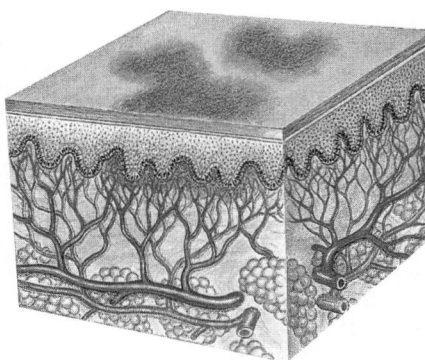

Spider angioma—red central body with radiating spiderlike legs that blanch with pressure to the central body Cause: Liver disease, vitamin B deficiency, idiopathic

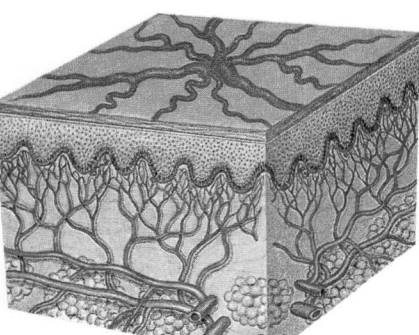

Venous star—bluish spider, linear or irregularly shaped; does not blanch with pressure Cause: Increased pressure in superficial veins

Petechiae—red-purple nonblanchable discoloration less than 0.5 cm diameter Cause: Intravascular defects, infection

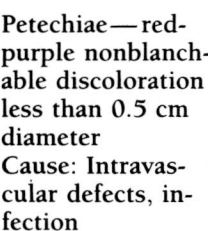

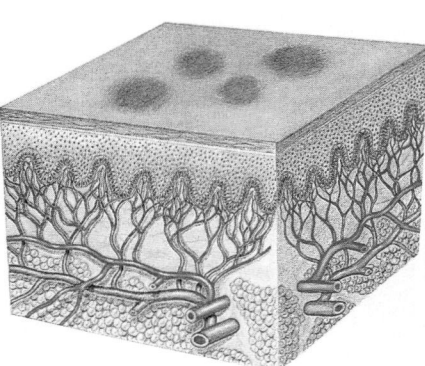

Telangiectasia—fine, irregular red line Cause: Dilation of capillaries

Ecchymoses—red-purple nonblanchable discoloration of variable size Cause: Vascular wall destruction, trauma, vasculitis

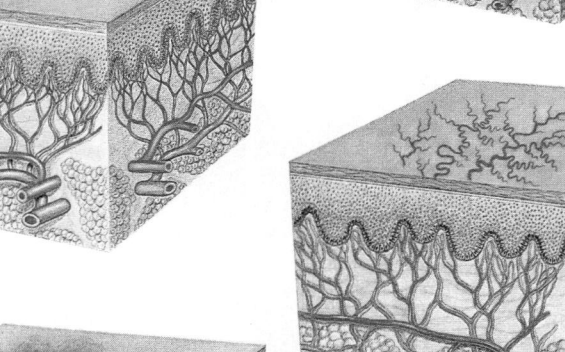

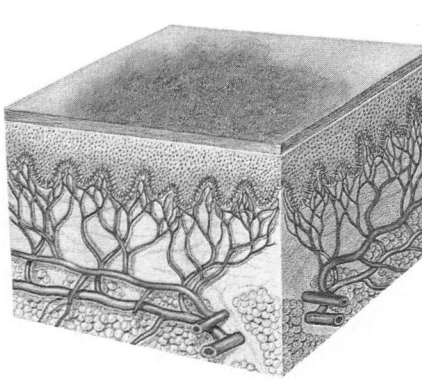

Capillary hemangioma (nevus flammeus)—red irregular macular patches Cause: Dilation of dermal capillaries

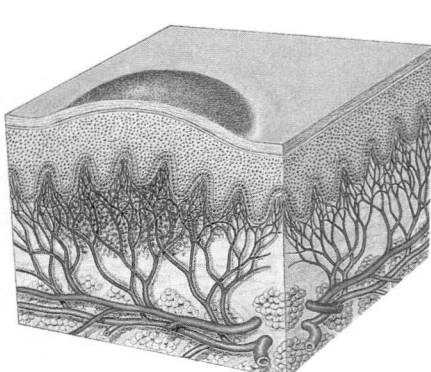

FIGURE 9-9 Characteristics and causes of vascular lesions. (From Seidel and others: *Mosby's guide to physical examination,* ed 2, St. Louis, 1991, Mosby—Year Book.)

TABLE 9-4

Stages of Dermatitis

Stage	Lesions
Acute	Erythema, edema, vesicles, exudate, crusting
Subacute	Erythema, residual crusting, scaling
Chronic	Scaling, hyperpigmentation, lichenification, fissuring

TABLE 9-5

Alopecia—Hair Loss

Type of alopecia	Description
Androgen (in female)	Thinning of scalp hair, male pattern, hirsutism on body
Areata	Circumscribed bald areas; sudden onset, usually reversible
Chemical	Hair brittle, breaks off
Cicatricial	Permanent localized loss of hair associated with scarring
Drug or radiation	Generalized loss of hair caused by antineoplastic agents, such as gold, thallium, and arsenic, or by radiation
Male pattern	Receding of anterior hairline, temples, and vertex; hereditary
Mucinosis	Erythmatous papules or plaques without hair
Syphilitic	Generalized thinning of hair or baldness; mucous patches without hair

will help you monitor the progression or resolution of the lesion. The term used to describe a lesion will vary with its size. For example, a vesicle is a fluid-filled lesion and is less than 1 cm in diameter. If it is greater than 1 cm, it is called a bulla.

Gently palpate lesions to determine the texture and firmness of the individual lesion and in some instances to determine the actual shape of the lesion. Always wear gloves when palpating a skin lesion.

4. Color—Describe the color of the individual lesion. There may be no discoloration, or you may see many colors. For example, with ecchymosis the initial dark-red and dark-blue fades and a yellow color appears. Lesions may be well defined with the color changes limited to the borders of the lesion. These lesions are referred to as "circumscribed." Lesions may have "diffuse" borders which are undefined with the color changes spread over a large area. You can use diascopy to observe for color changes of a lesion when pressure is applied. Place a transparent slide against the skin to express blood from the capillaries and superficial venules. Telangiectases will blanch, whereas petechial or purpuric lesions will not.

Hair

Inspection and palpation. Examine the hair over the entire body to determine the distribution, quantity, and quality.

Distribution. Hair may be present on the scalp, lower face, nares, ears, neck, axillae, anterior chest, back and shoulders, arms, legs, buttocks and pubic area, and around the nipples. Coarse terminal hair occurs on the scalp, on the pubic and axillary areas, and in the male's beard. The body is covered with fine vellus hair. A normal male or female hair pattern evolves after puberty. The pattern of hair distribution in the male genital area is diamond-shaped, while the pattern of hair distribution in the female genital area is an inverted triangle. A deviation may indicate an endocrine problem.

Quantity. Changes in the quantity of the hair are also important. **Hirsutism,** increased hair growth, oc-

curs in conditions such as Cushing's syndrome, polycystic ovary disease, and acromegaly. Decreased hair growth or loss of hair may be associated with hypopituitarism or a **pyogenic** infection. Patterns of hair loss may also be hormonally regulated as with "male-pattern" baldness (Figure 9-10). Table 9-5 lists types of **alopecia,** or hair loss.

Texture. Hair in the pubic and axillary areas is coarse. Scalp hair may be thick or thin, coarse or fine, straight, curly, or kinky. It should be shiny, smooth, and resilient. This characteristic may be affected by the use of beauty products such as rinses, hair straighteners,

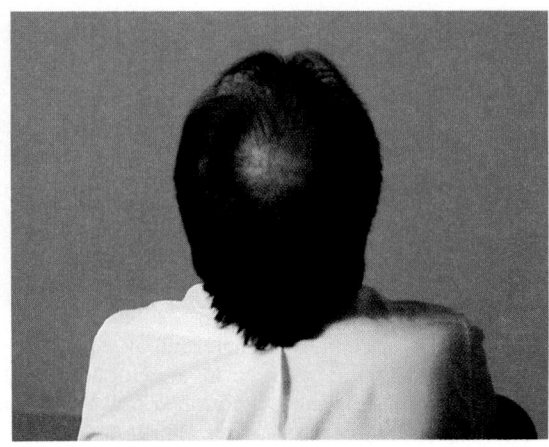

FIGURE 9-10 Male-pattern baldness.

dyes, or permanents. Texture may also change with systemic illnesses. For example, changes in texture of hair associated with hypothyroidism include dryness and coarseness, and changes associated with hyperthyroidism include increased silkiness and fineness. Texture and color determine the quality of the hair. Palpate the hair for texture and the scalp for dryness.

Color. Hair color may vary from light blond to black. Changes in color such as graying occur normally with aging. Premature graying may be indicative of underlying disease such as pernicious anemia. Patchy gray hair may develop following nerve injuries. Hair color may also change as the result of malnutrition. Use of dyes, rinses, or permanents will also influence hair color.

Nails

Inspection and palpation. The assessment of the nails is important to determine not only their condition but also possible evidence of systemic diseases. Examine the nails for shape, normal dorsal curvature, adhesion to the nail bed, regularity of the nail surface, color, cleanliness, and thickness. Examine the skinfolds around the nails for any color changes, swelling, increased temperature, or tenderness (Figure 9-2). Complete absence of the nail or **anonychia** is usually congenital.

Curvature. The nail surface is usually flat or slightly curved. The nail edges should be rounded and smooth. The normal angle of the nail base is 160°. **Clubbing,** which is associated with respiratory and cardiovascular problems, cirrhosis, colitis, and thyroid disease, occurs when the angle of the nail base exceeds 180° (Figure 9-11). With clubbing, the nail becomes thickened, hard, shiny, and curved at the free end. In advanced cases the entire nail is pushed away from the base at an angle greater than 180° and feels "spongy."

Nail adhesion. The nail should be firmly adherent to the nail bed, and the nail base should be firm to palpation. To test for adherence, gently squeeze the nail between your thumb and the pad of your finger (Figure 9-12). Examine the nail folds for swelling, redness, pus, warts, or tumors. **Paronychia** is an inflammation of the folds of tissue surrounding the nails leading to erythema, with inflammation, swelling, and induration of the nail fold accompanied by pain and tenderness (Figure 9-13). It is the most common complaint related to the nails.

Nail surface. The nail surface should be smooth and flat. Inspect for grooves, depressions, pitting, and ridging. Longitudinal ridging may be a normal variant (Figure 9-14) or may occur with **lichen planus** (Figure

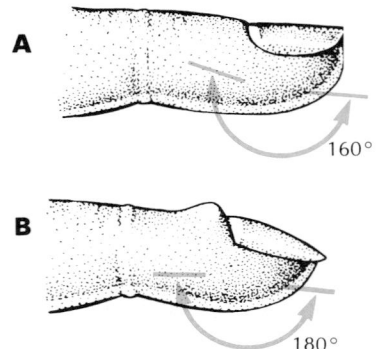

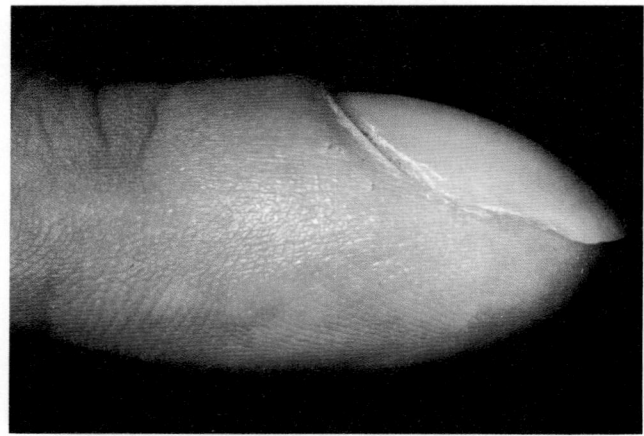

FIGURE 9-11 Finger clubbing. **A,** Normal angle of the nail. **B,** Abnormal angle of the nail seen in late clubbing. **C,** The distal phalanges are enlarged to a rounded bulbous shape. The nail enlarges and becomes curved, hard, and thickened. (From Habif TP: *Clinical dermatology,* ed 2, St. Louis, 1990, Mosby–Year Book.)

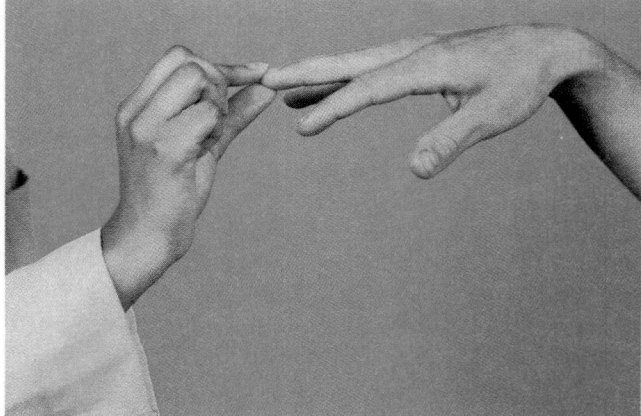

FIGURE 9-12 Palpate the nail to test for adherence.

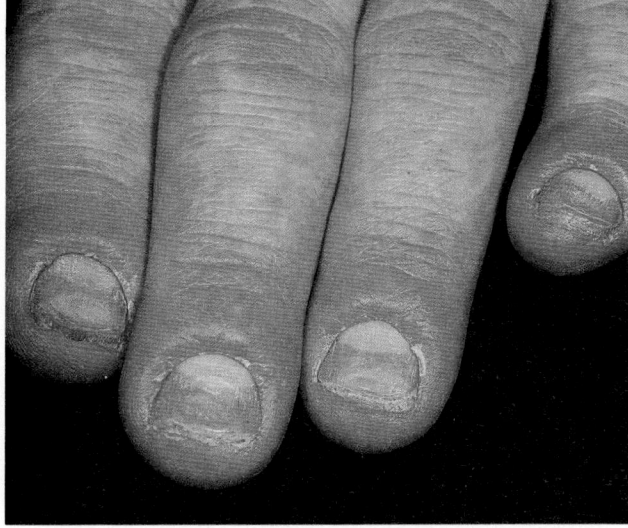

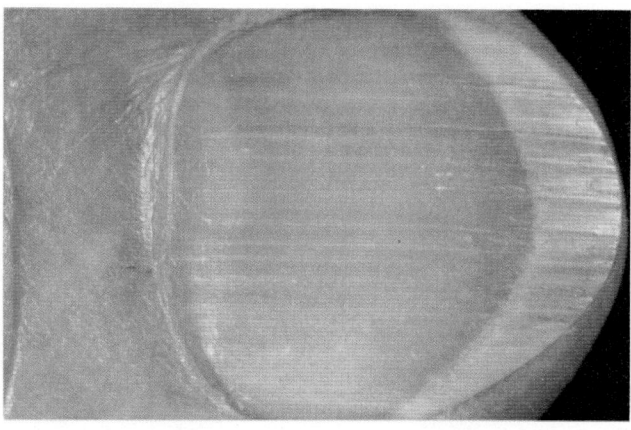

FIGURE 9-14 Longitudinal ridging. Parallel elevated nail ridges are a common aging change and do not indicate any deficiency. (From Habif TP: *Clinical dermatology,* ed 2, St. Louis, 1990, Mosby–Year Book.)

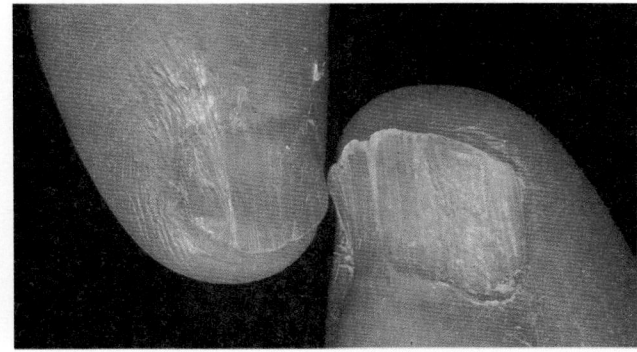

FIGURE 9-13 Paronychia. **A,** Acute paronychia. Erythema and purulent material occur at the proximal nail fold. **B,** Chronic paronychia. Erythema and swelling of the nail folds. The cuticle is absent. Chronic inflammation has caused horizontal ridging of the nails. (From Habif TP: *Clinical dermatology,* ed 2, St. Louis, 1990, Mosby–Year Book.)

FIGURE 9-15 Lichen planus. Inflammation of the matrix results in adherence of the proximal nail fold to the scarred matrix. (From Habif TP: *Clinical dermatology,* ed 2, St. Louis, 1990, Mosby–Year Book.)

9-15). The client may have transverse grooves related to repeated injury to the nail, such as picking.

Nail color. Nail color should be pink, although pigment bands may normally be present in the nail beds of dark-skinned individuals (Figure 9-16). Sudden appearance of a pigment band in white individuals may indicate melanoma.

Nail thickness. Thickening or hypertrophy of the nail is generally caused by trauma. The nail of the small toe is often the only one affected; it takes on a clawlike shape. Thickening of the nails has been associated with psoriasis, fungal infection, defective vascular supply, and trauma. Thinning of the nail has been linked to defective peripheral circulation and nutritional anemias. Brittleness of the nails is a common sign. Systemic diseases associated with brittle nails are nutritional anemias and impaired peripheral circulation. Prolonged exposure to water and alkaline substances also has been associated with brittle nails.

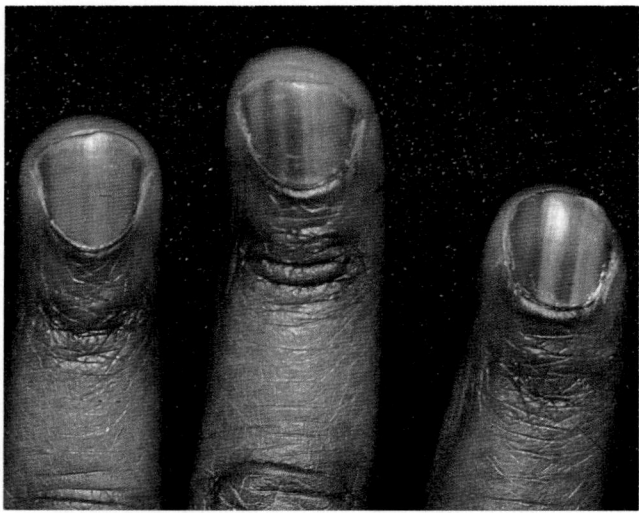

FIGURE 9-16 Pigmented bands occur as a normal finding in over 90% of black individuals. (From Habif TP: *Clinical dermatology*, ed 2, St. Louis, 1990, Mosby–Year Book.)

Sebaceous glands. The sebaceous glands, which are more numerous over the face and scalp areas, normally become more active during adolescence, resulting in increased oiliness of the skin. A sudden increase in the oil of the skin at other ages would not be normal and may suggest an endocrine problem.

SCREENING TESTS AND PROCEDURES

Fungal Exam

To confirm the presence of a fungal infection, take fungal scrapings from scaling and vesicular lesions. Using a scalpel, collect scales from the edge of a lesion. Place them on a glass slide. Cover the scrapings with 10 to 20% KOH (potassium hydroxide) solution and a coverslip. Gently heat the slide for 20 to 30 seconds and then cool it for 10 minutes. Examine the slide with a microscope using both high and low power. If a fungal infection exists, hyphae and spores will be visible as refractile tubules and oval bodies.

To assess for tinea capitis (ringworm of the scalp), use a Wood's lamp. Darken the room and then shine the light on the suspected area. Tinea capitis will fluoresce a characteristic bright blue-green. Tinea versicolor fluoresces a golden yellow.

VARIATIONS FROM HEALTH

The particular manifestations of the many skin problems that you may find in practice are too numerous

STEP-BY-STEP

Examination Step-by-Step

Skin
1. Perform an overall inspection of the entire body
2. Inspect each area of the body for:
   Color
   Symmetry
   Uniformity
   Thickness
   Pigmentation
   Lesions
3. Palpate the skin in each area of the body for:
   Moisture (dry, sweaty, oily, scaly)
   Temperature
   Thickness
   Mobility/turgor
4. Inspect and palpate lesions for:
   Size
   Color
   Surface texture (flat, raised, indurated)
   Pattern
   Location and distribution
   Exudates

Hair
1. Inspect the hair for the following:
   Quantity
   Distribution
   Pattern of loss
   Color
2. Palpate the hair for:
   Texture

Nails
1. Inspect the nails for:
   Angle
   Contour
   Color
   Ridges
   Symmetry
   Cleanliness
2. Palpate the nail plate for:
   Texture
   Consistency
   Thickness
   Adherence to the nail bed

to discuss here. This section presents a few examples of skin problems commonly seen in practice. For more specific details, consult a textbook on dermatology.

Tables 9-6 and 9-7 provide an overview of common skin lesions. Figures 9-17 to 9-43 illustrate common skin lesions and common problems of the hair and nails.

Text continued on p. 268.

TABLE 9-6

Common Lesions of the Skin

Condition	Lesion	Location
Actinic keratosis	Macule; scaling; red	Areas exposed to sunlight; scalp; ears
Atopic dermatitis	Dry, scaling inflammation; pruritus; excoriated lichenification; abnormally sensitive to environmental irritants	Forehead; cheeks; flexure regions; may be generalized
Contact dermatitis	Erythema; pruritus resulting from environmental irritant	Area of contact
Discoid lupus erythematosus	Discrete with hyperkeratotic plugs; scaling; central atrophy; scarring, red	Paranasal area; eyebrows; upper midback
Eczema		
Allergic	Erythema to exudate	Scalp; nose; forehead; eyelids; neck (from shampoo or hair dye); feet (from shoes); ears (from hearing aids or glasses); hands (from rubber gloves)
Chronic hereditary	Laminated silvery scales, tiny bleeding spots if scale pulled off	Points of trauma; genitalia
Nummular	Round lesions; moist surface; crusting; excoriation	Extensor surfaces of arms and legs
Intertrigo	Moist patches or erosions; borders well demarcated; red; associated with friction; macerated	Skinfolds (warm and moist); breasts; axilla; inguinal regions, between toes, marked in obesity
Pityriasis rosea (unknown cause)	Macules; scaling, oval shape; long axis follows lines of cleavage; red	Herald patch; then generalized
Psoriasis	Early lesion discrete; deep red patches; scaling; later discrete or confluent patches; plaques; gray-white thick scale; scale may appear shiny (disorder of keratin synthesis, hereditary)	May arise in one skin area or may appear as generalized skin involvement
Rosacea	Papules; pustules; oiliness; erythema; telangiectasia may be present	Face
Seborrhea	Noninflammatory dryness and scaling "dandruff" or oiliness	Scalp; face
Seborrheic dermatitis	Inflammation; dryness; scaling (loose, flaky); oiliness; pruritus; may be crushed; eczematous	Scalp; ears; face (nasolabial fold, temples, eyelids); shoulders; navel; perianal region
Seborrheic keratosis	Early lesion—tan macule; progresses to papules, plaques; surface brown, rough	Any area; common on trunk
Scleroderma	Indurated; atrophic; shiny; skin appears tight, fastened down; hyperpigmentation or depigmentation	Generalized; tight facies; claw fingers
Systemic lupus erythematosus	Purpuric lesions; erythema; telangiectasia	Malar prominence; over joints
Vascular		
Nevus flammeus (port wine stain)	Plaque; plexus of capillaries may have rough surface; red or purple	Present at birth; 50% on nuchal area
Nevus vasculosus	Capillary hemangioma; single tumor; rough surface; bright or dark red	75% in head region; appear in first or second month; most disappear by age 7
Spider nevus (arteriolar spider or spider angioma)	Small branching arteriole; red; blanches on pressure	Any area; most common on face, neck, arms, and upper trunk
Telangiectasia	Capillary dilatation; red; blanches on pressure	Lips, tongue, nose, palms, and fingers

Continued.

TABLE 9-6—cont'd

Common Lesions of the Skin

Condition	Lesion	Location
Extravasation of blood		
Senile purpura	Ecchymoses; large areas blue-black, then green-yellow, then yellow; lesions do not blanch	Usually occurs on the dorsum of the hand or forearm
Neoplasia		
Paget's disease	Crusted dermatitis; moist verrucous surface; pruritus	Nipple and areola (manifestation of deeper intraductal malignancy)
Kaposi's sarcoma (associated with AIDS*)	Reddish brown plaques and nodules often associated with lymphedema	Most commonly seen on lower extremities
Scar		
Striae	Linear; depressed; red-blue first, then silvery white	Abdomen, buttocks, or breasts; less often on thighs, upper arms, and back
Bacterial infection		
Erysipelas	Acute; edematous; red; tender	Face; limbs; abdomen
Impetigo	Yellow crusts; erythematous base; rapid spreading	Facial area; may be localized or may spread
Leprosy	Macules—tan to pink; nodules—yellowish; may ulcerate; incubation about 3 years	
Scarlet fever	Confluent, diffuse, blanching dermatitis; erythematous 1-7 days after—sore throat, fever	Generalized
Syphilis (secondary)	Macules; papules; lymphadenopathy; malaise, myalgia; low-grade fever	Mucous membranes; palms; soles
Syphilitic chancre	Small, round, red macule; erodes to indurated ulcer (1-2 cm); regional lymphadenopathy	Breast, vulva; penis
Trichomona infection		
Trichomoniasis	Granular vaginal mucosa; bright red; petechiae may be present; discharge "foamy"	Vagina, labia
***Candida* infection**		
Candida	Patch borders well demarcated; flaccid pustules; patches creamy white; erythematous base; curdlike white discharge, pruritus patches; erythema	Inguinal region, vagina; glans penis
Viral infection		
Rubella, rubeola, roseola	Macules; discrete; erythematous; fever; lymphadenopathy (rubella); Koplik's spots (rubeola); 2- to 3-week incubation (rubella); then malaise, fever	Appear on trunk first; spread peripherally
Varicella (chickenpox)	Papule; vesicle; erythematous base; first clear fluid, then turbid; crusting on fourth day; 2-week incubation; 24-hour fever; malaise	First on chest and back; then face, arms, and legs
Variola (smallpox)	Macules; erythematous; progress to umbilicated lesions; then pustules, firm, round; then crusting; 2- to 3-week incubation; 5-day prodromal; toxic myalgia; fever	More lesions on face, extremities

*AIDS, acquired immunodeficiency syndrome.

TABLE 9-6—cont'd

Common Lesions of the Skin

Condition	Lesion	Location
HIV† infection	Variety of dermatoses (macules, papules, nodules, plaques): bacterial, fungal, parasitic, viral; worsening of psoriasis, seborrheic dermatitis; herpes simplex, herpes zoster, oral candidiasis	Anywhere on body, including all mucosal surfaces
Fungal infection		
Tinea corporis (ringworm)	Scaling; red with pale center; vesicular border; pruritic	Face; neck; extremities
Tinea cruris	Scaling; crescentic; red-brown	Axilla; inguinal region
Tinea pedis (fungal infection of foot)	Scaling; circular; vesicular border; red; chronic hyperkeratotic	Feet
Infestations		
Pediculosis capitis	Pruritus; white concretions on hair—nits	Hair of scalp
Variation in pigmentation		
Hyperpigmentation		
Café au lait spots	Patches; light tan (six or more larger than 1.5 cm indicative of neurofibromatosis)	Anywhere on the skin
Freckle (ephelis)	Discrete; macule; tan to brown	Pigmenting increased in areas exposed to sun
Lentigo		
Juvenile	Discrete macule; brown	Not affected by sun exposure
Senile	Single macule; scaling; yellowish-brown; may be dark brown	Exposed surfaces, forehead, cheeks, extensor surfaces of limbs
Malignant	Mottled; irregular macule; enlarging; tan-brown, black-white; may ulcerate—then red	Face, also eyelids, conjunctiva, lips, penis, axilla
Mongolian spots	Patch; irregular; dark blue or purple (chromophobe-like cell in skin)	Sacrum; present at birth; more common with darker pigmented individuals; disappear spontaneously by age 4
Nevus	Macule; pigmented or nonpigmented; may be present at birth or arise later	
Peutz-Jeghers syndrome	Brown spots; abdominal pain	Lips; fingers; toes
Depigmentation		

Vitiligo
  Addison's disease
  Pernicious anemia
  Thyrotoxicosis
	Circumscribed patch(es) of depigmentation	Face, neck, axillae, groins, anogenital area, eyelids, hands, and wrist

†HIV, human immunodeficiency virus, HIV has been implicated as the cause of AIDS.

TABLE 9-7

Common Raised Lesions

Condition	Lesion	Location
Acne vulgaris	Comedones; papules; pustules; cysts; scars	Face; back; shoulders; upper arms
Dermatitis herpetiformis (chronic)	Macules; papules; vesicles; excoriated vesicles; pruritus (intense); residual hyperpigmentation; hereditary	Scalp; interscapular; sacral
Leukoplakia	Plaque; thick; indurated; white	Mucous membrane; mouth; labia; vagina
Lichen planus (unknown cause)	Maculopapular lesion; deep red to purple; pruritus; hyperkeratotic	Flexor surfaces of wrists; palms; soles; ankles; abdomen; sacrum
Lichen simplex (chronic)	Plaque; dry; lichenification; hyperpigmentation	Scalp; labia
Seborrheic keratosis	Single plaque; soft lesion with rough surface; brown	Back, chest, scalp, face, backs of hands, and external surfaces of forearms
Lipid disorder		
Xanthelasma	Papules or plaques; yellow; lipid deposits	Eyelids
Cysts		
Epidermoid and sebaceous cysts	Fluctuant, globular lesions	Scalp, face, back, or scrotum
Milia	Pinhead (1-2 mm) white, sebaceous cyst	Infraorbital skin; nose; chin; common in newborn
Neoplasia		
Acrochordon (skin tag)	Pedunculated skin tag; skin color	Neck; axilla; groin
Basal cell carcinoma	Nodular—rolled edge; tendency to ulcerate in center	Face, scalp, ears, or neck
Basal cell epithelioma	May follow actinic keratosis; papule or nodule—rolled edge; ulcer—nonhealing	Face, scalp, upper back
Squamous cell carcinoma	Nodule; indurated; ulcer—nonhealing; history of overexposure to sun, x-ray films; often opaque	Often on head (75%); hands (15%)
Dermatofibroma	Tumor; discrete; dome-shaped; brown; less than 1 cm	Usually legs
Lipoma	Fatty tumor; soft	Trunk, nuchal area, arms, and thighs
Malignant melanoma	Arises from pigmented nevus; indurated; may be flat or elevated, eroded, or ulcerated	Any area of skin or mucous membrane
Neurofibroma	Pedunculated; soft; flaccid lesion; skin color black, brown, rose, white	Anywhere on the skin, including the palms and soles
Pigmented nevus	Single or multiple dome-shaped lesions; may be hairy; brown to black; present at birth	Anywhere on the skin
Vascular		
Angioma (sometimes called senile angioma)	Papule; vascular; cherry red; pinhead (1-3 mm); most adults after climacteric	Usually on trunk
Hyperkeratosis		
Clavus (corn)	Hyperkeratosis; hard; tender; shape—inverted cone	Dorsum of toes; most common on fifth toe
Cutaneous horn	Horn projection of hyperkeratotic lesion	Face, arms, scalp, and dorsum of the hand

TABLE 9-7—cont'd

Common Raised Lesions

Condition	Lesion	Location
Wheals		
Dermographism	Wheal in response to scratch or pressure; (histamine easily released)	Anywhere on the skin
Erythema multiforme (varied causes)	Wheal like; round, darker, depressed center (target appearance)	Arms and legs first; then on body
Urticaria	Wheal; pale on erythematous base; pruritus; transient	Usually trunk but may appear anywhere on body
Bullae		
Pemphigus	Bullae; flaccid, moist, fluid-filled rupture easily bleeds; erythematous base; from lack of mucopolysaccharide protein for intercellular cement	Skin—all parts mucous membrane
From bacterial infection		
Chancroid	Vesicopustule; ulcer; ragged, undermined edges; shallow; may be multiple; red; lymphadenopathy	Genitalia—male and female
Folliculitis	Discrete perifollicular papules and pustules; erythematous	Any hairy area
Furuncle	Swelling becomes pustular; red; tender; painful	Any hairy site but most common on neck, buttocks, wrists, and ankles
From viral infection		
Herpes simplex	Vesicles; grouped; may be recurrent	Lips; anywhere on face
Herpes zoster	Tenderness; burning; pruritus; vesicles later crusting; erythematous base; hypersensitivity; localized lymphadenopathy	Pathway of a peripheral nerve, may have postherpetic neuralgia
Molluscum contagiosum	Multiple, discrete globules; waxy depression in center	Trunk
Verruca acuminata	Papillary (cauliflower-like); red; soft	Penis; vulva; perianal area
Verruca plantaris (plantar wart)	Circumscribed callus; surrounded by hyperkeratosis; black dots; tender	Plantar surface of foot or toes
Verruca vulgaris (wart)	Single or multiple; tan	Hands
From infestation		
Pediculosis corporis (body lice)	Wheal; central hemorrhagic spot; linear excoriations; later dry, scaly pigmentation	Trunk; can be generalized
Pediculosis pubis (pubic lice)	Papules; discrete; excoriated; gray-white dots at base of hair—nits; lice may be seen at base of hairs	Genital region; lower abdomen; chest; axillae; eyebrows; eyelashes
	Gray-blue macules	May be present on abdomen; chest; axillae; eyebrows; eyelashes
Scabies	Vesicles; papules; pruritus	Skinfolds

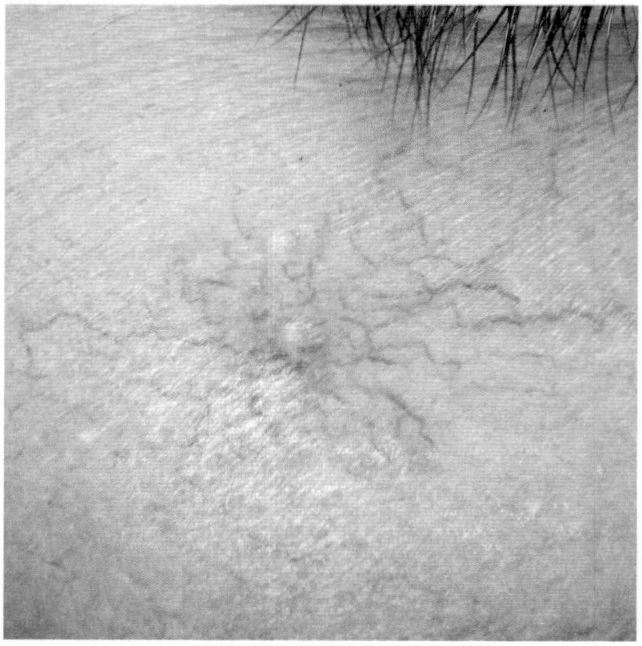

FIGURE 9-17 Vascular lesions. **A,** Cherry angioma. **B,** Nevus flammeus. **C,** Telangiectasias. **D,** Strawberry hemangioma (Courtesy American Academy of Dermatology and Institute for Dermatologic Communication and Education, Schaumburg, Illinois.) **E,** Spider angioma (Courtesy American Academy of Dermatology and Institute for Dermatologic Communication and Education, Evanston, Illinois.) (From Habif TP: *Clinical dermatology,* ed 2, St. Louis, 1990, Mosby–Year Book.)

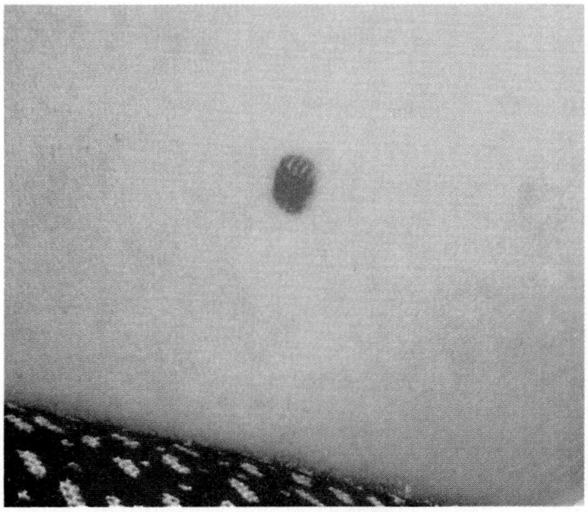

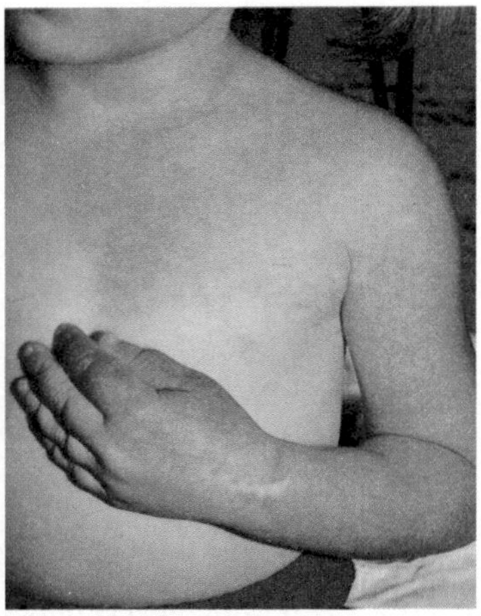

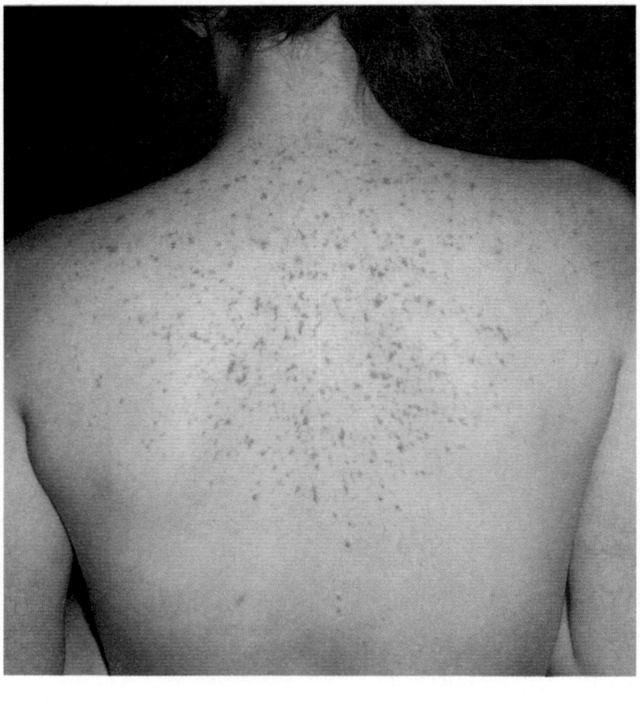

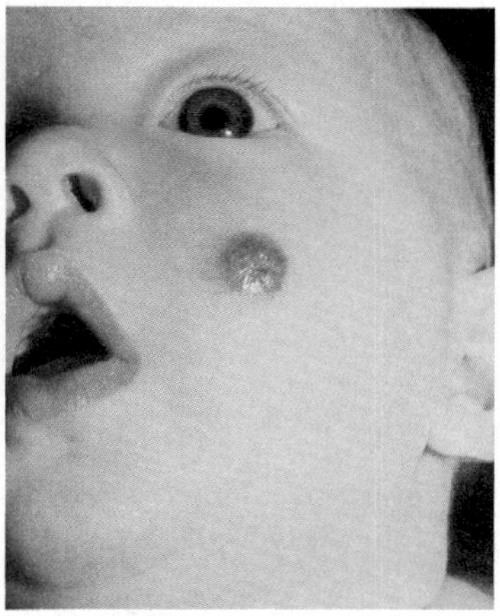

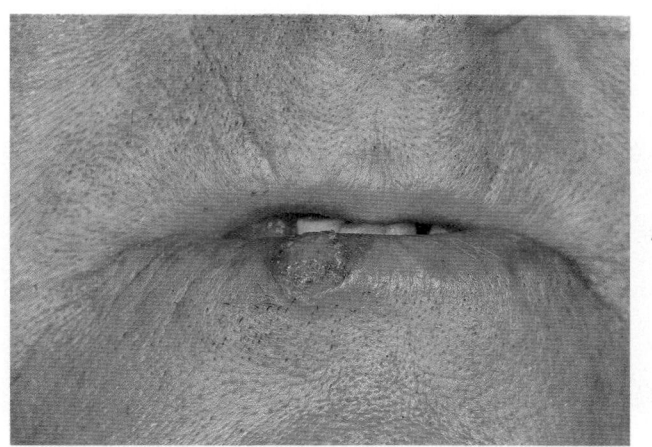

A

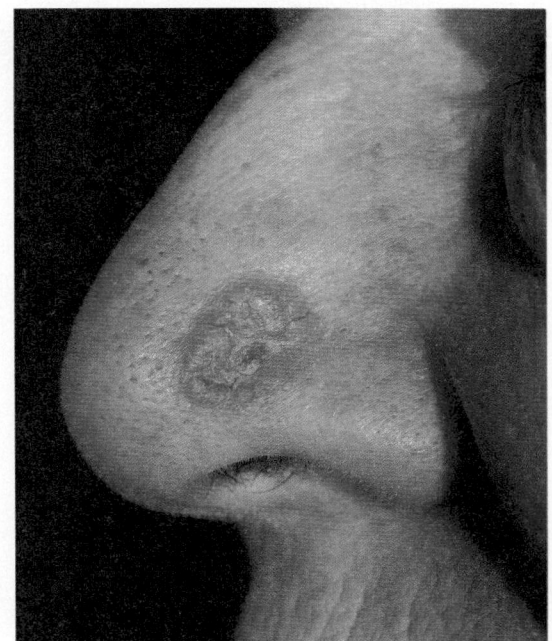

B

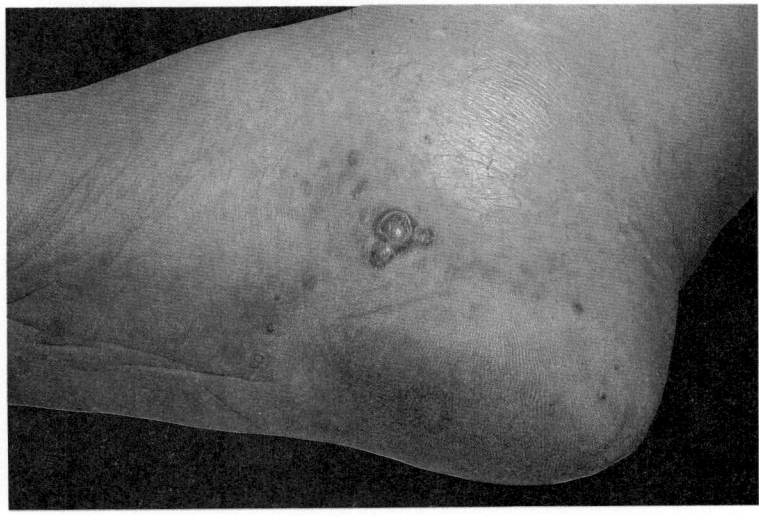

C

FIGURE 9-18 Neoplasias. **A,** Basal cell carcinoma. **B,** Squamous cell carcinoma. **C,** Kaposi's sarcoma. (From Habif TP: *Clinical dermatology,* ed 2, St. Louis, 1990, Mosby–Year Book.)

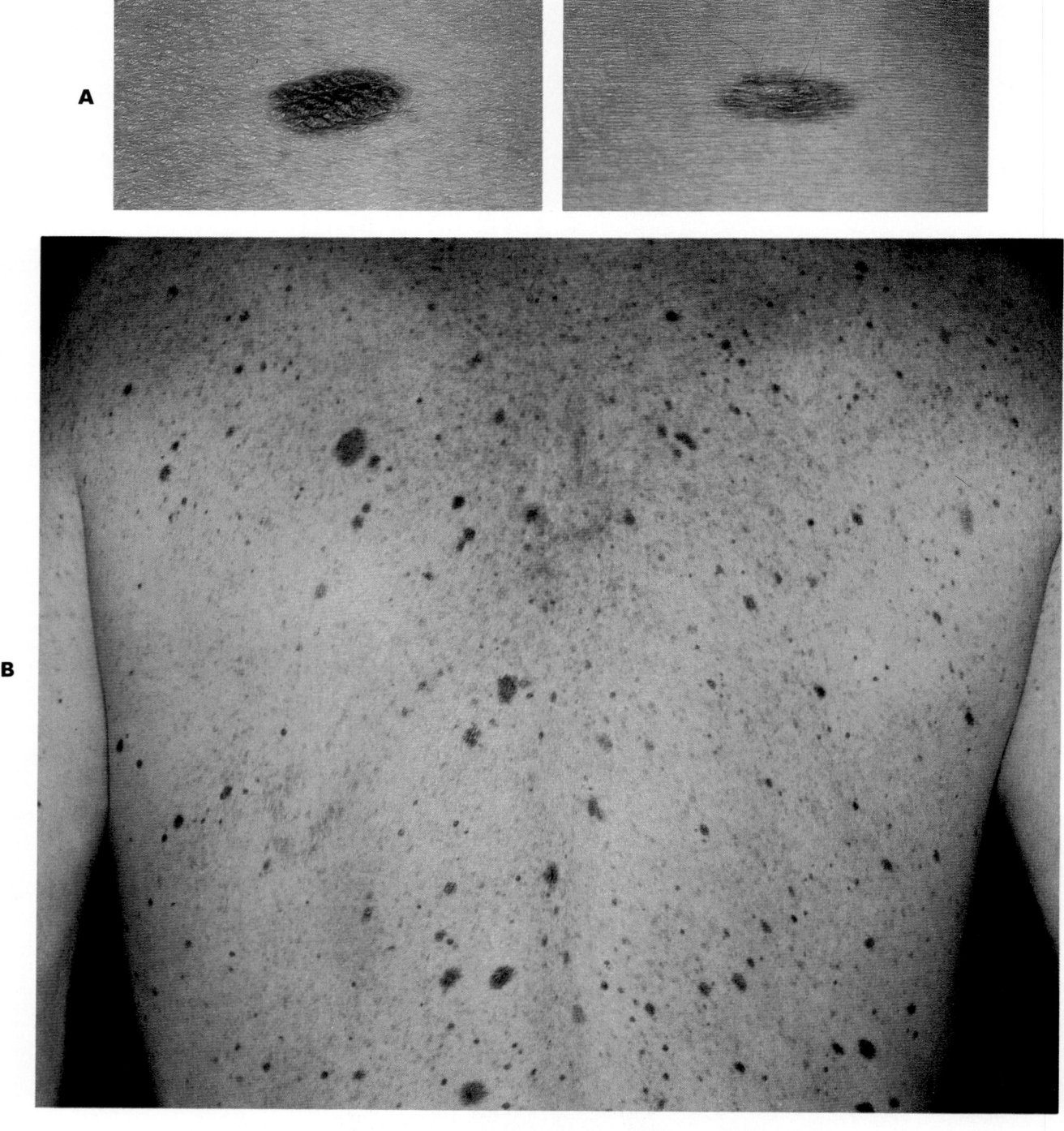

FIGURE 9-19 Melanocytic growths. **A,** Common Typical Moles. Junction nevus. Flat, black, and uniform. Compound nevus. Center is elevated. **B,** Dysplastic Nevi. There are numerous large nevi present. (From Habif TP: *Clinical dermatology,* ed 2, St. Louis, 1990, Mosby–Year Book.)

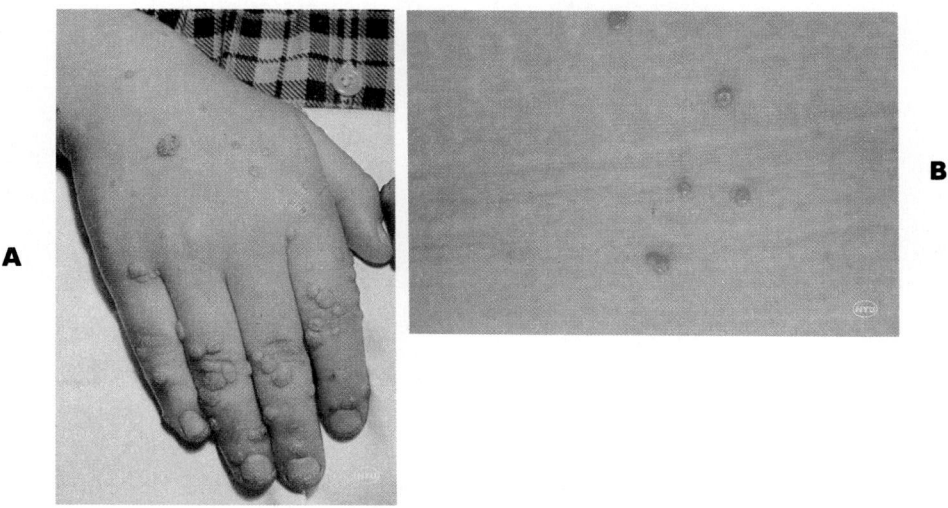

FIGURE 9-20 Warts. **A,** Verruca vulgaris. **B,** Molluscum contagiosum. (Courtesy American Academy of Dermatology and Institute for Dermatologic Communication and Education, Schaumburg, Illinois.)

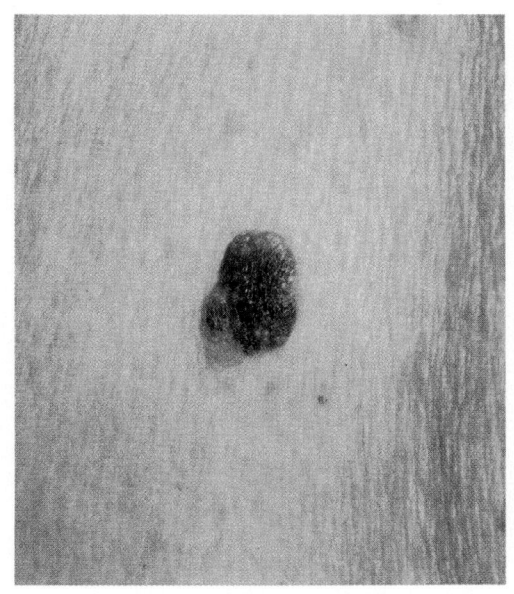

FIGURE 9-21 Seborrheic keratosis.

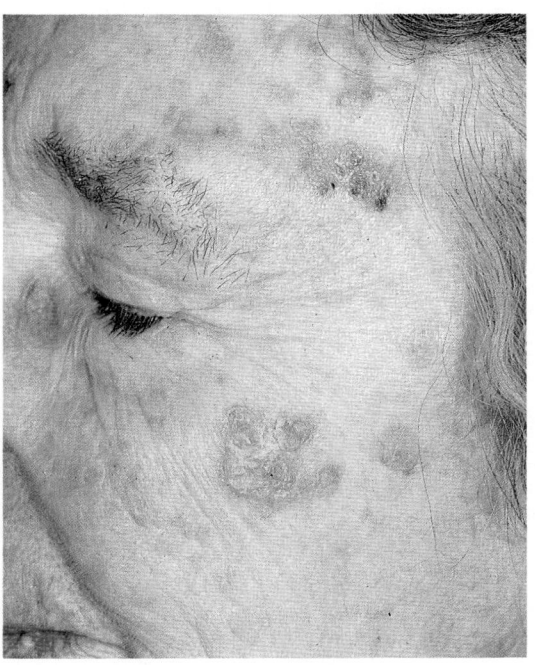

FIGURE 9-22 Actinic keratosis. Early lesions are present on the forehead. A more advanced lesion with yellow scale is on the cheek. (From Habif TP: *Clinical dermatology*, ed 2, St. Louis, 1990, Mosby–Year Book.)

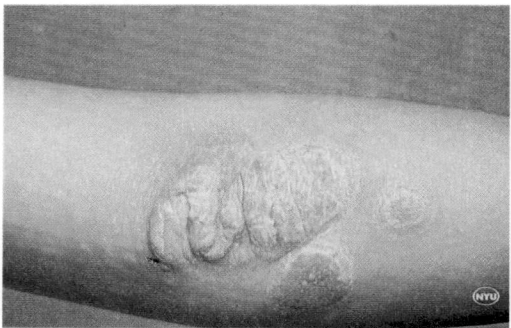
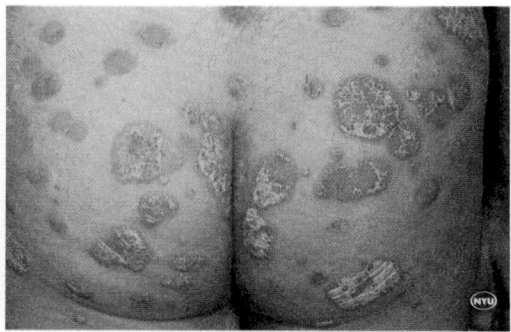

FIGURE 9-23 Psoriasis (Courtesy American Academy of Dermatology and Institute for Dermatologic Communication and Education, Schaumburg, Ill.)

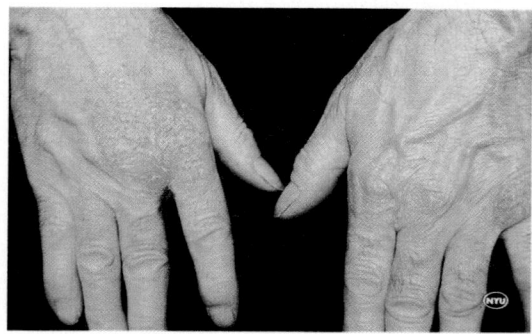

FIGURE 9-24 Nummular eczema. (Courtesy American Academy of Dermatology and Institute for Dermatologic Communication and Education, Schaumburg, Ill.)

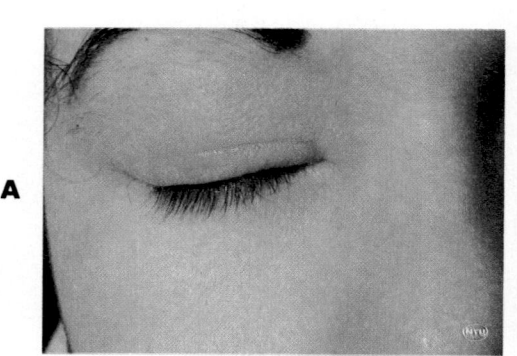
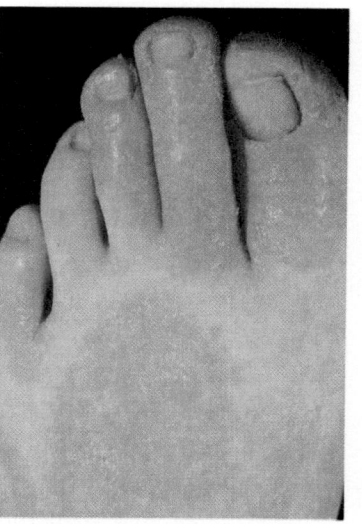

FIGURE 9-25 Contact dermatitis. **A,** From shampoo. **B,** From shoes. (Courtesy American Academy of Dermatology and Institute for Dermatologic Communication and Education, Schaumburg, Ill.)

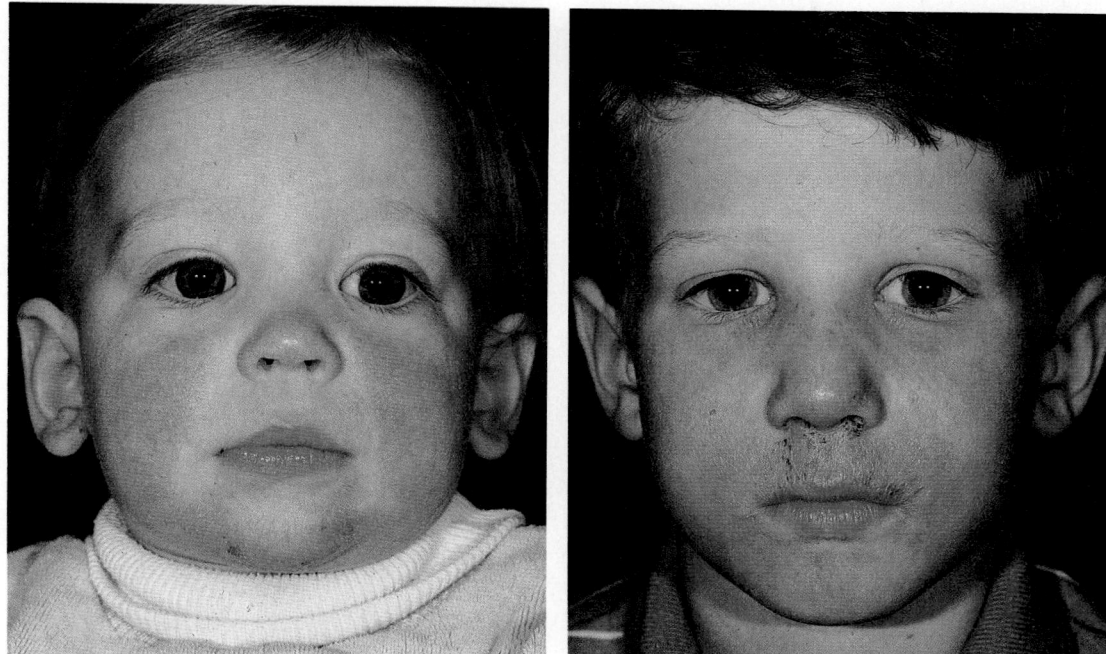

FIGURE 9-26 Atopic dermatitis (From Habif TP: *Clinical dermatology*, ed 2, St. Louis, 1990, Mosby–Year Book.)

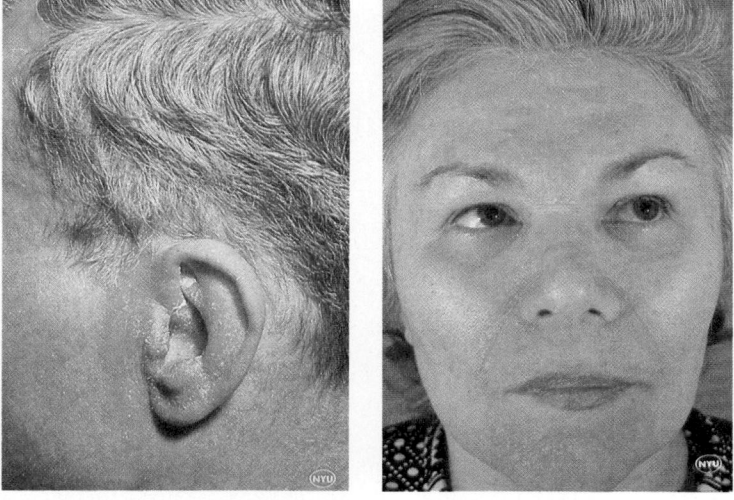

FIGURE 9-27 Seborrheic dermatitis. (Courtesy American Academy of Dermatology and Institute for Dermatologic Communication and Education, Schaumburg, Ill.)

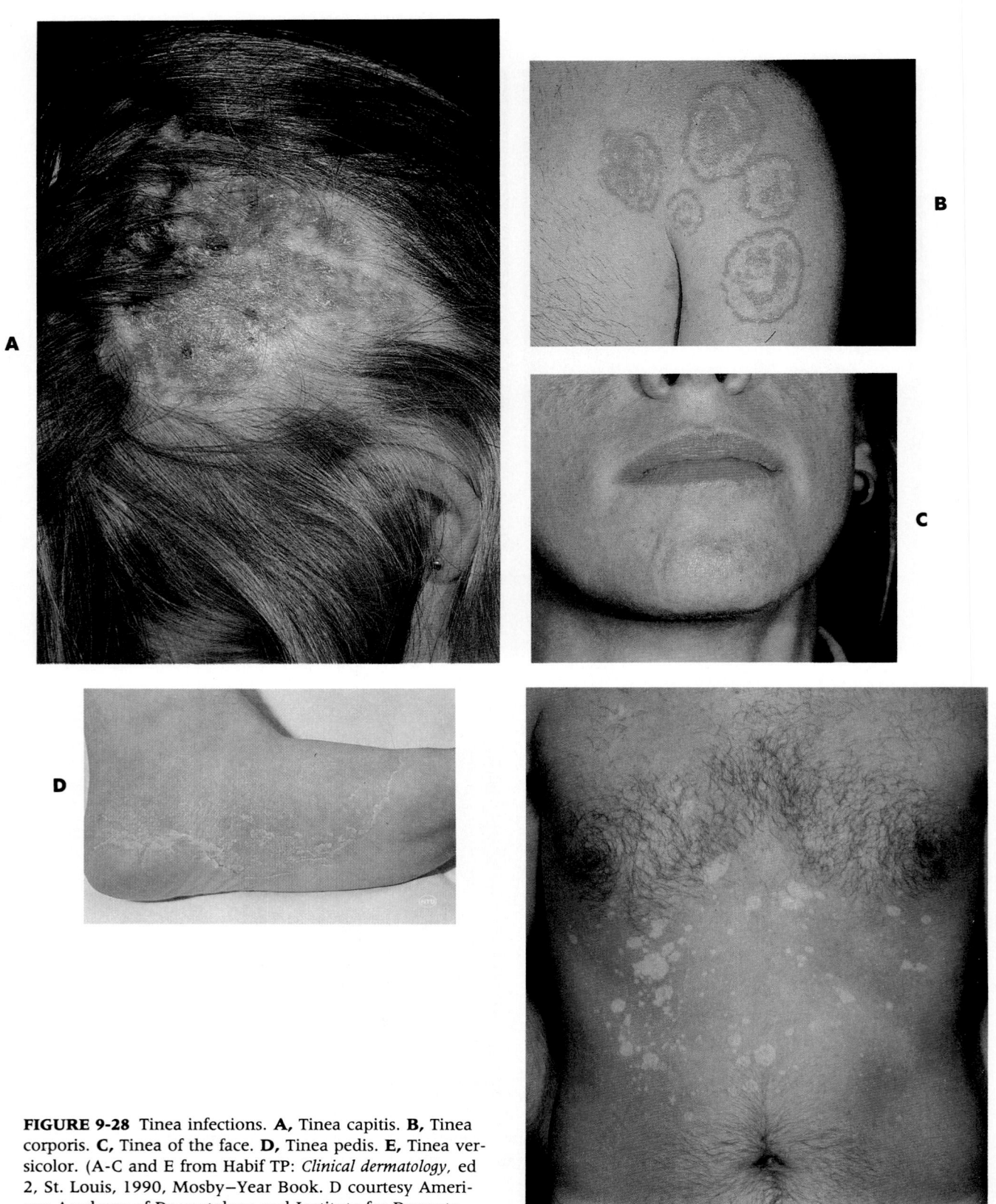

FIGURE 9-28 Tinea infections. **A,** Tinea capitis. **B,** Tinea corporis. **C,** Tinea of the face. **D,** Tinea pedis. **E,** Tinea versicolor. (A-C and E from Habif TP: *Clinical dermatology,* ed 2, St. Louis, 1990, Mosby–Year Book. D courtesy American Academy of Dermatology and Institute for Dermatologic Communication and Education, Schaumburg, Ill.)

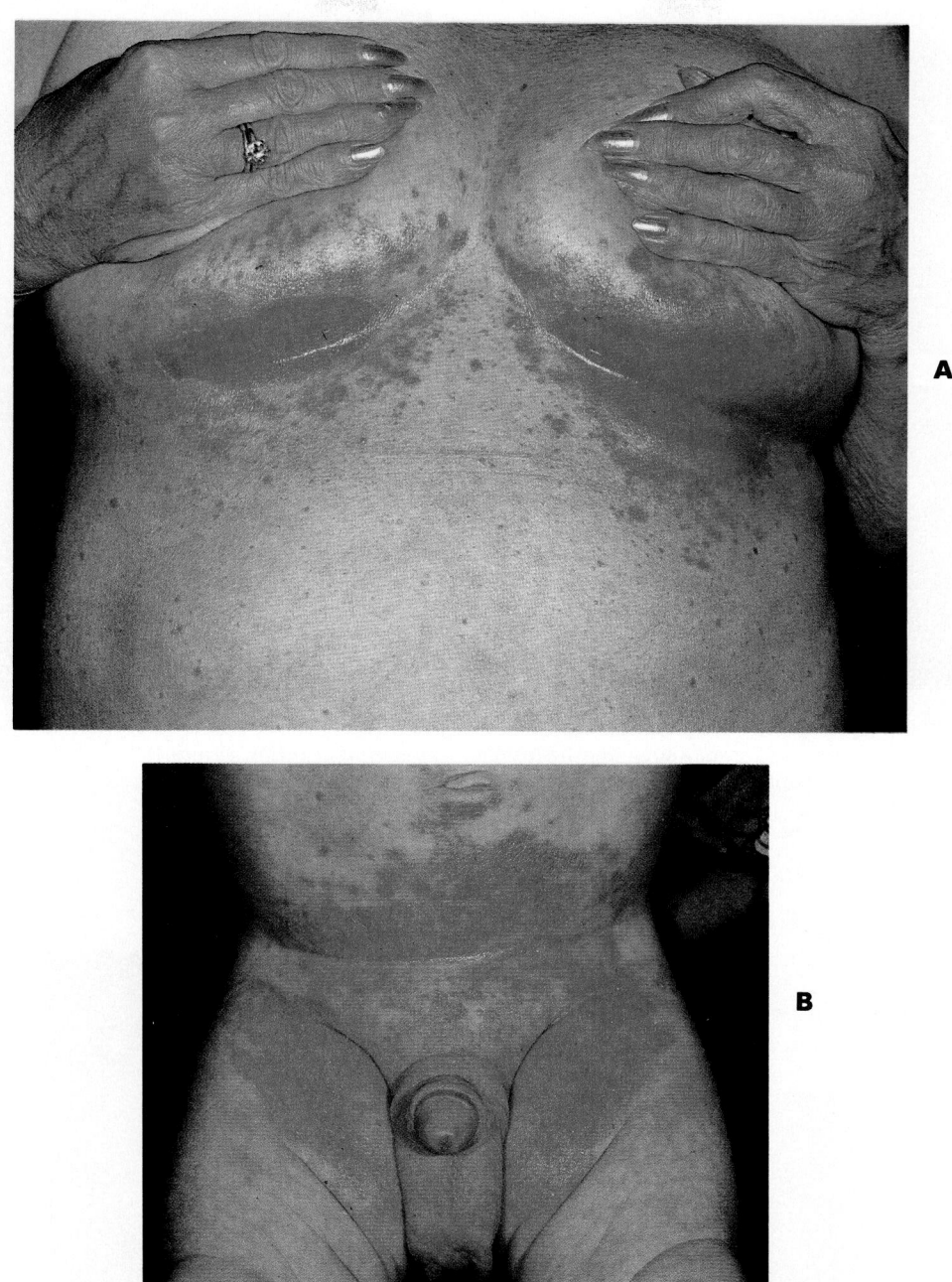

FIGURE 9-29 Candidiasis. **A,** Candida intertrigo. **B,** Diaper candidiasis. (From Habif TP: *Clinical dermatology*, ed 2, St. Louis, 1990, Mosby–Year Book.)

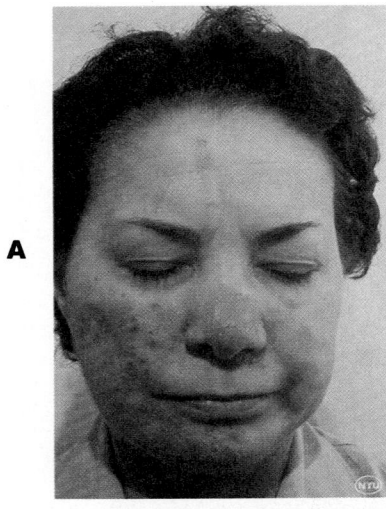

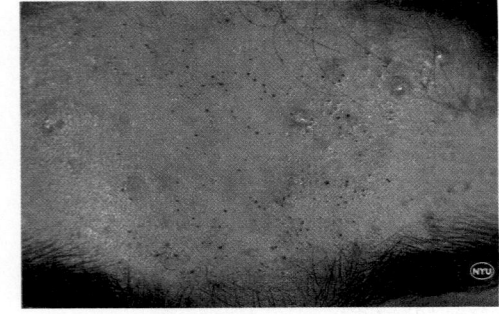

FIGURE 9-30 Acne. **A,** Acne rosacea. **B,** Acne vulgaris. (Courtesy American Academy of Dermatology and Institute for Dermatologic Communication and Education, Schaumburg, Illinois.)

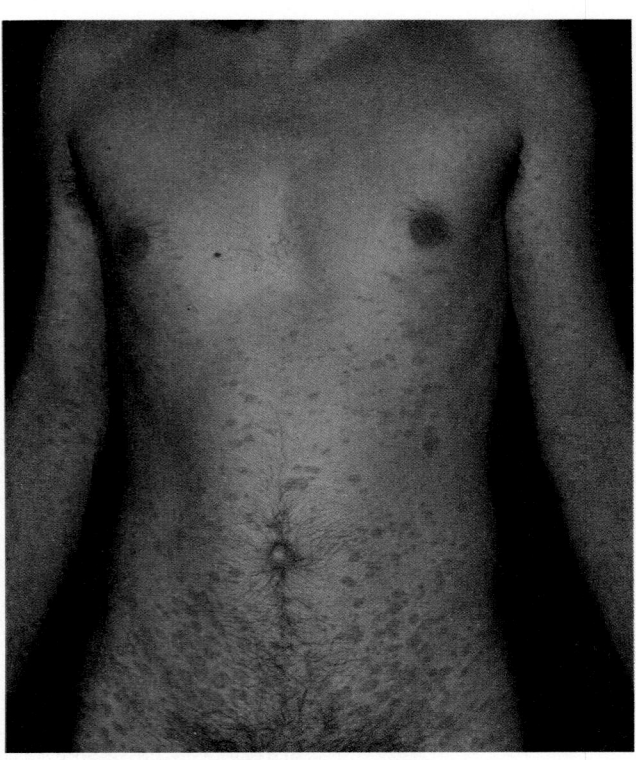

FIGURE 9-31 Pityriasis rosea. The fully evolved eruption 2 weeks after onset. (From Habif TP: *Clinical dermatology,* ed 2, St. Louis, 1990, Mosby—Year Book.)

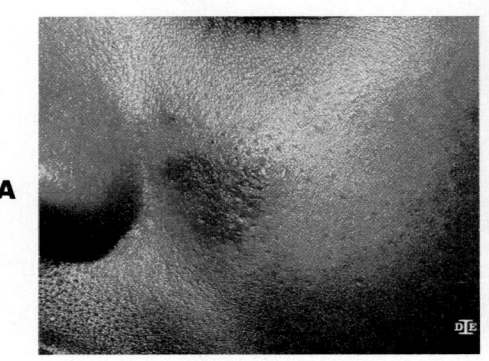

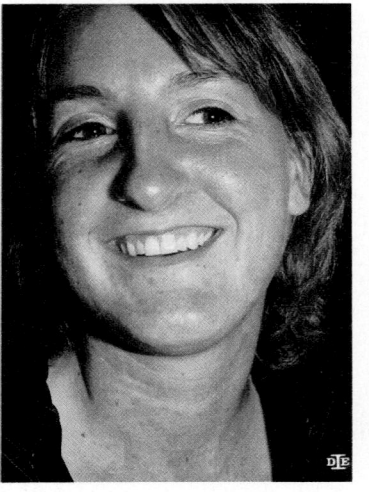

FIGURE 9-32 Lupus. **A,** Discoid lupus erythematosus. **B,** Systemic lupus erythematosus. (Courtesy American Academy of Dermatology and Institute for Dermatologic Communication and Education, Schaumburg, Illinois.)

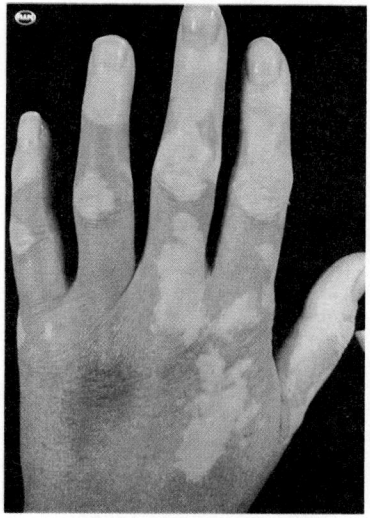

FIGURE 9-33 Vitiligo. (Courtesy American Academy of Dermatology and Institute for Dermatologic Communication and Education, Schaumburg, Ill.)

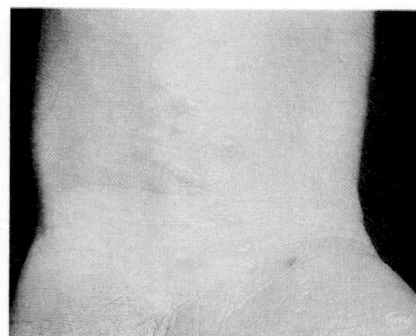 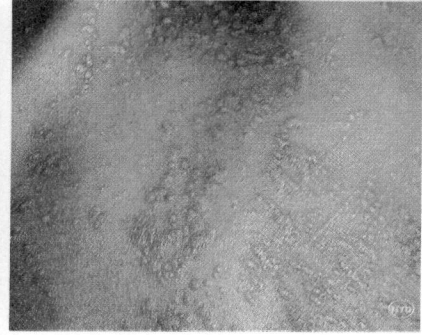

FIGURE 9-34 Lichen planus. (Courtesy American Academy of Dermatology and Institute for Dermatologic Communication and Education, Schaumburg, Ill.)

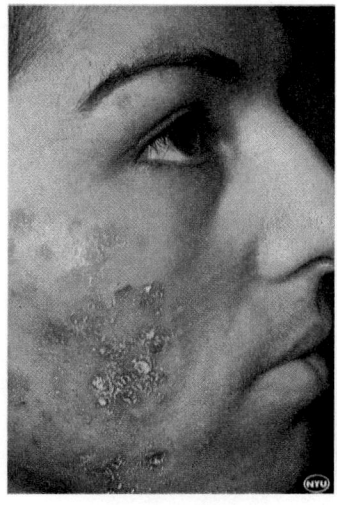 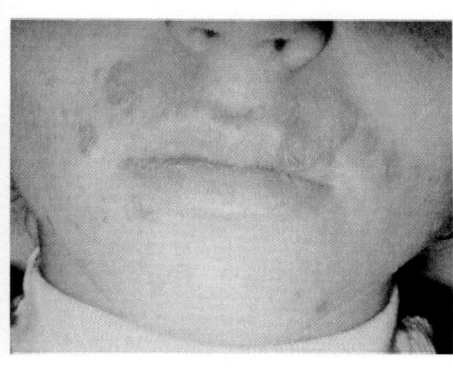 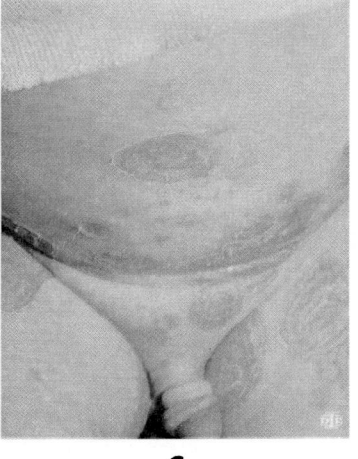

A   **B**   **C**

FIGURE 9-35 Impetigo. **A,** Impetigo contagiosa. **B,** Impetigo (bullous). **C,** Impetigo (bullous). (Courtesy American Academy of Dermatology and Institute for Dermatologic Communication and Education, Schaumburg, Illinois.)

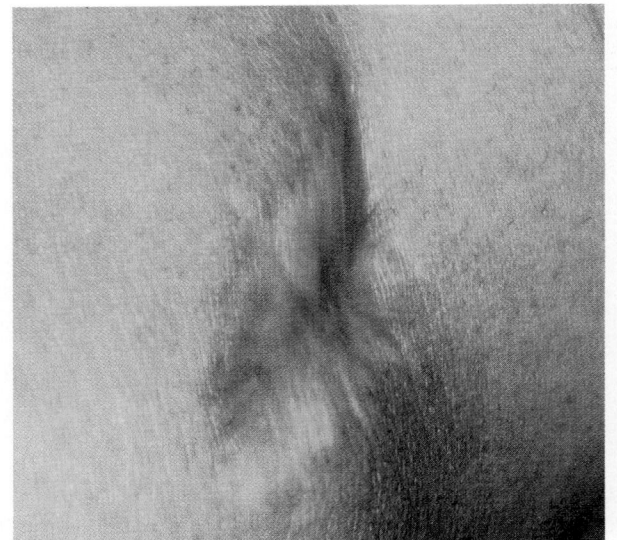
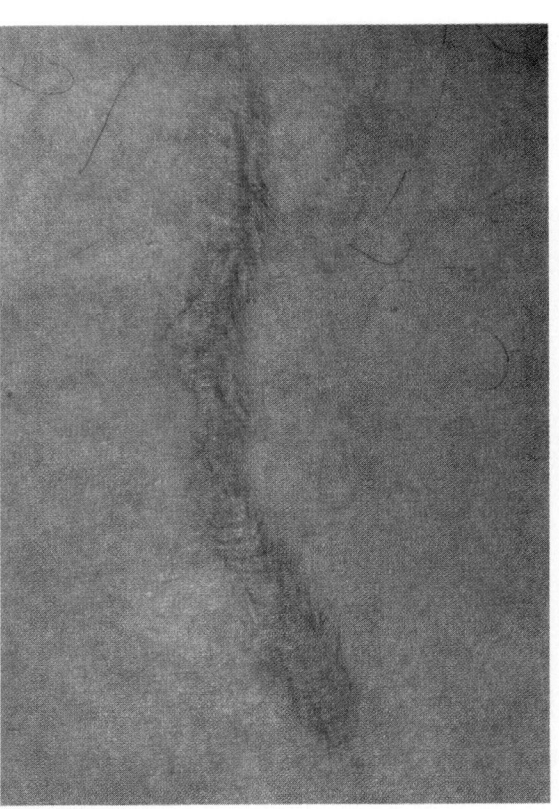

FIGURE 9-36 Scars. **A,** Scar on the knee. **B,** Scar from a second-degree burn on the leg.

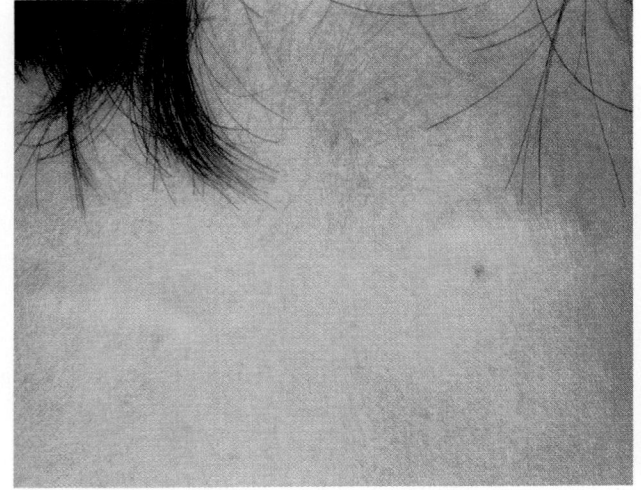
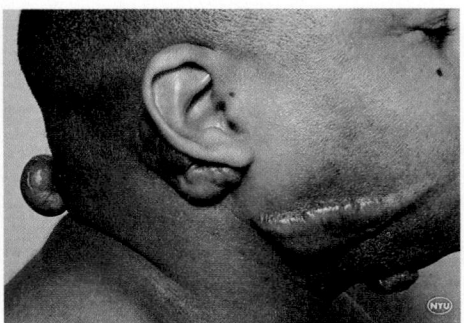

FIGURE 9-37 Keloids A, B. (Courtesy American Academy of Dermatology and Institute for Dermatologic Communication and Education, Schaumburg, Ill.)

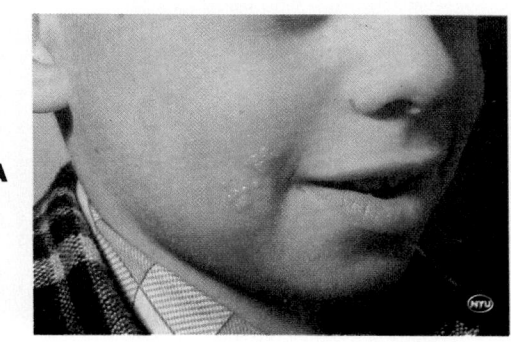
A

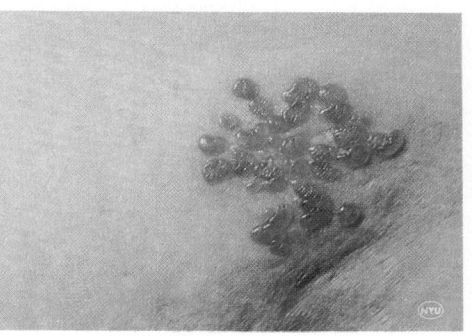
B

FIGURE 9-38 Herpes. **A,** Herpes simplex. **B,** Herpes zoster. (Courtesy American Academy of Dermatology and Institute for Dermatologic Communication and Education, Schaumburg, Illinois.)

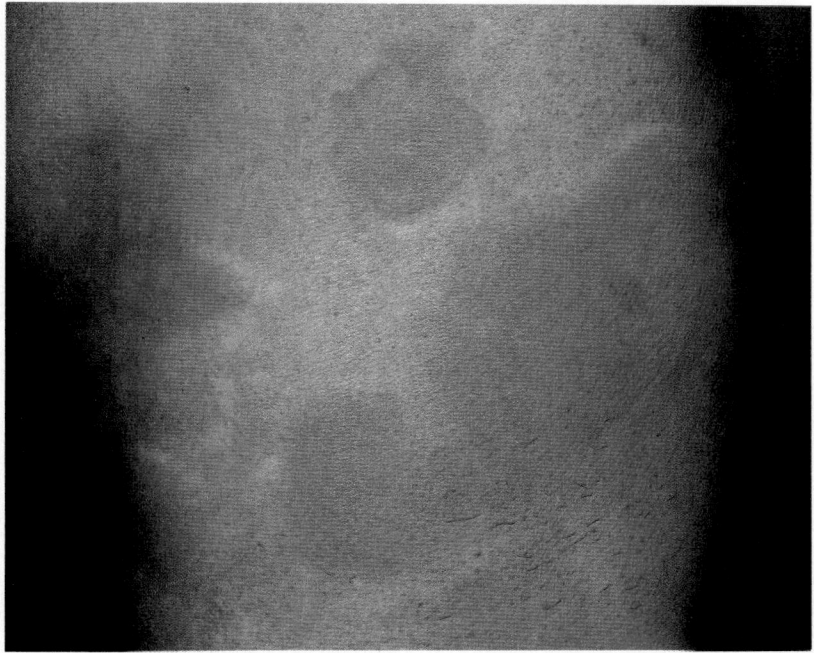

FIGURE 9-39 Hives. The most characteristic presentation is uniformly red edematous plaques surrounded by a white halo. (From Habif TP: *Clinical dermatology,* ed 2, St. Louis, 1990, Mosby–Year Book.)

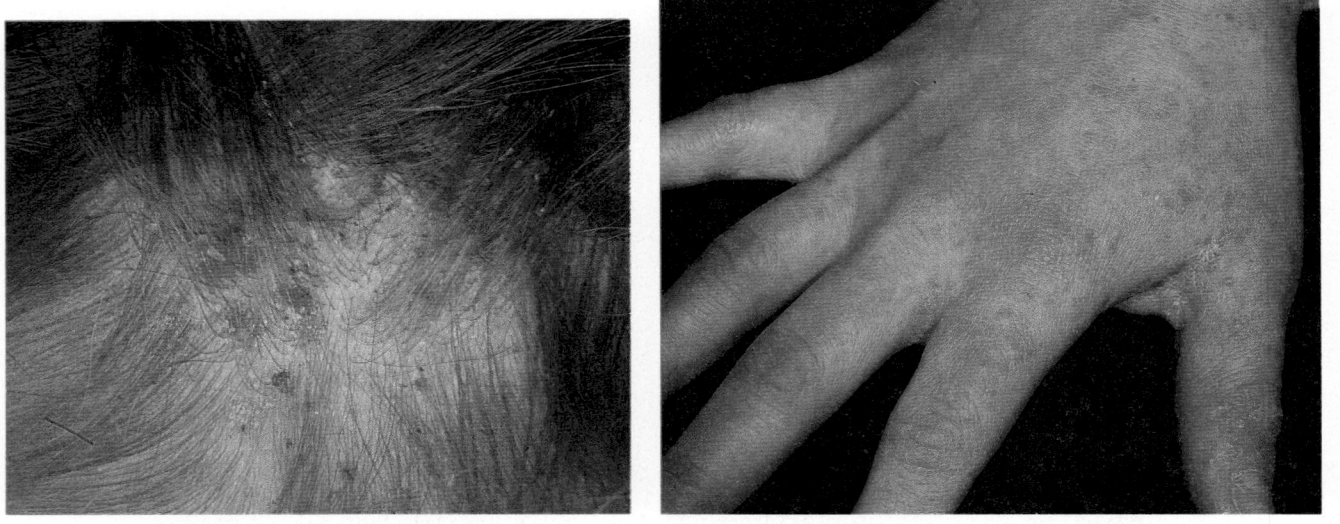

FIGURE 9-40 Infestations. **A,** Lice. **B,** Scabies. (From Habif TP: *Clinical dermatology,* ed 2, St. Louis, 1990, Mosby–Year Book.)

FIGURE 9-41 Hair disorders. **A,** Alopecia areata. **B,** Trichotillomania. **C,** Folliculitis. **D,** Hirsutism. (A and C courtesy American Academy of Dermatology and Institute for Dermatologic Communication and Education, Schaumburg, Illinois. B and D from Habif TP: *Clinical dermatology,* ed 2, St. Louis, 1990, Mosby–Year Book.)

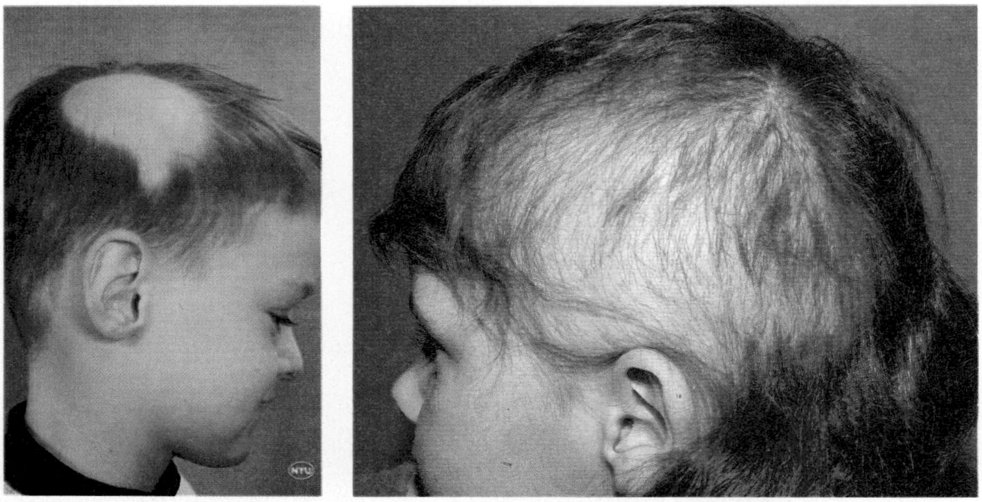

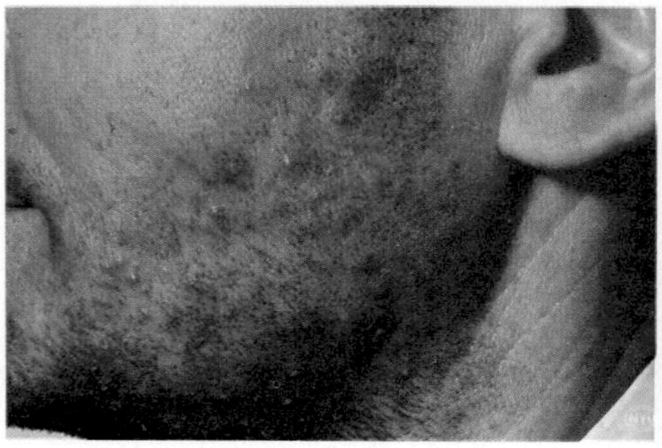

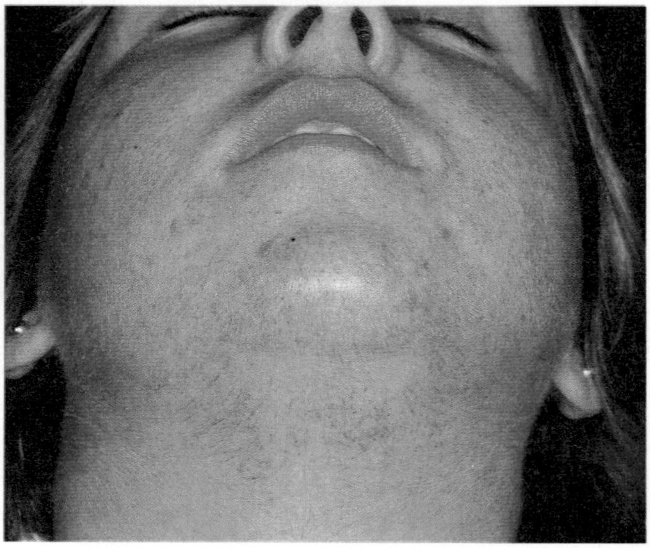

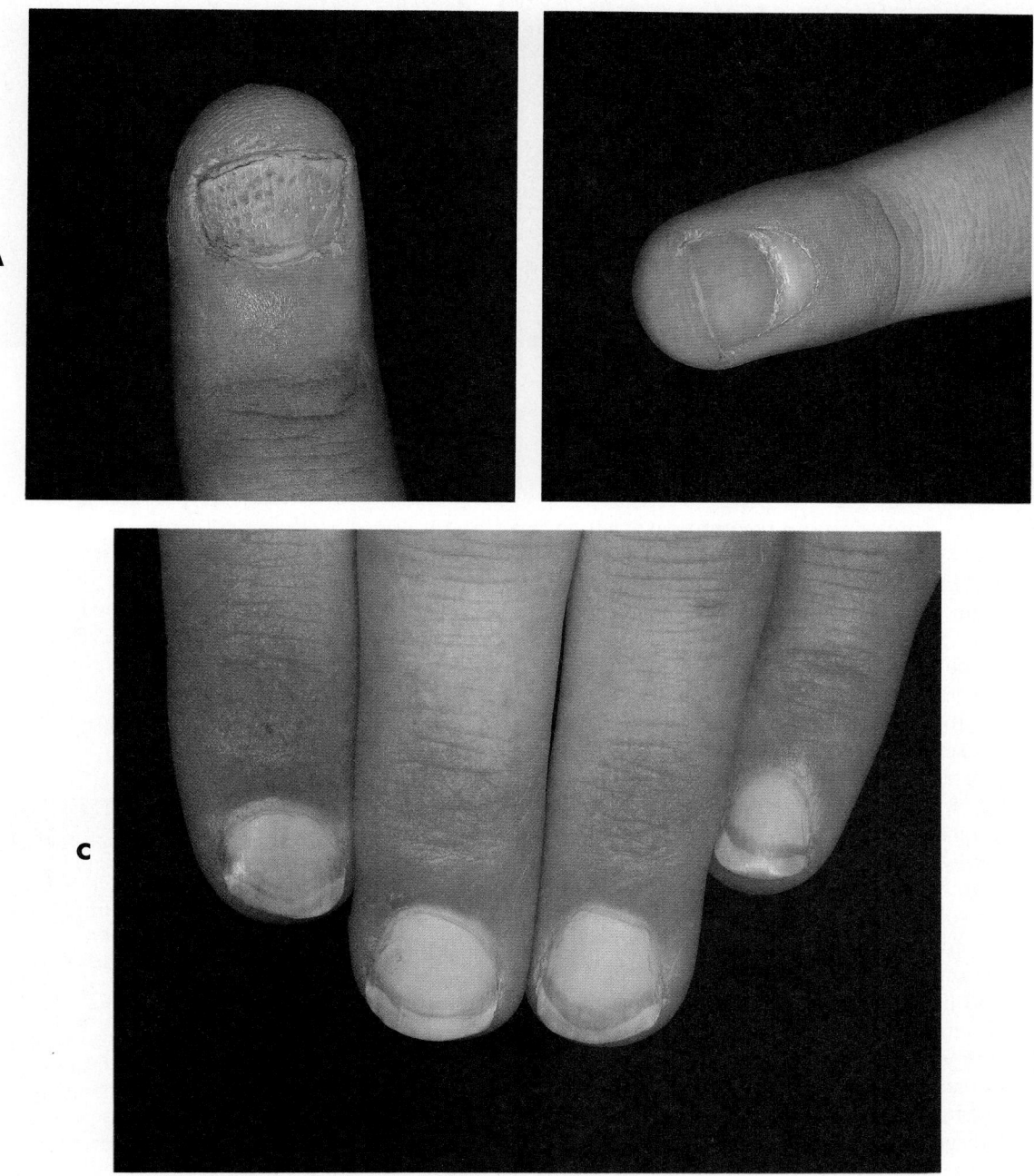

FIGURE 9-42 Nail changes associated with systemic disease. **A,** Psoriasis. Pitting is the most common change found in psoriasis. **B,** Beau's nails. A transverse depression of the nails occurs several weeks after certain illnesses. **C,** Terry's nails. The nail bed is white with only a narrow area of pink at the distal end. Findings are associated with cirrhosis, congestive heart failure, diabetes mellitus, and aging. (From Habif TP: *Clinical dermatology,* ed 2, St. Louis, 1990, Mosby–Year Book.)

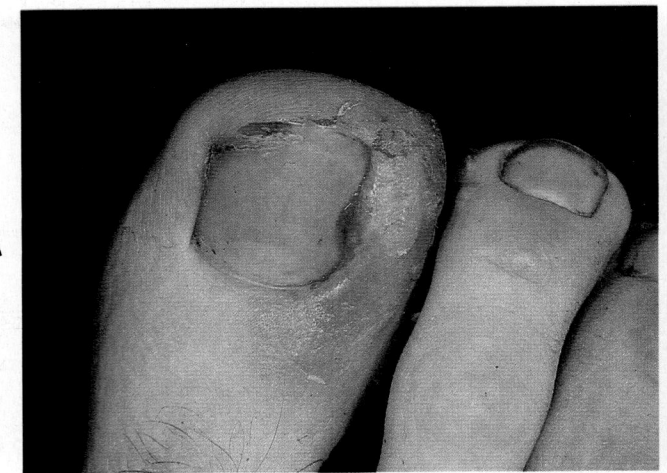 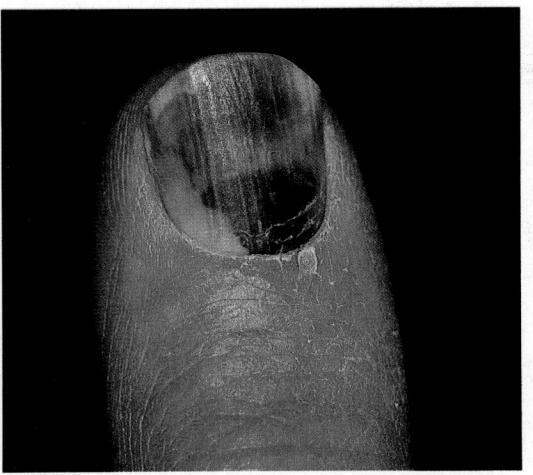

FIGURE 9-43 Nail changes associated with injury or infection. **A,** Ingrown toenail. **B,** Subungual hematoma.

TEACHING SELF-ASSESSMENT

Several professional organizations recommend teaching the client to do regular, monthly (ideally), self-examination of the skin for abnormal lesions, in addition to annual complete skin examinations by a health care provider. The U.S. Preventative Services Task Force finds no evidence for or against skin self-examination. However, there is agreement that individuals at high risk for melanoma (see Risk factor box, p. 231) can benefit from close monitoring and self-examination. In addition, organizations such as the American Academy of Dermatology and the U.S. Preventative Services Task Force (1989) recommend that individuals limit their exposure to sunlight, use sunscreen preparations (rated at least 15 SPF), and wear protective clothing when exposed to the sunlight.

Suggestions for individuals for performing self-examination (from the National Cancer Institute):

- Use a good light: adjust position to avoid glare.
- Use a full-length mirror and hand-held mirrors to examine your back and other hard-to-see areas. If possible, ask a relative or close friend to help inspect areas you are unable to see.
- Begin with your face and scalp and work your way down your body.
- Concentrate on areas where dysplastic nevi are most common—the shoulders and back, and least common—scalp, breasts, buttocks. Make sure to check between your toes and the soles of your feet.
- Keep a record, or take pictures, of moles, birthmarks, and other lesions. Note their location, size, and appearance.
- Compare photographs or your information about your moles to see if there is any change in appearance.

- Consult your health care provider promptly if you notice:
  - Any of the ABCDs of Melanomas (see Risk factor box, p. 231)
  - Existing moles that have changed in other ways, such as bleeding, or development of an ulcer or nodule
  - New moles
  - Sores that do not heal
  - Persistent swelling or lumps

DOCUMENTATION

Sample Documentation

Mr. J. states that 2 days ago he noticed that mole at back waistline had changed color (from brown to blue-black) and bled slightly yesterday. States waist band aggravates mole. Is concerned about skin cancer and has monitored mole for past few years. Past measurement of mole (approximately 2 months ago) was 5 mm in diameter, round, flat, brown in color. Denies any skin reactions or other lesions. Denies any pain or pruritus. Denies any change in scalp/body hair or excessive sun exposure. Denies any previous history of atypical moles or skin cancer, denies any family history of melanoma or skin cancer. States has been in good health with no other problems.

Physical Exam: 50-year-old, white male, appears quite anxious about change in mole. Skin: fair/pink, cool, smooth, elastic turgor, hyperpigmented macules noticed across shoulders, 5 mm round, raised nevus noted at waistline. Blue-black in color, excoriation with some crusting noted at the edges. Hair: Normal distribution and texture, Nails: No clubbing, deformities, no change in color, nail beds pink, brisk capillary refill.

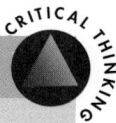

CRITICAL THINKING

Nursing Diagnosis *THE NEXT STEP—cont'd*

High risk for infection related to inadequate primary defenses (broken on coccyx).

Defining Characteristics (risk factors)
- Open area on coccyx
- Poor overall circulation
- Capillary refill >4 sec.
- Poor skin turgor
- Running a low-grade temperature

GLOSSARY

alopecia Partial or complete lack of hair resulting from normal aging, endocrine disorder, drug reactions, skin disease, and other causes.

anonychia Complete absence of the nail.

clubbing Proliferation of soft tissue of terminal phalanges, generally associated with relative hypoxia of peripheral tissues, loss of the angle between the skin and nail base, and sponginess of the nail base.

erythema Dilatation of capillaries, resulting in redness of the skin.

hirsutism Excessive hairiness, especially in females.

intertriginous Areas where two skin surfaces come together, like the groin area or the folds between large, pendulous breasts.

lichen planus A nonmalignant, chronic, pruritic skin condition characterized by small, flat, purplish papules or plaques. The cause is unknown.

nevus Well-demarcated, pigmented, congenital skin blemish that is usually benign but may become cancerous.

paronychia Inflammation and infection of the folds of tissue surrounding a fingernail.

pruritus Itching.

pyogenic A substance that tends to cause a rise in body temperature.

BIBLIOGRAPHY

Fitzpatrick TB and others: *Dermatology in general medicine,* ed 4, New York, 1987, McGraw-Hill.

Gordon M: *Manual of nursing diagnosis, 1991-1992,* St Louis, 1993, Mosby–Year Book.

Gordon M: *Nursing diagnosis: process and application,* ed 2, St Louis, 1987, Mosby–Year Book.

Habif TP: *Clinical dermatology,* ed 2, St. Louis, 1990, Mosby–Year Book.

The NIH Consensus Development Panel on Melanoma. Diagnosis and treatment of early melanoma, *JAMA* 268:1314-1319, 1992.

Pariser RJ, editor: Diagnostic and therapeutic techniques for evaluation and treatment of skin disorders, *Primary Care* 16(3): 823-846, 1989.

Samman PD: *The nails in disease,* ed 4, London, 1986, William Heinemann Medical Books.

Sauer GC: *Manual of skin diseases,* ed 6, Philadelphia, 1991, JB Lippincott.

Sawaya ME, Stough DB: Untangling misconceptions about hair, *Patient Care,* May 15, 1992, pp. 193-213.

US Preventive Services Task force: *Guide to clinical preventive services,* Baltimore, 1989, Williams and Wilkins.

Face, Head, and Neck

PURPOSE OF EXAMINATION

Facial expression and appearance are likely to be the first observations that a practitioner will make about a client. The initial examination of the client routinely begins with the face, head, and neck. The head and neck provide the protective casing for the special sense organs, brain, and upper spinal column. Many structures and portions of body systems are located in this region, including structures for sensation and expression; skin and hair; and musculoskeletal, vascular, lymphatic, and glandular components.

This chapter focuses on the elements and factors to be considered in assessment, including the face: appearance, expression, and landmarks; the head: bony structures, position, and scalp; and the neck: muscles, trachea, thyroid gland, and cervical vertebrae. The beginning practitioner will gradually learn to incorporate all these components into the examination.

For assessment of other structures of the face, head, and neck, see Chapters 11, 12, 18, and 19.

ANATOMY AND PHYSIOLOGY

Face

As an individual grows and develops from infancy throughout mature adulthood, the facial appearance changes. The distribution of underlying fat undergoes modification, nasal cartilage enlarges, and the features become more pronounced.

The external portions of the special sense organs of the face and head are generally symmetrical. These include the eyes, nose, mouth, and ears. The palpebral fissures and the nasolabial folds are also symmetrical. The **palpebral fissures** are the openings between the margins of the upper and lower eyelids. The **nasolabial folds** are the creases in the skin extending from the angle of the nose to the corner of the mouth (Figure 10-1).

Two cranial nerves mediate the sensation and motion of the face. The **trigeminal nerve,** cranial nerve (CN) V, carries sensation of the face (Figure 10-2). The tri-

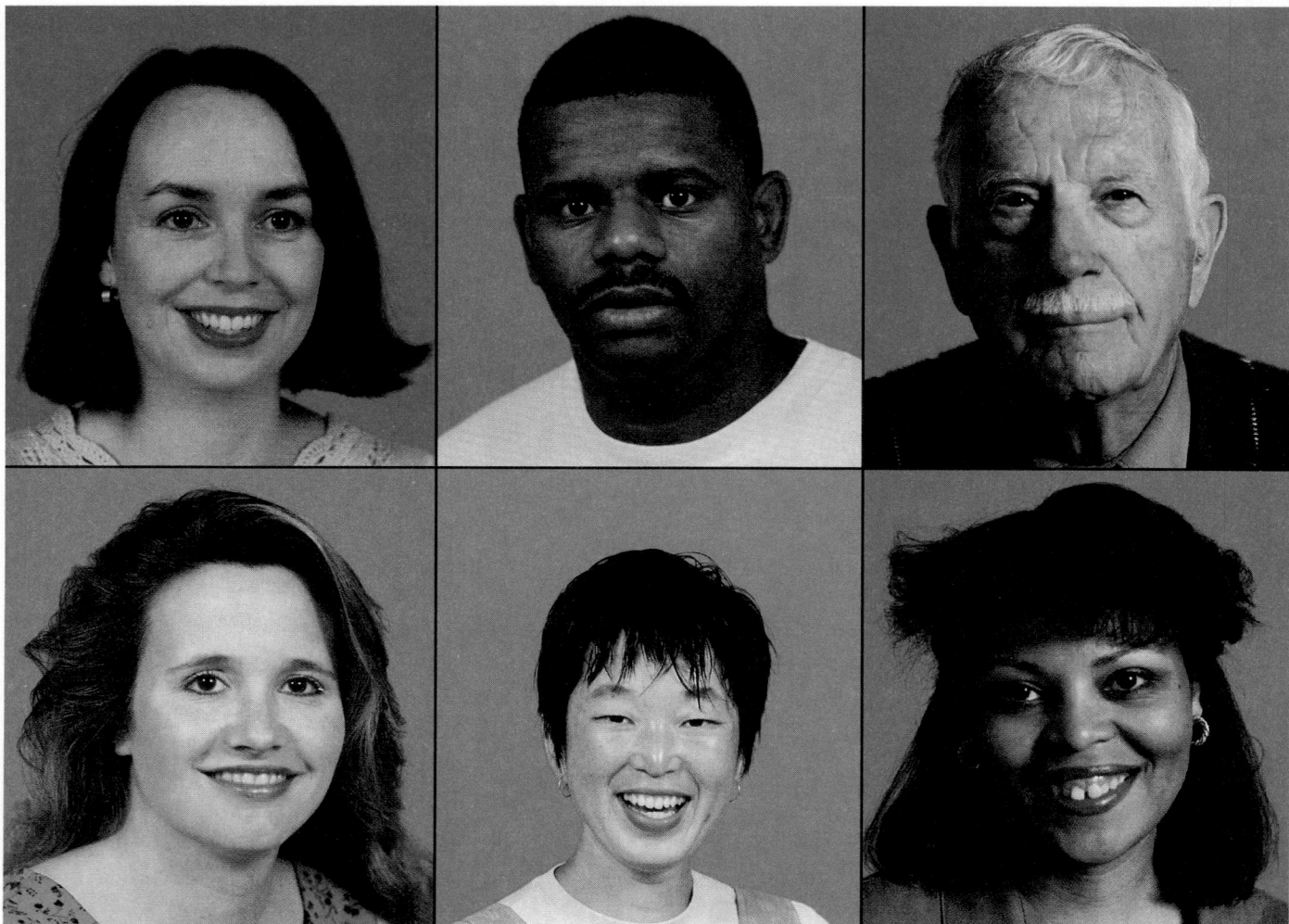

geminal nerve has three sensory branches: ophthalmic, maxillary, and mandibular. The **facial nerve,** CN VII, innervates the muscles of facial expression.

The artery accessible to examination on the face is the **temporal artery,** which runs anterior to the ear over the temporal bone and onto the forehead (Figure 10-3).

Head

The skull protects the sensitive structures of the brain. In infancy the cranial bones that compose the skull are soft and separated along suture lines, but by adulthood they have become fused along these suture lines (Figure 10-4). These cranial bones are made up of the following:

- Frontal
- Parietal
- Temporal
- Occipital

The facial bones give the face its contours, allow jaw mobility, and offer protection for the special sense organs. The fused bones of the face include the following:

- Frontal
- Nasal
- Zygomatic
- Lacrimal
- Sphenoid
- Maxilla

The mandible, or lower jaw bone, is not fused. It is connected to the temporal bone of the skull at the temporomandibular joint.

In assessment the bones should be used as landmarks to identify the regions of the head and their overlying structures.

The skin that overlies the skull, except on the face, is called the scalp. The scalp is normally covered with hair, although some clients, particularly adult males, may have a pattern of hair loss known as **alopecia.**

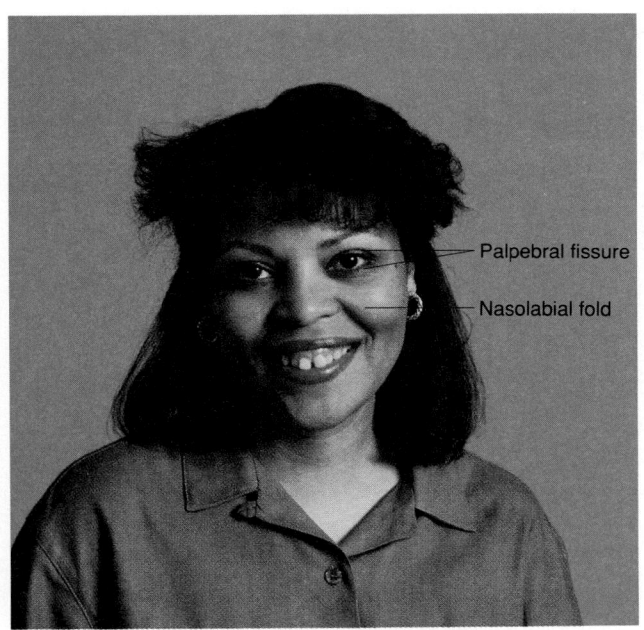

FIGURE 10-1 Palpebral fissures and nasolabial folds.

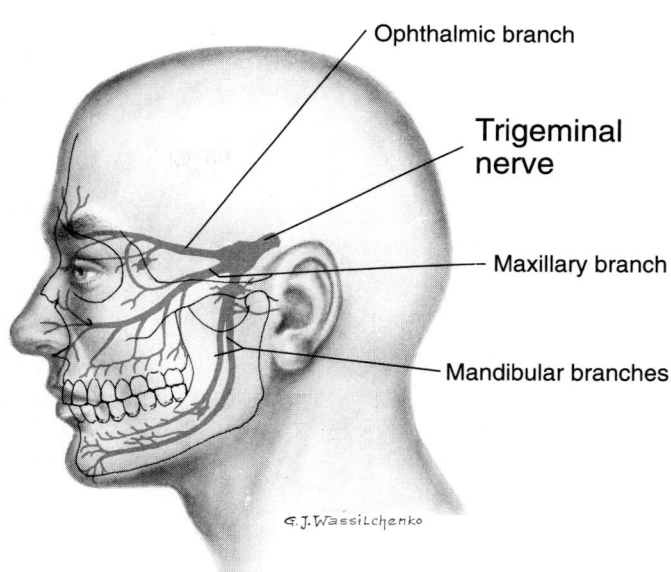

FIGURE 10-2 Trigeminal nerve with innervation to the face by ophthalmic, maxillary, and mandibular branches. (From Rudy EB: *Advanced neurological and neurosurgical nursing,* St. Louis, 1984, Mosby–Year Book.)

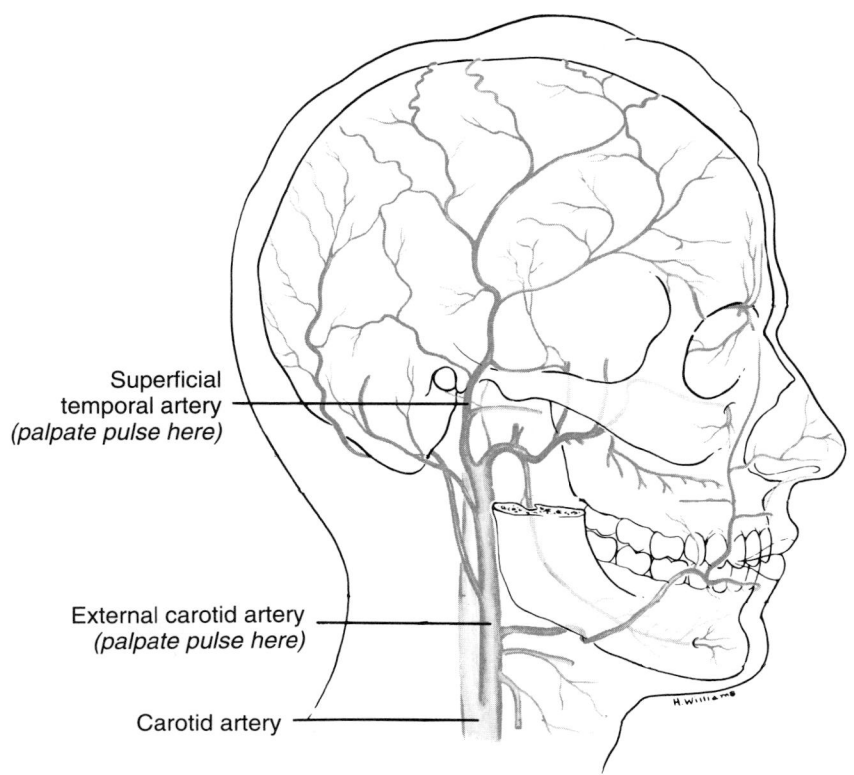

FIGURE 10-3 Temporal artery. (Modified from Francis CC, Martin AH: *Introduction to human anatomy,* ed 7, St. Louis, 1975, Mosby–Year Book.)

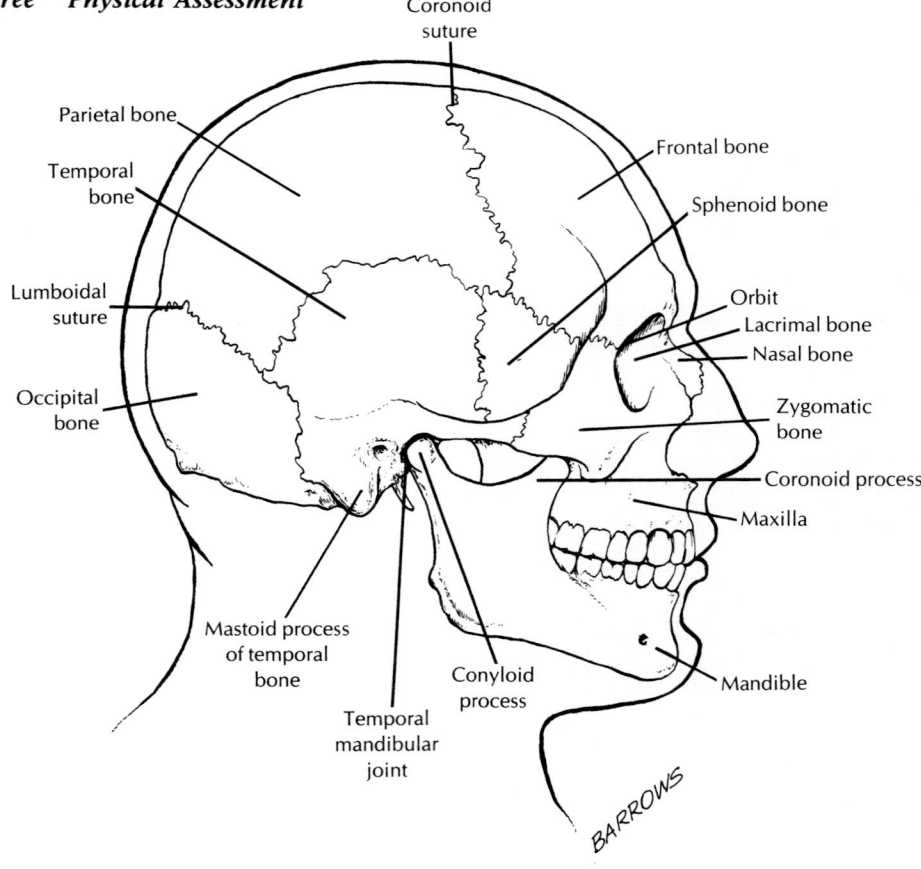

FIGURE 10-4 Bones of the head.

Neck

The following components are the major structures of the neck:

- sternocleidomastoid and trapezius muscles
- trachea
- thyroid gland
- carotid arteries and jugular veins
- cervical lymph nodes
- cervical vertebrae

Neck muscles. The two major muscles of the neck are the **sternocleidomastoid muscle** and the **trapezius muscle** (Figures 10-5 and 10-6). These symmetrical muscles provide support and allow movement of the neck, enabling it to flex, extend, rotate, and turn laterally. They are innervated by the **spinal accessory nerve,** CN XI. Both sets of muscles and their position in relation to adjacent bones can be used to describe anatomical landmarks and physical findings. Each sternocleidomastoid muscle extends from the upper sternum and the proximal portion of the clavical to the **mastoid process** of the temporal bone behind the ear.

This pair of muscles provides for turning and lateral flexion of the head.

The two trapezius muscles (see Figure 10-6) are large, flat, and triangular. Each one extends from the cervical and thoracic vertebrae and from the spine of the scapula to the occipital bone of the skull. The trapezius muscles are involved in the movements of shrugging the shoulders, pulling the scapulae downward and toward the vertebral column, rotating the head to the side, and extending the head backward.

For the purpose of describing findings, each side of the neck can be divided into two triangles called the **anterior and posterior triangles** (see Figure 10-5). Forming the anterior triangle are the edge of the mandible (superiorly), the sternocleidomastoid muscle (laterally), and the midline of the trachea (medially). Composing the posterior triangle are the sternocleidomastoid muscle (laterally), the trapezius muscle (posteriorly), and the clavicle (inferiorly).

Within the anterior triangle are the anterior cervical lymph nodes, the carotid artery, and the internal jugular vein. Several groups of lymph nodes lie within the posterior triangle.

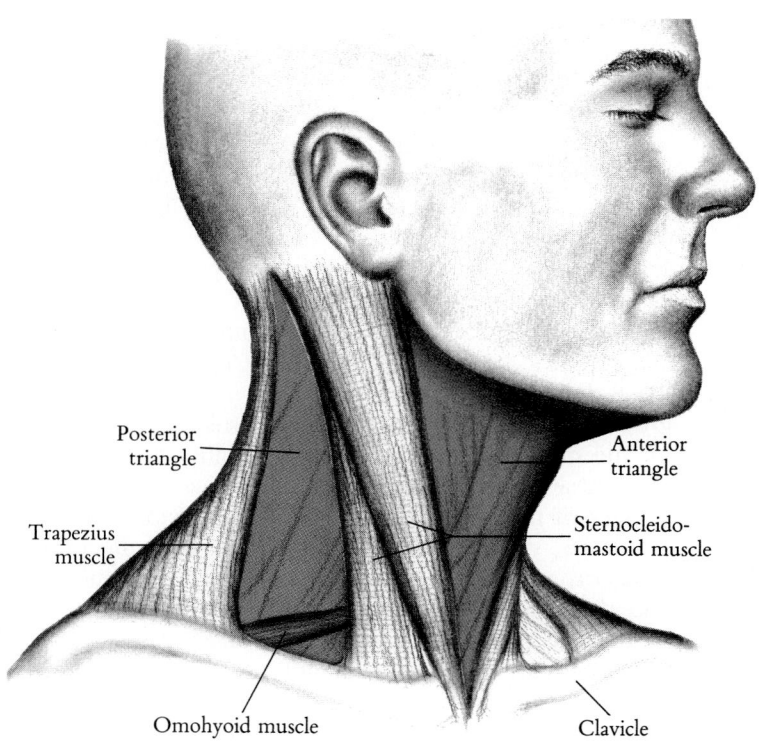

Posterior triangle

Anterior triangle

Trapezius muscle

Sternocleido-mastoid muscle

Omohyoid muscle

Clavicle

FIGURE 10-5 Sternocleidomastoid and trapezius muscles. Anterior and posterior triangles. (From Seidel HM, and others: *Mosby's guide to physical examination*, ed 2, St. Louis, 1991, Mosby—Year Book.)

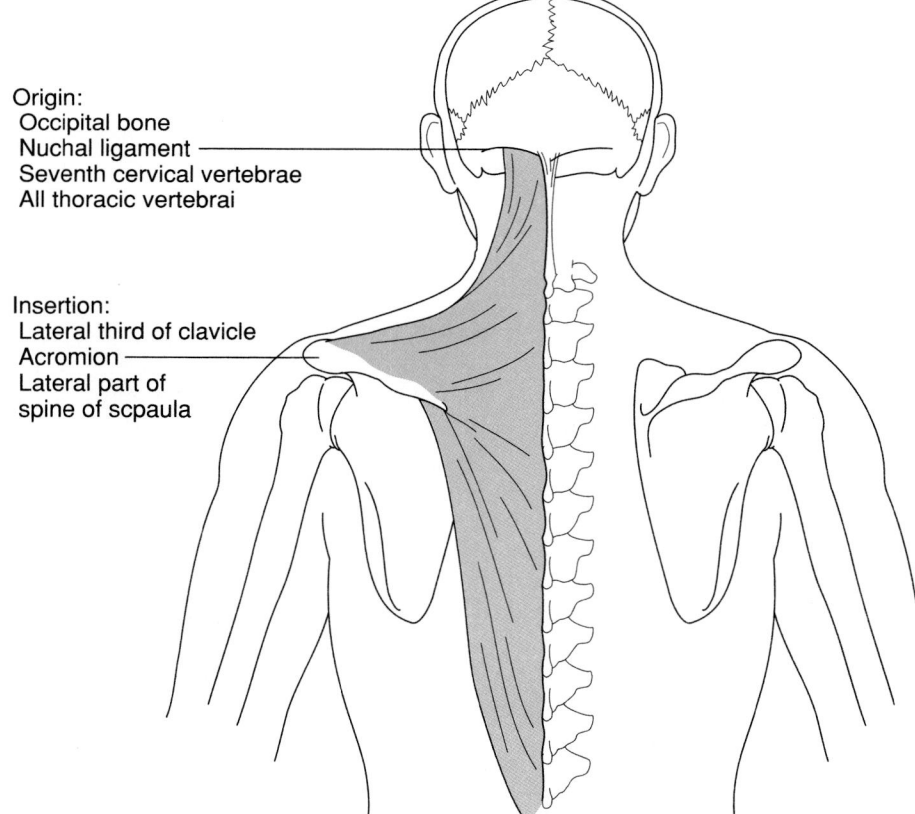

Origin:
 Occipital bone
 Nuchal ligament
 Seventh cervical vertebrae
 All thoracic vertebrai

Insertion:
 Lateral third of clavicle
 Acromion
 Lateral part of
 spine of scpaula

FIGURE 10-6 Trapezius muscle.

Midline neck structures. As shown in Figure 10-7, the anterior midline neck structures include the following:

- Hyoid bone
- Thyroid cartilage
- Cricoid cartilage
- Tracheal rings
- Isthmus of the thyroid gland

The hyoid bone lies just below the mandible at the angle of the floor of the mouth. The thyroid cartilage is shaped like a shield, with a notch at the upper edge that marks the level of bifurcation, or division, of the common carotid artery into the internal and external carotid arteries. The thyroid is the largest of the cartilaginous structures of the neck. The cricoid cartilage, the uppermost ring of the trachea, lies just below the thyroid cartilage. The isthmus of the thyroid gland is found across the trachea and below the cricoid cartilage. The cartilaginous trachea is located below the cricoid cartilage. It continues to the lungs, where it divides into two bronchi.

Thyroid gland. The **thyroid gland** (Figures 10-7 and 10-8) is the largest endocrine gland in the body and the only one that is accessible to direct physical examination. It is butterfly-shaped with a lobe on each side of the trachea. A connecting isthmus joins the lower part of the lobes just below the cricoid cartilage. The lobes curve posteriorly and are largely covered by the sternocleidomastoid muscles. Each lobe, which is somewhat irregular and cone-shaped, is approximately 5 cm long, 3 cm in diameter, and 2 cm thick. The normal consistency of the thyroid can be described as "meaty" or "rubbery." The thyroid arteries supply the highly vascular thyroid tissue.

The thyroid gland produces two hormones: thyroxine (T_4) and triiodothyronine (T_3). The functions of these hormones are essential for normal physical growth and development in infancy and childhood and for the maintenance of metabolic stability throughout life. These hormones influence the concentration and activity of numerous enzymes and the metabolism of substrates, vitamins, and minerals. They also affect the secretion and degradation rates of all other hormones and their target tissue responses. Thus thyroid hormones affect virtually all the tissues and organ systems of the body. It is important to note that changes due to altered thyroid function can occur in other body systems even when there is no change in the thyroid gland that is detectable on physical examination. Thyroid tissue

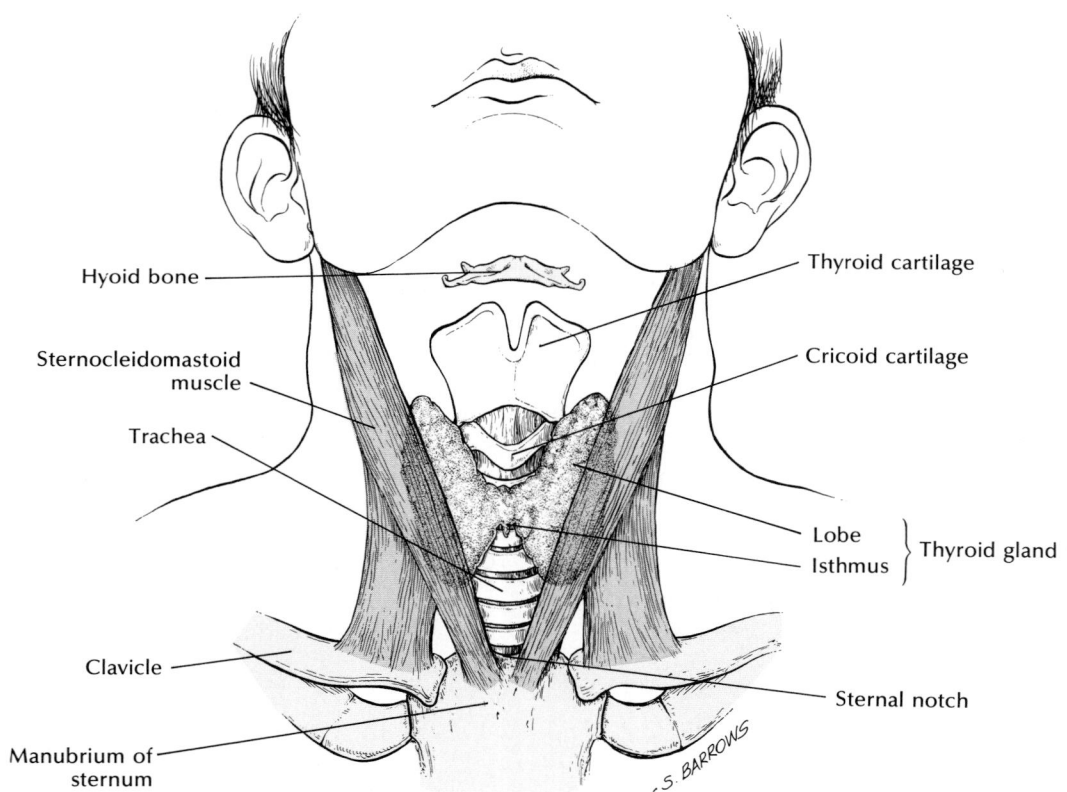

FIGURE 10-7 Anterior midline neck structures.

ANTERIOR   POSTERIOR

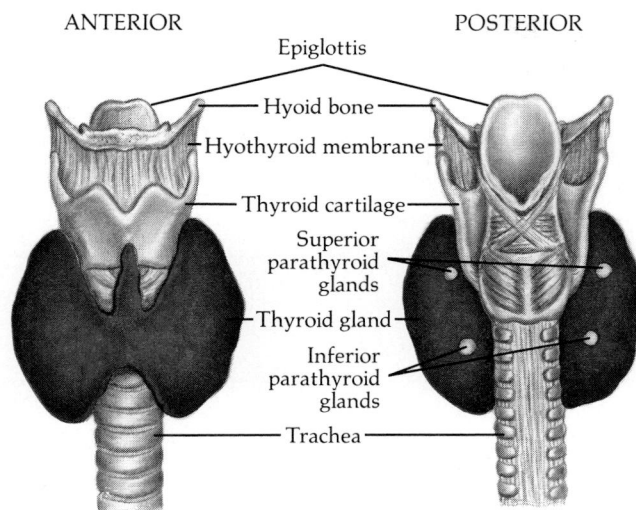

FIGURE 10-8 Thyroid gland. (From Thompson JM, Mc-Farland GK, Hirsch JE, and others: *Mosby's manual of clinical nursing,* ed 2, St. Louis, 1989, Mosby—Year Book.)

may enlarge retrosternally or in areas that are not accessible to palpation. If a thyroid disorder is suspected, clinical assessment must include other body systems, such as the cardiovascular, gastrointestinal, integumentary, and neurological systems.

Posterior bony structures. The seven cervical vertebrae with their spinous processes are located in the posterior neck.

EXAMINATION

Health History
General considerations, life-style, and health history
1. Home living environment: Includes potential risks for injury, such as use of handrails, presence of electrical cords, loose rugs.
2. Employment: Risk of head injury, use of helmet, protective eye shields, exposure to toxins, chemicals.
3. Participation in activities with potential for risk of injury, such as active sports.
4. Stress, tension, demands at home, work, school.
5. Nutrition: Eating habits, food intolerances, recent weight gain or loss.
6. Use of alcohol or drugs.
7. Medications: Analgesics, anticonvulsants, cardiac preparations, thyroid preparations, oral contraceptives.
8. History of trauma, injury, surgery, tumor, seizure disorder.

Headache
1. Type or types of headache and extent of time over which they have been occurring.
2. Onset: Time of day or night, gradual or abrupt.
3. Duration: Minutes, hours, days, weeks.
4. Frequency and timing: Occasional, clustering, headache-free periods.
5. Location: Entire head, unilateral, one spot, sinus region, behind eyes, "hatband" distribution, neck.
6. Character of pain: (a) Throbbing, pounding, boring, shocklike, dull, sharp, nagging, constant, intermittent; (b) effect of motion; (c) change in level of consciousness as pain increases.
   Severity: Same or different with each event. A graded scale of 1 to 5 or 1 to 10 may be useful in assessing this factor.
   Visual prodromal event(s): **Scotoma** (a defect of vision in a defined area) hemianopia; distortion of size, shape, or location of objects.
7. Pattern: Description of headache over course of day, worse or better as day progresses, occurrence during sleep.
8. Associated symptoms: Gastrointestinal symptoms such as nausea, vomiting, diarrhea; visual disturbances such as **photophobia** (abnormal sensitivity to light); increased tearing; difficulty falling asleep; nasal discharge; tinnitus; paresthesias; impaired mobility.
9. Precipitating factors: Fever, fatigue, stress, food or food additives, fasting, alcohol, seasonal allergies, menstrual cycle, intercourse, oral contraceptives, feelings of anxiety or depression. Inquiry should be made about client's activities during 24 hours preceding onset.
10. Efforts to treat: Medication(s), including analgesics, vasodilators, bronchodilators, oral contraceptives, and stimulants such as caffeine; sleep; meditation; other approaches.
11. Family history of headaches.
12. Diet: Include sensitivity to chemicals in food and beverages, alcohol intake.
13. Life-style: Includes use of tobacco, allergies.

A sample headache record, such as the one shown in Table 10-1, is useful in helping the client to record the pattern of headaches for a certain amount of time. The record helps to assess the type of headaches that the client is experiencing.

Head injury
1. History of traumatic event: State of consciousness, duration of unconsciousness, behaviors after event, other **sequelae.** It may be useful to have an observer's description of the event in addition to the client's account.

TABLE 10-1

Sample Headache Record

Date	Time of onset	Duration	Location	Severity 1 = mild 10 = severe	Efforts to relieve	Results	Possible precipitating factors

2. Predisposing factors: Visual changes, light-headedness, fainting, seizure disorder.
3. Associated symptoms: Blurred or double vision, change in level of consciousness, change in breathing pattern, discharge from nose or ears, gastrointestinal symptoms, head or neck pain, laceration, local tenderness.

Neck pain

1. History of neck injury or strain, head injury, swelling of neck, surgery.
2. Duration of symptoms.
3. History of bacterial or viral infection or other illnesses.
4. Character: Effect of movement on pain; limitation of motion; point of maximum pain; character of pain: burning, cramping, dull, sharp, throbbing; point of origin and radiation patterns to shoulders, arms, and back.
5. Neurological symptoms: Clumsiness, numbness, weakness, bowel or bladder dysfunction.
6. Emotional stress.
7. Efforts to treat and effectiveness of treatment: Heat, cold, medication, movement.

Thyroid function

1. History of thyroid dysfunction, radiation, or surgery.
2. Change in temperature preference: Altered sensitivity to heat or cold, wearing more or less clothing.
3. Swelling in neck; interference with swallowing; redness; pain with touch, swallowing, or hyperextension of neck.

4. Change in texture of hair, skin, or nails; increased pigmentation of skin at pressure points.
5. Change in emotional stability: Alteration in usual energy level, irritability, nervousness, lethargy, disinterest.
6. Increased prominence of eyes, puffiness in periorbital area, blurred or double vision.
7. Cardiorespiratory changes: Dyspnea on exertion, tachycardia, palpitations, cardiac irregularity.
8. Change in menstrual pattern.
9. Change in appetite, bowel habits, thirst, or frequency of urination; weight loss.
10. Family history of thyroid disorders.

RISK FACTORS

Headache: Exposure to stressful conditions and situations.

Head injury: Exposure to potentially traumatic situations in the home, at work, while traveling, or while participating in high-risk sports. If indicated, counsel client on measures to reduce the risk of household, environmental, and motor vehicle injuries.

Thyroid disease: Screening for congenital hypothyroidism is recommended for all neonates during the first week of life. Routine screening for thyroid disorders is otherwise not warranted in asymptomatic adults or children. Persons with a history of upper body irradiation may benefit from regular physical examination of the thyroid.

Adapted from *Guide to clinical preventive services: an assessment of the effectiveness of 169 interventions, Report of the U.S. Preventive Services Task Force*, Baltimore, 1989, Williams & Wilkins.

Preparation for Examination: Client and Environment

The examination room should provide the client with privacy, and the room temperature should be comfortable for the client. The room should be well lighted and quiet.

Technique for Examination and Normal Findings

Face. The techniques of inspection and palpation are used to perform a complete examination of the face.

Inspection. To begin, observe the client's facial expression and appearance. Facial expression is frequently a guide to a person's feelings because it communicates a message. However, it is important to remember that cultures vary in the degree and style of facial expression. Persons from certain cultures use pronounced facial expressions along with hand gestures and words. Those from other cultures are less expressive, particularly with strangers.

Inspect the color and condition of the facial skin and the shape and symmetry of the facial features, including the eyebrows, eyes, palpebral fissures, mouth, and nasolabial folds. The head is normally upright and still. The facial features should be symmetrical at rest and with a change of expression, although a slight degree of asymmetry is common.

Test facial muscular and neurological function by asking the client to elevate and lower the eyebrows, frown, close the eyes tightly so that the examiner cannot open them, puff the cheeks, show the teeth, and smile. This test is used to evaluate the function of the facial nerve, CN VII.

Palpation. Palpate the temporal arteries bilaterally just anterior to and slightly above the tragus of the ear (Figure 10-9). Note any thickening, hardness, or tenderness of the vessel. Use the bell of the stethoscope to auscultate the temporal artery for a **bruit,** which is a soft blowing sound of blood flowing through a stenosed (narrowed) vessel. A bruit is not normally present.

Palpate the **temporomandibular joint.** To locate this joint, place your fingertips just anterior to the tragus of the ear. Rest your fingertips over this area, and ask the client to open and close the mouth and move the joint from side to side. The temporomandibular joint should move smoothly up and down and to the right and left.

Head. The techniques of inspection and palpation are used for examination of the head.

Inspection. Observe the head for size, shape, symmetry, position, and any unusual movements. To inspect the scalp, part the hair in several areas. Hair con-

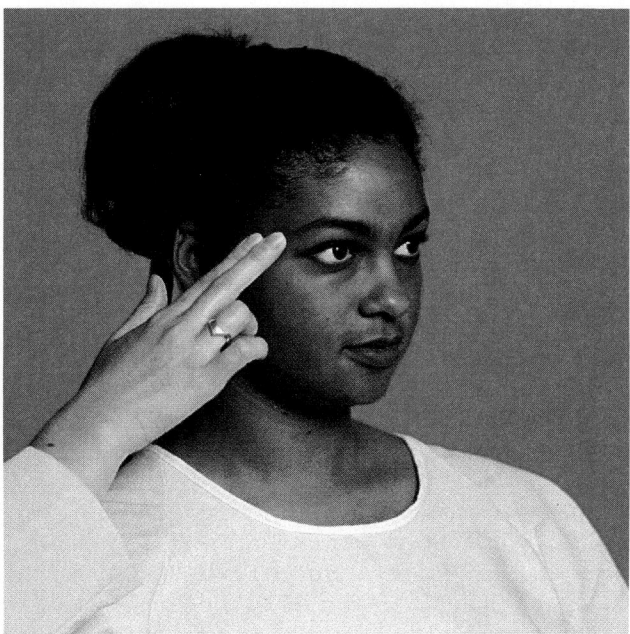

FIGURE 10-9 Palpation of the temporal artery.

dition and styling may be useful indicators of the client's social group identification, emotional status, and personal hygiene.

Palpation. If the client wears a wig or other hairpiece, ask him or her to remove it. Palpate the scalp in several areas with a gentle rotary motion. The scalp should move freely over the skull. Depressions, swelling, and tenderness are not normal findings. Inspect the distribution and texture of the hair, and note the use of coloring or lubricating agents.

Neck. *In a case involving traumatic neck injury, do not manipulate or examine the cervical spine. Stabilize the spine until further studies can be performed.*

The techniques of inspection, palpation, and auscultation are used for examination of the structures of the neck.

Inspection. Inspect the neck for symmetry and stability in normal position. Normally no masses, muscular

PREPARATION

Preparation for the Examination

Equipment

Item	Purpose
Stethoscope	Auscultation of thyroid
Glass of water	Observation and palpation of thyroid

asymmetries, scars, discolorations, or lesions are present. The neck muscles should be symmetrical, with no masses or swelling noted. To assess muscle function, ask the client to perform range of motion by flexing the chin to the chest (Figure 10-10, *A*), turning the head in lateral rotation (Figure 10-10, *B*), and *slightly* hyperextending the neck backward (Figure 10-10, *C*). These motions should be smooth and should not cause pain or dizziness. Inspect the midline cartilages, including the thyroid and cricoid cartilages and the tracheal rings, assessing for symmetry. The trachea should be centered and equidistant from each sternocleidomastoid muscle. Inspect the posterior aspect of the neck. The cervical vertebrae should be in alignment. The neck should be symmetrical, and no masses or swelling should be present.

Palpation. When you test the strength of the neck muscles, you are also assessing CN XI, the spinal accessory nerve. Test the sternocleidomastoid muscle by having the client turn the head to one side and then to the other against the resistance of your hand. Test for trapezius muscle strength by asking the client to shrug the shoulders against the resistance of your hands. If the client has pain, palpate the sternocleidomastoid for tenderness, spasm, swelling, and trigger points. (The neurological examination of these muscles and their innervation is discussed in Chapter 19.) Gently palpate the midline cartilages. They should be smooth and nontender. Palpate the occipital area, the mastoid process, and the spinous processes of the cervical vertebrae. These should be symmetrical, without tenderness, pain, or swelling.

Thyroid gland. The techniques used to examine the thyroid gland include inspection, palpation, and auscultation. The thyroid is assessed for enlargement, tenderness, nodules, and bruits. The normal thyroid gland is not visible or palpable (or only slightly so). Examining the thyroid is easy if the neck is long and slender. If the neck is short or thick, or if the client has had neck surgery, examination may be difficult. Note that determination of thyroid function includes more than assessment of the neck. Since effects of thyroid activity are widespread, observations of behavior, appearance, skin, eyes, hair, and cardiovascular status are also important.

INSPECTION. To inspect the thyroid gland, stand in front of the client and observe the lower half of the neck—first in normal position, next in slight extension, and then while the client swallows a sip of water (Figure 10-11). The movements of the cartilages are fairly easy to observe. Note any unusual bulging of thyroid tissue in the midline or of the lobes behind the sternocleidomastoid muscles; normally, none is seen.

PALPATION. Following inspection, palpate the neck for the presence of an enlarged thyroid, for consistency of the gland, and for any nodules. The lobes of the normal thyroid gland are generally not palpable. In a thin neck the isthmus is occasionally palpable. The thyroid is also sometimes palpable during pregnancy. In a short, stocky neck, even an enlarged gland may be difficult to palpate. Palpation may be done with the examiner standing either in front of or behind the client. Although several techniques can be used for palpation of the thyroid, the underlying principles for each technique include the following:

A   **B**   **C**

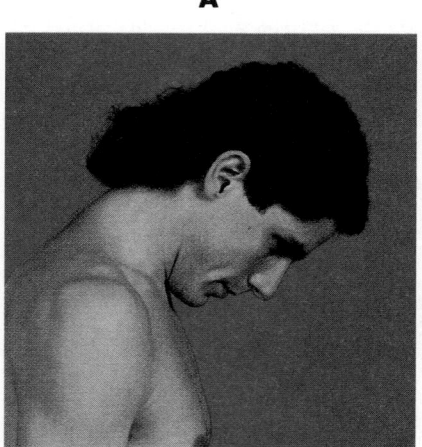   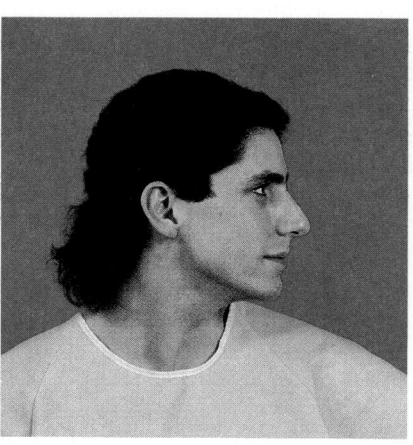   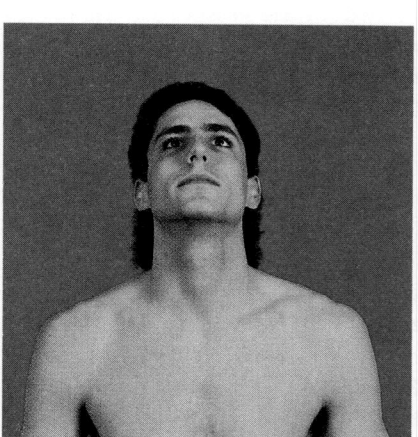

FIGURE 10-10   A, Flexion of the neck. **B,** Lateral rotation of the neck. **C,** Extension of the neck.

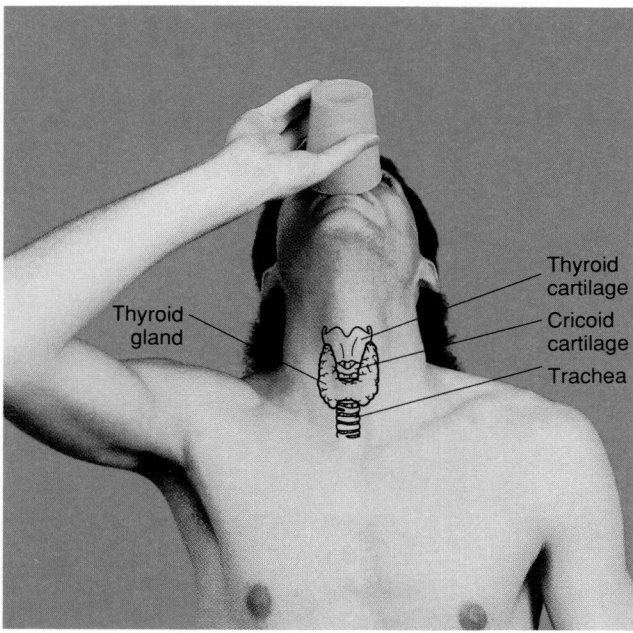

FIGURE 10-11 Inspection of the neck for enlargement of the thyroid gland.

1. Movement of the gland while the client swallows
2. Adequate exposure of the gland by tilting the head to one side to relax the muscles
3. Manual displacement of surrounding structures to better expose the gland
4. Comparison of one side of the gland with the other

Since the sternocleidomastoid muscles are strong and large, it is important to relax them. The thyroid gland is fixed to the trachea and rises during swallowing. This feature distinguishes the thyroid from other neck structures. Palpate the area where the isthmus and lobes are located to determine the gland's size, consistency, degree of enlargement, presence of nodules, and surface characteristics.

POSTERIOR APPROACH. The posterior approach is easier and less awkward for the practitioner than the anterior approach. Stand behind the client, who is seated on a chair or examining table. Ask the client to lower the chin to relax the sternocleidomastoid muscles. Curve your fingers anteriorly so that your fingertips rest on the lower half of the neck over the trachea below the cricoid cartilage (Figure 10-12). Ask the client to swallow a sip of water while you palpate for any enlargement of the thyroid isthmus. Next, in order to examine each lobe separately, ask the client to lower the chin and turn the head slightly to the right. With the fingers of your left hand, gently displace the thyroid cartilage slightly to the right while you use the fingers of your right hand to palpate the area next to the midline cartilage where the thyroid lobe lies (Figure 10-13). This procedure is then repeated with the client turning the chin to the left while you palpate with the fingers of your left hand. Having the client swallow a sip of water during this procedure may be helpful.

ANTERIOR APPROACH. Stand in front of the seated client. Using the fingertips of your index and middle fingers, palpate below the cricoid cartilage for the thyroid isthmus as the client swallows a sip of water. As in the procedure used for the posterior approach, ask the client to flex the head and turn it slightly to one side and then the other. Palpate the left lobe by displacing the thyroid cartilage slightly toward that lobe with the left hand and examining the thyroid with the right hand. This area can be more deeply palpated by hooking the thumb and fingers around the sternocleidomastoid muscle (Figure 10-14). Measure palpable masses or nodules, and describe their location, tenderness, size, shape, consistency, surface characteristics, and fixation to surrounding tissue.

AUSCULTATION. If enlargement of the gland is detected or suspected, perform auscultation over the lobes of the thyroid by using the bell of the stethoscope (Figure 10-15). Increased blood flow to the thyroid gland produces vibrations that may be heard as a soft rushing sound or bruit.

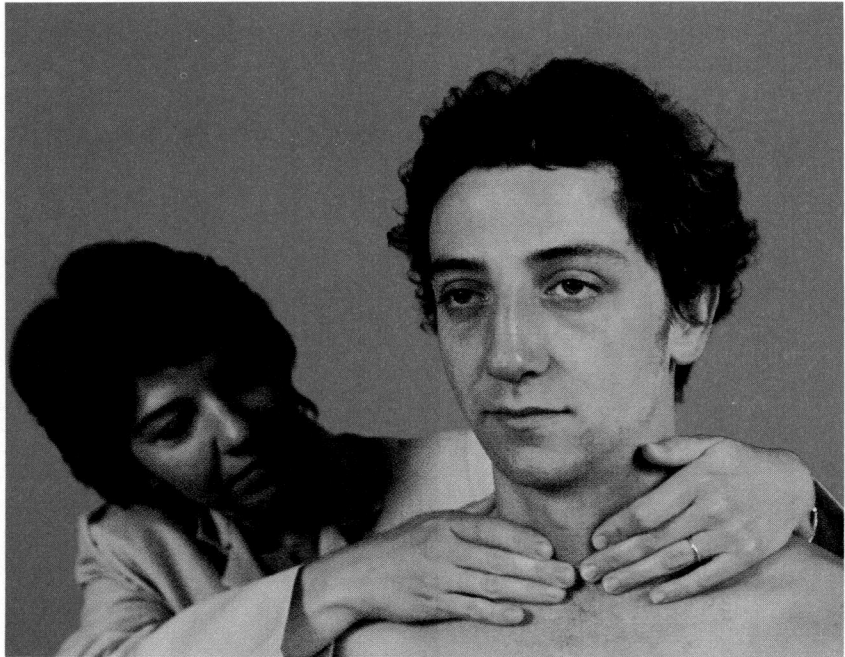

FIGURE 10-12 Palpation of the thyroid: posterior approach.

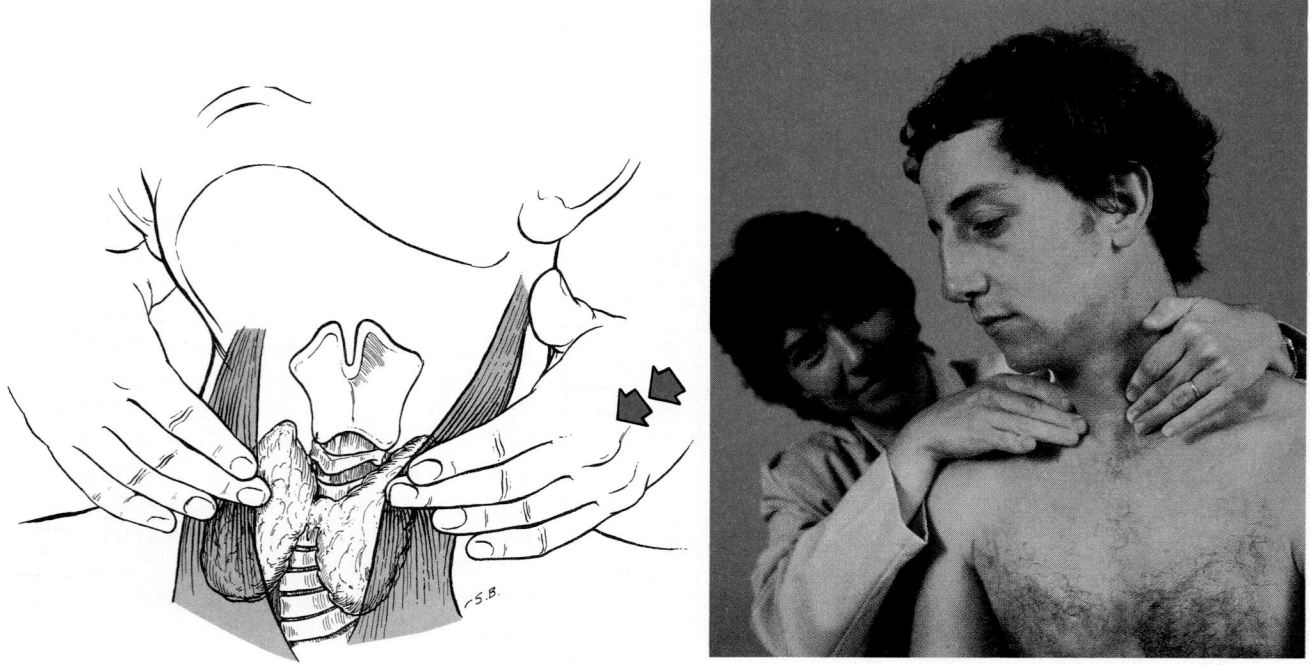

FIGURE 10-13 Posterior approach to thyroid examination. To examine the right lobe of the thyroid gland, the examiner displaces the trachea slightly to the right with the fingers of the left hand and palpates for the right thyroid lobe with the fingers of the right hand.

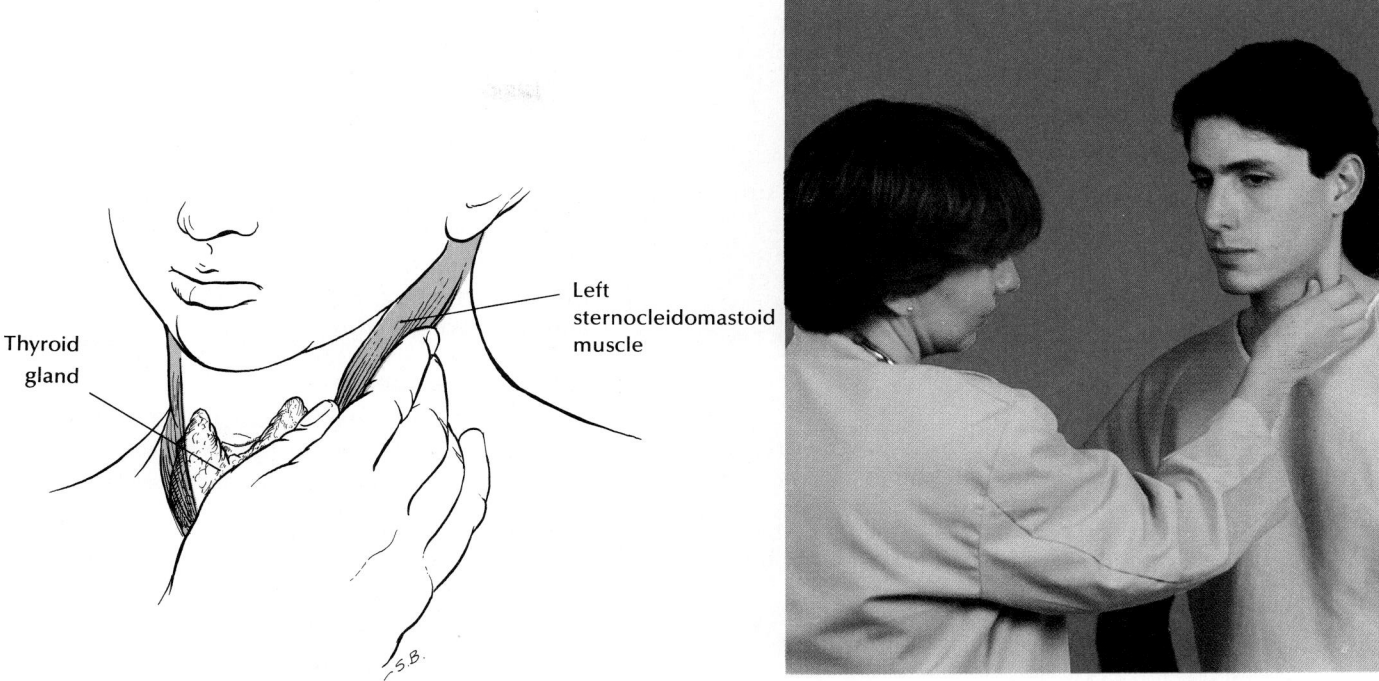

FIGURE 10-14 Anterior approach to thyroid examination. The examiner grasps around the left sternocleidomastoid muscle with the right hand to palpate for an enlarged left thyroid lobe.

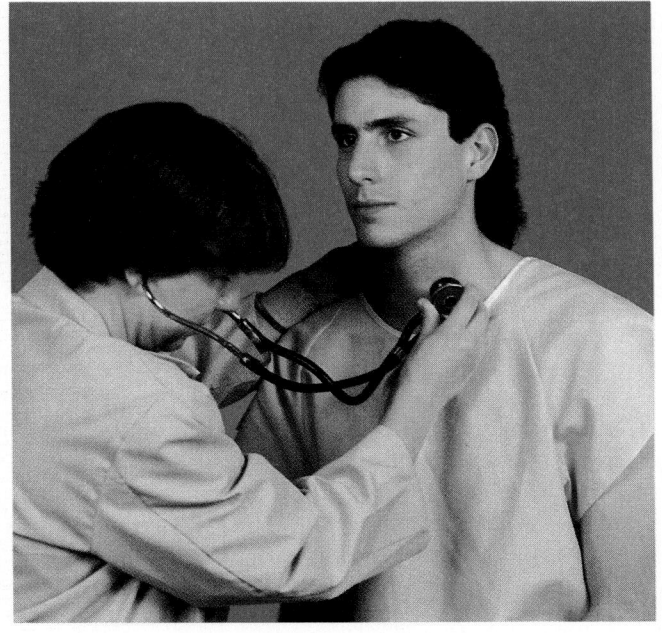

FIGURE 10-15 Auscultation over the thyroid gland.

Screening Tests and Procedures

Listed below are common laboratory tests used to help evaluate the client who has signs and symptoms of thyroid dysfunction. Since values differ among laboratories, the normal value range for the specific laboratory that provides the results needs to be determined.

Screening laboratory tests

Test	Significant abnormal findings	Possible related causes of abnormal findings
Thyroxine	Elevated	Hyperthyroidism
	Lowered	Congenital hypothyroidism
Thyroid-stimulating hormone	Elevated	Hypothyroidism
	Lowered	Hyperthyroidism

STEP-BY-STEP

EXAMINATION STEP-BY-STEP

Make sure that the examination room has good lighting, a comfortable temperature, and privacy for the client. Have the necessary equipment—a stethoscope and a glass of water—ready.

Inspection

1. Face: appearance, expression, symmetry of structure and features, skin color, movements
2. Head: size, shape, symmetry, condition of skin, hair (distribution, texture, quantity), and scalp (deformities, lesions), unusual movements
3. Neck: symmetry, mobility, range of motion, neck vessels

Palpation

1. Head: scalp (tenderness, deformities, lesions), hair (if indicated), temporal artery pulses, temporomandibular joint, lymph nodes
2. Neck: anterior midline neck structures, thyroid gland, carotid artery pulses, lymph nodes, muscle strength, cervical vertebrae

Auscultation

1. Neck: carotid arteries and thyroid gland for bruits

VARIATIONS FROM HEALTH

Face

Changes in coloration

1. Cyanosis: Occurs with poor circulation to local structures or when the amount of unsaturated hemoglobin in the body tissues is increased, as may occur with cardiac or pulmonary disease. Lips, nose, cheeks, ears, and oral mucosa may become bluish.
2. Pallor: Results from decreased vascular supply, as in shock.
3. Jaundice: Results from decreased liver function or obstruction and increased bilirubin deposits in the skin. Before the yellow color of jaundice is evident in the skin, it may be observed in the sclera and mucous membranes of the mouth.
4. Lupus erythematosus: An erythematous discoloration in a butterfly pattern bridges the cheeks and nose.
5. Other: Localized color changes from acne, moles, or scar tissue.

Changes in shape

1. Edema: Excess accumulation of fluid in the tissues may result from cardiovascular or renal disease. Often initially evident in the eyelids, where it is called periorbital edema, this condition can involve the entire face.

2. Protrusion of eyeballs (exophthalmos) and elevation of upper lids: Result of hyperthyroidism, gives face a staring or startled expression.
3. Puffiness with dry skin and coarse features: Result of hypothyroidism, called myxedema facies.
4. Face rounded, cheeks red: Result of increased adrenal hormone production (Cushing's syndrome) or secondary to intake of synthetic adrenal hormones, called moon facies.
5. Face sunken, skin rough and dry: Prolonged illness, dehydration, or starvation may produce this cachectic face. Eyes, cheeks, and temples appear sunken, and nose appears sharp.

Changes in symmetry

1. Asymmetry, abnormal movements, or both may result from facial nerve lesions or from central nervous system lesion such as a cardiovascular accident.
2. Paralysis of CN VII, or Bell's palsy, causes changes on affected side; eyelid does not close completely, lower eyelid and corner of mouth droop, and nasolabial fold disappears.

Changes in hair distribution

1. For women in some ethnic groups, increased facial hair, often above the upper lip, is a normal finding.
2. Excessive hair growth in moustache, sideburn, and chin areas results from elevated production of adrenal hormones.
3. Thinning of scalp hair and eyebrows is a result of increased thyroid activity.

Pain

1. Trigeminal neuralgia (tic douloureux). This neurological abnormality is caused by degeneration of or pressure on one or all of the three divisions of the trigeminal nerve, CN V (see Figure 10-2 for distribution pattern of this nerve):
   - Ophthalmic (first division): pain around eyes and over forehead
   - Maxillary (second division): pain in nose, cheek, and upper lip
   - Mandibular (third division): pain in lower lip and side of tongue

   The pain is aching, burning, flashing, or stablike, and attacks cause the person to wince with facial contractions. Pain attacks may occur spontaneously or may be evoked by pressure on a trigger zone, cold air, a light touch, biting, swallowing, chewing, laughing, talking, yawning, or sneezing. The pain may last from a few seconds to a few minutes. Cycles of pain and abatement may continue for hours. Trigeminal neuralgia affects persons in middle to late adulthood.

2. **Herpes zoster** may affect any sensory nerve, but the virus typically tends to invade the posterior root ganglia associated with the thoracic and trigeminal nerves. The pain may be constant or intermittent, superficial or deep.
3. Sinus tenderness results from inflammation of one or more of the paranasal sinuses. The client may experience pressure and pain in the area of the sinuses, headache, fever, and local tenderness to palpation.
4. Temporomandibular joint pain dysfunction syndrome is an abnormal condition marked by painful jaw movement and mandibular dysfunction. The joint may snap, lock, or "pop." The pain may be referred to other points on the face and neck.

Head

Changes in size

1. Abnormally large head in children: Caused by accumulation of fluid in the ventricles of the brain (hydrocephalus).
2. Large head in adults: Results from osteitis deformans (Paget's disease) or acromegaly, which causes an increase in thickness of the skull, lengthening of mandible, prominence of nose and forehead, coarsening of the facial features.

Changes in shape

1. Sebaceous cysts on scalp: Result from occlusion of sebaceous gland ducts; palpable as smooth rounded nodules attached to the scalp.
2. Trauma or surgical removal of a portion of the skull alters shape.

Changes in hair

1. Coarse, dry, brittle: Results from hypothyroidism.
2. Fine, silky, soft: Results from hyperthyroidism.
3. Thinning or hair loss (alopecia): May be hereditary (especially in men), a side effect of chemotherapy, or a result of prolonged illness or emotional stress.
4. Hair and scalp should be checked for dandruff and parasites.

Pain. Headaches are one of the most common symptoms experienced, resulting more often from tension or emotional distress than from organic disease. They may also be the presenting symptom of an injury or severe illness, such as cerebral hemorrhage, brain tumor, or meningitis. Whatever their cause, headaches are often intense and debilitating. In addition, individuals may suffer from more than one type of headache at a time.

Headaches can be classified in numerous ways. One approach is to divide them into three main groups: (1) muscle contraction or tension headaches, (2) **migraine** headaches; and (3) cluster headaches (Table 10-2).

Another group includes traction and inflammatory headaches, which are caused by disease or injury, such as sinus inflammation, cranial hemorrhage, or brain tumor, to some structure of the head or neck (e.g., brain, meninges, arteries, veins, eyes, ears, teeth, nose, paranasal sinuses, jaw, neck joints). The nature of the headache depends on the underlying disorder.

Sinus headaches are the most common type in this category of headaches. They are caused by inflammation of one or more of the paranasal sinuses. These headaches may be a complication of a respiratory infection, dental infection, allergy, or change in atmosphere (air travel, swimming) or may result from a structural defect. Swelling of the nasal mucous membranes obstructs the openings from the sinuses to the nose, resulting in an accumulation of secretions. This situation may cause tenderness, pressure, and headache.

Neck

If traumatic neck injury has occurred, the neck should not be moved.

Neck muscles. Common variations from health of the neck muscles include stiffness and pain caused by tension, cervical arthritis, or meningitis.

Temporomandibular joint disease. Pain in the area of the temporomandibular joint results from dislocation of the condyle, osteoarthritis, rheumatoid arthritis, or a myofacial pain syndrome. Pain is often localized to the neck and ear in the area adjacent to the joint. The client has limited motion of the jaw, muscle tenderness, and, occasionally, joint crepitus.

Polymyalgia rheumatica. This syndrome is characterized by an aching pain, tenderness, and stiffness in the neck and shoulders, which may extend to the upper arms, forearms, hips, and legs. Aching is increased with motion.

Thyroid gland: hyperthyroidism and hypothyroidism. Thyroid dysfunction, either hyperthyroidism or hypothyroidism, cannot be determined by the size of the gland alone. If thyroid dysfunction is suspected, thyroid function studies are necessary.

The thyroid gland may have diffuse or local enlargement. Symmetrical enlargement may occur with dietary iodine deficiency. Localized or nodular enlargement consists of one or more nodules and may be noted in the lobes or the isthmus. Solitary nodules suggest carcinoma, particularly in younger people. The clinical findings of hyperthyroidism in the elderly, such as anorexia, weight loss, weakness, and tremor, are subtle and viewed as a result of other changes associated with aging.

The effects of excessive or inadequate amounts of thyroid hormones on body structures and systems are presented in Table 10-3.

TABLE 10-2

Classification of Headaches

	Muscle contraction or tension headaches	Migraine headaches	Cluster headaches
Age at onset	Adolescence through adulthood	Childhood, adolescence, or young adulthood	Young to middle adulthood
Sex distribution	Males and females approximately equally	More frequent in females	More frequent in males
Typical onset	Gradual, often following stress	Begins as dull ache, progresses to intense pain, occurs anytime during day	Sudden, reaches peak intensity in several minutes, often occurs during evening or night, may awaken client
Location	"Hatband" distribution, may radiate to occipital area and around eyes	Generally unilateral, may be frontal around eye or cheek, may alternate from side to side with subsequent attacks, or may be bilateral	Unilateral, involving facial area from neck to temple, may be around eye
Character of pain	Dull, bandlike, constricting, persistent, with occasional episodes of severe pain	Intense, pulsating, throbbing	Sharp, intense, deep, burning, boring, stabbing, excruciating
Duration	Hours to days or months	Several hours to several days	Several minutes to several hours
Frequency	Varies	Varying intervals from several times per month to several times per year, may have a pattern, as with menstrual cycle	May be daily for several weeks in repetitive clusters several times per year
Associated symptoms	Neck stiffness, shoulder ache, nausea	Photophobia, nausea, vomiting	Tearing of eye and stuffiness of nostril on affected side, facial flushing; modified Horner's syndrome with mild **ptosis** (drooping of upper eyelid) and **miosis** (constriction of pupil) on affected side
Precipitating factors	Fatigue, stress, or no obvious precipitant	Fatigue, prolonged hunger, menstruation, birth control pills, stress, bright sunlight, foods or drugs containing vasoactive chemicals	Alcohol, vasodilators
Other factors	Most common type of head pain; may result from depression or anxiety or from organic problems such as cervical arthritis	Familial	
Prodromal events		Complex of neurological events that may precede the migraine include: paresthesias, aura, visual changes such as flashing lights, scotomata (blind spots), **hemianopsia** (loss of vision on one side), distorted perception of size and shape of objects	

TABLE 10-3

Effects of Hyperthyroidism and Hypothyroidism on Body Systems and Structures

Body system or structure	Hyperthyroidism	Hypothyroidism
General		
Weight	Loss	Gain
Temperature intolerance	Heat	Cold
Sleep	Insomnia	Sleepiness
Skin	Warm, moist; increased sweating; smooth texture; diffuse pigmentation; erythema; brittle nails	Cool, pale, dry, coarse, rough, scaly, itchy, doughy consistency
Hair	Fine texture, loss, inability to hold a permanent	Poor growth, loss, dryness
Cardiovascular/pulmonary	Increased cardiac output, increased blood pressure, wide pulse pressure, tachycardia, atrial arrhythmias, systolic murmur, palpitations, angina, dyspnea, edema, increase in rate or depth of respirations, bruit over thyroid	Congestive heart failure, angina, slow pulse, pericardial or pulmonary effusion
Gastrointestinal	Indigestion, anorexia, polyphagia, diarrhea, increased appetite	Decreased appetite, constipation
Renal	Polydipsia, polyuria, urgency	Decreased output
Nervous	Restlessness, irritability, anxiety, memory loss, easy distractability, decreased ability to concentrate, emotional liability, panic attacks, hyperreflexia, tremor	Decreased relaxation phase of deep tendon reflexes, depression
Muscular	Weakness, tremulousness	Stiffness, aching
Eyes	Lid lag and lid retraction (startled look), tearing, conjunctival irritation	Periorbital puffiness
Voice		Deep, hoarse
Hearing		Acuity may diminish
Reproductive		
Women	Hypomenorrhea, amenorrhea	Menorrhagia
Men	Loss of libido, decreased potency	Decreased libido, decreased potency

DOCUMENTATION

SAMPLE DOCUMENTATION

Past health history

Twenty-five-year-old female graduate student gives history of headaches occurring with increasing frequency.

Headaches begin late morning to early afternoon every 1 to 2 weeks for the past 5 months. Client describes them as "a tight band around my head with throbbing on the sides." Pain and stiffness develop at the base of the head and in the neck and shoulders. Pain is gradual in onset and is typically dull and nagging. Occasionally it becomes so severe that she must stop working for 1 to 2 hours. Associated symptoms include occasional slight nausea. No other GI symptoms and no photophobia, changes in vision, or paresthesias. Client uses aspirin or acetaminophen q 3 to 4 hours with some relief. She is not allergic to any food or drugs, does not smoke, drinks a glass of wine about twice a month. States she is very concerned about the increasing frequency of the headaches. She is a full-time graduate student and works about 30 hours per week.

Physical findings

Client appears tired and has an anxious expression; facial features are symmetrical. Scalp is clear of lesions and hair is normally distributed. Temporal artery pulse palpable, rhythm regular, no thickening or tenderness.

Eyes: Vision 20/20 in each eye using Snellen, visual fields intact, PERRLA, extraocular movements (EOMs) intact.

Neck: Thyroid not palpable, trapezius muscles stiff and tender, trapezius and sternocleidomastoid strength good bilaterally.

Neurological: Cranial nerves II-XII intact.

CRITICAL THINKING

Nursing Diagnosis *THE NEXT STEP—cont'd*

Nursing diagnoses that could apply to assessment and alterations of the face, head, and neck include, but are not limited to, the following:

PAIN The state in which an individual experiences and reports the presence of severe discomfort or an uncomfortable sensation.

Defining Characteristics

- Facial mask of pain in which the eyes lack luster, the pupils may be dilated
- Expression may have a "beaten look" or be a grimace
- Alteration in muscle tone
- Moaning/crying

Related Factors

- Injuring agents (biological, chemical, physical, psychological)

CHRONIC PAIN The state in which an individual experiences pain that continues for more than 6 months.

Defining Characteristics

- Verbal report or observed evidence of pain experienced for more than 6 months
- Fear of reinjury
- Physical and social withdrawal
- Altered ability to continue previous activities
- Anorexia
- Weight changes
- Changes in sleep patterns
- Facial masks
- Guarded movement

Related Factors

- Chronic physical/psychosocial disability

BODY IMAGE DISTURBANCE Disruption in the way one preceives one's body image.

Defining Characteristics

- Verbalized actual or perceived change in structure and/or function of body or body part
- Verbalized change in life-style because of negative feelings or perception of body
- Verbalized fear of rejections by others
- Repeated verbalizations focusing on past strengths, function, or appearance
- Verbalized negative feelings about body (dirty, big, small, unsightly)
- Verbalized feelings of helplessness, hopelessness, powerlessness in relation to the body
- Preoccupation with change in body or loss of part
- Personalization of part or loss by name
- Guilt, shame
- Refusal to verify actual change in body or body part
- Hiding or overexposing body part
- Not touching/looking at body part
- Change in social involvement or social relationships
- Emphasis on remaining strengths or heightened achievement

Related Factors

- Nonintegration of change in body characteristics, function, or limits; and perceived developmental imperfections

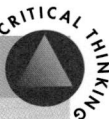

Nursing Diagnosis   *THE NEXT STEP—cont'd*

Clinical Application

Ms. T. is a 30-year-old female who has come into the clinic with new onset of left-sided facial drooping. She voices her biggest concern. "Did I have a stroke?" Her speech is slightly slurred. Further assessment reveals upward movement of the eyeball on the left side when she closes her eye; disappearance of nasolabial fold; lower left eyelid droops slightly; a slight lag time of left eye closure when compared to the right eye; and left side of mouth droops. She complains of pain when the left side of her face is palpated. She is worried about whether this will be permanent and how it looks. The diagnosis is Bell's palsy.

SUBJECTIVE DATA: Client complains of:
• Anxiety concerning "a stroke"
• Permanency of this facial drooping
• What her face looks like
• Pain upon palpation

OBJECTIVE DATA:
• Left eyelid does not close completely
• Left eyelid droops
• Left eyelid closes slightly behind right
• Left side of mouth droops
• Disappearance of nasolabial fold
• Slightly slurred speech

NURSING DIAGNOSES

Body image disturbance related to biophysical change.

Defining Characteristics
   • Verbal response to actual changes in facial structure negative feelings about her body
   • Pain related to cranial nerve VII damage

Pain related to cranial nerve VII damage

Defining Characteristics
   • Subjective communication of pain
   • Self-focusing
   • Narrow focus—withdrawal from social contact
   • Facial mask of pain

GLOSSARY

alopecia Partial or complete lack of hair resulting from normal aging, endocrine disorder, drug reaction, anticancer medication, or skin disease.

anterior triangle Landmark on the neck formed by the edge of the mandible (superiorly), the sternocleidomastoid muscle (laterally), and the midline of the trachea (medially). Used to describe the location of physical findings.

bruit Blowing sound heard over peripheral vessels on auscultation.

facial nerve (CN VII) Cranial nerve that innervates the scalp, forehead, eyelids, muscles of facial expression, cheeks, and jaw.

hemianopsia Defective vision or blindness in one half of the visual field.

herpes zoster Acute infection caused by the varicella-zoster virus, affecting mainly adults and characterized by the development of painful vesicular skin eruptions that follow the underlying route of cranial or spinal nerves inflamed by the virus.

mastoid process Bony prominence of the posterior portion of the temporal bone, located posterior to the lower part of the auricle, serving as the attachment for various muscles, including the sternocleidomastoid.

migraine Recurring vascular headache characterized by a prodromal aura, unilateral onset, severe pain, photophobia, and autonomic disturbances during the acute phase, which may last for hours or days.

miosis Constriction of the pupil.

nasolabial fold Crease in the skin extending from the angle of the nose to the corner of the mouth.

palpebral fissure Opening between the margins of the upper and lower eyelids.

photophobia Abnormal sensitivity to light.

posterior triangle Landmark on the neck formed by the sternocleidomastoid muscle (laterally), the trapezius muscle (posteriorly), and the clavical (inferiorly) used to describe the location of physical findings.

ptosis Drooping of the upper eyelid.

scotoma Defect of vision in a defined area in one or both eyes.

sequela Any abnormal condition that follows and results from a disease, treatment, or injury.

spinal accessory nerve (CN XI) Function of this nerve is essential for speech, swallowing, and certain movements of the head and shoulders.

sternocleidomastoid muscles Symmetrical muscles of the neck extending from the upper sternum and proximal portion of the clavicle to the mastoid process of the temporal bone behind the ear.

temporal artery Artery on the head that runs anterior to the ear over the temporal bone and onto the forehead.

temporomandibular joint One of two joints connecting the mandible of the jaw to the temporal bone of the skull.

thyroid gland Endocrine gland at the front of the neck, consisting of bilateral lobes connected in the middle by a narrow isthmus. Secretes thyroxine, which is essential for growth and metabolic stability.

trapezius muscles Symmetrical, large, flat triangular muscles of the shoulder and upper back. They extend from the occipital bone, the ligamentum nuchae, and the spinous processes of the seventh cervical and all the thoracic vertebrae. These muscles act to rotate the scapula, raise the shoulder, and abduct and flex the arm.

trigeminal nerve (CN V) Cranial nerve that mediates sensation of the face. It has three branches: ophthalmic, maxillary, and mandibular.

BIBLIOGRAPHY

Cummings C and others: Age: a clue in neck mass diagnosis, *Patient Care* 24:1, 38-47, 1990.

DeGroot LJ and others: *The thyroid and its diseases*, New York, 1984, John Wiley.

Derman H: Migraine headache: precision in diagnosis and improved therapeutic prospects, *Consultant* 31:5, 57-63, 1991.

Diamond S: Headaches common, but not ordinary [interview], *Emerg Med* 16:13, 32-44, 1984.

Diamond S, Dalessio DJ, editors: *The practicing physician's approach to headache*, ed 4, Baltimore, 1986, Williams & Wilkins.

Giger JN, Davidhizar RE: *Transcultural nursing*, St Louis, 1991, Mosby–Year Book.

Gilbert R, Warfield C: Evaluating and treating the patient with neck pain, *Hosp Pract* 22:8, 223-232, 1987.

Gordon M: *Manual of nursing diagnosis 1993-1994*, St Louis, 1993, Mosby–Year Book.

Haase GR and others: When facial pain is the problem, *Patient Care* 24:12, 119-124, 1990.

Lamb C, editor: Causes of neck masses in young adults, *Patient Care* 18:7, 30-37, 1984.

Peatfield R: *Headache*, Berlin, 1986, Springer-Verlag.

Purath J: Assessing headache pain, *RN* 54:10, 26-31, 1991.

Schleper J: Prevention, detection and diagnosis of head and neck cancers, *Semin Oncol Nurs* 5:3, 139-149, 1989.

Smith LS: Evaluation and management of the muscle contraction headache, *Nurse Pract* 13:1, 20-27, 1988.

Solomon DH: Clinical examination of the thyroid. In Van Middlesworth L, editor: *The thyroid gland: a practical clinical treatise*, Chicago, 1986, Mosby–Year Book.

Thompson JM and others, editors: *Mosby's manual of clinical nursing*, St Louis, 1993, Mosby–Year Book.

US Preventive Services Task Force: *Guide to clinical preventive services: an assessment of the effectiveness of 169 interventions*, Baltimore, 1989, Williams & Wilkins.

Whitney CM: New headache classification: implications for neuroscience nurses, *Neurosci Nurs* 22:6, 385-388, 1990.

PURPOSE OF THE EXAMINATION

Vision is one of our most important mechanisms for experiencing the world. The eyes are complex and delicate structures. They receive visual stimuli and transmit it to the visual cortex in the brain. The optic nerve (cranial nerve [CN] II) directly connects the eye and the brain. Six of the twelve cranial nerves are involved with the eyes. The eyes are balanced and held in place by six sets of extraocular muscles.

A thorough examination of the eyes can reveal a wealth of information about both local and systemic health and about variations from the healthy state.

In conjunction with observation of facial expression and body posture, observation of the eyes frequently provides information about the client's emotional status.

The examination of the eyes includes measurement of visual acuity, evaluation of visual fields, testing of ocular movements, inspection of ocular structures, testing of nerve reflexes, and the ophthalmoscopic examination.

ANATOMY AND PHYSIOLOGY

The eyes are located within the bony orbital cavity. The anterior aspect of the eye is exposed, and the remainder is protected within the skull. The structures of the eye described in this chapter include the following:

Eyelids and eyelashes
Conjunctiva
Sclera
Cornea
Anterior chamber
Lacrimal apparatus
Iris
Pupils
Lens
Vitreous body
Retina
Ocular muscles
Optic nerve

Portions of the retina that are described here include the following:

Optic disc
Retinal vessels
Macula
Retinal background

The structures of the eyelid and the globe of the eye are illustrated in Figures 11-1 through 11-3.

Ocular Structures

Eyelids and eyelashes. The eyelashes are distributed along the margin of each eyelid and curve outward. The eyelids **(palpebrae)** serve a protective function, covering the anterior aspect of the eye and distributing tears across the surface of the eye to keep it moist and lu-

bricated. The eyelids also limit the amount of light that enters the eyes and protect the eyes from foreign objects. When the eyes are open, the upper eyelid normally covers a small portion of the iris and the cornea overlying it, located about midway between the **limbus** and the pupil. The margin of the lower eyelid lies at or just below the limbus. The limbus is the junction line of the cornea and the sclera. The distance between the upper and the lower eyelid margin is called the **palpebral fissure.** The tarsal plates are thin strips of connective tissue that lie within the eyelid and give it form and consistency.

Conjunctiva. The **conjunctiva** lines the eyelids and covers the anterior portion of the eyeball. This continuous transparent lining is divided into two portions: palpebral and bulbar. The palpebral portion lines the eyelids; it appears shiny pink or red because it overlies the fleshy vascular structures of the lids. The bulbar portion lies over the sclera. The palpebral conjunctiva recesses into the folds of the eyelids and is continuous with the bulbar conjunctiva, which rests loosely over the sclera to the limbus, where it merges with the corneal epithelium. This portion of the conjunctiva is normally clear; the white color comes from the sclera below. The bulbar portion does, however, contain many small blood vessels. These vessels are normally visible and may become dilated, producing varying degrees of redness. A small fleshy elevation, the **caruncle,** is located in the nasal corner of the conjunctiva. Yellowish triangular deposits, called **pinguecula,** may occur in the bulbar conjunctiva near the limbus. These essentially normal senile changes are caused by a hyaline degeneration of fibrous tissue. The **meibomian**

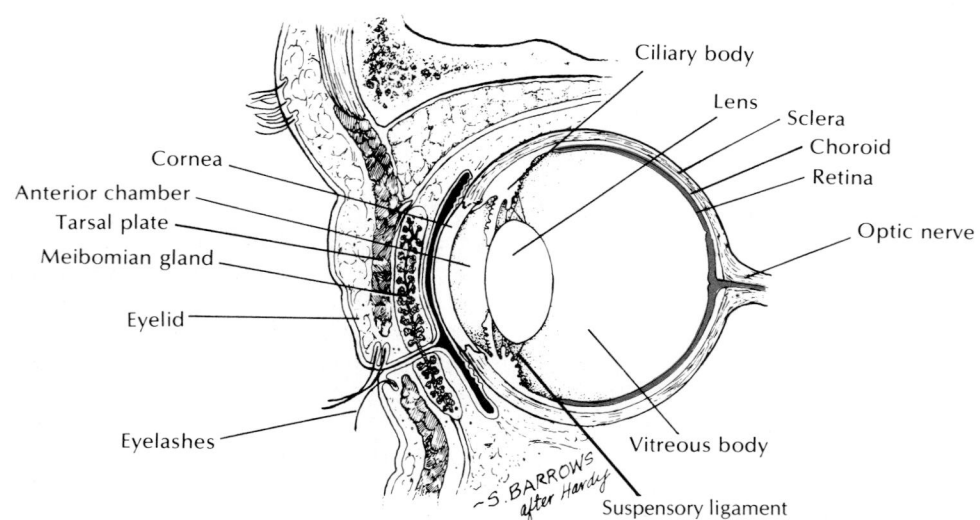

FIGURE 11-1 Structures of the eyelid and globe of the eye.

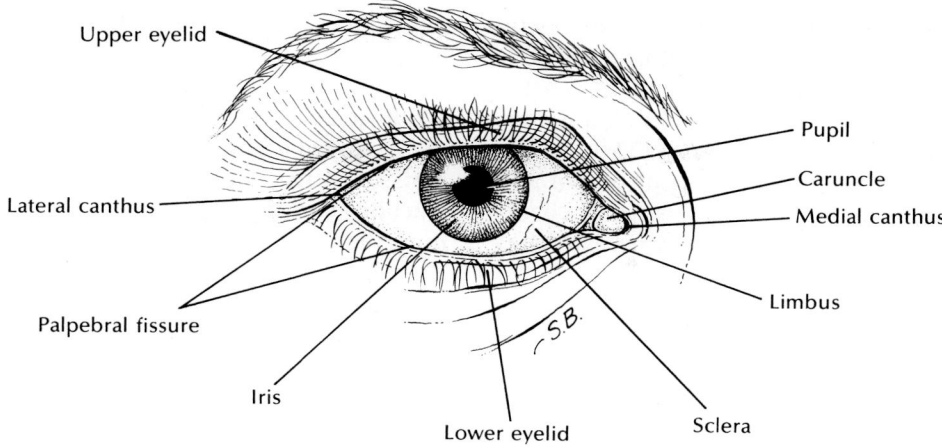

FIGURE 11-2 Anterior view of the eye.

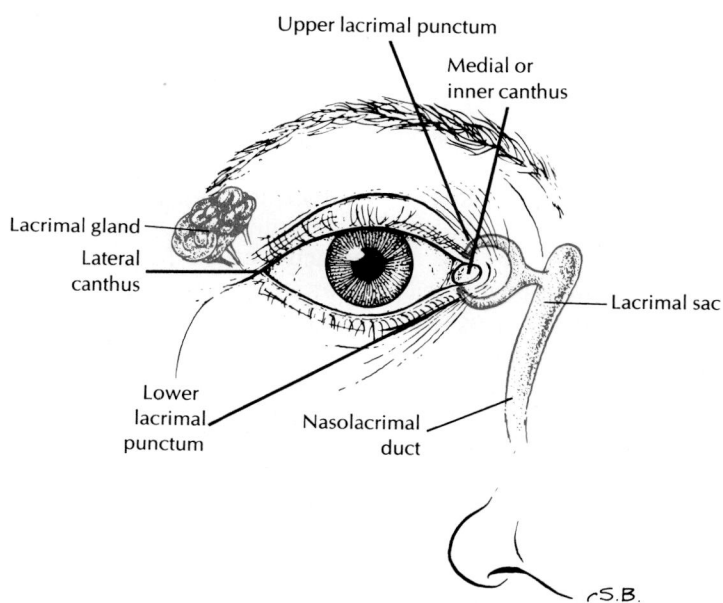

FIGURE 11-3 Lacrimal system.

glands, which secrete an oily lubricating substance, appear as vertical yellow striations on the palpebral conjunctiva.

Sclera. The globe of the eye is surrounded by three coats: **sclera, choroid,** and **retina.** The sclera is the outer fibrous layer. It is visible anteriorly as the white portion of the eye. Several small, distinct conjunctival vessels lie over the sclera, particularly around the periphery. In some dark-skinned persons, small dark-pigmented dots are located on the sclera near the limbus.

Cornea. The **cornea** is a smooth, moist tissue that covers the area over the pupil and the iris. It is continuous with the sclera. Like the bulbar conjunctiva, the cornea is transparent and permits the passage of light inward toward the retina. The cornea merges with the conjunctiva at the limbus. It separates fluid from the anterior chamber from the external environment. The cornea is sensitive to touch. This sensation is transmitted by the ophthalmic branch of the trigeminal nerve (CN V).

Anterior chamber. The anterior chamber lies posterior to the cornea. It is bounded anteriorly by the cornea, laterally by the sclera and the **ciliary body,** and posteriorly by the iris and that portion of the lens that is within the pupillary opening. The anterior chamber is filled with **aqueous humor,** a fluid that is continuously produced by the ciliary body. The relation between the rate of production of aqueous humor and the resistance to aqueous outflow at the anterior chamber angle determines the intraocular pressure, which is normally 15 mm Hg ± 3 mm Hg.

Lacrimal apparatus. The components of the lacrimal apparatus are the following:

Lacrimal gland
Lacrimal puncta
Lacrimal sac
Nasolacrimal duct

The lacrimal gland is located above and slightly lateral to the eye. It produces tears, which moisten and lubricate the conjunctiva and the cornea. The tears wash across the eye and drain through the upper and lower lacrimal **puncta,** which are small openings located at the nasal side of both the upper and lower eyelid margins. The tears then pass into the nasolacrimal sac, which is located medial to the eye. From the nasolacrimal sac, the tears pass into the nasolacrimal duct and the nasal meatus. Tearing is also referred to as **lacrimation.**

Iris. The iris is the circular disc containing pigmented fibrils that give the eye its distinctive color. It is located in front of the lens and behind the anterior chamber. The iris, the ciliary body, and the suspensory ligament form the interior portion of the choroid layer of the eye. Posterior to the layer of fibrils are two groups of muscles, dilator and sphincter muscles. These muscles function in a manner similar to the diaphragm of a camera within the image-forming portion of the eye.

Pupil. The **pupil** is the opening in the iris through which light passes. The size of the pupil is determined by the amount of light entering the eye and the closeness of the object being visualized. It is regulated by the constriction and dilation of the muscles of the iris. This muscular activity is controlled by the autonomic nervous system. Stimulation of the parasympathetic fibers leads to constriction of the pupils; stimulation of the sympathetic fibers produces dilation of the pupils. The amount of light that is present influences the size of the pupil. Increasing the amount of light causes pupillary constriction. Diminishing the light causes dilation. These changes represent **adaptation.** The pupils also constrict in response to **accommodation,** which is the change in focus from a distant to a near object.

The constricting response of the pupils to a bright direct light is a pupillary reflex. This reflex consists of two aspects: the direct reaction and the **consensual reaction,** or the consensual lift reflex. The direct reaction refers to the constriction of the pupil receiving the increased illumination. The constriction of the pupil that is not receiving increased light is the consensual reaction. The optic nerve (CN II) transmits the stimulus from the eye to the brain. The oculomotor nerve (CN III) transmits the reflex from the brain to both eyes. The presence of both direct and consensual responses indicates the functioning of these two cranial nerves.

Lens. The **lens** is located directly behind the iris at the pupillary opening. It is the center of the refracting system of the eye. The lens is composed of epithelial cells within an elastic membrane, the lens capsule. The lens is transparent and has no blood vessels, nerves, or connective tissue. The thickness of the lens is controlled by the muscles of the ciliary body. Changes in lens thickness enable the eye to focus on near and distant objects. The coordinated function of the muscles of the iris and the muscles of the ciliary body acting on the lens controls the amount of light permitted to reach the retina and the focusing of objects on the retina.

Vitreous humor. The **vitreous humor** is a transparent fluid that occupies the area posterior to the lens, which is called the posterior chamber. The vitreous humor is surrounded by the retinal layer of the globe of the eye.

Retina and retinal structures. The retina is the inner coat of the globe of the eye. It contains the neurosensory elements that transform light impulses into the electrical impulses that are carried to the visual cortex by way of the optic nerve and the optic tract. Several important structures are located on the retina, including (1) the optic disc, which is the head of the optic nerve; (2) four sets of retinal vessels, which emerge from the optic disc and travel medially and laterally around the retina; and the **macula,** where central vision is concentrated (Figure 11-4).

Optic disc and physiologic cup. The optic disc is located on the nasal half of the retina. This round structure is approximately 1.5 mm in diameter. It is creamy yellow to pink and is lighter than the surrounding retina. The color of both the disc and the retinal background vary from one individual to another; it is somewhat lighter in fair-complected, light-haired people and slightly darker in dark-complected, dark-haired people.

The **physiologic cup (physiologic depression)** is a small depression within the disc just temporal to the center of the disc. It is yellowish-white and slightly lighter in color than the rest of the disc. The physiologic

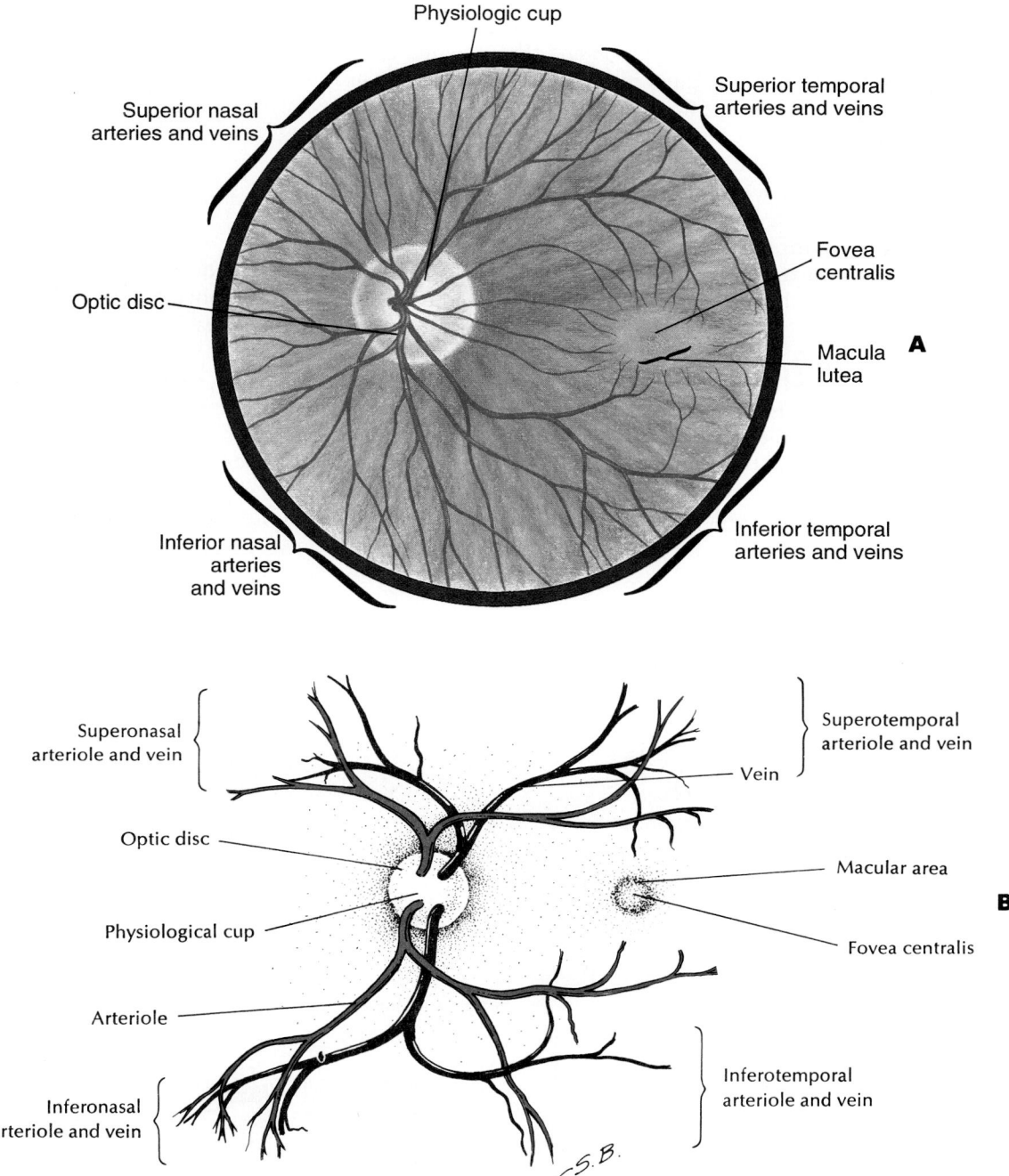

Physiologic cup

Superior nasal
arteries and veins

Superior temporal
arteries and veins

Optic disc

Fovea
centralis

Macula
lutea

A

Inferior nasal
arteries
and veins

Inferior temporal
arteries and veins

Superonasal
arteriole and vein

Superotemporal
arteriole and vein

Vein

Optic disc

Macular area

B

Physiological cup

Fovea centralis

Arteriole

Inferotemporal
arteriole and vein

Inferonasal
arteriole and vein

S.B.

FIGURE 11-4 A, Retinal structures of the left eye. **B,** Optic disc, physiologic cup, and
retinal vessels of the left eye. (**A** modified from Seidel HM and others: *Mosby's guide to
physical examination,* ed 2, St Louis, 1991, Mosby–Year Book.)

cup does not extend to the disc margins; it occupies
one fourth to one third of the area of the disc.

Retinal vessels. Four sets of retinal vessels emerge
from the optic disc and extend outward, becoming
smaller at the periphery. Each set of vessels, which includes an arteriole and a vein, is named according to
the quadrant of the disc in which it is located: superior

nasal, inferior nasal, superior temporal, and inferior
temporal. The arterioles are brighter red than the veins
because they carry oxygenated blood. The veins are
darker red because they carry deoxygenated blood.
Since the arterioles are approximately 25% smaller than
the veins, there is an arteriole-vein ratio (A:V ratio) of
about 2:3 or 4:5.

Macula and retinal background. The rods and the cones are neurosensory elements located in the retina. The rods mediate black-and-white vision, and the cones mediate color vision. At a point temporal to the optic disc at the posterior pole of the eye, the retina has a slight depression called the **fovea centralis.** The cones are most heavily concentrated in this area, making it the point of central vision and most acute color and daylight vision. The retinal area immediately around the fovea centralis is called the macula. The retinal background is reddish-orange.

Extraocular muscles and cranial nerves. Six muscles of each eye, working in a coordinated, or yoked, fashion with those of the other eye, control eye movement. The movements of the two eyes normally occur in conjugate, parallel fashion except during **convergence.** The eyes converge, or come toward each other, when the person focuses on a very close object. The six extraocular muscles (Figure 11-5) are the following:

Superior rectus
Inferior rectus
Lateral rectus
Medial rectus
Superior oblique
Inferior oblique

The parallel movement of the eyes makes it possible to have single-image binocular vision. The yoked muscles are the muscles in each eye that work together to move the eyes in parallel motion to any position of gaze (see Figure 11-5, *A*). For example, the left lateral rectus and the right medial rectus are yoked muscles that work concurrently to move the gaze to the left.

The six eye muscles are innervated by three cranial nerves. The oculomotor nerve (CN III) supplies four muscles: the superior, inferior, and medial rectus mus-

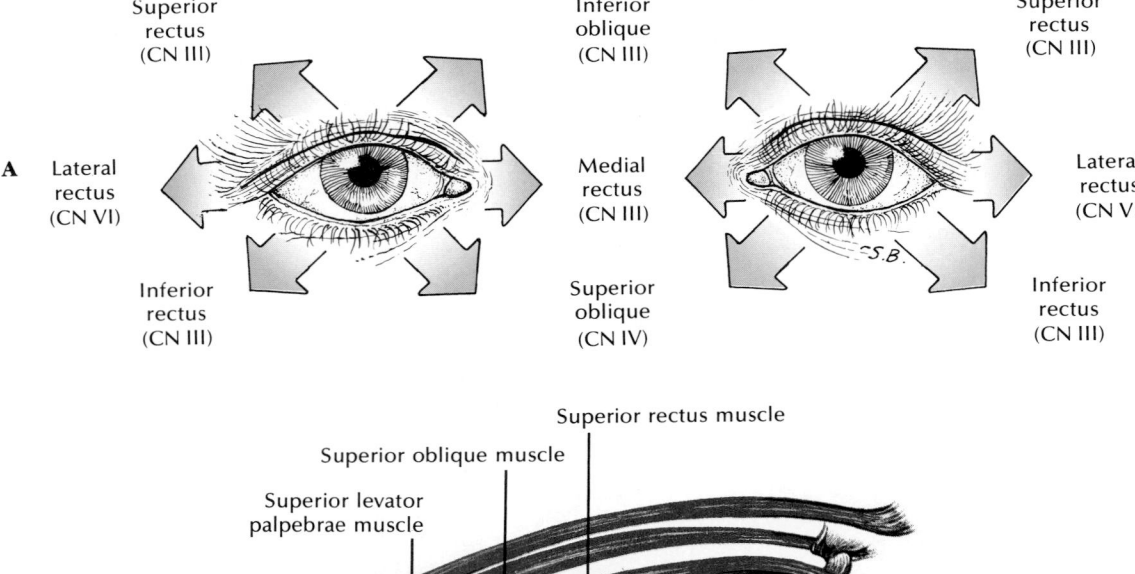

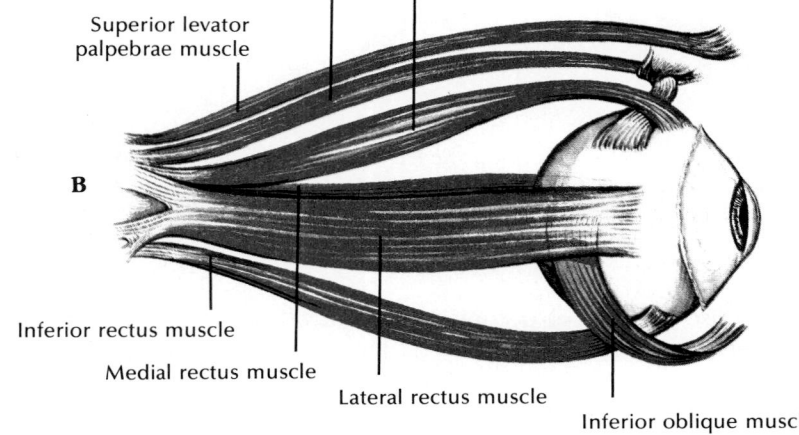

FIGURE 11-5 A, Movement of the eyes related to the six sets of extraocular muscles. **B,** Extraocular muscles of the right eye. (**B** from Thibodeau GA: *Anthony's textbook of anatomy and physiology,* ed 13, St Louis, 1990, Mosby–Year Book.)

cles and the inferior oblique muscle. The trochlear nerve (CN IV) innervates the superior oblique muscle. The abducens nerve (CN VI) supplies the lateral rectus muscle.

> **Helpful Hint:** *A mnemonic device useful for remembering the innervation of the six eye muscles is LR_6SO_4. The lateral rectus is innervated by CN VI, and the superior oblique is innervated by CN IV. The four remaining eye muscles are innervated by CN III.*

Six of the 12 cranial nerves and portions of the cerebral hemispheres are involved in the total neurological innervation of the eye and related structures. Table 11-1 summarizes the relationship of the six cranial nerves to the eye structures and their functions.

Physiology of Vision

For someone to perceive a clear visual image, light reflected from an object must pass through several transparent structures: cornea, anterior chamber, lens, and vitreous fluid. Then the light must focus on the retina, where the neural receptors, the rods and cones, are activated and carry the impulse along the optic nerve and tract to the visual cortex of the brain.

Formation of retinal image. Four processes lead to the formation of a clear image on the retina:

1. Refraction, or bending, of the light rays
2. Accommodation, or change in curvature, of the lens
3. Constriction of the pupil
4. Convergence of the eyes

Refraction is the bending or deflecting of light rays that occurs when the rays pass obliquely from one transparent medium into another of a different density. In the eye these media are the cornea, the aqueous humor, the lens, and the vitreous humor. All these structures work in conjunction to bring an object into focus on the retina (Figure 11-6).

Accommodation for near vision enables the eye to focus on near objects by increasing the curvature of the lens, constriction of the pupils, and convergence of the eyes. Light rays from close objects are divergent and must be bent to focus on the retina. The curvature of the lens increases to accomplish this result. Contraction of the ciliary muscle causes the elastic lens to bulge.

The pupils constrict as a result of contraction of the circular fibers of the iris. This constriction prevents divergent light rays from coming into the eye through the peripheral portions of the cornea and the lens. The pupil constricts both for near vision and in the presence of bright light.

Convergence is the movement of the eyes inward to bring together the visual axes on the object being viewed. Single binocular vision requires that light rays from an object fall on corresponding points of the two retinas so that a person sees one object instead of two. The extraocular muscles hold the visual axes of the two eyes parallel.

Visual pathways and visual fields. The images formed on the retina are reversed right to left and are

TABLE 11-1

Relationship of Cranial Nerves to Eye Structures and Functions

Cranial nerve		Function
II	Optic	Mediates vision
III	Oculomotor	Innervates medial, superior, and inferior rectus muscles, inferior oblique muscle, muscles elevating the eyelid (levator palpebrae), and muscles of the iris and ciliary body
IV	Trochlear	Innervates superior oblique muscle
V	Trigeminal (ophthalmic division)	Innervates sensory portion of corneal reflex
VI	Abducens	Innervates lateral rectus muscle
VII	Facial	Innervates lacrimal glands and muscles involved in lid closure (orbicularis oculi)

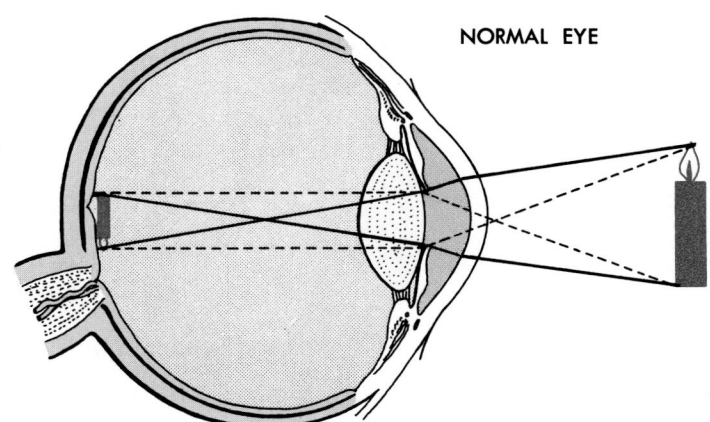

NORMAL EYE

FIGURE 11-6 Formation of a retinal image. In the normal eye, light rays from an object are refracted by the cornea, aqueous humor, lens, and vitreous humor; those rays converge on the fovea of the retina, where an inverted image is clearly formed. (From Thibodeau GA: *Anthony's textbook of anatomy and physiology*, ed 13, St Louis, 1990, Mosby–Year Book.)

upside down. Thus an object in the upper nasal **field of vision** is formed on the lower temporal quadrant of the retina. The field of vision is the area that can be visualized when the eye is not moving. Light stimulates neuron impulses that are conducted through the retina, the optic nerve, and the optic tract to the visual cortex of the occipital lobes.

The arrangement of the nerve fibers in the retina is continued in the optic nerve: temporal (lateral) fibers follow the lateral side of the nerve, and nasal (medial) fibers run along the medial portion of the nerve. At the optic chiasm, however, the nasal or medial fibers cross over and join the temporal fibers of the opposite optic tract. Thus the left optic tract contains fibers from only the left half of each retina or only the right half of each field of vision. The right optic tract contains fibers from only the right half of each retina or only the left half of each field of vision. This sequence of pathways and events produces vision. The relationship of visual pathways and fields of vision is illustrated in Figure 11-7.

EXAMINATION

Health History
Present health status
a. Adequacy of vision in each eye, use of corrective lenses, date of last eye examination, and results of that examination
b. Difficulty with vision
   1. Near or distant
   2. Central, peripheral, or specific area
   3. Constant or intermittent
   4. Day or night
   5. Presence of floaters, halos around lights
   6. Double vision
   7. Abnormal movements
c. Pain
   1. In or around eye
   2. Superficial or deep
   3. Onset: abrupt or gradual
   4. Associated symptoms: itching, burning, photophobia, injection, erythema, other sensations
d. Abnormal secretions
   1. Color
   2. Consistency
   3. Onset and duration
   4. Excessive or decreased tearing
e. Use of eye medications: type and purpose, frequency and duration of use
f. Trauma or foreign body

Past health history
a. Trauma, injury to eye(s)
   1. History of incident
   2. Structures damaged
   3. Efforts to correct damage and degree of success
b. Eye surgery
   1. Condition(s) requiring surgery
   2. Date surgery performed
   3. Outcome
c. Variations from health that may affect the eyes
   1. Hypertension
   2. Diabetes
   3. Thyroid disorder
   4. Glaucoma
   5. Cataract
   6. Eye infection

Family health history
a. Nearsightedness (myopia), farsightedness (hyperopia), strabismus

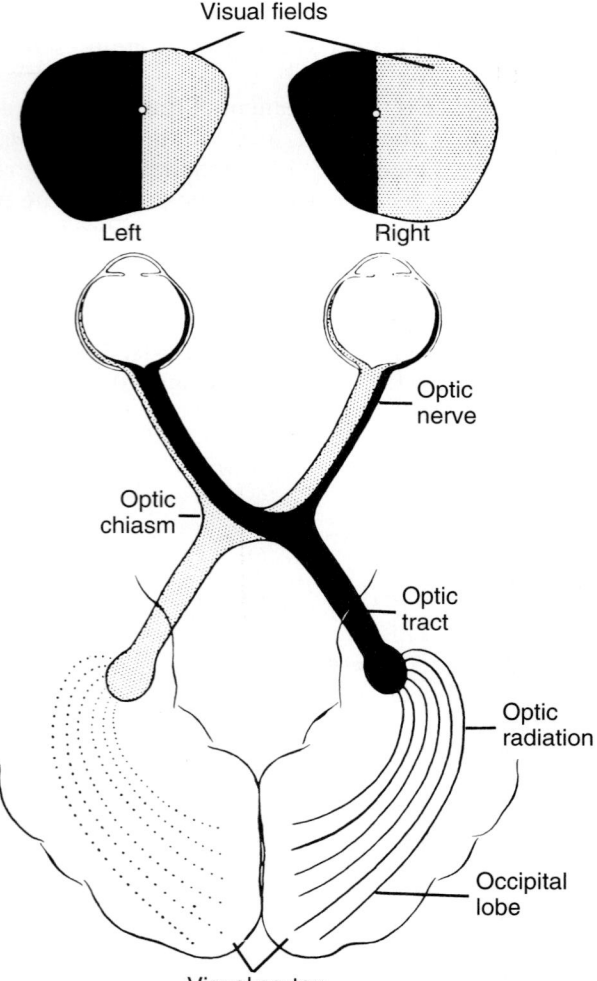

FIGURE 11-7 Representation of the visual field in the optic pathways. (From Havener WH: *Synopsis of ophthalmology,* ed 6, St Louis, 1984, Mosby–Year Book.)

b. Retinoblastoma (cancer of the retina)
c. Color blindness, cataracts, glaucoma, retinitis pigmentosa, macular degeneration, diabetes, hypertension, thyroid disorder
d. Conditions similar to that of client

General considerations

a. Exposure to irritating chemicals, gases
b. Activities: participation in sports that could endanger the eyes
c. Use of protective devices when participating in activities that could endanger the eyes

RISK FACTORS FOR GLAUCOMA

Glaucoma is the second leading cause of new cases of blindness in the United States. Open-angle glaucoma is the most common form. When symptoms are not present, it may progress until irreversible visual field loss occurs.

Risk factors for glaucoma include diabetes mellitus, myopia, and a family history of glaucoma. African Americans are at increased risk for glaucoma, which is the leading cause of blindness in this group. The elderly, those over age 75, are also at increased risk for glaucoma.

Clients who are at risk for glaucoma should be referred to an eye specialist for further assessment.

Preparation for Examination: Client and Environment

The examination should be conducted in a room where the lighting can be controlled. A well-lighted room is needed for the visual acuity tests, and it must be possible to darken the room to assess the pupillary reflexes and to perform the ophthalmoscopic examination. A room or hallway where the client can be 20 feet away from the Snellen chart is required for testing visual acuity.

The eye examination involves multiple components, which should be learned in a thorough and efficient arrangement. The order in which the examination is performed should focus on completeness and the comfortable positioning of the client. The client will remain seated during most of the examination. The assessment begins with visual acuity, ocular function, and visual fields. Then the external eye structures are examined. The ophthalmoscopic examination is done last.

Examination Technique and Normal Findings

In the eye examination, the range of normal findings is broad and variations are numerous. Much time, patience, and practice are needed to learn assessment of the many structures and functions of the eyes. Inspection is the main technique used to examine the eye. Palpation should be done only if a symptom or sign requires further investigation, such as palpating the lacrimal sac if blockage or infection is suspected. A description of the procedures that involve palpation is integrated into the discussion of inspection that follows.

Inspection. The components of the examination that involve inspection include the following:
Visual acuity
Visual fields
Extraocular muscle function
External ocular structures
Ophthalmoscopic examination

Preparation for the Examination

PREPARATION

Equipment

Item	Purpose

Visual acuity charts
   Snellen (for distant vision)
   Rosenbaum (for near vision)
	To assess visual acuity

Opaque card or eye cover	To assess visual acuity, visual fields, and muscle function
Penlight	To assess pupillary light reflex and external structures of eye
Cotton-tipped applicator	To evert upper eyelid
Ophthalmoscope	To assess transparent ocular media and perform retinal examination

Client and environment

The examination room must have lighting that can be controlled and comfortable seating for the client. An area for testing visual acuity is needed that allows the client to be 20 feet from the Snellen chart.

OPHTHALMOSCOPE

The ophthalmoscope (Figures 11-8 and 11-9) is an instrument designed to permit evaluation of certain internal structures of the eye. These structures include the lens, the vitreous humor, and the retinal structures. The ophthalmoscope contains a bright light and lenses of varying magnification can be used to bring the various structures of the eye into focus.

Bring the structures into focus by rotating the lens selector dial until the image becomes clear. You can hold and focus the instrument with one hand (see Figure 11-8). Look through the viewing aperture near the top of the ophthalmoscope to focus on the eye structures. Below the viewing aperture is another aperture that shows the number of the lens. The lens numbers go from 0 to +40 when you rotate the lens-selection dial clockwise. (These numbers appear in black.) The numbers go to −25 when you rotate the lens-selection dial counterclockwise. (These numbers appear in red.) The plus and minus lenses can compensate for nearsightedness or farsightedness in both the examiner and the client. The lens-selection dial is located on the side of the ophthalmoscope head. Of the several different apertures, the large full circle of light is used most frequently because it works best for illuminating most of the structures of the eye. (Other apertures that are used less frequently are described in Table 11-2.)

TABLE 11-2

Apertures of the Ophthalmoscope

Aperture	Description
Full aperture	Used most frequently because it provides a wide field of light for the retinal examination
Small aperture	Especially useful for examining the retina through a small pupil
Red-free filter	A green beam of light is used to examine the optic disc for pallor and the retina for small hemorrhages
Grid 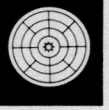	Used to estimate the size of retinal lesions
Slit 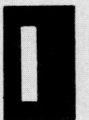	Used to examine the anterior portion of the eye and to determine the elevation of retinal lesions

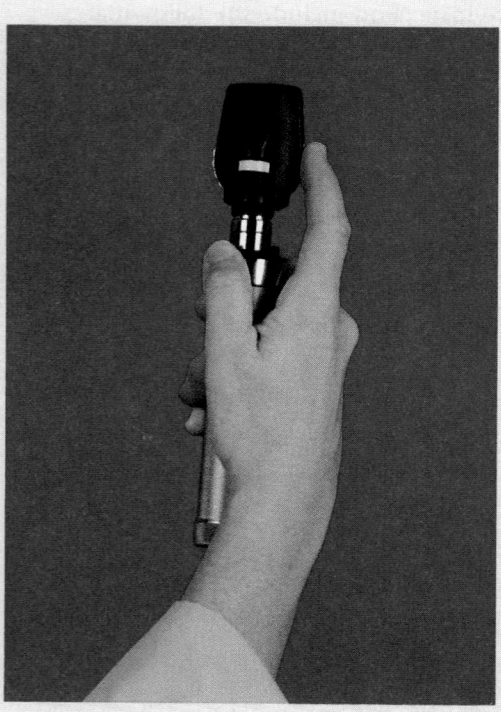

FIGURE 11-8 Holding the ophthalmoscope.

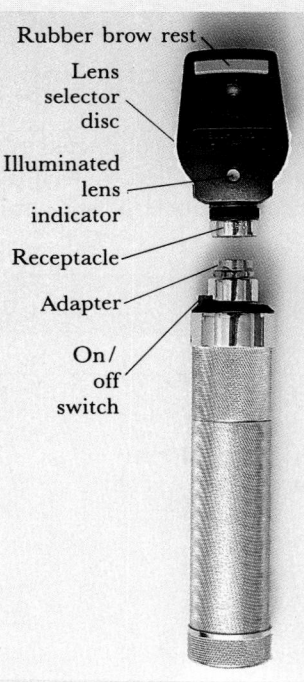

FIGURE 11-9 Ophthalmoscope. (From Seidel HM and others: *Mosby's guide to physical examination*, ed 2, St Louis, 1991, Mosby—Year Book.)

Visual acuity. The assessment of visual acuity is a simple and rewarding test of ocular function. Findings in the normal range of visual acuity give an indication of the clarity of the transparent structures (cornea, anterior body, lens, and vitreous humor), the adequacy of macular (central) vision, and the functioning of the nerve fibers from the macula to the occipital cortex.

The Snellen alphabet chart (Figure 11-10, *A*), which has various sizes of letters, is traditionally used to test visual acuity. For clients who are illiterate or those who are unfamiliar with the English alphabet, the E chart is useful. The letter E is shown in different directions, and the client can state or point to which side is open (Figure 11-10, *B*).

The Snellen chart has standardized numbers at the end of each line of letters. These numbers indicate the

A
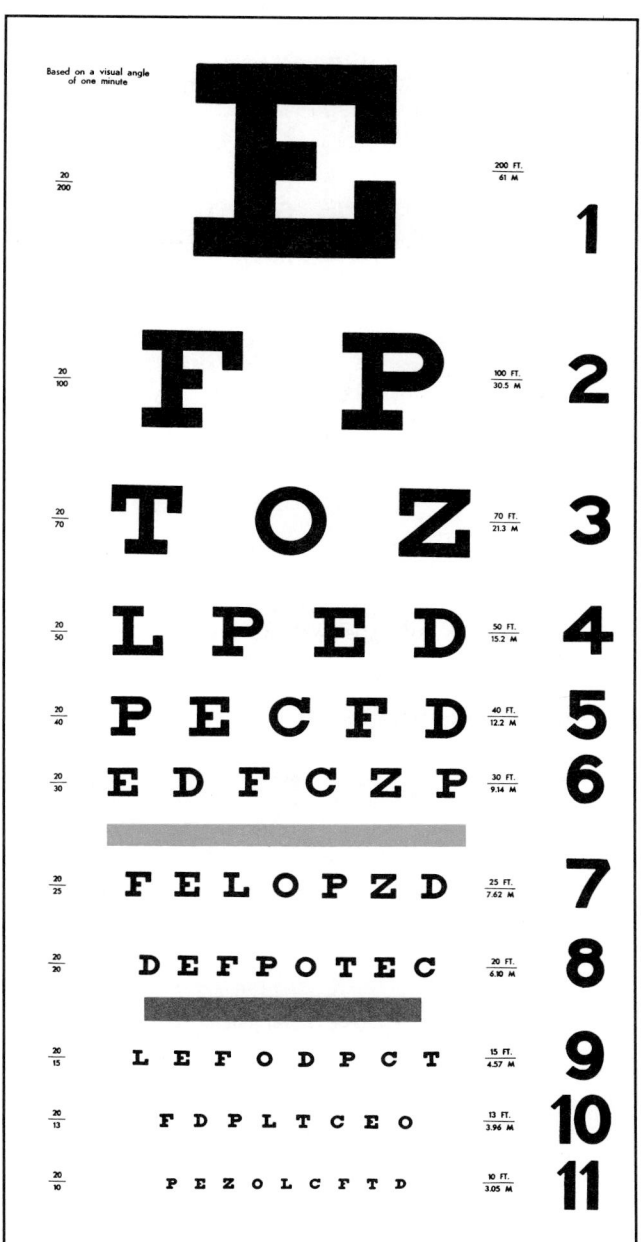

B
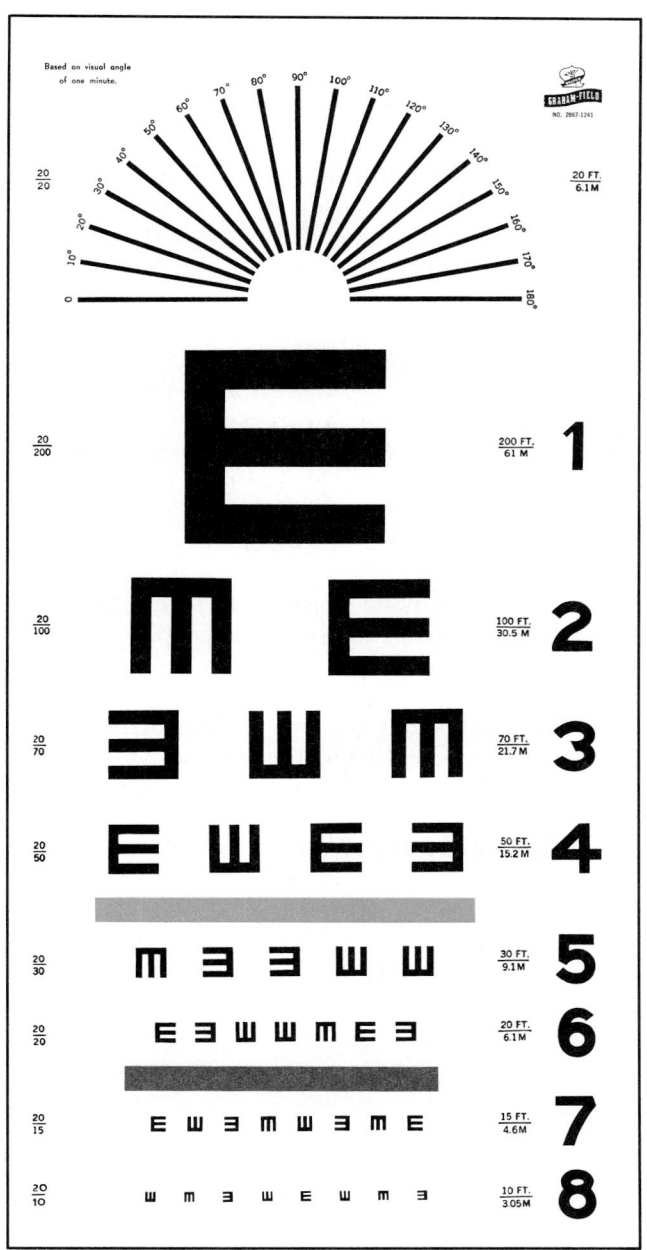

FIGURE 11-10 A, Snellen chart for testing distance vision. **B,** E chart for testing distance vision. (From Seidel HM and others: *Mosby's guide to physical examination,* ed 2, St Louis, 1991, Mosby–Year Book.)

degree of visual acuity demonstrated when the client reads the chart from a distance of 20 feet. The number above the line or to the left of it is 20, the distance in feet between the chart and the client. This amount is the standard testing distance. The number below the line or to the right of it is the distance from which the normal eye can read the letters on a particular line. The higher the number below the line or to the right, the poorer the visual acuity. For example, 20/20 vision is better than 20/40 vision.

Measurement of 20/20 vision in a client indicates normal visual acuity and a functional optic pathway. Measurement of less than 20/20 vision indicates either a refractive error or some other optic disorder.

Be sure that the room is well lighted for the visual acuity test. Have the client stand or sit 20 feet from the Snellen chart. The chart should be located approximately at eye level. To assess visual acuity, initially test only one eye at a time. Cover the other eye with an opaque card or an eye cover. Do not let the client use his or her fingers to cover the eye. Alternatively, both eyes may be tested together since binocular vision is the client's functional vision. Test a client who wears corrective lenses both with and without them. This approach allows for an assessment of the adequacy of correction. Since reading glasses blur distant vision, the client should not wear them for this test.

If a client cannot see the largest letter on the chart (20/200), check to see if he or she can perceive the movement of your hand at about 12 inches from the eyes or can perceive the light of a penlight directed into the eyes.

Perform a gross assessment of near vision for the client who has difficulty reading. Ask the client to read the letters on a Rosenbaum chart (Figure 11-11) or a newspaper with various sizes of print. Have the client hold the reading material at a distance of approximately 12 to 14 inches (Figure 11-12).

Visual fields confrontation test. The assessment of visual acuity indicates the functioning of the macular area, the area of central vision. It does not test the sensitivity of the other areas of the retina, which perceive the peripheral stimuli. The visual fields confrontation test (Figure 11-13) provides a gross assessment of peripheral vision. In this test you use your own visual fields to make comparisons with the client's visual fields. For this test to be useful, your own visual fields must be normal.

You and the client sit or stand opposite each other about 1½ to 2 feet apart with your eyes at the same horizontal level (see Figure 11-13). The client covers one eye with an opaque card or eye cover, and you cover your own eye that is opposite the client's covered

ROSENBAUM POCKET VISION SCREENER

		distance equivalent
95		20/800
874		20/400

			Point	Jaeger	
2 8 4 3			26	16	20/200
6 3 8 E Ш Ǝ X O O			14	10	20/100
8 7 4 5 Ǝ m Ш O X O			10	7	20/70
6 3 9 2 5 m E Ǝ X O X			8	5	20/50
4 2 8 3 6 5 Ш E m O X O			6	3	20/40
3 7 4 2 5 8 Ǝ Ш Ǝ X X O			5	2	20/30
9 3 7 8 2 6 Ш m E X O O			4	1	20/25
4 2 8 7 3 9 E Ш m O O X			3	1+	20/20

Card is held in good light 14 inches from eye. Record vision for each eye separately with and without glasses. Presbyopic patients should read thru bifocal segment. Check myopes with glasses only.

DESIGN COURTESY J. G. ROSENBAUM, M.D.

PUPIL GAUGE (mm.)

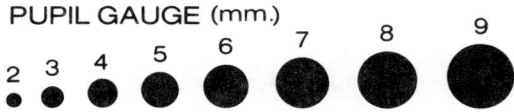

2 3 4 5 6 7 8 9

FIGURE 11-11 Rosenbaum chart for testing near vision. (From Seidel HM and others: *Mosby's guide to physical examination*, ed 2, St Louis, 1991, Mosby—Year Book.)

eye. For example, if the client's right eye is covered, then your left eye is covered. This method leaves the same field of vision open for assessment. You and the client stare directly into each other's open eye. Tell the client not to look at the object approaching from the periphery. Hold a small object, such as a penlight or a pen, and gradually move it in from the periphery toward the center from eight directions: right and left, above and below, and at the midpoints between each of these directions. At first, the object should be outside the field of vision. Hold the object equidistant between yourself

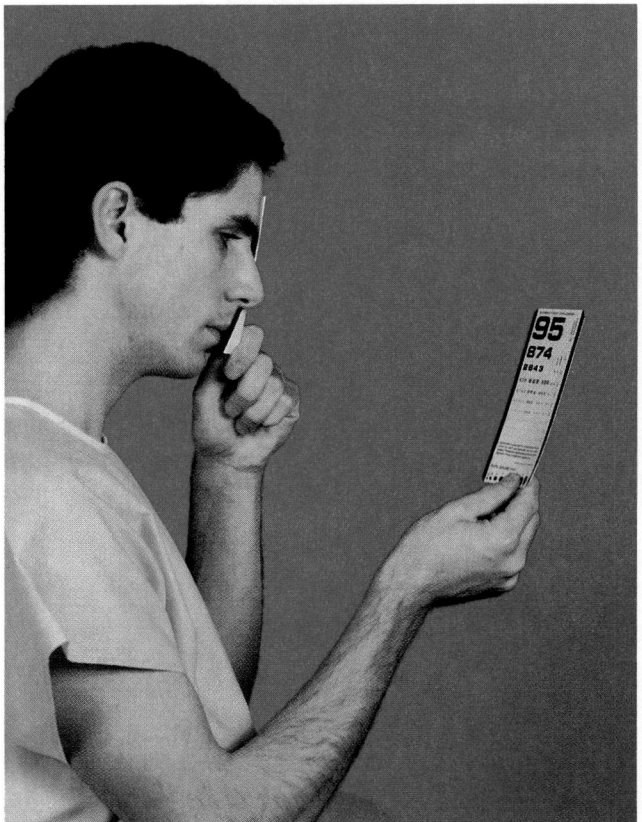

FIGURE 11-12 Assessing a client's near vision with the Rosenbaum chart.

and the client. Bring it in gradually toward the center. You and the client should be able to see the object enter the field of vision at the same time.

Helpful Hint: *You may find it difficult to move the test object out far enough in the temporal field so that neither you nor the client can see it. If this happens, hold the object slightly closer to the client than to yourself initially, and move it toward a line equidistant between you as you bring the object toward the center.*

This test provides only a crude estimate of visual fields. Although it may demonstrate large field defects, it does not usually detect small changes. Therefore clinical use of this test is limited. If you suspect decreased peripheral vision or loss of vision in certain areas, refer the client to an eye specialist for further testing.

Extraocular muscle function. The assessment of extraocular muscle function has these three components:

Six cardinal positions of gaze
Corneal light reflex
Cover-uncover test

Basic to each of these components is the observation of the parallelism of the eyes and ocular movements.

SIX CARDINAL POSITIONS OF GAZE. To assess the six cardinal positions of gaze (Figure 11-14, *A*), stand in front of the client and ask him or her to watch your finger or a small object as you move it through the six cardinal positions of gaze. Ask the client to hold the head still and to move only the eyes. Move your finger or the object clockwise to each of the six positions shown in Figure 11-14, *B*. Ask the client to hold the gaze briefly at each position. Observe for parallel movements and for slight oscillating movements of the eyes, called **nystagmus.** A small amount of end-position lateral nystagmus is normal. However, in any other position, nystagmus is abnormal. The eyes should move together in parallel fashion to each position.

After you have examined the extraocular muscles in the six cardinal positions, ask the client to look straight up and then down without moving the head. Observe the relationship of the upper eyelid to the iris as the client's gaze moves. The upper eyelid should overlap the iris slightly throughout this movement. No sclera should show between the iris and the upper eyelid (see Figure 11-2).

CORNEAL LIGHT REFLEX. You can assess the parallelism of the anterior and posterior axes of the two eyes by observing the reflection of light from the cornea. Ask the client to stare straight ahead while you shine a penlight toward the bridge of the nose from a distance of 12 to 15 inches. The bright dot of light reflected from the shiny surface of the corneas should be located symmetrically, for example, at the 12 o'clock position in both eyes. If the reflected dot of light is not symmetrical, perform the cover-uncover test.

COVER-UNCOVER TEST. Maintenance of parallelism of the eyes is a result of the fusion reflex that makes binocular vision possible. Normally, both eyes are aligned and centrally fixed and there is no movement of the eyes when they are covered or uncovered. If a muscle imbalance is present and the fusion reflex is blocked when one eye is covered, this weakness can be observed.

Ask the client to look at a specific fixed point, such as the corner of a picture or doorframe. Then cover one of the client's eyes with an opaque card or eye cover; while doing so, observe the uncovered eye to see if it moves to fix on the object (Figure 11-15, *A*). Then remove the cover and observe for any movement of the eye that was just uncovered (Figure 11-15, *B*). When an eye is covered, the appearance of an object on that retina is suppressed. The eye relaxes; if there is a weakness in one of the extraocular muscles, the eye drifts to

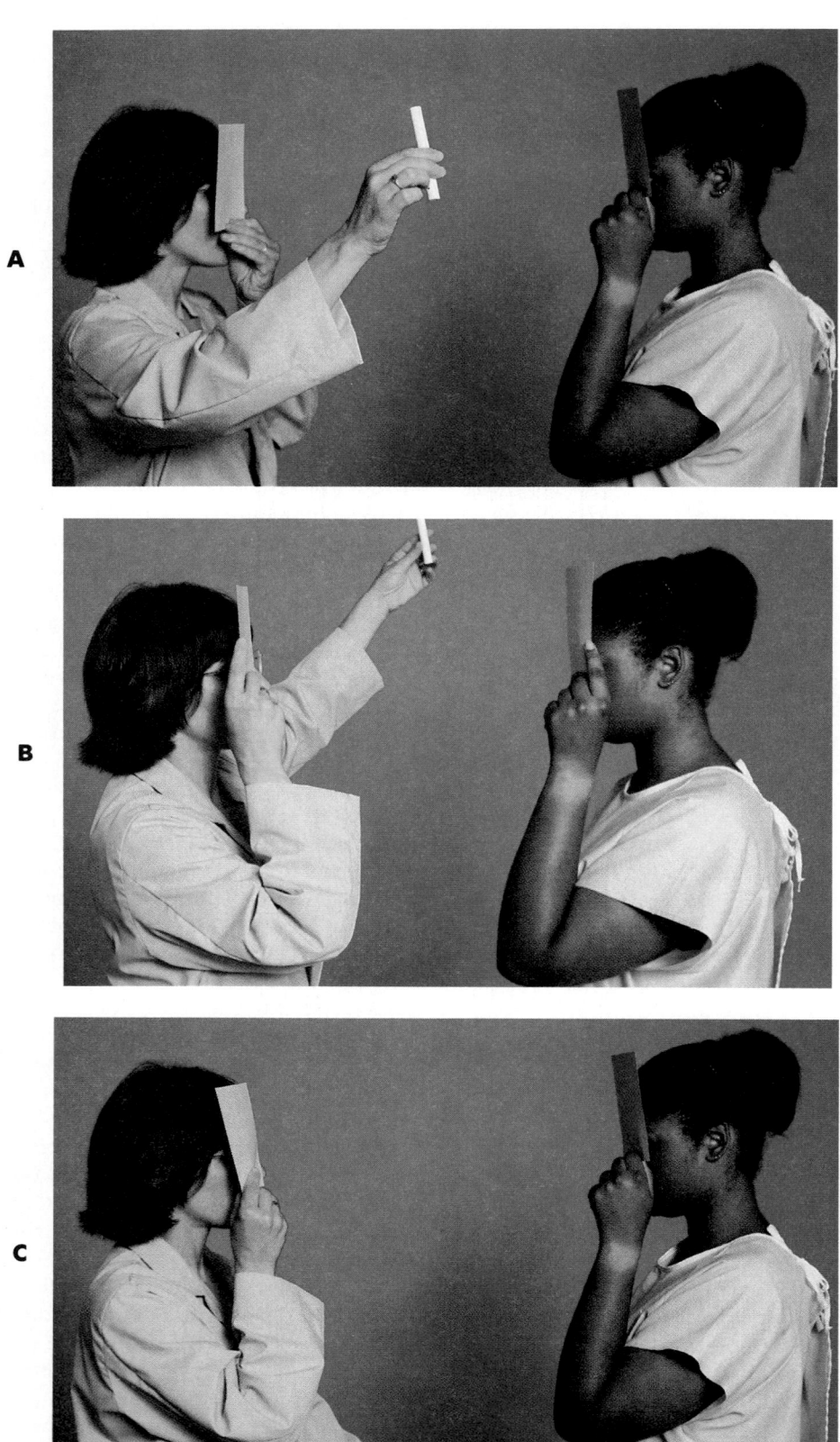

FIGURE 11-13 Visual fields confrontation test. Examiner assesses client's right field of vision from the nasal direction **(A)**, superior direction **(B)**, and inferior direction **(C)**. (Also tested but not shown: temporal direction.)

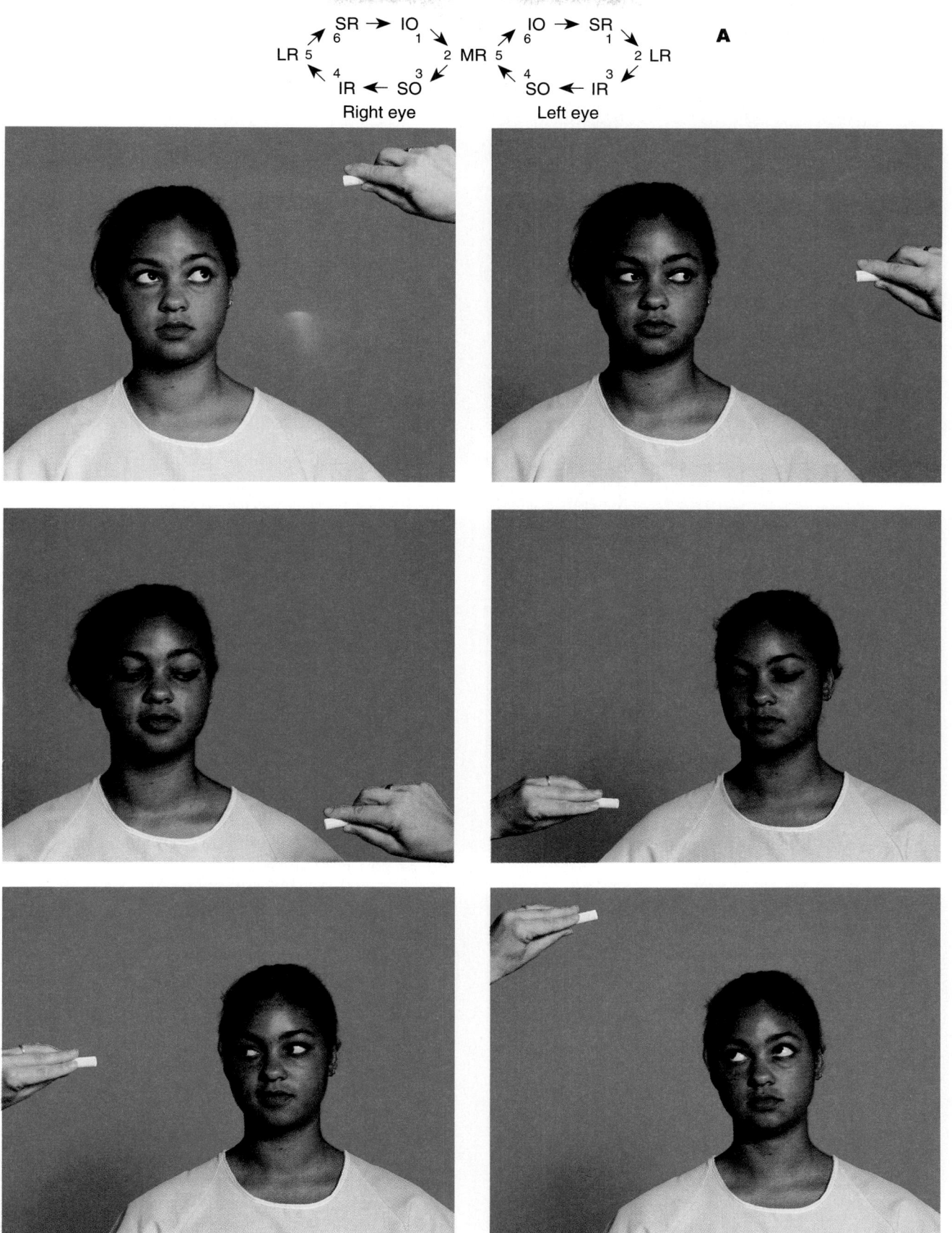

FIGURE 11-14 A, Six cardinal positions of gaze. **B,** Examination of the six cardinal positions of gaze.

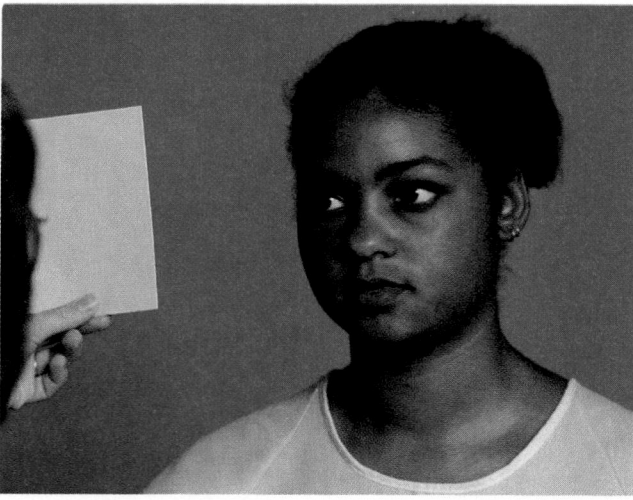

FIGURE 11-15 Cover-uncover test.

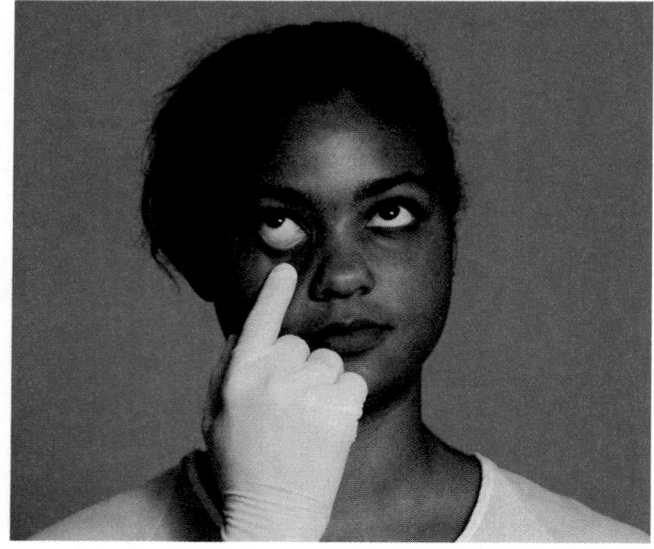

FIGURE 11-16 Examination of the conjunctiva.

another resting position. Then, when the eye is uncovered, it pulls back into alignment. Perform this procedure on both eyes.

External eye structures

EYELIDS AND EYELASHES. Inspect the eyelashes to see that they are present and curve outward. The palpebral fissures (distance between the upper and lower lids) should be equal. The margin of the upper eyelid is normally between the margin of the upper pupil and the margin of the upper limbus. Check to see that the client can close the lids completely. Note the position of the globe of the eye: normal, prominent, or sunken. Raised yellow plaques, or **xanthelasma,** may appear on the lids near the inner canthi. These plaques can be normal variations that grow slowly and may disappear spontaneously.

CONJUNCTIVA. Inspect the bulbar and palpebral portions of the conjunctiva by separating the eyelids widely and having the client look up, down, and to each side. When separating the eyelids, do not exert pressure against the eyeball. Hold the eyelid against the ridge of the bony orbit surrounding the eye (Figure 11-16). Normally, many small blood vessels are visible through the clear conjunctiva. The white sclera is visible through the bulbar conjunctiva.

Although **eversion** of the upper eyelid is not a necessary part of the physical examination, you should learn a careful technique for performing the procedure. It may be indicated, for example, when you suspect a foreign body in the upper eyelid. Explain the entire procedure to the client before you begin, and provide reassurance as you do it. If you do not show gentleness and care and give reassurance, the client is very likely to become tense when you manipulate the eyelid. When you are everting the eyelid, be aware of those techniques that promote relaxation rather than contraction of the muscles. Perform eversion of the upper eyelid (Figure 11-17) in the following way:

1. Ask the client to look down but keep the eyes slightly open. This maneuver relaxes the levator muscle. Closing the eyes contracts the orbicularis muscle, preventing lid eversion.
2. Gently grasp the upper eyelashes and pull them gently downward. Do not pull the lashes outward or upward since this action causes muscle contraction.
3. Place a cotton-tipped applicator about 1 cm above the eyelid margin and gently push downward with the applicator while still holding the lashes. This maneuver everts the lid.
4. Hold the lashes of the everted eyelid against the upper ridge of the body orbit, just beneath the eyebrow. Do *not* push against the eyeball.
5. Inspect the eyelid for a foreign object, lesion, swelling, or infection.

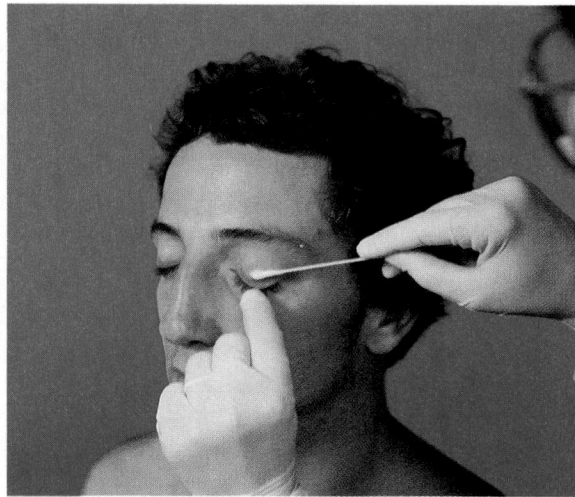

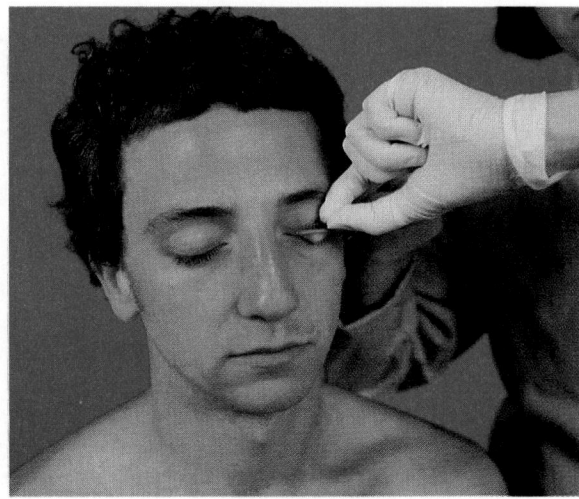

FIGURE 11-17 Eversion of the eyelid.

6. To return the eyelid to its normal position, move the lashes slightly forward and ask the client to look up and then blink. The lid should return easily to a normal position.

SCLERA. Inspect the sclera while you are inspecting the bulbar conjunctiva. The sclera is normally white. However, some pigmented deposits are within the ranges of normal findings.

CORNEA. Inspect the cornea by directing the light of a penlight at it obliquely from several positions. The cornea should be transparent, smooth, shiny, and bright. The surface should have no irregularities. The features of the iris should be fully visible through the cornea. In older persons the appearance of **arcus senilis** may be considered normal. Arcus senilis is a white ring that is located around the periphery of the cornea.

ANTERIOR CHAMBER. Inspect the anterior chamber while you are inspecting the cornea. Use the oblique light from a penlight to assess the anterior chamber (or use the light of the ophthalmoscope). The anterior chamber is a transparent structure. Any visible material is abnormal. Assess the depth of the anterior chamber, which is the distance between the cornea and the iris. Look at the eye from the side, rather than from directly in front, and shine the light across the eye from the opposite side. From a side view, the iris should appear flat and should not be bulging forward (Figure 11-18).

LACRIMAL APPARATUS. Of the several components of the lacrimal apparatus (lacrimal gland, puncta, lacrimal sac, and nasolacrimal duct), you can normally inspect only the puncta. These pinpoint openings are located near the inner canthus on the upper and lower eyelid margins. They should be just barely visible, with no swelling or redness noted. Check for blockage of the nasolacrimal duct by pressing against the lacrimal sac with your index finger or with a cotton-tipped applicator. Press in toward the lower inner orbital rim, not against the side of the nose (Figure 11-19). Then pull the lower lid down gently over the lower margin of the orbital rim to check for regurgitant material. Normally, there is no regurgitation of material through the puncta.

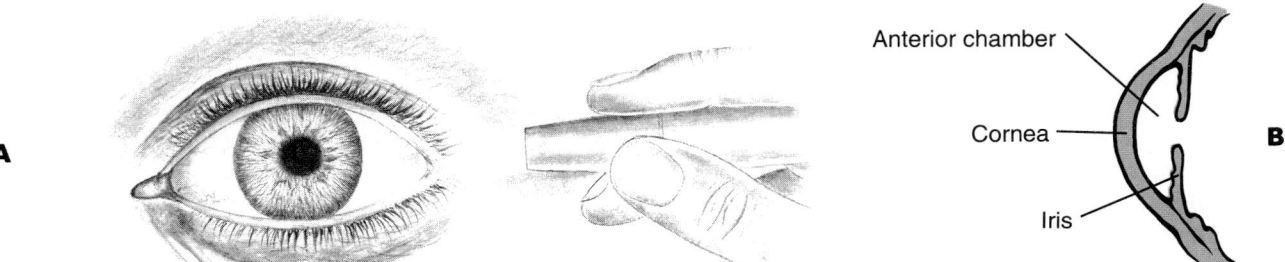

FIGURE 11-18 A, Anterior view of anterior chamber. **B,** Cross section showing normal anterior chamber. (**A** from Seidel HM and others; *Mosby's guide to physical examination,* ed 2, St Louis, 1991, Mosby–Year Book.)

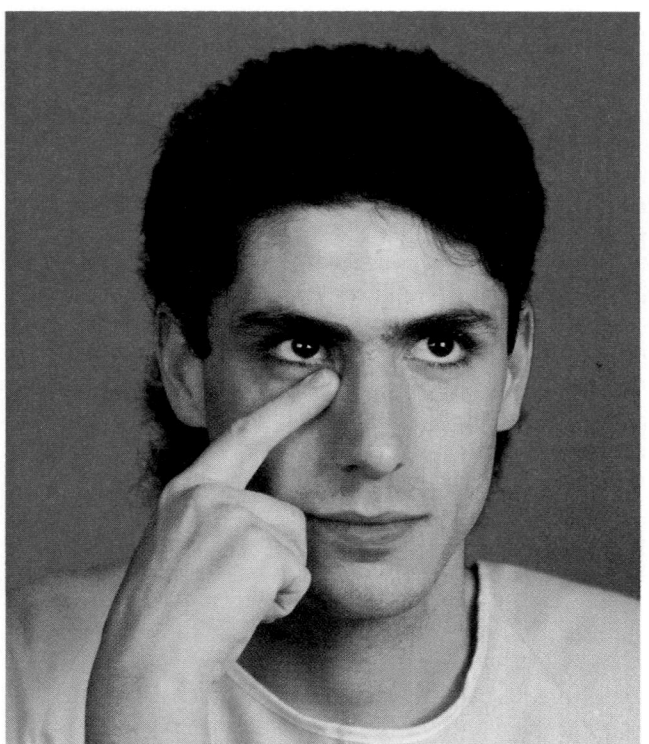

FIGURE 11-19 Examination of the nasolacrimal sac.

IRIS. Inspect the iris for regular round shape. As noted in the discussion of the anterior chamber, the iris should be flat, not bulging into the anterior chamber.

PUPIL. Inspection of the pupils includes the following four components:

Assessment of size
Assessment of shape
Reaction to light
Reaction of accommodation

The pupils are normally round and equal in size. Approximately 5% of people do have a slight but noticeable difference in the size of their pupils. Inequality in the size of the pupils is called **anisocoria.** Although this condition may be normal, regard the finding with some suspicion until you have completely assessed the health status of the client's eyes. The normal pupil is between 2 and 6 mm in diameter. The size of the pupils does vary among individuals exposed to the same amount of light. The pupils tend to be smaller in infancy and older age. Nearsighted persons tend to have larger pupils, whereas farsighted persons tend to have smaller pupils. Pupils of less than 2 mm in diameter are called miotic. Those that are more than 6 mm in diameter are called mydriatic.

To assess the pupillary response to light, bring the beam of a penlight in from the side of the client's head and direct it at one eye at a time. First observe the pupil toward which you are directing the light. Then glance quickly at the pupil of the other eye. Perform this assessment on each eye. The pupils normally constrict in response to light. There are two pupillary responses to light: direct and consensual. The pupil toward which the light is directed should constrict; this reaction is the direct pupillary response to light. The other pupil should also constrict; this reaction is the consensual response to light. Observe each eye for both direct and consensual response. Normally, both responses are present. The rapidity with which the pupils respond varies among individuals.

> **Helpful Hint:** *If you are having difficulty seeing the pupillary response, darken the room for a few moments so that the client's pupils will dilate. Shining the light into the client's eye should then show the pupillary constriction more clearly. A bright, sunny room makes it difficult to see the pupils constrict.*

The accommodation response of the pupils consists of convergence of the eyes and constriction of the pupils as the client shifts the glance from a distant to a near object. Ask the client to stare for several moments at an object across the room or at your finger held several feet away from the client. Visualizing a distant object normally causes the pupils to dilate. Then ask the client to switch the gaze to your finger, which you have placed about 6 inches from the client's nose. The normal response is pupillary constriction and convergence of the eyes. The rapidity of the pupillary response varies; it is slower in older persons.

Ophthalmoscopic examination. You can inspect the lens, vitreous humor, and retina with the ophthalmoscope. Darken the room so that the client's pupils will dilate (this lighting change will make the examination easier to perform). If the client wears corrective lenses, they may be left in place or removed. Try both ways to see which works most effectively for you.

Explain this portion of the examination to the client before you begin. The client's cooperation is essential since you will be asking him or her to hold the gaze constant and, for part of the examination, to stare into the bright light of the ophthalmoscope.

Ask the client to stare at a fixed point at eye level over your shoulder, such as a light switch or the corner of a picture. Staring at a distant object also helps to dilate the pupils. Tell the client that it is all right to blink, but no more than necessary. If blinking becomes

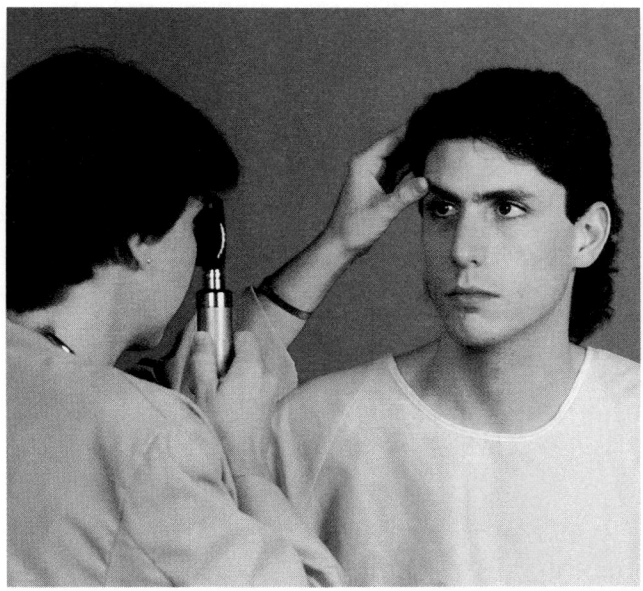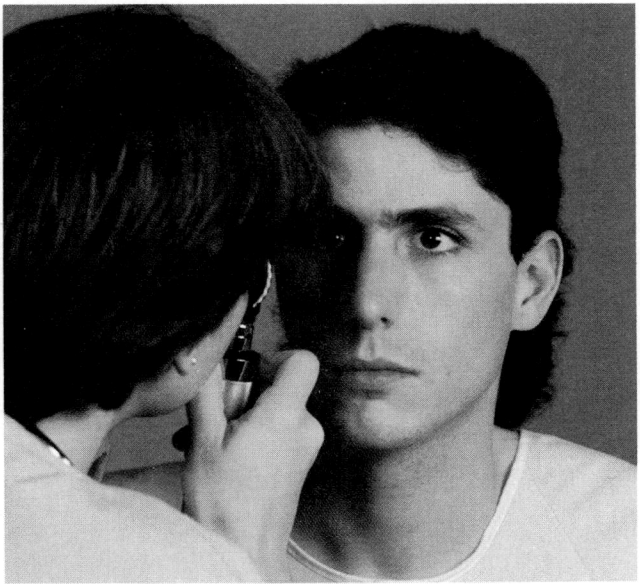

A

B

FIGURE 11-20 A, Ophthalmoscopic examination: finding the red reflex. **B,** Ophthalmoscopic examination: examining the retinal structures.

too frequent, you may need to elevate the upper lid and hold it against the upper orbital rim with your free hand. If you elevate the lid, do so for only a few seconds because the cornea can become dry, causing the client discomfort.

Turn on the ophthalmoscope light. Set the lens on 0 diopters. Begin by holding the ophthalmoscope in your right hand with your right index finger on the selector wheel. Hold the aperture of the ophthalmoscope up to your right eye. At a distance of about 12 inches, direct the light toward the client's right eye (Figure 11-20, *A*). When the beam of light falls on the client's pupil, you will see a red reflex, which is a reflection of the color of the retina.

> **Helpful Hint:** *If you lose sight of the red reflex, you are no longer directing the light through the pupil. Instead, you are directing it on the iris or sclera or away from the eye. If this situation occurs, move your head back from the ophthalmoscope, redirect the beam of light to the pupil, and bring your eye back to the aperture.*

Gradually move in closer to the client's eye until the ophthalmoscope is just a few inches away from the client's eye (Figure 11-20, *B*). Keep the red reflex in your line of vision while turning the selector wheel clockwise toward the positive numbers. This approach

enables you to focus on the more anterior structures, the lens and the vitreous body. Both structures should be clear, with no opacities or clouding. Gradually rotate the selector wheel counterclockwise toward the negative numbers. Look for a structure on the retina, such as the disc or a vessel. When you have found a certain structure, turn the wheel until it is in focus and you can visualize that structure clearly. With a nearsighted person, whose eyeball is more elongated than normal, you will need the more negative lenses in order to focus farther back. With a farsighted client, rotate the wheel toward 0. Focusing has individual variations and depends on the refractive state of both you and the client. If you locate the optic disc first, begin your inspection there. If you find a vessel first, follow that vessel in toward the optic disc. Examine the retinal structures in this order:

1. Optic disc
2. Retinal vessels
3. Retinal background
4. Macular area

OPTIC DISC. Examine the optic disc for size, shape, color, distinctness of its margins, and the physiologic cup. The disc is normally approximately 1.5 mm in diameter and round or slightly oval. It ranges in color from creamy yellow to pink and is lighter than the surrounding retina (see Figure 11-4). The color varies somewhat from one individual to another. The margins of the optic disc are usually sharp and clearly demarcated from the surrounding retina. However, several normal variations occur. Dense pigment deposits may be situated around the disc margins, particularly in dark-complected people. A whitish to grayish crescent of scleral tissue may be located immediately adjacent to the disc, particularly on the temporal side.

The physiologic cup, or physiologic depression, is a small depression just temporal to the center of the optic disc. It normally occupies about one third of the optic disc and is slightly lighter than the remainder of the disc.

The optic disc is a standard measurement device for findings on the retina. For example, a finding can be described as being 2 disc diameters away from the disc itself. Also, the size of the finding can be described in terms of the disc diameter. For example, an abnormality may measure one half of the disc diameter (Figure 11-21).

RETINAL VESSELS. Use the light from the ophthalmoscope to follow each of the four sets of vessels out from the optic disc to the periphery. Inspect the retinal vessels for the following four characteristics:

Color
Arteriolar light reflex
Arteriole-vein (A:V) ratio
Arteriovenous crossing changes

The arterioles are a brighter red than the veins and are approximately 25% smaller than the veins. The A:V ratio is about 2:3 or 4:5. Usually, the arterioles will have a narrow light reflex from the center line of the vessel. Veins do not show a light reflex. Normally, both arterioles and veins show a gradually and regularly diminishing diameter as they go from the disc to the periphery. They normally cross and intertwine, but where the vessels cross one another, there should be no change in the course or caliber of either vessel. Pulsations are sometimes visible in the veins near the optic disc.

> **Helpful Hint:** *To follow the course of the retinal vessels out to the periphery and to see more of the retinal background, ask the client to shift the gaze upward, downward, and to each side. This maneuver brings more of the retina into view.*

RETINAL BACKGROUND. Inspect the retinal background. It is normally fairly regular in color. Look for any areas that are darker or lighter.

MACULAR AREA. Inspection of the macular area should be done at the end of the ophthalmoscopic examination. Ask the client to stare directly at the bright light of the ophthalmoscope. You will then be looking at the macular area. The macula may be so similar in color to the rest of the retinal background that it will be difficult to visualize it as a separate structure; or it

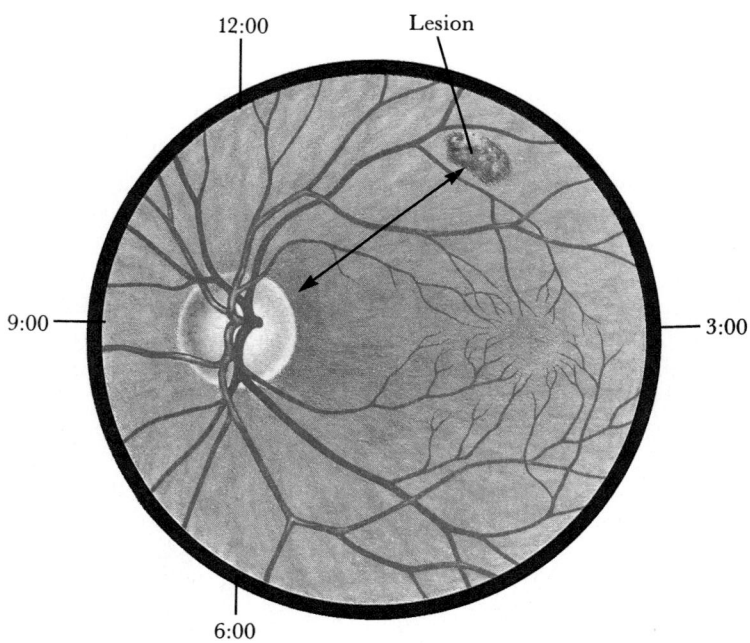

FIGURE 11-21 Method of describing retinal lesion in terms of the diameter of the optic disc. (From Seidel HM and others: *Mosby's guide to physical examination,* ed 2, St Louis, 1991, Mosby–Year Book.)

may be slightly darker. Learn to do this portion of the retinal examination quickly because the client may feel quite uncomfortable as you direct the bright light at the area of most acute color vision.

The macular area, which is approximately 1 disc diameter in size, is located about 2 disc diameters temporal to the optic disc. At the center of the macula is the fovea centralis. The macula appears as a regularly colored area with no large vessels visible. A bright spot of light may be reflected from the fovea centralis.

The retina appears reddish-orange because of its deep vascular supply and deeply pigmented layers. The pigment in the posterior layers of the retina also accounts for its slightly stippled appearance. Normally, the color of the retina is uniform, with no patches of light or dark discoloration present.

The macular area usually has no visible retinal vessels. It is nourished by choroidal vessels and appears slightly darker than the rest of the retinal background.

Screening Tests and Procedures

Screening for diminished visual acuity.* Approximately 2% to 5% of children in the United States suffer from **amblyopia** ("lazy eye") and **strabismus** (ocular misalignment), and nearly 20% have simple refractive errors by age 16. Vision screening is recommended for all children once before entering school, preferably at age 3 or 4 years. Routine vision testing is

*Data from Report of the U.S. Preventive Services Task Force: *Guide to clinical preventive services: an assessment of the effectiveness of 169 interventions,* Baltimore, 1989, William & Wilkins.

STEP-BY-STEP

Examination Step-by-Step

Perform examination of the eyes with the client sitting or standing.

Equipment needed includes:
Snellen chart
Rosenbaum chart or newspaper
Opaque card or eye cover
Penlight
Cotton-tipped applicator
Wisp of cotton
Ophthalmoscope

1. Measure visual acuity (CN II)
   a. Distant vision using Snellen chart
   b. Near vision using Rosenbaum chart or newspaper
2. Assess visual fields (CN II)
   a. Visual fields confrontation test
3. Assess extraocular muscle function (CN III, IV, VI)
   a. Six cardinal positions of gaze
   b. Corneal light reflex
   c. Cover-uncover test
4. Inspect external eye structures
   a. Position of globe: normal, protruding, or sunken
   b. Eyelids and eyelashes
      1. Position of eyelids and eyelashes, palpebral fissures
      2. Ability to close lids
      3. Redness, swelling, lumps
   c. Conjunctiva and sclera
      1. Clarity
      2. Eversion of eyelid, if indicated
      3. Redness, discharge
   d. Cornea
      1. Light reflex
      2. Arcus senilis

   e. Anterior chamber
      1. Clarity
      2. Depth
   f. Lacrimal apparatus
      1. Puncta
      2. Swelling or redness
      3. Regurgitation of material from lacrimal sac
   g. Iris
      1. Shape
      2. Fluttering movements
   h. Pupil
      1. Size
      2. Shape
      3. Response to light and accommodation
   i. Ophthalmoscopic examination
      1. Red reflex
      2. Optic disc
         a. Size and shape
         b. Color
         c. Margins
         d. Physiologic cup
      3. Retinal vessels
         a. Color
         b. Arteriolar light reflex
         c. Arteriole-vein ratio
         d. Arteriovenous crossing characteristics
      4. Retinal background
         a. Regularity
         b. Color
         c. Presence of microaneurysms, hemorrhages, exudates
      5. Macula and fovea centralis
         a. Regularity
         b. Color

not recommended as a component of the periodic health examination of asymptomatic school children. However, practitioners should be alert for signs of ocular misalignment when examining all infants and children. Vision screening of adolescents and adults is not recommended, but it may be appropriate in the elderly.

(*Note:* There are differences of opinion on the efficacy of vision screening for school children. In many settings vision screening with the Snellen chart is performed as part of the school physical at required intervals.)

Screening for glaucoma.* There is insufficient evidence to recommend routine performance of tonometry by primary care practitioners as an effective screening test for **glaucoma.** It may be clinically prudent, however, to advise clients at high risk, such as those aged 65 and older, to be tested periodically for glaucoma by an eye specialist.

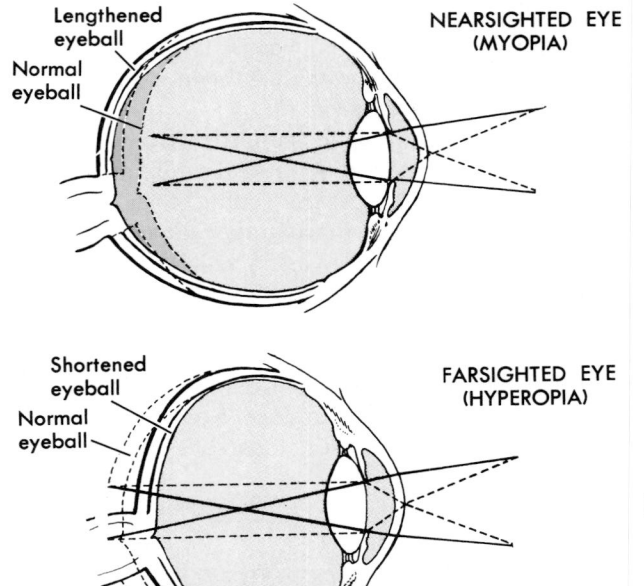

FIGURE 11-22 A, Nearsighted, or myopic, eye focuses the image in front of the retina. This condition may occur when the eyeball is too long or the lens is too thick. **B,** The farsighted, or hyperopic, eye can focus the image only at a hypothetical distance behind the retina. This condition may occur when the eyeball is too short or the lens is too thin. (From Thibodeau GA: *Anthony's textbook of anatomy and physiology,* ed 13, St Louis, 1990, Mosby–Year Book.)

VARIATIONS FROM HEALTH

Variations of Visual Function

Changes in visual function include the following:
1. Diminished visual acuity
2. Decreased vision
3. Blindness
4. Defects in color vision
5. Diplopia (double vision)
6. Faulty adaptation to the dark
7. Visualization of objects within eye
8. Iridescent vision

Diminished visual acuity. An error of refraction is a common variation from normal vision. It is an inability to focus rays of light on the retina. Common errors of refraction include nearsightedness (myopia), farsightedness (hyperopia), and astigmatism.

Nearsightedness (myopia). In **myopia** the eye focuses the image in front of the retina. This situation can occur when the eyeball is too long or the lens is too thick (Figure 11-22, *A*). Nearsighted individuals can see objects that are nearby, but not objects that are far away.

Farsightedness (hyperopia). In **hyperopia** the eye focuses the image at a hypothetical distance behind the retina. This situation can occur when the eyeball is too short or the lens is too thin (Figure 11-22, *B*). Farsighted individuals can see objects that are far away but not those that are nearby. As people age, they typically

*Data from Report of the U.S. Preventive Services Task Force: *Guide to clinical preventive services: an assessment of the effectiveness of 169 interventions,* Baltimore, 1989, William & Wilkins.

become farsighted as the lens of the eyes becomes more rigid, losing its elasticity. The ciliary muscles also become weaker, and the lens cannot bulge to accommodate for near vision. This condition is known as **presbyopia.**

Astigmatism. **Astigmatism** occurs with uneven curvature of the cornea. Vision is blurred, and use of the eyes may cause discomfort.

Decreased vision. Defects in the field of vision may be caused by lesions of the retina, along the optic nerve, at the optic chiasm (where portions of each nerve cross over to the opposite side), along the optic tract, or in the occipital lobes (Figure 11-23). The resulting defect in vision may be central, peripheral, or specific to portions of the visual fields (depending on the nature and location of the lesion). Visual field defects are described according to their location: temporal, nasal, superior, or inferior. The visual field reflects the visual function in the opposite areas of the retina involved. For example, a temporal visual field defect reflects a defect of

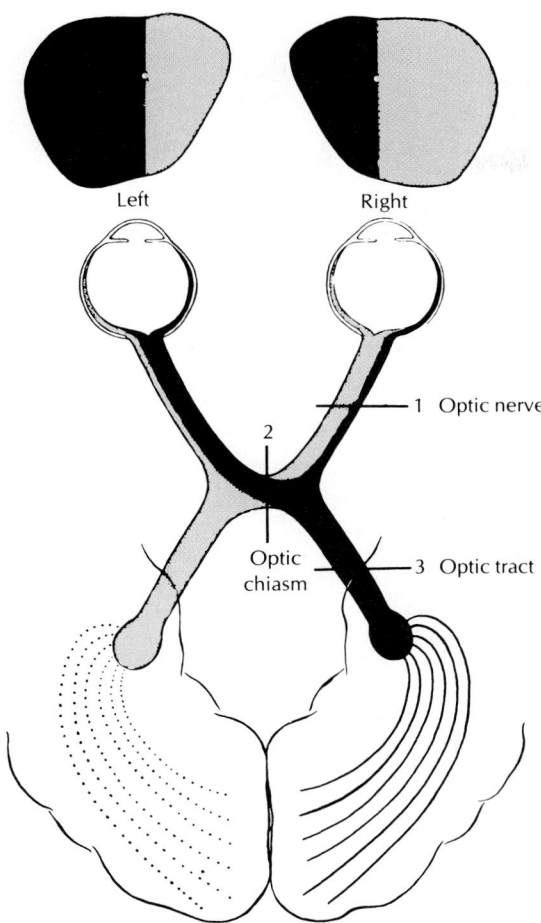

FIGURE 11-23 Visual field defects. *1,* Blind right eye. *2,* Bitemporal hemianopia: no temporal vision. *3,* Left homonymous hemianopia: no vision in left field of either eye. (Modified from Havener WH: *Synopsis of ophthalmology,* ed 6, St Louis, 1984, Mosby—Year book.)

the nasal retina. A superior field defect reflects an inferior retinal defect. Likewise, an inferior nasal retinal defect would cause a defect in the superior temporal field of vision. The effect of such lesions on the field of vision are illustrated in Figure 11-24.

Monocular visual defects. If the lesion is located in the retina of one eye or along one optic nerve anterior to the optic chiasm, it affects the vision in that eye.

Bitemporal hemianopsia. Lesions that are found at the optic chiasm, along the optic tract, or in the occipital lobes affect the visual fields of both eyes. This situation occurs because of the crossing and mixing of fibers from both eyes at the chiasm. A lesion at the optic chiasm may be caused by a pituitary tumor. A tumor would produce a loss of vision from the nasal portion of each

retina, resulting in a loss of both temporal fields of vision. This condition is called **bitemporal hemianopsia.**

Homonymous hemianopsia. Nerve fibers from both eyes mingle behind the chiasm in the optic tracts and in the brain. Lesions along the optic tract or in the temporal, parietal, or occipital lobes will impair the same half of the field of vision in both eyes. For example, a lesion of the right optic tract or the right side of the brain results in visual field defects in the right nasal field and in the left temporal field. Called **homonymous hemianopsia,** this condition may be caused by occlusion of the middle cerebral artery.

The location of disease on the retina determines the type of resultant visual field defects. Macular defects lead to a central blind area. Localized damage in other areas of the retina causes a loss of vision corresponding to the involved area. A blind spot is called a **scotoma.** It is an area of blindness surrounded by an area of vision. Advanced diabetic retinopathy may cause macular damage, resulting in a loss of central vision. Increased intraocular pressure, commonly associated with glaucoma, causes decreased peripheral vision. As glaucoma advances, it may also cause a loss of central vision. A retinal detachment causes loss of vision from that portion of the retina where the detachment occurs.

Blindness. A person is considered legally blind when the best visual acuity that can be achieved with corrective lenses in the better eye is 20/200 or less, or when the peripheral visual field is constricted to within 20 degrees. Major causes of blindness in North America are glaucoma, unoperated cataracts, and retinal disorders (mainly diabetic retinopathy and macular degeneration).

Defects in color vision. A variety of conditions may disturb color vision, including diseases of the optic nerve, diseases of the fovea centralis and macular area (where the cones are most concentrated), and nutritional disturbances. In macular degeneration, the decrease in color vision parallels the loss of visual acuity. The person who is deficient in color vision is unable to see the figures on color plates, which are easily recognizable to the person with normal color vision.

Diplopia. Diplopia, or double vision, occurs whenever the visual axes, the parallel lines of vision, are not directed simultaneously at the same object. It is a cardinal sign of weakness of one or more of the extraocular muscles. Diplopia can be a sign of pressure from a brain tumor or of increased intracranial pressure.

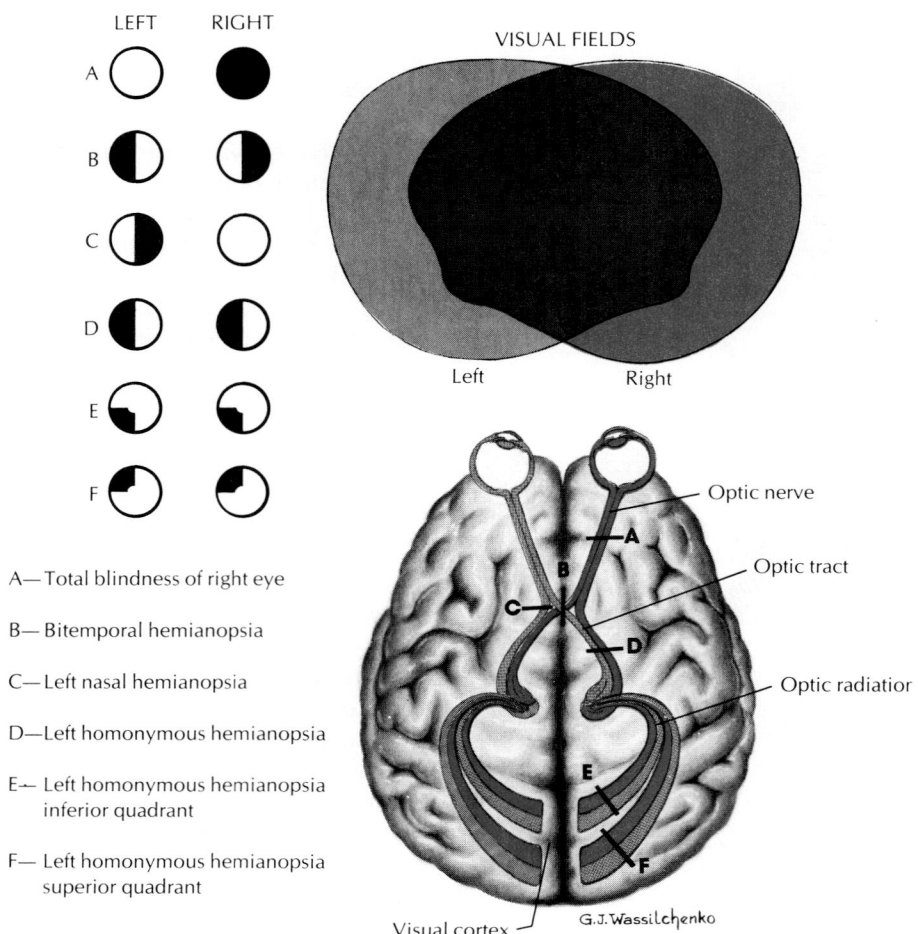

A—Total blindness of right eye

B—Bitemporal hemianopsia

C—Left nasal hemianopsia

D—Left homonymous hemianopsia

E—Left homonymous hemianopsia
inferior quadrant

F—Left homonymous hemianopsia
superior quadrant

FIGURE 11-24 Visual fields and examples of visual field defects along the optic nerve, optic chiasm, optic tracts, and optic radiations in the cortex. (From Rudy EB: *Advanced neurological and neurosurgical nursing,* St Louis, 1984, Mosby–Year Book.)

Faulty adaptation to dark. Night blindness is caused by pigmentary degeneration of the retina, optic nerve disease, glaucoma, or vitamin A deficiency. Deficiency in vitamin A may occur because of inadequate nutrition or cirrhosis of the liver. A client may experience slow recovery of vision during nighttime driving after the headlights of a passing car shine in the eyes.

Visualization of objects within eye. Translucent specks of various shapes and sizes that float across the visual field and are visible only when the eye is open are called **floaters.** They are small remnants of the hyaloid vascular system in the vitreous humor. Floaters are visualized as small dots that appear to dart away as the client tries to look at them. Many people experience occasional floaters that have no pathological significance. However, sudden showers of floaters may occur in the periphery of the visual field with vitreous hemorrhage. This occurrence may be the initial symptom of hole formation that precedes retinal separation. The location of the floaters may be helpful in finding the retinal tear. The sudden appearance of a moderately large floater is the main symptom of vitreous detachment. It is important to note that any sudden appearance of floaters is cause for immediate referral to an eye care specialist.

Iridescent vision. Iridescent vision is a term that describes the halos or rainbows that a client sees surrounding bright lights when he or she has corneal edema. This condition may follow a rapid increase in intraocular pressure with acute glaucoma, after prolonged wearing of hard contact lenses, with corneal abrasion, and with cataracts.

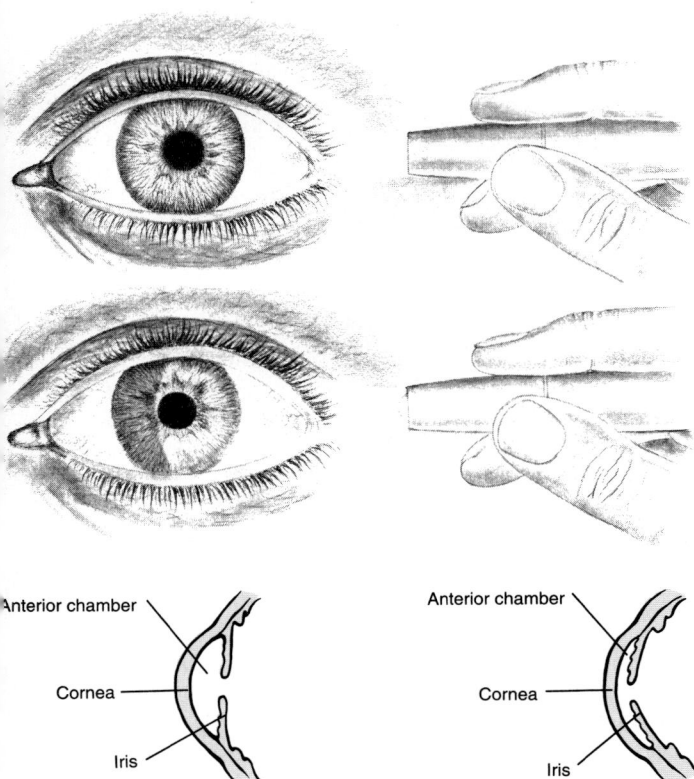

FIGURE 11-34 A, Anterior view of normal *(top)* and shallow *(bottom)* anterior chamber. **B,** Cross section of normal *(top)* and shallow *(bottom)* anterior chamber. (**A** from Seidel HM and others: *Mosby's guide to physical examination,* ed 2, St Louis, 1992, Mosby–Year Book.)

Hypopyon. An accumulation of purulent material in the anterior chamber is called **hypopyon.**

Iris

Iritis. **Iritis** is an inflammation of the iris. Associated findings include circumcorneal injection (a deep pink to red flush around the cornea), a bulging iris, inequality in the size of the pupils, throbbing pain, photophobia, visual blurring, and a constricted or irregularly shaped pupil. The affected client should be referred to an eye care specialist immediately.

> **Helpful Hint:** *With iritis a red flush is present around the iris and cornea. With conjunctivitis a red flush extends from the periphery toward the iris and cornea.*

Fluttering motion of iris. Removal of the lens takes away the normal support of the iris, leaving it with a tremulous or fluttering motion.

Pupils

Abnormalities of the pupils include alterations in size, shape, and reflexes.

Variations in size and shape

ANISOCORIA. A difference in the size of the pupils is called anisocoria. Approximately 5% of the population has a slight but noticeable difference in pupil size. Although this finding may be normal, until the cause is known, it should be regarded with some suspicion because it can be an indication of central nervous system disease.

DYSCORIA. Dyscoria is a congenital abnormality affecting the shape of the pupils.

MYDRIASIS. Mydriasis is an enlargement of the pupils that may result from emotional influences, recent or old trauma, acute glaucoma, a systemic reaction to parasympatholytic or sympathomimetic drugs, or the local use of dilating drops. A unilateral fixed and enlarged pupil may be caused by local trauma to the eye or the head. Oculomotor nerve damage (CN III) results in a pupil that is dilated and fixed; the eye deviates downward and laterally, and the eyelid droops. Fixed dilation of both pupils occurs with deep anesthesia, central nervous system injury, and circulatory arrest.

MIOSIS. Miosis is constriction of the pupils that is associated with iritis, the use of narcotics, and the use of pilocarpine drops for the treatment of glaucoma.

Variations in reflexes

ARGYLL ROBERTSON PUPIL. This condition is a failure of the pupils to react to light with preservation of the accommodation response. It is associated with chronic alcoholism, meningitis, and brain tumor.

ADIE'S PUPIL. With this condition, the pupil is dilated and constricts little to light and accommodation. It is often associated with absent deep tendon reflexes in the extremities. The cause of this condition is unknown.

HORNER'S SYNDROME. This condition involves sympathetic paralysis of the eye, which includes constriction of the pupil, drooping of the eyelid, and lack of tearing. The paralysis is caused by interruption of the cervical sympathetic chain.

MONOCULAR BLINDNESS. In monocular blindness, when light is directed at the blind eye, there is no response to light in either eye. However, when the seeing eye receives illumination, both pupils constrict; this situation occurs because the efferent pupil constriction stimulus via the oculomotor nerve is distributed to both eyes.

Lens

Cataract. A **cataract** is a gray-white opacity within the lens (Figure 11-35). On ophthalmoscopic exami-

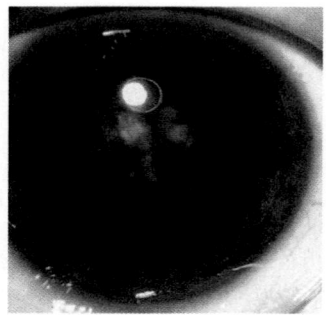

FIGURE 11-35 Cataract. (From Donaldson DD: *Atlas of diseases of the eye, vol V, The crystalline lens,* St Louis, 1976, Mosby—Year Book.)

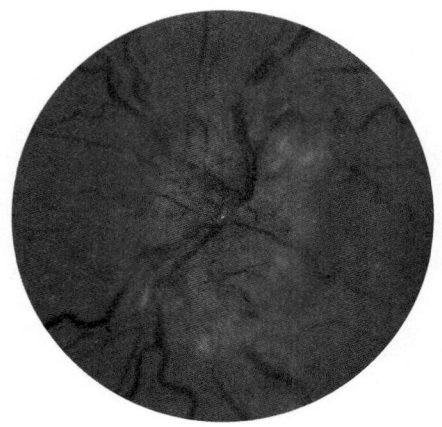

FIGURE 11-36 Papilledema. (Modified from Newell FW: *Ophthalmology: principles and concepts,* ed 7, St Louis, 1992, Mosby—Year Book.)

nation, the cataract is seen as a dark shadow or black spots within the red reflex or as an absent red reflex because the opacity prevents light from being reflected back to the examiner's eye. Cataracts vary in appearance. They may look like pieces of coral or crystals, or they may have a starlike (stellate) appearance. Cataract formation may accompany aging, or it may be associated with systemic disorders or congenital syndromes.

Senile cataracts occur as a result of various degenerative processes within the lens. These cataracts are the most common type and occur most often after 50 years of age. The tendency to develop cataracts is inherited.

In cataracts associated with diabetes mellitus, the metabolic disturbance results in formation of abnormal lens fiber. These cataracts occur more frequently in young people, are bilateral, progress rapidly, and have a classic snowflake appearance.

Congenital cataracts are usually hereditary. However, they may be caused by viral infection during the first trimester of gestation.

Typical symptoms of cataracts include blurred or cloudy vision, sensitivity to bright light, and, later, distorted or double vision. Untreated cataracts lead to loss of vision.

Retinal structures

Optic disc

PAPILLEDEMA. Papilledema is a condition characterized by swelling of the optic nerve head that causes the margins of the disc to become blurred and indistinct (Figure 11-36). It is a sign of increased intracranial pressure. This pressure causes decreased venous drainage from the eye and accumulation or leakage of fluid. Papilledema is associated with malignant hypertension, eclampsia of pregnancy, brain tumor, and hematoma.

The nerve head appears to be out of focus with the surrounding retina. The degree of elevation of the optic disc can be assessed by focusing first on the disc and then on the surrounding retina and noting the difference in diopters on the ophthalmoscope.

CUPPING OF OPTIC DISC. The increased intraocular pressure of glaucoma gradually exerts pressure posteriorly against the optic disc. This pressure causes **cupping,** an increased posterior curvature of the disc. It may also produce an increase in the cup-disc ratio. The cup may enlarge to more than one half the disc diameter. The pressure of glaucoma may also cause pallor of the disc, a sign of optic atrophy.

On ophthalmoscopic examination, cupping may be observed by following carefully the course of the vessels as they emerge over the margin of the optic disc. The increased intraocular pressure causes a vessel to seem to disappear from sight at the disc rim and then to reappear at a slightly different site just past the rim (Figure 11-37).

Cupping of the optic disc and optic atrophy are both late findings of glaucoma. If there is any suspicion of the disease, the client should be referred to an eye care specialist for further testing.

OPTIC ATROPHY. Death of the optic nerve fibers leads to the disappearance of the tiny disc vessels that give the disc its normal pinkish color. The affected disc is seen as pale and white, either in a portion of or throughout the disc.

> **Helpful Hint:** *The scleral crescent, a normal finding, is a pale crescent-shaped area around the rim of the disc only. Do not mistake it for disc atrophy.*

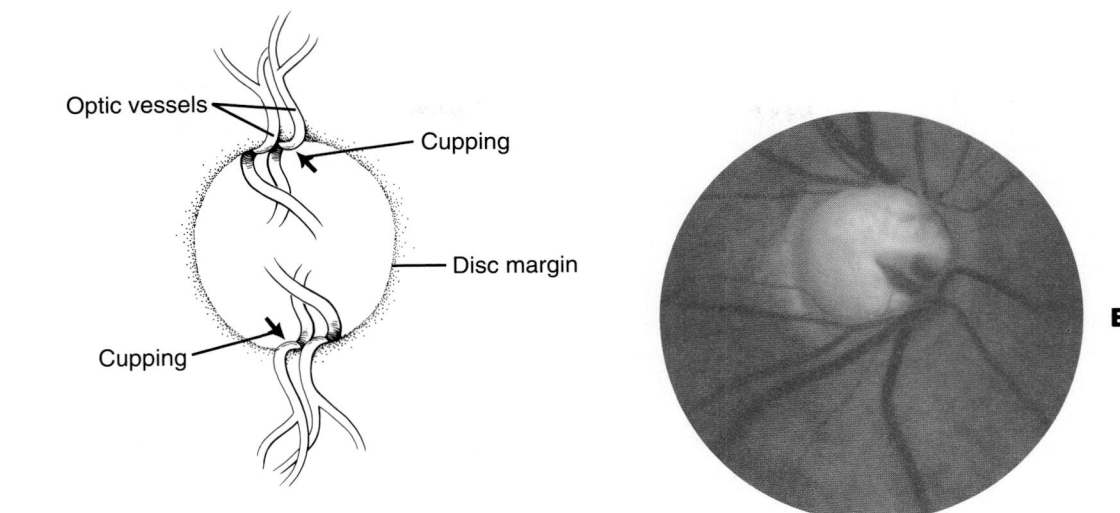

FIGURE 11-37 A, Glaucomatous cupping. **B,** Advanced glaucomatous optic atrophy with cupping of the disc and nasal displacement of the retinal vessels. (**B** from Newell FW: *Ophthalmology: principles and concepts,* ed 7, St Louis, 1992, Mosby—Year Book.)

Retinal vessels

VARIATION IN CALIBER. Variation in the caliber of retinal vessels may occur with hypertension. Since caliber changes may not be evenly distributed along the course of the vessel, it is necessary to follow the vessels out from the disc to the periphery. Arterioles are normally about two thirds to three fourths of the diameter of the corresponding veins. With hypertension, the arterioles may decrease in diameter so that they are only about one half the size of the corresponding vein.

VARIATION IN COLOR. Normally the color of the vessel is determined by the color of the blood within it. With hypertension, the arterioles may develop sclerotic or sheathing changes, causing them to become opaque and lighter. With arteriosclerosis the width of the light reflex from the arteriolar wall also increases to one third or more of the width of the vessel. In advanced stages the vessels may appear as fine, silvery lines.

VESSEL CROSSING VARIATIONS. Changes at arteriovenous crossings include an apparent narrowing or blocking of the vein, called **nicking,** at the point where an arteriole crosses over it (Figure 11-38). This appearance, which is the result of some degree of concealment of the underlying veins by an abnormally opaque arteriole wall, occurs with long-standing hypertension. It is initially apparent as a narrowing or tapering of the vessel at the crossing. Later it appears as a more complete interruption of the vessel.

An embolus in a retinal vessel abruptly impedes the flow of blood and results in the sudden narrowing of an arteriole or dilation of a vein.

RETINAL BACKGROUND VARIATIONS

MICROANEURYSMS. Microaneurysms are outpouchings in the walls of the capillaries that appear as tiny bright-red dots on the retina (Figure 11-39). They are frequently associated with diabetes mellitus.

RETINAL EXUDATES. Retinal exudates are whitish-yellow infiltrates on the retina (Figures 11-39, 11-40, and 11-41). Both "soft" and "hard" exudates exist. The soft exudates, which look somewhat like a cumulus cloud, are also called "cotton-wool" patches or exudates. Hard exudates have more distinct edges. Retinal exudates are associated with systemic diseases, including diabetes mellitus and hypertension. In addition, they may be associated with inflammatory or degen-

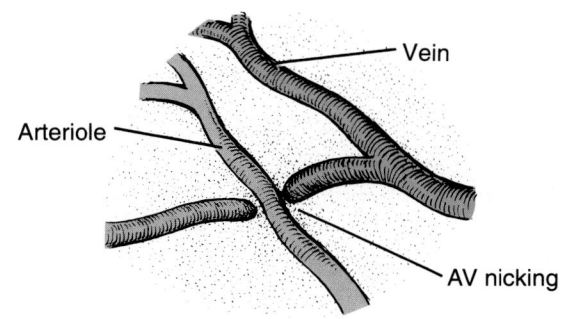

FIGURE 11-38 Arteriovenous nicking.

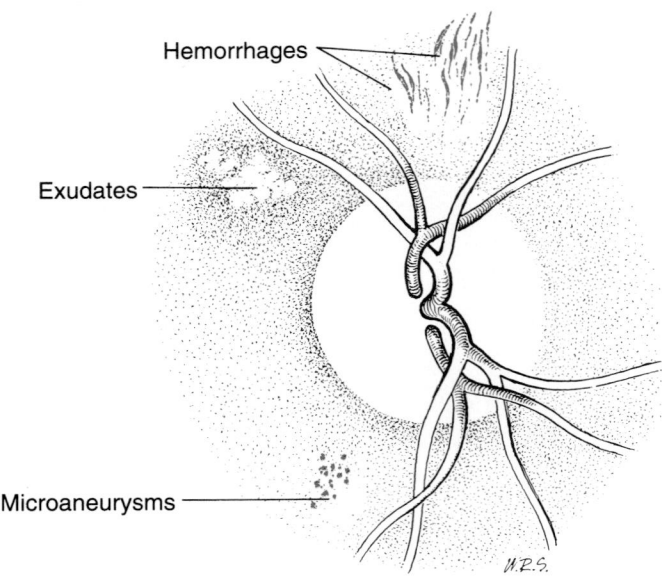

FIGURE 11-39 Microaneurysms.

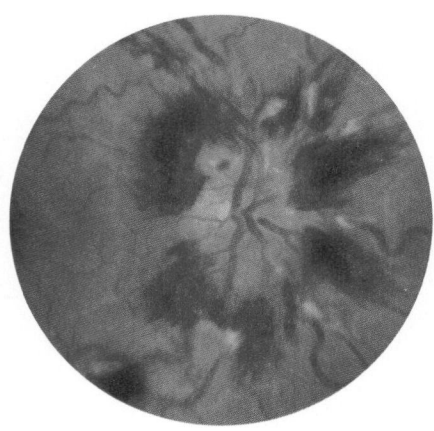

FIGURE 11-40 Flame-shaped hemorrhages and cotton-wool patches. (Modified from Newell FW: *Ophthalmology: principles and concepts*, ed 7, St Louis, 1992, Mosby–Year Book.)

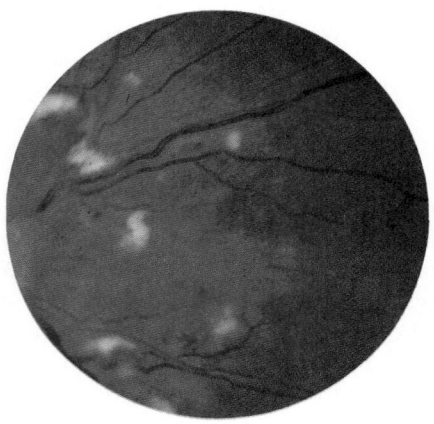

FIGURE 11-41 Cotton-wool patches, or exudates, in severe vascular hypertension. (Modified from Newell FW: *Ophthalmology: principles and concepts*, ed 7, St Louis, 1992, Mosby–Year Book.)

erative diseases of the retina. Some exudates are resorbed over time.

HEMORRHAGES ON RETINA. Retinal hemorrhages are bright to dark red. They may be small and round, as commonly occur with diabetes, or linear and flame-shaped, as noted with hypertension (see Figures 11-39 and 11-40).

TEARS, HOLES, OR RETINAL DETACHMENT. These variations may develop on the retina. Retinal detachment is a serious condition in which the retinal layer pulls away from the choroid.

Retinal changes may affect any part of the retinal background, including the macular area. Changes in central or peripheral vision depend on the location of the lesion.

Variations in Comfort

Numerous relatively minor ocular variations are accompanied by itching, burning, or discomfort of the eyes. These symptoms may result from fatigue, allergy, conjunctivitis, or inadequately corrected refractive error.

Superficial eye pain may be caused by any of the following factors:

Lesion in the eyelid

Foreign body on the cornea or conjunctiva

Loss of corneal or conjunctival epithelium

Deep, severe pain within the eye may result from either of these two conditions:

Inflammation of the iris or ciliary body

Rapid increase in intraocular pressure

Findings accompanying deep eye pain include redness and decreased vision. Immediate referral to an ophthalmologist is required.

Variation in Intraocular Pressure: Glaucoma

Acute glaucoma occurs with a sudden increase in intraocular pressure caused by blocked drainage of aqueous fluid from the anterior chamber.

Findings associated with acute glaucoma include the following:

Intense pain

Circumcorneal redness

Dilated pupil

Shallow anterior chamber

Visualizing halos around lights

The affected client should be referred to an eye care specialist immediately.

Glaucoma may also be a chronic condition. In this situation symptoms are absent, except for the gradual loss of peripheral vision over a long period of time.

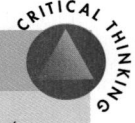

Sample Documentation

Health history
A 75-year-old woman noticed a bright-red spot over the sclera of her right eye. She has no pain, itching, inflammation, drainage, or redness (other than this area). She has no problems with her vision; wears corrective lenses for nearsightedness. History of mild hypertension for 20 years, controlled by medication.

Physical examination
—Visual acuity with correction: left eye, 20/20; right eye, 20/20. Near vision is normal with correction.
—Visual fields: intact on confrontation test.
—Extraocular muscles: EOMs intact, no nystagmus. Corneal light reflex: symmetrical. Cover-uncover test: eyes aligned, no deviation.
—External eye:
  —Palpebral fissures equal, lids and lashes normal
  —Conjunctiva: left eye: clear; right eye: bright-red area—4 mm in diameter, lower temporal side beneath conjunctiva, margins sharp
  —Sclera: white, except for few small blood vessels at cornices

—Cornea: clear, bright; arcus senilis present
—Lacrimal apparatus: no excessive tearing, no regurgitation of material from lacrimal sac
—Anterior chamber: normal depth, iris flat
—Pupils: equal, round, react to light and accommodation (PERRLA), though response is somewhat slow
—Ophthalmoscopy:
—Full red reflex present bilaterally
—Lens and posterior chamber clear
—Optic disc: round, yellowish-pink, margins distinct
—Vessels: arterioles—silver-wire appearance; slight nicking of superior temporal vessels—left eye, two disc diameters from optic disc; A:V ratio: 2:4
—Retinal background: color regular, no hemorrhages or exudates

Nursing Diagnosis *THE NEXT STEP*

Nursing diagnoses that could apply to assessment and alterations in the visual system include, but are not limited to, the following ones.

SENSORY/PERCEPTUAL ALTERATIONS (VISUAL) The state in which an individual experiences a change in the amount or patterning of incoming stimuli accompanied by a diminished, exaggerated, distorted, or impaired response to such stimuli.

Defining Characteristics
- Alert with periodic disorientation, general confusion, or nocturnal confusion
- Hallucinations (visual, auditory)
- Apathy
- Visual, reality-orienting, or time-orienting input reduced or absent
- Limited proprioceptive input
- Presence of uncompensated visual deficits

Related Factors
- Restricted environment
- Uncompensated visual loss
- Eye patches
- Compresses
- Medication

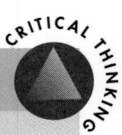

Nursing Diagnosis   *THE NEXT STEP—cont'd*

IMPAIRED PHYSICAL MOBILITY The state in which an individual experiences a limitation of ability for independent physical movement.

Defining Characteristics

- Inability to move purposefully within the physical environment
- Decreased muscle strength, control
- Impaired coordination
  Levels:
  I. Requires use of equipment or device
  II. Requires help from another person(s): assistance, supervision, or teaching
  III. Requires help from another person(s) and equipment or device
  IV. Is dependent and does not participate in movement

Related Factors

- Decreased visual stimuli; inability to visualize surroundings
- Pain, discomfort
- Uncompensated perceptual-cognitive impairment
- Uncompensated musculoskeletal impairment
- Uncompensated neuromuscular impairment

SELF-CARE DEFICIT (TOTAL) The state in which the individual experiences impaired ability to perform or complete any or all activities of daily living (ADLs).

Defining Characteristics

- Observation or valid report of inability to eat, bathe, toilet, dress, groom self independently
  Levels:
  I. Requires use of equipment or device
  II. Requires help from another person(s): assistance, supervision, or teaching
  III. Requires help from another person(s) and equipment or device
  IV. Is dependent and does not participate in self-care

Related Factors

- Intolerance of activity; decreased strength and endurance (decreased activity tolerance)
- Pain, discomfort
- Uncompensated perceptual-cognitive impairment
- Uncompensated neuromuscular impairment
- Uncompensated musculoskeletal impairment
- Severe anxiety
- Depression

DIVERSIONAL ACTIVITY DEFICIT The state in which an individual experiences a decreased stimulation from or interest or engagement in recreational or leisure activities.

Defining Characteristics

- Report of boredom
- Daytime napping
- Usual hobbies or activities cannot be undertaken
- Expressed wish for something to do, to read, etc.
- Inability to read newspaper or identify objects

Related Factors

- Long-term hospitalization—apathy
- Environmental lack of diversional activity
- Sensory input deficit—visual

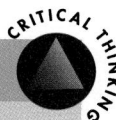

IMPAIRED HOME MAINTENANCE MANAGEMENT Inability to independently maintain a safe growth-promoting immediate environment.

Defining Characteristics

- Household members describe outstanding debts or financial crises
- Unwashed or unavailable cooking equipment, clothes, or linen
- Overtaxed family members (e.g., exhausted, anxious family members)
- Repeated hygienic disorders, infestations, or infections
- Disorderly surroundings
- Accumulation of dirt, food wastes, or hygienic wastes
- Offensive odors
- Inappropriate household temperature
- Lack of necessary equipment or aids
- Presence of vermin or rodents

Related Factors

- Inadequate support system
- Unfamiliarity with neighborhood resources
- Insufficient finances
- Disease or injury affecting vision

ALTERED ROLE PERFORMANCE Disruption in the way one perceives one's role performance.

Defining Characteristics

- Denial of role
- Change in self-perception of role
- Change in others' perception of role
- Change in physical capacity to resume role
- Unwillingness to discuss limitations
- Denial of loss of visual acuity
- Apathy
- Increasing dependence on others
- Refusal to take responsibility

Related Factors

- Visual (sensory) alteration
- Neurological alteration (i.e., cerebrovascular accident)
- Surgery (glaucoma, cataract, detached retina)
- Pain
- Trauma

SOCIAL ISOLATION Aloneness experienced by an individual and perceived as imposed by others and as a negative or threatened state.

Defining Characteristics

- Expresses feelings of aloneness imposed by others, rejection, or feelings of difference from others
- Perceived inadequacy of significant purpose in life or absence of purpose in life
- Seeks to be alone
- Sad, dull affect
- Uncommunicative, withdrawn, no eye contact
- Projects hostility in voice, behavior
- Preoccupation with own thoughts, repetitive meaningless actions
- Absence of supportive significant other(s): family, friends, group

Related Factors

- Alteration in physical appearance or mental status
- Unacceptable social behavior or values
- Altered state of wellness
- Inability to engage in satisfying personal relationships

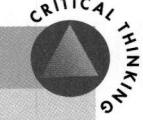

Nursing Diagnosis   *THE NEXT STEP—cont'd*

IMPAIRED SOCIAL INTERACTION The state in which an individual participates in an insufficient or excessive quantity or ineffective quality of social exchange.

Defining Characteristics

- Verbalized or observed discomfort in social situations
- Verbalized or observed inability to receive or communicate a satisfying sense of belonging, caring, interest, or shared history
- Observed use of unsuccessful social interaction behaviors
- Dysfunctional interaction with peers, family, and/or others
- Family report of change of style or patterns of interaction

Related Factors

- Knowledge/skill deficit (ways to enhance mutuality)
- Communication barriers
- Self-concept disturbance
- Absence of available significant others/peers
- Limited physical mobility due to visual impairment
- Environmental barriers
- Altered thought processes

Clinical Application

Mr. X. is a 52-year-old male admitted to the hospital for cardiac catheterization. He is one day post-procedure and is complaining of tearing and itching of both his eyes. Further assessment reveals redness of the conjunctiva, frequent tearing, and small amount of white-colored exudate on the lid margin and the inner aspects of each eye. Further questioning of patient reveals he has been treated before for conjunctivitis due to his many allergies during the spring season each year.

SUBJECTIVE DATA: Patient complains of:
Itching of both eyes
Frequent tearing of both eyes
Past treatment for conjunctivitis
Many allergies
Blurred vision

OBJECTIVE DATA: External Eye Physical Assessment:
Palpebral fissures equal, lids and lashes normal—slight amount of white exudate noted on top lashes of both eyes
Conjunctiva: LE: reddened; RE: reddened; engorgement of conjunctiva vessels noted on outer corners of both eyes; margins sharp.
Sclera: white except for a few small blood vessels at cornices.
Lacrimal apparatus: excessive tearing of both eyes; regurgitation of white flaky and sticky exudate from lacrimal sac.
Anterior chamber: normal depth; iris flat.
Pupils: equal round, react to light and accommodation (PERRLA).

NURSING DIAGNOSES

Sensory/perceptual alterations (visual) related to uncompensated visual loss.

Defining Characteristics

- Frequent tearing
- Frequent itching
- Blurred vision due to excessive tearing

Impaired physical mobility related to perceptual impairment (visual).

Defining Characteristics

- Blurred vision due to excessive tearing

GLOSSARY

accommodation Process by which the refractive power of the lens of the eye is increased through contraction of the ciliary muscle, which causes increased thickness and curvature of the lens. The accommodation response of the pupils consists of convergence of the eyes and constriction of the pupils as the gaze shifts from a distant to a near point.

adaptation Process by which the eye becomes more sensitive to either reduced or increased illumination.

amblyopia Reduced visual acuity in an eye that appears to be structurally normal.

anisocoria Condition in which the pupils of the two eyes are of unequal size.

aqueous humor Fluid secreted in the ciliary body, which is found in the anterior chamber of the eye.

arcus senilis Gray to white opaque ring that surrounds the cornea; generally occurs in individuals older than 50 years.

astigmatism Condition involving irregularity of the spherical curve of the cornea in which light rays cannot be focused in a point on the retina.

bitemporal hemianopsia Loss of vision in both temporal fields of vision.

blepharitis Inflammation of the eyelid margins.

caruncle Small, fleshy projection located at the inner canthus of the eye.

cataract Opacity of the lens of the eye.

chalazion Sebaceous cyst on the eyelid that is formed by distention of a meibomian gland.

choroid Thin, highly vascular membrane covering the posterior five-sixths of the eye located between the retina and the sclera.

ciliary body Thickened part of the vascular tunic of the eye that joins the iris with the anterior portion of the choroid; produces aqueous humor and regulates its outflow.

conjunctiva Mucous membrane that lines the inner surfaces of the eyelids and the anterior part of the sclera.

conjunctivitis Inflammation of the conjunctiva.

consensual reaction Constriction of the pupil of one eye when the other eye is being stimulated by light.

convergence Coordinated medial movement of the eyes in fixing on a near object.

cornea Convex, transparent anterior part of the eye that comprises one sixth of the outermost tunic of the eye bulb.

cupping Increased posterior curvature of the optic disc caused by the increased intraocular pressure of glaucoma, which gradually exerts pressure posteriorly against the optic disc.

dacryoadenitis Inflammation of the lacrimal gland.

dacryocystitis Inflammation of the lacrimal sac.

diplopia Double vision; simultaneous perception of two images for a single object.

dyscoria Abnormality in the shape of the pupil.

ectropion Turning outward of the margin of the eyelid.

enophthalmos Recession of the globe of the eye within the orbit.

entropion Inward turning of the eyelid.

epiphora Tearing that results from faulty drainage of the eyes.

esophoria Deviation of the visual axis of one eye toward that of the other eye that occurs in the absence of visual stimuli for fusion.

esotropia Strabismus characterized by an inward deviation of one eye relative to the other eye.

eversion Turning outward, as of the eyelid.

exophoria Deviation of the visual axis of one eye away from that of the other eye that occurs in the absence of visual stimuli for fusion.

exophthalmos Abnormal protrusion of one eye or both eyes.

exotropia Strabismus characterized by the outward deviation of one eye relative to the other.

field of vision Area simultaneously visible to a motionless eye.

floaters Spots that appear to drift in front of the eye and are caused by a shadow cast on the retina by vitreous debris.

fovea centralis Central spot of color vision on the retina that contains only cones and no rods.

glaucoma Ocular disease in which increased intraocular pressure causes atrophy and excavation of the optic nerve, producing visual field defects.

hemianopsia Defective vision or blindness in one half of the visual field.

homonymous Having the same name.

homonymous hemianopsia Blindness or defective vision in the right half or the left half of the visual field of both eyes.

hordeolum Inflammation of a sebaceous gland of the eyelid; sty.

hyperopia Farsightedness.

hyphema Blood in the anterior chamber of the eye.

hypopyon Purulent material in the anterior chamber of the eye.

iridescent vision Perception of halos around lights, particularly with corneal edema.

iritis Inflammation of the iris.

lacrimation Production of tears, especially in excess.

lens Transparent biconvex structure located behind the pupil and in front of the vitreous body.

lid lag Condition in which the eyelid margin is above the limbus and some sclera is visible; it may indicate thyroid disease.

limbus Edge of the cornea at the point where it meets the sclera.

macula Area of the retina where the receptors for color vision are most concentrated; located temporal to the optic disc.

meibomian gland One of several sebaceous glands that secrete sebum from their ducts on the posterior margin of each eyelid. The glands are embedded in the tarsal plate of each eyelid.

microaneurysm Outpouching in the wall of a capillary that appears as a red dot on the retina.

miosis Constriction of the pupil.

mydriasis Dilation of the pupil.

myopia Nearsightedness; condition in which parallel rays of light come to focus in front of the retina.

nicking Appearance of indentation of an optic vein where an arteriole crosses it.

night blindness Slow adjustment from bright to dim light.

nystagmus Involuntary rhythmic motion of the eye; may be horizontal, vertical, rotary, or mixed.

palpebra Eyelid.

palpebral fissure Opening between the upper eyelid and the lower eyelid when the eye is open.

papilledema Edema of the optic disc.

periorbital edema Accumulation of fluid in the eyelids and other tissues surrounding the eye.

phoria Mild weakness of the extraocular muscle(s); appears as deviation of the eye when fusion is suspended.

photophobia Abnormal intolerance of light.

physiologic cup (physiologic depression) Small depression just temporal to the center of the optic disc.

pinguecula Small, yellowish-white subconjunctival elevation located between the corneoscleral limbus and the canthus.

presbyopia Reduced capacity of the optic lens to accommodate; a condition that develops with advancing age.

pterygium Abnormal triangular thickening of the bulbar conjunctiva on the cornea, with the apex directed toward the pupil.

ptosis Drooping, as of the eyelid.

puncta Tiny apertures in the margins of each eyelid that open into the lacrimal ducts.

pupil Aperture in the iris that allows for the passage of light.

retina Delicate nervous tissue membrane of the eye that is continuous with the optic nerve; receives images of external objects and transmits visual impulses through the optic nerve to the brain.

retinal exudates White or yellow infiltrates that develop on the retina.

sclera Tough, inelastic opaque membrane that covers the posterior five sixths of the eye bulb; maintains the size and form of the bulb and attaches to muscles that move the bulb.

scotoma Islandlike area of blindness in the field of vision.

strabismus Condition in which the eyes are not simultaneously directed to the same object.

sty Inflammation of a sebaceous gland of the eyelid; also called hordeolum.

tropia Permanent deviation of the axis of an eye; strabismus.

vitreous humor Transparent substance contained in the posterior chamber of the eye.

xanthelasma Soft yellow spot or plaque that usually occurs in groups on the eyelids.

BIBLIOGRAPHY

Apple DJ, Rabb MF: *Ocular pathology: clinical applications and self-assessment,* ed 4, St Louis, 1991, Mosby–Year Book.

Arffa RC: *Grayson's diseases of the cornea,* ed 3, St Louis, 1991, Mosby–Year Book.

Boyd-Monk H: Assessing acquired ocular diseases, *Nurs Clin North Am* 25:4, 811-822, 1990.

Gordon M: *Manual of nursing diagnosis* 1993–1994, St Louis, 1993, Mosby–Year Book.

Hoskins HD, Kass MA: *Becker-Shaffer's diagnosis and therapy of the glaucomas,* ed 6, St Louis, 1989, Mosby–Year Book.

Lawlor MC: Common ocular injuries and disorders. I. Acute loss of vision, *J Emerg Nurs* 15:1, 32-43, 1989.

Newell FW: *Ophthalmology: principles and concepts,* ed 7, St Louis, 1992, Mosby–Year Book.

Sapira JD, Schneiderman H: The funduscopic examination: how to make the most of it, *Consultant* 30:6, 22-27, 1990.

Schneiderman H, Garibaldi RA: Physical examination of HIV-infected patients: head and neck, eyes, mouth and throat, and lymph nodes, *Consultant* 30:1, 42-51, 1990.

Small RG: Five steps toward a differential diagnosis, *Consultant* 31:7, 29-32, 1991.

Ears, Nose, Mouth, and Throat

PURPOSE OF EXAMINATION

The examination of the ears, nose, mouth, and throat is an important part of every physical examination because it provides the opportunity to inspect, directly or indirectly, most parts of the upper respiratory system and the first division of the digestive system. Examination of these body orifices provides information about the client's general health and the presence of any local disease. This chapter focuses on three areas: ears, nose and paranasal sinuses, and mouth and oropharynx.

ANATOMY AND PHYSIOLOGY

Ears

The ear is a sensory organ that functions both in hearing and in equilibrium. It is composed of three parts: the external ear, the middle ear, and the inner ear. Figure 12-1 illustrates the structures of the ear.

External ear. The external ear has two divisions, the flap called the **auricle,** or **pinna,** and the canal called the external auditory canal, or **meatus.** Stretching across the proximal portion of the canal is the **tympanic membrane** (eardrum), which separates the external ear from the middle ear. The auricle is composed of cartilage and skin. The main components of the auricle are the **helix,** anthelix, crus of helix, **lobule, tragus,** antitragus, and **concha** (Figure 12-2). The **mastoid process** is not part of the external ear; it is a bony prominence found posterior to the lower part of the auricle.

The external auditory canal, which is approximately 2.2 cm long, has a skeleton of cartilage in its outer third and a skeleton of bone in its inner two thirds. In adults, this skeleton curves slightly with the outer one third of the canal and is directed upward and toward the back of the head; the inner two thirds is directed downward and forward. The skin of the outer portion of the au-

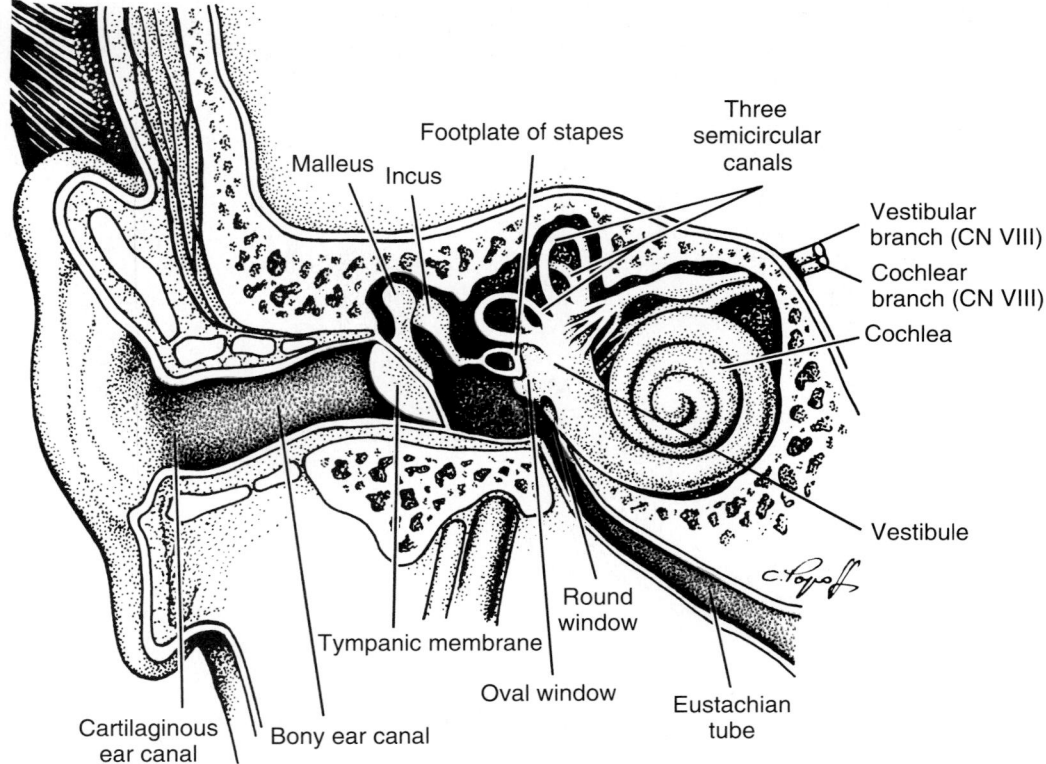

FIGURE 12-1 External auditory canal, middle ear, and inner ear.

ditory canal is hairy and contains **cerumen** (wax)-producing glands. The skin of the inner portion of the canal is very thin and sensitive.

Tympanic membrane. The tympanic membrane, which covers the proximal end of the auditory canal, is made up of layers of skin, fibrous tissue, and mucous membrane (Figure 12-3). The mucous membrane is

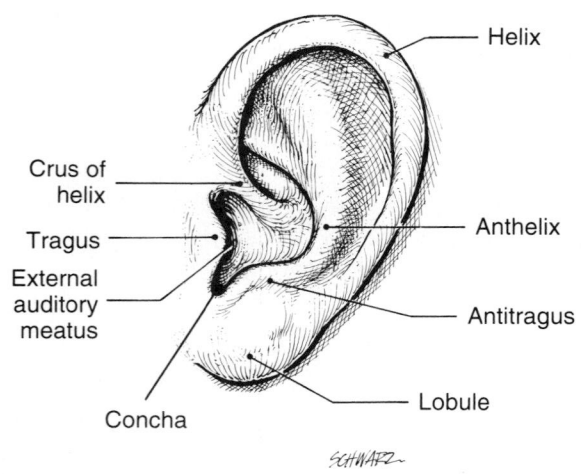

FIGURE 12-2 Structures of the external ear (pinna).

shiny, translucent, and pearl gray. The position of the eardrum is oblique with respect to the ear canal. The anteroinferior quadrant is most distant from the examiner. This positioning results in a reflex of light when a light is directed into the ear. This cone of light is located at the 5 o'clock position in the right ear and at the 7 o'clock position in the left ear.

The tympanic membrane, which is slightly concave, is pulled inward at its center by one of the ossicles of the middle ear called the **malleus.** The short process of the malleus protrudes into the eardrum superiorly, and the handle of the malleus extends downward from the short process to the umbo, the point of maximum concavity. Most of the tympanic membrane is taut and is known as the **pars tensa.** A small part located superiorly is less taut and is called the **pars flaccida.** The dense fibrous ring surrounding the tympanic membrane, except for the anterior and posterior malleolar folds superiorly, is the **annulus.**

Middle ear. The middle ear is an air-filled cavity located in the temporal bone. It contains three small bones called the **auditory ossicles:** malleus, **incus,** and **stapes.** The middle ear cavity contains several openings. One, which is from the external auditory meatus, is covered by the tympanic membrane. The two

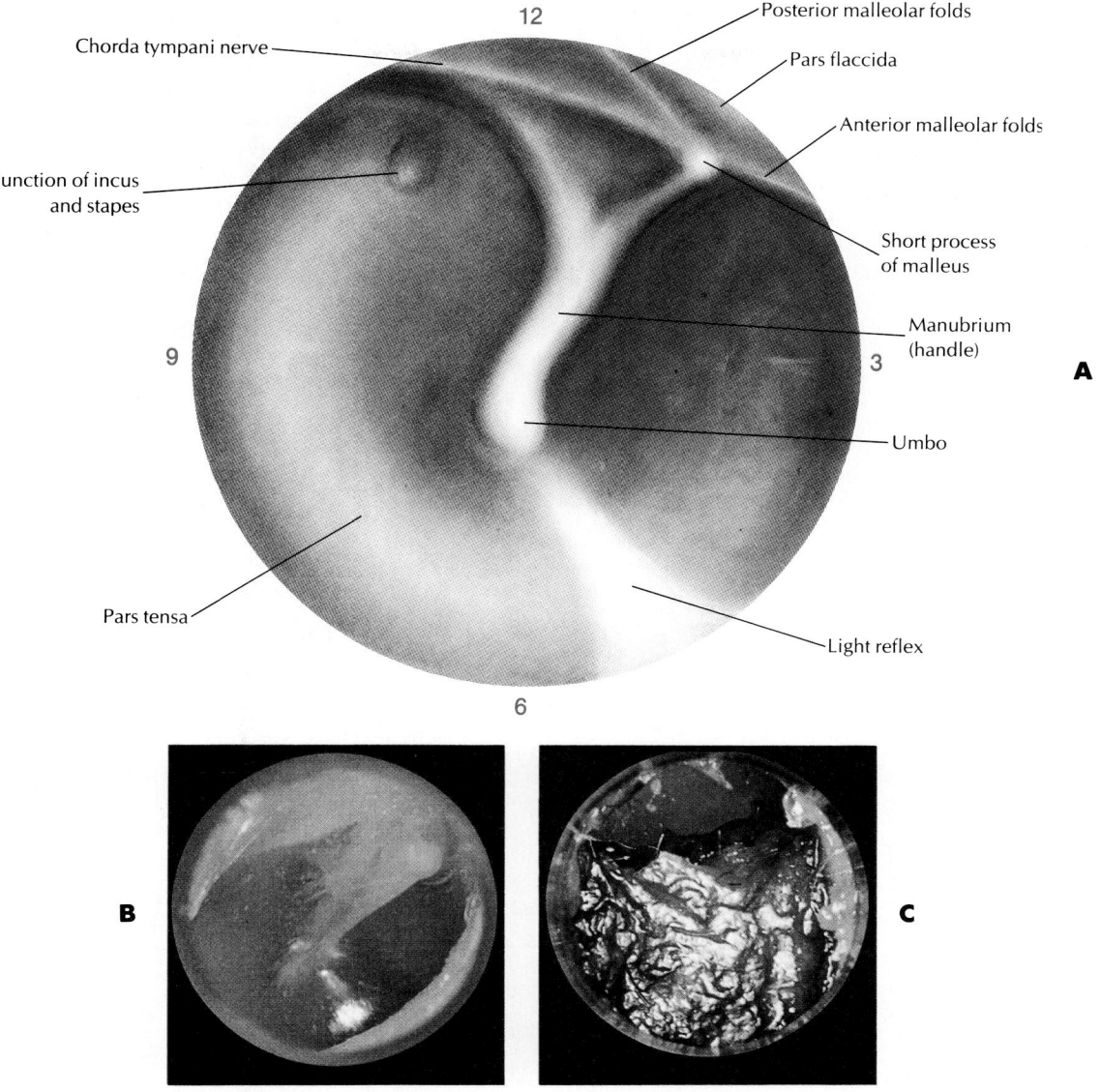

FIGURE 12-3 A, Usual landmarks of right tympanic membrane with "clock" superimposed.
B, Normal (right) tympanic membrane. **C**, External ear canal partially occluded with cerumen.
(A from Whaley LF, Wong DL: *Nursing care of infants and children,* ed 4, St Louis, 1991,
Mosby—Year Book. B and C courtesy Dr. Richard A. Buckingham, Clinical Professor, Otolaryn-
gology, Abraham Lincoln School of Medicine, University of Illinois, Chicago, Ill.)

openings into the inner ear are the oval window, into
which the stapes fits, and the round window, which is
covered by a membrane. Another opening connects the
middle ear with the **eustachian tube**.

The middle ear performs the following three functions:

1. Transmits sound vibrations across the ossicle
   chain to the inner ear's oval window.
2. Protects the auditory apparatus from intense vibrations.

3. Equalizes the air pressure on both sides of the
   tympanic membrane to prevent the membrane
   from being ruptured.

Inner ear. The two components of the inner ear are
the bony labyrinth and, inside this structure, a membranous labyrinth. The bony **labyrinth** consists of three
parts: **vestibule**, semicircular canals, and **cochlea**. The
vestibule and the semicircular canals comprise the organs of **equilibrium**. The cochlea is the organ of hear-

ing. A coiled structure that contains the organ of Corti, the cochlea transmits stimuli to the cochlear branch of the auditory nerve (cranial nerve [CN] VIII).

Pathways of hearing. Hearing occurs when sound waves enter the external auditory canal and strike the tympanic membrane, causing it to vibrate. The auricle does not direct or amplify sound. Its major function is to help perceive the direction of the source of sound (i.e., from behind or ahead). The vibrations are transmitted through the auditory ossicles of the middle ear to the oval window. From the oval window the vibra-

tions travel through the fluid of the cochlea, eventually reaching the round window, where they are dissipated. The vibrations of the membrane cause the delicate hair cells of the organ of Corti to beat against the membrane of Corti, acting as stimuli for impulses carried by the sensory endings of the cochlear branch of the auditory nerve (CN VIII) to the brain.

Nose and Paranasal Sinuses

The nose is the sensory organ for smell. It also warms, moistens, and filters the inspired air. The **paranasal**

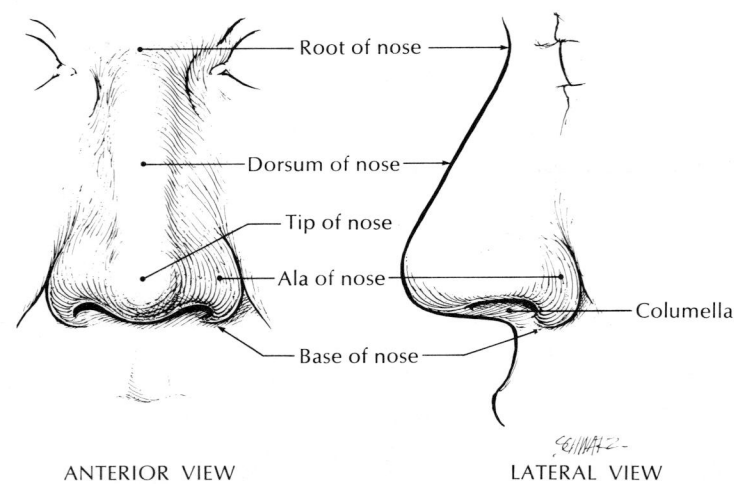

FIGURE 12-4 External structure of the nose.

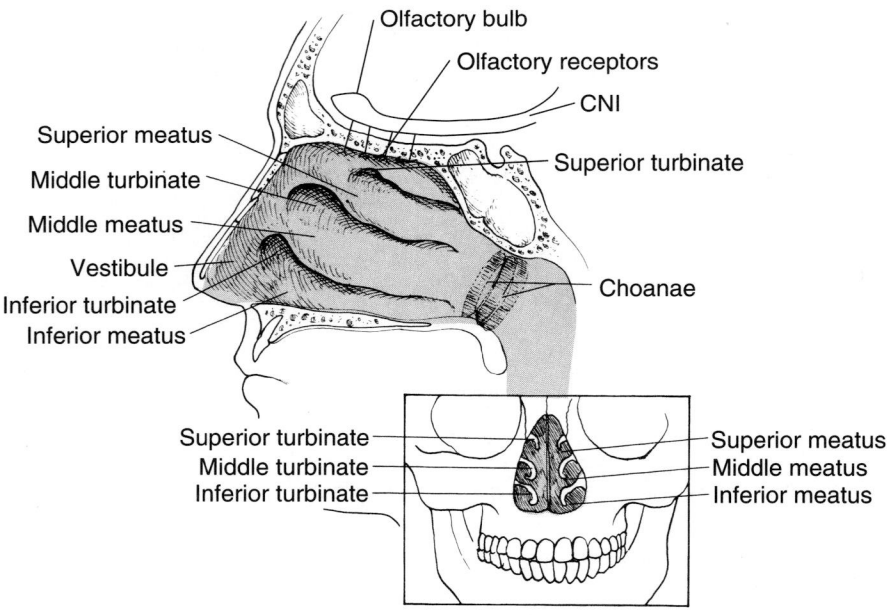

FIGURE 12-5 Lateral view of the left nasal cavity.

sinuses are air-filled cavities that make the skull lighter than it would otherwise be and perform the same functions as the nose—warming, moistening, and filtering air. These sinuses also aid in voice resonance.

The nose is composed of two parts, external and internal (nasal cavity) (Figure 12-4). The upper third of the nose is bone, and the remainder is cartilage. The nasal cavity is divided into two narrow cavities by the septum (Figure 12-5). The cavities have two openings. The anterior opening, which is the vestibule where the naris is located, is thickly lined with small hairs. The posterior opening, or **choana,** leads to the throat. The nasal septum forms the medial walls. The lateral walls are divided into the inferior, middle, and superior turbinate bones, which protrude into the nasal cavity. A highly vascular mucous membrane covers the turbinates. Below each turbinate is a meatus named according to the turbinate above it. The nasolacrimal duct drains into the inferior meatus, and most of the paranasal sinuses drain into the middle meatus. A plexus of blood vessels is located in the mucosa of the anterior nasal septum, which is a common site for **epistaxis** (nosebleeding).

The receptors for smell are located in the olfactory area, which is in the roof of the nasal cavity and the upper third of the septum. The receptor filament cells pass through openings of the cribriform plate, becoming the olfactory nerve (CN I), which transmits neural impulses for smell to the temporal lobe of the brain.

The paranasal sinuses are paired extensions of the nasal cavities within the bones of the skull. They are the frontal, maxillary, ethmoidal, and sphenoidal sinuses (Figure 12-6). Their openings into the nasal cavity are narrow and easily obstructed. The frontal sinuses are located in the anterior part of the frontal bone. The maxillary sinuses, the largest of the paranasal sinuses, are located in the body of the maxilla. The ethmoidal sinuses are small and occupy the ethmoidal labyrinth between the orbit of the eye and the upper part of the nasal cavity. The sphenoidal sinuses are found in the body of the sphenoid.

Mouth and Oropharynx

Mouth. The mouth is the first division of the digestive system and an entry site to the respiratory system. The oropharynx conducts air to and from the larynx and food from the mouth to the esophagus. The structures of the mouth and the oropharynx are illustrated in Figure 12-7. The boundaries of the mouth are the lips (anteriorly) and the soft palate and uvula (posteriorly). The mandibular bone, which is covered by loose, mobile tissue, forms the floor of the mouth. The hard and soft palates comprise the roof of the oral cavity. The soft palate is pink, and the hard palate is lighter. The **uvula** is a muscular organ that hangs down from the posterior margin of the soft palate. The muscles of **mastication** (chewing) are innervated by two main nerves: the trigeminal nerve (CN V) and the facial nerve (CN VII). The mouth contains the tongue, gums, teeth, and salivary glands.

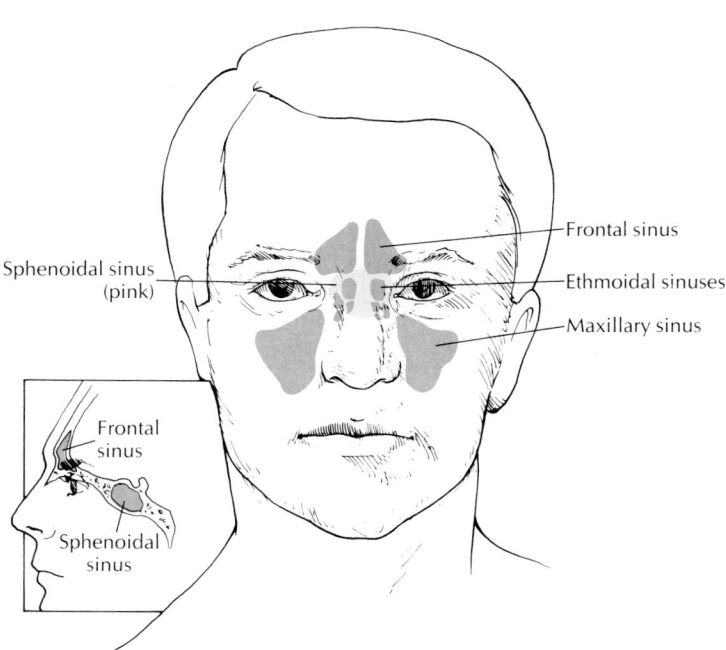

FIGURE 12-6 Anterior view of the frontal and maxillary sinuses.

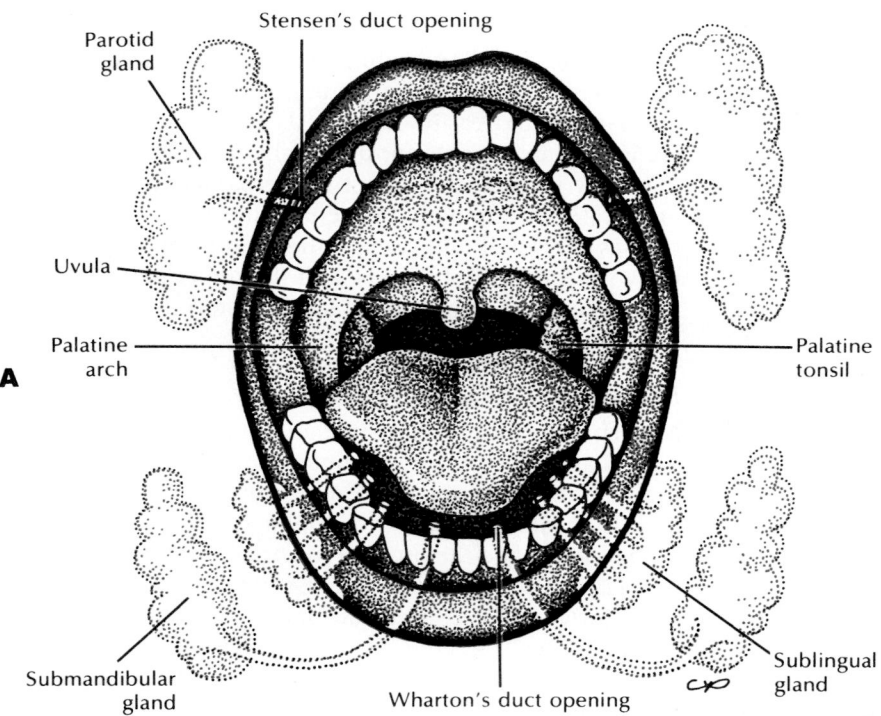

Parotid gland

Stensen's duct opening

Uvula

Palatine arch

A

Palatine tonsil

Submandibular gland

Wharton's duct opening

Sublingual gland

FIGURE 12-7 A and **B**, Structures of the mouth. **C**, The mouth and oropharnyx.

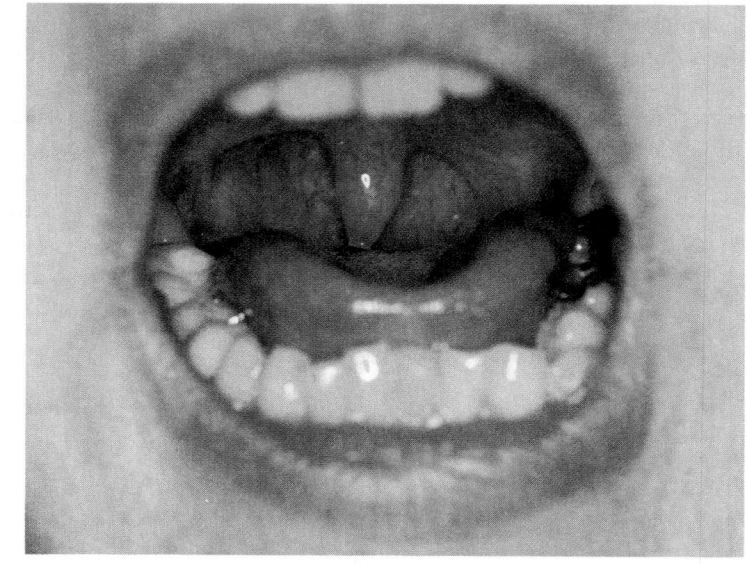

C

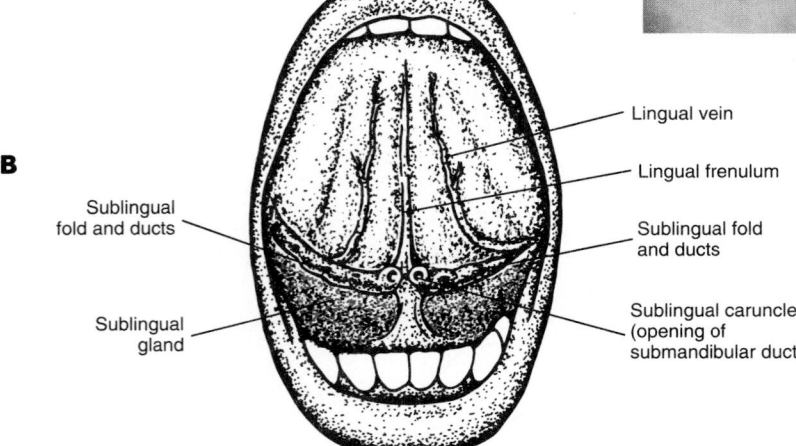

B

Lingual vein

Lingual frenulum

Sublingual fold and ducts

Sublingual fold and ducts

Sublingual gland

Sublingual caruncle (opening of submandibular duct)

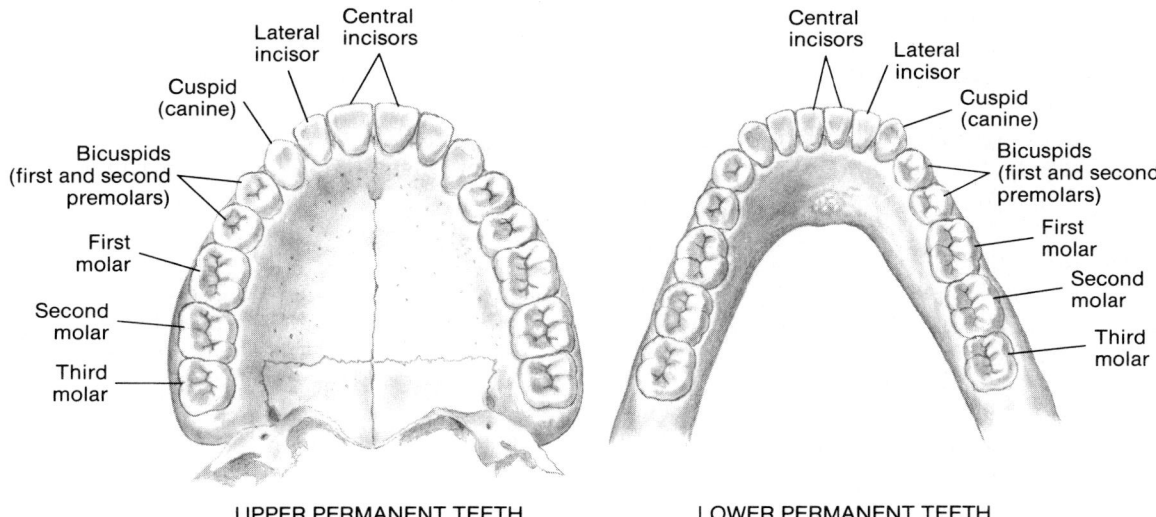

UPPER PERMANENT TEETH   LOWER PERMANENT TEETH

FIGURE 12-8 Upper and lower permanent teeth (From Seidel HM and others: *Mosby's guide to physical examination,* St. Louis, 1987, Mosby–Year Book.)

Tongue. The tongue is composed of a mass of striated muscles interspersed with fat and many glands. The dorsal surface is rough because of the presence of papillae. The ventral surface toward the floor of the mouth is smooth and shows large veins. The fold of mucous membrane that joins the tongue to the floor of the mouth is called the **frenulum.** The tongue is innervated by the hypoglossal nerve (CN XII). The sensory receptors for taste are the glossopharyngeal nerve (CN IX) for the posterior third of the tongue and the facial nerve (CN VII) for the anterior two thirds of the tongue.

Gums and teeth. The gums, fibrous tissue covered with a smooth mucous membrane, are attached to the alveolar margins of the jaws and to the necks of the teeth. An adult normally has 32 teeth, 16 in each arch (Figure 12-8).

Salivary glands. Three pairs of salivary glands secrete into the oral cavity. They are the parotid, submandibular, and sublingual salivary glands. The largest is the parotid gland, which lies in front of and below the external ear. The parotid (Stensen's) duct opens into the **buccal** membrane opposite the second molar. The submandibular gland lies below and in front of the parotid gland. The submandibular (Wharton's) duct opens at the side of the frenulum on the floor of the mouth. The sublingual gland, the smallest salivary gland, lies in the floor of the mouth and covers its superior surface to form the sublingual fold. The sublingual gland has numerous small openings, which open onto the sublingual fold (see Figure 12-7, *A-B*).

Oropharynx. The **oropharynx** is the section of the pharynx that is posterior to the oral cavity and most accessible to examination (see Figure 12-7, *C*). The nasopharynx lies behind the nasal cavities and is superior to the oropharynx. The laryngopharynx is inferior to the oropharynx. Along both lateral walls of the oropharynx are two palatine arches, and between these arches lie the tonsils. The tonsils are usually the same color as the surrounding tissue and do not normally extend beyond the pillars. Tonsillar tissue in children enlarges until puberty, when it shrinks back into the folds of the arches. Consequently, a child's tonsils may normally be larger than an adult's. The posterior pharyngeal wall that is visible during the clinical examination may show many small blood vessels and small areas of pink or red lymphoid tissue.

EXAMINATION

Health History

Throughout the health history interview, record the following data about a symptom or problem: (1) onset (specific date, sudden or gradual), (2) duration, (3) frequency, (4) precipitating factors, (5) aggravating or alleviating factors, (6) treatment received or self-care given, and (7) outcome.

1. Present health status
   a. Hearing loss
   b. Pain or discomfort: in ears, nose, mouth, or throat; pain or pressure around eyes, cheeks, or forehead
   c. Drainage from ears or nose
   d. Seasonal allergies or allergies to medications or food

e. Condition of teeth and gums: presence of dentures or braces, bleeding gums, ability to chew
f. Reduced ability to smell or presence of unusual odors
g. Unusual tastes or reduced ability to taste
h. Difficulty swallowing
i. Dental hygiene practices; frequency of dental checkups
j. Ear wax buildup
2. Past health history
    a. Any injury to nose, ears, mouth, or teeth
    b. Previous surgery of ears, nose, mouth, or teeth, including tonsillectomy
    c. Ringing in ears or dizziness
    d. History of frequent nosebleeds
    e. History of ear infections
3. Family health history
    a. Family history of hearing loss
4. Other considerations
    a. Exposure to loud noise
    b. Exposure to fumes or dust
    c. Use of protective gear for work or hobbies: earwear, safety goggles, face mask

Preparation for Examination: Client and Environment

The methods of examination for the ears, nose, mouth, and throat are primarily inspection and palpation.

The client should be seated for this examination. The examiner's head should be at approximately the same level as that of the client. A good light source, such as a gooseneck lamp with a 100- to 150-watt bulb, is helpful.

Tuning fork tests are useful in determining whether the client has a conductive or a perceptive (sensorineural) hearing loss. A fork with frequencies of 512 to 1024 hertz (Hz) is used because it provides an estimate of hearing loss in the speech frequencies of roughly 300 to 3000 Hz. The tuning fork should be held by the base without the fingers touching either of the two prongs. The sound vibrations are softened or stopped entirely when the prongs of the fork are touched or held. The fork is activated by stroking it between the thumb and index finger (Figure 12-9, *A*) or by tapping the tines on the knuckles of the opposite hand (Figure 12-9, *B*). The fork should be made to ring softly.

A
B

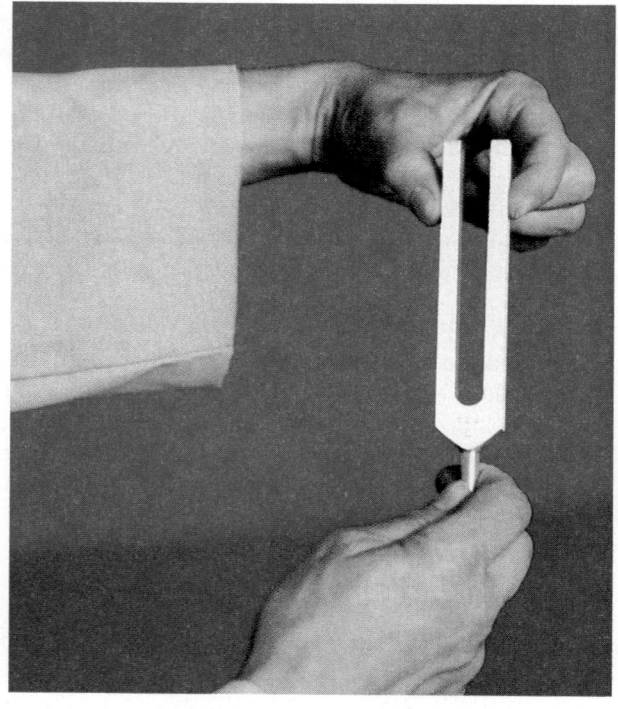
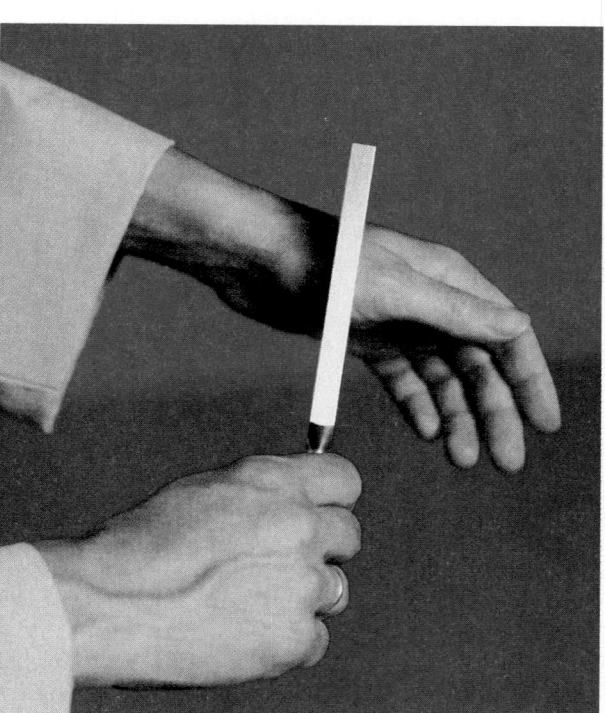

FIGURE 12-9 Activating the tuning fork. **A,** Stroking the fork. **B,** Tapping the fork on the knuckle.

Preparation for Examination

Equipment

Item	Purpose
Otoscope with various size speculums	Inspection of tympanic membrane; external auditory canal
Tongue blade	To help visualize oropharynx
4 x 4–inch gauze sponges	To grasp tongue for inspection
Disposable latex gloves (see Safety First box, Chapter 7)	For palpation of mouth
Tuning fork (512 cycles/sec [cps])	To assess hearing
Penlight	To visualize mouth, nasal turbinates, and oropharynx

Optional Equipment

Item	Purpose
Dental mirror	To visualize teeth
Nasal speculum	To visualize nasal turbinates

Client and Environment

Client should be seated, preferably near a good light source.

Examination Technique and Normal Findings

Ears

External ear. Begin the examination of the external ear with an inspection of both auricles to determine their horizontal and vertical position, size, and symmetry. The helix should be at or slightly above a line extending from the eye to the occipital area. Next inspect the lateral and medial surfaces of each auricle and the surrounding tissues for skin color and the presence of deformities, lesions, or nodules. Palpate the auricles and mastoid areas for evidence of swelling, tenderness, or nodules.

Manipulation of the auricle can be helpful in detecting tenderness. Ordinarily the client with otitis media has no discomfort. If pressure on the tragus or gently pulling on the auricle causes pain, the client may have external otitis. Although fairly simple, this part of the examination is frequently neglected (Figure 12-10, *A*).

External auditory canal. Examination of the external auditory canal and tympanic membrane requires an otoscope for additional lighting. Before inserting the speculum in the client's ear, carefully inspect the opening of the auditory canal for erythema (redness), swelling, narrowing of the canal, a foreign body, or discharge. Describe the appearance and odor of any discharge. A putrid odor may indicate mastoid disease involving bone destruction. After this inspection, insert the speculum.

> **Helpful Hint:** *For the otoscope to be effective, the batteries should be changed or recharged frequently to ensure good light.*

Inspect the auditory canal for cerumen, erythema, foreign bodies, or swelling. The appearance of the normal canal varies in diameter, shape, and growth of hairs (Figure 12-10, *B*).

Evaluate cerumen, which is produced by the sebaceous glands and the apocrine (sweat) glands in the outer third of the external auditory canal. A small amount of cerumen will not interfere with the examination. You can look past it and visualize the tympanic membrane. However, if cerumen is excessive, removing it may be necessary.

> **Helpful Hint:** *Racial variations in color of cerumen occur. Black or brown cerumen will be noted in the client with dark skin coloring. The color of fresh cerumen is light yellow or even pink as compared with older, drier cerumen, which is a darker yellowish-brown.*

Tympanic membrane. The examination of the tympanic membrane (see Figure 12-3, *A*) requires a careful assessment of the color of the membrane and the identification of landmarks. The membrane is usually translucent pearl gray, but when disease is present, it may be yellow, white, red, or dull gray. Some membranes have white flecks or dense white plaques, which are the result of healed inflammatory disease.

Identify landmarks, beginning with the light reflex, which is a triangular cone of reflected light seen in the anteroinferior quadrant of the membrane. This landmark is at the 5 o'clock position on the right tympanic membrane and at the 7 o'clock position on the left. At the top point of the light reflex toward the center of the membrane is the **umbo**, the inferior point of the handle of the malleus. Anterior and superior to the umbo lies the long process of the malleus, which appears as a whitish line extending from the umbo to the malleolar folds, where the short process of the malleus can be seen. The malleolar folds and the pars flaccida, the relaxed portion of the membrane, are superior and lateral to the short process, respectively. Finally, observe the

STEPS IN USING AN OTOSCOPE

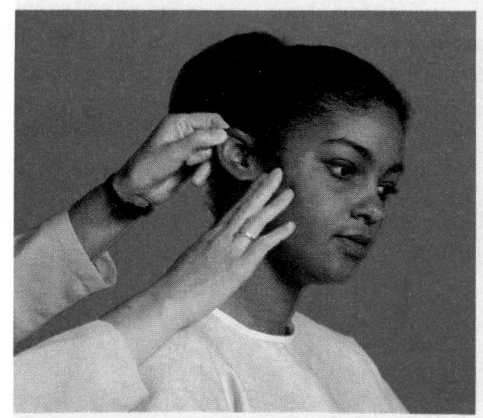

1. Use the largest speculum that can be inserted in the ear without causing pain.
2. Tip the client's head away from you for easy examination of the canal and the tympanic membrane.
3. In adults, straighten the ear canal by pulling the auricle upward and backward. In young children and infants, straighten the canal by pulling the auricle downward (Figure 12-10).
4. The inner two thirds of the external meatus is very sensitive to pressure. Insert the speculum gently to minimize discomfort.
5. Vary the angle at which you insert the speculum into the meatus to obtain the best view of the tympanic membrane.

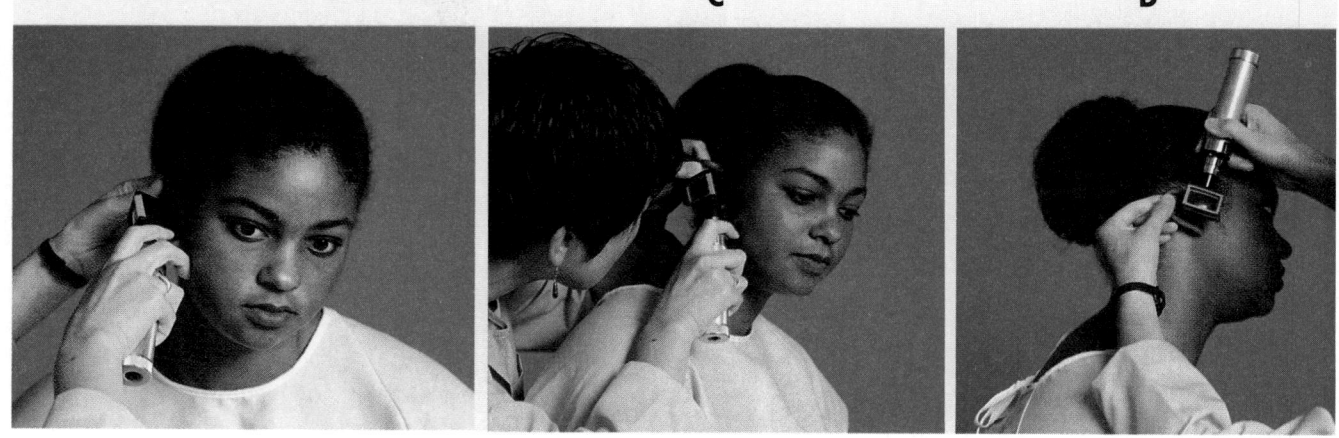

FIGURE 12-10 Examination of the ear with the otoscope. **A**, Inspection of the meatus. **B**, Client's head is tipped toward the opposite shoulder. **C** and **D**, Two ways of holding the otoscope.

periphery of the pars tensa. Perforations are frequently noted in the areas close to the annulus.

Normal tympanic membranes vary in size, shape, and color. By examining many normal, healthy membranes, an examiner acquires the ability to recognize the abnormal membrane.

Testing auditory function. Testing of auditory function starts early in the physical examination. Because the client's understanding of the spoken word is the principal use of hearing, an impairment of auditory function may become apparent during the interview. Specific testing of auditory function should be delayed until the end of the examination, after any obvious problems related to hearing have been identified. Al-

though the precise measurement of hearing requires the use of the audiometer, a good estimate of hearing during the physical examination can be made by using the tests discussed in the following sections.

AUDITORY ACUITY. Simple assessment of auditory acuity requires that only one ear be tested at a time. Therefore it is necessary to mask the hearing in the ear not being tested. Occlude (or have the client occlude) one of the client's ears by gently placing a finger against the opening of the auditory canal.

Voice tests are frequently used to estimate the client's hearing. Begin testing with a very low whisper. Your lips should be 30 to 60 cm (1 or 2 feet) away from the client's unoccluded ear. Softly whisper numbers that the client is to repeat. If necessary, increase the intensity of the whispered voice. To prevent lip-reading during the voice tests, stand behind the client. If being in front of the client is more convenient, ask the client to close his or her eyes.

The terms *bone conduction* and *air conduction* must be clearly understood (see following discussion of tuning fork tests). Air conduction is the transmission of sound through the ear canal, tympanic membrane, and ossicles to the cochlea and the auditory nerve. Sound transmitted through the bones of the skull to the cochlea and the auditory nerve is bone conduction. The client with normal auditory function will hear sound twice as long by air conduction, when the tuning fork is held near the external meatus, than by bone conduction, when the base of the tuning fork is placed on the mastoid bone. Explain these tests to the client before the examination so that he or she can fully cooperate.

TUNING FORK TESTS. To conduct the **Weber test**, which makes use of bone conduction, place the base of the vibrating tuning fork on the vertex of the skull or on the forehead (Figure 12-11). Ask the client if the sound is clearer in one ear or in the other. In a normal Weber test, the client reports hearing sound equally in both ears. In lateralization, sound is detected differently in each ear. In conductive deafness, the sound is lateralized (heard louder) to the deafer ear. This situation occurs because extraneous sounds in the environment will not disturb the cochlea on the weaker side; these

sounds are not transmitted because of a problem or defect in the ear canal or middle ear. In sensorineural hearing loss, the sound lateralizes to the better ear because the cochlea or auditory nerve is functioning more effectively.

The **Rinne test** makes use of air conduction and bone conduction. The tuning fork is used to compare the conduction of sound through the mastoid bone and the auditory meatus (Table 12-1). The client who has no conductive hearing loss will hear the sound twice as long by air conduction (AC) as by bone conduction (BC). This normal pattern is called a positive Rinne test (AC > BC) (Figure 12-12). To perform the Rinne test, place the activated tuning fork against the mastoid bone until the client can no longer hear the sound. Then move the fork close to the auditory meatus. The client with no conductive hearing loss will continue to hear the sound by air conduction. A negative Rinne test, a finding in conductive hearing loss, occurs when the client hears sound through bone conduction as long or longer than air conduction (AC = BC or AC < BC). The examiner can also time the duration in seconds or by the ratio of sound perceived by air and bone conduction (AC:BC 2:1).

Data from both tests need to be considered together to determine conductive or sensorineural loss. Tuning fork test results are difficult to interpret when hearing loss is mixed.

Nose and paranasal sinuses. Inspect the external portion of the nose for any deviations in shape, size, or color. Check the nares for flaring or discharge. Palpate the ridge and soft tissues of the nose for displacement of the bone and cartilage and for tenderness or masses (Figure 12-13).

Examination of the nasal function includes determination of the ability to smell and the patency of the nasal cavities. To determine patency, ask the client to breathe in through the nose while you occlude one naris with a finger. Repeat the procedure to determine the patency of the opposite naris. To determine the ability to smell, ask the client to close the eyes. Occlude one naris again. Place an aromatic substance, such as coffee or alcohol, close to the client's nose and ask the client to identify the odor. Test each side separately. Olfaction is not routinely tested in a screening examination unless a client describes a change or loss in the ability to smell.

To examine the nasal cavities, use an otoscope with the short, broad nasal speculum. Alternatively, use a penlight to shine a light while using your nondominant thumb to push the tip of the nose upward. The second method is easier to perform and more comfortable for the client (Figure 12-14).

Examination of the nasal cavity through the anterior naris is limited to the vestibule, the anterior portion of

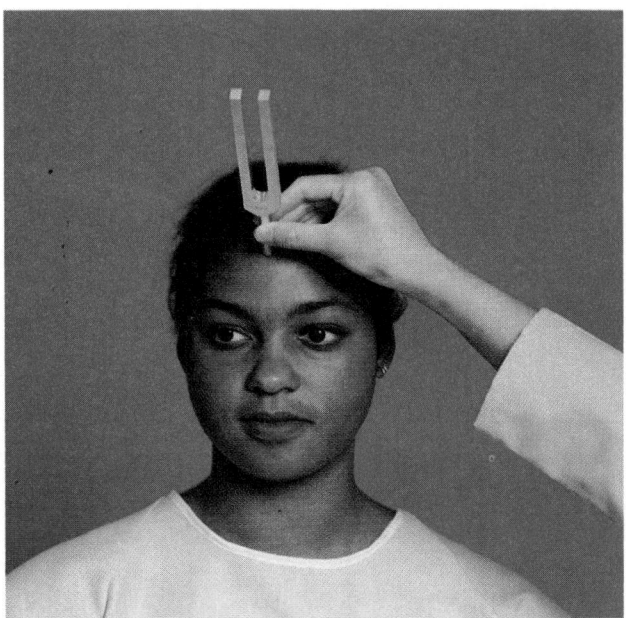

FIGURE 12-11 Weber test.

TABLE 12-1

Hearing Tests Using Tuning Fork

Hearing	Weber (bone conduction)	Rinne (air and bone conduction)

Normal

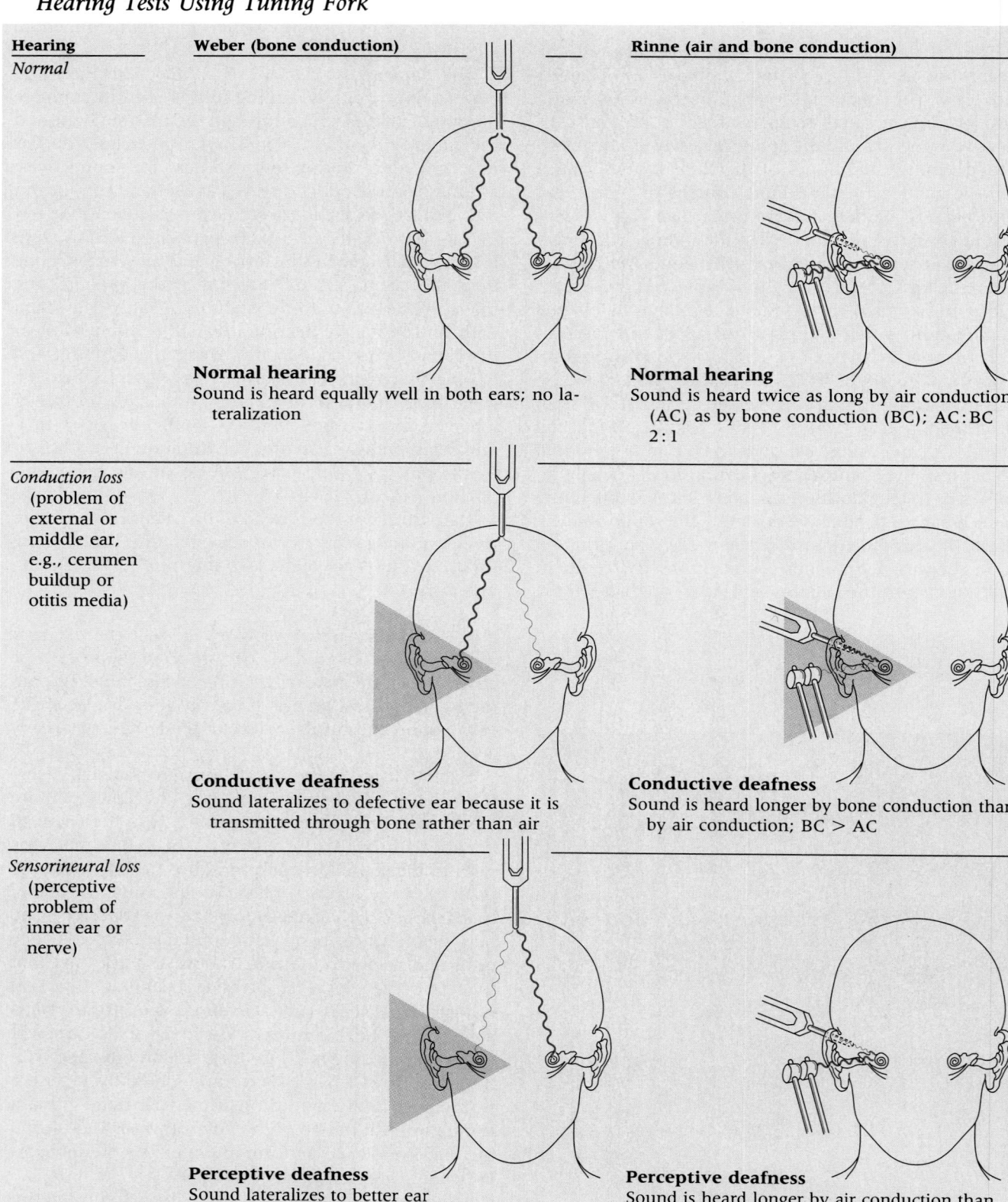

Normal hearing
Sound is heard equally well in both ears; no lateralization

Normal hearing
Sound is heard twice as long by air conduction (AC) as by bone conduction (BC); AC:BC 2:1

Conduction loss (problem of external or middle ear, e.g., cerumen buildup or otitis media)

Conductive deafness
Sound lateralizes to defective ear because it is transmitted through bone rather than air

Conductive deafness
Sound is heard longer by bone conduction than by air conduction; BC > AC

Sensorineural loss (perceptive problem of inner ear or nerve)

Perceptive deafness
Sound lateralizes to better ear

Perceptive deafness
Sound is heard longer by air conduction than by bone conduction (AC > BC) but for a shorter duration than with normal hearing

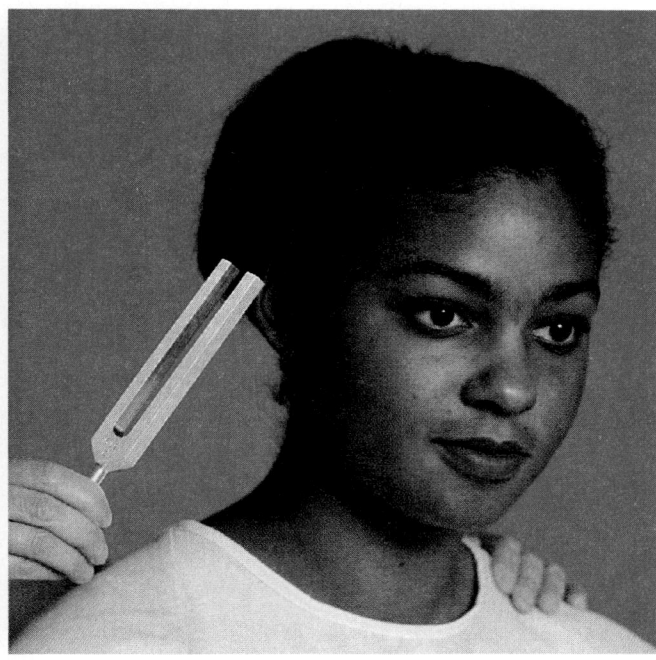

FIGURE 12-12 Rinne test. **A**, Bone conduction. **B**, Air conduction.

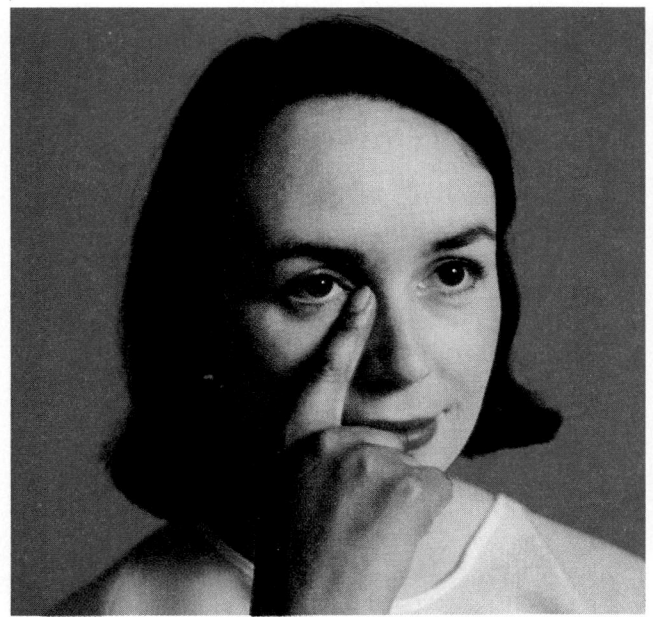

FIGURE 12-13 Palpation of external nose.

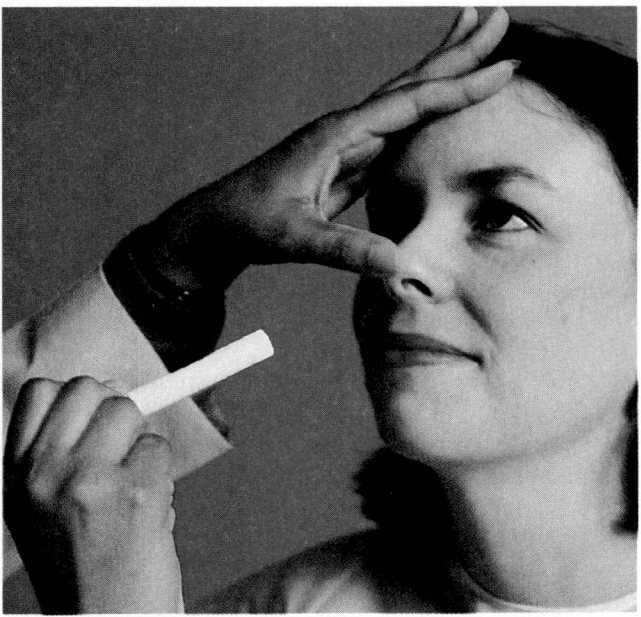

FIGURE 12-14 Examination of the anterior nasal cavity. Examiner thumb pressure on tip of the nose enhances visualization.

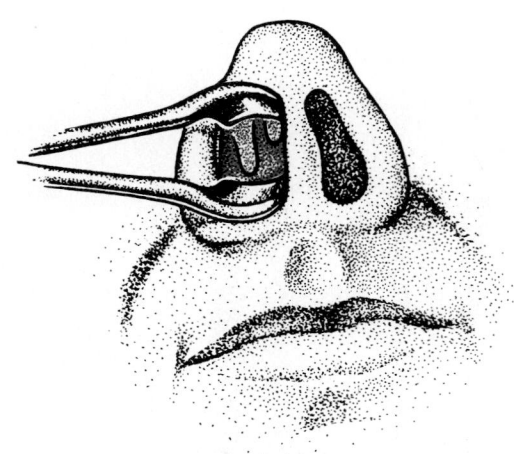

FIGURE 12-15 Examination of the anterior nasal cavity. View of the inferior and middle turbinates.

the septum, and the inferior and middle turbinates. When the client's head is tipped back, the inferior and middle turbinates can be seen (Figure 12-15). Inspect the septum for deviation, exudate, and perforation. Asymmetry of the nasal septum is normal. Examine the lateral walls of the nasal cavities and the inferior and middle turbinates for polyps, swelling, exudate, and color. The nasal mucosa is normally redder than the oral mucosa. Increased redness indicates infection. Pale turbinates are typical of allergy, whereas redness with edema may indicate localized irritation.

Describe any drainage from the middle meatus, which drains several of the paranasal sinuses. Carefully inspect the floor of the vestibule for evidence of a foreign body. Note the character of nasal secretions. The normal nasal secretion is mucoid. Watery secretions may indicate an acute upper respiratory infection or an allergic rhinitis. Purulent, crusty, or bloody secretions are abnormal.

Examination of the paranasal sinuses is performed indirectly. Inspection, percussion, and palpation of the overlying tissues and transillumination are used. Only the frontal and maxillary sinuses are accessible for examination. Palpate or percuss the maxillary sinuses over the maxillary areas of the cheeks to elicit any tenderness. By palpating both cheeks simultaneously, it is possible to determine differences in tenderness. Palpate the frontal sinuses by applying finger pressure below the eyebrows (Figure 12-16). Then percuss both the maxillary and the frontal sinuses for tenderness by lightly tapping the area with the index finger.

Mouth and oropharynx. Inspect the lips for symmetry, color, edema, or surface abnormalities. Ask the client to open and close the mouth to demonstrate the

mobility of the mandible and the occlusion of the teeth. While the client's mouth is opened wide and then closed, palpate the temporomandibular joint for tenderness, **crepitus**, or deviation (Figure 12-17). Pressure applied to the joint during closing of the mouth may result in referred pain to the ear, often caused by malocclusion. Palpate the lips for induration.

> **Helpful Hint:** *Conduct the examination from the anterior to the posterior areas of the mouth. Begin with the external components of the mouth and jaw.*

A good source of additional light is essential for examination of the mouth and throat. If the client wears dentures, ask him or her to remove them for the remainder of the examination.

The oral mucosal surfaces are normally light pink and moistened by saliva. Examine the surfaces systematically to ensure that you inspect all areas (Figure 12-18). Use a tongue depressor or your fingers as retractors. With the client's mouth partially open, inspect the mucosa in the anteroinferior area between the lower lip and gum. With the client's mouth wide open, examine the buccal mucosa and Stensen's duct (the opening to the parotid gland, opposite the upper second molar) of each cheek for patency or inflammation. Next examine the maxillary mucobuccal fold between the upper lip and gum.

Inspect the tongue for swelling, variation in size or color, coating, or ulceration. To test the function of the hypoglossal nerve (CN XII), ask the client to extend the tongue and observe for deviation, tremor, or limitation of movement. To inspect the posterior and lateral areas of the tongue, hold the extended tongue with a gloved hand (Figure 12-19). A 4 x 4–inch piece of gauze wrapped around the tip will make this step easier. Move the tongue to each side to inspect the lateral borders. Release the tongue and ask the client to touch the tip of the tongue to the palate. Observe the ventral surface for swelling or varicosities. Inspect the floor of the mouth for abnormalities or swelling. Identify Wharton's ducts (the openings of the submandibular glands), the frenulum, and the sublingual ridge. Because some abnormalities cause little change in the surface and can be detected only by palpation, use a gloved hand to palpate the entire tongue and floor of the mouth carefully.

The examination of the teeth and gums is not a substitute for a dental examination, but it should reveal gross problems that need attention. Use a dental mirror to reflect the surfaces of the teeth and gums that are not readily visible. Systematically inspect the teeth for decay (**caries**), missing teeth, and malocclusions so that each tooth of one arch is visualized before those of the

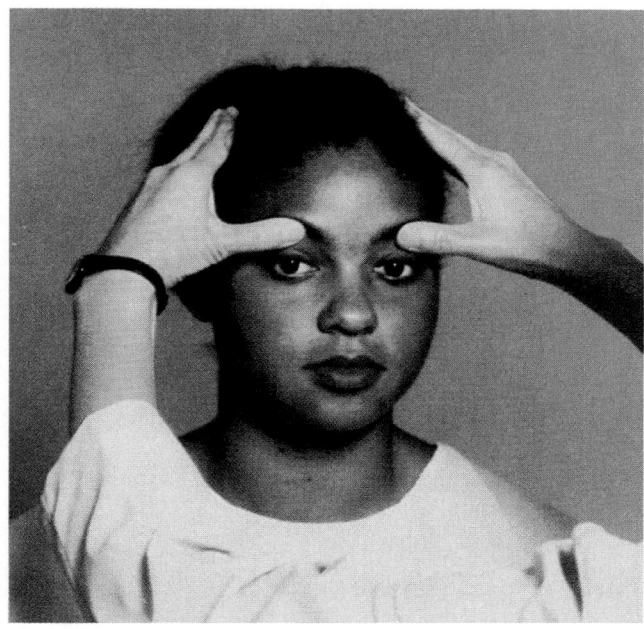
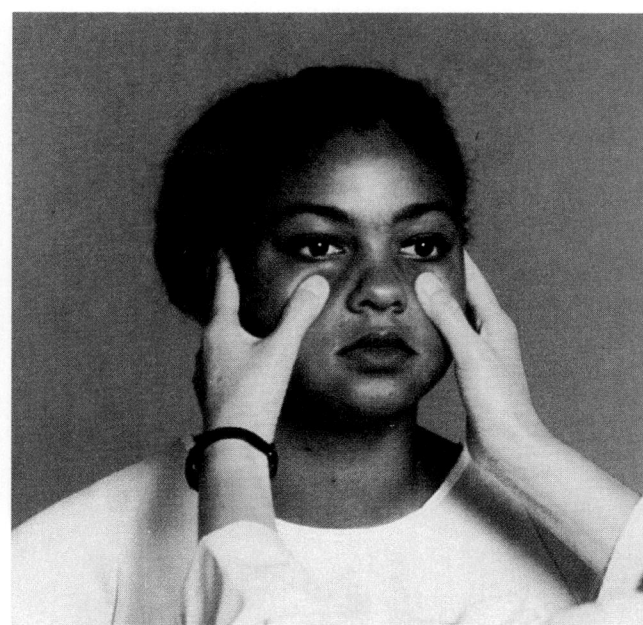

A

B

FIGURE 12-16 Palpation of the frontal **(A)** and maxillary **(B)** sinuses.

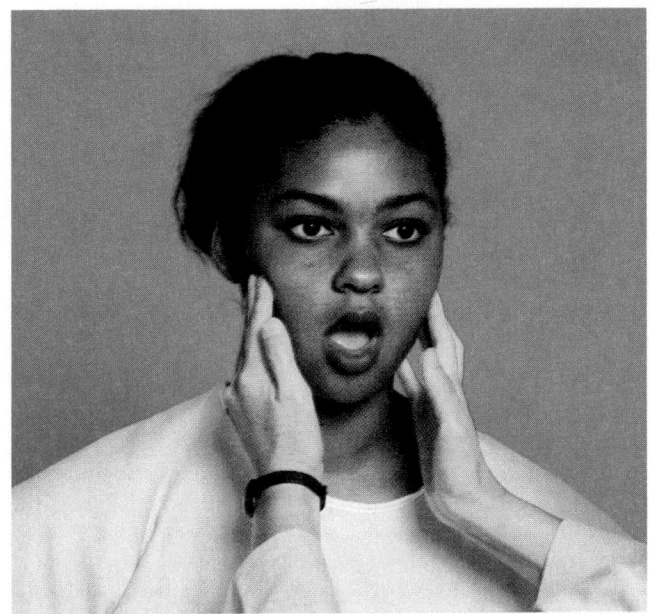

FIGURE 12-17 Palpation of the temporomandibular joint.

other arch are inspected. Any soft discolorations on the crown of a tooth should be suspected as carious. Inspect the gums for signs of inflammation and hemorrhage (**gingivitis**). With the client's head tipped back, inspect the palate and the uvula. Depressing the base of the tongue with a tongue blade may be necessary to visualize these structures better. Note the difference in color of the hard and the soft palate and any abnormality of architecture. Ask the client to say "ah," and note the rise of the soft palate and uvula. Any lack of, or asymmetry of, movement indicates impairment of the vagus nerve (CN X) or the glossopharyngeal nerve (CN IX).

> **Helpful Hint:** *When examining the throat, ask the client to open wide and say "ah" with the tongue extended. Most people will be able to lower the tongue and open sufficiently to allow visualization of the pharynx. Use a tongue blade only if necessary because many clients will involuntarily gag when an object is placed in the mouth. Ask a child to take a deep breath with the mouth open to flatten the tongue.*

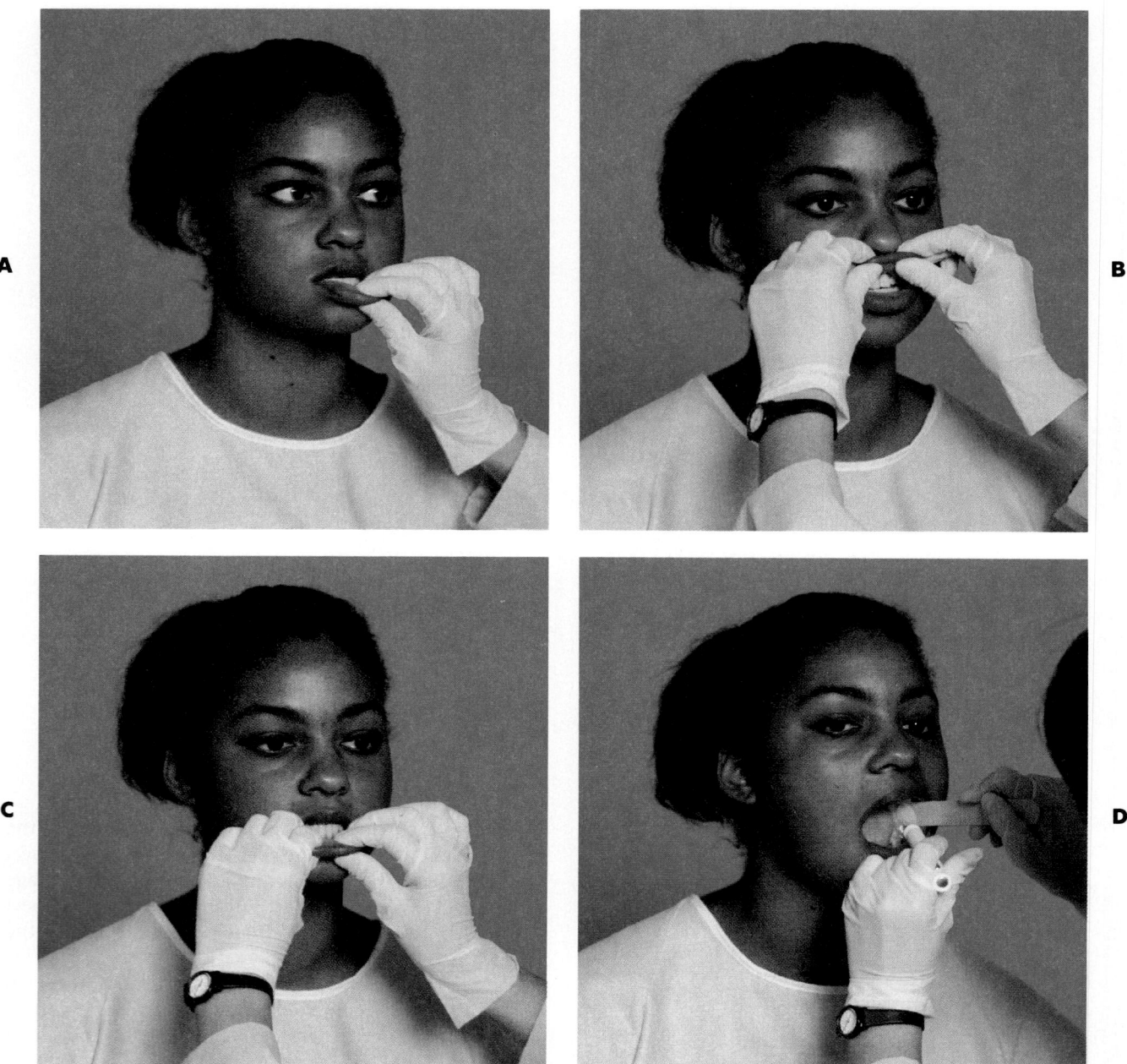

FIGURE 12-18 Examination of the lips and oral mucosa. **A**, Palpation of the lips. **B** and **C**, Inspection of the mucosa of the upper and lower anterior area. **D**, Inspection of mucosa of each cheek with identification of Stensen's duct opening.

Inspect the oropharynx while the client's head is tilted back, and gently depress the base of the tongue with a tongue depressor. Inspect the anterior palatine arches and the posterior arches for inflammation or swelling. Describe the size of the tonsils and note any exudate or postnasal discharge. Note the color of the posterior wall of the oropharynx. Test the glossopharyngeal nerve and the vagus nerve by either (1) having the client say "ah" and observing the uvula and soft palate rise symmetrically, or (2) touching the posterior wall of the pharynx on each side. The normal response to the second method is a gag reflex.

Throughout the examination of the mouth and throat, note any mouth odors, which may result from systemic or oral disease.

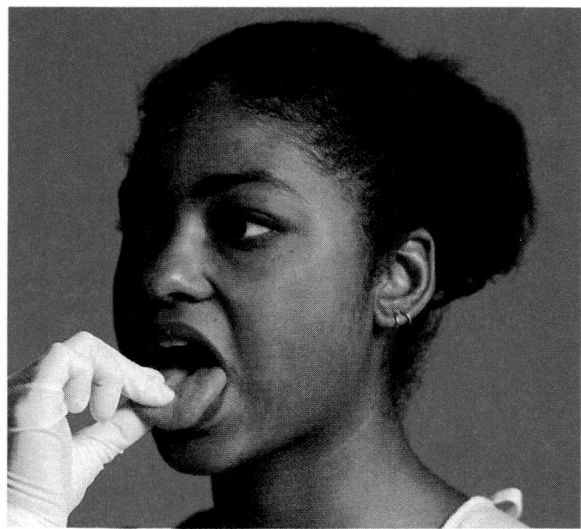

FIGURE 12-19 Examination of the tongue.

Special maneuvers

Cerumen removal. The methods for removing cerumen (earwax) buildup are curettage and irrigation. Curettage is indicated if the cerumen is soft or if the tympanic membrane might be perforated. However, this maneuver should be done only by a skilled clinician using an instrument called a curette or a cerumen spoon. The closeness of blood vessels and nerves to the surface of the auditory canal makes it easy to cause bleeding and pain. The risk also exists of perforating the tympanic membrane if the client moves or if the curette is used too vigorously. Use irrigation when the cerumen is dry and hard, but do not irrigate if the tympanic membrane might be perforated. Use lukewarm water for the irrigation, which is done by repeatedly injecting the water from a syringe toward the posterosuperior canal wall. This procedure may make the client feel dizzy. A dental irrigation system can also be used for cerumen removal.

Nasal speculum. To use a nasal speculum for inspection of the nasal mucosa and the turbinates, hold the instrument in the nondominant hand and place the index finger on the side of the client's nose to stabilize the position of the speculum. Use the dominant hand to position the client's head and hold the light. Be careful not to apply pressure on the nasal septum because of its great sensitivity. However, open the blades of the nasal speculum as far as possible (see Figure 12-15). Ask the client to hold the head erect and then tilt it back. This change in position increases visualization of the middle turbinate.

Examination Step-by-Step

Ears
Inspection

1. Observe position and shape of auricle.
2. Whisper in each ear separately at distance of 30 to 60 cm, and have client repeat what you whispered.
3. Apply vibrating tuning fork to middle of forehead, asking the client to identify in which ear the sound or vibration is heard louder (Weber test) or if it is heard equally in both ears.
4. Apply vibrating tuning fork to mastoid process, and instruct client to tell you when the sound stops. Then move the tuning fork close to the auditory meatus. Time the duration in seconds or the ratio of sound perceived by bone and air conduction (Rinne test). For example, if the bone conduction was heard for 30 seconds and air conduction was heard for 60 seconds, record "AC:BC 2:1 or AC > BC."

Palpation

1. Palpate pinna, tragus, and mastoid processes for tenderness, lesions, or masses.

Otoscopic examination

1. Observe condition of auditory canal.
2. Note color of tympanic membrane.
3. Locate landmarks on tympanic membrane (e.g., cone of light reflex, umbo, long and short processes of malleus, pars tensa, pars flaccida, and annulus.

Nose and paranasal sinuses
Inspection: Observe face for symmetry, swelling from a front and profile view.

Percussion: Directly percuss over maxillary areas of both cheeks and over middle of each eyebrow to assess tenderness.

Palpation: Apply pressure over maxillary areas of both cheeks and below eyebrows to assess tenderness.

Mouth and throat
Inspection: Using a tongue blade, penlight, and gloves, inspect lips, gums, teeth, buccal mucosa, sublingual areas, tongue, parotid duct openings, hard palate, pharnyx, and tonsils for color, condition, and presence of lesions. Observe movement of soft palate and uvula when the client says "ah."

Palpation: With gloved hands, palpate with fingers over lips and sublingual area to assess for tenderness or lumps.

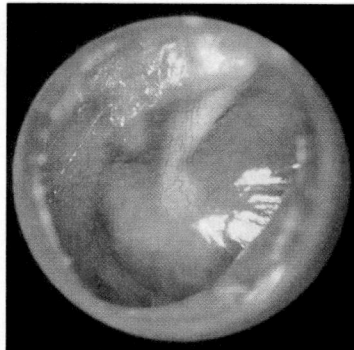 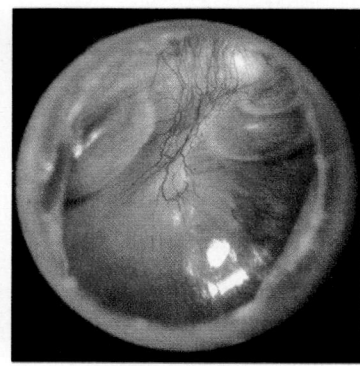

FIGURE 12-20 Secretory otitis. **A**, Middle ear filled with serous fluid. **B**, Air fluid levels in upper middle ear. (Courtesy Dr. Richard A. Buckingham, Clinical Professor, Otolaryngology, Abraham Lincoln School of Medicine, University of Illinois, Chicago, Ill.)

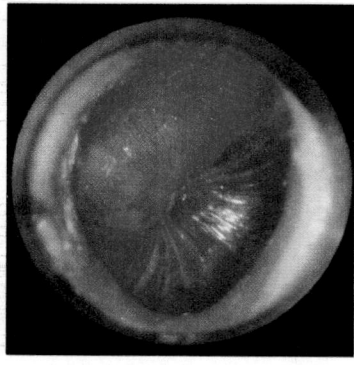 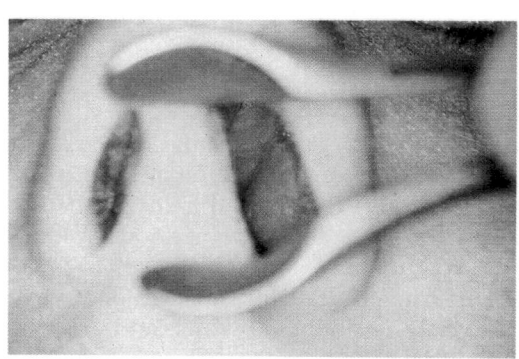

FIGURE 12-21 Acute otitis media—red, nonmobile tympanic membrane with loss of bony landmarks and light reflex. (Courtesy Dr. Richard A. Buckingham, Clinical Professor, Otolaryngology, Abraham Lincoln School of Medicine, University of Illinois, Chicago, Ill.)

FIGURE 12-22 Allergic rhinitis.

VARIATIONS FROM HEALTH

Hearing Loss

Although several types of hearing loss occur, most types can be classified under one of three headings: conductive hearing loss, sensorineural (perceptive) hearing loss, or mixed hearing loss.

Conductive hearing loss. Conductive hearing loss occurs with external or middle ear disorders such as impacted cerumen, perforation of the tympanic membrane, serum or pus in the middle ear, or a fusion of the ossicles. Since the vibrations are not adequately transmitted to the inner ear through the ear canal, tympanic membrane, middle ear, and ossicles, a partial loss of hearing occurs.

Sensorineural hearing loss. Sensorineural, or **perceptive, hearing loss** is noted with disorders of the inner ear, the auditory nerve, or the brain. Vibrations are transmitted to the inner ear, but an impairment of the cochlea or the auditory nerve attenuates the nervous impulses from the cochlea to the brain.

Mixed hearing loss. Mixed hearing loss is a combination of conductive and sensorineural loss in the same ear.

Tympanic Membrane

Fluid in the middle ear may sometimes be identified by air bubbles or a fluid level seen through the tympanic membrane (Figure 12-20).

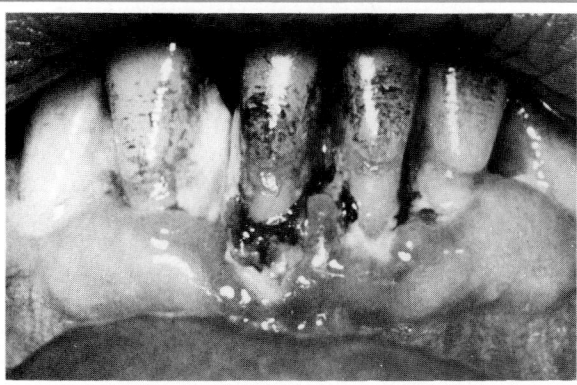

FIGURE 12-23 Advanced pyorrhea. (From DeWeese DD, Saunders WH, Schuller DE, Schleuning AJ II: *Otolaryngology—head and neck surgery*, ed 7, St. Louis, 1988, Mosby—Year Book.)

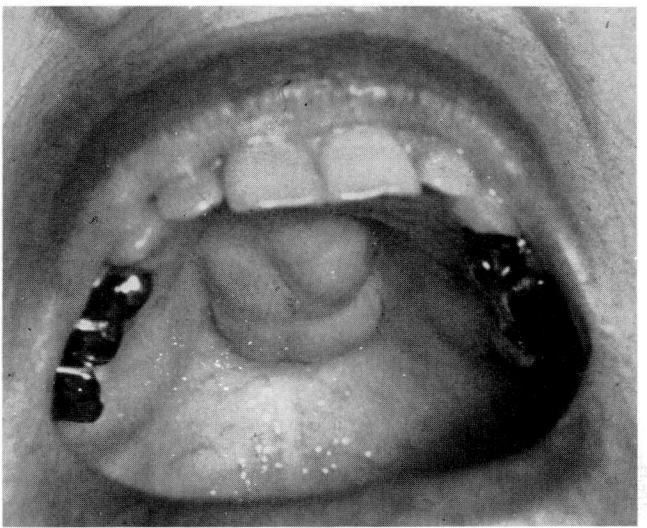

FIGURE 12-24 Exostosis. (From Prior JA, Silberstein JS, Stang JM: *Physical diagnosis: the history and examination of the patient*, ed 6, St. Louis, 1981, Mosby—Year Book.)

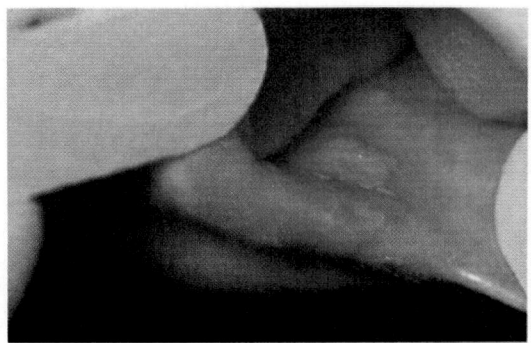

FIGURE 12-25 Herpes zoster. (Courtesy Dr. Edward L. Applebaum, Head, Department of Otolaryngology, University of Illinois Medical Center, Chicago, Ill.)

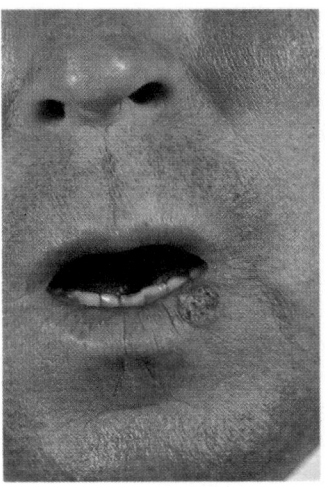

FIGURE 12-26 Epidermal carcinoma—lip. (Courtesy Dr. Edward L. Applebaum, Head, Department of Otolaryngology, University of Illinois Medical Center, Chicago, Ill.)

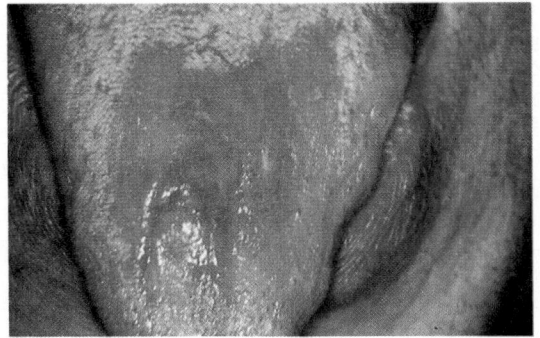

FIGURE 12-27 Drug reaction—tongue. (Courtesy Dr. Edward L. Applebaum, Head, Department of Otolaryngology, University of Illinois Medical Center, Chicago, Ill.)

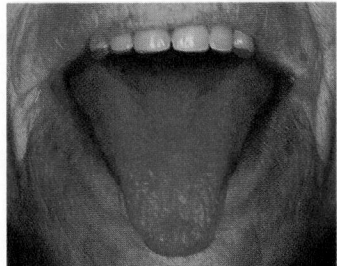

FIGURE 12-28 Smooth tongue resulting from vitamin deficiency. (From Seidel HM and others: *Mosby's guide to physical examination*, ed 2, St. Louis, 1991, Mosby—Year Book.)

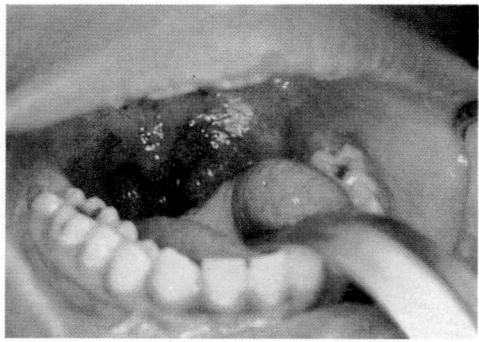

FIGURE 12-29 Acute viral pharyngitis. (Courtesy Dr. Edward L. Applebaum, Head, Department of Otolaryngology, University of Illinois Medical Center, Chicago, Ill.)

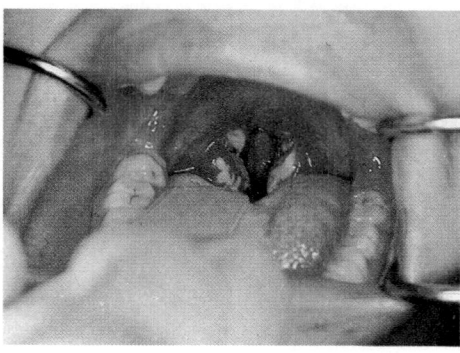

FIGURE 12-30 Tonsillitis, pharyngitis. (Courtesy Dr. Edward L. Applebaum, Head, Department of Otolaryngology, University of Illinois Medical Center, Chicago, Ill.)

Bulging of the tympanic membrane may occur when fluid forms in the middle ear. The pressure increases, and the membrane may bulge outward in one part, or the entire membrane may bulge, obliterating some or all of the landmarks. The light reflex may be lost or displaced, and the membrane appears amber or a dull blue-gray. The cause of this fluid may be pus from otitis media or serum from serous otitis media (Figure 12-21).

Retraction of the tympanic membrane occurs when pressure is reduced from obstruction of the eustachian tube, usually associated with an upper respiratory system infection or allergies. The retraction of the membrane accentuates the landmarks. The light reflex may appear less prominent.

Nose
(Figure 12-22)

Mouth

Pyorrhea is a serious periodontal disease involving the bones and ligaments that anchor the tooth in its socket (Figure 12-23). Note stains, tartar (calculus), or loose teeth as signs of periodontal disease.

Malocclusion is present when two teeth occupy the space for one, teeth overlap, and/or missing teeth create wide spaces. As a result, the lower front teeth are positioned outside the upper front teeth (underbite) or the upper front teeth protrude and hang over the lower front teeth (overbite). Normal occlusion or malocclusion can be demonstrated at oral examination while palpating the temporomandibular joint during opening and closing of the mouth.

An **exostosis** (torus palatinus) is frequently found in the midline of the posterior two thirds of the hard palate (Figure 12-24). This smooth, symmetrical bony structure results from the down-growth of the palatine processes. This type of growth is benign.

The uvula may be bifid and part of a submucosal cleft palate.

Additional variations from health noted in the mouth are shown in Figures 12-25 through 12-28.

Pharynx

Pharyngitis is an inflammation of the mucous membranes of the pharynx, usually of viral or bacterial origin. The posterior pharnyx is erythematous and sometimes has a white coating (exudate). Tonsils, if present, are enlarged (Figures 12-29 and 12-30).

Paranasal Sinuses

Sinusitis is an infection or inflammation of one or more of the paranasal sinuses. Examination reveals tenderness to palpation or percussion over one or more of the sinuses. The nasal mucosa is swollen, pale, or dull red.

SAMPLE DOCUMENTATION

Health history

Mr. Smith, a 19-year-old black male, complains of experiencing a sore throat for the past 2 days. The discomfort is described as a dull ache that increases in intensity with swallowing. Client has also noticed clear mucus draining from nose since yesterday. He has taken acetaminophen 650 mg prn for symptoms but without relief. Discomfort is slightly relieved with throat lozenges. Denies earaches, otorrhea, lethargy, or cough. Reports that his girlfriend has had similar symptoms for the past week.

Physical examination

Ears: Auricles properly positioned without lesions or tenderness on palpation. Able to hear whispered voice bilaterally at 15 feet. Weber and Rinne tests not done.

Otoscopic examination reveals small amount of yellow cerumen in each ear, tympanic membranes pearly gray, and cone of light in proper position.

Nose: Nasal septum slightly deviated to left. Nostrils patent bilaterally. Mucosa of inferior and middle turbinates pale pink with clear liquid mucus present. Frontal and maxillary sinuses nontender to percussion and palpation.

Mouth and throat: Lips dry and cracked. Gums pink and firm. Teeth in good repair and alignment. Tongue midline with thin white coating, no lesions. Buccal mucosa pink without lesions. Parotid and submaxillary gland orifices without swelling. Tonsils absent. Soft palate rises symmetrically on phonation. Uvula midline. Oropharynx reveals erythematous mucosa. No exudate visible.

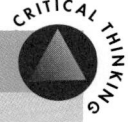

CRITICAL THINKING

Nursing Diagnosis   *THE NEXT STEP*

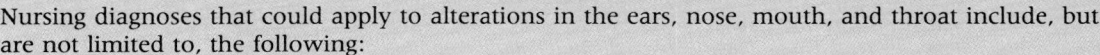

Nursing diagnoses that could apply to alterations in the ears, nose, mouth, and throat include, but are not limited to, the following:

HIGH RISK FOR INFECTION The state in which an individual is at increased risk for being invaded by pathogenic organisms.

Defining Characteristics (risk factors)

- Inadequate primary defenses (broken mucous membranes, change of pH of secretions)
- Inadequate secondary defenses (suppressed inflammatory response)
- Immunosuppression
- Insufficient knowledge to avoid exposure to pathogens
- Tissue destruction and increased environmental exposure
- Chronic disease
- Invasive procedures
- Malnutrition
- Pharmaceutical agents

ALTERED ORAL MUCOUS MEMBRANE The state in which an individual experiences disruptions in the tissue layers of the oral cavity.

Defining Characteristics

- Verbalization or signs of pain or discomfort in oral mucous membranes
- Decrease in or lack of saliva
- Coated tongue; xerostomia (dry mouth)
- Halitosis
- Edema of membranes; hyperemia
- Oral lesions: ulcers, desquamation, vesicles, hemorrhage, gingivitis, leukoplakia
- Stomatitis
- Oral plaque
- Carious teeth

Continued.

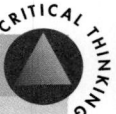

Related Factors

- Ineffective oral hygiene
- Malnutrition
- Dehydration
- Mouth breathing
- Decreased or absent saliva
- Chemical irritants
- Mechanical irritants (ill-fitting dentures, braces, surgery)
- Trauma
- Infections

IMPAIRED SWALLOWING The state in which an individual has decreased ability to voluntarily pass fluids and/or solids from the mouth to the stomach.

Defining Characteristics

- Observed evidence of difficulty in swallowing: stasis of food in oral cavity, coughing/choking when swallowing
- Presence of mechanical obstruction (i.e., tumor)
- Regurgitation of fluids/foods through mouth or nose
- Complaints of pain when swallowing
- Decreased gag reflex
- Edema of oropharyngeal cavity

Related Factors

- Decreased or absent gag reflex
- Decreased strength of muscles of mastication
- Perceptual impairment
- Mechanical obstruction
- Fatigue
- Limited awareness
- Irritated oropharyngeal cavity

INEFFECTIVE AIRWAY CLEARANCE The state in which an individual is unable to clear secretions or obstructions from the respiratory tract to maintain airway patency.

Defining Characteristics

- Cough (effective/ineffective; with or without sputum)
- Cyanosis

Related Factors

- Excess thick secretions
- Fatigue
- Altered level of consciousness
- Pain
- Obstruction
- Trauma

PAIN The state in which an individual experiences and reports the presence of severe discomfort or an uncomfortable sensation.

Defining Characteristics

- Communication (verbal or coded) of pain descriptors
- Guarding behavior—protective
- Self-focusing
- Narrowed focus (altered time perception, withdrawal from social contact, impaired thought process)
- Distraction behavior (moaning, crying)
- Facial mask of pain (eyes lack luster, "beaten look," fixed or scattered movement, grimace)
- Autonomic responses not seen in chronic, stable pain (diaphoresis, pupillary dilation)

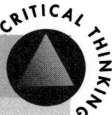

Related Factors

- Knowledge deficit (pain management techniques)
- Injuring agents (biological, chemical, physical, psychological)

SENSORY/PERCEPTUAL ALTERATIONS (AUDITORY, OLFACTORY, GUSTATORY) The state in which an individual experiences a change in the amount or patterning of incoming stimuli accompanied by a diminished, exaggerated, distorted, or impaired response to such stimulation.

Defining Characteristics

Auditory
- Alert with periodic disorientation, general confusion, or nocturnal confusion
- Hallucinations
- Apathy
- Auditory, reality-orienting, or time-orienting input reduced or absent
- Limited proprioceptive input
- Presence of uncompensated hearing deficits
- Inability to identify whispered sounds or normally voiced words
- Fear

Olfactory
- Diminished sense of smell
- Hypersensitivity of odor
- Distortion of odor

Gustatory
- Increased taste sensitivity
- Diminished sense of taste
- Altered taste sense
- Loss of appetite

Related Factors

- Trauma
- Infection
- Surgery
- Environmental exposure

HIGH RISK FOR ASPIRATION The state in which an individual is at risk for entry of gastric secretions, oropharyngeal secretions, or exogenous food or fluids into tracheobronchial passages due to dysfunction or absence of normal protective mechanisms.

Defining Characteristics (risk factors)

- Reduced level of consciousness
- Depressed cough and gag reflexes
- Presence of tracheotomy or endotracheal tube
- Overinflated tracheotomy/endotracheral tube cuff
- Inadequate tracheotomy/endotracheal tube cuff inflation
- Gastrointestinal tubes
- Bolus tube feedings/medication administration
- Situations hindering elevation of upper body
- Increased intragastric pressure
- Increased gastric residual
- Decreased gastrointestinal mobility
- Delayed gastric emptying
- Impaired swallowing
- Facial/oral/neck surgery or trauma
- Wired jaws

Continued.

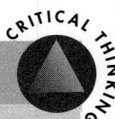

Nursing Diagnosis *THE NEXT STEP—cont'd*

Clinical Application

Mr. Coe is a 22-year-old male college student, seeking care for "sore throat and runny nose for the past 4 days." He reports a temperature of 38.3° C (101° F), swollen glands in his neck, occasional shaking chills, and extreme fatigue despite "sleeping a lot." He has treated himself with Tylenol and over-the-counter decongestants, with no change in his condition. Today all symptoms remain with the addition of a cough productive of green sputum. He states, "I can't eat the last 2 days because my throat burns so much." He does say that he drinks 4-5 glasses of fluids per day. He does not smoke.

SUBJECTIVE DATA:
Sore throat and runny nose
New onset of coughing with green sputum production
Unable to eat; throat burns

OBJECTIVE DATA:
Tympanic membranes pearl gray with landmarks intact
Small amount thick green colored nasal discharge
Nasal mucosa pink, slight swelling
Oral mucosa and gingivae pink, no lesions
Tonsils enlarged with white exudate
Pharyngeal wall bright red with white exudate
Enlarged anterior cervical nodes bilaterally, painful to palpation
Breath sounds clear throughout anterior and posterior thorax
No adventitious breath sounds.

NURSING DIAGNOSES

Impaired swallowing related to irritated oropharyngeal cavity.

Defining Characteristics

- Observed evidence of difficulty in swallowing
- Complaints of pain when swallowing
- Edema of oropharyngeal cavity

Ineffective airway clearance related to excess thick secretion.

Defining Characteristics

- Cough effective with sputum

Pain related to biological injuring agent of oropharyngeal cavity (pharyngitis).

Defining Characteristics

- Communication of pain when swallowing

GLOSSARY

annulus Dense, fibrous ring surrounding the tympanic membrane.

auditory ossicles Series of three small bones (malleus, incus, stapes) that extend across the middle ear.

auricle The external ear, also called pinna.

buccal Pertaining to the cheek.

caries Decay of the calcified protein of teeth.

cerumen Earwax produced by the apocrine and sebaceous glands within the ear canal.

choana A funnel-shaped channel.

cochlea Conical bony structure of the inner ear, perforated by numerous apertures for passage of the cochlear division of the acoustic nerve.

concha Body structure that is shell-shaped, such as the cavity in the external ear that surrounds the external auditory meatus.

conductive hearing loss Diminished ability to hear caused by the inability of vibrations to travel to or through the inner ear to an intact auditory nerve.

crepitus A dry crackling sound that occurs (1) in the joints, when dry synovial surfaces rub together, and (2) in the skin, when air is present subdermally.

epistaxis Bleeding or hemorrhage from the nose.

equilibrium Ongoing process of maintaining the orientation and position of the body in relationship to the ground and in space.

eustachian tube Cartilaginous and bony passage between the nasopharynx and the middle ear that allows equalization of air pressure between the middle ear and the external environment.

exostosis Abnormal benign growth on the surface of a bone.

frenulum Restraining portion or structure. An example is the sublingual frenulum.

gingivitis Inflammation of the papillary and marginal gingiva.

helix Superior and posterior free margin of the ear.

incus One of the three ossicles of the inner ear, resembling an anvil. It communicates sound vibrations from the malleus to the stapes.

labyrinth Intricate communicating passageway, such as the bony and membranous labyrinths of the inner ear.

lobule Small lobe, such as the soft, pendulous lower part of the external ear.

malleus One of the three ossicles of the middle ear, resembles a hammer, connected to the tympanic membrane.

mastication Act of chewing.

mastoid process Bony prominence found posterior to the lower part of the auricle.

meatus Passage or opening, especially at the external portion of a canal.

mixed hearing loss Combination of conductive and sensorineural loss in the same ear.

oropharynx One of the three anatomical divisions of the pharynx. It extends behind the mouth from the soft palate (above) to the level of the hyoid bone (below) and contains the palatine tonsils and the lingual tonsils.

paranasal sinus One of the air cavities in various bones around the nose. Examples are the frontal sinus in the frontal bone lying deep to the medial part of the superciliary ridge and the maxillary sinus within the maxilla between the orbit, the nasal cavity, and the upper teeth.

pars flaccida Less taut portion of the tympanic membrane.

pars tensa Taut portion of the tympanic membrane.

pinna Projecting part of the external ear; the auricle.

pyorrhea Purulent inflammation of the gums.

Rinne test Test comparing air conduction and bone conduction through the use of a tuning fork. In normal hearing, air conduction sounds are heard longer than bone conduction sounds (positive Rinne).

sensorineural hearing loss Diminished ability to hear caused by the inability of the acoustic nerve to transmit nervous impulses from the middle ear to the brain. Also called perceptive hearing loss.

stapes One of the three ossicles of the middle ear, resembling a tiny stirrup. It transmits sound vibrations from the incus to the internal ear.

tragus Projection of the cartilage of the auricle at the opening of the external auditory meatus.

tympanic membrane Eardrum; membranous structure separating the external ear from the middle ear.

umbo Landmark on the tympanic membrane created by the attachment of the membrane to the malleus.

uvula The small cone-shaped process, suspended in the mouth from the middle of the posterior border of the soft palate.

vestibule Space or cavity that serves as the entrance to a passageway.

Weber test Test of bone conduction through the use of a tuning fork placed on the top of the skull or middle forehead. A normal result occurs when the client reports that the sound is heard equally in both ears. The sound lateralizes when hearing loss is present.

BIBLIOGRAPHY

Bates B: *A guide to physical examination and history taking*, ed 5, Philadelphia, 1991, JB Lippincott.

DeWeese DD and others: *Otolaryngology-Head and Neck Surgery*, ed 7, St Louis, 1988, Mosby—Year Book.

Gordon M: *Manual of nursing diagnosis 1993-1994*, St Louis, 1993, Mosby—Year Book.

Koufman JA: *Core otolaryngology*, Philadelphia, 1990, JB Lippincott.

Lee KJ: *Textbook of otolaryngology and head and neck surgery*, New York, 1989, Elsevier.

Netter, FH: *CIBA collection of medical illustrations*, vol 3, *Digestive system Part I: upper digestive tract*, 1983.

Potter PA, Perry AG: *Basic nursing theory and practice*, ed 2, St Louis, 1991, Mosby—Year Book.

Riley MAK: *Nursing care of the client with ear, nose and throat disorders*, New York, 1987, Springer Publishing.

Seidel H and others: *Mosby's guide to physical examination*, ed 2, St Louis, 1991, Mosby—Year Book.

Serra AM: *Ear, nose and throat nursing*, Boston, 1986, Blackwell Scientific Publications.

Lymphatic System

PURPOSE OF THE EXAMINATION

The purpose of this chapter is to describe the structure and functions of the lymphatic system, and the techniques used in examination. Normal findings and some of the more common variations from health are covered.

The lymphatic system is a complete circulatory system separate and distinct from the blood circulatory system, but closely linked to it. It is one of the key security systems of the body and has a critical role in fluid balance, in immune surveillance and antibody production, and recognition by lymphocytes of foreign antigens. It provides resistance to viral infections and some bacterial infections with an antibody component to the host defense.

This system is not generally accessible to examination in healthy people. Variations in findings in the lymphatic system more often indicate illness elsewhere rather than within the system itself. *Acquired immune deficiency syndrome (AIDS)*, a result of infection by the human immune virus (HIV), affects the lymphatic system, resulting in some of the early physical findings of this disease.

ANATOMY AND PHYSIOLOGY

General

The lymphatic system consists of a network including:

1. Lymph fluid	4. Spleen
2. Collecting ducts	5. Thymus
3. Lymph nodes	6. Tonsils

Lymph vessels and nodes are widely spread throughout the body. Lymphatic vessels originate as microscopic, open-ended tubules or capillaries that merge to form large collecting ducts. These collect interstitial fluid and drain to specific lymph nodes. Ducts from the lymph nodes then empty into two main trunks, which drain into the venous system at the subclavian veins. The **right lymphatic duct** drains into the right subclavian vein. This trunk receives the lymphatic fluid from the right side of the head and neck, right arm, and right side of the chest wall. The **thoracic duct** drains the rest of the body and empties into the left subclavian vein (Figure 13-1). The lymphatic system contains a

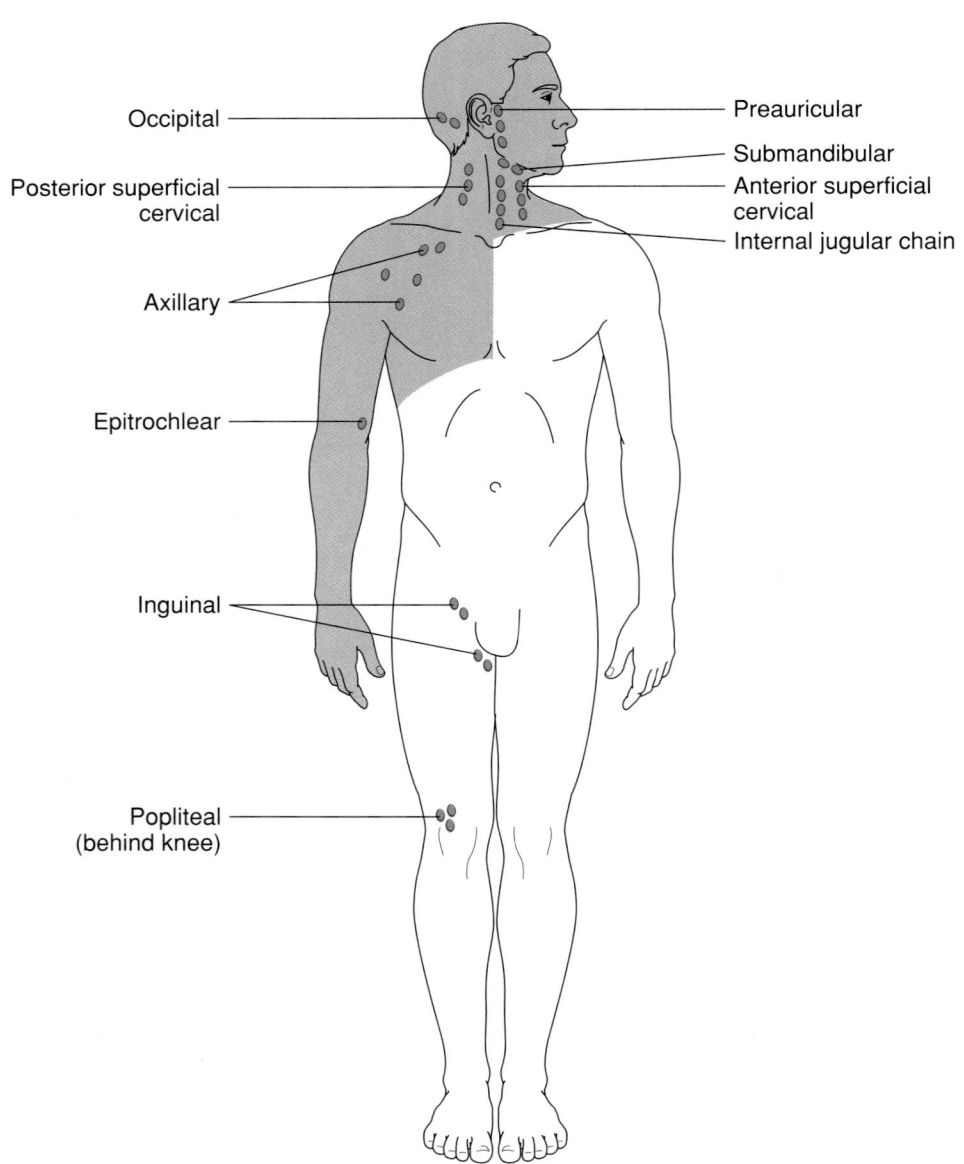

Occipital

Posterior superficial cervical

Axillary

Epitrochlear

Inguinal

Popliteal (behind knee)

Preauricular

Submandibular

Anterior superficial cervical

Internal jugular chain

FIGURE 13-1 Lymph node locations and drainage pattern.

series of valves. Flow is one-way from the small capillaries to the right lymphatic duct and the thoracic duct.

The lymphatic system has no pumping device of its own. Its movement is much slower than that of the blood circulatory system. Factors affecting the movement of lymph include:

1. Arteriolar pulsation
2. Compression of lymphatic vessels by contracting skeletal muscles
3. Contraction of the smooth muscles in the walls of the lymphatic vessels, lymph nodes, and collecting ducts
4. Pressure changes due to respiration

These pumping devices and a series of valves in the lymph ducts prevent backflow.

The lymphatic and cardiovascular systems are closely related. The fluid and proteins that compose the lymphatic fluid move originally from the vascular system to the interstitial spaces. Here they are collected by the microscopic lymphatic tubules, which in turn return the various fluids and proteins to the cardiovascular system. The lymphatic capillary system is very extensive. Many of the lymphatic vessels lie close to the vessels of the cardiovascular system. All tissues supplied with blood vessels also possess lymphatic vessels, except the central nervous system and the cornea.

Lymph is the clear or opalescent to yellow-tinged fluid containing lymphocytes of all sizes and degrees of maturity. Two types of lymph cells are the B lymphocytes and the T lymphocytes. They enable the immune system to recognize "self" from "nonself" cells or foreign antigens. The number of lymphocytes increases in response to most viral infections and some bacterial infections.

The main functions of the lymphatic system are to:

1. Return fluid, proteins, and electrolytes from tissue spaces to the blood
2. Absorb nutrients, particularly fat, from the gastrointestinal tract
3. Filter and engulf bacteria, red blood cells, or toxins in the lymph nodes
4. Provide a defensive immunity network against microorganisms and abnormal cells

Regional Nodes

Lymph nodes are small oval clumps of lymphatic tissue occurring in groups at intervals along the vessels. The superficial nodes lie in the subcutaneous connective tissues; the deeper nodes are beneath the muscular fascia or in various body cavities. Some nodes have a diameter of 0.5 cm, but most are smaller. Normally, lymph nodes cannot be felt or seen. With local infection, the lymph nodes adjacent to the area will enlarge and become tender as the lymphocytes enlarge and proliferate. When the superficial lymph nodes are enlarged, they are accessible to physical examination by observation or palpation.

Other tissues in the lymphatic system are the spleen, oropharyngeal and nasopharyngeal tonsils, and the thymus. The spleen is located in the left upper quadrant of the abdomen. In early childhood, it is a blood-forming organ. In adulthood it has four functions:

1. Storage of red blood cells
2. Destruction of old red blood cells
3. Production of antibodies
4. Filtration of microorganisms from the blood

The spleen may manufacture blood when the bone marrow is severely compromised. (See Chapter 17: Assessment of the Abdomen for further information on the spleen.)

The oropharyngeal tonsils are located between the palatine arches on either side of the larynx, just beyond the base of the tongue. They are composed mostly of lymphoid tissue and covered with mucous membrane. The nasopharyngeal tonsils, or adenoids, are located at the nasopharyngeal border. The tonsils tend to be large in the child and smaller after puberty.

The thymus is a gland located in the superior mediastinum behind the sternum. It is relatively large in the infant and young child, but atrophies after puberty. The thymus is important in developing the T lymphocytes of the immune system in children. Its role in adults is not certain.

Lymph nodes are widely distributed throughout the body. Only those that are fairly near the surface are accessible to physical examination, and then only when a client is experiencing some variation from health. Those groups of nodes that are accessible to examination are described by body region below.

The head, neck, and axilla are richly supplied with lymph nodes. The nodes in these areas have been classified a number of ways. One commonly used system of terms appears in this text with other fairly common terms in parentheses.

Head (Figure 13-2)

1. Preauricular—in front of the ear
2. Mastoid (or postauricular)—behind the ear slightly anterior to the mastoid process
3. Occipital—at the base of the skull posteriorly
4. Parotid—near the angle of the jaw
5. Submandibular—midway between the angle of the jaw and the tip of the mandible
6. Submental—in the midline of the face and neck posterior to the tip of the mandible

Neck

The neck is divided into anterior and posterior triangles by the sternocleidomastoid muscle (Figure 13-3). There are four main groups of neck nodes.

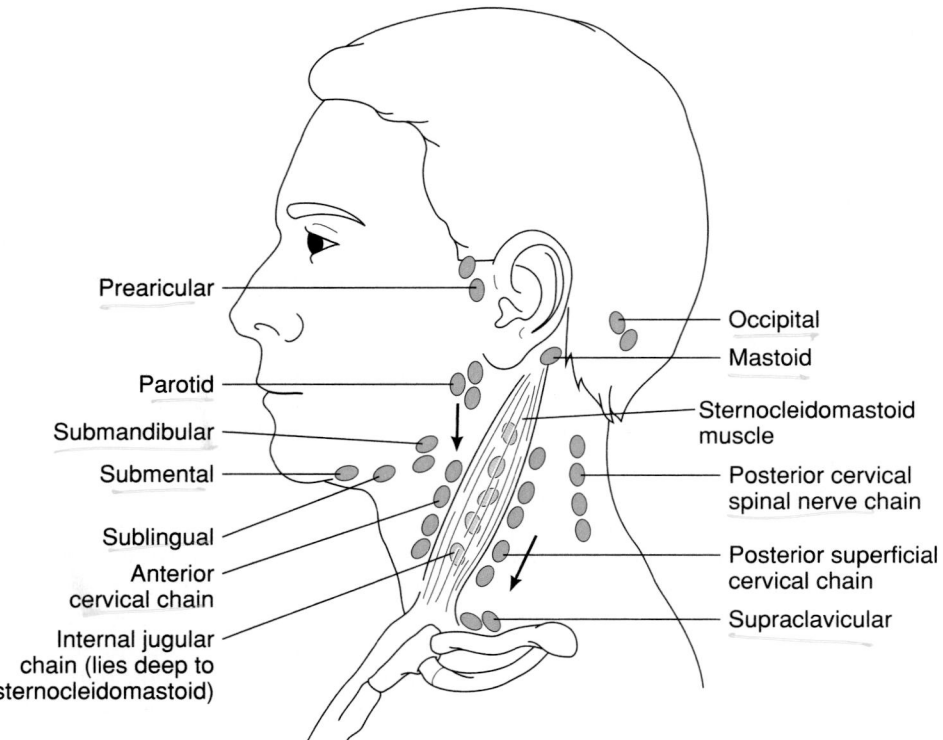

FIGURE 13-2 Lymph nodes of the head and neck.

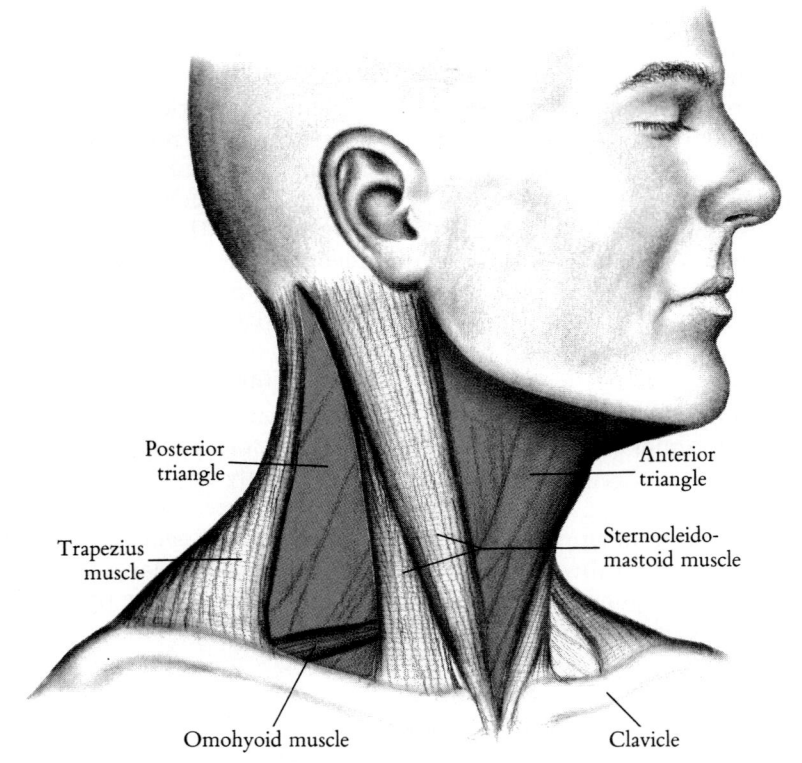

FIGURE 13-3 Anterior and posterior triangles. (From Seidel HM and others: *Mosby's guide to physical examination,* ed 2, St. Louis, 1991, Mosby–Year Book.)

1. Anterior cervical chain—over and anterior to the sternocleidomastoid muscle, in the anterior triangle
2. Posterior cervical chain—along the anterior edge of the trapezius, in the posterior triangle
3. Deep cervical chain—(scalene) deep to the sternocleidomastoid, at the border of the triangles. This chain is largely obscured by the sternocleidomastoid muscle
4. Supraclavicular—in the angle formed by the clavical and the sternocleidomastoid muscle

Axilla (Figure 13-4)

Five groups of lymph nodes are located in the axillary fossa. All drain upward and medially toward the main lymph-collecting channels. The central axillary nodes are the most frequently palpable. Nomenclature commonly used describes either the area of the axilla in which the nodes are located or their location in relation to one of the adjacent bones or blood vessels.

1. Lateral axillary (brachial) nodes lie along the humerus, inside the upper arm. They receive lymph from the upper extremity, deltoid region, and anterior wall of the chest, including part of the breast.
2. Posterior axillary (subscapular) nodes lie in the posterior aspect of the axilla along the lateral

edge of the scapula. They drain the posterior wall of the chest and the lower posterior aspect of the neck.
3. Central axillary (intermediate) nodes lie high in the middle of the axilla over the ribs. They receive ducts from the anterior axillary (pectoral), lateral axillary (brachial), and posterior (subscapular) lymph nodes draining the chest wall, breast, and arm. Lymph drains from them into the infraclavicular and supraclavicular nodes.
4. Anterior axillary (pectoral) nodes lie in the anterior aspect of the axilla and include a superior group of several nodes found in the region of the third rib and the second and third intercostal spaces and an inferior group located over the fourth to sixth ribs. The ducts entering these nodes are from the breast and front and side of the chest wall, and from the skin and muscles of the abdominal wall above the umbilicus. They lie along the lateral edge of the pectoralis major muscle, just inside the anterior axillary fold.
5. Apical axillary (infraclavicular or subclavian) nodes lie below the clavicle and receive ducts from the arm, breast, and chest wall. (These are sometimes examined and recorded along with the neck node group.)

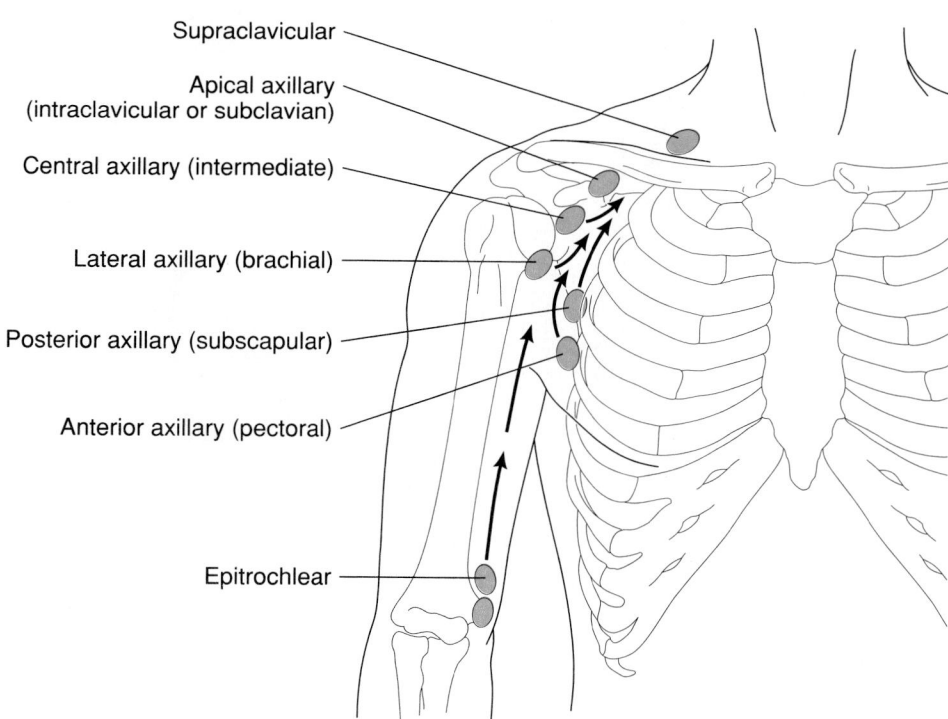

FIGURE 13-4 Axillary lymph nodes and epitrochlear nodes.

Breast (Figure 13-5)

(See Chapter 14: Assessment of the Breasts.) Lymph drainage from the breast goes to numerous groups of nodes; most of it goes to the axillary nodes. Drainage flows from the central axillary nodes into the apical axillary (infraclavicular) and supraclavicular nodes. A small amount of lymphatic drainage goes directly to the apical axillary (infraclavicular) nodes, deep into the chest or abdomen, or directly across to the opposite breast.

Depending on the location of a lesion in the breast tissue, drainage may go to the axillary nodes, the infraclavicular nodes, into deep channels in the chest or abdomen, or even to the opposite breast. Some are deep and not accessible to examination. Only the more superficial ones will be discussed here. Six of these groups are in the lower neck and axilla and are described above.

1. Anterior axillary (pectoral) nodes
2. Posterior axillary (subscapular) nodes
3. Lateral (brachial) nodes
4. Central axillary (intermediate) nodes
5. Apical axillary (infraclavicular) nodes
6. Supraclavicular nodes

Other groups that receive lymphatic drainage from the breast include:

7. Interpectoral (Rotter's or mammary) nodes lie within the pectoral muscle above the breast.
8. Parasternal (internal thoracic) nodes lie next to the sternum.

Arm (see Figure 13-4)

The only nodes palpable in the arm are the epitrochlear nodes. These are located on the medial surface of the arm above the elbow. They are above and posterior to the medial condyle of the humerus. They drain the ulnar surface of the forearm, the little and ring finger, and adjacent surface of the middle finger. The rest of the arm sends lymphatics directly to the axillary nodes.

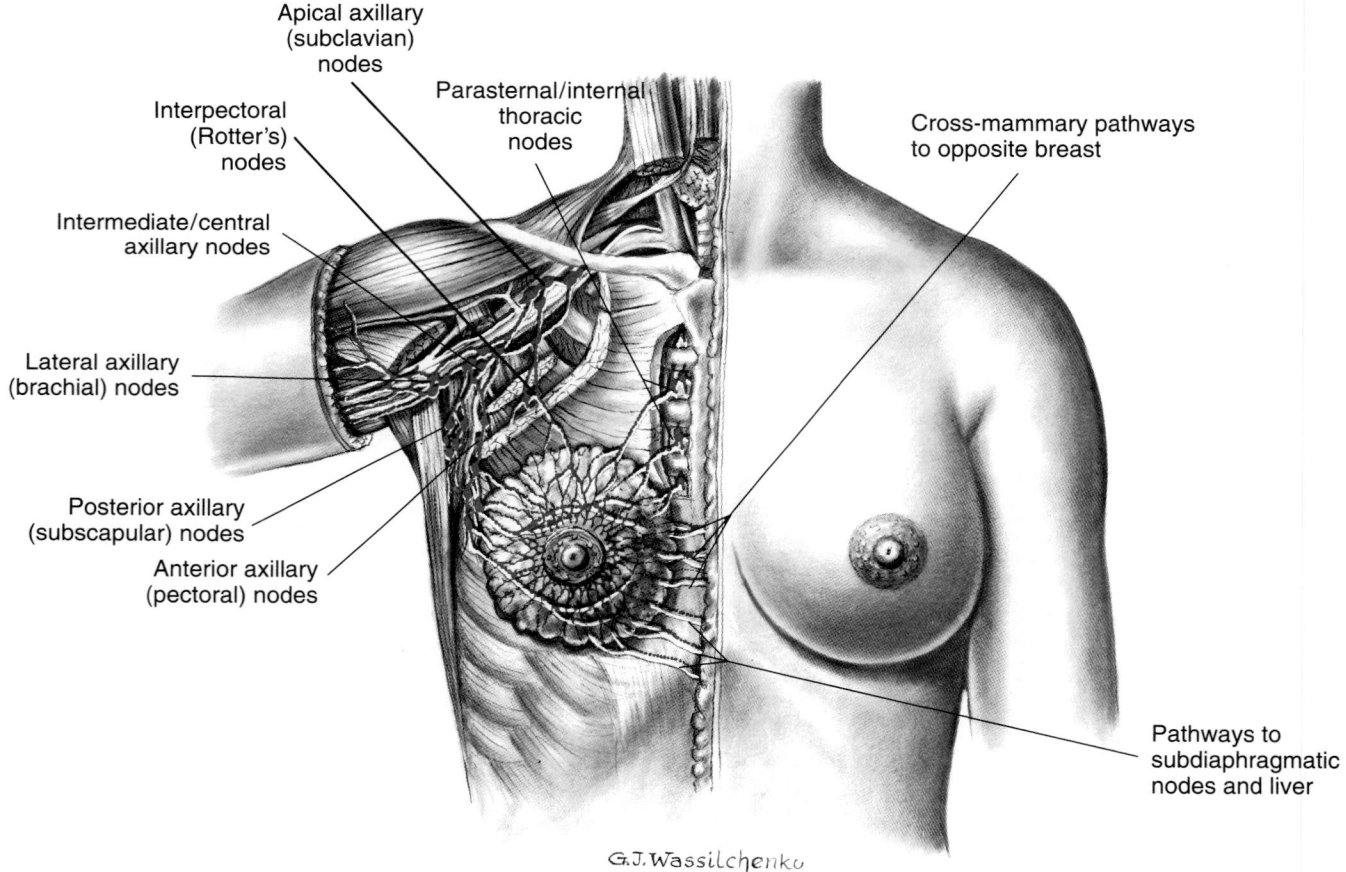

G.J. Wassilchenko

FIGURE 13-5 Lymph nodes of the breast. (From Bobak IM, Jensen MD, Zalar MK: *Maternity and gynecologic care: the nurse and the family,* ed 4, St. Louis, 1989, Mosby—Year Book.)

Inguinal area (see Figure 13-13)

The two groups of superficial nodes in the inguinal area are the superior and inferior inguinal nodes. These receive most of the lymph drainage from the legs. The superior inguinal nodes lie somewhat horizontally along the inguinal ligament. They receive drainage from the abdominal wall below the umbilicus, the external genitalia (excluding the testes), the anal canal, the vulva and lower one third of the vagina, the gluteal area, and the inferior inguinal nodes. Lymph from around the internal female genitalia drains into deeper nodes, which are not accessible to palpation. The inferior group lies somewhat vertically below the junction of the saphenous and femoral veins. This is a group of large lymph nodes that receives lymph from the superficial regions of the leg and foot. In males, lymph from the penile and scrotal surfaces drains to the inguinal nodes, but lymphatic drainage from the testes is deep into the abdomen.

Leg (Figure 13-6)

The popliteal nodes lie on the posterior surface of the leg behind the knee. They receive lymph from the medial portion of the lower leg.

EXAMINATION

Health History

Present health status. First obtain client's own description of her or his health status including any health problems.

1. Enlarged nodes (client may describe as lumps, bumps, kernels, or swollen glands)
   a. Characteristics: location, onset, duration, number, consistency, tenderness
   b. Associated symptoms: pain, fever, redness, warmth, red streaks, itching, ulceration, bleeding (note site and character), fatigue, weakness, weight gain or loss

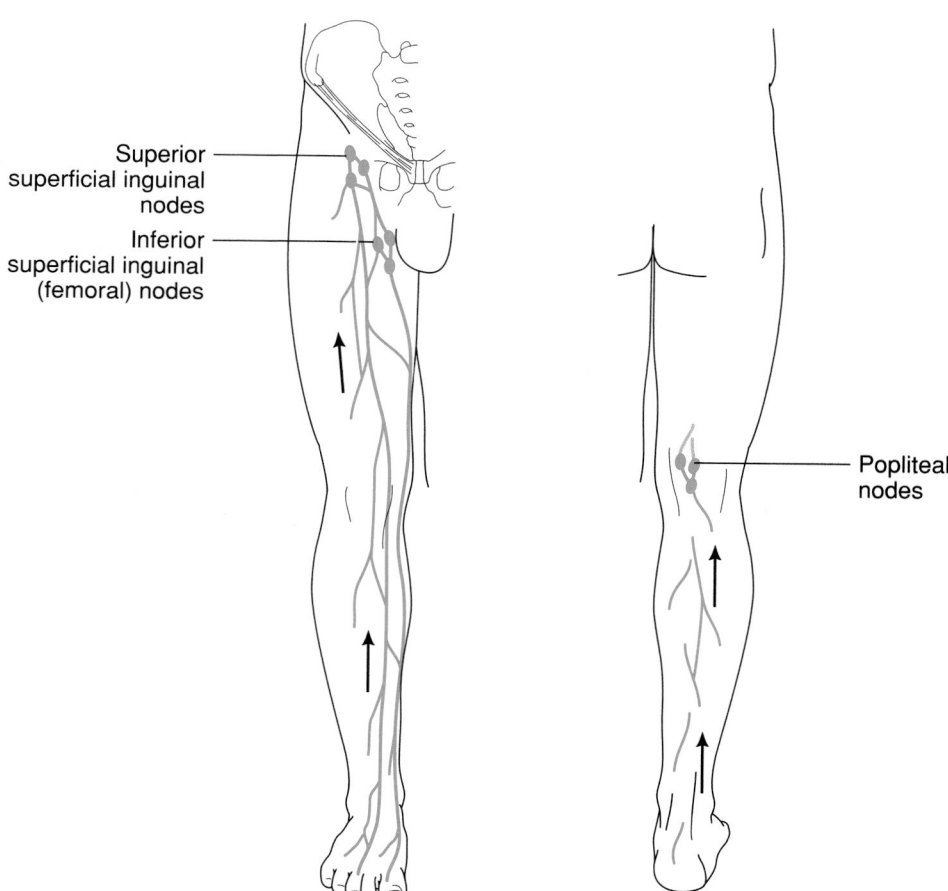

FIGURE 13-6 Inguinal and popliteal lymph nodes.

c. Predisposing factors: infection, surgery, trauma
2. Swelling
   a. Location
   b. Unilateral or bilateral, intermittent or constant, pitting or nonpitting, variations during the day, duration
   c. Predisposing factors: cardiac or renal disorder, surgery, infection, trauma, venous insufficiency
   d. Associated symptoms: warmth, redness or discoloration, ulceration, fatigue, weakness, weight gain or loss
   e. Treatment efforts and effect: support stocking, elevation

Past health history

1. Hodgkin's or other lymphoma
2. Other cancer
3. Chronic illness: cardiac, renal, tuberculosis
4. Medications including antibiotics and chemotherapy
5. Surgery: purpose, time, result, residual effects including trauma to regional lymph nodes
6. Recurrent infections including infectious mononucleosis
7. Blood transfusions
8. Environmental exposure to radiation, toxic chemicals, infections
9. Use of IV drugs
10. Sexual practices
11. Diagnosis of Acquired Immune Deficiency Syndrome (AIDS) or AIDS Related Complex (ARC)

Family health history

1. Malignancy
2. Anemia
3. Recent infections
4. Tuberculosis
5. Agammaglobulinemia
6. Hemophilia

Other considerations

1. Environmental exposure to radiation, toxic chemicals, infection (including HIV)
2. Travel to sites of infectious outbreaks

Preparation for the Examination: Client and Environment

Because examination of the lymphatic system involves examination of the body from the head to the knees, a space that provides privacy and a comfortable room temperature for the client are important. Explain the examination to the client before you begin and as you proceed, if needed.

RISK FACTORS FOR INFECTIONS THAT COULD AFFECT THE LYMPHATIC SYSTEM INCLUDE:

1. Inadequate primary defenses such as broken skin or stasis of body fluids
2. Inadequate secondary defenses such as suppressed inflammatory response
3. Immunosuppression
4. Chronic disease
5. Malnutrition
6. Risk factors for those cancers that involve the lymph nodes, such as lymphomas, breast cancer, lung cancer, and prostatic cancer

---

PREPARATION

Preparation for the Examination

Equipment

Item	Purpose
Ruler	Measure enlarged lymph nodes
Tape measure	Measure extremities for swelling

Client and Environment

A room that provides privacy, good lighting, and a comfortable temperature.

Technique for Examination and Normal Findings

The techniques of inspection and palpation are used to examine the lymphatic system. The beginning practitioner will need to develop an organized approach to lymph node examination, usually from head to knees. Eventually the practitioner will integrate the examination of the lymph nodes into the full body examination.

Inspection. In the healthy client, lymph nodes are not visible. If the client has signs or symptoms of infection or neoplasm, nodes may become visible. Inspect the areas where the superficial lymph nodes are located and observe any swelling, *edema,* skin lesions, erythema, and red streaks on the skin. Often the enlargement is subtle, so observation is based on a careful history and is carefully integrated with palpation. Inspect each area where lymph nodes may be visible as shown in Figure 13-1.

Palpation. To palpate the lymph nodes use the pads of the second, third, and fourth fingers in a gentle circular motion. Move the skin lightly over the underlying tissues rather than moving the examining fingers over the skin. Press lightly at first, increasing the pressure gradually, if needed. Heavy pressure can push the nodes into the deeper soft tissues so that their presence may be missed.

Although in the healthy client no nodes are palpable, some people have a few discrete (meaning separate or distinct), mobile, small (less than 1 cm in diameter) nodes that are not clinically significant. These are often referred to as "shotty" nodes. If any nodes are detected, describe them according to:

1. Location and symmetry
2. Size
3. Shape
4. Number of nodes
5. Surface characteristics
6. Consistency
7. Tenderness
8. Mobility or fixation to surrounding tissues
9. Discreteness or matting (This describes whether the nodes are palpated as separate from or connected to each other.)

Helpful Hint: *The groups of lymph nodes are not always as distinctive as the drawings indicate. If you are not certain which group you are palpating, describe them by location as precisely as possible. (See material in left column for terms commonly used to describe some of the characteristics of enlarged nodes.)*

Nodes enlarged because of infection are likely to be tender and matted. Nodes enlarged because of a malignancy are likely to be hard, discrete, asymmetric, and not tender. When you find enlarged lymph nodes, explore the areas drained by those nodes for signs of infection or malignancy.

Helpful Hint: *Whenever a lesion is present, look for involvement of the regional lymph nodes that drain it. Whenever a node is enlarged or tender, look for a source of infection or neoplastic growth in the area that it drains.*

Palpate the lymph nodes from head to knees in the order described in the section on anatomy and physiology. Generally you will examine each set of nodes one side at a time. For example, you will palpate the axillary nodes one side at a time. You may be able to palpate both sides of the head and neck nodes simultaneously.

TERMS USED TO DESCRIBE THE CHARACTERISTICS OF ENLARGED LYMPH NODES

Location:	Use imaginary body lines, such as the midclavicular line; bony prominences, such as the mandible; or muscles, such as the sternocleidomastoid, to describe specific location
Size:	Measure in cm
Shape:	Usually oval
Surface characteristics:	Smooth, nodular, irregular, singular or matted (in groups)
Consistency:	Soft, firm, hard, rubbery, spongy, cystic
Mobility/fixation:	Describe whether node moves freely or is attached to adjacent structure or underlying tissue
Tenderness:	Describe whether node is painful without palpation and/or tender with palpation
Signs of inflammation:	Erythema, increased warmth

Head
Assess the lymph nodes of the head:
Preauricular (Figure 13-7)
Mastoid (postauricular)
Occipital
Parotid
Submandibular
Submental
Use a gentle rotary motion to move the skin over the bony structures underlying the areas of the nodes.

Neck
Assess the lymph nodes of the neck:
Anterior cervical (Figure 13-8)
Posterior cervical
Deep cervical (scalene) (Figure 13-9)
Supraclavicular
Infraclavicular
When examining the neck nodes, ask the client to bend her or his head slightly forward and toward the side you are examining (see Figure 13-8). This position reduces muscle tension and enhances accurate palpation.

Examine the anterior and posterior cervical chains by palpating first superficially and then more deeply into the soft tissues of the anterior and posterior triangles of the neck.

The deep cervical chain is difficult to examine, particularly if pressed too heavily. Probe gently with thumb

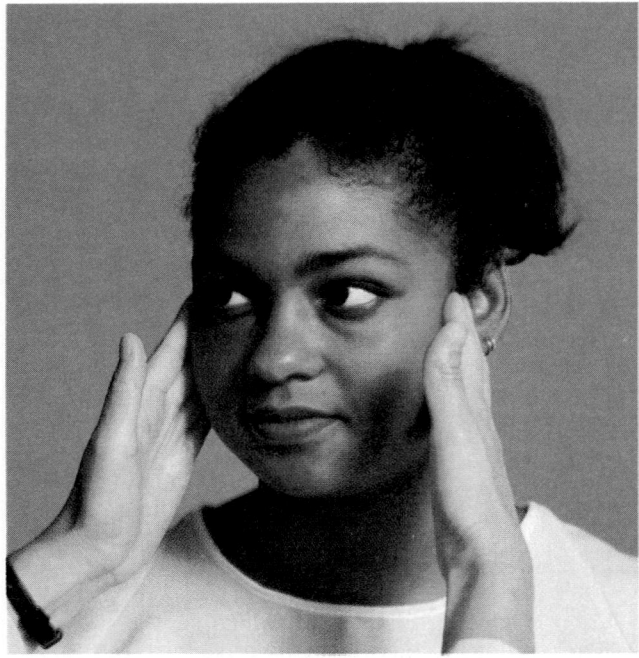

FIGURE 13-7 Palpation of preauricular lymph nodes.

and fingers around the sternocleidomastoid muscle (see Figure 13-9).

To examine the supraclavicular nodes, palpate into the soft tissue just above the clavicle (Figure 13-10, *A*). As with the other neck nodes, it is helpful to ask the client to tilt the chin slightly downward and toward the side being examined. This reduces the muscle tension in the area (Figure 13-10, *B*).

Axilla

Assess the lymph nodes of the axilla:
Lateral axillary (brachial)
Posterior axillary (subscapular)
Central axillary (intermediate)
Anterior axillary (pectoral)
Apical axillary (infraclavicular or subclavian)

To examine the axillary nodes, support the client's arm with your own and use your free hand to palpate the axilla (Figure 13-11). Use the pads of your fingertips. (If your fingernails are long, this examination will be very uncomfortable for the client!) First palpate superficially and then more deeply into the soft tissue of the axilla. This portion of the lymphatic examination can be difficult because the client may be ticklish or sensitive in this area. Develop a routine system, such as starting with the lateral nodes, then moving to the anterior, central, posterior, and apical nodes. Examining the apical nodes last is usually best because they are located more deeply and require more pressure from the examiner's fingers.

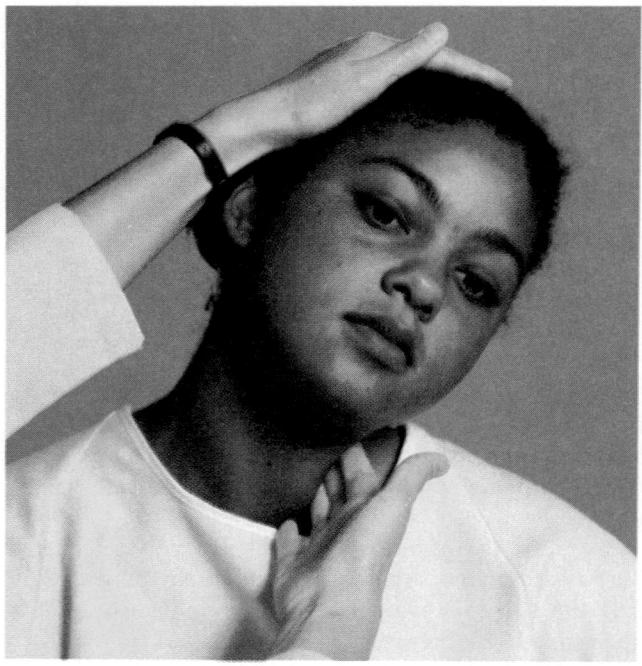

FIGURE 13-8 Palpation of anterior cervical lymph nodes.

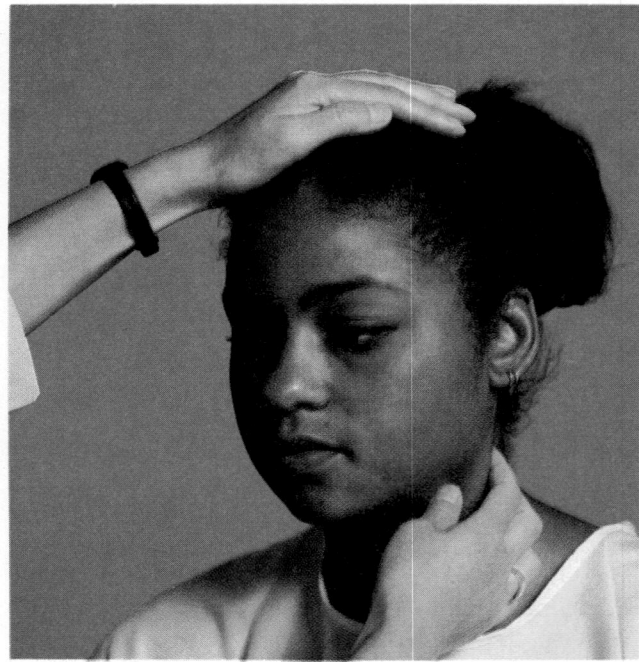

FIGURE 13-9 Palpation of deep cervical lymph nodes.

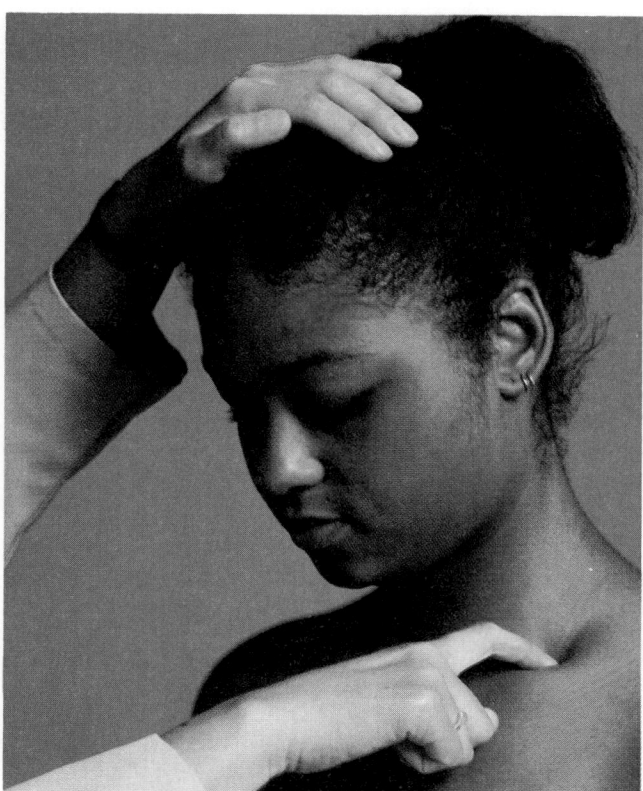

A

B

FIGURE 13-10 Palpation of the supraclavicular lymph nodes.

Breast

Assess the lymph nodes of the breast:
Anterior axillary
Posterior axillary
Lateral axillary
Anterior axillary
Apical axillary
Supraclavicular

The nodes draining the breast are listed here separately to indicate completeness of the lymphatic examination. See Chapter 14: Breasts, for a complete description of the breast examination.

Arm

Assess the lymph node of the arm:
Epitrochlear

Flex the client's arm to a 90° angle and palpate above the elbow on the medial aspect of the arm (Figure 13-12).

Inguinal area (Figure 13-13)

Assess the lymph nodes of the inguinal area:
Superior inguinal
Inferior inguinal

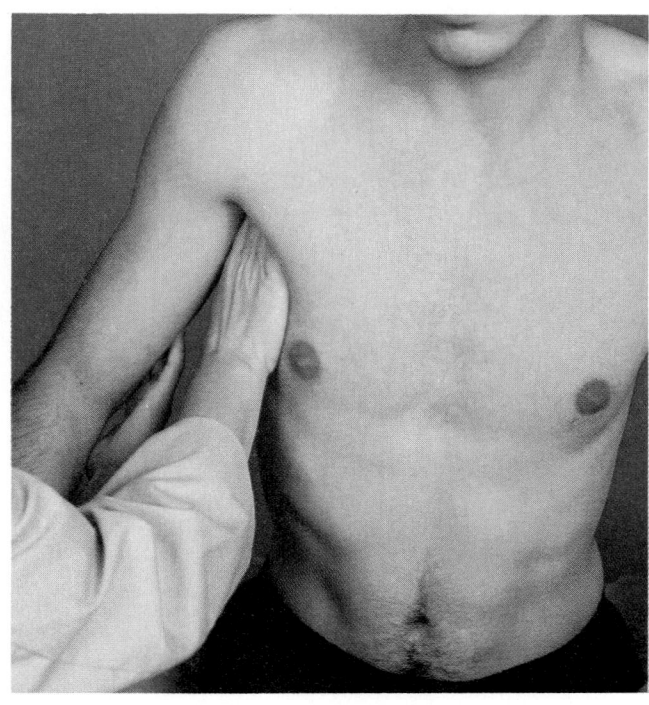

FIGURE 13-11 Palpation of the axillary lymph nodes.

The client must be lying down for the examination of the inguinal nodes. Flex the client's leg at the knee to relax the muscles of the inguinal area. Abduct the leg slightly: you may see a shallow, hollow space. Begin your palpation here, lightly at first, and then more deeply.

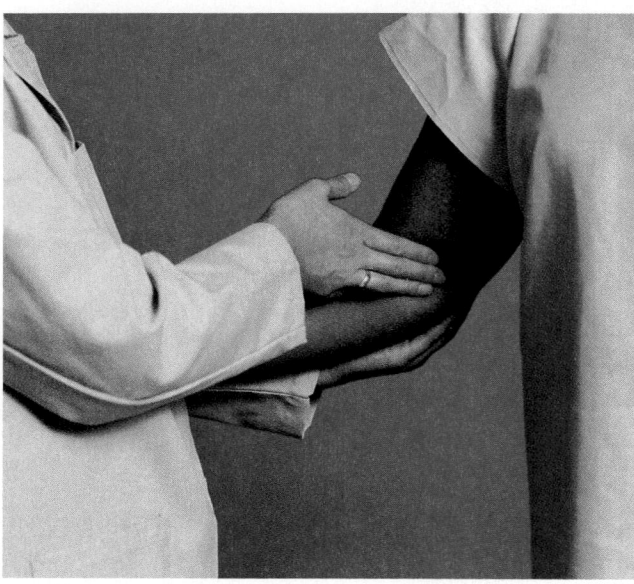

FIGURE 13-12 Palpation of the epitrochlear lymph nodes.

Leg (Refer to Figure 13-6)
Assess the lymph node of the leg:
Popliteal

The client may be sitting or lying down during palpation of the popliteal nodes. As with the inguinal nodes, flex the client's leg at the knee to relax the surrounding structures. Palpate the area on the dorsal aspect of the leg behind the knee cap.

VARIATIONS FROM HEALTH

Edema

Edema is an excessive accumulation of fluid in the tissue spaces resulting from a disturbance in the mechanisms of fluid exchange. Edema is a symptom of a primary condition. Factors that can cause edema include:

Obstruction of the lymph channels, as may occur with neoplasms

Mechanical obstruction of the veins as with cirrhosis of the liver

Surgical removal of lymph nodes

Reduction in the protein concentration of plasma

Rise in capillary blood pressure

Increased permeability of the capillary membrane

Increase in the filtering surface when the capillaries dilate

Congestive heart failure

Renal disease, as with nephrotic syndrome

Malnutrition

Toxic substances

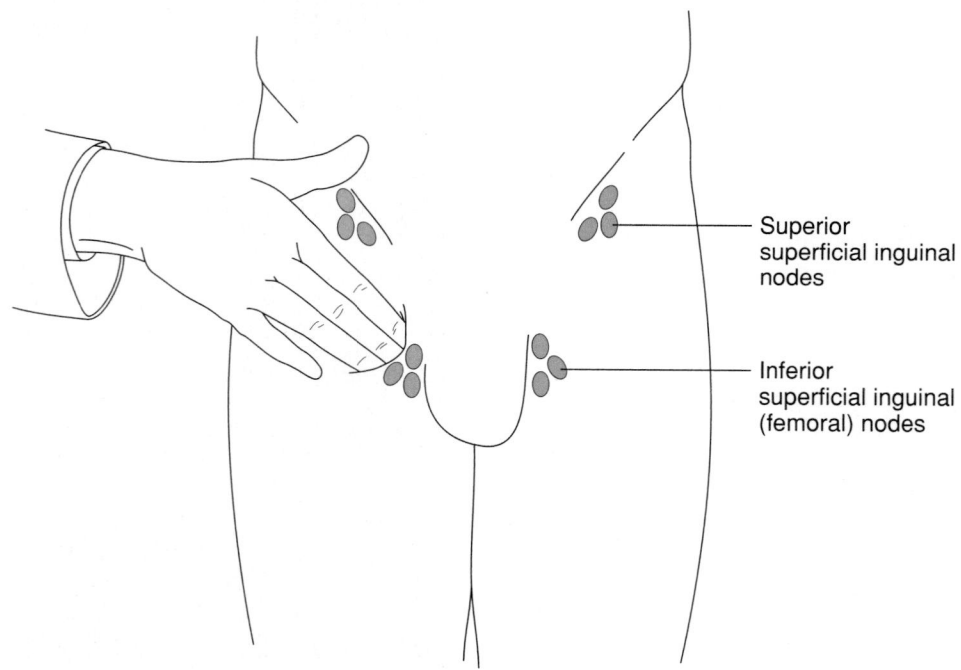

Superior superficial inguinal nodes

Inferior superficial inguinal (femoral) nodes

FIGURE 13-13 Palpation of the inguinal lymph nodes.

STEP-BY-STEP

Examination Step-by-Step

1. Preparation
   a. Assemble needed equipment—ruler and tape measure
   b. Make sure room provides privacy and comfortable temperature
   c. Explain examination to the client
2. Inspection—observe superficial lymph node as listed below for swelling, erythema, red streaks on skin.
3. Palpation—using pads of second, third, and fourth fingers, palpate with a gentle rotary motion all the superficial node areas listed below. Describe any nodes palpated in terms of location, size, shape, consistency, surface characteristics, symmetry, fixation or mobility, warmth, and tenderness.

Head:
  Preauricular
  Mastoid
  Occipital
  Parotid
  Submandibular
  Submental
Neck:
  Anterior cervical
  Posterior cervical
  Deep cervical
  Supraclavicular
  Infraclavicular
Axilla:
  Lateral axillary
  Posterior axillary
  Central axillary
  Anterior axillary
  Apical axillary
Breast:
  Axillary nodes
Arm:
  Epitrochlear
Leg:
  Superior inguinal
  Inferior inguinal
  Popliteal

Lymphedema. **Lymphedema** is the excessive collection of fluid in the tissues due to inadequate lymph drainage. Several factors can cause lymphedema. Lymph channels may be congenitally abnormal. Ac-

quired lymphedema results from trauma to the ducts of regional lymph nodes. Surgery, radiation, infection, fibrosis, inflammation, or neoplastic growth can cause lymphedema. The lymphatic channels may be blocked, absent, or not patent. Fluid transport is insufficient resulting in swelling. Except in the early phases, lymphedema is characteristically nonpitting.

Acute Infections

Acute infections may cause lymph nodes to be firm, tender, matted, or discrete. For example, common infection associated with enlarged neck nodes are bacterial infections such as streptococcal pharyngitis and viral infections like viral pharyngitis and infectious mononucleosis.

Lymphangitis. Lymphangitis is an inflammation of one or more lymphatic vessels, usually resulting from an acute streptococcal infection of an extremity. Fine red streaks extend from the infected area to the axilla or groin. It may be accompanied by fever, chills, and headache.

Lymphadenitis. Lymphadenitis is an inflammatory condition of the lymph nodes resulting from neoplastic disease, bacterial infection, or other inflammatory conditions. The nodes may be enlarged, hard, tender, smooth, or irregular. The overlying skin may become edematous, red, and warm. The site of the affected node indicates the site of the origin of the disease.

Streptococcal pharyngitis. Symptoms of streptococcal pharyngitis, a common condition, usually include a sore throat and runny nose and may include headache, fatigue, myalgias, and abdominal discomfort. Anterior cervical nodes are commonly felt and tend to be firm, discrete, mobile, and tender.

Epstein-Barr virus mononucleosis. Epstein-Barr virus mononucleosis (infectious mononucleosis) is most common in adolescents and young adults. Early symptoms include pharyngitis, fever, swollen lymph glands, fatigue, and malaise. Splenomegaly, hepatomegaly, and a rash may develop. Node enlargement may be generalized but is most common in the anterior and posterior cervical chains. Nodes vary in firmness, are generally discrete, and may be a bit tender.

Metastatic Disease

The first clinical sign of **metastatic** disease is the involvement of lymph nodes in the region draining the site of neoplastic growth. The lymph nodes may be hard, fixed to surrounding tissue, and nontender. Malignant **lymphomas,** including Hodgkin's disease, cause nodes to be large, discrete, nontender, and firm to rubbery. Such nodes may be localized to any area but are occasionally generalized. Chronic lymphocytic leukemia causes **lymphadenopathy** with the same characteristics as lymphoma, but the findings are usually generalized. Lymph nodes of metastatic cancer are nontender, have a firm to hard consistency, may be discrete or matted, and tend to be localized initially.

The various lymphomas differ in degree of cellular differentiation and content, but the manifestations are similar in all types. Characteristically, the appearance of a painless, enlarged lymph node or nodes in the neck is followed by weakness, fever, weight loss, and anemia. With widespread involvement of lymphoid tissue, the spleen and liver usually enlarge. GI disturbances, malabsorption, and bone lesions frequently develop.

Hodgkin's disease is a malignant disorder characterized by painless, progressive enlargement of lymphoid tissue, usually first evident in cervical lymph nodes, splenomegaly, and atypical macrophages. Symptoms include anorexia, weight loss, generalized pruritus, low-grade fever, night sweats, anemia, and leukocytosis. Non-Hodgkin's lymphoma (lymphosarcoma) is any kind of malignant lymphoma except Hodgkin's disease.

AIDS and AIDS-Related Complex

AIDS is a disease involving a defect in cell-mediated immunity. This syndrome is caused by the human immunodeficiency virus (HIV). It is characterized by the loss of T4 cells, which leads to the progressive loss of immune system competency with development of opportunistic infections, impairment of the central nervous system, chronic wasting, and often malignancy. It is manifested clinically as the development of recurrent, often severe, opportunistic infections. Initial symptoms include lymphadenopathy, extreme fatigue, intermittent fever, chills, night sweats, enlarged spleen, anorexia, diarrhea, weight loss, apathy, and depression. As the disease progresses, general malnourishment, decreased energy, and recurrent infections develop. Common opportunistic infections associated with AIDS are *Pneumocystis carinii* pneumonia, cytomegalovirus (CMV), herpes simplex, herpes zoster, *Candida albicans*, *Cryptococcus* organisms, *Toxoplasma gondii*, *Cryptosporidium* organisms, *Mycobacterium avium-intracellulare*, and tuberculosis. Most people with the disorder are susceptible to malignant **neoplasms,** especially Kaposi's sarcoma and non-Hodgkin's lymphoma.

AIDS-related complex (ARC) involves immunosuppression in a person who has HIV antibodies but has not yet developed recurrent infections and neoplastic disease associated with full-blown AIDS. Signs and symptoms of ARC may include weight loss, fever, malaise, severe fatigue, lethargy, weakness, persistent lymphadenopathy, arthralgias, oral thrush, and persistent diarrhea. ARC may remain in a mild form or may progress to AIDS.

TEACHING SELF-ASSESSMENT

Although examining the lymph nodes is not a self-care procedure routinely taught to clients, certain clients may be interested in learning to examine some areas of the body such as the neck, axilla, and groin for enlarged nodes in themselves and in their children. Clients can be taught to use the same techniques used by the examiner described in the section on examination techniques in this chapter.

DOCUMENTATION

Sample Documentation

Health History

A 20-year-old white female college student reports several days of malaise and "feeling a little sweaty" for the past week. For the past 2 days, she has had a sore throat, a fever of 38.1° C to 38.6° C (100° to 101° F), slight soreness in the neck, mild nausea, and urine slightly darker than usual. No known exposure to any infectious diseases, no chronic illnesses, malignancy, or surgery, does not use street drugs, not sexually active at this time. No family history of malignancy, blood diseases, or other chronic illnesses, other than father with mild hypertension, managed by diet. She has been taking aspirin, which provides temporary relief of symptoms.

Physical Examination

On examination she appears tired, has a temperature of 38.3° C (100.4° F). Her throat is slightly infected, no exudate. Anterior cervical nodes are enlarged bilaterally, several palpable, measuring 2 × 1 ½ cm, firm, rubbery, tender, mobile. Also has small anterior axillary nodes bilaterally, less than 1 cm. No other nodes palpable. Slight tenderness in the left and right upper quadrants of the abdomen.

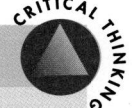

Nursing Diagnosis   *The Next Step*

Nursing diagnoses that could apply to alterations in the lymphatic system include, but are not limited to:

HIGH RISK FOR INFECTION The state in which an individual is at increased risk for being invaded by pathogenic organisms.

Defining Characteristics (risk factors)

- Inadequate primary and secondary defenses
- Immunosuppression
- Inadequate acquired immunity
- Insufficient knowledge to avoid exposure to pathogens
- Tissue destruction and increased environmental exposure
- Chronic disease
- Invasive procedures
- Malnutrition
- Pharmaceutical agents

FLUID VOLUME EXCESS The state in which an individual experiences increased fluid retention and edema.

Defining Characteristics

- Edema, effusion, anasarca
- Sudden weight gain
- Intake greater than output, oliguria, specific gravity changes
- Abnormal breath sounds (crackles, rales), change in respiratory pattern: dipphea, shortness of breath, orthoshea
- Pulmonary congestion by chest x-ray examination
- Blood pressure, venous pressure, pulmonary artery pressure changes
- Hemoglobin and hematocrit decreased
- Electrolytes altered, azotemia

Related Factors

- Compromised regulatory mechanisms

HIGH RISK FOR ACTIVITY INTOLERANCE The state in which an individual is at risk of experiencing insufficient physiological or psychological energy to endure or complete required or desired daily activities.

Defining Characteristics (risk factors)

- Deconditioned status
- Intention, or need, to engage in energy-consuming body movement

BODY IMAGE DISTURBANCE Disruption in the way one perceives one's body image.

Defining Characteristics

- Verbalized actual or perceived change in structure and/or function of body or body part
- Verbalized change in lifestyle because of negative feelings or perception of body
- Verbalized fear of rejection or reaction by others
- Repeated verbalizations focusing on past strength, function or appearance
- Verbalized negative feelings about body (dirty, big, small, unsightly)
- Verbalized feelings of helplessness, hopelessness, powerlessness in relation to the body
- Preoccupation with change in body
- Extension of body boundary to incorporate environmental objects (e.g., machines, oxygen, respirator)

Continued.

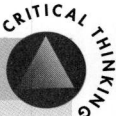

Nursing Diagnosis   *THE NEXT STEP—cont'd*

- Guilt, shame
- Emphasis on remaining strengths or heightened achievement
- Repeated expressions of negative feeling about loss of body fluids, addition of body fluids, or machines
- Trauma to nonfunctioning part (intentional or nonintentional)
- Change in social involvement or social relationships
- Hiding or overexposing body part

Related Factors

- Nonintegration of change and perceived imperfections

Clinical Application

Mr. M. is a 22-year-old male college student admitted into the hospital with a low grade fever, complaint of sore throat, fatigue, and headache for the past 5 days. Today he woke up with left side abdominal pain and a fine maculopapular rash over his trunk. The pain and the rash scared him into coming to the hospital. "I can't stop itching, I look horrible, and my left side hurts when I move." He expresses concern about missing school and his girlfriend. Vital signs: Temperature 39° C (102.2°F), pulse 88 beats/min., respirations 20 breaths/min, blood pressure 122/70. Physical assessment revealed: Throat: no tonsils, pharyngeal wall bright red with small amount white exudate. Enlarged anterior and posterior cervical nodes bilaterally, several palpable. Left upper quadrant abdominal pain tender to touch.

SUBJECTIVE DATA: Patient complains of:
Fever
Sore throat
Fatigue
Itching
Left-sided abdominal pain

OBJECTIVE DATA:
Temperature 102.2° F
Throat: pharyngeal walls bright red with small amount white exudate.
Skin: redden maculopapular rash all over trunk.
Neck: enlarged anterior and posterior cervical nodes bilaterally, painful to palpation, several palpable, measuring 1.5 × 1.5 cm, firm, rubbery, and mobile. Has large anterior axillary nodes bilaterally approximately 2 cm firm, rubbery, and mobile.
Abdomen: tenderness in left upper quadrant of abdomen, enlarged spleen noted.
Laboratory results: White blood cell count (WBC) with differential reveals 18,000/mm³; 50% are lymphocytes and monocytes; 20% are atypical lymphocytes. Monospot test positive.
Medical diagnosis of infectious mononucleosis.

NURSING DIAGNOSES

High risk for activity intolerance related to generalized weakness from infectious process.

Defining Characteristics

- Verbal report of fatigue
- Pain upon movement
- Itching upon movement

Body image disturbance related to verbalized actual change in body—red rash all over trunk.

Defining Characteristics

- Patient complains of red rash on body and looking horrible
- Patient complains of itching
- Patient complains of pain upon movement
- Patient complains of fatigue—not being able to maintain college and social life

GLOSSARY

acquired immune deficiency syndrome (AIDS) A disease involving a defect in cell-mediated immunity that has a long incubation period, follows a protracted and debilitating course, is manifested by various opportunistic infections and often by malignant neoplasms, and has a poor prognosis.

AIDS related complex (ARC) A subclinical form of acquired immune deficiency syndrome (AIDS). Signs and symptoms may include weight loss, fever, malaise, lethargy, oral thrush, and immunologic abnormalities characteristic of AIDS.

edema Excessive accumulation of fluids in the tissue spaces due to a disturbance in the mechanisms of fluid interchange.

lymphadenitis Inflammatory condition of the lymph nodes, usually the result of systemic neoplastic disease, bacterial infection, or other inflammatory condition. The location of the affected node is indicative of the site or origin of disease.

lymphadenopathy Disorder of the lymph nodes or lymph vessels.

lymphangitis An inflammation of one or more lymphatic vessels, usually resulting from an acute streptococcal infection of one of the extremities. Characterized by fine red streaks extending from the infected area to the axilla or groin, and by fever, chills, headache, and myalgia.

lymphedema Edema caused by obstruction of the lymph vessels; may be acquired as a result of cancer, scars, or surgical removal of the lymph nodes. A rare form is congenital.

lymphoma Neoplasm of lymphatic tissue.

metastasis The process by which tumor cells are spread to distant parts of the body. Because malignant tumors have no enclosing capsule, cells may escape, become emboli, and be transported by the lymphatic circulation or the bloodstream to implant on lymph nodes and other organs far from the primary tumor.

neoplasm Any abnormal growth of new tissue, benign or malignant; tumor.

right lymphatic duct One of two main trunks of the lymphatic system that drains lymphatic fluid from the right side of the head and neck, right arm, and right side of the chest wall. It drains into the right subclavian vein.

thoracic duct One of two main trunks of the lymphatic system that drains lymphatic fluid from all parts of the body except those areas drained by the right lymphatic duct.

BIBLIOGRAPHY

Baird SB and others: *Cancer nursing: a comprehensive textbook*, Philadelphia, 1991, WB Saunders.

Brady LW and others: Causes of neck masses in young adults, *Patient Care* 18:30, 1984.

Brady LW and others: When an older adult develops a neck mass, *Patient Care* 18:56, 1984.

Gordon M: *Manual of nursing diagnosis 1993–1994*, St. Louis, 1993, Mosby–Year Book.

Groenwald SL and others: *Cancer nursing: principles and practice*, ed 2, Boston, 1990, Jones and Bartlett Publishers.

Kim MJ and others: *Pocket guide to nursing diagnosis*, ed 5, St. Louis, 1993, Mosby–Year Book.

Longe RL and others: Peripheral vascular and clinical pharmacy, lymphatic systems, *Drug Intell Clin Pharm* 19:4, 252–258, 1985.

McConnell EA: Getting the feel of lymph node assessment, *Nursing 88* 18:54–57, 1988.

Netter FH: *Atlas of human anatomy*, Summit, NY, 1989, Ciba-Geigy Corporation.

West JB, editor: *Best and Taylor's physiological basis of medical practice*, ed 12, Baltimore, 1990, Williams & Wilkins.

Breasts

PURPOSE OF EXAMINATION

Breast examination is part of the assessment of sexual development and reproductive function. Because cancer of the breast is a major cause of morbidity and mortality in women, and because early detection and treatment of breast cancer improves survival rates, the breast examination is an important component of screening for cancer and an opportunity to teach breast self-examination.

The currently recommended guidelines for breast screening of women without signs and symptoms of breast disease are as follows (Dodd, 1992):

1. Clinical examination of the breast and mammography are the basic detection methods. The examinations are complementary, and both are necessary to achieve maximum detection rates.
2. The screening process should begin by 40 years of age and should consist of annual clinical ex-

aminations with screening mammography performed at 1- to 2-year intervals.
3. Beginning at age 50, both clinical examination and mammography should be performed on an annual basis.

In 1989 the U.S. Preventive Services Task Force issued a somewhat different set of guidelines for women at low risk for breast disease. This task force recommended an annual clinical breast examination for women age 40 and older and mammography every 1 to 2 years beginning at age 50 and concluding at approximately age 75.

Screening for breast cancer is the focus of one of the national health promotion and disease prevention objectives proposed in *Healthy People 2000* (U.S. Department of Health and Human Services, 1991). The objective is to increase (1) to at least 80% the proportion of women age 40 and older who have ever received a clinical breast examination and a mammogram, and (2) to at least 60% those age 50 and older who have received these screening tests within the preceding 1 to 2 years. (Baseline: 36% of women age 40 and older "ever" in 1987; 25% of women age 50 and older "within the preceding 2 years" in 1987.)

Although current research does not demonstrate that the initiation of dedicated screening programs for breast cancer detection *before age 40* is cost-effective for the early identification of breast cancer in populations, breast examination and the teaching of breast self-examination are essential components of health assessments for all women after puberty. Breast examination offers an excellent opportunity for breast and reproductive health education and for the identification of minor problems, which would be amenable to early intervention, and the uncommon breast cancers in young women.

ANATOMY AND PHYSIOLOGY

The breast is a modified sebaceous gland that is paired. It is located on the anterior chest wall between the second and third ribs (superiorly), the sixth and seventh costal cartilages (inferiorly), the anterior axillary line (laterally), and the sternal border (medially). Subcutaneous and retromammary fat compose much of the bulk of the breast. The breast, which is fairly mobile, is supported by a layer of subcutaneous connective tissue and by **Cooper's ligaments** (Figure 14-1, *B*). The latter are multiple fibrous bands that begin at the breast's subcutaneous connective tissue layer, run through the breast, and are attached to muscle fascia.

The functional components of the female breast are the **acini** (milk-producing glands), a ductal system, and a nipple (Figure 14-1, *A*). The glandular tissue units, called **lobes**, are situated in a circular, spokelike fashion around the nipple. Each breast has 15 to 25 lobes. A lobe is composed of 20 to 40 lobules, each containing 10 to 100 acini. Lactiferous ducts drain milk or other fluid from the lobes to the surface of the nipples. The nipples, composed of epithelium intertwined with circular and longitudinal smooth muscle fibers, are located centrally on the breasts. These muscle fibers contract in response to tactile, sensory, and autonomic stimuli, producing erection of the nipple and emptying of any material in the lactiferous ducts. The nipples are round, hairless, pigmented, protuberant structures. Their size and shape vary among women and in an individual woman, depending on the state of contraction. Usually nipples are directed, "pointing" slightly upward and laterally. This position of the nipples places them in an ideal angle for breast-feeding an infant.

Inversion of the nipple is an invagination or depression of its central portion. Inversion can occur congenitally or as a response to an invasive process. The **areolae** are pigmented areas surrounding the nipples. Their color varies from pink to brown, and their size differs greatly among individuals. Several to many sebaceous glands, termed **Montgomery's glands (also called tubercles or follicles)**, appearing as small bumps, may be present on the areolar surface.

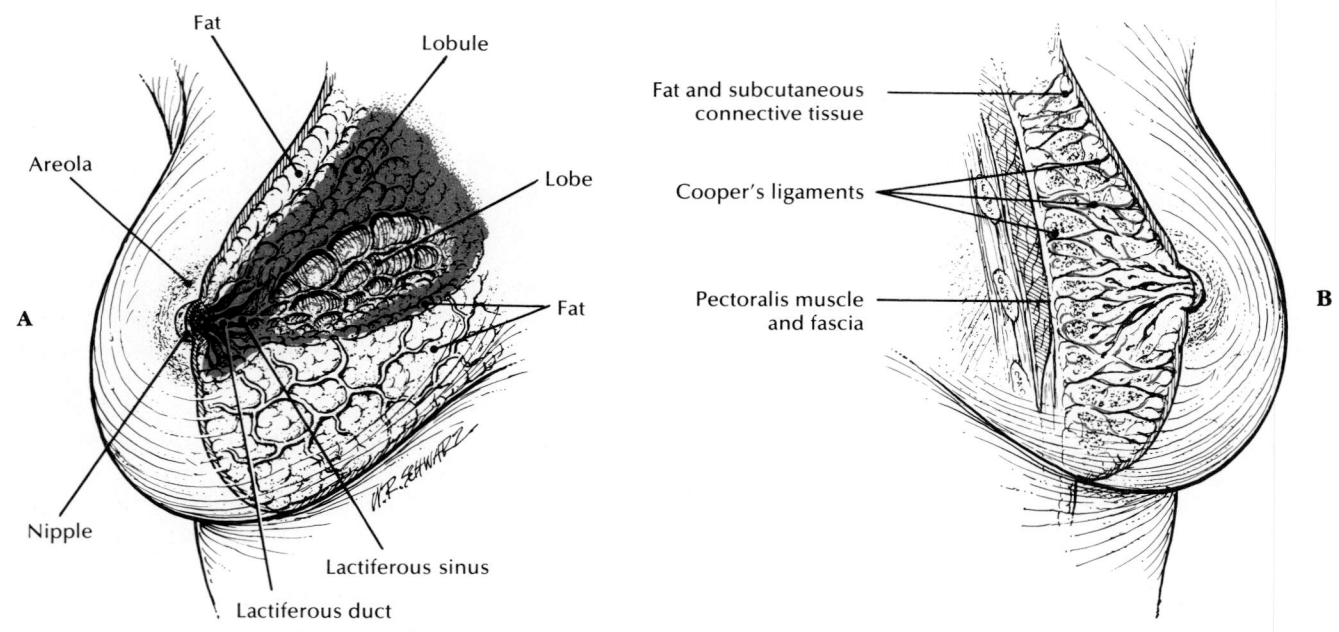

FIGURE 14-1 Female breasts. **A,** Internal structures. **B,** Supportive tissue structures.

During early embryonic development, longitudinal ridges appear, extending from the axilla to the groin. Called "milk lines" (Figure 14-2), these ridges usually atrophy, except at the level of the pectoral muscles, where a breast will eventually develop. In some women the ridges do not entirely disappear, and portions of the milk lines persist. This occurrence is manifested in the presence of a nipple, a nipple and a breast, or glandular breast tissue only. This congenital anomaly is called a supernumerary breast or nipple.

Knowledge of the lymphatic drainage of the breast is important because of the common metastasis of breast cancer throughout this system. Lymph drainage from the breast is directed toward numerous groups of nodes with most of the drainage routed to the axillary nodes. However, depending on the site of the lesion, drainage might also be directed into the infraclavicular nodes, the chest, the abdomen, or the opposite breast. (See Chapter 13 for a thorough discussion of the assessment of the lymphatic system.) The following three general types of lymphatic drainage from the breast occur (Figure 14-3).

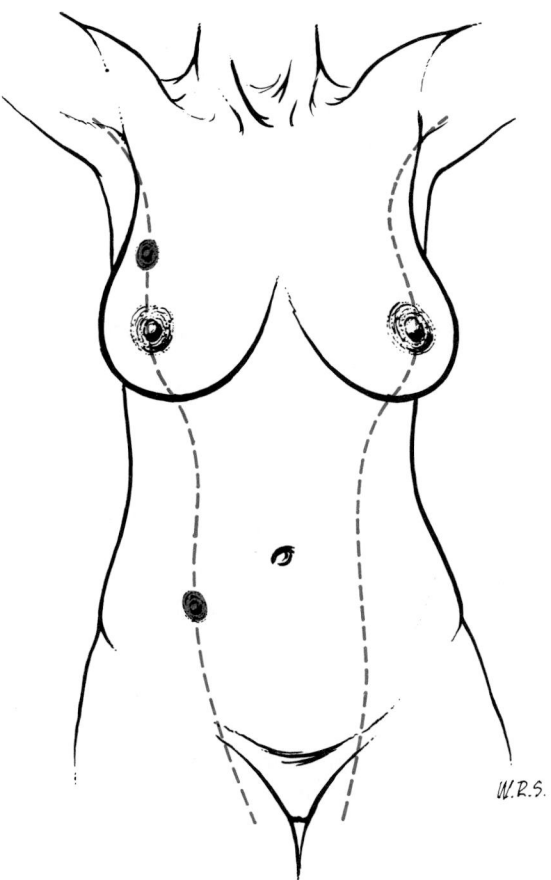

FIGURE 14-2 Milk lines.

Cutaneous lymphatic drainage occurs from the skin of the breast, excluding the areolar and nipple areas. The lymph flows into the ipsilateral axillary nodes (subscapular, brachial, and intermediate). Fluid from the medial cutaneous breast area may flow to the opposite breast. Lymph from the inferior portion of the breast can reach the lymphatic plexus of the epigastric region and subsequently may extend to the liver and other abdominal regions and organs.

Areolar lymphatic drainage involves lymph formed in the areolar and nipple areas of the breast. This lymph flows into the anterior axillary group of nodes (pectoral nodes).

Deep lymphatic drainage originates from the deep mammary tissues. This lymph flows into the anterior axillary nodes. Some of this fluid also flows into the apical, supraclavicular, and infraclavicular nodes. In addition, lymph from the retroareolar areas, medial glandular breast tissue areas, and lower glandular breast tissue areas communicates with lymphatic systems that drain into the thorax and the abdomen.

The largest portion of glandular breast tissue is found in the upper lateral quadrant of each breast. From this quadrant there is an anatomical projection of breast tissue into the axilla. This projection is termed the **axillary tail of Spence** (Figure 14-4). The majority of breast tumors are located in the upper lateral breast quadrant and in the tail of Spence.

On general appearance, the normal breasts are reasonably symmetrical in size and shape, although they are not usually absolutely identical. This symmetry remains constant at rest and with movement. The skin of the breast is the same as that of the abdomen or back. A small number of hair follicles may be scattered around the areola. In light-complected persons a horizontal or vertical vascular pattern may be observed. This pattern, when normally present, is symmetrical.

The gross appearance and size of the normal female breast vary both among individuals and for an individual at various phases of development. The following paragraphs describe breast development throughout a woman's life span (Figure 14-5).

1. *Appearance before age 10.* Gross appearance of male and female breasts differs little. The nipples are small and slightly elevated. No palpable glandular tissue or areolar pigmentation exists.

2. *Appearance between age 10 and 14.* The mammary tissues adjacent to and beneath the areola grow, resulting in an increased diameter of the areola and the formation of a "mammary bud." The nipple and breast protrude as a single mound. Breast development may begin normally or may occur unilaterally. Next, the general mammary growth and increases in diameter and pigmentation of the areola continue, resulting in further elevation of the breasts. The nipple begins to

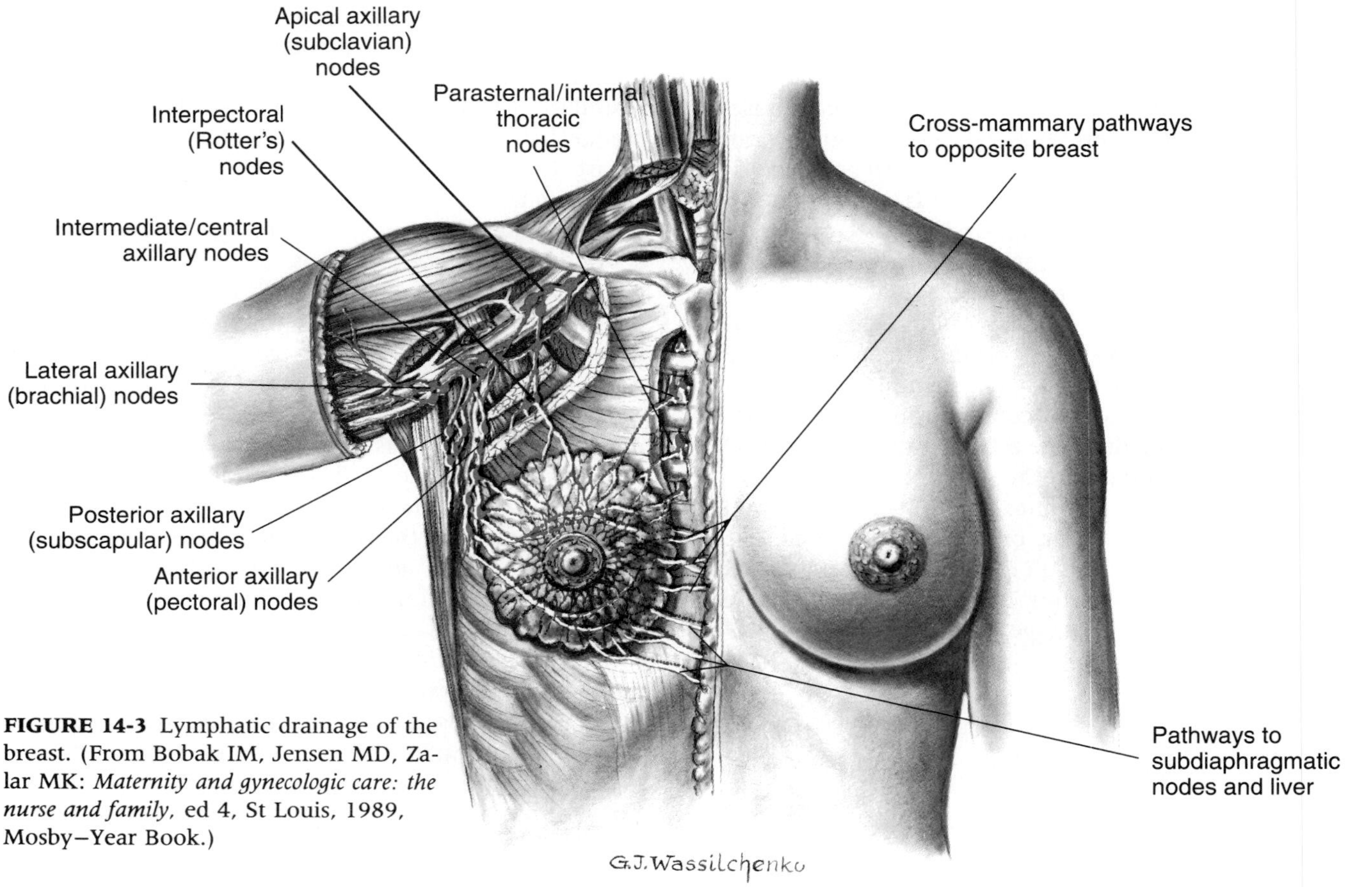

Apical axillary
(subclavian)
nodes

Interpectoral
(Rotter's)
nodes

Parasternal/internal
thoracic
nodes

Intermediate/central
axillary nodes

Cross-mammary pathways
to opposite breast

Lateral axillary
(brachial) nodes

Posterior axillary
(subscapular) nodes

Anterior axillary
(pectoral) nodes

Pathways to
subdiaphragmatic
nodes and liver

G.J.Wassilchenko

FIGURE 14-3 Lymphatic drainage of the breast. (From Bobak IM, Jensen MD, Zalar MK: *Maternity and gynecologic care: the nurse and family,* ed 4, St Louis, 1989, Mosby—Year Book.)

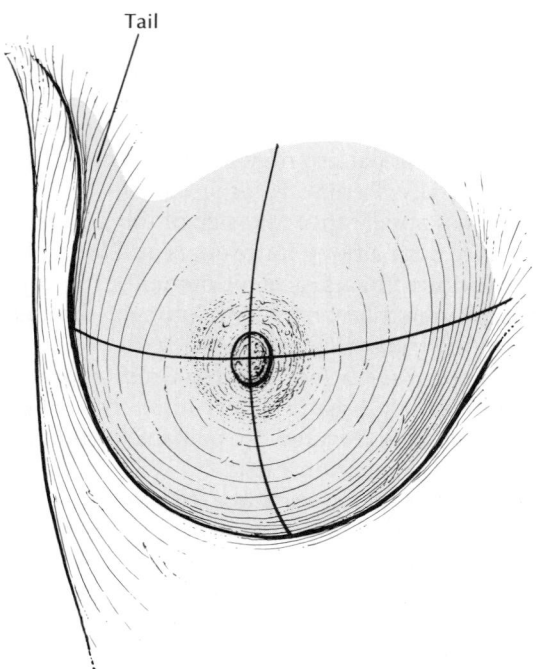

Tail

FIGURE 14-4 Four breast quadrants and the axillary tail of Spence.

separate from the areola. Growth continues in the mammary tissues. The nipple and areola form a mound that is distinct from the globular shape of the rest of the breast.

3. *Appearance after age 14.* The shape of the adult female breast gradually forms. The areola recedes into the general contour of the breast, and only the nipple protrudes. Heredity, individual sensitivity to hormones, and nutrition influence the size of the adult female breast.

4. *Appearance during reproductive years.* In response to hormonal changes during the menstrual cycle, a cyclic pattern of breast size change, nodularity, and tenderness occurs. These changes are maximal just before menses. The breast is smallest in days 4 through 7 of the menstrual cycle. Three to 4 days before the onset of menses, many women experience mammary tenseness, fullness, heaviness, tenderness, and pain because of hormonal changes and fluid retention. Total breast volume is significantly increased at this time.

5. *Changes in pregnancy.* The breast increases in size, sometimes reaching two to three times the usual size. The areolae and nipples become more prominent and more deeply pigmented. The veins become engorged, the Montgomery's glands become more apparent, and striae often develop.

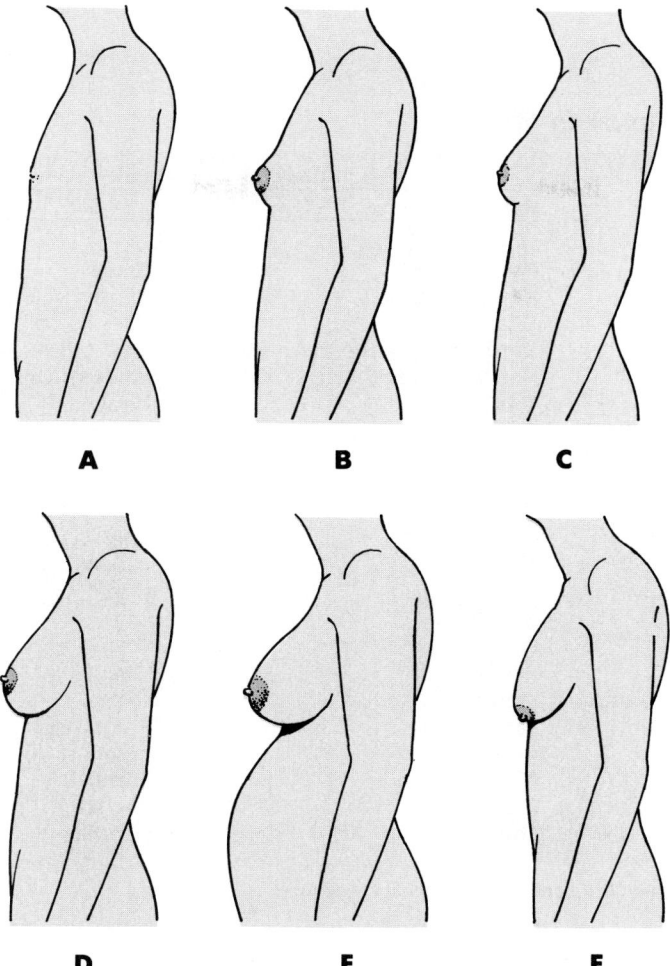

FIGURE 14-5 Appearance of the female breast in various life periods. **A,** Appearance before age 10. **B** and **C,** Appearance between ages 10 through 14. **D,** Appearance of the nulliparous, adult breast. **E,** Appearance of the breast during pregnancy. **F,** Appearance of the breast after menopause.

6. ***Menopausal changes.*** After menopause the breast's glandular tissue gradually involutes, and fat is deposited in the breasts. The breast formation becomes flabby and flattened.

The male breast contains a nipple and an areola. Beneath the nipple is a small amount of breast tissue, which usually cannot be clinically differentiated from the other subcutaneous tissues.

EXAMINATION

Health History

The foci of the health history are self-examination practices and identification of problems that require assessment. Throughout the health history, the following data about a symptom or problem are recorded: (1) onset (specific date, sudden or gradual), (2) duration, (3) frequency, (4) precipitating factors, (5) aggravating or alleviating factors, (6) treatment received or self-care given, and (7) outcome.

Present health status

1. Breast self-examination
   a. Frequency
   b. Timing with menstrual cycle
2. Changes in breast characteristics and their relationship to menstrual cycle: pain, tenderness, heaviness, swelling, lumps, discharge, and changes in appearance, size, or shape
3. Mammography
   a. Age at first mammography
   b. Date of last mammography and findings
4. Risk factors for breast cancer (Table 14-1)

TABLE 14-1

Risk Factors for Breast Cancer in Women

Factor	Differentiation of risk		Strength of factor
	High risk	**Low risk**	
Demographic factors			
Age	Old	Young	Strong
Marital status	Never married	Married young	Weak
Race	White	Black	Weak
Residence: country	North America, northern Europe	Asia, Africa	Strong
Residence: U.S. location	Northern United States	Southern United States	Weak
Residence: type	Urban	Rural	Weak
Socioeconomic status	Upper	Lower	Moderate
Personal history			
Age: menarche	Early	Late	Weak
Age: menopause	Late	Early	Weak
Age: first term pregnancy	>30 yr	<30 yr	Moderate
Family history: bilateral breast cancer	Present	Absent	Strong
Family history: breast cancer	Present	Absent	Moderate
History: cancer in one breast	Present	Absent	Strong
History: fibrocystic disease	Present	Absent	Moderate
History: cancer in ovary or endometrium	Present	Absent	Moderate
History: chest radiation	Large doses	Low exposure	Moderate
Oophorectomy	None	Present	Moderate
Premenopausal body build	Obese	Thin	Moderate
Diet	High fat	Low fat	Moderate
	Low fiber	High fiber	Moderate

Modified from Marchant DJ: *Breast disease*, New York, 1986, Churchill Livingstone.

Present illness*

1. Breast discomfort
   a. Pattern
   b. Onset
   c. Duration
   d. Severity
   e. Character
   f. Associated symptoms
   g. Contributory and alleviating factors
2. Swelling and lumps
   a. Location
   b. Size
   c. Changes in the surface characteristics of breast
   d. Mobility
   e. Time when first noted
   f. Changes over time
   g. Changes related to menses
   h. Associated symptoms
3. Discharge
   a. Color
   b. Consistency
   c. Amount

   d. Odor
   e. Factors associated with onset, recent injuries
   f. Reproductive status
4. Current medications

Past health history

1. Previous diagnoses of breast disease
2. Previous breast surgeries
3. Lactation history
4. **Mastitis**
5. Cancers in other sites

Associated systems

1. Reproductive and menstrual history
2. Medication history, especially hormones
3. Nutrition history, especially caffeine intake

Family health history

1. Breast cancer
2. Benign breast disease

Preparation for the Examination: Client and Environment

Some girls and women are embarrassed while undergoing a breast examination. Their reasons for embar-

*Common symptoms are listed.

Preparation for Examination

Equipment

Item	Purpose
Small pillow or folded towel	For placement under back of side being examined to spread breast tissue more evenly on chest
Centimeter ruler	To measure position and size of any masses located
Glass slide and cytological fixative	To prepare specimen of any abnormal drainage for microscopic examination. (Drainage; which is often thin and acellular, is most effectively collected on a frosted or albumin-coated slide to prevent runoff.)

Client and Environment

Setting

Well lit
Private
Warm

Client

Stripped to waist
Seated for first portion of examination, lying down for second portion

Examiner

Standing at front of examiner for first portion, at right side of client for second portion

---

rassment may include a sense of modesty or dissatisfaction with their breast development. The examiner should take care to ensure privacy during the examination and avoid unnecessary exposure of the breasts. It is also important to avoid making comments about the client's breast development that could be misinterpreted. Explaining the components of the examination helps to relieve the client's discomfort and provides important health education.

During the health history preceding the physical examination, the examiner should assess the woman's level of knowledge and practice regarding breast self-examination. The examination provides an excellent opportunity for reviewing the client's technique and for teaching breast self-examination.

Many adolescent or adult male clients may not have had a breast examination previously and may be concerned that the examiner will notice a problem. Explaining to male clients that breast lesions are possible in men and that the breast examination is a routine component of a complete health assessment will help to alleviate any worry and embarrassment. Some male clients have perspiration in the axilla and may be embarrassed when an examiner palpates this dampened area; it is helpful to offer the male client a tissue for drying the area before the examination is begun.

Technique for Examination and Normal Findings
Inspection

Inspection and palpation are the techniques used to examine the breast. For initial inspection, the client is seated on the side of the examination table and is uncovered to the waist. If the client reports that she has noticed a lump or a change in one of the breasts, ask her to point out the area and demonstrate the technique she used to feel the lump or change. Take special note of that area during the examination.

Observe the breasts, including the nipples and areolae, for symmetry of shape and size, surface characteristics, and abnormal amount or distribution of hair. As with inspection of all paired organs, use the client as her own control and compare both breasts to determine what is "normal" for that individual and to detect any unusual findings for a given individual. Lack of symmetry always indicates a need for additional assessment.

Symmetry of shape and size. Normal female breasts are bilaterally similar in shape and size. However, frequently one breast is somewhat smaller than the other (Figure 14-6). In males, the breasts are normally even with the chest wall, except for obese men, whose breasts

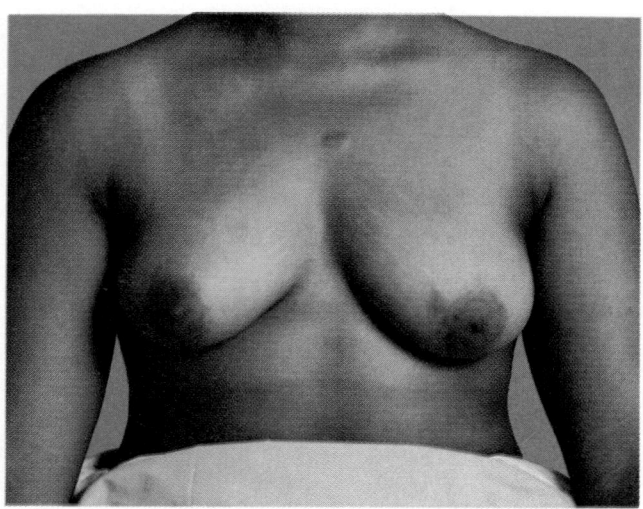

FIGURE 14-6 Observation of the breasts. These breasts have several characteristics that are deviations within normal limits: (1) the left breast is slightly larger than the right; (2) the nipples are directed in slightly different directions; (3) the left breast has a superficial skin lesion appearing as a dark area medial to the areola; and (4) both breasts have striae.

assume a bilaterally convex shape similar to that of female breasts.

Surface characteristics. The surface characteristics of breasts may include hyperpigmentation, moles and nevi, edema, retraction, dimpling, focal vascularity, and lesions. The skin of the breasts appears smooth, and the surface contour should appear even and uninterrupted. Normally, only the areola and the nipple are hyperpigmented. Other portions of the breast are normally a color that is uniform with the individual's skin in other covered parts of the body. Focal hyperpigmentation is an abnormal finding. Moles and nevi are common. The client should be questioned about changes or problems with any common skin lesion noted.

Edema of the breast, usually caused by blocked lymph drainage, produces exaggeration of the skin pores, creating an orange-peel appearance called **peau d'orange** (Figure 14-7, *B*).

Retraction, or **dimpling**, appears as a depression or pucker on the skin (Figure 14-7, *A*). It usually is caused by the fibrotic shortening and immobilization of Cooper's ligament by an invasive process.

Vascular patterns should be diffuse and symmetrical. Hypervascular patterns may be noted in pregnant, obese, and very fair skinned individuals. Focal or unilateral patterns are abnormal and may be produced by dilated superficial veins from increased blood flow to a malignancy (see Figure 14-7, *A*).

The elastic fibers of the dermis may be damaged whenever the skin of the breasts is stretched rapidly, and observable striae, or stretch marks, are produced. Newly created striae are reddish, but they become white with age.

Areolar area and nipple characteristics. The areolar area can range from light pink to dark brown, depending on the client's genetic skin color and hormonal influences. In pregnancy, the areolae enlarge and darken. The areolar area is normally round or oval and bilaterally similar. Irregular placement of Montgomery's tubercles is common and normal.

After puberty, women may normally have a scattering of coarse, curly hair on the breasts, mostly near the areola. After puberty, males often have a dense mass of chest hair around the areola. Male hair patterns in female clients are abnormal. The areolar areas should be inspected for size, shape, symmetry, color, surface characteristics, bulging, and lesions. Size, shape, and color can normally vary greatly in symmetrical patterns. Any asymmetry, mass, or lesion should be considered abnormal.

If the breasts are symmetrical, both nipples should be pointing laterally in the same way. The nipples should be inspected for size, shape, ability to become erect, color, discharge, and lesions. The nipples should be round, equal in size, homogeneous in color, and have convoluted surfaces, which produce a wrinkled appearance. They should appear soft and smooth and have no crusting, cracks, or discharge.

Inversion of one or both nipples, if present from puberty, is normal. However, this condition may interfere with breast-feeding. Recent inversion of the nipple is probably retraction (see Figure 14-7, *A*) and should be investigated.

Supernumerary nipples and areolae may appear along the milk lines (see Figure 14-4). These lesions can vary in size. They are the color of the individual's actual areolae and are often mistaken for moles. Occasionally glandular tissue may accompany these lesions.

Paget's disease, a malignant condition requiring prompt therapy, appears as a red glandular erosion of the nipple or as a nipple that is dry, scaly, or friable. The areola may also be affected.

Breast secretions are normal in pregnancy or lactation. Other causes of discharge are mechanical nipple stimulation, drug influence, hypothalamic and pituitary disorders, and malignant and benign breast lesions. The discharge can be milky, watery, purulent, serous, or bloody. The method for determining the origin of discharge production is discussed in the section on palpation.

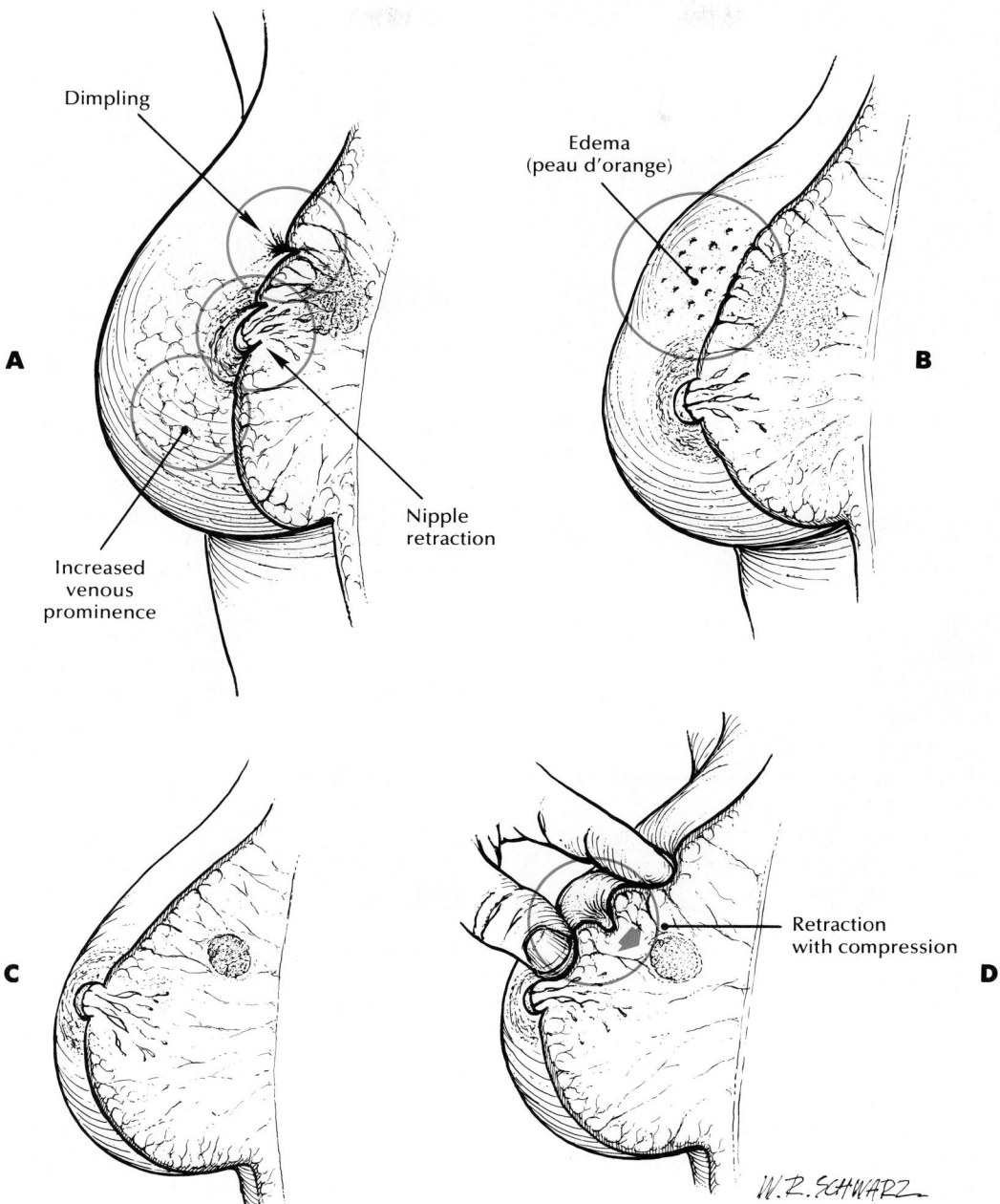

FIGURE 14-7 Abnormalities of the breast. **A,** Breast with dimpling, nipple retraction, and increased venous prominence. **B,** Breast with edema (peau d'orange or pigskin appearance). **C,** Breast with tumor; no retraction is apparent. **D,** Breast with tumor; retraction is apparent with compression.

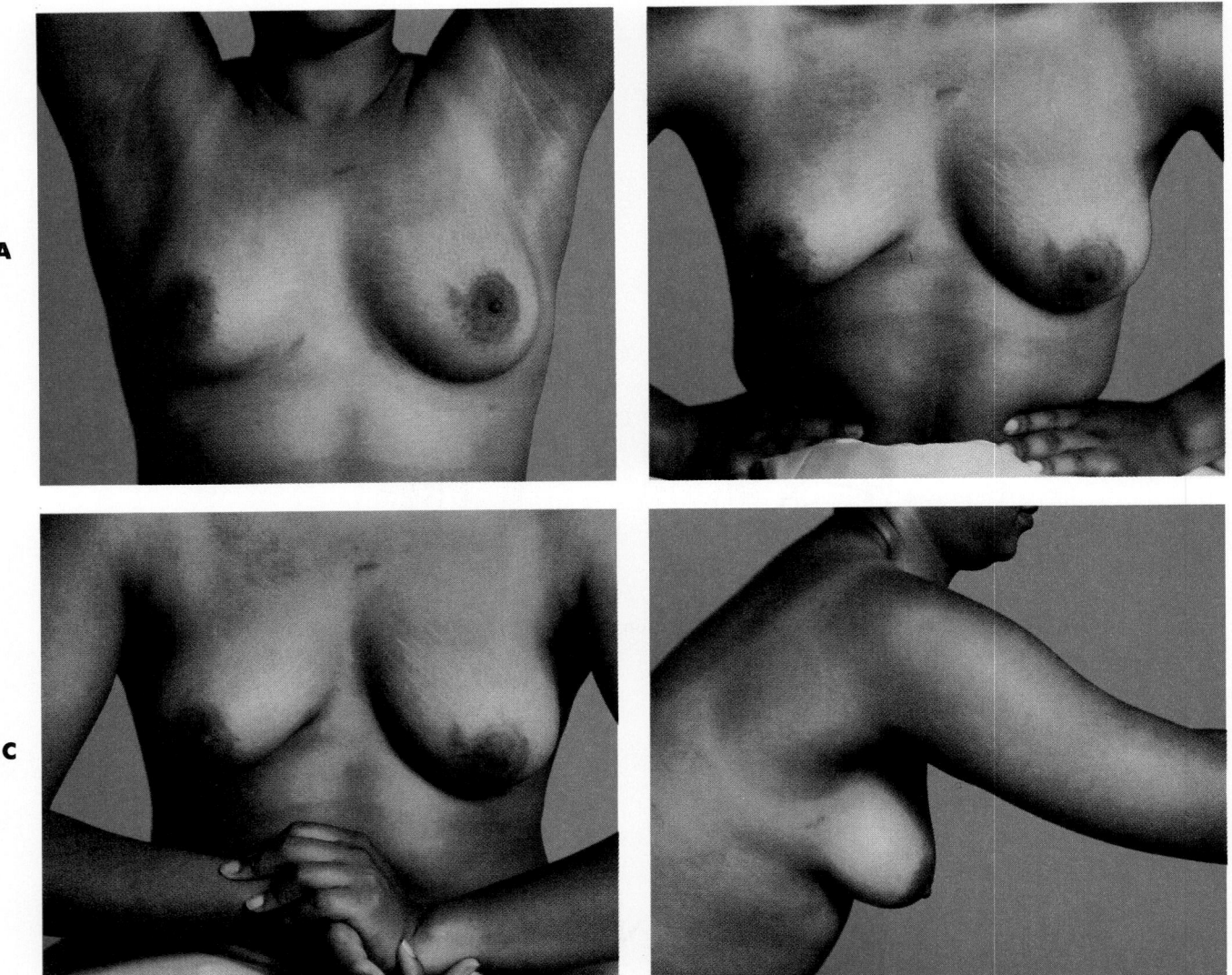

FIGURE 14-8 Observation of the breasts in several positions. **A,** Observation with client's arms overhead. **B,** Observation with client contracting pectoral muscles by pressing hands into waist. **C,** Alternate method of observing client with pectoral muscle contraction—hands pressed together in front of client. **D,** Observation with client leaning forward.

Sitting positions for breast inspection. There are four basic sitting positions used for breast inspection. Every adult female client should be examined in each position:

1. *Client is seated with arms at sides* (see Figure 14-6). Observe the breasts at rest and without movement to establish a baseline for comparison. Observe men in this position only, unless they have unusually large breasts, in which case the other inspection positions are also used.

2. *Client is seated with arms abducted over head* (Figure 14-8, *A*). This maneuver creates tension on the suspensory ligaments and may accentuate asymmetry, retraction, and fixation.

3. *Client is seated and pushes hands into hips* (or pushes palms together) (Figure 14-8, *B-C*). This action contracts the pectoral muscles and can reveal dimpling and deviations in symmetry.

4. *Client is seated and leans over* (Figure 14-8, *D*). The examiner assists in supporting and balancing the client during this maneuver. The breasts should hang evenly and symmetrically. This approach is especially useful in examining the movement and contour of large breasts.

A   **B**

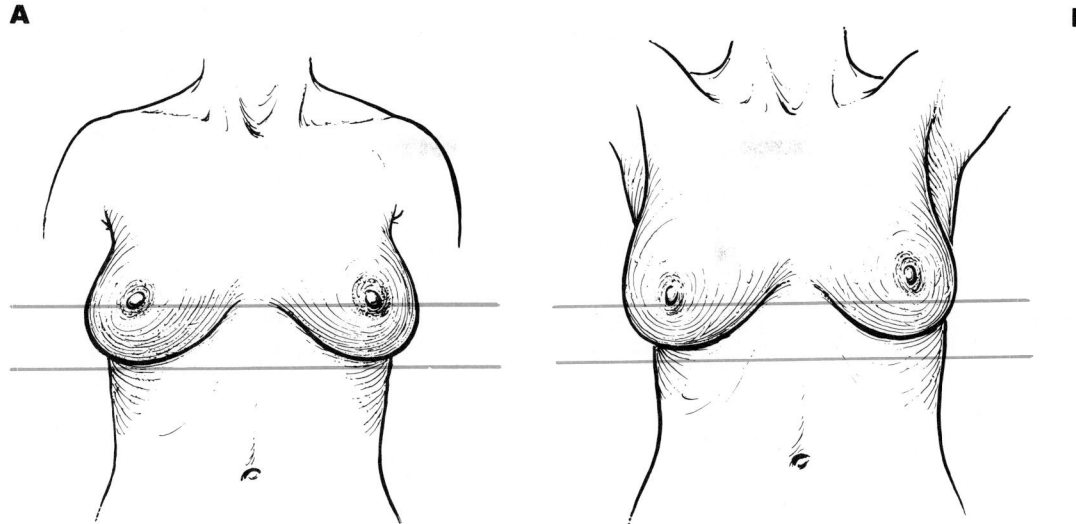

FIGURE 14-9 A, Breasts appear symmetric at rest. **B,** Breasts do not move symmetrically with arm elevation. The right breast is immobilized.

While the client is performing these maneuvers, carefully observe the breasts for symmetry, bulging, retraction, and fixation. An abnormality may not be apparent in the breasts at rest (Figure 14-9, *A*), but a mass may cause a breast, through invasion of suspensory ligaments, to fix, preventing it from upward or forward movements (Figure 14-9, *B*). Tension in the breasts through contraction of the pectoral muscles assists in eliciting dimpling if a mass has infiltrated and shortened suspensory ligaments.

Finally, observe the breasts while the client is lying down, before performing palpation.

Palpation

This portion of the breast examination begins with palpation for axillary, subclavicular, and supraclavicular lymph nodes. This step is most effectively performed with the client in a sitting position. The location and palpation of the axillary, subclavicular, and supraclavicular nodes are described in Chapter 13. To emphasize the importance of an adequate axillary area examination being done with each breast examination, this procedure is reviewed here.

To examine the axilla, the tissues can be best appreciated if the area muscles are relaxed. Contracted muscles may obscure slightly enlarged nodes. To achieve this relaxation while abducting the arm, support the **ipsilateral** arm (Figure 14-10). Visualize the axilla as a four-sided pyramid and thoroughly palpate the following areas:

1. *Lateral axillary nodes* (brachial) along the inside of the humerus (upper arm)
2. *Anterior axillary nodes* (pectoral) lying in the an-

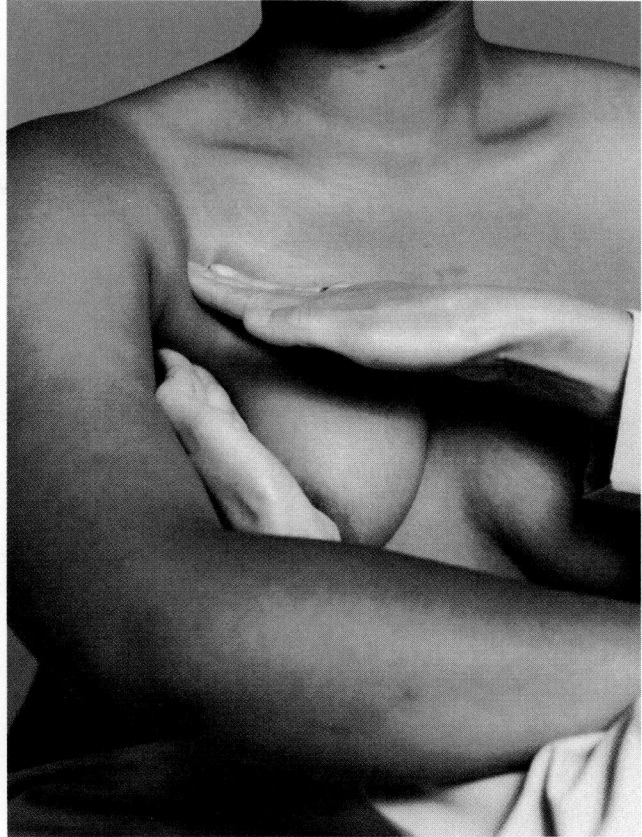

FIGURE 14-10 Palpation of the axillary lymph nodes. (Note that the client's arm is supported on the examiner's arm.)

A

B

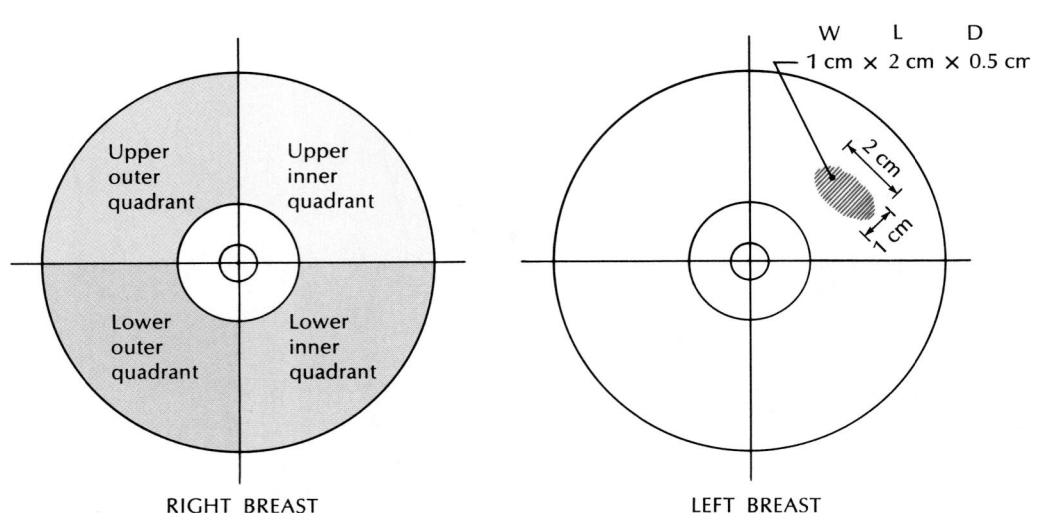

FIGURE 14-11 **A,** The four quadrants of the breast. **B,** Diagram of a mass within a breast.

ASSESSMENT OF BREAST MASSES

1. *Location:* Masses are designated according to the quadrant in which they lie: upper outer, lower outer, upper inner, or lower inner (Figure 14-11, *A*). To describe the mass in the client's record, it may be helpful to draw the mass within a diagram of the breast (Figure 14-11, *B*). Another method of describing location is to visualize the breast as the face of a clock with the nipple at center. A mass can be designated, for example, as being "5 cm from the nipple in the 8 o'clock position."

2. *Size:* The size should be approximated in centimeters in all its planes. For example, a mass may be ovoid, 3 cm wide, 2 cm long, and 1 cm thick.

3. *Shape:* The shape may be round, ovoid, irregular, or matted. Matting occurs in the presence of multiple lesions.

4. *Consistency:* The palpable consistency of a breast lesion may be soft, hard, solid, or cystic. One way to evaluate the consistency of a breast lesion is to palpate over the lesion with the pads of the index and middle fingers of the palpating hand (Figure 14-12, *A*).

5. *Discreteness:* The borders of a mass are assessed to determine if they are sharp and well defined or irregular. To assess discreteness, an attempt is made to palpate all the borders of the mass with the thumb and index finger of the palpating hand (Figure 14-12, *B*).

6. *Mobility:* The movability of the mass within the breast is assessed as freely movable or fixed. To assess mobility, the thumb and index finger of the examining hand are used to "hold" the mass, and then the mass is moved in all directions possible (Figure 14-12, *C*).

7. *Tenderness:* The client is questioned regarding any discomfort with palpation.

8. *Erythema:* The area of skin overlying the mass is inspected for erythema.

9. *Dimpling over the mass:* The tissue over the mass is compressed to determine if this maneuver produces dimpling (Figure 14-7, *D*).

10. *Depth of mass:* The location of the mass is determined in reference to the surface of the breast. Is the mass close to the surface at midlevel or deep against the chest wall?

terior aspect of the axilla and including several nodes found in the region of the third rib and the second and third intercostal spaces and over the fourth and sixth ribs

3. *Central axillary nodes* (intermediate) lying high in the middle of the axilla over the ribs
4. *Posterior axillary nodes* (subscapular) lying in the posterior aspect of the axilla along the lateral edge of the scapula
5. *Apical axillary nodes* (infraclavicular or subclavian) located below the clavicle

Develop a routine system for axillary node examination. Palpate the apical nodes last since their deep location will require extra pressure in examination. Normally, nodes should not be palpable.

The primary purpose of the palpation of the breasts is to discover masses. If a mass is discovered, assess it according to the characteristics noted in the box on p. 386 and shown in Figures 14-11 and 14-12.

The range of normal breast consistency is wide. The normal breast feels somewhat granular and "lumpy." This granularity is generalized and becomes more prominent with age. Breast lumpiness results from the configuration of the breast lobes, the fat and connective tissue between and supporting the lobes and other structures, and the irregular density of lobules. Thus the consistency of breasts is not uniform. However, this variation in consistency should be noted uniformly throughout the breasts of an individual client.

The breasts feel relatively homogeneous in the young adolescent. After menarche, the presence of progesterone in pregnancy and premenstrually causes the breasts to feel generally nodular. Hormonally induced nodularity is bilateral and diffuse.

The breasts are palpated most effectively with the client in a supine position. Because of time constraints on most physical examinations, it is not advised that all clients also undergo palpation in a sitting position. However, certain groups of clients should also have breast palpation done in the sitting position: women with present or past complaints of breast masses, women at high risk of breast cancer, and women with large and/or pendulous breasts.

If the breasts are to be examined with the client in a sitting position, small breasts can be examined by using one hand to support the breast and the other hand to palpate the tissue against the chest wall. For palpation of pendulous breasts, use a bimanual technique (Figure 14-13). Support the inferior portion of the breast in one hand while using the other hand to palpate breast tissue against the supporting hand.

With the client lying down, palpate the breasts while they are flattened against the rib cage. If the breasts are large, several methods can be used to enhance flattening. A small pillow or a rolled towel can be placed under

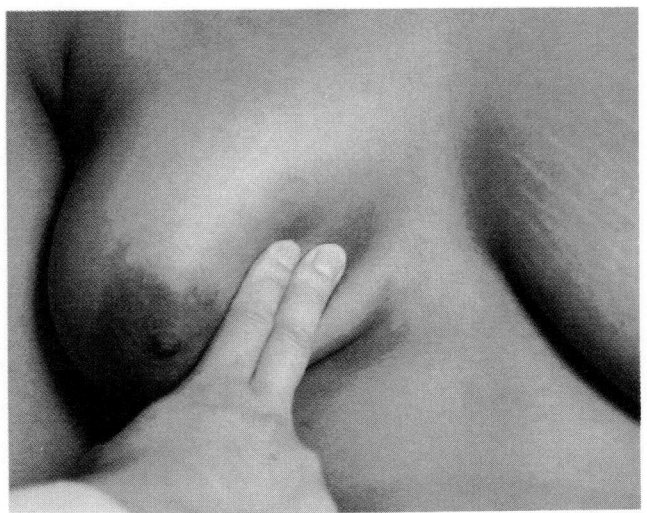

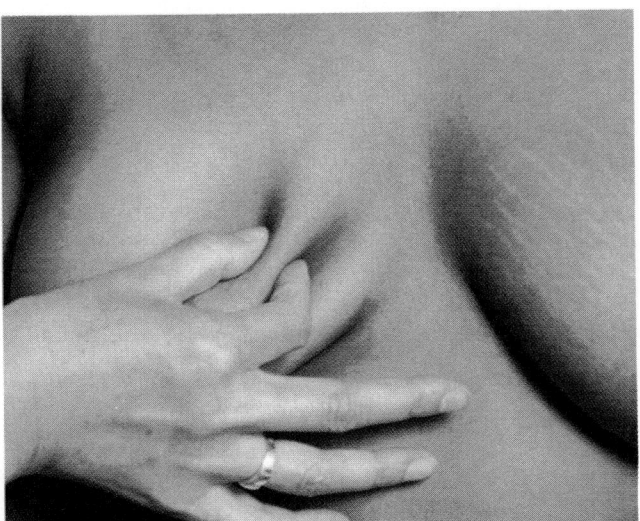

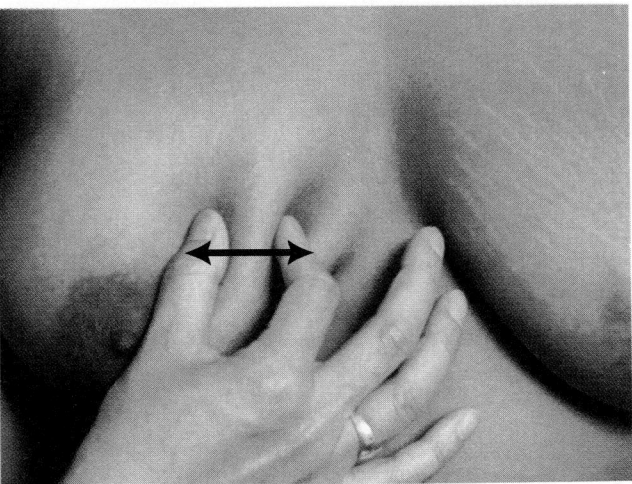

FIGURE 14-12 A, Palpating for consistency of breast lesion. **B,** Palpating for delineation of borders of breast mass. **C,** Palpating for mobility of breast mass.

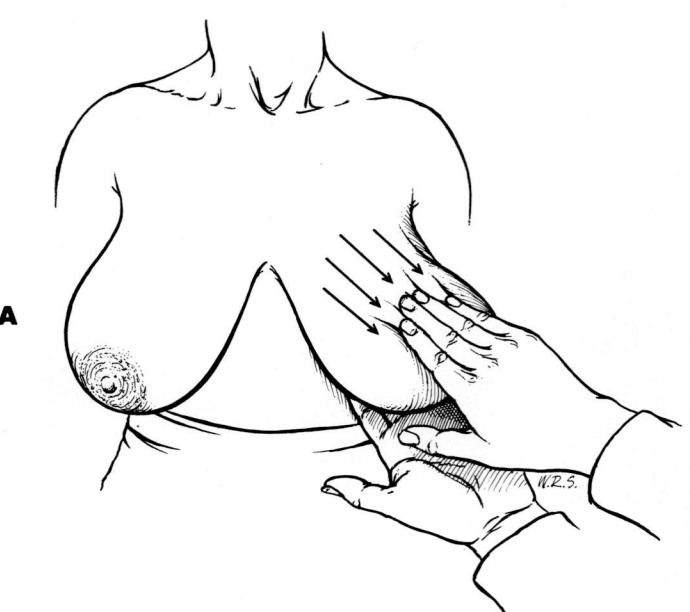

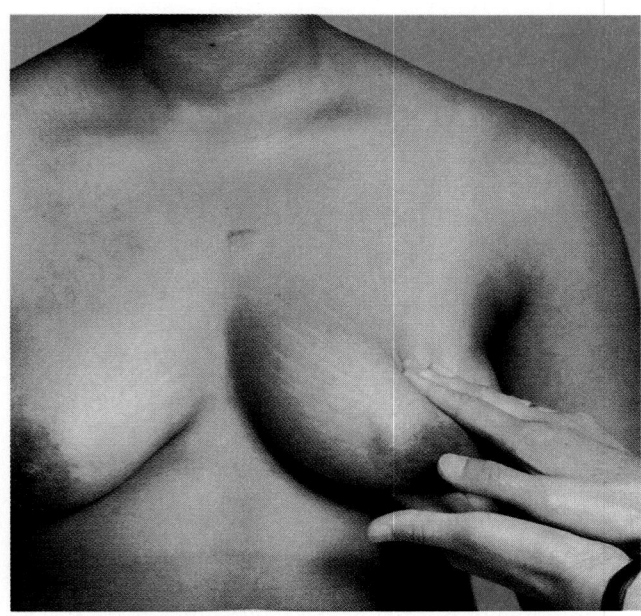

FIGURE 14-13 Bimanual palpation of the breasts.

the ipsilateral upper back, or the client can abduct the ipsilateral arm and place her hand under her neck (Figure 14-14). Both maneuvers shift the breast medially. For all clients, the humerus should be at least slightly abducted to allow for thorough palpation of the tail of Spence.

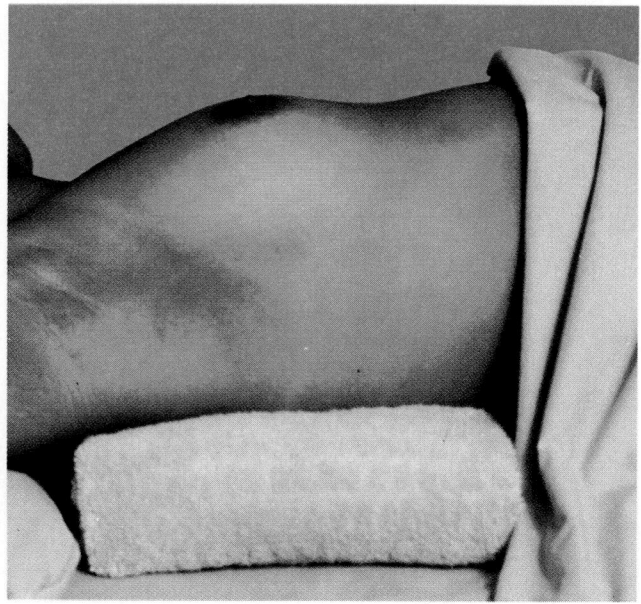

FIGURE 14-14 Use of a towel to shift breast tissue evenly over the chest for effective palpation.

Thoroughly palpate the breasts and the tail of Spence areas with the palmar surfaces of the three middle fingers held together (Figure 14-15, *A*). The movements should be smooth and should be done in a back-and-forth or circular motion. Press firmly enough to fully appreciate the underlying tissue, but not so firmly that the tissue is compressed against the rib cage.

Develop a system of breast examination and habitually start and end at a fixed point on the breasts. The important principle is development of a system that ensures a thorough examination of all breast tissues. Several examination patterns have been recommended:

1. The breast is visualized as a round wheel with multiple spokes. Palpation is done along each spoke until the breast has been thoroughly surveyed (Figure 14-16, *A*).
2. The breast is viewed as a group of concentric circles with the nipple as the center. Palpation is performed along the circumferences of the circle, starting at the outermost circle, until the total breast area has been adequately surveyed (Figure 14-16, *B*).
3. Palpation of the breast is done in vertical or horizontal sections, starting immediately below the clavicle at the sternal border and proceeding downward and upward or parallel to the sternal border or back and forth until the entire breast has been surveyed.

Whatever system and sequence of examination is used, a thorough examination of all breast tissue and the tail of Spence is critical. Special attention should be

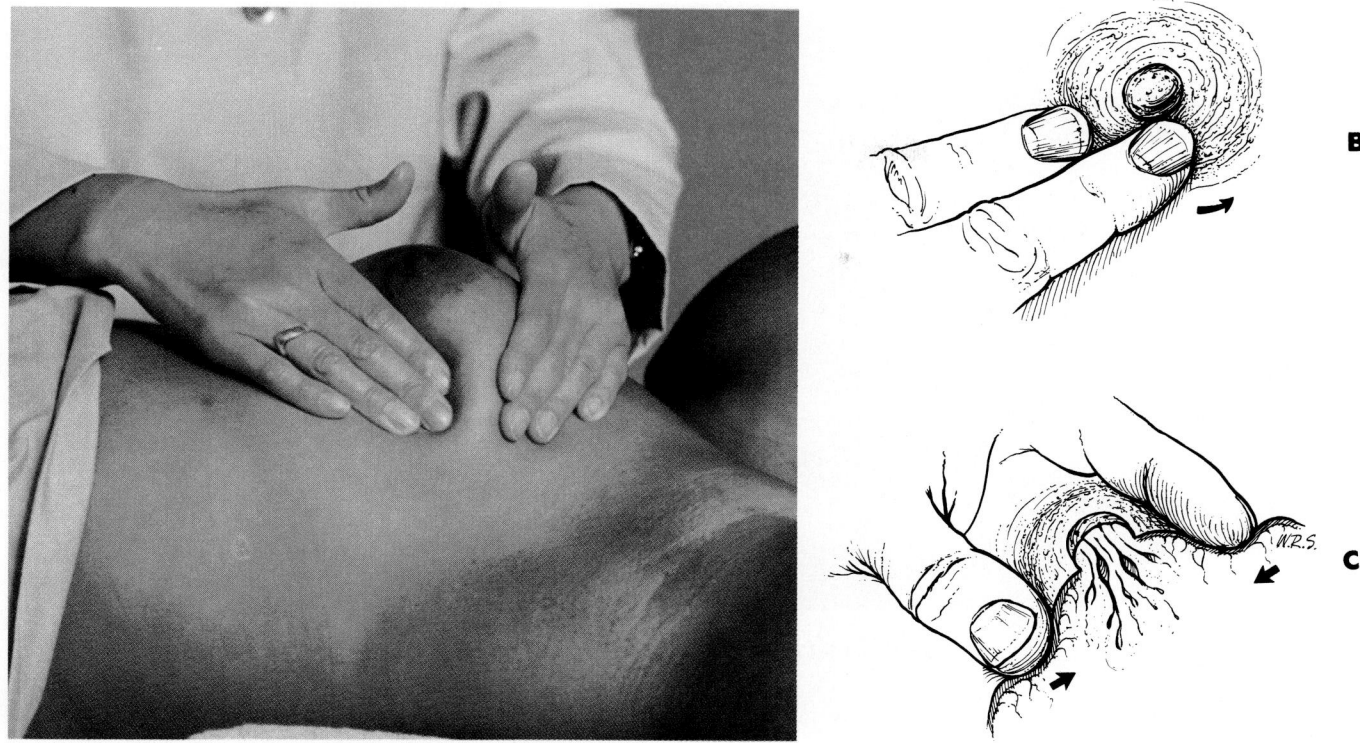

FIGURE 14-15 Palpation of breasts. **A,** Glandular areas. **B,** Areolar area. **C,** Compression of nipple.

FIGURE 14-16 Two methods of systematic breast palpation. **A,** Palpation in wedge sections from breast periphery to center. **B,** Palpation along concentric circles from periphery to center.

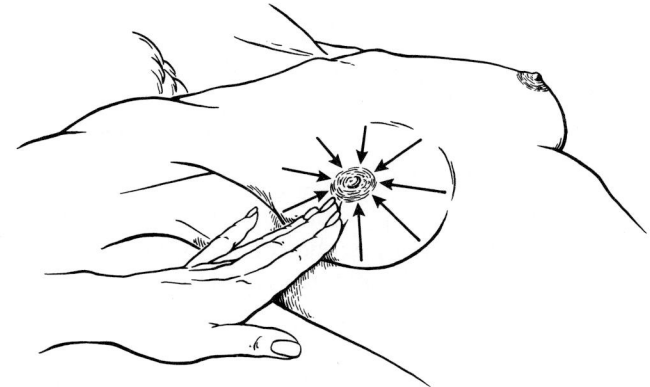

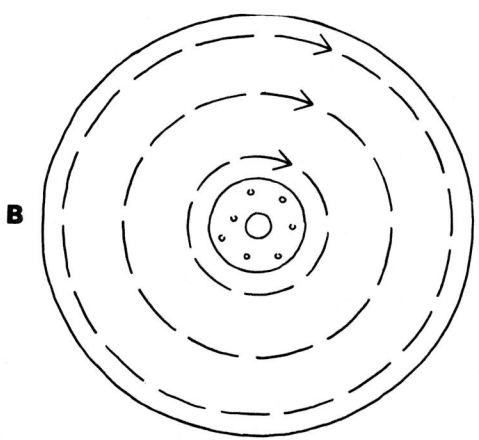

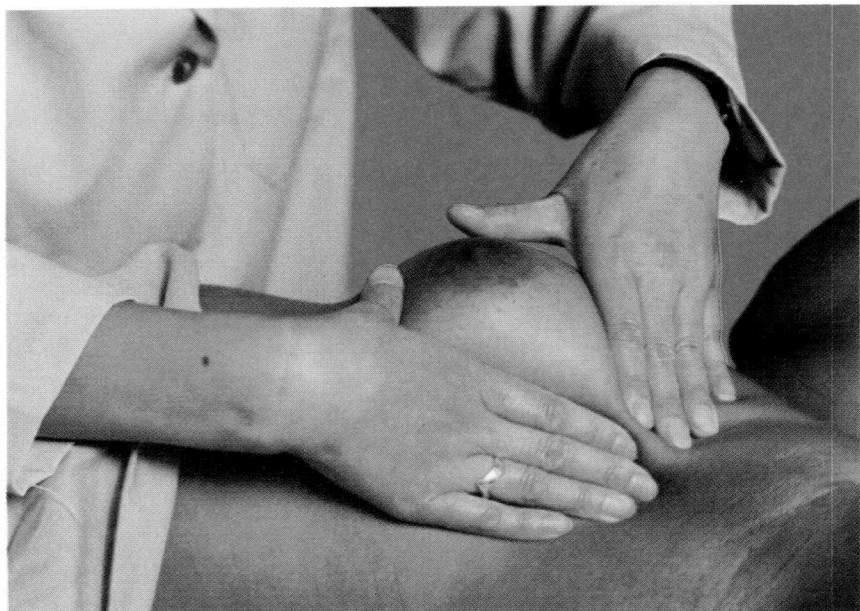

FIGURE 14-17 Palpation of the axillary tail of Spence.

focused on the upper outer quadrant area and the tail of Spence because approximately half of all breast cancers develop there (Figure 14-17).

Carefully palpate the areolar areas to determine the presence of underlying masses (see Figure 14-15, *B*). Gently compress each nipple to assess for the presence of masses and discharge (see Figure 14-15, *C*). If discharge is noted, milk the breast along its radii to identify the lobe from which the discharge is originating. Compression of the discharge-producing lobe will cause discharge to exude from the nipple. If the nipple discharge is not associated with normal changes in pregnancy or the postpartum period, collect a specimen of the discharge on a slide. Nipple discharge, which is often thin and cellular, is most effectively collected on a frosted or albumin-coated slide to prevent runoff. When discharge is present on the nipple, bring the slide in contact with the nipple and rub it across the nipple, allowing the discharge to collect across the slide.

If a client reports a breast mass, examine the "normal" breast first so that the baseline consistency of that breast will serve as a control for palpation of the reportedly abnormal one.

Mammary folds, or crescent-shaped ridges of breast tissue found at the inferior portions of very large or pendulous breasts, may be confused with breast masses, but they are nonpathological.

The complete sequence of the breast examination is illustrated in Figure 14-18.

Special breast examinations

The male breast. The routine male breast examination consists of the following steps:
1. Inspection of the breasts while the client is in a sitting position
2. Palpation of the axillary nodes
3. Palpation of the breasts while the client is lying down

Observe the breast with the client sitting. The specific sitting positions used with the woman are unnecessary unless the man has large breasts. Perform the axillary examination using the same technique as described for women. Palpate the breasts, nipples, and areolae while the client is supine, as with the female client.

Occurring most frequently in the areolar area, male breast cancer accounts for approximately 1% of all breast cancers. Every male client should be given a thorough breast examination with an adaptation of the technique used for female clients.

Gynecomastia, or enlargement of the male breast, is a frequently occurring, multicausal condition. Causes include pubertal changes, hormonal administration, cirrhosis, leukemia, thyrotoxicosis, and drugs.

Client who has had a mastectomy. The client who has had a mastectomy has special examination needs. This client may be embarrassed about the condition of the surgical site and apprehensive about the examination of the remaining breast. Perform the inspection

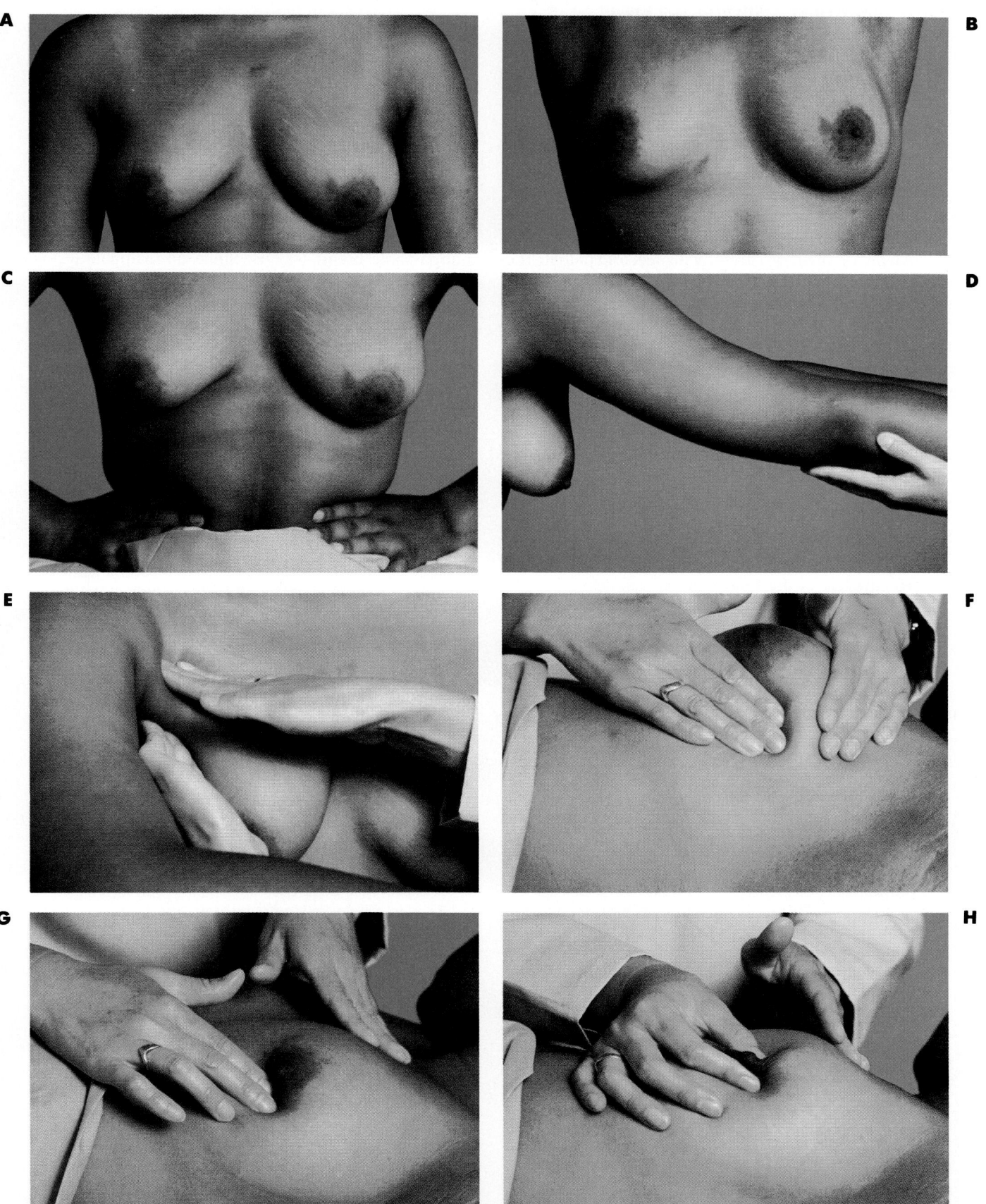

FIGURE 14-18 Sequence of the breast examination. **A,** Observation of the breasts at rest.
B, Observation with client's arms overhead. **C,** Observation with client contracting pectoral
muscles by pressing hands into waist. **D,** Observation with client leaning forward. **E,** Palpation
of axillary nodes. **F,** Palpation of the glandular area. **G,** Palpation of areolar area. **H,** Palpation
of nipple.

and palpation portions of the examination on the unaffected side as described for the routine examination. Palpate the scar with the palmar surface of two fingers of the examining hand with a back-and-forth or circular motion to detect any swelling, lumps, and tenderness. Then systematically and thoroughly palpate the axillary and chest tissue. Emphasize the importance of breast self-examination with these clients.

For the client who has had a mastectomy without reconstructive surgery, carefully inspect and palpate the scar and the remaining chest and axillary tissue on the surgical side to detect any swelling, lumps, redness, color changes, or lesions. Note the extent of muscle mass and edema and the general appearance and condition of the scar.

Client who has had breast reconstruction, augmentation, or lumpectomy. Examine the breasts in the usual manner, giving special attention to scars. Emphasize the need for breast self-examination with these clients.

Screening Tests and Procedures

Further evaluation of breast masses is accomplished through the use of the following techniques:

1. **Mammography** is a technique of breast examination that involves low-energy radiography.
2. **Xeromammography** is mammography done with a xerographic plate instead of film. The advantages of this technique are that radiation doses are smaller than with conventional mammography and the images produced are more distinct.

Mammography is the major method of detecting nonpalpable breast lesions. Since nonpalpable lesions are generally early, small, and local, survival rates are increased through early detection. The performance and interpretation of mammograms require specialized skill.

During the past 10 years, mammographic techniques have been improved tremendously in terms of safety and effectiveness. Often mammography is offered through a community-based screening program.

Since the initiation of mammographic screening services, recommended schedules for mammography have changed as research has produced new knowledge related to the detection of breast cancer. The following are recommendations of the Report of the U.S. Preventive Services Task Force (1989, p. 44):

Mammography every one to two years is recommended for all women beginning at age 50 and concluding at approxi-

STEP-BY-STEP

Examination Step-by-Step

Client: Seated and uncovered to waist
Examiner: Standing in front of client

Inspection

1. Skin of anterior thorax
2. Breast size, configuration, symmetry, and surface characteristics
3. Nipple configuration and plane
4. Symmetry of movement when arms are raised over head
5. Retraction of breast tissue when pectoral muscles are contracted by pushing arms into hips or pushing hands together
6. Symmetry of movement and retraction when woman leans forward
7. Skin of axilla

Palpation

1. Axillary nodes: Begin along inner aspect of arm and proceed to chest wall, anterior axilla, posterior axilla, and apex of axilla. (Supraclavicular and infraclavicular nodes are often palpated in conjunction with the axillary nodes. See the examination outline in Chapter 13.)
2. Palpate breasts (1) if unusual symptoms or inspection findings are noted, (2) if client is at risk for breast disease, or (3) if breasts are unusually large.

Client: Lying on back
Examiner: To right of client

Inspection

1. Skin of thorax
2. Surface characteristics of breasts

Palpation

1. Palpate breasts to determine consistency of tissue and presence of masses
2. Palpate areolar areas for masses
3. Palpate nipples to determine presence of discharge

Review client's technique of breast self-examination or teach breast self-examination.

mately age 75 unless pathology is detected. For the special category of women at high risk because of a family history or premenopausally diagnosed breast cancer in first degree relatives, it may be prudent to begin regular clinical breast examination and mammography at an earlier age (e.g., age 35).

Other authorities recommend initiation of mammograms at age 40 and a schedule of repeat mammograms every 1 to 2 years. New knowledge about the development of breast cancer and safe mechanisms for early detection and treatment may affect future guidelines for mammography screening schedules. The practitioner working with adult women clients should be alert to possible changes in screening guidelines.

VARIATIONS FROM HEALTH

The most common variations in breast health are noted in the form of breast lumps. The various causes of breast lumps are listed in Table 14-2, and the most common causes are discussed in this section.

Breast Cancer

Although certain breast lesions have characteristic findings on inspection and palpation, diagnosis is not made by clinical examination but by surgical procedures and laboratory examinations. Therefore the practitioner is encouraged to learn the distinguishing characteristics of breast lesions but not to rely on them for diagnosis.

The lesions of breast cancer are often solitary, unilateral, solid, hard, irregular, poorly delineated, nonmobile, painless, nontender, and located in the upper outer quadrants. Breast cancer is a leading cause of death in women in the United States and also a leading cause of cancer morbidity. On average, 1 of every 9 to 10 women will develop breast cancer. Knowledge of the factors indicating that a woman is at a higher than

TABLE 14-2

Causes of Breast Lumps

Origin	Lesion type	Frequency
Normal structures	Nodularity	Common
	Prominent fat lobule	Less common
	Prominent rib	Less common
	Intramammary lymph node	Rare
	Edge of biopsy wound	Less common
	Accessory breast	Rare
Aberrations of normal development and involution	Fibroadenoma	Common
	Cyclical nodularity	Common
	Cyst	Common
	Galactocele	Rare
	Sclerosing adenosis	Less common
	Stromal fibrosis	Rare
Inflammatory processes	Chronic infected abscess	Rare
	Fat necrosis	Rare
	Foreign body granuloma	Rare
	Mondor's disease	Rare
Benign tumor	Duct papilloma	Less common
	Giant fibroadenoma	Rare
	Lipoma	Rare
	Granular cell myoblastoma	Rare
Intermediate tumor	Phyllodes tumor	Rare
	Carcinoma in situ	Less common
Malignant tumor	Primary tumor	Common
	Secondary tumor	Rare
Lesions of nipple and areola	Squamous papilloma	Less common
	Leiomyoma	Rare
	Retention cyst	Rare
	Papillary adenoma	Rare
Skin lesions	Sebaceous cyst	Less common
	Hidradenitis	Rare
	Benign and malignant skin tumors	Rare

Modified from Hughes LE, Mansel RE, Webster DJT: *Benign disorders and diseases of the breast*, London, 1989, Baillière Tindall, p. 41.

usual risk of cancer can assist in making decisions about screening programs and the frequency of general physical examinations.

A summary of risk factors for breast cancer in women is presented in Table 14-1. For women at increased risk, monthly self-examination should be emphasized. Such women should receive a thorough breast screening examination at least once a year.

Benign Lesions

Benign lesions account for approximately 70% to 80% of breast operations. The most commonly seen benign breast lesions are those associated with fibrocystic disease and **fibroadenomas.**

Fibrocystic disease, noted as an exaggeration of the normal changes in the breasts during the menstrual cycle, is eventually characterized by the formation of single or multiple cysts in the breasts. Fibrocystic disease develops in three stages:

1. The first stage, called mazoplasia, occurs in the late teens and early twenties. It is characterized by painful, tender, premenstrual breast swelling (chiefly in the axillary tails) that subsides after menses.
2. The second stage occurs in the late twenties and early thirties. The breasts exhibit multinodular changes, and sometimes a dominant mass occurs, which is usually described as a thickness rather than a lump.
3. The third stage involves the development of cysts. The onset of cyst formation is often preceded by a sudden dull pain, a full feeling, or a burning sensation in the breast.

The lesions of fibrocystic disease are commonly bilateral, multiple, painful, tender, well delineated, and slightly mobile. The associated tenderness and the size of the lesions increase premenstrually.

Fibroadenomas are benign lesions that contain both fibrous and glandular tissues. They are usually solitary and unilateral. In general, they are palpated as mobile, solid, firm, rubbery, regular, well-delineated, nontender, painless lumps. Fibroadenomas are usually found in women between the ages of 15 and 35 and do not change with the menstrual cycle.

BREAST SELF-EXAMINATION

Despite improved mammographic techniques and their availability, a substantial portion of malignant breast lesions are found by women themselves. Women who perform regular self-breast examinations become very familiar with the inspection and palpatory findings within their own breasts and can note any changes immediately. Therefore the health-oriented examiner should assess each client's level of knowledge and practice related to monthly breast self-examination. During examination of the breasts, the examiner describes the steps of the examination and the rationale for each step. A return demonstration by the client on her own breasts reinforces the client's learning and memory of the procedure.

TEACHING BREAST SELF-EXAMINATION

The following points should be emphasized in the teaching of breast self-examination:

1. The majority of breast lumps are not cancerous.
2. The majority of cancerous breast lesions are curable.
3. Breasts should be examined each month between the fourth through the fourteenth day of the menstrual cycle, when the breasts are least congested for that individual. If, for any reason, menses are not present, a specific date of each month should be chosen for the monthly breast examination, for example, the date of the client's birthday.
4. Visual inspection and palpation should be done.
5. Visual inspection should be done in four arm positions with the woman stripped to the waist and looking at herself in a mirror. The four arm positions are: arms at rest, hands on hips and pressed into hips contracting chest muscles, hands over head, and arms forward with torso leaning forward.
6. Many women prefer to do palpation in the shower because the soap and water assist the hands to glide easily over the skin. However, the examination of large breasts and the axilla are better done in a supine than a standing position; therefore an examination done in the supine position is recommended in addition to the examination done in the bath or shower.
7. Each entire breast should be examined in a systematic way.
8. Specific examination of the nipple (through compression for discharge) and the areola (through palpation) should not be forgotten.
9. Any change should be reported to a health care provider as soon as possible.

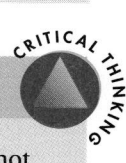

Sample Documentation

History

40-year-old white female noted a small lump in areolar area of right breast 2 weeks ago in breast self-examination, routinely done on day 7 of menstrual cycle. No change in lump since discovery. Has not noted any pain, swelling, change in appearance of breast, or discharge. No history of breast lesions. No hormonal medications taken. Last clinical breast examination 9 months ago. Has never had a mammogram. Menses regular, onset at age 13. Two pregnancies, delivered at full term 7 and 5 years ago and successfully breast-fed for 6 months. One aunt had breast cancer at age 50.

Examination

Inspection: Right breast slightly larger than left breast. Bilaterally similar in surface characteristics, plane of nipple, and mobility. Skin smooth with no unusual vascular patterns. No lesions, erythema, dimpling, or retraction.

Palpation: *Right breast*: A regular, round, movable mass, approximately 0.25 x 0.25 x 0.25 cm palpated in the LLQ at 5 o'clock position approximately 1 cm from the center of the nipple. Borders are well defined and mass is soft and cystic. Appears to be very close to the skin surface. Not tender on palpation or movement. *Left breast*: Breast soft, slightly nodular throughout. No masses or tenderness.

Nursing Diagnosis   *THE NEXT STEP*

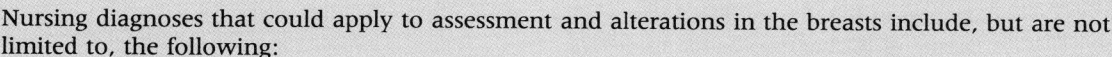

Nursing diagnoses that could apply to assessment and alterations in the breasts include, but are not limited to, the following:

ALTERED HEALTH MAINTENANCE Inability to identify, manage, and/or seek help to maintain health.

Defining Characteristics

- Demonstrated lack of knowledge regarding basic health practices (breast self-exam, clinical exam, mammography)
- Demonstrated lack of adaptive behaviors to internal or external changes (lumps, nodules, tenderness, etc.)
- Reported or observed lack of finances for health maintenance
- History of lack of health-seeking behavior

Related Factors

- Alteration or lack of communication skills
- Inability to make deliberative and thoughtful judgments
- Perceptual-cognitive impairment, complete or partial lack of gross or fine motor skills, ineffective coping
- Disabling spiritual distress
- Lack of material resources, unachieved developmental tasks
- Unachieved developmental tasks
- Dysfunctional grieving

BODY IMAGE DISTURBANCE Disruption in the way one perceives one's body image.

Defining Characteristics

- Verbalized actual or perceived change in structure and/or function of body or body part
- Verbalized change in life-style because of negative feelings or perception of body
- Verbalized fear of rejections by others
- Repeated verbalizations focusing on past strengths, function, or appearance
- Verbalized negative feelings about body (dirty, big, small, unsightly)
- Verbalized feelings of helplessness, hopelessness, powerlessness in relation to the body
- Preoccupation with change in body or loss of part

Continued.

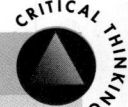

Nursing Diagnosis   *THE NEXT STEP—cont'd*

- Personalization of part or loss by name
- Guilt, shame
- Refusal to verify actual change in body or body part
- Hiding or overexposing body part
- Change in social involvement or social relationships
- Emphasis on remaining strengths or heightened achievement

Related Factors

- Nonintegration of change in body characterisitics, function, or limits; and perceived developmental imperfections

SELF-ESTEEM DISTURBANCE Negative self-evaluation/feelings about self or self-capabilities, which may be directly or indirectly expressed.

Defining Characteristics

- Self-negating verbalizations
- Lack of eye contact
- Expressions of shame/guilt
- Rationalization/rejection of positive feedback
- Exaggerations of negative feedback about self
- Hesitation to try new things/situations
- Denial of problems obvious to others
- Rationalization of personal failures
- Hypersensitivity to criticism
- Grandiosity
- Projection of blame/responsibility for problems
- Evaluations of self as unable to deal with events

Related Factors

- Self-negating verbalizations
- Lack of eye contact
- Expressions of shame/guilt
- Evaluations of self as unable to deal with events
- Rationalizations
- Rejections of positive feedback
- Exaggerations of negative feedback about self
- Hesitation to try new things/situations
- Denial of problems obvious to others
- Projection of blame/responsibility for problems
- Rationalization of personal failures
- Hypersensitvity to criticism
- Grandiosity

INEFFECTIVE BREASTFEEDING The state in which a mother, infant, and/or family experiences dissatisfaction or difficulty with the breastfeeding process.

Defining Characteristics

- Actual/perceived inadequate milk supply
- Infant inability to attach to maternal breast correctly
- No observable signs of oxytocin release
- Observable signs of inadequate infant intake
- Nonsustained/insufficient opportunity for suckling at the breast
- Insufficient emptying of each breast per feeding
- Persistence of sore nipples beyond the first week of breastfeeding

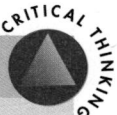

Nursing Diagnosis   *THE NEXT STEP—cont'd*

- Infant exhibiting fussiness and crying within first hour after breastfeeding; unresponsive to comfort measures
- Infant arching and crying at the breast; resisting latching on
- Previous history of breastfeeding failure

Related Factors

- Knowledge deficit
- Interrupted breast-feeding
- Maternal anxiety
- Prematurity of infant anomaly
- Maternal breast anomaly
- Previous breast surgery
- Poor infant sucking reflex
- Nonsupportive partner/family

EFFECTIVE BREASTFEEDING The state in which a mother-infant dyad/family exhibits adequate proficiency and satisfaction with breastfeeding process.

Defining Characteristics

- Mother able to position infant at breast to promote a successful latch-on response
- Infant is content after feeding
- Regular and sustained suckling/swallowing at the breast
- Appropriate infant weight patterns for age
- Effective mother/infant communication patterns (infant cues; maternal interpretation and response)
- Signs/symptoms of oxytocin release (let down or milk ejection reflex)
- Eagerness of infant to nurse
- Maternal verbalization of satisfaction with the breastfeeding process

Related Factors

- Basic breastfeeding knowledge
- Normal breast structure
- Normal infant oral structure
- Infant gestational age >34 weeks
- Support sources
- Maternal confidence

Clinical Application

Ms. L. is a 35-year-old single female who noted a small lump "the size of a nickel" in the areolar area of her left breast 4 weeks ago in a breast self-examination. She has not noted any pain, swelling, change in appearance of breast or discharge. She has a history of mild fibrocystic disease; no prior breast lesions. No hormonal medication taken. Has never has a mammogram and last clinical breast examination was 5 years ago. Mother has fibrocystic disease; aunt has had breast cancer. Ms. L. appears anxious and in a trembling and almost crying voice asks, "Is this breast lump serious? Will I have to have surgery?" Her sitting posture is stiff and rigid during the entire examination.

SUBJECTIVE DATA:
Patient complains of small lump in left breast; size of nickel
Concerned that lump is serious and may need surgery

Continued.

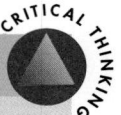

Nursing Diagnosis *THE NEXT STEP—cont'd*

OBJECTIVE DATA:
Appears anxious
Holds posture stiff and rigid throughout examination
Voice trembling and almost crying
PALPATION: Left breast: regular, round, movable mass, approximately 1 cm × 1 cm × 1 cm mass in the right lower quadrant at the 5:00 position, approximately 1.5 cm from the center of the nipple. Borders are well defined and mass soft and cystic. Appears to be very close to surface of skin. No tenderness on palpation or movement. Right breast: Soft, slightly nodular throughout. No masses, tenderness, or discharge.

NURSING DIAGNOSES

Altered health maintenance related to ineffective coping.

Defining Characteristics:

- Demonstrates lack of knowledge regarding basic health practices of yearly clinical exams and mammography
- Demonstrates lack of adaptive behaviors to internal changes (lumps)
- History of lack of health-seeking behavior

Body image disturbance related to cognitive-perceptual factors.

Defining Characteristics

- Nonverbal response to perceived changes in structure/function of breasts
- Feelings of helplessness
- Feelings of hopelessness

Self-esteem disturbance related to cognitive-perceptual factors.

Defining Characteristics

- Evaluation of self as unable to deal with an event such as loss of breast

GLOSSARY

acini Small saclike dilatations found in various glands.

areolae Pigmented areas surrounding the nipples. Their color varies from pink to brown.

axillary tail of Spence Anatomical projection of breast tissue into the axilla.

Cooper's ligaments Suspensory ligaments of the breast.

fibroadenoma Benign tumor composed of dense epithelial and fibroblastic tissue. A fibroadenoma of the breast is nontender, encapsulated, round, movable, and firm.

gynecomastia Hypertrophy of breast tissue in a male subject.

inversion Invagination or depression of the nipple's central portion. Can occur congenitally or as a response to an invasive process.

ipsilateral Pertaining to the same side of the body.

lobes Glandular tissue units in the breast situated in a circular, spokelike fashion.

lumpectomy Surgical excision of a tumor without removal of large amounts of surrounding tissue or adjacent lymph nodes.

mammary folds Crescent-shaped ridges of breast tissue found at the inferior portions of very large or pendulous breasts. May be confused with breast masses but are nonpathological.

mammography Radiography of the soft tissues of the breast to allow identification of various benign and malignant neoplastic processes.

mastitis Inflammation of breast tissue.

Montgomery's glands Small sebaceous glands located on the areola.

peau d'orange Orange-peel appearance of the breast caused by edema of the breast and resultant blocked lymph drainage.

retraction (dimpling) Appears as a depression or pucker on the skin. It usually is caused by the fibrotic shortening and immobilization or Cooper's ligament by an invasive process.

xeromammography Done with a xerographic plate instead of film

BIBLIOGRAPHY

Annonier C: *Female breast examination*, Berlin, 1986, Springer-Verlag.

Baines CJ: Breast self-examination, *Cancer Suppl* 69:1942, 1992.

Baines CJ, Miller AB, Bassett AA: Physical examination: its role as a single screening modality in the Canadian National Breast Screening Study, *Cancer Suppl* 63:1816, 1992.

Barth V, Prechtel K, Heywang SH: *Atlas of breast diseases*, Philadelphia, 1991, BC Decker.

Bland KI, Copeland EM: *The breast: comprehensive management of benign and malignant diseases*, Philadelphia, 1991, WB Saunders.

Champion V: Role of breast self-examination in breast cancer screening, *Cancer Suppl* 69:1985, 1992.

Dodd GD: American Cancer Society guidelines on screening for breast cancer, *Cancer Suppl* 69:1885, 1992.

Foster RS and others: Clinical breast examination and breast self-examination, *Cancer Suppl* 69:1992.

Gordon M: *Manual of nursing diagnosis 1993-1994*, St Louis, 1993, Mosby−Year Book.

Gordon M: *Nursing diagnosis: process and appiication*, ed 2, St Louis, 1987, Mosby−Year Book.

Hindle WH: *Breast disease for gynecologists*, Norwalk, Conn, 1990, Appleton & Lange.

Hughes LE, Mansel RE, Webster DJT: *Benign disorders and diseases of the breast*, London, 1989, Bailliere Tindall.

Isaacs JH: *Textbook of breast disease*, St Louis, 1992, Mosby−Year Book.

Leucht W: *Teaching atlas of breast ultrasound*, Stuttgart, 1992, Georg Thieme Verlag.

Love SM: *Dr. Susan Love's breast book*, East Norwalk, Conn, 1990, Addison-Wesley.

Mettlin C: Breast cancer risk factors, *Cancer Suppl* 69:1904, 1992.

Mitchell GW, Bassett LW: *The female breast and its disorders*, Baltimore, 1990, Williams & Wilkins.

Pagana KD, Pagana TJ: *Mosby's diagnostic and laboratory test reference*, St Louis, 1992, Mosby−Year Book.

Smallwood JA, Taylor I: *Benign breast diseases*, Baltimore, 1990, Urban & Schwarzenberg.

US Department of Health and Human Services: *Healthy people 2000*, Washington, DC, 1991, DHHS.

US Preventive Services Task Force: *Guide to clinical preventive services: an assessment of the effectiveness of 169 interventions*, Baltimore, 1989, Williams & Wilkins.

Respiratory System

PURPOSE OF EXAMINATION

The purpose of the respiratory examination is to assess the organs and structures of the respiratory system and the functioning of the system as a whole. Because the respiratory system functions in close relationship with the cardiovascular system, these systems are often examined together. The examination is accomplished through various methods, including inspection, percussion, palpation, and auscultation.

ANATOMY AND PHYSIOLOGY

The major functions of the respiratory system are to supply the body with oxygen and to eliminate carbon dioxide. These tasks are accomplished through the complex cooperation of many body systems that, in wellness, act in harmony. The actual transfer of oxygen and carbon dioxide between environmental gas and body liquid occurs in the **alveoli**, which are not accessible to clinical examination. However, assessment of respiratory efficiency is accomplished by direct and indirect appraisal of structures that support alveolar function.

The thoracic cage is a semirigid structure consisting of a skeleton of 12 thoracic vertebrae, 12 pairs of ribs, the sternum, the diaphragm, and the intercostal muscles (Figure 15-1). The skeletal components of the thoracic cage are the ribs, the sternum, and the vertebrae. The ribs are paired. Anteriorly, the costal cartilages of the first seven ribs articulate with the body of the sternum. The costal cartilages of the eighth to the tenth ribs are attached to the costal cartilages immediately superior to the ribs. The eleventh and twelfth ribs, the "floating ribs," are unattached anteriorly. The tips of the eleventh ribs are located in the lateral thorax; the tips of the twelfth ribs are found in the posterior thorax. Posteriorly, all ribs articulate with the thoracic vertebrae.

In the adult, the sternum is approximately 17 cm

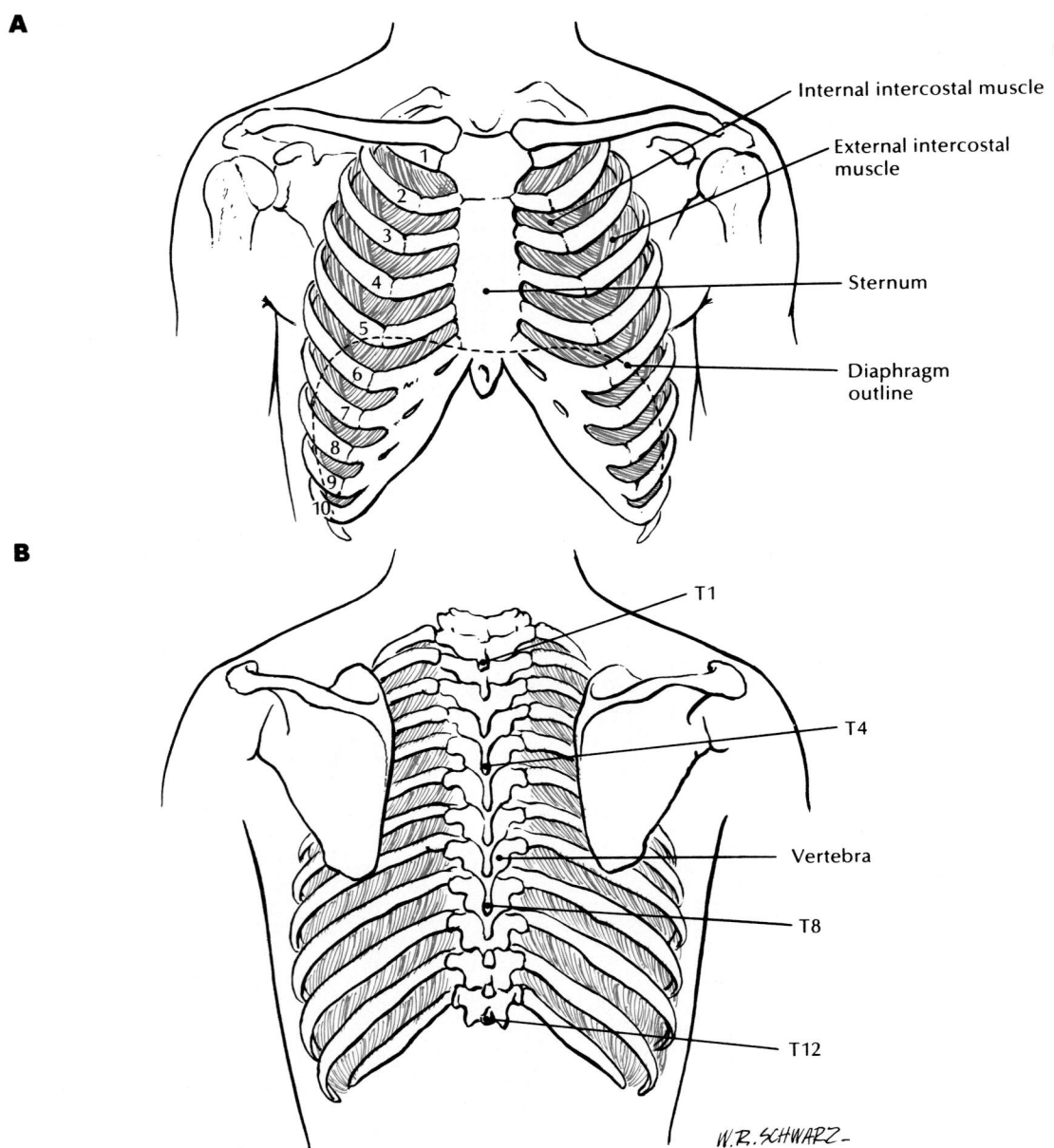

A

Internal intercostal muscle

External intercostal muscle

Sternum

Diaphragm outline

1
2
3
4
5
6
7
8
9
10

B

T1

T4

Vertebra

T8

T12

W.R. SCHWARZ

FIGURE 15-1 Thoracic cage. **A,** Anterior thorax. **B,** Posterior thorax.

long and consists of three parts: the manubrium, the body, and the **xiphoid** process. The manubrium of the sternum articulates with and supports the clavicle. The manubrium and the body of the sternum articulate with the first seven ribs. None of the ribs articulates with the xiphoid. An important anatomical landmark, the angle of Louis, is the junction of the manubrium and the body of the sternum (manubriosternal junction). The second rib attaches to the sternum at the angle of Louis.

The spaces between the ribs are termed **intercostal spaces**. Each space is named according to the rib im-

mediately superior to it; for example, the space between the second and third ribs is designated as the second intercostal space.

The thoracic cavity is divided into two distinct (right and left) pleural cavities, which are separated by the mediastinum, which contains the heart and the other structures that connect the head with the abdomen. The pleural cavities are lined by serous membranes, the parietal and visceral pleurae. The parietal pleura lines the chest wall and the diaphragm; the visceral pleura covers the outside of the lung. The potential space between

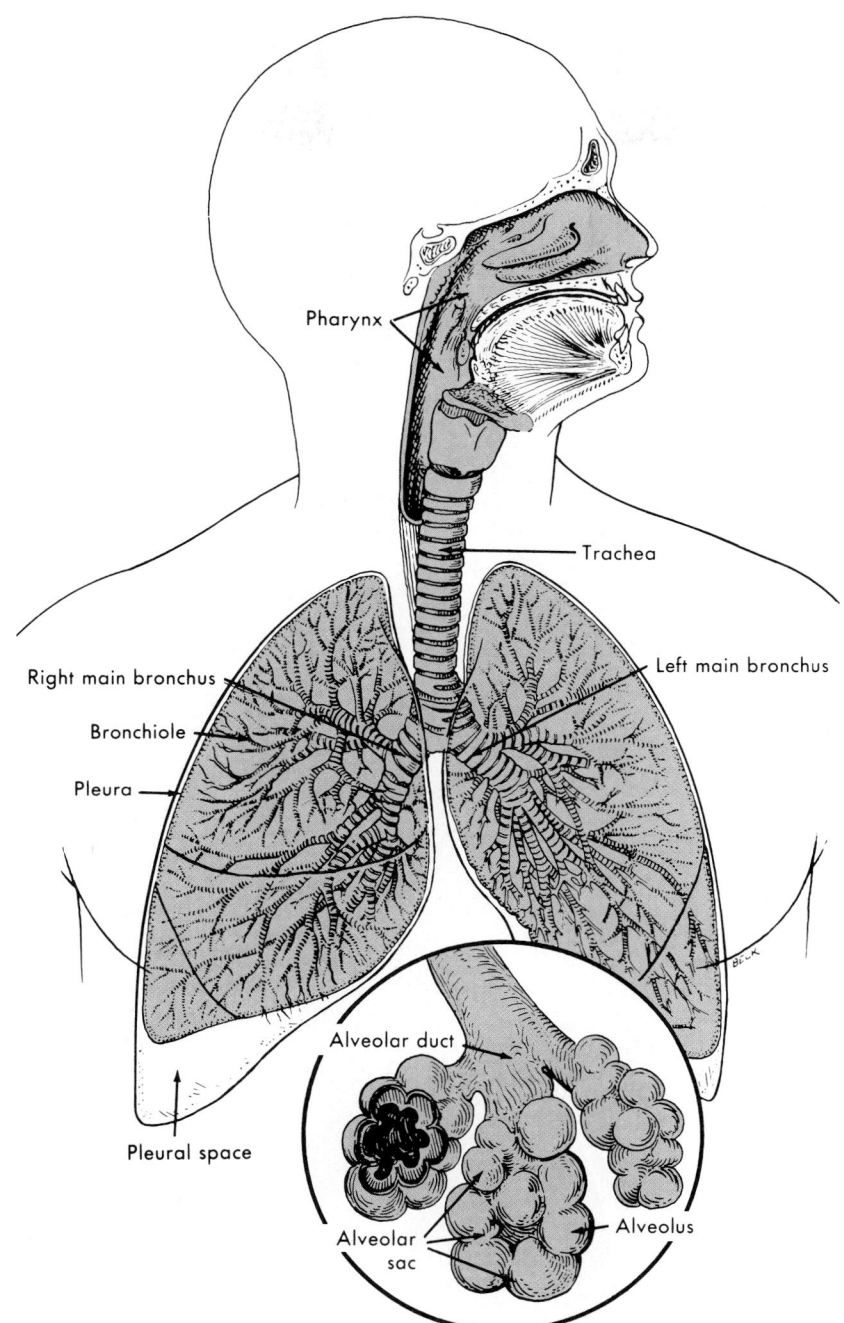

Pharynx

Trachea

Right main bronchus

Left main bronchus

Bronchiole

Pleura

Alveolar duct

Pleural space

Alveolar sac

Alveolus

FIGURE 15-2 Pharynx, trachea, and lungs. Alveolar sacs in inset. (From Thibodeau GA: *Anthony's textbook of anatomy and physiology,* ed 13, St Louis, 1990, Times Mirror/Mosby College Publishing.)

the pleurae contains a small amount of lubricating fluid.

The lungs are paired, asymmetrical, conical organs that conform to the shape of the thoracic cavity. The right lung contains three lobes, and the left lung has two lobes.

Air reaches the lungs through a system of flexible tubes. It enters through the mouth or the nose, passes through the respiratory portion of the larynx, and reaches the trachea. The trachea, approximately 10 to 11 cm long in the adult, begins at the lower border of the cricoid cartilage in the neck and divides into a left

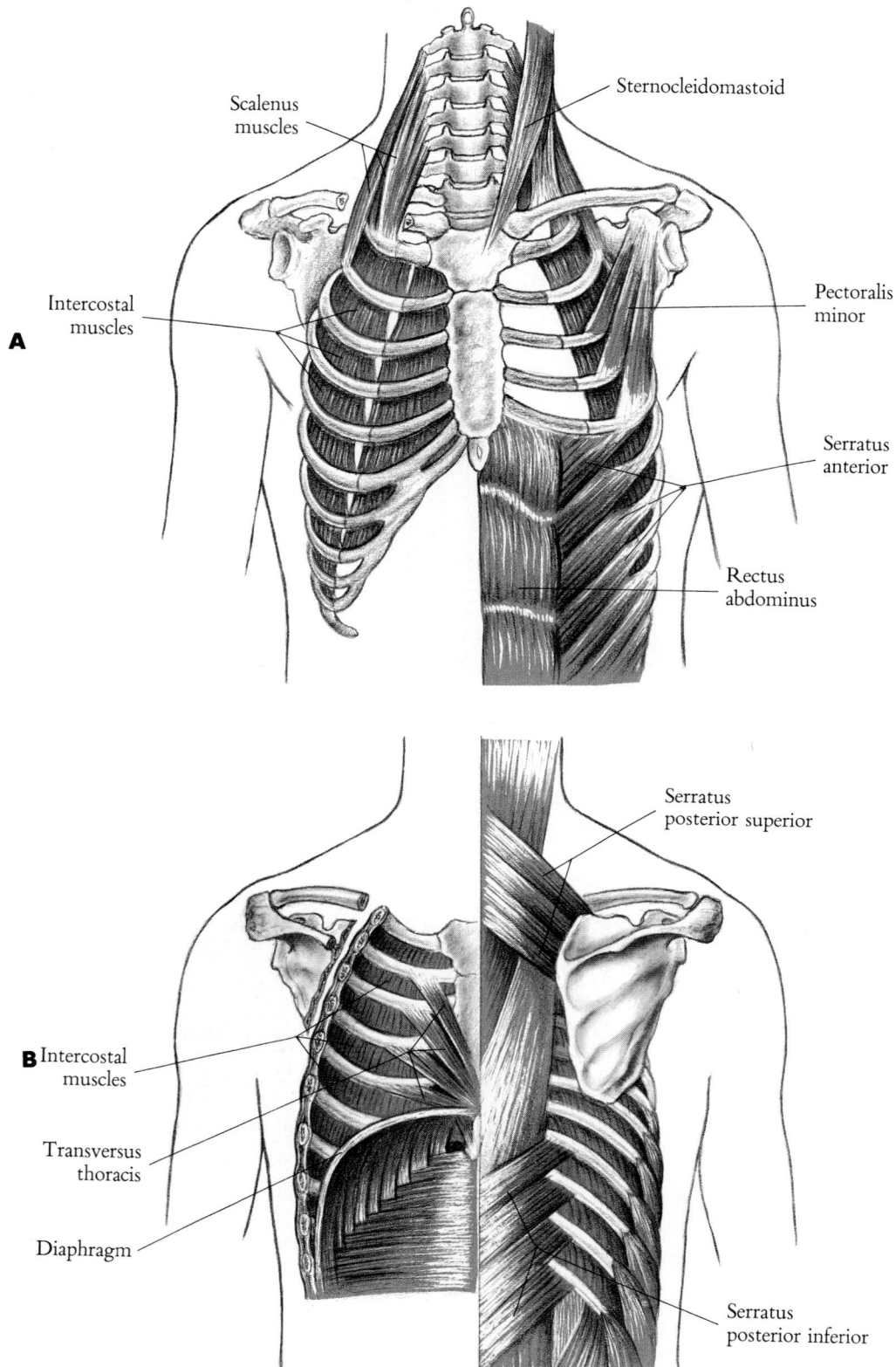

FIGURE 15-3 Muscles of ventilation. **A,** Anterior view. **B,** Posterior view. (From Seidel HM and others: *Mosby's guide to physical examination,* ed 2, St Louis, 1987, Mosby−Year Book.)

and right bronchus, usually at the level of T4 or T5 posteriorly and slightly below the manubriosternal junction anteriorly.

The right bronchus is shorter, wider, and more vertical than the left bronchus. The bronchial structures are subdivided into increasingly smaller bronchi and **bronchioles**. Each bronchiole opens into an alveolar duct from which multiple alveoli radiate (Figure 15-2). In the adult, the lungs contain approximately 300 million alveoli.

The bronchi have both transport and protective purposes. They form the pathway through which air is transported into and out of the lungs. In addition, they protect the respiratory system by filtering the air. The bronchial cavities contain mucus, which entraps foreign particles. This mucus is continuously swept into the throat by **ciliary movement** and then is eliminated.

Two types of muscles are used in respiration: primary and accessory (Figure 15-3). The diaphragm and the external intercostal muscles are the primary muscles of respiration. The accessory muscles of respiration can be used to facilitate or increase inspiration (i.e., to assist in raising the ribs and the sternum) or to force expiration in both health and disease. The accessory muscles of respiration are the scalene muscles and the parasternal intercostal muscles.

The thoracic cage is perpetually moving throughout the inspiratory and expiratory phases of respiration (Figure 15-4). During inspiration, the diaphragm descends and flattens and the intercostal muscles contract. Both the diameter and the length of the thorax are increased. These maneuvers produce differences in pressure among the areas of the mouth, the alveoli, and the pleural cavities, and air moves into the lungs. The intrathoracic pressure is decreased, the lungs are expanded, and the ribs flare, increasing the diameter of the thorax. The second to the sixth ribs move around two axes in a motion commonly termed the "pump handle" movement. The lower ribs move in a "bucket handle" motion. Because of the length and positioning of the lower ribs and because the lower interspaces are wider, the amplitude of movement is greater in the lower thorax.

Expiration is a relatively passive phenomenon. At the completion of inspiration, the diaphragm relaxes and the elastic recoil properties of the lungs expel air and pull the diaphragm to its resting position.

Topographical Anatomy

The topographical, or surface, landmarks of the thorax are helpful in identifying the location of the internal underlying structures and in describing the exact location of physical findings (Figure 15-5).

Manubriosternal junction (angle of Louis). The manubriosternal junction is the articulation between the manubrium and the body of the sternum. It is an extremely useful aid in rib identification. Also called the angle of Louis, this junction is a visible and palpable angulation of the sternum.

The superior border of the second rib articulates with the sternum at the manubriosternal junction. Palpation

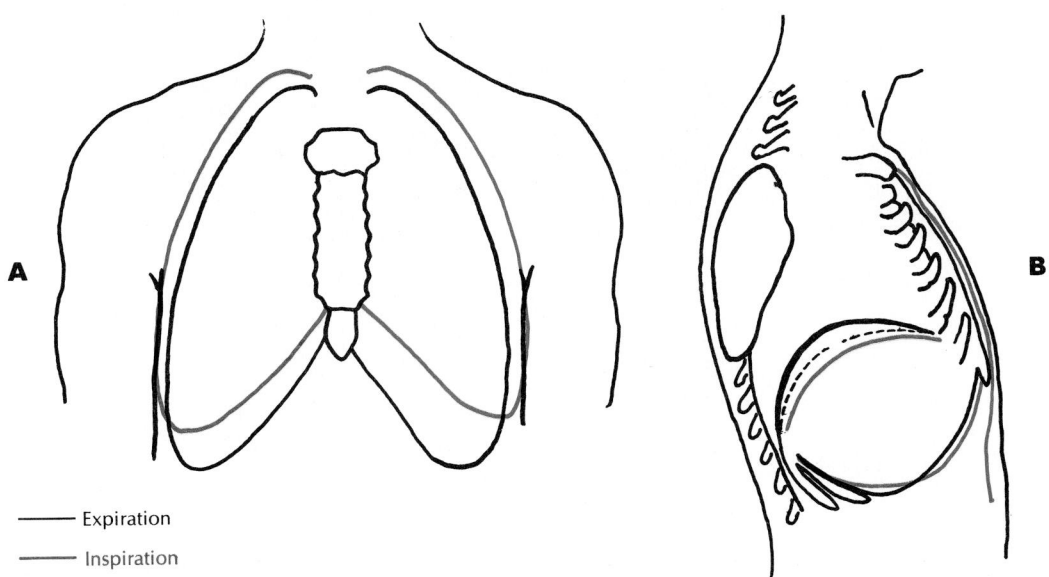

—— Expiration
—— Inspiration

FIGURE 15-4 Movement of the thorax during respiration. **A,** Anterior thorax. **B,** Lateral thorax.

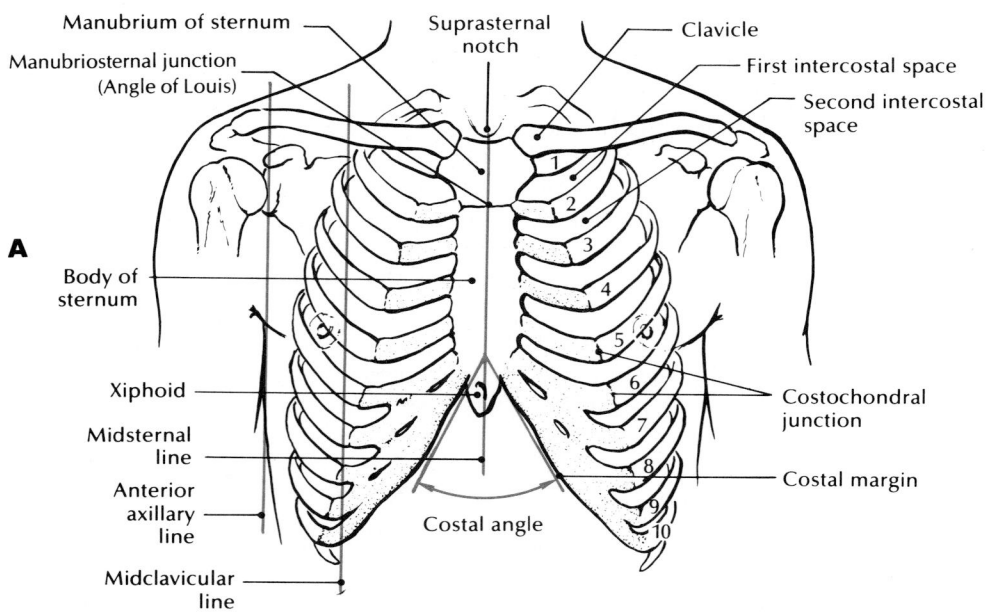

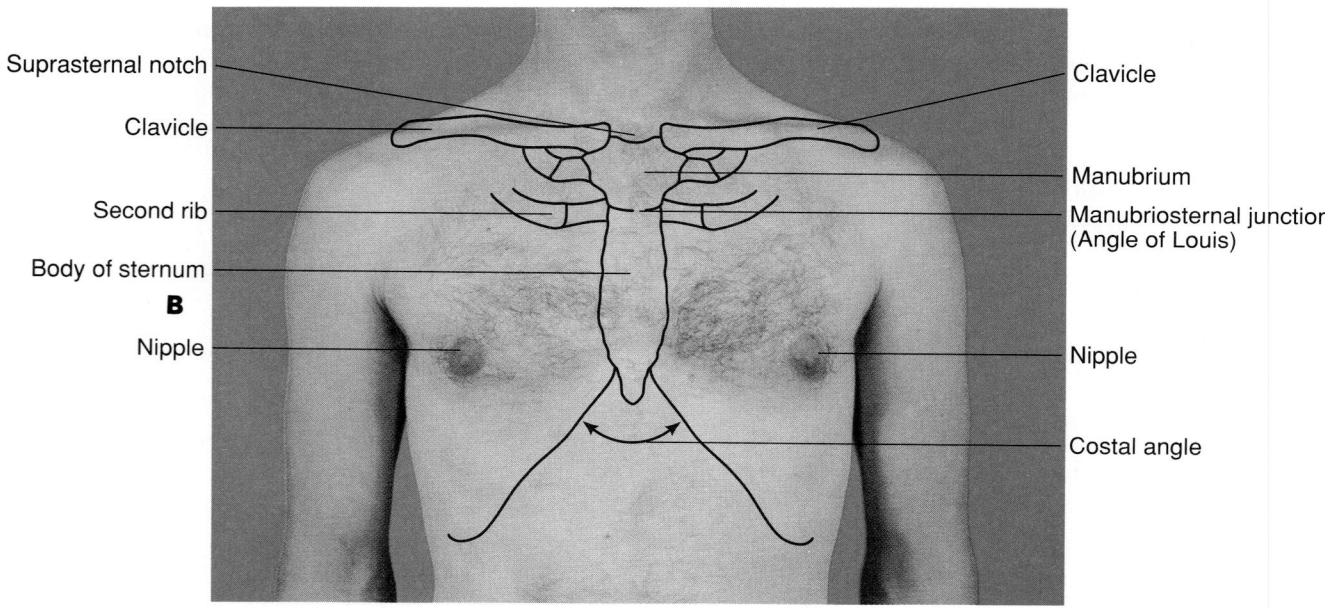

FIGURE 15-5 Topographic landmarks. **A** and **B,** Anterior thorax.

can be started at this junction, with distal ribs and rib interspaces counted from this point. As noted earlier, the number given to an intercostal space corresponds to the number of the rib immediately superior to that space. In palpation done for rib identification, the second intercostal space should first be identified at the sternum. Then palpation should be done along the midclavicular line, rather than at the sternal border, for the remaining ribs and interspaces. The rib cartilages are very close at the sternum and consequently are difficult to differentiate; the cartilages of only the first seven ribs attach directly to the sternum.

Suprasternal notch. The suprasternal notch is the depression above the manubrium.

Costal angle. The costal angle, which is formed by the intersection of the costal margins, normally measures 90 degrees or less.

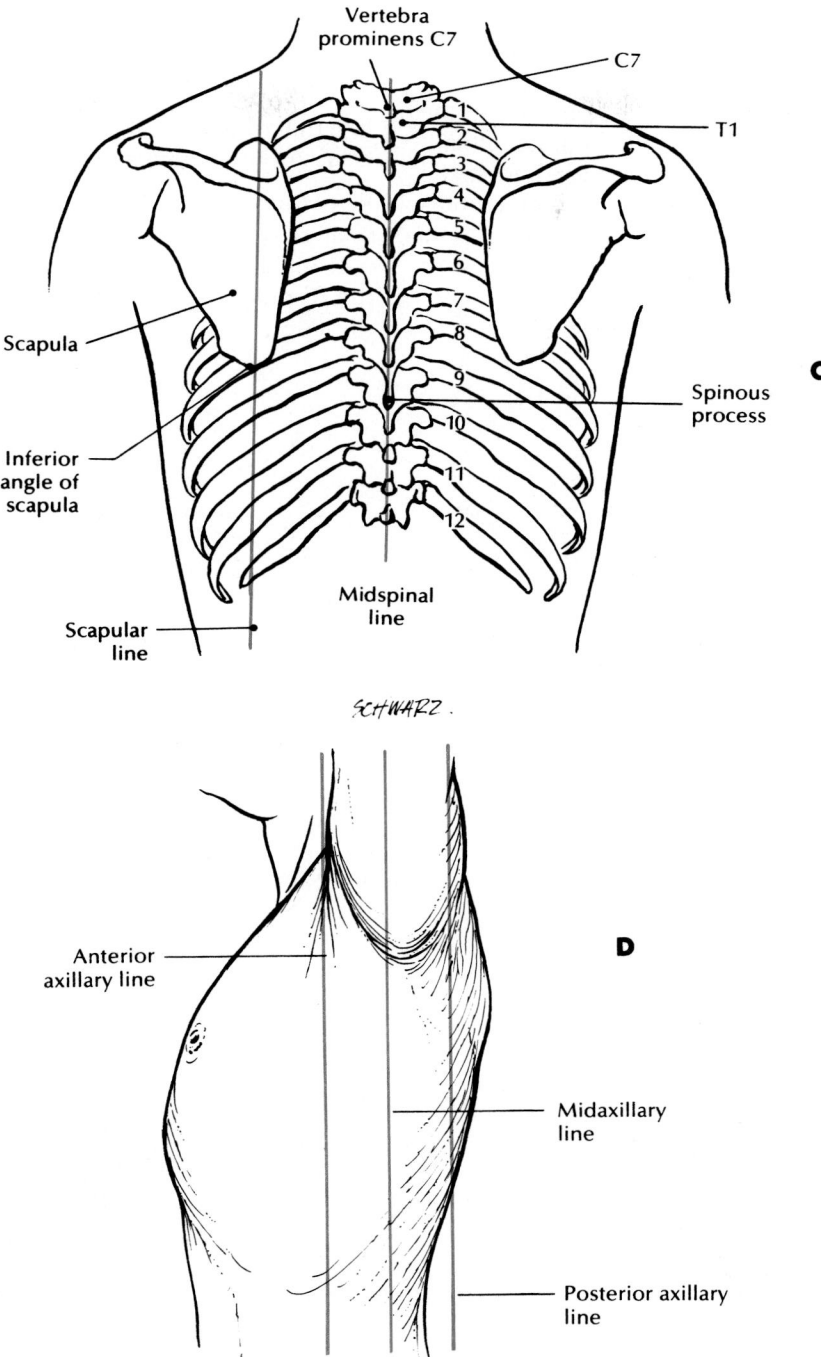

FIGURE 15-5, cont'd C, Posterior thorax. **D,** Lateral thorax.

Midsternal line. The midsternal line is an imaginary line drawn through the middle of the sternum.

Midclavicular lines. The midclavicular lines are left and right imaginary lines drawn through the midpoints of the clavicles and parallel to the midsternal line.

Anterior axillary lines. The anterior axillary lines are left and right imaginary lines drawn vertically from the anterior axillary folds, along the anterolateral chest, and parallel to the midsternal line.

Vertebra prominens (seventh cervical vertebra). When the client flexes the neck anteriorly and the posterior thorax is noted, a prominent spinous process can be observed and palpated. This structure is the seventh cervical vertebra. If two spinous processes are observed and palpated, the superior one is C7 and the inferior one is T1. The counting of ribs is more difficult on the posterior thorax than on the anterior thorax. The spinous processes of the vertebrae can be counted relatively easily from C7 to T4. From T4 the spinous processes project obliquely, causing the spinous process of the vertebra to lie over the rib below it rather than over its correspondingly numbered rib. For example, the spi-

nous process of the T5 lies over the body of T6 and is adjacent to the sixth rib.

Midspinal line. The midspinal line is an imaginary line that runs vertically along the posterior spinous processes of the vertebrae.

Scapular lines. The scapular lines are left and right imaginary lines that lie vertically and are parallel to the midspinal line. They pass through the inferior angles of the scapulae when the client stands erect with arms at the sides.

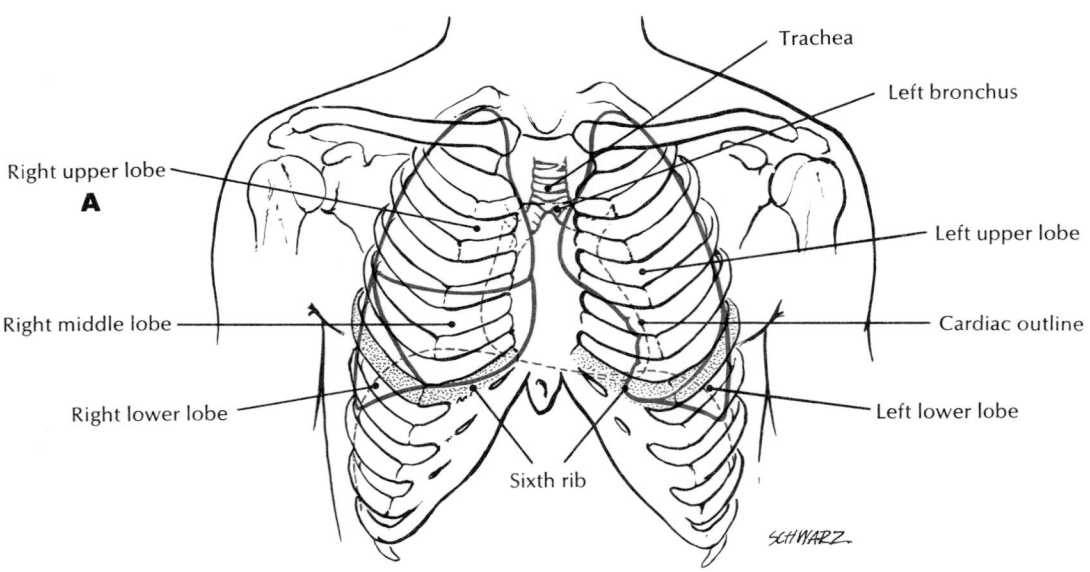

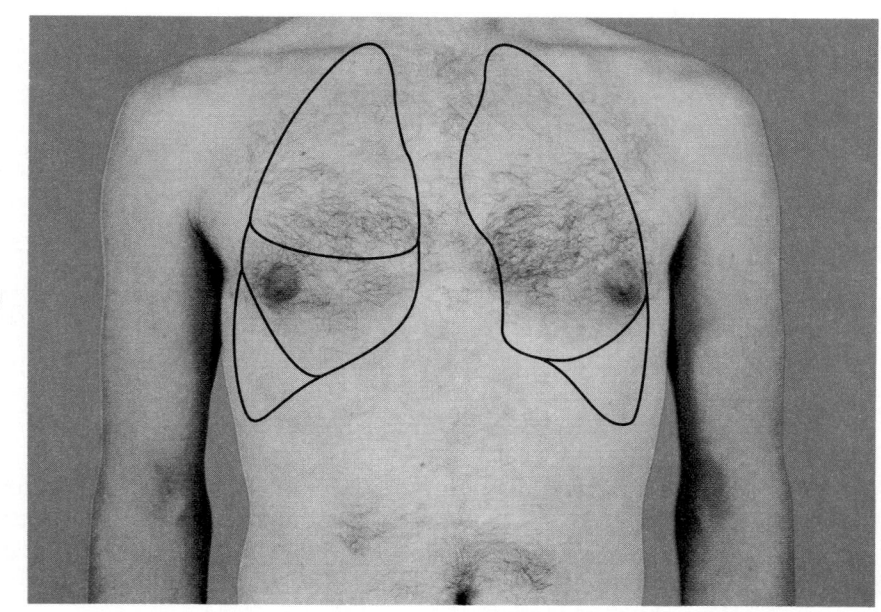

FIGURE 15-6 Anterior thorax. **A,** Internal organs and structures. **B,** Lung borders.

Posterior axillary lines. The posterior axillary lines are imaginary left and right lines drawn vertically from the posterior axillary folds along the posterolateral wall of the thorax when the lateral arm is abducted directly from the lateral chest wall.

Midaxillary lines. The midaxillary lines are imaginary left and right lines drawn vertically from the apices of the axillae. They lie approximately midway between

the anterior and the posterior axillary lines and run parallel to them.

Underlying Thoracic Structures

When examining the respiratory system, it is important to maintain a mental image of the placement of the organs and organ parts of the respiratory system and the other systems located in the thoracic area (Figures 15-6 through 15-9).

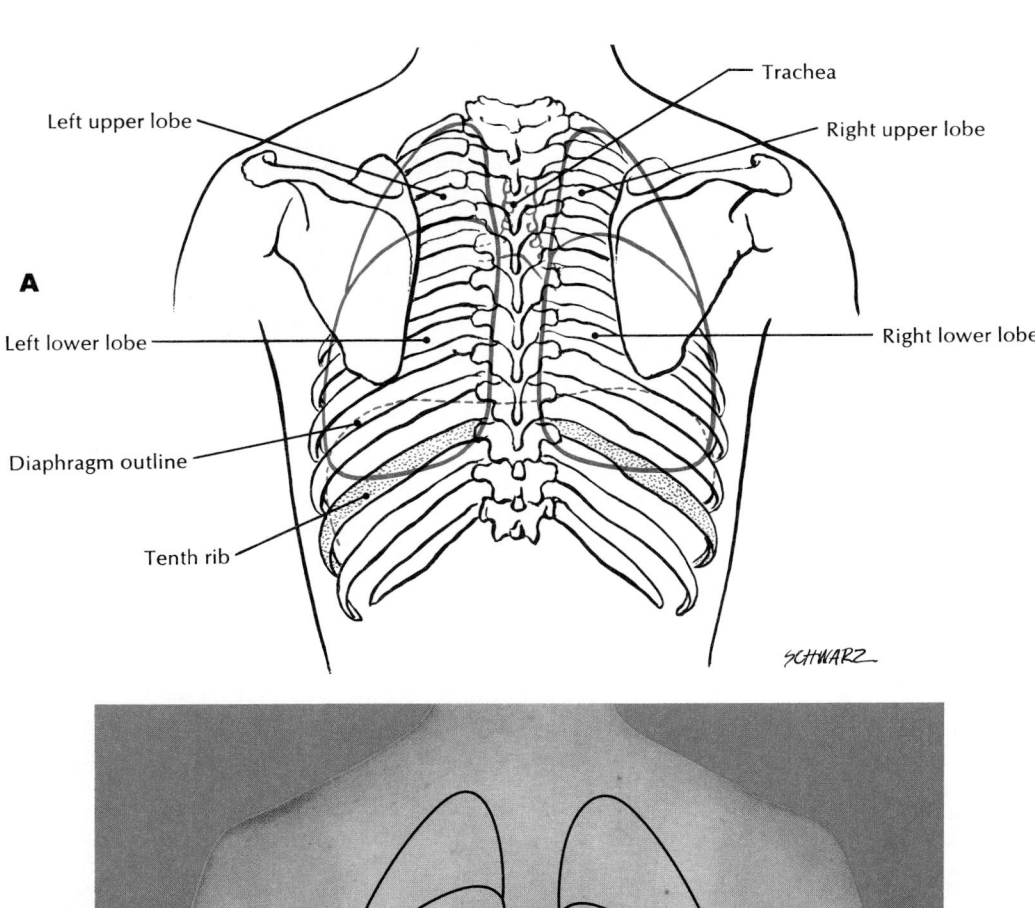

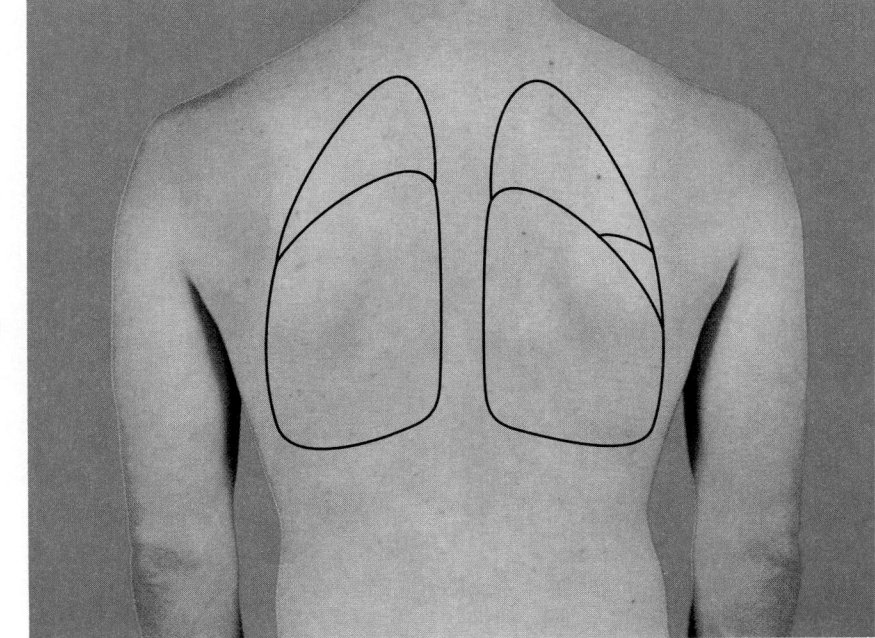

FIGURE 15-7 Posterior thorax. **A,** Internal organs and structures. **B,** Lung borders.

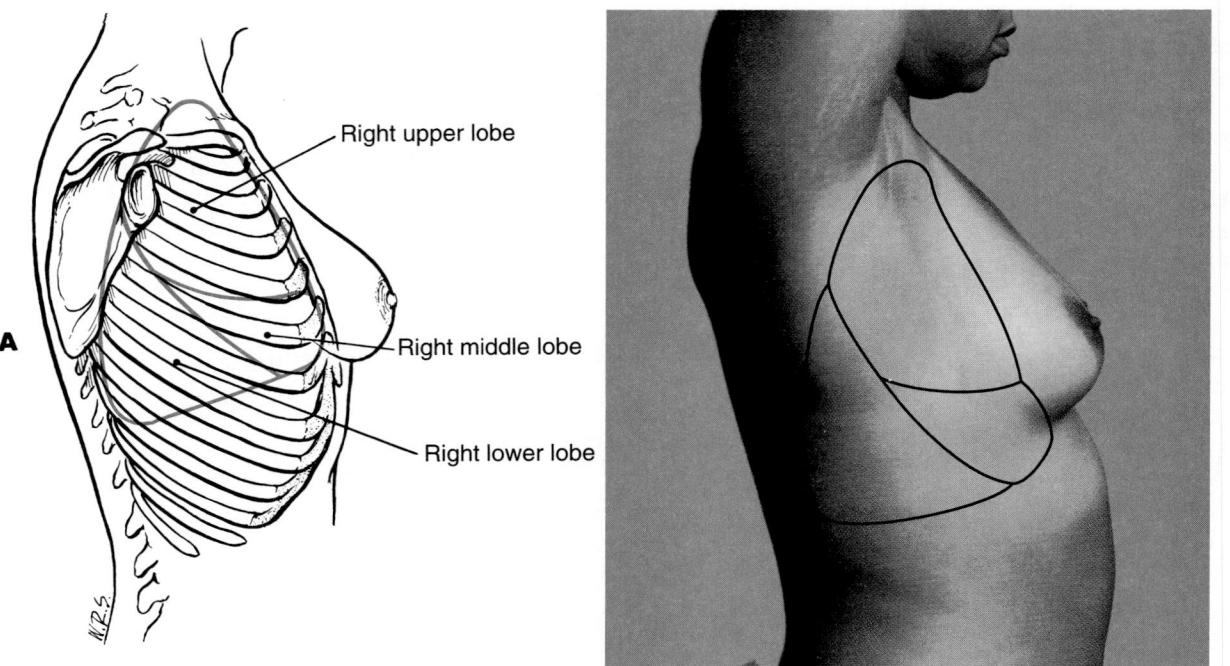

FIGURE 15-8 Right lateral thorax. **A,** Internal organs and chest structures. (Note the relationship of the breast to chest organs and structures.) **B,** Lung borders.

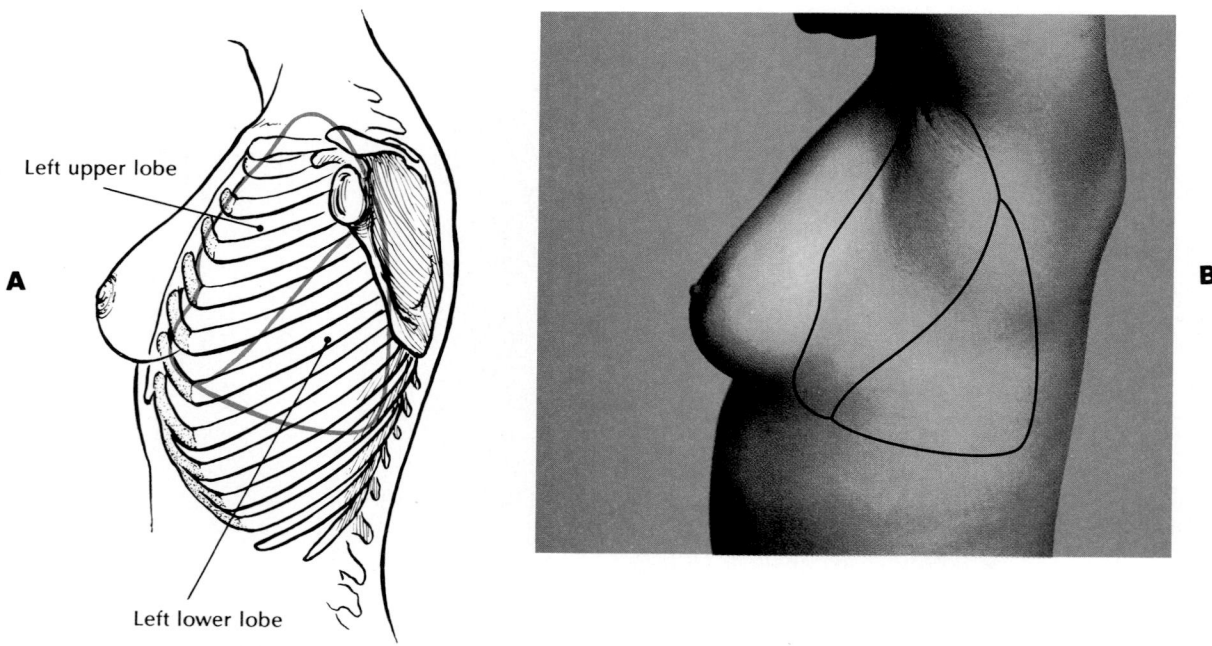

FIGURE 15-9 Left lateral thorax. **A,** Internal organs and chest structures. **B,** Lung borders.

Lung borders. In the anterior thorax, the apices of the lungs extend approximately 2 to 4 cm above the clavicles. The inferior borders of the lungs cross the sixth rib at the midclavicular line. In the posterior thorax, the apices extend to T1. The lower borders vary with respiration and usually extend from the spinous process of T10 on expiration to the spinous process of T12 on deep inspiration. In the lateral thorax, the lung extends from the apex of the axilla to the eighth rib of the midaxillary line.

Lung fissures. The right oblique (diagonal) fissure extends from the area of the spinous process of the third thoracic vertebra laterally and downward until it crosses the fifth rib at the right midaxillary line. It then continues anteriorly and medially to end at the sixth rib at the right midclavicular line. The right horizontal fissure extends from the fifth rib slightly posterior to the right midaxillary line and runs horizontally to the area of the fourth rib at the right sternal border. The left oblique (diagonal) fissure extends from the spinous process of the third thoracic vertebra laterally and downward to the left midaxillary line at the fifth rib. It continues anteriorly and medially until it terminates at the sixth rib in the left midclavicular line.

Border of diaphragm. Anteriorly, on expiration, the right dome of the diaphragm is located at the level of the fifth rib at the midclavicular line, and the left dome is situated at the level of the sixth rib. Posteriorly, on expiration, the diaphragm is at the level of the spinous process of T10; laterally, it is at the eighth rib at the midaxillary line. On inspiration, the diaphragm moves approximately 1.5 cm downward, with the right side being slightly higher than the left side because of the placement of the liver.

Trachea. The bifurcation of the trachea occurs approximately just below the manubriosternal junction anteriorly and at the spinous process of T4 posteriorly.

EXAMINATION

Health History

If a possible respiratory system problem is being investigated, the history of the respiratory system and the cardiovascular system should be taken together because of the symbiotic nature of the two systems, their sharing of the thoracic region of the body, and the potential effect that intervention directed at one system may have on the other system. However, the health history presented here focuses on the respiratory system.

Throughout the health history interview, record the following data about a symptom or problem: (1) onset (specific date, sudden or gradual), (2) duration, (3) fre-

quency, (4) precipitating factors, (5) aggravating or alleviating factors, (6) treatment received or self-care given, and (7) outcome.

Present health status

1. Allergies
2. Tobacco use
   a. Type of tobacco(s) smoked, age at which smoking was started, amount of smoking (packs per day), duration of habit (number of years). A smoking index can be determined by multiplying the number of years of smoking by the number of packs smoked per day.
   b. Exposure to smoke of others
3. Medications: Types and patterns of use
4. Use of aerosols or inhalants for any purpose
5. Recent screening or diagnostic assessments: Allergy test, skin test, chest x-ray examination
6. Nutritional data
   a. Sudden weight loss
   b. Obesity

Present illness*

1. Cough
   a. Type: Dry, moist, wet, productive, nonproductive, bubbling, hoarse, hacking, barking, whooping
   b. Onset: Sudden or gradual
   c. Duration
   d. Pattern: Regular or occasional; relationship to activities, time of day, weather, talking
   e. Severity: Effect on activities of daily living
   f. Associated symptoms: Shortness of breath, chest pain, fever, gagging, choking, changes in respiratory system
   g. Efforts to treat: Medications and other interventions, pattern of use and effectiveness
2. Sputum production
   a. Amount
   b. Color
   c. Presence of blood
   d. Odor
   e. Consistency
   f. Pattern of production
3. Shortness of breath (**dyspnea**)
   a. Onset: Sudden or gradual
   b. Frequency: Persistent or intermittent
   c. Pattern: Position when condition occurs; position most comfortable; relationship to exercise, other activity, time of day, eating
   d. Tolerance of activity: How many flights of stairs can be climbed before dyspnea occurs
   e. Differences between inhalation and exhalation

*Investigation of common symptoms is outlined.

f. Severity: Effect on activity during which short-ness of breath occurs and on activities of daily living

g. Associated symptoms: Anxiety, pain, discomfort, cough, fever

h. Response to treatment

i. Special situations

Orthopnea: Dyspnea that begins or increases when client lies down. Determine number of pillows that client uses.

Paroxysmal nocturnal dyspnea: Sudden onset of dyspnea after a period of lying down. Sitting upright helps to relieve the dyspnea.

Platypnea: Dyspnea that increases when client is upright.

4. Chest pain

a. Onset

b. Pattern

c. Severity

d. Duration

e. Associated symptoms: Trauma, coughing, infection, fever, anxiety, pain

Past health history

1. Respiratory infections and diseases: Type, frequency, pattern, and treatment. Specific inquiry should include past history of tuberculosis, **chronic obstructive pulmonary diseases** (e.g., **asthma, emphysema,** chronic **bronchitis**).

2. Trauma to respiratory system or area

3. Surgery to respiratory system or area

4. Chronic conditions of other systems: Cardiac diseases, malignancies, renal diseases

Family health history

1. Tuberculosis

2. Emphysema

3. Lung cancer

4. Allergies

RISK FACTORS

The following factors can differentially affect respiratory health:

Smoking: A major risk factor, contributing to a large portion of lung cancer cases

Sedentary life-style or recent immobilization

Age: Respiratory problems increase with aging

Environmental exposures: Especially occupational exposure to certain carcinogens

Extreme obesity

Weakened chest muscles for any reason

History of frequent respiratory infections for any reason

Other considerations

1. Employment and employment history: Place and nature of work can have a significant effect on the respiratory system. Determine client's exposure to chemicals, vapors, dust, allergens, animals, and other possible pulmonary irritants. Also ask client about presence of such possible irritants in the home environment; for example, types of heating, cooling, and ventilation may be important.

2. Current and past residence and travel to places where exposure to uncommon respiratory disease may have occurred

3. Hobbies that might involve exposure to respiratory irritants

Preparation for Examination: Client and Environment

Adequate respiratory examination requires a warm, well-lighted, quiet room. In addition to adequate room lighting, a mechanism for supplementary lighting is essential to aid in close inspection of specific areas.

Privacy is important because of the need to examine the entire chest area. Female clients may wish to have a gown or towel to cover their breasts while the posterior thorax is being examined. Tell them that you will be asking them to move their breasts to the side so that you will be better able to palpate, percuss, and auscultate the anterior thorax.

Preparation for the Examination

Equipment

Item	Purpose
Stethoscope with diaphragm	Auscultation of thorax
Marking pencil	Measurement of diaphragmatic excursion
Metric ruler	Measurement of diaphragmatic excursion

Client and environment
Client

Stripped to waist

Gown and sheet covering remainder of body

Covering available for female client to cover chest when not being examined

Instructed regarding breathing and position for examination of posterior thorax

Setting

Warm

Private

Before starting the examination, teach the patient now to sit and how to breathe during the auscultation of the posterior thorax. For examination of the posterior thorax, instruct the client to hunch forward slightly and cross the arms over the chest (see Figure 15-16) so that the greatest amount of lung surface is available for examination. Also, instruct the patient to breathe deeply and quietly, slowly inhaling and exhaling through the open mouth.

The client can be seated throughout the examination and stripped to the waist. Female clients can use a towel or gown to cover their breasts when the posterior and lateral portions of the chest are being examined.

The examination of the respiratory system generally is done in the traditional sequence—inspection, palpation, percussion, and auscultation.

Examination technique and normal findings

Inspection. Inspection is performed to (1) measure and assess the pattern of respirations and (2) assess the skin and the overall configuration, **symmetry**, and integrity of the thorax.

The approach to the physical examination is regional and integrated. The examination of systems is combined in body regions when appropriate. Because the client is uncovered to the waist during the examination, a large portion of skin and tissue is accessible to inspection. The observation of skin and underlying tissue provides information about the client's general nutritional state. Common thoracic skin findings are the spider nevi associated with cirrhosis and seborrheic dermatitis (see Chapter 9).

Lips and nails. Inspection of the respiratory system examination includes observation of lips and nailbeds for color and observation of the nails for clubbing. These techniques are discussed in Chapters 7 and 15.

Thoracic configuration. The first point of observation is the general shape of the thorax and its symmetry. Although no individual is absolutely symmetrical in both body hemispheres, most individuals are reasonably similar from side to side. Using the client as his or her own control whenever paired parts are examined is an excellent habit and often yields important findings. The anteroposterior diameter of the thorax in the normal adult is less than the transverse diameter at an approximate ratio of 1:2 to 5:7 (Figure 15-10). In the normal infant, in some adults with pulmonary disease, and in elderly adults, the thorax is generally round. This condition is called barrel chest. The barrel chest is characterized by horizontal ribs, slight kyphosis of the thoracic spine, and prominent sternal angle. The chest appears as though it is in continuous inspiratory position.

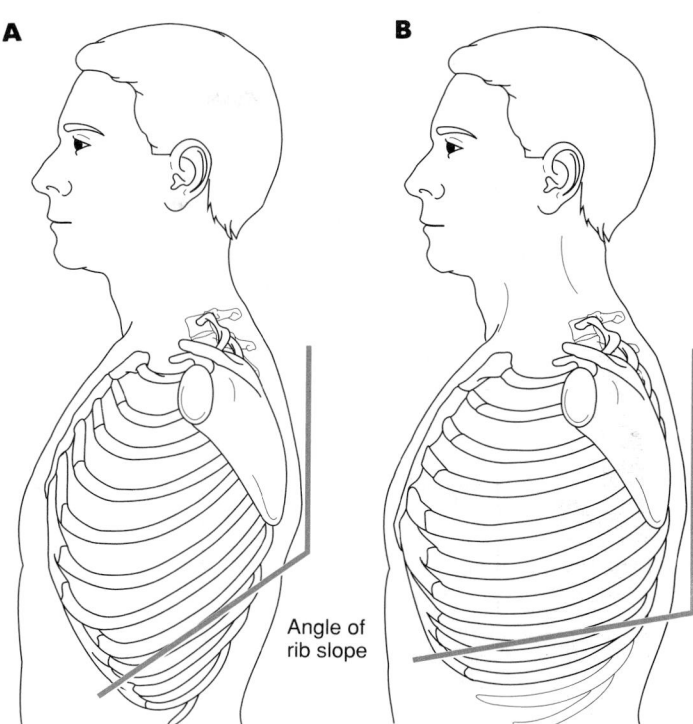

Angle of
rib slope

FIGURE 15-10 A, Normal thoracic configuration. **B,** Increased anteroposterior diameter. Note contrast in the angle of the slope of the ribs.

Other observed abnormalities of thoracic shape include the following:

1. *Retraction of thorax.* The retraction is unilateral, involving only one side.
2. *Pigeon or chicken chest (pectus carinatum).* Sternal protrusion anteriorly. The anteroposterior diameter of the chest is increased, and the resultant configuration resembles the thorax of a fowl.
3. *Funnel chest (pectus excavatum).* Depression of part or all of the sternum. If the depression is deep, it may interfere with both respiratory and cardiac function.
4. *Spinal deformities (scoliosis, kyphosis, lordosis).* The respiratory examination offers an excellent opportunity to initiate inspection of the spine. (See Chapter 18 for specific information on assessment of the spine.)

Ribs and interspaces. Retraction of interspaces on inspiration may indicate some obstruction of free air inflow. Bulging of interspaces on expiration occurs when air outflow is obstructed, or it may be the result of tumor, aneurysm, or cardiac enlargement.

Normally, the costal angle is less than 90 degrees, and the ribs are inserted into the spine at approximately

TABLE 15-1

Characteristics of Commonly Observed Respiratory Patterns

Type of respiration	Diagram	Discussion
Normal		2-20 respirations/min in adults; regular in rhythm; ratio of respiratory rate to pulse rate is 1:4
Hyperventilation or **Kussmaul respiration**		Increase in both rate and depth; hyperpnea is an increase in depth only
Periodic respiration		Alternating **hyperpnea,** shallow respiration, and apnea; sometimes called Cheyne-Stokes respiration; frequently occurs in the severely ill
Sighing respiration		Deep and audible; audible portion sounds like a sigh
Air trapping		Present in obstructive pulmonary diseases; air is trapped in the lungs; respiratory level rises, and breathing becomes shallow
Biot's breathing		Shallow breathing interrupted by **apnea;** seen in some CNS disorders and in healthy persons

a 45-degree angle (see Figure 15-1). In clients with obstructive lung disease, these angles are widened.

Pattern of respiration. Normally, men and children breathe diaphragmatically, and women breathe thoracically or costally. A change in this pattern might be significant. If the client appears to have labored respiration, it is important to observe for the use of the accessory muscles of respiration in the neck (sternocleidomastoid, scalenus, and trapezius muscles) and for supraclavicular retraction. Impedance to air inflow is often accompanied by retraction of the intercostal spaces during inspiration. An excessively long expiratory phase of respiration is characteristic of outflow impedance and may be accompanied by the use of abdominal muscles to aid in expiration.

In the normal adult, the resting respiratory rate is 12 to 20 breaths/min and is regular and unlabored. The ratio of respiratory rate to pulse rate normally is 1:4. **Tachypnea** is an adult respiratory rate of more than

20 breaths/min. **Bradypnea** is an adult respiratory rate of less than 10 breaths/min. Dyspnea is a subjective phenomenon of inadequate or distressful respiration. Many more abnormal patterns of respiration exist. Some of the commonly noted respiratory patterns are listed in Table 15-1.

Palpation. Palpation is performed to (1) further assess abnormalities suggested by the health history or by observation, such as tenderness, pulsations, masses, or skin lesions; (2) assess the skin and subcutaneous structures; (3) assess thoracic expansion; (4) assess **tactile fremitus;** and (5) assess tracheal position.

In examination of the thorax, four parts of the thorax need consideration: posterior chest, anterior chest, right and left lateral chest, and apices. During the examination, move from the area of one hemisphere to the corresponding area on the other side (right to left, left to right) until all four major parts have been surveyed. During palpation for assessment of fremitus and all sub-

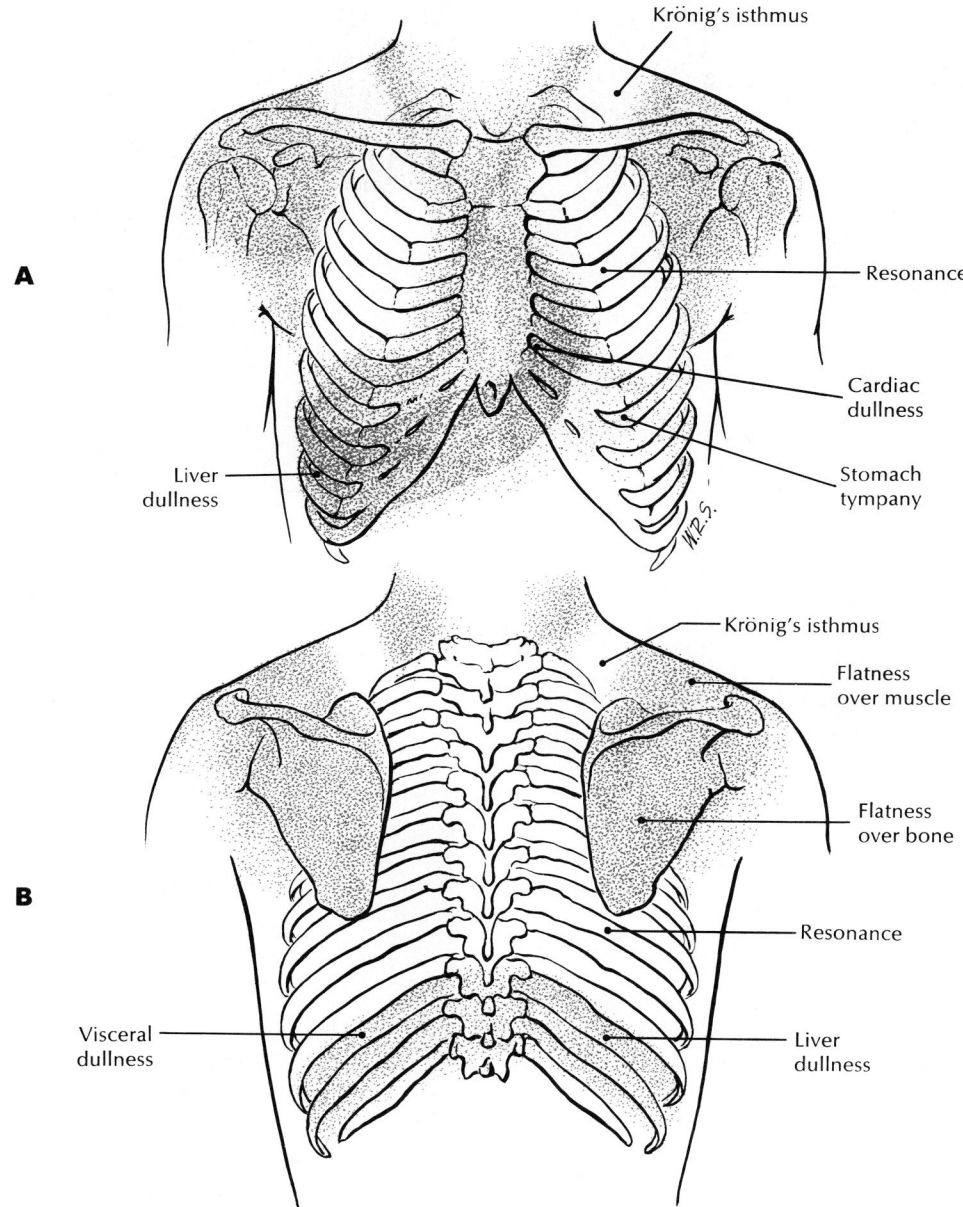

FIGURE 15-15 Percussion areas. **A,** Normal anterior chest. **B,** Normal posterior chest.

1. Instruct the client to inhale deeply and hold the breath in.
2. Percuss down the scapular line on one side, starting at T7 or at the end of the scapula, until the lower edge of the lung is identified. Sound will change from resonance to dullness.
3. Mark the point of change at the scapular line. This point is the edge of the diaphragm at full inhalation.
4. Instruct the client to take a few normal respirations.

5. Instruct the client to take a deep breath, exhale completely, and hold the breath at the end of the expiration.
6. Proceed to percuss upward from the marked point at the midscapular line. Mark the point where dullness of the diaphragm changes to the resonance of the lung. This point is the level of the diaphragm at full expiration. An alternate method of determining the level of the diaphragm at full exhalation is to percuss down along the scapular line and note where the res-

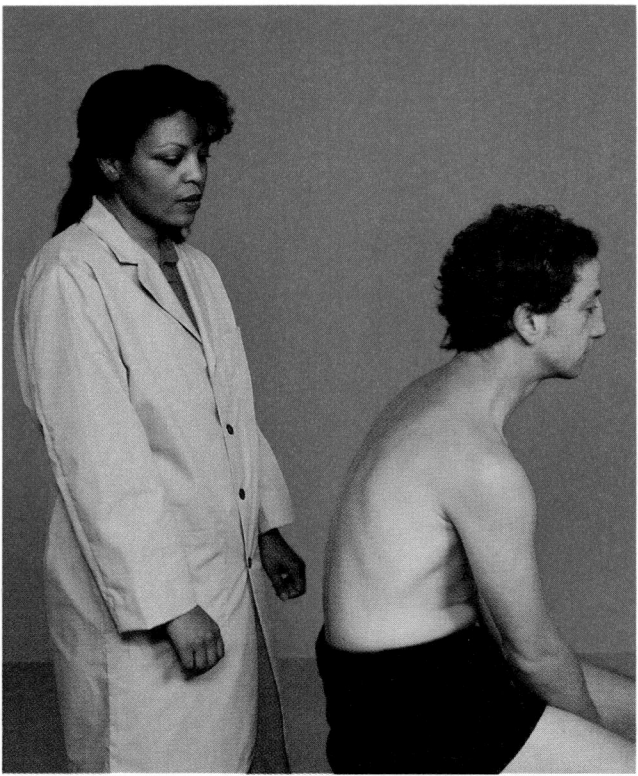

FIGURE 15-16 Position of the client for examination of the posterior thorax.

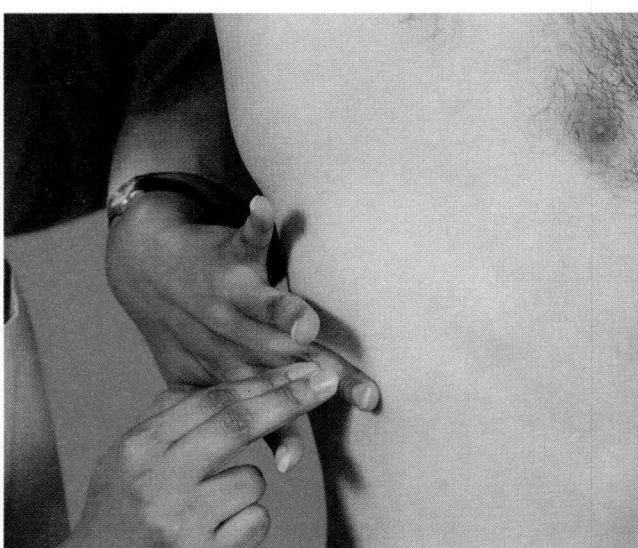

FIGURE 15-17 Position of the client for percussion of the lateral thorax.

onance of the lung changes to the dullness of the diaphragm.

7. Repeat the procedure on the opposite side.
8. Measure and record the diaphragmatic excursion, the distance between the upper and lower marks in centimeters for each side of the thorax.

The diaphragm is usually slightly higher on the right side because of the location of the liver on that side. Diaphragmatic excursion which is normally 3 to 5 cm bilaterally, is usually measured only on the posterior chest (Figure 15-18).

In the actual examination, the apices and the posterior and lateral chest would be examined before percussion of the anterior chest is done. A recommended sequence for the examination of the posterior, lateral, and anterior thoracic areas is illustrated in Figure 15-19.

Auscultation. Through auscultation, information can be obtained about the functioning of the respiratory system and about the presence of any obstruction in the passages. For auscultation of the lungs, a stethoscope is used. The diaphragm of the stethoscope is com-

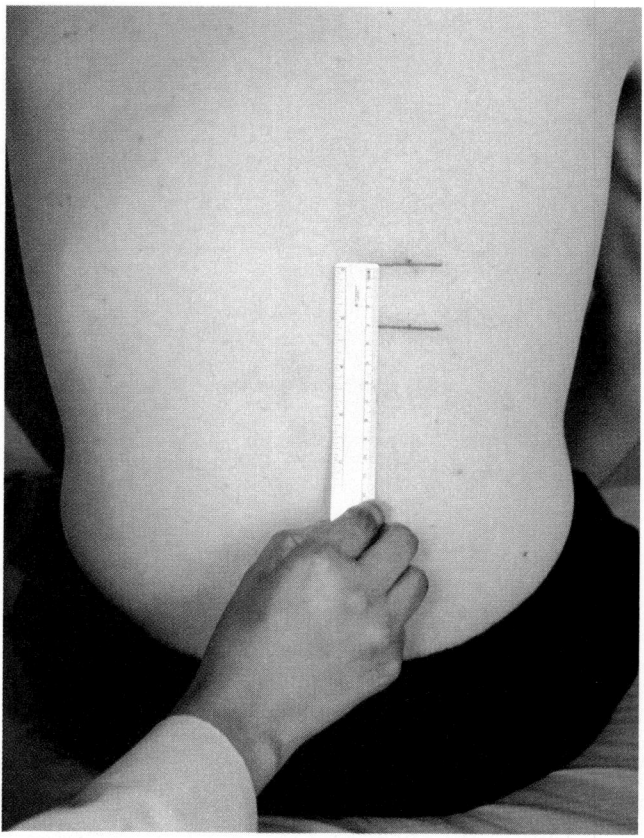

FIGURE 15-18 Assessment of diaphragmatic excursion.

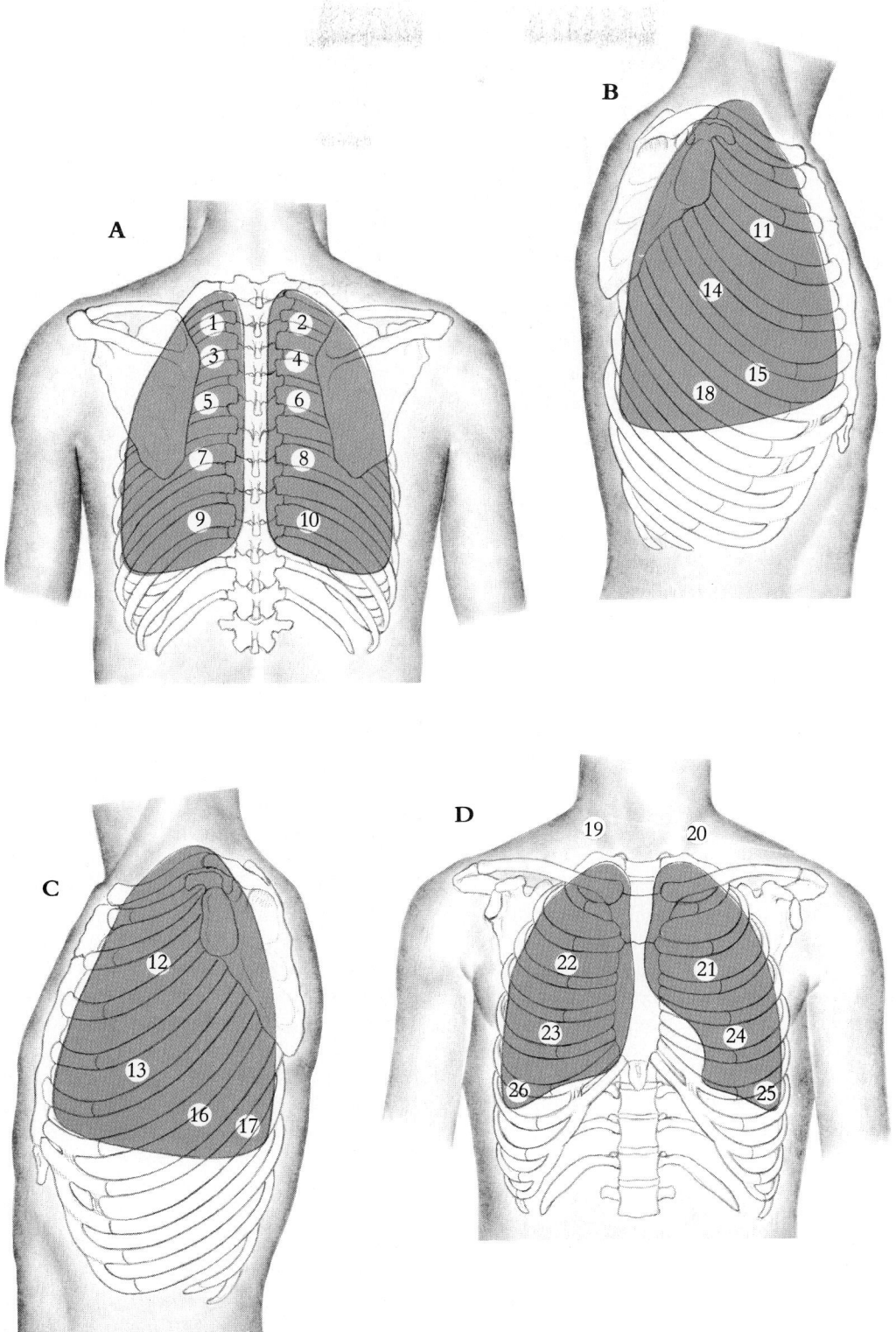

FIGURE 15-19 Routine for systematic percussion and auscultation of the thorax. Numbers indicate a recommended sequence for percussion and auscultation during a routine screening examination. **A,** Posterior thorax. **B,** Right lateral thorax. **C,** Left lateral thorax. **D,** Anterior thorax. (From Seidel HM, Ball JW, Dains JE, and Benedict GW: *Mosby's guide to physical examination,* ed 2, St Louis, 1991, Mosby–Year Book.)

TABLE 15-4

Characteristics of Breath Sounds

Sound	Duration of inspiration and expiration	Diagram of sound	Pitch	Intensity	Normal location	Abnormal location
Vesicular	Inspiration > expiration 2.5:1		Low	Soft	Peripheral lung	Not applicable
Bronchovesicular	Inspiration = expiration 1:1		Medium	Medium	First and second intercostal spaces at sternal border anteriorly; posteriorly at T4 medial to scapulae	Peripheral lung
Bronchial (tubular)	Inspiration < expiration 1:2		High	Loud	Over trachea	Lung area

monly used for the thoracic examination because it covers a larger surface than does the bell. Also, the diaphragm is designed to transmit the usually higher pitch of abnormal breath sounds.

Place the stethoscope firmly, but not tightly, on the skin. Avoid client or stethoscope movement because movements of muscle under the skin or movements of the stethoscope over hair produce confusing extrinsic sounds.

The auscultatory assessment includes (1) analysis of breath sounds, (2) detection of any abnormal sounds, and (3) examination of the sounds produced by the spoken voice. As with percussion, use a zigzag approach, comparing the finding at each point with the corresponding point on the opposite hemithorax.

Before beginning auscultation, instruct the client to breathe through the mouth and more deeply and more slowly than in usual respiration. Then, systematically auscultate the apices and the posterior, lateral, and anterior chest (see Figure 15-19). At each application of the stethoscope, listen to at least one complete respiration. Observe the client for signs of **hyperventilation** and alter the procedure if the client becomes lightheaded or faint.

Breath sounds. Breath sounds are produced by the movement of air through the tracheobronchoalveolar system. These sounds are analyzed according to pitch, intensity, quality, and relative duration of inspiratory and expiratory phases. Table 15-4 outlines the types of sounds heard over the normal lung and the abnormal lung.

The sounds heard over normal lung **parenchyma** are called vesicular breath sounds. The inspiratory phase of the vesicular breath sounds is heard better than the expiratory phase and is about 2.5 times longer. These sounds have a low pitch and soft intensity.

Bronchovesicular breath sounds are normally heard in the areas of the major bronchi, especially in the apex of the right lung and at the sternal borders anteriorly and posteriorly between the scapula. Bronchovesicular breath sounds are characterized by inspiratory and expiratory phases of equal duration, moderate pitch, and moderate intensity. When bronchovesicular breath sounds are heard over the peripheral lung of an adult, an underlying pathological condition is likely to be present.

Bronchial breath sounds are normally heard over the trachea and indicate a pathological condition if heard over lung tissue. They are high-pitched, loud sounds associated with shortened inspiratory and lengthened expiratory phases. A gap of silence audibly separates the inspiratory and expiratory phases.

Figure 15-20 shows the various areas for assessing breath sounds of the anterior and posterior thorax. Absent or decreased breath sounds can occur in (1) any condition that causes the deposition of foreign matter in the pleural space, (2) bronchial obstruction, (3) emphysema, or (4) shallow breathing.

Increased breath sounds, as from vesicular to bronchovesicular or bronchial, can occur in any condition that causes a consolidation of lung tissue.

Abnormal or adventitious sounds. Adventitious sounds are not alterations in breath sounds but abnormal sounds superimposed on breath sounds. Classification of these sounds varies among authorities; consequently, the nomenclatures are somewhat inconsistent. The commonly used terms for adventitious sounds are described in Table 15-5.

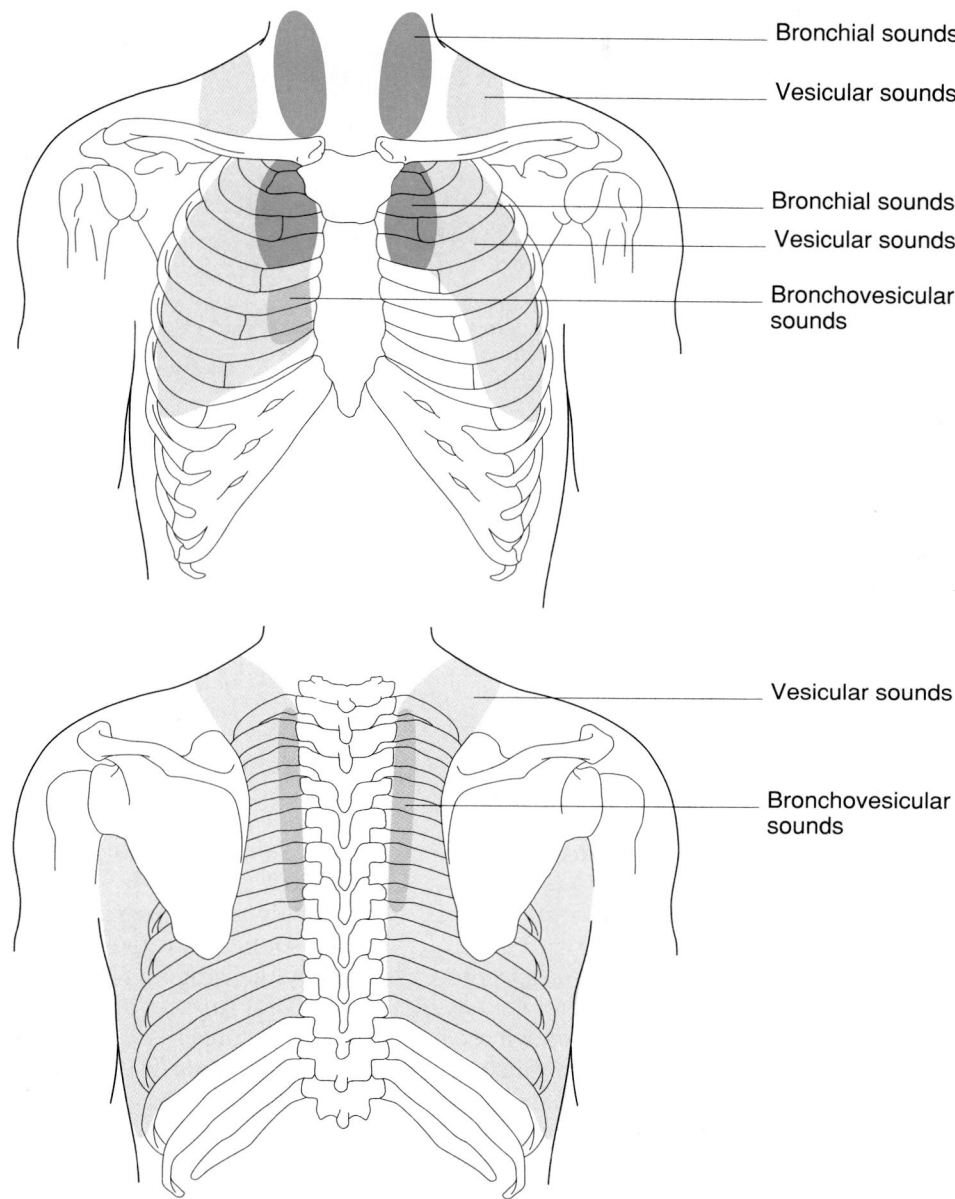

Bronchial sounds

Vesicular sounds

Bronchial sounds

Vesicular sounds

Bronchovesicular sounds

Vesicular sounds

Bronchovesicular sounds

FIGURE 15-20 Areas for assessing breath sounds of the anterior and posterior thorax. Areas more darkly colored indicate normal point for the auscultation of bronchial and bronchovesicular breath sounds.

A **crackle** (or *rale,* a term used in older texts) is a short, discrete, interrupted, crackling or bubbling sound that is most commonly heard during inspiration. The sound of crackles is similar to that produced by hairs being rolled between the fingers while close to the ear. The exact mechanism by which crackles are produced is not fully understood. Crackles are thought to be produced by air passing through moisture in the bronchi, bronchioles, and alveoli or by air rushing through passages and alveoli that were closed during expiration and abruptly opened during inspiration. The pitch and location in the inspiratory phase of the crackles are thought to indicate their site of production. Low-pitched, coarse crackles occurring early in inspiration are thought to originate in the bronchi, as in bronchitis. Medium-pitched crackles in midinspiration occur in

TABLE 15-5

Origin and Characteristics of Adventitious Sounds

Sound	Diagram of sound	Origin	Characteristics
Crackles*—fine to medium		Air passing through moisture in small air passages and alveoli	Discrete, discontinuous; inspiratory; have a dry or wet crackling quality; not cleared by coughing; sound is simulated by rolling a lock of hair near the ear
Crackles*—medium to coarse		Air passing through moisture in the bronchioles, bronchi, and trachea	As above; louder than fine crackles
Wheezes—sonorous		Air passing through air passages narrowed by secretions, swelling, tumors, and so on	Continuous sounds; originate in large air passages; may be inspiratory and expiratory but usually predominate in expiration; low-pitched, moaning or snoring quality; coughing may alter sounds
Wheezes—sibilant		Same as sonorous wheezes	Continuous sounds; originate in the small air passages; may be inspiratory and expiratory but usually predominated in expiration; high-pitched, wheezing sounds
Friction rubs		Rubbing together of inflamed and roughened pleural surfaces	Creaking or grating quality; superficial sounding; inspiratory and expiratory; heard most often in the lower antero-lateral chest (area of greatest thoracic expansion); coughing has no effect

*Crackles are also called rales or crepitations.

diseases of the small bronchi, as in **bronchiectasis**. High-pitched, fine crackles are found in diseases affecting the bronchioles and alveoli and occur late in inspiration.

Wheezes (rhonchi) are continuous sounds produced by the movement of air through narrowed passages in the tracheobronchial tree. Sonorous wheezes predominate in expiration because bronchi are shortened and narrowed during this respiratory phase. However, they can occur in both the inspiratory and the expiratory phase of respiration, suggesting that lumina have been narrowed during both respiratory phases. As with crackles, the pitch and location of sonorous wheezes in the expiratory phase are thought to indicate their origins. Low-pitched sonorous wheezes are usually heard in early expiration and probably originate in the larger bronchi. High-pitched, sibilant wheezes orig-

inate in small bronchioles and often occur in late expiration.

A pleural **friction rub** is a loud, dry, creaking or grating sound indicative of pleural irritation. It is produced by the rubbing together of inflamed and roughened pleural surfaces during respiration (e.g., in **pleurisy**). Therefore it is heard best during the latter part of inspiration and the beginning of expiration. Because thoracic expansion is greatest in the lower anterolateral thorax, pleural friction rubs are most often heard there.

If the client has crackles, listen for several respirations in the areas in which the crackles are heard to determine the effects of deep breathing. Also, ask the client to cough and note the changes in adventitious sounds after coughing. Crackles do not usually change with coughing, but ronchi will often do so.

If the client has complained of respiratory difficulty

VOICE SOUND ASSESSMENT TECHNIQUES

Client vocalization	Normal auscultatory finding	Abnormal auscultatory finding
"Ninety-nine" spoken	Muffled, nondistinct sound	"Ninety-nine": bronchophony
"e- e- e" spoken	Muffled, nondistinct sound	"a- a- a": egophony
"Ninety-nine" whispered	Barely audible, nondistinct sound	"Ninety-nine": whispered pectoriloquy

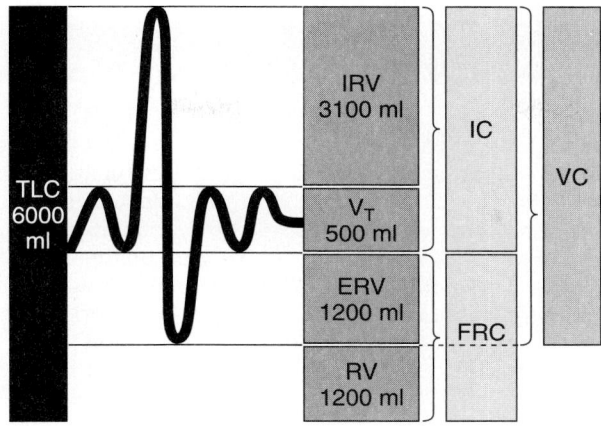

TLC = Total lung capacity	IRV = Inspiratory reserve volume	IC = Inspiratory capacity
	V_T = Tidal volume	FRC = Functional residual capacity
	ERV = Expiratory reserve volume	VC = Vital capacity
	RV = Residual volume	

FIGURE 15-21 Components of lung capacity. (From Wilson SF and Thompson JM: *Respiratory disorders*, St. Louis, 1990, Mosby–Year Book.)

and no adventitious sounds are heard, ask him or her to cough; often adventitious sounds are noted after coughing.

Vocal resonance. The same mechanism that produces tactile fremitus produces vocal resonance. Resonance is the transmission of voice sounds as heard through the stethoscope placed on the chest wall. Normal vocal resonance is heard as muffled, nondistinct sounds. It is loudest medially and is less intense at the periphery of the lung.

Vocal resonance should be assessed if any respiratory system abnormality has been detected on observation, palpation, percussion, or auscultation. The routine is the same systematic one previously used in assessing tactile fremitus (see Figure 15-13). The client says "one, two, three" or "ninety-nine" while the examiner does an auscultatory survey of the thorax

Bronchophony is an increase in loudness and clarity of vocal resonance. Special vocal resonance techniques are used when resonance is increased. These include tests for **whispered pectoriloquy** and **egophony**.

Whispered pectoriloquy is exaggerated bronchophony. The client is instructed to whisper a series of words. The words as heard through the stethoscope on the chest wall are distinct and understandable.

In egophony, the intensity of the spoken voice, as heard through the stethoscope applied to the chest wall, is increased and the voice has a nasal or bleating quality. If the client says "e- e- e," the transmitted sound will be "a- a- a."

Decreased vocal resonance occurs in the same clinical situations in which tactile fremitus is decreased and breath sounds are absent. Vocal resonance is increased and whispered pectoriloquy and egophony may be present in any condition that causes a consolidation of lung tissue.

Screening Tests and Procedures

A variety of radiological, functional, and chemical diagnostic tests are used in assessing respiratory health. It is beyond the capabilities of this text to describe these various tests fully. However, some of the major ones are listed here.

Chest x-ray examination. The chest x-ray is a common test used to determine the health of lung parenchyma.

Pulmonary function tests. Pulmonary function tests are procedures requiring some respiratory effort by the client. The effort includes blowing air into a spirometer designed to measure lung volumes and flow rates. This assessment is generally done by specialized technicians in a designated laboratory. Spirometry readings are commonly expressed in volumes and capacities. Volumes are single compartments in the lung. The addition of two or more volumes together results in a capacity. Volumes and capacities are expressed as a percentage of normal. Generally the normal range is plus or minus 20% of the predicted value of all volumes and capacities (Figure 15-21).

The following are common spirometric assessments:

STEP-BY-STEP

Examination Step-by-Step

The examination described here is for a client who is able to sit during the procedure. The approach would need to be adapted for a client who is unable to sit during the examination. In general, the examiner moves around the client, completing one aspect of assessment before initiating the next. Traditional organization of inspection, palpation, percussion, and auscultation is followed.

The client is stripped to the waist and seated so that all areas of the thorax are visible.

1. Inspect all areas of the thorax, noting especially:
   a. Breathing rate, pattern, inspiratory-expiratory ratio, audible adventitious sounds
   b. Use of accessory muscles of respiration
   c. Condition of skin and underlying structures
   d. Presence of bulging
   e. Skin color and superficial venous patterns
   f. Size, shape, and symmetry of thorax
2. Examine the posterior, lateral, and apical thorax
   a. Palpate the thorax
      1. General assessment of skin tone, temperature, tenderness, unusual sensations
      2. Thoracic expansion
      3. Tactile fremitus
   b. Percuss the thorax
      1. Percussion survey of thorax, including assessment of appropriateness of various tones for their location
      2. Diaphragmatic excursion
   c. Auscultate with the diaphragm of the stethoscope from apex to base, from side to side
      1. Appropriateness of type of breath sound for location
      2. Adventitious sounds
      3. Vocal resonance
3. Examine the anterior thorax
   a. Palpate the thorax
      1. General assessment of skin tone, temperature, tenderness, unusual sensations
      2. Position of trachea
      3. Thoracic expansion
      4. Tactile fremitus
   b. Percuss the thorax: Percussion survey of thorax includes assessment of appropriateness of various tones for their location
   c. Auscultate with the diaphragm of the stethoscope from apex to base, from side to side
      1. Appropriateness of type of breath sound for location
      2. Adventitious sounds
      3. Vocal resonance

---

1. *Tidal volume:* Volume of air exhaled or inhaled during quiet breathing.
2. *Minute volume:* Volume of gas expired over 1 minute.
3. *Total lung capacity:* Sum of the vital capacity and the residual volume.
4. *Vital capacity:* Maximum amount of air a person can exhale. Usually measured after forceful exhalation and termed *forced vital capacity.*
5. *Residual volume:* Amount of gas left in the lung after exhaling all that is physically possible. This measurement is expressed as a ratio of total lung capacity to vital capacity.
6. *Expiratory reserve volume:* Volume that can be maximally exhaled following a passive exhalation.
7. *Functional residual capacity:* Sum of the residual volume and the expiratory reserve volume.
8. *Forced expiratory volume in 1 second* (FEV_1): Measurement of the maximum volume of air exhaled during the first second of expiration.
9. *FEV_1/FVC:* Ratio of forced expiratory volume in 1 second and forced vital capacity.
10. *Peak flow:* Measurement of the maximum flow rate achieved during the forced vital capacity maneuver.
11. *Diffusing capacity:* Ability of gas to diffuse across the alveolar-capillary membrane.

Arterial blood gases. The measurement of arterial blood gases provides valuable information about the physiological functioning of the respiratory system. Some of the commonly used tests are listed here.

Oxygenation status is measured by the following values:

1. Pao_2: Partial pressure of oxygen in arterial blood.
2. Sao_2: Percent of saturation of oxygen on hemoglobin in arterial blood.
3. Cao_2: Content of oxygen in arterial blood expressed in ml/100 ml of blood.
4. Pvo_2: Partial pressure of oxygen in mixed venous blood.

Acid-base balance is measured by the following values:

1. pH: Hydrogen ion concentration in the blood.
2. Pco_2: Partial pressure of carbon dioxide in arterial blood.
3. HCO_3: Plasma bicarbonate concentration.
4. Base excess.

Sputum examination. Sputum contains exfoliated cells and organisms that are being expelled from the lungs. Therefore examination of sputum can be a valuable component of the respiratory assessment. Sputum specimens can be examined with Gram stain, cultures, and culture sensitivity tests for the presence of various organisms and by cytological examination for the presence of malignancies.

VARIATIONS FROM HEALTH

Despite the heavy reliance on laboratory and x-ray findings in the diagnosis of respiratory problems, reasonably sound diagnostic probabilities can be derived by compiling and analyzing the physical assessment data. Table 15-6 outlines the usual assessment findings in a variety of common lung conditions.

DOCUMENTATION

Sample Documentation

Health history

This is a regular health-monitoring clinic visit for a 65-year-old black male with the chief complaint of low energy. Emphysema diagnosed 3 years ago. Is always short of breath, but has been worse for the past 2 days during the hot, humid days. Staying at home with fans, but apartment is not air conditioned. No chest pain, fever, or change in sputum production. Is unable to climb stairs without resting. Has difficulty walking on flat ground for one block. Uses oxygen at home at 2 L/min after meals, at night, and during physical exertion. Has moist cough several times daily that produces white or yellow sputum. When sputum is yellow, takes ampicillin as directed. Color of sputum has cleared after medication. Sputum has been white for the past several months. Smoked 2 to 3 packs of cigarettes a day for 50 years, but stopped 3 years ago when emphysema was diagnosed. Denies allergies and exposure to lung irritants. Denies TB, cancer, familial lung disease, allergies, heart disease, and renal disease.

Physical Assessment

Inspection: Respirations regular at 21 breaths/min. Respirations deep. Chest is barrel-shaped. Thorax moves symmetrically; no bulges or retractions.
Palpation: Trachea midline. Thoracic expansion symmetrical at 3 cm. No areas of bulging or tenderness. Percussion tones resonant and symmetric. Tactile fremitus decreased.
Percussion: Diagrammatical excursion 2 cm bilaterally. Percussion sounds hyperresonant throughout thorax.
Auscultation: Diminished vesicular breath sounds throughout peripheral lung. Expiration sometimes prolonged. Fine crackles and occasional ronchi noted throughout right and left lungs.
Note: Condition of thoracic skin would be assessed, but recording would be under the skin heading.

TABLE 15-6

Assessment Findings Frequently Associated with Common Lung Conditions

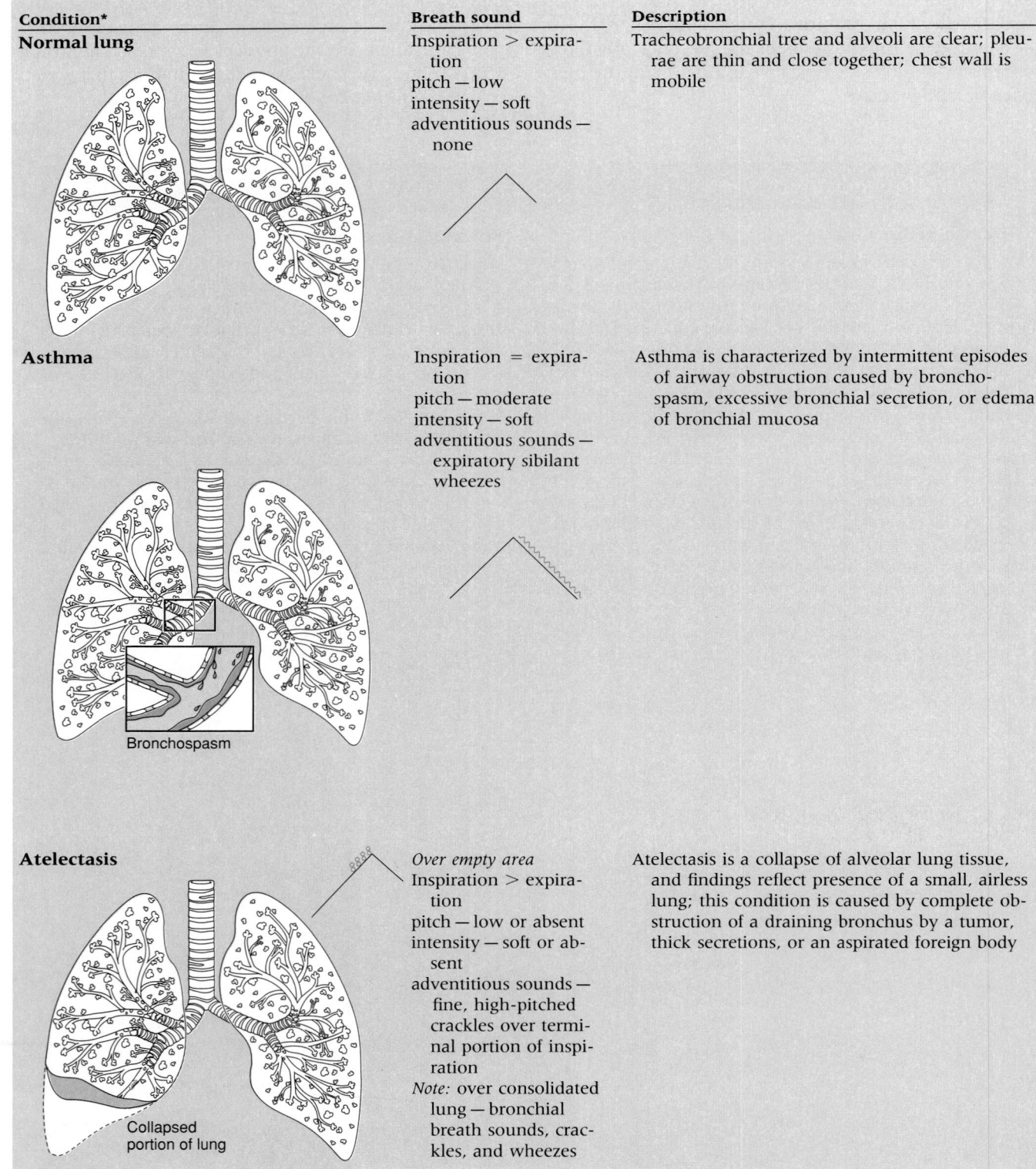

Condition*	Breath sound	Description
Normal lung	Inspiration > expiration pitch — low intensity — soft adventitious sounds — none	Tracheobronchial tree and alveoli are clear; pleurae are thin and close together; chest wall is mobile
Asthma	Inspiration = expiration pitch — moderate intensity — soft adventitious sounds — expiratory sibilant wheezes	Asthma is characterized by intermittent episodes of airway obstruction caused by bronchospasm, excessive bronchial secretion, or edema of bronchial mucosa
Atelectasis	*Over empty area* Inspiration > expiration pitch — low or absent intensity — soft or absent adventitious sounds — fine, high-pitched crackles over terminal portion of inspiration *Note:* over consolidated lung — bronchial breath sounds, crackles, and wheezes	Atelectasis is a collapse of alveolar lung tissue, and findings reflect presence of a small, airless lung; this condition is caused by complete obstruction of a draining bronchus by a tumor, thick secretions, or an aspirated foreign body

Bronchospasm

Collapsed portion of lung

*Although some disease conditions are bilateral, one diseased lung and one normal lung are illustrated for each condition to provide contrast. When an abnormality is illustrated, the pathological condition is illustrated on the left side and the normal lung is on the right side of the illustration.

Inspection	Palpation	Percussion	Auscultation
Good, symmetrical rib and diaphragmatic movement	Trachea — midline Expansion — adequate Tactile fremitus — moderate Diaphragmatic excursion — 3 to 5 cm	Resonant	Breath sounds — vesicular Vocal resonance — muffled Adventitious sounds — none, except for a few transient crackles at bases
Cyanosis Air trapping with audible wheezing Use of accessory muscles of respiration	Tactile fremitus — decreased	Hyperresonant	Breath sounds — distant Vocal resonance — decreased Adventitious sounds — wheezes
Less chest motion on affected side Affected side retracted, with ribs appearing close together Cough Rapid, shallow breathing	Trachea — shifted to affected side Expansion — decreased on affected side Tactile fremitus — decreased or absent	Dull to flat over collapsed lung Hyperresonant over remainder of affected hemithorax	Breath sounds — decreased or absent Vocal resonance — varies in intensity, usually reduced or absent on affected side Adventitious sounds — fine, high-pitched crackles may be heard over terminal portion of inspiration

Continued.

TABLE 15-6 — cont'd

Assessment Findings Frequently Associated with Common Lung Conditions

Condition*	Breath sound	Description
Bronchiectasis	Inspiration > expiration pitch — low intensity — soft adventitious sounds — crackles (sometimes disappear after coughing)	Bronchiectasis is abnormal dilation of bronchi or bronchioles or both
Dilated bronchi		
Bronchitis — acute	Inspiration > or = expiration pitch — low intensity — soft adventitious sounds — localized crackles, expiratory sibilant wheezes	Acute bronchitis is an inflammation of bronchial tree characterized by partial bronchial obstruction and secretions or constrictions; it results in abnormally deflated portions of lung
Bronchial inflammation and constriction		
Emphysema	Inspiration = expiration pitch — low to very low intensity — soft to very soft adventitious sounds — occasional sonorous and/or sibilant wheezes; fine inspiratory crackles	Emphysema is a permanent hyperinflation of lung beyond terminal bronchioles, with destruction of alveolar walls
Abnormally distended alveoli		

Inspection	Palpation	Percussion	Auscultation
If mild, respirations are normal If severe, tachypnea Less expansion of affected side Cough with purulent sputum	Trachea — midline or deviated toward affected side Expansion — decreased on affected side Tactile fremitus — increased	Resonant or dull	Breath sounds — usually vesicular Vocal resonance — usually muffled Adventitious sounds — crackles
If severe, tachypnea and cyanosis Rasping cough with mucoid sputum	Tactile fremitus — normal to increased	Resonant	Breath sounds — vesicular Vocal resonance — moderate Adventitious sounds — localized crackles, sibilant wheezes
Dyspnea with exertion Barrel chest Tachypnea Use of accessory muscles of respiration	Expansion — limited Tactile fremitus — decreased	Resonant to hyper-resonant Diaphragmatic excursion — decreased	Breath sounds — decreased intensity; often prolonged expiration Vocal resonance — muffled or decreased Adventitious sounds — occasional wheezes; often fine crackles in late inspiration

Continued.

TABLE 15-6 — cont'd

Assessment Findings Frequently Associated with Common Lung Conditions

Condition*	Breath sound	Description
Pleural effusion and thickening 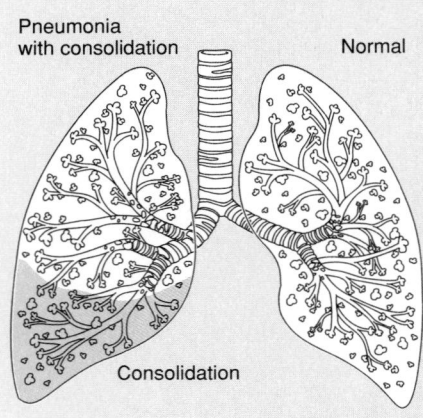	Inspiration > expiration pitch — low to absent intensity — soft to absent adventitious sounds — occasional pleural friction rub 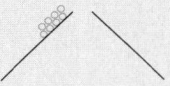	Pleural effusion is a collection of fluid in pleural space; if pleural effusion is prolonged, fibrous tissue may also accumulate in pleural space; clinical picture depends on amount of fluid or fibrosis present and rapidity of development; fluid tends to gravitate to most dependent areas of thorax, and adjacent lung is compressed
Pneumonia with consolidation	Inspiration = expiration pitch — high intensity — loud adventitious sounds — inspiratory crackles in terminal third of inspiration	Pneumonia with consolidation occurs when alveolar air is replaced by fluid or tissue; physical findings depend on amount of parenchymal tissue involved
Pneumothorax 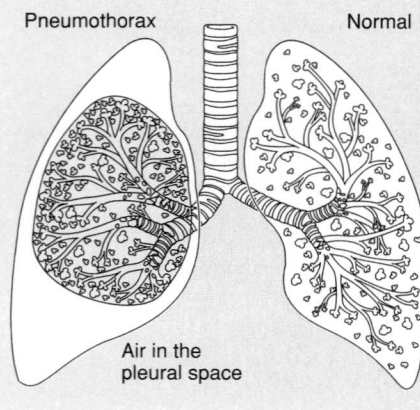	Inspiration > expiration pitch — low to absent intensity — soft to absent adventitious sounds — none 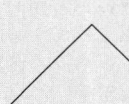	Pneumothorax implies air in pleural space There are three types of pneumothorax: (1) closed — air in pleural space does not communicate with air in lung; (2) open — air in pleural space freely communicates with air in lung; air in pleural space is atmospheric; and (3) tension — air in pleural space communicates with air in lungs only on inspiration; air pressure in pleural space is greater than atmospheric pressure Physical signs depend on the degree of lung collapse and presence or absence of pleural effusion

Labels in figures: Pleural effusion and thickening / Normal / Pleural effusion and thickening / Fluid in the pleural space / Pneumonia with consolidation / Normal / Consolidation / Pneumothorax / Normal / Air in the pleural space

Inspection	Palpation	Percussion	Auscultation
Tachypnea Decrease in definition of intercostal spaces on affected side	Trachea — deviation toward normal side Expansion — decreased on affected side Tactile fremitus — decreased or absent	Dull to flat	Breath sounds — decreased or absent Vocal resonance — muffled or absent; if fluid compresses lung, sounds may be bronchial over compression, and bronchophony, egophony, and whisper pectoriloquy may be present Adventitious sounds — pleural friction rub sometimes present
Tachypnea Guarding and less motion on affected side	Expansion — limited on affected side Tactile fremitus — usually increased, but may be weak if a bronchus leading to affected area is plugged	Dull to flat	Breath sounds — increased in intensity; bronchovesicular or bronchial breath sounds over affected area Vocal resonance — increased bronchophony, egophony, whisper pectoriloquy present Adventitious sounds — inspiratory crackles terminal third of inspiration
Restricted lung expansion If large, tachypnea Bulging in intercostal spaces on affected side Cyanosis	Trachea — deviated toward normal side Expansion — decreased on affected side Tactile fremitus — absent	Hyperresonant	Breath sounds — usually decreased or absent; if open pneumothorax, have an amorphous quality Vocal resonance — decreased or absent Adventitious sounds — none

Continued.

TABLE 15-6 — cont'd

Assessment Findings Frequently Associated with Common Lung Conditions

Condition*	Breath sound	Description
Pulmonary fibrosis — diffuse 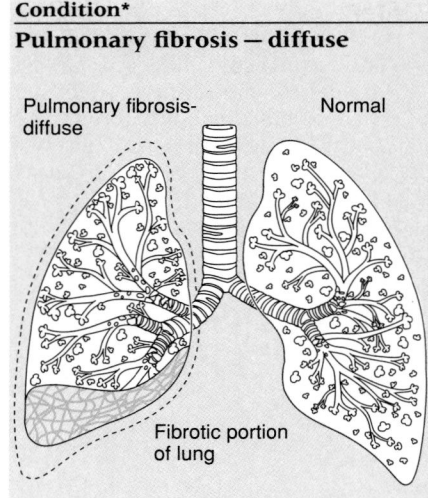	Inspiration = expiration pitch — low to absent intensity — soft to absent adventitious sounds — crackles	Pulmonary fibrosis is presence of an excessive amount of connective tissue in lungs; consequently, lungs are smaller than normal and less compliant; lower lobes are usually affected most

Nursing Diagnosis *THE NEXT STEP*

Nursing diagnoses that could apply to assessment and alterations in the respiratory system include, but are not limited to, the following:

ACTIVITY INTOLERANCE The state in which an individual has insufficient physiological or psychological energy to endure or complete required or desired daily activities.

Defining Characteristics

- Verbal report of fatigue or weakness
- Dyspnea
- Abnormal responses to activity (heart rate, blood pressure, or EKG changes reflecting ischemia or arrhythmias, pallor, cyanosis, vertigo, fatigue)
  Level I:
    Walk, regular pace, on level indefinitely; one flight or more but more short of breath than normally.
  Level II:
    Walk one city block 500 feet on level; climb one flight slowly without stopping.
  Level III:
    Walk no more than 50 feet on level without stopping; unable to climb one flight of stairs without stopping.
  Level IV:
    Dyspnea and fatigue at rest.

Related Factors

- Immobility
- Sedentary life-style
- Imbalance between oxygen supply and demand
- Generalized weakness

Inspection	Palpation	Percussion	Auscultation
Dyspnea on exertion Tachypnea Thoracic expansion diminished Cyanosis	Trachea — deviated to most affected side	Resonant to dull	Breath sounds — reduced or absent, bronchovesicular or bronchial Vocal resonance — increased, whisper pectoriloquy may be present Adventitious sounds — crackles on inspiration

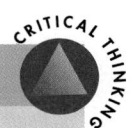

Nursing Diagnosis   *THE NEXT STEP—cont'd*

INEFFECTIVE AIRWAY CLEARANCE The state in which an individual is unable to clear secretions or obstructions from the respiratory tract to maintain airway patency.

Defining Characteristics

- Abnormal breath sounds (rales, crackles, rhonchi, wheezes)
- Cough (effective/ineffective, productive/nonproductive)
- Tachypnea
- Dyspnea (exertion/rest)
- Cyanosis
- Abnormal respiratory rate, rhythm, or depth
- Diaphoresis

Related Factors

- Excess thick secretions
- Decreased energy
- Fatigue
- Altered level of consciousness
- Pain
- Obstruction
- Tracheobronchial infection
- Trauma
- Perceptual/cognitive impairment

INEFFECTIVE BREATHING PATTERN The state in which an individual's inhalation and/or exhalation pattern does not enable adequate ventilation.

Defining Characteristics

- Dyspnea, shortness of breath
- Use of accessory muscles

Continued.

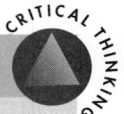

Nursing Diagnosis   *THE NEXT STEP—cont'd*

- Altered chest excursion
- Tachypnea
- Cough
- Nasal flaring
- Respiratory depth changes
- Pursed lip breathing/prolonged expiratory phase
- Increased anteroposterior diameter
- Fremitus
- Abnormal ABG's
- Cyanosis
- Orthopnic position

Related Factors

- Neuromuscular impairment
- Musculoskeletal impairment
- Perceptual/cognitive impairment
- Anxiety
- Decreased energy
- Fatigue
- Pain

IMPAIRED GAS EXCHANGE   Impaired gas exchange is the state in which an individual experiences an imbalance between oxygen uptake and carbon dioxide elimination at the alveolar-capillary membrane gas exchange areas.

Defining Characteristics

- Decreased hemoglobin saturation
- Increased Pco_2 Po_2 as determined by arterial blood gas testing
- Pursed lip breathing
- Tendency to assume three-point position
- Cyanosis
- Confusion
- Somnolence
- Hypoxia
- Restlessness
- Irritability
- Inability to move secretions
- Hypercapnia

Related Factors

- Ventilation-perfusion imbalance

VENTILATION, INABILITY TO SUSTAIN SPONTANEOUS   A state in which the response pattern of decreased energy reserves results in an individual's inability to maintain breathing adequate to support life.

Defining Characteristics

- **Major**
  Dyspnea
  Increased metabolic rate
- **Minor**
  Increased restlessness
  Apprehension
  Increased use of accessory muscles
  Decreased tidal volume
  Increased heart rate
  Decreased Po_2

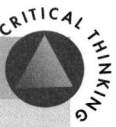

Nursing Diagnosis   *THE NEXT STEP—cont'd*

   Increased P_{CO_2} level
   Decreased cooperation
   Decreased S_{aO_2} level

Related Factors

- Metabolic factors
- Respiratory muscle fatigue

ANXIETY   A vague, uneasy feeling, the source of which is often nonspecific or unknown to the individual.

Defining Characteristics

- Subjective
  - Increased tension
  - Apprehension
  - Increased helplessness
  - Uncertainty
  - Fear
  - Feeling of being scared
  - Feeling of inadequacy
  - Shakiness
  - Fear of unspecific consequences
  - Regretfulness
  - Overexcitedness
  - Feeling of being rattled
  - Distress
  - Jitteriness
- Objective
  - Sympathetic stimulation—cardiovascular excitation, superficial vasoconstriction, pupil dilation
  - Restlessness
  - Insomnia
  - Glancing about
  - Poor eye contact
  - Trembling; hand tremors
  - Extraneous movements—foot shuffling; hand, arm movements
  - Expressed concern regarding changes in life events
  - Worry
  - Anxiety
  - Facial tension
  - Voice quivering
  - Focus on self
  - Increased wariness
  - Increased perspiration

Related Factors

- Unconscious conflict about essential values and goals of life
- Threat to self-concept
- Threat of death
- Threat to or change in health status
- Threat to or change in socioeconomic status
- Threat to or change in role functioning
- Threat to or change in environment
- Threat to or change in interaction patterns
- Situational and maturational crises
- Interpersonal transmission and contagion
- Unmet needs

Continued.

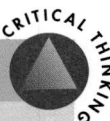

Nursing Diagnosis   *THE NEXT STEP—cont'd*

Clinical Application

Mr. M. is a 65-year-old, thin white male, retired mailman. His chief complaint is "increasing short-ness of breath and fatigue in the last month or so. I used to be able to walk 2 or 3 blocks without any difficulty." Unable to climb 1 flight of stairs or walk greater than 2 blocks without resting. Has 2 pillow orthopnea. Wakes 1-2 times during the night. Morning cough productive of 1 to 2 table-spoons thin white sputum. No complaints of chest pain, night sweats, hemoptysis. Denies allergies, TB, cancer, familial lung diseases, heart disease, or renal disease. Smoked 2 packs of cigarettes a day for 45 years.

SUBJECTIVE DATA: Patient complains of:
Shortness of breath
Fatigue
Unable to walk 2 blocks without resting
Unable to climb 1 flight of stairs without resting
Unable to sleep without 2 pillows
Waking up 1 or 2 times each night with shortness of breath
Morning cough

OBJECTIVE DATA:
Inspection: respirations resting 24 breaths/min; with exercise 30 breaths/min
Respirations shallow with prolonged expirations
Increased use of accessory muscles
Thorax movement symmetrical; no bulges or retractions
Palpation: Trachea midline. Minimal but symmetrical thorax expansion
No areas of bulging or tenderness
Tactile fremitus decreases.
Percussion: Diaphragmatical excursion is 1 cm bilaterally
Percussion sounds hyperresonant throughout thorax
Auscultation: Diminished vesicular breath sounds throughout all lung fields
Fine crackles noted throughout all lung fields
Arterial blood gases (ABG) reveal: pH 7.38 PaO_2 75, $PaCO_2$ 50 HCO_3 45
Patient diagnosis of emphysema.

NURSING DIAGNOSIS

Activity intolerance related to imbalances between oxygen supply and demand.

Defining Characteristics

- Patient complains of shortness of breath walking > 2 blocks or 1 flight of stairs
- Sleep orthopnea
- ABG at rest slight hypoxemia PaO_2 75

Ineffective breathing pattern related to decreased lung expansion.

Defining Characteristics

- Dyspnea on exertion
- Tachypnea with activity
- Tactile fremitus decreased
- Prolonged expiratory phase
- Increasing anteroposterior diameter
- Use of accessory muscles
- Altered chest excursion

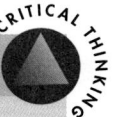

Nursing Diagnosis *THE NEXT STEP—cont'd*

Ineffective airway clearance related to tracheobronchial restriction.

Defining Characteristics

- Abnormal breath sounds—crackles throughout all lung fields
- Shallow frequent respiration
- Tachypnea especially with exercise
- Dyspnea

Impaired gas exchange related to alveolar-capillary membrane changes.

Defining Characteristics

- Hypoxemia Pao_2 on room air 75
- Hypercapnia $Paco_2$ on room air 50

Anxiety related to change in health status

Defining Characteristics

- Restlessness
- Insomnia
- Expressed concern regarding changes in life events

GLOSSARY

alveoli Small, thin-walled sacs through which gas exchange takes place between alveolar air and pulmonary capillary blood.

apnea Cessation of breathing in the end expiratory position.

asthma Paroxysmal dyspnea (wheezing) resulting from obstruction of the bronchi or spasm of smooth muscle.

atelectasis Incomplete expansion of a lung compromised since birth; collapse of the adult lung.

bradypnea Abnormally slow rate of breathing.

bronchiectasis Chronic dilation of one or more bronchi.

bronchioles Small airways of the respiratory system extending from the bronchi into the lobes of the lungs.

bronchitis Inflammation of one or more bronchi; condition may be chronic or acute.

bronchophony Sound of the voice as heard with abnormally increased clarity and intensity through the stethoscope over the lung parenchyma in an area of consolidation.

bronchovesicular Related to breath sounds from bronchial tubes and alveoli.

chronic obstructive pulmonary disease General term for disease involving airway obstruction, such as chronic bronchitis, emphysema, or asthma.

ciliary movement Waving motion of the hairlike processes projecting from the epithelium of the respiratory tract.

consolidation Process in which liquid or solid replacement of lung parenchyma as exudate from an inflammatory condition is amassed.

crackles Discrete, noncontinuous sound resembling fine crackling, radio static, or hairs being rubbed together as heard through a stethoscope; generally produced by air bubbling through an exudate.

crepitation Dry, crackling sound in (1) the lung, when air passes through abnormally accumulated moisture; (2) the joints, when dry synovial surfaces rub together; and (3) the skin, when air is present subdermally. Also called crepitus.

dyspnea Difficult or labored respiration; shortness of breath.

egophony Voice sound of a nasal or bleating quality as heard through a stethoscope; often defined by asking the client to say "ee," which sounds like "ay" in an area of consolidation.

emphysema Condition involving entrapment of air within tissue, either interstitial or pulmonary. *Pulmonary emphysema*, or chronic obstructive pulmonary disease, results from permanent dilation or enlargement of the passages peripheral to the terminal bronchiole, which causes increased resistance to airflow. *Interstitial emphysema* is the presence of air in the subcutaneous tissue mediastinum or connective tissue of the lung resulting from air leakage through a damaged portion of the respiratory passages or alveoli; may result in swelling of tissue or a distinctive crackling sound called crepitation.

fremitus Palpable vibration.

friction rub Crackling, grating sound as heard through a stethoscope when two inflamed, roughened surfaces rub together.

hyperpnea Increased depth of respiration with or without an increase in rate.

hyperventilation Increase in rate and depth of respiration.

intercostal space Space between two ribs.

Kussmaul respiration Rapid and deep respiratory cycles resulting from stimulation of the medullary respiratory center in metabolic acidosis; associated with pH less than 7.2 in diabetic ketoacidosis.

mediate (indirect) percussion Middle finger of one hand is used to strike the middle finger of the other hand to emit a sound or vibration.

orthopnea Dyspnea that begins or increases when client lies down.

parenchyma Tissue of an organ as distinguished from supporting or connective tissue.

paroxysmal nocturnal dyspnea Sudden onset of dyspnea after a period of lying down. Sitting upright helps relieve the dyspnea.

percussion Technique used to evaluate the size, borders, and consistency of certain internal organs and to determine the presence of and evaluate the amount of air and fluid in a body cavity.

platypnea Respiratory distress that increases when a person is upright.

pleural effusion Fluid of any kind in the pleural cavity.

pleurisy Pleural inflammation accompanied by pain.

rhonchus Wheezing or snoring sound produced by airflow across a partially constricted air passage. *Sibilant rhonchus:* High-pitched wheeze produced in a small air passage. *Sonorous rhonchus:* Low-pitched wheeze produced in a large air passage.

symmetry Similarity in size, shape, and position of body parts on both sides of the body.

tachypnea Rapid respiratory rate.

tympany Drumlike note produced by percussion done over an air-filled region.

wheeze Form of rhonchus characterized by a high-pitched musical quality. Caused by a high-velocity flow of air through a narrowed airway, it is heard during both inspiration and expiration.

whispered pectoriloquy Increased resonance of the whispered voice as heard through a stethoscope in an area of consolidation.

xiphoid Lowest portion of the sternum; composed of bone and cartilage.

BIBLIOGRAPHY

Burton GG, Hodgkin JE, Ward JJ: *Respiratory care: a guide to clinical practice*, ed 3, Philadelphia, 1991, JB Lippincott.

Dettenmeier PA: *Pulmonary nursing care*, St Louis, 1992, Mosby−Year Book.

Forster II and others: *The lung: physiologic basis of pulmonary function tests*, ed 3, Chicago, 1986, Mosby−Year Book.

George RB and others: *Chest medicine: essentials of pulmonary and critical care medicine*, Baltimore, 1990, Williams & Wilkins.

Gordon M: *Manual of nursing diagnosis 1993-1994*, St Louis, 1993, Mosby−Year Book.

Gordon M: *Nursing diagnosis: process and application*, ed 2, New York, 1987, McGraw-Hill.

Loudon RG: The lung exam, *Clin Chest Med* 8:265-2721987.

Martin L: *Pulmonary physiology in clinical practice: the essentials for patient care and evaluation*, St. Louis, 1987, Mosby−Year Book.

Mitchell RS, Petty TL, Schwarz MI: *Synopsis of clinical pulmonary disease*, ed 4, St Louis, 1989, Mosby−Year Book.

Mosby's medical, nursing, and allied health dictionary, ed 3, St Louis, 1990, Mosby−Year Book.

Nunn JF: *Applied respiratory physiology*, ed 3, London, 1987, Butterworth.

Op't Holt TB: *Assessment based respiratory care*, New York, 1986, John Wiley.

Pagana KD, Pagana TJ: *Mosby's diagnostic and laboratory test reference*, St Louis, 1992, Mosby−Year Book.

US Preventive Services Task Force: *Guide to clinical preventive services: an assessment of the effectiveness of 169 interventions*, Baltimore, 1989, Williams & Wilkins.

Weinberger SE: *Principles of pulmonary medicine*, ed 2, Philadelphia, 1992, WB Saunders.

Wilkins RL Hodgkin JE, Lopez B: *Lung sounds: practical guide*, St Louis, 1988, Mosby−Year Book.

Wilkins RL, Sheldon RL, Krider SJ: *Clinical assessment in respiratory care*, ed 2, St Louis, 1990, Mosby−Year Book.

CHAPTER 16

Cardiovascular System

Outline

PURPOSE OF THE EXAMINATION

The purpose of the examination of the cardiovascular system is to assess the function of the heart, the carotid arteries and jugular veins in the neck, and the peripheral vessels, including both arteries and veins. The heart, including its system of chambers and valves, is assessed for its effectiveness as a pump. The vessels closest to the heart that are accessible to clinical examination are the carotid arteries and the jugular veins. These vessels are assessed for local health status and cardiac function. The peripheral vessels are examined for their effectiveness in transporting blood and its nutrients and waste products to and from the tissues of the body.

ANATOMY AND PHYSIOLOGY

The cardiovascular system is composed of the heart and an extensive system of blood vessels. The heart is a muscular pump that circulates the blood continuously throughout two major loops: the systemic loop and the pulmonary loop. The systemic loop includes the cir-culation of blood to and from the entire body except for the lungs. The pulmonary loop involves circulation of blood to and from the lungs.

The area of the chest that overlies the heart and the great vessels is called the **precordium.** In the anatomical description of the heart and the major vessels and in subsequent examination and description of findings, several anterior chest wall landmarks (Figure 16-1) are important, including the following:

Midsternal line (MSL)
Midclavicular line (MCL)
Anterior, middle, and posterior axillary lines (AAL, MAL, PAL)
Suprasternal notch
Ribs and intercostal spaces (spaces between ribs) (ICS)

The heart occupies the space from the second to the fifth intercostal space and from the right edge of the sternum to the left midclavicular line. The following description of the cardiovascular system is divided into these components: (1) heart and great vessels; (2) neck vessels; and (3) peripheral vessels.

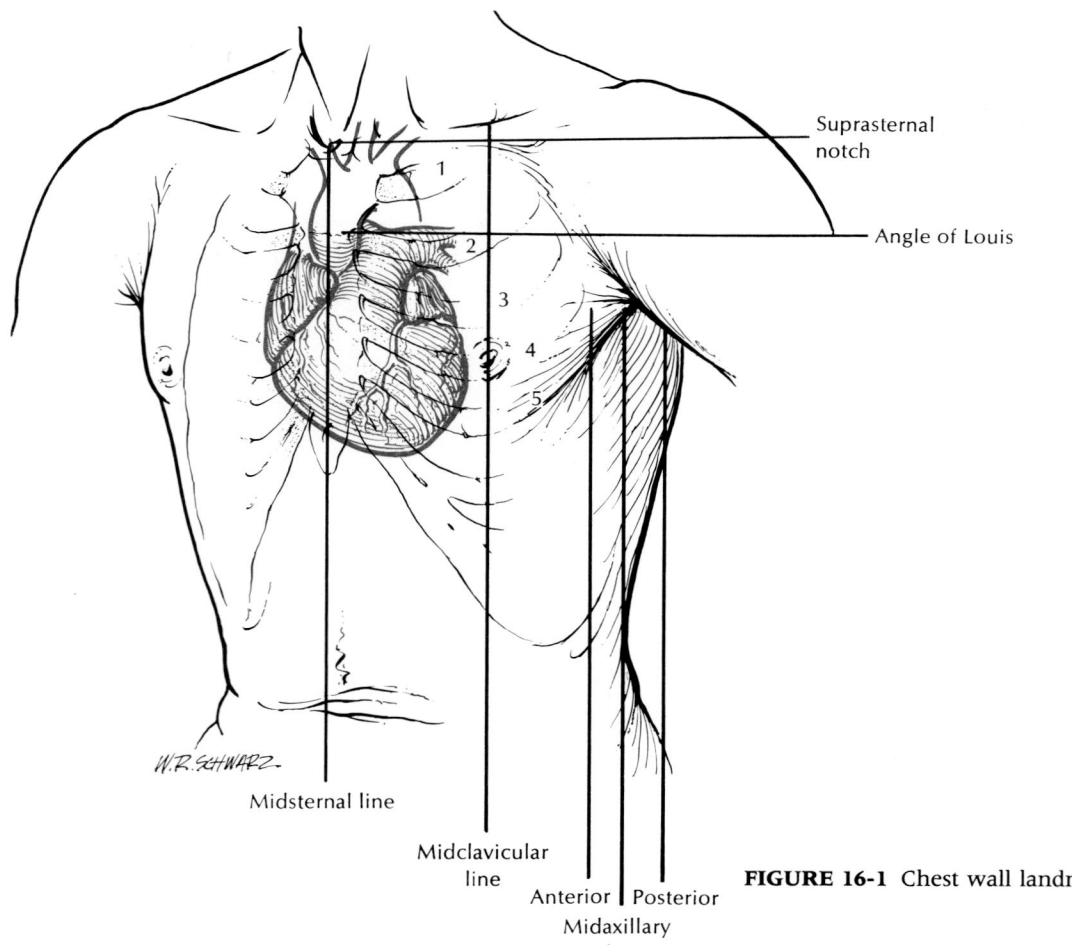

Suprasternal notch

Angle of Louis

Midsternal line

Midclavicular line

Anterior | Posterior
Midaxillary lines

W.R. SCHWARZ

FIGURE 16-1 Chest wall landmarks.

Heart and Great Vessels

The heart is a pump composed of four chambers. It lies in the thoracic cavity behind the sternum and between the lungs within an area called the **mediastinum.** Of the four chambers, two are **atria,** which receive blood from the body and the lungs, and two are **ventricles,** which pump blood out to the body and the lungs. The upper portion of the heart, consisting of both atria, lies behind the upper portion of the sternum. The lower portion of the heart, composed of both ventricles, is directed downward and toward the left.

The shape of the heart is somewhat like an inverted triangle. The upper portion is wider and forms the base of the heart. The lower left portion, the apex, is narrower. The great vessels, including the aorta, the vena cava, and the pulmonary arteries and veins, are located around the base, or upper portion, of the heart (Figure 16-2).

Heart wall. The heart wall has three main layers: *pericardium, myocardium,* and *endocardium.* The **pericardium** is a tough fibrous sac that surrounds the heart and the roots of the great vessels. A small amount of pericardial fluid surrounds the pericardium, permitting smooth, low-friction movement of the heart. The **myocardium** is the muscular wall that forms the bulk of the heart. This layer is the contractile tissue that pumps the blood. The **endocardium** is the thin layer of epithelial tissue that lines the inner surfaces of the heart.

Heart chambers. As previously noted, the heart is composed of four chambers (see Figure 16-2). The two atria receive blood from the body and the lungs, and the two ventricles pump blood out to the body and the lungs. Within the mediastinum, the heart is rotated so that the right ventricle composes most of the anterior surface and the left ventricle forms most of the posterior aspect. The right ventricle lies behind the sternum and extends to the left of it. The left ventricle is located posterior to the right ventricle and extends farther to the left, forming the left anterior border of the heart and making up a small portion of the anterior cardiac surface. The right atrium lies slightly above and to the right of the right ventricle, and the left atrium occupies a posterior portion of the heart. The contraction and thrust of the left ventricle during ventricular **systole** produces the **apical impulse.**

Heart valves (Figure 16-3, *A*). Valves located between the atria and the ventricles and between the ventricles and the great vessels prevent the backflow of blood during its circulatory journey. The closure of these valves produces the normal heart sounds. The atria and the ventricles are separated by the **atrioventricular (AV) valves.** The ventricles are separated from the great vessels by the **semilunar valves.**

The right AV valve is the **tricuspid valve.** The left AV valve is the bicuspid valve, or **mitral valve.** During ventricular systole, the cusps of these two valves meet and close to form a seal so that no blood regurgitates into the atria. The valve cusps are anchored by the *chordae tendineae* (strands of tendon) to the papillary muscles, which are attached to the ventricles. The chordae tendineae prevent prolapse of the AV valves into the atria during ventricular contraction.

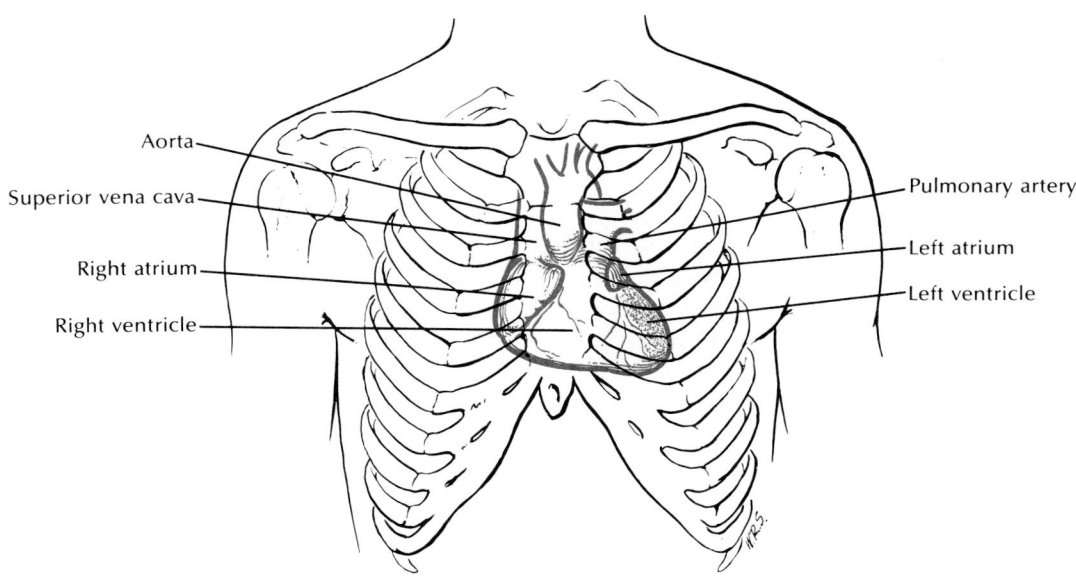

Aorta

Superior vena cava

Right atrium

Right ventricle

Pulmonary artery

Left atrium

Left ventricle

FIGURE 16-2 Position of the heart and great vessels.

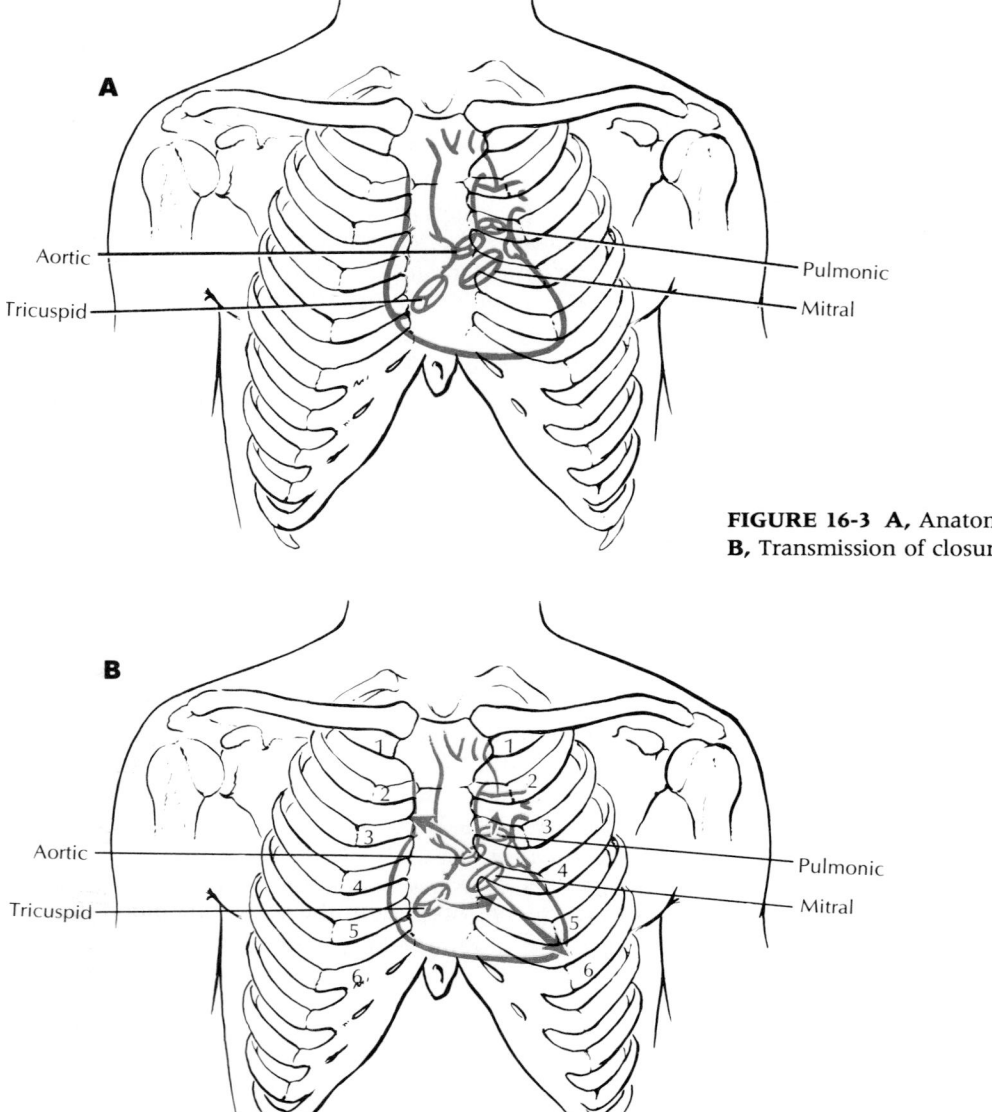

FIGURE 16-3 A, Anatomical location of the heart valves. **B,** Transmission of closure sounds from the heart valves.

The semilunar valves are located between the ventricles and the great arteries. On the right, the **pulmonic valve** separates the right ventricle from the pulmonary artery. On the left, the **aortic valve** separates the left ventricle from the aorta. During ventricular systole, these valves open to permit flow of the blood out from the heart. During ventricular **diastole,** when the ventricles are filling with blood, these valves are closed.

Transmission of sound from heart valves (Figure 16-3, *B*). Although the four heart valves are located close to one another in a small area behind the sternum, the areas on the chest wall where their closure sound is most audible are not located directly over the valves but rather in the direction of the flow of blood. The following list describes where the sound produced by the closure of each valve can normally be heard best:

Valve	Area where closure sound is heard best
Mitral	Apex, fifth left intercostal space at midclavicular line
Tricuspid	Left sternal border at fourth left intercostal space
Pulmonic	Second left intercostal space at sternal border
Aortic	Second right intercostal space at sternal border

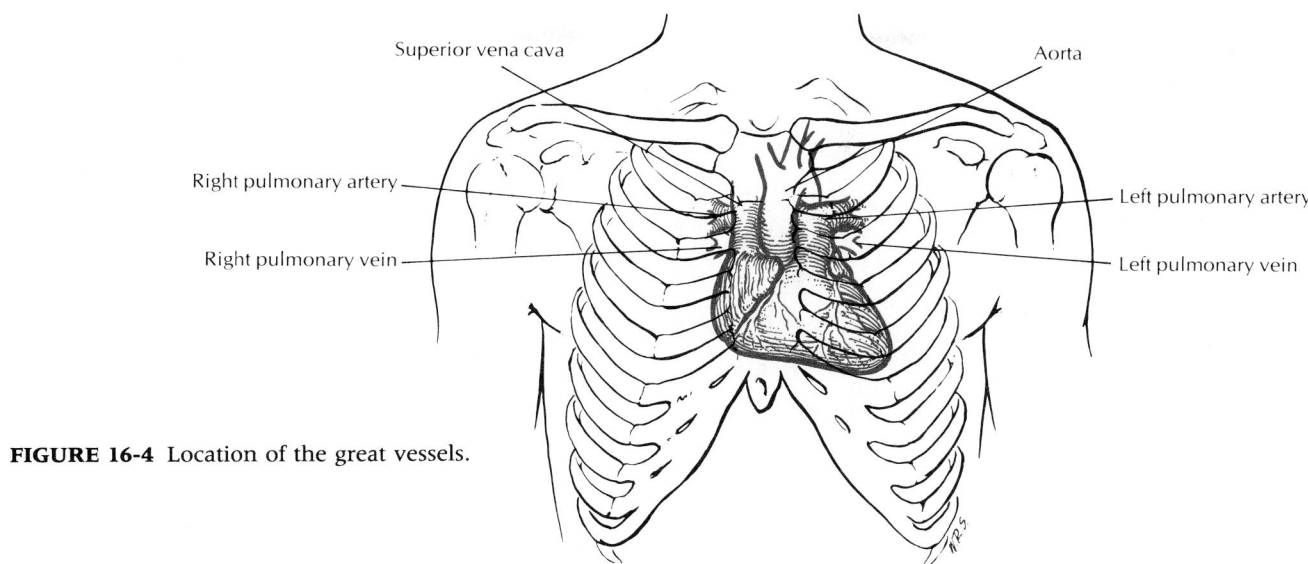

Superior vena cava

Aorta

Right pulmonary artery

Left pulmonary artery

Right pulmonary vein

Left pulmonary vein

FIGURE 16-4 Location of the great vessels.

Great vessels (Figure 16-4). The great vessels lie in a cluster at the top (base) of the heart. The superior and inferior vena cavae return unoxygenated blood from the body to the right atrium. The pulmonary artery leaves the right ventricle, bifurcates almost immediately, and carries the unoxygenated blood from the right ventricle to both lungs. The pulmonary veins return the oxygenated blood from the lungs to the left atrium. The aorta receives the blood from the left ventricle and carries it to the body. The aorta ascends from the left ventricle, arches back at the level of the sternal angle, and descends behind the heart. Several major arteries branch off along the aortic arch.

Variable position of heart. The position of the heart varies considerably, according to body build, chest configuration, and diaphragm level. In persons of average build, the heart lies obliquely: one third of it lies to the right of the midsternal line, and two thirds is found to the left of this line. In short, stocky persons, the heart is usually positioned more horizontally. In tall, slender individuals, it is placed more vertically. In the rare condition of **dextrocardia,** the position of the heart is reversed and the apex is on the right side of the chest.

Blood circulation (Figure 16-5). When blood is ejected from the ventricles, it flows through two circulatory systems: pulmonary and systemic. Blood returning from circulation throughout the body (systemic circulation) passes through the superior and inferior vena cavae and enters the heart at the right atrium. From there, it crosses the tricuspid valve and enters the right ventricle. When the right ventricle contracts, the blood

flows over the pulmonic valve and enters the pulmonary artery. The pulmonary circulation carries blood to the lungs, where it releases carbon dioxide and is reoxygenated. The blood returns to the heart through the pulmonary veins and enters the left atrium. From there, it flows across the mitral valve and into the left ventricle. When the left ventricle contracts, the blood crosses the aortic valve and enters the aorta. The arterial system carries the blood throughout the body. The blood then returns through the venous vasculature to the superior and inferior vena cavae and to the right atrium.

Cardiac cycle. The heart contracts and relaxes rhythmically, permitting it to fill and then to eject blood. The cardiac cycle begins with the return of blood from the upper and lower body by way of the superior and inferior vena cavae to the right atrium. Following ventricular systole, during which blood is ejected from the ventricles, the AV valves open, allowing blood that has collected in the atria to flow into the ventricles. This period is ventricular diastole, a passive filling phase during which blood flows past the AV valves from the atria into the ventricles (Figure 16-6). Toward the end of ventricular diastole, the atria contract, ejecting the blood that remains in them into the ventricles. At this point the ventricles are full of blood, and ventricular contraction begins. This phase is ventricular systole (Figure 16-7). As the intraventricular pressure increases, the AV valves are forced closed, preventing regurgitation of blood into the atria. The closure of the AV valves (mitral and tricuspid) produces the first heart sound, S_1. During the early part of contraction, the volume of blood in the ventricle remains the same. This

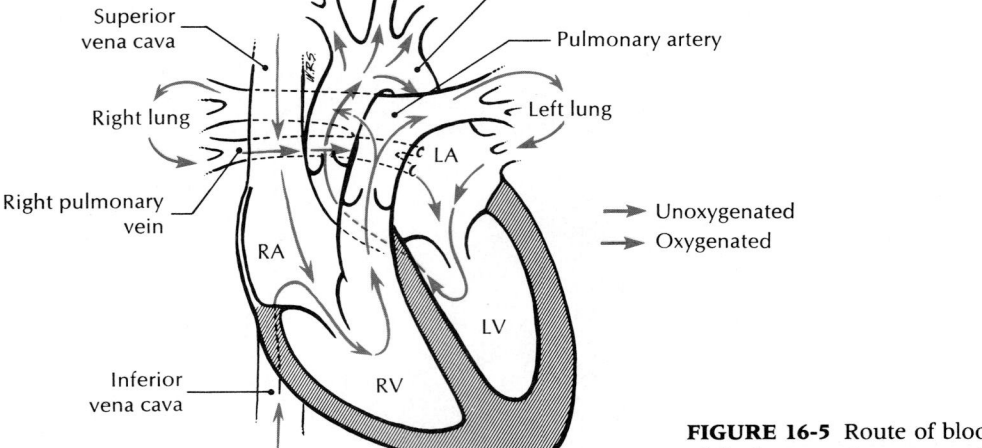

FIGURE 16-5 Route of blood flow through the chambers of the heart and great vessels.

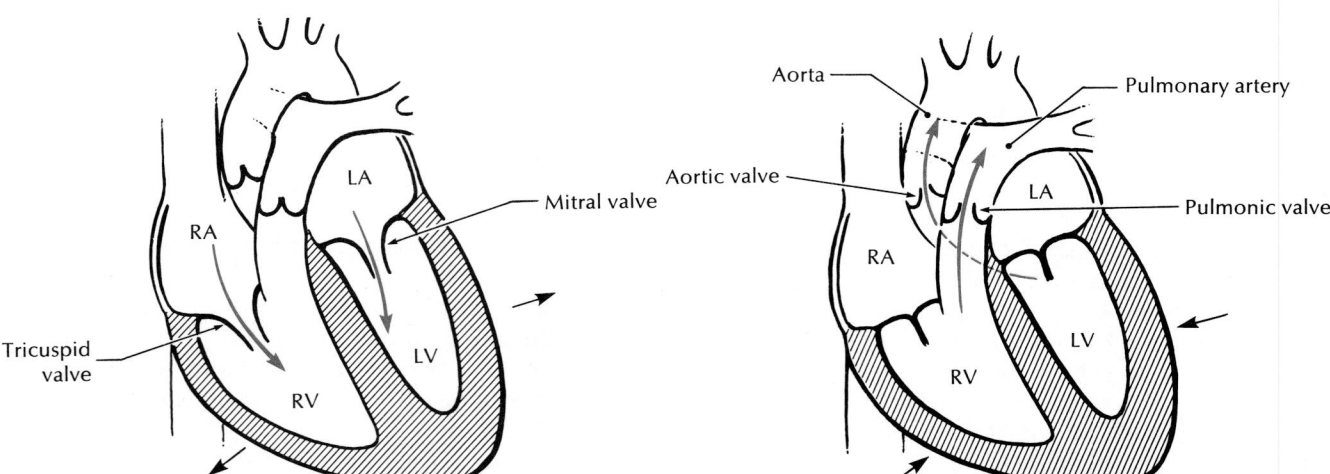

FIGURE 16-6 Ventricular diastole. The ventricles relax and the mitral and tricuspid valves open, allowing blood to flow from the atria to the ventricles.

FIGURE 16-7 Ventricular systole. The ventricles contract, forcing the aortic and pulmonic valves to open; blood flows into the aorta and the pulmonary artery.

phase is called the period of isovolumic (same volume) contraction.

As the pressure continues to rise during ventricular contraction, a point is reached when the pressure in the left ventricle exceeds the pressure in the aorta. The semilunar valves between the ventricles and the great arteries are forced open, and blood is ejected from the left ventricle into the aorta and from the right ventricle into the pulmonary artery. At the end of ventricular systole, the ventricles relax. The pressure in the ventricle drops below the pressure in the aorta and pulmonary artery, and the semilunar valves close, producing the second heart sound, S_2. The two components of S_2 are the aortic second sound (A_2) and the pulmonary second sound (P_2). A_2 is produced by aortic valve closure, and P_2 results from pulmonic valve closure.

In summary, both normal heart sounds are produced by valve closure: S_1 by closure of the AV valves, and S_2 by closure of the semilunar valves. The opening of the valves is normally silent.

During the time that the ventricles are contracting, the atria are filling with blood returning from the body and lungs. As the ventricles relax, ventricular pressure drops. The AV valves open, once again permitting the flow of blood into the ventricles. Atrial emptying and ventricular filling occur simultaneously, and atrial filling and ventricular systole take place simultaneously.

The relationships of the left ventricular pressure curve, the heart sounds, and the electrocardiogram (ECG) are illustrated in Figure 16-8.

Electrical stimulation of heart. Electrical discharges stimulate and coordinate the mechanical events just described. An electrical impulse activates each cardiac cycle (Figure 16-9). The electrical discharge originates at the sinoatrial (SA) node located in the right atrium. This electrical impulse flows through the atria, producing atrial contraction. The impulse travels to the AV node, located in the atrial septum. It proceeds through the bundle of His and its branches and then reaches the Purkinje fibers in the ventricular myocardium, thus stimulating ventricular contraction. The SA node is the cardiac pacemaker. It normally discharges between 60 and 100 electrical impulses per minute.

The passage of the electrical impulse as traced by the ECG is illustrated in Figure 16-10. The relationship of each segment of the ECG to the cardiac cycle is as follows:

ECG segment	Correlating component of cardiac cycle
P wave	Spread of impulse through atria (atrial depolarization)
PR interval	Passage of impulse from SA node, through atria and AV node, to ventricles; time from initial stimulation of atria to initial stimulation of ventricles
QRS complex	Spread of impulse through ventricles (ventricular depolarization)
ST segment and T wave	Ventricular muscle returns to resting state (ventricular repolarization)

The electrical stimulation briefly precedes the mechanical response of the myocardium. Because of the pattern in which cardiac depolarization occurs, events on the left side of the heart normally take place slightly before those on the right side of the heart. Therefore, in the production of S_1, mitral valve closure briefly precedes tricuspid valve closure. Similarly, in the production of S_2, aortic valve closure precedes pulmonic valve

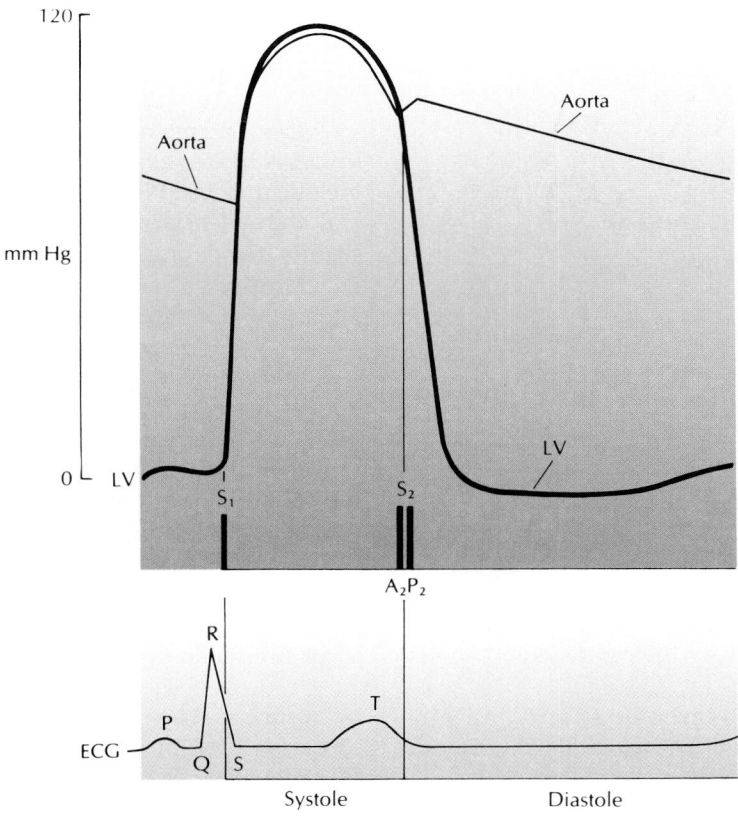

FIGURE 16-8 Pressure curves of the left ventricle and aorta, S_1 and S_2, and the ECG.

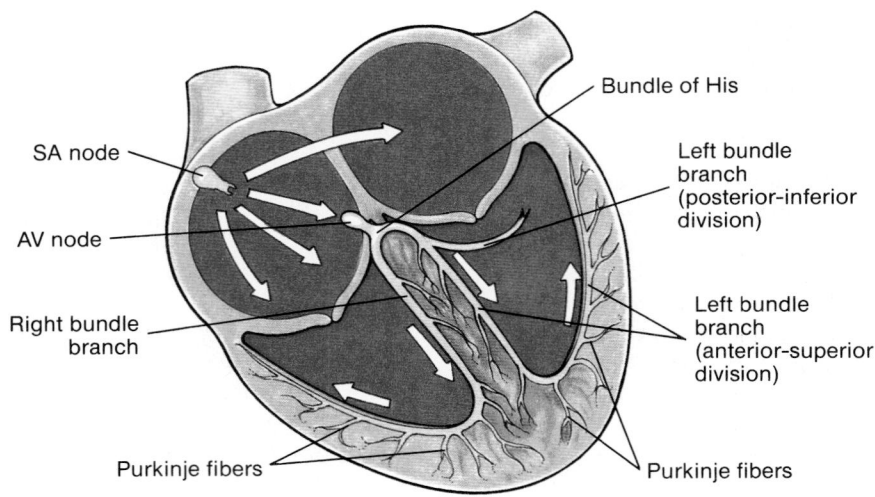

FIGURE 16-9 Cardiac electrical conduction. (From Canobbio MM: *Cardiovascular disorders, Mosby's clinical nursing series,* vol 1, St Louis, 1990, Mosby–Year Book.)

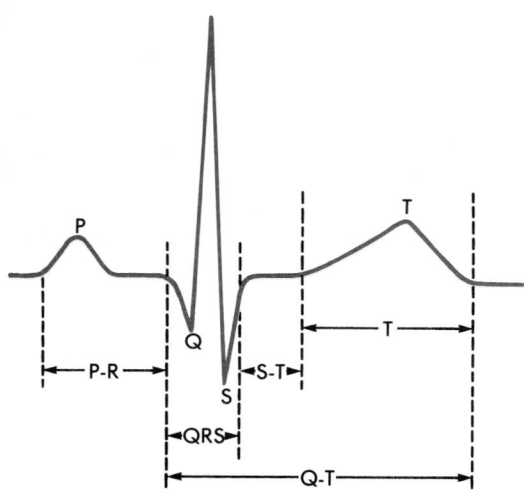

FIGURE 16-10 Normal ECG waveform. (From Berne RM, Levy MN: *Physiology,* ed 3, St Louis, 1993, Mosby–Year Book.)

> **Helpful Hint:** *All cardiovascular sounds are quiet and of relatively low pitch. A quiet room and focused concentration are essential as you begin to listen to these sounds.*

closure. The amount of pressure is also different on the two sides of the heart. Pressures are higher on the left side of the heart and lower on the right side.

Characteristics of cardiovascular sound.
All cardiovascular sounds have the following characteristics:
- Pitch (frequency)
- Loudness (intensity)
- Duration
- Timing in cardiac cycle

Pitch. The pitch is the frequency or tone at which a sound is heard. Examples of heart sounds of low pitch include the diastolic murmur of **mitral valve stenosis** and a **third heart sound (S_3).** The normal S_2 is of a slightly higher pitch, and the diastolic murmur of aortic or pulmonic valve **insufficiency** is of an even higher pitch.

Loudness. The loudness of cardiovascular sounds is widely variable. The range extends from quiet sounds, which can be heard only with great concentration, to louder sounds, which can be heard when the edge of the stethoscope is barely touching the chest wall. The loudness of the sound is modified by the amount of tissue and/or space that lies between the sound at its point of origin and the outer chest wall. The heart sounds seem diminished and distant in the client who is very muscular or overweight or who has emphysema.

Duration. The duration of most cardiovascular sounds is very brief, usually much less than 1 second. In cardiac auscultation, both the duration of sounds and the periods of silence are important. Normally, S_1 and S_2 are very brief, lasting only a fraction of a second. The intervals of silence, systole and diastole, are longer than the normal heart sounds. Diastole is longer than systole at a heart rate less than 120 beats/min. At faster rates, the duration of diastole is diminished, and systole and diastole become approximately equal in duration.

Timing. The timing of any additional cardiac sounds is designated as occurring during either systole or diastole. Systole lasts from S_1 to S_2; diastole lasts from S_2 to S_1. Cardiac sounds that take place during systole include systolic murmurs and **ejection clicks.** Cardiac sounds that occur during diastole include diastolic murmurs and the mitral valve opening snap (see discussion in variations from health.)

Illustration of heart sounds. Heart sounds are illustrated by vertical bars. The height of the bar indicates the relative loudness of the sound, and the width of the bar represents the duration of the sound. For example, S_1 and S_2, as heard at the base and the apex of the heart, are illustrated in Figure 16-11. S_2 is louder at the base and therefore has the longer vertical line. S_1 is quieter at the base and has the shorter vertical line. The situation is reversed at the apex. Here S_2 is normally quieter and has the shorter vertical line. S_1 is louder and has the longer vertical line.

Neck Vessels

Carotid arteries. The carotid arteries lie in the neck close to the heart (Figure 16-12). They are located in the groove between the trachea and the sternocleidomastoid muscle, just lateral to the trachea and medial to the sternocleidomastoid muscle. The **pulse** wave in the carotid artery results from the ventricular systole, which sends a pulse wave throughout the arterial system. Because of their close proximity to the heart, the carotid arteries are the easiest to palpate, and the carotid pulse wave is sometimes visible.

The normal carotid pulse consists of a single positive wave followed by a **dicrotic notch** (Figure 16-13). The curve of the wave is a reflection of left ventricular

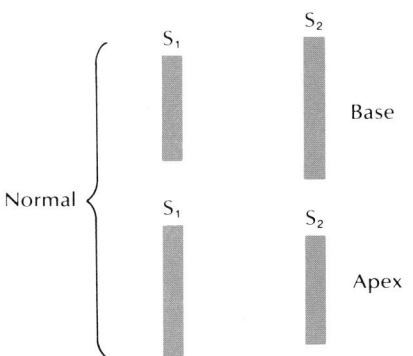

FIGURE 16-11 Relative loudness of S_1 and S_2 as heard over the base and the apex of the heart.

activity. The upstroke is smooth and rapid, the summit is dome-shaped, and the downstroke is less steep than the upstroke. The peak occurs just after the first heart sound. The size and amplitude of the carotid pulse, as with all the peripheral pulses, are determined by a variety of factors, including left ventricular stroke volume and ejection rate, peripheral resistance, vessel distensibility, and pulse pressure.

Jugular veins. The two sets of jugular veins are the internal jugulars and the external jugulars (see Figure 16-16). Blood from both sets of these veins flows directly into the superior vena cava: no valves separate the superior vena cava from the right atrium. The jugular veins reflect activity on the right side of the heart and provide an indication of the competency of right-side heart function. They reflect changes in right atrial volume and filling pressure.

The external jugular veins lie superficially and are visible bilaterally above the clavicle, close to the insertion of the sternocleidomastoid muscles. In the middle and lower neck, the internal jugular veins are located beneath the sternocleidomastoid muscle, lateral to the carotid artery. They are less accessible to inspection, but reflection of their activity may be visible on the overlying skin of the lower neck.

The external jugular veins are smaller, more discrete, more superficial, and located more laterally, than the internal jugular veins. Because of their superficial location, the external veins are often easier to see and may be particularly prominent in patients who have chronic elevation of venous pressure.

Jugular venous pulse (Figure 16-14). Venous pulsations are low-pressure impulses or waves that reflect the cardiac activity of the right atrium. Normal jugular venous pulsations are the result of a series of interruptions in the returning flow of venous blood to the right atrium. These interruptions are the contractions and relaxations of the atria and the ventricles. Because the return flow is interrupted, there is a temporary increase in the volume of blood in the veins. The normal jugular venous pulsation consists of two major upward waves and two descent slopes. The upward waves are the a and v waves. The c wave follows the a wave as the downward x slope begins. The two downward slopes are the x and y descents. The x descent follows the a and c waves, and the y descent follows the v wave. The a wave is larger than the v wave, and the x descent is more prominent than the y descent.

The a wave is the highest part of the total pulse wave. It results from a brief backflow of blood to the vena cava during right atrial contraction. It peaks just before the first heart sound.

The c wave is partly caused by transmitted carotid

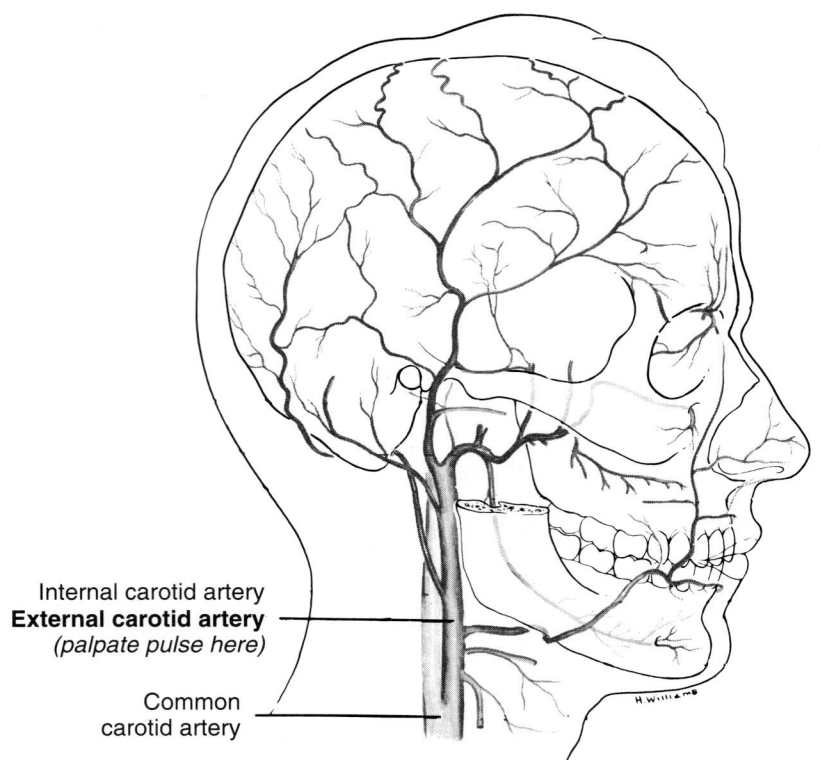

FIGURE 16-12 Carotid artery. (Modified from Francis CC, Martin AH: *Introduction to human anatomy*, ed 7, St Louis, 1975, Mosby—Year Book.)

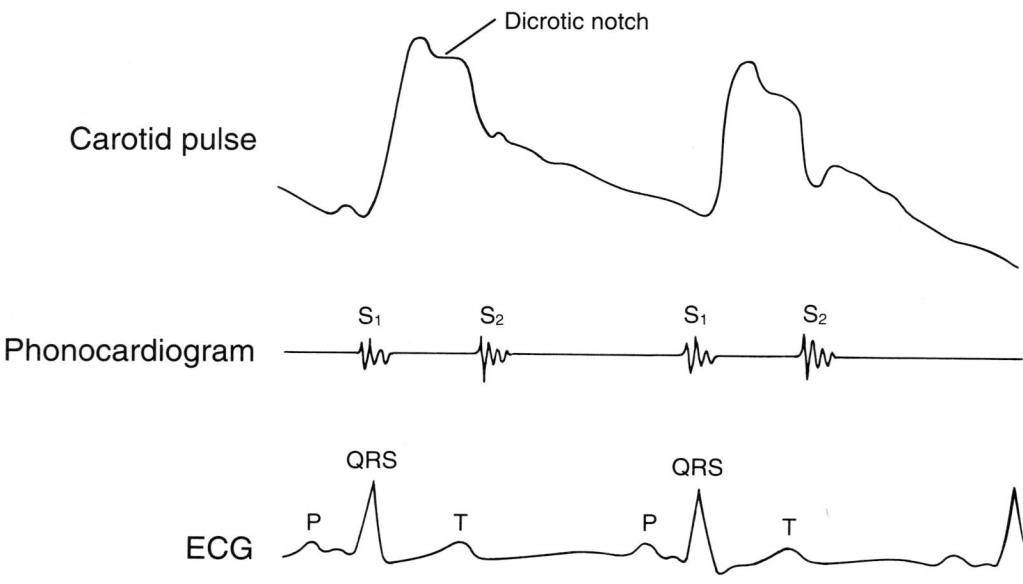

FIGURE 16-13 Carotid pulse wave in relation to S_1 and S_2 and the ECG.

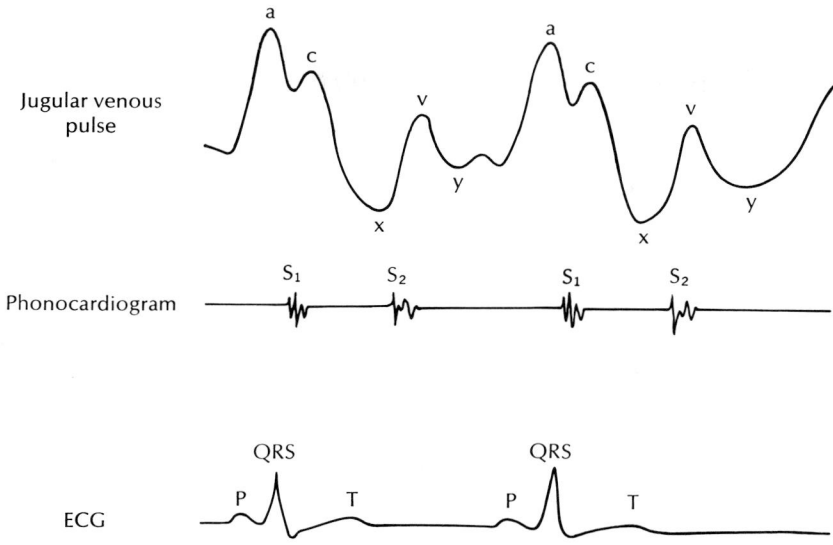

FIGURE 16-14 Jugular venous pulse waves in relation to S₁ and S₂ and the ECG.

artery pulsations and partly the result of upward displacement of the tricuspid valve early in systole. Except in individuals with forceful carotid arterial pulses, the c wave is difficult to recognize. It occurs at the end of S₁.

The x descent is produced by atrial diastole and a downward pull on the atria as the ventricles contract during systole.

The v wave is caused by continuous venous return to the right atrium during systole, a time when the tricuspid valve is closed. As the atria fill, pressure increases. The v wave ends when right atrial pressure falls after the opening of the tricuspid valve. The v wave peaks just after S₂.

The y descent following the v wave is initiated by the fall of right atrial pressure after the opening of the tricuspid valve, when the blood from the atria flows into the ventricles during ventricular diastole.

Jugular venous pressure. Jugular venous pressure is the level at which the jugular veins appear full. In a client with normal right heart function, any filling of the jugular veins is not evident until the person is nearly in a supine position. If the jugular veins appear full when you elevate the client's head to a higher position, this sign indicates less competent function of the right side of the heart.

Peripheral Vessels (Figures 16-15 and 16-16)

Arteries and veins differ somewhat in their structure, which is a reflection of their function. The arteries, which are subject to higher pressure, are tougher and less distensible. The venous system involves lower pressure, and the vein walls are less tough and more distensible. They also contain valves to prevent the backflow of blood. If blood volume increases, the veins can become distended and hold some of the excess blood.

Peripheral arteries. The peripheral arterial pulse is a pressure wave transmitted by left ventricular systole to the peripheral vessels. The nature of the peripheral pulse gives an indication of cardiac function and perfusion of the peripheral tissues. The normal heart rate is between 50 and 100 beats/min. The slowest rate is

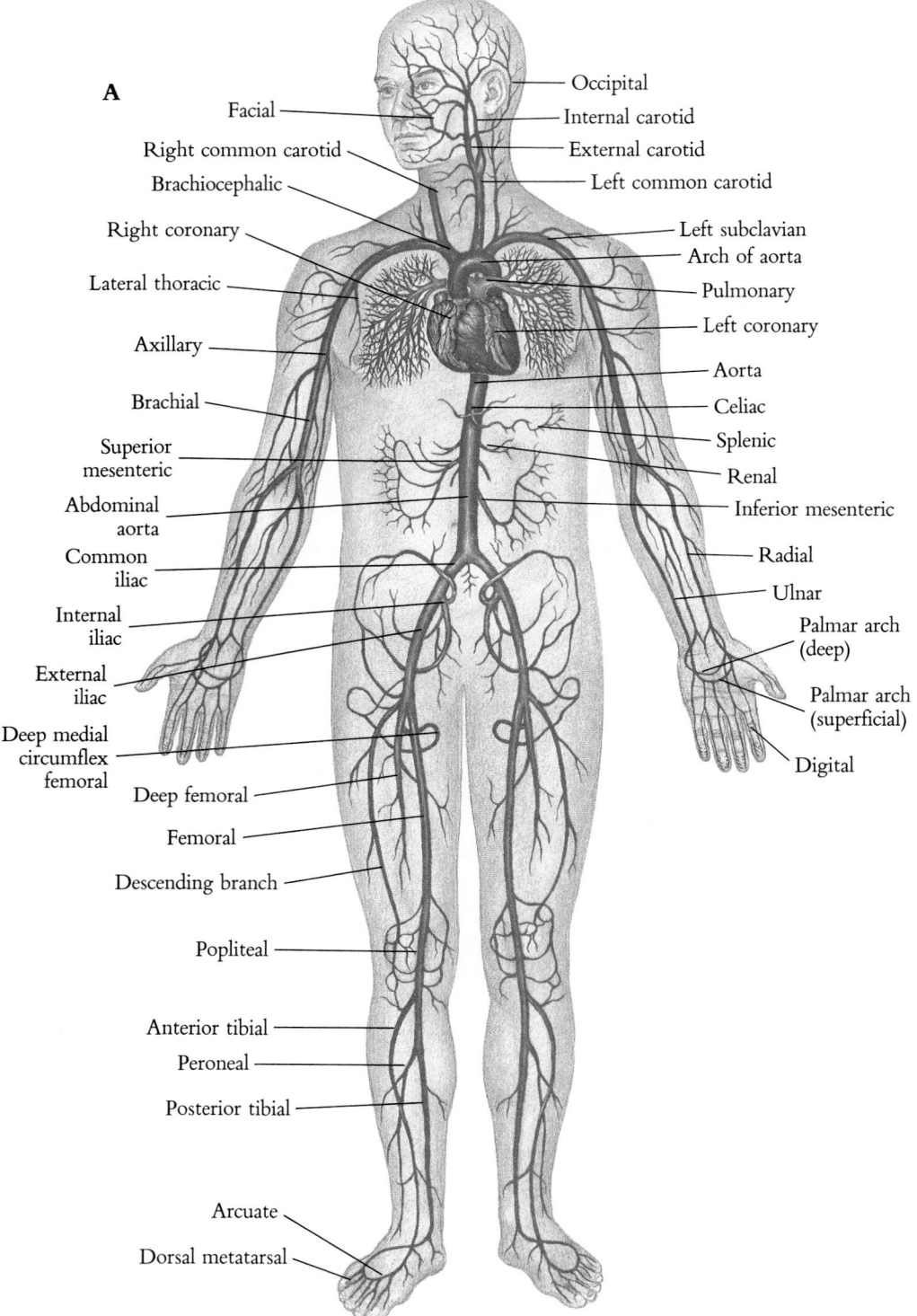

A

Facial
Right common carotid
Brachiocephalic
Right coronary
Lateral thoracic
Axillary
Brachial
Superior mesenteric
Abdominal aorta
Common iliac
Internal iliac
External iliac
Deep medial circumflex femoral
Deep femoral
Femoral
Descending branch
Popliteal
Anterior tibial
Peroneal
Posterior tibial
Arcuate
Dorsal metatarsal

Occipital
Internal carotid
External carotid
Left common carotid
Left subclavian
Arch of aorta
Pulmonary
Left coronary
Aorta
Celiac
Splenic
Renal
Inferior mesenteric
Radial
Ulnar
Palmar arch (deep)
Palmar arch (superficial)
Digital

FIGURE 16-15 Systemic circulation: arteries. (From Seidel HM and others: *Mosby's guide to physical examination*, ed 2, St Louis, 1991, Mosby–Year Book.)

Fig. 10-2 continued on p. 316.

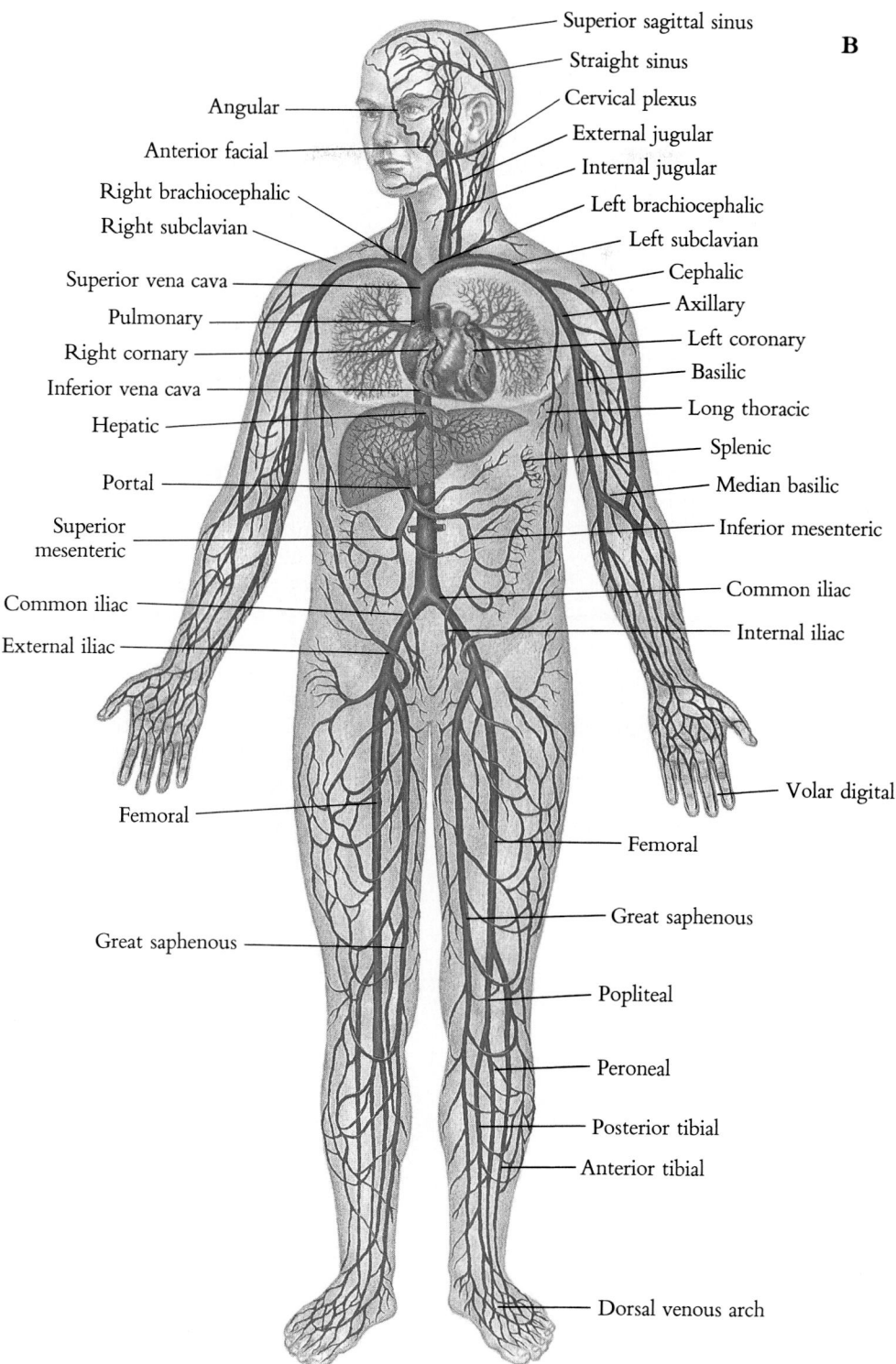

B

Superior sagittal sinus
Straight sinus
Cervical plexus
External jugular
Internal jugular
Left brachiocephalic
Left subclavian
Cephalic
Axillary
Left coronary
Basilic
Long thoracic
Splenic
Median basilic
Inferior mesenteric
Common iliac
Internal iliac
Volar digital
Femoral
Great saphenous
Popliteal
Peroneal
Posterior tibial
Anterior tibial
Dorsal venous arch

Angular
Anterior facial
Right brachiocephalic
Right subclavian
Superior vena cava
Pulmonary
Right cornary
Inferior vena cava
Hepatic
Portal
Superior mesenteric
Common iliac
External iliac
Femoral
Great saphenous

FIGURE 16-16 Systemic circulation: veins. (From Seidel HM, and others: *Mosby's guide to physical examination,* ed 2, St Louis, 1991, Mosby–Year Book.)

seen in the early morning hours, and the most rapid rates occur in the late afternoon and evening. Chronologically, the pulse rate decreases from infancy through the middle years and tends to increase again in the elderly.

The following peripheral pulses are assessed during the physical examination:

Temporal
Carotid
Brachial
Radial
Femoral
Popliteal
Dorsal pedal
Posterior tibial

Peripheral veins. As noted earlier, the veins are less tough and more distensible than the arteries. In contrast to the arteries, the veins contain valves that prevent backflow.

EXAMINATION

Health History

For each symptom, describe the following characteristics in the health history:

Character
Onset
Duration
Location
Associated symptoms
Aggravating factors
Efforts to relieve and effectiveness

Special features of the particular cardiovascular problems are included in the history outline that follows.

Always try to have the client explain or describe the situation in her or his own words before suggesting descriptive terms of your own.

Present health status

Chest pain

1. Character: aching, sharp, tingling, burning, heavy pressure, stabbing, crushing; note client's use of the clenched fist to describe the pain
2. Onset: sudden or gradual; related to eating, exercise, unusual physical exertion, emotional experience, or cold temperature
3. Duration
4. Location and radiation to arm(s), neck, scapula, jaws, teeth
5. Severity: degree of interference with activity, need to stop all activity, sleep disruption
6. Associated symptoms: anxiety; **dyspnea;** diaphoresis; dizziness; nausea and/or vomiting; **palpita-**

tions; faintness; cold, clammy skin; **cyanosis** of lips, ears, nailbeds; pallor
7. Efforts to relieve and effectiveness: rest, position change, nitroglycerin (number of tablets)

Shortness of breath: dyspnea (at rest or with exertion), orthopnea, paroxysmal nocturnal dyspnea

1. Amount of activity or exertion required to cause shortness of breath now, amount required 3 to 6 months ago (e.g., How many stairs is client able to climb before experiencing shortness of breath?)
2. Interference with activities of daily living
3. Constant or intermittent
4. Interference with sleep
5. Number of pillows required to sleep

Cough

1. Characteristics: dry, hacking, productive (if productive, describe: color, odor, amount, whether blood-tinged)
2. Duration
3. Frequency and relationship to time of day
4. Effect of activity, exercise
5. Efforts to treat and effectiveness: rest, change in position, medication(s)

Fatigue

1. Onset and duration
2. Inability to keep up with family, co-workers
3. Limitation of usual activities
4. Bedtime earlier than customary, naps
5. Associated symptoms: dyspnea on exertion, chest pain, palpitations, orthopnea, anorexia, nausea, vomiting

Edema

1. Location
2. Duration
3. Changes over 24-hour period
4. Weight gain

Leg pain or cramps

1. Onset: with activity or rest
2. Location
3. Duration
4. Character of pain, any radiation
   a. Continuous burning in toes, pain when pointing toes, pain in thighs or buttocks, charley horses, aching, pain over specific location
   b. Skin changes: cold skin, pallor, hair loss, sores, redness or warmth over vein, visible veins
   c. Fatigue or limping: occurs with walking, improves with walking
   d. Waking up at night with pain or cramps

Past health history

1. Chronic illness(es): **hypertension, coronary artery disease, hyperlipidemia,** diabetes, congenital heart defect, heart **murmur,** bleeding disorder

2. Cardiac surgery or hospitalization for cardiac disorder
3. Rheumatic fever, unexplained fever, swollen joints

Family health history

1. Heart disease
2. Stroke
3. Diabetes mellitus
4. Hyperlipidemia
5. Hypertension
6. Congenital heart defects
7. Sudden death, particularly of young and middle-aged relatives

Other considerations

1. Employment: physical demands, environmental hazards such as heat, chemicals, dust, sources of emotional stress
2. Nutritional status
   1. Usual diet: proportion of fat, use of salt, intake of caffeine products, food preference
   2. Weight: loss or gain, history of dieting
3. Tobacco use: type (cigarettes, cigars, pipe, chewing tobacco, snuff), duration, amount, age started, efforts to quit
   (*Note:* Pack-years of smoking are calculated by multiplying the number of years of smoking by the number of packs smoked each day.)
4. Alcohol consumption: amount, frequency, duration of current intake
5. Personality assessment: intensity, hostile attitudes, inability to relax, compulsive behavior

6. Work and relaxation habits
   1. Job, routine activities
   2. Hobbies
   3. Exercise: type, amount, frequency, intensity
7. Medications: antihypertensives, beta-blockers, digoxin, diuretics, oral contraceptives, aspirin/anticoagulants, over-the-counter drugs, street drugs; dosage, frequency, when began and why, compliance

Preparation for the Examination: Client and Environment

A quiet environment is essential for a thorough examination of the cardiovascular system. All heart sounds are quiet and of relatively low pitch. They are very difficult to hear when any extraneous noises are present. A room temperature that is comfortable for the client is also important to prevent chilling and subsequent interference with hearing the heart sounds. Good lighting in the room is required for inspecting the subtle motions of the precordium and the neck vessels. Good standard examination room lighting plus a light that can be directed at an angle across the precordium and neck vessels are both necessary.

Assess the client's cardiovascular system with the client in the sitting, supine, and left lateral recumbent positions (lying on the left side). Respect the client's needs for privacy. Provide a drape, and uncover only those portions of the body that are necessary as the examination proceeds.

Preparation for the Examination

PREPARATION

Equipment

Item	Purpose
Stethoscope with diaphragm and bell	Auscultation of heart and vessels
Sphygmomanometer	Measurement of blood pressure
Penlight or lamp with movable arm	Tangential lighting for inspection of precordium and jugular venous pulsations
Metric ruler	Measure distance of apical impulse from midclavicular line, height of jugular venous pressure
Examining table large enough for client to change positions easily	Client needs to be able to move to left lateral recumbent position for auscultation of heart

Client and environment

Quiet room
Room temperature comfortable for client
Good lighting
Privacy (provide drape for client)

Technique for Examination and Normal Findings

Complete examination of the cardiovascular system involves assessment of the entire body from the area of the chest wall overlying the heart to the vessels extending to the head and feet. Use the techniques of inspection, palpation, and auscultation. Examine the client in the sitting, supine, and left lateral recumbent positions. (Occasionally, if standing blood pressure measurement is indicated, you will need to have the client stand.) Because different positions are required of the client, you should learn a system of organizing the cardiovascular examination in such a way that you can perform all components in each of the three positions so that the client does not need to move around unnecessarily.

Measurement of blood pressure is an essential part of the cardiovascular examination. This technique is covered in Chapter 8, General Assessment.

The following description of the examination is divided into three parts: heart, neck vessels, and peripheral vessels.

Heart. To examine the precordium, the area of the chest wall overlying the heart and the great vessels, stand on the right side of the client. For complete assessment of the heart, you must examine the client in the sitting, supine, and left lateral recumbent positions. Perform inspection and palpation primarily with the client in the sitting and supine positions. To perform thorough auscultation, examine the client in all three positions. Have the client lean forward in the sitting position and lie in the left lateral recumbent position to bring various parts of the heart closer to the chest wall, enhancing certain auditory findings.

Inspection. Perform inspection and palpation of the precordium before applying the stethoscope to the chest wall. Although you may be tempted to use the stethoscope as the only means of assessing the heart, you can gain much valuable information by using visual and tactile assessment procedures. Findings from these procedures also give clues to use during auscultation.

With the client in the supine or sitting position, inspect the chest wall. You will need a tangential light for observing the subtle movements of the chest. Observe the chest first for size and symmetry and then for any pulsations, retractions, heaves, or lifts. Note the location and timing of all impulses.

APICAL IMPULSE. The thrust of the contracting left ventricle may produce a visible pulsation in the area of the midclavicular line in the fifth left intercostal space. This pulsation is the normal apical impulse. It occurs nearly synchronously with the carotid pulse, and simultaneous palpation of a carotid artery is helpful in identifying it. When visible, the apical impulse helps to identify an area very near the cardiac apex, thus giving some indication of cardiac size.

> **Helpful Hint:** *The apical impulse is visible in approximately half of the adult population.*

RETRACTION. A retraction is a pulling in of some of the tissues on the precordium related to the position and activity of the heart. A slight retraction of the chest wall just medial to the midclavicular line in the fifth interspace is a normal finding. It is more evident when the chest wall is thin.

LIFT. A lift is a slightly more sustained thrust than is normal.

HEAVE. A heave is an excessive thrust of the heart against the chest wall.

Lifts and heaves may be present with left ventricular hypertrophy.

Palpation. The technique of palpation builds on and expands the findings derived from inspection. Take time to "tune in" to movements over the precordium. Most of these movement are subtle and are perceived only after watching the precordium for a while before palpation. Pulsations should be described in relation to their timing in the cardiac cycle. This observation can be facilitated by simultaneously palpating the carotid pulsation with the left hand and the precordium with the right hand. All pulsations should be described in terms of their location in relation to an intercostal space and to the midclavicular, midsternal, or axillary lines. The shape and thickness of the chest wall are important variables. A thicker chest wall makes palpation more difficult.

Palpate the entire precordium methodically, starting at the apex (Figure 16-17, *A*), moving to the left sternal border (Figure 16-17, *B*), and then to the base of the heart (Figure 16-17, *C*). Use your fingers and the palmar surface of your right hand. Begin at the fifth left intercostal space in the midclavicular line, where the apical impulse is normally located. You will feel this as a slight, short-duration "tap" against the fingers. This pulsation is approximately 2 cm in diameter. On occasion, the apical impulse is located lateral to the midclavicular line, for example, in association with a high diaphragm, as occurs with pregnancy. The outward movement of the normal impulse is not very forceful and is palpable only during the first part of systole. The amplitude of the apical impulse may seem to be increased in normal individuals with thin chest walls. Move next to the left sternal border and then to the base of the heart. You may palpate other areas, if indicated, including the left

A **B** **C**

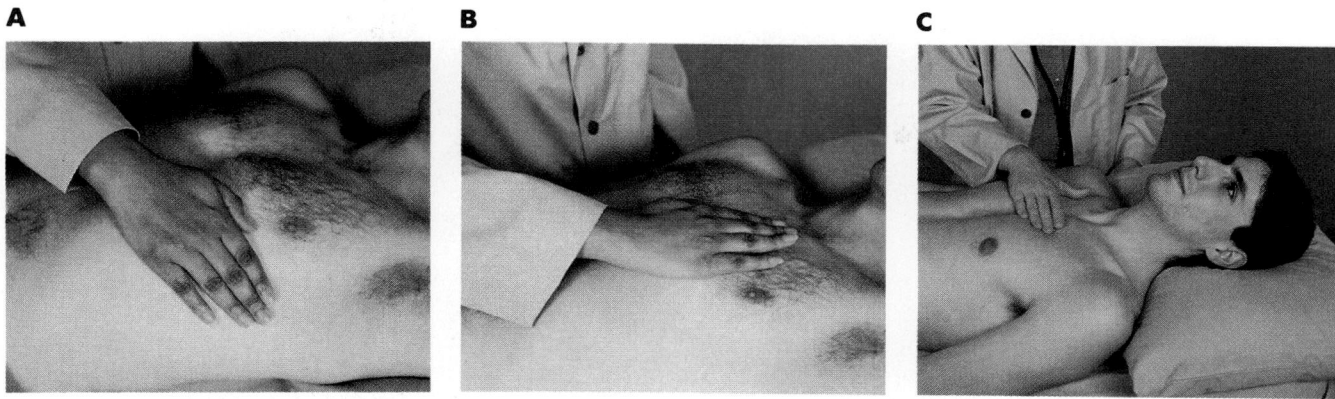

FIGURE 16-17 Palpation of the precordium. **A,** Apex. **B,** Left sternal border. **C,** Base.

anterior axillary area, the epigastrium, and the right sternal border. Also palpate for any abnormal heaves, retractions, or **thrills.**

> **Helpful Hint:** *A thrill is described as a palpable murmur. It is the palpation of blood flowing through the heart or an artery. A thrill is often likened to the feeling transmitted to the fingers when they are placed over the neck of a purring cat.*

Auscultation. Although heart sounds are described as being "high pitched" or "low pitched," these terms are relative. All heart sounds are low pitched and in a range that is difficult for the human ear to hear. A quiet room and careful use of the stethoscope make it possible to hear the sounds of the heart.

Review the material on the use of the stethoscope in Chapter 7. Use both the diaphragm and the bell of the stethoscope to auscultate heart sounds. Use the diaphragm to listen to the high-pitched sounds, such as S_1 and S_2. Use the bell to listen to the low-pitched sounds, such as S_3 and S_4.

> **Helpful Hint:** *If you apply too much pressure to the bell of the stethoscope, the underlying skin becomes tight and the skin itself then acts as a diaphragm. Place the bell very lightly on the chest wall, with just enough pressure applied to seal the edge.*

The client may be in the sitting or the supine position when you begin auscultation. A systematic method of auscultation is essential. Focus attention on each heart sound and the silences in between. Begin at the fifth

left intercostal space in the midclavicular line (Figure 16-18, *A*). Inch the stethoscope toward the lower left sternal border (Figure 16-18, *B*) and up along the border to the base of the heart. Listen at the base of the heart and at both the second left intercostal space at the sternal border (Figure 16-18, *C*) and the second right intercostal space at the sternal border (Figure 16-18, *D*). Repeat this pattern by using first the diaphragm and then the bell of the stethoscope. If any sounds radiate beyond the standard area of auscultation, follow them with the stethoscope. For example, sounds may radiate to the area of the anterior axillary line or up to the carotid arteries.

In each area listen selectively to each component of the cardiac cycle. As with palpation, this step usually requires a period of "tuning in." First, note the rate and rhythm of the heartbeat. Next, at each auscultatory area, focus initially on S_1, noting its intensity, any variations, possible duplication, and the effects of respiration. Then, focus on S_2, again listening for intensity, splitting, effects of respiration, and any variations. After listening to the first and second heart sounds, focus on the normally silent periods of systole and diastole. Then listen for any extra sounds or murmurs. Listen while the client holds his or her breath and during normal breathing.

> **Helpful Hint:** *Listen selectively to each component of the cardiac cycle:* sounds *and* silences. *It is impossible to listen for everything at once.*

If you perform the initial part of the examination with the client supine, ask the client to roll to the left

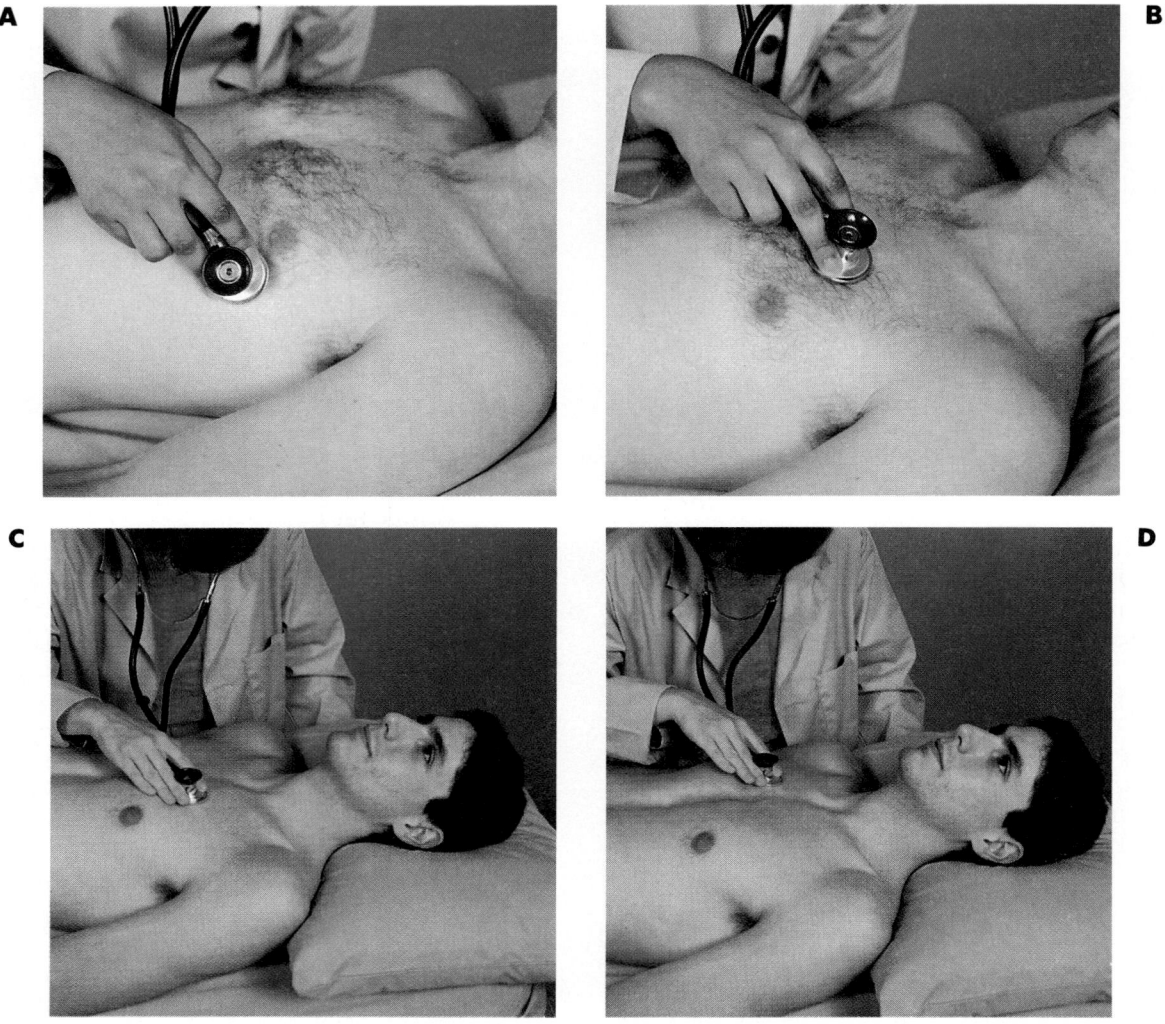

FIGURE 16-18 Auscultation of the precordium. **A,** Apex. **B,** Left sternal border. **C,** Second left intercostal space. **D,** Second right intercostal space.

side. Apply the bell of the stethoscope lightly at the apex and listen for any low-frequency diastolic sounds, such as a filling sound (S_3) or a mitral valve murmur (Figure 16-19). If the client has been in the sitting position, ask him or her to lean slightly forward. Press the diaphragm of the stethoscope firmly against the client's chest and listen at both the second left and the second right intercostal spaces at the sternal border to detect any high-pitched diastolic murmurs of aortic or pulmonic valve insufficiency (Figure 16-20). Listen during normal respiration, and then ask the client to hold his or her breath in deep expiration.

> **Helpful Hint:** *When you are first learning to listen to heart sounds, try to obtain an audiocassette that gives a detailed description of the sounds as you listen to them and can slow the sounds down, making it easier to distinguish each component (see this chapter's Bibliography).*

NORMAL HEART SOUNDS. The normal heart sounds you will hear in healthy clients are S_1, the first heart sound, and S_2, the second heart sound. A third heart sound, S_3, is a normal finding in some clients but a

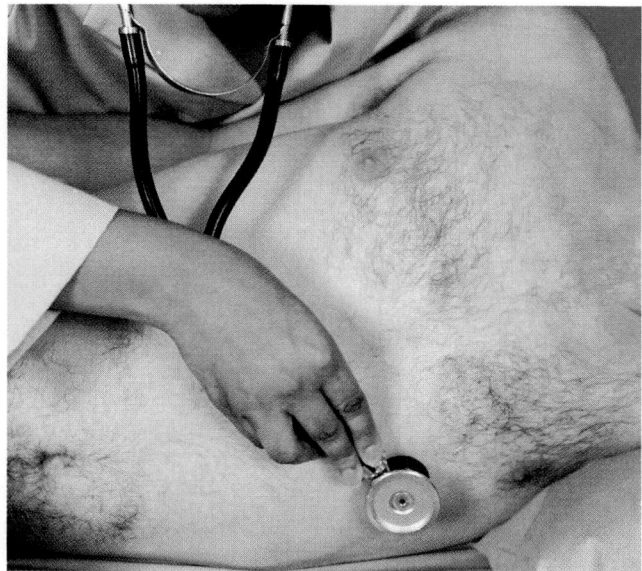

FIGURE 16-19 Auscultation at the apex of the heart with client in left lateral recumbent position.

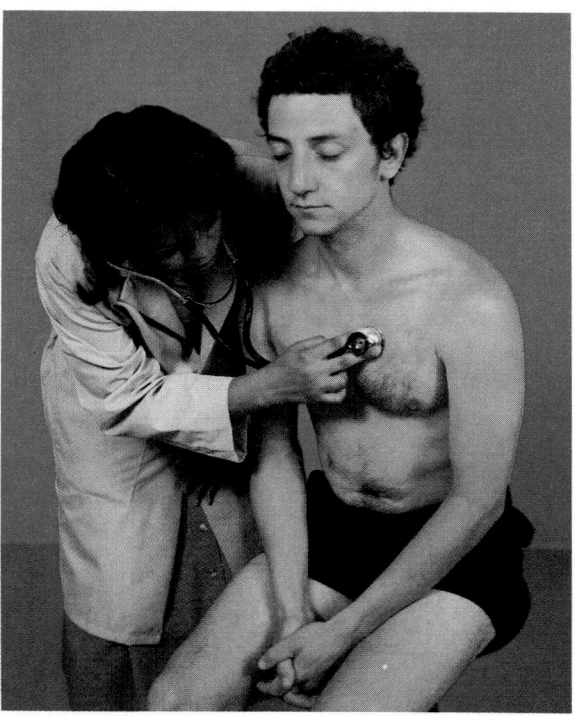

FIGURE 16-20 Auscultation at the base of the heart with client leaning forward.

variation from health in others. The normal heart sounds are described here. Variations in S_1, S_2, and S_3; extra heart sounds; and murmurs are included in the discussion of variations from health.

FIRST HEART SOUND (S_1). The first heart sound results from the closure of the AV valves. As ventricular pressure rises during ventricular systole, the AV valves are forced closed, producing S_1. Because depolarization occurs slightly earlier on the left side of the heart and because pressure is higher on the left side, mitral valve closure takes place slightly before tricuspid valve closure. You can hear S_1 over the entire precordium, but you will hear it best at the apex; it is usually louder than S_2 there (Figure 16-21). At the base of the heart, S_1 is usually louder on the left side than on the right; on both sides it is quieter than S_2. Usually you will hear both components of S_1, mitral and tricuspid valve closure, as one sound. As a result of slight asynchrony in valve closure, however, a split S_1 may be audible and you may hear it in the area where tricuspid valve closure is best transmitted, around the fourth left intercostal space at the sternal border. Splitting of S_1 is neither as commonly nor as easily heard as splitting of S_2.

> **Helpful Hint:** *A helpful method for distinguishing S_1 and S_2 and thus differentiating systole and diastole is to palpate the carotid pulse while auscultating the heart. The carotid pulsation and S_1 are very nearly synchronous: S_1 briefly precedes the carotid impulse.*

SECOND HEART SOUND (S_2). When ventricular systole is completed, pressure in the aorta and pulmonary artery exceeds ventricular pressure and the semilunar valves are forced closed. S_2 is audible over the entire precordium, but you will hear it best at the base of the heart, where it is louder that S_1 (see Figure 16-21). At the apex of the heart, S_2 is quieter than S_1. S_2 marks the beginning of diastole, normally the longer interval between heart sounds. S_2 is slightly higher in pitch and longer in duration than S_1.

Vibrations produced by closure of the aortic and pulmonic valves are responsible for the second heart sound. Aortic valve closure is referred to as A_2, and pulmonic valve closure is referred to as P_2. Pressure on the left side is higher than on the right, making aortic valve closure louder that pulmonic valve closure. Closure of the aortic valve is the loudest component of S_2 at both the right and the left second intercostal spaces. Normally you can hear the sound produced by the pulmonic valve only in a small area centering around the second left intercostal space. You can hear P_2 separately from A_2 when splitting of S_2 occurs.

In the *splitting of S_2* (Figure 16-22), the electrical stimulus that causes depolarization occurs slightly earlier on the left side of the heart than on the right. Also, right ventricular systolic ejection time is slightly longer

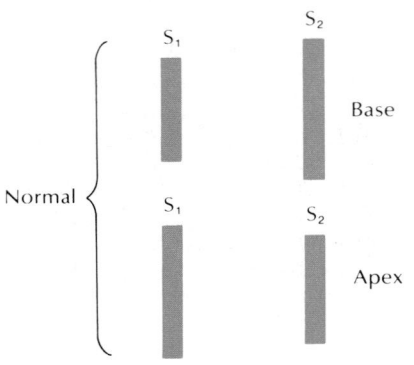

FIGURE 16-21 Relative loudness of S_1 and S_2 as heard over the base and the apex of the heart.

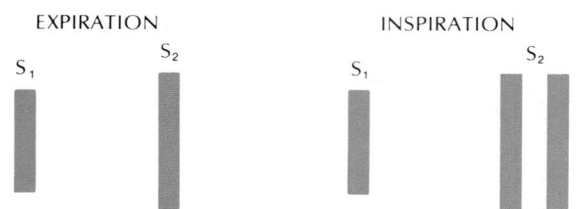

FIGURE 16-22 Normal splitting of S_2. Heard best at second left intercostal space.

than left ventricular systolic ejection time. Therefore pulmonic valve closure, which marks the end of right ventricular ejection, occurs slightly later than aortic valve closure. This action is known as normal physiological splitting of the second heart sound. This normal asynchrony of valve closure increases during inspiration because of the decrease in intrathoracic pressure, which facilitates increased venous return to the right side of the heart. This increased return further delays pulmonic valve closure: A_2 and P_2 are farther apart and more distinct. During expiration, the disparity between left and right ejection times is decreased and splitting becomes less pronounced or nonexistent. The valves close nearly synchronously, producing a single sound. Inspiratory splitting is commonly most marked at the peak of the inspiratory phase of respiration. Listen for splitting during normal respiration. If you have the client hold his or her breath in inspiration, the ejection times of both ventricles become approximately equal again and the split sound becomes single.

Helpful Hint: *You will hear splitting of S_2 only where both pulmonic and aortic valve closure are audible—around the second left intercostal space.*

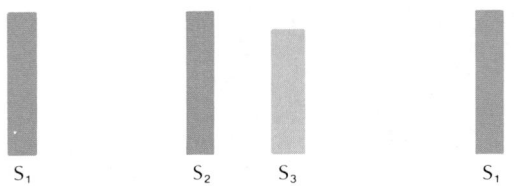

FIGURE 16-23 S_3, an early diastolic sound.

The degree of normal physiological splitting varies among individuals. In some people two distinct sounds are quite clear, although very close in sequence; the splitting may seem more like two parts of a single sound. In others splitting will not be heard. In some clients clear splitting is audible during inspiration, and a very slight degree of splitting is also audible during expiration.

THIRD HEART SOUND (S_3) (FIGURE 16-23). Two phases of rapid ventricular filling occur during diastole. The first, which takes place early in diastole, is a passive, rapid filling phase. When the AV valves open after the second heart sound, the blood stored in the atria flows rapidly into the ventricles. This rapid distention of the ventricles causes vibrations of the ventricular walls. These vibrations may produce a third heart sound, S_3. They are low in pitch and loudness and can be heard best at the apex with the bell of the stethoscope. To accentuate this sound, have the client assume the left lateral recumbent position. This sound is common in children and young adults, and in such instances it is known as a physiological S_3.

Helpful Hint: *As you gain proficiency in listening to heart sounds, alternating the application of light and heavy pressure to the bell of the stethoscope may be a helpful maneuver when listening to low-pitched sounds and trying to differentiate them from high-pitched sounds.*

Neck Vessels. The vascular structures of the neck that are accessible to examination are the carotid arteries and the jugular veins. Examination of these vessels provides information about the vessels themselves and also the activity of the heart. Use the techniques of inspection, palpation, and auscultation to examine the carotid arteries. Use the technique of inspection to examine the jugular veins.

Carotid arteries

INSPECTION. Inspect the neck for the amplitude of the carotid pulsation. Note unusually large, bounding pulsations or small, weak pulsations.

PALPATION. Use your fingertips to palate the carotid pulse just below and medial to the angle of the jaw (Figure 16-24). Palpate only one carotid artery at a time to avoid excessive carotid sinus massage, which can slow the pulse rate. Ask the client to turn his or her head slightly toward the side being examined to relax the sternocleidomastoid muscle. Since S_1 and the carotid pulse are nearly simultaneous, auscultation of the heart at the same time may be helpful in identifying the carotid pulse.

AUSCULTATION. Use the bell of the stethoscope to listen for **bruits** over the carotid arteries (Figure 16-25). A bruit is a blowing sound heard over an artery that indicates either increased flow through the artery or stenosis of the artery.

Jugular veins

Inspection

JUGULAR VENOUS PULSE. Examine the jugular venous pulse by using the technique of inspection only. Tangential lighting will be required because the wave forms are subtle. Direct the light at an angle across the neck where the jugulars are located (Figure 16-26). The jugular venous pulse can be recognized by its location in the neck and by its characteristic pulsation. However, the distinct a, c, and v waves described in the discussion of anatomy and physiology are not always clearly visible. The normal jugular venous pulse may appear as a gentle, undulant wave. Also, in the person with a healthy cardiovascular system, the venous pulse will not be visible until he or she is in, or nearly in, the supine position. To evaluate the jugular venous pulse, place the client in an optimum position, which varies according to the venous pressure. Raise or lower the client's head and thorax until the venous pulsations are optimally visible.

Because the jugular venous pulsations lie so close to the carotid artery pulsations, being able to distinguish them is important. Note the following five ways in which you can distinguish venous pulsations from arterial pulsations.

CHARACTER OF PULSE. The venous pulse waves are more undulating than the brisk arterial waves. The carotid pulse has one upstroke, whereas the venous pulse wave has two or three upstrokes, although these pulses may be somewhat difficult to distinguish. Palpating the carotid pulse on one side of the neck while observing the jugular venous pulse on the other may be helpful in differentiating the two pulses.

EFFECT OF POSITION. Arterial pulsations do not change as the client's position changes. Venous pulsations are present or absent, depending on the client's position.

EFFECT OF RESPIRATION. Venous pulsations change with respiration. With inspiration, intrathoracic pressure decreases, blood flow into the right atrium increases, and the level of the pulse wave in the neck veins descends. The opposite occurs during expiration. Arterial pulsations do not change with respiration.

EFFECT OF VENOUS COMPRESSION. You can easily eliminate the pulsation of the jugular veins by applying gentle pressure over the vein at the base of the neck above the clavicle. This maneuver blocks the retrograde transmission of the venous pulse wave, leaving only the arterial pulsations.

EFFECT OF ABDOMINAL PRESSURE. If you apply moderate pressure over the upper right quadrant of the abdomen for about 30 seconds, a slight rise in venous

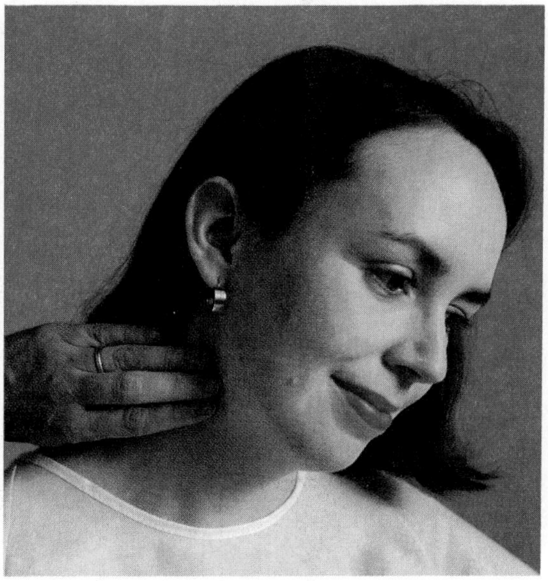

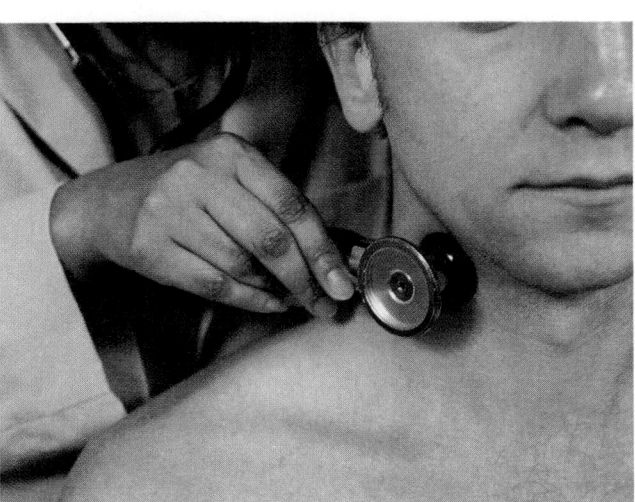

FIGURE 16-24 Palpation of carotid artery pulse.

FIGURE 16-25 Auscultation of carotid artery.

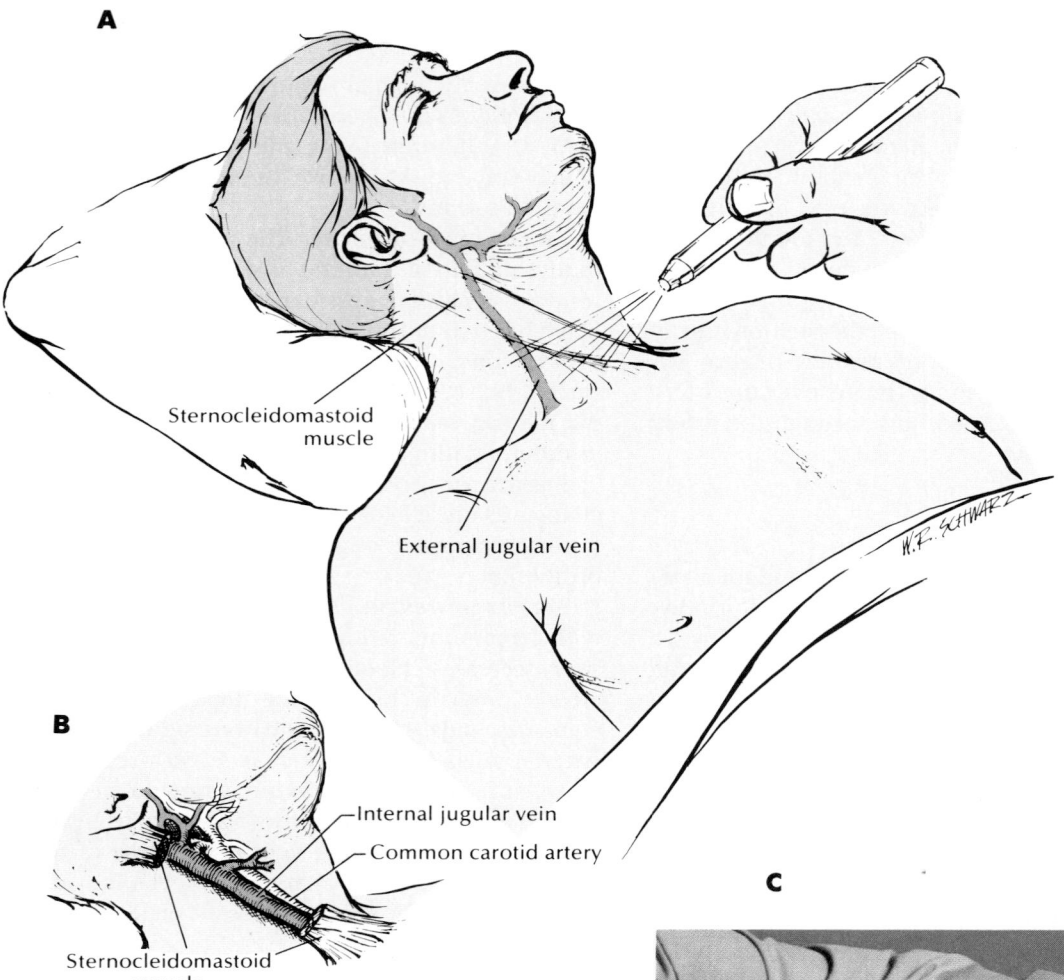

A

Sternocleidomastoid muscle

External jugular vein

W.R. SCHWARZ

B

Internal jugular vein

Common carotid artery

Sternocleidomastoid muscle

C

FIGURE 16-26 **A** and **C,** Inspection of external jugular vein, directing the light across the neck in order to see the venous pulse wave. **B,** Location of internal jugular vein and common carotid artery.

pulsation may occur in the normal client. With right-sided heart failure, the jugular venous pulsations and distention of the veins may markedly increase as venous return to the heart increases. This maneuver does not change the carotid pulsation.

VENOUS PRESSURE. Examine the jugular venous pressure by using the technique of inspection. The level of the column of blood in the jugular veins reflects the volume and pressure on the right side of the heart. Inspection of the neck veins provides a gross estimate of right heart pressure. When a healthy client lies in the supine position, full neck veins are normally visible. As you elevate the client's thorax, the venous pulses disappear. Only with greatly elevated venous pressure are the veins evident when the client is in the upright position.

One method of measuring the height of the venous column with the angle of the sternum is illustrated in Figure 16-27. Use the sternal angle, also called the angle of Louis, as a reference point. Measure the vertical distance between the sternal angle and the highest level of the jugular pulsations and record it in centimeters. The lower you must place the client's head before the pulsations are visible, the lower the pressure; the higher you must place the client's head before you can identify the upper level of the pulsations, the higher the venous pressure. Note the level to which you observe distention and the position of the client.

Peripheral vessels

Arterial pulses. You will feel pressure changes in the wall of the artery through the overlying skin and subcutaneous tissue as the arterial pulse.

Use the technique of palpation to examine the peripheral pulses. Pulses that are close to the surface of the body are easiest to palpate (Figure 16-28). With the pads of your fingers, apply enough pressure at the pulse points to gather information on the pulse rate, rhythm, amplitude, and symmetry; the elasticity of the arterial wall; and an estimate of pulse volume. Do not press so hard that the artery is occluded. If you have difficulty finding a pulse, move your fingers carefully in the area and vary the pressure that you are exerting with your fingertips. Excess tissue or fluid between your finger and the pulse site, such as fat or edema, makes feeling the pulse difficult. In the extremities palpate the most distal pulse first. This approach gives you an assessment of circulation at the farthest palpable point.

Table 16-1 lists the pulses assessed as part of the complete physical examination and their locations.

Brachial pulse assessment by auscultation is a part of the blood pressure evaluation (see Chapter 8). The radial pulse is most frequently used as an initial indication of the rate and rhythm of pulsation, the pattern of pulsation, and the consistency of the arterial wall. The pulse is easily accessible, and its evaluation causes little inconvenience to the client.

RATE. Assess the pulse rate by counting the pulsation for 60 seconds. In the healthy client, counting the rate for 30 seconds and multiplying by two is acceptable. However, for the new client or one in whom there is obvious irregularity or potential cardiovascular dysfunction, counting for the full 60 seconds enables you to assess the rate and other aspects of the pulse more fully.

RHYTHM. Check for a regular rhythm.

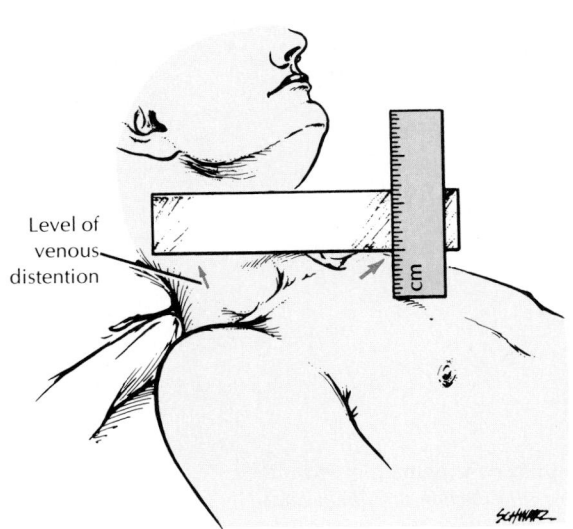
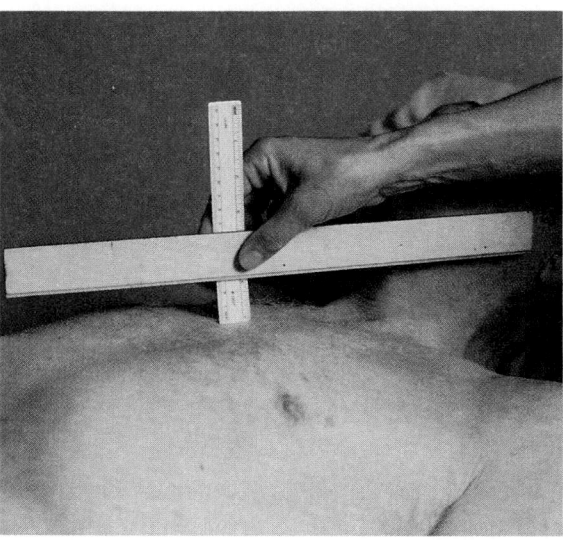

FIGURE 16-27 Measurement of jugular venous pressure. Arrows indicate the height of the jugular venous pressure in centimeters.

AMPLITUDE. The strength of the left ventricular contraction and the volume of blood is reflected in amplitude of the pulsation. There are various scales for recording the pulse force. Note which scale you are using when you record the measurement. Following is a three-point scale:

3+	Bounding, hyperkinetic
2+	Normal
1+	Weak, thready, hypokinetic
0	Absent

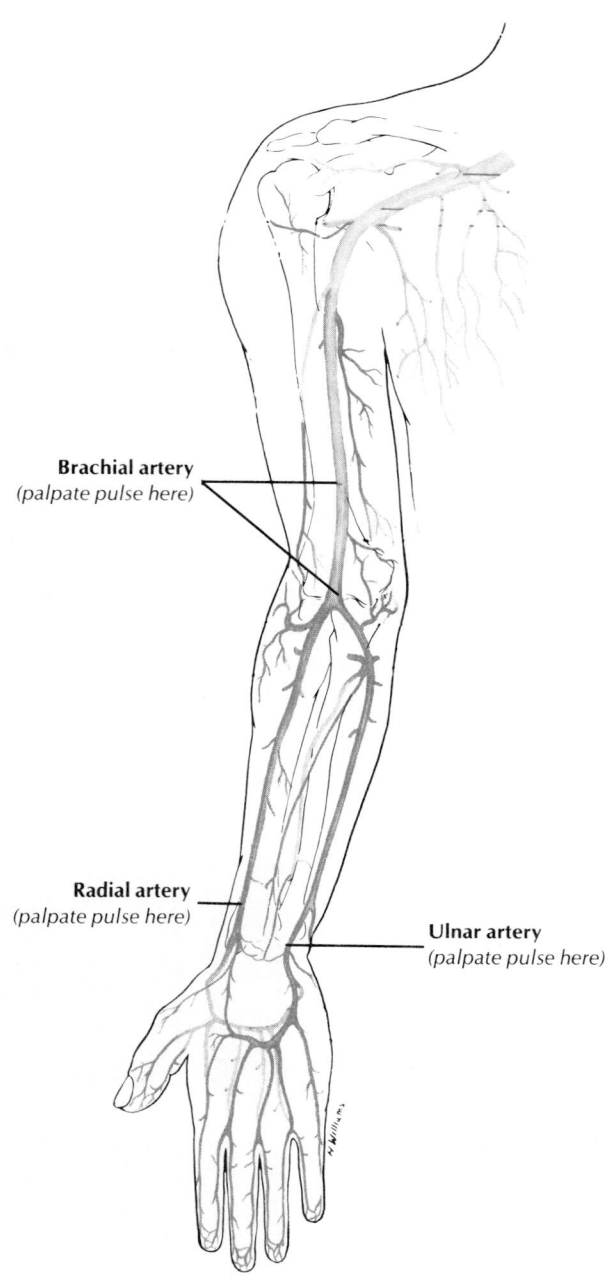

Brachial artery
(palpate pulse here)

Radial artery
(palpate pulse here)

Ulnar artery
(palpate pulse here)

FIGURE 16-28 Location of pulses for palpation. (Modified from Francis CC, Martin AH: *Introduction to human anatomy,* ed 7, St Louis, 1975, Mosby—Year Book.)

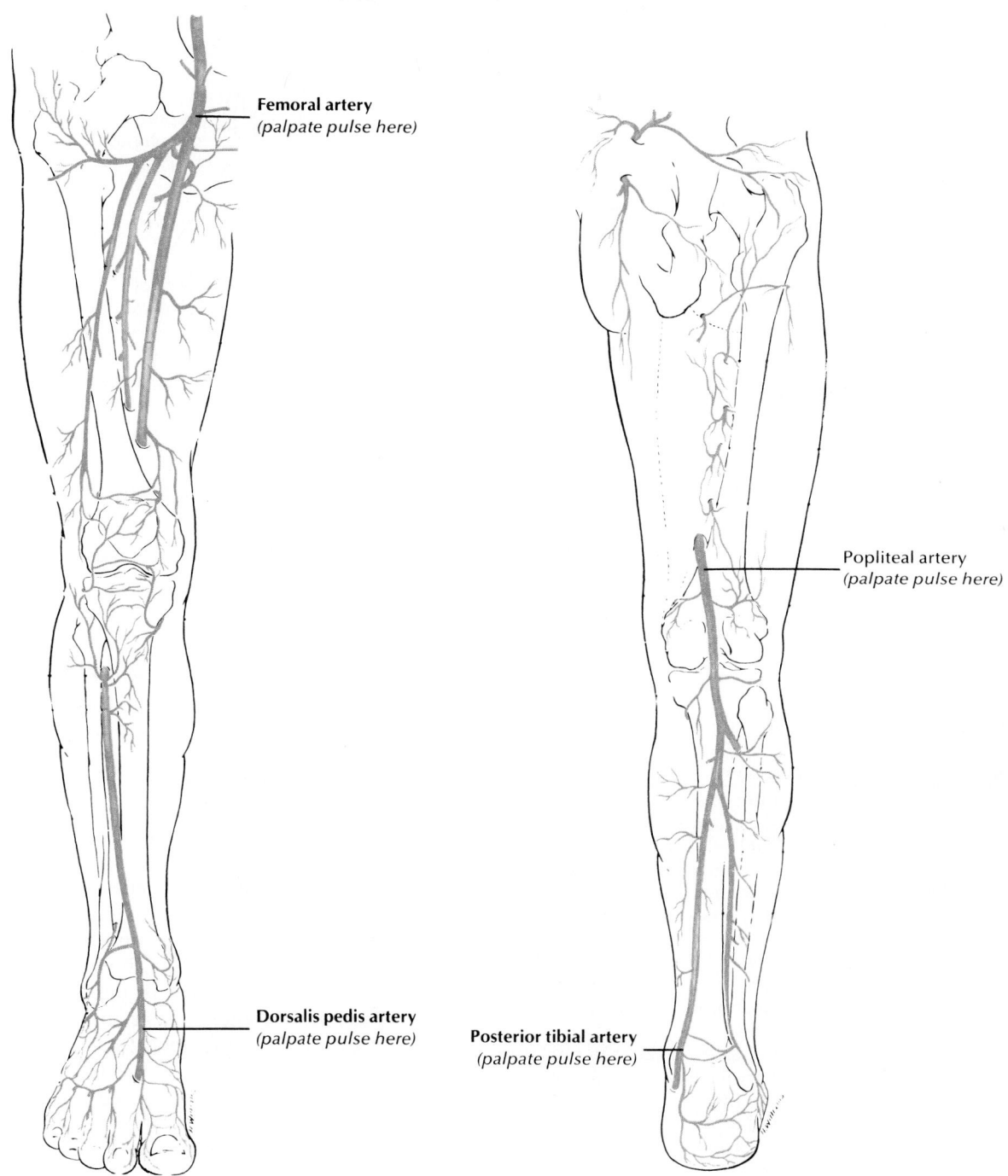

Femoral artery
(palpate pulse here)

Popliteal artery
(palpate pulse here)

Dorsalis pedis artery
(palpate pulse here)

Posterior tibial artery
(palpate pulse here)

FIGURE 16-28, cont'd   For legend, see opposite page.

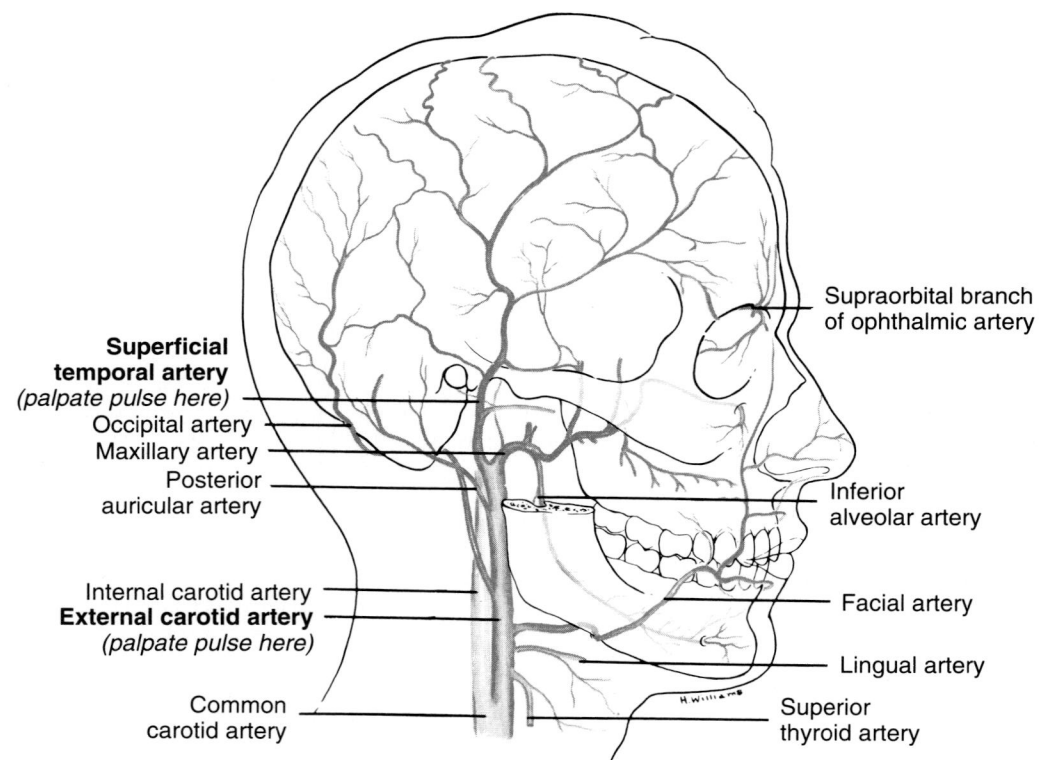

Superficial
temporal artery
(palpate pulse here)

Occipital artery

Maxillary artery

Posterior
auricular artery

Internal carotid artery
External carotid artery
(palpate pulse here)

Common
carotid artery

Supraorbital branch
of ophthalmic artery

Inferior
alveolar artery

Facial artery

Lingual artery

Superior
thyroid artery

FIGURE 16-28, cont'd For legend, see p. 464.

TABLE 16-1

Palpable Pulse Sites

Pulse	Location
Temporal (Figure 16-29, *A*)	In front of and slightly above tragus of ear and upward toward forehead
Brachial (Figure 16-29, *B*)	Upper half of cubital fossa at midline of ventral surface of elbow joint
Radial (Figure 16-29, *C*)	Medial and ventral aspect of wrist
Femoral (Figure 16-29, *D*)	Below and medial to inguinal ligament, midway between anterior superior iliac spine and symphysis pubis
Popliteal (Figure 16-29, *E*)	Dorsal aspect of knee in popliteal fossa (bend knee and press deeply into fossa)
Dorsal pedal (dorsalis pedis) (Figure 16-29, *F*)	Dorsal aspect of foot about midway between ankle and toes (flex foot). *Note:* This pulse may be absent in healthy individuals.
Posterior tibial (Figure 16-29, *G*)	Behind and slightly below medial malleolus of ankle (flex foot). *Note:* This pulse may be absent in healthy individuals.

ELASTICITY OF ARTERIAL WALL. Elasticity of the arterial wall is reflected by the expansibility of the artery as your fingers palpate it. The normal artery is soft and pliable, whereas the sclerotic vessel may be more resistant or even hard and cordlike.

Peripheral veins. Normally, the venous pattern is fairly flat and barely visible. Inspect the extremities for symmetry, color, and varicosities. They should be symmetrical without swelling, edema, discoloration, or atrophy. Palpate the hands and feet for temperature; they should be warm. Note, however, that a cool examining room can affect this finding. To test for deep phlebitis, flex the client's knee and gently compress the calf muscle against the tibia (Homan's sign) or sharply dorsiflex the foot while the knee is bent. This maneuver should not cause pain in the healthy client.

Cardiovascular diseases are major causes of morbidity and mortality in our population. Because of this situation, it is important to consider the risk factors while obtaining the health history and performing the physical examination, and later in the nursing process, while planning and implementing nursing interventions (see box).

Risk Factors: Diseases of Cardiovascular System*

Coronary artery disease
Principal modifiable risk factors include:
Elevated serum **cholesterol** (greater than 200 mg/dl) and **high-density lipoprotein (HDL)** (less than 35 mg/dl)
Smoking
Hypertension
Obesity (20% more above desirable body weight)
Excessive dietary intake of calories and fat, especially saturated fat
Diabetes mellitus
Sedentary life-style
Personality characteristics: intense, compulsive, hostile
Principal nonmodifiable risk factors include:
Increasing age
Sex (males are at greater risk)
Family history of cardiovascular disease, diabetes, hyperlipidemia, hypertension
Hypertension
Modifiable risk factors for hypertension include:
Obesity
Smoking
Excessive dietary intake of sodium
Nonmodifiable risk factors for hypertension include:
Family history of hypertension
Increasing age
African American descent
Hypertension is a leading risk factor for:
Coronary artery disease
Congestive heart failure
Stroke
Renal disease
Retinopathy

Cerebrovascular disease
Risk factors for cerebrovascular disease include:
Hypertension
Obesity
Smoking
Coronary artery disease
Atrial **fibrillation**
Diabetes mellitus
Increased age
Peripheral arterial disease
Risk factors for peripheral arterial disease include:
Smoking
Diabetes mellitus
Age over 50
Hypercholesterolemia
Risk factors for hypercholesterolemia include:
Obesity
Excessive dietary intake of fat, especially saturated fat
Hypercholesterolemia is a risk factor for:
Coronary artery disease
Hypertension
Cerebrovascular disease
Chronic venous insufficiency:
Risk factors include:
Prolonged standing or sitting
Obesity
Prolonged bedrest
History of congestive heart failure, varicosities, or thrombophlebitis

*Modified from Report of the U.S. Preventive Services Task Force: *Guide to clinical preventive services: an assessment of the effectiveness of 169 interventions,* Baltimore, 1989, Williams & Wilkins.

CULTURAL INFLUENCES AND FACTORS: HEART DISEASE AND STROKE

Heart disease and stroke are two of the major causes of death among people from various cultural backgrounds. Among Native American young adults, death from heart disease is approximately twice as high as that for all other Americans. A strikingly high incidence of diabetes exists among many Native American tribes.

African American males are twice as likely to die from stroke as are white males. Among African Americans ages 20 to 64 years, death from coronary artery disease is higher than among other Americans. This group also experiences a higher incidence of hypertension and diabetes.

Puerto Ricans, Cubans, Mexicans, and Filipinos all have a higher incidence of hypertension than whites do.

Life situations involving high stress, little stability, low educational levels, and inadequate coping mechanisms also contribute to high blood pressure.

A

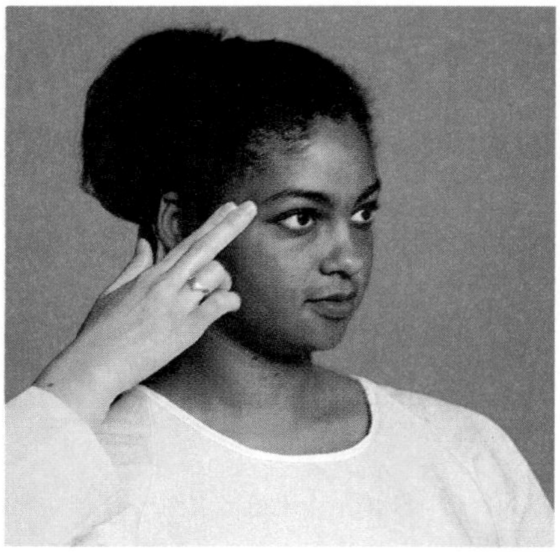

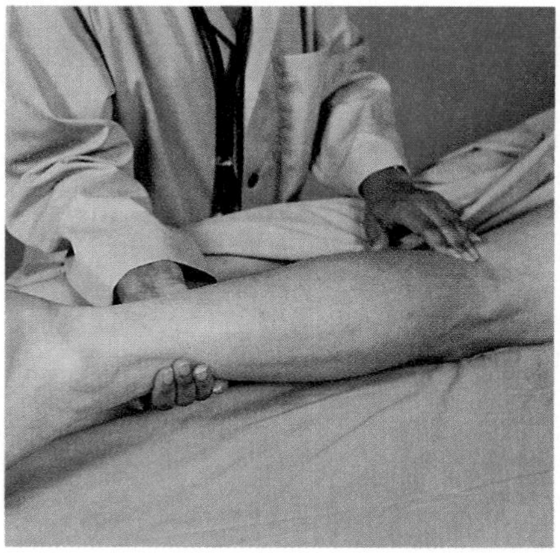

B

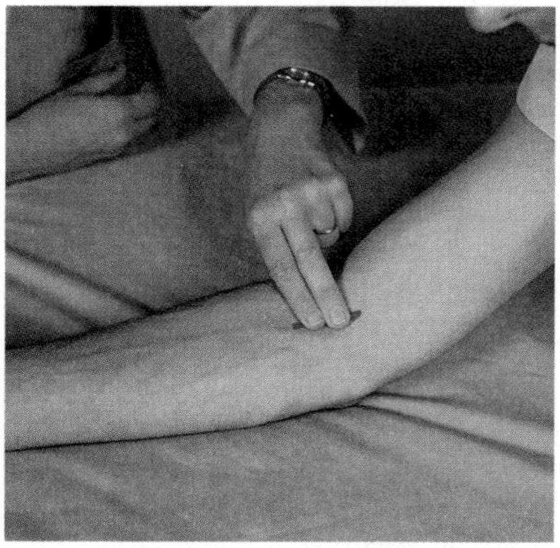

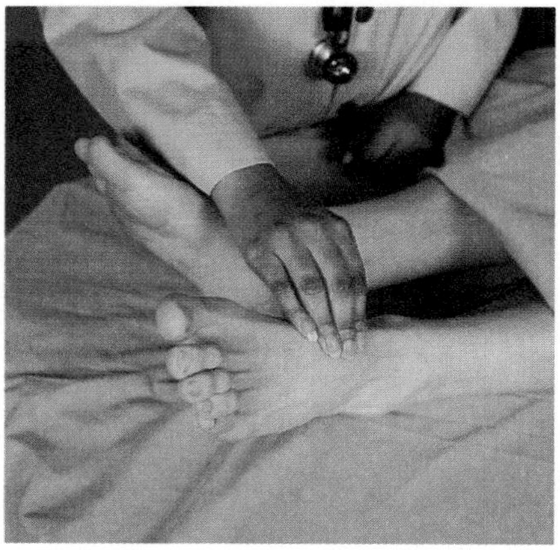

C

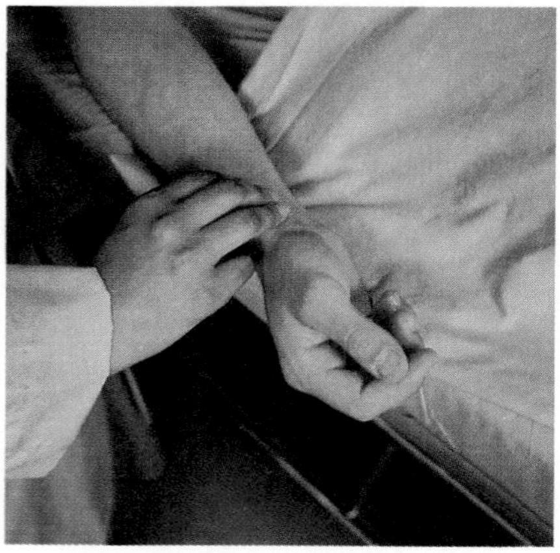

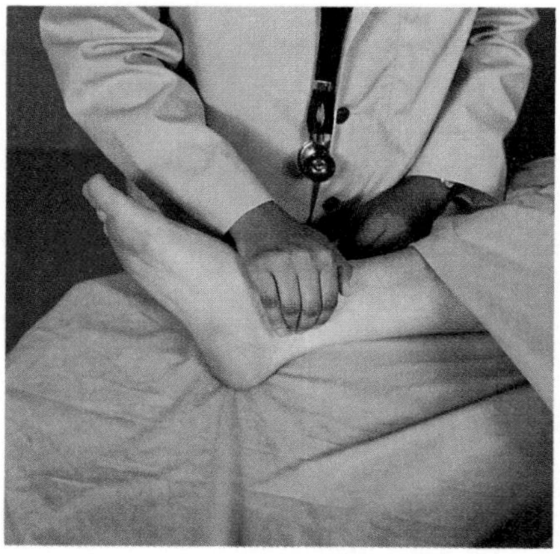

D

E

F

G

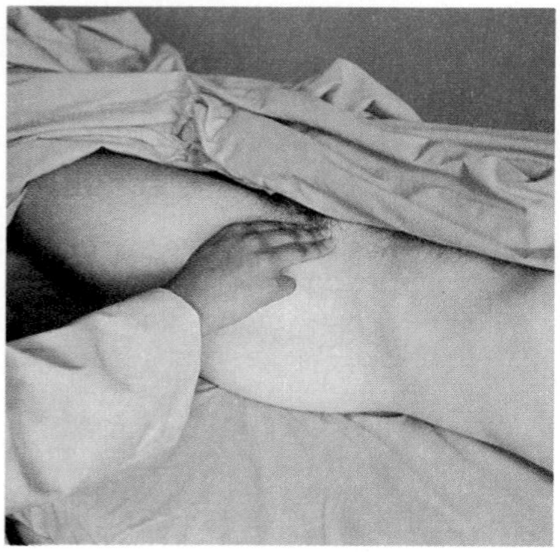

FIGURE 16-29 Palpation of various pulses. **A,** Temporal pulse. **B,** Brachial pulse. **C,** Radial pulse. **D,** Femoral pulse. **E,** Popliteal pulse. **F,** Dorsal pedal pulse. **G,** Posterior tibial pulse.

Screening Tests and Procedures
Screening for asymptomatic coronary artery disease (CAD)

1. Measure for high blood pressure
2. Check serum cholesterol for elevated levels
3. Investigate behavioral risk factors, such as:
    Tobacco use
    Excessive dietary intake of fat and cholesterol
    Inadequate physical activity

Screening for symptomatic coronary artery disease

In addition to the screening tests for asymptomatic CAD, perform the following test:
    Resting and exercise ECGs

Screening for high blood cholesterol. Periodic measurement of the total serum cholesterol level is most important for middle-aged men, and it may also be clinically prudent for young men, women, and the elderly. The National Heart, Lung, and Blood Institute recommends cholesterol testing in all adults aged 20 and older at least once every 5 years. All clients should receive periodic counseling regarding dietary intake of fat (especially saturated fat) and cholesterol.

Serum cholesterol levels normally undergo substantial physiological fluctuations related to gender, stress, and season. Therefore a single blood test may not be representative. Levels of elevated blood cholesterol include the following:
    High blood cholesterol: 240 mg/dl and above
    Borderline high cholesterol: 200 to 239 mg/dl
    Serum HDL cholesterol less than 35 mg/dl

Screening for hypertension. Blood pressure should be measured regularly in all persons aged 3 years and older.

The optimum interval for blood pressure screening has not been determined, but current expert opinion is that persons thought to be normotensive should receive blood pressure measurements at least once every 2 years if their last diastolic and systolic blood pressure readings were below 85 mm Hg and 140 mm Hg, respectively, and annually if their last diastolic blood pressure was 85 to 89 mm Hg or above.

Examination Step-by-Step

Before beginning the examination, be sure that the room is quiet, the temperature is comfortable for the client, and the equipment is ready. You will need a stethoscope with both a bell and a diaphragm, a good light source that can be directed tangentially, a small metric ruler, and a sphygmomanometer. The examining table must be large enough for the client to change positions easily. With the healthy client, perform the portions of the examination that require the sitting position first, the supine position next, and the left lateral recumbent position last. In this way the integrated examination moves from the head and shoulders to the chest and on to the extremities. Check the peripheral pulses while the client is sitting or supine.

Precordium and neck vessels

1. Inspection
    a. Precordium: pulsations, heaves, retractions
    b. Neck vessels
        (1) Carotid arteries: amplitude of pulsations
        (2) Jugular veins: pulsations and pressure level
2. Palpation
    a. Precordium at fifth left intercostal space in midclavicular line, left sternal border, and at second left and right intercostal space: apical impulse, lifts, heaves, thrills
    b. Carotid artery pulses (check each separately).

3. Auscultation
    a. Precordium at fifth left intercostal space, left sternal border, left intercostal space, and right intercostal space: normal heart sounds, extra heart sounds, murmurs. Auscultate the precordium with the client in the sitting, supine, and left lateral recumbent positions. Use both the diaphragm and the bell of the stethoscope at each area.
    b. Carotid arteries: bruits

Peripheral vascular system

1. Inspect the venous vasculature.
2. Palpate the peripheral arterial pulses, including:
    Temporal
    Brachial
    Radial
    Femoral
    Popliteal
    Dorsal pedal (dorsalis pedis)
    Posterior tibial
3. Inspect the skin and the peripheral tissues for adequate vascular delivery of nutrients and clearance of metabolic by-products and fluids.

STEP-BY-STEP

A single elevated reading does not indicate a diagnosis of hypertension. Elevated readings should be confirmed through more than one reading at each of the three separate visits.

Screening for cerebrovascular disease. Auscultation of the carotid arteries should be included in the physical examination of patients with established risk factors for cerebrovascular or cardiovascular disease.

Patients with carotid artery stenosis are at substantially increased risk for stroke and myocardial infarction. The risk is even greater for persons with neurological symptoms such as a **transient ischemic attack.**

VARIATIONS FROM HEALTH

Heart

Variations on inspection. Cardiac variations assessed by inspection reflect changes in left and right ventricular function.

Finding	Explanation
Apical impulse located more laterally and/or inferiorly (e.g., in sixth left intercostal space lateral to midclavicular line)	Occurs with left ventricular hypertrophy or dilation or both; may be seen with systemic hypertension
Apical impulse appears more forceful against chest well, apical thrust, or rocking motion	Left ventricular hypertrophy
Retraction of tissues around apical impulse	Pericardial disease
Heave or lift along left sternal border	Workload or forcefulness of right ventricle is increased

Variations on palpation

Finding	Explanation
Apical impulse larger and/or more forceful	Left ventricular hypertrophy, dilation; associated with volume overload and increased peripheral resistance
Heave or lift along left sternal border	Increased workload on right ventricle; right ventricular hypertrophy; associated with pulmonary valve disease, pulmonary hypertension, chronic lung disease
Apical impulse not palpable	Hypovolemia, pericardial effusion, (apical impulse is also not palpable in many healthy persons or if chest

	wall is thick because of muscle or fat)
Thrill	Heart murmur (sensation like purring of a cat transmitted to the fingers); present with murmurs of grade 4 or greater

Changes associated with left ventricular hypertrophy can be summarized as follows:
1. Forceful and sustained outward movement of the apical impulse during ventricular systole; thrust or rocking motion.
2. Apical impulse may be larger, lower, and more lateral to the midclavicular line, for example, in the sixth intercostal space 4 cm lateral to the midclavicular line, 4 cm in diameter.

The degree of displacement of the apical impulse generally correlates with the extent of cardiac enlargement. Displacement tends to be maximal when both hypertrophy and dilation of the ventricle are present. Conditions associated with volume overload, such as mitral and aortic **regurgitation** and left-to-right shunts, tend to produce hypertrophy and dilation.

Variations on auscultation. Variations that are audible with auscultation include changes in heart sounds, extra heart sounds, and murmurs.

Variations in heart sounds. The variations in heart sounds include changes in the loudness of S_1 and S_2 and changes in the splitting pattern of S_2.

VARIATIONS IN S_1

Change	Explanation
Faint/diminished S_1	As a result of rheumatic fever, mitral valve may become so fibrosed and calcified that only limited motion is possible
Loud/accentuated S_1	Increased blood velocity produces increased closing pressure and more abrupt closure; occurs with hyperkinetic states: exercise, fever, anemia, hyperthyroidism
	Mitral valve stenosis in which valve leaflets are still mobile; greater ventricular pressure is needed to overcome increase in atrial pressure: increased closing pressure and more abrupt closure result
Varying S_1	Incomplete heart block in which P-R interval is changing, atria and ventricles beat independently, and position of valves is changing from beat to beat

VARIATIONS IN S₂

Variations in S_2 include changes in loudness and splitting.

Change	Explanation
Loud/accentuated S_2	Louder closure sounds result from higher closing pressure; in systemic hypertension, S_2 may have a ringing sound
	Exercise and excitement increase pressure in aorta, producing an increase in A_2 component of S_2
	Conditions associated with pulmonary hypertension (e.g., mitral valve stenosis, and congestive heart failure) may produce an increase in P_2 component of S_2
	Semilunar valves that are injured but still flexible
Faint/diminished S_2	Decrease in systemic blood pressure, as occurs with shock, results in diminished A_2
	Injured valves that are thickened and calcified

VARIATIONS IN SPLITTING OF S₂ (FIGURE 16-30)

Wide splitting	Conditions causing delayed electrical stimulation of right ventricle (e.g., right bundle branch block) cause a delay in pulmonic valve closure; wide splitting of S_2 exists with expiration; with inspiration, splitting is even wider
Fixed splitting	Associated with atrial septal defect; pulmonic closure is delayed because with each beat right ventricle is ejecting a larger volume than is left ventricle; right-side filling cannot be further increased by inspiration, so split sound remains fixed
Paradoxical splitting	Delayed closure of aortic valve in left bundle branch block results in narrowed splitting or splitting where normal sequence of sounds is reversed: pulmonic closure precedes aortic closure; paradoxically, inspiration results in the two sounds coming closer together and even fusing into a single sound, and expiration results in more widely separated sounds

Extra heart sounds. The extra heart sounds described here include: S_3, S_4, the **opening snap** of the mitral valve, the ejection click of the semilunar valves, and the pericardial friction rub. S_3, S_4, and the opening snap all occur during diastole, the ejection click takes place during systole, and the pericardial friction rub may occur during both systole and diastole.

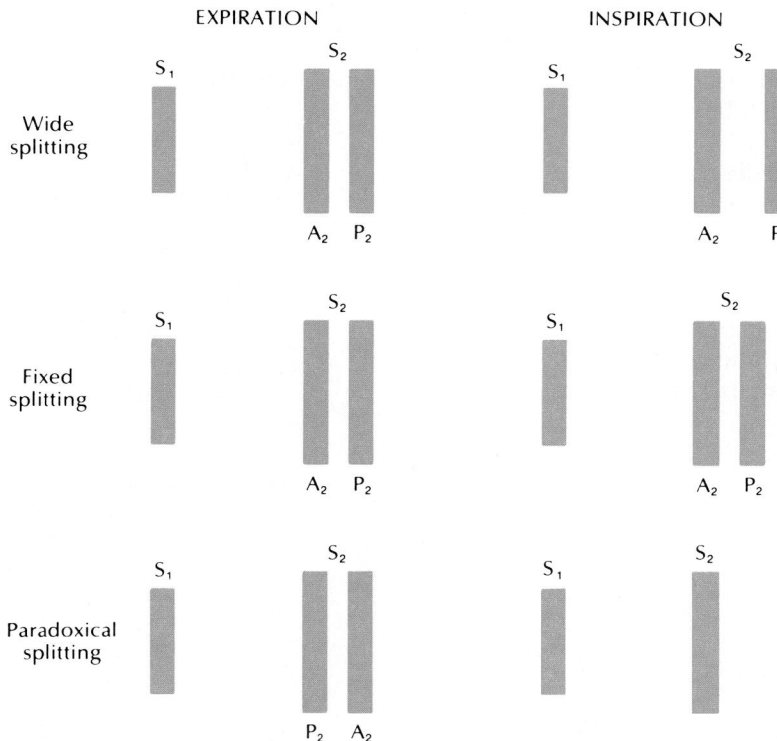

FIGURE 16-30 Variations in splitting of S_2.

THIRD HEART SOUND (S_3). S_3 is a ventricular filling sound that occurs in early diastole (see Figure 16-23). It is a low-pitched, soft sound. Have the client lie in the left lateral position. Auscultate at the apex, placing the bell of the stethoscope lightly against the skin, with just enough pressure to form a seal. The pathological S_3 indicates decreased compliance of the ventricles, as in congestive heart failure. This sound may be an early sign of heart failure. S_3 may also occur with conditions of volume overload, such as with mitral, tricuspid, or aortic valve regurgitation. It is important to remember that S_3 may also occur in high cardiac output conditions in which no heart disease exists, such as with anemia and hyperthyroidism, in healthy young adults, and during pregnancy.

The differences between an S_3 and a split S_2 can be summarized in the following way:

S_3	Split S_2
Heard best at apex or lower left sternal border	Heard best at base
Does not vary with respiration	Varies with respiration
Heard best with bell of stethoscope	Heard best with diaphragm of stethoscope

FOURTH HEART SOUND (S_4). In late diastole, when the atria contract to eject blood into the ventricle, the second active, rapid ventricular filling phase occurs immediately before S_1 (Figure 16-31). The inflow of this phase may cause vibrations of the valves, supporting structures, or ventricular walls, resulting in a late diastolic filling, or fourth heart sound, S_4. This soft, low-pitched sound can be heard best by using the bell of the stethoscope and having the client in the left lateral position.

A physiological S_4 may be heard in middle-aged adults with thin-walled chests, especially after exercise. However, it is less likely to be found in a well client than is a physiological S_3.

An abnormal S_4 results from (1) an increased resistance to filling secondary to decreased compliance of the ventricle, as occurs with cardiomyopathy and coronary artery disease, and (2) systolic overload, includ-

ing obstruction to outflow from the ventricle, as occurs with aortic stenosis and systemic hypertension.

SUMMATION GALLOP. When both phases of rapid ventricular filling become audible events as S_3 and S_4, a quadruple rhythm **(gallop rhythm)** with four audible components results. S_3 is an early diastolic (protodiastolic) sound, and S_4 is a late diastolic (presystolic) sound. If the heart rate increases and diastole becomes shorter, S_3 and S_4 come closer together and they may be heard as one sound in diastole. Three cardiac sounds may follow: S_1, S_2, and the summation sound of S_3 and S_4. The last, known as a summation gallop, resembles a galloping sound. It may be louder than S_1 and S_2.

OPENING SNAP, EJECTION CLICK, AND PERICARDIAL RUB. Two of the extra heart sounds always indicate an abnormality. Both sounds are produced by the opening of diseased valves. They are the opening snap of the mitral valve and the ejection click of a semilunar valve. A pericardial friction rub also produces an abnormal extra cardiac sound. Use the diaphragm to listen for each of these sounds.

OPENING SNAP OF MITRAL VALVE (FIGURE 16-32, A)**.** The opening of the mitral valve is normally a silent event. It is audible if the valve becomes thickened or altered by a disease such as rheumatic heart disease. This sound occurs early in diastole. It is high pitched and brief and has a snapping or clicking quality. Usually you can hear it best medial to the apex and toward the lower left sternal border; it may radiate toward the base. S_1 is strong and may be accentuated. It can be differentiated from an S_3 because it occurs earlier. (The mitral valve must open before ventricular filling can begin.) It is higher pitched than S_3 and radiates more widely.

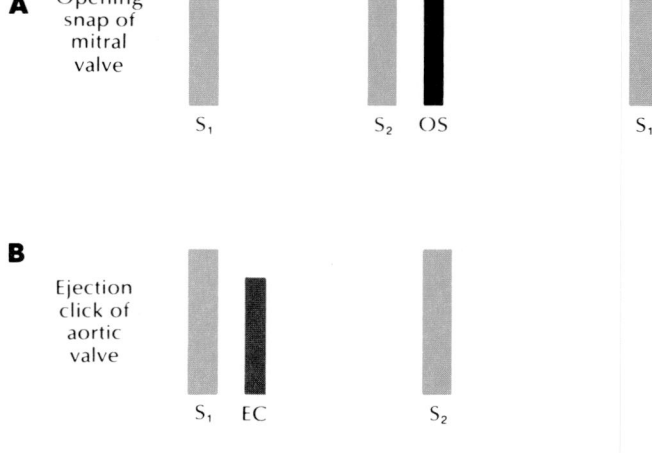

A, Opening snap of mitral valve

S_1 S_2 OS S_1

B, Ejection click of aortic valve

S_1 EC S_2

FIGURE 16-32 A, Opening snap of the mitral valve following S_2. **B,** Ejection click of the aortic valve following S_1.

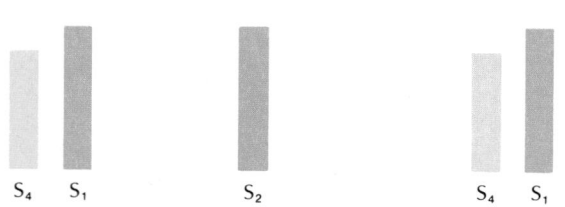

S_4 S_1 S_2 S_4 S_1

FIGURE 16-31 S_4, a late diastolic sound.

The following are the characteristics of the opening snap of the mitral valve:

Timing: early diastole
Pitch: high (higher than S_3)
Duration: brief
Best heard: medial to apex, toward lower left sternal border

The differences between an opening snap and a split S_2 can be summarized in the following way:

Opening snap	S_2
Best heard at apex and lower left sternal border	Best heard at second left intercostal space, sternal border
Does not vary with respiration	Varies with respiration

EJECTION CLICK (FIGURE 16-32, B). Alterations in the semilunar valves (aortic and pulmonic) may also be associated with an opening sound. Normally, the semilunar valves open silently. Stenosis of either valve may result in sound production. An ejection click occurs early in systole at the end of isovolumic contraction when the semilunar valves open. An ejection click, which is a short, high-pitched sound, can be heard best with the diaphragm of the stethoscope. An aortic valve ejection click is more common than a pulmonic valve ejection click. An aortic ejection click can be heard at both the base and the apex. It does not change with respiration. A pulmonic valve ejection click can be heard best at the second left intercostal space. It changes in loudness with respiration, increasing with expiration and decreasing with inspiration. The characteristics of ejection clicks are the following:

Timing: early systole
Pitch: high (use diaphragm of stethoscope)
Duration: short
Best heard: aortic valve ejection click: base to apex
pulmonic valve ejection click: second left intercostal space

PERICARDIAL FRICTION RUB. Inflammation of the pericardial sac causes the parietal and visceral surfaces of the roughened pericardium to rub against each other. This action produces an extra cardiac sound having a to-and-fro character and both systolic and diastolic components. This sound is high pitched and can be heard best with the diaphragm of the stethoscope. It resembles the sound of squeaky leather and is often described as grating, scratching, or rasping. The sound seems very close to the ear and may seem louder than (or may even mask) the other heart sounds. Pericardial friction rubs can usually be heard best between the apex and the sternum, where the pericardium comes in close contact with the chest wall, but the sound may be widespread. It is common after a myocardial **infarction.**

The characteristics of a pericardial friction rub are the following:

Pitch: high
Timing: systole and diastole
Heard best: between apex and lower left sternum
Quality of sound: to-and-fro grating, scratching, or rasping like squeaky leather

Heart murmurs. Heart murmurs are abnormal sounds that occur during systole or diastole. They are produced mainly by an increase in blood flow or by the crossing of blood through defective heart valves. Blood flow that becomes diminished or increased sets up vibrations within the heart or in the walls of the large vessels. A murmur can be heard around the area of sound transmission from the valve responsible for its production.

Murmurs can be illustrated by the way that they appear in a phonocardiogram, with a series of vertical lines either in systole (between S_1 and S_2) or in diastole (between S_2 and S_1). These lines are drawn to indicate the loudness (intensity) of the sound, the increase or decrease in the sound, and the duration of the sound. See Figures 16-33 through 16-42 for examples of murmur illustration.

MECHANISMS OF MURMUR PRODUCTION. Four main factors are related to murmur production (Figure 16-33):

1. Increased flow rate of blood across a normal valve (Figure 16-33, A)
2. Forward flow through a stenotic valve or into a dilated vessel or chamber (Figure 16-33, B)
3. Backflow, or regurgitant flow, through an incompetent, or insufficient, valve (Figure 16-33, C) (the terms *incompetent* and *insufficient* are used interchangeably)
4. Flow through an abnormal opening, such as a septal defect or a patent ductus arteriosus (Figure 16-33, D).

These factors may be combined.

HEART VALVE ALTERATIONS. Adequate opening and closing of the valves and the opening size determine the characteristics of murmurs. Heart valves that are functioning normally and competently permit forward flow of blood and prevent backflow, or regurgitation. To understand murmurs, it is necessary to understand the positions and movements of the valves and the flow of blood during the cardiac cycle.

The positions of valves during ventricular systole are:
Mitral and tricuspid valves close, preventing backflow to the atria
Aortic and pulmonic valves open, permitting forward flow into the aorta and pulmonary artery

The position of valves during ventricular diastole are:
Mitral and tricuspid valves are open, permitting blood flow from the atria to the ventricles
Aortic and pulmonic valves are closed, preventing backflow from the aorta and pulmonary artery into the ventricles

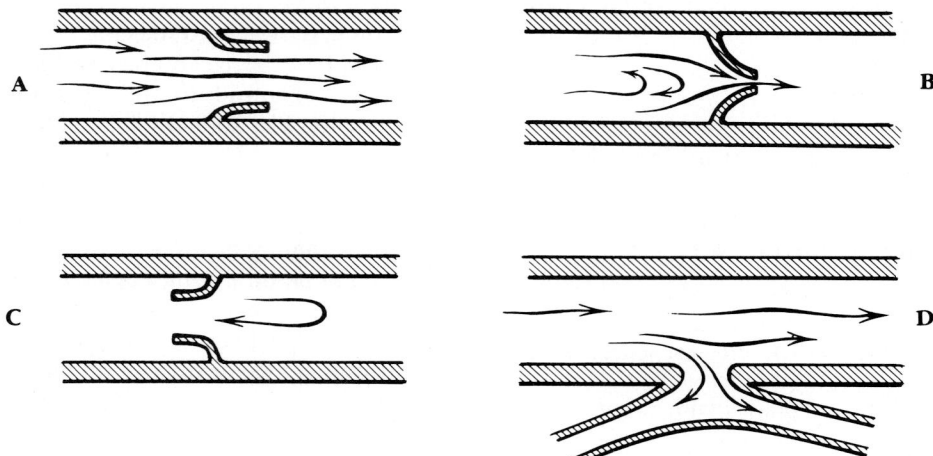

FIGURE 16-33 Mechanisms of murmur production. **A,** Increased flow across a normal valve. **B,** Forward flow through a stenotic valve. **C,** Backflow (regurgitation) through an incompetent valve. **D,** Flow through an abnormal opening such as a septal defect or an arteriovenous fistula (patent ductus arteriosus).

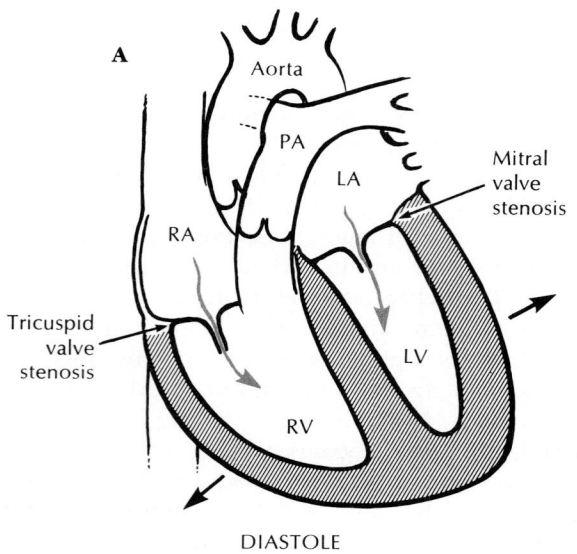

DIASTOLE

FIGURE 16-34 Mitral or tricuspid valve stenosis produces a diastolic murmur.

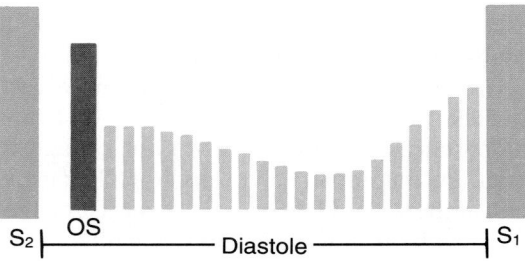

S_2 OS —————— Diastole —————— S_1

FIGURE 16-35 Diastolic murmur of mitral valve stenosis.

A stenotic mitral valve or tricuspid valve interferes with the forward flow of blood from the atrium to the ventricle during ventricular diastole (Figure 16-34). Mitral or tricuspid valve stenosis produces a diastolic murmur (Figure 16-35).

Stenotic valves are constricted or narrowed. They prevent adequate forward flow of blood. Incompetent or insufficient valves do not close completely during the phase of the cardiac cycle when their leaflets should form a tight seal. They leave an opening through which blood flows inappropriately back from the ventricles to the atria or from the aorta or pulmonary artery back to the ventricles. This difficulty with forward flow or inappropriate backflow of blood produces turbulence of the bloodstream and vibrations of the valve and myocardium that result in murmurs.

TYPE OF MURMUR IN RELATION TO DEFECT	
Valve defect	**Type of murmur**
Mitral stenosis	Diastolic
Mitral insufficiency	Systolic
Tricuspid stenosis	Diastolic
Tricuspid insufficiency	Systolic
Aortic stenosis	Systolic
Aortic insufficiency	Diastolic
Pulmonic stenosis	Systolic
Pulmonic insufficiency	Diastolic

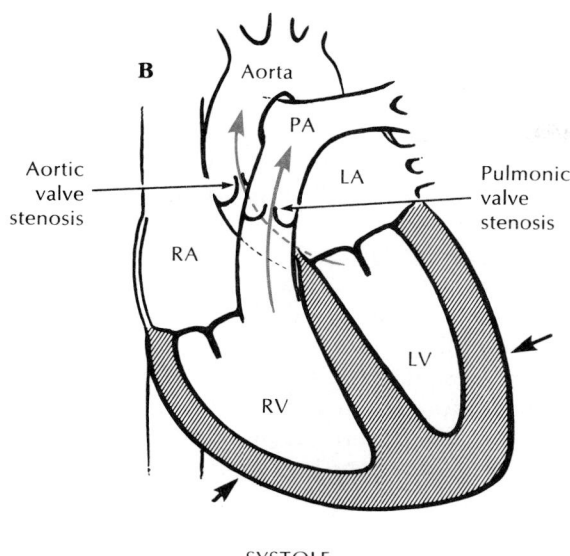

SYSTOLE

FIGURE 16-36 Aortic or pulmonic valve stenosis.

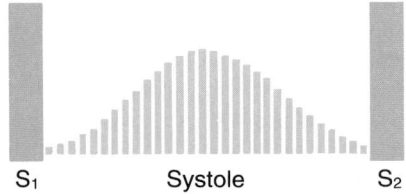

S₁   Systole   S₂

FIGURE 16-37 Murmur of aortic valve stenosis.

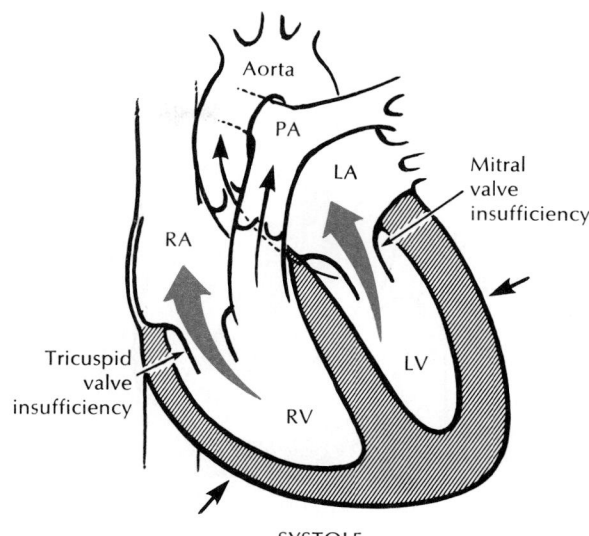

SYSTOLE

FIGURE 16-38 Mitral or tricuspid valve insufficiency.

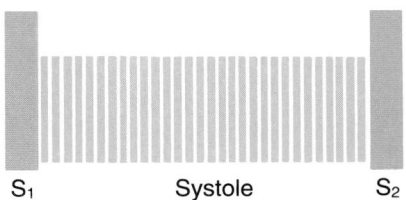

S₁   Systole   S₂

FIGURE 16-39 Holosystolic regurgitant murmur of mitral or tricuspid valve insufficiency.

A stenotic aortic or pulmonic valve prevents adequate forward flow of blood from the ventricles to the aorta or pulmonary artery during ventricular systole (Figure 16-36). Aortic stenosis produces a midsystolic ejection murmur (Figure 16-37).

An incompetent mitral or tricuspid valve permits the inappropriate backflow of blood from the ventricle to the atrium during ventricular systole (Figure 16-38). This backflow is referred to as regurgitation. Mitral or tricuspid valve incompetency produces a holosystolic murmur, a murmur that occurs throughout all of systole (Figure 16-39).

An incompetent aortic or pulmonic valve permits the backflow of blood from the aorta or pulmonary artery to the ventricle (Figure 16-40). Aortic valve incompetency produces a diastolic murmur (Figure 16-41).

CHARACTERISTICS OF MURMURS. Murmurs are described and classified according to the following characteristics:

Timing (systolic or diastolic)
Pitch (frequency)
Loudness (intensity)
Location

Radiation
Quality
Effect of respiration

TIMING. Record the timing of murmurs, as occurring during systole or diastole, or both. Timing can be further characterized according to how much of systole or diastole a murmur occupies. A murmur may last the entire phase of systole or diastole, or it may occur during the early, middle, or late component of the cycle. Murmurs that last throughout the entire cycle are called holosystolic (pansystolic) or holodiastolic (pandiastolic). Early diastolic murmurs are referred to as protodiastolic, and late diastolic murmurs are called presystolic.

In general, systolic murmurs are caused by stenotic aortic or pulmonic valves or by incompetent mitral or tricuspid valves, and diastolic murmurs are produced by stenotic mitral or tricuspid valves or by incompetent aortic or pulmonic valves.

PITCH (FREQUENCY). The pitch of murmurs varies from high to low. The main determining factor is the velocity of blood flow. Generally, when the rate of flow is rapid, a high pitch results; when the velocity is slower,

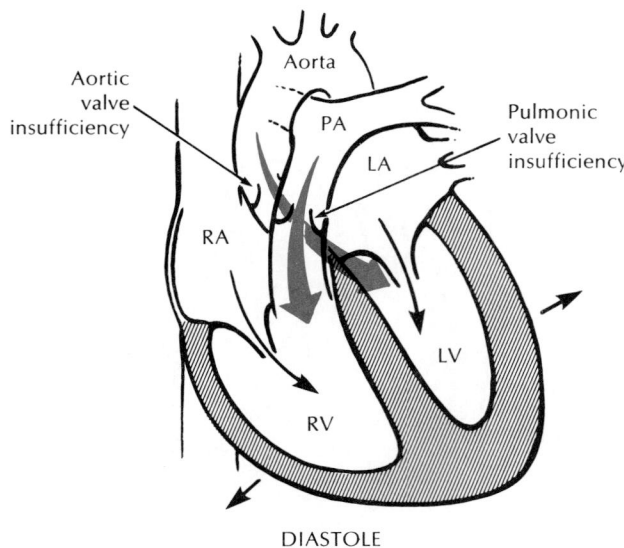

FIGURE 16-40 Aortic or pulmonic valve insufficiency.

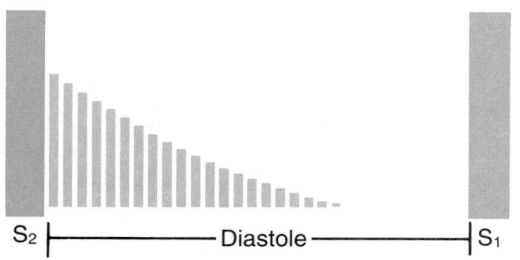

FIGURE 16-41 Diastolic murmur of aortic valve insufficiency.

the pitch is low. The pitch of a murmur should be described as high, medium, or low.

LOUDNESS (INTENSITY). Describe the loudness of a murmur on a scale of one to six: one is the softest and six is the loudest. The description of each level is as follows:

Grade I — Very faint, barely audible; can be heard only with special effort

Grade II — Quiet but clearly audible

Grade III — Moderately loud

Grade IV — Loud; thrill may be present

Grade V — Very loud; may be heard with stethoscope partly off the chest wall; thrill palpable

Grade VI — Loudest possible; audible with the stethoscope just removed from contact with the chest wall; thrill palpable

Note: Although grading the loudness of a murmur is helpful, it is also a subjective description. Differences in the hearing and experience of examiners affect the grade assigned.

The terms *crescendo* and *decrescendo* are used to describe the pattern of loudness that reflects changes in the blood flow rate. A crescendo murmur increases from quiet to louder. A decrescendo murmur decreases from louder to quieter. A crescendo-decrescendo murmur increases from quiet to louder and then decreases again. An example of a crescendo-decrescendo murmur is the murmur of aortic stenosis (see Figure 16-37). It increases, reaches a peak, and then decreases. An example of a decrescendo murmur is the diastolic murmur of aortic insufficiency, which begins loud and tapers off (see Figure 16-41).

LOCATION. Describe the location of a murmur by using the anatomical landmarks of the area where you can best hear it. Some murmurs are localized to small areas; others are heard over large portions of the precordium. Usually you can hear a murmur originating from a diseased valve best in the area to which sounds from that valve are transmitted. For example, the murmur of aortic valve stenosis is most audible in the area of the second right intercostal space.

RADIATION. The sound of a murmur may radiate beyond the area where you can hear it best. Factors affecting radiation include the direction of the bloodstream, the velocity of bloodflow, and the sound transmission through various tissues. For example, you can hear the diastolic murmur of aortic insufficiency best at the second right intercostal space with radiation along the left sternal border.

QUALITY. Several descriptive terms are traditionally used to describe a murmur. These include *musical, harsh, blowing,* and *rumbling.* For example, the murmur of aortic valve stenosis may be harsh, that of mitral insufficiency may be blowing, and that of mitral valve stenosis may be rumbling.

EFFECT OF RESPIRATION. As discussed earlier, events on the right side of the heart are affected by respiration. This effect is a result of intrathoracic pressure changes and subsequent right-sided filling changes. Murmurs that originate on the right side of the heart are also subject to influence by these factors. For example, the murmur of tricuspid insufficiency may increase with inspiration when the volume of return blood flow increases.

SYSTOLIC AND DIASTOLIC MURMURS. The more common murmurs that occur during systole or diastole are described here.

SYSTOLIC MURMURS. Murmurs occurring during ventricular systole result from any of the following factors:

1. Increased blood flow across a normal valve
2. Blood flow across an altered valve
3. Septal defect

Systolic ejection murmurs may occur within a normal cardiovascular system or may be caused by stenosis of

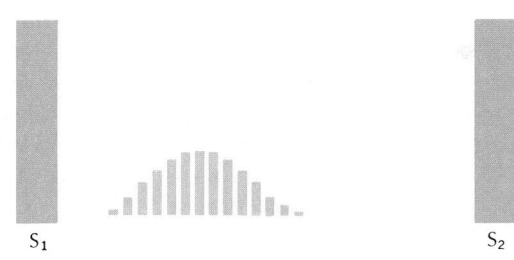

S_1 S_2

FIGURE 16-42 Midsystolic ejection murmur.

the aortic or pulmonic valve. Those occurring within a normal cardiovascular system are called *innocent systolic ejection murmurs*. These murmurs are common in children and adolescents. They may also occur with other high cardiac output states, including pregnancy, anxiety, anemia, fever, and thyrotoxicosis. They reflect the contractile force of the heart that results in greater blood flow velocity during early systole or midsystole. Because a short time interval exists between the closing of the AV valves (S_1) and the opening of the semilunar valves, systolic ejection murmurs begin after the first heart sound, reflecting the ejection of blood during ventricular contraction. They end before the second heart sound. Because of this pattern, they are called midsystolic ejection murmurs (Figure 16-42). You can hear innocent systolic ejection murmurs best by placing the bell of the stethoscope lightly against the chest in the area of the second left intercostal space and along the left sternal border. These murmurs tend to be short, rarely extending throughout systole. They are quieter than grade III murmurs, are of medium pitch, and have a blowing quality. They increase when expiration is held, may change with position, and may be most clearly audible when the client is in the recumbent position. S_1 and S_2 remain unchanged.

Stenotic aortic or pulmonic valves make it difficult for the blood to flow from the ventricles to the aorta and pulmonary artery during ventricular systole (see Figure 16-36). Stenosis of these valves results in midsystolic ejection murmurs (see Figure 16-37). The murmur of aortic valve stenosis begins after the first heart sound, when the pressure in the ventricle is high enough to open the aortic valve, and it ends before the aortic valve closes. This murmur has a crescendo-decrescendo pattern. The murmur is medium-pitched and harsh. It may be faint to loud. You can hear it best with the diaphragm of the stethoscope placed at the first or second right intercostal space with the client sitting up and leaning forward and holding the breath in expiration. If the murmur is loud, you may hear it over the entire thorax; it is often accompanied by a thrill. Other findings associated with the systolic murmur of aortic stenosis include a palpable thrill, the sustained thrusting apical impulse of left ventricular hypertrophy, a diminished second heart sound, an early ejection click, a slowly rising carotid pulse wave, and narrow pulse pressure.

Systolic regurgitant murmurs result from incompetent AV valves that do not prevent backflow of the blood from the ventricles to the atria during ventricular systole. They reflect the flow of blood from a high pressure to a low pressure area, and they last as long as there is a sufficient pressure gradient across the incompetent valve. Those murmurs that last throughout systole are called holosystolic, or pansystolic, regurgitant murmurs (see Figure 16-39). The murmur of **mitral regurgitation** is usually loudest at the apex and often radiates to the left axilla. It has a blowing quality. This murmur does not increase with respiration. The first heart sound varies according to the condition of the mitral valve. The second sound may be normal or accentuated. A third heart sound may be present.

The systolic murmur resulting from a ventricular septal defect reflects the flow of blood from a high pressure area to a low pressure area: from the left ventricle to the right ventricle. This type of murmur is most audible at the fourth, fifth, and sixth intercostal spaces at the left sternal border. It is high-pitched and harsh and may be accompanied by a thrill.

DIASTOLIC MURMURS. Diastole is normally free of murmurs, and therefore a diastolic murmur indicates a diseased valve. Causes of diastolic murmurs include incompetent aortic or pulmonic valves and stenotic mitral or tricuspid valves. An incompetent aortic or pulmonic valve permits backflow of blood from the aorta or the pulmonary artery into the ventricle during ventricular diastole (see Figure 16-40). Mitral or tricuspid valve stenosis prevents the adequate forward flow of blood from the atria into the ventricles during ventricular diastole (see Figure 16-34). Diastolic murmurs may occur during early, middle, or late diastole. Early diastolic murmurs are usually produced by aortic or pulmonic valve insufficiency. Middle and late diastolic murmurs are usually caused by mitral or tricuspid valve stenosis.

The diastolic regurgitant murmur of aortic valve insufficiency begins with the aortic component of the second heart sound, A_2. As the pressure in the aorta falls and the ventricles fill, the murmur decreases in loudness (see Figure 16-41). It is a high-pitched, blowing, decrescendo murmur. You can hear it best with the diaphragm of the stethoscope placed in the area of the second right intercostal space. Have the client lean forward and hold his or her breath in deep expiration.

The diastolic murmur of mitral valve stenosis reflects a narrowed valve opening that interferes with the flow of blood from the left atrium to the left ventricle (see Figure 16-34). This middiastolic murmur is loudest after the opening snap of the mitral valve (see Figure 16-

35). As the degree of stenosis increases, atrial contraction may force more blood across the valve at the end of ventricular diastole, immediately before the first heart sound. This murmur is low-pitched and rumbling or harsh. You can hear it best at the apex or just medial to and above the apex with the client in the left lateral position. Use the bell of the stethoscope, touching it lightly to the skin. Heavy pressure on the bell may obliterate the sound of a faint diastolic murmur.

Coronary artery disease. Coronary artery disease results from **atherosclerosis** of the coronary arteries. It is characterized by inadequate perfusion, or ischemia, of a portion of the myocardium. Atherosclerosis is a disorder of lipid metabolism characterized by deposits of fat-containing substances along the inner walls of blood vessels and by smooth muscle cell proliferation. Advanced atherosclerosis of the coronary arteries always leads to ischemic heart disease, but lesser amounts of atherosclerotic changes in the coronary arterial walls may exist without producing disease of the myocardium. The location and degree of atherosclerotic lesions are important in determining whether clinically evident ischemia will develop. The extent of collateral circulation to the myocardium is another factor in the development of ischemic heart disease.

An inadequate blood supply to the myocardium results in mechanical and electrical alterations. Contractility of the myocardium is impaired. If it is limited to the ischemic portion, an asymmetrical, inefficient pattern of contraction occurs. The affected portion bulges out while the rest of the ventricle contracts. Ventricular wall compliance may decrease, impairing filling of the ventricle. Early electrical changes are in the repolarization process, which appear as inverted T waves and later by displacement of the ST segment. An additional significant consequence of an ischemic myocardium is ventricular irritability, which can result in premature ventricular systole, ventricular tachycardia, and **ventricular fibrillation.** Most sudden deaths from ischemic heart disease are from ventricular **arrhythmias.**

Angina pectoris is a clinical syndrome characterized by chest pain. The majority of individuals affected by angina pectoris are men in their fifties and sixties. A complete and detailed history of the anginal attacks is essential in assessment of the client since the physical examination of individuals with angina pectoris typically reveals little about changes in the heart. The attacks typically follow a meal, exertion, or strong emotions.

The client may describe the chest symptoms as painful, aching, tightness, pressure, heaviness, burning, choking, or squeezing. The sensations may feel like indigestion or heartburn. Anginal pain is not described as knifelike or sharp. Most individuals indicate the lo-cation as retrosternal or slightly to the left of the sternum. The pain may radiate to the left shoulder and upper arm and may travel to the inner aspect of the left arm, elbow, jaw, or epigastric area. The client may experience pain only in the area of radiation and not in the substernal area. Anginal attacks usually last several minutes, but they may continue for 15 to 20 minutes if precipitated by extreme anger or a heavy meal. The relationship of angina to exertion and emotion is significant since these factors produce the discomfort and rest relieves it. Nitroglycerin also relieves the pain. Other symptoms that may accompany anginal pain include digestive disturbances, dizziness, dyspnea, faintness, pallor, palpitations, and sweating.

Myocardial infarction is an obstruction of circulation to some portion of the heart that may be caused by coronary artery disease, an **embolus** in the coronary artery, or spasm of the arteries supplying the heart. It is characterized by severe pain that usually involves the central area of the chest and may radiate to the arms, abdomen, back, jaw, and/or neck. Some myocardial infarcts, however, are without pain. Associated symptoms may include sweating, weakness, nausea, vomiting, dyspnea, light-headedness, restlessness, coolness of the extremities, and anxiety.

Physical examination findings vary but may include the following:

Tachycardia (although some individuals develop bradycardia of 40 to 50 beats/min)

Normal or diminished heart sounds

An extra heart sound (S_4 is the most common extra heart sound; S_3 is less common)

At the apex, a systolic murmur of mitral regurgitation resulting from papillary muscle dysfunction

Pericardial friction rub

Hypertension. Systemic hypertension is a sustained or intermittent elevation of the blood pressure above 140/90 mm Hg. It is often called the "silent disease" because persons with hypertension may have no symptoms. Even those persons who are aware of their condition may not receive adequate treatment or may not comply with the treatment prescribed. Persons with a blood pressure between 140/90 and 160/95 are considered borderline hypertensive. A single elevated reading does not indicate a diagnosis of hypertension; it means that further assessment is necessary. Blood pressure does vary with both physical and emotional activity.

Hypertension is classified according to type as systolic or diastolic and according to cause as primary (essential) or secondary. Systolic pressure represents the greatest pressure exerted by the blood against the arterial walls following ventricular contraction. With systolic hypertension only the systolic component is elevated. This elevation is associated with increased cardiac output and increased pulse pressure, which can result from a loss of elastic tissue and arteriosclerotic changes that occur in the arterial system with advancing age. Systolic hypertension can also be associated with anxiety, fever, hyperthyroidism, anemia, aortic regurgitation, and complete **atrioventricular (AV) block.**

Diastolic pressure represents the amount of pressure exerted on the arterial walls during the phase of ventricular relaxation. Diastolic hypertension (diastolic pressure greater than 90 mm Hg) can result from decreased space within the arterioles caused by atherosclerosis or vasoconstriction.

Primary, or essential, hypertension is the most common form, accounting for approximately 90% of persons with this health problem. Its cause remains unknown. Two mechanisms, however, are probably involved in its development: (1) an overactive sympathetic nervous system that accelerates cardiovascular function, and (2) sodium and water retention by the kidneys. In primary hypertension both systole and diastole are elevated.

Secondary hypertension results from numerous conditions, including kidney, endocrine, or central nervous system disorders or coarctation of the aorta. It may also be drug-induced.

The symptoms associated with hypertension vary. Many individuals have no symptoms. Some affected persons may experience headaches, dizziness, tinnitus, vague precordial discomfort, or palpitations. However, symptoms are not a reliable indicator of elevated blood pressure.

Physical examination findings vary with the degree of hypertension and the duration of the problem. During the early stages the physical examination may reveal nothing more than blood pressure elevation. If the disease has progressed, several organs may be affected. On palpation, the apical impulse may be forceful and displaced lateral to the left midclavicular line and lower than the fifth left intercostal space. On auscultation, an accentuated second sound may be heard at the base of the heart. Other auscultatory changes may include a systolic murmur. The client may have an apical systolic murmur caused by dilation of the subvalvular structures of the mitral valve, producing mitral regurgitation. Or the client may have an aortic systolic murmur resulting from dilation of the aortic valve ring or rapid flow of blood through a dilated aorta.

The pathological changes associated with untreated hypertension increase over time. The left ventricle develops hypertrophy and dilation because of increased peripheral resistance. These changes may lead to coronary insufficiency and myocardial infarction if the enlarged heart muscle exceeds its blood supply. Other systems that can be affected include the eyes, kidneys, and brain.

Heart failure. Heart failure is a condition in which the heart cannot pump enough blood in relation to the venous return or in relation to the metabolic requirements of the body. It may result from some defect in the heart or in the rhythmicity pattern. Heart failure may be predominantly left-sided or right-sided. Peripheral edema develops with right-side heart failure. Pulmonary congestion and dyspnea develop with left-side heart failure. Pulmonary hypertension can lead to right heart hypertrophy and right ventricular failure. This condition is known as **cor pulmonale.** The dysfunction of the heart produces changes in other organs, including the lungs, kidneys, and liver. On physical examination, changes may be found related to cardiac function and/or the effects on the other organs. Cardiac findings associated with heart failure may include heaves, lifts, or displacement of the apical impulse caused by ventricular hypertrophy; an audible S_3; and distention of the jugular veins. Findings in other organs include edema, ascites, enlargement of the liver, moist rales, and bronchial wheezing.

Neck Vessels
Variations of jugular venous pulse wave

Variations in a wave. The a wave, the highest or most pronounced of the venous waves, is increased when it becomes more difficult for the contracting right atrium to empty into the right ventricle. This development occurs with tricuspid valve stenosis. The most common cause of a prominent a wave is decreased compliance of the right ventricle secondary to right ventricular hypertrophy. Irregularly enlarged a waves result from complete AV block. When the atrium contracts against a closed tricuspid valve, giant, or cannon, a waves are produced.

Variations in x descent and c and v waves. An incompetent tricuspid valve permits backflow of blood from the right ventricle to the right atrium during ventricular systole. This increased backflow obliterates the x slope, which is replaced by an enlarged combined c-v wave. With severe disease, the wave may become as large as a bounding carotid pulsation.

Variations of y descent. The tricuspid valve opens shortly after S_2, and the rapid filling phase of ventricular diastole begins. The characteristics of the y descent depend on right-sided pressure and volume and on resistance to flow across the tricuspid valve. Tricuspid stenosis produces a slow y descent because it obstructs right atrial emptying. In clients with severe heart failure in whom the venous pressure is extremely high, an exaggerated y wave is produced.

Variations of jugular venous pressure. Jugular veins that are distended when the client is not supine or only slightly elevated indicate increased central venous pressure. This increased pressure occurs with right-side congestive heart failure, constrictive pericarditis, or obstruction of the superior vena cava. Applying pressure over the abdomen that results in jugular venous distention indicates right-side heart failure. This maneuver is the hepatojugular reflex.

Venous hum. The venous hum is a continuous, low-pitched humming sound heard over the major veins at the base of the neck in many children and in some adults. It usually has no pathological significance. It is produced by turbulent blood flow in the internal jugular veins. The venous hum is most audible over the supraclavicular spaces, more commonly in the right supraclavicular space (Figure 16-43). Auscultation can be improved by turning the client's head away and slightly upward from the side being auscultated. The hum is loudest during diastole. Because it is produced by blood flow in the jugular veins, the hum can be stopped by applying gentle pressure over the internal jugular vein in the neck between the trachea and the sternocleidomastoid muscle at approximately the level of the thyroid cartilage.

Variations of carotid pulse. The carotid pulse, like all other pulses in the body, may vary in rate, rhythm, and amplitude. The variations in the pulse are covered in the discussion of variations in the peripheral arterial

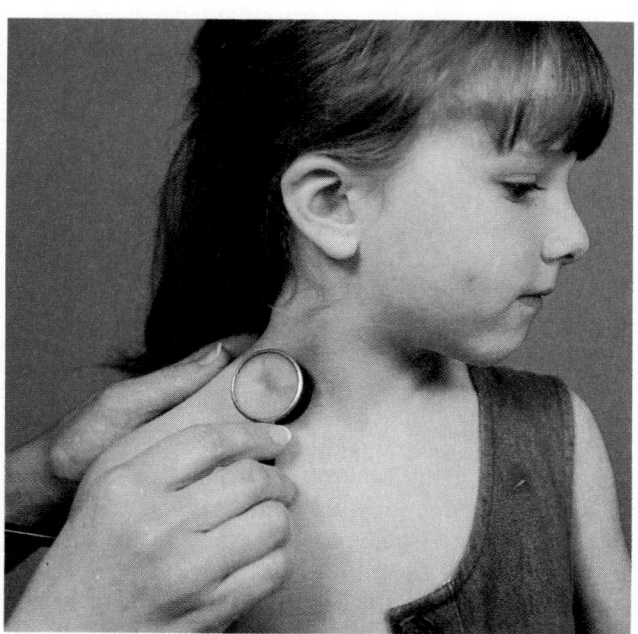

FIGURE 16-43 Venous hum. A continuous, low-pitched hum noted over the neck in many children, it is often best heard over the right supraclavicular space.

pulse. All these variations, except for **pulse deficit,** are assessed in carotid arteries. The **pulsus bisferiens** can be determined best at the carotid arteries.

A bruit heard over the carotid artery on auscultation indicates turbulence having a local vascular cause such as atherosclerotic narrowing. (A bruit is a sound similar to a murmur that is heard over an artery.) Some aortic valve murmurs radiate to the neck and may also be audible over the carotid arteries.

Peripheral Vessels

Variations of arterial pulse. Peripheral arterial pulses can vary in rate, rhythm, and amplitude. Exaggerated or bounding pulses are referred to as hyperkinetic. Diminished, thready, or weak pulses are referred to as hypokinetic. On palpation, an impression of variations can be sensed in the amplitude and changes in the upstroke and downstroke.

Tachycardia. Tachycardia is a heart rate greater than 100 beats/min. In the healthy client, tachycardia can be the result of exercise, anger, anxiety, or fear. Rates persistently greater than 100 beats/min suggest some abnormality. Heart rate is increased during fever, anemia, hypoxia, and low-volume states (shock).

The various types of tachycardia include the following:

Atrial flutter: rapid, regular, uniform atrial contraction caused by AV block; ventricular rhythm varies with the degree of blockage

Atrial tachycardia: arrhythmia caused by the atria; rapid, regular beat of the entire heart

Ventricular tachycardia: arrhythmia caused by the ventricles; rapid, relatively regular heartbeat

Bradycardia. A slow heart rate of fewer than 50 beats/min is known as **bradycardia.** The well-trained athlete normally has cardiac rates of fewer than 50 beats/min. Slow rates may indicate stimulation of the parasympathetic system or failure in the electrical conduction system of the heart. In addition, bradycardia may result from digitalis overdose.

For variations in the pulse discussed in the following seven sections, see Figure 16-44.

Weak, thready (hypokinetic) pulse. A weak pulse accompanies conditions in which there is a diminished stroke volume of the left ventricle, increased peripheral vascular resistance, narrowed pulse pressure, or resistance to flow across the cardiac valves. It may occur with left ventricular failure caused by myocardial infarction, constrictive pericarditis, and aortic valve stenosis. With aortic valve stenosis, the pulse has a slow upstroke and a delayed peak. This type of pulse may be difficult to palpate, with a tendency to fade out or

NORMAL PULSE

POSSIBLE CAUSE

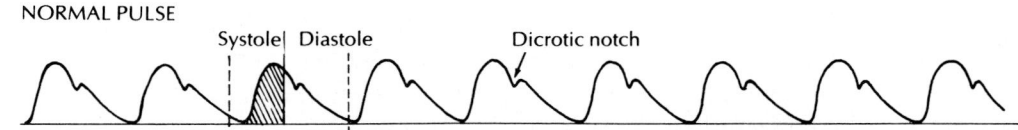

Partial arterial occlusion
Myocardial infarction
Myocarditis
Pericardial effusion shock
Stenosis of valyes: aortic,
mitral, pulmonic, tricuspid

Graphic recording of pulse pressure as obtained from electrical transducer. The normal pulse is easily palpable but may be obliterated by pressure. The wave of a single pulsation rises in systole, reaches a summit, and descends more slowly in diastole. The secondary rise in pressure, noted in diastole, is associated with closure of the aortic valve. The point at which the increase in pressure changes the downward slope is known as the dicrotic notch. This may not be palpable. The difference in pressure from the endpoint of diastole to the summit is the amplitude. Normal amplitude (30-40 mm Hg) is recorded as 2 + . A pulse of greater amplitude is called strong, and one of lesser amplitude is weak or faint.

SMALL, WEAK PULSE

Hypovolemia
Physical obstruction to
left ventricular output,
e.g., aortic stenosis

A weak pulse may be difficult to feel, and the vessel may be obliterated easily by the fingers. The pulse may "fade out" (be impalpable). This pulse is recorded as 1 + . The pulsation is slower to rise, has a sustained summit, and falls more slowly than the normal. A pulse that is weak and variable in amplitude is called thready.

LARGE, BOUNDING PULSE

Exercise
Anxiety
Fever
Hyperthyroidism
Aortic rigidity or
atherosclerosis

The large, bounding (also called hyperkinetic or strong) pulse is readily palpable. It does not "fade out" and is not easily obliterated by the examining fingers. This pulse is recorded as 3 + .

WATER-HAMMER PULSE

Patent ductus arteriosus
Aortic regurgitation

The water-hammer pulse (also known as collapsing) has a greater amplitude than the normal pulse, a rapid rise to a narrow summit, and a sudden descent.

PULSUS ALTERNANS

Left ventricular failure
More significant if pulse
slow

Pulsus alternans is characterized by alternation of a pulsation of small amplitude with the pulsation of large amplitude while the rhythm is normal.

FIGURE 16-44 Variations in arterial pulse.

BIGEMINAL PULSE

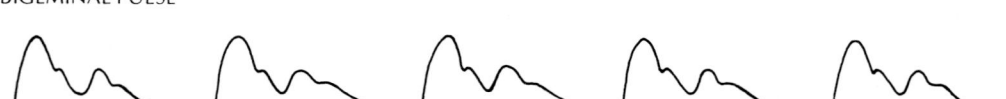

Bigeminal pulsations result from a normal pulsation followed by a premature contraction. The amplitude of the pulsation of the premature contraction is less than that of the normal pulsation.

PULSUS PARADOXUS

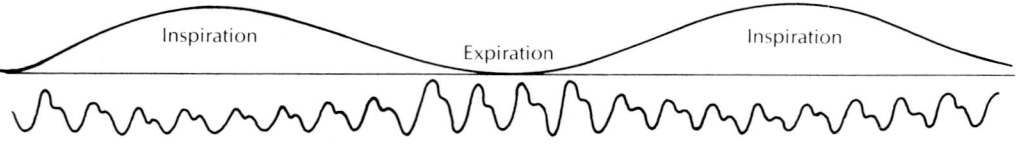

Pulsus paradoxus is characterized by an exaggerated decrease (>10 mm Hg) in the amplitude of pulsation during inspiration and increased amplitude during expiration. (See text for measurement with sphygmomanometer.)

PULSUS BISFERIENS

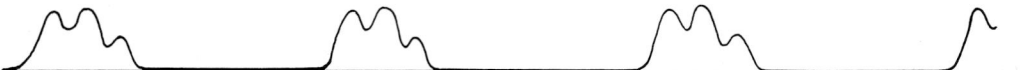

Pulsus bisferiens is best detected by palpation of the carotid artery. This pulsation is characterized by two main peaks. The first is termed percussion wave and the second, tidal wave. Although the mechanism is not clear, the first peak is believed to be the pulse pressure and the second, reverberation from the periphery.

IRREGULAR PULSE RHYTHM

Pulse deficit means that the number of pressure waves palpable at the peripheral vessel is less than the cardiac contractions.

POSSIBLE CAUSE

Disorder of rhythm

Premature cardiac contraction

Tracheobronchial obstruction
Bronchial asthma
Emphysema
Pericardial effusion
Constrictive pericarditis

Aortic stenosis combined
with aortic insufficiency

Cardiac arrhythmia
Atrial fibrillation
Atrial flutter with block
Second-degree heart block
Irregular sinus depolarization
Premature complexes
Weak, premature ventric-
ular contractions

FIGURE 16-44, cont'd; For legend, see p. 481.

disappear with touch; in fact, it can be easily obliterated with pressure.

Bounding (hyperkinetic) pulse. A bounding pulse is large and strong with a normal contour. It is associated with normal high-output states such as pregnancy, exercise, and anxiety, and with hyperthyroidism, fever, and anemia.

Water-hammer pulse. Water-hammer pulse has a greater amplitude than normal. It is characterized by a rapid rise to a narrow summit followed by a sudden descent. Also known as a collapsing pulse, water-hammer pulse is associated with aortic valve insufficiency and patent ductus arteriosus.

Pulsus alternans. With **pulsus alternans (alternating pulse),** the rhythm is regular but the ampli-

tude alternates between strong and weak beats. When the variation is marked, the alternation from weak to strong beats is palpable. However, to determine minor variations, it may be necessary to measure the blood pressure. The alternation of loud and soft sounds can be heard. Pulsus alternans is produced by left ventricular failure in which the contractile force varies.

Bigeminal pulse. A **bigeminal pulse** alternates in amplitude from beat to beat. A normal strong beat is followed by a premature small beat. The strong pulse occurs after a long diastolic filling phase that follows the premature beat. The pulse is irregular. This condition can be identified by simultaneously palpating the radial pulse and listening at the precordium. It is associated with a conduction disturbance such as premature atrial or ventricular contractions.

***Pulsus paradoxus.* Arterial pressure** fluctuates with the respiratory cycle, falling with inspiration and rising with expiration. With **pulsus paradoxus (paradoxical pulse)** beats have weaker amplitude with inspiration and stronger amplitude with expiration. The variation in arterial pressure can be determined best by measuring the blood pressure. When you hear the first *Korotkoff sound*, allow the pressure to decrease very slowly until the sound can be heard throughout the respiratory cycle. The decrease in arterial pressure during inspiration in the normal individual may be 10 ± 5 mm Hg. A difference greater than 15 mm Hg indicates pulsus paradoxus. This condition is associated with cardiac tamponade and constrictive pericarditis.

Pulsus bisferiens. In pulsus bisferiens each pulse has two strong peaks with a dip between them. This pulse is associated with combined aortic valve stenosis and insufficiency. The carotid artery is the best location to assess it.

Pulse deficit. A pulse deficit exists when the number of pressure waves palpable at the peripheral pulse point is less than the actual number of muscular contractions of the heart. Pressure waves initiated by weak, premature ventricular contractions may not be transmitted to the periphery. Simultaneous auscultation at the precordium and palpation at a peripheral pulse point reveal this deficit (Figure 16-45).

Peripheral atherosclerotic disease (arterial insufficiency). Lack of blood supply to the extremities may be caused by atherosclerotic plaques in the arteries and arterioles. Signs of an insufficient arterial supply to the peripheral tissues include decreased pulses or no pulses, pallor of an extremity, cutaneous ischemia, pain, aching or cramping (intermittent claudication) after exercise, skin ulcers, tissue death, or gangrene. Severe occlusion leads to pain in the leg or foot even at rest.

Arterial aneurysm. An **aneurysm** is a localized dilation of an artery resulting from weakness of the arterial wall. The aorta is the most common site for an aneurysm, but an aneurysm may also occur in other peripheral vessels. A bruit, thrill, or visible pulsation may be present over the site of the aneurysm.

Coarctation of aorta. Coarctation is a localized narrowing of the aorta. It results in increased pressure proximal to the narrowing and decreased pressure distal to the narrowing. Other symptoms and signs include dizziness, headaches, fainting, epistaxis, reduced or absent femoral pulses, and muscle cramps in the legs. Blood pressure in the arms will be higher than in the legs.

Temporal arteritis. Arteritis is an inflammatory condition of one or more layers of the arterial wall. Temporal arteritis usually affects individuals older than 50 years and is characterized by flulike symptoms, polymyalgia, ocular symptoms, and headache. The skin over the temporal artery becomes red, swollen, and tender. The temporal pulse may be strong, weak, or absent.

Raynaud's phenomenon. In **Raynaud's phenomenon**, intermittent spasm of the arterioles causes ischemia of the extremities, especially the fingers, toes, ears, and nose. Severe blanching may occur, followed by cyanosis, then redness. This condition may be accompanied by numbness, tingling, burning, and pain. The attack may last from minutes to hours. The skin may eventually become smooth, shiny, and tight, and ulcers may appear on the fingertips. Raynaud's phenomenon occurs most frequently in young, otherwise healthy women.

Edema. Edema is an accumulation of fluid in the tissues that changes the shape of the area affected. Inspect the lower extremities for edema by pressing your index finger over a bone such as the tibia or the medial malleolus of the ankle for several seconds. A depression in the skin that does not refill quickly indicates pitting (orthostatic) edema. Right-side heart failure leads to increased fluid volume, which, in turn, leads to edema in dependent parts of the body. Edema caused by congestive heart failure is bilateral. Pitting edema is not usually accompanied by thickening or pigmentation of the overlying skin. Edema accompanied by some thickening and ulceration of the skin is associated with deep venous obstruction or valvular incompetence. This type of edema occurs in the affected extremity.

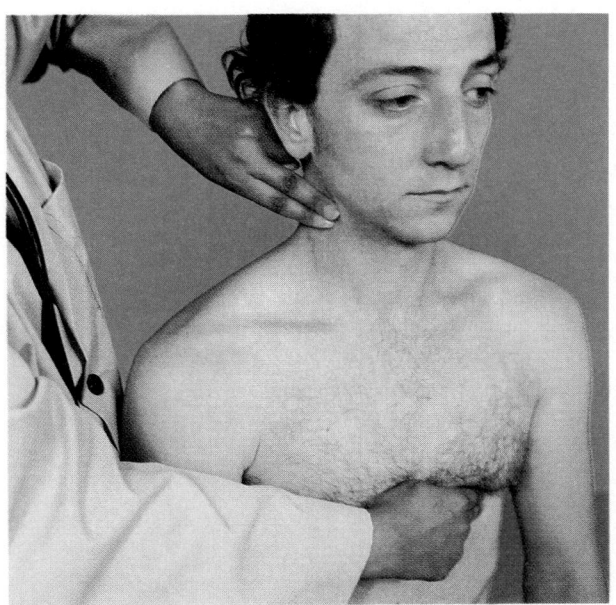

FIGURE 16-45 Testing for pulse deficit.

The degree of edema can be graded on a scale of 1 + to 4 + as follows:

1 +   Slight pitting; no visible change in the shape of the leg

2 +   Somewhat deeper pitting; no marked change in the shape of the leg

3 +   Pitting is deep; leg is full and swollen

4 +   Pitting is very deep; leg is very swollen

It is important to note the degree of edema and the scale that you are using.

Varicose veins. Varicose veins may result from a weakened vessel wall, incompetent venous valves, or an obstruction in a proximal vein. Inside the veins there is a decreased flow rate and an increased intravenous pressure. Superficial varicosities are readily visible on inspection, especially when the client is standing. The veins appear dilated, swollen, and tortuous.

Deep venous thrombosis. This condition is characterized by the presence of a clot in a vein. Thrombosis can occur gradually or suddenly. The symptoms vary. Tenderness along the affected vessel, swelling of the legs, or ankle edema may be noted. Measure both legs at the same distance from the patella, and test for a positive Homan's sign.

Homan's sign is positive when compressing the calf muscle or sharply dorsiflexing the foot causes pain. A positive Homan's sign is noted with both deep venous thrombosis and superficial thrombophlebitis, but it is also found with other conditions that affect the lower leg.

Thrombophlebitis. Thrombophlebitis, the inflammation of a vein, is often accompanied by formation of a clot. It occurs most commonly as a result of trauma to the vessel wall; hypercoagulability of the blood; infection; chemical irritation; postoperative venous stasis; prolonged sitting, standing, or immobilization; or a long period of intravenous catheterization. Thrombophlebitis of a superficial vein has the following characteristics:

The vessel feels hard and thready or cordlike and is extremely sensitive to pressure.

The surrounding area may be erythematous, edematous, and warm to the touch.

The entire limb may be pale, cold, and swollen.

TEACHING SELF-ASSESSMENT

Clients can be taught the skills of pulse assessment and blood pressure measurement. These skills may be particularly important for clients whose blood pressure needs to be monitored frequently and for those taking digitalis preparations or other cardiac medications that regulate the heart rate. Digital blood pressure kits are readily available for purchase. Clients with hypertension should be instructed to take their blood pressure not only when they think it is elevated but also on a regular schedule. Clients should be taught how to check their own pulse rate at either the carotid or the radial pulse site. They should be cautioned (1) not to put pressure on the carotid sinus, and (2) not to put pressure on both carotid pulses at the same time.

DOCUMENTATION

Sample Documentation

Present health status

White female, 80 years old, requests to have her "blood pressure and heart checked." She reports that she is generally in good health, not overweight, has been on various diuretics for about 25 years, which have controlled her hypertension. Currently on hydrochlorothiazide (50 mg daily). She states that she has no chest pain, shortness of breath, or cough. No edema or leg cramps. She experiences fatigue only "when I try to do too much," such as working in the garden, cleaning house, or attending more community meetings than usual.

Past health history

She reports no chronic illnesses other than hypertension. Smoked cigarettes during her 30s and 40s, but stopped about 35 years ago. Did have one transient ischemic attack about 15 years ago that lasted for about 1 minute while she was attending a movie. Angiogram performed that week showed that carotids were clear. No similar episodes since then. Blood lipids have always been within normal limits.

Family health history

Parents both died of stroke in their 80s. Father had diabetes controlled by diet.

Other considerations

She is active as a volunteer in the community, watches her weight, consumes some alcohol (1 to 2 glasses of wine per week), lives alone in her own home, reads, gardens, and visits with friends.

Physical examination

BP: 144/86 RAS (right arm, sitting)
   144/88 LAS (left arm, sitting)

Pulse: 82 (radial); full, regular rhythm; normal amplitude

Heart: no lifts, heaves, or retractions over precordium; apical impulse visible and palpable just lateral to MCL, 5th LICS, 2 cm in diameter

S_1 loudest at base; S_2 increased at apex; no S_3, S_4, extra sounds, or murmurs. Rhythm regular.

Neck vessels: jugular venous pulse wave normal, veins not distended. No bruits over carotids.

Pulses: temporal artery firm, nontender; radial, brachial, femoral, popliteal—all +2 (on scale of 3). Dorsal pedal and posterior tibial pulse not palpable. No signs of arterial or venous insufficiency in lower extremities.

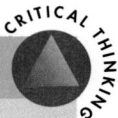

Nursing Diagnosis *THE NEXT STEP*

Nursing diagnoses that could apply to assessment of and alterations in the cardiovascular system include, but are not limited to, the following ones.

PAIN The state in which an individual experiences and reports the presence of severe discomfort or an uncomfortable sensation.

Defining Characteristics

- Subjective
  Communication (verbal or coded) of pain descriptors
- Objective
  Guarding behavior; protective
  Self-focusing
  Narrowed focus (altered time perception, withdrawal from social contact, impaired thought process)
  Distraction behavior (moaning, crying, pacing, seeking other people and/or activities, restlessness)
  Facial mask of pain (eyes lack luster, "beaten look," fixed or scattered movement, grimace)
  Alteration in muscle tone (may span from listless to rigid)
  Autonomic responses not seen in chronic, stable pain (diaphoresis, blood pressure and pulse rate change, pupillary dilation, increased or decreased respiratory rate)

Related Factors

- Injuring agents
  Biological
  Chemical
  Physical
  Psychological

CHRONIC PAIN The state in which an individual experiences pain that continues for more than 6 months.

Defining Characteristics

- Verbal report or observed evidence of pain experienced for more than 6 months
- Fear of reinjury
- Physical and social withdrawal
- Altered ability to continue previous activities
- Anorexia
- Weight changes
- Changes in sleep patterns
  Facial masks
  Guarded movement

Related Factor

- Chronic physical/psychosocial disability

HIGH RISK FOR FLUID VOLUME DEFICIT The state in which an individual is at risk of experiencing vascular, cellular, or intracellular dehydration.

Defining Characteristics (risk factors)

- Loss of blood volume through injury
- Deviations affecting access to fluids, such as physical immobility or unconsciousness
- Factors influencing fluid requirements, such as hyperthermia
- Knowledge deficit related to fluid volume needs
- Medications, such as diuretics

Continued.

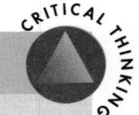

Nursing Diagnosis   *THE NEXT STEP—cont'd*

FLUID VOLUME DEFICIT The state in which in individual experiences vascular, cellular, or intracellular dehydration

Defining Characteristics
- Change in urine output or concentration
- Decreased venous filling
- Hypotension; decreased pulse volume/pressure
- Increased pulse rate
- Sudden weight loss
- Change in serum sodium concentration
- Weakness
- Lethargy
- Confusion
- Change in mental status

Related Factors
- Failure of regulatory mechanisms
- Active loss of body fluid

FLUID VOLUME EXCESS The state in which an individual experiences increased fluid retention and edema.

Defining Characteristics
- Edema, anasarca, effusion
- Sudden weight gain
- Change in mental status
- Intake greater than output, specific gravity changes, oliguria
- Shortness of breath, dyspnea, orthopnea
- Jugular venous distention
- Abnormal breath sounds (crackles, rales), changes in respiratory pattern
- Pulmonary congestion (on x-ray film)
- Decreased hemoglobin and hematocrit
- Electrolyte imbalance, azotemia
- Taught, shiny skin
- Restlessness and anxiety

Related Factors
- Compromised regulatory mechanisms
- Excess fluid or sodium intake

IMPAIRED TISSUE INTEGRITY The state in which an individual experiences damage to mucous membrane or corneal, integumentary, or subcutaneous tissue.

Defining Characteristics
- Damaged or destroyed tissue (integumentary or subcutaneous)

Related Factors
- Altered circulation
- Fluid excess/deficit
- Impaired mobility
- Knowledge deficit
- Nutritional deficit/excess
- Irritants

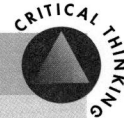

Nursing Diagnosis   *THE NEXT STEP—cont'd*

ACTIVITY INTOLERANCE The state in which an individual has insufficient physiological or psychological energy to endure or complete required or desired daily activities.

Defining Characteristics

- Verbal report of fatigue or weakness
- External discomfort or dyspnea
- Abnormal responses to activity: heart rate, blood pressure, or ECG changes reflecting ischemia or arrhythmias)
  Level I
    Walk, regular pace, on level indefinitely; one flight or more but more short of breath than normally
  Level II
    Walk one city block 500 feet on level; climb one flight slowly without stopping
  Level III
    Walk no more than 50 feet on level without stopping; unable to climb one flight of stairs without stopping
  Level IV
    Dyspnea and fatigue at rest

Related Factors

- Bedrest
- Immobility
- Sedentary life-style
- Imbalance between oxygen supply and demand
- Generalized weakness

FATIGUE An overwhelming sense of exhaustion and decreased capacity for physical and mental work regardless of adequate sleep.

Defining Characteristics

- Verbalization of unremitting and overwhelming lack of energy
- Inability to maintain usual routines
- Lethargy
- Listlessness
- Decreased performance (accident prone); perceived need for additional energy to accomplish routine tasks

Related Factors

- Altered body chemistry due to cardiovascular medications

IMPAIRED PHYSICAL MOBILITY The state in which an individual experiences a limitation of ability for independent physical movement.

Defining Characteristics

- Inability to move purposefully within physical environment (bed mobility, transfers, ambulation)
- Imposed restrictions of movement (mechanical or medical protocols)

Related Factors

- Intolerance to activity due to diminished cardiovascular performance

Continued.

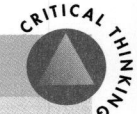

Nursing Diagnosis   *THE NEXT STEP—cont'd*

DECREASED CARDIAC OUTPUT   The state in which the blood pumped by an individual's heart is sufficiently reduced to the extent that it is inadequate to meet the needs of the body's tissues.

Defining Characteristics

- Cough, frothy sputum
- Variations in blood pressure reading
- Jugular vein distention
- Decreased peripheral pulses
- Arrhythmias
- Changes in skin color and temperature
- Restlessness
- Changes in mental status
- Rales
- Orthopnea
- Dyspnea
- Edema
- Gallop rhythm
- Syncope, vertigo
- Cold, clammy skin
- Oliguria

Related Factors

- Cardiac and extracardiac dysfunction or injury
- Electrical or mechanical dysfunction
- Structural alterations

ALTERED TISSUE PERFUSION: CEREBRAL, CARDIOPULMONARY, RENAL, GASTROIN-TESTINAL, PERIPHERAL   The state in which an individual experiences a decrease in nutrition and oxygenation at the cellular level due to a deficit in capillary blood supply.

Defining Characteristics

- Changes in mental status
- Cool extremities
- Oliguria
- Diminished arterial pulsations
- Angina
- Dyspnea
- Decreased peristalsis
- Claudication
- Bruits
- Slow-healing wounds/gangrene
- Lack of lanugo hair
- Shiny skin surfaces
- Changes in skin color and temperature
- Nausea/vomiting
- Edema
- Tachycardia
- Loss of sensory functions
- Extremities blue or purple when dependent; pale on elevation or color does not return on lowering leg
- Blood pressure changes in extremities

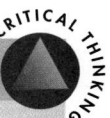

Nursing Diagnosis   *THE NEXT STEP—cont'd*

Related Factors

- Interruption of arterial flow
- Interruption of venous flow
- Exchange problems
- Hypovolemia
- Hypervolemia

ANXIETY A vague, uneasy feeling, the source of which is often nonspecific or unknown to the individual.

Defining Characteristics

- Subjective
    - Increased tension
    - Apprehension
    - Increased helplessness
    - Uncertainty
    - Fear
    - Feeling of being scared
    - Feeling of inadequacy
    - Shakiness
    - Fear of unspecific consequences
    - Regretfulness
    - Overexcitedness
    - Feeling of being rattled
    - Distress
    - Jitteriness
- Objective
    - Sympathetic stimulation—cardiovascular excitation, superficial vasoconstriction, pupil dilation
    - Restlessness
    - Insomnia
    - Glancing about
    - Poor eye contact
    - Trembling; hand tremors
    - Extraneous movements—foot shuffling; hand, arm movements
    - Expressed concern regarding changes in life events
    - Worry
    - Anxiety
    - Facial tension
    - Voice quivering
    - Focus on self
    - Increased wariness
    - Increased perspiration

Related Factors

- Unconscious conflict about essential values and goals of life
- Threat to self-concept
- Threat of death
- Threat to or change in health status
- Threat to or change in socioeconomic status
- Threat to or change in role functioning
- Threat to or change in environment
- Threat to or change in interaction patterns
- Situational and maturational crises
- Interpersonal transmission and contagion
- Unmet needs

Continued.

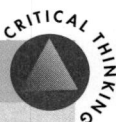

Nursing Diagnosis *THE NEXT STEP—cont'd*

Clinical Application

A 69-year-old male who has just transferred out of the cardiac intensive care unit. He is 4 days post inferior myocardial infarction. He is complaining of being tired all the time, short of breath when he gets up to the bedside commode, light-headed when he stands up, dark-colored urine, and a racing heart off and on.

SUBJECTIVE DATA: Patient complains of:
Fatigue and dyspnea with exertion
Dizziness and light-headedness when changing body positions
Dark-colored urine
Palpitations intermittently

OBJECTIVE DATA:
BP lying 100/60, standing 88/50
Heart rate at rest 110, with activity 150
Respirations are 24/minute at rest with 32/minute with activity
Cardiac monitor shows occasional premature ventricular contractions (PVCs)
Heart auscultation reveals S_3 at apical area
Lung auscultation reveals wet crackles bibasilar
Palpation of the dorsalis pedis pulses reveals trace or +1 diminished bilaterally
Capillary refill time >4 seconds bilaterally
24-hour intake 2200 ml and output 800 ml

NURSING DIAGNOSES

Decreased cardiac output related to cardiac injury (left ventricular infarction)

Defining Characteristics:
- Variation in blood pressure readings—low baseline BP, with orthostatic changes
- Decreased peripheral pulses
- Dysrhythmias
- Bibasilar crackles
- Dyspnea on exertion
- Vertigo
- Poor capillary refill

Altered peripheral tissue perfusion related to exchange problems

Defining Characteristics:
- Oliguria
- Diminished arterial pulsations
- Dyspnea
- Tachycardia
- Blood pressure changes in extremities

Fluid volume excess related to compromised regulatory mechanism, altered cardiopulmonary circulation.

Defining Characteristics:
- Intake greater than output
- Oliguria
- Shortness of breath
- Dyspnea on exertion
- Abnormal breath sounds (crackles in bibasilar lobe

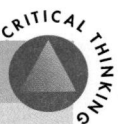

Nursing Diagnosis *THE NEXT STEP—cont'd*

Activity intolerance related to imbalance between oxygen supply and demand.

Defining Characteristics:

- Complaints of fatigue all the time—Level IV
- Change in blood pressure—orthostatic hypotension
- Dyspnea with exertion
- Heart rate increases significantly with activity
- Respirations increase significantly with activity

GLOSSARY

aneurysm Localized dilation of an artery. Most prominent and significant in the aorta but also occurs in peripheral vessels.

angina pectoris Pain that is substernal and/or radiating to the left arm, neck, or jaw; frequently correlated with myocardial ischemia. May be accompanied by a feeling of suffocation or impending death. Attacks are often related to exertion, emotional stress, or exposure to intense cold.

aortic valve Heart valve separating the left ventricle from the aorta.

apical impulse Pulsation of the apex of the heart against the chest wall, normally at the fifth left intercostal space in the midclavicular line.

arrhythmia Any deviation from the normal pattern of the heartbeat. Kinds of arrhythmias include atrial fibrillation, atrial flutter, heart block, premature atrial contraction, and sinus arrhythmia.

arterial insufficiency Inadequate supply of blood by way of the arteries to peripheral areas.

arterial pressure Force exerted by the blood against the arterial walls.

arteriosclerosis Common arterial disorder characterized by hardening, thickening, loss of elasticity, and calcification of arterial walls, resulting in a decreased blood supply, especially to the cerebrum and the lower extremities.

arteritis Inflammatory condition of the inner layers or the outer coat of one or more arteries.

atherosclerosis Type of arteriosclerosis characterized by deposits (atheromas) of cholesterol, lipoid material, and lipophages in the walls of large arteries and arterioles. This condition usually occurs with aging and is often associated with obesity, hypertension, and diabetes.

atrioventricular (AV) block Impairment of impulse conduction from the atria to the ventricles that occurs at the AV node or the bundle of His (or its branches).

atrioventricular (AV) valves Valves in the heart through which blood flows from the atria to the ventricles. The left AV valve is the mitral valve. The right AV valve is the tricuspid valve.

atrium (plural; atria) One of the two upper chambers of the heart. The right atrium receives deoxygenated blood from the superior and inferior vena cavae. The left atrium receives oxygenated blood from the pulmonary veins.

bigeminal pulse Abnormal pulse in which two beats in close succession are followed by a pause during which no pulse is felt.

bradycardia Circulatory condition in which the myocardium contracts steadily but at a rate of less than 50 beats/min.

bruit Murmur or blowing sound heard over the peripheral vessels indicating increased flow or stenosis of the vessel.

cholesterol Fat-soluble crystalline steroid alcohol found in animal fat, oil, and egg yolk. Increased levels of serum cholesterol may be associated with the pathogenesis of atherosclerosis.

chordae tendineae Strands of tendon attaching the atrioventricular valves to the papillary muscles at the heart.

claudication Weakness of the legs accompanied by cramplike pains in the calves caused by poor circulation of the blood to the leg muscles. This condition is exacerbated by walking.

coarctation Stricture or contraction of the walls of a vessel such as the aorta.

coronary artery disease Any one of the abnormal conditions that may affect the arteries of the heart and produce various pathological effects, especially the reduced flow of oxygen and nutrients to the myocardium.

cor pulmonale Right-side heart hypertrophy and right ventricular failure resulting from pulmonary hypertension.

cyanosis Bluish discoloration of the skin and mucous membranes caused by an excess of deoxygenated hemoglobin in the blood or a structural defect in the hemoglobin molecule.

dextrocardia Rare condition in which the position of the heart is reversed and lies on the right side of the chest.

diastole Time between contractions of the atria or the ventricles during which blood enters the relaxed chambers.

dicrotic notch The interval between the two peaks of a dicrotic pulse.

dicrotic pulse Presence of two sphygmographic waves to one beat of the pulse.

dyspnea Difficult or labored respiration.

edema Abnormal increase in the quantity of interstitial fluid.

ejection click High-pitched clicking sound produced by the forceful opening of a diseased aortic or pulmonic valve heard soon after the first heart sound.

embolism Sudden obstruction of an artery by a clot or other foreign substance. Symptoms vary with the degree of occlusion that the embolism causes, the character of the embolus, and the size, nature, and location of the occluded vessel.

embolus Foreign object, quantity of air or gas, bit of tissue or tumor, or piece of thrombus that circulates in the bloodstream until it becomes lodged in a vessel.

endocardium Lining of the heart chambers.

extrasystole Cardiac contraction that is abnormal in timing or in origin of impulse; premature contraction of the heart.

fibrillation Fine, continuous twitching caused by contraction of a single muscle or group of fibers. Fibrillation of a chamber of the heart results in inefficient random contraction of that chamber and disruption of the normal sinus rhythm of the heart. This condition is usually described by the part that is contracting abnormally (e.g., atrial fibrillation or ventricular fibrillation).

gallop rhythm Heart rate characterized by three sounds.

high-density lipoprotein (HDL) Plasma protein containing about 50% protein with cholesterol and triglycerides. It may serve to stabilize very low-density lipoprotein. Called "good" cholesterol, it is involved in transporting cholesterol and other lipids from the plasma to the tissues.

hypercholesterolemia Condition in which greater than normal amounts of cholesterol are present in the blood. High levels of cholesterol and other lipids may lead to the development of atherosclerosis.

hyperlipidemia Excess of lipids in the plasma.

hypertension Common, often asymptomatic disorder characterized by elevated blood pressure that persistently exceeds 140/90 mm Hg.

infarction Obstruction of circulation followed by ischemic necrosis.

insufficiency Inadequate closure of a heart valve resulting in backflow of blood into the ventricles or atria.

jugular venous pulse Pulse wave in the jugular veins reflecting cardiac activity on the right side of the heart.

Korotkoff sounds Turbulent sounds heard during auscultation done to determine blood pressure.

low-density lipoprotein (LDL) Plasma protein containing relatively more cholesterol and triglycerides than protein. Called "bad" cholesterol, it is involved with the formation of atherosclerotic plaques.

mediastinum Portion of the thoracic cavity in the middle of the thorax, between the pleural sacs that contain the two lungs.

mitral regurgitation Backward flow of blood from the left ventricle to the left atrium associated with an incompetent mitral valve.

mitral valve Left atriovertricular valve.

mitral valve stenosis Fibrosis and thickening of the cusps of the mitral valve with narrowing of the aperture between the left atrium and the left ventricle.

murmur Low-pitched blowing or humming sound caused by turbulence of blood flow; heard through the stethoscope over the heart or the great vessels.

myocardial infarction Occlusion of a coronary artery caused by atherosclerosis or thrombosis resulting in damage to the myocardium.

myocardium Thick, contractile middle layer of the heart; composed of muscle tissue that forms the bulk of this organ.

opening snap Snapping sound produced by the opening of a diseased mitral or tricuspid valve. It is an early diastolic sound heard soon after the second heart sound.

palpitation Pulsations of the heart and arteries that are perceptible to the client and are associated with normal emotional responses and certain heart disorders.

pericardium Fibrous sac that surrounds the heart and the roots of the great vessels.

precordium Area of the anterior chest wall overlying the heart and the great vessels.

pulmonic valve Heart valve separating the right ventricle from the pulmonary artery.

pulse Palpable rhythmic expansion of an artery caused by ejection of blood from the left ventricle during systole.

pulse deficit Condition that exists when the peripheral pulse count is less than the ventricular rate taken at the apex of the heart. It indicates a lack of peripheral perfusion for some of the heart contractions.

pulsus alternans (alternating pulse) Pulse characterized by a regular alternation of weak and strong beats without a change in the length of the cycle.

pulsus bisferiens Arterial pulse that has two palpable peaks, the second of which is slightly stronger than the first.

pulsus paradoxus (paradoxical pulse) Abnormal decrease in systolic pressure and pulse-wave amplitude during inspiration. The normal fall in pressure is less than 10 mm Hg. An excessive decline may be a sign of precordial tamponade, adhesive pericarditis, severe lung disease, advanced heart failure, or other conditions.

Raynaud's phenomenon Intermittent attacks of ischemia of the extremities, especially the fingers, toes, ears, and nose.

regurgitation Backward flow of blood through a defective heart valve.

S_1 First heart sound in the cardiac cycle. It is associated with closure of the mitral and tricuspid valves and is synchronous with the apical pulse. Auscultated at the apex, it is louder, longer, and lower than the second sound (S_2), which follows it.

S_2 Second heart sound in the cardiac cycle. It is associated with closure of the aortic and pulmonary valves immediately before ventricular diastole. Auscultated at the base of the heart, the second sound is louder than the first.

S_3 Third heart sound; related to early ventricular filling. Normally, this sound is audible only in children and physically active young adults. In older people it is an abnormal finding and usually indicates myocardial failure.

S_4 Fourth heart sound; related to late ventricular filling. This sound occurs late in diastole on contraction of the atria. Rarely heard in normal clients, it indicates an abnormally increased resistance to ventricular filling, as in hypertensive cardiovascular disease, coronary artery disease, myocardiopathy, and aortic stenosis.

semilunar valves Valves with half-moon–shaped cusps located between the ventricles and the great vessels. The left semilunar valve is the aortic valve. The right semilunar valve is the pulmonic valve.

systole Contraction of the heart.

tachycardia Rapid heart rate (more than 100 beats/min). Types of tachycardia include:

  atrial flutter Rapid, regular, uniform atrial contraction caused by AV block; ventricular rhythm varies with the degree of AV block.

  atrial tachycardia Arrhythmia caused by the atria; rapid, regular beat of the entire heart.

  ventricular tachycardia Arrhythmia caused by the ventricles; rapid, relatively regular heartbeat.

thrill Fine vibration accompanying turbulent blood flow in the heart or the great vessels. It is palpable when the examiner's fingers are placed over the site of the altered blood flow.

thrombophlebitis Inflammation of a vein.

thrombus Aggregation of platelets, fibrin, clotting factors, and the cellular elements of the blood attached to the interior wall of a vein or artery that sometimes occludes the lumen of the vessel.

transient ischemic attack Occlusion of a central nervous system vessel that results in a focal neurological disturbance.

tricuspid valve Right atrioventricular valve.

varicose Dilated, distended, or bulging. This term is used particularly to describe a vein.

ventricle One of two muscular pumping chambers of the heart. The left ventricle pumps blood into the aorta. The right ventricle pumps blood into the pulmonary artery.

ventricular fibrillation Cardiac arrhythmia marked by rapid, disorganized depolarizations of the ventricular myocardium.

ventricular tachycardia Tachycardia that usually originates in the ventricular Purkinje system.

BIBLIOGRAPHY

Andreoli KG and others: *Comprehensive cardiac care,* ed 6, St Louis, 1987, Mosby—Year Book.

Dennison R: Cardiopulmonary assessment, *Nursing 86* 16:4, 34—40, 1986.

Erickson B: *Heart sounds and murmurs: a practical guide,* ed 2, St Louis, 1991, Mosby—Year Book [book and audiocassette].

Ewy GA: Evaluation of the neck veins, *Hosp Pract* 22:3, 72—80, 1987.

Gordon M: *Manual of nursing diagnosis, 1993-1994,* St Louis, 1993, Mosby—Year Book.

Gordon M: *Nursing diagnosis: process and application,* ed 2, New York, 1987, McGraw-Hill.

Guzzetta CE, Dosey BM: *Cardiovascular nursing: body-mind tapestry,* St Louis, 1984, Mosby—Year Book.

Handerhan B: How to measure jugular venous distension, *Nursing 87* 17:9, 48—9, 1987.

Harris R: *Clinical geriatric cardiology,* ed 2, Philadelphia, 1986, JB Lippincott.

Heart sounds and common murmurs, *Am J Nurs* 88:12, 1679-1689, 1983.

Report of the US Preventive Services Task Force: *Guide to clinical preventive services: an assessment of the effectiveness of 169 interventions,* Baltimore, 1989, Williams & Wilkins.

Tobin MB: Cardiovascular assessment, *Orthop Nurs* 5:5, 35-41, 1986.

Yacone-Morton L: Cardiac assessment, *RN* 54:12, 28-35, 1991.

Abdomen

PURPOSE OF THE EXAMINATION

Because the abdominal cavity contains many of the body's vital organs, the abdominal examination provides information about a variety of systems. It yields direct and indirect information about the functioning of the gastrointestinal system and the genitourinary system. The examination may also reveal specific vascular anomalies, such as an aortic aneurysm, and inflammatory processes affecting various organs.

The screening examination includes a general survey of the organs for signs of tenderness, enlargement, masses, and other indications of dysfunction. Specific maneuvers allow the examiner to determine the source of symptoms such as abdominal pain and to delineate more clearly the characteristics of masses and other abnormal findings. Although directly examining many of the abdominal organs is difficult, some of the examination techniques provide indirect information about organ function. When abnormal findings are present,

further diagnostic studies and laboratory tests need to be conducted.

This chapter focuses on the abdominal portion of the gastrointestinal system. Chapter 12 addresses the mouth and throat examination and Chapter 22 describes assessment of the anus and rectum.

ANATOMY AND PHYSIOLOGY

The abdomen, the largest body cavity, extends from the diaphragm to the lesser pelvis. It is bounded anteriorly by the abdominal muscles, the costal border, and the superior border of the pelvis and posteriorly by the vertebral column and the lumbar muscles. The abdomen contains many of the body's vital organs: stomach, small and large intestines, liver, gallbladder, pancreas, spleen, kidneys, bladder, adrenal glands, uterus (in women), and major blood vessels (Figure 17-1). Because many major body organs are contained in this single cavity, susceptibility to organ dysfunction is in-

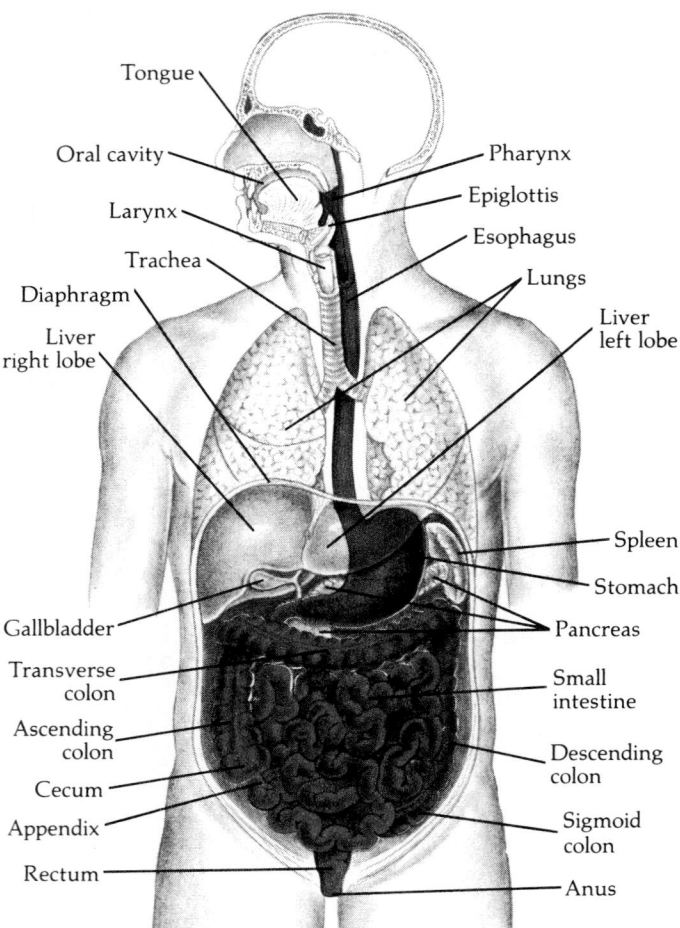

FIGURE 17-1 Anatomy of gastrointestinal system. (From Thompson JM, McFarland GK, Hirsch JE, and others: *Mosby's manual of clinical nursing*, ed 2, St. Louis, 1989, Mosby–Year Book.)

creased. Methodical and systematic evaluation is vital to distinguish variations from the norm.

Stomach

The stomach is located in the left upper quadrant of the abdomen, directly below the diaphragm. It is separated into three areas: (1) the fundus, located above and to the left of the cardiac sphincter; (2) the body, found directly below the fundus; and (3) the pyloric antrum, positioned proximal to the pyloric sphincter.

Two sphincters regulate the flow of substances into and out of the stomach. The cardiac sphincter controls the inflow of food from the esophagus into the stomach. The pyloric sphincter regulates the outflow of chyme to the duodenum.

The primary functions of the stomach are to store food, to mix digestive enzymes and hydrochloric acid, and to liquify food into chyme. Protein breakdown is initiated with the conversion of protein to peptones.

Intestines

The small intestine fills a major section of the abdominal cavity and extends from the pyloric sphincter to the ileocecal valve. It consists of three segments: the duodenum, the top portion; the jejunum, the middle portion; and the ileum, the lower portion. At the duodenum, bile and pancreatic secretions are received from the common bile duct for digestion. Absorption then takes place through the walls of the small intestine.

The large intestine extends from the ileocecal valve to the anus. It is composed of three segments: the cecum (with the vermiform appendix), the colon, and the rectum.

The cecum is located in the lower right quadrant of the abdomen. The vermiform appendix is a process extending from the lower part of the cecum. It is subject to infection and inflammation that can cause a rupture, expelling bacteria-laden substances into the abdominal cavity.

The colon frames the abdominal cavity. The ascending colon advances upward on the right side to the hepatic flexure. The transverse colon passes along the top of the abdominal cavity anterior to the liver and the stomach. The colon curves downward at the splenic flexure. The descending colon progresses to the brim of the pelvis, where it unites with the sigmoid colon and proceeds to the rectum and anus.

Liver

The liver lies primarily within the right hypochondrium and epigastrium, with a small portion situated in the left hypochondriac region. It is situated beneath the diaphragm. The rib cage covers a substantial part of the liver, with only the lower margin left exposed. The liver spans the upper quadrant of the abdomen from the fifth intercostal space to slightly below the costal margin.

The liver performs the following functions:
1. Produces and secretes bile.
2. Plays a major role in regulating blood glucose levels.
3. Maintains an important part in protein, carbohydrate, and lipid metabolism.
4. Stores vitamins—A, B_{12} and other B-complex vitamins, and D—and various minerals such as iron and copper.
5. Synthesizes most plasma proteins, such as serum albumin, serum globulin, fibrinogen, and blood-clotting factors.
6. Is instrumental in the detoxification of many substances, including drugs.

Gallbladder

The gallbladder is located on the inferior surface of the liver. A pear-shaped sac, it acts as a reservoir for bile secreted from the liver. The gallbladder concentrates the bile by absorbing excess water through its walls.

The gallbladder is drained by the cystic duct. The cystic duct unites with the hepatic duct to form the common bile duct, which passes downward into the duodenum.

Pancreas

Immediately below the liver lies the pancreas. The pancreas is situated posterior to the greater curvature of the stomach in front of the first and second lumbar vertebrae.

The pancreas has both an exocrine and an endocrine function. The endocrine secretions from the islets of Langerhans produce insulin, glucagon, and gastrin, which are used in carbohydrate metabolism. The exocrine secretions from the acinar cells produce bicarbonate and pancreatic enzymes necessary for digestion and absorption in the small intestine.

Spleen

Located to the left of the stomach and directly above the kidney in the left upper abdominal quadrant is the spleen. The spleen has numerous functions, but its four primary ones are as follows:

1. Acts as a blood reservoir for 1% to 2% of the red blood cell mass.
2. Removes old or agglutinated red blood cells and platelets.
3. Is partially responsible for iron metabolism.
4. Helps produce erythrocytes outside the bone marrow in the fetus and during bone marrow depression.

Kidneys, Ureters, and Bladder

Covered by peritoneum and embedded in fat, the kidneys are located in the dorsal part of the abdomen between the twelfth thoracic and third lumbar vertebrae. The right kidney is slightly lower than the left one. The kidneys measure approximately 11 cm long, 5 to 7.5 cm wide, and 2.5 cm thick.

The nephron is the working unit of the kidney. Its structure consists of the glomerulus and the tubular system. Filtration occurs at the glomerular membrane, whereas reabsorption and secretion of essential materials takes place in the tubular system.

The kidneys are drained by the ureters and empty into the bladder. The ureters pass anteriorly along the psoas major muscles toward the pelvis. These tubes enter the bladder at the posterolateral aspect. Peristaltic action propels the urine downward to the bladder.

Located behind the symphysis pubis in the anterior half of the pelvis is the bladder, which has a maximum storage capacity of 1000 to 1800 ml. Moderate distention is felt when the bladder contains approximately 250 ml of urine, and discomfort is experienced with 400 ml. When distended, the bladder will rise above the level of the pubic bone.

Peritoneum

The peritoneum is a serous membrane that covers and protects the abdominal cavity. It is divided into two layers, the parietal and the visceral peritoneum. The parietal peritoneum lines the abdominal wall, and the visceral peritoneum covers the organs in the abdomen. The mesentery and the omentum are two folds of the peritoneum. The mesentery encircles the jejunum and the ileum and attaches them to the posterior abdominal wall. In addition, it supports blood vessels, lymphatic vessels, lymph nodes, and nerves. The greater omentum is connected to the upper border of the duodenum, to the lower edge of the stomach, and to the transverse colon. Its function is to protect and insulate. The lesser omentum is attached between the liver and the stomach.

Peritonitis is an inflammation of the peritoneum, often associated with rupture of an intraabdominal viscus such as the appendix.

EXAMINATION

Health History

The health history related to the abdominal examination focuses on concerns related to the digestive system. The interviewer needs to ask both general questions about the client's health and specific questions that will vary according to the client's symptoms and the organs affected. Determining the client's primary concern is important because it guides the interview and will also influence the client's receptiveness to care. Because a client's nutritional practices, habits, and level of stress influence many gastrointestinal complaints, eliciting information about the client's life-style, perceived level of stress, and means of coping with stress is also important.

Chief complaint. The chief complaint is the client's immediate concern, the problem that he or she wants dealt with at this time.

Present health status

1. Nutrition: Appetite, recent change in eating pattern, recent (intentional or unintentional) weight loss or gain, food preferences, food intolerances, cultural influences on eating (foods commonly served or forbidden), life-style influences on intake, special diets, 24-hour dietary recall.

2. Allergies (food, medications).
3. Alcohol intake: Usual amounts, frequency.
4. Medications: Prescription and over-the-counter drugs, laxatives, antiemetics, stool softeners, antidiarrheal agents, antacids, high doses of aspirin, acetaminophen, or nonsteroidal antiinflamatory agents, corticosteroids, diuretics, or antihypertensives.
5. Cigarette smoking (number of packs/day and number of years of habit).
6. Stool characteristics: Frequency, consistency, color, odor.
7. Urinary characteristics: Frequency, urgency, color, odor, pain (dysuria, suprapubic, flank), ease of starting stream, force of stream, ability to empty bladder, dribbling, or episodes of incontinence.
8. Exposure to infectious diseases: Flu, hepatitis, gastroenteritis, family members or companions with similar symptoms, travel history.
9. Recent stressful life events: Social, psychological, and physical changes.
10. Possibility of pregnancy: Date of last menstrual period, use of contraceptives, unprotected intercourse.

Specific problems

Abdominal pain
1. Onset and duration: Specific date, sudden or gradual, persistent or recurrent, specific time of day or unpredictable.
2. Character: Burning, knifelike, cramping, aching.
3. Location: Radiation, change in location.
4. Quality: How bad is pain on a scale of 1 to 10 (with 10 being the worst pain)? Does it interfere with daily activities?
5. Course: Getting better or worse.
6. Associated symptoms: Vomiting, diarrhea, constipation, flatulence, belching, jaundice, fever, weight loss.
7. Alleviating or precipitating factors: Efforts to treat, medications or other interventions, patterns and effectiveness.

Nausea
1. Onset and duration: Related to particular stimuli (odors, time of day), relationship to food intake, date of last menstrual period.
2. Associated symptoms: Vomiting, dizziness, headache.

Vomiting
1. Onset and duration: Sudden or preceded by nausea, time elapsed since last meal, frequency.

2. Character: Nature of emesis (coffee grounds or fresh blood, color, undigested food), quantity, ability to keep fluids or solids in stomach, force (projectile).
3. Associated symptoms: Nausea, fever, headache, previous meal, weight loss, abdominal pain.
4. Exposures: Any family members or companions experiencing similar symptoms.

Indigestion
1. Onset: Relationship to meals, time of day or night, sudden or gradual.
2. Character: Bloated feeling after eating, excessive belching or flatulence, heartburn, loss of appetite, severe pain.
3. Location: General or localized, radiation to shoulders or arms.
4. Associated symptoms: Vomiting, headache, diarrhea.
5. Alleviating or precipitating factors: Association with type or quantity of food, response to antacids, rest, activity, other self-care measures.

Diarrhea
1. Onset and duration: Gradual or sudden, frequency of stools, number per day, any change in usual pattern of bowel movements.
2. Characteristics: Watery; explosive; color; presence of mucus, blood, undigested food, or fat; odor.
3. Course: Improving or getting worse.
4. Associated symptoms: Fever, chills, weight loss, abdominal pain, thirst, recent course of antibiotics.
5. Alleviating or precipitating factors: Follows a specific pattern related to food intake or stressful encounters; self-care measures attempted and their effectiveness.

Constipation
1. Onset and duration: Recent occurrence or long-standing problem, sudden or gradual, last bowel movement.
2. Character: Dry, hard stools; number of bowel movements per week; change in size or pattern of stools; black or tarry or associated with bright blood; accompanied by abdominal or rectal pain, alternating with diarrhea.
3. Associated symptoms: Abdominal pain, depression.
4. Course: Continuous or intermittent problem.
5. Alleviating or precipitating factors: Diet (recent change in intake, increase or decrease in fiber, fluid intake); use of enemas, laxatives, or stool softeners; response to self-care measures.

Dysuria

1. Onset: Gradual or sudden.
2. Character: Pain or burning; at start of stream, at midstream, or throughout stream; force of stream; frequency; urgency; color; presence of blood (internal or external).
3. Course: Improving or increased discomfort.
4. Associated symptoms: Abdominal pain, flank pain, fever, chills, labial or scrotal pain.

Urinary incontinence

1. Character: Amount, frequency, constant or intermittent, dribbling vs. saturation.
2. Course: Associated with sneezing, exertion, urgency, continuous vs. intermittent.
3. Associated symptoms: Fever, chills, dysuria, frequency.

Past health history

1. Previous gastrointestinal problems, such as peptic ulcer, ulcerative colitis, polyps, intestinal obstruction, pancreatitis, gallbladder disease, hepatitis, or cirrhosis of the liver.
2. Abdominal or urinary tract surgery or injury.
3. Past history of urinary tract infections (number, how many in the past year, treatment), or renal calculi (number, treatment).
4. History of major illnesses, such as cancer (type), arthritis (specify steroid or aspirin use), kidney disease, cardiac disease, respiratory disease (steroid use).

Family health history

1. Kidney problems.
2. Colon cancer.
3. Malabsorption syndromes (cystic fibrosis, celiac disease).
4. Gallbladder disease.
5. Colitis.

RISK FACTORS TO CONSIDER

Colon cancer

Age older than 50. (Risk increases markedly after age 40, but 90% of cancers occur after age 50.)

First-degree family member (parent or sibling) with colorectal cancer.

Personal history of endometrial, breast, or ovarian cancer.

Previous diagnosis of inflammatory bowel disease, adenomatous polyps, or colorectal cancer.

Hepatitis B

According to the Centers for Disease Control Guidelines (1991), the following individuals are at risk and should consider vaccination against hepatitis B virus (HBV):

Persons with occupational risk, such as health care workers and public safety workers who may be exposed to blood or other body fluids.

Clients and staff in institutions for the developmentally disabled.

Hemodialysis patients.

Recipients of blood or blood products.

Household contacts and sexual partners of persons with an active or ongoing case of HBV or HBV carriers.

Adoptees from countries where HBV is endemic (e.g., China, Southeast Asia).

International travelers, particularly those visiting regions where HBV is endemic.

Injecting drug users.

Sexually active homosexual and bisexual men.

Sexually active heterosexual men and women with a history of (1) more than one partner in 6 months, (2) sexually transmitted diseases, or (3) prostitution.

Inmates of long-term correctional facilities.

Preparation for Examination: Client and Environment

Helping the client to relax is an important prerequisite to performing a thorough examination of the abdomen. The client should have an empty bladder before the examination begins. He or she needs to be in a comfortable supine position with arms at the sides. To help the client to relax the stomach muscles, place a small pillow under the head and ask the client to flex the knees slightly. A pillow can also be placed behind the knees to support them in a slightly flexed position. The examination room should be warm enough so that the client will not shiver (thereby tensing the abdomen). The abdomen must be fully exposed. For both warmth and modesty, drape the client's chest and groin area.

Have the client breathe quietly and slowly through the mouth. Your hands and the diaphragm of the stethoscope should be warm and your fingernails should be short. Talk to the client in a slow and gentle manner. Avoid any sudden movements. Explain what you will be doing during the examination. Have the client point to any tender areas and tell the client that you will examine those areas last. Observe the client's facial expression as you conduct the examination. The stoic client may not admit to discomfort, but his or her facial expression may show when that person feels tenderness. You can then confirm this observation with the client and modify your examination accordingly.

PREPARATION

Preparation for Examination

Equipment

Item	Purpose
Stethoscope (with bell and diaphragm)	To listen to bowel and vascular sounds
Metric ruler	To measure liver span
Marking pen	To mark borders of organs
Small pillows	To position client

Client and environment

1. Assemble needed equipment (stethoscope, ruler, marking pen, pillows).
2. Make sure that the room is comfortably warm.
3. Explain the steps of the examination to the client.
4. Position the client in a comfortable supine position with arms at the sides, head supported by a pillow, and knees slightly flexed.
5. Completely expose the abdomen from the costal border to the symphysis pubis, draping the client's chest and pubic area for modesty and warmth.
6. Ask the client to point to any tender areas and reassure the person that you will examine those areas last.
7. Watch the client's facial expressions for signs of discomfort during the examination.

Examination Techniques and Normal Findings

The physical assessment of the abdomen includes all four methods of examination (inspection, auscultation, percussion, and palpation). However, in the abdominal examination, auscultation is done before percussion and palpation because stimulation by pressure on the bowel can alter bowel motility and heighten bowel sounds. Palpation is the technique most useful in detecting pathological conditions of the abdomen.

Anatomical mapping. In order to describe clearly the location of organs and the areas of pain or tenderness, the abdomen can be divided into either four quadrants (Figure 17-2) or nine regions (Figure 17-3). The most frequently used method is division into four quadrants. An imaginary vertical line is drawn from the sternum down to the pubic bone through the umbilicus, and a second line is drawn perpendicular to the first line through the umbilicus. In general, abdominal structures will be located in one of these quadrants (see Figure 17-2). Loops of the small bowel are found in all four quadrants. The bladder and the uterus are located at the lower midline.

The second, less frequently used, method of establishing zones of the abdomen involves nine sections (see Figure 17-3). This division is accomplished by drawing two imaginary vertical lines from the midclavicle to the middle of Poupart's (inguinal) ligament, analogous to the lateral borders of the rectus abdominis muscles. At right angles to these lines, two imaginary parallel lines cross the border of the costal margin and the anterosuperior spine of the iliac bones. Essentially, the abdominal structures correlate with the zones shown in Figure 17-3, *B*.

Certain anatomical structures are used as landmarks to facilitate the description of abdominal signs and symptoms (Figure 17-4). The following landmarks are useful for this purpose: the ensiform (xiphoid) process of the sternum, the costal margin, the midline (drawn from the tip of the sternum through the umbilicus to the pubic bone), the umbilicus, the anterosuperior iliac spine, Poupart's (inguinal) ligament, and the superior margin of the pubic bone.

Abdominal structures protected by the rib cage that are examined in health assessment are the liver, stomach, and spleen (Figure 17-5). These structures are evaluated by palpation and percussion.

Inspection. A good source of light is necessary for inspection of the abdomen. Direct the light at a right angle to the long axis of the client, or focus the light lengthwise over the client, shining it from the foot to the head. Assume a sitting position, *generally at the right side of the client.* To enhance shadows, your head should be only slightly higher than the client's abdomen. Shadows highlight small changes in contour, thus increasing the likelihood of detecting a pathological condition.

Note the position that the client assumes voluntarily. The individual with abdominal pain frequently draws up the knees to reduce tension on the abdominal muscles and to alleviate intraabdominal pressure. The client with generalized **peritonitis** lies almost motionless with the knees flexed. Marked restlessness has been associated with biliary and intestinal colic, renal colic, and intraperitoneal hemorrhage.

Familiarity with the normal topography of the abdomen is important to avoid identifying normal contours as masses (Figure 17-6). Carefully focus attention on the abdomen to describe accurately the presence or absence of symmetry, distention, masses, visible peristaltic waves, and respiratory movements. If the presence of peristalsis is in question, carefully study the abdomen for several minutes.

To detect masses, such as an enlarged liver or spleen, ask the client to take a deep breath. This action forces the diaphragm downward and decreases the size of the abdominal cavity, which makes masses become more obvious.

The rectus muscles (Figure 17-7) are prominent landmarks of the abdominal wall. **Diastasis recti ab-**

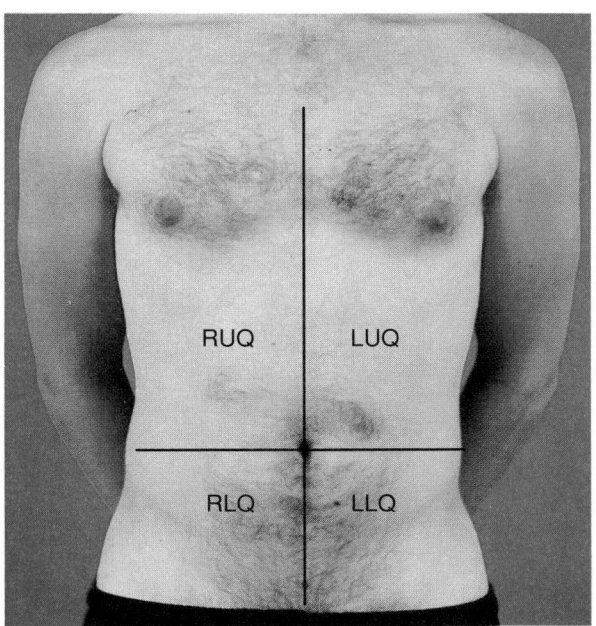

FIGURE 17-2 Four quadrants of the abdomen.

ANATOMIC CORRELATES OF THE FOUR QUADRANTS OF THE ABDOMEN

Right upper quadrant

Liver and gallbladder
Pylorus
Duodenum
Head of pancreas
Right adrenal gland
Portion of right kidney
Hepatic flexure of colon
Portions of ascending and transverse colon

Left upper quadrant

Left lobe of liver
Spleen
Stomach
Body of pancreas
Left adrenal gland
Portion of left kidney
Splenic flexure of colon
Portions of transverse and descending colon

Right lower quadrant

Lower pole of right kidney
Cecum and appendix
Portion of ascending colon
Bladder (if distended)
Ovary and salpinx
Uterus (if enlarged)
Right spermatic cord
Right ureter

Left lower quadrant

Lower pole of left kidney
Sigmoid colon
Portion of descending colon
Bladder (if distended)
Ovary and salpinx
Uterus (if distended)
Left spermatic cord
Left ureter

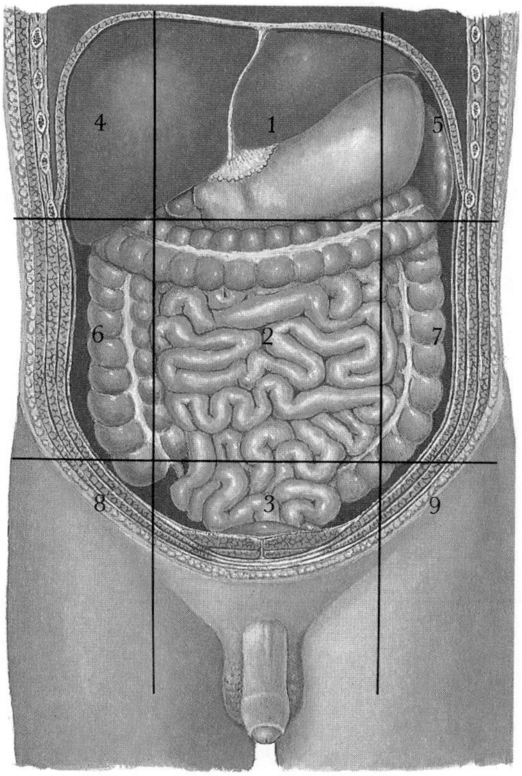

FIGURE 17-3 Nine regions of the abdomen. **1,** Epigastric. **2,** Umbilical. **3,** Hypogastric (pubic). **4** and **5,** Right and left hypochondriac. **6** and **7,** Right and left lumbar. **8** and **9,** Right and left inguinal. (Left or top from Seidel HM and others: *Mosby's guide to physical examination,* St. Louis, 1991, Mosby–Year Book.)

ANATOMIC CORRELATES OF THE NINE REGIONS OF THE ABDOMEN

Right hypochondriac

Right lobe of liver
Gallbladder
Portion of duodenum
Hepatic flexure of colon
Portion of right kidney
Suprarenal gland

Epigastric

Pyloric end of stomach
Duodenum
Pancreas
Portion of liver

Left hypochondriac

Stomach
Spleen
Tail of pancreas
Splenic flexure of colon
Upper pole of left kidney
Suprarenal gland

Right lumbar

Ascending colon
Lower half of right kidney
Portion of duodenum and jejunum

Umbilical

Omentum
Mesentery
Lower duodenum
Jejunum and ileum

Left lumbar

Descending colon
Lower half of right kidney
Portions of jejunum and ileum

Right inguinal

Cecum
Appendix
Ileum (lower end)
Right ureter
Right spermatic cord
Right ovary

Hypogastric

Ileum
Bladder
Uterus (in pregnancy)

Left inguinal

Sigmoid colon
Left ureter
Left spermatic cord
Left ovary

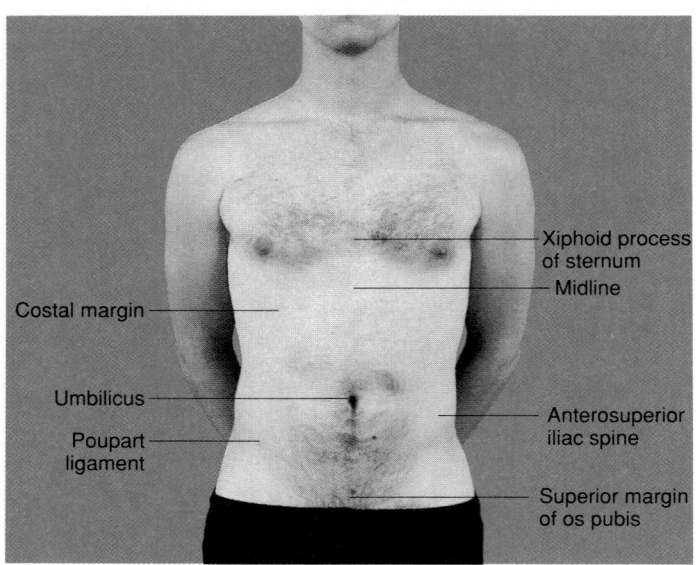

FIGURE 17-4 Landmarks of the abdomen.

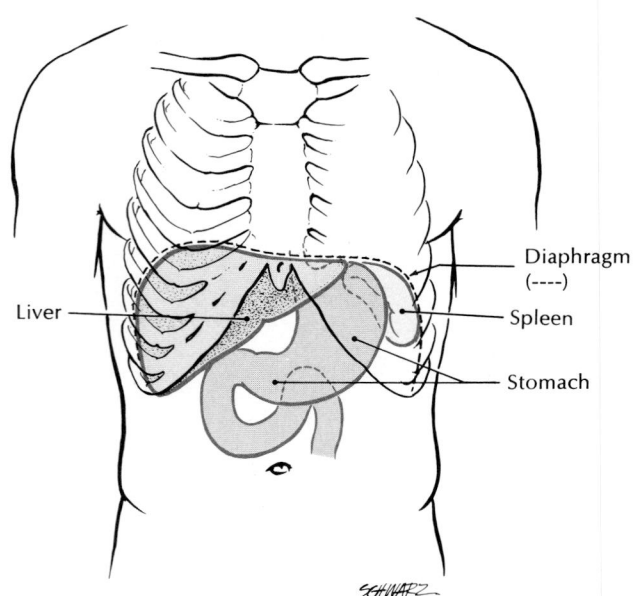

FIGURE 17-5 Abdominal structures protected by the rib cage. The liver, stomach, and spleen are examined by palpation and percussion.

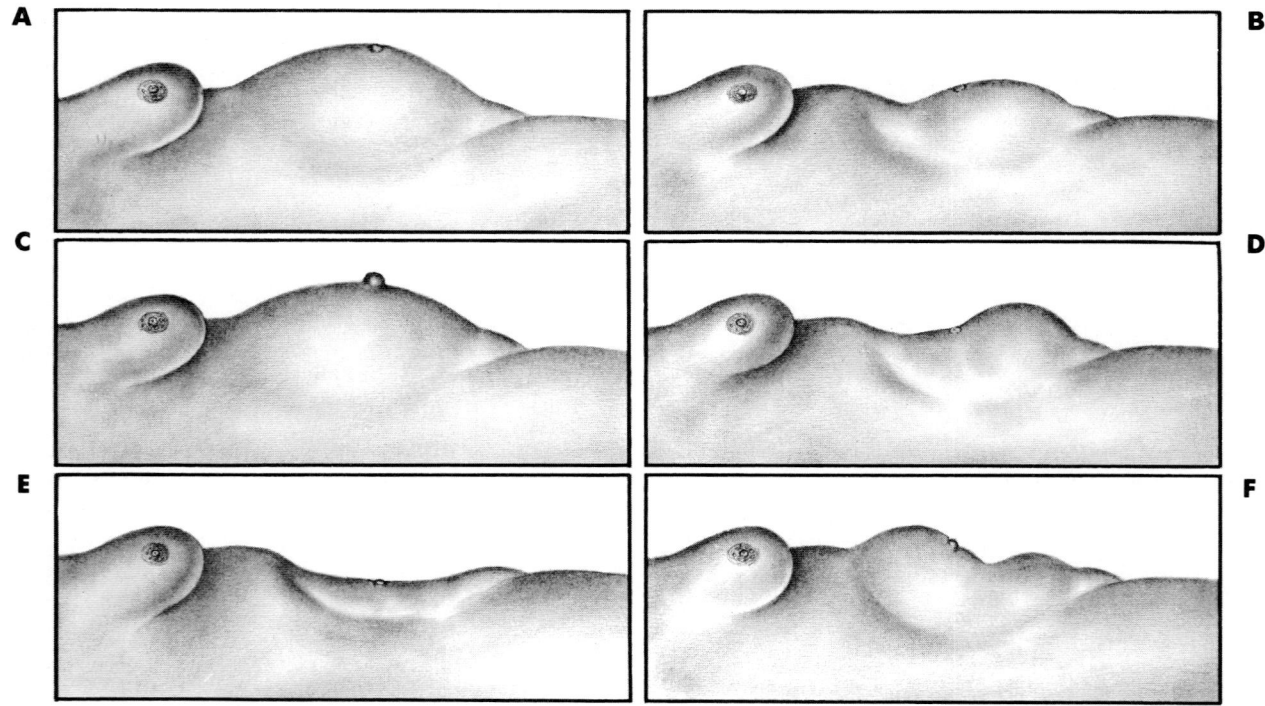

FIGURE 17-6 Abdominal profiles. **A,** Fully rounded or distended, umbilicus inverted. **B,** Distended lower half. **C,** Fully rounded or distended, umbilicus everted. **D,** Distended lower third. **E,** Scaphoid. **F,** Distended upper half. (From Seidel HM and others: *Mosby's guide to physical examination,* ed 2, St. Louis, 1991, Mosby–Year Book.)

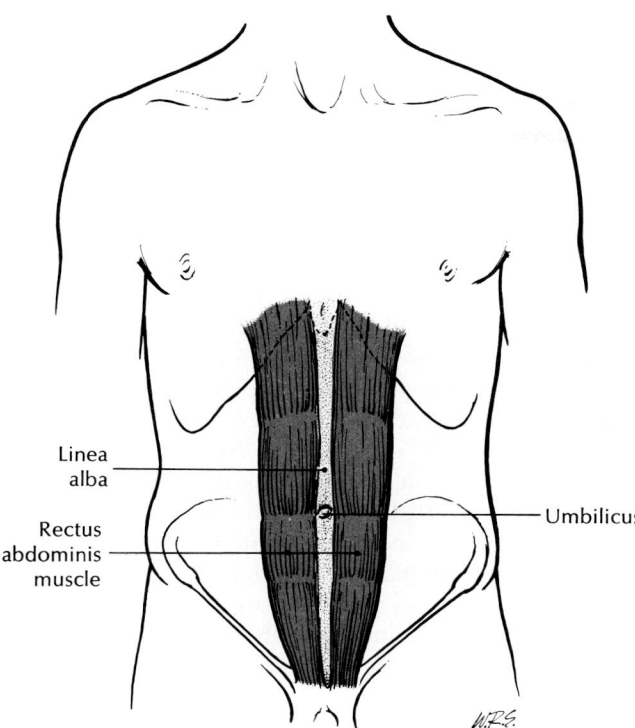

Linea
alba

Rectus
abdominis
muscle

Umbilicus

FIGURE 17-7 Rectus abdominis muscles. Separation of these muscles is called diastasis recti and may be detected by observation or palpation.

dominis is a separation of the rectus abdominis muscles. The separation may be palpated and may be observed as a ridge between the muscles when the intraabdominal pressure is increased by raising the head and shoulders. This defect does not pose a threat to the functions of the abdominal structures. Diastasis recti abdominis generally occurs as a result of pregnancy or marked obesity.

Next, inspect the abdomen from a standing position at the foot of the bed or examining table. Asymmetry of the abdominal contour may be more readily detected from this position.

Skin. The abdomen is an especially valuable area for dermatological observation because it encompasses a relatively large expanse of skin. Inspection of the abdominal skin for pigmentation (particularly jaundice), lesions, striae, scars, dehydration, general nutritional status, venous patterns, and the condition of the umbilicus can yield valuable information about the client's general state of health.

PIGMENTATION. Because clothing frequently protects the skin of the abdomen from the sun, abdominal skin may serve as a baseline for comparison with the pigmentation of the more tanned areas. Jaundice is more readily observed in this less exposed skin. Irregular patches of faint tan pigmentation may be a result of **von Recklinghausen's disease**.

LESIONS. The observation of skin lesions is of particular significance because gastrointestinal alterations are frequently associated with skin changes. Although the presence of small, hard, painless nodules over a wide area of the abdomen may be caused by metastasis of a malignancy, the nodules are generally not the result of carcinoma of the abdominal viscera. Tense and glistening skin is often correlated with ascites or edema of the abdominal wall.

STRIAE. Lineae albicantes (striae) are atrophic lines or streaks that may be seen in the skin of the abdomen following rapid or prolonged stretching that disrupts the elastic fibers of the reticular layer of the cutis. Striae of recent origin are pink or blue but progress to silvery white. Striae occurring as a result of Cushing's disease, however, remain pink-purple. The stretching of abdominal skin may occur as a result of pregnancy *(striae gravidarum)* (Figure 17-8), an abdominal tumor, **ascites**, or obesity.

SCARS. Inspection of the abdomen for scars may yield valuable data concerning previous surgery or trauma. The size and shape of scars are best described through the use of a drawing of the abdomen on which the landmarks or quadrants are shown and the dimensions are noted in centimeters.

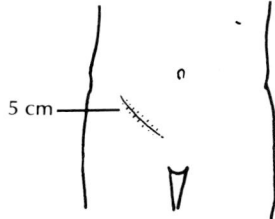

5 cm

If the cause of the scar is not elicited through the history, this information should be sought through inspection. The fact that the client has experienced a previous surgery should alert the examiner to the possibility that adhesions may be present.

Deep, irregular scars may indicate burns. Some individuals produce a dense overgrowth or hypertrophy of fibrous tissue in the healing process. This overgrowth, which is called a **keloid**, consists of large essentially parallel bands of dense collagenous material separated by bands of cellular fibrous tissue. Keloid formation most frequently occurs following a traumatic injury or burn. Increased prevalence of keloid formation has been noted in African-American individuals and those of Asian extraction.

VEINS. A fine venous network is often seen in the abdominal wall. Dilated veins are observed in vena cava obstruction that is usually related to congested portal circulation.

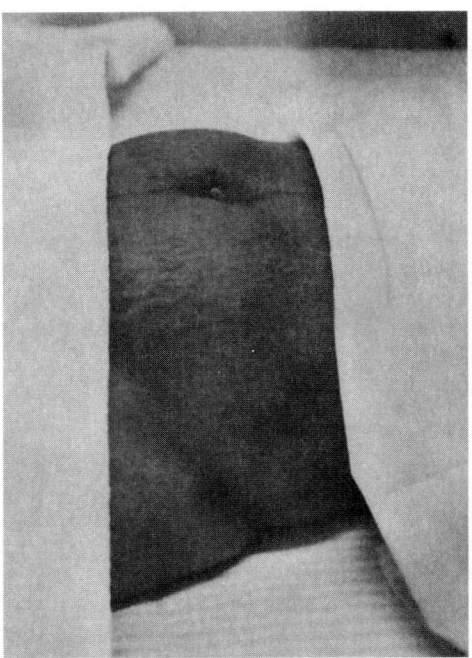

FIGURE 17-8 Striae of the abdominal wall resulting from stretching of the skin from pregnancy (striae gravidarum).

UMBILICUS. The umbilicus should be observed for signs of vena cava obstruction (dilated veins), umbilical hernia, metastatic carcinoma, and dampness or the smell of urine (patent urachus).

Contour. Contralateral areas of the normal abdomen are symmetrical in contour and appearance. The contour is determined by the abdominal profile from the rib margin to the pubic bone as viewed from a right angle to the umbilicus with the client in a recumbent position (see Figure 17-6). The contour of the normal abdomen is described as flat, rounded, or scaphoid.

A flat contour is seen in the muscularly competent and well-nourished individual. A rounded or convex contour is normal in the infant or toddler, but in the adult it is generally caused by poor muscle tone, excessive subcutaneous fat deposits, or both. The rounded abdomen is often called the "spare tire" or "bay window" of middle age (see Figure 17-6, *A*). A scaphoid, or concave, contour may be seen in thin clients of all ages. This type of contour reflects a decrease in fat deposits in the abdominal wall and relaxed or flaccid abdominal musculature (see Figure 17-6, *E*).

Distention is the term used for unusual stretching of the abdominal wall. Abdominal distention may result from fat (obesity), feces or flatus (constipation or intestinal obstruction), fetus (pregnancy), fluid (ascites), fibroid tumor, or fatal tumor. The presence of distention generally implies disease and therefore warrants further investigation. **Asymmetrical distention** of the abdominal wall may be caused by hernia, tumor, cysts, or bowel obstruction. A mnemonic device for classifying the six most common causes of distention are fluid, **flatulence**, fat, feces, fibroid tumor, and fetus—the six Fs.

Generalized, or *symmetrical, distention* of the abdomen with the umbilicus in its normal inverted position is generally a result of obesity or recent pressure of fluid or gas within the hollow viscera. If the umbilicus is in an everted position (umbilical hernia), ascites or underlying tumor may be the cause (see Figure 17-6, *C*). Ovarian tumor, distended bladder, or pregnancy may be suspected if the distention is confined to the area between the umbilicus and the symphysis pubis (see Figure 17-6, *B*). Distention of the lower third of the abdomen suggests ovarian tumor, uterine fibroid tumor, pregnancy, or bladder enlargement (see Figure 17-6, *D*). Possible causes of distention of the upper half of the abdominal wall include pancreatic cyst or tumor and gastric dilation (Figure 17-6, *F*).

Movement
RESPIRATORY MOVEMENT. Observation of respiratory movement has more significance in the male client because men exhibit predominantly abdominal movement with respiration. Women exhibit mainly costal movement. Therefore limited abdominal respiratory action in the male client may be indicative of peritonitis or other abdominal infection or disease. Abdominal breathing is also common in a child less than 6 or 7 years old. The presence of abdominal respiratory movements in an older child may indicate respiratory problems. The absence of abdominal respiratory movements in the child who is younger than 6 years suggests peritoneal irritation. Retraction of the abdominal wall on inspiration, called Czerny's sign, is associated with certain central nervous system diseases such as chorea.

VISIBLE PERISTALSIS. In lean individuals motility of the stomach and intestines may be seen as movement of the abdominal wall even in the absence of disease. However, when strong contractions are visible through an abdominal wall of average thickness, the possibility of bowel obstruction should be investigated. Sit at the client's side and gaze across the abdomen for several minutes. Percussing the abdomen may augment weak peristalsis. Peristaltic waves of the stomach and small intestine may be seen as elevated oblique bands in the upper left quadrant that move downward to the right. Several of these peristaltic waves occurring in rapid succession may produce a series of parallel bands or a "ladder effect."

Reverse peristalsis, observed in the upper abdomen in an infant, is seen as an undulation moving from left to right. This observation indicates the presence of pyloric stenosis or, less commonly, duodenal stenosis or malrotation of the bowel.

PULSATION. In thin persons pulsation of the abdominal aorta is visible throughout most of its length. However, in most persons it is visible in the epigastrium.

Auscultation. Auscultation of the abdomen precedes percussion because bowel motility, and thus bowel sounds, may be increased by palpation and percussion. Both the stethoscope and the examiner's hands should be warm. If they are cold, they may initiate a contraction of the abdominal muscles.

Auscultatory findings of diagnostic significance are those sounds originating from the viscera, the arterial system, the venous system, muscular activity, or parietal friction rubs. Gently place the stethoscope on the abdomen to auscultate (Figure 17-9). Light pressure on the stethoscope is sufficient to detect bowel sounds and bruits. Use the diaphragm of the stethoscope, which accentuates the higher-pitched sounds, to listen to the relatively high-pitched abdominal intestinal sounds. Use the bell of the stethoscope to listen for low-pitched arterial bruits and venous hums.

Peristaltic sounds. Normal bowel sounds are high-pitched, gurgling noises that occur approximately every 5 to 15 seconds. Some authorities suggest that the number is as high as 15 to 20 per minute, or roughly one bowel sound for each breath sound. The duration of a single sound may be less than 1 second or may extend over several seconds. The frequency of sounds is related

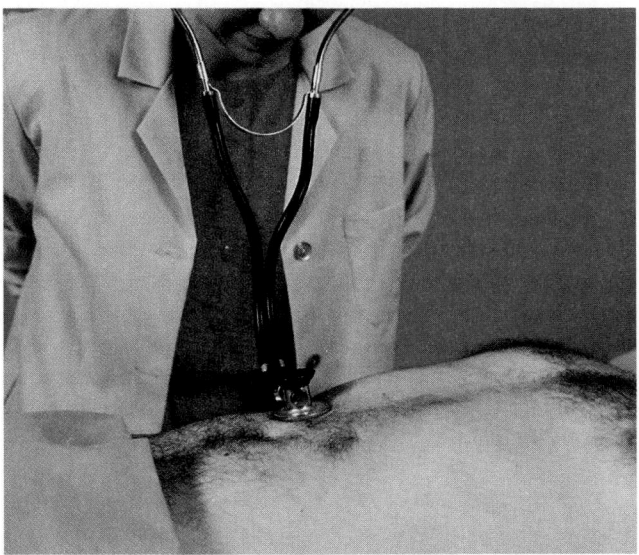

FIGURE 17-9 Auscultation for bowel sounds. The diaphragm of the stethoscope is used to listen to the relatively high-pitched intestinal sounds.

to the presence of food in the gastrointestinal tract or to the state of digestion. Because the passage of fluids and gases through the intestine causes bowel sounds, uninterrupted bowel sounds may be heard over the ileocecal valve 4 to 7 hours following a meal. A silent abdomen (i.e., the absence of bowel sounds) indicates the arrest of intestinal motility. Flicking the abdominal wall with a finger (direct percussion) will stimulate peristalsis. Because peristaltic sounds may be quite irregular, listening for at least 5 minutes is essential before concluding that no bowel sounds are present. When evaluating for absence of sounds, it is important to auscultate each of the four quadrants for at least 1 minute so that no sounds will be missed and so that specific sounds can be localized.

The two significant alterations in bowel sounds are (1) the absence of any sound or extremely soft and widely separated sounds; and (2) increased sounds with a characteristically high-pitched, loud, rushing sound **(borborygmi)**.

DECREASED BOWEL SOUNDS. Diminished or absent bowel sounds accompany inhibition of bowel motility. Decreased motility occurs with inflammation, gangrene, or paralytic ileus. Decreased peristalsis frequently accompanies peritonitis, electrolyte disturbances, the aftermath of surgical manipulation of the bowel, and late bowel obstruction. In addition, diminished bowel sounds are often correlated with lower lobe pneumonia.

INCREASED BOWEL SOUNDS. Loud, gurgling borborygmi accompany increased motility of the bowel, such as with diarrhea. Sounds of loud volume also are heard over areas of a stenotic bowel. Sounds from an early bowel obstruction are high pitched. These may be splashing sounds, similar to the emptying of a bottle into a hollow vessel. Fine, metallic, tinkling sounds are emitted as tiny gas bubbles break through the surface of intestinal juices. Increased motility may be caused by the use of a laxative or by gastroenteritis. Common pathological conditions associated with increased bowel sounds are gastroenteritis and subsiding ileus.

Vascular sounds

ARTERIAL SOUNDS. Bruits are heard when an artery is partially obstructed, causing turbulent flow. A bruit that is heard with the bell of the stethoscope held lightly against the abdomen while the client is in a variety of positions may indicate a dilated, tortuous, or constricted vessel (Figure 17-10). Loud bruits detected over the aorta suggest the presence of an aneurysm. Auscultation of the aorta should be done superior to the umbilicus. The locations of the aorta, renal arteries, and iliac arteries are illustrated in Figure 17-11. Soft, medium- to low-pitched murmurs resulting from renal arterial stenosis may be heard over the upper midline or toward the flank.

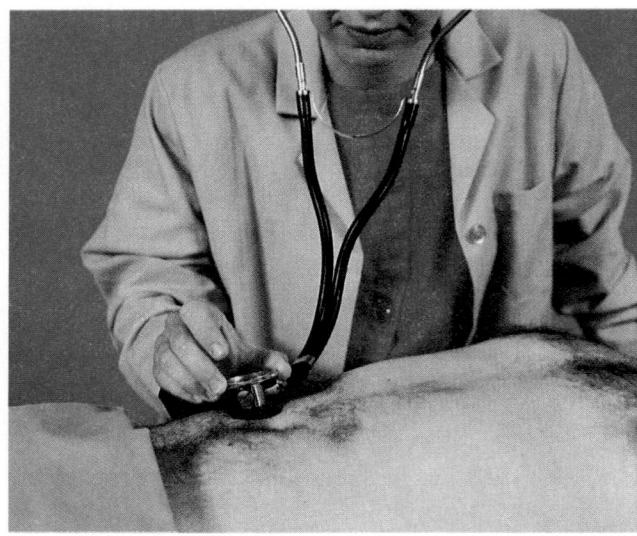

FIGURE 17-10 Auscultation for bruits is performed with the bell of the stethoscope held lightly against the abdomen.

FIGURE 17-11 Sites to auscultate for bruits: renal arteries, iliac arteries, aorta, and femoral arteries.

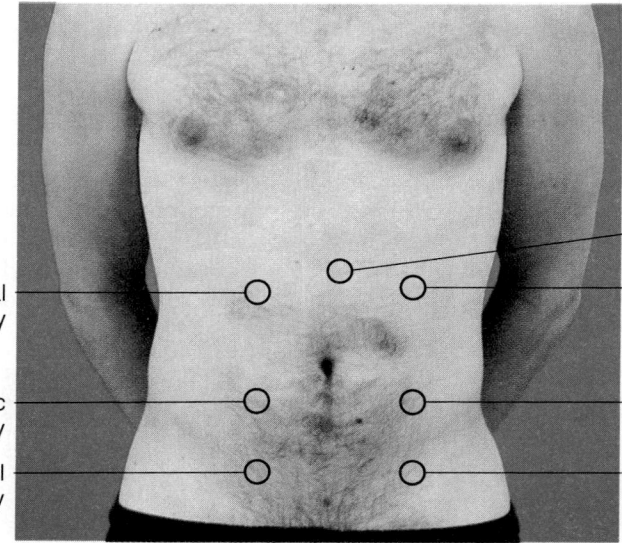

Right renal artery

Right Iliac artery

Right femoral artery

Aorta

Left renal artery

Left Iliac artery

Left femo artery

For the hypertensive client, listen carefully over the center epigastrium and posterior flank for a bruit in the arterial tree. An epigastric bruit radiating laterally suggests renal artery stenosis.

VENOUS HUMS. A normal hum originating from the inferior vena cava and its large tributaries is continuously audible with a stethoscope. Its tone is medium pitched and is similar to a muscular fibrillary hum. In the presence of obstructed portal circulation, as from a cirrhotic liver, an abnormal venous hum may be detected in the periumbilical region. Pressure on the bell may obscure the hum. A palpable thrill may accompany the hum.

Another pathological hum accompanies the dilated periumbilical circulation of Cruveilhier-Baumgarten disease. This hum may be detected near the midline between the umbilicus and the xiphoid process. Hepatic angiomas may produce hums that can be auscultated over the liver.

Peritoneal friction rub. Peritoneal friction rub creates a rough, grating sound that resembles two pieces of leather being rubbed together. Because the liver and the spleen have large surface areas that are in contact with the peritoneum, these two structures are most often the originating sites of peritoneal friction rubs.

Common causes of friction rubs include splenic infection, abscess, and tumor. These sounds are heard best over the lower rib cage in the anterior axillary line. Deep respiration may emphasize the sound. Metastatic disease of the liver and abscess are the usual causes of peritoneal friction rubs located over the lower right rib cage.

Muscular activity sounds. A fibrillating muscle produces a hum that can be heard with a stethoscope. Both voluntary and involuntary contractions (e.g., muscle guarding of a painful area) produce this sound. Palpation of the tender area often accentuates the hum.

Percussion. Percussion of the abdomen is done to detect fluid, gaseous distention, and masses and to assess the position and size of solid structures within the abdomen. Percussion can be done independently or in conjunction with palpation. For example, in a client with a tumor, percussion should be done before deep palpation in order to establish a sense of the size and location of the enlarged organ.

Lightly percuss the entire abdomen for a general picture of the areas of tympany and dullness. Tympany will predominate because of the presence of gas in the large bowel and the small bowel. Solid masses will percuss as dull, as will organs such as a distended bladder. To lessen the chance of omitting any portion of the examination, establish a systematic pattern or route to use each time you percuss abdominal structures (Figure 17-12).

Assessment of the liver span. To determine the size of the liver, begin percussion in the right midclavicular line at a level below the umbilicus (Figure 17-13, *A*). Start percussion over a region of gas-filled bowel (tympany) and progress upward toward the liver. The first dull percussion note indicates the lower border of the liver. (Be careful not to confuse the costal border with the liver border. Both are dull, but the costal border is easily palpable.) Mark the lower border on the abdomen. To determine the upper border of liver dullness, start percussion in the midclavicular line and examine from an area of lung resonance down to the first dull percussion note (generally the fifth to seventh interspace [Figure 17-13, *B*]). Mark this spot and measure the distance between the two marks in centimeters (Figure 17-13, *C*). Other sites for percussion and measurement when the liver appears enlarged are the anterior axillary line and the midsternal line.

The descent of the liver can also be assessed. Ask the client to take a deep breath and hold it while you percuss upward from the abdomen to detect the lower liver border. The liver will normally descend 2 to 3 cm with inspiration. This maneuver can help to guide placement of your hands for palpating the liver border.

The suggested ranges of normal values are 6 to 12 cm in the midclavicular line and 4 to 8 cm in the midsternal line (Figure 17-14). A direct correlation exists between body size (lean body mass) and liver span. It is important to remember that men have larger livers than women. The mean midclavicular liver span in men

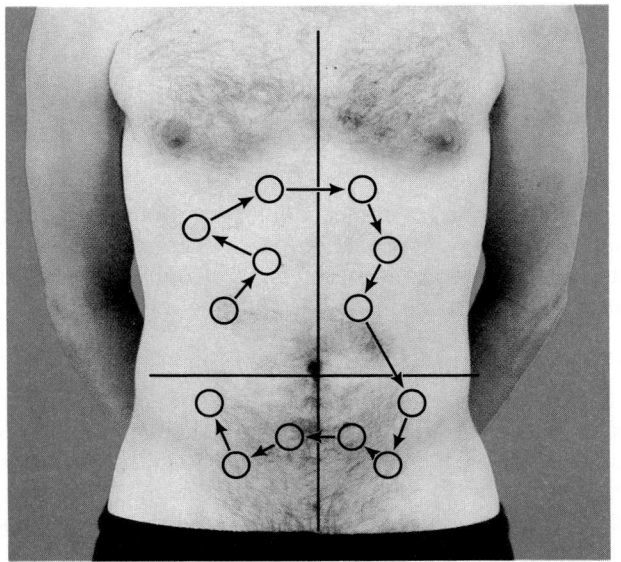

FIGURE 17-12 Systematic route for abdominal percussion.

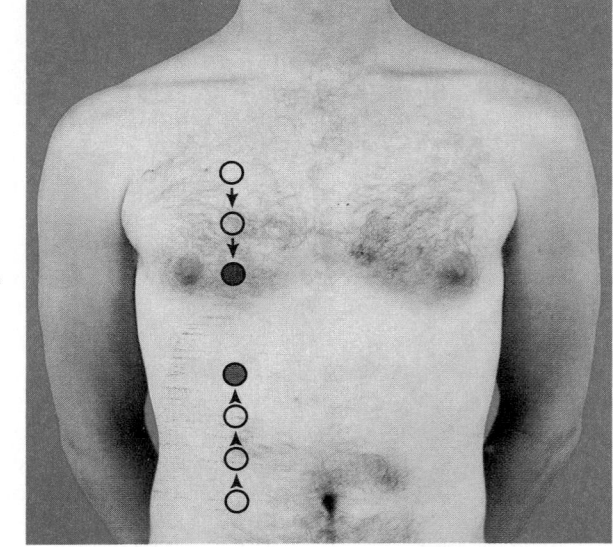

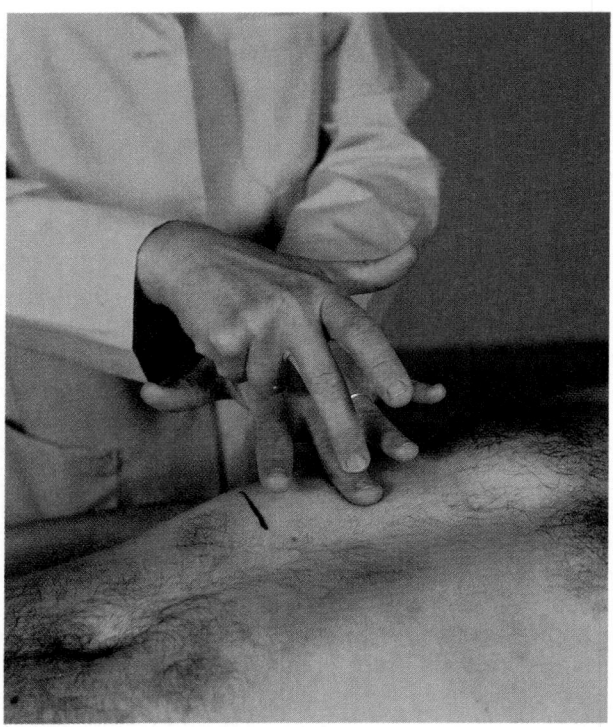

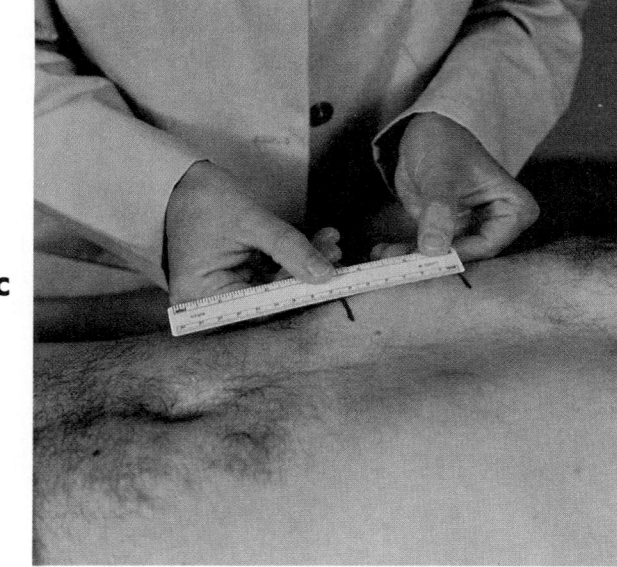

FIGURE 17-13 A, Liver percussion route. **B,** Percussion method of estimating the size of the liver in the mid-clavicular line. Lower border percussion is begun over a region of air- or gas-filled bowel and carried upward to the dull percussion note of the liver. The spot is marked. Upper border percussion is performed over the midclavicular line from an area of lung resonance to the first dull percussion note (generally the fifth to seventh interspace). The spot is marked. **C,** The distance between the two marks measured in estimating the liver span in the midclavicular line is normally 6 to 12 cm.

is 10.5 cm, whereas it is 7 cm in women. A midclavicular liver span of 11 cm may indicate **hepatomegaly** in a 5-foot, 100-pound woman, but it may be within normal limits for a man.

Error in estimating the liver span can occur when pleural effusion or lung consolidation obscures the upper liver border or when gas in the colon obscures the lower border. On inspiration, the diaphragm moves downward. This movement shifts the normal span of liver dullness inferiorly 2 to 3 cm. Pulmonary edema may also displace the liver downward. Ascites, massive tumors, or pregnancy may push the liver upward. The liver assumes a more square configuration in **cirrhosis**

of the liver, and the midclavicular and midsternal measurements may approach equality. Percussion of liver dullness is important in detecting atrophy of the liver, such as might occur in acute fulminating hepatitis.

Percussion for tympany and dullness

SPLEEN. Splenic dullness can be percussed from the level of the seventh to the eleventh rib just posterior to or at the midaxillary line on the left side. Begin percussion at the tenth rib just posterior to the midaxillary line. Percuss in several directions from dullness to resonance or tympany to outline the edges of the spleen (Figure 17-15). The span of normal splenic dullness

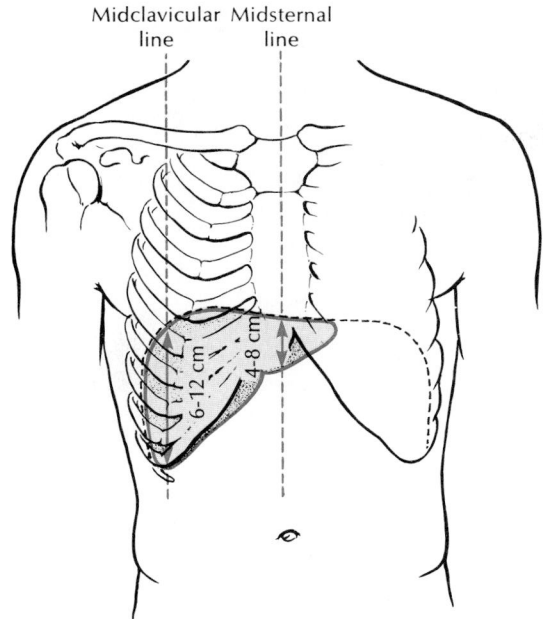

FIGURE 17-14 The range of liver span in the midclavicular and midsternal lines. The size of the liver shows a direct correlation to lean body mass. Thus, the mean clavicular liver span is 10.5 cm in men and 7.0 cm in women.

does not exceed 7 cm. When the spleen has normal dimensions, resonance may be percussed over the lowest left intercostal space between the anterior and midaxillary lines during both inspiration and expiration. However, a finding of resonance on expiration and dullness on inspiration probably denotes splenic hypertrophy. A full stomach, an enlarged kidney, or a colon packed with feces may elicit dullness and therefore can mimic splenic enlargement. Gastric or colonic air may also obscure normal splenic dullness.

STOMACH. The percussion note of the gastric air bubble is lower pitched tympany than that of the intestine. Percuss in the area of the left lower anterior rib cage and in the left epigastric region to define the area occupied by the bubble (Figure 17-16). The percussion sounds of the stomach vary with the time the last meal was eaten.

Fist percussion. Another percussion method used in the abdominal examination is fist percussion, which causes the tissue to vibrate rather than to produce sound (Figure 17-17). Place the palm of the left hand over the region of liver dullness and strike a light blow to the left hand with the fisted right hand. Tenderness elicited by this method is usually associated with hepatitis or cholecystitis. Fist percussion done at the costovertebral angle (CVA) is also used to assess renal tenderness. Common causes of tenderness are pyelonephritis and renal calculi.

Palpation. Palpation is the most important part of the abdominal examination. It is used to substantiate find-

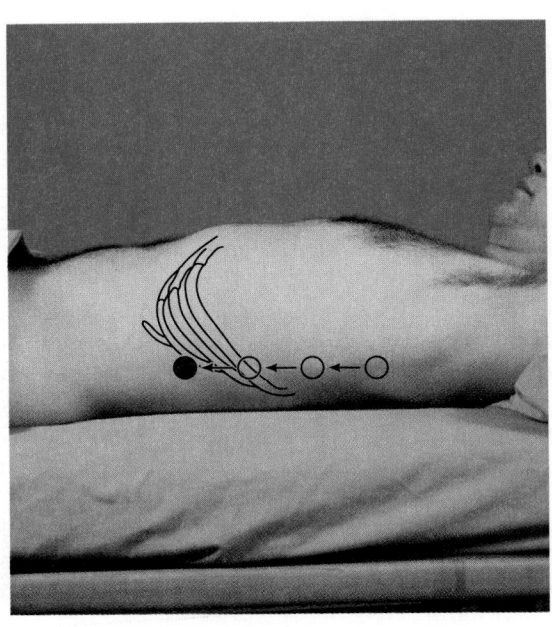

FIGURE 17-15 Spleen percussion route.

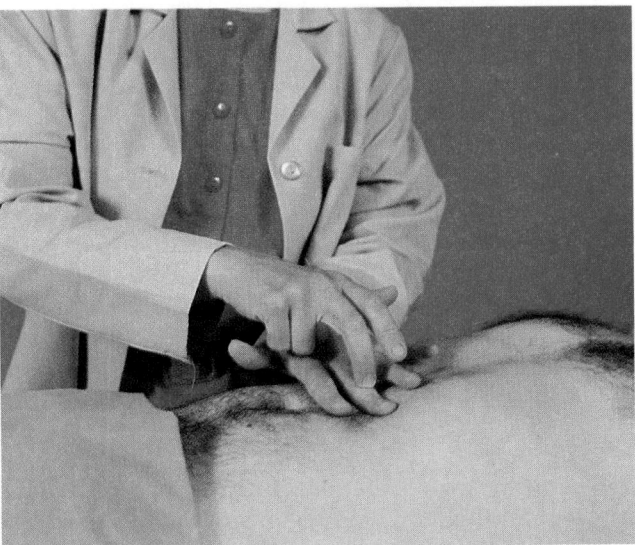

FIGURE 17-16 Percussion of the abdomen for evaluation of fluid, gaseous distention, and masses within the abdominal cavity.

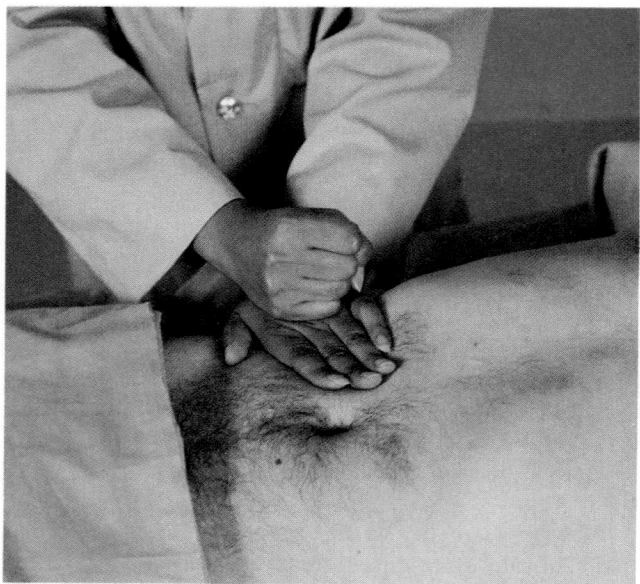

FIGURE 17-17 Fist percussion of the liver. The palm of the hand is placed over the region of liver dullness and a light blow is struck with the fisted right hand. Tenderness elicited by this method is usually a result of hepatitis or cholecystitis.

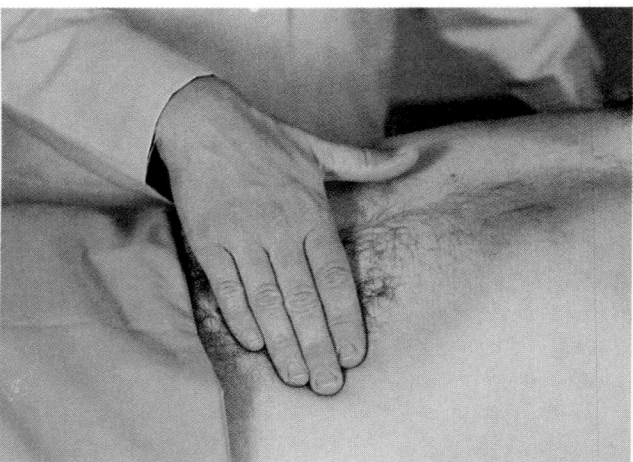

FIGURE 17-18 Light palpation is performed with the hand parallel to the floor and the fingers approximated. The fingers depress the abdominal wall about 1 cm. This method of palpation is recommended for eliciting slight tenderness, large masses, and muscle guarding.

ings noted from careful inspection, auscultation, and percussion and to explore the abdomen further. Palpation allows for evaluation of the major organs of the abdomen in terms of shape, position, mobility, size, consistency, tenderness, and tension. Thorough and systematic screening is performed to detect areas of tenderness, muscular spasm, masses, or fluid.

Make sure that the client is comfortable and that your hands are warm. The client's abdominal muscles should be relaxed. You may need to use relaxation techniques to help the client achieve the appropriate level of relaxation. If the client is unable to relax the abdominal muscles despite these maneuvers, try exerting downward pressure on the lower sternum with the left hand while palpating with the other hand. The deeper inspiration that results inhibits abdominal muscle contraction. You can also ask the client to put his or her hand on the abdomen so that you can palpate on top of the client's hand.

Light palpation. Light palpation is gentle exploration performed while the client is in the supine position. It is helpful in identifying regions of tenderness, large or superficial masses, and muscle guarding. Frequently, an enlarged or distended structure may be noted through a sense of resistance. Areas of tenderness or guarding, or both, should alert you to proceed with caution in more vigorous manipulation of these structures during deep palpation.

Begin palpation at a site distant from areas described as painful or expected to be tender. Elicitation of pain may result in the client's refusing further examination. Stand at the client's right side. Place the palm of your hand lightly on the client's abdomen with your fingers extended and approximated (Figure 17-18). Press the fingertips gently into the abdominal wall approximately 1 cm. Use a light dipping motion (avoid a digging action). Move systematically from one quadrant to another. The abdomen should feel smooth and soft. Watch the client's face for signs of pain elicited by palpation and confirm this verbally with the client.

Tensing of the abdominal musculature may occur because (1) the examiner's hands are too cold or are pressed too vigorously or deeply into the abdomen, (2) the client is ticklish or guards involuntarily, or (3) a subjacent, generally inflammatory, pathological condition exists. If resistance occurs, try to determine whether it is an involuntary spasm or voluntary tensing by feeling for the rectus muscle, which should normally relax as the client exhales. If the rigidity remains unaltered, it is probably an involuntary response to localized or generalized rigidity. Rigidity is a boardlike hardness of the abdominal wall overlying peritoneal irritation. In generalized peritonitis, rigidity may be constant and hard.

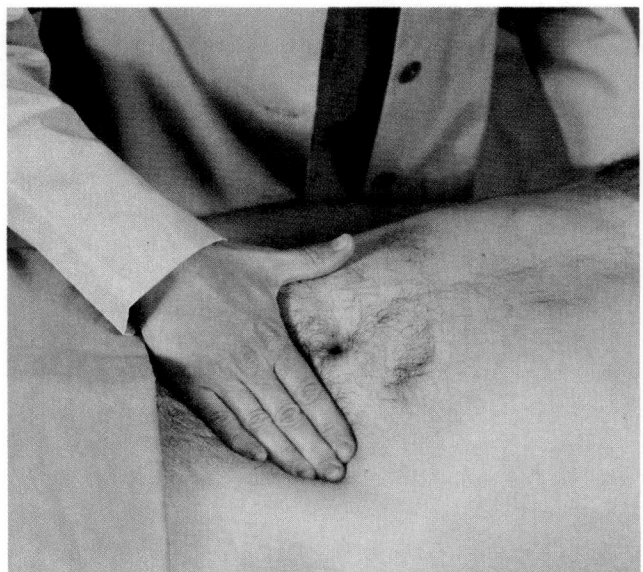

FIGURE 17-24 Deep palpation. Press palmar surfaces of the extended fingers deeply and evenly into the abdominal wall.

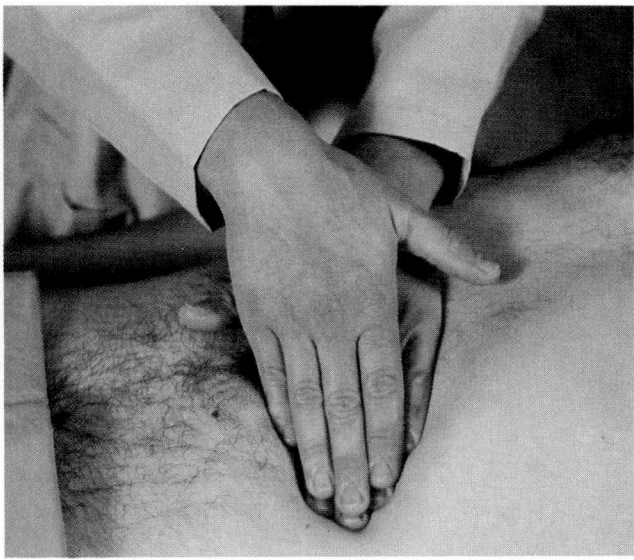

FIGURE 17-25 Deep bimanual palpation. Apply pressure with upper hand while concentrating on feeling structures with lower hand.

aorta. Pulsation may also be felt in a mass held between the hands. This palpatory finding indicates that the structure being felt is pulsating rather than transmitting pulsation.

Examination of specific abdominal structures. Palpation is a useful technique for identification and assessment of the specific abdominal structures. Use a systematic approach, always beginning at the same area, so that you do not skip any part of the abdomen. Because you are approaching the client from the right, the liver may be the most convenient structure to palpate first.

Liver. Two types of bimanual palpation are recommended for examination of the liver. In the first method, place your left hand beneath the client at the level of the eleventh and twelfth ribs. Apply upward pressure with your left hand to throw the liver forward, toward your right hand. Place the examining hand below the costal margin and palpate for the liver border with deep inspiration. There are two methods of positioning your right hand. Either place the palmar surface of your right hand parallel to the right costal margin (Figure 17-26, *A*) or place your right hand on the abdomen, with the fingers pointing toward the head and extended along the right midclavicular line below the level of liver dullness (Figure 17-26, *B*). Ask the client to breathe normally for two or three breaths and then to breathe deeply. The diaphragm is exerted downward on inspiration and will push the liver toward the examining hand (see Figure 17-26, *A*).

The liver usually cannot be palpated in the normal adult. However, in extremely thin but otherwise well individuals, it may be felt at the costal margin on inspiration. When the normal liver margin is palpated, it feels smooth, regular in contour, and somewhat sharp. Descriptions of the abnormal liver are listed in Table 17-1.

In the second technique, frequently referred to as the "hooking technique" or "Middleton's technique," place your hands side by side on the client's right costal margin below the border of liver dullness. Stand on the right side facing the client's feet. Press in with your fingers and up toward the costal margin. Ask the client to take a deep breath. As the client inspires, the liver may be felt to descend toward your fingers (Figure 17-26, *C*). Regardless of the technique that is chosen, palpation of the liver should be done slowly, carefully, and gently so that the liver margin is not missed.

To demonstrate tenderness over the liver, place the palm of one hand over the lateral costal margin and deliver a blow to that hand with the ulnar surface of the other hand, which has been curled into a fist (fist percussion) (see Figure 17-17).

SCRATCH TEST. The scratch test is useful when the usual techniques for determining the lower liver border have been unsuccessful. This test makes use of the difference in sound over solid as opposed to hollow organs. Actually a percussion technique, the scratch test can be used to assess the size of the liver. Place the stethoscope over the liver while using the opposite hand to scratch lightly over the abdominal surface with short

A   **B**   **C**

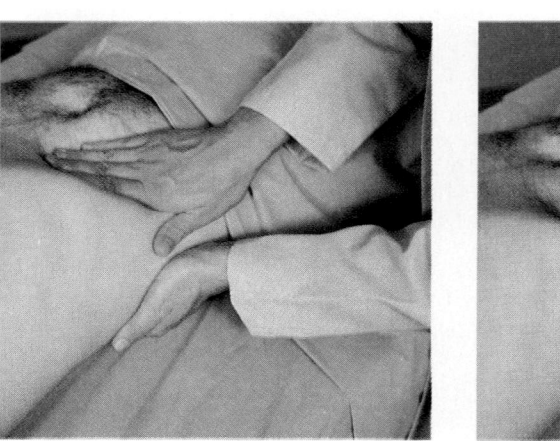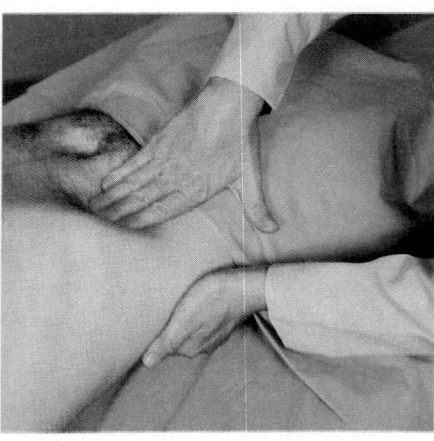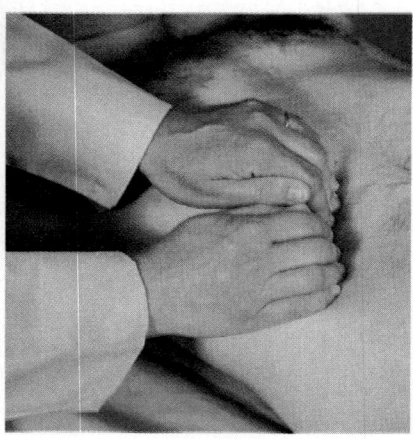

FIGURE 17-26 **A,** Palpating the liver with fingers parallel to the costal margin. **B,** Palpating the liver with fingers extended along the right midclavicular line. **C,** Palpating the liver with fingers "hooked" over the costal margin.

TABLE 17-1

Characteristics of Hepatomegaly Related to Common Pathological Conditions

Description of liver	Possible pathological condition
Smooth, nontender	Portal cirrhosis
	Lymphoma
	Passive congestion of liver
	Portal obstruction
	Obstruction of vena cava
	Lymphocytic leukemia
	Rickets
	Amyloidosis
	Schistosomiasis
Smooth, tender	Acute hepatitis
	Amebic hepatitis or abscess
	Early congestive cardiac failure
Nodular	Late portal cirrhosis
	Tertiary syphilis
	Metastatic carcinoma
Hard	Carcinomatosis

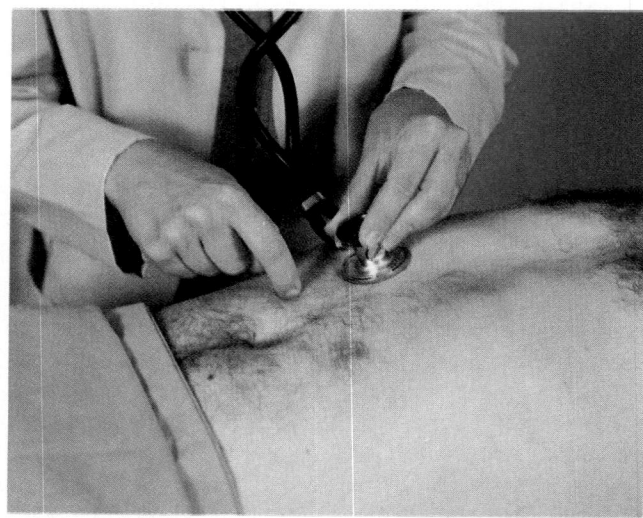

FIGURE 17-27 Scratch test in assessment of liver size. Place the stethoscope over the liver while the other hand scratches lightly over the abdominal surface with short, transverse strokes; when the scratch is done over the liver, the sound is magnified.

transverse strokes (Figure 17-27). When the scratch is done over the liver, the sound is magnified. Although this test is of questionable accuracy, it may be of some value in assessing the individual with abdominal distention or spastic abdominal muscles.

Spleen. The spleen is not usually palpable in the normal adult because it is normally soft and is located in the retroperitoneal area. If the spleen is palpable, it is probably enlarged. Turning the client on the right side (to gain gravitational advantage) brings the spleen downward and forward and thus closer to the abdom-

inal wall, and therefore this position is often employed in the examination.

While standing at the supine client's right side, extend your left hand and place it beneath the client's left costovertebral angle. Exert an upward pressure with your left hand to displace the spleen anteriorly. Feel for the spleen by pressing your right hand gently under the left anterior costal margin (Figure 17-28). Have the client take a deep breath, and palpate as the client ex-

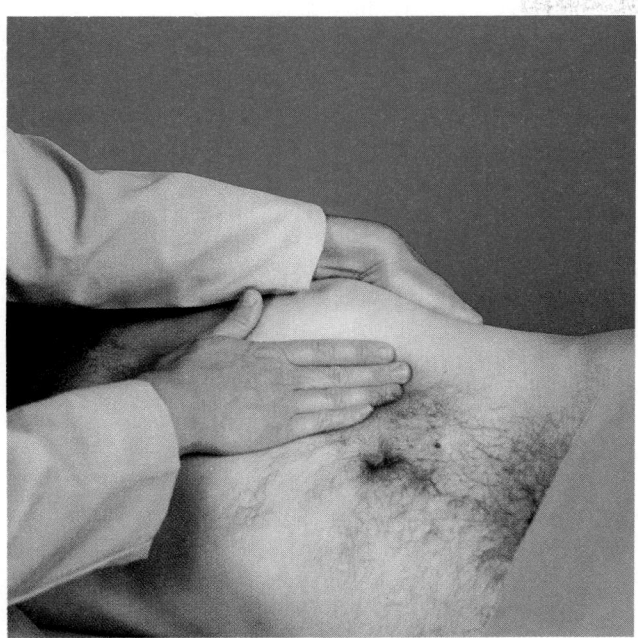

FIGURE 17-28 Palpation of the spleen.

hales. Repeat the examination with the client lying on the right side with hips and knees slightly flexed. It is important to remember that the enlarged spleen can rupture with vigorous palpation. If splenic enlargement is suspected, first percuss the splenic area and then palpate very gently and carefully.

Splenic enlargement is described by the number of centimeters that the spleen extends below the costal margin: (1) slight: 1 to 4 cm below the costal margin, (2) moderate: 4 to 8 cm below the costal margin, and (3) great: more than 8 cm below the costal margin. As previously mentioned, the spleen may be percussed to assess enlargement. Normally, splenic dullness may be percussed from the seventh to the eleventh rib in the midaxillary line or posterior to the line.

To best describe splenic enlargement, draw the anterior abdomen, indicating the relative size and shape of the spleen in relation to the costal border and the umbilicus (Figure 17-29).

Gallbladder. The normal gallbladder cannot be felt. However, a distended gallbladder can be palpated below the liver margin at the lateral border of the rectus muscle. The cystic nature of the mass helps to identify the gallbladder. However, the location of the left border varies greatly. It may be found either more medially or more laterally.

An enlarged, tender gallbladder indicates cholecystitis, whereas a large but nontender gallbladder suggests obstruction of the common bile duct. **Murphy's sign**, elicited through a bimanual technique, is helpful in de-

termining the presence of cholecystitis. While performing deep palpation, ask the client to take a deep breath. As the descending liver brings the gallbladder in contact with the examining hand, the client with cholecystitis will experience pain and will stop the inspiratory movement. Pain may also occur in the client with hepatitis.

Pancreas. The pancreas cannot be palpated in the normal client because of its small size and retroperitoneal position. However, a pancreatic mass may occasionally be felt as a vague sensation of fullness in the epigastrium.

Urinary bladder. The urinary bladder is not palpable in the normal client unless it is distended with urine. A distended bladder is felt as a smooth, round, and rather tense mass. Percussion can be used to define the outline of the distended bladder, which may extend upward as far as the umbilicus.

Umbilicus. Observe the umbilicus for its relationship to the skin surface, hernia, inflammation, or signs of bleeding. The normal umbilicus is recessed below the skin surface.

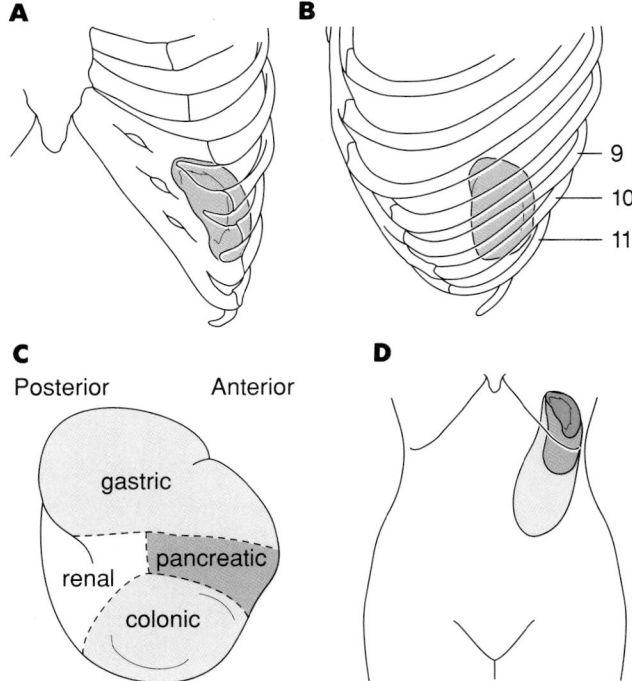

FIGURE 17-29 Normal **(A, B, C)** and enlarged **(D)** spleen. **A,** Anterior view. **B,** Left lateral view. **C,** Regions of spleen (anterior view) that touch other viscera. **D,** Directions of splenic enlargement. (Redrawn from *G.I. Series: physical examination of the abdomen,* Chapter 2, Palpation, Richmond, Va, 1981, AH Robins Co.)

UMBILICAL HERNIA. The umbilical hernia noted in children is seen directly at the umbilical opening, which is centrally located in the linea alba. In the adult, this defect is often apparent above an incomplete umbilical ring and is referred to as paraumbilical. Examine for an umbilical hernia by pressing your index finger into the navel. The fascial opening may feel like a sharp ring with a soft center. The umbilicus may be everted by marked intraabdominal pressure from masses, pregnancy, or large amounts of ascitic fluid.

Abdominal reflexes. To elicit the abdominal reflex, use a key, the base end of an applicator, or your fingernail to stroke the abdominal skin gently over the lateral borders of the rectus abdominis muscles toward the midline (Figure 17-30). Repeat this maneuver in each quadrant. With each stroke, observe contraction of the rectus abdominis muscles, coupled with pulling of the umbilicus to the stimulated side. The abdominal reflex may be weak or absent in the individual who has sustained a good deal of stretching of the abdominal musculature. Thus you may be unable to obtain the abdominal reflex in the multiparous or obese client. In addition, the reflex may be absent in the normal aging

client. Its absence may also indicate a pyramidal tract lesion. Absence of the upper abdominal reflex suggests problems at the spinal levels of T7, T8, and T9. Absence of lower abdominal reflexes indicates problems at the spinal levels of T10 and T11.

Aorta. With the client in a supine position, press firmly and deeply in the upper abdomen slightly to the left of midline and palpate for aortic pulsations. In an older individual (over age 50), try to assess the width of the aorta to screen for an aneurysm. Press deeply in the upper abdomen with one hand on either side of the aorta (Figure 17-31). The normal aorta is approximately 2.5 to 4 cm wide, whereas an aneurysm is much broader.

As noted previously, a bruit is generally heard over an aneurysm. The most common physical finding in clients with an abdominal aneurysm is the presence of an expanding, pulsating mass. More than 95% of such masses are located below the renal arteries but generally at or above the umbilicus. Femoral pulses are usually present but are markedly damped in amplitude. Since more than half of clients with abdominal aneurysms are asymptomatic, the mass may be discovered during a screening physical examination. Although more than 80% of abdominal aneurysms can be palpated, small aneurysms in the markedly obese client may not be felt.

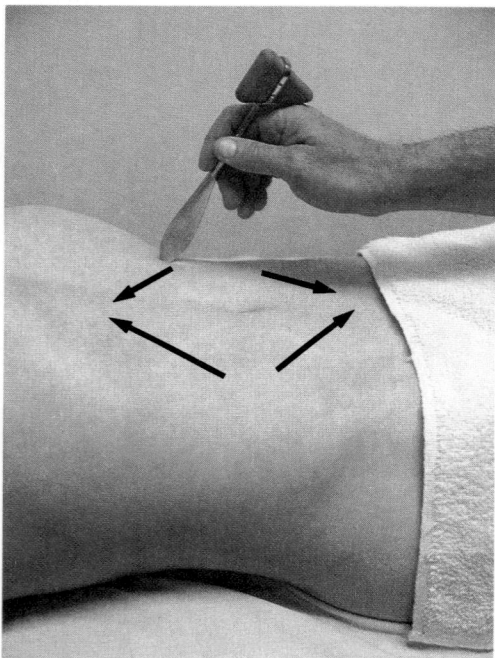

FIGURE 17-30 Examination of the superficial abdominal reflexes. One of several approaches is illustrated. Stroke the upper abdominal area upward, away from the umbilicus, and the lower abdominal area downward, away from the umbilicus. (From Seidel HM and others: *Mosby's guide to physical examination,* ed 2, St. Louis, 1991, Mosby–Year Book.)

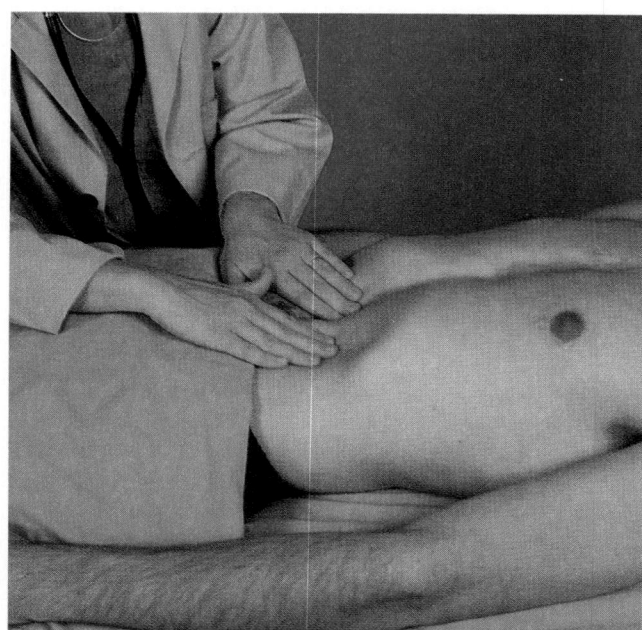

FIGURE 17-31 Palpation of the aorta. Press fingers deeply with one hand on either side of the aorta and feel for pulsation.

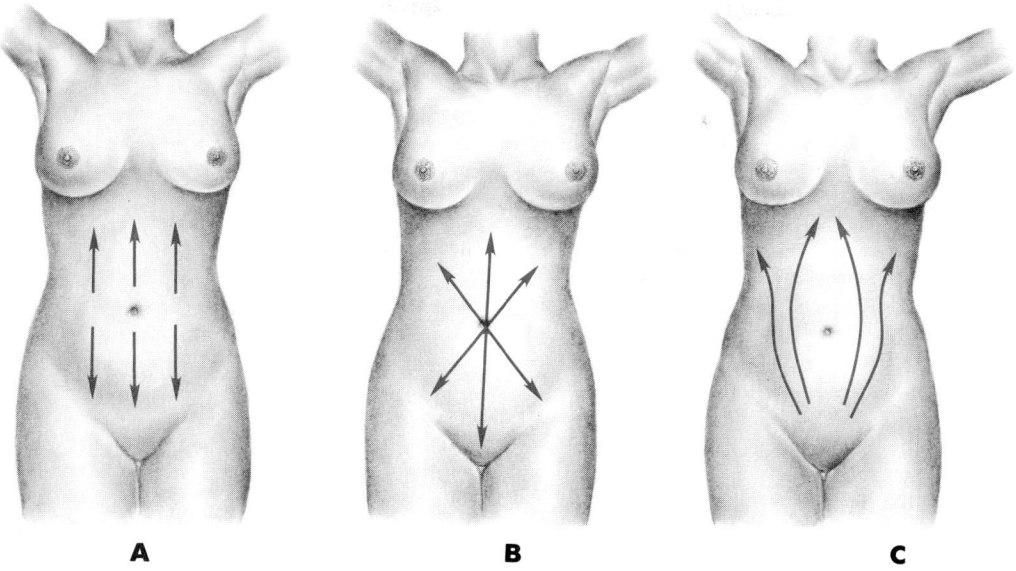

FIGURE 17-32 Abdominal venous patterns. **A,** Normal. **B,** Portal hypertension. **C,** Inferior vena cava obstruction. (From Seidel HM and others: *Mosby's guide to physical examination,* ed 2, St. Louis, 1991, Mosby—Year Book.)

Changes in vascular patterns: venous engorgement. In a healthy person, the veins of the abdominal wall are not prominent. However, in the malnourished individual, the veins are more easily visible because of decreased adipose tissue. The venous return to the heart is cephalad in the veins above the umbilicus and caudal below the navel. The visibility of veins is not useful. However, the direction of flow in visible veins can be helpful to assess obstruction of the vena cava (Figure 17-32). To demonstrate the direction of flow, place the index fingers side by side over a vein, pressing laterally and separating the fingers. A section of the vein may be emptied. Remove one finger and measure the time for filling. "Milk" the blood from a short section of the vein, remove the other index finger, and measure the time for filling from this side. The flow of venous blood is in the direction of the faster filling side.

Reversal of flow or an upward venous flow in the veins below the umbilicus accompanies obstruction of the inferior vena cava. Superior vena cava obstruction promotes downward flow in the veins above the navel. A pattern of engorged veins around the umbilicus, called caput medusae, is occasionally seen as an accompaniment to emaciation or to obstruction of the superior or inferior vena cava, the superficial vein, or the portal vein.

Kidney. When palpating the kidneys, stand at the client's right side with the client in a supine position. To examine the left kidney, reach across the client with your left arm and place your hand behind the client's

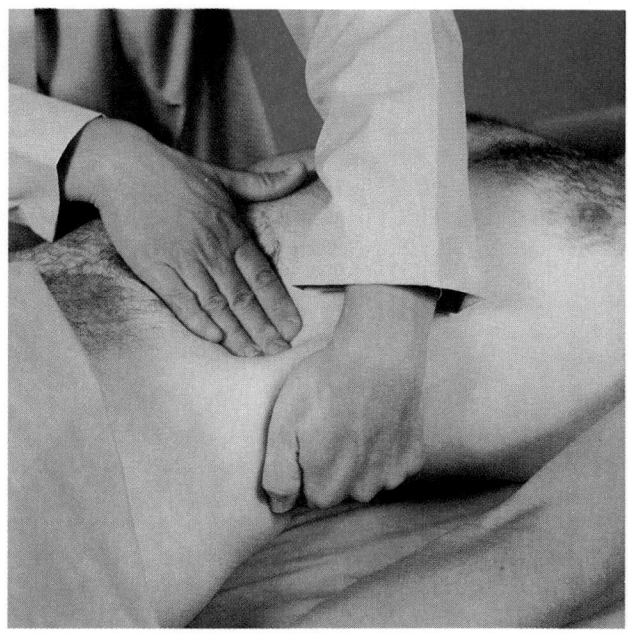

FIGURE 17-33 Palpation of left kidney.

left flank (Figure 17-33). Elevate the left flank with your fingers, displacing the kidney anteriorly. Then use the palmar surface of your right hand to palpate the kidney deeply.

To examine the right kidney, remain on the client's right side. Elevate the right flank with the left hand.

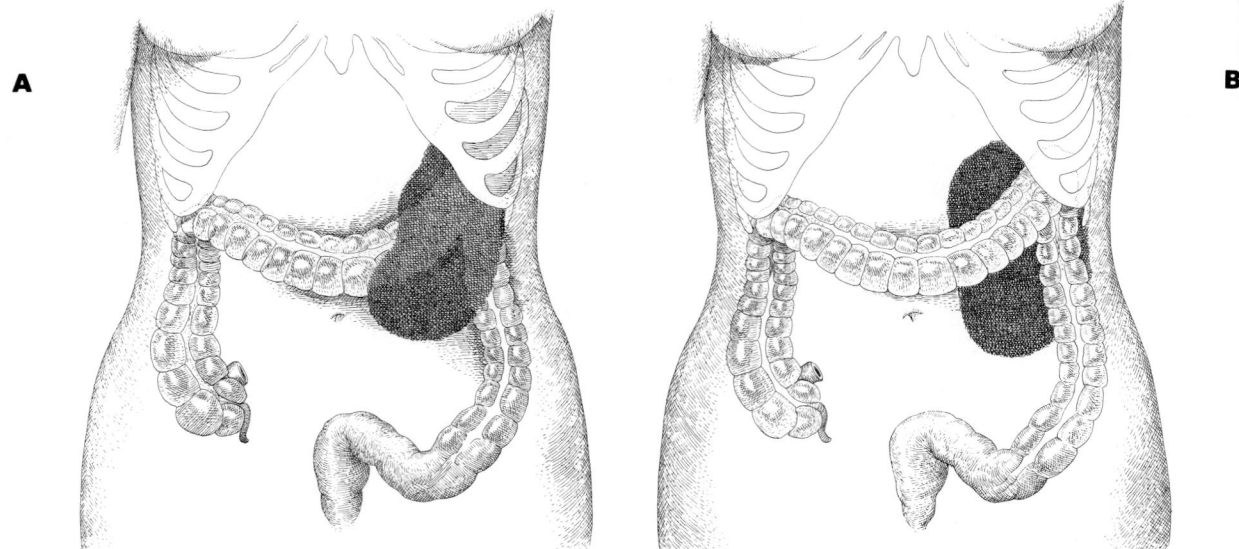

FIGURE 17-34 Differentiation of enlarged spleen **(A)** from enlarged left kidney **(B)**. (From *G.I. Series: physical examination of the abdomen,* Chapter 3, Percussion, Richmond, Va, 1981, AH Robins Co.)

Use the right hand to palpate the right kidney deeply. The lower pole of the right kidney may be felt as a smooth, rounded mass that descends on inspiration.

The kidneys are usually not palpable in the normal adult. In very thin persons, only the lower pole of the right kidney can be felt. In the elderly, as muscle tone decreases and elastic fibers are lost, the kidneys may be more readily palpated. The left kidney is generally not palpable.

Percussion may be used to differentiate between splenic and left kidney enlargement. The percussion note over the spleen is dull because the bowel is displaced downward. Resonance is heard over the kidney because it is located behind the bowel (Figure 17-34). In addition, the free edge of the spleen is sharp in contour and tends to enlarge caudally and to the right.

Back. The final step in the abdominal examination includes inspection and fist percussion of the back for renal problems. The client should be in the sitting position for this portion of the examination. In the normal individual, the flanks are symmetrical. Fullness or asymmetry may be a result of renal disorders. Ecchymoses of the flanks **(Grey Turner's sign)** are associated with retroperitoneal bleeding and may indicate hemorrhagic pancreatitis. Unilateral flank pain or tenderness suggests renal or ureteral disease such as stone, tumor, infection, or infarct.

Fist percussion in each costovertebral angle is done to evaluate kidney tenderness. Figure 17-35 demon-

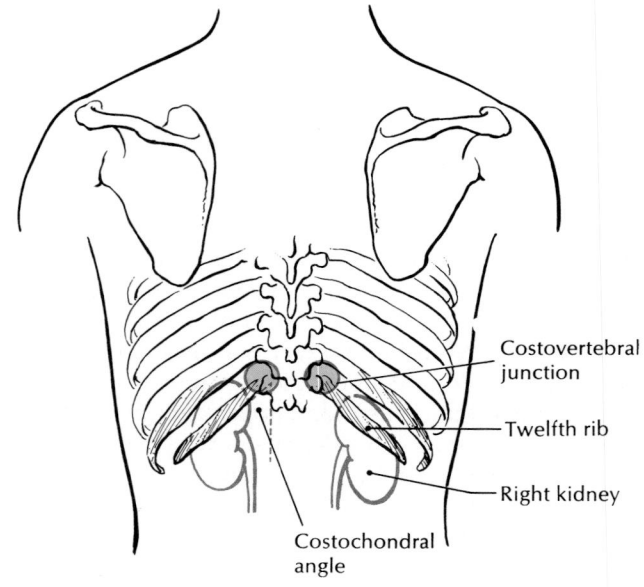

FIGURE 17-35 Relationship of the kidney to the 12th rib. Note the costovertebral junction.

strates the relationship of the kidney to the costovertebral junction. For indirect percussion, place the palm of one hand in the costovertebral angle and strike it with the ulnar surface of the fist of your other hand (Figure 17-36, *A*). Direct percussion is demonstrated in Figure 17-36, *B*. In either type of percussion, use

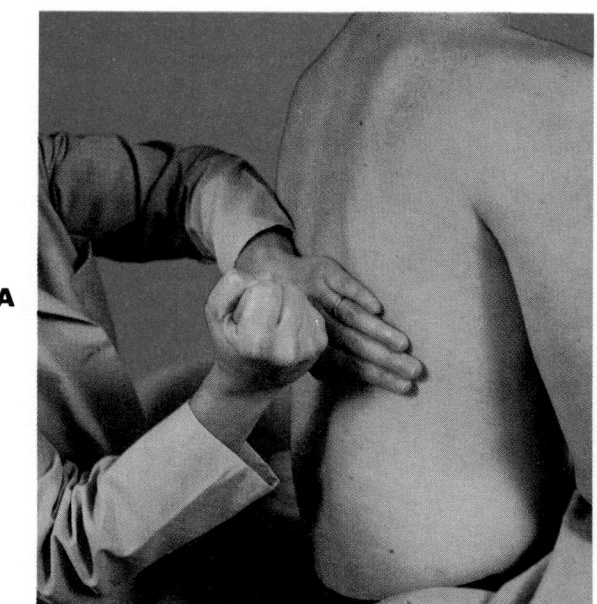 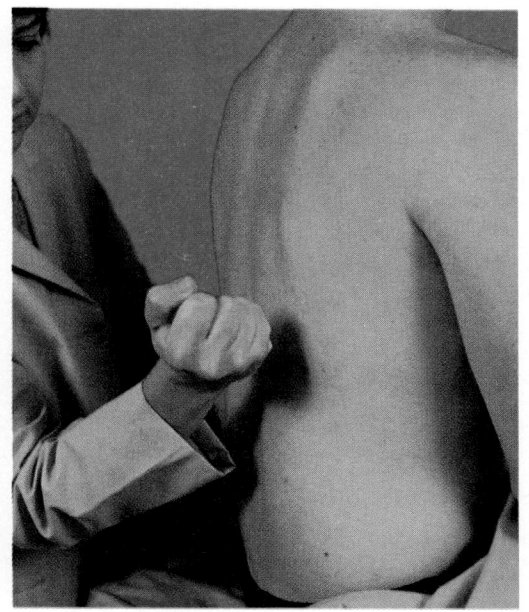

FIGURE 17-36 A, Indirect percussion of the costovertebral angle to elicit tenderness related to the kidney. **B,** Direct percussion of the costovertebral angle to elicit tenderness related to the kidney.

enough force for the client to perceive a painless jarring or a thud. Fist percussion should not cause pain in the normal person. Pressure from your fingertips in the costovertebral angle may be enough to reveal tenderness in the client with a kidney infection. Frequently, this maneuver is integrated into the back examination, or it is done at the end of the posterior lung examination for increased efficiency and client comfort.

Special maneuvers

Evaluation of ascites (free fluid). Ascites should be considered in the client with a protuberant abdomen and bulging flanks. This condition is caused by (1) diseases of the liver, such as cirrhosis and hepatitis; (2) diseases of the heart, such as congestive failure and constrictive pericarditis; (3) pancreatitis; (4) cancer, such as peritoneal metastases and ovarian tumors; (5) tuberculous peritonitis; and (6) hypoalbuminemia.

A technique for differentiating ascites from cysts or edema fluid in the abdominal wall is the percussion test for shifting dullness. Palpation of a fluid wave is another method to assess for ascites.

SHIFTING DULLNESS. Place the client in the supine position. Percuss for areas of dullness and resonance. Ascites will sink with gravity and will produce a dull percussion note in dependent areas (Figure 17-37, *A*). Gas-filled loops of bowel will rise to the upper areas and have a resonant note. Mark the borders between tympany and dullness. Next, test for shifting dullness

(see Figure 17-37, *B*). After marking the borders, ask the client to turn on one side. The ascites will flow with gravity to shift the line of dullness closer to the umbilicus on the client's lying side. Percuss and mark a new line and measure the change in centimeters. In a person without ascites, the borders will remain relatively constant. A volume of free fluid in the peritoneal cavity greater than 2 L can be detected by methods of shifting dullness.

FLUID WAVE. The presence of large amounts of fluid within the peritoneal cavity allows the elicitation of a fluid wave (Figure 17-38). To test for the presence of a fluid wave, place the client in a supine position. Ask the client or an assistant to place the edge of one hand and lower arm firmly in the vertical midline of the client's abdomen. This maneuver will help to stop vibrations that might otherwise be transmitted through fat. Place the palmar surface of one of your hands firmly against the lateral abdominal wall and tap the other side with your other hand. An easily felt fluid wave suggests ascites. However, this sign is often negative until ascites becomes obvious. The fluid wave may sometimes be felt in individuals without ascites.

Ballottement. **Ballottement** (Figure 17-39) is an advanced palpation technique used to assess a floating object. Fluid-filled tissue is pushed toward the examining hand so that the object will float against the examining fingers. This technique is used to determine by

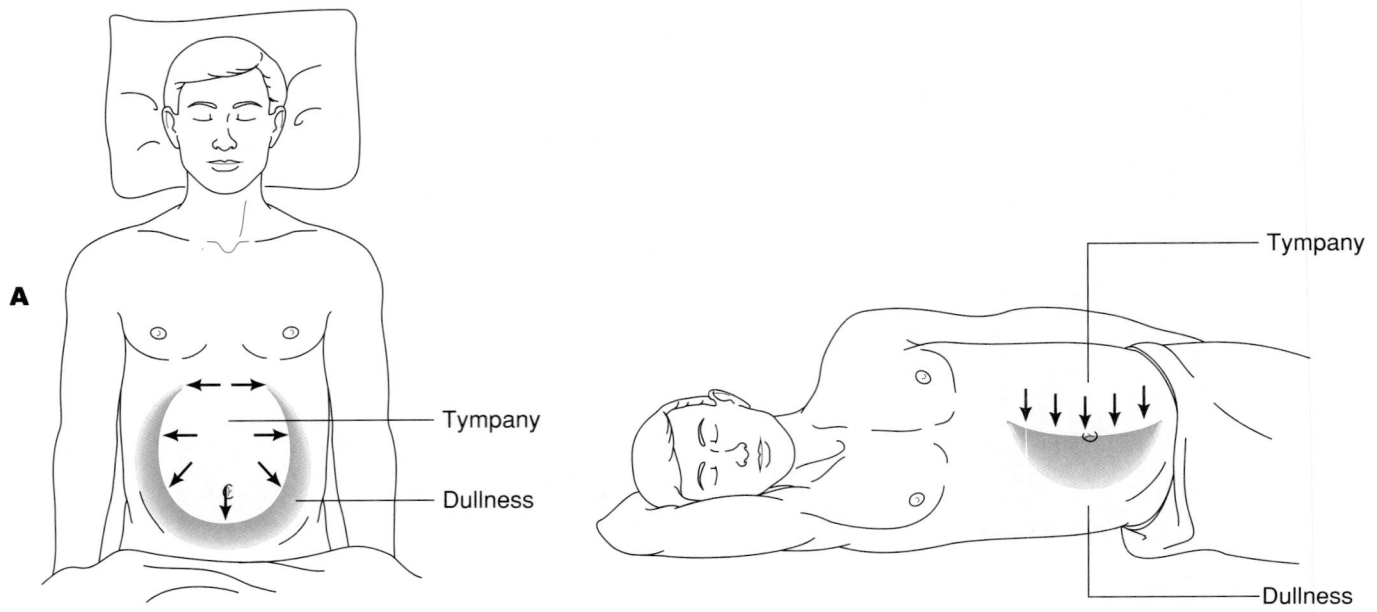

FIGURE 17-37 Assessment of ascites. **A,** In the supine client, ascites fluid will sink with gravity and give a dull percussion note. Mark borders between tympany and dullness. **B,** To test for shifting dullness, ask the client to turn on one side. Ascites fluid will flow with gravity. Dullness shifts to the dependent side while tympany shifts to the top. Percuss and mark new line and measure change.

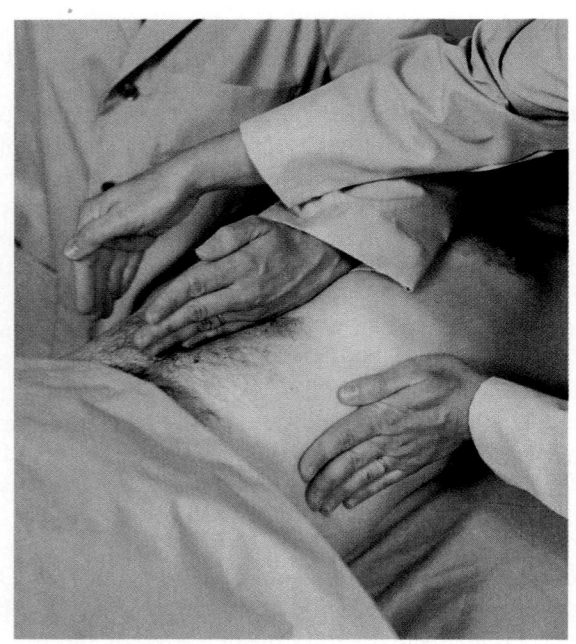

FIGURE 17-38 Testing for fluid wave. Place palmar surface of one hand against abdominal wall and tap the other side with other hand. Easily felt fluid wave suggests ascites.

abdominal palpation whether the head or the breech of the fetus is in the fundus of the uterus (Leopold's maneuver).

SINGLE-HANDED BALLOTTEMENT. Single-handed ballottement is performed with the fingers extended in a straight line with the forearm and positioned at a right angle to the abdomen. Move the fingers quickly toward the mass or organ to be examined and hold them there. As fluid or other structures are displaced, the mass will move upward and be felt at the fingertips. Some examiners prefer this technique for examination of the spleen.

BIMANUAL BALLOTTEMENT

To perform bimanual ballottement, use one hand to push on the anterior abdominal wall to displace the contents to the flank while the other hand receives the mass or structure pushed against it and feels its dimensions.

Palpation to elicit rebound tenderness. Rebound tenderness is a symptom of peritoneal irritation. To provoke rebound tenderness, hold your hand with the fingers extended at a 90-degree angle. Push your fingers gently but deeply in a region remote from the area of suspected tenderness and then rapidly remove them. The maneuver, when performed over **McBurney's point** (as illustrated in Figure 17-40), may elicit re-

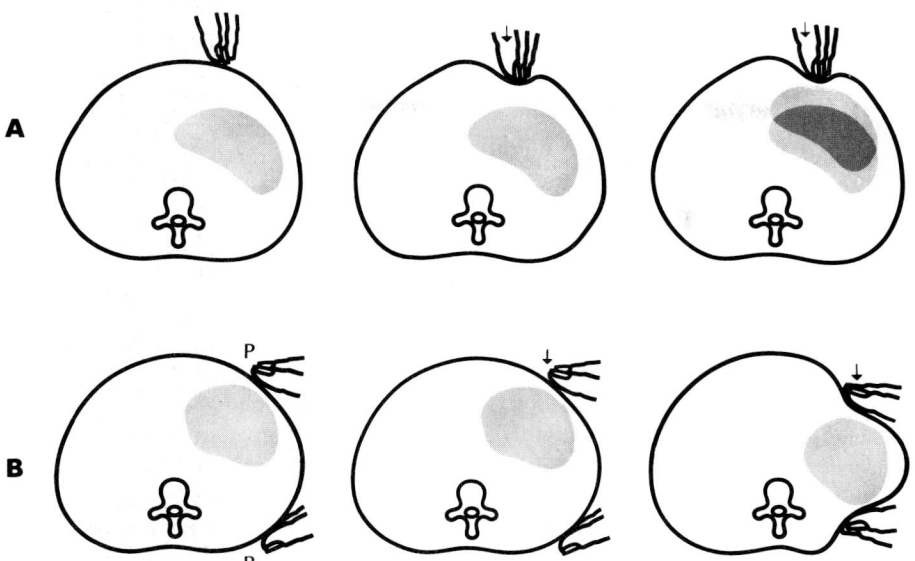

FIGURE 17-39 Ballottement. **A,** Single-handed ballottement: **B,** Bimanual ballottement: *P,* Pushing hand; *R,* receiving hand. (From *G.I. Series: physical examination of the abdomen,* Chapter 2, Palpation, Richmond, Va, 1981, AH Robins Co.)

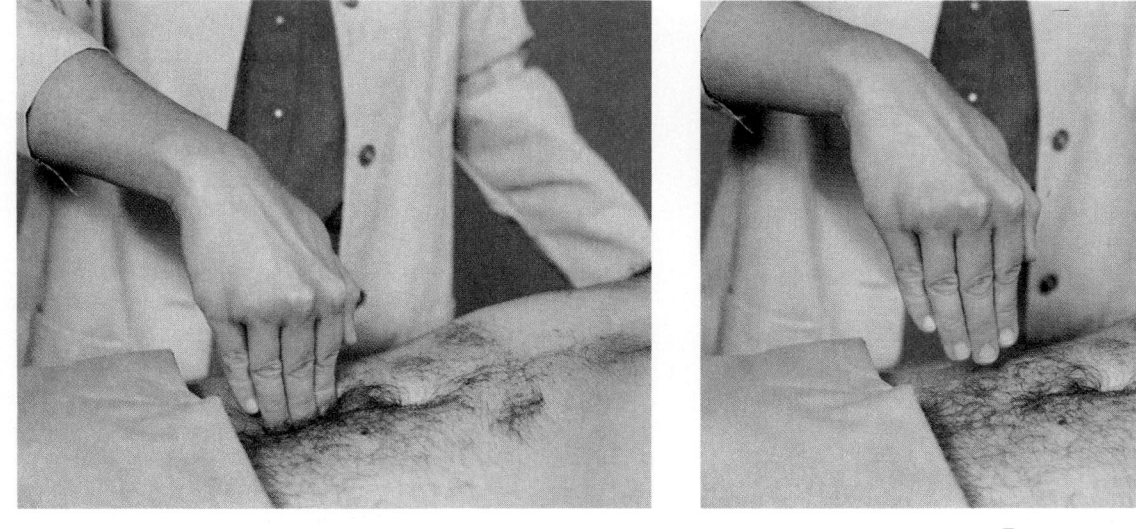

FIGURE 17-40 Palpation to elicit rebound tenderness. **A,** Deep pressure is applied to the abdominal wall. **B,** On release of pressure, a sensation of pain would indicate peritoneal irritation. This is a test for appendicitis.

bound tenderness related to appendicitis. The rebound of the structures indented by palpation causes a sharp, stabbing sensation of pain on the side of the inflammation. This sensation following the withdrawal of pressure is a sign of peritoneal irritation. The test may be repeated on the side of the suspected disease. It is best performed near the conclusion of the examination because the production of severe pain or muscle spasm may interfere with subsequent examination. Voluntary coughing by the client may produce the same results.

Many examiners consider the elicitation of rebound tenderness by palpation to be a crude and painful technique. The resultant severe pain and muscle spasm not only interfere with subsequent examination but also may adversely affect the element of trust in the client-physician relationship. Light percussion can be used to produce vibration, which causes a mildly uncomfortable response in the presence of peritoneal inflammation. This technique is reputed to be able to localize very small areas of peritoneal inflammation, in some instances an area as small as a quarter.

Palpation for abdominal masses. One of the goals of abdominal palpation is to determine the presence of abdominal masses. (Palpation techniques have been described in detail in the preceding sections.) Once a mass has been found, carefully describe its characteristics. Of particular importance are consistency, regularity of contour movement with respiration, tenderness, and mobility (Table 17-2). A sketch of the anterior abdominal wall with all its bony landmarks and the umbilicus may be the most efficient way to convey location, shape, and size.

To determine whether a palpable mass is located in the anterior abdominal wall or is situated in an intraabdominal position, ask the client to raise the head and shoulders from a supine position or to flex the abdominal muscles. Masses in the subcutaneous tissue will continue to be palpable, whereas those in the peritoneal cavity will be more difficult to feel or will be pushed out of reach altogether.

TABLE 17-2

Characteristics of Abdominal Masses Related to Common Pathological Conditions

Description of mass	Possible pathological condition
Descends on inspiration	Liver, spleen, or kidney mass
Pulsatile mass	Abdominal aneurysm, tortuous aorta
Movable from side to side, not head to foot	Mesenteric or small bowel mass
Complete fixation	Tumor of pancreatic or retroperitoneal origin

Normal abdominal structures that are occasionally mistaken for masses are the following (Figure 17-41):

1. Lateral borders of rectus abdominis muscles
2. Uterus
3. Feces-filled ascending colon
4. Feces-filled descending colon and sigmoid colon
5. Aorta
6. Common iliac artery
7. Sacral promontory

PALPABLE BOWEL SEGMENTS. The presence of feces within the bowel frequently contributes to the examiner's ability to palpate the cecum, ascending colon, descending colon, and sigmoid colon. The feces-filled cecum and ascending colon produce a sensation suggestive of a soft, boggy, rounded mass. The client may complain of cramps resulting from stimulation of the bowel by the movements of palpation.

Tests for irritation resulting from appendicitis

ILIOPSOAS MUSCLE TEST. An inflamed or perforated extrapelvic appendix may cause contact irritation of the lateral iliopsoas muscle. To elicit an indication of involvement, place the client in a supine position. Ask the client to flex the lower extremity at the hip. As the client is flexing, simultaneously exert a moderate downward pressure over the lower thigh (Figure 17-42). With psoas muscle inflammation, the client will describe pain in the lower quadrant. A more sensitive test of psoas muscle irritation is performed with the client lying on the left side. Pain is elicited through all positions of full extension of the right lower limb at the hip.

OBTURATOR MUSCLE TEST. A perforated intrapelvic appendix or a pelvic abscess adjacent to it can cause irritation of the internal obturator muscle. This pain is demonstrated with the client in the supine position. Ask the client to flex the right extremity at the hip and at the knee to 90 degrees. Grasp the ankle and rotate it internally and externally (Figure 17-43). A complaint of hypogastric pain indicates obturator muscle involvement.

TEST FOR DIASTASIS RECTI OR ABDOMINAL HERNIA. If an umbilical or incisional hernia or diastasis recti abdominis is suspected, instruct the client to raise the head from the pillow, thus increasing the intraabdominal pressure, which may cause the hernia to protrude. Asking the client to cough will also cause a hernia to bulge outward. When the client raises the head from the pillow, the rectus muscles contract and will reveal a separation of the muscles. Diastasis recti may be congenital or may be acquired as a result of weakening of the muscles by conditions such as pregnancy and obesity.

Assessment of muscle spasticity. Involuntary muscle contraction or spasticity may indicate peritoneal irritation. Further palpation is done to determine whether

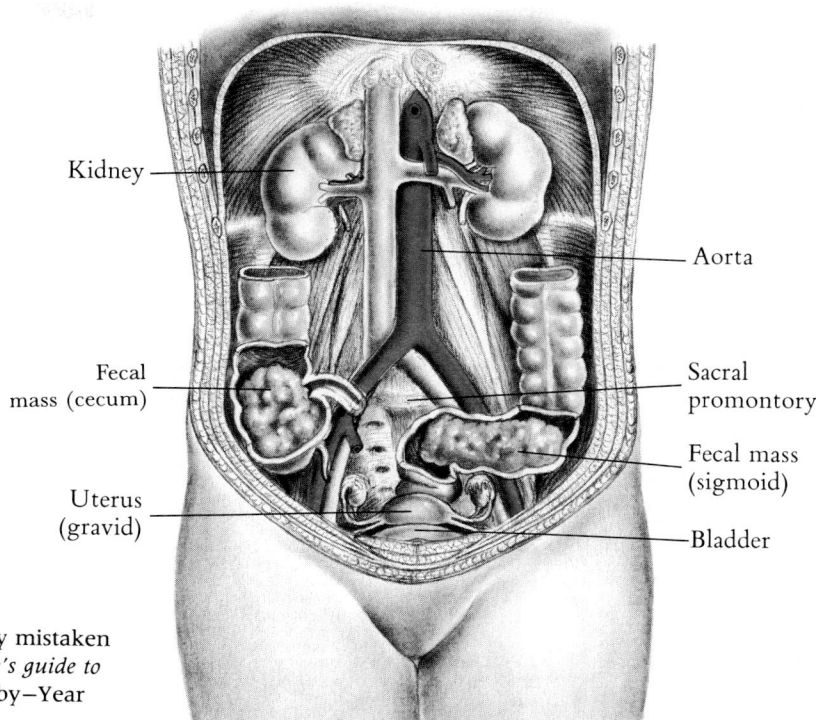

FIGURE 17-41 Abdominal structures frequently mistaken for masses. (From Seidel HM and others: *Mosby's guide to physical examination,* ed 2, St. Louis, 1991, Mosby–Year Book.)

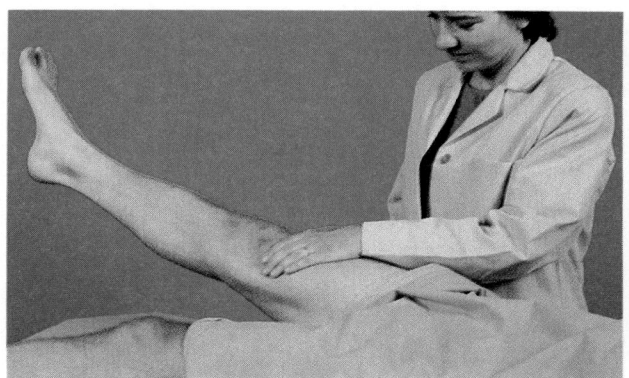

FIGURE 17-42 Iliopsoas muscle test.

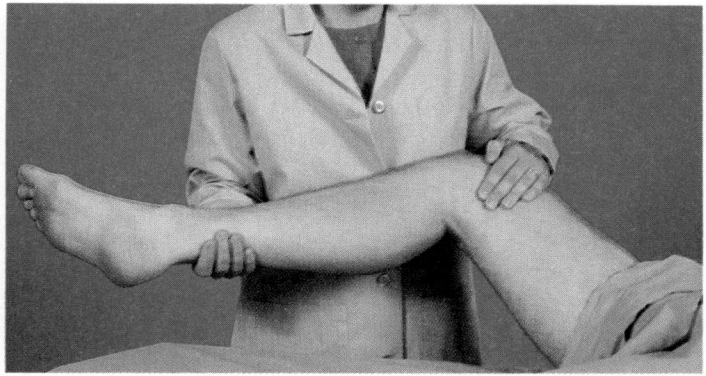

FIGURE 17-43 Obturator muscle test.

the spasticity is unilateral or present on both sides of the abdomen. Generalized and boardlike contraction is thought to be typical of peritonitis. Ask the client to raise the trunk from a horizontal position without arm support. The experience of unilateral pain in response to this maneuver may further pinpoint the areas of spasticity. This mechanism may also help to differentiate muscle contraction from abdominal mass. As the head is raised, the examining hand would be moved away from an abdominal mass. Rigidity and tenderness over McBurney's point, and in some cases over the entire right side, strongly suggest appendicitis. Acute cholecystitis is frequently accompanied by rigidity of the right hypochondrium.

Examination Step-by-Step

Preparation

1. Assemble needed equipment (stethoscope, ruler, marking pen).
2. Make sure that the room is comfortably warm.
3. Explain the examination to the client.
4. Position the client in a comfortable supine position with arms at the sides, head supported by a pillow, and knees slightly flexed (and supported by a pillow, if available).
5. Completely expose the abdomen from just above the costal margin to the symphysis pubis, draping the client's chest and pubic area for modesty and warmth.
6. Ask the client to point to any tender areas and reassure the person that you will examine those areas last.
7. Watch the client's facial expressions for signs of discomfort during the examination.

Inspection

Observe the surface of the abdomen for the following factors:
1. Skin color
2. Scars
3. Venous network
4. Umbilicus—placement, contour, surface characteristics
5. Symmetry (view from right side at eye level and from behind the client's head)
6. Contour
7. Surface characteristics
8. Surface motility—peristalsis, pulsations

Auscultation

1. Listen to all four quadrants and the epigastrium using the diaphragm of the stethoscope; note timing and quality of sounds.
2. Listen for arterial vascular sounds (abdominal aorta, renal and femoral arteries). Use the bell of the stethoscope to pick up low-pitched sounds such as a venous hum.
3. Listen for a friction rub, most commonly heard over the liver or the spleen.

Percussion

1. Lightly percuss all four quadrants.
2. Percuss liver borders at the midclavicular and midsternal lines. Mark upper and lower borders with a pen and measure liver span.
3. Percuss spleen at the left midaxillary line.
4. Percuss "gastric bubble" at the left lower rib cage.

Palpation

1. Use light palpation with pads of fingertips to survey all four quadrants for tenderness, muscle tone, masses.
2. Use moderate palpation with the flat and the sides of the hands to continue to assess all four quadrants for tenderness, muscle tone, masses, and general location of major structures.
3. Use deep palpation to survey all four quadrants for tenderness, masses, and location of deeper structures.
4. Palpate specific organs:
   a. Liver: Deeply palpate by placing the left hand under the eleventh and twelfth ribs and the right hand parallel to the right costal margin. Have the client breathe normally and then take a deep breath.
   b. Spleen: While standing on the client's right side, extend your left hand and place it beneath the client's left costovertebral angle. Feel for the spleen by pressing your right hand gently under the left anterior costal margin. Have the client take a deep breath and palpate as the client exhales. Repeat the examination with the client lying on the right side with hips and knees slightly flexed.
   c. Aorta: With the client in the supine position, deeply palpate slightly to the left of midline to feel for the aortic pulsation.
   d. Palpate the umbilicus with the fingertips for bulges, nodules, and the umbilical ring.
   e. Kidneys: With the client supine, palpate each kidney. *Left kidney:* Extend the left hand across the client to elevate the left flank (left kidney is usually not palpable). Then deeply palpate the kidney with the right hand. *Right kidney:* Place the left hand under the right flank and palpate deeply with the right hand.

To assess kidney tenderness, have the client sit up and use fist percussion at the right and left costovertebral angles.

VARIATIONS FROM HEALTH

Tables 17-3 through 17-6 list the history, signs, and symptoms of various conditions associated with the abdomen. The signs and symptoms of intestinal obstruc-tion and of peritoneal irritation are shown in the boxes on p. 527.

Abdominal Pain

Tables 17-7 and 17-8 list possible pathological condi-tions based on descriptions of abdominal pain and its onset.

TABLE 17-3

Conditions Associated with the Right Lower Quadrant of the Abdomen

Condition	History	Symptoms	Signs
Appendicitis	Children (except in-fants) and young adults	Anorexia Nausea Pain: early vague epigas-tric, periumbilical, or generalized pain after 12-24 hours; RLQ at McBurney's point	Signs may be absent early Vomiting Localized RLQ guarding and tenderness after 12-24 hours Rovsing's sign: pain in RLQ with pressure RLQ, iliop-soas sign Obturator sign White blood cell count 10,000 mm^3 or shift to left Low-grade fever Cutaneous hyperesthesia in RLQ Signs are highly variable
Mesenteric adenitis	Young person with his-tory of respiratory in-fection	Lower abdominal pain May have normal appetite	Tenderness in RLQ Peritoneal irritation signs rare
Perforated duodenal ulcer	Prior history	Abrupt onset pain in epi-gastric area or RLQ	Tenderness in epigastric area or RLQ Signs of peritoneal irritation Heme-positive stool Increased white blood cell count
Cecal volvulus	Seen most frequently in the elderly	Abrupt severe abdominal pain	Distention Localized tenderness Tympany
Strangulated hernia	Any age Women: femoral Men: inguinal	Severe localized pain If bowel obstructed, gen-eralized pain	If bowel obstructed, distention

Ectopic pregnancy (1% of all pregnancies)	Woman of child-bearing age
	Previous tubal preg-nancy or pelvic in-flammatory disease
	Missed menstrual period
	Spotting
		Symptoms of pregnancy (i.e., breast changes)
		Lower abdominal pain
		Referred pain to shoulder
		Nausea
			Unruptured
			  Tenderness: cervical
			  Mass: adnexal or cul-de-sac
			Ruptured
			  Shock
			  Distention
			  Rigidity
			Mass: cul-de-sac
			Fever

Pelvic inflammatory dis-ease	Woman
	
	Exposure to infection
		Lower abdominal pain
		
		Dyspareunia
			Tenderness: adnexal and cer-vical (chandelier sign)
			Cervical discharge
			Endocervical smear
			  Gonococcus in one third to one half of cases
			  Chlamydial and anaerobic bacteria cause remainder

Tubal abscess	Woman Exposure to infection Dyspareunia	Lower abdominal pain Mass: adnexal	Fever

TABLE 17-4

Conditions Associated with the Right Upper Quadrant of the Abdomen

Condition	History	Symptoms	Signs
Liver hepatitis	Any age, often young blood product user	Fatigue Malaise Anorexia	Hepatic tenderness Hepatomegaly Bilirubin elevated Jaundice
	Drug addict	Pain in RUQ Low-grade fever May have severe fulminating disease with liver failure	Lymphocytosis in one third of cases Liver enzymes elevated Hepatitis A or B or antibodies to the viruses may be found
Acute hepatic congestion	Usually elderly with congestive heart failure Pericardial disease Pulmonary embolism	Symptoms of congestive heart failure	Hepatomegaly Congestive heart failure
Biliary stones, colic	"Fair, fat, forty" (90%) but can be 30 to 80 years of age	Anorexia Nausea Pain severe in RUQ or epigastric area Episodes last 15 minutes to hours	Tenderness in RUQ Jaundice
Acute cholecystitis	"Fair, fat, forty" (90%) but may be 30 to 80 years of age	Severe RUQ or epigastric pain Episodes prolonged up to 6 hours	Vomiting Tenderness in RUQ Peritoneal irritation signs Increased white blood cell count
Perforated peptic ulcer	Any age	Abrupt RUQ pain	Tenderness in epigastrium and/or right quadrant Peritoneal irritation signs Free air in abdomen

TABLE 17-5

Conditions Associated with the Left Upper Quadrant of the Abdomen

Condition	History	Symptoms	Signs
Splenic trauma	Blunt trauma to LUQ of abdomen	Pain: LUQ pain of the abdomen often referred to the left shoulder (Kehr's sign)	Hypotension Syncope Increased dyspnea X-ray studies show enlarged spleen
Pancreatitis	Alcohol abuse Pancreatic duct Obstruction Infection Cholecystitis	Pain in LUQ or epigastric region radiating to the back or chest	Fever Rigidity Rebound tenderness Nausea Vomiting Jaundice Cullen's sign Turner's sign Abdominal distention Diminished bowel sounds
Pyloric obstruction	Duodenal ulcer	Weight loss Gastric upset Vomiting	Increasing dullness in LUQ Visible peristaltic waves in epigastric region

TABLE 17-6

Conditions Associated with the Left Lower Quadrant of the Abdomen

Condition	History	Symptoms	Signs
Ulcerative colitis	Family history Jewish ancestry	Chronic, watery diarrhea with blood, mucus Anorexia Weight loss Fatigue	Fever Cachexia Anemia Leukocytosis
Colonic diverticulitis	Over age 39 Low-residue diet	Pain that recurs in LUQ	Fever Vomiting Chills Diarrhea Tenderness over descending colon

TABLE 17-7

Nature of Abdominal Pain

Description of pain	Possible pathological condition
Burning	Ulceration (peptic)
Cramping	Biliary colic
Severe cramping (colic)	Appendicitis with fecalith
Aching	Appendiceal inflammation
Knifelike	Pancreatitis
Radiation of pain	See Figure 17-44

TABLE 17-8

Onset of Abdominal Pain

Description of onset	Possible pathological condition
Gradual onset	Infection
Acute onset	
Awakening client from sleep	Duodenal ulcer
Loss of consciousness	Acute pancreatitis Perforated ulcer Ruptured ectopic pregnancy Intestinal obstruction (strangulated)

SIGNS AND SYMPTOMS OF INTESTINAL OBSTRUCTION

General signs

Distention
Hyperactive bowel sounds of high-pitched, tinkling
  character
Minimum rebound tenderness
Pain

Signs of proximal obstruction

Acute onset
Vomiting (marked)
Frequent bouts of pain
Distention (minimal)

Signs of distal obstruction

Onset may be more gradual
Less marked vomiting
Less frequent bouts of pain
Distention (marked)

SIGNS AND SYMPTOMS OF PERITONEAL IRRITATION

Boardlike, increased rigidity of abdominal wall
Silent bowel sounds
Tenderness and guarding
Severe focal pain
Palpable abdominal rigidity
Positive obturator test
Positive iliopsoas test
Nausea, vomiting
Shock-diaphoresis (requires emergency attention)
Hypotension

Referred Pain or Somatic Pain from Intraabdominal Structures

Pain related to abdominal structures may be sensed in remote body surface regions (Table 17-9). The explanation for this phenomenon is that, as pain is intensified, increased afferent impulses lower the client's pain threshold and excite secondary sensory neurons in the spinal cord. Thus contact may be established between afferent visceral fibers and somatic nerves of the same embryological dermatome. An example of this phenomenon is pain sensed in the top of the shoulder that is caused by abdominal lesions or peritonitis. The diaphragm, which is irritated in this situation, originates in the region of the fourth cervical nerve and derives its nerve supply from the third, fourth, and fifth cervical nerves. The shoulder is innervated by the fourth cervical nerve. Thus shoulder pain may be a valuable clue in diagnosing perforated ulcer, hepatic abscess, pancreatitis, cholecystitis, ruptured spleen, pelvic inflammation, and hemorrhage into the peritoneum. Other examples of referred pain are noted in Figure 17-44.

TABLE 17-9

Symptoms or Signs Elicited in Other Systems that May Focus the Abdominal Examination

Symptom or sign	Possible pathological condition	Symptom or sign	Possible pathological condition
Shock	Acute pancreatitis, ruptured tubal pregnancy	Flank tenderness	Renal inflammation, pyelonephritis
Mental status deficit	Hemorrhage—duodenal ulcer Abdominal epilepsy		Renal stone Renal infarct
Hypertension	Aortic dissection Abdominal aortic aneurysm Renal infarction Glomerulonephritis Vasculitis	Leg edema	Renal vein thrombosis Iliac obstruction, pelvic mass Renal disease Renal vein thrombosis
Orthostatic hypotension	Hypovolemia—blood loss, fluid loss	Lymphadenopathy	Hepatitis Lymphoma Mononucleosis
Pulse deficit	Aortic dissection Aortic aneurysm or thrombosis	Jaundice	Liver-biliary disease Excessive hemolysis
Bruits	Aortic dissection Aortic aneurysm Dissection or aneurysm of arteries—splenic, renal, or iliac	Dark yellow to brown urine	Liver-biliary disease Blood resulting from kidney stone, infarct, glomerulonephritis, or pyelonephritis
Low-output cardiac symptoms Atrial fibrillation	Ischemia of mesentery	Fever (103° F) and chills	Peritonitis Pelvic infection Cholangitis Pyelonephritis
Valvular disease, congestive heart failure	Embolus	White blood cell count >10,000 mm³ or shift to left (more than 80% polymorphonuclear cells) >20,000 mm³	Appendicitis (95%) Acute cholecystitis (90%) Localized peritonitis Bowel strangulation Bowel infarction
Pleural effusion	Esophageal rupture Pancreatitis Ovarian tumor		

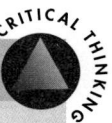

Nursing Diagnosis *THE NEXT STEP—cont'd*

Palpitation: tenderness over epigastric area; slight tenderness over all four abdominal quadrants. No organomegaly; no costovertebral angle tenderness; negative Murphy's sign; negative McBurney's sign.

NURSING DIAGNOSES

Pain related to irritation of gastric mucosa.

Defining Characteristics

- Subjective communication of pain
- Grimacing of face when abdomen palpated
- Guarding behavior of upper abdomen

Altered nutrition: less than body requirement related to nausea, vomiting, and pain.

Defining Characteristics

- Abdominal pain
- Aversion to eating at the present time
- Lack of interest in food at the present time

Diarrhea related to irritation of gastric mucosa.

Defining Characteristics

- Abdominal pain
- Cramping
- Increased frequency of bowel movements
- Increased frequency of bowel sounds

GLOSSARY

ascites Abnormal accumulation of fluid within the abdominal cavity.

ballottement Palpation technique used to assess a floating object. Fluid-filled tissue is pushed toward the examiner's hand so that the object will float against the examiner's fingers.

borborygmi Audible bowel sounds, generally caused by gas propulsion through the intestine.

bruit Murmur (blowing sound) heard over peripheral vessels.

cirrhosis Disease characterized by destruction of liver parenchyma. The affected liver is characterized by fibrous tissue and yellow-tan nodules.

diastasis recti abdominis Separation of the rectus muscles of the abdominal wall. May occur as a result of pregnancy or obesity.

flatulence Presence of an excessive amount of gas in the gastrointestinal tract.

Grey Turner's sign Bruising of the flank skin.

hepatomegaly Abnormal enlargement of the liver, usually a sign of liver disease.

keloid Scar formation caused by a dense overgrowth of fibrous tissue, usually raised and thickened.

lineae albicantes (striae) Atrophic lines or streaks that differ in texture and color from the surrounding skin and are caused by disrupted elastic fibers of the reticular layer of the skin.

McBurney's point Anatomical landmark located approximately 2 inches above the right anterosuperior iliac spine on a line between the umbilicus and the spine.

Murphy's sign Sign noted by a maneuver done during deep palpation in the approximate location of the gallbladder. On deep inspiration, the liver descends, bringing the gallbladder in contact with the examiner's hand. Pain is elicited in the presence of cholecystitis.

peritonitis Inflammation of the peritoneum.

striae gravidarum Atrophic, pinkish or purplish scarlike lesions observed on the breasts, thighs, abdomen, and buttocks during pregnancy; lesions later become silvery white.

von Recklinghausen's disease Also known as neurofibromatosis, this congenital condition is characterized by fibrous tumors of the nerve tissue (neurofibromas), café-au-lait spots on the skin, and, in some cases, developmental anomalies of the muscles, bones, and viscera.

BIBLIOGRAPHY

Bowers AC, Thompson JM: *Clinical manual of health assessment*, ed 4, St Louis, 1992, Mosby—Year Book.

Centers for Disease Control: Hepatitis B virus: a comprehensive strategy for eliminating transmission in the United States through universal childhood vaccination—recommendations of the Immunization Practices Advisory Committee (ACIP), *MMWR* 40(No. RR-13), 1991.

Christensen J: *Bedside logic in diagnostic gastroenterology*, New York, 1987, Churchill Livingstone.

Gordon M: *Manual of nursing diagnosis 1993-1994*, St Louis, 1993, Mosby—Year Book.

Gordon M: *Nursing diagnosis: process and application*, ed 2, St Louis, 1987, Mosby—Year Book.

Johnson LR: *Gastrointestinal physiology*, ed 4, St Louis, 1991, Mosby—Year Book.

Seidel HM and others: *Mosby's guide to physical examination*, ed 2, St Louis, 1991, Mosby—Year Book.

Thompson JM and others: *Mosby's manual of clinical nursing*, ed 2, St Louis, 1989, Mosby—Year Book.

US Preventive Services Task Force: *Guide to clinical preventive services*, Baltimore, 1990, Williams & Wilkins.

Musculoskeletal System

PURPOSE OF THE EXAMINATION

The purpose of the musculoskeletal examination is to perform a systematic functional assessment of the musculoskeletal system as it relates to activities of daily living and detection of common dysfunctions.

The musculoskeletal system provides support for the body, protection for the internal organs, mobility to engage in physical activities, production of red blood cells, and storage of minerals. It includes bones, muscles, ligaments, tendons, cartilage, and joints. Because the central nervous system coordinates muscle and bone function, understanding how these two systems interrelate is important. The neurological examination is detailed in Chapter 19.

Musculoskeletal concerns vary at different ages. Injuries, however, are the most common musculoskeletal disorders seen in clinical practice, particularly in children and young adults. Middle-aged and older adults (and to a lesser degree children) are also affected by inflammatory, degenerative, and rheumatic conditions. In addition, neurological problems may also affect the musculoskeletal system. A particular symptom, such as difficulty walking, may be caused by a musculoskeletal injury or a cerebellar defect.

ANATOMY AND PHYSIOLOGY

Skeleton

The skeleton is made up of 206 bones that are shaped according to their function (Figure 18-1). Bones provide support, allowing the individual to stand erect. They protect the tissues and the internal organs (e.g., skull, rib cage, and pelvis). They assist movement in coordination with muscles and joints. Bones provide storage areas for minerals and serve as sites for the formation of red blood cells (hematopoiesis).

The appendicular skeleton consists of the bones of the shoulders, arms, legs, and pelvis. The axial skeleton is composed of the bones of the face, skull, auditory ossicles, hyoid bone, vertebrae, ribs, and sternum (Figures 18-2 and 18-3).

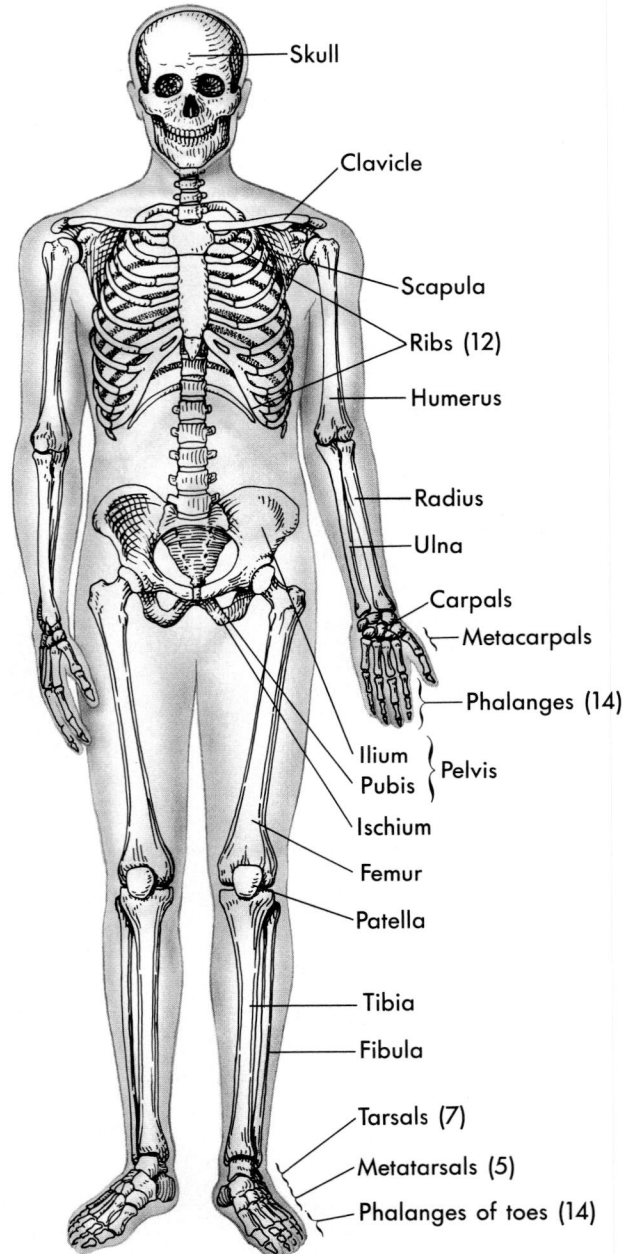

FIGURE 18-1 Bones that compose the skeleton. (From Mourad LA: *Orthopedic disorders,* St Louis, 1991, Mosby–Year Book.)

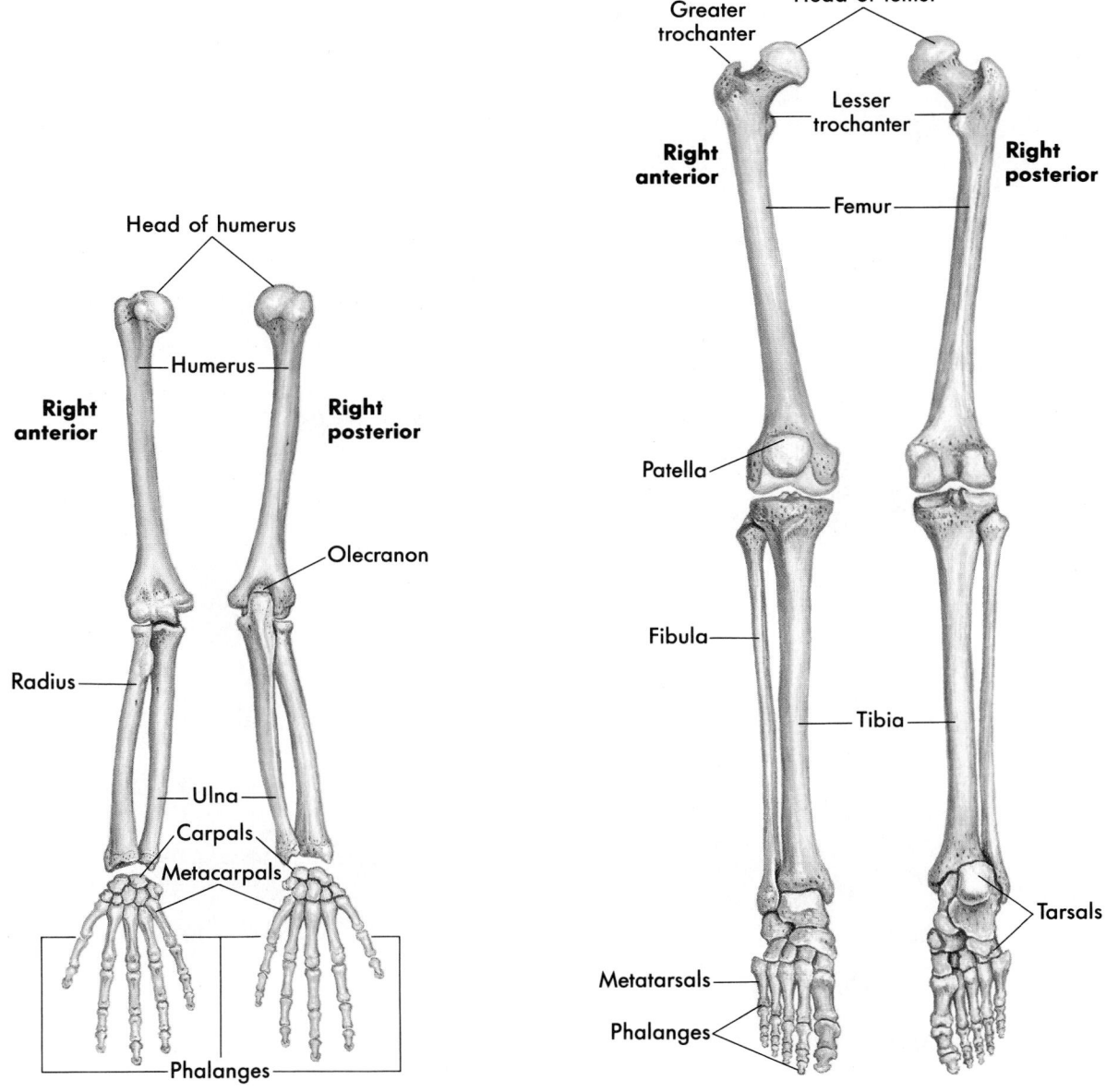

FIGURE 18-2 Bones of the upper and lower extremities. (From Mourad LA: *Orthopedic disorders*, St Louis, 1991, Mosby–Year Book.)

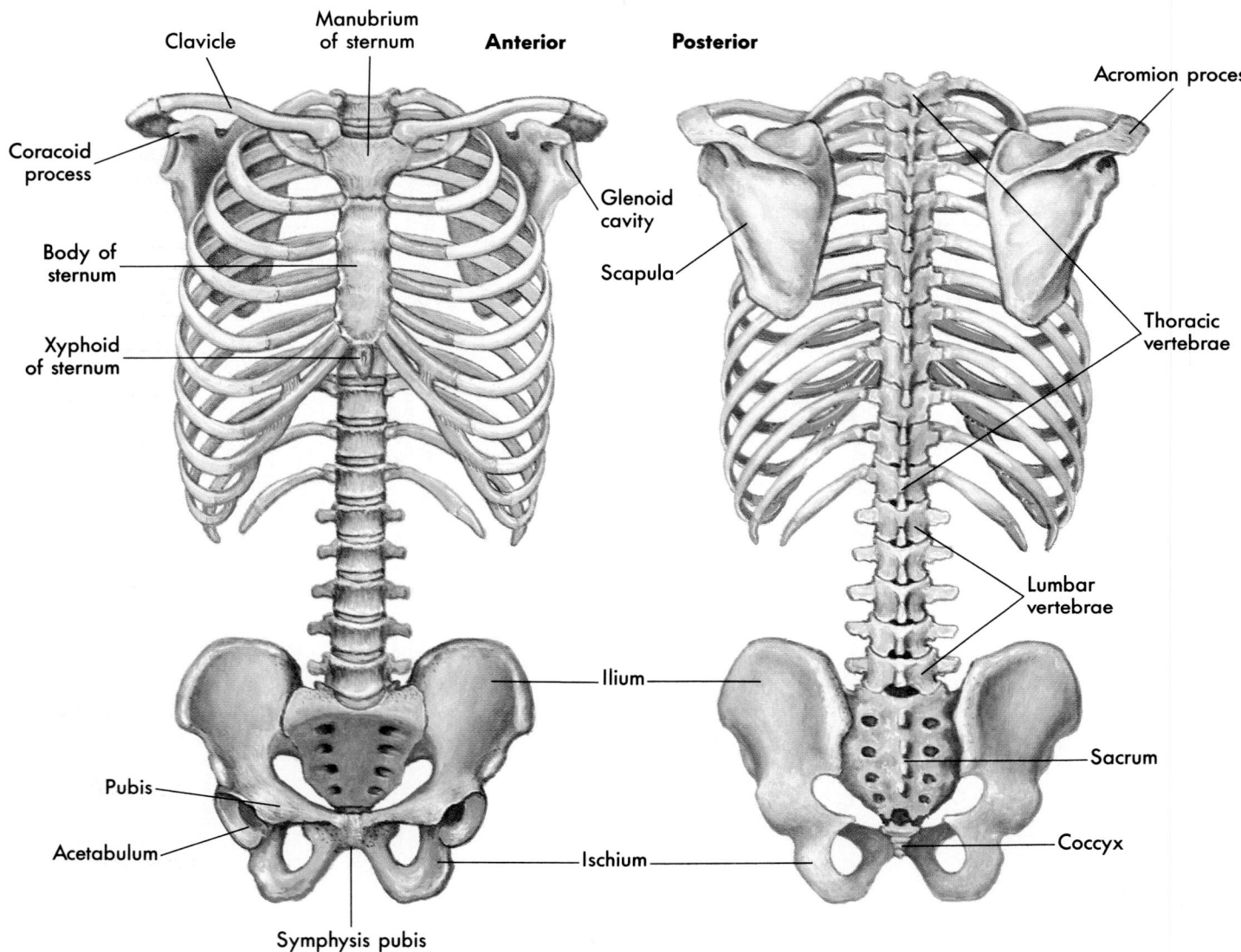

FIGURE 18-3 Bones of the trunk and pelvis. (From Mourad LA: *Orthopedic disorders,* St Louis, 1991, Mosby–Year Book.)

Muscles

The musculoskeletal system is composed of more than 600 voluntary, or striated, muscles (Figure 18-4). It constitutes the principal organ of movement and is a repository for metabolites. There are three types of muscles: visceral (smooth, involuntary), cardiac, and skeletal (striated, voluntary). This discussion concerns only skeletal muscle. Skeletal muscle mass accounts for 40% to 45% of body weight. The partial contracture of skeletal muscle makes possible all the characteristic postures of human beings, including the upright position that distinguishes the anthropoid. Muscles are attached at each end to a bone, tendon, ligament, or fascia. The fixed end of the muscle is called the origin. The more movable end is known as the muscle insertion. Muscles are normally full and supple. Aging may bring a loss of muscle fiber and an increase in connective tissue that causes loss of muscle strength. Nutrition, exercise, gender, and genetic constitution account for variations in muscle strength among individuals.

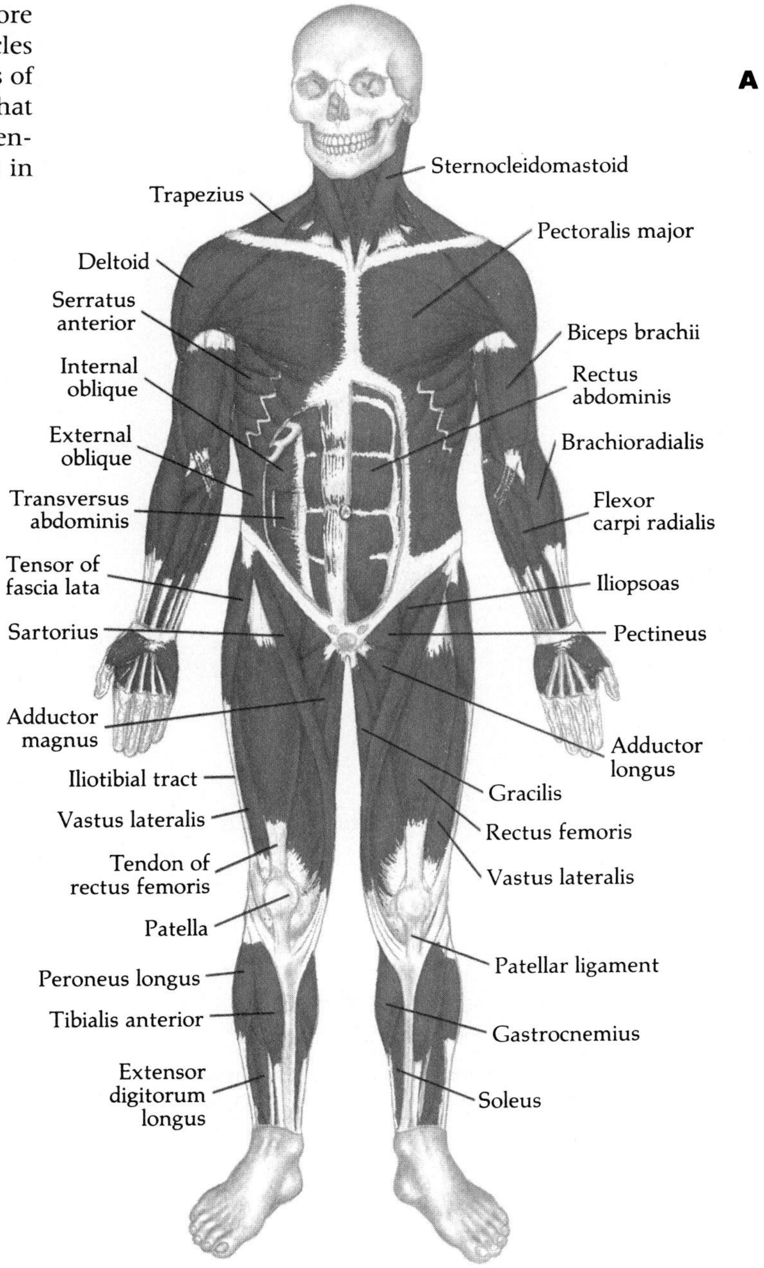
A
Sternocleidomastoid
Trapezius
Pectoralis major
Deltoid
Serratus anterior
Biceps brachii
Internal oblique
Rectus abdominis
External oblique
Brachioradialis
Transversus abdominis
Flexor carpi radialis
Tensor of fascia lata
Iliopsoas
Sartorius
Pectineus
Adductor magnus
Adductor longus
Iliotibial tract
Gracilis
Vastus lateralis
Rectus femoris
Tendon of rectus femoris
Vastus lateralis
Patella
Patellar ligament
Peroneus longus
Tibialis anterior
Gastrocnemius
Extensor digitorum longus
Soleus

FIGURE 18-4 Muscles of the body. **A,** Anterior view.

Continued.

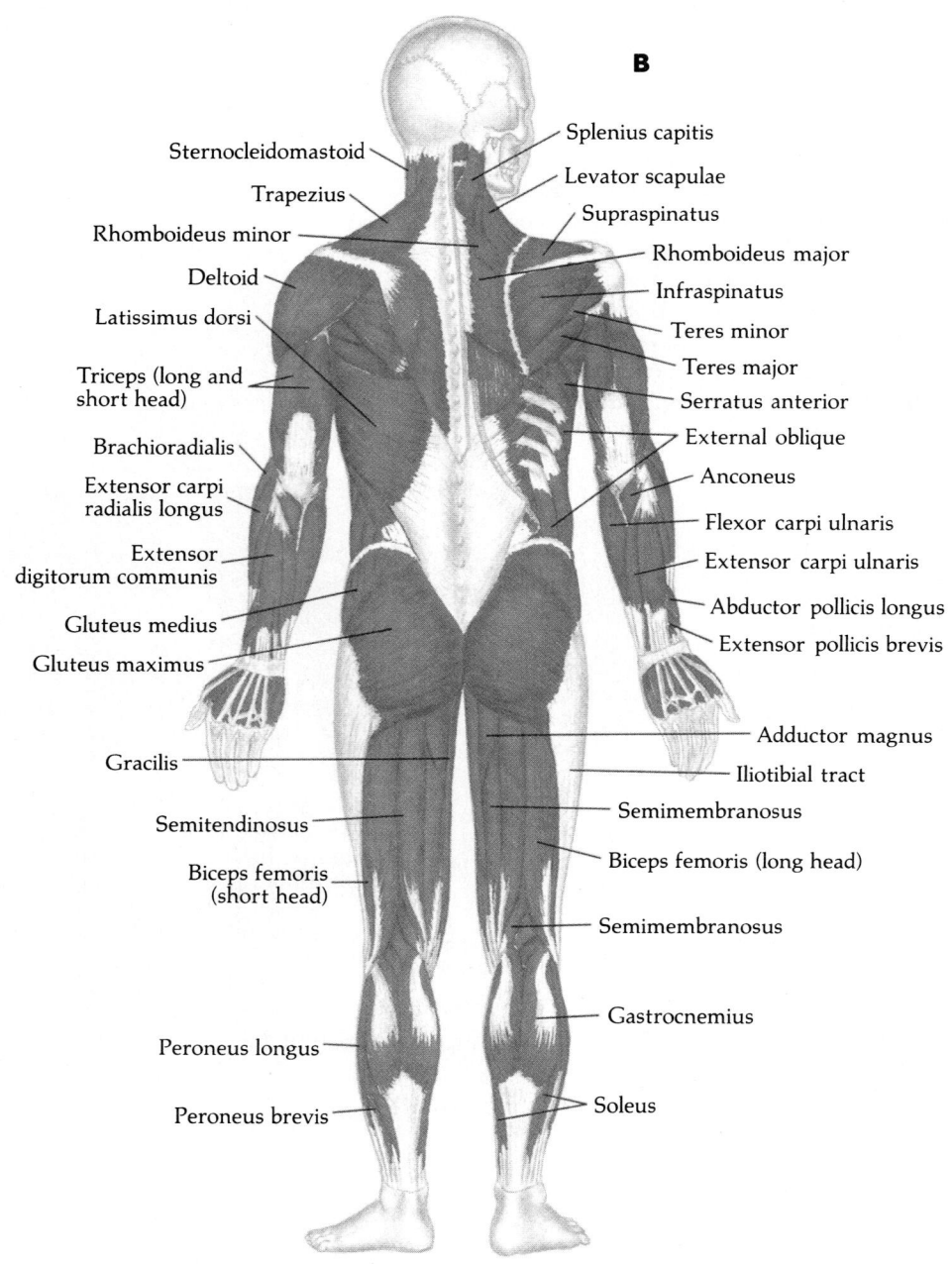

B

Sternocleidomastoid
Trapezius
Rhomboideus minor
Deltoid
Latissimus dorsi
Triceps (long and short head)
Brachioradialis
Extensor carpi radialis longus
Extensor digitorum communis
Gluteus medius
Gluteus maximus
Gracilis
Semitendinosus
Biceps femoris (short head)
Peroneus longus
Peroneus brevis

Splenius capitis
Levator scapulae
Supraspinatus
Rhomboideus major
Infraspinatus
Teres minor
Teres major
Serratus anterior
External oblique
Anconeus
Flexor carpi ulnaris
Extensor carpi ulnaris
Abductor pollicis longus
Extensor pollicis brevis
Adductor magnus
Iliotibial tract
Semimembranosus
Biceps femoris (long head)
Semimembranosus
Gastrocnemius
Soleus

FIGURE 18-4, cont'd B, Posterior view. (From Thompson JM and others: *Mosby's clinical nursing*, ed 3, St Louis, 1993, Mosby–Year Book.)

Ligaments

Ligaments are strong, dense, flexible bands of connective tissue that join bones to one another. They may add strength and stability to a joint by encircling it, as with the hip joint, or they may hold on to the joint obliquely or lie parallel to the ends of bones across the joint, as with the knee joint (Figure 18-5). Ligaments allow movement in some directions and restrict movement in other directions. They may be injured by partial tears (sprains), or they may become detached from the bones (avulsion).

Tendons

Tendons are strong, dense bands of connective tissue at the end of muscles. They attach muscles to the periosteum, the fibrous membrane that covers the bone (see Figure 18-5). Tendons enable bones to move when skeletal muscles contract. They are capable of transmitting great force from the contractile muscles to the bone or cartilage without being injured themselves. Most tendons are small (2 to 3 cm in length). The Achilles tendon is the longest and largest in the body (10 to 14 cm long).

Cartilage

Cartilage is a semismooth layer of elastic, gel-like supporting tissue found at the ends of bones. It forms a cap over the ends of bones to protect and support the bone during weight-bearing activities. The outer layer of cartilage is avascular and receives its nourishment from synovial fluids forced into it during movement and weight-bearing activity. Cartilage must have weight-bearing activity and joint movement to remain healthy. It may fray or wear unevenly if joints are abnormally shaped or unstable.

Joints

Joints are locations where two surfaces of bone come together or where two bones are joined to each other. There are three types of joints, classified by their degree of movement and the material that separates them. *Synarthrotic joints* are immovable. This type of joint separates bones with a thin layer of cartilage. An example is the cranial suture. *Amphiarthrotic joints* are slightly movable and separate bones with cartilage, such as the symphysis pubis or the manubriosternal joint, or with a fibrocartilaginous disk, such as the joints between the vertebral bodies (Figure 18-6, *A*). *Diarthrotic joints* are freely movable. They are lined with a synovial membrane that secretes a lubricating synovial fluid. Diarthrotic joints, which are frequently called synovial joints, include the ankle, wrist, knee, hip, or shoulder joints. Most joints are freely movable, or synovial, joints. These joints are supported by a casing that surrounds them, called the joint capsule. Ligaments also add strength by encasing the capsule (Figure 18-6, *B*).

Range of Motion

The degree of movement of a joint is called its range of motion. Diarthrotic, or freely movable, joints are the only joints that have one or more ranges of motion (Figure 18-7). Seven types of joint motion have been defined as follows:

Flexion is the bending forward of the joint to decrease the angle between the bones that it connects.

Extension is the straightening of a limb to increase the joint angle.

Abduction is the movement of a limb away from the midline of the body.

Adduction is the movement of a limb toward the central axis of the body or beyond it.

Internal rotation is the turning of the body part inward toward the central axis of the body.

External rotation is the turning of the body part away from the midline.

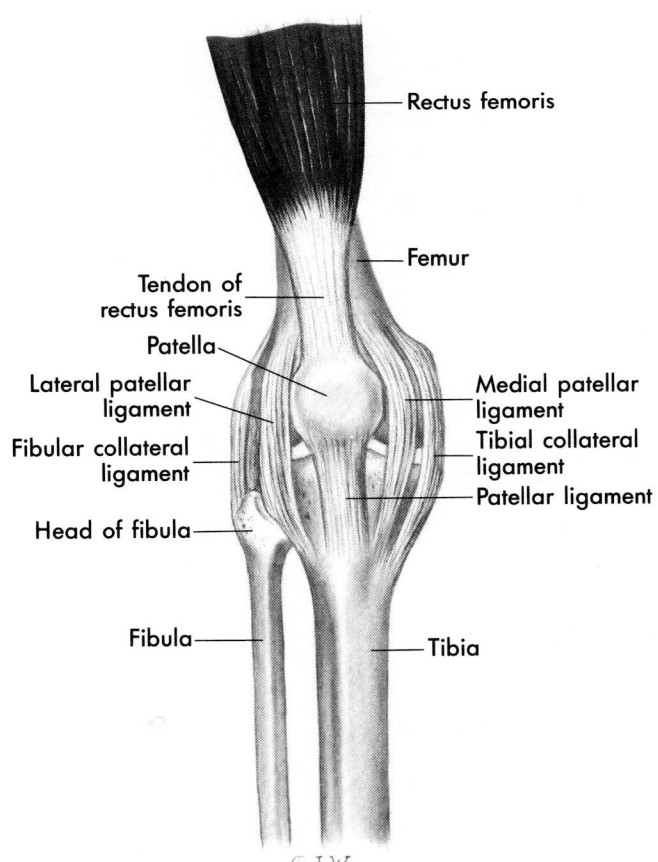

Labels: Rectus femoris — Femur — Tendon of rectus femoris — Patella — Lateral patellar ligament — Fibular collateral ligament — Head of fibula — Fibula — Medial patellar ligament — Tibial collateral ligament — Patellar ligament — Tibia

G.J.W.

FIGURE 18-5 Ligaments and tendons of the knee joint. (From Mourad LA: *Orthopedic disorders,* St Louis, 1991, Mosby–Year Book.)

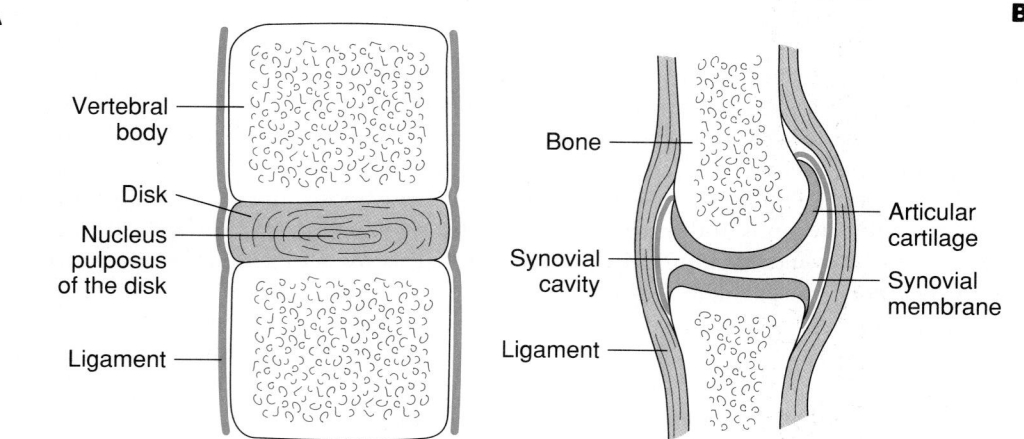

FIGURE 18-6 Structure of a joint. **A,** Intervertebral joint. **B,** Synovial joint.

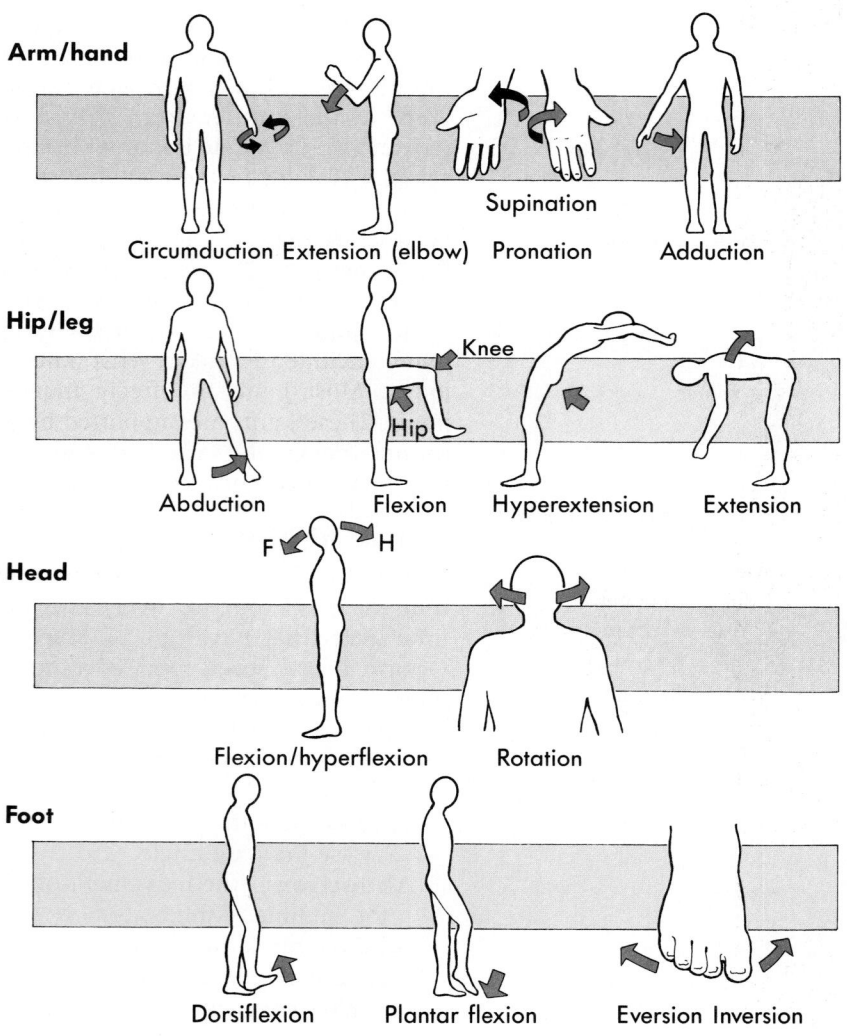

FIGURE 18-7 Body movements provided by synovial (diathrotic) joints. (From Mourad LA: *Orthopedic disorders,* St Louis, 1991, Mosby–Year Book.)

Circumduction is the movement of a body part in a circular pattern. It is not a singular motion but a combination of motions.

Muscles are categorized according to the type of joint movement produced by their contraction. Therefore they are called flexors, extensors, adductors, abductors, internal rotators, external rotators, or circumflexors. Muscles shorten on contraction and in so doing exert pull on the bones to which they are attached. This action moves them closer together. Most muscles attach to two bones that articulate at an intervening joint. Generally, one bone moves while the other is held stable. This effect is caused by simultaneous shortening of other muscles. The body of the muscle that produces movement of an extremity generally lies proximal to the bone that is moved.

EXAMINATION

Health History

The health history for the musculoskeletal system includes information about the client's current concerns, general health, and specific life-style factors that may affect his or her physical condition. Life-style factors include information about employment, activity level, and any recent or past injuries. Common complaints include pain, loss of mobility, deformity, swelling, inflammation, and weakness. The client's chief complaint may indicate the direction for emphasis in the physical assessment. The individual with a chief complaint of body deformity, paralysis, weakness, or pain associated with movement causes the examiner to focus attention on the bones, joints, and muscles as the possible sites of disorder.

Pain is the symptom that most frequently causes the client to seek help. Understanding the character of the pain may be helpful in determining its cause and in guiding the physical assessment of the involved joints. The client should be encouraged to try to recall those events that occurred before the onset of pain. Most individuals tend to forget minor injuries or unusual physical activity in the weeks before the pain began. The client also is unlikely to correlate symptoms and signs of infection in the preceding months with current joint pain. The nature of the onset of pain also needs to be determined. For example, rheumatoid symptoms begin gradually, whereas gout-related attacks are characterized by sudden onset that frequently awakens the client from sleep.

A client frequently has difficulty in localizing the pain associated with joint disease. The client's description may involve large areas of the body, for example; "my neck" (while moving the hand from the head to the thoracic vertebra), "my back," or "all down my arm."

This difficulty in localizing the pain may be related to whether the pain is deep or superficial and whether a nerve is involved.

The location or distribution of the pain may also provide valuable information. Rheumatoid involvement is migratory, that is, involving first one joint, which improves, then another. On the other hand, most infectious arthritis is confined to one joint. The joint involvement in rheumatoid arthritis tends to be symmetrical, whereas that of gout, psoriatic arthritis, and Reiter's syndrome tends to occur initially in one or two joints but becomes polyarticular in the later stages. Spondylitis is first detected in the spine and then spreads to peripheral joints (centrifugal spread), whereas rheumatoid arthritis starts peripherally in the hands and feet and then involves the large joints of the hips, shoulders, and spine in the later stages of the disease (centripetal spread).

The time that pain occurs may also be diagnostic. The individual with osteoarthritis generally reports that the pain is worsened by increased use of the affected joint; therefore the affected person frequently has pain later in the day or when tired. The individual with rheumatoid arthritis generally reports that stiffness and pain occur early in the morning and notes some improvement after exercising the part.

Ask the client to describe any referred pain. Individuals frequently feel spinal nerve root involvement in peripheral tissues. For instance, the client may experience lumbosacral nerve root irritation (**sciatica**) as pain in the thigh or the knee on the involved side. The area of referred pain corresponds with the segmental innervation of the structures. The description of this type of pain may include words associated with paresthesias, such as "prickling," "like an electric shock," "pins and needles," and "numbing." The client may describe pain of muscle origin as "pulled" or "charley horse." Joint pain descriptions may range along a spectrum from dull, aching, or stiff to excruciating and intolerable.

Note also those measures that are known to alleviate the pain, for example, exercise for rheumatoid arthritis and rest for osteoarthritis.

Present health status

1. Chief complaint: concern(s) client wants to deal with at this time
2. Current and previous employment: risk of accidental injury, lifting, repetitive motion activities, safety precautions
3. Activities of daily living: ability to perform personal care (bathing, dressing, grooming, eating, elimination), household tasks, walking, shopping, communication
4. Exercise: walking, specific regimen of exercise or

sports activity (type, frequency, duration, special equipment, safety measures), overall conditioning
5. Weight: recent changes, overweight or underweight
6. Nutrition: calcium and vitamin D intake
7. Cigarette smoking (number of packs/day/number of years)
8. Alcohol intake
9. Medications: calcium supplements, nonsteroidal antiinflammatory agents, muscle relaxants, hormone replacement therapy

Specific complaints

1. Joint
   a. Character: which joint(s) affected, number of joints involved, pain or ache, stiffness or limitation of movement, redness, increased warmth, or swelling
   b. Onset: specific date of first episode (or age when it occurred), sudden or gradual
   c. Duration: length of episode
   d. Frequency: change in pattern, similar episodes in the past
   e. Precipitating factors: specific movements, prolonged activity, rest, injury, weather, time of day, specific foods, medications (e.g., diuretics), alcohol intake
   f. Alleviating factors: rest, movement
   g. Associated symptoms: fever, weight loss, fatigue, malaise, rash, chronic diarrhea
   h. Efforts to treat and their effectiveness: medications, heat and/or ice, exercise, weight reduction, splints, home remedies
2. Skeletal
   a. Character: pain associated with particular movement or weight-bearing, localized tenderness, swelling, **crepitus,** limping, numbness, tingling or pressure, deformity or change in skeletal contour
   b. Onset: specific date, sudden or gradual
   c. Duration: length of episode
   d. Frequency: change in pattern, similar episodes in the past
   e. Precipitating factors: injury, sudden movement, repetitive movement, stress
   f. Alleviating factor: rest
   g. Associated symptoms or conditions: fever, weight loss, fatigue, malaise, past history of cancer, circulatory problems
   h. Efforts to treat and their effectiveness: medications, heat and/or ice, exercise, weight reduction, splints, home remedies
3. Muscular
   a. Character: Localized or generalized pain, weakness, limitation of movement, paralysis, spasms, wasting, tremor
   b. Onset: specific date, sudden or gradual
   c. Duration: length of episode
   d. Frequency: change in pattern, similar episodes in the past
   e. Precipitating factors: injury, muscle contraction, sudden movement, repetitive movement, stress
   f. Alleviating factor: rest
   g. Associated symptoms or conditions: fever, malaise
   h. Efforts to treat and their effectiveness: medications, heat and/or ice, exercise, weight reduction, splints, home remedies
4. Injury
   a. Mechanism of injury: what happened—direct trauma, overuse, overstretching, fall
   b. Character: location of pain; any noise with injury (popping, click, tearing); numbness; tingling; loss of sensation, strength, or mobility; warmth or coldness; swelling (immediate or gradual)
   c. Onset: sudden, gradual
   d. Duration: length of episode
   e. Frequency: similar episodes in the past
   f. Precipitating factors: sudden movement, repetitive movement, stress
   g. Alleviating factors: rest, position of comfort
   h. Associated symptoms or conditions: loss of consciousness, other injuries
   i. Efforts to treat and their effectiveness: medications, heat and/or ice, splints, immobilization, home remedies

---

RISK FACTORS: OSTEOARTHRITIS AND OSTEOPOROSIS

Osteoarthritis

Age over 40
Family history of osteoarthritis
Obesity
Joint abnormality
History of trauma, rheumatoid arthritis, or other degenerative process

Osteoporosis

Advanced age
Gender (female)
Family history of osteoporosis
Estrogen deficiency due to menopause, surgical removal of the ovaries, or anorexia accompanied by amenorrhea
Small stature
Race (white)
Northern European descent
Heavy cigarette and/or alcohol use
Poor diet with low calcium intake
Periods of immobilization
Use of steroids
Sedentary life-style

Preparation for the Examination

Equipment

Item	Purpose
Nonstretchable tape measure	To measure length of extremities and limb circumference
Goniometer	To measure joint range of motion

Client and environment

Provide a warm room with adequate lighting.

Protect the client's sense of modesty while exposing as fully as possible the areas to be examined.

Explain each procedure before beginning to perform it.

Use short, clear instructions.

Arrange for extra examination time for older or debilitated clients.

Stabilize the joints by having the client sit or lie down.

Properly sequence the examination to minimize position changes from sitting to lying.

Preparation for the Examination: Client and Environment

Thorough assessment of the musculoskeletal system requires appropriate exposure of the client. Have the ambulatory individual wear shorts or underwear, which will allow the extremities and the spine to be available for examination. Allow the female client to wear a bra or some other abbreviated form of chest cover. Make an effort to protect the client's sense of modesty, but recognize that you cannot accurately examine a fully clothed client.

For each examination, position the client in a way that provides the greatest stability for the joints.

Technique for Examination and Normal Findings

The examination of neuromuscular coordination begins when you first meet and observe the client. It continues as the client advances into the room, sits, rises from a sitting position, climbs onto the examining table, lies down, and rolls over. Note the client's speed, coordination, and strength of motion. In particular note any clumsy, awkward, or involuntary movements and tremor or fasciculation. Assess the client's handshake to gain an estimate of muscle strength.

Explore the structure and function of the body's equipment for movement through the techniques of inspection and palpation of the joints and muscles, assessment of active and passive ranges of motion, and tests for muscle strength.

Use the cephalocaudal (head-to-toe) organization for examination of the bones, joints, and muscles. This organization provides order and aids in avoiding omissions. Use side-to-side comparison as the basic criterion for assessment. When injury or discomfort is involved, examine the unaffected side first.

Inspection. General inspection of the musculoskeletal system includes a visual scanning for **symmetry,** contour, size, involuntary movement of the two sides of the body (**tremors** or **fasciculations**), gross deformities, areas of swelling or edema, and ecchymoses or other discoloration (Figure 18-8). Inspect the muscles for symmetry of size and contour. Measure asymmetry, noted as hypertrophy or atrophy, for verification.

Examine the posture, or stance, and body alignment from both in front of and behind the client. Note the structural relationships of the feet to the legs and the hips to the pelvis. For the upper extremities, compare the shoulder girdle and the upper trunk.

A deformity is an abnormality in appearance. **Varus** and **valgus** are terms used to describe an angular deviation from the normal structure of an extremity. The reference point is the midline of the body. Genu varum (bowleg) is the lateral deviation of the leg from the midline (Figure 18-9). Genu valgum (knock-knee) is deviation of the leg toward the midline (Figure 18-10).

Palpation. Palpate all joints, bones, and associated muscles. Palpate joints for the presence of tenderness, swelling, increased temperature, and crepitation. Gently palpate painful and tender joints and always examine the pain-free side first. Palpate muscles to detect swelling, localized temperature changes, tone, and marked changes in shape. Note the consistency or tone of the muscle on palpation.

Measurement of extremities. The musculoskeletal examination frequently includes measurement of the extremities for length and circumference. Take length measurements to verify the symmetry of two limbs or to determine whether the limbs are in the normal range. Take measurements with the client lying relaxed on a hard surface (examining table) with the pelvis level and the hips and knees fully extended and with both hips equally adducted. Frequently, apparent discrepancies in limb size are a result of position.

The length of the upper extremity is the distance from the tip of the acromion process to the tip of the middle finger; the shoulder is adducted, and the other joints are at neutral zero (anatomical position: limb in extension). The length of the lower extremity is the distance from the lower edge of the anterosuperior iliac spine to the tibial malleolus (Table 18-1).

Measurement of muscle mass. Examine the muscles for gross hypertrophy or atrophy. Only in the mark-

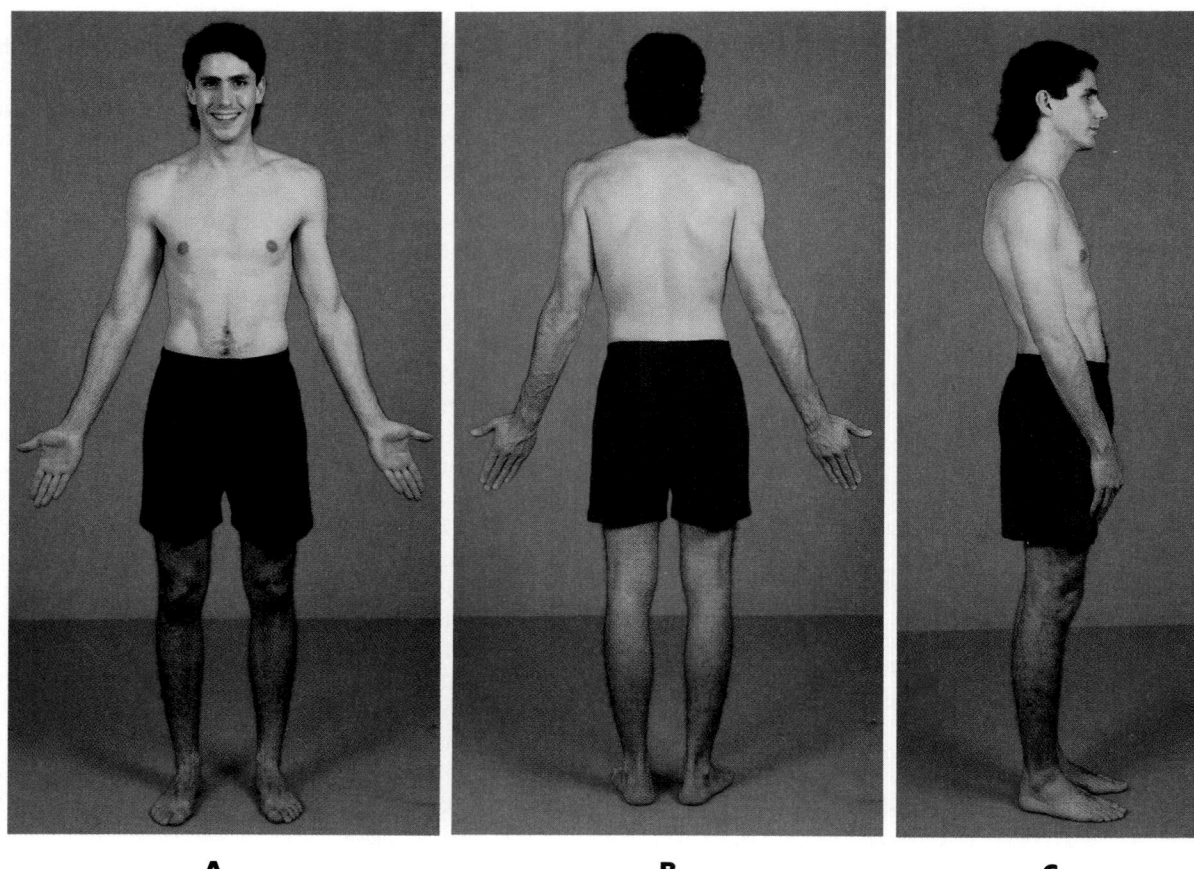

A   B   C

FIGURE 18-8 Inspection of overall body posture for symmetry of contour and size, gross deformities, swelling, alignment of extremities. **A,** Anterior view. **B,** Posterior view. **C,** Lateral view.

TABLE 18-1

Anatomical Guideposts for Measuring Extremities

Area	From	To
Entire upper extremity	Tip of acromion process	Tip of middle finger
Upper arm	Tip of acromion process	Tip of olecranon process
Forearm	Tip of olecranon process	Styloid process of ulna
Entire lower extremity	Lower edge of anterosuperior iliac spine	Tibial malleolus
Thigh	Lower edge of anterosuperior iliac spine	Medial aspect of knee joint
Lower leg	Medial aspect of knee	Tibial malleolus

edly obese client are changes in muscle mass difficult to assess. The difference between the firm, hypertrophic muscle of the athlete and the limp, atrophic muscle of the paralytic is obvious both on inspection and on palpation with the finger. Although muscle size is largely a function of use or disuse of the muscle fibers, changes in the size of muscles may indicate disease. Malnutrition and lipodystrophy tend to reduce muscle size and markedly weaken the strength of contraction. Lack of neural input resulting from lesions of the spinal cord or the peripheral motor neuron may reduce muscle size by as much as 75% of the normal volume. Such a decrease may occur over as short a time as 3 months. Measuring limbs at their maximal circumference may provide a baseline for comparison when swelling or atrophy is suspected on subsequent routine examination.

Make sure that the limbs are in the same position and the muscles are in the same state of tension each time you take measurements. Several corresponding

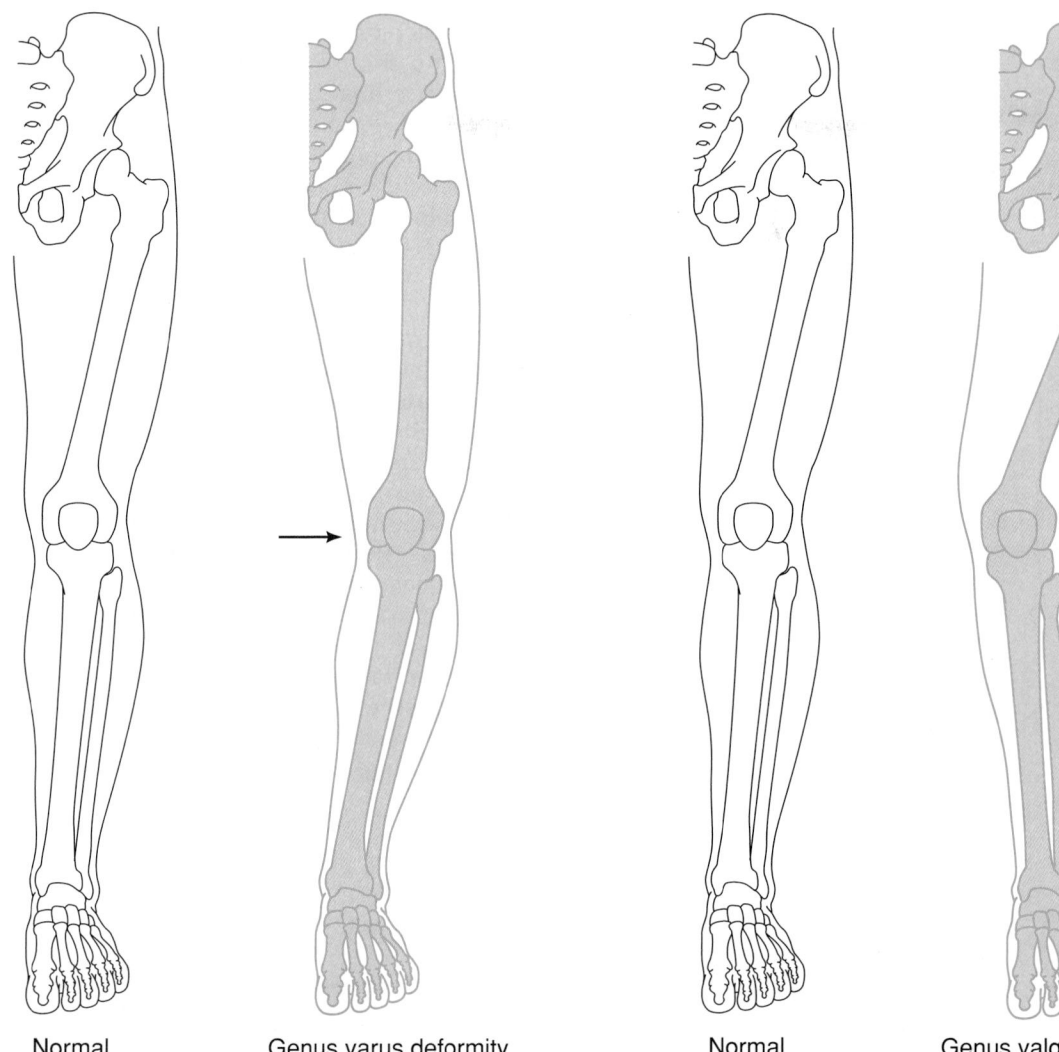

Normal	Genus varus deformity

FIGURE 18-9 Varus deformity of the leg: lateral deviation from the midline (bowleg).

Normal	Genus valgus deformity

FIGURE 18-10 Valgus deformity of the leg: deviation of the leg toward the midline (knock-knee).

points may be measured above and below the patella and the olecranon process. To provide uniformity, some clinics routinely measure at 10 cm below and at points 10 and 20 cm above the middle patella. Regardless of the points you select, draw a small diagram showing the points measured (Figure 18-11) in order to ensure consistency in future measures. Differences in symmetry or variations in limb size of less than 1 cm, noted at different times, are not significant (Figure 18-12). The dominant side is usually slightly larger than the nondominant side.

Measurement of range of joint motion. A standardized method for measuring and recording joint mo-

tion has been published by the American Academy of Orthopaedic Surgeons (1965). This method describes the range of motion in degrees of deviation from a defined neutral zero point for each joint. The position of neutral zero is that of the extended extremity or the anatomical position.

Goniometry and *arthrometry* are terms that describe the measurement of joint motion. It is important to learn to use the **goniometer** to measure the range of motion and to communicate findings to other health team professionals.

The two arms of the goniometer are a protractor and a pointer that are joined at the zero point of the protractor (Figure 18-13). The hinge should provide suf-

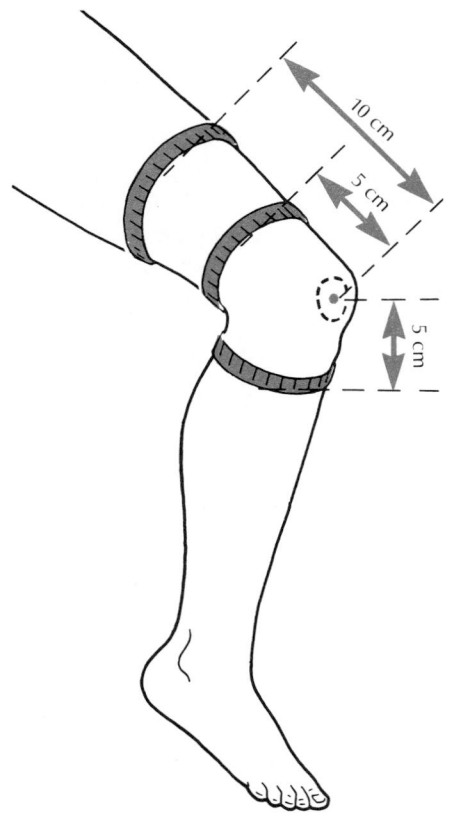

FIGURE 18-11 Sites at which a limb is measured are carefully noted to establish accurate location for future comparative measurements.

ficient friction so that the instrument remains in position when you pick it up to read it after placing it against the joint. You should be able to read the scale easily from a distance of 18 inches. Some goniometers have full-circle scales, whereas others have half-circle scales. For the sake of portability, the length of the arms is generally about 6 inches.

Describe range of motion as active when the client moves the joint and as passive when you provide the motion.

Active motion. In **active range of motion,** the joint movement is smooth and painless through its complete range and generally indicates the absence of any advanced lesion. Less muscle tension and joint compression are produced by the voluntary movement of the joints through their range of motion than when the joints are moved against resistance, as in the strength tests. Therefore range of active motion should be assessed before muscle strength because the more marked contraction may induce pain in the client, which may skew the test results.

If the active range of motion of a given joint is less than the **passive range of motion,** further investigation should focus on true weakness, joint stability, pain, malingering, or hysterical weakness as possible causes.

Passive motion. Move the relaxed joint through the limits of its movement. When the range of motion is

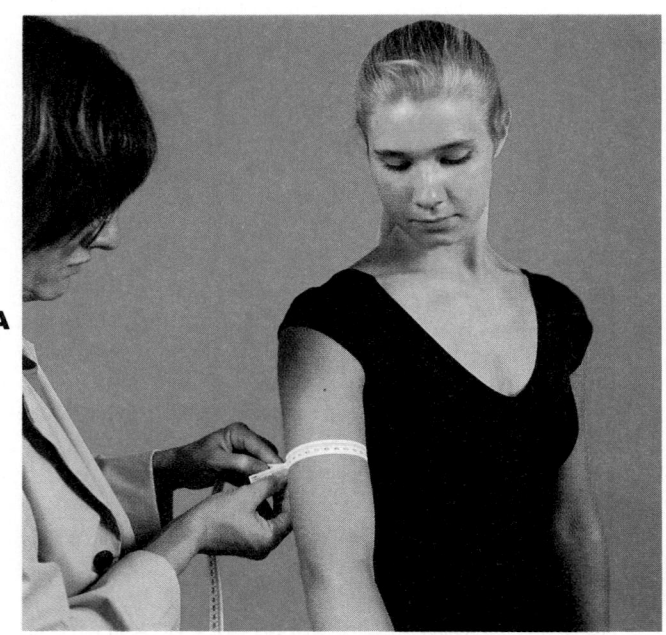

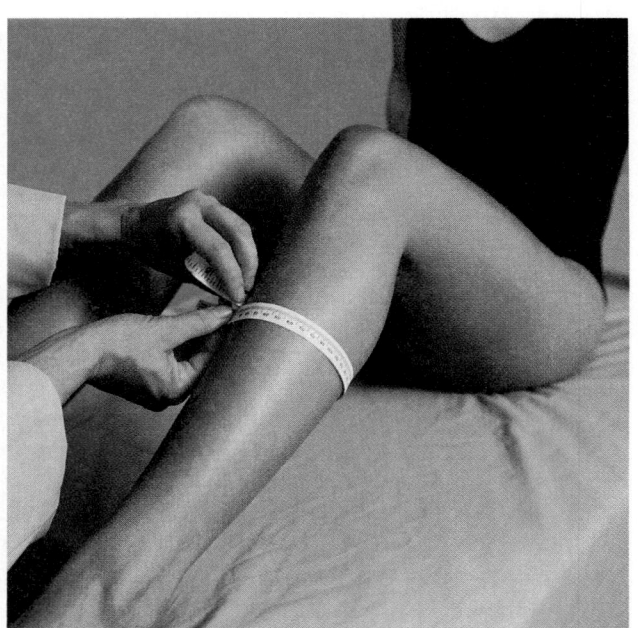

FIGURE 18-12 A, Measurement of upper midarm circumference. **B,** Measurement of midgastrocnemius circumference.

limited, explore further to determine whether: (1) excess fluid is within the joint; (2) loose bodies, such as pieces of cartilage, are present in the joint; or (3) joint surface irregularity or contracture of the muscle, ligaments, or capsule exists. Moving the joint through the range of its motion may also reveal hypermobility of the joint. In such a situation further examination should be directed toward differentiating among (1) a connective tissue disruption, such as the relaxation of the ligaments that occurs in Marfan's syndrome; (2) a ligamentous tear; and (3) an intraarticular fracture. An example of how this information might aid in diagnosis is a joint that can be flexed to a smaller angle with passive movement than with active **flexion.** Such a finding probably indicates a problem related to the musculature rather than a problem within the joint that causes a block in the flexion.

Recording range of motion. The box on p. 552 summarizes joint movements and the maximal expected angles of movement. Record limited joint movement from the angle of the starting position to the maximal angle reached during movement (i.e., from 20 degrees to 50 degrees).

Screening Examination

Assessment of the full range of motion may not be part of the screening examination unless the history or other parts of the physical examination indicate that muscular or neural dysfunction is a possible problem for the client. Note that movement of the neck and the trunk may be examined by functional groups, rather than by individual joints, to determine joint range of motion and muscle strength.

In the screening examination, carry joints actively through the ranges of motion and describe the results as full range of motion. In joints that do not exhibit full range of motion, measure with the goniometer and record the results. Expect limitations in full range of motion in older individuals.

Examination of bones, joints, and muscles

Bones. Examine bones for deformity and tumors. Also examine bones for integrity by testing resistance to a deforming force. Palpate the bone to assess the presence of pain or tenderness. Tenderness of a bone may indicate tumor, inflammation, or the aftermath of a trauma. Frequently, traumatic injuries are associated with damage to both bone and nerve. Paralysis of the ulnar and median nerves in the hand is frequently the result of a hand injury and may result in a clawlike posture of the hand.

Joints

SIGNS AND SYMPTOMS OF DISORDERS. Pain, tenderness, swelling, partial or complete loss of mobility, stiffness, weakness, and fatigue are the signs and symptoms most frequently associated with disorders of the joints. Joint disease may be indicated by skin that feels warm, is red, has lesions, or is ulcerated. In psoriatic arthritis, skin lesions and pitting of the nails are involved in approximately 50% of cases. Pitting is the most commonly recognized change. Isolated pitting of a single nail may occur or the pitting may be *uniformly* distributed across the nails.

LIMITATION OF RANGE OF MOTION. The client may voluntarily limit the motion of a joint in response to pain. Spasm of the muscles involved in the movement of a joint may limit its motion. Mechanical obstruction to movement may accompany bony overgrowth and scar tissue. Limitation of motion in a joint is accompanied by weakness and atrophy of the muscles that are involved. Decreased range of motion occurs in joints in which there is inflammation of surrounding tissues, arthritis, fibrosis, or bony fixation **(ankylosis).**

DEFORMITY. Deformities of the joint include absorption of tissues, flexion contracture, and bony overgrowth. Absorption may produce a flail joint, which makes the joint move erratically. Deformities result from scarring phenomena following inflammation and infection.

SWELLING. The amount of swelling of the joint may range from difficult to detect to visually evident fluid within the joint (i.e., visible or palpable as a bulging of the joint capsule). Pressure on the sac at one point

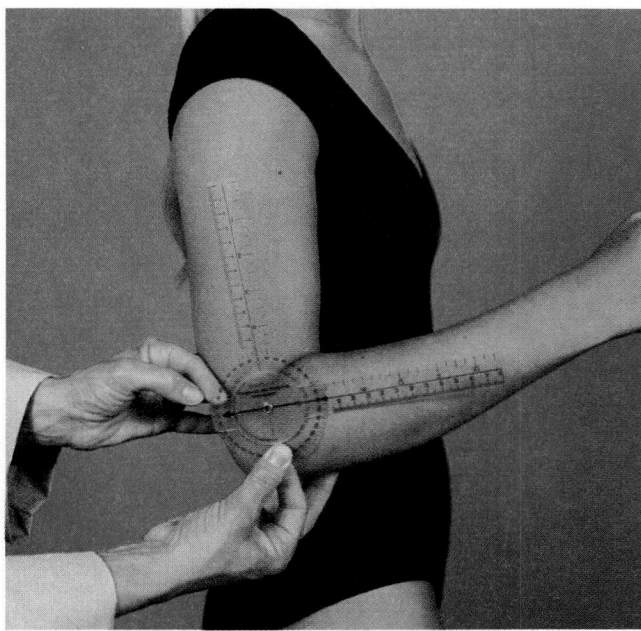

FIGURE 18-13 Use of goniometer to measure range of motion of a joint.

RECORDING RANGE OF MOTION IN DEGREES

Cervical spine		Fingers	
Flexion	45	Flexion—distal interphalangeal joint	90
Extension	50	Flexion—proximal interphalangeal joint	100
Rotation (right)	70	Flexion—metacarpophalangeal joint	90
Rotation (left)	70	Extension—metacarpophalangeal joint	45
Lateral bending (right)	40	Hyperextension—distal interphalangeal joint	10
Lateral bending (left)	40	Abduction (measure from tips of fingers)	Varies
Spine		Adduction	Varies
Forward flexion (C7 to S1 = 4 in)	70	Hip	
Extension (standing)	30	Flexion (knees bent)	110-120
Extension (lying)	20	Extension	30
Rotation (right)	45	Abduction	45
Rotation (left)	45	Adduction	30
Lateral bending (right)	35	Internal rotation (hip and knee flexed)	40
Lateral bending (left)	35	External rotation (hip and knee flexed)	45
Shoulder		Knee	
Forward flexion	180	Flexion-extension	135
Backward extension	60	Hyperextension	10
Horizontal flexion	130-135	Ankle	
Horizontal extension	40	Dorsiflexion	20
Abduction	180	**Plantar flexion**	50
Adduction	50	Inversion hind foot (passive)	5
Internal rotation	90	Eversion hind foot (passive)	5
External rotation	90	Inversion	30
Elbow		Eversion	20
Flexion-extension	150	Abduction forefoot (passive)	10
Hyperextension	0-15	Adduction forefoot (passive)	20
Forearm (elbow and wrist)		Great toe	
Pronation	80-90	Flexion—metatarsophalangeal joint	45
Supination	80-90	Extension—metatarsophalangeal joint	70
Wrist		Flexion—interphalangeal joint (passive)	90
Extension	80	Lateral four toes	
Flexion	70	Flexion—distal interphalangeal joint	60
Radial deviation	20	Extension—distal interphalangeal joint	30
Ulnar deviation	30	Flexion—proximal interphalangeal joint	35
Thumb		Flexion—metatarsophalangeal joint	40
Abduction	50	Extension—metatarsophalangeal joint	40
Flexion—interphalangeal joint	80	Abduction	Varies
Flexion—metacarpophalangeal joint	50	Adduction	Varies
Flexion—carpometacarpal joint	15		
Opposition to tip or base of little finger			

causes the fluid within it to shift and may lead to bulging at another site. The sac may vary from soft to tense, and the involvement may be symmetrical or unilateral. Frequently, the swelling is fusiform. Redness, warmth, swelling, and pain in a joint are the classic descriptors of an inflammatory process. The inflammation may be within the joint itself or in the soft tissue surrounding it. Swelling may also result from intraarticular effusion, synovial thickening, or bony overgrowth. In addition, swelling may result from the deposition of fat in the region adjacent to the joint. The synovial membrane is not palpable in normal joints. The palpation of a "boggy" or "doughy" consistency generally indicates a thickened or otherwise abnormal synovial membrane.

TENDERNESS. Injury and inflammatory processes cause joints to be tender. **Arthritis,** tendonitis, **bursitis,** and osteomyelitis are associated with tenderness in and around a joint. Therefore it is important to attempt to determine the anatomic structure that is tender.

INCREASED TEMPERATURE. Heat noted over a joint indicates inflammation and suggests rheumatoid or septic arthritis. Compare symmetrical joints for temperature when one joint is hot. Use the backs of the fingers when comparing temperature.

REDNESS. Vasodilation or inflammation occurs in the skin overlying a tender joint that is affected by septic arthritis and gouty arthritis.

CREPITATION. Crepitation (crackling or grating sounds) produced by motion of the joint is caused by irregularities of the articulating surfaces. The coarseness of the surface may involve the cartilage or the bony capsule.

INSPECTION AND PALPATION. Either make a systematic assessment of individual joints during the performance of the head-to-toe physical examination, or examine all the joints at a preselected time during the examination. As with all bilateral structures, compare the paired joints.

The sequence for performing the examination of the joints is inspection, palpation, active range of motion, passive range of motion, and muscle strength testing. Use this sequence in a coordinated examination of each joint.

Begin the assessment with inspection of the joint for swelling, redness, deformity, subcutaneous nodules, or tumors. Let the presence of any observed abnormalities guide you in palpation. Palpate joints for the presence of pain with movement, tenderness, swelling, increased temperature, and crepitation. Palpate painful and tender joints lightly.

Give special consideration to the temporomandibular, sternoclavicular, manubriosternal, shoulder, elbow, wrist, hip, knee, and ankle joints.

RECORDING JOINT PROBLEMS. To conveniently summarize the results of examination of the joints, circle the joint involved on a diagram (Figure 18-14) and briefly note any pathological condition.

Muscles. Examine muscles in symmetrical pairs, that is, first one and then the other, for equivalence in size, contour, tone, and strength. Position the contralateral, matching muscle pairs uniformly while you examine them. Examine the muscles both at rest and in a state of contraction.

The assessment sequence is inspection, palpation, and testing of muscle strength. You may incorporate the examination of functional muscle groups into the examination of the joints.

INSPECTION AND PALPATION. Inspect the muscles for symmetry of size and contour. Measure asymmetry, noted as hypertrophy or atrophy, for verification.

Use palpation to detect swelling, localized temperature changes, and marked changes in shape. Note the consistency of the muscle on palpation.

Muscle tone is the tension present in the resting muscle. You will also notice it in the slight resistance you

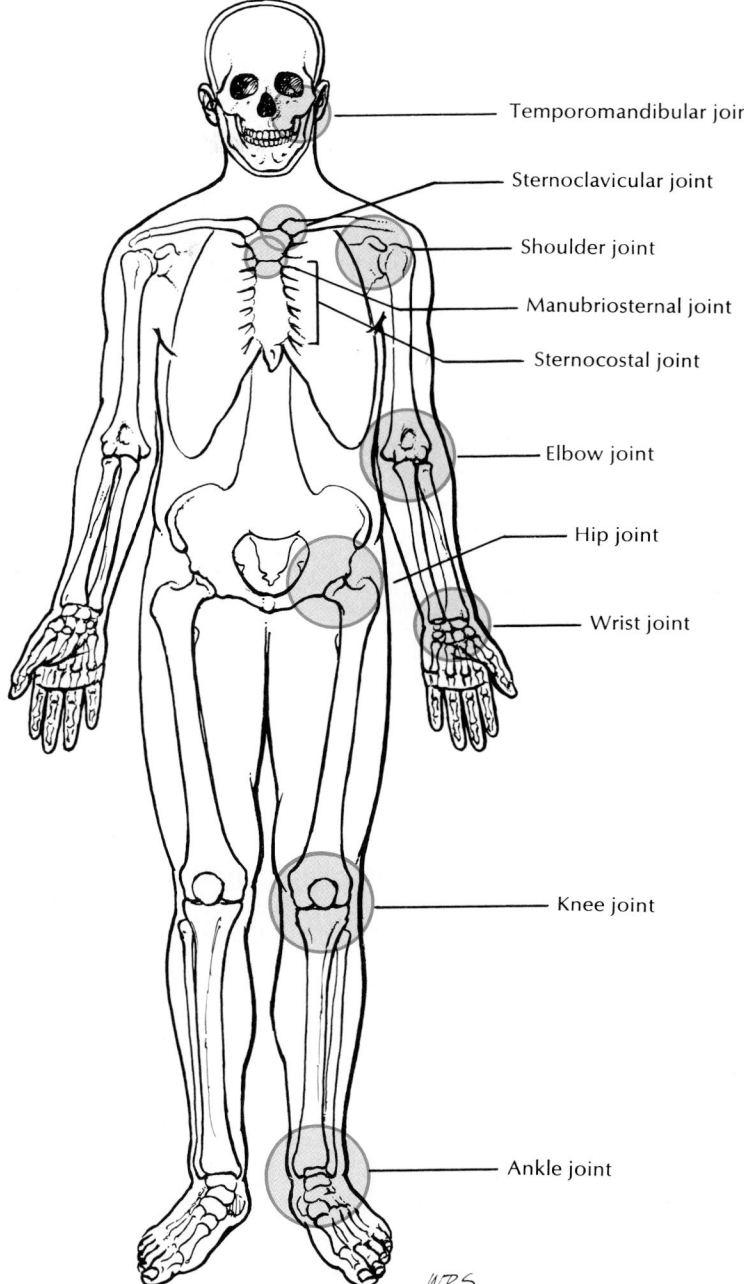

FIGURE 18-14 Results of the examination of joints may be summarized by circling on a diagram the joints involved and briefly noting the pathological condition.

feel when you passively move the relaxed limb. While palpating the muscle, be alert to fasciculations, which are involuntary contractions or twitching of groups of muscle fibers.

Ask the client to tell you of any sensation while you feel the muscles and tendons. Then record the client's descriptions of pain or tenderness on palpation.

TABLE 18-2

Criteria for Grading and Recording Muscle Strength

Functional level	Lovett scale	Grade	Percent of normal
No evidence of contractility	Zero (0)	0	0
Evidence of slight contractility	Trace (T)	1	10
Complete range of motion with gravity eliminated	Poor (P)	2	25
Complete range of motion with gravity	Fair (F)	3	50
Complete range of motion against gravity with some resistance	Good (G)	4	75
Complete range of motion against gravity with full resistance	Normal (N)	5	100

Tendon stretch reflexes, described in Chapter 19, are generally altered in muscle disease, especially if the peripheral nerves are involved. For instance, the tendon reflexes are diminished in muscular dystrophy and polymyositis in proportion to the loss of muscle strength. A lengthened reflex cycle is characteristic of hypothyroidism, whereas a shortened period indicates the hypermetabolic state.

RECORDING MUSCLE STRENGTH. Examiners frequently use the criteria in Table 18-2 for recording the grading of muscle strength.

Some examiners prefer to use simple descriptive words such as *paralysis, severe weakness, moderate weakness, minimum weakness,* and *normal.* Disability is considered to exist if (1) the muscle strength is less than grade 3; (2) external support may be required to make the involved part functional, and (3) activity of the part cannot be achieved in a gravity field.

Muscle strength is expected to be greater in the dominant arm and leg. Movements should be coordinated and painless.

The examiner performs only a musculoskeletal screening test unless he or she suspects a musculoskeletal problem.

TABLE 18-3

Screening Test for Muscle Strength

Muscles tested	Client activity	Examiner activity	Muscles tested	Client activity	Examiner activity
Ocular musculature			Biceps	Flex arm	Pull to extend arm
			Triceps	Extend arm	Push to flex arm
Lids	Close eyes tightly	Attempt to resist closure	Wrist musculature	Extend hand	Push to flex
				Flex hand	Push to extend
Yoke muscles	Track object in six cardinal positions		Finger muscles	Extend fingers	Push dorsal surface of fingers
Facial musculature	Blow out cheeks	Assess pressure in cheeks with fingertips		Flex fingers	Push ventral surface of fingers
	Place tongue in cheek	Assess pressure in cheek with fingertips		Spread fingers	Hold fingers together
			Hip musculature	In supine position raise extended leg	Push down on leg above knee
	Stick out tongue, move it to right and left	Observe strength and coordination of thrust and extension	Hamstring, gluteal, abductor, and adductor muscles of leg	Sit and perform alternate leg crossing	Push in opposite direction of crossing limb
Neck muscles	Extend head backward	Push head forward	Quadriceps	Extend leg	Push to flex leg
	Flex head forward	Push head backward	Hamstring	Bend knees to flex leg	Push to extend leg
	Rotate head in full circle	Observe mobility, coordination	Ankle and foot muscle	Bend foot up (dorsiflexion)	Push to plantar flexion
	Touch shoulders with head	Observe range of motion		Bend foot down (plantar flexion)	Push to dorsiflexion
Deltoid	Hold arms upward	Push down on arms	Antigravity muscles	Walk on toes Walk on heels	

SCREENING TEST FOR MUSCLE STRENGTH. Muscle weakness in adults is generally mild and transitory. However, it may be the outcome of musculoskeletal, neurological, metabolic, or infectious problems. Therefore an evaluation is necessary.

Although you can assess muscle strength throughout the full range of motion for each muscle or group of muscles, there are several simple screening tests that will allow you to find muscle or reflex abnormalities. One brief but effective approach is to observe the client carefully as he or she walks into the examining room and undresses. Watch for cues to neurological and motion deficit. This approach may also help you ascertain whether physical evidence can verify the chief complaint. Table 18-3 gives an example of a formal screening examination.

The usual method of testing is manual and subjective. Place the client in the position that best allows movement through the full range. Apply resistance to the muscles. Grade the muscle contractions according to your judgment of the client's responses. The test allows for a systematic testing of muscle groups from head to toe.

Specific Joints and Muscles

TEMPOROMANDIBULAR JOINT. The temporomandibular joint is the articulation between the mandible and the temporal bone (Figure 18-15). The joint is divided into two cavities as a fibrocartilaginous disk. Swelling appears as a tumescence over the joint, but it must be considerable to be visible. Palpate the joint by placing the fingertips anterior to the external meatus of

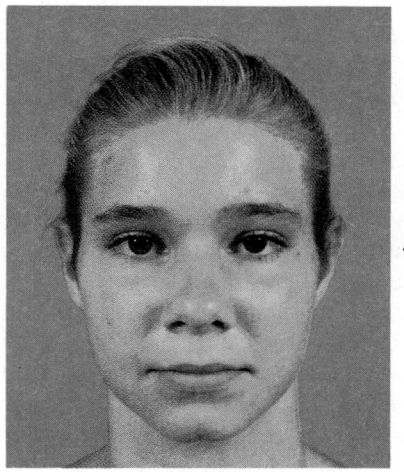
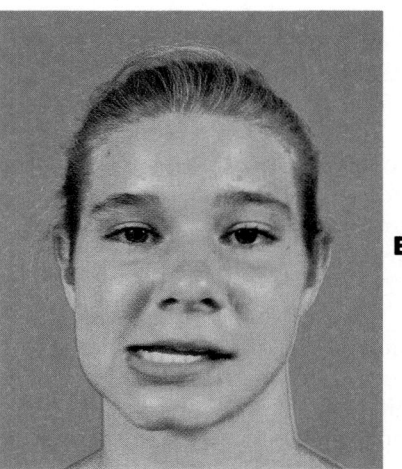
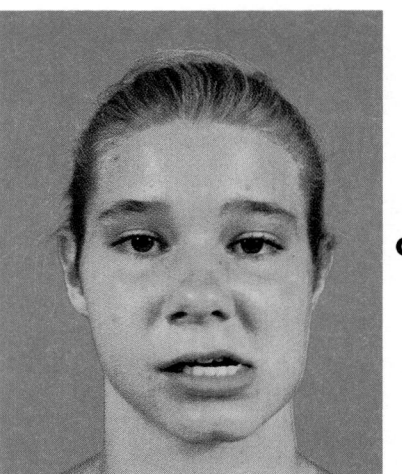

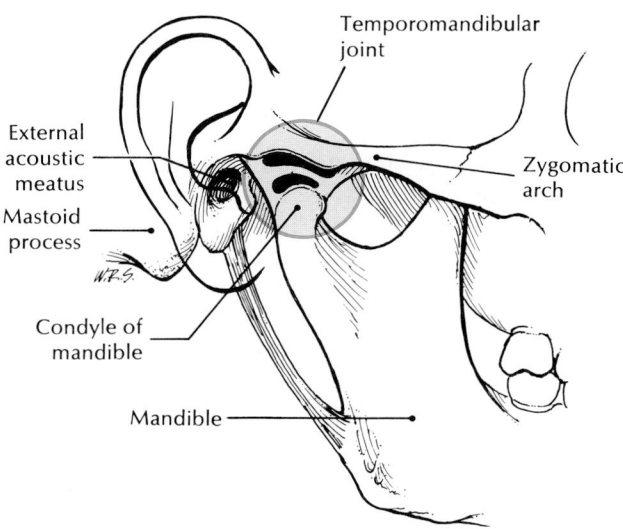

FIGURE 18-15 Temporomandibular joint. A fibrocartilaginous disk divides the articulation point into two synovial cavities. Note the proximity at this joint to the external acoustic meatus.

FIGURE 18-16 Lateral motion is determined by asking the client to move the lower jaw from side to side. Distance measured is the amount that the midline of the lower lip deviates in each direction. Midline of the stationary upper lip may be used as the baseline.

the ear. In the normal joint there is a depression over the joint. Swelling may make this indentation difficult to feel. Palpate the jaw while the client moves it through its range of motion.

To test range of motion, ask the client to:
1. Open and close the mouth
2. Project the lower jaw (jutting of jaw)
3. Move the jaw from side-to-side (Figure 18-16)

The normal range of distance between the upper and lower incisors is 3 to 6 cm. Measure lateral motion of the jaw when the client projects the jaw and moves it from side to side. Measure the distance that the midline of the lower lip deviates in each direction. The normal range of motion is 1 to 2 cm. Audible "clicks" on movement may be heard and are considered normal.

To test muscle strength, ask the client to:
1. Bite down hard while you palpate the masseter muscles.
2. Clench the teeth while you apply downward pressure on the chin.

These maneuvers also test the motor function of cranial nerve (CN) V.

STERNOCLAVICULAR JOINT. The sternoclavicular joint is located at the juncture of the clavicle and the manubrium of the sternum. This joint is divided into two synovial cavities by a disk of cartilage and fibrous material. The joint is reinforced by a fibrous capsule and ligaments (Figure 18-17). The obtuse angle formed by the junction of the manubrium and the body of the sternum, called the angle of Louis, is used as a landmark for counting the ribs. Inspection of this joint is easy because little tissue overlies it. Swelling, redness, bony overgrowth, and dislocation are not difficult to see.

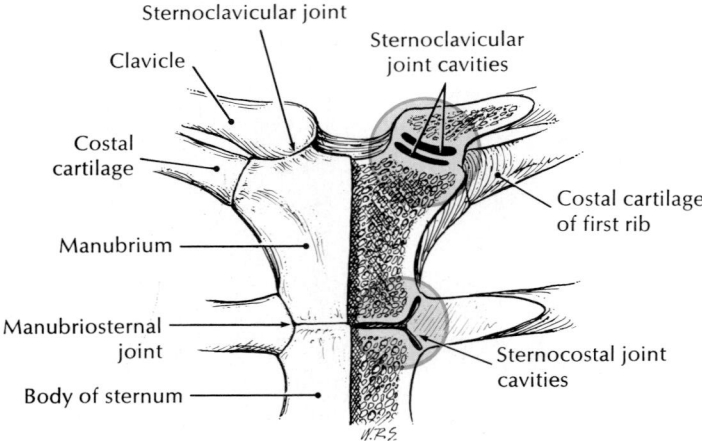

Sternoclavicular joint
Sternoclavicular joint cavities
Clavicle
Costal cartilage
Costal cartilage of first rib
Manubrium
Manubriosternal joint
Body of sternum
Sternocostal joint cavities

FIGURE 18-17 Sternoclavicular joint is divided into two synovial cavities. Movement of the shoulder girdle may cause pain when these joints are diseased. Manubriosternal joint examination is done largely by inspection and palpation since these joints move minimally.

Swelling of the joint appears as a smooth, round bulge. Although this joint is often overlooked, it is frequently involved in problems following surgery of the neck.

Palpate the joint with your fingertips. Movements of the shoulder depend on the normal function of this joint. Inflammation of the sternoclavicular joint may result in pain on movement of the shoulder girdle.

CERVICAL SPINE. The cervical vertebrae are the most mobile of the spinal vertebrae. Flexion and extension occur between the skull and C1. Rotation occurs between C1 and C2. Inspect the neck from both an anterior and a posterior position for deformities or abnormal posture. Note the alignment of the head with the shoulders. The cervical spine should be straight with the head erect. The normal spinal curvature should be concave in the cervical area.

Palpate the spinous processes of the cervical spine including the trapezius, paravertebral, and sternocleidomastoid muscles. There should be symmetry in size, good tone, and no tenderness or muscle spasm.

To evaluate range of motion, ask the client to:
1. Touch the chin to the chest.
2. Extend the head backward as far as possible (Figure 18-18, *A*).
3. Bend the head laterally toward each shoulder (touch ear to shoulder without raising shoulder) (Figure 18-18, *B*)
4. Rotate head from side to side (pointing chin toward each shoulder) (Figure 18-18, *C*)

To evaluate muscle strength, ask the client to:
1. Push the cheek against your hand (right and left sides). This maneuver also tests the motor function of CN XI (sternocleidomastoid muscle) (Figure 18-19, *A*)
2. Push the forehead against your hand (Figure 18-19, *B*)
3. Push the head back against your hand (Figure 18-19, *C*)

SHOULDERS. The shoulder joint is a ball-and-socket joint that is the articulation of the humerus and the glenoid fossa of the scapula (Figure 18-20). The joint is protected by the muscles and the ligaments. A fibrous capsule surrounds the joint completely. Overlying these structures is the subacromial **bursa**. The portion of the bursa that lies beneath the deltoid is called the subdeltoid bursa. The clavicle and the acromion process of the scapula are articulated by the acromioclavicular joint.

Inspect the shoulders, including the muscles and the acromioclavicular joint, with the client standing with his or her back to you. Look for equality of shoulder height and contour and shape of the shoulders. Inspect the scapulae and related muscles. Inspection may reveal anterior dislocation of the shoulder as a flattening of its lateral aspect. Swelling of the joint resulting from fluid collection may be visible only when the amount of fluid

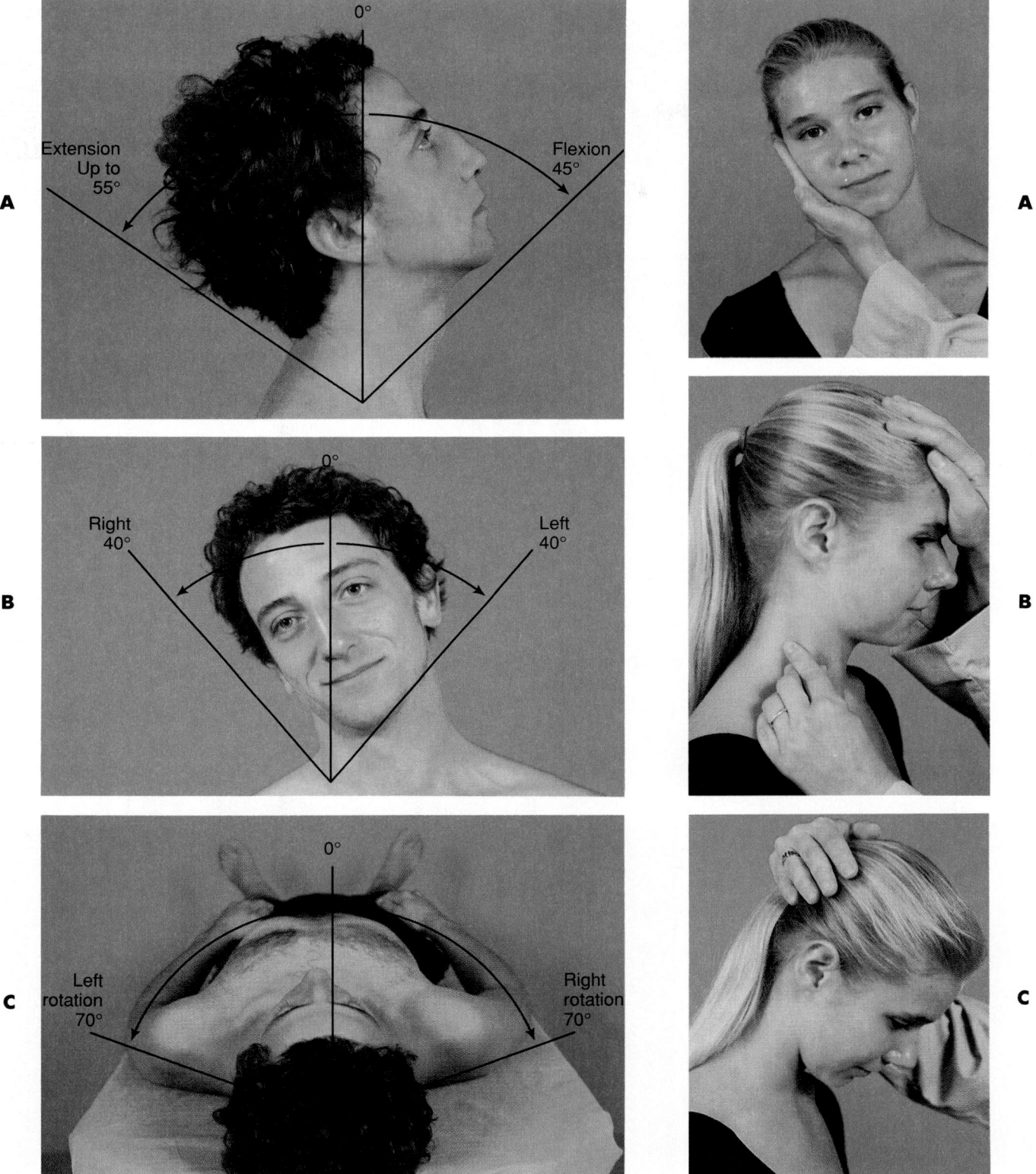

FIGURE 18-18 Range of motion of the cervical spine. **A,** Flexion and hyperextension. **B,** Lateral bending. **C,** Rotation.

FIGURE 18-19 Examining the strength of the sternocleidomastoid and trapezius muscles. **A,** Rotation against resistance. **B,** Flexion with palpation of the sternocleidomastoid muscle. **C,** Extension against resistance.

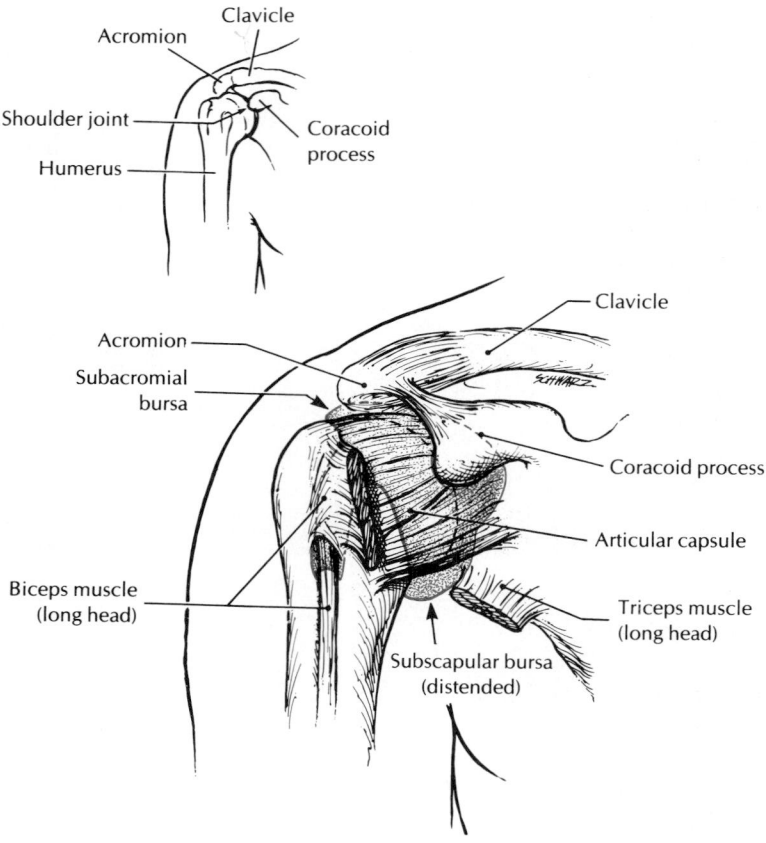

FIGURE 18-20 Shoulder joint.

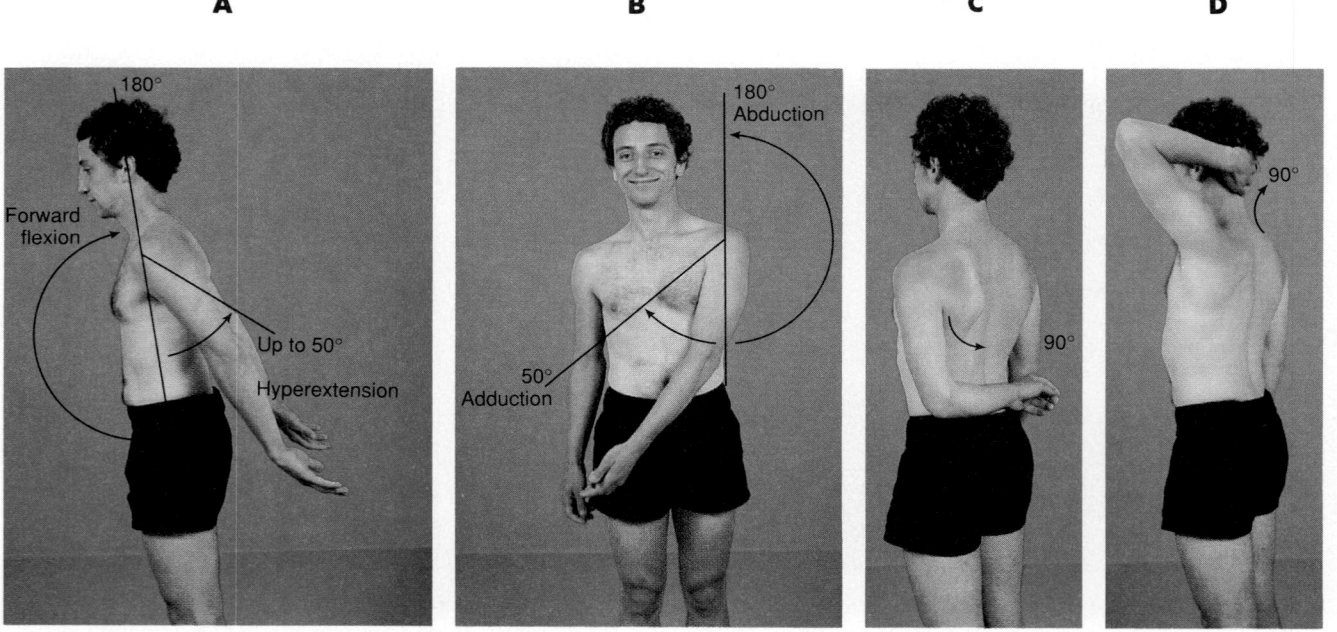

FIGURE 18-21 Range of motion of the shoulder. **A,** Forward flexion and hyperextension. **B,** Abduction and adduction. **C,** Internal rotation. **D,** External rotation.

is moderate to large. Visible swelling generally appears over the anterior aspect of the shoulder. Palpate the joint and the bursal sites. Sites to palpate include the acromium process, clavicle, scapulae, acromioclavicular joint, greater tubercle of the humerus, sternoclavicular joint, biceps groove, and area muscles. If you suspect neoplasia or infection, palpate the axilla for lymph nodes. Give special attention to the tendons of the teres minor and infraspinatus muscles (rotator cuff). Palpate these tendons for swelling, nodes, tears, and pain.

To test for range of motion, ask the client to (Figure 18-21):

1. Extend both arms forward (forward flexion).
2. Extend both arms backward (hyperextension).
3. Put the hands behind the back as if one were going to reach up to touch the shoulder blade (internal rotation).
4. Put the hands behind the head (external rotation).

To test for muscle strength, ask the client to:

1. Hold the arms upward while you try to push them down (deltoid muscles).
2. Extend the arms and then try to flex them while you try to pull them into extension (biceps muscle) (Figure 18-22).
3. Flex the arms and then extend them while you attempt to push them into a flexed position (triceps muscle) (Figure 18-23).
4. Shrug the shoulders while you try to push down on them (CN XI, trapezius muscle) (Figure 18-24).

ELBOW. The elbow is the articulation of the humerus, the radius, and the ulna (Figure 18-25). The three articulating surfaces are enclosed in a single synovial cavity. The synovial membrane is generally palpable only on the posterior aspect of the joint. Radial and ulnar ligaments provide protection to the joint. The olecranon bursa is the largest bursa of the elbow, although several smaller bursae are present. Swelling and redness are easily visible over the posterior aspect of the elbow.

Inspect the size and contour of the elbow in flexion and extension. Note deviations in the carrying angle of the arm while the arm is passively extended with the palm facing forward (Figure 18-26). The carrying angle is between 5 and 15 degrees in adults. Variations in the carrying angle are cubitus valgus (forearm farther outward than the arm) and cubitus varus (forearm carried more inwardly). These variations can be caused by acute injury, posttraumatic arthritis, or other forms of arthritis.

With the client's arm flexed to approximately 70 degrees, palpate the elbow with the tips of the fingers while applying pressure on the opposite side of the joint with the thumb of the dominant hand. Support the arm

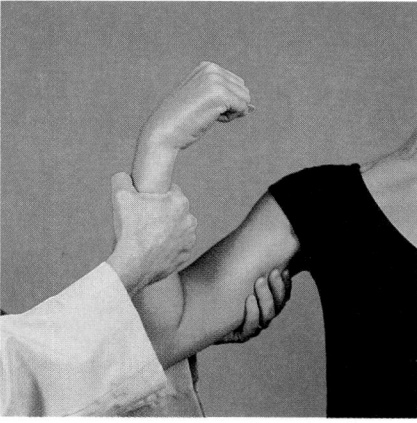

FIGURE 18-22 Assessment of biceps muscle strength. Client flexes her arm while examiner attempts to pull the arm into extension.

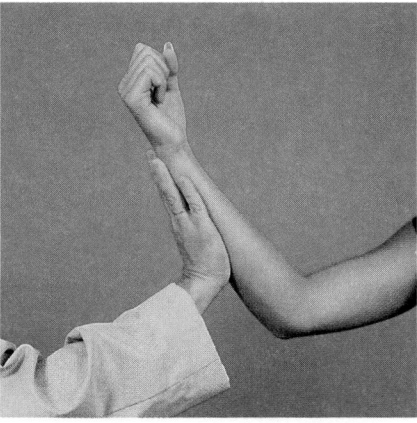

FIGURE 18-23 Assessment of triceps muscle strength. Client attempts to extend her arm while examiner tries to push the arm into a flexed position.

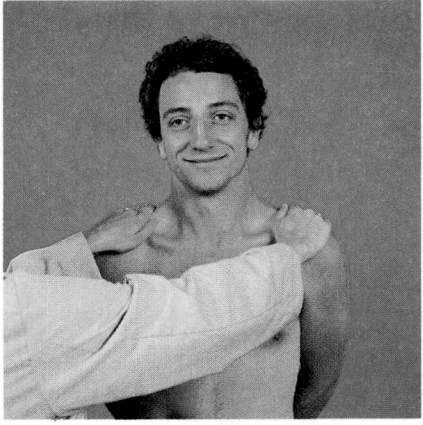

FIGURE 18-24 Assessment of trapezius muscle strength. Client shrugs his shoulders while examiner attempts to push them down.

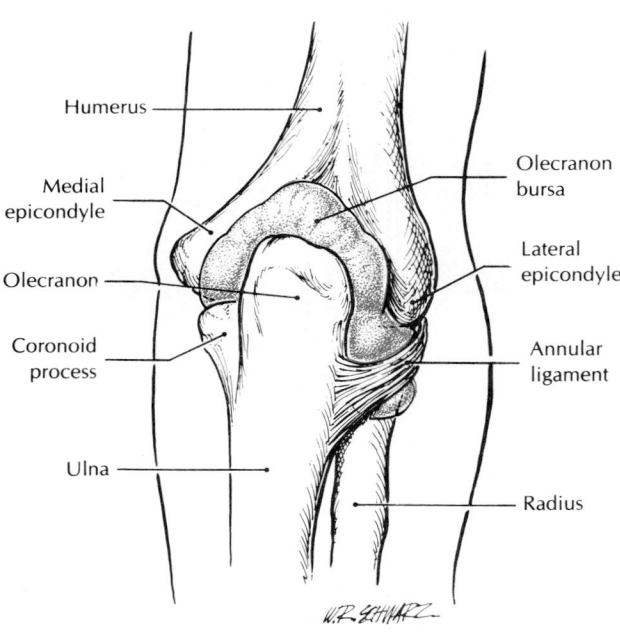

FIGURE 18-25 Elbow joint (posterior view).

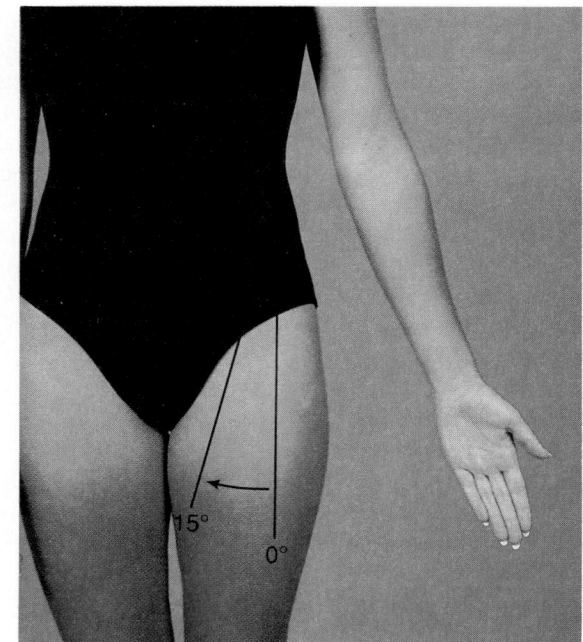

FIGURE 18-26 Expected carrying angle of the arm is between 5 and 15 degrees in the adult.

A

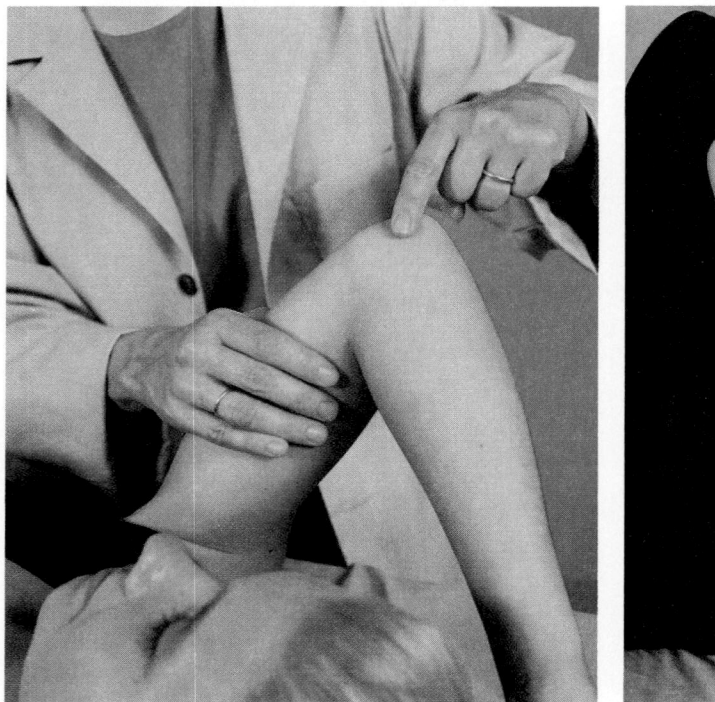

B

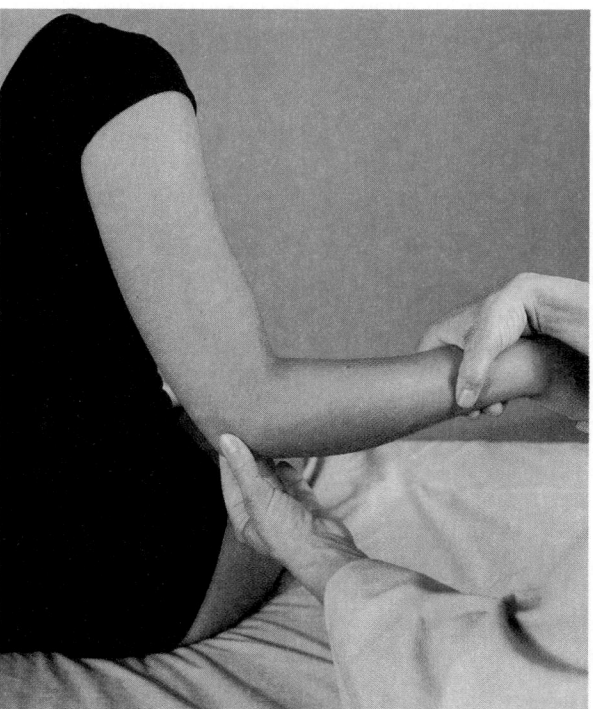

FIGURE 18-27 A, Examination of the extensor surface of the elbow with client in the supine position. **B,** Examination of the extensor surface of the elbow joint with client in the sitting position.

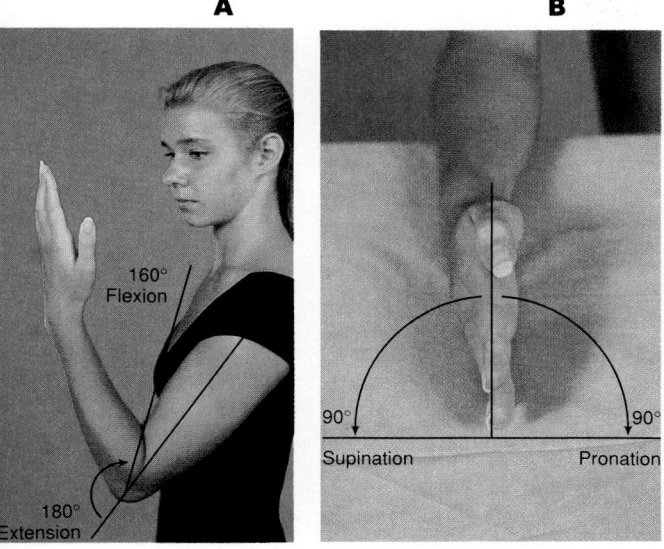

FIGURE 18-28 Range of motion of the elbow. **A,** Flexion and extension. **B,** Pronation and supination.

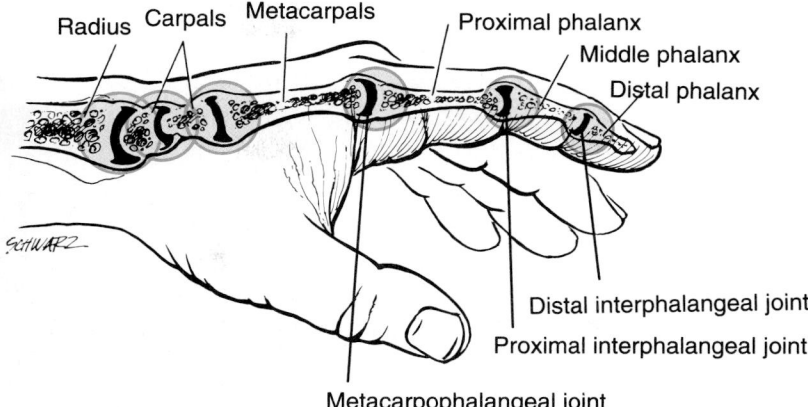

FIGURE 18-29 Joints articulating the bones of the wrist and hand.

with your other hand. Palpate the lateral and medial condyles, the olecranon process, and the grooves on either side of the olecranon process. Joint swelling is most often palpable in the medial groove (Figure 18-27).

To test range of motion (Figure 18-28), ask the client to:
1. Bend and straighten the elbow.
2. Turn the hand face up (supination); face down (pronation).

To test muscle strength, use the tests for the biceps and triceps muscles described in the section on shoulders.

WRISTS, HANDS, AND FINGERS. The wrist joint contains the points of articulation between the distal radius and the proximal portions of the following carpal bones: scaphoid (navicular), lunate, and triangular (Figure 18-29). An articular disk divides the radius from the ulnar bone and also separates the radius from the wrist joint. The wrist joint is protected by a fibrous capsule and ligaments. The joint is lined by synovial membrane.

Inspect the wrist and the hands for position, contour, symmetry, smoothness, edema, atrophy or hypertrophy, and deformity. Swelling of the wrist joint most frequently appears on the dorsal surface distal to the ulnar tip. Swelling is easily visible over the dorsal surface of the hand because little tissue covers the joints.

Use two hands for palpation of the wrist so that the thumbs and the index fingers are opposed on either side of the wrist. Apply enough pressure to outline bony

and soft tissue structures. Palpate the joints between the carpal, metacarpal, and phalangeal bones. Use your thumbs and index fingers to palpate each of these joints (Figure 18-30).

To test range of motion of the hands and wrist (Figure 18-31), ask the client to:
1. Spread the fingers apart and bring them back again.
2. Make a fist.
3. Touch the thumb to each fingertip and to the base of the little finger.
4. Bend the fingers up and down at the metacarpophalangeal joint.
5. Bend the hand up and down at the wrist.
6. With the palm facing down, turn the hand to the right (radial deviation) and to the left **(ulnar deviation).**

To assess wrist strength, ask the client to:
1. Maintain wrist flexion while you try to extend the wrist.
2. Try to extend the wrist as you try to flex it (Figure 18-32).

To assess grip strength, ask the client to squeeze your first two fingers as hard as he or she can (Figure 18-33). If you cross your fingers, you will not feel as much discomfort if the client is exceptionally strong.

To assess finger strength, ask the client to:
1. Extend the fingers while you push down on the dorsal surface.
2. Flex the fingers while you push up on the ventral surface.
3. Spread the fingers as far apart as possible while you try to push them together (Figure 18-34).
4. Push the fingers as close together as possible while you try to pull them apart.

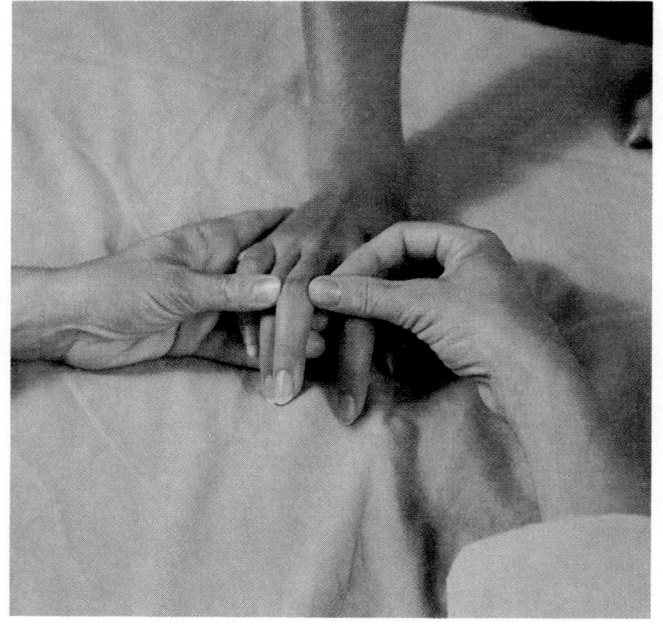

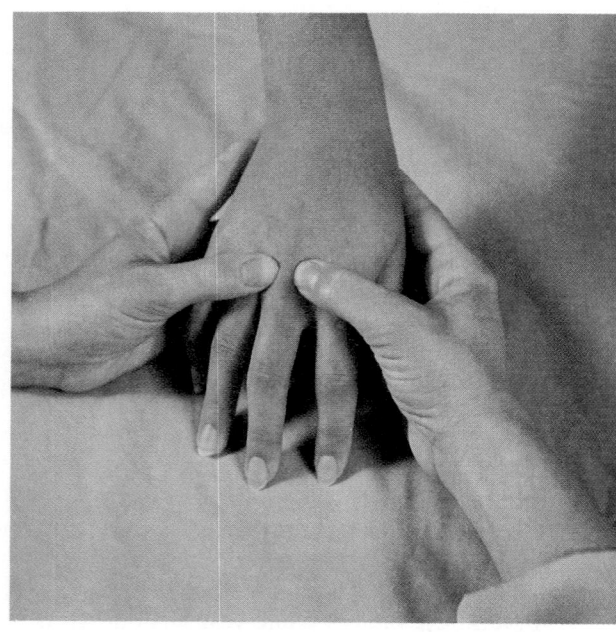

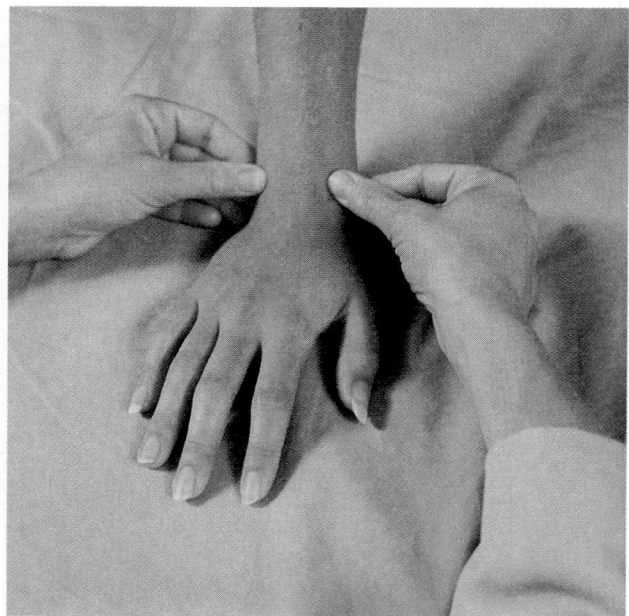

FIGURE 18-30 Palpation of joints of the hand and wrist. **A,** Interphalangeal joints.
B, Metacarpophalangeal joints. **C,** Radiocarpal groove and wrist.

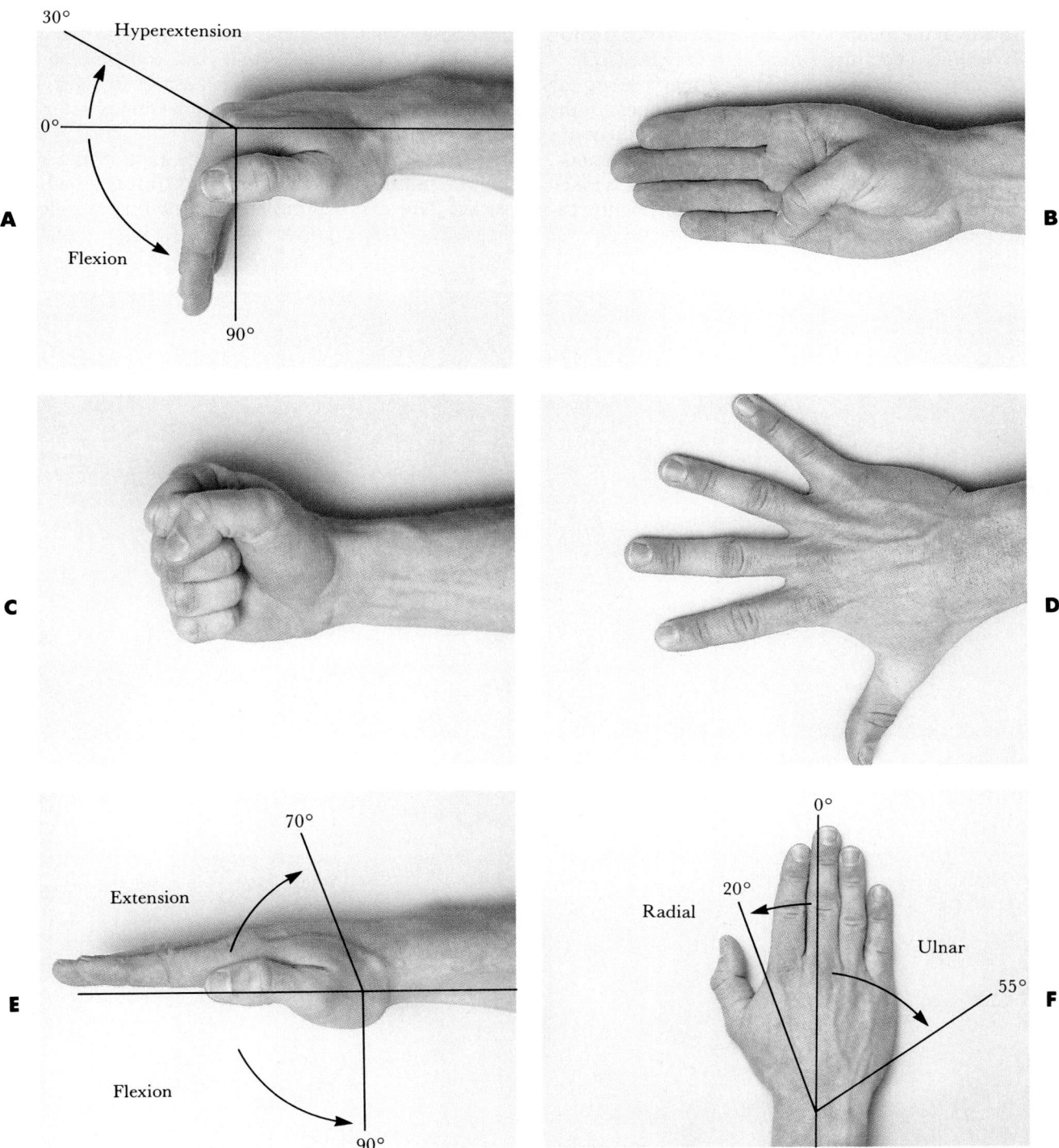

FIGURE 18-31 Range of motion of the hand and wrist. **A,** Metacarpophalangeal flexion and hyperextension. **B,** Finger flexion: thumb to each fingertip and to base of little finger. **C,** Finger flexion: fist formation. **D,** Finger abduction. **E,** Flexion and hyperextension of wrist. **F,** Radial and ulnar movement of wrist. (From Seidel HM and others: *Mosby's guide to physical examination,* St Louis, 1991, Mosby–Year Book.)

Many tendons cross the wrist and hands to their insertions on the fingers. Thickening of the flexor tendon sheath of the median nerve (seen in **carpal tunnel syndrome**) is a common problem. It may lead to feelings of numbness, burning, and paresthesia along the distribution of the median nerve. The thickness of the sheath may be visible on the palmar surface of the wrist. Two tests may elicit these altered sensory phenomena. In the first of these tests, Phalen's test, the client is asked to maintain palmar flexion for 1 minute (Figure 18-35). The experience of numbness and paresthesia over the palmar surface of the hand and the first three fingers and part of the fourth is called Phalen's sign. The symptoms resolve quickly after the hand returns to the resting position. The second test, Tinel's test, consists of tapping over the median nerve (palmar aspect of wrist). The client's sensation of tingling or prickling is known as Tinel's sign (Figure 18-36).

HIPS. The hip joint is the articulation of the acetabulum and the femur (Figure 18-37). It is a ball-and-socket joint that is protected by a fibrous capsule and ligaments. Three bursae reduce friction in the hip:

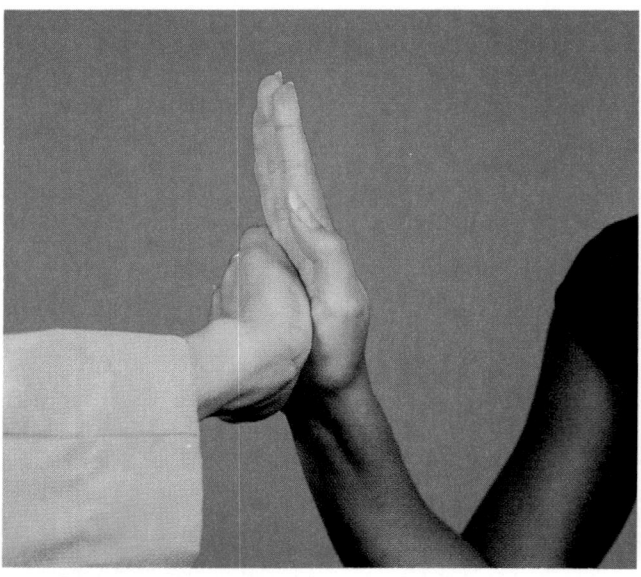

FIGURE 18-32 To assess wrist strength, client attempts to extend her wrist while examiner tries to flex it.

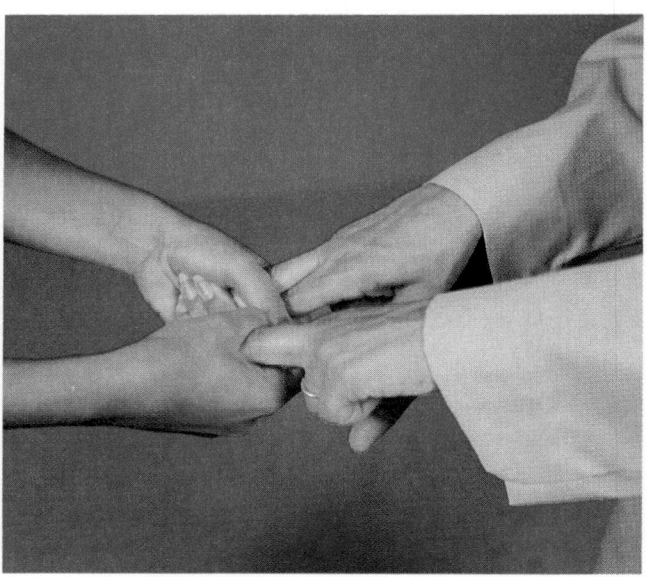

FIGURE 18-33 Assessment of grip strength.

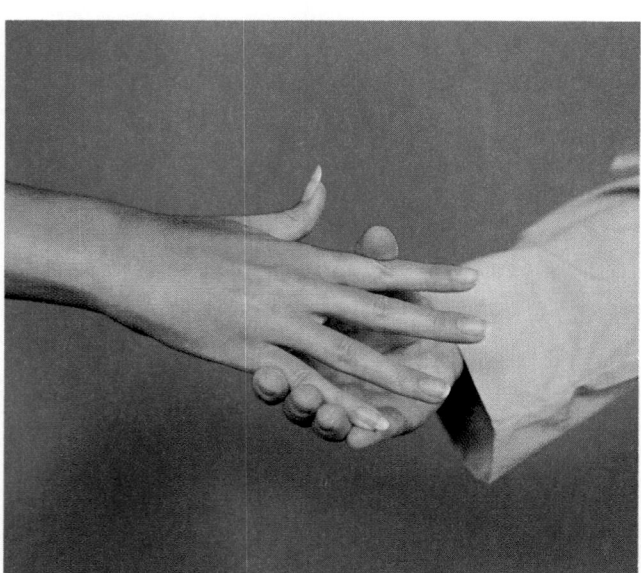

FIGURE 18-34 Assessment of finger strength.

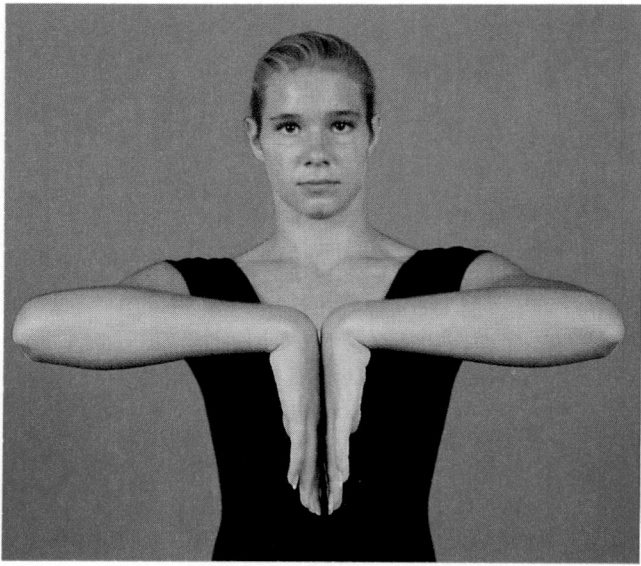

FIGURE 18-35 Phalen's test for carpal tunnel syndrome.

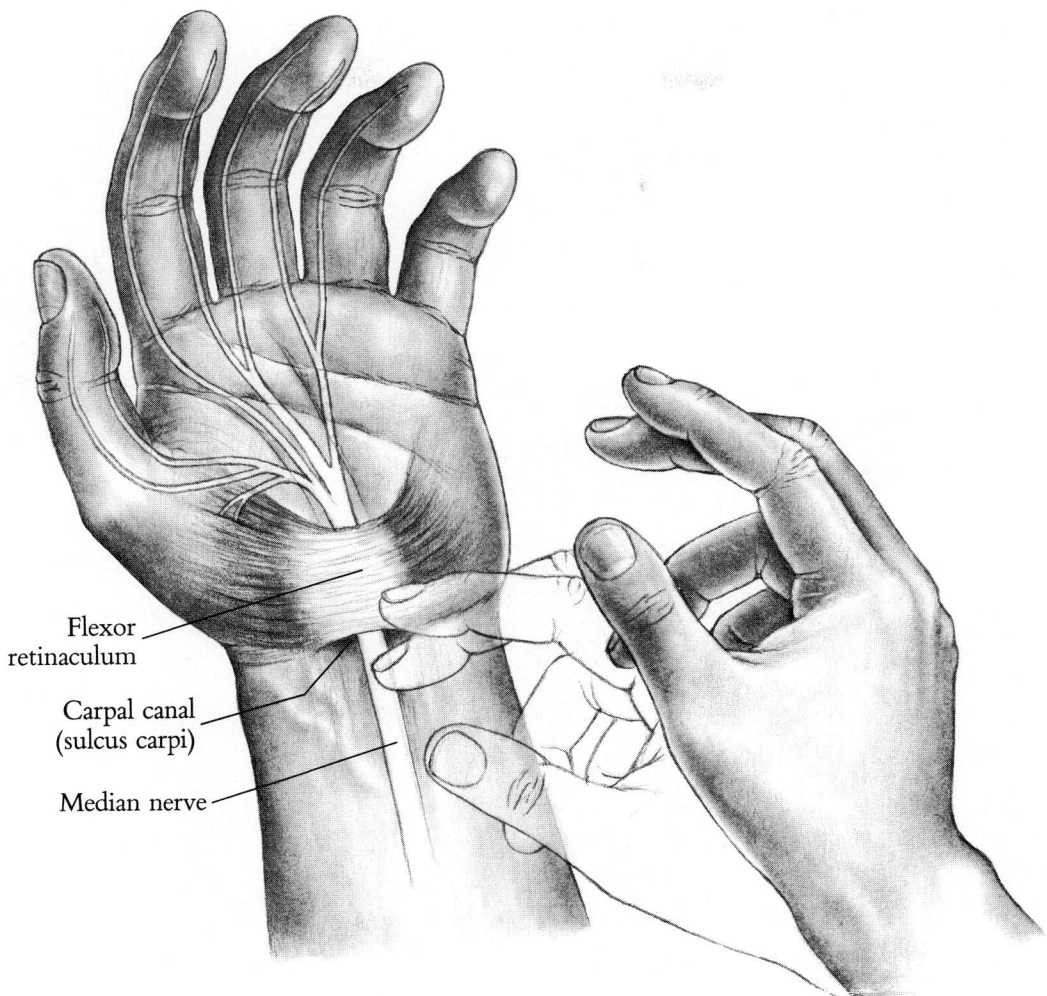

Flexor
retinaculum

Carpal canal
(sulcus carpi)

Median nerve

FIGURE 18-36 Elicitation of Tinel's sign. (From Seidel HM and others: *Mosby's guide to physical examination,* St Louis, 1991, Mosby–Year Book.)

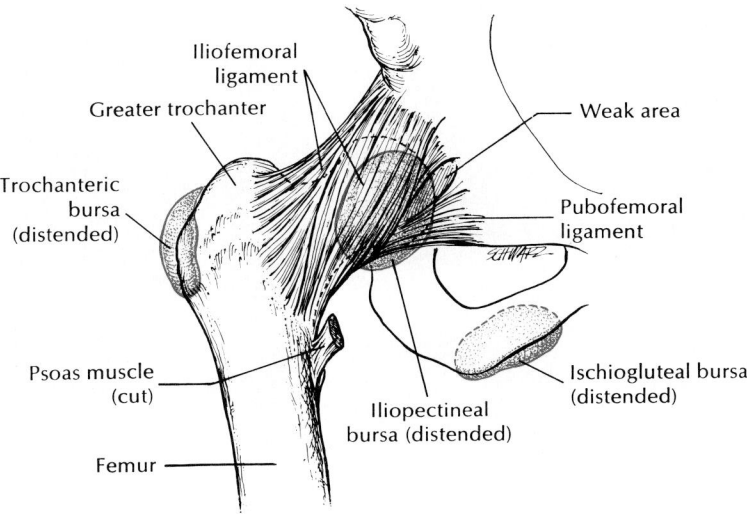

Iliofemoral
ligament

Greater trochanter

Weak area

Trochanteric
bursa
(distended)

Pubofemoral
ligament

Psoas muscle
(cut)

Ischiogluteal bursa
(distended)

Iliopectineal
bursa (distended)

Femur

FIGURE 18-37 Hip joint.

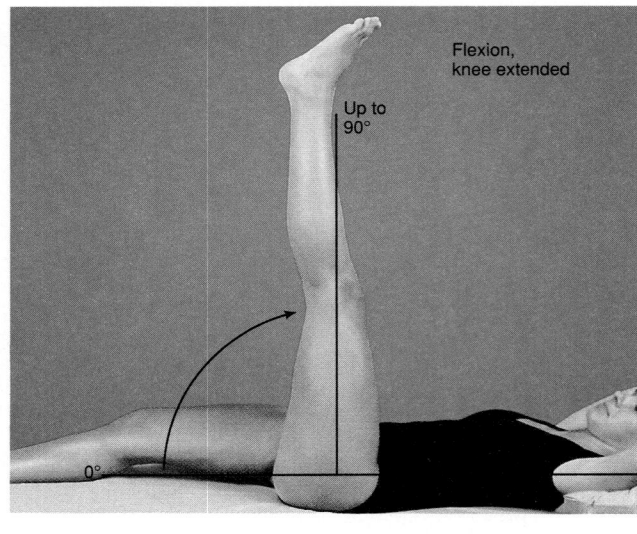

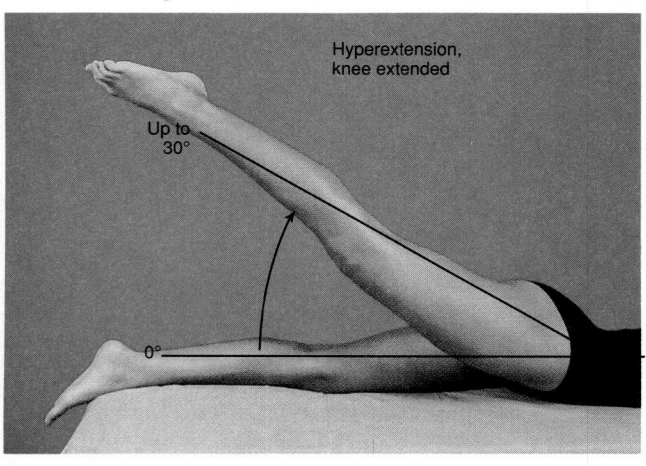

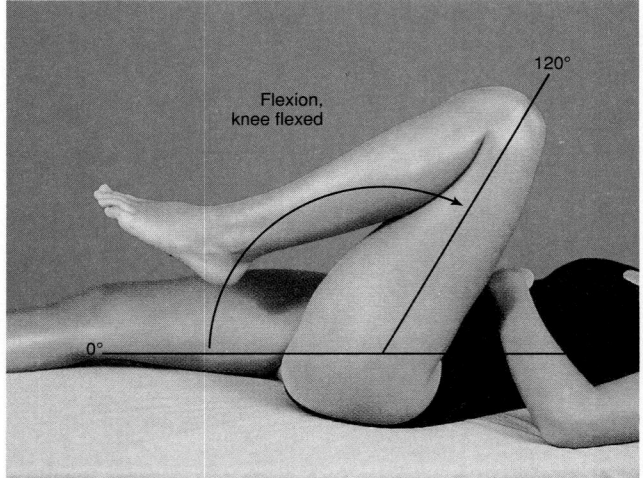

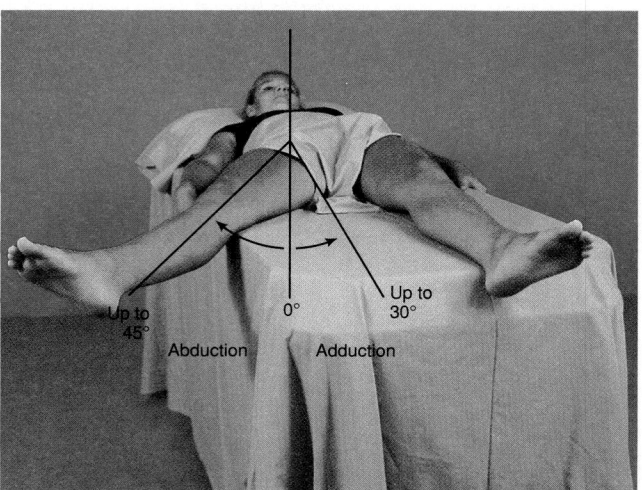

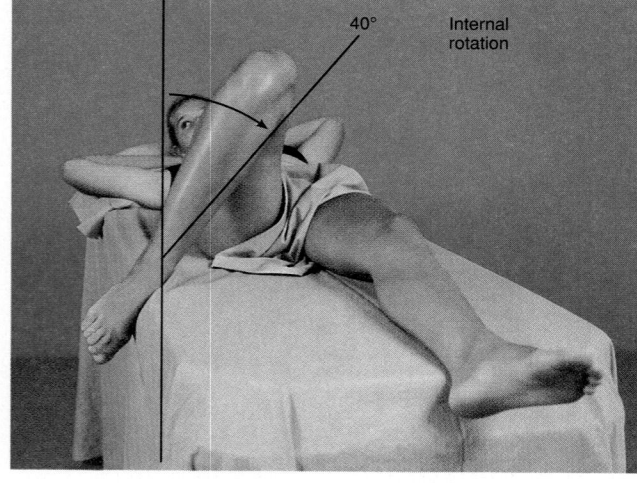

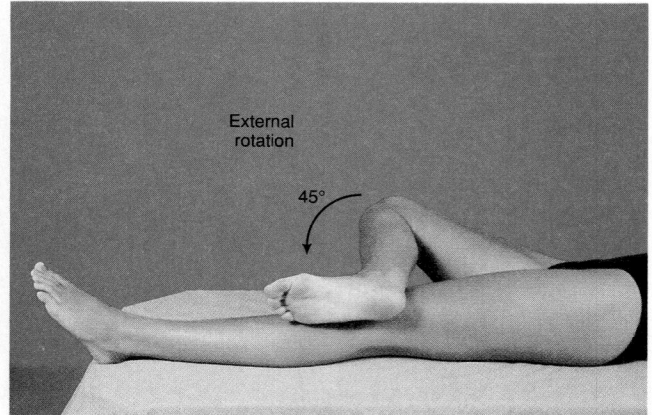

FIGURE 18-38 Range of motion of the hip. **A,** Hip flexion, leg extended. **B,** Hip hyperextension, knee extended. **C,** Hip flexion, knee flexed. **D,** Abduction. **E,** Internal rotation. **F,** External rotation.

(1) the trochanteric, between the posterolateral greater trochanter and the gluteus maximus; (2) the iliopectineal, between the anterior surface of the joint and the iliopsoas muscle; and (3) the ischiogluteal, situated over the ischial tuberosity.

Inspect the hips anteriorly and posteriorly while the client stands. Look for symmetry in iliac crest height, size of the buttocks, and number and level of gluteal folds. Inspection of the hip joint includes an assessment of gait. A smooth and even gait indicates equal leg length and functional hip motion. Antalgic limp is characteristic of disease that produces pain in a hip joint; the body tilts toward the involved diseased hip in such a way that the weight of the body is directly over the hip. This limp decreases the need for abductor muscle movement and thus may alleviate muscle spasm. If the abductor muscles are weak, that is, unable to support the pelvis, the unaffected hip may move downward in such a way that the weight is borne on that side. This condition is called Trendelenburg's limp.

With the client supine, palpate the hips and the pelvis for stability, tenderness, or crepitus. The bursae are not palpable unless they are swollen. Swelling and tenderness are the diagnostic findings of pathological conditions of these structures.

To test range of motion of the hips (Figure 18-38), ask the client to:
1. While supine, raise the leg above the body with the knee extended.
2. While supine, bring the knee to the chest while keeping the other leg straight.
3. While supine, swing the leg laterally and medially while keeping the knee straight.
4. While supine, place the side of the foot on the opposite knee and move the flexed knee down toward the examining table (external rotation).
5. While supine, flex the knee and rotate the leg so that the flexed knee moves inward toward the opposite leg (internal rotation).
6. While either prone or standing, swing the straightened leg behind the body.

To test muscle strength in the hips, ask the client to:
1. While in a supine position, raise the extended leg while you attempt to hold it down.
2. While in a supine position, with your hands placed on the bed on either side of the client's knees, push both legs against your hands.
3. While in a supine position, with your hands placed on the bed between the client's knees, bring both legs together.

To assess muscle strength in the hamstring, gluteal, abductor, and adductor muscles, ask the client to sit and perform alternate leg crossing (Figure 18-39).

KNEE. The knee joint is the articulation of the femur, the tibia, and the patella (Figure 18-40). The lining of

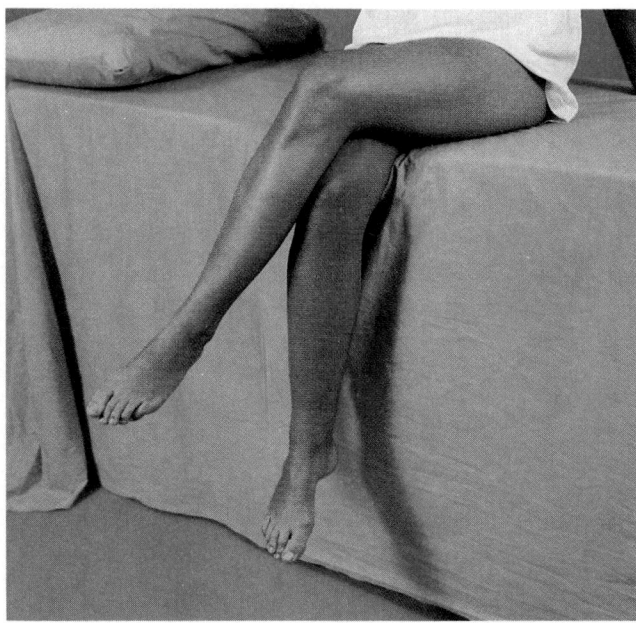

FIGURE 18-39 Alternate leg crossing for assessment of hamstring, gluteal, abductor, and adductor muscle strength.

the joint is a fibrous membrane. Synovial membrane covers the articular surface of the femur and the tibia with folds to the patella. The medial and lateral menisci are fibrocartilaginous disks whose outside edges (horns) are attached to the tibia and are continuous with the articular capsule. The medial convexity of the femur rotates with the inner portion of the meniscus that is attached to it. A spiral distortion of the menisci occurs on rotation, making these disks susceptible to rupture. The surfaces of the menisci have no synovial membrane. They are thought to aid the spread of synovial fluid, and this function may account for their existence. An anterior pouch in the knee joint that separates the patella and quadriceps tendon and muscle from the femur is called the suprapatellar pouch.

The bursae of the knee are numerous. On the anterior knee the prepatellar bursa lies immediately in front of the patella. The superficial infrapatellar bursa lies anterior to the patellar ligament, and the deep infrapatellar bursa is behind the ligament. The bursae of the posterior knee include the two gastrocnemius bursae, one of which separates the lateral head of the gastrocnemius muscle from the articular capsule and the other of which divides the medial head of the gastrocnemius muscle from the articular capsule. In addition, a large bursa separates the medial head of the gastrocnemius muscle from the semimembranous muscle.

Inspect the knee with the client walking (to observe gait), sitting, and supine with knees extended. Be familiar with the normal contour of the knee because loss

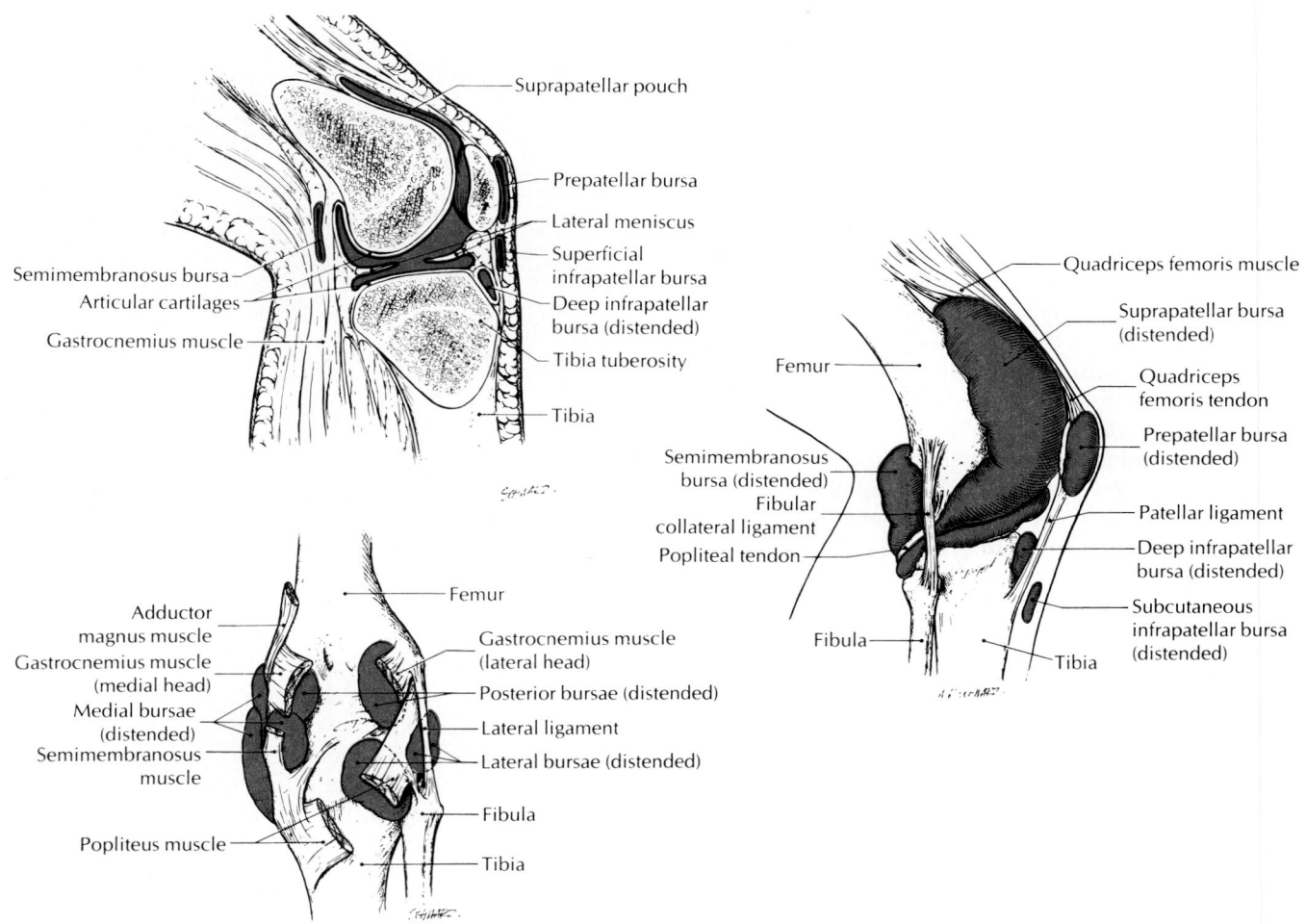

FIGURE 18-40 Knee joint.

of contour may occur with swelling. The client may voluntarily maintain the knee at 15 to 20 degrees of flexion because the knee joint is at maximal capacity at this angle and thus pain is reduced. Swelling as a result of synovitis is most apparent at the suprapatellar pouch. Swelling caused by meniscal cysts appears at the lateral or the medial joint surface. Popliteal swelling is more obvious when the knee is extended. Swelling of the knee observed on the anterior aspect of the knee is called prepatellar bursitis or "housemaid's knee."

Palpate the knee with the client in the sitting or supine position, whichever affords more comfort for the client. Apply downward pressure over the suprapatellar pouch to localize the synovial fluid in the lower portion of the articular cavity. Use the examining hand to palpate the lateral and medial joint surfaces with the fingers while using the thumb for stability (Figure 18-41).

In a second procedure for the examination of the knee, palpate the suprapatellar pouch with the thumb and the fingers of one hand while the other hand pushes the contents of the articular cavity upward. To do this, place your thumb on one side of the patella with the rest of your fingers on the other side to form an arch below the patella. Apply an inward and upward pressure to move any fluid upward into the suprapatellar bursa. Place the examining hand about 10 cm above the patella and move it gradually toward the patella.

A test for small effusions in the knee joint is called the *bulge sign*. Take the ball of your hand and firmly milk the medial aspect of the knee upward two to three times to displace fluid. Then press or tap behind the lateral margin of the knee (Figure 18-42). A positive bulge sign will show a swelling or bulge of fluid in the hollow area medial to the patella. The bulge sign is useful for assessing small effusions, but it may be absent in large effusions.

When considerable fluid is present in the suprapatellar pouch, **ballottement** of the patella may be pos-

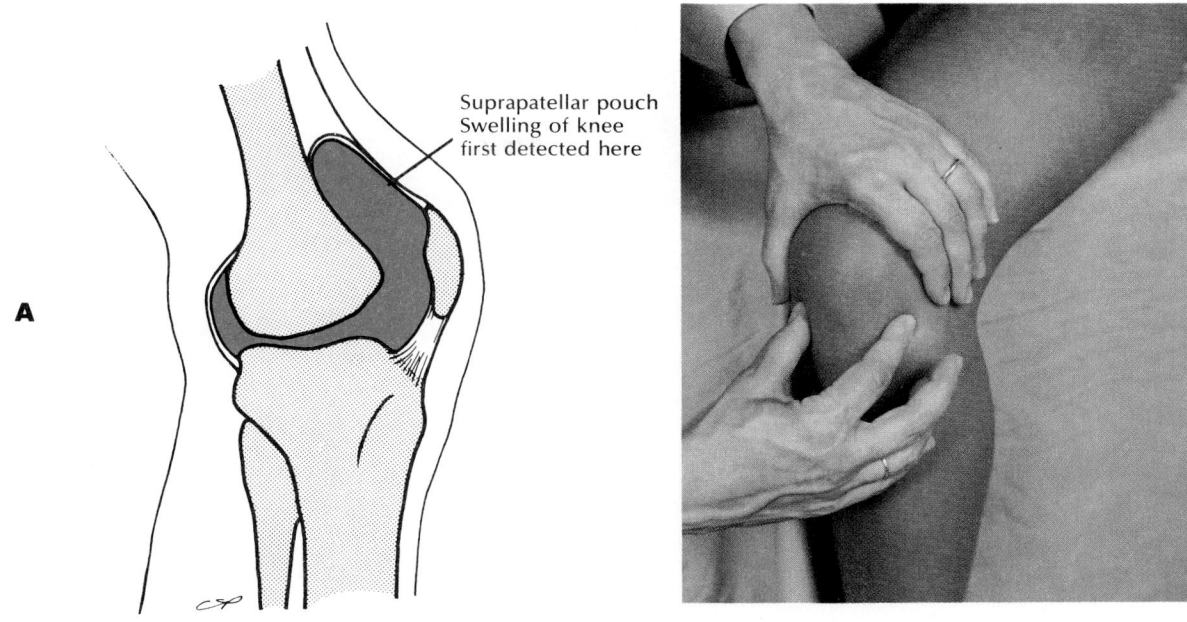

FIGURE 18-41 **A,** Knee effusion. **B,** Examination of the knee.

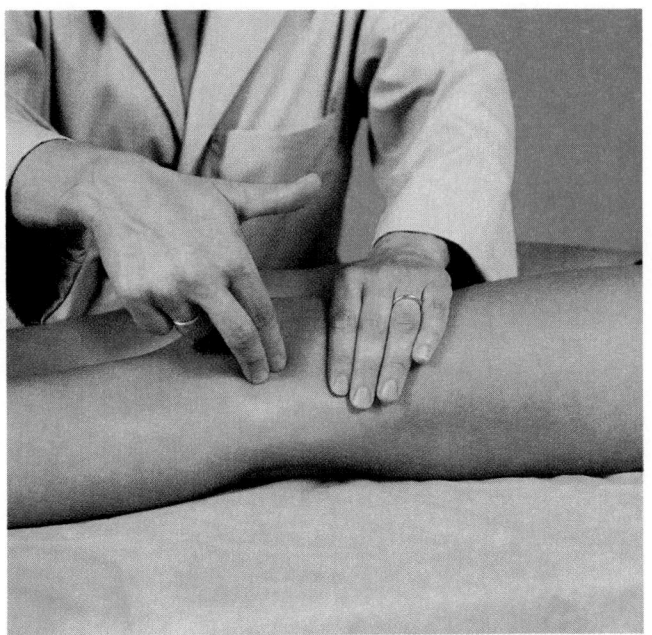

FIGURE 18-42 Testing for the bulge sign. After milking the medial aspect of the knee, the lateral side of the patella is tapped.

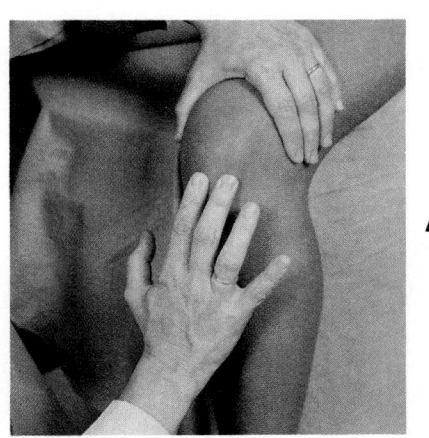

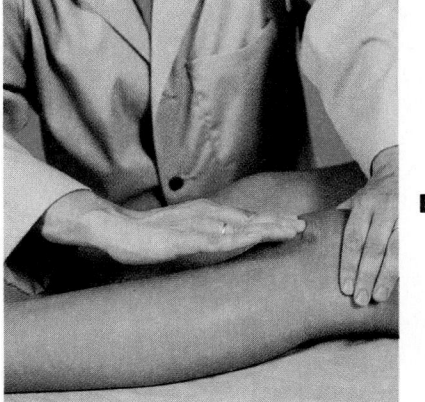

FIGURE 18-43 Ballottement of the patella. **A,** Sitting. **B,** Supine.

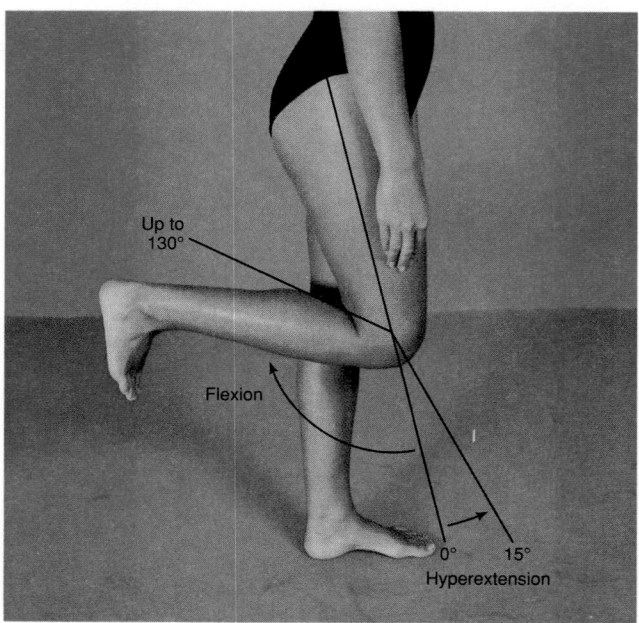

FIGURE 18-44 Range of motion of the knee: flexion and extension.

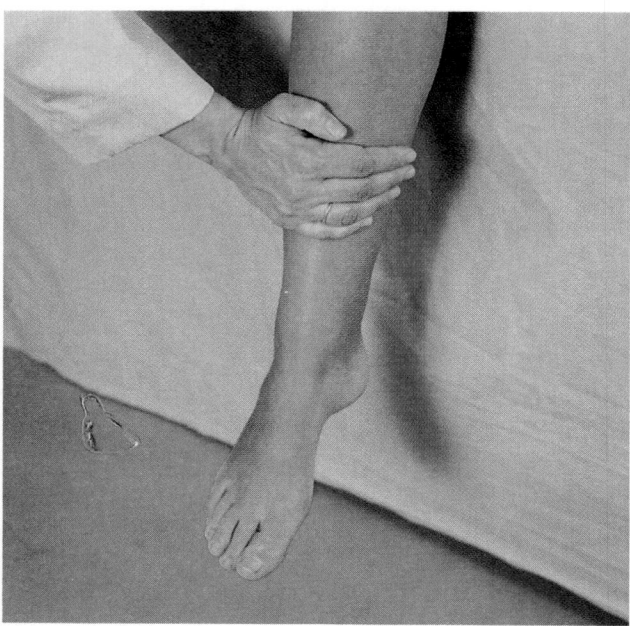

FIGURE 18-45 Assessment of quadriceps muscle strength. Client attempts to straighten the leg while examiner tries to flex it.

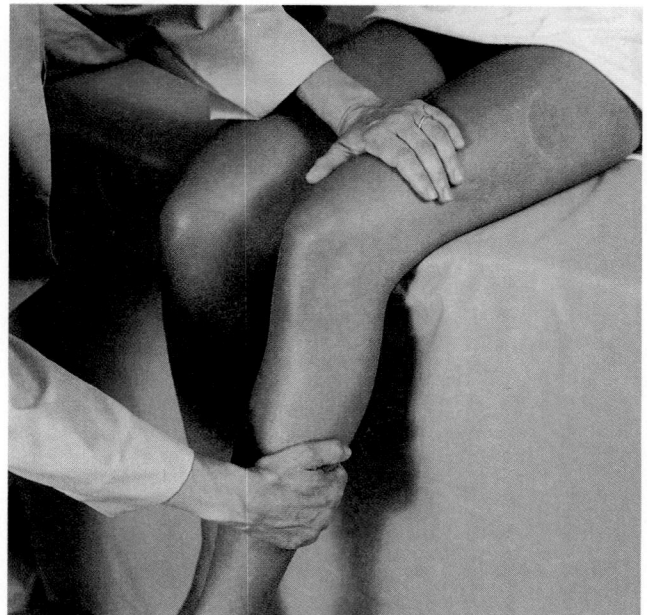

FIGURE 18-46 Assessment of hamstring muscle strength. Client flexes his knees while examiner tries to straighten them.

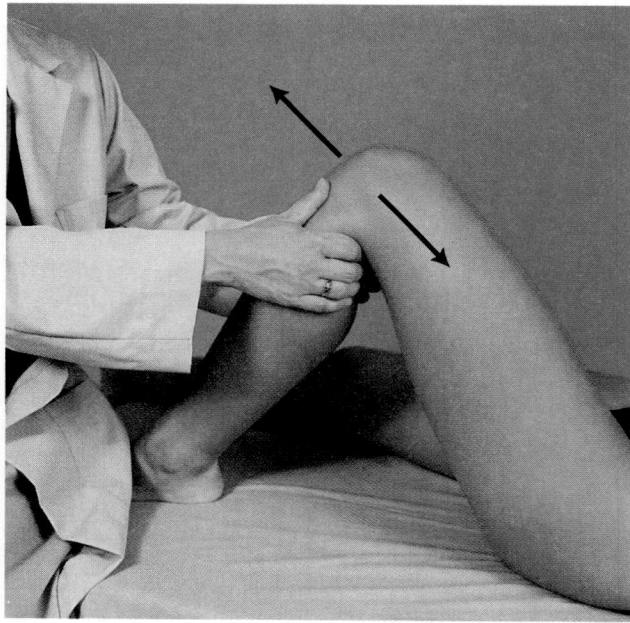

FIGURE 18-47 Examination of the knee with the drawer test for anterior and posterior stability.

sible (Figure 18-43). Ballottement involves applying downward pressure with one hand while pushing the patella backward against the femur with a finger of the opposite hand. Examine the popliteal region with the client in the prone position or while standing. Swelling of the joint in the popliteal region, which is called **Baker's cyst,** is generally an extension of the articular cavity.

To test range of motion of the knee (Figure 18-44), ask the client to:

1. Bend the knee.
2. Straighten and stretch the leg.

To test muscle strength in the knee, ask the client to:

1. Extend the leg as you try to bend it (quadriceps muscle strength) (Figure 18-45).
2. Bend the knees as you try to straighten them (hamstring muscle strength) (Figure 18-46).

Sprains or tears of the ligaments are the most common injuries of the knee. Two sets of ligaments play a role in movement of the knee. They are the anterior and posterior cruciate ligaments and the medial and lateral collateral ligaments. The anterior cruciate ligament limits extension and rotation, whereas the posterior cruciate ligament stabilizes the femur against forward dislocation. The collateral ligaments prevent lateral and medial dislocation of the knee. Abnormal movements of the knee may indicate dislocation. You may be able to palpate the tears in the assessment of the knee.

To test the stability of the anterior and posterior cruciate ligaments, use the drawer test (Figure 18-47) or the Lachman test (if you are assessing the anterior ligament). For the drawer sign, have the client lie in a supine position with the knee flexed to 90 degrees and the foot flat on the examining table. Position yourself on the edge of the table so that you can stabilize the foot by sitting on it. Cup your hands around the tibia. To test the stability of the anterior cruciate ligament, pull the tibia toward you. If it slides forward from under the femur, the drawer test is positive and suggests a tear in the anterior ligament. To test the posterior cruciate ligament, push the tibia posteriorly. If it moves backward, the ligament is probably damaged. This test is usually performed in one continuous motion. Test the other knee to compare findings.

The Lachman test is thought to be a better indicator of injury to the anterior cruciate ligament (Magee, 1992). Have the client lie in a supine position with the involved leg beside you. Place the client's knee between 20 and 30 degrees of flexion (close to the functional position of the knee). Stabilize the femur with one hand while you move the proximal aspect of the tibia forward with the other hand. If there is a soft or "mushy" feel and the infrapatellar slope disappears when the tibia is moved forward on the femur, the Lachman test is positive. This sign indicates damage to the anterior cruciate ligament, especially the posterolateral band. Test the other knee to compare findings.

TESTS FOR MENISCUS DAMAGE. Indications of pathological conditions of meniscus include (1) pain or tenderness on the lateral surfaces of the knee joint; (2) popping, snapping, or grating sounds with movement; and (3) inability to fully extend the knee ("locking"). The medial meniscus is more often injured than is the lateral. The two tests commonly used to aid in the diagnosis of a torn meniscus are the Apley test and the McMurray test.

Attempt to elicit **Apley's sign** (Figure 18-48) in the client you suspect of having a loose object in the knee joint or one who has given a history of knee joint locking. Have the client assume the prone position with the suspected knee flexed to 90 degrees. Exert downward pressure on the foot so that the tibia is firmly opposed to the femur. Rotate the leg externally and internally. Locking of the knee, pain with the maneuver, or the sound of clicks is a positive sign and may indicate that a loose body, such as torn cartilage, is trapped in the articulation. Clicks or popping sounds are generated as the object escapes. Repeat the maneuver using distraction rather than downward pressure (compression) on the foot. If the pain is worse when rotation plus compression are used, there is probably a meniscus injury. Pain that is worse when rotation plus distraction are used is probably ligamentous.

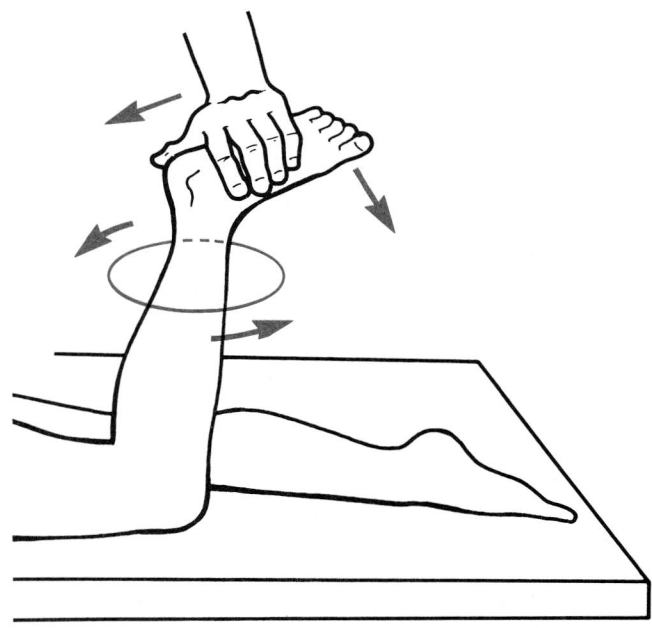

FIGURE 18-48 Elicitation of Apley's sign with compression.

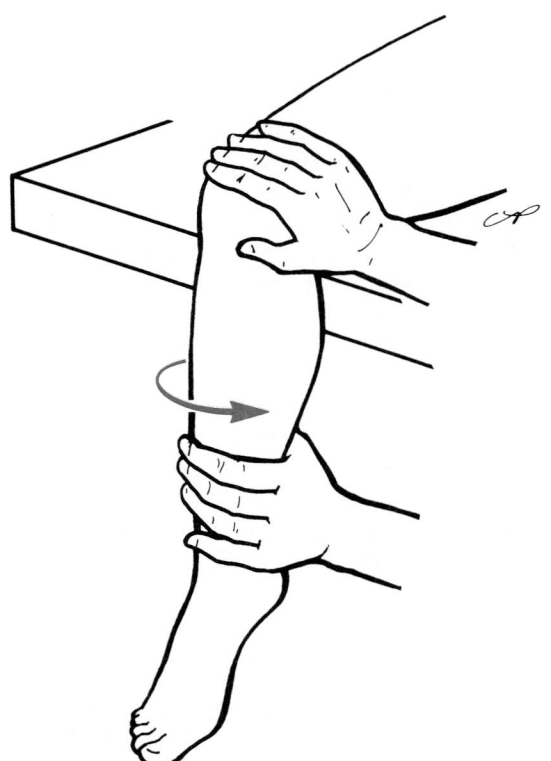

FIGURE 18-49 Elicitation of McMurray's sign to test the lateral meniscus.

When the client states that he "feels something in the knee joint" or complains that "sometimes it just won't bend,"attempt to elicit **McMurray's sign** (Figure 18-49). Perform this test with the client in the sitting position with the knee flexed to 90 degrees or in the supine position. Have the client internally rotate the leg while you slowly extend it with one hand. Use the other hand to provide resistance at the medial aspect of the knee. This maneuver tests the medial meniscus. Extension of the knee may not be possible (positive sign) if a loose body impedes its movement. Repeat the procedure by employing external rotation and applying resistance to the lateral aspect of the knee. This maneuver tests the lateral meniscus.

ANKLES AND FEET. The ankle joint is the articulation of the tibia, the fibula, and the talus (Figure 18-50). The capsule is lined with synovia. The ankle joint is protected by ligaments on the medial and lateral surfaces but not on the anterior or posterior surfaces. The joint between the talus and the calcaneus bones is called the talocalcaneal, or subtalar, joint. The forward extension of the joint cavity is the articulation of the talus and the navicular bones. Articular capsules lined with synovial membrane separate the remainder of the tarsal, metatarsal, and phalangeal bones of the foot.

Inspect the ankle and the foot with the client standing, walking, and sitting (not bearing weight). To best evaluate for swelling, examine the dorsal aspect of the foot because there is less tissue over the bone. Hallux valgus is a lateral deformity of the great toe in which it may lie above or below the second toe. The metatarsophalangeal joint is distorted in such a way that the first metatarsal bone is angled medially. A callus or bursal distention generally occurs at the joint. Hammer toe is a result of hyperextension of the metatarsophalangeal joint and flexion of the proximal phalangeal joint (Figure 18-51).

Palpate the anterior aspect of the ankle joint with your thumbs to assess for bogginess, swelling, or tenderness. Palpate the Achilles tendon for tenderness and nodules (Figure 18-52). Palpate the metatarsal and phalangeal joints with the fingers on the anterior surface and the thumb on the sole of the foot. Note any tenderness.

To test range of motion of the ankle and foot (Figure 18-53), ask the client to:
1. Point the foot up toward the ceiling.
2. Point the foot down toward the floor.
3. With the foot bent at the ankle, point the medial side of the foot toward the floor **(inversion)** and repeat with the lateral side **(eversion)**.
4. Rotate the ankle in order to turn the foot away from and then toward the other foot.

To test muscle strength in the ankle and foot, ask the client to:
1. Flex the foot upward against your hand.
2. Push the foot down against your hand (Figure 18-54).

THORACIC AND LUMBAR SPINE. Inspect the shape of the spine and its structural relationship to the shoulder girdle, thorax, and pelvis. The normal spinal curvatures are concave at the cervical area, convex at the thoracic area, and concave at the lumbar area. Note any differences in heights of the shoulders and the iliac crests. Unusual heights of the iliac crests suggest uneven leg lengths. Variations in spinal curvature may indicate a structural problem.

Scoliosis is a deformity of the spine that appears as a lateral deviation (Figure 18-55). This angling of the spine produces a downward slant of the thoracic cage on the affected side and an upward tilt of the pelvis on the contralateral side. A rotary deformity of the rib cage also occurs. The ribs protrude posteriorly on the convex side of the spine. A hump or "razorback" may be visible. The protrusion may become more obvious when the client bends over.

To assess for scoliosis, ask the client to stand with the feet approximately 6 inches apart and bend over slowly to touch the toes. Stand behind the client and

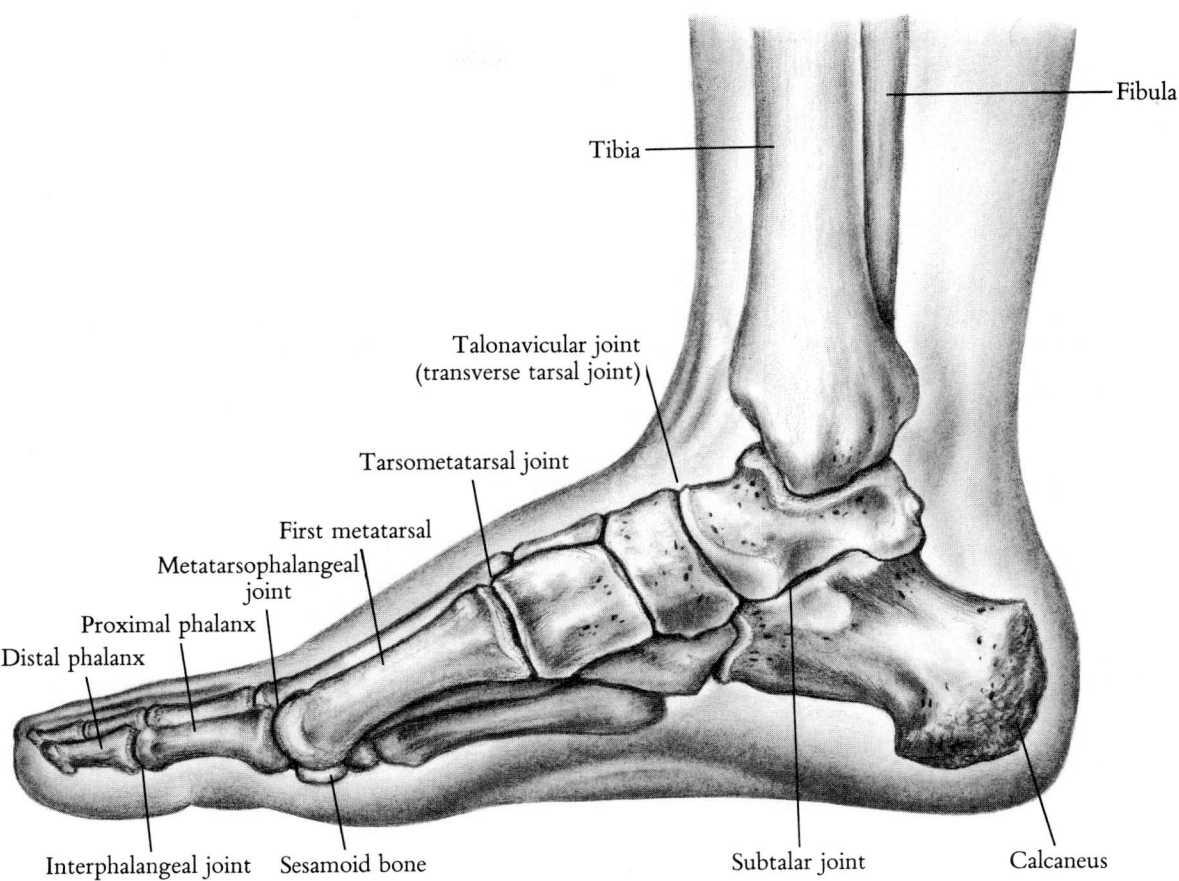

FIGURE 18-50 Bones and joints of the ankle and foot. (From Seidel HM and others: *Mosby's guide to physical examination,* St Louis, 1991, Mosby–Year Book.)

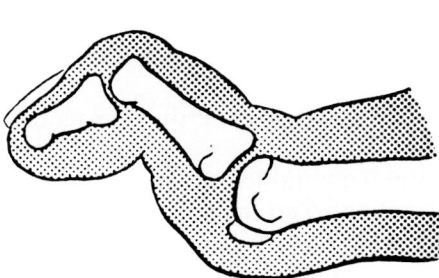

FIGURE 18-51 Hammer great toe. (From Mann RA: *DuVries's surgery of the foot,* ed 5, St Louis, 1984, Mosby–Year Book.)

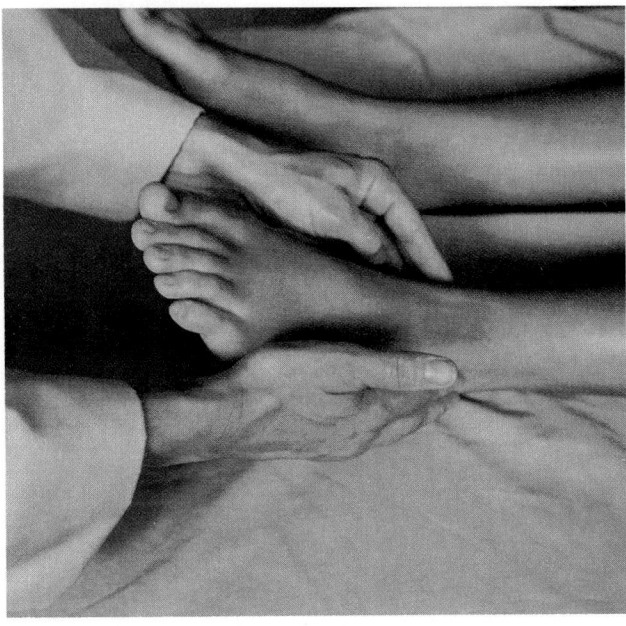

FIGURE 18-52 Examination of the ankle joint.

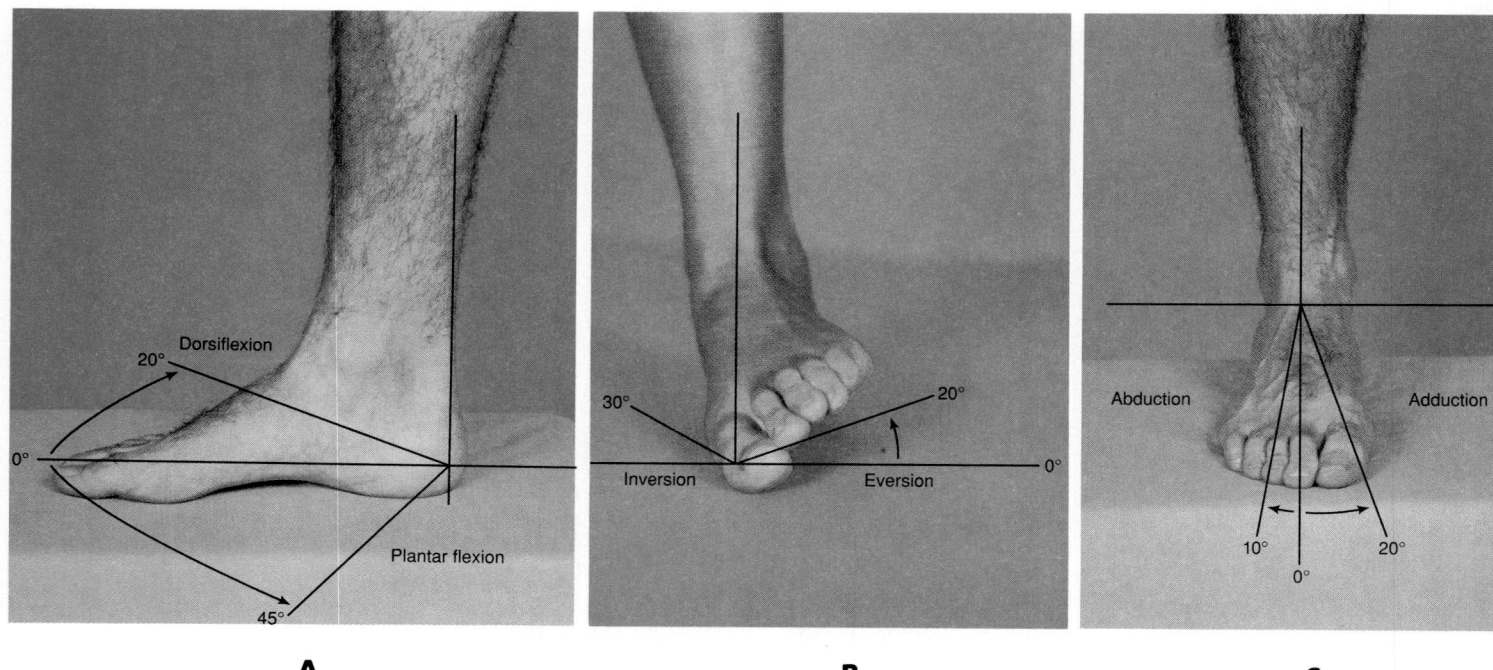

FIGURE 18-53 Range of motion of the ankle and foot. **A,** Dorsiflexion and plantar flexion. **B,** Inversion and eversion. **C,** Abduction and adduction.

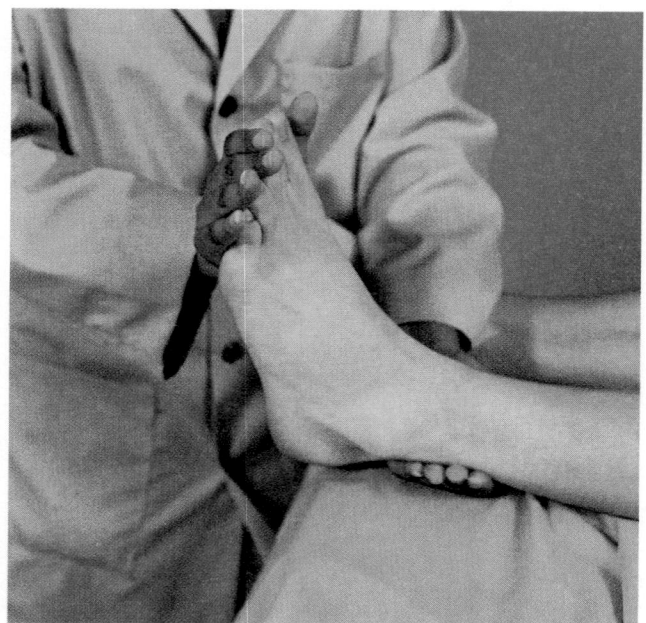

FIGURE 18-54 Testing muscle strength in the ankle and foot.

observe the movement of the spine as the client bends and comes back to an upright position (Figure 18-56). This maneuver provides a "skyline" view of the spine. Structural scoliosis, which is caused by vertebral rotation, tends to become more prominent as the client bends forward. Functional scoliosis, which compensates for structural abnormalities other than those associated with the vertebral column, disappears when the client bends forward. Also note symmetry of the muscles, movement, protrusions, or sharp angulation.

Kyphosis (humpback) is a flexion deformity (Figure 18-57, *B*). When the angle of the defect is sharp, the apex is called a gibbus.

Lordosis (swayback) is an extension deviation of the spine, commonly in the lumbar area (Figure 18-57, *C*).

To assess range of motion of the spine (Figure 18-58) ask the client to:
1. Bend back as far as possible (hyperextend the spine).
2. Bend to the right and left side as far as possible (lateral bending). You may need to stabilize the client's pelvis.
3. Turn to the right and left in a circular motion (while you stabilize the pelvis).
4. Slowly bend forward at the waist and try to touch the toes (while you watch from behind the client and observe for signs of scoliosis).

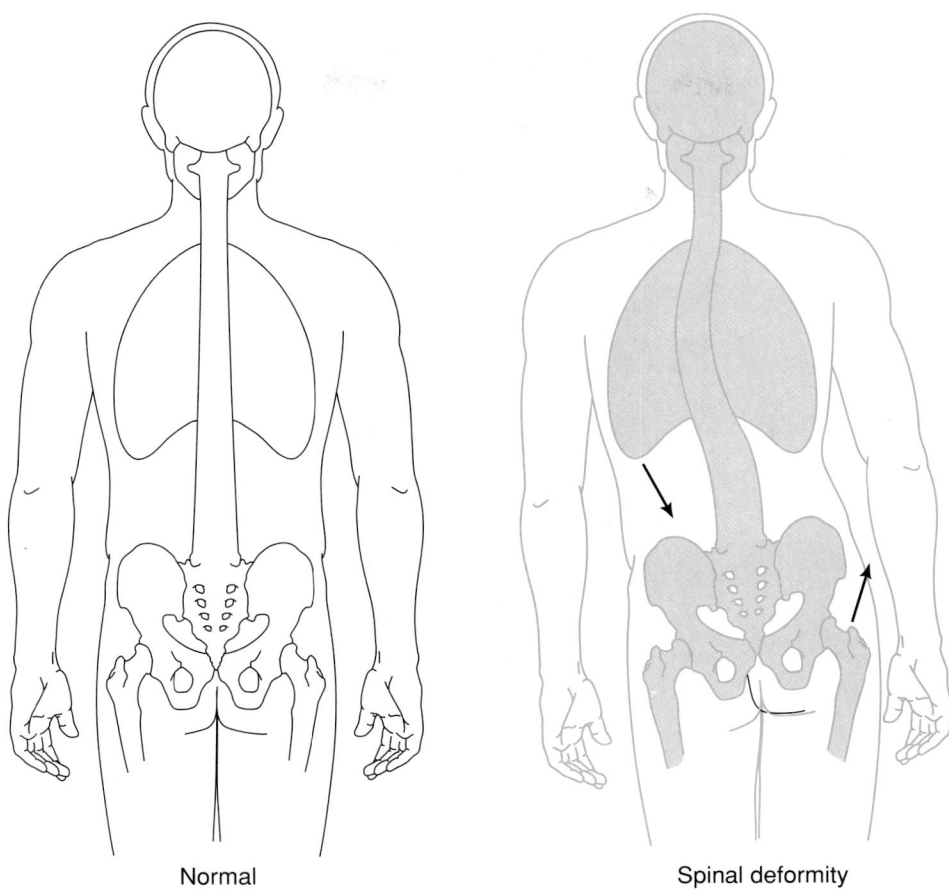

Normal   Spinal deformity

FIGURE 18-55 Deformity of the spine. Scoliosis is a lateral deviation of the spine. Arrows indicate direction of thoracic and pelvic tilt.

Palpate the spinal processes as the client bends over to touch the toes (Figure 18-59). Palpate paravertebral muscles for symmetry, tenderness, and spasm. You may want to percuss for tenderness over the spinous process.

ASSESSMENT OF GAIT. Evaluate **gait** in both phases, stance and swing, for rhythm and smoothness (Figure 18-60). *Stance* is considered to consist of three processes: (1) heel strike—the heel contacts the floor or ground; (2) midstance—the body weight is transferred from the heel to the ball of the foot; and (3) push-off—the heel leaves the ground (see Chapter 8).

The *swing* phase also consists of three processes: (1) acceleration; (2) swing-through—the lifted foot travels ahead of the weight-bearing foot; and (3) deceleration—the foot slows in preparation for the heel strike.

To describe the client's gait, include *phase* (conformity), *cadence* (symmetry, regular rhythm), *stride length* (symmetry, length of swing), *trunk posture* (related to

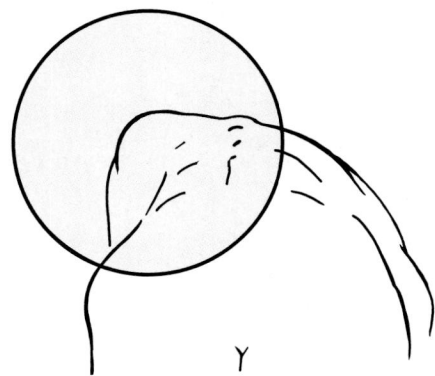

FIGURE 18-56 Rotary deformity of scoliosis produces a humpback or "razorback" deformity. This deviation is best demonstrated by asking the client to bend at the waist.

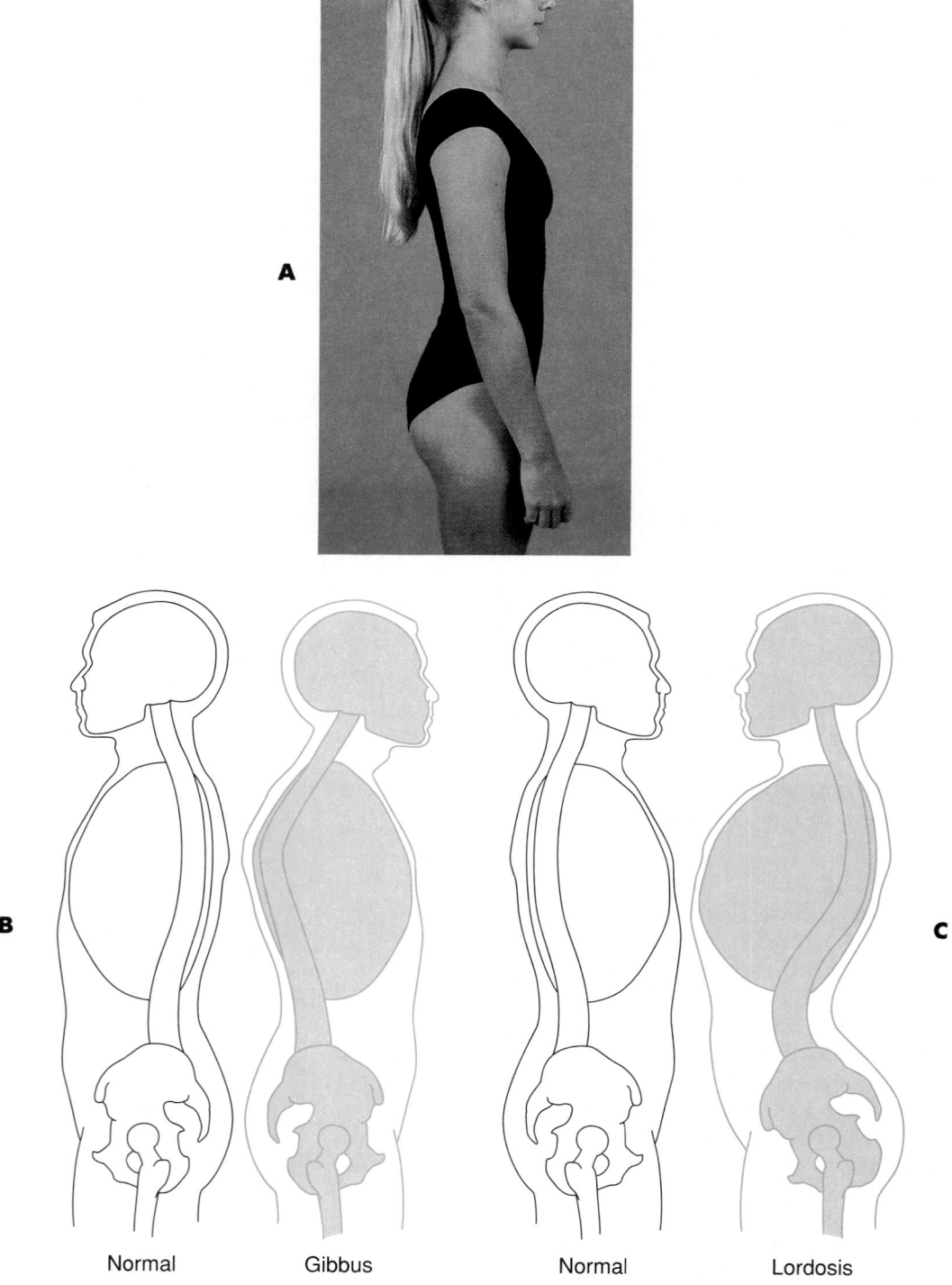

Normal   Gibbus   Normal   Lordosis

FIGURE 18-57 A, Normal curvature of the spine. **B,** Kyphosis, a flexion deformity of the spine. **C,** Lordosis, an extension deformity of the spine.

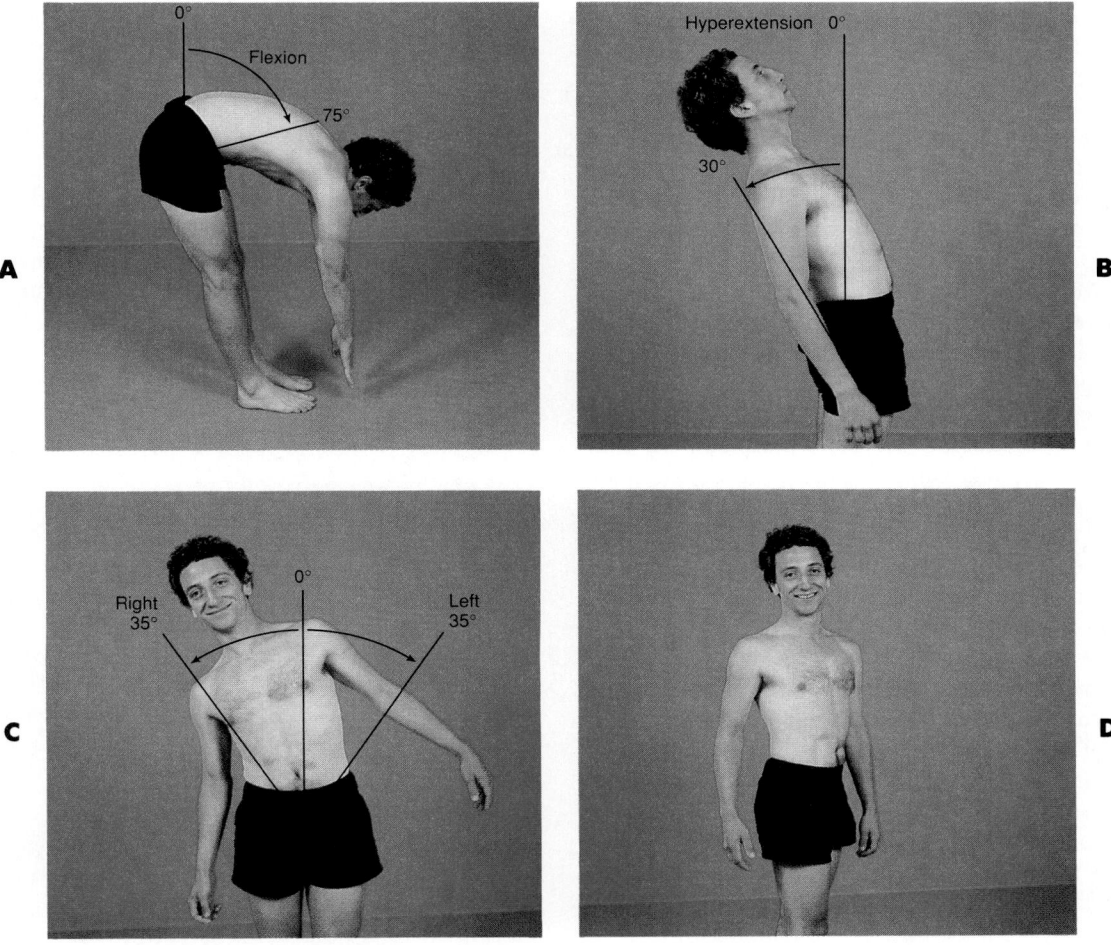

FIGURE 18-58 Range of motion of the thoracic and lumbar spine. **A,** Flexion. **B,** Hyperextension. **C,** Lateral bending. **D,** Rotation of the upper trunk.

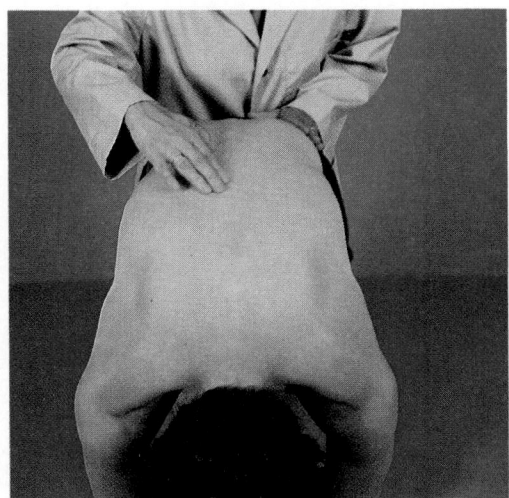

FIGURE 18-59 Palpation of spinal processes as client bends over.

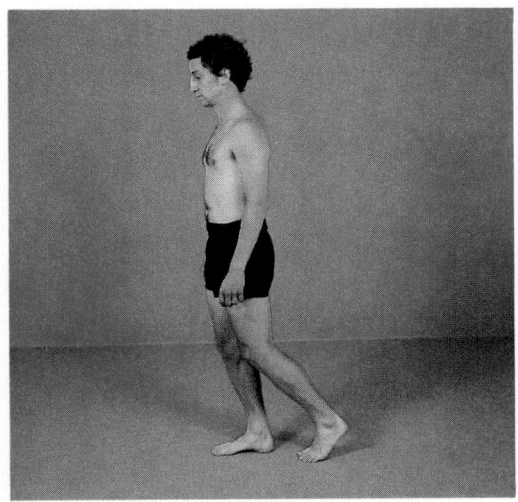

FIGURE 18-60 Assessment of gait.

phases), *pelvic posture* (related to phases), and *arm swing* (symmetry, length of swing).

If pain is present, describe it in relation to the phases of gait.

To assess gait, ask the client to walk naturally for a short distance so that you can observe the gait (if you have not already done so). Then ask the client to take a few steps on the toes and a few steps on the heels.

Special Maneuvers

STRAIGHT LEG-RAISING TEST. The straight leg-raising test, which is also known as Lasègue's test (Figure 18-61), is useful in determining herniated lumbar disk as the cause of sciatic nerve pain. Perform the test for clients who complain of low back pain or pain that radiates down the leg. Have the client lie on the back on a firm surface with the leg and thigh as relaxed as possible. Slowly raise the foot, keeping the knee straight until the client complains of pain. Then dorsiflex the foot. A positive test includes the following responses: (1) pain is produced before 70 degrees is reached; (2) **dorsiflexion** aggravates the pain; and (3) pain relief occurs with flexion of the knee. Pain induced in this manner is caused by pressure on the dorsal roots of the lumbosacral nerves and is characteristic of herniated disk. Repeat this maneuver with the other leg and compare the results. Nerve root irritation is suggested by pain in lumbar, hip, or posterior leg or by muscle spasm. If one leg is raised and pain is felt in the opposite side, then a large herniated disk is likely.

THOMAS TEST. The Thomas test evaluates flexion contractures of the hip. With the client in the supine position, ask the client to pull one knee up toward the chest as far as possible (Figure 18-62, *A*). In the individual with normal hip function, when the hip is flexed, the opposite leg remains flat on the examination table. For the individual with an immobile hip, the opposite hip and leg flex in response to flexion of the leg. Approximate the extent of the flexion contracture by noting the degree of flexion of the opposite leg (the angle between the client's leg and the table) (Figure 18-62, *B*).

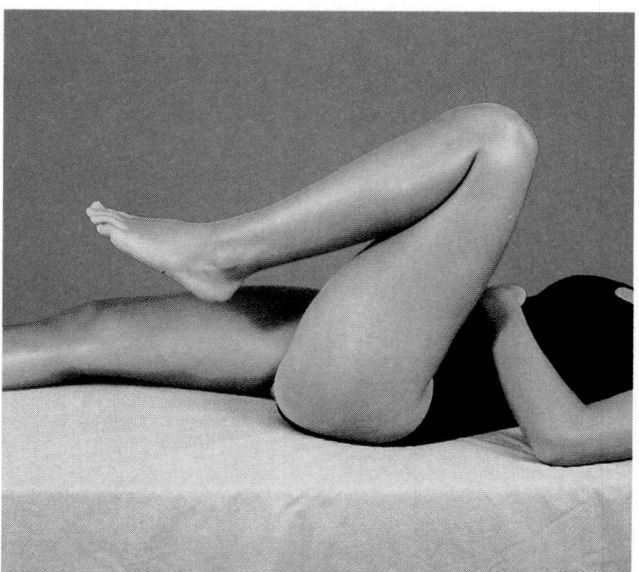

A

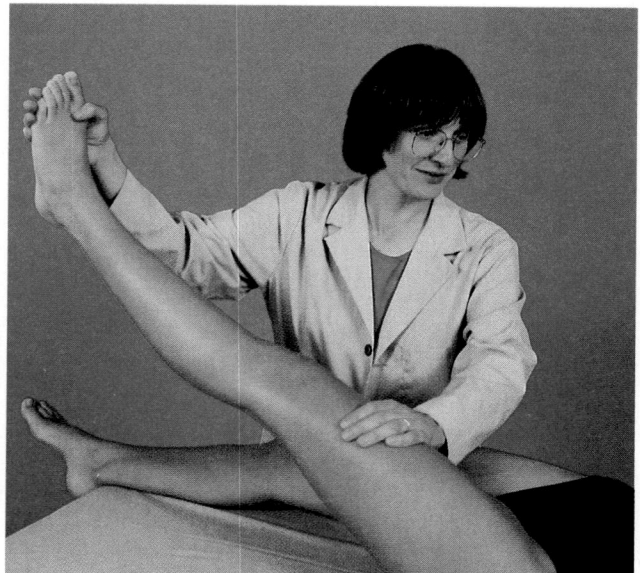

FIGURE 18-61 Straight leg-raising test.

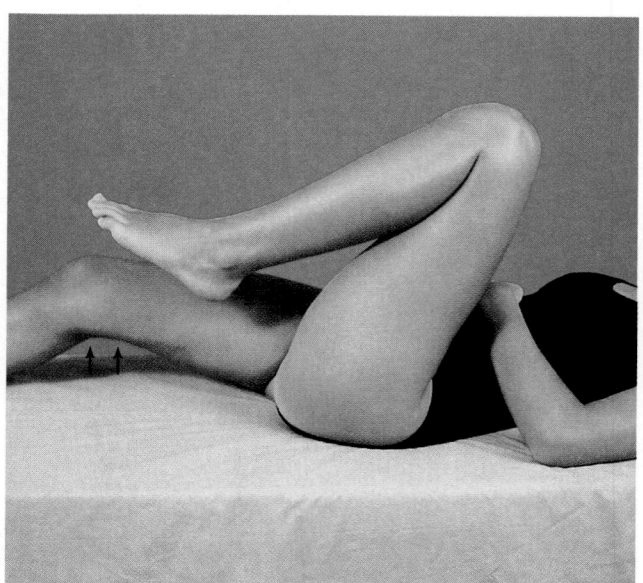

B

FIGURE 18-62 Thomas test. **A,** Negative. **B,** Positive.

Examination Step-by-Step

1. Observe the client for gait, ease of movement, ability to change positions, and signs of discomfort as the client enters the room and interacts during the examination.
2. Observe body alignment and stature with the client standing erect (front, back, and side). Note any deformities, spinal curvatures, atrophied or hypertrophied limbs, and age-related variations in posture and body size.

With the client sitting on the examination table, examine the following:

3. Head

   Inspect the musculature for facial symmetry of skinfolds, muscles, and wrinkles.

   Palpate the temporomandibular joint while the client opens and closes the mouth.

   To test range of motion, ask the client to:
   a. Open and close the mouth.
   b. Project the lower jaw.
   c. Move the jaw from side to side.

   To test muscle strength, ask the client to:
   a. Bite down hard while you palpate the masseter muscles (CN V).
   b. Clench the teeth while you apply downward pressure on the chin.

4. Cervical Spine

   Inspect the neck for alignment and symmetry of skinfolds and muscles.

   Palpate the cervical spine.

   To evaluate range of motion, ask the client to:
   a. Touch the chin to the chest.
   b. Extend the head backward as far as possible.
   c. Bend the head laterally to each shoulder (touch the ear to the shoulder without raising the shoulder).
   d. Rotate the head from side to side (pointing the chin toward each shoulder).

   To evaluate muscle strength, ask the client to:
   a. Push the cheek against your hand (right and left sides) (test CN XI).
   b. Push the forehead against your hand.
   c. Push the head back against your hand.

5. Shoulders

   Inspect the shoulders, including the muscles and the acromioclavicular joint, for contour and equality.

   Palpate the shoulders and the bursal sites.

   To test for range of motion, ask the client to:
   a. Extend both arms forward (forward flexion).
   b. Extend both arms backward (hyperextension).
   c. Put your hands behind your back as if you were going to reach up to touch your shoulder blade (internal rotation).
   d. Put your hands behind your head (external rotation).

   To test for muscle strength, ask the client to:
   a. Hold the arms upward while you try to push them down (deltoid muscles).
   b. Extend the arms and then try to flex them while you try to pull them into extension (biceps muscle).
   c. Flex the arms and then try to extend them while you attempt to push them into a flexed position (triceps muscle).
   d. Shrug the shoulders while you try to push down on them (trapezius muscle, CN XI).

6. Elbows

   Inspect the elbows in both flexed and extended positions for carrying angle and contour.

   Palpate the extensor surface of the ulna for nodules, the olecranon process and grooves, and the lateral epicondyles of the humerus for tenderness.

   To test range of motion, ask the client to:
   a. Bend and straighten the elbow.
   b. Turn the hand face up (**supination**) and face down (**pronation**).

7. Hands and Wrists

   Inspect the dorsal and palmar surfaces of the hands for position, shape, contour, and number and completeness of digits. Inspect the wrists.

   Palpate the hand and wrist joints.

   To test range of motion of the hands and wrist, ask the client to:
   a. Spread the fingers apart and bring them back again.
   b. Make a fist.
   c. Touch the thumb to each fingertip and to the base of the little finger.
   d. Bend the fingers up and down at the metacarpophalangeal joint.
   e. Bend the hand up and down at the wrist.
   f. With the palm facing down, turn the hand to the right and to the left.

   To test strength in the muscles of the hands and wrist, ask the client to:
   a. Maintain wrist flexion while you try to extend the wrist.
   b. Try to extend the wrist as you try to flex it.
   c. Squeeze your first two fingers as hard as he or she can.
   d. Extend the fingers while you push down on the dorsal surface.
   e. Flex the fingers while you push up on the ventral surface.
   f. Spread the fingers apart while you try to push them together.
   g. Push the fingers together while you try to pull them apart.

Continued.

Examination Step-by-Step—cont'd

8. Hips

Inspect the hips for symmetry in iliac crest height and level of gluteal folds.

Palpate the hips and the pelvis for stability, tenderness, and crepitus.

To test range of motion of the hips ask the client to:
   a. While supine, raise the leg above the body with the knee extended.
   b. While supine, bring the knee to the chest while keeping the other leg straight.
   c. While supine, swing the leg laterally and medially while keeping the knee straight.
   d. While supine, place the side of the foot on the opposite knee and move the flexed knee down toward the examination table (external rotation).
   e. While supine, flex the knee and rotate the leg so that the flexed knee moves inward toward the opposite leg (internal rotation).
   f. While either prone or standing, swing the straightened leg behind the body.

To test muscle strength in the hips, ask the client to:
   a. While in a supine position, raise the extended leg while you attempt to hold it down.
   b. While in a supine position with your hands placed on the bed on either side of the client's knees, push both legs against your hands.
   c. While in a supine position with your hands placed on the bed between the client's knees, bring both legs together.

To assess muscle strength in the hamstring, gluteal, abductor, and adductor muscles, ask the client to sit and perform alternate leg crossing.

9. Knees

Inspect the knees for natural concavities and swelling.

Palpate the joint space and the popliteal space.

To test range of motion of the knee, ask the client to:
   a. Bend the knee.
   b. Straighten and stretch the leg.

To test muscle strength in the knee, ask the client to:
   a. Extend the leg as you try to bend it (quadriceps muscle strength).
   b. Bend the knees as you try to straighten them (hamstring muscle strength).

10. Ankles and Feet

Inspect the ankles and the feet during weight-bearing and non–weight-bearing for position, size, contour, and number of toes.

Palpate the ankle joint, Achilles tendon, and metatarsophalangeal joints.

To test range of motion of the ankle and foot, ask the client to:
   a. Point the foot up toward the ceiling.
   b. Point the foot down toward the floor.
   c. With the foot bent at the ankle, point the medial side of the foot toward the floor (inversion) and repeat with the lateral side (eversion).
   d. Rotate the ankle in order to turn the foot away from and then toward the other foot.

To test muscle strength in the ankle and foot, ask the client to:
   a. Flex the foot upward against your hand.
   b. Push the foot down against your hand.

11. Thoracic and Lumbar Spine

Inspect the spine for alignment.

Palpate the spinous processes and the paravertebral muscles for tenderness and spasm.

To assess range of motion of the spine, ask the client to:
   a. Bend back as far as possible (hyperextend the spine).
   b. Bend to the right and to the left side as far as possible (lateral bending) (you may need to stabilize the client's pelvis).
   c. Turn to the right and to the left in a circular motion (while you stabilize the pelvis).
   d. Slowly bend forward at the waist and try to touch the toes and then return to an upright position (watch from behind the client, take a "skyline view" of the spine, and observe for signs of scoliosis).

VARIATIONS FROM HEALTH

Osteoarthritis

Osteoarthritis is a degenerative joint disease characterized by a progressive loss of articular cartilage and formation of new bone at the joint surfaces and subchondral area. It occurs primarily in people older than 50 years, and the onset of signs and symptoms is insidious.

Bony overgrowths that feel like hard, nontender nodules frequently occur in the fingers. When located in the distal interphalangeal joints, they are called **Heberden's nodes (nodules)** (Figure 18-63). When located in the proximal interphalangeal joints, they are called Bouchard's nodes (see Figure 18-63). Bony spurs, particularly in the knees, are also typical of osteoarthritis. Most symptoms are related to weight bearing and are relieved by rest.

Rheumatoid Arthritis

Rheumatoid arthritis is a chronic, systemic, inflammatory disorder that affects individuals of all ages, although its onset is most common in the thirties and forties age group. It affects symmetrical joints. Deformities are related to inflammatory destruction of the joint with marginal bone erosion. Systemic complaints include fatigue and malaise in addition to joint pain. Joint inflammation is common, with marked edema, tenderness, pain, and limitation of movement. Stiffness early in the day is common. On palpation, joints will feel "boggy." Common deformities related to rheumatoid arthritis are de-

viation of the fingers, swan neck, and boutonnière deformities of the fingers (Figure 18-64).

Gout

Gout is a crystal-induced arthritis related to abnormalities in purine metabolism that result in prolonged hyperuricemia and subsequent deposition of uric acid crystals in the joint space. It can be caused by an overproduction of uric acid or an interference in uric acid excretion. It most commonly occurs in men older than 40 years. Joint involvement is usually monarticular. Classically, the proximal phalanx of the great toe is the joint affected (Figure 18-65). However, joints of the foot, ankle, and knee may also be affected. Pain is typically constant and severe (often called "exquisite") during an acute attack and is characterized by marked erythema, swelling, warmth, and tenderness. Tophi or urate crystal deposits may also occur on the ears and in the joints.

Osteoporosis

Osteoporosis is a systemic condition in which a decrease in bone mass occurs because bone resorption exceeds bone deposition. The bones become fragile, and fractures may occur even with minor trauma or during routine activities. The hips, vertebrae, and wrists are the most common fracture sites. Osteoporosis is most common in women (4:1, women:men). A decrease in calcium intake, decrease in estrogen production in women, lack of weight-bearing activities and exercise, and sedentary life-style are among the contributing factors (see box, p. 546).

Muscle Weakness

The client who has difficulty in walking up steps or getting up from a sitting position or the client who is able to rise only by pushing off with the hands and arms or by pulling up by grasping some nearby furniture may have a problem involving the shoulder or hip girdle musculature. Further tests are necessary to ascertain the presence of muscular dystrophy, myasthenia gravis, parkinsonism, or polymyositis.

Myasthenia gravis should be strongly suspected if the following are true: (1) the client who has difficulty rising can rise easily after being instructed to sit back and relax for a few minutes, (2) the client is a woman in her twenties or a man in his fifties or sixties, (3) muscle atrophy is not present, and (4) the client has ptosis or extraocular muscle weakness resulting in diplopia.

The presence of myasthenia gravis in the client with ptosis can be conclusively determined by the use of the Tensilon test, which is performed in the following manner. The examiner injects 2 mg of edrophonium chloride (Tensilon) while watching the client's eyelids. If no change occurs after a minute, the examiner injects

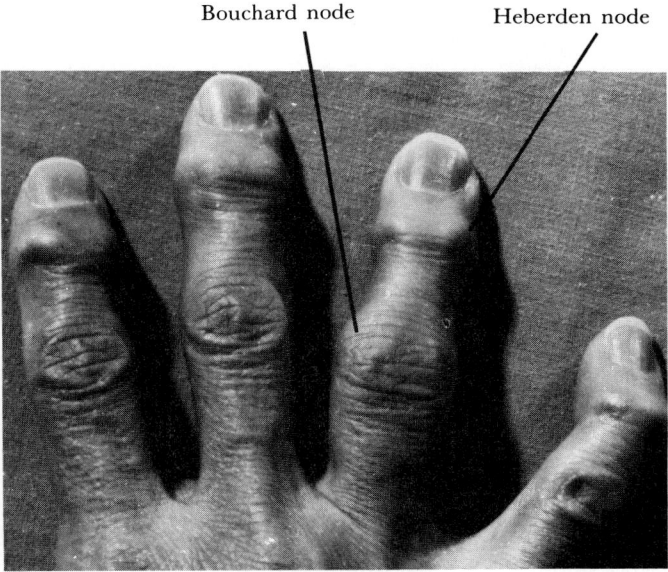

Bouchard node   Heberden node

FIGURE 18-63 Nodules of the hand associated with osteoarthritis. (From Swanson AB: *Flexible implant resection arthroplasty in the hand and extremities,* St Louis, 1973, Mosby–Year Book.)

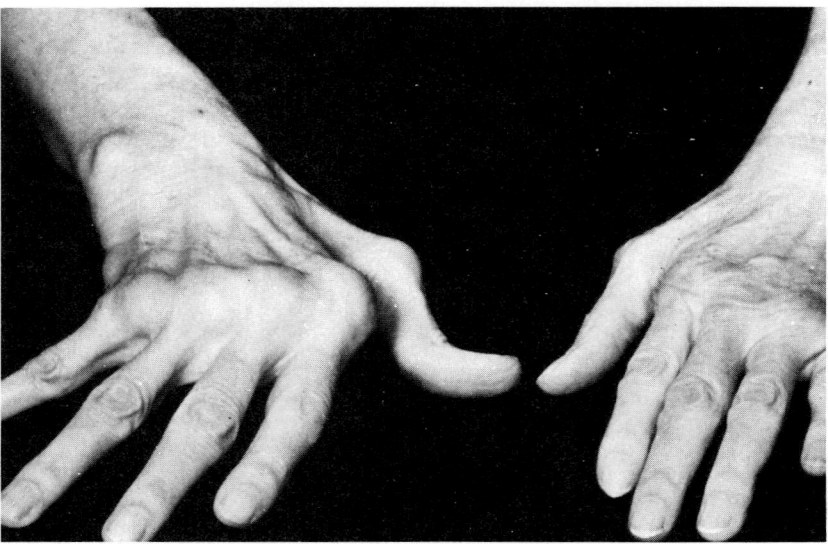

FIGURE 18-64 Unilateral ulner deviation of the metacarpophalangeal joints of the right hand secondary to rheumatoid arthritis. (From Prior JA, Silberstein JS, Stang JM: *Physical diagnosis: the history and examination of the patient,* ed 6, St Louis, 1981, Mosby–Year Book.)

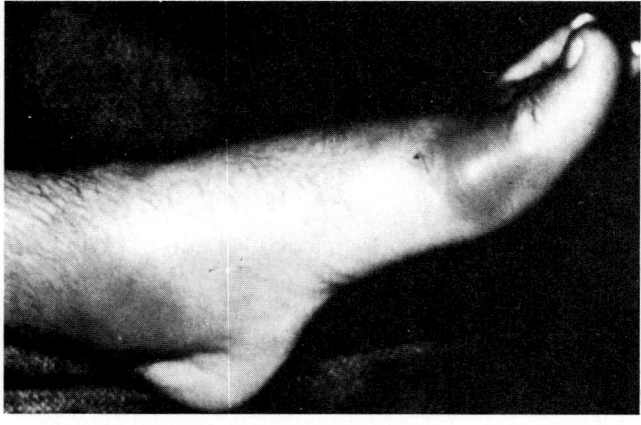

FIGURE 18-65 Inflammatory response of acute gout of the great toe. (From Prior JA, Silberstein JS, Stang JM: *Physical diagnosis: the history and examination of the patient,* ed 6, St Louis, 1981, Mosby–Year Book.)

another 8 mg. In 90% of clients who have myasthenia gravis, the ptosis is markedly improved since muscle strength increases following the injection.

Polymyositis is a progressive inflammatory disease that occurs in children and adults. It involves progressive symmetrical weakness of the limb girdles, neck, and pharynx. The client who has polymyositis may have pain, muscle atrophy, or a rash, particularly around the eyelids, and low-grade fever.

Parkinsonism may be the underlying cause when the aging client has difficulty rising from a chair. This impression is substantiated if the client says stiffness is a problem. In such a case it is important to be alert for signs of flexion posture, slow and intermittent movement, frequent tremor, masked facies, or movement of several joint units at one time because these signs are also characteristic of Parkinson's disease.

Viral upper respiratory tract infection should be suspected in the individual who has a mild elevation in temperature and whose chief complaint reveals that he or she had no symptoms only a day or so earlier but currently feels weak, almost unable to move. If the initial examination fails to demonstrate muscular or neural disease, the possibility of fatigue should be considered.

The client who complains of intermittent bouts of muscle weakness requires methodical and careful investigation for ischemic attacks, disorders of glucose metabolism (diabetes), anemia, and serum electrolyte disturbances, particularly of potassium or calcium ion concentrations.

Transient ischemic attacks may cause a focal episode of motor dysfunction related to vascular disease, such as arteriosclerosis or essential hypertension. Listening for bruits over the neck vessels in the elderly client with muscle weakness is particularly important since these bruits might strengthen the impression of vascular disease.

Clinical correlation of signs of muscle weakness and disease entities have shown that each neuromuscular disease has a general predilection for a particular group

TABLE 18-4

Topographical Patterns of Muscle Palsy

Muscle weakness or paralysis	Signs	Possible cause
Ocular	Diplopia	Myasthenia gravis
	Ptosis	Thyroid disease
	Strabismus	Ocular dystrophy and botulism
Bifacial	Inability to smile	Myasthenia gravis
	Inability to expose teeth	Facioscapulohumeral dystrophy
	Inability to close eyes	Guillain-Barré syndrome
Bulbar	Dysphonia	Myasthenia gravis
	Dysarthria	Myotonic dystrophy
	Dysphagia	Botulism
	Hanging-jaw facial weakness (may or may not be present)	Diphtheria
		Poliomyelitis
		Early polymyositis
Cervical	Inability to lift head from pillow (hanging-head syndrome)	Polymyositis
		Dermatomyositis
	Weakness of posterior neck muscles	Progressive muscular dystrophy
Bibrachial	Weakness, atrophy, and fasciculations of hands, arms, and shoulders (hanging-arm syndrome)	Amyotrophic lateral sclerosis
Bicrural	Lower leg weakness	Diabetic polyneuropathy
	Floppy feet	
	Inability to walk on heels and toes	
Limb-girdle	Inability to raise arms	Polymyositis
	Inability to rise from sitting position	Dermatomyositis
	Difficulty in climbing stairs without use of arms	Progressive muscular dystrophy
	Waddling gait	
Distal limb	Foot-drop with steppage gain	Familial polyneuropathy
	Weakness of all leg muscles	
	Wrist-drop—weakness of handgrips ("claw hand") (later sign)	
Generalized or universal	Limb and cranial muscle weakness (acute in onset and periodic)	Electrolyte imbalance
		Hypokalemia
		Hypocalcemia
		Hypomagnesemia
	Slow onset and progressive paralysis	Motor system disease
	Atrophy	
	Fasciculations of limb and trunk muscles	
	No sensory loss	
	Paralysis developing over several days	Guillain-Barré syndrome
	Mild degree of generalized weakness	Glycogen storage diseases
		Vitamin D deficiency
Single muscles or groups of muscles	Inability to contract affected muscles	Thyrotoxic myopathy (almost always neuropathic)

of muscles. A given pattern of weakness, then, suggests the possibility of a certain disease and excludes others. An example lies in the adage that peripheral muscle involvement in the extremities is of muscular origin, whereas distal disease is of neuropathic origin. Further explanation of the correlation of assessment data with underlying disease processes is presented in Table 18-4.

Hypokalemia

Since the ratio of the concentrations of potassium ion of the intracellular environment to the extracellular fluid determines the rate of cell firing, a deficit of this ion is accomplished by disorders of structure and function in muscular and neural tissues. Both skeletal and smooth muscles are affected by hypokalemia. The client complains of varying degrees of weakness and lassitude. Extreme hypokalemia may be accompanied by muscular paralysis. Some other signs that will help confirm hypokalemia as the cause of muscle weakness are abnormalities in motor and secretory activities of the gastrointestinal tract, changes in electrocardiograms, and dilute urine. Some of the conditions known to be correlated with a deficiency of potassium ion are diarrhea, excessive losses in the urine resulting from the use of chlorthiazide, mercurial diuretics, or steroid hormones; Cushing's syndrome; and primary aldosteronism.

Age-related Muscle Weakness

Wasting of muscles and a decrease in muscle strength have been traditionally attributed to the aging process. Histologically, the muscle tissue shows increased amounts of collagen initially, followed by fibrosis of connective tissue.

Involuntary Contraction of Skeletal Muscles

Fasciculations. Fasciculations are the visible, spontaneous contraction of a number of muscle fibers supplied by a single motor nerve filament. Visible dimpling or twitching may occur, although there is usually insufficient power generated to move the joint.

Fasciculations that occur during muscular contraction (twitching) are associated with conditions of irritability that result in poorly coordinated contraction of small and large motor units. Benign fasciculation occurs in the normal individual and is characterized by normal muscle strength and size. Rarely, myokymia, a rippling appearance of the muscle occasioned by numerous fasciculations, is noted in a normal individual.

Fascicular twitches noted during rest in a client with exaggerated muscular weakness and atrophy are characteristic of a peripheral motor neuron disorder. Generalized fascicular twitching that occurs in a progressive, wavelike pattern over an entire muscle and progressing to complete paralysis is characteristic of certain types of poisoning (organic phosphate) and of poliomyelitis.

Cramps and spasm. Muscular spasm, or tremor (Table 18-5), may occur at rest or with movement and may be noted in the normal individual with metabolic and electrolyte alterations. Cramping is a common complaint following excessive sweating and with hyponatremia, hypocalcemia, hypomagnesemia, and hyperuricemia. Diseases that magnify these alterations are correlated with the presence of muscle spasm. A continuous spasm that is heightened by attempts to move the affected muscles occurs in tetanus and following the bite of the black widow spider. Paravertebral muscle spasm is often responsible for low back pain.

Tetany. Hypocalcemia and hypomagnesemia may cause the involuntary spasms of skeletal muscle that resemble cramping. The calcium deficit causes depolarization of the distal segments of the motor nerve. Furthermore, a change occurs within the muscle fibers themselves since nerve section or block does not prevent these tetanic contractions. Tetanic cramps can be elicited by percussing the motor nerve leading to a muscle group at frequencies of 15 to 20/sec. **Chvostek's sign** is the spasm of the facial muscles produced by tapping over the facial nerve near its foramen of exit. The instability of the neuromuscular unit is heightened by hyperventilation (alkalosis) and hypoxia (ischemia). **Trousseau's sign** is the production of tetany of the carpal muscles following occlusion of the blood supply to the arms by a tourniquet. The client may also describe tingling and prickling paresthesia resulting from the stimulation of sensory nerve fibers. Electromyographical tracings show fast-frequency doublets and triplets of motor unit potentials. Tetany in its mildest form affects the distal musculature in the form of carpopedal spasm, but it may involve all the muscles of the body except those of the eye.

TABLE 18-5

Tremor Classification

Cause	Type and rate of movement	Description
Anxiety	Fine, rapid, 10 to 12/sec	Irregular, variable
		Increased by attempts to move part; decreased by relaxation of part
Parkinsonism	Fine, regular, or coarse, 2 to 5/sec	Occurs at rest
		May be inhibited by movement
		Involves flexion of finger and thumb "pill rolling"
		Accompanied by rigidity, "cogwheel" phenomena, bradykinesia
Cerebellar tremor	Variable rate	Evident only on movement (most prominent on finger-to-nose test)
		Dysmetria (seen when client is asked to pat rapidly; pats are of unequal force and do not all arrive at same point)
Essential or senile	Coarse, 3 to 7/sec	Involves the jaw, sometimes the tongue, and sometimes the entire head
		Disappears on complete relaxation or in response to alcohol
Metabolic		Variable
		Client is obviously ill; if illness is a result of hepatic failure, client will have other signs, such as palpable liver, spider nevi

Muscle cramp. Muscle **cramp** frequently occurs after a day of vigorous exercise. As the feet cool, a sudden movement may trigger a strong contraction of the foot and leg. The musculature is visible, and the muscle feels hard on palpation. The spasm will cease in response to stretch of the fibers. In the case of the gastrocnemius muscle, the stretch can be achieved by dorsiflexion of the foot. Occasionally, massage is helpful in relaxing the spasm. Fasciculations frequently appear before and after the cramp, and they are further evidence of the hyperexcitability of the neuromuscular unit.

Electromyogram recordings show high-frequency action potentials during the cramp. These muscle spasms have greater frequency when the client is dehydrated or sweating and in the pregnant client.

The cause of the pain associated with muscle cramp has not been determined but some believe its causes to be the increased metabolic needs of the hyperactive muscles and the collection of the metabolic waste products, such as lactic acid, within the muscle.

Elevated Muscle Enzyme Levels

Destructive diseases of striated muscle fibers result in the loss of enzymes from the intracellular compartment of the muscle. The enzymes enter the blood and can be measured. The usual laboratory analysis of serum enzymes includes alkaline phosphatase, lactic dehydrogenase (LDH), serum glutamic oxaloacetic transaminase (SGOT), and creatine phosphokinase (CPK). Enzymes are found in all tissues. Since high concentrations of these enzymes occur in the heart and liver, elevated serum level values may result from myocardial infarction or hepatitis. However, CPK, although present in the heart and the brain, is most concentrated in striated muscle. The level may rise from a normal range of 0 to 65 IU to more than 1000 IU in clients with destructive lesions of the striated muscles.

Myalgia

"I hurt all over" is frequently the chief complaint of the client with diffuse muscle pain that accompanies many types of systemic infection, for example, influenza, measles, rheumatic fever, brucellosis, dengue fever, or salmonellosis. Soreness and aching are other descriptions given for this type of involvement. Little is known of the cause of myalgia. **Fibromyositis** is inflammation of the fibrous tissue in muscle, fascia, and nerves. The client may complain of pain and tenderness in a muscle after exposure to cold, dampness, or minor trauma.

Firm, tender zones, occasionally several centimeters in diameter, may be found on palpation. Palpation, active contraction, or passive stretching increases the pain. Intense pain localized to a smaller group of muscles may be a result of epidemic myalgia, also called pleurodynia, "painful neck," or "devil's grip." Intense pain

at the beginning of neurological involvement may occur in poliomyelitis and herpes zoster.

The pain of poliomyelitis is described as marked during the initial involvement of the nerve, whereas the later sensation of the paralyzed muscle is one of aching. The segmental pattern of the intense pain of herpes zoster is caused by the inflammation of spinal nerves and dorsal root ganglia that occurs 3 to 4 days before the skin eruption.

The initial symptoms of rheumatoid arthritis may be diffuse muscular soreness and aching, which may antedate the joint involvement by weeks or months. The muscles are tender, and the client describes the pain as occurring not at the time of activity but hours later. An increased sedimentation rate or a positive latex fixation test may support the conclusion of rheumatoid involvement.

DOCUMENTATION

Sample Documentation

Health history

Ms. S. complains of dull, bilateral, lower back pain that radiates down her right leg. Sharp lower back pain began 2 weeks ago after she fell from a curb. Pain improved with rest, but radiation of pain was noted down right leg when standing. Is worse when walking up stairs. Is having difficulty with ADLs; requires assistance with bathing and household chores. Has had severe muscle spasm and increased weakness in right leg muscles. Today developed a burning sensation in right foot. Denies paresthesias. No hip, knee, or ankle pain. Notes slight improvement when lying down with head elevated and knees flexed. Ibuprofen 600 mg, every 4 to 6 hr, provides some relief. Denies other medications or treatments. Denies history of spinal injuries or other systemic illnesses. No family history of osteoporosis or arthritis. Has had difficulty going to job as a shop clerk since must stand for long periods.

Physical examination

55-year-old, white female who moves with difficulty and appears quite uncomfortable. MS exam: Gait—walks with stiffness, no limp. Back—loss of lumbar lordosis. ROM intact. Paraspinal muscles—exquisitely tender to right of L-5/S-1 and tense on palpation. Straight leg raising—positive in supine position at 45 degrees. Neuro exam (would be included for above complaint [see Chapter 19]).

Nursing Diagnosis *THE NEXT STEP*

Nursing diagnoses that could apply to assessment of and alterations in the musculoskeletal system include, but are not limited to, the following ones.

ACTIVITY INTOLERANCE The state in which an individual has insufficient physiological or psychological energy to endure or complete required or desired daily activities.

Defining Characteristics

- Verbal report of fatigue or weakness
- External discomfort or dyspnea
- Abnormal responses to activity: heart rate, blood pressure, or ECG changes reflecting ischemia or arrhythmias

Level I:
  Walk, regular pace, on level indefinitely; one flight or more but more short of breath than normally.

Level II:
  Walk one city block 500 feet on level; climb one flight slowly without stopping.

Level III:
  Walk no more than 50 feet on level without stopping; unable to climb one flight of stairs without stopping.

Level IV:
  Dyspnea and fatigue at rest.

Related Factors

- Bed rest
- Immobility
- Sedentary life-style
- Generalized weakness
- Imbalance between oxygen supply and demand

HIGH RISK FOR ACTIVITY INTOLERANCE The state in which an individual is at risk of experiencing insufficient physiological or psychological energy to endure or complete required or desired daily activities.

Defining Characteristics (risk factors)

- Prolonged inactivity
- Circulatory or respiratory problems
- History of previous activity intolerance
- Need to engage in energy-consuming body movement

IMPAIRED PHYSICAL MOBILITY The state in which an individual experiences a limitation of ability for independent physical movement.

Defining Characteristics

- Inability to move purposefully within the physical environment (bed mobility, transfer, ambulation)
- Limited active joint range of motion
- Decreased muscle strength, control, and/or mass
- Impaired coordination

Level I:
  Walk, regular pace, on level indefinitely; one flight or more; more short of breath than normally.

Level II:
  Walk one city block 500 feet on level; climb one flight slowly without stopping.

Level III:
  Walk no more than 50 feet on level without stopping; unable to climb one flight of stairs without stopping.

Level IV:
  Dyspnea and fatigue at rest.

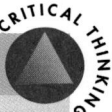

Nursing Diagnosis   *THE NEXT STEP—cont'd*

Related Factors

- Decreased muscle strength and endurance
- Pain
- Uncompensated musculoskeletal or neurological impairment
- Depression
- Uncompensated perceptual-cognitive impairment

HIGH RISK FOR DISUSE SYNDROME The state in which an individual is at risk for deterioration of body systems as the result of prescribed or unavoidable inactivity.

Defining Characteristics (risk factors)

- Paralysis
- Prescribed immobilization
- Mechanical immobilization
- Altered level of consciousness
- Severe pain

HIGH RISK FOR INJURY The state in which an individual is at risk of injury as a result of environmental conditions interacting with the individual's adaptive and defensive resources.

Defining Characteristics (risk factors)

Multiple possible behaviors with the potential for traumatic injury, such as:
- Impaired sensory function
- Faulty judgment
- Slippery floors
- Unsafe housing conditions
- Driving at excessive speeds
- Nonuse of safety devices such as seatbelts or bicycle helmets

PAIN The state in which an individual experiences and reports the presence of severe discomfort or an uncomfortable sensation.

Defining Characteristics

- Verbal communication of pain descriptors
- Narrowed focus (altered time perception, withdrawal from social contact, impaired thought processes)
- Distraction behavior (moaning, crying, pacing, seeking out other people and/or activities, restlessness)
- Facial mask of pain (eyes lack luster, "beaten look," fixed or scattered movement, grimace)
- Alteration in muscle tone (may range from listlessness to rigidity)
- Autonomic responses not seen in chronic, stable pain (diaphoresis, blood pressure and pulse rate change, pupillary dilation, increased or decreased respiratory rate)
- Fatigue/weakness
- Immobilization of painful area
- Clutching of painful area
- Rigidity of painful area
- Guarding of painful area

Related Factors

- Pain subsequent to trauma
- Diagnostic tests
- Chemical irritants
- Immobility or improper positioning
- Knowledge deficit in relation to pain management techniques

Continued.

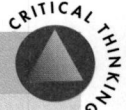

Nursing Diagnosis   *THE NEXT STEP—cont'd*

CHRONIC PAIN The state in which an individual experiences pain that continues for more than 6 months.

Defining Characteristics

- Verbal report or observed evidence of pain experienced for more than 6 months
- Facial masks (of pain)
- Guarded movement
- Fear of reinjury
- Physical and social withdrawal
- Altered ability to continue previous activities

Related Factors

- Inflammation
- Overactivity
- Arthritis
- Stress
- Chronic physical/psychosocial disability

Clinical Application

Mrs. W. is a 50-year-old female executive secretary who is complaining of swelling and burning in her hands off and on for the past 2 weeks. "My hands hurt and the swelling is so bad in the morning I can hardly type!" She says she takes Ibuprofen for relief of pain. The pain is worse in the morning, due to stiffness, lasting about 1-2 hours. Joints in hands feel warm, swollen, and tender. Patient also mentions "I have no energy. I become tired more easily especially in the early afternoon." Physical assessment completed. Patient grimaces when touching her hands, tends to pull away and guard both hands.

SUBJECTIVE DATA: Patient complains of:
Hands hurting
Hands stiff and swollen so bad can't type
Tiring easily especially in early afternoon

OBJECTIVE DATA:
Physical assessment:
Body joints within normal limits except for joints of wrists and hands.
Both hands are warm to touch veins engorged with spindle-shaped swelling of proximal interphalangeal joints, third digits both hands; ulnar deviation of metacarpophalangeal joints.
Serum blood counts:
Rheumatoid factor positive
Erythrocyte sedimentation rate (ESR) elevated at 25 mm/hr
White blood cell count with differential mildly elevated
Red blood cell count slightly decreased (normocytic anemia)
Nutritional assessment:
No report of weight loss or changes in eating habits.

NURSING DIAGNOSIS

Pain related to inflammatory process

Defining Characteristics

- Subjective communication of pain
- Self focusing
- Guarding behavior
- Grimaces in pain

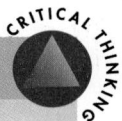

Nursing Diagnosis *THE NEXT STEP—cont'd*

Activity intolerance related to anemia and disease state

Defining Characteristics
- Verbal reports of fatigue and weakness especially in early afternoon
- Verbal reports of loss of energy

Impaired physical mobility related to joint and systemic involvement

Defining Characteristics
- Limited range of motion of hands
- Decreased muscle strength and control of hands and wrist
- Impaired coordination of hands

GLOSSARY

abduction Movement of a body part away from the median plane.

active range of motion Purposeful joint movement performed by the client without assistance from the examiner.

adduction Movement toward the axial line (for a limb) or the median plane (for the digits).

ankylosis Rigidity and consolidation of a joint.

Apley's sign Pain, locking of the knee, or clicking evoked with rotation of flexed knee. Positive sign is indicative of a loose object in the knee (cartilage) that occurs with a torn meniscus.

arthritis Inflammation of a joint.

Baker's cyst Swelling in the popliteal space resulting from herniation of the synovial membrane of the knee.

ballottement Palpation technique used to assess a floating object. Fluid-filled tissue is pushed toward the examiner's hand so that the object will float against the examiner's fingers.

bursa Sac or saclike cavity filled with fluid and located in sites where friction would otherwise develop, as in a joint or over a bony prominence.

bursitis Inflammation of a bursa.

carpal tunnel syndrome Entrapment of the median nerve in the carpal tunnel resulting in paresthesia, pain, and muscle weakness.

Chvostek's sign Spasm of the facial muscle evoked by tapping branches of the facial nerve; may be caused by hypocalcemia or hypomagnesemia.

circumduction Circular movement.

cramp Involuntary, painful skeletal muscle contraction.

crepitus (crepitation) Dry, crackling sound in (1) the lung, when air passes through abnormally accumulated moisture; (2) the joints, when dry synovial surfaces rub together; and (3) the skin, when air is present subdermally.

dorsiflexion Backward bending.

eversion Turning outward or inside out.

extension Straightening of a limb so that the joint angle is increased.

external rotation Turning of a body part away from the central axis or midline of the body.

fasciculation Rapid, fine twitching movements resulting from contraction of a fasciculus (bundle of muscle fibers) served by one anterior horn cell; usually does not cause movement of a joint.

fibromyositis Any one of a large number of disorders in which the common element is stiffness and joint or muscle pain accompanied by localized inflammation of the muscle tissues and of the fibrous connective tissues.

flexion Bending of a joint so that the joint angle is decreased.

gait Manner of progression in walking. In *ataxic gait* the foot is raised high and the sole strikes down suddenly.

goniometer Instrument used to measure joint angles.

gout Disease caused by deposition of crystals of monosodium urate; characterized by a disorder in purine metabolism and associated with exacerbations of arthritis of a single joint.

Heberden's nodes (nodules) Small, hard nodules of the terminal interphalangeal joints associated with osteoarthritis.

internal rotation Turning of the body part toward the central axis or midline of the body.

inversion Turning inward.

kyphosis Increased posterior convexity of the spine (humpback).

lordosis Anterior concavity of the lumbar spine (swayback, saddleback).

luxation Dislocation.

McMurray's sign Inability to extend flexed knee may indicate loose object in knee (cartilage) due to torn meniscus

passive range of motion Joint movement of the client that is produced by the examiner.

plantar flexion Bending of the foot toward the floor.

pronation (1) Assumption of the prone (face down) position; (2) turning the forearm so that the palm is posterior; or (3) eversion and abduction of the foot.

sciatica Pain, weakness, or paresthesias associated with the course of the sciatic nerve; may affect the posterior aspect of the thigh and the posterolateral and anterolateral aspects of the leg into the foot.

scoliosis Lateral deviation of the spine.

supination Assumption of the supine (lying down) position.

symmetry Similarity in size, shape, and position to the body part on the opposite side.

tophi Deposits of monosodium urate, associated with gout.

tremor Involuntary, somewhat rhythmic, oscillatory quivering of muscles caused by alternating contraction of opposing groups of muscles. *Cerebellar tremor:* Occurs during intentional movement, becoming more pronounced near the end of the movement; associated with lesions of the dentate nucleus. *Coarse tremor:* Slow rate and large amplitude movements.

Essential (familial) tremor: Usually initially appears around age 50 with fine tremors of the hands; aggravated by intentional movement; commonly affects the head, jaws, lips, or voice. *Fine tremor:* Rapid (10 to 20 oscillations/sec) and low amplitude movements, usually in the fingers and hands. *Moderate tremor:* Medium rate and medium amplitude movements. *Passive tremor:* present at rest; may improve during intentional movement (e.g. pill-rolling tremor or Parkinson's disease.) *Physiological tremor:* Experienced by healthy people in fatigue, cold, and stress. *Toxic tremor:* Caused by endogenous (thyrotoxicosis, uremia) or exogenous toxins (alcohol, drugs).

Trousseau's sign Carpopedal spasm elicited by compression of the upper arm with a tourniquet or blood pressure cuff; is associated with hypocalcemic tetany.

ulnar deviation Turning the wrist away from the midline of the body.

valgus Angulation of an extremity toward the midline. *Genu valgum:* Condition in which the knees are abnormally close together, knock-knee.

varus Angulation of an extremity away from the midline. *Genu varum:* Condition in which the knees are abnormally separated; bowleg.

BIBLIOGRAPHY

American Academy of Orthopaedic Surgeons: *Joint motion: method of measuring and recording,* Chicago, 1965, The Academy.

Ausenhus MK: Osteoporosis: prevention during the adolescent and young adult years, *Nurse Pract* 13:19-24, 1988

Beetham W, Polley H: *Rheumatologic interviewing and physical examination of the joints,* ed 2, Philadelphia, 1978, WB Saunders.

Collo MC, and others: Evaluating arthritic complaints, *Nurse Pract* 16:9-20; 1991.

Daniels L, Worthingham C: *Muscle testing: techniques of manual examination,* ed 5, Philadelphia, 1986, WB Saunders.

Gordon M: *Manual of nursing diagnosis, 1991-1992,* St Louis, 1991, Mosby—Year Book.

Gordon M: *Nursing diagnosis: process and application,* ed 2, St Louis, 1987, Mosby—Year Book.

Hoppenfield S: *Physical examination of the spine and extremities,* New York, 1976, Appleton-Century-Crofts.

Magee DJ: *Orthopedic physical assessment,* ed 2, Philadelphia, 1992, WB Saunders.

Mann RA, editor: *DuVries' surgery of the foot,* ed 5, St Louis, 1986, Mosby—Year Book.

McCarty DJ, editor: *Arthritis and allied conditions,* ed 11, Philadelphia, 1989, Lea & Febiger.

Mercier LR: *Practical orthopedics.* St Louis, 1987, Mosby—Year Book.

Mourad LA: *Orthopedic disorders,* St Louis, 1991, Mosby—Year Book.

CHAPTER 19

Neurological System, Including Mental Status

Outline

PURPOSE OF THE EXAMINATION

The neurological system integrates all the functions of the body. The cells of the central nervous system depend on an adequate supply of glucose for their metabolic processes. This supply can be maintained only when peripheral tissues function well. The neurological system controls cognitive and voluntary behavioral processes as well as subconscious and involuntary body functions. The major functions of the neurological system are reception (sensory), integration, and adaptation; that is, the normal nervous system receives stimuli from the environment, compares the adaptive processes necessary to adjust body functions to the environment, and effects changes to ensure homeokinesis, or survival.

The **mental status examination** is an integral part of the neurological examination. In the context of the total health assessment, this appraisal begins at the initial contact with the client. Most examiners make assessments of mental status while obtaining the client's history and perform special tests of cognitive function immediately afterward.

For the purpose of facilitating learning of this complex system, this chapter is organized with the physical assessment portion of the neurological examination presented first, followed by techniques for examination of mental status. This organization, however, is not the usual order for conducting the assessment; in practice, the mental status examination begins when the practitioner first encounters the client (see Chapter 1).

ANATOMY AND PHYSIOLOGY

All components of the neurological system are highly interconnected and integrated in function. Maturation of the nervous system continues throughout childhood until early adolescence. For instructional purposes the nervous system is divided into two major parts: (1) the central nervous system, which consists of the brain and spinal cord, and (2) the peripheral nervous system, which is composed of (a) the cranial nerves, (b) 31 pairs of spinal nerves that emerge from the spinal cord, and (c) the **autonomic nervous system**. The autonomic nervous system is divided into the sympathetic (thoracolumbar) and parasympathetic (craniosacral) nervous systems. It is considered part of the peripheral nervous system because in most parts of the body innervated by these systems, their structures appear together.

Central Nervous System

Brain. The brain is made up of gray and white matter. Gray matter contains cell bodies, and white matter includes myelinated nerve fibers. The brain consists of the **cerebrum**, the largest part of the brain, which is composed of two hemispheres; the **brainstem** (midbrain, pons, and medulla); the diencephalon; and the **cerebellum** (Figure 19-1). The left side of the brain controls language, whereas the right side is the nonverbal, or perceptual, hemisphere. Ninety percent of the population has a dominant left hemisphere, and these individuals are right-handed. The cerebral functions in-

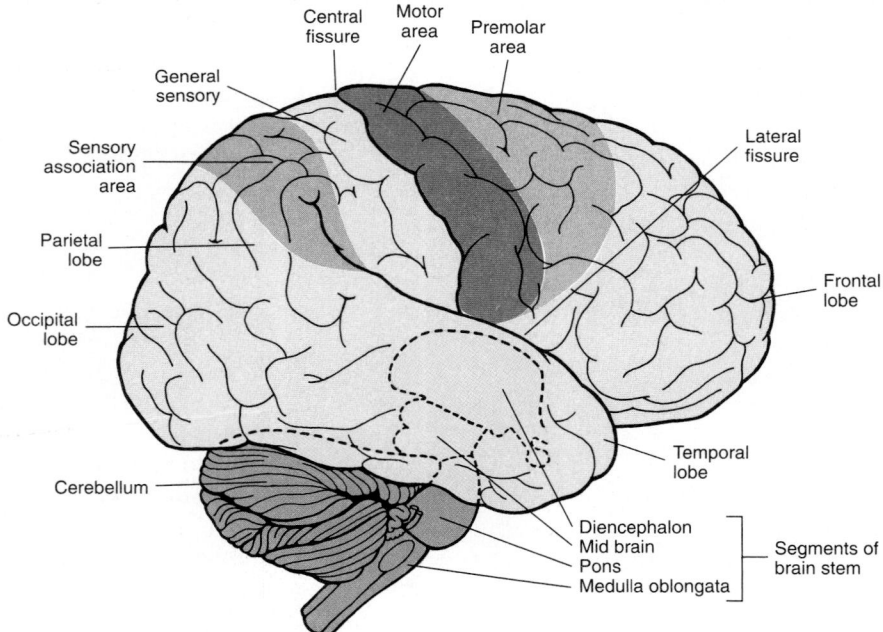

FIGURE 19-1 Lateral view of the brain. (Modified from Smith CG: *Serial dissections of the human brain,* Baltimore, 1981, Urban and Schwarzenberg.)

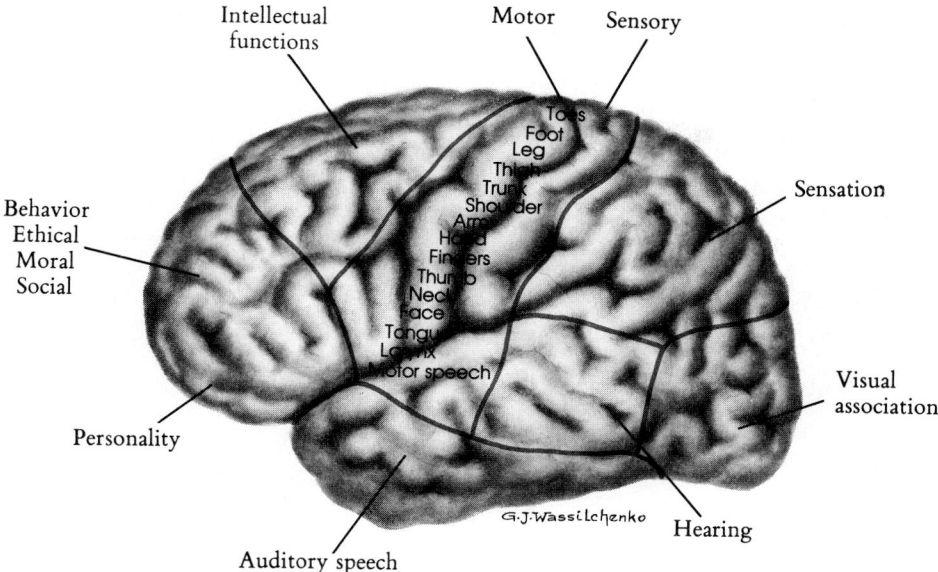

FIGURE 19-2 Functional subdivisions of the cerebral cortex.

teract with the **reticular activating system**, located in the upper brainstem and diencephalon, to control conscious movement, thought, and perception. The major cerebellar functions influence mechanisms of equilibrium, muscle tone, and coordinated movement, such as control of gait (Figure 19-2).

Approximately 20% of the oxygen consumed by the body is used to provide energy to the brain. Since the brain depends totally on glucose for metabolism, a lack of oxygen for 2 to 5 minutes can result in irreversible brain damage. The circle of Willis, located at the base of the brain, is an arterial communication between the right and the left cerebral circulation. Its function is to equalize blood flow to various parts of the brain. Superficial and deep veins drain into the system of sinuses of the dura mater, which empties into the internal jugular vein.

Spinal cord. A cross section of the spinal cord reveals H-shaped gray matter surrounded by white matter. The gray matter is made up of cell bodies, **axons** and **dendrites**. The gray matter also contains posterior (dorsal) and anterior (ventral) **horns**. The actual shape and extent of the white and gray matter vary at different levels of the cord. Figure 19-3 shows a cross section of the spinal cord, with a labeling scheme of laminae (layers) from I to X, as described by Rexed, to show the major longitudinal columns. The columns are identified according to similarity in appearance and function. For example, lamina V receives dorsal root afferent fibers from sensory fibers such as those that transmit pain, temperature, and light touch (spinothalamic tract).

Motor and sensory pathways. Neurons that transmit impulses can be motor, sensory, or mixed. Motor neurons, or **efferent neurons**, carry impulses from the central nervous system to effectors, located in muscles, organs, and glands. Sensory neurons, or **afferent neurons**, carry impulses from receptors to the central nervous system. General sensory afferent fibers involve conscious sensation, such as pain and light touch. General visceral afferent fibers carry sensory impulses from the viscera.

The dorsal roots carry sensory impulses from receptors to the dorsal root **ganglia**, in which cell bodies of the sensory nerves are located, to the spinal cord. Ventral roots carry efferent (motor) impulses from the spinal cord to the body.

In the spinal cord, descending tracts (pyramidal and extrapyradmidal) carry motor impulses away from the brain. Ascending tracts (dorsal columns or spinothalamic) carry sensory impulses to the brain.

Motor pathways

PYRAMIDAL SYSTEM. The pyramidal system (corticospinal tracts) consists of neurons of spinal cord white matter arranged in long columns, or fiber tracts, lateral to the gray matter. The majority of these columns cross to the contralateral side at the level of the medulla. Those that do not cross in the medulla continue as the anterior corticospinal tract and cross over at the cervical or thoracic level of the cord. The pyramidal tract uniquely transmits stimuli concerned with voluntary movements and temporal (time) and spatial qualities (e.g., perceiving change over time).

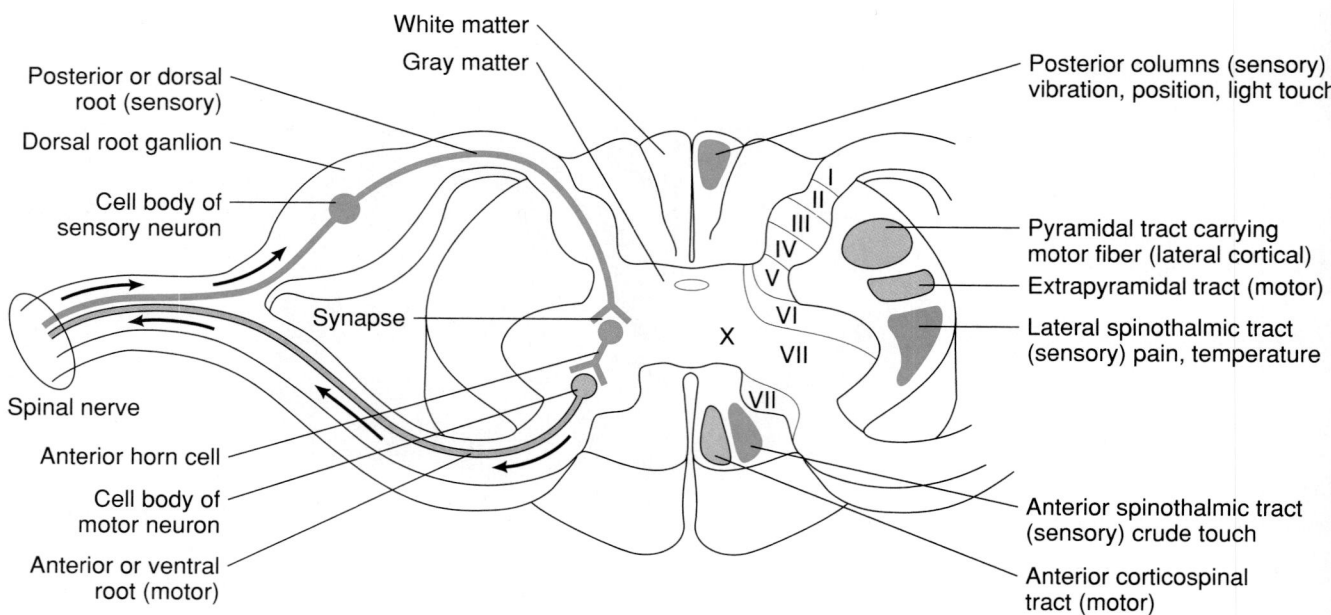

FIGURE 19-3 Cross section of the spinal cord. Spinal nerve roots and their neurons appear on the left side. Spinal nerve tracts appear in the white matter on the right side. All tracts and nerves are bilateral.

UPPER AND LOWER MOTOR NEURONS. A model of a two-neuron chain is used here to simplify understanding of the basic structure of the **pyramidal tract**. The chain begins in the motor area of the cerebral cortex, located anterior to the central **sulcus**. The size of the cortical area correlates with the degree of skilled function carried out by a particular body part (Figure 19-4). Note that the face and hands cover the largest areas. This neural chain travels to skeletal muscle and is contained in one of the many ascending and descending pathways in the spinal cord.

The **upper motor neuron** cell bodies are located in the cerebral cortex, and their axons cross over to the opposite side (contralateral) at the level of the medulla to **synapse** with the **lower motor neuron** cell body in the cranial nerve motor nuclei or the anterior horn of the spinal cord (Figure 19-5). The axon of the lower motor neuron becomes the peripheral nerve. Because upper motor neurons affect motor activity only through the lower motor neurons, the latter are referred to as the final common pathway. Damage to a lower motor neuron will cause motor impairment on the same (ipsilateral) side of the body, whereas damage to an upper motor neuron leads to motor impairment on the contralateral side. For example, the facial nerve (CN VII) is a lower motor neuron. Damage to the motor portion of the right facial nerve results in impaired movement of the right side of the face. However, if a stroke damages the right upper motor neuron that synapses with

the right facial nerve, the result would be impaired motor function of the left face, primarily its lower portion.

Lower motor neurons are either (1) alpha type, which when included with all muscle fibers supplied are called motor units, or (2) gamma type, which supply the muscle fibers of the **neuromuscular spindle** and control length and tension receptors for the stretch **reflex** and proprioception.

EXTRAPYRAMIDAL SYSTEM. The **extrapyramidal system** is more complex than other motor pathways. It includes all the motor neurons originating in the motor cortex and the cerebellum outside the pyramidal tracts, in addition to the sensory (spinothalamic) tracts. The extrapyramidal tract integrates input from many sources and modifies the motor impulses of the pyramidal system, especially those needed to maintain posture, balance, and slow movement. Since the sensory tracts are located close to the corticospinal tracts in the spinal cord, it is common for both sensory and motor deficits to occur with spinal cord damage.

Sensory pathways. Sensory impulses travel from the receptors through afferent fibers in the peripheral nerve, through the dorsal root, and to the spinal cord. Various types of receptors are stimulated by pain and temperature, position and movement, or visceral sensations of fullness or cramping. In the spinal cord sensory impulses travel via two major pathways to higher levels of the nervous system, the posterior columns or the

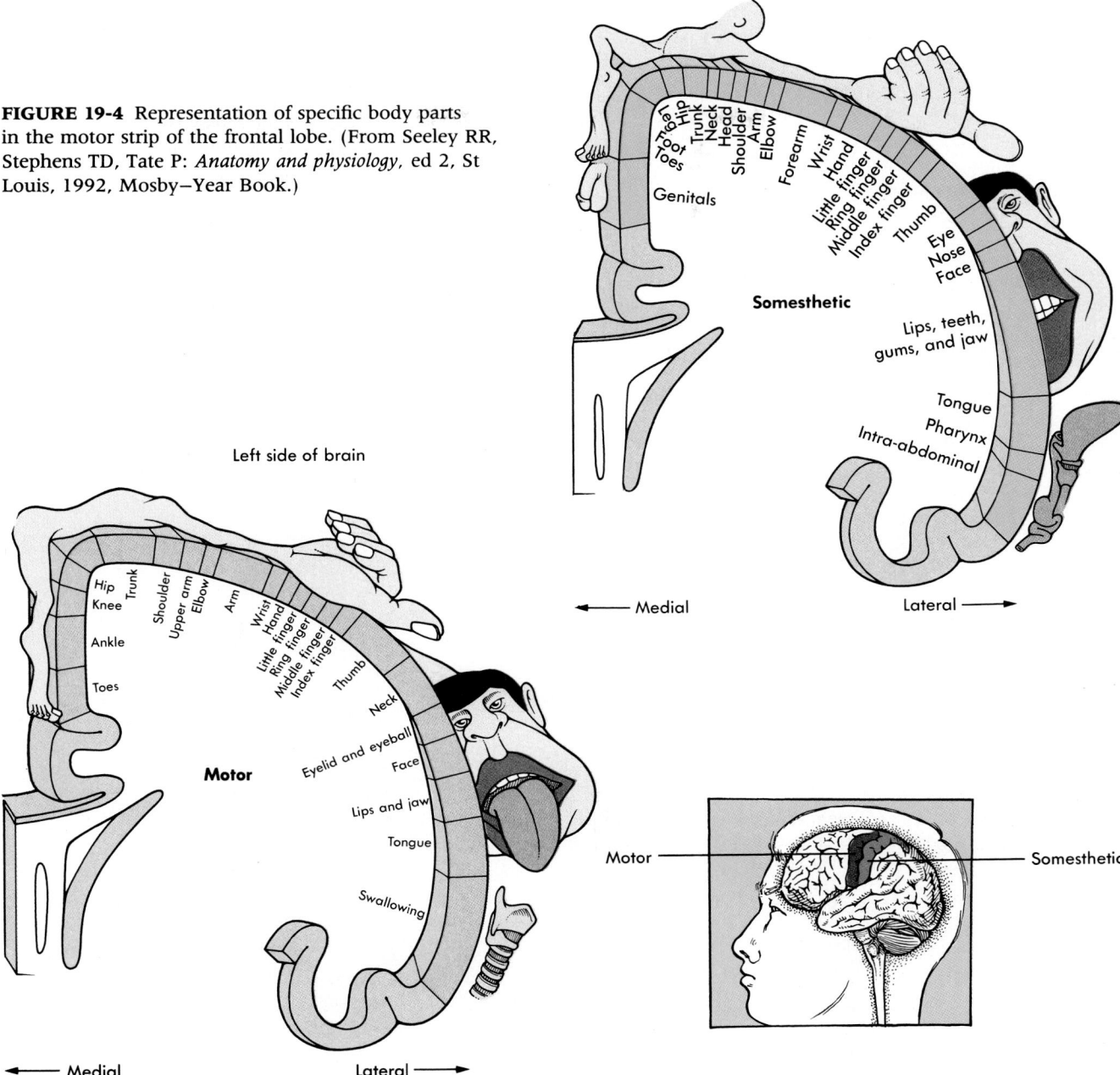

FIGURE 19-4 Representation of specific body parts in the motor strip of the frontal lobe. (From Seeley RR, Stephens TD, Tate P: *Anatomy and physiology*, ed 2, St Louis, 1992, Mosby–Year Book.)

spinothalamic tract. The lateral spinothalamic tract contains sensory fibers that transmit the sensations of pain, temperature, and light touch. Fibers in the posterior columns transmit stimuli involved with position, vibration, and manipulation with digits, such as stereognosis and graphesthesia (see Figure 19-3).

Peripheral Nervous System

Spinal nerves. Each spinal cord nerve segment communicates with specific parts of the body through 31 pairs of spinal nerves, both afferent and efferent, at that level (8 cervical, 12 thoracic, 5 lumbar, 5 sacral, and 1 coccygeal). Each nerve is designated by a letter and a number to indicate its location. For example, C8 is the eighth cervical nerve. Each spinal nerve has a dorsal root, which carries afferent (sensory) impulses to the cord, and a ventral root, which carries efferent (motor) impulses away from the cord. Sensory fibers (dorsal root) from a single spinal nerve that serve a particular skin surface are collectively called a **dermatome** (Fig-

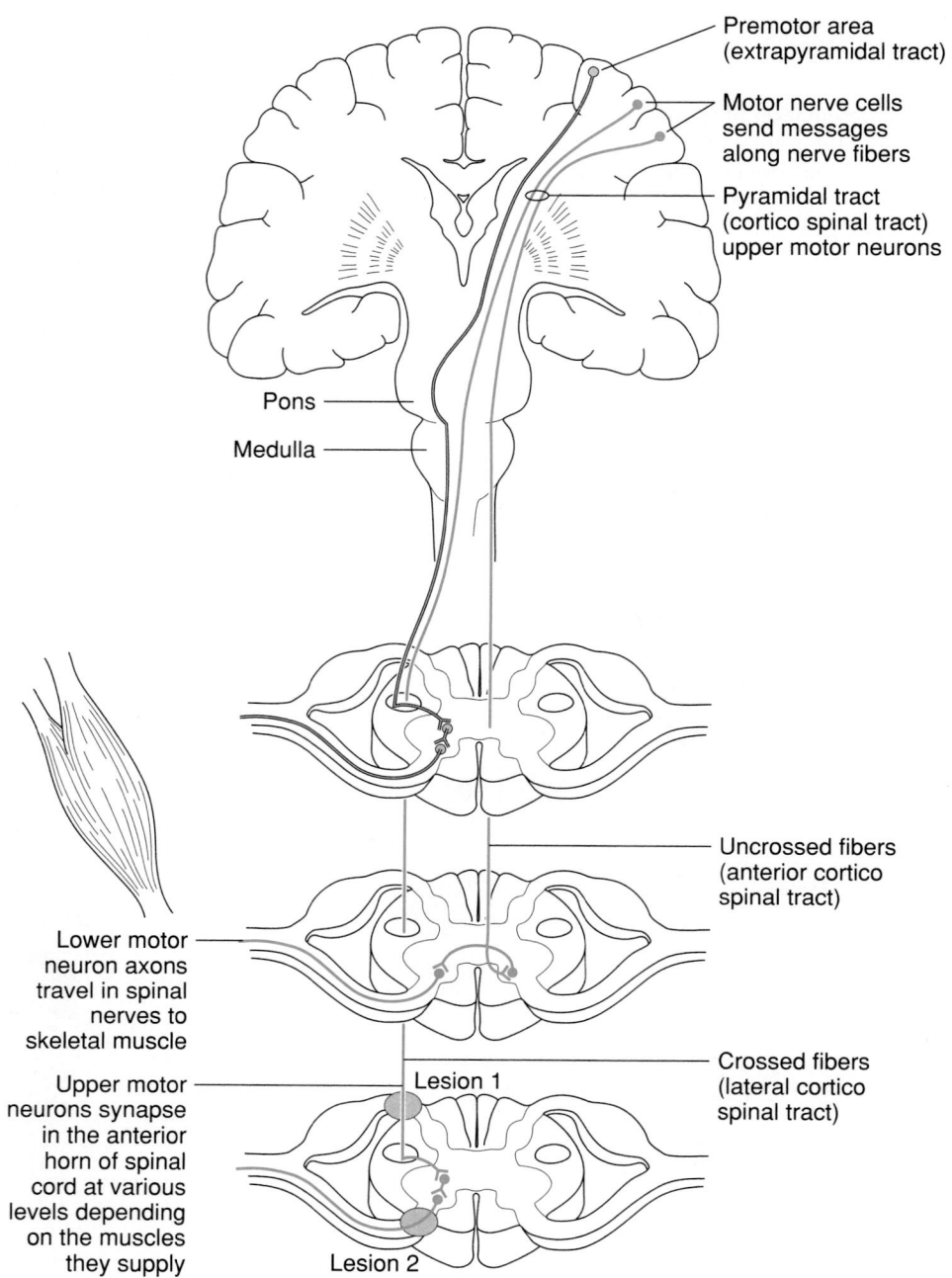

FIGURE 19-5 Major motor pathways between the cerebral cortex and lower motor neurons in the spinal cord.

ure 19-6). Because of considerable overlap between adjacent dermatome areas, sensory loss results only if a number of dermatomes are damaged.

Reflex arc. Reflexes are part of the motor system. They control automatic responses to stimuli at the level of the spinal cord (segmental response), freeing the cortex from involvement in most muscle movements that oc-

cur in the body. Reflexes provide rapid responses, such as withdrawal from painful stimuli. The simplest reflex arc is monosynaptic, in which the sensory fiber interacts directly with the motor neuron (see Figure 19-7).

Skeletal muscles contract when they are stretched by contraction of the antagonistic muscle, the pull of gravity, or external manipulation. The muscles also contract when their tendons are stretched. Deep tendon reflexes,

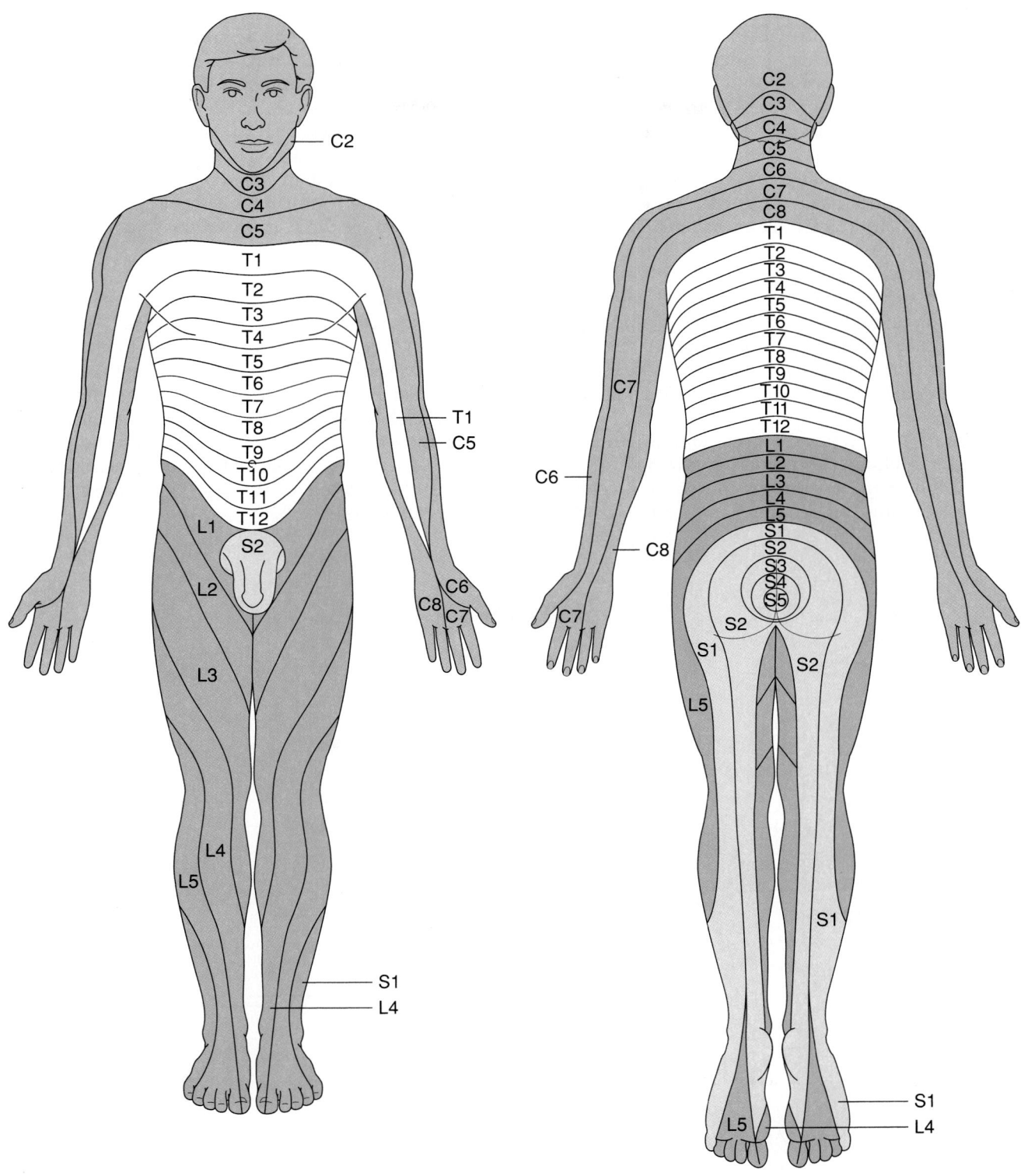

FIGURE 19-6 Dermatomes of the body. Each dorsal (sensory) spinal root innervates one dermatome. The first cervical nerve usually has no cutaneous distribution. The trigeminal nerve (CN V) supplies most of the general somatic sensory innervation to the anterior part of the head. (Modified from Rudy EB: *Advanced neurological and neurosurgical nursing,* St Louis, 1984, Mosby–Year Book.)

or muscle stretch reflexes, are segmental responses elicited by striking a tendon with a reflex hammer. This stimulus stretches the neuromuscular spindles of the muscle group.

Muscle spindles (gamma fibers), which are abundant in skeletal muscles, especially antigravity muscles, are attached to muscle by connective tissue. The spindles are capsules surrounding specialized muscle cells known as intrafusal fibers. Both ends of the intrafusal fiber consist of contractile tissue, whereas the central portion, the nuclear bag, is expanded and nucleated. Primary afferent fibers are stimulated when the bag is stretched to carry impulses to the spinal cord, where alpha motor neurons are activated. The alpha motor neuron impulses terminate at the endplates of the skeletal muscle, and gamma efferent impulses terminate in the muscle spindle, stimulating both tendon and muscle contraction.

Figure 19-7 illustrates the deep tendon reflex, with the patellar tendon reflex used as an example. The patellar tendon of the quadriceps muscle is attached to the tibia. Tapping this tendon with a reflex hammer causes the muscle to be stretched, activating the muscle spindles and thereby the femoral (primary afferent) nerve, to the spinal cord. In the spinal cord the sensory neurons synapse with the alpha motor nerve in the cord segment (L3 and L4). The alpha efferent fibers carry impulses back to the muscle, resulting in contraction of the quadriceps muscle and extension of the leg. Dysfunction of the tendon reflex, therefore, could result from problems in the thigh muscle, the femoral nerve, or the segment of the spinal cord being tested.

Superficial reflexes. Superficial reflexes are reactions that can be elicited by stroking the skin or muscle. Examples of these reflexes include the abdominal reflex, which tests spinal cord levels T8 through T12; the cremasteric reflex, observed in males (T12-L2) when stroking of the skin of the inner upper thigh results in testicular movement on the same side; and the plantar reflex (L4-L5, S1-S2), elicited by firmly stroking the lateral surface of sole of the foot to stimulate plantar flexion of the toes.

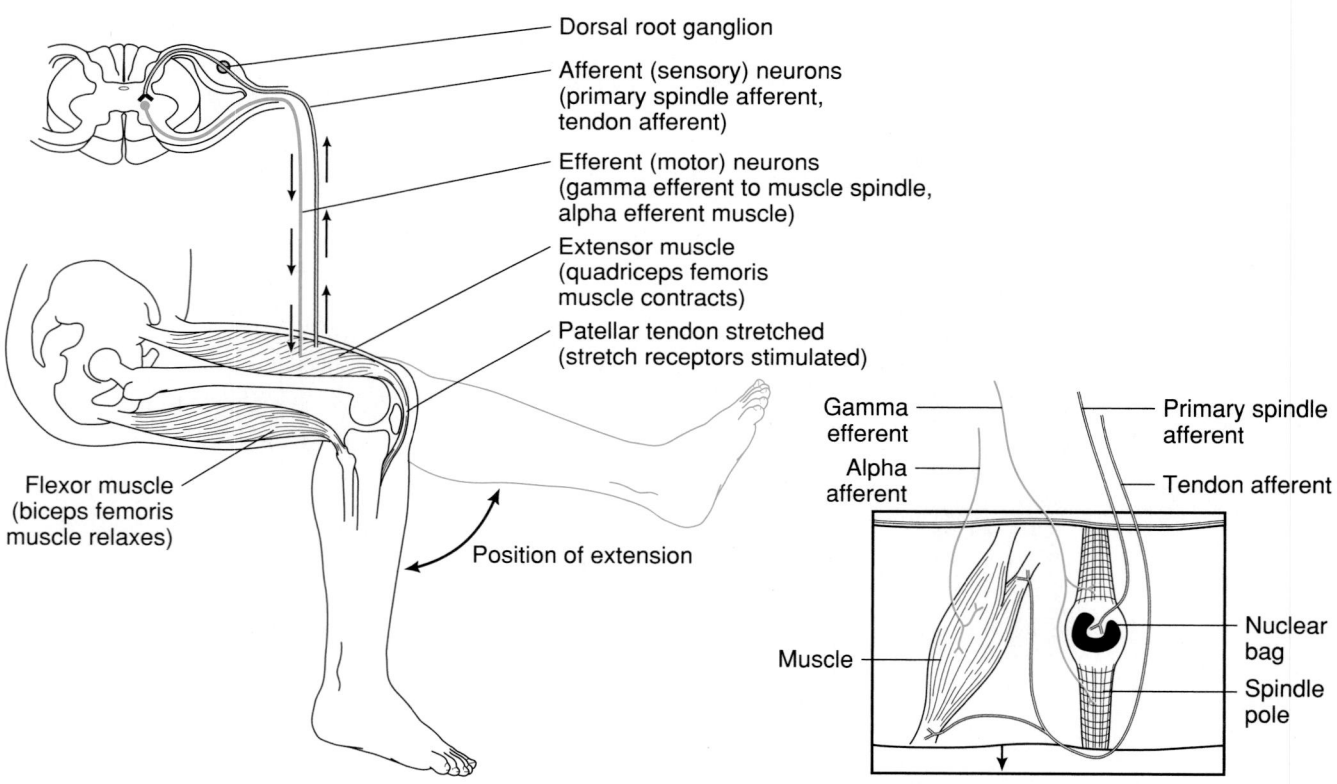

FIGURE 19-7 Deep tendon (stretch) reflex (knee-jerk or patellar tendon reflex). Inset shows afferent fibers from muscle spindle and tendon organs and efferent fibers to muscle and spindle. Note that patellar tendon of extensor muscle attaches to tibia below the knee.

Cranial nerves. Twelve pairs of cranial nerves emerge from the brain or brainstem. Cranial nerves consist of fibers that have sensory (afferent) and motor (efferent) functions as well as special sensory afferent functions such as vision, hearing, and equilibrium. Cranial nerves also contain special visceral efferent nerve fibers for voluntary motor function; special visceral afferent fibers carry visceral sensation such as taste and smell (Figure 19-8).

CN I: Olfactory nerve. The olfactory nerve is sensory for smell. The peripheral neurons of the olfactory nerve penetrate the nasal mucosa in the roof of the nose, the upper septum, and the medial wall of the superior nasal **concha.** Unless the individual sniffs or inspires deeply, most of the inspired air does not contact the olfactory epithelium; during normal respiration, inspired air does not rise that high in the nares (see Figure 12-5).

CN II: Optic nerve. The optic nerve, sensory for sight, is described in Chapter 11 (see the discussions of examination of visual acuity, visual fields, retinal fields, and the optic disc).

CN III: Oculomotor nerve, CN IV: Trochlear nerve, CN VI: Abducens nerve. The oculomotor, trochlear, and abducens nerves, which control movement of the eyeball, elevation of the eyelid, and pupillary constriction, are always tested together. These cranial nerves are also described in Chapter 10 (note the sections on neuromuscular and extraocular muscle function and tests of eye movement).

CN V: Trigeminal nerve. The trigeminal nerve is motor to the muscles of mastication and sensory to the cornea, mucosa of the nose and mouth, and skin of the face and forehead in perceiving touch, temperature, and

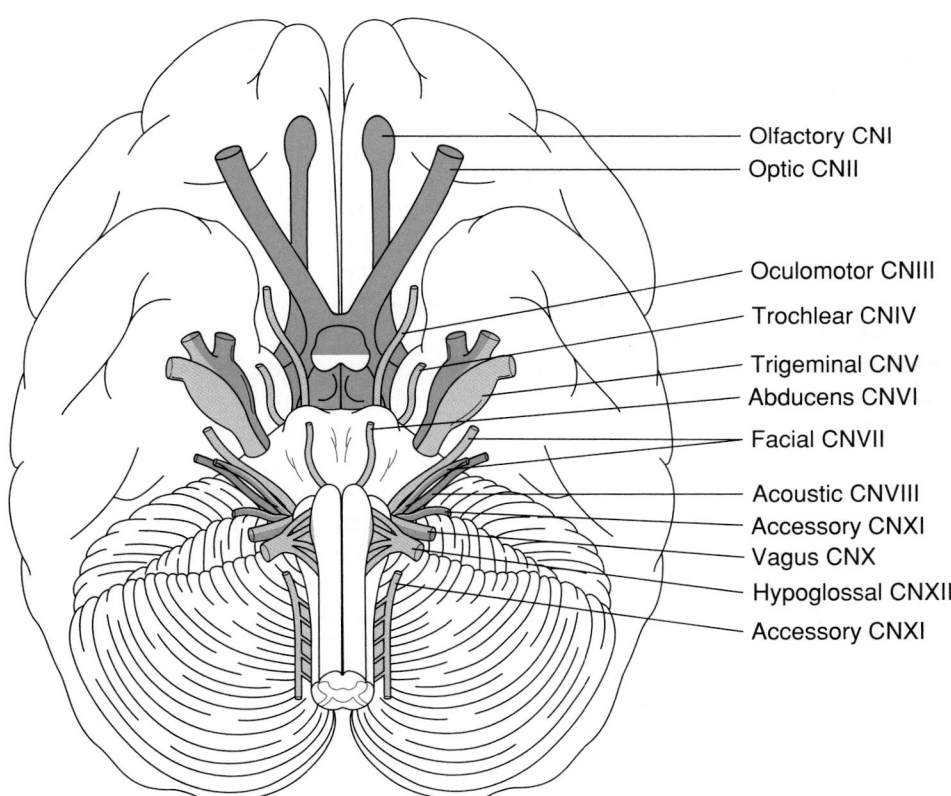

Olfactory CNI
Optic CNII

Oculomotor CNIII
Trochlear CNIV
Trigeminal CNV
Abducens CNVI
Facial CNVII
Acoustic CNVIII
Accessory CNXI
Vagus CNX
Hypoglossal CNXII
Accessory CNXI

FIGURE 19-8 Diagram of base of brain showing entrance or exit of the cranial nerves. Right column indicates anatomical location of the connection of each cranial nerve to the central nervous system.

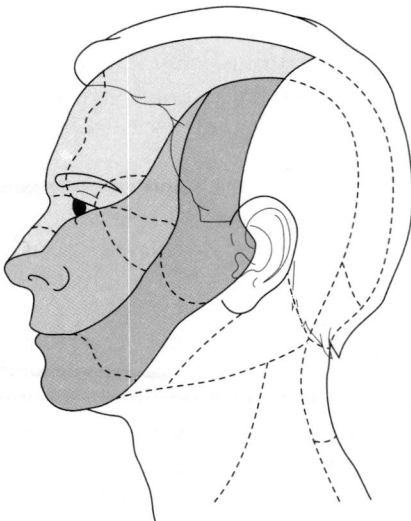

FIGURE 19-9 Cutaneous fields of head and upper part of neck. Shaded areas show location of sensory loss in face following resection of trigeminal nerve. Cutaneous fields of the three branches of the trigeminal nerve are identified as: *I,* ophthalmic; *II,* maxillary; and *III,* mandibular.

MAJOR AREAS OF NEUROLOGICAL EXAMINATION

1. Mental status (performed first during the interview, but in this chapter discussed after the other areas of examination)
2. Cranial nerves
3. Proprioception and cerebellar function
4. Motor function (see Chapter 18)
5. Sensory function
6. Deep tendon reflexes

pain. The sensory fibers are contained in one of the three divisions of the nerve: ophthalmic, maxillary, or mandibular (Figure 19-9).

CN VII: Facial nerve. The facial nerve is motor to the facial muscles and sensory to taste on the anterior two thirds of the tongue. Visceral sensation from the salivary glands and mucosa of the mouth and pharynx is also conducted by CN VII. In addition, the facial nerve carries parasympathetic fibers that stimulate secretion of the salivary glands, the lacrimal glands, and the mucosa of the nose, palate, and nasopharynx.

CN VIII: Acoustic nerve. The acoustic nerve is composed of two divisions, the cochlear and the vestibular.
COCHLEAR DIVISION. The cochlear division is sensory for hearing. Tests for cochlear function are described in Chapter 12.
VESTIBULAR DIVISION. Tests for vestibular functions, or equilibrium, are *not* routine in the physical examination. One method used to test vestibular function by producing changes in the flow of **endolymph** is the caloric test. In the caloric test, the examiner irrigates the client's ear with ice water; a normal reaction includes nausea, dizziness, and nystagmus.

CN IX: Glossopharyngeal nerve, CN X: Vagus nerve. The glossopharyngeal and vagus nerves are closely related both anatomically and physiologically, and they are tested as a unit. The glossopharyngeal nerve contains sensory and motor fibers. The sensory component is taste on the posterior third of the tongue and sensation from the tonsillar and pharyngeal mucosa. CN IX also has sensory fibers for the carotid sinus and body. The motor function of this nerve innervates the pharynx and parotid glands to control swallowing, gagging, and salivation.

The vagus nerve is sensory for the external ear and pharynx. It functions as a motor nerve to the soft palate, pharynx, larynx, and esophagus. CN X provides parasympathetic control to smooth and cardiac muscle and abdominal organs.

CN XI: Spinal accessory nerve. The spinal accessory nerve supplies the sternocleidomastoid and trapezius muscles with motor innervation.

CN XII: Hypoglossal nerve. The hypoglossal nerve provides motor fibers to the muscles of the tongue, making possible articulation of lingual speech sounds and swallowing.

Autonomic nervous system. The autonomic nervous system is made up of motor neurons called general visceral efferent neurons. The function of this system is to maintain a stable internal environment for the body. The sympathetic nervous system, also called the thoracolumbar division, is activated during stress and brings about widespread responses, such as increased heart rate, vasodilation in skeletal muscle, reduction in gastric secretions, and dilation of bronchioles. These "fight or flight" responses enable us to be physically prepared to handle potential danger. Sympathetic (thoracolumbar) preganglionic fibers emerge from T1 to L2 levels of the spinal column.

The parasympathetic system, also called the craniosacral division, is associated with conservation, restoration, and maintenance of normal body functions, such as decreasing the heart rate and increasing gastrointestinal motility. Parasympathetic (craniosacral) preganglionic fibers emerge from the cranial nerves (III, VI, IX, X) and S1 through S4 segments of the spinal cord.

EXAMINATION OF THE NEUROLOGICAL SYSTEM

Health History

Clues to areas of abnormality may be evident during the client's history, such as orientation, speech, and ability to interact with the examiner. The presence of certain symptoms in a client who appears normal may indicate neurological problems. If any symptom is present, it is important to obtain further information about onset, duration, intensity, frequency, aggravating and alleviating factors, and effects on the client's activity (see Chapter 1).

Present health status
   a. Numbness, tingling or loss of feeling
   b. Difficulty with speaking, vision, or hearing
   c. Any physical disability
   d. Medications
   e. Problems with coordination or balance
   f. Change in ability to remember
   g. Shakiness or tremors of the hands or leg
   h. Presence of anxiety or depression
   i. Recent changes in self, such as alterations in sleep habits, changes in sexual activity, unexplained weight gain or loss, difficulty in performing usual daily activities

Past health history
   a. Seizures, fainting spells, or dizzy spells
   b. Headaches
   c. History of head injury or major trauma

Preparation for Examination: Client and Environment

The neurological examination begins as soon as you, the examiner, and the client are introduced. Begin to form an overall impression and continue to make general observations before focusing on problem areas. Conduct the interview and examination in a quiet, private room without interruption. Perform the mental status examination with both you and the client comfortably seated. Conduct the remainder of the neurological examination with the client seated on the edge of the examination table or standing. Ask the client to remove shoes, socks, and outer clothing that covers the extremities. Give the client a loose-fitting gown to wear.

> **Helpful Hint:** *Be cautious about interpreting results whenever a client does not do something you have instructed. It may be simply a misunderstanding of directions and not a neurological defect. An isolated abnormal finding is very difficult to interpret.*

Examination Technique and Normal Findings

Cranial nerves. Table 19-1 summarizes the cranial nerves, including their functions, structures innervated, test, and normal findings.

CN I (olfactory). Do not test CN I during a screening examination unless the history suggests a problem. Before testing the olfactory nerve, examine the nares for any signs of obstruction. Ask the client, with eyes closed, to sniff familiar odors such as coffee, cigarettes, or chocolate. Test each side separately (Figure 19-10).

PREPARATION

Preparation for Examination

Equipment

Item	Purpose
Cottonball, safety pin	Light touch, pain sensation, and localization
Tongue blade	Tongue strength, gag reflex
Tuning fork (512 cps)	Vibration sense
Ophthalmoscope	Optic nerve, pupil constriction
Calipers	Two-point discrimination
Reflex hammer	Deep tendon reflexes
Pencil and paper	Fine coordinated movements
Printed material	Reading and comprehension
Optional:	
Test tubes for cold and warm water	Temperature sensation
Aromatic substances	Olfaction
Sweet, sour substances	Taste

Client and the Environment

Client clothed in loose-fitting gown over underwear	Comfortable chairs
Quiet private room	Examination table

TABLE 19-1

The Cranial Nerves

Nerve	Function	Structure innervated	Test	Normal findings
I Olfactory	Sensory Smell	Olfactory epithelium in nasal cavity	Apply simple odors to one nostril at a time	Correct identification of odor
II Optic	Sensory Vision	Retina of eye	Visual acuity using Snellen chart Visual fields using a confrontation test Ophthalmoscopic examination	Correct identification of letters No visual fields defects Normal fundus
III Oculomotor	Motor Upward, downward, medial eye movement	Superior, medial, inferior rectus, inferior oblique, and levator palpebrae superior muscles	Flash light in one eye at a time EOM: Ask client to follow an object while you move it to left, then up and down left of midline; to right, then up and down right of midline	Direct and consensual light reflex Both eyes follow object in parallel
	Lid elevation		Observe lids	Palpebral fissures equal
	Pupil constriction			Pupils constrict
IV Trochlear	Motor Downward, medial eye movement	Superior oblique muscle	EOM	Same as EOM of CN III
V Trigeminal	Sensory Face Scalp Nasal mucosa Buccal mucosa Jaw muscles	Skin and mucosa of face and head via ophthalmic, maxillary, and mandibular divisions	Test tactile and pain sensation of all three divisions	Normal sensory perception from entire face
	Motor Masseter muscle Temporal muscle Digastric muscle		Feel two masseter muscles as client bites down	Equal contraction of masseters and no deviation of mandible
			Corneal reflex	Blinking of eye
VI Abducens	Motor Lateral eye movement	Lateral rectus muscle	EOM	Same as EOM of CN III
VII Facial	Sensory External ear Taste: anterior two thirds of tongue Deep facial	Taste buds of anterior two thirds of tongue Lacrimal, sublingual, and submandibular glands; other minor glands and mucosal surfaces	Apply small amount of sugar or salt to anterior two thirds of tongue	Correct identification of substance

TABLE 19-1—cont'd

The Cranial Nerves

Nerve	Function	Structure innervated	Test	Normal findings
VII Facial— cont'd	Motor			
	Facial movement Scalp muscle Auricular muscle Stylohyoid muscle Digastric posterior belly	Facial, stapedius, sty-lohyoid, and poste-rior digastric muscles Middle ear External ear	Ask client to wrinkle forehead, close eyes, show teeth, whistle	Normal execution of movements
	Parasympathetic Salivation: sub-maxillary glands, sublin-gual glands Lacrimation: lacri-mal glands Mucous membrane Nasopharynx			
VIII Acoustic	Sensory			
	Cochlear: hearing	Spiral organ of cochlea	Hearing acuity using a watch or a whis-per	Normal and bilater-ally symmetrical hearing
			Rinne test (tuning fork on mastoid process)	Air conduction greater than bone conduction
			Weber test (tuning fork on center of forehead)	Heard in both ears equally
			Otoscopic examina-tion	Normal tympanic membrane
	Vestibular: equilib-rium	Ampullae of semicircu-lar ducts and macu-lae of saccule and utricle	Romberg test*	Able to maintain balance with eye closed
			Caloric	Nystagmus
IX Glosso-pharyn-geal	Sensory External ear Taste: posterior third of tongue Carotid: reflexes, baroreceptors and chemore-ceptors, sinus, body	Taste buds of posterior third of tongue Parotid gland Pharynx (gag reflex), carotid sinus, poste-rior third of tongue, auditory tube, and middle ear Stylopharyngeus muscle External ear		
	Motor Pharynx: gag re-flex, swallowing, pharyngeal mus-cles Parotid gland: sali-vation		Touch pharynx with cotton applicator	Gag reflex Able to swallow
X Vagus	Sensory External ear Pharynx	External ear Carotid and aortic bodies; muscles of soft palate, phar-ynx, larynx, and esophagus	Listen to person talk	Lack of hoarseness

*Also a test of proprioception sense.

Continued.

TABLE 19-1—cont'd

The Cranial Nerves

Nerve	Function	Structure innervated	Test	Normal findings
X Vagus— cont'd	Motor Swallowing, gag reflex Pronation Cardiac slowing Bronchocon- striction Gastric secretion Peristalsis	Epiglottis	Ask person to say "ah"	Both sides of soft palate contract and uvula remains in midline
	Parasympathetic Thoracic and ab- dominal viscera Aortic arch Chemoreceptors Baroreceptors	Smooth and cardiac muscles and glands of thoracic and ab- dominal organs through transverse colon		
XI Accessory	Motor Swallowing pha- ryngeal muscles Turning of head: sternocleidomas- toid muscles Elevation of shoul- ders: trapezius muscles	Larynx and pharynx (with CN X)	Ask client to turn head to each side and shrug shoul- ders while you re- sist the movements	Strong contractions of sternocleido- mastoid and tra- pezius muscles
XII Hypo- glossal	Motor Muscles that move tongue: hypo- glossus, genio- glossus, stylo- glossus	Extrinsic and intrinsic muscles of tongue	Ask client to protrude tongue fully Move client's tongue side to side against resistance with tongue blade	Tongue protrudes in midline Good tongue strength

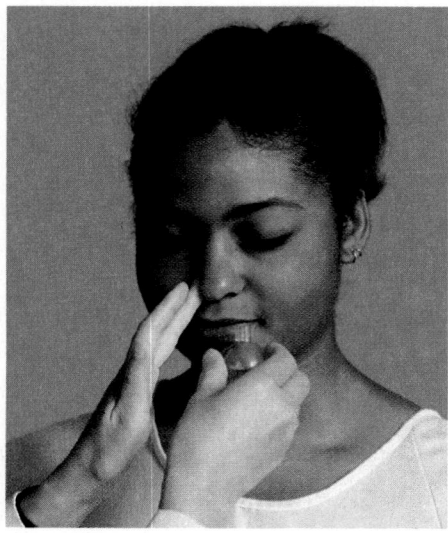

FIGURE 19-10 Testing for the ability to smell. Examiner asks client to sniff while placing a test tube containing the test substance beneath the nostril. Examiner holds the other nostril closed.

CN II (optic), III, IV, and VI (extraocular movements). See Chapter 11 for specific examination techniques.

CN V (trigeminal). With the client's eyes closed, test for the presence of several types of sensation, comparing both sides and testing areas innervated by the three branches of the trigeminal nerve (Figure 19-11). Check whether the client perceives sensation equally on both sides. Test the corneal reflex only on an unconscious client by touching a wisp of cotton lightly to the cornea and observing a blink response. Test for light touch by using a wisp of cotton and asking the client to localize where the sensation is perceived. By alternating the sharp and dull end of a safety pin, test for pain sensation; discard the safety pin after use. The sharp edge of a broken tongue blade can also be used. Test each branch on both sides of the face with a pain (sharp) stimulus. Testing for temperature sensation is not routine since pain and temperature are both carried by the lateral spinothalamic tract.

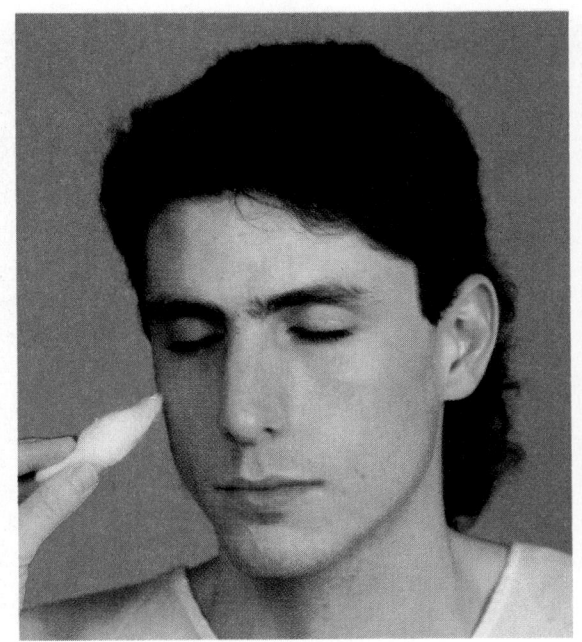
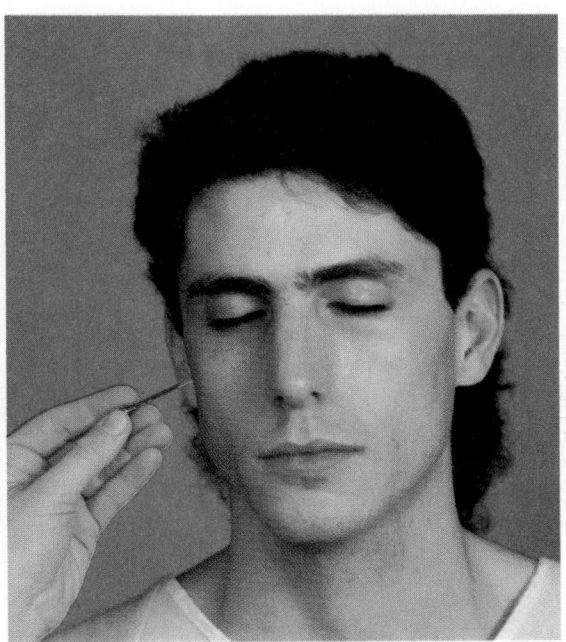

FIGURE 19-11 Testing sensation of light touch **(A)** and pain **(B)**. Examiner applies a wisp of cotton just firmly enough to stimulate the sensory nerve endings. To test superficial pain, examiner uses the sharp point of a safety pin alternating with the dull end of the pin.

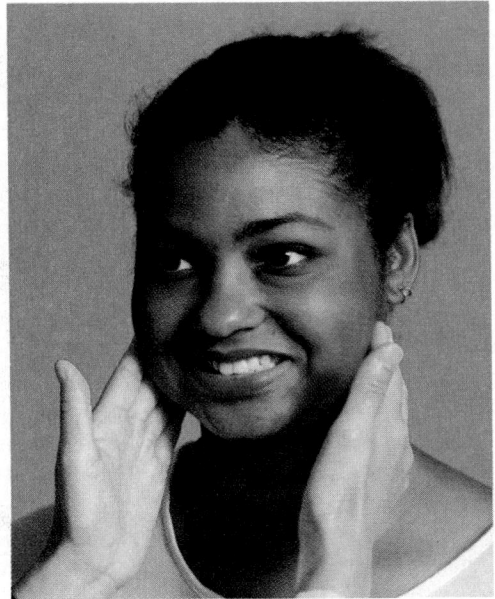

FIGURE 19-12 Palpation of the masseter muscles for size, strength, and symmetry to test CN V (trigeminal nerve).

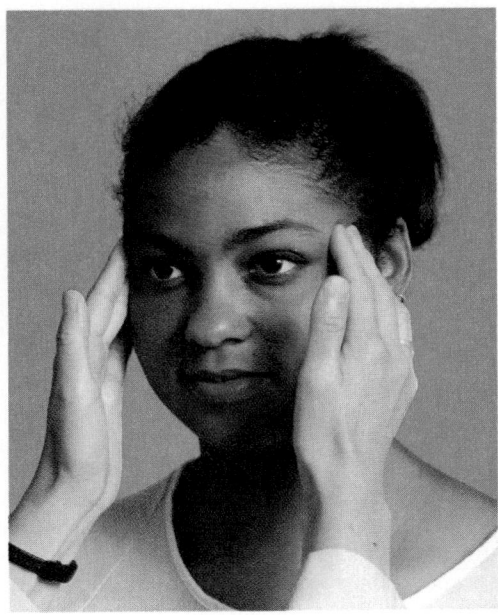

FIGURE 19-13 Palpation of the temporal muscles for size, shape, and symmetry to test CN V (trigeminal nerve).

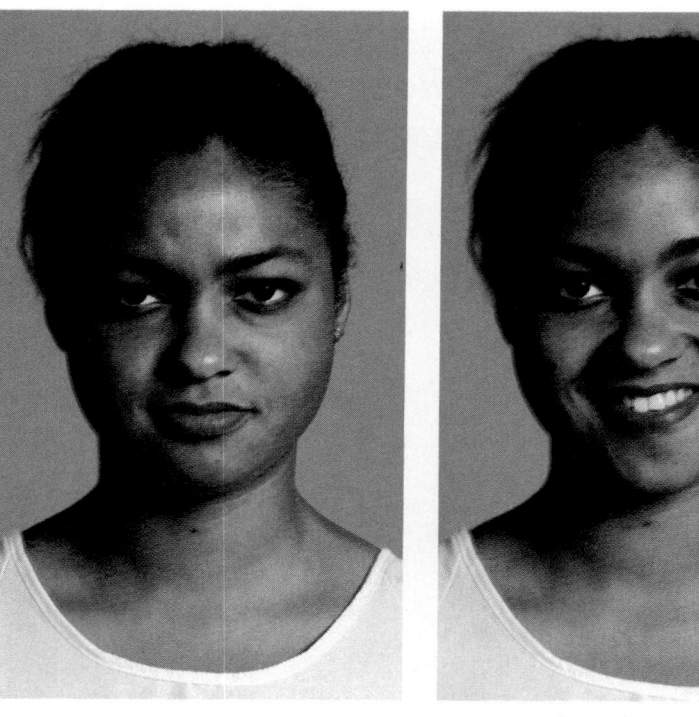
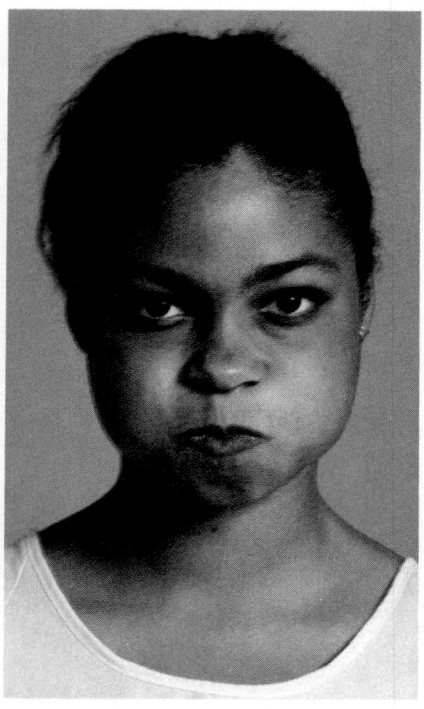

A   **B**   **C**

FIGURE 19-14 Testing motor function of CN VII (facial nerve). Examiner inspects client's ability to frown **(A)**, smile **(B)**, and puff out cheeks **(C)**.

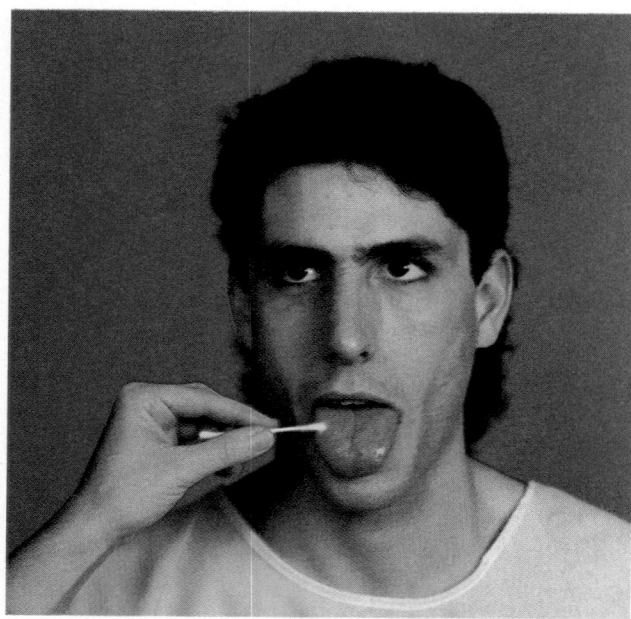

FIGURE 19-15 Testing taste sensation (CN VII [facial nerve] and CN IX [glossopharyngeal nerve]). Examiner applies to the anterior two thirds of the tongue salty or sweet solutions; and to the posterior one third of the tongue sour or bitter solutions. Right and left sides of the tongue are tested while the client's tongue is projected.

Test muscles of **mastication** and the motor functions of the trigeminal nerve by palpating the masseter muscles (Figure 19-12) and the temporal muscles (Figure 19-13) while asking the client to bite down hard. Test jaw strength against resistance by applying downward pressure on the chin while asking the client to resist opening the mouth.

CN VII (facial). Inspect the client's face for symmetrical movement when he or she looks at the ceiling, wrinkles the forehead, frowns, smiles, puff out cheeks, and raises eyebrows (Figure 19-14). Ask the client to close the eyes, first lightly and then tightly, while you try to open them. In infants, evaluate the facial muscles during crying. Evaluate tone and note any atrophy and **fasciculations**, or twitching, of a muscle group.

Testing for taste, salivation, and lacrimation is generally not part of the routine physical examination. When it is appropriate to test taste sensation, use an applicator to apply salty or sweet solutions to the anterior of each side of the tongue. Use a different applicator for each substance, and allow the client a sip of water between tests to avoid mixing tastes. Have the client leave the tongue protruded until he or she identifies the taste. To avoid spreading the test substance over the tongue, give the client a card with the words salty, sweet, sour, and bitter (the vagus nerve innervates sour and bitter taste on the posterior tongue) and ask the client to point to the one that best describes the solution on the tongue (Figure 19-15). Record the number of correct responses.

CN VIII (acoustic). See Chapter 12.

CN IX (glossopharyngeal) and X (vagus). Testing of cranial nerves IX and X focuses on the musculature of the palate, pharynx, and larynx. Inspect the soft palate for symmetry. Identify the uvula and record any deviation from the midline. Test the gag reflex by touching the posterior wall of the pharynx with an applicator or a tongue blade; check for elevation of the palate and contraction of the pharyngeal muscles.

Note that the vagus nerve is functioning normally if the client can swallow and speak clearly without hoarseness. Ask the client to say "ah," and note whether the palate rises symmetrically. (See Chapter 12.)

CN XI (spinal accessory). To test the spinal accessory nerve, evaluate the symmetry, size, and strength of the muscles. Ask the client to turn the head to one side against the resistance of your hand while you palpate the opposite sternocleidomastoid muscle (Figure 19-16).

To assess the trapezius muscles, ask the client to shrug the shoulders while you exert downward pressure. Evaluate the muscles for strength and symmetry (Figure 19-17).

CN XII (hypoglossal). Inspect the tongue for size (atrophy), symmetry, and fasciculations. Ask the client to stick out the tongue as far as possible. Note the client's ability to stick the tongue straight out and the strength of the movement against lateral resistance produced with a tongue blade. Test the client's muscle strength by asking him or her to push out the cheek with the tongue while you push against it from the outside (Figure 19-18).

Proprioception and cerebellar function. The proprioceptive system of the nervous system maintains posture, balance, and coordination. The neural structures involved in proprioception are the posterior columns of the spinal cord, the cerebellum, and the vestibular apparatus. The posterior columns of the spinal cord carry stimuli from the proprioceptors in tendons and joints in addition to fibers for touch and two-point discrimination. Lesions affecting the posterior column impair muscle and position sense. The cerebellum in-

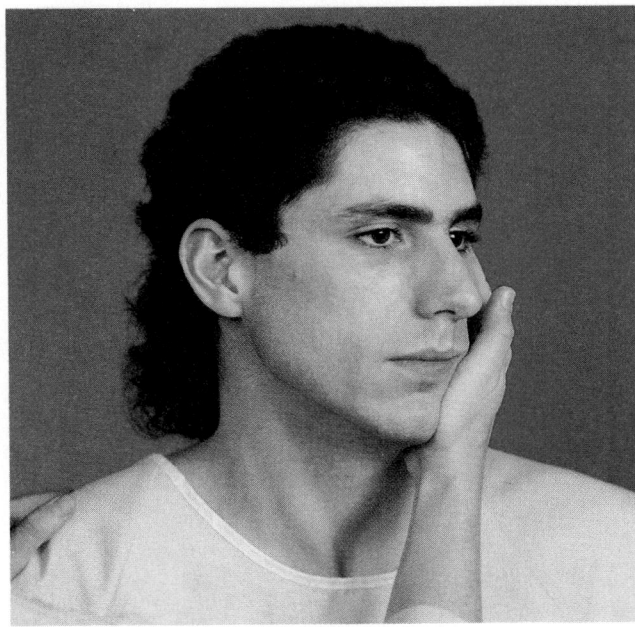

FIGURE 19-16 Assessing the symmetry, size, and strength of the sternocleidomastoid muscle in test of CN XI (spinal accessory nerve). Client is asked to turn the head to one side against the resistance of examiner's hand. Contralateral sternocleidomastoid muscle will stand out as it contracts. Examiner palpates the visible muscle to assess tension.

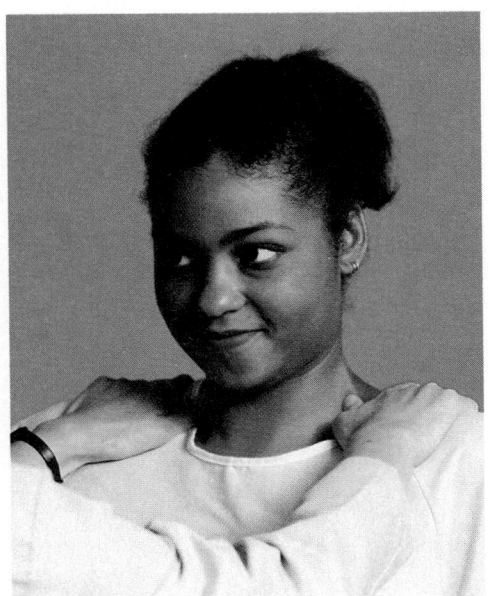

FIGURE 19-17 To test CN XI (spinal accessory nerve), trapezius muscle strength, client shrugs the shoulders against the resistance of examiner's hands.

tegrates muscle contractions to maintain posture. Lesions affecting the cerebellum impair balance and coordination.

The vestibular system is concerned with correcting movements. Vestibular disease is characterized by **vertigo**, nausea, and vomiting. Vertigo is the illusion of movement of the individual or the environment. Nausea and vomiting frequently accompany this condition.

The following examination techniques are used to assess proprioception and cerebellar functions:

Finger-to-nose movements. Ask the client to touch his or her nose with the index finger of one hand and then the other, first with the eyes open and then with the eyes closed (Figure 19-19). A normal finding is the ability to accurately target the nose.

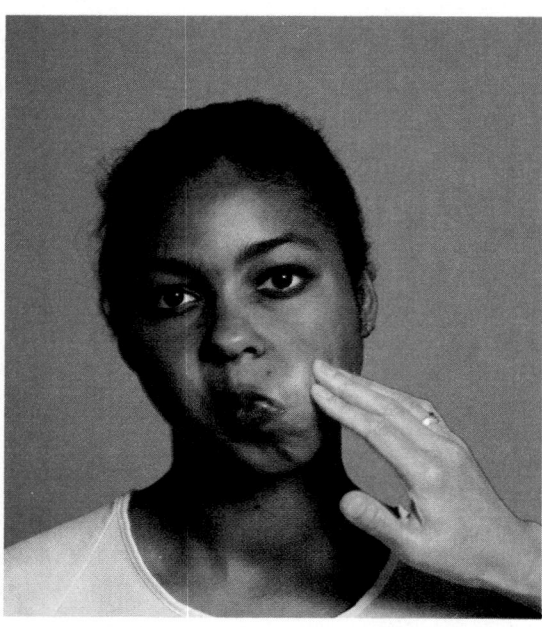

FIGURE 19-18 Assessing the strength of the tongue. Examiner asks the client to push against the inner surface of the cheek with as much strength as possible. Examiner palpates the external surface of the cheek simultaneously.

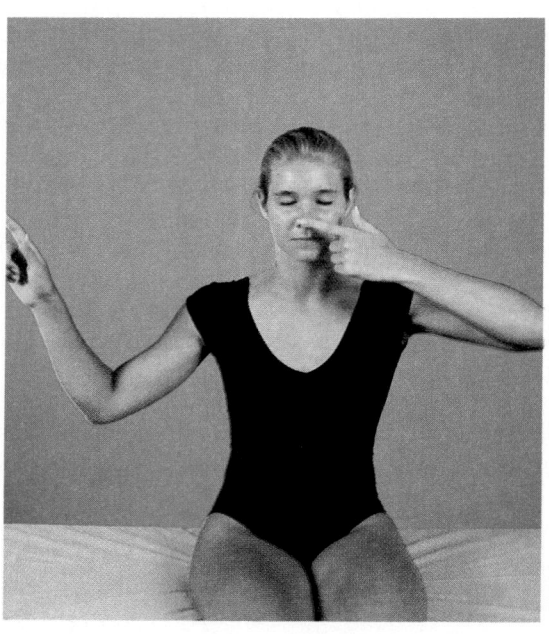

FIGURE 19-19 Testing of cerebellar function. Client attempts to alternately touch the nose with the index finger of each hand, repeating the motion with increasing speed.

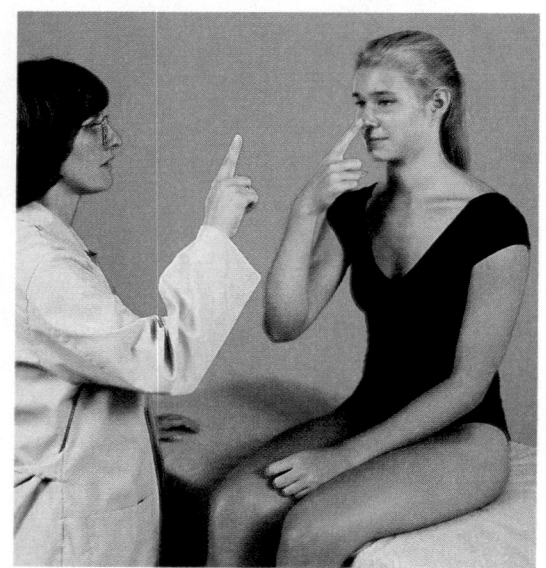

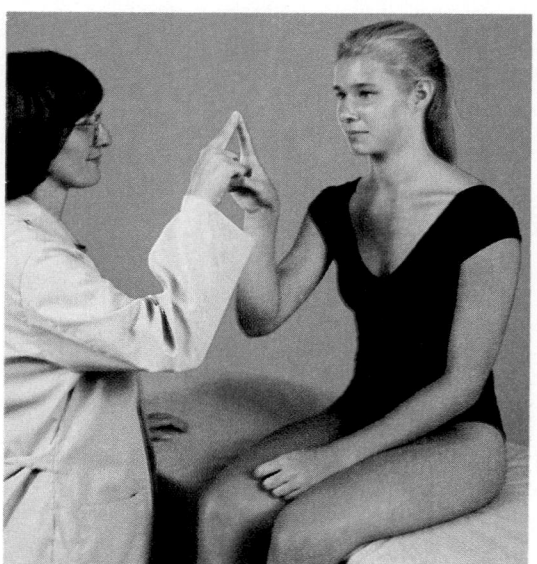

FIGURE 19-20 Testing cerebellar function. Client attempts to move finger from nose, **(A)**, to examiner's finger, **(B)**, rapidly. Examiner's index finger is about 18 inches from client's eye and moves the position of the finger target.

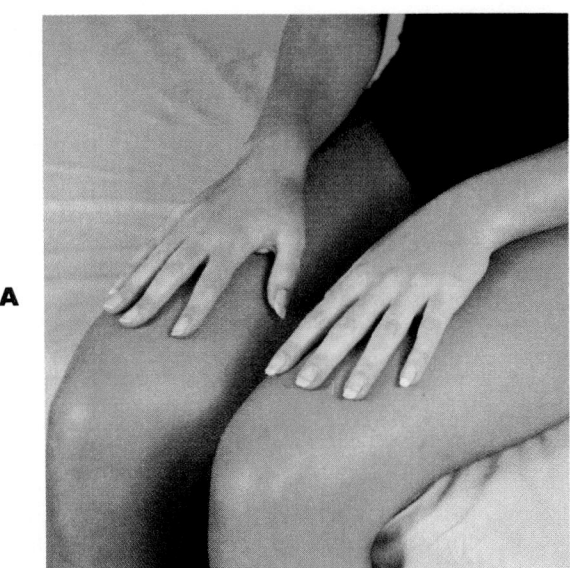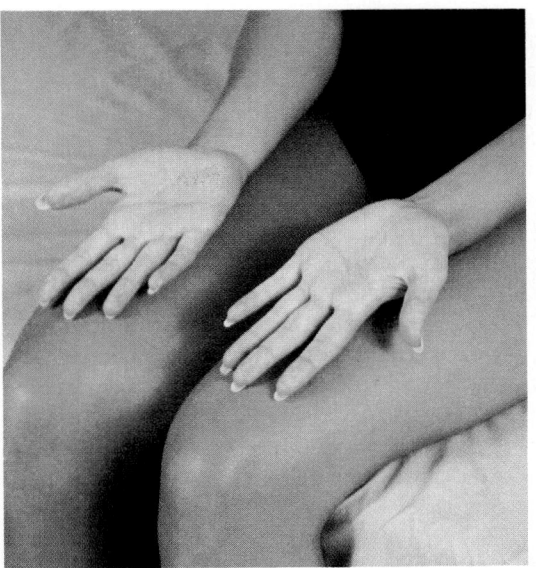

FIGURE 19-21 Testing cerebellar function: pronation **(A)** and supination **(B)** of the hands, with progressively more rapid movement.

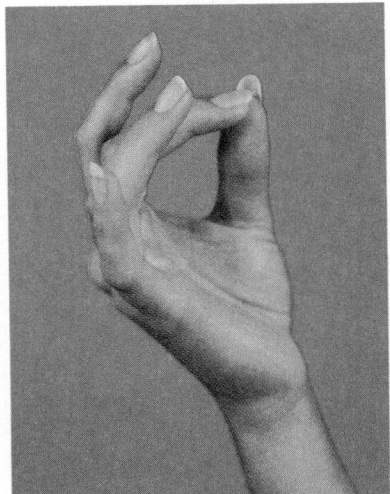

FIGURE 19-22 Testing cerebellar function. Examiner instructs client to touch each finger to the thumb as rapidly as possible.

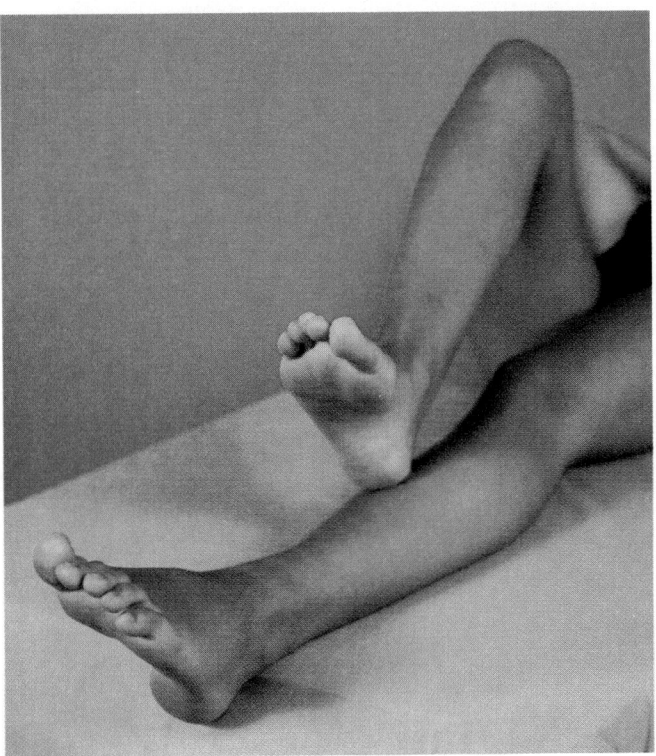

FIGURE 19-23 Testing cerebellar function. Examiner asks client to run the heel of each foot down the opposite shin.

Finger-nose-finger movements. Ask the client, with eyes open, to touch his or her nose and then your finger at a distance of approximately 45 cm. Have the client increase the speed as you move your finger (Figure 19-20). Test each hand separately. Note the speed and accuracy of movement.

Rapid alternating movements. Ask the client to pat his or her knees with the palms of the hands followed by the backs of the hands at an ever-increasing rate (Figure 19-21). Then have the client perform thumb-to-finger opposition by touching each finger of one hand to the thumb of the same hand as rapidly as possible (Figure 19-22).

Heel to shin. Ask the client to run the heel of each foot down the opposite shin (Figure 19-23).

Romberg test. Ask the client to stand with feet together, first with eyes open and then with the eyes closed (Figure 19-24). Slight swaying is normal. Stand close enough to the client to prevent falling. The normal client is able to do this for about 5 seconds with the eyes closed.

Coordination. After the client opens the eyes, ask him or her to walk naturally, then in a heel-to-toe fashion (Figure 19-25), and then to stand on each foot (Figure 19-26). If the client does this without difficulty, ask him or her to hop on one foot, then the other (Figure 19-27), and to do a deep knee bend (Figure 19-28). Since shoes can interfere with balance, have the client perform these tests without shoes.

Sensory function. Although evaluating sensation over the entire skin surface is not necessary, stimuli should be applied strategically to test the dermatomes and the major peripheral nerves. A minimal number of test sites includes areas on the forehead, cheek, hand, and foot. In the screening examination, assume the nerve to be intact if sensation is normal at its most distal area. When there is evidence of dysfunction, localize

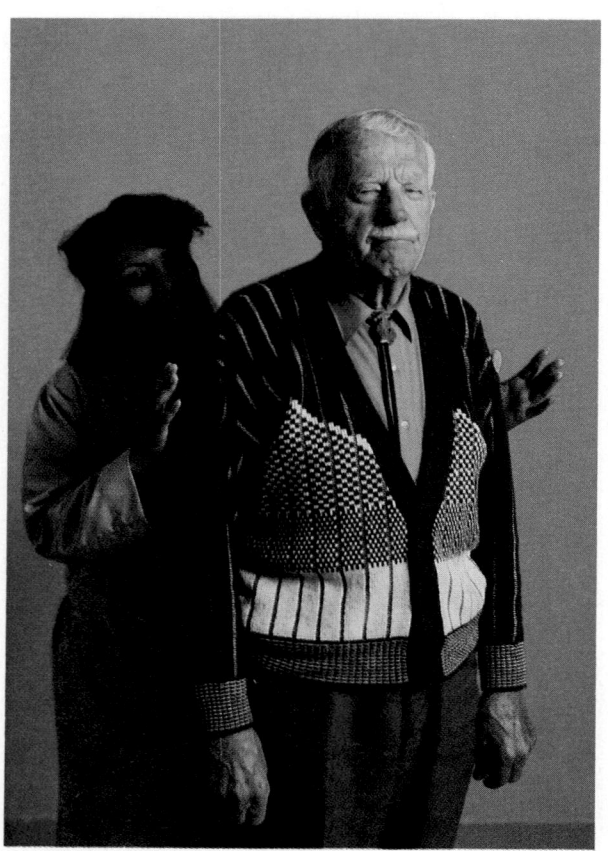

FIGURE 19-24 Testing the proprioceptive system. Romberg test: client should be able to stand with eyes closed and feet together without swaying for approximately 5 seconds.

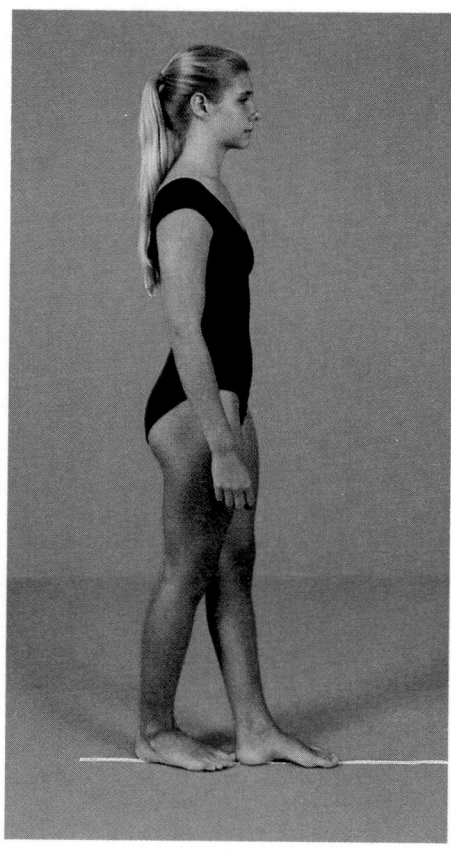

FIGURE 19-25 Testing the proprioceptive system. Client attempts to walk a straight line placing heel to toe.

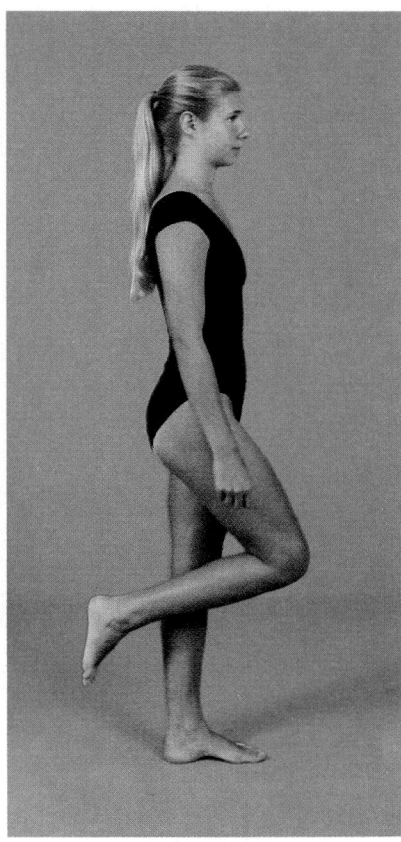

FIGURE 19-26 Testing the proprioceptive system. Client attempts to stand on one foot and then the other.

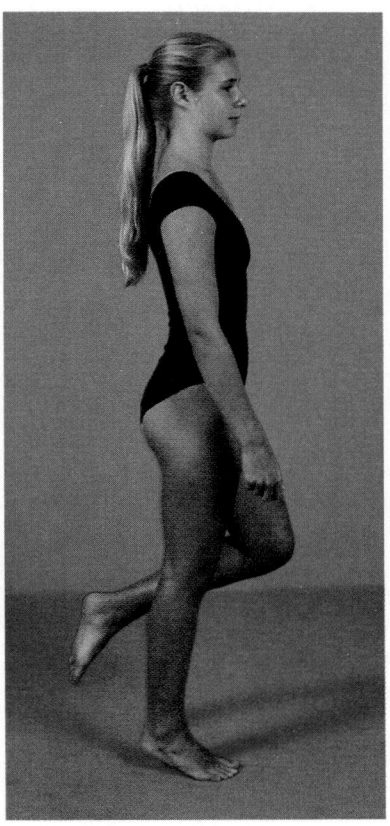

FIGURE 19-27 Testing the proprioceptive system. Client attempts to hop in place on one foot and then the other.

the site of the dysfunction and map the boundaries. Sketch the region involved and describe the sensory change.

Variation in sensitivity of skin areas is normal. Use a stronger stimulus over the back, the buttocks, and areas where the skin is heavily cornified. Establish symmetry of sensation by checking first one spot and then the same area on the opposite side of the body.

Instruct the client to close the eyes during evaluation of sensory modalities. A client who is able to see the stimulus applied may be influenced by visual cues rather than responding to the specific sensory modality being tested.

> **Helpful Hint:** *Ensure that both you and the client are rested because fatigue may result in errors. Otherwise, you may interpret inattention or low motivation as a sensory loss. Also, in order to avoid predictability, vary the testing sites and the timing in applying the stimulus.*

The following terms are useful in describing and recording sensory dysfunction:

Anesthesia—the absence of normal sensation

Hyperesthesia—an extreme sensitivity of one of the body's senses

Hypoesthesia—an abnormal weakness of sensation in response to sensory stimulation

Paresthesia—any subjective sensation, experienced as numbness, tingling, or a "pins and needles" feeling

Light touch sensation. Light touch and pain are mediated by different nerve endings. Sensory fibers for light touch enter the spinal cord and travel upward in the anterior spinothalamic tracts to the thalamus. Both anterior spinothalamic tracts must suffer destruction before transmission of light touch is lost.

Test light touch by contacting the skin with a wisp of cotton (see Figure 19-11, *A*). Does the client feel the touch of a wisp of cotton? Instruct the client to say "yes" or "now" when the touch is felt. If desired, combine this test with localization (a higher cortical func-

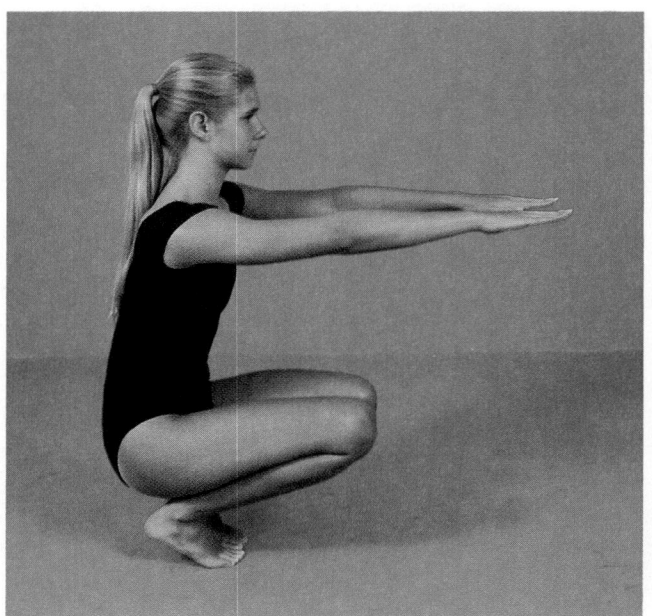

FIGURE 19-28 Testing the proprioceptive system. Client attempts a knee bend without support.

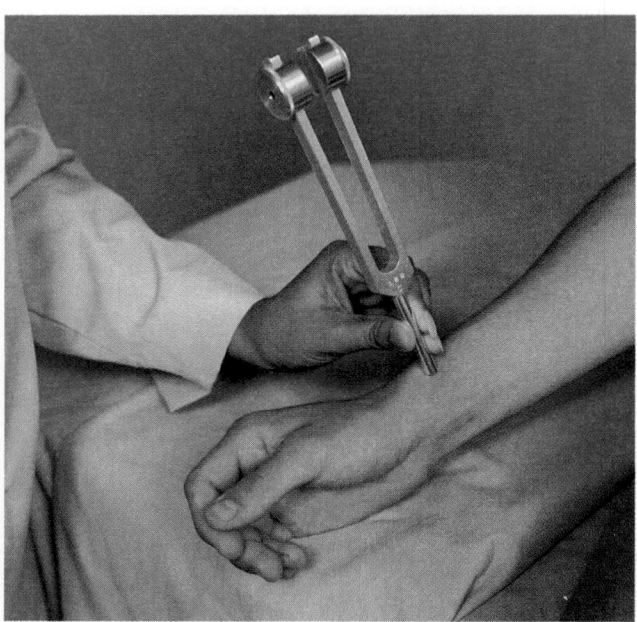

FIGURE 19-29 Testing sensitivity to vibration. Examiner applies the base of the vibrating tuning fork to a bony prominence such as the wrist.

tion) by asking the client to state where he or she is touched. Compare each side of the body. Record areas of anesthesia or hyperesthesia.

Pain and temperature sensation. Pain and temperature fibers both travel in the lateral spinothalamic tract. A screening examination does not include temperature assessment unless pain sensation is abnormal. To test temperature sensation, roll tubes filled with warm and cold water against the client's skin over dermatome areas. (First test the stimuli on your own skin to avoid burning the client and to provide a comparison.) Ask the client to say "hot," "cold," or "can't tell."

Evaluate the sensory perception of superficial pain by using the sharp and dull points of a safety pin (see Figure 19-11, *B*). Compare each side of the body in the same locations as you test tactile sensation. To avoid any risk of infection, discard the safety pin after use. Instruct the client to say "sharp" or "dull" when touched. Remember that each area examined must be touched with a sharp stimulus because dull touch simply validates light touch perception.

Vibration sensation. The normal client can perceive vibration as a buzzing or tingling sensation when a bony prominence, such as the wrist, elbow, or ankle, touches the base of a vibrating tuning fork. With the client's eyes closed, test vibratory sensation by applying the vibrating tuning fork to the wrists, elbows, knees, and ankles (Figure 19-29). Ask the client to say "yes" or "now" (1) when first feeling the vibrations and (2) when the vibrations stop. Dampen the vibrations of the tuning fork to move along more rapidly. Compare sensitivity from side to side and proximal to distal parts of the extremities. Apply the tuning fork to the most distal point of the extremity since normal vibratory perception, or intactness of posterior columns, decreases from a proximal to a distal point.

A normal finding in the older client (older than 65 years) is diminished vibratory sensation, particularly in the extremities.

Tactile discrimination. Tactile discrimination requires interpretation by the cerebral cortex. Three types of tactile discrimination that are tested clinically are (1) stereognosis, (2) two-point discrimination, and (3) extinction.

Stereognosis is the ability to recognize objects by touching and manipulating them. Test stereognosis with universally familiar objects, such as a key, safety pin, or coin (Figure 19-30). Test **graphesthesia** by asking the client to identify letters or numbers written on each palm with a blunt point. The normal client can correctly identify the letters or numbers inscribed (Figure 19-31).

Two-point discrimination is the ability to sense whether one or two areas of the skin are being stimulated by pressure. There is considerable variability of perceptual ability over the different parts of the body.

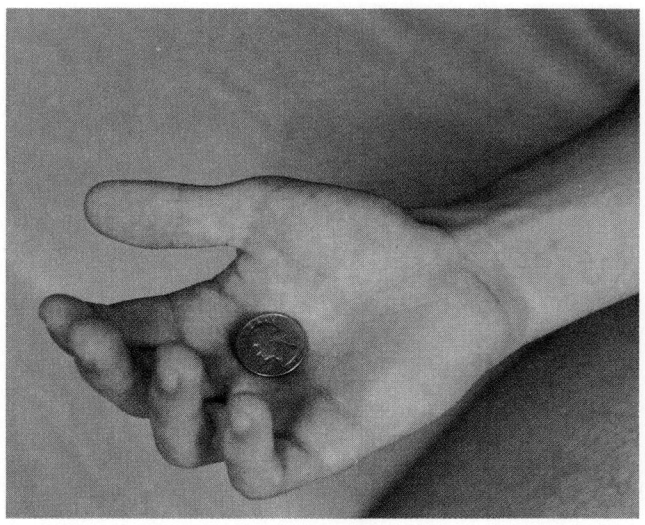

FIGURE 19-30 Testing for stereognosis. Normal client can identify a familiar object (coin, key) by touching and manipulating it.

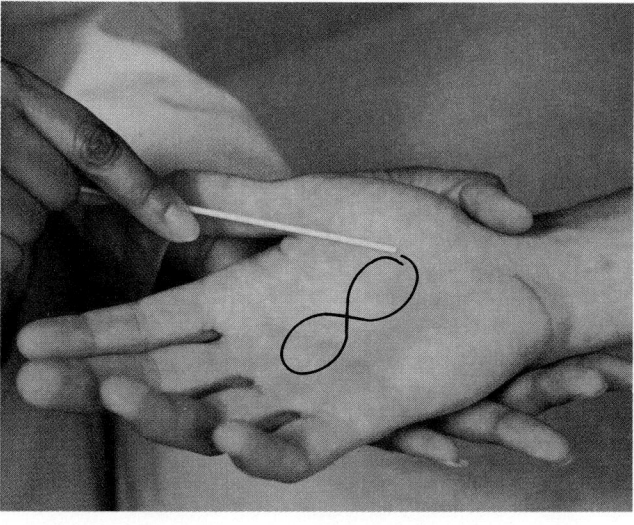

FIGURE 19-31 Testing for graphesthesia. Normal client can identify a number or letter written on the palm.

The following are minimal distances between the two points of the calipers at which the normal adult can sense simultaneous stimulation:

Tongue: 1 mm
Fingertips: 2.8 mm
Palms of hands: 8 to 12 mm
Chest, forearms: 40 mm
Back: 40 to 70 mm
Upper arms, thighs: 75 mm

To test two-point discrimination, apply pins (or calipers) to the skin simultaneously. Ask the client if he or she feels one or two pinpricks (Figure 19-32).

To test for **extinction**, touch the skin on the same areas on both sides of the body. Failure to perceive touch on one side is called the extinction phenomenon.

Position sense. Position sense **(kinesthetic sensation)** is facilitated by proprioceptive receptors in the muscles, tendons, and joints. Perception of the position, orientation, and motion of limbs and body parts is obtained from kinesthetic sensations.

With the client's eyes closed and the joint in a neutral position, and with your fingers placed on each side of the client's digit (finger or toe), slightly move the position of the client's digit. Be careful not to touch other digits during this maneuver. Ask the client to describe how the position of the finger changes. Always move the digit to a neutral position before moving it again (Figure 19-33).

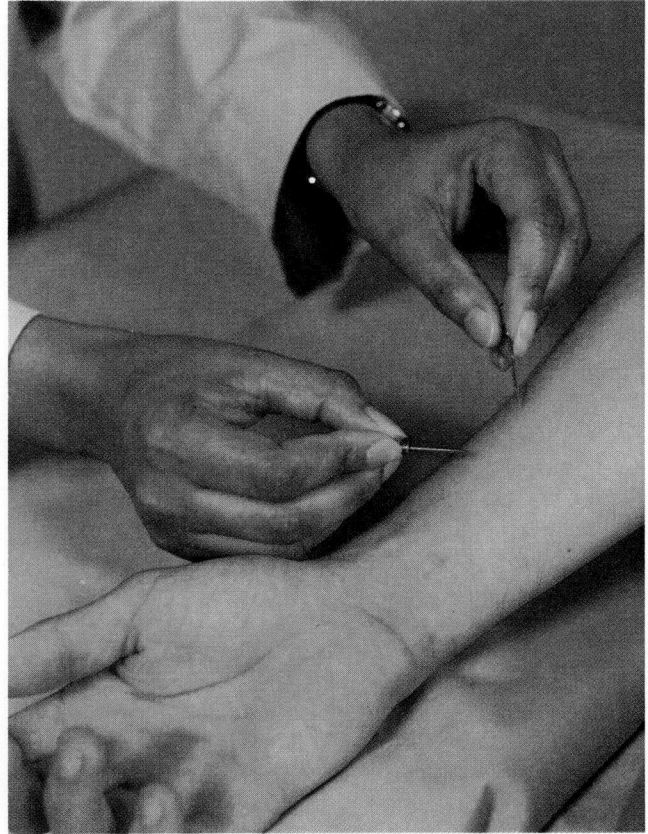

FIGURE 19-32 Testing for two-point discrimination. Pins, calipers, or paper clips bent into a ∪ shape can be used.

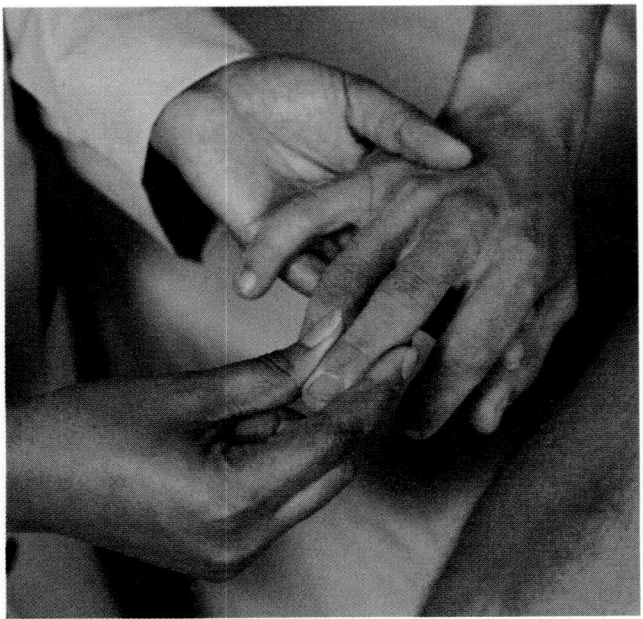

FIGURE 19-33 Testing position sense. With client's eyes closed, examiner slightly changes the position of a digit up or down. Client describes how the position was changed.

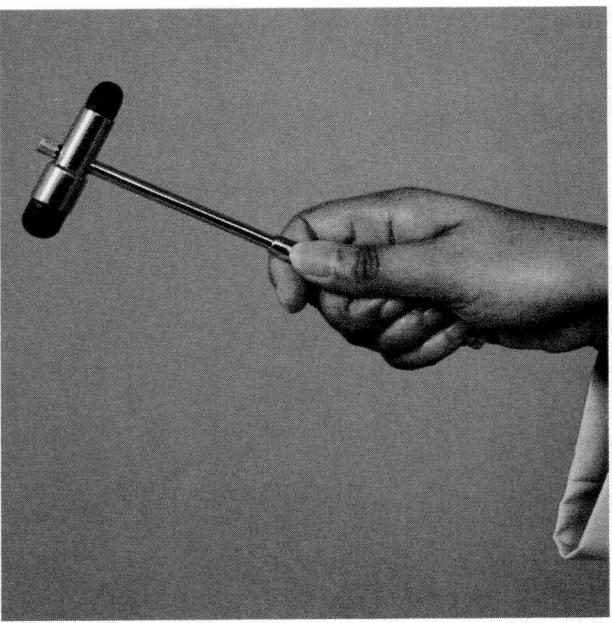

FIGURE 19-34 Examiner holds the reflex, or percussion, hammer in the dominant hand between the thumb and index finger and uses a striking motion to assess the deep tendon reflex.

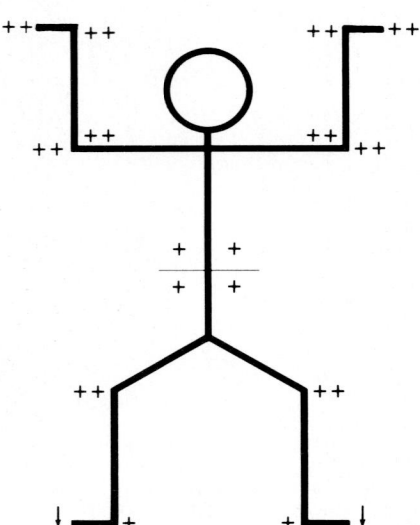

FIGURE 19-35 Stick-figure drawing for recording reflexes. These are the reflexes usually tested in the screening examination; " + + " values shown here are normal.

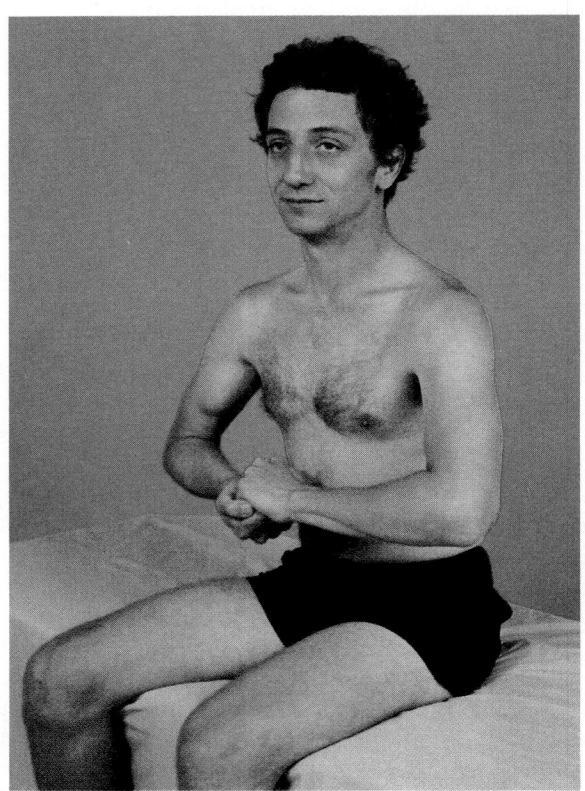

FIGURE 19-36 Augmentation maneuver for deep tendon reflexes.

TABLE 19-2

Reflexes Commonly Tested in the Physical Examination and Segmental Levels of the Central Nervous System Involved

Deep tendon reflexes	Segmental level	Superficial reflexes	Segmental level
Biceps	C5, 6	Pharyngeal (gag)	Medulla
Triceps	C6, 7, 8	Abdominal (upper)	T7, 8, 9
Brachioradialis	C5, 6	Abdominal (lower)	T12; L1
Patellar	L2, 3, 4	Cremasteric	L1, 2, 3
Ankle (Achilles)	S1, 2	Gluteal	L4, 5
		Plantar	L4, 5; S1, 2

Reflexes

Deep tendon reflexes. Assess deep tendon reflexes to obtain information about the function of the reflex arcs and the spinal cord segments (Table 19-2). Elicit deep tendon reflexes by deforming (tapping) a tendon with a reflex hammer (Figure 19-34). Grade reflexes for the record as follows:

4⁺   Brisk, hyperactive, clonus of tendon associated with disease

3⁺   More brisk than normal, not necessarily indicative of disease

2⁺   Normal

1⁺   Low normal, slightly diminished response

0   No response

Record the symmetry of the reflex from one side of the body to the other. A succinct method of recording the reflex findings is the stick-figure representation (Figure 19-35). To obtain the best muscle contraction, test when the muscle is slightly stretched before the tendon is stretched (tapped with the reflex hammer).

Augmentation of the reflex is done by asking the client to isometrically tense muscles not directly involved in the reflex arc being tested. For example, ask the client to clench the fists or to lock the fingers together and pull the hands apart (Figure 19-36) as you assess lower extremity reflexes. To reinforce the reflex arcs of the upper extremities, ask the client to clench the jaw or to tense the quadriceps. Document that augmentation was used to elicit the deep tendon reflex.

BICEPS REFLEX (FIGURE 19-37). To check the biceps reflex, have the client flex the arm at the elbow. Place your thumb firmly over the biceps tendon to augment the tendon stretch. The thumb is struck with the reflex hammer. The normal response is flexion of the arm at the elbow.

> **Helpful Hint:** *Compare reflexes bilaterally for symmetry, degree and speed of response, and recovery to original position. To accurately compare reflexes, make sure that each limb is in the same position.*

TRICEPS REFLEX (FIGURE 19-38). Tap the triceps tendon (above the olecranon process) with the reflex hammer. The normal response is extension of the elbow. Begin with the client's arm flexed at the elbow and resting in the client's lap. Alternatively, you can start with the client's arm flexed at the elbow and abducted while you hold it in position. The latter position sometimes allows for better viewing of the normal response of extension of the elbow.

BRACHIORADIALIS REFLEX (FIGURE 19-39). To test the brachioradialis reflex, begin with the client's arm in a relaxed position. Strike the styloid process of the radius with the hammer while palpating the tendon 3 to 5 cm above the wrist. The normal response is flexion of the elbow and pronation of the forearm. The fingers of the hand may also flex.

PATELLAR REFLEX (FIGURE 19-40). For this test the client's legs should be hanging freely over the side of the bed or chair or the client should be resting in a supine position. Palpate the muscle above the patella

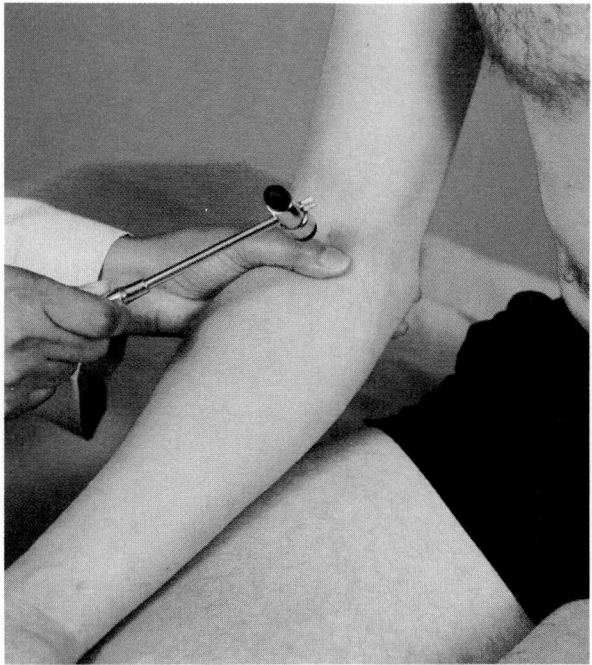

FIGURE 19-37 Eliciting the biceps reflex. With client's arm flexed, examiner places the thumb over the biceps tendon and strikes the thumb with the reflex hammer.

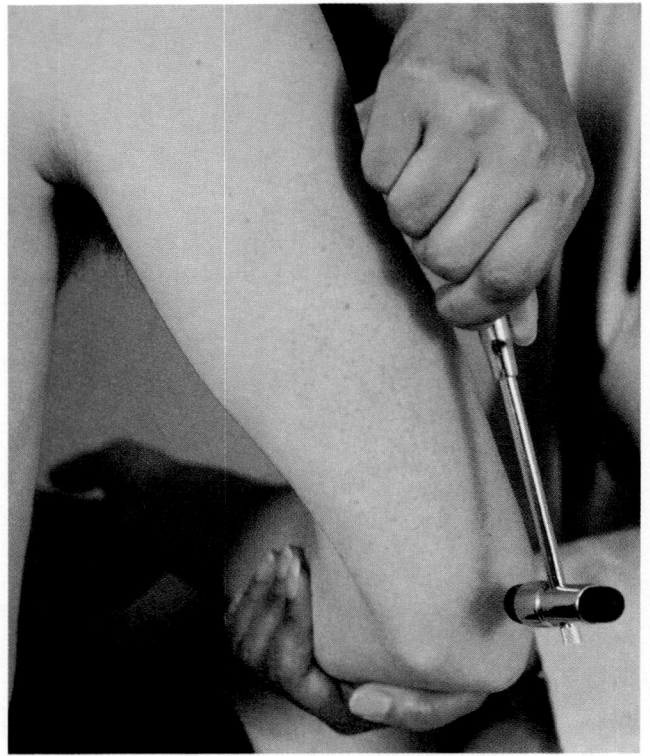

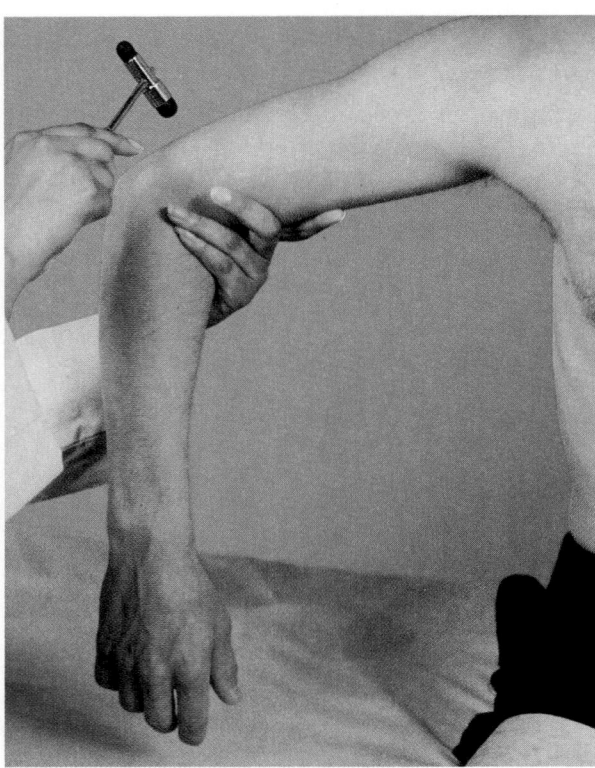

A

B

FIGURE 19-38 Eliciting the triceps reflex. **A,** With arm flexed at elbow, examiner taps the triceps tendon. **B,** Examiner holds flexed arm in position. Normal response is straightening or extension of the arm.

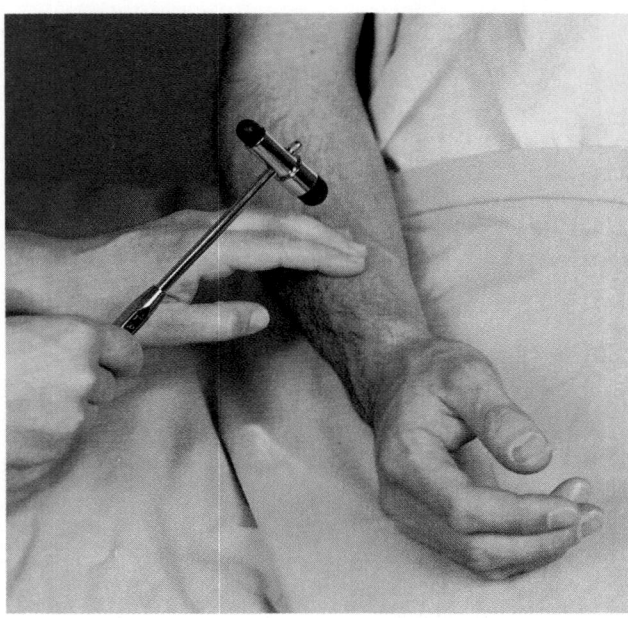

FIGURE 19-39 Eliciting of the brachioradialis reflex. Normal response is flexion of the arm at the elbow, pronation of the wrist, or slight flexion of the fingers.

with one hand while striking the tendon with the reflex hammer directly below the patella. The normal response is extension or kicking of the leg as the quadriceps muscle contracts.

ANKLE (OR ACHILLES) REFLEX (FIGURE 19-41). Hold the client's foot in a slightly dorsiflexed position with one hand and strike the Achilles tendon with the reflex hammer. The normal response is plantar flexion of the foot.

Superficial reflexes. Superficial, or cutaneous, reflexes are obtained by stimulating the skin.

PLANTAR REFLEXES (FIGURE 19-42). Plantar reflexes are superficial reactions. Use a pin, the sharp edge of a broken tongue blade, or the handle portion of the reflex hammer to elicit the reflex. Apply the stimulus to the lateral border of the client's sole, starting at the heel and continuing across the ball of the foot and ending beneath the great toe. The normal response is flexion of the toes (Figure 19-43). Extension or dorsiflexion of the great toe and fanning of the others, which is abnormal, is called the Babinski reflex. Before a child can walk, fanning and extension of the toes are the normal response.

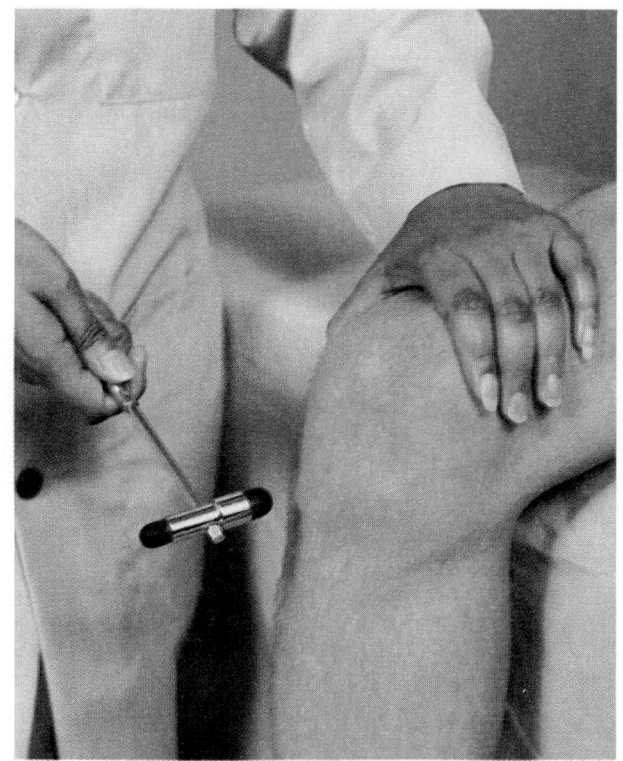
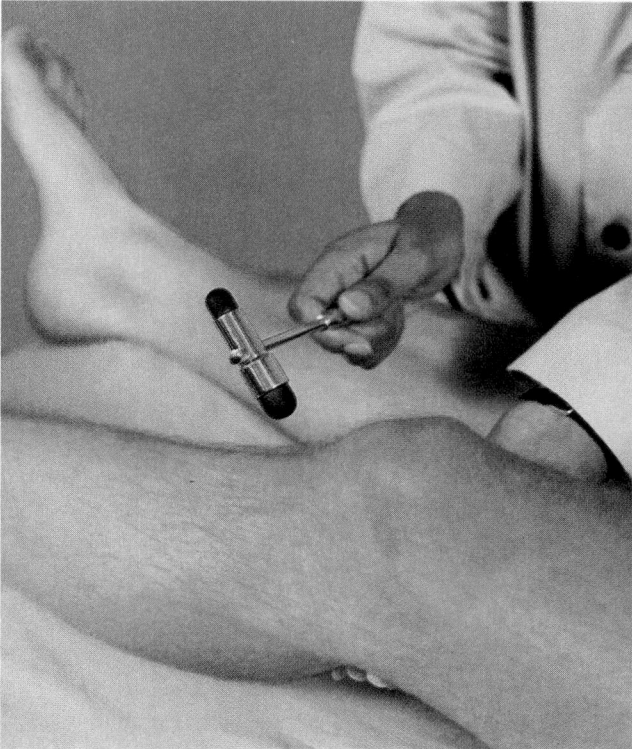

FIGURE 19-40 Eliciting the patellar reflex. With client's legs hanging freely **(A)** or with client in a supine position **(B),** examiner strikes the tendon below the patella. Normal response is extension of the leg.

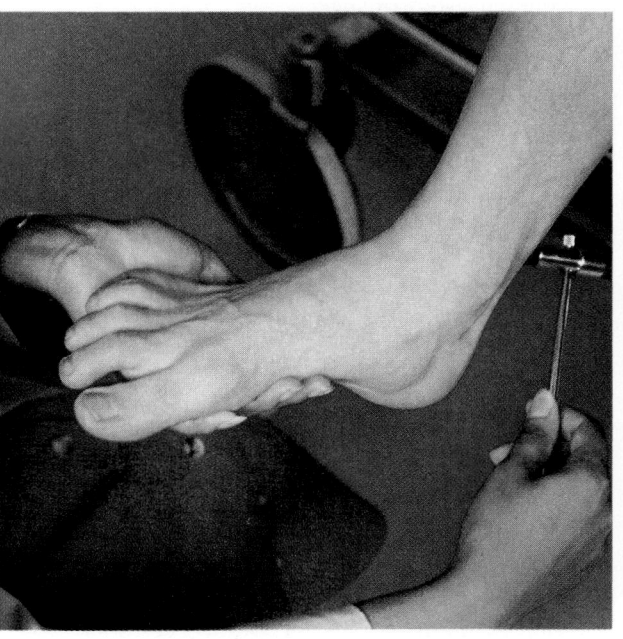
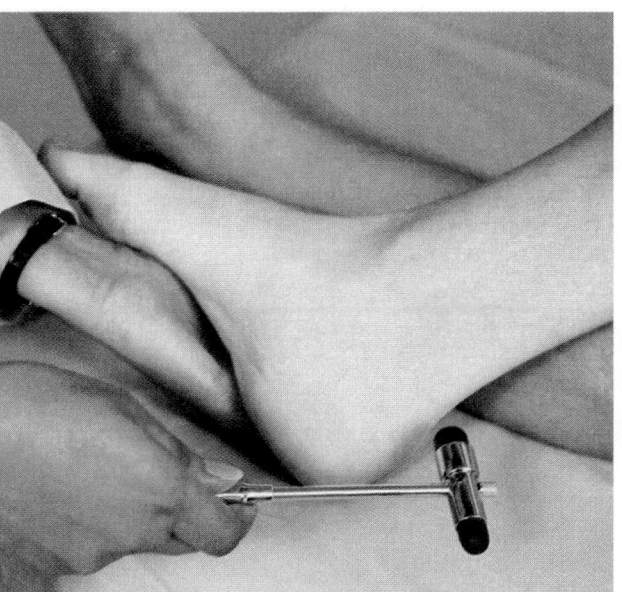

FIGURE 19-41 Eliciting the ankle reflex. **A,** Sitting. **B,** Lying down. Examiner strikes the Achilles tendon with the reflex hammer while holding the foot in a slightly dorsiflexed position. Normal response is plantar flexion of the foot.

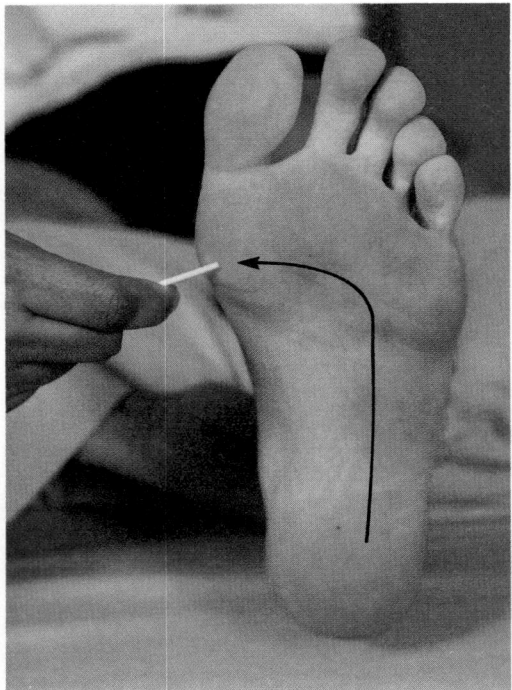

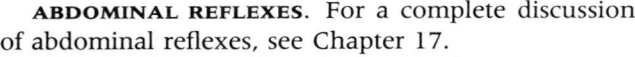

FIGURE 19-42 Eliciting the plantar reflex. Examiner applies a hard object along the lateral surface of the sole, starting at the heel and moving along the ball of the foot, ending beneath the great toe.

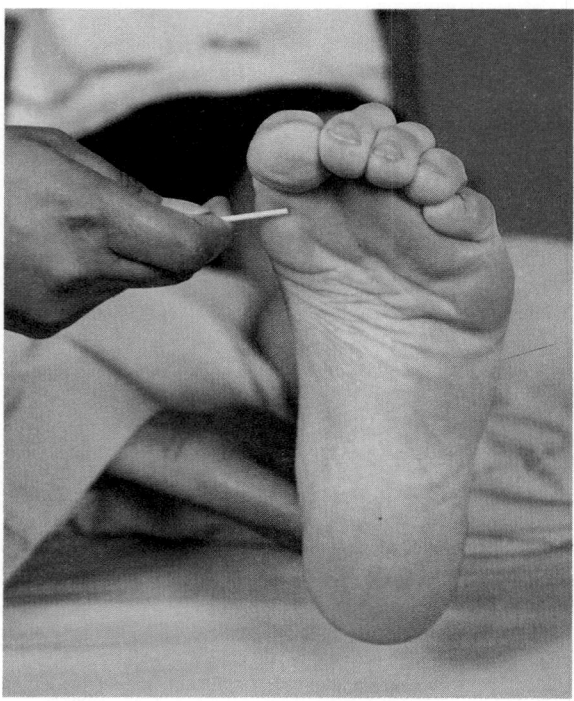

FIGURE 19-43 Normal response to plantar stimulation: flexion of all the toes.

ABDOMINAL REFLEXES. For a complete discussion of abdominal reflexes, see Chapter 17.

CREMASTERIC REFLEX. Stimulate the male client's inner thigh with a sharp object, such as the stick end of an applicator. The expected response is retraction (elevation) of the scrotum on the same side as the cremaster muscle contracts.

GLUTEAL REFLEX. Spread the client's buttocks and stimulate the perianal area. The normal response is contraction of the anal sphincter.

MENTAL STATUS EXAMINATION

Purpose of the Examination

The purpose of the mental status examination is to assess the client's current emotional and mental capacity and functioning. The mental status examination provides a baseline for a client's psychological state and specific information that helps to establish a nursing diagnosis. The examination includes the description of the client's:

General appearance
Behavior

Mood or **affect**
Characteristics of speech
Orientation
Thought processes
Insight and judgment
Memory and learning
Perceptions and attitudes

The examiner focuses on assessing the client's ability to interact with the environment. Responses elicited during a single interview are only samples of the individual's thoughts and feelings. Fears regarding illness, family responsibilities, attitudes of others, and financial worries are some factors that can alter a client's feelings and behaviors. Considering the effects of prescription and illicit drugs on the client's mental processes and behaviors is important.

Assessment of Mental Status

Health history. Assessment of mental status includes interviewing and inspection or observation. During the interview, make an overall assessment of whether the client is cooperative, friendly, or hostile. Obtain information about the client's educational and physical development; occupation; economic status; relationships; responsibilities felt toward family, work, or school;

stressors (actual or perceived); goals (attainable and unrealistic); and support systems (individuals and affiliations).

Use therapeutic communication skills (see Chapter 2). Focus on obtaining data about symptoms, including how the client views these symptoms and how disruptive they are to the client and others. Compare and contrast your observations with the client's perceptions. Document a client's behaviors and words accurately, succinctly, and in *measurable*, descriptive terms. Use short, direct quotes only when doing so enhances the client's meaning or clarifies the situation:

Correct: Client smoked ½ pack of cigarettes in 30 minutes. He paced across the room 4 to 5 times and stated "I'm really feeling nervous" twice.

Incorrect: Client chain-smoked during interview. He appeared agitated and verbalized his anxiety.

Preparation for the examination: client and environment. Equipment needed to conduct a mental status examination includes a pencil, paper, and reading material. The setting should be quiet and should provide privacy. Communication barriers related to age or culture can often be bridged through the use of qualified interpreters, friends, or family members. When information is obtained from sources other than the client, the examiner must understand the relationship of these individuals to the client.

General appearance. Carefully observe the client's general physical appearance, grooming, manner of dress, facial expression, and body posture as a measure of mental function. Do not focus too early on obvious abnormalities since the subtle clues may be missed.

Grooming and manner of dress. Observe the client's clothing to determine its appropriateness to time, place, age, and life-style. Grooming of hair and nails and general cleanliness should be noted. A disheveled appearance in someone who was previously well groomed is especially significant.

Posture. Posture is important in providing clues to the client's feelings. The client who walks slowly into the room, barely lifting the feet, and who slumps in the chair while avoiding the examiner's glance may be showing a lack of affect or depression.

Coordination. Assess general coordination of movement by observing the client's gait (see Chapter 8). To

TABLE 19-3

Levels of Consciousness (Responsiveness)

Level	Behaviors
Consciousness	Appropriate response (rate and quality) to external stimuli; oriented to time, place, and person
Confusion	Inappropriate response to stimuli and decreased attention span and memory; reactions to simple commands
Lethargy (hypersomnia)	Drowsiness or increased sleep time; can be aroused; responds appropriately; may fall asleep again immediately
Delirium	Confusion, disorder perception, and decreased attention span; motor and sensory excitement; inappropriate reactions to stimuli; marked anxiety
Coma	Loss or lowering of consciousness
Stage I (stupor)	Arousable for short periods to verbal, visual, or painful stimuli; simple motor and verbal response to stimuli; slow responses; corneal and pupillary reflexes sluggish; deep tendon and superficial reflexes unaffected; pathological reflexes may be obtained
Stage II (light coma)	Simple motor and verbal (moaning) response to painful stimuli; mass motor movement or flexion (avoidance) response
Stage III (deep coma)	Decerebrate posturing to painful stimuli (extension of body and limbs and pronation of arms)
Stage IV	Flaccid muscles; pupillary reflex absent; apneic; on ventilator; superficial and some deep tendon reflexes present
Brain death	Two EEG tracings 24 hours apart indicate absence of brain waves; cerebral function absent for 24 hours; failure of cerebral perfusion; expert opinion rules out hypothermia or drug toxicity (*Note:* All these behaviors must be present.)
Syncope	Temporary loss of consciousness (partial or complete) associated with increased rate of respiration, tachycardia, pallor, perspiration, and coolness of skin
Fugue state	Dysfunction of consciousness (hours or days) in which the individual carries on purposeful activity that he or she does not remember afterward
Amnesia	Memory loss over time or for specific subjects; individual affected responds appropriately to external stimuli

evaluate the complex coordination, give the client simple phrases to write and simple geometric figures to draw.

Behavior

Level of consciousness. Consciousness is awareness of one's thoughts and feelings and of the environment. The levels of consciousness (responsiveness) are generally described according to the behavior exhibited by the individual. Table 19-3 includes a useful categorization of the levels of consciousness. Response to pain may be the only indication of sensory stimulation. Stimuli used to assess response to pain include pinching of skin, pricking with a pin, pressure over supraorbital notches, or squeezing muscle masses or tendons, particularly the calf muscle. The client may respond by extension of limbs, facial grimacing, or withdrawal. Flexion responses are considered withdrawal responses and therefore purposeful. Nonpurposeful responses are mass reactions or extension of limbs.

Mood or affect. Affect is the observable manifestation of the internally experienced emotion or feeling state. In general, it is possible to estimate the client's emotional status or affective state from verbal and nonverbal behaviors. Affects may be described as **labile** if moods rapidly and abruptly shift. Observe the *appropriateness* and degree of affect to a given idea as well as the range of affect.

To understand the client's perspective and to bring out the feelings of clients who resist offering information spontaneously, try the interview protocol described in the accompanying box.

Characteristics of speech. Evaluate the client's comprehension of and ability to use the spoken language.

INTERVIEW PROTOCOL

How would you describe the problem that has brought you here?

What do you think is causing your problem?

Why do you think it happened to you?

Why do you think it started when it did?

How have your spirits been lately?

How do you feel life has been treating you?

Have you told anyone else about your feelings or problems?

Have you ever considered hurting yourself? If yes: Did you follow through and actually harm yourself? If yes: How did you do it?

Do you have any plans to harm yourself now? If yes: What are your plans?

Do you think about dying? If yes: How often?

The client's manner of speech may offer clues about his or her thought processes. The mentally healthy individual answers questions frankly. Responses to your questions and instructions give valuable information about the client's comprehension and willingness to cooperate. Note failure to answer a question, other evasive replies, and unwarranted criticism of you as the examiner.

Facial expression. Facial expression should be consistent with and appropriate to the topic. In some Southeast Asian cultures, direct eye contact is avoided, especially by women, since the examiner is considered to hold a position of respect. In many Asian cultures, an open display of one's distress is not considered appropriate behavior.

Cognitive functions. Assess the client's orientation, attention, memory, use of language, and intellectual skills. The Mini–Mental Status Examination (MMSE) is a simplified and practical 11-question instrument used to assess orientation, memory, concentration, calculation, and language abilities (see discussion of special screening tests).

Orientation. Assess orientation from the client's awareness of person, place, and time. The following questions can help in obtaining this information:

Person

What is your name? Address? Telephone number?

Do you know who I am?

Do you know what my job is?

Place

Tell me where you are. What is the name of this place?

Do you know the name of the town you are in?

Who brought you here?

Time

Do you know what day this is? Month? Year?

Record the degree of **disorientation**. Time is the orientation most frequently disordered in clients with mental disease. A disturbance of place orientation may accompany organic mental disorders or schizophrenia. An individual may not be oriented to another person in the aftermath of cerebral trauma or seizures.

Attention span. An appraisal of the individual's attention span includes the client's ability to maintain interest and to concentrate. Attention span is one of the first functions of the sensorium to become affected in individuals who are fatigued, anxious, or chemically impaired.

Memory. Memory is a function of general cerebral function. Impairment of memory occurs in both neurological and psychiatric disorders. Some general questions that may help to elicit a disorder in memory are as follows:

Have you noticed any loss of memory?

Do you remember those things that happened years ago best or those that happened today or yesterday?

IMMEDIATE MEMORY. Immediate memory is verbalized remembering immediately after presentation. Test immediate memory by digit recall. Two sample tests follow.

To test your memory skills, I'd like you to repeat four series of numbers after me:

7, 4

9, 6, 5, 3

8, 9, 4, 1, 5

3, 8, 7, 4, 1, 6

I will say some numbers. You say them backward. For instance, I say *8, 2;* you say *2, 8:*

3, 8

7, 2, 0

5, 9, 2, 7

The average individual can generally repeat five to seven digits forward and four to six digits backward.

RECENT MEMORY. Recent memory is verbalized after several minutes to an hour. Examples of questions and exercises for assessing recent memory are as follows:

How long have you been here?

What were you doing before you came here?

What time did you get up today?

What did you eat for breakfast today?

REMOTE MEMORY. Remote memory is verbalized after hours, days, or years. At the beginning of the interview, give the client three to five unrelated words to remember. Other examples of questions for assessing remote memory are as follows:

Where were you born?

Tell me the name of the high school you attended.

What was your mother's maiden name?

In testing for memory, do not ask questions for which the answers cannot be verified. Memory loss in organic dementia may involve disorders for immediate and recent events; however, affected individuals may be able to recall events from childhood with accuracy.

Intellectual functioning

ABSTRACTION ABILITY. To assess abstraction ability, ask the client to give the meaning of familiar proverbs:

A bird in the hand is worth two in the bush.

People who live in glass houses shouldn't throw stones.

Don't count your chickens before they hatch.

A rolling stone gathers no moss.

Helpful Hint: *Interpretation of abstraction ability must take into consideration a client's cultural orientation, age, and educational level. Some proverbs may be culturally bound or more familiar to clients of a certain age group.*

ABILITY TO LEARN (COMPREHENSION). The ability to learn includes abilities in perception, retention, association (interpretation), and recent memory. Give the client an address or a sentence that is not familiar and ask him or her to remember the content verbatim:

Listen to me carefully. I am going to give you an address that I want you to remember. Later on, I will ask you to repeat it for me: Apartment 13, Dover Hill Building.

COMPUTATION. The following exercise is useful in assessing the client's computational abilities:

Ask the client to subtract 7 from 100. Have the client continue subtracting 7 from the resulting remainder for several more calculations.

The normal client is able to complete the computation in 1½ minutes with fewer than four errors. Computation skills may be impaired by fatigue, depression, or anxiety.

ABILITY TO READ. Use a copy of a current newspaper to determine the client's reading skills. Be certain that the client is wearing corrective lenses if they are needed for reading. Impairment of the ability to read is called **dyslexia.**

GENERAL KNOWLEDGE. Assessment of general knowledge may include an estimate of what the client has learned in school and his or her awareness of current events. Match inquiries to the educational, sociocultural, and life experiences of the client. Ask questions about presidents, capitals of countries, names of oceans, or current events in newspaper headlines.

INSIGHT AND JUDGMENT. Insight is the client's understanding of and beliefs about the cause and nature of his or her illness. Simple questions such as "Why did you decide to come here [name of health care facility] at this time?" allow clients to explain in their own words a comprehension of their own health status. An example of an interview protocol designed to elicit information about the client's mental representation or beliefs about his or her health or illness follows:

When did you first notice the problem?

What do you think this problem does to you?

How severe do you think this problem is?

What do you feel is causing the problem?

Have you noticed any troubling symptoms or feelings?

What do you think is the best treatment for this problem?

MINI–MENTAL STATUS EXAMINATION

Maximum Score	Score	
		Orientation
5	( )	What is the (year)(season)(date)(day)(month)?
5	( )	Where are we:(state)(country)(town)(hospital)(floor)?
		Registration
3	( )	Name three objects: 1 second to say each. Then ask the client after you have said them. Give 1 point for each correct answer. Then repeat them until all three are learned. Count trials and record.
		Attention and calculation
5	( )	Serial 7's. 1 point for each correct. Stop after five answers. Alternatively spell "world" backward.
		Recall
3	( )	Ask for three objects repeated above. Give 1 point for each correct.
		Language
9	( )	Name a pencil and a watch (2 points)
		Repeat the following: "No ifs, ands, or buts" (1 point)
		Follow a three-stage command:
		"Take a paper in your right hand, fold it in half, and put it on the floor" (3 points)
		Read and obey the following:
		Close your eyes. (1 point)
		Write a sentence. (1 point)
		Copy design. (1 point)
30		Total score

ASSESS level of consciousness along a continuum

Alert	Drowsy	Stupor	Coma

Instructions for administration of mini–mental state examination
Orientation

(1) Ask for the date. Then ask specifically for parts omitted, for example, "Can you also tell me what season it is?" One point for each correct.

(2) Ask in turn "Can you tell me the name of this hospital (etc.)?" One point for each.

Registration

Ask the client if you may test memory. Then say the names of three unrelated objects, clearly and slowly, about 1 second for each. After you have said all three, ask the client to repeat them. This first repetition determines the score (0-3), but keep saying them until all three are repeated, up to six trials. If all three cannot be learned, recall cannot be meaningfully tested.

Attention and calculation

Ask the client to begin with 100 and count backward by 7. Stop after five subtractions (93, 86, 79, 72, 65). Score the total number of correct answers. If the client cannot or will not perform this task, ask him or her to spell the word "world" backward. The score is the number of letters in correct order, e.g., dlrow = 5, dlorw = 3.

Recall

Ask the client to recall the three words you previously asked him or her to remember. Score 0-3.

From Folstein MF, Folstein SE, McHugh PR: "Mini–mental state": a practical method for grading the cognitive state of patients for the clinician, *J Psychiatr Res* 12:189-198, 1975.

MINI–MENTAL STATUS EXAMINATION—cont'd

Language

Naming: Show the client a wristwatch and ask what it is. Repeat for pencil. Score 0-2.

Repetition: Ask the patient to repeat the sentence after you. Allow only one trial. Score 0 or 1.

Three-stage command: Give the client a piece of plain blank paper, and repeat the command. Score 1 point for each part correctly executed.

Reading: On a blank piece of paper, print the sentence "Close your eyes" in letters large enough for the client to see clearly. Ask the client to read it and do what it says. Score 1 point only if the client actually closes his or her eyes.

Writing: Give the client a blank piece of paper, and ask him or her to write a sentence for you. Do not dictate a sentence; it is to be written spontaneously. It must contain a subject and verb and be sensible. Correct grammar and punctuation are not necessary.

Copying: On a clean piece of paper, draw intersecting pentagons, each side about 1 inch, and ask the client to copy it exactly as it is. All 10 angles must be present and 2 must intersect to score 1 point. Tremor and rotation are ignored.

Estimate the client's level of sensorium along a continuum, from alert on the left to coma on the right.

Judgment is a skill necessary for evaluation, assessment, and decision-making, particularly in those situations in which two or more experiences are related to one another. The individual who is able to evaluate a situation and determine the appropriate reaction(s) is said to have good judgment or reasoning ability. Assess judgment through the client's expressed attitudes to his or her social, physical, occupational, and domestic status and plans for the future.

Judgment may be impaired in highly charged emotional states, mental retardation, organic mental disorder, schizophrenia, effects of drugs and alcohol, and anxiety. Two examples of questions that elicit judgment skills follow:

What would you do if you were in a theater when fire broke out?

What would you do if you found four stamped, addressed envelopes?

THOUGHT PROCESSES. Verbal and nonverbal expressions are used to assess the client's ability to think logically and coherently and in a goal-directed sequence.

Screening Tests

Mini–mental status examination. Using the Mini–Mental Status Examination (MMSE) (see box on p. 622), ask the client the 11 questions. Score items so that a score of 30 indicates optimal function. The test takes about 10 minutes to administer to a client with normal mental status functioning.

Glasgow Coma Scale. The Glasgow Coma Scale is an assessment tool that rates level of consciousness by assigning a numerical score to three behavioral evaluations: eye opening, verbal response, and motor re-

ponse. The score is the sum of these ratings (Table 19-4). A person with normal consciousness would obtain a score of 14.

Special Tests and Procedures

Data from psychological tests to assess brain damage are more reliable than behavioral observations, although both examine the same functions, such as the

TABLE 19-4

Glasgow Coma Scale—Record of Individual Recovering from Coma

	Score		Day 1	2	3	4	5
Eye opening response	Spontaneous opening	4					x
	To verbal stimuli	3				x	
	To pain	2	x	x	x		
	None	1					
Most appropriate verbal response	Oriented	5					x
	Confused	4					
	Inappropriate words	3				x	
	Incoherent	2		x	x		
	None	1	x				
Most integral motor response (arm)	Obeys commands	5				x	x
	Localizes pain	3					
	Flexion to pain	4		x	x		
	Extension to pain	2	x				
	None	1					
TOTAL SCORE			5	8	8	11	14

From Teasdale G, Jennett B: *Lancet* 2:81, 1974.

Examination Step-by-Step

There is no one method for conducting the neurological examination. Each examiner may develop his or her own method. If abnormalities are found, a more complete examination of that area is necessary. The order below is a logical one for performing the complete mental status and neurological examination.

1. During the interview, assess cerebral function:
   —Observe appearance and behavior for appropriateness to the situation.
   —Assess mental status for orientation to person, place, and time; attention span; and calculation.
   —Assess recent and remote memory and abstract reasoning.
   —Assess emotional status, observing affect, mood, thought content, and expression of ideas.
   —Assess communication skills; ability to express oneself and to listen; clarity of expression.
2. With the client standing:
   —Observe gait.
   —Assess Romberg's sign (standing with feet slightly apart, eyes closed).
   —Observe heel-to-toe walking (tandem gait, toe-walking, heel-walking).
   —Test standing on one foot, then the other; hopping on each foot.
   —Assess deep knee bend (optional).
3. With the client sitting, examine the following regions in a head-to-toe direction:

Head and face:
   —Observe facial symmetry (CN VII).
   —Have client frown, smile, puff cheeks, close eyes tightly, and resist examiner opening eyes.
   —Ask client, with eyes closed, to indicate when and where he or she is touched with a cotton wisp on three areas of the face innervated by CN V.
   —Ask client, with eyes closed, to indicate "sharp" or "dull" sensation when touched with a pin on three areas of the face innervated by CN V.

Eyes:
   —Observe symmetry of lids, palpebral fissures (CN III).
   —Observe symmetry of pupillary light reflex and pupil response (direct and consensual) to light and accommodation.
   —Test extraocular movements (CN III, IV, VI) for six fields of gaze.

   —Assess visual acuity using Snellen chart (CN II).
   —Test visual fields by confrontation, having client indicate when examiner's fingers come into peripheral vision in eight visual fields.
   —Use ophthalmoscope to examine CN II.

Ears:
   —Test hearing acuity using Weber and Rinne tests (CN VIII).

Nose:
   —Test smell (CN I) (not done in screening examination).

Mouth and throat:
   —Observe symmetrical rise of soft palate with "ah" swallow (CN IX and X).
   —Assess jaw strength and symmetry (CN V).
   —Assess tongue strength (CN XII).
   —Test taste sensations (CN VII and IX) (not done in screeening examination).

Neck:
   —Test trapezius and sternocleidomastoid strength (CN XI)
4. Assess cerebellar function and proprioception:
   —Observe rapid alternating movements (upper and lower extremities).
   —Perform finger-to-nose test.
   —Perform finger-to-thumb test.
   —Perform heel-down-shin test.
5. Test sensory function with client's eyes closed:
   —Assess light touch and pain on each extremity from distal to proximal.
   —Test position sense.
   —Check vibration sense.
   —Test stereognosis.
   —Test graphesthesia.
   —Assess two-point discrimination.
6. Assess deep tendon reflexes:
   —Test biceps reflex.
   —Assess brachioradialis reflex.
   —Test triceps reflex.
   —Assess patellar reflex.
   —Assess ankle jerk reflex.
   —Assess plantar reflex.
   Not tested in a screening examination:
Extinction
Reflexes: corneal, abdominal, cremasteric, gluteal

speed of response, level of comprehension, and use of language. Neuropsychological testing assesses visual memory and psychomotor skills in depth by using a wide range of standardized tests. Testing is performed by a skilled clinician specifically trained to administer and interpret these tests.

VARIATIONS FROM HEALTH

Variations in Sensory Function

Anosmia is the loss of the sense of smell. **Hyposmia** is an impaired sense of smell. In hyposmia, flavor perception is also impaired since it is a synthesis of smell, taste, and perceptions from stimulation of end organs in the mouth and pharynx. The individual with CN I (olfactory) involvement may complain only of loss of the sense of taste.

Ageusia is the loss of taste or the lack of ability to discriminate sweet, sour, salty, and bitter tastes.

Shingles (herpes zoster) is caused by the herpes varicella-zoster virus, the same virus that causes chickenpox. The virus may remain dormant in the dorsal root ganglia of some spinal nerves. With increasing age the immune system may not be as effective in keeping it inactive, and the reactivated virus causes shingles. Shingles appears on the skin as a painful papulovesicular rash that follows the course of peripheral, and sometimes cranial, nerves. No specific treatment is available and these lesions may ulcerate and **keratinize**. Neuralgia or anesthesia may remain after the rash disappears.

Variations in Motor Function

Multiple sclerosis (MS) is a demyelinating disease that involves deterioration of myelin sheaths of neurons in the central nervous system. Without the myelin, nerve impulses become short-circuited and do not reach their intended destinations. Evidence exists that this is an autoimmune disease triggered by a virus.

Symptoms of MS first appear between the ages of 20 to 40 years. The disease may progress rapidly or slowly. Symptoms vary but may include muscle weakness or paralysis, partial loss of sensation, visual changes, loss of bowel and bladder control, and loss of spinal cord reflexes. Some individuals experience remissions, when symptoms disappear for an unpredictable period of time. No cure exists for MS at present.

Table 19-5 summarizes the causes and characteristics of upper and lower motor neuron lesions.

Bell's palsy is a facial nerve palsy of acute onset and unknown cause. Evidence of this lower motor neuron disorder, which results in paralysis of an entire side of the face, is the closing of only one eye when the client attempts to close both eyes. When the client tries to raise the eyebrows, the eyebrow on the affected side does not rise and the forehead does not wrinkle. The client may exhibit overflow of tears or be unable to hold fluids orally because of a sagging mouth.

Neck trauma is the most frequent cause of dysfunction of the spinal accessory nerve (CN XI). Torticollis is a condition of intermittent or constant contraction of the sternocleidomastoid muscle in which the head is flexed forward and the chin is rotated away from the affected side.

A cerebrovascular accident (CVA), or stroke, is damage to a blood vessel in the brain that results in lack of oxygen to that part of the brain. Either a blood clot (thrombosis) or hemorrhage, often from the rupture of an aneurysm, causes the interruption in circulation. The symptoms depend on the part of the brain affected. Onset of symptoms may be slow if a clot formation decreases blood flow before complete occlusion occurs. In the case of a ruptured aneurysm, however, onset may be sudden. Recovery from a CVA depends largely on its location and the extent of damage. In many individuals, especially those who begin rehabilitation early, the brain is able to establish new pathways to compensate for damaged areas.

TABLE 19-5

Deep Tendon Reflex and Muscle Changes in Upper and Lower Motor Neuron Lesions

Lesion	Common cause	Characteristics
Upper motor neuron lesion (corticospinal tract)	Cerebral vascular occlusion	Hyperreflexia
	Cerebral neoplasm	Paralysis of voluntary movement
Spasticity		
Usually includes damage to parallel pathways	Trauma	Babinski's sign present
		Minimal muscle atrophy
Lower motor neuron lesion (anterior horn cell, somatic motor part of cranial nerves)	Poliomyelitis	Muscle weakness
	Neoplasm	Paralysis
	Trauma	Muscle atrophy
		Hyporeflexia or absent reflexes
		Fasciculations

Lesions of the Dominant Cerebral Hemisphere

Aphasia, the inability to comprehend or use language symbols, is caused by a lesion in the cortical areas necessary for speech or by neural connections in the cerebral hemisphere dominant for speech. The most common cerebral pathological condition associated with aphasia is vascular disease. Data show that 95% of persons who are right-handed and have a language deficit have lesions of the left cerebral hemisphere, whereas 70% of left-handed individuals with language impairment also have a lesion of the left cerebral hemisphere.

If the motor cortex for speech is involved, the person can understand written and spoken words but cannot contract the muscles used for speech to form words properly. Damage to the interpretation area of the cortex for speech results in the inability to comprehend the meaning of spoken words. Aphasia often accompanies **agnosia,** the inability to recognize once-familiar objects.

Lesions of Nondominant Cerebral Hemisphere

A disturbance in the ability to perform a purposeful act when comprehension is intact is termed **apraxia.** For example, if given a fork, the client may be unable to use it to eat; or the client may be unable to dress or button a shirt.

COMPARISON OF DISORDERS OF CEREBELLUM, POSTERIOR COLUMNS, AND VESTIBULAR APPARATUS

Cerebellar dysfunction

Ataxia present with eyes opened or closed
Clumsiness
Poor coordination
Tremor
Hypotonia
Nystagmus

Posterior column dysfunction

Ataxia made worse with eyes closed
Positive Romberg's sign (swaying with eyes closed)
Inability to recognize limb position
Loss of two-point discrimination
Astereognosis
Loss of vibratory sense

Vestibular apparatus dysfunction

Nystagmus
Nausea
Vomiting
Ataxia present with eyes opened and closed

Variations in Cerebellar Function

The client with cerebellar disease has difficulty with rapid patting and supination-pronation alterations. The problem involves both smooth control of muscles and the starting and stopping of motion. Clumsiness of movement and irregular timing are characteristic of affected individuals.

Dyssynergia (impairment of muscle coordination or of the ability to perform movements smoothly) is loss of cerebellar function and results in intention tremor, or hypotonia.

Abnormalities of muscle tone, gait, speech, and nystagmus in lateral gaze may also indicate cerebellar dysfunction. Disturbances in the timing of movements may also be evident.

Ataxia is the impairment of position sense.

The client with a cerebellar gait walks with a wide base; the trunk and head are held rigidly; the legs bend at the hips; arm movements are not coordinated with the stride; the client lurches and reels, frequently falling.

The client with cerebellar speech has slow, hesitant, or dysarthric verbalization.

Pathological Reflexes

Reflexes may be altered in pathophysiological changes involving the sensory pathways from the tendons and muscles or the motor component.

Babinski reflex. The Babinski reflex is dorsiflexion of the great toe and fanning of the other toes. Lesions of the pyramidal tract or motor nerves may be present in the client with a Babinski reflex.

Grasp reflex (Figure 19-44). This reflex, while present in individuals with widespread brain damage, is normal in infants less than 4 months of age. To test the grasp reflex, place your index finger and middle finger in the client's palm, entering between the client's thumb and the index finger. Gently withdraw your fingers, pulling them across the skin of the client's palm. A positive response consists of the client's grasping of your fingers.

Lesions of Corticospinal Tract

Clients with lesions of the corticospinal tract perform fine movements of the hands, such as picking up coins or pencils, slowly. Also, they are able to perform thumb-to-finger opposition less rapidly.

Signs of meningeal irritation. Meningeal irritation most commonly results from infection or intracranial hemorrhages. **Nuchal rigidity** (stiff neck) is a common sign of meningitis and may be demonstrated by flexing the cervical spine, which produces discomfort in the posterior neck. In addition, the client cannot touch his or her chin to chest.

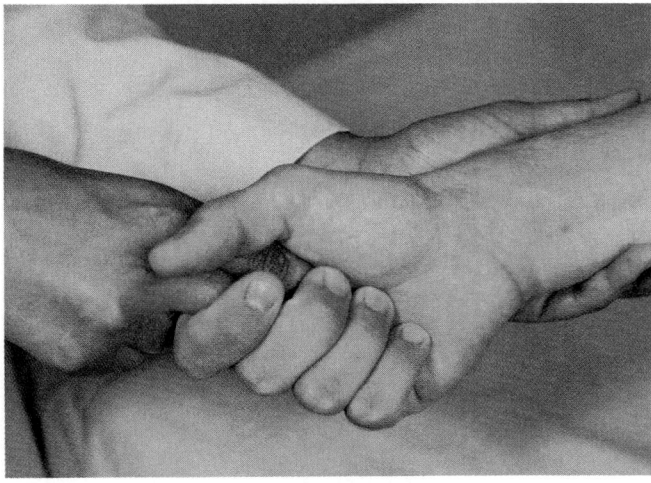

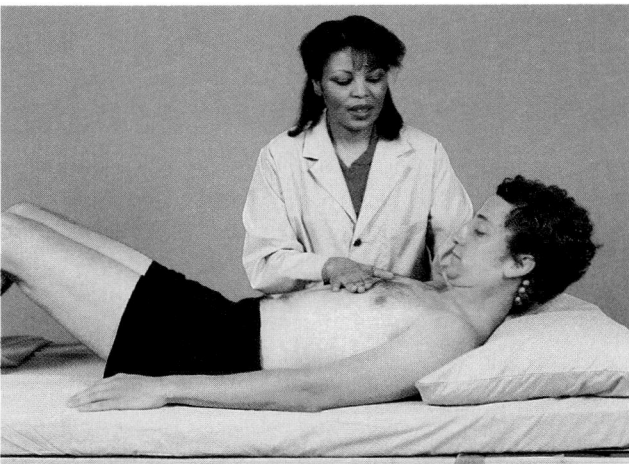

FIGURE 19-45 Eliciting Brudzinski's sign. With meningeal irritation, pain is elicited when the head is flexed.

FIGURE 19-44 Eliciting the grasp reflex. **A,** Examiner places the index and middle finger in client's palm and gently withdraws them. **B,** Positive response consists of client grasping the examiner's fingers.

Brudzinski's sign (Figure 19-45) is elicited with the client supine. Lift the client's head toward the sternum. The person with meningeal irritation will resist the movement and may flex the hips and knees. The movement is commonly accompanied by pain in the spine.

Variations in Mental Status

Confabulation is an attempt by the client to "fill in the gaps" with fabricated answers when he or she is unable to remember.

A client who rapidly skips from one complete idea to another without any relationship to the preceding idea may be manifesting **flight of ideas.**

It is important to carefully observe the client's affect to see whether it is congruent with the individual's verbal content. For example, a client who expresses little or no emotion while verbalizing the desire for self-harm or harm to others is demonstrating an incongruence between affect and verbal content.

Organic brain syndromes. Organic brain syndrome describes a symptom complex that causes an impairment of orientation, memory, or regulation of emotions. Affective symptoms, **delusions,** hallucinations, and obsessions may also be present. An acute brain syndrome **(delirium)** is one of short duration that is usually reversible. A chronic brain syndrome **(dementia)** is long-standing and often progressive in nature, with a less favorable prognosis.

Alzheimer's disease is a progressive, incurable form of mental deterioration that usually affects the elderly. Although the cause is not known, certain environmental factors bring out a genetic predisposition to this disease. Symptoms include confusion, forgetfulness, and loss of ability to execute simple tasks. As the disease progresses, a total loss of memory occurs. On autopsy the cerebral cortex shows structural changes, including increased fibrous tissue.

Affective (mood) disorders. The client with an affective disorder runs the gamut from depression to exaggerated **euphoria,** or mania. The highs and lows show little correlation with the person's life situation.

A **bipolar disorder** is diagnosed when mania is present or is indicated by the health history, whether or not depression occurs. Depression that occurs in the absence of mania is known as major **depression** (unipolar).

Schizophrenic disorders. Hallucinations and delusions are the diagnostic signposts of schizophrenia. Delusions are false beliefs that are improbable in nature. Hallucinations are visual perceptions for which no external stimuli can be ascertained. Hallucinations may be suspected in the person who appears preoccupied.

Anxiety. The client who demonstrates symptoms of severe anxiety has recurrent periods of abrupt onset anxiety that end without intervention. The client com-

plains of fright without a known object. The autonomic nervous system is activated, possibly resulting in such signs and symptoms as palpitations, breathlessness, dizziness, feeling of impending doom, headache, fatigue, nausea and vomiting, and diarrhea.

Phobia. Phobia is a highly disturbing, recurring, and unrealistic fear that may relate to any situation or object.

Sample Documentation

DOCUMENTATION

Health history

Client states wife died 3 months ago after a short illness and since then he has felt sad and lonely. He feels tired and listless all day. Admits to sleeping 2 to 3 hours per night. Reports a 10-pound weight gain in the past 2 months, which he attributes to increased intake of "junk" food, drinking 4 to 6 cans of beer per evening, and reduced physical activity. He works on the assembly line and reports no job absences or injuries in the last 5 years. Denies any history of mental illness, suicidal thoughts, or serious depression. Reports no sensory, motor, or coordination changes.

Physical examination

Mental status: Appears well-groomed, appropriate dress, slightly slumped posture. Gazing at the floor

through most of the interview. Responds to questions appropriately. Oriented, alert, and cooperative throughout the exam. Recent and remote memory intact.

CN II-XII: Intact (CN I not tested).

Cerebellar: Finger-to-nose, heel-to-shin, alternating rhythms done easily but slowly. Romberg negative. Able to stand on each foot, hop, do deep knee bend, heel-to-toe walk without difficulty.

Face and extremities sensitive to light touch, localization, and pain. Vibration and position sense intact in each extremity. Stereognosis: able to identify safety pin.

DTRs: Bilaterally symmetrical, 1+, plantar reflex present.

Nursing Diagnosis   *THE NEXT STEP*

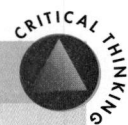

CRITICAL THINKING

Nursing diagnoses that could apply to assessment of and alterations in the neurological system include, but are not limited to, the following ones.

HIGH RISK FOR ASPIRATION The state in which an individual is at risk for entry of gastric secretions, oropharyngeal secretions, or exogenous food or fluids into tracheobronchial passages due to dysfunction or absence of normal protective mechanisms.

Defining Characteristics (risk factors)

- Reduced level of consciousness
- Depressed cough and gag reflex
- Situations hindering elevation of upper body

ALTERED NUTRITION: LESS THAN BODY REQUIREMENTS The state in which an individual experiences an intake of nutrients insufficient to meet metabolic needs.

Defining Characteristics

- Twenty percent or more under ideal body weight
- Reported or observed inadequate food intake relative to minimum daily requirements
- Weight loss (with or without adequate intake)
- Fatigue
- Muscle weakness

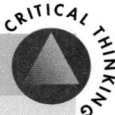

Nursing Diagnosis   *THE NEXT STEP—cont'd*

Related Factors

- Altered taste sensation
- Inability to prepare/procure food
- Knowledge deficit of daily requirements
- Emotional stress
- Muscle weakness (mastication and swallowing)
- Social isolation

HIGH RISK FOR IMPAIRED SKIN INTEGRITY The state in which an individual's skin is at risk of being adversely altered.

Defining Characteristics (risk factors)

- Physical immobilization
- Excretions/secretions on skin
- Altered sensation/consciousness
- Psychogenic factors
- Hypothermia/hyperthermia
- Decreased fatty tissue
- Skeletal prominence

BOWEL INCONTINENCE The state in which an individual experiences a change in normal bowel habits characterized by involuntary passage of stool.

Defining Characteristics

- Involuntary passage of stool

Related Factors

- Loss of sphincter control
- Cognitive/perceptual impairment

TOTAL INCONTINENCE (URINARY) The state in which an individual experiences a continuous and unpredictable loss of urine.

Defining Characteristics

- Constant flow of urine at unpredictable times without distention (or uninhibited bladder contractions/spasms)
- Unsuccessful incontinence refractory treatments
- Nocturia
- Lack of perineal or bladder filling awareness
- Unawareness of incontinence

Related Factors

- Neuropathy (preventing transmission of reflex indicating bladder fullness)
- Neurological dysfunction (triggering micturation at unpredictable times)
- Independent contraction of detrusor reflex (resulting from surgery)
- Trauma (affecting spinal cord)

IMPAIRED PHYSICAL MOBILITY The state in which an individual experiences a limitation of ability for independent physical movement.

Defining Characteristics

- Inability to purposefully move within the physical environment (bed mobility, transfers, ambulation)
- Limited active joint range of motion
- Decreased muscle strength, control, and/or mass

Continued.

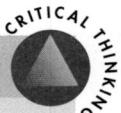

Nursing Diagnosis *THE NEXT STEP—cont'd*

- Impaired coordination
- Imposed restriction of movement (mechanical or medical protocol restrictions)
- Level I: requires use of equipment or device
- Level II: requires help from another person(s): assistance, supervision, or teaching
- Level III: requires help from another person(s) and equipment or device
- Level IV: is dependent and does not participate in movement

Related Factors

- Intolerance to physical activity
- Pain
- Uncompensated perceptual-cognitive, musculoskeletal, or neuromuscular impairment
- Depression
- Anxiety

DIVERSIONAL ACTIVITY DEFICIT The state in which an individual experiences a decreased stimulation from or interest or engagement in recreational or leisure activities.

Defining Characteristics

- Boredom
- Desire for something to do, to read, etc.
- Usual hobbies cannot be undertaken in hospital

Related Factors

- Environmental lack of diversional activity
- Long-term hospitalization
- Frequent, lengthy treatments

SELF-CARE DEFICIT, BATHING/HYGIENE The state in which one experiences an impaired ability to perform or complete bathing/hygiene activities for oneself.

Defining Characteristics

- Inability to wash body or body parts
- Inability to obtain or get to water source
- Inability to regulate temperature or flow
- Level I: requires use of equipment or devices
- Level II: requires help from another person(s): assistance, supervision, teaching
- Level III: requires help from another person(s) and equipment or device
- Level IV: is dependent and does not participate in self-bathing/hygiene

Related Factors

- Intolerance to activity
- Pain
- Uncompensated perceptual-cognitive, musculoskeletal, or neuromuscular impairment
- Depression
- Anxiety

SELF-CARE DEFICIT, DRESSING/GROOMING The state in which one experiences an impaired ability to perform or complete dressing and grooming activities for oneself.

Defining Characteristics

- Impaired ability to put on or take off necessary items of clothing
- Impaired ability to obtain or replace articles of clothing, fasten clothing, and maintain appearance at a satisfactory level
- Specify degree of deficit described in Levels I-IV (see preceding section)

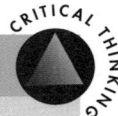

Nursing Diagnosis   *THE NEXT STEP—cont'd*

Related Factors

- Intolerance to activity
- Pain
- Uncompensated perceptual-cognitive, musculoskeletal, or neuromuscular impairment
- Depression
- Anxiety

SENSORY-PERCEPTUAL ALTERATIONS (VISUAL, AUDITORY) The state in which an individual experiences a change in the amount or patterning of incoming stimuli accompanied by a diminished, exaggerated, distorted, or impaired response to such stimuli.

Defining Characteristics

- Alert with periodic disorientation, general confusion, or nocturnal confusion
- Hallucination
- Apathy
- Auditory, visual, reality-orienting, or time-orienting input reduced or absent
- Limited proprioceptive input
- Presence of uncompensated visual or hearing deficits

Related Factors

- Isolation (restricted environment)
- Therapeutic environmental restriction (isolation, bedrest, confining illness)
- Socially restricted environment (institutionalization, homebound)
- Uncompensated visual or hearing deficit
- Impaired communication

UNILATERAL NEGLECT The state in which an individual is perceptually unaware of and inattentive to one side of the body.

Defining Characteristics

- Consistent inattention to stimuli on affected side
- Inadequate self-care of affected side
- Lack of positioning and/or safety precautions in regard to affected side
- Does not look toward affected side
- Leaves food on plate on affected side

Related Factors

- Effects of disturbed perceptual abilities (e.g., one-sided blindness or neurological damage)

ANXIETY A vague, uneasy feeling, the source of which is often nonspecific or unknown to the individual.

Defining Characteristics

- Verbalizes apprehension, uncertainty, fear, distress, worry
- Verbalizes painful and persistent feelings of increased helplessness, inadequacy, regret
- Overexcited, rattled, jittery, scared
- Restlessness, focus on self, insomnia, increased perspiration
- Increased wariness, glancing about, poor eye contact, facial tension, voice quivering
- Increased tension, foot shuffling, hand/arm movements, trembling, hand tremor, shakiness

Related Factors

- Perceived threat to self-concept, health status, socioeconomic status, role functioning, interaction patterns, or environment
- Perceived threat of death

Continued.

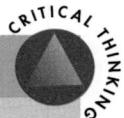

Nursing Diagnosis   *THE NEXT STEP—cont'd*

- Unconscious conflict (essential values, life goals)
- Intepersonal transmission/contagion

HOPELESSNESS The subjective state in which an individual sees limited or no alternatives or personal choices available and is unable to mobilize energy on own behalf.

Defining Characteristics

- Passivity
- Decreased verbalization
- Decreased affect
- Verbalization of despondent or hopeless content (e.g., "I can't," sighing)
- Lack of initiative
- Decreased response to stimuli
- Lack of involvement in care/passively allowing care
- Turning away from speaker
- Closing eyes
- Shrugging in response to speaker
- Decreased appetite
- Increased sleep

Related Factors

- Prolonged activity restriction (creating isolation)
- Failing or deteriorating physiological condition
- Long-term stress
- Abandonment

BODY IMAGE DISTURBANCE Disruption in the way one perceives one's body image.

Defining Characteristics

- Verbalized actual or perceived change in structure and/or function of body or body part
- Verbalized fear of rejection or reaction by others
- Repeated verbalizations focusing on past strengths, function, or appearance
- Verbalized negative feelings about body (dirty, big, small, unsightly)
- Verbalized feelings of helplessness, hopelessness, powerlessness in relation to body
- Preoccupation with change in body or loss of part
- Depersonalization of part or loss by impersonal pronoun
- Extension of body boundary to incorporate environmental objects (e.g., machines, oxygen, respirator)
- Refusal to verify actual change in body or body part
- Guilt, shame
- Emphasis on remaining strengths or heightened achievement
- Repeated expressions of negative feeling about loss of body fluids, addition of body fluids or machines
- Change in ability to estimate spatial relationship of body to environment

Related Factors

- Nonintegration of change (in body characteristics, function, or limits)
- Perceived developmental imperfections

SOCIAL ISOLATION Aloneness experienced by an individual and perceived as imposed by others and as a negative or threatened state.

Defining Characteristics

- Expresses feelings of aloneness imposed by others, rejection, or feelings of difference from others
- Expresses values acceptable to subculture but unacceptable to dominant cultural group

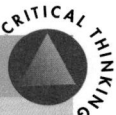

Nursing Diagnosis *THE NEXT STEP—cont'd*

- Perceived inadequacy of significant purpose in life or absence of purpose in life
- Perceived inability to meet expectations of others or insecurity in public
- Observed or expressed interests/activities inappropriate to the developmental age/stage
- Shows behavior unaccepted by dominant cultural group
- Seeks to be alone or to exist in a subculture
- Sad, dull affect
- Uncommunicative, withdrawn, no eye contact
- Projects hostility in voice, behavior
- Preoccupation with own thoughts; repetitive, meaningless actions
- Absence of supportive significant other(s): family, friends, group
- Apathy
- Verbalization of isolation from others
- Low contact with peers
- Absent or limited contact with community
- Lack of contact with or absence of significant others
- Seclusion

Related Factors

- Impaired mobility
- Therapeutic isolation
- Sociocultural dissonance
- Insufficient community resources
- Body image disturbance
- Fear (environmental hazards, violence)

IMPAIRED VERBAL COMMUNICATION The state in which an individual experiences a decreased or absent ability to use or understand language in human interaction.

Defining Characteristics

- Speaks or verbalizes with difficulty
- Does not, or cannot, speak
- Stuttering
- Slurring
- Difficulty forming words or sentence
- Difficulty expressing thought verbally
- Inappropriate verbalization
- Dyspnea
- Disorientation

Related Factors

- Decrease in circulation to the brain
- Physical barrier (brain tumor, tracheostomy, intubation)
- Psychological barrier (psychosis, lack of stimuli)
- Developmental or age-related

SEXUAL DYSFUNCTION The state in which an individual experiences a change in sexual function that is viewed as unsatisfying, unrewarding, or inadequate.

Defining Characteristics

- Verbalizations of problem in sexuality
- Alterations in achieving perceived sex role
- Actual or perceived limitation imposed by disease and/or therapy
- Alteration in achieving sexual satisfaction
- Inability to achieve desired sexual satisfaction

Continued.

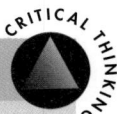

Nursing Diagnosis   *THE NEXT STEP—cont'd*

Related Factors

- Physical or psychosocial abuse
- Lack of privacy
- Misinformation
- Lack of significant other
- Altered body structure or function (disease processes, trauma)

INEFFECTIVE COPING (INDIVIDUAL) Impairment of adaptive behaviors and problem-solving abilities of a person in meeting life's demands and roles.

Defining Characteristics

- Verbalization of inability to cope
- Inability to ask for help
- Anxiety, fear, anger, irritability, tension
- Presence of life stress
- Inability to meet role expectations
- Inability to meet basic needs
- Alteration in societal participation
- Destructive behavior toward self and others
- Inappropriate or ineffective use of defense mechanisms
- Change in usual communication patterns
- High rate of accidents
- Verbal manipulation
- Excess food intake, alcohol consumption; smoking
- Digestive, bowel, appetite disturbance: chronic fatigue or sleep-pattern disturbance

Related Factors

- Situational crises
- Maturational crises
- Personal vulnerability
- Knowledge deficit
- Problem-solving skills deficit

Clinical Application

Mrs. W. a 60-year-old female, visits her doctor complaining of tension headaches. She states they have become more frequent in the last month, since her husband died. Sometimes they last for 2-3 days and are accompanied by fatigue and dizziness. "All I can do is stay in bed." She denies head injuries, seizures, or tremors. No weakness, numbness or tingling, difficulty swallowing, or speaking. Has no past history of cerebral vascular incidents, transient ischemic attacks, spinal cord injury, meningitis, or alcoholism. Denies any history of mental illness, suicidal thoughts, or serious depression. A physical exam is completed.

SUBJECTIVE DATA: Client complains of:
Headaches that last 2-3 days
Nausea and dizziness
Being unable to leave bed when experiencing a headache
No prior neurological history

OBJECTIVE DATA:
Weight: 125 lbs
Client's previous weight 1 year ago 145 lbs
Mental status: Appears well groomed, behavior and speech appropriate
Alert and oriented × 3
Answers all questions appropriately and cooperatively throughout the exam
Recent and remote memory intact

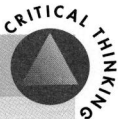

Nursing Diagnosis *THE NEXT STEP—cont'd*

Cranial nerves:

II Vision 20/150 OS, 20/100 OD, wears glasses for nearsightedness, peripheral fields intact, fundi normal

III, IV, VI EOMs intact, no ptosis or nystagmus, pupil equal, round, react to light and accommodation (PERRLA)

V Sensation intact and equal bilaterally, jaw strength equal bilaterally

VII Facial muscle intact and symmetrical

VIII Whispered words heard bilaterally, Weber midline, Rinne positive—(AC > BC)

IX, X Swallowing intact, gag reflex intact, uvula rises in midline on phonation

XI Shoulder shrug and head movement strong and equal bilaterally

XII Tongue midline, no tremors

Cerebellar: Finger-to-nose, heel-to-shin, alternating rhythms done easily, but slowly. Rhomberg negative. Gait normal. Able to stand on each foot, hop, and do deep knee bend.

Sensory: Extremities sensitive to light touch, localization, and pain. Vibration and position sense intact bilaterally upper and lower extremities. Stereognosis: able to identify a paper clip. DTRs: Bilaterally symmetrical, 1+, plantar reflex present.

NURSING DIAGNOSES

Altered nutrition: less than body requirement related to emotional stress.

Defining Characteristics

- Twenty percent or more under ideal body weight
- Weight loss of 20 lbs recently
- Fatigue

Anxiety related to perceived threat to role functioning.

Defining Characteristics

- Verbalized apprehension and uncertainty about the future
- Focuses on self by complaint of headaches

Hopelessness related to prolonged activity restriction (creating isolation).

Defining Characteristics

- Lack of initiative
- Decreased appetite
- Increased sleep

Ineffective coping (individual) related to situational crisis (death of spouse).

Defining Characteristics

- Anxiety, fear of future
- Presence of life stress
- Alteration in societal participation

GLOSSARY

affect Outwardly manifested emotional range attached to ideas. *Appropriate affect:* emotional tone in harmony with the accompanying idea, thought, or verbalization. *Blunted affect:* disturbance manifested by a severe reduction in the intensity of affect. *Flat affect:* absence or near-absence of any signs of affective expression. *Inappropriate affect:* incongruence between the emotional feeling tone and the idea, thought, or speech accompanying it. *Labile affect:* rapid changes in emotional feeling tone that are unrelated to external stimuli.

afferent neuron Any neuron that transmits nerve impulses from the periphery toward the central nervous system (sensory).

ageusia Loss of the sensation of taste or of the ability to discriminate sweet, sour, salty, and bitter tastes.

agnosia Inability to discriminate sensory stimuli. *Acoustic or auditory agnosia:* impaired ability to recognize familiar sounds. *Tactile agnosia:* impaired ability to recognize familiar objects by touch or feel. *Visual agnosia:* impaired ability to recognize familiar objects by sight. *Somatagnosia:* disturbance in recognition of body parts.

anesthesia Absence of normal sensation, especially sensitivity to pain, as induced by an anesthetic substance or hypnosis or as occurs with traumatic or pathophysiological damage to nerve tissue.

anosmia Inability to smell.

aphasia Dysfunction or loss of the ability to express thoughts by speech, writing, symbols, or signs. *Fluent aphasia:* ability to produce words but with frequent errors in the choice of appropriate words or in the creation of words. *Nonfluent aphasia:* inability to produce words, either in spoken or written form.

apraxia Impairment of the ability to carry out purposeful movement (although muscle and sensory apparatus are intact), such as an inability to draw or construct forms of two or three dimensions.

ataxia Impairment of coordination of muscular activity.

augmentation Technique used to reinforce expression of deep tendon reflexes. The individual isometrically tenses muscles not directly involved in the reflex arc.

autonomic nervous system Part of the peripheral nervous system that regulates involuntary vital function, including the activity of the cardiac muscle, the smooth muscle, and the glands. It has two divisions: (1) the sympathetic nervous system accelerates heart rate, constricts blood vessels, and raises blood pressure; (2) the parasympathetic nervous system slows heart rate, increases intestinal peristalsis and gland activity, and relaxes sphincters.

axon Cylindrical extension of a nerve cell that conducts impulses away from the neuron cell body.

bipolar disorder Affective or mood disorder characterized by periods of mania alternating with periods of depression, with normal mood intervals occurring between the two.

brainstem Portion of the brain that comprises the medulla oblongata, the pons, and the mesencephalon. It performs motor, sensory, and reflex functions and contains the corticospinal and the reticulospinal tracts. The 12 pairs of cranial nerves arise mainly from the brainstem.

cerebellum Part of the brain located in the posterior cranial fossa behind the brainstem. Its functions are concerned with coordinating voluntary muscular activity.

cerebrum Largest part of the brain, consisting of the right and left cerebral hemispheres. Its many functions include movement, sensation, learning, and memory.

concha Body structure that is shell-shaped, such as the cavity in the external ear that surrounds the external auditory canal meatus.

confabulation Fabrication of facts or events in response to questions about situations that are not recalled because of memory impairment.

delirium Clouded state of consciousness; reduction in clarity of awareness of environment accompanied by a reduced capacity to shift, focus, and sustain attention to environmental stimuli.

delusion False belief that is improbable in nature; not influenced by contrary experience or related to the client's cultural and educational background.

dementia Loss of cognitive abilities of sufficient magnitude to interfere with social or occupational functioning. It involves impairment of memory, abstract thinking, or judgment or other disturbance of high cortical function.

dendrite Branching process that extends from the cell body of a neuron. Each neuron usually possesses several dendrites, which receive impulses that are conducted to the cell body.

depression Term used to define (1) a mood, (2) a syndrome, and (3) an illness. The mood of depression is described as dejection and lowering of functional activity; it is a normal experience that may be incurred in response to frustration and loss. The syndrome of depression includes a depressed mood in combination with one or more of the following symptoms: inability to concentrate, anorexia, weight loss, and suicidal ideas. The illness of depression is characterized by the syndrome of depression but lasts longer. Related functional impairment may include the inability to carry on daily activities, particularly work.

dermatome Area on the surface of a body innervated by afferent fibers from one spinal root.

disorientation Lack of awareness as to time, place, or person.

dyslexia Disturbance in understanding the written word; difficulty in reading.

dyssynergia Inability to perform movements smoothly or an impairment in muscle coordination.

efferent neuron Any neuron that transmits nerve impulses from the central nervous system toward the periphery (motor).

endolymph Fluid found in the membranous labyrinth of the internal ear.

euphoria False sense of elation or well-being; pathological elevation of mood. This condition is most notable in clients who are experiencing the manic phase of bipolar disorder.

extinction Loss of touch perception on one side of the body.

extrapyramidal system Tract of motor nerves from the brain to the anterior horns of the spinal cord, except for the fibers of the pyramidal tract. It controls and coordinates the postural, static, supporting, and locomotor mechanisms and causes contractions of muscle groups in sequence or simultaneously.

fasciculation Observable, localized, uncoordinated, uncontrollable twitching of a single muscle group innervated by a single motor nerve fiber or filament.

flight of ideas Nearly continuous flow of rapid speech with abrupt changes from topic to topic. This condition is noted most frequently in organic mental disorders, schizophrenia, and psychotic disorders and as a reaction to stress.

ganglia A type of nerve cell, chiefly collected in groups outside the central nervous system. Individual cells and very small groups abound in association with alimentary organs.

graphesthesia Ability to identify letters or numbers inscribed with a blunt object on the palm of the hand, back, or other areas. Higher cortical integration is required to perform this function.

horn Projection or protuberance of a body structure. Examples include the gray horns of the spinal cord, horn of the hyoid bone, and iliac horn.

hyperesthesia Extreme sensitivity of one of the body's sense organs, such as pain or touch receptors in the skin.

hypoesthesia Abnormal weakness of sensation in response to stimulation of the sensory nerves.

hyposmia Diminished sense of smell.

keratinization Process by which epithelial cells exposed to the external environment lose their moisture and are replaced by horny tissue.

kinesthetic sensation Feeling facilitated by the proprioceptive receptors in the muscles, tendons, and joints.

labile Readily altered, unstable.

lower motor neuron Peripheral neuron with a motor (efferent) function. Its cell body is located in the anterior horns of the spinal cord or brainstem nuclei, and it terminates in skeletal muscles.

mastication Chewing, tearing, or grinding food with the teeth while it becomes mixed with saliva.

mental status examination Record of current findings that includes a description of a client's appearance, behavior, motor activity, speech, alertness, mood, cognition, intelligence, reactions, views, and attitudes.

neuromuscular spindle Any one of a number of small bundles of delicate muscular fibers, enclosed by a capsule, in which sensory nerve fibers terminate. Spindles vary in length from 0.8 to 5 mm, accommodating as many as four large myelinated nerve fibers that pierce the capsule and lose their myelin sheaths.

nuchal rigidity Pertaining to limited range of motion of the cervical spine, usually associated with pain. The term *nuchal* refers to the nape of the neck.

orientation Conscious awareness of person, place, and time.

paresthesia Any subjective sensation, experienced as numbness, tingling, or a "pins and needles" feeling.

perception Awareness of objects and relations that follows stimulation of peripheral sense organs.

pyramidal tract Pathway composed of groups of nerve fibers in the white matter of the spinal cord through which motor impulses are conducted to the anterior horn cells from the opposite side of the brain. These descending fibers regulate the voluntary and reflex activity of the muscles through the anterior horn cells.

reflex Involuntary functioning or movement of any organ or part of the body in response to a particular stimulus. The function or action occurs immediately, without the involvement of the will or consciousness.

reticular activating system Functional system in the brain that is essential for wakefulness, attention, concentration, and introspection. A network of nerve fibers in the thalamus, hypothalamus, brainstem, and cerebral cortex contribute to the system.

stereognosis Faculty of perceiving and understanding the form and nature of objects by the sense of touch. Higher cortical integration is required to perform this function.

stressor Stimulus perceived by the individual or the organism as challenging, threatening, or damaging.

sulcus Shallow groove, depression, or furrow on the surface of an organ, such as one that separates the convolutions of the cerebral hemisphere.

synapse Joining; point of contact between two neurons or between a neuron and an effector organ, across which nerve impulses are transmitted through the action of a neurotransmitter, such as acetylcholine or norepinephrine.

two-point discrimination Ability to sense the simultaneous stimulation of two areas of skin. Higher cortical integration is required to perform this function.

upper motor neuron Long neurons with cell bodies in the motor portion of the cerebral cortex and axons that extend down the spinal cord, terminating at segmental levels of the spinal cord. They transmit impulses to lower motor neurons.

vertigo Illusion of movement, with imagined rotation of one's self *(subjective vertigo)* or of one's surroundings *(objective vertigo)*.

BIBLIOGRAPHY

Alspach JG: *Core curriculum for critical care nursing,* ed 4, Philadelphia, 1991, WB Saunders.

Bates B: *A guide to physical examination and history taking,* ed 5, Philadelphia, 1991, JB Lippincott.

Bowers AC, Thompson JM: *Clinical manual of health assessment,* ed 4, St Louis, 1992, Mosby—Year Book.

DeJong RN and others: *Essentials of the neurological examination,* Philadelphia, 1978, SmithKline Corporation.

Hickey JV: *The clinical practice of neurological and neurosurgical nursing,* ed 3, Philadelphia, 1992, JB Lippincott.

Jones D: *Health assessment manual,* New York, 1986, McGraw-Hill.

Lewis SM, Collier IC: *Medical-surgical nursing: assessment and management of clinical problems,* ed 3, St Louis, 1992, Mosby—Year Book.

Matthews PJ, Carlson CE: *Spinal cord injury: a guide to rehabilitation nursing,* Rockville, Md, 1987, Aspen Publications.

Potter P: *Pocket guide to physical assessment,* ed 2, St Louis, 1990, Mosby—Year Book.

Rudy EB, Gray VR: *Handbook of health assessment,* ed 3, Norwalk, Conn, 1991, Appleton & Lange.

Scanlon VC, Sanders T: *Essentials of anatomy and physiology,* Philadelphia, 1991, FA Davis.

Seidel H and others: *Mosby's guide to physical examination,* St Louis, 1991, Mosby—Year Book.

Snyder M: *A guide to neurological and neurosurgical nursing,* ed 2, Albany, NY, 1991, Delmar Publishers.

Sparks SM, Taylor CM: *Nursing diagnosis reference manual,* Springhouse, Pa, 1991, Springhouse Corporation.

Stuart GW, Sundeen SJ: *Principles and practice of psychiatric nursing,* ed 3, St Louis, 1987, Mosby—Year Book.

Teasdale G, Jennett B: Assessment of coma and impaired consciousness: a practical scale, *Lancet* 2:81, 1974.

Thompson JM and others: *Mosby's manual of clinical nursing,* ed 2, St Louis, 1989, Mosby—Year Book.

Watson C: *Basic human neuroanatomy: an introductory atlas,* ed 4, Boston, 1991, Little, Brown.

Male Genitalia

PURPOSE OF THE EXAMINATION

The purpose of the examination of the male genitalia is to assess the health of the male genital organs. The examination also provides an opportunity for teaching the client about genital area self-examination.

ANATOMY AND PHYSIOLOGY

The male genitalia (Figure 20-1) include the penis, scrotum, testes, epididymides, vas deferens, seminal vesicles, and prostate.

The shaft of the penis is formed by three columns of erectile tissue bound together by heavy fibrous tissue to form a cylinder. The dorsolateral columns are called the corpora cavernosa. The ventromedial column, which contains the urethra, is called the corpus spongiosum. Distally the penis terminates in a cone-shaped

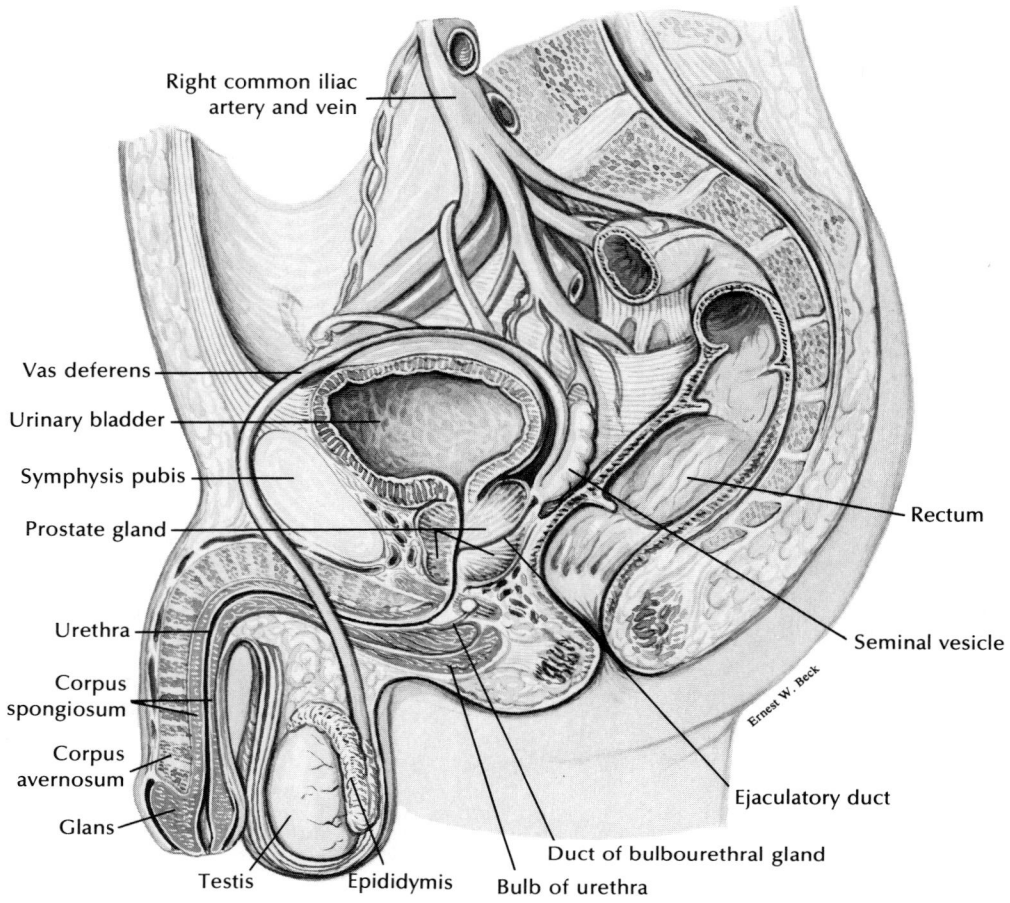

FIGURE 20-1 Male genitalia. (From Thibodeau GA: *Anatomy and physiology,* St Louis, 1987, Mosby–Year Book.)

Right common iliac artery and vein

Vas deferens

Urinary bladder

Symphysis pubis

Prostate gland

Urethra

Corpus spongiosum

Corpus avernosum

Glans

Testis

Epididymis

Bulb of urethra

Duct of bulbourethral gland

Ejaculatory duct

Seminal vesicle

Rectum

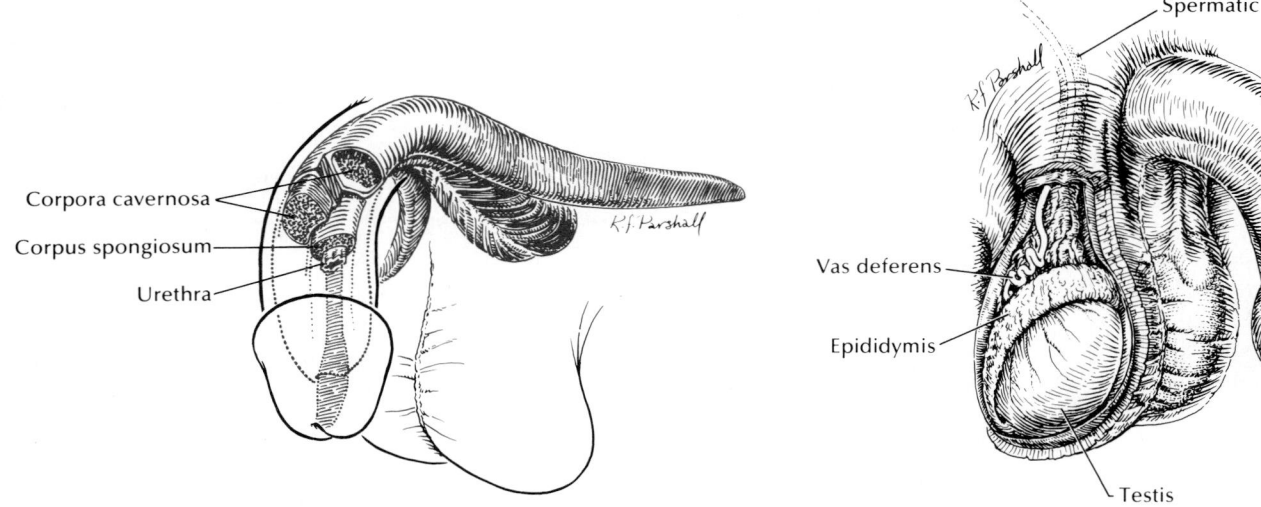

Corpora cavernosa

Corpus spongiosum

Urethra

FIGURE 20-2 Circumcised penis.

Spermatic cord

Vas deferens

Epididymis

Testis

FIGURE 20-3 Scrotum and scrotal contents.

entity called the **glans** penis. The glans penis is formed by an extension and expansion of the corpus spongiosum penis, which fits over the blunt ends of the corpora cavernosa penis. The corona is the prominence formed where the glans joins the shaft. The urethra traverses the corpus spongiosum, and the external urethral orifice is a slitlike opening located slightly ventrally on the tip of the glans.

The skin of the penis is thin, hairless, darker than the other skin on a person's body, and only loosely connected to the internal parts of the organ. At the area of the corona, the skin forms a free fold, called the **prepuce,** or foreskin. When allowed to remain, this flap covers the glans to a variable extent. Often the prepuce is surgically removed through circumcision (Figure 20-2).

The penis serves as the terminal excretory organ for urine and, with erection, as the means of ejaculating sperm. The physiological process of erection occurs when the two corpora cavernosa become engorged with approximately 20 to 50 ml of blood through decreased venous outflow and increased arterial dilation. Orgasm is a major pleasurable sensation accompanying emis-

sion of secretions from the epididymides, vas deferens, seminal vesicles, prostate, and penis.

The scrotum is a deeply pigmented cutaneous pouch that contains the testes and parts of the spermatic cords (Figure 20-3). This sac is formed by an outer layer of thin, rugous skin overlying a tight muscle layer (cremaster muscle). The left side of the scrotum is often lower than the right side because the left spermatic cord is usually longer. Internally, the scrotum is divided into halves by a septum; each half contains a testis and its epididymis and part of the spermatic cord. The testes are ovoid and are suspended vertically, slightly forward; they lean slightly laterally in the scrotum. The mediolateral surfaces are flattened. Each testis is approximately 4 to 5 cm long, 3 cm wide, and 2 cm thick.

The testes produce both spermatozoa and testosterone. The epididymides serve as receptacles for storage, maturation, and transmission of sperm. The vas deferens serves as a mechanism of transit from each epididymis to the seminal vesicles. The prostate produces the bulk of ejaculatory fluid. The dartos muscle of the scrotum controls the temperature of the testes by adjusting the distance of the scrotum, and consequently

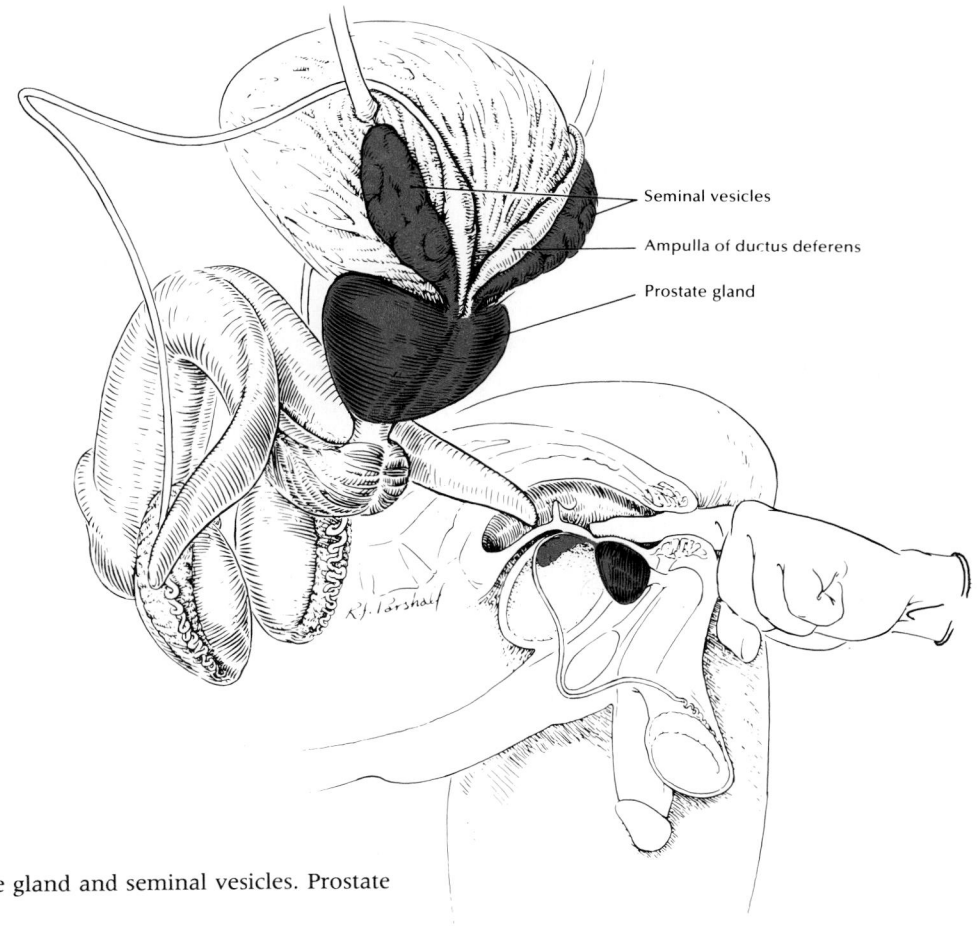

Seminal vesicles

Ampulla of ductus deferens

Prostate gland

FIGURE 20-4 Prostate gland and seminal vesicles. Prostate examination.

the testes, from the body. **Spermatogenesis** requires temperatures below 37° C. Therefore the scrotum appears low in hot weather and high in cold weather.

The epididymis is a comma-shaped structure that is curved over the posterolateral surface and upper end of the testis. It creates a visual bulge on the posterolateral surface of the testis. The ductus deferens (vas deferens) begins at the tail of the epididymis, ascends the spermatic cord, travels through the inguinal canal, and eventually descends on the **fundus** of the bladder (see Figure 20-1).

The prostate, a slightly conical gland, lies under the bladder, surrounds the urethra, and measures approximately 4 cm at its base (or uppermost) part, 3 cm vertically, and 2 cm in its anteroposterior diameter. The prostate gland is roughly the size and shape of a chestnut. It has three lobes, left and right lateral lobes and a median lobe. These lobes are not well demarcated from one another. The median lobe is the part of the prostate that projects inward from the upper posterior area toward the urethra. Enlargement of this lobe causes urinary obstruction in benign prostatic hypertrophy.

The posterior surface of the prostate lies in close contact with the rectal wall and is the only portion of the gland that is accessible to examination. Its posterior surface is slightly convex. A shallow median furrow divides all except the upper portions of the posterior surface into right and left lateral lobes.

The seminal vesicles are a pair of convoluted pouches, 5 to 10 cm long, that lie along the lower posterior surface of the bladder, anterior to the rectum (Figure 20-4).

EXAMINATION

Health History

The health history of the male reproductive system is integrated with the urinary system history and the sexual history. The client may need some explanation about the reasons for the exploration of the sexual history and reassurance that such information is important in assessing overall health.

Throughout the health history, the following data about a symptom or problem should be recorded: (1) onset (specific date, sudden or gradual), (2) duration, (3) frequency, (4) precipitating factors, (5) aggravating or alleviating factors, (6) treatment received or self-care given, and (7) outcome. An outline for a regional history of the male genitourinary system follows.

Present health status

1. Changes in urination: frequency, urgency, **nocturia, dysuria,** straining, difficulty in starting stream, incontinence. If present, describe frequency, amount of voidings, difficulty starting stream, changes in color or odor of urine, pain or burning with urination.
2. Satisfaction with sexual functioning
3. Sexual partners: sex, number, and their health
4. Use of contraceptives
5. Problems with sexual functioning: pain, difficulty in obtaining or maintaining an erection, premature ejaculation. If present, investigate frequency, characteristics associated with intercourse, including partners, medications, and use of alcohol.
6. Pattern of scrotal self-examination
7. Penile discharge: If present, determine color, amount, odor, associated symptoms, treatment, diagnoses.
8. Penile lesions: appearance, associated symptoms, treatment, diagnoses
9. Scrotal and groin masses, swelling, tenderness, pain, treatment, diagnoses
10. Enlargements or hernias in the inguinal area: intermittent or constant, association with activity involving staining, groin pain, use of truss or similar device

Past health history

1. Urinary tract infections, kidney disease, kidney stones, flank pain, prostate problems
2. Reproductive history: number of children and current health
3. Sexually transmitted diseases
4. Reproductive or hernia surgery
5. Trauma to genitourinary system

RISK FACTORS: MALE GENITALIA
For injury to genital area:
Employment in which there is risk of trauma to reproductive organs
Involvement in contact sports without wearing of protective devices
For sexually transmitted diseases:
Intercourse with multiple partners or with persons having multiple partners
For testicular cancer:
Age 20 to 35
History of undescended testes, groin hernia, or testicular swelling with mumps
Family history of testicular cancer
White race
History of maternal use of oral contraceptives or diethylstilbestrol during pregnancy
Higher social class
Never married or married late

Associated conditions

1. Diabetes
2. Exposure to mumps after puberty

Family health history

1. Cancer of prostate or testes
2. Infertility problems
3. Mother's use of hormones during pregnancy or exposure to radiation during pregnancy

Preparation for the Examination: Client and Environment

Both the client and the practitioner usually perceive the examination of the genital organs as being different from the examination of other body parts. Characteristically the genital and rectal examinations are the last

---

Helpful Hints for an Effective Examination: *Have the client void before the abdominal and pelvic area examination so that he will be more comfortable during palpation.*

Examination by a female practitioner:

A female practitioner should feel emotionally comfortable with the examination. If she does not, she should routinely refer this part of the physical examination to a male practitioner. If she is comfortable with the examination, she must accept the fact that the male client may be reluctant to have a woman examine his genitalia. Cajoling a client into an uncomfortable procedure may destroy further rapport; the client's wishes in the situation should be respected. In most clinical settings, a male practitioner is available for a few minutes to examine the male genitalia. Our experience has been that most male clients are agreeable to examination by a woman; discomfort, if it exists, is usually on the examiner's part. It is therefore recommended that the beginning female examiner critically analyze her own feelings, fears, and beliefs; attempt male genital examination under supervision and with several cooperative clients; and then reexamine her feelings.

Conversation during examination:

The client may perceive questioning about sexual activity or performance while the genitalia are being handled as evaluative or provocative.

Erection during examination:

Erection can occur. If it does, reassure the client that an erection sometimes happens during the genital examination. Proceed with the examination without additional comment about the erection unless the client brings up the subject.

Preparation for Examination

Equipment

Item	Use
Disposable latex gloves	Protect examiner from infection
Flashlight	**Transillumination** of observed scrotal mass
Material to take slide or culture	In case of abnormal discharge

Client and environment
Client

Explain purpose and procedure
Uncovered from the waist down
Lying or standing

Environment

Warm
Private

---

portions of the physical assessment. The practitioner precedes the examination with a thorough history of the urinary system and a history of sexual functioning. The examiner should generally take the sexual history during the history-taking portion of the assessment while the client is dressed.

In preparation for the physical assessment, advise the client of its purpose and the procedures involved in the examination. Assemble the needed equipment.

The client may be lying down (with the examiner standing) or standing (with the examiner sitting or standing for various portions of the examination). Trousers and shorts should be removed. Put on rubber gloves before initiating the examination and wear them throughout the examination.

Examination Technique and Normal Findings

Inspection of genital area and penis. The techniques of inspection and palpation are used to examine the male genitalia. Inspection and palpation are done consecutively for each portion of the genitalia. After the inguinal and genital areas have been exposed, inspect the skin, hair, and gross appearance of the penis and scrotum (Figure 20-5). General examination of the skin and hair is discussed in Chapter 9. Assess the size of the penis and the secondary sex characteristics in relationship to the client's age and general development.

The onset of the appearance of adult sexual characteristics is extremely variable. Pubic hair appears and the testes enlarge between the ages of 12 and 16 years. Penile enlargement and the onset of seminal emission

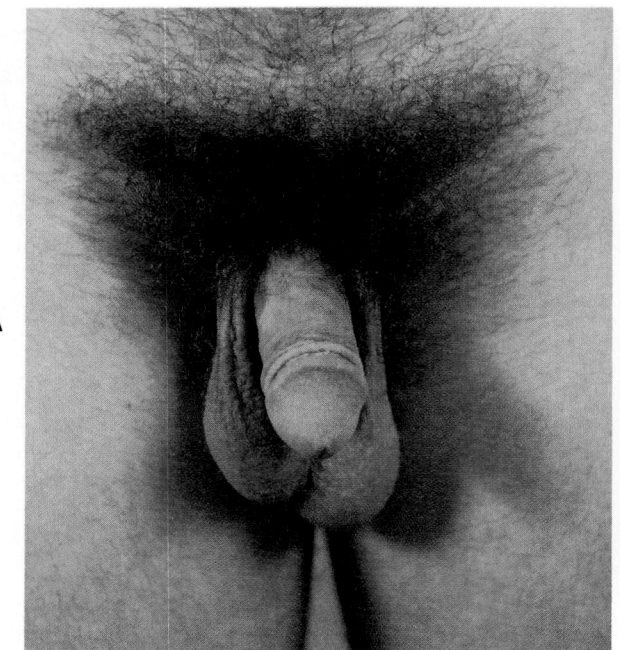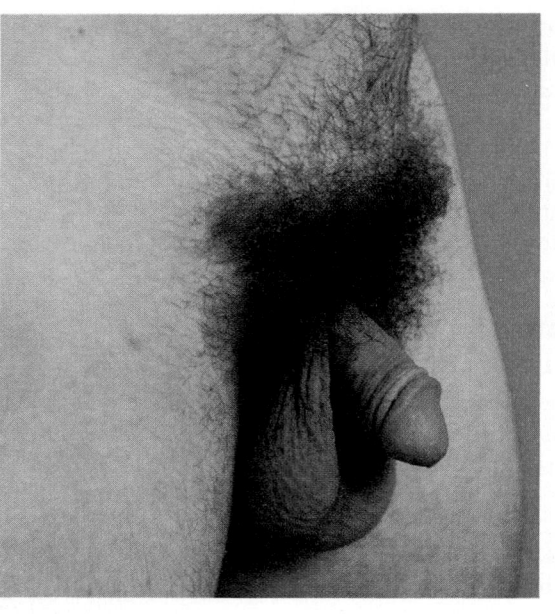

FIGURE 20-5 Normal appearance of male genitalia. **A,** Frontal view. **B,** Lateral view.

normally occurs between the ages of 13 and 17 years. Table 20-1 contains a summary of developmental changes in the male genital system.

Genital hair is coarser than scalp hair. It is similar in color and appearance to axillary and chest hair. In the adult male, pubic hair will be abundant in the pubic region and will extend in a diamond pattern narrowing upward toward the umbilicus. The penis is hairless, and the scrotum may have a sparse distribution of hairs.

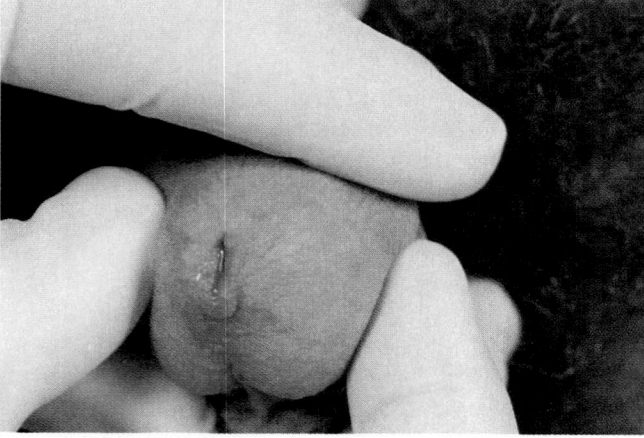

FIGURE 20-6 Usual position and appearance of urethral meatus.

An ambulatory, cooperative client can assist in the examination by handling the penis and scrotum during inspection. The examiner must do all the handling for the debilitated client. It is important to examine all the surfaces, including the posterior surfaces, of the male genitalia.

The color of the penis ranges from pink to light brown in whites and from light brown to dark brown in blacks. A prominent dorsal vein is often noted. Observe the entire penis for lesions, nodules, swelling, inflammation, and discharge. Then observe the glans and the urethral **meatus** for lesions and inflammation (Figure 20-6). If the client is uncircumcised, ask him to retract the prepuce from the glans, and carefully examine the glans and foreskin. If the uncircumcised client has retracted the foreskin for examination of the glans, remind him to return the foreskin to its usual position after the glans has been inspected.

If any discharge is present, obtain a smear and culture for gonorrhea and possibly chlamydia (see Chapter 21 for a discussion of procedures for obtaining smears and cultures). If the client has reported a discharge but none is present, request him to strip the penis from the base to the urethra. If a discharge is then present, make a culture. The procedure for stripping the penis is as follows:

1. Grasp the base of the penis with the thumb and fingers, with the thumb at the front and the fingers behind.

TABLE 20-1

Developmental Changes in Appearance of the Male Genital Organs

Developmental time	Pubic hair	Appearance Penis	Testes and scrotum
Stage 1 Sexual maturity	None except for fine body hair as on the abdomen	Size proportional to body size as in childhood	Size proportional to body size as in childhood
Stage 2 Sexual maturity	Sparse, long, slightly pigmented, thin hair at the base of the penis	Slight enlargement	Enlargement of testes and scrotum; reddened pigmentation; texture more prominent
Stage 3 Sexual maturity	Darkens, becomes more coarse and curly; growth extends over symphysis	Elongation	Enlargement continues

Stage 1　　　　Stage 2　　　　Stage 3

Developmental time	Pubic hair	Penis	Testes and scrotum
Stage 4 Sexual maturity	Continues to darken, thicken, and become coarser and more curly; growth extends laterally, superiorly, and inferiorly	Breadth and length increase; glans develops	Enlargement continues; skin pigmentation darkens
Stage 5 Sexual maturity	Adult distribution and appearance; growth extends to inner thighs, umbilicus, and anus and is abundant	Adult appearance	Adult appearance
Elderly clients	Hair sparse and gray	Decrease in size	Testes hang low in scrotum; scrotum appears pendulous

Stage 4　　　　Stage 5　　　　Stage 6

Illustrations modified from Tanner JM: *Growth at adolescence,* ed 2, Oxford, 1962, Blackwell Scientific Publications.

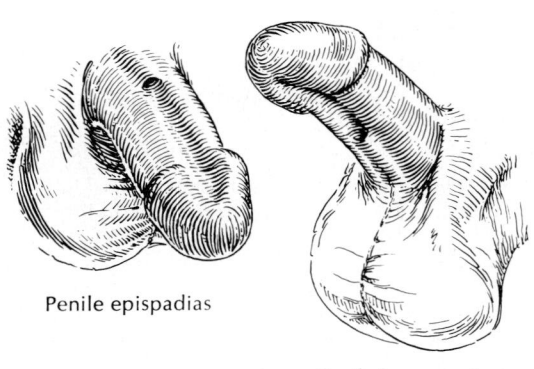

Penile epispadias

Penile hypospadias

FIGURE 20-7 Hypospadias, a malpositioning of urethral meatus.

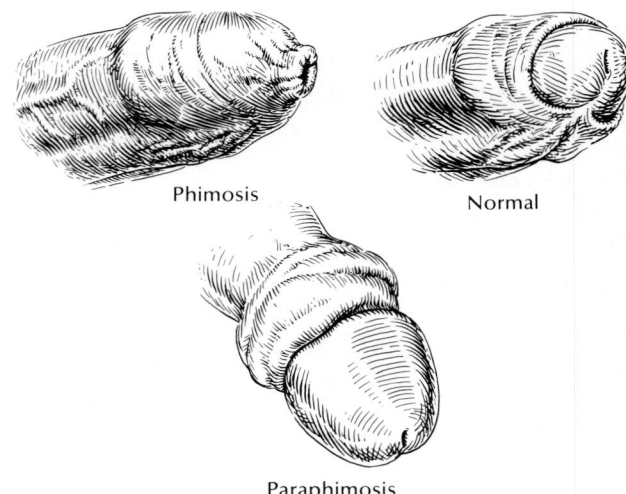

Phimosis

Normal

Paraphimosis

FIGURE 20-8 Phimosis, normal retraction of prepuce, and paraphimosis.

2. While applying a moderate amount of consistent pressure, move the thumb and the fingers slowly from the base to the tip of the penis.

The urethral meatus should appear pink and slitlike and should be positioned rather centrally on the glans. When the distal urethral **ostium** occurs on the ventral corona or at a more proximal and ventral site on the penis or perineum, the condition is called **hypospadias** (Figure 20-7). **Epispadias** is a similar malpositioning of the urethral meatus in the dorsal area.

When hypospadias or epispadias is noted, describe the location of the urethral meatus as precisely as possible. Hypospadias is classified as being glandular, penile, penoscrotal, or perineal. Epispadias is classified as being glandular, penile, or complete. Glandular refers to a location somewhere between the normal position and the junction of the glans with the body of the penis. Penile refers to a location on the penile shaft. Penoscrotal hypospadias indicates a positioning of the meatus along the anterior margin of the scrotum. Perineal hypospadias indicates an urethral orifice located on the perineum; in this condition, the scrotum is bifid. Epispadias is described as complete when the urethral orifice is located anterior to and off the penis.

The prepuce, if present, should be easily retractable from the glans and returnable to its original position. **Phimosis** exists when **retraction** cannot occur (Figure 20-8). This condition presents problems with cleanliness and prevents observation of the glans and interior surfaces of the prepuce. If the foreskin has been partially retracted but has impinged on the penis so that it cannot be returned to its usual position, the condition is called **paraphimosis**.

Palpation of the penis. Carefully palpate the penile shaft with the thumb and the first two fingers of the examining hand. The penis should feel smooth and

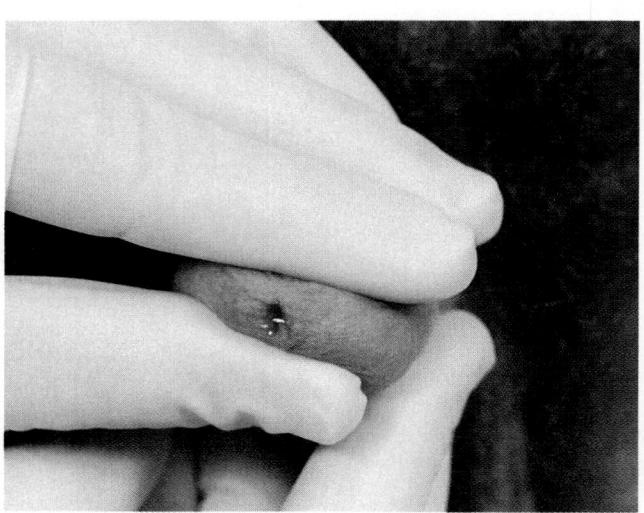

FIGURE 20-9 Compression of glans to open urethral meatus.

semifirm. The overlying skin appears slightly wrinkled and feels somewhat movable over the underlying structures. Note any swelling, nodules, and induration as possibly abnormal findings. Occasionally, hard, nontender subcutaneous plaques are palpated on the dorsomedial surface. The client with this condition, called **Peyronie's disease,** may report penile bending with erection and painful intercourse.

Either compress the tip of the glans, or ask the client to compress the glans anteroposteriorly (Figure 20-9). This maneuver opens the distal end of the urethra for

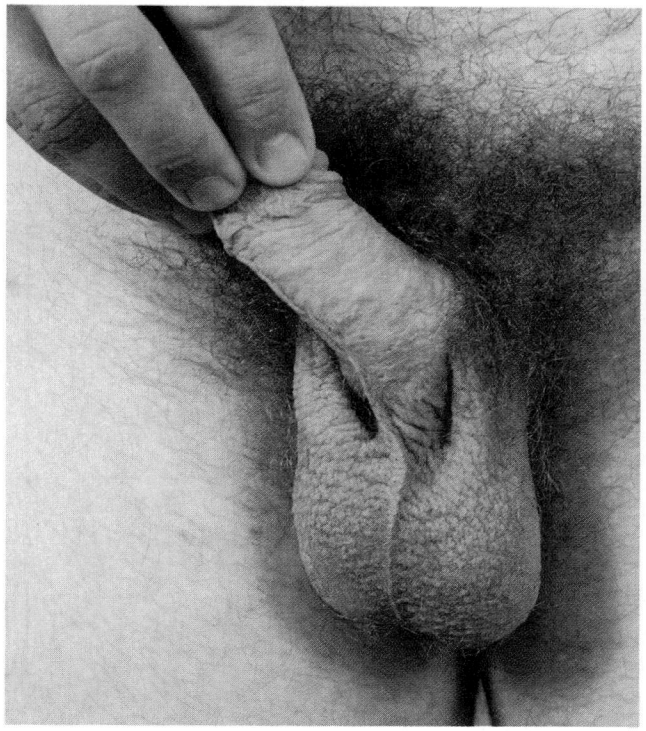

FIGURE 20-10 Normal appearance of scrotum in the adult.

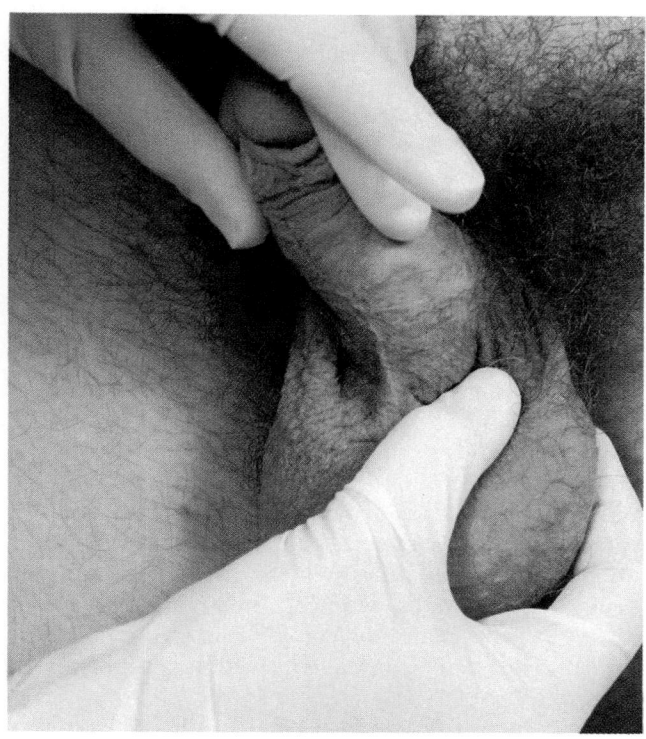

FIGURE 20-11 Palpation of scrotal contents.

inspection. Observe for evidence of neoplastic lesions or inflammatory processes.

Inspection of the scrotum. Instruct the client to hold the penis out of the way, and observe the general size, superficial appearance, and symmetry of the scrotum (Figure 20-10). The scrotum normally appears asymmetrical because the left testis is generally lower than the right testis. Also, the tone of the dartos muscle determines the size of the scrotum; this muscle contracts when the area is cold and relaxes when the area is warm. In advanced age, the dartos muscle is somewhat **atonic** and the scrotum may appear pendulous.

The scrotal skin is more darkly pigmented than that of the rest of the body. To observe the scrotal skin, spread its **rugated** surface. Also, remember to inspect the posterior and posterolateral and anterior and anterolateral skin areas. A common abnormality, occurring as a single lesion or as multiple lesions, is that of sebaceous cysts. These are firm, yellow to white, nontender cutaneous lesions measuring up to 1 cm in diameter.

Palpation of the scrotum. Palpate the contents of each half of the scrotal sac (Figure 20-11). Both testes should be present in the scrotum at birth. If not present,

determine their location by retracing their course of descent back into the abdomen.

Palpate both testes with the first two fingers. Determine their consistency, size, shape, and response to pressure. The testes should be smooth, homogeneous in consistency, regular, equal in size, freely movable, and slightly sensitive to compression. If possible, palpate both testes simultaneously to allow for comparison between them.

Next, palpate each epididymis. The epididymides are located in the posterolateral area of the testes in 93% of the male population. In approximately 7%, the epididymides lie in the anterolateral or anterior areas. Palpate them and note their size, shape, consistency, and tenderness. They should feel smooth, discrete, larger cephalad, and nontender. Then palpate each of the spermatic cords by bilaterally grasping each between the thumb and the forefinger, starting at the base of the epididymis and continuing to the inguinal canal. The vasa deferentia feel similar to smooth cords and are movable. The arteries, veins, lymph vessels, and nerves feel like indefinite threads along the side of the vas.

If swelling, irregularity, or nodularity is noted in the scrotum, an attempt should be made to transilluminate it by darkening the room and placing a lighted flashlight behind the scrotal contents. Transillumination is noted by a red glow. Serous fluid will transilluminate; tissue and blood will not. On transillumination, the normal scrotum and epididymis will appear as dark masses with regular borders. Small areas of transilluminated space appear around the testes, with a larger transilluminated space superior to the testes. The amount of transilluminated space superior to the testes is dependent on the amount of scrotal relaxation. Because of concern about the transmission of disease, a disposable flashlight or a flashlight with a disposable plastic cover should be used.

The scrotum can be edematous, and palpation may produce pitting. Edema of the scrotum can occur in any condition that causes edema in the lower trunk, for example, cardiovascular disease.

Palpation of the prostate. With an ambulatory client, executing the rectal and prostate examination is done most satisfactorily with the client standing, hips flexed, toes pointed toward each other, and upper body resting on the examining table. This position flattens the buttocks, deters gluteal contraction, and makes the anus and rectum more accessible to evaluation. A debilitated client may be examined in the left lateral or lithotomy position. If the left lateral position is used remind the client to flex his right knee and hip and to have his buttocks close to the edge of the examining table. The general procedure for the anal and rectal examination is described in Chapter 22. Perform the general rectal examination first. Then palpate the prostate gland and seminal vesicles with the pad of the index finger (Figure 20-12, *A*). The prostate gland is located on the anterior rectal wall but should not be protruding into the rectal lumen.

Prostatic enlargement, or protrusion of the prostate gland into the rectal lumen, is commonly described in grades:

Grade I: Encroaches less than 1 cm into the rectal lumen

Grade II: Encroaches 1 to 2 cm into the rectal lumen

Grade III: Encroaches 2 to 3 cm into the rectal lumen

Grade IV: Encroaches more than 3 cm into the rectal lumen

The gland should be approximately 3 cm long, approximately 4 cm across at its base, symmetrical, movable, and of a rubbery (like a pencil eraser) consistency. Its median **sulcus** normally can be felt. The lateral margins of the prostate gland should be discrete, and a moderate degree of mobility can be noted when the tip of the index finger is hooked over the upper border of the gland and the gland is pulled down gently.

The proximal portions of the seminal vesicles can sometimes be palpated as corrugated structures above

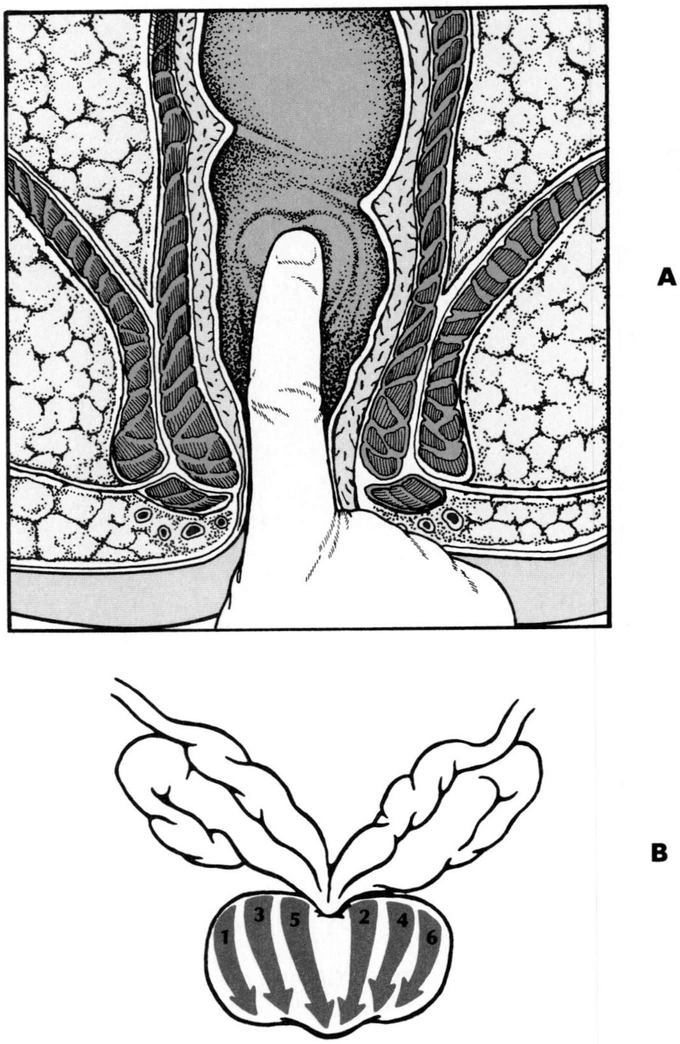

FIGURE 20-12 Palpation of prostate. **A,** Position of examiner's finger. **B,** Prostatic massage. Arrows indicate areas of the prostate that are massaged and sequence and direction of the massage.

the lateral to the midpoint of the gland. Normally they are too soft to be palpated. Attempt to examine all available surfaces of the prostate gland and the entire area of the seminal vesicles. Significant abnormalities of the prostate gland or seminal vesicles include protrusion into the rectal lumen; hard, nodular areas; bogginess; tenderness; and asymmetry (see accompanying box, p. 649).

The prostate gland can be massaged centrally from its lateral edges to force secretions into the urethra (Figure 20-12, *B*). Stroke the prostate from its distal to proximal areas, with the order of strokes indicated in the figure. Secretions at the urethral opening can be

Helpful Hints for prostate examination: *Consider the following questions about the prostate:*
Surface: *Smooth or nodular?*
Consistency: *Rubbery, hard, boggy, soft, or fluctuant?*
Shape: *Rounded or flat?*
Size: *Normal, enlarged, or atrophied?*
Sensitivity: *Tender or not?*
Movability: *Movable or fixed?*

Examination Step-by-Step

Inspect the condition of the skin and hair in the pubic region.
Inspect the pubic hair distribution. Assess the consistency of findings with the client's age.
Inspect the penis:
  Ask client to retract foreskin (if present).
  Glans—inflammation
  Condition and position of urethral meatus
  Condition of skin—color, lesions, swelling
Palpate the penis:
  Compression of glans—inflammation, discharge
  Shaft of penis—tenderness, induration (anterior and posterior surfaces)
  Strip urethra for discharge (if symptomatic).
Inspect the scrotum:
  Client holds penis out of way.
  Condition of skin and surface—color, symmetry, swelling
Palpate the scrotum:
  Spread rugae to examine surface—consistency, size, tenderness, masses.
  Each spermatic cord—consistency, size, tenderness, masses
  Palpate testes.
  Palpate epididymides.
  Transilluminate any masses present.
Palpate the prostate gland (in conjunction with rectal examination):
  Assess extension into lumen, size, contour, consistency, tenderness, and mobility.

examined and cultured. It is important that all areas of the prostate available for palpation be massaged.

Screening Tests and Procedures

The U.S. Preventive Services Task Force (1989) recommendation about screening for testicular cancer is as follows:

Periodic screening for testicular cancer by testicular examination is recommended for men with a history of **cryptorchidism, orchiopexy,** or testicular atrophy. There is insufficient evidence of clinical benefit or harm to recommend for or against routine screening of other asymptomatic men.

Because this recommendation is somewhat ambiguous and since the self-examination is easily and quickly done during a bath or a shower, consider teaching it to every client and recommending that it be done monthly on some target date.

The U.S. Preventive Services Task Force (1989) recommendation about screening for prostate cancer is as follows:

There is insufficient evidence to recommend for or against routine digital rectal examinations as an effective screening test for prostate cancer in asymptomatic men. Transrectal ultrasound and serum tumor markers are not recommended for routine screening in asymptomatic men [p. 63].

VARIATIONS FROM HEALTH

Penis

Among the more common penile lesions are syphilitic chancre, condylomata acuminata, and cancer. The syphilitic chancre is the primary lesion of syphilis. It begins as a single papule that eventually erodes into an oval or round red ulcer with an indurated base that discharges serous material. It is usually painless.

Condylomata acuminata are wart-appearing growths. They are caused by human papillomavirus and may be seen occurring singly or in multiple cauliflower-like patches on the penis and throughout the genital area. They can be transmitted to a partner via sexual intercourse.

Carcinoma of the penis occurs most frequently on the glans and the inner lip of the prepuce. It may appear dry and scaly, ulcerated, or nodular. It is usually painless.

Scrotum

The common abnormalities of the scrotum are described and illustrated in Table 20-2. All scrotal masses should be described by their placement, size, shape, consistency, and tenderness and by whether they transilluminate.

Prostate

A hard single or multiple lesion on a firm and fixed prostate gland may indicate cancer. The initial lesion of carcinoma is frequently on the posterior lobe and can be easily identified during the rectal examination. A soft, symmetrical, boggy, nontender prostate gland may indicate benign prostatic hypertrophy, a condition very

TABLE 20-2

Description of Scrotal Abnormalities

Abnormality	Definition/causation	Basis for diagnosis
Hydrocele	Accumulation of serous fluid between the visceral and parietal layers of the tunica vaginalis	Transilluminates; fingers can get above the mass
Scrotal hernia	Hernia within the scrotum	Bowel sounds auscultated; does not transilluminate; fingers cannot get above the mass
Varicocele	Abnormal dilation and tortuosity of the veins of the pampiniform plexus; often described as a "bag of worms" in the scrotum*	Complaints of a dragging sensation or dull pain in the scrotal area; feels like a soft bag of worms; collapses when the scrotum is elevated and increases when the scrotum is dependent; more commonly present on the left side; usually appears at puberty
Spermatocele	Epididymal cyst resulting from a partial obstruction of the spermatic tubules*	Transilluminates; round mass, feels like a third testis; painless

Hydrocele   Scrotal hernia   Varicocele   Spermatocele

Epididymal mass   Epididymitis   Torsion of the spermatic cord   Testicular tumor

Abnormality	Definition/causation	Basis for diagnosis
Epididymal mass or nodularity	May be result of benign or malignant neoplasms, syphilis, or tuberculosis	Nodules are not tender; in tuberculosis lesions, vas deferens often feels beaded
Epididymitis	An inflammation of the epididymis, usually resulting from *Escherichia coli*, *Neisseria gonorrhoeae*, or *Mycobacterium tuberculosis* organisms*	Spermatic cord often thickened and indurated; pain relieved by elevation
Torsion of the spermatic cord	Axial rotation or volvulus of the spermatic cord, resulting in infarction of the testicle	Elevated mass; pain not relieved by further elevation; more common in childhood or adolescence; history of extreme pain and tenderness of the testis, followed by hyperemic swelling and hydrocele
Testicular tumor	Multiple causes	Usually not painful; hydroceles may develop as a result of a tumor; if a testis cannot be palpated, fluid may need to be aspirated so that the testis can be accurately evaluated

*From Betesh S, editor: *Diseases of the urinary tract and male genital organs*, Geneva, 1974, Council for Internal Organizations for Medical Sciences, pp 86-90.

common in men over 50 years of age. In the later stages of this condition, the median sulcus may be obliterated. A boggy, fluctuant, or tender prostate gland may indicate acute or chronic **prostatitis.**

TEACHING SELF-ASSESSMENT

Genital self-examination is a means of early identification of scrotal cancer and sexually transmitted diseases. Individuals with malignant testicular tumors, the most common neoplasms in men, typically have the following characteristics:

Aged 20 to 34

History of undescended testes

White race

History of maternal use of oral contraceptives or diethylstilbestrol during early pregnancy

History of maternal abdominal or pelvic x-ray examination during pregnancy

Higher social class

Never married or late marriage

Clients with the following characteristics are at risk for sexually transmitted diseases: (1) more than one sexual partner and (2) intercourse with person(s) having multiple partners

At the initiation of the teaching, assess the male client's level of knowledge about genital self-examination, reinforce the importance of a monthly self-examination, and provide instruction for the examination. The following outline can be used for the health teaching along with pictures of the anatomy of the male genitalia:

1. Cancer of the testes is one of the most curable forms of cancer when detected early. The cure rate is approximately 90%.
2. Cancer of the testes can affect males of any age but is most common between ages 15 to 35. It is much more likely in men whose testicles descended after infancy or never descended at all.
3. Men can have normal sexual relations after being treated for cancer of the testicle.
4. Examine the genitalia once a month.
5. Do the self-examination following a shower or warm bath, when the testes are relaxed, descended, and accessible for palpation.
6. Examine the penis for lesions and discharge:
   a. Inspect the head of the penis—retract foreskin (if present).
   b. Examine the entire shaft.
   c. Inspect the urethral meatus for discharge (Figure 20-13, *A*).
7. Examine the skin and pubic hair for lesions and parasites.
8. Examine the scrotum:
   a. Use the thumbs and the index and middle fingers for examination, with the thumbs placed on the top and the fingers on the underside of the scrotum (Figure 20-13, *B*).
   b. Gently roll the contents of the scrotum between your thumbs and fingers. The normal

A 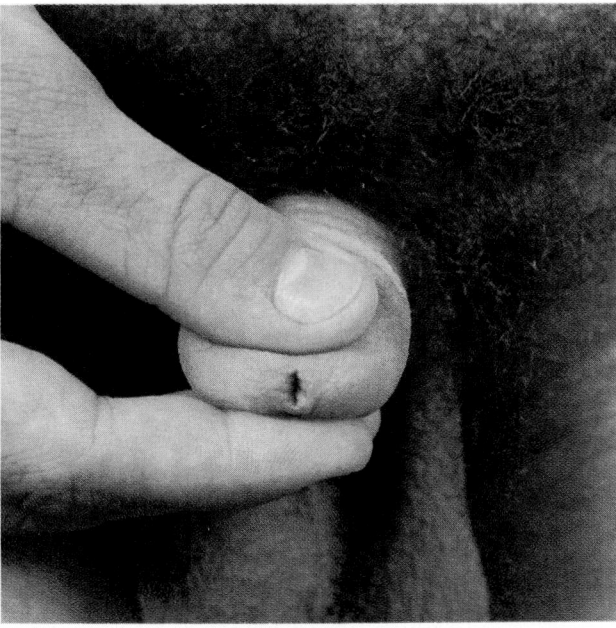   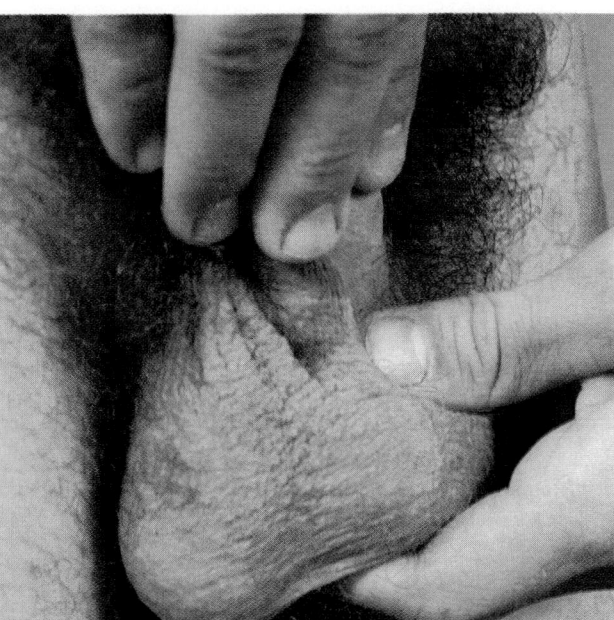 **B**

FIGURE 20-13 Male genital self-examination. **A,** Examination of urethral meatus. **B,** Scrotal assessment.

testicle is about 1½ to 2 inches long. It feels smooth, rubbery, and firm but not hard. The epididymis is the storage tube found behind each testicle. Each should feel soft and spongy and sometimes slightly tender. The spermatic cords extend from the bottom of the epididymides and up into the pelvis. They should feel like smooth, firm tubes.

c. The examination should be painless unless the pressure is too hard or some problem exists. A small amount of tenderness may be noticed during the palpation of the testes and the epididymides; this is normal.

d. Any lump or change in texture, whether painful or not, should be reported to and assessed by a health care provider as soon as possible.

ASSESSMENT OF INGUINAL AREA FOR HERNIAS

PURPOSE OF THE EXAMINATION

The purpose of the inguinal area assessment for **hernias** is to determine the presence of inguinal and femoral hernias. This examination is addressed in conjunction with the male genital examination because most kinds of hernias are more common in males than in females. However, this discussion pertains to the physical examination of both sexes.

ANATOMY AND PHYSIOLOGY

The inguinal ligament **(Poupart's ligament)** extends from the anterosuperior spine of the ilium to the pubic tubercle. The inguinal canal is a flattened tunnel between two layers of abdominal muscle, measuring approximately 4 to 6 cm in the adult. Its internal ring is located 1 to 2 cm above the midpoint of the inguinal ligament. The spermatic cord traverses this internal ring, passes through the canal, exits the canal at its external (subcutaneous) ring, and then moves up and over the inguinal ligament and into the scrotum (Figure 20-14).

Hesselbach's triangle is the region superior to the inguinal canal, medial to the inferior epigastric artery, and lateral to the margin of the rectus muscle.

DOCUMENTATION

Sample Documentation

Health history

Swelling of the scrotum started 2 weeks ago. No pain, but clothing uncomfortable. An athletic support alleviates some discomfort. No previous swelling noted. Unable to identify precipitating factors—no trauma to the area. Denies penile discharge and lesions. No changes in urination. Has had no reproductive system or hernia surgery. Denies exposure to infectious process. No family history of cancer. Sexually active with wife for 4 years. Denies other sex partners during that time.

Physical examination

Pubic hair pattern in adult male distribution. Skin clear of lesions. Circumcised penis with no lesions, induration, or discharge. Urethral meatus on ventral surface at tip of glans—no inflammation or discharge. Right side of scrotum swollen to about three times the normal size. Testes difficult to feel, but a large cystic mass felt on the right epididymis. Mass does transilluminate. Left testis and epididymis without tenderness, swelling, or masses. Inguinal areas smooth. Inguinal canals without masses, bulging, or tenderness.

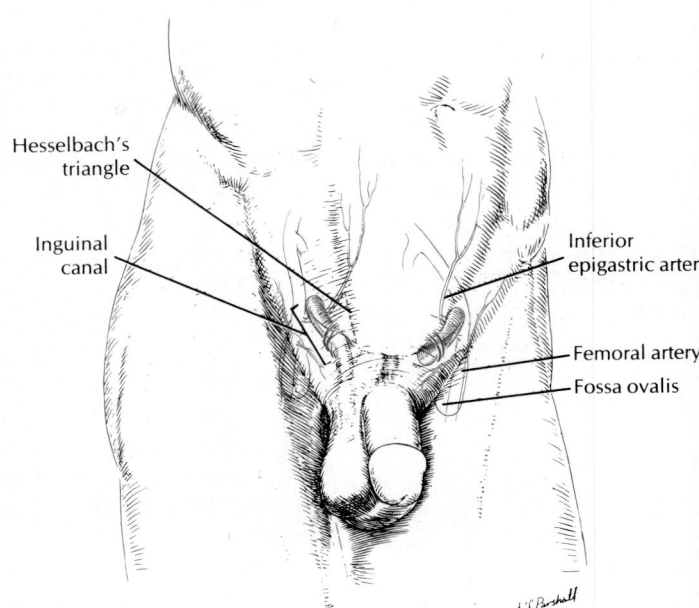

Hesselbach's triangle
Inguinal canal
Inferior epigastric artery
Femoral artery
Fossa ovalis

FIGURE 20-14 Superficial anatomy of anterior pelvic area.

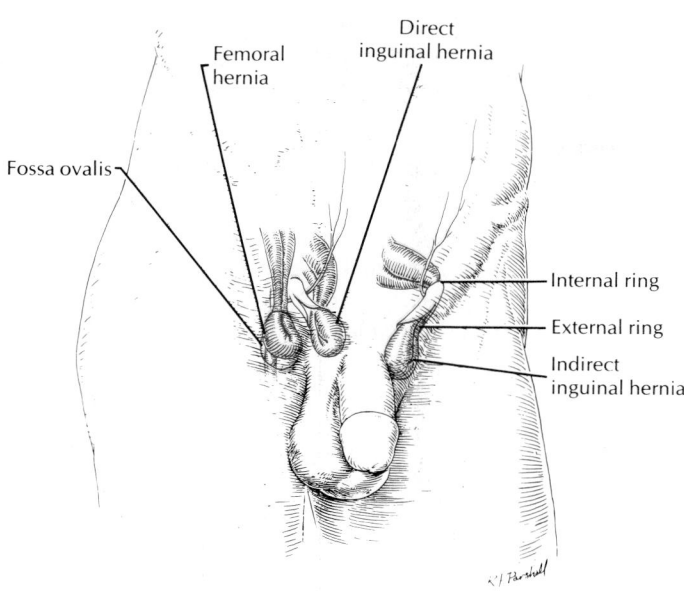

FIGURE 20-15 Three common pelvic area hernias.

The femoral canal is a potential space just inferior to the inguinal ligament and 3 cm medial and parallel to the femoral artery. When the examiner's right hand is placed on the client's right anterior thigh with the index finger over the femoral artery, the femoral canal will be under the examiner's ring finger.

The three main types of pelvic area hernias are shown in Figure 20-15. In the indirect inguinal hernia, the hernial sac enters the internal inguinal canal, and its tip is located somewhere in the inguinal canal or beyond the canal. In men, indirect inguinal hernias may descend into the scrotum. The direct inguinal hernia emerges directly from behind and through the external inguinal ring. The femoral hernia emerges through the femoral ring, the femoral canal, and the fossa ovalis. The characteristics of the three main types of hernias are compared in Table 20-3.

EXAMINATION

Health History

Throughout the health history interview, the following data should be recorded about a symptom or problem: (1) onset (specific date, sudden or gradual), (2) dura-

TABLE 20-3

Comparison of Inguinal and Femoral Hernias

| | Inguinal hernia | | Femoral hernia |
	Indirect	Direct	
Course	Sac emerges through the internal inguinal ring, lateral to the inferior epigastric artery; can remain in the canal, exit the external ring, or pass into the scrotum	Sac emerges directly from behind and through the external inguinal ring; located in the region of Hesselbach's triangle	Sac emerges through the femoral ring, the femoral canal, and the fossa ovalis; observed medial to the femoral artery
Incidence	More common in infants under 1 year and in young men 16 to 20 years; more common in men than in women at a ratio of approximately 4:1, 60% of all hernias	Most often observed in men over 40 years of age; rarer than the indirect hernia	Less common than inguinal hernias; seldom seen in children; more common in women; 4% of all hernias
Cause	Congenital or acquired	Congenital weakness exacerbated by (1) lifting, (2) atrophy of abdominal muscles, (3) ascites, (4) chronic cough, or (5) obesity	Acquired; may be caused by (1) stooping frequently, (2) increased abdominal pressure, (3) loss of muscle substance
Clinical symptoms and signs	Soft swelling in the region of the internal inguinal ring—swelling increases when client stands or strains, is sometimes reduced when client reclines; pain during straining	Abdominal bulge in the area of Hesselbach's triangle, usually in the area of the internal ring; usually painless; easily reduced when client reclines; rarely enters scrotum	Right side more commonly affected; pain may be severe; strangulation frequent; sac may extend into the scrotum, into the labium, or along the saphenous vein

tion, (3) frequency, (4) precipitating factors, (5) aggravating or alleviating factors, (6) treatment received or self-care given, and (7) outcome.

Present health status

1. Enlargement in the inguinal area
   a. Frequency: intermittent or constant
   b. Presence of pain: character, location, association with lifting or straining
   c. Association with straining or lifting
   d. Change in size
   e. Reducibility
   f. Use of truss or other treatment

Past health history

1. Surgery to the inguinal area

Family health history

1. Hernias

Preparation for Examination: Client and Environment

If a client has an inguinal or groin area hernia, he or she will probably complain of a swelling or bulging in that area, especially during abdominal straining. As part of the routine physical examination, all clients should be screened for inguinal and femoral hernias, even if they do not complain of groin swelling.

No special equipment is needed for the examination. The examiner should wear rubber gloves.

Examination Technique and Normal Findings

Inspection. Inspection and palpation are the techniques used for assessment of the inguinal area. When-

ever possible, perform the examination for hernias with the client standing. However, if the client is debilitated or especially tense, perform the examination while he or she is lying down on a flat surface.

First, expose the areas of inguinal and femoral hernias and observe them with the client at rest and while the client holds his or her breath and exerts abdominal pressure with the diaphragm. Straining is preferred to coughing because a more sustained pressure is elicited. Sometimes the impulse of coughing can be confused with the impulse of a hernia. Often, small hernias in women and children are more easily observed than felt because of the fatty tissue in the area.

Palpation. Palpate for a direct inguinal hernia by placing two fingers over each external inguinal ring and instructing the client to bear down. The presence of a hernia will produce a palpable bulge in the area.

To determine the presence of an indirect inguinal hernia, ask the client to flex the ipsilateral knee slightly while you attempt to direct your index or little finger into the path of the inguinal canal. When the finger has traversed as far as possible, ask the client to strain. A hernia will be felt as a mass of tissue meeting the finger and then withdrawing. To examine the client's left side, use the index or little finger of the left hand with palm side out. For the client's right side, use the right hand. In women, the canal is narrow, and the finger cannot be inserted far, if at all. In men, the finger invaginates scrotal skin into the inguinal canal (Figure 20-16).

In both men and women, each fossa ovalis area is palpated while the client is straining (Figure 20-17). The femoral hernia will be felt as a soft tumor at the fossa, below the inguinal ligament and lateral to the pubic tubercle.

Occasionally, the client may complain of the symptoms of hernia although none can be palpated. In such cases a load test is suggested. The client lifts a heavy object while the inguinal area is observed. A previously unobserved bulge may become prominent.

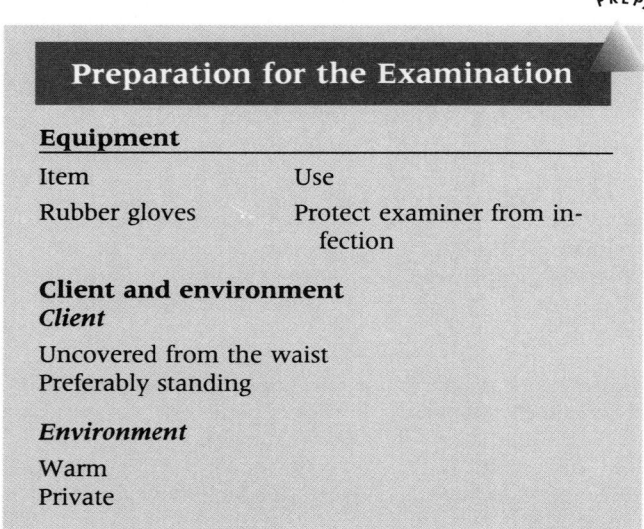

PREPARATION

Preparation for the Examination

Equipment

Item	Use
Rubber gloves	Protect examiner from infection

Client and environment
Client

Uncovered from the waist
Preferably standing

Environment

Warm
Private

STEP-BY-STEP

Examination Step-by-Step

Inspect the inguinal area for bulges at rest and with straining.
Palpate the inguinal canals for direct hernia—bilaterally at rest and with straining.
Palpate the inguinal canals for indirect hernia—bilaterally at rest and with straining.
Palpate the femoral areas at rest and with straining.

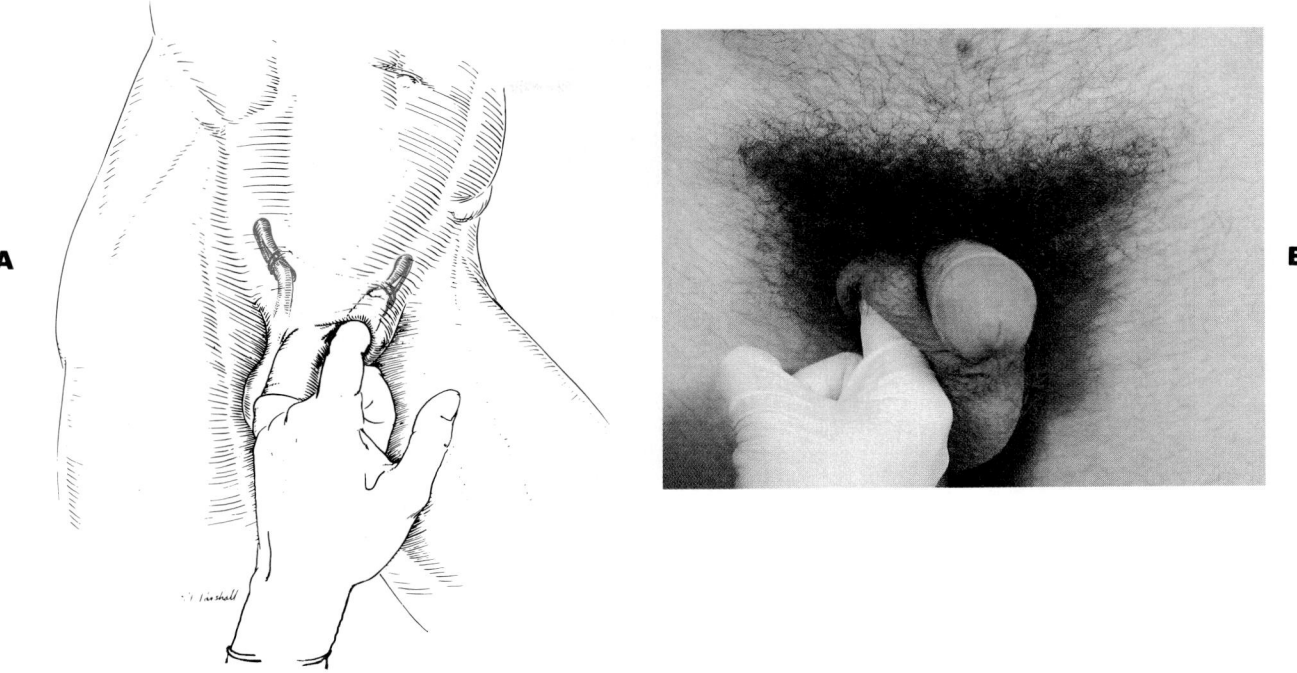

FIGURE 20-16 Examination of a male client for indirect inguinal hernia.

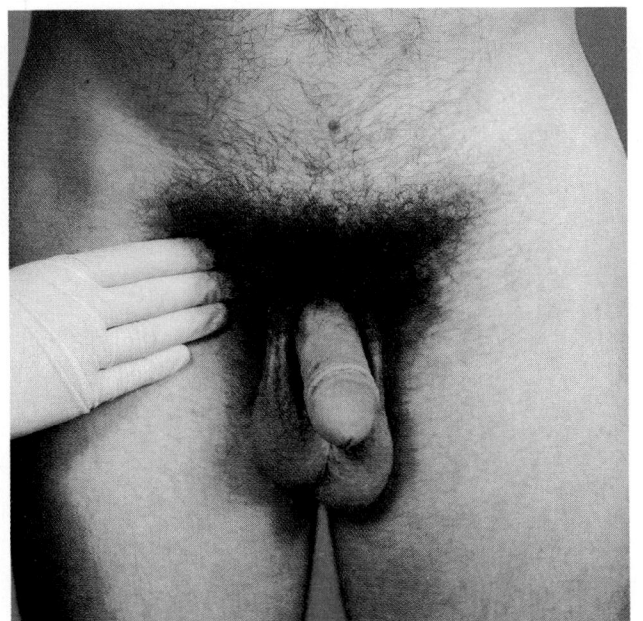

FIGURE 20-17 Palpation for femoral hernia.

Sample Documentation

Health history

No history of hernias. Denies pain or swelling in inguinal area.

Physical examination

Inguinal and femoral canal areas are without masses, bulging, or tenderness.

Nursing Diagnosis *THE NEXT STEP*

Nursing diagnoses that could apply to assessment and alterations in the male reproductive system include, but are not limited to, the following ones.

SEXUAL DYSFUNCTION The state in which an individual experiences a change in sexual function that is viewed as unsatisfying, unrewarding, or inadequate.

Defining Characteristics
- Verbalizations of problem in sexuality
- Alterations in achieving perceived sex role
- Actual or perceived limitation imposed by disease and/or therapy (impotence)
- Conflicts involving values (cultural/religion)
- Alteration in achieving sexual satisfaction
- Inability to achieve desired sexual satisfaction
- Frequent seeking of confirmation of desirability
- Alteration in relationship with significant others
- Change in interest in self and others

Related Factors
- Ineffectual or absent models
- Physical abuse
- Psychosocial abuse
- Vulnerability
- Misinformation or lack of knowledge
- Values conflict
- Lack of privacy
- Lack of significant other
- Altered body structure or function

ALTERED SEXUALITY PATTERNS The state in which an individual expresses concern regarding his/her sexuality.

Defining Characteristics
- Reported difficulties, limitations, or changes in sexual behaviors or activities

Related Factors
- Knowledge skill deficit
- Altered body function or structure
- Illness or medical treatment
- Lack of privacy
- Lack of significant other
- Ineffective or absent role models
- Conflicts with sexual orientation or variant preferences
- Fear
- Impaired relationship with significant other

STRESS INCONTINENCE The state in which an individual experiences a loss of urine of less than 50 ml occurring with increased abdominal pressure.

Defining Characteristics
- Reported or observed dribbling with increased abdominal pressure
- Urinary urgency
- Urinary frequency (more often than every 2 hours)

Related Factors
- Incompetent bladder outlet
- Age-related degenerative changes in pelvic muscles and structural supports

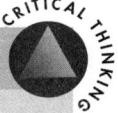

Nursing Diagnosis *THE NEXT STEP—cont'd*

- Weak pelvic muscles and structural supports
- High intraabdomial pressure
- Overdistention between voidings

ANXIETY A vague, uneasy feeling, the source of which is often nonspecific or unknown to the individual.

Defining Characteristics

- Subjective
  Increased tension
  Apprehension
  Uncertainty
  Fear
  Feeling of being scared
  Feeling of inadequacy
  Shakiness
  Fear of unspecific consequences
  Regretfulness
  Feeling of being rattled
  Distress
  Jitteriness
- Objective
  Insomnia
  Glancing about
  Poor eye contact
  Trembling; hand tremors
  Extraneous movements—foot shuffling; hand, arm movements
  Expressed concern regarding changes in life events
  Worry
  Facial tension
  Voice quivering
  Focus on self
  Increased wariness
  Increased perspiration

Related Factors

- Threat to self-concept
- Threat to or change in health status
- Threat to or change in role functioning
- Threat to or change in interaction patterns
- Situational and maturational crises
- Interpersonal transmission and contagion
- Unmet needs

Clinical Application

B.D. is an 18-year-old college freshman who has come into the college health clinic complaining of "painful urination." "I always feel like I have to go and I void almost every hour in small amounts." He has also noted a thick white penile discharge. Temperature 37.5° C, pulse 72, respirations 16, blood pressure 120/72. Denies fever, side pain, abdominal pain or genital rash. No known allergies. No history of genitourinary disease. No prior history of STD. Physical assessment completed. While being examined, B.D. voices concern about a recent episode of unprotected sexual intercourse approximately 10 days ago. He questions, "Could I have gotten an infection during sex?"

SUBJECTIVE DATA: Patient complains of:
Painful urination

Continued.

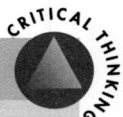

Nursing Diagnosis *THE NEXT STEP—cont'd*

Voiding frequently in small amounts
Always feeling like he has to void
Thick white penile discharge
Concern over acquiring an infection with recent unprotected sexual intercourse

OBJECTIVE DATA:
Afebrile, vital signs stable
Physical assessment:
Purulent clear white discharge from urethra
Inflammation around the meatus
Slight pain upon palpation of genitalia
Testes symmetrical without masses
No lymphadenopathy

NURSING DIAGNOSES

Altered sexuality patterns related to effects of infection-pain.

Defining Characteristics

- Decreased ability to have sexual intercourse due to genital pain
- Penile discharge
- Voiced concern about previous unprotected sexual encounter

Anxiety related to threat to and/or changes in sexual health status.

Defining Characteristics

- Uncertainty of health status
- Voiced worry over whether he has STD

Urinary retention related to infection of unknown origin.

Defining Characteristics

- Small frequent voiding
- Sensation of bladder fullness

GLOSSARY

atonic Lacking normal muscle tone.
cryptorchidism Failure of one or both of the testicles to descend into the scrotum.
dysuria Painful urination.
epispadias Congenital anomaly in which the urethra opens on the dorsum of the penis.
fundus The base or the deepest part of an organ.
glans Small, rounded mass. *Glans penis:* Caplike, conical tip of the penis that covers the end of the corpora cavernosa penis and the corpus spongiosum.
hernia Abnormal protrusion of an organ or tissue through an opening. *Incarcerated hernia:* Protrusion of abdominal contents through a weakness in the abdominal wall so that the contents cannot be returned to the abdominal cavity. *Direct inguinal hernia:* Protrusion of abdominal contents through a weakness in the abdominal musculature in the region of

Hesselbach's triangle. *Indirect inguinal hernia:* Protrusion through an internal inguinal ring hernia descending beside the spermatic cord. *Scrotal hernia:* Protrusion (generally indirect) of abdominal contents into the scrotal sac. *Strangulated hernia:* Hernia in which the blood supply to the protruded tissue is obstructed.
hydrocele Circumscribed collection of fluid, particularly in the scrotum.
hypospadias Developmental anomaly in which the urethra opens on the underside of the penis.
meatus Opening or tunnel through any part of the body.
nocturia Excessive urination at night.
orchiopexy Operation performed to mobilize an undescended testis, bring it into the scrotum, and attach it so that it will not retract.

ostium Orifice.

paraphimosis Condition characterized by an inability to replace the foreskin in its normal position after it has been retracted behind the glans penis.

Peyronie's disease Disease of unknown cause resulting in fibrous induration of the corpora cavernosa of the penis. The chief symptom is painful erection.

phimosis Difficulty in retraction of the foreskin of the penis.

Poupart's ligament Inguinal ligament; the fibrous band that runs from the anterior superior iliac spine to the pubic spine.

prepuce Foreskin.

prostatitis Acute or chronic inflammation of the prostate gland, generally in conjunction with cystitis and urethritis. Symptoms include low back and perineal pain, fever, urinary frequency, and dysuria.

retraction Condition of being drawn back.

rugated Having ridges or folds.

spermatogenesis Process of development of spermatozoa.

transillumination Passage of light through a solid or liquid substance.

sulcus Shallow groove.

varicocele Distention of the veins of the spermatic cord.

BIBLIOGRAPHY

Blandy JP, Lytton B: *The prostate,* London, 1986, Butterworth.

Blesch KS: Health beliefs about testicular cancer and self-examination among professional men, *Oncol Nurs Forum* 13:29-33, 1986.

Gillenwater JY and others: *Adult and pediatric urology,* St Louis, 1991, Mosby–Year Book.

Gordon M: *Manual of nursing diagnosis, 1993-1994,* St Louis, 1993, Mosby–Year Book.

Gordon M: *Nursing diagnosis: process and application,* ed 2, New York, 1987, McGraw-Hill.

Mayhew HE, Selman SH: Genitourinary problems in the male patient, *Prim Care* 16:857-1068, 1989.

Mosby's medical, nursing, and allied health dictionary, ed 3, St Louis, 1990, Mosby–Year Book.

Nyhus LM, Condon RE: *Hernia,* ed 3, Philadelphia, 1989, Lippincott.

Ostwald SK, Rothenberger J: Development of a testicular self-examination program for college men, *J Am Coll Health* 33:234, 1985.

Pagana KD, Pagana TJ: *Mosby's diagnostic and laboratory test reference,* St. Louis, 1992, Mosby–Year Book.

Sherwood MJ and others: *Determining nursing diagnosis through assessment,* Baltimore, 1988, Williams & Wilkins.

Stanford J: Testicular self-examination, *Prof Nurse* 1:132-133, 1986.

Stanford J: Testicular self-examination: teaching, learning and practice by nurses, *J Adv Nurs* 12:13-19, 1986.

U.S. Preventive Services Task Force: *Guide to clinical preventive services: an assessment of the effectiveness of 169 interventions,* Baltimore, 1989, Williams & Wilkins.

Vogt HB, McHale MS: Testicular cancer, *Postgrad Med* 93:93-96 +, 1992.

Female Genitalia

Outline

PURPOSE OF THE EXAMINATION

The purpose of the examination of the female genitalia is to assess the health of the female reproductive system and to screen for various sexually transmitted diseases and cervical cancer. The regional examination of the female genital system consists of (1) the abdominal examination, (2) inspection of the external genitalia, (3) palpation of the external genitalia, (4) the **speculum** examination, (5) obtaining specimens, (6) the bimanual vaginal examination, and (7) the rectovaginal examination.

ANATOMY AND PHYSIOLOGY

External Genitalia

The external female genitalia are termed the **vulva** or **pudendum** (Figure 21-1). The symphysis pubis is covered by a pad of fat called the mons pubis or mons

661

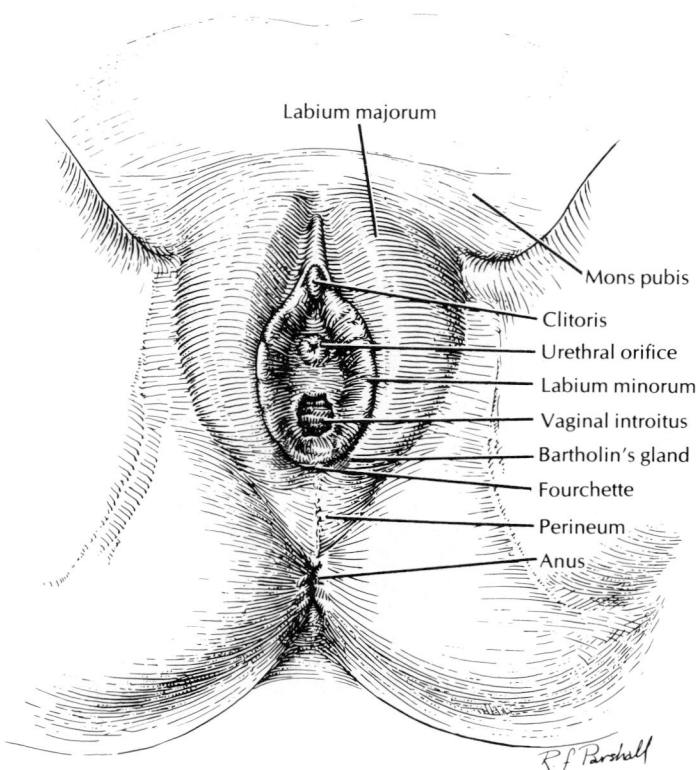

FIGURE 21-1 Female external genitalia.

veneris. In the postpubertal female the mons is covered by a patch of coarse, curly hair that extends to the lower abdomen. The abdominal portion of the female escutcheon is flat and forms the base of an inverted triangle of hair.

The labia majora are two bilobate folds of adipose tissue extending from the mons to the perineum. After puberty, their outer surfaces are covered with hair and their inner surfaces are smooth and hairless. The labia minora are two folds of skin that are thinner and darker than the labia majora. The labia minora lie within the labia majora and extend from the clitoris to the **fourchette**. Anteriorly, each labium minus divides into a medial and a lateral part. The lateral parts join posteriorly to form the prepuce of the clitoris, and the medial parts join anterior to the clitoris to form the **frenulum** of the clitoris. The clitoris is composed of erectile tissue, homologous to the corpus cavernosum of the penis. Its body is normally about 2.5 cm long; the length of its visible portion is 2 cm or less.

The vestibule is the boat-shaped anatomic region between the labia minora. It contains the urethral and vaginal **orifices.** The urethral orifice is located approximately 2.5 cm posterior and inferior to the clitoris and is visualized as an irregular, vertical slit or an inverted "V." The vaginal orifice, or **introitus,** lies immediately

behind and inferior to the urethral orifice and can be observed as a thin vertical slit or as a large orifice with irregular skin edges, depending on the condition of the hymen. The hymen is a membranous, annular, or crescentic fold at the vaginal opening. When unperforated, it is usually a continuous membrane but on occasion may be **cribiform**. After perforation, small rounded fragments of hymen attach to the introital margins; these are called hymenal caruncles.

The ducts of two types of glands open on the vulva. Skene's glands are multiple, tiny organs located in the paraurethral area. Their ducts, numbering approximately 6 to 31, lie inside and just outside of the urethral orifice and are usually not visible. These ducts open laterally and slightly posterior to the urethral orifice in approximately the 5 and 7 o'clock positions. The urethral orifice is the center of the clock. Bartholin's glands are small, ovoid organs located lateral and slightly posterior to the vaginal orifice, partially behind the bulb of the vestibule. Their ducts are approximately 2 cm long and open in the groove between the labia minora and the hymen in approximately the 5 and 7 o'clock positions. These ducts are also usually not visible.

The perineum consists of the tissues between the introitus and the anus.

The pelvic floor consists of a group of muscles at-

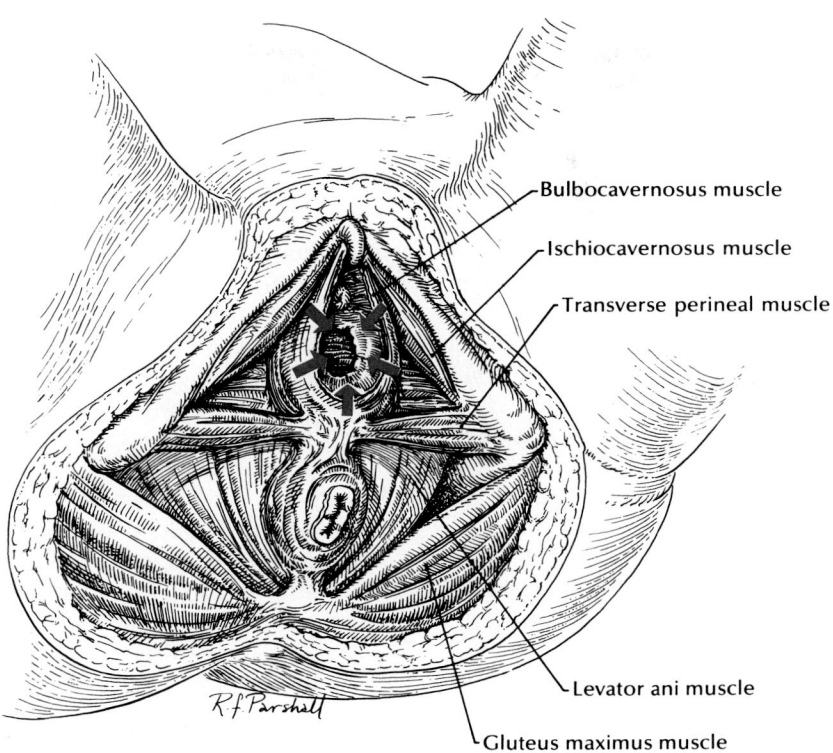

FIGURE 21-2 Muscles of the pelvic floor. Arrows illustrate the direction of contraction of the bulbocavernosus muscle.

tached to points on the bony pelvis (Figure 21-2). These muscles form a suspended sling that assists in holding the pelvic contents in place. The muscles are pierced by the urethral, vaginal, and rectal orifices and function both passively as a pelvic support and actively in voluntary contraction of the vaginal and anal orifices.

Internal Genitalia

Figure 21-3 illustrates the internal genitalia. The vagina is a pink, transversely **rugated**, collapsed tube that in the adult is approximately 9 cm long posteriorly and 6 to 7 cm long anteriorly. It inclines posteriorly at approximately a 45-degree angle with the vertical plane of the body. The vagina is highly dilatable, especially in its superior portion and anteroposterior dimension. When collapsed, it is roughly H-shaped in transverse section. Superiorly and usually anteriorly, the vagina is pierced by the uterine cervix. The recess between the portion of the vagina adjacent to the cervix and the cervix is called the vaginal **fornix**. Although it is actually continuous, the fornix is anatomically divided into anterior, posterior, and lateral fornices.

The uterus is an inverted, pear-shaped, muscular organ that is flattened anteroposteriorly. It is usually found inclined forward 45° from the vertical plane of

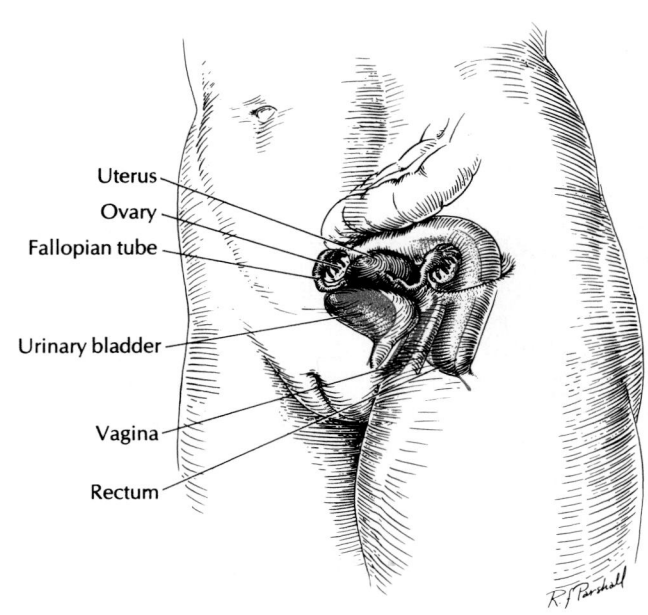

FIGURE 21-3 Internal female genitalia.

the erect body and is approximately 5.5 to 8 cm long, 3.5 to 4 cm wide, and 2 to 2.5 cm thick. The uterus of the **parous** client may be normally enlarged an additional 2 to 3 cm in any of the three dimensions. The uterus is divided into two main parts: the body and the cervix. The body in turn is composed of three parts: the fundus, the prominence above the insertion of the fallopian tubes; the body, or main portion, of the uterus; and the isthmus, the constricted lower portion of the uterus, which is adjacent to the cervix. The cervix extends from the isthmus into the vagina.

The uterine cavity communicates with the vagina through an **ostium**, the cervical os. The os is a small, depressed, circular opening in the **nulliparous** client. In women who have borne children, the os is enlarged and irregularly shaped. The position of the uterus is not fixed; it is a relatively movable organ. The uterus may be anteverted, anteflexed, retroverted, or retroflexed in position; or it may be in midposition. (See Table 21-2 for illustrations of these positions.) In the normal adult with an empty bladder the uterus is usually anteverted and slightly anteflexed in position.

The ovaries are a pair of oval organs; each is approximately 3 cm long, 2 cm wide, and 1 cm thick. They are usually located near the lateral pelvic wall, at the level of the anterosuperior iliac spine. The two fallopian tubes insert in the upper portion of the uterus, are supported loosely by the broad ligament, and run laterally to the ovaries. Each tube is approximately 10 cm long.

The uterus, ovaries, and tubes are supported by four pairs of ligaments: the cardinal, uterosacral, round, and broad ligaments (Figure 21-4).

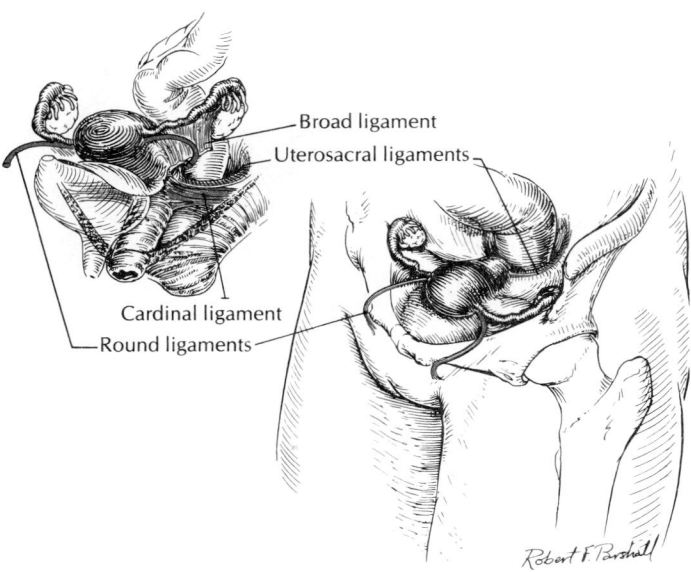

FIGURE 21-4 Ligaments of the internal female genitalia.

The rectouterine pouch, or Douglas' cul-de-sac, is a deep recess formed by the peritoneum as it passes over the intestinal surface of the rectum. It is the lowest point in the abdominal cavity.

EXAMINATION

Health History

The reproductive health history is fairly extensive. For a follow-up encounter in a health care system, much of the historical information will probably be on the record, and the focus of the interval history will be on the health need or problem. The gynecological and obstetrical regional history for a new adult client will be, out of necessity, somewhat lengthy (see below). Throughout the health history interview, record the following data about a symptom or problem: (1) onset (specific date, sudden or gradual); (2) duration; (3) frequency; (4) precipitating factors; (5) aggravating or alleviating factors; (6) treatment received or self-care given; and (7) outcome.

A. Menstrual history
1. Age initiated **(menarche)**
2. Date of last menstrual period [LMP = last menstrual period]
3. Date of last normal menstrual period [LNMP] Note: This date may the same or different from the LMP. Discrepancies may be clinically significant.
4. Pattern—frequency (days), duration (days), and amount of bleeding (in total number of tampons and/or pads used), presence of clots (size; e.g., size of a quarter)
5. Associated symptoms **(dysmenorrhea)**—pain, cramping, distention, weight gain, irritability, mood swings, breast engorgement
6. Intermenstrual bleeding or spotting
7. Changes in cycle: **metrorrhagia, oligomenorrhea**

B. Self-care
1. Pattern of douching (including solution used, strength of solution, and frequency)
2. Use of feminine hygiene sprays
3. Type of material in underpants and pantyhose
4. Planning for pregnancy, if applicable
5. Use of protection against sexually transmitted diseases

C. Gynecologic history
1. Date and results of last Pap smear
2. Gynecological diagnoses, procedures, and surgeries
3. Pregnancies—dates, durations, complications, condition of infant if live birth, and other relevant outcomes (include abortions [spontaneous, elective, therapeutic], and **ectopic pregnancies**)

4. If postmenopausal—history of hot flashes, headaches, palpitations, sweats, mood swings, vaginal dryness and itching, other signs and symptoms
5. Sexually transmitted diseases—diagnoses and treatment
   a. Gonorrhea
   b. Herpes
   c. Vaginitis
   d. HIV
   e. Syphilis
6. Infertility—diagnosis and treatment
D. Medications—contraceptive, hormonal, or other prescribed for management of reproductive system problems
   1. Name
   2. Dosage
   3. Purpose
   4. Frequency
   5. Duration
   6. Side effects
   7. Compliance
E. Sexual history
   1. Date of first intercourse
   2. Pattern and number of partners
   3. Health of partners
   4. Number and health of partners' partners
   5. Satisfaction with intercourse
   6. Current satisfaction with partner and opportunities for intercourse
   7. **Dyspareunia**
F. Present health/present illness (examples of history for common problems)
   1. *Abdominal/pelvic pain*
      a. Onset
      b. Related factors
      c. Character—sharp, dull, aching, burning, knifelike
      d. Location
      e. Frequency
      f. Intensity
      g. Associated symptoms—malaise, fever, nausea, vomiting, constipation
      h. Relief measures
   2. *Vaginal bleeding*
      a. Onset
      b. Related factors
      c. Color—pink, red, dark red, brown, other
      d. Character—thin, thick, watery, mixed with mucus. If clots, how many and how large
      e. Amount—what size of saturation on underwear or saturation of how many pads or tampons in a specific time period
      f. Frequency and relationship to menstrual cycle

g. Associated symptoms or events (e.g., cramping, injury)
3. *Vaginal discharge*
   a. Onset
   b. Color—white, yellow-green, gray, other
   c. Character—thin, curd-like, purulent, other
   d. Odor—"fishy," foul, other
   e. Associated symptoms—vulvar itching, vaginal itching, rash, pain with intercourse
   f. Relief measures
   g. Previous experiences with the same symptoms
4. *Urinary problems*
   a. Character
   b. Frequency
   c. Previous diagnoses
   d. Description of urine
   e. Associated symptoms—fever, chills, flank pain, urgency, frequency, dysuria, hematuria
   f. Relationship of problems to changes in sexual intercourse frequency, technique, or partner

RISK FACTORS

Cervical cancer

Age—between 40 and 50 years
History—cervical **dysplasias, condylomata acuminata** lesions, herpes infection
First coitus—early age
Sex partners—multiple or partner with multiple partners
Pregnancies—multiple
History—exposure to diethylstilbestrol, smoking

Endometrial cancer

Age—postmenopausal
Menarche—early
Menopause—late
Parity—low or infertility
Body weight—obese
History—hypertension, diabetes, endometrial **hyperplasia**, liver disease
Estrogen—history of replacement
Family history—endometrial, breast, or colon cancer

Ovarian cancer

Age—between 40 and 60
History—ovarian dysfunction, spontaneous abortions, cancer of breast or endometrium, irradiation of pelvic organs, **endometriosis**
Family history—ovarian or breast cancer
Environment—exposure to talc or asbestos

G. Associated conditions
1. Diabetes
2. Hypertension
3. Genitourinary problems
4. Cancer
H. Family history
1. Reproductive problems
2. Cancer (See the box on page 665 for risk factors for cancer.)
3. Diabetes
4. Mother's use of hormones during pregnancy

Preparation for the Examination: Client and the Environment

Most female clients perceive the examination of their reproductive organs as being different from the examination of other body parts. Past admonitions of "do not touch" and "keep it covered" have created a population of anatomically unaware and sometimes inappropriately "modest" women who are often unnecessarily difficult to examine. This is particularly true of older women and members of certain ethnic groups. Most practitioners believe that they can obtain a great amount of information about a female client by examining the genital area and performing screening tests. However, because of their experience with fearful and tense reactions of many clients, practitioners have sometimes routinely omitted the examination of the genital organs or have referred their clients to gynecologic specialists for routine examinations.

One cause of the female client's tenseness during an examination of the genital area may be fear of discovery. During the history investigate areas of anatomic and physiological function and dysfunction. The review of systems on all clients should include a sexual history. If you have skillfully accomplished this portion of the history and if the client has been cooperative, she should not be apprehensive about the possible discovery of sexual "secrets."

Other causes of tenseness during the pelvic examination include fear of discovery of disease and the memory of previous, uncomfortable pelvic examinations. Many clients are not knowledgeable regarding the anatomy of the pelvic area. Determine the client's need for basic information regarding the structure of the genital organs and provide this instruction before the pelvic examination, along with a demonstration of the instruments and an explanation of the procedure. Show the speculum to the client and demonstrate the mechanism used to open and close it. Advise the client about the clicking sounds normally made by a speculum as it is opened and closed. A relatively short amount of time taken to inform and orient all female clients at their first examinations provides long-term benefits in preventing anxiety and increasing cooperation. See the box

> **Hints to Help the Client Relax During a Pelvic Examination**: *Teaching the client a relaxation technique will often make an examination shorter in length, and, in the case of a very tense client, possible at all.*
>
> *One successful relaxation technique is the following: instruct the client to:*
> *Place her hands on her chest at about the level of the diaphragm*
> *Breathe deeply and slowly through her mouth*
> *Concentrate on the rhythm of breathing*
> *Relax all body muscles with each exhalation*
> *The tense client is apt to hold her breath and tighten. Even the coached client may forget and hold her breath. A gentle reminder, advising her to keep breathing, usually enables the client to maintain relaxation. This technique is particularly helpful in the adolescent or virginal client, whose introitus may be especially small.*
>
> *Additional relaxation or, more specifically, distraction technique, is the placement of a sign or mobile above the examining table. Some clients appreciate having something to look at, and their attention is constructively diverted from the examiner's activities.*

above for hints to help the client relax during a pelvic examination.

Most clients find it difficult to engage in lengthy conversations while in a **lithotomy** position. They do appreciate explanations and reassurances from examiners but prefer not to have to respond to questions until they are again upright and at eye level with the examiner. Questioning a client extensively during the pelvic examination is apt to make her tense.

Environmental conditions are also important in enhancing cooperation during examination of the genital area. The environment and the client should be warm. The examining area should be private and safe from unexpected intrusion. The room, the examiner's hands, and all materials touching the client should be warm.

Clients should be advised not to douche or use vaginal medications or other inserts during the 24 hours preceding the pelvic examination and reminded to empty their bladders immediately before the examination.

Materials needed for the examination should be assembled and readily available before the client is put in the lithotomy position. See the box on page 667.

Some clients have difficulty assuming the lithotomy position, especially moving their buttocks sufficiently downward to the edge of the table. The practitioner can assist the client by asking the client to raise her buttocks (while the client is lying on the table with heels in the

Preparation for the Examination

Equipment

Item	Purpose
Disposable latex gloves	Protect examiner and client from transfer of infectious organisms
Speculums of various sizes	Inspection of internal genitalia
Sterile cotton swabs	Cleanse internal genitalia
	Obtain specimens for examination
Lubricant* (water soluble)	Facilitate insertion of speculum and fingers for examination
Cotton balls	Cleanse tissues
Sponge forceps	Insert cotton or gauze to cleanse tissues
Cytology fixative	Fix Pap smear
Floor examination light	Visualization of internal structures
Ayre spatulas	Obtain cell samples for Pap smear
Cervical brushes	Obtain **endocervical** specimens for Pap smears
Culture media	Inoculation of specimens from cervical and vaginal areas
Glass slides	For Pap smears and for preparing a sample of vaginal discharge for examination
Hand mirror	Enable client to visualize internal genitalia
Normal saline	Prepare discharge on slides to assess for presence of specific organisms
Potassium hydroxide	Prepare discharge on slides to assess for presence of specific organisms

*An amount of lubricant, sufficient for the examination, should be placed on a piece of paper or gauze. The examiner should avoid handling the tube of lubricant during the examination, since it might be contaminated during handling and become a mechanism of infection transmission. Also, single-use tubes of lubricant are available.

Client

Explain procedure
Empty bladder right before examination
Assist client to assume lithotomy position

1. Instruct the client to lie down on the examination table and assist her to put her heels into the stirrups and to stabilize them. Some clients are more comfortable leaving shoes and/or socks on.
2. Retract the end of the table if it is still extended.
3. Assist the client to bring her buttocks to the very bottom edge of the table. Gently guide the client or advise her to feel and aim for the end of the table herself.
4. Redrape the client so that the knees and symphysis pubis are covered. Depress the drape between the knees so you can see the client's face for responses during the examination.
5. Reposition upper torso so head and shoulders are slightly elevated to increase client comfort and assist relaxation of abdominal muscles.

Environment

Warm
Well lit with additional light available to assist the visualization of internal genitalia
Private

Examiner

Gloved throughout the examination
Standing and sitting (on a wheeled stool) between the client's legs during various parts of the examination
Monitoring client's face throughout examination

stirrups) and by guiding the client's buttocks downward from a position at the client's side or from a position at the foot of the table. Clients usually feel more comfortable wearing shoes and/or socks when their feet are in the stirrups, rather than supporting their weight with bare heels against the hard, cold metal of the stirrups.

The client and the examiner assume several positions for the examination. For the abdominal examination, the client is lying supine on the examination table and the examiner is facing the client's right side. For the inspection and palpation of the external genitalia and the speculum examination, the client is in the lithotomy position (Figure 21-5) and the examiner is seated on a stool, facing the client's genitalia. For the bimanual ex-

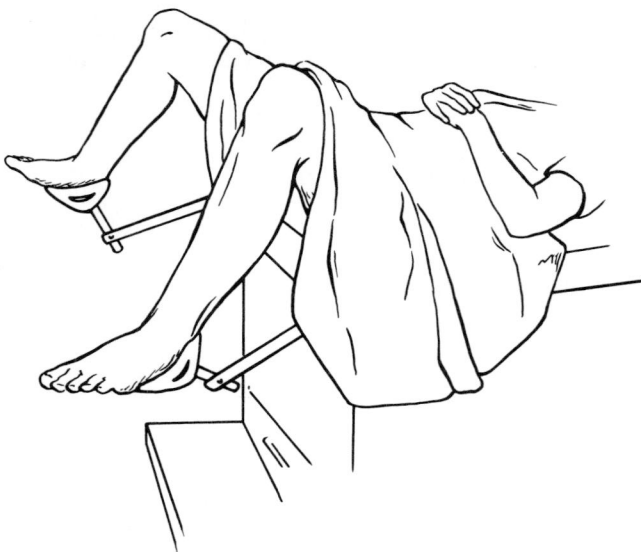

FIGURE 21-5 Lithotomy position for the female genital examination.

amination and the rectovaginal examination, the client remains in the lithotomy position, and the examiner is standing.

The abdominal examination is discussed in Chapter 17 on assessment of the abdomen. The examination of the female genital system should be preceded by a thorough examination of the abdomen.

Always wear gloves on both hands for the genital area examination. If infection is suspected, double gloves may provide additional protection for the examiner. Also, double gloving facilitates changing of gloves between the vaginal examination and the rectovaginal examination. The top pair can be shed right before the rectovaginal examination. However in the case of infection or suspected infection, the examiner may want to double glove throughout the examination.

Technique for Examination and Normal Findings

Inspection of the external genitalia. With the client in lithotomy position, sit on a stool, facing the external genitalia. Ask the client to relax and spread her legs. First, observe the skin and hair distribution. Adult female hair distribution should be approximately shaped as an inverse triangle. Some abdominal hair is normal and may be hereditary. Male hair distribution patterns (diamond-shaped) in women are abnormal.

In the adolescent client, assess sexual maturity by observing breast growth and pubic hair growth. Table 21-1 outlines and illustrates sexual maturity ratings for the appearance of the female genitalia. Along with changes in pubic hair, the following occur:

1. Increase in prominence in labia majora
2. Enlargement of the labia minora
3. Increase in size of the clitoris
4. Increase in elasticity of vaginal tissue
5. Enlargement of vagina and ovaries

Skin and hair. Although the client knows she will be touched, she may startle when the fingers are placed on the genitalia at the initiation of the palpation. To enable the client to accommodate to the touching, touch her first on the inner thigh with the back of a hand before touching any part of the genitalia. Tell the client you will be placing your hand against her thigh. Then place it gently, but firmly there. This helps relax the client and enables the examiner to assess the degree of relaxation.

Inspect the total skin area for lesions and parasites. Use the gloved fingers of one hand to spread the hair and labia so that all skin surfaces can be adequately visualized. The skin should be the same color as the remainder of the body or slightly darker. The hair is normally coarse in texture and somewhat to very curly. **Sebaceous cysts** are often seen on the labia.

Labia. The labia are flat in childhood, plump during adulthood, and atrophic in old age. Estrogen influences fat deposition, which causes a round, full appearance of the labia. The labia majora of the nulliparous client will be in close approximation covering the labia minora and the vestibule area. After a vaginal delivery, the labia may appear slightly shriveled and gaping. Regardless of general appearance, the labia should appear reasonably symmetric. The mucous membranes are normally dark pink in color and moist in appearance. The skin of the vulvar area is a slightly darker pigment than the skin of the rest of the body.

Clitoris. Examine the clitoris for size and examine the adjacent area for lesions. The visible portion of the clitoris should not exceed 2 cm in length and 1 cm in width. The area of the clitoris particularly is a common site for chancres of syphilis in the younger client and for cancerous lesions in the older client.

Urethral orifice. The urethral orifice appears slitlike, stellate, or as an inverted "V" and is of the same color as the membranes surrounding it. The openings of the paraurethral (Skene's) glands are not usually visible. Erythema or a polyp located in this area or a discharge from the urethra or gland ducts is abnormal.

Glandular areas. The examiner next observes the area of Bartholin's glands and their ducts for tenderness, swelling, erythema, duct enlargement, or discharge. The presence of any of these conditions is abnormal.

TABLE 21-1

Developmental Changes in the General Appearance of Female Genitalia

Developmental stage	Description	Developmental stage	Description
Stage 1 sexual maturity (preadolescence)	No pubic hair, except for fine body hair	Stage 4 sexual maturity	Texture and curl of pubic hair as in adult but not as thick and not spread over the thighs (usually seen between ages 13 and 14)
Stage 2 sexual maturity	Sparse growth of long, slightly pigmented, fine pubic hair, which is slightly curly and located along the labia (usually seen at ages 11 to 12)	Stage 5 sexual maturity	Adult appearance in quality and quantity of pubic hair; growth is spread onto the inner aspect of the upper thighs
Stage 3 sexual maturity	Pubic hair becomes darker, curlier, and spreads over the symphysis (usually seen at ages 12 to 13)	Elderly	Pubic hair is thin, sparse, brittle, and gray

Perineum. Inspect the perineum for lesions and evidence of an **episiotomy** and its healing. Also inspect the anus at this time (see Chapter 22 on assessment of the anus and rectum).

Palpation of the external genitalia

Labia. Use one hand to spread the labia open while the other hand is used to palpate the labia majora and labia minora. The labia should feel soft, and the texture should be homogeneous. Palpate any areas of observed abnormality below the skin surface to determine size, shape, consistency, movability, and tenderness.

Glands. Insert approximately half the index finger of the palpating hand into the vagina. First, gently milk the urethra and area of Skene's duct openings from about the level of 4 cm on the anterior vaginal wall down to the orifice (Figure 21-6). This procedure should not normally cause pain or discharge. If a discharge is present, a specimen is obtained with a swab and placed onto a Thayer-Martin culture plate. Then rotate the hand without removing the finger and palpate the area of Bartholin's glands and their ducts for swelling or tenderness (Figure 21-7). Palpate this area using the intravaginal finger and the thumb of that same

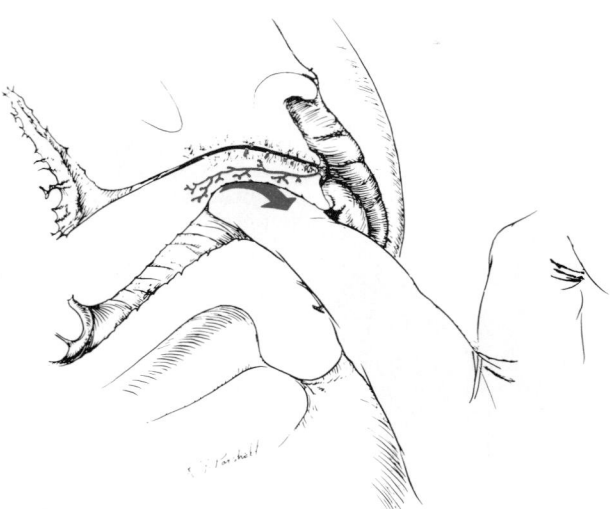

FIGURE 21-6 Palpation of Skene's glands.

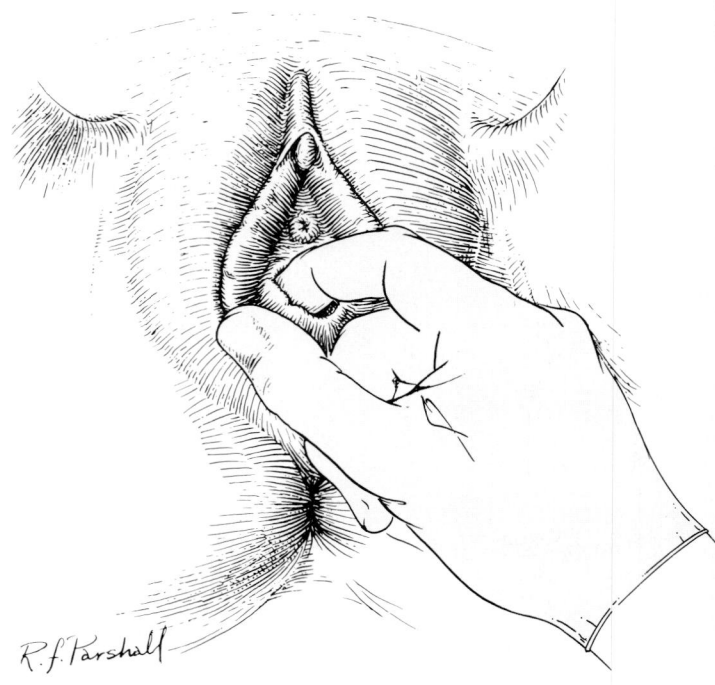

R.f. Parshall

FIGURE 21-7 Palpation of Bartholin's glands.

hand on the external surface. Normally Bartholin's glands are not palpable.

Perineum and musculature of the vaginal introitus. While the finger is in the vagina, perform several maneuvers to assess the integrity of the pelvic musculature. Palpate the perineal area between the finger inside the vagina and the thumb of that same hand. In the nulliparous client the perineum is felt as a firm, muscular body. After an episiotomy has healed, the perineum feels thinner and more rigid because of scarring. If this area is very thin and if the palpating fingers can almost approximate, ask the client about bowel or sexual problems.

Ask the client to constrict her vaginal orifice around the examiner's finger while placed in the vagina. A nulliparous client will demonstrate a high degree of tone; a **multiparous** client, less tone.

Presence of cystocele, rectocele, enterocele, and uterine prolapse. Place the index and middle fingers in the vagina, spread them laterally, and ask the client to push down against them. The presence of urinary stress incontinence, cystocele, rectocele, enterocele, or uterine prolapse can be observed if present. **Cystocele** is the prolapse into the vagina of the anterior vaginal wall and the bladder. Clinically, a pouching would be seen on the anterior wall as the client strains. **Rectocele** is the prolapse into the vagina of the posterior vaginal wall and the rectum. Clinically, a pouching would be seen on the posterior wall as the client strains. **Enterocele** is a hernia of the pouch of Douglas into the vagina. Clinically, a bulge would be seen emerging from the posterior fornix. If this is observed, the client should

be additionally examined by assessing the effect of straining (1) during the speculum examination with the inserted speculum, half opened, three fourths of its length into the vagina; and (2) during the bimanual examination with the intravaginal fingers in the posterior fornix.

There are three degrees of uterine prolapse. In first-degree prolapse, the cervix appears at the introitus when the client strains. In second-degree prolapse, the cervix is outside the introitus when the client strains. In third-degree prolapse, the whole uterus is outside the introitus, and the vagina is essentially turned inside out when the client strains.

Inspection of the internal genitalia—Speculum examination. You will have obtained clues regarding the most appropriate type and size of speculum to use in the speculum examination through the history and inspection of the external genitalia. The two basic types of speculums are the Graves speculum and the Pederson speculum (Figure 21-8). The Graves speculum is one of the most commonly used in examination of the adult female client. It is available in lengths varying from 3½ to 5 inches and in widths from ¾ to 1½ inches. The Pederson speculum is both narrower and flatter than the Graves speculum and is used with virgins, nulliparous clients, or clients whose vaginal orifices have contracted postmenopausally.

ABOUT SPECULUMS

A vaginal speculum consists of two blades, a handle, and some mechanism to open the distal end of the blades. There are two basic types: reusable metal and disposable plastic. Each basic type is available in various sizes. The two general speculum designs are the Graves speculum, the commonly used type, and the Pederson speculum, with blades flatter and narrower than the Graves. The Pederson speculum is used with women having narrow vaginal openings.

Metal and plastic speculums operate somewhat differently, although both have (1) levers that, when depressed, open the distal ends of the blades; (2) mechanisms that allow for separation of the proximal ends of the blades; and (3) locking mechanisms. Metal speculums have two positioning devices: depression of the lever opens the distal end of the blades, and fixing the screw on the lever locks the blades open at that point. In addition, the opening at the proximal end (and consequently the distal end) of the blades can be widened and locked wide by loosening and then lifting a plate attached to both the handle of the speculum and the upper blade.

The distal and proximal blade-opening mechanisms are connected in the plastic speculum. As the plastic lever is depressed in the plastic speculum, the distal end of the blades open. If the lever is fully depressed and then pushed upward on the handle, the proximal ends of the blades also widen. The lever fixes automatically into grooves on the handle of the speculum. The clicking sound of the plastic speculum is loud, sharp, and sometimes perceived as alarming to some clients, who think the speculum is breaking inside of them. Anticipatory warning about the sound of the plastic mechanism is advised. Plastic speculums also tend to get locked into position and are sometimes hard to release.

Because each type of speculum operates somewhat differently, the beginning examiner should practice with the mechanisms apart from examination and before use with clients.

Warm metal speculums before insertion. An effective way to do this is to run warm water over it. The warm water also assists in lubricating both the metal and plastic speculums and should be used as the method of lubrication if cultures and smears are to be taken. Gel lubricant is bacteriostatic and also distorts cells on Papanicolaou (Pap) smears. Therefore, do not use lubricant if cultures or smears are to be obtained.

Use the following procedure for speculum insertion:
1. Place the index finger and middle finger of one hand about 2 cm into the vagina.
2. Spread the fingers and exert pressure toward the posterior vaginal wall. Advise the client that she will feel intravaginal pressure and ask her to relax the muscles you are pushing against.
3. Hold the speculum in the opposite hand with the blades between the index and middle fingers.
4. Ask the client to bear down. This maneuver helps to open the vaginal orifice and relax perineal muscles.
5. Insert the speculum blades obliquely along the top of the intravaginal fingers, taking advantage of the H configuration of the relaxed vagina (Figure 21-9, *A*).
6. Continue to insert the speculum at a plane parallel to the examining table until the end of the speculum has reached the tips of the fingers in the vagina. Then withdraw the intravaginal fingers (Figure 21-9, *B*).
7. Rotate the speculum to a transverse position, and alter the plane in adaptation to the plane of the vagina, approximately one of a 45-degree angle with the examining table (Figure 21-9, *C*). Insert the speculum until it touches the end of the vagina.
8. Depress the lever of the speculum; this opens the blades and allows visualization. Ideally, the cervix is seen between the blades (Figure 21-9, *D*). Sometimes, however, especially for the beginning examiner, it is not. In such cases the speculum is either anterior (usually the situation) or posterior to the cervix. If this occurs, withdraw the speculum halfway and redirect it into a different plane. Be careful not to pinch the patient because the blades can catch tissue between them as they are being closed and rotated.
9. After the entire cervix is in view, fix the depressed lever in an open position.

If the client is tense and is resisting insertion of the speculum, do not withdraw the speculum but stop the insertion, leaving the speculum in its position. Remind the client to use relaxation techniques, and continue the examination when relaxation has occurred.

Cervix. Observe the cervix for color, position, size, projection into the vaginal vault, shape, general symmetry, surface characteristics, shape and patency of the os, and discharge:

COLOR: The normal color of the cervix is pink. The cervix is normally pale after menopause and cyanotic in pregnancy. Cyanosis can occur with any condition that causes systemic hypoxia or regional venous congestion. Hyperemia may indicate inflammation. An additional cause of pallor is anemia.

POSITION: The position of the cervix is related to the position of the uterus. The cervix is usually midline and

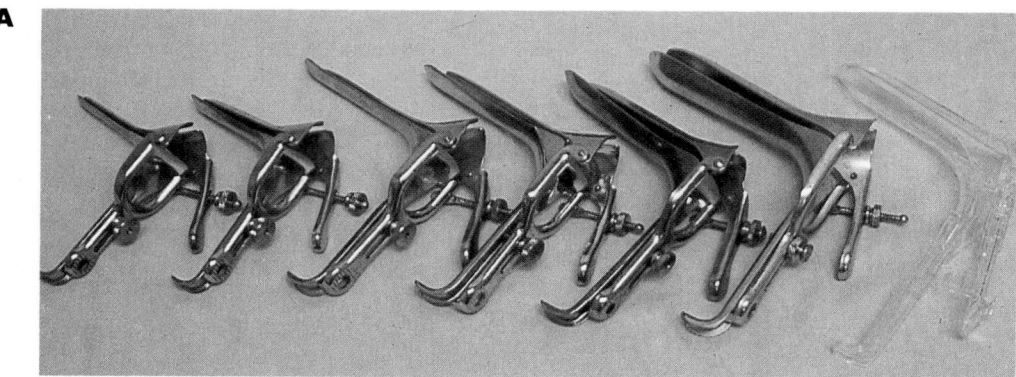

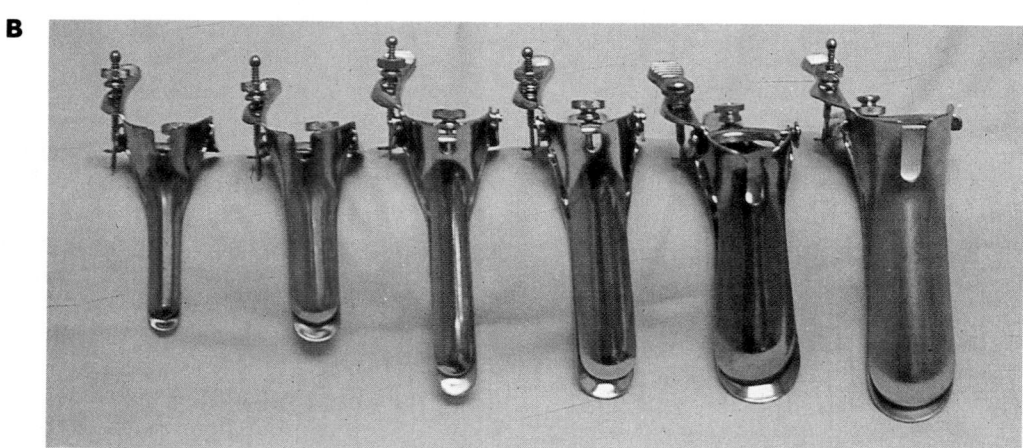

FIGURE 21-8 Vaginal specula. From left to right. **A,** Short-billed pediatric, pediatric, small Pederson, Pederson, small Graves, large Graves, plastic Graves. **B,** Short-billed pediatric, pediatric, small Pederson, Pederson, small Graves, large Graves. (From Seidel HM and others: *Mosby's guide to physical examination,* ed 2, St Louis, 1991, Mosby–Year Book.)

extends approximately 2 cm into the vagina. A cervix projecting more deeply than 3 cm into the vaginal vault may indicate uterine prolapse. A cervix situated on a lateral vaginal wall may indicate tumor or adhesion of a superior structure.

SIZE: The cervix of women of childbearing age is usually 2 to 3 cm in diameter. A cervix larger than 4 cm in diameter is hypertrophied, and the presence of inflammation or tumor should be considered.

SURFACE CHARACTERISTICS: The cervix should look smooth and firm. Lesions and polyps are commonly seen on the cervix and require more than visual assessment to determine if a pathological condition exists. Any irregularity or **nodularity** of the cervical surface should be considered possibly abnormal (Figure 21-10). One relatively benign condition is the presence of **nabothian** cysts, which appear as smooth, round, small (less than 1 cm in diameter), yellow or grayish-white lesions. Nabothian cysts are caused by obstruction of the cervical gland ducts.

When the **squamocolumnar junction** is on the ectocervix, the columnar epithelium will appear as a red, relatively symmetric circle around the os. This condition may be a normal variation of the placement of the squamocolumnar junction or may be caused by the separation by speculum blades of a cervix whose external os has been altered and enlarged by childbirth. This condition is termed *eversion* or *ectropion.* Erosions appear similar to eversions but are usually irregular, rough, and friable. Erosions frequently indicate pathologic conditions and require further assessment and treatment. Because of the occasional presence of the squamocolumnar junction on the ectocervix and its visual similarity to erosions and other lesions, the differential assessment of a normal cervix from an abnormal cervix using inspection alone is impossible.

Diffuse punctuate hemorrhages, colloquially referred to as "strawberry spots," are occasionally observed in association with trichomonal infections.

DISCHARGE: The character of the normal cervical mucus varies in the menstrual cycle. Normal discharge is always odorless and nonirritating. Its color and con-

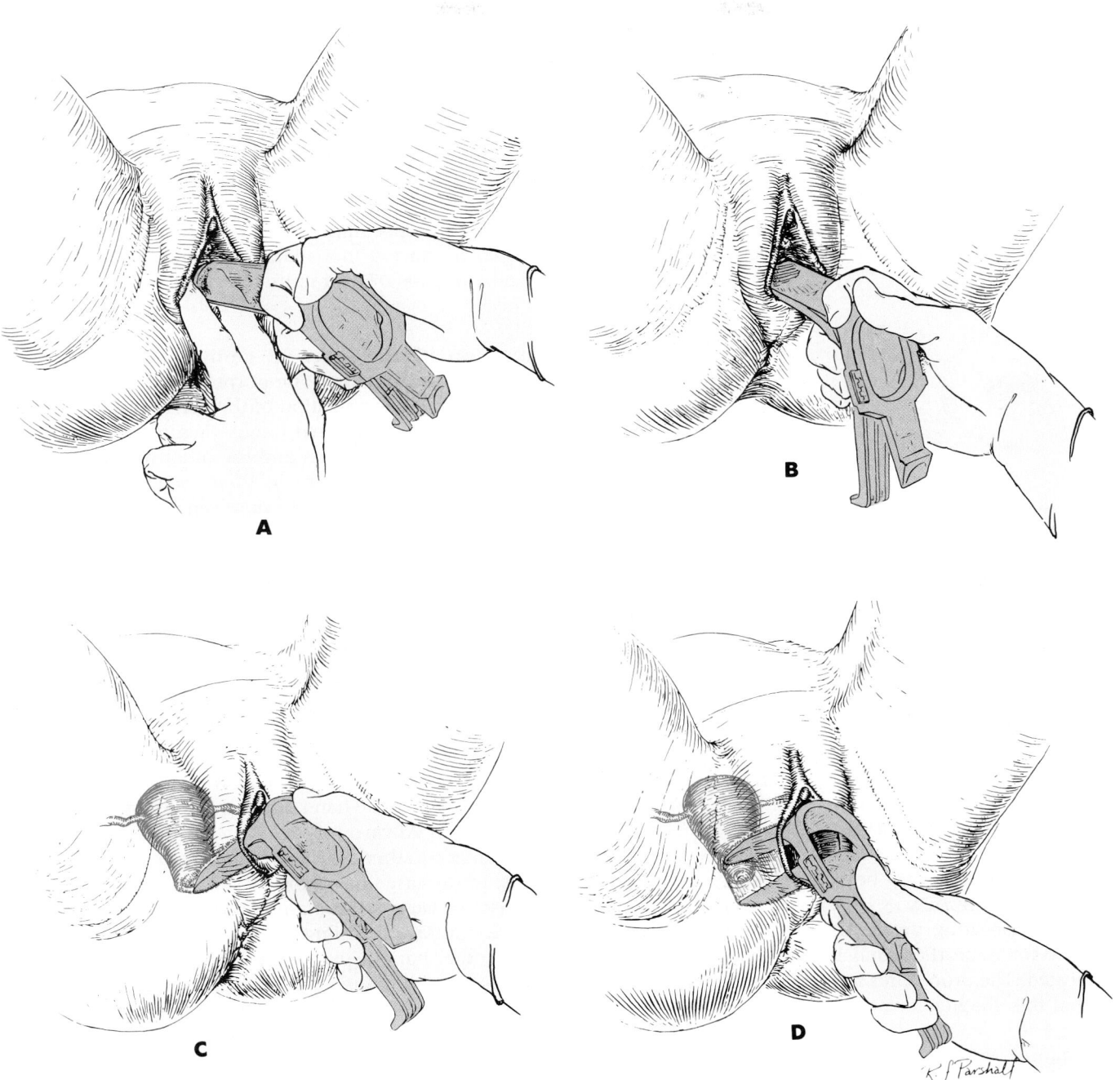

FIGURE 21-9 Procedure for vaginal examination. **A,** Opening of the introitus. **B,** Oblique insertion of the speculum. **C,** Final insertion of the speculum. **D,** Opening of the speculum blades.

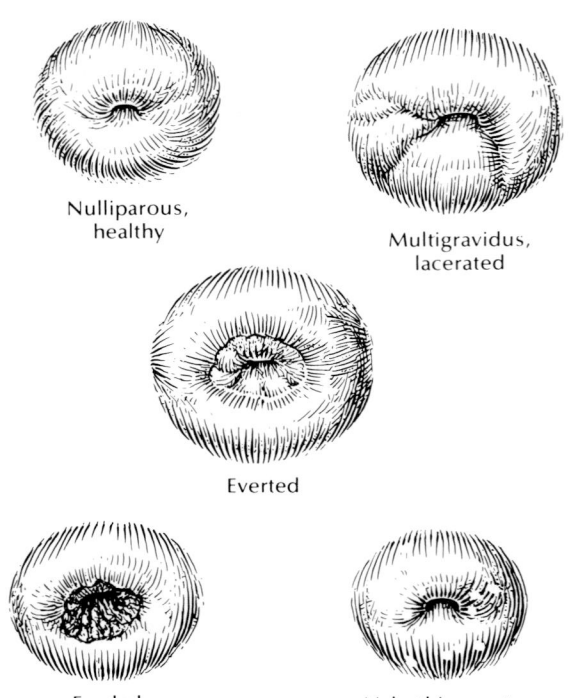

Nulliparous,
healthy

Multigravidus,
lacerated

Everted

Eroded

Nabothian cysts

FIGURE 21-10 Common appearances and lesions of the cervix.

sistency may vary from clear to white and from thin to thick and stringy. Colored, malodorous, or purulent discharges exuding from the os or present in the area of the cervix are probably abnormal.

SHAPE OF THE OS: The cervical os of the nulliparous client is small and evenly round. The cervical os of a parous client who has had a vaginal delivery shows the effects of the stretching and laceration of childbirth and is irregular in shape.

Many clients have not seen their cervices. The client should be asked if she wishes to see her cervix. This visualization can easily be accomplished through the use of a hand mirror.

After inspecting the cervix, obtain the Pap smear, culture for gonorrhea, and hanging drop specimen if indicated. The procedures for these are described at the end of this chapter.

Vagina. Next, inspect the vagina. This step is done during speculum insertion, while the speculum is open, and during its removal. Note the color and condition of the vaginal mucosa and the color, odor, consistency, and appearance of vaginal secretions. Pallor, cyanosis, and hyperemia may be present for the same reasons as described for the cervix. **Leukoplakia** may also occur on vaginal mucosa.

As with cervical discharge, vaginal discharge is nor-

mally odorless, nonirritating, thin or mucoid, and clear or cloudy. Also, the presence of some whitish, creamy material (**leukorrhea**) is normal. Describe any other vaginal discharge according to its color, odor, consistency, amount, and appearance.

After the inspection of the vagina, slowly withdraw the speculum. As it is withdrawn, loosen the nut, or catch, and control the lever again with the thumb. Slowly close the blades as they are withdrawn, and carefully rotate the speculum so that all areas of vaginal tissue are inspected. As the blades are closed, be careful to prevent pinching of tissue or the catching of hairs between the blades.

Inspect the speculum for odors and either discard it (plastic) or place it in a soaking solution (metal). See the box on page 671 for more information about speculums.

Palpation of the internal genitalia—Bimanual vaginal examination. The purpose of the bimanual examination is the palpation of the pelvic contents between the examiner's two hands (Figures 21-11 and 21-12): one in the vagina and the other on the lower abdomen. Examiners vary in their preference of the placement of the dominant, more sensitive hand. The beginning examiner should attempt alternating hands for examinations and then decide on a routine that is most individually workable.

The client remains in the lithotomy position. Stand between the client's legs. The vaginal examining hand assumes the obstetric position: index and middle fingers extended and together, thumb abducted, and fourth and little fingers folded on the palm of the hand. Lubricate the vaginal examining fingers. Spread the labia with the thumb and index finger of the opposite hand. Insert the lubricated fingers into the vagina with the palmar surface of the hand directed toward the anterior vaginal wall. Always palpate with the palmar surface of the fingers rather than with the less sensitive tips or backs. In the case of a young or old client with a small and narrow vagina, the examination may be performed with one intravaginal finger.

The other hand is placed on the abdomen and used to press the abdominal and pelvic contents toward the intravaginal hand. If the glove on this hand has been soiled by excessive discharge during the external genital inspection or speculum insertion, the glove on this hand should be changed.

Movement of both the intravaginal and abdominal hands should be slow and firm. To palpate adequately, the client must be relaxed. If the client becomes tense, stop the procedure and help the client relax; however, leave the examining hands in position.

Locate the cervix and assess it for size, contour, surface characteristics, consistency, position, patency of the

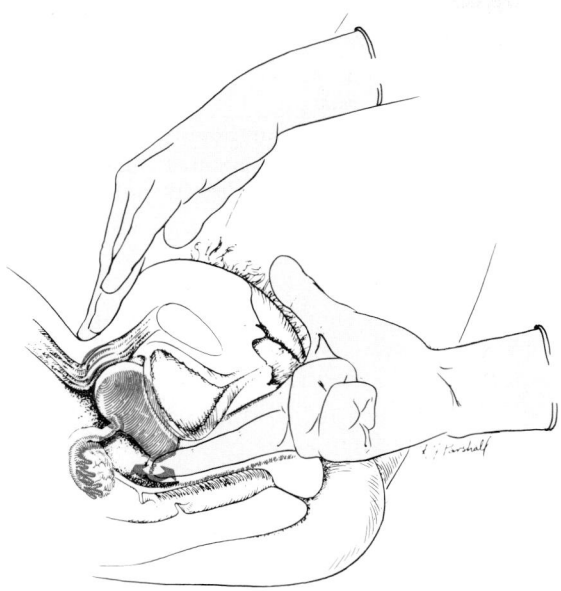

FIGURE 21-11 Bimanual palpation of the uterus.

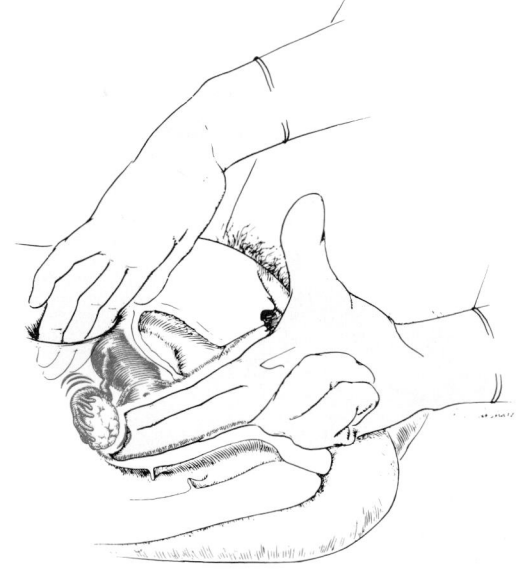

FIGURE 21-12 Bimanual palpation of the adnexa.

os, and mobility. Use the palmar surfaces of both fingers to completely palpate the cervix and fornices. Gently place a fingertip into the external os to assess its patency. Determine on which vaginal wall the cervix is placed and if the cervix is approximately midline. Place the fingers in the lateral fornices, and move (wag) the cervix back and forth between the fingers for 1 to 2 cm in each direction to assess for CMT (cervical motion tenderness). The cervix and uterus should be freely movable and should move without tenderness. An immobile or tender cervix and uterus are abnormal.

The surface of the cervix normally feels smooth. Nabothian cysts, tumors, or lesions will make it feel nodular or irregular. The consistency of the cervix is firm and slightly resilient and feels analogous to the tip of the nose. The cervix softens in pregnancy and hardens with tumors. The cervix is normally located on the anterior wall in the midline or on the posterior wall. A laterally displaced cervix may indicate tumor or adhesion. The external os in the nonpregnant client should admit a finger for about 0.5 cm. It should be open and firm. A stenosed external os is abnormal.

Assess the size, shape, surface characteristics, consistency, position, mobility, and tenderness of the uterine body and fundus. First, determine the position of the uterus because techniques used to assess the uterine body and fundus will vary with the uterine position in the client (Table 21-2). The uterus is in one of the three basic positions: anteversion, midposition, or retroversion. Version in this context indicates deflection, specifically the relationship of the long axis of the uterus

to the long axis of the body. If the axis of the uterus is deflected anteriorly, the uterus is said to be anteverted; if the uterus is deflected posteriorly, the uterus is said to be retroverted; and if the long axis of the uterus is roughly parallel to that of the total body, the uterus is in midposition. When the long axis of the uterus is not straight but is bent on itself, the uterus is said to be flexed. Thus, the anteverted or retroverted uterus can be flexed, or bent on itself, to produce two additional variations of position: anteflexion and retroflexion.

The position of the cervix provides clues of the uterine position. A cervix on the anterior wall may indicate an antepositioned or retroflexed uterus; a centrally located cervix probably indicates a uterus in midposition; and a cervix on the posterior vaginal wall suggests a retroverted uterus.

Because approximately 85% of uteri are in anteposition (i.e., anteverted or anteflexed), first attempt palpation of the uterus anteriorly. Place the intravaginal fingers in the anterior fornix. Place the hand on the abdomen flat on the midline and in a position approximately halfway between the symphysis pubis and the umbilicus. This hand acts as a resistance against which the intravaginal fingers palpate the pelvic organs. With the fingers in the anterior fornix, gently lift the tissues against the hand on the abdomen. If the uterus is in anteposition, it will be palpated between the hands. If the uterus is not palpated anteriorly, place the fingers in the posterior fornix and again raise them forward toward the hand on the abdomen. If the uterus is in retroversion, only the isthmus will be felt between the

TABLE 21-2

Findings in Bimanual Vaginal and Rectovaginal Examination

Position of uterus		Bimanual	
		Position of the cervix	Body and fundus
Anteverted 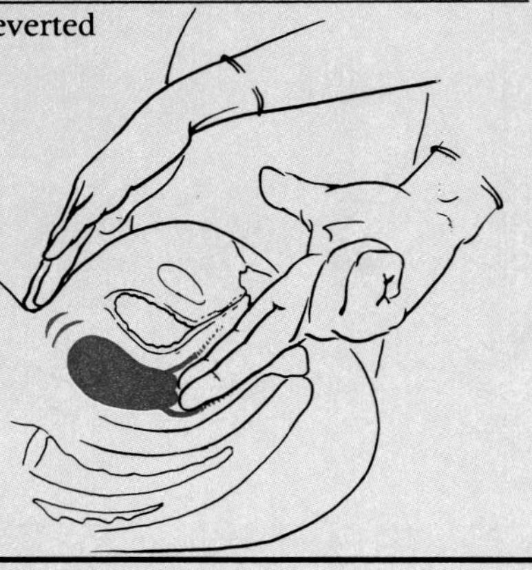	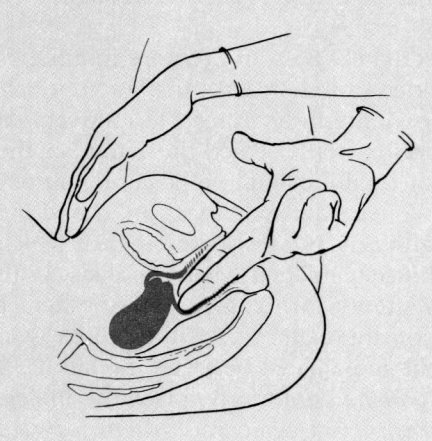	Anterior vaginal wall	Palpable by one hand on the abdomen and the fingers of the other in the vagina
Midposition 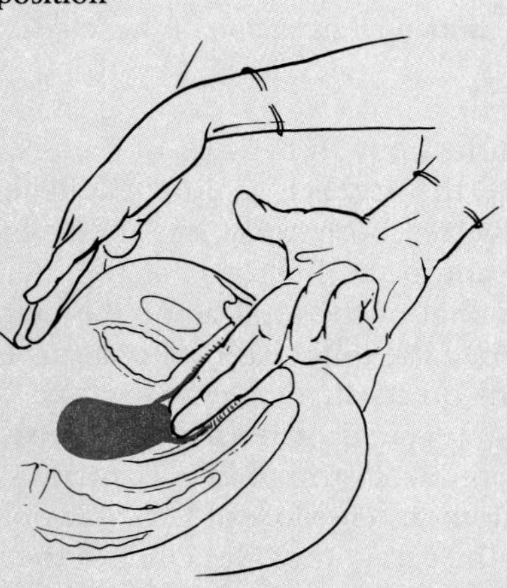		The apex of the vagina	May not be palpable
Retroverted		Posterior vaginal wall	Not palpable

Anterior and posterior portion of uterus	Rectovaginal	
	Cervix	**Body and fundus**
Palpable as the uterus is rotated even more anteriorly	Palpable through the rectovaginal septum	Not palpable by fingers in the rectum

May not be palpable	Posterior portion felt through the rectovaginal septum	May not be palpable

Posterior portion may be palpable by fingers in the posterior fornix	May not be palpable by fingers in the rectum	Body easily palpable by fingers in the rectum; fundus may not be palpable

Continued.

TABLE 21-2—cont'd

Findings in Bimanual Vaginal and Rectovaginal Examination

	Bimanual	
Position of uterus	**Position of the cervix**	**Body and fundus**
Anteflexed	Anterior vaginal wall or apex	Easily palpable; angulation of the isthmus may be felt in the anterior fornix
Retroflexed	Anterior or posterior vaginal wall or apex	Not palpable

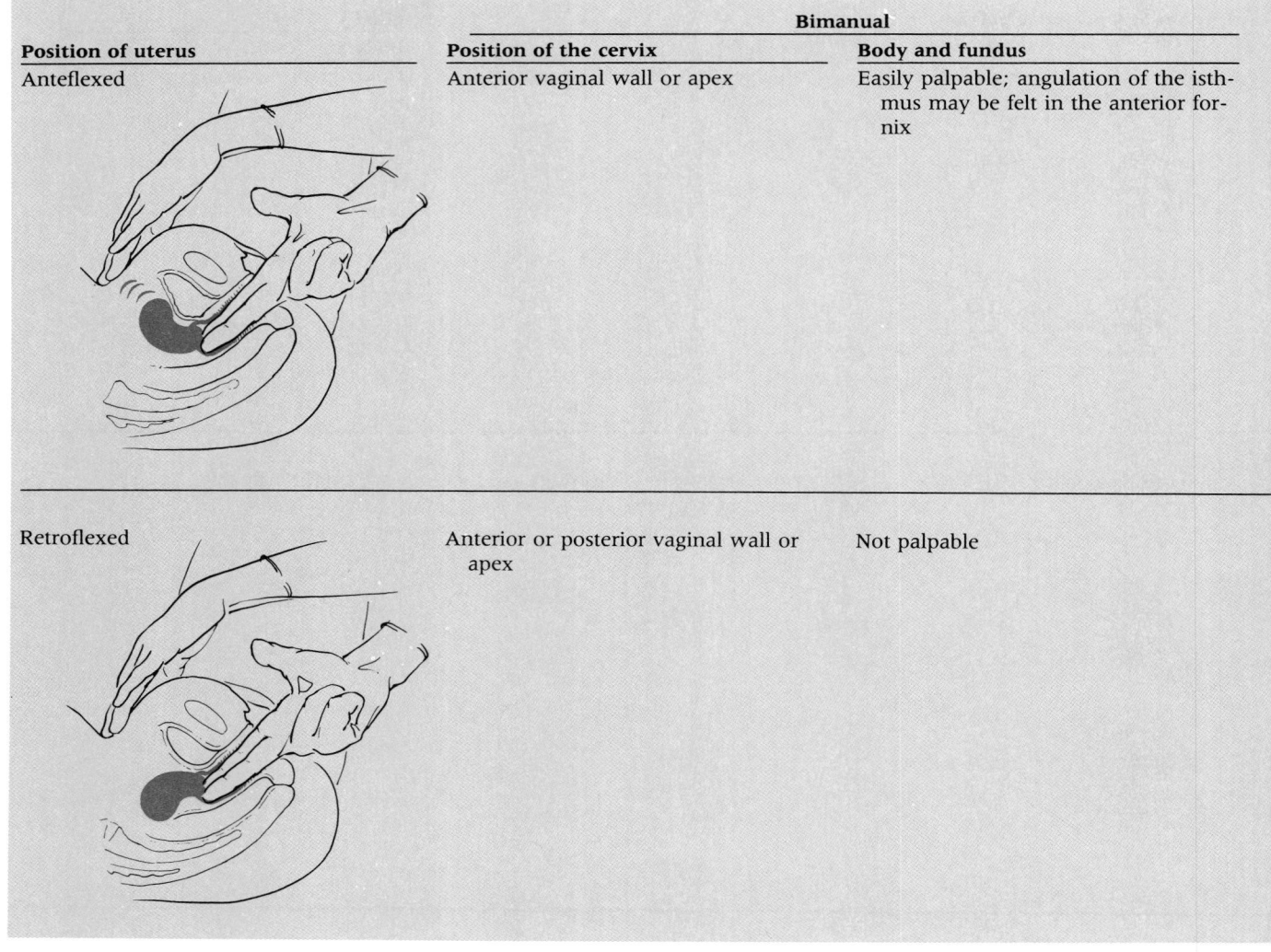

hands, and the corpus may be felt with the backs of the intravaginal fingers. A retroverted uterus is felt best during the rectovaginal examination.

If the uterus is identified as being in anteposition or midposition, attempt to palpate all its anterior and posterior surfaces by maneuvering its position and by "walking up" its surface with the intravaginal fingers.

After palpating the uterus, examine the **adnexal** areas. The adnexal areas are those structures and spaces surrounding the uterus, including the fallopian tubes and ovaries. The structures in these areas are of a size, consistency, and position that they may not be specifically palpated. If you have appropriately examined the area and no masses larger than the normal-size ovaries are identified, assume that no masses are present.

Palpate each of the adnexal areas, left and right. Place the index and middle finger of the intravaginal hand in one of the lateral fornices; place the hand on the abdomen on the ipsilateral iliac crest; and bring the hands together, moving in an inferior and medial direction, allowing the tissues lying between the two hands to slip between them (see Figure 21-12). The hand on the abdomen acts as resistance, and the intravaginal hand palpates the organs between the hands. Frequently, no specific organ is palpated in this maneuver.

If normal ovaries are palpated, they are smooth, firm, slightly flattened, ovoid, and no larger than 4 to 6 cm in their largest dimension. Ovaries of prepubertal girls or postmenopausal women are normally smaller than 4 cm in their largest dimension. The ovaries are sensitive

Anterior and posterior portion of uterus	Rectovaginal	
	Cervix	**Body and fundus**
Easily palpable	Same as anteverted	Same as anteverted

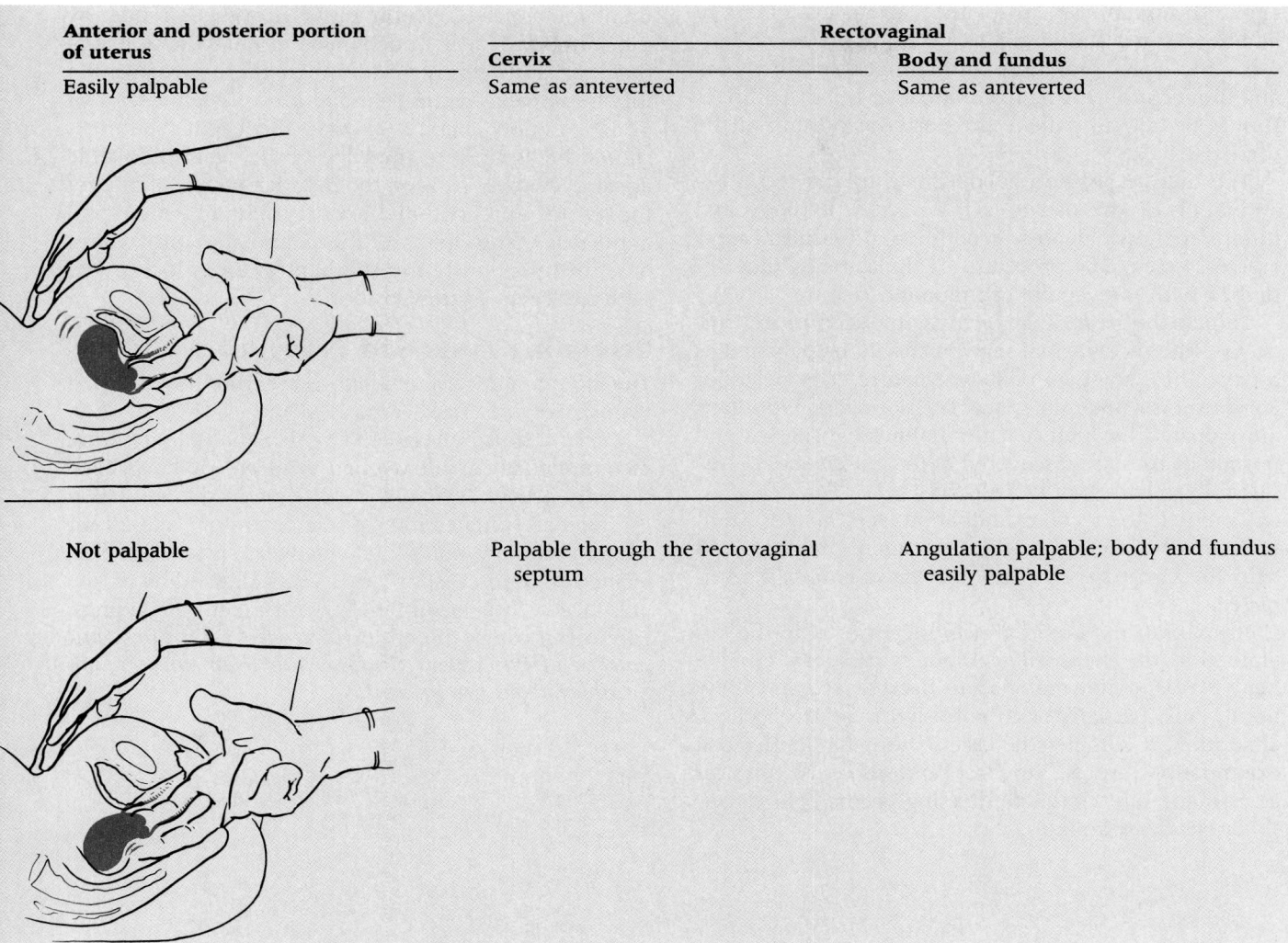

Not palpable	Palpable through the rectovaginal septum	Angulation palpable; body and fundus easily palpable

to touch but are not tender. They are highly movable and will easily slip between the palpating hands. Normal fallopian tubes are not palpable. One clue to an ectopic pregnancy is the presence of arterial pulses in the adnexal areas.

Cordlike structures that are sometimes palpable are round ligaments.

Rectovaginal examination. The rectovaginal examination is uncomfortable for most women. However, because it enables examination not possible through the vaginal examination alone, it is recommended in all complete pelvic examinations. The rectovaginal examination allows for greater depth (approximately 2 cm higher) than the vaginal examination alone and

enables assessment of the posterior portion of the uterus and pelvic cavity. Because the examination is uncomfortable, prepare the client for it by instruction regarding its purpose and anticipatory guidance about the possible feeling of urgency for bowel movement.

After completing the vaginal examination, withdraw the intravaginal hand, change the glove on the internal examining hand to prevent the possible transfer of infection from the vagina into the rectum, and lubricate the index and middle fingers. Advise the client that the next procedure is the last part of the pelvic examination and remind her to cooperate by relaxing the muscles. Next, ask the client to bear down. Then, place the index finger into the vagina in the posterior fornix of the cervix, and place the middle finger into the rectum. (See

Chapter 22 for detailed explanation of the method for inserting examining finger into the rectum.) Both fingers are inserted as far as possible. Place the other hand above the symphysis, as for the vaginal examination, and depress the abdominal hand. Bring the pelvic contents into closer proximity to the fingers in the vagina and the rectum. During this maneuver the rectal finger should be able to palpate the posterior portion of the uterus.

The uterine position is confirmed by the rectal examination. If the uterus is retroverted, its body and fundus are now palpated. In addition, the adnexal areas are reassessed. The procedure is the same as that described with the vaginal examination (Figure 21-13).

Palpate the areas of the rectovaginal septum and cul-de-sac. The rectovaginal septum should be palpated as a firm, thin, smooth, pliable structure. The posterior cul-de-sac is a potential space. The normal pelvic organs are palpated through it. Often, abnormal masses and normal ovaries are discovered in the cul-de-sac. Uterosacral ligaments may be palpable.

Complete the rectal examination (see Chapter 22 on assessment of the anus and rectosigmoid region), and help the client sit up when the examination is completed.

Because of the amount of lubricant used in the examination, the client will feel somewhat sticky. Provide her with disposable materials to clean herself and allow her to dress partially or completely (if the physical examination is completed). Often the pelvic and rectal examinations are the very last portions of the physical assessment, and complete dressing occurs before consultation about findings.

Special maneuvers

Examination of clients who are unable to assume the lithotomy position. The lithotomy position is optimal for a pelvic examination. However, it may be difficult for a very ill or debilitated client to assume and maintain a lithotomy position. An alternative position for the female genital examination is a left lateral or Sims' position (Figure 21-14). The client's buttocks should be as close to the edge of the examining table as safety allows. Position the right leg on top of or over the left leg and bend and abduct it. Stand behind and at the side of the client. All the examination procedures described previously in this chapter can be performed with the client in this position.

Screening Tests and Procedures

The following recommendations are from the U.S. Preventive Services Task Force (1989):

Cervical cancer. Regular Papanicolaou (Pap) tests are recommended for all women who are or have been sexually active. Testing should begin at the age when the woman initiates intercourse or around age 20 for women who are not sexually active. Pap tests are performed at an interval of 1 to 3 years, depending on the presence of risk factors, history, and clinical findings. Pap smears can be discontinued at age 65 *if the previous pattern of Pap smear findings has been normal and no risk factors are present*.

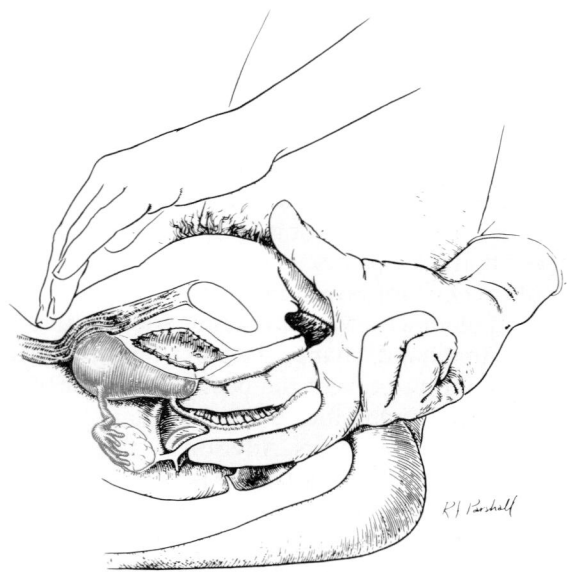

FIGURE 21-13 Rectovaginal palpation.

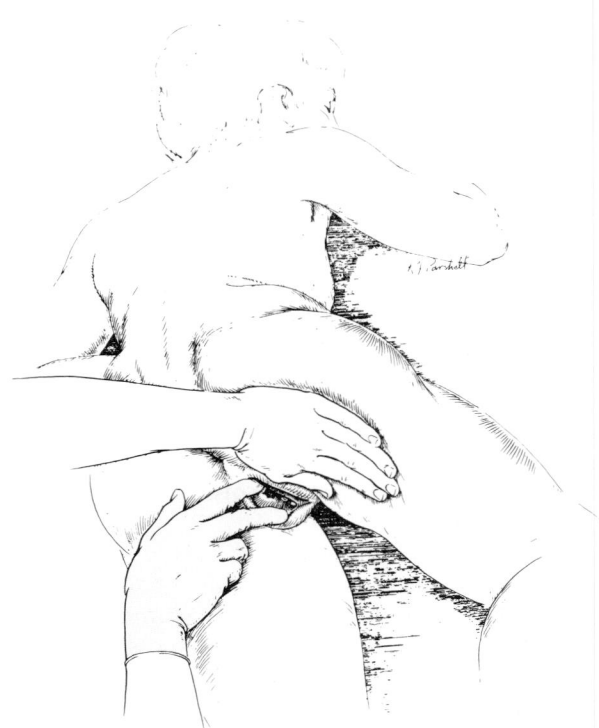

FIGURE 21-14 Left lateral position for genital examination.

Chlamydial infection. Routine testing for *Chlamydia trachomatis* is recommended for the following groups of clients:

—asymptomatic persons who attend clinics for sexually transmitted diseases.

—having specific risk factors for chlamydial infection: less than 20 years of age, multiple sexual partners, or sexual partner with multiple sexual contacts.

—recent sexual partners of persons with positive cultures.

—pregnant women in high risk group at the first prenatal visit and at later visits if the risk for infection is high.

Gonorrhea. Routine cultures for gonorrhea are recommended for the following groups:

—asymptomatic persons in high-risk groups: prostitutes, persons with multiple sexual partners

—sexual contact with person diagnosed with gonorrhea

—persons with a history of repeated episodes of gonorrhea

—pregnant women at the first prenatal visit and at a later visit if risk for infection is high

Cervical Papanicolaou smear. The Papanicolaou (Pap) smear is taken to detect neoplastic cells in cervical and vaginal secretions. Normal and abnormal cervical and endometrial cells are shed onto the cervix and into the vagina and intermix with the normal secretions. The Pap smear is very accurate (95%) in detecting cervical cancer but only moderately effective in detecting endometrial cancer.

The client is in the lithotomy position, and the speculum has been inserted. All materials listed earlier in the chapter are assembled. If a cervical mucus plug is present, remove it with a cotton ball held with forceps. There are many variations among laboratories regarding the areas from which cell samples are to be obtained, the mixing of cells from two or more areas, and the fixing of cells. One procedure is described here. However, variations are acceptable, and the practitioner should consult with the cytopathologist reading the smears for locally recommended procedures. The following paragraphs describe methods for obtaining samples from the endocervix, the cervix, and the vaginal pool.

Endocervical specimen. Figure 21-15 illustrates a procedure for obtaining a sample of cells from the endocervix:

1. Insert a sterile cotton-tipped applicator, moistened with normal saline, approximately 0.5 cm into the cervical os. Rotate it 360° and leave it in 10 to 20 seconds to ensure saturation. The moistening with normal saline prevents the absorption of cells into the applicator and the

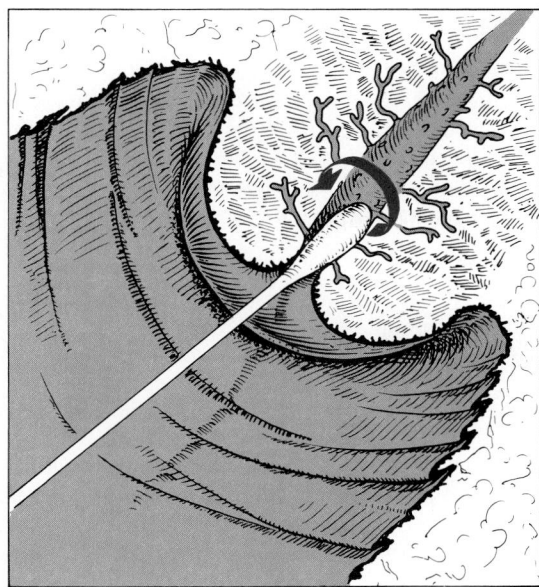

FIGURE 21-15 Endocervical specimen.

shedding of cotton filaments onto the specimen collection slide.

2. Spread the endocervical smear on a slide labeled *"endocervix."* Rotate the swab so that all sampled areas are smeared on the slide. Avoid smearing thick areas on the slide as the cells would be difficult to visualize microscopically. The slide is immediately fixed by a spray fixative or immersion into a fixative solution.

Use of brushes. Several new products are available to facilitate the collection of Pap smears. The cylindric-type brush is used to collect endocervical cells. This brush is used in the same way the cotton swab would be used (described above), but does not need to be moistened with saline. Insert the brush into the os until only the bristles closest to the handle are seen, and then rotate the brush. A paintbrush-type brush has also been developed to collect simultaneously both endocervical and ectocervical cells and is used as one would use the Ayre spatula as described below.

Cervical specimen. Figure 21-16 illustrates the procedure for a cervical specimen:

1. Insert the larger humped end of the Ayre spatula into the cervical os so that the cervix fits comfortably into the groove created by the two humps. With moderate pressure, rotate the spatula 360 degrees, scraping the entire cervical surface and the squamocolumnar junction.

2. Spread the material from both sides of the spatula on a slide marked "cervix."

3. Fix the slide immediately.

ABOUT PAP SMEARS

Client preparation

No douching, use of vaginal medications or other topical inserts, or tub baths for 24 hours before the procedure
Defer if menstrual flow or infection
Do not use lubricating jelly on the speculum

Findings

Results are reported in classes or in cervical intraepithelial neoplasia (CIN) levels:

Class 1: Benign: absence of atypical or abnormal cells (normal finding).
Class 2: Benign with inflammation: atypical cells, but no evidence of malignancy.
Class 3: Mild *dysplasia:* cytologic findings suggestive of but not conclusive of malignancy (must receive prompt follow-up).
Class 4: Carcinoma in situ: cytologic findings strongly suggestive of malignancy.
Class 5: Invasive cancer: cytologic changes conclusive of malignancy.

CIN 1: mild and mild-to-moderate dysplasia (similar to classes 2 and 3)
CIN 2: moderate and moderate-to-severe dysplasia (similar to class 3)
CIN 3: severe dysplasia and carcinoma in situ (similar to classes 3 and 4)

Important

Secretions must be fixed before they dry. Drying will distort the cells and make interpretation difficult.

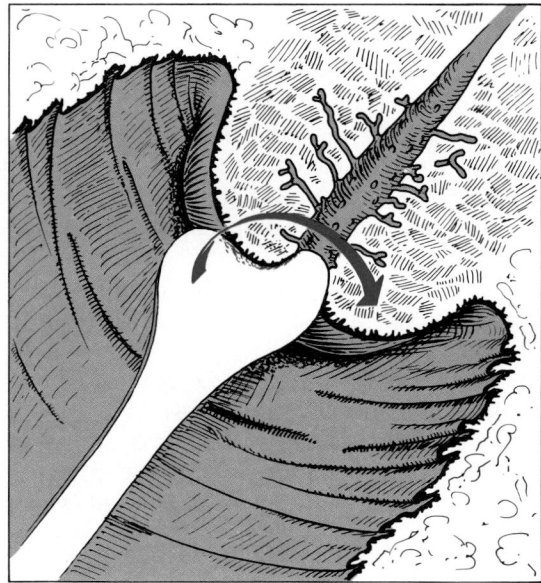

FIGURE 21-16 Cervical specimen.

The female client is in the lithotomy position with a speculum inserted. The male is in a supine position to prevent possible falling if vasovagal syncope occurs with the introduction of the specimen-collecting instrument into the urethra.

ENDOCERVICAL CULTURE

1. Obtain a specimen from the endocervical canal with a sterile cotton applicator. The technique is the same as that described for the Pap smear. Leave the applicator in the os for at least 30 seconds.
2. Inoculate a special culture plate or place the specimen in a special culture container as soon as possible.
3. If a Thayer-Martin culture plate is used, have the medium at room temperature, roll the swab in a large Z pattern on the culture plate; simultaneously rotate the swab as it is creating the Z so that all swab surfaces will be inoculated (Figure 21-17). Incubate the culture plate within 15 minutes of its inoculation in a warm, anaerobic environment. Place the culture plate, medium side up, in a candle jar, light the candle, tightly secure the cover of the jar, and leave the jar in a warm area until specimens can be placed in an incubator. In some clinics the inoculation is immediately cross-streaked with a sterile wire loop. Usually, however, this step is done in the laboratory, not in the examining room.
4. If another type of culture medium is used, fol-

VAGINAL POOL SMEAR

1. With the paddle or handle end of the Ayre spatula, scrape the area of the posterior cervical fornix.
2. Spread the material on the spatula in the area marked "vaginal pool."
3. Fix the slide immediately by spraying or immersion into a fixative solution.

See the box above for more information about Pap smears.

Gonorrheal culture. Cultures for gonorrheal infection are performed on men and women at risk for the infection. Additionally, all pregnant women should be screened for gonorrhea because of possible fetal complications. Cervical cultures are done for women, urethral cultures for men, and rectal and oral cultures for persons engaged in rectal or oral sex. Bacterial cultures use a special medium, such as Thayer-Martin, specifically designed for the cultivation of gonorrhea organisms.

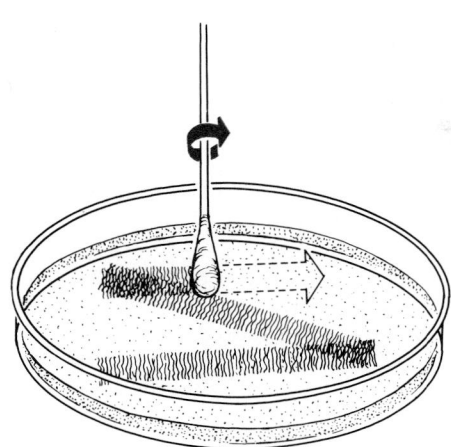

FIGURE 21-17 Inoculation of the Thayer-Martin culture.

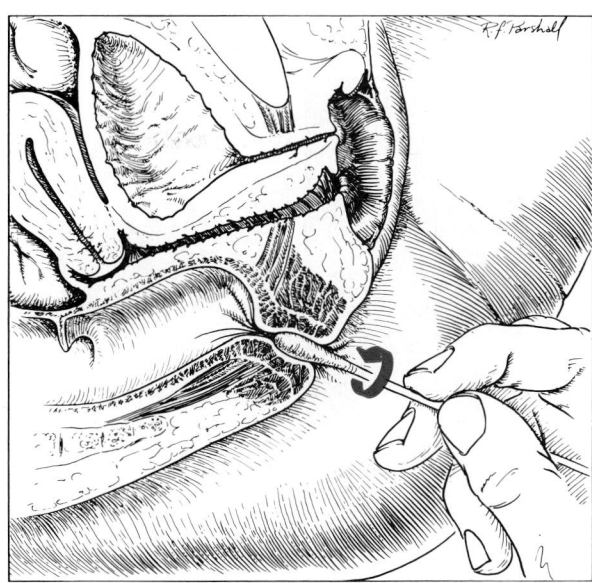

FIGURE 21-18 Anal specimen.

low instructions for specimen collection and handling.

ANAL CULTURE

Figure 21-18 illustrates the procedure for an anal culture:

1. Insert a sterile cotton-tipped applicator into the anal canal. Rotate the applicator 360 degrees and move it from side to side. Leave it in for 10 to 30 seconds to allow for absorption of secretion and organisms. If the swab contains feces, discard it and take another specimen.
2. Inoculate the culture plate and incubate it as described previously, using a separate culture plate labeled by source of specimen.

OROPHARYNGEAL CULTURE

1. Obtain a specimen of secretion from the oropharynx with a sterile swab.
2. Inoculate the medium and incubate as described for endocervical specimens.

See the box below for more information about gonorrheal cultures.

ABOUT GONORRHEA CULTURES

Client preparation—females

No douching, topical vaginal inserts, or tub baths for 24 hours

No lubricant on speculum

Avoid taking specimens during menses—menses alter results

Client preparation—males

No voiding within 1 hour of specimen collection—voiding washes out the organisms

---

Chlamydial culture. *Chlamydia trachomatis* is a common sexually transmitted disease. Detecting is important because the organism causes trachoma, an eye disease resulting in the most common form of preventable blindness. Obtain vaginal and urethral specimens in the same manner described for the gonorrhea culture. Special culture material is inoculated with the specimen.

Smears for Trichomonas vaginalis, Candida albicans, and Gardnerella vaginalis

1. Obtain a specimen of vaginal secretions directly from the vagina or from material in the inferior speculum blade. For *Trichomonas vaginalis,* mix the secretions with a drop of normal saline solution on a glass slide. For *Candida albicans,* mix the secretions with a drop of 10% potassium hydroxide (KOH) solution on a slide. For *Gardnerella vaginalis* (formerly and also called *Hemophilus vaginalis*), the secretions are mixed with a 10% potassium hydroxide solution.
2. Place a glass cover slip on the slide.
3. If *G. vaginalis* is suspected, perform a "whiff" test as the slide is being prepared with the KOH. If *G. vaginalis* is present an unpleasant, "fishy" odor will be noted after the drop of KOH is added. Immediately observe the slide under a microscope (Figure 21-19). If positive for *T. vaginalis*, trichomonads will be seen. These are single-cell flagellates somewhat larger than a white blood cell, but smaller than a vaginal squamous epithelial cell. If positive for *C.*

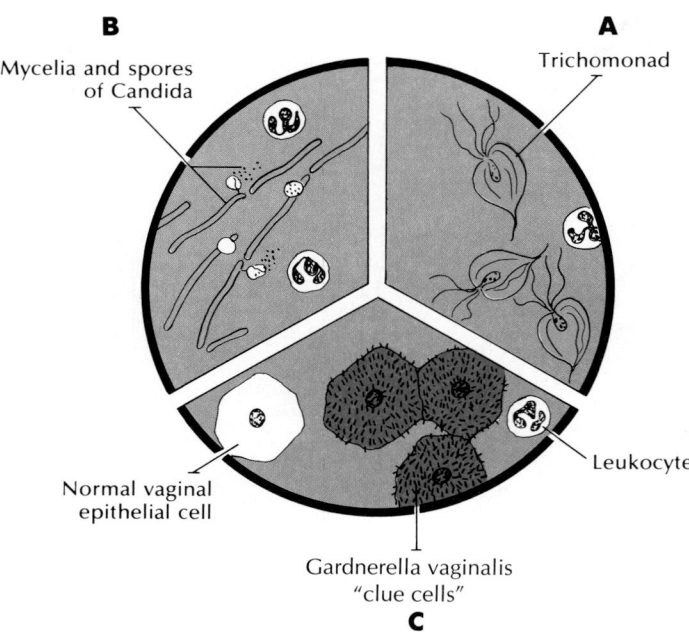

B
Mycelia and spores
of Candida

A
Trichomonad

Leukocyte

Normal vaginal
epithelial cell

Gardnerella vaginalis
"clue cells"

C

FIGURE 21-19 Microscopic appearance of vaginal microorganisms. **A,** *Trichomonas.* **B,** Mycelia and spores. **C,** Epithelial cells stippled by *Gardnerella vaginalis* bacteria.

albicans, **mycelia** and spores are seen. If positive for *G. vaginalis,* characteristic "clue cells" are seen.

VARIATIONS FROM HEALTH

Skin and Labia

Common abnormalities of the skin and labia include parasites, skin lesions of all types, areas of leukoplakia, varicosities, hyperpigmentation, erythema, depigmentation, and swelling.

—*Parasites.* Excoriations and erythematous areas are noted on the skin. Lice appear as dark spots on the skin and their eggs (nits) are adherent to the pubic hair near the roots.

—*Skin lesions.* Commonly seen skin lesions are those of herpes progenitalis, appearing as small, shallow vesicles with surrounding erythema; and condylomata acuminata, which appear in single or multiple cauliflower-like patches.

—*Leukoplakia.* This appears as white, adherent patches on the skin; it may be likened to spots of dried white paint.

Vaginal Discharges

Vaginal discharges may result from various conditions of the uterus, cervix, and vagina. Causes include fungal,

Examination Step-by-Step

Inspect external genitalia

Skin color, condition, integrity
Hair characteristics and distribution
Labia majora—symmetry, color, inflammation, lesions, inflammation
Clitoris—size
Labia minora
Urethral opening—discharge and inflammation
Vaginal opening—size and condition
Perineum—condition, inflammation, lesions
Anus

Palpate external genitalia

Place hand on inner thigh to prepare client for palpation
Labia
Skene's glands
Bartholin's glands

Assess support of the pelvic musculature

Palpate perineum
Test vaginal introitus musculature
Assess for rectocele, cystocele, enterocele, and uterine prolapse

Speculum examination

Insert speculum
Inspect the cervix and os—color, position, size, surface characteristics, discharge, shape
Obtain specimens for cervical and vaginal smears and cultures if needed
Inspect the vaginal wall—color, surface characteristics, discharge

Bimanual palpation

Vaginal wall—smoothness and lesions
Cervix and fornices—size, shape, position, mobility, patency of os, surface characteristics, tenderness
Uterus—location, size, position, shape, mobility, tenderness
Ovaries—size, shape, consistency, tenderness
Adnexal areas—masses and tenderness
Cul-de-sac—masses and tenderness

Rectovaginal palpation

Anus
Rectovaginal septum—thickness, tone, nodules
Rectum—masses, tone
Uterus and adnexae
Cul-de-sac

EXAMINATION OF A CLIENT WHO HAS HAD A HYSTERECTOMY

Determine to the extent possible the details of the procedure, especially the extent of the procedure.

On speculum examination the cervix will be absent. An identifiable suture line will be present. Take a Pap smear at the suture line with the blunt end of the spatula. Label the Pap smear requisition form with the fact of the hysterectomy.

The vaginal walls may appear as they would after menopause without replacement therapy—decrease in rugae and secretions.

In bimanual palpation, the uterus will obviously not be present, but the adnexal areas should be palpated as in the usual examination.

protozoal, viral, bacterial, spirochetal, and parasitic infections; benign and malignant neoplasms; chemical irritations; foreign bodies; fistulas; or poor hygiene. Full discussion of the various causes of discharges is beyond the scope of this text. However, clinical signs and symptoms accompanying common vaginal infections producing discharges are described:

—*Candida albicans*—Candida albicans is a fungus that causes approximately 20% of vaginal infections. Common symptoms are vulvovaginal itching; vulvar redness and swelling; and thick, white, curdy (similar to cottage cheese) discharge. On examination the vulva and the vagina are frequently erythematous and edematous; curdy white discharge may be present in labial folds and in the vagina; and the vagina and cervix may appear edematous and covered with adherent, thrush-like patches.

—*Trichomonas vaginalis*—This infection is caused by trichomonads, parasitic protozoans having motile flagella. Clients complain of watery, bubbly, profuse, yellowish-green, malodorous discharge, which is generally most severe immediately after menses. On physical examination, the vulva may appear erythematous, and a yellow-green, foul-smelling discharge is present at the introitus and in the vagina. In addition, the vagina may be erythematous, and the vagina may have red, raised papules and petechiae.

—*Gardnerella vaginalis*—This is a bacterial vaginosis that is thought to account for 50% to 60% of vaginal infections. Clients complain of increased, watery, gray, malodorous vaginal discharge. Findings characteristic of the physical examination include little to no vulvar edema, and a thin, creamy, gray-white, malodorous discharge covering the vagina and cervix.

TEACHING SELF-ASSESSMENT

The teaching of genital self-examination may be indicated for clients in the following situations:

1. Clients using barrier or intrauterine contraceptive devices. The clients need to check the placement of devices.
2. Clients who have recurring vaginal infections.
3. Clients at risk for sexually transmitted diseases.

The teaching session is initiated with a thorough presentation of the anatomy of the female genitalia and the normal appearance and feel of organs, structures, and discharge.

The following steps are recommended in teaching self-examination:

1. Find a comfortable position that will allow for viewing of the external genitalia with a mirror. A source of light from a nearby lamp is often necessary.
2. Inspect the condition of the hair and skin over the genitalia. Spread the hairs and inspect all the surfaces of the labia. Look for bumps, sores, warts, and blisters.
3. Spread the labia and look at the clitoris for bumps, blisters, sores, and warts.
4. Look at the urethral opening and the area of the Bartholin's glands for swelling or redness.
5. Insert a finger into the vagina and feel the consistency of normal tissue and get used to the plane of the vagina.
6. Insert a finger deep into the vagina and locate the cervix. Feel the os and then feel the entire surface by circling it with the finger.
7. Look carefully at the type of discharge that is on the finger when it is taken out.

Some women's self-help groups teach self-examination by vaginal speculum. This is not recommended because of the difficulty of this maneuver on oneself and because professional judgment is needed for adequate assessment.

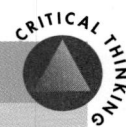

Sample Documentation

Health history (client with a problem)

Complains of constant, dull, aching pain in the lower abdomen and lower back and feeling tired and weak. Discomfort started 5 to 6 weeks ago following a 100° fever for 2 days. No alleviating or aggravating factors noted; no treatment or consultation with health care provider. Menses began at age 13. Denies change in menses, which are regular (every 30 days) with moderate flow (uses a total of approximately ten tampons and three pads across 4 days). Has had foul smelling vaginal discharge for last 4 weeks. Discharge thin and yellow in color. Has worn one to two mini pads per day between menses to collect the discharge—pads are about half saturated. Has had no pregnancies or miscarriages. Has used oral contraceptives for the last 4 years. Denies known exposure to sexually transmitted diseases—has had two partners in the last 4 years, her husband only for the last year. Denies diabetes and has no family history of reproductive cancer or diabetes. Last Pap smear 6 months ago: results, class 1.

Physical examination

Female hair distribution. No masses, lesions, or swelling on labia, area of clitoris, and perineum. No redness, swelling, or discharge around urethral orifice or Bartholin's glands. No scars on perineum. Demonstrates strong vaginal musculature when asked to squeeze muscles on finger. No prolapses or incontinence noted on straining.

Vaginal mucosa slightly reddened, a moderate amount of thin, yellow discharge covers vaginal mucosa. Discharge malodorous, but not "fishy." Cervix pink, smooth, midline, no lesions; os is in shape of a lateral slit. Os admits a fingertip without difficulty.

Bimanual palpation somewhat uncomfortable. Uterus—midline, movable, anteverted, firm, approximately 8 cm long. Cervix smooth, without lesions, somewhat tender on movement.

Left and right ovaries palpable—approximately 3 cm × 2 cm × 1 cm. No masses. No masses palpated in adnexal or cul-de-sac areas.

Rectovaginal septum intact without lesions. Some tenderness during this examination as well. Cervix palpated through rectal wall.

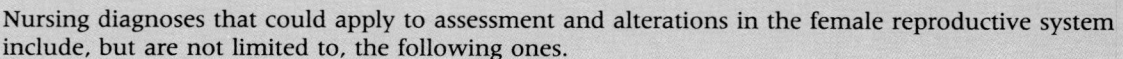

Nursing Diagnosis *THE NEXT STEP*

Nursing diagnoses that could apply to assessment and alterations in the female reproductive system include, but are not limited to, the following ones.

STRESS INCONTINENCE The state in which an individual experiences a loss of urine of less than 50 ml occurring with increased abdominal pressure.

Defining Characteristics

- Reported or observed dribbling with increased abdominal pressure
- Urinary urgency
- Urinary frequency (more often than every 2 hours)

Related Factors

- Incompetent bladder outlet
- Age-related degenerative changes in pelvic muscles and structural supports
- Weak pelvic muscles and structural supports
- High intraabdominal pressure
- Overdistention between voidings

SEXUAL DYSFUNCTION The state in which an individual experiences a change in sexual function that is viewed as unsatisfying, unrewarding, or inadequate.

Defining Characteristics

- Verbalizations of problem in sexuality
- Alterations in achieving perceived sex role
- Actual or perceived limitation imposed by disease and/or therapy

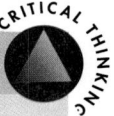

Nursing Diagnosis   *THE NEXT STEP—cont'd*

- Conflicts involving values (cultural/religion)
- Alteration in achieving sexual satisfaction
- Inability to achieve desired sexual satisfaction
- Frequent seeking of confirmation of desirability
- Alteration in relationship with significant other
- Change of interest in self and others

Related Factors

- Ineffectual or absent models
- Physical abuse
- Psychosocial abuse
- Vulnerability
- Misinformation or lack of knowledge
- Values conflict
- Lack of privacy
- Lack of significant other
- Altered body structure or function

ALTERED SEXUALITY PATTERNS The state in which an individual expresses concern regarding his/her sexuality.

Defining Characteristics

- Reported difficulties, limitations, or changes in sexual behaviors or activities

Related Factors

- Knowledge skill deficit
- Altered body function or structure
- Illness or medical treatment
- Lack of privacy
- Lack of significant other
- Ineffective or absent role models
- Conflicts with sexual orientation or variant preferences
- Fear
- Impaired relationship with significant other

RAPE TRAUMA SYNDROME Forced, violent sexual penetration against the victim's will and consent. The trauma syndrome that develops from this attack or attempted attack includes an acute phase of disorganization of the victim's life-style and a long-term process of reorganization of life-style.

Defining Characteristics

Acute Phase
- Report of forced, violent, sexual penetration
- Anger
- Embarrassment
- Fear of physical violence and death
- Humiliation
- Revenge
- Self-blame/guilt
- Multiple physical symptoms (e.g., gastrointestinal irritability, genitourinary discomfort, increased muscle tension, sleep-pattern disturbance)
- Denial
- Mistrust
- Change in sexual behavior

Long-Term Phase
- Changes in life-style (changes in residence, dealing with repetitive nightmares or phobias, seek-

Continued.

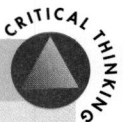

Nursing Diagnosis   *THE NEXT STEP—cont'd*

ing social network support)
- Anxiety
- Depression

ANXIETY A vague, uneasy feeling, the source of which is often nonspecific or unknown to the individual.

Defining Characteristics

- Subjective
  Increased tension
  Apprehension
  Uncertainty
  Fear
  Feeling of being scared
  Feeling of inadequacy
  Shakiness
  Fear of unspecific consequences
  Regretfulness
  Feeling of being rattled
  Distress
  Jitteriness
- Objective
  Insomnia
  Glancing about
  Poor eye contact
  Trembling; hand tremors
  Extraneous movements—foot shuffling; hand, arm movements
  Expressed concern regarding changes in life events
  Worry
  Facial tension
  Voice quivering
  Focus on self
  Increased wariness
  Increased perspiration

Related Factors

- Threat to self-concept
- Threat to or change in health status
- Threat to or change in role functioning
- Threat to or change in interaction patterns
- Situational and maturational crises
- Interpersonal transmission and contagion
- Unmet needs

Clinical Application

Mrs. D. is a 65-year-old female in for her annual gynecologic checkup. "In the past 2 months I have been feeling pressure down there all the time. I feel like I have to urinate all the time. Every time I cough, laugh, or sneeze I dribble urine. I'm so embarrassed. I have not had sex with my husband, I'm afraid I'll urinate."

Menarche age 14, cycle usually every 30 days, duration 6 days, flow moderate to heavy, no dysmenorrhea, LMP 15 years ago. Gravida 3/para 3/abortion 0. Gyne checkups yearly. Last Pap test 1 year ago Class 1. Internal and external exam completed.

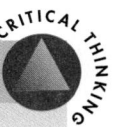

Nursing Diagnosis   *THE NEXT STEP—cont'd*

SUBJECTIVE DATA: Patient complains of:
feeling pressure in vagina all the time
feeling like she has to urinate all the time
dribbling urine every time she sneezes, coughs, or laughs
unwilling to have sex for fear of urinating

OBJECTIVE DATA:
External genitalia: no swelling, lesions, or discharge.
Internal exam: vaginal wall has 2 cm soft round anterior bulge, cervix pale and glistening with no lesions.
Bimanual: no pain on moving cervix, uterus feels small and firm, ovaries unable to palpate.
Rectal: no hemorrhoids, fissures, lesions, masses, or tenderness.

NURSING DIAGNOSES

Stress incontinence related to prolapsed bladder.

Defining Characteristics

- reported dribbling with increased abdominal pressure
- urinary frequency
- urinary urgency

Sexual dysfunction related to altered body structure and/or function (bladder prolapse into vagina).

Defining Characteristics

- Verbalization of fear of sex due to incontinence
- embarrassed about stress incontinence

Altered sexuality patterns related to altered body structure and/or function.

Defining Characteristics

- Verbalization of fear of sex due to incontinence

GLOSSARY

adnexal Being next to or near another, related structure, the ovaries in the case of female genitalia.

condyloma (also, condylomata acuminata) Hyperkeratotic exophytic lesions of stratified squamous epithelium; these develop as small, elevated, soft nodules that enlarge and coalesce to become cauliflower-like excrescences.

cribiform Perforated, like a sieve.

cystocele Herniation of the urinary bladder into the anterior vaginal wall.

dysmenorrhea Painful menstruation.

dyspareunia Difficult or painful sexual intercourse in women.

dysplasia Any abnormal development of tissues or organs.

ectocervix The outside portion of the cervix.

ectopic pregnancy Abnormal pregnancy in which the conceptus implants outside the uterine cavity.

endocervical Pertaining to the inside of the cervix.

endocervix The membrane lining the canal of the uterine cervix.

endometriosis Presence of endometrial stroma and glands in ectopic locations such as the ovaries, pelvic peritoneum, or colon.

enterocele A herniation of the intestine into the vagina.

episiotomy A surgical procedure in which an incision is made in a woman's perineum to enlarge her vaginal opening for delivery.

fornix An archlike structure of space.

fourchette A tense band of mucous membranes at the posterior angle of the vagina connecting the posterior ends of the labia minora.

frenulum A restraining portion or structure.

hirsutism Excessive hairiness, especially in females.

hyperplasia An increase in the number of cells in a body part.

intraepithelian Within the epithelium.

introitus An entrance or orifice to a cavity or a hollow tubular structure of the body.

leukoplakia A disease appearing as white, thickened patches on mucous membranes.

leukorrhea White discharge from the vagina.

lithotomy position The position assumed by the patient lying supine with the hips and the knees flexed and the thighs abducted and rotated externally.

menarche The first menstruation and the commencement of cyclic menstrual function.

menorrhagia Excessive menstruation.

metrorrhagia Irregular and/or dysfunctional uterine bleeding.

multiparous Having delivered one or more viable infants.

mycelia Masses of interwoven, branched threadlike filaments that make up most fungi.

nabothian cysts Cystlike formations of the mucosa of the uterine cervix resulting from an accumulation of retained secretion in occluded glands.

neoplasia The new and abnormal development of cells that may be benign or malignant.

nodularity Lumpiness.

nulliparous Not having delivered a viable infant.

oligomenorrhea Decreased frequency of menstruation with an interval of 38 to 90 days.

orifice An opening.

ostium Orifice.

parous Having borne one or more viable offspring.

rectocele Herniation of the rectum into the posterior vaginal wall.

rugated Having ridges or folds.

salpingitis Inflammation of the fallopian tubes as a result of infection. Leukorrhea, adnexal tenderness, abdominal pain, and fever may be present.

sebaceous Pertaining to or secreting sebum, an oily secretion composed of fat and epithelial debris.

sebaceous cyst Retention of the fatty secretion of the sebaceous gland.

speculum A device made of two narrow blades or a hollow tube, used to assist in opening a body cavity.

squamocolumnar junction The area of the cervix where the membranes covered by squamous cells of the vaginal portion of the cervix meet the membranes of the columnar portion of the cervix.

BIBLIOGRAPHY

Barber HRK, Fields DH, Kaufman SA: *Quick reference to ob gyn procedures,* ed 3, Philadelphia, 1990, JB Lippincott.

Clarke-Pearson DL, Dawood MY: *Green's gynecology,* ed 4, Boston, 1990, Little, Brown.

Gordon M: *Manual of nursing diagnosis: 1993-1994,* St. Louis, 1993, Mosby–Year Book.

Gordon M: *Nursing diagnosis: process and application,* ed 2, New York, 1987, McGraw Hill.

Herbst AL, Mishell DR, Stenchever MA, Droegemueller W: *Comprehensive gynecology,* ed 2, St Louis, 1992, Mosby–Year Book.

Lichtman R, Papera S: *Gynecology: well-woman care,* Norwalk, Conn, 1990, Appleton & Lange.

Mackay EV, Beischer NA, Pepperell RJ, Wood C: *Illustrated textbook of gynaecology,* ed 2, Sydney, 1992, Harcourt Brace Jovanovich.

Mosby's medical, nursing, and allied health dictionary, ed 3, St. Louis, 1990, Mosby–Year Book.

Olsson HM, Gullberg MT: Role of the woman patient and fear of the pelvic examination, *West J Nurs Res* 9:357-367, 1987.

Pagana KD, Pagana TJ: *Mosby's diagnostic and laboratory test reference,* St. Louis, 1992, Mosby–Year Book.

Ryan RJ, Berkowitz R, Barbieri RL: *Kistner's gynecology,* ed 5, Chicago, 1990, Year Book Medical Publishers.

Seidel, HM, Ball JW, Dains JE, Benedict GW: *Mosby's guide to physical examination,* ed 2, St. Louis, 1991, Mosby–Year Book.

Stenchever MA: *Office gynecology,* St. Louis, 1992, Mosby–Year Book.

Sherwood MJ, Szczech PC, Glasgow GM, Munoz CC: *Determining nursing diagnosis through assessment,* Baltimore, 1988, Williams & Wilkins.

U.S. Preventive Services Task Force: *Guide to clinical preventive services: an assessment of the effectiveness of 169 interventions,* Baltimore, 1989, Williams & Wilkins.

Willson JR, Carrington, ER: *Obstetrics and gynecology,* ed 9, St. Louis, 1991, Mosby–Year Book.

Anus and Rectosigmoid Region

PURPOSE OF THE EXAMINATION

The purposes of the rectal examination include assessment of anorectal status, the accessible pelvic viscera, and the male prostate gland and seminal vesicles and additional assessment of the female genitalia. The methods used to carry out this examination are inspection and palpation.

The rectal examination is an important component of every comprehensive physical examination. This type of examination is also indicated whenever the client is at risk for problems of the anorectal region or complains of symptoms that may indicate a problem or dysfunction of the region.

Because of the nature of the rectal examination, it is usually done at the end of the physical examination, which allows the client to clean himself or herself and dress on completion.

ANATOMY AND PHYSIOLOGY

The terminal gastrointestinal tract, which is called the rectosigmoid region, includes the anus, the rectum, and the caudal portion of the sigmoid colon.

The anal canal is the final segment of the colon. It is 2.5 to 4 cm long and opens into the perineum (Figure 22-1). The anal canal slants forward in a general line toward the umbilicus and forms a right angle with the rectum. The tract is surrounded by the external and internal sphincters, which keep it closed except when flatus and feces are passed. These sphincters are arranged in concentric layers. The striated external muscular ring is under voluntary control, whereas the internal smooth-muscle sphincter is under autonomic control. The internal sphincter is innervated from the pelvic plexus. Sympathetic stimulation contracts the sphincter; parasympathetic stimulation relaxes it. The

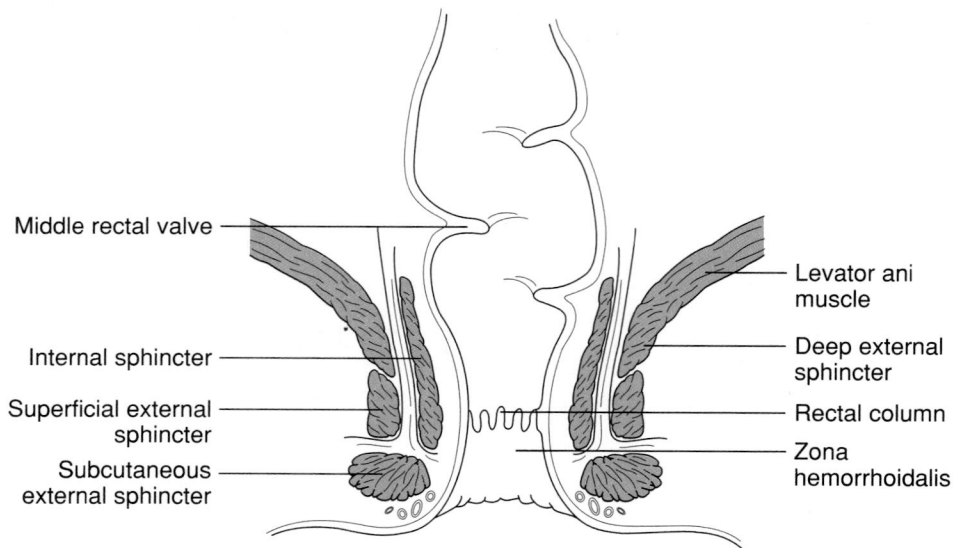

Middle rectal valve

Internal sphincter

Superficial external
sphincter

Subcutaneous
external sphincter

Levator ani
muscle

Deep external
sphincter

Rectal column

Zona
hemorrhoidalis

FIGURE 22-1 Anus and rectum.

anal canal, unlike the adjacent rectum, contains numerous somatic sensory nerves. Thus sensation in the canal is very keen. The distal portion of the external sphincter extends past the internal sphincter and may be palpated by the examining finger.

The stratified squamous epithelial lining of the anus is visible to inspection because it extends beyond the sphincters, where it merges with the skin. This junction is characterized by pigmentation and the presence of hair. From an internal view of the anal canal, columns of mucosal tissue, which extend from the rectum and terminate in papillae, can be identified. These anal columns, called the columns of Morgagni, fuse to form the pectinate, or dentate, line. The spaces between these columns are called crypts. The anal columns are invested with cross channels of **anastomosing** veins, which form mucosal folds known as anal valves. These anastomosing veins form a ring termed the zona hemorrhoidalis. When dilated, these veins are called **internal hemorrhoids**. The lower section of the anal canal contains a venous plexus, which has only a minor connection with the zona hemorrhoidalis and drains downward into the inferior rectal veins. Varicosed veins of this plexus are known as **external hemorrhoids**. Thus internal hemorrhoids occur superior to the pectinate line and are characterized by the moist, red epithelium of the rectum. External hemorrhoids are located inferior to the pectinate line and have the squamous epithelium of the anal canal or skin as their surface tissue.

The rectum is the portion of the gastrointestinal tract that is superior to the anal canal. Approximately 12 cm long, the rectum is lined with columnar epithelium.

Superiorly, the rectum has its origin at the third sacral vertebra and is continuous with the sigmoid colon. Its distal end dilates to form the rectal **ampulla**, which contains flatus and feces. Four semilunar transverse folds, the valves of Houston, extend across half the circumference of the rectal lumen. The purpose of these valves is not clear. They may serve to support feces while allowing flatus to pass.

The sigmoid colon has its origin at the iliac flexure of the descending colon and terminates in the rectum. Approximately 40 cm long, it is accessible to examination with the sigmoidoscope. Flexible fiberoptic instruments have made possible inspection of the mucosal surfaces of the entire sigmoid colon and of the other portions of the colon.

EXAMINATION

Health History

In practice, the history of the anus and rectum is integrated into that of the gastrointestinal system. The regional history outlined here focuses on the distal portion of the gastrointestinal system. Throughout the health history interview, the following data are recorded about a symptom or problem: (1) onset (specific date, sudden or gradual), (2) duration, (3) frequency, (4) precipitating factors, (5) aggravating or alleviating factors, (6) treatment received or self-care given, and (7) outcome. A regional history of the entire abdominal area is required for an adequate history of the anus and rectum. (See Chapter 17 for a discussion of history-taking of the abdominal area.)

Present health status

1. Diet
   a. Focus on fiber content and fluids
   b. Presence of lactose intolerance
2. Bowel habits
   a. Frequency
   b. Color
   c. Consistency
   d. Patterns of **diarrhea** and **constipation**
   e. Use of laxatives and enemas
3. Rest and activity patterns
4. Medications: focus should be on those intended to treat bowel problems and those medications with intestinal tract side effects
5. Sexual practices involving anus and rectum

Present illness*

1. Bowel movement pattern changes
   a. Nature of change
   b. Type of stool: color, consistency, presence of matter other than feces, odor
   c. Frequency of bowel movements
   d. Presence of **incontinence**
   e. Onset: association with diet, illness, changes in daily pattern, stress, travel, other events
   f. Accompanying symptoms: flatus, nausea, vomiting, distention, cramping, **colic**
   g. Corrective measures taken and results
2. Anal region discomfort
   a. Description of type of discomfort: location; amount of itching, pain, burning, discharge
   b. Association with body position: sitting, standing, walking, lying down
   c. Association with defecation or straining of stool
   d. Presence of blood, mucus, or other unusual substance in or on stool
   e. Corrective measures taken and results
3. Rectal bleeding
   a. Color of blood: bright red, dark red, or red-black
   b. Amount: blood on tissue, spotting in toilet, or active bleeding
   c. Location: blood on stool or in stool
   d. Relationship to defecation and changes in stool and bowel habits
   e. Associated gastrointestinal and regional symptoms
   f. Duration
4. Discharge
   a. Type
   b. Pattern
   c. Incontinence

*Current signs or symptoms of problems in region or in gastrointestinal tract.

d. History of trauma
e. Pattern
5. Rectal pain
   a. Timing related to bowel function and activity
   b. Character
   c. Location

Past health history

1. Past history of problems in region
2. Surgeries in region
3. Trauma to region
4. Recent travel to countries where exposure to parasitic diseases could have occurred

Family health history

1. Family history of cancer in region or in gastrointestinal tract

Preparation for Examination: Client and Environment

Most clients experience a significant amount of embarrassment and apprehension about the rectal examination. They may be concerned about the cleanliness of the area, the exploration of troubling symptoms, or pain. These fears can cause spasms of the anal sphincters and buttocks, which make the examination unnecessarily uncomfortable. The following interventions can be used to alleviate anxiety and facilitate client cooperation so that a thorough and comfortable examination can be performed:

1. Teach the client relaxation techniques. Remind the client to continue slow, deep breathing during the examination.
2. Advise the client that unusual sensations may occur during the examination, especially the feeling that defecation is imminent; reassure the client that defecation is unlikely. Tell the client that sometimes flatus is passed during the examination, and should not be a cause for embarrassment. Remind clients that they may feel an urge to void when the prostate is palpated.

RISK FACTORS: ANORECTAL PROBLEMS

Anal sexual practices
Travel to countries where parasitic and tropic diseases are common
Diabetes
Cardiac conditions
Malignancies
Family history of cancer, Crohn's disease, ulcerative **colitis**

3. If the client has fecal incontinence, protect the client and the examination area with appropriate padding.

4. Proceed with the examination in a sympathetic but confident manner.

5. Maintain gentleness in approach, avoiding undue force and allowing time for relaxation but not withdrawing the examining hand until the examination has been completed. However, if the client experiences extreme pain that persists, discontinue the examination.

6. Drape the client to avoid unnecessary exposure of the genitalia.

Technique for Examination and Normal Findings

Examine the client in one of the following positions, as shown in Figure 22-2:

Rectal exam position

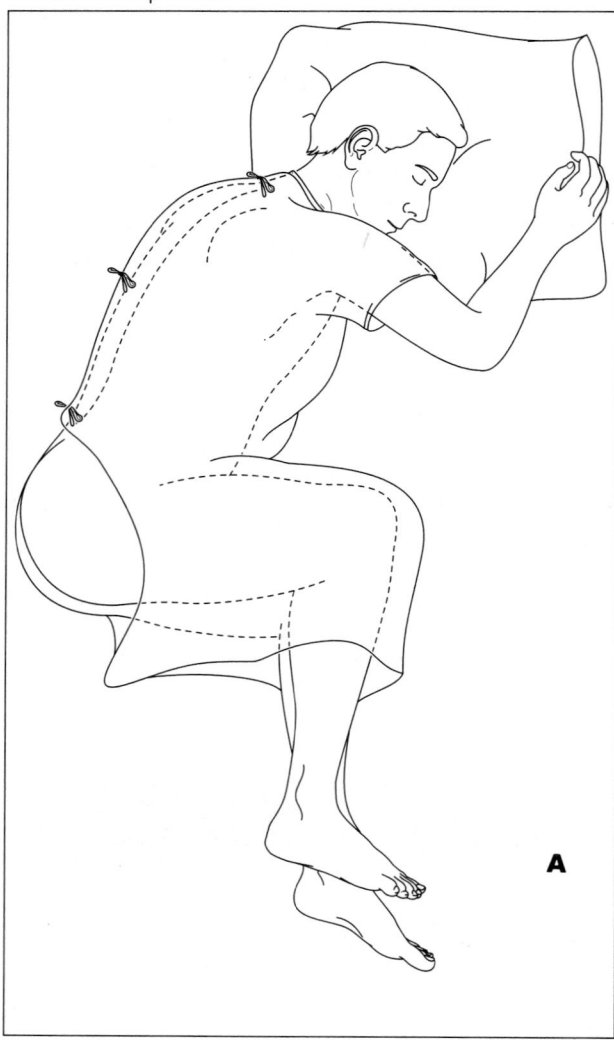

A

PREPARATION

Preparation for Examination

Equipment

Item	Purpose
Water-soluble lubricant	To enable more comfortable digital insertion and examination
Disposable gloves	To protect examiner's hands from feces and infection
Penlight	To observe skin of anus
Material for testing stool	To determine presence of occult blood

Client and environment

Provide a warm, private room with adequate lighting
Explain examination
Teach relaxation
Reassure about sensations
Position comfortably
Drape adequately

Knee-chest (genupectoral) position

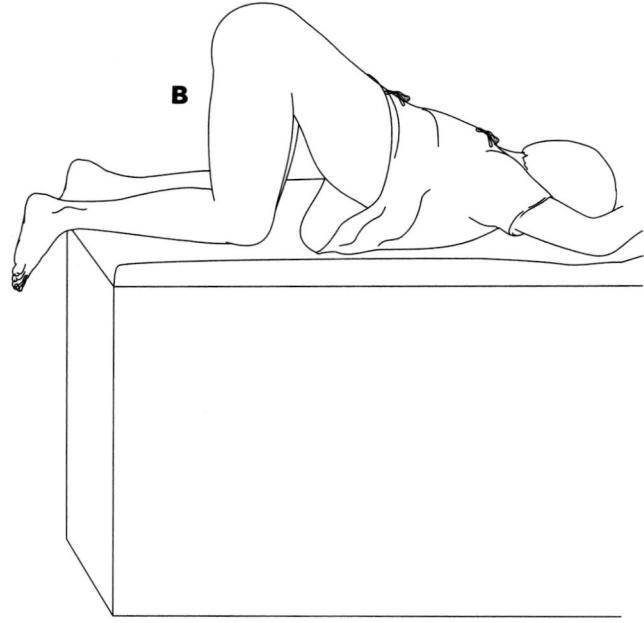

B

FIGURE 22-2 Positions for rectal exam. **A,** Left lateral or Sims' position. **B,** Knee-chest position.

1. Left lateral or Sims' position. The client lies on the left side with the superior thigh and knee flexed, bringing the knee close to the chest. The client's left hip should rest on a small, firm pillow or sandbag placed immediately adjacent to the side of the examination table, allowing the buttocks to be elevated and to project slightly over the edge of the table. The client's trunk should lie obliquely across the table top so that the head rests on a pillow near the opposite edge. The hips should be flexed to an angle slightly less than 90 degrees, with the lower leg placed close to the opposite side of the table and parallel to its edge. The right side of the body should be displaced slightly forward. In this position the rectal ampulla is pushed down and posteriorly and thus is advantageously aligned for the detection of rectal masses. However, the upper rectum and the pelvic structure tend to fall away in this position. This examination position is good for bed-bound clients, for males, and for females who are not receiving a pelvic examination during this assessment.

2. Knee-chest position. The client kneels on the examining table with the shoulders and head in contact with the examining table. The knees are positioned more widely apart than the hips. The angle at the hip is 75 to 80 degrees. The size of the prostate gland is best assessed with the client in this position. However, this position is an uncomfortable and embarrassing for many clients.

3. Standing position. The client stands over the examining table with the hips flexed and the trunk resting on the table. This position is commonly used for examination of the prostate gland.

4. Lithotomy position. This position is used with female clients for a screening rectal examination following a pelvic examination. The client is supine with knees flexed and feet elevated and supported in stirrups.

5. Squatting position. The client squats on a firm, flat surface with the examiner behind the client. Rectal prolapse frequently can be noted when the client is in this position, and some lesions of the rectosigmoid region and pelvis can be felt especially well in this position.

For all rectal examinations, the examiner should wear gloves on both hands throughout the entire procedure. If a risk of infection exists, two gloves should be worn on each hand for additional protection. Thorough hand-washing after degloving is recommended.

Inspection.   The manner in which the client sits throughout the preceding portions of the assessment provides some evidence of discomfort in the anal region. A client who continuously changes position during the examination may be having some anal discomfort.

Spread the buttocks carefully with both hands to examine the anus and the tissue immediately surrounding it. This skin is more pigmented and coarser than the rest of the perianal skin and is moist and hairless.

C

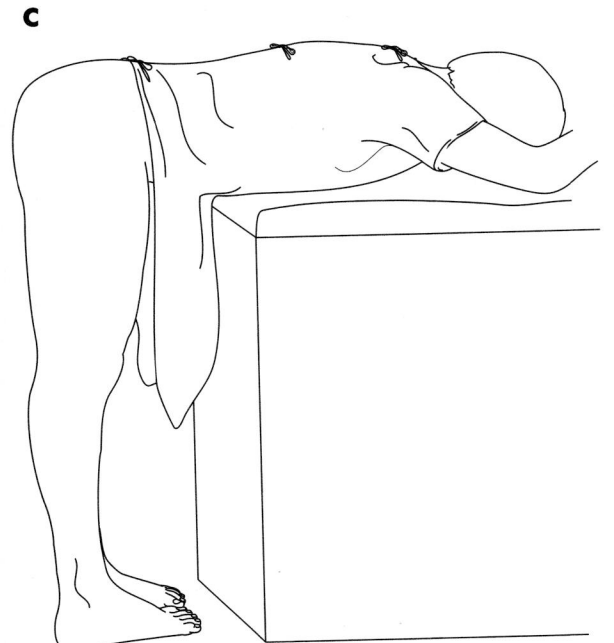

D

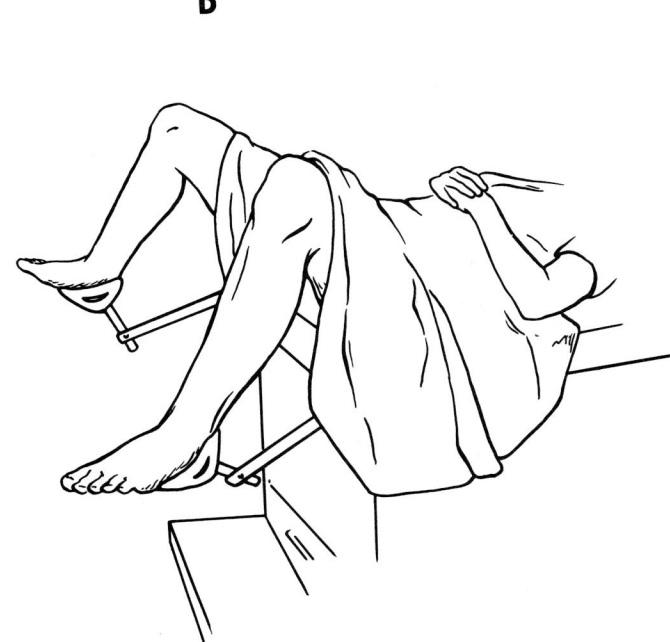

FIGURE 22-2, cont'd   C, Standing position. **D,** Lithotomy position. (Squatting position is not shown because it is infrequently used.)

Visually assess the perianal region for any lesions. Skin tags, scars, inflammation, perirectal abscesses, fissures, sentinel piles from rectal fissures, external hemorrhoids, fistula openings, condylomata acuminata (viral warts), tumors, and rectal prolapse may be observed through this inspection.

After the initial inspection, ask the client to strain downward, as though defecating, and inspect the anus during straining. With this maneuver, it is possible to identify rectal prolapse, polyps, or internal hemorrhoids. Describe any abnormal findings in terms of clock position, with the 12 o'clock position being the apex of the anus (point closest to symphysis pubis).

Inspect the sacrococcygeal area for pilonidal cyst or sinus. Normally, this area appears smooth and the overlying skin is healthy. Inspect the pilonidal area (at tip of coccyx) for dimples, sinus openings, or signs of inflammation. Also palpate the pilonidal area at this time for tenderness, induration, or swelling.

The skin over a pilonidal sinus may have abundant hair growth. The accumulation of secretions within the sinus often leads to infection, which is generally accompanied by foul-smelling discharge and local tenderness.

Next examine the skin of the entire perineal area for lesions and inflammation.

Palpation. Spread the buttocks with the nondominant hand. If the sphincter tightens, instruct the client to relax and reassure the client. Then, when the sphincter has relaxed, continue the examination. Occasionally, painful lesions or bleeding may prevent completion of the examination unless a local analgesic agent is administered.

Lubricate the pad of the gloved index finger of the hand to be used for palpation. Instruct the client to strain downward against this finger. Then gently place the lubricated index finger of the examining hand against the anal verge. Exert firm pressure until the rectal sphincter begins to yield; then slowly insert the finger into the anal canal in the direction of the umbilicus as the sphincter relaxes (Figure 22-3). Ask the client to tighten the sphincter around the examining finger to provide a measurement of muscle strength of the anal sphincter. Hypertonicity of the external sphincter may occur with anxious voluntary or involuntary contraction or as a result of an anal fissure or other local pathological condition. A relaxed or hypotonic sphincter is seen occasionally after rectal surgery, or it may be caused by a neurological deficiency.

The anal canal is short. The distance from the anal verge to the anorectal junction is less than 3 cm, which is roughly equivalent to the distance from the fingertip

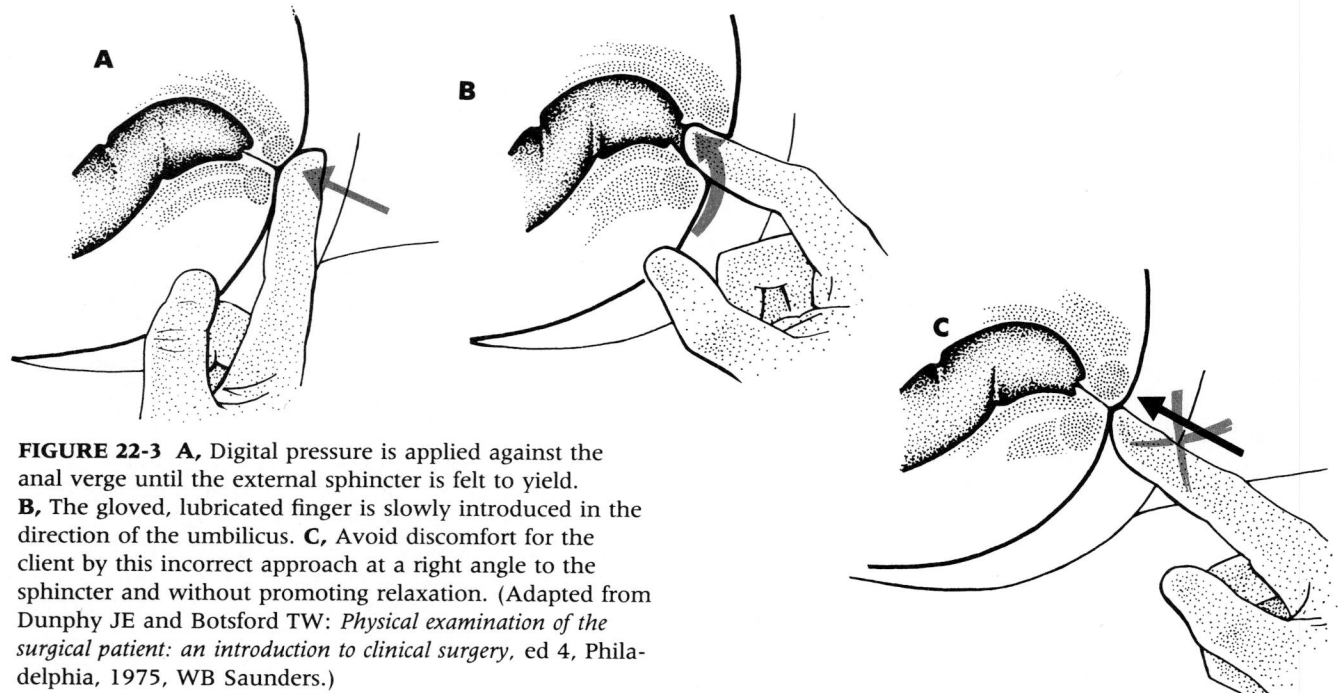

FIGURE 22-3 A, Digital pressure is applied against the anal verge until the external sphincter is felt to yield. **B,** The gloved, lubricated finger is slowly introduced in the direction of the umbilicus. **C,** Avoid discomfort for the client by this incorrect approach at a right angle to the sphincter and without promoting relaxation. (Adapted from Dunphy JE and Botsford TW: *Physical examination of the surgical patient: an introduction to clinical surgery,* ed 4, Philadelphia, 1975, WB Saunders.)

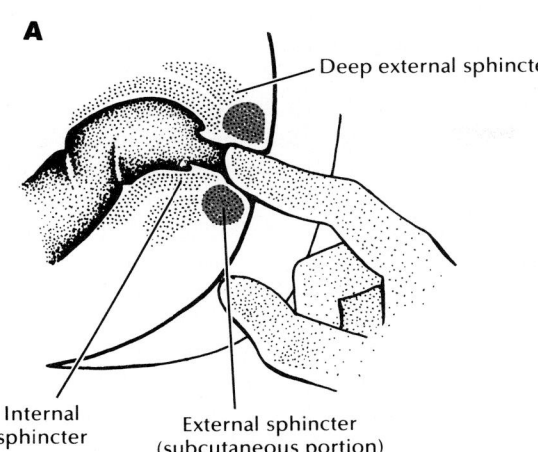

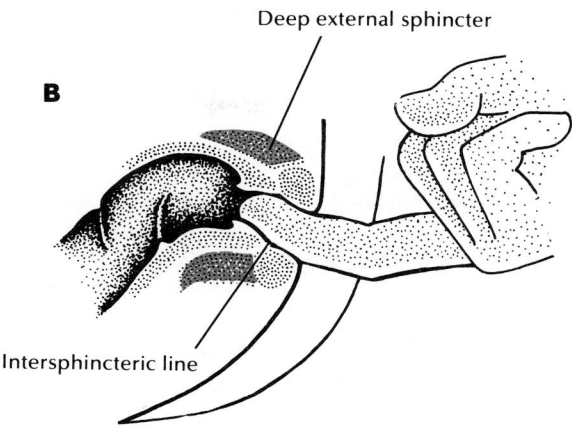

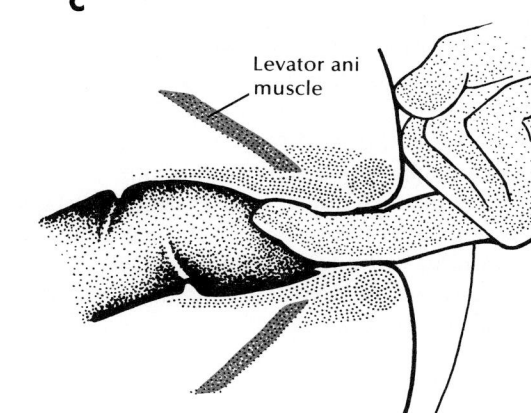

FIGURE 22-4 The subcutaneous portion of the external sphincter is palpated, **A,** followed by digital exploration of the deep external sphincter, **B. C,** Palpation of the levator ani muscle. (Adapted from Dunphy JE and Botsford TW: *Physical examination of the surgical patient: an introduction to clinical surgery,* ed 4, Philadelphia, 1975, WB Saunders.)

to the interphalangeal joint. Palpate the subcutaneous portion of the external sphincter on the inner aspect of the anal verge. Rotate the palpating finger to examine the entire muscular ring. A palpable indentation marks the intersphincteric line. Palpate the deep external sphincter through the lower part of the internal sphincter, which it surrounds. Bidigital palpation of the sphincter area may yield more information than would be obtained by probing with the index finger alone. For bidigital palpation, press the thumb of the examining hand against the perianal tissue and move the examining index finger toward it. This technique is useful for detecting a perianal abscess and for palpating the bulbourethral (Cowper's) glands.

To assess the levator ani muscle, palpate laterally and posteriorly the area where the muscle is attached to the rectal wall on one side and then the other (Figure 22-4). Palpate the mucosa of the anal canal for tumors and polyps. Palpate the coccyx to determine its mobility and sensitivity. To assess muscular structures and the coccyx, perform bimanual examination with the index finger and the thumb.

The posterior wall of the rectum follows the curve of the coccyx and the sacrum and feels smooth to the palpating finger. The examining finger is able to palpate a distance of 6 to 10 cm of the rectal canal. To palpate the lateral walls of the rectum, rotate the index finger along the sides of the rectum. The ischial spines and the sacrotuberous ligaments can be identified through palpation. Rectal valves may be misinterpreted as protruding intrarectal masses, especially when they are well developed.

Because the prostate gland is situated anterior to the rectum, palpation through the mucosa of the anterior wall of the rectum allows for assessment of the size, shape, tenderness, surface characteristics, mobility, and consistency of the prostate gland. Ask the client to bear down so that an otherwise unreachable mass may be pushed downward into the range of the examining finger.

The prostate gland, a bilobed structure, has a normal diameter of approximately 4 cm at its widest part. The palpating finger is used to identify the smooth lateral lobes separated by a central groove. The prostate, which is approximately 3 cm long, should protrude about 1 cm into the rectum, should feel rubbery and smooth, and should be slightly movable. The prostate should be nontender to palpation. (Ask the client specifically to report any tenderness to touch.) Note the presence of nodules. (For a complete discussion of the prostate examination see Chapter 20.)

The normal cervix can be felt as a small round mass through the anterior wall of the rectum. In addition, a vaginal tampon or a retroverted uterus can be palpated through the rectal wall. (See Chapter 21 for a complete discussion of the assessment of the female genitalia.)

At the termination of the examination, assist the client to a more comfortable position and offer tissues to remove any lubricant remaining around the anal opening.

Examination of Stool. After the examining finger has been withdrawn, examine the nature of any feces clinging to the glove (Table 22-1). Note the presence of pus or blood.

Next, test a small quantity of the feces for the presence of occult blood. This determination is made through a standard chemical test, as described later in this discussion. Small abrasions of the gastrointestinal tract are thought to be responsible for a blood loss of 1 to 3 ml daily in the feces. The loss of more than 50 ml from the upper gastrointestinal tract will produce melena. To detect quantities of blood less than 50 ml or to determine whether black stools actually do contain blood, any of several reagents may be used.

Various factors other than bowel disease may contribute to occult blood in the stools. For example, the following factors might contribute to a positive test:

1. Bleeding gums following a dental procedure or resulting from another reason.
2. Ingestion of red meat within 3 days of the test.
3. Ingestion of fish, turnips, and horseradish.
4. Drugs that cause gastrointestinal bleeding, such

as anticoagulants, aspirin, colchicine, iron preparations, nonsteroidal antiarthritics, and steroids.
5. Other substances that might cause false-positive results for various reasons, such as oxidizing drugs, rauwolfia derivatives, and vitamin C.

Tests for occult blood in the feces rely on substances that detect peroxidase as an indication of hemoglobin content demonstrated through color change in the stool specimen tested. Various reagent substances are used to detect occult blood. Their sensitivity varies as follows:

1. Orthotoluidine (Hematest, Occultest) — 10 times more sensitive than benzidine.
2. Benzidine — 10 (or more) times more sensitive than guaiac.
3. Guaiac (Hemoccult) — the least sensitive reagent.

A single positive test result does not necessarily confirm the presence of gastrointestinal bleeding. A positive result is an indication to repeat the test at least three times while the client follows a meatless high-residue diet.

The various commercially prepared screening tests for occult blood are packaged with complete instructions for use. Since the steps of the various tests are similar, the following instructions for the Hematest are presented as an example:

1. After the digital examination, wipe a bit of the feces on the glove of the examining finger on a square of filter paper supplied with the kit.
2. Place the filter paper with the stool smear on a glass slide.
3. Place a reagent tablet in the center of the smear on the filter paper.
4. Place one drop of water on the tablet, and allow the water to soak into the tablet for 5 to 10 seconds. Then add a second drop of water, which should run from the tablet onto the specimen and the filter paper.

TABLE 22-1

Assessment of Stool Characteristics

Description of stool	Possible explanation
Yellow or green	Severe diarrhea, sterilization of bowel by antibiotics, diet high in chlorophyll-rich vegetables, and use of the drug calomel
Light tan, gray	Absence of bile pigments, as may be found in blockage of the common bile duct, pancreatic insufficiency, obstructive jaundice, and diets high in milk or fat and low in meat
Black, tarry	Bleeding into the upper gastrointestinal tract, ingestion of iron compounds or bismuth preparations, and high proportions of meat in the diet
Red	Bleeding from the lower gastrointestinal tract; some foods such as beets
Translucent mucus on stool	Spastic constipation, nucleus colitis, emotional disturbance, and excessive straining
Bloody mucus	Neoplasm or inflammation of the rectal canal
Mucus with pus and blood	Ulcerative colitis, bacillary dysentery, ulcerating cancer of the colon, and acute diverticulitis
Fat in stool	Malabsorption syndromes, enteritis and pancreatic diseases, surgical removal of a section of the intestine, **steatorrhea,** and chronic pancreatic disease

5. After 2 minutes, the filter paper will turn blue if the test is positive. The color on the tablet itself or color appearing after 2 minutes is irrelevant.

If the screening test is positive, the client is retested after 48 to 72 hours. Instruct the client to refrain from eating meat, poultry, fish, turnips, and horseradish during the next testing period. In addition, the client may need to temporarily discontinue the use of the following substances: iron preparations, bromides, iodides, rauwolfia derivatives, indomethacin, colchicine, salicylates, phenylbutazone, oxyphenylbutazone, bismuth compounds, steroids, and ascorbic acid.

Screening Tests and Procedures

Screening for colorectal cancer is done through fecal occult blood testing and sigmoidoscopy. However, the U.S. Preventive Services Task Force (1989) has found insufficient evidence to recommend either for or against such screening tests in asymptomatic persons. The report of this task force states that it may be clinically prudent to offer screening to persons aged 50 and older who have first-degree relatives with colorectal cancer; a personal history of endometrial, ovarian, or breast cancer; or a previous diagnosis of inflammatory bowel disease, adenomatous polyps, or colorectal cancer. Periodic colonoscopy is recommended for all persons with a family history of familial polyposis coli or cancer family syndrome (p. 51).

The presence of a pathological condition detected by digital examination may be further explored by one of the procedures shown in the box below.

Examination Step-by-Step

Inspection

Spread the client's buttocks.
Observe the perianal region for inflammation, lesions, hemorrhoids, and fissures.
Observe the sacrococcygeal area.

Palpation

Lubricate the examining finger.
Insert the finger into the anus.
Place the pad of the finger gently along the anal verge.
Feel the sphincter tense and then relax. When the sphincter has relaxed, flex the tip of the finger and slowly insert it into the anal canal in the direction of the umbilicus.
Rotate the finger and palpate the entire muscular ring.
Assess tone by asking the client to contract the muscles.
Assess the perianal tissue, muscular structures, and mobility of the coccyx through bidigital palpation.
Assess the remaining rectal wall.
Men: Palpate the prostate gland and the seminal vesicles on the anterior wall.
Women: Perform the rectovaginal examination.

Assessment of stool

Withdraw the examining finger.
Examine the feces on the gloved finger.
Test the stool for occult blood.

OTHER INVESTIGATIVE TECHNIQUES

Anoscopy

Use of an anoscope for a more complete examination of the anal canal and the internal hemorrhoidal zone.

Proctoscopy

Use of a proctoscope to visualize the anus and the lower rectum. Approximately 9 to 15 cm of the lower intestinal tract can be visualized. The warmed and lubricated instrument is passed with the obturator for its full length. The obturator is removed, and the proctoscope is removed slowly while the examiner observes for ulcers, inflammation, strictures, or the cause of a palpable mass. Biopsy may be performed through the tube.

Sigmoidoscopy

Visual examination of the upper portion of the rectum, an area that cannot be felt with the examining finger, is possible with a sigmoidoscope, which allows direct visualization of the lower 24 cm of the gastrointestinal tract. This examination is particularly important since half of all carcinomas occur in the rectum and colon. The early detection of polyps and malignant lesions may result in early and successful treatment of an otherwise fatal disease.

Manometry

This technique measures intraluminal pressure by a balloon probe attached to a catheter that is connected to a pressure transducer and a polygraph.

Sphincter electromyography

Needle or surface electrodes are used to detect the contractile activity of striated muscle and to obtain separate recordings from the external sphincter and from the puborectalis muscle.

Defecography and balloon proctography

These radiological investigations are designed to image the rectum and the pelvic floor at rest and during contraction and defecation.

VARIATIONS FROM HEALTH

Bright-red blood, in small or large amounts, may originate in the large intestine, the sigmoid colon, the rectum, or the anus. The stool is likely to be red-black if the bleeding is coming from the ascending colon. Colonic bleeding should be suspected when blood is mixed with the feces. Rectal bleeding is probably occurring when blood is observed on the surface of the stool. The presence of a good deal of blood in the stool may be associated with marked malodor.

A black, tarry stool (melena) may result from bleeding in the stomach or the small intestine; the blood is partially digested during its passage to the rectum. On the other hand, the black color may result from ingested iron compounds and bismuth preparations.

Pilonidal Cyst and Sinus

A pilonidal cyst is a hairy sac that develops in the sacral region of the skin. A pilonidal sinus is an abnormal channel that contains a tuft of hair and is most frequently situated over or close to the tip of the coccyx. Even though it is thought to be a congenital lesion, pilonidal sinus is commonly first diagnosed between the ages of 15 and 30 years. It is located superficial to the coccyx, or lower sacrum. The sinus opening may look like a dimple, with another very small opening found in the midline. In other cases of pilonidal sinus, a cyst can be observed and palpated. In more advanced conditions, a sinus tract can be palpated. The affected area may become edematous, erythematous, and tender, and a tuft of hair may be observed. The ingrowth of the hairs is probably the cause of infection, cyst, and fistula formation. These cysts and fistulas are generally removed surgically.

Pruritus Ani

Pruritus ani is a common chronic condition characterized by itching of the perianal skin. Excoriated, thickened, and pigmented skin may result from chronic inflammation associated with this condition. The itching and burning of the rectal area are most often traceable to pinworms in children and to fungal infections in adults. Clients with diabetes are particularly vulnerable to fungal infections. A dull, grayish-pink color of the perianal skin is characteristic of fungal infections. The radiating folds of skin may appear enlarged, and the skin may be cracked or fissured. Pruritus ani that is characterized by dry and brittle skin is thought to be related to psychosomatic disease.

Rectal Tenesmus

Rectal **tenesmus** is painful straining at stool associated with spasm of the anal and rectal muscles. The chief complaint is a distressing feeling of urgency. The client should be questioned concerning the nature of the stool. A hard, dry stool indicates constipation. A bloody, diarrheal stool might indicate ulcerative colitis. When the client's stools are normally constituted, rectal fissure may be the cause of tenesmus. The client with a perirectal inflammation, such as prostatitis or **proctitis,** may also experience tenesmus.

The client who complains of constant rectal pain should be examined carefully for thrombosed rectal hemorrhoids.

Fecal Impaction

Fecal impaction is the accumulation and dehydration of fecal material in the rectum. When motility of the rectum is inhibited, the normal progression of feces does not occur and excessive amounts of water are reabsorbed through the bowel wall. The feces become hard and difficult to pass, and the accumulation may lead to complete obstruction. Fecal impaction is observed in individuals with chronic constipation and in those who have retained barium following gastrointestinal x-ray examination. The client complains of a sense of rectal fullness or urgency. Frequent small liquid-to-loose stools may occur in incomplete obstruction. The dehydrated fecal mass is easily felt on palpation.

Anal Fissure

Anal fissure is a linear ulceration or laceration of the skin of the anus. A thin tear of the superficial anal mucosa, generally weeping, may be identified by asking the client to bear down as though straining to evacuate stool. The fissure is most commonly (in more than 90% of affected patients) found in the posterior midline of the anal mucosa and less frequently in the anterior midline (Figure 22-5). Anal fissure usually results from trauma, such as that associated with the passage of a large, hard stool or with anal intercourse. The client may complain of local pain, itching, or bleeding. Pain generally accompanies the passage of stool, and blood may be observed on the stool or on the toilet tissue. The inspection finding may include a sentinel skin tag or ulcer through which the muscles of the internal sphincter may be visible at the base. Because the examination is painful to the client, which makes it difficult to relax the anal muscle, the use of a local anesthetic may be necessary.

Fistula-in-Ano

Fistula-in-ano is an abnormal opening on the cutaneous surface near the anus. It usually results from a local crypt abscess but is also common in Crohn's disease. A tract from an anal fissure or infection that terminates in the perianal skin or other tissue is termed an anorectal fistula. This type of fistula usually originates from local crypt abscesses. The fistula is a chron-

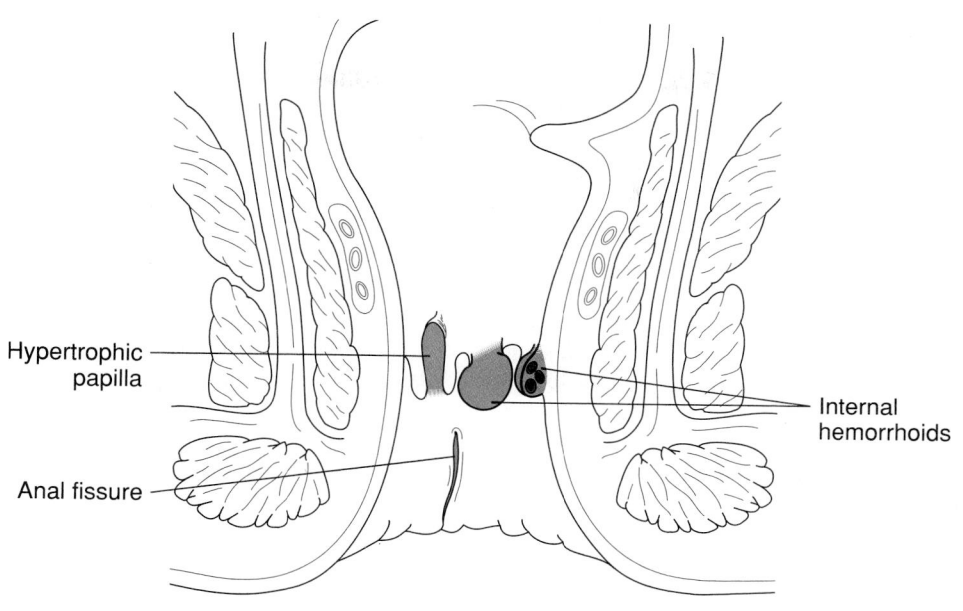

FIGURE 22-5 Common problems of the anus and rectum.

TABLE 22-2		
Location of Fistula Site Related to the External Opening		
	External opening	**Location in anus**
Goodsell's rule	Posterior to a line between the ischial tuberosities	Posterior
	Radial from drainage site	Anterior
Salmon's law	Posterior to anus or more than 2.5 cm anterior or lateral	Posterior
	Anterior or less than 2.5 cm lateral	Anterior

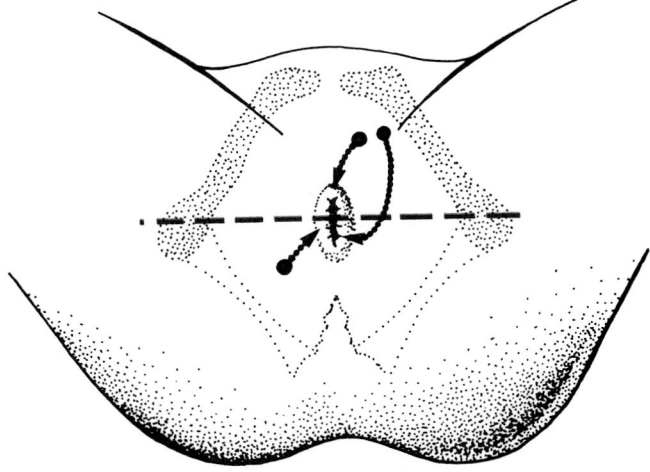

FIGURE 22-6 Salmon's law. Fissure location related to the aperture of the fistula. (Adapted from Dunphy JE and Botsford TW: *Physical examination of the surgical patient: an introduction to clinical surgery,* ed 4, Philadelphia, 1975, WB Saunders.)

ically inflamed tube, made up of fibrous tissue surrounding granulation tissue, that frequently can be palpated. The external opening is generally visible as a red elevation of granulation tissue. Local compression may result in the expression of serosanguineous or purulent drainage. Bidigital palpation is best accomplished with a finger in the anorectal cavity that compresses the tissue against the thumb on the skin surface. The fistulous tract feels like an indurated cord.

The site from which drainage from an anal infection occurs can be identified by relating the location of the external opening of the fissure to the anus (Table 22-2 and Figure 22-6).

Hemorrhoids

Hemorrhoids are dilated, congested veins. Hemorrhoidal swelling is associated with increased hydrostatic pressure in the portal venous system. The pressure associated with hemorrhoids correlates positively with pregnancy, straining at stool, chronic liver disease, and sudden increases in intraabdominal pressure. Bowel habits also play a role: for example, hemorrhoids frequently occur with diarrhea or incomplete bowel emptying. Local factors such as abscess or tumor may also contribute to venous stasis.

Hemorrhoidal skin tags are ragged, flaccid skin sacs located around the anus. They cover connective tissue sacs and are the locus of resolved external hemorrhoids. Clients describe these tags as painless. Internal hemorrhoids occur proximal to the pectinate line (Figure 22-5), whereas external hemorrhoids are those that are seen distal to this boundary. External hemorrhoids are covered by skin or anal squamous tissue.

External hemorrhoids are often painful, particularly if an increase in stool mass stretches the skin. Because the mass is located near the sphincter muscles, spasm is not uncommon. External hemorrhoids often cause itching and bleeding on defecation. These dilated veins may not be apparent at rest; however, they may appear as bluish, swollen areas at the anal verge when thrombosed. A thrombosed hemorrhoid is one in which blood has clotted, both within and outside the vein.

Internal hemorrhoids generally do not cause pain unless they are complicated by thrombosis, infection, or erosion of overlying mucosal surfaces. Discomfort is increased if the hemorrhoids prolapse through the anal opening. Bleeding may occur from the internal hemorrhoids with or without defecation. **Proctoscopy** is generally necessary for their identification.

Rectal Polyps

Rectal polyps, which feel like soft nodules, are encountered frequently. They may be pedunculated (on a stalk) or sessile (irregularly moundlike, growing from a relatively broad base, and closely adherent to the mucosal wall). Because of their soft consistency, rectal polyps may be difficult or impossible to identify by palpation. Proctoscopy is usually necessary for identification, and a biopsy is performed to identify malignant lesions. A pedunculated rectal polyp occasionally prolapses through the anal ring.

Rectal Prolapse

Internal hemorrhoids are the most common type of tissue protrusion through the anal ring. The pink-colored mucosa is described as appearing like a doughnut or rosette. In the older client, however, protruding mucosa may herald eversion or prolapse of the rectum. Incomplete prolapse involves only mucosa, whereas complete rectal prolapse also is associated with the sphincters.

The client describes the prolapse of tissue through the anal ring as occurring with exercise or while straining at stool. Frequently, the client is able to push the mass back in with digital pressure. Inspection reveals a red, bulging mucosal mass protruding through the anal ring.

Anal Incontinence

Loss of the voluntary ability to control defecation is called incontinence. It may range from the involuntary passage of flatus to complete loss of sphincter tone. The loss of fecal gases or liquids may also occur in the presence of a normal sphincter in hyperdynamic bowel states.

Abscesses

Abscesses of the lower gastrointestinal tract that can be identified by physical examination (Figure 22-7) include the following type:

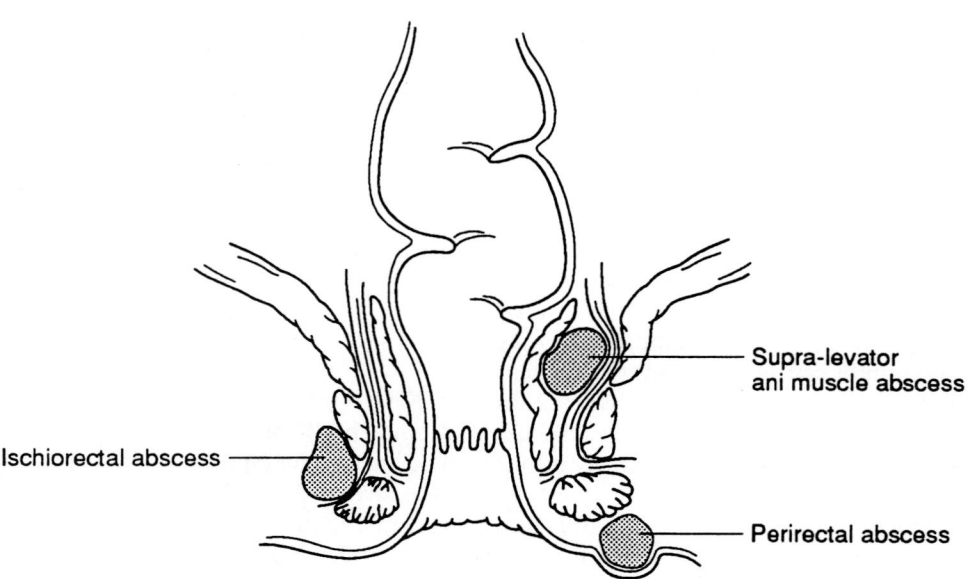

FIGURE 22-7 Common sites of abscess formation in the lower gastrointestinal tract.

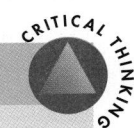

1. *Perirectal abscess*: May be palpated as a tender mass adjacent to the anal canal. The increased temperature of the mass may be helpful in identifying the inflammatory process.
2. *Ischiorectal abscess*: May be palpated as a tender mass protruding into the lateral wall of the anal canal.
3. *Supra–levator ani muscle abscess*: May be felt by the examining finger as a tender mass in the lateral rectal wall.

Masses

The presence of a mass in the rectum deserves special attention because nearly half of the rectal masses discovered are malignant. The client frequently denies pain or other symptoms. Early lesions are felt as small elevations or nodules with a firm base. Ulceration of the center of the lesion results in a crater that may be palpated. An ulcerated carcinoma may be identified through palpation by its firm, nodular rolled edge. The lesion of carcinoma is described by including annular or tubular shape, degree of fixation, and distance from the anus. The consistency of the malignant mass is often stony and hard, and the contour is irregular. Extension of metastatic carcinoma from the peritoneum to the pelvic floor is described as a rectal shelf. It is palpated as a hard nodular ridge.

Sample Documentation

Health history

Diagnosis of hemorrhoids several months ago by a physician in another state. Was advised to use over-the-counter hemorrhoid preparations and constipation prevention. Continues to have mild rectal discomfort and itching, almost continuously. Small amounts of bright-red blood in stools for several bowel movements every 2 to 3 weeks. Stools are hard and sometimes gray. Denies abdominal pain and changes in sleep, activity, and dietary patterns. No fecal incontinence. Has frequent constipation and strains to produce stool. Has 2 to 3 stools per day. Denies history of rectal infections, traumas, and surgeries. Is on a high-fiber diet supplemented with prescribed stool softeners and drinks 6 to 8 glasses of fluid per day. Negative family history for cancer, hemorrhoids, colon disease.

Physical examination

Perianal area clean—no fissures or lesions. Area around anus edematous with erythema and tender with palpation. Large sphincter tone good with no prolapses noted. Rectal walls smooth without masses or tenderness. Stool—soft, brown, formed. Guiac—negative.

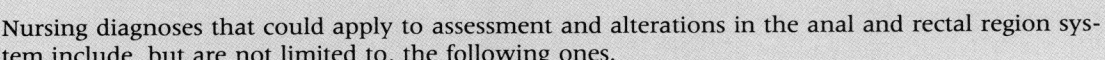

Nursing Diagnosis   *THE NEXT STEP*

Nursing diagnoses that could apply to assessment and alterations in the anal and rectal region system include, but are not limited to, the following ones.

CONSTIPATION The state in which an individual experiences a change in normal bowel habits characterized by a decrease in frequency and/or passage of hard, dry stools.

Defining Characteristics

- Frequency less than normal pattern
- Hard formed stools, decreased quantity
- Palpable mass
- Reported feeling of pressure in rectum
- Feeling of rectal fullness
- Straining at stool

Related Factors

- Low-roughage diet
- Low fluid intake
- Decreased activity level
- Absence of time routines
- Routine use of enemas or laxatives

Continued.

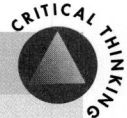

Nursing Diagnosis   *THE NEXT STEP—cont'd*

PERCEIVED CONSTIPATION The state in which an individual makes a self-diagnosis of constipation and ensures a daily bowel movement through use of laxatives, enemas, and suppositories.

Defining Characteristics

- Expectation of daily bowel movements with the resulting overuse of laxatives, enemas, and/or suppositories
- Expected passage of stool at the same time daily

Related Factors

- Cultural and family health beliefs
- Faulty appraisal
- Impaired thought processes

DIARRHEA The state in which an individual experiences a change in normal bowel habits characterized by the frequent passage of loose, fluid, unformed stools.

Defining Characteristics

- Loose, fluid stools
- Cramping, abdominal pain
- Frequent bowel movements
- Hyperactive bowel sounds
- Urgency
- Change in color of stools

Related Factors

- Food intolerance

BOWEL INCONTINENCE The state in which an individual experiences a change in normal bowel habits characterized by involuntary passage of stool.

Defining Characteristics

- Involuntary passage of stool

Related Factors

- Loss of sphincter control
- Cognitive/perceptual impairment

PAIN The state in which an individual experiences and reports the presence of severe discomfort or an uncomfortable sensation.

Defining Characteristics

- Subjective
  Communication (verbal or coded) of pain descriptors
- Objective
  Guarding behavior; protective
  Self-focusing
  Narrowed focus (altered time perception, withdrawal from social contact, impaired thought process)
  Distraction behavior (moaning, crying, pacing, seeking other people and/or activities, restlessness)
  Facial mask of pain (eyes lack luster, "beaten look," fixed or scattered movement, grimace)
  Alteration in muscle tone (may span from listless to rigid)
  Autonomic responses not seen in chronic, stable pain (diaphoresis, blood pressure and pulse rate change, pupillary dilation, increased or decreased respiratory rate)

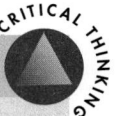

Nursing Diagnosis   *THE NEXT STEP—cont'd*

Related Factors

- Injuring agents
  Biological
  Chemical
  Physical
  Psychological

Clinical Application

Mrs. P. is a 35-year-old female complaining of burning and itching sensation in the rectal area, especially after having a bowel movement. Mrs. P. has noted a small amount of blood on her toilet tissue occasionally after a bowel movement. Mrs. P. has had a history of hemorrhoids after her last pregnancy 3 years ago, but has not had previous problems until this past month. Further questioning of Mrs. P. reveals she has not moved her bowels regularly in the past month. She has been taking a laxative every 2 to 3 days. When she does have a bowel movement it is hard and she has mild pain (dyschezia), followed by burning and itching. Mrs. P. reveals she has just started working outside her home so she does not eat as nutritiously as she used to, nor does she exercise at all. A physical assessment is completed.

SUBJECTIVE DATA: Patient complains of:
Burning and itching sensation after each bowel movement
Occasional blood on toilet tissue after bowel movement
Pain during bowel movements

OBJECTIVE DATA:
Abdomen: flat, bowel sounds normal and heard in all four quadrants. No organomegaly or tenderness to palpation.
Rectal: Small 1 cm × 1 cm blue-red swollen mass noted below the anorectal junction. Sphincter tone good. Rectal wall smooth, slight tenderness upon palpation of posterior wall unable to feel any masses. Stool brown, guaiac negative.

NURSING DIAGNOSES

Constipation related to low roughage diet and low fluid intake.

Defining Characteristics

- Frequency less than normal pattern
- Hard formed stools, decreased quantity
- Straining at stool

Colonic constipation related to less than adequate fluid intake, dietery intake, and physical activity.

Defining Characteristics

- Decreased frequency
- Hard stool
- Straining at stool
- Painful defecation

Pain related to constipation.

Defining Characteristics

- Verbal communication that defecation is painful

GLOSSARY

ampulla Rounded, saclike dilatation of a duct, canal, or any tubular structure.

anastomosing Joining.

colic Acute abdominal pain associated with smooth muscle contraction of the gastrointestinal tract.

colitis Inflammation of the colon.

constipation Infrequent or difficult evacuation of feces; often associated with drying and hardening of the stool.

diarrhea Increased frequency and liquid content of fecal evacuation.

hemorrhoid Dilatation of a part of the venous hemorrhoidal plexus in the mucosal membrane of the rectum. A hemorrhoid may occur as a result of increased hydrostatic pressure in the venous system, as in pregnancy, or from disease that causes portal hypertension and straining at stool. *Internal hemorrhoids:* Varicosity of superior or middle hemorrhoidal veins below the anal mucosa; may result in bleeding. *External hemorrhoids:* Varicosity of the inferior hemorrhoidal vein under the anal skin; may cause pain and swelling around the anal sphincter and itching and bleeding.

incontinence Failure of control of excretory functions.

obstipation Severe constipation.

proctitis Inflammation of the rectal mucosa.

proctoscopy Examination of the rectum with a short cylindrical instrument called a proctoscope.

steatorrhea Abnormal increase of fat in the feces.

tenesmus Persistent, ineffectual spasms of the rectum accompanied by the desire to empty the bowel.

BIBLIOGRAPHY

Beahrs OH, Higgins GA, Weinstein JJ: *Colorectal tumors*, Philadelphia, 1986, JB Lippincott.

Cherry DA, Rothenberger DA: Pelvic floor physiology, *Surg Clin North Am* 68:1217-1230, 1988.

Ger R: Surgical anatomy of the pelvis, *Surg Clin North Am* 68:1202-1216, 1988.

Gordon PH: The anorectum: anatomic and physiologic considerations in health and disease, *Gastroenterol Clin North Am* 16(1):1-15, 1987.

Gordon M: *Nursing diagnosis: process and application*, ed 2, New York, 1987, McGraw-Hill.

Gordon M: *Manual of nursing diagnosis, 1993-1994*, St. Louis, 1993, Mosby–Year Book.

Kirsner JB, Shorter RG, editors: *Diseases of the colon, rectum, and anal canal*, Baltimore, 1988, Williams & Wilkins.

Localio SA, Eng K, Coppa GF: *Anorectal, presacral, and sacral tumors: anatomy, physiology, pathogenesis, and management*, Philadelphia, 1987, WB Saunders.

Marti MC, Givel JC: *Surgery of anorectal diseases*, Berlin, 1990, Springer-Verlag.

Mosby's medical, nursing, and allied health dictionary, ed 3, St. Louis, 1990, Mosby–Year Book.

Pagana KD, Pagana TJ: *Mosby's diagnostic and laboratory test reference*, St Louis, 1992, Mosby–Year Book.

Payne JE: Symptoms and the diagnosis of bowel cancer: a critical view, *Med J Aust* 148:505-507, 1988.

Raufmann JP, Straus EW: Endoscopic procedures in the AIDS patient: risks, precautions, indications, and obligations, *Gastroenterol Clin North Am* 17:495-506, 1988.

Schrock TR: Diseases of the anorectum. In Sleisenger MH, Fordtran JS: *Gastrointestinal disease*, ed 4, Philadelphia, 1986, WB Saunders.

Sherwood MJ, and others: *Determining nursing diagnosis through assessment*, Baltimore, 1988, Williams & Wilkins.

Smith LE, editor: *Practical guide to anorectal testing*, New York, 1990, Igaku-Shoin.

US Preventive Services Task Force: *Guide to clinical preventive services: an assessment of the effectiveness of 169 interventions*, Baltimore, 1989, Williams & Wilkins.

*U*nit IV, Assessing Special
Populations, contains thorough
discussions of the application of
history and physical assessment
techniques to special populations
often served by nursing practitioners: specifically, pregnant women,
children, elderly clients, and clients
with functional limitations. The
content of these chapters assumes
some mastery of the basic history
taking and physical examination
skills described in the previous
chapters. The emphasis in these
chapters is the measurement of
health for the purposes of health
promotion and health maintenance
care.

Assessing Special Populations

Pregnant Clients

PURPOSE OF THE EXAMINATION

This chapter focuses on the assessment of healthy pregnant women. It assumes and builds on knowledge of and skill in the physical examination of the adult client. The emphasis of this chapter is on the effects of the pregnant state on examination findings and the special techniques used to assess the health of the fetus and the woman's ability to deliver vaginally. To obtain complete information about the management of care for pregnant women, additional references are necessary.

PHYSICAL CHANGES IN PREGNANCY

A number of physical changes occur normally in pregnant women, many of which are noted in the physical assessment. All the physiological changes of pregnancy are directly or indirectly initiated by the hormones produced by the fetal **chorionic** tissues and the placenta. In early pregnancy the fetal **trophoblast** produces large amounts of human chorionic gonadotropic (HCG) hormone, which provides the basis for biological pregnancy testing. HCG is present in amounts detectable by immunological tests performed 8 to 10 days after conception.

Large amounts of estrogens and progesterone are produced during pregnancy. Estriol, an estrogen, is produced in large amounts during middle and late pregnancy. It is the basis for biological tests of placental and fetal well-being because a well-functioning placenta, a healthy fetus, and an intact fetal circulation are prerequisites for the continuous production of this hormone. The estrogens and progesterone maintain the **decidua** of pregnancy and cause the growth and hyperemia of the uterus, other pelvic organs, and the breasts.

In more than 50% of prenatal clients, the thyroid gland is symmetrically enlarged as a result of hyperplasia of glandular tissue, new follicle formation, and increased vascularity. The basal metabolic rate is increased, largely because of increased growth and oxygen consumption by the pregnant uterus, the fetus, and the placenta.

Uterus, Cervix, and Vagina

Changes in the uterus include the development of the decidua, hypertrophy of muscle cells, increased vascularity, formation of the lower uterine segment, and softening of the cervix. During pregnancy the overall size of the uterus increases five to six times, its weight increases about 20 times, and its capacity increases from approximately 2 to 5000 ml.

Hormones supply the initial stimulus for uterine hypertrophy. During the first 6 to 8 weeks of pregnancy, the uterus will increase in size whether the pregnancy is uterine or extrauterine. In early pregnancy the uterus is a pelvic organ and only internally palpable. At approximately 10 to 12 weeks' gestation, the growing uterus is double its nonpregnant size and reaches the top of the symphysis, where it is palpable abdominally. The uterine **fundus** lies approximately halfway between the symphysis and the umbilicus at about 16 weeks' gestation and reaches the umbilicus at about 20 to 22 weeks' gestation. After the 20 weeks' gestation, the average upward growth of the uterus is about 3.75 cm per month (1 cm per week). At approximately 36 weeks' gestation, the uterus reaches the xiphisternum. In the last month of pregnancy, the fundus of the uterus may drop several centimeters if the fetal head descends deep into the pelvis.

The position of the uterus changes during gestation. In early gestation an exaggerated anteflexion is common. As the uterus ascends into the abdomen, a slight dextrorotation develops. In early pregnancy the uterus changes from a flattened pear shape to a globular shape. The globular shape continues until approximately 20 to 24 weeks, when a definite ovoid shape develops and continues until delivery.

At approximately 6 to 8 weeks' gestation, the uterine isthmus becomes softened and easily compressible, and the cervix, on palpation, seems almost detached from the uterine fundus. At about 8 weeks' gestation, the entire uterus softens.

During pregnancy the uterus contracts intermittently. Painless contractions, called **Braxton-Hicks contractions**, begin in early pregnancy and are first noted by the client and the examiner at about 24 weeks' gestation. These contractions can be stimulated by palpation of the uterus. If a contraction occurs during the abdominal examination, the examiner should wait until the contraction ends to continue palpation and subsequently palpate more gently.

Three major changes occur in the cervix: (1) hypertrophy of the glands in the cervical canal, (2) softening of the cervix, and (3) bluish discoloration. These changes begin early in pregnancy—at about 6 weeks' gestation. Because of changes in the cervical epithelium, commonly a portion of the squamous epithelium is replaced by an outward extension of the columnar epithelium, producing an observable cervical ectropion or eversion of the cervical canal. This condition usually persists throughout pregnancy but disappears soon after the delivery.

The increase in pelvic vascularity causes a bluish discoloration of the cervix, vagina, and vulva at about 6 to 8 weeks' gestation. In addition, the vaginal mucosa thickens, the connective tissue becomes less dense, and the muscular areas hypertrophy. These changes are reflected in palpatory findings of softening and relaxation. The hypertrophied glands secrete more mucus. The total vaginal discharge is increased and more acidic than normal.

Breasts

Breast changes begin at about week 8 of pregnancy with enlargement of the breasts. Shortly afterward the nipples become larger and more erectile, the areolae become more darkly pigmented, and the sebaceous glands (Montgomery's tubercles) in the areolae hypertrophy. Sometimes an irregular secondary areola develops, extending from the primary areola. Hypertrophy of the breasts often causes a slight tenderness. In women with well-developed axillary breast tissue, the hypertrophy may produce symptomatic lumps in the axillae. Colostrum can be expressed from the breast at about week 24 of pregnancy. The colostrum appears clear and yellowish at first but becomes cloudy later.

Stretching of the skin on the breast may produce **striae gravidarum,** and increased vascular supply may visibly engorge superficial breast veins.

Abdomen

The muscles of the abdominal wall stretch to accommodate the growing uterus, and the umbilicus becomes flattened or protrudes. The rapid stretching of abdominal skin may cause the formation of striae gravidarum, which appear pink or red during pregnancy and become silvery white after delivery. In the third **trimester** of pregnancy, the rectus abdominis muscles are under considerable stress, and their tone is diminished. A wide permanent separation of these muscles, called **diastasis recti abdominis**, may occur. This condition allows the abdominal contents to protrude into the midline of the abdomen but requires no intervention.

In pregnancy, peristaltic activity is reduced, resulting in decreased bowel sounds. Smooth muscle relaxation, or **atony,** contributes to a variety of changes in gastrointestinal function. These changes include a high incidence of pregnancy-associated nausea and vomiting, heartburn, and constipation. In addition, the increased regional blood flow to the pelvis and venous pressure contribute to hemorrhoids, a source of discomfort in late pregnancy. Nausea and vomiting usually do not persist beyond the third month, but heartburn, constipation, and hemorrhoids are more characteristic and troublesome in late pregnancy.

Less frequently noted gastrointestinal symptoms include ptyalism, or excessive salivation, and pica, a craving for substances of little or no food value. Pica is often an expression of the folkways of some cultural groups. It becomes a concern when it interferes with good nutrition.

The enlarging uterus displaces the colon laterally, upwardly, and posteriorly. Since this displacement changes the anatomical situation of the appendix, signs of appendicitis during pregnancy are not localized in McBurney's point of the right lower quadrant.

Skin, Mucous Membrane, and Hair

The **melanocytes** in all portions of the skin are extremely active in pregnancy. There is a tendency toward generalized darkening of all skin, especially in skin that is hyperpigmented in the nonpregnant state. In some women a brownish-black pigmented streak may appear in the midline of the abdomen. This line of pigmentation is called the **linea nigra**. Some women develop a darkly pigmented configuration on the face that has been characteristically called the "mask of pregnancy," or **chloasma**. Scars and moles may also darken during pregnancy from the influence of melanocyte-stimulating hormone. Palmar erythema and spider nevi on the face and upper trunk also may accompany pregnancy.

Many pregnant women observe hypertrophy of the gums or **epulis,** resulting from hormonally induced, increased vascularity.

The hair of pregnant women may straighten and change in oiliness. Some women experience hair loss, especially in the frontal and parietal areas. Occasionally, increases in facial and abdominal hair, resulting from increased androgen and **corticotropic** hormone, are noted.

Cardiovascular System

Many changes, too numerous to discuss adequately here, occur in the maternal circulatory system during pregnancy. However, several major changes that alter the physical examination findings are summarized as follows.

Blood volume is increased up to 45% and cardiac output is increased up to 30% in pregnancy compared with the prepregnant state. Blood volume and cardiac output changes contribute to auscultatory changes that are common in pregnancy. Heart sounds are accentuated, and a low-grade systolic murmur (usually grade 2) is often noted.

As pregnancy advances, the heart is displaced upwardly and laterally. The apical impulse is displaced to a point 1 to 1.5 cm lateral to its location in the non-pregnant client. The pulse rate increases about 10 beats/min from the prepregnancy rate, and palpitations may be noticed during pregnancy. The blood pressure is unchanged or may decrease in the second trimester.

A progesterone-induced generalized relaxation of the smooth muscle, arteriolar dilation, and increased capacity of the vascular compartment occur. The systolic blood pressure remains the same or slightly lower during midpregnancy. There is no change in venous pressure in the upper body, but venous pressure increases in the lower extremities when the client is supine, sitting, or standing because of the pressure of the gravid uterus. This situation predisposes the woman to varicosities of the legs and the vulva and to edema.

Respiratory System

During pregnancy, tidal volume increases and respiratory rate increases slightly. Alveolar ventilation increases, and a more efficient exchange of lung gases occurs in the alveoli. Oxygen consumption rises by almost 20%, and plasma carbon dioxide content decreases.

As the uterus enlarges, it pushes the thoracic cage and the diaphragm upward and the thorax widens at the base. Physical assessment may reveal a change in respiration from abdominal to costal. In addition, dyspnea is a common complaint, especially in the last trimester, and deep respirations and sighing may be more frequent.

The tissue of the respiratory tract, sinuses, and nasopharynx manifests hyperemia and edema. This situation may contribute to engorgement of the turbinates, nasal stuffiness, and mouth breathing. Some women note increased nasal and sinus secretion and nosebleeds. Vocal cord edema may cause voice changes. Increased vascularity of the tympanic membranes and blockage of the eustachian tubes may contribute to decreased hearing, a sense of fullness in the ears, or earaches.

Musculoskeletal System

The pelvic joints exhibit slight relaxation in pregnancy as a result of some unknown mechanism. This relaxation is maximal from about the seventh month onward. Because the gravid uterus has caused the pregnant client's weight to be thrust forward, the muscles of the spine are used to achieve a temporary new balance. The pregnant client throws her shoulders back and straightens her head and neck. The lower vertebral column is hyperextended (Figure 23-1).

The musculoskeletal changes are often reflected in postural and gait changes, lower backache, and fatigue. Often the pregnant woman's gait is described as waddling, and her balance is less stable from about week 24 onward.

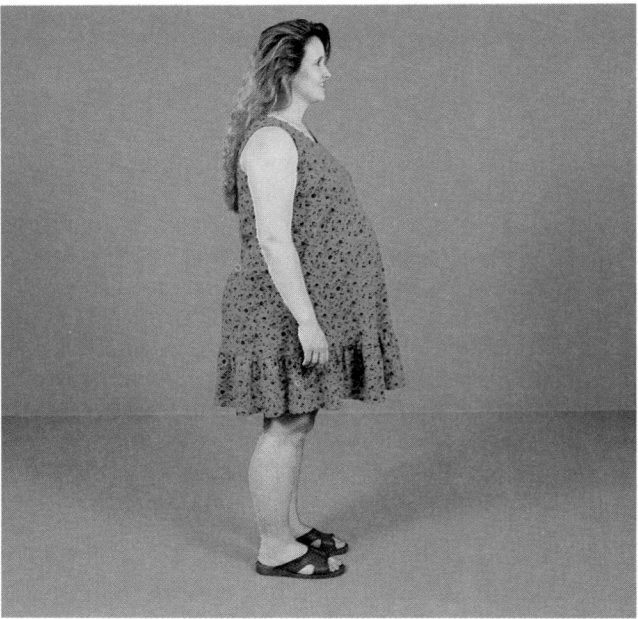

FIGURE 23-1 Posture of a pregnant woman.

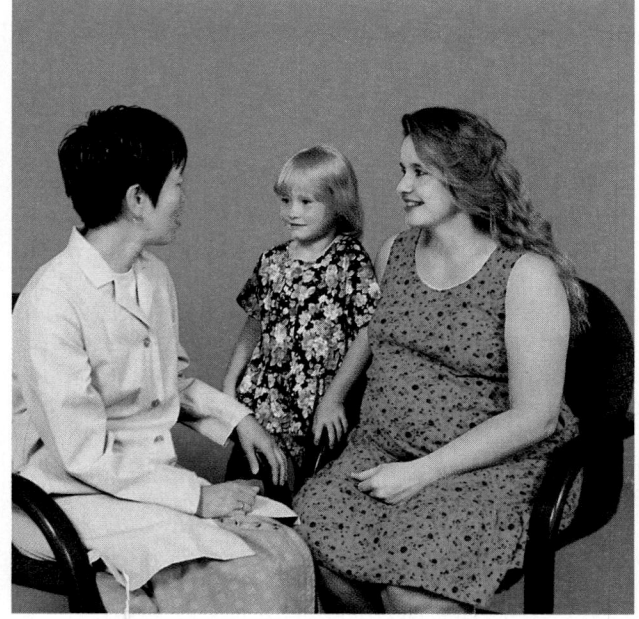

FIGURE 23-2 Interview with a pregnant woman and another family member.

EXAMINATION

Prenatal Health History

A complete health history is an essential component of the initial visit for prenatal care (Figure 23-2). The structure of the health history is the same as that described for the adult client, with special attention given to the reproductive system and to the physical, social, and emotional readiness of the woman to incorporate a new child in her life.

The health history is important in pregnancy because information derived from it assists the practitioner in differentiating the client who is essentially normal and who will be expected to deliver a full-term, healthy baby from the high-risk expectant mother whose pregnancy is likely to affect her own or her fetus's health negatively. High-risk clients are given special care in most health care systems. The early identification of risk factors and their effective management enable the prenatal care to achieve maximal benefit for the mother, family, and infant.

The health history for the obstetrical client follows the same basic protocol as that presented for all adults in Chapter 2. However, in prenatal care the following areas of history-taking should receive special and complete attention:

Biographical information
1. Age
2. Race and/or ethnic background
3. Marital status and support network
4. Educational status

Sexual history
1. Pattern of sexual activity
2. Satisfaction with sexuality and sexual activity
3. Partners—number and health
4. Contraception use

Past obstetrical history
1. Gravidity and parity
   a. A five-number code with the abbreviation G-T-P-A-L is often used to summarize gravity and parity information.
      First digit = Total number of pregnancies, including current one (if applicable) (G)
      Second digit = Number of full-term births (T)
      Third digit = Number of **preterm births** (i.e., those between 21 and 37 weeks' gestation) (P)
      Fourth digit = Number of abortions (i.e., those terminated at or before 20 weeks' gestation (A)
      Fifth digit = Number of living children (L)
      Thus, for example, the gravidity/parity 5-2-1-1-3 indicates that: the client is pregnant for the fifth time, she has three living children, two of whom were delivered after full-term gestation and one of whom was premature; and she has had one abortion.
      Alternate methods of indicating parity include two-digit, three-digit, and four-digit codes.

Two-digit codes: The first digit indicates gravidity, defined as the total number of pregnancies. The second digit represents parity, the number of live births (G-P). In the preceding example this code would be recorded as 5-3.

Three-digit codes: The first digit indicates gravidity, the second digit represents parity, and the third digit indicates abortions (G-P-A).

Four-digit codes: The first digit indicates gravidity, the second digit represents parity, the third indicates abortion, and the fourth represents the number of living children (G-P-A-L).

Note: The term **nullipara** describes a woman who has not given birth to a viable offspring.

b. The following information is obtained for every past pregnancy:
   1. Date of delivery
   2. Duration of gestation
   3. Significant problems or complications
   4. Manner in which labor started, specifically whether labor was spontaneous or induced. If labor was induced, the reason for induction is noted. Type of abortion: spontaneous (S), induced (I), or elective (E).
   5. Length of labor
   6. Complications of labor
   7. Presentation of infant at delivery
   8. Type of delivery—vaginal or cesarean; if cesarean, the reason is noted
   9. Type of anesthesia used at delivery
   10. Condition of infant(s) at birth and birth weight
   11. Postpartum problems, especially infection, hemorrhage, and thrombophlebitis
   12. Problems like jaundice, respiratory distress, infection, and **congenital** anomalies
   13. Type of infant feeding
   14. Current health of child

Present obstetrical history

1. Last normal menstrual period
   An important task during the prenatal history is to estimate the expected date of confinement (EDC). Because the exact date of conception is unknown for the majority of prenatal clients, the EDC is calculated according to the first day of the last normal menstrual period (LNMP). The EDC is determined by counting backward 3 calendar months from the LNMP and adding 7 days (Nägele's rule). The year, of course, may change. For example, if the LNMP were 10-15-84, the EDC would be 7-22-85. If the client has a history of irregular menses, the EDC can be more accurately estimated by physical examination than by using the LNMP. Critical features that aid in determination or validation of the EDC are the date of quickening (when the mother first notices fetal movement, usually at about 18 weeks), and the time at which the fetal heart tones can be auscultated (at 10 to 12 weeks for a Doppler instrument and at 16 to 20 weeks for a fetoscope). Because of the variation that characterizes these events, ultrasonic measurement of fetal size and growth is being used more frequently to date pregnancy and assess fetal growth, along with measurement of the progressive enlargement of the uterus.
2. Symptoms of pregnancy
3. Feelings about pregnancy, especially determination if pregnancy was planned or unplanned
4. Bleeding since LNMP
5. Date when fetal movements were first felt
6. Fetal exposure to infections, radiation, and drugs (including oral contraceptives and spermacides)

Current and past medical gynecological history

1. Urinary tract infections
2. Sexually transmitted diseases
3. Bacterial and viral infections
4. Diabetes
5. Hypertension
6. Heart disease
7. Endocrine disorders
8. Anemia
9. Genital tract history, especially:
   a. Anomaly
   b. Cervical incompetence
   c. Myomas
   d. Contracted pelvis
   e. Ovarian mass
   f. Vaginal infections
   g. Surgery
   h. Abnormal Pap test results
   i. Use of hormones (e.g., birth control pills)
   j. Menstrual history and functioning
   k. Endometriosis
10. Medication history—over the counter and prescribed drugs
11. Current or past habitual use of alcohol, tobacco, mood-altering drugs or other nonprescribed drugs

Family health history. Features of the family history that have special significance in pregnancy include diabetes, renal or hematological disorders, hypertension, multiple pregnancy, and congenital defects and retardation. It is important to learn if the primigravida's mother had preeclampsia or high blood pressure during pregnancies, especially if she convulsed.

PRENATAL RISK FACTORS

The following factors have been associated with increased morbidity and mortality of mothers and infants. The examiner should take special note of these factors during the health history interview and its recording.

Habits

Smoking
Alcohol consumption
Drug addiction
Violent life-style

Maternal characteristics

Age: younger than 18 or older than 40
Poverty
Single status
Family disorganization
Conflict about pregnancy
Height less than 5 ft
Weight less than 100 lbs
Inadequate diet
Low educational level

Reproductive history

More than one previous abortion
Perinatal death
Infant weighing less than 2500 g
Infant weighing more than 4000 g
Infant with isoimmunization or ABO incompatibility
Infant with major congenital or perinatal disease
Uterine anomaly
Myomas
Ovarian masses
Sexually transmitted diseases

Medical problems

Hypertension
Renal disease
Diabetes mellitus
Heart disease
Sickle cell disease
Anemia
Pulmonary disease
Endocrine disorder

Present pregnancy

Bleeding
Premature rupture of membranes
Anemia
No prenatal care
Preeclampsia or eclampsia
Hydramnios
Multiple pregnancy
Breech, transverse, or abnormal fetal position
Low or excessive weight gain
Hypertension (blood pressure greater than 140/90, a 30 mm Hg systolic increase, or a 15 mm Hg diastolic increase from baseline readings)
Abnormal fasting blood sugar
Rh-negative sensitized
Exposure to teratogens
Viral infections
Sexually transmitted diseases
Bacterial infections
Protozoal infections
Postmaturity

A scoring system is useful in estimating the level or extent of risk for maternal or fetal illness or prematurity. Table 23-1 presents a tool for quantifying the risk of a prenatal client by using data collected through the history. Local populations may require adaptation of the content, the scoring mechanism, or the weighting of factors on this tool or any other tool selected. However, such a summarization of risk factors is usually helpful in the care of both individuals and a total clinic population.

Emotional, psychological, and developmental status. Pregnancy is an important developmental event in a woman's life. The developmental tasks of pregnancy are incorporation of the fetus and differentiation and, eventually, separation from the fetus. These tasks roughly coincide with the three trimesters of pregnancy.

During the first trimester, the gravida is involved with the process of accepting the fetus as a fact and a part of her body. Most women initially experience some ambivalence about their pregnancy and a resultant increase in anxiety. Many body changes occur that cause increased somatic awareness and inward focus. Relationships with key persons, especially the child's father and the gravida's mother, become especially important. Unresolved feelings and conflicts undergo reexamination. Feelings of dependency and vulnerability occur and can be additional causes of anxiety.

In the second trimester, the fetus develops a separate identity. The gravida has had some time to become accustomed to her body changes and often feels better physically because the nausea has ceased. The fetus's movements are an important event, confirming the presence of the fetus and reminding the woman of the independence of the fetal movements from her control. The woman begins to think about the infant and their future. Worries about the possibility of producing an abnormal infant are common.

In the last trimester of pregnancy, the gravida prepares for her separation from the fetus and her entrance into a new relationship with the newborn. This time is occupied with preparatory activities, such as attending parents' classes and buying clothing and equipment for the newborn. Concerns about labor and delivery and the physical discomforts of late pregnancy contribute to the woman's readiness for separation from the fetus and her movement toward the tasks of parenthood.

Social, economic, and cultural status. Because pregnancy and birth are important events in the de-velopment of any family and because the quality of the family affects the infant's health, the interviewer must assess the circumstances relating to the pregnancy and the family environment. The following are several important areas of exploration in the social history.

1. Client's desire for and feelings about this pregnancy
2. Feelings of significant others regarding this pregnancy
3. Client's personal and culturally derived health beliefs about pregnancy
4. Client's knowledge regarding pregnancy and parenting
5. Amount of support and assistance provided by family and significant others (including father of child and siblings)
6. Economic burdens imposed on client or family by pregnancy
7. Condition of the family's physical and emotional environment
8. Presence of physical abuse

TABLE 23-1

Rating Scale of Prenatal Risk Factors

	Factors			
Score	**Socioeconomic**	**Past history**	**Habits**	**Current pregnancy**
1	Two children at home	First trimester abortion × 1 <1 year since last birth	Work outside home	Unusual fatigue
2	<20 years >40 years Single parent	First trimester abortion × 2	>10 cigarettes/day >6 cups coffee/day	<12 lbs weight by 32 weeks Albuminuria Hypertension Bacteriuria
3	Low socioeconomic status Malnourished Less than 5 ft Less than 100 lb	First trimester abortion × 3	Unusual anxiety Heavy work Long, tiring trip Long commuting distance	Breech at 32 weeks Weight loss of 2 kg Head engaged before 34 weeks Febrile illness Leiomyomas
4	Less than 18 years	Pyelonephritis		Uterine bleeding after 12 weeks Effacement or dilation of cervix before 36 weeks Uterine irritability
5		Uterine anomaly Second trimester abortion DES exposure		Placenta previa Hydramnios
10		Premature delivery Repeated second trimester abortion		Twins Abdominal surgery

Modified from Zuspan FP, Quilligan EJ: *Practical manual of obstetric care,* St Louis, 1982, Mosby—Year Book.
Total score is computed by adding the scores for the total set of factors present for given client. 0 to 5 points, minimal risk; 6 to 9 points, moderate risk; >10 points, high risk.

PREPARATION

Preparation for Examination

Equipment

In addition to all the equipment needed for a comprehensive physical examination that includes a pelvic examination, the following items are needed for the prenatal examination.

Item	Purpose
Long measuring tape	To assess growth of uterus
Doppler instrument or fetoscope	To auscultate fetal heart tones

Client and environment

Provide a warm, private room.

Make sure that the patient is adequately gowned and draped throughout the examination.

Help the patient to assume various positions throughout the examination, as required by the assessment techniques.

Avoid allowing the client to lie on her back for extended periods because of the negative effects of the gravid uterus on the abdominal organs, the vessels, and the back. The most comfortable backlying position is with the head elevated to about 45 degrees (Figure 23-3) and the knees slightly bent.

General Physical Examination

A complete physical examination should be performed on the first prenatal visit because (1) the examination may reveal problems that need special or immediate attention, and (2) initial data provide the baseline against which changes that occur later in pregnancy can be compared. The initial general physical examination of the prenatal client is the same as for other clients, except for special emphasis on the diagnosis of pregnancy, the assessment of pelvic adequacy, and the assessment of fetal growth and well-being.

Several signs unrelated to the reproductive system may be normally altered in pregnancy. Such alterations of physical findings are listed in the box below.

Diagnosis of Pregnancy

The diagnosis of pregnancy takes into account both the history of subjective symptoms noticed by the client and the objective signs noted by the examiner. In addition, laboratory tests are especially helpful in confirming early pregnancy.

Traditionally, the signs and symptoms of pregnancy have been categorized as (1) presumptive symptoms, (2) probable signs, and (3) positive signs. Presumptive symptoms are those concerns that the prenatal client identifies in the present illness and chief complaint portions of the history and several additional general physical signs. They include the subjective data that may

---

PHYSICAL FINDINGS ALTERED IN PREGNANCY

Respiratory system

Change in breathing from abdominal to costal
Shortening and widening at the base of the thoracic cage
Elevation of the diaphragm
Increase in respiratory rate

Cardiovascular system

Displacement of the apical impulse laterally 1 to 1.5 cm
Grade 2 systolic murmur
Increase in pulse rate
Slight fall in blood pressure in the second trimester

Musculoskeletal system

Slight instability of pelvis
Alteration of standing posture and gait to compensate for gravid uterus

Abdominal region

Contour changes because of gravid uterus
Striae gravidarum
Decrease in muscle tone
Linea nigra
Reduced peristaltic activity

Skin and mucous membranes

Chloasma
Linea nigra
Hyperpigmentation of skin and bony prominences
Palmar erythema
Spider nevi on face and upper trunk
Striae gravidarum on breasts and abdomen
Gum hypertrophy

Breasts

Enlargement
Large, erect nipples
Darkening of areolar pigment
Development of secondary areola
Hypertrophy of sebaceous glands in the areola
Formation of colostrum
Tenderness on palpation
Striae gravidarum
Engorgement of superficial veins

Other alterations

Straightening of hair
Loss of hair over frontal and parietal regions
Enlarged thyroid

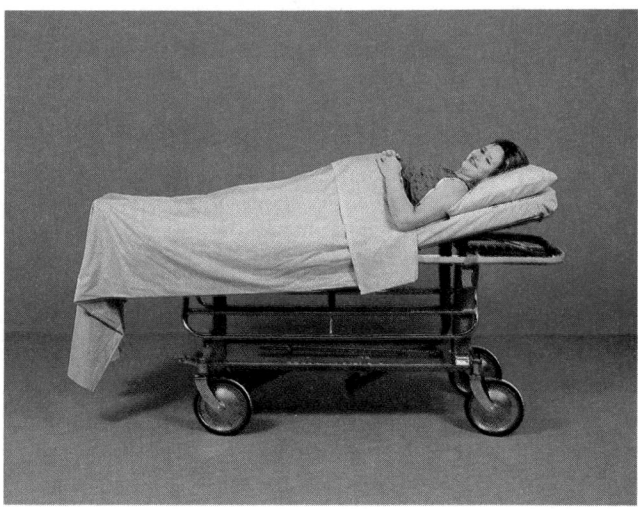

FIGURE 23-3 Elevation of head and shoulders for a prenatal examination.

LABORATORY SCREENING TESTS

In addition to the appropriate screening test for relevant risk factors, the following laboratory tests are characteristically included in the initial prenatal assessment:

Complete blood count
Blood type and Rh identification
General antibody screening test
VDRL (Veneral Disease Research Laboratory) test
Rubella titer
Clean-catch urinalysis for glucose, albumin, and ketones and a microscopic examination
Papanicolaou smear
Cervical smear for gonorrhea

The following additional tests are done as indicated for high-risk groups:

Cervical smear for *Chlamydia trachomatis*
Tine test for PPD (purified protein derivative) for tuberculosis
Antibody screening for *Toxoplasma gondii*, cytomegalovirus, herpes simplex virus, human immunodeficiency virus (HIV), and hepatitis B surface antigen
Hemoglobin electrophoresis for all black women

At 24 to 28 weeks' gestation, the following tests are often done:

Repeat hemoglobin and hematocrit
Repeat antibody screen
Serum glucose screen and a mini–glucose tolerance test that consists of a fasting reading and a 1-hour glucose determination after a 50 g load

At 32 to 36 weeks' gestation, the following tests are often repeated:

Hemoglobin and hematocrit
VDRL
Cervical smear for gonorrhea

have led the client to seek confirmation of pregnancy. *Presumptive symptoms* include (1) absence of menses 10 or more days after the expected date of onset, (2) **morning sickness**, nausea, or appetite change, (3) frequent urination, (4) soreness or a tingling sensation in the breasts, (5) Braxton Hicks contractions, (6) quickening, (7) abdominal enlargement, and (8) bluish discoloration of the vagina.

The following are *probable signs* of pregnancy: (1) progressive enlargement of the uterus, (2) softening of the uterine isthmus (Hegar's sign), (3) asymmetrical, soft enlargement of one uterine **cornu** (Piskacek's sign), (4) bluish or cyanotic color of the cervix and upper vagina (Chadwick's sign), (5) softening of the cervix (Goodell's sign), (6) internal **ballottement**, (7) palpation of fetal parts, and (8) positive test results for HCG in urine or serum. These signs are termed "probable" because clinical conditions other than pregnancy can cause any of them. However, if they occur together, a strong case can be made for pregnancy.

The *positive signs* of pregnancy are those that prove the presence of a fetus: (1) documentation of a fetal heartbeat by auscultation, electrocardiogram, or Doppler instrument, (2) palpation of active fetal movements, and (3) radiological or ultrasonographic demonstration of fetal parts. Ultrasonographic techniques can demonstrate the presence of a gestational sac as early as 6 weeks' gestation. Doppler instruments can detect a fetal heartbeat as early as 10 to 12 weeks' gestation.

Currently, clinical diagnosis of pregnancy is made by using laboratory tests in conjunction with the probable signs of pregnancy. Technology and marketing have made available reliable, low-cost home and in-clinic pregnancy tests that, in conjunction with clinical findings, can confirm the diagnosis of pregnancy early in the first trimester. The commonly used immunological pregnancy tests are the hemagglutination inhibition test and the latex agglutination test. These tests depend on an antigen-antibody reaction between HCG and an antiserum obtained from rabbits immunized against this antigen. These tests are available for use by both health professionals and laypersons and are very sensitive. Most commercial tests use standardized anti-HCG rabbit serum and dead cells or standardized latex particles coated with HCG. Anti-HCG serum is mixed first with a sample of the client's urine; then HCG-coated red blood cells or particles are added. The lack of agglutination is a positive test because urine that contains HCG has neutralized the HCG antibodies. If the urine sample contains no HCG, agglutination occurs, indicating a negative test for pregnancy.

Pregnancy tests based on the presence of HCG in the urine can be reliably performed from 2 days after the first missed menses through 16 weeks' gestation. During this time the production of HCG is at its peak. Currently, home pregnancy testing is widely available to women and is becoming a common method of self-assessment. Home pregnancy tests vary in accuracy and instructions. Although the techniques are relatively simple and straightforward, mistakes are possible, and a careful clinical assessment is always an important component of the diagnosis of pregnancy.

Several early clinical findings are used in conjunction with laboratory tests to diagnose pregnancy. In pregnancy, a pelvic examination done approximately 6 to 8 weeks after the last normal menses shows uterine enlargement. The uterus first enlarges in the pelvis. By 12 weeks' gestation, the examiner can palpate the uterus abdominally just above the symphysis pubis. In addition to enlarging, the uterus becomes globular and then ovoid.

The uterus softens during pregnancy because of its increased vascularity. The isthmus of the uterus is the first part to soften. At about 6 to 8 weeks' gestation, the softened isthmus produces a dramatic palpatory finding. On palpation, the enlarged globular uterus feels almost detached from the cervix, which is still not completely softened, because the isthmus feels so indistinct (Figure 23-4). This phenomenon is called Hegar's sign.

By 7 or 8 weeks' gestation, the cervix and the uterus can be easily flexed at their junction (McDonald's sign). Speculum examination shows cyanosis of the cervix as early as 6 to 8 weeks' gestation, a change that results from the increased vascularity in the area.

Often uterine enlargement does not progress symmetrically. Rather, the area of placental development enlarges more rapidly. This imbalance produces a palpatory asymmetrical enlargement of one uterine cornu, called Piskacek's sign (Figure 23-5).

The timetable for physical signs of pregnancy is presented in Table 23-2. This table also includes an outline of fetal development during pregnancy.

Technique for Examination and Normal Findings

Prenatal assessments include examination of both the mother and the developing fetus. After the initial assessment, examinations of the prenatal client are done at regular intervals. Reexamination schedules vary among clients. However, a common schedule includes examinations done approximately every 3 to 4 weeks during the first 28 weeks of pregnancy, then every 2 to 3 weeks until 36 weeks, and weekly thereafter.

At each prenatal revisit, the examiner usually assesses the following:

1. Interval history
2. Weight gain
3. Blood pressure
4. Urine for glucose, albumin, and ketones
5. Legs for edema
6. Abdomen
   a. Determination of uterine growth
   b. Determination of fetal presentation and position (beginning at 28 weeks and continuing to full term)
   c. Measurement of fetal heart rate

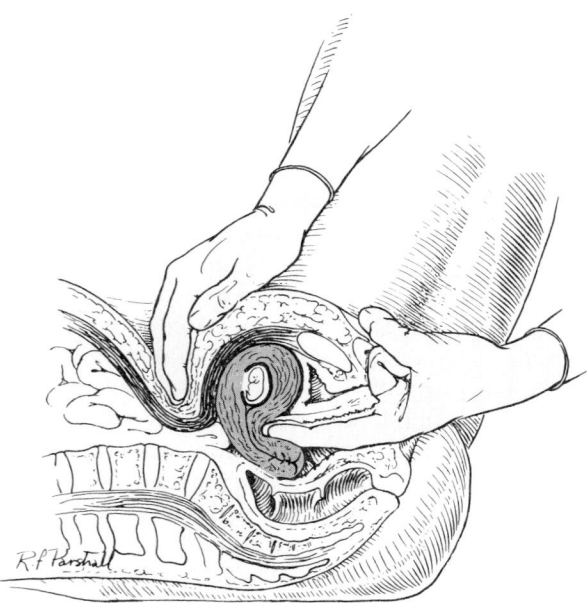

FIGURE 23-4 Hegar's sign, softening of the lower uterine segment.

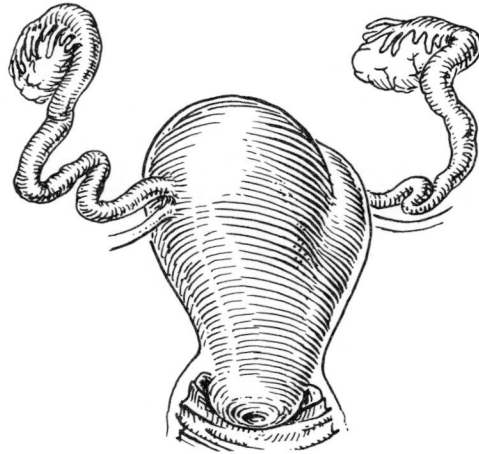

FIGURE 23-5 Piskacek's sign, asymmetric enlargement of the uterine fundus.

TABLE 23-2

Physical Signs of Pregnancy and Corresponding Stage of Fetal Development

Sign	Approximate gestation (weeks since last menses)		Fetal development
Amenorrhea.	2	0-4	Fertilization occurs. Blastocyst implants. Placental circulation established. Organogenesis initiated. Development of nervous system and vital organs initiated. Anatomical structures and systems are in rudimentary form. Size: 0.25 in by fourth week.
Softening of cervix (Goodell's sign).	4-6		
Softening of cervicouterine junction (Ladin's sign).	5-6	5-8	All major organs in rudimentary form.
Gestational sac may be noted by ultrasonography.	6		Fingers are present.
Compressibility of the lower uterine segment (Hegar's sign).	6-8		Ears and eyes are formed. Heart complete and functioning.
Dilation of breast veins.			Development of muscles is initiated.
Pulsation of uterine arteries in lateral fornices (Oslander's sign).			Size: 1.25 in by eighth week.
Flexing of fundus of cervix (McDonald's sign).	7-8		
Asymmetrical softening and enlarging of uterus (Piskacek's sign).			
Uterus changes from pear to globular shape.			
Bluish coloration of vagina and cervix (Chadwick's sign).	8-12	9-12	Organs forming and growing. Swallowing and sucking reflexes present.
Detection of fetal heartbeat with a Doppler instrument.	10-12		Body movements increase. Size: 3 in, 0.5 oz by 12th week.
Uterus palpable just above symphysis pubis.	12	13-16	Circulatory system is established.
Ballottement of fetus possible by abdominal and vaginal examination.	16		Size: 6 in, 4 oz by 16th week.
Uterus palpable halfway between symphysis and umbilicus.			
Fetal movements noted by mother (quickening).	16-20	17-20	Rapid growth.
Pigment change may occur.			Size: 8 in, 8 ounces by 20th week.
Uterine fundus at lower border of umbilicus.	20	21-24	Meconium present in intestines.
Fetal heartbeat auscultated with fetoscope.			Size: 11 in, 1-1.5 lbs by 24th week.
Fetus palpable.	24		
Mother begins to notice Braxton Hicks contractions.	24-26	25-28	Nervous system can control breathing and temperature.
Uterus changes from globular to ovoid shape.			Size: 12 in, 2-3 lbs by 28th week.
Fetus easily palpable, very mobile, and may be found in any lie, presentation, or position.	28	29-32	Fat deposits under skin. Size: 13 in, 3-5 lbs by 32nd week.
Uterus is approximately half the distance from the umbilicus to the xiphoid.			
Fetus usually lies longitudinally with a vertex presentation.	32	33-36	Primitive reflexes are present. Size: 14 in, 5-6 lbs by 36th week.
Uterine fundus is approximately two thirds the distance between the umbilicus and the xiphoid.			
Uterine fundus is just below the xiphoid.	34		
Vertex presentation may engage in the pelvis.	36-40	37-40	Less active because of crowding. Size: 19-21 in, 6-8 lbs by 40th week.

Interval history. At each visit, it is important to ask the client about new symptoms and signs and to update information about any health problems or issues noted in the initial history. Sometimes flow sheets with common signs and symptoms are used to facilitate documentation. Commonly reviewed areas include presence and character of fetal movements, vaginal discharge or bleeding, cramps, pelvic pressure, and signs and symptoms of urinary tract infection.

Weight gain. At term, the infant, uterine contents, and other changes in the body account for approximately 20 pounds of weight. Optimal weight gain during pregnancy, based on the lowest rate of complications and optimal birth weight of infants, is 24 to 27.5 lb (a wider range is 20 to 30 lbs). High prepregnancy weight correlates significantly with an increased risk of preeclampsia. Women with a low prepregnancy weight who gain little weight during pregnancy are more likely to have low-birth-weight infants (i.e., infants weighing 2500 g or less). Sudden weight gain, especially in the third trimester, usually indicates fluid retention, and this change should be evaluated in conjunction with maternal blood pressure. Apart from this transient cause of weight gain, many women tend to add to their body fat stores during pregnancy, and this weight gain may not be entirely lost after delivery. The gain in weight should occur gradually, averaging 1½ to 2 lbs per month during the first 24 weeks and ½ to 1 lbs a week during the remainder of pregnancy.

Blood pressure. Mean systolic blood pressure and mean diastolic blood pressure are essentially unchanged during pregnancy, except for a mild and transient decrease during the middle trimester in a normal pregnancy. Hypertension, however, contributes significantly to prenatal morbidity and mortality, and pregnancy-induced hypertension is a disease peculiar to pregnancy. This disorder typically develops after week 24 of pregnancy and is characterized by some combination of the following factors:

1. Systolic blood pressure of at least 140 mm Hg or a rise of 30 mm Hg or more above the usual level in two readings done 6 hours apart
2. Diastolic pressure of 90 mm Hg or more or a rise of 15 mm Hg above the usual level in two readings done 6 hours apart
3. Proteinuria
4. Edema of the face or hands
5. Excessive weight gain (≥2.5 lbs per week)
6. Hyperreflexia

Assessment of edema and extremities. Ankle swelling and edema of the lower extremities occur in two thirds of women during late pregnancy. Women notice this swelling late in the day after they have been standing for some time. Sodium and water retention caused by steroid hormones, an increased hydrophilic property of intracellular connective tissue, and increased venous pressure in the lower extremities during pregnancy contribute to this edema. Assessment includes palpation of the ankles and pretibial areas to determine the extent of the edema and observation for hand, face, or generalized edema. Generalized edema may be manifested by pitting in the sacral area or by the appearance of a depression on the gravid abdomen from the rim of the fetoscope after it has been pressed against the abdomen to auscultate the fetal heart rate.

In addition to assessment for edema formation, examination of the legs includes inspection for varicose veins and dorsiflexion of the foot with the legs extended to check for Homans' sign and thrombophlebitis. In the presence of an elevated or a borderline elevated blood pressure, deep tendon reflexes should be assessed. Hyperreflexia and clonus, combined with other signs, may indicate preeclampsia.

Leg cramps during pregnancy may accompany extension of the foot and sudden shortening of leg muscles. This cramping may be caused by an elevation of serum phosphorus with a diet that includes a large quantity of milk.

Many discomforts and sensations in the legs result from compression of nerves caused by the pressure of the enlarging uterus. These include numbness in the lateral femoral area, resulting from compression of that nerve beneath the inguinal ligament. Medial thigh sensation may result from the compression of the obturator nerve against the side walls of the pelvis. Periodic numbness of the fingers occurs in at least 5% of gravidas. This is apparently caused by a brachial plexus traction syndrome from drooping shoulders. Drooping is associated with the increased weight of the breasts as pregnancy advances. Finger movement may be impaired by compression of the median nerve in the arm and hand caused by physiological changes in the fascia, tendons, and connective tissue during pregnancy. This impairment, known as carpal tunnel syndrome, is characterized by a paroxysm of pain, numbness, tingling, or burning in the sides of the hands and fingers—particularly the thumb, second, and third fingers and the side of the fifth finger.

Abdominal examination. As pregnancy progresses, the uterus enlarges steadily. The height of the uterine fundus serves as a rough guide to fetal gestation and overall fetal growth. Figure 23-6 shows the expected fundal height at various gestational ages. At the week 12 of pregnancy, the fundus is palpable just above the symphysis. At 16 weeks, the fundus is approximately halfway between the symphysis and the umbilicus. At week 20, the fundus usually reaches the lower border of the umbilicus. After week 20, the uterus increases

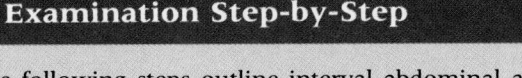

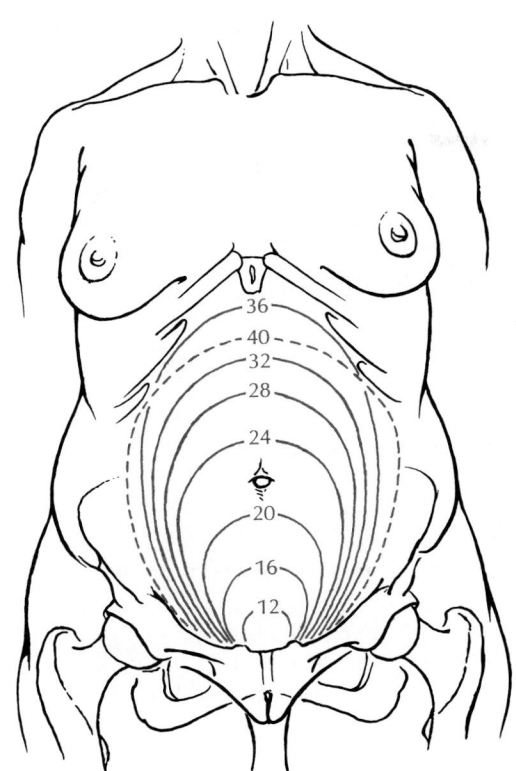

FIGURE 23-6 Approximate levels of the uterine fundus at various gestational points. Numbers indicate weeks of gestation.

in height at approximately 3.75 cm per month (or about 1 cm per week) until weeks 34 to 36, when the fundus almost reaches the xiphoid. Then, in approximately 65% of gravidas, the fetal head drops further into the pelvis with "lightening." If this occurs, the fundal measurement at 36 weeks may be greater than that noted later in pregnancy. These benchmarks are averages, and it should be noted that the length of the torso and the position of the umbilicus are highly variable among clients. In prenatal assessment, the client serves as her own control for assessment of adequate progress of fundal growth.

Unless the fetal head drops into the pelvis, the fundal height between weeks 37 and 40 will stay approximately the same. During this period the fetus is growing, but the amount of amniotic fluid decreases.

The abdominal examination consists of the following components:

1. Inspection
2. Measurement of fundal height
3. Assessment of fetal position
   a. Fundal palpation
   b. Lateral palpation
   c. Pawlik's palpation
   d. Deep pelvic palpation
4. Auscultation of fetal heartbeat

Examination Step-by-Step

The following steps outline interval abdominal assessment for the pregnant client:
Measurement of fundal height
Palpation of the abdomen to determine fetal position using Leopold's maneuvers:
  Fundal palpation
  Lateral palpation
  Pawlik palpation
  Deep pelvic palpation
Auscultation of fetal heart tones

Inspection. In addition to the observations that are made during assessment of the abdomen (e.g., skin and scars), for the pregnant client the examiner observes the size and configuration of the enlarging uterus.

Normally, the uterine size should relate to the estimated gestational age. Any discrepancy between observed size and estimated gestational age requires further exploration. A uterus larger than expected may indicate incorrect gestational age estimation, multiple pregnancy, or polyhydramnios. A smaller uterus may indicate a poorly growing fetus or gestational miscalculation.

Observation of the abdomen may provide the first clues to fetal presentation and position. An asymmetrical appearance or distention in width versus longitudinal enlargement may suggest a transverse or oblique fetal lie that palpation can verify. After approximately week 28, fetal movements may be seen.

Measurement of fundal height. Measurement of the height of the fundus provides a general assessment of the development of the pregnancy. Therefore such measurements should be taken at each prenatal visit. Before the fundal measurement is done, calculate the estimated gestational age based on the last normal menstrual period and use the estimate of age as a benchmark against which fundal growth is assessed. Between 20 and 31 weeks' gestation, the fundal height in centimeters is approximately equal to the gestational age in weeks. In general, a 1 cm increase per week is a normal pattern.

The procedure for measuring the fundal height is as follows:

1. Determine the top of the fundus (Figure 23-7).
   a. Stand at the right side of the supine client, facing her head.
   b. Place your hands on each lateral side of the uterus midway between the symphysis and the fundus.
   c. Move the uterus from side to side between your hands with gentle pressure.
   d. Palpate up the sides of the uterus to the fundus, being sure to stay on the sides of the uterus.

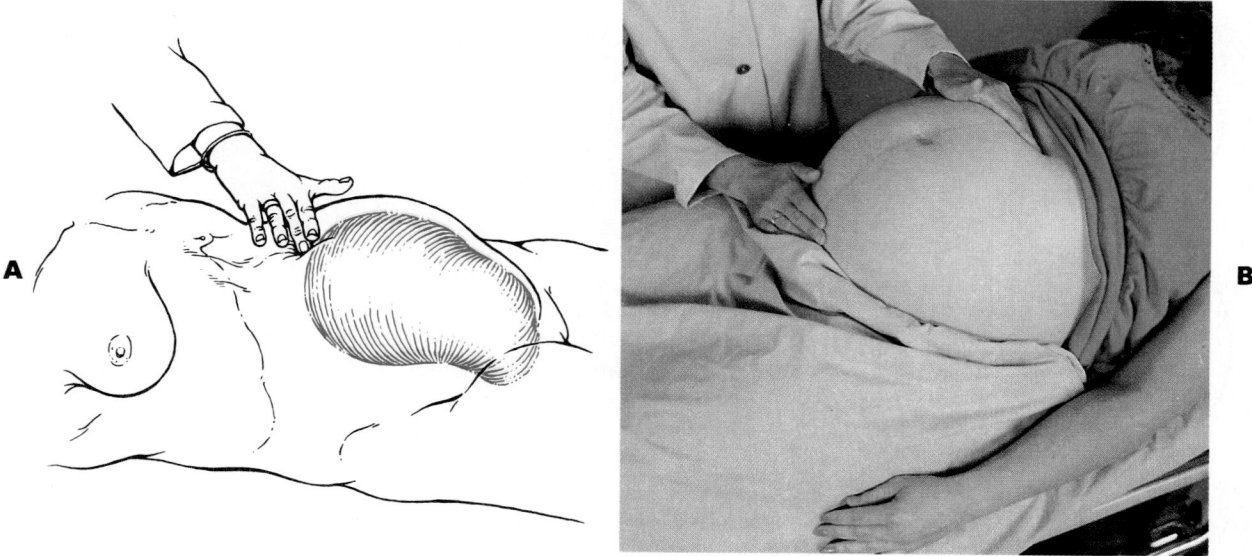

FIGURE 23-7 Palpation to determine height of the uterine fundus.

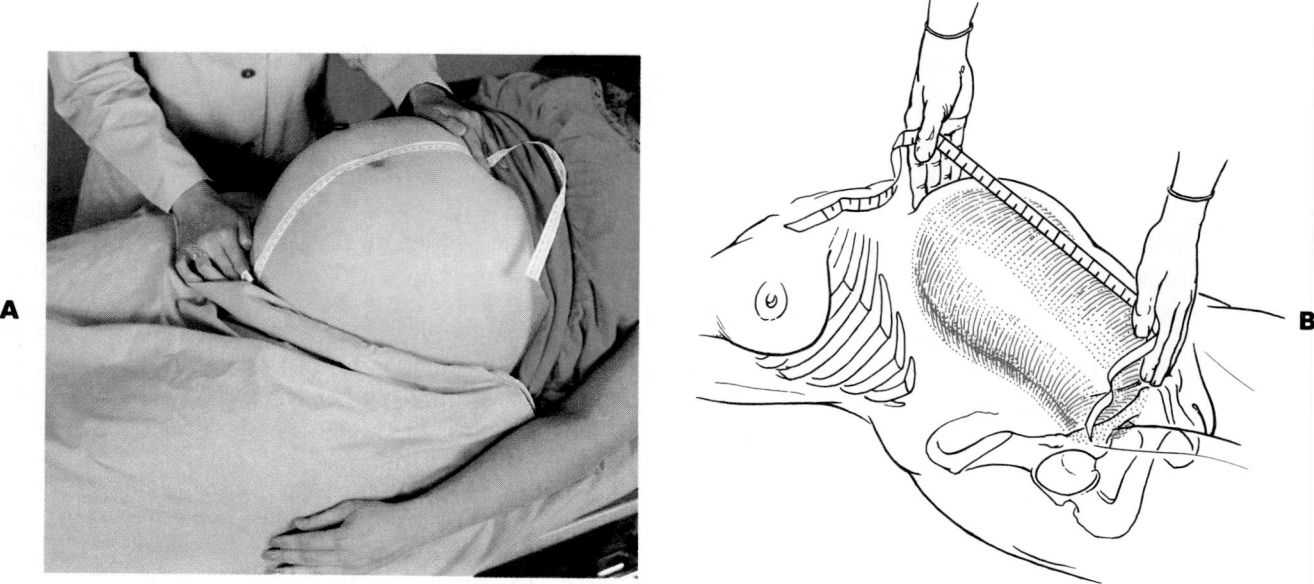

FIGURE 23-8 Measurement of fundal height.

e. As you come near the fundus, your hands will come together, meeting at the top of the fundus.

2. Measure the distance to the fundal edge from the upper border of the symphysis with a measuring tape. Place the zero point of the tape at the top of the symphysis and measure the distance to the top of the fundus (Figure 23-8).

3. When the fundus is below the umbilicus, record the measurement in centimeters above the symphysis (preferable) or below the umbilicus. When the measurement is above the umbilicus, record the measurement in centimeters above the symphysis.

The measurement of fundal height is approximate, and estimates of fundal height measurement may vary 1 to 2 cm among examiners. However, measurement, if done consistently by one examiner or a team of examiners within a clinical situation, should provide an excellent picture of fetal growth with each visit. If fundal height is <4 cm less than expected, additional assessments of menstrual history or fetal status are indicated.

Assessment of fetal position. Next, palpate the abdomen to determine fetal lie, presentation, position, attitude, and size.

The lie is the relationship of the long axis of the fetus to the long axis of the uterus. The lie can be longitudinal, oblique, or transverse (Figure 23-9).

The presentation of the fetus is that fetal part that is most dependent. The presentation can be vertex, brow, face, shoulder, or breech (Figure 23-10).

The position is the relationship of a specified part of the fetal presentation, the denominator, to a particular part of the maternal pelvis (Figure 23-11). The denominator in a vertex presentation is the occiput (O); in a breech presentation, it is the sacrum (S); in a face presentation, it is the mentum (M), or chin; in a brow presentation, it is the frontum (F); and in a transverse lie presentation, it is the scapula (S). The position is standardly abbreviated according to the left or right of the pelvis, the denominator, and the pelvic portion as follows:

Side of pelvis	Denominator	Pelvic portion
L = Left	O = Occiput	A = Anterior
R = Right	S = Sacrum	P = Posterior
	M = Mentum	T = Transverse
	F = Frontum	
	S = Scapula	

For example, if the occiput were presenting closest to the left anterior portion of the pelvis, the fetal position would be LOA.

The fetal attitude is the relationship of the fetal head and limbs to its body (Figure 23-12). The fetus may be fully flexed, poorly flexed, or extended. When the fetus is fully flexed, the spine is flexed, the head is flexed on the chest, and the arms and legs are crossed over the chest and abdomen.

Engagement occurs when both the biparietal and suboccipitobregmatic diameters of the fetal head pass into the inlet of the pelvis (Figure 23-13). When this occurs, the fetal head can be felt at the level of the ischial spines on vaginal palpation.

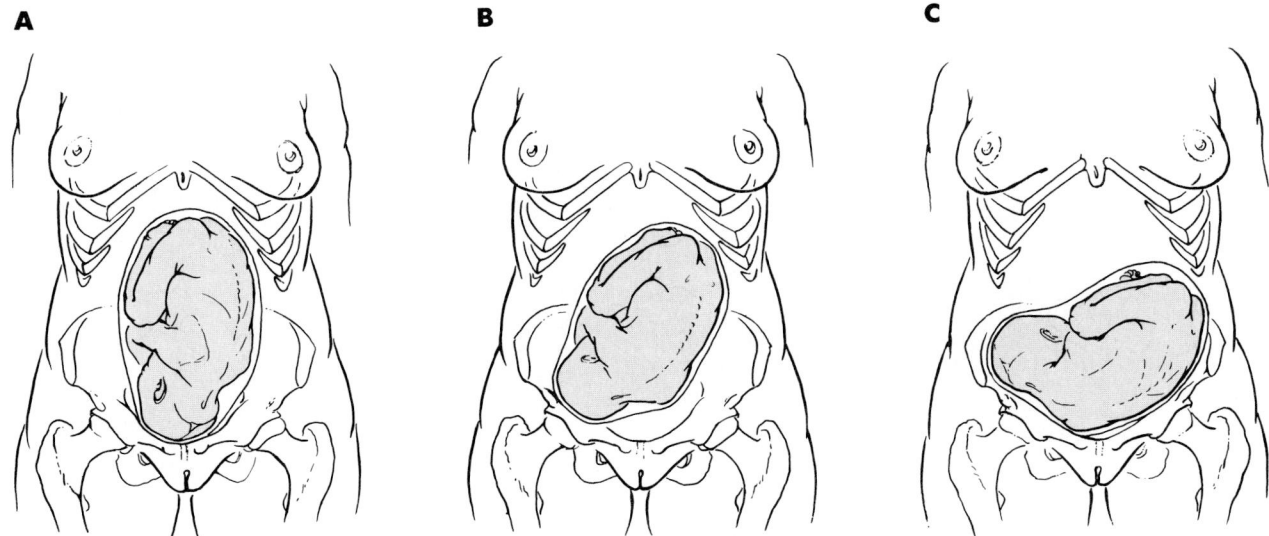

A **B** **C**

FIGURE 23-9 Examples of fetal lie. **A,** Longitudinal lie. **B,** Oblique lie. **C,** Transverse lie.

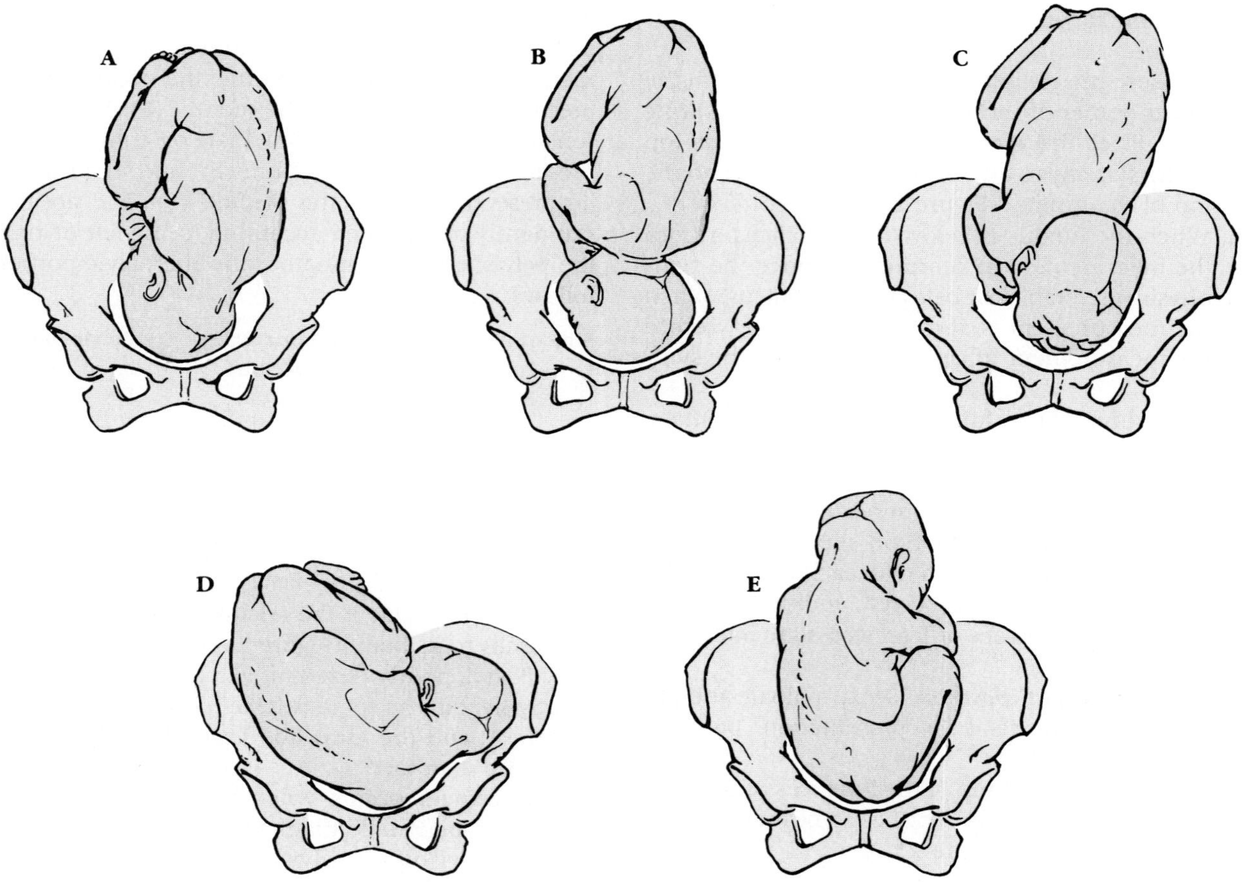

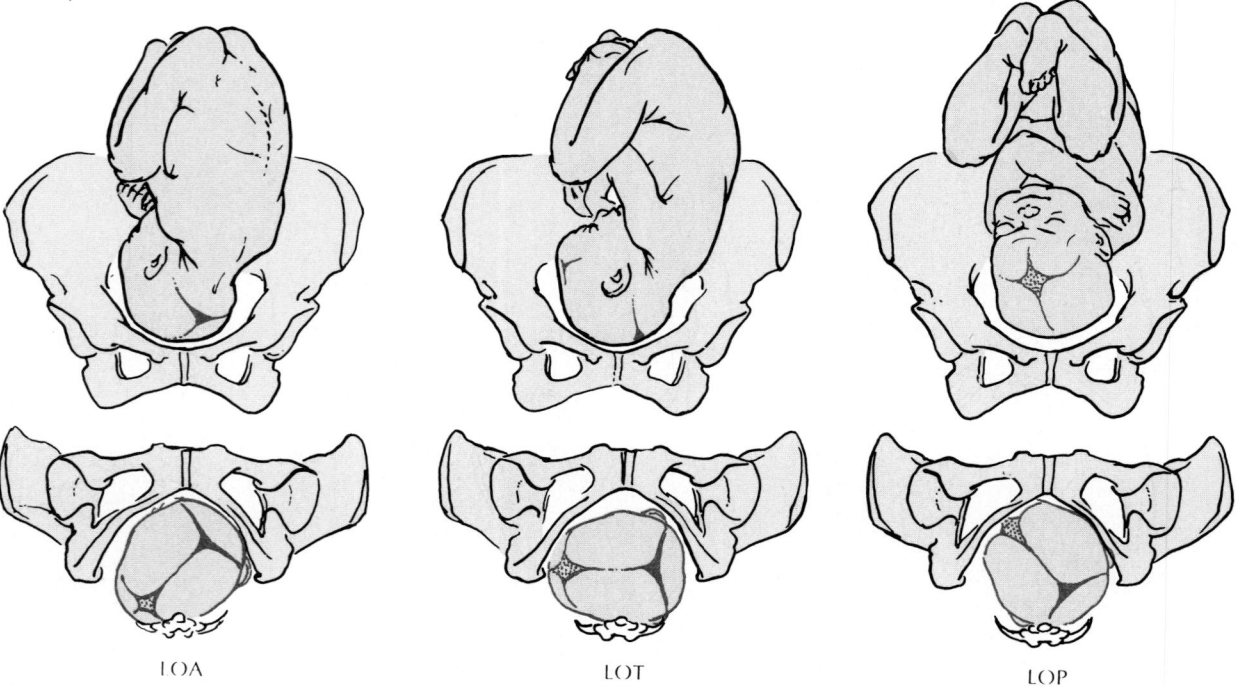

FIGURE 23-10 Examples of fetal presentation, **A,** Vertex. **B,** Brow. **C,** Face. **D,** Shoulder. **E,** Breech.

LOA   LOT   LOP

FIGURE 23-11 Examples of fetal position.

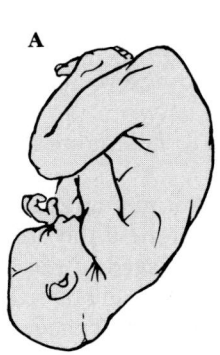 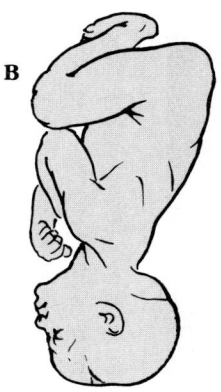 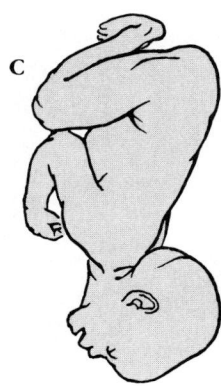

FIGURE 23-12 Fetal attitude. **A,** Fully flexed. **B,** Poorly flexed. **C,** Extended.

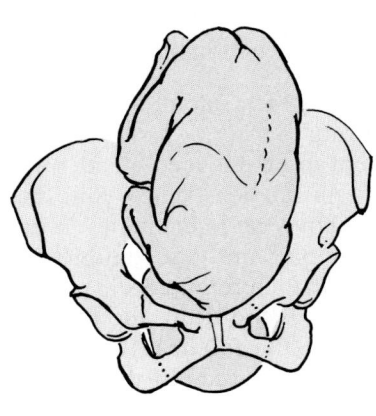 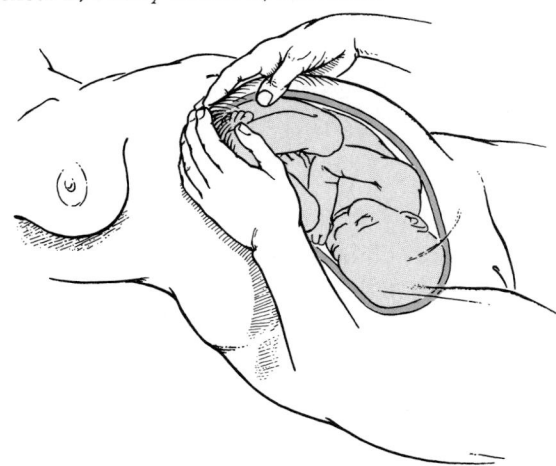

FIGURE 23-13 Engagement. Both the biparietal and suboccipitobregmatic diameters of the fetal head have passed into the inlet of the pelvis.

Abdominal palpation determines fetal lie, presentation, position, attitude, and size. Systematically palpate the abdomen using Leopold's maneuvers in the four sequential steps as follows:

1. Fundal palpation
2. Lateral palpation
3. Pawlik's palpation
4. Deep pelvic palpation

Leopold's maneuvers are usually not especially productive until 26 to 28 weeks' gestation, when the fetus is large enough for its parts to be differentiated through abdominal and uterine structures.

For this examination the client is supine. Elevating the client's head and shoulders and bending the knees may assist in decreasing tension of the abdominal muscles and in making the examination more comfortable for the client.

Helpful Hints in Doing Leopold's Maneuvers:

Use the palmar surface of the fingers for palpating.
Keep the fingers of the hand together.
Apply firm, smooth, steady pressure as necessary to determine needed information.
Avoid jabbing or poking movements.
If uterine contraction occurs, wait for it to pass and then palpate less strongly.
Have the client bend the knees to facilitate her comfort.
Review findings with the client and teach her to recognize the fetal parts.

FUNDAL PALPATION

1. Stand at the client's right side, facing her head.
2. Place the palmar surface of both hands on the uterine fundus to determine what part of the fetus is occupying the fundus (Figure 23-14).

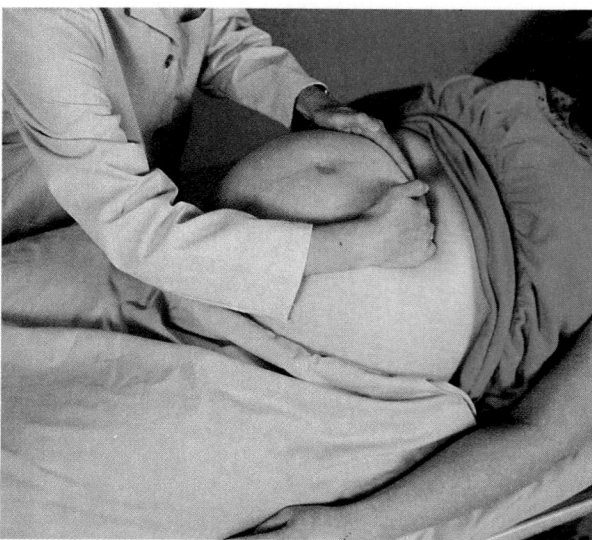

FIGURE 23-14 Palpation to determine the contents of the uterine fundus.

Usually the buttocks of the fetus are in the fundus; they are felt as a soft, irregular, and slightly movable mass. The lower limbs are felt adjacent to the buttocks. If the head is in the fundus, it is felt as smooth, round, hard, and ballottable. The groove of the neck is felt between the trunk and the upper limbs. The head is freely movable in contrast to the buttocks, which can move only sideways and with the trunk.

LATERAL PALPATION (FIGURE 23-15)
1. While you are still facing the client's head, move both of your hands to either side of the uterus to determine the side on which the fetal back is located.
2. Support the fetus with one hand on one side while the other hand palpates the fetus on the other side.
3. Then reverse the procedure to palpate each side of the uterus.

The fetal back is felt as a continuous, smooth, firm object, whereas the fetal limbs, or small parts, are felt as small, irregular, sometimes moving objects. On each side, palpate the flank to the midline, making special note of the edge of the fetal back as a landmark in determining the fetal position.

PAWLIK PALPATION
1. Perform this procedure with the right hand only to determine what fetal part lies over the pelvic inlet. Place the right hand over the symphysis so that the fingers are on the left side of the uterus and the thumb is on the right side (Figure 23-16). The hand should be approxi-

mately around the fetal presenting part, usually the head.
2. Palpate the presenting part gently to determine its form and consistency.
3. Grasp and gently move the presenting part sideways back and forth between the thumb and fingers several times to determine its movability.

This palpation is done to confirm impressions about the presenting part and to determine if the presenting part (usually the fetal head) is engaged. If the fetal head is movable above the symphysis, it is not engaged. If the head is not movable, it may be engaged. The only method of confirming engagement is pelvic examination to determine if the biparietal diameter of the fetal head is level with the ischial spines.

DEEP PELVIC PALPATION
1. Change position (Figure 23-17). Remain on client's right side but turn and face her feet.
2. Place a hand on each side of the uterus near the pelvic brim.
3. Ask the client to take a deep breath and to exhale slowly. As she does, allow your fingers to sink deeply above the pubic bones to palpate the presenting part and to determine the location of the cephalic prominence.

If the presenting part is the head, the location of the cephalic prominence (the forehead) helps determine the fetus's position and attitude. If the head is flexed, the occiput lies deeper in the pelvis, is flatter, and is less defined than the forehead, which is more prominent and on the same side as the small parts. If the head is not well flexed, the cephalic and occipital prominences are palpated at the same level, and the occipital portion, on the same side as the back, may be more prominent.

Throughout these maneuvers, assess the congruence of the size of the fetus with the gestational age.

Following is a series of questions that you, as the examiner, should mentally ask about each client during abdominal assessment and an indication of the procedures that assist in answering the questions.

Question	Source of evidence to answer question
What is the fetal lie?	Abdominal inspection Lateral abdominal palpation
What is the fetal presentation?	Fundal palpation Pawlik's palpation Deep pelvic palpation
What is the fetal position?	Lateral palpation Deep pelvic palpation
What is the fetal attitude?	Deep pelvic palpation
Is the fetal growth congruent with gestational age?	Fundal height measurement All Leopold's maneuvers

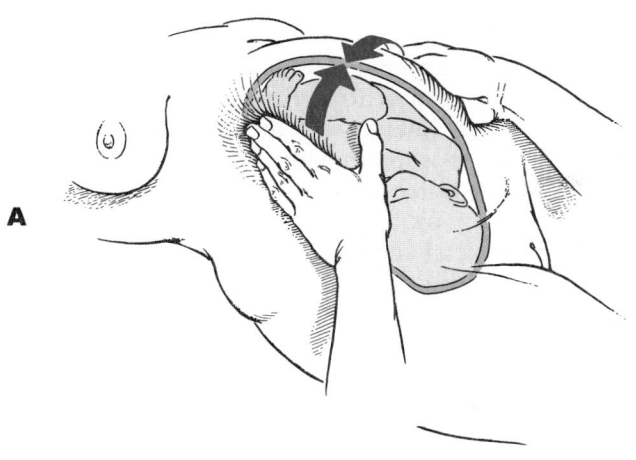
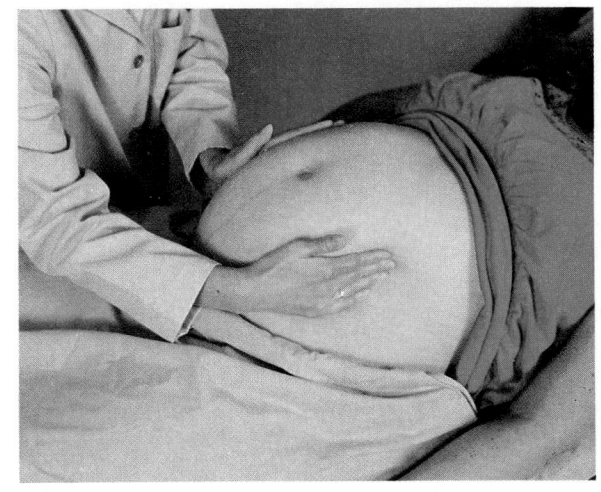

FIGURE 23-15 Palpation of lateral uterine fundus to determine the position of the back and extremities of the fetus.

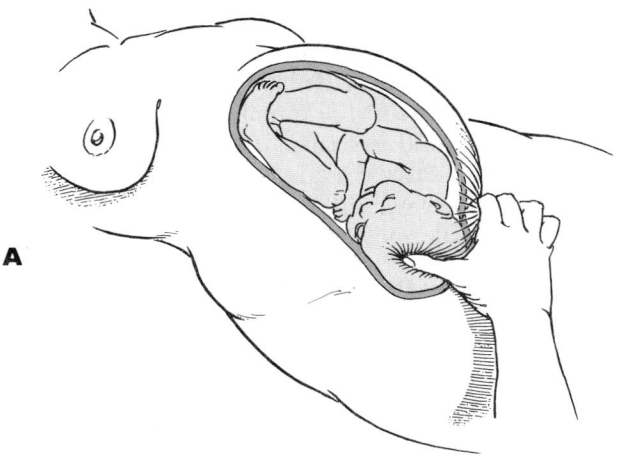
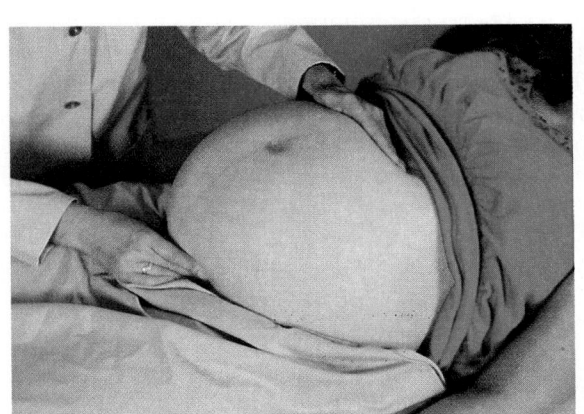

FIGURE 23-16 Pawlik's palpation to determine fetal presenting part.

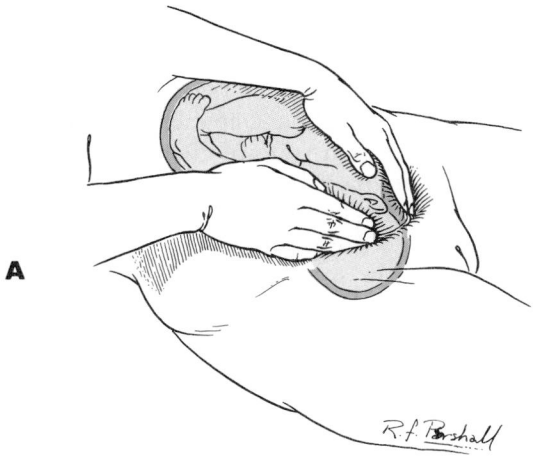
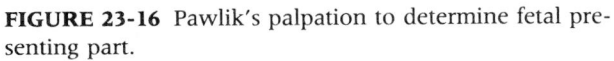
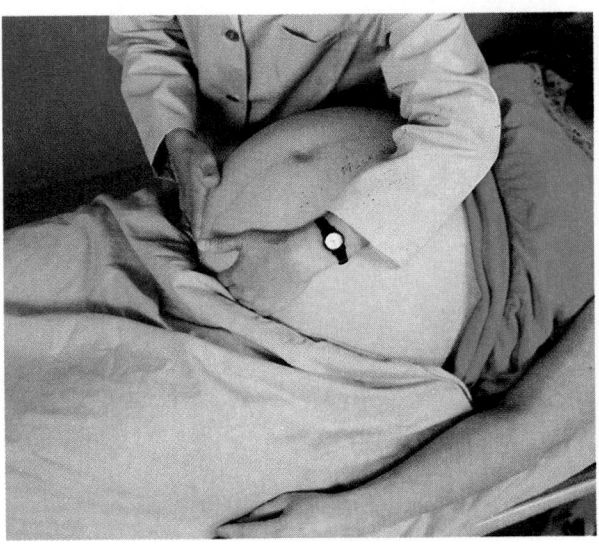

FIGURE 23-17 Deep pelvic palpation to determine fetal attitude and descent.

Auscultation. The fetal heart rate is an indicator of fetal health status and requires monitoring throughout pregnancy. Auscultate the fetal heart rate with a special stethoscope called a fetoscope or a Doppler instrument. The Doppler instrument can be used to monitor the fetal heart rate after about 10 to 12 weeks' gestation as the fundus rises beyond the symphysis pubis. If you do not hear fetal heartbeats by Doppler monitoring after 12 to 14 weeks, reevaluate the gestational age estimate or fetal status. With a fetoscope, the fetal heart rate can first be heard between 16 and 20 weeks' gestation.

The use of the fetoscope is demonstrated in Figure 23-18. The fetal heart rate is rapid and soft. The use of a fetoscope avoids noises produced by fingers on the stethoscope and takes advantage of the benefits of both air and bone conduction. The bell of an ordinary stethoscope can be used to auscultate fetal heart tones, but it is less effective than a fetoscope in transmitting fetal heartbeats, especially around 20 weeks.

The fetal heart rate is normally between 120 and 160 beats/min, and the heartbeats resemble the sound of a watch's ticking heard through a pillow. These sounds are best heard through the fetal back. When the fetus is large enough for its position to be determined, place the bell of the fetoscope or the Doppler head on the fetus's posterior thorax. When the fetus is less than 20 weeks' gestation, the heart rate is often best heard at the midline, just above the pubic hairline.

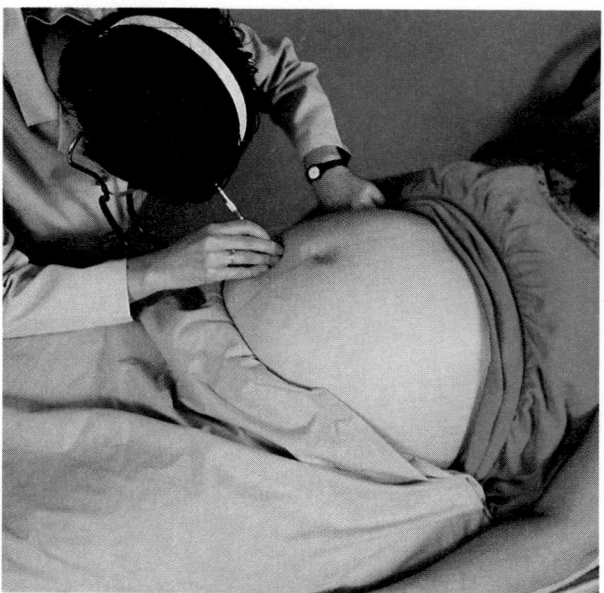

FIGURE 23-18 Use of the fetoscope to auscultate the fetal heart. Note: The hand on the bell of the fetoscope is used to adjust it. When the fetal heartbeats are actually being measured, the hand should be removed.

Count the fetal heart rate for at least 15 seconds, and record it in number of beats per minute according to location of maximal intensity (by the abdominal quadrant in which it is most prominent). The fetal heart rate is normally much faster than the maternal heart rate, and therefore it can usually be well differentiated from it. Moreover, the fetal and maternal heart rates are not synchronous. Differentiate the maternal rate by palpating the mother's pulse while auscultating the abdomen.

Sounds other than the maternal and fetal heart tones can be heard in the uterus. Blood rushing through the placenta is uterine souffle. The uterine souffle is a soft, blowing sound that is synchronous with the maternal pulse. The intensity of the souffle has been interpreted as an indicator of uterine blood flow and placental function. A loud uterine souffle has been associated with high levels of urinary estriol and a soft or absent souffle with lower estriol levels. Thus a soft or absent uterine souffle may indicate poor uterine blood flow and placental function, particularly in late pregnancy. Occasionally the blood flow in the umbilical artery can be auscultated. The sound is similar to a bruit and, as a rule, the rate is equal to the fetal heart tones. However, the sound does not have distinct heart sounds; rather it is similar to the uterine souffle.

Examination of Bony Pelvis

The purpose of the examination of the bony pelvis is to determine if the pelvic cavity is large enough to allow for passage of a full-term infant **(term infant).** Clinical pelvimetry is a gross estimate of the adequacy of the pelvis for delivery of a fetus. It is not uncommon for clients whose pelvises have been assessed to be of borderline adequacy to deliver full-term infants vaginally. If the clinical assessment in early pregnancy indicates a possible inadequacy, the pelvis needs to be reassessed clinically and possibly by x-ray in late pregnancy and in relationship to the size of the infant at term. This examination is performed on the initial prenatal evaluation; it need not be repeated if the pelvis is of adequate size. However, if findings indicate that the pelvis is of borderline adequacy or if you are unable to adequately perform the examination on the initial visit because of the client's tenseness and subsequent muscular contraction, repeat the examination at approximately 36 weeks' gestation. In the third trimester, the pelvic joints and ligaments relax, and the client is more accustomed to examination. Thus you can more thoroughly and accurately accomplish examination of the bony pelvis at that time.

The examination of the bony pelvis is done not so much to diagnose the type of pelvis but to determine its configuration and size. Because the examiner does not have direct access to the bony structures and because the bones are covered with variable amounts of soft tissue, estimates are approximate. X-ray examination can provide precise bony pelvis measurements. However, x-rays are not needed or indicated for the vast majority of prenatal clients.

The assessment of the bony pelvis must be put in the perspective of the capacity necessary to accommodate a full-term fetus. When the head of a full-term fetus is well flexed, the two largest presenting diameters are the biparietal and the suboccipitobregmatic, each measuring approximately 9.5 cm (Figure 23-19).

The pelvis consists of four bones: the two innominate bones, the sacrum, and the coccyx. Each innominate bone consists of three bones that fuse after puberty. These three bones are the ilium, the ischium, and the os pubis (Figure 23-20). The innominate bones form the anterior and lateral portions of the pelvis.

The sacrum and the coccyx comprise the posterior portion of the pelvis. The sacrum is composed of five fused vertebrae. Its upper anterior portion is called the sacral promontory, which forms the posterior margin of the pelvic brim. The coccyx is composed of three to five fused vertebrae and articulates with the sacrum.

The pelvis is divided by the brim into two parts: the false pelvis and the true pelvis. The false pelvis is that part above the brim and is of no obstetrical interest.

The brim and the area below it constitute the true pelvis. The true pelvis is divided into three parts: inlet or brim, midpelvis or cavity, and outlet. The inlet is formed anteriorly by the upper margins of the pubic bones, laterally by the iliopectineal lines, and posteriorly by the anterior upper margin of the sacrum, the sacral promontory. The cavity is formed anteriorly by the posterior aspect of the symphysis pubis, laterally by the inner surfaces of the ischial and iliac bones, and posteriorly by the anterior surface of the sacrum. The outlet, which is diamond-shaped, is formed anteriorly by the inferior rami of the pubic and ischial bones, laterally by the ischial tuberosities, and posteriorly by the inferior edge of the sacrum (if the coccyx is movable).

Each of the pelvic portions can be imagined as a series of planes: the plane of the brim (or pelvic inlet), the planes of the midpelvis, and the plane of the outlet. These planes are illustrated in Figure 23-21.

The plane of the inlet in an average female pelvis measures approximately 11 to 13 cm in the anteroposterior diameter and 13 to 14 cm in the transverse diameter. The anteroposterior diameter of the inlet, measured from the middle of the sacral promontory to the superior posterior margin of the symphysis pubis, is called the true conjugate and is an important obstetrical measurement. However, only radiographic methods can be used to directly assess this measurement. The true conjugate can be estimated by measuring the diagonal conjugate, which is the distance between the inferior border of the symphysis pubis and the sacral promontory. The diagonal conjugate is approximately 1 to 2 cm longer than the true conjugate, depending on the height and inclination of the symphysis. The clinical measurement of the diagonal conjugate, the most valuable single measurement of pelvic adequacy, is discussed later in this section.

The midpelvis contains the planes of greatest and least pelvic dimensions. The plane of least pelvic dimensions is bounded by the junction of the fourth and fifth sacral vertebrae, the symphysis, and the ischial spines. The average dimensions of this plane are 12 cm (anteroposterior diameter) and 10.5 cm (transverse diameter). The transverse diameter is the distance between the ischial spines.

The pelvic outlet is composed of two triangular planes, having a common base in the most inferior portion of the transverse diameter between the ischial tu-

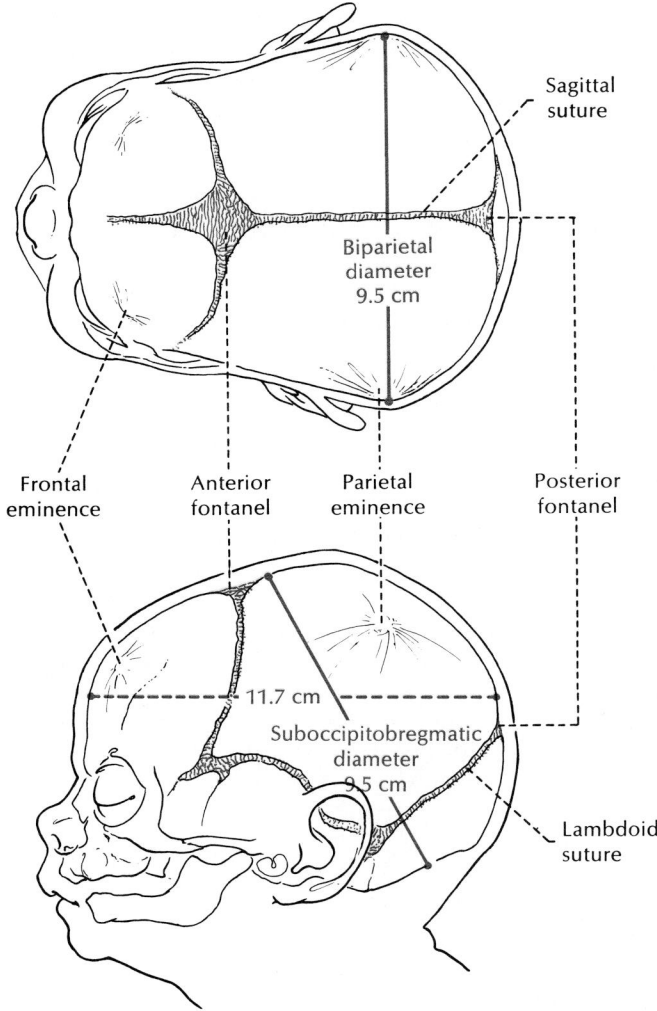

FIGURE 23-19 Various diameters of the fetal head at term.

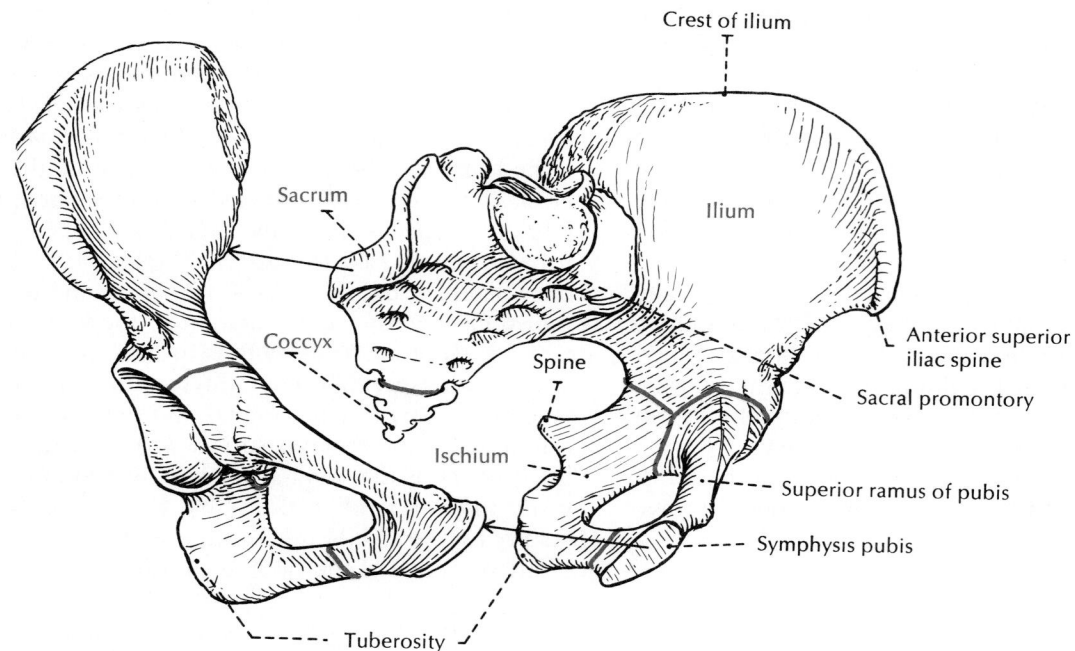

FIGURE 23-20 Bones of the pelvis.

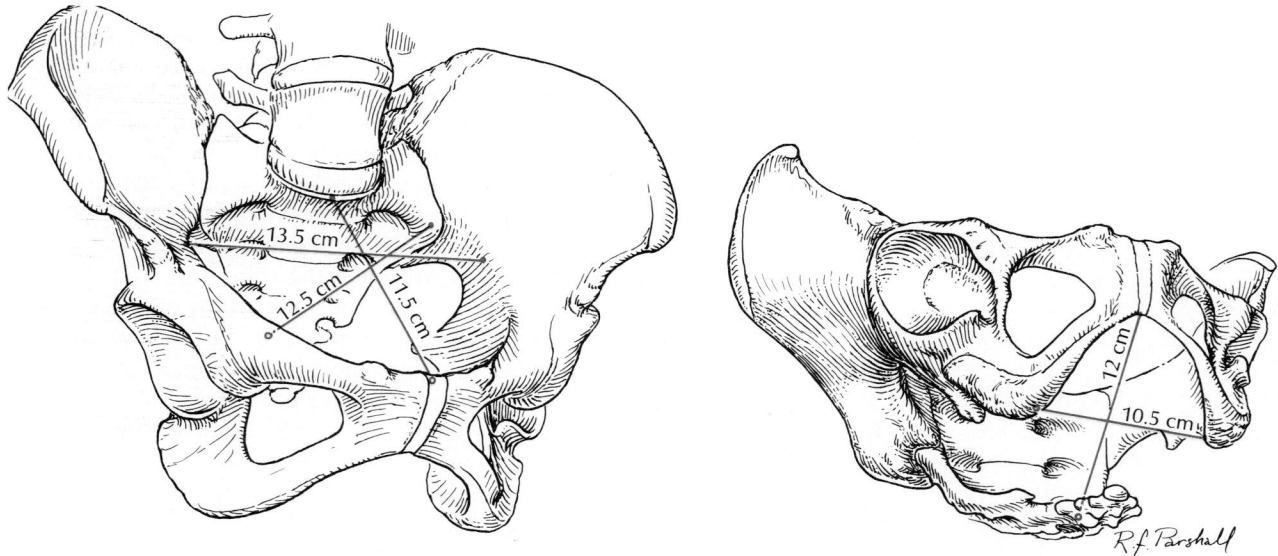

FIGURE 23-21 Planes of the pelvic inlet and midpelvis. (Measurements are averages within normal limits.)

berosities. The obstetrical anteroposterior diameter of the outlet is the distance between the inferior edge of the symphysis pubis and the edge of the sacrum (if the coccyx is movable). This measurement is usually 11.5 cm.

The transverse diameter of the outlet is the distance between the inner surfaces of the ischial tuberosities and usually measures approximately 11 cm (Figure 23-22).

Although there is a characteristic shape of the adult female pelvis that is different from the characteristically male pelvis, a female client may have any one of four types of human pelvises or a mixture of these types. In addition, the shape of the pelvis may have been distorted congenitally or by disease.

The four basic pelvic types, as originally classified by Caldwell and colleagues (1939) are: (1) gynecoid, (2) android, (3) anthropoid, and (4) platypelloid.

The typical female pelvis is the gynecoid pelvis, which is found in approximately 40% to 50% of adult women. This pelvis is characterized by a rounded inlet, except for a slight projection of the sacral promontory; a deep posterior half made possible by a wide sacrosciatic notch and concave sacrum; and a wide anterior half made possible by a wide, subpubic angle.

The android pelvis is found in approximately 15% to 20% of adult women. This pelvic type is roughly wedge- or heart-shaped, with the transverse diameter of the inlet approximately equal to the anteroposterior diameter but with the widest transverse diameter located closer to the sacrum. Other characteristics of the android pelvis include the following:

1. Narrow subpubic arch
2. Convergent side walls
3. Large encroaching spines
4. Short sacrosciatic notch and sacrospinous ligament
5. Short interspinous diameter
6. Straight sacrum
7. Short intertuberous diameter

The anthropoid pelvis has an elongated anteroposterior diameter and is found in approximately 25% to 35% of women. It is characterized by the following:

1. Narrow subpubic arch
2. Prominent ischial spines
3. Wide sacrosciatic notch and long sacrospinous ligaments
4. Deeply curved sacrum

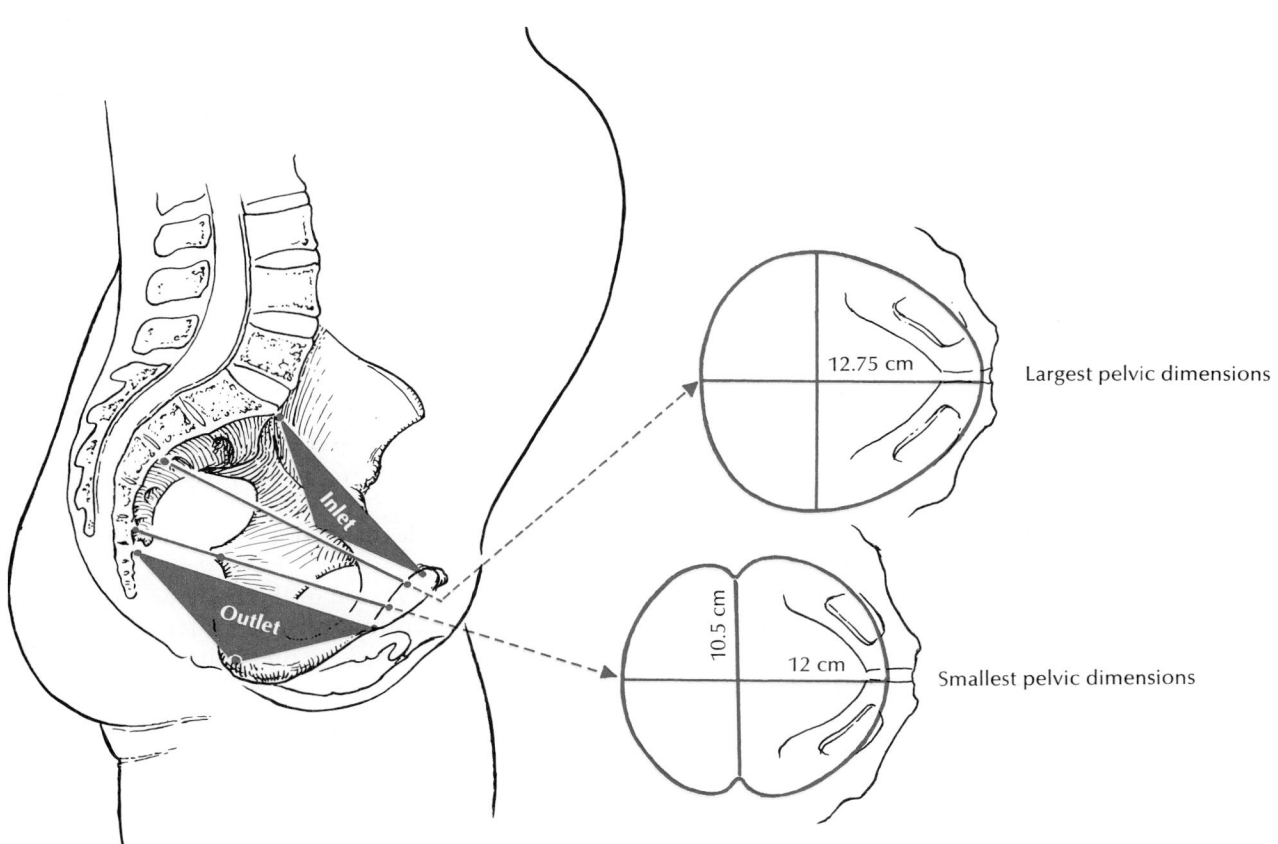

FIGURE 23-22 Pelvic outlet.

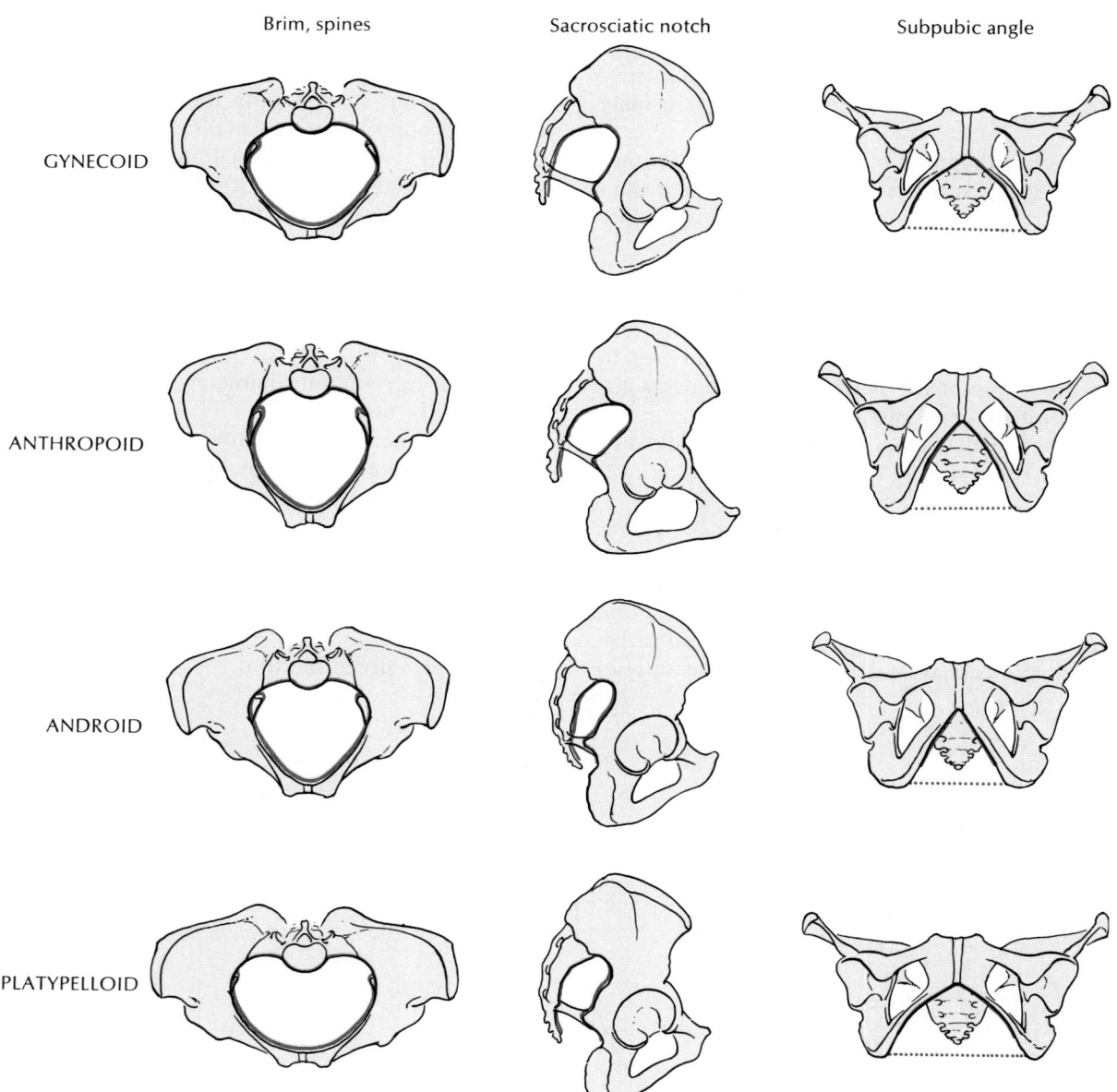

Brim, spines	Sacrosciatic notch	Subpubic angle

GYNECOID

ANTHROPOID

ANDROID

PLATYPELLOID

FIGURE 23-23 Comparisons of various portions of the four basic pelvic types.

The platypelloid pelvis has a flattened anteroposterior dimension with a relative widening of the transverse diameter. This pelvic type is seen in approximately 5% of women. The platypelloid pelvis is characterized by the following:

1. Wide subpubic arch
2. Flat ischial spines
3. Wide sacrosciatic notch and long sacrospinous ligaments
4. Straight sacrum

The various dimensions of the four basic pelvic types are compared and contrasted in Figure 23-23. Pure pelvic types are unusual; most pelves are mixtures of two pelvic types, with the characteristics of one type predominating.

Because examination of the bony pelvis can be uncomfortable, perform it after the internal examination of the soft pelvic organs. In preparing the client, include an explanation of the procedure, the client's emptying of her bladder, and instructions on relaxation.

A standard procedure for the bony pelvis examination is recommended. Begin with examination of the anterior pelvis, proceed to lateral examination on one side, compare the initially examined side with the opposite side, and conclude with examination of the posterior and inferior portions.

The following bony pelvis parts and landmarks are especially important in examining the pelvis:

1. Subpubic arch
2. Symphysis pubis
3. Side walls
4. Ischial spines
5. Sacrosciatic notch
6. Sacrum
7. Coccyx
8. Sacral promontory
9. Ischial tuberosities

The following is a recommended procedure for assessment of the bony pelvis:

1. Palpate the width of the subpubic arch, and estimate its angle. Normally both examining fingers should fit comfortably in the arch, which optimally forms an angle that measures slightly greater than a right angle (90-degree angle) (Figure 23-24).

2. Estimate the length and inclination of the symphysis pubis by sweeping the examining fingers under the symphysis (Figure 23-25). Also, palpate the retropubic curve of the forepelvis and envision its configuration. Measurement difficulties created by a large amount of soft tissue in the area and reliability with slope measurements preclude a precise estimation of the length and inclination of the symphysis. Essentially, you are screening for an unusually long or steeply inclined symphysis pubis and for an angular rather than a rounded forepelvis.

3. Examine the right or the left lateral pelvic area. First, palpate the side walls to determine if they are straight, convergent, or divergent. Assess the splay of the side walls by following a line from the point of origin of the widest transverse diameter of the inlet downward to the inner aspect of the **tuberosity**. Another method for assessing the side walls is to place the examining fingers on the base of the ischial spine as a landmark and then to palpate above and below the landmark to determine the inclination.

4. Examine the ischial spine and the sacrospinous ligament on that same side. Assess the spines as being blunt, prominent, or encroaching. Outline the sacrosciatic notch with palpating fingers, if possible, and determine its width in centimeters or fingerbreadths. Often tracing the entire notch is difficult, and the sacrospinous ligament is useful in estimating the width of the notch (Figure 23-26).

5. Examine the other side of the pelvis in the manner previously described to determine overall pelvic symmetry. Attempt to do this part of the examination with the palm of the hand up, rather than rotating the hand so that the palm is down.

6. Estimate the interspinous diameter by moving the examining fingers in a straight line from one spine across to the other (Figure 23-27). You may need to pronate the hand for this estimation. Calculate the estimate in centimeters. The usual measurement is 10.5 cm.

7. Next examine the sacrum and the coccyx. Sweep the fingers down the sacrum, noting whether it is straight, curved, or hollow and if its inclination is forward or backward. Examine the coccyx gently because it may be tender on movement. Gently press the coccyx backward to determine if it is movable or fixed. Note its tilt as anterior or posterior.

8. Assess the diagonal conjugate last because this assessment can be uncomfortable for the client. A moderate amount of constant pressure is necessary to de-

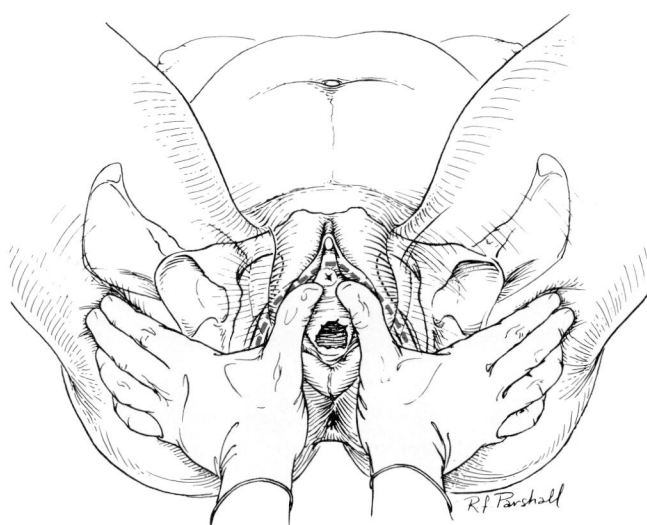

FIGURE 23-24 Method of estimating the angle of the subpubic arch.

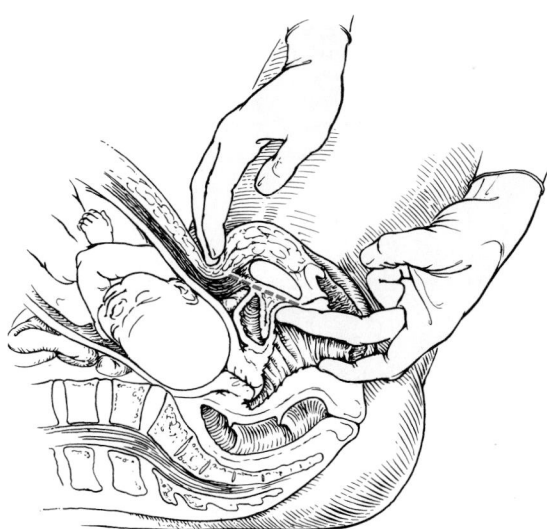

FIGURE 23-25 Estimation of the length and inclination of the symphysis pubis.

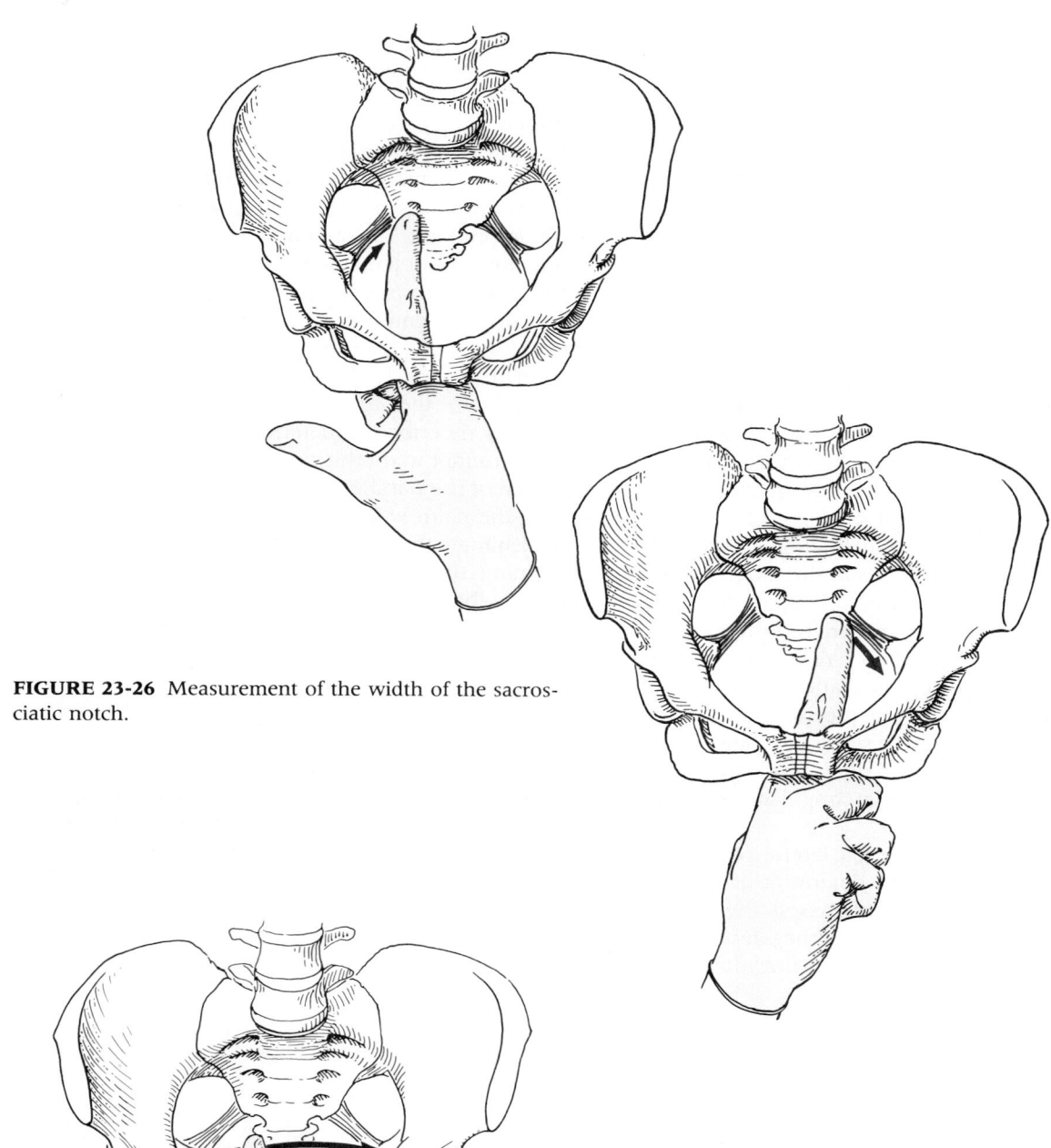

FIGURE 23-26 Measurement of the width of the sacrosciatic notch.

FIGURE 23-27 Measurement of the interspinous diameter.

press the perineum adequately. Exert pressure with your body rather than with the hand and forearm. Place your foot (the one on the same side as the examining hand) on a stool and the elbow of the examining arm on your thigh or hip. Then apply the needed pressure, controlling it with your body. For this examination, make sure that your fingers and wrist form a straight line with your forearm.

Locate the sacrum with the examining fingers, and with the middle finger "walk" up the sacrum until you reach the promontory or until you can no longer touch the sacrum. Mark the point where the client's symphysis touches your hand with the thumb of the opposite hand, and measure the distance in centimeters with a ruler (Figure 23-28). In obstetrical examining rooms, a ruler is often fixed to the wall for this measurement.

Often, you will not reach the sacral promontory. Become familiar with the "reach" of your examining fingers and record the findings as greater than (>) the centimeters of this reach. Normally the diagonal conjugate is >12.5 cm.

9. Withdraw the examining hand from the vagina, and measure the intertuberous diameter. With both thumbs, externally trace the descending rami down to the tuberosities. Then make a fist and attempt to insert the fist between the tuberosities to measure the transverse diameter of an outlet (Figure 23-29). The intertuberous diameter is usually 10 to 11 cm. Again, know the span of your own fist and estimate the intertuberous diameter accordingly.

In summary, the areas of bony pelvic examination and the assessment descriptors for these areas follow:

Sequence of areas of bony pelvic examination	Assessment descriptors
1. Subpubic arch	*Inclination*: less than 90 degrees, more than 90 degrees
2. Side walls	*Direction*: parallel, convergent, divergent
3. Ischial spines	*Size*: small, average, large *Prominence*: blunt, prominent, encroaching
4. Sacrosciatic notch Sacrospinous ligament	*Length*: estimated width or length in centimeters (usual length = 3 to 4 cm)
5. Opposite pelvic side	*Symmetry*: symmetrical, asymmetrical
6. Interspinous diameter	*Length*: estimated length in centimeters (usual length = 10.5 cm)
7. Sacrum	*Shape*: concave, straight, convex
8. Coccyx	*Position*: straight, projects anteriorly, projects posteriorly *Movability*: movable, fixed
9. Diagonal conjugate	*Length*: actual length or length greater than the measurement that the examiner can reach (usual length = 12.5 cm)
10. Intertuberous diameter	*Length*: actual length in centimeters if Thom's pelvimeter is used or an estimated length using a closed fist (usual length is 10 to 11 cm)

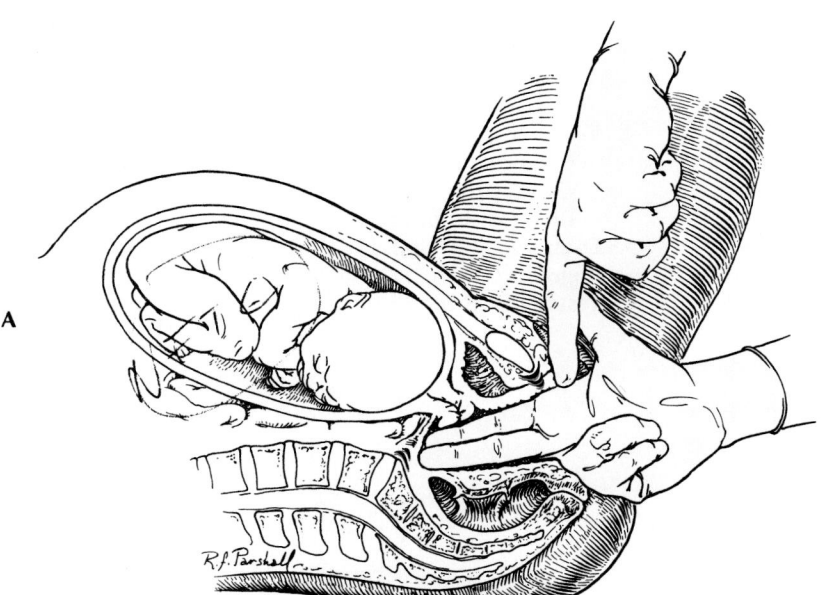

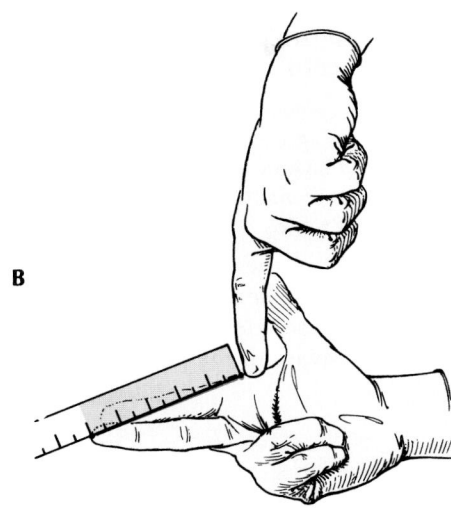

FIGURE 23-28 Measurement of the diagonal conjugate. **A,** Internal palpation. **B,** Use of a ruler to specify estimation in centimeters.

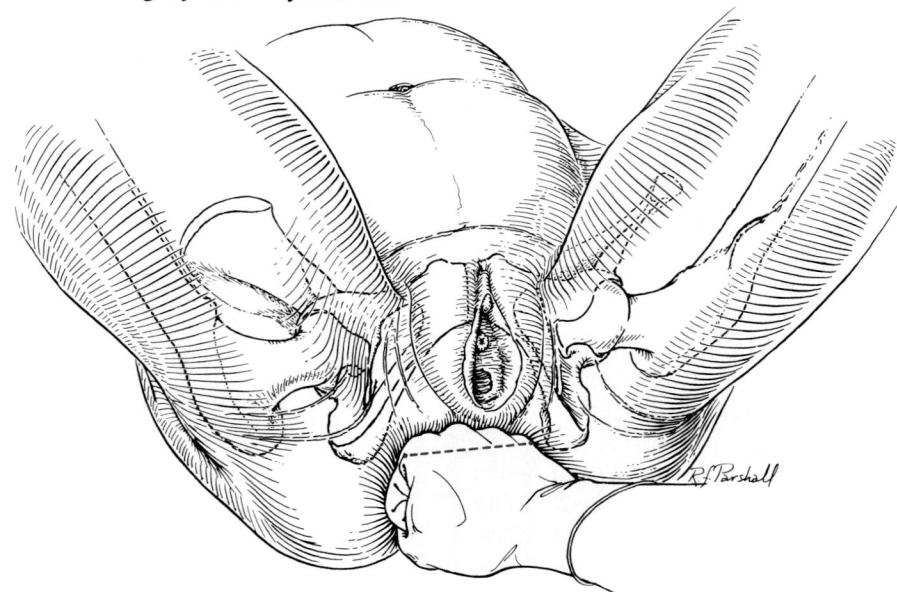

FIGURE 23-29 Use of a fist to estimate the intertuberous diameter.

Special Screening Tests

Fetal Assessment during Pregnancy. Earlier in this chapter, several prenatal screening tests were listed. The tests involved, for the most part, assessment of various maternal specimens to assess the health of both the mother (directly) and the fetus (indirectly). Currently, a number of options exist for direct assessment of the fetus. These tests are used in various situations as indicated (see box, p. 719). The following recommendation (U.S. Preventive Services Task Force, 1989, p. 229) provides some guidelines for the use of fetal assessment screening tests:

Amniocentesis for karyotyping should be offered to pregnant women aged 35 and older. Counseling before the procedure should include a comparison of the risks to the fetus from the procedure and the probability of a chromosomal defect at the patient's age.

Neither the scope nor the size of this textbook are appropriate for the discussion of specialized fetal evaluation tests. However, the beginning practitioner needs to be aware of the developments in the field and to be prepared to integrate such assessments into practice since they may become common screening tests.

TYPES OF FETAL EVALUATION TESTS

1. Tests to evaluate fetal morphology or genetic structure:
   Karotyping
   Fetal sex determination
2. Alpha-fetoprotein (AFP) determination
3. Biochemical tests of fetal well-being:
   Estriol measurement
   Human placental lactogen (HPL) measurement
4. Functional tests of fetal well-being:
   Nonstress test (NST)
   Contraction stress test (CST)
   Biophysical profile
5. Evaluation of fetal size and growth by ultrasonography
6. Tests of fetal maturity

Assessments near term. Two additional assessments of changes are done near the expected date of delivery: estimation of the length and dilation of the cervix and determination of the fetal station. Figure 23-30 displays a method of measuring the length of the cervix. Before 34 to 36 weeks' gestation, the cervix should maintain its usual length of 1.5 to 2 cm. During the last 4 weeks of gestation, the cervix shortens as the fetal head descends and the internal cervical os softens and opens and is pulled upward and incorporated into the isthmus of the uterus. When the cervix shortens (effaces), it also begins to dilate. Cervical dilation is estimated by the diameter of the cervical os and measured in centimeters—from 0 cm when closed to 10 cm when completely opened.

The degree of descent of the fetal presenting part, usually the head, is measured by the station. Station refers to the relationship of the presenting part to the plane of the ischial spines. If the lowest portion of the presenting part is at the level of the spines, it is at station 0. Other stations of the fetal presenting part are the following:

Minus 3	At the pelvic inlet
Minus 2	One third of the distance from the inlet to the spines
Minus 1	Two thirds of the distance from the inlet to the spines
Station 0	At the level of the ischial spines
Plus 1	One third of the distance between the spines and the pelvic floor
Plus 2	Two thirds of the distance between the spines and the pelvic floor
Plus 3	At the pelvic floor

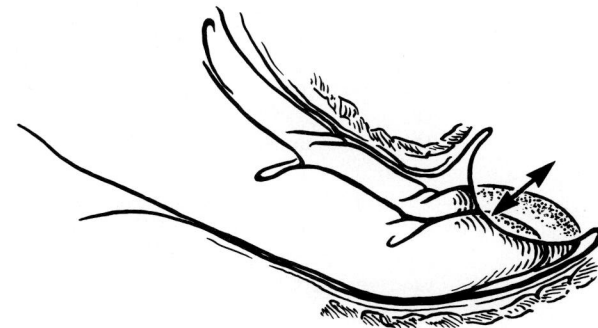

FIGURE 23-30 Measurement of cervical length.

DOCUMENTATION

Sample Documentation

(Return visit for a primigravid patient)

Health history

Has been feeling well during the 1 month since last visit. Nausea and vomiting have ceased and diet and dietary patterns have returned to normal. Experiencing a mild amount of lower abdominal and leg discomfort at the end of the day, relieved by rest with legs elevated. Client and husband have started to set up a nursery. Both continue to be enthusiastic about the baby and supportive of each other. Plans to work until labor starts and take a 3 month leave postpartum. Fetal movements being felt every day—increasing in intensity. Occasional, mild, Braxton Hicks contraction noticed. No vaginal bleeding or discharge or other changes or problems noted.

Physical examination

Urine—negative for glucose, albumin, and ketones
Weight—156 pounds (prepregnant = 140); 4-pound gain in 4 weeks since last visit
BP—118/76
Extremities—no edema
Abdominal assessment: Fundus at umbilicus (consistent with estimated 20-week gestation), measuring 19 cm. Fetal position uncertain because of small fetal size. Fetal heart tones heard in midline, regular at 158 beats/min.

Nursing Diagnosis   *THE NEXT STEP*

Nursing diagnoses that could apply to assessment of pregnant women include, but are not limited to, the following ones.

PAIN The state in which an individual experiences and reports the presence of severe discomfort or an uncomfortable sensation.

Defining Characteristics

- Subjective
  Communication (verbal or coded) of pain descriptors
- Objective
  Guarding behavior; protective
  Self-focusing
  Narrowed focus (altered time perception, withdrawal from social contact, impaired thought process)
  Distraction behavior (moaning, crying, pacing, seeking other people and/or activities, restlessness)
  Facial mask of pain (eyes lack luster, "beaten look," fixed or scattered movement, grimace)
  Alteration in muscle tone (may span from listless to rigid)
  Autonomic responses not seen in chronic, stable pain (diaphoresis, blood pressure and pulse rate change, pupillary dilation, increased or decreased respiratory rate)

Related Factors

- Injuring agents
  Biological
  Chemical
  Physical
  Psychological

BODY IMAGE DISTURBANCE Disruption in the way one perceives one's body image.

Defining Characteristics

Either the following A or B must be present to justify the diagnosis of body image disturbance:
  A. Verbal response to actual or perceived change in structure and/or function
  B. Nonverbal response to actual or perceived change in structure and/or function
The following clinical manifestations may be used to validate the presence of A or B:
- Objective
  Actual change in structure and/or function
  Not looking at body part
  Not touching body part
  Hiding or overexposing body part (intentional or unintentional)
  Change in social involvement
  Negative feelings about body
  Feelings of helplessness, hopelessness, or powerlessness
- Preoccupation with change or loss
- Emphasis on remaining strengths, heightened achievement
- Extension of body boundary to incorporate environmental objects
- Refusal to verify actual change

Related Factors

- Biophysical
- Cognitive perceptual
- Psychosocial
- Cultural or spiritual

CRITICAL THINKING

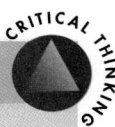

Nursing Diagnosis   *THE NEXT STEP—cont'd*

CONSTIPATION The state in which an individual experiences a change in normal bowel habits characterized by a decrease in frequency and/or passage of hard, dry stools.

Defining Characteristics

- Frequently less than usual pattern
- Hard formed stools
- Reported feeling of rectal fullness
- Palpable mass
- Straining at stool
- Decreased bowel sounds
- Reported feeling of adbominal or rectal fullness or pressure
- Less than usual amount of stool
- Nausea

Other Possible Defining Characteristics

- Abdominal pain
- Back pain
- Headache
- Interference with daily living
- Use of laxatives
- Decreased appetite
- Appetite impairment

Related Factors

- Less than adequate intake
- Less than adequate dietary intake and bulk
- Less than adequate physical activity or immobility
- Personal habits
- Medications
- Chronic use of medication and enemas
- Gastrointestinal obstructive lesions
- Neuromuscular impairment
- Musculoskeletal impairment
- Pain on defecation
- Diagnostic procedures
- Lack of privacy
- Weak abdominal musculature
- Pregnancy
- Emotional status

SLEEP PATTERN DISTURBANCE Disruption of sleep time causes discomfort or interferes with desired life-style

Defining Characteristics

- Verbal complaints of difficulty falling asleep
- Awakening earlier or later than desired
- Interrupted sleep
- Verbal complaints of not feeling well rested
- Changes in behavior and performance
  Increasing irritability
  Restlessness
  Disorientation
  Lethargy
  Listlessness

Continued.

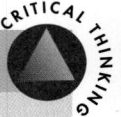

Nursing Diagnosis   *THE NEXT STEP—cont'd*

- Physical signs
  Mild, fleeting nystagmus
  Slight hand tremor
  Ptosis of eyelid
  Expressionless face
- Thick speech with mispronunciation and incorrect words
- Dark circles under eyes
- Frequent yawning
- Changes in posture
- Not feeling well rested

Related Factors

Sensory alterations
- Internal factors
  Illness
  Psychological stress
- External factors
  Environmental changes
  Social cues

ACTIVITY INTOLERANCE The state in which an individual has insufficient physiological or psychological energy to endure or complete required or desired daily activities.

Defining Characteristics

- Verbal report of fatigue or weakness
- Abnormal heart rate or blood pressure response to activity
- Exertional discomfort or dyspnea
- Electrocardiographic changes reflecting arrhythmias or ischemia

Related Factors

- Generalized weakness
- Sedentary life-style
- Imbalance between oxygen supply and demand
- Bed rest or immobility

ALTERED ROLE PERFORMANCE Disruption in the way one perceives one's role performance.

Defining Characteristics

- Change in self-perception of role
- Denial of role
- Change in others' perception of role
- Conflict in roles
- Change in physical capacity to resume role
- Lack of knowledge of role
- Change in usual patterns or responsibility

Related Factors

- Changes in values and beliefs
- Inadequate role socialization
- Developmental transitions
- Negative self-perception
- Situational transitions
- Cultural discrepancies
- Health-illness transition

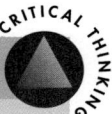

Nursing Diagnosis *THE NEXT STEP—cont'd*

- Physical limitations
- Incompatible prescribed behaviors from two or more roles
- Major disruptions in life-style
- Inadequate knowledge
- Lack of opportunity to practice role
- Threat to self-concept
- Incompatible role expectation from others

HIGH RISK FOR ALTERED PARENTING The state in which the ability of nurturing figure(s) to create an environment that promotes the optimal growth and development of another human being is altered or at risk.

Defining Characteristics (risk factors)

- Unavailable or ineffective role model
- History of physical or psychosocial abuse
- Support system deficit
- Unmet social, emotional, developmental needs
- Interruption in bonding process
- Unrealistic expectation
- Perceived threat to own survival
- Physical impairment
- Physical or mental illness
- Presence of stress
- Knowledge of skill deficit
- Limited cognitive functioning
- Lack of role identity
- Lack of appropriate response of child to relationship
- Social isolation
- Fear

IMPAIRED PHYSICAL MOBILITY The state in which an individual experiences a limitation of ability for independent physical movement.

Defining Characteristics

- Inability to purposefully move within physical environment, including bed mobility, transfer, and ambulation
- Reluctance to attempt movement
- Limited range of motion
- Decreased muscle strength, control, and/or mass
- Imposed restrictions of movement, including mechanical; medical protocol
- Impaired coordination

Related Factors

- Intolerance to activity; decreased strength and endurance
- Pain and discomfort
- Perceptual or cognitive impairment
- Neuromuscular impairment
- Musculoskeletal impairment
- Depression; severe anxiety

Continued.

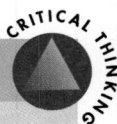

Nursing Diagnosis   *THE NEXT STEP—cont'd*

Clinical Application

Mrs. K. is a 24-year-old primigravid client in for her second trimester (20 weeks) checkup. Has been feeling better since last visit 1 month ago. Nausea and vomiting have disappeared and diet has returned to normal. Complaining of mild pain in breasts and a mild amount of lower abdominal and leg discomfort at night. She has experienced frequent urination at night and usually only gets up 2 to 3 times each night. Mrs. K. and her husband are getting more and more enthusiastic about the baby and are supportive of each other. Mrs. K. will continue to work until the baby is born, then will take 6 to 8 weeks leave postpartum. She has just begun to feel fetal movement. Occasional, mild, Braxton Hicks contractions noted. No vaginal bleeding or discharge noted. No other problems noted.

SUBJECTIVE DATA: Client complains of:
Mild pain in breasts
Mild amount lower abdominal discomfort
Mild amount of leg discomfort
Frequent urination at night

OBJECTIVE DATA:
Urine-negative for glucose, albumin, and ketones
Weight-165 pounds (prepregnant weight 140; up 6 pounds in 4 weeks since last visit)
Breast assessment:
Areolae of nipple darker in color, diameter about 5 cm, blue veins prominent over the surface.
Slight secretion of thin watery fluid may be expelled from both nipples.
Abdominal assessment:
Fundus at umbilicus (consistent with estimated 20-week gestation), measuring 20 cm.
Fetal position uncertain due to small fetal size.
Fetal heart tones, heart in midline, regular at 162 beats/minute.

NURSING DIAGNOSES

Altered nutrition: high risk for more than body requirements related to weight gain > 25 pounds in 20 weeks

Defining Characteristics

- Weight 10% to 20% over ideal for height and frame

Pain related to physical body changes during pregnancy (breast enlargement, lower abdominal pressure, and leg pressure).

Defining Characteristics

- Complains of pain in breasts
- Complains of pressure in lower abdomen and legs

Sleep pattern disturbances related to frequent urination at night.

Defining Characteristics

- Interrupted sleep 2 to 3 times each night to urinate

GLOSSARY

atony Weak; lacking normal tone.

ballottement Palpation technique used to assess a floating object; fluid-filled tissue is pushed toward the examiner's hand so that the object will float against the examiner's fingers.

Braxton Hicks contraction Irregular tightening of the uterus that begins in the first trimester and increases in frequency, duration, and intensity as the pregnancy advances.

chorionic Pertaining to the chorion, a fetal membrane composed of trophoblast that forms the fetal portion of the placenta.

chloasma Tan or brown pigmentation, particularly of the forehead, cheeks, and nose.

congenital Present at birth.

cornu Any horn-shaped structure.

corticotropic Of or pertaining to stimulation of the adrenal cortex.

decidua Endometrium during pregnancy that is shed in the postpartum period.

diastasis recti abdominis Separation of the two rectus muscles along the median line of the abdominal wall.

epulis Any tumor or growth on the gingiva.

fundus The base or deepest part of any organ.

linea nigra Pigmentation of the linea alba, the tendinous median line on the anterior abdominal wall, during pregnancy.

melanocyte Body cell capable of producing melanin.

morning sickness Nausea and vomiting occurring from the fifth or sixth week through the fourteenth to sixteenth week of pregnancy.

nullipara Woman who has not given birth to a viable offspring.

preterm infant Infant born before 37 weeks' gestation.

striae gravidarum Atrophic, pinkish or purplish scarlike lesions observed on the breasts, thighs, abdomen, and buttocks during pregnancy. The lesions later become silvery white.

term infant Infant born between 37 and 41 weeks' gestation.

trimester Period of 13 weeks.

trophoblast Peripheral cell layer of the blastocyst that attaches the fertilized ovum to the uterine wall and becomes the placenta and the membranes.

tuberosity An elevation or protuberance, especially of a bone.

BIBLIOGRAPHY

Andolsek KM: *Obstetric care: standards of prenatal, intrapartum, and postpartum management,* Philadelphia, 1990, Lea & Febiger.

Barber HRK, Fields DH, Kaufman SA: *Quick reference to ob-gyn procedures,* ed 3, Philadelphia, 1990, JB Lippincott.

Caldwell WE, Maloy HC, Swenson PC: The use of the roentgen ray in obstetrics: anatomical variations in the female pelvis and their classification according to morphology, *Am J Roentgenol* 41:505, 1939.

Gabbe SG, Niebyl JR, Simpson JL: *Obstetrics: normal and problem pregnancies,* ed 2, New York, 1991, Churchill Livingstone.

Gordon M: *Manual of nursing diagnosis: 1993-1994,* St Louis, 1993, Mosby–Year Book.

Gordon M: *Nursing diagnosis: process and application,* ed 2, New York, 1987, McGraw-Hill.

James, DK, Stirrat, GM (editors): *Pregnancy and risk: the basis for rational management.* Chichester; New York: 1988, Wiley.

Lichtman R, Papera S: *Gynecology: well-woman care,* Norwalk, Conn, 1990, Appleton & Lange.

Merkatz IR, Thompson JE, *New perspectives on prenatal care,* New York, 1990, Elsevier.

Mosby's medical, nursing, and allied health dictionary, ed 3, St Louis, 1990, Mosby–Year Book.

Nagey DA: The content of prenatal care, *Obstet Gynecol* 74:516, 1989.

Oxorn H: *Oxorn-Foote human labor and birth,* Norwalk, Conn, 1986, Appleton-Century-Crofts.

Pagana KD, Pagana TJ: *Mosby's diagnostic and laboratory test reference,* St Louis, 1992, Mosby–Year Book.

Pernoll ML: *Current obstetric and gynecologic diagnosis and treatment,* ed 7, Norwalk, Conn, 1991, Appleton & Lange.

Sherwood MJ and others: *Determining nursing diagnosis through assessment.* Baltimore, 1988, Williams & Wilkins.

Suonio S and others: Clinical assessment of the pelvic cavity and outlet, *Arch Gynecol* 329:11, 1986.

Tucker S: *Pocket guide to fetal monitoring,* St Louis, 1992, Mosby–Year Book.

U.S. Preventive Services Task Force: *Guide to clinical preventive services: an assessment of the effectiveness of 169 interventions,* Baltimore, 1989, Williams & Wilkins.

Varney H: *Nurse-midwifery,* ed 2, Boston, 1987, Blackwell Scientific Publications.

Willson JR and others: *Obstetrics and gynecology,* ed 9, St Louis, 1991, Mosby–Year Book.

Pediatric Clients

PURPOSE OF THE EXAMINATION

Pediatric care is, to a large extent, health care aimed at promoting the health of the child and preventing illness and disability through early identification of problems, anticipatory guidance to help parents deal with physical and developmental issues before they become problems, and early and ongoing intervention for health care needs.

Ideally the practitioner performs the examination of the child over an extended time in a planned sequential pattern. The dynamic changes that occur throughout the child's normal growth and development require that the practitioner assess certain aspects carefully: increments in growth; changes in physiological function; and development of cognitive, social, and motor skills of the child during each examination.

The health of the child is determined by comparing the individual child's current growth achievements and parameters of health with those found in his or her previous examinations, and with norms for children in the same age range. The practitioner should see the child frequently, usually every 2 to 3 months for well-child care during infancy, when growth changes are most rapid and dramatic. The practitioner should assess the older child at regular, but less frequent, intervals for well-child care.

In order to provide holistic care to the child, it is also important to consider the needs and concerns of the child's primary caretaker(s), usually the parents. The adults responsible for the child's care often have questions and concerns about the child's development and about their own ability to manage care. The practitioner needs to encourage them to express their concerns and to discuss their needs in addition to the needs of the child. The examiner should have a sense of the parent as a person. What are the stresses and issues that the parents are dealing with? What impact do these factors have on their ability to parent? Parents who feel that their questions and concerns are being heard and that they are receiving support and respect will be better able to care for their children (Figure 24-1).

A part of each well-child assessment (and sick-child visit, if that is the only time that the family comes in for care, or if the potential for problems is apparent during an acute care visit) should address anticipatory guidance. Anticipatory guidance involves teaching parents what to expect in terms of their child's physical, cognitive, emotional, and social development. The goal of anticipatory guidance is to promote positive parent-child relationships and prevent the development of emotional and behavioral disturbances related to difficulties in parent-child interactions. Frequently problems develop because parents or caregivers are unaware that "problem" behaviors are in fact normal stage-specific behaviors related to development. Examples include the "stranger anxiety" demonstrated when a

9-month-old is picked up by his grandmother whom he sees infrequently or the "negativism" of the 2-year-old. Helping the parent identify what is normal development versus abnormal or problem behavior can help parents feel more secure in their ability to respond to their children. For example, the 9-month-old will still cry when picked up by the "stranger," his grandmother, but his parents will be able to identify this reaction as a normal (although embarrassing) behavior rather than a reflection of being "spoiled" by the parents.

Anticipatory guidance also involves helping the parent identify and problem-solve around problematic areas. Examples include talking with a parent about how to deal with negativism or temper tantrums and anticipating what to do if the child has a tantrum in the grocery store, or helping parents who are planning to bring their 9-month-old child to a family reunion consider ways to introduce their child to relatives in a nonthreatening manner. Anticipatory guidance can also be used to help new parents address issues such as differences in attitudes toward discipline or the role each parent plays in child care activities before these differences become a source of family conflict.

Assessing the quality of the parent-child relationship is crucial. The practitioner should support positive interactions (Figure 24-2). Receiving recognition for their parenting skills is especially helpful for parents. The practitioner also should be alert to any signs of stress between the parent and the child. A mother who is concerned, anxious, or angry about a child's behavior or physical condition may be showing evidence of stress that can interfere with the mother-child relationship

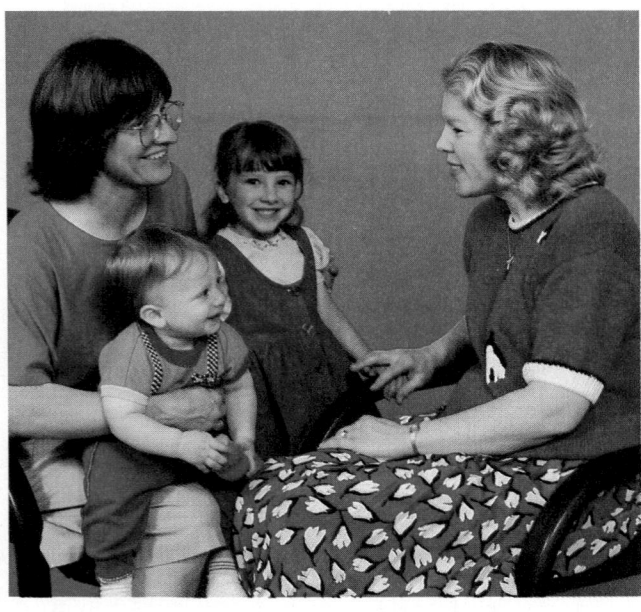

FIGURE 24-1 Attention to the concerns of both the parent and the child is an important component of the assessment.

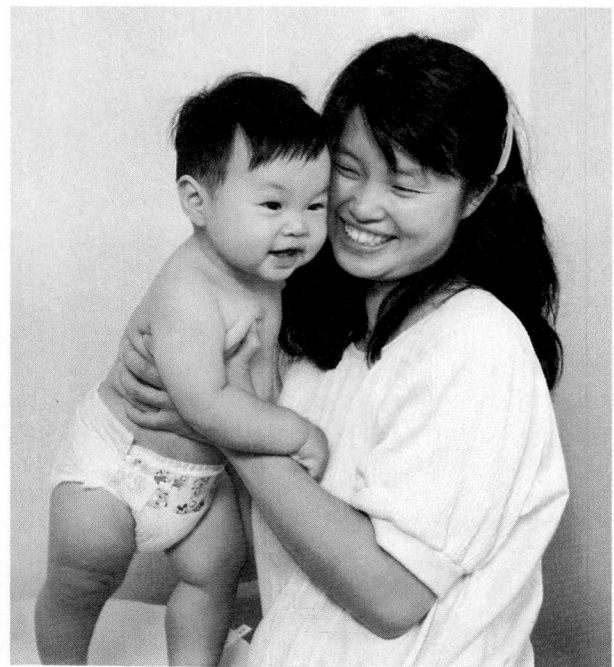

FIGURE 24-2 Quality of the parent-child interactions needs to be assessed and positive attitudes should be supported.

and ultimately with the child's development. The practitioner can identify difficulties in the parent-child interaction and initiate early interventions to promote better interactions. This issue emphasizes the importance of considering needs of the parent or other adults caring for the child in addition to those of the child.

The practitioner should always demonstrate respect for both the child and the parent, be willing to listen to problems, and help in finding adequate solutions. Both the child and the parent will be aware of the practitioner's attitudes and will respond according to their impressions. In essence, it is important to be sensitive to the child as a growing, developing human being who is always changing.

This chapter discusses approaches to the child and the parent and some techniques used to obtain health information and to assess the child's health. In addition, it covers some of the physical differences between the child and the adult. Because it is not possible to include a survey of all the components of child development that are assessed, the reader is referred to Chapter 3 and standard pediatric texts for assistance in understanding the parameters of normal development and health of children.

GUIDELINES FOR HEALTH SUPERVISION

Much of the care given to children focuses on health promotion and the prevention of disease. The American Academy of Pediatrics (1988) suggests the schedule of well-child care shown in Table 24-1 for the care of children who (1) are receiving competent parenting, (2) have no manifestations of any important health problems, and (3) are growing and developing in a satisfactory fashion. The following situations may warrant additional visits:

1. Firstborn or adopted children or those not with natural parents
2. Parents with a particular need for education and guidance
3. Families from a disadvantaged social or economic environment
4. Presence or possibility of perinatal disorders (e.g., prematurity, low birth weight, **congenital** defects, or familial diseases)
5. Children with acquired illness or previously identified diseases or problems

EXAMINATION

Pediatric History

The pediatric history provides the opportunity to interview both child and parent to gather information about the child's health, development, relationships with others, and care. It also offers the opportunity for the child to become acquainted with the practitioner before being examined. The pediatric history is an adaptation of the model used for the adult history. It incorporates areas uniquely pertinent to the child, such as the history of the mother's health during the pregnancy, the history of birth and the neonatal period, and specific areas related to the child's psychosocial development (e.g., stage-related behaviors, school performance, peer relationships).

Cultural differences and individual parental beliefs about child-rearing and health influence the care of the infant and child and are revealed in the history of the child's care. The practitioner should respect these differences and make culturally sensitive decisions with regard to content and approaches in counseling.

The informant for the history may be a parent, a relative, a caretaker, and/or the child. Identify the informant and indicate the reliability of the information obtained. Commonly the child, even the young child, participates in the interview and volunteers useful information. Indicate the information gained from the child as such in the history.

The comprehensive health history described in Chapter 2 is adapted for the pediatric client by making certain changes in format. The following developmental and nutritional data should be gathered before the review of systems since these data are usually critical to the present health status of the infant or child:

1. Biographical information
2. Chief complaint or client's request for care
3. Present illness or present health status
4. Past health history
5. Developmental data
6. Nutritional data
7. Family health history
8. Review of systems
   a. Physical systems
   b. Sociological system
   c. Psychological system
9. Anticipatory guidance

Biographical information. The following information needs to be obtained in the biographical category. It is essentially the same as for the adult client with the addition of the parents' information.

1. Full name
2. Address
3. Birth date
4. Sex
5. Race
6. Religion
7. Birthplace
8. Parents' names

TABLE 24-1

Guidelines for Health Supervision

	Infancy						Early childhood				
Age[2]	By 1 mo	2 mo	4 mo	6 mo	9 mo	12 mo	15 mo	18 mo	24 mo	3 yr	4 yr
History											
Initial/interval	●	●	●	●	●	●	●	●	●	●	●
Measurements											
Height and weight	●	●	●	●	●	●	●	●	●	●	●
Head circumference	●	●	●	●	●	●					
Blood pressure										●	●
Sensory screening											
Vision	S	S	S	S	S	S	S	S	S	S	○
Hearing	S	S	S	S	S	S	S	S	S	S	○
Developmental/behavioral assessment[4]	●	●	●	●	●	●	●	●	●	●	●
Physical examination[5]	●	●	●	●	●	●	●	●	●	●	●
Procedures[6]											
Heredity/metabolic[7] screening	●										
Immunization[8]		●	●	●			●	●			
Tuberculin test[9]						●			●		
Hematocrit or hemoglobin[10]					●				●		
Urinalysis[11]				●					●		
Anticipatory guidance[12]	●	●	●	●	●	●	●	●	●	●	●
Initial dental referral[13]										●	

Adapted from American Academy of Pediatrics Committee on Psychosocial Aspects of Child and Family Health, 1988.

1. Adolescent-related issues (e.g., psychosocial, emotional, substance usage, and reproductive health) may necessitate more frequent health supervision.
2. If a child comes under care for the first time at any point on the schedule, or if any items are not accomplished at the suggested age, the schedule should be brought up to date at the earliest possible time.
3. At these points, history may suffice; if a problem is suggested, a standard testing method should be employed.
4. By history and appropriate physical examination; if suspicious, by specific objective developmental testing.
5. At each visit a complete physical examination is essential, with infant totally unclothed, older child undressed and suitably draped.
6. These may be modified, depending on entry point into schedule and individual need.
7. Metabolic screening (e.g., thyroid, PKU, galactosemia) should be done according to state law.
8. Schedule(s) per Report of Committee on Infectious Disease, *1991 Red Book.*
9. For low-risk groups, the Committee on Infectious Diseases recommends the following options: (1) no routine testing or (2) testing at three times—infancy, preschool, and adolescence. For high-risk groups, annual TB skin testing is recommended.

9. Parents' marital status
10. Parents' ages
11. Source of referral
12. Usual source of health care
13. Source and reliability of information
14. Date of interview

Chief complaint or client's request for care. The chief complaint statement gives the reason for making the visit and should be recorded in the words of the informant. The informant could be the parent or the child. Elicit this information with a neutral question ("How may I help you today?") since the visit may be for routine health care rather than for treatment of a health problem. The chief complaint statement for routine health care may be "It is time for his checkup" or "Well-baby check."

When the visit is for a well-child examination, you may want to ask: "Before we begin the examination, are there any particular questions or concerns that you

Age[2]	Late childhood					Adolescence[1]			
	5 yr	6 yr	8 yr	10 yr	12 yr	14 yr	16 yr	18 yr	20 + yr
History									
Initial/interval	●	●	●	●	●	●	●	●	●
Measurements									
Height and weight	●	●	●	●	●	●	●	●	●
Head circumference									
Blood pressure	●	●	●	●	●	●	●	●	●
Sensory screening									
Vision	○	○	○	S	○	○	S	○	○
Hearing	○	S[3]	S[3]	S[3]	○	S	S	○	S
Developmental/behavioral assessment[4]	●	●	●	●	●	●	●	●	●
Physical examination[5]	●	●	●	●	●	●	●	●	●
Procedures[6]									
Heredity/metabolic[7] screening									
Immunization[8]	●					●			
Tuberculin test[9]								●	
Hematocrit or hemoglobin[10]			●					●	
Urinalysis[11]			●					●	
Anticipatory guidance[12]	●	●	●	●	●	●	●	●	●
Initial dental referral[13]									

10. Present medical evidence suggests the need for reevaluation of the frequency and timing of hemoglobin or hematocrit tests. One determination is therefore suggested during each time period. Performance of additional tests is left to the individual practice experience.
11. Present medical evidence suggests the need for reevaluation of the frequency and timing of urinalysis. One determination is therefore suggested during each time period. Performance of additional tests is left to the individual practice experience.
12. Appropriate discussion and counseling should be an integral part of each visit for care.
13. Subsequent examinations as prescribed by dentist.
NOTE: *Special chemical, immunological, and endocrine testing* are usually carried out on specific indications.
Testing other than newborn (e.g., inborn errors of metabolism, sickle disease, lead) are discretionary with the physician.
Key: ● = to be performed; S = subjective, by history; ○ = objective, by a standard testing method.

would like to discuss?" This question encourages the client, parent, or child to raise issues that may not be addressed in the health history format and reinforces the idea that their questions and concerns are important.

Present illness or present health status. The present illness or present health status section incorporates the same categories of information obtained in the adult health history and includes a statement about the client's usual health; a description of the current concern, including the onset and chronological story; any relevant family history; any negative information; and

a disability assessment. You may want to ask an open-ended question ("How has the baby been since you were last here?") to get a general picture of how things have been going (interval history). Also ask the parent the reason for seeking help at this time. Usually something significant has occurred that motivates the person to come for an evaluation. Physical changes in the child's condition, family stresses that make the problem more difficult to handle, or issues such as a similar problem in a friend or relative may have triggered the visit. Understanding these concerns will help in making your assessment of the situation and planning effective interventions.

Past health history. The past health history of infants, young children, and any child with a possible developmental deficiency should include the following information:

1. Prenatal history
   a. Health of the mother while pregnant with this child
   b. Mother's feelings about the pregnancy
   c. Amount of prenatal care and when initiated
   d. History of complications (excessive weight gain, hypertension, vaginal bleeding, nausea and vomiting, urinary problems, or infections such as rubella, cytomegalovirus, or venereal disease)
   e. Medications or drugs prescribed or used during pregnancy
   f. Use of alcohol, cigarettes, and other drugs (e.g., cocaine, heroin) during the pregnancy
2. Birth history
   a. Date of birth
   b. Hospital where child was born
   c. Duration of the pregnancy
   d. Parity of the mother
   e. Nature and duration of the labor
   f. Type of delivery
   g. Use of sedation or anesthesia
   h. Birth weight of the baby
   i. State of the infant at birth and use of any *special* procedures
   j. Apgar score, if known (Table 24-2)
3. Postnatal history
   a. Any problems during the first days of life (including skin color, bleeding, seizures, respiratory distress, congenital anomalies or birth injuries, difficulty in sucking, rashes, or poor weight gain during the first days and weeks after birth)
   b. Age of infant at discharge from hospital after birth

The past health history of *all* children includes the following information:

1. Past illnesses
   a. Childhood illnesses (including communicable diseases such as chickenpox and rubeola)
   b. Injuries
   c. Hospitalizations
   d. Operations
   e. Other major illnesses
   f. Frequency of infections
2. Allergies
   a. Environmental
   b. Food
   c. Drug
   d. Other
3. Immunizations (including booster inoculations) (Tables 24-3 through 24-5)
4. Habits
   a. Sleep: Does child sleep through the night? Note naps, number of hours of sleep at night, bedtime routines
   b. Elimination: urination and bowel movements, toilet training, occurrence of accidents
   c. Exercise: types of activities, frequency, organized sports
   d. Behavior patterns (e.g., fussiness, response to frustration, thumb sucking, nail biting): What is your child like? Does he or she have a particularly fussy time during the day?, etc.
   e. Use of alcohol, tobacco, drugs, coffee, tea, colas
   f. Discipline: methods used, success, failure, concerns
   g. Sexuality: inquisitiveness about girl-boy differences and pregnancy; parental responses and sex education offered; concerns and

---

TABLE 24-2

The Apgar Scoring System for Newborns

Clinical sign	Assigned score		
	0	**1**	**2**
Heart rate	Absent	Slow (<100 beats/minute)	>100 beats/minute
Respiratory effort	Apnea	Slow and irregular	Immediate, strong
Muscle tone	Flaccid	Some flexion of arms and legs	Active movement
Reflex irritability*	No response	Grimace or cry	Crying vigorously
Color	Pale, blue	Body pink, extremities blue	Pink all over

*Reaction when soft rubber catheter is inserted into the external nares.
A score of 8 to 10 is excellent, 4 to 7 is guarded, and 0 to 3 is critical.

TABLE 24-3

1992 Childhood Immunization Schedule

Age	Hepatitis B vaccine*	DTP	TOPV	HbCV†	MMR	Td
Birth (first visit)	Hepatitis B vaccine 1					
1-2 months	Hepatitis B vaccine 2 (or vaccine 1)					
2 months (earliest age)		DTP 1 (6 weeks)	TOPV 1 (6 weeks)	HbCV 1 (6 weeks)		
4 months (minimal interval)	(or vaccine 2)	DTP 2 (4 weeks after first dose)	TOPV 2 (6 weeks after first dose)	HbCV 2 (4 weeks after first dose)		
6 months (minimal interval)		DTP 3 (4 weeks after second dose)		HbCV 3 (only if HbOC is used; 4 weeks after second dose)		
6-18 months (minimal interval)	Hepatitis B vaccine 3‡ (2 months)					
12 months (minimal interval)				HbCV 3 (only if PRP-OMP is used; 2 months after second dose and 12 months old)†		
15 months (earliest age or minimal interval)		DTP 4 (do not give earlier than 15 months and 6 months after third dose); usually give at 18 months	TOPV 3 (do not give earlier than 15 months and 6 weeks after second dose); usually give at 18 months	HbCV 4 (if HbOC is used, 2 months after third dose and 15 months old)†	MMR 1 (12 months in high-risk areas only)	
4-6 + years (minimal interval)		DTP 5§	TOPV 4‖		MMR 2 (1 month after first dose and 4 to 14 years old)	
14-16 years						Td 1
Usual number of doses in series	3	5	4	4 (3 if PRP-OMP is used)	2	N/A
Dose	IM	0.5 ml IM	0.5 ml oral	0.5 ml IM	0.5 ml SQ	0.5 ml IM

From Zimmerman R, Giebink G: Childhood immunizations: a practical approach for clinicians, *Am Fam Physician* 45:1759-1776, 1992.

NOTE: Use Td, not DTP, for series at age 7 years or later. Do not give split doses of DTP. Except in special circumstances, HbCV is not given at age 5 years or later; IM doses should be given in the anterolateral thigh for infants. For children, hepatitis B vaccine is given in the deltoid muscle.

DTP = diphtheria, tetanus, and pertussis; TOPV = trivalent oral poliovirus vaccine; HbCV = *Haemophilus B* conjugate vaccine; MMR = measles, mumps, and rubella; HbOC = diphtheria CRM$_{197}$ protein conjugate; PRP-OMP = meningococcal protein conjugate; IM = intramuscularly; SQ = subcutaneously.

*Children under 7 years of age should receive 2.5 μg (0.25 ml) doses of Recombivax HB or 10 μg doses of Engerix-B as part of universal childhood immunization. Offspring of hepatitis B carriers should receive hepatitis B immunoglobulin at birth and the hepatitis B vaccine series with Recombivax HB at the 5.0 μg (0.5 ml) dose or Engerix-B at the 10 μg dose.

†See Table 24-4 for HbCV vaccine schedules when starting series late.

‡If hepatitis B vaccine 2 is late, give hepatitis B vaccine 3 at 3 to 5 months after hepatitis B vaccine 2.

§This dose is not needed if the fourth dose is given after the fourth birthday.

‖This dose is not needed if the third dose is given after the fourth birthday.

Based on recommendations from the Immunization Practices Advisory Committee, American Academy of Pediatrics and American Academy of Family Physicians.

TABLE 24-4

Number of Doses of Haemophilus B *Conjugate Vaccine Needed for Children Who Are Behind Schedule*

Age when series started and number of previous doses	Number of additional doses needed by current age of child and vaccine				
	7-11 months		12-14 months		15-59 months
	HbOC	PRP-OMP	HbOC	PRP-OMP	Any product
6 months 1 previous dose	2 + 15-month booster	1 + 12-month booster	1 + 15-month booster	1 + booster	1
2 previous doses	1 + 15-month booster	12-month booster	1 + 15-month booster	Booster	1
11 months 1 previous dose	1 + 15-month booster	1 + 12-month booster	1 + 15-month booster	1 + 15-month booster	1
2 previous doses	15-month booster	12-month booster	15-month booster	15-month booster	1
12 to 14 months 1 previous dose			15-month booster	15-month booster	1
2 previous doses			0	0	0*
Not yet begun HbCV series None	2 + 15-month booster	2 + 15-month booster	1 + 15-month booster	1 + 15-month booster	1

From Zimmerman R, Giebink G: Childhood immunizations: practical approach for clinicians, *Am Fam Physician* 45:1759-1776, 1992.

NOTE: To vaccinate infants who have fallen behind in the Hib vaccine schedule, refer to the child's current age and the age at which vaccine was initiated to determine the number of additional doses needed, as in Table 24-3. Except in special circumstances, HbCV is not given at or beyond the age of 5 years. Children with chronic illnesses associated with an increased risk of Hib disease, such as asplenia or chemotherapy for Hodgkin's lymphoma, should receive HbCV even if they are older than 5 years of age. Booster doses should be given at least 2 months after the preceding dose. HbOC = diphtheria CRM$_{197}$ protein conjugate; PRP-OMP = meningococcal protein conjugate; HbCV = *Haemophilus B* conjugate vaccine; Hib = *H. influenzae* type b.

*Provided the 15-month booster was given.

Adapted from the schedule of immunizations developed by the Minnesota Department of Health, 1991.

TABLE 24-5

Immunization Schedule for Children 7 Years of Age or Older Who Were Not Immunized in Infancy

Immunization timing	Td (adult dose)*	TOPV†	MMR
First visit	Td 1	TOPV 1	MMR 1
2 months after Td 1 (minimal interval)	Td 2 (4 weeks)	TOPV 2 (6 weeks)	MMR 2 (1 month)
6-12 months after Td 2 (minimal interval)	Td 3 (6 months)	TOPV 3 (6 weeks)	
10 years after Td 3	Td		
Number of doses in basic series	3	3	2

From Zimmerman R, Giebink G: Childhood immunizations: a practical approach for clinicians, *Am Fam Physician* 45:1759-1776, 1992.

Td = tetanus and diphtheria toxoids; TOPV = trivalent oral poliovirus vaccine; MMR = measles, mumps, and rubella; DTP = diphtheria, tetanus, and pertussis; DT = diphtheria and tetanus.

*DTP or DT doses given before age 7 years should be counted toward the three needed doses; the third dose should be given at least 6 months after the second dose and after the seventh birthday.

†Routine poliovirus immunization is not recommended for adults 18 years of age or older who are residing in the United States. If vaccine is indicated, adults should usually receive enhanced inactivated poliovirus vaccine.

TABLE 24-6

Developmental/Behavioral Milestones

Age	Expectations	Age	Expectations
Newborn	Demonstrate the newborn's ability to fix and follow a human face and alert toward a human voice Observe for: Consolability Self-quieting Cuddlesomeness Tendency to startle	6 months, cont'd	Turns to sounds that originate from out of his immediate sight and changes his activity Shows signs of stranger anxiety; appears able, on the basis of facial and body gestures, to distinguish between angry and friendly voice patterns Laughs, squeals, takes the initiative in vocalizing and babbling at others; blows bubbles; imitates such things as a cough, a "raspberry"; may play at making sounds while alone or with others
1 month	At this age the typical infant: Raises her head slightly when lying prone Fixes on a face or object and follows movement with her eyes	9 months	At this age the typical child: Sits well Crawls, creeps on her hands, hitches on her bottom Pulls to a stand; cruises and has parachute reflex
2 months	At this age the typical child: Holds his head temporarily erect but unsteadily when held upright, until 3 months of age Grasps a rattle when placed in his hand Holds a rattle briefly Exhibits a social smile—an important developmental milestone Coos; reciprocally vocalizes Regards one's face when it is in his direct line of vision; begins to distinguish and respond more to his parents than to others Responds to loud sounds		Uses inferior pincer grasp; pokes with the index finger Finger-feeds partially Imitates vocalization; demonstrates monosyllabic and possibly polysyllabic babbling (e.g., may say "dada" or "mama" in a nonspecific way) Responds to her own name, to questions such as "Where is mama or dada?" or to familiar objects when named Understands a few words: "no-no," "bye-bye" Enjoys social games with adults, such as peek-a-boo and pat-a-cake Reacts to strangers with soberness, anxiety, or even fear Has a concept of object permanence; retrieves a toy hidden by a cloth
4 months	At this age the typical child: Holds her head high and raises her body on her hands when lying prone Maintains steady head control when held upright; no head lag when pulled to sit Rolls from prone to supine position Opens hands while at rest; can play with hands, hold a rattle Looks at a mobile and activates her arms Follows parent(s) and objects with her eyes through a 180° range Initiates social contact by smiling, cooing, laughing, squealing; may be displeased or cry when a parent moves away Recognizes preparations for feeding and is able to wait a short time	12 months	At this age the typical child: Pulls to stand; cruises; walks with support; may take a few steps alone Shows a precise pincer grasp; points; bangs two blocks together; can put one object inside another May say one to three meaningful words besides using "mama" and "dada" correctly; imitates vocalization Has a concept of object permanence (e.g., looks for a dropped or hidden object) Plays social games (e.g., peek-a-boo, pat-a-cake, so-big); waves bye-bye May cooperate in dressing and in feeding himself; uses a cup
6 months	At this age the typical child: Rolls over Shows no head lag when pulled to a sitting position Sits with support or leans forward on his hands when placed in a sitting position; begins to demonstrate the right- and left-side parachute reflex Bears some weight on the lower extremities Reaches for and grasps objects; by the end of 6 months, transfers objects from hand to hand May be able to hold his own bottle to feed Looks at and may approach tiny objects with a raking movement Plays with his feet	15 months	At this age the typical child: Walks alone, stops and starts, stoops, explores Self-feeds with fingers; drinks well from a cup Has a three- to six-word vocabulary; uses jargon and gestures Scribbles spontaneously Points to one or two body parts on request; understands simple commands Pats a picture in a book and attends to a story being read

Adapted from American Academy of Pediatrics: *Guidelines for health supervision II,* Chicago, 1988, The Association.

Continued.

TABLE 24-6—cont'd

Developmental/Behavioral Milestones

Age	Expectations	Age	Expectations
15 months, cont'd	Indicates wants by pulling, pointing, grunting, or vocalizing Stacks two blocks Gives and takes a toy Hugs	3 years	At this age the typical child: Jumps in place, kicks a ball, balances and stands briefly on one foot Pedals a tricycle Alternates feet when ascending stairs Opens doors Builds a tower of nine cubes; imitates a bridge made of three cubes Demonstrates speech that is mostly intelligible. (The child who fails to speak in sentences or whose speech is unintelligible to strangers should be referred for speech, language, and hearing evaluation.) Knows his name, age, and sex May comprehend "cold," "tired," "hungry," and may understand the prepositions "on" and "under"; differentiates "bigger" and "smaller"; can convey the use of a ball, scissors, key, and pencil Copies a circle, may imitate a cross, and begins to visually discriminate colors Describes action in picture books Puts on some clothing and shoes Feeds himself
18 months	At this age the typical child: Walks fast, may run stiffly, walks up stairs with one hand held, walks backward, sits in a small chair, climbs into an adult chair, kicks and throws a ball Stacks three or four blocks; may place rings on a cone, then dump them and try again Turns single pages in book or magazine; looks selectively at pictures and names some objects Uses a vocabulary of 4 to 10 words with specificity; may combine two-word phrases; understands and follows some simple directions; may voice two or more wants; shows an imitative vocabulary greater than his vocabulary of spontaneously used words; identifies (points to) some body parts on request Pulls a toy Feeds himself, uses a spoon appropriately, holds and drinks from a cup adequately Imitates a crayon stroke on paper May dump a raisin from a bottle without previous demonstration Holds and "loves" a doll or stuffed animal; may use a household-type toy (e.g., toy telephone) functionally Puckers lips and kisses parent on the cheek		
24 months	At this age the typical child: Climbs and descends steps alone, one step at a time, holding the stair rail or the parent's hand Opens doors, climbs on furniture, uses a spoon and cup well, kicks a ball, throws overhand Stacks five or six cubes and aligns two or three blocks after demonstration May have a vocabulary of at least 20 words, although language development shows great variability at this age; makes two-word phrases with pronouns; refers to herself by name (If speech is unintelligible or delayed, consider referral for developmental assessment including speech and hearing evaluations.) Responds to two-part verbal commands Spontaneously makes or imitates horizontal and circular strokes with a crayon Shows interest in bowel and bladder control Enjoys imitating adults Shows interest in helping the parent dress her; washes and dries hands Uses a toy appropriately (e.g., hammers pegs in a cobbler's bench)	4 years	At this age the typical child: Alternates feet when descending stairs, hops, jumps forward, can stand on one foot for 3 to 5 seconds Climbs a ladder Rides a tricycle Can walk on tiptoes Holds and uses a pencil with good control Builds a tower of ten or more cubes Has the ability to cut and paste Engages in conversational give-and-take Asks why, when, how, and inquires about the meaning of words May name three or four primary colors Counts from 1 to 5; can sing a song Enjoys jokes Washes and dries hands and brushes teeth Dresses and undresses with supervision except for handling laces and buttons, if allowed sufficient time to dress; may begin to be selective about clothes Initiates dramatic make-believe and dressing-up play in which the child assumes a specific role Is imaginative and intensely curious Has formed gender identification Copies a cross and a circle Draws a person with two to three parts Enjoys the companionship of other children, plays cooperatively, and shows interest in other children's bodies Meets the challenges of kindergarten class

TABLE 24-6—cont'd

Developmental/Behavioral Milestones

Age	Expectations	Age	Expectations
5 years	At this age the typical child: Skips, walks on tiptoes, broad jumps Can cut and paste Names four or five colors and can identify coins Tells a simple story and knows several nursery rhymes Defines at least one word (e.g., "ball," "shoe," "chair," "table," "dog") Dresses and undresses without supervision Copies a triangle from an illustration Recognizes most letters of the alphabet Draws a person with a head, body, arms, and legs Begins to understand right and wrong, fair and unfair Engages in dramatic make-believe and dressing-up play, in which the child assumes a specific role; engages in domestic role-playing Enjoys the companionship of other children; plays cooperatively Has formed gender identification ("Are you a boy or a girl?")	6 years, cont'd	Rides a bicycle Ties her shoelaces Counts up to 10, prints her first name, prints numbers up to 10 Knows right from left Draws a person with six body parts, with the figure depicted wearing clothing
		8 years	At this age the typical child: Can tell time (although this may be a 9-year achievement) Can read for pleasure and use a library card Has a sense of humor ("Do you know any good jokes? What's your favorite joke?") Is concerned about rules and good (fair) vs. bad (unfair) Cares for room and belongings; can take responsibility for home chores
6 years	At this age the typical child: Bounces a ball four to six times, throws and catches Skates	10 years	At this age, the child may be expected to: Display self-confidence with a sense of mastery and pride in school and extracurricular activities Make a few friends and participate in group activities Understand and comply with most rules at home and at school Assume reasonable responsibility for health, schoolwork, and chores

questions parents/child may have about masturbation, menstruation, nocturnal emissions, development of secondary sex characteristics, dating, and sexual urges and activity
5. Medications taken regularly
   a. By practitioner's prescription
   b. By self-prescription (over-the-counter or use of prescription medications)

Developmental data. Chapter 3 discusses the assessment of the development of the child in detail. The history of the child's development is a component of that assessment and should provide clues that indicate when a more formal assessment is indicated. Table 24-6 summarizes developmental milestones from birth to age 10 years. The initial history should include the following information:
1. Age at which the child attained specific developmental achievements:
   a. Held head erect
   b. Rolled over
   c. Sat alone
   d. Walked alone
   e. Said first words
   f. Used sentences
   g. Controlled feces
   h. Learned urinary continence
2. Current developmental performance. Assess developmental performance by asking specific questions related to expected abilities for the child's age range (see Table 24-6). You may want to ask a broad question ("What new things have you noticed your child doing since the last visit?") followed by a more specific question ("Has he rolled over yet?"). You may also determine development by use of a screening tool such as the Denver Developmental Screening Test II (see Figure 3-1).
3. Any periods of decreased or increased growth. Was this area evaluated? Were there any known or suspected causes for such growth

(family stress, illness, etc.)? These questions can be asked either during the nutritional assessment or at this time.

4. Questions concerning developmentally appropriate activities (e.g., peer relationships, school achievement, dating) may be covered in the review of systems but are also appropriate to address here.

Nutritional data. Questions regarding nutrition vary according to the child's age. More detailed and specific information may be obtained for the infant, who is growing rapidly, than for the older child.

Early infancy (birth to 6 months)
1. Type of feeding (breast-feeding, brand of commercial formula, or home-prepared formula)
2. Frequency of feedings
3. Amount consumed with each feeding and during a 24-hour period. Be specific in terms of number of ounces per feeding, number and size of cans of formula used per day, type of formula and how formula is prepared (add water to concentrate versus ready to pour from can), and number of times and length of breast-feeding sessions per day
4. Any changes in feeding (e.g., from breast-feeding to bottle-feeding or addition of a supplementary bottle if breast-feeding, date of change, introduction of solids)
5. Any problems observed with feeding (e.g., colic or spitting up)
6. How long the mother plans to continue breast-feeding or bottle-feeding
7. Vitamin, iron, or fluoride supplements (including name of the preparation, when it was started, amount given, and method of administration)
8. Solid foods, including type (commercially prepared or home prepared), amount given, how they are given (by spoon or in bottle), and frequency

---

EXAMPLES OF MEDICANTS, FOODS, AND SUNDRIES THAT ARE EXCRETED IN BREAST MILK AND MAY BE CONTRAINDICATED DURING BREAST-FEEDING*

Analgesics
  Codeine in habituated doses
  Heroin in habituated doses
  Meperidine in habituated doses
  Morphine in habituated doses
  Propoxyphene in IV
  Sodium salicylate in high doses
Antihistamines
Antimicrobials
  Ampicillin
  Chloramphenicol
  Metronidazole
  Penicillin
  Sulfonamides
  Tetracyclines
Depressants
  Barbiturates
    Long-acting, hypnotic doses
    Short-acting, hypnotic doses
  Others
    Alcohol
    Bromides, hypnotic doses
    Chloral hydrate
    Diazepam
    Reserpine
Diuretics
  Hydrochlorothiazide, chlorothiazide

Hormonal compounds
  Iodides
  Oral contraceptives
  Pregnane beta-diol
  Propylthiouracil
  Thyroid
Anthraquinone derivatives
  Cascara
  Danthron
Social drugs (legal)
  Caffeine
  Tobacco
Social drugs (illegal)
  Cocaine and other abuse drugs: stimulants, depressants, narcotics, psychedelics in high doses
Miscellaneous
  Amethopterin
  Anticoagulants, oral
  Cimetidine
  Cyclophosphamide
  DDT
  Ergotrate maleate
  Fluorides
  Foods: white navy beans, corn, egg white, chocolate, unripe fruit, pickles, peanuts, cottonseed, and wheat
  Gold salts
  Radiopharmaceuticals

Data from Levin R: In Herfindal ET, Hirschman J, editors: *Clinical pharmacy and therapeutics,* Baltimore, 1975, Williams & Wilkins; and from Committee on Drugs: *Pediatrics* 72:375, 1983.
*Refer questions to physician.

9. Water, including amount given, frequency offered, whether given plain or with a sweetener

10. Infant's appetite and reaction to eating

If the infant is breast-feeding, obtain the following information about the mother:

1. How the mother feels she is doing with breast-feeding

2. Any questions or concerns about herself or the baby

3. Any problems with her breasts (discomfort, blisters, chafing, tenderness, etc.)

4. How the mother cares for her breasts

5. Mother's program of daily exercise, rest, diet, and fluid intake

6. Medications being taken (specify name, frequency, purpose, and effectiveness) (see box on p. 758 for a list of drugs known to be excreted in human milk and to have side effects in breast-fed infants)

7. Support she receives from her spouse, family members, and/or friends

8. How long she plans to breast-feed and when (or if) she wants to introduce bottle-feeding

9. If using supplementary bottles, is she expressing breast milk or using formula? What kind of formula? How is she storing breast milk? Any problems with expressing milk?

10. Is there any other information that the mother would like (e.g., resources, support groups, lactation consultation)

To determine if the baby is getting enough breast milk, ask the mother:

1. How often the infant wets his or her diaper (should have at least eight wet diapers in a 24-hour period)

2. To describe the baby's bowel movements (should be large amount of yellow stool; may have bowel movements several times a day or every few days)

If the infant is receiving bottle-feedings, ask if he or she is held for all feedings or if the bottle is propped. The infant who receives a bottle of milk or juice at bedtime or naptime, to be used in much the same way as a pacifier, is at risk for dental caries and destruction of the anterior maxillary teeth (referred to as "baby bottle syndrome" [Figure 24-3]). This practice also puts the child at risk for aspiration of fluids and middle ear infections.

Later infancy (6 to 12 months)

During this period the infant is beginning to vigorously manipulate his or her body and the environment. In addition to the questions outlined for the period of early infancy, ask questions regarding the infant's developing skills:

1. Has the infant started using a cup, finger-feeding, or using a spoon?

2. Does the infant receive coarser foods such as junior foods or table foods?
   a. What foods does he or she like?
   b. Has there been any problem (diarrhea, rash) after eating any particular food?
   c. How often does the infant eat solids (meals and snacks)?

3. How does the mother feel about the infant's developing independent feeding behaviors? What are her expectations of the child (e.g., should not make a mess, should be able to use a spoon)?

4. Have there been any feeding problems?

Toddlerhood

During this stage the child's rapid growth rate slows. In addition, the child is experiencing an increased sense of independence and has the ability to feed himself or herself. This is a time when parents often become concerned about decreased food intake and "battles" over feeding can develop. Therefore it is important to ask questions to determine the adequacy of food intake (recognizing that toddlers require smaller amounts of food than most parents realize) and the existence or signs of development of feeding problems.

1. What does the child eat during a typical day?
   a. What foods does he or she like?
   b. Has there been any problem (diarrhea, rash) after eating any particular food?
   c. How often does he or she eat meals and snacks? What are the amounts (e.g., tablespoonfuls number of crackers)
   d. How does he/she feed himself (fingers, spoon, fork, holds cup, is still fed by parent)?

2. How do the parents feel about the toddler's feeding behaviors? What are their expectations

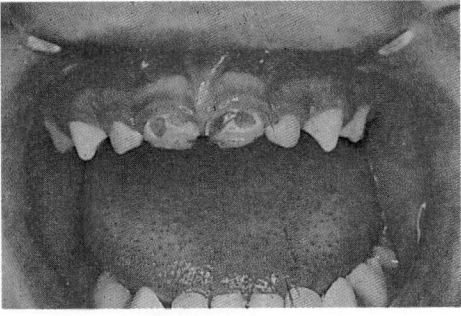

FIGURE 24-3 Nursing-bottle caries in a 20-month-old child. Note extensive carious involvement of the maxillary primary incisors and first molars (Courtesy Drs. Abelson and Cameron, Lutherville, Md.)

of the child (should not make a mess, should be able to use a spoon, fork, etc.)?
3. Have there been any feeding problems?
   a. Have there been any "hunger strikes" (typical of an 18-month-old child)?
   b. Does the child go on "food jags" in which he or she will eat only one type of food?
   c. Is he or she a "picky eater"?
   d. Have there been many struggles for control (parent trying to make the child eat) over eating and how do these resolve?

Preschool age, school age, and adolescence. Chapter 4 discusses the *24-hour recall method* and the *dietary history method,* which are appropriate for obtaining information about the diet and eating habits of the child. A sample form for gathering nutritional data is included at the end of Chapter 4. Find out about the parents' attitudes toward eating and the child's eating pattern and the parents' response to any eating problems that might exist. Pay special attention to preadolescents' and adolescents' concerns about being "overweight." Assess for possible eating disorders and crash dieting in addition to general nutrition patterns.

Family health history. The family medical history of the child is similar to the history obtained for the adult client (see Chapter 2). It includes the health and age of the grandparents, maternal and paternal aunts and uncles, parents, and siblings and the age at death and cause of death for deceased relatives. In addition, the pediatric family history should include information about miscarriages and stillbirths, congenital defects, and familial diseases.

Outline the family history information (or put it in

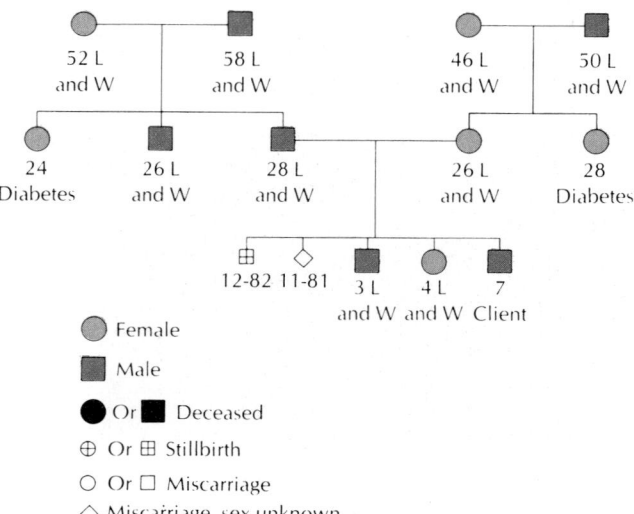

24 Diabetes | 26 L and W | 28 L and W | 26 L and W | 28 Diabetes

● Female
■ Male
● Or ■ Deceased
⊕ Or ⊞ Stillbirth
○ Or □ Miscarriage
◇ Miscarriage, sex unknown

FIGURE 24-4 Family tree used in a pediatric history.

the form of a family tree) to identify any illnesses or problems that may have implications for the child's future health and current health. The family tree, which is similar to the pedigree used in a genetic study, allows a study of the patterns of distribution of genetic traits in kindred people. When the information obtained in the family history reveals suspected genetic problems, refer the child and the parents to a specialist in genetics for diagnosis and counseling. Figure 24-5 illustrates a family tree for a pediatric client.

Review of systems. The review of systems is essentially the same as that for the adult history (see Chapter 2) except for age-appropriate modifications. The general format remains the same.

Physical systems
General (additional questions)
Recent and significant gain or loss of weight, failure to gain weight appropriate for age, or failure to increase in height
Changes in behavior
Behavior changes such as increased crying, irritability, nervousness, or withdrawal or changes in sleep patterns. These questions are usually found under the review of the central nervous system in the adult history. However, behavior changes in children may represent the first symptoms of a problem in any physical system or may indicate psychosocial problems, including abuse and neglect.
Skin (additional questions)
Birthmarks, rashes, acne
Head
Injuries, headaches
Eyes (additional questions)
Strabismus, discharge, vision disturbance (ask about behaviors that might be indicative of problems, such as sitting very close to the television, writing with head near the desk, rubbing the eyes)
Ears (additional questions)
Ear infections, earaches, hearing loss (note loud speech, delayed speech, need to repeat questions), previous hearing tests
Nose (additional questions)
Constant or frequent runny or stuffy nose (unilateral or bilateral), type of rhinorrhea
Mouth and throat (additional questions)
Age of eruption of teeth, cleft lip or cleft palate
Number of teeth at 1 year, thrush
Neck and nodes (additional questions)
Limitation of movement, enlarged nodes
Breasts (deletions and additional questions)
In the newborn there may be breast enlargement secondary to maternal hormones that resolves spontaneously (but may be of concern to the parents).

Stage	Breast development		Development description
1			Preadolescent
2			Breast and papilla elevated as small mound; areolar diameter increased
3			Breast and areola enlarged; no contour separation
4			Areola and papilla form secondary mound
5			Mature; nipple projects areolar part of general breast contour

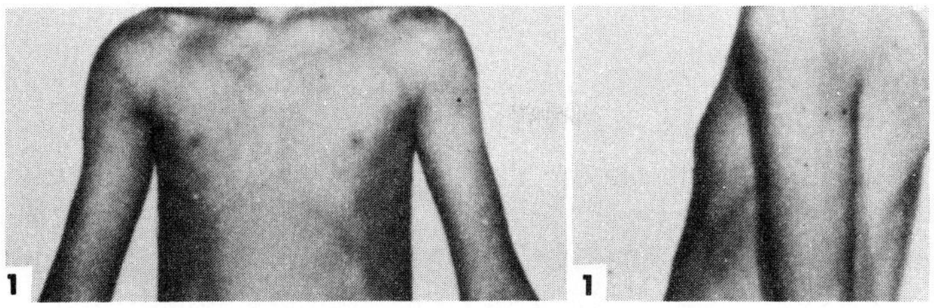

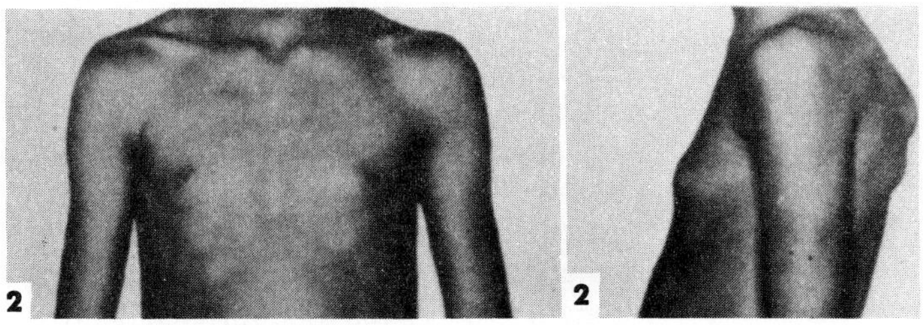

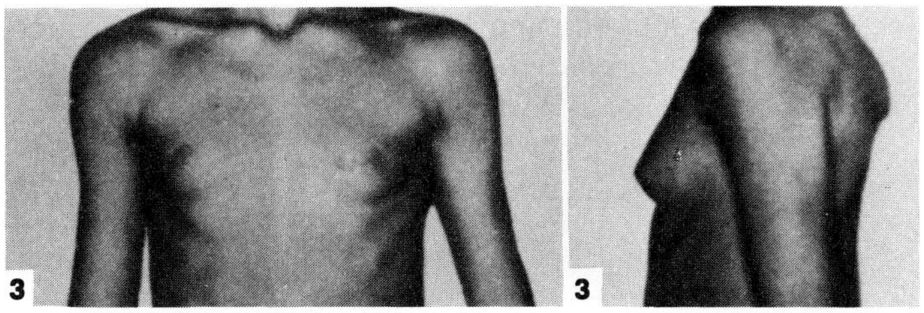

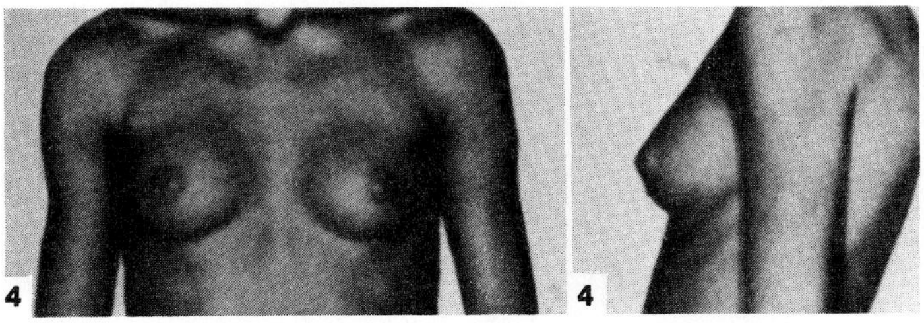

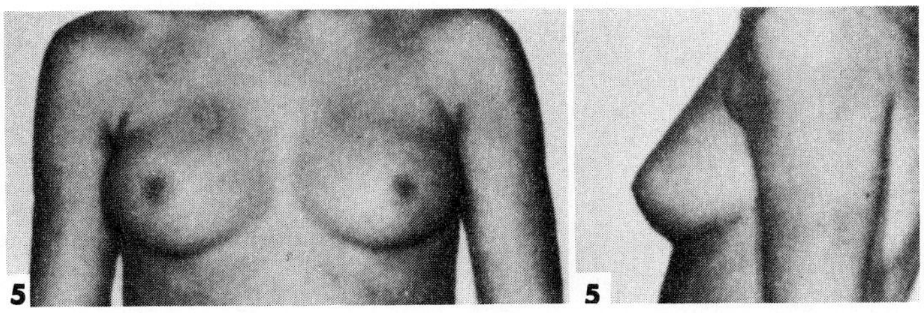

FIGURE 24-5 Maturational sequence in girls. (From Tanner JM: *Growth at adolescence,* ed 2, Oxford, 1962, Blackwell Scientific Publications.)

Ask the preadolescent and the adolescent boy or girl if he or she has noticed changes in the breasts. (Figure 24-5 describes the normal stages of breast development in girls. Boys may experience some degree of transient gynecomastia during puberty.)

Ask about individual concerns regarding breast development, such as comparisons made with peers or the unequal development of the breasts. This subject may be approached by acknowledging that such concerns are common at this age and stating that you would be happy to answer any questions the adolescent may have. For girls, teach self-breast examination once breast buds have begun to develop.

Respiratory (additional questions)

Stridor, wheezing, episodes of croup, frequent colds, nighttime coughing, reduced exercise tolerance. Does child play as actively as other children or curtail strenuous exercise?

Cardiovascular systems (additional questions)

History of heart murmur and any evaluation and follow-up if murmur is present, fatigue on exertion

Gastrointestinal system

Abdominal pain, constipation, diarrhea, change in continence, toilet training and "accidents"

Genital system (deletions and additional questions)

Male

Ask the preadolescent and adolescent male questions about the development of the secondary sex characteristics (Figures 24-6 and 24-7 describe normal changes). This discussion also provides an opportunity to teach about the normal changes that have or are going to occur and to reassure the client that what he is experiencing is normal. Characteristics to ask about include the following:

Appearance of hair on face and body
Appearance of axillary hair
Appearance of pubic hair
Increase in size of testes
Testicular self-examination (teach client)

Ask about individual concerns regarding sexual development. An effective approach is to universalize concerns. For example, say: "Many boys your age have questions about.... What questions would you like me to answer?" Delete the question about impotence until it is determined that the young man is sexually active.

Development	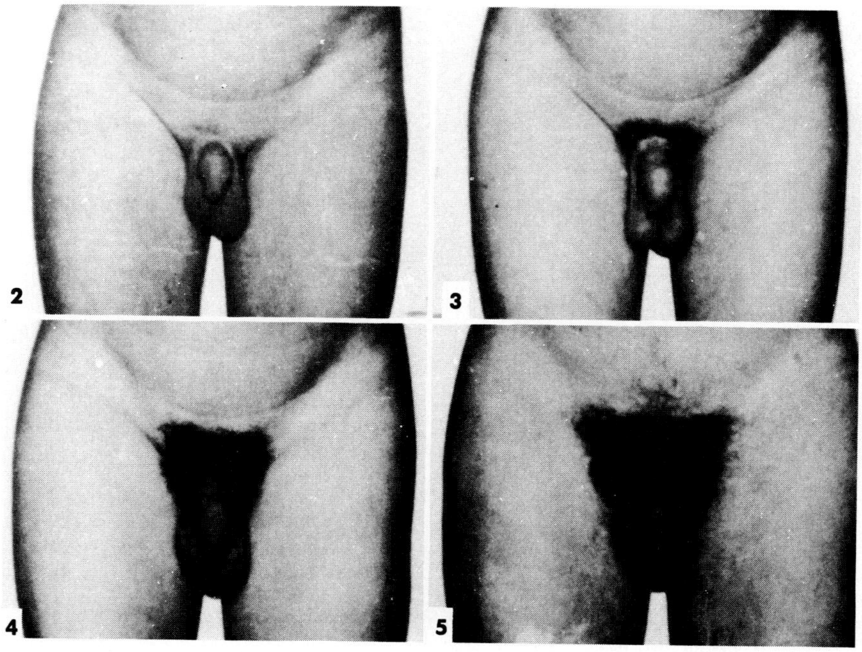	Stage	Description
		1	None; preadolescent
		2	Scant, long, slightly pigmented
		3	Darker, starting to curl small amount
		4	Resembles adult, but less quantity; coarse, curly
		5	Adult distribution, spread to medial surface of thighs

FIGURE 24-6 Pubic hair development in males. (From Tanner JM: *Growth at adolescence,* ed 2, Oxford, 1962, Blackwell Scientific Publications.)

Female

Ask the preadolescent and adolescent female questions about the development of the secondary sex characteristics (Figure 24-8 describes normal changes). This discussion also offers the chance to teach about the normal changes that have or are going to occur and to reassure the client that what she is experiencing is normal. Characteristics to ask about include the following:

Onset of menses (if menarche has occurred): determine if periods are painful

Appearance of axillary hair

Appearance of pubic hair

Ask about individual concerns regarding sexual development. Again, universalizing the question will make it more comfortable for the teenager to respond: "Many girls your age have questions about. . . . What questions would you like me to answer?"

Delete the questions about obstetrical history until you determine that the girl is sexually active.

Delete the question about Pap tests until the girl is 15 years of age unless you determine that (1) the girl younger than 15 years is sexually active or (2) was exposed to DES (diethylstilbestrol) before birth and has begun to menstruate.

Both sexes

You should ask questions about sexual activity and sexually transmitted diseases once the child is about 10 years old. Explain the reason that the questions must

Development	Stage	Description
	1	Penis, testes, and scrotum preadolescent
	2	Enlargement of scrotum and testes, texture alteration; scrotal sac reddens; penis usually does not enlarge
	3	Further growth of testes and scrotum; penis enlarges and becomes longer
	4	Continued growth of testes and scrotum; scrotum becomes darker; penis becomes longer; glans and breadth increase in size
	5	Adult in size and shape

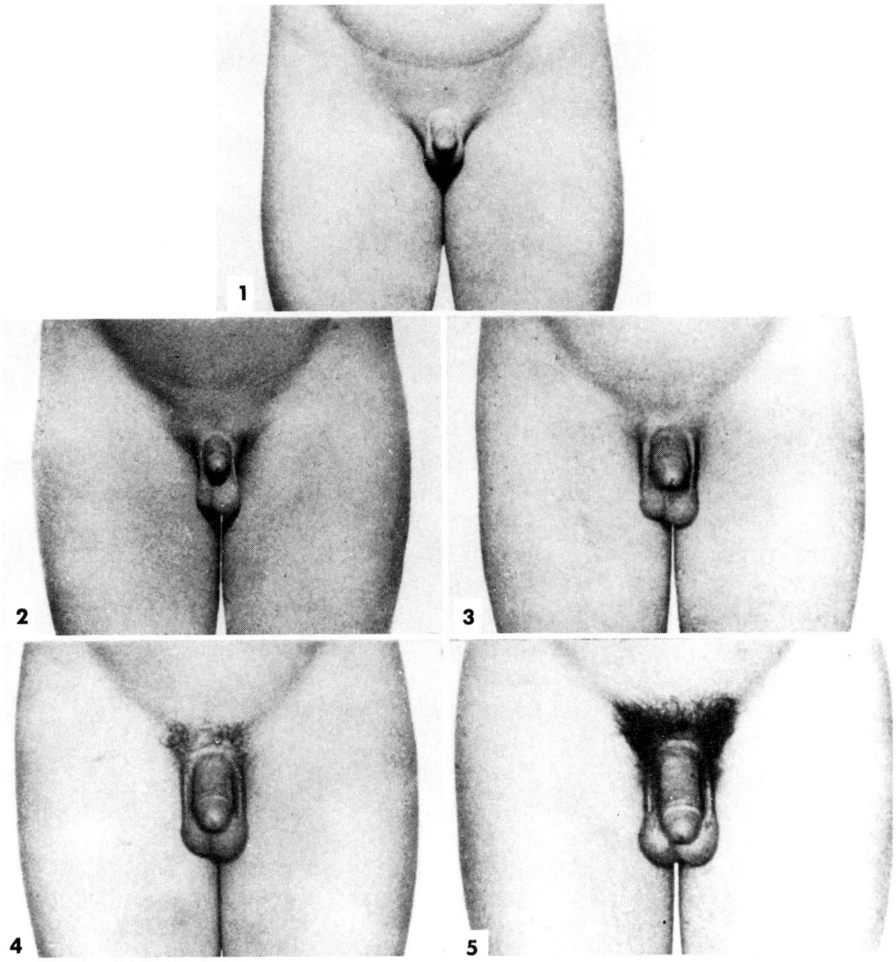

FIGURE 24-7 Penis and testes/scrotum development in males. (From Tanner JM: *Growth at adolescence*, ed 2, Oxford, 1962, Blackwell Scientific Publications.)

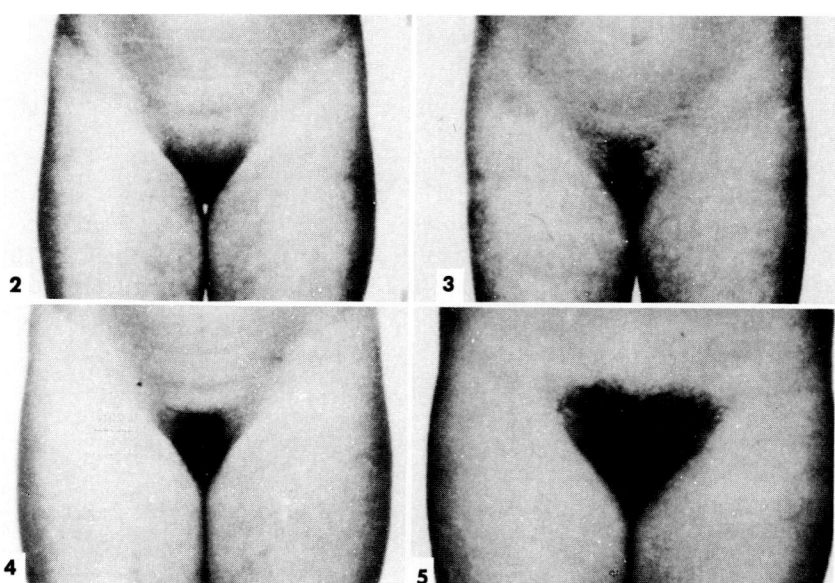

1	None; preadolescent
2	Sparse, lightly pigmented, straight along medial border of labia
3	Darker, beginning to curl, increased amount
4	Coarse, curly, abundant amount but less than adult
5	Adult female triangle, spread to medial surface of thighs

FIGURE 24-8 Pubic hair development in females. (From Tanner JM: *Growth at adolescence*, ed 2, Oxford, 1962, Blackwell Scientific Publications.)

be asked. Discuss "safer" sexual practices, contraception, and the option of abstinence, particularly if the client is sexually active.

Extremities and musculoskeletal system (additional questions)

"Growing pains"
Postural deformities or changes
Changes in gait
Injuries to muscles or joints

Central nervous system (additional questions)

Ability to concentrate, hyperactivity, headaches
Additional information about this system will be obtained in the developmental history and social history.

Sociological system

1. Relationship with family and significant others (can be done in the form of a family tree or genogram)
   a. Client's position in the family (birth order), natural child or adopted *(addition)*
   b. Person(s) with whom client lives
   c. Persons with whom client relates (Who is the primary caretaker? What are arrangements for baby-sitters? Does the child have special friends?)
   d. Recent family crises or changes (should include history of parental divorce, separation, or remarriage and birth or adoption of siblings)
2. Environment
   a. Home (Heated? Adequate hot water? Well or city water? Number of rooms, toilets, cooking facilities? Where does child play?)
   b. Neighborhood: safety issues, play areas, sense of community
   c. Recent changes in environment
   d. To what degree are cultural and religious practices observed?
3. Occupational history (if appropriate)
   a. Jobs held
   b. Satisfaction with present and past employment
   c. Current place of employment
   d. Future goals concerning occupation, career, etc.
4. Economic status and resources
   a. Parents' occupations and sources of income
   b. Parents' perception of adequacy or inadequacy of income
   c. Arrangements for child care while parent(s) are at work; type of care (baby-sitter, child care center, relatives, after-school program),

satisfaction with care, concerns about child care
  d. Effect of child's illness on parents' economic status; plans for "sick child" care if both parents work outside the home
5. Educational level (this area may also be covered in the developmental assessment section)
  a. Name of child's school
  b. Current grade level. Has child ever been held back?
  c. Judgment of intellect relative to age (parent may be asked to make this judgment by asking how this child performs compared with siblings or other children of the same age)
  d. Satisfaction with school, relationships with teacher, etc.
  e. Concerns about school performance
6. Daily profile
  a. Sleep, rest, activity patterns
  b. Social activities (play activities)
  c. Special weekend activities
  d. Recent changes in daily activities

  e. Parental concerns and management of any specific behavior, such as masturbation, thumb-sucking, nail-biting, temper tantrums, or bed-wetting
7. Patterns of health care
  a. Private and public primary care agencies
  b. Dental care
  c. Preventive care
  d. Emergency care

Psychological system. The outline for the psychological system review provided in Chapter 2 (and repeated here) is appropriate for use with the child and parent with the addition of information about the child's personality style. Include both the parent and the child because it will be the parent who is primarily responsible for the child's care during the childhood years. The adolescent child will be more responsible for self-care but will continue to need direction and support from an informed, understanding parent.

You can describe personality in general terms such as outgoing or shy. One way of describing personality that practitioners have found useful in working with families is to identify the child's behavioral or temperament style. Temperament refers to the way an indi-

ATTRIBUTES OF TEMPERAMENT

Activity—level of physical motion during activity, such as sleep, eating, play, dressing, and bathing.

Rhythmicity—regularity in the timing of physiological functions, such as hunger, sleep, and elimination.

Approach-withdrawal—nature of initial responses to a new stimulus, such as people, situations, places, foods, toys, and procedures. *Approach* responses are positive, displayed by activity or expression; *withdrawal* responses are negative expressions or behaviors.

Adaptability—ease or difficulty with which the child adapts or adjusts to new or altered situations.

Threshold of responsiveness (sensory threshold)—amount of stimulation, such as sounds or light, required to evoke a response in the child.

Intensity of reaction—energy level of the child's reactions, regardless of quality or direction.

Mood—amount of pleasant, happy, friendly behavior compared with unpleasant, unhappy, crying, unfriendly behavior exhibited by the child in various situations.

Distractibility—ease with which a child's attention or direction of behavior can be diverted by external stimuli.

Attention span and persistence—length of time a child pursues a given activity *(attention)* and the continuation of an activity in spite of obstacles *(persistence).*

From Whaley LF, Wong DL: *Nursing care of infants and children,* ed 4, St Louis, 1991, Mosby—Year Book.

BEHAVIOR PROFILES

Easy child

Easygoing children are even-tempered, regular, and predictable in their habits and have a positive approach to new stimuli. They are open and adaptable to change and display a mild to moderately intense mood that is typically positive.

Difficult child

Difficult children are highly active, irritable, and irregular in their habits. Negative withdrawal responses are typical, and they require a more structured environment. These children adapt slowly to new routines, people, or situations. Mood expressions are usually intense and primarily negative. They exhibit frequent periods of crying, and frustration often produces violent tantrums.

Slow-to-warm-up child

Slow-to-warm-up children typically react negatively and with mild intensity to new stimuli and, unless pressured, adapt slowly with repeated contact. They respond with only mild but passive resistance to novelty or changes in routine. They are quite inactive and moody but show only moderate irregularity in functions.

From Whaley LF, Wong DL: *Nursing care of infants and children,* ed 4, St Louis, 1991, Mosby—Year Book.

vidual deals with new situations and life in general. Chess and Thomas (1986) have identified nine temperament categories (box, p. 765) that can be combined to form three behavior profiles—the easy child, the difficult child, and the slow-to-warm-up child (box, p. 765). These patterns appear to exist over long periods and may affect the child's adjustment to a variety of childhood situations. Chess and Thomas emphasize that the style itself is not problematic; it is the degree of "fit" between the child's style and his or her environment, in particular the parents, that determines the degree of difficulty experienced. Direct interventions at helping parents to understand their child's style and to work with it rather than against it.

In assessment of the adolescent client (age 12 years and older), it is important to explore some additional areas, including depression and suicide potential, involvement with drugs and alcohol, and sexuality. The boxes on this page and Table 24-7 give suggestions for what to cover and how to get the most information in the adolescent interview. Always inform teenage clients that the information that they share will be kept confidential unless they or someone else is in danger of physical harm. At the same time, encourage teens to talk with their parents about these issues.

SUICIDE RISK/DEPRESSION SCREENING

1. Sleep disorders (usually induction problems; also early/frequent waking or greatly increased sleep and complaints of increasing fatigue)
2. Appetite/eating behavior change
3. Feelings of "boredom"
4. Emotional outbursts and highly impulsive behavior
5. History of withdrawal/isolation
6. Hopeless/helpless feelings
7. History of past suicide attempts, depression, psychological counseling
8. History of No. 7 in family or peers
9. History of drug/alcohol abuse, acting-out/crime, recent change in school performance
10. History of recurrent serious "accidents"
11. Psychosomatic symptomatology
12. Suicidal ideation (including significant current and past losses)
13. Decreased affect on interview, avoidance of eye contact—depression posturing
14. Preoccupation with death (clothing, music, media, art)

From Goldenring JM, Cohen E: Getting into adolescent heads, *Contemp Pediatr* 5:75-86, 1988.

THE HEADS PSYCHOSOCIAL INTERVIEW FOR ADOLESCENTS

Home

Who lives with patient? Where?
Own room?
What are relationships like at home?
What do parents and relatives do for a living?
Ever institutionalized? Incarcerated?
Recent moves? Running away?
New people in home environment?

Education and employment

School/grade performance—any recent changes? any dramatic past changes?
Favorite subjects—worst subjects? (include grades)
Any years repeated/classes failed?
Suspension, termination, dropping out?
Future education/employment plans/goals?
Any current or past employment?
Relations with teachers, employers—school/work attendance?
Recent change of schools—number of schools in last 4 years?

Activities

With peers (what do you do for fun? where and when?)
With family or clubs?
Sports—regular exercise?

Church attendance, clubs, projects?
Hobbies—other home activities?
Reading for fun—what?
TV—how much weekly—favorite shows?
Favorite music?
Does patient have car, use seat belts?
History of arrests—acting-out—crime?

Drugs

Use by peers? Use by patient? (include alcohol/tobacco)
Use by family members? (include alcohol/tobacco)
Amounts, frequency, patterns of use/abuse, and car use while intoxicated?
Source—how paid for?

Sexuality

Orientation?
Degree and types of sexual experience and acts?
Number of partners?
Masturbation? (Normalize)
History of pregnancy/abortion?
Sexually transmitted diseases—knowledge and prevention?
Contraception? Frequency of use?
Comfort with sexual activity, enjoyment/pleasure obtained?
History of sexual/physical abuse

From Goldenring JM, Cohen E: Getting into adolescent heads, *Contemp Pediatr* 5:75-86, 1988.

TABLE 24-7

Opening Lines—Good and Bad

	Poor	Better	Reason
Home	Tell me about mom and dad.	Where do you live, and who lives there with you?	Parent(s) may have died or left the home. Open-ended question enables one to collect "environmental" as well as personal history.
Education	How are you doing in school?	What are you good at in school? What is hard for you? What grades do you get?	Poor questions can be answered "okay." Good questions ask for information about strengths and weaknesses and allow for quantification/objectification.
Activities	Do you have any activities outside of school?	What do you do for fun? What things do you do with friends? What do you do with your free time?	Good questions are open-ended and allow patient to express himself.
Drugs	Do you do drugs?	Many young people experiment with drugs, alcohol, or cigarettes. Have you or your friends ever tried them? What have you tried?	Good question is an expression of concern with specific follow-up. With younger teens, it is best to begin by asking about friends.
Sexuality	Have you ever had sex? Tell me about your boyfriend/girlfriend.	Have you ever had a sexual relationship with anyone? Most young people become interested in sexual relationships at your age. Have you had any with boys, girls, or both? Tell me about your sex life.	What does the term "have sex" really mean to teenagers? Asking only about heterosexual relationships closes doors at once.

From Goldenring JM, Cohen E: Getting into adolescent heads, *Contemp Pediatr* 5:75-86, 1988.

1. Personality: How does the parent describe the child's general characteristics? What are his or her temperament characteristics (see box, p. 765)? How does this influence the child's interactions with family, friends, peers, etc.?
2. Cognitive abilities (for the child, this information may be included in the developmental assessment)
   a. Comprehension
   b. Learning patterns
   c. Memory
3. Response to illness and health
   a. Reaction to illness
   b. Coping patterns
   c. Value of health
   d. Use of well-child and health promotion services
4. Response to care
   a. Perceptions of the caregivers
   b. Compliance
5. Cultural implications for care
   a. Patterns of therapy
   b. Beliefs about child care and child-rearing
   c. Patterns of illness response

Anticipatory guidance. As noted earlier in the chapter, anticipatory guidance should be addressed at each visit. This area includes evaluating the parents' understanding of child development and education, upcoming developmental changes, and questions or issues of concern. The focus should be individualized to the family's needs. In addition, information about child safety (e.g., child-proofing the home, use of bicycle helmets, seat belts) (Figure 24-9) needs to be communicated. This information is most effective when it is offered just before a developmental change is about to occur. The boxes on pp. 768-769 and 770 provide guidelines for such information.

Anticipatory guidance information may be most easily integrated into other parts of the health history. For example, when you are getting information about the child's current developmental achievements, you can tell the parent what to look for over the next few months. For example, "Now that your baby has started to crawl, you can expect that he will start to explore new and potentially dangerous areas of your home." This approach can lead to a discussion of safety concerns that the parent will need to consider related to the child's mobility and ability to get into things (e.g., safety gates, plugs for electrical outlets, door/cupboard latches, need for syrup of ipecac).

Preparation for the Examination: Client and Environment

How you conduct the interview and physical examination will vary according to the child's age, develop-

ANTICIPATORY GUIDANCE TOPICS

Prenatal and newborn

Prenatal visit

Health: pregnancy course, worries, tobacco, alcohol, drug use, hospital and pediatric office procedures
Safety: infant care seat, crib safety
Nutrition: planned feeding method
Child care: help after birth, later arrangements
Family: changes in relationships (spouse, siblings), supports, stresses, return to work

Newborn visits

Health: jaundice, umbilical cord care, circumcision, other common problems, when to call the physician's office
Safety: infant car seat, smoke detector, choking, keeping tap water temperature below 120° F
Nutrition: feeding, normal weight loss, spitting, vitamin and fluoride supplements
Development/behavior: individuality, "consolability," visual and auditory responsiveness
Child care: importance of interaction, parenting books, support for primary caregiver
Family: postpartum adjustments, fatigue, "blues," special time for siblings

First year

0 to 6 months

Health: immunizations, exposure to infections
Safety: falls, aspiration of small objects or powder, entanglement in mobiles with long strings, curtain cords
Nutrition: supplementation of breast milk or formula, introduction of solids, iron
Development/behavior: crying/colic, irregular schedules (eating, sleeping, eliminating), responding to infant cues, reciprocity, interactive games, beginning eye-hand coordination
Child care: responsive and affectionate care, caregiving schedule
Family: return to work, the nurturing of all family relationships (spouse and siblings)

12 months

Safety: locks for household poisons and medications, gates for stairs, ipecac, poison center telephone number; outlet safety covers; avoid dangling cords or tablecloths; safety devices for windows/screens, toddler car seat at 20 pounds; avoid toys with small detachable pieces; supervise child in tub or near water
Nutrition: discourage use of bottle as a pacifier or while in bed; offer cup and soft finger foods (with supervision); introduce new foods one at a time
Development/behavior: attachment, basic trust versus mistrust, stranger awareness, night waking, separation anxiety, bedtime routine, transitional object
Child care: prohibitions few but firm and consistent across caregiving settings; discipline defined as "learning" (not punishment)
Family: spacing of children

Second year

2 years

Health: immunizations
Safety: climbing and falls common; supervise outdoor play; ensure safety caps on medicine bottles; note dangers of plastic bags, pan handles hanging over stove, and space heaters
Nutrition: avoid feeding conflicts (decreased appetite common); period of self-feeding, weaning from breast or bottle; avoid sweet or salty snacks
Development/behavior: autonomy versus shame/doubt, ambivalence (independence/dependence), tantrums, negativism, getting into everything, night fears, readiness for toilet training, self-comforting behaviors (thumb sucking, masturbation), speech, imaginative play, no sharing in play, positive reinforcement for desired behavior
Child care: freedom to explore in safe place; day care; home a safer place to vent frustrations; needs show of affection, language stimulation through reading and conversation
Family: sibling relationships

ANTICIPATORY GUIDANCE TOPICS—CONT'D

Preschool

2 to 5 years

Health: tooth brushing, first dental visit

Safety: needs close supervision near water or street; home safety factors include padding of sharp furniture corners, fire escape plan for home, and locking up power tools; should have car lap belt at 40 pounds and bike helmet; should know (a) name, address, and telephone number, (b) not to provoke dogs, and (c) to say "no" to strangers

Nutrition: balanced diet; avoid sweet or salty snacks; child should participate in conversation at meals

Development/behavior: initiative versus guilt; difficulty with impulse control and sharing; developing interest in peers, high activity level; speaking in sentences by age 3; speech mostly intelligible to stranger by age 3, reading books; curiosity about body parts; magical thinking, egocentrism

Child care/preschool: needs daily special time with parent(s), bedtime routine; talk about day in day-care; limit TV and watch with child, reprimand privately, answer questions factually and simply; adjustment to preschool, kindergarten readiness

Family: chores, responsibilities

Middle childhood

5 to 10 years

Health: appropriate weight; regular exercise; somatic complaints (limb and abdominal pain, headaches); alcohol, tobacco, and drug use; sexual development; physician and child dealings (more direct)

Safety: bike helmets and street safety; car seat belts; swimming lessons; use of matches, firearms, and power tools; fire escape plan for home; saying "no" to strangers

Nutrition: balanced diet, daily breakfast, limited sweet and salty snacks, moderate fatty foods

Development/behavior: industry versus inferiority, need for successes, peer interactions, adequate sleep

School: school performance, homework, parent interest

Family: more time away but continuing need for family support, approval, affection, time together, and communication; family rules about bedtime, chores, and responsibilities; guidance in using money; parent(s) should encourage reading; limit TV watching and discuss programs seen together

Other activities: organized sports, religious groups, other organizations, use of spare time

Adolescence

Discuss with adolescent

Health: alcohol, tobacco, and drug use, dental care, physical activity, immunizations

Safety: bike and skateboard helmet and safety, car seat belts, driving while intoxicated, water safety, hitchhiking, risk-taking

Nutrition: balanced diet, appropriate weight, avoidance of junk foods

Sexuality: physical changes, sex education, peer pressure for sexual activity, sense of responsibility for self and partner, OK to say no, prevention of pregnancy and sexually transmitted diseases, breast and testes self-examination

Development/relationships: identity versus role confusion, family, peers, dating, independence, trying different roles

School: academics, homework

Other activities: sports, hobbies, organizations, jobs

Future plans: school, work, relationships with others

Discuss with parent

Communication: let adolescent participate in discussion and development of family rules; needs frequent praise and affection, time together, interest in adolescent's activities

Independence: parent and child ambivalence about independence; expect periods of estrangement; promote self-responsibility and independence; still needs supervision

Role model: actions speak louder than words—parents provide model of responsibile, reasonable, and compassionate behavior

From Foye HR: Anticipatory guidance. In Hoekelman R and others: *Primary pediatric care,* ed 2, St Louis, 1992, Mosby–Year Book.

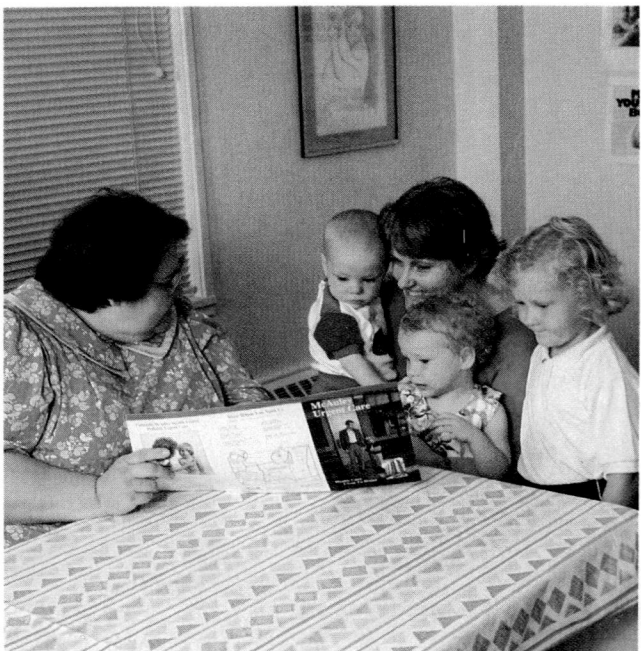

FIGURE 24-9 Anticipatory guidance needs to be addressed at each visit and should be individualized to the family's needs.

PERTINENT INFORMATION FOR ANTICIPATORY GUIDANCE

A. Information about the *child*
   1. Concerns—expressed by parent or child
   2. Health—current status and follow-up of past problems
   3. Routine care—feeding, sleep, and elimination
   4. Development—evaluated by school performance or with standardized tests (e.g., Denver Developmental Screening Test,[6] Early Language Milestone Scale[3])
   5. Behavior—temperament and interaction with family, peers, and others
B. Information about the *child's environment*
   1. Family composition (at home)
   2. Caregiving schedule—who and when
   3. Family stresses—e.g., work, finances, illness, death, move, marital, and other relationships
   4. Family supports—relatives, friends, organizations, material resources
   5. Stimulation in the home
   6. Stimulation/activities outside the home, e.g., preschool/school, peers, organizations
   7. Safety

From Foye Jr HR: Anticipatory guidance. In Hoekelman R and others: *Primary pediatric care,* ed 2, St Louis, 1992, Mosby–Year Book.

ment, and behavior and the type of setting in which the care is being provided. If you do not give consideration to the child's age and development, the examination likely will be incomplete. If the child is fearful or fatigued, you will need to be more creative, patient, and selective (if possible) in performing the examination.

In carrying out a pediatric examination, keep in mind that each visit for health care is a learning experience for the child and the parent(s). The experience may result in increased confidence in themselves and others, or it may produce feelings of failure and distrust toward the professionals who are caring for them. Thus it is important to provide opportunities to develop positive relationships during the visits for routine health care (Figure 24-10). Also, remember that any separation of the child from the parent may provoke anxiety in both parties and may increase their level of fear and distrust. Encourage parents to participate in the examination and support their young child. This participation may be done by holding the child during the examination or by soothing the child in other ways. The older child may be able to participate more freely without the parent present. Most parents will recognize the older child's need to develop independence and encourage the child to participate alone. Finally, prepare the child and the parent for any new or painful procedures. An appre-

ciation for the feelings of children and parents will make them more cooperative.

Developmental approach to examination of child. Conduct the physical examination of the child in an organized and systematic manner, taking into account differences between an adult and a pediatric examination. Perform distressing parts of the examination at the end if you believe that the child will be unable to cooperate. You can alter the order of the examination to accommodate the individual child's behavior, for example, listening to the heart and lungs early in the examination before crying starts or becomes more vigorous. Similarly, you may begin the examination of a child with a body part that is least likely to interfere with developing a sense of trust and confidence, for example, the hands or the eyes. Table 24-8 presents a summary of the different approaches used for the physical examination at different developmental stages.

Infant. Usually little difficulty is encountered in performing the physical examination of the infant in the first 6 months of life since the infant has little fear of

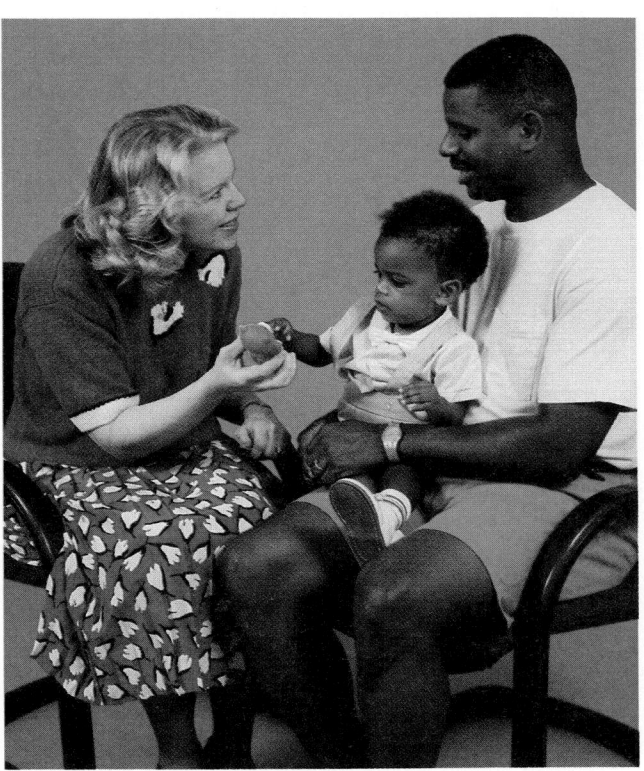

strangers. The parent or the examiner can distract the infant with repetitive vocal sounds and smiles. However, since the examination of the ears and mouth may cause distress, this area should be saved for the end of the examination. Take advantage of the opportunities that are offered. If the infant is quiet or sleepy, start with the auscultation of the chest and do so while the caretaker is still holding the infant. If the infant is playful and active, start with the extremities and wait for a quieter moment to examine the chest.

During the last half of the first year of life, the infant experiences an increasing fear of strangers. In this situation conduct the entire examination while the infant is held on the parent's lap (Figure 24-11). Even under the best of circumstances, creating an ideal situation may not be possible. The infant may remain resistant throughout the examination. If this happens, you need to be efficient in carrying out the examination in the least amount of time and with minimal restraint of the infant. The parent often experiences discomfort or embarrassment because of the infant's behavior and will need reassurance that the infant is behaving normally. The situation is ideal for helping the parent to understand normal development and the needs of the infant at this age.

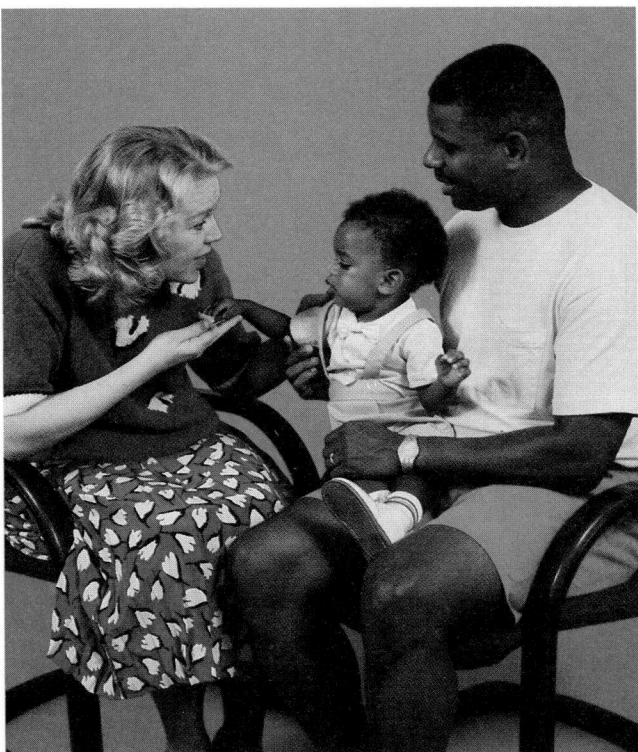

FIGURE 24-10 The physical examination can be a learning experience for both the parent and the child. It is important to listen to the parent's concerns and to assess the child's needs during the interview.

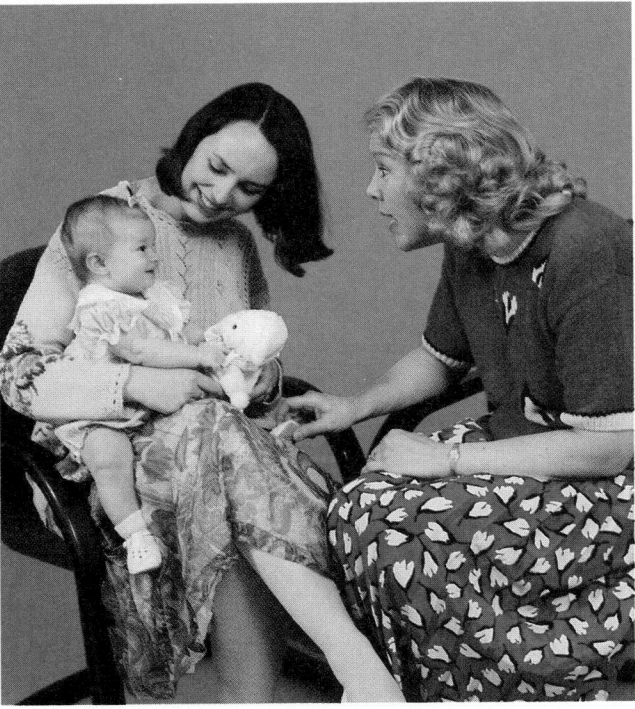

FIGURE 24-11 The interview is a time for the child to become familiar with the examiner as well as a time to gather information.

TABLE 24-8

Developmental Approach to the Pediatric Examination

Age (approximate)	Developmental stage	Position	Sequence	Preparation
Infant 0-6 months	Symbiotic (not fearful of strangers)	Before sits alone: supine or prone, preferably in parent's lap; before 4 to 6 months; can place on examining table After sits alone: use sitting in parent's lap whenever possible If on table, place with parent in full view	If quiet, auscultate heart, lungs, abdomen Record heart and respiratory rates Palpate and percuss same areas Proceed in usual head-toe direction Perform traumatic procedures last (eyes, ears, mouth [while crying], rectal temperature [if taken]) Elicit reflexes as body part examined Elicit Moro reflex last	Completely undress if room temperature permits Leave diaper on male Gain cooperation with distraction, bright objects, rattles, talking Smile at infant; use soft, gentle voice Pacify with bottle of sugar water or feeding Enlist parent's aid for restraining to examine ears, mouth Avoid abrupt, jerky movements
Toddler 6 months-3 years	Separation-individuation (fear of strangers initially followed by toddler clinging to parent)	Sitting or standing on/by parent Prone or supine in parent's lap	Inspect body area through play: "count fingers," "tickle toes" Use minimal physical contact initially Introduce equipment slowly Auscultate, percuss, palpate whenever quiet Perform traumatic procedures last (same as for infant)	Have parent remove outer clothing Remove underwear as body part examined Allow to inspect equipment; demonstrating use of equipment usually ineffective If uncooperative, perform procedures quickly Use restraint when appropriate; request parent's assistance Talk about examination if cooperative; use short phrases Praise for cooperative behavior
Preschool child 3-6 years	Preschool age: age of initiative (period of fantasy play and increasing verbal ability)	Prefers standing or sitting Usually cooperative prone/supine Prefers parent's closeness	If cooperative, proceed in head-toe direction If uncooperative, proceed as with toddler	Request self-undressing Allow to wear underpants if shy Offer equipment for inspection; briefly demonstrate use (may demonstrate on parent) Make up "story" about procedure: "I'm seeing how strong your muscles are" or "I am going to give your arm a hug with this special cloth" (blood pressure) Use paper-doll technique Give choices when possible Expect cooperation; use positive statements: "Open your mouth"

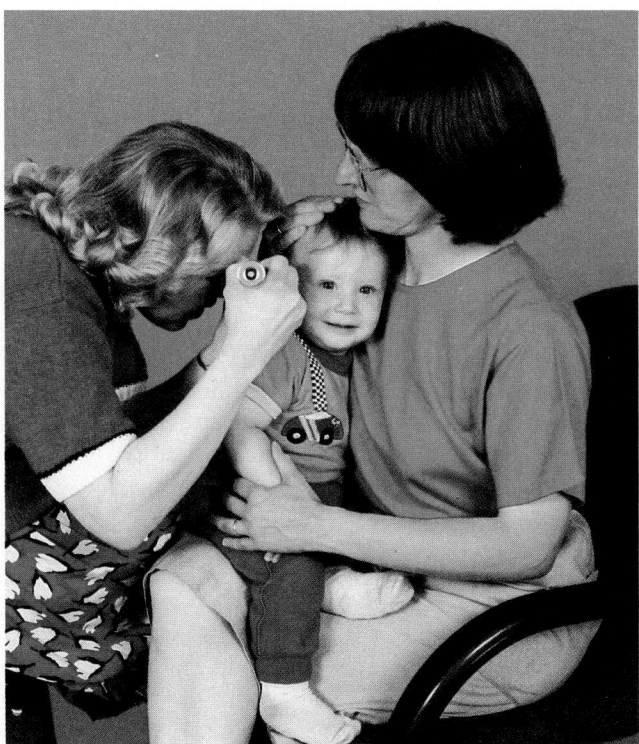

FIGURE 24-16 Restraint using the "hug" restraint.

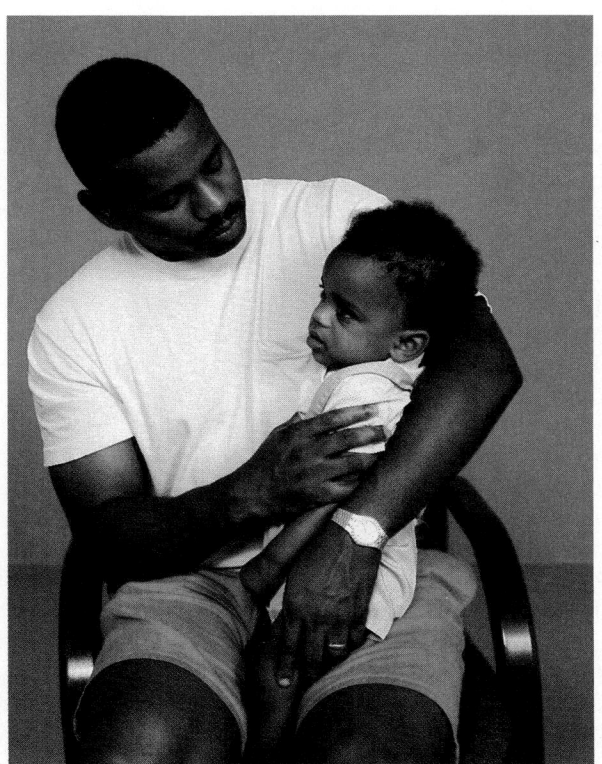

FIGURE 24-17 Restraint of the older child using the leg restraint.

Another method for the older child is sometimes called the "hug." Have the child sit on the parent's lap with the legs to the side and one arm tucked under the parent's arm while the parent holds the child's other arm securely (Figure 24-16). Obtain greater immobility of the child by having the parent place the child's legs between his or her own (Figure 24-17). If the parent is uncomfortable about assisting with restraint, you may ask another adult to help. However, the child usually feels less threatened if the parent does the holding.

Measurements. Take measurements of the temperature, pulse rate, respiratory rate, blood pressure (for children over age 3 years), height, and weight as part of the physical examination of the child. In addition, note the measurements of the head circumference for the child who is less than 3 years of age. Comparing the physical measurements of a child with those of other healthy children over time makes it possible to determine if the child is progressing within normal parameters or if significant deviations exist.

Assessment of vital signs

Temperature. The body areas commonly used for obtaining temperature measurements—the mouth, the axilla, and the rectum, and a more recent approach, the ear canal and tympanic membrane—and types of thermometers are discussed in detail in Chapter 3, General Assessment, and are briefly reviewed here. The child's ability to cooperate and the health status determine the method selected.

AXILLARY TEMPERATURE. You can obtain an axillary temperature on any child. This method reduces the risk of injury and is less intrusive than rectal or oral reading. Use the axillary route, whenever possible, to obtain the newborn infant's temperature. This approach may also be preferable for toddlers and preschoolers. Consider using an axillary temperature when the child objects to the rectal temperature and the oral temperature is not appropriate. Many practitioners recommend using the axillary method first and confirming an elevated temperature with a rectal or oral reading. Place the thermometer tip deep into the axilla and hold the arm close to the body for at least 5 minutes (a digital thermometer reading will be faster). Restrain the child by using the "hug" if necessary.

RECTAL TEMPERATURE. Obtaining a rectal temperature has been a common practice during the first few years of a child's life. However, many now recommend using this method only when no other route can be used. The main drawbacks are the danger of perforation of the rectum in the newborn and young infant and the increased discomfort for the young child, who experiences this as an intrusive procedure. Do not use this method with children who cannot tolerate this kind of stimulus to the CNS, as is the case with some children who have epilepsy, or on children who are on chemotherapy that affects the gastrointestinal mucosa.

A safe restraint method for taking a rectal temperature of a young infant is to lay the child face down on the parent's lap or on a padded table. Have the adult place the left forearm firmly across the child's hip area, so that the child cannot raise the buttocks off the adult's lap or the table. Use the thumb and forefinger of the non-dominant hand to separate the buttocks, and gently insert the lubricated thermometer with the dominant hand. Do not insert the thermometer any farther than 1 in. (2.5 cm). Deeper insertion increases risk of perforation since the colon curves posteriorly at a depth of 1¼ in. (3 cm). The temperature registers within 3 to 4 minutes on a glass thermometer (a digital thermometer reading is much quicker).

The infant's rectum is quite short; therefore insert the thermometer only a short distance. Three considerations help to determine sufficient entry: noting that the column of mercury is rising steadily, inserting no more than 1 in. (2.5 cm), and observing a decrease in the child's effort to push against the thermometer. It is normal for the child to push against the thermometer as the rectal sphincter muscles contract in response to the stimulus. Wait until the sphincter relaxes before continuing to insert. Hold the thermometer firmly enough to keep the child from pushing it out. Use care to hold the thermometer firmly but not to push it in further. Also, hold the child securely to prevent jerking and pushing the thermometer further into the rectum.

ORAL TEMPERATURE. Generally reserve oral temperature reading (with a glass thermometer) for children who are 5 to 6 years of age and older. Younger children may be able to use a digital thermometer. The child must be able to understand not to bite on the glass or digital thermometer and to keep the mouth closed during the procedure. Place the thermometer under the tongue for at least 5 minutes, it can take up to 7 minutes to reach the maximum temperature (for a glass thermometer, a digital thermometer will be much quicker). Sometimes the child's health condition interferes with being able to use this method, for example, mouth breathing or limited intellectual functioning.

TYMPANIC THERMOGRAPHY. A more recent method for taking temperatures is tympanic thermography (see Chapter 8). The tympanic thermometer is placed in the ear canal and uses an infrared sensor to detect the temperature of blood flowing through the eardrum. It registers within 2 seconds. The ease and speed of this approach is making it the preferred method for use in many health care settings.

Temperature regulation is less exact in children than in adults. The rectal temperature is normally higher in infants and younger children, and the average temperature is above 99° F (37.2° C) until age 3 years. When a temperature is being recorded, it is important to indicate the route of measurement (rectal, oral, axillary, tympanic). However, do not add or subtract degrees based on route since there is disagreement as to how much variability in temperature exists. The increase in temperature with even a minor infection is usually greater in infants and young children than in adults. However, young infants with a severe infection may have a normal or subnormal temperature.

Pulse and respiration. Apprehension, crying, and physical activity, as well as the examination procedure itself, can alter a child's heart and respiratory rates. Thus, if possible, take these measurements while the child is at rest, either sleeping or lying quietly. If the child has been active, delay taking the measurement until the child has relaxed for about 5 to 10 minutes. If you must measure the respiratory rate and the heart rate while the child is crying or agitated, note this information next to your recording of the rate.

Examine the child's pulse for rate, rhythm, quality, and amplitude, just as for an adult. Auscultation of the heart—measuring the apical pulse—is the most easily obtained pulse in a young infant. The average heart rate of the infant at birth is 140 beats/min. At 2 years of age the child's heart has adjusted downward to 110. At 10 years the rate is 85, and by the time the child reaches age 18, the pulse may have lowered to 82. A child, usually an adolescent, who engages in exercise regularly, such as swimming laps, may exhibit a much slower rate, that is, in the 60s.

TABLE 24-10

Average Heart Rate for Infants and Children at Rest

Age	Average rate
Birth	140
1st mo	130
1-6 mo	130
6-12 mo	115
1-2 yr	110
2-4 yr	105
6-10 yr	95
10-14 yr	85
14-18 yr	82

TABLE 24-11

Amplitude, Quality of Heart Rate, and Site as They Relate to Differential Diagnosis of Heart Dysfunction in Young Infants and Children

Amplitude, quality, site	Cardiac dysfunction
Narrow, thready	Congestive heart failure
	Severe aortic stenosis
Bounding	Patent ductus arteriosus
	Aortic regurgitation
Pulsation in supra-sternal notch	Aortic insufficiency
	Patent ductus arteriosus
	Coarctation of the aorta
Palpable thrill in suprasternal notch	Aortic stenosis
	Valvular pulmonary stenosis
	Coarctation of aorta, occasionally patent ductus arteriosus

Data from Kempe CH and others: *Current pediatric diagnosis and treatment,* ed 9, Los Altos, Calif, 1987, Lange Medical Publications.

TABLE 24-12

Variations in Respiration with Age

Age	Rate/minute
Premature	40-90
Newborn	30-80
1 yr	20-40
2 yr	20-30
3 yr	20-30
5 yr	20-25
10 yr	17-22
15 yr	15-20
20 yr	15-20

Data from Lowrey GH: *Growth and development of children,* ed 8, St. Louis, 1986, Mosby–Year Book.

Table 24-10 lists the average heart rates for children from birth to 18 years. Heart rhythm in children is not always regular. Often the rate will change in relation to the respiratory cycle. The heart rate accelerates during inspiration because of the increase in pressure in the thoracic cavity and decreases during expiration. This phenomenon, which is called sinus arrhythmia, is considered normal in children. Palpation of the brachial and femoral pulses is an essential step in the examination of the young infant. Irregularities often are the first signs of serious heart dysfunction. The amplitude and rhythm of the femoral pulse are expected to equal those of the brachial pulse. Absence or weakness of the femoral pulse indicates the possibility of **coarctation** of the aorta in the young infant. Table 24-11 compares some differences in amplitude, quality, and site and how they may relate to the differential diagnosis of heart disorders in children.

Obtain the respiratory rate by inspection or auscultation. In infants, respiratory movements are primarily diaphragmatic and are observed by abdominal movement. Since these movements are frequently irregular, you need to count them for a full minute for accuracy. The average range of normal respirations is 30 to 80/min in the newborn period compared with 20 to 30/min in the 2-year-old. By 10 years of age, the respiratory rate has adjusted to 17 to 22/min, and by age 20 it averages 15 to 20/min. Table 24-12 shows variations in respiration with age.

Blood pressure. The levels of systolic and diastolic blood pressure gradually increase during childhood,

and normally a considerable variation exists in a child's pressure. The systolic pressure of the child may be raised by crying, vigorous exercise, or anxiety. Therefore choose a time when the child is quiet and comfortable to obtain this measurement.

The National Task Force on Blood Pressure Control in Children recommends that children 3 years or older have their blood pressure measured annually as part of their regular health care. The child of this age is usually able to cooperate when you explain the procedure for obtaining a blood pressure measurement. Routinely measuring the blood pressure of the child less than 3 years of age is unnecessary unless there are indications of underlying problems such as renal or cardiac disease.

The most common method of measuring the blood pressure of the child is still auscultation with a mercury

---

Helpful Hints for Taking Children's Blood Pressures:

1. *Child should be seated. Take pressure routinely in the right arm held at heart level.*
2. *Do not press too hard with the stethoscope.*
3. *If no pediatric cuff is available, use an adult cuff around the child's thigh and place stethoscope over the popliteal area (behind knee) to hear Korotkoff sounds. This measurement averages about 10 mm Hg higher than blood pressure taken in the arm.*
4. *Refer a child with abnormally high serial readings to a physician.*
5. *Significant hypertension is blood pressure persistently between the 95th and 99th percentile for age and sex.*
6. *Severe hypertension is blood pressure persistently at or above the 99th percentile for age and sex.*

or aneroid sphygmomanometer. The selection of the cuff size and the method of measuring the blood pressure are described in detail in Chapter 8. The size of the cuff is important because a cuff that is too small causes falsely elevated values. Pediatric cuffs are available in several sizes for newborns, infants, and children. A pediatric stethoscope with a small diaphragm is also essential when measuring the blood pressure of a young child. The systolic pressure is recorded as that point at which the Korotkoff sounds are initially heard. The diastolic pressure is recorded for the point at which the fourth-phase Korotkoff sound is heard, when the sound first becomes muffled. The fifth phase Korotkoff sound is the disappearance of all sound. In young children the fourth and fifth sounds frequently occur simultaneously, and sometimes the Korotkoff sounds are heard all the way to zero.

The Doppler instrument, although relatively expensive, is useful with young infants and children. It measures systolic blood pressure, which is the first sound heard. The Doppler device is useful for systolic measurement, but it has not been found to be reliable for diastolic pressure measurement.

If a Doppler instrument is unavailable, you can use the flush method to approximate the mean blood pressure. (This method is rarely used, but it is helpful to know it for situations in which advanced technology is unavailable.) Elevate the extremity, with the uninflated cuff in place. Stroke or milk the arm from the hand to the elbow. Inflate the cuff to a point above the estimated systolic blood pressure. Slowly release the pressure. A sudden reddening or "flush" of the extremity (as compared with the other extremity) will occur at a point about halfway between the systolic and diastolic pressures.

Record the blood pressure measurements on appropriate blood pressure charts, such as those developed by the Second National Task Force on Blood Pressure Control in Children, which were based on studies supported by the National Heart, Lung and Blood Institute. These charts allow you to record the blood pressure measurements in serial fashion, determine how the child compares with other children of the same age, and observe a trend or pattern for the child over time. Hypertension can be diagnosed only after serial readings have been taken. Table 24-13 gives parameters for hypertension classification at different ages.

Growth measurements. The routine measurement of growth is a screening procedure rather than a diagnostic procedure. Yet such measurement can provide clues to serious health problems. Growth is a continuous process that the practitioner must evaluate over time. Successive serial measurements plotted on a standardized growth chart provide objective information about the individual child's rate and pattern of growth

TABLE 24-13

Classification of Hypertension by Age Group

Age group	Significant hypertension (mm Hg): >95%	Severe hypertension (mm Hg): >99%
Newborns (7 d)	Systolic BP ≥96	Systolic BP ≥106
(8-30 d)	Systolic BP ≥104	Systolic BP ≥110
Infants	Systolic BP ≥112	Systolic BP ≥118
(<2 yr)	Diastolic BP ≥74	Diastolic BP ≥82
Children	Systolic BP ≥116	Systolic BP ≥124
(3-5 yr)	Diastolic BP ≥76	Diastolic BP ≥84
Children	Systolic BP ≥122	Systolic BP ≥130
(6-9 yr)	Diastolic BP ≥78	Diastolic BP ≥86
Children	Systolic BP ≥126	Systolic BP ≥134
(10-12 yr)	Diastolic BP ≥82	Diastolic BP ≥90
Adolescents	Systolic BP ≥136	Systolic BP ≥144
(13-15 yr)	Diastolic BP ≥86	Diastolic BP ≥92
Adolescents	Systolic BP ≥142	Systolic BP ≥150
(16-18 yr)	Diastolic BP ≥92	Diastolic BP ≥98

Modified from the Report of the Second Task Force on Blood Pressure Control in Children–1987, *Pediatrics* 79:1-25, 1987.

in comparison with the general population. This information is useful in providing reassurance to parents and professionals regarding the child who is growing normally, in assessing the nutritional status of the child, and in identifying the child who may have abnormalities that are affecting the various growth parameters. Examples of abnormalities that could impair growth include growth-hormone deficiency, inflammatory bowel disease, and cardiac and renal disorders.

The three parameters of growth that are routinely measured during each examination of the child less than 3 years of age are recumbent length, body weight, and head circumference. For the child older than 3 years of age, it is sufficient to obtain standing height and weight measurements. Assessment of body segments, skinfold thickness, bone age, and dentition may be useful for further study of body growth, but it is not usually included in the routine physical examination.

Growth charts published by, or based on data from, the National Center for Health Statistics (NCHS) are most commonly used to record growth measurements (Figure 24-18). They are based on large, nationally representative samples of children. Two groups of charts were developed from the data: the first for the age interval from birth to 36 months and the second for the interval from 2 to 18 years. The charts for infants (birth to 36 months) were developed separately for boys and girls and include graphs for head circumference, recumbent length by age, weight by age, and weight by length. The charts for children 2 to 18 years are in separate versions for boys and girls and include graphs for stature

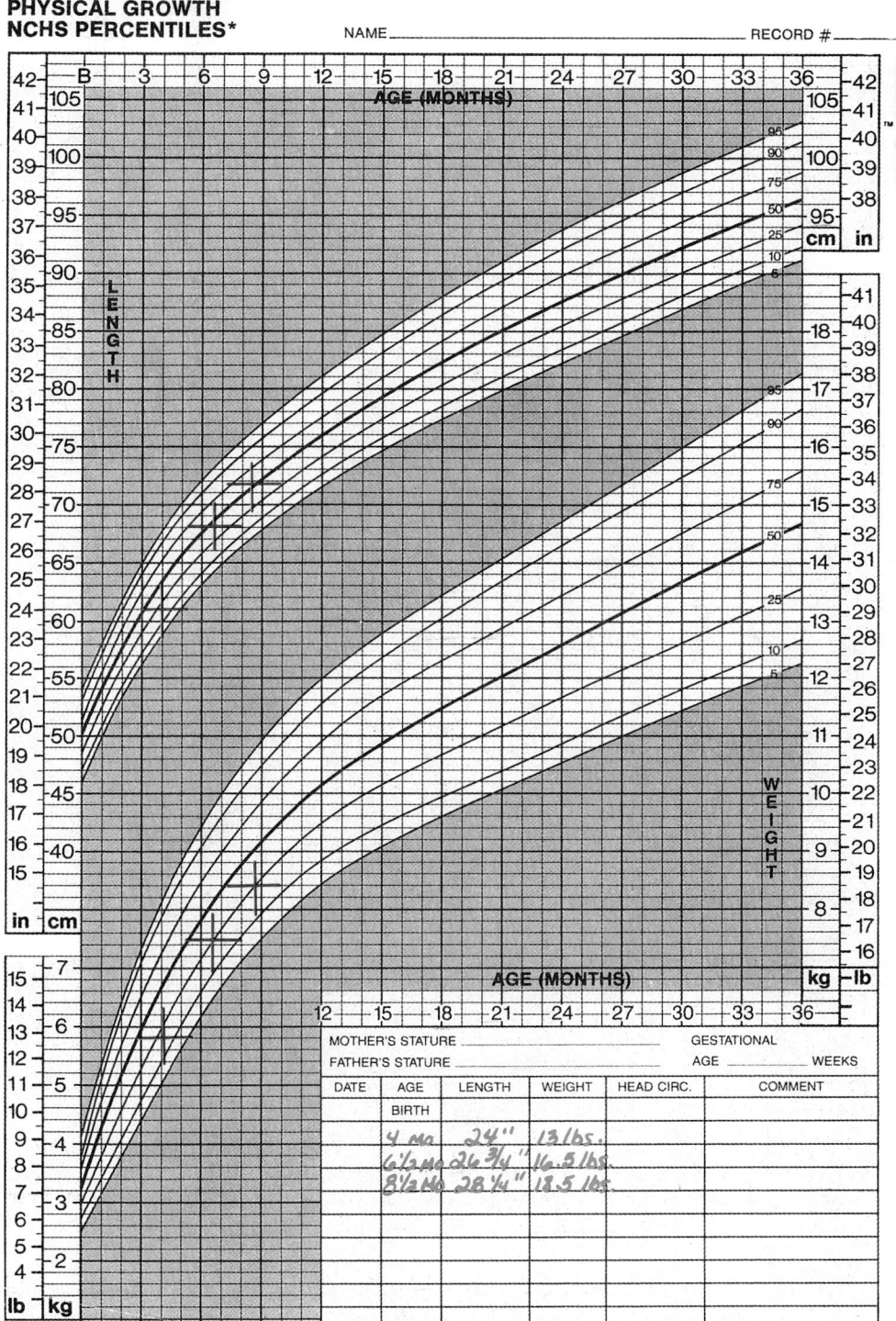

FIGURE 24-18 Samples of physical growth charts for children. **A,** Boys: birth to 36 months, for length. (Courtesy Ross Laboratories).

BOYS: BIRTH TO 36 MONTHS
PHYSICAL GROWTH
NCHS PERCENTILES*

NAME ______________________ RECORD # ____________

B

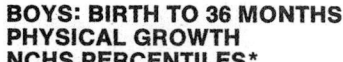

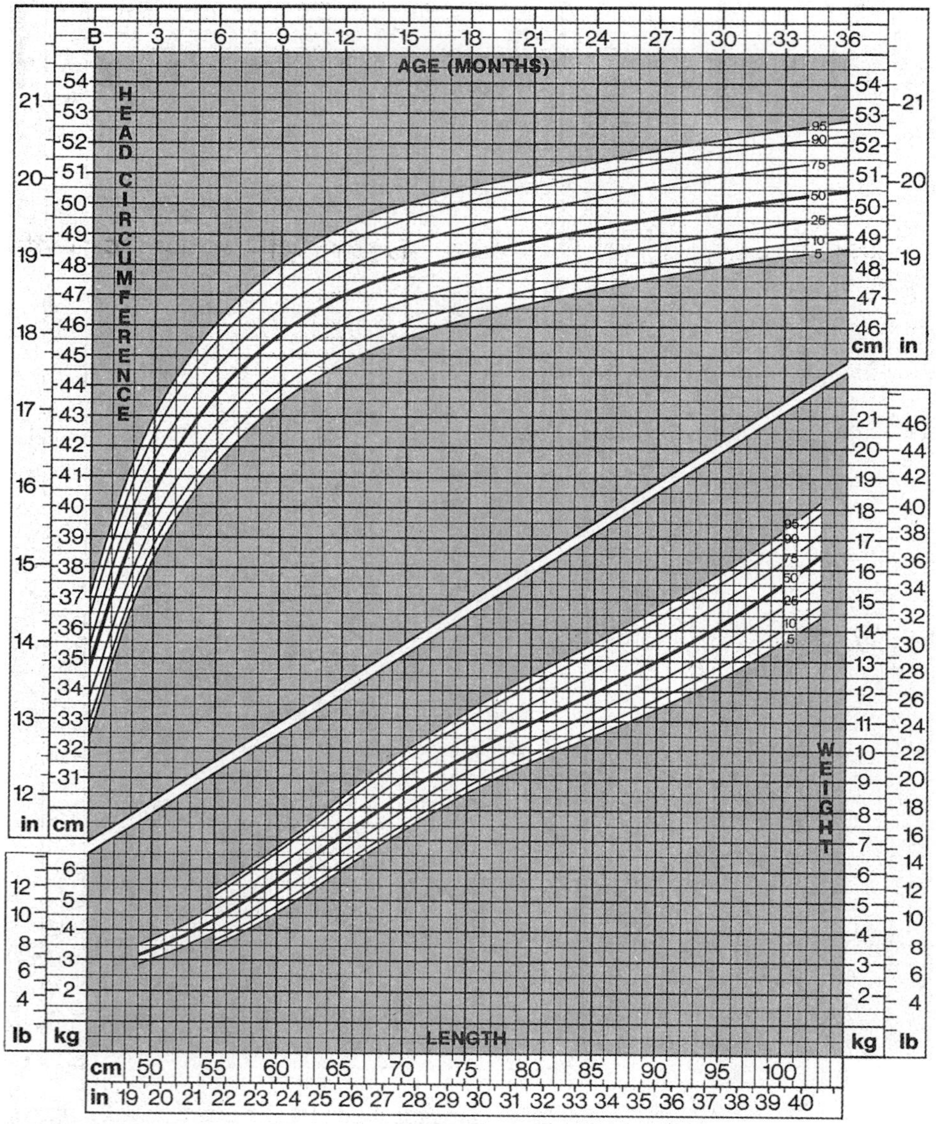

DATE	AGE	LENGTH	WEIGHT	HEAD CIRC.	COMMENT

*Adapted from: Hamill PVV, Drizd TA, Johnson CL, Reed RB, Roche AF, Moore WM: Physical growth: National Center for Health Statistics percentiles. AM J CLIN NUTR 32:607-629, 1979. Data from the Fels Research Institute, Wright State University School of Medicine, Yellow Springs, Ohio.

ROSS LABORATORIES
COLUMBUS, OHIO 43216
Division of Abbott Laboratories, USA

FIGURE 24-18, cont'd B, Boys: birth to 36 months, for head circumference. (Courtesy Ross Laboratories.)

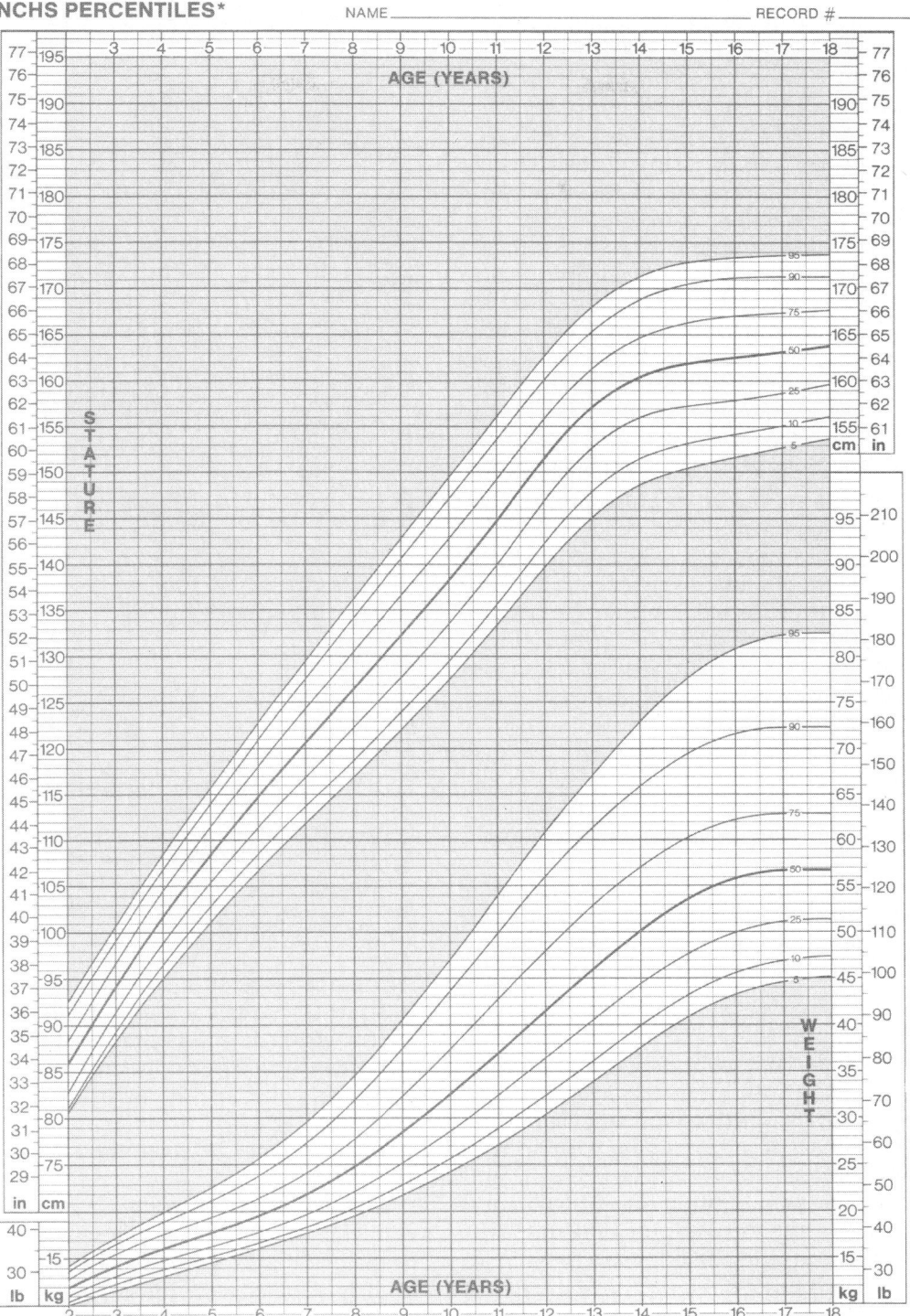

FIGURE 24-18, cont'd C, Girls: ages 2 through 18 years, for height and weight. (Courtesy Ross Laboratories.)

(standing height) by age, weight by age, and weight by stature of prepubescent children.

The appropriate use of the charts requires that consistent measurement techniques be used at each point in time. For instance, do not record standing height or stature on the birth-to-36 months chart since the infant will appear shorter than if the recumbent length were used. There can be a difference of up to 1 inch between recumbent and standing measures of the same child. Record standing height on the 2-to-18 year chart.

To interpret growth measurements, you need to take into account several factors. First, children whose weight and height fall between the 5th and 95th percentiles are likely to be growing normally. Evaluate and follow closely, however, those who fall below the 5th or above the 95th percentile. Consider the size of the parents and also the ethnic and racial background of the child. If both parents are small or large, their children's growth likely will be similar. Differences from the norm, which was determined for middle-class Caucasian children, have been noted for children of different ethnic groups. For example, based on standards from China, Chinese children's average weight and height fall in the 10th percentile on the NCHS charts rather than the 50th percentile. However, when investigators studied these children's growth patterns over time, their growth was normal (Whaley and Wong, 1991). This example emphasizes that the overall pattern of growth is more important than any single measure.

The relationship between height and weight is also significant. Pay specific attention to children who have a disparity between these two measures. For example, a child whose height falls in the 75th percentile but whose weight falls in the 25th percentile needs more in-depth evaluation and monitoring. Other areas of concern are a child's failure to show expected increases in height and weight, particularly during peak growth periods such as infancy and adolescence, and sudden changes in height or weight from the child's growth curve (e.g., sudden increases or decreases).

Length or height. Measure recumbent length (birth to 3 years) with the child in the supine position with the legs extended. To measure length, facilitate the procedure by having two people participate. The parent is usually available and interested in providing this assistance. If you use a measuring board, place the infant's head against the fixed headboard, and have the parent hold it in the midline while you gently push on the infant's knees until the legs are fully extended and both heels are firmly touching the movable footboard. If a measuring device is not available, follow the same procedure, placing the child on a paper-covered flat surface and marking the paper at the top of the child's head and at the bottom of the heels (Figure 24-19, *A*). Mea-

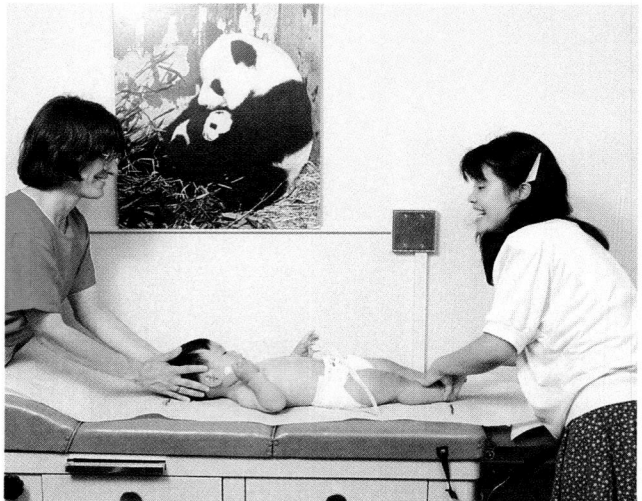

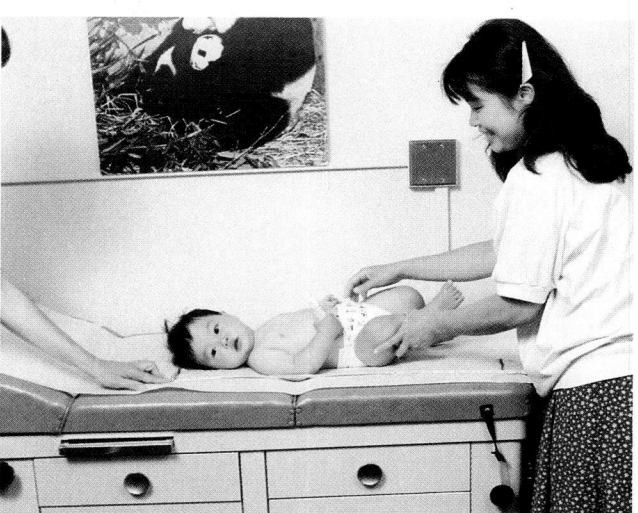

FIGURE 24-19 A, Measuring recumbent length with parent's assistance. Child is placed on a paper-covered flat surface and marks are made at the head and feet. **B,** Distance between the two marks is measured while the child relaxes.

sure the distance between the two points (Figure 24-19, *B*).

Measure standing height or stature (2 to 18 years) with the shoes off. Ask the child to stand as tall as possible and look straight ahead so that the top of the head is parallel with the ceiling. The feet should be together, and the shoulders, buttocks, and heels should be touching the wall without any flexion of the knees (Figure 24-20). Bring a block, squared at right angles against the wall, or a measuring board to the top of the child's head. When a measuring device is not available, you can make a mark on the wall at the top of the child's head and measure the distance from the floor.

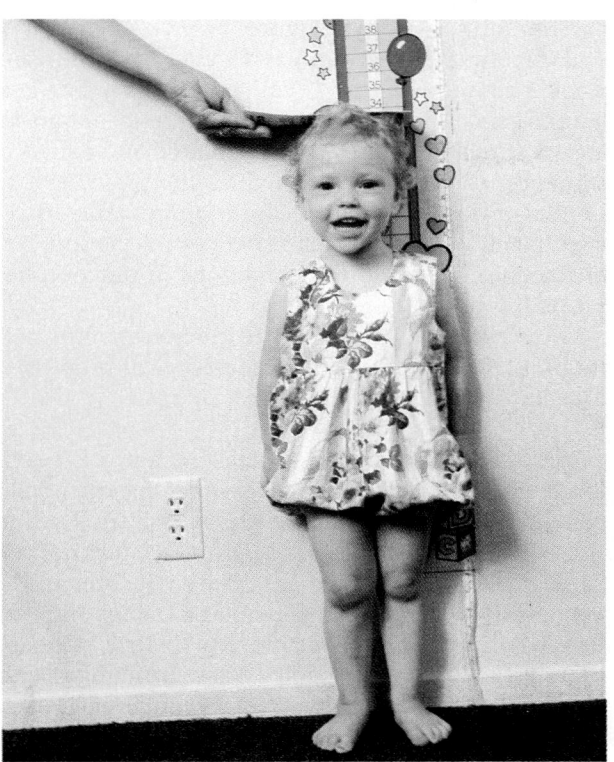

FIGURE 24-20 Measurement of standing height.

Weight. To weigh the child, use an appropriately sized beam scale with nondetachable weights. Two scales are suggested: one for infants and small children, which measures weights to the nearest 0.5 oz or 10 g, and one for older children and adults, which measures weights to the nearest 0.25 lb or 100 g. Before weighing the child, check the scale to determine if it is balanced. Return the weights to the zero setting and make sure that the balance is resting in the middle.

When infant growth charts (birth to 36 months) are used, weigh the child naked on the infant scale (Figure 24-21). With the charts for older children (2 to 18 years), use the upright adult scale, ideally with the child dressed only in underpants or a light gown (Fig. 24-22).

Head circumference. Measure the head circumference during each examination between birth and 36 months of age and in any child whose head size is questionable. Pass a nonstretchable tape measure over the most prominent part of the occiput and just above

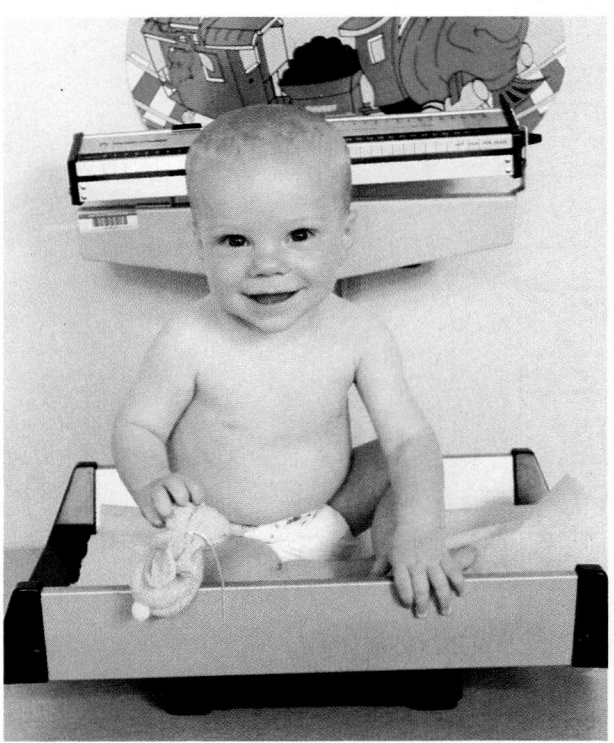

FIGURE 24-21 Weighing the young infant.

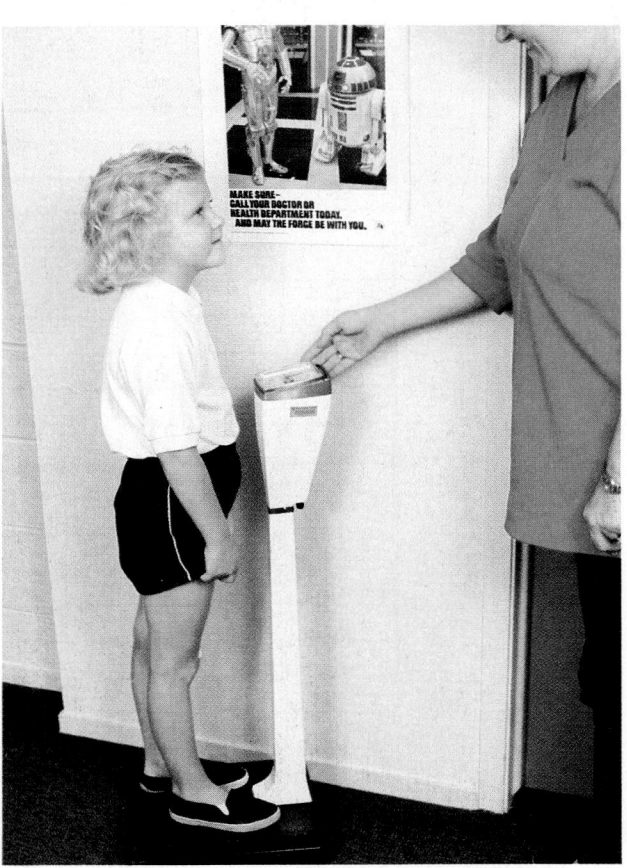

FIGURE 24-22 Weighing the older child. Ideally, the child would be dressed only in underwear or a light gown with shoes removed.

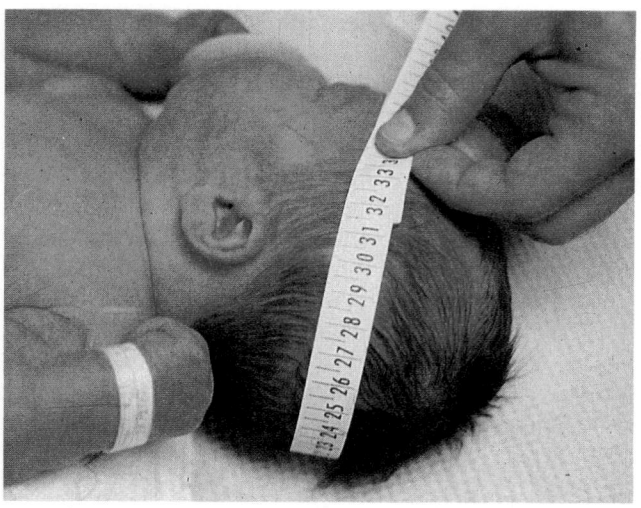

FIGURE 24-23 Appropriate placement of the measuring tape to obtain the head circumference. (From Seidel HM and others: *Mosby's guide to physical examination*, ed 2, St Louis, 1991, Mosby–Year Book.)

the supraorbital ridges (Figure 24-23). The average head circumference at birth is 35 cm (14 inches) and by age 2 has increased to 49 cm (19.2 inches). The head circumference is an important measure to obtain because it is related to intracranial volume and allows an estimation of the rate of growth of the brain. Plot sequential measurements on the appropriate NCHS growth chart. Check any discrepancy or deviation, with consideration given to the conditions of microcephaly and hydrocephaly.

Always measure the head circumference of the child who is suspected of having a neurological problem or a developmental delay, regardless of age.

Chest circumference. The measurement of the circumference of the chest at delivery and in early infancy has become significant in that it may indicate birth injury, congenital anomalies, or system dysfunction, for example, cardiac enlargement. Otherwise, measuring the chest circumference on a regular basis beyond early infancy is unnecessary. Exceptions to this might include observed body disproportion or malformation of the thoracic cage. Measure the chest circumference of the child by placing a nonstretchable cloth tape measure at

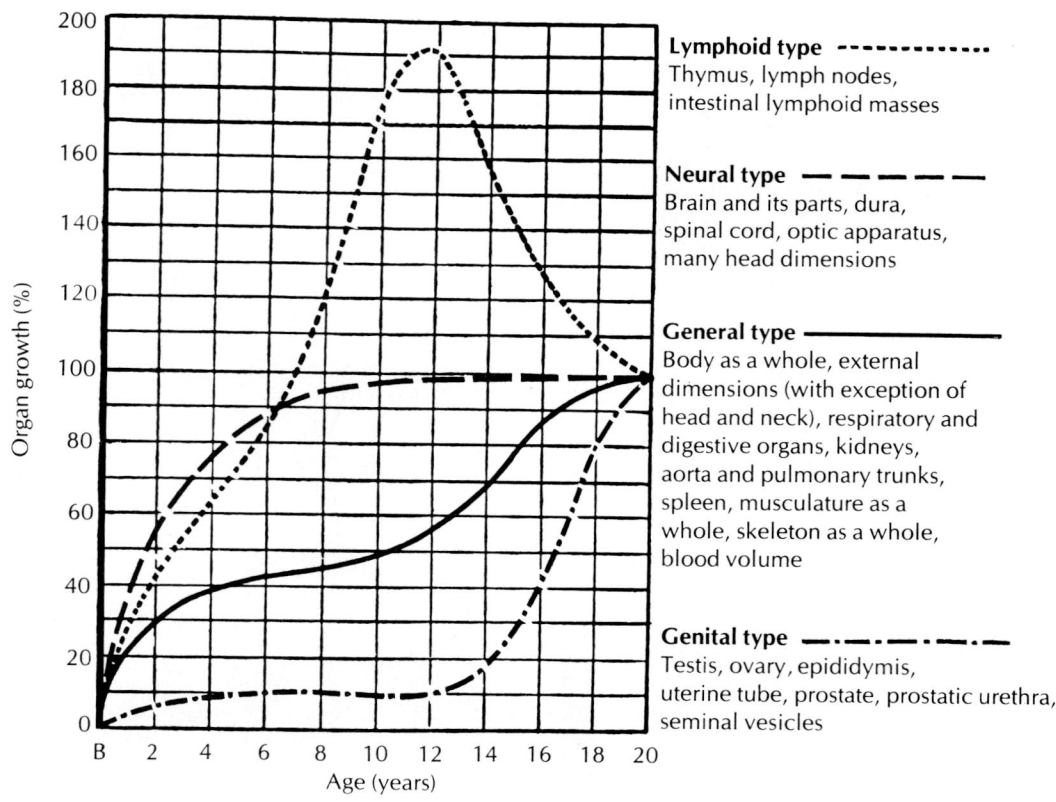

FIGURE 24-24 Differential organ growth curves. (From Harris JA and others: *The measurement of man*, Minneapolis, 1930, University of Minnesota Press.)

the level of the nipple, with the child in a supine position. Take the measurement midway between inspiration and expiration.

Growth curves of the body as a whole and of three types of tissue—lymphoid, neural, and genital—demonstrate the age ranges when children are expected to exhibit growth spurts (Figure 24-24).

> **Helpful Hints for Using Pediatric Growth Charts:** *Age- and sex-specific growth charts are readily available from the major formula manufacturers and from the makers of growth hormone. These charts have been standardized by using data from thousands of children so that comparisons can be made. Proper documentation of height and weight onto growth charts is as important as proper assessment. On the sample growth chart (see Figure 24-18), note that crossed lines are drawn with a straight edge to ensure that the child's age and measurements are recorded exactly. If the child is 9 years and 9 months old, the vertical line is drawn in a different place than if the child is 9 years and 2 months old. This distinction can make a big difference as to the percentile into which the child's height, weight, or head circumference falls.*
>
> *If a child is born prematurely, use the "corrected age" on growth charts and developmental assessments until the child is 2½ years old. To calculate "corrected age," subtract the number of weeks the child was born prematurely from the child's chronological age. Example: One would expect a 15-month-old child born 6 weeks prematurely to be in the same growth and developmental range of normal as a 13½-month-old.*

General inspection. The general inspection of the child includes observations similar to those of the adult examination (see Chapter 8). These include changes in facies, posture, and body contour; hygiene; and changes in gait. Also keep in mind those physical and behavioral characteristics that are expected for the individual child at the present chronological age (Figure 24-25). Chapter 3 describes the normal physical and behavioral changes that occur during the child's development. Table 24-6 also summarizes these changes. Observations made about the child's development during the interview and examination may indicate the need for a more formal assessment.

Observe and describe the child's behavior during the visit. Is this a quiet, shy child or an active, restless child? Is this child comfortable during the visit, or anxious and afraid? Does the child respond to the parent or other adults in an appropriate way?

Each child is a unique being, and it is a challenge to observe and record a description of any child's behavior. Keep in mind that behavior observed during a visit for health care may not be typical for that child.

Skin, hair, and nails. Assess the skin for color, texture, temperature, moisture, turgor, and any rashes or lesions. Observe the hair for color, texture, quality, and distribution. Assess the nails for color, shape, texture, and quality.

The examination of the skin provides valuable information about the general health of the child and evidence of specific skin problems. Inspect and palpate the skin of the entire body at each examination. Since the normal condition of the skin changes with age, it is important to become familiar with those changes seen in children, as described in the following sections.

Newborn and infant. The skin of the newborn is soft and smooth and appears almost transparent. The superficial vessels are prominent, giving the skin its red color. Use natural daylight to assess for jaundice. A mild degree of jaundice is frequently present after the second or third day in normal infants. If the jaundice is severe or occurs within the first 24 hours, however, you should consider the presence of a serious problem.

Small papular patches, called nevus flammeus, may be present over the occiput, forehead, and upper eyelids in the newborn period; these patches usually disappear by the end of the first year of life. The nose and cheeks

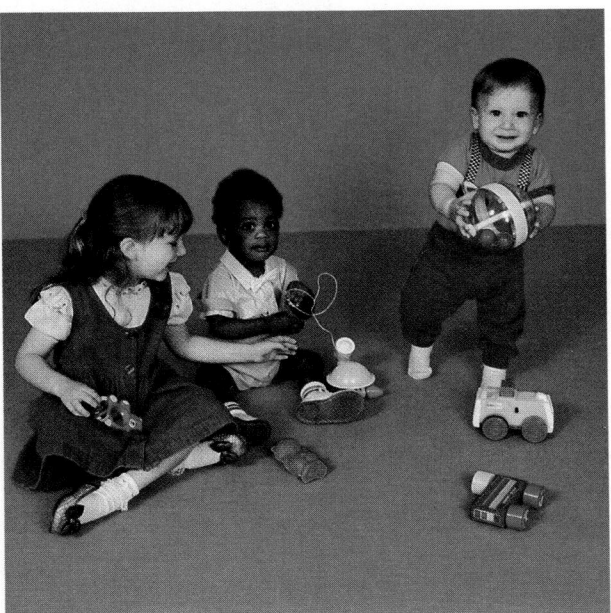

FIGURE 24-25 Observations of children at play in the waiting area, as well as during the examination, can provide helpful information about their behavioral styles and development.

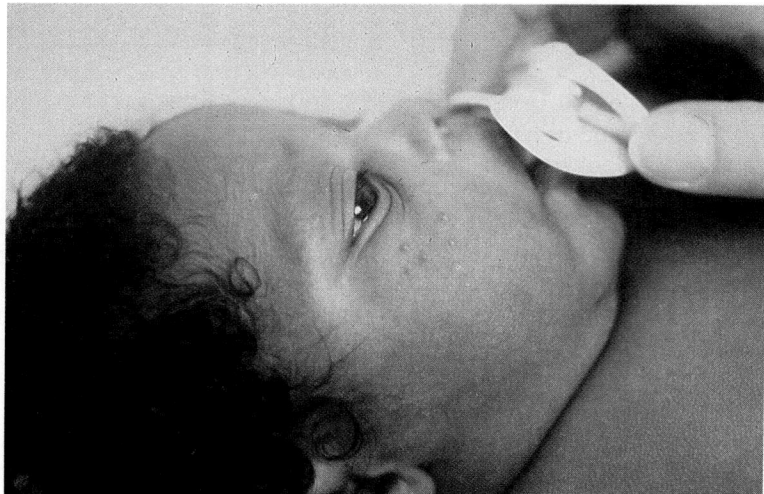

FIGURE 24-26 Milia in an infant. (From Seidel HM and others: *Mosby's guide to physical examination,* ed 2, St Louis, 1991, Mosby—Year Book.)

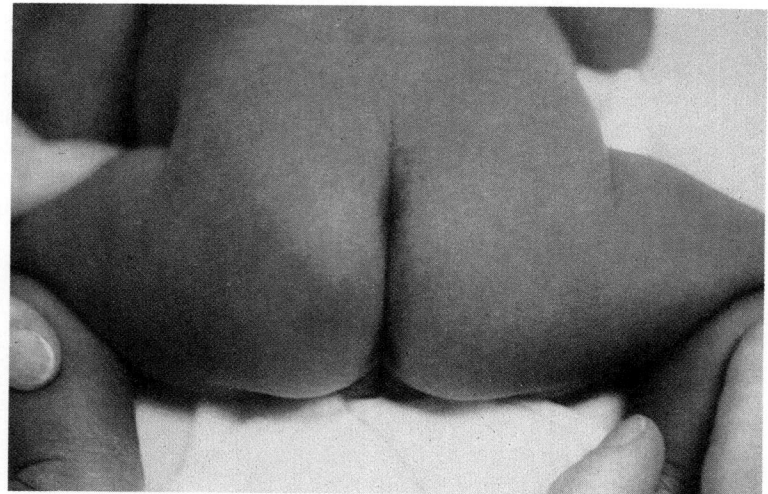

FIGURE 24-27 Mongolian spots are common in infants with dark skin. (From Seidel HM and others: *Mosby's guide to physical examination,* ed 2, St Louis, 1991, Mosby—Year Book.)

are frequently covered by small white papules called milia (Figure 24-26), caused by plugging of the sebaceous glands during the neonatal period. Both sweat and sebaceous glands are present in the newborn, but they do not function until the second month of life. Some desquamation is common during the first weeks and varies in individual babies. Mongolian spots, which are blue or bluish-brown, irregularly shaped, flat areas, occur in the sacral and buttocks area of some infants, usually those who have darkly pigmented skin (Figure 24-27). These spots usually disappear by the end of the first or by the second year, but occasionally they persist for a longer time. A considerable amount of fine hair, called lanugo, covers the body of the newborn, and is lost during the first weeks of life. The nails of the full-term newborn are well formed and firm in contrast to those of the premature infant, which are imperfectly formed.

During the first year of life, the proportion of subcutaneous fat continuously increases and raw areas re-

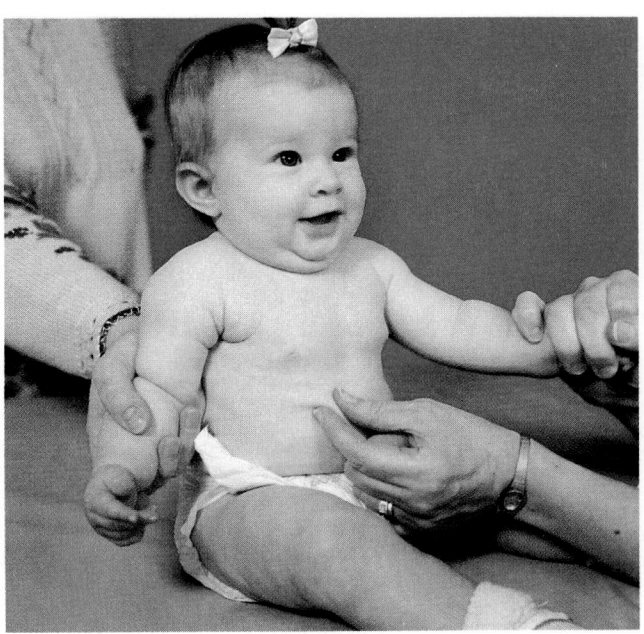

FIGURE 24-28 Checking skin turgor in an infant.

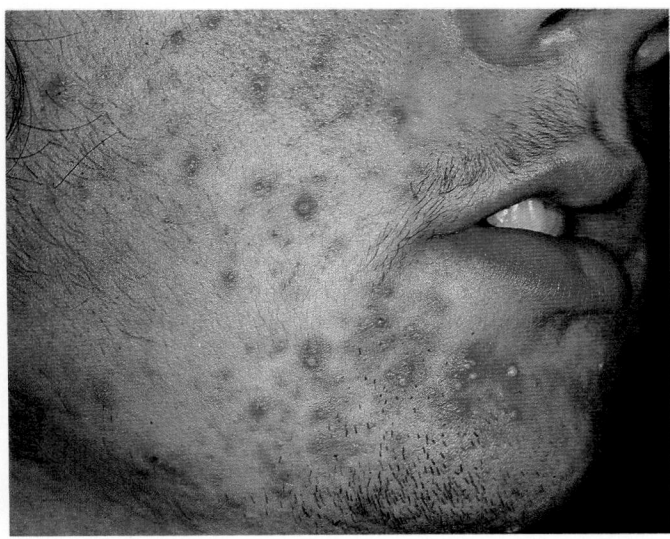

FIGURE 24-29 Acne in an adolescent. (From Habif TP: *Clinical dermatology: a color guide to diagnosis and therapy,* ed 2, St Louis, 1990, Mosby–Year Book.)

sulting from skin rubbing against skin are more prevalent in young obese infants. This condition is called **intertrigo.** During the second year of life, the proportion of subcutaneous fat decreases and intertrigo is less common. Skin turgor is a good indicator of hydration status. Check skin turgor by grasping the skin on the abdomen between your thumb and index finger, releasing it, and observing how quickly it returns to its normal shape (Figure 24-28).

Older child and adolescent. After the first year of life, the normal child shows little change in the skin until the onset of puberty, when considerable development of both sweat and sebaceous glands occurs. Associated with the development of the sebaceous glands is acne vulgaris, which is so common in its mildest forms that it is sometimes considered a normal physiological change. Early evidence of acne is the occasional comedo, or blackhead, on the nose and chin. At age 13 or 14 years, papules and small pustules may begin to appear (Figure 24-29). However, by age 16, many children will have recovered completely. Changes in the amount and distribution of hair also occur. Hair growth becomes heavier; the appearance of pubic, axillary, and most of the more prominent body hair is influenced by sexual development during adolescence.

Lymph nodes. Inspect and palpate the lymph nodes for size, mobility, temperature, and tenderness.

Lymph nodes in children have the same distribution as those in adults, but the nodes are usually more prom-

inent until puberty (Figure 24-30). The amount of lymphoid tissue is considerable at birth and increases steadily until after puberty. Shotty, discrete, movable, small, nontender nodes are common in the occipital, postauricular, anterior and posterior cervical, parotid, submaxillary, sublingual, axillary, epitrochlear, and inguinal areas in the normal healthy child. Examine lymph nodes during the examination of each part of the body.

Head and neck. Inspect the head for shape and symmetry. Palpate the fontanels in the infant and young child.

Newborn and infant. The shape of the newborn's head is often asymmetrical as a result of the molding that occurs during the passage through the birth canal. It may be a few days or weeks before the normal shape is restored. The newborn has a skull that molds easily because the bones of the cranium are not fused, which allows for some overlapping of the bones. Trauma may result in caput succedaneum or cephalhematoma. **Caput succedaneum** is an edematous swelling of the superficial tissues of the scalp manifested by a generalized soft swelling not bounded by suture lines. This condition is temporary and is usually resolved within the first few days of life. **Cephalhematoma** occurs as a result of bleeding into the periosteum and results in swelling that does not cross the suture line. Most cephalhematomas are absorbed within 2 weeks to 3 months. Flattening of the head often occurs in normal

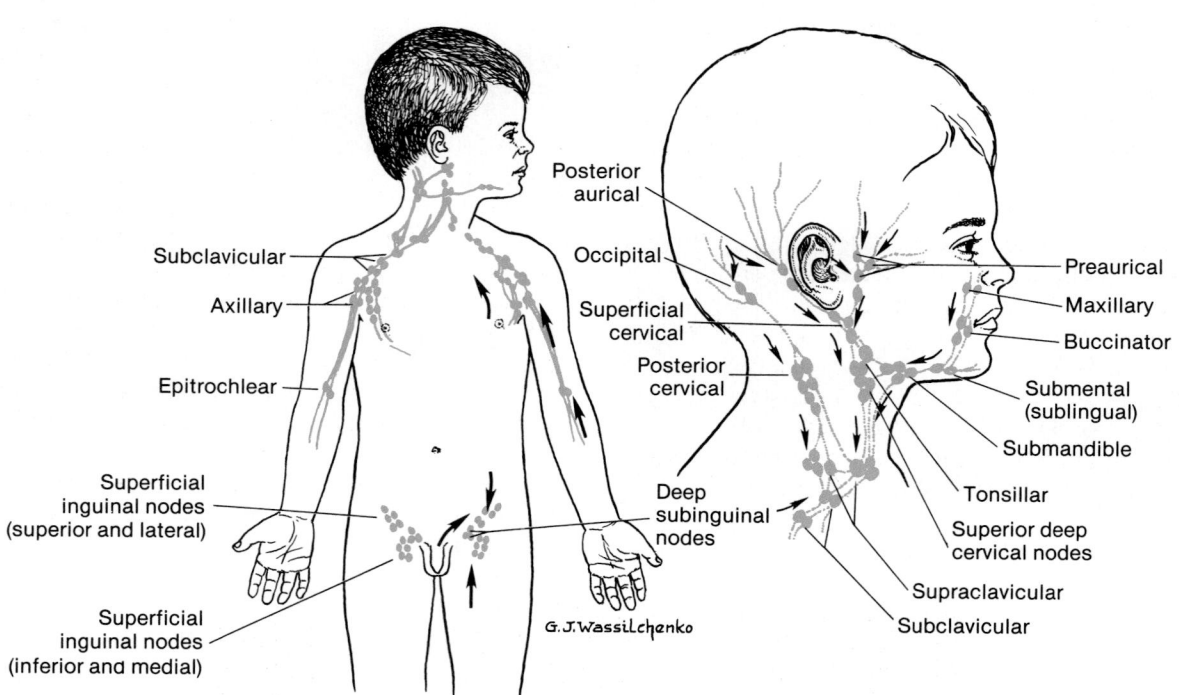

FIGURE 24-30 Location of superficial lymph nodes, Arrows indicate directional flow of lymph. (From Whaley LF, Wong DL: *Nursing care of infants and children,* ed 4, St Louis, 1991, Mosby—Year Book.)

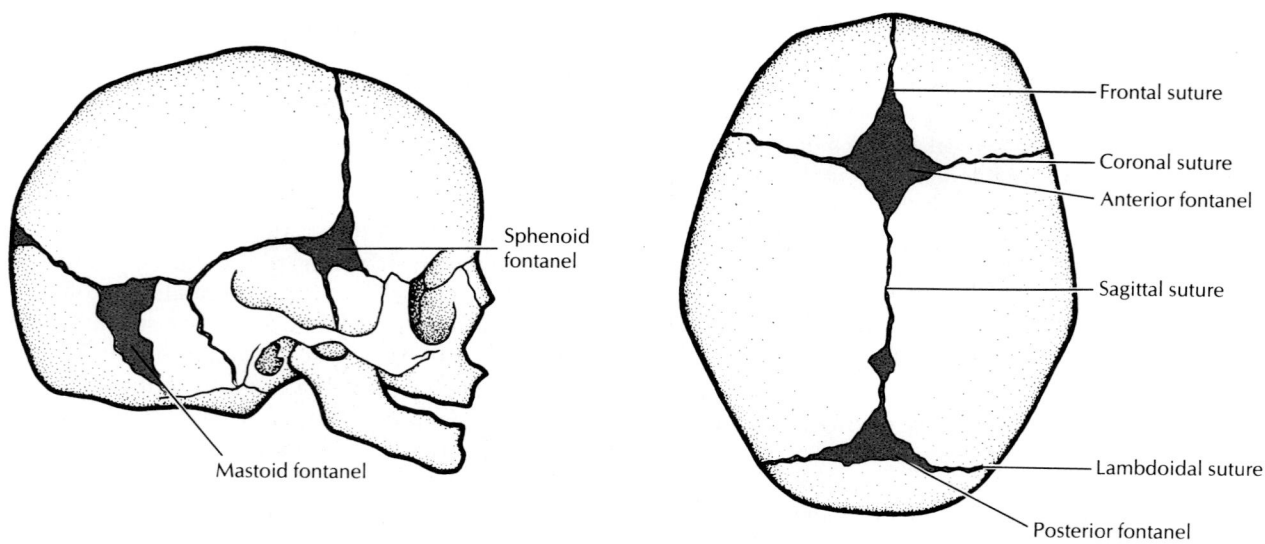

FIGURE 24-31 Skull bones of the infant, showing fontanels and sutures.

children, but it can also indicate problems such as mental retardation or rickets.

Palpate the sutures of the skull, which can usually be felt as ridges until the age of 6 months. Palpate the fontanels during each examination of the infant and young child to determine the size, shape, and presence of any tenseness or bulging. Normally, the posterior fontanel closes by 2 months of age and the anterior fontanel closes by the end of the second year (Figure 24-31). Tenseness or bulging of the fontanel is most easily detected when the child is in a sitting position and should be assessed when the child is quiet. Bulging may occur with increased intercranial pressure (or when the child is crying). The fontanel may be depressed when the infant is dehydrated or malnourished. Note early closure or delayed closure of the fontanel. Early closure can result from microcephaly and delayed closure from prolonged intracranial pressure.

The importance of measuring the head circumference of the child up to 3 years of age has already been discussed.

Transillumination of the skull is a useful procedure in the initial examination of the infant and for any infant with an abnormal head size. Perform transillumination in a completely darkened room with an ordinary flashlight equipped with a rubber adaptor. Place the light against the infant's head. If the cerebrum is absent or greatly thinned, as from increased intracranial pressure, the entire cranium lights up. Often, defects transilluminate in a more limited way. Auscultation of the skull may reveal bruits, which are commonly found in normal children up to 4 years of age. After the age of 4 years, bruits are evidence of problems such as aneurysms or increased intracranial pressure.

Inspect the young infant's scalp for evidence of crusting, which often results from a seborrheic dermatitis commonly called "cradle cap" (Figure 24-32).

Inspect the shape of the face. A facial paralysis is most easily observed when the child cries or smiles and the asymmetry is increased. An abnormal or unusual facies may indicate a chromosomal abnormality such as Down's syndrome.

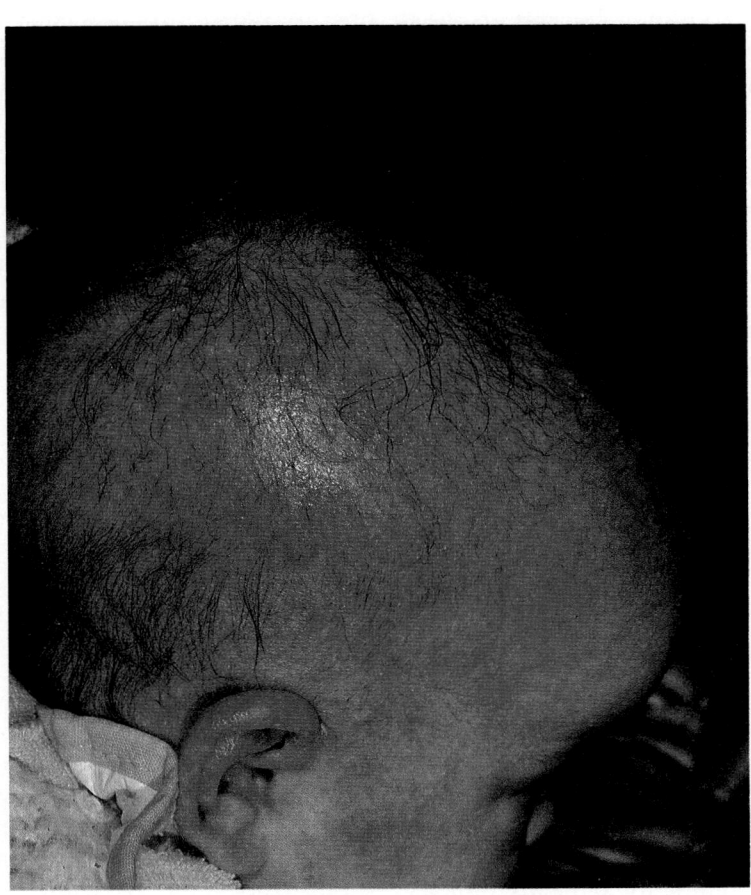

FIGURE 24-32 Seborrheic dermatitis of the scalp in an infant. (From Habif TP: *Clinical dermatology: a color guide to diagnosis and therapy*, ed 2, St Louis, 1992, Mosby–Year Book.)

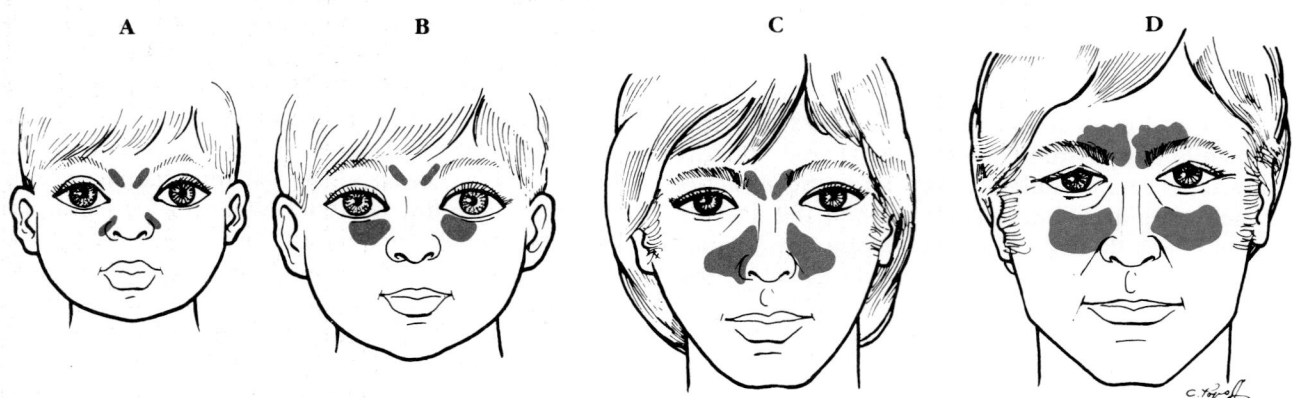

A   B   C   D

FIGURE 24-33 Development of the frontal and maxillary sinuses. **A,** Early infancy. **B,** Early childhood, **C,** Adolescence. **D,** Adulthood.

Older child and adolescent. Percuss the frontal and maxillary sinuses by the direct method and palpate them in the child who is over 2 or 3 years of age. Until that age the sinuses are too small and poorly developed for percussion or palpation (Figure 24-33).

Palpate the submaxillary and sublingual glands in the same way as in the adult examination. Check for local swelling of the parotid gland by observing the child in the sitting position with the head raised and the neck extended and by noting any swelling below the angle of the jaw. You can feel the swollen parotid gland by palpating downward from the zygomatic arch. Unilateral or bilateral swelling of the parotid gland usually indicates mumps.

Examine the neck with the child lying flat on the back. Note the size of the neck. The neck of the infant normally is short. It lengthens at about 3 or 4 years of age. Palpate the lymph nodes, thyroid glands and trachea. Carefully palpate the sternocleidomastoid muscle. A mass on the lower third of the muscle may indicate a congenital **torticollis**. Finally, determine the mobility of the neck by lifting the child's head and turning it from side to side or bringing the chin forward to touch the chest. Any resistance to flexion may indicate meningeal irritation.

Eyes. Examination of the eyes is most easily accomplished when the child is able to cooperate. The school-age child can participate in the adult format for the eye examination (see Chapter 11). The infant and young child are much more of a challenge to the examiner.

Visual function at birth is limited, but it improves as the structures develop. Vision can be tested grossly in the very young infant by noting the pupillary response to light. This is one of the most primitive visual functions and is normally found in the newborn. The blink reflex is also present in normal newborns and young infants.

The infant will blink the eyes when a bright light is introduced. It is important to make sure that the infant has a full red reflex in each eye. A white reflex could indicate cataract or retinoblastoma.

At 5 or 6 weeks of age, the child should be able to fixate and give some evidence of following a bright toy or light. When 3 or 4 months old, the infant begins to reach for objects at different distances. At 6 to 7 months of age, the infant can have a funduscopic examination, although it is not routinely performed at this early an age. For children 3 to 6 years of age, a Snellen E chart can be used. Ask the child to hold the fingers in the same direction as the fingers of the E. You can also use Allen picture cards. The child identifies pictures, such as a tree, a telephone, a car, a house, and a teddy bear on an Allen card from a distance of 15 feet. Familiarizing the child with the procedure before testing may be helpful (Figure 24-34). The young child is normally farsighted and does not achieve visual acuity of 20/20 until the age of 7 years.

Tests for **strabismus** (squint, cross-eye), an imbalance of the extraocular muscles, are important because strabismus can lead to **amblyopia**, a type of blindness in the affected eye. Early recognition is essential to restore binocular vision since the prognosis for a successful outcome for the child over 6 years of age is poor. An easy method for detecting strabismus is the corneal reflex test (or Hirschberg's test). Shine a bright light from a flashlight or ophthalmoscope directly into the eyes from about 16 inches (40.5 cm). In normal eyes the reflection of the light should fall symmetrically within each pupil. Any deviation warrants further evaluation. Another, more accurate, test to assess muscle imbalance is the cover-uncover test described in Chapter 10. You can use this test in both younger and older children. Have the child focus on an object. Cover one eye with your hand, a card, or specially designed eye-

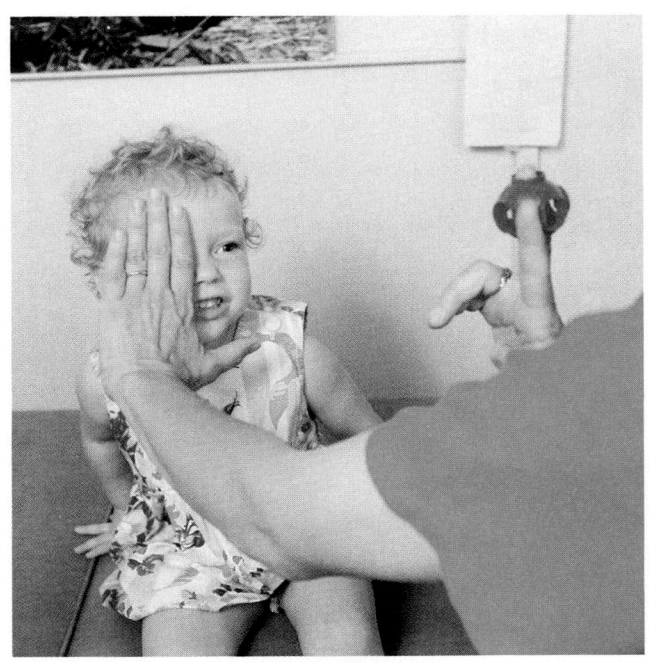

FIGURE 24-34 Preparing the child for participation in testing of visual acuity.

wear and observe the uncovered eye for movement (Figure 24-35, *A*). Then uncover the eye and observe the recently covered eye for movement (Figure 24-35, *B*). If movement is noticed in either or both eyes, strabismus is present. The type of strabismus is determined by the combination of movements. Repeat the test to examine the other eye. Transient strabismus is common during the first months of life. If it persists beyond 6 months of age, however, or becomes fixed at an earlier age, the child should be referred to an ophthalmologist.

Test extraocular movements during the first weeks of life, as soon as the child is able to demonstrate following of movement. You can also at least partially examine the visual fields in infants and young children by having the child sit on the parent's lap with the head in the midline and one eye covered. As the light or bright object is brought into the visual field, the child will look at it or reach for it.

Inspect the outermost structures of the eyes in the same way as in the adult examination. The ophthalmoscopic examination depends on the child's ability to cooperate and the examiner's efficiency in observing as much as possible in a limited time. Attempts to restrain the child and force the eyes to remain open prove unsuccessful. If possible, direct the child's attention toward an object or light while you approach without touching the child. The appearance of the red reflex alone is important information for ruling out opacities of the cornea and lens and cataracts. Attempt to use the oph-

A 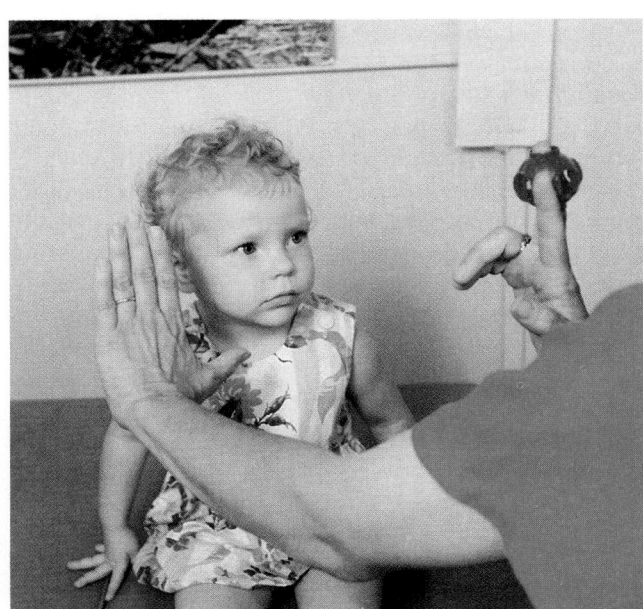 **B**

FIGURE 24-35 Cover-uncover test for strabismus. **A,** Have the child look at an object (preferably a brightly colored toy) and cover one eye. Observe the uncovered eye for movement. **B,** While the child is still focused on the object, uncover the eye and observe it for movement.

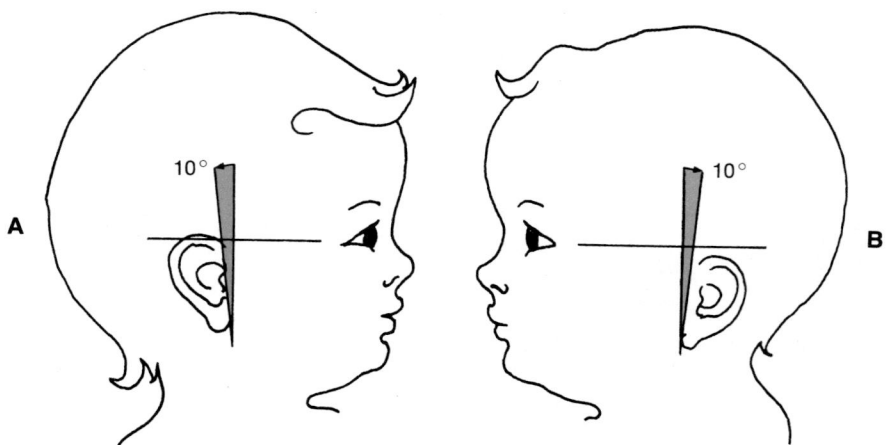

FIGURE 24-36 Ear alignment. **A,** Normal. **B,** Abnormal. (From Whaley LF, Wong DL: *Nursing care of infants and children,* ed 4, St Louis, 1991, Mosby–Year Book.)

thalmoscope to observe the red reflex at each examination of the infant and child beginning in the first weeks of life.

Ears. Examination of the ears is often difficult; however, it is important because the immature structure of the young child's ears makes them more prone to infection. In the infant the eustachian tube is shorter and wider than in the adult. It is also in a more horizontal position than in the adult, which makes it easier for pathogens to infect the middle ear.

Inspect and palpate the external ear and the posterior mastoid areas for any obvious deformities. Note the position and size of the ears. Normally the top of the ear is on a horizontal line with the inner and outer canthus of the eye (Figure 24-36).

Next, use the otoscope. This examination becomes more difficult as the infant grows older. It is usually helpful to spend some time preparing the child by letting him or her see the light and by inserting the speculum

gently for only a few seconds and then removing it to assure the child that the procedure does not hurt (Figure 24-37). When restraint is necessary, have the parent firmly hold the child (Figure 24-38). Before inserting the otoscope, inspect the meatus for evidence of a foreign body or external otitis. In infancy and early childhood, the auditory canal is directed upward: pull the pinna of the ear down and back to aid in visualization (Figure 24-39). Hold the otoscope so that the hand holding it rests firmly on the head; the top of the spec-

> **Helpful Hints for the Ear Examination:**
> *Pneumotoscopy is an important technique to learn, especially when working with children. It involves blowing air into the ear canal (either with a rubber squeeze bulb or gently blowing or sucking with the end of the rubber tube in the examiner's mouth). The normal tympanic membrane will move in and out as positive and negative pressures are applied. In the presence of infection there is fluid behind the tympanic membrane and therefore a decrease in mobility when pressure is applied.*

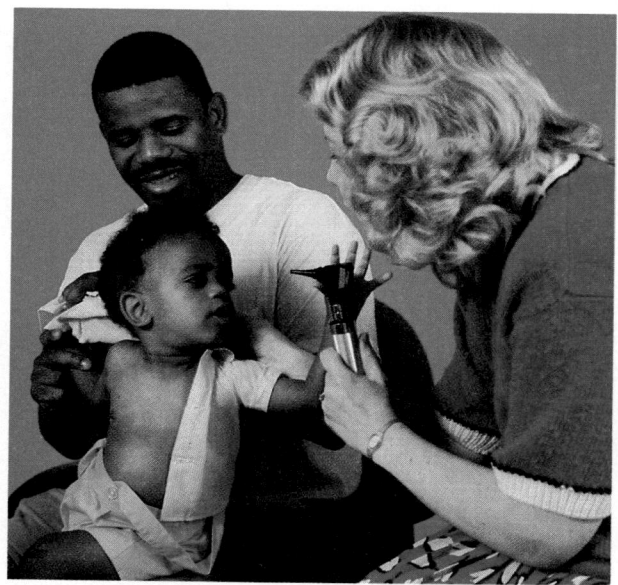

FIGURE 24-37 It is helpful to let the child see the speculum and examine it in preparation for the otoscopic examination.

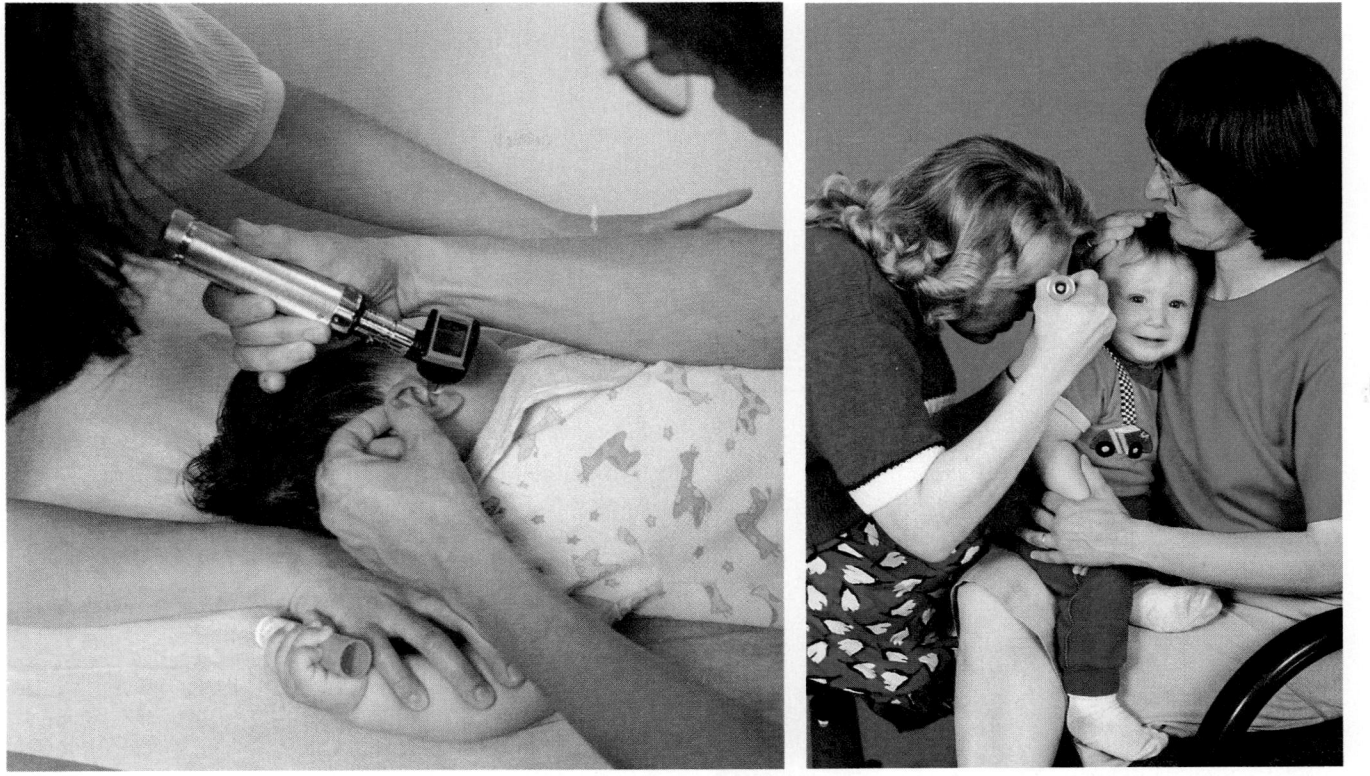

FIGURE 24-38 Positioning for restraining the child for an ear examination. **A,** Supine. **B,** Restraint using the hug.

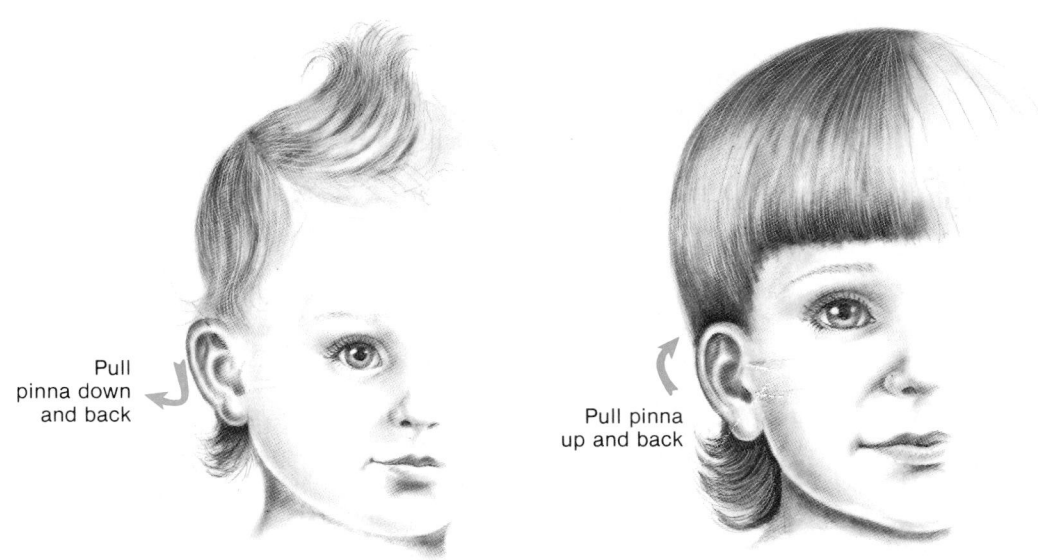

FIGURE 24-39 Straightening the ear canal in the infant, **(A)** and the child over 3 years of age **(B).** (From Whaley LF, Wong DL: *Nursing care of infants and children,* ed 4, St Louis, 1991 Mosby–Year Book.)

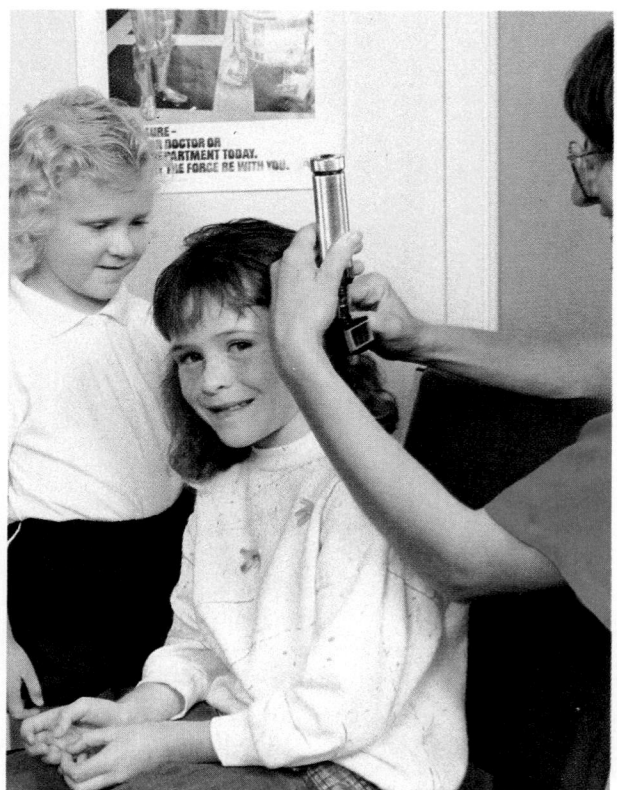

FIGURE 24-40 Examination of the ear in an older child.

procedures to remove the cerumen. Avoid discomfort so that the child will not become conditioned to expect pain with future ear examinations.

In the infant, test hearing by asking an assistant to stand behind the child and make a noise, such as a hand slap, several inches away from the child's ear while you observe the child for an eye blink. This test is often inaccurate since the child may be responding to air movement. In the young child, hearing can be grossly tested with the whispered voice. Stand behind the child, occlude one ear with your hand, and whisper the child's name. The child will usually turn when his or her name is heard. Repeat this step to test the other ear.

Nose. Purulent secretions are common with any nasal infection, including the common upper respiratory infection. Children with redness, discharge, and crusting on the outer edges of the alar may have a beta-hemolytic streptococcal infection. Watery nasal secretions may indicate foreign bodies, the common cold, or an allergy.

Note any unusual shape of the nose, flaring of the nostrils, and the character and amount of discharge.

Examine the septum, turbinates, and vestibule by pushing the tip of the nose upward with the thumb of the nondominant hand and shining a light into the naris. A speculum is usually not necessary for adequate visualization, and it might cause the child to be apprehensive.

ulum is inserted only ¼ or ½ in into the canal to avoid any unnecessary discomfort. For the older child, pull the pinna up and back to visualize the tympanic membrane (Figure 24-40). Before you examine the tympanic membrane, carefully inspect the canal for evidence of furuncles or redness. Inspect the tympanic membrane for color, light reflex, and the usual landmarks of the bony prominences of the middle ear. If you suspect that fluid is present behind the tympanic membrane, you may want to use pneumotoscopy or a tympanogram.

If the canal is filled with cerumen, occasionally you may need to remove the cerumen by irrigation or curettage. The irrigation procedure is unpleasant, may cause vomiting, and is not done unless necessary. Never do this procedure if you suspect a perforation of the tympanic membrane. Avoid removing the cerumen with a curette unless you are skillful in doing so. The procedure may cause pain and bleeding and may result in increased crying, which only exacerbates the redness of the membrane. Flexible plastic curettes are now available and seem easier for many children to tolerate. Often cerumen that is not dry but fairly soft will move during the examination. Visualization of the membrane then becomes possible without the need for any special

Mouth and oropharynx. The mouth and oropharynx area can be examined last since this examination is often fear-provoking to the child. However, it is helpful to some children to do this examination first. For example, the child who is anticipating discomfort may be relieved to have it accomplished and then can cooperate with the rest of the examination. Deciding on this approach requires knowledge about the individual child's behavior and responses. This information may be obtained during the history or in discussion with the parent.

The procedures are the same as in the adult examination. However, the young child will probably need to be restrained by the parent (Figure 24-41, *A*). The older child is usually able to cooperate (Figure 24-41, *B*). The examination findings are different from those of adults. The number of deciduous and permanent teeth and the pattern of eruption are determined by the child's age and development. There are 20 deciduous teeth, and their eruption is completed by the age of 2½ years. The first permanent molar and the lower incisor erupt at 6 years of age (Figure 24-42). The tonsils are normally larger in children than in adults, and they usually extend beyond the palatine arch until the age

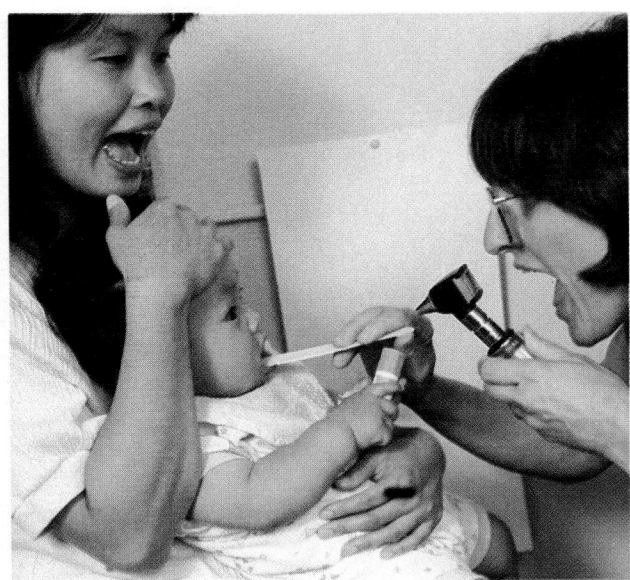
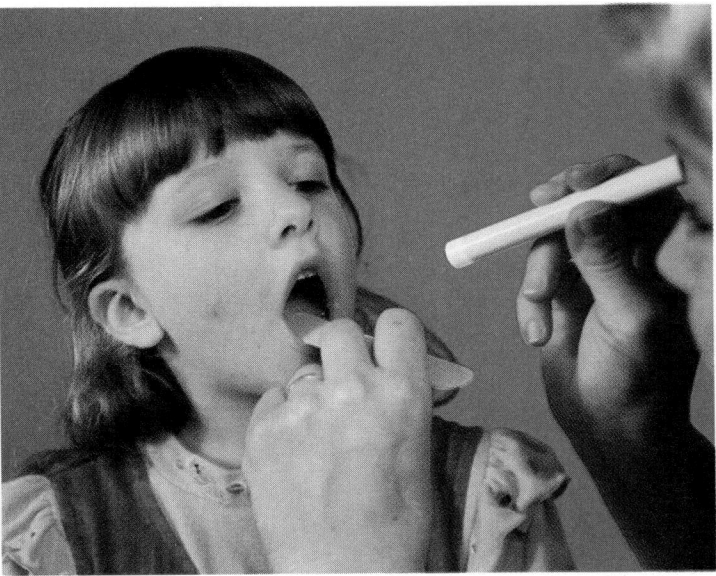

A   **B**

FIGURE 24-41 Positioning the child for examination of the mouth. **A,** The young child often requires restraint by the parent and encouragement from both parent and examiner. **B,** The older child is usually cooperative.

of 11 or 12 years. Inspect the palate for a cleft. A bifid uvula may indicate a submucous cleft palate (a cleft covered by membrane), which cannot be identified by inspection alone.

Chest. Begin the examination of the chest with an inspection of its general shape and circumference. In infancy the chest is almost round; the anteroposterior diameter equals the transverse diameter (i.e., barrel chest). This shape changes as the child grows from preschool to school age. The chest circumference is normally the same as, or slightly less than, the head circumference until age 2 years. Respiratory activity is abdominal and does not become primarily thoracic until age 7 years. Little intercostal motion is seen in infants and young children. Therefore, if you observe intercostal motion in the young child, suspect lung disease.

You can perform palpation and evaluate tactile fremitus while the child is crying. Perform percussion of the chest by using either the direct or the indirect method. The child's chest is normally more resonant than that of the adult. Breath sounds will seem much louder because of the thinness of the chest wall and are almost all bronchovesicular (Figure 24-43).

Heart. A quiet child and environment are necessary for accurate assessment of the heart (Figure 24-44). Therefore making this the first part of the examination is a good idea. The examination of the cardiovascular system (see Chapter 16) applies to the examination of the child; however, some cardiac findings of normal children are not considered normal in adults.

The pulse rate in children of different ages is discussed earlier in this chapter. The palpation of pulses in all the extremities is a part of the cardiovascular examination. The pulses in the lower extremities, especially the femoral pulses, are of special importance in children. Their absence or diminution may indicate coarctation of the aorta.

During infancy the position of the heart is more nearly horizontal and has a larger diameter in comparison with the total diameter of the chest than it does in the adult (Figure 24-45). The apex is one or two intercostal spaces above that considered normal for the adult. Therefore the apical impulse in young children is normally felt in the fourth intercostal space immediately to the left of the midclavicular line. This location changes gradually, and by 7 years of age the apical impulse is normally found in the fifth intercostal space at the midclavicular line.

Sinus arrhythmia is a normal finding in infants and children. The degree of arrhythmia is less in the young infant and greatest in the adolescent. The heart sounds are louder because of the thinness of the chest wall. They are also of a higher pitch and shorter duration than those of the normal adult. A splitting of the second heart sound can be heard in the second left intercostal space in most infants and children. The physiological

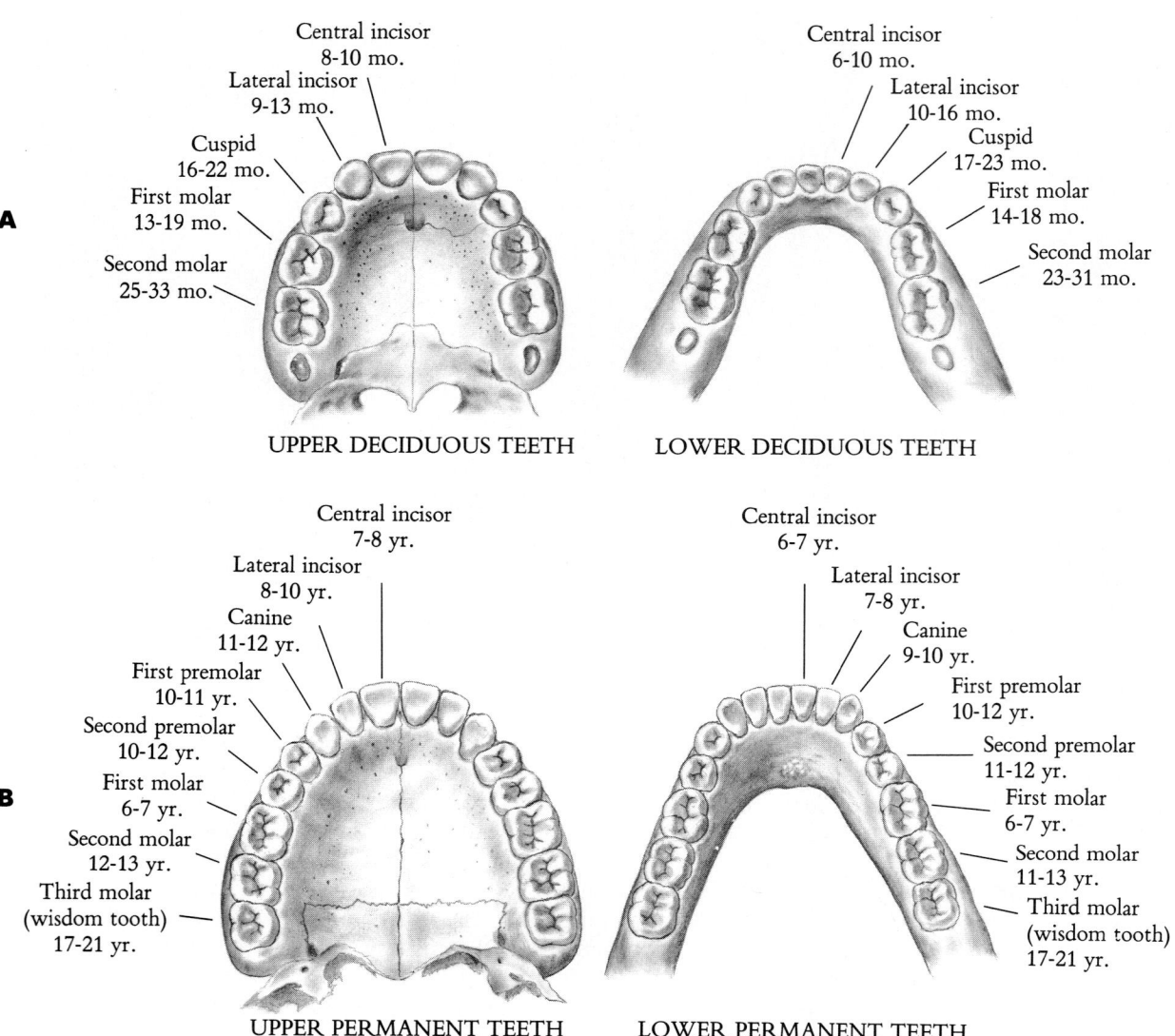

UPPER DECIDUOUS TEETH

LOWER DECIDUOUS TEETH

UPPER PERMANENT TEETH

LOWER PERMANENT TEETH

FIGURE 24-42 A, Dentition of deciduous teeth and their sequence of eruption. **B,** Dentition of permanent teeth and their sequence of eruption. (From Seidel HM and others: *Mosby's guide to physical examination,* ed 2, St Louis, 1991, Mosby–Year Book.)

split normally widens with inspiration. A third heart sound is present in approximately one third of all children and is best heard at the apex.

Many children have murmurs without heart disease. The significance of a murmur may be difficult to determine. Innocent murmurs are characteristically systolic in timing; are grade 1 or 2 in intensity; have a soft, blowing quality; and are not transmitted to other areas. It is not always possible to determine whether the murmur is innocent or pathological by auscultation alone, although murmurs of grade 3 or louder usually indicate heart disease. A venous hum is commonly present in children. It is a continuous, low-pitched sound origi-

nating in the internal jugular vein that is heard either above or below the clavicles. It is accentuated in the upright position and disappears when the child is lying down. Because it is not pathologically significant, a venous hum should be differentiated from a murmur. Refer any murmur that is symptomatic (i.e., accompanied by chest pains or palpitations) to a physician.

Abdomen. The abdomen is somewhat easier to examine in the child than in the adult because of the client's less well developed abdominal wall. To gain the child's cooperation, several approaches may be helpful. For example, a nursing bottle may calm the infant, or

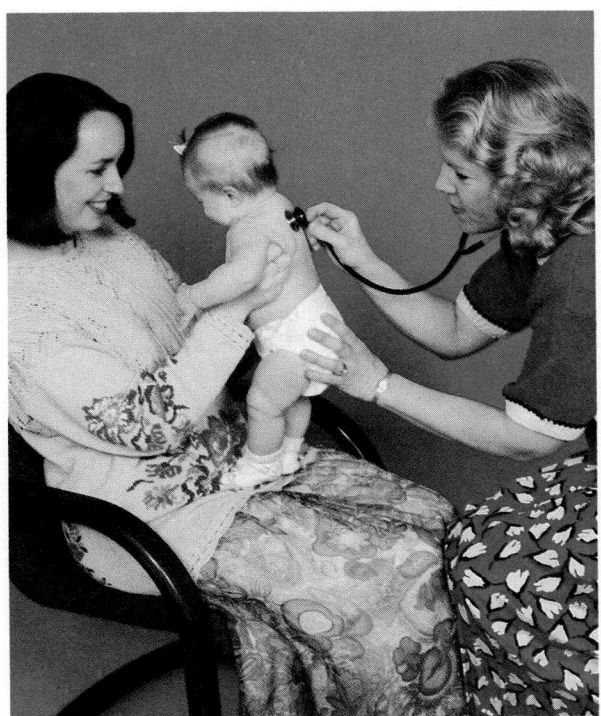

FIGURE 24-43 Examination of the lungs. The young child is more comfortable and cooperative on the parent's lap.

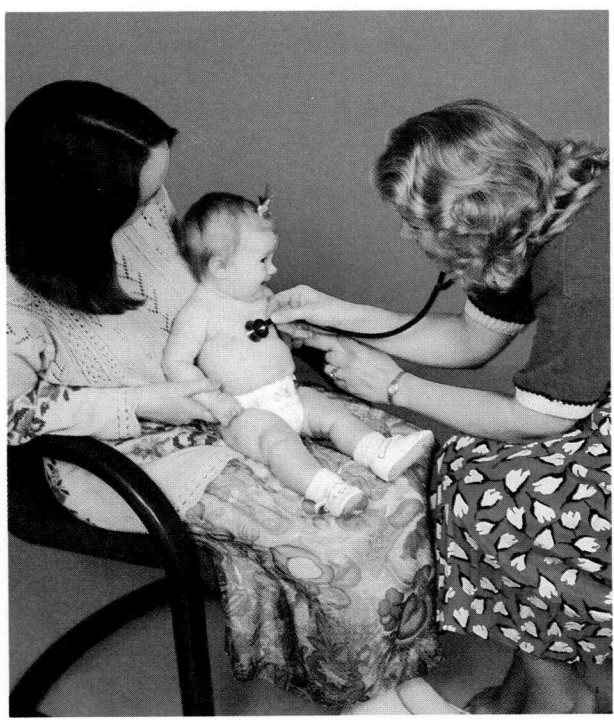

FIGURE 24-44 Auscultation of the heart requires a quiet child. Doing the examination on the parent's lap increases the child's comfort and cooperation.

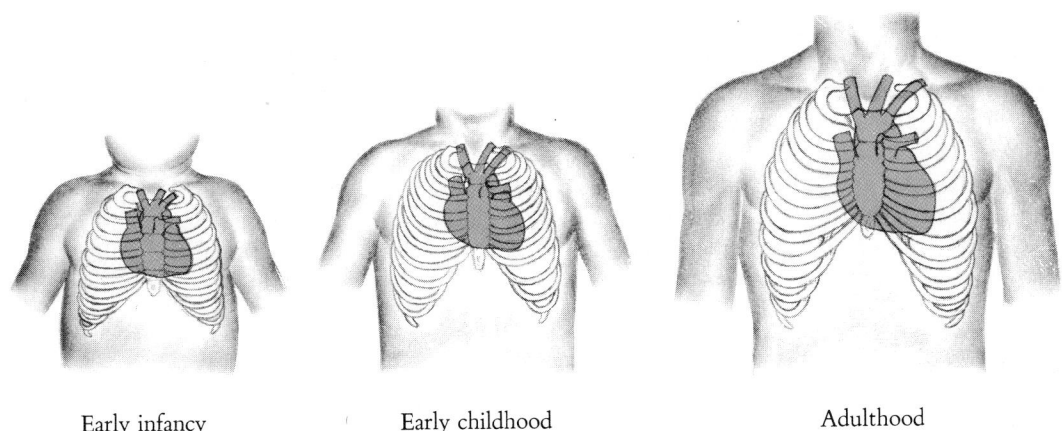

Early infancy   Early childhood   Adulthood

FIGURE 24-45 Position of the heart at various ages. (From Seidel HM and others: *Mosby's guide to physical examination*, ed 2, St Louis, 1991, Mosby–Year Book.)

the young child may be more comfortable and relaxed if examined while sitting on the parent's lap. Find the approaches that are most productive in particular situations (Figure 24-46).

The order of the abdominal examination procedures for the young child should be inspection, auscultation, percussion, palpation. First, inspect the abdomen. The abdomen is larger than the chest in children less than 4 years of age and appears pot bellied in both supine and sitting positions. The child up to 13 years of age will have a pot belly in the standing position. This normal shape must be differentiated from true distention caused by enlargement of organs or the presence of tumors, cysts, or ascites. A depressed abdomen may

> **Helpful Hints on Abdominal Assessment:** *In a relaxed child the abdomen is somewhat easier to examine than in the adult because the abdominal wall is less well developed and (usually) less adipose tissue is present. If a child's muscles become tense, however, the task becomes quite difficult.*
>
> *Many children become anxious or very ticklish during this part of the examination. To help the child relax, make sure he or she keeps the knees bent while lying on the back, and have the child keep a hand over yours as you palpate. You can also have the child's hand under your examining fingers during palpation.*

result from dehydration or malnutrition. Respirations are largely abdominal in children up to 7 years of age. Any splinting or loss of movement may indicate peritonitis, appendicitis, or other acute problems. The umbilicus is normally closed, but umbilical hernias are common in Caucasian children up to 2 years of age and for longer periods in black children (Figure 24-47). Also, observe the abdomen for peristaltic waves (indicating pyloric stenosis) and dilated veins (indicating liver disease).

Carry out auscultation of the abdomen in the same manner as described in the examination of the adult—before percussion and palpation. Percussion may be useful in obtaining the boundaries of the liver, spleen, and any tumors. Children may be intrigued by the percussion sounds, especially the gastric bubble. Having the child listen for the gastric bubble sound is one way to make the examination seem less threatening.

Perform palpation in the same way as in the examination of the adult except for the modifications in approach and in the positions of the child. Light palpation enables you to determine the tenseness of the abdominal muscles, the presence of superficial masses, and the presence of tenderness. The child is not able to pinpoint the area of tenderness, and only by watching the facial expressions can you determine the point of maximal tenderness. The liver is palpable 1 to 2 cm below the right costal margin in the first year of life. If it extends more than 2 cm below the costal margin, investigate further. The spleen is normally palpable 1 to 2 cm below the left costal margin in the first weeks of life. Note any increase in size. Any evidence of tenderness may indicate serious blood dyscrasias or other problems. Determine tissue turgor by grasping a few inches of skin and subcutaneous tissue over the abdomen, pulling it up, and then quickly releasing it (see Figure 24-28). If the creases formed do not disappear immediately, dehydration is present. Do deep palpation in all four quadrants by single-hand or bimanual meth-

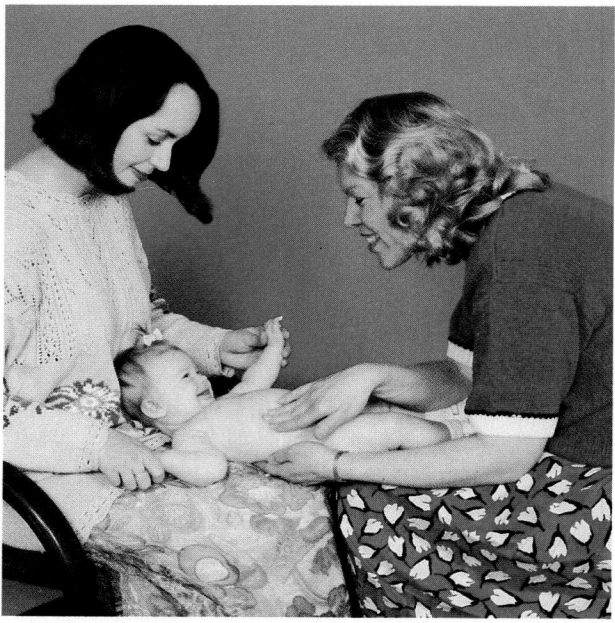

FIGURE 24-46 Examination of the abdomen in an infant.

ods. Palpate the inguinal and femoral regions for hernias, lymph nodes, and femoral pulses (Figure 24-47).

Genitalia. The examination of the genitalia of both male and female children is usually carried out by inspection and palpation.

As part of the genital examination, you need to consider the child's or the adolescent's stage of pubertal development. The Sexual Maturity Rating (SMR) scale developed by Tanner (1962) is composed of five classes, which are based on pubic hair and breast development in females (see Figures 24-5 and 24-8) and pubic hair and genitalia in males (see Figures 24-6 and 24-7). This information is important for identifying abnormal puberty and also for reassuring the adolescent that he or she is normal. Record the SMR, or Tanner stage, at the initial visit and yearly thereafter.

Male genitalia. In the male child two primary areas are examined: the penis and the scrotum. First examine the foreskin of the penis. The foreskin of the uncircumcised infant is normally tight for the first 2 or 3 months of life and does not retract easily. If the tightness persists beyond this period, it is called **phimosis.** Determine whether this condition causes any interference with urination. Do any retraction of the foreskin carefully since the delicate membranes attached to the foreskin may be easily torn, resulting in adhesions. Next, examine the meatus to determine its position and the presence of any ulceration. The meatus is normally located at the

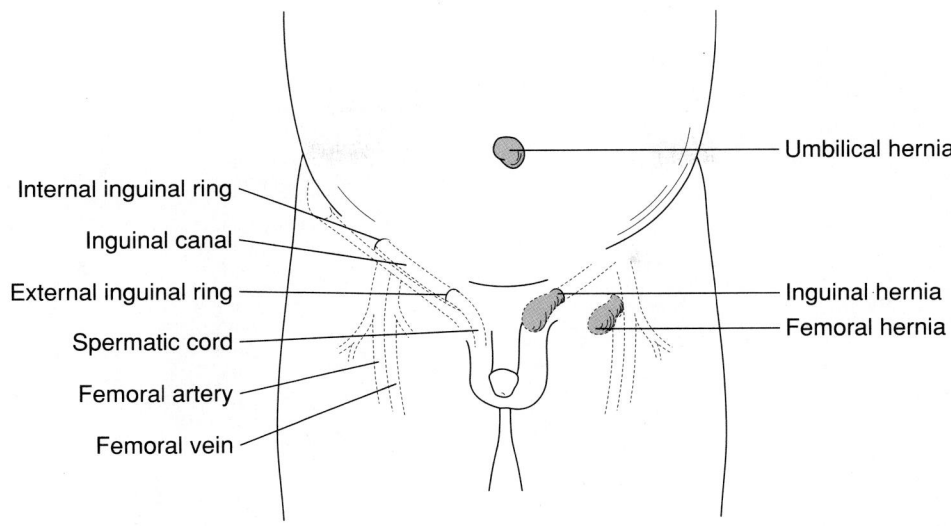

Internal inguinal ring

Inguinal canal

External inguinal ring

Spermatic cord

Femoral artery

Femoral vein

Umbilical hernia

Inguinal hernia

Femoral hernia

FIGURE 24-47 Location of hernias.

tip of the shaft. An abnormal location of the meatus on the ventral surface is called **hypospadias**; an abnormal location on the dorsal surface is called **epispadias**.

Inspect the scrotum for evidence of enlargement. An enlarged scrotum may be indicative of a hernia or hydrocele. Palpate the scrotum to determine if the testes are descended (Figure 24-48). Use your index finger to block the inguinal canal and gently push toward the scrotum. Use the finger and thumb of the opposite hand to palpate the scrotum and grasp the testes as they are pushed downward into the scrotum. If you cannot easily palpate the testes in an older boy, have him sit in a chair with his legs apart, his heels on the seat of the chair, and his arms around his knees. This procedure interrupts the cremasteric reflex and creates pressure by flexing the abdomen and the thigh. You will feel the testes as a soft mass about 1 cm in diameter. They are normally descended if you can palpate them in the scrotum even if retraction into the inguinal canal occurs immediately. In an infant, block the inguinal canals with the nondominant hand and palpate the testes as soon as the diaper is removed before the cold room air causes retraction.

For the adolescent male, follow the same procedure as for the adult male (see Chapter 20).

Female genitalia. Inspect the genitalia of the female child by separating the labia majora with the thumb and the forefinger to expose the labia minora, urethral meatus, and vaginal orifice (Figure 24-49). Examine the young infant in a supine position on the mother's lap with the knees held in a flexed position and separated. Sit facing the mother and child. The older child can help by spreading back her labia with her hands

(Figure 24-50). Urethral discharges are pathological and indicate infection somewhere in the urinary tract. A bloody vaginal discharge during the first month of life (secondary to residual maternal hormones) is normal but not common. Purulent or mucoid vaginal discharges indicate infection or the presence of a foreign body. Inspect the labia and the clitoris for any abnormality in size or for evidence of adhesion or infection. Inspect the vaginal area; usually it is not palpated. An imperforate hymen may be apparent if there is fluid behind it.

The vaginal examination is usually omitted for the child. If concerns or symptoms require such an examination, an experienced clinician or a gynecologist should examine the child. Vaginal examinations should be done on the adolescent who is sexually active, has been sexually assaulted, is considering contraception, requests such an examination, or has indications of an infection or other pelvic disorder (Lichtman and Papera, 1990). The age at which the first pelvic examination is recommended varies, but a commonly accepted age is 16 years.

Musculoskeletal system. The skeleton of the infant and young child is made up largely of cartilaginous tissues, which accounts for the relative softness and malleability of the bones. It is also the reason that many defects identified early in life can be corrected with more ease than in later years.

Conduct much of the musculoskeletal examination while watching the child or while playing with the child. Since the infant or younger child is not able to understand directions, you can perform much of the examination by helping the child passively go through

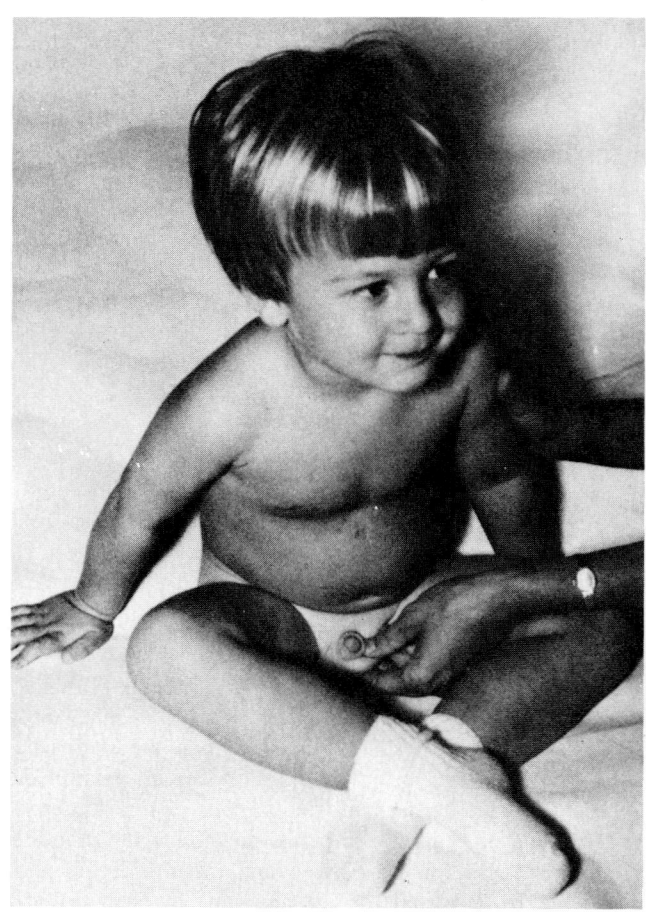

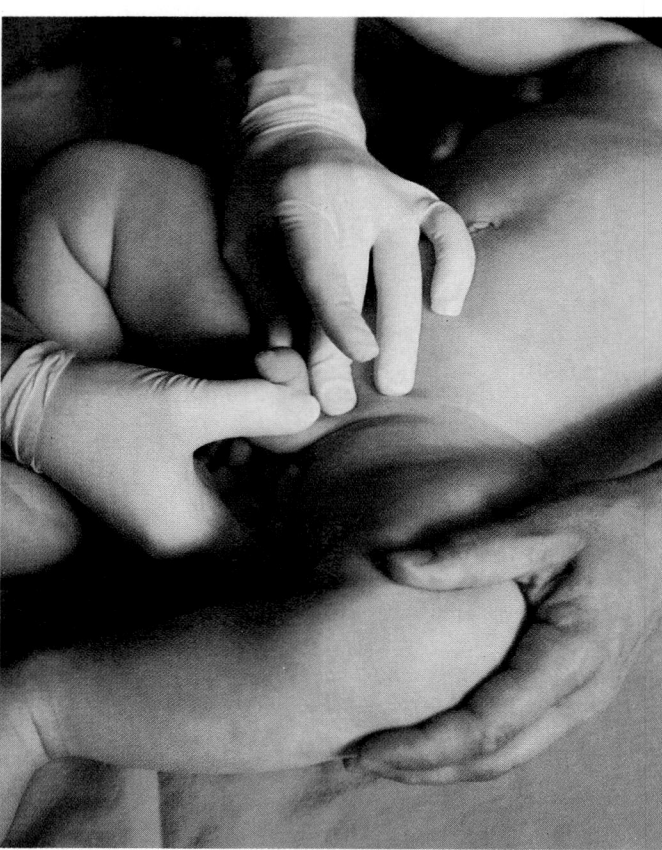

A

B

FIGURE 24-48 A, Preventing cremasteric reflex by having child sit in "tailor" position. **B,** Palpation of the scrotum to determine if the testes are descended, blocking the inguinal canal. (**A** from Whaley LF, Wong DL: *Nursing care of infants and children,* ed 4, St Louis, 1991, Mosby—Year Book.)

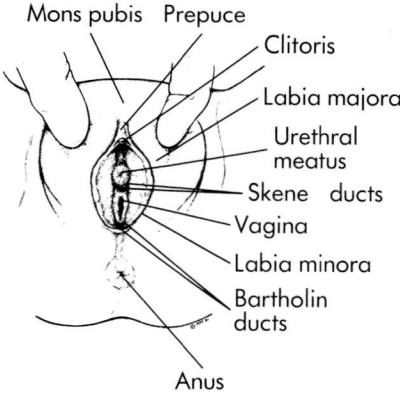

Mons pubis Prepuce
Clitoris
Labia majora
Urethral
meatus
Skene ducts
Vagina
Labia minora
Bartholin
ducts
Anus

FIGURE 24-49 External structures of the genitalia in a prepubertal female. Labia are spread to reveal deeper structures material. (From Whaley LF, Wong DL: *Nursing care of infants and children,* ed 4, St Louis, 1991, Mosby—Year Book.)

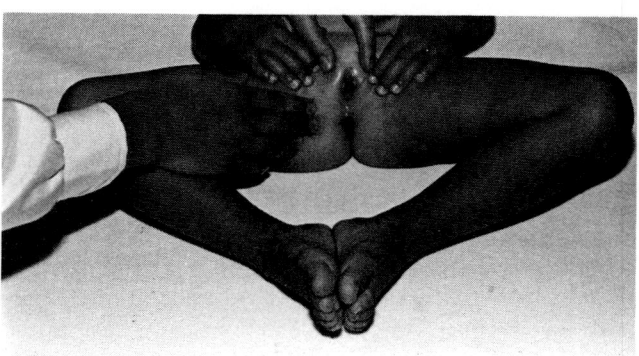

FIGURE 24-50 Postition for examining the genitalia in a female child. (From Whaley LF, Wong DL: *Nursing care of infants and children,* ed 4, St Louis, 1991, Mosby—Year Book.)

TABLE 24-14

Four Primary Deformities of the Foot in Relation to the Position of the Heel, Forefoot, and/or Toes

Primary deformity	Heel	Forefoot	Toes
Varus	Inverted	Adducted inverted (sole in)	
Valgus	Everted	Abducted everted (sole out)	
Equinus	Plantar flexed		At level lower than heel
Calcaneus	Dorsiflexed		At level higher than heel
Combinations			
Equinovarus	Plantar flexed inverted	Adducted inverted (sole in)	At level lower than heel
Equinovalgus	Plantar flexed everted	Abducted everted (sole out)	At level lower than heel
Calcaneovarus	Dorsiflexed inverted	Adducted inverted (sole in)	At level higher than heel
Calcaneovalgus	Dorsiflexed everted	Abducted everted (sole out)	At level higher than heel

Data from Swanger R: Common problems of toddlers and preschoolers, lecture, 1972.

range-of-motion movements. An older child is able to follow directions, and you can complete a routine musculoskeletal examination.

Inspect the neck, extremities, hips, and spine for symmetry, increased or decreased mobility, and anatomical defects.

The newborn at rest assumes the position maintained in utero and the feet are rarely straight. They are usually held in the varus (forefoot turned in) or valgus (forefoot turned out) position and simulate the clubfoot. To determine whether this is a true abnormality or a transient position, scratch the outside border and the inside border of the foot. The normal foot will usually assume a right-angle position with the leg. If this is a fixed deformity or it is difficult to bring the foot to the neutral position, refer the infant for an orthopedic evaluation (Table 24-14 and the box at right).

Infants generally have bowlegs until 12 to 18 months. When they begin walking, their gait is wide based. Some children tend to evert their feet so that they bear weight on the inner aspects of the feet, and this is normal. The young child also has a fat pad under the arch of the foot and may appear flat-footed until about 3 to 4 years of age. The child's bowlegged appearance changes as the gait improves, and then the child becomes mildly knock-kneed (Figure 24-51). The normal configuration of the legs develops by age 6 or 7 years.

Intoeing may result from metatarsus varus (forefoot turned in); medial tibial torsion, in which the entire foot turns in while the knee remains straight; or medial femoral torsion, in which the entire leg turns in with the foot and knee turned medially. A child who has intoeing as a result of a fixed deformity of the forefoot that cannot be corrected to neutral should be referred for orthopedic care. The problems of medial tibial tor-

ORTHOPEDIC DISORDERS COMMON TO VARIOUS AGE GROUPS OF CHILDREN

Neonate

Oligohydramnios
  Compressed face
  Limb deformities
  Thoracic compression
  Lung hypoplasia
Prolonged breech position
Dislocation of hip
Deformations of knee
Hyperextension of knee
Dislocation of knee
Foot deformities
  Calcaneovalgus
  Metatarsus adductus
  Equinovarus
  Overlapping toes
Craniofacies
  Compressed face
    Molding of calvaria
    Mandibular asymmetry
  Torticollis
Dislocated hip(s)
Postural scoliosis

Preschooler

Postural-orthopedic abnormalities of the foot
Abnormalities of the toenail
Disorders of the skin
Deviations in gait
Poor foot hygiene
Inadequate footgear

School-age child

Idiopathic adolescent scoliosis
Other types of scoliosis
Kyphosis
Lordosis
Alignment problems of lower extremity
Juvenile arthritis
Athletic injuries
  Unstable knee
  Upper extremity, elbow clean
  Epiphyseal injuries

Young adult

Disabling low back pain
Osteoarthritis
Athletic injuries
  Jogging-related injuries

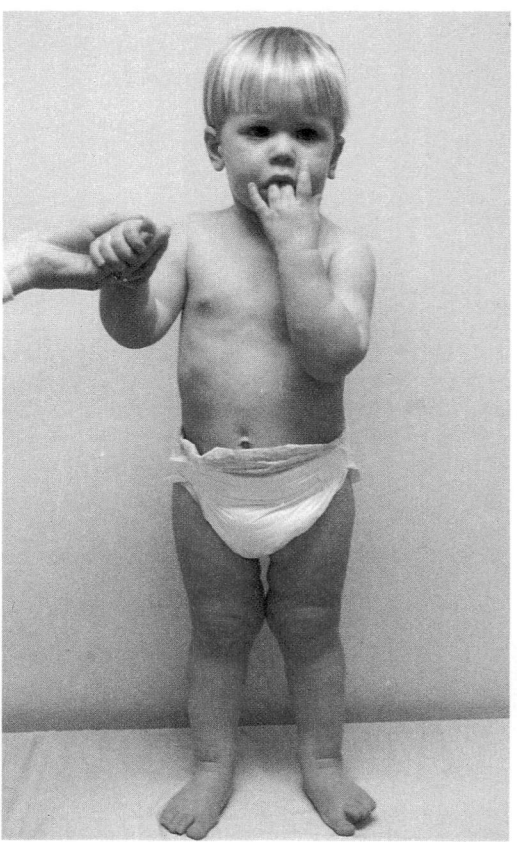

FIGURE 24-51 Genu valgum (knock-knee) in the young child. (From Seidel HM and others: *Mosby's guide to physical examination,* ed 2, St Louis, 1991, Mosby–Year Book.)

sion and medial femoral torsion are more cosmetic than functional and usually disappear by age 4 or 5 years.

Examine the hips for congenital dislocation or subluxation at every routine visit during the first year of life. In congenital dislocation the head of the femur is found outside the acetabulum, and relocation may or may not be possible. **Subluxation** means that the capsule is lax enough to allow the femoral head to be displaced but not dislocated. Clinical signs of an abnormal hip may be asymmetry of the skinfolds, creases on the dorsal surfaces, and an apparent leg length inequality (Figure 24-52). However, these signs may not be apparent in the young infant who has a hip that is susceptible to dislocation rather than a dislocated hip. The examination of the hips is done with the infant in the supine position. Flex the infant's hips and knees, and then **abduct** the hips fully. In the newborn each thigh should abduct to almost 90 degrees (Figure 24-53). Any limitation in the abduction of either or both hips may indicate dislocation.

To check the stability of the individual hip, place your middle finger over the greater trochanter (Figure 24-54) with your thumb placed medially. **Adduct** the thigh while still in the flexed position and apply pressure along the long axis of the femur in the direction of the posterior lip of the acetabulum. As dislocation occurs, you will feel the click of exit (Barlow's test). You will feel a similar click or "clunk" when you reverse the maneuver by abducting the hip and the head of the femur slips back into the joint (Ortolani maneuver). When you feel lateral movement of the head of the

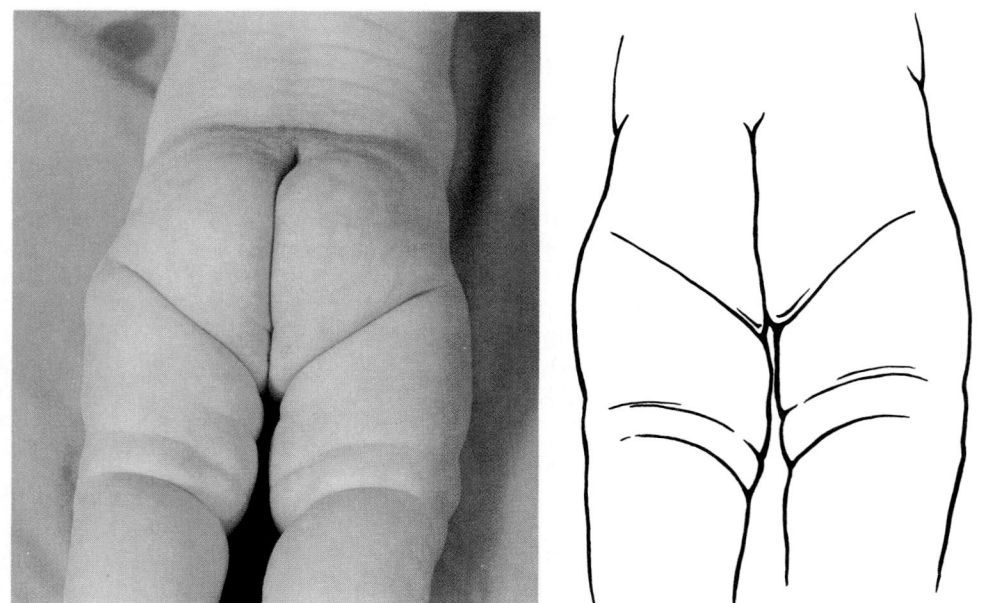

FIGURE 24-52 Examination of the hips. **A,** Normal gluteal folds. **B,** Abnormal gluteal folds.

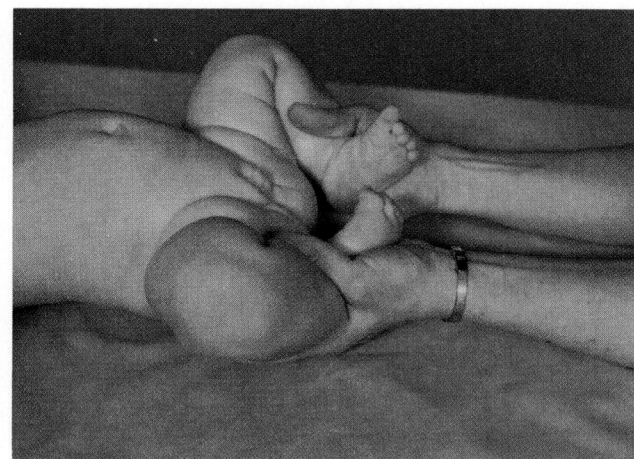

FIGURE 24-53 Examination of the hips for dislocation: abduction.

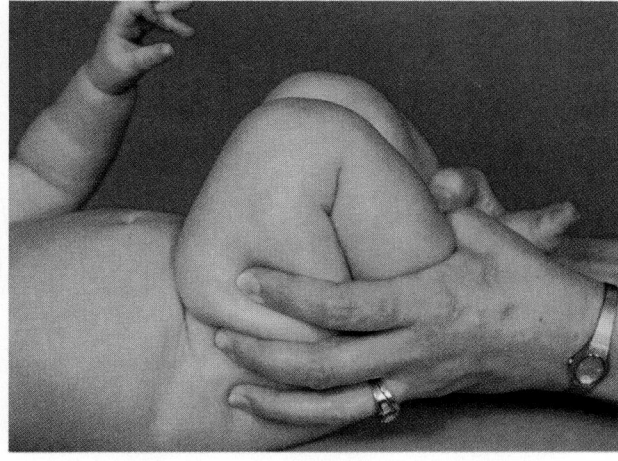

FIGURE 24-54 Examination of the hips for dislocation: adduction.

femur without dislocation, the hip is subluxed. Most dislocated hips in the newborn will relocate naturally. However, an unstable hip may become fixed in the dislocated position during the first weeks of life and the Ortolani maneuver cannot be done to replace the head. Dislocated hips can resolve spontaneously, but there is no way to be sure this will happen. Refer the infant suspected of having a dislocation to an orthopedist without delay since treatment is far more effective at an early age.

All children should have a spinal examination during each health visit. In the young infant and child, a tuft of hair or small dimple usually located toward the distal portion of the spine, but which may appear anywhere from the coccyx to the skull, may indicate underlying spina bifida or may be only a superficial anomaly. If a dimple is apparent, note its interior and depth. A dimple often indicates a dermoid cyst, which may become a site of infection. The young infant and child should be examined for congenital scoliosis, whereas the child of 10 years or older should be examined for idiopathic scoliosis. The method of examination is the same as for the adult (Figure 24-55). Observe the shoulders for symmetry in the standing position. Ask the child to bend the shoulders forward with the arms hanging freely and the head down. In this position you can observe any prominence of one side of the rib cage. Examine the young infant in a sitting position while bending the child forward on your hand. If a scoliosis is suspected, refer the child to an orthopedist.

Athletic injuries are becoming more common with the increase in organized sports activities for preadolescents and adolescents. The growing child is at risk for epiphyseal fractures where the least resistance to stress is found. Stress fractures of the tibia or the femur

occur frequently, and the affected child complains of pain in the proximal region of the tibia or distal portion of the femur. A painful knee may be caused by a dislocation of the patella. The history of the child's recent activities will give some indication of the kind of injury sustained. Refer the child for evaluation by an orthopedist.

Neurological system. Although you must adapt the formal neurological examination of the infant or child to the age of the individual, at all times a complete examination consists of an assessment of the cranial nerves and special senses, the motor system, coordination and cerebellar function, sensation, and both superficial and deep reflexes. In children less than 2 years of age, the neurological assessment is closely related to the increasing myelinization and maturation of the neural system. In this age group you can only estimate the degree of maturation rather than quantify it.

In the newborn, infant, and child older than 2 years, the primary mode of examination is one of observation and inspection. This approach is usually reinforced by palpation and passive manipulation.

Observation of the child in the natural state and then with purposeful stimulation is often the examiner's most valuable tool. Such observation is the best opportunity to determine how the child's overall function and behavior meet age-related norms. Seven assessment areas include symmetry of spontaneous movements, appearance, positioning, posture, movement of extremities, seizure activity, and responsiveness to the parents and the environment.

A good tool for assessing neurological status in an infant and young child is the Denver Developmental Screening Test II (see Figure 3-1). Gross and fine motor

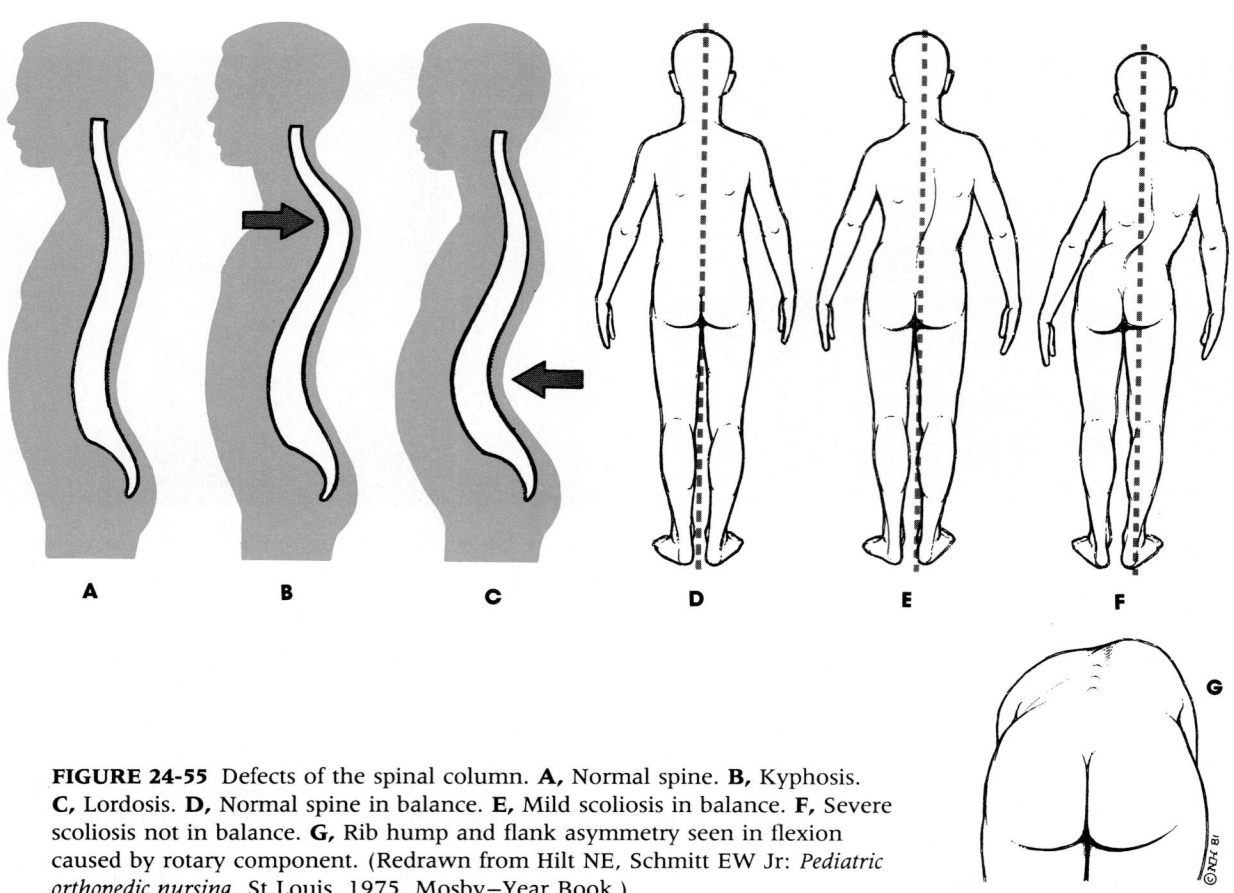

FIGURE 24-55 Defects of the spinal column. **A,** Normal spine. **B,** Kyphosis. **C,** Lordosis. **D,** Normal spine in balance. **E,** Mild scoliosis in balance. **F,** Severe scoliosis not in balance. **G,** Rib hump and flank asymmetry seen in flexion caused by rotary component. (Redrawn from Hilt NE, Schmitt EW Jr: *Pediatric orthopedic nursing,* St Louis, 1975, Mosby–Year Book.)

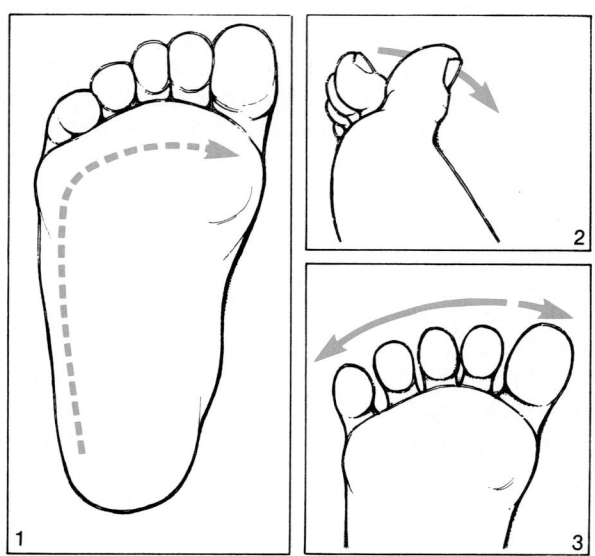

FIGURE 24-56 Babinski reflex. *1,* Direction of stroke. *2,* Dorsiflexion of big toe. *3,* Fanning of toes. (From Whaley LF, Wong DL: *Nursing care of infants and children,* ed 4, St Louis, 1991, Mosby–Year Book.)

skills, language skills, and social skills provide clues to neurological status when the child is compared with other children of the same age. The Denver II is a major revision of the Denver Developmental Screening Test (DDST). It was developed to address criticisms of cultural and gender bias in the DDST.

Because the neurological system affects every other system, the neurological examination should be integrated with other parts of the physical examination. For example, changes in the pigmentation of the skin, lesions of the skin, masses in the abdomen, abnormal size and shape of the head, gaps and protrusions in the spinal column, and limited range of motion can all reflect a disease, lesion, or injury to the nervous system. In addition, because a child is going through an intense period of development that is in part related to the increasing myelinization and maturation of the neural system, meticulous observation of the child's developmental progress is important. The quality, pitch, loudness, and duration of a child's cry; drowsiness; irritability; and social, adaptive, language, and motor skills are all measures of how well the neurological system is functioning.

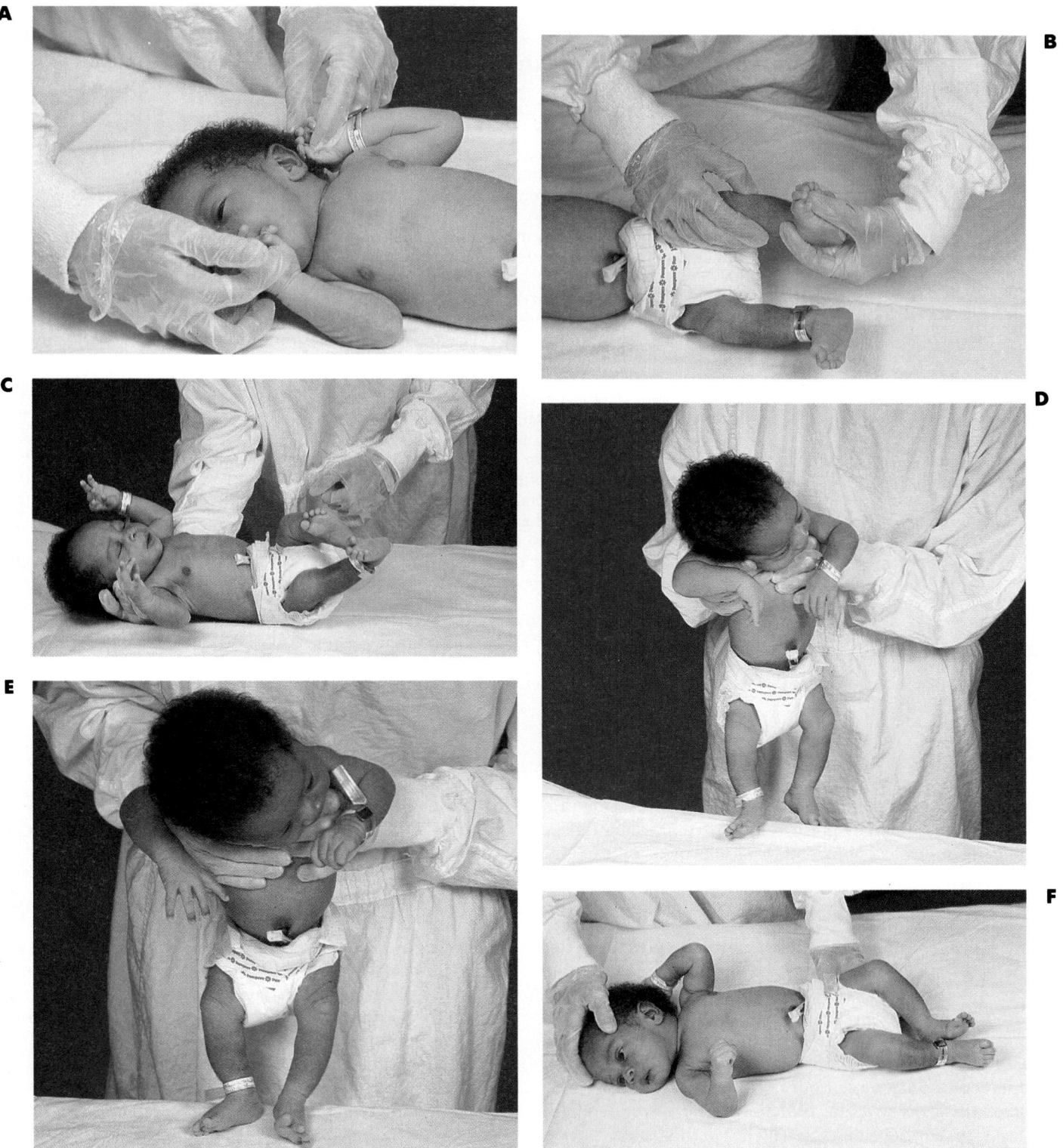

FIGURE 24-57 Elicitation of the primitive reflex. **A,** Palmar grasp. **B,** Plantar grasp. **C,** Moro reflex. **D,** Placing reflex. **E,** Stepping reflex. **F,** Tonic neck reflex. Proper positioning of the head and neck is shown, but this infant is too young for the reflex to be present. (From Seidel HM and others: *Mosby's guide to physical examination,* ed 2, St Louis, 1991, Mosby–Year Book.)

TABLE 24-15

Primitive Reflexes Routinely Evaluated: Procedure for Examination, Expected Findings, Time of Appearance and Disappearance

Reflex (appearance)	Procedure and findings
Palmar grasp (birth)	Making sure the infant's head is in midline, touch the palm of the infant's hand from the ulnar side (opposite the thumb). Note the strong grasp of your finger. Sucking facilitates the grasp. It should be strongest between 1 and 2 months of age and disappear by 3 months (Figure 24-57, *A*).
Plantar grasp (birth)	Touch the plantar surface of the infant's feet at the base of the toes. The toes should curl downward. It should be strong up to 8 months of age (Figure 24-57, *B*).
Moro (birth)	With the infant supported in semisitting position, allow the head and trunk to drop back to a 30-degree angle. Observe symmetrical abduction and extension of the arms; fingers fan out and thumb and index finger form a C. The arms then adduct in an embracing motion followed by relaxed flexion. The legs may follow a similar pattern of response. The reflex diminishes in strength by 3 to 4 months and disappears by 6 months (Figure 24-57, *C*).
Placing (4 days of age)	Hold the infant upright under its arms next to the table or chair. Touch the dorsal side of the foot to the table or chair edge. Observe flexion of the hips and knees and lifting of the foot as if stepping up on the table. Age of disappearance varies (Figure 24-57, *D*).
Stepping (between birth and 8 weeks)	Hold the infant upright under the arms and allow the soles of the feet to touch the surface of the table. Observe for alternate flexion and extension of the legs, simulating walking. It disappears before voluntary walking (Figure 24-57, *E*).
Tonic neck or "fencing" (by 2 to 3 months)	With the infant lying supine and relaxed or sleeping, turn its head to one side so the jaw is over the shoulder. Observe for extension of the arm and leg on the side to which the head is turned and for flexion of the opposite arm and leg. Turn the infant's head to the other side, observing the reversal of the extremities' posture. This reflex diminishes at 3 to 4 months of age and disappears by 6 months. Be concerned if the infant never exhibits the reflex or seems locked in the fencing position. This reflex must disappear before the infant can roll over or bring its hand to its face (Figure 24-57, *F*).

From Seidel HM and others: *Mosby's guide to physical examination,* ed 2, St Louis, 1991, Mosby–Year Book.

The automatic infant reflexes that are normal at birth disappear at approximately 4-6 months of age, as voluntary control begins to develop. They include the Moro reflex, palmar grasp reflex, plantar grasp reflex, placing reflex, stepping reflex, tonic neck reflex, and rooting reflex. Absence of these reflexes at birth may indicate a severe problem of the central nervous system. Persistence of these reflexes may be equally serious.

A positive Babinski reflex is normally present in the newborn and disappears by the age of 12 to 24 months or when the child begins to walk (Figure 24-56). Table 24-15 describes several reflexes found in full-term infants. Figure 24-57 illustrates these reflexes.

Examine the child who is 2 years of age or older with many of the same methods used for an adult. However, alter the conversation, directions, and developmental tasks to be more suitable to the child's interests and knowledge level. In a child of this age, more specific examination is possible, including auditory testing, funduscopic examination, and stereognosis testing. You can expand assessment to observe the quantity and quality of spontaneous voluntary motor activity, the ease in performing voluntary movements, lateral dominance, spontaneous drawing, articulation of sounds, and language acquisition. Also, note the child's auditory discrimination, memory, reading, speech, and calculation skills. Last, test the child for awareness of body parts, spatial orientation, and emotional lability.

Regardless of the child's age, if you suspect meningeal irritation during an illness episode, note the presence of paradoxical irritability, Kernig's sign, or Brudzinski's signs. In paradoxical irritability the child is not easily comforted when held by the parent, contrary to his or her usual behavior. To elicit Kernig's sign, have the child lie on the table, face up, with the leg bent at the knee. Attempt to extend the hip by raising the knee. If you encounter pain and resistance, the maneuver is positive for meningeal irritation. Obtain Brudzinski's sign by having the child lie supine on a table. Bend the neck gently. If the child's knees flex spontaneously, this sign is positive. Tables 24-16 and 24-17 give detailed information on techniques for evaluating cranial nerve function in infants and young children.

• • •

TABLE 24-16

Testing Procedures and Expected Behaviors for Indirect Cranial Nerve Evaluation in Newborns and Infants

Cranial nerves	Procedures and observations
CN II, III, IV, and VI	Optical blink reflex: shine a light at the infant's open eyes. Observe the quick closure of the eyes and dorsal flexion of the infant's head. No response may indicate poor light perception. Gazes intensely at close object or face. Focuses on and tracks an object with its eyes. Doll's eye maneuver: see CN VIII.
CN V	Rooting reflex: touch one corner of the infant's mouth. The infant should open its mouth and turn its head in the direction of stimulation. If the infant has been recently fed, minimal or no response is expected. Sucking reflex: place your finger in the infant's mouth, feeling the sucking action. The tongue should push up against your finger with a fairly good rate. Note the pressure, strength, and pattern of sucking.
CN VII	Observe the infant's facial expression when crying. Note the infant's ability to wrinkle its forehead and the symmetry of the smile.
CN VIII	Acoustic blink reflex: loudly clap your hands about 30 cm from the infant's head; avoid producing an air current. Note the blink in response to the sound. No response after 2-3 days of age may indicate hearing problems. Infant will habituate to repeated testing. Moves eyes in direction of sound. Freezes position with high-pitched sound. Doll's eye maneuver: hold the infant under the axilla in an upright position, head held steady, facing you. Rotate the infant first in one direction and then in the other. The infant's eyes should turn in the direction of rotation and then the opposite direction when rotation stops. If the eyes do not move in the expected direction, suspect a vestibular problem or eye muscle paralysis.
CN IX and X	Swallowing and gag reflex.
CN XII	Coordinated sucking and swallowing ability. Pinch infant's nose: mouth will open and tip of tongue will rise in a midline position.

From Seidel HM and others: *Mosby's guide to physical examination,* ed 2, St Louis, 1991, Mosby–Year Book.

TABLE 24-17

Cranial Nerve Examination Procedures for Young Children

Cranial nerves	Procedures and observations
CN II	If the child cooperates, the Snellen E or Picture Chart may be used to test vision. Visual fields may be tested, but the child may need the head immobilized.
CN III, IV, and VI	Have the child follow an object with the eyes, immobilizing the head if necessary. Attempt to move the object through the cardinal points of gaze.
CN V	Observe the child chewing a cookie or cracker, noting bilateral jaw strength. Touch the child's forehead and cheeks with cotton and watch the child bat it away.
CN VII	Observe the child's face when smiling, frowning, and crying. Ask the child to show the teeth. Demonstrate puffed cheeks and ask the child to imitate.
CN VIII	Observe the child turn to sounds such as bell or whisper. Whisper a commonly used word behind the child's back and have the child repeat the word. Perform audiometric testing.
CN IX and X	Elicit gag reflex.
CN XI and XII	Instruct older child to stick out the tongue and shrug the shoulders or raise the arms.

From Seidel HM and others: *Mosby's guide to physical examination,* ed 2, St Louis, 1991, Mosby–Year Book.

A thorough working knowledge of growth and development, combined with solid physical assessment skills, and an appreciation of the need to include the family in the assessment process will help the practitioner successfully assess pediatric clients and promote the health of children and their families.

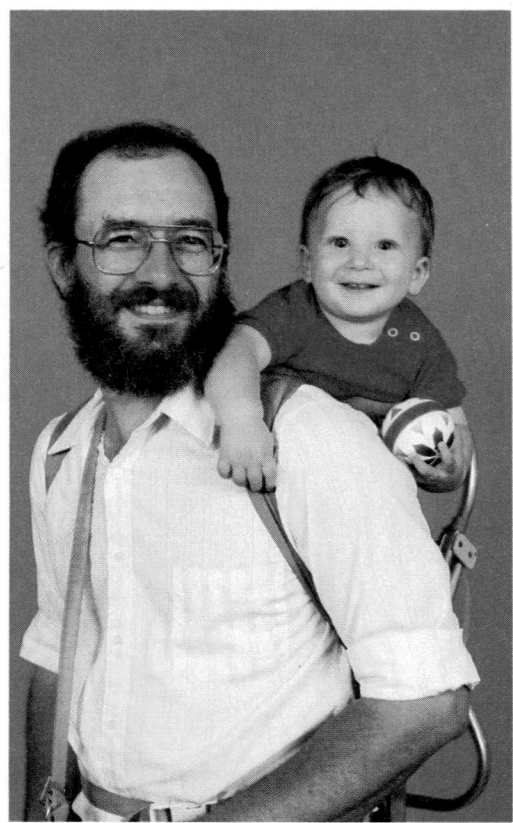

Sample Documentation

Health history

CC: 7-year-old white female brought to clinic by her mother for a sore throat and fever for the past day. Interval history: She has been in good health except for approximately four colds since her visit 1 year ago. She has no known allergies to any medications. HPI: Mother states that Debbie has had a fever up to 102.7° F (oral) since yesterday. The fever comes down with acetaminophen 320 mg. Her last dose of acetaminophen was about 3 hours ago. Debbie also complains of a sore throat. She has been drinking plenty of liquids, but her appetite has decreased since she has had the fever. Debbie denies any pain when bending her neck, abdominal pain, or pain with urination. Her mother states that Debbie is tired but alert and moderately active. She states that several of Debbie's classmates have strep throat and she is concerned that Debbie may also have strep throat. No one in her family is sick.

Developmental history: Debbie is in the second grade of the Urban elementary school. She states that she enjoys school but thinks her teacher "is too hard sometimes." Her mother says that all school reports are good and that Debbie has many friends in school and the neighborhood and has recently started "sleeping over" with her girl friends. Mother states that everyone in the family is fine, no major stresses or life changes.

Physical examination

Cooperative, pleasant, 7-year-old white female who appears flushed and feverish. Temp: 101.8° F (tympanic).

Eyes—clear, no discharge or redness. Ears—TMs pearly with landmarks visible. Nose—mucosa pink, slight clear discharge noted. Mouth—pink, no lesions. Throat—tonsils red, swollen 3+ with yellow-white exudate. Neck—enlarged and tender tonsilar nodes bilaterally. Chest—lungs clear, breath sounds normal anterior and posterior, resonant to percussion, no adventitious sounds.

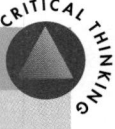

Nursing Diagnosis *THE NEXT STEP*

Nursing diagnoses that could apply to the pediatric client include, but are not limited to, the following ones

HIGH RISK FOR TRAUMA Accentuated risk of accidental tissue injury (e.g., wound, burn, fracture).

Defining Characteristics (risk factors)
- Impaired judgement related to immature age
- Muscle weakness, incoordination; balancing difficulties

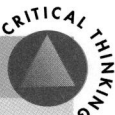

Nursing Diagnosis *THE NEXT STEP—cont'd*

- History of previous trauma, accidental injury (i.e., falling)
- Insufficient finances to purchase safety equipment or to make repairs
- Lack of parental safety precautions, safety education
- Excess alcohol-ingestion pattern (parental)
- Altered blood-clotting factors (bleeding tendency)
- Slippery, littered, or obstructed floors, stairs, walkways (water, snow, ice)
- Unanchored rugs, unsturdy or absent stair rails; unsteady chairs
- Bathtub without hand grips or anti-slip equipment
- Entering unlighted rooms
- Unanchored electric wires
- High beds
- Children playing without gates at top of stairs
- Unsafe window protection in homes with young children
- Parents smoking in bed or near oxygen
- Pot handles facing toward front of stove
- Bathing in very hot water; unsupervised bathing of young children
- Experimenting with chemicals or gasoline; contact with acid or alkali
- Play or work near vehicle pathways (driveways, laneways, railroad tracks)
- Children playing with matches, candles, cigarettes, fireworks, gunpowder, sharp-edged toys
- Inadequate stored combustible or corrosive materials (matches, oily rags, lye)
- Children riding in front seat of automobile; unrestrained babies riding in car
- Highly flammable children's toys or clothing
- Faulty electrical plugs; frayed wires
- Overexposure to sun
- Use of cracked dishware or glasses; knives stored uncovered
- Guns or ammunition stored unlocked
- Large icicles hanging from roof
- High-crime neighborhood
- Unsafe roads or road-crossing conditions
- Non-use or misuse of seat restraints, headgear for cyclists and passengers

HIGH RISK FOR POISONING Accentuated risk of accidental exposure to or ingestion of drugs or dangerous products in doses sufficient to cause poisoning.

Defining Characteristics (risk factors)

- Lack of safety or drug education
- Cognitive impairment
- Insufficient finances
- Large supplies of drugs in the house
- Medicines stored in unlocked cabinets accessible to children
- Availability of illicit drug potentially contaminated by poisonous additives
- Flaking, peeling paint or plaster in presence of young children
- Chemical contamination of food or water
- Unprotected contact with heavy metals or chemicals
- Paint, lacquer, etc., in poorly ventilated areas or without effective protection
- Presence of poisonous vegetation
- Presence of atmospheric pollutants

HIGH RISK FOR SUFFOCATION Accentuated risk of accidental suffocation (inadequate air available for inhalation).

Defining Characteristics (risk factors)

- Cognitive impairment
- Lack of safety education or safety precaution
- Pillow placed in an infant's crib
- Propped bottle placed in an infant's crib

Continued.

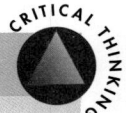

Nursing Diagnosis   *THE NEXT STEP—cont'd*

- Pacifier hung around an infant's head
- Children playing in plastic bags, inserting small objects into their mouths or noses
- Discarded or unused refrigerators; freezers without removed doors
- Children left unattended in bathtubs, pools
- Household gas leaks
- Use of fuel-burning heaters not vented to the outside
- Eating large mouthfuls of food

CONSTIPATION The state in which an individual experiences a change in normal bowel habits characterized by a decrease in frequency and/or passage of hard, dry stools.

Defining Characteristics

- Frequency less than usual pattern
- Hard formed stools, decreased quantity
- Palpable mass
- Straining at stool
- Abdominal pain, cramps
- Appetite impairment
- Headache
- Use of laxatives
- Nausea, vomiting
- Irritability
- Abdominal distention

Related Factors

- Eating habits
- Decreased activity
- Use of enemas

DIARRHEA The state in which an individual experiences a change in normal bowel habits characterized by the frequent passage of loose, fluid, unformed stools.

Defining Characteristics

- Loose, fluid stools
- Abdominal pain, discomfort
- Cramping
- Frequent bowel movements
- Increased frequency of bowel sounds
- Urgency
- Change in color of stools (greenish)

Related Factors

- Stress
- Food intolerance

ALTERED URINARY ELIMINATION The state in which an individual experiences a disturbance in urine elimination.

Defining Characteristics

- Dysuria
- Frequency
- Hesitancy
- Nocturia
- Retention
- Incontinence
- Urgency

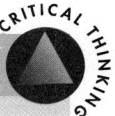

Nursing Diagnosis *THE NEXT STEP—cont'd*

Related Factors

- Urinary tract infection
- Incontinence
- Spinal cord injury
- Other medical problems

ALTERED GROWTH AND DEVELOPMENT The state in which an individual demonstrates deviations in norms from his/her age-group.

Defining Characteristics

- Delay or difficulty in performing skills (motor, social, or expressive) typical of age group
- Altered physical growth
- Inability to perform self-care or self-control activities appropriate for age.

Related Factors

- Inadequate caretaking
- Separation from significant others
- Environmental and stimulation difficulties

SLEEP PATTERN DISTURBANCE Disruption of sleep time causes discomfort or interferes with desired life-style.

Defining Characteristics

- Verbal complaints of difficulty falling asleep (sleep onset)
- Early awakening
- Interrupted sleep
- Sleep pattern reversal
- Verbal complaints of not feeling well rested
- Increasing irritability
- Restlessness
- Lethargy
- Listlessness
- Mild, fleeting nystagmus
- Ptosis of eyelids
- Dark circles under eyes
- Frequent yawning
- Nightmares

Related Factors

- Environmental or habit changes
- Personal or family stress
- Physical discomfort
- Fear

SELF-ESTEEM DISTURBANCE Negative self-evaluation/feelings about self or self-capabilities, which may be directly or indirectly expressed.

Defining Characteristics

- Self-negating verbalizations
- Lack of eye contact; head flexion; shoulder flexion
- Expressions of shame/guilt
- Exaggerations of negative feedback about self
- Hesitation to try new things/situations
- Projection of blame/responsibility for problems
- Rationalization of personal failures
- Hypersensitivity to a slight or to a criticism

Continued.

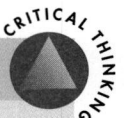

Nursing Diagnosis *THE NEXT STEP—cont'd*

<u>Related Factors</u>

- Related factors to be developed

IMPAIRED SOCIAL INTERACTION The state in which an individual participates in an insufficient or excessive quantity or ineffective quality of social exchange.

Defining Characteristics

- Verbalized or observed discomfort in social situations
- Verbalized or observed inability to receive or communicate a satisfying sense of belonging, caring, interest, or shared history
- Observed use of unsuccessful social interaction behaviors
- Dysfunctional interaction with peers, family, and/or others
- Family report of change of style or patterns of interaction
- Does not speak in sentences
- Infrequent verbalization
- Unable to work out social interaction through play—does not talk with dolls/toys
- Unwilling to share "mine"

Related Factors

- Sociocultural dissonance
- Environmental barriers
- Absence of available significant others or peers
- Knowledge or skill deficit
- Communication barriers

Clinical Application

T.J. is a 3-year-old male brought into the clinic by his mother. T.J. has been running a low grade temperature of 101° F (axillary) for the past 2 days and is coughing and sneezing, has a runny nose and is pulling at his left ear. He refuses to eat or drink anything saying, "throat hurt." Last night he woke twice, coughing and crying. His mother is worried because T.J. usually is so active but all he has done this morning is sleep. Physical assessment is completed.

SUBJECTIVE DATA: Mother states the following about client:
Temperature of 101° F for 2 days
Coughing
Sneezing
Runny nose
Pulling at left ear
Refusing to eat or drink
Lethargic, sleeping increased during the day
Waking up several times during the night

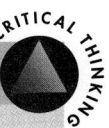

Nursing Diagnosis *THE NEXT STEP—cont'd*

OBJECTIVE DATA:
Temperature 101.2° (tympanic)
Pulse 105/min.
Respirations 26 breaths/min.
Blood pressure 90/58
Left ear, canal, TM normal
Right ear, canal normal
Right TM retracted, with multiple air bubbles
Drum color is yellow/amber
No sinus tenderness
Nose: turbinates injected and swollen, mucopurulent discharge
Throat: tonsils 3 +, pharyngeal wall bright red with yellow-white exudate, exudate on both tonsils
Neck: enlarged anterior cervical nodes bilaterally, painful to palpation
Chest: resonant to percussion throughout, breath sounds scattered wheezes throughout, some clear with coughing

NURSING DIAGNOSES

Ineffective airway clearance related to tracheobronchial secretion

Defining Characteristics

- Abnormal breath sounds, scattered wheezes
- Cough effective with sputum
- Fever

Pain related to ear infection and sore throat

Defining Characteristics

- Crying unrelieved by usual comfort measures
- Pulling at left ear
- Verbal expression of sore throat
- Decreased activity, self-imposed

Sleep pattern disturbances related to coughing and fever

Defining Characteristics

- Interrupted sleep
- Increased irritability
- Increased lethargy

Altered nutrition: less than body requirements related to sore throat (refusal to eat or drink anything).

Defining Characteristics

- Reported inadequate food or drink intake
- Lack of interest in food
- Sore inflamed throat

GLOSSARY

abduction Movement away from the axial line (for a limb) or the median plane (for the digits).

adduction Movement toward the axial line (for a limb) or the median plane (for the digits).

amblyopia Reduced vision in an eye that appears structurally normal on ophthalmoscopic examination.

caput succedaneum Localized pitting edema in the scalp of a newborn that may overlie the sutures of the skull.

cephalhematoma Swelling caused by subcutaneous bleeding and accumulation of blood in the scalp of a newborn; usually the result of birth trauma.

coarctation Tightening or compression of the walls of a vessel, producing a narrowed lumen.

congenital Present at birth.

epispadias Congenital anomaly in which the urethra opens on the dorsum of the penis.

hypospadias Developmental anomaly in which the urethra opens on the underside of the penis.

intertrigo Erythematous irritation in areas where two skin surfaces come together, such as the groin area or the folds between large, pendulous breasts.

phimosis Narrowness of the opening of the prepuce that causes difficulty in retraction of the foreskin of the penis.

strabismus Disparity in the anteroposterior axes of the eyes; the optic axes cannot be directed to the same object because of lack of muscular coordination.

subluxation Partial dislocation.

torticollis Abnormal condition in which the contraction of neck muscles causes the head to be inclined to one side. This condition may be congenital or acquired.

BIBLIOGRAPHY

American Academy of Pediatrics: *Report of the committee on infectious diseases*, ed 22, Elk Grove Village, Ill, 1991, The Academy.

American Academy of Pediatrics: *Guidelines for health supervision II*, ed 2, Elk Grove Village, Ill, 1988, The Academy.

Chess S, Thomas A: *Temperament in clinical practice*, New York, 1986, Guilford Press.

Daniels SR: Primary hypertension in childhood and adolescence, *Pediatr Ann* 21:224-234, 1992.

Dixon SD, Stein M: *Encounters with children*, ed 2, St Louis, 1992, Mosby–Year Book.

Goldenring JM, Cohen E: Getting into adolescent heads, *Contemp Pediatr* 5:75-86, 1988.

Hoekelman R and others: *Primary pediatric care*, ed 2, St Louis, 1992, Mosby–Year Book.

Lichtman R, Papera S: *Gynecology: well woman care*, Norwalk, Conn, 1990, Appleton & Lange.

Lowrey GH: *Growth and development of children*, ed 8, St Louis, 1986, Mosby–Year Book.

National Heart, Lung and Blood Institute: Report of Second Task Force on Blood Pressure Control in Children–1987, *Pediatrics* 79:1-25, 1987.

Satter E: *Child of mine: feeding with love and good sense*, Palo Alto, Calif, 1991, Bull Publishing.

Schwartz MW and others: *Pediatric primary care: a problem-oriented approach*, ed 2, St Louis, 1990, Mosby–Year Book.

Seidel HM and others: *Mosby's guide to physical examination*, ed 2, St Louis, 1991, Mosby–Year Book.

Strassburger V, Brown R: *Adolescent medicine: a practical guide*, Boston, 1991, Little, Brown.

Tanner JM: *Growth at adolescence*, ed 2, Oxford, 1962, Blackwell Scientific Publications.

US Department of Health, Education and Welfare: *NCHS growth curves for children birth to 18 years*, Hyattsville, Md, 1977, National Center for Health Statistics.

US Department of Health and Human Services, Public Health Service: *Healthy people 2000: national health promotion and disease prevention objectives*, DHHS No 91-50213, Washington, DC, 1990.

Whaley LF, Wong DL: *Nursing care of infants and children*, ed 4, St Louis, 1991, Mosby–Year Book.

Zimmerman R, Giebink G: Childhood immunizations: a practical approach for clinicians, *Am Fam Physician* 45:1759-1776, 1992.

Zitelli B, Davis H: *Atlas of pediatric physical diagnosis*, New York, 1987, Gower Medical Publishing.

Aging Clients

Outline

PURPOSE OF THE EXAMINATION

This chapter highlights areas of the health history and physical exam that may differ in the older adult. The increased number of older adults who are living longer presents several challenges to health care professionals.

Demographics

The percentage of the American population over the age of 65 has tripled from 1900 to 1990. Approximately 12.6% of the current population is over 65 and by 2030, when the baby boom generation has aged, about 22% of the population will be over 65. While the actual maximum life span has not increased (approximately 110 years), the number of older persons living into their 80s and 90s has increased. The fastest growing segment of the American population is the group of individuals 85 years and older.

While the majority of older adults live active lives, most have at least one chronic disease, and many have multiple chronic diseases. The extent to which these

MAJOR CHRONIC CONDITIONS IN OLDER ADULTS

- Arthritis
- Hypertension
- Hearing impairments
- Heart disease
- Cataracts
- Orthopedic impairments
- Sinusitis
- Diabetes
- Visual impairments
- Varicose veins

chronic diseases cause illness and functional disability depends on the type and severity of the diseases, co-existing diseases, environmental factors such as financial and social resources, and the individual's perception of health and coping styles or coping strategies. The major chronic conditions in the older population are outlined by order of prevalence in the box above.

USE AND COST OF HEALTH CARE

Data reported by the American Association of Retired Persons and the Administration on Aging (1991) indicate that older individuals account for a disproportionate number of hospital stays and, once in the hospital, the average length of stay is longer for older than younger individuals, 8.9 days versus 5.3 days, respectively. Noninstitutional older adults also had more physician contacts than younger persons. About 1% of the population 65 to 74 years of age live in nursing homes, and by age 85, about 25% of older adults live in nursing homes. One third of the country's total personal health care dollars pay for health care for those over 65 years. Medicare and Medicaid cover about two thirds of these expenses. In addition, Medicare does not cover dental care. Many older adults must pay significant out-of-pocket health care expenses. This fact is important since almost 20% of those over 65 are considered poor or near poor. Lack of financial resources can cause people to ration their medications and/or delay seeking care. This behavior may lead to worsening health conditions and lengthy, expensive hospital stays that might otherwise be controlled.

Nurses are likely to care for older clients in a variety of settings. And, since after age 65 there are 149 women to 100 men, a majority of these clients are likely to be women.

EXAMINATION

Health History

Older adults are likely to have different types of problems than younger and middle-aged adults. This section discusses the presentation of conditions that are more likely to occur in an older population. These conditions are sometimes referred to as "geriatric syndromes" and include falls, incontinence, delirium, inappropriate medication use, mental status and mood impairment, functional impairment, and poor nutrition. While conditions are not diseases, these conditions place the client at risk for functional decline, morbidity, and mortality.

Altered clinical presentation. Diseases associated with "classic" symptoms in young and middle aged adults may be associated with more general symptoms in later life. For example, a myocardial infarction may present with mental confusion, a fall, or nausea and vomiting, as opposed to crushing substernal pain radiating down the left arm. In addition, the presence of one condition may mask another. For example, a person with severe chronic obstructive lung disease may not be active enough to bring about the symptoms of angina despite the presence of severe ischemic heart disease.

Concomitant disease. Since multiple medical problems are common in older adults, an examination directed at one symptom may uncover more than one problem. When examining the client for a complaint of recurrent falls, the examiner may discover that the falls are related to hurrying to the bathroom to avoid an incontinent episode.

Accumulated life history. Intelligence does not decline with age. Therefore, treat older adults with respect for their intelligence, wisdom, and accumulated life experiences. Remember that the person has lived with his or her body a long time and may be able to detect subtle changes in health status better than the health professional. The older adult may have a long history of medical problems, and the interview may become lengthy. Whenever necessary, gently redirect the conversation to obtain the most pertinent history while at the same time avoiding giving the client the impression that offered information is not valued. To redirect the interview say, "This is valuable information that I would like to hear about at some later point in time, but right now I need to focus on your problem of dizziness."

The following impairments are more frequently encountered in older adults. Awareness of these conditions will assist you in focusing questions on specific signs and symptoms.

DSM III-R DEMENTIA CRITERIA
1. Loss of intellectual abilities of sufficient severity to interfere with social or occupational functioning 2. Memory impairment 3. One or more of the following • Impaired abstract thinking • Impaired judgment • Disturbances of higher cortical function such as apraxia or agnosia • Personality change

DSM-IIIR DEPRESSION CRITERIA
Presence of at least five of the following symptoms: 1. Changes in appetite and weight 2. Disturbed sleep 3. Motor agitation or retardation 4. Fatigue and loss of energy 5. Depressed or irritable mood 6. Loss of interest or pleasure in usual activities 7. Feelings of worthlessness, self-reproach, excessive guilt 8. Suicidal thinking or attempts 9. Difficulty with thinking or concentration

Mental status and mood impairment

Dementia. Dementia is a clinical condition characterized by a decline in memory and intellectual functioning. Several different diseases may cause dementia. The most common cause of dementia is Alzheimer's disease, a disease in which neuron loss and a decrease in chemical transmitters occurs in certain areas of the brain. Other causes of dementia include multiple strokes, alcohol abuse, and Parkinson's disease, Huntington's disease, and acquired immunodeficiency disease. The box below lists the criteria from the revised third edition of the Diagnosis and Statistical Manual of Mental Disorders (DSM-IIIR) required to make a diagnosis of dementia.

Older clients are more likely to present with dementia symptoms since the prevalence of dementia increases with age. At age 65, about 1.5% of the population has dementia; this percentage increases to about 50% at 90 years. If dementia is suspected, refer the client to a physician for a complete evaluation.

The answers to the following questions may provide information about the client's mental status:
- Did the client come to the appointment alone or accompanied by someone?
- Is the client appropriately dressed?
- Is the client having difficulty answering questions?

Not all clients need a formal assessment of their mental status. If, however, the examiner suspects some impairment in mental status, he or she can use a number of standardized assessment instruments to evaluate mental status. The Mini-Mental Status Examination (MMSE) is a commonly used 30-item questionnaire that assesses orientation, registration, attention and calculation, recall, and language (see p. 622). A score of 23 or less suggests some type of mental status impairment. The MMSE, however, is only a screening exam and *no diagnosis is made or excluded solely on the basis of the exam score.* Dementia may be present with a score greater than 23.

Depression. Depression is the most common mood disorder in late life. The 1991 Consensus Development Conference on the Diagnosis and Treatment of Depression in Late Life defines depression as a syndrome that includes physiological, affective, and mental symptoms. The box above outlines the DSM-IIIR criteria for depression.

Depression is not more common in late life than in earlier life. About 3% of community-dwelling elderly suffer from major depression. In nursing homes, however, as many as 25% of residents may have depression. Some of the symptoms of depression, such as weight loss, sleep disturbances, and fatigue, may be associated with other conditions, and the examiner may miss a diagnosis of depression in the older adult. Simply asking the client, "Do you feel sad, blue, or depressed much of the time?" provides insight into the client's mood. Assessing for depression is an important part of the health history for older adults, particularly for males, because older white males are at the highest risk for suicide of any age group.

A number of questionnaires are available to look for depressive symptoms. The Geriatric Depression Scale (GDS) is a 30-item questionnaire designed specifically to screen for depression in the elderly. Similar to the MMSE, the GDS score does not diagnose or exclude depression. Refer a client scoring high on the GDS to a physician or psychologist for further evaluation of a possible depression. Also, if the history suggests depression even in the absence of a high GDS score, refer the client for further evaluation.

Delirium. **Delirium** is an acute change in mental status with symptoms meeting the DSM-IIIR criteria outlined in the box on the next page.

Delirium usually occurs during an acute medical illness, and studies have reported that 5% to 35% of hospitalized elderly develop delirium during their hospi-

DSM-IIIR DELIRIUM CRITERIA

1. Reduced ability to attend to external stimuli
2. Disorganized thinking
   At least two of the following:
   a. reduced level of consciousness
   b. perceptual disturbances
   c. disturbance of sleep-wake cycle
   d. altered psychomotor activity
   e. disorientation
   f. memory impairment
3. Abrupt onset with fluctuating course
4. One of the following:
   a. evidence of a specific etiological factor
   b. in the absence of above, no nonorganic factor mental disorder accounting for symptoms

ACTIVITIES OF DAILY LIVING

Dressing
Transferring
Feeding
Bathing
Toileting
Bowel control
Bladder control
Walking
Climbing stairs
Grooming

INSTRUMENTAL ACTIVITIES OF DAILY LIVING

Telephoning
Reading
Leisure
Medication management
Money management
Transportation
Shopping
Meal preparation
Laundering
Housekeeping
Home maintenance

talization. Delirium may develop in a few hours, and the client may have periods of clear thinking alternating with disorientation. Delirium is distinguished from dementia by its rapid onset. Delirium most often occurs in clients who had normal mental status before surgery or before developing an acute illness. Almost any acute disorder that affects brain function, such as hypoxia, fever, arrhythmias, and anemia, can cause delirium. One of the major causes of delirium in the older adult is medications. While delirium is most prevalent in hospitals, acutely ill older clients may be brought into a clinic accompanied by family members who report sudden and dramatic changes in the elderly person's mental status. These mental status changes may be the first sign of an acute illness.

Functional impairment. The older client's ability to maintain independence depends on his or her ability to meet basic physical and daily life management needs or to secure these needs through community resources. Basic physical needs are referred to as **activities of daily living** (ADLs) and life management needs are called **instrumental activities of daily living** (IADLs) (see the boxes). One or more physical and psychological impairments can greatly affect the client's ability to perform ADLs or IADLs. Assess ADL and IADL function in the older client.

The most accurate assessment of ADL and IADL function is direct observation of the client performing each specific task. This, however, is not practical in the clinic or hospital setting. Instead, ask clients whether they can perform the various ADL and IADL tasks alone or with assistance. If assistance is required, find out who provides the assistance and with what frequency. In addition, simply observe the client entering the room, sitting in a chair and undressing for the exam for clues

about several ADL functions. One quick and easy assessment of mobility is the timed get-up-and-go test. Time the client getting up from a chair, walking 10 feet, turning around, walking back to the chair, and sitting back down (Figure 25-1). Use a standard arm chair with a seat height of about 46 cm. While the time required to perform this test varies with clients, highly mobile, independent older adults can perform this test in about 10 seconds. Detect changes over time by repeating this test at subsequent visits.

Standardized assessment questionnaires are also available for evaluating ADL and IADL tasks. These are described in detail in Chapter 26. The Katz Index of ADL and the Barthel Index are two examples of such questionnaires. The Barthel Index provides a score from 0 (total dependence) to 100 (total independence), which is useful for following changes over time. The Assessment of Living Skills and Resources (ALSAR) is a form that assesses both the client's ability to perform IADLs and available resources.

Incontinence. Between 15% and 30% of older adults living at home and up to 50% of nursing home residents

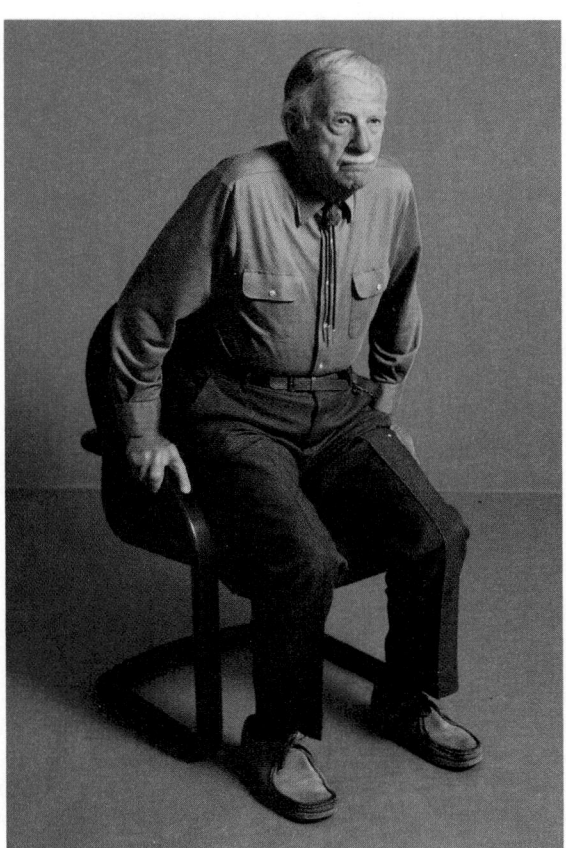

FIGURE 25-1 The timed "get-up-and-go" test measures the time it takes the client to rise from a chair, walk 10 feet, turn around, return to the chair, and sit down.

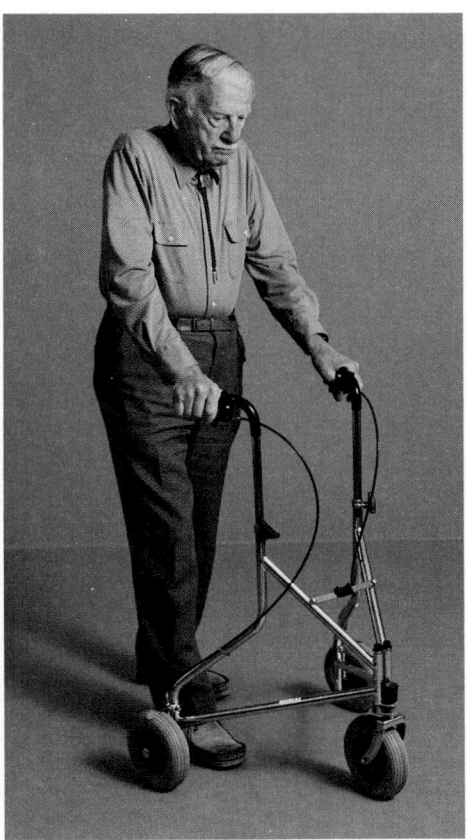

FIGURE 25-2 Many older clients use assistive devices, such as a Delta walker, to provide additional stability when ambulating.

have incontinence. **Incontinence** is an involuntary loss of urine with or without warning. The incontinent older adult may experience physical, psychological, and financial burdens. For example, fear of an accident may lead to restriction of outside activities and contribute to social isolation.

Incontinence may be transient or established. Transient incontinence is acute in onset and is often related to a change in health status such as a urinary tract infection, medications, stool impaction, delirium, polyuria, or restricted mobility. Often several of these factors are present during hospitalization, and it is not uncommon for older adults to develop incontinence when hospitalized.

Established incontinence occurs when leakage of urine persists after treating suspected causes (i.e., decreasing a dose of diuretic). Established incontinence is caused by a problem either with bladder muscle activity or with the bladder outlet. The bladder muscle, the **detrusor,** may be either overactive or underactive (Table 25-1). Detrusor overactivity is the most common

cause of incontinence in older adults and may result from stroke, Parkinson's disease, or Alzheimer's disease. This type of incontinence is also called urge incontinence, characterized by little warning before voiding large amounts of urine. A client may state, "I just can't seem to get to the bathroom on time." Detrusor underactivity is less frequent and is caused by injury to the nerves of the bladder or to autonomic neuropathy, which may occur in diabetes. In this type of incontinence, the bladder contracts reflexively.

Stress incontinence is the second most common cause of incontinence in older women and is the result of bladder outlet incompetence. Relaxation of the pelvic floor muscles allows the proximal portion of the urethra and bladder neck to be displaced into the urogenital diaphragm with increased abdominal pressure. Stress incontinence causes involuntary loss of urine when abdominal pressure increases such as when the woman coughs, laughs, lifts, or suddenly stands up. The amount of urine lost may vary from a few drops to a large quantity. Outlet obstruction, the second most common

TABLE 25-1

Common Causes of Incontinence

Urologic dysfunction	Cause	Symptoms
Detrusor muscle problem		
Overactivity	Stroke, dementia, Parkinson's disease	Urgency, little warning before voiding, usually large amounts of urine
Underactivity	Diabetes, bladder nerve injury	Bladder contracts reflexively without warning
Bladder outlet problem		
Incompetence	Relaxation of pelvic floor muscles	Involuntary loss of urine with increased abdominal pressure, such as coughing, sneezing, lifting, standing
Obstruction	Prostatic hypertrophy	Overflow of urine from distended bladder

type of incontinence in older men, is due to prostatic enlargement, tumor, or urethral stricture. With outlet obstruction the bladder becomes distended with urine and eventually leaks urine from overflow.

Detrusor underactivity and overactivity and outlet incompetence and obstruction are dysfunctions of the lower urinary tract that cause incontinence. Functional incontinence results from a variety of environmental and personal factors that impede getting to the bathroom before voiding occurs. Restricted mobility, bathroom location, and decreased manual dexterity or balance may cause incontinence in the absence of any urinary tract dysfunction or may exacerbate preexisting incontinence.

Clients are often reluctant to volunteer information about incontinence symptoms. Some individuals have the mistaken belief that incontinence is a normal part of aging that must be tolerated. State the following to help the client relate incontinence symptoms, if present. "Some older people have a problem with leakage of urine at inappropriate times. This is not something that normally happens with aging and can often be treated. Do you ever have problems with leakage of urine?" Asking the question in this way informs the client that other people have a similar problem, it is not normal, and it may be treatable. If a client is experiencing symptoms, question about the frequency and amount of the incontinence, associated activities, medications, eating and drinking habits, and current management of the problem by the client. Instruct the client on how to complete a voiding diary. The diary is an account of the frequency and amount voided, incontinent episodes, and associated activities.

Falls. Falls are a common occurrence in the older population. As many as one third of older adults living at home fall each year. This increases to about 50% by age 80. Accidents are the sixth leading cause of death for individuals over age 65; falls are the leading type of accident in this age group. About 5% of falls result in a fracture, with the most common fracture sites being the humerus, wrist, pelvis, ankle, and hip.

Risk factors for falls include sensory impairment such as visual changes, proprioceptive and vestibular dysfunction; neurological disorders resulting in gait impairment or mental status impairment; musculoskeletal disorders affecting strength and mobility; cardiovascular conditions, particularly orthostatic hypotension; and medications. Situational factors such as acute illness or an unfamiliar environment may precipitate a fall in individuals with or without predisposing risk factors. Falls are sometimes nonspecific signs of acute illness. For example, a nursing home resident falls and in the course of the post-fall assessment, the nurse measures a temperature of 102°, and a subsequent diagnosis of pneumonia is made.

Ask clients whether they have fallen in the past 6 months. Obtain a detailed history about any reported falls including risk factors for falls, frequency of falls, activity at the time of the fall, a description of the environment in which the fall occurred, and any injuries associated with the fall. For clients who live alone, always ask whether they were able to get up from the fall or whether they had to wait for help. The physical exam for clients who report a fall should include a neurological, musculoskeletal, and cardiovascular exam to assess for visual, balance, and gait impairment, muscle weakness, arrhythmias, and postural changes in blood pressure.

Inappropriate medication use. Older adults are the largest consumers of prescription drugs and also purchase many nonprescription medications. Several factors place the older client at risk for the ingestion of inappropriate medication including multiple diseases, multiple health care providers, nonprescription medication use, sharing medications, and rationing medications. Older adults who see several different physicians for different problems may accumulate multiple medications, some of which may facilitate or impair the effect of others. Due to limited financial resources, the older adult may only purchase a portion of prescribed medications or may ration the medication such as taking a pill once a day that is prescribed three times a day.

Medication dosage for some drugs may be altered for older clients due to age-related changes in the responsiveness of receptor cells to certain drugs, the distribution of drugs, and the metabolism and excretion of drugs. Since variability exists among older clients, consider medication dosages on an individual basis.

Instruct the client to bring all prescribed and nonprescribed medications to the examination, whether the client is currently taking them or not (people often stockpile unused medications at home). Using the last refill date on the bottle and the dose schedule, calculate the number of pills that should remain. Compare this to the actual number of pills remaining to determine if the client is using the medication as ordered. Assess the number and type of medications in relation to the client's physical problems. Question the client about medications that do not seem to correspond to information obtained during the health history. For instance, a client might bring in a bottle of thyroid medication and fail to mention any thyroid problem. Conversely, the client may relate a diagnosis of hypertension and not have any antihypertensive medication. If you notice a discrepancy between the way in which a medication was prescribed and the way in which the client takes the medication, explore reasons for this discrepancy.

The greater the number of medications prescribed, the greater the likelihood that not all will be ingested. Clients may have difficulty opening the medication bottles, reading the labels, or remembering to take their medications. Advise clients that they can request easy opening pill bottles from their pharmacist. Suggest medication reminder boxes, which have compartments for both the days of the week and different times of the day. Medications can be sorted into these compartments either by the client, a family member, or a community nurse.

Poor nutrition. Nutritional status depends on the amount and type of food in the diet. Energy needs or caloric intake, in part, is based on the basal metabolic rate (BMR). The BMR depends on the amount of lean body mass. Since lean body mass declines with age, the BMR also declines. A declining BMR suggests that the older adult, in general, needs fewer calories with increasing age. You must consider, however, activity level and the presence of any acute or chronic illnesses when determining energy needs.

Since the client may need fewer calories with increasing age, the type of food the client eats becomes relatively more important to ensure adequate nutrient intake and to prevent poor nutritional status. The nutritional history should focus on both caloric needs and the types of food consumed.

Poor nutritional status, as defined by the 1991 Nutrition Screen Initiative Consensus Conference, includes nutritional deficiencies as well as dehydration, undernutrition, nutritional imbalances, obesity, and excesses such as alcohol abuse. This consensus conference developed a plan for self-screening and professional nutritional screening for older adults. The client self-assessment screen is called the *Checklist To **DETERMINE** Nutritional Health*. This screening form asks the client to answer questions about the following nutritional risk factors:

- **D**isease, chronic or acute
- **E**ating habits
- **T**ooth loss
- **E**conomic hardship
- **R**educed social contact
- **M**ultiple medications or drugs
- **I**nvoluntary weight loss or gain
- **N**eeded assistance with self-care
- **E**ighty years of age or greater

The purpose of this self-screening is to encourage clients to examine their nutritional intake and to seek professional help if they appear to be at risk.

The Nutrition Screen Initiative recommends two levels of professional nutritional screening. Level I screening identifies those individuals who either need preventive interventions such as assistance with meals or who need a more in-depth nutritional assessment. Level I screening includes obtaining the client's height and weight history. Height may be difficult to obtain in some older clients due to kyphosis, inability to stand, or inability to maintain balance. When the client cannot stand, estimate height by measuring the length from the bottom of the foot to the anterior knee with the ankle and knee at a 90° angle.

- Male height = $64.19 - (0.04 \times$ age in years$)$ $+ (2.02 \times$ knee height [cm]$)$
- Female height = $84.88 - (0.24 \times$ age in years$)$ $+ (1.83 \times$ knee height [cm]$)$

The weight history includes questions about unintentional weight gain or loss in the past 6 months. Significant weight loss occurs if 5% or more of prior body weight is lost in 1 month, 7.5% in 3 months, or 10%

or more in 6 months. Inquire about where the person eats, how often meals are skipped, usual intake, facilities available for food preparation, resources available to purchase food, and ability to perform activities of daily living. A 3-day diet record provides a good indication of food consumption, and many computer programs are available to calculate the energy and nutrient intake based on this 3-day record. You can mail this record, along with instructions for use, to clients before their appointment.

Perform Level II screening, a more thorough nutritional assessment, when the client has an unintentional weight gain or loss in the past 6 months or appears underweight or overweight. Focus history questions on special dietary needs (i.e., is the client on a restricted sodium diet?); clinical symptoms such as sore mouth, difficulty chewing or swallowing; history of fractures; mood; mental status; and medications. Do laboratory screening for albumin level and serum cholesterol.

Comprehensive Geriatric Assessment (CGA). It is apparent that the health assessment of the geriatric client may be complex and time-consuming. Older clients with multiple complex problems benefit from a comprehensive geriatric assessment. Such an assessment by team members from a variety of disciplines improves the accuracy of assessment, discharge planning and placement, and functional status. In addition, studies suggest that when geriatric teams provide care, prolonged survival, reduced medical care costs, reduced hospitalizations, decreased nursing home use, decreased medications, and increased use of home health services result.

In 1987 the National Institutes of Health convened a consensus conference on geriatric assessment. CGA was defined as the multidisciplinary evaluation in which the multiple problems of older persons are uncovered, described, and explained, if possible, and in which the resources and strengths of the person are catalogued, need for services assessed, and a coordinated care plan developed to focus interventions for the person's problems (1988, p. 342). The various domains covered by CGA are physical, mental, social, economic, functional, and environmental status. In recent years more inpatient units and outpatient clinics offer comprehensive geriatric assessment. This type of thorough assessment generally takes several hours during which a core team—consisting of at least a physician, nurse, and social worker—sees and examines the client. Many teams also include physical and occupational therapists, a pharmacist, and a nutritionist. Often, the members of the various disciplines use standardized screening questionnaires, such as those mentioned previously, as they perform their assessment of the client. CGA is a time-consuming and costly evaluation, and not all older

---

QUESTIONS TO TARGET POTENTIAL AGE-RELATED IMPAIRMENTS

1. Do you ever have a problem with urine leaking?
2. Have you fallen in the past 6 months?
3. Do you often feel sad, blue, down in the dumps, or depressed?
4. Do you often travel places away from home alone?
5. Do you have enough money to purchase your medications?
6. Do you sometimes skip your medications?
7. Do you skip meals often?

---

clients require this type of extensive evaluation. Those clients likely to benefit most from CGA are those over the age of 75 with potentially reversible functional disabilities.

Preparation for the Examination: Client and the Environment

Examiner-client interaction. Older adults may be accompanied to the examination by a spouse, adult child, or other relative or friend. Notice whether the client is able to come into the exam room by himself or herself. An inability to independently present oneself to the exam room may indicate some type of sensory, functional, or mental status impairment. Sometimes relatives accompany independent and competent older adults into the exam room. Determine the client's wishes regarding the presence of others in the exam room. If the client requests that a relative or friend remain in the room, pay careful attention to who is answering questions and spontaneously providing information. A relative answering questions for the client may indicate that the client has some type of cognitive impairment and cannot answer. Politely but firmly inform the relative or friend that the client should be allowed to answer the questions first and that any additional information the relative or friend can supply will be welcomed after the client speaks.

Ask whether the client needs help in getting undressed for the exam or getting dressed after the exam. Clients may need extra time and assistance in getting on and off the exam table. Some clients may fatigue quickly during the exam. If this occurs, adjust the sequence of the exam to include the most relevant assessments based on the presenting problem.

Sensory impairment. The loss of auditory acuity is the most common sensory loss among aging individuals and may impede history taking. Face the client directly since many people with a hearing impairment rely to some extent on lip reading. Use simple, direct questions and avoid shouting. Shouting obscures the consonant sounds, sounds that are lost with hearing impairment in late life. Lowering the voice and speaking slightly louder may help. Amplification devices may assist in communication and will be discussed later in this chapter.

Techniques for Examination and Normal Findings

General inspection. The physical changes that highlight the aging process are graying hair and wrinkling of skin. Due to loss of connective tissue, body contours may appear sharper and hollows deeper, such as the orbits of the eyes and the axilla.

Skin

Age changes. Heredity, changes in the connective and epithelial tissues, endocrine alterations, and vascular changes all influence aging changes of the skin. Excessive exposure to sun accelerates these changes. The skin epidermis decreases in thickness. The melanocytes lose some of their ability to protect the skin from ultraviolet light. With chronic sun exposure, some melanocytes may be destroyed, resulting in hypopigmentation, or white spots, on the skin. Sun exposure can also stimulate melanocytes to produce hyperpigmented areas called **lentigines.** Lentigines are flat, tan to brown macules and are usually located on sun-exposed surfaces. They may be as large as 1 or 2 cm.

The dermis decreases in thickness and as a result, the skin takes on a thin, translucent appearance. Sun exposure changes the structure of the dermal layer and contributes to sagging and wrinkling of the skin. With thinning of the dermis, less support exists for capillary walls, and blood vessel walls dilate. Visible dilated vessels are called **telangiectasias.** Skin capillaries are also more fragile. A bump to the skin can cause blood to leak through the capillaries into the dermis resulting in bruising known as **senile purpura.** Ask the client how bruising occurred since bruising may indicate a recent fall. A client unaware of bruising may have decreased sensory perception.

Subcutaneous fat decreases with age. While sebaceous glands may increase in size, their ability to function decreases. This decrease in function, together with water loss from the skin, contributes to dry skin or xerosis, a frequent complaint in older clients.

Lesions. Various skin lesions are common with increasing age. **Seborrheic keratoses** are benign, raised, warty-type lesions usually located on the face, shoulders, and trunk. The borders are irregular and the surface scaly. These lesions have a "pasted-on" greasy appearance. Early lesions may be yellowish to tan with the color changing to dark brown or black over time. Although benign, some people request their removal for cosmetic purposes.

Skin tags are soft, flesh-colored lesions and are attached to the skin by a stalk. They vary in size from a pinhead to a pea and are most commonly found on the vertical and lateral surfaces of the neck and the axillary area. Like seborrhea keratoses, these lesions have little clinical importance but may be removed if they are irritated by clothing or for cosmetic reasons.

Cherry angiomas are another type of benign skin lesion occurring with increased frequency in older adults. These lesions are caused by proliferation and dilation of the superficial capillaries of the skin. They are bright red, soft, and dome-shaped with a diameter of 1 mm or greater.

Actinic keratoses are pink to slightly red, dry lesions with indistinct borders. Rough adherent scales cover the lesions. These lesions occur over sun exposed areas such as the face, ears, and dorsal surfaces of the hands and arms. A small percentage of these actinic keratoses will transform into squamous cell skin cancers. Therefore, these lesions are generally removed.

Basal cell skin cancer is the most common of all cancers. Look for lesions that are nodular with rolled borders, translucent, and pearly in appearance. Telangiectasias are frequent inside the nodule. These lesions, which may be ulcerating, are most often located on sun-exposed body surfaces (Figure 25-3). Basal cell skin cancer is locally invasive and destructive but does not

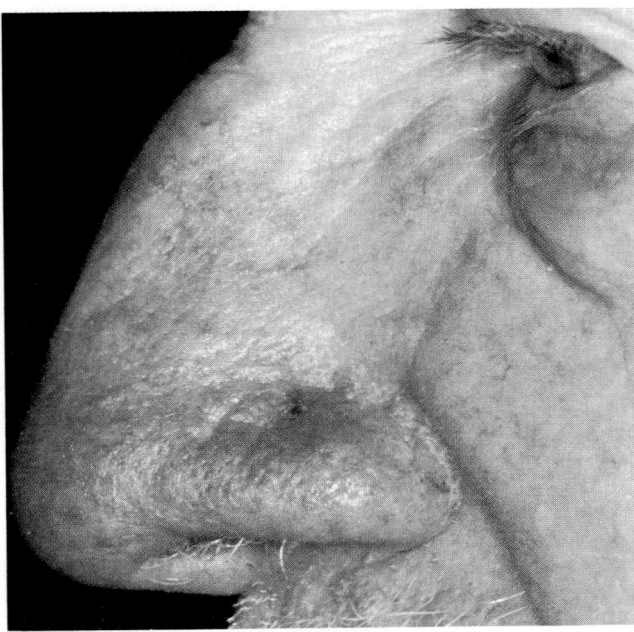

FIGURE 25-3 Basal cell cancer on the nose.

metastasize. Several techniques are available to remove these lesions depending on the patient and the size and location of the cancer.

Hair and nails. Hair and nail growth change with age. Scalp, axillary, and pubic hair thins and decreases. Eyebrow, nostril, and ear hair becomes coarser, and some older women develop an increase in facial hair. A loss of hair pigment contributes to the universal graying of hair. Nail growth slows and nails may yellow and lack luster. Some nails may become thin and split while others, especially the toenails, may thicken.

Head and Neck

Eyes. The cells responsible for lubricating the conjunctiva decrease and "dry eye syndrome" may develop, characterized by a scratchy sensation with chronic irritation. Observe for an **arcus senilis,** the accumulation of calcium and cholesterol salts at the limbus of the eye. This appears as a grayish to gray-white arc or halo and has no association with elevated serum cholesterol or other system illness. The cornea tends to become hazy. Pupils decrease in size, react more slowly to light, and dilate more slowly in the dark. As a result, the older adult requires more time adapting to a dark room. Restriction of upward movement of the pupil occurs with age and the client may have to tip the head back further to look up.

LIDS. Loss of fat from the orbit of the eye causes a sunken appearance. A decrease in strength of the muscles allowing the lids to shut tightly may result in an **ectropion.** This is the turning out of the lower lid exposing the punctum of the lower lid. If this occurs, tears do not drain properly and the client may complain of excess tearing. The opposite condition, **entropion,** is a turning inward of the lower lid caused by muscle spasm. The eyelashes of the lower lid contact the conjunctiva and cornea. If chronic irritation occurs, surgical correction may be necessary. The muscles that hold the upper lid open may weaken, causing lid droop or **ptosis.** The lid droop may hamper vision and can be corrected with surgery. Tear production may decrease and contribute to complaints of dry eyes.

VISION. The ability to accommodate decreases progressively with age. This condition is called **presbyopia** and increases with frequency after age 40. Assess for presbyopia by checking near vision with a hand-held reading card or newspaper. The ophthalmoscopic exam may be more difficult due to smaller pupil size. Look for mildly narrowed vessels, granular pigment in the macula, and a loss of bright macular and foveal reflexes. The fundus itself lacks luster and may appear more yellow.

Cataract, glaucoma, and **age-related macular degeneration** (AMD) are eye problems occurring more frequently in the older client. A cataract is an opacity in the lens, which gradually impairs vision. A client who complains about glare from headlights when driving a car at night may have a cataract. The most common type of glaucoma in the older adult is open-angle glaucoma. Measuring intraocular pressures on a regular basis helps to detect glaucoma early. Age-related macular degeneration, a loss of central vision, is one of the leading causes of blindness in the elderly. Laser therapy is one method of treatment for AMD. Clients with AMD may also be referred to low vision specialists for assessment of magnification aids.

Ears. OUTER EAR. Aging changes begin to appear in the outer ear between ages 30 and 50. The skin becomes dry and less resilient, and connective tissue is lost. Pruritis may occur in the external auditory canal leading to scratching. Remind clients not to use cotton tip applicators to relieve itching. Hair growth may be visible along the periphery of the helix, antihelix, and tragus of the pinna. The hairs are coarse and wirelike. The pinna increases in both length and width, and the earlobes are elongated. There is a decrease in cerumen production, and this reduction correlates with an increased dryness in cerumen. This may contribute to the increased tendency toward cerumen impactions.

MIDDLE EAR. Degenerative changes in the joints of the bones of the middle ear occur with increasing age. These changes, however, do not appear to have an appreciable effect on sound transmission.

INNER EAR. The specialized cells of the auditory pathways have a limited ability to regenerate. Approximately 24% of individuals between ages 65 and 74 and 39% over age 75 have hearing loss. A variety of genetic and environmental factors contribute to this age-related hearing loss called **presbycusis.** Two common types of presbycusis are sensory and neural presbycusis. Sensory presbycusis is associated with degeneration of the organ of Corti and involves the inability to hear high-frequency sounds. Neural presbycusis is primarily a loss of speech discrimination. Neural presbycusis is associated with a decrease in the cochlear neurons, while the organ of Corti remains functional.

A mild loss of speech frequency may pose little problem for the older person when listening to normal, clearly spoken conversation in a quiet room. In rooms with environmental noise such as a churches, restaurants, or movie theaters, a mild hearing loss may present greater hearing problems.

If you suspect hearing loss, check for and remove any cerumen impactions. If hearing problems persist, refer the client to an audiologist. Several aids are available for amplification of sound. The purpose of a hearing aid is to increase the intensity of the sound with as little distortion as possible. Several types of hearing aids

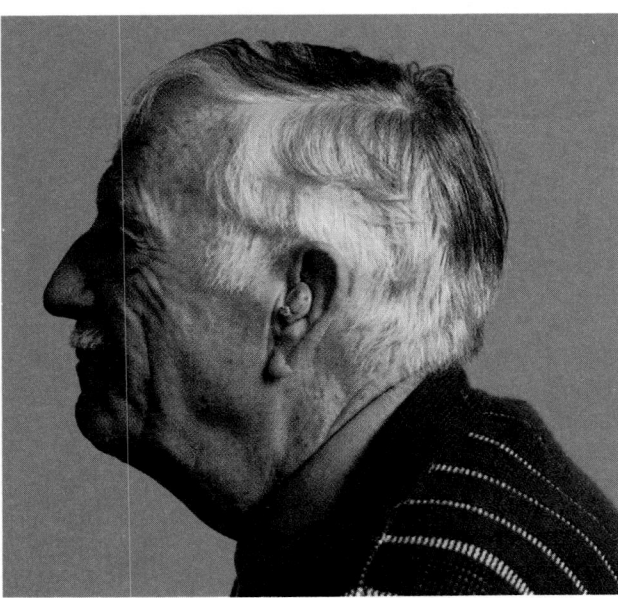

FIGURE 25-4 In-the-ear hearing aid.

are available: behind-the ear; eyeglass with aid; in-the-ear; in-the-canal; and body aids (Figure 25-4). The older adult may fear the social stigma associated with hearing aids. Successful adjustment to an aid depends largely on the client's motivation in wanting to use the aid.

Situation-specific assistive listening devices (ALDS) amplify speech for the hearing-impaired (Figure 25-5). An ALD is the size of a small transistor radio. A microphone is placed near the sound source while the listener places earphones in the ears. Sound travels to the earphones via infrared, audio loop, FM radio, or direct audio input. The sound is enhanced and extraneous noise reduced. Many theaters, churches, and lecture halls have such devices. They may also be used in exam rooms or hospital rooms.

Nose. Olfactory function decreases with age, and many older adults have a decreased ability to correctly identify odors. Although smell is not routinely assessed in the physical exam, question the client about altered smell since failure to detect the smell of smoke or gas can be life-threatening. In addition, a decreased sense of smell may contribute to decreased food intake.

Mouth. The number of taste buds does not decline with aging. There is no age-related deterioration in the ability of healthy older adults to taste sweet, sour, salty,

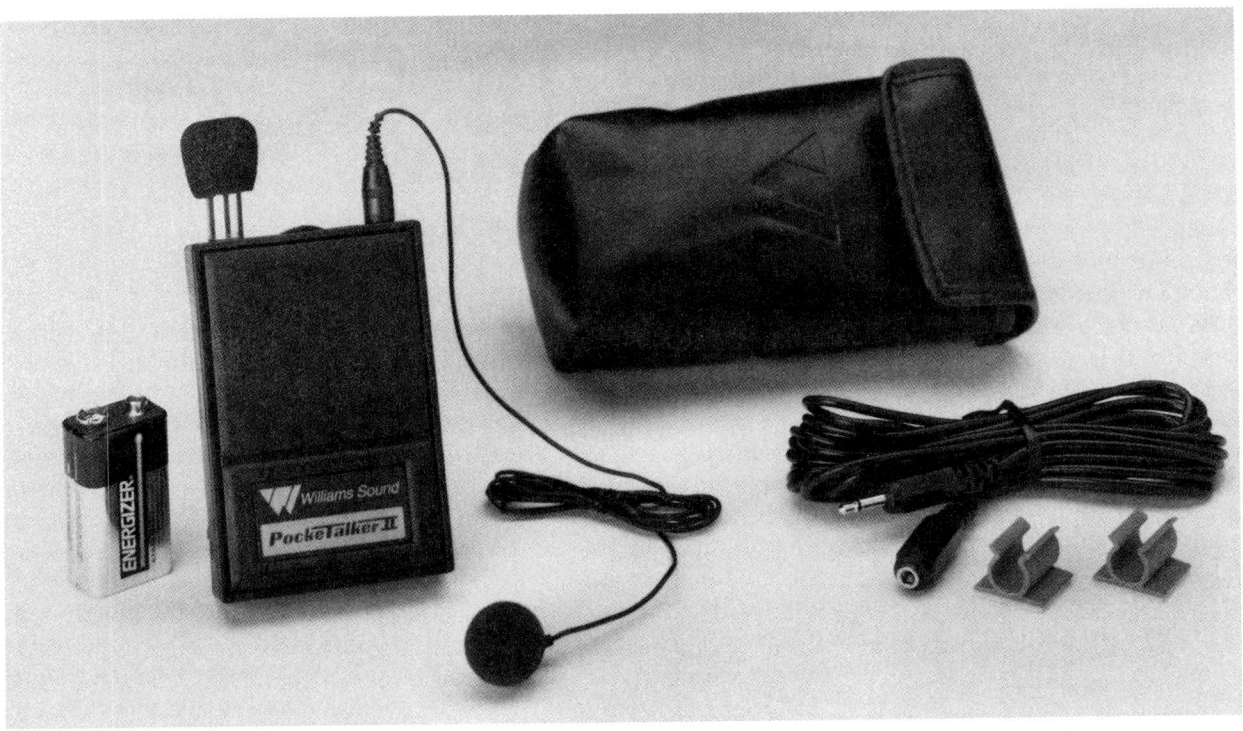

FIGURE 25-5 Assistive listening device.

CLASSES OF MEDICATIONS KNOWN TO CAUSE XEROSTOMIA

- anticholinergics
- antidepressants
- antihistamines
- antihypertensives
- antispasmodics
- decongestants
- antiparkinsonians
- antipsychotics
- diuretics

and bitter at usual concentrations. Older adults are retaining more of their teeth longer. When tooth loss occurs, it is due to two major causes: dental caries and periodontal disease. Periodontal disease is the major cause of tooth loss in the older adult. Dental caries in older adults tend to develop at the root or bottom of the tooth along the gum where gingival recession or periodontal disease causes exposure of the root surface.

Healthy adults do not have diminished saliva production. Decreased salivary function does, however, occur commonly as a side effect of medications with anticholinergic effects. Decreased salivary function causes dry mouth or **xerostomia** (see box above). Xerostomia is also caused by irradiation of the salivary glands or salivary tumors. Observe for dry oral mucous membranes and dry tongue. Saliva has many functions including antibacterial and antifungal activity, oral lubrication, buffering of bacteria-produced acids, mechanical cleansing, remineralization of teeth and as an aid in mastication. Decreased saliva may contribute to caries formation. Instruct clients with xerostomia to brush their teeth after every meal and to avoid moistening their mouth with candy unless it is sugar-free. A variety of salivary lubricants are available to moisten the mouth in clients who have xerostomia.

The majority of oral cancers develop after age 40. Individuals with a history of tobacco and/or alcohol abuse are particulary at risk for developing an oral cancer. Carefully inspect the oral mucosa for red or white lesions. Remove any dentures during the examination, since poorly-fitting dentures can cause trauma to the oral mucosa. In addition, oral candidiasis may be present on areas of the mucosa where the dentures rest.

Breasts. With increasing age, the amount of fat in the breast increases as the glandular tissue atrophies. Breast consistency and shape change and are often described as pendulous. The incidence of breast cancer in the United States increases with age; therefore the detection of a lump is significant and requires evaluation. Most

recommendations suggest yearly mammograms for women between ages 50 and 59 and every 2 years after age 60.

Respiratory system. Calcification occurs in the costochondral joints of the ribs, and the chest wall becomes less compliant. Skeletal changes in the spine may cause an increase in the anterior-posterior diameter of the chest. If this occurs, breath sounds may be more difficult to hear during auscultation.

Cardiovascular system

Age-related changes. Diseases of the cardiovascular system are common in the elderly and are the leading cause of death in this age group. Maximal heart rate decreases with age. Despite a decrease in heart rate, healthy older adults can maintain a normal cardiac output during exercise by increasing their stroke volume. While healthy older adults maintain normal cardiac output, many older clients do have cardiac disorders and do have decreased cardiac output and decreased activity tolerance.

BLOOD PRESSURE. Isolated systolic hypertension and orthostatic hypotension are two problems commonly associated with changes in blood pressure in older adults.

Systolic blood pressure increases with age due to increased stiffness of the aorta and its branches. **Isolated systolic hypertension** occurs when the systolic blood pressure is greater than 160 mmHg in the presence of a normal diastolic pressure. Isolated systolic hypertension occurs more frequently in older adults and is associated with an increased risk for strokes and fatal cardiovascular events. Research has shown that treating isolated systolic hypertension in older adults reduces the likelihood of strokes.

Postural or **orthostatic hypotension** occurs when the systolic blood pressure drops 20 mmHg or greater when the client goes from a lying or sitting position to a standing position. Baroreceptor sensitivity remains intact in healthy older adults and is not a likely cause of postural hypotension. One common cause of postural hypotension is medications, particularly antihypertensive medications, diuretics, and medications with anticholinergic effects.

In older clients, measure blood pressure in both arms with the client lying and standing or sitting and standing. Have the client lying or sitting at rest at least 15 minutes before taking the initial blood pressure reading. Then have the client stand and take the blood pressure immediately. If you record a drop in the standing blood pressure, retake the blood pressure again in 1 minute. A drop in blood pressure upon rising places the older client at risk for lightheadedness and falls. If these symptoms occur, refer the client to a physician for further

toms occur, refer the client to a physician for further evaluation. In addition, instruct the client to sit on the edge of the bed or chair for a couple of minutes before standing and have a firm object such as a heavy chair close by to use for support if needed.

HEART. Precordial palpation may be difficult in those elderly who have an increased anterior-posterior diameter. **Kyphosis,** often occurring in the older client, may cause a downward dislocation of the cardiac apex.

With age, there is an increase in fibrosis and calcification of the aortic valve cusps, a condition called aortic sclerosis. The thickening of these valves, together with dilatation of the aorta, may cause a systolic murmur. Aortic sclerosis is of little clinical significance unless the sclerosed valve progresses to aortic stenosis. The aortic sclerosis murmur is best heard at the right base. It is low in intensity and short in duration, and it peaks early in systole. The differential diagnosis of aortic stenosis versus aortic sclerosis is difficult and best made by an echocardiogram. A fourth heart sound (S_4) is common with increased age and is often heard along with an aortic sclerotic murmur. An S_4 in the older client is most likely due to decreased ventricular compliance. **Abdomen.** In some older clients, the general loss of fibroconnective tissue and muscle wasting may make the abdominal wall slacker, thinner, and easier to palpate. In other clients, increased fat deposits around the abdomen may make palpation more difficult.

Reproductive system

Female client. Cells of the reproductive tract and the breasts are estrogen-dependent for growth and function. The decline of estrogen production starting at menopause is responsible for many changes in the tissues of older female clients.

The ovaries, uterus, and cervix decrease in size. The ovaries may not be palpable. The vagina narrows and shortens. The vaginal epithelium atrophies; the surface is thin, pale, fragile, and easily traumatized; intercourse may be painful. The frequency of intercourse in older women depends on the availability of a partner, physical health, previous sexual activity, and desire. Table 25-2 lists changes in the phases of intercourse in the older woman. Vaginal estrogen creams often provide relief for painful symptoms associated with atrophic vaginitis. Observe for vaginal erosions, ulcerations, and adhesions.

Male client. Testosterone declines in older males. This decline occurs later than the decline in estrogen in the female. Testes decrease in size and are less firm on palpation. While sperm production either remains the same or decreases slightly, sperm motility decreases and size changes. The prostate gland is enlarged, and secretion is impaired. The seminal fluid is reduced in amount and viscosity.

These changes do not necessarily mean a decrease in libido or a loss in the sense of satisfaction from intercourse. Most men over 60 reported having intercourse one or two times a week. Table 25-3 notes changes in the phases of intercourse in the older man.

Musculoskeletal system. With increasing age, thinning of the intervertebral discs and shortening or collapse of the intervertebral bodies result in loss of height. Changes in the spine also contribute to the development of kyphosis and an increase in AP diameter.

Muscle mass and strength decrease with age. You can easily see atrophy of muscle by observing the back

TABLE 25-2

Changes in the Four Phases of Intercourse in the Aging Female Client

Phase	Alteration
Excitement	• Delay in production of vaginal secretion and lubrication
Plateau	• Reduction in vaginal length and width expansion
	• Decreased uterine elevation
	• Labia majora flaccid and do not elevate and flatten against perienum
	• Labia minora do not undergo sex color change from pink to burgundy or become congested
	• Clitoral size decreases after 60 years of age
Orgasm	Shorter than in younger persons
Resolution	Occurs more rapidly

TABLE 25-3

Changes Observed in the Four Phases of Intercourse in the Aging Male Client

Phase	Alteration
Excitement	• Slower increment in excitement
	• Sex flush less in duration and intensity
	• Diminished involuntary spasms
	• Increased time to obtain erection
	• Lessened testicular elevation and scrotal sac vasocongestion in erection
Plateau	• Longer duration
	• Increase in penile diameter due to less preejaculatory fluid emission
Orgasm	• Shorter duration
	• Fewer contractions in expulsion of semen bolus
Resolution	• Lasts 12 to 24 hours
	• Loss of erection may take only a few seconds

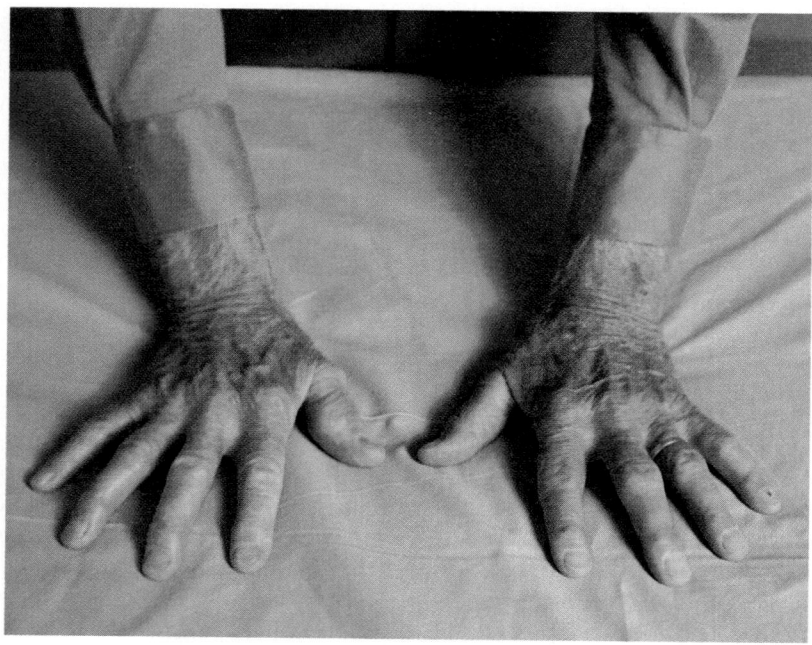

FIGURE 25-6 Heberden's and Bouchard's nodes.

of the hands where grooves are present between the bones.

Osteoarthritis is a common age-related condition involving joints throughout the body, particularly the spine, knees, hips, and fingers. Most clients over 60 will have osteoarthritic changes in the spine. Accumulated injuries to the cartilage over time cause slow but progressive deterioration of the joint. With loss of cartilage, bony overgrowths protrude from the bone into the joint capsule. These overgrowths can cause angular deformities, pain, and limited mobility. In the spine, these overgrowths are called osteophytes. Bony enlargement of the dorsolateral and dorsomedial aspects of the distal and proximal joints of the fingers are called Heberden's nodes and Bouchard's nodes, respectively (Figure 25-6).

Nervous system. The assessment of mental status and cranial nerves has been previously discussed. Motor strength may decrease slightly with age. Investigate further any asymmetry of strength. Vibratory sensation decreases with age, especially in the feet and ankles. Posture may become stooped. Changes in gait, including decreased stride length, anteroflexion of the upper torso, flexion of the arms and knees, and diminished arm swing, may contribute to postural unsteadiness. Deep tendon reflexes remain intact in healthy elderly people although they may be more difficult to elicit. In many older clients, ankle jerks may be diminished or absent.

Summary

History taking is especially important in preparing for the physical examination of the older adult. Asking the following questions will help you to know if you need to seek additional information about potential problems that occur more frequently in older clients:

1. Do you ever have a problem with urine leaking?
2. Have you fallen in the past 6 months?
3. Do you often feel sad, blue, down in the dumps, or depressed?
4. Do you often travel places away from home alone?
5. Do you have enough money to purchase your medications?
6. Do you sometimes skip your medications?
7. Do you skip meals often?

Observe the client entering the exam room and note whether he or she walks slowly, uses a cane or walker, or is in a wheelchair. Watch how the client sits down in the chair. During the interview, determine if the client appears to have problems with memory, ambulation, and/or dressing. If the client has limitations in any of these areas, determine what assistance you will need to provide the client both in undressing for the exam, getting on and off the exam table, and redressing. The procedure for performing the physical exam on the older adult is similar to that outlined in previous chapters for each body system. As with all clients, make sure the exam room is quiet and the temperature is comfortable.

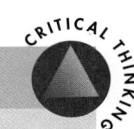

Sample Documentation

Health history

Mrs. Peterson, an 80-year-old woman who lives alone, complains of lightheadedness when getting out of bed in the morning and when rising from a chair in the afternoon. Yesterday morning she lost her balance getting out of bed and started to fall. She was able to break the fall by holding on to a chair next to the bed. She denies vertigo or any unsteadiness when she walks. One week ago her doctor ordered Enalaprin 5 mg two times a day for hypertension. Her blood pressure at that time was 185/80 sitting. She had taken the medication as prescribed.

Physical examination

Well groomed, appropriately dressed, and able to provide history without hesitation.
Oral temperature 37.1° C (98.8° F).

Lying blood pressure in right arm: 150/70; left arm 146/72. Immediate standing blood pressure: right arm 128/68; left arm 132/70. After one minute, blood pressure right arm, 146/80; left arm, 150/78.
Lungs: Breath sounds vesicular without crackles or wheezes.
Heart: 80/min. lying; 86/min. standing. Regular rate and rhythm.
Lower extremities: bilateral posterior tibial and pedal pulses 2+/4. Muscle strength 4/5 bilaterally. Knee and ankle reflexes 2+ bilaterally
Gait slow and slightly wide based. Rhomberg negative. Rising from a chair after sitting 15 minutes caused lightheadedness and slight swaying.

Nursing Diagnosis   *THE NEXT STEP*

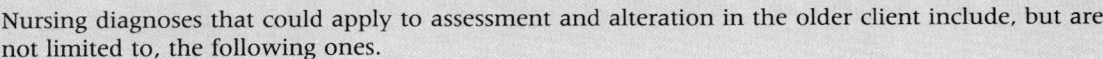

Nursing diagnoses that could apply to assessment and alteration in the older client include, but are not limited to, the following ones.

ALTERED NUTRITION: LESS THAN BODY REQUIREMENTS The state in which an individual experiences an intake of nutrients insufficient to meet metabolic needs.

Defining Characteristics

- Twenty percent or more under ideal body weight
- Reported or observed inadequate food intake relative to minimum daily requirements
- Weight loss (with or without adequate intake)
- Capillary fragility
- Pale conjunctiva and mucous membranes
- Fatigue
- Excessive hair loss; poor muscle tone
- Hyperactive bowel sounds; abdominal cramping, pain
- Diarrhea
- Decreased serum albumin, total protein, cholesterol
- Poor skin turgor
- Lack of interest in food
- Confusion
- Inability to feed self
- Fixed, limited income
- Social isolation

Related Factors

- Buccal cavity discomfort/pain
- Pain with mastication
- Altered taste sensation
- Inability to prepare/procure food
- Diarrhea, steatorrhea

Continued.

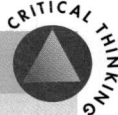

Nursing Diagnosis   *THE NEXT STEP—cont'd*

- Knowledge deficit
- Financial limitations
- Edentulous
- Social isolation
- Anorexia, setophobia, early satiety
- Chemical dependency
- Emotional stress
- Food faddism, dieting practices
- Weakness of the muscles of mastication/swallowing

HIGH RISK FOR IMPAIRED SKIN INTEGRITY The state in which an individual's skin is at risk of being adversely altered.

Defining Characteristics (risk factors)

- Reddened skin area
- Verbalized pain or discomfort in local area
- Presence of shearing forces, pressure, friction
- Physical immobilization
- Excretions/secretions on skin
- Altered sensation, consciousness
- Alterations in nutritional state
- Altered metabolic state, anemia
- Altered circulation, edema, arteriosclerosis
- Psychogenic factors
- High humidity, environmental temperature
- Hyper-hypothermia
- Medication
- Altered pigmentation
- Decreased fatty tissues, skeletal prominence
- Alteration in skin turgor
- Immunologic factors
- Radiation

STRESS INCONTINENCE The state in which an individual experiences a loss of urine of less than 50 ml occurring with increased abdominal pressure.

Defining Characteristics

- Reported or observed dribbling of urine with increased abdominal pressure
- Urinary urgency
- Urinary frequency (more than every 2 hours)
- Loss of urine in standing position

Related Factors

- Incompetent bladder outlet
- Age-related degenerative changes in pelvic muscles and structural supports
- Weak pelvic muscles and structural supports
- High intraabdominal pressure
- Overdistention between voidings

URGE INCONTINENCE The state in which an individual experiences involuntary passage of urine occurring soon after a strong sense of urgency to void.

Defining Characteristics

- Urinary urgency
- Frequency (voiding more often than every 2 hours)

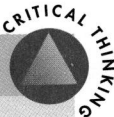

Nursing Diagnosis *THE NEXT STEP—cont'd*

- Bladder contracture/spasm
- Nocturia (greater than 2 times per night)
- Voiding in small amounts (less than 100 ml) or in large amounts (more than 550 ml)
- Inability to reach toilet in time
- Cloudy urine

Related Factors

- Decreased bladder capacity
- Bladder spasm
- Alcohol
- Caffeine
- Increased fluids
- Increased urine concentration
- Overdistention of bladder

IMPAIRED PHYSICAL MOBILITY The state in which an individual experiences a limitation of ability for independent physical movement.

Defining Characteristics

- Inability to purposefully move within the physical environment (bed mobility, transfer, ambulation)
- Limited active joint range of motion
- Decreased muscle strength, control, and/or mass
- Impaired coordination
- Imposed restrictions of movement (mechanical or medical protocol restrictions)
- Hemiplegia, paraplegia

Related Factors

- Intolerance to activity
- Decreased strength and endurance
- Pain
- Discomfort
- Uncompensated perceptual-cognitive impairment
- Uncompensated musculoskeletal impairment
- Uncompensated neuromuscular impairment
- Depression
- Severe anxiety

IMPAIRED HOME MAINTENANCE MANAGEMENT Inability to independently maintain a safe growth-promoting immediate environment.

Defining Characteristics

- Household members express difficulty in maintaining their home in a comfortable fashion
- Household members describe outstanding debts or financial crises
- Unwashed or unavailable cooking equipment, clothes, or linen
- Overtaxed family members (e.g., exhausted, anxious family members)
- Repeated hygienic disorders, infestations, or infections
- Household members request assistance with home maintenance
- Disorderly surroundings
- Accumulation of dirt, food wastes, or hygienic wastes
- Offensive odors
- Inappropriate household temperature
- Lack of necessary equipment or aids
- Presence of vermin or rodents

Continued.

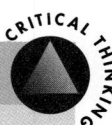

Nursing Diagnosis *THE NEXT STEP—cont'd*

Related Factors

- Individual/family member disease or injury
- Insufficient family organization/planning
- Insufficient finances
- Unfamiliarity with neighborhood resources
- Impaired cognitive or emotional functioning
- Knowledge deficit
- Lack of role modeling and inadequate support system

DYSFUNCTIONAL GRIEVING The state in which actual or perceived object loss (object loss is used in the broadest sense) exists. Objects include people, possessions, a job, status, home, ideals, parts and processes of the body, etc.

Defining Characteristics

- Verbal expression of distress at loss or denial of loss
- Expression of guilt
- Expression of unresolved issues
- Anger
- Sadness
- Crying
- Difficulty in expressing meaning of loss
- Alterations in eating habits
- Alterations in activity level or socialization
- Altered libido
- Idealization of lost object
- Reliving past experiences
- Interference with life functioning
- Developmental regression
- Labile affect
- Alterations in concentration and/or pursuits of tasks
- Continued indicators of grieving beyond expected time for cultural group

Related Factors

- Loss or perceived loss/change
- Unavailable support systems

CAREGIVER ROLE STRAIN A caregiver's felt difficulty in performing the family caregiver role.

Defining Characteristics

Caregiver's Report
- Inadequate resources to provide required care
- Difficulty providing specific caregiving activities
- Worry about the care receiver (e.g., care receiver's health and emotional state, having to put the care receiver in an institution, and/or who will care for the care receiver if something should happen to the caregiver)
- Feeling that caregiving interferes with other important roles in caregiver's life
- Feeling of loss because the care receiver is "like a different person" compared with before caregiving began
- Family conflict around issues of providing care
- Stress or nervousness in caregiver's relationship with the care receiver
- Depression
- Anxiety
- Knowledge deficit
- Noncompliance with prescribed treatment regimens

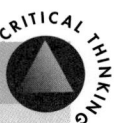

Nursing Diagnosis *THE NEXT STEP—cont'd*

Related Factors

- Illness severity
- Unpredictable course of illness
- Unstable health
- Caregiver health impairment
- Addition/codependency

HIGH RISK FOR INJURY The state in which an individual is at risk of injury as a result of environmental conditions interacting with the individual's adaptive and defensive resources.

Defining Characteristics (risk factors)

Internal
- Biochemical
  Regulatory function
    Sensory dysfunction
    Integrative dysfunction
    Effector dysfunction
  Tissue hypoxia
  Malnutrition
  Immune-autoimmune
  Abnormal blood profile
- Physical
  Broken skin
  Altered mobility
- Psychological
  Affective
  Orientation
External
- Biological
  Immunization level of community
  Microorganism
- Chemical
  Pollutants
  Poisons
  Drugs
    Pharmaceutical agents
    Alcohol
    Caffeine
    Nicotine
- Physical
  Design, structure, and arrangement of community, building, and/or equipment
  Mode of transport/transportation
  Nosocomial agents

SLEEP PATTERN DISTURBANCE Disruption of sleep time causes discomfort or interferes with desired life-style.

Defining Characteristics

- Verbal complaints of difficulty in falling asleep
- Awakening earlier or later than desired
- Interrupted sleep
- Verbal complaints of not feeling well rested

Continued.

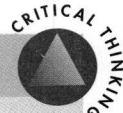

Nursing Diagnosis   *THE NEXT STEP—cont'd*

- Changes in behavior and performance
  Increasing irritability
  Restlessness
  Disorientation
  Lethargy
  Listlessness
- Physical signs
  Mild, fleeting nystagmus
  Slight hand tremor
  Ptosis of eyelid
  Expressionless face
- Thick speech with mispronunciation and incorrect words
- Dark circles under eyes
- Frequent yawning
- Changes in posture
- Not feeling well rested

Related Factors

Sensory alterations
- Internal factors
  Illness
  Psychological stress
- External factors
  Environmental changes
  Social cues

Clinical Application

Mr. B. is a 78-year-old retired farmer, admitted to the Alzheimer unit at East Park long-term care facility with the medical diagnosis of senile dementia Alzheimer. During the admission interview, Mr. B.'s wife tells the nurse she can no longer care for him at home. "He usually thinks I'm his mother or sister, not his wife," she says. The main problems Mrs. B. describes are problems with toileting, verbal and physical aggression, and wandering. Mr. B. wears adult diapers because "he doesn't use the bathroom when he needs to." Mr. B. sleeps only briefly and has become increasingly restless. He sleeps a lot during the day and has taken to wandering around the house at night. He even refuses to sit down to eat. Recently Mr. B. has become physically aggressive, especially when the television or radio is playing.

SUBJECTIVE DATA: Mrs. B. states that client:
Doesn't know who she is
Is incontinent all of the time
Is verbally and physically abusive
Sleeps during the day and wanders at night
Refuses to sit down and eat

OBJECTIVE DATA:
Vital signs: axillary temperature 37° C (98.0° F), pulse 80 beats/min and regular, respirations 18 breaths/min and nonlabored, sitting blood pressure right arm 132/86.
Height: 183 cm (72 in)
Weight: 65.8 kg (145 lbs). He is thin and pale, and has dark circles under his eyes.
Cardiovascular: S_1 and S_2 heard. No murmurs, no extra sounds.
Peripheral pulses present 1+ dorsalis pedis and radial bilaterally; skin turgor poor; capillary refill > 4 seconds; noted numerous bruises on extremities, in various stages of resolution.
Abdomen: Hyperactive bowel sounds heard in all 4 quadrants; no tenderness noted.
Cranial nerves: I—not tested. Taste sensation not tested. II-XII intact. CN VIII—Difficulty hearing spoken voice. Uses glasses for reading.

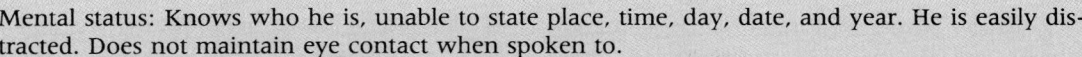

Nursing Diagnosis   *THE NEXT STEP—cont'd*

Mental status: Knows who he is, unable to state place, time, day, date, and year. He is easily distracted. Does not maintain eye contact when spoken to.

Cerebellar: Refused to cooperate with full exam. Decreased muscle tone in both upper and lower extremities.

Sensation to light touch and pain: Refused to cooperate.

Laboratory values: Decreased Hematocrit, Hemoglobin, iron binding capacity and serum albumin.

NURSING DIAGNOSES

Altered nutrition: less than body requirements related to inability to ingest food (client too restless to sit and eat).

Defining Characteristics

- Body weight greater than 20% under ideal body weight
- Inadequate food intake
- Anemia-hemoglobin and hematocrit decreased
- Decreased serum albumin
- Decreased iron binding capacity
- Refuses to sit down to eat
- Hyperactive bowel sounds
- Poor muscle tone

Sleep pattern disturbances related to psychological and environmental changes.

Defining Characteristics

- Dark circles under eyes
- Irritable
- Interrupted sleep
- Napping during the day

Altered urinary elimination: functional incontinence related to inability to recognize the need to void.

Defining Characteristics

- Loss of urine before reaching bathroom
- Unpredictable voiding pattern

High risk for trauma related to mental status changes.

Defining Characteristics (risk factors)

- History of previous trauma
- Cognitive difficulties
- Lack of safety precautions—wandering and aggressiveness
- Decreased hearing
- Lack of sleep

Caregiver role strain related to cognitive impairment of care receiver.

Defining Characteristics

- Unpredictable course of Alzheimer disease
- Patient's aggressive behavior—both physically and verbally

GLOSSARY

actinic keratoses Pink to slightly red, dry, scaly lesions with indistinct border and malignant potential.

activities of daily living Basic physical needs of dressing, transferring, feeding, bathing, toileting, bowel and bladder control, walking, climbing stairs, grooming.

age-related macular degeneration Degeneration of the macula leading to decreased central vision.

agnosia Inability to identify or recognize objects.

apraxia The inability to carry out purposeful skilled acts despite an intact sensory and motor system.

arcus senilis Grayish to gray-white arc or halo around limbus of eye.

basal cell skin cancer Nodular, translucent lesions with small blood vessels often seen inside nodule.

cataract Opacity in the lens that gradually impairs vision over time.

cherry angiomas Benign, bright red, small, dome-shaped skin lesion.

detrusor Bladder muscle.

entropion Turning inward of the lower lid of the eye.

ectropion Turning outward of the lower lid of the eye.

glaucoma Increased intraocular pressure that damages the optic nerve and retinal blood vessels resulting in vision loss.

incontinence Involuntary loss of urine with or without warning.

instrumental activities of daily living Life management skills of telephoning, reading, leisure, medication management, money management, transportation, shopping, meal preparation, laundering, housekeeping, home maintenance.

isolated systolic hypertension Systolic blood pressure greater than 160 mmHg and normal diastolic blood pressure.

kyphosis Rounding of the thorax.

lentigines Flat, tan to brown macules located in sun-exposed surfaces.

orthostatic hypotension Drop of 20 mmHg or more in systolic blood pressure upon rising from a lying or sitting position.

presbycusis Age-related hearing loss.

presbyopia Decreased ability to accomodate to near vision with increasing age.

ptosis Drooping of the upper eyelid often interfering with vision.

seborrheic keratoses Benign, raised, wart-like skin lesions appearing with increasing age.

senile purpura Skin bruising due to leakage of blood through fragile skin capillaries.

skin tags Benign, soft, flesh-colored skin lesions.

telangiectasias Visible dilated capillaries located in skin.

xerostomia Dry mouth usually caused by medications or radiation therapy.

BIBLIOGRAPHY

A profile of older Americans, Program Resources Department, American Association of Retired Persons and the Administration of Aging, US Department of Health and Human Services, Washington, DC, 1991.

American Psychiatric Association: *Diagnosis and statistical manual of mental disorders,* ed 3, Washington, DC, 1987, The Association.

Cassel, CK and others: *Geriatric medicine,* ed 2, New York, 1990, Springer-Verlag.

Consensus conference differential diagnosis of dementing diseases, *JAMA* 1987;258:3411-3416.

Dwyer J: *Screening older Americans' nutritional health: current practices and future possibilities,* Washington, DC, 1992, Nutritional Screening Initiative.

Folstein, M, Folstein, SE, McHugh, PR: Mini-mental state: a practical method for grading the cognitive state of patients for the clinician, *J Psychiatr Res* 12:189-198, 1975.

Gordon M: *Manual of nursing diagnosis* 1993-1994, St. Louis, 1993, Mosby—Year Book.

Hirsch CH and others: The natural history of functional morbidity in hospitalized older patients. *Am Geriatr Soc* 38:1296-1303, 1990.

Katz S, Ford AB, Moskowitz RW and others: Studies of illness in the aged: the Index of ADL: a standard measure of biologic and psychosocial function, *JAMA* 185:914-919, 1963.

Levkoff SE and others: Delirium: the occurrence and persistence of symptoms among elderly hospitalized patients, *Arch Intern Med* 152:334-340, 1992.

Mahoney FI, Barthel DW: Functional evaluation: the Barthel Index, *Maryland State Med J* 14:61-65, 1965.

Podsiadlo D, Richardson S: The timed "up & go": a test of basic functional mobility for frail elderly persons, *J Am Geriatr Soc* 39:142-148, 1991.

Schor JD and others: Risk factors for delirium in hospitalized elderly, *JAMA* 267:827-831, 1992.

Williams JH and others: Development and testing of the assessment of living skills and resources (ALSAR) in elderly community-dwelling veterans, *Gerontologist* 31:76-83, 1991.

Yesavage JA and others: Development and validation of a geriatric depression screening scale: preliminary report, *J Psychiatr Res* 17:37-49, 1983.

Clients with Functional Limitations

PURPOSE OF THE FUNCTIONAL ASSESSMENT

The various components of the physical examination and health history provide an indication of the health of a client's body systems and data about the relationship of the client with the environment, defined broadly. For most clients, the data also implicitly provide information about self-care and overall functional abilities. For special populations, however, including the elderly and handicapped, the usual components of

the health assessment may be insufficient in providing adequate information regarding the client's capabilities and activities (i.e., a functional assessment). This chapter presents and discusses several approaches to measuring functional assessment and guidelines to incorporate a functional assessment into the routine health assessment.

In practice with a given client group, a practitioner may choose to use standardized tools for all clients or to integrate functional assessment questions and techniques into the routine health assessment as individual

ADVANTAGES AND DISADVANTAGES—TWO MAIN FUNCTIONAL ASSESSMENT APPROACHES	
Approach *Integration into general assessment*	**Evaluation** *Advantages* Flexible Individualized Focus on variables of interest
	Disadvantages Can be incomplete Lack of standardized terminology Generally unsuitable for statistical analyses
Standardized tools	*Advantages* Objective Explicit Standardized
	Disadvantages May include irrelevant items Issues of validity and reliability

situations may indicate. Either method has advantages as well as disadvantages. (See the box above.) Because standardized tools are devised to yield comparable numerical scores, they are useful in situations where information must be summarized for communication across systems and providers, or when client, program, or other outcome evaluation is desired for general planning or discharge planning purposes. However, standardized tools often are not fully applicable across all groups and may include items not relevant for specific clients or client groups.

The examiner can integrate appropriate functional assessment parameters into the client's health assessment. Such integration can be effective if the examiner takes a highly individualized approach to the health history and physical examination and if sufficient time is available to add items. However, difficulty in obtaining reliable data in vulnerable populations may foster neglect in obtaining functional assessment information that could influence choice and scope of intervention.

Pinholt and colleagues (1987) compared the sensitivity and specificity of routine assessments and comprehensive functional assessment instruments. They found that physicians and nurses could identify severe impairments with routine approaches, but more prevalent and less prominent impairments were poorly recognized. The authors recommended the use of functional assessment instruments to detect moderate impairments, especially those remediable through early intervention.

INTRODUCTION TO KEY TERMS AND DEFINITIONS

Several conceptual definitions are useful for understanding the discussion in this chapter and other literature in the area of functional assessment. The World Health Organization (WHO) (1980) developed the following definitions to standardize terminology and facilitate communication in this area:

Impairment: An impairment is any loss or abnormality of psychological, physiological, or anatomical structure or function. An impairment is independent of its etiology and does not necessarily mean that a disease is still present. An example of an impairment is loss of a limb.

Disability: A disability is any restriction or lack of ability to perform an activity in the manner or within the range considered normal for a person of the same age and similar circumstances. A disability may be temporary or permanent and can occur in any component of human functioning. Different impairments may result in similar disabilities, and the same impairments do not necessarily result in similar disabilities. Not all impairments result in disability. An example of a disability is inability to climb stairs.

Handicap: A handicap is a disadvantage for a given individual, resulting from an impairment or a disability, that limits or prevents the fulfillment of a role that is normal for that individual. A handicap is characterized by a difference between what an individual appears to be able to do and the expectations of the particular group of which he is a member. The state of being handicapped is strongly influenced by existing societal values.

Functional Status: Functional status refers to the normal or characteristic performance of the individual. Functional status can be conceptualized into four categories:

1. Physical function: sensory-motor performance.
2. Mental function: intellectual, cognitive, or reasoning capabilities of the individual.
3. Emotional function: affect and effectiveness in coping psychologically with life stresses.
4. Social function: performance of social roles or obligations.

The following additional definitions are derived from legislative practice (NH Rev Stat Ann 464-A:2 [VII], [XI] [1983]. Cited in Nolan, 1984, p. 213):

Incapacity means a legal, not a medical, disability and shall be measured by functional limitations. It shall be construed to mean or refer to any person who has suffered, is suffering, or is likely to suffer substantial harm due to an inability to provide for his personal needs for food, clothing, shelter, health care, safety, or an inability to manage his or her property or financial affairs.

Functional limitations means behavior or conditions in an individual that impair his or her ability to participate in and perform minimal activities of daily living that secure and maintain proper food, clothing, shelter, health care, or safety for himself or herself.

The following models by Granger and colleagues (1987), based on the work of Nagi (1975) and Wood (1975), provide insight into the relationships among disease, impairment, and handicap.

Nagi Model

Pathologic → Impairment → Functional → Disability
condition   limitations

Wood Model

Disease or
disorder   → Impairment   → Disability   →   Handicap
(Intrinsic) → (Exteriorized) → (Objectified) → (Socialized)

INTEGRATING FUNCTIONAL ASSESSMENT INTO THE ROUTINE EXAMINATION

Functional Assessment Variables

Functional assessment can include a broad range of areas for examination. In practice, the examiner chooses those assessment areas relevant to a particular client or client group. For example, basic and instrumental activities of daily living would be important for assessment of a residential geriatric population, whereas the examiner would choose other assessment parameters for a rehabilitation unit accepting transfers from intensive care units. The following is a list of general categories of functional assessment topics:

Basic Activities of Daily Living (ADL)
  Grooming and personal hygiene
  Skin care
  Bathing
  Dressing and undressing
  Managing brace
    or prosthesis
  Going to the toilet
  Eating and feeding

Instrumental Activities of Daily Living (IADL)
  Managing personal finances
  Managing business affairs
  Shopping
  Cooking
  Preparing balanced meals
  Using problem-solving skills
  Managing medications
Mobility
  Capability of upper and lower extremities
  Body movement
  Bed activities: turning, sitting, shifting
  Transferring: between bed and wheelchair, wheelchair and chair, or chair and toilet
  Operating a wheelchair
  Walking on level surface
  Ascending and descending stairs
  Traveling
Medical condition
  Amount of medical supervision needed
  Continence—bowels and bladder
  Speech
Communication
  Reading
  Auditory comprehension
  Language expression (verbal)
  Language expression (gestural)
  Writing (motor)
  Written language expression
Senses
  Hearing
  Vision
Mental capability
  Orientation
  Understanding
  Communication
  Reading
  Writing
  Attention span
  Memory
  Judgment and reasoning
  Ability to play games and work on hobbies
  Awareness of current events
  Ability to comprehend movies and books
  Memory of appointments and commemorations
  Ability to manage travel instructions
Resources
  Significant others
  Social support
  Social interaction
Behavior problems
  Presence of emotional or psychiatric disorders
  Amount of supervision required
  Cooperation
  Depression

FIGURE 26-1 Assessing a client in his own surroundings allows for a full evaluation of the client's capabilities. These several photographs show a man with quadriplegia who is able to work and manage a number of activities of daily living quite independently in his home. **A, B,** Using the computer to work at home. **C,** Adapting a telephone to enable full use of this resource. **D, E,** Using a board to transfer frozen meals into and out of a microwave oven for independent food preparation.

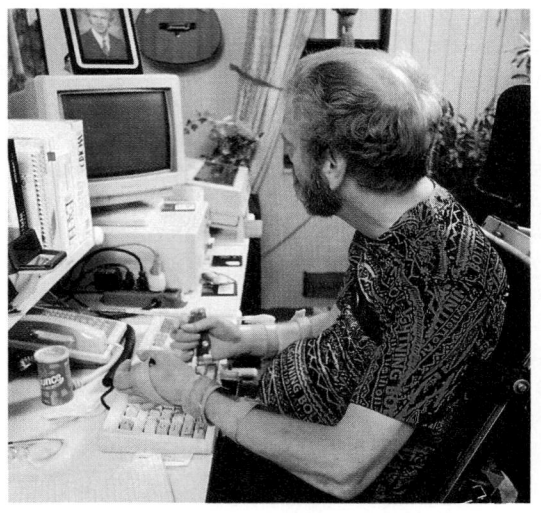

A

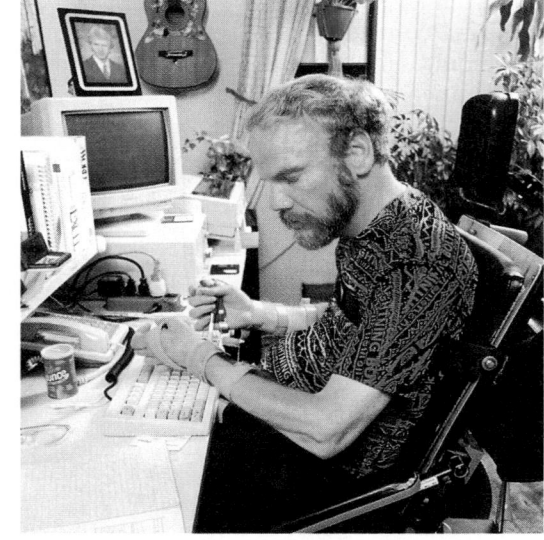

B

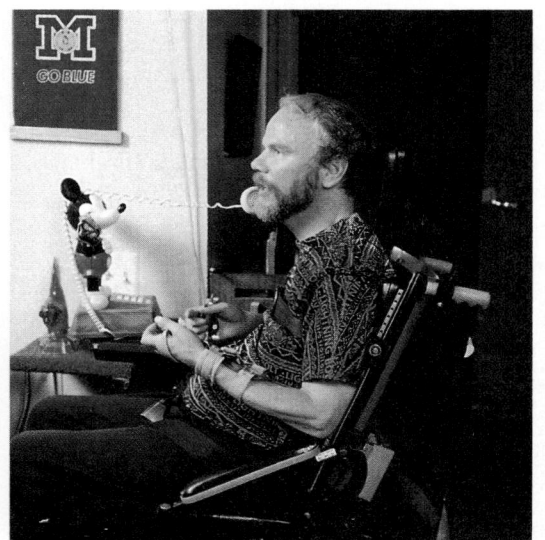

C

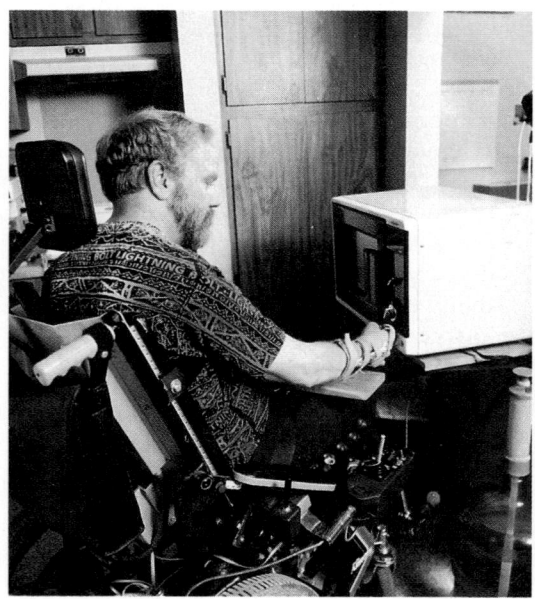

D

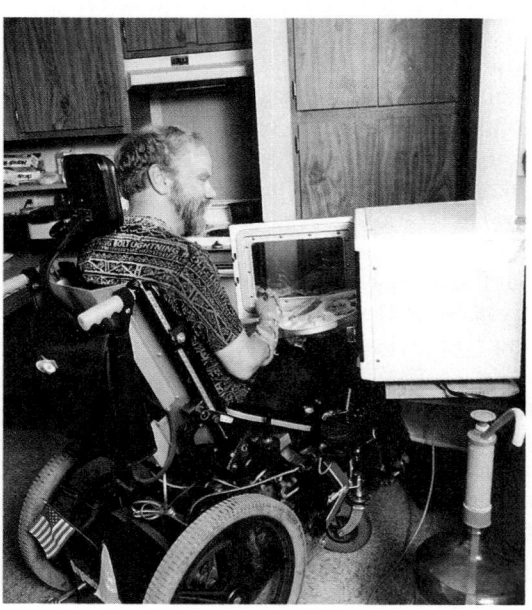

E

General Assessment with Emphasis on Functional Status

You can perform the functional assessment at any time during the routine health assessment. If you are using a standardized tool, this assessment is probably most logical at the end of the history and before the examination. Findings may provide guidance for particular follow-up during the physical examination.

The functional assessment requires no equipment in addition to that used in a comprehensive examination; most of the approaches require only interview and observation. Be prepared, however, to verify responses to various questions as needed. For example, you may want to ask the client to demonstrate operation of a wheelchair or ability to climb stairs. The best location for functional assessment is often the client's own surroundings, where environmental adaptations enable a full range of independent activities (Figure 26-1, *A* to 26-1, *E*). Table 26-1 outlines the major components of the history and physical examination and identifies the areas in which an assessment, focused on functional status, would require special emphases.

FUNCTIONAL ASSESSMENT TOOLS

Choosing and Administering Functional Assessment Tools

If you choose to use standardized tools to measure functional assessment in a given population, first determine the variables of primary interest and then match those variables with items on extant tools. When examining potential screening and assessment tools, examine both the content of the items and the scope of measurement. For example, you may want to determine whether a certain functional disability exists, the extent to which the functions are enabled by human or mechanical assistance, or both.

Desirable characteristics of a functional assessment tool include the following:

1. *Applicability*: appropriate for the client population.
2. *Continuity*: applicable to the client population across phases of treatment.
3. *Ease in administration*: can be administered by various health care professionals.
4. *Efficiency*: balance between comprehensiveness and time required for administration.
5. *Reliability*: demonstration of good test-retest and inter-rater reliability.
6. *Validity*: findings consistent with other assessment data.
7. *Sensitivity*: ability to differentiate among clients in general and a given client during various stages of treatment.

Although numerous tools have been developed to measure functional status, this chapter presents only some of the extant tools based on their perceived applicability to a health assessment framework. Criteria for selection include length of the tool, broad applicability to the elderly or the handicapped, ability to complement the usual components of a history and physical examination, ease of administration, and published data about the tool's conceptual bases, validity, reliability, usability, and quality.

The functional assessment tools in this chapter generally are designed to be administered by health care professionals. Sometimes the care provider may wish the client or client caregiver to administer the tools, for example, after hospital discharge and between clinic visits. However, findings from various studies, comparing client self-report with professional and caregiver assessments, indicate that the type of rater may influence scores. McGinnis and others (1986) compared the use of a modified Barthel Index by clients and health care professionals. Findings indicated that assessments were significantly different between groups, with providers rating clients higher in abilities than they rated themselves at a time immediately before discharge.

Rubenstein and others (1984) compared the ratings of hospitalized elderly by various groups using three instruments: the Lawton Personal Self-Maintenance Scale (PSMS), the Instrumental Activities of Daily Living Scale (IADL), and the Katz Activities of Daily Living Scale (ADL). Comparisons of ratings by the clients themselves, the clients' nurses, and clients' significant others revealed that the PSMS scores by clients were significantly higher than those of significant others, that the clients' IADL scores were significantly higher than scores by the nurses and the significant others, and that client scores for the ADL were significantly higher than the nurses' scores. The authors concluded that clients may overestimate their abilities and that significant others may underestimate clients' functional abilities as compared with professional nursing assessments.

Another issue regarding functional assessment is the relative reliability of various forms of client self-report. Spiegel and associates (1985) observed that clients with arthritis are more willing to admit difficulties with self-care activities in a self-administered questionnaire than in a personal interview.

Specific Functional Assessment Tools

This discussion presents a number of standardized functional assessment tools that may be useful with populations commonly seen in ambulatory and long-term

TABLE 26-1

Functional Assessment Emphases in the History and Physical Examination

Areas of assessment	Special emphases
History	
Present illness	Determine how present illness interferes with the client's ability to carry out self-care, work, and execute roles appropriate for age and social situation.
Past health history	Gain knowledge of abilities before incapacitating illness or situation in order to understand expectations and set rehabilitation goals.
Family health history	Note genetically transmitted disabling conditions.
Review of systems	Determine capabilities of the systems unaffected by the disability. These strengths will support rehabilitation. Complete review of affected and likely to be affected systems.
Social history	Describe in detail relationships and living arrangements and the adequacy of those relationships and living arrangements. For a hospitalized client after an unanticipated traumatic event, the accessibility of the living arrangements and the willingness of family and significant others to assist are important.
Employment history	Note the nature of the client's work and the client's ability to continue to manage that work or return to that work.
Physical examination	
Neurological evaluation	Mental Status
	Orientation to time, place, and person
	Memory
	Attention span
	Ability to perform calculations
	Abstract thinking
	Behavior
	Ability to follow commands
	Judgment
	Insight
	Mood
	Motor System
	Atrophy
	Spontaneous muscle activity
	Tone
	Increases in spasticity or rigidity
	Hypotonia or flaccidity
	Sensory Status—complete assessment
	Reflexes—complete assessment
	Vision
	Hearing
	Swallowing
	Speech and language
	Gait and mobility
	Use of assistive devices
	Ability to transfer
	Demonstration of methods of mobility and transfer
Musculoskeletal, soft tissue, and joint evaluation	Inspection—symmetry, postural attitudes, scars, edema, atrophy, masses, skin changes
	Palpation—muscles, bones, joints for local and general spasm, masses, swelling, or tenderness
	Measurement of active and passive range of motion with a goniometer
	Shoulder range of motion
	Finger flexion
Cardiac status	Complete assessment
Respiratory status	Adequacy of ventilation
	Ability to clear tracheobronchial secretions
	Physical endurance or capacity
	Psychological reaction to breathing difficulties
Skin	Condition of pressure areas—**ischial,** sacral, and **trochanteric** prominences
Bladder function	If incontinence or retention, extensive urological evaluation
	If intermittent self-catheterization or Foley used, review of technique
Bowel function	Review pattern and interventions used to achieve regular pattern
Pain	Quality, location, temporal characteristics, provocative factors, alleviating factors

A

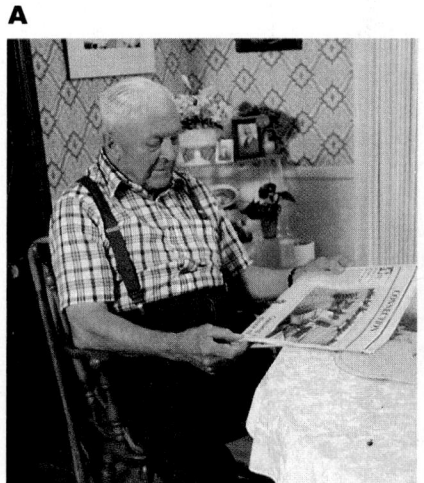

B

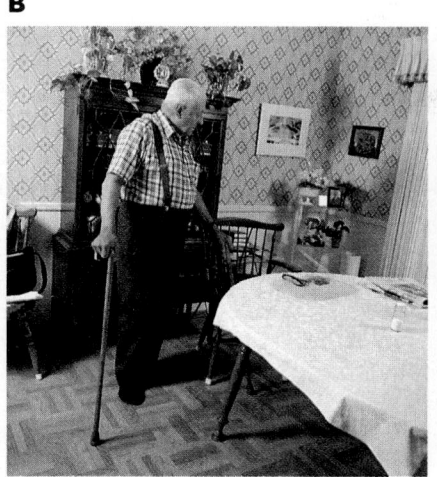

C

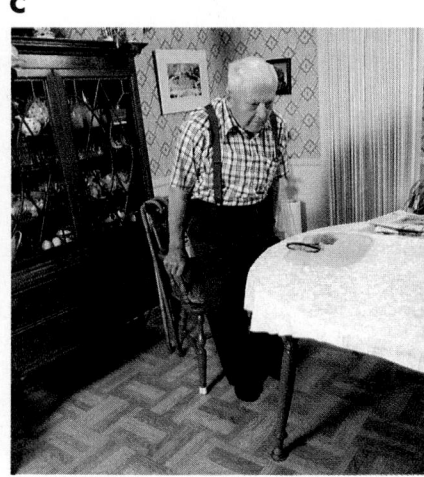

The elderly enjoy being able to sit in familiar surroundings and engage in activities they have enjoyed all of their lives. **A,** This elderly man with a walking disability enjoys sitting at the kitchen table and reading the daily newspapers in several languages. **B,** He demonstrates his method of walking with the use of two canes. **C,** He demonstrates his method of lowering and lifting himself up from his chair.

This man with paraplegia works outside his home each day and engages in a number of other outside activities. **A,** He demonstrates use of a mobile chair designed for his needs. **B,** He demonstrates his mobility in getting around his apartment building with a walker.

A

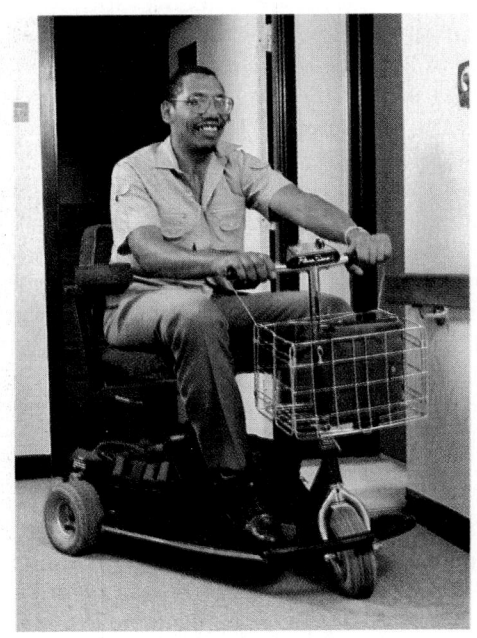

B

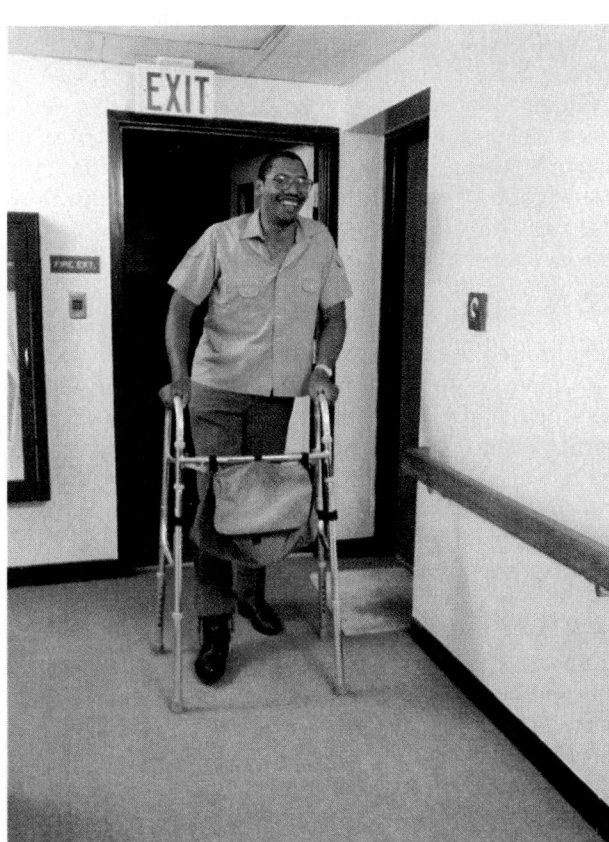

care settings. Numerous other tools exist; see McDowell and Newell (1987) or Rothstein (1985) for additional information about the tools presented in this chapter and for information about tools designed for special populations and for research applications.

Katz ADL Index (Revised Version 1976)

The original Katz ADL (activities of daily living) tool was among the earliest tools to standardize functional assessment. Both the original and revised versions focus on several basic activities of daily living and are very easy to administer and score (Katz and associates, 1963; Katz and Akpom, 1976). The revised version of the Katz ADL Index (Table 26-2) measures self-care and mobility, specifically the following activities:

Bathing
Dressing
Using the toilet
Transfer
Continence
Feeding

The examiner rates each activity as 1 or 0, 1 indicating performance of the activity without human help and 0 indicating performance of the activity with human assistance or that the activity is not performed at all. The scores form an ordinal or Gunman scale as noted on the top portion of Table 26-2.

The original Katz tool has been adapted for scoring by a Likert-type scale, using a scale range of 0 to 3 (0, complete independence; 1, use of a device; 2, use of human assistance; 3, complete dependence). No category exists for clients who use both a device and human assistance. The examiner adds the scores to obtain an overall score. A community-based version of the Katz adds items of walking and grooming but excludes continence. Brorsson and Saber (1984) have judged the reliability and validity of the tool as good.

The Katz tool is a general measure of self-care and a very limited measure of mobility. It is probably most applicable with populations in which a level of disability is assumed or already established (e.g., individuals with chronic illness). The tool is short and very easy to administer; therefore, the examiner could easily include a version on a printed history form. Its scoring approaches allow for comparison of a given individual over time or compilation across client groups.

PULSES Profile

The PULSES Profile was developed by Moskowitz and McCann (1957) to assess the functional independence of chronically ill, elderly persons. The PULSES instrument (Table 26-3) measures impairment, and the title of the tool is an acronym for its assessment components:

P = Physical condition
U = Upper limb functioning
L = Lower limb functioning
S = Sensory components
E = Excretory function
S = Support factors

The examiner scores each dimension using an ordinal scale from 1 to 4, with 1 representing essential intactness and 4 representing total dependence. The six categories are equally weighted, and the examiner sums the scores to produce a total score ranging from 6 to 24. Scores over 12 imply serious impairment, and scores over 16 usually reflect severe disability.

Several authors have reviewed the reliability and validity evidence for the scale (McDowell and Newell, 1987; Jetty, 1985) and they have assessed it as acceptable.

The main limitations of the tool are the general focus on a broad array of categories and redundancy with items commonly measured in a routine history and physical examination. The instrument was designed for use in a rehabilitation setting and is probably most applicable in situations where changes in levels of impairment are anticipated.

Barthel Index

The Barthel Index (BI) (Maine and Barthel, 1965; Granger, 1982) (Table 26-4) is a weighted index for assessing dependence in various areas of self-care, mobility, and continence. The original scale contains 10 items that the examiner scores with a weighted rating of 15, 10, 5, or 0, depending on the amount of help the client needs to perform the function. Total scores range from 0 (total dependence) to 100 (total independence) and are intended to indicate the amount of assistance a client requires. A score of 60 indicates the threshold between independence and dependence; a score of 40 or below indicates severe dependence; and a score of 20 or below reflects total dependence in self-care and mobility. Granger and associates (1979) reported the test-retest reliability and inter-rater agreements as 89% and 95%, respectively.

Forties and associates (1981) modified the original BI (Table 26-5). The modified BI contains 15 items and the following changes: two items of dressing (i.e., upper and lower body) rather than one general item; addition of items for use (brace or prosthesis), transfer to toilet, transfer to tub or shower; and differentiation of the walking and wheelchair propelling items.

Advantages of the BI include its widespread use, the clarity of scoring, and completeness of the set of items.

Instrumental ADL Scale

The Instrumental ADL Scale (Lawton, 1972) (Table 26-6) measures behaviors that are more cognitively and less directly physically oriented than the other self-care scales. The tool includes eight items measuring ability

TABLE 26-2

The Index of Independence in Activities of Daily Living: Scoring and Definitions

The index of Independence in Activities of Daily Living is based on an evaluation of the functional independence or dependence of patients in bathing, dressing, going to toilet, transferring, continence, and feeding. Specific definitions of functional independence and dependence appear below the index.

A—Independent in feeding, continence, transferring, going to toilet, dressing and bathing.

B—Independent in all but one of these functions.

C—Independent in all but bathing and one additional function.

D—Independent in all but bathing, dressing, and one additional function.

E—Independent in all but bathing, dressing, going to toilet, and one additional function.

F—Independent in all but bathing, dressing, going to toilet, transferring, and one additional function.

G—Dependent in all six functions.

Other—Dependent in at least two functions, but not classifiable as C, D, E, or F.

Independence means without supervision, direction, or active personal assistance, except as specifically noted below. This is based on actual status and not on ability. A patient who refuses to perform a function is considered as not performing the function, even though he is deemed able.

Bathing (sponge, shower, or tub)

Independent: assistance only in bathing a single part (as back or disabled extremity) or bathes self completely

Dependent: assistance in bathing more than one part of body; assistance in getting in or out of tub or does not bathe self

Dressing

Independent: gets clothes from closets and drawers; puts on clothes, outer garments, braces; manages fasteners; act of tying shoes is excluded

Dependent: does not dress self or remains partly undressed

Going to toilet

Independent: gets to toilet; gets on and off toilet; arranges clothes; cleans organs of excretion (may manage own bedpan used at night only and may or may not be using mechanical supports)

Dependent: uses bedpan or commode or receives assistance in getting to and using toilet

Transfer

Independent: moves in and out of bed independently and moves in and out of chair independently (may or may not be using mechanical supports)

Dependent: assistance in moving in or out of bed and/or chair; does not perform one or more transfers

Continence

Independent: urination and defecation entirely self-controlled

Dependent: partial or total incontinence in urination or defecation; partial or total control by enemas, catheters, or regulated use of urinals and/or bedpans

Feeding

Independent: gets food from plate or its equivalent into mouth (precutting of meat and preparation of food, as buttering bread, are excluded from evaluation)

Dependent: assistance in act of feeding (see above); does not eat at all or parenteral feeding

Adapted from Katz S, Downs TD, Cash HR, Grotz R: The index of independence in activities of daily living, progress in development of the index of ADL, *Gerontologist* 10:23, 1970.

to use a telephone, shop, prepare food, keep house, do laundry, use public transportation, take responsibility for one's medications, and handle finances. The examiner scores each item on a 3-, 4-, or 5-point scale reflecting the amount of assistance used or limitation in performing the activity.

The Instrumental ADL Scale expands the concept of self-care beyond specific and basic physical ability by measuring performance in the usual household maintenance activities. The examiner could use this scale with community-based populations and individuals whose mobility is compromised or who are at risk of progressive debilitation (e.g., the frail elderly).

TABLE 26-3

The PULSES Profile

	P **Physical condition** Cardiovascular pulmonary and other visceral disorders	**U** **Upper extremities** Shoulder girdles, cervical and upper dorsal spine	**L** **Lower extremities** Pelvis, lower dorsal and lumbosacral spine	**S** **Sensory function** Vision, hearing, speech	**E** **Excretory functions** Bowel and bladder	**S** **Social and mental status** Emotional and psychiatric disorders
NORMAL	1 Health maintenance	1 Complete function	1 Complete function	1 Complete function	1 Continent	1 Compatible with age
MILD	2 Occasional medical supervision	2 No assistance required	2 Fully ambulatory despite some loss of function	2 No appreciable functional impairment	2 Occasional stress incontinence or nocturia	2 No supervision required
MODERATELY SEVERE	3 Frequent medical supervision	3 Some assistance necessary	3 Limited ambulation	3 Appreciable bilateral loss or complete unilateral loss of vision or hearing. Incomplete aphasia	3 Periodic incontinence or retention	3 Some supervision necessary
SEVERE	4 Total care Bed or chair confined	4 Nursing care	4 Confined to wheelchair or bed	4 Total blindness Total deafness Global aphasia or aphonia	4 Total incontinence or retention (including catheter and colostomy)	4 Complete care in psychiatric facility

Adapted from McDowell I, Newell C: The presentation of the PULSES profile as published in Functional disability and handicap, *Measuring health: a guide to rating scales and questionnaires*, New York, 1987, Oxford University Press, pp 46-47.

P. *Physical* condition including diseases of the viscera (cardiovascular, pulmonary, gastrointestinal, urologic, and endocrine) and cerebral disorders which are not enumerated in the lettered categories below.
  1. No gross abnormalities considering the age of the individual.
  2. Minor abnormalities not requiring frequent medical or nursing supervision.
  3. Moderately severe abnormalities requiring frequent medical or nursing supervision yet still permitting ambulation.
  4. Severe abnormalities requiring constant medical or nursing supervision confining individual to bed or wheelchair.

U. *Upper* extremities including shoulder girdle, cervical and upper dorsal spine.
  1. No gross abnormalities considering the age of the individual.
  2. Minor abnormalities with fairly good range of motion and function.
  3. Moderately severe abnormalities but permitting the performance of daily needs to a limited extent.
  4. Severe abnormalities requiring constant nursing care.

L. *Lower* extremities including the pelvis, lower dorsal and lumbosacral spine.
  1. No gross abnormalities considering the age of the individual.
  2. Minor abnormalities with a fairly good range of motion and function.
  3. Moderately severe abnormalities permitting limited ambulation.
  4. Severe abnormalities confining the individual to bed or wheelchair.

S. *Sensory* components relating to speech, vision, and hearing.
  1. No gross abnormalities considering the age of the individual.
  2. Minor deviations insufficient to cause any appreciable functional impairment.
  3. Moderate deviations sufficient to cause appreciable functional impairment.
  4. Severe deviations causing complete loss of hearing, vision, or speech.

E. *Excretory* function, i.e., bowel and bladder control.
  1. Complete control.
  2. Occasional stress incontinence or nocturia.
  3. Periodic bowel and bladder incontinence or retention alternating with control.
  4. Total incontinence, either bowel or bladder.

S. *Mental and emotional status*.
  1. No deviations considering the age of the individual.
  2. Minor deviations in mood, temperament, and personality not impairing environmental adjustment.
  3. Moderately severe variations requiring some supervision.
  4. Severe variations requiring complete supervision.

TABLE 26-4

Original Barthel Index

	With help	Independent
1. Feeding (if food needs to be cut up = help)	5	10
2. Moving from wheelchair to bed and return (includes sitting up in bed)	5-10	15
3. Personal toilet (wash face, comb hair, shave, clean teeth)	0	5
4. Getting on and off toilet (handling clothes, wipe, flush)	5	10
5. Bathe self	0	5
6. Walking on level surface (or if unable to walk, propel a wheelchair)	10	15
	0[a]	5[a]
7. Ascend and descend stairs	5	10
8. Dressing (includes tying shoes, fastening fasteners)	5	10
9. Controlling bowels	5	10
10. Controlling bladder	5	10

From Mahoney FI, Barthel DW: Functional evaluation: the Barthel index, *Maryland State Med J* 14:61, 1965. Used with permission.
[a]Score only if unable to walk.
Instructions for scoring the Barthel Index (Note: A score of zero is given when the patient cannot meet the defined criterion):

1. Feeding
   10 = Independent. The patient can feed himself a meal from a tray or table when someone puts the food within his reach. He must put on an assistive device if this is needed, cut up the food, use salt and pepper, spread butter, etc. He must accomplish this in a reasonable time.
   5 = Some help is necessary (when cutting up food, etc., as listed above).
2. Moving from wheelchair to bed and return
   15 = Independent in all phases of this activity. Patient can safely approach the bed in his wheelchair, lock brakes, lift footrests, move safely to bed, lie down, come to a sitting position on the side of the bed, change the position of the wheelchair, if necessary, to transfer back into it safely, and return to the wheelchair.
   10 = Either some minimal help is needed in some step of this activity or the patient needs to be reminded or supervised for safety of one or more parts of this activity.
   5 = Patient can come to a sitting position without the help of a second person but needs to be lifted out of bed, or if he transfers with a great deal of help.
3. Doing personal toilet
   5 = Patient can wash hands and face, comb hair, clean teeth, and shave. He may use any kind of razor but must put in blade or plug in razor without help as well as get it from drawer or cabinet. Female patients must put on own make-up, if used, but need not braid or style hair.
4. Getting on and off toilet
   10 = Patient is able to get on and off toilet, fasten and unfasten clothes, prevent soiling of clothes, and use toilet paper without help. He may use a wall bar or other stable object of support if needed. If it is necessary to use a bed pan instead of a toilet, he must be able to place it on a chair, empty it, and clean it.
   5 = Patient needs help because of imbalance or in handling clothes or in using toilet paper.
5. Bathing self
   5 = Patient may use a bathtub, a shower, or take a complete sponge bath. He must be able to do all the steps involved in whichever method is employed without another person being present.
6. Walking on a level surface
   15 = Patient can walk at least 50 yards without help or supervision. He may wear braces or prostheses and use crutches, canes, or a walkerette but not a rolling walker. He must be able to lock and unlock braces if used, assume the standing position and sit down, get the necessary mechanical aides into position for use, and dispose of them when he sits. (Putting on and taking off braces is scored under dressing.)
   10 = Patient needs help or supervision in any of the above but can walk at least 50 yards with a little help.
6a. Propelling a wheelchair
   5 = If a patient cannot ambulate but can propel a wheelchair independently. He must be able to go around corners, turn around, maneuver the chair to a table, bed, toilet, etc. He must be able to push a chair at least 50 yards. Do not score this item if the patient gets score for walking.
7. Ascending and descending stairs
   10 = Patient is able to go up and down a flight of stairs safely without help or supervision. He may and should use handrails, canes, or crutches when needed. He must be able to carry canes or crutches as he ascends or descends stairs.
   5 = Patient needs help with supervision of any one of the above items.
8. Dressing and undressing (Women need not be scored on use of a brassiere or girdle unless these are prescribed garments.)
   10 = Patient is able to put on and remove and fasten all clothing, and tie shoe laces (unless it is necessary to use adaptations for this). The activity includes putting on and removing and fastening corset or braces when these are prescribed. Such special clothing as suspenders, loafer shoes or dresses that open down the front may be used when necessary.
   5 = Patient needs help in putting on and removing or fastening any clothing. He must do at least half the work himself. He must accomplish this in a reasonable time.
9. Continence of bowels
   10 = Patient is able to control his bowels and have no accidents. He can use a suppository or take an enema when necessary (as for spinal cord injury patients who have had bowel training).
   5 = Patient needs help in using a suppository or taking an enema or has occasional accidents.
10. Controlling bladder
   10 = Patient is able to control his bladder day and night. Spinal cord injury patients who wear an external device and leg bag must put them on independently, clean and empty bag, and stay dry day and night.
   5 = Patient has occasional accidents or cannot wait for the bed pan or get to the toilet in time or needs help with an external device.

TABLE 26-5

Modified Barthel Index Scoring

Independent		Dependent			Independent		Dependent		
I Intact	II Limited	III Helper	IV Null		I Intact	II Limited	III Helper	IV Null	
10	5	0	0	Drink from cup/feed from dish	15	15	7	0	Transfer, chair
					6	5	3	0	Transfer, toilet
5	5	3	0	Dress upper body	1	1	0	0	Transfer, tub or shower
5	5	2	0	Dress lower body	15	15	10	0	Walk on level 50 yards or more
0	0	−2	0	Don brace or prosthesis					
					10	10	5	0	Up and down stairs for one flight or more
5	5	0	0	Grooming					
4	4	0	0	Wash or bathe	15	5	0	0	Wheelchair/50 yards— only if not walking
10	10	5	0	Bladder continence					
10	10	5	0	Bowel continence					
4	4	2	0	Care of perineum/ clothing at toilet					

Adapted from the presentation of the Modified Barthel Index in Fortinsky RH, Granger CV, Seltzer GB: The use of functional assessment in understanding home care needs, *Med Care* 19:489, 1981.

TABLE 26-6

The Instrumental Activities of Daily Living Scale

A. Ability to use telephone
   1. Operates telephone on own initiative—looks up and dials numbers, etc.
   2. Dials well-known numbers.
   3. Answers telephone but does not dial.
   4. Does not use telephone at all.
B. Shopping
   1. Takes care of all shopping needs independently.
   2. Shops independently for small purchases.
   3. Must be accompanied on any shopping trip.
   4. Completely unable to shop.
C. Food preparation
   1. Plans, prepares, and serves adequate meals independently.
   2. Prepares adequate meals if supplied with ingredients.
   3. Heats and serves prepared meals, or prepares meals but does not maintain adequate diet.
   4. Needs to have meals prepared and served.
D. Housekeeping
   1. Maintains house alone or with occasional assistance.
   2. Performs light daily tasks such as dishwashing, bedmaking.
   3. Performs light daily tasks but cannot maintain acceptable level of cleanliness.
   4. Needs help with all home maintenance tasks.
   5. Does not participate in any housekeeping tasks.
E. Laundry
   1. Does personal laundry completely.
   2. Launders small items—rinses socks, stockings, etc.
   3. All laundry must be done by others.

F. Mode of transportation
   1. Travels independently on public transportation or drives own car.
   2. Arranges own travel by taxi but does not otherwise use public transportation.
   3. Travels on public transportation when assisted or accompanied by another.
   4. Travel limited to taxi or automobile with assistance of another.
   5. Does not travel at all.
G. Responsibility for own medications
   1. Is responsible for taking medications in correct dosages at correct time.
   2. Takes responsibility if medications are prepared in advance in separate dosages.
   3. Is not capable of dispensing own medications.
H. Ability to handle finances
   1. Manages financial matters independently (budgets, write checks, pay rent, bills, go to bank), collect and keep track of income.
   2. Manages day-to-day purchases but needs help with banking, major purchases, etc.
   3. Incapable of handling money.

From Brody E, Lawton M Powell: Philadelphia Geriatric Center, 5301 Old York Road, Philadelphia, PA 19141. Used with permission.

The Physical Self-Maintenance Scale

The Physical Self-Maintenance Scale (PSMS) (also known as the Lawton and Brody Scale, 1969) (Table 26-7) includes six items of self-care and mobility that the examiner rates using a unique Gunman scale for each item. The six items are toileting (including continence), feeding, dressing, grooming, physical ambulation, and bathing. The examiner may use either of two scoring methods: a count of the number of items for which disability is noted, or a severity scale summing the response codes for each item, resulting in a summary score ranging from 6 to 30.

This tool demonstrates good reliability and validity (McDowell and Newell, 1987). The scale is probably most applicable to homebound or institutionalized populations. Administration is easy and rapid.

The Functional Activities Questionnaire

The Functional Activities Questionnaire (FAQ) (Pfeffer and associates, 1984) (Table 26-8) is a screening tool for assessing independence in daily activities. It is designed to measure universal skills among older adults and is completed by the client's significant other. The FAQ consists of 10 items relating to tasks necessary for independent living. For each activity, the respondent rates the client based on four levels, ranging from dependence (score = 3) to independence (score = 0). For activities the client does not usually perform, the respondent specifies whether the person would be unable to undertake the task if requested (score = 1). The total score is the sum of individual items, with higher scores reflecting greater dependency.

The authors of the FAQ are in the process of revising

TABLE 26-7

The Physical Self-Maintenance Scale

A. Toilet
1. Cares for self at toilet completely, no incontinence.
2. Needs to be reminded, or needs help in cleaning self, or has rare (weekly at most) accidents.
3. Soiling or wetting while asleep more than once a week.
4. Soiling or wetting while awake more than once a week.
5. No control of bowels or bladder.

B. Feeding
1. Eats without assistance.
2. Eats with minor assistance at meal times and/or with special preparation of food, or help in cleaning up after meals.
3. Feeds self with moderate assistance and is untidy.
4. Requires extensive assistance for all meals.
5. Does not feed self at all and resists efforts of others to feed him.

C. Dressing
1. Dresses, undresses, and selects clothes from own wardrobe.
2. Dresses and undresses self, with minor assistance.
3. Needs moderate assistance in dressing or selection of clothes.
4. Needs major assistance in dressing but cooperates with efforts of others to help.
5. Completely unable to dress self and resists efforts of others to help.

D. Grooming (neatness, hair, nails, hands, face, clothing)
1. Always neatly dressed, well-groomed, without assistance.

2. Grooms self adequately with occasional minor assistance, e.g., shaving.
3. Needs moderate and regular assistance or supervision in grooming.
4. Needs total grooming care, but can remain well-groomed after help from others.
5. Actively negates all efforts of others to maintain grooming.

E. Physical ambulation
1. Goes about grounds or city.
2. Ambulates within residence or about one block distant.
3. Ambulates with assistance of (check one) a ( ) another person, b ( ) railing, c ( ) cane, d ( ) walker, e ( ) wheelchair.
   1 _____ Gets in and out without help.
   2 _____ Needs help in getting in and out.
4. Sits unsupported in chair or wheelchair, but cannot propel self without help.
5. Bedridden more than half the time.

F. Bathing
1. Bathes self (tub, shower, sponge bath) without help.
2. Bathes self with help in getting in and out of tub.
3. Washes face and hands only, but cannot bathe rest of body.
4. Does not wash self but is cooperative with those who bathe him.
5. Does not try to wash self and resists efforts to keep him clean.

Adapted from the presentation of the Physical Self-Maintenance scale in Lawton MP, Brody EM: Assessment of older people: self-maintaining and instrumental activities of daily living, *Gerontologist* 9-180, 1969.

TABLE 26-8

The Functional Activities Questionnaire

Activities questionnaire to be completed by spouse, child, close friend, or relative of the participant.

Instructions: The following pages list 10 common activities. *For each activity,* please read all choices, then choose the *one* statement which best describes the *current* ability of the participant. Answers should apply to *that persons's* abilities, not your own. Please check off a choice for *each* activity; do not skip any.

1. Writing checks, paying bills, balancing checkbook, keeping financial records
   _____ A. Someone has recently taken over this activity completely or almost completely.
   _____ B. Requires frequent advice or assistance from others (e.g., relatives, friends, business associates, banker), which was *not previously necessary.*
   _____ C. Does without any advice or assistance, but more difficult than used to be or less good job.
   _____ D. Does without any difficulty or advice.
   _____ E. Never did and would find quite difficult to start now.
   _____ F. Didn't do regularly but can do normally now with a little practice if they have to.

2. Making out insurance or Social Security forms, handling business affairs or papers, assembling tax records
   _____ A. Someone has recently taken over this activity completely or almost completely, and that someone did not used to do any or as much.
   _____ B. Requires more frequent advice or more assistance from others than in the past.
   _____ C. Does without any more advice or assistance than used to, but finds more difficult or does less good job than in the past.
   _____ D. Does without any difficulty or advice.
   _____ E. Never did and would find quite difficult to start now, even with practice.
   _____ F. Didn't do routinely, but can do normally now should they have to.

3. Shopping alone for clothes, household necessities, and groceries
   _____ A. Someone has recently taken over this activity completely or almost completely.
   _____ B. Requires frequent advice or assistance from others.
   _____ C. Does without advice or assistance, but finds more difficult than used to or does less good job.
   _____ D. Does without any difficulty or advice.
   _____ E. Never did and would find quite difficult to start now.
   _____ F. Didn't do routinely but can do normally now should they have to.

4. Playing a game of skill such as bridge, other card games or chess, or working on a hobby such as painting, photography, woodwork, stamp collecting
   _____ A. Hardly ever does now or has great difficulty.
   _____ B. Requires advice, or others have to make allowances.
   _____ C. Does without advice, or assistance, but more difficult or less skillful than used to be.
   _____ D. Does without any difficulty or advice.
   _____ E. Never did and would find quite difficult to start now.
   _____ F. Didn't do regularly, but can do normally now should they have to.

5. Heat the water, make a cup of coffee or tea, and turn off the stove
   _____ A. Someone else has recently taken over this activity completely or almost completely.
   _____ B. Requires advice or has frequent problems (for example, burns pots, forgets to turn off stove).
   _____ C. Does without advice or assistance but occasional problems.
   _____ D. Does without any difficulty or advice.
   _____ E. Never did and would find quite difficult to start now.
   _____ F. Didn't usually, but can do normally now, should they have to.

6. Prepare a balanced meal (e.g., meat, chicken, or fish, vegetables, dessert)
   _____ A. Someone else has recently taken over this activity completely or almost completely.
   _____ B. Requires frequent advice or has frequent problems (for example, burns pots, forgets how to make a given dish).
   _____ C. Does without much advice or assistance, but more difficult (for example, switched to TV dinners most of the time because of difficulty).
   _____ D. Does without any difficulty or advice.
   _____ E. Never did and would find quite difficult to do now even after a little practice.
   _____ F. Didn't do regularly, but can do normally now should they have to.

7. Keep track of current events, either in the neighborhood or nationally
   _____ A. Pays no attention to, or doesn't remember outside happenings.
   _____ B. Some idea about *major* events (for example, comments on presidential election, major events in the news, or major sporting events).
   _____ C. Somewhat less attention to, or knowledge of, current events than formerly.
   _____ D. As aware of current events as ever was.
   _____ E. Never paid much attention to current events, and would find quite difficult to start now.
   _____ F. Never paid much attention, but can do as well as anyone now when they try.

Adapted from the presentation of the functional activities questionnaire in McDowell I, Newell C: *Functional disability and handicap. Measuring health: A guide to rating scales and questionnaires,* New York, 1987, Oxford University Press, pp. 86-87.
Continued.

TABLE 26-8—cont'd

The Functional Activities Questionnaire

8. Pay attention to, understand, and discuss the plot or theme of a one-hour television program; get something out of a book or magazine
   _____ A. Doesn't remember, or seems confused by, what they have watched or read.
   _____ B. Aware of the *general idea,* characters, or nature while they watch or read, but may *not recall* later; may *not grasp theme* or have opinion about what they saw.
   _____ C. Less attention, or less memory than before, less likely to catch humor, points which are made quickly, or subtle points.
   _____ D. Grasps as quickly as ever.
   _____ E. Never paid much attention to or commented on T.V., never read much and would probably find very difficult to start now.
   _____ F. Never read or watch T.V. much, but read or watch as much as ever and get as much out of it as ever.
9. Remember appointments, plans, household tasks, car repairs, family occasions (such as birthdays or anniversaries), holidays, medications
   _____ A. Someone else has recently taken this over.
   _____ B. Has to be reminded some of the time (more than in the past or more than most people).

   _____ C. Manages without reminders but has to rely heavily on notes, calendars, schemes.
   _____ D. Remembers appointments, plans, occasions, etc. as well as they ever did.
   _____ E. Never had to keep track of appointments, medications, or family occasions, and would probably find very difficult to start now.
   _____ F. Didn't have to keep track of these things in the past, but can do as well as anyone when they try.
10. Travel out of neighborhood: driving, walking, arranging to take or change buses and trains, planes
   _____ A. Someone else has taken this over completely or almost completely.
   _____ B. Can get around in own neighborhood but gets lost out of neighborhood.
   _____ C. Has more problems getting around than used to (for example, occasionally lost, loss of confidence, can't find car, etc) but usually OK.
   _____ D. Gets around as well as ever.
   _____ E. Rarely did much driving or had to get around alone and would find quite difficult to learn bus routes or make similar arrangements now.
   _____ F. Didn't have to get around alone much in past, but can do as well as ever when has to.

and testing a new version of this tool that includes the addition of four items on activities of daily living and one item on initiative.

McDowell and Newell (1987) have reviewed the evidence regarding validity and reliability of the original tool and concluded that the initial findings were very promising.

Linn Rapid Disability Rating Scale

The Rapid Disability Rating Scale-2 (Linn and Linn, 1982) (Table 26-9) is an 18-item global disability scale measuring assistance needed with activities of daily living, disability, and special problems according to the assistance required, degree of disability, or degree of special problems. Each item is briefly defined and has options of four scale points. The total scores range from 18 to 72, with higher values indicating greater disability.

The scale demonstrates high reliability in use (McDowell and Newell, 1987; Rothstein, 1985), and the initial results of validity examination are positive.

This tool contains several items that the examiner would include in the routine health assessment (e.g.,

hearing, sight, diet, medication), and it may be most appropriate for screening situations.

The Functional Status Rating System

The Functional Status Rating System (Fore, 1981) (Table 26-10) measures the amount of assistance needed in self-care and mobility and the amount of impairment in communication, psychosocial adjustment, and cognitive function. It is unusually comprehensive for a functional assessment tool, covering 30 items under five topics. Although the tool may in small part duplicate portions of the health assessment, most of the items measure new assessment factors.

The amount of currently available psychometric information about the tool is limited.

Functional Independence Measure (FIM) and FIM Expanded

A recent innovation in the field of rehabilitation medicine is the proposal of a uniform, national data system for functional assessment. This standardized database would establish a uniform language and set of defini-

TABLE 26-9

The Rapid Disability Rating Scale-2

Directions: Rate what the person *does* to reflect current behavior. Circle one of the four choices for each item. Consider rating with any aids or prostheses normally used. None = completely independent or normal behavior. Total = that person cannot, will not or may not (because of medical restriction) perform a behavior or has the most severe form of disability or problem.

Assistance with activities of daily living

Eating	None	A little	A lot	Spoon-feed: intravenous tube
Walking (with cane or walker if used)	None	A little	A lot	Does not walk
Mobility (going outside and getting about with wheel-chair, etc., if used)	None	A little	A lot	Is housebound
Bathing (include getting sup-plies, supervising)	None	A little	A lot	Must be bathed
Dressing (include help in se-lecting clothes)	None	A little	A lot	Must be dressed
Toileting (include help with clothes, cleaning, or help with ostomy, catheter)	None	A little	A lot	Uses bedpan or unable to care for ostomy/catheter
Grooming (shaving for men, hairdressing for women, nails, teeth)	None	A little	A lot	Must be groomed
Adaptive tasks (managing money/possessions; tele-phoning; buying newspaper, toilet articles, snacks)	None	A little	A lot	Cannot manage

Degree of disability

Communication (expressing self)	None	A little	A lot	Does not communicate
Hearing (with aid if used)	None	A little	A lot	Does not seem to hear
Sight (with glasses, if used)	None	A little	A lot	Does not see
Diet (deviation from normal)	None	A little	A lot	Fed by intravenous tube
In bed during day (ordered or self-initiated)	None	A little (<3 hrs)	A lot	Most/all of time
Incontinence (urine/feces, with catheter or prosthesis, if used)	None	Sometimes	Frequently (weekly +)	Does not control
Medication	None	Sometimes	Daily, taken orally	Daily: injection (+ oral if used)

Degree of special problems

Mental confusion	None	A little	A lot	Extreme
Uncooperativeness (combats ef-forts to help with care)	None	A little	A lot	Extreme
Depression	None	A little	A lot	Extreme

Adapted from the presentation of the Rapid Disability Rating Scale-2 as published in Linn MW, Linn BS: The rapid disability rating scale-2, *J Am Geriatr Soc* 30:380, 1982.

tions for communicating disability and rehabilitation information. Toward this end the major researchers in the field have developed the minimum data set for the field, the Functional Independence Measure (FIM) tool. The FIM tool measures 18 items in the categories of self-care, mobility, locomotion, communication, and social cognition. The seven-point rating scale is de-signed to assess the patient's level or degree of inde-pendence, the amount of assistance required, use of adaptive or assistive devices, and the percentage of a given task completed successfully. The FIM requires 15 to 20 minutes for administration and can be performed by a variety of health care professionals.

The staff of the Santa Clara Medical Center has ex-
Text continued on p. 868.

TABLE 26-10

The Functional Status Rating System

Functional status in self-care

A. *Eating/feeding:* Management of all aspects of setting up and eating food (including cutting of meat) with or without adaptive equipment.

B. *Personal hygiene:* Includes set up, oral care, washing face and hands with a wash cloth, hair grooming, shaving, and makeup.

C. *Toileting:* Includes management of clothing and cleanliness.

D. *Bathing:* Includes entire body bathing (tub, shower, or bed bath).

E. *Bowel management:* Able to insert suppository and/or perform manual evacuation, aware of need to defecate, has sphincter muscle control.

F. *Bladder management:* Able to manage equipment necessary for bladder evacuation (may include intermittent catheterization).

G. *Skin management:* Preformance of skin care program, regular inspection, prevention of pressure sores, rashes, or irritations.

H. *Bed activities:* Includes turning, coming to a sitting position, scooting, and maintenance of balance.

I. *Dressing:* Includes performance of total body dressing except tying shoes, with or without adaptive equipment (also includes application of orthosis and prosthesis).

Functional status in mobility

A. *Transfers:* Includes the management of all aspects of transfers to and from bed, mat, toilet, tub/shower, wheelchair, with or without adaptive equipment.

B. *Wheelchair skills:* Includes management of brakes, leg rests, maneuvering and propelling through and over doorway thresholds.

C. *Ambulation:* Includes coming to a standing position and walking short to moderate distances on level surfaces with or without equipment.

D. *Stairs and environmental surfaces:* Includes climbing stairs, curbs, ramps or environmental terrain.

E. *Community mobility:* Ability to manage transportation.

Functional status in communication

A. *Understanding spoken language*

B. *Reading comprehension*

C. *Language expression (non-speech/alternative methods):* Includes pointing, gestures, manual communication boards, electronic systems.

D. *Language expression (verbal):* Includes grammar, syntax, and appropriateness of language.

E. *Speech intelligibility*

F. *Written communication (motor)*

G. *Written language expression:* Includes spelling, vocabulary, punctuation, syntax, grammar, and completeness of written response.

Functional status in psychosocial adjustment

A. *Emotional adjustment:* Includes frequency and severity of depression, anxiety, frustration, lability, unresponsiveness, agitation, interference with progress in therapies, motivation, ability to cope with and take responsibility for emotional behavior.

B. *Family/significant others/environment:* Includes frequency of chronic problems or conflicts in patient's relationships, interference with progress in therapies, ability and willingness to provide for patient's specific needs after discharge, and to promote patient's recovery and independence.

C. *Adjustment to limitations:* Includes denial/awareness, acceptance of limitations, willingness to learn new ways of functioning, compensating, taking appropriate safety precautions, and realistic expectations for long-term recovery.

D. *Social adjustment:* Includes frequency and limitation of social contacts, responsiveness in one to one and group situations, appropriateness of behavior in relationships, and spontaneity of interactions.

Functional status in cognitive function

A. *Attention span:* Includes distractability, level of alertness and responsiveness, ability to concentrate on a task, ability to follow directions, immediate recall as the structure, difficulty and length of the task varies.

B. *Orientation*

C. *Judgment reasoning*

D. *Memory:* Includes short- and long-term.

E. *Problem-solving*

Summary of rating scales

Self-care and mobility items

1.0 = Unable—totally dependent
1.5 = Maximum assistance of 1 or 2 people
2.0 = Moderate assistance
2.5 = Minimal assistance
3.0 = Standby assistance
3.5 = Supervised
4.0 = Independent

Communication, psychosocial, and cognitive function items

1.0 = Extremely severe
1.5 = Severe
2.0 = Moderately severe
2.5 = Moderate impairment
3.0 = Mild impairment
3.5 = Minimal impairment
4.0 = No impairment

Adapted from the presentation of the Functional Status Rating System as published in McDowell C, Newell C: *Functional disability and handicap. Measuring health: A guide to rating scales and questionnaires,* New York, 1987, Oxford University Press, pp 69-70, 1987.

TABLE 26-11

Functional Assessment Measures (FAM)

The 7-point Rating Scale is as follows:

Independent	Another person is not required for the activity (NO HELPER).
7	**Complete Independence**—All of the tasks described as making up the activity are typically performed safely without modification, assistive devices, or aids and within reasonable time.
6	**Modified Independence**—Activity requires any one or more of the following: an assistive device, more than reasonable time, or there are safety (risk) considerations.
Dependent	Another person is required for either supervision or physical assistance in order for the activity to be performed, or it is not performed (REQUIRES HELPER).
	MODIFIED DEPENDENCE—The subject expends half (50%) or more of the effort. The levels of assistance required are:
5	**Supervision or Setup**—Subject requires no more help than standby, cuing or coaxing, without physical contact. Or, helper sets up needed items or applies orthoses.
4	**Minimal Contact Assistance**—With physical contact the subject requires no more help than touching, and subject expends 75% or more of the effort.
3	**Moderate Assistance**—Subject requires more help than touching, or expends half (50%) or more (up to 75%) of the effort.
	COMPLETE DEPENDENCE—The subject expends less than half (less than 50%) of the effort, maximal or total assistance is required, or the activity is not performed. The levels of assistance required are:
2	**Maximal Assistance**—Subject expends less than 50% of the effort, but at least 25%.
1	**Total Assistance**—Subject expends less than 25% of the effort.

Each item is operationally defined in terms of these seven levels on the following pages.

Self-care items

1. FEEDING

Includes use of suitable utensils to bring food to mouth, chewing and swallowing, once meal is appropriately prepared. Opening containers, cutting meat, buttering bread and pouring liquids are *not* included as they are often part of meal preparation.

No helper

7	**Complete Independence**—Eats from a dish and drinks from a cup or glass presented in the customary manner on a table or a tray. Uses ordinary knife, fork, spoon.
6	**Modified Independence**—Uses an adaptive or assistive device such as a straw, spork, rocking knife or requires more than a reasonable time to eat.

Helper

5	**Supervision or Setup**—Requires supervision (e.g., standby, cuing, or coaxing) or setup (application of orthoses).
4	**Minimal Contact Assistance**—Subject performs 75% or more of feeding tasks.
3	**Moderate Assistance**—Performs 50% to 74% of feeding tasks.
2	**Maximal Assistance**—Performs 25% to 49% of feeding tasks. Or, the individual does not eat or drink full meals by mouth, but relies in part on other means of alimentation, such as parenteral or gastrostomy feedings, then he/she administers the feedings him/herself.
1	**Total Assistance**—Performs less than 25% of feeding tasks. Or, the individual does not eat or drink full meals by mouth but must rely in part on other means of alimentation, such as parenteral or gastrostomy feedings, and does not administer the feedings him/herself.

2. GROOMING

Includes oral care, hair grooming, washing hands and face, and either shaving or applying makeup.

No helper

7	**Complete Independence**—Cleans teeth or dentures, combs or brushes hair, washes hands and face, shaves or applies makeup, including all preparations.
6	**Modified Independence**—Uses specialized equipment or takes more than a reasonable time, or there are safety considerations.

TABLE 26-11—cont'd

Functional Assessment Measures (FAM)

2. GROOMING—cont'd

Helper

5	**Supervision or Setup**—Requires supervision (e.g., standby, cuing, or coaxing) or setup (application of orthoses, setting out specialized grooming equipment, and initial preparation such as apply toothpaste to brush, opening makeup containers).
4	**Minimal Contact Assistance**—Subject performs 75% of grooming tasks.
3	**Moderate Assistance**—Performs 50% to 74% of grooming tasks.
2	**Maximal Assistance**—Performs 25% to 49% of grooming tasks.
1	**Total Assistance**—Performs less than 25% of grooming tasks.
3. BATHING	Includes bathing the body from the neck down (excluding the back), either tub, shower or sponge/bed bath.

No helper

7	**Complete Independence**—Bathes and dries the body.
6	**Modified Independence**—Uses specialized equipment or takes more than a reasonable time or there are safely considerations.

Helper

5	**Supervision or Setup**—Requires supervision (e.g., standby, or cuing or coaxing) or setup (setting out specialized bathing equipment, and initial preparation such as preparing the water or washing materials).
4	**Minimal Contact Assistance**—Subject performs 75% or more of bathing tasks.
3	**Moderate Assistance**—Performs 50% to 74% of bathing tasks.
2	**Maximal Assistance**—Performs 25% to 49% of bathing tasks.
1	**Total Assistance**—Performs less than 25% of bathing tasks.
4. DRESSING—UPPER BODY	Includes dressing above the waist as well as donning and removing prosthesis or orthosis when applicable.

No helper

7	**Complete Independence**—Dresses and undresses including obtaining clothes from their customary places such as drawers and closets; manages bra, pull-over garment, and front-opening garment; manages zippers, buttons, and snaps; dons and removes prosthesis or orthosis when applicable.
6	**Modified Independence**—Uses special adaptive closure such as Velcro, or assistive device, or takes more than a reasonable time.

Helper

5	**Supervision or Setup**—Requires supervision (e.g., standby, cuing, or coaxing) or setup (application or orthoses, setting out clothes or specialized dressing equipment).
4	**Minimal Contact Assistance**—Subject performs 75% or more of dressing tasks.
3	**Moderate Assistance**—Performs 50% to 74% of dressing tasks.
2	**Maximal Assistance**—Performs 25% to 49% of dressing tasks.
1	**Total Assistance**—Performs less than 25% of dressing tasks, or is not dressed.
5. DRESSING—LOWER BODY	Includes dressing from the waist down as well as donning or removing prosthesis or orthosis when applicable.

No helper

7	**Complete Independence**—Dresses and undresses including obtaining clothes from their customary places such as drawers and closets; manages underpants, slacks, skirt, belt, stockings, and shoes; manages zippers, buttons, and snaps; dons and removes prosthesis or orthosis when applicable.
6	**Modified Independence**—Uses special adaptive closure such as Velcro, or assistive device, or takes more than a reasonable time.

Functional Assessment Measures developed by the staff of the Santa Clara Valley Medical Center, Santa Clara, Calif. *Continued.*

TABLE 26-11—cont'd

Functional Assessment Measures (FAM)

5. DRESSING—LOWER BODY—cont'd

Helper

5   **Supervision or Setup**—Requires supervision (e.g., standby, cuing, or coaxing) or setup (application or orthoses, setting out clothes or specialized dressing equipment).

4   **Minimal Contact Assistance**—Subject performs 75% or more of dressing tasks.

2   **Maximal Assistance**—Performs 25% to 49% of dressing tasks.

1   **Total Assistance**—Performs less than 25% of dressing tasks, or is not dressed.

6. TOILETING   Includes maintaining perineal hygiene and adjusting clothing after toileting.

No helper

7   **Complete Independence**—Cleanses self after voiding or bowel movement; puts on sanitary napkins/inserts tampons; adjusts clothing after using toilet.

6   **Modified Independence**—Uses specialized equipment or takes more than reasonable time or there are safety considerations.

Helper

5   **Supervision or Setup**—Requires supervision (e.g., standby, cuing, or coaxing) or setup (application of adaptive devices or opening packages).

4   **Minimal Contact Assistance**—Performs 75% or more of toileting tasks.

3   **Moderate Assistance**—Performs 50% or 74% of toileting tasks.

2   **Maximal Assistance**—Performs 25% or 49% of toileting tasks.

1   **Total Assistance**—Performs less than 25% of toileting tasks.

Comment: If subject requires assistance with sanitary napkins (usually 3-5 days per month) level of assistance is 5, supervision or setup.

7. SWALLOWING   Ability to safely eat a regular diet by mouth.

Helper

7   **Complete Independence**—Able to eat a regular diet of choice in a reasonable period of time.

6   **Modified Independence**—Able to eat a regular diet by mouth. May require excessive time for eating. May require assistive devices or multiple swallows to clear food.

No helper

5   **Supervision** (Modified Dependence)—Able to take all nourishment by mouth. May need modified diet. Supervision required for cueing, coaxing. May need assistance with food choices.

4   **Minimal Assistance** (Modified Dependence)—Able to take primary nourishment by mouth. May require diet restrictions. Minimal assistance required to monitor speed and amount of food intake. Subject performs 75% of the activity.

3   **Maximal Assistance** (Modified Dependence)—Able to take some nourishment by mouth. May require diet restrictions and modifications. May require moderate assistance to monitor speed and amount of food intake. Subject performs 50%-74% of the activity.

2   **Maximal Assistance** (Dependent)—Unable to receive adequate nourishment via oral feedings. Tube feedings provide primary nutrition. Oral feedings are limited and require maximal assistance. Subject performs 25%-49% of the activity.

1   **Unable** to take anything by mouth. Nutrition is *provided via tube feedings*.

Sphincter control

8. BLADDER MANAGE-MENT   Includes complete intentional control of urinary bladder and use of equipment or agents necessary for bladder control.

No helper

7   **Complete Independence**—Controls bladder completely and intentionally and is never incontinent.

TABLE 26-11—cont'd

Functional Assessment Measures (FAM)

8. BLADDER MANAGEMENT—cont'd

6   **Modified Independence**—Requires a catheter, urinary collecting device, or urinary diversion or uses medication for control; if catheter is used, the individual instills or irrigates catheter without assistance; cleans, sterilizes, and sets up the equipment for irrigation without assistance. If the individual uses a device, he/she assembles and applies condom drainage or an ileal appliance without assistance of another person; empties, puts on, removes, and cleans leg bag or empties and cleans ileal appliance bag. No accidents.

Helper

5   **Supervision or Setup**—Requires supervision (e.g., standby, cuing, or coaxing) or setup of catheterization equipment to maintain a satisfactory voiding pattern or to maintain an external device; or because of the lapse of time to get to bed pan or the toilet the individual may have occasional bladder accidents, but less often than *monthly.*

4   **Minimal Contact Assistance**—Requires minimal contact assistance to maintain an external device; the individual performs 75% or more of bladder management tasks; or may have occasional bladder accidents, but less often than *weekly.*

3   **Moderate Assistance**—Requires moderate assistance to maintain an external device; the individual performs 50% to 74% of bladder management tasks; or may have occasional bladder accidents, but less often than *daily.*

2   **Maximal Assistance**—Despite assistance, the individual is wet on a frequent or almost daily basis, necessitating wearing diapers or other absorbent pads, whether or not a catheter or ostomy device is in place. The individual performs 25% to 49% of bladder management tasks.

1   **Total Assistance**—Despite assistance, the individual is wet on a frequent or almost daily basis, necessitating wearing diapers or other absorbent pads, whether or not a catheter or ostomy device is in place. The individual performs less than 25% of bladder management tasks.

Comment: The functional goal of bladder management is to open the bladder sphincter only when that is needed and to keep it closed the rest of the time. This may require devices, drugs or assistance in some individuals. This item, therefore, deals with two variables: 1) level of success in bladder management and 2) level of assistance required. Usually the two follow each other. e.g., when there are more accidents usually more assistance is required. However, should the two levels not be exactly the same, always record the *lower* level.

9. BOWEL MANAGEMENT   Includes complete intentional control of bowel movement and use of equipment or agents necessary for bowel control.

No helper

7   **Complete Independence**—Controls bowels completely and intentionally and is never incontinent.

6   **Modified Independence**—Uses digital stimulation or stool softeners, suppositories, laxatives, or enemas on a regular basis, or uses other medications for control. If the individual has a colostomy, he/she maintains it. No accidents.

Helper

5   **Supervision or Setup**—Requires supervision (e.g., standby, cuing, or coaxing) or setup of equipment necessary for the individual to maintain a satisfactory excretion pattern or to maintain an ostomy device; or the individual may have occasional bowel accidents, but less often than *monthly.*

4   **Minimal Contact Assistance**—Requires minimal contact assistance to maintain a satisfactory excretion pattern by using suppositories or enemas or an external device; the individual performs 75% or more of bowel management tasks; or may have occasional bowel accidents, but less often than *weekly.*

3   **Moderate Assistance**—Requires moderate assistance to maintain a satisfactory excretory pattern by using such means as suppositories or enemas or to maintain an external device; the individual performs 50% to 74% of bowel management tasks; or may have occasional bowel accidents, but less often than *daily.*

Continued.

TABLE 26-11—cont'd

Functional Assessment Measures (FAM)

9. BOWEL MANAGEMENT—*cont'd*

2   **Maximal Assistance**—Despite assistance, the individual is soiled on a frequent or almost daily basis, necessitating wearing diapers or other absorbent pads, whether or not an ostomy device is in place. The individual performs 25% to 49% of bowel management tasks.

1   **Total Assistance**—Despite assistance, the individual is soiled on a frequent or almost daily basis, necessitating wearing diapers or other absorbent pads, whether or not an ostomy device is in place. The individual performs less than 25% of bowel management tasks.

Comment: The functional goal of bowel management is to open the anal sphincter only when that is needed and to keep it closed the rest of the time. This may require devices, drugs or assistance in some individuals. This item, therefore, deals with two variables: 1) level of success in bowel management and 2) level of assistance required. Usually the two follow each other. e.g., when there are more accidents usually more assistance is required. However, should the two levels not be exactly the same, always record the *lower* level.

Mobility items

10. TRANSFERS: BED, CHAIR, WHEELCHAIR   Includes all aspects of transferring to and from bed, chair, or wheelchair, or coming to a standing position, if walking is the typical mode of locomotion.

No helper

7   **Complete Independence**—If *walking*, approaches, sits down and gets up to a standing position from a regular chair; transfers from bed to chair. Performs safely.

If *in a wheelchair*, approaches a bed or chair, locks brakes, lifts foot rests, removes arm rests if necessary, and performs either a standing pivot or sliding transfer and returns. Performs safely.

Modified Independence—Uses adaptive or assistance device such as a sliding board, a lift, grab bars, or special seat or chair or brace or crutches; takes more than reasonable time or there are safety considerations.

Helper

5   **Supervision or Setup**—Requires supervision (e.g., standby, cuing, or coaxing) or setup (positioning sliding board, moving foot rests, etc.)

4   **Minimal Contact Assistance**—Subject performs 75% or more of transferring tasks.

3   **Moderate Assistance**—Performs 50% to 74% of transferring tasks.

2   **Maximal Assistance**—Performs 25% to 49% of transferring tasks.

1   **Total Assistance**—Performs less than 25% of transferring tasks.

11. TRANSFERS: TOILET   Includes getting on and off a toilet.

No helper

7   **Complete Independence**—*If walking,* approaches, sits down on and gets up from a standard toilet. Performs safely.

If *in a wheelchair,* approaches toilet, locks brakes, lifts foot rests, removes arm rests if necessary and does either a standing pivot or sliding transfer and returns. Performs safely.

6   **Modified Independence**—Uses adaptive or assistive device such as a sliding board, a lift, grab bars, or special seat; takes more than reasonable time or there are safety considerations.

Helper

5   **Supervision or Setup**—Requires supervision (e.g., standby, cuing, or coaxing) or setup (positioning sliding board, moving foot rests, etc).

4   **Minimal Contact Assistance**—Subject performs 75% or more of transferring tasks.

3   **Moderate Assistance**—Performs 50% to 74% of transferring tasks.

2   **Maximal Assistance**—Performs 25% to 49% of transferring tasks.

1   **Total Assistance**—Performs less than 25% of transferring tasks.

TABLE 26-11—cont'd

Functional Assessment Measures (FAM)

12.	TRANSFERS: TUB OR SHOWER	Includes getting into and out of a tub or shower stall.

No helper

7   **Complete Independence**—*If walking*, approaches, enters and leaves a tub or shower stall. Performs safely.

If in a wheelchair, approaches tub or shower, locks brakes, lifts foot rests, removes arm rests if necessary and does either a standing pivot or sliding transfer and returns. Performs safely.

6   **Modified Independence**—Uses adaptive or assistive device such as a sliding board, a lift, grab bars, or special seat; takes more than reasonable time or there are safety considerations.

Helper

5   **Supervision or Setup**—Requires supervision (e.g., standby, cuing, or coaxing) or setup (positioning sliding board, moving foot rests, etc).

4   **Minimal Contact Assistance**—Subject performs 75% or more of transferring tasks.

3   **Moderate Assistance**—Performs 50% to 74% of transferring tasks.

2   **Maximal Assistance**—Performs 25% to 49% of transferring tasks.

1   **Total Assistance**—Performs less than 25% of transferring tasks.

13. **CAR TRANSFERS**   The activity includes approaching the car, managing the car door and lock, getting on or off the car seat and managing the seat belt. If a wheelchair is used for mobility, the activity includes loading and unloading the wheelchair.

7   **Complete Independence**—The patient is able to complete the activity without assistive devices, or aids, and within a reasonable amount of time.

6   **Modified Independence**—The patient requires an assistive device or aid, requires more than a reasonable amount of time or there is a safety risk in completing the activity.

5   **Supervision** (Modified Dependence)—The patient requires cueing, but no physical assistance, to complete the activity.

4   **Minimal Assistance** (Modified Dependence)—The patient performs at least 75% of the activity, requiring contact assistance with less than 25% of the activity.

3   **Moderate Assistance** (Modified Dependence)—The patient performs 50%-75% of the activity, requiring more than contact guard with 25%-50% of the activity.

2   **Maximal Assistance** (Complete Dependence)—The patient performs only 25%-50% of the activity and requires heavy assistance for 50%-75% of the activity.

1   **Total Assistance** (Complete Dependence)—The patient performs less than 25% of the activity and requires heavy assistance for more than 75% of the activity.

LOCOMOTION

14. **WALKING/WHEEL-CHAIR**   Includes walking, once in a standing position, or using a wheelchair, once in a seated position, indoors.

Check most frequent mode of locomotion. If both are about equal, check W *and* C.

(   ) W = *Walking*   (   ) C = wheelchair

No helper

7   **Complete Independence**—*Walks* with a minimum of *150* feet without assistive devices. Does not use a wheelchair. Performs safely.

6   **Modified Independence**—*Walks* with a minimum of *150* feet but uses a brace (orthosis) or prosthesis on leg, special adaptive shoes, cane, crutches, or walkerette; takes more than reasonable time or there are safety considerations.

If not walking, operates manual or electric wheelchair independently for a minimum of *150* feet; turns around; maneuvers the chair to a table, bed, toilet; negotiates at least a 3 percent grade; maneuvers on rugs and over door sills.

Continued.

TABLE 26-11—cont'd

Functional Assessment Measures (FAM)

14. WALKING/WHEEL-CHAIR—cont'd

Helper

5   **Supervision or Setup**—*If walking,* requires standby supervision, cuing or coaxing to goal minimum of *150* feet, *or* walks independently only short distances (a minimum of *50* feet). *If not walking,* requires standby supervision, cuing, or coaxing to go a minimum of *150* feet in wheelchair, *or* operates manual or electric wheelchair independently only short distances (a minimum of *50* feet).

4   **Minimal Contact Assistance**—Subject performs 75% or more of locomotion effort to go a minimum of *150* feet.

3   **Moderate Assistance**—Performs 50% to 74% of locomotion effort to go a minimum of *150* feet.

2   **Maximal Assistance**—Performs 25% to 49% of locomotion effort to go a minimum of *50* feet. Requires assistance of one person only.

1   **Total Assistance**—Performs less than 25% of effort, or requires assistance of two people, or does not walk or wheel a minimum of *50* feet.

Comment: There are several ways to estimate percent of effort. For instance, a disabled individual who can walk *unassisted* for 75 feet (that is 50% (½) of the 150 feet) then requires assistance for the remaining 75 feet, would be at level 4 if steadying was required, or level 3 if full support of one person was required the rest of the way.

15. STAIRS   Goes up and down 12 to 14 stairs (one flight) indoors.

No helper

7   **Complete Independence**—Goes up and down at least one flight of stairs without any type of handrail or support. Performs safely.

6   **Modified Independence**—Goes up and down at least one flight of stairs using side support or handrail, cane, or portable supports; takes more than reasonable time or there are safety considerations.

Helper

5   **Supervision or Setup**—Requires standby supervision, cuing, or coaxing to go up and down one flight.

4   **Minimal Contact Assistance**—Performs 75% or more of stair climbing effort.

3   **Moderate Assistance**—Performs 50% to 74% of stair climbing effort.

2   **Maximal Assistance**—Performs 25% to 49% of stair climbing effort. Requires the assistance of one person only.

1   **Total Assistance**—Performs less than 25% of the effort or requires the assistance of two people, or does not go up and down one flight of stairs, or is carried.

Comment: Note that 6 steps equals 25% (¼) of 12 steps up and down (24 total steps).

16. COMMUNITY   Ability to manage transportation including planning a route, time management, paying
    MOBILITY   fares, and anticipating access barriers (excluding car transfers).

No helper

7   **Complete Independence**—The patient independently uses public transportation (bus, van or taxi) or is able to drive a car.

6   **Modified Independence**—The patient uses adaptive devices to drive, must keep trips to a short distance due to needed rest periods; or there are safety considerations in using public transportation.

Helper

5   **Supervision** (Modified Dependence)—The patient requires cueing to use public transportation or ride in a car.

4   **Minimal Assistance** (Modified Dependence)—The patient is able to use public transportation or rides in a car, but needs assistance for up to 25% of the activity.

3   **Moderate Assistance** (Modified Dependence)—The patient uses public transportation or rides in a car, but needs assistance for 25%-50% of the activity.

TABLE 26-11—cont'd

Functional Assessment Measures (FAM)

16. COMMUNITY MOBILITY—cont'd

2   **Maximal Assistance** (Complete Dependence)—The patient may use public transportation or ride in a car but needs assistance for 50%-75% of the activity.

1   **Total Assistance** (Complete Dependence)—The patient is unable to use public transportation or ride in a car without heavy assistance for more than 75% of the activity.

Communication items

17. COMPREHENSION   Includes comprehension of either auditory or visual communication. This means understanding linguistic information by the spoken or written word.

Check and evaluate the most usual mode of comprehension. If both are about equally used, check A *and* V.

( ) A = Auditory   ( ) V = Visual

No helper

7   **Complete Independence**—Understands spoken or written directions (such as three-step commands) or conversation that is complex or abstract; comprehends either spoken or written native language.

6   **Modified Independence**—Understands spoken or written directions (such as three-step commands) or conversation that is complex or abstract with mild difficulty. May require a hearing or visual aid, other assistive device, or extra time to understand the information.

Helper

5   **Standby Prompting**—Understands conversation or reading material about every day situations more than 90% of the time. Requires prompting less than 10% of the time.

4   **Minimal Prompting**—Understands conversation or reading material about everyday situations 75% to 90% of the time.

3   **Moderate Prompting**—Understands conversation or reading material about everyday situations 50% to 74% of the time.

2   **Maximal Prompting**—Understands conversation or reading material about every day situations 25% to 49% of the time. Needs prompting more than half the time.

1   **Total Assistance**—Understands conversation or reading material about every day situations less than 25% of the time or does not understand or may not respond appropriately or consistently despite assistance.

18. EXPRESSION   Includes clear expression of verbal or nonverbal language. This means expressing linguistic information verbally or graphically with appropriate and accurate meaning and grammar.

Check and evaluate the most usual mode of expression. If both are about equally used, check V *and* N.

( ) V = Verbal   ( ) N = Nonverbal

No helper

7   **Complete Independence**—Expresses complex or abstract ideas intelligibly and fluently, verbally or nonverbally, including either signing or writing.

6   **Modified Independence**—Expresses complex or abstract ideas with mild difficulty. May require an augmentative communication device or system.

Helper

5   **Standby Prompting**—Expresses basic needs and ideas about everyday situations more than 90% of the time. Requires prompting less than 10% of the time.

4   **Minimal Prompting**—Expresses basic needs and ideas about everyday situations 75% to 90% of the time.

3   **Moderate Prompting**—Expresses basic needs and ideas about everyday situations 50% to 74% of the time.

2   **Maximal Prompting**—Expresses basic needs and ideas 25% to 49% of the time. Needs prompting more than half the time.

Continued.

TABLE 26-11—cont'd

Functional Assessment Measures (FAM)

18. EXPRESSION—cont'd

1   **Total Assistance**—Expresses basic needs and ideas less than 25% of the time or does not express basic needs appropriately or consistently despite assistance.

19. READING

7   **Complete Independence**—Completely able to read and understand complex, lengthy paragraphs (newspapers, books, etc).

6   **Modified Independence**—Able to read and understand complex sentences or short paragraphs. May demonstrate reduced speed or retention problems.

5   **Standby Prompting**—Able to read and understand short, simple sentences but shows increased difficulty with length or complexity.

4   **Minimal Prompting**—Able to recognize single words and familiar short phrases.

3   **Moderate Prompting**—Able to recognize letters, objects, forms, etc. Able to match words to pictures (under 50% accuracy).

2   **Maximal Prompting**—Able to match identical objects, forms, letters (under 50% accuracy) but may require cues.

1   **Total Assistance**—Unable to consistently match or recognize identical letters, objects, or forms.

20. WRITING

7   **Complete Independence**—Able to write with complete average accuracy in spelling, grammar, syntax, punctuation, and completeness.

6   **Modified Independence**—Able to accurately write sentences and form short paragraphs. May have occasional spelling or grammatical errors.

5   **Standby Prompting**—Able to write phrases or simple sentences. Evidences spelling, grammar, syntax errors.

4   **Minimal Prompting**—Able to write simple words, occasional phrases to express ideas. Spelling errors and reduced legibility are evident.

3   **Moderate Prompting**—Able to write name (cuing may be required) and some familiar words. Legibility is poor.

2   **Maximal Prompting**—Able to write some letters spontaneously. Able to trace or copy letters and numbers.

1   **Total Assistance**—Unable to copy letters or simple shapes.

21. SPEECH INTELLIGIBILITY

7   **Complete Independence**—Able to converse with well-articulated, well-modulated articulation and voice. No difficulty understanding what is being said.

6   **Modified Independence**—Evidence of minor sound distortions but generally adequate intelligibility. Speaking rate may be reduced.

5   **Standby Prompting**—Speech intelligibility is always reduced. Articulation is consistently distorted. May attempt self-corrections.

4   **Minimal Prompting**—Able to intelligibly produce single words and simple phrases. General conversation intelligibility.

3   **Moderate Prompting**—Can produce single syllable words with adequate intelligibility. Listener burden evident for sentences or longer verbalization.

2   **Maximal Prompting**—Can produce vowels, some consonants. Can imitate some single words but productions may require listener guessing.

1   **Total Assistance**—No intelligible speech.

Psychosocial adjustment items

22. SOCIAL INTERACTION   Includes skills related to getting along and participating with others in therapeutic and social situations. It represents how one deals with one's own needs and the needs of others.

7   **Complete Independence**—Interacts appropriately with staff, other patients, and family members (e.g., controls temper, accepts criticism, is aware that words and actions have an impact on others).

TABLE 26-11—cont'd

Functional Assessment Measures (FAM)

22. SOCIAL INTERACTION—cont'd

6   **Modified Independence**—Interacts with staff, other patients, and family members in structured situations or modified environments.

Helper

5   **Supervision**—Requires supervision (e.g., standby, cuing, or coaxing) only under stressful or unfamiliar conditions, but no more than 10% of the time.

4   **Minimal Direction**—Interacts appropriately 75% to 90% of the time.

3   **Moderate Direction**—Interacts appropriately 50% to 74% of the time.

2   **Maximal Direction**—Interacts appropriately 24% to 49% of the time. May need restraint occasionally.

1   **Total Assistance**—Interacts appropriately less than 25% of the time. May need restraint continuously.

Examples of socially inappropriate behaviors: temper tantrums, loud, foul, or abusive language, excessive laughing, crying, physical attack.

23. EMOTIONAL ADJUSTMENT   Includes frequency and severity of depression, anxiety, frustration, lability, unresponsiveness, agitation, interference with progress in therapies and/or home life, ability to cope with and take responsibility for emotional behavior.

7   **Complete Independence**—Patient rarely exhibits depression, anxiety, frustration, lability and/or agitation and is effectively able to control this behavior reflecting self responsibility and involvement in treatment and home life.

6   **Modified Independence**—Patient may exhibit occasional but minimal depression, anxiety, frustration, lability, and/or agitation. Coping skills are adequate to keep distress within manageable limits. Behavior does not interfere with progress in therapies and/or home life.

5   **Supervision**—Patient exhibits occasional and mild depression, anxiety, frustration, lability, and/or agitation. Patient has assumed responsibility for most of this behavior and is learning to cope with his/her condition. This behavior does not significantly interfere with progress in therapies.

4   **Minimal Direction**—Patient exhibits frequent and moderate depression, anxiety, frustration, lability, and/or agitation. Patient is assuming more responsibility for this behavior and it interferes with progress in therapies and/or home life less than 25% of the time.

3   **Moderate Direction**—Patient exhibits frequent and moderate depression, anxiety, frustration, lability, and/or agitation. Patient is beginning to assume responsibility for some behavior but this behavior still interferes with progress in therapies and/or home life 25% to 50% of the time.

2   **Maximal Direction**—Patient exhibits constant and severe depression, anxiety, frustration, lability, and/or agitation. Patient is rarely able to control this behavior and this behavior interferes with progress in therapies and/or home life 50 to 75% of the time.

1   **Total Assistance**—Patient exhibits constant and severe depression, anxiety, frustration, lability, unresponsiveness, and/or agitation. Patient is unaware and unable to control this behavior which continually interferes with progress in therapies and/or home life more than 75% of the time.

24. ADJUSTMENT TO LIMITATIONS   Includes denial/awareness, acceptance of limitations, willingness to learn new ways of functioning, compensating, taking appropriate safely precautions, and realistic expectations for long-term recovery.

7   **Complete Independence**—Patient demonstrates ability to compensate for limitations which are the result of the patient's disease or injury, exercises safe judgment in ADL's, and has realistic expectations for long-term recovery.

6   **Modified Independence**—Patient may have some denial of physical, emotional, or social limitations, but this denial does not interfere with progress in therapy and/or home life. Patient compensates for most of these limitations and has learned new ways of functioning. Patient may have some unrealistic expectations for long-term recovery. Patient exercises safe judgment in ADLs most of the time.

Continued.

TABLE 26-11—cont'd

Functional Assessment Measures (FAM)

24. ADJUSTMENTS TO LIMITATIONS—cont'd

5   **Supervision**—Patient's denial of physical, emotional, and social limitations interferes with progress in therapies less than 25% of the time. Patient is beginning to compensate for some of these limitations and is willing to learn new ways of functioning. Patient may still have unrealistic expectations for long-term recovery. Patient exercises safe judgment in ADLs 75% of the time.

4   **Minimal Direction**—Patient's denial of limitations interferes with progress in therapies and/or home life 25%-50% of the time. Patient resists compensating for limitations and learning new ways of functioning.

3   **Moderate Direction**—Patient may have some awareness of physical, emotional, or social limitations which are the result of the patient's disease or injury. Denial of limitations interferes with progress in therapies and/or home life 50% to 75% of the time.

2   **Maximal Direction**—Patient may have limited awareness of physical, emotional, or social limitations which are the result of the patient's injury or disease. Denial of limitations interferes with progress in therapies and/or home life 75% to 100% of the time.

1   **Total Assistance**—Patient has no awareness of physical, emotional, or social limitations which are the result of the patient's disease or injury. Patient's denial of these limitations continually interferes with progress in therapies and/or home life.

25. VOCATIONAL RE-ENTRY

The term employed as used in this scale represents a job in one or more of the following categories:
- in the regular workforce
- in a sheltered workshop
- as a student
- as a homemaker
- as a community service volunteer

Score to be assessed on the basis of a combination of the above if patient is involved in more than one activity.

7   **Complete Independence**—Patient is successfully employed full time.

6   **Modified Independence**—Patient is employed part time, with an adjusted workload, requires an assistive device, requires more than a reasonable time to do the job, or there are safety considerations.

5   **Supervision**—Patient is involved in a retraining program to develop necessary skills for employment (i.e., vocational retraining, O.T. for homemaking training) and requires supervision.

4   **Minimal Assistance**—Patient is involved in a retraining program and requires minimal assistance.

3   **Moderate Assistance**—Patient is involved in a retraining program and requires moderate assistance.

2   **Maximal Assistance**—Patient is able to participate in a retraining program on a limited basis, has made the necessary contacts but has not actively enrolled and requires maximal assistance with job-related tasks.

1   **Total Assistance**—Patient is unable to regain employment or develop necessary employment skills and requires total assistance.

Cognitive function items

26. PROBLEM SOLVING

Includes skills related to solving problems of daily living. This means making reasonable, safe, and prudent decisions regarding financial, social, and personal affairs and initiating, sequencing, and self-correcting tasks and activities to solve the problems.

No helper

7   **Complete Independence**—Consistently makes appropriate decisions, initiates and carries out a sequence of steps to solve problem until task is completed, and self-corrects if errors are made.

6   **Modified Independence**—Has some difficulty deciding, initiating, sequencing, or self-correcting in unfamiliar situations.

TABLE 26-11—cont'd

Functional Assessment Measures (FAM)

26. PROBLEM SOLVING—cont'd

Helper

5   **Supervision or Setup**—Requires supervision (e.g., cuing, or coaxing) to solve problems only under stressful or unfamiliar conditions, but no more than 10% of the time.

4   **Minimal Contact Assistance**—Solves problems 75% to 90% of the time.

3   **Moderate Assistance**—Solves problems 50% to 74% of the time.

2   **Maximal Assistance**—Solves problems 25% to 49% of the time. Needs direction more than half the time.

1   **Total Assistance**—Solves problems less than 25% of the time or does not effectively solve problems.

Examples: Adapting to a change in hospital schedule. Getting food into the house either by shopping or arranging to have food or meals brought in.

27. MEMORY   Includes skills related to awareness in performing daily activities in an institutional or community setting. It includes ability to store and retrieve information, particularly verbal and visual. A deficit in memory impairs learning as well as performance of tasks.

No helper

7   **Complete Independence**—Recognizes people frequently encountered and remembers daily routines; executes requests of others without need for repetition.

6   **Modified Independence**—Has some difficulty recognizing people, remembering daily routines and requests of others. May use self-initiated or environmental cues, prompts, or aids.

Helper

5   **Supervision**—Requires prompting (e.g., cuing, or coaxing) only under stressful or unfamiliar conditions, but no more than 10% of the time.

4   **Minimal Prompting**—Recognizes and remembers 75% to 90% of the time.

3   **Moderate Prompting**—Recognizes and remembers 50% to 74% of the time.

2   **Maximal Prompting**—Recognizes and remembers 25% to 49% of the time. Needs prompting more than half the time.

1   **Total Assistance**—Recognizes and remembers less than 25% of the time or does not effectively recognize and remember.

28. ORIENTATION   Includes consistent orientation to person, place, time, and situation.

7   **Complete Independence**—Completely oriented to person, place, time, and situation 100% of the time without cues.

6   **Modified Independence**—Patient may require more than a reasonable amount of time but without cues.

5   **Supervision**—Patient requires cuing less than 25% of the time.

4   **Minimal Prompting**—Patient requires minimal assistance and is oriented 75% of the time.

3   **Moderate Prompting**—Patient requires moderate assistance and is oriented 50% to 75% of the time.

2   **Maximal**—Patient requires maximal assistance and is oriented 25% to 50% of the time.

1   **Total Assistance**—Patient is consistently disoriented to person, place, time, and situation. Total assistance is required. Patient is oriented less than 25% of the time.

29. ATTENTION SPAN   Includes distractibility, level of alertness and responsiveness, ability to concentrate on a task, ability to follow directions, immediate recall as the structure, difficulty, and length of task varies.

7   **Complete Independence**—Patient is able to concentrate on complex tasks for 1 hour or more without structure. Patient can independently initiate and complete most tasks.

6   **Modified Independence**—Patient is able to concentrate on more complex tasks for longer periods of time (30 to 40 minutes), but still requires some structure. Patient may be distracted occasionally but can resume the task. Patient is able to immediately recall most past activities.

Continued.

TABLE 26-11—cont'd

Functional Assessment Measures (FAM)

29. ATTENTION SPAN—cont'd

5 **Supervision**—Patient exhibits differentiated and purposeful responses to environmental stimuli 75%-100% of the time. Selected attention to tasks may be impaired especially with difficult or unstructured tasks, but is now functional for common daily activities (20 to 30 minutes). Patient is mildly distractible and immediate recall is somewhat impaired.

4 **Minimal Direction**—Patient exhibits differentiated and purposeful responses to environmental stimuli 50%-75% of the time. Patient appears alert and is able to respond to simple commands fairly consistently. As the difficulty or length of the task increases, patient is more easily distracted and requires frequent structure or redirection back to the task. Patient is able to concentrate on simple tasks for 10 to 20 minutes. Patient's immediate recall of activities is limited.

3 **Moderate Direction**—Patient's attention span is easily aroused and patient exhibits differentiated and purposeful responses to environmental stimuli 25%-50% of the time. Patient is able to concentrate on simple tasks for less than 10 minutes. Patient is able to follow one- or two-step directions, but as the difficulty and length of the task increase, patient is more easily distracted and responses are delayed. Frequent cues may be necessary to maintain patient's attention.

2 **Maximal Direction**—Patient inconsistently exhibits differentiated and purposeful responses to environmental stimuli. Patient may be able to concentrate on simple tasks, follow one-step directions for short periods of time with delayed responses. Continuous cues may be necessary to maintain patient's attention for short periods of time (1 to 2 minutes).

1 **Total Assistance**—Patient exhibits nonpurposeful and undifferentiated responses to environmental stimuli. Patient is unable to concentrate on a task or follow directions, and is easily and continually distracted.

panded the FIM to a 29-item scale, titled the Functional Assessment Measures (FAM) (Table 26-11). The expanded tool uses the same rating scheme and requires 20 to 25 minutes for administration. The summary rating scale for the FAM is in Table 26-12. Comprehensive tools like the FIM and FAM are likely to be used in long term care rehabilitation programs.

SUMMARY

Use of an organized functional assessment is recommended for all clients whose daily activities may be affected by impairments or disabilities; the elderly and the handicapped are the more obvious examples of such groups. The literature has shown that health care providers often do superficial assessments of this assessment area and may not appreciate the client's capabilities or limitations. This lack of appreciation may cause inappropriate or insufficient treatment, lack of support, and neglect of problems that may be treatable.

The approaches and tools presented in this chapter have applicability across the range of settings and circumstances in which practitioners perform health assessments. Because the functional assessment is not a routine component of the health assessment, an approach standardized across practitioners does not exist for general populations. Therefore, the practitioner is advised to explore the assessment options and to select and use, as indicated, the most applicable and useful approaches and tools.

TABLE 26-12

Functional Assessment Worksheet

Rating Scale: 7 Complete Independence (Timely, safely)
6 Modified Independence (Extra time, device)
5 Supervision
4 Minimal Assist (subject 75% of task)
3 Moderate Assist (50%-74% of task)
2 Maximal Assist (25%-49% of task)
1 Total Assist (subject 25% of task)

Self-care items

1. Feeding   Adm _____ Goal _____ D/C _____ F/U _____
2. Grooming   Adm _____ Goal _____ D/C _____ F/U _____
3. Bathing Technique _____   Adm _____ Goal _____ D/C _____ F/U _____
4. Dressing Upper Body   Adm _____ Goal _____ D/C _____ F/U _____
5. Dressing Lower Body   Adm _____ Goal _____ D/C _____ F/U _____
6. Toileting   Adm _____ Goal _____ D/C _____ F/U _____
* 7. Swallowing   Adm _____ Goal _____ D/C _____ F/U _____

Sphincter control

8. Bladder Management   Adm _____ Goal _____ D/C _____ F/U _____
9. Bowel Management   Adm _____ Goal _____ D/C _____ F/U _____

Mobility items
Transfers technique _____

10. Bed, Chair, Wheelchair   Adm _____ Goal _____ D/C _____ F/U _____
11. Toilet   Adm _____ Goal _____ D/C _____ F/U _____
12. Tub or Shower   Adm _____ Goal _____ D/C _____ F/U _____
*13. Car Transfers   Adm _____ Goal _____ D/C _____ F/U _____

Locomotion

14. Walking/Wheelchair   Adm _____ Goal _____ D/C _____ F/U _____
15. Stairs   Adm _____ Goal _____ D/C _____ F/U _____
*16. Community Mobility   Adm _____ Goal _____ D/C _____ F/U _____

Communication items

17. Comprehension   Adm _____ Goal _____ D/C _____ F/U _____
18. Expression   Adm _____ Goal _____ D/C _____ F/U _____
*19. Reading   Adm _____ Goal _____ D/C _____ F/U _____
*20. Writing   Adm _____ Goal _____ D/C _____ F/U _____
*21. Speech Intelligibility   Adm _____ Goal _____ D/C _____ F/U _____

Psychosocial adjustment items

22. Social Interaction   Adm _____ Goal _____ D/C _____ F/U _____
*23. Emotional Adjustment   Adm _____ Goal _____ D/C _____ F/U _____
*24. Adjustment to Limitations   Adm _____ Goal _____ D/C _____ F/U _____
*25. Vocational Re-entry   D/C _____ F/U _____

Cognitive function

26. Problem Solving   Adm _____ Goal _____ D/C _____ F/U _____
27. Memory   Adm _____ Goal _____ D/C _____ F/U _____
*28. Orientation   Adm _____ Goal _____ D/C _____ F/U _____
*29. Attention   Adm _____ Goal _____ D/C _____ F/U _____

*Added to the FIM (Functional Independent Measure) tool. D/C = at discharge: F/U = at follow-up.

Nursing Diagnosis   *THE NEXT STEP*

Nursing diagnoses that could apply to functional assessment and alterations include, but are not limited to, the following ones.

ALTERED HEALTH MAINTENANCE Inability to identify, manage, and/or seek help to maintain health.

Defining Characteristics

- Demonstrated lack of knowledge regarding basic health practices
- Demonstrated lack of adaptive behaviors to internal or external changes
- Reported or observed inability to take responsibility for meeting basic health practices in any, or all, functional pattern areas
- Reported or observed lack of equipment, finances, or other resources for health maintenance
- History of lack of health-seeking behavior
- Expression of interest in improving health behaviors

Related Factors

- Alteration or lack of communication skills
- Inability to make deliberative and thoughtful judgments
- Perceptual-cognitive impairment
- Complete or partial lack of gross-fine motor skills
- Ineffective coping
- Disabling spiritual distress
- Lack of material resources
- Unachieved developmental tasks
- Dysfunctional grieving

HIGH RISK FOR INJURY The state in which an individual is at risk of injury as a result of environmental conditions interacting with the individual's adaptive and defensive resources.

Defining Characteristics (risk factors)

- Disorientation
- Impaired judgment
- Muscle weakness, paralysis, uncoordination, balancing difficulties, mobility impairment
- Sensory-perceptual deterioration, history of previous trauma, accidental injury
- Insufficient finances to purchase safety equipment or effect repairs
- Lack of safety precautions, safety education
- Excess alcohol-ingestion pattern
- Altered blood clotting factors
- Slippery, littered, or obstructed floors, stairs, walkways
- Unanchored rugs, unsteady or absent stair rails, unsteady ladders or chairs
- Bathtub without hand grips or anti-slip equipment
- Entering unlighted rooms, unanchored electric wires
- High beds
- Smoking in bed or near oxygen, inappropriate call-for-aid mechanisms for bed-resting client
- Pot handles facing toward front of stove
- Bathing in very hot water
- Potential igniting gas leaks
- Use of thin or worn potholders or mitts

IMPAIRED SWALLOWING The state in which an individual has decreased ability to voluntarily pass fluids and/or solids from the mouth to the stomach.

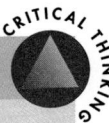

Nursing Diagnosis *THE NEXT STEP—cont'd*

Defining Characteristics

- Observed evidence of difficulty in swallowing: stasis of food in oral cavity (cheek pocket), coughing/choking when swallowing
- Evidence of aspiration

Related Factors

- Neurological impairment
- Decreased or absent gag reflex
- Decreased strength or excursion of muscles involved in mastication
- Perceptual impairment
- Facial paralysis
- Mechanical obstruction
- Edema
- Tracheotomy tube
- Tumor
- Fatigue
- Limited awareness

IMPAIRED SKIN INTEGRITY The state in which an individual's skin is adversely altered.

Defining Characteristics

- Disruption of skin surface
- Destruction of skin layers
- Invasion of body structures

Related Factors

- Altered circulation, metabolic state
- Hyperthermia or hypothermia
- Physical immobilization
- Humidity
- Alteration in turgor
- Altered nutritional status
- Altered sensation, immunological deficit
- Medication
- Developmental factors
- Psychogenic factors

TOTAL INCONTINENCE The state in which an individual experiences a continuous and unpredictable loss of urine.

Defining Characteristics

- Constant flow of urine at unpredictable times without distention or uninhibited bladder contractions/spasms
- Unsuccessful incontinence refractory treatments
- Nocturia
- Lack of perineal or bladder filling awareness
- Unawareness of incontinence

Related Factors

- Neuropathy
- Neurological dysfunction
- Independent contraction of detrusor reflex
- Trauma
- Disease
- Anatomic alterations

Continued.

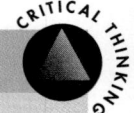

Nursing Diagnosis   *THE NEXT STEP—cont'd*

IMPAIRED PHYSICAL MOBILITY The state in which an individual experiences a limitation of ability for independent physical movement.

Defining Characteristics

- Inability to purposefully move within the physical environment (bed mobility, transfer, ambulation)
- Limited active joint range of motion
- Decreased muscle strength, control, and/or mass
- Impaired coordination
- Imposed restrictions of movement (mechanical or medical protocol restrictions)

Level I:
 Requires use of equipment or device
Level II:
 Requires help from another person(s): assistance, supervision, teaching
Level III:
 Requires help from another person(s) and equipment or device
Level IV:
 Is dependent and does not participate in movement

Related Factors

- Intolerance to activity
- Decreased strength and endurance
- Pain
- Discomfort
- Uncompensated perceptual-cognitive impairment
- Uncompensated neurological impairment
- Depression
- Severe anxiety

HIGH RISK FOR DISUSE SYNDROME The state in which an individual is at risk for deterioration of body systems as the result of prescribed or unavoidable inactivity.

Defining Characteristics (risk factors)

- Paralysis
- Mechanical immobilization
- Prescribed immobilization
- Severe pain
- Altered level of consciousness

TOTAL SELF-CARE DEFICIT The state in which one experiences an impaired ability to perform or complete bathing/hygiene, dressing/grooming, feeding, and toileting activities for oneself.

Defining Characteristics

- Observation or valid report of inability to eat, bathe, toilet, dress, groom self-independently

Level I:
 Requires use of equipment or device
Level II:
 Requires help from another person(s): assistance, supervision, teaching
Level III:
 Requires help from another person(s) and equipment or device
Level IV:
Is dependent and does not participate in self-care

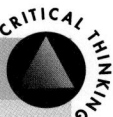

Nursing Diagnosis   *THE NEXT STEP—cont'd*

Related Factors

- Intolerance to activity
- Decreased strength and endurance
- Pain
- Discomfort
- Uncompensated perceptual-cognitive impairment
- Uncompensated neurological impairment
- Uncompensated musculoskeletal impairment
- Severe anxiety
- Depression

IMPAIRED HOME MAINTENANCE MANAGEMENT Inability to independently maintain a safe growth-promoting immediate environment.

Defining Characteristics

- Household members describe outstanding debts or financial crises
- Unwashed or unavailable cooking equipment, clothes, or linen
- Overtaxed family members (e.g., exhausted, anxious family members)
- Repeated hygienic disorders, infestations, or infections
- Household members request assistance with home maintenance
- Disorderly surroundings
- Accumulation of dirt, food wastes, or hygienic wastes
- Offensive odors
- Inappropriate household temperature
- Lack of necessary equipment or aids
- Presence of vermin or rodents

Related Factors

- Individual/family member disease or injury
- Insufficient family organization/planning
- Insufficient finances
- Unfamiliarity with neighborhood resources
- Impaired cognitive or emotional functioning
- Knowledge deficit
- Lack of role modeling
- Inadequate support system

CHRONIC PAIN The state in which an individual experiences pain that continues for more than 6 months.

Defining Characteristics

- Verbal report or observed evidence of pain experienced for more than 6 months
- Facial masks (of pain)
- Guarded movement
- Fear of reinjury
- Physical and social withdrawal
- Altered ability to continue previous activities
- Anorexia
- Weight changes
- Changes in sleep pattern

Related Factors

- Chronic physical/psychosocial disability

Continued.

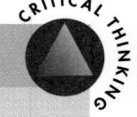

Nursing Diagnosis *THE NEXT STEP—cont'd*

SENSORY-PERCEPTUAL ALTERATIONS The state in which an individual experiences a change in the amount or patterning of incoming stimuli accompanied by a diminished, exaggerated, distorted, or impaired response to such stimuli.

Defining Characteristics

- Alert with periodic disorientation, general confusion, or nocturnal confusion
- Hallucinations
- Apathy
- Auditory, visual, reality-orienting, or time-orienting input reduced or absent
- Limited proprioceptive input
- Presence of uncompensated visual or hearing deficits

Related Factors

- Isolation
- Therapeutic environment restriction
- Socially restricted environment
- Uncompensated visual or hearing deficit
- Impaired communication

ALTERED THOUGHT PROCESSES The state in which an individual experiences a disruption in cognitive operations and activities.

Defining Characteristics

- Impaired attention span, distractibility
- Inappropriate behavior; nonreality-based thinking
- Impaired recall ability
- Impaired ability to grasp ideas (conceptualize) or order ideas (reason and reflection)
- Impaired perception, judgment, decision making
- Increased self-concern (egocentricity)
- Hypovigilance or hypervigilance

Related Factors

- Developmental lag
- Sensory overload (environmental complexity)

POWERLESSNESS Perception that one's own action will not significantly affect an outcome; a perceived lack of control over a current situation or immediate happening.

Defining Characteristics

Severe
- Verbalization of having no control (situation, outcome, or self-care)
- Depression over physical deterioration (occurring despite compliance with regimes)
- Apathy

Moderate
- Nonparticipation in care of decision making when opportunities provided
- Expressed dissatisfaction or frustration over inability to perform previous tasks/activities
- Expressed doubt regarding role performance
- Passivity
- Does not monitor progress, seek information regarding care, or defend self-care practices when challenged
- Dependence on others that may result in irritability, resentment, anger, and guilt
- Reluctance to express true feelings, fearing alienation from caregivers

Low Passivity
- Expressed uncertainty about fluctuating energy levels

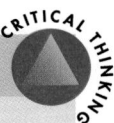

Nursing Diagnosis   *THE NEXT STEP—cont'd*

Related Factors

- Illness-related regime
- Health care environment
- Interpersonal interaction
- Life-style of helplessness

BODY IMAGE DISTURBANCE Disruption in the way one perceives one's body image.

Defining Characteristics

- Verbalized actual or perceived change in structure and/or function of body or body part
- Verbalized change in life-style because of negative feelings or perception of body
- Verbalized fear of rejection or reaction by others
- Repeated verbalizations focusing on past strength, function, or appearance
- Verbalized negative feelings about body (dirty, big, small, unsightly)
- Verbalized feelings of helplessness, hopelessness, powerlessness in relation to body
- Preoccupation with change in body or loss of part
- Personalization of part, or loss, by name
- Depersonalization of part or loss by impersonal pronoun
- Extension of body boundary to incorporate environmental objects (e.g., machines, oxygen, respirator)
- Refusal to verify actual change in body or body part
- Guilt, shame
- Emphasis on remaining strengths or heightened achievement
- Repeated expressions of negative feeling about loss of body fluids, addition of body fluids or machines
- Change in ability to estimate spatial relationship of body to environment
- Trauma to nonfunctioning part (intentional/nonintentional)
- Change in social involvement or social relationships
- Hiding or overexposing body part
- Not touching body part
- Not looking at body part
- Missing body part
- Actual change in structure and/or function of body or body part

Related Factors

- Nonintervention of change
- Perceived developmental imperfections

ALTERED ROLE PERFORMANCE Disruption in the way one perceives one's role performance.

Defining Characteristics (risk factors)

- Denial of role
- Conflict in roles
- Change in self-perception of role
- Change in others' perception of role
- Change in physical capacity to resume role
- Lack of knowledge of role
- Change in usual patterns of responsibilities

SOCIAL ISOLATION Aloneness experienced by an individual and perceived as imposed by others and as a negative or threatened state.

Continued.

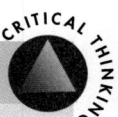

Nursing Diagnosis   *THE NEXT STEP—cont'd*

Defining Characteristics

- Apathy
- Verbalization of isolation from others
- Low contact with peers
- Absent or limited contact with community
- Lack of contact with or absence of significant others
- Seclusion

Related Factors

- Impaired mobility
- Therapeutic isolation
- Sociocultural dissonance
- Insufficient community resources
- Body image disturbance
- Fear

IMPAIRED SOCIAL INTERACTION The state in which an individual participates in an insufficient or excessive quantity or ineffective quality of social exchange.

Defining Characteristics

- Verbalized or observed discomfort in social situations
- Verbalized or observed inability to receive or communicate a satisfying sense of belonging, caring, interest, or shared history
- Observed use of unsuccessful social interaction behaviors
- Dysfunctional interaction with peers, family, and/or others
- Family report of change of style or patterns of interaction

Related Factors

- Knowledge/skill deficit
- Communication barriers
- Self-concept disturbance
- Absence of available significant others/peers
- Limited physical mobility
- Therapeutic isolation
- Sociocultural dissonance
- Environmental barriers
- Altered thought processes

IMPAIRED VERBAL COMMUNICATION The state in which an individual experiences a decreased or absent ability to use or understand language in human interaction.

Defining Characteristics

- Unable to speak dominant language
- Speaks or verbalizes with difficulty
- Does not, or cannot, speak
- Stuttering
- Slurring
- Difficulty forming words or sentences
- Difficulty expressing thought verbally
- Inappropriate verbalization
- Dyspnea
- Disorientation

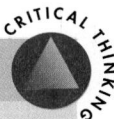

Nursing Diagnosis   *THE NEXT STEP—cont'd*

Related Factors

- Decrease in circulation to brain
- Anatomical defects
- Cultural difference
- Physical barrier
- Psychological barrier

Clinical Application

Mr. K., a 59-year-old plumber who owns his own business, has just been transferred from the neurologic intensive care unit onto the medical floor to stabilize his condition before transfer to the rehabilitation center. It is 6 days after a cerebrovascular accident and he has a diagnosis of left hemiplegia and aphasia. Because of Mr. K.'s speech dysfunction, his history was provided by his wife. Mr. K. was admitted 6 days ago unconscious after he did not awaken to the alarm clock. He was noted to respond only to deep pain; his left arm and leg were limp. Two days later, he regained consciousness, was unable to move his left side arm or leg, was unable to speak clearly or swallow or perform any activities of daily living (ADLs).

SUBJECTIVE DATA: Wife states patient unable to:
Move left arm or leg
Speak clearly
Swallow
Do own ADLs

OBJECTIVE DATA:
Mental status: Patient lying in bed, body slumps slightly to the left side, appears alert but has difficulty maintaining eye contact. Speech slow, requires much effort and garbled. Hard to determine if appropriate. Seems to understand all language spoken to him. Follows requests slowly but appropriately within limits of motor weakness.
Cranial nerves:
I not tested.
II acuity normal, fields by confrontaion—left homonymous hemianopia, fundi normal.
III, IV, VI EOMs intact, slight left side ptosis, no nystagmus, pupil equal round react to light and accommodation (PERRLA).
V sensation intact to pinprick and light touch. Jaw strength weak on left.
VII flat nasolabial fold on left, motor weakness on left lower face. Unable to wrinkle forehead bilaterally, unable to smile on left side.
VIII hearing intact.
IX, X no swallowing or gag reflex present, uvula rises slightly to right on phonation.
XI shoulder shrug, head movement weaker on left.
XII tongue protrudes slightly to right, no tremors.
Cerebellar: Unable to move left hand or leg, unable to support weight. Spasticity in left arm and leg. Unable to stand and walk unassisted. Unable to perform finger-to-nose or heel-to-shin on left side. Right side intact but slow.
Sensory: Pinprick and light touch present but decreased on left arm and leg. Vibration intact. Position sense decreased on left, intact on right. Stereognosis intact.
DTRs: Right side intact 1 + , left side 0, Babinski present left side. Plantar reflex absent left side, intact on right side.

NURSING DIAGNOSES

Impaired swallowing related to neuromuscular impairment (absent gag reflex).

Defining Characteristics

- Observed evidence of difficulty swallowing
- Observed coughing/choking when swallowing
- Assessed no gag or swallowing ability

Continued.

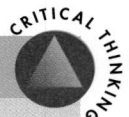

Nursing Diagnosis   *THE NEXT STEP—cont'd*

Altered nutrition: less than body requirement related to muscle weakness (mastication and swallowing).

Defining Characteristics

- Inability to swallow
- No gag reflex
- Observed inadequate food intake

High risk for impaired skin integrity related prolonged immobility.

Defining Characteristics

- Physical immobility—cannot move left side
- Incontinence of both bladder and bowel—excretion on skin

Bowel incontinence related to cognitive/perceptual impairment.

Defining Characteristics

- Involuntary passage of stool
- Inability to communicate need (aphasia)

Total incontinence related to cognitive/perceptual impairment.

Defining Characteristics

- Lack of perineal or bladder filling awareness
- Unaware of incontinence
- Inability to communicate need (aphasia)

Impaired physical mobility related to neuromuscular impairment.

Defining Characteristics

- Inability to purposefully move within the physical environment
- Decreased muscle strength
- Impaired coordination
- Level IV—is dependent and at this time does not participate in movement

Total self-care deficit related to neuromuscular impairment.

Defining Characteristics

- Inability to wash body or body parts
- Inability to obtain or get to water source
- Inability to regulate temperature or flow of water
- Impaired ability to put on or take off necessary items of clothing
- Impaired ability to obtain or replace articles of clothes, fasten clothing, and maintain appearance at a satisfactory level
- Level IV—is dependent and does not participate in self-care at this time

Sensory-perceptual alterations (kinesthetic) related to neuromuscular impairment.

Defining Characteristics

- Measured change in sensory acuity
- Altered communication patterns
- Inability to sit or stand
- Motor incoordination

Unilateral neglect related to neuromuscular impairment, inability to move left side.

Defining Characteristics

- Consistent inattention to stimuli on affected side
- Lack of positioning and/or safety precautions regarding left side
- Does not look toward affected side

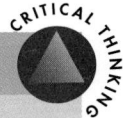

Nursing Diagnosis   *THE NEXT STEP—cont'd*

Body image disturbance related to nonintegration to change in body function and limitations.

Defining Characteristics
- Verbalized fear of rejection or reaction by others
- Verbalized feelings of powerlessness in relation to body
- Depersonalization of part or loss by impersonal pronoun
- Refusal to verify actual change in body
- Change in ability to estimate spatial relationship of body to environment

Impaired verbal communication related to neuromuscular impairment.

Defining Characteristics
- Speaks or verbalizes with difficulty
- Difficulty forming words
- Difficulty expressing thoughts verbally

Impaired social interaction related to communication barrier and limited physical mobility.

Defining Characteristics
- Observed discomfort in social situations
- Observed inability to communicate a satisfactory sense of belonging

GLOSSARY

atrophy Wasting; decrease in the size of a cell, tissue, organ, or body part.

contractures An abnormal, usually permanent condition of a joint, characterized by flexion and fixation and caused by atrophy and shortening of muscle fibers or loss of the normal elasticity of the skin.

hypotonia Decrease in body tonus.

ischial spines The two relatively sharp bony projections into the pelvic outlet from the ischial bones that form the lower border of the pelvis.

trochanteric Pertaining to the two bony projections on the proximal end of the femur that serve for the attachment of various muscles.

BIBLIOGRAPHY

Boies AH: Activities of daily living, *Home Healthcare Nurse* 5:40-41, 1987.

Bower FN, Patterson J: A theory-based nursing assessment of the aged, *Top Clin Nurs* 8:22-32, 1984.

Brorsson B, Asberg KH: Katz index of independence in ADL: reliability and validity in short-term care, *Scand J Rehabil Med* 16:125-132, 1984.

Buchanan B: Functional assessment: measurement with the Barthel Index and PULSES profile, *Home Healthcare Nurse* 4:11-17, 1986.

Dittmar SS: *Rehabilitation nursing: process and application*, St. Louis, 1989, Mosby–Year Book.

Forer SK: *Revised functional status rating instrument*, Glendale, Calif: 1981, Rehabilitation Institute, Glendale Adventist Medical Center.

Fortinsky RH, Granger CV, Seltzer GB: The use of functional assessment in understanding home care needs, *Med Care* 19:489-497, 1981.

Fuhrer MJ, editor: *Rehabilitation outcomes: analysis and measurement*, Baltimore, 1987, Brookes.

Golden RR, Teresi JA, Gurland BJ: Development of indicator scales for the comprehensive assessment and referral evaluation (CARE) interview schedule, *J Gerontol* 39:138-146, 1984.

Goodgold J: *Rehabilitation medicine*, St. Louis, 1988, Mosby–Year Book.

Gordon M: *Manual of nursing diagnosis: 1993-1994*, St. Louis, 1993, Mosby–Year Book.

Gordon M: *Nursing diagnosis: process and application*, ed 2, New York, 1987, McGraw Hill.

Granger CV: Health accounting—functional assessment of the long-term patient. In Kottke FJ, Stillwell GK, Lehmann JF, editors: *Krusen's handbook of physical medicine and rehabilitation*, ed 3, Philadelphia, 1982, WB Saunders.

Granger CV, Albrecht GL, Hamilton BB: Outcome of comprehensive medical rehabilitation: measurement by PULSES profile and the Barthel Index, *Arch Phys Med Rehabil* 60:145-154, 1979.

Granger CV, Gresham G, editors: *Functional assessment in rehabilitation medicine*, Baltimore, 1984, Williams & Wilkins.

Granger CV and others: Advances in functional assessment for medical rehabilitation, *Topics Clin Rehabil* 1:59-74, 1986.

Granger CV, Seltzer GB, Fishbein CF: *Primary care of the functionally disabled: assessment and management*, Philadelphia, 1987, JB Lippincott.

Gulick EE: The self-assessment of health among the chronically ill, *Top Clin Nurs* 8:74-82, 1986.

Gurland B and others: The comprehensive assessment and referral evaluation (CARE)—rationale, development and reliability, *Int J Aging Human Develop* 8:9-42, 1977.

Gurland B and others: The SHORT-CARE: an efficient instrument for the assessment of depression, dementia, and disability, *J Gerontol* 39:166-169, 1984.

Hamilton GG and others: A uniform national data system for medical rehabilitation. In Fuhrer MJ, editor: *Rehabilitation outcomes: analysis and measurement*, Baltimore, 1987, Brookes, pp. 137-147.

Hertanu JS and others: Stroke rehabilitation: correlation and prognostic value of computerized tomography and sequential functional assessments, *Arch Phys Med Rehabil* 65:505-508, 1984.

Jacelon CS: The Barthel index and other indices of functional ability, *Rehab Nurs* 11:9-11, 1986.

Jette AM: State of the art in functional status assessment. In Rothstein JM: *Measurement in physical therapy*, New York, 1985, Churchill Livingstone, pp. 137-168.

Katz S, Akpom CA: Index of ADL, *Med Care* 14:116-118, 1976.

Katz S and others: Studies of illness in the aged. The index of ADL: a standardized measure of biological and psychosocial function, *JAMA* 185:914-919, 1963.

Keith RA: Functional assessment measures in medical rehabilitation: current status, *Arch Phys Med Rehabil* 65:74-78, 1984.

Keith RA and others: The functional independence measure: a new tool for rehabilitation. In Eisenberg MG, Grzesiak RC, editors: *Advances in clinical rehabilitation*, New York, 1987, Spring, pp. 6-18.

Lawton MP: Assessing the competence of older people. In Kent D, Kastenbaum R, Sherwood S, editors: *Research, planning and action for the elderly*, New York, 1972, Behavioral Publications.

Lawton MP, Brody EM: Assessment of older people: self-maintaining and instrumental activities of daily living, *Gerontologist* 9:180, 1969.

Linn MW, Linn BS: The rapid disability rating scale-2, *J Am Geriatr Soc* 30:378-382, 1982.

Mahoney FI, Barthel DW: Functional evaluation: the Barthel index, *Maryland State Med J* 14:61, 1965.

McDowell I, Newell C: *Measuring health: a guide to rating scales and questionnaires*, New York, 1987, Oxford University Press.

McGinnis GE and others: Program evaluation of physical medicine and rehabilitation departments using self-report Barthel, *Arch Phys Med Rehabil* 67:123-125, 1986.

Mosby's medical, nursing, and allied health dictionary, ed 3, St. Louis, 1990, Mosby—Year Book.

Moskowitz E, McCann CB: Classification of disability in the chronically ill and aging, *J Chronic Dis* 5:342-346, 1957.

Moskowitz E: PULSES Profile in retrospect, *Arch Phys Rehabil* 66:647-648, 1985.

Nagi S: *Disability, concepts and prevalence*. Unpublished paper presented at the First Mary Switzer Memorial Seminar, Cleveland, Ohio, May 1975.

Ninos M, Makohon R: Functional assessment of the patient, *Geriatric Nurs* 6:139-142, 1985.

Nolan BS: Functional evaluation of the elderly in guardianship proceedings, *Law, Medicine and Healthcare* 12:210-218, 1984.

O'Toole DM, Goldberg RT, Ryan B: Functional changes in vascular amputee patients: evaluation by Barthel, PULSES profile and ESCROW scale, *Arch Phys Med Rehabil* 66:508-511, 1985.

Pfeffer RI, Kurosaki TT, Chance JM and others: Index in older adults: reliability, validity, and measurement of change over time, *Am J Epidemiol* 120:922-935, 1984.

Pinholt EM and others: Functional assessment of the elderly: a comparison of standard instruments with clinical judgment, *Arch Int Med* 147:484-488, 1987.

Rothstein JM: *Measurement in physical therapy*, New York, 1985, Churchill Livingstone.

Rubenstein LZ and others: Systematic biases in functional status assessment of elderly adults: effects of different data sources, *J Gerontol* 39:686-691, 1984.

Sheikh K and others: Repeatability and validity of a modified Activities of Daily Living (ADL) index in studies of chronic disability, *Int Rehab Med* 1:51, 1979.

Sherwood MJ, and others: *Determining nursing diagnosis through assessment*, Baltimore, 1988, Williams & Wilkins.

Spiegel JS, Hirshfield MS, Spiegel TM: Evaluation of self-care activities: comparison of a self-reported questionnaire with an occupational therapist interview, *Br J Rheumatol* 24:357-361, 1985.

Teresi JA, Golden RR, Gurland BJ: Concurrent and predictive validity of indicator scales developed for the comprehensive assessment and referral evaluation interview schedule, *J Gerontol* 39:158-165, 1984.

Teresi JA and others: Construct validity of indicator scales developed from the comprehensive assessment and referral evaluation interview schedule, *J Gerontol* 39:147-157, 1984.

U.S. Preventive Services Task Force. *Guide to clinical preventive services: an assessment of the effectiveness of 169 interventions*, Baltimore, 1989, Williams & Wilkins.

Wood P: *Classification of impairments and handicaps*, Geneva, 1975, World Health Organization.

World Health Organization: *International classification of impairments, disabilities, and handicaps*, Geneva, 1980, The Organization.

*U*nit V, The Complete Health
and Physical Assessment, contains
two summative and linking
chapters. Chapter 27, The Complete
Health and Physical Assessment:
Step by Step, provides a detailed
outline for an integrated physical
examination. This chapter is
designed to assist the beginning
practitioner to "pull it all together"
in an efficient and effective manner.
Chapter 28, Clinical Decision
Making for Determining Health
Status, is designed to link the
knowledges and skills of health
assessment to the next steps in the
nursing and care processes—
conclusions about health status, and
decision making regarding care
planning interventions.

The Complete Health and Physical Assessment

The Complete Health and Physical Assessment: Step by Step

PERFORMANCE OF INTEGRATED PHYSICAL EXAMINATION

This chapter includes three sections: description of and outline for the performance of a comprehensive, integrated physical examination, description of the documenting of the comprehensive physical examination, and a worksheet for documenting a physical examination.

After practicing and acquiring proficiency in the performance of regional examinations, it is important to develop a systematic pattern for performing an integrated physical examination. In practice, practitioners perform both regional examinations, such as in acute care settings, as well as comprehensive multisystem examinations, such as in health maintenance programs.

In developing a personal routine for a complete examination, consider factors of efficiency and client comfort. The examiner who performs procedures systematically and efficiently conserves time and is less likely to forget a procedure or a part of the body than is the examiner who performs the examination haphazardly.

Clients who are ill or debilitated lose energy quickly. A system of examination involving the fewest number

PREPARATION

Preparation for the Examination

Equipment

The equipment needed for a complete physical examination include the following (the purposes and uses of all the listed items have been explained in the preceding chapters):

Cotton balls
Cotton-tipped swabs or applicator sticks
Flashlights—both large and penlight
Gauze squares
Glass of water
Gloves—latex, disposable examination
Marking pencil or pen
Materials to test pain and light touch sensation (pin, cotton ball)
Measuring tape
Nasal speculum (optional)
Odoriferous substances for cranial nerve examination
Ophthalmoscope
Otoscope
Printed material for visual acuity and comprehension examination
Reflex (percussion) hammer
Ruler
Scale
Snellen eye chart
Sphygmomanometer
Stethoscope with diaphragm and bell heads
Substances for taste sensation evaluation
Thermometer
Tongue blades
Tuning forks (one 500-1000 cycles per second [CPS] for testing auditory function; and one 100-400 CPS for testing vibratory sense)

Watch that records seconds
If a pelvic or a rectal examination is to be done, add the following equipment and supplies:
Lubricant (water-soluble)
Materials to prepare vaginal secretions or specimens for laboratory examination
Materials to examine fecal material for occult blood
Mirror
Vaginal speculums

Client and the environment

The physical examination should occur in a comfortable room that provides privacy, adequate lighting, and a reasonable amount of space for client and examiner movement. The recommended equipment for an examination room includes the following:

Desk with two chairs
Examination lamp
Examining table
Scale
Sink
Stand or counter to hold supplies
Stool

In preparation for the examination, the following procedures are recommended:

Check for availability of needed materials within easy reach
Review examination procedure with client
Have client empty bladder
Have client undress and put on gown

---

of client position changes enhances acceptability and decreases the number of examinations and portions of examinations deferred because of client intolerance.

The manner in which the examiner conducts the physical examination can enhance or compromise rapport developed during the history-taking interview. A disorganized examiner who leaves the room to obtain missing equipment, who changes positions several times in a short time period, or who has the client change positions frequently may lose the client's confidence.

The outline presented in the section of this chapter entitled "Technique for examination" is a suggested format for performing the physical examination. It is intended as a guide for the beginning practitioner to use in practice sessions. In actual client care situations, this outline may require adapting because of the client's age or disability, examination protocols and priorities of the care agency, or examiner preference. The suggested for-

mat is designed to avoid excessive client and examiner movement. The approach integrates body systems into the examination of body regions.

Technique for Examination

The client enters the examination room, the examiner and *client* greet each other, and the examiner observes the client (Figure 27-1).

Inspect general appearance
1. Skin color
2. Consistency of general appearance with age
3. General state of nutrition
4. Hygiene
5. Obvious physical deformities, limitations, use of assistive devices

Inspect stature and movement
1. Symmetry
2. Posture

3. Body build
4. Gait
5. Mobility

Inspect demeanor

1. Facial expression
2. Composure
3. Speech
4. Orientation and mental status
5. Disposition
6. Eye contact

Take the health history

At this point in a comprehensive assessment, the examiner takes the health history (Figure 27-2). The comprehensive health history is discussed in Chapter 2. The student is referred to that chapter for review as needed. Allow the client to remain in street clothes for the history taking interview. Just before starting the physical examination, have the client change from street clothes into the examination gown.

Take measurements

1. Measure weight
2. Measure height
3. Measure temperature
4. Palpate pulses (radial and brachial)
5. Measure blood pressure (both arms)
6. Measure respiratory rate

Client is sitting on the bed or examination table. Examiner is facing client (Figure 27-3).

Inspect and palpate upper extremities

1. Examine skin (color, temperature, vascularity, lesions, hydration, turgor, texture, edema, masses), muscle mass, and skeletal configuration
2. Examine nails (color and condition)

Examine head p273

1. Inspect configuration of skull
2. Inspect condition of skin, scalp, and hair (masses, parasites, lesions)
3. Inspect hair distribution
4. Inspect face—appearance, expression, symmetry of structure and features, movements
5. Inspect head—size, shape, symmetry, extra movements
6. Inspect movements of head and face
7. Palpate skull, hair, and face (deformities, tenderness, lesions, texture, distribution, quantity)
8. Palpate and percuss paranasal sinus areas (tenderness)
9. Palpate temporomandibular joint (tenderness, crepitations)

Examine eyes

1. Inspect eyebrows, eyelids, eyelashes, conjunctiva, cornea, sclera, iris, pupil, and palpebral fissures
2. Measure visual acuity (cranial nerve [CN] II)
3. Assess visual fields (CN II)
4. Determine alignment of eyes (perform cover test and corneal light reflex)

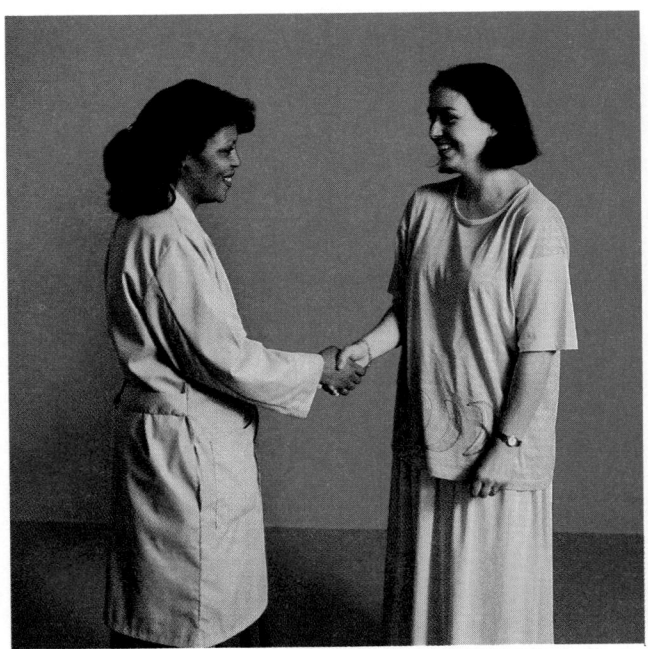

FIGURE 27-1 Examiner greeting the client.

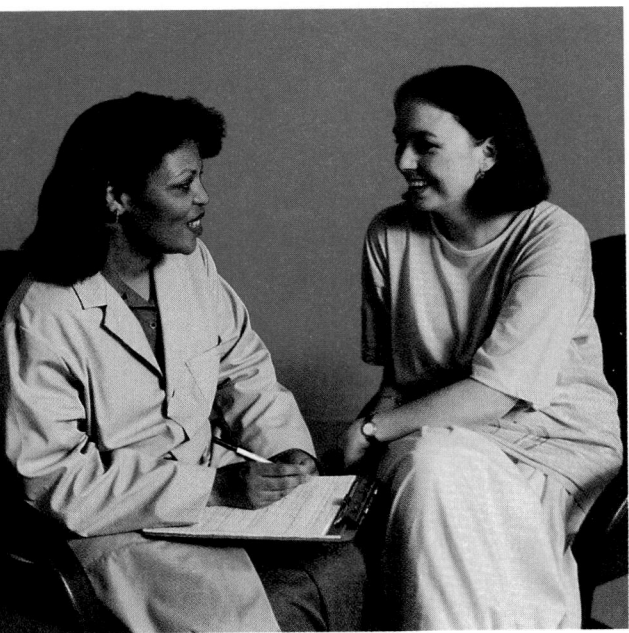

FIGURE 27-2 Interview for the health history.

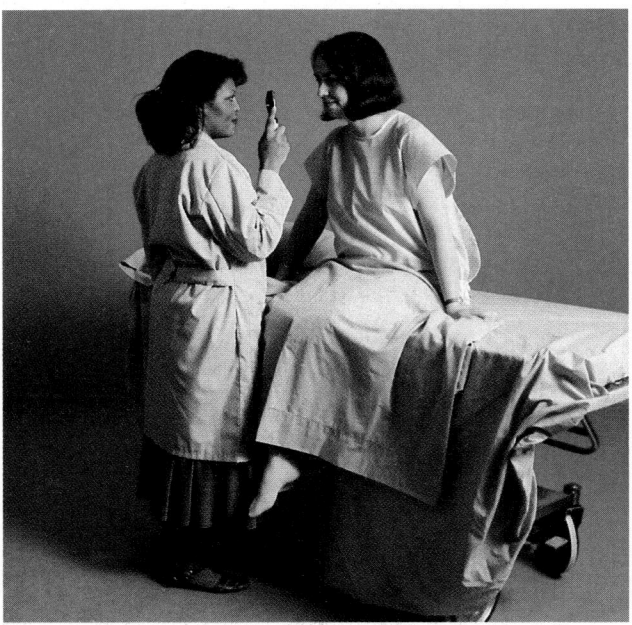

FIGURE 27-3 Client gowned and seated; examiner facing client.

5. Test extraocular movements (CN III, CN IV, CN VI)
6. Palpate lacrimal sac
7. Test pupillary responses (light and accommodation) (CN III)
8. Perform ophthalmoscopic examination of lens, media, and retina (CN II)
9. Test corneal reflex (CN V, CN VII)

Examine ears
1. Inspect auricle (masses, lesions, tenderness)
2. Palpate auricle (masses, lesions, tenderness)
3. Perform otoscopic examination (Inspect canals and tympanic membranes.)
4. Determine auditory acuity (CN VIII)
5. Perform Weber and Rinne tests

Examine nose
1. Inspect alignment of septum and surface characteristics
2. Determine patency of each nostril
3. Test for olfaction (CN I)
4. Inspect mucosa, septum, and turbinates (inflammation, allergy, lesions, epistaxis)

Examine mouth and pharynx
1. Inspect lips, total buccal mucosa, teeth, gums, tongue, sublingual area, roof of mouth, tonsillar area, and pharynx (as appropriate, for presence, condition, color, symmetry, surface characteristics, movement)
2. Note mouth odor

3. Test glossopharyngeal nerve (CN IX) and vagus nerve (CN X) ("ah" and gag reflex)
4. Test hypoglossal nerve (CN XII) (tongue movement)
5. Test taste (CN VII)

Complete examination of cranial nerves.
1. Test trigeminal nerve (CN V) (jaw clenching, lateral jaw movements, pain, and light touch to face)
2. Test facial nerve (CN VII) (Client smiles, raises eyebrows, shows teeth, puffs cheeks, keeps eyes closed against resistance.)
3. Test spinal accessory nerve (CN XI) (trapezius and sternocleidomastoid muscles)

Complete examination of the head and examine neck
1. Inspect range of motion of the head and neck
2. Palpate nodes (preauricular, posterior auricular, mastoid, occipital, tonsillar, parotid, submaxillary, submandibular, submental, anterior cervical, posterior cervical, supraclavicular, and infraclavicular nodes)
3. Palpate carotid arteries
4. Palpate for position of trachea
5. Palpate thyroid gland
6. Auscultate carotid arteries and thyroid gland for bruits

Client is sitting on the bed or examining table, total chest uncovered if male, breasts covered if female (Figure 27-4). Examiner is standing behind client.

Examine back
1. Inspect spine
2. Palpate spine
3. Inspect skin and thoracic configuration
4. Palpate muscles and bones
5. Palpate costovertebral area, asking client about tenderness

Examine lungs (apices and lateral and posterior areas). NOTE: Apical, posterior, and lateral lung regions can usually be examined from a position behind client
1. Inspect respiration (depth, rhythm, pattern) and posterior and lateral thorax
2. Palpate for thoracic expansion and tactile fremitus
3. Percuss systematically
4. Determine diaphragmatic excursion
5. Auscultate systematically (breath sounds and adventitious sounds).
6. Auscultate for vocal resonance

Client is sitting on the bed or examining table, uncovered to the waist. Examiner is facing client (Figure 27-5)

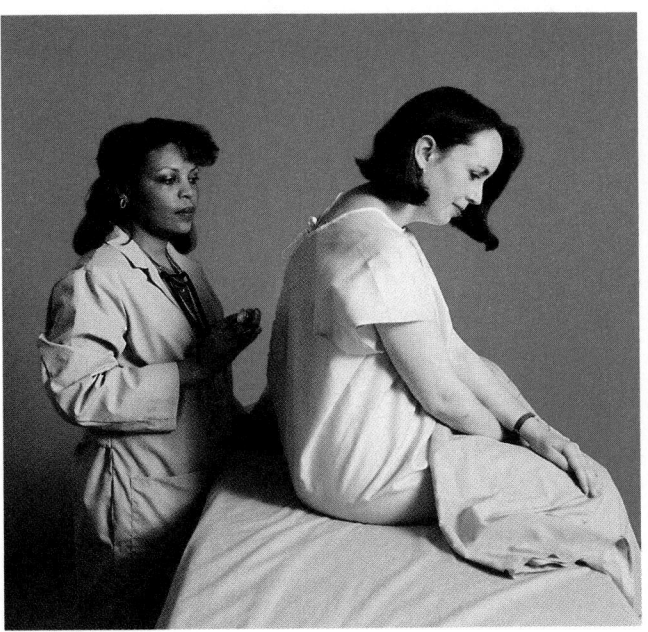

FIGURE 27-4 Client seated; examiner behind client.

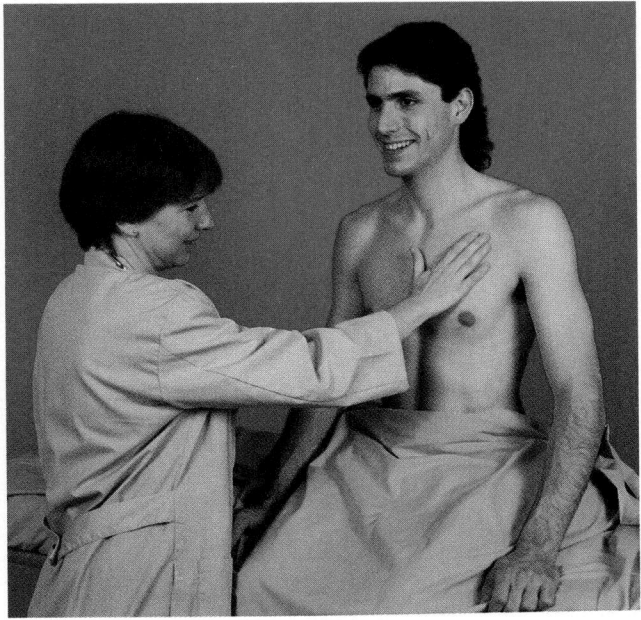

FIGURE 27-5 Client seated and stripped to waist; examiner facing client.

Examine lungs (anterior areas)
1. Inspect configuration and skin
2. Palpate for tactile fremitus
3. Percuss systematically
4. Auscultate lungs systematically
5. Auscultate for vocal resonance

Examine heart
1. Inspect precordium (pulsations and heaving)
2. Palpate precordium (apical impulse, thrills, heaves, pulsations)
3. Auscultate precordium (aortic area, pulmonic area, left sternal border, apical area)
4. Inspect jugular venous pulses and pressure

Examine breasts (female client and men with gynecomastia)
1. Inspect breasts with client's arms and hands at the side; above the head; and pressed into the hips, eliciting pectoral contraction
2. Inspect breasts with client leaning forward
3. If lesions are suspected or client is at risk for other reasons, palpate breasts in all four quadrants
4. If large breasts, perform a bimanual examination

Complete palpation of nodes in the upper body
1. Axillary nodes (lateral axillary, posterior axillary, central axillary, anterior axillary, and apical axillary)
2. Epitrochlear nodes

Client is supine. Examiner is at the right side of client (Figure 27-6)

Examine breasts (male and female)
1. Palpate breasts systematically in all four quadrants and the tail of Spence
2. Attempt to express secretion from the nipples

Examine heart
1. Inspect precordium
2. Palpate precordium (apical impulse, thrills, heaves, pulsations)
3. Auscultate precordium (supine and on left side)
4. Inspect jugular venous pulses and pressure
5. Measure supine blood pressure (both arms)

Examine abdomen
1. Inspect abdomen at rest (skin characteristics, scars, contour, pulsations, movement)
2. Examine abdomen with head raised for integrity of abdominal musculature
3. Auscultate bowel sounds, aorta, renal arteries, and femoral arteries
4. Percuss abdomen
5. Percuss and measure liver
6. Percuss spleen
7. Palpate all four quadrants lightly (tenderness, masses, organomegaly)
8. Palpate all four quadrants deeply (tenderness, masses, organomegaly)

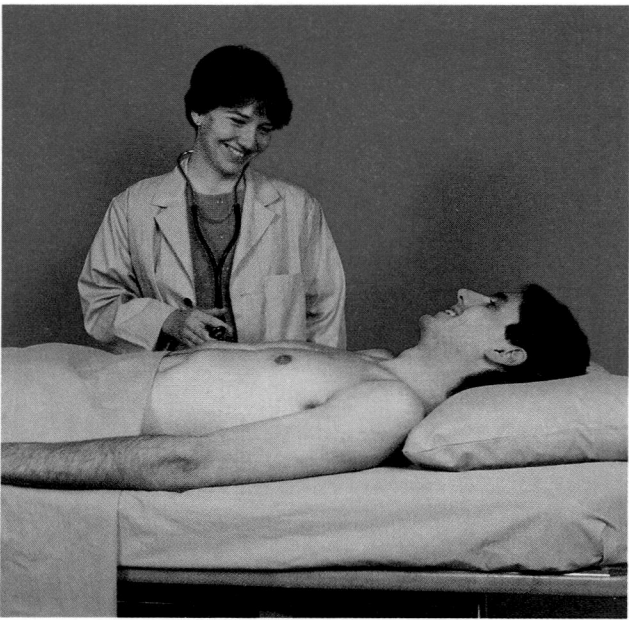

FIGURE 27-6 Client supine; examiner standing at right side of client.

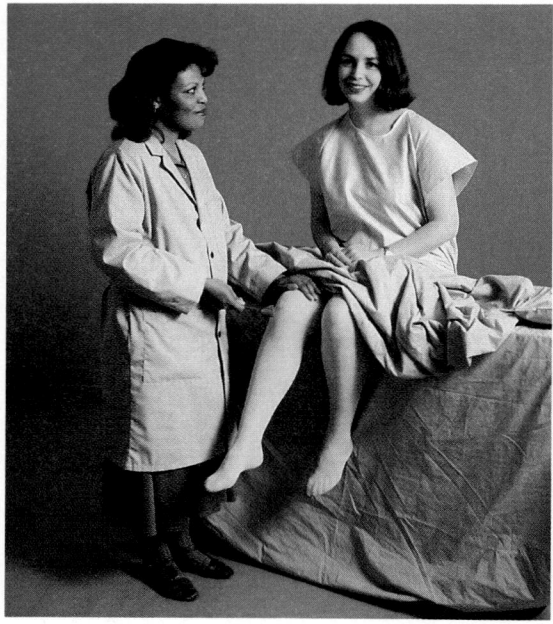

FIGURE 27-7 Client seated; examiner facing client.

9. Palpate liver, spleen, inguinal and femoral node and hernia areas, and femoral pulses
10. Test abdominal reflexes

Examine lower extremities
1. Inspect skin, hair distribution, muscle mass, and skeletal configuration
2. Palpate for temperature, texture, edema, popliteal pulses, posterior tibial pulses, and dorsal pedal pulses
3. Test range of motion (toes, feet, ankles, knees, hips)
4. Test strength (toes, feet, ankles, knees, hips)
5. Test hips for stability
6. Test sensation (pain, light touch, and vibration)
7. Test position sense

Client is sitting on the bed or examining table. Examiner is standing in front of client (Figure 27-7).

Assess neural system
1. Elicit deep tendon reflexes (biceps, triceps, brachioradialis, patellar, and Achilles reflexes)
2. Test for Babinski's reflex bilaterally
3. Test for coordination of upper and lower extremities (cerebellar function)
   a. Touch nose with rapidly alternating index fingers
   b. Touch thumb with rapidly alternating fingers

c. With index finger alternately touch own nose and examiner's rapidly moving finger
   d. Run heel down tibia of opposite leg
   e. Alternately and rapidly cross leg over knee
   f. Perform figure "8" in air with leg
4. Test sensory function (face and arms)
5. Test two-point discrimination—palms, thighs, back
6. Test stereognosis, graphesthesia

Test upper extremities
1. Strength
2. Range of motion
3. Sensation
4. Vibration
5. Position sense

Client is standing. Examiner is standing next to and then behind client (Figure 27-8).

Measure standing blood pressure in both arms
Examine spine and sacral area
1. Inspect with client bending over
2. Test for range of motion—hyperextension, lateral bending, rotation of upper trunk
3. Inspect sacrococcygeal and perianal areas

Assess neural system
1. Inspect gait (tandem, heel walking, toe walking, usual)

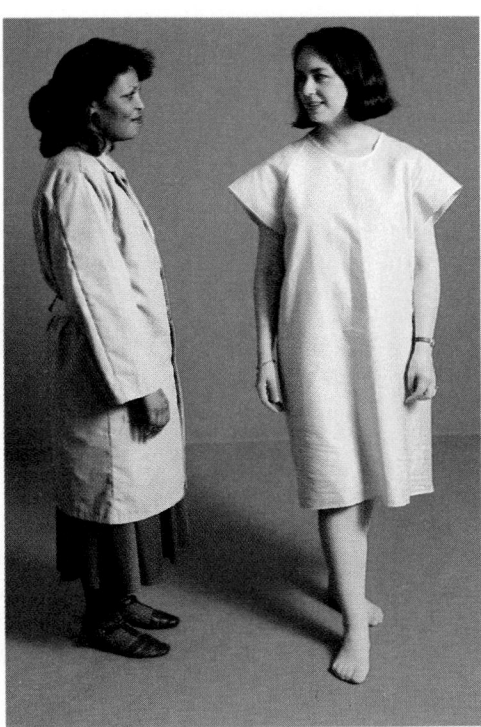

FIGURE 27-8 Client standing; examiner standing next to client.

2. Test for proprioception and cerebellar function
   a. Perform Romberg test
   b. With eyes closed, stand on one foot and then the other
   c. Hop in place on one foot and then the other
   d. Observe deep knee bends

Male client *is standing. Examiner is standing next to the client.*

Examine external genitals
1. Inspect penis, urethral opening, pubic hair distribution, and scrotum
2. Palpate penis
3. Palpate scrotal contents

Assess for presence of hernias
1. Observe for inguinal and femoral hernias at rest and with straining
2. Palpate bilaterally for femoral hernias
3. Palpate bilaterally for inguinal hernias

Rectal examination (client leans over examination table)
1. Palpate rectum (sphincter tone and characteristics)
2. Palpate prostate and seminal vesicles
3. Inspect characteristics of stool on gloved finger when removed

Female client *is in lithotomy position, genital area uncovered. Examiner is sitting, facing the genital area*

Examine genitalia
1. Inspect genitalia (pubic hair condition and distribution, labia, clitoris, urethral opening, perineum, perianal area, and anus)
2. Palpate external genital area (labia, Bartholin's and Skene's glands)
3. Perform speculum examination (inspect vagina and cervix)
4. Take smears and cultures
5. Perform bimanual vaginal examination (vagina, cervix, uterus, tubes, ovaries, muscle tone)

Examine rectum
1. Perform bimanual rectovaginal examination (sphincter tone, rectovaginal septum, ligaments, uterus, tubes, ovaries, cul-de-sac)
2. Inspect appearance of feces on gloved finger when removed

Teaching Self-Assessment

While the client is still gowned, teach or review self-examinations appropriate to the situation. Generally, it is most effective to teach self-examinations during the corresponding portion of the examiner's examination. However, there may be reasons to defer teaching until the end of the examination.

Completion of the Examination

When the examination and the teaching of self-examinations are completed, provide the client with disposable materials to clean areas where lubricant may remain. Then leave the examination room; allow the client privacy for dressing. Return to discuss findings and complete care.

EXAMINATION OF THE BEDRIDDEN CLIENT

The regional and integrated examinations presented in this book are focused on clients who are able to sit and stand. For bedridden patients, the examination is adapted. A suggested sequence is: (1) examination of the head, neck, anterior chest, and abdomen while the client is supine or supported in a sitting position on the bed; (2) examination of the back, posterior thorax, and skin while the client is rolled to the side; (3) completion of the examination with the client supine.

DOCUMENTING THE PHYSICAL EXAMINATION

The record should describe what the examiner saw, heard, palpated, and percussed. Whenever appropriate, write the exact description. Avoid evaluations such as "normal," "good," or "poor" or use them judiciously. Too frequently, examiners describe a major system, such as the cardiovascular system, in one word, "normal." This description is limited because it does not indicate what components of that system were assessed or the examiner's parameters of normal.

In documenting the physical examination, continuously attempt to achieve a balance between conciseness and comprehensiveness. To be concise, use outlines, phrases, and abbreviations. Sacrifice full sentences and write only essential words. Using a form for recording the physical examination is helpful. A form provides an outline into which data can be entered. Forms also serve as reminders for completeness, and they save time. If all members of a health care system use the same forms systematically, they become extremely useful indexes for rapid information retrieval.

As recommended in the recording of the history (see Chapter 2 on the health history), the beginning practitioner should record as many details as possible, including all findings from the examination. With increased skill and discrimination regarding the significance of findings, the practitioner will be able to weed out irrelevant information and consolidate significant data.

GUIDELINES FOR DOCUMENTING THE PHYSICAL EXAMINATION

Be specific

Be concise

Be complete

Avoid using vague terms such as "negative," "normal," or "good"

Specify portions of the examination omitted or deferred, if the plan is to do it at a later time

Use agreed-on and understood abbreviations

Record exact size or placement of lesions—draw a picture or diagram

Use illustrations when appropriate

Table 27-1 is a guideline designed to assist the beginning recorder (see also the box above). The first column indicates the body systems or regions that are examined. The second column contains a list of the areas of recording. These areas should be described for most clients. The third column is a partial list of areas to be recorded if abnormalities are identified in the examination of that system. The fourth column contains examples of recording for each body system or area. The examples of recording do not relate to one client; therefore, the fourth column should not be read as an example of the composite physical examination of one person. A sample worksheet for recording a physical examination can be found in the last section of this chapter.

Helpful Hints for Performing the Integrated Physical Examination

Warm hands and instruments

Keep fingernails short and smooth

Assure a quiet, private setting

Adapt to the circumstances

Position the examining table away from a wall to enable maximum movement for yourself

Explain what you are doing and observing during the examination

Avoid vague or evaluative statements that the client may misunderstand

Advise the patient of specific, possible discomfort and unusual sensations

Ask the client to tell you about unusual sensations or pain elicited during the examination

Expose the area to be examined fully to assure a complete assessment, but drape all areas not being examined appropriately

TABLE 27-1

Areas and Examples of Documentation for the Physical Examination

Area of examination	Descriptions usually recorded	Descriptions recorded in detail if abnormalities are present (partial listing only)	Examples of documentation
Vital signs	Temperature: oral or rectal Pulse Respiration Blood pressure; both arms in at least two positions (lying and sitting recommended) Weight: indicate if client is clothed or unclothed Height: without shoes	Blood pressure in standing position and in both thighs	T: 98.6° F (oral) P: 76/min—strong and regular: R: 16/min BP: Lying: R, 110/70/60; L, 112/68/60 Sitting: R, 116/74/67; L, 120/76/65 Wt: 130 lbs, unclothed Ht: 5 ft 3 in
General health	Appearance as relative to chronological age Apparent state of health Awareness Personal appearance Emotional status Nutritional status Affect Response Cooperation	Handshake Speech Respiratory difficulties Gross deformity Movements Unusual behavior	Slightly obese, alert, white male who looks younger than his stated age of 45. Moves without difficulty; no gross abnormalities apparent. Appears healthy and in no acute distress; is neatly dressed, responsive, and cooperative. Responds appropriately; smiles frequently.
Skin and mucous membranes	Color Edema Moisture Temperature Texture Turgor	Discharge Drainage Lesions: distribution, type, configuration Superficial vascularity Mobility Thickness	*Skin:* Uniformly brown in color; soft, warm, moist, elastic, of normal thickness. No edema or lesions. *Mucous membranes:* Pink, moist, slightly pale.
Nails	Color of beds Texture	Lesions Abnormalities in size or shape Presence of clubbing	Nail beds pink, texture hard, no clubbing.
Hair and scalp	Quantity Distribution Color Texture	Lesions Parasites	*Hair:* Normal male distribution; thick, curly; black color with graying at temples. *Scalp:* Clean, no lesions.
Cranium	Contour Tenderness	Lesions	Normocephalic, no tenderness.
Face	Symmetry Movements Sinuses CN V CN VII	Tenderness Edema Lesions Parotid gland	Symmetric at rest and with movement. Jaw muscles strong, no crepitations or limitation in movement of temporomandibular joint. Sinus areas not tender. Sensory: pain and light touch intact.

Continued.

TABLE 27-1—cont'd

Areas and Examples of Documentation for the Physical Examination

Area of examination	Descriptions usually recorded	Descriptions recorded in detail if abnormalities are present (partial listing only)	Examples of documentation
Eyes	Visual acuity Visual fields Alignment of eyes Alignment of eyelids Movement of eyelids Conjunctiva Sclera Cornea Anterior chamber Iris Pupils: size, shape, symmetry, reflexes (PERRLA may be used for "Pupils, equally round, react to light and accommodation") Lens Lacrimal apparatus Ophthalmologic examination (disc, vessels, retina, macular areas)	Eyebrows Tonometry Lesions Exophthalmia	Vision (distant with glasses): R, 20/40; L, 20/30; can read newspaper at 18 in. Visual fields full. Alignment: no deviation with cover test; light reflex equal; palpebral fissure normal. Extraocular movements: bilaterally intact; no nystagmus, ptosis, lid lag. Conjunctiva: clear, slightly injected around area of R inner canthus. Sclera: white. Cornea: clear, arcus senilis, R eye. Anterior chamber: not narrowed. Iris: blue, round. Pupils: PERRLA. Lens: clear. Funduscopic examination: normal veins and arteries; disc round, margins well defined, color yellowish pink; macular areas visualized; no arteriovenous (AV) nicking, hemorrhages, or exudates. Lacrimal system: no swelling or discharge. Corneal reflex: present.
Ears	Auricle Canal Otoscopic examination (color, presence of landmarks) Rinne and Weber tests	Position Discharge Pathologic alterations present on otoscopic examination Lesions Mastoid tenderness General tenderness	Auricle: no lesions, canal free of cerumen. Otoscopic examination: drum intact, color pearly gray, landmarks and light reflex in proper positions. Hearing: finger rub heard in both ears at 3 ft. Rinne and Weber tests heard equally in both ears, AC 2 × > BC.
Nose	Patency of each nostril Olfaction Turbinates and mucous membranes	External nose Vestibule Transillumination of sinuses	Nostrils patent, odors identified. Septum: slightly deviated to R. Turbinates and membranes: pink, moist, no discharge.
Oral cavity	Buccal mucosa Gums Teeth (decayed, missing, filled) Floor of mouth Hard and soft palate Tonsillar areas Posterior pharyngeal wall Taste Tongue position and movement	Breath odor Lips Lesions Laryngoscopic examination Palpation of mouth Parotid duct	Membranes: pink and moist, no lesions. Gums: no edema or inflammation. Teeth: in good repair. Palate: intact, moves symmetrically with phonation, gag reflex present. Tonsils: present, not enlarged. Pharynx: pink and clean. Tongue: strong, midline, moves symmetrically. Taste: able to differentiate sweet and sour.

TABLE 27-1—cont'd

Areas and Examples of Documentation for the Physical Examination

Area of examination	Descriptions usually recorded	Descriptions recorded in detail if abnormalities are present (partial listing only)	Examples of documentation
Neck	Movements: rotation and lateral bend Symmetry Thyroid gland Tracheal position Glands and nodes	Postural alignment Tenderness Tone of muscles Lesions Masses	Full ROM, strong symmetrically, thyroid not palpable, trachea midline, no enlargement of head and neck regional nodes.
Breasts	Axillary nodes Supraclavicular nodes Infraclavicular nodes Breasts: observation and palpation Nipples and areolar areas Discharge Masses	Retraction Dimpling	No nodes palpable—axillary, infraclavicular, or supraclavicular; no masses, retraction, or discharge; L breast slightly larger than R breast, otherwise symmetrical at rest and with movement. Nipples symmetrically positioned.
Chest and respiratory system	Shape of thorax Symmetry of thorax Respiratory movements Respiratory excursion Palpation: tactile fremitus, tenderness, masses Percussion notes Diaphragmatic excursion and level Auscultation: breath sounds, adventitious sounds	Deformity Use of accessory muscles of respiration Vocal resonance Egophony, bronchophony, whispered pectoriloquy	Thorax oval, AP diameter < lateral diameter; symmetrical at rest and with movements; excursion equal bilaterally; tactile fremitus equal bilaterally; no masses or tenderness; percussion tones resonant, diaphragmatic excursion 5 cm bilaterally between T10 and T12; vesicular breath sounds bilaterally; no adventitious sounds.
Central cardiovascular system	Position in which the heart was examined; lying, sitting, left lateral, recumbent Inspection: bulging, depression, pulsation (precordial and juxtaprecordial) Palpation: thrusts, heaves, thrills, friction rubs Apical impulse Auscultation: rate and rhythm, character of S_1, character of S_2, comparison of S_1 in aortic and pulmonic areas, comparison of S_1 and S_2 in major auscultatory areas, presence or absence of extra sounds—if present, description	Murmur or extra sound: whether systolic or diastolic; intensity; pitch; quality; site of maximum transmission; effect of position, respiration, and exercise; radiation	Examined in sitting and lying positions; no abnormal pulsations or lifts observed; PMI in the 5th ICS, slightly medial to the LMCL; no abnormal pulsations palpated. Apical pulse: 72, regular; Heart sounds; S_1 single sound; S_2 splits with inspiration; S_1 heard loudest at apex, S_2 heard loudest at base; no murmurs or other sounds.

Continued.

TABLE 27-1—cont'd

Areas and Examples of Documentation for the Physical Examination

Area of examination	Descriptions usually recorded	Descriptions recorded in detail if abnormalities are present (partial listing only)	Examples of documentation
Arterial pulses	Radial pulse: rate, rhythm; consistency and tenderness of arterial wall Amplitude and character of peripheral pulses: superficial temporal, brachial, femoral, popliteal, posterior tibial, dorsal pedal Carotid pulses: equality, amplitude, thrills, bruits	Any abnormality: analysis of type	Radial pulse: bilaterally equal, regular, strong; no tenderness or thickening of vessels; 76/min. Peripheral pulses:
Venous pulses and pressures	Jugular venous pulsations, presence of waves a, c, and v Venous pressure: distention present at 45 degrees	Hepatojugular reflex Analysis of jugular venous waves	Jugular venous distention, 5 cm with client at 45 degrees.

Abdomen	Inspection: scars, size, shape, symmetry, muscular development, bulging, movements
	Auscultation: peristaltic sounds—present or absent; vascular bruits—present or absent
	Palpation
	  Masses
	  Tenderness (local, referred, rebound), tone of musculature
	  Liver: size, contour, character of edge, consistency, tenderness
	  Kidney (indicate if palpable or not)
	  Costovertebral area: tenderness
	Percussion: liver size at MCL, spleen, masses
		Diastasis
		Distention
		Mass or bulging: specific description
		Palpable spleen: indication of size, surface contour, splenic notch, consistency, tenderness, mobility
		Palpable kidney: indication of location, size, shape, consistency
		Distention of urinary bladder
		Fluid wave
		Flank dullness
		Shifting dullness
		Aorta
		Gallbladder
			Healed scar RLQ (appendectomy); slightly obese, protuberant; symmetrical, no bulging; bowel sounds present, no bruits; no abnormal movements, symmetric; no masses; no tenderness; liver 11 cm in RMCL; no CVA tenderness; no organs palpated; muscle tone lax.
			Area of midline diastasis: 6 cm × 2 cm inferior and superior to the umbilicus.

Peripheral pulses:

	Right	Left
Temporal	2	2
Brachial	3	3
Femoral	2	2
Popliteal	0	0
Posterior tibial	2	2
Dorsal pedal	1	1

Carotid pulses: equal, strong, no bruits.

3 cm

TABLE 27-1—cont'd

Areas and Examples of Documentation for the Physical Examination

Area of examination	Descriptions usually recorded	Descriptions recorded in detail if abnormalities are present (partial listing only)	Examples of documentation

Neural system	Orientation
	Intellectual performance
	Emotional status
	Insight
	Memory
	Cranial nerves
	Coordination
	Sensory: touch, pain, position, vibration
	Babinski's sign
	Romberg test
		Thought content
		Speech
		Sensory: hot, cold, two-point discrimination
		Stereognosis
		Involuntary movements
			Alert, oriented ×3; mood appropriate and stable; remote and recent memory intact; several calculations by 6 accurate; insight normal; cranial nerves I-XII intact, examined and recorded in head and neck regions; all movement coordinated; able to perform rapid coordinated movements with upper and lower extremities.
			
			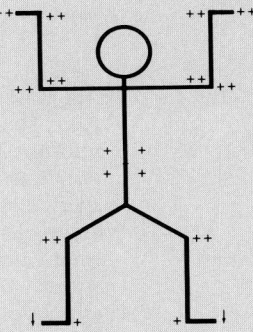
			
			Deep tendon reflexes (0 to 4 +)
			    0 = absent
			    + (or 1 +) = decreased
			    + + (or 2 +) = normal
			    + + + (or 3 +) = hyperactive
			    + + + + (or 4 +) = clonus
			Sensory: Able to detect light touch, pain, and vibration to face, trunk, and extremities bilaterally and symmetric; walks with coordination, able to maintain standing position with eyes closed.

Extremities and musculoskeletal system	Both upper and lower extremities: general assessments—size, shape, mass, symmetry, hair distribution, color; temperature; edema; varicosities; tenderness; epitrochlear lymph nodes Bones and joints: range of motion, tenderness, gait Muscles: size, symmetry, strength, tone, tenderness, consistency Back: posture, tenderness; movement—extension, lateral bend, rotation	Lesions Deformities Color and temperature—changes on elevation and dependency Homans' sign Redness Heat Swelling Deformity Crepitations Contractures Muscle spasms Tenderness Atrophy Hypertrophy	Muscular development and mass normal for age; arms and legs symmetrical; skin warm, soft, male hair distribution on arms, legs, and feet; no edema, varicosities, or tenderness; no nodes palpated; joints nontender, not swollen; full ROM; good muscle tone and strength equal bilaterally; back—full ROM; no tenderness or deformities.

Continued.

TABLE 27-1—cont'd

Areas and Examples of Documentation for the Physical Examination

Area of examination	Descriptions usually recorded	Descriptions recorded in detail if abnormalities are present (partial listing only)	Examples of documentation
Anus and rectum	Anal area Skin Hemorrhoids Sphincter tone Rectum Tumors Stool color Occult blood	Lesions Fissures Pilonidal sinus Condition of perineal body Tenderness Proctoscopic examination	Skin clean, no lesions; sphincter tone good; no hemorrhoids or masses noted; stools brown, guaiac negative.
Inguinal area	Hernia: inguinal, femoral Nodes	Size, shape, consistency, tenderness, reducibility of hernia or nodes	Hernias not present; no enlargement of nodes noted
Male genitalia	Penis: condition of prepuce, skin Scrotum: size, skin, testes, epididymides, spermatic cords Prostate gland: size, shape, symmetry, consistency, tenderness Seminal vesicles: size, shape, consistency	Scars Lesions Structural alterations Masses Swelling Nodules	Penis: circumcised, clean, no lesions. Scrotum and contents: normal size, no masses or tumors noted. Prostate and inferior portions of seminal vesicles: palpated, normal consistency, nontender. Prostate: not enlarged, rubbery, not tender. Seminal vesicles: not palpable.
Female genitalia	External: hair distribution; labia; Bartholin's glands, urethral meatus, Skene's glands (BUS); hymen; introitus Vaginal observation: presence or absence of rectocele, urethrocele, cystocele; tissue; discharge (smears or cultures taken); cervix Bimanual examination: cervix, uterus, adnexa Rectovaginal examination; uterus, cul-de-sac, septum	Lesions Tumors Prolapses	Normal female hair distribution; no lesions or masses. BUS: no tenderness, redness, or discharge. Hymen: present in caruncles. Labia: pink, no lesions. Introital tone: good; no prolapses; no scars, perineum thick. Vagina: pink, discharge—small amount, thin, clean, nonodorous. Cervix: pink, nulliparous, firm, not tender, movable, midline. Uterus: pear-shaped, movable, normal size, firm, no masses. Tubes: not palpable. Ovaries: palpable, movable, not tender, approximately 2 × 3 × 2 cm; smooth surface, no lesions, firm consistency. Rectovaginal septum: thick and firm; no masses palpated in rectum or cul-de-sac.

WORKSHEET FOR DOCUMENTING A PHYSICAL EXAMINATION

Vital signs

Temperature _____ Respiration _____ /min   BP (L) Arm   (R)

_____ Supine _____

_____ Sitting _____

_____ Standing _____

Height _____ ft _____ in Weight _____ lbs (stripped or clothed)

General inspection

Skin, hair, nails, mucous membranes

Head

Scalp _____

Face _____

(CNs V, VII) _____

_____

Sinus areas _____

Nodes _____

Cranium _____

Eyes

Visual acuity _____

Visual fields _____

Ocular movements (CNs III, IV, VI) _____

Convergence _____

Lids, lacrimal organs _____

Conjunctiva, sclera _____

Cornea (CN V) _____

Lens and media _____

Pupils: Pupillary reflexes (CN III) _____

Light, direct and consensual _____

Accommodation _____

Fundi (CN II) _____

Continued.

WORKSHEET FOR DOCUMENTING A PHYSICAL EXAMINATION—CONT'D

Ears

External structures _____

Canal _____

Tympanic membranes and landmarks _____

Hearing (CN VIII) _____

Nose

External structure _____

Septum _____

Mucous membranes _____

Patency _____

Olfactory sense (CN I) _____

Oral cavity

Lips _____

Buccal mucosa and ducts _____

Gums _____

Teeth _____

Palates and uvula (CNs IX, X) _____

Tonsillar areas _____

Tongue (CN XII) _____

Floor _____

Voice _____

Breath _____

Taste (CN VII, IX) _____

Neck

General structure _____

Trachea _____

Thyroid _____

Nodes _____

Muscles (CN XI) _____

Breasts and area nodes (axillary, supraclavicular, infraclavicular)

Inspection _____

Palpation _____

WORKSHEET FOR DOCUMENTING A PHYSICAL EXAMINATION—CONT'D

Chest, respiratory system

Chest shape _____

Type of respiration _____

Expansion _____

Fremitus _____

General palpation _____

Percussion _____

_____   Diaphragmatic excursion: (R) _____ cm (L) cm

Breath sounds _____

_____

_____

Adventitious sounds _____

_____

Cardiovascular system

Rate and rhythm: Radial (palpation) _____

Apical (auscultation) _____

Precordium: Inspection _____

Palpation _____

Auscultation _____

S_1 _____

S_2 _____

Other sounds _____

Murmur(s): Systolic _____

Diastolic _____

Carotid arteries _____

Jugular venous distention _____

Description of peripheral pulses

Brachial	Radial	Femoral	Popliteal	Dorsal pedal	Post. tibial
R					
L					

Continued.

WORKSHEET FOR DOCUMENTING A PHYSICAL EXAMINATION—CONT'D

Abdomen and inguinal areas

Contour, tone _____

Scars, marks _____

Auscultation _____

_____

Liver _____ Span _____ cm at RMCL

Spleen _____

Kidneys _____ CVA tenderness _____

Bladder _____

Hernias _____

Masses _____

Palpation _____

_____

Percussion _____

Genitalia and area nodes

_____

_____

_____

Rectal examination

Musculoskeletal system

Gait _____

Upper extremities _____

Lower extremities _____

Deformities _____

Joint evaluation _____

_____

Muscle strength _____

_____

Muscle mass _____

Nodes _____

Range of motion _____

Continued.

WORKSHEET FOR DOCUMENTING A PHYSICAL EXAMINATION—CONT'D

Spine

Contour _____

Position _____

Motion _____

_____

Nervous system

Mental status _____

Language _____

Cranial nerves (summarize) _____

Motor: Coordination: Upper extremities _____

Lower extremities _____

Involuntary movements _____

Deep tendon reflexes:

Note: +s denote finger jerks, brachioradialis, biceps, triceps, reflexes, 4-quadrant abdominal scratch reflexes, patellar Achilles reflexes, and plantar reflexes. Abdominal reflexes are recorded as 0 or +. Scale: 0-4 (+ + + +); normal = 2 (+ +).

Sensory

Light touch _____

Pain (pinprick) _____

Vibration _____

Position _____

Clinical Decision Making for Determining Health Status

The preceding chapters have presented methods to collect data when performing a general health assessment. The examiner uses these data to formulate conclusions about the client's health status. To reach a conclusion, or diagnosis, the practitioner uses a process known as diagnostic reasoning, or decision making. This chapter discusses the process of decision making and its relationship to nursing process and nursing diagnosis. In addition, it presents some methods for facilitating decision making.

THE DECISION-MAKING PROCESS

Process of Gathering Information

The first step in clinical decision-making is gathering information. The general health assessment provides the data or information needed to formulate a diagnosis and eventually a plan of treatment and evaluation. The data gathering process includes:

1. Data collection
2. Data validation
3. Data organization
4. Pattern identification

Data collection. Data include information gathered from the first encounter with the client and during the health interview and physical examination. Laboratory data, if applicable, are also considered. These components of a data base are part of a general health assessment. In later follow-up with a client, the practitioner focuses the assessment by collecting data on a specific problem or concern.

Data are collected using a system or framework. In the physical examination, the examiner can collect data using several organizing principles: head-to-toe, regional areas of the body (e.g., pelvic examination), or body systems (e.g., the cardiovascular or neurological). Each of these methods provides a logical, organized framework for collecting physical assessment data. The practitioner's decision about which method to use is influenced by both priority needs of the client and personal preference. For example, if you see a client for a periodic health examination, you would use a head-to-toe approach. However, if a client who appears in acute distress stated she had just injured her hand, you would begin the assessment by focusing on the body region affected.

As you develop expertise as a practitioner, you will develop your own approach to data collection that is appropriate to the circumstances, such as the client's age, sex, emotional state, and acuity of the health problem or concern. Whatever approach is used, you must think about the the range of possibilities and develop a sensitivity to the possible meaning of all signs and symptoms.

Data validation. *Validation* is a process of making sure the data collected are accurate. Data obtained using an instrument with a measurement scale can be validated by repeating the measure. For example, if a weight on the clinic scale indicates a 10-pound weight loss since the last visit, you can repeat the weight to validate this measure. Verify information with the client by direct observation or interview. Preferably validate information yourself, rather than relying on information obtained by others, especially if it involves subjective data open to interpretation. Strategies to validate data include the following:

1. Recheck your own data. Go back to an area of the physical exam that you need to palpate or observe again.
2. Be sure other factors did not influence the accuracy of the data (e.g., while in a hurry to obtain a blood pressure, you used the wrong size blood pressure cuff).
3. Always recheck information that is grossly abnormal. For example, repeat a systolic blood pressure reading of 260 mmHg.
4. Ask someone, preferably more experienced, to collect the same data. If you hear a grade III systolic heart murmur on physical exam, have another clinician also listen to the heart.
5. Recheck previous documentation yourself or with other clinicians to see if abnormal findings were previously recorded.

Data organization. Data are organized by clustering. The ability to do this efficiently depends on the examiner's knowledge, skill, and preference. Theoretical frameworks help to organize data and are discussed in more detail later in this chapter. The earlier chapters in this book have presented various frameworks for health assessment. For example, Chapter 16 presents a systems approach (cardiovascular). Chapters 3 and 25 present a developmental approach that modifies the health history and physical exam for the client's age.

Pattern identification. The examiner analyzes the data to determine if gaps exist or if more data are needed to make a diagnosis. For example, if a client states he has a loss of appetite, obtaining a weight is critical to determine if weight loss occurred. You would compare the current weight to previous weights to determine if a pattern of weight change is evident. If no previous weights were recorded, you and the client would plan to obtain weight data at a designated frequency over the next month. You would then assess these data to detect any pattern of weight change.

Medical Diagnostic Reasoning Processs

Many investigators have studied how physicians diagnose illness. By comparison, few studies concern nursing decision making. However, some of the research that has been done suggests that physicians and nurses use similar decision-making processes. This conclusion seems reasonable, since researchers have suggested both tradition and necessity require nurses to make both medical and nursing judgments.

The medical decision-making process includes four major steps (Table 28-1).

Cue recognition. In the first phase of decision making, the practitioner must recognize that a **cue** is significant. A cue is a piece of information. It can consist of either subjective or objective data. For example, a subjective cue might be the client's statement, "I feel

---

TABLE 28-1

Stages of Diagnostic Reasoning or Decision Making

Stage	Example
Cue recognition	Look at client's face—notice cyanosis as abnormal
Hypothesis formulation	Client is experiencing impaired gas exchange
Hypothesis testing	Arterial blood gas result: pH 7.32, pCO_2, 55m pO_2 65. The client appears restless and confused. Weak cough effort
Hypothesis evaluation	Do enough data exist to confirm the diagnosis of impaired gas exchange? If yes, then diagnosis is made. Impaired gas exchange related to . . .

nervous." In contrast, an objective cue might be a client's hand tremor.

Whether a cue is considered significant depends on the practitioner's ability to distinguish between normal and abnormal behavior, physical characteristics, and diagnostic findings. This ability, in turn, depends on the examiner's knowledge base and expertise. You must stay attuned to even slight variations of normal findings since they may have a significance that is not at first obvious. A knowledgeable and experienced practitioner, for example, might note the slight pallor of a client's nail beds and consider the diagnosis of anemia. In contrast, an inexperienced student might not even notice the subtle change in nail bed color.

In summary, during the first phase of decision making, **cue recognition,** the practitioner receives thousands of pieces of information. Next, he or she begins to sort the data, keeping some pieces of information and ignoring others. This process of sorting information is called clinical judgment. The remaining data or cues serve as a more efficient resource for the next step in the process, hypothesis formulation.

Hypothesis formulation. During the second phase of decision making the practitioner decides on possible explanations for the cues recognized in the previous step. This phase is often referred to as hypothesis formulation. **Inference** is the process of perceiving and interpreting a cue. The examiner must be a critical observer to pick up all cues available. Before making any conclusions, the examiner first clusters or links the cues to determine any patterns. One cue, in isolation, is rarely enough to suggest a particular hypothesis or diagnosis. Rather, the presence of several cues that are usually or always associated with a specific problem helps indicate what other further information is necessary before arriving at a conclusion.

As in the first phase, an examiner's knowledge and expertise strongly influence the decision-making process. The practitioner's knowledge influences the interpretation and relative importance of the remaining cues. Often the novice jumps to early and erroneous conclusions caused by misinterpreting cues, focusing on only one cue, or failing to efficiently eliminate irrelevant cues from the cues considered. As a practitioner gains knowledge and experience, he or she builds associations between cues and clinical situations. These associations enable the examiner to cluster cues into meaningful groups and formulate hypotheses.

The formulation of hypotheses or tentative conclusions helps focus further data collection efforts on a manageable group of possibilities. However, the examiner must be careful not to limit further investigation to only one hypothesis, since the likelihood of an accurate final diagnosis increases when several explanations are considered. The examiner must think about the more likely problems, since common problems occur with more frequency, while at the same time entertaining the probability that a rare problem might be presenting itself.

Hypothesis testing. During the third stage of diagnostic reasoning, the practitioner focuses on gathering data to support or reject the previously generated hypotheses. This phase is called **hypothesis testing.** Examiners use many different data collection strategies during this stage. Tables 28-2 and 28-3 list methods of continued inquiry. One or more of these techniques may be appropriate for a given clinical situation. In addition, the practitioner may be more comfortable using some methods rather than others.

Throughout the hypothesis testing phase the practitioner needs to guard against having biases about hypotheses. Some of these biases may lead to prematurely accepting a possible explanation or prematurely rejecting an explanation (Table 28-4).

TABLE 28-2

General Strategies for Hypothesis Testing

Approach	Explanation	Example
Cue-based	Explore each aspect of initial cues until all facets are covered	Facial cyanosis—mucous membranes, ears, skin color
Hypothesis-driven	Investigate the defining characteristics to confirm their presence or absence	Hypoxia? Hypercapnia? Restlessness? Confusion? Irritability? Inability to move secretions?
Systematic	Review body systems	Start with respiratory system, then move to cardiovascular system, etc.
Hit and miss	No recognizable strategy	Ask client when last bowel movement took place

TABLE 28-3

Hypothesis Testing Strategies Used by Experts

Strategy	Explanation
Confirmation	Seek data to confirm hypothesis
Elimination	Eliminate hypothesis based on absence of key signs and symptoms (defining characteristics)
Discrimination	Investigate defining characteristics that separate diagnoses with similar signs and symptoms (i.e., look for those characteristics that are different)
Exploration	Consider investigation of diagnoses with similar manifestations

TABLE 28-4

Biases Affecting Diagnosis

Bias	Explanation
Frequency of occurrence	If the diagnosis being considered has been made frequently, it has a higher probability of being chosen.
Recency of experience	If the clinician has made the considered diagnosis in the recent past, the clinician may be more familiar with this diagnosis than with other related diagnoses.
Profoundness of memory	Vivid impressions of cases in which a certain diagnosis was made can influence decision making in favor of this diagnosis.

Helpful Hints: *To minimize bias in hypothesis testing*
- *Don't maintain a narrow focus*
- *Don't jump to conclusions*
- *Do explore alternative explanations*
- *Do keep an open mind*
- *Do take your time*

Hypothesis evaluation. After the practitioner has investigated all reasonable explanations for the initial set of cues, he or she must evaluate each hypothesis in light of the new evidence collected and reach a final diagnosis or conclusion. Hypothesis evaluation requires synthesis of all data that have been collected, since information obtained to refute one hypothesis may support another. You might also find that the data suggest that more than one problem exists.

Careful recording of data collected is crucial. Failure to document data fully increases the chance that information necessary to evaluate the hypothesis will be lost or forgotten. Missing data, in turn, can lead to erroneous conclusions. Chapter 27 contains an example of one form that can be used to record data during the assessment process.

During this phase of decision making, the practitioner determines which explanation has the most supporting data and chooses this hypothesis as the diagnosis. In some cases, however, the examiner can merely eliminate hypotheses until only the one with the highest probability remains.

THE INFLUENCE OF THEORETICAL FRAMEWORKS ON DECISION MAKING

Although nurses and physicians seem to use the same general decision making process, these two groups of professionals reach conclusions that are quite different. The reason for this difference stems from each profession's focus of concern.

Medical and Nursing Concerns

The focus of medicine is the diagnosis and treatment of disease. The knowledge base physicians use is derived, in part, from cell and germ theories. The organizing framework for the biomedical model is biochemical or biophysical systems. As a result, physicians concentrate their investigations on biological abnormalities and identifying the cause of such disorders. Traditionally, the role of how human psychosocial and socioeconomic factors have an impact on health has not been a focus of medicine.

In contrast, nursing's primary focus is the diagnosis of human responses to actual or potential health problems. These responses may result in health problems but may not be disease states. Nursing assessment focuses on the client's physical, psychological, and spiritual reactions to illness and the environment. Nurses use many theoretical frameworks to explain these phenomena. Some examples are Roy's adaptation model, Orem's self-care model, and the unitary person framework proposed by the North American Nursing Diagnosis Association (NANDA).

Theory-Based Decision Making: the Unitary Person Framework

Using a framework to guide assessment and decision making is beneficial because it helps organize knowledge and provides direction for further investigation of initial cues. A framework also provides practitioners with specific terminology, which facilitates more effective communication between members of the same discipline. NANDA has been instrumental in providing a common language to communicate nursing findings and a common framework to explain the phenomena nurses observe. The language provided by NANDA consists of **nursing diagnoses** arranged in a **taxonomy**, or meaningful pattern, called Taxonomy I Revised, based on the unitary person framework.

Taxonomy I Revised—A Nursing Classification System

Taxonomy I Revised is a nursing diagnosis classification system arranged in a hierarchy from the general to the specific based on the unitary person framework. The unitary person framework suggests that a person's health status is manifested by observable phenomena that can be classified into nine human response patterns. The most general concept of the system is the unitary person. A slightly more specific concept is health. Health, in turn, is determined by functioning within the nine human response patterns. The nine response patterns have subcategories that identify specific human patterns and behaviors within each particular response pattern (Figure 28-1). These nine human response patterns act as the major categories for the NANDA Taxonomy I Revised (see box).

The next level of this system consists of nursing diagnoses and other subcategory headings that NANDA's

Taxonomy Committee has determined to be related to a particular pattern. The boxed material on pp. 911-912 shows diagnoses arranged according to the nine human response patterns of the unitary person framework.

NANDA Taxonomy I can be used to guide clinical decision making. A practitioner can select the general response pattern and assess for signs and symptoms associated with that response pattern. Response patterns are broad and can be further defined.

For example, the examiner wishing to evaluate the exchanging pattern might start by assessing the client's elimination, since "Altered Elimination" is one diagnosis found in this pattern.

The examiner then decides which type of elimination to evaluate first, bowel or urinary. He or she chooses bowel elimination.

Next, the examiner looks for signs and symptoms of diarrhea, constipation, or incontinence. Nursing diagnoses have been defined and determined to have certain signs and symptoms called **defining characteristics.** These defining characteristics most often serve as cues for decision making.

Occasionally, the examiner can make even more specific diagnoses, for example, Colonic Constipation (see Figure 28-1). If the defining characteristics for one of these disorders exists, the examiner can make a nursing diagnosis.

A practitioner can also use Taxonomy I Revised to investigate a specific finding, such as an abdomen that is firm to palpation. Other cues may be associated with this finding, for example, the client's complaint of a feeling of abdominal fullness. Based on these cues, the examiner makes a tentative diagnosis of constipation. The practitioner then tests this diagnosis by searching for the presence of its other defining characteristics, such as client reports of no bowel movement for 3 days. If several of these signs and symptoms are present, the examiner can make the diagnosis of "Constipation."

The predictive relationships between defining characteristics and nursing diagnoses are not perfect. These relationships are initially based on the observations of experienced clinicians who propose new nursing diagnoses. Much research is currently being conducted to validate the defining characteristics of the diagnoses accepted by NANDA. Although the association of a cluster of signs and symptoms with a nursing diagnosis may be strong, no single group of characteristics ever absolutely indicates a particular nursing diagnosis.

Using the Taxonomy I Revised method of assessment and decision making may be difficult at first, since nurses traditionally have not been taught to organize their thinking in this manner. As more nursing diagnoses are developed, defined, and verified, the taxonomy will continue to be refined. This, in turn, will make the nursing diagnosis process easier.

NINE HUMAN RESPONSE PATTERNS OF THE UNITARY PERSON FRAMEWORK

1. Exchanging: mutual giving and receiving
2. Communicating: Sending messages
3. Relating: Establishing bonds
4. Valuing: Assigning worth
5. Choosing: Selection of alternatives
6. Moving: Activity
7. Perceiving: Reception of information
8. Knowing: Meaning associated with information
9. Feeling: Subjective awareness of information

From Sparks SM, Taylor CM: *Nursing diagnosis reference manual,* Springhouse, Pa, 1991, Springhouse Corporation.

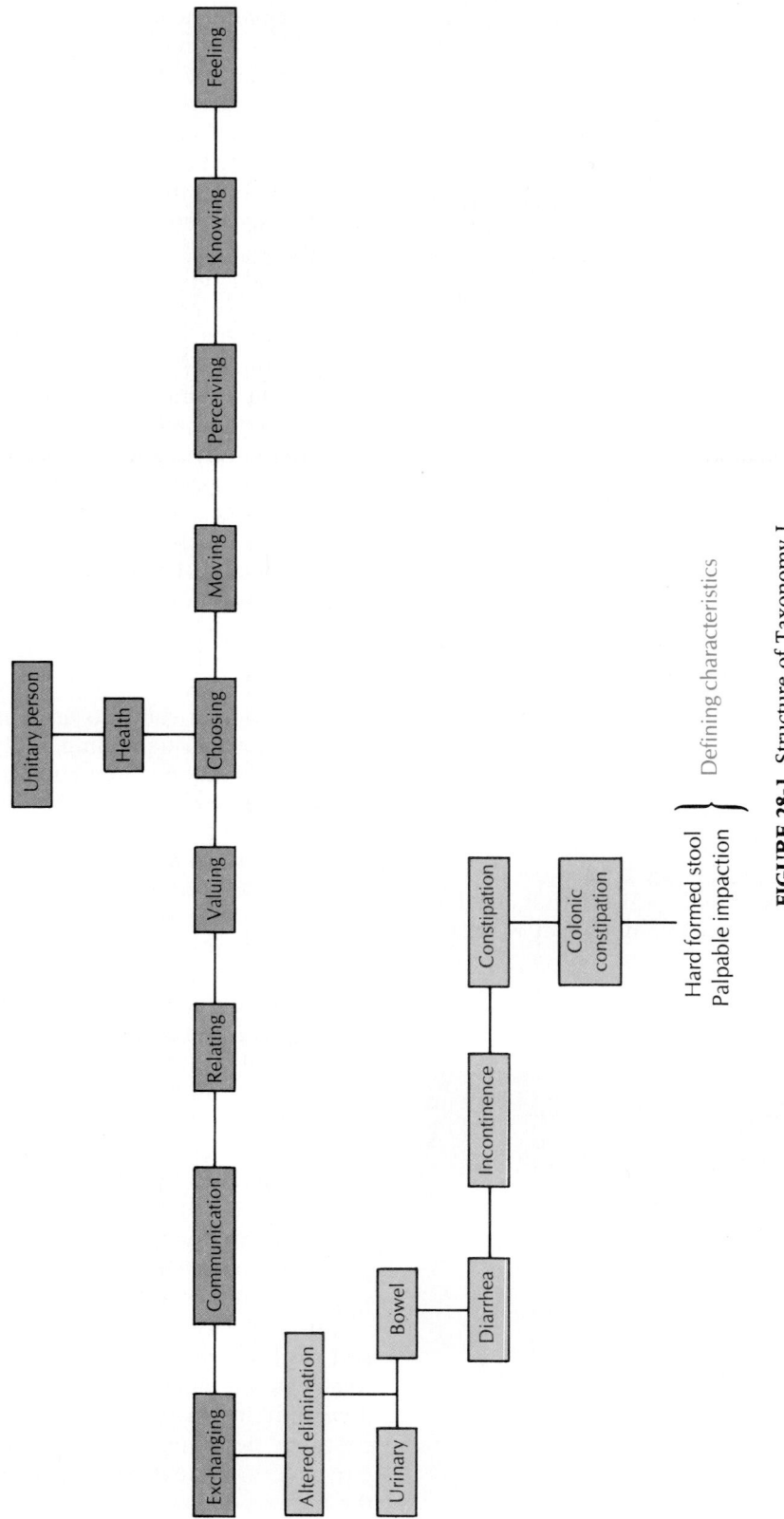

FIGURE 28-1 Structure of Taxonomy I.

CLASSIFICATION OF NURSING DIAGNOSES BY HUMAN RESPONSE PATTERNS (NANDA TAXONOMY I—REVISED)

Exchanging

Altered nutrition: more than body requirements
Altered nutrition: less than body requirements
Altered nutrition: high risk for more than body requirements
High risk for infection
High risk for altered body temperature
Hypothermia
Hyperthermia
Ineffective thermoregulation
Dysreflexia
Constipation
Perceived constipation
Colonic constipation
Diarrhea
Bowel incontinence
Altered urinary elimination
Stress incontinence
Reflex incontinence
Urge incontinence
Functional incontinence
Total incontinence
Urinary retention
Altered tissue perfusion (specify type) (renal, cerebral, cardiopulmonary, gastrointestinal, peripheral)
Fluid volume excess
Fluid volume deficit
High risk for fluid volume deficit
Decreased cardiac output
Impaired gas exchange
Ineffective airway clearance
Ineffective breathing pattern
Inability to sustain spontaneous ventilation
Dysfunctional ventilatory weaning response
High risk for injury
High risk for suffocation
High risk for poisoning
High risk for trauma
High risk for aspiration
High risk for disuse syndrome
Altered protection
Impaired tissue integrity
Altered oral mucous membrane
Impaired skin integrity
High risk for impaired skin integrity

Communicating

Impaired verbal communication

Relating

Impaired social interaction
Social isolation
Altered role performance
Altered parenting
High risk for altered parenting

Sexual dysfunction
Altered family processes
Caregiver role strain
High risk for caregiver role strain
Parental role conflict
Altered sexuality patterns

Valuing

Spiritual distress (distress of the human spirit)

Choosing

Ineffective individual coping
Impaired adjustment
Defensive coping
Ineffective denial
Ineffective family coping: disabling
Ineffective family coping: compromised
Family coping: potential for growth
Ineffective management of therapeutic regimen (individuals)
Noncompliance (specify)
Decisional conflict (specify)
Health-seeking behaviors (specify)

Moving

Impaired physical mobility
High risk for peripheral neurovascular dysfunction
Activity intolerance
Fatigue
High risk for activity intolerance
Sleep pattern disturbance
Diversional activity deficit
Impaired home maintenance management
Altered health maintenance
Feeding self-care deficit
Impaired swallowing
Ineffective breastfeeding
Interrupted breastfeeding
Effective breastfeeding
Ineffective infant feeding pattern
Bathing/hygiene self-care deficit
Dressing/grooming self-care deficit
Toileting self-care deficit
Altered growth and development
Relocation stress syndrome

Perceiving

Body image disturbance
Self-esteem disturbance
Chronic low self-esteem
Situational low self-esteem
Personal identity disturbance
Sensory/perceptual alterations (specify) (visual, auditory, kinesthetic, gustatory, tactile, olfactory)

Continued.

CLASSIFICATION OF NURSING DIAGNOSES BY HUMAN RESPONSE PATTERNS (NANDA TAXONOMY I—REVISED)—cont'd

Unilateral neglect
Hopelessness
Powerlessness

Knowing

Knowledge deficit (specify)
Altered thought processes

Feeling

Pain
Chronic pain

Dysfunctional grieving
Anticipatory grieving
High risk for violence: self-directed or directed at others
High risk for self-mutilation
Post-trauma response
Rape-trauma syndrome
Rape-trauma syndrome: compound reaction
Rape-trauma syndrome: silent reaction
Anxiety
Fear

USING A CLASSIFICATION SYSTEM TO FACILITATE DECISION MAKING

Classification systems such as Taxonomy I Revised serve as road maps for diagnostic reasoning. From any given location in the classification scheme, a practitioner can investigate in the direction of either a more general or a more specific conclusion, whichever is appropriate for the situation.

Body Systems Approach

One classification system frequently used in physical assessment is the body systems approach. Using a body systems approach, an examiner might choose to evaluate the gastrointestinal system. This is a general category that consists of several organs and tissues. After choosing the system to assess, the practitioner focuses on evaluating the functioning of the various organs and tissues. With an abnormal finding, the examiner then searches for additional signs and symptoms known to be associated with this finding to make a diagnosis.

Examiners can also use the body systems approach to move from a specific complaint or finding to an evaluation of the functioning of one or more systems. For example, a practitioner investigating tachycardia might first search for other cardiac-related signs and symptoms. However, during this search, the practitioner observes that the client has abdominal distress and difficulty concentrating, and describes a smothering sensation. The diagnostic process might then involve assessing environmental variables for other data to confirm the tentative nursing diagnosis of anxiety related to situational crisis.

Theoretical Frameworks

Nurses, as well as physicians, have traditionally used the body systems approach to assessment. However, this approach does not always facilitate the formulation of nursing diagnoses. To ease the process of making nursing diagnoses, nurses must use a theory-based approach to assessment and decision making.

Maslow's hierarchy of needs. Maslow's hierarchy of needs is a system of classifying human needs based on the idea that lower-level physiological needs must be met before higher-level abstract needs can be met. By considering categories of needs, the nurse can provide more holistic care. Nursing diagnoses can be related to each of the categories in Maslow's hierarchy:

1. Physiological needs—oxygen, food, elimination, temperature control, sex, movement, rest, comfort
2. Safety and security—safety from physical or psychological threat; protection, continuity, stability, lack of danger
3. Love and belonging—affiliation, affection, intimacy, support, reassurance
4. Self-esteem—sense of self-worth, self-respect, independence, dignity, privacy, self-reliance
5. Self-actualization—recognition and realization of one's potential, growth, health, autonomy

Orem's universal self-care demands. For humans to function they must be able to perform universal self-care demands. If a person is not able to meet these demands, a self-care deficit occurs. In Orem's theory, the goals of nursing include helping the client to overcome circumstances that interfere with or cause self-care deficits.

Gordon's functional health patterns. The most widely used organizing framework for nursing diagnoses is based on functional health patterns described by Marjory Gordon. The 11 health patterns allow for easy organization of basic nursing information obtained during an initial health assessment. Gordon's functional health patterns are listed below:

1. Health-perception—health-management pattern
2. Nutritional-metabolic pattern
3. Elimination pattern
4. Activity-exercise pattern
5. Sleep-rest pattern
6. Cognitive-perceptual pattern
7. Self-perception—self-concept pattern
8. Role relationship pattern
9. Sexuality-reproductive pattern
10. Coping-stress-tolerance pattern
11. Value-belief pattern

DECISION MAKING AND THE NURSING PROCESS

Assessment and Decision Making

The nursing process consists of four phases: assessment, planning, implementation, and evaluation. The assessment phase includes history taking and physical examination and ends with the determination of actual or potential nursing diagnoses. This definition implies that some form of decision making has occurred.

Assessment occurs before and during the decision making process. During the initial phase of decision making, the practitioner performs a cursory initial assessment for significant cues. This initial assessment can be as simple as eliciting the client's presenting complaint and making general observations concerning the client's appearance. After clustering the initial cues and formulating tentative hypotheses, the examiner performs a second, more focused assessment. Thus, assessment and decision making are intertwined.

Nursing Diagnoses and Decision Making

Nursing diagnoses are actual or potential problems that can be prevented, resolved, or reduced through independent nursing interventions. The nursing focus is holistic and includes comfort as well as cure. The culmination of nursing assessment and decision making is the formulation of nursing diagnoses.

According to NANDA's recommendations, a nursing diagnosis should be stated in a problem-etiology-signs and symptoms (P-E-S) format. This format also conveniently summarizes the key decision-making factors or defining characteristics leading to the final diagnosis.

Following is a sample nursing diagnosis:

Problem (P)—Impaired physical mobility

Etiology(E)—"related to" a fractured tibia; status after cast application

Signs and Symptoms(S)—"as manifested by"; client states "I can't walk without help. I feel clumsy using crutches." The client requires stand-by assistance when ambulating to the bathroom; is observed to position crutches correctly during ambulation.

Diagnostic statement: Impaired physical mobility related to a fractured tibia after cast application manifested by statements that she cannot walk without help and feels clumsy, and observation that she needs stand-by assistance when using crutches correctly.

> **Helpful Hints:** *A nursing diagnosis is **not***
> - *A diagnostic test (schedule for mammogram)*
> - *A nursing problem (difficulty visualizing cervix)*
> - *A medical diagnosis (fractured tibia)*
> - *A nursing goal (teach breast self-examination)*

When nursing diagnoses are recorded in this manner, any nurse reading the diagnostic statement is able to determine how this decision was reached. In addition, nursing diagnoses written in P-E-S format provide clues about possible nursing interventions by indicating which defining characteristics are present and therefore require intervention. In this way, nursing diagnoses can also assist in the planning phase of the nursing process. For example, the diagnosis in Figure 28-2 suggests planning interventions that would allow the client to ventilate feelings regarding the loss of a leg. Another suggested intervention would be fostering the client's independence by encouraging self-care and personal decision making.

Planning and Clinical Management

Prioritize diagnoses. Whenever you develop more than one diagnosis, assign priority to each diagnosis to plan care. In your plan, first address the diagnoses with the highest priority. Some needs may be emergency needs such as:

High risk for violence: self-directed related to suicide attempt manifested by repeated statements: "I want to shoot myself" and possession of a handgun.

You may prioritize other needs as intermediate. Low priority needs do not directly relate to a specific current problem. An organizing framework, such as Maslow's hierarchy of needs, will help you assign priorities.

Establish outcomes or goals. Establish goals to let others know what is to be accomplished and when. The examiner must also assess the client's preferences and

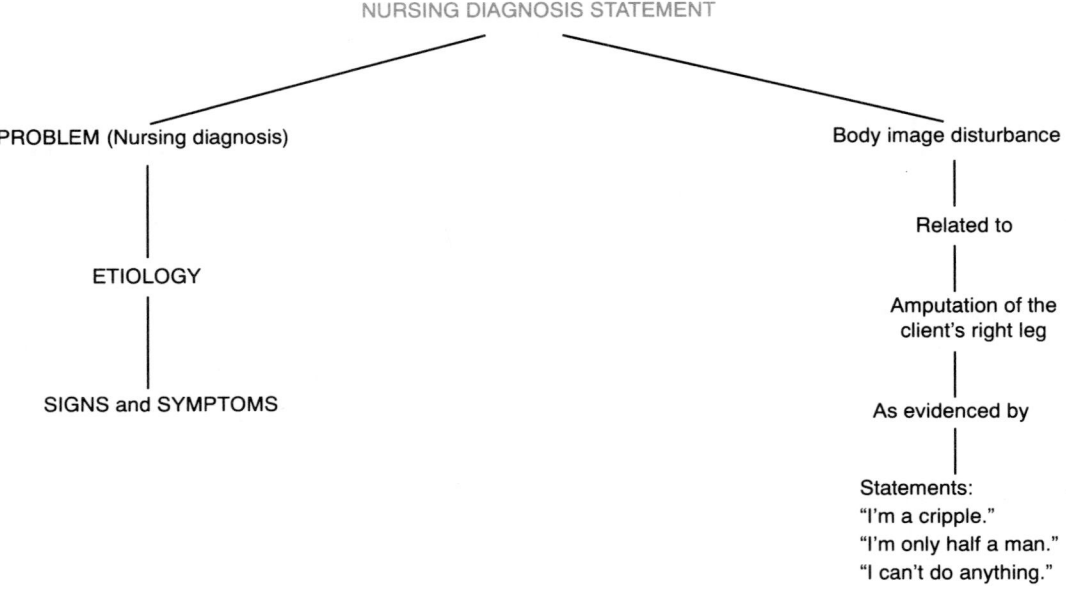

FIGURE 28-2 Nursing diagnosis statement.

expectations before establishing goals. Short-term goals are those that can be met relatively quickly (days or weeks), and long-term goals can be met over months or years. For example, a short-term goal for a client would be "Increase skill in breast self-examination." The long-term goal would be "Client incorporates monthly breast self-examination into life-style habits."

Outcomes are the specific measurable events associated with each goal, including a time frame by which the expected outcomes should be accomplished. The client outcome is a statement of behavior that demonstrates an improvement in, or resolution of, the problem.

To continue with the previous example, the client outcome related to the short-term goal would be "The client will be able to perform a breast self-examination after observing a demonstration." The outcome related to the long-term goal would be "At 1-year follow-up the client will report performing monthly breast self-examination." Each of these outcomes is stated in measurable terms, one verified by practitioner observation and one by data obtained in an interview.

Intervention

Once you have prioritized and identified client outcomes, record a plan of action and specific nursing strategies for meeting the goals. The etiology of a problem or response pattern guides selection of the specific interventions. When listing nursing interventions, include when the action should be done; who should be in-

volved; and the frequency, quantity, and method to be used. For example, "The employee health nurse will offer on site 1 hour classes twice yearly on breast self-examination technique to all female employees." Methods of intervention include assessing, teaching, counseling, consulting, and referring.

When implementing nursing interventions, determine the difference between nursing diagnoses and collaborative problems. Nursing diagnoses relate to health problems or potential problems that nurses can independently treat. Independent nursing interventions are within the legal scope of nursing practice and require no supervision or direction by others.

On the other hand, collaborative interventions involve direction from or collaboration with an appropriate and legally designated health professional. Collaborative problems can be prevented, resolved, or reduced through collaborative or interdependent nursing interventions.

Each time you identify a problem or potential problem, ask yourself "Can I initiate the treatment independently?" If the answer is no, another licensed health professional, usually a physician, must provide collaboration or direction.

Evaluation

The criteria for evaluation are the same as the goals or outcomes identified during planning. To evaluate goal achievement, compare the documented outcome criteria with the client's actions or behaviors. Once you have determined whether the client has achieved the outcomes, gather data to analyze what factors contributed to success or failure. Factors that may contribute to unsuccessful outcomes might be:

- New problems developed
- The original problem changed
- The interventions were not appropriate
- The goals were unrealistic
- The intervention did not fit the client

After you have evaluated the goals and outcomes, develop a revised plan of care with new goals, outcomes, and interventions. Work with the client on all phases of this process, including how to revise the care plan. This evaluation process is ongoing as long as the practitioner has a role in caring for the client.

SUMMARY

In conclusion, decision making is an integral part of the nursing process. All four phases of the decision-making process occur during nursing assessment. The end products of nursing assessment and decision making are nursing diagnoses. The NANDA taxonomy provides a classification system and a language for communicating. Using a nursing framework to guide assessment and decision making facilitates the formulation of nursing diagnoses. In addition, nursing diagnoses written in the P-E-S format contribute useful information to the rest of the nursing process.

Nursing diagnostic categories require further work and further clinical testing. Revisions will occur as diagnoses are used to organize assessment data, as a basis for care planning, and as a focus for nursing documentation.

GLOSSARY

cue Something that is noted by using the five senses (taste, touch, smell, sight, and hearing). A cue can be either subjective data or objective data.

defining characteristics Signs and symptoms that help to confirm a diagnosis.

inference How one perceives or interprets a cue.

nursing diagnosis A statement that describe's a client's health state, or response to illness, treatable by a nurse.

taxonomy A framework for classifying and organizing information according to hierarchical categories.

validation The process of making sure the information or data you have collected is factual or true.

BIBLIOGRAPHY

Alfaro R: *Application of nursing process: a step-by-step guide,* Philadelphia, 1986, JB Lippincott.

Carroll-Johnson R, editor: *Classification of nursing diagnoses: proceedings of the ninth conference,* NANDA, Philadelphia, 1991, JB Lippincott.

Engle GL: The need for a new medical model: a challenge for biomedicine, *Science* 196:129-196, 1970.

Gordon M: *Nursing diagnoses: process and application,* New York, 1987, McGraw-Hill.

Gordon M: *Manual of nursing diagnosis 1993-1994,* St. Louis, 1993, Mosby–Year Book.

Guzzetta CE, Bunton SD, Prinkey LA and others: *Clinical assessment tools for use with nursing diagnoses,* St Louis, 1989, Mosby–Year Book.

Maslow A: *Motivation and personality,* New York, 1970, Harper & Row.

Orem DE: *Nursing: concepts of practice,* ed 3, New York, 1985, McGraw-Hill.

Sparks SM, Taylor SM: *Nursing diagnosis reference manual,* Springhouse, Pa, 1991, Springhouse.

Yura H, Walsh MB: *The nursing process: assessing, planning, implementing, and evaluating,* ed 4, New York, 1983, Appleton-Century-Crofts.

Index